W9-CTS-582

UNIT VII:

Scientific Basis for Nursing Practice

UNIT VIII:

Basic Physiological Needs

UNIT IX:

Clients With Special Needs

CANADIAN Fundamentals *of* Nursing

CANADIAN Fundamentals of Nursing

FOURTH EDITION

PATRICIA A. POTTER
RN, MSN, PhD, FAAN
Research Scientist
Barnes-Jewish Hospital
Siteman Cancer Center at Washington University School of Medicine
St. Louis, Missouri

ANNE GRIFFIN PERRY
RN, EdD, FAAN
Professor and Chair
Department of Primary Care and Health Systems Nursing
School of Nursing, Southern Illinois University
Edwardsville, Illinois

SECTION EDITORS

AMY HALL, RN, BSN, MS, PhD
Chair
Department of Nursing and Health Sciences
Associate Professor of Nursing
University of Evansville
Evansville, Indiana

PATRICIA A. STOCKERT, RN, BSN, MS, PhD
Professor and Associate Dean
Undergraduate Program
Saint Francis Medical Center College of Nursing
Peoria, Illinois

CANADIAN EDITORS

JANET C. ROSS-KERR, RN, BScN, MS, PhD
Professor Emeritus
Faculty of Nursing
University of Alberta
Edmonton, Alberta

MARILYNN J. WOOD, BSN, MSN, DrPH
Professor Emeritus
Faculty of Nursing
University of Alberta
Edmonton, Alberta

CANADIAN SECTION EDITORS

BARBARA ASTLE, RN, PhD
Faculty of Nursing
University of Alberta
Calgary, Alberta

SONYA GRYPMA, RN, PhD
Associate Professor
School of Nursing
Trinity Western University
Langley, British Columbia

NICOLE LETOURNEAU, RN, PhD
Canada Research Chair in Healthy Child Development
Peter Lougheed/CIHR New Investigator (honourary)
Professor
Faculty of Nursing and Research Fellow CRISP
University of New Brunswick
Fredericton, New Brunswick

MOSBY
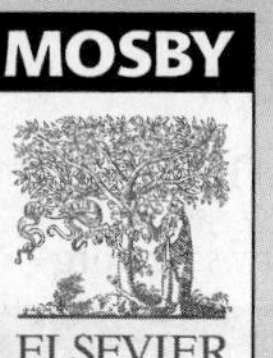
ELSEVIER

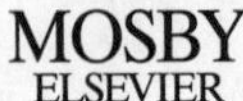

Copyright © 2009 Elsevier Canada, a division of Reed Elsevier Canada, Ltd.

Adapted from *Fundamentals of Nursing,* 7th edition, by Patricia A. Potter and Anne Griffin Perry. Copyright © 2009, 2005, 2001, 1997, 1993, 1989, 1985 by Mosby, Inc., an affiliate of Elsevier Inc.

All rights reserved. No part of this publication may be reproduced or transmitted in any form or by any means, electronic or mechanical, including photocopy, recording, or any information storage and retrieval system, without permission in writing from the publisher. Reproducing passages from this book without such written permission is an infringement of copyright law.

Requests for permission to make copies of any part of the work should be mailed to: College Licensing Officer, Access Copyright, 1 Yonge Street, Suite 1900, Toronto, ON, M5E 1E5. Fax: (416) 868-1621. All other inquiries should be directed to the publisher.

Every reasonable effort has been made to acquire permission for copyright material used in this text and to acknowledge all such indebtedness accurately. Any errors and omissions called to the publisher's attention will be corrected in future printings.

Notice

Knowledge and best practice in this field are constantly changing. As new research and expertise broaden our knowledge, changes in practice, treatment, and drug therapy may become necessary or appropriate. Readers are advised to check the most current information provided (i) on procedures featured or (ii) by the manufacturer of each product to be administered and to verify the recommended dose or formula, the method and duration of administration, and contraindications. It is the responsibility of practitioners, relying on their own experience and knowledge of the client, to make diagnoses, to determine dosages and the best treatment for each individual patient, and to take all appropriate safety precautions. To the fullest extent of the law, neither the Publisher nor the Authors assumes any liability for any injury and/or damage to persons or property arising out of or related to any use of the material contained in this book.

The Publisher

Library and Archives Canada Cataloguing in Publication

Potter, Patricia Ann

Canadian fundamentals of nursing / Patricia A. Potter, Anne Griffin Perry; [Canadian editors] Janet C. Ross-Kerr, Marilynn J. Wood—4th ed.

Includes bibliographical references and index.
ISBN 978-0-7796-9993-3

1. Nursing–Textbooks. 2. Nursing–Canada–Textbooks. I. Kerr, Janet C., 1940– II. Perry, Anne Griffin III. Wood, Marilynn J. IV. Title.

RT41.P68 2009 610.73 C2008-905528-4

ISBN-13-978-0-7796-9993-3
ISBN-10-0-7796-9993-9

Vice President, Publishing: Ann Millar
Developmental Editor: Toni Chahley
Managing Developmental Editor: Martina van de Velde
Managing Production Editor: Lise Dupont
Copy Editor: Anne Ostroff
Cover, Interior Design: Christine Rae, Interrobang Graphics, Inc.
Typesetting and Assembly: Jansom
Printing and Binding: Transcontinental

Elsevier Canada
905 King Street West, 4th Floor
Toronto, ON, Canada M6K 3G9
Phone: 1-866-896-3331
Fax: 1-866-359-9534

Printed in Canada

1 2 3 4 5 13 12 11 10 09

Working together to grow
libraries in developing countries
www.elsevier.com | www.bookaid.org | www.sabre.org
ELSEVIER BOOK AID International Sabre Foundation

Contents

Preface to the Student

Canadian Fundamentals of Nursing provides you with all of the fundamental nursing concepts and skills you will need in a visually appealing, easy-to-use format. As you begin your nursing education, it is very important that you have a resource that includes all the information required to prepare you for lectures, classroom activities, clinical assignments, and examinations. We've designed this text to meet all of those needs.

Check out the following special learning aids featured in *Canadian Fundamentals of Nursing*:

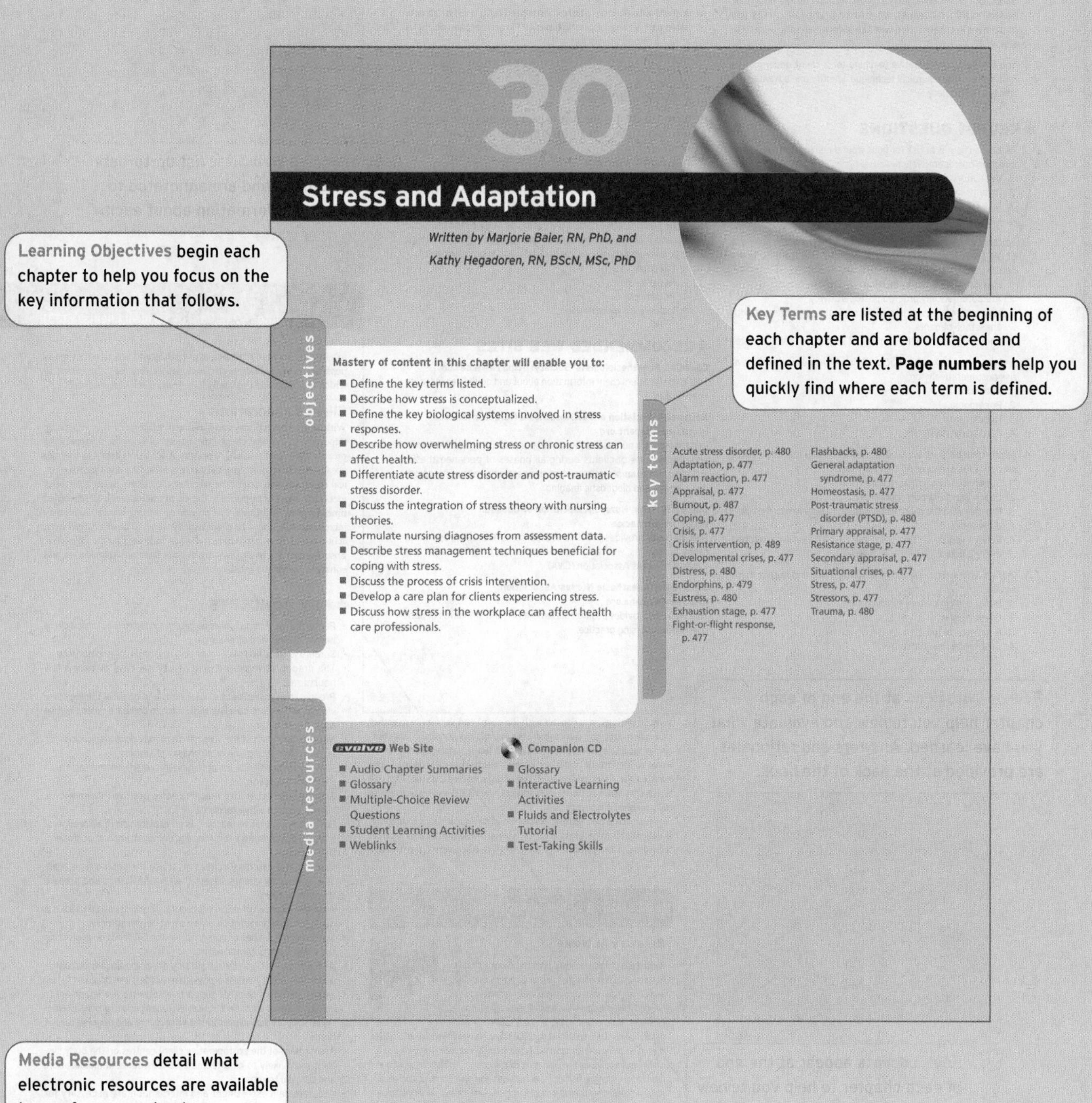

✻ CRITICAL THINKING EXERCISES

1. An 82-year-old client is admitted for surgery on a fractured hip caused by a fall. What postoperative complications are typical in the older client undergoing this type of surgery?
2. Mr. B. is a 52-year-old client who will undergo thoracic surgery. He has smoked one pack of cigarettes per day for 30 years. What type of pulmonary preventive measures would you expect Mr. B to need postoperatively?
3. Mrs. C. was admitted for ambulatory surgery for an inguinal hernia repair. What discharge criteria would be used for Mrs. C., and what discharge instructions would she require?
4. Your client is scheduled for abdominal hysterectomy at 2:00 p.m. Based on NPO guidelines, what fasting schedule should you implement in collaboration with the surgeon and the anaesthesiologist?
5. You are doing preoperative teaching for a client undergoing a minimally invasive surgical technique. Identify one advantage of this type of surgery.

✻ REVIEW QUESTIONS

1. An obese client is at risk for poor wound healing and for wound infection postoperatively because:
   1. Ventilatory capacity is reduced
   2. Fatty tissue has a poor blood supply
   3. Risk for dehiscence is increased
   4. Resuming normal physical activity is delayed
2. You should ask each client preoperatively for the name and dose of all prescription and over-the-counter medications taken before surgery because they:
   1. May cause allergies to develop
   2. Are automatically ordered postoperatively
   3. May create greater risks for complications or interact with anaesthetic agents
   4. Should be taken on the morning of surgery with sips of water
3. A client who smokes two packs of cigarettes per day is most at risk postoperatively for:
   1. Infection
   2. Pneumonia
   3. Hypotension
   4. Cardiac dysrhythmias
4. Family members should be included when you teach the client preoperative exercises so that they can:
   1. Supervise the client at home
   2. Coach the client postoperatively
   3. Practise with the client while waiting to be taken to the operating room
   4. Relieve you by getting the client to do his or her exercises every 2 hours
5. In the postoperative period, measuring input and output helps assess:
   1. Renal and circulatory function
   2. Client comfort
   3. Neurological function
   4. Gastrointestinal function
6. In the PACU, one measure taken to maintain airway patency is to:
   1. Suction the pharynx and bronchial tree
   2. Give oxygen through a mask at 10 L/minute
   3. Position the client so that the tongue falls forward
   4. Ask the client to use an incentive spirometer
7. Which one of the following measures promotes normal veno[us] return and circulatory blood flow?
   1. Suctioning artificial airways and the oral cavity
   2. Monitoring fluid and electrolyte status during every shift
   3. Having the client use incentive spirometry
   4. Encouraging the client to perform leg exercises at least once an hour while awake
8. A client with an international normalized ratio (INR) or an activated partial thromboplastin time (APTT) greater than normal is at risk postoperatively for:
   1. Anemia
   2. Bleeding
   3. Infection
   4. Cardiac dysrhythmias
9. When the client is engaging in deep breathing and coughing exercises, it is important to have the client sitting because this position:
   1. Is more comfortable
   2. Facilitates expansion of the thorax
   3. Increases the client's view of the room and is more relaxi[ng]
   4. Helps the client to splint with a pillow
10. In the postoperative period, if a client has unexpected tachyca[r]dia and tachypnea; jaw muscle rigidity; body rigidity of limbs, abdomen, and chest; or hyperkalemia, you should suspect:
    1. Infection
    2. Hypertension
    3. Pneumonia
    4. Malignant hyperthermia

✻ RECOMMENDED WEB SITES

Canadian Anesthesiologists' Society: http://www.cas.ca
This Web site offers client information about and guidelines for using anaesthesia.

National Association of PeriAnesthesia Nurses of Canada: http://www.napanc.org
Perianaesthesia nurses are registered nurses with advanced knowledge in the care of clients during all phases of perianaesthesia, including, for example, nurses in postanaesthetic care units, same-day surgery, and diagnostic imaging.

Operating Room Nurses Association of Canada: http://www.ornac.ca
This Web site provides practice standards for Canadian operating room nurses, as well as information on certification with the Canadian Nurses Association (CNA).

Ontario PeriAnesthesia Nurses Association: http://www.opana.org
This Web site provides position statements on and standards of perianaesthesia nursing practice.

Critical Thinking Exercises encourage you to think creatively and effectively to apply essential content.

Recommended Web Sites list up-to-date online resources and are annotated to give you some information about each.

Review Questions at the end of each chapter help you review and evaluate what you have learned. Answers and rationales are provided at the back of the book.

surgical settings, you consult with the client and the family to gather evaluation data. You can evaluate the ambulatory surgical client's outcomes via a telephone call to the client's home, asking specific questions to determine whether complications have developed and whether the client understands restrictions or medications. This call is usually placed 24 hours after surgery, which allows you to evaluate the progress of recovery.

In an acute care setting, evaluation of a surgical client is ongoing. If a client fails to progress as expected, you revise the client's care plan according to the priorities of the client's needs. Every effort is made

✻ BOX 49-8 FOCUS ON PRIMARY HEALTH CARE

Recovery at Home

Regardless of the length of time the client spends in hospital, it is essential that you ensure that the client and family have the appropriate information and skills needed to continue a successful recovery at home. However, time is often very limited, especially with the move toward preadmission units and short hospital stays. A comprehensive approach is needed to ensure continuity of care from hospital to home. A client often has to continue dressing care, follow activity restrictions, continue medication therapy, and observe for signs and symptoms of complications on returning home. In addition, the client needs someone to be present for the first 24 hours to ensure that there is no delayed reaction from the anaesthesia, such as difficulty breathing. A referral to home care assists clients who are unable to perform self-care activities. Close association with home care services is required for some clients if dressing changes or physiotherapy is needed. It is useful to have a case management nurse in attendance at discharge to convey what tasks a client can perform effectively.

Key Concepts appear at the end of each chapter to help you review important content.

to assist the client in returning to as healthy and functional a state as possible. Your evaluation also includes determining the extent to which the client and the family have learned self-care measures.

Client Expectations

With short hospital stays and ambulatory surgery, it is especially important to evaluate client expectations early in the postoperative process. Pain relief is usually a priority. Asking the client if everything possible has been done to alleviate pain, including nonpharmacological measures, can determine whether the client's needs have been met. Timeliness of response to the client's needs, such as scheduled times for pain medication and prompt answering of a call light, may increase satisfaction. The client usually wants to be discharged from acute care as soon as possible and when indicated by the physician. Ensuring that discharge plans are in place facilitates that process and enhances the client's satisfaction with care.

✻ KEY CONCEPTS

- Perioperative nursing is nursing care provided to the surgical client before, during, and after surgery.
- Surgery is classified by level of severity, urgency, and purpose.
- The preoperative period may be several days or only a few hours long.
- Preoperative assessment of vital signs and physical findings provides an important baseline with which to compare postoperative assessment data.
- Nursing diagnoses of the surgical client may pose implications for nursing care during one or all phases of surgery.
- Primary responsibility for obtaining informed consent rests with the client's surgeon.
- Structured preoperative teaching has a positive influence on a client's postoperative recovery.
- Basic to preoperative teaching is an explanation of all preoperative and postoperative routines and demonstration of postoperative exercises.
- In ambulatory surgery, nurses must use the limited time available to educate clients, assess their health status, and prepare them for surgery.
- A routine preoperative (preprocedure) checklist can be used as a guide for final preparation of the client before surgery.
- Many responsibilities of nurses within the OR focus on protecting the client from potential harm.
- All medications taken before surgery are automatically discontinued after surgery unless a physician reorders the drugs.
- Family members or other supportive networks are important in assisting clients with any physical limitations and in providing emotional support during postoperative recovery and ongoing care at home.
- Assessment of the postoperative client centres on the body systems most likely to be affected by anaesthesia, immobilization, and surgical trauma.
- Accurate pain assessment and intervention are necessary for healing
- Nurses in the postoperative surgical unit provide the discharge education required so that the client and the family can manage at home.

❖Evaluation

Client Care

To evaluate outcomes and response to nursing care, measure the effectiveness of all interventions. The actual outcomes are compared with the outcomes selected during planning. Evaluate specific interventions designed to promote body alignment, improve mobility, and protect the client from the hazards of immobility. Client and family teaching to prevent future risks to body alignment and hazards of immobility is also evaluated (Figure 46–34). The evaluation enables you to determine whether new or revised therapies are required and if new nursing diagnoses have developed.

Client Expectations

Clients who are immobile and dependent on others for some or all of their needs can become overly dependent or try to do too much themselves too early. Finding the balance between independence and dependence is a difficult task. Clients will want control over their mobility that is personally satisfactory. For the client who is completely dependent on others for care, control over how and when things are done may be very important. Do clients feel they are treated with dignity? Do caregivers treat them as adults? Are they given opportunities to make meaningful choices?

✻ KEY CONCEPTS

- Body mechanics are the coordinated efforts of the musculoskeletal and nervous systems as the person moves, lifts, bends, stands, sits, lies down, and completes daily activities.
- Balance is assisted through nervous system control by the cerebellum and inner ear.
- Range-of-motion (ROM) exercises include one or all of the body joints and can be active or passive.
- Body alignment is the condition of joints, tendons, ligaments, and muscles in various body positions.
- Balance is achieved when a wide base of support is present, the centre of gravity falls within the base of support, and a vertical line falls from the centre of gravity through the base of support.
- Developmental stages influence body alignment and mobility; the greatest impact of physiological changes on the musculoskeletal system is observed in children and older adults.
- The risk of disabilities related to immobilization depends on the extent and duration of immobilization and the client's overall level of health.
- Immobility may result from illness or trauma or may be prescribed for therapeutic reasons (bed rest).
- Immobility presents hazards in the physiological, psychological, and developmental dimensions.
- Use the nursing process and critical thinking synthesis to provide care for clients who are experiencing or are at risk for the adverse effects of impaired body alignment and immobility.
- After identifying nursing diagnoses, plan and implement interventions to prevent or minimize the hazards and complications of impaired body alignment and immobilization.
- Clients with weakness and impaired function of the nervous, skeletal, or muscular system often require nursing assistance to attain proper body alignment while in bed or sitting and to transfer from a bed to a chair.

Knowledge
- Effects of improved mobility status on physiological systems and clients' psychosocial and developmental status

Experience
- Previous client responses to planned mobility interventions

Evaluation
- Evaluate the client for signs and symptoms of improved or decreased mobility status
- Ask for the client's perception of mobility status after intervention
- Ask if the client's expectations of care are being met

Standards
- Use established expected outcomes (e.g., lung fields remain clear) to evaluate the client's response to care

Attitudes
- Display humility when identifying those interventions that were not successful
- Use creativity when redesigning new interventions to improve the client's mobility status

The unique **Critical Thinking Model** clearly shows how the nursing process and critical thinking come together to help you provide the best care for your clients.

Concept Maps show you the association among multiple nursing diagnoses and their relationship to medical diagnoses.

The five-step **Nursing Process** provides a consistent framework for presentation of content in clinical chapters.

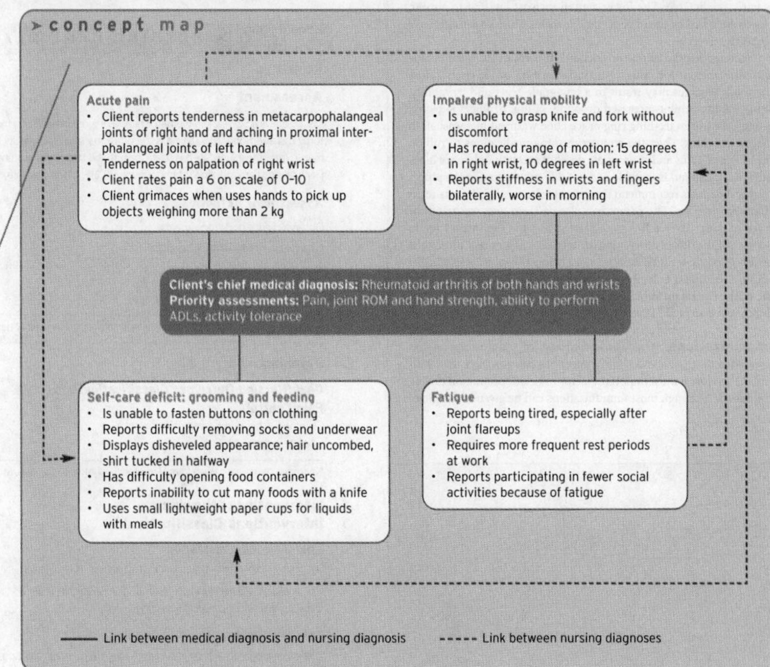

Figure 42-10 Concept map for client with pain related to rheumatoid arthritis.

pain in affected areas. Occupational therapists can devise splints to support painful body parts. Clergy members can help clients resolve spiritual pain. The family should also be involved in the care plan because they may need to administer care in the home after discharge. If the pain management plan is not successful, you should talk with the physician about changing the plan. Consultation with pain experts might be necessary.

❖Implementation

The nature of the pain and how much it affects well-being determines the choice of interventions. Pain therapy requires an *individualized* approach, perhaps more so than any other client problem. You, the client, and the family must be partners in using pain-control measures. Administer and monitor pain treatments ordered by a physician, but consider using other complementary comfort measures. Client remedies are often most successful, especially when the client has already had experience with pain. Generally, the least invasive or safest therapy should be tried first.

Health Promotion

The Ottawa Charter for Health Promotion (https://www.who.int/healthpromotion/conferences/previous/ottawa/en/) defines health promotion as the process of enabling individuals to gain control over and to improve their health and well-being (World Health Organization, 1990). Chronic pain and suffering diminishes quality of life; thus, relieving pain and promoting self-control becomes important. Once pain is controlled to an acceptable level, provide clients and their families with education and information about pain so that they can participate in the pain care decision-making process. This will help reduce anxiety and increases a client's sense of control. For example, clients who are in hospital for the first time may know that they require tests, but do not understand them. As a result, they may become anxious and fearful. Fear increases the perception of painful stimuli. Remember, however, that health promotion goes beyond teaching. Using pain management techniques from the Ottawa

Research Highlight boxes provide abstracts of current nursing research studies and explain the implications for your daily practice.

BOX 23-5 RESEARCH HIGHLIGHT

Breastfeeding

Research Focus

Success in breastfeeding largely depends on the woman's self-confidence in her ability to breastfeed. You can play an important role in assisting new mothers to feel more confident in their ability to breastfeed by being aware of some of the factors that promote successful breastfeeding.

Research Abstract

Kingston et al. (2007) explored some of the factors that enhanced women's self-efficacy in breastfeeding 48 hours and 4 weeks after the birth of their babies. Kingston et al. examined such influences as previous successful breastfeeding experiences, professional assistance with breast-feeding, watching other mothers breastfeed, watching videos of other women breastfeeding, giving positive feedback and consistent advice, receiving praise from family members and friends, encouraging mothers to continue breastfeeding, and encouraging mothers to think positively about the breastfeeding experience, as well as physiological influences on breastfeeding such as pain, fatigue, and feeling overwhelmed. Self-efficacy was measured by the Breastfeeding Self-Efficacy Scale–Short Form. The study was performed with a small sample of mothers ($N = 65$) in a hospital in central Canada. The researchers found that self-efficacy was significantly higher in women who had seen videotapes of women breastfeeding as part of their breastfeeding education or had received praise from their partners or own mothers. Women who reported pain or received help with breastfeeding from professionals had significantly lower scores. Women receiving more help would have a greater need for assistance, and this might affect self-efficacy.

Evidence-Informed Practice

- Assess the breastfeeding self-efficacy of new mothers.
- Examine the educational material used with clients, and show clients videos of successful breastfeeding.
- Consider the physiological condition of the mother, and address issues such as pain.
- Include the mother's partner and, if possible, the woman's own mother in supporting and offering praise to the breastfeeding mother.
- Examine other factors that increase or decrease the mother's self-confidence in her ability to breastfeed.

References: Kingston, D., Dennis, C.-L., & Sword, W. (2007). Exploring breast-feeding self-efficacy. *Journal of Perinatal and Neonatal Nursing, 21*, 207–215.

dietary habits through feeding experiences mutually satisfying for the parents and infant. Eating habits are frequently affected by the family's sociocultural background. Because some cultures consider a fat baby to be a sign of good mothering, any suggestion to limit intake or slow weight gain may be seen as a threat. It is important for you to develop an understanding of the cultural influences to develop effective nursing interventions.

Dentition. The average age at which the first tooth erupts is 7 months, but considerable variation exists among infants because of their genetic endowment. An occasional infant is born with a tooth, whereas others remain toothless at 1 year. The order of tooth eruption is fairly predictable: The lower central incisors are first to appear, closely followed by the upper central incisors. Most 1-year-olds have six teeth.

Teething may result in considerable discomfort for some infants and little or none for others. The inflammation of the gums before the tooth emerges may result in a low-grade fever and irritability. Some infants exhibit increased drooling, biting, or finger sucking. Biting on a frozen teething ring or ice cube wrapped in a washcloth may be soothing. Over-the-counter teething medications to rub on the inflamed gums and appropriate doses of acetaminophen are helpful when the infant is irritable and has difficulty eating or sleeping.

Most dentists recommend that parents cleanse their infant's teeth after each feeding. The parent can place a clean, wet washcloth or piece of gauze over a finger and use it to wipe the infant's teeth. Because of the risk of developing dental caries, discourage prolonged breast- or bottle-feeding, especially just before the infant goes to sleep because the infant is likely to leave milk in the mouth and around the teeth. The infant should never go to bed with a bottle of juice or milk (Behrman et al., 2008).

Immunizations. The widespread use of immunizations has resulted in the dramatic decline of infectious diseases since the 1950s and is therefore a most important factor in health promotion during childhood. Although most immunizations can be given to people of any age, the Public Health Agency of Canada (2006) recommended that the administration of the primary series begin soon after birth and be completed during early childhood (Table 23–2). Minor side effects may occur, but serious reactions are rare. Parents must receive instructions regarding the potential side effects of immunizations. High fever and extreme irritability should be reported to their health care professional.

As a result of complacency and fear regarding the side effects of certain vaccines, especially diphtheria and tetanus toxoids and pertus-

Nursing Care Plans feature a format that helps you understand the process of assessment, the relationship between assessment findings and nursing diagnoses, the identification of goals and outcomes, selection of interventions, and the process for evaluating care.

BOX 14-4 NURSING CARE PLAN

Acute Pain

Assessment

Ms. Devine is a 52-year-old woman who was injured in a fall two months ago that caused rupture of a lumbar disc. She is scheduled for a lumbar laminectomy this afternoon. Ms. Devine is the office manager for a realty business she runs with her husband. She was not able to work regularly over the first month after the injury. She has sciatic pain that is sharp and burning, radiating down from her right hip to her right foot. The pain worsens when she sits. Her vital signs are as follows: temperature, 99.2°F; blood pressure, 138/82 mm Hg; pulse, 84 beats per minute; and respirations, 24 breaths per minute.

Assessment Activities	*Findings and Defining Characteristics**
Observe client's body movements	Client limps **slightly with right leg. Turns** in bed **slowly.**
Observe client's facial expression	Client **grimaces** when she attempts to sit down.
Ask client to rate pain at its worst	Client **rates pain on a scale of 0 to 10 at an 8 or 9 at its worst.**

*Defining characteristics are in boldface type.

Nursing Diagnosis: Acute pain related to pressure on spinal nerves

Planning

Goal (Nursing Outcomes Classification)†	*Expected Outcomes†*
Pain Control	**Knowledge of Treatment Procedures**
Client will achieve improved pain control before surgery.	Client's self-report of pain will be 3 or less on a scale of 0 to 10 Client's facial expressions reveal less discomfort when turning and repositioning.

†Outcomes classification labels from Moorhead S, Johnson, M., & Maas, M. (2008). *Nursing Outcomes Classification (NOC)* (3rd ed). St. Louis, MO: Mosby.

Interventions (Nursing Interventions Classification)‡	**Rationale**
Analgesic Administration	
Set positive expectations regarding effectiveness of analgesics.	Optimizes client's response to medication (Bulechek et al., 2008).
Give analgesic 30 minutes before turning or positioning client and before pain increases in severity.	Medication will exert peak effect when client attempts to increase movement.
Pain Management	
Reduce environmental factors in client's room (e.g., noise, lighting, temperature extremes).	Pleasurable sensory stimuli reduce pain perception.
Offer client information about any procedures and efforts at reducing discomfort.	Information satisfies client's interests and enables client to evaluate and communicate pain (McCaffery & Pasero, 1999).
Progressive Muscle Relaxation	
Direct client through progressive muscle relaxation exercise.	Relaxation techniques enable self-control when pain develops, reversing
Coach client through exercise.	the cognitive and affective–motivational component of pain perception.

‡Intervention classification labels from Bulechek, G. M., Butcher, H. K., & Dochterman, J. M. (2008). *Nursing Interventions Classification (NIC)* (4th ed.). St. Louis, MO: Mosby.

Evaluation

Nursing Actions	*Client Response and Finding*	*Achievement of Outcome*
Ask client to report severity of pain 30 minutes after analgesic administration.	Ms. Devine reports pain at a level of 5 on a scale of 0 to 10.	Pain is reduced, necessitates further nonpharmacological intervention to achieve outcome.
Observe client's facial expressions.	Ms. Devine is observed to have a relaxed facial expression.	Client's level of comfort is improving.

Rationales for each of the interventions in the care plans help you to understand why a specific step or set of steps is performed.

Evaluation explains how to evaluate and determine whether the outcomes have been achieved.

Evidence-Informed Practice Guideline boxes provide examples of recent state-of-the-science guidelines for nursing practice.

Client Teaching boxes highlight what and how to teach clients and how to evaluate learning.

BOX 44-13 CLIENT TEACHING

Pelvic Floor Muscle Exercises (Kegels)

Objectives

The client who is cognitively alert and motivated will achieve continence or experience fewer episodes of incontinence through increased pelvic floor muscle tone and strength.

Teaching Strategies

- Explain the method used to identify proper muscle contraction: female client sits on toilet with knees apart and tightens muscles to stop the flow of urine; male client tries to stop the flow of urine midstream.
- After muscle is identified, instruct the client to lie down with knees bent and apart, or to sit.
- Instruct the client to contract the pelvic floor muscle gradually and hold for 3 to 10 seconds without tensing muscles of legs, buttocks, back, or abdomen. Remind the client to breathe during the exercise.
- Instruct the client to relax the muscle gradually for an equal time period between each contraction.
- The client should repeat this exercise at least two or three times, and work up to 10 repetitions as it becomes easier. The client should do this exercise two or three times a day, or as often as possible.
- Explain that within the first week of exercises, the client and nurse can assess whether proper muscle contraction is occurring by placing two fingers in the vagina (or, for men, one finger in the rectum) while contracting the pelvic floor muscle. The client should feel tightening in the vagina or anus during the contraction.
- Teach the client and the caregiver to keep a 24- to 72-hour urinary diary to identify changes in patterns of urinary elimination.

Evaluation

- Ask the client if he or she has identified pelvic floor muscle via finger insertion.
- During vaginal or rectal (male) bimanual examination, ask the client to do exercises and assess muscle tone.
- Monitor the client's urinary diary.
- Ask the client and the caregiver about degree of satisfaction related to the control achieved over urinary elimination.

BOX 44-14 EVIDENCE-INFORMED PRACTICE GUIDELINE

Prompted Voiding for People with Urinary Incontinence

- Approach the client at scheduled prompted voiding times.
- Wait five seconds for the client to initiate a request to toilet.
- Ask the client if he or she is wet or dry.
- Physically assess the client to determine continence status.
- Provide positive feedback if the client is dry.
- Prompt the client to toilet.
- Offer assistance with toileting.
- Provide feedback.
- Inform the client of the next scheduled prompted voiding session.
- Encourage the client to self-initiate requests to toilet.
- Record the result of the prompted voiding session.

Adapted from Wyman, J. (2008). Prompted voiding. In B. Ackley, B. Swan, G. Ludwig, & S. Tucker (Eds.), *Evidence-based nursing care guidelines. Medical–surgical interventions* (pp. 696–698). St. Louis, MO: Mosby.

The first step in bladder training is establishing a baseline. The client or caregiver completes a urinary diary to assess maximum voiding intervals. It is not uncommon for the client with frequency or an overactive bladder to void small amounts hourly or more often. An initial training schedule for such a client might involve a voiding schedule of every 75 minutes while awake, increasing every 1 to 3 weeks by 15-minute increments toward a 3-hour schedule. The rate of incremental changes will depend on the client's progress and on his or her ability to adhere to a rigid schedule. Urge-suppression techniques, such as counting backward from 100 when the urge to void is felt and performing pelvic floor muscle contractions, are helpful. You must be aware that the client who has experienced an episode of incontinence in public will be particularly hesitant to deter voiding for even brief periods.

Habit Retraining and Prompted Voiding. Habit retraining and **prompted voiding** are useful strategies for clients with cognitive or physical impairment, or both, who rely on caregiver assistance. Habit retraining involves assessment of a client's normal pattern of voiding to establish a toileting schedule that pre-empts incontinence (Ostaszkiewicz et al., 2008). Such individualized toileting schedules have demonstrated effectiveness but are labour-intensive. You should help the client to the bathroom before episodes of incontinence occur. Fluids and medications are timed to prevent interference with the toileting schedule. When combined with positive reinforcement, this approach is also called prompted voiding (Box 44–14).

Self-Catheterization. Some clients with chronic disorders such as spinal cord injury learn to perform self-catheterization. The client must be physically able to manipulate equipment and assume a position for successful catheterization. You must teach the client the structure of the urinary tract, the clean versus sterile technique, the importance of adequate fluid intake, and the frequency of self-catheterization. In general, the goal is to have clients perform self-catheterization every six to eight hours, but the schedule should be individualized.

❖Evaluation

Client Care

The client is the best source of evaluation of outcomes and responses to nursing care (Figure 44–18). However, you will also evaluate the effectiveness of nursing interventions through comparisons with baseline data. You should evaluate for changes in the client's voiding pattern, the presence of urinary tract alteration, and the client's physical condition. Actual outcomes are compared with expected outcomes to determine the client's health status. Continuous evaluation allows you to determine whether new or revised therapies are required or if any new nursing diagnoses have developed.

Client Expectations

If you have developed a trust relationship with the client, indications of the client's degree of satisfaction with his or her care will be evident. The client may smile or nod in appreciation. However, you need to confirm whether the client's expectations have been met to full satis-

Older Adults. The cardiac and respiratory systems undergo changes throughout the aging process (Box 39–3). The changes are associated with calcification of the heart valves, SA node, and costal cartilages. The arterial system develops atherosclerotic plaques. Osteoporosis leads to changes in the size and shape of the thorax.

The trachea and large bronchi become enlarged from calcification of the airways. The alveoli enlarge, decreasing the surface area available for gas exchange. The number of functional cilia is reduced, causing a decrease in the effectiveness of the cough mechanism, putting the older adult at increased risk for respiratory infections (Meiner & Leuckenotte, 2006). Ventilation and transfer of respiratory gases decline with age because the lungs are unable to expand fully, leading to lower oxygenation levels.

Lifestyle Risk Factors

Lifestyle modifications that influence cardiopulmonary functioning are frequently difficult because a client is being asked to change a habit or behaviour that may be enjoyed, such as cigarette smoking or eating certain foods; however, these changes can be achieved with encouragement, support, and time (Box 39–4). Risk factor modification is important, including smoking cessation, weight reduction, a low-cholesterol and low-sodium diet, management of hypertension, and moderate exercise. Although it may be difficult to get older adults to change long-term behaviour, developing healthy behaviours can slow or halt the progression of their cardiopulmonary disease (Meiner & Leuckenotte, 2006).

Poor Nutrition. Nutrition affects cardiopulmonary function in several ways. Severe obesity decreases lung expansion, and the increased body weight increases oxygen demands to meet metabolic needs. The malnourished client may experience respiratory muscle wasting, resulting in decreased muscle strength and respiratory excursion. Cough efficiency is reduced secondary to respiratory muscle weakness, putting the client at risk for retention of pulmonary secre-

ciency of the myocardial muscle (JNC, 2003).

Smoking. Cigarette smoking is associated with a number of diseases, including heart disease, chronic obstructive lung disease, and lung cancer. Cigarette smoking can worsen peripheral vascular and coronary artery diseases (JNC, 2003). Inhaled nicotine causes vasoconstriction of peripheral and coronary blood vessels, increasing blood pressure and decreasing blood flow to peripheral vessels. Women who take birth control pills and smoke cigarettes are at increased risk for cardiovascular problems such as thrombophlebitis and pulmonary emboli.

BOX 39-3 FOCUS ON OLDER ADULTS

- The tuberculin skin test is an unreliable indicator of tuberculosis in older clients. They frequently display false-positive or false-negative skin test reactions.
- Older clients are at an increased risk for reactivation of dormant organisms that have been present for decades, as a result of age-related changes in the immune system.
- The standard 5-TU Mantoux test is given and repeated or repeated with the 250-TU strength to create a booster effect.
- If the older client has a positive reaction, a complete history is necessary to determine any risk factors.
- Older adults have more atypical signs and symptoms of coronary artery disease (Meiner & Leuckenotte, 2006).
- The incidence of atrial fibrillation increases with age and is the leading contributing factor for stroke in the older adult (Meiner & Leuckenotte, 2006).
- Mental status changes are often the first signs of respiratory problems and may include forgetfulness and irritability.
- Older adults may not complain of dyspnea until it affects the activities of daily living that are important to them.
- Changes in the older adult's cough mechanism may lead to retention of pulmonary secretions, airway plugging, and atelectasis if cough suppressants are not used with caution.

BOX 39-4 FOCUS ON PRIMARY HEALTH CARE

Positive Lifestyle Practices for Cardiopulmonary Health Promotion

As part of a primary health care focus, it is important to educate young to older adults about the following lifestyle practices that promote cardiopulmonary health:

- Maintain ideal body weight.
- Eat a low-fat, low-salt, calorie-appropriate diet.
- Engage in regular aerobic exercise of 1 hour daily.
- Use a filter mask when exposed to occupational hazards.
- Use stress-reduction techniques.
- Reduce exposure to secondary infections.
- Be smoke free.
- Avoid second-hand smoke and other pollutants.
- Have annual visits with a health care professional.
- Monitor blood pressure.
- Monitor cholesterol and triglyceride levels.
- Get an annual influenza vaccine if at risk for the development of influenza.
- Get a pneumococcal vaccine if appropriate.

Focus on Older Adults boxes prepare you to address the special needs of older adults.

Focus on Primary Health Care boxes draw attention to principles of primary health care and their application.

➤ SKILL 38-4 Performing Mouth Care for an Unconscious or Debilitated Client video

Delegation Considerations

The skill of brushing teeth of an unconscious or debilitated client can be delegated to an unregulated care provider. You must first assess the client for the gag reflex and determine whether the person providing assistance can safely use oral suctioning for clearing the client's oral secretions (see Chapter 39). When delegating tasks to an unregulated care provider it is important to instruct him or her about the following:

- The proper way to position the client for mouth care
- How to safely use oral suctioning for clearing oral secretions (see Chapter 39)
- To report to any bleeding of the mucosa or gums, any painful reaction by the client, or excessive coughing or choking

Equipment

- Anti-infective solution (e.g., commercial diluted hydrogen peroxide solution) that loosens crusts
- Small soft-bristled toothbrush
- Sponge swab (e.g., Toothette swab) or tongue blade wrapped in a single layer of gauze
- Oral airway
- Padded tongue blade
- Face towel
- Paper towels
- Emesis basin
- Water glass with cool water
- Water-soluble lip lubricant
- Small-bulb syringe (optional)
- Suction equipment
- Disposable gloves

Video Icons indicate video clips associated with specific skills that are available on the free CD *Companion and Evolve Student Learning Resources.*

Delegation Considerations guide you in delegating tasks to assistive personnel.

Procedure

STEPS	RATIONALE
1. Assess client's risk for oral hygiene problems (see Table 38–5).	• Oral care is provided frequently to intubated clients who also have a nasogastric tube and who are at risk of aspiration, which can lead to pneumonia (Smeltzer & Bare, 2004).
2. Explain procedure to client.	• Allows debilitated client to anticipate procedure without anxiety. Unconscious clients retain ability to hear.
3. Test for the presence of a gag reflex by placing a tongue blade on back half of the client's tongue.	• Reveals whether client is at risk for aspiration.
Critical Decision Point: Clients with an impaired gag reflex require oral care as well. You must determine the type of suction apparatus needed at the bedside to protect the client's airway against aspiration.	
4. Raise bed to the appropriate height; lower head of the bed and then lower the side rail.	• Allows use of good body mechanics and reduces the risk of injury.
5. Pull curtain around the bed, or close the room door.	
6. Perform hand hygiene and put on disposable gloves.	
7. Place paper towels on an overbed table and arrange equipment. If needed, turn on a suction machine and connect tubing to the suction catheter.	
8. Position client on side (Sims' position) with head turned well toward dependent side. Move client close to side of the bed. Raise the side rail.	
9. Place a towel under client's head and an emesis basin under the chin.	
10. Carefully separate upper and lower teeth with padded tongue blade by inserting blade, quickly but gently, between back molars. Insert blade when client is relaxed, if possible. Do not use force (see Step 10 illustration).	
Critical Decision Point: Never use fingers to separate the client's teeth.	
11. Inspect condition of the oral cavity (see Chapter 32).	
12. Clean mouth using brush or sponge Toothette swabs moistened with chlorhexidine solution if client condition can tolerate it; otherwise, moisten with water. Clean chewing and inner and outer tooth surfaces. Swab roof of mouth, gums, and inside cheeks. Gently swab or brush tongue, but avoid stimulating gag reflex (if present). Moisten clean swab or Toothette swab with water to rinse. (Bulb syringe may also be used to rinse.) Repeat rinse several times.	
13. Suction secretions as they accumulate, if necessary.	

Nursing Skills are presented in a clear, two-column format that includes Steps and Rationales to help you learn how and why a skill is performed.

➤ SKILL 38-4 Performing Mouth Care for an Unconscious or Debilitated Client *continued*

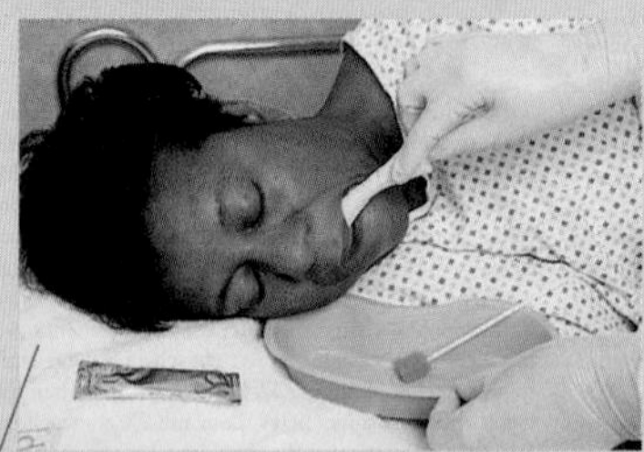

Step 10 Separate upper and lower teeth with padded tongue blade.

Step 14 Application of water-soluble moisturizer to lips.

STEPS	RATIONALE
15. Inform client that procedure is completed.	• Provides meaningful stimulation to unconscious or less responsive client.
16. Put on clean gloves, and inspect oral cavity.	• Determines efficacy of cleansing. Once thick secretions are removed, underlying inflammation or lesions may be revealed.
17. Ask debilitated client whether mouth feels clean.	• Evaluates level of comfort.
18. Reposition client comfortably, raise side rail as appropriate or as ordered, and return the bed to original position.	• Maintains client's comfort and safety. Raising all four side rails may be considered a restraint, and a physician's order is needed.
19. Clean equipment and return to its proper place. Place soiled linen in the proper receptacle.	• Proper disposal of soiled equipment prevents the spread of infection.
20. Remove and discard gloves. Perform hand hygiene.	• Reduces the transmission of microorganisms.
21. Assess client's respirations on an ongoing basis.	• Ensures early recognition of aspiration.

Unexpected Outcomes and Related Interventions

Secretions or Crusts Remaining on Oral Mucosa, Tongue, or Gums

- Increase frequency of oral hygiene.
- Try using a pediatric-size toothbrush—it may provide better hygiene.

Localized Inflammation of Gums or Mucosa

- Increase frequency of oral hygiene with a soft-bristled toothbrush.
- Apply moisturizing gel on the oral mucosa.
- Chemotherapy and radiation can cause stomatitis. To provide relief and promote oral hygiene, topical anti-inflammatories and anaesthetics may be prescribed (Smeltzer & Bare, 2004).

Aspiration of Secretions

- Suction oral airway.
- Perform tracheal bronchial suctioning.
- Notify the physician.

Recording and Reporting

- Record the procedure, including pertinent observations (e.g., the presence of bleeding gums, dry mucosa, ulcerations, or crusts on the tongue).
- Report any unusual findings to the person in charge or the physician.

Home Care Considerations

- Cavity should be irrigated with bulb syringe.
- Mouth care should be given at least twice a day. Caregivers can buy nonprescription oral care solutions (e.g., chlorhexidine solutions) at most pharmacies.
- Have caregivers demonstrate positioning of the client to prevent aspiration.

Critical Decision Points alert you to critical steps within a skill to ensure safe and effective client care.

Clear, close-up photos and illustrations show you how to perform important nursing techniques.

Recording and Reporting sections provide guidelines for what to chart and report with each skill.

Home Care Considerations explain how to adapt skills for the home setting.

BOX 30-5 CULTURAL ASPECTS OF CARE

Cultural context shapes the types of environmental stimuli that produce stress. For example, diverse cultures address developmental transitions and life's turning points differently. How a person leaves the parental home, experiences health crises or chronic illness, cares for the family, or becomes disabled or dependent are all culturally bound. Furthermore, how a person appraises stress is also dependent on the person's culture. Coping strategies are also influenced by culture. According to Aldwin (1992), cultures vary in their emotion-focused and problem-focused coping strategies. According to some cultures, emotions should be controlled; according to others, they should be expressed. *Problem-focused coping* refers to controlling or managing stress. In addition, cultures provide different institutions for coping with stress. These include the legal system for conflict resolution, advice givers or support groups, and rituals.

Implications for Practice

- Realize that stressors and coping styles vary with different cultures.
- Use introspection to examine your own perceptions of stress and coping in a cultural context.
- Assess the influence of culture on a client's appraisal of stress.
- Determine the available resources within a client's culture that may facilitate coping.

From Aldwin, C. M. (2000). *Stress, coping and development: An integrative perspective* (pp. 30–22). New York: Guilford Press.

Nursing Process

❖Assessment

When assessing a client's stress level and coping resources, you must ask the client to share personal and sensitive information. Therefore, you must first establish a trusting nurse–client relationship. By asking open-ended questions, listening carefully, observing the client's nonverbal behaviour, and observing the client's environment, you learn about the client's stress. You use critical thinking skills to synthesize and analyze information (Figure 30–3). Often clients have difficulty expressing what is troubling them until they have the opportunity to talk with someone who has time to listen.

Subjective Findings

When assessing a client's level of stress and coping resources, you arrange a nonthreatening physical environment, without a desk as a barrier, for the interaction (Varcarolis, 2002). You assume the same height as the client, arranging the interview environment so that eye contact can be comfortably maintained or avoided. By placing chairs at a 90-degree angle or side by side, you can reduce the intensity of the interaction (Varcarolis, 2002). You use the interview to determine the client's view of the stress, past successful coping resources, any possible maladaptive coping, and adherence to prescribed medical recommendations, such as medication or diet (Monat & Lazarus, 1991; Table 30–1). If the client is using denial as a coping mechanism, you must be alert to whether he or she is overlooking necessary information. Other clients may state that they feel overwhelmed and unable to cope, but with help, they can reduce their multiple interacting stressors to manageable pieces. As in all interactions with the client, you must respect the confidentiality and sensitivity of the information shared.

safety alert Medical conditions such as sleep apnea and thyroid dysfunction that are common in older adults can initially cause symptoms that mimic stress-related symptoms. For this reason, a thorough physical assessment of an older adult who appears stressed or anxious is necessary to rule out potentially serious medical disorders. In addition, in older adults, signs of stress and crisis must be differentiated from emerging dementia and also from acute confusion, a condition that can be life-threatening.

Objective Findings

You obtain further findings about stress and coping by observing the client's appearance and nonverbal behaviour during the interview, including grooming and hygiene, handshake and gait, body language, speech quality, eye contact, and attitude. Before or at the end of the interview, depending on the client's anxiety level, you take basic vital signs to assess for physiological signs of stress, such as elevated blood pressure, heart rate, or respiratory rate (Figure 30–4).

Client Expectations

It is crucial that you understand the meaning the client attaches to the precipitating event and how stress is affecting the client's life. You must allow the client time to express priorities for coping. For example, if a woman has just been told that a breast mass was identified on a routine mammogram, you must discern what the client wants and needs most from you. Some clients identify an immediate need for information about biopsy or mastectomy; others need guidance and support on how to share the news with family members. In some cases, when nothing can be done to change or improve the situation, allowing the client to use denial as a coping mechanism can be help-

Knowledge
- Basic stress response

Experience
- Caring for clients whose

Safety Alerts indicate techniques you can use to ensure client and nurse safety.

Cultural Aspects of Care boxes prepare you to care for clients of diverse populations and suggest actions needed to meet different cultural needs and preferences.

Procedural Guidelines provide streamlined, step-by-step instructions for performing basic skills.

Nursing Story boxes tell a real-life story concerning one or more topics in the chapter.

BOX 45-9 Procedural Guidelines

Digital Removal of Stool

Delegation Considerations: The digital removal of stool procedure should not be delegated to unregulated care providers.

Equipment

- Bath blanket
- Waterproof pad
- Disposable gloves
- Lubricant
- Towel
- Washcloth
- Soap and water
- Bedpan

Procedure

1. Explain the procedure to the client.
2. Perform hand hygiene. Take baseline vital signs prior to the procedure. Help the client to lie on the left side with knees flexed and back toward you.
3. Drape the trunk and lower extremities with a bath blanket and place a waterproof pad under the buttocks. Keep a bedpan next to the client.
4. Apply disposable gloves and lubricate the index finger of your dominant hand with lubricating jelly.
5. Gently insert the gloved index finger into the rectum and advance the finger slowly along the rectal wall toward the umbilicus.
6. Gently loosen the fecal mass by massaging around it. Work the finger into the hardened mass.
7. Work the feces downward toward the end of the rectum. Remove small pieces at a time and discard into the bedpan.
8. Reassess the client's vital signs and look for signs of fatigue. Stop the procedure if the heart rate drops significantly or if the heart rhythm changes.
9. Continue to remove feces and allow the client to rest at intervals.
10. After completion, wash and dry the buttocks and anal area.
11. Remove the bedpan and dispose of the feces. Remove gloves by turning them inside out, and then discard.
12. Assist the client to the toilet or position the client on a clean bedpan if the urge to defecate develops.
13. Perform hand hygiene. Record results of the removal of the impaction by describing the fecal characteristics.
14. Follow the procedure with enemas or cathartics as ordered by physician.
15. Reassess the client's vital signs and level of comfort.

BOX 45-10 NURSING STORY

Disimpaction Is a Painful Stimulus

The first time I, as a newly hired nursing instructor, took fourth-year students to a clinical experience, we attended a small (8-bed) neurological intensive care unit. One client, a young man in his late teens who was conscious but still confused, was recovering from a motorbike accident. The student who was assigned to this client read the doctor's order for rectal disimpaction (the client's bowels had not moved since the accident five days previously). The student and I discussed in great detail the procedure and came to a disagreement about the highest priority for the client after safety. I said that the student required assistance, but she said no the greater need was for the client's privacy. As I hovered near the curtains, she explained the procedure to the young man, assessed his vital signs, prepared the bedpan, put on her gloves, lubricated her index finger, and drew the curtains ever tighter. She then attempted to insert her gloved, lubricated finger into the rectum. To the young man, this was a startling procedure (although it had been verbally explained to him). I heard a loud yell from the client and the clatter of a bedpan bouncing across the floor, and then a bedraggled nursing cap sailed under the curtains. I rushed behind the curtains to rescue the student from the flailing arms of the strong young man. No harm was done and the student gratefully accepted assistance from the orderly.

Lesson learned: disimpaction is a strong, noxious stimulus and the client's reactions may be unpredictable. In an older adult client, the reaction may even be pathological, such as a cardiovascular response or increased heart rate and blood pressure from sympathetic stimulation. In very ill clients, the crash cart should be present at the bedside because a cardiac arrest could ensue.

As a footnote to the story, this student and I had a several further disagreements that year. Several years later, however, I received a note from this woman, who was now teaching nursing herself. She apologized for her behaviour. She had taught several students who had reminded her of herself when she was a student, she said; and now she wondered how I ever put up with her behaviour.

TABLE 45-6 Purposes of Nasogastric Intubation

Purpose	Description	Type of Tube
Decompression	Removal of secretions and gaseous substances from the gastrointestinal tract to prevent or relieve abdominal distension	Salem sump, Levin, Miller-Abbott
Feeding (i.e., gavage; see Chapter 43)	Instillation of liquid nutritional supplements or feedings into the stomach for clients unable to swallow fluid	Duo, Dobhoff, Levin
Compression	Internal application of pressure by means of an inflated balloon to prevent internal esophageal or gastrointestinal hemorrhage	Sengstaken-Blakemore
Lavage	Irrigation of the stomach in cases of active bleeding, poisoning, or gastric dilation	Levin, Ewald, Salem sump

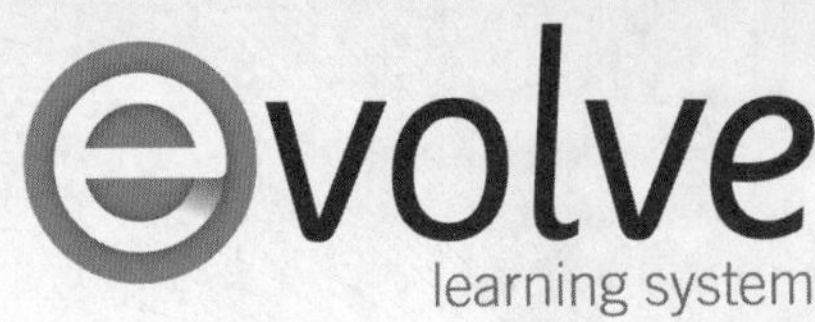

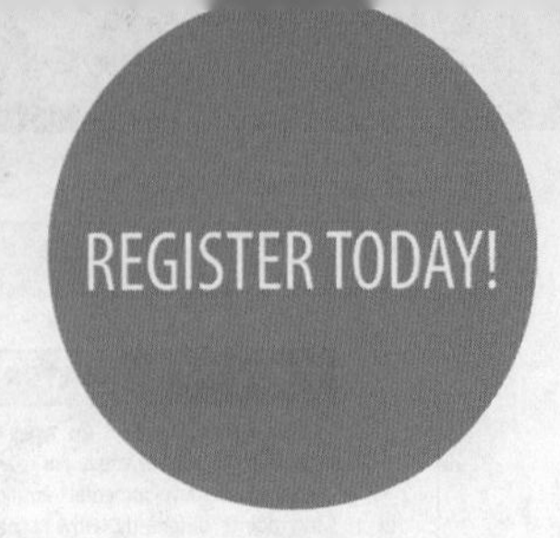

Evolve provides online access to free learning resources and activities designed specifically for the textbook you are using in your class. The resources will provide you with information that enhances the material covered in the book and much more.

Visit the Web address listed below to start your learning evolution today!

http://evolve.elsevier.com/Canada/Potter/fundamentals/

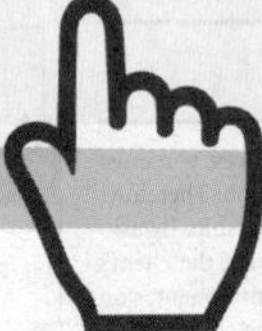

Evolve® Student Learning Resources for Potter & Perry,* Canadian Fundamentals of Nursing, 4th Edition, *offer the following features:

Student Resources

- **Audio Summaries for each chapter are downloadable to an MP3 device or CD.**
- **Student Learning Activities include Hangman, Match Its, and Drag and Drop exercises.**
- **Animations feature exciting images related to various chapters in the textbook.**
- **Video Clips demonstrate important aspects of various nursing skills described in the textbook.**
- **Web links are a useful resource that allows you link to hundreds of Web sites carefully chosen to supplement the content of the textbook.**
- **Content Updates include the latest information from the authors of the textbook to help you keep abreast of recent developments in select areas of study.**

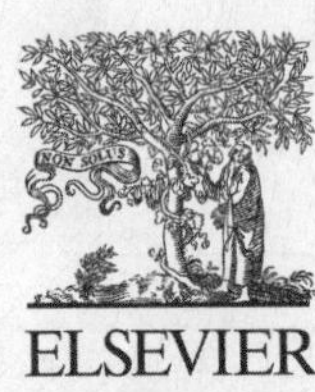

Preface to the Instructor

The future of nursing in Canada looks promising. Dynamic change and ongoing development of the discipline point to the need for extensive and wide-ranging knowledge as the foundation of good care. The nurses of tomorrow will need to practise outstanding nursing and demonstrate its importance in maintaining and improving the health of Canadians. Nursing practice will be characterized by critical thinking, client advocacy, excellence in clinical decision making, and client teaching within a broad spectrum of health services.

Canadian Fundamentals of Nursing is designed for beginning students in all types of professional nursing programs. The text provides comprehensive coverage of fundamental nursing concepts, skills, and techniques required for safe and competent nursing practice.

The fourth edition of *Canadian Fundamentals of Nursing* has been extensively revised and thoroughly edited for easier reading and understanding. Across its 49 chapters, the text is more concise than in the previous edition. All chapters have been written or revised so that they reflect Canadian standards, traditions, research, and practice. The text is organized to indicate the order in which topics are usually taught. For example, foundational chapters such as "The Development of Nursing in Canada" and "Research as a Basis for Practice" appear in Unit I.

Canadian Fundamentals of Nursing includes content covering the entire scope of primary, acute, and restorative care. The focus is on the central role of primary health care in all areas of nursing practice. Emphasis is also placed on evidence-informed practice in skills and care plans to foster understanding of how research findings should guide clinical decision making. The book includes concept maps that demonstrate the relationships among nursing assessment, diagnosis, planning, intervention, and evaluation. In the form of Nursing Stories, first-person accounts of issues that have arisen in nursing practice are designed to engage the student's attention and encourage more detailed reading and understanding.

New to this edition is an **Editorial Advisory Board** comprising three prominent Canadian nurses who are leaders in nursing education in Canada. For this task, we chose three accomplished individuals from diverse regions of the country: Dr. Sally Thorne, Director and Professor of the School of Nursing at the University of British Columbia, is well known as a researcher and theoretician in nursing. Her research has focused upon applying conceptual knowledge to nursing practice, critical thinking, nursing theory and the philosophy of nursing science. Dr. Shirley Solberg, Associate Professor, School of Nursing, Memorial University of Newfoundland, researches women's health, health promotion and education, primary care, and cancer care. Dr. Ann Tournageau, Associate Professor, Faculty of Nursing, University of Toronto and Adjunct Scientist, Institute for Clinical Evaluative Studies in Ontario, holds a Career Scientist award from the Ontario Ministry of Health and Long-Term Care. Her research and teaching centre on nursing outcomes, in which she evaluates the contribution of nursing care and nursing work environments to client and organizational outcomes. Moreover, our Editorial Advisory Board consulted with us to ensure that all aspects of the book are current and attuned to the needs of beginning nursing students across the country.

One of the many issues about which we consulted our board was our choice of terminology. For this edition, we have chosen not to use the familiar term "evidence-based practice." We have chosen instead to use **evidence-*informed* practice** because although "evidence-based policy" is used in the literature, it largely relates to one type of evidence only: research. Using the term "evidence-influenced" or "evidence-informed" reflects the need to be context sensitive and to consider use of the best available evidence in dealing with everyday circumstances. A variety of distinct pieces of evidence and sources of knowledge inform policy, such as histories and experience, beliefs, values, competency or skills, legislation, politics and politicians, protocols, and research results.

This textbook is the result of the combined efforts of many talented professionals committed to excellence. Expert contributors from across Canada approached the revision with enthusiasm, and worked hard to ensure that the content is current and reflects the Canadian health care system, Canadian health and social organizations, and uniquely Canadian health care issues. Reviewers scrutinized the chapters and made many helpful suggestions. We appreciate the conscientiousness and enthusiasm of all these dedicated professionals.

Classic Features

- **Comprehensive** coverage and readability of all fundamental nursing content are provided.
- **Full-colour** text is used to enhance visual appeal and instructional value.
- **Primary health care and health promotion** issues are discussed throughout the text.
- **Focus on Primary Health Care** boxes highlight how the principles of primary health care can be applied to the topic of the chapter; the context of each of these boxes pertains uniquely to Canadian health care.
- **Health promotion, acute and tertiary care,** and **restorative care** are covered in order to address today's practice in various settings.
- **Cultural diversity** is presented in Chapter 10, stressed in clinical examples throughout the text, and highlighted in special boxes.
- **Research Highlight** boxes are integrated throughout the text to provide current nursing research studies and explain the implications for daily practice; many of these present Canadian research.
- **Client education** is stressed in boxes that list teaching objectives, strategies, and evaluation for clinical topics throughout the text.
- **Evidence-informed practice** is discussed throughout the text.
- **Evidence-Informed Practice Guidelines** boxes provide examples of recent state-of-the-science guidelines for nursing practice.
- **Gerontological nursing** principles are addressed in Chapter 25, as well as in special **Focus on Older Adults** boxes throughout the text.
- **Health Assessment and Physical Examination** (Chapter 32) provides students with important background in this important area of practice.
- **Diverse clinical settings,** including clinics, long-term-care facilities, and the home, as well as acute care settings, are described.
- **Historical boxes** entitled **"Milestones in Canadian History"** provide information about nursing leaders and critical events in Canadian nursing history.

- **Critical thinking** in clinical chapters is presented through a dimensional **critical thinking model** that visually demonstrates the ongoing assimilation of knowledge, critical thinking attitudes, intellectual and professional standards, and experience in relationship to clinical decision making and the nursing process.
- **Nursing Care Plans** guide students on how to conduct an assessment and analyze the defining characteristics that indicate nursing diagnoses. The plans include Nursing Interventions Classification (NIC) and Nursing Outcomes Classification (NOC) to familiarize students with this important nomenclature. The evaluation sections of the plans show students how to determine the expected outcomes and evaluate the results of care.
- Important nursing skills are presented in a clear, two-column format with a rationale for all steps; whenever possible, rationales are based on the most current research evidence.
- **Unexpected Outcomes and Related Interventions** are highlighted within discussions of nursing skills.
- **Critical pathways** address collaborative care in home and acute care settings.
- **Concept maps** demonstrate the relationship between nursing assessment, diagnosis, planning, intervention, and evaluation.
- **Procedural Guidelines** boxes provide streamlined, step-by-step instructions about how to perform basic skills.
- **Video Icons** indicate video clips associated with specific skills that are available on the free CD-Companion and Evolve Student Learning Resources.
- **End-of-chapter review questions** help students review and evaluate what they have learned. Answers and rationales are provided at the end of the book.
- The annotated **Recommended Web Sites** sections at the end of each chapter direct the student to current Web-based resources, most of which are Canadian.

New Features

- New chapter on **Nursing Informatics** (Chapter 17), written by leading Canadian nursing authorities, helps students to understand the growing dimensions of computerization in nursing practice.
- New chapter on **Caring for the Cancer Survivor** (Chapter 5) helps students support clients and families facing cancer.
- Extensively revised **Community Health Nursing Practice** chapter (Chapter 4) now includes discussions of home care and rural health care.
- **Nursing process content** has been condensed and is presented in Chapters 13, 14, and 15, making key concepts clearer for students.
- **Nursing Story** boxes present first-person accounts of issues in relation to chapter content.
- **References** have been updated throughout to include Canadian research and practice standards, such as the best nursing practice guidelines of Health Canada, Statistics Canada, the Canadian Nurses Association, and the Registered Nurses Association of Ontario. References have been organized by chapter and compiled at the end of the text.
- **Media Resources** boxes detail available electronic resources.
- Free **CD Companion** in each text has been enhanced to include Test-Taking Skills, in addition to Butterfield's Fluids and Electrolytes program, interactive exercises, and a glossary.
- Updated **Practical Nursing in Canada** appendix (Appendix A) provides important information on this nursing role in Canada.
- New **Laboratory Values** appendix (Appendix B) is a concise, up-to-date source of current laboratory values for use in clinical practice.

Ancillaries

For the Student

Free Companion CD-ROM in each text includes Test-Taking Skills and Review Questions, in addition to Butterfield's Fluids and Electrolytes program, interactive learning activities, and an audio glossary.

Evolve Course Web site enables students to access downloadable audio and video clips for on-the-go learning with portable media devices, plus review questions, Mosby's Nursing Skills video clips, audio chapter summaries, a searchable Spanish–English audio glossary, Butterfield's Fluids and Electrolytes Tutorial, test-taking tips, and chapter-specific Web links.

Study Guide and Skills Performance Checklists provide ideal supplements to help students understand and apply the content of the text. Each chapter includes multiple sections:

- Preliminary reading includes a chapter assignment from the text.
- Comprehensive understanding provides a variety of activities to reinforce the topics and main ideas from the text.
- Review questions are multiple-choice, requiring students to provide rationales for their answers. Answers and rationales are provided in the answer key.
- Clinical chapters include critical thinking models that expand the case study from the chapter's care plan; students are asked to develop a step in the model on the basis of the actions of the nurse and client in the scenario. This helps students learn to apply both content learned and the critical thinking synthesis model.
- Skills performance checklists are included so that students can evaluate skill competency.

Clinical Companion is a concise, portable guide that features all of the facts and figures that students need to know in their early clinical experiences.

Virtual Clinical Excursions is a workbook and CD-ROM package that provides a hands-on learning experience in which students care for a variety of clients on a multifloor virtual hospital.

Nursing Skills Online focuses on the skills that are most difficult to teach and those that pose the greatest risk to client safety; this one-of-a-kind, interactive, and evaluative online course engages students in media-rich learning modules with realistic, case-based lessons to help students review and evaluate their competency before performing skills in the clinical setting.

For the Instructor

Integrated lesson plans give you everything you need to deliver effective lectures, engage student learning, and provide application opportunities, including live links to teaching resources and classroom teaching strategies.

Evolve Online Courseware includes secure access to integrated lesson plans, an ExamView computerized test bank, an electronic image collection, PowerPoint slides, and all student online resources.

Mosby's Nursing Video Skills on DVD helps you show your students how to perform nursing skills safely. Version 3.0 includes all-new footage and an exciting, interactive format on basic, intermediate, and advanced DVDs. Sold separately.

Acknowledgements

Developing a nursing text for the Canadian market is an enormous undertaking, and in this fourth Canadian edition, every chapter has been written by expert Canadian nurses. We acknowledge the contributions of each of our Canadian authors, who developed and wrote outstanding material in a short time frame. Their dedication and expertise is evident throughout, and we thank them for the extraordinary effort they put forward to make this book a success.

The Editorial Advisory Board, composed of three experts—Dr. Shirley Solberg, Dr. Sally Thorne, and Dr. Ann Tourangeau—provided outstanding direction for the fourth Canadian edition. In addition, the appointment of section editors was a new feature of this edition. The individuals who served in this capacity, providing support to the authors and editors, were Dr. Barbara Astle, Dr. Sonya Grypma, and Dr. Nicole Letourneau.

Toni Chahley, Developmental Editor, provided excellent leadership and capable organization of all parts of the developmental process and has been extremely supportive of all the authors and editors. We are grateful to her for her skill, hard work, and dedication to the task. We would also like to thank Lise Dupont, Managing Production Editor, Elsevier Canada.

Ann Millar, Publisher, Elsevier Canada, is a visionary leader who was highly involved in the development of the fourth Canadian edition of *Canadian Fundamentals of Nursing*. We thank her for all her efforts; without her, this edition would not have been possible.

Janet C. Ross-Kerr
Marilynn J. Wood

Canadian Contributors

CANADIAN EDITORS

Janet C. Ross-Kerr, RN, BScN, MS, PhD
Professor Emeritus
Faculty of Nursing
University of Alberta
Edmonton, Alberta

Marilynn J. Wood, BSN, MSN, DrPH
Professor Emeritus
Faculty of Nursing
University of Alberta
Edmonton, Alberta

CANADIAN SECTION EDITORS

Barbara Astle, RN, PhD
Faculty of Nursing
University of Alberta
Calgary, Alberta

Sonya Grypma, RN, PhD
Associate Professor
School of Nursing
Trinity Western University
Langley, British Columbia

Nicole Letourneau, RN, PhD
Canada Research Chair in Healthy Child Development
Peter Lougheed/CIHR New Investigator (honourary)
Professor
Faculty of Nursing and Research Fellow CRISP
University of New Brunswick
Fredericton, New Brunswick

CANADIAN EDITORIAL ADVISORY BOARD

Shirley M. Solberg, RN, PhD
Professor
School of Nursing
Memorial University of Newfoundland
St. John's, Newfoundland and Labrador

Sally Thorne, RN, PhD
Professor and Director
School of Nursing
University of British Columbia
Vancouver, British Columbia

Ann Tourangeau, RN, PhD
Associate Professor and Career Scientist
The Lawrence S. Bloomberg Faculty of Nursing
University of Toronto
Toronto, Ontario

CANADIAN CONTRIBUTORS

Marion Allen, RN, PhD
Professor Emeritus
University of Alberta
Edmonton, Alberta

Marjorie C. Anderson, RN, PhD
Associate Professor (Retired)
University of Alberta
Edmonton, Alberta

Colleen Astle, RN, MN
Nurse Practitioner, Nephrology
University of Alberta Hospital, Grey Nuns Hospital
Edmonton, Alberta

Maureen A. Barry, RN, MScN
Senior Lecturer
Lawrence S. Bloomberg Faculty of Nursing
University of Toronto
Toronto, Ontario

Sylvia S. Barton, RN, PhD
Associate Professor
University of Alberta
Edmonton, Alberta

Yvonne G. Briggs, RN, BScN, MN
Faculty, School of Nursing
Grant MacEwan College
Edmonton, Alberta

Ann Brokenshire, RN, BScN, MEd
Instructor
Daphne Cockwell School of Nursing
Ryerson University
Toronto, Ontario

Phyllis Castelein, RN, MN
Faculty Lecturer
University of Alberta
Edmonton, Alberta

Marion Clauson, RN, MSN
Senior Instructor
School of Nursing
University of British Columbia
Vancouver, British Columbia

Rene A. Day, RN, PhD
Professor
University of Alberta
Edmonton, Alberta

Wendy Duggleby, RN, PhD
Professor
University of Saskatchewan
Saskatoon, Saskatchewan

Susan Duncan, RN, PhD
Dean
School of Nursing
Thompson Rivers University
Kamloops, British Columbia

Kaysi Eastlick Kushner, RN, PhD
Associate Professor
University of Alberta
Edmonton, Alberta

Nancy Edgecombe, RN-NP, BN, MN, PhD
Assistant Professor
School of Nursing
Dalhousie University
Halifax, Nova Scotia

Frances Fothergill-Bourbonnais, RN, PhD
Full Professor
School of Nursing, Faculty of Health Sciences
University of Ottawa
Ottawa, Ontario

Jo-Ann E.T. Fox-Threlkeld, RN, BN, MSc, PhD
Professor Emeritus
McMaster University
Hamilton, Ontario

Nancy Goddard, RN, PhD
Nursing Instructor
Red Deer College
Red Deer, Alberta

Kathryn J. Hannah, RN, PhD
President
HECS Inc.
and
Professor (ADJ)
Department of Community Health Science
Faculty of Medicine
University of Calgary
Calgary, Canada

Giuliana Harvey, RN, MN
Lecturer
University of Toronto
Toronto, Ontario

Kathy Hegadoren, RN, PhD
Professor
University of Alberta
Edmonton, Alberta

Deborah Hobbs, RN, BScN, CIC
Infection Control Practitioner
University of Alberta Hospital
Edmonton, Alberta

Jim Hunter, RN, MSN
Program Head, Year 2
British Columbia Institute of Technology
Burnaby, British Columbia

Kathleen F. Hunter, RN, NP, PhD GNC(C)
Assistant Professor
Faculty of Nursing, University of Alberta
and
Nurse Practitioner
Capital Health Specialized Geriatric Services
Edmonton, Alberta

Darlaine Jantzen, RN, MA, PhD(c)
University of Alberta
Nursing Faculty
Camosun College
Victoria, British Columbia

Willy Kabotoff, RN, BScN, MN
Faculty Lecturer
University of Alberta
Edmonton, Alberta

Anne Katz, RN, PhD
Adjunct Professor
University of Manitoba
Winnipeg, Manitoba

Margaret Ann Kennedy, RN, PhD
President
Kennedy Health Informatics Inc.
Merigomish, Nova Scotia

Rosemary Kohr, RN, PhD, ACNP(cert)
Advanced Practice Nurse
London Health Sciences Centre
and
Assistant Professor
Faculty of Health Sciences
University of Western Ontario
London, Ontario

Francis Loos, RN, MN, CNCC(C)
Clinical Nurse–Post Anesthetic Care Unit
Regina Qu'Appelle Health Region
Regina, Saskatchewan

Jeannie McClennon-Leong, RN, MN, APNP
ADN Instructor
Northeast Wisconsin Technical College
Green Bay, Wisconsin

Jill Milne, RN, PhD
Research Associate, Adjunct Assistant Professor
Faculty of Medicine
University of Calgary
Calgary, Alberta

Anita E. Molzahn, RN, MN, PhD
Professor and Dean
Faculty of Nursing
University of Alberta
Edmonton, Alberta

Judee E. Onyskiw, RN, BScN, MN, PhD
Educator, and Research and Scholarship Advisor
Faculty of Health and Community Studies
MacEwan College
Edmonton, Alberta

Jan Park Dorsay, RN(EC), MN, NP, CON(C)
Advanced Practice Nurse,
Rehabilitation
Hamilton Health Sciences
and
Assistant Clinical Professor
School of Nursing
McMaster University
Hamilton, Ontario

Barb Pesut, RN, PhD
Assistant Professor
School of Nursing
University of British Columbia Okanagan
Kelowna, British Columbia

Pammla Petrucka, RN, PhD
Associate Professor
University of Saskatchewan (Regina Site)
Regina, Saskatchewan

Shelley Raffin Bouchal, RN, PhD
Associate Professor
Faculty of Nursing
University of Calgary
Calgary, Alberta

Linda Reutter, RN, PhD
Professor
Faculty of Nursing
University of Alberta
Edmonton, Alberta

Daria Romaniuk, RN, BN, MN, PhD(c)
Assistant Professor
Daphne Cockwell School of Nursing
Ryerson University
Toronto, Ontario

Donna M. Romyn, RN, PhD
Director and Associate Professor
Centre for Nursing and Health Studies
Athabasca University
Athabasca, Alberta

Cheryl Sams, RN, MSN
Professor
Seneca College
Toronto, Ontario

Brett Sanderson, BScPT
Physiotherapist
Hamilton Health Sciences
Henderson Hospital
Hamilton, Ontario

Carla Shapiro, RN, MN
Instructor II
University of Manitoba
Winnipeg, Manitoba

D. Lynn Skillen, RN, PhD
Professor Emerita
University of Alberta
Edmonton, Alberta

Kathryn A. Smith Higuchi, RN, PhD
Assistant Professor
School of Nursing
University of Ottawa
Ottawa, Ontario

Shirley M. Solberg, RN, PhD
Professor
Memorial University of Newfoundland
St. John's, Newfoundland and Labrador

Tracey C. Stephen, RN, MN
Faculty Lecturer
University of Alberta
Edmonton, Alberta

Sally Thorne, RN, PhD
Professor and Director
University of British Columbia
Vancouver, British Columbia

Jill E. Vihos, RN, BScN, MN, PhD(c)
Faculty Lecturer
University of Alberta
Edmonton, Alberta

Fay F. Warnock, RN, PhD
Michael Smith Foundation for Health Research Scholar
Nurse Scientist, Children's and Women's Health Centre of British Columbia
and
Assistant Professor
School of Nursing
University of British Columbia
Vancouver, British Columbia

Kathryn Weaver, RN, PhD
Associate Professor
Faculty of Nursing
University of New Brunswick
Fredericton, New Brunswick

US Contributors

Marjorie Baier, RN, PhD
Associate Professor
School of Nursing
Southern Illinois University
Edwardsville, Illinois

Sylvia K. Baird, RN, BSN, MM
Manager of Nursing Quality
Spectrum Health
Grand Rapids, Michigan

Karen Balakas, RN, PhD, CNE
Associate Professor
Goldfarb School of Nursing at Barnes-Jewish College
St. Louis, Missouri

Lois Bentler-Lampe, RN, MS
Instructor
Saint Francis Medical Center College of Nursing
Peoria, Illinois

Sheryl Buckner, RN-BC, MS, CNE
Academic and Staff Developer and Clinical Instructor
College of Nursing
University of Oklahoma
Oklahoma City, Oklahoma

Jeri Burger, RN, PhD
Assistant Professor
College of Nursing and Health Professions
University of Southern Indiana
Evansville, Indiana

Janice C. Colwell, RN, MS, CWOCN, FAAN
Clinical Nurse Specialist
University of Chicago Hospitals
Chicago, Illinois

Eileen Costantinou, RN, MSN, BC
Consultant
Center for Practice Excellence
Barnes-Jewish Hospital
St. Louis, Missouri

Margaret Ecker, RN, MS
Director, Nursing Quality
Kaiser Permanente Los Angeles Medical Center
Los Angeles, California

Susan J. Fetzer, RN, PA, BSN, MSN, MBA, PhD
Associate Professor
College of Health and Human Services
University of New Hampshire
Durham, New Hampshire

Victoria N. Folse, APRN, BC, LCPC, PhD
Assistant Professor
School of Nursing, Illinois Wesleyan University
Bloomington, Illinois

Steve Kilkus, RN, MSN
Faculty
Edgewood College School of Nursing
Madison, Wisconsin

Judith Ann Kilpatrick, RN, MSN, DNSc
Assistant Professor
Widener University School of Nursing
Chester, Pennsylvania

Lori Klingman, RN, MSN
Faculty
School of Nursing
Ohio Valley General Hospital
McKees Rocks, Pennsylvania

Anahid Kulwicki, RN, DNS, FAAN
Deputy Director
Wayne County Department of Health and Human Services
and
Professor
Oakland University
School of Nursing
Rochester, Michigan

Annette Lueckenotte, RN, MS, BC, GNP, GCNS
Gerontologic Clinical Nurse Specialist
Barnes-Jewish West County Hospital
Creve Coeur, Missouri

Barbara Maxwell, RN, BSN, MS, MSN, CNS
Associate Professor of Nursing
Ulster Department of Nursing
The State University New York
Stone Ridge, New York

Elaine Neel, RN, BSN, MSN
Nursing Instructor
Graham Hospital School of Nursing
Canton, Illinois

Wendy Ostendorf, BSN, MS, EdD
Associate Professor
Neumann College
Aston, Pennsylvania

Patsy Ruchala, RN, DNSc
Director and Professor
Orvis School of Nursing
University of Nevada–Reno
Reno, Nevada

Lynn Schallom, MSN, CCRN, CCNS
Clinical Nurse Specialist
Surgical Critical Care
Barnes-Jewish Hospital
St. Louis, Missouri

Ann Tritak, BS, MS, EdD
Dean of Nursing
School of Nursing
Saint Peter's College
Jersey City, New Jersey

Janis Waite, RN, MSN, EdD
Professor of Nursing
Saint Francis Medical Center College of Nursing
Peoria, Illinois

Jill Weberski, RN, MSN, PCCN, CNS
Instructor
Saint Francis Medical Center College of Nursing
Peoria, Illinois

Mary Ann Wehmer, RN, MSN, CNOR
Nursing Faculty
College of Nursing and Health Professions
University of Southern Indiana
Evansville, Indiana

Joan Wentz, RN, MSN
(Retired) Assistant Professor of Nursing
Goldfarb School of Nursing at Barnes-Jewish College
St. Louis, Missouri

Katherine West, BSN, MSEd, CIC
Infection Control Consultant
Infection Control/Emerging Concepts, Inc.
Manassas, Virginia

Rita Wunderlich, RN, MSN(R), PhD
Chair, Baccalaureate Nursing Program
St. Louis University School of Nursing
St. Louis, Missouri

Valerie Yancey, RN, PhD
Associate Professor
Southern Illinois University
Edwardsville, Illinois

Reviewers

Catherine Aquino-Rusell, BScN, MN, PhD
Associate Professor, Faculty of Nursing
University of New Brunswick
Moncton, New Brunswick

Heidi Matarasso Bakerman, RN, BA, MScN
Nursing Instructor
Vanier College
St. Laurent, Quebec

Lisa Barrett, RN, MN, RPN
Faculty Lecturer, Faculty of Nursing
University of Alberta
Edmonton, Alberta

Kathleen Barrington, RN, MEd
Coordinator, PN Program
Centre for Nursing Studies
St. John's, Newfoundland and Labrador

Maureen Barry, RN, MScN
Senior Lecturer, Lawrence S. Bloomberg Faculty of Nursing
University of Toronto
Toronto, Ontario

Zoraida DeCastro Beekhoo, RN, MA
Lecturer, Lawrence S. Bloomberg Faculty of Nursing
University of Toronto
Toronto, Ontario

Arleigh Bell, RN, BSN, MN
BSN Faculty
Kwantlen Polytechnic University
Surrey, British Columbia

Christine Boyle, RN, BScN, MA
Faculty
Mount Royal College
Calgary, Alberta

Roni Clubb, RN, BScN, MScN
Faculty, Practical Nursing Program
Saskatchewan Institute of Applied Science and Technology
Regina, Saskatchewan

Mary Jane Comiskey, RN, BScN, BEd
Professor, Nursing
School of Health and Community Services
Lambton College of Applied Arts and Technology
Sarnia, Ontario

Michelle Connell, BScN, MEd
Professor and Coordinator, Collaborative Nursing Degree Program
Centennial College
Scarborough, Ontario

Donna Cooke, RN, BSN, MN
Faculty, Nursing Education Program
Saskatchewan Institute of Applied Science and Technology
Regina, Saskatchewan

Fiona D'Costa-Box, RN, BA (Hons.), BScN, MScN
Professor, Nursing
School of Health and Community Services
Lambton College of Applied Arts and Technology
Sarnia, Ontario

Julie Duff Cloutier, RN, BScN, MSc
Assistant Professor, School of Nursing
Laurentian University
Sudbury, Ontario

Lynne Esson, RN, BSN
Lecturer, School of Nursing
University of British Columbia
Vancouver, British Columbia

Wendy Fostey, RN, BHScN, MHScN
Professor, Nursing
NEOCNP Collaborative BScN Program
Sault College
Sault Ste. Marie, Ontario

Marla Fraser, RN, BSN
Faculty, Practical Nursing Program
Saskatchewan Institute of Science and Technology
Regina, Saskatchewan

Jacalynne Glover, RN, MN, IBCLC
Faculty, Nursing Education in Southwestern Alberta (NESA)
Lethbridge College
Lethbridge, Alberta

Jackie Halliday, RN, BSN, MN
Instructor, Faculty of Community and Health Studies BSN Program
Kwantlen Polytechnic University
Surrey, British Columbia

Rae Harwood, RN, BN, MA
Clinical Course Leader, Faculty of Nursing
University of Manitoba
Winnipeg, Manitoba

Vicki Holmes, RN, BScN, MScN
Assistant Professor, School of Nursing
Thompson Rivers University
Kamloops, British Columbia

Kerri L. Honeychurch, RN, BScN, MEd
Coordinator and Professor, School of Health Sciences
Seneca College of Applied Arts and Technology
Toronto, Ontario

Jean Jackson, RN, MEd
Professor, School of Health and Community Services
Durham College
Oshawa, Ontario

Lynda Johnston, RN, BSN, MEd
Program Faculty, BSN Program
Douglas College
Coquitlam, British Columbia

Jo-Ann MacDonald, RN, BScN, MN, PhD(c)
Assistant Professor, Faculty of Nursing
University of Prince Edward Island
Charlottetown, Prince Edward Island

M. Star Mahara, RN, BSN, MSN
Assistant Professor, School of Nursing
Thompson Rivers University
Kamloops, British Columbia

Claire Marshall, RN, CMH, BTSN
Instructor, Practical Nursing Program
Vancouver Island University
Nanaimo, British Columbia

Karey D. McCullough, BScN, MScN, PhD(c)
Assistant Professor, School of Nursing
Nipissing University
North Bay, Ontario

Florence Melchior, RN, PhD
Nursing Instructor, Health Studies
Medicine Hat College
Medicine Hat, Alberta

Barbara Morrison, RN, HBScN, MEd
Professor, Nursing
Confederation College
Thunder Bay, Ontario

Enid Muirhead, RN, BScN, MEd
Clinical Associate
University of British Columbia
Vancouver, British Columbia

Denise Newton-Mathur, RN, BA, MA
Assistant Professor, School of Nursing
Laurentian University
Sudbury, Ontario

Wanda Pierson, BSN, MSN, MA, PhD
Chair, Nursing Department
Langara College
Vancouver, British Columbia

Joanne Profetto-McGrath, RN, BScN, BA Psych, MEd, PhD
Associate Professor, Faculty of Nursing
and
Associate Dean, Executive and Partnership Development
University of Alberta
Edmonton, Alberta

Michael Scarcello, RN, HBScN, MA(N)(c)
Professor, Practical Nursing Program
School of Health and Community Services
Confederation College
Thunder Bay, Ontario

Candide Sloboda, BN, MEd
Faculty Lecturer, Faculty of Nursing
University of Alberta
Edmonton, Alberta

Lynne Thibeault, RN(EC), BScN, MEd, DNP(c)
Professor, Nursing
Confederation College
Thunder Bay, Ontario

Wendy Wagner, RN, BScN, MA, CACE, RYT
Nursing Instructor
Malaspina University-College
Nanaimo, British Columbia

Molly Westland, RN, BScN, MN, CCHN(c)
Program Coordinator, Trent/Fleming School of Nursing
Trent University
Peterborough, Ontario

Lucille Wittstock, RN, MN
Associate Director, Undergraduate Student Affairs
School of Nursing
Dalhousie University
Halifax, Nova Scotia

Pat Woods, BSN, MSN
Student and Curriculum Coordinator, Department of Nursing
Langara College
Vancouver, British Columbia

1

Health and Wellness

Written by Linda Reutter, RN, PhD,
and Kaysi Eastlick Kushner, RN, PhD

objectives

Mastery of content in this chapter will enable you to:

- Define the key terms listed.
- Discuss ways that definitions of health have been conceptualized.
- Describe key characteristics of medical, behavioural, and socioenvironmental approaches to health.
- Identify factors that have led to each approach to health.
- Discuss contributions of the following Canadian publications to conceptualizations of health and health determinants: *Lalonde Report, Ottawa Charter, Epp Report, Strategies for Population Health, Toronto Charter.*
- Discuss key health determinants and their interrelationships and how they influence health.
- Contrast distinguishing features of health promotion and disease prevention.
- Describe the three levels of disease prevention.
- Identify the five health promotion strategies discussed in the *Ottawa Charter.*
- Analyze how the nature and scope of nursing practice are influenced by different conceptualizations of health and health determinants.

key terms

Behavioural approach, p. 3
Behavioural risk factors, p. 4
Determinants of health, p. 6
Disease, p. 2
Disease prevention, p. 10
Health, p. 2
Health as actualization, p. 2
Health as actualization and stability, p. 2
Health as stability, p. 2
Health disparities, p. 6
Health field concept, p. 3
Health promotion, p. 10
Health promotion strategies, p. 10
Illness, p. 2
Medical approach, p. 3
Physiological risk factors, p. 3
Population health approach, p. 5
Prerequisites for health, p. 4
Psychosocial risk factors, p. 4
Social determinants of health, p. 6
Socioenvironmental approach, p. 4
Socioenvironmental risk conditions, p. 4
Wellness, p. 2

media resources

evolve Web Site

- Audio Chapter Summaries
- Glossary
- Multiple-Choice Review Questions
- Student Learning Activities
- Weblinks

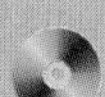
Companion CD

- Glossary
- Interactive Learning Activities
- Fluids and Electrolytes Tutorial
- Test-Taking Skills

Concepts of health and what determines health have changed significantly since the 1970s. This conceptual change has major implications for Canadian nursing in the twenty-first century because how you perceive health—and what determines it—influences the nature and scope of nursing practice. The importance of health to nursing is reflected in nursing models and frameworks, in which health is one of the four "metaparadigm" concepts along with *person, environment,* and *nursing* (see Chapter 6). In each framework, health concepts are congruent with the assumptions and focus of the model.

Conceptualizations of Health

Discussion about the nature of health revolves around its relationship to *disease, illness,* and *wellness.* Often, debates focus on whether health is defined in negative or positive terms. When health is negatively defined as the absence of disease, health and illness are represented on a continuum, with maximum health at one end and death at the other. When health is positively defined, however, health and illness are viewed as distinct but interrelated concepts. Therefore, a person can have disease, such as a chronic pathological condition, and have healthy characteristics as well.

Many people use the words *illness* and *disease* interchangeably. Others suggest that **disease** is an objective state of ill health, the pathological process of which can be detected by medical science, whereas **illness** is a subjective experience of loss of health (Jensen & Allen, 1993; Labonte, 1993; Naidoo & Wills, 1994). Figure 1–1 shows the relationships among health, illness, and disease.

Definitions of health beyond the absence of disease usually have multidimensional components, including physical, mental, social, and spiritual health (e.g., the widely accepted biopsychosocial conceptualization of health put forward by Engel in 1977). Although some scholars have considered this broad definition of health to be synonymous with wellness (Labonte, 1993; Pender et al., 2006), others have argued that health and wellness are different concepts. That is, others have argued that **health** is an objective process characterized by functional stability, balance, and integrity, whereas **wellness** is a subjective experience (Jensen & Allen, 1993; Orem, 1995).

The word *health* is derived from the Old English word *hoelth*, meaning whole of body. Historically, physical wholeness was important for social acceptance, and people with contagious or disfiguring diseases were often ostracized. Good health was considered natural, whereas disease was considered unnatural. As science progressed, disease was regarded less negatively because it could be countered by scientific medicine. After World War II, the World Health Organization (WHO, 1947) in its constitution defined health as "a state of complete physical, mental and social well-being, and not merely the absence of disease or infirmity." This is still the most commonly cited definition of health.

Classifications of Health Conceptualizations

Pender et al. (2006) classified health in three ways:

- **Health as stability.** Health is defined as the maintenance of physiological, functional, and social norms, and it relates to concepts of adaptation and homeostasis.
- **Health as actualization.** Health is defined as the actualization of human potential. Scholars and researchers who adhere to this definition often use the terms *health* and *wellness* interchangeably.
- **Health as actualization and stability.** Both actualization and stabilization concepts are incorporated in the definition of health as "the actualization of inherent and acquired human potential through goal-directed behaviour, competent self-care and satisfying relationships with others, while making adjustments as needed to maintain structural integrity and harmony with relevant environments" (Pender et al., 2006, p. 23).

In 1984, the WHO updated its conceptualization of health as follows:

> "... *the extent to which an individual or group is able, on the one hand, to realize aspirations and satisfy needs; and, on the other hand, to change or cope with the environment. Health is, therefore, seen as a resource for everyday life, not the objective of living; it is a positive concept emphasizing social and personal resources, as well as physical capacities.*" (*p. 3*)

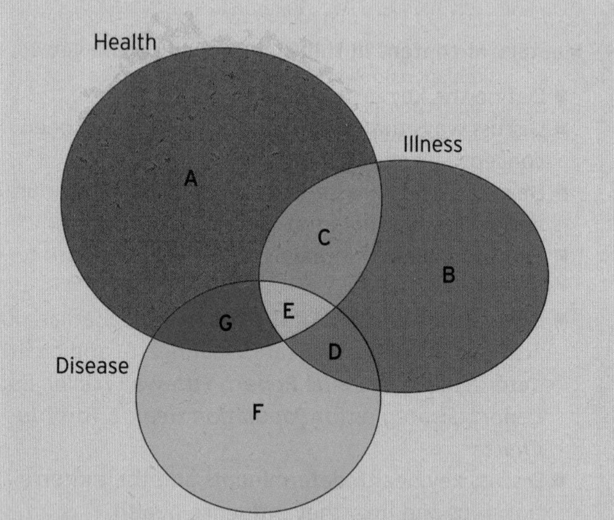

Legend

Circle A represents health or wellness, the clear area being experiences such as feeling vital, enjoying good social relationships, having a sense of purpose in life, and experiencing a connectedness to "community."

Circle B represents experiences of illness, the clear area representing illness that cannot be explained by conventional biomedical concepts and research.

Shaded area C is feeling "so-so," where little is required to tip one into wellness or illness.

Shaded area D is where a diagnosed pathology objectively validates and explains the subjective experience of illness.

Shaded area E represents feeling "so-so," being diagnosed with a pathology, and becoming sick.

Circle F represents diagnosed pathology, the clear area being undiagnosed or silent pathology, such as hypertension, CVD, congenital diseases, or cancers.

Shaded area G represents being diagnosed with a pathology, but still reporting oneself as feeling well or healthy.

Figure 1-1 Health, illness, and disease. **Source:** From Labonte, R. (1993). *Issues in health promotion series. 3. Health promotion and empowerment: Practice frameworks* (p. 18). Toronto, ON: Centre for Health Promotion, University of Toronto, & ParticipACTION.

Rather than viewing health as an ideal state of well-being (as in the 1947 WHO definition), this definition, incorporating both actualization and stability dimensions, suggests that people in a variety of situations—even those with physical disease or nearing death—could be considered healthy.

Labonte (1993) developed a multidimensional conceptualization of health that reflects both actualization and stability perspectives. Aspects include the following qualities:

- Feeling vitalized and full of energy.
- Having satisfying social relationships.
- Having a feeling of control over one's life and living conditions.
- Being able to do things that one enjoys.
- Having a sense of purpose.
- Feeling connected to community.

Using the WHO dimensions of physical, mental, and social well-being, Labonte (1993) categorized these characteristics into a Venn diagram (Figure 1–2). The diagram clearly depicts the concept of holism, whereby health is more than the sum of the component parts in that the interrelationships between and among different components result in different aspects of health.

Nurse scholars use nursing frameworks to conceptualize health in different ways (see Chapter 6). For example, the McGill model concept of health as coping and development is very congruent with the WHO (1984) definition (Gottlieb & Rowat, 1987). Jones and Meleis (1993) articulated health as empowerment: "health is being empowered to define, seek, and find conditions, resources, and processes to be an effective agent in meeting the significant needs perceived by individuals" (p. 12). This conceptualization is congruent with Labonte's (1993) focus and reflects the essence of health promotion, to be discussed later. In a review of the concept of health, Raeburn and Rootman (2007) suggested that in view of current realities of the

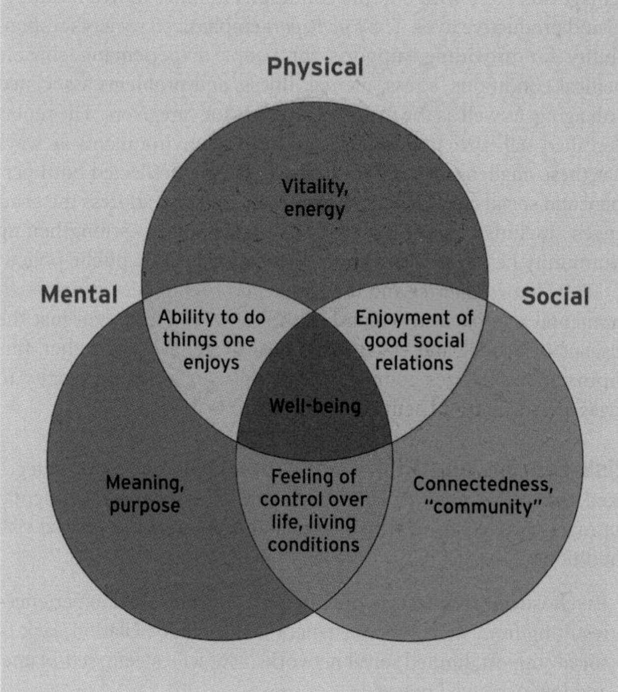

Figure 1-2 Dimensions of health and well-being. **Source:** From Labonte, R. (1993). *Issues in health promotion series. 3. Health promotion and empowerment: Practice frameworks* (p. 20). Toronto, ON: Centre for Health Promotion, University of Toronto, & ParticipACTION.

twenty-first century, a definition of health needs to be positive (not based on pathology or deficit), comprehensive (with a broad set of determinants), particularly attentive to the mental health dimension, and inclusive of quality of life and spirituality.

Historical Approaches to Health in Canada

Definitions of health emerge from different contexts. In modern times, the three major approaches to health have been medical, behavioural, and socioenvironmental (Labonte, 1993). These approaches offer a useful framework for examining the evolution of health orientations in Canada.

Medical Approach

The **medical approach**, which represents a stability orientation to health, dominated Western thinking for most of the twentieth century. It emphasizes that medical intervention restores health. Health problems are defined primarily as **physiological risk factors**—physiologically defined characteristics that are precursors to or risk factors for disease. Examples include hypertension, hypercholesterolemia, genetic predispositions, and obesity. The biopsychosocial view of health (Engel, 1977) includes psychological and social elements; however, in practice, a medical focus on pathology was retained (Antonovsky, 1987). In the medical approach, an adequate health care system is paramount to ensuring that populations remain healthy.

Focusing on treatment of disease was strongly supported after World War II, when new technological and scientific medical advances facilitated the medical approach. In Canada, postwar economic growth increased funding to build new hospitals. National health insurance was created to remove financial barriers to care. Many people believed that scientific medicine could solve most health problems and that accessible and quality health care (or, more correctly, illness care) would improve the health of Canadians. Within this approach, less emphasis was given to health promotion and disease prevention.

Behavioural Approach

By the early 1970s, increasingly large amounts of money were spent on health care, but the health status of the population did not improve proportionately. To better understand what contributed to illness and death, the Minister of Health and Welfare, Marc Lalonde, commissioned a study that resulted in the 1974 report *A New Perspective on the Health of Canadians*. This so-called *Lalonde Report* shifted emphasis from a medical to a **behavioural approach** to health. The report concluded that the traditional medical approach to health care was inadequate and that "further improvements in the environment, reductions in self-imposed risks, and a greater knowledge of human biology" were necessary to improve the health status of Canadians (p. 6). The *Lalonde Report* was the first modern government document in the Western world to acknowledge the inadequacy of a strictly biomedical health care system.

The *Lalonde Report* broadly defined health determinants as *lifestyle, environment, human biology,* and the *organization of health care*. This **health field concept** was widely used, modified, and expanded by other countries, and its release was a turning point in broadening Canadians' attitudes about factors that contribute to health, along with the role of government in promoting health (Health Canada, 1998). Of the four determinants, lifestyle received the most attention, perhaps because lifestyle behaviours contributed to chronic diseases (such as cancer and heart disease) and to injuries—both of which are the leading causes of morbidity and mortality in Canada (Labonte, 1993). In addition, greater understanding of behavioural social psychology revealed factors that motivated individuals to engage in healthy or unhealthy behaviours. In 1978, the Canadian government established the Health Promotion Directorate in the Department of National Health and Welfare, the first official health promotion undertaking of its kind. Its aim was to decrease **behavioural risk factors** such as smoking, substance abuse, lack of exercise, and an unhealthy diet. Public health programs such as Operation Lifestyle and ParticipACTION were developed through this department.

The behavioural approach places responsibility for health on the individual, thereby favouring health promotion strategies such as education and social marketing. Strategies are often based on the assumption that if people know the risk factors for disease, then they will engage in healthy behaviours. Indeed, health-enhancing practices among Canadians increased during this time. With the ParticipACTION initiative, for instance, many people increased their physical activity. Antismoking campaigns led to a substantial decrease in tobacco use.

Socioenvironmental Approach

By the mid-1980s, however, the behavioural approach to health and illness prevention fell into disfavour. Studies showed that lifestyle improvements were made primarily by well-educated, well-employed, and higher income Canadians.The *Lalonde Report* was criticized for deflecting attention from the environment and for how environment and lifestyle were defined. Lifestyle was viewed as being within an individual's control, with health risks as "self-imposed" behaviours. This supported "victim-blaming" and views that health was largely an individual responsibility. Critics suggested that health-related behaviours could not be separated from the social contexts (environments) in which they occurred. For example, living and working conditions were perceived as barriers to engaging in healthy behaviours (Labonte, 1993).

In the **socioenvironmental approach**, health is closely tied to social structures. For example, poverty and unhealthy physical and social environments, such as air pollution, poor water quality, and workplace hazards, are recognized as influencing health directly. Thus, Canadian public health professionals expanded Lalonde's (1974) health field concept to emphasize the social context of health and the relationship between personal health behaviours and social and physical environments (Hancock & Perkins, 1985).

Internationally, more attention was also given to the social context of health. The WHO Regional Conference in Europe produced a discussion paper identifying the social conditions that influence health (WHO, 1984). Just as Canada led the behavioural approach to health with the *Lalonde Report*, it was now instrumental in focusing on social and environmental conditions. In 1986, the First International Conference on Health Promotion was held in Ottawa, sponsored by the WHO, the Canadian Public Health Association (CPHA), and Health and Welfare Canada. It produced a watershed document—the *Ottawa Charter for Health Promotion*—that supported a socioenvironmental approach. This document has since been translated into more than 40 languages.

Ottawa Charter. The *Ottawa Charter for Health Promotion* (WHO, 1986) identified **prerequisites for health** as peace, shelter, education, food, income, a stable ecosystem, sustainable resources, social justice, and equity. These prerequisites clearly go beyond lifestyles or personal health practices to include social, environmental, and political contexts. They place responsibility for health on society rather than only on individuals. The *Charter's* focus on social justice and equity also incorporated the concept of *empowerment*—a person's ability to define, analyze, and solve problems—as an important goal for health care professionals (Registered Nurses Association of British Columbia, 1994). Indeed, Wallerstein (1992) contended that powerlessness could be the underlying health determinant influencing other risk factors. Consequently, health promotion literature emphasizes the concept of empowerment. The *Ottawa Charter* incorporated the then-new 1984 WHO definition of health (discussed previously), which identified health as having both social and individual dimensions, emphasized its dynamic and positive nature, and viewed it as a fundamental human right (Naidoo & Wills, 1994). The *Charter* outlined five major strategies to promote health: building healthy public policy, creating supportive environments, strengthening community action, developing personal skills, and reorienting health services (detailed later in this chapter).

Achieving Health for All. Concepts from the *Ottawa Charter* were incorporated into another important Canadian document, *Achieving Health for All: A Framework for Health Promotion* (Epp, 1986). This report, developed under the leadership of Jake Epp, Minister of National Health and Welfare from 1984 to 1989, became Canada's blueprint for achieving the WHO goal of "Health for All 2000" (Figure 1–3).

Epp's (1986) report identified three major health challenges: reducing inequities, increasing prevention, and enhancing coping mechanisms. It acknowledged disparities in health, particularly between low- and high-income people, and that living and working conditions were critical determinants of health. It emphasized the need for effective ways to prevent injuries, illnesses, chronic conditions, and disabilities. Enhancing coping was an acknowledgment that the dominant diseases in Canada were chronic conditions that could not be cured. Therefore, the challenge is assisting people to manage and cope with chronic conditions in order to live meaningful and productive lives. The *Epp Report* emphasized society's responsibility for providing supports for people experiencing chronic medical conditions, stress, mental illness, and problems associated with aging, as well as the need for supports for caregivers. The report identified self-care, mutual aid, and healthy environments as ways that these challenges could be addressed, which reflected both personal and social responsibility. Specific strategies to address the challenges included fostering public participation, strengthening community health services, and coordinating healthy public policy.

The *Ottawa Charter* and the *Epp Report* each reflect a socioenvironmental approach in which health is seen as more than just the absence of disease and engaging in healthy behaviours; rather, this approach emphasizes connectedness, self-efficacy, and capacity to engage in meaningful activities (see Figure 1–2).

Risk Factors and Risk Conditions. Labonte (1993) categorized the major determinants of health in a socioenvironmental approach as psychosocial risk factors and socioenvironmental risk conditions:

- **Psychosocial risk factors** are complex psychological experiences resulting from social circumstances that include isolation, lack of social support, limited social networks, low self-esteem, self-blame, and low perceived power.
- **Socioenvironmental risk conditions** are social and environmental living conditions that include poverty, low educational or occupational status, dangerous or stressful work, dangerous physical environments, pollution, discrimination, relative political or economic powerlessness, and inequalities of income or power.

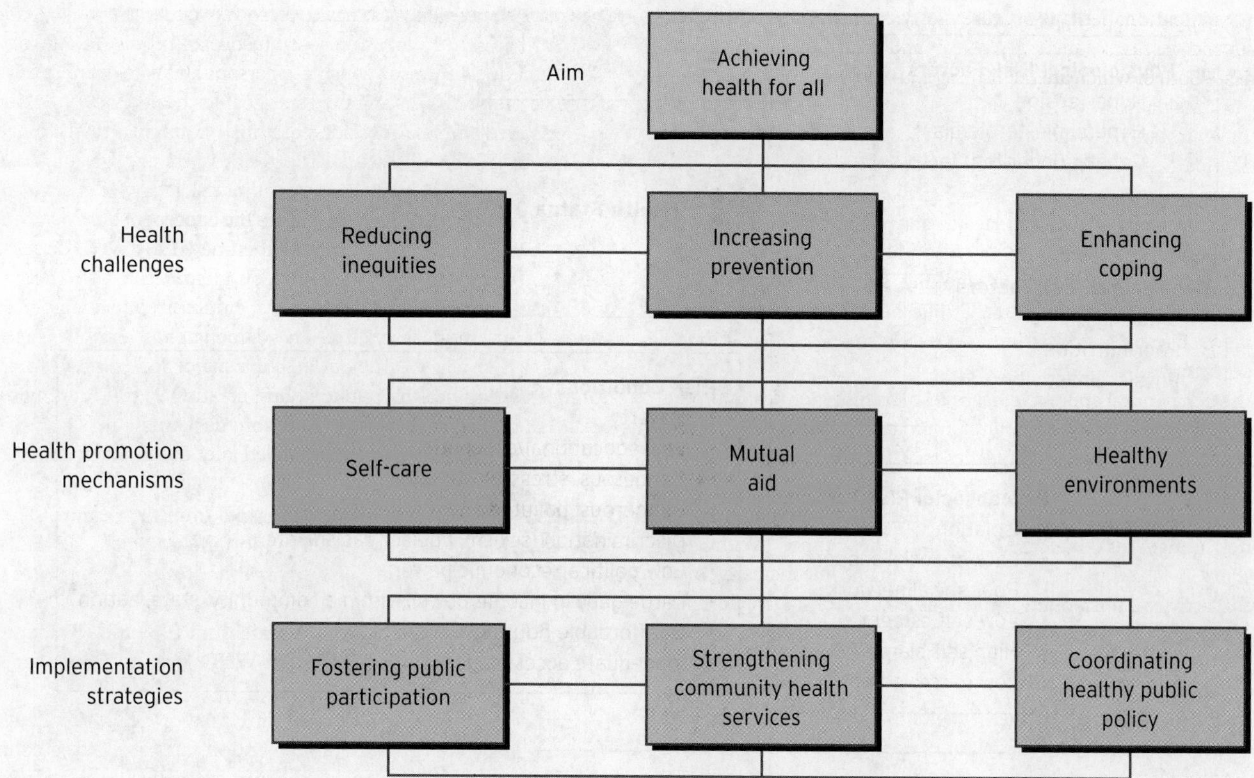

Figure 1-3 Achieving health for all: A framework for health promotion. **Source:** From Epp, J. (1986). *Achieving health for all: A framework for health promotion* (p. 8). Ottawa, ON: Health and Welfare Canada. Reproduced with the permission of the Minister of Public Works and Government Services Canada, 2005.

According to a socioenvironmental approach to health, political, social, and cultural forces affect health and well-being both directly and indirectly through their influence on personal health behaviours. Socioenvironmental risk conditions can contribute to psychosocial risk factors, which can then result in unhealthy behaviours (Figure 1–4). This means that health care professionals should recognize the influence of environment on personal behaviours and that "health-inhibiting" behaviours could be coping strategies for managing the stress created by living and working conditions that decrease access to resources. In other words, "to change behaviour it may be necessary to change more than behaviour" (Wilkinson, 1996, p. 64). For example, in addition to working "downstream" to assist people who are experiencing the negative health effects of socioenvironmental conditions, nurses need to work "upstream" by advocating for policies that ensure affordable housing, financial support to clients with low incomes, and safe, fulfilling work environments.

Strategies for Population Health. In Canada, the determinants of health have been further emphasized through the **population health approach**. This approach, initiated by the Canadian Institute for Advanced Research, was officially endorsed by the federal, provincial, and territorial ministers of health in the report titled *Strategies for Population Health: Investing in the Health of Canadians* (Federal, Provincial, and Territorial Advisory Committee on Population Health [ACPH], 1994). In a population health approach, "the entire range of known individual and collective factors and conditions that determine population health status, and the interactions among them, are taken into account in planning action to improve health" (Health Canada, 1998). The population health approach emphasizes the use of epidemiological data to determine the etiology of health and disease.

The key health determinants identified in the *Strategies for Population Health* report are as follows:

- Income and social status.
- Social support networks.
- Education.
- Employment and working conditions.
- Physical environments.
- Biology and genetic endowment.
- Personal health practices and coping skills.
- Healthy child development.
- Health services.

In 1996, Health Canada added *gender, culture,* and *social environments* to this list. Note that the list includes determinants at the individual level (personal health practices and coping skills; biology and genetic endowment) and at the population level (education, employment, and income distribution).

Jakarta Declaration. *The Jakarta Declaration on Health Promotion into the 21st Century* (WHO, 1997) emerged from the 4th International Conference on Health Promotion, the first to be held in a developing country and to involve the private sector. The *Jakarta Declaration* affirmed the *Ottawa Charter* prerequisites for health; added four other prerequisites (*empowerment of women, social security, respect for human rights, and social relations*); and declared poverty to be the greatest threat to health. The Declaration identified the following priorities for action: promoting social responsibility for health in public and private sectors; increasing investments for health in all sectors; consolidating and expanding partnerships for health to all levels of government and the private sector; increasing community capacity and empowering the individual; and securing adequate infrastructure for health promotion.

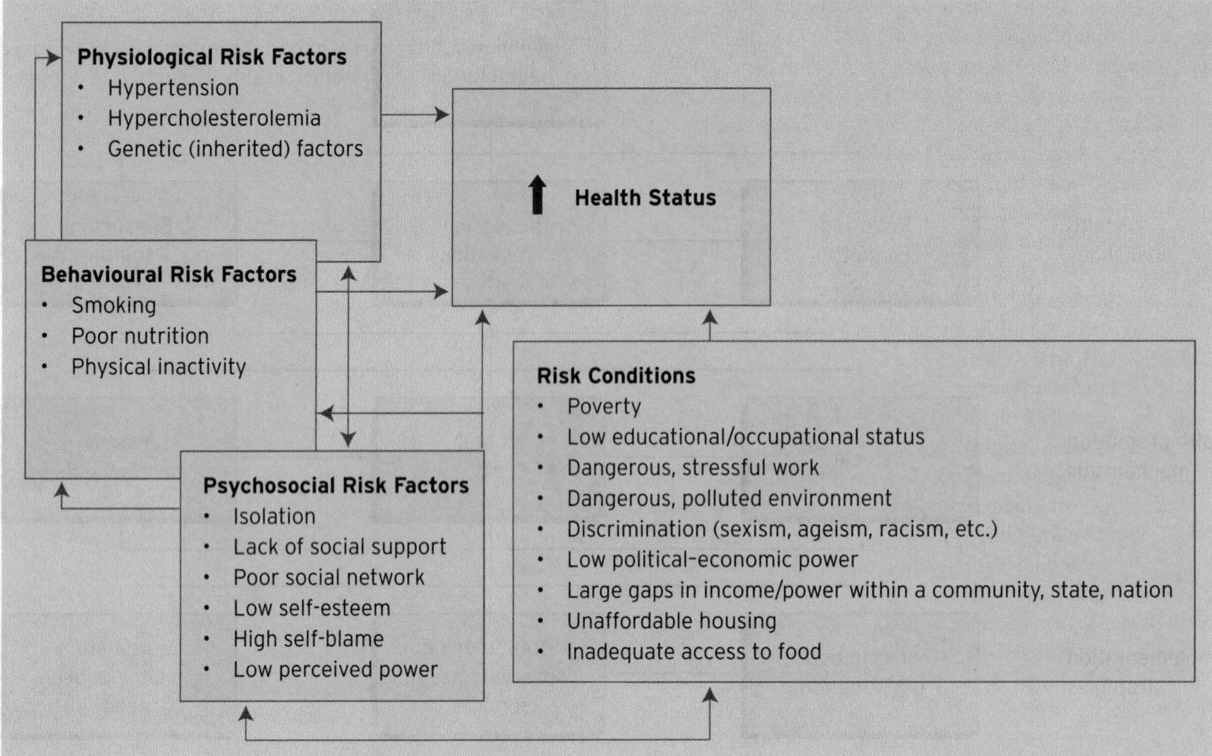

Figure 1-4 Socioenvironmental approach to health. **Source:** From Labonte, R. (1993). *Issues in health promotion series. 3. Health promotion and empowerment: Practice frameworks* (p. 11). Toronto, ON: Centre for Health Promotion, University of Toronto, & ParticipACTION.

Bangkok Charter. The *Bangkok Charter for Health Promotion in a Globalized World* (WHO, 2005) affirmed health as a human right and emphasized mental and spiritual well-being as important elements. It identified critical factors influencing health, such as the increasing inequalities within and between countries, global environmental change, and urbanization. The *Charter* emphasized strong political action and sustained advocacy, empowering communities with adequate resources, and corporate sector commitment to healthy workplaces and ethical business practices.

Toronto Charter. In the early to middle 1990s, Canadian social and health policies resulted in increased social and economic inequalities (Bryant, 2002; Raphael et al., 2004) and health disparities. These concerns culminated in the *Toronto Charter on the Social Determinants of Health*, which identified the following social determinants as particularly important for health: early childhood development, education, employment and working conditions, food security, health care services, housing shortages, income and its equitable distribution, social safety nets, social exclusion, and unemployment and employment security. **Social determinants of health** can be defined as "the *economic and social conditions* that influence the health of individuals, communities, and jurisdictions as a whole . . . [and] determine the extent to which a person possesses the physical, social, and personal resources to identify and achieve personal aspirations, satisfy needs, and cope with the environment" (Raphael, 2004, p. 1; italics ours). This conceptualization of health determinants emphasizes *societal* responsibility for reducing health disparities because it focuses on how a society distributes economic and social resources through its economic and social policies.

Concern about **health disparities** (i.e., differences in health status among different population groups) has been raised worldwide. The WHO Commission on Social Determinants of Health (WHO, 2006) was charged with developing strategies to narrow health disparities through action on the social determinants of health. Nationally, the Health Disparities Task Group (2005), commissioned by the Public Health Agency of Canada (PHAC), identified socioeconomic status, Aboriginal identity, gender, and geographic location as the most important factors related to health disparities. Health disparities are associated with inequitable access (unfair or unjust lack of access) to health determinants, resulting from economic and social policies. You will see how some of these factors play out in the discussion of determinants in the following sections.

Determinants of Health

The following section introduces you to some of the major determinants of health affecting Canadians (Health Canada, 1996). Although each determinant contributes individually to health (enhances or inhibits health), the determinants are also interrelated and influence each other.

Income and Social Status (Income Distribution)

Income and social status is the greatest **determinant of health** (Canadian Institute for Health Information [CIHI], 2004; Raphael et al., 2004). According to Statistics Canada pretax low-income cut-offs in 2004, 16% of Canadians lived in poverty, with much higher rates among single mothers (47%) and unattached individuals younger than 65 years (38%) (National Council of Welfare, 2007) and among Aboriginal peoples (34%), Canadians of colour (28%), people with disabilities (23%), and recent urban immigrants (43%) (Canadian Council on Social Development, 2007).

Poverty exerts its effect on health through lack of material resources that support health, through higher levels of psychosocial stress, and through health-threatening behaviours to cope with limited resources and stress (Raphael, 2004). Low-income Canadians are more likely to die early and to suffer from most diseases, regardless of age, sex, race, culture, or place of residence. It is estimated that 23% of Canadians' premature loss of life can be accounted for by income differences (Raphael, 2004). People with lower incomes are more likely to have chronic health problems, particularly cardiovascular disease and type II diabetes (Raphael et al., 2003; Raphael & Farrell, 2002; Wilkins et al., 2002); lower self-esteem, lower sense of mastery and coherence; and higher levels of depression (Federal, Provincial, and Territorial ACPH, 1999).

Low birth weight, an important marker for subsequent poor child and adult health, has a 43% higher incidence in poor neighbourhoods than in higher income neighbourhoods (Wilkins et al., 2002). Children living in poverty are more likely to have chronic diseases such as asthma, to visit emergency rooms, and to die from injuries (Canadian Institute on Children's Health, 2000) and are at greater risk for cognitive difficulties, delayed vocabulary development, and behavioural problems (CIHI, 2004).

With each step up the economic ladder, Canadians' health status improves. This suggests that ill health is related to more than absolute material deprivation. Social deprivation may also influence health, perhaps through its effects on personal control and uncertainty (Wilkinson & Marmot, 1998).

Income inequality (i.e., the increasing gap between the rich and the poor [Dunn, 2002; Phipps, 2003]), also influences population health, and some academics have suggested that it is the greatest threat to the well-being of Western societies (Kawachi & Kennedy, 1997). Countries with economic inequality have higher levels of poverty, fewer public services, weaker social safety nets (Raphael, 2004), and lower overall health and life expectancies (Dunn, 2002; Wilkinson, 1996).

Social Support Networks

Social support affects health, health behaviours, and health care utilization (Carpiano, 2007; Stewart, 2000) through practical, emotional, informational, and affirmational support (House, 1981). Indeed, some experts believe that relationships may be as important to health as established risk factors such as obesity, smoking, and high blood pressure (Federal, Provincial, and Territorial ACPH, 1999). A strong body of research links social support with positive health outcomes (Berkman, 1995; Carpiano, 2007; Cohen, 1992; Tomaka et al., 2006).

In general, Canadians have reported high levels of support (Federal, Provincial, and Territorial ACPH, 1999). Four of five Canadians reported they had someone to confide in, whom they could count on in a crisis or for advice, and who made them feel loved and cared for. Nevertheless, men, single parents, and lower income Canadians generally reported less support than did their respective counterparts. Support from families and friends and from informal and formal groups can provide practical aid during times of crisis and emotional support in times of distress and change. Social support can decrease stress (Kosteniuk & Dickinson, 2003). Social support also assists coping and behavioural changes and can help individuals solve problems and maintain a sense of mastery and control over their lives. A survey of young parents in Alberta identified spouses, family, and friends as major sources of support in encouraging healthy behaviours (exercise, diet) by providing emotional, affirmational, and practical support, including child care and financial assistance (Reutter et al., 2001). In another study, a support intervention helped mothers of very preterm infants gain confidence in their parenting skills and understand their infants' medical conditions (Preyde, 2007).

Education and Literacy

Education and literacy are important influences on health status because they affect many other health determinants. Literacy can influence health both directly (e.g., medication use, safety practices) and indirectly through use of services, lifestyles, income, work environments, and stress levels. For example, people with low literacy skills are more likely to be unemployed, earn minimum wages in unskilled jobs, and make less use of preventive services (Rootman & Ronson, 2005). Education increases job opportunities and income security, which provide knowledge and skills to solve problems and gain a sense of control (PHAC, 2004). People with higher education levels tend to smoke less, be more physically active, and have access to healthier foods and physical environments (Federal, Provincial, and Territorial ACPH, 1999).

Employment and Working Conditions

Employment and working conditions significantly affect physical, mental, and social health. Paid work provides financial resources, a sense of identity and purpose, social contacts, and opportunities for personal growth (CPHA, 1996a). Unemployed people have reduced life expectancy and experience significantly more health problems than do employed people (Bartley et al., 1999).

Working conditions themselves can support health or pose health hazards. Healthy workplaces include job and employment security, safe physical conditions, reasonable work pace, low stress, opportunities for self-expression and individual development, participation, and work–life balance (Jackson, 2004). Temporary employees, part-time workers, and people working in low-wage jobs have high levels of job insecurity and frequent periods of unemployment. Often such jobs do not provide benefits or pensions, which can lead to uncertainty and stress (Menendez et al., 2007; Tompa et al., 2007). In 2000, more than one in four Canadian workers believed that their place of work was not healthy (Canadian Policy Research Networks, 2008). One third of Canadian workers in 2003 reported high stress at work, with even higher rates (45%) for health care workers (Wilkins, 2007). Indeed, the concern regarding negative workplace conditions in the health sector is considerable; nurses have had the highest or second-highest rates of absenteeism of all workers in Canada since the early 1990s (Villeneuve & MacDonald, 2006). Workplace stress is linked to increased risk of physical injuries, high blood pressure, cardiovascular disease, depression, and increases in tobacco and alcohol use (Jackson, 2004). In 2003, almost 10% of Canadian workers in trades, transport, and equipment operation sustained on-the-job injuries, which is more than four times the rate among workers in the "white-collar" sector (Wilkins & Mackenzie, 2007).

Physical Environments

Housing, indoor air quality, and community planning are important determinants of health. Contaminants in air, water, food, and soil also adversely affect health, sometimes contributing to cancer, birth defects, respiratory illness, and gastrointestinal ailments. Children from low-income families, who often live in substandard housing and in neighbourhoods near highways and industrial areas, are particularly likely to be exposed to these contaminants (Federal, Provincial, and Territorial ACPH, 1999). Asthma, which is characterized by high sensitivity to airborne contaminants, is the most common chronic respiratory disease among children, accounting for 25% of all school absenteeism (Canadian Council on Social Development, 2006); children in poverty are particularly vulnerable to this disease (Lethbridge & Phipps, 2005).

Involuntary exposure to tobacco smoke (second-hand smoke) has received considerable attention in Canada. Children exposed to tobacco smoke are at increased risk for sudden infant death syndrome

(SIDS), acute respiratory infections, ear problems, and reduced lung development, and exposure of adults to second-hand smoke can lead to coronary heart disease and lung cancer (US Department of Health and Human Services, 2006). Municipalities throughout Canada have incorporated smoking bans in public places, which has reduced exposure to second-hand smoke. In 2005, 23% of nonsmokers reported regular exposure in at least one venue (public place, home, or vehicles), and children were at highest risk for exposure (Shields, 2007).

Another important aspect of the environment is affordable and adequate housing. Homelessness in Canada is increasing, in part because of reduced government funding of social housing and lack of affordable rental accommodation (Bryant, 2004; Khandor & Mason, 2007). The number of working poor homeless is also on the rise, particularly in areas experiencing economic boom, such as Alberta. Homeless populations are at greater risk for a variety of health problems, including mental illness, substance abuse, suicide, tuberculosis, injuries and assaults, chronic medical conditions (e.g., respiratory and musculoskeletal), and poor oral and dental health, and for early death (Frankish et al., 2005; Khandor & Mason, 2007). Whereas inadequate housing can affect health directly, lack of affordable housing can also *indirectly* affect health through its influence on other determinants (Bryant, 2004). Spending a disproportionate amount of income on rent, for example, reduces the amount of money that families can spend on food, clothing, recreation, and health care.

The determinant of physical environment also includes the effects of climate change on the health of populations and the planet itself. The Canadian Nurses Association and Canadian Medical Association (2005) developed position statements on ecosystem health and environmentally responsible activity in the health sector. The need for sustainable ecosystems, included as a prerequisite for health in the *Ottawa Charter*, is becoming more critical.

Biological and Genetic Endowment

Heredity is strongly influenced by social and physical environments, and considerable effort has been expended to prevent congenital defects through monitoring and improved preconception and prenatal care (Federal, Provincial, and Territorial ACPH, 1999). This effort has led to substantial decreases in anomalies at birth.

Age is also a strong determinant of health. Many older people develop chronic diseases, although disability can be reduced with healthy aging (Healthy Aging and Wellness Working Group, 2006). Indeed, 70% of older people in Canada report good overall health, including good functional health and independence in activities of daily living (Shields & Martel, 2006). Nurses need to consider how much of the decline associated with aging is related to biological aging versus other determinants such as socioeconomic status, social support, and individual health practices.

Individual Health Practices and Coping Skills

Effective coping skills help people face challenges without resorting to risk behaviours such as substance abuse. Many so-called risk behaviours may, in fact, be coping strategies for stress and strain caused by living circumstances. For example, considerable evidence reveals that low-income women use smoking as a coping strategy (Stewart et al., 2004). Three risk behaviours with major detrimental health consequences are physical inactivity, poor nutrition, and tobacco use.

Physical inactivity is a major risk factor for some types of cancer, diabetes, cardiovascular disease, osteoporosis, obesity, hypertension, depression, stress, and anxiety. In 2004, just over half (52%) of Canadians aged 12 and older were at least moderately active during their leisure time (equivalent to walking at least 30 to 60 minutes a day). Those who were active were more likely to rate their health as excellent or very good and to report lower levels of stress and were less likely to be overweight, obese, or hypertensive (Gilmour, 2007).

Poor nutrition, particularly overconsumption of fats, sugars, and salt, is linked to such diseases as some cancers, cardiovascular diseases, type 2 diabetes, hypertension, osteoarthritis, and gallbladder disease and to functional limitations and disabilities (Tjepkema, 2006). Obesity is now considered a major public health problem. The 2004 Canadian Community Health Survey (CCHS) revealed that 23% of adult Canadians were obese (body mass index [BMI] of 30 or more) and 36% were overweight (Shields 2006); as BMI increased, so did the likelihood of reporting high blood pressure, diabetes, and heart disease. About 26% of children (aged 2–17 years) were overweight or obese (Shields, 2006). The 2004 CCHS (Nutrition section) revealed that 70% of children aged 4–8 years ate fewer than the minimum five servings of vegetables and fruit daily. Moreover, 25% of Canadians overall (and one third of teenagers aged 14–18) had eaten at fast-food outlets the previous day (Garriguet, 2007), which feature foods high in fats and salt. Several factors influence food consumption patterns, including household income, food advertising, and availability of nutritious choices. Food insecurity (the limited or uncertain availability of nutritious foods) is a growing problem in Canada. In 2004, more than 40% of households with low or lower middle incomes reported food insecurity (Ledrou & Gervais, 2005); those receiving social assistance were particularly vulnerable. Food insecurity is significantly associated with multiple chronic conditions, obesity, distress, and depression (Che & Chen, 2001; Tarasuk, 2004).

Tobacco use remains the leading preventable cause of death, disease, and disability (Makamowski Illing & Kaiserman, 2004). Smoking is linked to many diseases, such as cancer, cardiovascular disease, and respiratory illnesses, and it reduces the health of smokers in general (US Department of Health and Human Services, 2004). The smoking rate in Canada in 2007 was 19% (Health Canada, 2008). People most likely to smoke are men and women in their 40s, those living in poverty (Physicians for a Smoke-free Canada, 2005), and Aboriginal people (Health Canada, 2007) People with mental illness are twice as likely as the general population to smoke tobacco and to smoke more heavily (Lasser et al., 2000).

Clearly, many factors influence individual health behaviours (e.g., income, education, gender, culture, and social support). Resources to develop and maintain health-enhancing behaviours need to include not only health education but also social policies such as income security and anti-smoking legislation to make healthy choices the "easy" choices.

Healthy Child Development

All determinants influence child development, but healthy child development is a separate determinant because of its importance to lifelong health. Increasing evidence reveals that events during conception and through the age of 6 years influence children's health for the rest of their lives (CIHI, 2004). Three conditions for healthy child development are adequate and equitable income, effective parents and families, and supportive community environments (CIHI, 2004; Stroick & Jenson, 1999).

From conception to birth, two significant health risks are low birth weight and maternal tobacco, alcohol, and drug use (Steinhauer, 1998). Low birth weight contributes to perinatal illness and death; is associated with higher rates of long-term health problems, including cerebral palsy and learning difficulties, and with more frequent hospitalizations (Canadian Institute on Children's Health, 2000); and is related to development of chronic diseases in adulthood, especially heart disease and type II diabetes (Raphael et al., 2003; Raphael & Farrell, 2002). From birth through the toddler years, family environment is important, particularly establishing attachment to a primary caregiver during the first two years of life (Steinhauer, 1998). Throughout the toddler, preschool, and school-aged years, meeting a child's development needs is crucial. Family conflict, violence, and poverty threaten healthy child development. Schools in which students feel secure, respected, challenged, and cared for help ensure that children succeed academically. Community support is also important (Steinhauer, 1998).

Quality early childhood education and care are particularly important in early child development, so much so that they have been singled out by some researchers as a combined social determinant of health (Friendly, 2004). High-quality programs promote cognitive development and social competence and support parents in education and employment. Canada has acknowledged the importance of early childhood intervention through its Early Childhood Development Initiative (Health Council of Canada, 2006); however, Canada lacks a national child care program.

Health Services

Approximately 25% of a population's health status is attributed to the quality of health care services (Saskatchewan Public Health Association, 1994). Quality, accessible acute-care treatment, long-term care, home care, and preventive services are therefore important. More funding is given to acute-care services than to health promotion and disease prevention, and yet the latter services contribute even more to population health. Prenatal care, well-child and immunization clinics, education services about healthy lifestyles, and services that maintain older adults' health and independence are important examples of preventive and primary health care services (discussed further in Chapters 2 and 4) that Canadians should continue to develop. Canada's national health insurance scheme is considered a hallmark of society. Principles of the *Canada Health Act*—universality, portability, accessibility, comprehensiveness, and public administration—apply to the provision of medically insured services. Increasingly, the trends in health care service provision are from institutionalized care to community-based care, toward decision making that is based on the best available evidence, and toward more regional administration. In Canada, considerable monies have been invested in initiatives that incorporate principles of primary health care; however, the progress in this regard has been relatively slow.

Gender

Gender is "the array of society-determined roles, personality traits, attitudes, behaviours, values, relative power, and influence that society ascribes to the two sexes on a differential basis" (PHAC, 2004). Many health issues are a function of gender-based social roles, and gender can influence health status, behaviours, and care (Spitzer, 2005). In Canada, men are more likely than women to die prematurely, largely as a result of heart disease, unintentional fatal injuries, cancer, and suicide. Women, however, are more likely to suffer from depression, stress (often resulting from efforts to balance work and family life), chronic conditions such as arthritis and allergies, and injuries and death from family violence (Federal, Provincial, and Territorial ACPH, 1999). Moreover, gender influences men's and women's experience of sex-specific health concerns (e.g., pregnancy, prostate cancer, presentation of cardiovascular signs and symptoms), exposure to potential risk conditions (e.g., caregiving demands as traditionally women's responsibility), and interactions with health care professionals (e.g., gender stereotypes, medicalization of health experience) (Pederson & Raphael, 2006).

Culture

Cultural and ethnic factors influence people's interactions with a health care system, their participation in prevention and health promotion programs, their access to health information, their health-related lifestyle choices, and their understanding of health and illness (Health Canada, 1996). Cultural factors also influence whether and how determinants are met (see Chapter 10). For example, among immigrants and refugees, unmet expectations and challenges to successful social integration negatively impact individual health (Simich et al., 2003, 2005). Language differences can lead to isolation and decreased social support networks. Prejudice can cause individuals to be denied opportunities for education, employment, and access to housing (Health Canada, 1996). First Nations people are much more likely to suffer ill health; however, it is important to acknowledge the intersection of culture with other health determinants such as social support and income.

Social Environments

Social environments are defined as "the array of values and norms of a society [that] influence in varying ways the health and well-being of populations. In addition, social stability, recognition of diversity, safety, good working relationships, and cohesive communities provide a supportive society that reduces or avoids many potential risks to good health" (PHAC, 2004). The social environment is clearly related to other factors and expands on the social support determinant by incorporating broader community characteristics, norms, and values. Healthy social environments include freedom from discrimination and prejudice—particularly for people marginalized by income, age, gender, activity limitations, ethnicity, and sexual orientation. The determinant of social environment is also evident in the *Jakarta Declaration's* prerequisites of human rights, social security, and social relations (WHO, 1997). These prerequisities relate to social exclusion—the process by which people are denied opportunities to participate in many aspects of cultural, economic, social, and political life (Galabuzi, 2004). People most likely to be excluded are poor citizens, Aboriginal people, New Canadians, and members of racialized or nonwhite groups. Social exclusion limits people's access to the resources that support health and their participation in community life (Stewart et al., 2008).

Another important aspect of the social environment is the absence of violence, both in the home and in the community. In 2004, 7% of Canadians aged 15 years and older had experienced spousal violence in the previous 5 years; Aboriginal people were at a three-fold greater risk, and women were more likely to suffer from serious types of violence. Children accounted for 21% of cases of physical assault and 61% of cases of sexual assault, and close to 40% of elderly women suffered some kind of assault from family members (Canadian Centre for Justice Statistics, 2005). The health effects of family violence are devastating, for those experiencing or exposed to violence and for the perpetrators, and include psychological, physical, behavioural, academic, sexual, interpersonal, self-perceptual, or spiritual consequences, which may appear immediately or over time (Department of Justice Canada, 2008).

Violence is also experienced in other venues, particularly schools and workplaces. More than one third (36%) of Canadian students in grades 6–10 reported being victims of bullying. Victimized children are at risk for anxiety, depression, loss of self-esteem, and somatic complaints; perpetrators are also at risk for long-term problems such as antisocial behaviour and substance use (Craig & Edge, 2008). Health care workers, including nurses, have experienced violence perpetrated by clients, family members, and coworkers (Duncan et al., 2001).

Strategies to Influence Health Determinants

Health Promotion and Disease Prevention

The understanding that health is qualitatively different from disease has led to a differentiation of the concepts of health promotion and disease prevention, although they are interrelated. Pender et al. (2006) differentiated between health promotion and disease prevention as follows: **health promotion** is "directed toward increasing the level of well-being and self-actualization" (p. 37); **disease prevention** (particularly primary prevention) is "action to avoid illness/disease" (p. 36). On the other hand, other researchers consider health promotion as one aspect of primary prevention (Leavell & Clark, 1965; Neuman, 1995) and not necessarily disease specific (Leavell & Clark, 1965). In contrast, the *Ottawa Charter* views health promotion as the overarching concept, defined as "the process of enabling people to increase control over, and improve, their health" (WHO, 1986). The following more comprehensive definition was offered by Nutbeam (1998):

> *"Health promotion represents a comprehensive social and political process, it not only embraces actions directed at strengthening the skills and capabilities of individuals, but also action directed towards changing social, environmental and economic conditions so as to alleviate their impact on public and individual health. Health promotion is the process of enabling people to increase control over the determinants of health and thereby improve their health. Participation is essential to sustain health promotion action."* (p. 351)

Three levels of disease prevention correspond to the natural history of disease:

- *Primary prevention* activities protect against a disease before signs and symptoms occur (prepathogenesis stage of disease). Examples include immunization (to prevent infectious diseases) and reduction of risk factors (such as inactivity, smoking, and exposure to air pollution).
- *Secondary prevention* activities promote early detection of disease once pathogenesis has occurred, so that prompt treatment can be initiated to halt disease and limit disability. Examples include preventive screening for cancer (e.g., mammography, testicular self-examination); blood pressure screening to detect hypertension; and blood glucose screening to detect diabetes.
- *Tertiary prevention* activities are initiated in the convalescence stage of disease and are directed toward minimizing residual disability and helping people to live productively with limitations. An example is a cardiac rehabilitation program after a myocardial infarction.

Nursing strategies guided by a prevention framework focus on assessment and alleviation of risk factors for disease. On the other hand, health promotion may be viewed more broadly than disease prevention (Laffrey & Craig, 2000) inasmuch as it emphasizes enhancing personal competencies and capacities and is committed to empowerment and community-based health planning (Robertson, 1998). Health promotion strategies, therefore, are often political because they emphasize addressing structural and systemic inequities and have a strong philosophy of social justice. Health promotion is guided by the following principles (CPHA, 1996b):

- Health promotion addresses health issues in context.
- Health promotion supports a holistic approach.
- Health promotion requires a long-term perspective.
- Health promotion is multisectoral.
- Health promotion draws on knowledge from social, economic, political, environmental, medical, and nursing sciences, as well as from first-hand experiences.

Health Promotion Strategies

The *Ottawa Charter* identified five broad strategies to enhance health. The following is a brief introduction to each of these **health promotion strategies.**

1. Build Healthy Public Policy. Advocating healthy public policies is a priority strategy for health promotion in Canada. Indeed, some academics have suggested that this strategy is the foundation of all others because policies shape how money, power, and material resources are distributed to society (CPHA, 1996b). Advocating healthy public policy is a collaborative effort to identify the most important areas in which policy can make a difference. As a nurse, you might work with others to develop policy options, encourage public dialogue, persuade decision makers to adopt the healthiest option, and follow up to make sure the policy is implemented (CPHA,

BOX 1-1 NURSING STORY

Cathy Crowe: Advocating Healthy Public Policy

Cathy Crowe is a Toronto street nurse who has advocated for policies related to a variety of social determinants. Her work as an outreach street nurse in Toronto since the 1980s exemplifies nursing's role not only in attending to immediate health needs of people who are homeless but also advocating for policies that will provide more adequate and affordable housing to alleviate the root causes of these health problems. Ms. Crowe cofounded the Toronto Disaster Relief Committee (TDRC) in 1998, which declared homelessness a national disaster in Canada. The Committee advocated a "1% solution," calling on the federal, provincial, and territorial governments to allocate an additional 1% of their budget to fully fund a national affordable housing program. The efforts of the TDRC increased awareness, both in large cities in Canada and at the United Nations, of Canada's housing problem. This awareness led to the appointment of a federal minister responsible for homelessness and federal emergency relief monies (e.g., for shelter beds, food banks, programs for homeless youth). Although monies were also made available to provide housing, the goal of a fully funded national housing strategy has not yet been realized, and homelessness continues to increase across Canada.

Ms. Crowe has fostered numerous coalitions and advocacy initiatives, working with homeless people and other organizations. The TDRC was involved in fighting the evictions of Toronto's Tent City in 2002 and succeeded in eventually securing housing for many residents. Ms. Crowe is currently on the Board of Directors of a nonprofit organization that is building affordable housing in Toronto. To raise awareness about children who are homeless, she is currently producing a film set in several Canadian cities. As part of this initiative, a children's forum on homelessness was organized to provide children the opportunity to voice their concerns to the United Nations Special Rapporteur on Adequate Housing when he visited Canada. Ms. Crowe has also written a book, *Dying for a Home,* co-authored with activists who are homeless themselves.

Ms. Crowe has received numerous awards for her advocacy work. She sees advocacy as a critical nursing role and responsibility. You are encouraged to view her many speeches and activities on the TDRC Web site at http://www.tdrc.net or at http://tdrc.net/index.php?page=cathy-crowe.

1996b). Cathy Crowe, a Toronto "street nurse," is an excellent example of a nurse who advocates for healthy public policy: she works to reduce homelessness (Box 1–1).

The CPHA recommends that more emphasis be placed on policies that create healthy living conditions and enable people who are least powerful to express their concerns. This priority is also reflected in the *Toronto Charter on the Social Determinants of Health*, discussed earlier, which focuses specifically on determinants that have policy implications. Because the determinants of health are broad, healthy public policy necessarily extends beyond traditional health agencies and government health departments to other sectors such as agriculture, education, transportation, labour, social services, energy, and housing. Therefore, policymakers in all government sectors and organizations should ensure that their policies have positive health consequences.

Increasingly, policy advocacy is incorporated into nursing role statements (e.g., Community Health Nurses Association of Canada, 2003; International Council of Nurses, 2001) and nursing education curricula (Rains & Barton-Kriese, 2001; Reutter & Duncan, 2002; Reutter & Williamson, 2000). You should think about what policies have contributed to health problems, what policies would help alleviate the problem, and how you can champion public policies. For example, how do current welfare incomes, which are lower than poverty "lines" (low-income cut-offs), influence recipients' abilities to obtain adequate food and shelter and participate meaningfully in Canadian society? Cohen and Reutter (2007) outlined several ways that nurses can engage in policy advocacy in relation to child and family poverty.

2. Create Supportive Environments. The *Ottawa Charter* (WHO, 1986) states that "the overall guiding principle . . . is the need to encourage reciprocal maintenance, to take care of each other, our communities and our natural environment" (p. 2). This strategy helps ensure that physical environments are healthy and safe and that living and working conditions are stimulating and satisfying. Creating supportive environments also means protecting the natural environment and conserving natural resources (WHO, 1986).

An excellent example of an initiative that helps create supportive environments is the Comprehensive School Health Initiative, which focuses on improving school environments by providing health instruction, social support, support services, and positive physical environments (Mitchell & Laforet-Fliesser, 2003). Other examples of supportive environments include flexible workplace policies and quality child care programs that support early child development and parental employment.

3. Strengthen Community Action. Strengthening communities is a requisite for successful health promotion and for community health nursing practices in Canada (Community Health Nurses Association of Canada, 2003; CPHA, 1996b). In this strategy, often referred to as *community development,* communities identify issues and work together to make changes that will enhance health. In a community development approach, health professionals help community groups identify important issues and organize and implement plans and strategies to resolve these issues, often partnering with other community organizations (see Chapter 4). Public participation in all phases of community programming is key to community development (Labonte, 1993).

4. Develop Personal Skills. This strategy, which is probably most familiar to nurses, helps clients develop personal skills, enhance coping strategies, and gain control over their health and environments so that they can make healthy lifestyle choices. Personal skills development includes health education, but it also emphasizes adequate support and resources. Some examples of interventions to enhance personal skills include early intervention programs for children, home visiting by public health nurses, and parenting classes. School health education focusing on developing interpersonal skills and health practices is another example.

5. Reorient Health Services. Health system reform has two objectives: to shift emphasis from treating disease to improving health and to make the health care system more efficient and effective (CPHA, 1996b). A proactive approach to health requires improved access to primary health care services, increased community development, improved community-based care services, increased family-based care, and public participation. In Canada, there is considerable emphasis on developing the primary health care model, which nursing associations have advocated for many years (Reutter & Ogilvie, in press).

Population Health Promotion Model: Putting It All Together

This chapter has presented two major approaches to health: health promotion and population health. Hamilton and Bhatti (1996) integrated these two concepts into one model that shows their relationship to each other (Figure 1–5). Aimed at developing actions to improve health, the model explores four major questions: "On *what* can we take action?"; "*How* can we take action?"; "With *whom* can we act?"; and "*Why* take action?" (Saskatchewan Health, Population Health Branch, 2002).

The document *Strategies for Population Health* (Federal, Provincial, and Territorial ACPH, 1994) indicates health determinants actions that could be taken (the "what"). The *Ottawa Charter* provides a comprehensive set of five strategies to enhance health (the "how"). Together, these documents suggest that to enhance population health, action must be taken on a variety of levels (the "who"). Clearly, nurses must direct these strategies toward individuals and families, communities, individual sectors of society (such as health or environmental sectors), and society as a whole. For example, to promote the health of lower income clients, you can help them access resources and supports that will enhance their personal skills. Community programs such as school lunch programs, recreational activities, collective kitchens, and support groups can be provided. You can lobby government sectors responsible for housing and employment to implement healthy public policies pertaining to affordable housing, job creation, child care, income security, and financially accessible health services. On a societal level, nurses can raise awareness about the negative effects of poverty on health and well-being and can advocate for policies that will decrease poverty. The population health promotion model shows how evidence-informed decision making is a foundation to ensure that policies and programs focus on the right issues, take effective action, and produce successful results (Hamilton & Bhatti, 1996), the "why" of action (Saskatchewan Health, Population Health Branch, 2002). Evidence is informed by research, experiential learning, and evaluation of programs, policies, and projects. Values and assumptions that are the foundation of the model include the following:

- Stakeholders representing the various determinants must collaborate to address health determinants.
- Society is responsible for its members' health status.
- Health status is a result of people's health practices and their social and physical environments.

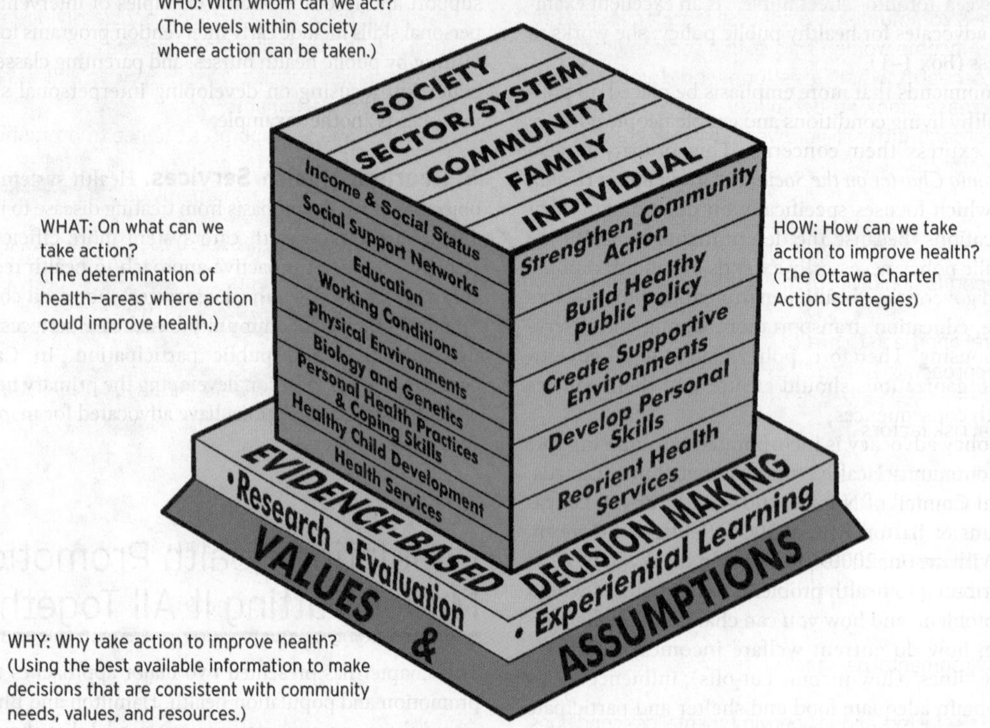

Figure 1-5 Population health promotion model. **Source:** From Hamilton, N., & Bhatti, T. (1996). *Population health promotion: An integrated model of population health and health promotion.* Ottawa, ON: Health Promotion Development Division, Health Canada. Copyright 1996 © by Minister of Public Works and Government Services Canada.

- Opportunities for healthy living are based on social justice, equity, and relationships of mutual trust and caring, rather than on power and status.
- Health care, health protection, and disease prevention complement health promotion.
- Active participation in policies and programs is essential.

Summary

This chapter has introduced you to different ways of viewing health and health determinants, including the historical development of these concepts within the Canadian context. The content of the chapter challenges you to approach health situations broadly by identifying the myriad determinants that influence health. An increased understanding of health determinants should enable you to provide more sensitive care at the individual level and to consider strategies at the community and policy levels that will address the root causes of health situations.

✻ KEY CONCEPTS

- Health conceptualizations and determinants influence the nature and scope of professional practice.
- Definitions of health can be classified in several ways; recent definitions reflect a multidimensional perspective and a positive orientation.
- Three recent approaches to health are medical, behavioural, and socioenvironmental.
- Behavioural approaches focus primarily on health practices.
- Socioenvironmental approaches emphasize psychosocial factors and socioenvironmental conditions.
- Health determinants are interrelated.
- Canada is a leader in ever-changing views of health and health determinants.
- Health promotion differs from disease prevention.
- Three levels of disease prevention are primary (protection against disease), secondary (activities that promote early detection), and tertiary (activities directed toward minimizing disability from disease and helping clients learn to live productively with their limitations).
- The *Ottawa Charter* identifies five major categories of health promotion strategies: building healthy public policies; creating supportive environments; strengthening community action; developing personal skills; and reorienting health care services.

✻ CRITICAL THINKING EXERCISES

1. Describe your current level of health. What criteria did you use? Which definition of health discussed in this chapter best matches your understanding of health? Consider another definition of health discussed in this chapter. Does your current level of health change on the basis of this definition? How might your nursing practice differ depending on which conceptualization of health you choose to guide your practice? How might your definition of health change as you experience different life transitions (e.g., aging, parenthood)?

2. What do you consider to be the three most important health problems facing Canadians today? What are the major determinants of these problems? Which health promotion strategies would you consider the most appropriate to address them?

3. Imagine you are a community health nurse working in an area where many low-income women smoke. In a socioenvironmental approach to health, what questions would you need to address to decrease smoking behaviour in your area? How would your approach differ if you were using a behavioural approach to health?

✻ REVIEW QUESTIONS

1. The *Lalonde Report* is significant in that it was the first to emphasize
   1. A behavioural approach to health
   2. A medical approach to health
   3. A socioenvironmental approach to health
   4. Physiological risk factors
2. The "watershed" document that marked the shift from a lifestyle to a socioenvironmental approach to health was the
   1. *Lalonde Report*
   2. National Forum on Health (1997)
   3. *Toronto Charter*
   4. *Ottawa Charter*
3. From a socioenvironmental perspective, the major determinants of health are
   1. Psychosocial risk factors and socioenvironmental risk conditions
   2. Physiological risk factors and behavioural risk factors
   3. Behavioural and psychosocial risk factors
   4. Behavioural and socioenvironmental risk factors
4. The main reason that intersectoral collaboration is a necessary strategy to reach the goal of "Health for All" is
   1. The determinants of health are broad
   2. Intersectoral collaboration is cost-effective
   3. Intersectoral collaboration encourages problem solving at a local level
   4. Intersectoral collaboration is less likely to result in conflict
5. Providing immunizations against measles is an example of
   1. Health promotion
   2. Primary prevention
   3. Secondary prevention
   4. Tertiary prevention
6. Which one of the following statements does *not* accurately characterize health promotion?
   1. Health promotion addresses health issues within the context of the social, economic, and political environment.
   2. Health promotion emphasizes empowerment.
   3. Health promotion strategies focus primarily on helping people develop healthy behaviours.
   4. Health promotion is political.
7. The belief that health is primarily an individual responsibility is most congruent with the ______________ approach to health.
   1. Medical
   2. Behavioural
   3. Socioenvironmental
   4. Public health
8. All of the following statements accurately describe the Population Health Promotion Model *except*
   1. The model suggests that action can address the full range of health determinants
   2. The model incorporates the health promotion strategies of the *Ottawa Charter*
   3. The model focuses primarily on interventions at the societal level
   4. The model attempts to integrate population health and health promotion concepts
9. Which of the following is the most influential health determinant?
   1. Personal health practices
   2. Income and social status
   3. Health care services
   4. Physical environment
10. Health promotion activities are aimed at
    1. Providing protection against disease
    2. Increasing the level of well-being
    3. Avoiding injury or illness
    4. Teaching clients to learn to live with their limitations

✻ RECOMMENDED WEB SITES

Canadian Institute for Health Information (CIHI): http://secure.cihi.ca/cihiweb/dispPage.jsp?cw_page=home_e
The CIHI is a not-for-profit Canadian organization working to improve the health of Canadians and the health care system. One of its goals is to generate public awareness about factors affecting good health. This Web site offers current information and numerous links to government health reports.

Public Health Agency of Canada: http://www.phac-aspc.gc.ca
The Web site of the Public Health Agency of Canada provides excellent information on many aspects of public health, including the population health approach and the determinants of health.

Population Health: Determinants of Health: http://www.phac-aspc.gc.ca/ph-sp/determinants/determinants-eng.php#income
This Web page also provides links to health promotion research and documents.

World Health Organization publications: http://www.who.int/pub/en/
This Web site provides links to the publications of the World Health Organization, including the *World Health Report*.

WHO Commission on Social Determinants of Health: http://www.who.int/social_determinants/en/
This Web page provides many excellent papers pertaining to several determinants of health and provides a global perspective.

2

The Canadian Health Care System

Written by Pammla Petrucka, RN, BSc, BScN, MN, PhD

objectives

Mastery of content in this chapter will enable you to:

- Define the key terms.
- Discuss the evolution of Canada's social safety net and Medicare program.
- Identify and define the principles of the *Canada Health Act* and significant legislations related to the Canadian health care system.
- Discuss principal factors influencing health care reform and the current health care system.
- Discuss clients' rights to health care.
- Discuss multiple roles of nurses and challenges faced by them in different health care settings.
- Describe five levels of health care and the types of services aligned with each.
- Identify various settings and models of care delivery in the Canadian health care system.
- Identify initiatives related to enhancing the quality of the Canadian health care system.

key terms

Accessibility, p. 16
Acute care, p. 22
Adult day care centres, p. 24
Assisted-living facilities, p. 23
Comprehensiveness, p. 16
Continuity of care, p. 20
E-health, p. 25
Evidence-informed practice, p. 26
Health promotion, p. 19
Home care, p. 15
Hospice, p. 24
Inpatients, p. 16
Insured residents, p. 16
Levels of health care, p. 24
Long-term care facility, p. 15
Medicare, p. 15
Nursing informatics, p. 25
Outpatients, p. 22
Palliative care, p. 19
Parish nursing, p. 24
Portability, p. 16
Primary health care, p. 17
Primary health care centre, p. 21
Public administration, p. 16
Quality care, p. 25
Regional Health Authorities, p. 19
Rehabilitation, p. 18
Rehabilitation centre, p. 22
Respite care, p. 25
Secondary care, p. 22
Self-care, p. 25
Social safety net, p. 15
Supportive care, p. 25
Tertiary care, p. 22
Universality, p. 16
Voluntary agencies, p. 16

media resources

evolve Web Site

- Audio Chapter Summaries
- Glossary
- Multiple-Choice Review Questions
- Student Learning Activities
- Weblinks

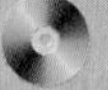

Companion CD

- Glossary
- Interactive Learning Activities
- Fluids and Electrolytes Tutorial
- Test-Taking Skills

Nurses are an essential part of the Canadian health care system, constituting the largest employment group within the health care system and recognized as invaluable to the health of Canadians. Nursing services are necessary for virtually every client seeking care of any type. In 2006, there were 252,948 registered nurses (77.8% of the regulated nursing workforce), 67,300 (20.7%) licensed practical nurses, and 5051 (1.6%) registered psychiatric nurses, which reflected an overall increase of 1.3% in the 2005 numbers (Canadian Institute for Health Information [CIHI], 2007a, 2007b, 2007c; see Box 2–1). Since the late 1990s, the size of the Canadian nursing workforce has remained relatively stable, despite a 9.1% increase in the general population, which means a decrease in the number of nurses per capita (CIHI, 2004a, 2004b). *Building the Future* (2005) was the first national study endorsed by stakeholder groups to outline a long-term strategy for ensuring adequate nursing human resources in Canada. The nursing workforce is challenged by the aging of its workers, a high retirement rate, and a lack of full-time positions.

Nursing is an integral part of the health care system, and so you must understand the system and the issues that affect how care is provided to clients. As a practicing nurse, you must appreciate the complexities of a health care system faced with rising costs, human resource challenges, and lack of availability of quality services. Financial pressures have forced hospitals and other institutions to shift priorities and to control costs by cutting the workforce and support services. Nursing professionals can help restructure delivery systems and achieve excellence in health care. The role of nurses in client advocacy is crucial for ensuring that everyone's health care needs are served. The success of health care depends on the participation of nurses to create systems that deliver quality, cost-effective care. Nurses must lead the way, advocating, reinforcing, and retaining its values for safe, quality, and **evidence-informed** client care.

➤ BOX 2-1 Facts About Nursing in Canada, 2007

- Of all registered nurses, 33% were degree-prepared; 13.9% had a baccalaureate degree when they entered practice.
- Nearly half (46.3%) of post-2000 registered nurses entered practice with a baccalaureate degree.
- Of the registered nurse workforce, 7.7% were foreign graduates; 1.8% of licensed practical nurses were foreign graduates.
- Of all registered nurses, 63.2% practiced in the hospital sector; 11.1%, in **long-term care;** 13.8%, in community and **home care;** and 11.9%, in other settings.
- Of all licensed practical nurses, 45.2% practiced in hospitals and 39.3% in long-term care.
- Of all registered nurses, 94.5% were female and 5.5% were male; of licensed practical nurses, 93.0% were female and 7% were male.
- Average age of registered nurses was 45; that of licensed practical nurses was 44.1; and that of registered psychiatric nurses was 47.2.
- Of all registered nurses, 20.8% were aged 55 years or older; 8.0% were aged 60 years or older; and 1.9% were aged 65 years or older. There were more Canadian registered nurses aged 55–59 than there were aged 25–29.
- More than 50% of the registered nurses had graduated more than 20 years earlier.
- Of all licensed practical nurses, 35.9% were aged 50 years or older.

Sources: Canadian Institute for Health Information (CIHI). (2007a). *Workforce trends of licensed practical nurses in Canada, 2006.* Ottawa, ON: Author; CIHI. (2007b). *Workforce trends of registered nurses in Canada, 2006.* Ottawa, ON: Author; and CIHI. (2007c). *Workforce trends of registered psychiatric nurses in Canada, 2006.* Ottawa, ON: Author.

Evolution of the Canadian Health Care System

Despite significant changes since the 1960s, a network of national provincial, and territorial social programs, referred to as the **social safety net**, is still needed to protect the most vulnerable members of Canadian society. Most programs are targeted to specific populations (e.g., elderly persons, children), but a few are universally accessible to all Canadians. For example, provincial social assistance programs provide income support to clients who are unemployed for a long time, and the federal Employment Insurance program provides income support for those with short-term interruption of employment. A key component of Canada's social safety net for citizens is the provision of hospital and medical insurance, known as **Medicare**, which is funded by general taxation.

Although often referred to as a "national" program, Medicare is, in fact, an interlocking set of 10 provincial and three territorial insurance schemes that provide "free" access to medically necessary hospital and physician services to all citizens, landed immigrants, and permanent residents (Health Canada, 2006a). Medicare is a source of significant national pride as a Canadian commitment to the well-being of its citizens, as well as a source of national debate regarding its costs, effectiveness, and sustainability. Few issues are as important and controversial to Canadians as health care.

Early Health Care in Canada

Europeans who came to Canada in the fifteenth century brought infectious diseases that flourished under conditions of poor sanitation. Settlements enacted public health laws to control the spread of diseases. For years, government care was limited to essential services (i.e., care of insane persons and epidemics). Permanent boards of health did not exist; families, churches, and local communities were expected to be self-reliant in handling all other medical and social problems. The first Canadian nurses were nuns from religious orders, such as the legendary Marguerite d'Youville (see Box 2–2).

Canada became a self-governing colony with the passage of the *British North America Act* (also known as the *Constitution Act*) in 1867 which united three colonies into the original four provinces of

➤ BOX 2-2 Moments in Canadian Nursing History*

Throughout Canada's history, nurses have been meeting the health care needs of individuals, families, and communities. As nurses encountered changing practice environments, such as World Wars or the Great Depression in the 1930s, they transformed their practices and skills to meet the new situations. During English–French hostilities from 1756 to 1760, the Grey Nuns cared for sick and wounded soldiers, including British prisoners of war. This order was known for its excellent hospitals, offering care regardless of race, colour, creed, or financial status. By the middle of the twentieth century, nursing transformed from a predominately spiritual vocation to a secular profession (Mansell, 2004). Most nurses worked in hospitals and communities but were also present in nursing and health care organizations such as the Red Cross, the Victorian Order of Nurses, military or navy service, tuberculosis sanatoria, professional nursing associations, and nursing unions. Although "the practice of nursing is perceived as an integral part of health care services in Canada" (Mansell, 2004, p. 204), the struggle for professionalism and recognition has not been an easy one.

*Section Contributor: S. L. Bassendowski, RN, EdD

Ontario, Quebec, Nova Scotia, and New Brunswick. This Act accorded certain powers to the national (federal) government and certain powers to the provincial governments. Responsibility for health, education, and social services was accorded to the provinces; the federal government retained jurisdiction for parts of these public policies (Storch, 2006). For example, health care for Canada's Aboriginal peoples and pharmaceutical safety remain federal responsibilities, but regulation of hospitals is a provincial jurisdiction.

As Canada's population grew and became more urban and industrial, crowded living conditions, poor housing, and sanitation led to more disease. Provinces enacted public health acts to establish local boards of health to hire medical health officers and sanitation inspectors. The nurses working directly in the community and with the poor were the first public health nurses.

By 1920, health and social programs had expanded, and **voluntary agencies** formed; the latter included the Children's Aid Society (formed in 1891), the Red Cross (in 1896), the Victorian Order of Nurses (in 1897), and the Canadian Mental Health Association (in 1918). Municipalities organized services for the poor and established hospitals. Clients who could not pay depended on charity (Figure 2–1). Fraternal societies (e.g., Knights of Columbus) and unions created trusts that members could access when ill, injured at work, or unemployed. Such programs were precursors of modern employment insurance.

As urbanization continued, rural communities had difficulty attracting and paying physicians. The federal *Municipality Act* of 1916 gave communities the power to levy taxes to pay for physicians. The Great Depression during the 1930s dramatically affected the health care system. Many families could not pay their medical bills, and hospital stays caused financial ruin. As needs increased, it became apparent that many provinces did not have the tax base to fund these services and to ensure that they were similar in scope across the country.

These hardships inspired the Canadian provincial governments to create a prepaid medical and hospitalization insurance plan. In 1947, Premier Tommy Douglas of Saskatchewan introduced a public, universal hospital insurance plan. This program became the basis of the first major federal initiative to expand hospital insurance across the country with the passage of the *Hospital Insurance and Diagnostic Services Act* (*HIDSA*) in 1956. For provinces that agreed to set up universal hospital insurance, *HIDSA* provided federal funds to cover approximately half of service cost. By 1961, all provinces and territories were in agreement to provide coverage for **inpatient** hospital care.

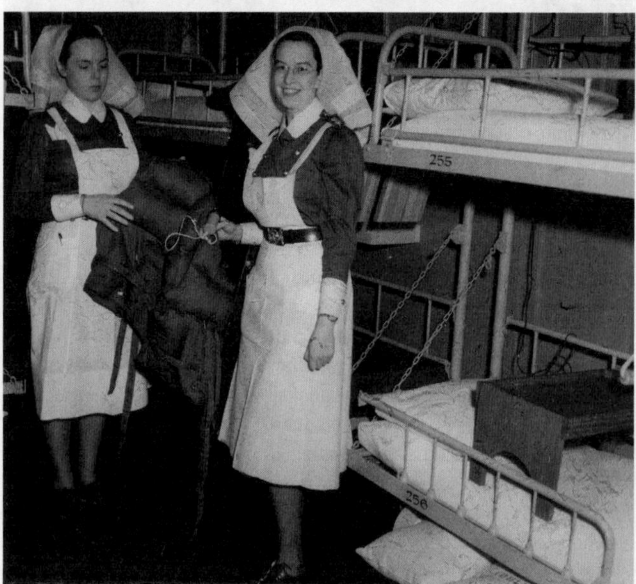

Figure 2-1 Military nurses. **Source:** Photo courtesy of WJR Bateman.

The next step was to ensure medical services outside hospitals. Again, Saskatchewan took the lead. Because the federal government now covered half of the cost of hospital insurance in the province, Saskatchewan could now afford to provide medical insurance, and in 1962, the *Medical Care Insurance Act* was passed. The legislation was opposed by the province's physicians, who went on a 23-day strike. They eventually reached a compromise with the government in which the physicians' autonomy to practice as they wished was preserved in exchange for agreeing to a single-payer insurance system to fund their services.

In 1964, the Royal Commission on Health Services was appointed to study the provision of hospital and medical care to all Canadians and concluded that "strong federal government leadership and financial support for medical care" was needed (Wilson, 1995). The *Hall Commission Report*, named after lead commissioner, Justice Emmett Hall, called for the expansion of the Saskatchewan model across the country on a cost-shared basis similar to that of *HIDSA* (Royal Commission on Health Services, 1964, 1965).

On the basis of these recommendations, the federal government passed the *Medical Care Act* in 1966. Federal grants were awarded on a cost-sharing basis with the provinces if programs provided universal, comprehensive, portable, and publicly administered coverage of hospital and physician services. The federal, provincial, and territorial governments agreed to share health care expenses equally. By 1972, all provincial and territorial insurance plans had extended their coverage to include medical services provided outside hospitals. Thus began modern Medicare, inasmuch as all Canadians now had free access to hospital and medical care, regardless of personal wealth.

Although programs prospered, cost sharing did not last. In 1977, the Canadian government enacted the *Federal Provincial Fiscal Arrangements and Established Programs Financing Act* to replace cost sharing with block transfers of funds and a complicated formula of transferring tax points from the federal government to the provinces and territories. These block transfers resulted in decreased federal contributions. To make up this shortfall, some provinces allowed the so-called extra billing of clients by hospitals and provider groups over the amount that the universal insurance program covered. These charges were seen by Medicare's defenders as a threat to the universality of Canada's medical insurance scheme and as a violation of the principle that care should be accessible on the basis of need and not on the ability to pay.

The federal government's response was to enact the *Canada Health Act* in 1984, which amalgamated the previous acts of *HIDSA* and *Medical Care Act* and effectively banned extra billing and user fees. The *Canada Health Act* added the principle of **accessibility** to the principles of **public administration, comprehensiveness, universality,** and **portability** (see Table 2–1). These principles apply to all **insured residents** (i.e., eligible residents) of a province or territory but exclude members of the Canadian Forces, Royal Canadian Mounted Police (RCMP), veterans, and inmates of federal penitentiaries. First Nations and Inuit health services receive special consideration, which is discussed later in this chapter. Under previous acts, access to services was through physician gatekeepers. Revisions to the *Canada Health Act* allowed multiple points of access and insurance for care providers other than physicians. Although opposition to the *Canada Health Act* arose, all provinces and territories were following its principles by 1987 (Health Canada, 1992). According to the *Canada Health Act*, the primary objective of Canadian health care policy is ". . . to protect, promote and restore the physical and mental well

➤ TABLE 2-1 Principles of the Canada Health Act of 1984

Public administration	A public authority administers and operates the plan on a nonprofit basis; it is responsible to the provincial and territorial governments for decision making on benefit levels and services and is subject to financial audits.
Comprehensiveness	The plan covers all medically necessary hospital and physician services and, as the province or territory permits, services of other health care practitioners. The palette of services publicly funded for each province and territory varies, which is controversial and under review (e.g., Commission on the Future of Health Care in Canada [Romanow, 2002]; Ontario Health Services Restructuring Commission, 2000).
Universality	Insured residents are entitled to health care services provided by the plan on uniform terms and conditions. Universality negates discrimination based on race, gender, income, ethnicity, or religion (Health Canada, 2006b; Romanow, 2002).
Portability	Insured residents can access health care services in another province or territory without cost or penalty. Personal coverage must be maintained when an insured person moves or travels within Canada or travels outside of Canada.
Accessibility	Insured residents have reasonable access to medically necessary hospital and physician services, regardless of income, age, health status, gender, or geographical location. Additional charges for insured services are not permitted, and *essential* health care services must be available to all Canadians on the basis of need (Romanow, 2002).

Adapted from Health Canada. (2007c). *Canada Health Act: Introduction*. Retrieved March 31, 2008, from http://www.hc-sc.gc.ca/hcs-sss/pubs/cha-lcs/2006-cha-lcs-ar-ra/intro-eng.php

being of residents of Canada and to facilitate reasonable access to health services without financial or other barriers"(Health Canada, 2007a).

The *Canada Health Act* is a major piece of legislation that influences the delivery of health care services across Canada. A wide array of other legislation (see Table 2–2) at the federal level influences health and health services for the people of Canada in areas such as tobacco use, environmental health, and health research.

Aboriginal Health Care

Another major source of legislation is the *Indian Act* of 1985, which identifies the federal government's role in providing health care services to First Nations and Inuit people (Department of Justice Canada, 2003). First Nations and Inuit Health (FNIH), a part of Health Canada, and Indian and Northern Affairs Canada (INAC) share responsibility for ensuring that health care services are provided to Canada's First Nations and Inuit people (Health Canada, 2006a; INAC, 2004). Treaties with so-called Indian bands in Canada were signed before Confederation with the British government and after Confederation with the government of Canada (Natural Resources Canada, 2003). These treaties outlined agreements regarding land, services, and relationships; some (such as Treaty 6) included a provision for health care services to be provided by the government to the First Nations communities, often referred to as the "medicine chest" clause (INAC, 2004). These treaties have enabled direct delivery of services to First Nations and Inuit peoples, regardless of where they live in Canada, including **primary health care** (PHC) and emergency services on remote and isolated reserves where provincial or territorial

➤ TABLE 2-2 Relevant Health-Related Legislation*

Legislation and Date Passed	Purpose
Canadian Environmental Protection Act, 1999	Regulates pollution prevention; environmental protection and human health contribute to sustainable development
Canadian Institutes of Health Research Act, 2000	Strategizes and funds health-related research
Controlled Drugs and Substances Act, 1996	Controls certain drugs, their precursors, and related substances
Emergency Preparedness Act, 1988	Develops and implements civil emergency plans by facilitating and coordinating among government institutions and with provincial and territorial governments, foreign governments, and international organizations
Food and Drugs Act, 1985	Regulates food, drugs, cosmetics, and therapeutic devices
Quarantine Act, 1985	Controls introduction and spread of infectious or contagious diseases
Tobacco Act, 1997	Regulates manufacture, sale, labelling, and promotion of tobacco products

*Section contributor: T. McIntosh, PhD.

services are not readily available; community-based health programs both on reserves and in Inuit communities; and noninsured health benefits programs (e.g., pharmaceuticals, dental, vision, and medical transportation). All three levels of government (federal, provincial and territorial, and Aboriginal) are working together to improve and integrate health service delivery (Health Canada, 2006a). Aboriginal self-governance has been enabled through the "inherent right of self-government" under Section 35 of the *Canadian Constitution Act* of 1982. As self-governance models emerge, health care, as part of the palette of services and programs within Aboriginal jurisdiction, will challenge health care professionals to be "responsive to their particular political, economic, legal, historical, cultural, and social circumstances" (INAC, 2008).

The Organization and Governance of Health Care

Under the Canadian constitution, administration and delivery of health care services are primarily provincial or territorial responsibilities. The federal government has a role in health care financing, enforcement of the *Canada Health Act,* delivery of services to previously described targeted groups, and setting national agendas such as those relating to public health and safety, pharmaceuticals, and biomedical and health services research.

Federal Jurisdiction

The federal government accomplishes the following tasks:

- Sets and administers national principles for the health care system through the *Canada Health Act.*
- Assists in financing of provincial and territorial health care services through transfer payments (i.e., transferring tax money to share cost of health care services) on the basis of adherence to the *Canada Health Act* principles.
- Delivers health services for targeted groups, including First Nations and Inuit people, military veterans, federal inmates, and the RCMP.
- Provides national policy and programming to promote health and prevent disease, such as healthy environment and consumer safety programs and public health programs.

Provincial and Territorial Jurisdiction

Each provincial and territorial government accomplishes the following tasks:

- Develops and administers its own health care insurance plan.
- Manages, finances, and plans insurable health care services and delivery, in alignment with *Canada Health Act* principles (see Table 2–1).
- Determines organization and location of hospitals or long-term care facilities; the mix of health care professionals employed in hospitals or health care facilities; and the amount of money dedicated to health care services.
- Reimburses physician and hospital expenses; provides some **rehabilitation** and long-term care services, usually on the basis of copayments with individual users.

Each provincial and territorial plan is unique, and what is covered and by how much varies across the country. For example, coverage for drugs taken outside of hospitals, ambulance services, and home care varies widely by province and territory. Marchildon (2006) reviewed what is and is not covered by each province and territory. To offset costs for services not covered by provincial or territorial insurance, Canadians can buy private health insurance or participate in employer-offered individual or group insurance plans.

Professional Jurisdiction

Most health professions (i.e., medicine, nursing, pharmacology) in Canada are self-regulated, which means they determine standards, competencies, codes of ethics, and disciplinary actions for their respective members. Some professions are regulated through governments (e.g., emergency medical technicians in British Columbia, Manitoba, Ontario, and Saskatchewan) or other regulatory mechanisms (e.g., osteopathic physicians in Alberta and British Columbia). In some cases, so-called omnibus legislations regulate several professions simultaneously (e.g., *Alberta's Health Disciplines Act* of 2000).

Health Care Spending

"Canadians pay, directly or indirectly, for every aspect of our health care system through a combination of taxes, payments to government, private insurance premiums, and direct out-of-pocket fees of varying types and amounts" (Romanow, 2002, p. 24). In a 2005 Commonwealth Fund International Health Policy Survey, Schoen et al. (2005) found that Canadians are dissatisfied with their health care system; 78% asserted that fundamental change or a complete overhaul was needed. This dissatisfaction exists despite steady growth in health care costs since the late 1950s—faster on average than the economy as a whole.

In 2006, Canada spent an estimated $148 billion on health services, more than three times what was spent in 1975, adjusted for inflation (CIHI, 2006). Overall, in Canada, about $4548 per person was spent on health care in 2006, in comparison with $3572 in 2002 (CIHI, 2006). In addition, the average Canadian household expended $1870 (Statistics Canada, 2008) for health care, an amount up 6% from that of the previous year. Furthermore, per capita spending is higher for children and older adults than for younger adults. Although older adults constitute 12.6% of the population, they account for approximately 50% of hospital costs (CIHI, 2004b). In 2006, health care spending as a share of Canada's gross domestic product was 10.3% (CIHI, 2006), in comparison with 16% in the United States (National Coalition on Health Care, 2008) or 9.4% in Sweden (Vårdguiden, 2007). In 2006, hospital and health care institutions (30%), retail drug sales (17%) and physician services (13%) accounted for more than half of health care spending. In 2005, this translated to hospital expenditures of $40.35 billion, drug expenditures of $23.34 billion, and physician services expenditures of $18.34 billion, in contrast to $8.46 billion for public health services and $15.21 billion for other health care professionals' services. Despite these significant expenditures, Canada ranks 8th of 17 industrialized countries in the Organization for Economic Cooperation and Development (Conference Board of Canada, 2007) on a series of indicators such as life expectance, perceived health status, disease specific mortality rates, and lifestyle behaviours (e.g., smoking, obesity).

Trends and Reforms in Canada's Health Care System

Since the 1980s, rapid and significant changes in health care delivery, technology, and public expectations have challenged the Canadian federal, provincial, and territorial governments to reconstruct a health care system that balances current and future political, legal, economic, and social realities (Petrucka, 2005). In most provinces, restructuring has become entrusted to **regional health authorities**, which are led by appointed or elected community representatives and whose mandates, roles, and responsibilities are guided by provincial legislations (Lewis & Kouri, 2004). Regionalization was intended to streamline health services, to reduce fragmentation, to respond to local needs, to improve public participation, and to address the continuum of health care services from disease prevention and health promotion to curative, supportive, restorative, and **palliative** treatments (Lewis & Kouri, 2004). Although these principles were initially attractive and promising, the process has not lived up to its potential; instead, it has become primarily a fiscal exercise rather than a philosophical or health-motivated reform (Petrucka, 2005).

According to Armstrong (1999), health reform ***concerns primarily continuity and integration, quality and accountability, and disease prevention and health promotion. Framed within the determinants of health literature, the reforms are intended to deliver better quality and more appropriate care at lower cost, primarily by adopting managerial strategies from the business sector.*** Numerous federally and provincially sponsored reports have made recommendations for reforming the health care system. Two influential national reports on Canada's health care system include the *Kirby Report* (Kirby, 2002) and the report of the Romanow Commission (Romanow, 2002; see Box 2–3).

Many experts claim that Canadians' current rate of health care expenditures is unsustainable. As discussed previously, health care spending has continued to grow exponentially, and some academics have predicted that by 2020, it will near $250 billion (Conference Board of Canada, 2007). Because health care costs are rising faster than government revenues, some Canadian citizens and decision makers believe that spending on health care will eventually crowd out spending on other programs in the social safety net and will consume 100% of all monies (MacKinnon, 2004). If health care spending absorbs all available monies, the future of education programs, social services, transportation safety, and environmental protection—all of which have a profound impact on health—will be uncertain.

The Canadian Nurses Association (CNA) is a strong proponent of a health care system that continues to respect the principles of the *Canada Health Act* and acknowledges the advancement of nursing as a primary access point to health care (see CNA, 2005; Smadu, 2006).

Role of Nurses in Health Care Policy

Nurses play a key role in health care policy, both as leaders at the political and community level and in their everyday work lives. Individually and collectively, nurses are integral to policy development (Falk-Raphael, 2005; Hart, 2004). For most of the years since the late 1950s, the position of a senior or chief nurse has existed at the federal government level, and many provincial governments employ nurses in similar positions. These nurses bring the nursing perspectives to health policy decisions, present government perspectives to nurses and clients, and articulate the potential impact of policy decisions to politicians and other stakeholders. Referring to a broader level, Villeneuve and MacDonald (2006) stated that all nurses can be at the forefront of the coming changes, setting the agenda to create a health care system that truly serves and reflects the priorities of Canadians. Falk-Rafael (2005) stated that "nurses . . . are ideally situated and morally obligated to include political advocacy and efforts to influence health public policy in their practice" (p. 212). Health care across the country needs a coordinated, integrated approach by nurses if they are to inform policy decisions and help shape the country's health care systems (Villeneuve & MacDonald, 2006).

➤ BOX 2-3 Influential Health Care Reports

The Romanow Commission

Romanow (2002) concluded that Medicare is sustainable and must be preserved because it represents Canadians' core values. His top priority was to modernize the *Canada Health Act* through appropriate funding and to initiate the following changes:

- Create a new diagnostic service fund
- Build information technology infrastructure
- Improve access (e.g., in rural and remote areas and for Aboriginal peoples)
- Ensure and measure quality
- Improve and expand PHC
- Strengthen and expand home care
- Offer catastrophic drug coverage
- Create a National Health Council responsible for indicators, benchmarks, and performance measures

Romanow (2002) did not attach a specific cost to any of his recommendations, but he did stress accountability for funding and services provided.

The *Kirby Report*

Kirby (2002) concluded that the current Medicare system is not sustainable. He advocated stronger private sector involvement in health care delivery. Although Kirby did not address the core values or recommend changes to the *Canada Health Act,* he clarified the impact of spiraling health care costs on other social programs. Kirby recommended the following priorities:

- Shift funding for hospitals to a service-based model
- Grant more responsibility to regional health authorities for delivering publicly insured health services, contracting out these services, or both
- Reform PHC
- Offer a health care guarantee to Canadians (e.g., time limits for wait times; if the wait time is exceeded, the government pays for care provided elsewhere)

Like Romanow (2002), Kirby (2002) emphasized accountability for services and funding. Instead of a National Health Council (as recommended by Romanow), he suggested an appointed council with limited advisory functions.

Based on Romanow, R. J. (2002). *Building on values: The future of health care in Canada—Final report.* Ottawa, ON: Commission on the Future of Health Care in Canada; and Kirby, M. J. L. (2002). *The health of Canadians—The federal role. Vol. 6: Recommendations for reform.* Ottawa ON: Standing Senate Committee on Social Affairs, Science and Technology, retrieved August 8, 2008, from http://www.parl.gc.ca/37/2/parlbus/commbus/senate/com-e/soci-e/rep-e/repoct02vol6-e.htm

Right to Health Care

The consensus in Canada is that everyone has a right to health care. Upon entering the health care system, a person becomes a client with certain rights. In general, consumers have a right to determine what kind of health care should be available to them. However, the *Canadian Charter of Rights and Freedoms* of 1982 does not explicitly include health care as a right; therefore, federal and provincial legislation must prove legal entitlement. (Only Quebec has health care rights in its legislation.) The *Canada Health Act* influences rights by setting conditions for federal funding, giving insured persons the right to have health care costs covered, but the right to health care itself is not guaranteed in the Act.

Rights Within the Health Care System

Sutherland and Fulton (1992) articulated a number of rights that Canadian health care workers expect: namely, the right to reasonable working conditions, including safety and absence of discrimination. The Commission on the Future of Health Care in Canada called for the adoption of a health covenant that would specify the rights, obligations, and expectations of governments, citizens, and health care professionals (Romanow, 2002), but, to date, governments have shown little interest in ratifying this kind of arrangement. Although, in practice, no statutory requirement exists in Canada to include client advocacy (or other stakeholder) groups in the policymaking process, a number of national groups (e.g., Canadian Cancer Society, Canadian Diabetes Association), as well as disease-specific client groups, are involved. These groups often share information, endorse, report on, or criticize health care policy decisions (Health Consumer Powerhouse AB & Frontier Centre for Public Policy, 2008).

Primary Health Care

PHC is a foundation of Canada's health care system, providing entry point of contact into the health care system, as well as the vehicle for **continuity of care** (Health Council of Canada, 2008). Rooted in a 1974 document by then–Minister of Health and Welfare Marc Lalonde, who advocated a broad strategy, PHC involves addressing nonmedical determinants of health in order to improve the health of citizens (Health Canada, 2006a). The report outlined the connection between health status and the social determinants of health, including employment, poverty, lifestyle, environment, and genetic endowment. Other documents, such as the Alma-Ata declaration on PHC (World Health Organization [WHO], 1978) and the *Ottawa Charter for Health Promotion* (Lalonde, 1986), built the framework that has informed population health and **health promotion** approaches globally. The WHO has continued its focus on population health, and Canadian federal, provincial, and territorial health departments have established units or branches that focus on and fund programs and services to promote this approach.

According to the CNA, PHC is a philosophy and a model for improving health that supports essential health care services (promotive, preventive, curative, rehabilitative, and supportive), with a strong emphasis on the principles of health promotion and disease prevention. Most definitions of PHC recognize the importance of placing stronger emphasis on the determinants of health and strategies to advance individual and population health (Health Council of Canada, 2008). PHC is cited as the key to health care reform and sustainability. In June 2002, Romanow stated, "PHC is the single most important basis from which to renew the health care system" (CNA, 2003).

PHC, as an integrated approach, refers to health and a related spectrum of services external to the traditional health care system. These services represent health in its broadest sense, such as income, housing, education, and environment (Health Canada, 2006b). The PHC model (see Figure 2–2) focuses on collaboration among health professionals, community members, and others working in multiple sectors, emphasizing health promotion, development of health policies, and prevention of diseases for all individuals. According to the National Primary Health Care Awareness Strategy [NPHCAS] (2006a), PHC accomplishes the following:

- Prevents people from becoming ill or injured.
- Enables clients to manage chronic conditions.
- Optimizes use of health care professional expertise.
- Enables health care workers to treat acute and episodic illness.
- Coordinates for efficiency and access.
- Enables individuals to participate fully in their health care.
- Recognizes factors external to the health care system that affect individual and community health.

Throughout this book, "Focus on Primary Health Care" boxes highlight the vital role that nurses play in providing PHC. Box 2–4 links health care situations to PHC principles.

Barriers to Primary Health Care

The meaning of PHC has caused confusion among health care consumers and even health care professionals. The distinction between PHC and **primary care (PC)** is difficult to understand. Access to PC is a key element of PHC, but it is only one component. PC focuses on personal health services, whereas PHC extends beyond PC to include health education, proper nutrition, maternal and child health care, family planning, immunizations, and control of locally endemic diseases. This broader concept of PHC proposed for Canada relates to the continuum of care by interprofessional teams of providers working with the client as the driver (Annapolis Valley Health, 2007).

Challenging the adoption of PHC is an underlying concern that "Many Canadians see the health system as an 'illness care' system that will be there when they need it" (CNA, 2003). Some experts fear that if monies are dedicated to PHC priorities and implementation, benefits will be limited, at least in the near term. PHC is a sensible approach to health care that is cost-effective and benefits people most in need. It offers vulnerable people the chance for a healthy life. For example, by attending a community health program on infant and child care, parents learn the importance of recognizing signs and symptoms of urinary tract infection (UTI) in children and the importance of seeking medical treatment if they suspect their child has a UTI. With this knowledge, parents may prevent long-term serious complications of untreated UTIs, such as kidney damage and distress, as well as reduce health care costs.

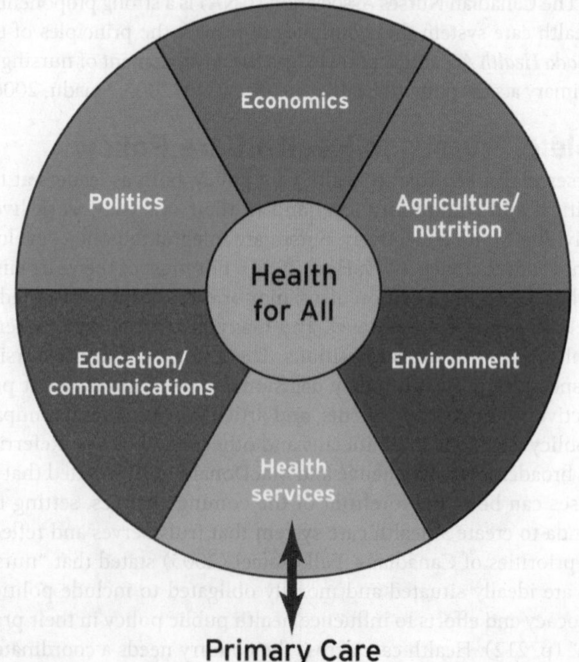

Figure 2-2 Primary health care model: A multisectoral or intersectoral approach. **Source:** From Shoultz, J., & Hatcher, P. A. (1997). Looking beyond primary health care: An approach to community-based action. *Nursing Outlook, 45*(1), 24. © 1996 by P. Hatcher, J. Shoulz, and W. Patrick.

The Canadian Health Services Research Foundation (2005) stated that clients seeking interdisciplinary care "in addition to their PC physicians fare at least as well as those receiving care from their doctors alone, and many studies find significant improvements." Despite this finding, some professionals do not support a PHC model, which requires interdisciplinary collaboration and flexible boundaries between health care professions. Smadu (2005) stated that many health care professionals are socialized to believe—and act as if—they alone must have all the answers and provide all the direction for their clients. In response, Health Canada (2007b) introduced the Interprofessional Education for Collaborative Patient-Centred Practice strategy, which provided interprofessional education opportunities across Canada aimed at improving socialization, decision making, respect, understanding, and competencies related to enhancing collaborative practice. This program strives to highlight changes in the way health care professionals are educated with the knowledge and skills to work interprofessionally and to be responsive in achieving health care change.

BOX 2-4 FOCUS ON PRIMARY HEALTH CARE

The Four Pillars of Primary Health Care*

A number of models for PHC have been described. The NPHCAS (2006b) described four pillars of PHC as follows: teams, access, information, and healthy living.

Teams

PHC requires a team of health care providers working together to improve continuity of care, reduce duplication, and ensure access to appropriate health care professionals (Mang, 2005). Of importance is that clients are at the centre of the team and are empowered to make decisions about their own care (Smadu, 2005).

West Winds Primary Health Centre (WWPHC) in Saskatoon is a **PHC centre** addressing the health care needs of men, pregnant and nonpregnant women, adolescents, children, new immigrants, First Nations and Métis peoples, and older adults. WWPHC functions as a partnership with the University of Saskatchewan and the Saskatoon Health Region to deliver PHC in a community setting. WWPHC offers outstanding research and program evaluation opportunities for students in the health sciences, including medicine. Transdisciplinary, intersectoral collaboration is evolving at WWPHC, providing a full range of services that include but are not limited to health promotion, chronic disease prevention and management, the Healthy Mother Healthy Baby program, maternal mental health, the Food for Thought program, mental health and addiction services, diabetes education, public health services, and dental clinics. Staff includes physicians, nutritionists, clinical health psychologists, clinic nurses, nurse practitioners, occupational therapists, physical therapists, speech-language pathologists, pharmacists, social workers, public health nurses, and clinical researchers. A community participation working group and a collaborative practice resource group provide direction and support development of evidence-informed programs.

Access

PHC is rooted in ensuring that Canadians have greater access to the appropriate services when and where they are needed. According to Mang (2005), PHC recognizes the need for advice, information, and care outside of office hours. PHC improves access in three ways: It provides faster entry into the health care system, maximizes scopes of practice for all health professionals, and reduces demands for heath care by making clients healthier (Rachlis, 2005).

In urban settings, teams of nurses, physicians, social workers, counsellors, nutritionists, and other professionals bring PHC to the streets. They seek out the vulnerable groups—people who are in poor health (often with addictions, human immunodeficiency virus [HIV] infection or acquired immunodeficiency syndrome [AIDS], and hepatitis C), homeless, and malnourished and who lack support—to assess and monitor the health status and provide care "in place." Nurses on "PHC street teams" care for individuals who are in need, as well as for the needs of entire communities. For example, one nurse visits a 17-year-old prostitute who is 8 months pregnant, is addicted to crack, and lives within a boxcar community. The nurse also runs a community program called "Having Healthy Babies" for young, vulnerable women, which is located at a centre near the train tracks, to increase accessibility.

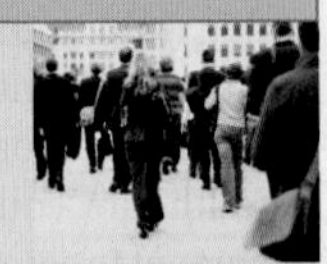

Information

PHC is about sharing and increasing access to information between health care professionals and Canadians who use the health care system or seek health care advice (NPHCAS, 2006b). Tools (e.g., electronic health records; diagnostic equipment) and skills (e.g., telehealth) are needed to facilitate quality, access, and coordination of information. An appropriate technology is the telephone triage systems now used successfully in many provinces and territories. Individuals dial a toll-free number and are immediately connected to a qualified nurse who can answer their health questions. This technology has addressed access to health care, especially in rural and remote areas. For example, nurses in the New Brunswick program have responded to the questions and concerns of almost 75% of callers.

Canada Health Infoway (Infoway) is a federally funded, independent, not-for-profit organization with representation from 14 federal, provincial, and territorial health ministries. Infoway fosters and accelerates development and adoption of electronic health information systems with compatible standards and communications technologies on a pan-Canadian basis. The vision is of a high-quality, sustainable, and effective infostructure that provides Canadians and health care professionals with timely, appropriate, and secure access to the appropriate information when and where they enter into the health care system. This infostructure further empowers clients by providing a cumulative personal health history that provides health care professionals with accurate health information (Alvarez, 2005).

Healthy Living

PHC, with its wellness focus, embraces strategies of prevention, management of chronic illness, and self-care. It recognizes that factors outside the health care system (e.g., social, economic, environmental) influence individual and community health. At the individual level, healthy living means making positive choices; at a broader level, it addresses factors that influence people's health and their ability to make healthy choices (Harvey, 2005).

A case in point is the story of a public health nurse in southern Ontario who was running a program that educated low-income mothers about nutrition, child development, and community action. The women shared their ideas about how to meet their family's nutritional requirements on tight budgets. They were alarmed to learn that a national bakery was closing its local day-old–bread outlet. The nurse coached the women to call a local newspaper reporter, who, in turn, contacted the bakery's president, and persuaded the owner to keep the outlet open. The nurse's health promotion activities resulted in a decision that benefited the community.

*Section contributor: V. R. Ramsden, RN, PhD.

Source: Canadian Nurses Association. (2003). Primary health care—The time has come. *Nursing Now, 16*, 1–4.

Future of Primary Health Care

In a restructured health care system that emphasizes PHC, programs necessarily will cross sectors. For example, trauma programs will have health promotion activities (road safety education), preventive programming (helmet legislation), **secondary** and **tertiary care** (emergency transportation), and rehabilitation (head injury–related recovery programs). Programs will cover multiple sites, may be defined by a particular disease or population group (e.g., children), and will comprise multiple disciplines and sectors of society (e.g., health care, education, justice systems). Nursing will have a significant role in every aspect of a PHC-integrated program.

Because of its integrated approach, PHC may hold the key to Canada's looming health care crisis. If Canadians stay healthier because more money is spent on PHC, they will need less medical care, and the proportion of money going to medical care will decline. If health care, education, social services, and the voluntary sector have integrated programs, competition among the various sectors for government monies may decline. This integration requires each sector to think beyond its own boundaries (see Box 2–5). If the PHC agenda in Canada is to progress, a number of resources and strategies are considered necessary, including the following (Health Canada, 2006b):

- An adequate supply of health care human resources.
- A team approach focused on client needs, to ensure that the greatest number of appropriate providers work collectively to optimize outcomes.
- Information technology (i.e., electronic health records).
- Governance and funding models that support team-based care.
- Links to public health.
- A culture of accountability, performance measurement, and quality improvement.

Settings for Health Care Delivery

Although health care organization and delivery varies across Canada, three types of delivery agencies are comparable: institutional agencies, formal community agencies, and voluntary and private sector agencies.

Institutional Sector

The institutional agencies include hospitals, long-term care facilities, psychiatric facilities, and **rehabilitation centres**. All offer health care services to inpatients (clients who stay at an institution for diagnosis, treatment, or rehabilitation). Most offer services to **outpatients** (clients who visit an institution for these services).

BOX 2-5 CASE STUDY

Primary Health Care

During a community meeting in a core area of a small city, parents, educators, health care professionals, and volunteers agreed to pilot an integrated program to prevent obesity in children. Social services and volunteers run a breakfast program. Fruits and vegetables for twice-daily snacks are donated by a local grocery store. Nutritionists and kinesiologists educate the teachers to integrate nutrition and physical fitness into the curriculum. Schools commit to having students and teachers participate in activities for at least 15 minutes every day and establish rules for school lunches (e.g., no soda pop). Nurse practitioners arrange visits with the parents of children identified as being overweight or at risk. If only 10% of the children in the program develop a healthier lifestyle, future savings to the health care system will pay for program costs.

Hospitals. Hospitals have traditionally been considered major health care agencies, most specializing in **acute care** services. Hospital services may include emergency and diagnostic, inpatient, surgical intervention, intensive care, outpatient, and rehabilitation services. The numbers of hospitals, hospital beds, and admissions in Canada have decreased significantly since the 1990s; the results are a higher proportion of clients with more acute needs and rapid turnover of clients in hospitals, in turn creating more intense, specialized, and increased workloads for health care providers (CIHI, 2007a, 2007b, 2007c). Hospitals strive to provide the highest quality of care possible and to facilitate early client discharge safely to the home, community, or a facility that can adequately manage remaining health care needs. Acute care is health care delivered for a short time (usually days to weeks, typically less than 3 months) in which an immediate health problem is diagnosed, treated, or both.

Hospitals are distinguished by their size (e.g., community hospitals), service provision (e.g., cancer care hospitals), and connection to academic institutions (e.g., university health science centres), as well as by public or private status. Public hospitals are financed and operated by a government agency at the local, provincial, or national level and constitute the largest group of health employers in Canada. Private hospitals are owned and operated by groups such as churches, corporations, and charitable organizations. Military hospitals, although limited in Canada, provide medical services to members of the military and their families. Veterans' hospitals provide residential, extended care, and rehabilitation to aging, injured, and disabled military veterans.

Roles and functions of hospitals and hospital-based health care professionals have rapidly evolved in this era of health care reform. Hospital nurses use critical thinking skills (see Chapter 12), apply the nursing process (see Chapter 13), coordinate and delegate care elements (see Chapter 11), and stress client teaching and postdischarge self-care (see Chapter 21). A trend is currently emerging toward evidence-informed practice when client interventions are determined. Nurses participate in discharge planning as a critical interdisciplinary coordination strategy in the continuity of care for clients, ensuring the smooth and safe transitions of clients between levels of care and the community. Many hospital nurses specialize as clinical nurse specialists, for example, in caring for clients with specific needs (e.g., palliative) or specific diseases (e.g., cardiovascular). Other hospital roles include nurse manager, infection control coordinator, clinical educator, and clinical nurse researcher.

Long-Term Care Facilities. A long-term care (extended care) facility provides accommodations and 24-hour intermediate and custodial care (e.g., nursing, rehabilitation, dietary, recreational, social, and spiritual services) for residents of any age with chronic or debilitating illnesses or disabilities. Most residents are frail, older adults with multiple health issues (see Chapter 25). Some are younger adults with severe, chronic health conditions (see Chapter 24). A long-term care facility functions as the resident's temporary or permanent home; therefore, the surroundings should be as homelike as possible. The philosophy of care is to provide a planned, systematic, and interdisciplinary approach that helps residents reach and maintain their highest level of function. Long-term care facilities are not part of the insured services bundle within the *Canada Health Act,* although many provincial and territorial plans do provide some coverage. In these settings, nurses plan and coordinate resident care, manage chronic illnesses, and conduct rehabilitation programs. Nursing roles involving education (see Chapter 21), communication (see Chapter 18), and family-related interventions (see Chapter 20) are prevalent in this setting.

Psychiatric Facilities. Located in hospitals, independent outpatient clinics, or mental health clinics, psychiatric facilities offer inpatient and outpatient services. Mental health is often seen as one of the "orphan children of Medicare," never being fully integrated into the health care system (Romanow, 2002). Nurses in these facilities collaborate with doctors, psychologists, social workers, and therapists to make plans that enable a client to return to the community. At discharge from inpatient facilities, clients are usually referred for follow-up through community-based agencies. Nurses working in these settings are especially skillful in communication skills (see Chapter 18) and client safety (see Chapter 37).

Rehabilitation Centres. A rehabilitation centre is a residential institution that provides therapy and restorative training, the goal being to decrease clients' dependence on care. Many centres offer programs that teach the client, the client's family, or both to achieve maximum function after a stroke, head or spinal cord injury, or other impairment. Drug rehabilitation centres help clients withdraw from drug dependence and return to the community. Nurses in rehabilitation centres collaborate closely with physical and occupational therapists, psychologists, and social workers. They work with clients experiencing stress and adaptation (see Chapter 30) and those who are at risk of challenges to mobility (see Chapter 46) and to safety (see Chapter 37).

Community Sector

Community services are directed at primary and secondary care, described later in this chapter, and should be accessible to clients in locations where they live, work, play, and engage. The focus in the community sector is on empowerment and community development opportunities that effect change at the broadest social level (Health Canada, 2006c). Community health nurses oversee and participate in outreach programs that provide services and locate clients who might not seek care at traditional health care centres. Community health care agencies include physicians' offices, clinics, community health centres, home health care agencies, and crisis intervention centres. Nurses practicing in the community sector are involved in community-based nursing (see Chapter 4) and caring throughout the lifespan (see Unit V).

Public Health. Public health is committed to ensuring conditions and circumstances in which people can be healthy through appropriate screening, assessment, development, monitoring, and support (i.e., public policy). Whether it concerns environmental, biological, or disease issues, public health differs from many clinical practice settings in its focus on entire populations rather than on individual clients.

Activities related to pandemic planning, severe acute respiratory syndrome (SARS), West Nile virus, and global surveillance have put public health into the forefront (refer to the *Canadian Pandemic Influenza Plan for the Health Sector* [Public Health Agency of Canada, 2006]) in terms of protection and promotion efforts. Public health nurses work closely with a range of health care professionals, including medical health officers, environmental and public health inspectors, psychologists, nutritionists, and therapists. Nurses are the primary professionals in public health clinics offering well-baby clinics, school health programs, sexually transmitted infections surveillance, and screening programs, as well as health promotion (e.g., tobacco reduction) and disease prevention programs. For example, during an outbreak of a communicable disease such as meningitis, the public health care system mobilizes to detect cases early and prevent transmission, often through mass vaccination, communication, and public education.

Physician Offices. Physician offices offer PC and tend to focus on the diagnosis and treatment of specific illnesses rather than on health promotion. The majority of physicians function as private contractors within the publicly funded health care system, working on a fee-for-service basis. In this setting, nurses record vital signs, prepare clients for examination, and collaborate with physicians to conduct physical examinations, document histories, offer health education, and recommend therapies.

Community Health Centres (CHCs) and Clinics. Staff at these centres plan, manage, and deliver comprehensive services to designated geographic areas or specific at-risk populations. CHCs typically offer a variety of health and social services, including family medicine, social work, counselling, health promotion, and community development programs. CHCs are cost-effective, reduce hospitalization, and function interprofessionally (Yalnizyan & Macdonald, 2005). Increasingly, nurse practitioners and nurses are managing CHCs, with the intention of enabling clients to assume more responsibility for their health. Nurse practitioners have become CHC team members focused on prevention and supportive services rather than on family practitioner–driven curative and rehabilitative care.

Assisted Living. Assisted living facilities are community-based residential facilities where adults live and receive a range of support services, including personalized assistance in achieving a level of independence. Personal assistance services are "designed to promote maximum dignity and independence," including meal preparation, personal hygiene practice, mobility, and socialization. These facilities usually have a combination of professional and nonprofessional staff available on a round-the-clock basis.

Home Care. Canadian health care is shifting from an institution-based system to one in which community care is playing a greater role (see Chapter 4). Home care is the provision of health care services and equipment to clients and families in their homes and is offered in all jurisdictions in Canada. Home care is not included in the *Canada Health Act* as a medically necessary service, and so the range of public funding varies significantly among jurisdictions (Health Canada, 2006a). All provinces and territories fund assessment and case management, nursing care, and support services for eligible clients. Clients may pay for extra professional or support services through insurance programs or pay-for-service arrangements. The federal government delivers home care services to First Nations people on reserves and Inuit people in designated communities, to members of the armed forces and the RCMP, to federal inmates, and to eligible veterans.

Home care involves primarily nursing care but also includes other professional and nonprofessional services, such as physiotherapy; social work; nutrition counselling; and occupational, respiratory, and speech therapy. Support services are nonmedical services and include personal care, assistance with activities of daily living, and assistance with home management.

Home care was created to provide individualized care for people after hospital discharge but has increasingly included clients in a range of ages from very young to very old; those with mental, physical or developmental challenges; and those needing recovery to end-stage care. A cost-effective alternative to institutional care, home care assists clients in maintaining health and independence longer (Hollander & Chappell, 2001). Nurses working in home care have experience with all levels of care occurring within the home setting (see "Levels of Care" section), as well as complex caseloads. Home care nurses must respond to issues of cultural diversity (see Chapter 10), family nursing (see Chapter 20), and client safety (see Chapter 37).

Adult Day Care Centres. Adult day care centres are associated with a hospital or long-term care facility or exist as independent centres. Frequently, rather than hospitalization, continuous health care services are needed for specific clients (e.g., those with dementia, those needing physical rehabilitation or counselling, or those with chemical dependency). These centres enable family members to participate in providing care, while maintaining employment and other activities (Meiner & Lueckenotte, 2006). Nurses in adult day care centres provide continuity between the care delivered at home and care delivered in the centre. For instance, nurses administer treatments, encourage clients to adhere to prescribed medication regimens (see Chapter 34), link clients with community resources (see Chapter 4), and provide counselling services (see Chapter 20).

Community and Voluntary Agencies. National, provincial, and regional voluntary agencies (e.g., the Heart and Stroke Foundation of Canada; Canadian Diabetes Association) meet specific needs. Most voluntary agencies offer programs to educate about, prevent, and detect specific conditions, rather than treat them. Voluntary agencies depend on the help of professional volunteers (e.g., Victorian Order of Nurses) and lay volunteers (e.g., Meals on Wheels); financial support for training physicians and nurses is often derived from fundraising and donations.

Occupational Health. More than 2000 members of the Canadian Occupational Health Nurses Association (2008) deliver integrated occupational health and safety services to individual and communities of workers. Nurses certified in occupational health have met specific eligibility requirements, have passed a written examination, and have met a national standard of competency. Occupational health nurses often work with physiotherapists, occupational therapists, and psychologists for large corporations in broad-based programs that encompass the range of promotion, maintenance, and restoration of health and prevention of illness and injury.

Hospice and Palliative Care. A hospice is a family-centred care system that enables a person to live in comfort, with independence and dignity, while living with a life-threatening illness. Hospice care is palliative, not curative (see Chapter 29). Its multidisciplinary approach involving physicians, nurses, social workers, pharmacists, and pastoral care staff is crucial. Hospice nurses work in hospitals, free-standing structures called *hospices,* or the client's home, caring for the client and family during the terminal phase of illness and at the time of death. They may offer continued services in the form of bereavement counselling to the family after the client's death.

Parish Nursing. Parish nursing is becoming more popular as faith-based communities promote and maintain members' health. According to the Canadian Association for Parish Nursing Ministry [CAPNM] (2007), a parish nurse is a registered nurse with specialized knowledge who is called to ministry and affirmed by a faith-based community to promote health, healing, and wholeness. Currently, more than 200 members of the CAPNM promote the integration of faith and health through advocacy, counselling, education, and linkages to health and intersectoral services (Caiger, 2006; CAPNM, 2007).

Levels of Care

Five levels of health care exist: promotive, preventive, curative (diagnosis and treatment), rehabilitative, and supportive (including home care, long-term care, and palliative care) (CNA, 2003; WHO, 1978).

Level 1: Health Promotion

The first level of health care, health promotion, focuses on "the process of enabling people to increase control over, and to improve their health" (Health Canada, 2006b). Examples of this process include the provision of wellness services, antismoking education, promotion of self-esteem in children and adolescents, and advocacy for healthy public policy.

Health promotion takes place in many settings. For example, community clinics offer prenatal nutrition classes that promote the health of the woman, fetus, and infant. The *Ottawa Charter for Health Promotion* (Lalonde, 1986) lists five action strategies for health promotion: building healthy public policy, creating supportive environments, strengthening community action, developing personal skills, and reorienting health care services. The *Ottawa Charter for Health Promotion* details how health care professionals can enable clients to make decisions that affect their health. Furthermore, it states that the foundation of health promotion consists of "the fundamental conditions and resources for health [which] are peace, shelter, education, food, income, a stable ecosystem, sustainable resources, social justice, and equity" (see Chapter 1).

Level 2: Disease and Injury Prevention

The second level of health care delivery includes illness prevention services to help clients, families, and communities reduce risk factors for disease and injury (see Chapter 4). Prevention strategies include clinical actions (screening, immunizing), behavioural aspects (lifestyle change, support groups), and environmental actions (societal pressure for a healthy environment)(see Chapter 1).

Level 3: Diagnosis and Treatment

Diagnosis and treatment, which are the services most often used, focus on recognizing and treating clients' existing health problems. Within this level of care, three sublevels exist: primary, secondary, and tertiary care. These typically refer to health care activities aimed at individuals, rather than at families or communities.

- PC is the first contact of a client with the health care system that leads to a decision regarding a course of action to resolve any actual or potential health problem. PC providers include physicians and nurse practitioners in practice settings such as physicians' offices, nurse-managed clinics, schools, and occupational settings. The focus is on early detection and routine care, with emphasis on education to prevent recurrences. (Recall and note the difference from PHC.)
- Secondary care, which occurs usually in hospital or home settings, involves provision of a specialized medical service by a physician specialist or a hospital on referral from a PC practitioner. Secondary care deals with clients seeking definitive diagnosis or requiring further diagnostic review.
- Tertiary care is specialized and highly technical care in diagnosing and treating complicated or unusual health problems. Clients requiring tertiary care have an extensive, often complicated pathological condition. Tertiary care occurs in regional, teaching, university, or specialized hospitals that house sophisticated diagnostic equipment and perform complex therapeutic procedures.

Level 4: Rehabilitation

Rehabilitation is the restoration of a person to his or her fullest physical, mental, social, and vocational functioning possible (Clemen-Stone et al., 2002). Clients require rehabilitation after a physical or mental illness, injury, or chemical addiction. Initially, rehabilitation may focus on preventing complications from the illness or injury. As a condition stabilizes, rehabilitation is necessary until clients return to their previous level of function or reach a new level of function limited by their illness or disease. The goal is to assist a client in regaining maximal functional status, thereby enhancing quality of life while promoting independence and self-care.

Rehabilitation nurses work closely with physiotherapy, occupational and speech therapy, and social services. Ideally, rehabilitation begins the moment a client enters a health care setting for treatment. For example, some orthopedic programs have clients undergo physiotherapy exercises before major joint repair so as to enhance their recovery (see Chapter 36). Nurses have a key role in the continuity of care aspects of rehabilitation, which occurs in many health care settings, including institutions, outpatient settings, and the community.

Level 5: Supportive Care

Clients of all ages with illnesses or disabilities that are chronic (i.e., are long-term) or progressive (i.e., worsen over time) may require supportive care. **Supportive care** consists of health, personal, and social services provided over a prolonged period to people who are disabled, who do not function independently, or who have a terminal disease. The need for supportive care is evolving. People are living longer; chronic conditions are becoming more common; and care settings (i.e., institutional, community, and home) are becoming more diverse.

Palliative care is a component of supportive care. Palliative care is services for people living with progressive, life-threatening illnesses or conditions. *Palliate* means to soothe or relieve. The goal of palliative care is to meet the physical, emotional, social, and spiritual needs of the client and family. Palliative care can be provided in hospitals, hospices, or homes.

Respite care is another component of supportive care that provides short-term relief or time off for family caregivers. Adult day care is one form of respite care. However, respite care can be provided within the home by health care professionals and trained volunteers.

Challenges to the Health Care System

Canada's health care system is faced with many issues and challenges, which can be categorized either as cost accelerators or as costs associated with trying to provide equal care and access to care for all.

Cost Accelerators

Technologies. New technologies, such as new-generation antibiotics, diagnostic imaging equipment, and specialized beds, have become integral in the treatment of diseases and disabilities. The effectiveness of these technical advances have contributed to reductions in mortality and morbidity rates; however, costs have increased with these innovations.

The overarching term **e-health** is used to describe the application of information and communications technologies in the health care sector (see Chapter 17). As part of this strategy, there is an emphasis on developing a national health infostructure to support direct care, telehealth, and the maintenance of electronic health records. For nurses, the area of **nursing informatics** is an emerging area of practice that "integrates nursing science, computer science, and information science to manage and communicate data, information, and knowledge in nursing practice. Nursing informatics facilitates the integration of data, information, and knowledge to support clients, nurses, and other providers in their decision-making in all roles and settings" (Canadian Nursing Informatics Association, 2008).

Demographics. As the population ages, chronic and age-related diseases are increasing in frequency, largely because older people are more likely to become ill and disabled. They require more treatment and drugs, which results in higher costs to the health care system. According to a Statistics Canada (2007) report titled *Canada's Population by Age and Sex*, "nationally, 13.4 per cent of Canada's population was comprised of seniors aged 65 and over, up from 12.7 per cent in 2002 . . . . This number should increase for another 20 years, when people born during the peak of the baby-boom generation reach retirement age. At that time, more than half a million will turn 65 each year" (Corbella, 2008).

Another demographic that has resulted in higher health care costs is maternal age, the average of which has risen steadily since the mid-1980s.

Consumer Involvement. Canadians are better informed than ever about their health care options and demand **high-quality care** for their tax dollars. For example, clients might ask a physician to order an expensive diagnostic test such as magnetic resonance imaging (MRI), whereas previously they would have been satisfied with an X-ray film.

There is a growing presence of and demand for **self-care**, which Health Canada (2006d) described as one of the pillars of health care and health care reform. According to the CNA (2002) and Health Canada (2006d), self-care is a range of activities (e.g., information exchange, decision making, networking) undertaken to improve health with the involvement of informal and family caregivers.

Equality and Quality

The Canadian health care system strives to provide equal care and access to care for all.

Income Status. Income assistance programs for older adults and social assistance recipients cover some health care expenses not covered by Medicare, such as optometric, dental, and pharmaceutical care. However, Canadians with low wages may experience poorer access and, consequently, poorer health status. Lower income Canadians visit dentists less often than do middle- or upper income Canadians and are less likely to seek preventive eye care.

Cultural Competence. Canada is a country of diversity; regardless of the health status and needs of Aboriginal peoples or of newcomers, it is apparent that the health care system and its providers are challenged to be responsive and respectful (see Chapter 10). As discussed earlier, the federal government has a key role in the provision of health care services to First Nations and Inuit people. Since 1986, a movement to transfer responsibility and control for health services to First Nations and Inuit governance has emerged (Health Canada, 2003). The shift in the health structures and PHC seem to hold the promise of aligning with Aboriginal peoples' beliefs, especially in terms of holism and integration.

Immigration has shaped Canada's population historically and currently. Between 2001 and 2006, newcomers represented two thirds of the population growth, with significant influxes in urban centres and neighbouring municipalities (Chui et al., 2007). Linguistic and cultural diversity is immense, more than 70% of newcomers having reported a mother tongue other than English or French (mostly Chinese) (Chui et al., 2007). Variations in the health status of the newcomers are based on their reasons for immigration, place or circumstances of origin, and social supports (Wayland, 2006). Issues of income, psychological well-being, and ethnic support are identified as important aspects of adjustment and risk reduction (Wayland, 2006).

Evidence-Informed Practice. Nursing practice is constantly evolving, and nurses must remain responsive to new developments, innovations, and information. **Evidence-informed practice** has become the gold standard in clinical decision making that is informed by *both* best available research evidence and clinical considerations (e.g., experience and client preferences) (Melnyk & Fineout-Overholt, 2005).

Evidence-informed practice resources are available on CNA's portal called NurseONE/INF-Fusion (http://www.nurseone.ca/). NurseONE is a personalized, interactive web-based resource providing a gateway for nurses and nursing students to resources to enhance client care, manage their careers, pursue life-long learning opportunities, and connect to colleagues (Bassendowski et al., 2008).

Quality and Client Safety. According to the International Society for Quality in Health Care (ISQua, 2007), quality practice and performance improvement underpin the work of the health care team across the continuum of care. Quality and safety in health care involve health facilities and providers, clinicians, and other professionals, providing the right care for the right people at the right first time and in the right amount (ISQua, 2007). The ISQua reported that consumers consistently rank quality and safety of their care high among their concerns.

According to Baker and Norton (2004), approximately 70,000 preventable adverse events occur annually in Canadian hospitals, which translated to between 9000 and 24,000 deaths in 2000. One per nine clients contracts an infection while in hospital, and the same number experiences a medication-related error (Baker et al., 2004). The Canadian Patient Safety Institute (2005) is charged with providing leadership in building and advancing a safer health care system.

Quality Workplaces. According to Law et al. (2007), the health of health care workers and healthy workplaces is a critical aspect of health care sustainability and a target for investment in the Canadian health care system. Health care has the most diverse range of work environments, which further challenges addressing quality issues and potentially affects recruitment and retention.

Privatization of Services. Governments are struggling to maintain the principle of universality against the benefits and challenges of privatization. At present, not all health care services are available and accessible to all Canadians. For example, some infertility treatments and laser eye surgical procedures are performed in private offices and are available to only to clients who can pay for them. Discussions continue about what constitutes "medically necessary services" and what core services should be available and accessible to everyone. Many experts contend that Medicare can be saved only by privatizing more parts of the health care system.

Health Care Human Resources. According to Chui et al. (2007), in 2006, more than 1 million people (about 6% of the total workforce) in Canada worked directly in health-related occupations. Despite these numbers, accessibility to health care services is compromised by shortages of physicians, nurses, and other health care professionals. According to Health Canada (2007b), health and human resources planning must occur within the context of the broader health care system and must recognize the systemic challenges of wait times, client safety, and bed closures.

Aboriginal peoples are significantly under-represented in health care roles. In response, Health Canada established a five-year initiative, known as the Aboriginal Health Human Resources Initiative (AHHRI), which focuses on increasing representation of Aboriginal peoples in health care and retention of health care providers who work with Aboriginal peoples.

Nursing's Future in the Emerging Health Care System

This chapter has included an extensive discussion about restructuring and challenges within the Canadian health care system. In response to this context, nursing roles continue to evolve and diversify. In the future, nurses will increasingly be regarded as critical stakeholders, partners, and providers within the emerging health care system. Nurses will continue to draw on their historical legacy, forge ahead, and use evidence to inform their pursuit of excellence and quality in care, while advocating and innovating for the benefit of their clients.

* KEY CONCEPTS

- Medicare is a key component of Canada's social safety net.
- Government plays a major role in the Canadian health care system by funding national health insurance and by setting health care policy according to the principles of the *Canada Health Act.*
- The *Canada Health Act* forbids extra billing and user fees and stresses the principles of public administration, comprehensiveness, universality, portability, and accessibility.
- Health care services are provided in institutional and community settings, across all age groups, and for individual, family, group, community, and population clients.
- The five levels of health care are as follows: promotive, preventive, curative, rehabilitative, and supportive.
- Escalating costs are driving health care reform efforts, challenging health care institutions to deliver quality care more efficiently.
- Issues of equality, access, and continuity of care challenge the health care system.
- To achieve continuity of care when a client is discharged from a hospital, the staff nurse must anticipate and identify the client's continuing needs and then work with all members of the multidisciplinary team to develop a plan that transfers the client's care from the hospital to another environment.
- The rise of PHC and home care is a result of reforms to the health care system.
- Successful health promotion and disease prevention programs, such as those found in community health centres, schools, and community clinics, are designed to help clients acquire healthier lifestyles and achieve a decent standard of living.
- Home care is one of the fastest growing components of the health care system partly because clients are sent home from hospital sooner than they used to be.
- Demographic, geographical, and technological realities affect the functioning of the Canadian health care system.
- The existence of sufficient and qualified health human resources is a key challenge to the Canadian health care system.
- Enhancing the health of Aboriginal peoples in Canada is a significant challenge to society and to the health care system.
- Nurses must continually seek out information and evidence to remain responsive to providing quality and safe client care.

* CRITICAL THINKING EXERCISES

1. Debate the following issues in relation to the future of the Canadian health care system: escalating costs, privatization, continuity of care, accessibility.
2. Consider and describe how the national economy, changes in the population, and technology have changed the Canadian health care system. Identify what implications these changes have for nursing practice.

3. Consider Mr. W., a 68-year-old widower with no immediate family supports, who is scheduled to have major surgery to replace the joint in his hip. He is generally in good health otherwise and lives in a seniors-only apartment complex in the centre of town. After surgery, he will need extensive therapy in order to walk normally again. Describe the type of health care services and client safety issues that might become involved in his care.

* REVIEW QUESTIONS

1. Canada contributes 10.3% of its gross domestic product to health care. Which one of the following countries contributes a greater percentage to its health care system?
   1. United Kingdom
   2. United States
   3. Japan
   4. Sweden
2. Which of the following people are insured under the *Canada Health Act*?
   1. Aboriginal peoples
   2. RCMP members
   3. Members of military services
   4. Persons in transit between provinces
3. Public health focuses on
   1. Treatment
   2. Promotion
   3. Intervention
   4. Institutionalization
4. The *Canada Health Act* embraces the following five principles:
   1. Public administration, comprehensiveness, universality, portability, accessibility
   2. Social justice, equity, acceptability, efficiency, effectiveness
   3. Accountability, equality, economy, collaboration, coordination
   4. Insured health services, compensation for providers, hospital services, community care, and prescription drugs
5. An adult day care centre is an example of
   1. A home care organization
   2. An institutional agency
   3. A community agency
   4. An ambulatory care centre
6. What are the five levels of health care services?
   1. Promotive, preventive, curative, rehabilitative, supportive
   2. Prevention, protection, diagnosis, treatment, palliative care
   3. Promotion, prevention, treatment, PHC, diagnosis
   4. Assessment, diagnosis, planning, implementation, evaluation
7. The largest share of health expenditures in Canada goes to
   1. Physicians
   2. Home care
   3. Prescription drugs
   4. Hospitals
8. Which is *not* a cause of Canada's increasing health care costs?
   1. Workplace injuries
   2. Aging of the population
   3. New technologies and drugs
   4. Chronic and new diseases
9. A nurse organizes a blood pressure screening program. This is an example of
   1. Health promotion
   2. Disease prevention
   3. Continuing care
   4. Rehabilitation
10. The provision of specialized medical services by a physician specialist or a hospital is known as
    1. PC
    2. PHC
    3. Secondary care
    4. Tertiary care

* RECOMMENDED WEB SITES

Canadian Health Services Research Foundation: Research Theme: Primary Health Care: http://www.chsrf.ca/research_themes/ph_e.php
This site addresses initiatives of the Foundation that relate to PHC reform and research.

Canadian Institute of Health Information: http://www.cihi.ca
This is a not-for-profit organization seeking to improve the health care system and the health of Canadians by providing health information.

Canadian Public Health Association: http://www.cpha.ca
This is a national, not-for-profit association seeking excellence in public health nationally and internationally.

Commission on the Future of Health Care in Canada: http://www.hc-sc.gc.ca/hcs-sss/hhr-rhs/strateg/romanow-eng.php
This site provides an overview of the Romanow Commission and access to the full report.

Health Canada: http://www.hc-sc.gc.ca
This Web site provides links to information about the Canadian health care system, including a link to the *Canada Health Act* (http://www.hc-sc.gc.ca/hcs-sss/medi-assur/cha-lcs/index-eng.php), legislation, federal reports, and related publications.

Canadian Patient Safety Institute: http://www.patientsafetyinstitute.ca
This Institute was established in 2003 to build and advance a safer health care system for Canadians. This site reports on activities in leadership role across health sectors and health care systems, highlights promising practices, and raises awareness with stakeholders and the public about client safety.

Health Quality Council (Saskatchewan): http://www.hqc.sk.ca
The Saskatchewan Health Quality Council was established in 2002 through provincial legislation to improve health care in Saskatchewan by encouraging the use of best evidence.

Health Council of Canada: http://www.healthcouncilcanada.ca/en/
This council fosters accountability and transparency by assessing progress in improving quality, effectiveness, and sustainability of the health care system. The Web site reports monitoring and facilitates informed discussion regarding barriers and facilitators to health care renewal and the well-being of Canadians.

3

The Development of Nursing in Canada

Written by Janet C. Ross-Kerr, RN, BScN, MS, PhD

objectives

Mastery of content in this chapter will enable you to:

- Define the key terms listed.
- Discuss the historical development of professional nursing.
- Discuss the historical development of nursing education in Canada.
- Describe educational programs available for professional nurses.
- Identify the roles and career opportunities for nurses.
- Discuss the role of professional nursing organizations and practice acts.
- Describe trends affecting nurses' roles and responsibilities.

key terms

Clinical nurse specialist, p. 35
Code of ethics, p. 37
Continuing education, p. 35
In-service education, p. 35
International Council of Nurses (ICN), p. 29
Nurse administrator, p. 35
Nurse educator, p. 35
Nurse practitioner, p. 35
Nurse researcher, p. 35
Professional organization, p. 36

media resources

evolve Web Site

- Audio Chapter Summaries
- Glossary
- Multiple-Choice Review Questions
- Student Learning Activities
- Weblinks

Companion CD

- Glossary
- Interactive Learning Activities
- Fluids and Electrolytes Tutorial
- Test-Taking Skills

Over the centuries, the goals of nursing have been to help people maintain their health and to provide comfort and care to the sick. Modern nursing is a professional discipline with a unique body of knowledge applied to the needs of individuals and families. The foundations of professional practice emerge from historical and philosophical traditions in nursing and health care, social policy and practice, and ongoing research in nursing. It is interesting to explore the origins of nursing because they have contributed to modern nursing. The evolution of nursing has brought the profession to a challenging and exciting time in its history. There are tremendous opportunities to improve the health and quality of life of clients and communities with advances in professional knowledge and practice.

The philosophical and theoretical basis of the profession provides the necessary foundation for practice (see Chapter 6). Henderson's (1966) famous definition of nursing was adopted by the **International Council of Nurses (ICN)** in 1973 and continues to be the primary description of the role of the nurse:

> *"The unique function of the nurse is to assist the individual, sick or well, in the performance of those activities contributing to health [and] its recovery, or to a peaceful death that the client would perform unaided if he had the necessary strength, will, or knowledge. And to do this in such a way as to help the client gain independence as rapidly as possible." (p. 15)*

As a profession, nursing is committed to public service. The practice of nursing requires specialized knowledge that must be acquired and carries a high degree of responsibility. Nursing has practical and theoretical components, is motivated by altruism, and is based on ethical standards. The profession evolves as society, health care, and social policies change. This chapter traces the roots of the nursing profession over many centuries to its establishment and development in Canada. Although there has been a dramatic increase in the nature and extent of knowledge and skills required for nursing, the professional mandate has remained relatively constant over time and continues to be an inspiring force for the profession. The transformation of the profession to the modern era is highlighted.

Highlights of World Nursing History

Nursing's historical roots are deep and honourable and can be traced over many centuries. In the sixteenth century B.C., the ancient Egyptians recognized the importance of preventing illness and maintaining health. They understood that a good diet was important in maintaining health, and consumed a reasonably well-balanced diet of fruits, vegetables, fish, milk, legumes, seeds, and oil. Priest-physicians ministered to the people, using herbs to relieve pain and a variety of treatments for illness that were based on spiritual or mythological beliefs about its causation. The Papyrus Ebers and the Edwin Smith Papyrus, came to light in Thebes (now Luxor) in 1862 and document the Egyptians' knowledge of disease and treatment. These ancient manuscripts have helped modern scholars understand how they dealt with health and illness as far back as 3300–1500 B.C.

The theories of health and illness of the ancient Egyptians provided a framework for the development of medicine in ancient Greece. Although the early Greeks believed in the spiritual causes of disease, Hippocrates (circa 460–370 B.C.) was the first to make observations of patients and develop treatments on the basis of symptoms. He founded a school of medicine on the island of Cos and wrote numerous books on disease. Hippocrates is considered the father of scientific medicine and Western medical ethics; he developed methods of treating disease and establishing ethical principles upon which practice was based. Through his influence, medicine developed into a science. Galen (circa A.D. 130–203), another Greek physician-scientist, made important contributions to the field of physiology through research on animals and also wrote a number of books, eventually moving to Rome and becoming physician to the gladiators. Knowledge acquired through Galen and other Greek physicians had a significant influence on the Romans.

The Romans recognized the importance of fresh water and hygiene for public health. As their cities grew and the water supply became inadequate, Roman engineers developed aqueducts in Rome between 312 B.C. and 226 A.D. to carry fresh water from distant springs. They also developed public baths and constructed public toilets and sewers, which greatly improved the health of the population.

The ancient Hebrews believed in a spiritual basis of illness and that following the Ten Commandments promoted health. They also recognized the importance of nutrition and developed dietary laws that protected the public by prescribing what foods could or could not be eaten together, or eaten at all, as well as guidelines for safely eating the meat of slaughtered animals. Nurses cared for the sick in the home and community and served as midwives during childbirth.

During the early Christian period, with the emphasis of Christianity on love for others, nursing became a caring service undertaken by women. The Benedictine Order originated with St. Benedict of Nursia in A.D. 529 and is the oldest of the Catholic nursing orders. Fabiola, a well-to-do Christian woman in Rome, offered respite to ill and fatigued pilgrims travelling to the Holy Land. Later, during the twelfth and thirteenth centuries, hospitals were built to provide care for the sick. The Knights Hospitallers of the Order of St. John of Jerusalem emerged from the Benedictine nursing tradition to become one of a number of religious orders formed during the Crusades (eleventh to thirteenth centuries) that were committed to caring for and defending pilgrims. Hospices were constructed for pilgrims. When the Protestant Reformation took hold in Europe after the Crusades, monasteries were disbanded, and the hospitals and other institutions where monks and nuns cared for the sick and weary were closed. When new hospitals were built, untrained and unsuitable individuals were responsible for nursing patients. Conditions deteriorated as lack of sanitation prevailed and disease spread rapidly.

During the seventeenth century, conditions began to improve and there was greater emphasis on nursing. St. Vincent de Paul founded the Sisters of Charity in 1633 to care for the sick, poor, and orphaned. Because this order was noncloistered (the first such order), the nuns were able to go into the community to care for people. For the most part, women who entered convents to become nurses came from the upper classes and were well educated. In Germany, Pastor Theodore Fliedner established his now rather famous Institute of Deaconesses at Kaiserwerth in 1836 to prepare women to serve as nurses.

Nineteenth Century and Florence Nightingale

The movement to improve standards of nursing care in the mid-nineteenth century was spearheaded by Florence Nightingale, who is considered the founder of modern nursing. Brought up in a wealthy family, Nightingale railed against the customs of her time that did not allow middle- and upper class women to work outside the home: "Why have women passion, intellect, moral activity—these three—and a place in society where no one of the three can be exercised?" (Nightingale, 1872/1979). She was well educated and, against the wishes of her family, sought to prepare herself for nursing in 1850 by travelling to Kaiserwerth, Germany, where she worked with the German deaconesses under Pastor Fliedner. She later worked in

France with nuns in the French nursing orders. Then, in 1853, she accepted the post of superintendent at Harley Street Hospital in London and developed the nursing services there. When reports reached London of the appalling conditions for British wounded soldiers, Nightingale was asked to organize a group of nurses to go to the Crimea in 1854.

Nightingale and her staff of nurses made every possible attempt to care for the wounded and make them comfortable in ways that would foster their recovery. These women were able to achieve dramatic reductions in morbidity and mortality rates, saving the lives of thousands of wounded British soldiers by applying principles of cleanliness and comfort to nursing care. Accounts of Nightingale's work were distributed to the British press by a reporter covering the war. She achieved worldwide fame because of her success in reducing morbidity and mortality through exemplary nursing care. Nightingale helped to elevate the status of nursing so that it became accepted as a suitable field of work for women outside the home. At the same time, remarkable advances in health care and the expansion in the number and importance of hospitals created a need for nurses, and the nursing profession became one of the most significant avenues of work for women in the nineteenth century. Nursing thus became an instrument of women's emancipation against the prevailing middle-class restrictions on women working outside the home.

After her remarkable service during the Crimean War, Nightingale was plagued by continuing ill health. She became an advocate for the health of people, reform of the health care system of the British army, and educational preparation for nursing. She made her views known through her voluminous writings and lobbied members of parliament and acquaintances to support and act on her views. She drew her conclusions from health data that she collected and analyzed. She thus became known as the first health statistician. Nightingale is the subject of a large, ongoing scholarly writing project spearheaded by McDonald (2008) that incorporates the most significant analyses of her work to date.

Early History of Nursing in Canada

The roots of nursing and health care in North America may be found in the values and ideals of the European settlers in New France. At a time when knowledge of disease was primitive, technology was virtually nonexistent, and a few herbal remedies were the only medicines available, the practice of nursing developed as an integral part of the emerging health care system. Nursing care was often the sole weapon in fighting infectious disease. Its importance is underscored in accounts of the devastating epidemics of smallpox, diphtheria, cholera, and other infectious diseases that continually ravaged the population (Paul & Ross-Kerr, in press).

A long-established indigenous society existed in North America before the arrival of the first settlers. At the time of the first sustained contact with European people, the estimated number of indigenous people in North America was about 500,000, although this is acknowledged as probably a conservative number (Royal Commission on Aboriginal Peoples, 1996). The Aboriginal peoples also had health care knowledge of their own, including the use of herbal remedies.

The First Nurses and Hospitals in New France

In 1608, Samuel de Champlain selected Quebec as the site for a colony of settlers to support the growing fur trade. For the next two decades, the first colonists in New France provided their own health care. The first laywoman to provide nursing care in New France was Marie Rollet Hébert. She and her husband, Louis Hébert, who was a surgeon-apothecary, emigrated with their three children at the request of Champlain in 1617. Mme Hébert became the first woman to emigrate to the new world from France and cared for Native people and settlers alike. Her husband's apothecary and agricultural skills helped prevent starvation and mitigate illness (Brown, 2002). Although she was a layperson, Madame Hébert extended care to Aboriginal people and settlers who were ill, just as she would for ill family members, the latter being a customary role for women at the time.

The first nurses to tend the sick in a type of health care centre were male attendants at a "sick bay" established at the French garrison in Port Royal in Acadia in 1629 (Gibbon & Mathewson, 1947). The Jesuit priests, who were missionary immigrants to New France, also served as nurses. They found that in order to carry out their mission to convert the Aboriginal people to Christianity, they had to minister to the sick. Many religious orders and laypersons came to New France voluntarily to assist the Jesuits. Most of the women who came to New France were motivated by Christian ideals of educating Native children and caring for the sick. Although small in number, these women led the young colony's efforts in health care and teaching. They proved remarkably resilient as they battled smallpox epidemics and tended to people injured in the Iroquois wars.

The first nursing mission was established in 1639 at Sillery, outside the citadel of Quebec, by three Augustinian nuns who were Hospitalières de la Miséricorde de Jésus. As a result of the Iroquois wars, the nuns abandoned this mission in 1644 and opened another mission inside the citadel, where they nursed French settlers. This mission later became known as Hôtel-Dieu, Quebec's first hospital. In 1641, Jeanne Mance came to New France to found a hospital in the yet unsettled region of Ville Marie (later Montreal); Mance and her fellow travellers were not warmly received. Their intentions to care for the sick were viewed with suspicion by the settlers. When she arrived at Ville Marie in 1642, Mance was the only person with health care knowledge in the new settlement. She was a leader in the community and became an inspiration for later generations of nurses (Box 3–1).

A Canadian order of nuns, the Sisters of Charity of Montreal, formed in 1737 by Marguerite d'Youville (see Chapter 2), became the first visiting nurses in Canada. They began as a small group of women who pooled their possessions to form a refuge for the poor and needy (Gibbon & Mathewson, 1947). Because some colonists doubted their charitable intentions, the women were called "les soeurs grises," a derogatory term meaning both "the grey nuns" and "the tipsy nuns." However, the goodness of their intentions was clear, and they were respected for their work. They proudly referred to themselves as the "Grey Nuns" from then on, and were given a charter to take over the General Hospital of Montreal. To meet their hospital expenses, these resourceful women made military garments and tents, started a brewery and a tobacco plant, and operated a freight and cartage business (Paul & Ross-Kerr, in press).

Nursing During the British Regime

During the war between the British and the French in 1756, the Grey Nuns designated a ward of the General Hospital of Montreal for the care of English soldiers, thus caring for soldiers on both sides of the conflict. The status of nursing and the quality of care provided at this time differed markedly between Canada and Great Britain. Nursing in Britain had fallen into disrepute after Henry VIII's renunciation of the Catholic Church. The nursing orders of nuns, which had previously provided the nursing services in the large London hospitals, were replaced by women of questionable morals and little knowledge. However, nursing remained strong in early Canada because of the influence of France, where nursing was performed at a highter standard.

BOX 3-1 Milestones in Canadian Nursing History

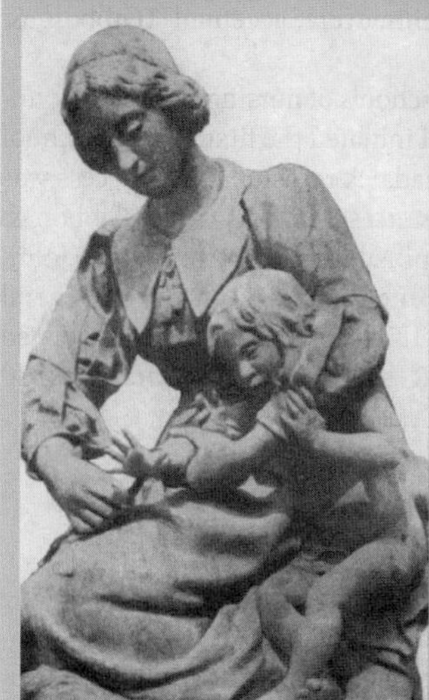

Jeanne Mance, 1606–1673

Jeanne Mance was born in a wealthy family in Langres, France, in 1606. She was the daughter of a wealthy legal advisor to the court of the King of France and decided early to devote her life to God. She learned about New France from a cousin, a Recollet priest who had served there. She gained nursing knowledge and skills in Langres, where an epidemic of plague occurred and many people were wounded in the Thirty Years' War. Supported by a wealthy widow who wanted to finance a hospital at Ville Marie, Jeanne Mance sailed to New France with Paul de Chomédey, Sieur de Maisonneuve, and his band of 40. Maisonneuve's mission was to establish a settlement at Ville Marie, but arriving in Quebec after a 2-month voyage, the settlers learned that the governor was suspicious of their mission, and he tried to dissuade them from it.

They decided that it was too late in the summer to try to build the colony, and so they remained in Quebec, involving themselves in the community. Mance spent time learning about nursing and health care in New France from the Augustinian nuns in their hospital.

In the spring, the settlers set out for Ville Marie in three boats and immediately began building houses and the Hôtel-Dieu. The next year, during an attack by the Iroquois, several settlers were killed, and others were taken hostage. The remaining settlers managed to finish the hospital and build a stockade around their colony. However, the attacks increased, and Mance was kept busy caring for both wounded settlers and Aboriginal people. By 1649, the settlers' funds were low, and the colony was close to having to disband. Mance sailed to Paris, where she raised money and recruited settlers. Over the next few years, relations with the Iroquois continued to be poor. A guard was placed at the hospital and Mance slept within the fort. In 1650, the Iroquois killed 30 of 70 settlers.

Maisonneuve went to France in 1651 to gain further support and did not return for 2 years. This period was difficult, but Mance held the colony together during his absence. After a truce reached between the French and the Iroquois in 1654, Mance was able to move back to the Hôtel-Dieu. In 1657, Mance fell on the ice, and fractured her right arm in two places, and dislocated her wrist, and she experienced continuing disability. She decided to make another trip to France to ask the order of nuns at La Flèche to come and help her in the hospital. While in Paris during prayer at the Seminary of Saint Sulpice, she discovered she could move her arm without pain, and it healed miraculously. She made her last trip to France in 1663, again to solicit funding for the colony because it was, again, close to bankruptcy. En route back, she contracted typhus and nearly died. She was shocked to find upon her return that Maisonneuve had been replaced as governor. In declining health, Mance was less able to help at the hospital. She died peacefully in her sleep in 1673.

As well as founding and managing the Hôtel-Dieu, Mance asssisted Maisonneuve in running the colony as confidant, advisor, and accountant. She is hailed as a founder of the city of Montreal. Today, the Canadian Nurses Association (CNA) awards its highest honour in the name of this courageous pioneer.

Infectious diseases carried by immigrants and travellers spread rapidly in the British colonies. The increasing populace and continuing epidemics created a need for more health care facilities. In areas not served by the French-Canadian nursing orders, institutions were established with standards similar to those in Britain at the time (CNA, 1968). Laywomen offered their services and organized groups to provide proper care, but because they lacked knowledge and skill, these efforts were largely unsuccessful. The established French-Canadian orders expanded their services, and new English-speaking orders were founded to help the sick and the poor.

Opening of the West and the Grey Nuns

In 1844, four Grey Nuns embarked on a perilous canoe journey from Montreal to St. Boniface, Manitoba, where their mission was to care for the sick. Soon after their arrival, a series of epidemics began. The nuns visited the sick at home, where they cared for people with measles, dysentery, and smallpox and treated them with medicines and local herbs.

In 1859, another group of Grey Nuns travelled from Montreal by rail through the United States and then North to St. Boniface. After resting for a time, they set off by ox cart over rough terrain to arrive in what is now Alberta to establish their first mission in Lac Ste. Anne, where they visited clients in their homes and cared for them in the convent. Arriving before most of the settlers, the sisters established systems of health care to care for the sick. Demand from the populace was such that they later built a separate hospital building. Later, they established small missions in what is now northern Saskatchewan and the Northwest Territories to provide health care in Native settlements. In 1895, they were asked to construct a hospital in Edmonton (the General Hospital) because settlement was burgeoning there.

Nursing Education in Canada

In 1860, Florence Nightingale established a financially independent school of nursing in association with St. Thomas's Hospital in London, England. Interest in the new school was high. Soon hospital training schools for nurses were established throughout Europe and North America.

Unfortunately, the educational model of the Nightingale school was missing from the new hospital schools. This was largely because the new schools had no financing and required students to provide nursing service to the hospital in return for their education and living expenses, which enabled hospitals to provide nursing services at minimal cost. The race to establish hospitals in the early 1890s was undoubtedly spurred on by the financial benefits of establishing associated schools of nursing. The early hospitals were challenged financially because they did not charge poor clients. Services thus had to be of high enough quality to attract paying clients, and a training school attached to a hospital ensured a higher standard of care than one without a school (Young, 1994).

The First Canadian Nursing Schools

The first hospital diploma school in Canada, the St. Catharines Training School, opened in 1874 at the St. Catharines General and Marine Hospital. Admission standards were "plain English education, good character, and Christian motives" (*St. Catharines Annual Report*, cited by Healey, 1990). At that time, nursing was still considered an undesirable vocation for a refined lady in Canada, the only acceptable profession being teaching (Healey, 1990). Students learned chemistry, sanitary science, physiology, anatomy, and hygiene. They were taught to observe patients for changes in temperature, skin condition, pulse, respirations, and functions of organs and to report "faithfully" to the attending physician (Healey, 1990).

The School for Nurses at the Toronto General Hospital was established in 1881; Mary Agnes Snively was appointed superintendent in 1884 (Box 3–2). Although work and living conditions were poor, Miss Snively worked hard to improve the program. In 1896, she introduced a 3-year course with 84 hours of practical nursing and 119 hours of instruction by the medical staff (Gibbon & Mathewson, 1947).

In Montreal, after several unsuccessful attempts, The School for Nurses at the Montreal General Hospital was established in 1890 under the direction of Nora Livingston. Conditions were deplorable, but Livingston quickly made improvements. The popularity of the school increased rapidly. Livingston reported 169 applications in the first year, from which 80 students were accepted (Gibbon & Mathewson, 1947).

The move to establish hospital schools of nursing swept the country. The Winnipeg General Hospital initiated the first Training School for Nurses in 1887 in western Canada. A measure of its success was that 134 of its graduates served as nurses in World War I (Gibbon & Mathewson, 1947). By 1890, hospitals in Fredericton, Saint John, Halifax, and Charlottetown had opened schools. Vancouver General Hospital began a school in 1891, and in Alberta, a school was opened in Medicine Hat in 1894. By 1930, there were approximately 330 schools of nursing in Canada (CNA, 1968; Box 3–3).

BOX 3-2 Milestones in Canadian Nursing History

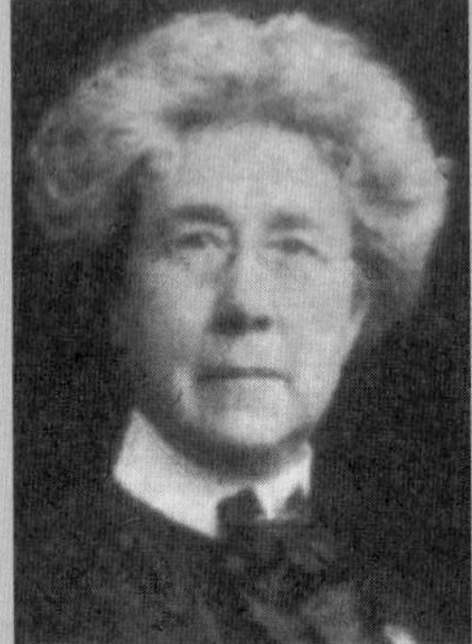

Mary Agnes Snively, 1847–1933

Born in St. Catharines, Ontario, Mary Agnes Snively was a teacher before she was a nurse. Upon graduation from the school of nursing at Bellevue Hospital, New York, in 1894, she was appointed Lady Superintendent of Nurses at Toronto General Hospital and director of the school of nursing. The school, founded along with the hospital 3 years earlier, was in a state of disorganization.

Students provided most of the nursing care at Toronto General Hospital at little cost to the hospital. Snively found no organized plan for classes or clinical experience, nor was there a residence (students were housed in various locations in the hospital). Written records of nursing care, medical orders, and client histories were also lacking. Recruiting desirable applicants was difficult because students in the school faced so many hardships that parents were reluctant to allow their daughters to seek admission.

Snively rectified all these deficiencies. A residence was soon built; she developed a curriculum plan, including nursing theory and practice; and she lengthened the education period to 3 years. By the end of her tenure in 1910, the Toronto General Hospital school was thriving as the largest school of nursing in Canada with hundreds of graduates, a full complement of students, and many more seeking admission. All parental skepticism had been overcome, and Toronto General Hospital served as a model for others across the country.

Snively achieved acclaim for her organizational work. She helped found the first nurses' alumnae association in Canada at Toronto General Hospital in 1894. She also attended the historic 1899 founding meeting of the ICN in London, England and was elected first honorary treasurer of the ICN, even though Canada did not have the necessary national nursing association to become an ICN member at the time. In 1907, Snively established the Canadian Society of Superintendents of Training Schools of Nursing, and, recognizing that an organization that would include all nurses would be needed for Canada to become a member of the ICN, she was the driving force behind the 1908 founding of the Provisional Organization of the Canadian National Association of Trained Nurses (later the CNA), becoming its first president. She shepherded the entry of the fledgling Canadian organization to membership in the ICN and served later as ICN vice president.

Sources: Gibbon, J. M., & Mathewson, M. S. (1947). *Three centuries of Canadian nursing.* Toronto, ON: Macmillan; and Riegler, N. (1997). *Jean I. Gunn, nursing leader.* Markham, ON: Associated Medical Services with Fitzhenry and Whiteside.

The Impact of Nursing Organizations on Nursing Education

At the same time that hospital training schools for nurses were being established, nurses began to advocate for improved educational standards and passage of legislation for their profession. Women's associations were instrumental in the public health care crusade in Canada and in the rise of nursing organizations. The National Council of Women under the presidency of Lady Ishbel Aberdeen, wife of the governor general of Canada, approved the formation of thse Victorian Order of Nurses (VON) in 1898. Lady Aberdeen had conceived the idea of establishing the VON after she discovered the plight of women in Western Canada who had to give birth in remote locations with no assistance. The formation of the VON signified a professional standard of education for Canadian nurses that recognized the need not only for altruism and compassion but also for nursing knowledge.

Nurses from around the world were beginning to form organizations, inspired by the leadership of women such as Ethel Gordon Bedford Fenwick. Editor of the *British Journal of Nursing,* she attended the 1893 Congress of Charities, Corrections, and Philanthropy in Chicago, where she spoke of British struggles to achieve registration for nurses. Her North American colleagues had similar concerns. After the Congress, they formed the American Society of Superintendents of Training Schools for Nurses of the United States and Canada, later to become the National League for Nursing Education, whose goal was to raise standards of nursing education. Soon afterward in 1896, the Nurses' Associated Alumnae of the United States and Canada was formed, becoming the American Nurses Association in 1911. A major goal was to secure legislation to differentiate between trained and untrained nurses (CNA, 1968).

In 1899, Bedford Fenwick founded the ICN, with Britain, Germany, and the United States as member organizations. Nations without national nursing organizations could not become members. As mentioned previously, although Canada did not yet have a national nursing organization, Mary Agnes Snively, Superintendent of Nurses at Toronto General Hospital, was elected the first honourary treasurer of the ICN in 1899 (CNA, 1968).

The Origins of the Canadian Nurses Association and Provincial Nursing Associations. The Canadian Society of Superintendents of Training Schools for Nurses was formed in 1907. The next year, the Provisional Society of the Canadian National Association of Trained Nurses (CNATN) was formed. Mary Agnes Snively served as founding president of both organizations (CNA, 1968). Membership in this new national organization was through affiliated societies in the provinces. At the ICN meeting in 1909, Canada became a full-fledged member of the organization. Later, the CNATN streamlined its organization when registration of nurses was established through legislation in each province. Its name was

> BOX 3-3 **Milestones in Canadian Nursing History**

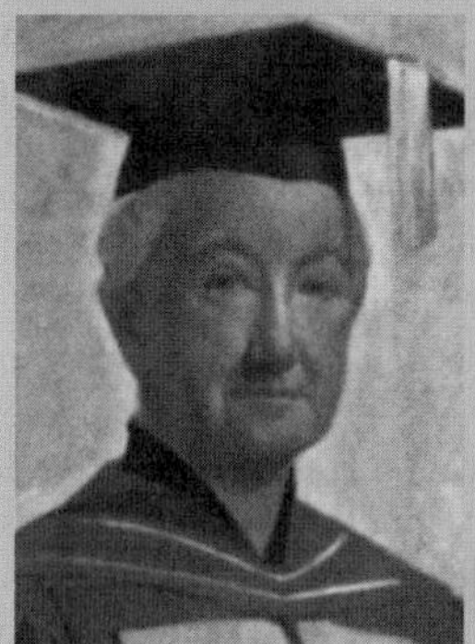

Jean I. Gunn, 1882–1941

Born in 1882 in Belleville, Ontario, Jean I. Gunn completed teacher training studies at Albert College in Belleville; her father was not in favour of her pursuing a career in nursing. Assisted by her mother, she went to New York to visit her sister and investigate nursing schools there. She then enrolled in the School of Nursing at Presbyterian Hospital, New York, graduating in 1905. After experience at her alma mater and in community nursing, Gunn was appointed superintendent of nurses at the Toronto General Hospital in 1913. In this position, she was also responsible for the school of nursing.

Gunn recruited outstanding nursing administrators to assist her and became involved in provincial, national, and international health care and nursing organizations. She was a tireless worker and served with many organizations. Gunn was very supportive of the Toronto General Hospital alumnae association that in 1904 helped establish the Graduate Nurses' Association of Ontario (later the Registered Nurses Association of Ontario) and pressed for legislation for the registration of nurses. She became secretary of the Canadian National Association of Trained Nurses in 1914 and president in 1917. She served on the executive of the National Council of Women and became very involved in the Canadian Red Cross Society, in which she chaired a committee on surgical dressings during World War II. In this role, she oversaw production of millions of dressings by female civilian volunteers.

Nurses were in short supply during this time. With most men in the armed forces, many industrial jobs were now open to women and at wages far surpassing those of nurses. In 1917, Gunn pressed for the establishment of a permanent cadre of trained nurses for national service. She continued to work for the registration of nurses, which came to fruition in Ontario in 1922.

Gunn advocated for nursing and nurses on many fronts. She castigated hospital boards for reviewing costs of hospital services while ignoring the savings that accrued from educating a nurse. She was passionately interested in improving standards of nursing education. She decried the

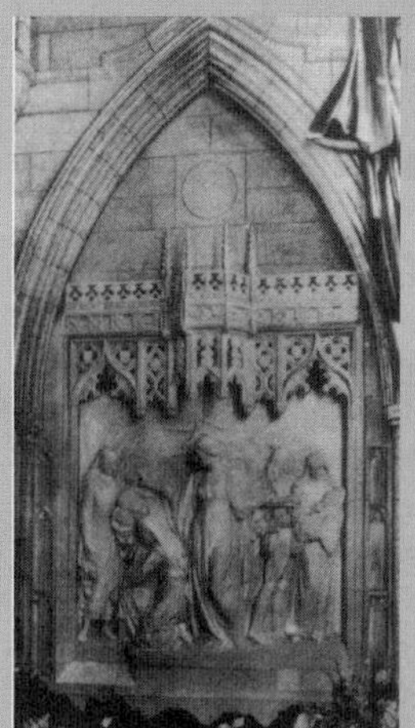

exploitation of nurses in schools of nursing and worked with other nursing leaders to establish the Weir study of nursing and nursing education, jointly sponsored by the CNA and the Canadian Medical Association. The 1932 Weir report confirmed the deficiencies that she and other nursing leaders had publicized for so long, and she campaigned for the implementation of its recommendations.

Gunn also envisioned university degree programs in nursing and in 1914 arranged for the Department of Social Service at the University of Toronto to give lectures to third-year Toronto General Hospital students. In 1917, a course in chemistry taught by university instructors was implemented. The following year, field experience in public health nursing was introduced, and Gunn organized centralized lectures among Toronto schools of nursing held at the University of Toronto.

Gunn is perhaps best remembered for her work toward the Nurses' War Memorial, which recognized the service of military nurses during World War I. She lobbied politicians and other health care organizations extensively and raised money from 10,000 nurses and their organizations from all over Canada. The result was a bas-relief sculpture in white Carrara marble that was unveiled in 1924 in a prominent position in the Centre Block of the Parliament Buildings, located in the Hall of Honour, separating the House of Commons from the Senate. In 1932, Gunn was responsible for having the crest of the CNA added to the sculpture.

In recognition of her outstanding service to nursing and health care throughout her life, Gunn received a number of honours in her final years, including a King's Jubilee Medal in 1935 and a Doctor of Laws degree from the University of Toronto in 1938. Jean Gunn was a leader among leaders in nursing and an individual who was able to inspire nurses to contribute to the common good.

Source: Riegler, N. (1997). *Jean I. Gunn, nursing leader.* Markham, ON: Associated Medical Services with Fitzhenry and Whiteside.

changed to the *Canadian Nurses Association* in 1924, and it became a federation of provincial associations in 1930.

The struggle for women's rights helped nurses to secure laws to regulate their profession. Nurses formed provincial nurses' associations and sought legislation that would set educational standards and improve nursing care. The first province to gain legislation was Nova Scotia, where a voluntary registration act was passed in 1910. It also allowed nongraduate nurses to register. Initial acts passed in other provinces contained more restrictive standards. Admission criteria and curricula were set for nursing schools, as were rules governing the registration and discipline of practising nurses.

All provinces and two territories eventually secured mandatory registration, requiring that all practising nurses register with the regulatory body approved by the provincial nursing act (Canadian Institute for Health Information, 2006). The distinguishing feature of mandatory rather than permissive legislation is a statute containing a definition of the scope of nursing practice, as well as protecting the use of the title of *registered nurse.* Permissive legislation only protects the title of *registered nurse* (Wood, in press). Licensure laws are designed to protect the public against unqualified and incompetent practitioners.

The First University Programs

The devastating consequences of World War I and the influenza pandemic of 1918 led to support for public health programs and new patterns of health care delivery. Community health care was promoted, and nurses were seen as central participants who needed university-level education. To this end, the Canadian Red Cross Society awarded grants to a number of Canadian universities to develop postgraduate courses in public health nursing: University of Toronto, McGill University, University of British Columbia, University of Alberta, Dalhousie University, and University of Western Ontario (Canadian Red Cross Society, 1962).

The first Canadian undergraduate nursing degree program was established at the University of British Columbia in 1919, with Ethel Johns as director. The operating costs of the new department were to be borne by the hospital, an incentive for the university to support the program. The program was nonintegrated—that is, "the university assumed no responsibility for the two or three years of nursing preparation in a hospital school of nursing" (Bonin, 1976, p. 7).

Several new 5-year, nonintegrated degree programs began at Canadian universities in the 1920s and 1930s: the University of

Western Ontario, the University of Alberta, l'Institut Marguerite d'Youville, the University of Ottawa, and St. Francis Xavier University. The religious order associated with the University of Ottawa launched what was essentially a hospital diploma program in 1933.

From the Depression to the Post-World War II Years

When nursing schools were established, women's education was a low priority. Nursing students were exploited in the hospital-based programs: in effect, subsidizing hospital operations. Nursing leaders fought to improve education at nursing schools and limit service, developing a standard curriculum that they urged schools to use. To eliminate weak programs, they encouraged the closure of hospital schools with insufficient beds. In 1932, the Weir report confirmed what nurses already knew about nursing schools: The conditions were deplorable, the health of students was in jeopardy, and education was secondary to hospital service (Weir, 1932).

The Great Depression "brought unemployment and hardship to nurses" (Allemang, 1974, p. 172). Clients could no longer afford to employ private-duty nurses, which had been the most promising area of employment for graduate nurses (Gunn, 1933). During the Depression, Canadian universities faced reduced revenues, staff layoffs, and difficult working conditions. The Depression was especially hard on McGill University, which depended on funds from private sources. During the Depression, raising private funds became next to impossible. Leaders of McGill's nursing school had fought unsuccessfully for years for a degree program. Once the university's finances began to deteriorate, the Board of Governors threatened to close the school altogether. The school's director, Bertha Harmer, gave up her salary, the faculty bought books for the library, and nursing alumnae groups all over the country raised funds to ensure the survival of the McGill nursing school (Tunis, 1966).

During World War II, health education became a priority as doctors and nurses were needed to care for military personnel, as well as civilians. Nurses who held critical positions as administrators, supervisors, teachers, and public health nurses were recruited for military service and left their positions. A shortage of nurses soon developed.

During and after the war, a new interest in nursing education led to increased external university funding, more scholarships and bursaries from private foundations, the growth of existing schools, and the founding of new programs. Programs were initiated at Queen's and McMaster Universities in 1941, followed by the University of Manitoba in 1943, Mount Saint Vincent University in 1947, and Dalhousie University in 1949. At McGill, new funds flowed in, and in 1944, supporters of the school were rewarded with a 5-year nonintegrated degree program.

Most nonintegrated programs offered a 2- to 3-year apprenticeship-based hospital diploma program sandwiched between 2 years of university study. The nonintegrated degree pattern with its stepladder approach to nursing education was well established, and the hospital programs on which this approach depended had been entrenched for many years. However, the new interest in nursing education led to exciting innovations.

In 1942, the University of Toronto introduced an integrated basic degree program. Under the leadership of Edith Kathleen Russell (see Chapter 4), courses in arts and sciences were taught concurrently with nursing courses to enhance student development. Also, university instructors supervised student clinical practice in the health care agencies. Four years after the introduction of the University of Toronto basic degree program, a second basic degree program was developed at McMaster University under Gladys Sharpe's direction.

Expansion in the 1950s and 1960s

In the 1960s, existing nursing degree programs expanded, and new programs emerged in other universities. The first master's degree program in nursing was established at the University of Western Ontario in 1959, followed in the 1960s and 1970s by similar programs in universities across the country. In 1962, the Canadian Nurses Foundation was established as an entity separate from the CNA, to provide scholarships, bursaries, and fellowships for graduate study in nursing.

Nursing schools' financial dependence left them at the mercy of hospital administrators. "The lack of nursing instructors and of other graduate nurses on patient care units meant that there were few role models for students for observation, questions and general discussion. In most cases senior students were left in charge of teaching junior students, and this with very limited supervision" (Paul, 1998, pp. 133–134). Many authorities have suggested that this was not a true apprenticeship model because it lacked the "master craftsman" to guide the students (Chapman, 1969).

Nursing leaders called for better faculty preparation, more integrated programs, and more university-based opportunities for students, such as student placements and increased enrolments. The movement to separate nursing education programs from the authority of hospitals began in earnest. Studies of nursing education identified persistent problems. Helen K. Mussallem found that hours on duty for students in hospital schools of nursing were too long, nursing instructors were too few, and the instructors were not qualified (CNA, 1965). In a 1965 survey, 65% of hospital schools reported that clinical assignments were based on the service needs of the patient care units, not on the students' educational needs (CNA, 1965).

Universities resisted introducing basic integrated degree programs because of the costs associated with the low student–teacher ratios required for clinical nursing. It was cheaper for them to let hospitals finance clinical education, but this meant that universities granted degrees for work over which they had no control. In 1964, the Royal Commission on Health Services castigated universities for this practice. By the late 1960s, the basic integrated degree program modeled on the program at the University of Toronto finally became the prototype for the establishment of integrated programs in nursing in universities across the nation.

From the 1970s to 2000

In 1975, the Alberta Task Force on Nursing Education proposed a postion on entry to practice, a radical proposal at the time, that recommended that all new nursing graduates be qualified at the baccalaureate level by 1995. Provincial governments gradually accepted the proposal and increased the capacity of degree-granting nursing education programs to accommodate all students studying nursing at the undergraduate level (CNA, 1991). Most provincial and regulatory bodies have now made the baccalaureate degree a requirement for the practice of nursing (CNA & Canadian Association of Schools of Nursing, 2004).

Throughout the 1970s and 1980s, university faculties and schools of nursing developed research resources so that they could offer graduate programs first at the master's level and then at the doctoral level. The first doctoral nursing program was established at the University of Alberta Faculty of Nursing on January 1, 1991, and others quickly followed.

The CNA has developed a position statement on promoting nursing history (CNA, 2008d), noting that learning from the lessons of history is "critical to advancing the profession in the interests of the Canadian public." This statement outlined the responsibilities of nurses across the whole gamut of roles and settings to promote nursing history.

Nursing Education Today

With continuing expansion of health care knowledge and technology, beginning practitioners require a broad educational foundation. New curricula and collaborative baccalaureate programs across the country attest to the profession's commitment to maintaining high standards of health care and responding to society's changing health care needs. The Internet, computerized learning programs, shared faculty through teleconferencing, and weekend and evening courses provide practising nurses with many options to complete degrees. The CNA's nursing portal, NurseOne, has made database information available to nurses across the country. Some universities have innovative programs at the baccalaureate level, including accelerated programs in which candidates hold baccalaureate degree in other fields. Baccalaureate programs, master's degree programs, and some courses in doctoral programs are also offered through distance education.

Standards for nursing education are monitored by each province to ensure that educational programs are of appropriate quality and respond to changes in health care. As professionals, nurses must acquire, maintain, and continuously enhance the knowledge, skills, attitudes, and judgment necessary to meet client needs in an evolving health care system. The responsibility for educational support for competent nursing practice is shared among individual nurses, professional nursing organizations, educational institutions, and governments (Wood, in press).

The need for nurses with graduate degrees is rising, along with the need for research. A master's degree in nursing is necessary for nurses seeking positions as clinical nurse specialists, nurse practitioners, nurse administrators, or nurse educators. Most master's programs in Canada now offer a concentration in advanced nursing practice for clinical nurse specialists and nurse practititioners. This provides advanced preparation in nursing science, theory, and practice, with emphasis on evidence-based clinical practice. Nurses with doctorates can undertake research that advances knowledge and evidence-based practice in clinical settings (see Chapter 7). This research enhances the quality of nursing care and improves Canadians' health outcomes. Today, there are 30 master's programs and 12 doctoral programs in nursing in Canada.

Continuing and In-Service Education

Nurses need to continually update their skills and knowledge to practise in a constantly changing health care environment. **Continuing education** includes formal, organized, and educational programs offered by provincial associations and educational and health care institutions. In addition, health care agencies and institutions offer **in-service education** programs, designed to increase the knowledge, skills, and competencies of nurses and other health care professionals employed by the institution. A growing number of professional associations are developing continuing competence programs in which nurses must provide evidence that they are taking steps to update their knowledge and skills.

Professional Roles and Responsibilities

Contemporary nursing requires that the nurse possess knowledge and skills for a variety of professional roles and responsibilities. In the past, the principal role of nurses was to provide care and treatment, as well as comfort. This role has grown to include increased emphasis on health promotion and on concern for clients and families. The role of the nurse in primary health care (see Chapter 1) is an evolving and important one because nurses are involved with assisting clients and families to learn as much as possible about their health and health care in order to ensure health and well-being. Nurses also help clients make the transition from home to the health care agency, or vice versa, as seamless as possible.

As advanced knowledge and technology are being rapidly incorporated into care, nursing roles have also been evolving. Thus, nursing offers expanded roles and a broad range of career opportunities (Figure 3–1). Examples of career roles include those as nurse educators, managers or **administrators**, **researchers**, quality improvement nurses, consultants, and even business owners. Many nurses are employed in the areas of education and administration.

Since the late 1980s, there have been significant developments in the expansion of nursing roles, specifically in advanced nursing practice. *Advanced nursing practice* is an umbrella term that refers to two advanced nursing roles in Canada: namely, the clinical nurse specialist and the nurse practitioner. The CNA (2008c) developed a national framework intended to guide the development of advanced nursing practice in Canada in which it defined core competencies in five areas: clinical nursing, research, leadership, collaboration, and change agency. It also stipulated a graduate degree in nursing as the minimum educational requirement and recommended that regulation of practice be part of the current scope of nursing practice and regulation.

The **clinical nurse specialist** role is one that involves a high level of nursing practice in a specialized area such as oncology or gerontology, and this role has been integrated into health care. The difference between the roles of nurse practitioners and clinical nurse specialists is an important one. **Nurse practitioners** provide mainly primary care, whereas clinical nurse specialists function in a more consultative way as expert clinicians and educators. Although nurse practitioners have

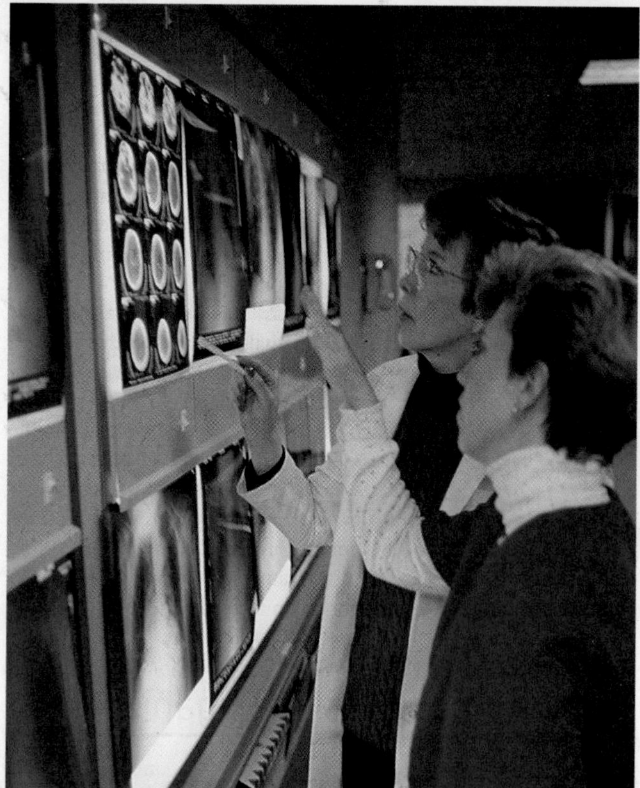

Figure 3-1 Nurse specialists consult on a difficult case.

been practising in Ontario since the 1970s, this was the culmination of a movement that began a decade previously. Furthermore, legislation to govern their practice in primary health care settings has more recently been developed as part of existing legislation in all jurisdictions (MacDonald et al, 2005). Although there is variation from one jurisdiction to another, the nurse practitioner may prescribe medications with certain exclusions and treat health problems within the scope of nursing practice. Developments in the educational programs for and licensing of nurse practitioners have been taking place at a rapid pace and have greatly extended the scope of practice for this group of nurses. There have been discussion and some controversy about advanced practice roles that could be developed in Canada, including roles such as nurse anesthetist and nurse midwife (Schreiber & MacDonald, 2008).

Gender and Diversity in Nursing

Nursing is a profession in transition from one that has been predominantly female in character to one that is gender balanced. Traditional societal values that negate nurturing roles for men have been changing. However, even though the number of men employed in nursing in Canada has increased, the current proportion of male nurses represents only 5.6% of the total nurse population, a slight increase over the 4.7% it represented in 2000 (CNA, 2006). This is remarkable at a time when the proportion of women in traditionally male-dominated professions has increased at a phenomenal rate. O'Lynn and Tranbarger (2006) pointed to communication problems, reverse discriminatory practices, and gender-based barriers for male students in nursing. However, although many factors have deterred men from pursuing careers in nursing, some of the negative influences are slowly beginning to change.

Canadian society has also become multicultural. The increase in racial, ethnic, and cultural diversity has meant that individuals of different races, ethnic descent, and cultural backgrounds are present in every major population and occupational group. The benefit to Canada of this new diversity is inestimable and provides a far richer background for local, national, and international relationships. Some groups have historically been underrepresented in certain professions, including nursing, in comparison with their representation in the population. Recognition of the contributions of different ethnic and cultural groups, including Aboriginal groups, to the cultural mosaic in Canadian society has been slow in coming.

Villeneuve (2002–2003) decried the fact that the majority of nurses in Canada remain white and female, a situation that is common in the health care professions. Gates (2007) found that the greater the perceived increased difference in status between a staff nurse and others in the setting, the weaker was the nurse's intent to remain on the job. There has been pressure for the profession to enhance and improve programs in order to encourage nurses with minority cultural and racial backgrounds to enter programs and remain committed to their choices. The development of shared value systems, along with defined strategies to enhance recruitment, retention, and management, has been seen as crucial for retaining staff (Gates, 2007).

Professional Nursing Organizations

A **professional organization** deals with issues of concern to people practising in the profession. Professional nursing organizations establish educational and practice standards for nurses, carry out the regulatory functions of registration and licensure, and discipline members who do not meet the standards. Most of these organizations have continuing competence programs to ensure that their members maintain competence through continuing education. The terms *registration* and *licensure* have different meanings, although they are often used interchangeably. *Registration* refers to the listing of a member in good standing on the membership roster of an organization, whereas *licensure* refers to the exclusive right to practise a profession, granted by a government body to a member in good standing. In most provinces and territories (except Ontario), governments entrust administration of the legislation to the professional nursing association.

Nursing associations at the provincial or territorial level are organizations that serve as official representatives of the nursing profession and interact with provincial or territorial government officials on issues concerning the health of the populace and the roles of nurses. In most provinces, these organizations perform the regulatory functions of registration and professional conduct. Professional organizations are concerned with standards of practice and education. They present education programs, publish journals or newsletters, and work to increase public understanding of nursing and nursing outcomes on the health of individuals, families, and communities. They also collaborate with other health care professions on matters of mutual interest. Some professional organizations and special interest groups focus on specific areas such as critical care, nursing administration, or research. Examples include the Canadian Gerontological Nursing Association, the Canadian Association of Neuroscience Nurses, and the Aboriginal Nurses Association of Canada. These organizations seek to improve the standards of practice, to expand nursing roles, and to foster the welfare of nurses within the specialty areas. In some provinces or territories, "colleges" of registered nurses have been established through new legislation to replace existing nursing legislation. Although the primary mandates in these "colleges" are registration, professional conduct, and standards of practice and education, the degree of involvement in professional association matters varies. For example, in British Columbia (personal communication, Laurel Brunke, May 22, 2008) and Ontario, the respective "colleges" are concerned solely with matters pertaining to registration, professional conduct, and standards of education and practice. However, in other jurisdictions, such as Alberta (personal communication, Kim Campbell, June 11, 2008), Manitoba, and Nova Scotia, the "college" assumes regulatory functions in addition to those of a professional association speaking for and representing nurses on issues and concerns of the profession.

Nurses form a large and very powerful group and have made important contributions to public health through the leadership provided by their professional organizations. The CNA works at the national level for the improvement of health standards and the availability of health care services for all people, fosters high standards of nursing, stimulates and promotes the professional development of nurses, and advances their economic and general welfare. As the national voice of professional nurses, the CNA represents nurses across the country to the federal government and national organizations (Box 3–4). It regularly presents briefs to the House of Commons on areas such as taxation, poverty, health care, unemployment insurance, employment opportunities, part-time work, economic and social affairs, science and technology, and federal and provincial fiscal arrangements, including funding for health care. The CNA also collaborates with other national nursing and health organizations on issues related to practice, education, and research, and it holds regular meetings and discussions with government officials to ensure that the federal government is aware of CNA positions on health care and policy issues.

The CNA also gives individual nurses a collective means to influence health care policy at the national level. For example, in February 2000, after extensive lobbying by the CNA, the federal government

> **BOX 3-4 Canadian Nurses Association: Vision and Mission Statement**
>
> CNA is the national professional voice of registered nurses, supporting them in their practice and advocating for public health policy and a quality, publicly funded, not-for-profit health care system.
>
> In pursuit of its vision and mission, CNA (2008e) has established the following goals:
>
> - Advancing the discipline of nursing in the interest of the public.
> - Advocating public policy that incorporates the principles of primary health care (access; interdisciplinary practice; patient and community involvement; health promotion, including determinants of health and appropriate technology, roles, or models) and respects the principles, conditions, and spirit of the *Canada Health Act*.
> - Advancing the regulation of registered nurses in the interest of the public.
> - Working in collaboration with nurses, other health care providers, health care system stakeholders, and the public to achieve and sustain quality practice environments and positive client outcomes.
> - Advancing international health care policy and development in Canada and abroad to support global health care and equity.
> - Promoting awareness of the nursing profession so that the roles and expertise of registered nurses are understood, respected, and optimized within the health care system.
>
> Adapted from Canadian Nurses Association. (2008). *Vision and mission statement.* Ottawa, ON: Author.

committed $2.5 billion to the Canada Health and Social Transfer, earmarking a substantial portion of that amount for nursing. After the 2004 federal election, the CNA lobbied federally for its *Common Vision for the Canadian Health System* on health care in order to develop an agreement with the provinces to ensure "an adequate supply of health providers, pan-Canadian benchmarks and real targets for timely access to care, the expansion of the continuum of care and sufficient, on-going and predictable federal long-term funding" (*Media Statement*, 2004).

Unions

Nursing unions represent nurses in job-related negotiations with their employers. The primary interest of the unions is the economic welfare of the nurses they represent, but bargaining covers a broad area, including benefits, working conditions, and responsibilities.

A movement to establish a national voice for unionized nurses began in the early 1960s, when nurses pressed their professional associations to become involved in collective bargaining for them. Thus, professional organizations initially were responsible for collective bargaining. However, the 1973 Supreme Court decision in the appeal of the Saskatchewan case *Service Employees International Union [SEIU] v. Nipiwan District Staff Nurses Association* (in which the Staff Nurses Association was a unit of the Saskatchewan Registered Nurses Association) led to the separation of professional associations across the country (SEIU Local 333, 1973). The Staff Nurses Association had applied to be certified as a bargaining unit, but certification was denied on the basis of the potential conflict of interest in determining salaries of registered nurses because the Staff Nurses Association's Board of Directors could include nurse managers. Within a decade, every province had both a separate nursing association and a union. Some nursing unions represent both registered nurses and registered practical nurses (licensed practical nurses).

In 1981, the National Federation of Nurses' Unions was formed to represent the interests of nurses in both watchdog and lobbying activities. This organization became the Canadian Confederation of Nurses' Unions (CCNU) and by 2004 all provinces except Quebec were members. Nursing unions have lobbied for professional responsibility clauses in union contracts and are the representatives of nurses in particular provinces or territories when new contracts are negotiated. The CCNU has been active in raising the issues for nurses concerning current and projected nursing shortages and in arguing the case for public health care.

Standards of Nursing Practice

As a self-regulating profession, nursing sets its own standards of practice, which serve as objective guidelines for nurses to provide and evaluate care. Standards are based on research and clinical evidence and help assure clients that they are receiving high-quality care. Quality assurance programs incorporate measures to ensure high standards of practice. Because health is a provincial responsibility, each professional nursing organization is responsible for developing its own standards of nursing practice. In Table 3–1, the nursing practice standards developed for the province of Ontario by the College of Nurses of Ontario (2002) are presented as an example.

Ethical Standards of Practice

Ethical standards that guide practice are fundamental to all professions. Normally, these standards are expressed as "codes" of ethics; they emerged as a result of the Nuremberg Code, developed in 1947 from the post–World War II war crimes investigation of experimentation on human beings. The first **code of ethics** for nursing was developed by the ICN in 1953. The CNA adopted the ICN code the next year and in 1980 developed its first code of ethics. The *Code of Ethics for Registered Nurses* was most recently updated (CNA, 2008b). The Code of Ethics provides nurses with direction for ethical decision making and practice in everyday situations. Because nursing in Canada is a provincial responsibility, each province and territory is responsible for its code of ethics. Therefore, each provincial statute regulating nursing incorporates a code of ethics. Many provinces use the CNA Code of Ethics in their statutes (see Chapter 8).

Registration and Licensure

Because constitutional responsibility for education and health falls under the purview of the provinces and territories, each has a nursing practice act to regulate the licensure and practice of nursing. The scope of nursing practice is defined within the legislation in each province and territory. Provincial and territorial nursing practice acts are revised regularly to reflect changes in nursing practice. In all provinces except Ontario and Quebec, provincial and territorial nursing associations assume responsibility for defining and monitoring standards. In addition, nurses working in hospitals and other health care agencies also practice according to hospital or agency policies. These policies are more detailed and are specific to the nature of the care provided in the the particular health setting. In most jurisdictions, to be eligible for registration, students must complete a prescribed course of study from a nursing program approved by the body legislatively responsible for the regulation of nursing. The legislation governing nursing in all Canadian jurisdictions has been amended since the 1990s to allow for licensing of nurse practitioners (CNA, 2004).

Certification

With the development of highly specialized knowledge in a variety of discrete areas of nursing, there arose a need to ensure that clients received care from nurses who had developed the necessary knowledge and skills to work in particular specialized areas. The CNA

TABLE 3-1 Standards of Professional Practice

The following are broad descriptions of the expectations of nurses and apply to all nurses in every area of practice. Although written by the College of Nurses of Ontario for nurses in Ontario, the general themes are relevant for nurses across the country.

Accountability *Each nurse is accountable to the public and responsible for ensuring that her/his practice and conduct meets legislative requirements and the standards of the profession.*	Nurses are responsible for their actions and the consequences of those actions. Part of this accountability includes conducting themselves in ways that promote respect for the profession. Nurses are not accountable for the decisions or actions of other care providers when there was no way of knowing about those actions.
Continuing Competence *Each nurse maintains and continually improves her/his competence by participating in the College of Nurses of Ontario's Quality Assurance (QA) Program.*	Competence is the nurse's ability to use her / his knowledge, skill, judgment, attitudes, values and beliefs to perform in a given role, situation and practice setting. Continuing competence ensures the nurse is able to perform in a changing health environment. Continuing competence also contributes to quality nursing practice and increases the public's confidence in the nursing profession. Participation in the College's QA Program assists nurses to engage in activities that promote or foster lifelong learning. The program helps nurses to maintain and improve their competence and is a professional requirement.
Ethics *Each nurse understands, upholds, and promotes the values and beliefs described in the College's ethics practice standard.*	Ethical nursing care means promoting the values of client well-being, respecting client choice, assuring privacy and confidentiality, respecting sanctity and quality of life, maintaining commitments, respecting truthfulness, and ensuring fairness in the use of resources. It also includes acting with integrity, honesty, and professionalism in all dealings with the client and other health team members.
Knowledge *Each nurse possesses, through basic education and continuing learning, knowledge relevant to her/his professional practice.*	RNs and RPNs study from the same body of nursing knowledge. RPNs study for a shorter period of time, resulting in a more focused or basic foundation of knowledge in clinical practice, decision making, critical thinking, research, and leadership. RNs study for a longer period of time for a greater breadth and depth of knowledge in clinical practice, decision making, critical thinking, research utilization, leadership, health care delivery systems, and resource management. All nurses add to their basic education and foundational knowledge throughout their careers by pursuing ongoing learning.
Knowledge Application *Each nurse continually improves the application of professional knowledge.*	The quality of professional nursing practice reflects nurses' application of knowledge. Nurses apply knowledge to practice using nursing frameworks, theories and/or processes. This includes the performance of clinical skills because the technical and cognitive aspects of care are closely related and cannot be separated.
Leadership *Nurses demonstrate [their] leadership by providing, facilitating and promoting the best possible care/service to the public.*	Leadership requires self-knowledge (understanding one's beliefs and values and being aware of how one's behaviour affects others), respect, trust, integrity, shared vision, learning, participation, good communication techniques, and the ability to be a change facilitator. The leadership expectation is not limited to nurses in formal leadership positions. All nurses, regardless of their positions, have opportunities for leadership.
Relationships *Each nurse establishes and maintains respectful, collaborative, therapeutic, and professional relationships.*	Relationships include therapeutic nurse–client relationships and professional relationships with colleagues, health team members and employers. ***Therapeutic Nurse-Client Relationships*** The client's needs are the focus of the relationship, which is based on trust, respect, intimacy, and the appropriate use of power. Nurses demonstrate empathy and caring in all relationships with clients, families, and significant others. It is the responsibility of the nurse to establish and maintain the therapeutic relationship. ***Professional Relationships*** Professional relationships are based on trust and respect, and result in improved client care.

Adapted from College of Nurses of Ontario. (2002). *Professional Standards, Revised 2002.* Toronto, ON: Author. For links to indicators of each standard, see http://www.cno.org/docs/prac/41006_ProfStds.pdf

passed a resolution at its convention in 1980 to explore the feasibility of developing certification examinations in major nursing specialties. As a first step, the CNA Testing Service developed a certification examination for the Canadian Council of Occcupational Health Nurses. The CNA then developed policies for a voluntary certification program, and the Canadian Association of Neuroscience Nurses became the first to sponsor such a program in conjunction with the CNA. As of 2008, the CNA, along with national nursing specialty organizations, offered certification in 18 specialties: cardiovascular care, community health care, critical care, critical care–pediatrics, emergency care, gastroenterology, gerontology, hospice palliative care, nephrology, neuroscience, occupational health care, oncology, orthopedics, perinatal care, perioperative care, psychiatric or mental health care, rehabilitation, and enterostomal therapy (CNA, 2008a). The CNA certification program has been highly successful, inasmuch as it has provided a means of recognizing the specialized knowledge and skills necessary in a great number of areas of practice. It is likely that even more specialty groups will apply to be part of the certification program in the future.

Conclusion

Organized nursing has been a part of the social setting in Canada since the early days of the European settlement at Quebec, a period of more than three and a half centuries. The first nurses who came to found hospitals and to provide care for Aboriginal people and settlers were motivated by altruism and serve as excellent role models for nurses today. Altruism, a hallmark of any profession, remains an important characteristic of the nursing profession despite vast difference between the health care settings of the early days and those of today.

A fundamental and guiding principle of the French-Canadian hospitals that survived largely intact into the twentieth century was that care was available to all people regardless of their background, status in life, or ability to pay. This continues to be a principle for which nurses, through their professional organizations, have argued for determinedly in national debates on the nature and continuing direction of Canada's national health care insurance program. In the presence of pressure to reshape Medicare, nurses have continued to strongly resist calls for privatization of more aspects of the health system. They have also repeatedly called for all health care professionals to be remunerated on a salary or contract basis (Ross-Kerr, in press).

Multidisciplinary teams are an integral component of the health care organization in the community. However, nurses are the primary health care professionals both in home care and in community health settings. Thus, expanded and enhanced educational systems for nurses that incorporate knowledge and skills for community health and home care nursing are essential to meet the health needs of the populace today.

Nursing today requires a vast range of knowledge and skills, and thus educational programs to prepare nurses for the health systems of today and the future are demanding. Nurses have unlimited opportunities for fulfilling careers in a vast array of general and specialty areas. Numerous educational opportunities are open to nurses throughout their careers to enhance knowledge and skills and to move into new areas if desired. In nursing practice, nurses carry more responsibility than ever before. Nurse educators have challenging opportunities in practice, education, and research. Nursing scientists are leaders in health research, and the results of their investigations have changed health practices around the world.

The transformation of the nursing profession and of the educational programs that support it since the nineteenth century has been truly remarkable. Despite monumental obstacles, nurses have demonstrated the value of their service, the integrity of their goals, the quality of their educational programs, and the strength of their commitment. Although developments through the twenty-first century are as yet unknown, it is certain that the nursing profession will continue to evolve in the interest of providing a high quality of nursing care to the populace.

* KEY CONCEPTS

- Nursing has responded to the health care needs of society, influenced over time by economic, social, and cultural factors.
- Nursing in Canada is rooted in the traditions of good nursing that developed in New France.
- Florence Nightingale revolutionized nursing as an acceptable profession for women as lay nurses in the late 1800s and early 1900s.
- The development of a system of nursing education in Canada emerged from the early nursing sisterhoods and from schools of nursing associated with hospitals.
- Baccalaureate entry to practice is almost fully implemented in Canada.
- Basic nursing education is acquired in college, collaborative college-university, or university programs.
- Nurses have a variety of career opportunities and roles, including those of clinical nurse, clinical nurse specialist, nurse practitioner, educator, administrator, and researcher.
- The ranks of the profession are moving toward gender balance and a racial, ethnic, and cultural mix that reflects the Canadian population.
- Professional nursing organizations establish standards of education and practice for nurses, perform the regulatory functions of registration and professional conduct, deal with issues of concern to nurses and specialist groups within the nursing profession, and empower nurses to influence health care policy and practice.
- Nursing sets its own standards of practice—from scientific research and the work of nurse clinical experts—to ensure high-quality care.

* CRITICAL THINKING EXERCISES

1. Explain the importance of Florence Nightingale's work to establish nursing as a profession.
2. Identify some of the enduring values that have emerged from the history of nursing in Canada.
3. Observe various levels of nursing practice, such as a staff nurse, nurse practitioner, and nurse educator. Identify similarities and differences in their roles and educational preparation.
4. Outline some career objectives for yourself after completing your nursing program. Think about what you want to do as a professional nurse, and then outline strategies for achieving these goals.

* REVIEW QUESTIONS

1. The founder of modern nursing is
   1. Hippocrates
   2. Florence Nightingale
   3. Jeanne Mance
   4. Mary Agnes Snively

2. The founder of the Sisters of Charity of Montreal, which later became known as the Grey Nuns, is
   1. Marie Rollet Hébert
   2. St. Vincent de Paul
   3. Marguerite d'Youville
   4. Lady Ishbel Aberdeen
3. The first doctoral nursing program in Canada was established in
   1. 1890
   2. 1933
   3. 1975
   4. 1991
4. Nurse practitioners in Canada
   1. Work in university health settings
   2. Are able to function independently
   3. Are licensed under nursing legislation in jurisdictions
   4. Function as unit directors in health agencies
5. Nursing has a code of ethics that professional registered nurses follow, which
   1. Defines the principles of nursing care
   2. Ensures identical care to all clients
   3. Protects the client from harm
   4. Improves self-health care
6. Which of the following is *not* a function of a professional nursing organization?
   1. Regulating registration and professional conduct
   2. Monitoring unregulated care providers
   3. Collaborating with other health care organizations on matters of mutual interest
   4. Establishing standards of education and professional practice
7. The practice of nursing is regulated by
   1. The CNA
   2. Nursing practice acts
   3. Best practice guidelines
   4. Hospital administrators
8. Some of the professional standards outlined by the College of Nurses of Ontario include
   1. Accountability, ethics, leadership
   2. Administering medications, personal hygiene and grooming
   3. Care of vulnerable populations
   4. Care of people in financial crises
9. Except for Ontario and Quebec, minimum standards for nursing education are set by
   1. The nursing school
   2. The provincial or territorial nursing association
   3. The Canadian Nurses Association
   4. The Canadian Nurses Federation
10. A role of a nursing union is to
    1. Devise ethical standards to guide practice
    2. Set the standards of practice for nursing
    3. Represent nurses in bargaining for new contracts
    4. Carry out registration and licensure

* RECOMMENDED WEB SITES

Canadian Association for the History of Nursing (CAHN): http://www.cahn-achn.ca/

An affiliate group of the CNA, the CAHN offers information about Canadian nursing history and promotes historical research.

Canadian nursing organizations: http://www.canadianrn.com/directory/assoc.htm

This site offers a list of current Canadian nursing organizations, including contact information.

4

Community Health Nursing Practice

Written by Kaysi Eastlick Kushner, RN, PhD

objectives

Mastery of content in this chapter will enable you to:

- Define the key terms listed.
- Explain the relationship between community health nursing and primary health care.
- Discuss the roles and functions of the community health nurse.
- Differentiate between public health nursing and home health (community-based) nursing.
- Explain the characteristics of clients from vulnerable populations that influence a nurse's approach to care.
- Describe the roles and competencies important for success in community health nursing practice.
- Describe elements of a community assessment.

key terms

Community, p. 42
Community-based nursing, p. 45
Community health nursing, p. 43
Community health nursing practice, p. 42
Empowerment, p. 43
Harm reduction, p. 49
Home health nursing, p. 45
Population, p. 42
Population health, p. 44
Primary health care, p. 43
Public health, p. 44
Public health nursing, p. 43
Public health principles, p. 44
Vulnerable populations, p. 46

media resources

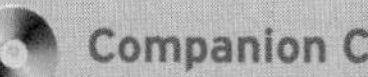

Web Site

- Audio Chapter Summaries
- Glossary
- Multiple-Choice Review Questions
- Student Learning Activities
- Weblinks

Companion CD

- Glossary
- Interactive Learning Activities
- Fluids and Electrolytes Tutorial
- Test-Taking Skills

Today's health care climate is rapidly changing in response to economic pressures, technological and medical advances, and client participation in health care. As a result, many clients are receiving care in the community rather than in hospital. There is a growing need to deliver health care where people live, work, and learn through a community health nursing practice model (Community Health Nurses Association of Canada [CHNAC], 2003). Community health nursing care focuses on health promotion, disease prevention, and restorative and palliative care. The goals of community health nursing are to keep individuals healthy, encourage client participation and choice in care, promote health-enhancing social environments, and provide in-home care for ill or disabled clients.

Promoting individual and community health has always been key to the holistic practice of nursing. In the 1730s, the Grey Nuns were established as Canada's first community nursing order. More than a century later, in England, Florence Nightingale articulated a nursing philosophy grounded in knowledge of environmental conditions. By the end of the century, the Victorian Order of Nurses was providing in-home nursing, often in outpost and remote regions. After World War I, community nursing responsibilities "extended to screening programs to detect disease at early stages, to helping to maintain a healthy environment, and to providing nursing care" (Ross-Kerr, 1996, p. 11).

Canadians such as Kate Brighty Colley (Box 4–1) and Edith Kathleen Russell (Box 4–2) pioneered community health nursing and public health nursing in Canada. Today, nursing is leading the way in assessing, implementing, and evaluating all types of public and community-based health services needed by clients. Community health nursing is essential for improving the health of the general public.

Promoting the Health of Populations and Community Groups

Nurses practising in the community face many challenges in promoting the health of populations and community groups. A **population** is a collection of individuals who have in common one or more personal or environmental characteristics (Maurer & Smith, 2005). Examples of populations include Canadians inclusively and, more specifically, high-risk infants, older adults, or a cultural group such as Aboriginal peoples. A healthy population is composed of healthy individuals, and the health status of individuals is considered an overall aggregate that reflects an average or general health status. To determine a population's health status, individual characteristics (such as occurrence of illness, disability, and death; lifespan; education; and living conditions) are considered. A **community** is a group of people who share a geographic (locational) dimension and a social (relational) dimension (Edwards & Moyer, 2000; Laverack, 2004). The social dimension—which comprises individual relationships, interactions among groups, and shared characteristics among members—distinguishes a community from a population. Examples of communities include geographic groupings (e.g., neighbourhoods) and shared interest groups (e.g., women's health networks). A healthy community consists of healthy individuals engaged in collective relationships that create a supportive living environment. Both individual and community characteristics are used to determine community health status. Key characteristics of a healthy community include a collective capacity to solve problems; adequate living conditions; a safe environment; and sustainable resources such as employment, health care, and educational facilities.

Community Health Nursing Practice

The scope of **community health nursing practice** includes population health promotion, protection, maintenance, and restoration; community, family, and individual health promotion; and individual rehabilitation or palliative care. Community health nursing promotes

➤ BOX 4-1 Milestones in Canadian Nursing History

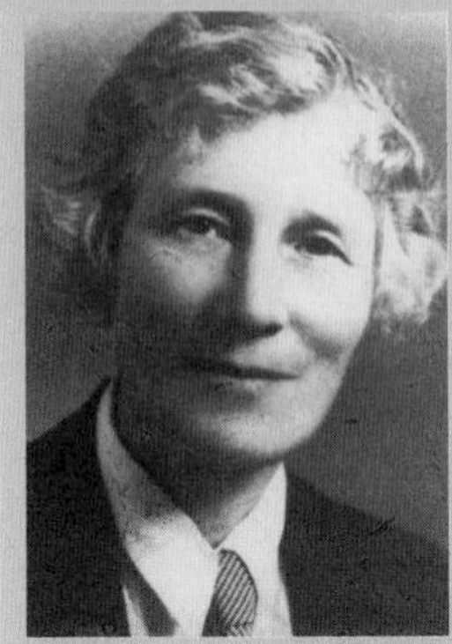

Kate Brighty Colley, 1883–1985

Born in England in 1883, Kate Brighty immigrated with her parents to Nova Scotia at the age of 3 years. She graduated from the Royal Alexandra Hospital School of Nursing in Edmonton in 1917, after which she enlisted with the Canadian Army Medical Corps in Calgary.

After completing a course in public health nursing at the University of Alberta in 1919, Brighty was one of the first nurses to be appointed to the staff of the new Alberta Department of Public Health. Soon afterward, the Alberta Department of Agriculture engaged her to teach home nursing, bedside care, and hygiene in Grande Prairie.

In the same year, Brighty was appointed matron of the second municipal hospital in Alberta, the Mission Hospital at Onoway. Because there were no physicians in the region, she and her two employees staffed the hospital and visited rural patients on horseback. In 1923, she returned to the Department of Public Health to establish a district nursing centre at Buck Lake near Pendryl, southwest of Edmonton—an area that had no roads at the time—and then another centre, farther north at Wanham, near the Peace River. Here she travelled by cutter to assist women in labour and those who were ill.

In 1925, Brighty took a postgraduate course in public health nursing at Columbia University, New York. Upon her return to Alberta in 1928, she was appointed director of the Department of Public Health Nursing. Her responsibilities were expanded a year later to include the post of inspector of hospitals.

In her new post, Brighty established a number of new district nursing centres. As a former district nurse, she understood the problems these nurses faced, and she travelled widely to visit staff. She expanded the health education program and gave talks on the radio on health, hygiene, nutrition, and child welfare. These broadcasts were important to residents of remote areas, where little formal health care was available.

Brighty was active in the Alberta Association of Registered Nurses (AARN) and, in 1936, was elected president of the organization. She wrote the first history of nursing in Alberta, the *AARN Blue Book* (Brighty, 1942).

After 24 years of service to the Department of Public Health Nursing, she retired in 1943 to Vancouver Island, where she contributed regularly to the *Halifax Chronicle, Atlantic Monthly,* and other magazines. She married W. H. Colley after her retirement, and in 1970, she published *While Rivers Flow: Stories of Early Alberta*, experiences and short stories based on her public health nursing practice.

Sources: Brighty, K. (1942). *Collection of facts for a history of nursing in Alberta: 1864–1942.* Edmonton, AB: Alberta Association of Registered Nurses; and Brighty Colley, K. (1970). *While rivers flow: Stories of early Alberta.* Saskatoon, SK: The Western Producer; and Stewart, I. (1979). *These were our yesterdays: A history of district nursing in Alberta.* Altona, MB: Friesen Printers.

and protects the health of individuals, families, groups, communities, and populations (CHNAC, 2003). It involves coordinating care and planning services, programs, and policies by collaborating with individuals, caregivers, families, other disciplines, communities, and governments (CHNAC, 2003). It combines knowledge of nursing theory, social sciences, and public health sciences.

Community health nursing includes public health nursing, home health (community-based) nursing, and community mental health nursing, as well as a variety of other specialities such as street health, telehealth, and parish nursing (CHNAC, 2003; see also Stamler & Yiu, 2008, and Stanhope et al., 2008, for in-depth descriptions of community health nursing roles in Canada). Occupational health nursing has emerged as a distinctive specialized practice, although it is arguably within the inclusive focus of community health nursing. The community health nursing focus is broader than that of public health nursing, emphasizing both the community's health and direct care to subpopulations within that community. By focusing on subpopulations, the community health nurse cares for the whole community and considers the individual to be one member of a group. The practice focus of various specialties within community health nursing can be compared to the shifting perspective of a camera lens: For example, home health nurses "zoom in" to focus on individual clients, then enlarge their view (wide angle) to consider family and community, whereas public health nurses more often shift from a "wide-angle" view of populations to a "close-up" view of specific vulnerable groups or families (CHNAC, 2003).

Regardless of specific role, function, or setting, community health nursing practice is guided by values and beliefs in caring, multiple ways of knowing, individual–community partnerships, primary health care, and empowerment (CHNAC, 2003). **Primary health care** focuses on education, rehabilitation, support services, health promotion, and disease prevention. It involves multidisciplinary teams and collaboration with other sectors, as well as with secondary and tertiary care facilities (see Chapter 2). Primary health care principles guide community health nurses to use empowerment-based models of community practice (Chalmers & Bramadat, 1996; CHNAC, 2003). **Empowerment** may be most simply described as a means by which people, individually and collectively in organizations and communities, exercise their ability to effect change to enhance control, quality of life, and social justice (CHNAC, 2003). Empowerment is both an outcome and a process by which that outcome is achieved. Empowerment exists in dynamic power relations among people, which from a health promotion perspective are expressed as "power-with" rather than "power-over" relations (Labonte, 1993). Although empowerment is commonly conceptualized as a process continuum from personal to small group to community organzation to partnership to social and political action (Laverack, 2004), Labonte's holosphere (Venn diagram) better depicts the interrelated and nonlinear dynamic of these empowering processes in practice. Criticisms that empowerment is often misinterpreted as increasing individual responsibility but overlooking power and control (Cooke, 2002) highlight the importance of action to ensure that adequate resources are available for individuals and for groups and communities collectively. Such action would be grounded in ethical commitment to inclusion, diversity, participation, social justice, advocacy, and interdependence as a complementary foundation to the Canadian Nurses Association (CNA) Code of Ethics intended to guide all nursing practice (Racher, 2007).

Empowerment-based skills of client advocacy, communication, and the design of new systems in cooperation with existing systems help make community health nursing practice effective. Figure 4–1 depicts the Canadian Community Health Nursing Practice Model. The model shows how community health nursing care encompasses action aimed at illness care; prevention of illness, disease, or injury; and health promotion. These actions complement one another, even as their underlying aims, approaches to care, and perceptions of clients differ.

Community health nursing practice requires a distinct set of skills and knowledge. Expert community health nurses understand the needs of a population or community through experiences with individuals, families, and groups. They think critically in applying a wide range of knowledge to find the best approaches for partnering with their clients. In 2006, the CNA introduced a certification process for nurses in community health nursing (CNA, 2006). Certification confirms practitioner competence in the specialty, recognizes nurses who meet the national standards of the specialty, and, most important, promotes excellence in nursing care for the Canadian population (see CNA, 2006, and CHNAC, 2003, for details about standards and certification procedures).

Public Health Nursing

Public health nursing merges knowledge from the public health sciences with professional nursing theories to safeguard and improve the health of populations in the community (Canadian Public Health Association, 1990; CHNAC, 2003). To understand public health

> **BOX 4-2 Milestones in Canadian Nursing History**
>
> 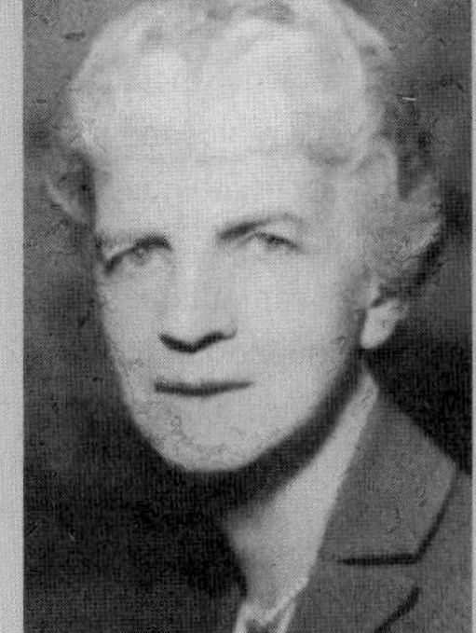
>
> ### Edith Kathleen Russell, 1886–1964
>
> Edith Kathleen Russell was born in Windsor, Nova Scotia, in 1886. She entered the Toronto General Hospital School of Nursing in 1915 and, after graduating, worked with the Department of Public Health in Toronto. In 1920, the Department of Public Health Nursing at the University of Toronto was established, and Russell was appointed its first director.
>
> Russell recognized the great need for improved nursing education. At the time, the norm was an apprenticeship system in hospital schools, in which students, rather than graduate nurses, fulfilled nursing tasks. The primary focus of the hospital school system was not education but hospital service; the incentive was mainly financial. Although public health nursing was her department's original focus, Russell turned her attention to hospital nursing. She gained the support of the University of Toronto and the Rockefeller Foundation for an experiment in basic nursing education and obtained a grant of more than $250,000. This was at the height of the Great Depression, when other university schools were fighting for their very existence.
>
> Russell's diploma program, begun in 1933, prepared nurses for hospital and public health nursing. In 1942, her program evolved into an integrated basic degree program controlled by the university, in which clinical practice was obtained at affiliated hospitals under supervision of university instructors. This program was the first of its kind in Canada and was hailed throughout the world as an important new system of nursing education. Today, hospital-based schools of nursing have largely given way to schools in the general educational system, either in community colleges or in universities, and most provinces are adopting the degree as the basic credential for nursing practice. Edith Kathleen Russell is widely recognized as the architect of the integrated degree nursing program.
>
> Source: Carpenter, H. (1982). *A divine discontent: Edith Kathleen Russell, reforming educator.* Toronto, ON: University of Toronto Faculty of Nursing. Photo: Reproduced by permission of Helen M. Carpenter (BS, MPH, EdD).

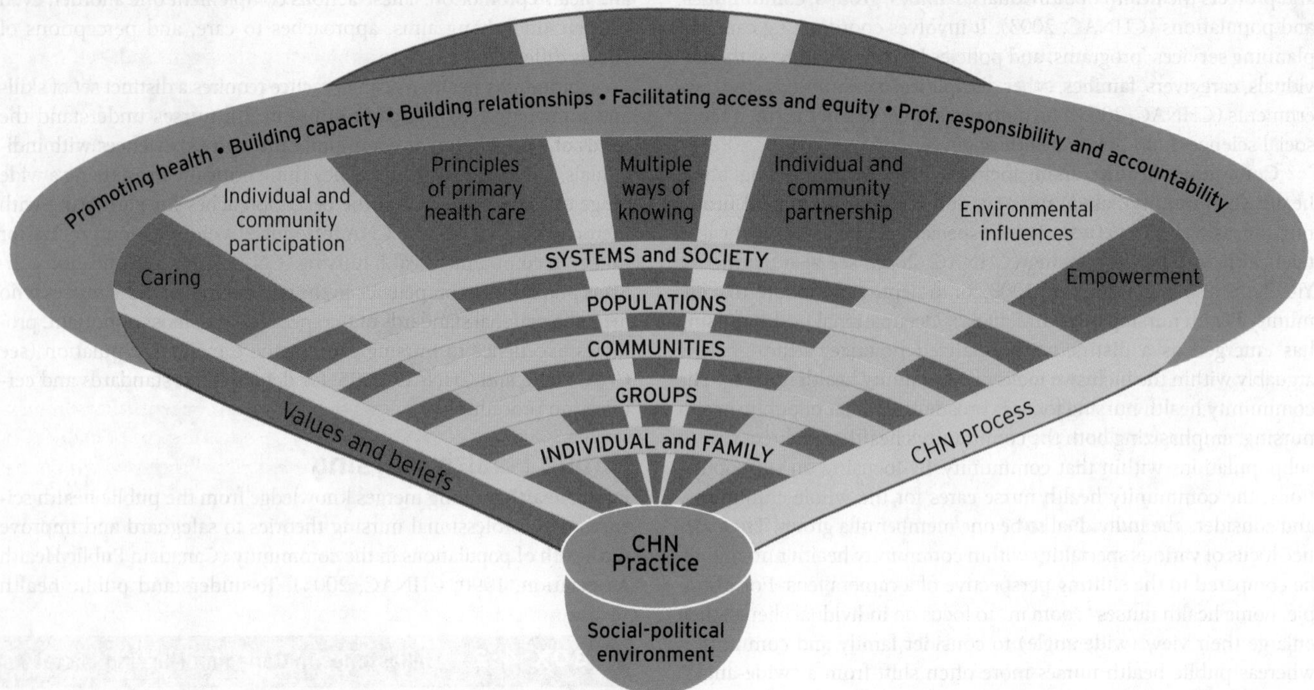

Figure 4-1 The canadian community health nursing practice model. The model illustrates the dynamic nature of community health nursing (CHN) practice, embracing the present and projecting into the future. The values and beliefs (*green* or *shaded*) ground practice in the present and yet guide the evolution of community health nursing practice over time. The community health nursing process (*pink* or *unshaded*) provides the vehicle through which community health nurses work with people, and supports practice that exemplifies the standards of community health nursing. The standards of practice revolve around both the values and beliefs and the nursing process, and the energies of community health nursing are always being focused on improving the health of the people in the community and facilitating change in systems or society in support of health. Community health nursing practice occurs not in isolation but rather within an environmental context, such as policies within nurses' workplace and the legislative framework applicable to their work. **Source:** Adapted from Community Health Nurses Association of Canada. (2008). *Canadian community health nursing standards of practice.* Retrieved September 10, 2008, from http://www.chnac.ca/images/downloads/standards/chn_standards_of_practice_mar08_english.pdf

nursing, it is necessary to know how public health works. The emphasis in **public health** is on the health of the entire population. Historically, government-funded agencies have supported public health programs that improve food and water safety and provide adequate sewage disposal. Public health policy has largely been responsible for the dramatic gain in life expectancy for North Americans during the past century (McKay, 2008; Shah, 2003). The goal of public health is to achieve a healthy environment for everyone. **Public health principles** of disease prevention, health promotion and protection, and healthy public policy (Canadian Public Health Association, 2008) can be applied to individuals, families, groups, or communities. Public health practice calls for competencies (i.e., knowledge, skills, attitudes) that cross the boundaries of specific disciplines and are independent of programs and roles (Public Health Agency of Canada, 2007). These competencies include "population health assessment, surveillance, disease and injury prevention, health promotion, and health protection" (Public Health Agency of Canada, 2007, p. 1).

A public health focus requires understanding the needs of a population. Focus may be narrowed to vulnerable populations, such as low-income families or recent immigrants. Public health professionals must understand factors influencing the health promotion and health maintenance of groups, trends and patterns influencing the occurrence of disease or risks within populations, environmental factors contributing to health and illness, and political processes used to influence public policy (see Chapter 1, "Determinants of Health" section).

As discussed in Chapter 1, **population health** emerged in Canada in the 1990s as an approach to public health care. The overall goals of a population health approach are to maintain and improve the health of the entire population and to eliminate health disparities (Health Canada, 1998). The population health promotion approach (Hamilton & Bhatti, 1996) provides a framework for thinking about health and for taking action to improve the health of populations. Action is directed primarily at community levels. Strategies address the determinants of health in order to improve population health and reduce risks (see Chapter 1). Most health determinants involve other sectors of society such as education, agriculture, business, and government. Multisectoral collaboration between the health sector and other sectors is essential in a population health approach. This approach further broadens the scope of nursing practice in the community. Population-based public health programs focus on disease prevention, health protection, and health promotion, which provide the foundation for health care services at all levels (see Chapter 2).

Public health nurses perceive value in their distinctive practice, which enables them to see "the big picture" as a result of their "broad health knowledge base, in-depth understanding of the community and community resources, and . . . appreciation of individual–family–community inter-relationships" (Reutter & Ford, 1996, p. 8). By using public health principles, the nurse is better able to understand the environments in which clients live, the factors that influence client health, and the types of interventions supportive of client health. Figure 4–2 illustrates a framework for public health programs that provides a means of organizing program development in public health practice (Edwards & Moyer, 2000).

Successful public health nursing practice involves empowerment-based strategies initiated by building relationships with the community and being responsive to changes within it (Canadian Public Health Association, 1990; CHNAC, 2003; Diekemper et al., 1999). For example, when increasing numbers of grandparents are caring for their grandchildren in a particular community, nurses can collaborate with local schools and agencies to create a program that might include opportunity for peer support and education about available resources. The public health nurse is responsive by being active in the community; knowing its members, needs, and resources; and working collaboratively to establish health promotion and disease prevention programs. This means developing and maintaining relationships with other professional systems and individuals and encouraging them to respond to a population's needs.

Home Health Nursing

Home health nursing, also known as **community-based nursing**, involves acute, chronic, and palliative care of individuals and their families that enhances their capacity for self-care and promotes autonomy in decision making (Ayers et al., 1999; CHNAC, 2003). Nursing takes place in community settings such as the home, a long-term care facility, or a clinic. The nurse's competence is based on critical thinking and decision making at the level of the individual client: assessing health status, selecting nursing interventions, and evaluating care outcomes. Because they provide care where clients live, work, and play, home health nurses need to be individual- and family-oriented and also need to appreciate a community's values (CHNAC, 2003; Zotti et al., 1996).

Components of home health nursing practice include self-care as a client and family responsibility; preventive care; care within the community context; continuity of care between home and health system services; and collaborative client care among health practitioners (CHNAC, 2003; Hunt & Zurek, 1997). Nurses use their clinical expertise to provide direct care (e.g., a case manager monitors clients recovering from stroke and provides rehabilitation services). Nursing supports and improves clients' quality of life. Illness is seen as one aspect of clients' everyday lives. Nursing tends to be problem focused, addressing client needs for primary, secondary, and tertiary prevention (CHNAC, 2003; Hunt, 1998).

A strong theoretical foundation for home health nursing is provided by the human ecological model, which conceptualizes human systems as open and interactive with the environment (Chalmers et al., 1998). In an ecological model, the individual is viewed within the larger systems of family, social network, community, and society, which can be depicted as four concentric circles: the innermost circle of the client and the immediate family, the second circle of people and settings that have frequent contact with the client and family, the third circle of the local community and its values and policies, and the outermost circle of larger social systems such as business and government (Ayers et al., 1999). A home health nurse must understand the interaction of all systems while caring for clients and families in their home environment. Nurses typically become involved in the domain of the first three circles. For example, as a home health nurse, you work closely with a client in whom diabetes

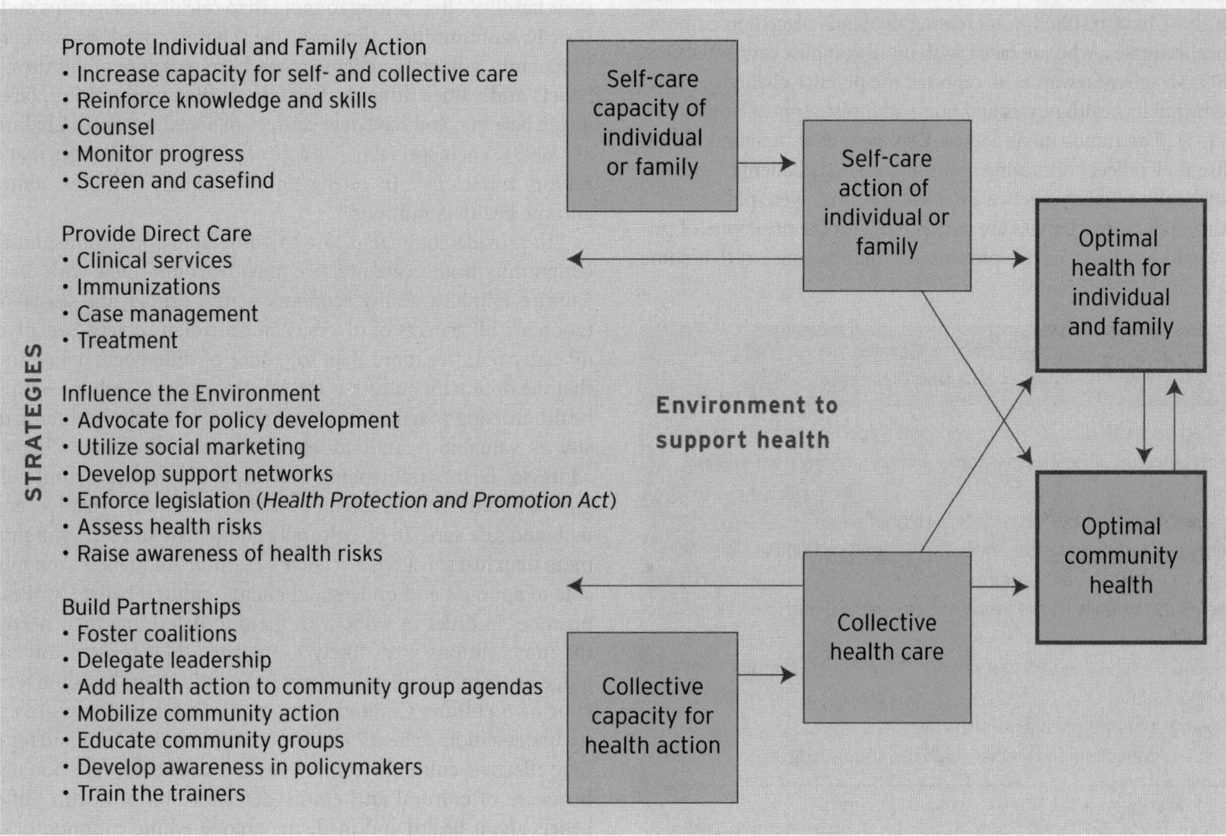

Figure 4-2 Framework for public health programs. **Source:** From N. Edwards et al. (1995). *Building and sustaining collective health action: A framework for community health practitioners.* Ottawa, ON: Community Health Research Unit, Pub. No. DP95-1, as cited by Edwards, N. C., & Moyer, A. (2000). Community needs and capacity assessment: Critical component of program planning. In M. J. Stewart (Ed.): *Community nursing: Promoting Canadians' health* (2nd ed., pp. 433), Toronto, ON: W. B. Saunders.

was recently diagnosed and with the family to establish a care plan. You use your observations of the client's lifestyle when considering an exercise schedule and meal routines. Knowing community resources (e.g., shops with glucose-monitoring supplies and local diabetes support groups) enables you to provide comprehensive support.

Home health nursing is family-centred care (Ayers et al., 1999; CHNAC, 2003). This care requires knowledge of family theory (see Chapter 20), cultural diversity (see Chapter 10), communication (see Chapter 18), and group dynamics. Empowerment-based strategies guide you to work in partnership with clients and families to support them and help them participate in their health care decisions (Toofany, 2007). The client and family are partners with you in planning, decision making, implementation, and evaluation of health care approaches.

The Changing Focus of Community Health Nursing Practice

Community health nursing practice has changed since the 1960s in response to social, economic, and political influences. Changes were documented by Chalmers et al. (1998), who interviewed community health nurse educators, administrators, and staff nurses who worked in public health agencies, home health services, and community health centres in Manitoba. The nurses noted shifts in practice focus from universal programs to programs directed to high-risk or vulnerable groups, from generalized to specialized practice, and from delivery of traditional public health services to more community-based acute care. These shifts have resulted in increasing demands placed on community health nurses, who are faced with more complex care situations. In 2005, Meagher-Stewart et al. reported the practice challenges articulated by public health nurses and nurse administrators in Nova Scotia (Box 4–3). The trends identified by Chalmers et al. remain relevant because they reflect continuing shifts and related challenges in community health nursing practice a decade after they were publicized.

Although many changes are consistent with the principles of primary health care and health promotion, there is concern that some changes put universal accessibility of public health nursing services at risk (Meagher-Stewart et al., 2005; Reutter & Ford, 1998). This concern also has emerged in home health practice, in which a policy agenda of increasing medicalization "stands in contrast to the principles of primary health care, and potentially leads to further marginalization of the most vulnerable" (Duncan & Reutter, 2006, p. 242). Home health care case managers expressed concern about limits on their practice arising from a conflict between professional discourse that guides practice and economic discourses that drive organizational priorities (Ceci, 2006).

➤ BOX 4-3 Challenges to Community Health Nursing Practice

- Pulled between documenting work and valued practice with clients
- Torn between prescribed programs and community partnership activities
- "Never enough time," especially for higher needs
- Increased task orientation, specialization, and working in silos
- Lack of evaluation of program effectiveness
- Increasing inequity of programs to rural, seniors, and low income populations
- Feeling stretched related to shortage of nursing and administrative support staff
- Staying current on health information
- Loss of connection and visibility with the community

From Meagher-Stewart, D., Aston, M., Edwards, N., Smith, D., Young, L., Woodford, E., et al. (2005). *The study of public health nurses in primary health care. Fostering citizen participation and collaborative practice: Tapping the wisdom and voices of public health nurses in Nova Scotia. Research Report* (p. 6). Halifax, NS: Dalhousie University. Retrieved August 12, 2008, from http://preventionresearch.dal.ca/pdf/PHN_study_Nov25.pdf

Vulnerable Populations

Community health nurses care for clients from diverse cultures and backgrounds and with various health conditions. However, because of changes in the health care delivery system, high-risk groups have become the nurses' principal clients.

Vulnerable populations of clients are those who are likely to develop health problems as a result of excessive risks, who experience barriers when trying to access health care services, or who are dependent on others for care. Vulnerability can be understood in relation to the determinants of health, particularly social determinants that compromise socioeconomic status, literacy, and social inclusion (see Chapter 1). People living in poverty, homeless people, people in precarious circumstances (such as women in abusive interpersonal relationships), people with chronic conditions and disabilities, and people who engage in stigmatizing risk behaviours (including substance abuse and unsafe sexual practices), as well as Aboriginal peoples and new immigrants and refugees, are examples of vulnerable populations (Beiser & Stewart, 2005). Vulnerable individuals and their families often belong to more than one of these groups and may live in communities that can be characterized as vulnerable. Frequently, vulnerable clients come from a variety of cultures, have beliefs and values different from the mainstream culture, face language barriers, and have few sources of social support (Chalmers et al., 1998). Their special needs contribute to the challenges that community nurses face in caring for increasingly complex acute and chronic health conditions.

To provide competent care to vulnerable populations, nurses in community health care practice must be comfortable with diversity. Culture, ethnicity, ability, economic status, gender, and sexual orientation are all aspects of diversity in Canadian society. Sensitivity to diversity requires more than tolerance of difference, which implies that the dominant culture is the reference point. Rather, community health nursing practice that is sensitive to diversity embraces diversity as valuable to individual and social well-being. Chapter 10 addresses factors influencing individual differences within cultural groups and the nurse's role in providing culturally sensitive, competent, and safe care. To be culturally competent and safe, you must be more than just sensitive to a client's cultural uniqueness. You must be able to appraise and understand clients' cultural beliefs, values, and practices in order to work with them to determine their needs and the interventions most likely to improve their health. You cannot judge or evaluate a client's beliefs and values about health in terms of your own culture. Communication and caring practices are crucial for understanding clients' perceptions of their problems and for planning effective, culturally competent, and safe health care. You need to be aware of cultural and ethnic determinants of health, differing beliefs about health and medicine among ethnic communities, and barriers to accessing care that affect members of ethnic minorities.

Vulnerable populations typically experience poorer health outcomes than do people with ready access to resources and health care services (Beiser & Stewart, 2005). Higher morbidity and mortality rates characterize members of ethnically and racially diverse minority groups (Barr et al., 2002; Hwang, 2000). Members of vulnerable groups frequently experience cumulative risk factors or combinations of risk conditions that make them more sensitive to the adverse effects of individual risk factors that others might overcome (Rew et al., 2001). Community health nurses must assess clients from vulnerable populations by considering multiple risk factors and the clients' ability to deal with stressors. Box 4–4 summarizes guidelines for assessing clients from vulnerable population groups.

Poor and Homeless People. People who live in poverty are more likely to live in hazardous environments, work at high-risk jobs, eat less nutritious foods, and experience multiple stressors. They face practical problems such as limited access to transportation, limited quality child care to support employment, and limited medication or dental coverage from supplementary health benefits. Low-income status is prevalent among lone-parent families, unattached older adults (mostly women), and Aboriginal families (Canadian Population Health Initiative, 2004). Homeless people have even fewer resources than do low-income people. Their vulnerability lies in their social condition, lifestyle, and environment, which diminish their ability to maintain or improve their health or access health care. Homeless people live on the streets or in temporary accommodation such as shelters and boarding houses. They may distrust health and social services as bureaucratic and judgemental, using them only when their health has deteriorated (Thibaudeau & Denoncourt, 2000). Chronic health problems worsen because of barriers to supportive self-care and medical care. Homeless people have a high incidence of mental illness and substance abuse. Nurses can help low-income and homeless people identify their capacities and resources, their eligibility for assistance, and interventions to help improve their health. For example, Cathy Crowe's work as a street nurse in Toronto includes direct care such as "dressing a wound under a highway overpass," "treating frostbite," and "providing intravenous rehydration to patients in shelters during a Nowalk virus outbreak," as well as advocacy such as "constantly seeking donations like Gatorade to counter dehydration" and "documenting police-inflicted injuries" (Crowe, 2007, p. 6).

People in Precarious Circumstances. Women are at greater risk for problems related to low income, violence, and the stressors associated with unpaid caregiving. Such risks are further complicated for some by geographically isolated settings that challenge women's resilience in maintaining their health (Leipert & Reutter, 2005). Community health nurses's work is guided by their recognition of the need to listen to, respect, and communicate with women in their communities (Leipert, 1999).

Physical, emotional, and sexual abuse, as well as neglect, are major public health problems, particularly affecting older adults, women, and children (Canadian Public Health Association, 1994; Sebastian, 2006). Abuse occurs in many settings, including the home, workplace, school, health care facility, and public areas, and is most often committed by an acquaintance of the victim (Canadian Public Health Association, 1994). When dealing with clients at risk for or who may have suffered abuse, you must provide protection for them. Interviews with clients should occur in private when the individual suspected of being the perpetrator is not present. Clients who have been abused often fear retribution if they discuss their problems with a health care professional. Most regions have reporting agencies or hotlines for notification when an individual has been identified as being at risk, and you can work with clients to reflect on concerns, identify acceptable alternatives, and make decisions about their situation.

Unintentional injuries, unemployment, depression, and suicide are a concern among youth, particularly young men and those in Aboriginal communities. "Community health nurses who are

➤ BOX 4-4 Guidelines for Assessing Members of Vulnerable Population Groups

Setting the Stage

- Create a comfortable, nonthreatening environment.
- Learn as much as you can about the culture of the clients you work with, so that you will understand traditions and values that influence their health care practices.
- Provide culturally competent assessment by understanding the meaning of language and nonverbal behaviour in the client's culture.
- Be sensitive to the fact that the individual or family may have priorities, such as financial or legal problems, that are more important to them than traditional health concerns. Within your scope as a nurse, you may need to help them deal with these priority concerns before you can address specific health concerns.
- Collaborate with others as appropriate; connect your client with someone who can help.

Nursing History of an Individual or a Family

- You may have only one opportunity to work with a vulnerable person or family. Try to document a history that provides essential information you need to help on that day. Organize what you need to ask, and be prepared to explain why the information is necessary.
- Use a modified comprehensive assessment form to focus on the special needs of the vulnerable group. Be flexible. With some clients, it is impractical and unethical to ask all questions on the form. If you expect to see the client again, ask less urgent questions at the next visit.
- Include questions about social support, economic status, resources for health care, developmental issues, current health problems, medication, and how the person or family manages health status. Your goal is to obtain information that will enable you to provide family-centred care.
- Determine whether the individual has any condition that compromises his or her immune status, such as human immunodeficiency virus (HIV) infection or acquired immunodeficiency syndrome (AIDS), or is receiving therapy that would result in immunodeficiency, such as cancer chemotherapy.

Physical Examination or Home Assessment

- Complete as thorough a physical examination (on an individual) or home assessment as you can. Collect only information you can use to work with the individual or family.
- Be alert for indications of mental or physical abuse, substance use, or differences from normal physical examination findings.
- Observe a family's living environment. Does the family have running water, functioning plumbing, electricity, and access to a telephone? Is perishable food left on tables and countertops? Are surfaces reasonably clean? Is paint peeling on the walls and ceilings? Are room ventilation and temperature adequate? Is the home next to a busy highway, exposing the family to high noise levels and automobile exhaust?

Adapted from Sebastian, J. G. (2006). Vulnerability and vulnerable populations: An overview. In M. Stanhope & J. Lancaster (Eds.), *Foundations of nursing in the community: Community-oriented practice* (pp. 403–417). St. Louis, MO: Mosby.

concerned with adolescent health promotion must consider the broad range of factors that affect adolescent health decisions and behaviours. Individual, family and environmental factors must be considered, together with many structural and societal factors" (Gillis, 2000, p. 257).

People with Chronic Conditions and Disabilities.

"Chronic conditions are impairments in function, development, or disease states that are irreversible or have a cumulative effect" (Ogden Burke et al., 2000, p. 211). There are physical and emotional aspects of living with chronic conditions. Societal trends toward greater family mobility, maternal employment, smaller families, and female-headed lone-parent low-income families are challenges for families caring for children with chronic conditions (Ogden Burke et al., 2000). Older adults experience more chronic conditions as they age (Health Canada, 1999). The shift in health care service delivery from institutional to community-based care places demands on families, particularly women, to provide caregiving in the community. You need to work with individuals, families, and communities to promote adequate support for family caregivers and access to resources and services.

For a client with a severe mental illness, multiple health and socioeconomic problems must be explored. Many such clients are homeless or marginally housed. Others are unable to work or provide self-care. They require medication therapy, counselling, housing, and vocational assistance. No longer hospitalized in long-term psychiatric institutions, clients with mental illness are offered resources within their community. However, many communities face continuing difficulties in the establishment of comprehensive, coordinated, and accessible community-based service networks (Health Canada, 2002; Shah, 2003). Many clients who lack functional skills are left with fewer and more fragmented services. An increasing number of young mentally ill people have only episodic hospital care. Collaboration among community resources is key to helping mentally ill people obtain health care. For example, the interdisciplinary Psychiatric Outreach Team of the Royal Ottawa Hospital provides mobile services to shelters and drop-in centres to initiate mental health care, assist in linking clients to community resources, and provide education and assistance in connecting with mental health and addiction treatment (Farrell et al., 2005).

With the increasing population of older adults, there is a corresponding increase in the number of clients with chronic disease and a greater demand for health care (Craig, 2000). You must view health promotion from a broad perspective, by understanding what health means to older adults and ways they can maintain their own health. Among individuals who feel empowered to control their own health, the incidence of disability from chronic disease is lower (Baas et al., 2002). You can help improve the quality of life for older adults.

People Who Engage in Stigmatizing Risk Behaviours.

Potentially stigmatizing risk behaviours include substance abuse and unsafe sexual practices. The social determinants of health provide a holistic perspective to address social and structural conditions that influence behaviour and to challenge the "unprecedented reliance on interventions that focus on addressing what is wrong with the individual" (Shoveller & Johnson, 2006, p. 56). *Substance abuse* is a general term for the use of illegal drugs and the abuse of alcohol and prescribed medications such as antianxiety agents and narcotic analgesics. Clients who abuse substances also frequently have health and socioeconomic problems. A substantial proportion of adult HIV and AIDS cases have been attributed to injection drug use (Geduld & Gatali, 2003). Substance abuse, particularly alcohol abuse, remains a serious problem among Canadian adolescents (Gillis, 2000). Socioeconomic problems often result from financial strain, employment loss, and family breakdown. The incidences of

BOX 4-5 RESEARCH HIGHLIGHT

AIDS Prevention Street Nurse Program

Research Focus

The AIDS Prevention Street Nurse Program in Vancouver provides outreach services for preventing HIV and sexually transmitted infection in vulnerable, high-risk clients (Hilton, Thompson, & Moore-Dempsey, 2000; Hilton, Thompson, Moore-Dempsey, & Hutchinson, 2000, 2001). The program was awarded the Provincial Health Officer's Award of Excellence in 2007 and acknowledged as symbolizing best nursing practices and organizational commitment. Community health nurses with the program use harm reduction and health promotion approaches in their work. Harm reduction includes needle exchange for injection drug use, education to promote safer drug use and sexual behaviour, and support to clients in addiction treatment programs. Nurses go where the clients are: clinics, drop-in centres, detoxification centres, jails, door-to-door in hotels, or on the street.

Research Abstract

The purpose of the program evaluation study was to describe the nurses' work and its impact on clients, the challenges that nurses faced, and the program fit with other services (Hilton, Thompson, Moore-Dempsey, & Hutchinson, 2001). Program nurses were interviewed, as were clients of the program, including youths living on the streets, sex trade workers, and injection drug users. Challenges facing nurses include building trust with clients, providing needed care or resources, and involving other health care professionals. Clients reported gaining knowledge, feeling better about themselves, being supported, and changing their behaviours to help themselves and others (Hilton, Thompson, Moore-Dempsey, & Hutchinson, 2000, 2001).

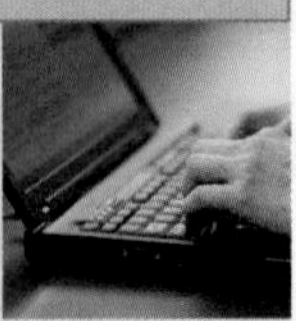

Evidence-Informed Practice

- Key strategies for reaching vulnerable populations include working with clients "at their location, on their own terms, and according to their own agenda" (Hilton, Thompson, Moore-Dempsey, & Hutchinson, 2001, p. 274) and encouraging and facilitating client participation and choice.
- Client empowerment can be promoted through nurses' nonjudgmental care, trust, and respect.
- Educating marginalized clients about health promotion and harm prevention increases their self-concept and encourages them to change their behaviour.

References: Hilton, A. B., Thompson, R., & Moore-Dempsey. L. (2000). Evaluation of the AIDS prevention street nurse program: One step at a time. *Canadian Journal of Nursing Research, 32*(1), 17–38; Hilton, A. B., Thompson, R., Moore-Dempsey, L., & Hutchinson, K. (2001). Urban outpost nursing: The nature of the nurses' work in the AIDS prevention street nurse program. *Public Health Nursing, 18*(4), 273–280; and Thompson, R., Hilton, A. B., Moore-Dempsey, L., & Hutchinson, K. (2000). AIDS prevention on the streets: Vancouver nurses are taking AIDS prevention to the streets. *Canadian Nurse, 96*(8), 24–28.

unsafe sexual practices and multiple risk-taking behaviours remain high among young people, particularly young men (Health Canada, 1999). Unsafe sex creates serious health and social risks, including the risks of unplanned pregnancy and acquiring sexually transmitted infections (e.g., HIV infection and AIDS). Unplanned adolescent pregnancy poses risks for both mothers and infants, including pregnancy complications (DiCenso & Van Dover, 2000), low income, low academic achievement, unemployment, violence (Gillis, 2000), and stigma (Fulford & Ford-Gilboe, 2004). You can partner with clients to assess the circumstances that contribute to substance use, unsafe sexual practices, and other high-risk behaviours and identify strategies to address the often multiple and interrelated concerns. For example, Steenbeek (2004) identified strategies such as peer leader training and self-advocacy skill development within an empowering health promotion framework to prevent sexually transmitted infections among Aboriginal youth. The AIDS Prevention Street Nurse Program (Box 4–5) and the Nursing Story (Box 4–6) illustrate **harm reduction**, an important but controversial approach to health promotion, that is based on user input and demand, compassionate pragmatism, and commitment to offer alternatives to reduce risk behaviour consequences, to accept alternatives to abstinence, and to reduce barriers to treatment by providing user-friendly access (Hilton, Thompson, Moore-Dempsey, & Janzen, 2001; Pauly et al., 2007; Shah, 2003).

Competencies, Roles, and Activities in Community Health Nursing

Nurses in community health practice must have a broad base of knowledge and skills in order to work with clients to meet their health care needs and develop community relationships. Primary health care and health promotion approaches help nurses recognize the interplay between individual experience and social conditions, the value of diversity, and the importance of building capacity to promote health-enhancing change. In community health nursing practice, "nurses are responsible for the maintenance of professional nursing standards and of public health standards by being accountable for the quality of their own practice, striving for excellence, ensuring that their knowledge is current and taking advantage of opportunities for life long learning" (Canadian Public Health Association, 1990, p. 5). Cradduck (2000) concluded that the "legacy of community health nursing is its multidimensional role, community orientation, and advocacy" (p. 367). The CHNAC (2003) identified five standards of practice for community health nurses: promoting health, building individual and community capacity, building relationships, facilitating access and equity, and demonstrating professional responsibility and accountability. These standards reflect the nursing process "of assessment, planning, intervention, and evaluation. Community health nurses enhance this process through individual or community participation in each component multiple ways of knowing awareness of the influence of the broader environment on the individual or community that is the focus of their care (e.g., the community will be affected by provincial or territorial policies, its own economic status and the actions of its individual citizens) (CHNAC, 2008, p. 9). A summary of key roles and practice dimensions identified by the Canadian Public Health Association (1990) and that remain relevant to current community health nursing practice is presented in the following sections.

Communicator. Communication skills support all other activities in community health nursing practice. Skill as an effective communicator is closely related to the leadership, enabling, and advocacy skills of the facilitator. As communicators, you may use negotiation and mediation to foster collaboration.

Facilitator. To facilitate is to promote. Community health nurses work within a participatory process to identify issues, develop goals for change, and implement strategies for action and evaluation of results. Leadership, enabling, and advocacy skills are key to these activities. Leadership focuses on supporting processes that build capacity among participants, rather than on directing or controlling decision making. Enabling encourages client participation and experiential learning. Advocacy fosters equity and accessibility of care, especially among vulnerable populations.

Collaborator. Collaboration is a way of working together that is characterized by recognition of interdependence, collective responsibility, and negotiated equity in relationships (Gray, 1989; Labonte, 1993). Collaboration involves more than linking or networking with others. Community health nurses participate in a collective process

BOX 4-6 NURSING STORY

Harm Reduction Nursing

Harm reduction initiatives, such as needle exchange programs now available in most Canadian provinces, exemplify community nursing practice guided by primary health care, health promotion, empowerment, and ethical principles. The leadership, creativity, and dedication of nurses have contributed significantly to the development of these initiatives. For example, Wood et al. (2003) successfully advocated for the establishment of a supervised injection site for injection drug users as part of the Day Program services provided by the Dr. Peter Centre in Vancouver's Downtown Eastside. Collaborating with local HIV and AIDS network members, researchers, and street nurses (see Box 4–4), they developed policies, procedures, and protocols to deliver harm reduction services to a highly vulnerable population in which stigmatizing risk behaviours were compounded by homelessness, precarious life circumstances, and chronic conditions and disabilities. In addition to the supervised injection site, nurses provide sterile drug injection supplies through a needle exchange program, teach about safe sex, offer condoms, talk with sex trade workers about safer ways of dealing with johns, counsel on addiction, support methadone maintenance regimens, and help when individuals are ready to enter detoxification programs or rehabilitation (Griffiths, 2002, p. 12). Serving the same population, Insite, North America's first dedicated legal supervised drug injection site, opened in 2003 and provides health care, counseling, education, and support from a multidisciplinary team that includes nurses. Since 1989, nurses with the Streetworks initiative in Edmonton have worked from several fixed daytime sites and from a mobile van for evening outreach to offer harm reduction strategies in partnership with agencies serving the inner city community. Nurses' work in these initiatives illustrates many of the role dimensions needed for community health practice, including activities as communicator, facilitator, collaborator, coordinator, educator, care or service provider, community developer, policy formulator, and researcher. "Using professional practice to create change, the passion and leadership of a few nurses are resulting in an innovative approach. If such an approach were adopted across Canada, the number of human lives and health care dollars saved would be monumental" (Wood et al., 2003, p. 24). You are encouraged to reflect on these nursing roles and activities by reading more about these and similar programs in communities across the country.

Web Sites

Dr. Peter Centre http://www.drpeter.org/
Insite http://www.vch.ca/sis/
StreetWorks http://www.streetworks.ca/pro/index.html

as a collaborator with clients, community members, agencies, and sectors. This process is supported by developing honest relationships and mutual respect, recognizing many forms of expertise, valuing diversity, and being organized and committed.

Coordinator. The coordinator's role has long been associated with nursing practice. Community health nurses work with clients and diverse agencies to coordinate or organize activities, resources, access, and care to promote client health. Coordinator activities complement activities as educator, direct care or service provider, community developer, and social marketer.

Consultant. As consultants, community health nurses rely on a broad knowledge base to provide information and to support participation in health activities. As a nurse, you involve not only clients but also community members, health care professionals, professionals from other disciplines, members of other sectors, policymakers, and government officials. You respond to inquiries about and make referrals to community resources. By developing collaborative relationships, you support client access to these resources.

Educator. Competence in client education with individuals and groups requires a broad knowledge base, as well as communication and learning process theory. Nurses provide information to support community, family, and individual decision making. You may participate in formal education sessions, such as prenatal classes, or in informal sessions, such as discussions with families during home visits. Clients need information to make decisions about health issues, but this is not enough to produce behavioural change. You support clients in applying information to their everyday lives.

Direct Care or Service Provider. Community health nurses act as direct care or service providers when they work with clients to promote and protect health and to prevent injury and illness. In many communities, home visiting remains integral to community health nursing practice, as do services such as health assessment and immunization clinics. Care may involve treating illness, monitoring risk conditions, educating or guiding informed decision making, and supporting client self-care.

Community Developer. As a community developer, community health nurses must support community participation. Participation encourages open identification of issues, shared decision making, egalitarian relationships, and collective ownership of action (Labonte, 1993). Participation and empowerment are closely linked.

Social Marketer. Social marketing is an approach to social change related to health behaviours in which marketing and change theory are used to design and manage programs (Kotler & Roberto, 1989). Interdisciplinary and intersectoral collaboration provides a broad base of expertise. Community health nurses may act as social marketers to promote public awareness of issues and available programs and to build support for social action initiatives.

Policy Formulator. Activities as a policy formulator include identifying the need for policy and program development; participating in program development, implementation, and evaluation; and helping establish policies to support their practice. Community health nurses can support the collective voice of their professional associations (e.g., CNA, CHNAC) to advocate for health-enhancing public policy.

Researcher. Research is used to generate information, identify issues, determine directions for action, consider strategies to promote change, and evaluate results. Community health nurses need to review research and apply knowledge to practice. They also engage in research projects as participants or investigators to support evidence-informed practice.

Community Assessment

As a community health nurse, you need to assess the community—the environment in which people live and work. Without an understanding of that environment, any effort to promote health and to support change is unlikely to succeed, whether you work with an individual, a family, a group, or a community as client.

The community can be seen as having three components: the locale or structure, the social systems, and the people. A complete assessment involves studying each component to understand the health status of the people and the health determinants that influence their health as a basis on which to identify needs for health policy, health program development, and service provision (see Chapter 1; for detailed descriptions of community assessment strategies, see also community health nursing textbooks such as Stamler & Yiu, 2008; Stanhope et al., 2008; and Vollman et al., 2008). To assess the locale or structure, you might travel around the community and observe the physical environment, the location of services, and the places where residents congregate (completing a windshield or walking survey). Information about social systems, such as schools, health care facilities, recreation, transportation, and government, may be acquired by visiting various sites and learning about their services (observing activities, interviewing key informants). Community statistics from a local library or health department can help assess a population's demographics and health status (reviewing population data). Discussion with community members is also helpful (interviewing key informants, holding focus groups) to identify priority issues within the community. It is essential to identify community resources and capacities, as well as issues and problems (Edwards & Moyer, 2000).

Recall the determinants of health as you consider the following scenario. As a community health nurse, you wish to familiarize yourself with the local area to help you begin to identify potential health concerns and available resources that will guide your work with the community. Your windshield and walking surveys reveal an older, high-density neighbourhood where pawn shops and bars outnumber grocery stores, schools, and community recreation facilities. You observe a culturally diverse population, including young families and older people, who interact with each other at community events sponsored by faith-based groups and social agencies. Your observations are reinforced in discussions as you develop relationships with community leaders and with health and social agency staff, whose perspectives are supported by census tract data and regional health statistics. Neighbourhood Watch members, however, alert you to tensions related to high unemployment, language barriers to services, and youth crime, particularly break-ins and vandalism. Once you have a good understanding of the community, you may then perform individual or family client assessment against that background. For example, consider assessment of an older couple's safety. Are windows in their apartment secure and intact? Is lighting along walkways and entryways operational? Do they feel comfortable calling on their neighbours for assistance if necessary? Are health and social services easy to reach when needed? How safe do they feel in the neighbourhood? No individual or family assessment should occur in isolation from the environment and conditions of the community setting. A collaborative approach to community assessment grounded in an empowerment process helps you establish working relationships, identify shared concerns, recognize collective capacities, and develop effective strategies to enhance health.

Promoting Clients' Health

The challenge for nurses in community health practice is how to promote and protect the health of clients, whether within the context of their community or with the community as the focus. You may bring together the resources necessary to improve the continuity of client care. In collaboration with clients, health care and social service professionals, and other community members, you coordinate health care services, locate appropriate social services, and develop innovative approaches to address clients' health issues.

Perhaps the key to being an effective community health nurse is the ability to understand clients' everyday lives. The foundation for this understanding is the establishment of strong, caring relationships with clients (see Chapters 18 and 19) that support empowerment as an active growth process rooted in cultural, religious, and personal belief systems (Falk-Rafael, 2001). The quasi-insider status of nurses in a community often enables them to identify local patterns and needs that can be addressed through programs, policies, and advocacy (SmithBattle et al., 2004) that are responsive, supportive, and effective. This is difficult because the time that nurses have to spend with clients continues to decline. However, the expert nurse is able to advise, counsel, and teach after being accepted into the client's family or the community and by understanding what makes clients unique. The day-to-day activities of family and community life and the cultural, economic, and political environment influence how you adapt nursing interventions. The time of day an individual client goes to work, the availability of the spouse and client's parents to provide child care, and the family values that shape views about health are just a few examples of the many factors you must consider in community health practice. Once you acquire an understanding of a client's life, interventions designed to promote health and prevent disease can be introduced. Similarly, understanding the relationships, activities, and concerns of client groups and communities is central to health promotion practice.

Community health nursing practice is influenced by trends that focus attention on consumer participation, aggregates and communities, independent and interdependent practice, health promotion (Stewart & Leipert, 2000), population health, and health and social system reform that emphasizes service delivery in the community. A continuing challenge articulated by Stewart and Leipert is "to translate all these trends into the everyday practice of community health nurses in Canada" (p. 609) in ways that respect and promote collective empowerment, as well as individual and family empowerment, to enhance health in everyday life.

* KEY CONCEPTS

- A successful community health nursing practice involves building relationships with the community members and being responsive to changes within the community.
- The principles of public health nursing practice aim at assisting individuals in acquiring a healthy environment in which to live.
- The public health nurse cares for the community as a whole and considers the individual or family to be one member of a population or potential group at risk.
- The home health nurse's competence is based on decision making at the level of the individual client.
- Within an ecological model of home health nursing, the individual is viewed within the larger systems of family, social network, community, and society.
- Vulnerable individuals and their families often belong to more than one vulnerable group.
- The special needs of vulnerable populations contribute to the challenges that nurses face in caring for these clients' increasingly complex acute and chronic health conditions.
- Exacerbations of chronic health problems are common among homeless people because they have few resources.
- An important principle in dealing with clients at risk for or who may have suffered abuse is protection of the client.
- Clients who engage in risk behaviours such as substance abuse may respond to a harm reduction approach.
- In community health practice, it is important to understand what health means to clients and the steps they can take to maintain their own health.
- A community health nurse must be competent in fulfilling a multidimensional role, including activities as communicator, facilitator, collaborator, coordinator, consultant, educator, care or service provider, community developer, social marketer, policy formulator, and researcher.
- Assessment of a community includes assessing population health status and relevant determinants of health in relation to three elements: locale or structure, the social systems, and the people.
- An important consideration in becoming an effective community health nurse is to strive to understand clients' lives.

* CRITICAL THINKING EXERCISES

1. You are working with the family of a severely disabled child and learn that no respite services to provide parental support, and only limited educational resources, are available in your community. What activities or roles of the community health nurse would be important to establish a special-education day care service, operated by volunteer educators?
2. Mr. Crowder is a 42-year-old man with diabetes mellitus and visual impairment. Your assessment reveals that he is homeless and spends nights in a local shelter. He is not able to buy medications or ensure adequate diet to control his blood glucose. What factors might you consider to support Mr. Crowder's self-care?
3. Conduct a community assessment of an area that you have visited infrequently. Observe the community locale by driving or walking through the more populated area. Look for the following services: hospital, clinic, pharmacy, grocery store, schools, park or playground, and police and fire departments.

* REVIEW QUESTIONS

1. The overall goals of a population health approach are to
   1. Maintain and improve the population's health and eliminate health disparities
   2. Gather information on incidence rates of certain diseases and social problems
   3. Assess the health care needs of individuals, families, or communities
   4. Develop and implement public health policies and improve access to acute care
2. Public health nursing merges knowledge from professional nursing theories and the
   1. Population sciences
   2. Public health sciences
   3. Environmental sciences
   4. Social sciences

3. Home health nursing involves acute, chronic, and palliative care of clients and families to enhance their capacity for
   1. Nursing care that promotes autonomy in decision making
   2. Improving their health care and self-care
   3. Self-care and autonomy in decision making
   4. Learning about their illnesses
4. Vulnerable populations are more likely to develop health problems as a result of
   1. Acute diseases, homelessness, and poverty
   2. Lack of transportation, dependence on others for care, and lack of initiative
   3. Poverty, lack of education, and mental illness
   4. Excess risks, barriers to health care services, and dependence on others for care
5. Which is *not* an aspect of competent care of vulnerable populations?
   1. Providing culturally appropriate care
   2. Creating a comfortable, nonthreatening environment
   3. Assessing living conditions
   4. Offering financial or legal advice
6. Major public health problems affecting older adults, women, and children are
   1. Prescribed medication abuse, poverty, sexual abuse
   2. Physical, emotional, and sexual abuse, as well as neglect
   3. Acute illnesses, neglect, substance abuse
   4. Financial strain, poverty, physical abuse
7. A successful community health nursing practice requires
   1. A graduate degree in health education or health promotion
   2. Building relationships with and responding to changes in the community
   3. Taking a passive role to allow the community to initiate change
   4. Subspecialty education in public health sciences
8. Teaching classes about infant care, cancer screening, and home safety adaptations for older people are examples of a nurse in the role of
   1. Consultant
   2. Collaborator
   3. Educator
   4. Facilitator
9. A community health nurse who is directing a client to community resources is an example of a nurse in the role of a
   1. Consultant
   2. Collaborator
   3. Coordinator
   4. Researcher
10. A community includes the following three elements, each of which must be assessed:
    1. Locale or structure, social systems, and people
    2. People, neighbourhoods, and social systems
    3. Health care systems, geographic boundaries, and people
    4. Environment, families, and social systems

* RECOMMENDED WEB SITES

Canadian Public Health Association: http://www.cpha.ca

The Canadian Public Health Association (CPHA) is a national, independent, not-for-profit, voluntary association representing public health care in Canada.

Community Health Nurses Association of Canada: http://www.chnac.ca/

The CHNAC is a national-level organization. It provides standards and information on community health nursing.

Fact Sheet: The Primary Health Care Approach: http://cna-aiic.ca/CNA/documents/pdf/publications/FS02_Primary_Health_Care_Approach_June_2000_e.pdf

This Canadian Nurses Association publication defines and describes primary health care in Canada.

Public Health Agency of Canada: Health Promotion: http://www.phac-aspc.gc.ca/hp-ps/index-eng.php

This federal Web site provides links to many useful health promotion resources and guides that will aid health professionals and community leaders.

Victorian Order of Nurses: http://www.von.ca/

The Victorian Order of Nurses (VON) is Canada's leading charitable organization addressing community health and social needs.

5

Caring for the Cancer Survivor

Original chapter by Patricia A. Potter, RN, MSN, PhD, GMAC, FAAN

Canadian content written by Willy Kabotoff, RN, BScN, MN

objectives

Mastery of content in this chapter will enable you to:

- Define the key terms listed.
- Discuss the concept of cancer survivorship.
- Describe the influence of cancer survivorship on clients' quality of life.
- Discuss the effects cancer has on the family.
- Explain the nursing implications related to cancer survivorship.
- Discuss the essential components of survivorship care.

key terms

Biological response modifiers (biotherapy), p. 54
Cancer-related fatigue, p. 55
Cancer survivor, p. 54
Chemotherapy, p. 54
Hormone therapy, p. 54
Lumpectomy, p. 56
Mastectomy, p. 56
Neuropathy, p. 55
Oncology, p. 61
Paresthesias, p. 55
Post-traumatic stress disorder (PTSD), p. 56
Radiation therapy, p. 54

media resources

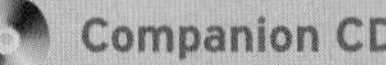

Web Site

- Audio Chapter Summaries
- Glossary
- Multiple-Choice Review Questions
- Student Learning Activities
- Weblinks

Companion CD

- Glossary
- Interactive Learning Activities
- Fluids and Electrolytes Tutorial
- Test-Taking Skills

Cancer survivors have not been recognized for the extent and nature of the health problems that they experience. Cancer has been diagnosed in approximately 833,100 Canadians at some time during the previous 15 years (Canadian Cancer Society [CCS], 2007). The number of survivors will continue to grow because more than 159,000 new cases of cancer are diagnosed each year (CCS, 2007). Cancer survivors' health care problems have largely been ignored or misunderstood because of the belief that for those who receive treatment, survive, and are given a "clean bill of health," their health problems are over. Such is not the case; different trajectories or courses for cancer survival exist (Box 5–1). With the advances made in diagnosis and treatment, more clients are becoming long-term survivors of cancer, whereas others with cancers such as lymphoma control the disease with ongoing or periodic treatment. The major forms of cancer therapy—surgery, **chemotherapy, hormone therapy, biological response modifiers (biotherapy)**, and **radiation therapy**—often create unwanted, long-term effects on tissues and organ systems that impair a person's health and quality of life in small and large ways (Institute of Medicine [IOM] & National Research Council [NRC], 2006). A diagnosis of cancer presents many physical, emotional, and spiritual challenges to clients, families, and other loved ones. Although many individuals who survive cancer continue to live productive and rewarding lives, these challenges may persist beyond the physical recovery of the cancer itself. A large number of Canadians living with the effects of cancer require repeated active treatment, as well as extensive use of rehabilitation and supportive care resources. This increased demand and the complexity of survivors' health care needs must be considered in the planning and development of interdisciplinary health care services (CCS, 2007).

Yabroff et al. (2004) offered one definition of a **cancer survivor**: "An individual is considered a cancer survivor from the time of diagnosis, through the balance of his or her life." Family members and friends should also be considered survivors, because they experience the effects that cancer has on their loved ones. Cancer truly is a life-changing event. One phase of cancer care is often neglected: the period following first diagnosis and initial treatment and before the development of a recurrence of the initial cancer or death (IOM & NRC, 2006). In this phase of their disease, survivors do not have consistent health care follow-up. Frequent contact with a cancer care professional often stops suddenly, and survivors' unique psychosocial needs often go unnoticed or untreated. Despite the incredible advances made in cancer care, many long-term survivors suffer unnecessarily and die as a result of delayed cancer diagnoses or treatment-related chronic disease.

As a nurse, you have the responsibility for better understanding the needs of cancer survivors and for providing the most current evidence-informed approaches to managing late and long-term effects of cancer and cancer treatment. As many as 75% of survivors have serious health deficits, both physical and psychological, that are related to their treatment (Aziz & Rowland, 2003). Disparities in health care among ethnic groups are related to a complex interplay of economic, social, and cultural factors, with poverty being a key factor (IOM & NRC, 2006). Being able to provide comprehensive care to a cancer survivor begins with recognizing the effects of cancer and its treatment and learning about the survivor's own meaning of health.

➤ BOX 5-1 The Phases of Cancer Survival

- **Acute survival:** Starts with the diagnosis of cancer. Diagnostic and therapeutic efforts dominate. Fear and anxiety are constant elements of this phase.
- **Extended survival:** Period during which a client's disease goes into remission or the basic, rigorous course of treatment has ended and a phase of watchful waiting begins. Client undergoes periodic examinations, intermittent therapy, or both. The fear of recurrence is common. This is usually a period of physical limitations. Diminished strength, fatigue, pain, nausea, reduced tolerance for exercise, or hair loss often occurs in the acute phase, but clients now have to deal with the effects of cancer at home, in the community, and in the workplace.
- **Permanent survival:** This phase is roughly equated with "cure," but the experience permanently affects the survivor. Problems with employment and insurance are common. The long-term secondary effects of cancer treatment on health represent an area in which permanent survivors are at risk.

Adapted from Mullan, F. (1985). Seasons of survival: Reflections of a physician with cancer. *New England Journal of Medicine, 313*(4), 270; and Hewitt, M., Greenfield, S., & Stovall, E. (Eds.). (2006). *From cancer client to cancer survivor: Lost in transition.* Washington, DC: National Academies Press.

The Effects of Cancer on Quality of Life

As people live longer after diagnosis and treatment for cancer, it becomes important to understand the types of distress that many survivors experience and how it affects their quality of life (Figure 5–1). Cancer survivors have poorer health outcomes than do similar individuals without cancer (Box 5–2). Cancer survivors report struggles to find a balance in their lives and a sense of wholeness and life purpose (Ferrell, 2006). Quality of life in cancer survivorship means having a balance between the experience of increased dependence while seeking both independence and interdependence. Of course, exceptions exist with regard to the level of distress that survivors face. For some, cancer becomes an experience that provides self-reflection and an enhanced sense of what life is about. Regardless of each survivor's journey with cancer, having cancer affects each person's physical, social, psychological, and spiritual well-being.

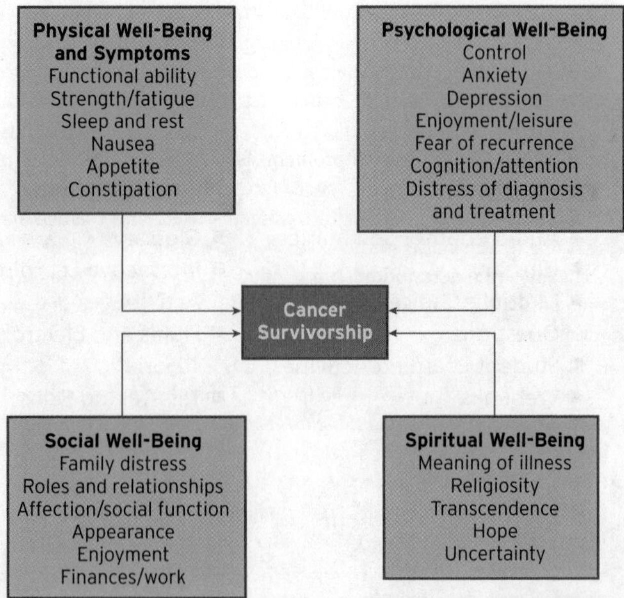

Figure 5-1 Dimensions of quality of life affected by cancer. **Source:** From Ferrell, B. (2006). *Introduction to cancer survivorship strategies for success: Survivorship education for quality cancer care.* Pasadena, CA: City of Hope National Medical Center.

BOX 5-2 EVIDENCE-INFORMED PRACTICE GUIDELINE

The Burden of Illness for Cancer Survivors

Evidence Summary

Yabroff et al. (2004) wanted to learn about the burden of illness among cancer survivors. The researchers studied more than 1800 cancer survivors, as well as individuals without cancer (the control group) who were matched with cancer survivors by age, sex, and educational attainment. The researchers examined several measures of burden or stress, including a person's sense of utility (feeling useful), a perception of overall health, and days lost from work. The results of the study showed that cancer survivors had poorer outcomes than did matched control subjects across all measures: lower sense of utility, higher levels of lost productivity, and more likelihood of reporting their health as fair or poor.

Application to Nursing Practice

As a nurse, you must learn to assess the many ways in which cancer affects the lives of clients who are survivors. Because cancer causes long-term effects, it is important for you to spend time assessing clients' symptoms, the effects of symptoms on lifestyle and self-care ability, the effects on client relationships, the clients' ability to remain productive and successful in their jobs, their economic security, and their physical well-being. When you attempt any intervention that requires the client to be motivated and involved, it is important to understand the client's self-perceptions.

Source: Yabroff, K. R., Lawrence, W. F., Clauser, S., Davis, W. W., & Brown, M. L. (2004). Burden of illness in cancer survivors: Findings from a population-based national sample. *Journal of the National Cancer Institute, 96*(17), 1322.

Physical Well-Being and Symptoms

Cancer survivors are at increased risk for developing a subsequent cancer (either a recurrence of the cancer for which they were treated or a secondary cancer) and for a wide range of treatment-related problems (IOM & NRC, 2006). The risk for developing a secondary cancer increases as a result of cancer treatment, genetic or other susceptibility, or an interaction between treatment and susceptibility. The risk for treatment-related problems is associated with the complexity of the cancer itself (e.g., type of tumour and stage of disease); the type, variety, and intensity of treatments used; and the age and underlying health status of the client.

The following description (Leigh, 2006) offers an example of how a cancer survivor's physical health problems can be so complex and burdensome.

> *Susan was an Army nurse, who learned 7 months after discharge from the Army that she had Hodgkin's disease. Hodgkin's is a malignancy of lymphoid tissue. Susan received an aggressive course of treatment, including surgery, 6 months of chemotherapy, and 3 months of total lymph node irradiation. It took many months for her bone marrow to heal and blood values to return to normal. After a few years she had bilateral mastectomies for treatment-related breast cancer. She also received 3 years of immunotherapy for cancer in situ (tumour not metastasized) of the bladder. She continues to experience many noncancer conditions: premature menopause, early osteoporosis, hypothyroidism, lung fibrosis, and atrophy of neck and upper chest muscles. (Leigh, 2006)*

Such a story is not unusual among survivors; it highlights the long disease course that many cancer survivors face. Numerous tissues and body systems are impaired as a result of cancer and its treatment (Table 5–1). Late effects of chemotherapy include osteoporosis, congestive heart failure, diabetes, amenorrhea in affected women, sterility in affected men and women, gastrointestinal motility problems, abnormal liver function, impaired immune function, **paresthesias**, hearing loss, and problems with thinking and memory (IOM & NRC, 2006). The cancer itself or its treatment often induces pain and **neuropathy** (Polomano and Farrar, 2006). **Cancer-related fatigue** and associated sleep disturbances are the most frequent and disturbing complaints of people with cancer (Barton-Burke, 2006). Certain conditions resolve over time, but irreversible tissue damage causes conditions to progress and persist indefinitely. Health care professionals do not always recognize these conditions as delayed problems. In many cases, conditions such as osteoporosis, hearing loss, or change in memory are instead considered to be age related. The problem for many survivors is that these conditions go undiagnosed and are never treated.

Cognitive changes are characterized by a set of physical symptoms very common in survivors that develop from the disease, treatment, the complications of treatment, underlying medical conditions, and psychological responses to the diagnosis of cancer (Nail, 2006). Cognitive changes can occur during all phases of the cancer experience, from small deficits in information processing to acute delirium. Often the cognitive impairments that survivors experience are not evident to someone else but are apparent to the person experiencing them, especially in relation to work performance with high cognitive demands (Anderson-Hanley et al., 2003). For example, clients report attention problems, loss of memory, and difficulty in recognizing and solving problems. Studies have revealed that systemic cancer treatment, including chemotherapy or biotherapy, has a generalized, subtle effect on cognitive function. In addition, systemic treatment causes both short-term and persistent cognitive impairment in a variety of cognitive domains. Researchers do not yet understand the effects of specific cognitive changes on survivors' daily lives (Nail, 2006).

The estimates for 2008 indicate that about 69% of new cancer cases will occur in Canadians over the age of 60 (CCS, 2007). The most common cancers in this age group are those of the prostate, lung, and colon. Often, health care professionals wrongly attribute the symptoms of cancer or those from the side effects of treatment to aging. This can lead to late diagnosis or a failure to provide aggressive and effective treatment of symptoms.

Cancer is a chronic disease because of the serious consequences and the persistent nature of some of its late effects (IOM & NRC, 2006). The effects that clients suffer are diverse. For example, a 46-year-old woman with early-stage melanoma on the right arm may undergo successful surgery, and the only effect is an inconspicuous scar. In contrast, Susan, the Canadian Forces nurse diagnosed with Hodgkin's disease, underwent intensive chemotherapy followed by an extended course of radiation. She faced serious and substantial long-term health problems from her treatment. The type of conditions that develop and the length of time the conditions persist vary significantly.

Numerous factors contribute to survivors' not receiving timely and appropriate treatment for the effects of their disease or treatment. Survivors are often reluctant to report symptoms because of a fear of being perceived as ungrateful for being disease-free or a fear of cancer recurrence (Polomano and Farrar, 2006). Survivors are not always aware that painful conditions or syndromes are common and frequently believe that pain relief is not possible (see Chapter 42) (Box 5–3). Health care professionals have limited awareness of the prevalence and incidence of pain and other symptoms among survivors, and education in symptom management is frequently limited. In the case of pain management, health care professionals often do not

TABLE 5-1 Examples of Late Effects of Surgery Among Adult Cancer Survivors

Procedure	Late Effect
Any procedure	Pain, psychosocial distress, impaired wound healing
Surgery involving brain or spinal cord	Impaired cognitive function; motor and sensory alterations; alterations in vision, swallowing, language, and bowel and bladder control
Head and neck surgery	Difficulties with communication, swallowing, and breathing
Abdominal surgery	Intestinal obstruction, hernia, altered bowel function
Lung resection	Difficulty breathing, fatigue, generalized weakness
Prostatectomy	Urinary incontinence, sexual dysfunction, poor body image

Modified from Institute of Medicine and National Research Council. (2006). *From cancer client to cancer survivor: Lost in transition* (M. Hewitt, S. Greenfield, & E. Stovall, Eds.). Washington, DC: National Academies Press.

acknowledge the potential for chronic pain after curative cancer therapies or fail to inform clients about potential long-term consequences of cancer treatment (Polomano and Farrar, 2006). Few health care settings track the health-related quality of life and symptoms of clients over time. Thus, limited evidence exists about the long-term patterns of symptoms most commonly associated with certain forms of cancer and its treatment

Research on breast cancer is extensive. Women with a history of breast cancer constitute the largest group of cancer survivors (IOM & NRC, 2006). After their primary treatment for breast cancer, women generally report decreased physical functioning but good emotional functioning, especially those who undergo **mastectomy** or receive chemotherapy (Ganz, 2004). Symptoms that persist one year after either **lumpectomy** or mastectomy to treat early-stage breast cancer often include numbness in the chest wall or axilla, tightness and a pulling sensation in the arm or axilla, fatigue, difficulty sleeping, and hot flashes (Shimozuma et al., 1999). By two to three years after surgery, breast cancer survivors report a quality of life more favourable than that reported by clients with other common medical conditions (Ganz et al., 1996). However, the same breast cancer survivors reported problems with sexual function, body image, and physical function after three years.

BOX 5-3 Examples of Chronic Pain Syndromes Associated With Cancer Treatments

Postoperative Pain Syndromes

Postmastectomy syndrome
Post–radical neck dissection pain
Postamputation pain
Fistula formation

Postradiation Pain Syndromes

Myelopathy
Enteritis or proctitis
Lymphedema
Brachial or lumbosacral plexopathy

Postchemotherapy Pain Syndromes

Peripheral neuropathy
Avascular necrosis of femur or humerus

Modified from Polomano, R. C., & Farrar, J. T. (2006). Pain and neuropathy in cancer survivors. *American Journal of Nursing, 106*(Suppl. 3), 39.

Psychological Well-Being

The physical effects of cancer and its treatment sometimes cause serious psychological distress (see Chapter 30). In the context of cancer, distress is defined as a multifactorial unpleasant emotional experience of a psychological, social, and or spiritual nature (see Chapter 28) that interferes with the ability to cope effectively with cancer, its symptoms, and its treatment (Wilkes, 2003). Survivors' feelings of distress range along a continuum from sadness to disabling depression (Vachon, 2006). The long-term presence of fatigue and sleep disturbances, for example, is often associated with anxiety and depression in many cancer survivors (Barton-Burke, 2006). Research has revealed an association between depression and decreased cancer survivorship. A study conducted by Brown et al. (2003) suggested that a cancer diagnosis and its effects predispose people to distress, which if maintained over time will enhance disease progression.

Another common psychological problem for survivors is **post-traumatic stress disorder (PTSD)**. PTSD is a psychiatric disorder characterized by an acute emotional response to a traumatic event or situation. Cancer survivors experience symptoms of PTSD (e.g., grief, nightmares, panic attacks, or fear) at a rate of 4% to 19%, as a result of their diagnosis, treatment, or a past traumatic episode (Kwekkeboom & Seng, 2002). Being female, being younger, being less educated, having a lower income, and having less social and emotional support increase the risk for PTSD. Results of studies of clients with PTSD suggest that the stress response of the hypothalamus–pituitary–adrenal system is abnormal (see Chapter 30). The same response—negative feedback inhibition of cortisol production, which results in alterations in cortisol level—also occurs in cancer (Yehuda, 2003).

The disabling effects of chronic cancer symptoms disrupt family and personal relationships, impair individuals' work performance, and often isolate survivors from normal social activities. Such changes in lifestyle create serious implications for a survivor's psychological well-being. When cancer changes a client's body image or alters sexual function, the survivor frequently experiences significant anxiety and depression with regard to interpersonal relationships. In the case of breast cancer survivors, studies have revealed that poorer self-ratings of quality of life are associated with poor body image, poor coping strategies, and a lack of social support (IOM & NRC, 2006).

The risk of a cancer survivor's having psychological problems is high because of a complex set of factors. Anderson (1993) developed a model for predicting the psychological well-being in women with gynecological cancer (Figure 5–2). The model has applications for other client groups as well. How well a survivor adapts to the cancer experience depends on predisposing factors (e.g., age, gender, race, income, prior psychiatric disorder, marital status, coping style, and social support), the client's current psychological status, and the presence of disruptive signs and symptoms. In a client who has few disruptive signs and symptoms and in which the cancer is less extensive, the risk of poor psychological well-being is low. In contrast, in a client who has numerous disruptive signs and symptoms, an advanced stage of cancer, and other health problems, the risk of psychological distress is high.

Certain factors help ease the psychological stress associated with having cancer. A survivor's appraisal of the cancer experience makes a difference. A survivor who sees cancer as a challenging experience and a controllable threat will have less stress (Jacobsen, 2006). Clients who use problem-oriented, active, and emotionally expressive coping processes also manage stress well (see Chapter 30). Survivors who have social and emotional support systems and maintain open communication with their treatment professionals are also likely to experience less psychological distress (Jacobsen, 2006).

Social Well-Being

Cancer affects all age groups (Figure 5–3). The developmental effects of cancer are perhaps best seen in the social impact that occurs across the lifespan. For adolescents and young adults, cancer seriously alters a young person's social skills, sexual development, body image, and the ability to think about and plan for the future (see Chapter 23). Cancer interrupts their lives, causing young survivors either to feel out of touch with the interests of their peers or to perceive those interests as superficial (Blum, 2006). In addition, because cancer makes them feel different, young survivors, out of fear of rejection, have difficulty dating and developing new relationships. The course of cancer or its treatment often causes young adults to delay leaving their parents. The natural separation that occurs when young adults finish school and look to start their careers is postponed or stopped. Often a young adult with cancer feels ill equipped to take on the real world.

Adults aged 30 to 59 who have cancer experience significant changes in their families. Once a member of the family receives a diagnosis of cancer, every family member's role, plans, and abilities change (Blum, 2006). The healthy spouse often takes on added job responsibilities to provide additional income for the family. A spouse, sibling, grandparent, or child often has to assume caregiving responsibilities for the client with cancer. The marriages of clients who experience changes in sexuality, intimacy, and fertility are affected; too often, this results in divorce. A history of cancer significantly affects employment opportunities and the ability of a survivor to obtain and retain health and life insurance (IOM & NRC, 2006). Often a survivor experiences health-related work limitations (Box 5–4) that necessitate a reduced work schedule or a complete change in employment. However, most cancer survivors who worked before the diagnosis return to work after the treatment (Spelten et al., 2002). The problem is that employers and supervisors often assume that persons with cancer are not able to perform job responsibilities as well as they did before the diagnosis; thus, job discrimination against cancer survivors is common. Cancer survivors report problems in the workplace,

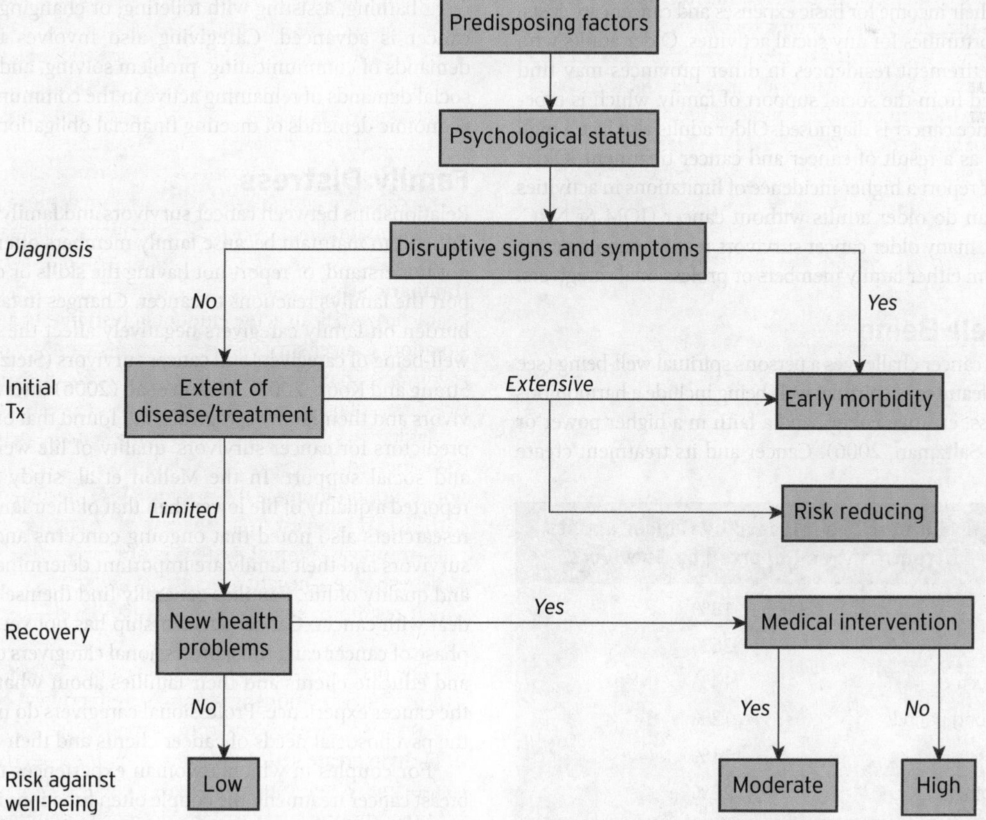

Figure 5-2 Predicting psychological well-being. **Source:** Modified from Anderson, B. L. (1993). Predicting sexual and psychologic morbidity and improving the quality of life for women with gynecologic cancer. *Cancer, 71*(Suppl. 4), 1678.

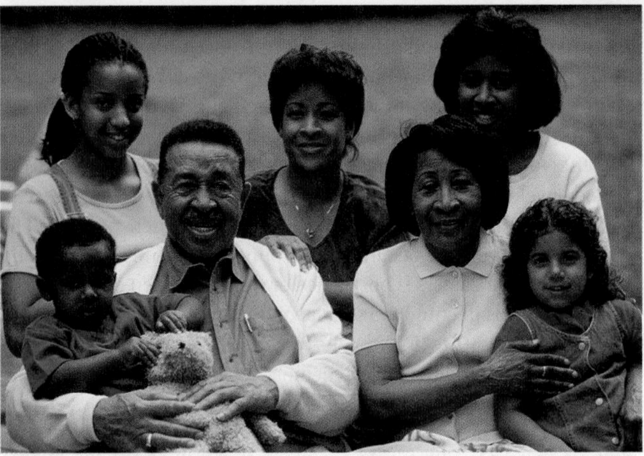

Figure 5-3 Photo of a family, representing young and old.

including dismissal, failure to hire, demotion, and denial of promotion. Many survivors also experience "job lock": A survivor will stay in an undesirable job or in one that has become difficult to perform in order not to lose insurance benefits.

The economic burden of cancer is enormous. If a survivor's illness affects his or her ability to work, the individual and family accrue less income. Also, there is usually an increase in high out-of-pocket expenses for prescription drugs, medical devices, and supplies (CCS, 2005). Some expenses may not be covered by provincial or private health insurance plans. Older adults face numerous social concerns as a result of cancer. The disease often causes clients to retire prematurely.

Many older adults have a fixed income. The older cancer survivors can see their retirement pensions erode away quickly. The survivors often have to use their income for basic expenses and cancer care costs, which limits opportunities for any social activities. Older adults who have moved to retirement residences in other provinces may find themselves isolated from the social support of family, which is especially important once cancer is diagnosed. Older adults also face a high level of disability as a result of cancer and cancer treatment. Older adults with cancer report a higher incidence of limitations in activities of daily living than do older adults without cancer (IOM & NRC, 2006). As a result, many older cancer survivors require ongoing caregiving support from either family members or professional caregivers.

Spiritual Well-Being

The experience of cancer challenges a person's spiritual well-being (see Chapter 28). Key features of spiritual well-being include a harmonious interconnectedness, creative energy, and a faith in a higher power or life force (Brown-Saltzman, 2006). Cancer and its treatment create physical and psychological changes that cause survivors to ask the question "Why me?" and to wonder whether perhaps the disease is some form of punishment. Survivors often experience a level of spiritual distress, a disruption in a person's spirit or life principle. Survivors most at risk for spiritual distress are those with energy-consuming anxiety, an inability to forgive, low self-esteem, maturational losses, and mental illness (Brown-Saltzman, 2006). Additional risk factors include poor relationships and situational losses (see Chapter 29).

Relationships, whether with a higher power, nature, family, or community, are crucial for cancer survivors. Cancer threatens relationships because it makes it difficult for survivors to maintain a connection and a sense of belonging with what is important to them. Cancer may isolate survivors from meaningful interaction and support, which then threatens their ability to maintain hope. The long courses of treatment, the reoccurrence of cancer, and the lingering side effects of treatment all create uncertainty for survivors.

➤ BOX 5-4 Limitations Imposed by Cancer and Its Treatment as Reported by Survivors

Physical tasks	18%
Lift heavy loads	26%
Stoop, kneel, crouch	14%
Concentrate for long periods	12%
Analyze data	11%
Keep pace with others	22%
Learn new things	14%

Adapted from Bradley, C. J., & Bednarek, H. L. (2002). Employment patterns of long-term cancer survivors. *Psycho-Oncology, 11*, 188.

Cancer and Families

A survivor's family takes different forms: the traditional nuclear family, the extended family, single-parent family, close friends, and the blended family (see Chapter 20). Once cancer affects a member of the family, it affects all other members as well. It is usually a member of the family who becomes the client's caregiver. Family caregiving is a stressful experience, depending on the relationship between client and caregiver and on the nature and extent of the client's disease. Many caregivers who are 30 to 50 years old must care for their own immediate family in addition to a parent with cancer. The demands are many, from providing ongoing encouragement and support and assisting with household chores to providing hands-on physical care (e.g., bathing, assisting with toileting, or changing a dressing) when cancer is advanced. Caregiving also involves the psychological demands of communicating, problem solving, and decision making; social demands of remaining active in the community and work; and economic demands of meeting financial obligations.

Family Distress

Relationships between cancer survivors and family members become difficult to maintain because family members often do not know, do not understand, or report not having the skills or confidence to support the family's reactions to cancer. Changes in family roles and the burden on family caregivers negatively affect the quality of life and well-being of caregivers and cancer survivors (Stetz and Brown, 2004; Strang and Koop, 2003). Mellon et al. (2006) interviewed cancer survivors and their family caregivers and found that one of the strongest predictors for cancer survivors' quality of life were family stressors and social support. In the Mellon et al. study, family caregivers reported a quality of life lower than that of their family members. The researchers also noted that ongoing concerns and problems facing survivors and their family are important determinants of adjustment and quality of life. Families generally find themselves ill prepared to deal with cancer. Cancer survivorship has not yet become a distinct phase of cancer care; thus, professional caregivers often fail to inform and educate clients and their families about what to expect during the cancer experience. Professional caregivers do not usually address the psychosocial needs of cancer clients and their families.

For couples in which a woman experiences the acute phase of breast cancer treatment, the couple often functions in a survival mode, during which competing demands from their jobs or other family members distract the couple from attending to each other's needs, thoughts, and feelings (Lewis, 2006). Many such couples struggle with interpersonal problem solving, because they do not have the communication or problem-solving skills to understand one another's views, concerns, or fears. Less is known about what happens to family relationships in long-term survivorship. Lewis (2006) suggested two possible outcomes: benefit-finding behaviour (identifying positive aspects in the cancer experience) and heightened interpersonal tension.

Families struggle to maintain core functions when one of their members is a cancer survivor. Core family functions include maintaining an emotionally and physically safe environment, interpreting and reducing the threat of stressful events (including the cancer) for family members, and nurturing and supporting the development of individual family members (Lewis, 2006). In child-rearing families, this means providing attentive parenting for children and providing information and support to children when their sense of well-being is threatened.

When a member of the family has cancer, these core functions become threatened. Women with cancer who were mothers of young and adolescent children reported the inability to be the parent they wanted to be during the treatment phase of the disease (Zahlis & Lewis, 1998). Spouses often do not know what to do to support the survivor, and they struggle with how to help. In the end, family functions become fragmented, and family members develop an uncertainty about their roles.

Implications for Nursing

Cancer survivorship creates many implications for nursing. As a professional nurse, you must play a leadership role in helping survivors plan for optimal lifelong health. Much needs to be done in conducting nursing research to find appropriate interventions for the effects of cancer and its treatment. Nurses are in a strong position to take the lead in improving public health care efforts to manage the long-term consequences of cancer. Improvement is also necessary in the education of nurses and survivors about the phenomenon of survivorship. As a nursing student, you too can make a difference. This section addresses approaches to incorporate cancer survivorship into your nursing practice.

Survivor Assessment

Knowing that there are many cancer survivors in the health care system, you can consider how to assess clients who report a history of cancer. It is important that assessment of cancer survivors' needs is a standard part of your practice. While you are documenting a health nursing history (see Chapter 32), explore with your clients their history of cancer, including the diagnosis and type of treatment they either are undergoing or have received in the past. You must be aware that some clients do not always report that they have had cancer. So, when a client tells you he or she has had surgery, ask whether it was cancer related. When a client reveals a history of chemotherapy, radiation, biotherapy, or hormone therapy, you need to refer to resources to help you understand how those therapies typically affect clients in both the short and long term. Once you do so, extend your assessment to determine whether these treatment effects exist for your client. Remember that you need to consider not only the effects of the cancer and its treatment but also how it will affect any other medical condition. For example, if a client also has heart disease, how will the fatigue related to chemotherapy affect this individual?

From a client's own story, you can achieve an understanding of the cancer experience. By asking a general question about the client's being a cancer survivor, you can encourage the client to reveal his or her story. For example, you might ask, "Having cancer is a journey for many. How does the disease most affect you right now?" or "What is the biggest problem that you are experiencing from cancer?" This type of question helps you focus on the area that is most important to the client. Communicate to clients your interest in their situation. Show a caring approach so that clients know that you hear their story (see Chapter 19). You might further ask, "What can I do to help you at this point?"

Symptom management is an ongoing problem for many cancer survivors. If cancer is their primary diagnosis, it will be natural for you will explore any presenting symptoms. Be sure to learn specifically how any symptoms are affecting the client. For example, is pain also causing fatigue, or is a neuropathy causing the client to walk with an abnormal gait? If cancer is secondary, then important symptoms must not go unrecognized. Ask the client, "Since your diagnosis and treatment of cancer, what physical changes or symptoms have you had?" and "Tell me how these changes affect you now." Depending on the symptoms that a client identifies, you will explore each one in order to gain a complete understanding of the client's health status (Table 5–2). Remember that some clients are reluctant to report or discuss their symptoms. Be patient, and once you identify a symptom, explore the extent to which the symptom is currently affecting the client.

Because you know that cancer affects a client's quality of life in many ways, be sure to explore the client's psychological, social, and spiritual needs and resources. Sometimes you will not be able to conduct a thorough assessment when you document an initial health

TABLE 5-2 Assessment Questions for Cancer Survivors

Category	Examples of Questions
Symptoms	• Have you had any pain or discomfort in the area where you had surgery or radiation; discomfort, pain, or unusual sensations in your hands or feet; weakness in your legs or arms; or problems moving around? • Do you experience fatigue, sleeplessness, or shortness of breath? If so, please describe them. • Sometimes people feel as if they are starting to have problems after chemotherapy, such as paying attention, remembering things, or finding words. Have you noticed any changes like these?
Psychosocial problems	• How distressed are you feeling at this point on a scale of 0 to 10, with 10 being the worst distress that you could imagine? • How do you think your family is dealing with your cancer? • What do you see in your family members' responses to your cancer that is a concern for you?
Sexuality problems	• If you have had sexual changes, what strategies have you tried to make things better? Have these strategies worked? • Would you be open to a health care professional who knows how to help you? • Since your cancer diagnosis, do you see yourself differently as a person?

nursing history. If this is the case, incorporate your assessment into your ongoing client care. Observe your client's interactions with family members and friends. When you are administering care to clients, talk about their daily lives and determine the extent to which cancer has changed their lifestyle.

One area that is often difficult for nurses to assess well is a client's sexuality. Sexuality is more than simply the physical ability to perform a sex act or conceive a child. It also includes a person's body image, sexual response (e.g., interest and satisfaction), and sexual roles and relationships (see Chapter 27). Surgery for many cancers is disfiguring, and chemotherapy and radiation often alter a client's sexual response. Cancer therapies have the potential to cause fatigue, apathy, nausea, vomiting, malaise, and sleep disturbances, all of which interfere with a client's libido (Pelusi, 2006).

It is important to realize that cancer often does influence the client's sexuality. This realization helps you develop a comfort level in acknowledging with clients that sexual changes are common at any age level. Ask a client, "Since your diagnosis and treatment of cancer, has your ability or interest in sexual activity changed? If so, how?" Clients will appreciate your sensitivity and interest in their well-being. When clients begin to discuss their sexual problems, you need to know the expert resources in your institution (e.g., psychologist or social worker) available for client referral.

Client Education

It is nurses' responsibility to educate survivors and their families about the consequences of cancer and cancer treatment. This means that when you care for a cancer survivor, you need to understand the nature of the client's particular disease and know the effects of each therapy that a client receives and the short- and long-term consequences. You play a key role in preparing a cancer survivor with the knowledge and resources needed for ongoing self-management. Lorig (2003) defined the purpose of self-management education as the provision of skills for clients to live an active and meaningful life with chronic disease. In designing education that promotes self-management in caregiving, plan activities on the basis of the caregiver's and cancer survivor's perceived disease-related problems, and assist them with problem solving and gaining the self-efficacy or confidence to deal with these problems. Client education helps survivors assume more healthy lifestyle behaviours that will then give them control of some aspects of their health and improve outcomes from cancer and chronic illness.

When caring for clients with an initial diagnosis of cancer, reinforce their health care professional's explanations of the risks related to their cancer and treatment, what they need to self-monitor (e.g., appetite, weight, and effects of fatigue and sleeplessness), and what to discuss with health care professionals in the future. If clients learn about the potential for adverse treatment effects such as pain, neuropathy, or cognitive change, they are more likely to report their symptoms. Survivors need to learn how to manage problems related to persistent symptoms. For example, survivors with neuropathy need to learn how to protect their hands and feet, prevent falls, and avoid accidental burns.

Because survivors are at increased risk for developing a secondary cancer, a chronic illness, or both, it is important for them to learn about lifestyle behaviours that will improve the quality of their lives. Health promotion education is timely after an initial cancer diagnosis, when many survivors become motivated to change their behaviour (Satia et al., 2004). Many survivors become interested in learning more about dietary supplements and nutritional complementary therapies to manage disease symptoms (IOM & NRC, 2006). Scientific evidence reveals several health promotion areas of interest to cancer survivors: smoking cessation, physical activity, diet and nutrition (see Chapter 43), and the use of complementary and alternative medicine (see Chapter 35). You can explore with clients useful strategies to promote their health. For example, behavioural interventions for increasing physical activity among cancer survivors have yielded positive and consistent effects on vigor, cardiorespiratory fitness, quality of life, fatigue, and depression (Holtzman et al., 2004).

Providing Resources

Numerous organizations and agencies provide resources to cancer survivors. The problem is that many survivors do not receive timely and appropriate referral to these resources. As a nurse, you will find that many people (e.g., friends, neighbours, and family members) ask for your advice about health care before they actually become clients. It is important to know that cancer-related hospital and ambulatory care are not standardized. For example, when a client with cancer is hospitalized, the availability of ancillary services for long-term care varies by care setting.

A designated cancer centre offers the most comprehensive and up-to-date clinical care. National Cancer Institute–designated centres also conduct important clinical trials to investigate the most up-to-date cancer therapies. Many clients benefit when they have the opportunity to participate in these trials. Your role is to tell clients about the different resources available so that clients are able to make informed choices.

A number of cancer-related community support services are available to survivors through voluntary organizations. Most offer their services at no cost. Many supportive services offer call centres and Internet-based information and discussion boards, in addition to direct service delivery (IOM & NRC, 2006). Health care professionals are not consistent in referring clients to these valuable services. In addition, although community-based services help most survivors, gaps exist in service provision for assistance with transportation, home care, child care, and financial assistance. Become knowledgeable about the services within your community. Several national agencies exist; these include the Canadian Cancer Society, National Cancer Institute of Canada, and the Public Health Agency of Canada.

Components of Survivorship Care

Once a cancer client's primary treatment ends, health care professionals must develop an organized plan for survivorship care. This does not always occur, however, because of inadequacies in the health care system, including a failure of any one health care professional to assume responsibility for coordinating care, fragmentation of care between specialists and general practitioners, and a lack of guidance about how survivors can improve their health outcomes (IOM & NRC, 2006). Clients with cancer often do not receive noncancer care (e.g., care for diabetes or heart conditions) when the cancer diagnosis shifts attention away from care that is routine but necessary. Follow-up of cancer care is also poor, even though recommended guidelines exist. For example, some women with a history of breast cancer do not undergo annual mammography, and some clients with colorectal cancer do not undergo regular colorectal examinations. The IOM and NRC (2006) made recommendations for four essential components of survivorship care: (1) prevention and detection of new cancers and recurrent cancer; (2) surveillance for cancer spread, cancer recurrence, or secondary cancers; (3) intervention for consequences of cancer and its treatment (e.g., medical problems, symptoms, and psychological distress); and (4) coordination between specialists and primary care professionals.

Survivorship Care Plan

Just as health care professionals must improve cancer survivorship care, a strategy for survivors' ongoing clinical care is also needed. The IOM and NRC (2006) recommended the provision of a "survivorship care plan" that should be written by the principal health care professional who coordinates the client's **oncology** treatment. Ideally, you would review a survivorship care plan with a client when he or she is formally discharged from a treatment program. The plan would become a guide for any future cancer-related care. Health care professionals would use the plan as a guide for client education. Survivors would use the plan to raise questions with physicians to prompt appropriate care during follow-up visits. Box 5–5 highlights the components of a survivorship care plan.

Few health care agencies provide survivorship care plans. Those that do are usually children's hospitals. Thus, nurses and other health care professionals need to become more vigilant in recognizing cancer survivors and attempting to link them with the support and resources they require. You can make a difference in considering the long-term issues that cancer survivors face after the time of diagnosis and in contributing to solutions to manage or relieve cancer-associated health problems. A strong multidisciplinary approach that includes nurses, oncology specialists, dietitians, social workers, pastoral care, and rehabilitation professionals is necessary. Together, a multidisciplinary team can provide a plan of care that addresses treatment-related problems and future health risks and offers a wellness focus to give clients a sense of hope as they enter their survivor experience.

BOX 5-5 Survivorship Care Plan

Upon discharge from cancer treatment, every client and his or her primary health care professional should receive a record of all care received and a follow-up plan incorporating available evidence-informed standards of care.

Care Summary

- Diagnostic tests performed and their results
- Tumour characteristics (e.g., site, stage, and grade)
- Dates when treatment started and stopped
- Type of therapy (surgery, chemotherapy, radiotherapy, transplant, hormonal therapy, or gene therapy) provided, including the specific agents used
- Psychosocial, nutritional, and other supportive services provided
- Full contact information about the treating institutions and key health care professionals
- Identification of a key point of contact and coordinator of care

Follow-Up Plan

- Likely course of recovery
- Description of recommended cancer screening and other periodic testing and examinations
- Information about possible late and long-term effects of treatment and the symptoms of such effects
- Information about possible signs of recurrence and secondary tumours
- Information about the possible effects of cancer on the marital or partner relationship, on sexual functioning, on work, and on parenting
- Information about the potential insurance-related, employment-related, and financial consequences of cancer and, as necessary, referral for counseling, legal aid, and financial assistance
- Specific recommendations for healthy behaviours
- Information about genetic counselling and testing as appropriate
- Information about known effective chemoprevention strategies for secondary prevention
- Referrals to specific follow-up health care professionals
- A listing of cancer-related resources and information

Adapted from President's Cancer Panel. (2004). *Living beyond cancer: Finding a new balance.* Bethesda, MD: National Cancer Institute; and Hewitt, M., Greenfield, S., & Stovall, E. (Eds.). (2006). *From cancer client to cancer survivor: Lost in transition.* Washington, DC: National Academies Press.

✻ KEY CONCEPTS

- The health care system has largely ignored or misunderstood cancer survivors' health care problems.
- The definition of *cancer survivor* includes family members, friends, and caregivers who are also affected by survivorship.
- The majority of cancer survivors have serious health deficits that are related to their treatments.
- Evidence reveals that cancer survivors have poorer health outcomes than do similar individuals without cancer.
- Survivors are often reluctant to report symptoms because of a fear of being perceived as ungrateful for being disease free or a fear of cancer recurrence.
- How well a survivor adapts to the cancer experience psychologically depends on predisposing factors, the person's current psychological status, the extent of the disease, and the presence of disruptive signs and symptoms.
- The developmental effects of cancer have a social impact that occurs across the lifespan.
- Relationships between cancer survivors and family members become difficult to maintain because family members often do not know, do not understand, or report not having the skills or confidence to support the family's reactions to cancer.
- As a nursing student, you should incorporate cancer survivorship care into your nursing practice through client assessment, education, and referral of clients to available resources.
- Because survivors are at an increased risk for developing a secondary cancer, chronic illness, or both, it is important to educate them about lifestyle behaviours that will improve the quality of their lives.
- Once a cancer client's primary treatment ends, health care professionals should develop an organized plan for survivorship care.
- A client's principal health care professional should write a survivorship care plan that coordinates the client's oncology treatment.
- Ideally, you would review a survivorship care plan with a client when he or she is formally discharged from a treatment program, and it would become a guide for any future cancer-related care.

✻ CRITICAL THINKING EXERCISES

1. Do you have a friend or family member who has cancer and is willing to talk about it? If so, ask the individual to tell you what the experience has been like and what he or she would recommend to help nurses provide better care for survivors.

2. Ms. Ritter is a 32-year-old woman who visits the medical outpatient clinic for her final course of chemotherapy to treat breast cancer. She is married and has one child, a daughter, who is six years old. She and her husband have hoped to have another child in the near future but now wonder whether that will be possible. She has shared with the nursing staff her concerns about the future and how cancer will affect her and her family. Her

case manager talks with her about a survivorship care plan before discharge from the clinic. Identify two follow-up care plan components that would be important when considering Ms. Ritter's role as a wife and parent.

3 Ms. Ritter tells her nurse, "This chemotherapy has made me feel so tired, and there are many nights I cannot sleep very well. I am looking forward to this going away." What is an appropriate response the nurse might give Ms. Ritter?

✻ REVIEW QUESTIONS

1. Cancer survivors are at risk for treatment-related problems. Which of the clients listed below has the greatest risk for developing such a problem?
   1. An 80-year-old woman undergoing surgery for removal of a basal cell carcinoma on the face
   2. A 71-year-old man receiving chemotherapy and radiation for an advanced-stage lymphoma
   3. A 26-year-old man receiving chemotherapy for testicular cancer that is localized to the testicle
   4. A 48-year-old woman receiving radiation for Hodgkin's disease that involves lymph nodes extending above and below the diaphragm
2. The nurse reviews the medical record of a new client admitted to her nursing unit. She notices in the history that the client had a history of bladder cancer three years ago. Which of the following factors should she consider when conducting an assessment of this client? (Select all that apply.)
   1. The number and type of cancer therapies given to the client
   2. The presence of other medical conditions affecting the client
   3. Use of an approach that encourages the client to tell his or her story
   4. The readiness of cancer survivors to report the symptoms they are experiencing
   5. Assessment of sexuality as to whether the client can perform a sexual act
3. A nurse working in a medicine clinic knows it is important to recognize cancer survivors who are most at risk for post-treatment symptoms. Which of the following clients is probably at greatest risk for post-treatment symptoms?
   1. A 50-year-old mother in whom breast cancer was diagnosed at late stage
   2. A 20-year-old male college student diagnosed with leukemia whose father had lung cancer
   3. A 32-year-old Cantonese woman with cervical cancer who does not have children and who does have supplemental health insurance.
   4. A 72-year-old First Nations retired Army captain who underwent surgical removal of his colon for cancer and who is now also receiving radiation
4. A 41-year-old man who underwent a craniotomy for the removal of a brain tumour two years ago comes to the clinic for his six-month follow-up visit. In planning your assessment, you anticipate that the client may possibly experience which of the following late effects of surgery? (Select all that apply.)
   1. Intestinal obstruction
   2. Difficulty breathing
   3. Blurred vision
   4. Poor attention span
5. In order to successfully assess whether a client is experiencing cognitive changes as a result of cancer treatment or complications of treatment, which of the following questions is probably be most relevant?
   1. "Can you describe for me your medication schedule?"
   2. "How distressed are you feeling right now, on a scale of 0 to 10?"
   3. "When did you first notice symptoms from your chemotherapy?"
   4. "What differences do you notice in your ability to get work done at your office?"

✻ RECOMMENDED WEB SITES

BC Cancer Agency: http://www.bccancer.bc.ca
This provincial Web site offers resources to the patient, the public, and the health care professional. Resources range from recommended books and pamphlets to online information regarding screening programs to detailed information about specific treatment protocols.

Canadian Breast Cancer Network: http://www.cbcn.ca
This organization is a survivor-directed national network of organizations and individuals. The site provides resources for all Canadians affected by breast cancer and those at risk. Topics include the use of alcohol, issues of beauty and personal care, best practices, and lymphedema.

Canadian Cancer Society: http://www.cancer.ca
This Web site contains French and English content for people affected by cancer (clients, families, and the general public). It presents up-to-date information about cancer prevention, research, and support services, as well as positions and perspectives on cancer-related issues such as tobacco and marijuana use, and occupational exposures.

The Wellness Community: http://www.wellness-community.org
This US site offers virtual as well as actual connections to other cancer survivors and caregivers. It also offers educational resources that range from those supplying general cancer information to those providing very diagnosis-specific information.

6

Theoretical Foundations of Nursing Practice

Written by Sally Thorne, RN, PhD, FCAHS

objectives

Mastery of content in this chapter will enable you to:

- Define the key terms listed.
- Appreciate the role of "theorizing" about the essence of nursing.
- Describe different theories of nursing practice and differentiate between them.
- Describe challenges inherent in theorizing about nursing practice.
- Appreciate the historical development of thought related to nursing practice.
- Recognize selected conceptual frameworks associated with nursing practice.
- Interpret current debates surrounding various theories of nursing practice.
- Describe relationships between theorizing and other forms of nursing knowledge.

key terms

Assumption, p. 64
Concept, p. 64
Conceptual framework, p. 64
Conceptualization, p. 64
Descriptive theory, p. 66
Grand theory, p. 66
Metaparadigm concepts, p. 66
Middle-range theory, p. 66
Models for nursing, p. 64
Nursing diagnosis, p. 64
Nursing process, p. 64
Nursing science, p. 64
Nursing theory, p. 64
Paradigms, p. 66
Philosophy of science, p. 64
Praxis, p. 72
Prescriptive theory, p. 66
Proposition, p. 64
Theoretical model, p. 65
Theory, p. 64
Ways of knowing, p. 67

media resources

evolve Web Site

- Audio Chapter Summaries
- Glossary
- Multiple-Choice Review Questions
- Student Learning Activities
- Weblinks

Companion CD

- Glossary
- Interactive Learning Activities
- Fluids and Electrolytes Tutorial
- Test-Taking Skills

Although certain nursing tasks can be mastered by most people trained to perform them, the hallmark of nursing practice is its unique body of knowledge, as well as the set of principles that guide the systematic application of this knowledge in an expanding array of contexts. **Nursing theory** aims to make sense of knowledge about nursing to enable nurses to use it in a professional and accountable manner (Beckstrand, 1978).

A **theory** is a purposeful set of **assumptions** or **propositions** that identify the relationships between **concepts.** Theories are useful because they provide a systematic view for explaining, predicting, and prescribing phenomena. A nursing theory tends to be not explicitly propositional but rather a **conceptualization** of nursing for the purpose of describing, explaining, predicting, or prescribing care (Meleis, 2007). Theories constitute one aspect of disciplinary knowledge and create vital linkages to how inquiry is approached (Fawcett et al., 2001). Nursing theories provide nurses with a perspective from which to view client situations, a way to organize data, and a method of analyzing and interpreting information to bring about coherent and informed nursing practice.

Early Nursing Practice and the Emergence of Theory

Nursing practices have been documented throughout history (Yura & Walsh, 1973). However, modern nursing practice, in which the knowledge and practice of nursing are formalized into a professional context, is often attributed to the work of Florence Nightingale, a visionary leader in Victorian England who created systems for nursing education and practice (see Chapter 3). Contemporary scholars now consider Nightingale's work as an early theoretical and conceptual **model for nursing.** Her descriptive theory provided nurses with a way to think about nursing practice in a frame of reference that focuses on clients and the environment.

Since Nightingale's era, the status of nursing practice has parallelled that of the authority of women in society. After World War II, major developments in science and technology had a powerful influence on health care, including nursing practice. **Nursing science** came into its own. No longer simply applying the knowledge of other disciplines, nurses now began to acquire a unique body of knowledge about the practice of nursing.

Since the 1960s, scientific knowledge has burgeoned across disciplines. In particular, knowledge about nursing has drawn from and contributed to developments in health sciences, basic physical sciences, social and biobehavioural sciences, social theory, ethical theory, and the **philosophy of science.** Each of these sources has relevance for the interpretation of nursing care and the synthesis of relevant facts and theories for application to practice.

Major developments in nursing theory occurred in the late 1960s (Meleis, 2007). The health care system was expanding and changing, influenced by scientific discoveries and technological applications. Disease intervention became more sophisticated and scientifically driven. The focus of society shifted from simply attending to sick and injured people toward the larger problem of curing and eradicating disease, which expanded physicians' influence over the structure of health care. For the first time, nurses realized the urgency of articulating exactly how their role differed from those of other health care professionals (Chinn & Kramer, 2004; Engebretson, 1997; Fawcett, 2005; Newman, 1972).

The drive for early theorizing about the practice of nursing was led by nursing educators, who noted that traditional ways of preparing professional nurses were rapidly becoming outdated. Until the 1960s, a nursing apprenticeship model, augmented by lectures offered by physicians, had seemed sufficient. Around this time, nursing educational leaders became inspired to theorize about nursing in order to structure and define what a curriculum oriented to nursing knowledge might contain (Dean, 1995; Orem & Parker, 1964; Torres, 1974). This meant grappling with large theoretical and philosophical questions, such as the following:

- What are the focus and scope of nursing?
- How is nursing unique and different from other health care professions?
- What should be the appropriate disciplinary knowledge for professional nursing practice?

To answer these questions, early theorists developed **conceptual frameworks,** in which they organized core nursing concepts and proposed relationships among these concepts. These conceptual frameworks were "mental maps" whose purpose was to make sense of the information and decisional processes that nurses needed to apply knowledge to nursing practice (Ellis, 1968; Johnson, 1974; McKay, 1969; Wald & Leonard, 1964). Expressing knowledge about nursing in scientific language created a context in which nursing science gained stature and flourished (Cull-Wilby & Peppin, 1987; Jones, 1997). However, these nursing theories were not the kind of scientific theories that could be proved or disproved with empirical evidence (Levine, 1995); rather, they represented ideas about how nurses might organize knowledge, as well as the processes by which they would apply it to unique practice situations. Table 6–1 defines some of the basic terms that are used in theorizing about scientific issues.

Nursing Process

Early nursing theorists sought to organize the knowledge about the practice of nursing that nurses draw upon to direct their approach to clinical encounters. However, theorists generally lacked ways of systematically explaining how nurses work with knowledge in new situations (Field, 1987). An important early step in the application of knowledge to nursing practice was Orlando's (1961) development of a problem-solving approach that came to be known as the **nursing process** (Yura & Walsh, 1973). This process originally involved four steps: assessment, planning, intervention, and evaluation, whereby each step represented a distinct way in which general nursing knowledge could be applied to unique and individual nurse–client situations (Carnevali & Thomas, 1993; Henderson, 1966; Meleis, 2007; Torres, 1986):

- Assessment phase: Nurses would gather information, including biological, sociocultural, environmental, spiritual, and psychological data, to create an understanding of the client's unique health or illness experience. Organizing the data would enable the nurses to interpret major issues and concerns (Barnum, 1998) and produce a **nursing diagnosis:** the nurses's perspective on the appropriate focus for the client (Durand & Prince, 1966).
- Planning phase: Nurses would prioritize the issues raised during assessment in relation to the nursing diagnoses, identify which issues could be supported or assisted by nursing intervention, and create a plan of care.
- Intervention phase: The plan of care would be carried out.
- Evaluation phases: The plan's success or failure would be judged both against the plan itself and against the client's overall health status; that is, it would be determined whether the intended outcomes had been achieved or whether the nursing intervention strategies required revision. The nursing process was intended as

TABLE 6-1 The Terminology of Scientific Theorizing

Term	Description	Example
Concept	A mental formulation of objects or events, representing the basic way in which ideas are organized and communicated.	Anxiety
Conceptualization	The process of formulating concepts.	Framing behavioural patterns as anxiety related
Operational definition	A description of concepts, articulated in such a way that they can be applied to decision making in practice. It links concepts with other concepts and with theories, and it often includes the essential properties and distinguishing features of a concept.	Differentiation and measurement of state and trait anxiety
Theory	A purposeful set of assumptions or propositions about concepts; shows relationships between concepts and thereby provides a systematic view of phenomena so that they may be explained predicted, or prescribed.	Social determinants of health
Assumption	A description of concepts or connection of two concepts that are accepted as factual or true; includes "taken for granted" ideas about the nature and purpose of concepts, as well as the structure of theory.	"Nursing exists to serve a social mandate"
Proposition	A declarative assertion.	"Clients who receive appropriate nursing care have better health outcomes"
Phenomenon	An aspect of reality that can be consciously sensed or experienced (Meleis, 2007); nursing concepts and theories represent the theoretical approach to making sense of aspects of reality of concern to nursing.	Pain
Theoretical model	Mental representation of how things work. For example, an architect's plan for a house is not the house itself but rather the set of information necessary to understand how all of the building elements will be brought together to create that particular house.	Biopsychosocial model of health
Conceptual framework	The theoretical structure that links concepts together for a specific purpose. When its purpose is to show how something works, it can also be described as a *theoretical model*. Nursing conceptual frameworks link major nursing concepts and phenomena to direct nursing decisions (e.g., what to assess, how to make sense of data, what to plan, how to enact a plan, and how to evaluate whether the plan has had the intended outcome). Conceptual frameworks are also often referred to as *nursing models* or *nursing theories* (Meleis, 2007).	Orem's (1971) self-care model for nursing

a sequence within which thoughtful interpretation always preceded action, and the effects of action were always evaluated in relation to the original situation.

The nursing process was widely accepted by nurses because it was a logical way to describe basic problem-solving processes in which knowledge was used effectively to guide nursing decisions (Henderson, 1982). Nurses quickly adopted the nursing process because it represented a continuous, rapid cycling of information through each of the phases. Although it was useful for organizing and applying knowledge to clinical practice (Meleis, 2007), some later theorists began to challenge the nursing process as being too linear and rigid for nursing's purposes (Varcoe, 1996).

In current practice, terms such as *clinical judgement* are used to refer to reasoning processes that rely on *critical thinking* and multiple ways of knowing; clinical judgement implies the systematic use of the nursing process to invoke the complex intuitive and conscious thinking strategies that are part of all clinical decision making in nursing (Alfaro-LeFevre, 2004; Benner & Tanner, 1987; Tanner, 1993).

Conceptual Frameworks

The conceptual framework builders of the late 1960s and after are usually referred to as the *nursing theorists*. All were fascinated with how effective nurses systematically organize general knowledge about nursing in order to understand an individual client's situation and determine which of many available strategies would work best to restore health and ameliorate or prevent disease (Orem & Parker, 1964). This reasoning process was different from linear, cause-and-effect reasoning, and it was what the nursing theorists understood to be the hallmark of excellence in nursing practice (Barnum, 1998; Meleis, 2007). Indeed, when effective nurses made intelligent clinical decisions, it was often difficult to determine the precise dynamics that explained how those nurses applied that knowledge (Benner et al., 1996).

The building of nursing models was an attempt to theorize how all nurses might be taught to organize and synthesize knowledge about nursing so that they would develop advanced clinical reasoning skills (Raudonis & Acton, 1997). Theorists who developed these frameworks and models sought to depict theoretical structures that would enable a nurse to grasp all aspects of a clinical situation within the larger context of available options for nursing care. Table 6–2 describes four types of theory: **grand theory, middle-range theory, descriptive theory,** and **prescriptive theory.**

Metaparadigm Concepts

Each conceptual framework was an attempt to define nursing by creating a theoretical definition for the substance and structure of the key bodies of knowledge that would be needed to understand clinical situations (Figure 6–1). This collective body of knowledge was called the **metaparadigm concepts** and included the concepts of person, environment, health care, and nursing care (Fawcett, 1992).

Client and Person

By the 1960s, professional leaders recognized that nurses did much more than simply care for hospitalized clients. Because of this, nursing theorists started to use the term *client,* rather than *patient,* to refer to the person at the centre of any nursing process. The term signified a range of health states, including both sickness and wellness, and a more interactive relationship between the nurse and the persons to whom care was directed. At the same time, nurses were becoming aware of their potential to deliver care beyond the individual—that is, to families, groups, and communities. Although theories to articulate the role of nursing care in families and communities also began to arise around this time, most early conceptual models focused on the individual.

To help nurses systematically organize and make sense of the vast amount of information that might be relevant to any particular client, most early models clearly defined the concept of the person. Theorists variously understood a person as a system of interacting parts, a system of competing human needs, or an entity with biological, psychological, social, and spiritual dimensions. Each framework drew attention to multiple aspects of human experience so that the nurse could understand each instance of wellness and illness for its uniqueness within the context of that individual's body, feelings, and situation. Each model depicted a way of thinking about a whole individual, with the aim of helping nurses understand how the implications of any action or intervention could be systematically individualized toward the benefit of all facets of that individual.

Environment

Each conceptual framework reflected an understanding that the person is part of and interacts with a complex environmental system. This environment may involve the person's family and social ties, the community, the health care system, as well as the geopolitical issues that affect health. The early conceptual frameworks helped shape nurses' increasing appreciation of how to work within a larger context of every experience of wellness and illness. In so doing, these frameworks led to a future in which nurses would spearhead advances in social and health care policy, health promotion, and community development.

Health

Because the practice of nursing has a social mandate to improve the health of both the individual and society, the early theorists struggled to articulate a goal for nursing. They defined health as much more than simply the absence of disease or injury but rather as an ideal state of optimal health or total well-being toward which all individuals could strive (see Chapter 1). This definition reflected a vision of

➤ TABLE 6-2 Types of Theory

Type of Theory	Description
Grand theory	Global, conceptual framework that provides insight into abstract phenomena, such as human behaviour or nursing science. Grand theories are broad in scope and therefore require further application through research before the ideas they contain can be fully tested (Chinn & Kramer, 2004). They are intended not to provide guidance for specific nursing interventions but rather to provide the structural framework for broad, abstract ideas about nursing. They are sometimes called **paradigms** because they represent distinct world views about those phenomena and provide the structural framework within which narrower-range theories can be developed and tested.
Middle-range theory	Encompasses a more limited scope and is less abstract. Middle-range theories address specific phenomena or concepts and reflect practice (administration, clinical, or teaching). The phenonoma or concepts tend to cross different nursing fields and reflect a variety of nursing care situations.
Descriptive theory	Describes phenomena (e.g., responding to illness through patterns of coping), speculates on why phenomena occur, and describes the consequences of phenomena. Descriptive theories have the ability to explain, relate, and in some situations predict phenomena of concern to nursing (Meleis, 2007). Descriptive nursing theories are designed not to direct specific nursing activities but rather to help explain client assessments and possibly guide future nursing research.
Prescriptive theory	Addresses nursing interventions and helps predict the consequences of a specific intervention. A prescriptive nursing theory should designate the prescription (i.e., nursing interventions), the conditions under which the prescription should occur, and the consequences (Meleis, 2007). Prescriptive theories are action oriented, which tests the validity and predictability of a nursing intervention. These theories guide nursing research to develop and test specific nursing interventions (Fawcett, 2005).

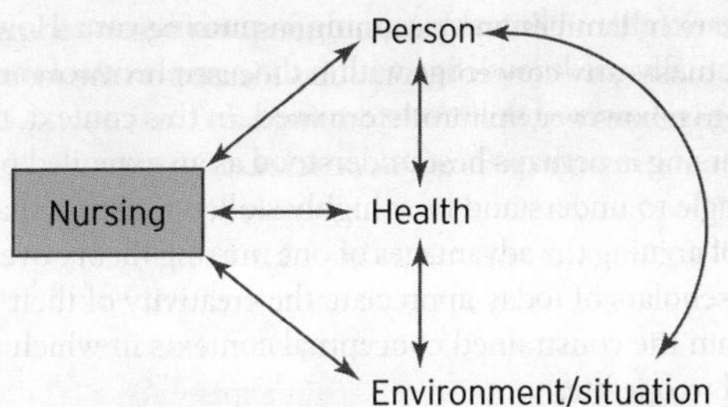

Figure 6-1 Nursing's metaparadigm concepts.

nursing care that applied to both the individual and society and to all clients, sick or well. It recognized that persons with chronic disease could strive for better health and that overall health could be compromised by psychosocial or spiritual challenges, even among the most physicially fit individuals. Although perfect health was not always achievable, this conceptualization guided nurses to help all clients reach outcomes that were productive and satisfying.

Nursing

Each early conceptual framework included a unique definition of nursing that linked a view of the client with an understanding of the person's environment, life, and health goals. Built on a distinct subset of knowledge, each conceptual framework presented a coherent and complete belief system about nursing practice, although each did so in different terms and with a different alignment of ideas. Because most nursing scholars of the era assumed that one model would eventually become dominant (Meleis, 2007), competition among the frameworks occurred. Over time, the application of the frameworks in practice became more rigid and codified. The focus, originally on guiding nurses to think systematically, had shifted to using language in particular ways and filling out assessment forms correctly. Many experienced nurses began to conclude that these frameworks actually inhibited their systematic thinking, and much debate ensued with regard to the utility of the models.

Philosophy of Nursing Science

When nursing theorists began developing their frameworks and models, nurses understood the process of building a knowledge base as a matter of science and discovery. In that context, theories were considered logical propositions that could be rigorously tested for their capacity to answer (or not answer) the hypothetical questions posed by a discipline. However, while creating frameworks for the complex reasoning in nursing practice, these early theorists were applying traditional scientific ways of understanding how knowledge works without fully appreciating the limitations of science, especially in relation to complex problems. As thinkers in all disciplines began to move beyond their traditional boundaries, other possibilities for the development of knowledge about the practice of nursing began to emerge.

Scientific Revolutions

Thomas S. Kuhn, a philosopher of science, created a way of thinking about science and knowledge that expanded thought in many disciplines. First published in 1962, his book, *The Structure of Scientific Revolutions,* became popular in the 1970s and 1980s as scholars began to realize the potential of its ideas to support new thinking about how knowledge is built. Kuhn challenged the traditional notion of science as a logical progression of discoveries, arguing that major scientific developments occurred only when scientists thought about problems in radically new ways. These ways of thinking departed from the traditional to such an extent that an entirely different world view, or "paradigm shift," developed. According to Kuhn, scientific advances happen when people think creatively and look beyond established norms. Such creative thinking could stimulate new undersandings of problems that were once considered irresolvable (e.g., quantum physics introduced the idea that the behaviour of very small particles could explain atomic behaviour in ways that defied explanation through conventional Newtonian physics). This new way of thinking about the philosophy of science led nurses to consider their theoretical frameworks as more than theoretical propositions about logical relationships among concepts, but as actual world views, or *paradigms,* that might help them grasp the complexities of nursing (Fry, 1995).

Complexity Science

A second major shift in scientific thinking occurred with the introduction of chaos theory (Gleick, 1987). Originating from observations in physics that predictable patterns existed among factors that could not be predicted scientifically, this theory created a new way of approaching complex situations. In rejecting the simple cause-and-effect relationships used in traditional science, chaos theory led to what has been termed *complexity science.* In this kind of science, dynamic and interactive phenomena are reduced to the smallest properties that can be observed within their natural context so that their interactions can be interpreted with as little interference as possible from prior assumptions. For example, chaos theory explains how, in sensitive weather systems, minor variations in initial conditions (e.g., barometric pressure) might explain large-scale physical patterns over time (e.g., hurricanes). These ideas created a new language to apply to scientific thinking. Because experiences of health and illness are difficult to understand out of their individual context, chaos theory offered a new way to approach nursing science (Coppa, 1993; Ray, 1998).

Ways of Knowing in Nursing Practice

As ideas shifted, nursing theorists also realized that science was just one of several forms of knowledge necessary for their practice discipline. In 1978, Carper published an influential paper in which she used the expression **ways of knowing** to refer to patterns of knowledge application in nursing practice. Carper articulated a critical role in nursing practice not only for empirical science but also for ethical, personal, and esthetic knowledge. Later theorists added sociopolitical knowledge (White, 1995) and critical thinking (see Chapter 12) to the list of central ways of knowing that are essential to the highest quality of clinical nursing. These ideas contributed to discussions emerging in other social and life sciences around *how* nurses know what they know (Chinn & Kramer, 2004; Kikuchi & Simmons, 1999).

Paradigm Debates Within Nursing

With the new philosophical approach to scientific knowledge, nurses struggled with how to define their work as both an art and a science and as both applied and practical (Donaldson, 1995; Johnson, 1991; Rodgers, 1991; Sarter, 1990). Ideas about the theoretical foundations of nursing practice shifted. Some scholars began to question conceptual models as a valid form of theorizing (Holden, 1990). The frustration resulting from overly formal and rigid approches to applying many of these models led to a period of what has been called *model bashing* (Engebretson, 1997). However, the question confronting the early theorists remained as follows: How does a nurse organize and make sense of all available knowledge and apply it intelligently to the challenges that arise in an individual clinical case?

In this context, many nurse scholars began to appreciate the original theories as being better understood as philosophical statements rather than scientific prescriptions. However, one group of theorists, considering some of the original theories to be overly simplistic and insufficiently holistic, began to categorize various nursing models as reflective of entirely different paradigms of thinking (Parse, 1987). That group of theorists depicted the majority of nursing's models and frameworks as old-fashioned and outdated and, coining the collective term *totality paradigm frameworks,* contended that these models reduced an understanding of the human person to fragmented parts out of context. These theorists identified a contrasting set of conceptual frameworks as radically different by virtue of being both holistic and philosophically sophisticated, and they termed these theories *simultaneity paradigm frameworks* (Parse, 1987). Advocates of simultaneity theories continue to depict the diverse universe of theorizing about nursing as reflecting these two mutually exclusive groupings, positioning one set of conceptual frameworks as philosophically and morally superior to what they understand the other to represent (Cody, 1995; Nagle & Mitchell, 1991; Newman, 1992).

Nursing Diagnosis

Another discussion about nursing theory centred on nursing diagnosis. The scholars who devised conceptual frameworks focused on models to assess and interpret data about individual client situations. However, the conceptual frameworks were less explicit about how to plan, implement, and evaluate nursing care. To fill this gap, nursing diagnosis emerged as an additional phase in that process. It became a discrete focus of theorizing about nursing care.

In the 1970s, scholars noted a need for precise language to categorize and document nursing diagnoses into a taxonomy (Warren & Hoskins, 1990). This resulted in the formation of the North American Nursing Diagnoses Association (NANDA) (see Chapter 14), which held a series of consensus conferences to establish a list of the common client problems addressed by practicing nurses. The nursing diagnosis movement led to considerable general debate on the merits of NANDA's fixed list of nursing diagnoses versus the theoretically infinite options for nursing care intended by the conceptual models (Fitzpatrick, 1990; Roy, 1982). Although it is recognized as practical rather than theoretical (Fitzpatrick, 1990), NANDA's list has become a popular device for organizing nursing care because it enables efficient categorization into electronic databases and the subsequent standardization of nursing care plans (Warren & Hoskins, 1990). Despite its popularity with health care administrators, NANDA's list is recognized by many nurses as a system that relies entirely upon an agreement about what constitutes average wellness and illness experiences. It can therefore create worrisome barriers to the individualized care of clients (Lee et al., 2006).

Reflections on Conceptualizing Nursing

The scientific and philosophical aspects of today's nursing practice is built on the foundation of early nursing theories about nursing. The history of "nursing theory" is the story of an enlightened attempt to articulate excellent clinical reasoning in nursing care. How effective nurses actually use knowledge within the complexity of their clinical reasoning is, however, still undetermined. In this context, theorizing about nursing is perhaps best understood as an extended philosophical struggle to understand how highly skilled nurses actually think. Instead of arguing the advantages of one nursing theory over another, nursing scholars of today appreciate the creativity of their predecessors within the constrained conceptual contexts in which they were expected to operate.

Major Theoretical Models

Some of the major theoretical models are summarized briefly in Table 6–3; the similarities and differences among them are illustrated. Note, however, that because many nursing theorists based their models on complex combinations of theories from many disciplines, the categorization used here is somewhat oversimplistic. It may be helpful to view the conceptual frameworks in terms of larger theories on which they have drawn, such as adaptation theory, systems theory, or human needs theory.

Practice-Based Theories

All conceptual models of nursing are designed to guide and shape practice. Although their theoretical inspiration is derived directly from the practice setting, many conceptual models do not capture all of what might be influencing that practice, such as societal and demographic changes, current health care belief models, and therapeutic strategies, as well as the political struggles inherent to health care delivery. The early practice theories, therefore, reflect the issues that were shaping the role and context of nursing during those specific timeframes.

Florence Nightingale. Whereas most later theorists drew on social and psychological theories, Nightingale was directly inspired by nursing practice. Writing *Notes on Nursing* in 1859, she described conditions necessary to promote health and healing. Her observations during the Crimean War led to the first set of principles for nursing practice, acknowledging the particular importance of the environment, including clean living areas, fresh air, and the presence of light. The role of nursing care included ensuring that wounded soldiers were warm, comfortable, and adequately fed. Torres (1986) noted that Nightingale demonstrated how to think about clients and their environment. By shifting the focus from disease processes toward an environment conducive to healing, Nightingale's conceptualization clearly differentiated the role of nursing from that of medicine.

The McGill Model. Dr. Moyra Allen (Box 6–1) conceived the McGill model, and she and her colleagues developed it (Gottlieb & Rowat, 1987). Systematically studying actual nursing situations, Allen and her colleagues created a way of thinking about nursing that focused on promoting health. They recognized that many clients' health concerns were best approached through changes in lifestyle. The McGill scholars focused on the individual in the context of the family and, like Nightingale, viewed nursing as complementary to medicine. The main features of the McGill model were "a focus on health rather than illness and treatment, on all family members rather than the patient alone, on family goals rather than on the nurse's, and on family strengths rather than their deficits" (Gottlieb & Feeley, 1999, p. 194). Over time, the model has been further developed to demonstrate its application within a range of clinical contexts and settings (e.g., Feeley & Gerez-Lirette, 1992; Feeley & Gottlieb, 1998).

TABLE 6-3 Milestones in the Development of Nursing Theory

1859	Florence Nightingale's *Notes on Nursing: What It Is and What It Is Not* was published (updated version published 1946)
1952	*Nursing Research* (the first peer-reviewed scientific journal about nursing care) was established
1952	Hildegard Peplau's text on *Interpersonal Relations in Nursing* was published
1955	Virginia Henderson's definition of nursing was first published in the 5th edition of Harmer and Henderson's (1955) basic nursing text
1961	Ida Orlando introduced the nursing process
1970	Martha Rogers' model was first published
1970	Callista Roy's model was first published
1971	Dorothea Orem's model was first published
1976	The North American Nursing Diagnosis Association (NANDA) list of nursing diagnoses was first published
1976	The University of British Columbia model of nursing practice was first published (Campbell et al., 1976)
1978	Barbara Carper's paper on fundamental patterns of knowing in nursing practice was published
1979	Evelyn Adam's model was first published (English version published 1981)
1981	Rosemarie Parse's model was first published
1987	The McGill model of nursing was first published (Gottlieb & Rowat, 1987)

Needs Theories

Many early theorists organized their thinking by conceptualizing the client as representing a collection of needs. This reflected a common orientation to studying the nature of people, popularized in the 1960s, in which needs, drives, and competencies were thought to hold potential for explaining human behaviour. Of these theories, Maslow's (1954) hierarchy of needs was one of the best known and most influential. The idea that complex human behaviour can be best explained as a response to the competing demands of various basic needs is featured prominently in many nursing models.

Virginia Henderson. Henderson (Harmer & Henderson, 1955) conceptualized the client as a compilation of 14 basic human needs: to breathe, eat and drink, eliminate waste products, move and maintain posture, rest and sleep, dress and undress, maintain body temperature, be clean, avoid danger, communicate, worship, work, play, and learn. Viewing the client in this way clearly defined the nurse's role. Accordingly, Henderson defined nursing practice as assisting the individual, sick or well, in the performance of activities that contribute to health, recovery, or a peaceful death. Henderson's model has remained popular in practice because its language is familiar and easily comprehensible and because it explains how a person's biological, psychological, social, and spiritual components combine to influence the way illness is experienced and health can be regained.

Dorothea Orem. Orem's (1971) self-care theory, the origins of which lay in Henderson's work, was used widely in both nursing practice and research. Orem's theory addressed the ways in which people are responsible for meeting the following universal self-care requisites:

- Maintaining sufficient intake of air, water, and food.
- Maintaining a balance between activity and rest and between solitude and interaction.
- Providing for elimination processes.
- Preventing hazards to life, functioning, and well-being.
- Promoting functioning and growth in social groups in accordance with human potential.

BOX 6-1 Milestones in Canadian Nursing History

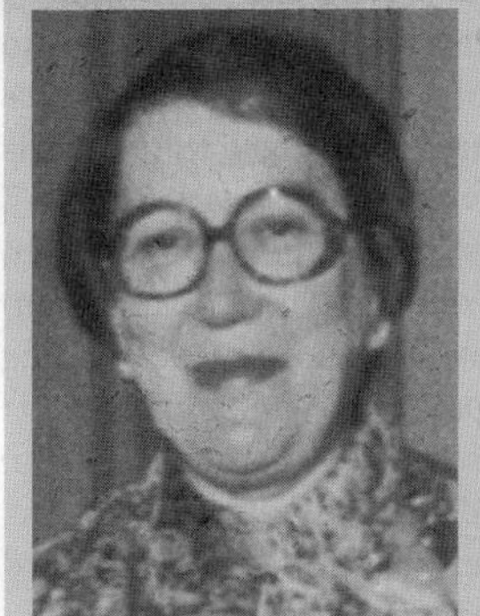

Moyra Allen, 1921–1996

A creative and independent thinker, Moyra Allen was one of the first Canadian nurses to earn a doctoral degree. She lobbied for collective bargaining rights for nurses and was the founding president of the United Nurses of Montreal. She was also the founder of *Nursing Papers*, later renamed the *Canadian Journal of Nursing Research*.

Dr. Allen was a founding member of the World Health Organization committee that developed the criteria for accreditation of nursing schools. She designed an evaluation model for nursing schools and evaluated schools in South America, India, and Ghana. She joined the faculty of the School of Nursing at McGill in 1954 and became professor emeritus in 1985 on her retirement.

In demonstrating her model of nursing, now known as the McGill model, Dr. Allen established The Health Workshop in 1977, a community health facility, in which she put into practice a developmental concept of health and nursing as a prototype of primary health care. The workshop, viewed as complementary to existing services, was staffed with nurses, a community development officer, and a health librarian. The workshop's purpose was to demonstrate the validity of a local health resource managed by nurses that focused on long-term family health. It proved to be an innovative means of improving the health status of families coping with illness and other problems.

Dr. Allen received numerous awards, including the Jeanne Mance Award, which recognizes major contributions to the health of Canadians. In 1987, she became a member of the Order of Canada for her outstanding contributions to Canadian nursing.

Drawing on both human need and developmental theory, Orem's theory focused on the individual's role in maintaining health. This theory emerged at a time when the passive role of the client was being questioned and the health care system was beginning to shift away from full responsibility for people's health. With increased understanding of illness patterns, Orem acknowledged the effects of multiple lifestyle factors such as smoking, diet, and exercise, reminding nurses that clients can look after their own health and that they must learn to care for themselves within their families and communities. Thus, the role of the nurse, according to Orem, was to act temporarily for the client until the client could resume a more independent role in self-care.

Interactionist Theories

Interactionist theories focused on the relationships between nurses and their clients. These theories defined more clearly the specific human communicative and behavioural patterns by which practitioners met their clients' needs. As the theorists reframed definitions of the nursing profession, they drew from the work of psychologists and psychoanalysts such as Harry Stack Sullivan, Abraham Maslow, and Sigmund Freud.

Hildegard Peplau. Peplau, a psychiatric specialist, defined the core of nursing care as the interpersonal relationship between the nurse and the client. Building upon the ideas of psychoanalyst Harry Stack Sullivan, Peplau depicted the practice of nursing as an interactive and therapeutic relationship. Peplau felt that such relationships allowed nurses to challenge the practice of long-term stays in large inpatient psychiatric hospitals and to envision supporting clients to achieve independent living. "The kind of person each nurse becomes makes a substantial difference in what each patient will learn as he is nursed through his experience with illness" (Peplau, 1952, p. vii). According to Peplau, a nurse was "an investigator, prober, interpreter, and reporter, using the rich data she extracts from the patient concerning his life. She develops insights, his and hers, into the meaning of a patient's behaviour and helps the patient recognize and change patterns that obstruct achievement of his goals" (Barnum, 1994, p. 217). An early advocate of an orderly and systematic approach to care, Peplau created a way of thinking about nursing care that directed nurses toward preventing illness and maintaining health.

Joyce Travelbee. Writing in the late 1960s and early 1970s, Travelbee also viewed nursing care as an interpersonal process. In contrast to Peplau's more psychoanalytic orientation, Travelbee drew on a form of thinking known as *existential philosophy* to guide her theorizing. Travelbee (1971) viewed the "client" as including not only the individual but also the client's family and community, and she articulated the role of the nurse as assisting clients to "prevent or cope with the experience of illness and suffering and, if necessary, to find meaning in these experiences" (p. 7). Travelbee emphasized that nurses must recognize the humanity of their clients, suggesting that even the term *patient* should be regarded as a stereotypical categorization. Recognizing the reciprocity of human interaction, Travelbee focused attention on the communication that occurs between nurses and their clients as an important vehicle for finding meaning in illness.

Evelyn Adam. Influenced by Dorothy Johnson, as well as by earlier interactionist theorists (George, 1995), Canadian theorist Evelyn Adam (1979, 1991) articulated the essence of nursing as a helping process. From her perspective, the nurse played a complementary–supplementary role in supporting the client's strength, knowledge, and will. Adam's model drew on Henderson's framework of basic human needs and extended it into a model that would explain not only how nurses conceptualized the client but also how they applied that knowledge in the context of a helping relationship characterized by empathy, caring, and mutual respect.

Systems Theories

In the 1970s and 1980s, as conceptual models of nursing became more sophisticated and structured, several theorists drew on general systems theory (von Bertalanffy, 1968) for guidance in conceptualizing the complexity of human health. The main appeal of systems theory was that it accounted for the whole of an entity (the system) and its component parts (subsystems), as well as the interactions between the parts and the whole. In this way, systems theory allowed theorists to expand the conceptualization of nursing practice through both structure and process, whereby the individual was viewed as an open system in constant interaction with his or her environment. Being outside the system, the nurse became one of the many forces to have an effect on that system. Using this perspective, nurses were encouraged to appreciate the interactions of a system with its component parts and with its environment. Systems approaches helped nurses recognize that intervention in any one part of a system would produce consequent reactions in other parts, as well as in the system as a whole. Regardless of how each theorist depicted the nature of the system, these general principles common to all living systems were featured in each of the nursing systems models.

Dorothy Johnson. Johnson's theoretical work was popularized in the early 1960s through class notes and speeches, but it remained unpublished until much later (Grubbs, 1980; Johnson, 1980). In her nursing model, Johnson identified the individual as a behavioural system with seven subsystems, each of which has a goal, a set of behaviours, and a choice. The notion of goals of the subsystems was based on the drives that were considered universal and applicable to all clients. However, the meanings attributed to each goal and the set of behaviours for achieving goals were seen as highly individual and unique to each client. Together with the choices made by the client in relation to meeting his or her behavioural system goals, each subsystem also had a function that could be considered analogous to the physiological function of a biological system (Meleis, 2007).

The University of British Columbia Model. The behavioural systems model developed at the University of British Columbia (UBC) School of Nursing was inspired by Johnson's model and developed by a committee led by Margaret Campbell that included several of Johnson's former students. Broadening the view of human experience on the basis of behavioural drives, the UBC model depicted the behavioural system as being composed of nine basic human needs, each of which is shaped by the psychological and sociocultural environment in which it is expressed (Campbell et al., 1976). Whereas needs were considered universal and therefore fundamental to human experience, the specific goals toward which needs-related human behaviour were directed and the strategies for achieving those goals were recognized as unique to individuals and their particular physiological, psychological, or social circumstances (Thorne et al., 1993). Thus, the UBC model provided a structure by which general knowledge about human health and illness could be combined with particular knowledge about each individual client. In accordance with the tenets of general systems theory, the goal of nursing practice was balance of the behavioural system. The nurse's role was to foster, protect, sustain, and teach (Campbell, 1987) and thereby bring about not only system balance but also stability and optimal health.

Betty Neuman. Neuman's approach to theorizing about nursing differed from that of other systems theorists in that it did not rely on concepts concerning needs and drives, nor did it break the system into any component parts. Neuman understood the person to be a physiological, psychological, sociocultural, developmental, and spiritual being (Meleis, 2007) and oriented the attention of the nurse to the client system in a health care–oriented and holistic manner (Neuman, 1982). Neuman considered the client system to have innate factors consistent with being human, as well as unique factors that characterized each individual person. According to Neuman, each client had a unique set of response patterns determined and regulated by a core structure. Neuman believed that because the person was vulnerable to environmental stressors, the role of the nurse ought to focus on actual and potential stressors. In this way, Neuman's model focused on prevention.

Sister Callista Roy. In contrast to most other systems theorists, Roy considered the client not as behavioural system but rather as an adaptive one. She viewed the person as a biopsychosocial being in constant interaction with a changing environment (Roy, 1984). Her model depicted four modes of adaptation: physiological needs, self-concept, role function, and interdependence (Roy, 1974). She saw the person as an adaptive system with two major internal processes by which to adapt: the cognator and the regulator subsystems (Roy & Andrews, 1999). Roy used these mechanisms to describe and explain the interconnectedness of all aspects of human adaptation and to conceptualize the role of the nurse in managing the stimuli that influence that adaptation (Meleis, 2007).

Simultaneity Theories

The theorists who identified their work as belonging to the simultaneity paradigm considered their theories to be radically different from the practice, needs, interactionist, and systems theories. Although simultaneity theories were first articulated long before the paradigm debate arose and before the terms *simultaneity* and *totality* were used to categorize the various theories, the language of simultaneity has become prominent in distinguishing this group of nursing theories from others. A characteristic feature of these theories is what Rogers (1970) called the *unitary human being*. Previous theorists had sought to identify aspects of the individual that could represent an abstract conceptualization of the whole but also provided an understanding of the person and his or her problems, needs, or goals. In contrast, the simultaneity theorists viewed the individual as an entirely irreducible whole, inherently and "holographically" connected with the universal environment (Parse, 2004). Thus, these theories represented a distinct way of articulating an understanding of the client of nursing and of nursing's role in relation to that client.

Martha Rogers. Martha Rogers's (1970) model was revolutionary in presenting the client not simply as a person but as an energy field in constant interaction with the environment, which itself was also an irreducible energy field, coextensive with the universe (Meleis, 2007). According to Rogers, who based her theory on her interpretations of evolving ideas in physics, the role of nursing was to focus on the life process of a human being along a time–space continuum (Rogers, 1970). An early proponent of pattern recognition, Rogers believed that pattern gave the energy field its identity and its distinguishing characteristics (Meleis, 2007). The objective of nursing practice became one of helping clients reach their maximum health potential in the context of constant change and and to develop what Rogers referred to as homeodynamic unity within diversity.

Rosemarie Parse. Parse's (1981) theory of "man–living–health," later termed *human becoming* (Parse, 1997), was another view of the individual as a unitary being who is "indivisible, unpredictable, and everchanging" and "a freely choosing being who can be recognized through paradoxical patterns cocreated all-at-once in mutual process with the universe" (Parse, 2004, p. 293). According to Parse's perspective, the caring presences of nurses and their particular patterns of relating support individuals in the human "becoming" process. Within Parse's nursing theory, the goal of nursing is articulated not in traditional definitions of health but rather as the notion of people in a continuous process of making choices and changing health priorities. According to Parse's theory, nurses engage with people in their process of "becoming" through the application of three core processes referred to as explicating, dwelling with, and moving beyond (Parse, 1999).

Jean Watson. Watson (1979) considered the individual to be a totality who can be viewed as a transpersonal self. According to Watson, in contrast to depictions of the individual as a body and an ego, it is more useful to understand the individual as "an embodied spirit; a transpersonal transcendent evolving consciousness; unity of mindbodyspirit; person–nature–universe as oneness, connected" (Watson, 1999, p. 129). Watson therefore believed that nurses must do far more than deal with physical illness: they must attend to their primary function, which is caring. From Watson's perspective, caring infuses all aspects of a nurse's role and draws attention to nursing acts as embodying an esthetic that facilitates both healing and growth (see Chapter 19).

Each of the models just described attracts continual analysis and implementation. In some instances, nurses draw on them holistically as a coherent approach to guide all of their practices. More often, nowadays, nurses consider themselves informed by the intellectual structure that any good model provides, but typically expand their thinking beyond the limitations of a single model as their practice develops and progresses.

Theorizing in the Future

Theoretical knowledge leads us to reflect on "the basic values, guiding principles, elements, and phases of a conception of nursing" (Meleis, 2007). The goals of theoretical knowledge are to stimulate thinking and create a broad understanding of the science and practice of the nursing discipline (King & Fawcett, 1997). Although nurses today can appreciate the inherent complexity of these objectives, the creativity and vision modeled by these early theorists continue to inspire theorizing about the essence of nursing.

Nursing is solidly established as a distinct health care discipline with its own unique science. In addition, current theorists draw heavily from philosophy to resolve some of nursing's theoretical challenges. However, as Kikuchi (1999) pointed out, much of the theorizing about the purpose of nursing has confused rather than clarified thinking. As nursing scholarship evolves to include stronger philosophical and scientific inquiry, nursing practice must be conceptualized with increasing clarity (Silva et al., 1995). Nurse philosophers, as well as scientists, are continuing to use new ways of tackling nursing's most complex theoretical feature, which is applying expanding, dynamic, and multiple sources of knowledge to a diverse range of client situations. This problem of understanding the general and applying it to the particular appears in the work of many contemporary nursing scholars.

Meleis (1987), a scholar of nursing theory, challenged nurses to direct their theorizing away from the processes by which nurses use knowledge and toward the equally challenging issues associated with the substance of that knowledge. In accepting this challenge, many nursing scholars have shifted their theorizing about nursing to include both theoretical and substantive knowledge. Liaschenko (1997; Liaschenko & Fisher, 1999) oriented this theorizing into three levels of abstraction: knowing the case, knowing the client, and knowing the person. Engebretson (1997) positioned nursing theory in relation not only to biomedicine but also to Eastern and holistic understandings of health and illness. Starzomski and Rodney (1997) worked toward articulating the link between definitions of health and more philosophical notions of the greater social good. Campbell and Bunting (1991) explored the possibilities of using critical social and feminist theories for emancipatory theorizing in nursing. Watson (1990; see also Brenwick & Webster, 2000) developed the idea of embedding "caring" as a moral component into nursing theory. Yeo (1989) considered the implications of ethical reasoning for nursing theory.

The interrelationships between theory and practice are of increasing interest to nursing scholars. A dialogue representing the dynamic interaction between theorizing and clinical practice (termed **praxis**) has started to emerge (Clarke et al., 1996; Mitchell, 1995; Reed & Ground, 1997; Reed, 1995; Thorne, 1997). This newer theorizing does not seek static truths about nursing practice; rather, it creates a foundation upon which nurses can build, challenge, and integrate an infinite range of new knowledge and new ideas. As Levine (1995) wrote, "Theory is the poetry of science" (p. 14). Hence, theorizing brings familiar concepts of nursing together into bold new configurations, making disconnected aspects of human experience part of a greater whole. In so doing, it makes the discipline of nursing come alive.

* KEY CONCEPTS

- The hallmark of nursing practice is its unique body of knowledge and the way nurses use it.
- Nursing science has evolved in a historical and social context.
- Nursing theory represents the attempts by nursing scholars to articulate ways in which knowledge from various sources can be systematically applied in a wide variety of ways to guide professional, accountable, and defensible nursing practice.
- Much of the early theorizing about nursing practice was specifically designed to guide nursing curriculum development so that nursing education would be focused on the knowledge unique to nursing care.
- The nursing process is the fundamental problem-solving process by which new situations are assessed, plans are developed, and interventions are performed and evaluated.
- Nursing care requires the application of general knowledge to an infinite range of unique situations. Nursing process and nursing theory represent strategies to guide the process of such application.
- The major components of nursing theory, sometimes called the *metaparadigm concepts*, are person, environment, health, and nursing.
- Nurses' understanding of the role of science has changed as more complex forms of science have been articulated by philosophers of science; science is no longer limited to simple relationships such as cause and effect but instead provides strategies for understanding much more complex relationships and phenomena.
- Nursing knowledge derives from various sources in addition to science, including esthetics, personal knowing, sociocultural understanding, and ethics.
- Nursing theorists based their conceptual frameworks on various ways of thinking about human behaviour and experience; some drew their ideas from what they observed in excellent nursing practice, whereas others drew from theories of human behaviour, such as needs, interaction, or systems.
- Nursing conceptual frameworks include those for understanding both the person as the nurse's client and the nurse's role in relation to that client.
- Although each framework may have attempted to organize nursing knowledge and systematic reasoning processes in a different way, each was aiming for a very similar ideal of excellent decision making in nursing practice.
- Although nursing theoretical frameworks are no longer considered useful as prescriptive models for practice, they provide a way of conceptualizing nursing's interests and of identifying researchable nursing problems.
- As the practice of theorizing about nursing care evolves, the role of philosophy in helping nurses understand their relationship to knowledge has become increasingly relevant.

* CRITICAL THINKING EXERCISES

1. How do you think that different ways of conceptualizing the client might influence the kinds of decisions that nurses might make in their practice? Consider how understanding the person in terms of needs, system theory, or interaction might lead you to notice certain things and not others.
2. What sorts of gaps in information or misunderstandings might occur if nurses failed to use a systematic way of thinking about each individual client in their care?
3. How do you think that conceptual frameworks and nursing theories might be used to generate research questions for developing knowledge for evidence-informed practice?
4. Why is it useful for nurses to question how they know what they think they know?

* REVIEW QUESTIONS

1. A theory is a set of assumptions or propositions that is useful because it
   1. Helps people meet their self-care needs
   2. Isolates concepts
   3. Helps the nurse implement care
   4. Provides a systematic view of explaining, predicting, and prescribing phenomena
2. The drive for early theorizing about nursing practice was derived from
   1. Physicians
   2. Political leaders
   3. Nursing educators
   4. Policymakers
3. The nursing process originally involved which four basic steps?
   1. Assessment, planning, intervention, evaluation
   2. Assessment, nursing diagnosis, planning, intervention
   3. Nursing diagnosis, planning, intervention, evaluation
   4. Planning, assessment, intervention, evaluation
4. The metaparadigm concepts included
   1. The person, environment, health, and nursing
   2. The theories of Thomas Kuhn
   3. Chaos theory and games theory
   4. The grounded theory approach

5. The main question confronting early nursing theorists was about
   1. How to differentiate between nursing theories and medical theories
   2. How to reconcile the generalizations of the North American Nursing Diagnoses Association with the unique situations of each client
   3. How to organize and make sense of general nursing knowledge and apply this knowledge to an individual clinical case
   4. Whether to use theories from other disciplines such as philosophy and to apply them to nursing

6. According to Kuhn, scientific advances happen when creative individuals
   1. Approach a problem in a new way
   2. Use the cause-and-effect model to solve problems
   3. Use the work of other scientists to solve problems
   4. Use empirical evidence to solve problems

7. The McGill model
   1. Focuses on health rather than on illness or treatment
   2. Accounts for holistic aspects of the individual, rather than component parts
   3. Views the person as an energy field in constant interaction with the environment
   4. Considers the human experience to be based on behavioural drives

8. Hildegard Peplau considered the essence of nursing to be
   1. The role of the individual in health maintenance
   2. The relationship between the nurse and client
   3. Advancing nursing theories
   4. Caring

9. Theorist Evelyn Adam articulated the essence of nursing as
   1. A collaboration with health care professionals
   2. A helping process
   3. The management of clients and health care systems
   4. All of the above

10. Systems theorists considered the human being to be
    1. An irreducible whole
    2. A whole and component parts
    3. An embodiment of mind, body, and spirit
    4. All of the above

11. Parse's theory relies on
    1. A traditional definition of illness and health
    2. The idea of people engaging in a continuing process of making choices
    3. The notion of nursing as a caring profession
    4. All of the above

* RECOMMENDED WEB SITES

Department of Nursing, Clayton State University School of Nursing, "Nursing Theory Link Page": http://healthsci.clayton.edu/eichelberger/nursing.htm

This collection offers links to a wide range of nursing theories, including theories of nursing in general and theories about substantive fields within nursing.

Hahn School of Nursing and Health Science, University of San Diego, "The Nursing Theory Page": http://www.sandiego.edu/academics/nursing/theory/

This site orients the student to most of the major nursing theorists and resources to expand an understanding of their contributions.

7

Research as a Basis for Practice

Original chapter by Patricia A. Potter, RN, MSN, PhD, GMAC, FAAN

Canadian content written by Marilynn J. Wood, BSN, MSN, DrPH

objectives

Mastery of content in this chapter will enable you to:

- Define the key terms listed.
- Differentiate evidence-informed practice from traditional practice
- Identify methods of locating research findings
- Discuss how to implement evidence-informed practice
- Identify the various ways to acquire knowledge.
- Discuss methods for developing new nursing knowledge.
- Define nursing research.
- Discuss Canadian nursing research priorities.
- Identify ethical principles important in undertaking research.
- Explain how the rights of human research subjects are protected.
- Explain how to organize information from a research report.

key terms

Empirical data, p. 82
Ethnography, p. 84
Evidence-informed practice, p. 75
Grounded theory, p. 85
Hypothesis, p. 82
Informed consent, p. 85
Nursing research, p. 80
Phenomenology, p. 85
Qualitative nursing research, p. 84
Quantitative nursing research, p. 83
Quasi-experimental research design, p. 84
Research process, p. 82
Scientific method, p. 82
Scientific nursing research, p. 83
Subjects, p. 83
Surveys, p. 84
True experiment, p. 83

media resources

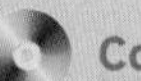 Web Site

- Audio Chapter Summaries
- Glossary
- Multiple-Choice Review Questions
- Student Learning Activities
- Weblinks

Companion CD

- Glossary
- Interactive Learning Activities
- Fluids and Electrolytes Tutorial
- Test-Taking Skills

Rick has been a nurse in the emergency department for more than five years. During that time, the nurses have followed a policy of restricting the presence of family members when clients experience critical events that necessitate resuscitation. This policy allows staff to attend to the client and administer life-saving care without family interference. The nurses have assumed that the experience of watching a loved one undergoing resuscitation is too traumatic for family members. However, Rick has noticed for some time that the families of resuscitated clients experience significant stress when they are unable to stay with their loved one. Later, after the resuscitation, the families may express anger or resentment toward staff. Rick raises a question with the other nurses in the department: "What if we allowed family presence during resuscitation. What would be the outcomes for the families? Is it possible that families can benefit?"

Rick and the other emergency nurses have been practising according to what they know from their education and experience, as well as the policies and practices of their hospital. This type of practice may not be based on up-to-date information. Current evidence in the scientific literature is that family presence during resuscitation may have distinct benefits. The considerable number of studies that have been done all demonstrate a positive outcome for the family. In spite of the evidence, however, health care practitioners continue to doubt the value of having families remain with the patient (Boudreaux et al., 2002; McGahey-Oakland et al., 2007). This doubt exemplifies the gap between research and practice.

Why Evidence?

Today, anyone can be an expert. The Internet opens up a world of information accessible to anyone. The public is more informed than ever before about individuals' own health and the issues facing society, as well as the types of errors that occur within health care insititutions across the country. Greater attention is paid to why certain health care approaches are used and which ones do and do not work. As a result, **evidence-informed practice** provides a safety net for nurses and other health professionals because it enables them to make accurate, timely, and appropriate clinical decisions. Evidence-informed practice is the integration of the most informative research evidence with evidence from expert clinical practice and other sources to produce the best possible care for clients.

Nursing knowledge must be expanded continuously to keep approaches to nursing care relevant and current. Without new knowledge, nursing cannot improve therapies such as infant care, pain management, grief counselling, or client education. The major source of new knowledge is research, which can provide a solid foundation for nursing practice. It is important to translate the best evidence into best practices at a client's bedside. Nurses need a sound knowledge base to support practice, and research is essential for building that knowledge.

Professional nurses must stay informed about current evidence. This is not easy to do. Students diligently read the assigned readings from texts and articles. A good textbook incorporates evidence into the practice guidelines it describes. However, it takes about two years for a book to be written, published, and in print; therefore, the scientific literature used in the book is often outdated by the time the book is published. Articles, particularly scientific ones, are more likely to be current, but the findings may not be easily applied. They may be inconclusive, or the particular practice may not have been studied yet. Moreover, these articles are not readily available to staff nurses at the bedside. It is a distinct challenge to obtain the best, most current evidence when you need it for client care.

The sources of information about evidence are well-designed, systematically conducted research studies, found in scientific journals; however, much of that evidence does not reach the bedside. Nurses currently have limited access to databases for scientific literature. When no evidence is available, tradition prevails.

Nonresearch evidence is another source of information to support practice. This includes quality improvement and risk management data; international, national, and local standards; infection control data; chart reviews; and clinical expertise. These sources can be valuable, but their value never approaches that of research evidence.

A third source of evidence that must be incorporated into good clinical decisions consists of individual clients and their values, beliefs, and experience. No efficacious clinical decision can be made without consideration of the uniqueness of the client.

Much current research focuses on ways to improve the use of new knowledge in practice. Steps to foster success are summarized in Box 7–1.

Researching the Evidence

Ask the Clinical Question

Clinical questions arise out of your practice and represent problems that you wonder about, or things that do not make sense to you. Titler et al. (2001) suggested using problem- and knowledge-focused triggers to think critically about clinical and operational nursing unit issues. A problem-focused trigger is a question you face while caring for a client or a trend you see on a nursing unit. For example, while caring for an unconscious client, you wonder, "What is the best cleaner to use when I provide mouth care to this client?" A problem-focused trend might be an increase in client falls or in the incidence of postoperative urinary tract infections. These trends lead you to ask, "How can I reduce falls on my unit?" or "What can I do to prevent urinary tract infections postoperatively?"

A knowledge-focused trigger is a question seeking new information available on a topic: for instance, "What is the current evidence to improve pain management in clients with migraine headaches?" Important sources of this type of information can be found in practice guidelines available from professional associations. All professions have focused on ensuring that service professionals understand practice guidelines. "Best practices" are guiding principles leading to the most appropriate courses of action in certain standard practice situations. They are based on the accumulated research findings, as

BOX 7-1 STEPS FOR SUCCESSFUL EVIDENCE-INFORMED PRACTICE

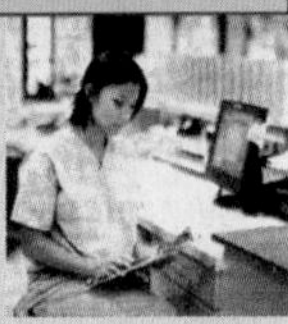

1. Ask a question that clearly presents the clinical problem.
2. Identify and gather the most relevant and best evidence.
3. Critically appraise the evidence.
4. Integrate all evidence with clinical expertise, clients' preferences, and clients' values to make a practice decision or change.
5. Evaluate the outcome of the practice decision or change.

From Melnyk, B. M, & Fineout-Overholt, E. (2005). *Evidence-based practice in nursing and health care. A guide to best practice*. Philadelphia: Lippincott Williams & Wilkins. Reprinted by permission of Lippincott Williams & Wilkins.

well as on evidence from practice. This sets best practices apart from the much more general nursing practice standards. Since 1999, the Ontario Ministry of Health and Long-Term Care has given substantial annual funding to the Registered Nurses Association of Ontario (RNAO) for a project to develop, vet, and disseminate "best practice guidelines" that identify actions in particular client situations. This is a multiyear project to assist nurses in providing informed and high-quality care (RNAO, 2008). These guidelines are available to all Canadian nurses (Box 7–2).

The questions you ask will eventually lead you to the evidence required for an answer. When you consult the scientific literature for an answer, you want to read the most informative four to six articles that address your practice question specifically, not be mired in hundreds of articles that might have some relationship to your question. This means that your question must be well stated and focused on just the relevant components of the issue. Unfocused questions ("What is the best way to reduce wandering?" "What is the best way to measure blood pressure?") are too vague and will lead to many irrelevant sources of information. Melnyk and Fineout-Overholt (2005) suggested using a "PICO" format to state your question. A PICO question has four components:

P = Patient population of interest: What are the age, gender, ethnicity, and disease or health problem of the clients?
I = Intervention of interest: What is the best intervention (treatment, diagnostic test, prognostic factor)?
C = Comparison of interest: What is the usual standard of care or current intervention used now in practice?
O = Outcome: What result (e.g., change in client behavior, physical finding) do you want to achieve as a result of the intervention?

Do not be satisfied with clinical routines if they do not improve the patient's quality of life. Always question and use critical thinking to consider better ways to provide client care. The questions you raise by using a PICO format help you identify knowledge gaps within a clinical situation and assist you in making sound clinical decisions for change.

Collect the Best Evidence

Once you have a clear and concise PICO question, you are ready to search for evidence. You can find the evidence you need in a variety of sources: agency policy and procedure manuals, quality improvement data, existing clinical practice guidelines, or bibliographical databases. Always ask for help to find appropriate evidence. Nursing faculty are always a key resource, as are advanced practice nurses, staff educators, and infection control nurses.

➤ BOX 7-2 Selected Nursing Best Practice Guidelines of the Registered Nurses Association of Ontario

Adult Asthma Care Guidelines for Nurses: Promoting Control of Asthma
Assessment and Device Selection for Vascular Access
Assessment and Management of Foot Ulcers for People with Diabetes
Assessment and Management of Pain
Assessment & Management of Stage I to IV Pressure Ulcers—Revised 2007
Assessment and Management of Venous Leg Ulcers
Best Practice Guideline for the Subcutaneous Administration of Insulin in Adults with Type 2 Diabetes
Breastfeeding Best Practice Guidelines for Nurses
Care and Maintenance to Reduce Vascular Access Complications
Caregiving Strategies for Older Adults with Delirium, Dementia and Depression
Client Centred Care
Crisis Intervention
Enhancing Healthy Adolescent Development
Establishing Therapeutic Relationships
Integrating Smoking Cessation into Daily Nursing Practice
Interventions for Postpartum Depression
Nursing Care of Dyspnea: The 6th Vital Sign in Individuals with Chronic Obstructive Pulmonary Diseases (COPD)
Nursing Management of Hypertension
Prevention of Constipation in the Older Adult Population
Prevention of Falls and Fall Injuries in the Older Adult
Primary Prevention of Childhood Obesity
Promoting Asthma Control in Children
Promoting Continence Using Prompted Voiding
Reducing Foot Complications for People with Diabetes
Risk Assessment and Prevention of Pressure Ulcers
Screening for Delirium, Dementia and Depression in Older Adults
Stroke Assessment Across the Continuum of Care
Supporting and Strengthening Families Through Expected and Unexpected Life Events
Woman Abuse: Screening, Identification and Initial Response

See http://www.rnao.org/Page.asp?PageID=1110&SiteNodeID=190 for links to the abovementioned guidelines.

➤ BOX 7-3 Searchable Scientific Literature Databases and Sources

Database Sources

Cumulative Index of Nursing and Allied Health Literature (CINAHL): http://www.cinahl.com
Includes studies in nursing, allied health, and biomedicine

MEDLINE: http://medline/COS.com/
Includes studies in medicine, nursing, dentistry, psychiatry, veterinary medicine, and allied health

EMBASE: http://www.embase.com
Includes biomedical and pharmaceutical studies

PsycINFO: http://www.apa.org/psycinfo/
Contains information in psychology and related health care disciplines

Cochrane Database of Systematic Reviews: http://www.cochrane.org/reviews
Contains full text of regularly updated systematic reviews prepared by the Cochrane Collaboration; includes completed reviews and protocols

National Guideline Clearinghouse: http://www.guideline.gov
Contains structured abstracts (summaries) about clinical guidelines and their development; also includes condensed version of guideline for viewing

PubMed: http://www.nlm.nih.gov
Health science library at the US National Library of Medicine; offers free access to journal articles

OnLine Journal of Knowledge Synthesis for Nursing
Electronic journal; contains articles that provide a synthesis of research and an annotated bibliography for selected references

NurseOne Portal: http://www.nurseone.ca
Offers free access to all major databases; available to members of the Canadian Nurses Association (CNA)

When you go to the literature for evidence, a librarian can help you to locate the appropriate databases (Box 7–3). The databases contain published scientific studies, including peer-reviewed research. An article that has undergone peer review has been reviewed by a panel of experts before publication. The search process requires you to come up with key words or phrases from your PICO question that most accurately describe what you want from the search. The librarian can help you find the language that yields the most informative results. You usually need to adjust the wording of your search criteria until you get the results you want.

The best-known databases for nursing literature are MEDLINE and CINAHL. These are comprehensive databases containing articles from most nursing and health journals. These are usually available at no cost to students through the university or college library. Members of the CNA have free access to these and other databases through the NurseOne Portal (see Box 7–3).

The pyramid in Figure 7–1 represents the hierarchy of available evidence. At the top of the pyramid are systematic reviews and meta-analyses. These reviews have been conducted by experts in the clinical area, who review the evidence about a specific clinical question or issue and summarize the state of the science. Of primary importance in these reviews are the randomized controlled trials (RCTs) that have been conducted on the topic. On occasion, they include other types of research as well. Later in this chapter, the research process is examined more carefully, and you will find that the majority of nursing research is not at the level of the RCT. Nevertheless, the RCT is considered the "gold standard" in scientific research, in which the effect of a specific treatment or intervention is tested through the use of experimental and control groups. A systematic review of RCTs in which an intervention (such as computerized interactive patient teaching) is used would answer a PICO question about the effectiveness of this intervention in managing the blood glucose levels of clients with newly diagnosed diabetes.

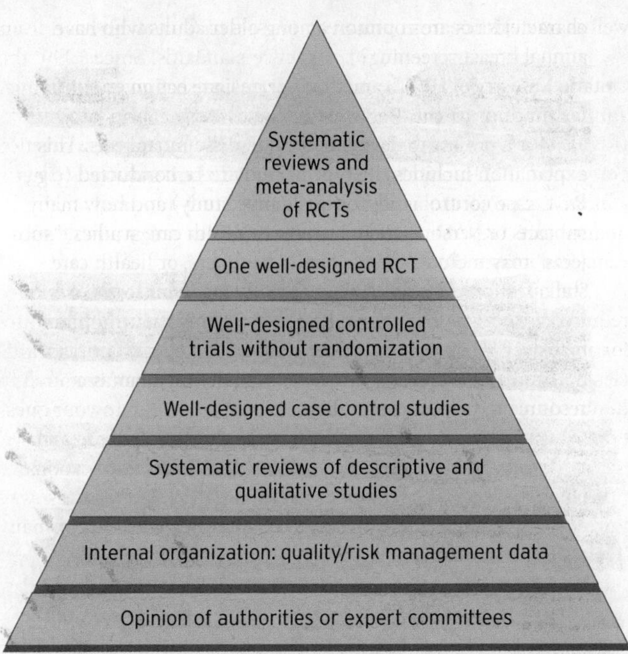

Figure 7-1 Hierarchy of evidence. RCT, randomized controlled trial. **Source:** Adapted from Guyatt, G., & Rennie, D. (2002). *User's guide to the medical literature.* Chicago: American Medical Association; and Melnyk, B. M., & Fineout-Overholt, E. (2005). *Evidence-based practice in nursing and healthcare: A guide to best practice.* Philadelphia: Lippincott Williams & Wilkins.

Critique the Evidence

The most difficult step in the evidence-informed practice process probably is critiquing or analyzing the available evidence. The critiquing of evidence involves determining its value, feasibility, and utility for changing practice. When you critique evidence, first evaluate the scientific merit and clinical applicability of each study's findings. Then, with a group of studies and expert opinion, determine what findings have a strong enough basis for use in practice. After critiquing the evidence, you will be able to answer the questions, Do the articles together offer evidence to explain or answer your PICO question? Do the articles show that the evidence is true and reliable? Can you use the evidence in practice? Because you are a student and new to nursing, it will take time to acquire the skills to critique evidence like an expert. When you read an article from the literature, do not let the statistics or technical wording cause you to stop reading the article. Know the elements of an article, and use a careful approach when you review each one. Evidence-informed articles include the following elements:

- *Abstract:* An abstract is a brief summary of the article that quickly tells you whether the article is research or clinically based. An abstract summarizes the purpose of the study or clinical query, the major themes or findings, and the implications for nursing practice.
- *Introduction:* The introduction contains information about the purpose of the article and the importance of the topic for the audience who reads the article. Brief supporting evidence is usually presented as to why the topic is important from the author's point of view. Together, the abstract and introduction tell you whether you want to read the entire article. You will know if the topic of the article is similar to your PICO question or related closely enough to provide you with useful information. Continue to read the next elements of the article:
- *Literature review or background:* A useful article has a detailed background of the existing level of science or clinical information about the topic of the article. Therefore, it offers an argument about what led the author to conduct a study or report on a clinical topic. This section of an article is valuable. Perhaps the article itself does not address your PICO question in the way you desire, but it may lead you to other articles that are more useful. A literature review of a research article indicates how past research led to the researcher's question. For example, an article about a study designed to test an educational intervention for older adult family caregivers reviews literature that describes characteristics of caregivers, the type of factors influencing caregivers' ability to cope with stressors of caregiving, and any previous educational interventions used with families.
- *Manuscript narrative:* "Middle sections," or narratives, of articles differ according to the type of evidence-informed article they are (Melnyk & Fineout-Overholt, 2005). A clinical article describes a clinical topic and often includes a description of a client population, the nature of a certain disease or health alteration, how clients are affected, and the appropriate nursing therapies. Some clinical articles explain how to use a therapy or new technology. A research article will contain several subsections within the narrative, including the following:
  - *Purpose statement:* A purpose statement explains the focus or intent of a study. It identifies what concepts were researched. This includes research questions or hypotheses: predictions made about the relationship or difference between study variables (concepts, characteristics, or traits that vary within subjects). An example of a research question is as follows: "What

characteristics are common among older adults who have annual breast screening?"

- *Methods or design:* The methods or design section explains how a research study is organized and conducted in order to answer the research question or to test the hypothesis. This explanation includes the type of study to be conducted (e.g., RCT, case control study, or qualitative study) and how many subjects or persons are in a study. In health care studies, "subjects" may include clients, family members, or health care staff. The language in the methods section is sometimes confusing because it contains details about how the researcher designs the study to minimize bias so as to obtain the most accurate results possible. Use your faculty member as a resource to help interpret this section.
- *Results or conclusions:* Clinical and research articles have a summary section. A clinical article explains the clinical implications for the topic presented, whereas a research article details the results of the study and explains whether a hypothesis is supported or how a research question is answered. If the study is quantitative, this section includes a statistical analysis . For a qualitative study, the article presents a thorough summary of the descriptive themes and ideas that arise from the researcher's analysis of data. Do not be stumped by the statistical analysis in an article. Read carefully, and ask whether the researcher describes the results and whether the results were significant. Have a faculty member assist you in interpreting statistical results. A helpful results section also discusses any limitations to a study. This information on limitations is valuable in helping you decide whether you want to use the evidence with your clients.
- *Clinical implications.* A research article includes a section that explains whether the findings from the study have clinical implications. This section also explains how to apply findings in a practice setting for the type of subjects studied. After you have critiqued each article for your PICO question, synthesize or combine the findings from all of the articles to determine the state of the evidence. Use critical thinking to consider the scientific rigor of the evidence and how well it answers your area of interest. Consider the evidence in view of your clients' concerns and preferences. Your review of articles offers a snapshot conclusion that is based on combined evidence about one focused topical area. As a clinician, judge whether to use the evidence for a particular client or group of clients, who usually have complex medical histories and patterns of responses (Melnyk & Fineout-Overholt, 2005). It is ethically important to consider evidence that benefits clients and does no harm. Decide whether the evidence is relevant, is easily applicable in your setting of practice, and has the potential for improving client outcomes.

Integrate the Evidence

Once you decide that the evidence is strong and applicable to your clients and clinical situation, incorporate the recommended evidence into practice. Your first step is to simply apply the research in your plan of care for a client. Use the evidence you find as a rationale for an intervention you plan to try. For instance, you learned about an approach for bathing older adults who are restless, and you decide to use the technique during your next clinical assignment. You use the bathing technique with your own assigned clients, or you work with a group of other students or nurses in revising a policy and procedure or in developing a new clinical protocol. In another example, after being concerned about the rate of intravenous catheter dislodgement, you consult the evidence to compare the efficacy of gauze dressings with that of transparent dressings. The literature suggests that fewer catheter dislodgements occur with transparent dressings on peripheral intravenous sites than with gauze dressings, with no increase in phlebitis or infiltration rates (Melnyk & Fineout-Overholt, 2005; Tripepi-Bova et al., 1997). As a result of your findings, you meet with the policy and procedure committee of your institution to recommend the use of transparent dressings routinely. You then implement the use of transparent dressings in the routine care of peripheral intravenous catheters.

Evidence is useful in a variety of ways in formulating teaching tools, clinical practice guidelines, policies and procedures, and new assessment or documentation tools. Depending on the amount of change needed to apply evidence in practice, it becomes necessary to involve a number of staff from a given nursing unit. It is important to consider the setting in which you want to apply the evidence: Do all staff members support the change? Does the practice change fit with the scope of practice in the clinical setting? Are resources (time, administrative support, and staff) available to make a change? When evidence is not strong enough to apply in practice, your next option is to conduct a pilot study to investigate your PICO question. A pilot study is a small-scale research study or a study that includes a quality or performance improvement project. As a nursing student integrating evidence, your study begins with searching for and applying the most useful evidence to improve the care you provide directly to your clients. The evidence available within nursing literature gives you an almost unlimited access to innovative and effective nursing interventions. Using an evidence-informed practice approach helps you improve your skills and knowledge as a nurse and improve outcomes for your clients.

Evaluate the Practice Decision or Change

After applying evidence in your practice, your next step is to evaluate its effect. How does the intervention work? How effective was the clinical decision for your client or practice setting? Sometimes your evaluation is as simple as determining whether the expected outcomes you set for an intervention are met. For example, after the use of a transparent intravenous dressing, does the catheter dislodge, or does the complication of phlebitis develop? When you use a new approach to preoperative teaching, does the client learn what to expect after surgery?

When an evidence-informed practice change occurs on a larger scale, an evaluation is more formal. For example, evidence of factors that contribute to pressure ulcers might lead a nursing unit to adopt a new skin care protocol. To evaluate the protocol, the nurses track the incidence of pressure ulcers over a course of time (e.g., six months to a year). In addition, the nurses collect data to describe both the clients who develop ulcers and those who do not. This comparative information is valuable for determining the effects of the protocol and whether modifications are necessary.

Support for Evidence-Informed Practice

Nursing practice is based on theory, professional values, and evidence. Nurses base decisions on these factors, as well on other influences such as individual values, ethics, legislation, client choice, and practice environments. The CNA recommends evidence-informed decision making as an essential component of providing quality nursing care that optimizes the outcomes for patients. The evidence to be used in practice is derived through scientific evaluation of practice. Types of evidence include experimental studies of nursing interventions, meta-analysis of groups of studies on a particular topic, nonexperimental or observational studies, expert opinion through consensus documents, and historical information (CNA, 2002).

Knowledge Development in Nursing

Knowledge that provides the rationale for nursing practice is organized in a variety of ways. In her classic article on patterns of knowing in nursing, Carper (1978) identified four patterns: "empirics," or the science of nursing; esthetics, or the art of nursing; personal knowing; and ethics, or the moral component. A fifth type of knowing, emancipatory knowing, was later added by Chinn and Kramer (2008) (Table 7–1). These different types of knowledge focus on the meaning and value of nursing expertise. With evidence-informed practice, the evidence can be derived from any of these sources of knowledge.

Empirics: The Science of Nursing

Carper (1978) described empirics as "knowledge that is systematically organized into general laws and theories for the purpose of describing, explaining and predicting phenomena of special concern to the discipline of nursing" (p. 14). This pattern of knowing implies an objective reality; by studying this, you can interpret the meaning of particular phenomena and develop understandings of other similar phenomena. Fundamental to this model is the rational stance in which you can generalize from a sample to a population. The theoretical or conceptual models and frameworks help explain particular phenomena in health and illness and identify important questions for nursing research. The goal of scientific research is to produce this type of knowledge.

Esthetics: The Art of Nursing

Nursing incorporates an artistic, expressive component, which involves knowledge and understanding. As Carper (1978) noted, "The art of nursing involves the active transformation of the patient's behavior into a perception of what is significant in it—that is, what need is being expressed by the behavior" (p. 17). She further stated that perception is beyond mere recognition and, as such, moves nursing activities into the esthetic realm. Qualitative research often explores this area.

Personal Knowledge

This pattern of knowing can be the most difficult to understand and to teach. The nature of the relationship formed with the client and the depth and quality of the interpersonal experience are fundamental to the realm of personal knowledge. As Carper (1978) stated, "Personal knowledge is concerned with the knowing, encountering and actualizing of the concrete, individual self" (p. 18). Many investigators have attempted to understand the nature of therapeutic relationships. Through the rapport established with the client, how does a nurse succeed in assisting that client to reach health goals? Perhaps "the nurse in the therapeutic use of self rejects approaching the patient–client as an object and strives instead to actualize an authentic personal relationship between two persons" (Carper, 1978, p. 19). The knowledge gleaned from experience belongs to this pattern.

Ethics: The Moral Component

Nurses are faced with ethical questions that centre on what ought to be done in particular situations. Ethics goes beyond ethical theories, principles, and codes of professional conduct to include dilemmas such as choosing the better of two or more somewhat unsatisfactory actions. Now that technology can prolong life, ethical dilemmas have become more frequent and complex. As Carper (1978) stated, "The ethical pattern of knowing in nursing requires an understanding of different philosophical positions regarding what is good, what ought to be desired, and what is right; of different ethical frameworks devised for dealing with the complexities of moral judgements; and of various orientations to the notion of obligation" (p. 21).

Emancipatory Knowing: The Social, Economic, and Political Component

Emancipatory knowing makes it possible to create social and structural change (Chinn & Kramer, 2008). It represents the ability to recognize social and political problems of injustice or inequity, to picture how things could be different, and to figure out how to change a difficult situation into one that improves the lives of people. Nurses have dealt with emancipatory knowledge since the nineteenth century, when Florence Nightingale wrote passionately about the inequities in society affecting women. As described by Chinn and Kramer, "Emancipatory knowing is the capacity not only to notice injustices in a social order, but also to critically examine why injustices seem not to be noticed or remain invisible, and to identify social and structural changes that are required to right social and institutional wrongs" (p. 78).

TABLE 7-1 Fundamental Patterns of Knowing in Nursing

Empirics: the science of knowledge development in nursing	Knowledge developed through systematic research to describe and explain phenomena
Esthetics: the art of nursing	Creativity, with an artistic or expressive component
Personal knowledge	Knowledge derived from the depth and power of the interpersonal relationship with the client
Ethics: the moral component	Knowledge that emerges from ethical dilemmas and is based on what ought to be done in particular situations
Emancipatory knowing: the social, economic, and political component	Knowledge that allows change to occur

From Carper, B. A. (1978). Fundamental patterns of knowing in nursing. *Advances in Nursing Science, 1*(1), 13; and Chinn, P., & Kramer, M. (2008). Integrated theory and knowledge development in nursing (p. 78). St. Louis, MO: Mosby/Elsevier.

Nurses benefit from all these ways of knowing. According to the concept of evidence-informed practice, evidence gained from any and all of these means guides nurses to make sound clinical decisions. The knowledge gained from empirics is but one pattern of knowledge, but with it, you can build strength and confidence as you pursue research into nursing questions.

The Development of Research in Nursing

Research is the primary means by which new knowledge is discovered and brought into practice to improve the care that nurses provide to their clients. It is a systematic process in which questions that generate knowledge are asked and answered. This knowledge becomes part of the scientific basis for practice and may be used to validate interventions.

Nursing research is a systematic examination of phenomena important to the nursing discipline, as well as to nurses, their clients, and families. Its purpose is to expand the knowledge base for practice by answering nurses' questions. Nursing research addresses a range of issues related to actual and potential client populations and to individual and family responses to health problems. Some research tests nursing theories; other research generates theory from findings. This "back-and-forth" relationship between theory and research is the way knowledge develops in any discipline (Wood & Ross-Kerr, 2006). In the current health care environment, nursing research is frequently undertaken in multidisciplinary teams, in which nurses examine factors relevant to nursing in the context of the larger health care picture. The scientific knowledge needed for nursing practice is discovered, tested, and enhanced through nursing research. The multidisciplinary nature of nursing challenges nurses not only to keep up with nursing research but also to know the status of research in other health disciplines, as well as in the behavioural, social, and physical sciences.

The International Council of Nurses (ICN; 2007) is a staunch supporter of nursing research as a means to improve people's health and welfare. Research is a way to identify new knowledge, improve education and practice, and use resources effectively. In 1983, the National Center for Nursing Research in the United States and the ICN established priorities for nursing research. These priorities were to promote the in-depth knowledge base for nursing practice, to recognize nursing research as an integral part of nursing practice and education, to facilitate cross-cultural research, to ensure adequate preparation of nurse researchers, and to encourage all national nursing associations to establish ethical research standards (National Center for Nursing Research/ICN, 1990). These priorities are updated regularly. In 1999, the ICN established the ICN Research Network. The Network provides a means for sharing of research ideas, results, and progress around the world. Network members communicate with one another through the ICN Web site, as well as at annual conferences.

In 1995, the CNA, the Canadian Association of Schools of Nursing, and the Canadian Association for Nursing Research developed research priorities. These priorities identified the need to expand the knowledge base for nursing practice in Canada, including the study of contextual issues such as the social, political, and environmental predictors of health; specific clinical populations; and a range of interventions from health promotion strategies to specific clinical measures (Canadian Association of Schools of Nursing, 1997) (Box 7–4).

> **BOX 7-4 Canadian Nursing Research Priorities**
>
> **Priority 1: Nursing Practice**
>
> - Context (including determinants of health, health reform, and ethical issues)
> - Populations (vulnerable groups, as well as specific clinical populations)
> - Interventions (wide range, from health promotion to comfort measures)
>
> **Priority 2: Outcomes**
>
> - Development of valid measures for multiple dimensions
> - Links with clinical judgement
>
> **Priority 3: Enhanced Links Between Research and Practice**
>
> - Development of body of nursing knowledge
>
> Data from Canadian Association of Schools of Nursing. (1997). *Canadian nursing research priorities, results of Phase III of National Nursing Research Symposium.* Ottawa ON: Author. Retrieved November, 2008, from http://www.CAUSN.ca/Research/research.htm

Nursing research improves nursing practice, raising the profession's standards. Involvement in research takes many forms, including designing studies, being on a research team, collecting data, and using research findings to change clinical practice, improve client outcomes, and contain health care costs (Titler et al., 2001). Promoting research and using it in practice increases the scientific knowledge base for nursing practice. Clients benefit from these improvements to practice.

The History of Nursing Research in Canada

During the Crimean War, Florence Nightingale's detailed and systematic observation of nursing actions and outcomes resulted in major changes in nursing practice (Box 7–5). Her work demonstrated the importance of systematic observational research to nursing practice.

In Canada, the establishment of university nursing courses starting in 1918, followed by master's degree programs in the 1950s and 1970s and by doctoral programs in the 1990s and 2000s, was key to the development of nursing research. The first master's degree program, established at the University of Western Ontario in 1959, highlighted the need for Canadian research capacity in nursing.

The first nursing research journal, *Nursing Research,* was launched in the United States in 1952. The first nursing research journal published in Canada, *Nursing Papers* (later the *Canadian Journal of Nursing Research*), was established at McGill University in 1969. Other journals were later established, and today, nurses publish their research, both within nursing and in interdisciplinary fields, in dozens of journals.

Since the 1970s and 1980s, the two major factors in the development of nursing research have been the establishment of research training through doctoral programs and the establishment of funding to support nursing research. Throughout the 1970s and 1980s, university faculties and schools of nursing built their research resources so that they could establish doctoral programs. The first provincially

BOX 7-5 Historical Milestones in the Development of Canadian Nursing Research

1858	Florence Nightingale published *Notes on Matters Affecting the Health, Efficiency and Hospital Administration of the British Army* and *Notes on Hospitals.*
1918	The University of British Columbia launched the first baccalaureate nursing program in Canada.
1952	The American Nurses Association first published the journal *Nursing Research.*
1959	First Canadian Nursing master's degree program was launched at the University of Western Ontario.
1964–1965	The first nursing research project was funded by a Canadian federal granting agency; the *International Journal of Nursing Studies* and *International Nursing Index* were launched.
1969–1970	*Nursing Papers,* forerunner of the *Canadian Journal of Nursing Research,* was published at McGill University; Lysaught's (1970) report, *An Abstract for Action,* recommending increased research in education and practice, was published.
1971	McGill University launched Centre for Nursing Research; first national Canadian conference was held on nursing research; both were financed by the Department of National Health and Welfare.
1975	Commission on Canadian Studies noted that the slow start of graduate programs in Canada, and inadequate funding, resulted in few studies in nursing.
1978	Heads of university nursing schools and deans of graduate studies attended the Kellogg National Seminar on Doctoral Education in Nursing.
1982	The Alberta Foundation for Nursing Research, first funding agency for nursing research, was established; the Working Group on Nursing Research was established by the Medical Research Council (MRC).
1985	Report of the Working Group on Nursing Research was released by the MRC.
1988	The MRC and the National Health Research and Development Program established a joint initiative to structure nursing research grants.
1990	Francine Ducharme was the first nurse to graduate with a PhD in nursing from a Canadian university, through a special case program at McGill University.
1991	First Canadian nursing PhD program was launched at University of Alberta, followed by one at University of British Columbia
1992–1994	PhD programs in nursing were launched at McGill University, University of Toronto, and McMaster University
1992	The MRC mandate was revised to include health research.
1999	The Nursing Research Fund was launched with a $25 million grant over 10 years; the Canadian Health Services Research Foundation administered the funds.
	PhD program in nursing was launched at the University of Calgary.
2003–2008	PhD programs in nursing were initiated at Dalhousie University, the University of Victoria, the University of Western Ontario, the University of Ottawa, l'Université Laval, and l'Université de Sherbrooke.
2004	Forum on doctoral education held in Toronto under the auspices of Canadian Association of Schools of Nursing to develop a national position paper on the PhD in nursing for Canada.

approved doctoral nursing program was established at the University of Alberta Faculty of Nursing in 1991. Another was established at the University of British Columbia School of Nursing later that year, and programs at McGill University and the University of Toronto followed in 1993. Between 1993 and 2008, other programs were launched, which brought the total across Canada to 12.

Growing awareness of the importance of nursing research gradually led to the availability of research funds. The year 1964 marked the first time that a federal granting agency funded nursing research in Canada (Good, 1969). In 1999, 14 years after the US government had established funding for nursing research under the National Institutes of Health, the Canadian government established the Nursing Research Fund, budgeting $25 million for nursing research ($2.5 million over each of the following 10 years); the funds were to be administered by the Canadian Health Services Research Foundation. The research areas targeted for support included nursing policies, management, human resources, and nursing care. A total of $500,000 each year is designated for the Open Grants Competition, $500,000 to the Canadian Nurses Foundation for research on nursing care, $750,000 for training (postdoctoral fellowships and student grants), and $250,000 for knowledge networks and dissemination activities. Five chairs in nursing research, representing excellence in nursing research across Canada, were funded by this initiative. The incumbents were to develop research capacity in a particular area of nursing:

- Dr. Lesley Degner, University of Manitoba: Development of Innovative Nursing Interventions to Influence Practice and Policy in Cancer Care, Palliative Care, and Cancer Prevention
- Dr. Alba Dicenso, McMaster University: Evaluation of Nurse Practitioner/Advanced Practice Nurse Roles and Interventions
- Dr. Nancy Edwards, University of Ottawa: Multiple Interventions in Community Health Nursing Care
- Dr. Janice Lander, University of Alberta: Evaluating Innovative Approaches to Nursing Care
- Dr. Linda O'Brien-Pallas, University of Toronto: Nursing Human Resources for the New Millennium

More information about these five chairs is available at http://www.chsrf.ca/cadre/chair_awards_lca_e.php.

Nursing research has focused progressively on evidence-informed practice in response to demands to justify care practices and systems by improving client outcomes and controlling costs. The scope of nursing research has also broadened to include historical and philosophical inquiry. The establishment of the Institute for Philosophical Nursing Research at the University of Alberta and the Nursing History Research Unit at the University of Ottawa exemplify this new direction.

Three new training centres funded by the Nursing Research Fund at the Canadian Health Services Research Foundation were mandated in order to increase research capacity in nursing and related disciplines:

- The Centre FERASI (http://www.ferasi.umontreal.ca) in Quebec is a joint initiative among l'Université de Montréal, McGill University, and l'Université Laval to build research capacity in the administration of nursing services. It focuses on developing partnerships with health care decision makers in order to provide training opportunities and insights into the decision-making environment. Funding is provided for student scholarships.
- The Ontario Training Centre in Health Services and Policy Research (http://www.otc-hsr.ca) involves six Ontario universities for the purpose of enhancing health services and policy research. The centre is located at McMaster University and involves collaboration with the University of Toronto, York University, the University of Ottawa, Laurentian University, and Lakehead University.
- The Centre for Knowledge Transfer was designed as a national training centre at the University of Alberta providing funding for students and offering courses in knowledge utilization and transfer. This centre is now closed.

Nursing Research

In a mature discipline, practitioners use multiple research methods to develop a unique knowledge base (Wood and Ross-Kerr, 2006). A person continuously acquires knowledge, using critical thinking to interpret and evaluate complex information. Current research can be classified into one of two ways of thinking: scientific or qualitative (interpretive). Both have a great deal to offer when you are seeking evidence to support your practice.

The Scientific Paradigm

The term *paradigm* was introduced by Kuhn (1970) and can be loosely defined as a way of thinking (see Chapter 6). According to Kuhn, a dominant research paradigm can be identified during any one era. Eventually, this paradigm no longer provides solutions to research problems and is challenged by new ideas. It is then replaced by a new paradigm, and the process continues. The dominant paradigm for most of the nineteenth and twentieth centuries has been positivism. Positivism emphasizes tested and systematized experience, rather than speculation, and focuses on the search for cause-and-effect relationships to explain phenomena. In this paradigm, the **scientific method** arose as the major research approach.

Researchers who use the scientific method pose research questions and collect and analyze data to find answers to the questions. The process is rigorous and systematic and is guided by scientific principles, the most important of which is empiricism, which means that only things that can be observed by the human senses can be called *facts*. The focus is on deductive reasoning, in which a **hypothesis** is tested experimentally to confirm or reject theoretical explanations of phenomena.

The scientific method is characterized by systematic, orderly procedures that, although not without fault, are intended to limit the possibility of error and minimize the likelihood that any bias or opinion by the researcher might influence the results of research and, thus, the knowledge gained. Wood and Ross-Kerr (2006) described the **research process** as follows: The process begins with a researchable question. If properly stated, the question guides the rest of the process; thus, asking the question is a crucial step. Three levels of questions exist, and the appropriate level is chosen based on how much is known about the research topic. Once an initial question has been formulated, the literature is searched to discover what is already known about the topic and to determine whether the question must be revised in light of prior knowledge. The level of the question determines the research design needed to answer it. Table 7–2 describes the basic steps in planning nursing research.

The research design provides the ground rules for data collection and analysis, ensuring that the research question will have a valid answer. The design steps are systematic and precise in order to control unwanted influences that might affect the answer. For example, in a study of the relationship between diet and heart disease, influences such as stress or smoking must be controlled because they are known to influence heart disease. The design also specifies the type of sample and sample selection techniques that will provide the most useful data for the study.

Evidence that is part of experience (**empirical data**) is gathered from the sample through measurement techniques that quantify the variables in the research question. Techniques include interviews, tests of knowledge, and physiological measures such as heart rate and blood pressure. When the evidence is analyzed, the result answers the original question and becomes the basis for discovering new knowledge.

A goal of scientific research is to understand phenomena so that the knowledge gained can be applied generally, not just to isolated cases. Researchers achieve this goal by studying a sample that represents a larger population; this increases the likelihood that the results will apply across that population. In the scientific paradigm, researchers conduct studies that contribute to the testing or development of theories, thereby advancing knowledge that can be applied in nursing practice.

The Qualitative (Interpretive) Paradigm

Positivism has been criticized by those academics who believe that reality and people's perception of reality are so intertwined that they cannot be separated. Interpretivism is an alternative to positivism, representing the view that people construct their own world as they strive to make sense of their social environments (Speziale & Carpenter, 2006). The research that is driven by interpretivism can be broadly designated *qualitative research*. Qualitative research avoids the empirical notion of the study of people as objects and strives instead to understand human behaviour in the context of the people being studied. A qualitative researcher studies the behaviours, experiences, perceptions, and motives of individuals in social and cultural settings (Speziale & Carpenter, 2006).

Several approaches to qualitative research exist, and each is very different from the others. Unlike the scientific approach, many qualitative approaches have their own unique philosophic base, which makes comparisons difficult. Speziale and Carpenter (2006, p. 21) identified the following six characteristics common to all qualitative research:

- Belief in multiple realities.
- Commitment to identifying an approach to understanding that will support the phenomenon studied.
- Commitment to the participant's point of view.
- Conduct of inquiry in a way that does not disturb the natural context of the phenomena of interest.
- Acknowledged participation of the researcher in the research.
- Conveyance of the understanding of phenomena by reporting in a literary style rich with participants' commentary.

The idea of multiple realities is a challenge to positivist thinking, which proposes that researchers are searching for one reality or truth. Interpretivists say that because the experience of each individual is unique, each individual can come to know the world differently, which implies that many truths exist, rather than one. This

TABLE 7-2 Basic Steps in Planning Nursing Research

Steps	Level I	Level II	Level III
Question	What?	What is the relationship?	Why?
Problem	Little known about topic	Conceptual base; variables have been studied before	Theoretical base
Purpose	Declarative statement	Question or hypothesis	Hypothesis
Design	Exploratory descriptive	Descriptive survey, correlational or comparative	Experiment
Sample	Convenience sample or total population	Probability sample	Random assignment to treatment and control groups
Methods	Qualitative, unstructured data; some quantitative descriptive data	Quantitative data collected by all methods	Quantitative data
Analysis	Content analysis; descriptive statistic	Correlation or tests of association; regression analysis	Differences between means: t test, analysis of variance (ANOVA)
Answer	Description of processes, concepts, or population	Explanation of relationship among variables	Test of theory

Adapted from Wood, M., & Ross-Kerr, J. (2006). *Basic steps in planning nursing research: From question to proposal*. Sudbury, MA: Jones & Bartlett. Copyright © 2006: Jones & Bartlett. Reprinted with permission.

belief leads qualitative researchers to seek multiple ways of understanding the world and to change methods and data collection strategies as needed, rather than following a single prescribed set of strategies. It follows that the participant's point of view would be the focus of the research and would guide the process. The researcher becomes a coparticipant in the process of understanding the participant's point of view.

Qualitative research is carried out in the participants' natural setting to maintain a natural context. The researcher is a participant and acknowledges that being a participant will affect the other participants and the setting. Objectivity is not a goal in qualitative research; rather, subjectivity from the participants' perspective is sought. Because of the nature of the data, rich with personal experience and example, the research is usually reported in a literary style, similar to storytelling. Liberal quotation from the participants adds to the detail of the report.

Research Designs

Nursing research approaches vary, depending on the specific problem to be studied. The paradigms of positivism and interpretivism lead to two research approaches, often categorized as quantitative (scientific method) and qualitative (interpretive). Neither is used exclusively in nursing research, although the scientific method is dominant. Nonetheless, interpretivism and qualitative methods have much to offer nursing research. The next section describes some common research designs in these two categories.

Scientific Nursing Research

Scientific nursing research (quantitative nursing research) is the investigation of nursing phenomena that can be precisely measured and quantified. Examples are pain severity, rates of wound healing, and body temperature changes. These designs fall within the scientific paradigm and provide rigorous, systematic, objective examination of specific concepts and their relationships. The goal is to test theory and use numerical data, statistical analysis, and controls to eliminate bias (Polit & Beck, 2004; Wood & Ross-Kerr, 2006).

Experimental Research. Experimental design is the hallmark of scientific research. Experiments are appropriate designs for questions at level III (see Table 7–2), which concern why one variable causes a predictable change in another variable. In a **true experiment**, the conditions under which the variables are studied are tightly controlled to provide objective testing of hypotheses, which predict cause-and-effect relationships. Experimental research requires that the data be collected and quantified in a prescribed manner.

The requirements of a true experiment are as follows:

- The study usually includes at least one control or comparison group, which does not receive the nursing treatment or intervention being investigated. The results for this group are compared with those of the experimental group, which is the group that receives the treatment or intervention. The **subjects**—people selected for the comparison and experimental groups—are randomly assigned to these groups, so that the groups are as similar as possible to each other before the intervention. Random assignment of subjects ensures that all subjects have the same chance to be in the control or experimental (treatment) group and that variables that could affect the outcome of the study are randomly distributed between the groups and therefore are no more likely to affect experimental subjects than to affect control subjects.
- An experimental variable must be manipulated by the researcher. For example, in a study of the effect of preoperative teaching on postoperative anxiety, the researcher manipulates preoperative teaching by providing it for the experimental group but not for

the control group. The expectation is that the differences in postoperative anxiety measures between the two groups can be attributed to the effect of preoperative teaching because all other factors are under control. However, the researcher cannot control subjects' prior experiences, such as hearing other clients' stories about surgery. Psychological factors, which cannot be controlled, may influence a subject's level of anxiety. If subjects are randomly assigned to the two groups, however, those with negative prior experiences should be distributed equally between the two groups, and these experiences would affect both groups equally. Thus, differences between the groups in postoperative anxiety can still be attributed to the preoperative teaching intervention.

- The researcher proposes theory-based and statistically tested hypotheses about the action of the variables to answer the research question. For example, in a study of preoperative teaching, the hypothesis might be as follows: "Clients who receive interactive preoperative teaching will have significantly lower postoperative anxiety levels than will clients who receive other teaching methods." The researcher must explain why a lower anxiety level is expected in a discussion of the theory behind the study.

A **quasi-experimental research design** is one in which groups are formed and the conditions are controlled, but the subjects are not randomly assigned to a control group or to treatment conditions. These designs also answer level III questions (Wood & Ross-Kerr, 2006). In many health care settings, assigning subjects randomly to experimental and control groups is not feasible. Quasi-experimental research is often carried out for practical reasons related to the subjects themselves. For example, to test the effect of a new intervention in the care of clients with Alzheimer's disease, carrying out two treatments on the unit at the same time might confuse the subjects. A quasi-experiment could entail the use of two care units: one as the experimental unit, in which all subjects receive the new intervention, and the second as the control group, in which subjects receive the usual care but not the new intervention. The two groups are compared before and after the intervention with regard to the outcome variable. The weakness in a quasi-experiment is that the researcher does not know whether the two groups were equivalent before the intervention. Unrecognized differences between the two units might exist that could influence the outcome of the study. For instance, subjects in one unit might have more cognitive impairment than do those in the other unit, and this difference could influence the outcome.

Descriptive Survey Designs. Surveys are designed to answer level II questions about relationships among variables. The research question that leads to a survey design begins with "What is the relationship between . . . ?" and addresses two or more variables (Wood and Ross –Kerr, 2006): for example, the relationship between ethnicity and suicide among university students.

In many types of research, investigators use surveys in which people in a group are compared with regard to two or more variables. The purpose is to discover relationships among variables in the population. In a survey design, the sample determines whether the survey yields informative or uninformative results. The sample should be representative of the population so that generalizations can be made on the basis of the sample data. Surveys contain three key elements: First, a random sample of the population must be drawn, from which inferences can be made about the population. Second, the population sampled should be large enough to keep sampling error to a minimum. Third, the measurement tools (e.g., questionnaires, interviews) must yield accurate measurements of the study variables.

Exploratory Descriptive Designs. Exploratory descriptive designs provide in-depth descriptions of populations or variables not previously studied. Level I (basic) questions are asked because not much is known about the topic. They typically begin with "what"; for example, "What are the health-promoting behaviours of older adults living in subsidized housing?" The results provide a detailed description of the variable or population. No relationships among variables are posited at this stage, although the results might indicate that relationships should be examined in subsequent research.

Data Analysis. Except for some exploratory descriptive studies in which the outcome is a verbal description, all quantitative studies entail the use of statistical analysis. In experimental designs, researchers must discover whether the experimental and control groups are significantly different from each other after the intervention has been applied. Statistical tests that provide a test of group means are generally used for experiments.

Descriptive survey designs entail the use of statistical techniques to test for significant relationships among the variables. In general, these are correlational tests that indicate whether one subject's score on one variable (e.g., blood pressure) is related to the same subject's score on another variable (e.g., weight). The results of a correlational analysis of these two variables would reveal how much influence increased body weight has on blood pressure.

Exploratory descriptive studies entail the use of several techniques to analyze data, depending on the type collected. Unstructured data that do not lend themselves to numerical form are summarized verbally. If quantitative measures are used to collect the data, they can be described both numerically and verbally. Descriptions usually include measures of central tendency (mean, median, or mode) and dispersion (range, standard deviation).

Qualitative Nursing Research

Qualitative nursing research poses questions about nursing phenomena that cannot be quantified and measured. Examples are the study of the experience of pregnancy and the culture of a long-term care facility. To answer questions about these phenomena, researchers must understand the perspective of the person in the situation. Researchers using qualitative methods can choose one of many design strategies. Examples of three qualitative designs (ethnography, phenomenology, and grounded theory) are discussed in the following sections, but keep in mind that many other qualitative approaches, such as participatory action research, interpretive descriptive research, and narrative inquiry, are used in nursing research. As with scientific research, the research question is the basis for the choice of design. In addition, each of the various qualitative methods has its own unique underlying philosophy. Ethnography is chosen if the research question leads to the study of behaviour within a specific group or culture, phenomenology if the question relates to the lived experience of the participants, and grounded theory if the question is about a social process.

Ethnography. Ethnography involves the observation and description of behaviour in social settings. It is derived from anthropology, and it provides the means to study the culture of groups of people. Anthropologists use participant observation as the major source of data collection, together with other sources such as artifacts and photographs. Nurse researchers use ethnography to study the behaviour of nurses and their clients in a variety of settings. The goal of ethnography is to understand the culture of the study population as the culture is practised in its own setting. The focus is on the cultural norms and social forces that shape behaviour in a given setting. The researcher becomes an accepted member of the community under study and collects data through repeated interviews of informants from the community. Data collection continues until understanding has been reached about why the members of the community behave as they do. Interview data are supplemented by other forms, such as artifacts and historical documents; the result is a detailed description of the culture. For example, Lauzon Clabo (2008) examined nursing pain assessment practice across two units, to seek variation that might exist and to examine the impact of the social context on pain assessment practice. The ethnographic analysis revealed a predominant pattern of pain assessment on each unit that was profoundly shaped by the social context of the unit.

Phenomenology. The focus of **phenomenology** is on the lived experience of a specific phenomenon from the perspective of the people who are in the situation. Phenomenology has its roots in German philosophy of the early twentieth century, stemming from the philosopher Edmund Husserl (1931/1962), who posited that only people who experience phenomena are capable of communicating these experiences. The researcher must learn to understand a phenomenon from the viewpoint of people experiencing it. For example, an investigator may want to study the impact of surrogate decision making regarding end-of-life decisions (Jeffers, 1998). The goal of this research is to describe fully the lived experience of surrogate decision makers, their perceptions of the surrogate role, the decision-making process, and the meaning of the decisions. The source of the data is the subject, and the data are the result of in-depth conversations. The units of analysis are the conversations, which are coded and analyzed to extract the meaning to the subjects of the phenomenon.

Grounded Theory. **Grounded theory** as a research method was developed by Glaser and Strauss (1967) as a means of generating hypotheses and theories about social processes inductively from the data. The grounded theory is "discovered," developed, and verified through a rigorous process of data collection and analysis. Glaser and Strauss advocated that researchers not review the literature before carrying out the study because they might be influenced by what others have found. The strength of the grounded theory approach comes from examining the situation afresh and opening up the possibility of a new perspective on an old problem.

For example, Mills et al. (2007) studied mentoring among rural nurses in the Australian workforce by using a grounded theory approach. The social process that was identified in this study was called "Live my work," stemming from the mentors' own histories of living and working in the same community. Personal strategies adapted to local context were the skills that these mentors passed on to neophyte nurses in rural areas through mentoring, which at the same time protected them through troubleshooting and translating local cultural norms.

Conducting Nursing Research

Nurses conduct research in a variety of settings. Student nurses and practitioners participate in investigations of client outcomes and nursing care, commonly called *quality assurance* or *improvement studies* (see Chapter 11). Data are collected to determine the influence of nurses on achievement of client care objectives in a particular clinical setting. Because the results usually apply only to one facility, this research is not scientific. However, it is important to the facility involved because the study can demonstrate the contributions made by nurses to client care and the facility can improve processes if necessary.

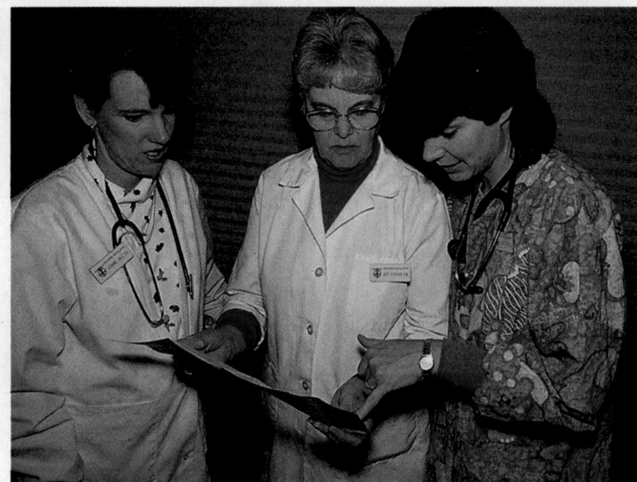

Figure 7-2 Nurses collaborating on research.

Clinical nursing research should be undertaken by nurses educated to conduct scientific investigations (Figure 7–2). An experienced researcher is usually more qualified than a beginner to undertake a complex, long-term project. Nurses new to research may, however, assist with data collection, conduct replication studies (studies previously performed elsewhere), or conduct less complex studies.

Ethical Issues in Research

Research must meet ethical standards in ways that respect the dignity and preserve the well-being of human research participants. In Canada, every health care facility and university receiving public funds for research must meet federal standards for protecting human research participants. The most recent standard is the *Tri-Council Policy Statement* (Canadian Institutes of Health Research et al., 2003), which requires that the institution have in place a research ethics board (REB) to review all research proposals to determine whether ethical principles are being upheld (Box 7–6). The REB focuses on **informed consent** and weighs benefits versus harms from the research. No research may be performed in a university or health care facility without the approval of the REB. All proposals are subject to review. However, if data collection processes (such as quality assurance studies) are a normal part of institutional business, performance reviews, or testing within normal educational requirements and are not for research purposes, they are exempt from REB review.

To refine existing knowledge and develop new knowledge, investigators in clinical research sometimes use new procedures whose outcome is doubtful or unknown. This research may seem to conflict with the purpose of nursing practice, which is to meet specific clients' needs. In such cases, the investigator must structure the research to avoid or minimize harm to the subjects. Although not all undesirable effects can be anticipated, investigators are obligated to inform everyone involved about the known potential risks. Other basic human rights must also be observed. These principles are set forth by the CNA (2008). Procedures for obtaining informed consent must be outlined in the study protocol. The consent form must describe in lay language the purpose of the study, the role of the subjects, types of data that are to be obtained, how the data are obtained, the duration of the study, subject selection, procedures, risks to the subject (including financial risks), potential benefits (including the possibility of no

BOX 7-6 Guiding Ethical Principles for Research in Canada

1. *Respect for human dignity:* This principle is designed to protect the multiple and interdependent interests of the person (i.e., their bodily, psychological, and cultural integrity).
2. *Respect for free and informed consent:* This principle presumes that individuals have the capability and right to make free and informed decisions.
3. *Respect for vulnerable persons:* Children, institutionalized people, or others who are vulnerable are entitled, on grounds of human dignity, caring, solidarity, and fairness, to special protection against abuse, exploitation, or discrimination.
4. *Respect for privacy and confidentiality:* Standards of privacy and confidentiality protect the access, control, and dissemination of personal information and thus help protect mental or psychological integrity. These standards are consonant with values underlying privacy, confidentiality, and anonymity.
5. *Respect for justice and inclusiveness:* The ethics review process should be independent and use fair methods, standards, and procedures. No segment of the population should be unfairly burdened with the harms of research. Investigators have particular obligations to protect vulnerable individuals unable to protect their own interests. Individuals and groups who may benefit from advances in research must neither be discriminated against nor be neglected.
6. *Balancing harms and benefits:* Research ethics require a favourable harms–benefit balance so that the foreseeable harms should not outweigh anticipated benefits.
7. *Minimizing harm:* Nonmaleficence (the duty to avoid, prevent, or minimize harms to others) is considered essential in research. No research subjects should be subjected to unnecessary risks of harm, and their participation in research must be essential to achieving important aims for science and for society.
8. *Maximizing benefit:* Beneficence, the duty to benefit others, in research ethics means a duty to maximize net benefits. In most research, the primary benefits produced are for society and for the advancement of knowledge, rather than for the individual research participant.

Adapted from Canadian Institutes of Health Research, the Natural Sciences and Engineering Research Council of Canada, & the Social Sciences and Humanities Research Council of Canada. (2003). *Tri-Council policy statement: Ethical conduct for research involving humans, 1998* (with 2000, 2002, and 2005 amendments). Retrieved August 20, 2008, from http://www.pre.ethics.gc.ca/english/policystatement/policystatement.cfm

benefit), alternatives to participation, and contact information concerning the principal investigator and local REB. The consent process gives subjects complete information regarding the study's risks, benefits, and costs so that they can make an informed decision.

The REB also determines whether the investigator has the necessary knowledge and skills to undertake the research, including familiarity with the clinical area in which the data will be collected and sufficient research training and experience. For example, a nurse planning a study of psychiatric clients should be familiar with psychiatric nursing principles and theory, as well as research procedures for data collection and analysis.

Rights of Other Research Participants

Student nurses and practising nurses may be asked to participate in research as data collectors or may be involved in the care of clients participating in a study. All participants, including health care professionals, have the right to be fully informed about the study, its procedures (including the consent process and risk factors), and physical or emotional injuries that clients could experience as a result of participation. Often, the physical risks are more obvious than the emotional risks. For example, clients may be asked to give highly personal, intrusive information; some may find this experience stressful. The researcher should prepare all participants, including nurses delivering care, for this possibility and assist them in coping with the effects. Participants also have the right to see review forms from the REB that certify approval of the study. Participants can refuse to perform research procedures if they are concerned about ethical aspects.

Applying Research Findings to Nursing Practice

Research evidence as a basis for scholarly, professional decision making in clinical practice is essential for providing competent, efficient, and state-of-the art nursing care (McCaughan et al., 2002). Advances in care through research are meaningless unless they are accessible to nurses at the point of care. You make links between research findings and nursing care by reading relevant literature, identifying appropriate clinical problems, and incorporating **evidence-informed practice** activities into the nursing practice of your nursing unit or agency (Box 7–7).

In a policy statement, the CNA (2002) stated that evidence-informed decision making by registered nurses is key to quality nursing practice. Nurses need not only skills to access and appraise existing research but also scientific knowledge and skills to change practice settings and to promote evidence-informed decisions about client care.

Evidence-informed nursing practice deemphasizes ritual, isolated, and unsystematic clinical experiences; ungrounded opinion; and tradition as bases for nursing practice. It stresses the use of research findings and, as appropriate, quality improvement data, other evaluation data, and the consensus of recognized experts and affirmed experience to support a specific practice (Stetler et al., 1998). Many aspects of health care are not justly served by the research in only one discipline. The expertise of several disciplines must be brought to bear on complex health issues. Just as nurses play a vital role on the health care team, so they are crucial to multidisciplinary health research. Policymakers in the broader arena of health care must account for nursing practice, which is so essential to client care. Nurses need a sound knowledge base to support practice, and research is essential for building that knowledge.

* KEY CONCEPTS

- Nursing knowledge has five patterns: empirics, esthetics, personal knowledge, ethics, and emancipatory knowledge.
- A scientific investigation is an orderly, planned, and controlled study of real-life situations that tests theories and whose results can be applied to general situations.
- In nursing research, physical or psychosocial responses of people of all ages in various states of health and illness are examined.

BOX 7-7 RESEARCH HIGHLIGHT

Comparison of Two Aerobic Training Programs on Outcomes for Women After a Cardiac Event

Research Focus

This study (Arthur et al., 2007) was carried out by a multidisciplinary team of researchers in cardiac rehabilitation, in an attempt to maximize the effect of exercise on the quality of life of women after myocardial infarction or cardiac surgery.

Research Abstract

The purpose of this study was to compare the effect and sustainability of a six-month combined aerobic and strength training program with those of aerobic training alone in women who had undergone coronary bypass graft surgery or who had experienced myocardial infarction. The primary outcome was improved health-related quality of life. Secondary outcomes were increases in perceived self-efficacy, strength, and exercise capacity.

The study was a two-group RCT. Ninety-two participants meeting the study criteria were randomly assigned to the two study groups. Measurements were taken at baseline, after two months, at the completion of the six-month exercise training program, and one year after discharge from the six-month program, which was 18 months after baseline measurements.

Participants were eligible to be in the study if (1) they were women, (2) they had undergone coronary artery bypass grafting or experienced myocardial infarction 8–10 weeks previously, (3) they were post-menopausal, (4) they were able to attend a supervised exercise program regularly, and (5) they were able to complete English-language questionnaires. Participants who exhibited negative responses to exercise were excluded from the study.

The study was approved by the Research Ethics Board of McMaster University and the Hamilton Health Sciences Centre.

Both groups attended an intitial eight-week session of twice-a-week aerobics classes. Both groups were expected to attend supervised exercise seeions (separately) twice per week for six months. The sessions included 10–15 minutes of warm-up exercises, followed by aerobic interval training with stationary bicycles, treadmills, arm ergometers, and stair climbers. The total exercise time for both groups was 40 minutes per session, followed by a cool-down period of 10–15 minutes. After the initial eight weeks, 20–25 minutes of strength training was implemented in the treatment group in addition to aerobic exercise.

Results revealed no important baseline differences between groups with regard to demographics, medical history, peak volume of oxygen consumption (VO_2), peak metabolic equivalents level, or strength. The main outcome, health-related quality of life, improved over the six months of exercise training in both groups. However, one year after the completion of the intervention, scores differed significantly, in favor of the group with combined aerobic-strength training. Both groups experienced significant increases from baseline in both self-efficacy and strength, but these levels were not statistically significant between groups.

These findings demonstrate that strength training may be an important exercise intervention for female cardiac patients, inasmuch as most activities performed by persons in later life, especially after a cardiac event, require strength, not endurance. Both physical and psychological gains are apparent with either form of exercise, but it is likely that sustained or continued improvements may be achieved most efficiently through combined strength and aerobic training in woman with coronary artery disease.

Implications for Practice

- Women who have experienced a cardiac event should be encouraged to attend a supervised aerobic exercise program as part of their rehabilitation.
- A combined aerobic and strength-training program is likely to most effectively prepare these women to resume independent activities of daily living.

References: Arthur, H. M., Gunn, E., Thorpe, K. E., Ginis, K. M., Mataseje, L., McCartney, N., & McKelvie, M. (2007). Effect of aerobic vs. combined aerobic-strength training on 1 year post-cardiac rehabilitation outcomes in women after a cardiac event. *Journal of Rehabilitation Medicine, 39*(9), 730–735.

- In an experimental research study, investigators control factors that could influence the results, include comparison and experimental treatment groups of subjects, and use random means for selecting study subjects.
- In a qualitative research study, investigators organize information in narrative format so that phenomena can be described and patterns of relationships can be discovered.
- When human subjects participate in research, the researcher must obtain informed consent of study subjects, must maintain the confidentiality of subjects, and must protect subjects from undue risk or injury.
- When summarizing data reported in a research study, the nurse should note when, how, where, and by whom the investigation was conducted and who and what were studied.
- A researchable clinical nursing problem is one that is not satisfactorily resolved by current nursing interventions, occurs frequently in a particular group, can be measured or observed, and has a possible solution within the realm of nursing practice.
- To determine whether research findings can be used in nursing practice, the nurse considers the scientific worth of the study by substantiating evidence from other studies, the similarity of the research setting to the nurse's own clinical practice setting, the status of current nursing theory, and factors affecting the feasibility of application.

✻ CRITICAL THINKING EXERCISES

1. The nurse is concerned about learning to properly treat a pressure ulcer. Explain the benefits to the client if the nurse learns how to treat the sore by drawing from information in the research literature rather than using the scientific method.
2. The research literature reflects many different methods for treating pressure ulcers. If you wished to determine the best method for doing this, what type of research design would you use?
3. The nurses working on an orthopedic unit decide to study the factors that commonly result in clients' falling in their unit. How could they design a study to answer their questions?

* REVIEW QUESTIONS

1. The first provincially approved doctoral program in nursing was established in
   1. 1969
   2. 1974
   3. 1982
   4. 1991
2. Empirics is described by Carper (1978) as
   1. The artistic expression of knowledge
   2. Knowledge derived from the interpersonal relationship with the client
   3. Knowledge derived from ethical dilemmas
   4. Knowledge systematically organized into general laws and theories
3. The scientific method is characterized by
   1. Systematic procedures that seek to limit error and eliminate bias
   2. Studies of behaviours, experiences, perceptions, and motives
   3. A commitment to the participants' point of view
   4. The use of the participants' natural setting
4. If the research question leads to the study of behaviour within a specific culture, the design chosen is
   1. Phenomenology
   2. Grounded theory
   3. Ethnography
   4. Quantitative research
5. Subjectivity is the goal of
   1. Positivism
   2. Qualitative research
   3. True experiments
   4. The scientific method
6. Which research method is quantitative?
   1. Grounded theory
   2. Phenomenology
   3. Ethnography
   4. Quasi-experimental research
7. A sample in a survey design
   1. Is the main component of qualitative research
   2. Should be representative of the population surveyed
   3. Should be small enough to keep sampling error to a minimum
   4. Should be no different from the control group
8. Procedures for obtaining informed consent do *not* include
   1. Describing the purpose of the study
   2. Describing the role of the subjects
   3. Giving the names of other participants in the study
   4. Describing the risks that the subject may incur
9. In a quasi-experimental research design, subjects are assigned to
   1. An empirical group
   2. An ethnographic group
   3. Either a control group or a treatment condition, but not randomly
   4. An experimental group
10. Evidence-informed practice
    1. Enables the transfer of clinical practice techniques into a positivist paradigm
    2. Requires that evidence be always research based
    3. Is synonymous with research-based practice
    4. Entails the use of knowledge based on research studies and takes into account a nurse's clinical experience and client preferences.

* RECOMMENDED WEB SITES

Canadian Nurses Association: http://www.cna-aiic.ca/cna/
This Web site contains information about policies and position statements for nursing research in Canada, as well as information about research funding.

Canadian Nurses Foundation: http://www.cnf-fiic.ca/
This Web site provides information about available research funding and about scholarships for students.

The Canadian Health Services Research Foundation: http://www.chsrf.ca
This Web site contains information about funding for health services research and about the Nursing Research Fund.

Canadian Institutes of Health Research (CIHR): http://www.cihr.ca
This Web site contains pages for all 13 CIHR institutes.

8

Nursing Values and Ethics

Original chapter by Margaret Ecker, RN, MS

Canadian content written by Shelley Raffin Bouchal, RN, PhD

objectives

Mastery of content in this chapter will enable you to:

- Define the key terms listed.
- Discuss the role of values in the study of ethics.
- Examine and clarify personal values.
- Discuss how values influence client care.
- Explain the relationship between ethics and professional practice.
- Describe some basic ethical philosophies relevant to health care.
- Apply a method of ethical analysis to a clinical situation.
- Identify contemporary ethical issues in nursing practice.

media resources

evolve Web Site

- Audio Chapter Summaries
- Glossary
- Multiple-Choice Review Questions
- Student Learning Activities
- Weblinks

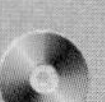

Companion CD

- Glossary
- Interactive Learning Activities
- Fluids and Electrolytes Tutorial
- Test-Taking Skills

key terms

Accountability, p. 92
Advance directives, p. 98
Adverse events, p. 99
Advocacy, p. 92
Answerability, p. 92
Autonomy, p. 93
Beneficence, p. 94
Bioethics, p. 93
Biomedical ethics, p. 93
Care theory, p. 94
Code of ethics, p. 90
Consequentialism, p. 93
Constrained moral agency, p. 93
Cultural values, p. 90
Deontology, p. 93
Embodiment, p. 95
Engagement, p. 95
Environment, p. 95
Ethical dilemma, p. 95
Ethics, p. 90
Feminist ethics, p. 94
Informed consent, p. 98
Justice, p. 94
Medical futility, p. 98
Moral distress, p. 99
Moral integrity, p. 99
Moral residue, p. 99
Morality, p. 91
Mutuality, p. 95
Nonmaleficence, p. 94
Relational ethics, p. 94
Responsibility, p. 92
Social justice, p. 94
Teleology, p. 93
Utilitarianism, p. 93
Value, p. 90
Values clarification, p. 90
Whistleblowing, p. 99

Values and ethics are inherent in all nursing acts. A **value** is a strong personal belief and an ideal that a person or group (such as nurses) strives to uphold. **Ethics** is the study of the philosophical ideals of right and wrong behaviour. The term also commonly refers to the values and standards to which individuals and professions strive to uphold (e.g., health care ethics, nursing ethics). In other words, ethics are a reflection of what matters most to people or professions. Nurses and other health care professionals agree to national codes of ethics that offer guidelines for responding to difficult situations that occur in practice and demonstrate to the public an overview of professional practice standards. For example, the Canadian Nurses Association (CNA; 2008) publishes a **code of ethics** that outlines nurses' professional values and ethical commitments to their clients and the communities they serve.

Because of their prominent and intimate role in the provision of health care, nurses continually make decisions about the correct course of action in different circumstances. In many situations, no answer or course of action is best. To manage such difficult situations, nurses need a keen awareness of their values and those of their clients, a good understanding of ethics, and a sound approach to ethical decision making. They also must be guided by a broader understanding of ethics through the application of philosophies, theories, and sets of principles.

Values

Values are at the heart of ethics. Values influence behaviour on the basis of the conviction that a certain action is correct in a certain situation. An individual's values reflect cultural and social influences, relationships, and personal needs. Values vary among people, and they develop and change over time. In the context of beliefs about morality, values generate rights and duties.

In nursing, value statements express broad ideals of nursing care and establish reasonable directions for practice. The CNA (2008) *Code of Ethics* is organized around seven values that are central to ethical nursing practice. These values include providing safe, compassionate, competent, and ethical care; promoting health and well-being; being accountable; and preserving dignity. Each provincial nursing association also has shared values, such as those held in position statements and practice standards. These standards reflect the values of the profession and clarify what is expected of you as a practising nurse.

Because of the intimacy of the nurse–client relationship, you must be aware of your personal values, as well as the values of clients, physicians, employers, or other groups. To understand the values of others, it is important to understand your own values: what they are, where they came from, and how they relate to others' values.

Values Formation

People acquire values in many ways, beginning in early childhood. Throughout childhood and adolescence, people learn to distinguish right from wrong and to form values on which to base their actions. This is known as *moral development* (see Chapter 23). Family experiences strongly influence value formation.

Values are also learned outside the family. A person's culture, ethnic background, and religious community strongly influences that person's values, as do schools, peer groups, and work environments. **Cultural values** are those adopted as a result of a social setting (see Chapter 10). A basic task of the young adult is to identify personal values within the context of the community. Over time, the person acquires values by choosing some values that are strongly upheld in the community and by discarding or transforming others. A person's experience as well as lack of experience also influences his or her values.

Values Clarification

Within the context of nursing, several layers of values inform the ethical questions and actions that you consider in your practice. Clarifying your values helps you articulate what matters most and what priorities are guiding your life and decision making. Values influence how you interpret confusing or conflicting information. As you mature and experience new situations, your values change. You may reorder your values or replace old values with new ones. As a result, you may modify your attitudes and behaviour. The willingness to change reflects a healthy attitude and an ability to adapt to new experiences.

To adopt new values, you must be aware of your existing values and how they affect behaviour. **Values clarification** is the process of appraising personal values (Box 8–1). It is not a set of rules, nor does it suggest that certain values should be accepted by all people; rather, it is a process of personal reflection. When you clarify your values, you make careful choices. The result of values clarification is greater self-awareness and personal insight.

By understanding your personal values, you will better understand your clients' and colleagues' values. In *value conflict*, personal values are at odds with those of a client, a colleague, or an institution. Values clarification plays a major role in resolving these dilemmas. In addition, you can better advocate for a client when you can identify your personal values and the values of the client.

➤ BOX 8-1 Values Clarification Questions

- Describe a situation in your personal or professional experience in which you felt uncomfortable, in which you believed that your beliefs and values were being challenged, or in which you believed your values were different from others.
- As you record the situation, mention how you felt physically and emotionally at the time you experienced the situation.
- Write down your feelings as you remember the situation. Are your current reactions any different from those when you were actually in the situation?
- What personal values do you identify in the situation? Try to remember where and from whom you learned these values. Do you completely agree with the values, or do you question some aspect of the values, or do you wonder about their validity?
- What values do you think were being expressed by others involved? Are they similar to or different from your own values?
- What do you think you reacted to in the situation?
- Can you remember having similar reactions in other situations? If you do, how were the situations similar or different?
- How do you feel about your response to the situation? If you could repeat the scenario, would you change something about it? Rewrite the scenario with the same changes. What might be the consequences of these same changes?
- How do you feel about the new scenario?
- What do you need to do to reinforce behaviours, ideals, beliefs, and qualities that you have identified as personal values in this situation? When and how can you do this?

From Burkhardt, M.A., & Nathaniel, A. K. (2007). *Ethics and issues in contemporary nursing* (3rd ed.). Albany, NY: Thomson Delmar Learning. © Delmar, a part of Cengage Learning, Inc. Reproduced by permission (www.cengage.com/permissions).

Once you master the skill of clarifying personal values, you can help clients identify their personal priorities, values, and emotions. This may help clients resolve conflicts between values and behaviours. The goal of values clarification with clients is effective nurse–client communication. As the client becomes more willing to express problems and feelings, you can collaborate with the client in developing an individualized plan of care.

Structured communication is a useful way in which to clarify values with a client. Simple strategies that promote the process of sharing feelings can be effective. For example, responding to a client by repeating the client's sentence as a question ("You wish you could be at home?") encourages the client to continue the story. Instead of asking questions that can be answered by only "yes" or "no," you can encourage the client to answer in greater detail. For example, rather than asking, "Do you want to live at home with your daughter?" the nurse might say, "Tell me how you feel about living at home with your daughter."

Your response can motivate the client to examine personal thoughts and actions. When you make a clarifying response, it should be brief and nonjudgemental. For example, when talking with a client who exercises only rarely, you might ask, "What is your understanding of the purpose of exercise?" An effective clarifying response encourages the client to think about personal values after the exchange is over and does not impose your own values onto the client. In this way, you respect the client's self-direction and avoid inappropriately introducing personal values into the conversation.

Values clarification plays a key role in communication. In particular, when the topic concerns issues of personal health, private habits, and quality of life, participants in a discussion benefit from clarity of values. In appreciating values, you can identify differences between personal opinion and the values that others embrace. Through values clarification, you can better serve the needs of clients, especially when values differ. By demonstrating respect for the client's differences and helping the client to clarify values, you are better able to teach and to heal.

Ethics

Ethics is the study of good conduct, character, and motives. It is concerned with determining what is good or valuable for all people. Often the terms *ethics* and *morals*, or *morality*, are used interchangeably (Johnstone, 2004), inasmuch as both words are derived from an original meaning of "custom or habit." Johnstone suggested that it is not incorrect to use these terms interchangeably and that the choice is a matter of personal preference rather than of philosophical debate. The classic textbook definition of *ethics* is a "generic term for various ways of understanding and examining the moral life" (Beauchamp & Childress, 2001, p. 1). Essentially, ethics requires you to be critically reflective exploring your values, behaviours, actions, judgements, and justifications (Beauchamp & Childress, 2001, p xii). In this chapter, the terms *ethics* and *morals* are used interchangeably.

Professional Nursing and Ethics

Codes of Ethics. A "code of ethics serves as a foundation for nurses' ethical practice" (CNA, 2008, p. 3) and is accepted by all members of a profession. The code is a statement of the ethical values of nurses and of nurses' commitments to clients with health care needs and clients who receive care. It is intended for nurses in all contexts and domains of practice and at all levels of decision making. The code is relevant for all nurses in their practices with individuals, families, communities, and public health care systems. The code developed by nurses for nurses serves the profession when questions arise about practising ethically and working through ethical challenges (CNA, 2008). The nursing code of ethics, as in other professions, sets forth ideals of conduct.

"The code provides guidance for ethical relationships, responsibilities, behaviours and decision-making and it is to be used in conjunction with professional standards, laws and regulations that guide practice" (CNA, 2008, p. 4). It does not provide rules of behaviour for every circumstance. Situations are unique to the context in which they occur. The environment or institution can greatly influence the values that you are encouraged to uphold. Furthermore, a code does not offer guidance as to which values should take priority or how to balance them in practice.

The CNA and the International Council of Nurses (2006) have established widely accepted codes for nurses that reflect the principles of responsibility, accountability, and advocacy (Boxes 8–2 and 8–3).

➤ BOX 8-2 Canadian Nurses Association Code of Ethics

The following is the CNA's statement of the seven values that must be upheld in nursing practice. The complete code of ethics also includes responsibility statements outlining how nurses can incorporate these values into their practice; it can be found on the CNA Web site (see the "Recommended Web Sites" section at the end of this chapter).

Providing Safe, Compassionate, Competent, and Ethical Care

Nurses provide safe, compassionate, competent, and ethical care.

Promoting Health and Well-Being

Nurses work with clients to enable them to attain their highest level of health and well-being.

Promoting and Respecting Informed Decision Making

Nurses recognize, respect, and promote a client's right to be informed and make decisions.

Preserving Dignity

Nurses recognize and respect the intrinsic worth of each client.

Maintaining Privacy and Confidentiality

Nurses recognize the importance of privacy and confidentiality, and they safeguard personal, family, and community information obtained in the context of a professional relationship.

Promoting Justice

Nurses uphold principles of justice by safeguarding human rights, equity, and fairness in promoting the public good.

Being Accountable

Nurses are accountable for their actions and answerable for their practice.

Adapted from Canadian Nurses Association. (2008). *Code of ethics for registered nurses.* Ottawa, ON: Author.

BOX 8-3 International Council of Nurses: The Code of Ethics for Nurses

Nurses have four fundamental responsibilities: to promote health, to prevent illness, to restore health, and to alleviate suffering. The need for nursing care is universal. Inherent in nursing care is respect for human rights, including cultural rights, the right to life and choice, the right to dignity, and the right to be treated with respect. Nursing care is respectful of and unrestricted by considerations of age, creed, culture, disability or illness, gender, sexual orientation, nationality, politics, race, economic status, or social status. Nurses render health services to the individual, the family, and the community, and they coordinate their services with those of related groups.

Nurses and People

The nurse's primary professional responsibility is to clients who require nursing care.

In providing care, the nurse promotes an environment in which the human rights, values, customs, and spiritual beliefs of the individual client, family, and community are respected.

The nurse ensures that the individual client receives sufficient information on which to base consent for care and related treatment.

The nurse keeps the client's personal information confidential, sharing it only with appropriate other professionals.

The nurse shares with society the responsibility for initiating and supporting action to meet the health and social needs of the public, particularly those of vulnerable populations.

The nurse also shares responsibility to sustain and protect the natural environment from depletion, pollution, degradation, and destruction.

Nurses and Nursing Practice

The nurse carries personal responsibility and accountability for nursing practice and for maintaining competence by continual learning.

The nurse maintains a standard of personal health in such a way that the ability to provide care is not compromised.

The nurse uses judgement regarding individual competence when accepting and delegating responsibility.

The nurse at all times maintains standards of personal conduct that reflect positively on the profession and enhance public confidence.

In providing care, the nurse ensures that the use of technology and scientific advances is compatible with the safety, dignity, and rights of clients.

Nurses and the Nursing Profession

The nurse assumes the major role in determining and implementing acceptable standards of critical nursing practice, management, research, and education.

The nurse is active in developing a core of research-based professional knowledge.

The nurse, acting through the professional organization, participates in creating and maintaining equitable social and economic working conditions in nursing.

Nurses and Coworkers

The nurse sustains a cooperative relationship with coworkers in nursing and other fields.

The nurse takes appropriate action to safeguard clients when their care is endangered by a coworker of the nurse or by any other person.

Adapted from International Council of Nurses. (2006). *ICN code of ethics for nurses.* Geneva, Switzerland: Author. Reprinted by permission of International Council of Nurses.

Responsibility. **Responsibility** refers to the characteristics of reliability and dependability. It implies an ability to distinguish between right and wrong. In professional nursing, responsibility includes a duty to perform actions adequately and thoughtfully. When administering a medication, for example, you are responsible for assessing the client's need for the drug, for administering it safely and correctly, and for evaluating the client's response to it. By agreeing to act responsibly, you gain trust from clients, colleagues, and society.

Nurses in all domains of practice uphold responsibilities related to all the values in the code of ethics. You are responsible in your interactions with individual clients, families, groups, populations, communities, and society, as well as with students, nursing colleagues, and other health care colleagues. These responsibilities serve as the foundation for articulating nursing values to employers, other health care professionals, and the public (CNA, 2008).

Accountability. **Accountability** means being able to accept responsibility or to account for one's actions and refers to being answerable to someone for something one has done. **Answerability** means being able to offer reasons and explanations to other people for aspects of nursing practice. You balance accountability to the client, the profession, the employer, and society. For example, you may know that a client who will be discharged soon is confused about how to self-administer insulin. The action that you take in response to this situation is guided by your sense of accountability. The client, the institution, and society rely on your judgement and trust you to take action in response to this situation. You may request more hospitalization to provide further teaching, or you may arrange home care to continue teaching at home. The goal is the prevention of injury to the client. Your sense of accountability guides actions that achieve this goal.

According to the CNA (2008), nurses who are enacting professional accountability are (1) keeping up with professional standards, laws, and regulations; (2) ensuring that they have the skill to provide these practices; (c) maintaining their fitness to practise, ensuring that they have the necessary physical, mental, and emotional capacity to practise safely and competently; (d) sharing their knowledge with other nurses through mentorship and giving feedback to other nurses when appropriate.

Professional accountability is also the mandate of professional associations. Professional associations both check unethical practice in a profession and support conscientious professionals who may be under pressure to act unethically or to overlook unethical activity by colleagues. Professional nursing associations have the authority to register and discipline nurses. They also set and maintain professional standards of practice and communicate them to the public. These standards, developed by nursing clinical experts, provide a basic structure against which nursing care is objectively measured. They do not eliminate the need for individualized care plans; rather, the nurse incorporates the standards into each client's care plan.

Advocacy. The ethical responsibility of **advocacy** means acting in behalf of another person, speaking for persons who cannot speak for themselves, or intervening to ensure that views are heard. The CNA

(2008) advises nurses to advocate for all clients in their care. This includes protecting the client's right to choice by providing information, obtaining informed consent for all nursing care, and respecting clients' decisions. Nurses should protect clients' right to dignity by advocating for appropriate use of interventions in order to minimize suffering, intervening if other people fail to respect the dignity of the client, and working to promote health and social conditions that allow clients to live and die with dignity. Nurses should protect a client's right to privacy and confidentiality by helping the client access his or her health records (subject to legal requirements), intervening if other members of the health care team fail to respect the client's privacy, and following policies that protect the client's privacy. According to the *Code of Ethics*, nurses should also advocate for the discussion of ethical issues among health care team members, clients, and families, and nurses should advocate for health policies that enable fair and inclusive allocation of resources.

Advocacy requires that you have a strong awareness of the context in which situations arise, as well as an understanding of the influence of power and politics on how you make decisions. If you experience **constrained moral agency**—that is, if you feel powerless to act for what you think is right, or if you believe your actions will not effect change—then you will have difficulty being an effective advocate.

Ethical Theory

Ethics concern the examination of the moral basis for judgements, actions, duties, and obligations. For centuries, moral philosophers have tried to answer two questions: "What is the meaning of right and good?" and "What is the morally right thing to do in a given situation?" You are mainly concerned with the second question because you are often in situations in which you must make decisions that affect client well-being.

Philosophical discussion about health care issues has progressed over time, just as developments in health care and society itself have progressed. The philosophical constructions that shape the discussions have also changed. Ethics began as a standard reference point for the determination of right action. It has grown into a field of study filled with differences of opinion, competing systems of values, and deeply meaningful efforts to understand human interaction through new technologies. Some knowledge of ethical theories that have shaped philosophical thinking is necessary to understand the development of nursing ethics. The following section introduces a variety of contemporary ethical theories. It is neither exclusive nor comprehensive.

Deontology. A traditional ethical theory, **deontology** is the system of ethics that is perhaps most familiar to practitioners in health care. Its foundations are often associated with the work of the eighteenth century philosopher Immanuel Kant (1724–1804). In deontology, actions are defined as right or wrong on the basis of their "right-making characteristics such as fidelity to promises, truthfulness, and justice" (Beauchamp & Childress, 2001). The essence of right or wrong is located within deontological principles. Deontologists specifically do not look to consequences of actions to determine rightness or wrongness. Instead, they critically examine a situation for the existence of essential rightness or wrongness. Ethical principles such as justice, allowing free choice (autonomy), and doing the greatest good (beneficence) serve to define right or wrong. If an act is just, respects autonomy, and provides good, then the act is ethical. The process depends on a mutual understanding and acceptance of these principles.

Difficulty arises when you must choose among conflicting principles, which is often the case in ethical dilemmas concerning health care. For example, applying the principle of respect for autonomy can be confusing when dealing with the health care of children. The health care team may recommend a treatment, but a parent may disagree with or refuse the recommendation. In discussion of the dilemma, you may refer to a guiding principle such as respect for autonomy. However, questions remain: Whose autonomy should receive the respect? The parent's? Who should advocate for the child's best interest? Society often struggles to understand who should be ultimately responsible for the well-being of children. A commitment to respect autonomy does not guarantee that controversy can be avoided.

Utilitarianism. According to a utilitarian system of ethics, the value of something is determined by its usefulness. This philosophy, **utilitarianism**, may also be known as **consequentialism** because its main emphasis is on the outcome or consequence of action. A third term associated with this philosophy is **teleology** (from the Greek word *telos*, meaning "end"), which is the study of ends or final causes. Its philosophical foundations were first proposed by John Stuart Mill (1806–1873), a British philosopher and social commentator. The greatest good for the greatest number of people is the guiding principle for determining the correct action in this system. As with deontology, this theory relies on the application of a certain principle, namely: measures of "good" and "greatest" (Beauchamp & Childress, 2001). The difference between utilitarianism and deontology is in the focus on consequences or outcomes. Utilitarianism concerns the effect that an act will have; deontology concerns the presence of principle, regardless of outcome.

Individuals or groups may have conflicting definitions of "greatest good." For example, research suggests that education regarding safer sex practices may reduce the spread of the human immunodeficiency virus. Some scholars argue, however, that education about sex should be provided by the family and that sex education in public schools diminishes the role and the value of the family. For them, the greater good is the preservation of family values and the protection of individual choices regarding sex education of children. For other scholars, however, the "greater good" is defined as educating the greatest number of people in the most effective way possible. The concepts of utilitarianism provide guidance, but they do not invariably provide for universal agreement.

Bioethics. In the 1970s, a group of ethics scholars concluded that then-current ethical theories were not sufficient for the health care field because they did not provide specific guidance for important moral questions that arose in the context of medicine. **Biomedical ethics** came to denote ethical reasoning for physicians, whereas **bioethics** became the general term for principled reasoning across health care professions. The central idea of bioethics is that moral decision making in health care should be guided by four principles: autonomy, beneficence, nonmaleficence, and justice. According to this theory, health care providers should examine each situation, determine which of the principles has priority, and use that principle to guide action.

Autonomy. **Autonomy** refers to your ability to make choices for yourself that should be based on full understanding, free of controlling influences (Beauchamp & Childress, 2001). Respect for another person's autonomy is fundamental to the practice of health care. It is the reason why clients should be included in all aspects of decision making regarding their care. The agreement to respect autonomy involves the recognition that clients have the right to be respected and supported by you with regard to their health care decisions. For example, the purpose of the preoperative consent that clients must read and sign before surgery is to ensure in writing that the health care team respects the client's independence by obtaining permission to proceed. The consent process implies that a client may refuse treatment, and in most cases, the health care team must agree to follow the client's wishes. Health care professionals agree to abide by a standard of respect for the client's autonomy.

Beneficence. **Beneficence** means doing or promoting good for others. It involves taking positive actions to help others. Commitment to beneficence helps guide difficult decisions concerning whether the benefits of a treatment may be challenged by risks to the client's well-being or dignity. For example, vaccination may cause temporary discomfort, but the benefits of protection from disease, both for the client and for society, outweigh the client's discomfort. The agreement to act with beneficence also requires that the best interests of the client remain more important than self-interest. For example, you do not simply follow medical orders; you act thoughtfully to understand client needs and then work actively to meet those needs.

Nonmaleficence. *Maleficence* refers to harm or hurt; thus **nonmaleficence** is the avoidance of harm or hurt. In health care ethics, ethical practice involves not only the will to do good but also the equal commitment to do no harm. The health care professional tries to balance the risks and benefits of a plan of care while striving to cause the least harm possible. This principle is often helpful in guiding discussions about new or controversial technologies. For example, a new bone marrow transplantation procedure may provide a chance for cure. The procedure, however, may entail long periods of pain and suffering. These discomforts should be considered in view of the suffering that the disease itself might cause and in view of the suffering that other treatments might cause. The commitment to provide least harmful interventions illustrates the term *nonmaleficence.* The standard of nonmaleficence promotes a continuing effort to consider the potential for harm even when it may be necessary to promote health.

Justice. **Justice** refers to fairness. The term is often used during discussions about resources: When competition for a scarce resource exists, justice mandates that decisions be fair and, to the greatest extent possible, unbiased. In decisions about which client receives an available lung for transplantation, for example, it is understood that the lung will be allocated as fairly as possible. Understandings of fairness depend on community values. In Canadian society, community standards dictate that the decision should not depend on who has the higher intellect or larger salary; instead, the decision must be based on need alone. Of course, the definition of need can be debated, and when two people have equal need, nothing in the theory helps health care professionals decide between them. These are ethical questions that require further exploration of values, principles, and priorities to guide decisions in resource allocation.

The literature also mentions other prevalent forms of justice that you need to understand, such as **social justice.** Social justice is often related to a concern for the eqitable distribution of benefits and burdens in society (Boutain, 2005) and has also been discussed as changing social relationships and institutions to promote equitable relationships (Drevdahl et al., 2001). According to the "Ethical Endeavours" section of the CNA (2008) *Code of Ethics,* your moral obligations extend to recognizing "the need for change in systems and societal structures in order to create greater equity for all. You should endeavour as much as possible, individually and collectively, to advocate for and work toward eliminating social inequities . . . ." (p. 16). This section of the *Code of Ethics* is somewhat visionary, inasmuch as its statements extend beyond just "what is" to "what ought to be" in nursing as a profession. It makes clear that if the status quo in health care is inefficacious, you must be an active participant in effecting change. This means you must recognize that part of your role is to work for change at the broader systems level, agitating for revisions to social policy, legislation, and institutional structures. This section of the *Code of Ethics* emphasizes the advocacy role for you and the need to work to bring about a system that is more focused on prevention, takes more account of the social determinants of health, is more accessible, and is more sustainable. This is a daunting task, but you have the educational preparation and theoretical base to assume a leadership role in making the reality of Canadian health care match the vision (Oberle & Raffin Bouchal, in press).

Feminist Ethics. Feminist ethicists consider their work a critique of conventional ethics, as well as a critique of social values. Their work focuses on continuing inequalities between people (Lindemann, 2006). They look to the nature of relationships between people for guidance in working out ethical dilemmas. The underlying values, according to a group of noted feminist nursing scholars, are social justice, relationships, and community (Peter et al., 2004).

Changes in attitudes toward women reflect new perspectives in women's relationship with family, with work, with science, and with society (Sherwin, 1992). For example, until the early 1980s, moral development was thought to reach the highest stages more often in men than in women. According to this thinking, moral development occurred in predictable stages. The most complex stage involved a sense of justice, and young girls did not reach this stage as often as did young boys (Kohlberg, 1981). Findings of research in the early 1980s disputed this conclusion. Gilligan (1982) proposed that Kohlberg's tools to measure moral development were gender biased. Gilligan went on to build a revised theory of moral development from her findings. She attempted to accommodate gender differences. Specifically, she concluded that young girls tend to pay attention to community and to individual circumstances and that young boys tend to process dilemmas through ideals or principles determined abstractly.

Feminist ethicists value the role of relationships and stories about relationships. They emphasize the importance of stories and the role of community over an attention to universal principles. In fact, they argue that it is impossible to be unbiased or not influenced by relationships to people. They propose that the natural human urge to be influenced by relationships is a positive value (Wolf, 1996).

This system of ethics also addresses issues of gender-based inequality. Feminists propose that an inequality of attention to women can be remedied by routinely asking, in the midst of any ethical dilemma, how bioethical decisions affect women (Sherwin, 1992). For example, in a discussion regarding the ethics of fetal surgery (surgical intervention in an unborn child), **feminist ethics** would propose that questions about the effects of the intervention on the mother are at least as important as questions about the effects on the fetus. Hilde Lindemann Nelson (2000), a noted feminist scholar in the United States, provided a history of the development of feminist ethics and bioethics. She noted that the feminist attention to gender and gender-related issues gave rise to an important perspective called **care theory,** which is about a type of virtue ethic that gives moral weight to caring for others (see Chapter 19). This was an important development in thinking about ethics because it moved attention away from the traditional masculine virtues towards those that had traditionally been considered more feminine.

Relational Ethics. It is becoming increasingly apparent that relationships are the basis of ethics in nursing. According to **relational ethics** theory, ethical understandings are formed in, and emerge from, a person's relationships with others, whether those others are clients, families, communities, or colleagues (Bergum, 2004; Bergum, & Dossetor, 2005; Hartrick Doane & Varcoe, 2007). Relational ethics refers not only to individual relationships but also to a person's relationships within an institutional structure. It is important that you understand the concept of relational ethics because many ethics scholars believe it is the foundation of your moral understanding of nursing. According to Bergum (2004), relational ethics is a way of "being," displayed in everyday interactions rather than a mode of decision making. It is how you insert a needle, how you enter into conversation, how you show respect, or how you behave with other people.

Relational ethics focuses on the role of relational context or the experience of the relationships in shaping moral choices (Bergum, 2004). In research on relational ethics, Bergum (2004) identified four themes: environment, embodiment, mutual respect, and engagement. **Environment** concerns critical elements or characteristics of the health care system within which you work and how the nature of the your relationships is affected by this system. Bergum encouraged nurses to consider the entire health care arena as a network or matrix, in which each part is connected, either directly or indirectly, to the other. An awareness of this connectedness encourages you to look beyond the immediate situation and to try to envision a broader context. It also makes you conscious of how power and politics affect your entire system of care (Oberle & Raffin Bouchal, 2009).

In relational ethics, **embodiment** means recognizing that the mind–body split is artificial and that healing for both client and family cannot occur unless "scientific knowledge and human compassion are given equal weight [and it is recognized that] emotion and feeling are as important to human life as physical signs and symptoms" (Bergum, 2004, p. 492). Such recognition requires you to become truly aware of what other people may be experiencing. You must make this awareness a part of your own experience. The nurse–client relationship requires that you value clients and treat them with respect. It goes far beyond just being "nice" to them; in addition, it requires a commitment to care about clients and their experience.

Within the nurse–client relationship, you use nursing knowledge to enhance the client's health and well-being. You always consider the unique needs of the client as an individual. Mutual respect is created, with attention to both your and the client's needs, wishes, expertise, and experience (Bergum & Dossetor, 2005). **Mutuality,** loosely defined as a relationship that benefits both you and the client and harms neither, requires your and the client's willingness to participate in a relationship that embraces the values and ideas of one other as a means of developing new understandings, rather than judging the other person's values and ideas.

Engagement means connecting with another person in an open, trusting, and responsive manner. Bergum (2004) suggested that it is through this connection that you develop a meaningful understanding of the other person's experience. Engagement takes skill and practice, inasmuch as it requires a commitment to keeping the relationship caring and respectful. Bergum asserted that engagement "does not ask for *selflessness* on the part of you, but for both you and the patient to be recognized as *whole beings*" (p. 498). Engagement requires that you connect with the client but, at the same time, set boundaries in such a way that the relationship remains on a professional level. Knowing how much to engage with another person is one of the greatest challenges in nursing.

How to Process an Ethical Dilemma

An **ethical dilemma** is a conflict between two sets of human values, both of which are judged to be "good" but neither of which can be fully served. Ethical dilemmas can cause distress and confusion for clients and caregivers. You may well be faced with ethical questions that have not been examined previously and for which no practical wisdom exists. You must be able to examine issues and apply experience and wisdom in each situation. The CNA (2008) *Code of Ethics* identified the responsibility of nurses to maintain their "fitness to practice" as having the "necessary physical, mental or emotional capacity to practice safely and competently" (p. 15). Such fitness requires you to be knowledgeable and skillful as you engage in problem solving. Ethical issues must be processed carefully and deliberately. An ethical decision is not based solely on emotions or on what people want and feel; however, the process promotes the free expression of feelings. Ethical decision making is a negotiating process that evolves over time, not in a straight line with a beginning and an end.

To resolve an ethical dilemma—in a committee setting, at the client's bedside, or in a family conference—you apply a careful, critical reflection of the dilemma. Resolving an ethical dilemma requires deliberate, critical, and systematic thinking. It also requires negotiation of differences (between beliefs, values, opinions, and so forth), incorporation of conflicting ideas, and an effort to respect differences of opinion. The process of negotiating ethical dilemmas may be in part the process of understanding ambiguities. You need to be knowledgeable and adept in making logical, fair, and consistent decisions. Ethical decision-making models offer a variety of methods for making informed conclusions (Box 8–4).

Each step in the processing of an ethical dilemma resembles steps in critical thinking. You begin by gathering information and move through assessment and identification of the problem, planning a solution, implementation of a solution, and evaluation of the results. The first step guides you in determining whether the problem is an ethical one. Not all problems are ethical in nature. You learn to distinguish ethical problems from questions of procedure, legality, or medical diagnosis. To distinguish an ethical problem from other problems, Curtin and Flaherty (1982) recommended that you decide whether the problem has one or more of the following characteristics:

- It cannot be resolved solely through a review of scientific data. To make this determination, you must gather detailed information about the situation. This information may come from medical records, health care literature, or consultation with colleagues or with the client and the client's family.
- It is perplexing. It is hard to think logically or make a decision about the problem, or you may disagree with a decision that other people are making, and the difference of opinion is perplexing.
- The answer to the problem is profoundly relevant to several areas of human concern.

A part of gathering information includes an examination of your own values as they relate to the issues. The distinction between personal opinion and the facts of the case, or the opinions of others, is essential for resolution to proceed. To clarify the true ethical issues in any situation, you need to be aware of personal responses.

After reviewing relevant information and personal values, a clear statement of the ethical problem becomes the groundwork to begin negotiation. Discussions are more likely to remain focused and constructive when all parties agree on the statement of the dilemma. The group then lists possible courses of action. Possibilities may occur at any time during deliberations. After alternatives are considered, people in an ethical conflict come to a point of resolution or agreement, and action is taken. Decisions are made that can be evaluated in an ongoing manner (Box 8–5).

Documentation of the ethical process can take a variety of forms. Whenever the process involves a family conference or results in a change in the plan of care, the process should be documented in the medical record. At some institutions, the ethics committee may use

BOX 8-4 Two Ethical Decision-Making Frameworks

Diagram on left: From Storch, J. L. (2004). Model for ethical decision making for policy and practice. In J. Storch, P. Rodney, & R. Starzomski (Eds.), *Toward a moral horizon: Nursing ethics for leadership and practice* (p. 515). Toronto, ON: Pearson Education. Diagram on right: From Alberta College and Association of Registered Nurses (1996). A model for questioning. In *Ethical decision-making for registered nurses in Alberta: Guidelines and recommendations* (p. 13). Edmonton, AB: Author. Reprinted by permission of College and Association of Registered Nurses of Alberta.

a formal consultation format whenever a request for discussion arises. If the ethical dilemma does not directly affect client care, however, discussion may be documented by minutes from a meeting or in a memorandum to affected parties. In the following case study, the nursing concerns and the family conferences would be recorded in the medical record and in nursing flow sheets.

On your unit, a 35-year-old woman has been hospitalized in the final stages of brain cancer. She is a single mother with two young children. Although she has been treated by both conventional and experimental treatments, the tumour continues to grow, and the medical team has agreed that further treatment would be futile. You have cared for this client during past hospital admissions, and during an especially open discussion, she expressed wishes to explore "do not resuscitate" (DNR) orders. During the current admission, her primary physician is out of town. The attending physician does not know the client personally, but he has spent time with her. He has reviewed the clinical data and agrees that the client is entering the terminal stage of the disease. In his opinion, however, the client is not ready to discuss end-of-life issues. He states that the client has declined to discuss DNR orders with him. You ask the physician to convene a family conference about the issues. He refuses, stating that he believes the client is not ready to participate.

Step 1: Is this an ethical dilemma? What may at first appear to be a question of ethics may be resolved by clarifying your knowledge base about clinical facts. A review of policy and procedure, or of standards of care, may reveal legal obligations that determine a course of action, regardless of personal opinion. If the question remains perplexing, and

BOX 8-5 How to Process an Ethical Dilemma

Step 1: Determine whether the issue is an ethical dilemma.
Step 2: Gather all the information relevant to the case.
Step 3: Examine and determine your own values on the issues.
Step 4: Verbalize the problem.
Step 5: Consider possible courses of action.
Step 6: Reflect on the outcome.
Step 7: Evaluate the action and the outcome.

the answer will be profoundly relevant to several areas of human concern, then an ethical dilemma may exist.

The single mother's situation meets the criteria for an ethical dilemma. Further review of scientific data will probably not contribute to a resolution of the dilemma, but it is important to review the data carefully to make this determination. The disagreement does not revolve around whether the client is in a terminally ill state, so further clinical information will not change the basic question: Should the client have an opportunity to discuss DNR orders at this time? The question is perplexing. Two professional team members disagree on an assessment of a client's readiness to confront the difficult issues related to dying. The answer to the question "Is this client ready to discuss end of life?" has important implications. If she is not ready, then raising the issue may cause anguish and fear in the client and her family. If she is ready and the team avoids discussion, she may suffer unnecessarily in silence. If she is very close to death, then in the absence of a DNR order, necessitate cardiopulmonary resuscitation (CPR) will be performed in a futile situation. You know that CPR can cause pain. If applied in a situation in which the client's life is unlikely to be extended or improved, then CPR could prolong her suffering and reduce her dignity.

Step 2: Gather as much information as possible that is relevant to the case. Because resolution to dilemmas may arise from unlikely sources, incorporate as much knowledge as possible at every step of the process. At this point, the information could include laboratory and test results, the clinical state of the client, and current literature about the diagnosis or condition of the client. It may include investigation of the psychosocial concerns of the client, as well as those of her significant others. The client's religious, cultural, and family orientations are part of the nurse's assessment.

You obtain all the clinical information that is pertinent to the question. It may be helpful to determine whether the client retains most cognitive functions, even though her tumour is aggressive. You review the chart and discuss this aspect with the physician, and you agree that the client is fully competent but afraid and overwhelmed by the prognosis. Because two professionals disagree on a client's state of mind, it may be helpful to reassess the client or request that an independent person assess the client's readiness to discuss end-of-life issues. Sometimes family members or significant others hold important clues to a client's state of mind.

Step 3: Examine and determine your own values on the issues. This step is important for all participants in the discussion. At this stage, you and the other participants practice values clarification, and you differentiate between your own values and the values of the client and of other health care team members. Essential parts of the goal are to form your own opinion and to respect others' opinions.

At this point, you stop to reflect on your own values. Your own religious practices may allow you to decide to forgo further treatment if you were in the client's condition. You also may not yet have family members who rely on you, such as children or elderly parents. This client's religious practices may be more strictly constructed than your own. Her religion discourages actions that diminish life in any way, and you realize that she may have come to see a DNR order as giving up, or as "acting like God." In addition, you understand that the attending physician has not had time to know this client as her own physician has or as you have. You continue to believe that the client would be capable of a discussion, despite her statements to the physician. In fact, you believe that she would benefit from a discussion, because perhaps the presence of an unfamiliar caretaker, combined with declining physical health, has silenced her, even though her fears and concerns persist.

Step 4: Verbalize the problem. Once all relevant information has been gathered, accurate definition of the problem may proceed. It is helpful to state the problem in a few sentences. By agreeing to a statement of the problem, the health care team, the patient, and the family can proceed with discussion in a focused way.

Here, the problem seems to be this: whether this client should discuss DNR at this time. Determine the benefits and risks of a DNR order at this time. Other important questions relate to the client's current state of mind: Is she afraid to speak? Is she feeling cut off from her normal network (a primary physician)? Are these feelings contributing to confusion about DNR decisions?

Step 5: Consider possible courses of action. What options are available within the context of the situation and the client's values?

Once you have asked the basic question, other questions and possible courses of action arise. Should you initiate a discussion with the client independently of the physician? Would you be outside your professional role if you facilitated a DNR order? What if your assessment were incorrect? Would you contribute not to the dignity but to the distress of the client? The answers to these questions may be elusive, because they depend on an understanding of the client's feelings and values that are not necessarily obvious. Even if the nurse cannot legally write a DNR order, the nurse can influence a physician's or client's decision regarding DNR; therefore, troubling questions remain.

Step 6: Reflect on the outcome. This is the most important and delicate step of the process. These negotiations may happen informally at the client's bedside or in the charting room, or a formal ethics meeting may be necessary. Your point of view represents a unique contribution to the discussion.

In an ethics committee meeting, the discussion is usually multidisciplinary. A facilitator or chairperson ensures that all points of view are examined and that all pertinent issues are identified. A decision or recommendation is the usual outcome of discussion and the result of a successful discussion. In the best of circumstances, participants discover a course of action that meets criteria for acceptance by all. On occasion, however, participants may leave the discussion disappointed or even opposed to the decision.

The discussion focuses on the disagreement between your assessment and the physician's regarding the client's readiness to discuss end-of-life issues. The principles involved during the discussion include beneficence and nonmaleficence: Which plan would provide the most good for this client—a DNR order or no order? A separate question addresses the client's point of view: Would a discussion with the client promote well-being or promote anguish? Furthermore, according to the principle of autonomy, a troublesome question remains: Does the client want something different from the desire she is expressing?

With several members of the health care team present, the discussion proceeds. You present your point of view. You continue to sense that the client is ready to discuss DNR orders but that she may be reluctant to trust the circumstances of this admission. But you also respect the attending physician and his analysis and continue to be concerned that the client may have experienced a change of mind between the last admission and this one. In the end, the team proposes the following: a formal meeting with the client, in which you, the attending physician, and a supportive family member are all present. You support this proposal because you sense that it will maximize the support of the client's existing network. In addition, you recognize that in a trusting environment, the client is more likely to express her fears, insecurities, and wishes. Team members agree to keep the discussion open ended and exploratory. You suggest that rather than asking whether the client wants a DNR order, perhaps the team could wait for her to bring up the issue. In this way, the team could be assured of her consent and willingness to participate in the discussion.

Step 7: Evaluate the action and the outcome.

At the meeting, the client in fact opens up. She expresses relief at the chance to explore her options and feelings. Pain management issues are clarified. She wants to discuss a DNR order but requests a visit from her priest before she must make a final decision.

Ethical Issues in Nursing Practice

With increased professional responsibility and accountability, and with changes in the workplace and health care system, you are increasingly facing a myriad of ethical issues. You face ethical issues daily while caring for clients and families, while relating to other health care professionals, institutions, and global societal issues. The following section explores current issues in which ethical issues arise.

Client Care Issues

Informed Consent. The intimacy and integrity of the nurse–client relationship mandate that you protect the rights of their clients. You achieve this mandate as you follow standards, policies, guidelines, and legislation regarding consent to treatment. **Informed consent** is consent to treatment on the basis of accurate and complete information (see Chapter 9). The goal of informed consent is to protect the client's right to autonomy. The CNA (2008) *Code of Ethics* (p. 11) asserts that to promote and respect informed decision making, some of the nurse's ethical responsibilities are as follows:

- Building trusting relationships to ensure that the client's choice is understood, expressed, and advocated.
- Providing the desired information and support so that clients can make informed decisions.
- Assisting clients in obtaining the most accurate current knowledge about their health condition.
- Being sensitive to the inherent power differentials between health care professionals and clients: nurses must not misuse power to influence decision making.
- Recognizing that the client has the right to refuse or withdraw consent.
- Respecting the informed choices of capable persons, including choice of lifestyles or of treatment not conducive to good health.

Many unethical scenarios can involve consent: a client's signing consent forms without understanding what treatment entails; a nurse's mistaken assumption that a physician has explained a medical procedure to a client before obtaining the client's consent; obtaining consent from a client who does not speak the health care team's language without the assistance of an interpreter; or a client's consenting to a procedure without knowing about associated risks or potential adverse side effects.

Although obtaining informed consent for medical procedures is not a nursing duty, you may witness the client's signature on the consent form. When you provide consent forms for clients to sign, your main responsibility lies with ensuring that the client fully understands the nature of the treatment or procedure. If not, notification of the physician must occur so that the physician can clarify or provide additional information.

Futile Care. In the early 1980s, issues such as enhanced life-sustaining technologies, clients rights movements, and growing concerns about using health care resources in a cost-effective and efficient manner led to academic discussions, debates, and practice policies on medical futility. **Medical futility** is defined as a medical treatment that is considered nonbeneficial because it is believed to offer no reasonable hope of recovery from or improvement in the client's condition (CNA, 2001). Clients often worry, in the event of their becoming incapacitated and unable to express their wishes, that they will be "hooked up to machines" and receive treatment that they do not desire (Figure 8–1). At issue is whether clinicians are sufficiently objective to establish that a given intervention is futile and that they are therefore authorized to withhold or withdraw its use (Callahan, 1991).

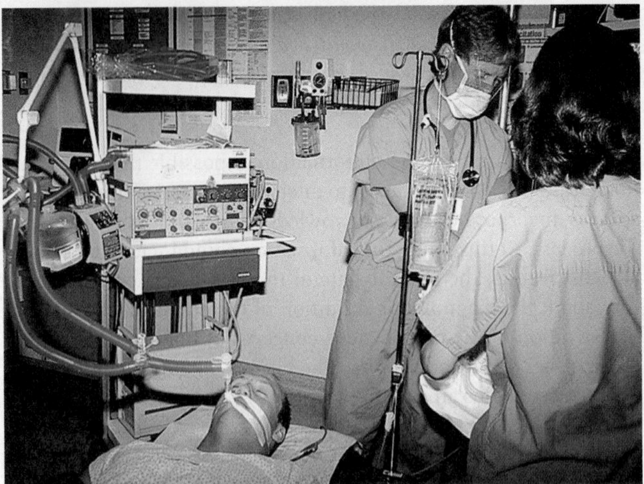

Figure 8-1 Nurses often struggle when clients are receiving care that they believe is prolonging their suffering and their life.

Although health care professionals are best equipped to determine the physical benefits of treatment, only the client or people who know the client best can determine whether treatment is advancing the client's overall well-being. Bennett Jacobs and Taylor (2005a) identified this issue as "qualitative" futility or subjective determination, in which not just medical facts but also values lead the client or the client's surrogate decision makers to conclude that the treatment has no benefit according to those values.

Achieving holistic outcomes of care must be based on an interplay of physical facts and subjective values. Taylor (1995) suggested the following four classifications of futility: (1) not futile: beneficial to both physical and overall well-being; (2) futile: nonbeneficial to either physical or overall well-being; (3) futile from the client's perspective: medically indicated but not valued by the client; and (4) futile from the clinicians' perspective and not medically indicated but valued by the client (p. 301). It is evident that these classifications have objective and subjective dimensions, as well as quantitative and qualitative dimensions, and constitute a more complete way of viewing the complex notion of futility.

The issue of who has priority in health care decision making remains complex and often troublesome. The potential for futility conflicts is high in situations of critically and chronically ill clients. What then, is your role? Taylor (1995) suggested that nurses play a leading role in working toward pursuing negotiated compromise between health care professionals and clients equally, for the best possible outcome for the particular client. She suggested that this may be accomplished "by identifying patients, families, and health care teams at risk of experiencing conflict about futile care, and then initiating dialogue that may prevent or resolve conflict" (p. 303).

Advance directives are one way to address this problem (see Chapter 9). They are "the means used to document and communicate a person's preferences regarding life-sustaining treatment in the event that they become incapable of expressing those wishes for themselves" (CNA, 1998, p. 1). Advance directives are commonly expressed in two ways: (1) an instruction directive, or living will, that identifies what life-sustaining treatment a client desires in certain situations, and (2) a proxy directive, or power or attorney for personal care, that explains who is to make health care decisions if the client becomes incompetent (CNA, 1998). A routine part of any admission to a hospital now usually includes inquiry about the client's advance directives; if they exist, they are included as part of the medical record. It has become necessary for nurses to be aware of the legal status of all types of advance directives in their province or territory.

You have several roles regarding advance directives. You may be involved in helping clients plan an advance directive by discussing its uses and helping clients to clarify their values and wishes for end-of-life treatment. Your role also includes following the advance directive, alerting other health care professionals to changes in the client's wishes, and advocating on behalf of the client or substitute decision maker if the client's wishes or advance directive are not being followed.

Withdrawal of Food and Hydration. Maintaining nutrition is a natural life-sustaining measure and common part of the nursing role. A change in the client's ability to drink and eat raises many issues. When food and hydration are administered for a prolonged period to a client whose condition is not expected to improve, some nurses may view this care as extraordinary or heroic, whereas others see this as humane.

Current literature suggests that fluids should not be routinely administered to dying individuals or automatically withheld from them; rather, they should be given on the basis of the goals of care and a careful assessment of the client's comfort. A position statement by the CNA (2001) on futility stresses the importance of the health care team to determine whether food and fluid are most beneficial or harmful to a client. The following questions may aid health care professionals in reflecting on the goals of care: Will the client's well-being be enhanced by administration of nutrition? Does the client have symptoms that could be relieved or aggravated by administration of nutrition? Could hydration enhance the client's mental status or level of consciousness? Will it prolong the client's life? Is that the wish of the client and family? (Bennett Jacobs & Taylor, 2005b; Ganzini, 2006).

Administration of hydration may raise dilemmas when its use is intended merely to maintain physical life (e.g., when the client is in a vegetative state or is near death). You should know that during the natural dying process, the body starts to "shut down," and the client may lose the desire for food and fluids. Force-feeding a dying client may sometimes do more harm than good. Withholding or withdrawing nutrition or hydration from a client is no different from the decision to forgo any other medical treatment that may prolong the dying process. It is considered appropriate to withhold or discontinue life-sustaining medical interventions if they are not benefiting the client or are contrary to the client's wishes. Furthermore, it is important to stress to families that dying individuals who are not receiving artificial nutrition or hydration will still be provided with adequate overall care.

Issues of Safety in the Work Environment

Nurses are responsible for providing safe, compassionate, competent, and ethical care (CNA, 2008). In ensuring safety, care must be such that harm is minimized. Lack of control over important aspects of the environment can lead to ethically ambiguous situations (Austin et al., 2003). Complex life-and-death events, multiple role responsibilities, loyalties and expectations, reduced numbers of skilled health care professionals, minimal clinical nursing leadership, interdisciplinary team conflict, and autocratic organizational decision making may create personal moral conflict for you (Aiken et al., 2002; Canadian Health Services Research Foundation, 2006).

Causing harm to clients in the form of pain and suffering from continuing treatment is a source of **moral distress** for nurses that they often believe could be avoided. "Moral distress arises when there is inconsistency betweens one's beliefs and one's actions" (Hardingham, 2004, p. 128). Sometimes nurses find it hard to care for a client when other health care professionals, usually physicians, make choices that nurses think are causing more harm than good. For example, the situation of a client in intensive care who is comatose but seems to experience great pain when turned over can be very upsetting for nurses. They may experience moral distress if they feel that they are, in effect, torturing the client each time they turn him or her over. Keeping clients safe from harm can be difficult, and sometimes it requires great ethical sensitivity to be aware of harms that are being caused. In these situations, nurses may lose their sense of **moral integrity** or "wholeness" when they are committed to certain values and beliefs that are not upheld because of situational constraints. If these situations continue and integrity is compromised, nurses may experience **moral residue**, a long-lasting discomfort that arises whenever they face moral distress (Webster & Baylis, 2000). Relational ethics helps you know what the client considers harm, and it is crucial to engage in discussions with your clients and colleagues.

Other kinds of harm can come to clients because of inadequate or inappropriate caregiving. Sometimes harm results from mistakes that can be explained; sometimes it results from carelessness or incompetence. For example, when you have a lot of very ill clients to care for and you have many demands on your time, medication errors can occur because you are distracted and feeling rushed. These kinds of errors are unfortunate, but they are not breaches of ethics as such. On the other hand, if you make a medication error because you have been out partying all night before your shift and you were not fit to practice that day, the error would be considered unethical. Either way, you need to monitor your own competence to practice, and you must admit to your mistakes. Regardless of the cause, if you make a mistake, not admitting it is considered unethical.

In a multidisciplinary environment, all health care professionals must take responsibility for the care that is provided (Box 8–6). You need to be aware of what other professionals are doing for and with their clients. If **adverse events** occur—that is, "unexpected, undesirable incidents resulting in injury or death that are directly associated with the process of providing health care or services to a person receiving care" (CNA 2008, p. 18)—then you must report them, regardless of who is responsible. The person who is most directly involved when an adverse event occurs should be the one to report it, but sometimes that does not happen. In that situation, if you observe the event, you must report it. It is your obligation to ensure client safety, but it is not easy because it can mean exposing the incompetence of a colleague. Imagine, for example, that you observe another nurse drop a frail elderly client during transfer. The client does not seem hurt, and the other nurse does not seem to plan to report the incident. Should you report it yourself? Your obligation is to speak to the other nurse and ensure that the incident is reported. If the nurse does not report it, then you must, inasmuch as this is a clear issue of client safety, and your obligations are clear. **Whistleblowing** (i.e., reporting a colleague's errors, incompetence, unsafe or negligent practice, or abuse of clients) is one of the most difficult actions you must take in ensuring that safe, compassionate, competent, and ethical care is met (Oberle & Raffin Bouchal, 2009).

BOX 8-6 RESEARCH HIGHLIGHT

Ethics in Nursing Practice

Research Focus

Rodney et al. (2006) were interested in exploring ethical nursing practice in a large emergency department and a medical oncology unit located in separate regions of British Columbia, Canada. Rodney et al.'s goal was to describe the moral climate of nurses' workplaces and how the nurses acted to improve it.

Research Abstract

This participatory action research study involved participant observation, interviews, focus groups, meetings, workshops, and everyday work in the two practice settings. The research team at each site included a team of staff nurses (clinical nurse researchers), academic investigators, and research assistants, all of whom worked in partnership. Qualitative data were collected in focus groups, interviews, and regular meetings with staff to discuss, debrief, and plan for change. The research process supported staff in initiating changes in their workplaces aimed at improving the environment for ethical practice.

Evidence-Informed Practice

- Strong evidence must influence the everyday practice of individual nurses and the moral climate in which nursing care takes place.
- Many factors influence nurses' difficulties in practising ethically: deficiencies in resources; how nurses feel about themselves; how they treat other nurses and health care professionals, clients, and clients' families; and how they are treated by other professionals who also adhere to the often unspoken values that reflect their practices.

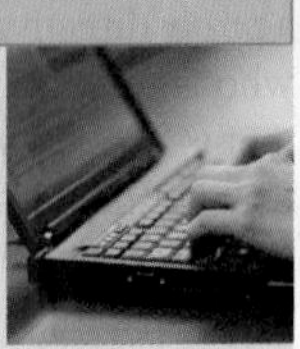

References: Rodney, P., Hartrick Doane, G., Storch, J., & Varcoe, C. (2006). Ethics in action: Strengthening nurses' enactment of their moral agency within the cultural context of health care delivery. *Canadian Nurse, 102*(8), 25–26.

BOX 8-7 FOCUS ON PRIMARY HEALTH CARE

How to Encourage Nurses Individually and Collectively to Work Toward Eliminating Social Inequities

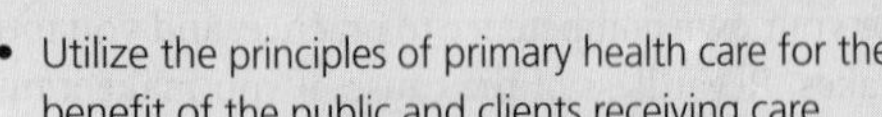

- Utilize the principles of primary health care for the benefit of the public and clients receiving care.
- Understand that some groups in society are systemically disadvantaged, which leads to poorer health and diminished well-being. Nurses work to improve the quality of lives of people who are part of disadvantaged and vulnerable groups and communities, and they take action to overcome barriers to health care.
- Recognize and work to address organizational, social, economic, and political factors that influence health and well-being within the context of your role in the delivery of care.

* KEY CONCEPTS

- Values clarification helps nurses explore personal values and feelings and to decide how to act on personal beliefs. It also facilitates nurse-client communication.
- Ethics is the study of philosophical ideals of what is beneficial or valuable for all.
- A code of ethics provides a foundation for professional nursing. Such a code promotes accountability, responsibility, and advocacy.
- Theories of bioethics refer to ethical issues specific to the delivery of health care. They are based on the principles of autonomy, beneficence, nonmaleficence, and justice.
- Relational ethics theory encompasses more than bioethics: It addresses the role of relationship in the ethical delivery of health care. It maintains that the nurse-client relationship is the foundation of nursing ethics.
- Ethical problems arise from differences in values, from technological advances, from end-of-life experiences, and from changes in work environments.

Reporting the wrongdoing of a colleague can be distressing. You worry about how to report or deal with unacceptable practice and still maintain healthy relationships with other colleagues. You need to examine the relative risks and benefits and then decide on appropriate action (Box 8–7). You must be prepared to struggle with difficult questions and reflect on the facts and your internal values and perspectives. Such concerns, in addition to having elements of a classic dilemma, reveal the complexity and effect of relational issues within the workplace. When positive professional relationships are absent, both the profession and the professionals suffer.

- A standard process for thinking through ethical dilemmas, including critical thinking skills, helps health care professionals resolve conflict or uncertainty about correct actions.

* CRITICAL THINKING EXERCISES

1. Complete the values clarification exercise (Box 8-1) with your classmates or others. Compare the answers and discuss the differences.
2. You are a clinic nurse in a small community clinic. A 17-year-old female client has been coming to the clinic for treatment for and support with a sexually transmitted disease. During recent months, she has lost her support from a close friend. In addition, her parents are divorced, and she has little contact with them. Her health and well-being are of concern. Her appearance is unkempt, her nutritional status is not balanced, and she has admitted to being depressed. She asks for your help in planning her suicide. Discuss your response to her request. Begin by acknowledging the laws related to assisted suicide in Canada. Examine your personal feelings about suicide. Include a discussion about your understanding of sexually transmitted diseases: Where do they come from? Who gets these diseases? Why do people get these diseases? What are your feelings and opinions about people with sexually transmitted diseases? Construct your response, keeping in mind the theory of relational ethics. Discuss your role in this situation. What are your possible courses of action?
3. You have been assigned the care of a 98-year-old woman who was recently admitted with a diagnosis of pneumonia. She has a history of cardiac disease and takes a number of medications. She had been fairly active until the past few days, when her cough worsened and a fever developed. You note that her pulse has become weak and threadlike and that her respirations are increasingly laboured. The client is now too weak to respond to you. When you mention to the family that you may need to call the physician and even take heroic lifesaving measures, the client's son and daughter become distraught, saying that they do not want their mother to be kept alive on "machines." They report that they have discussed this situation with their mother.

You find that her wishes have not been documented in her chart. The family members have not discussed this situation with the client's primary physician. What actions would you consider taking at this moment? Take into account the ethical principles of autonomy and beneficence and the idea of futile care. What are your personal values about interventions at the end of life?

* REVIEW QUESTIONS

1. Values clarification plays a major role in:
   1. Creating a set of rules for conduct
   2. Identifying values that should be accepted by all
   3. Resolving issues of "value conflict"
   4. Developing a code of ethics
2. In Canada, equitable access to health care means that all citizens have equal access to medically necessary services. Many jurisdictions have implemented private magnetic resonance imaging clinics. A discussion about the ethics of this situation would involve predominately the principle of
   1. Accountability
   2. Autonomy
   3. Relational ethics
   4. Justice
3. It may seem redundant when health care professionals, including professional nurses, agree to "do no harm" to their clients. The point of this agreement is to reassure the public that in all ways, not only will the health care team work to heal clients but they also agree to do this in the least painful and harmful way possible. The principle that describes this agreement is called
   1. Beneficence
   2. Accountability
   3. Nonmaleficence
   4. Respect for autonomy
4. Vaccination may cause temporary discomfort, but the benefits of protection from disease, both for the individual and for society, outweigh the client's discomfort. This involves the principle of
   1. Beneficence
   2. Fidelity
   3. Nonmaleficence
   4. Respect for autonomy
5. If a nurse assesses a client for pain and then offers a plan to manage the pain, the principle that encourages the nurse to monitor the client's response to the plan is
   1. Beneficence
   2. Justice
   3. Nonmaleficence
   4. Respect for autonomy
6. Including clients in decision making regarding their care and respecting their choices of treatment demonstrate the principle of:
   1. Beneficence
   2. Autonomy
   3. Justice
   4. Veracity
7. Nurses agree to be advocates for their clients. Practice of advocacy calls for the nurse to
   1. Seek out a nursing supervisor in situations involving conflict
   2. Work to understand the law as it applies to the client's clinical condition
   3. Assess the client's point of view and prepare to articulate this point of view
   4. Document all clinical changes in the medical record in a timely manner
8. Which of the following is *not* part of the nurse's role as client advocate?
   1. Intervening if other people fail to respect the client's dignity
   2. Protecting the client's right to confidentiality and privacy
   3. Making nursing care decisions for the client
   4. Advocating for appropriate use of interventions to minimize suffering
9. The philosophy of relational ethics suggests that ethical dilemmas can best be solved by attention to
   1. Relationships
   2. Ethical principles
   3. Clients
   4. Code of ethics for nurses
10. Ethical dilemmas often arise over a conflict of opinion. Once the nurse has determined that the dilemma is ethical, a critical first step in negotiating the difference of opinion is to
    1. Consult a professional ethicist to ensure that the steps of the process occur in full
    2. Gather all relevant information regarding the dilemma
    3. List the ethical principles that inform the dilemma so that negotiations agree on the language of the discussion
    4. Ensure that the attending physician has written an order for an ethics consultation to support the ethics process

* RECOMMENDED WEB SITES

Canadian Bioethics Society: http://www.bioethics.ca
Founded in 1988 through the amalgamation of the Canadian Society of Bioethics and the Canadian Society for Medical Bioethics. Members include health care administrators, lawyers, nurses, philosophers, physicians, theologians, and other professionals concerned with the ethical and humane dimensions of health care. The Web site offers information about the annual CBS conference, national and international ethics organization links, and relevant ethics journals from a variety of disciplines.

Canadian Nurses Association-Code of Ethics: http://www.cna-aiic.ca/CNA/documents/pdf/publications/Code_of_Ethics_2008_e.pdf
Provides a link to the CNA and the *Code of Ethics for Registered Nurses* (CNA, 2008).

W. Maurice Young Centre for Applied Ethics: http://www.ethics.ubc.ca
Established by the University of British Columbia in 1993; primarily an interdisciplinary research centre in which a variety of ethics topics are studied. The Web site has links to other ethics organizations and ethics resources. The centre's newsletter is also available on the Web site.

Nursing Ethics.ca: http://www.nursingethics.ca/
Has links to Canadian resources that support ethical nursing practice.

Provincial Health Ethics Network of Alberta (PHEN): http://www.phen.ab.ca/
Established as a society in 1995; provides information for all Albertans about ethics and access to health ethics resources. Its mission is to facilitate examination, discussion, and decision making with regard to ethical issues in health and health care.

9

Legal Implications in Nursing Practice

Written by Carla Shapiro, MN, RN

Based on the original chapter by Janis Waite, RN, MSN, EdD

objectives

Mastery of content in this chapter will enable you to:

- Define the key terms listed.
- Explain legal concepts that apply to nurses.
- Describe the legal responsibilities and obligations of nurses.
- List sources for standards of care for nurses.
- Define legal aspects of nurse–client, nurse–physician, nurse–nurse, and nurse–employer relationships.
- List the elements needed to prove negligence.
- Give examples of legal issues that arise in nursing practice.

key terms

Advance directive, p. 111
Adverse occurrence report, p. 112
Assault, p. 105
Battery, p. 105
Civil law, p. 103
Common law, p. 103
Euthanasia, p. 111
Incident report, p. 112
Informed consent, p. 107
Intentional torts, p. 105
Living will, p. 111
Negligence, p. 105
Nursing practice acts, p. 104
Risk management, p. 112
Standards of care, p. 103
Statute law, p. 103
Tort, p. 105

media resources

evolve Web Site

- Audio Chapter Summaries
- Glossary
- Multiple-Choice Review Questions
- Student Learning Activities
- Weblinks

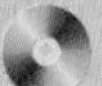 **Companion CD**

- Glossary
- Interactive Learning Activities
- Fluids and Electrolytes Tutorial
- Test-Taking Skills

Safe nursing practice includes knowledge of the legal boundaries within which nurses must function. Nurses must understand the law to protect themselves from liability and to protect their clients' rights. Nurses need not fear the law; rather, they should view it as representing what society expects from them. Laws are continually changing to meet the needs of the people they are intended to protect. As technology has expanded the role of the nurse, the ethical dilemmas associated with client care have increased and often become legal issues as well. As health care evolves, so do the legal implications for health care. Although federal laws apply to all provinces and territories, nurses must also be aware that laws do vary across the country. It is important for nurses to know the laws in their province or territory that affect their practice. Being familiar with the law enhances nurses' ability to be client advocates.

Legal Limits of Nursing

Nurses have a fiduciary relationship with their clients. A fiduciary relationship is one in which a professional (the nurse) provides services that, by their nature, cause the recipient (the client) to trust in the specialized knowledge and integrity of the professional. In the fiduciary relationship, nurses are obligated to provide knowledgeable, competent, and safe care.

Although legal actions against nurses were once rare, the situation is changing. The public is better informed now than in the past about their rights to health care and are more likely to seek damages for professional negligence. The courts have upheld the concept that nurses must provide a reasonable standard of care. Thus, it is essential that nurses understand the legal limits influencing their daily practice.

Sources of Law

The Canadian legal system can be divided into two main categories: public law and private law. Public law is chiefly concerned with relations between individuals and the state or society in general and includes constitutional, tax, administrative, human rights, and criminal law. Private law involves disputes between individuals and covers issues such as wills, contracts, marriage and divorce, and civil wrongs (e.g., negligence). Whereas public law is addressed in the same manner across the country, two systems deal with private law issues—**civil law** (based on Roman law) in Quebec and **common law** (based on British common law) throughout the rest of the country. These two systems differ primarily in their legal processes. In each system, courts interpret the rules made by the legislature in the context of specific disputes.

When either a civil or a criminal case goes to court, decisions are based on previous case rulings. How courts rule on the circumstances and facts surrounding the case is called a *precedent*. If a case is decided on the basis of certain facts, the court is bound to follow that decision in subsequent similar cases. Not every jurisdiction has case law on a given issue. For example, cases regarding a client's right to refuse treatment are not found in every province. In such situations, other jurisdictions are consulted for guidance. In general, breaches of private law result in the payment of money to compensate the aggrieved party for damages incurred. Violations of public law may result in a range of remedies, including fines or imprisonment.

Statute law is created by elective legislative bodies such as Parliament and provincial or territorial legislatures. Federal statutes apply throughout the country, and provincial and territorial statutes apply only in the province or territory in which they were created. Examples of provincial statutes are the *Regulated Health Professions Act* (1991) in Ontario and nursing practice acts throughout the country, which describe and define nursing practice within each province. Examples of federal statutes are the new *Assisted Human Reproduction Act* (2004), the *Controlled Drugs and Substances Act* (1996), and the *Food and Drugs Act* (1985).

Professional Regulation

Like all self-governing professions in Canada, nursing is regulated at the provincial or territorial level. Each province and territory has legislation that grants authority to a nursing regulatory body. These regulatory bodies are accountable to the public for ensuring safe, competent, and ethical nursing care. Regulatory bodies are responsible for granting certificates of registration, offering practice support, ensuring continuing competence of its members, investigating complaints against members' conduct, and disciplining members when necessary. Regulatory bodies are also responsible for developing codes of ethics, setting standards of practice, and approving nursing education programs (McIntyre et al., 2006).

Separate regulatory bodies exist for registered nurses and practical nurses. Some provinces also have regulatory bodies for registered psychiatric nurses. These regulatory bodies are called either the *provincial association* or the *college of nursing* (e.g., the Alberta Association of Registered Nurses; the College of Licensed Practical Nurses of Alberta; the College of Nurses of Ontario). The trend appears to be a move to the college model, with a stronger focus on regulation of practice and accountability to the public.

Nurses must be registered by the professional nursing association or college of the province or territory in which they practise. The requirements for registration (or licensure, as applicable) varies across the country, but most provinces and territories have minimum education requirements and require the nurse to pass an examination. All provinces and territories (except Quebec) use the Canadian Registered Nurse Examination. Quebec has created its own examination. Registration (or licensure) enables people to practise nursing and use the applicable nursing title and initials: registered nurse (RN) or registered practical nurse (RPN). All nurses' credentials must be verified, either by the listing of their names on a register or by their holding a valid licence to practise.

Registration can be suspended or revoked by the regulatory body if a nurse's conduct violates provisions in the registration statute. For example, nurses who perform illegal acts, such as selling controlled substances, jeopardize their registration status. Due process must be followed before registration can be suspended or revoked. *Due process* means that nurses must be notified of the charges brought against them and have an opportunity to defend themselves against the charges in a hearing. Such hearings do not occur in courts but are usually conducted by the regulatory body. If a nurse loses his or her professional licence, or if the nurse's name is removed from the provincial or territorial register, and if the case involves civil or criminal wrongs, then further legal consequences may follow.

Standards of Care

Standards of care are legal guidelines for nursing practice. Standards establish an expectation of nurses to provide safe and appropriate client care. If nurses do not perform duties within accepted standards of care, they may place themselves in jeopardy of legal action and, more important, place their clients at risk for harm and injury. Nursing standards of care arise from a variety of sources, including statutes and laws of broad application, such as the statutes and common law relating to human rights, privacy, and negligence; provincial statutes that specifically apply to health care professionals or nurses only; and the detailed regulations, practice standards, and codes of ethics that are generated by the professional associations. Nursing standards are also outlined in the written policies and procedures of employing institutions.

All provincial and territorial legislatures have passed health professions, **nursing practice acts,** or both that define the scope of nursing practice. These acts set educational requirements for nurses, distinguish between nursing and medical practice, and generally define nursing practice. The rules and regulations enacted by the provincial or territorial regulatory body help define the practice of nursing more specifically. For example, a nursing association may develop a rule regarding intravenous therapy. All nurses are responsible for knowing the provisions of the nursing practice act for the province or territory in which they work, as well as the rules and regulations enacted by the regulatory administrative bodies of their province or territory.

Professional organizations are another source for defining standards of care. The Canadian Nurses Association (CNA) has developed standards for nursing practice, policy statements, and similar resolutions. The standards delineate the scope, function, and role of the nurse in practice. Nursing specialty organizations also have standards of practice defined for certification of nurses who work in specific specialty areas, such as the operating room or the critical care unit. The same standards also serve as practice guidelines for defining safe and appropriate nursing care in specialty areas.

The Canadian Council on Health Services Accreditation requires that accredited health care institutions have nursing policies and procedures in writing that detail how nurses are to perform their duties. These internal standards of care are usually quite specific and are found in procedural manuals on most nursing units. For example, a procedure or policy that outlines the steps that should be taken when a dressing is changed or medication is administered gives specific information about how nurses are to perform these tasks. Nurses must know the policies and procedures of their employing institution because they all must follow the same standard of care. Institutional policies and procedures must conform to laws and cannot conflict with legal guidelines that define acceptable standards of care.

In a negligence lawsuit, these standards are used to determine whether the nurse has acted as any reasonably prudent nurse in a similar setting with the same credentials would act. A nursing expert is called to testify about the standards of nursing care as applied to the facts of the case (Box 9–1). The expert may be called to define and explain to the court what a reasonably prudent nurse would have been expected to do in view of the facts of the case in any similar setting around the country. It is recognized and understood that nursing practice differs according to the rural or urban nature of the institutional setting. In addition, home health care, occupational health nursing, and other community-based clinical settings require that the expert be familiar with the standards of care in these settings, as opposed to the traditional hospital or institutional setting. The expert must have the appropriate credentials, the appropriate experience, and an understanding of what the standard of care should have been in the specific case. The expert witness is distinguished from the fact witness. Staff nurses may testify in a court proceeding as fact witnesses if they have first-hand personal experience with the facts of the case. The expert witness evaluates the defendant's professional judgements and behaviour under the circumstances being reviewed.

General duty nurses are often legally responsible for meeting the same standards as other general duty nurses in similar settings. However, specialized nurses, such as nurses in a critical care unit or nurses who perform dialysis, are held to standards of care and skill that apply to all professionals in the same specialty. All nurses must know the standards of care that they are expected to meet within their specific specialty and work setting. Ignorance of the law or of standards of care is not a defence against negligence, nor is being asked by an employer to perform an out-of-scope procedure. The law as written overrules any agency policy or procedure.

> **BOX 9-1 Anatomy of a Lawsuit**
>
> **Pleadings: Statements of Claim and Defence**
>
> - The plaintiff outlines what the defendant or defendants did wrong and how that action caused injury.
> - The statement of claim is then issued by the court and served on the defendant or defendants.
> - Statements of claim are often very broad and may be served on the employer, institution, and all members of the health care team involved in the client's care at the relevant time.
> - The defendant or defendants must deliver a statement of defence to the allegations. The defendant or defendants can admit or deny each allegation in the petition.
>
> **Procedures of Discovery**
>
> Pretrial proceedings enable each side to gather legally relevant information from the other side and usually lead to a settlement between the parties before a trial.
>
> 1. *Examination for discovery:* The plaintiff's lawyer is permitted to question each defendant under oath. Examination for discovery usually takes place in private offices, with only the plaintiffs and defendants, their lawyers, and a reporter present to record a transcript of the testimony. Questioning can be wide-ranging and detailed in order to reveal useful information. Answers given to questions will be available for trial.
> 2. *Discovery of documents:* Each side can be forced to produce all documents relevant to the litigation. Medical records and nurses' notes may be of particular value.
> 3. *Independent medical examination of the plaintiff:* This examination is conducted to determine the extent of the plaintiff's injuries. Negligence cannot be charged without proof of damage.
> 4. *Discovery by interrogatories:* Similar to the examination for discovery, interrogatories involves a series of written questions, which must be answered under oath.
>
> **Expert Witnesses**
>
> An expert witness is an individual who, because of education, experience, or both, has knowledge that can assist decision makers in establishing whether the nursing care that was provided met the expected standard of practice. Each side usually selects experts to help explain and interpret the evidence as it emerges.
>
> **Pretrial Conference**
>
> The purpose of the pretrial conference is to identify points of contention, narrow down the issues, and encourage settlement out of court. In some jurisdictions, the pretrial conference may be mandatory. A pretrial conference is presided over by a judge and attended by counsel for the various parties. Most settlements take place without any admission of liability.
>
> **Trial**
>
> A trial usually occurs several years after the initial statement of claim is filed. Most nursing negligence cases are heard and decided by a judge alone. Damages are usually assessed at trial.

Legal Liability Issues in Nursing Practice

Torts

A **tort** is a civil wrong committed against a person or property. Torts may be classified as intentional or unintentional. **Intentional torts** are willful acts that violate another person's rights (Keatings & Smith, 2000). Examples are assault, battery, invasion of privacy, and false imprisonment. Negligence is example of an unintentional tort.

Intentional Torts

Assault. Assault is conduct (such as a physical or verbal threat) that creates in another person apprehension or fear of imminent harmful or offensive contact. No actual contact is necessary in order for damages for assault to be awarded (Fridman, 2003; Osborne, 2003). Threats by a nurse to give a client an injection or to restrain a client for an x-ray procedure when the client has refused consent constitute assault. The key issues are whether the client was afraid of being harmed in the situation and whether the client consented to a procedure. In a lawsuit wherein assault is alleged, the client's consent would negate the claim of assault against a nurse.

Battery. Battery is any intentional physical contact with a person without that person's consent. The contact can be harmful to the client and cause an injury, or it can be merely offensive to the client's personal dignity (Sneiderman et al., 2003). In the example of a nurse's threats to give a client an injection without the client's consent, if the nurse actually gives the injection, it is considered battery. Battery could even be life-saving, as in the Ontario case of *Malette v. Shulman* (1990). In that case, the plaintiff was unconscious and bleeding profusely. The physician determined that she needed a life-saving blood transfusion. Before the transfusion, a nurse found a signed card in the plaintiff's purse that identified the client as a Jehovah's Witness and stated that under no circumstances was she to receive blood. Despite this, the physician chose to administer the blood to preserve the client's life. The plaintiff survived, recovered from her injuries, and successfully sued the physician for battery (Sneiderman et al., 2003).

In some situations, consent is implied. For example, if a client gets into a wheelchair or transfers to a stretcher of his or her own volition after being advised that it is time to be taken for an x-ray procedure, the client has given implied consent to the procedure. A client has the right to revoke or withdraw consent at any time.

Invasion of Privacy. The tort of invasion of privacy protects the client's right to be free from unwanted intrusion into his or her private affairs. Clients are entitled to confidential health care. Nursing standards for what constitutes confidential information are based on professional ethics and the common law. The ideals of privacy and sensitivity to the needs and rights of clients who may not choose to have nurses intrude on their lives, but who depend on nurses for their care, guide the nurse's judgement. The nurse's fiduciary duty requires that confidential information not be shared with anyone else except on a need-to-know basis.

One form of invasion of privacy is the release of a client's medical information to an unauthorized person, such as a member of the press or the client's employer. The information that is contained in a client's medical record is a confidential communication. It should be shared with health care providers only for the purpose of medical treatment.

A client's medical record is confidential. The nurse should not disclose the client's confidential medical information without the client's consent. For example, a nurse should respect a wish not to inform the client's family of a terminal illness. Similarly, a nurse should not assume that a client's spouse or family members know all of the client's history, particularly with regard to private issues such as mental illness, medications, pregnancy, abortion, birth control, or sexually transmitted infections.

Confidentiality is not an absolute value, however, and in certain circumstances, breaching confidentiality is justifiable. At times, a nurse may be required by law (statutory duty) to breach confidentiality and disclose information to a third party. For example, each province and territory has laws that require health care workers to report suspected child abuse to a local child protection agency. Nurses may also be required to release information about a client when they receive a subpoena (a legal order) to testify in court.

Nurses are under no legal obligation to release confidential information to the police except in rare cases in which the life, safety, or health of the client or an innocent third party is in jeopardy (such as when a client tells a nurse that he or she intends to hurt or kill someone; Tapp, 1996). Such a statement should be reported to the authorities of the institution and to the police. Other admissions made by a client to a nurse about past or future criminal activity may not have to be disclosed unless the nurse is compelled to do so by a court of law. The conflict between confidentiality and risk of public harm is not always clear. When a nurse has serious concerns about the welfare of others (e.g., if a client is infected with human immunodeficiency virus [HIV] and admits to having unsafe sex or donating blood), the nurse should first suggest and strongly encourage the client to disclose this information. If the client refuses, then the nurse should seek consultation with professional colleagues and supervisors. A careful balancing of the need for privacy and confidentiality of privileged communication would need to be weighed carefully.

Computers and Confidentiality. Most health care facilities use computer systems to maintain client records. "Computerization in health care raises major legal concerns related to confidentiality of health records becauses of the potential for unauthorized access and data sharing" (Tapp, 2003). Access to confidential client information is generally controlled by means of a variety of technological safeguards, including magnetized cards and passwords. It is important that these security devices not be shared with other people and that access cards be used to retrieve files only when warranted. The improper use of a magnetized card and password to seek out confidential information could lead to legal repercussions or disciplinary action.

Likewise, the use of e-mail messages carries a potential legal risk because they are susceptible to unauthorized access by third parties. E-mail messages may also be introduced as evidence in any court or legal proceedings (Tapp, 2001).

False Imprisonment. The tort of false imprisonment serves to protect a person's individual liberty and basic rights. Preventing a client from leaving a health care facility voluntarily may constitute the tort of false imprisonment. The inappropriate or unjustified use of restraints (e.g., by confining a person to an area, or by using physical or chemical restraints) may also be viewed as false imprisonment. Nurses must be aware of their facility's policies and specific legislation in their jurisdiction (e.g., under the *Mental Health and Consequential Amendments Act*, 1998) relating to when and how restraints can be used (Canadian Nurses Protective Society [CNPS], 2004a).

Unintentional Torts

Negligence. When nurses are sued, most often the proceedings against them are for the tort of negligence, also referred to as *malpractice* (Sneiderman et al., 2003). **Negligence** in nursing is conduct that does not meet a standard of care established by law. No intent is needed for negligence to occur. It is characterized chiefly by inadvertence, thoughtlessness, or inattention. Negligence may involve carelessness, such as not checking an identification bracelet, which results in administration of the wrong medication. However, carelessness is not always the cause of misconduct. If nurses perform a procedure for which they have not been educated and do so carefully but still harm the client, a claim of negligence can be made. In general, courts define nursing negligence as the failure to use the degree of skill or learning ordinarily used under the same or similar circumstances by members of the nursing profession (Box 9–2).

Nurses can be found liable for negligence if the following criteria are established: (1) The nurse (defendant) owed a duty to the client (plaintiff); (2) the nurse did not carry out that duty; (3) the client was injured; and (4) the nurse's failure to carry out the duty caused the injury.

The ability to predict harm (i.e., the foreseeability of risk) is evaluated in negligence cases. The circumstances surrounding the injury are evaluated to determine whether it was likely that the injury or harm to the client could have been expected from the care that was or was not provided. The cause of the injury is also investigated through the evaluation of the actual and the nearest causes of the injury. Had it not been for what the nurse did or did not do, could an injury have been prevented?

The case of *Downey v. Rothwell* (1974) is an example of nursing negligence. This case involved a plaintiff who suffered a severe arm injury when she fell off an examining table while under the care of a nurse. The client, who had a history of epilepsy, informed the nurse that she was about to have a seizure. The nurse left the client unattended on an examining table while she left the room for a few moments. During this time, the client had a seizure, fell onto the floor, and broke her arm. The nurse should have anticipated that the client could have fallen during a seizure and ensured her safety either by moving her to the floor or by putting up guard rails on the examining table. This case involved an undertaking by the nurse to provide care, a reliance by the client on this nurse, and a foreseeable risk. The nurse was found negligent in this case, and her employers were held vicariously liable. "Vicarious liability is a legal doctrine that applies in situations where the law holds the employer legally responsible for the acts of its employees that occur within the scope and course of their employment" (CNPS, 1998).

In the case of *Granger v. Ottawa General Hospital* (1996), two nurses (a staff nurse and her team leader) were found negligent in the care they provided to a woman in labour. During labour, the plaintiff's fetal heart monitor strip showed deep, persistent, variable decelerations. The staff nurse did not appreciate that these were a sign of fetal distress and did not immediately report these findings to other members of the obstetrical team. The ensuing delay in care resulted in severe and permanent brain injury in the baby, leaving her severely disabled. In this case, the nurses breached their duty to exercise appropriate skill in making an assessment and to communicate the information to the physicians.

BOX 9-2 Common Negligent Acts

- Medication errors that result in injury to clients
- Intravenous therapy errors that result in infiltrations or phlebitis
- Burns caused by equipment, bathing, or spills of hot liquids and foods
- Falls resulting in injury to clients
- Failure to use aseptic technique as required
- Errors in sponge, instrument, or needle counts in surgical cases
- Failure to give a report, or giving an incomplete report, to an incoming shift of health care staff
- Failure to monitor a client's condition adequately
- Failure to notify a physician of a significant change in a client's status

Preventing Negligence. The best way for nurses to avoid being negligent is to follow standards of care; give competent health care; insist on appropriate orientation, continuing education, and adequate staffing; communicate with other health care providers; develop a caring rapport with the client; and document assessments, interventions, and evaluations fully.

The health care record, or "chart," is a permanent record of the nursing process. The courts consult the patient's chart for a chronological record of all aspects of care provided from admission to discharge. "Courts use nursing documentation at trial to reconstruct events, establish times and dates, refresh memories of witnesses and . . . resolve conflicts in testimony" (CNPS, 2007a). As a legal document, it is the most comprehensive record of the care provided. Careful, complete, and thorough documentation is one of the best defences against allegations of negligence or violations of nursing standards (see Chapter 16). The record can show that even in the event of an adverse patient outcome, the nursing care that was provided met the expected standards. An institution has a legal duty to maintain nursing records. Nursing notes contain substantial evidence needed in order to understand the care received by a client. If records are lost or incomplete, the care is presumed to have been negligent and therefore the cause of the client's injuries. In addition, incomplete or illegible records undermine the credibility of the health care professional.

In the case of *Kolesar v. Jeffries* (1976), the Supreme Court of Canada addressed the issue of poor record keeping. In that case, a client underwent major spinal surgery and was transferred to a surgical unit, where he was nursed on a Stryker frame. The client was found dead the following morning. No nursing notes were recorded from 2200 hours the previous evening until 0500 hours, when he was found dead. Although at trial several nurses and nursing assistants testified that they had tended to the client multiple times throughout the night, the court inferred that "nothing was charted because nothing was done." One of the nurses was held negligent for this client's death.

It is very important for documentation to be accomplished in a timely manner. Any significant changes in the client's condition must be reported to the physician and documented in the chart (see Chapter 16). Recording nursing care notes in a notebook and then transferring them to the chart at the end of the shift can be a dangerous practice. If this practice is followed, other health care professionals may administer medications or provide care to the client without up-to-date information. Harm may come to a client whose record is not accurate and current. Nurses must always follow the particular style of charting adopted by their employer (Phillips, 1999a).

Truthful documentation is also essential. If an error is made in the documentation, it is important to follow the policies and procedures of the institution to correct it. Obliterating or erasing errors may appear to be concealing misconduct and lead to charges of fraud. The credibility of a nurse who goes to court is negatively affected if it appears that the nurse's initial charting has been changed after an injury has occurred to a client. This scenario is exemplified in the case of *Meyer v. Gordon* (1981). Nurses did not adequately monitor a woman in labour, and their notes were sloppy and vague. The fetus experienced severe distress, required resuscitation on delivery, and was transferred to another hospital. When a nurse realized that the documentation was deficient, she altered it. However, the original chart had already been photocopied and sent to the second hospital. At trial, it was obvious that the original document had been tampered with. The court held that the nursing staff had been negligent in several ways, and the judge severely condemned the nurse's tampering with the evidence. The court commented as follows: "My criticism of the defendant hospital is not confined to the lack of care of its nursing staff. The hospital chart contains alterations and additions which compel me to view with suspicion the accuracy of many of the observations which are recorded."

Nurses should also be familiar with the current nursing literature in their areas of practice. They should know and follow the policies and procedures of the institution in which they work. Nurses should be sensitive to common sources of injury to clients, such as falls and medication errors. Nurses must communicate with the client, explain the tests and treatment to be performed, document that specific explanations were provided to the client, and listen to the client's concerns about the treatment.

Nurse–client relationships are very important not only in ensuring quality care but also in minimizing legal risks. Trust develops between a nurse and client. Clients who believe that the nurses performed their duties correctly and were concerned with their welfare are less likely to initiate a lawsuit against the nurses. Sincere caring for clients is an essential role of the nurse and is an effective risk-management tool. However, caring does not protect nurses completely if negligent practice occurs. When a client is injured, the investigation into the incident may implicate the nurses even if the client feels kindly toward them.

Criminal Liability

Although most nursing liability issues involve private law matters (e.g., torts), the criminal law is also relevant. Canadian nurses have been charged with criminal offences such as assault, administering a noxious substance, and criminal negligence that causes death (a category of manslaughter). The difference between the tort of negligence and criminal negligence charges is the degree to which the act deviated from the standard of a reasonably competent practitioner. For example, in the case of criminal negligence, the courts must prove that the nurse was extremely careless, indicating "wanton or reckless disregard for the lives or safety of other persons" (*Criminal Code*, 1985, Part VIII, Section 219 [1]).

Consent

A signed consent form is required for all routine treatment, procedures such as surgery, some treatment programs such as chemotherapy, and research involving clients. A client signs general consent forms when admitted to the hospital or other health care facility. The client or the client's representative must sign a special consent or treatment form before each specialized procedure or treatment. "If a person receiving care is clearly incapable of consent, the nurse respects the law on capacity assessment and substitute decision-making in his or her jurisdiction" (CNA, 2008, p.11; see also CNPS, 2004b). Provincial and territorial laws describe what constitutes the legal ability to give consent to medical treatment. Nurses should know the law in their own jurisdiction and be familiar with the policies and procedures of their employing institution with regard to consent.

In general, the following factors must be verified for consent to be legally valid:

- The client must have the legal and mental capacity to make a treatment decision.
- The consent must be given voluntarily and without coercion.
- The client must understand the risks and benefits of the procedure or treatment, the risks of not undergoing the procedure or treatment, and any available alternatives to the procedure or treatment.

If a client is deaf, is illiterate, or does not speak the language of the health care professionals, an official interpreter must be available to explain the terms of consent. A family member or acquaintance who is able to speak a client's language should not be used to interpret health information except as a last resort. A client experiencing the effects of a sedative is not able to clearly understand the implications of an invasive procedure. Every effort should be made to assist the client in making an informed choice.

Nurses must be sensitive to the cultural issues of consent. The nurse must understand the way in which clients and their families communicate and make important decisions. It is essential for nurses to understand the various cultures with which they interact. The cultural beliefs and values of the client may be very different from those of the nurse. It is important for nurses not to impose their own cultural values on the client (see Chapter 10).

Informed Consent.

"Nurses ensure that nursing care is provided with the person's informed consent. Nurses recognize and support a capable person's right to refuse or withdraw consent for care or treatment at any time." (CNA, 2008, p. 11).

Informed consent is a person's agreement to allow a medical action to happen, such as surgery or an invasive procedure, on the basis of a full disclosure of the likely risks and benefits of the action, alternatives to the action, and the consequences of refusal (Black, 1999). Informed consent creates a legal duty for the physician or other health care professional to disclose material facts in terms that the client can reasonably understand in order to make an informed choice (Sneiderman et al., 2003). The explanation should also describe treatment alternatives, as well as the risks involved in all treatment options. Failure to obtain consent in situations other than emergencies may result in a claim of battery. In the absence of informed consent, a client may bring a lawsuit against the health care professional for negligence, even if the procedure was performed competently. Informed consent requires the provision of adequate information for the client to form a decision and the documentation of that decision.

The following materials are required for informed consent (Sneiderman et al., 2003):

- A brief, complete explanation of the procedure or treatment.
- Names and qualifications of people performing and assisting in the procedure.
- A description of any possible harm, including permanent damage or death, that may occur as a result of the procedure.
- An explanation of therapeutic alternatives to the proposed procedure/treatment, as well as the risks of doing nothing. Clients also need to be informed of their right to refuse the procedure/treatment without discontinuing other supportive care and of their right to withdraw their consent even after the procedure has begun.

Informed consent is part of the physician–client relationship. Because nurses do not perform surgery or direct medical procedures, obtaining clients' informed consent is not usually one of nurses' duties. Even though the nurse may assume the responsibility for witnessing the client's signature on the consent form, the nurse does not legally assume the duty of obtaining informed consent. The nurse's signature witnessing the consent means that the client voluntarily gave consent, that the client's signature is authentic, and that the client appears to be competent to give consent (Sneiderman et al., 2003). When nurses provide consent forms for clients to sign, the clients should be asked whether they understand the procedures to which they are consenting. If they deny understanding, or if the nurse suspects that they do not understand, the nurse must notify the physician or nursing supervisor. Some consent forms also have a line for the physician to sign after explaining the risks and alternatives to a client. Such a form is helpful in a court case when a client alleges that consent was not informed. If a client refuses treatment, this rejection should also be written, signed, and witnessed.

If a client participates in an experimental treatment program or submits to use of experimental drugs or treatments, the informed consent form must be even more detailed and stringently regulated. An organization's institutional review board should review the information in the consent form for research involving human subjects. The client may withdraw from the experiment at any time (see Chapter 8).

Many procedures that nurses perform (e.g., insertion of intravenous or nasogastric tubes) do not require formal written consent; nonetheless, clients' right to give or refuse consent to treatment must be protected. Implied consent to treatment is often involved in nursing procedures. For example, when the nurse approaches the client with a syringe in hand and the client rolls over to expose the injection site, consent is implied. If the client resists the injection either verbally or through actions, the nurse must not proceed with the injection. Forcing or otherwise treating a client without consent could result in criminal or civil charges of assault and battery. Many advanced practice nurses are now autonomously treating clients. It is therefore likely that formal written consent for nursing procedures will also be expected for the treatment received from advance practice nurse specialists.

Parents are usually the legal guardians of pediatric clients, and, therefore, consent forms for treatment must be signed by parents. If the parents are divorced, the form must be signed by the parent with legal custody. On occasion, a parent or guardian refuses treatment for a child. In those cases, the court may intervene in the child's behalf. The practice of making the child a ward of the court and administering necessary treatment is relatively common in such cases.

The example of 13-year-old Tyrell Dueck from Saskatchewan illustrates such a case. The teenager received a diagnosis of cancer in 1998. He completed part of the chemotherapy treatment when he decided that he did not want more treatment or the recommended amputation of his leg, believing that he had been "cured by God" and that further treatment was unnecessary. His statements were consistent with his family's Christian value system. Following his parents' advice, the boy wished to undergo alternative therapy at a clinic in Mexico. The treating physicians maintained that without further conventional treatment, Tyrell would die within a year. A judge concluded that Tyrell had been given inaccurate information by his father about the benefits and risks of the proposed alternative therapy and, therefore, was unable to make an informed consent or refusal. Thus, the family's wishes to forgo conventional treatment were legally overruled, and the boy's grandparents were to take him for treatments. Before the enforced treatment could be started, however, tests revealed that the cancer had already spread and the treatment would no longer be helpful. The teenager was returned to the care of his parents, and he died a short time later.

In some instances, obtaining informed consent is difficult or simply not possible. If, for example, the client is unconscious, consent must be obtained from a person legally authorized to give consent on the client's behalf. Other surrogate decision makers may have legally been delegated this authority through proxy directives or court guardianship procedures. In emergency situations, if it is impossible to obtain consent from the client or an authorized person, the procedure required to benefit the client or save the client's life may be undertaken without liability for failure to obtain consent. In such cases, the law assumes that the client would wish to be treated. This is referred to as the *emergency doctrine*.

Clients with mental health problems and frail older adults must also be given the opportunity to give consent. They retain the right to refuse treatment unless a court has legally determined that they are incompetent to decide for themselves.

Nursing Students and Legal Liability

Nursing students must know their own capabilities and competencies and must not perform nursing actions unless competent to do so. "However, if a student nurse performs a nursing action which is one an RN would perform (e.g. administration of an I.M. [intramuscular] injection), that student will be held to the standard of an RN. Student nurses, like all other nurses, are accountable for their own actions" (Phillips, 2002). In a few reported cases in Canada, nursing students were sued for negligence in their care of patients. A nursing student in Nova Scotia who caused permanent injury in a client through an improperly administered intramuscular injection was found negligent, and the hospital was found vicariously liable for the student's actions (CNPS, 2007b; *Roberts v. Cape Breton Regional Hospital*, 1997). Thus, nursing students are liable if their actions cause harm to clients. However, if a client is harmed as a direct result of a nursing student's actions or lack of action, the liability is generally shared by the student, the instructor, the hospital or health care facility, and the university or educational institution. Nursing students should never be assigned to perform tasks for which they are unprepared, and they should be carefully supervised by instructors as they learn new skills. Although nursing students are not considered employees of the hospital, the institution has a responsibility to monitor their acts. Nursing students are expected to ensure that their student status is known to clients and to perform as professional nurses would in providing safe client care. Faculty members are usually responsible for instructing and observing students, but in some situations, staff nurses serving as preceptors may share these responsibilities. Every nursing school should provide clear definitions of student responsibility, preceptor responsibility, and faculty responsibility (Phillips, 2002).

When students are employed as nursing assistants or nurses' aides when not attending classes, they should not perform tasks that do not appear in a job description for a nurses' aide or assistant. For example, even if a student has learned to administer intramuscular medications in class, this task may not be performed by a nurses' aide. If a staff nurse overseeing the nursing assistant or aide knowingly assigns work without regard for the person's ability to safely conduct the task as defined in the job description, that staff nurse is also liable. If students employed as nurse's aides are requested to perform tasks that they are not prepared to complete safely, this information should be brought to the nursing supervisor's attention so that the needed help can be obtained.

The Web site of the CNPS (http://www.cnps.ca/ through its members-only section) is an excellent resource available to nursing students, providing information about legal risks nurses face in practice. However, nursing students are not entitled to receive legal consultation services or financial assistance from the CNPS; these services are provided only for the benefit of eligible registered nurses.

Professional Liability Protection

Most nurses in Canada are employed by publicly funded health care facilities that carry malpractice insurance. These facilities are considered employers and therefore are vicariously liable for negligent acts of their employees as long as the employees were working within the normal scope and course of practice (Keatings & Smith, 2000).

Because of this legal principle, if an employee is found liable in a civil lawsuit, the employer is generally ordered to pay the damages (CNPS, 1998). A nurse who exceeds the bounds of acceptable practice or is self-employed is fully liable for his or her own negligence. All nurses should be aware of their employment status and professional liability coverage.

The CNPS is a nonprofit society established in 1988 to provide legal support and liability protection to nurses. The services of CNPS are available free as a benefit of membership in a subscribing provincial or territorial professional association or college. The only two jurisdictions in Canada not included in CNPS are British Columbia and Quebec. Registered nurses in British Columbia are covered by their own insurance corporation, and those in Quebec have commercial insurance available through the Order of Nurses of Quebec. CNPS services are available to nurses in a variety of work settings, including independent practice and volunteer settings. Eligible nurses can obtain confidential assistance from a nurse lawyer by contacting the CNPS toll-free by telephone, Monday to Friday from 0845 to 1630 hours Eastern Standard Time or Eastern Daylight Time at 1-800-267-3390. A nurse providing emergency assistance at an accident scene would not be covered by an employer's insurance policy because the care given would not be the responsibility of the employer. However, some provinces have passed "Good Samaritan" laws (e.g., Alberta's *Emergency Medical Aid Act,* 2000) that prevent voluntary rescuers from being sued for wrongdoing unless it can be proved that they displayed gross negligence. Nurses must be familiar with these laws in their own province or territory (Phillips, 1999b).

Abandonment, Assignment, and Contract Issues

Short Staffing. During nursing shortages or periods of staff downsizing, the issue of inadequate staffing may arise. Legal problems may result if the number of nurses is insufficient or if an appropriate mix of staff to provide competent care is lacking. If assigned to care for more clients than is reasonable, nurses should bring this information to the attention of the nursing supervisor. In addition, a written protest such as a workload or staffing report form should be completed to document the nurse's concerns about client safety. Most provinces and territories have some reporting mechanism in place to document heavy workload or staffing situations. Although such a protest may not relieve nurses of responsibility if a client suffers injury because of inattention, it would show that they were attempting to act reasonably. Whenever a written protest is made, nurses should keep a copy of this document in their personal files. Most administrators recognize that knowledge of a potential problem shifts some of the responsibility to the institution.

Nurses should not walk out when staffing is inadequate, because charges of abandonment could be made. A nurse who refuses to accept an assignment may be considered insubordinate, and clients would not benefit from having even fewer staff available. It is important to know the institution's policies and procedures and the nursing union's collective agreement on how to handle such circumstances before they arise.

Floating. Nurses are sometimes required to "float" from the area in which they normally practise to other nursing units. Nurses must practise within their level of competence. Nurses should not be floated to areas where they have not been adequately cross-trained. Nurses who float should inform the nursing supervisor of any lack of experience in caring for the type of clients on the nursing unit. They should also request and be given orientation to the unit. A nursing supervisor can be held liable if a staff nurse is given an assignment he or she cannot safely perform. In one case (*Dessauer v. Memorial General Hospital,* 1981), a nurse in obstetrics was assigned to an emergency room. A client entered the emergency room, complaining of chest pain. The obstetrical nurse gave the client too high a dosage of lidocaine, and the client died after suffering irreversible brain damage and cardiac arrest. The nurse lost the negligence lawsuit.

Physicians' Orders. The physician is responsible for directing medical treatment. Nurses are obligated to follow physicians' orders unless they believe the orders are in error, violate hospital policy, or would harm clients. Therefore, all orders must be assessed, and if an order is found to be erroneous or harmful, further clarification from the physician is necessary. If the physician confirms the order and the nurse still believes it is inappropriate, the supervising nurse should be informed. A nurse should not proceed to perform a physician's order if harm to the client is foreseeable. The nursing supervisor should be informed of and given a written memorandum detailing the events in chronological order; the nurse's reasons for refusing to carry out the order should also be written, to protect the nurse from disciplinary action. The supervising nurse should help resolve the questionable order. A medical or pharmacy consultant may be called in to help clarify the appropriateness or inappropriateness of the order. A nurse carrying out an inaccurate or inappropriate order may be legally responsible for any harm suffered by the client.

In a negligence lawsuit against a physician and a hospital, one of the most frequently litigated issues is whether the nurse kept the physician informed of the client's condition. To inform a physician properly, nurses must perform a competent nursing assessment of the client to determine the signs and symptoms that are significant in relation to the attending physician's tasks of diagnosis and treatment. Nurses must be certain to document that the physician was notified and to document his or her response, the nurse's follow-up, and the client's response. For example, nurses noticed that a client with a cast on his leg was experiencing poor circulation in his foot. The nurses recorded these changes but did not notify the physician. Gangrene subsequently developed in the client, and an amputation was required. The hospital, physician, and nursing staff were all charged with negligence.

The physician should write all orders, including "do not resuscitate" (DNR) orders, which many physicians are reluctant to write out because they fear legal repercussions for criminal neglect or failure to act. The nurse must make sure that orders are transcribed correctly. Verbal orders are not recommended because they increase the possibilities for error. If a verbal order is necessary (e.g., during an emergency), it should be written and signed by the physician as soon as possible, usually within 24 hours. The nurse should be familiar with the institution's policy and procedures regarding verbal orders.

Dispensing Advice Over the Phone. Providing advice over the telephone is a high-risk activity because diagnosing over the phone is extremely difficult. The nurse is legally accountable for advice given over the phone. The most common allegations of negligence in this area are provision of inadequate advice, improper referrals, and failure to refer (CNPS, 1997). It is essential that nurses precisely follow institutional guidelines and policies and thoroughly document each call to avoid serious repercussions for all parties.

Contracts and Employment Agreements. In Canada, most nurses belong to unions or associations that engage in collective bargaining on behalf of a group. The collective agreements between employers and union members are written contracts that set out the conditions of employment (e.g., salary, hours of work, benefits, layoffs, and termination). Many laws, including labour laws, apply to nurses. For example, laws outline eligibility for and details of workers' compensation and maternity benefits. It is important for nurses to understand the employment laws in the province or territory where they work.

By accepting a job, a nurse enters into an agreement with an employer. The nurse is expected to perform professional duties competently, adhering to the policies and procedures of the institution. In return, the employer pays for the nursing services and ensures that facilities and equipment are adequate for safe care.

Legal Issues in Nursing Practice

Abortion

In the 1988 case of *R. v. Morgentaler*, the Supreme Court of Canada ruled that the *Criminal Code* (1985) regulations on legal access to abortion were unconstitutional. The *Criminal Code* had required a woman seeking abortion to secure the approval of a hospital-based committee before the procedure could be performed. By rejecting the *Criminal Code* provisions, the Supreme Court in effect referred the abortion issue to Parliament, but Parliament has not rewritten a criminal law policy on abortion. Abortion is thus unregulated by law, which is tantamount to its legalization. However, the legal entitlement to abortion does not mean abortion services are readily available. Because health care facilities are not obliged to offer abortions, many do not do so. Thus, access remains a continuing issue.

Drug Regulations and Nurses

Canadian law closely regulates the administration of drugs. Two federal acts control the manufacture, distribution, and sale of food, drugs, cosmetics, and therapeutic devices in Canada: the *Food and Drugs Act* (1985) and the *Controlled Drugs and Substances Act* (1996). The *Food and Drugs Act* lists the drugs that can be sold only by prescription (e.g., antibiotics) and drugs that are subject to stringent controls (e.g., barbiturates, amphetamines). The distribution of these drugs requires specific handling and record keeping. The *Controlled Drugs and Substances Act* controls the manufacture, distribution, and sale of narcotics (e.g., morphine, codeine). However, it also regulates other drugs that are controlled in the same manner as narcotics, such as cocaine and marijuana. Most institutions have policies about medication administration and record keeping, especially for controlled drugs and narcotics. Nurses must be aware of their employer's policies.

Nurses are not legally entitled to prescribe drugs. However, in several jurisdictions, nurse practitioners may prescribe certain non-narcotic drugs specific to their area of practice.

The administration of medications in accordance with a physician's prescription is a basic nursing responsibility. A competent nurse is expected to know the purpose and effect of any drug administered, as well as potential side effects and contraindications. It is also a nurse's responsibility to question any physician's orders that may be incorrect or unsafe. A nurse who follows a physician's order that is unclear or incorrect may be found negligent.

Communicable Diseases

The care of people with communicable conditions such as HIV infection, acquired immunodeficiency syndrome (AIDS), hepatitis, or severe acute respiratory syndrome (SARS) or during a possible influenza pandemic has legal implications for nurses. Health care workers are at risk for exposure to communicable diseases because of the nature of their work. Despite the best attempts to protect oneself against communicable diseases through the proper and consistent use of protective gear (e.g., latex gloves or masks), accidental needle-stick injuries or life-threatening illnesses such as SARS can occur. Nurses have an ethical and legal obligation to provide care to all assigned clients, and employers have an obligation to provide their employees with necessary protective gear. However, there may be "some circumstances in which it is acceptable for a nurse to withdraw from care provision or to refuse to provide care" (College of Registered Nurses of British Columbia [CRNBC], 2007, p. 1; see also College of Registered Nurses of Nova Scotia, 2006). "Unreasonable burden is a concept raised in relation to duty to provide care and withdrawing from providing or refusing to provide care. An unreasonable burden may exist when a nurse's ability to provide safe care and meet professional standards of practice is compromised by unreasonable expectations, lack of resources, or ongoing threats to personal well-being" (CNA, 2008; see also CRNBC, 2007, p. 1).

In all cases involving privacy, confidentiality, and disclosure, the rights of the clients with a communicable disease must be balanced with the rights of the public or of health care professionals. Both civil and criminal liability can result if private information is disclosed without authorization. Nurses must understand the reporting laws in the province or territory in which they practise. Courts can order disclosure of the records of clients with AIDS in situations that are not addressed by a statute, even without the client's consent. Whenever information about a client is requested by any third parties, including insurance companies or employers, nurses must obtain a signed release from the client before releasing confidential information. Not every health care professional who comes in contact with a client has a need to know the client's HIV status. Confidential information must be protected.

The courts have upheld the employer's right to fire a nurse who refuses to care for a client with AIDS. Nurses who flatly refuse to care for HIV-infected clients or possibly a client with SARS may be reprimanded or fired for insubordination. According to the CNA's (2008) *Code of Ethics for Registered Nurses*, nurses must not discriminate in the provision of nursing care on the basis of factors such as a person's sexual orientation, health status, or lifestyle (p. 13). One limitation outlined in the code regarding a nurse's right to refuse care to a client is that nurses are not obligated to comply with a client's wishes when those wishes are contrary to the law (e.g., assisting the client to commit suicide). If the care requested is contrary to the nurse's personal values, such as assisting with an abortion, the nurse must provide appropriate care until alternative care arrangements are arranged.

Nurses must be concerned with balancing the right to protect themselves with protection of the client's rights. Both are afforded protection against discrimination and protection of privacy by human rights legislation. Most current legal cases involving nurses and communicable diseases are related to the protection needed for nurses as employees. Strict compliance with standard precautions and routine practices and the use of transmission-based precautions (e.g., against airborne or droplet transmission) for clients known or suspected of having other serious illnesses is the nurse's wisest strategy (see Chapter 33).

Death and Dying

Many legal issues surround the event of death, including a basic definition of when a person is considered dead. The only province that has a statutory definition of death is Manitoba, which defines it as "the irreversible cessation of all brain function" (*Vital Statistics Act*, 1987). However, this "brain death" definition has become standard medical practice across Canada. Until the 1960s, death was defined as the irreversible cessation of cardiopulmonary function. However, two developments at that time necessitated a shift to consideration of the brain: (1) the emergence of artificial life-support devices that could maintain cardiopulmonary functioning in a brain-dead person and (2) the emergence of organ transplantation. Death had to be redefined so that organs could be donated.

Ethical and legal questions are raised by the related issues of euthanasia and assisted suicide. **Euthanasia** is an act undertaken by one person with the motive of relieving another person's suffering and the knowledge that the act will end the life of that person (Downie, 2004). In Canada, euthanasia is illegal. It is legally irrelevant whether the client has consented to the act because according to Section 14 of the *Criminal Code* (1985), "no person can consent to have death inflicted on him." Furthermore, according to Section 241 of the *Criminal Code*, it is an offence to "aid a person to commit suicide, whether suicide ensues or not."

On the other hand, the law draws a distinction between "killing" and "letting die." Euthanasia and assisted suicide are considered "killing." Withholding or withdrawing life-prolonging treatment is considered "letting die." The disease process causes the client to die a natural death. Thus, a mentally competent client has the legal right to refuse life-prolonging treatment. If, for example, such a client requests that a ventilator be disconnected, understanding that she will die as a result, her wishes must be honoured in accordance with the principle of "no treatment without consent."

In the case of *Nancy B. v. Hôtel-Dieu de Québec* (1992), a young, mentally competent client who was totally and permanently paralyzed by a neurological disease had twice asked that her ventilator be disconnected. After the second refusal, she sought a court order to enforce her will. The order was granted by the Quebec Superior Court, which ruled that as a mentally competent client, she could not be treated without consent. Also, even if a client has not asked for the termination of life-prolonging treatment (either directly or by way of an advance directive), physicians are still allowed, after consultation with family members, to terminate such treatment when it no longer offers any reasonable hope of benefit to the person.

When clients reject life-prolonging treatment, the nurse focuses on the goal of caring versus curing. Nurses have a legal obligation to treat the deceased person's remains with dignity (see Chapter 29). Wrongful handling of a deceased person's remains could cause emotional harm to the surviving family members and other loved ones.

Advance Directives and Health Care Surrogates

The **advance directive** is a mechanism enabling a mentally competent person to plan for a time when he or she may lack the mental capacity to make medical treatment decisions. It takes effect only when the person becomes incompetent to speak for himself or herself. The advance directive is a more sophisticated concept than that of the living will, although the two terms are often confused. A **living will** is a document in which the person makes an anticipatory refusal of life-prolonging measures during a future state of mental incompetence. An advance directive, in contrast, is not restricted to the rejection of life-support measures; its focus is on treatment preferences, which may include both requests for and refusals of treatment. The advance directive assumes two forms: the instructional directive (in which the maker of the document spells out specific directions for governing care, in more detail than is generally found in the living will); and the proxy directive (in which the person appoints someone as a health care agent to make treatment decisions in his or her behalf). Legislation in British Columbia, Alberta, Saskatchewan, Manitoba, Ontario, Prince Edward Island, Newfoundland and Labrador, and the Yukon gives full legal effect to both kinds of directives; the proxy directive is also recognized in Quebec and Nova Scotia. Even in provinces and territories that do not recognize an instructional directive, nothing prohibits a physician from following a directive.

If nurses know about the existence of a health care directive, they are required to follow it. Nurses are also required to follow the wishes of a validly appointed proxy (assuming these instructions are legal). A proxy has the right to receive all medical information concerning the client's condition and proposed plan of care. Failure to comply with a proxy's directions could result in charges of battery.

If a physician ignores the advance directive, the nurse must bring the advance directive to the physician's attention and document that he or she did so, along with the physician's response to this information. The nurse should also notify the nursing supervisor, who can then give direction regarding institutional policies and guidelines for such circumstances.

The psychiatric advance directive is a new type of advance directive. An individual with mental health problems completes this type of directive during periods of mental stability and competence. The directive outlines how the client wishes to be treated in the future if the underlying mental illness causes him or her to lose decision-making capacity. For example, it may specify preferences for and against certain interventions (e.g., electroconvulsive therapy) or medications. The psychiatric advance directive can also designate a surrogate decision maker to act on the person's behalf in the event of an incapacitating mental health crisis.

Organ Donation

Legally competent people are free to donate their bodies or organs for medical use. Every province and territory has human tissue legislation that provides for both the *inter vivos* (live donor) and post-mortem (cadaveric) donation of tissues and organs. For example, a mentally competent adult is allowed to donate a kidney, a lobe of the liver, or bone marrow. Statutes provide that adults may consent to organ donation after death. If the deceased has left no direction for post-mortem donation, then consent may be obtained from the person's family. In two provinces—Manitoba and Nova Scotia—the statutes contain "required request" provisions that take effect when a deceased person did not consent to organ removal but is considered a good donor candidate. In such an event, the physician is legally obliged to seek permission from the family. In many hospitals, a nurse transplantation coordinator performs this function.

Mental Health Issues

Treating clients with mental health problems raises legal and ethical issues. Provincial mental health legislation such as the *Mental Health and Consequential Amendments Act* (1998) provides direction for health care professionals, protects client autonomy, and recognizes that some individuals with severe mental health problems may lack the ability to appreciate the consequences of their health condition.

A client can be admitted to a psychiatric unit involuntarily or on a voluntary basis. Clients admitted on a voluntary basis should be treated no differently than any other client. They have the right to refuse treatment and the right to discharge themselves from hospital. However, provincial mental health legislation provides that if the client may cause harm to self or others, police officers (or other authorized parties) may bring the client to a health care facility for examination and treatment without the client's consent (Morris et al., 1999).

Potentially suicidal clients may be admitted to psychiatric units. If the client's history and medical records indicate suicidal tendencies, the client must be kept under supervision. A lawsuit may result if a client attempts suicide within the hospital. The allegations in the lawsuits would be that the institution failed to provide adequate supervision or safeguard the facilities. Documentation of precautions against suicide is essential.

Public Health Issues

It is important that nurses, especially those employed in community health settings, understand the public health laws. Public health acts, which have been enacted in all provinces and territories, are directed toward the prevention, treatment, and suppression of communicable disease (Sneiderman et al., 2003). Community health nurses have the legal responsibility to follow the laws enacted to protect the public health. These laws may include reporting suspected abuse and neglect, such as child abuse, elder abuse, or domestic violence; reporting communicable diseases; and reporting of other health-related issues enacted to protect the public's health.

Some provinces (e.g., Ontario and New Brunswick) have legislation that requires proof of immunization for school entry. In these provinces, however, exceptions are permitted on medical or religious grounds and for reasons of conscience (Health Canada, 1997). Although a signed consent form is not required for an immunization, nurses are advised to obtain some documentation (evidence) that they discussed the risks and benefits with the parent or legal guardian. Nurses should be aware of their employer guidelines for documentation.

Every province and territory has child abuse legislation that requires health care professionals, such as nurses, to report witnessed or suspected child abuse or neglect directly to child protection agencies. To encourage reports of suspected cases, the laws offer legal immunity for the reporter if the report is made in good faith. Health care professionals who do not report suspected child abuse or neglect maybe held liable for civil or criminal action. Several provinces and territories also have laws that require health care workers to report witnessed or suspected abuse of clients within facilities (e.g., *The Protection of Persons in Care Act*, 2000, in Manitoba). These reports must be made directly to a public authority. Even if public reporting is not required, nurses should report all suspicions of client abuse to their nursing supervisors. It is essential for nurses to know their provincial or territorial laws and employer policies regarding the reporting of abuse.

Risk Management

Risk management is a system of ensuring appropriate nursing care by identifying potential hazards and eliminating them before harm occurs (Guido, 2006). The steps involved in risk management include identifying possible risks, analyzing them, acting to reduce them, and evaluating the steps taken.

One tool used in risk management is the **incident report**, or **adverse occurrence report.** When a client is harmed or endangered by incorrect care, such as a drug error, a nurse completes an incident report (see Chapter 16). Such reports are analyzed to determine how future problems can be avoided. For example, if incident reports show that drug errors commonly involve a new intravenous pump, the risk manager must ensure that staff members have been properly trained in its use. In-service education may be all that is necessary to prevent future errors.

The underlying rationale for quality assurance in risk-management programs is the highest possible quality of care. Some insurance companies and medical and nursing organizations require the use of quality assurance and risk-management procedures. Quality care is the responsibility of both the employer and the individual provider.

Risk management requires sufficient documentation. The nurse's documentation can be the evidence of what actually was done for a client and can serve as proof that the nurse acted reasonably and safely. Documentation should be thorough, accurate, and performed in a timely manner. When a lawsuit is being evaluated, the nurse's notes are very often the first record to be reviewed by the plaintiff's counsel. If the nurse's credibility is questioned because of these documents, the risk of greater liability exists for the nurse. The nurse's notes are risk-management and quality assurance tools for the employer and the individual nurse.

Professional Involvement

Nurses must be involved in their professional organizations and on committees that define the standards of care for nursing practice. If current laws, rules and regulations, or policies under which nurses must practise do not reflect reality, nurses must become involved as advocates to see that the scope of nursing practice is accurately defined. Nurses must be willing to represent the nursing profession's perspective, as well as the client's perspective in the community. Nurses can be powerful and effective when the organizing focus is the protection and welfare of the public entrusted to their care.

* KEY CONCEPTS

- With increased emphasis on client rights, nurses in practice today must understand their legal obligations and responsibilities to clients.
- The civil law system is concerned with the protection of a person's private rights, and the criminal law system deals with the rights of individuals and society.
- A nurse can be found liable for negligence if the following criteria are established: the nurse (defendant) owed a duty of care to the client (plaintiff), the nurse did not carry out that duty, the client was injured, and the nurse's failure to carry out the duty caused the client's injury.
- Clients are entitled to confidential health care and freedom from unauthorized release of information.
- Under the law, practising nurses must follow standards of care, which originate in nursing practice acts and regulations, the guidelines of professional organizations, and the written policies and procedures of employing institutions.
- Nurses are responsible for confirming that the client has given informed consent to any surgery or other medical procedure before the procedure is performed.
- Nurses are responsible for performing all procedures correctly and exercising professional judgement as they carry out physicians' orders.
- Nurses are obligated to follow physicians' orders unless they believe the orders are in error or could be detrimental to clients.
- Staffing standards determine the ratio of nurses to clients, and if the nurse is required to care for more clients than is reasonable, a formal protest should be made to the nursing administration.
- Legal issues involving death include documenting all events surrounding the death and treating the deceased client's remains with dignity.
- A competent adult can legally give consent to donate specific organs, and nurses may serve as witnesses to this decision.
- All nurses should know the laws that apply to their area of practice.
- Depending on provincial statutes, nurses are required to report suspected child abuse and certain communicable diseases.
- Nurses are client advocates and ensure quality of care through risk management and lobbying for safe nursing practice standards.
- Nurses must file incident reports in all situations when someone could or did get hurt.

* CRITICAL THINKING EXERCISES

1. Nurse Rossi and Nurse Kao are getting on an elevator to go down to the cafeteria. Several visitors are present in the elevator, as are hospital personnel. Nurse Rossi and Nurse Kao are talking about a client who is in the intensive care unit who has just tested positive for HIV infection. They identify the client as "the man in Room 14B." One of the visitors on the elevator who overhears this information is a woman who is engaged to the client in Room 14B.
   a. Have Nurse Rossi and Nurse Kao breached a client's right to confidential health care?
   b. Would the client in Room 14B have any legal cause of action against the nurses?
   c. Even though the client's fiancée may have a right to know the HIV status of her future husband, do the nurses have any duty to disclose confidential information to the fiancée?
2. While transporting a client down the hall on a stretcher, Nurse Reyes stops to chat with an orderly. The side rails on the stretcher are down, and while Nurse Reyes has her back to the stretcher, the client rolls over, falls off the stretcher, and fractures his hip. In a lawsuit by the client against Nurse Reyes, what must the client establish to prove negligence against the nurse?

* REVIEW QUESTIONS

1. The nursing practice acts are an example of
   1. Statute law
   2. Common law
   3. Public law
   4. Criminal law
2. Treating a client without his or her consent is considered
   1. Battery
   2. Negligence
   3. Implied consent
   4. Expressed consent
3. The nurse restrains a client without the client's permission and without a physician's order. The nurse may be guilty of
   1. Assault
   2. False imprisonment
   3. Invasion of privacy
   4. Neglect
4. The situation in which a confused client fell out of bed because side rails were not used when they were ordered is an example of which type of liability?
   1. False imprisonment
   2. Assault
   3. Battery
   4. Negligence
5. What should you do if you think the client does not understand the procedure for which he or she is being asked to give consent?
   1. Do not be concerned if the consent is already signed.
   2. Notify the physician or nursing supervisor.
   3. Send the client for the procedure and discuss it afterward.
   4. Ask a family member to give consent.
6. When a client is harmed as a result of a nursing student's actions or lack of action, the liability is generally held by
   1. The student alone
   2. The student's instructor or preceptor
   3. The hospital or health care facility
   4. All of the above
7. When the nurse stops to help in an emergency at the scene of an accident, if the injured party files suit and the nurse's employing institution's insurance does not cover the nurse, the nurse would probably be covered by
   1. The nurse's automobile insurance
   2. The nurse's homeowner's insurance
   3. The Patient Care Partnership, which may grant immunity from suit if the injured party consents
   4. The Good Samaritan laws, which grant immunity from suit if no gross negligence is involved
8. The nurse is obligated to follow a physician's order unless
   1. The order is a verbal order
   2. The physician's order is illegible
   3. The order has not been transcribed
   4. The order is in error, violates hospital policy, or would be detrimental to the client
9. If a third party (e.g., insurance company of employer) requests health information on a client, the nurse must
   1. Provide the information
   2. Refuse to provide the information
   3. Obtain a signed release by the client before releasing the information
   4. Contact the client's family or lawyer

* RECOMMENDED WEB SITES

Canadian Nurses Association–Provincial/Territorial Members: http://www. cna-aiic.ca/CNA/about/members/provincial/default_e.aspx
This CNA site offers up-to-date Weblinks and contact information for all provincial and territorial nursing colleges and associations.

The Canadian Nurses Protective Society: http://www.cnps.ca
The Canadian Nurses Protective Society (CNPS) helps nurses manage their professional legal risks by offering legal support and liability protection. The members-only section of the Web site (the user name is the acronym of your professional association or college, and the password is "assist") provides information on a variety of legal topics affecting Canadian nursing practice.

The College of Licensed Practical Nurses of Nova Scotia: http://www.clpnns.ca/provincial_links/outofprovincelinks.html
This site provides links to all provincial licensing authorities.

Department of Justice Canada: http://laws.justice.gc.ca/en/
This site provides links to consolidated statutes, including the *Criminal Code* (1985) of Canada.

The Health Law Institute of Dalhousie University: The End of Life Project: http://as01.ucis.dal.ca/dhli/cmp_welcome/default.cfm
This site contains information about the Canadian law pertaining to various aspects of end-of-life care, including advance directives and withholding of life-sustaining treatment.

10

Culture and Ethnicity

Written by Barbara J. Astle, RN, PhD,

and Sylvia Barton, RN, PhD

Based on the original chapter by Anahid Kulwicki, RN, DNS, FAAN

objectives

Mastery of content in this chapter will enable you to:

- Describe the key terms listed.
- Describe the enthocultural diversity of the Canadian population.
- Define key cultural concepts related to health, illness, and ethnicity.
- Describe the historical development of transcultural nursing, cultural competence, and cultural safety in relation to nursing practice.
- Describe social and cultural influences on healing, well-being, and caring patterns.
- Analyze components of cultural assessment to understand the values, beliefs, and practices critical in the nursing care of people experiencing ethnocultural transitions.
- Apply selected components of cultural assessment to a particular cultural group as an example.
- Examine nursing obligations that underpin relational practice and the way in which relational inquiry can enhance contemporary nursing practice.
- Apply research findings to the provision of culturally competent care with considerations for cultural safety and relational practice.

key terms

media resources

evolve Web Site

- Audio Chapter Summaries
- Glossary
- Multiple-Choice Review Questions
- Student Learning Activities
- Weblinks

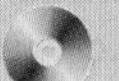

Companion CD

- Glossary
- Interactive Learning Activities
- Fluids and Electrolytes Tutorial
- Test-Taking Skills

Ethnocultural Diversity

Canada has always been a multicultural nation. At the time of Confederation, more than 50 Aboriginal groups—each with their own language and culture—lived in Canada, in addition to the founding, British and French settlers and other settlers migrating from primarily European countries. Canada is well known as a country that embraces ethnic diversity, relying heavily on immigration for population growth (Adams, 2007). As a result, the societal landscape changes continuously, integrating people from many ethnic groups who have migrated to this country and formed a cultural mosaic that is uniquely Canadian (Statistics Canada, 2007a, 2008b).

The ethnocultural profile of Canada is continually evolving. More than 200 ethnic orgins were reported by the total population in Canada in the 2006 census. After Canadian, the other most frequently reported origins in 2006, either alone or with other origins, were English, French, Scottish, Irish, German, Italian, Chinese, North American Indian, and Ukrainian. According to the 2006 census, visible minorities acccounted for 16.2% of Canada's total population, up from 13.4% in 2001 and 11.2% in 1996 (Statistics Canada, 2008b; Figure 10–1). Between 2001 and 2006, the visible minority population increased at a much faster rate than did the total population (Statistics Canada, 2008b). For the purposes of the 2006 census, the *Employment Equity Act* defines visible minorities as persons, other than Aboriginal peoples, who are non-Caucasian in race or nonwhite in colour (Statistics Canada, 2008b). The increase in the visible minority population was largely attributable to the high proportion of newcomers who belonged to visible minorities.

Figure 10–2 shows the most common visible minority groups in Canada. The three largest visible minority groups are South Asians, Chinese, and Blacks. South Asians surpassed Chinese as the largest visible minority group in 2006 (Statistics Canada, 2008b). Both the populations of South Asians and Chinese were well over 1 million. In Canada in 2006, South Asians represented 24.9% of all visible minorities and 4.0% of the total population; Chinese accounted for about 24.0% of the visible minority population and 3.9% of the total population; and Blacks accounted for 15.5% of the visible minority population and 2.5% of the total population (Statistics Canada, 2008b).

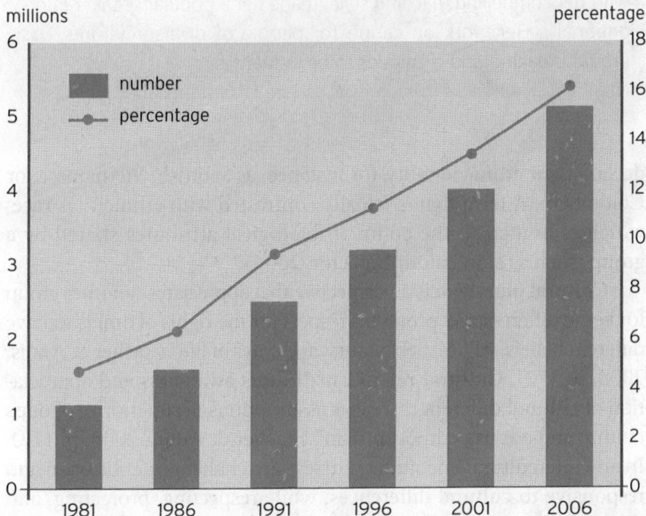

Figure 10-1 Number and share of visible minority persons in Canada, 1981–2008. **Source:** Adapted from Statistics Canada (2008b). *Canada's ethnocultural mosaic, 2006 census.* Retrieved April 2, 2008, from http://www12.statcan.ca/english/census06/analysis/ethnicorigin/index.cfm

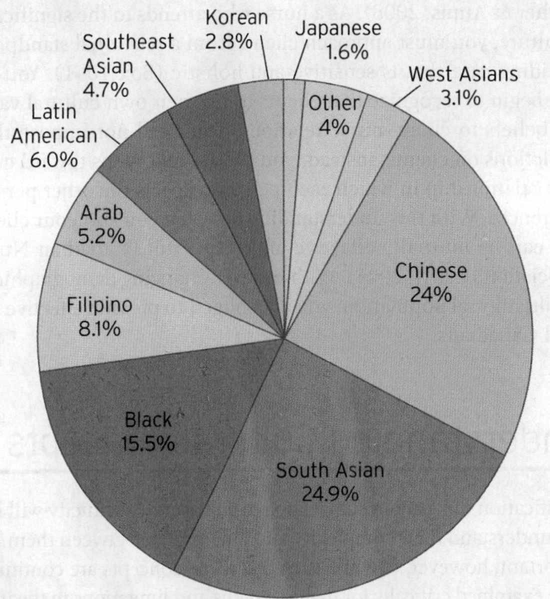

Figure 10-2 The composition of Canada's visible minority population, 2006. **Source:** Adapted from Statistics Canada (2008b). *Canada's ethnocultural mosaic, 2006 census.* Retrieved April 2, 2008, from http://www12.statcan.ca/english/census06/analysis/ethnicorigin/index.cfm

Immigration continues to play a pivotal role in shaping Canada's ethnocultural profile (Statistics Canada, 2007a). According to the 2006 census, approximately 19.8% (one per five) of Canada's total population were born outside of the country, reaching its highest level in 75 years (Statistics Canada, 2007a). For the purposes of the 2006 census, a *foreign-born population* is also known as an *immigrant population* and is defined as persons who are, or who have been, landed immigrants in Canada (Statistics Canada, 2007a). Canada ranks second only to Australia as the country with the highest proportion of foreign-born citizens. In addition, Canada per capita receives more immigrants than does the United States (Statistics Canada, 2007a). The largest groups of immigrants to Canada are from Asian and Middle Eastern countries; this fact has remained virtually unchanged since the 2001 census. In contrast, during 1971, only 12.1% of immigrants to Canada were born in Asian and Middle Eastern countries, and 61.6% were born in Europe. By 2006, 58.3% of recent immigrants were Asian and only 16.1% were European. Immigration has now outpaced the natural birth rate of the country, as revealed by Statistics Canada (2007a) between 2001 and 2006. It indicates that Canada's foreign-born population increased by 13.3%, which was four times higher than the increase in the Canadian-born population of 3.3%. Thus, immigrants and refugees come to Canada from many places, representing more than 200 ethnocultural groups across the country (Statistics Canada, 2007a).

Two other significant parts of Canada's cultural mosaic are the Aboriginal population and the population of French ancestry. In the 2006 census, more than 2 million people, representing 3.8% of the total population, reported having at least some Aboriginal ancestry (Statistics Canada, 2008a). Further details of the Aboriginal population are given later in this chapter. In the 2006 census, population by knowledge of official language by province and territory revealed that citizens who spoke only French totaled more than 4 million, of a total of more than 31 million Canadians (Statistics Canada, 2007b).

In response to Canada's ethnocultural mosaic, nurses require an understanding of difference in order to perceive, critically, the diversity influences that shape healing, well-being, and caring patterns

(Racher & Annis, 2008). As a nurse who attends to the significance of culture, you must approach clients from a relational standpoint, providing care that is sensitive and holistic (Box 10–1). You will then begin to recognize that clients bring their own cultural values and beliefs to client–nurse relations. You need not impose these restrictions on clients; instead, you should take steps toward creating a relationship in which each person respects the other person's differences. With this understanding between you and your clients, care can be mutually effective and respectful (Canadian Nurses Association [CNA], 2004). With the ever-changing demographics of a multicultural population, you are obliged to provide effective care to all Canadians.

> BOX 10-1 **Milestones in Canadian Nursing History**

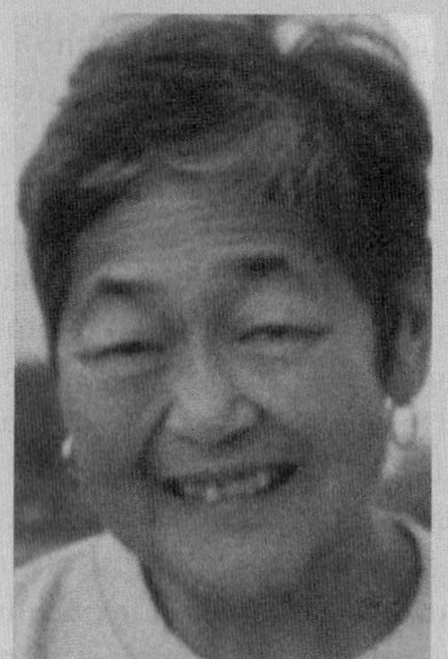

May Aiko Watanabe Yoshida, 1930–2000

Born in Vancouver, British Columbia, May Aiko Watanabe Yoshida was a clinical nurse, teacher, and researcher. She focused her professional life on the need to understand clients and their families in light of their cultural heritage. Not surprisingly, her respect for the cultures and traditions of others grew out of her early personal experiences of discrimination as a Japanese Canadian.

Racist attitudes toward Japanese were rampant in Canada from the time the first immigrants arrived in the late nineteenth century. Laws excluded Asians from most professions, the civil service, and teaching. All Japanese Canadians—including the Canadian-born children of immigrants—were denied the right to vote. Anti-Japanese feeling peaked after Japan attacked Pearl Harbor in 1941; the Canadian government used the *War Measures Act* to order the removal of all Japanese Canadians living within 160 km of the Pacific Coast. Approximately 21,000 men, women, and children of Japanese ancestry—75% of whom were Canadian citizens—were stripped of their property and transported to detention camps. May Watanabe Yoshida and her family were among them.

After the war ended in 1945, Japanese Canadians were forced to choose between deportation to Japan or dispersal east of the Rocky Mountains. May's family chose to relocate in southern Ontario. May, a brilliant student, entered the nursing program at McMaster University in Hamilton and graduated in 1953. She went on to earn a master's degree in 1959.

As a clinician, May Watanabe Yoshida was well known for her work with immigrant families. Specializing in parent–child nursing, she focused on the child-bearing and child-rearing practices of various ethnic groups. She came to believe that people's cultural traditions were central to their health and well-being. Professor May Watanabe Yoshida's many research projects on a range of cultural issues, together with her compelling teaching style, made her a popular speaker internationally. Her work on caring for people of diverse cultures was groundbreaking and continues to be influential.

Understanding Cultural Concepts

Clarification of key concepts related to culture and ethnicity will help you understand their complexity and differentiate between them. It is important, however, to emphasize that these concepts are continuing to be examined critically for their strengths and limitations in the interpretation of social reality (Gustafson, 2005). When you think critically, you analyze and evaluate thinking with the goal of improving it. The CNA (2004) describes **culture** broadly as shared patterns of learned values and behaviours that are transmitted over time and that distinguish the members of one group from another. Culture can include language, ethnicity, spiritual and religious beliefs, socioeconomic class, gender, sexual orientation, age, group history, geographic origin, education, as well as childhood and life experiences. According to the CNA's (2008) *Code of Ethics*, "When providing care, nurses do not discriminate on the basis of a person's race, ethnicity, **culture**, political and spiritual beliefs, social or marital status, gender, sexual orientation, age, health status, place of origin, lifestyle, mental or physical ability or socioeconomic status or any other attribute" (p. 14).

Culture has both **visible** (easily seen) and **invisible** (less observable) components. The invisible value and belief system of a particular culture is the major driving force behind visible practices. Although a Sikh man can be easily identified by visible symbols (uncut hair with wooden comb, beard, turban, steel bracelet, and steel dagger), for example, the meanings and beliefs associated with these artifacts are not readily apparent. These artifacts symbolize a devotee's allegiance to the pillars of Sikhism, and removal of them without expressed consent of the individual or his family is considered sacrilegious, violating the ethnoreligious identity of the person. Conversely, an Arab woman who wears a veil may not believe in the reasons for wearing it, but she does so because of her cultural norms.

Any society can be viewed traditionally as being more homogeneous, both linguistically and religiously, than the rest of the country (Adams, 2007). Issues of migration and pluralism, however, are present in each Canadian province. It is important to acknowledge that unique concerns and discussions that characterize the homogeneous societies' approach to new immigrants need to be examined critically. Although **subcultures** may have similarities with the homogeneous culture, their unique life patterns, values, and norms are maintained. In Canada, the prevalent cultures are Anglophones and Francophones with origins from Western Europe. Subcultures such as the Ukrainian and Acadian cultures represent various ethnic, religious, and other groups with characteristics distinct from those of the prevalent cultures. **Ethnicity** refers to groups whose members share a social and cultural heritage. Members of ethnic groups, for example, may share common values, language, history, physical characteristics, and geographical space. The most important characteristic of an ethnic group is that its members feel a sense of common identity. People may declare their ethnic identity, for instance, as Scottish, Vietnamese, or Colombian. A term that is usually contrasted with ethnicity is **race**, which is limited to the common biological attributes shared by a group, such as skin colour (Spector, 2004).

Cultural pluralism is a perspective that appreciates "another group for being different and promotes respect for the rights of others to have different beliefs, values, behaviours, and ways of life" (Racher & Annis, 2008, p. 172). **Cultural relativism** "fosters awareness and appreciation of cultural differences, rejects assumptions of superiority of one's culture and adverts ethnocentrism" (Racher & Annis, 2008, p. 172). In any intercultural encounter, nurses "are challenged to be open and responsive to cultural differences, while respecting, protecting, and promoting the rights and well-being of those people and groups with whom they work" (Racher & Annis, 2008, p. 172). As a nurse, for example, you may be baffled by a Korean woman's request for seaweed soup for her first meal after she gives birth. Your personal view of professional postpartum care may not include understandings of the

Korean culture, and so you may be unaware of the significance of the client's traditional cultural practices. Conversely, the Korean client who has an alternative view of Canadian professional care may assume that seaweed soup should be available in the hospital, because it cleanses the blood and promotes healing and lactation (*Korean Health Beliefs*, 2003). Unless you seek to learn your client's ethnocultural views, you are likely to offer inappropriate suggestions, such as another choice of soup.

The processes of enculturation and acculturation facilitate cultural learning. Socialization into one's primary culture during childhood is known as **enculturation**. The process of adapting to and adopting characteristics of a new culture is **acculturation** (Cowan & Norman, 2006). Acculturation outcomes may result in varying degrees of affiliation with the mainstream culture (Spector, 2004). **Assimilation** is a process whereby a minority group gradually adopts the attitudes and customs of the mainstream culture (Srivastava, 2007a).

In contrast to assimilation, **multiculturalism**, regarded as a fundamental characteristic of Canadian society, is a process whereby "many cultures co-exist in society and maintain their cultural differences. Multiculturalism also refers to the public policy of managing cultural diversity in a multi-ethnic society, emphasizing tolerance and respect for cultural diversity" (Srivastava, 2007b, p. 328). In 1971, Canada became the first country in the world to officially adopt a multiculturalism policy. Since then, various laws have been passed to protect and promote the rights of minorities in Canada (Box 10–2). As expressed in the spirit of the multicultural policy, citizens are able to retain their unique ethnnocultural traditions within a Canadian context.

Cultural Conflicts

Culture provides the context for valuing, evaluating, and categorizing life experiences. As values, morals, and norms are transmitted from one generation to another, members of ethnic groups may display **ethnocentrism**, a tendency to view their own way of life as more valuable than others'. Health care practitioners who do not understand cultural differences often resort to **cultural imposition**, in which they use their own values and ways of life as the absolute guides in providing services to clients and interpreting their behaviours. Hence, if a nurse believes that pain is to be borne quietly as a demonstration of strong moral character, that nurse may be annoyed by a client's insistence on being given pain medication and, in denying the client's discomfort, may exacerbate the client's pain.

Ethnocentrism is the root of stereotypes, biases, and prejudices against other people perceived to be different from the valued group. You must avoid **stereotypes**, which are generalizations about any particular group that prevent further assessment of unique characteristics. When a person acts on his or her prejudices, **discrimination**—treating people unfairly on the basis of their group membership—occurs. **Racism** involves specific actions and an attitude whereby one group exerts power over others on the basis of either skin colour or racial heritage; its effects are to marginalize and oppress some people and to endow others with privileges (Srivastava, 2007a). Often people do not realize that they are displaying prejudice or discrimination; such displays may be simply negative or fearful reactions to cultural differences (see Chapter 11, description of Ethel Johns's work on racism).

> **BOX 10-2 Legislation Recognizing Diversity in Canada**
>
> ***Official Languages Act* (1969; Updated 1988)**
>
> This act recognizes English and French equally as Canada's official languages. The 1988 amendment to this act outlines the obligations of Canadian federal institutions to be committed to promoting full recognition and use of both English and French in Canadian society, as well as supporting the development of the Anglophone and Francophone communities across the country.
>
> ***Canadian Constitution Act* (1982)**
>
> This act replaced the *British North America Act* as Canada's Constitution, outlining how Canada governs and structures its society. It also recognizes the Aboriginal peoples of Canada as Indians (Status and Non-Status), Inuit, and Métis.
>
> ***Canadian Charter of Rights and Freedoms* (1982)**
>
> Written into the Canadian Constitution in 1982, this charter is a statement of the basic human rights and freedoms of all Canadians.
>
> ***Canadian Multiculturalism Act* (1988)**
>
> In recognition of Canada's cultural diversity, this act enshrines the enhancement and preservation of multiculturalism in Canada.

Cultural Awareness

You must be tolerant and nonjudgemental about clients' beliefs and practices. It is important to realize that you will bring your own personal cultural perspectives to the nurse–client relationship and to be aware of how your own culture influences your provision of care (CNA, 2004; Vollman et al., 2008). A strategy for achieving **cultural awareness** is to conduct a self-assessment in order to reflect on your biases and feelings. A set of questions for personal reflection is suggested for this purpose in Box 10–3. Another strategy is to observe nurses who are considered to be exemplary relational practitioners and to notice the particular qualities or characteristics they display when handling of cultural aspects of relationships (Box 10–4).

Historical Development of the Nursing Approach to Culture

It is important to review historically the emergence of transcultural nursing in relation to shifts in thinking about the provision of culturally competent care and cultural safety. Framed primarily within the Canadian context, this history is also best discussed in terms of culturally appropriate nursing practice and education. The importance of being culturally sensitive and aware of a diverse society has been acknowledged by nurses and continues to evolve. Nurses became aware of the conceptual limitations of culture, partly by studying the complexities of race (Ramsden, 2002). Through a critical cultural analysis of the significance of power relations and structural constraints on health and health care, nurses are conceptualizing new ways to provide culturally competent and culturally safe care (Anderson et al., 2003; Browne & Varcoe, 2006; Ramsden, 2002; Smith et al., 2006). A critical historical view of transcultural nursing, cultural competence, and cultural safety is important for understanding the strengths and limitations of these approaches in nursing practice and education (Gustafson, 2005). Increasingly, nurse scholars are questioning whether the health needs of ethnocultural groups are being equitably met (Anderson et al., 2003; Baker, 2007; Smith et al., 2006). Equity may be considered one of the prerequisites and conditions for health. Mill et al. (2005) revealed how "nurses can provide valuable support to the realization of the goal of global health by becoming informed advocates and integrating these concepts, in nursing practice, education and research" (p. 22). Furthermore, in a second article (Ogilvie et al., 2005),

➤ BOX 10-3 Questions for Reflection and Building Awareness in Community Practice

Personal Self-Awareness

What is my ethnic background? How does my knowledge of my ethnicity affect my identity? What meaning do I ascribe to my ethnic origins? How have they shaped who I am today? What cultural groups do I belong to? What are the rules, customs, and rituals that have been passed on to me and that I will pass on to the next generation of my family? How were these passed on to me, and what meaning do I give to them now? How do the rules and customs passed on to me inform how I engage with others?

Professional Self-Awareness

In my work, how do I relate to others of different cultures? What taken-for-granted assumptions am I prepared to make in the name of efficiency and time constraints? What stereotypes do I hold? How do these beliefs influence my practice? How do I maintain an attitude of cultural attunement in my work with groups and organizations? How do I bridge the differences between ethnic backgrounds in my work? What action might I take to improve my cultural attunement?

Organizational Awareness

What are the values and principles of my organization for working cross-culturally? How does my organization reflect behaviours, attitudes, policies, and structures when working cross-culturally? How does my organization value diversity, manage the dynamics of difference, acquire and institutionalize cultural knowledge, and adapt to diversity and the cutural contexts of the communities it serves?

Community Awareness

How do the dynamics of the community, such as racial tensions, enter into my work with community groups and organizations? When does difference make a difference? How does this community influence feelings of belonging among its residents? What actions do we take to be inclusive? How do we celebrate and honour cultural diversity? What do we need to do differently to be more inclusive and generate feelings of belonging among residents from all cultures?

Adapted from Hoskins, M. L. (1999). Worlds apart and lives together: Developing cultural attunement. *Child and Youth Care Forum, 28*(2), 73–85; Kirkham, S. (2003). The politics of belonging and intercultural health care. *Western Journal of Nursing Research, 25*(7), 762–780; Goode, T. (2004). *Cultural competence continuum.* Washington, DC: National Center for Cultural Competence. Retrieved November 30, 2006, from http://www11.georgetown.edu/research/gucchd/nccc/projects/sides/dvd/continuum.pdf; and Racher, F. E., & Annis, R. C. (2008). Honouring culture and diversity in community practice. In A. R. Vollman, E. T. Anderson, & J. McFarlane (Eds.), *Canadian community as partner: Theory & multidisciplinary practice* (2nd ed., p. 185). Philadelphia, PA: Lippincott Williams & Wilkins.

the same scholars explained how "nurses can play a pivotal role by becoming informed advocates, challenging their organizations to incorporate a global health mandate and exercising their rights as citizens to influence policy" (p. 25).

The discipline of anthropology and seminal work by Leininger (2002a) relative to cultural nursing have highly influenced the establishment of a theoretical foundation of transcultural nursing (Glittenberg, 2004). Leininger defined **transcultural nursing** as a comparative study of cultures, an understanding of similarities (culture universal) and differences (culture specific) across human groups in order to provide meaningful and beneficial delivery of health care (Leininger,

➤ BOX 10-4 An Exemplary Relational Practitioner

1. *Identify* someone who you would say is "good at relationships." Why did you identify that person? What qualities or characteristics stand out?
2. Now *identify* someone who is a nurse and is good at relationships. Think of someone with whom you have worked—perhaps a fellow student, a colleague, an instructor. What makes [this person] good at relationships? How is this person perceived by his or her colleagues?
3. *Compare notes* with someone else. Talk to someone who has thought about this question, or talk to someone who knows the person or people you have identified. Do you both value similar attributes and qualities?

From Doane, G. H., & Varcoe, C. (2005). *Family nursing as relational inquiry: Developing health-promoting practice* (p. 192). Philadelphia, PA: Lippincott Williams & Wilkins.

2002a). According to Leininger, the goals of transcultural nursing are to provide *culturally congruent* and *culturally competent* care.

Culturally congruent care is "the use of sensitive, creative, and meaningful care practices to fit with the general values, beliefs, and lifeways of clients" (Leininger & McFarland, 2002, p. 12). In other words, you need to determine how to provide care that does not conflict with clients' valued life patterns and sets of meanings, which may be distinct from your own (Leininger, 2002b).

Leininger and McFarland (2002) defined **culturally competent care** as "the explicit use of culturally based care and health knowledge in sensitive, creative, and meaningful ways to fit the general lifeways and needs of individuals or groups for beneficial and meaningful health and well-being or to help them face illness, disabilities, or death" (p. 84). To provide culturally competent care, you must bridge cultural gaps in care, work with cultural differences, and enable clients and families to receive meaningful care. You need to exhibit specific ability, knowledge, sensitivity, openness, and flexibility toward the appreciation of cultural difference (Suh, 2004). You are then able to develop effective and meaningful interventions that promote optimal health for clients, families, and communities.

The work of Leininger in promoting culturally competent care with people from diverse cultures has been the prevailing model identified in the nursing literature. It has been used as a guide in nursing curricula and practice policies in North America for several decades. In addition, other scholars have developed models of cultural competency in which they have expanded Leininger's work. Davidhizar and Giger (1998; Giger & Davidhizar, 2004) developed a **transcultural assessment model** with a focus on cultural competency that is used in nursing practice. The underlying premise of their model is that each person is culturally unique and should be assessed according to six cultural phenomena: communication, space, social organization, time, environmental control, and biological variations. The model suggests that these phenomena are apparent in all cultural groups, but their application to practice settings varies. Giger and Davidhizar's transcultural assessment model offers a means for you to assess clients' unique health care needs, including their specific cultural health practices.

Campinha-Bacote (2002) further defined cultural competence as an ongoing process, whereby you continuously strive to work within the client's cultural context. As a result, you develop cultural competence rather than possess it. This ongoing process involves integrating cultural awareness, knowledge, skill, encounters, and desire, as depicted in Figure 10–3. *Cultural awareness* is insight into of your own background, and it involves an in-depth self-examination to recognize biases, prejudices, and assumptions about other people. *Cultural knowledge* is knowing about the client's culture. It involves learning about diverse groups, including their values, health beliefs, care practices, and world views. As a nurse assigned to a female Egyptian-Canadian client, for example, you decide to seek information about the Egyptian culture. Upon learning that female modesty and gender-congruent care are valued in the culture, you encourage the client's female relatives to assist with her hygiene needs. *Cultural skills* include assessment of social, cultural, and biophysical factors that influence client care. *Cultural encounters* involve engaging in cross-cultural interactions that can teach about other cultures. *Cultural desire* is the motivation and commitment to learn from other people, to accept the role as learner, to be accepting of cultural differences, and to build relationships based on cultural similarities.

Narayanasamy (2002), a nurse scholar in Britain, also developed a framework for cultural competence: the ACCESS model (A for assessment; C for communication; C for cultural negotiation and compromise; E for establishing respect and rapport; S for sensitivity; and S for safety). The focus of this model is on developing cross-cultural communication, cultural negotiations, diversity, and celebrations, and on fostering cultural safety (Narayanasamy & White, 2005).

In Canada, the CNA (2004) advocated in its position paper that culturally competent care can and should be practised in all clinical settings. Although nurses are responsible for providing culturally competent care, nursing regulatory bodies, professional associations, educational institutions, governments, health service agencies, and accreditation organizations share the responsibility of supporting culturally competent care. You are in a position to build partnerships with other health care professionals, clients, and funding agencies in order to establish culturally diverse practices that optimize clients' health outcomes.

The provision of culturally competent care has been promoted since the 1960s. Only since 2000, however, have Canadian nurse scholars begun to question the limitations of such an approach (Anderson et al, 2003; Kirkham, 2003) and to examine, critically, the concept of **cultural safety** as another approach to providing care to diverse groups, in contrast to the conceptual notion of transcultural nursing (Ramsden, 2002). The College of Registered Nurses of British Columbia's (2006) profile of newly graduated registered nurse practice focuses on the establishment and maintenance of therapeutic caring and culturally safe relationships between clients and health care team members. The cultural safety literature is framed within a critical social theory and postcolonial framework. The concept of cultural safety evolved over a number of years in New Zealand, as nurses tried to identify a way in which health care professionals could more effectively address the inequity in the health status of Maori people. This was combined with an analysis of the historicial, political, social, and economic situations influencing the health of Maori people (Ramsden, 2002). Cultural safety involves considering the redistribution of power and resources in a relationship. The notion "is based on the premise that the term 'culture' is used in its broadest sense to apply to any person or group of people who may differ from the nurse/midwife because of socio-economic status, age, gender, sexual orientation, ethnic origin, migrant/refugee status, religious belief or disability" (Ramsden, 2002, Chapter 8, p. 3). In contrast to transcultural nursing, the term *culture* refers to ethnicity. As a result, the philosophy of cultural care has shifted from a notion of cultural sensitivity underpinning the provisions of care irrespective of culture to one of cultural safety with the recognition of power imbalances, the understanding of the nature of interpersonal relationships, and the awareness of institutional discrimination (Browne, & Fiske, 2001; Polaschek, 1998) (Box 10–5).

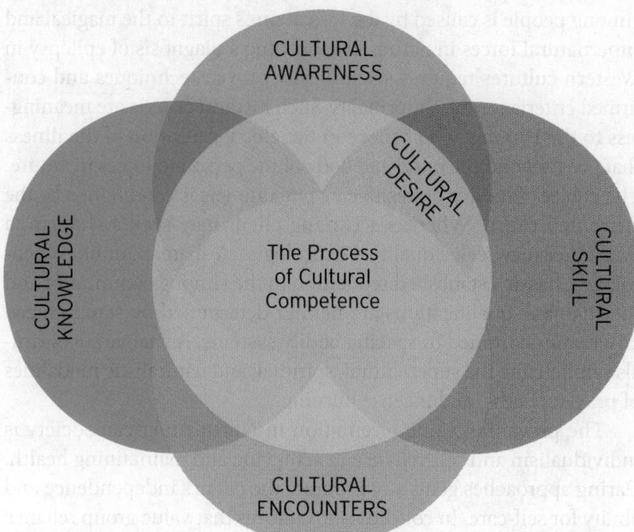

Figure 10-3 The process of cultural competence. **Source:** From Campinha-Bacote, J. (2002). The process of cultural competence in the delivery of healthcare services: A model of care. *Journal of Transcultural Nursing, 13*(3), 181. Printed with permission from Transcultural CARE Associates, Cincinnati, OH.

Ramsden (2002) articulated that *cultural awareness* and *cultural sensitivity* are separate concepts and that those terms are not interchangeable with *cultural safety*. Achieving cultural safety is a stepwise progression from cultural awareness through cultural sensitivity to cultural safety (see Figure 10–4). The outcome of cultural safety is that safe care, defined as such by clients who receive the care, is provided. According to Ramsden (2002), **cultural sensitivity** "alerts students to the legitimacy of difference and begins a process of self-exploration as the powerful bearers of their own life experience and realities which can have an impact on others" (Ramsden, 2002, Chapter 8, p. 4). *Cultural awareness* "is a beginning step toward understanding that there is difference. Many people undergo courses designed to sensitize them to formal ritual and practice rather than the emotional, social, economic and political context in which people exist" (Ramsden, 2002, Chapter 8, p. 4). In terms of achieving cultural safety in nursing practice, Ramsden stated that "the skill for nurses does not lie in knowing the customs or even the health related beliefs of ethno-specific groups. The step before that lies in professional acqusition of trust. . . . Rather than the nurse determining what is culturally safe, it is consumers or patients who decide whether they feel safe with the care that has been given, that trust has been established, and that difference between the patient, the nurse and the institutions that underpin them, can then be identified and negogiated" (Ramsden, 2002, Chapter 8, p. 4), as depicted in Figure 10–4.

Cultural Context of Health and Caring

Healing, well-being, and caring are phenomena embedded in a culture (Leininger, 2002a). Culture is the context in which groups of people interpret and define their experiences relevant to life transitions, such as birth, illness, and death. It is the system of meanings by which people make sense of their experiences. Culture is the framework used in defining social phenomena, such as when a person is healthy or requires medical intervention.

BOX 10-5 RESEARCH HIGHLIGHT

Globalization and the Cultural Safety of an Immigrant Muslim Community

Research Focus

The social health of Muslims who reside in smaller areas of Canada is not clearly understood by health care professionals. The concept of cultural safety has been used in studies of both Aboriginal peoples and immigrants to understand the health of Aboriginal peoples and immigrants in a large metropolitan centre, but the dichotomy between culturally safe and unsafe groups was found to be blurred. To further understand the concept of cultural safety, Baker (2007) focused on the social health of a small immigrant community of Muslims in a relatively homogeneous region of Canada after the terrorist attacks in the United States on September 11, 2001 ("9/11").

Research Abstract

Many Muslims living in North America and Western Europe were negatively affected by the events of 9/11. A qualitative approach based on the constructivist paradigm was used to guide the study, and 26 in-depth interviews were conducted with Muslims (10 women and 16 men) of Middle Eastern, Pakistani, or Indian origin. The participants resided in the province of New Brunswick, Canada, between 2002 and 2003. Data collection and analysis were conducted simultaneously. Steps of unitizing, categorizing, and pattern seeking were used to dissect the interviews until saturation was obtained. Many participants reported that after 9/11, their Islamic faith and experiences of being Muslim suddenly became significant to society at large. The research findings revealed that these participants talked about a sudden transition from cultural safety to cultural risk after 9/11. Their positive experiences of cultural safety included invisibility as a minority and a sense of social integration in the community. Cultural risk was found to stem from intensive international media attention that highlighted their now-visible minority status.

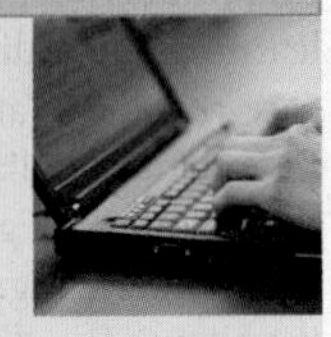

Evidence-Informed Practice

In this study, the findings indicated that globalization does not necessarily blur the distinction between culturally safe and culturally unsafe groups. Cultural risk may be generated by outside forces rather than by long-term inequities in relationships between groups within the community, which did not necessarily originate in historical events. Such findings suggest that you need to think about cultural safety in Muslims within the context of globalization. In addition, you should be cognizant about the cultural safety of your practice when providing care to members of socially disadvantaged cultural groups and how this may influence the heath care received.

References: Baker, C. (2007). Globalization and the cultural safety of an immigrant Muslim community. *Journal of Advanced Nursing, 57,* 296–305.

Table 10–1 provides comparative cultural contexts of health and illness in Western and non-Western cultures. As noted, attributed causes of illness are highly influenced by cultural beliefs. Among the Hmong refugees (a group of people who originated from the mountainous regions of Laos), for example, epilepsy is believed to be caused by wandering of the soul; hence, treatment includes intervention by a shaman who can perform the ritual to retrieve the client's soul (Helsel et al., 2005). The Hmong refugees' beliefs are distinct from those of the scientific community which determine that neurological abnormality causes seizures.

Cultural safety is an outcome of nursing education that enables safe service to be defined by those who receive the service.

Cultural sensitivity alerts nurses to the legitimacy of difference and begins a process of self-exploration as powerful bearers of their own realities which can have an impact on others.

Cultural awareness is a beginning step toward understanding that there is difference. Many people undergo courses designed to desensitize them to formal ritual and practice rather than the emotional, social, economic, and political context in which people exist.

Figure 10-4 Steps toward achieving cultural safety in nursing practice. **Source:** From De, D., & Richardson, J. (2008). Cultural safety: An introduction. *Paediatric Nursing, 20*(2), 42.

In the Hmong refugee example, the biomedical orientation of Western cultures, which emphasizes scientific investigation and views the human body as reduced into distinct parts, is in conflict with the holistic conceptualization of health and illness in non-Western cultures. Holism is evident in the belief of continuity between humans and nature and between human events and metaphysical and magical–religious phenomena. Hence, epilepsy as conceived by the Hmong people is caused by the loss of one's spirit to the magical and supernatural forces in nature. Establishing a diagnosis of epilepsy in Western cultures requires scientifically proven techniques and confirmed criteria for the abnormality. Such medical criteria are meaningless to the Hmong, who believe in the global causation of the illness that goes beyond the mind and body of the person to forces in nature. The choice of healers or health care practitioners is conditioned by the attributed cause. Whereas a Hmong client may seek a shaman, a Westerner may seek a qualified neurologist. A shaman, unlike a neurologist, has an established reputation in the Hmong community, and the shaman's qualifications are neither determined by standardized criteria nor confined to specific bodily systems. A shaman uses rituals symbolizing the supernatural, spiritual, and naturalistic modalities of prayers, herbs, and incense burning.

The prevailing value orientation in North American society is individualism and self-reliance in achieving and maintaining health. Caring approaches generally promote the client's independence and ability for self-care. In collectivistic cultures that value group reliance and interdependence, such as traditional South Asian culture, caring behaviours are manifested by actively providing physical and psychosocial support for family members. Adult clients are not expected to be solely responsible for their care and well-being; rather, family members are relied upon to make decisions and provide for the care

TABLE 10-1 Comparative Cultural Contexts of Health and Illness

Characteristic	Western Cultures	Non-Western Cultures
Cause of illness	Biomedical causes	Imbalance between humans and nature Supernatural Magical–religious
Method of diagnosis	Scientific, high-tech Specialty focused Organ-specific manifestations	Naturalistic, magical–religious Holistic Mixed (e.g., magical–religious, supernatural herbal, biomedical) Observation of global, nonspecific symptoms
Treatment	Specialty specific Pharmacological Surgery	Holistic Mixed
Practitioners/healers	Uniform standards and qualifications for practice	May be learned through apprenticeship Nonuniform criteria for practice Reputation established in community
Caring pattern	Self-care Self-determination	Caring provided by others Group reliance and interdependence

Data from Foster, G. (1976). Disease etiologies in non-Western medical systems. *American Anthropology, 78,* 773; Kleinman, A. (1979). *Patients and healers in the context of culture.* Berkeley, CA: University of California Press; and Leininger, M., & McFarland, M. (2002). *Transcultural nursing: Concepts, theories, research and practice* (3rd ed.). New York: McGraw-Hill.

of clients (Pacquiao, 2003). For example, an older Chinese woman's refusal to independently perform rehabilitation exercises after hip surgery, until her daughter is present to assist her, may be misconstrued by you as a lack of responsibility and motivation for self-care. In contrast, she may interpret your insistence on self-reliance as uncaring behaviour.

Cultural Healing Modalities and Healers

Foster (1976), an anthropologist, identified two distinct cross-cultural categories of healers. **Naturalistic practitioners** attribute illness to natural, impersonal, and biological forces that cause alteration in the equilibrium of the human body. Healing emphasizes naturalistic modalities with the use of herbs, chemicals, heat, cold, massage, and surgery. In contrast, **personalistic practitioners** believe that health and illness can be caused by the active influences of an external agent, which can be human (i.e., a sorcerer) or nonhuman (e.g., ghosts, evil, or a deity). Personalistic beliefs emphasize the importance of humans' relationships with other people, both living and deceased, and with their deities. A voodoo priest, for example, uses modalities that combine supernatural, magical, and religious beliefs through the active facilitation of an external agent or personalistic practitioner. A Haitian woman who believes in voodoo may attribute her illness to a curse that has been placed on her and may then seek the services of a voodoo priest to remove the curse. Personalistic approaches also include naturalistic modalities such as massage, aromatherapy, and herbs (see Chapter 35). Some clients seek both types of practitioners to achieve health and treat illness.

Because clients may use both healing systems simultaneously, you must avoid making judgements about clients' practices. To prevent cultural imposition, you need to gain knowledge and understanding of folk remedies used by clients. Many Southeast Asian cultures, for example, practise folk remedies such as coining, cupping, pinching, and burning to relieve aches and pains and to remove bad winds or noxious elements that cause illness. Other groups, including Eastern Europeans, also use cupping to treat respiratory ailments. These folk remedies leave peculiar visible markings on the skin in the form of ecchymosis, representing superficial burns, strap marks, or local tenderness. Cultural ignorance may lead a health care practitioner to call authorities for suspicion of abuse. Instead of dismissing the herbal therapy as dangerous and incompatible with Western medicine, you need to inquire further into whether the practice needs to be changed. By consulting and collaborating with herbalists and other naturalistic practitioners, you can prevent unwarranted distress for clients.

Culture and the Experience of Grief and Loss

Dying and death bring a resurgence of traditions that have been meaningful to groups of people most of their lives (see Chapter 29). Societies assign different meanings to death of a child, death of a young person, and death of an older adult. In Western cultures with strong time orientation toward the future and in which children are expected to survive their parents, death of a young person is devastating. In cultures in which infant mortality rates are high, however, the emotional distress over a child's death may be tempered by the reality of the commonly observed risks of growing up. Hence, the untimely death of an adult may be mourned more deeply.

In societies that hold a belief in the concept of reincarnation, such as those of devout Hindus and Buddhists, people may view death as a step toward rebirth. Hence, care of the dying is focused on supporting the client's preparation for a good death. The family may pray and read religious scriptures to the client to improve his or her chances for a good next life. Buddhists generally believe that suffering is a part of life and is mitigated when a person moves beyond the earthly desires and atones for past misdeeds. A dying Hindu man may prepare for a good death by refusing nourishment and medications, concentrating all his energies on the spiritual aspects of the journey for the next life cycle (Pacquiao, 2002).

Culture also strongly influences pain expression and need for pain medication. Whereas most people in Western culture desire freedom from pain and suffering, other groups accept discomfort. As a nurse, you should not assume that pain relief is valued equally across groups. Clients may experience cultural pain when their valued way of life is disregarded by practitioners (Leininger & McFarland, 2002). Because of limitations on the number of visitors allowed at a dying client's bedside. Orthodox Jews may not be permitted to pray in groups there, and this restriction can cause emotional pain to the client and family. Working with the family and its religious or spiritual leader facilitates culturally congruent care (Pacquiao, 2003).

Regulatory mandates and organizational policies intended to benefit clients should be implemented with sensitivity and understanding of clients' cultural life patterns. The high value that Western society places on personal autonomy and self-determination may be in direct conflict with the values of diverse groups. Advanced care directives, informed consent, and consent for hospice are examples of mandates that may violate clients' values. Informed consent and advanced care directives protect the right of the individual to know and make decisions, ensuring continuity of these rights even to the time when the person is incapacitated. Other cultures, however, are organized so that in these situations, the group assumes decision making for a family member and is trusted to make the right decision for the person. Indeed, some groups such as Asian Canadians and South Asian Canadians may expect their family to make decisions for them, and family members may prefer to protect the person from unnecessary suffering caused by knowing that death is imminent. These cultures value group interdependence and view personal autonomy as an unnecessary burden for a loved one who is ill (Pacquiao, 2002, 2003).

The meaning and expression of grief also vary among cultures. Among the usually reserved East Asians, the social position and status of the deceased reflects the extent to which mourners publicly express grief. Korean families, for example, sometimes hire people to lead the open grieving. Religious beliefs also affect attitudes toward cremation, organ donation, and the treatment of body parts. Devout Muslims may refuse an autopsy or organ donation for fear of desecrating the dead and because of their belief that one be whole to appear in front of the creator.

Cultural Assessment

A comprehensive cultural assessment is the basis for providing culturally competent care. A cultural assessment, combined with critical thinking skills, provides the knowledge necessary for transcultural nursing care (Andrews & Boyle, 2003). Cultural assessment is a systematic and comprehensive examination of the cultural care values, beliefs, and practices of individuals, families, and communities. The goal of cultural assessment is to generate from the clients themselves significant information that enables culturally congruent care (Leininger & McFarland, 2002). Several models of cultural assessment exist, each involving different levels of skill and knowledge. Leininger's Sunrise Model (Leininger & McFarland, 2002) depicted in Figure 10–5, demonstrates the inclusiveness of culture in everyday life and helps explain why cultural assessment must be comprehensive. According to the Sunrise Model, cultural care values, beliefs, and practices are embedded in the cultural and social structural dimensions of society, which include environmental contexts, language, and ethnohistory (i.e., significant historical experiences of a particular group). For older adults, for example, the experience of the Great Depression has sometimes resulted in a tendency to be frugal. You must encourage clients to share stories about their lives that reveal how they think and the cultural lifestyle they embrace. Leininger's model differentiates folk care, which is caring as defined by the people, from the health care professions, which is based on the scientific, biomedical system of care.

Whichever assessment model is used, you begin cultural assessment by knowing population demographic changes in the practice setting. You anticipate the client populations that use their own methods of care and gain some knowledge about their cultures before they come to the clinical setting. Background knowledge about a culture assists you in conducting a focused assessment when time is limited. Demographic information can be gathered from the local and regional census data, as well as from the clients themselves. Population demographic information might include the distribution of ethnic groups, education, occupations, and incidence of the most common illnesses. Comprehensive cultural assessment requires skill and time; hence, preparation and anticipation of needs are important.

A challenge in cultural assessment is the lack of ability to assess multiple perspectives of clients and to interpret the assessment information elicited. It helps to use open-ended questions (e.g., "What do you think caused your illness?"), focused questions (e.g., "Have you had this problem before?"), and contrast questions (e.g., "How different is this problem from the one you had previously?"). The aim is to encourage clients to describe values, beliefs, and practices that are significant to their care, which may be taken for granted unless otherwise revealed. Culturally oriented questions are by nature broad and require a lot of description. Table 10–2 provides a list of guiding questions (a **cultural assessment guide**) that focuses on social and cultural dimensions of assessment.

According to some health care professionals, the idea of a specific cultural assessment model or tool further marginalizes those from particular cultures by placing emphasis on the difficulties with difference. It is important to remember that the many questions used in the cultural assessment tool and culturally sensitive communication tool are just as suitable for Canadians within the dominant group, such as white Anglo-Saxons. The question to be raised is this: Why not just have one assessment tool for everyone? For instance, everyone might be asked what their preference for touch is or how they like to be addressed.

Selected Components of Cultural Assessment

Cultural assessment is important in the total care of any client. Over time, you will learn various skills needed to gather an accurate and comprehensive assessment. The following sections describe certain components of cultural assessment which provide information that can be useful in planning and providing nursing care. You may use the following information as a starting point to assess the similarities and differences of clients and families. However, you must not assume that because any two clients come from the same region or country, they share similar values, beliefs, attitudes, and experiences. Other elements to consider are socioeconomic, educational background, family heritage, work or occupation, length of time in Canada, urban or rural origin, and other individual characteristics, such as a disability, sexual orientation, and sociocultural identity (St. Hill et al., 2003).

Ethnohistory

Knowledge of a client's country of origin and its history and ecological contexts is significant to health care. Haitian immigrants, for example, have linguistic and communication patterns distinct from

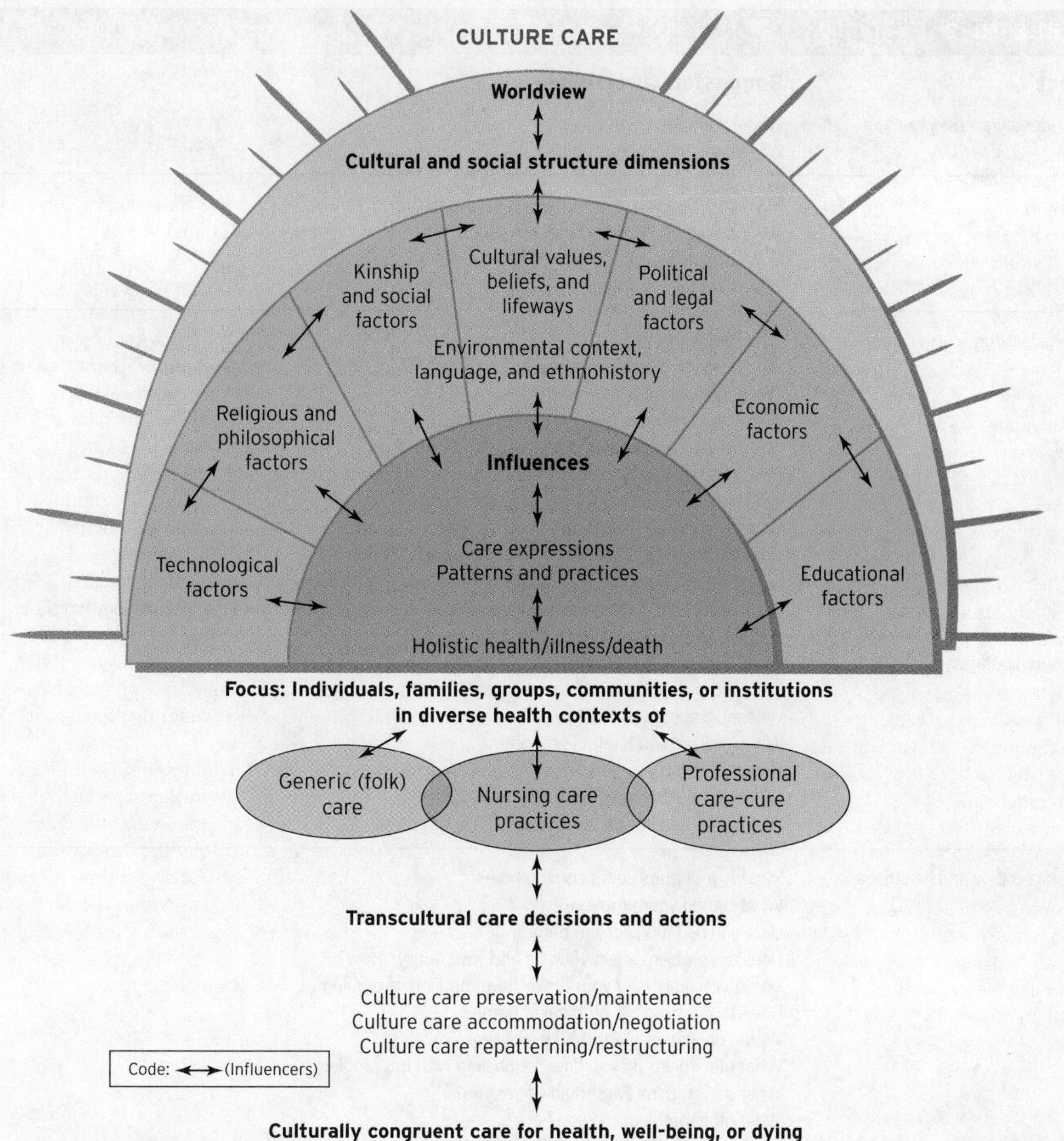

Figure 10-5 Leininger's culture care theory and Sunrise Model. **Source:** From Leininger, M. M., & McFarland, M. R. (2002). *Transcultural nursing: Concepts, theories, research and practice* (3rd ed., p. 80). New York: McGraw-Hill.

those of Jamaicans, even though both groups come from the Caribbean region and may have a common history of oppression. Differences can be traced to their colonial history and intermingling with the local indigenous people. Cultural characteristics of Hindu immigrants from Jamaica are different from those of Hindu immigrants from India because of the cultural contexts of the different regions. The nutritional, communication, and health patterns of Hindus from Jamaica may be more similar to those of African Jamaicans than to those of South Asian Hindus. When caring for a Hindu client of Indian descent who grew up in Jamaica, you may expect that he or she will interact more like a Jamaican, although he or she may look South Indian.

You should be aware that people immigrate to another country for various reasons and have different motivations for doing so. Refugees may be relocated without having chosen their new location, in contrast to immigrants who are able to choose where they live. Refugees tend to experience greater dislocation and deprivation than do immigrants who enter Canada with specialized skills and education and who have the option to return to their homeland. Age at immigration may determine the level of acculturation: Younger immigrants acculturate faster than do their older counterparts. Similarities shared by an immigrant group with the prevailing culture in society are strong predictors of how easily the members of that group adjust. Although acculturation and length of residence in the new country are related, outcomes may be affected by other factors, such as education, racial characteristics, and familiarity with language and religion. You may ask clients about the circumstances that brought them to Canada and how they believe they are adjusting. You need to understand, for instance, any problems the client may have (such as becoming comfortable with routines or the language used to arrange medical appointments), in order to make reasonable and appropriate adjustments to care.

TABLE 10-2 Cultural Assessment Guide

Subject	Suggested Questions
Cultural identity/ancestry/heritage	Where were you born? Where were your parents born?
Ethnohistory	How long have you or your parents resided in this country? What is your ethnic background or ancestry? How strongly are you influenced by your culture? Why did you leave your homeland?
Social organization	Who lives with you? Whom do you consider members of your family? Where do you live? Where do other members of your family live? How do you contact them? How often do you have contact with your family members? Who makes the decisions for you or your family? Whom do you go to outside of your family for support? What do you expect your family members to do for you? How different are your expectations of them now from your expectations at other times? What expectations do you have of your family members who are male, female, old, or young?
Socioeconomic status	What do you do for a living? What did you do back in your homeland? Where did you go to school? What level did you finish in school? How different is your life here from your life back in your homeland? Do you have a primary health care professional? What other health care professionals have you seen?
Biocultural ecology and health risks	What is your purpose for coming here? What caused your problem? Have you had this problem before? Does this problem affect your life and your family? How? Do other members of your family have this kind of problem? How do you treat this problem at home? Whom do you go to for this kind of problem? What other plans do you have for dealing with this problem? What do you think we should do for you? What other problems do you have? Have these problems occurred with any other member of your family?
Language and communication	What language(s) do you speak at home? What language(s) are you most comfortable speaking? In what language(s) can you read and write? How do you want us to talk to you? How should we address you, or what should we call you? What kinds of communication upset or offend you? What words would you use to describe how you feel? Do you need an interpreter? Would you prefer a female or male interpreter?
Religion/spirituality	What is your religion? Who is your religious or spiritual leader? Do you want to be in touch with your religious leader? How do we contact your spiritual leader? What are some of the things we need to do within your religion? How do you practise your religion? Do you follow specific dietary practices?

➤ TABLE 10-2 Cultural Assessment Guide *continued*

Caring beliefs and practices	What do you do to keep yourself well? What do you do to show someone you care? How does your family or you take care of sick family members? Which caregivers do you seek when you are sick? How do you decide when to go to a caregiver and which one to go to? How different is what we do from what your family does for you when you are sick? Are we doing what you think we should be doing for you? How should we give you care?
Experience with professional health care	Since you came to this country, have you had contact with doctors or hospitals? How do you compare your past health care experience is with those of the present? What were some of the problems that you encountered? How were they resolved? What were the positive experiences you had? What type of health care professional do you prefer? Why? If you have a choice, what changes do you wish to see?

You should also be aware that newly arrived immigrants and refugees, depending on the geographic location from which they originate, are vulnerable to a variety of health conditions, including tuberculosis, hepatitis B, anemia, dental caries, intestinal parasites, nutritional deficiencies, incomplete immunization, and mental and emotional concerns such as depression and post-traumatic stress disorder (Kemp, 2004). New immigrants and refugees also frequently experience language barriers, social isolation, separation from family, loss and grief, and a lack of information about available resources. It is important that you explore the historical and sociopolitical background of a client with regard to the specific immigrant community; this knowledge assists you in formulating a plan of care (Lo & Pottinger, 2007). Therefore, you should be aware of, and advocate for, primary health care programs in the community for these vulnerable clients (Box 10–6).

Social Organization

Cultural groups consist of units of organization delineated by kinship, status hierarchy, and appropriate roles for their members. In the prevailing Western society, the most common unit of social organization is the nuclear family, in which adult children are expected to establish residences separate from those of their parents. In collectivistic cultures, family composition may be extended to distant blood relatives across generations and non–blood-related kin. Kinship may be extended to both the father's and mother's side of the family (bilineal) or limited to the side of either the father (patrilineal) or the mother (matrilineal). Patrilineally extended families—in which a woman is expected to move into her husband's clan after marriage and kinship ties with her family of orientation (her own parents and siblings) are minimized—are observed among Chinese and Hindus. You must consider all options when determining a client's next of kin. This is especially relevant to new immigrants and refugees, who may have relocated without intact families. Collectivistic groups may regard members of their ethnic group as closest kin and might want to consult them for health care decisions, as well as permit them to speak on their behalf.

The status of a client within the social hierarchy is generally linked with qualities such as age and gender, as well as with achievements such as education and position. The mainstream culture in Canada emphasizes achievement as the determinant of status, whereas most collectivistic cultures give higher priority to age and gender. In many

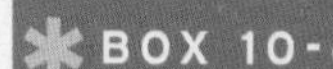

✱ BOX 10-6 FOCUS ON PRIMARY HEALTH CARE

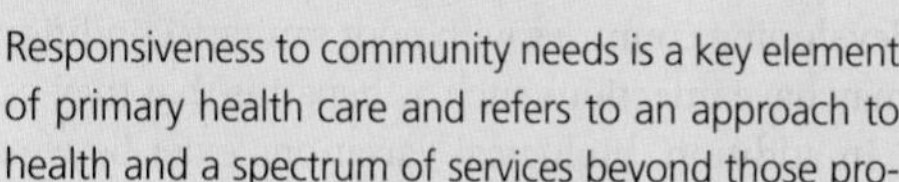

Providing Primary Health Care to Canadian Immigrants

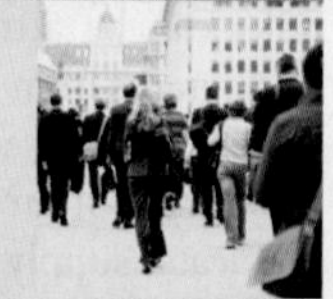

Responsiveness to community needs is a key element of primary health care and refers to an approach to health and a spectrum of services beyond those provided by the traditional health care system. New immigrants and refugees in Canada often need assistance overcoming the language, cultural, and information service barriers that prevent them from using health and social services. Across the country, many community health centres respond to these needs; for example, the New Canadian Clinic in Surrey (NCCS) is overcoming barriers to provide better primary health care access to immigrants who have recently arrrived in the lower mainland of British Columbia. The NCCS is an excellent example of innovation in action that is effectively addressing a pressing community need to ensure that all community members have access to timely and appropriate medical care. Its goal is to augment and integrate existing Fraser Health services with the social supports of the immigrant network in Surrey, British Columbia, in order to provide a coordinated continuum of care. The benefits of this new health care model include shorter lengths of stay in hospitals, fewer visits to emergency departments, and improvement in the overall health of immigrants.

The NCCS uses a multidisciplinary and multilingual team approach to assist new immigrants in integrating more quickly into the mainstream health care system. The team, led by a nurse practitioner, includes a nurse, a mental health counsellor, a medical office assistant, and a community health liaison worker, each of whom has the skills necessary to address the complex needs of recently arrived immigrants. The services of interpreters are readily used, and the clinical team focuses mainly on providing health management, education, and self-management support for new immigrants with multiple chronic diseases, such as heart disease, lung disease, diabetes, and renal disease.

Modified from Ministry of Health, Fraser Health, British Columbia. (2008, January 23). *Innovation helping to meet health needs of immigrants* [news release]. Retrieved September 4, 2008, from http://www2.news.gov.bc.ca/news_releases_2005-2009/2008HEALTH0006-000079.htm

Asian and African cultures, for instance, the eldest son is next in line after his father in terms of authority. Therefore, a Korean mother is subject to the authority of her oldest son in the absence of her husband. Older adults generally occupy higher status in some societies, so that grandparents may impose their decisions regarding the care of grandchildren over the decisions of their married children. You may be required to facilitate and support the negotiations for determining who has the responsibility for family decision making. Think of a nurse you have observed who acted as negotiator, advocator, and facilitator in a situation in which family roles needed to be clarified.

Role expectations of family members may be defined by culture and differentiated by gender. Devout female Muslims, for example, tend to be caregivers, and male Muslims tend to be providers and major decision makers. Some Muslim women may insist on staying at the bedside of an unwell child, in-laws, or husband, but the assumption that she can be relied on to make decisions independently as the primary caregiver may be unrealistic. An understanding of the social hierarchy of the family must be determined as soon as possible, in order to avoid offending clients and their families.

Socioeconomic Status, Biocultural Ecology, and Health Risks

The identification of health risks related to sociocultural and biological history can be assessed on admission of clients. Distinct health risks can be attributed to the ecological context of the culture. Immigrants from the region near the Nile River, for example, are generally predisposed to parasitic infestations endemic to that region. Immigrants from developing countries with poor sanitary conditions and water supply may have infections such as hepatitis that they can pass on to others. In addition, biological variations exist between people from different ethnic groups. As a result, some groups have greater risk of developing certain health conditions. Some genetic disorders, for example, are linked with specific groups, such as Tay-Sachs disease among Ashkenazi Jews and malignant hypertension among Black Canadians.

Language and Communication

Distinct linguistic and communication patterns are associated with different cultural groups. These patterns reflect the core cultural values of a society. In Western cultures that uphold individualism, assertive communication is valued because it demonstrates autonomy and self-determination. People are expected to say what they mean and to mean what they say. In collectivistic cultures, communication is shaped by the context of relationships among participants. Group harmony is the priority, so that participants interact on the basis of their expected positions and relationships within the social hierarchy. People are more likely to remain respectful and show deference to older adults or family leaders, even though they may disagree on an issue. Differences in status and position, age, and gender determine the content and process of communication (Box 10–7). Among Asian cultures, for example, face-saving communication promotes harmony by indirect, ambiguous communication and by conflict avoidance. Messages spoken may have little to do with their meanings. Saying "no" to a superior or older person may not be permitted; hence, an affirmative response of a subordinate may mean only "I heard you," rather than full agreement.

In cultural groups with distinct linear hierarchy, conflict is negotiated between people with the same level of position or authority. Identifying and working with family members of an established hierarchy may prevent miscommunication. In cultures with highly differentiated gender roles, some clients may place more value on the advice of a male nurse than on that of a female nurse. By recognizing and working within a particular cultural context, the nurse can become more effective in achieving appropriate outcomes.

> **BOX 10-7 FOCUS ON OLDER ADULTS**
>
> **Culturally Sensitive Communication**
>
> - Ask older adults how they like to be addressed. If you are in doubt, address them formally (e.g., "Mr. Lin").
> - Determine the client's preferences where touch is concerned. For example, US citizens often greet each other with a firm handshake. Many Native Americans, however, may see this as a sign of aggression, and touch outside of marriage is sometimes forbidden for older adults from the Middle East.
> - Investigate the client's preferences vis-à-vis silence. In general, silence is valued in Eastern cultures, whereas in Western cultures, people are uncomfortable with silence.
> - Be aware of the client's beliefs about eye contact during conversation. Direct eye contact in European American cultures may be a sign of honesty and truthfulness. However, eye contact with other groups, such as older Native Americans, may not be allowed. Older Asian adults sometimes avoid eye contact with authority figures because this is considered disrespectful, and direct eye contact between genders in Middle Eastern cultures is sometimes forbidden except between spouses.
>
> Data from Meiner, S. E., & Leuckenotte, A. G. (2006). *Gerontologic nursing* (3rd ed.). St. Louis, MO: Mosby.

Nonverbal communication is also shaped by communication. Culture influences the distance between participants in an interaction, the extent of touching, the degree of eye contact, and how much private information the client shares. Clients use less distance when speaking to trusted affiliates and persons of the same gender, age, and social position. Members of many ethnic groups tend to speak their own dialect with each other in order to feel ease and to secure privacy. To minimize the distance when communicating with clients, you need to consider taking up a relational approach to cultural nursing that greatly enhances the ability to know and respond to people (Hartrick Doane & Varcoe, 2005). A relational approach to nursing allows you not only to connect across differences but also to recognize cultural similarities and differences more intently. Such an approach provides opportunities "to attend to issues of meaning, experience, race, history, culture, health, and sociopolitical systems. In addition, as we relationally honor and attend to such differences the potential for growth, change, and knowledge development is enhanced" (Hartrick Doane & Varcoe, 2005, p. 9).

Religion and Spirituality

Religious and spiritual beliefs have major influences on the person's attitudes toward health and illness, pain and suffering, and life and death. The distinction between religion and spirituality is often blurred. It is advisable for you to understand the multiple perspectives of clients. Many cultures do not separate religion and spirituality, whereas many others have totally distinct concepts of the two. To a Hmong animist, spirits could be those of dead ancestors or forces external to the person. To an Anglo-Canadian, spirituality may mean an inner, personal relationship with a higher being. Although a discussion of religious and spiritual philosophies is difficult in a hospital setting, you must assess what is important to the spiritual well-being of clients and learn as much as possible about their spiritual and religious practices (see Chapter 28).

Caring Beliefs and Practices

Caring beliefs and practices incorporate a client's perception of his or her ability to control circumstances or factors in the environment. Specifically, it may refer to a client's perception of how he or she can influence causes of illness and use cultural healing modalities and healers. During cultural assessment, you should identify the health practices of the client and respect them (Box 10–8). Obtain information about folk remedies used and cultural healers employed by the client. Unless these practices are harmful, they should be incorporated into the client's plan of care.

Experience with Professional Health Care

All cultures have concepts of past, present, and future dimensions of time. An aspect of a client's experience with professional health care, for instance, may be your understanding of the client's orientation of time. This information can be useful in planning care, arranging appointments for procedures, and helping a client plan self-care activities at home. Differences exist in the concepts of time that cultures emphasize and in how time is expressed. Communication concerning time may be indirect and circular in order to avoid offending and disrespecting other people.

Present time orientation, for instance, may conflict with the policies of a health care institution that emphasizes punctuality and adherence to appointments. Improving clients' access to health services may be achieved by mutually negotiating schedules and by accommodating cultural patterns.

BOX 10-8 NURSING STORY

Identifying the Client's Health Care Practices

A Chinese immigrant who recently arrived in Canada has given birth to her first child. Once the newborn has been cared for and is resting, you ask the new mother if she would like to take a shower. The mother refuses politely. Her belief is that if she takes a shower, she could contract rheumatism in old age. Then the mother's food tray arrives, and she does not touch or eat anything. For this newcomer to Canada, the hospital food may seem different and served in an unfamiliar manner. Her family brings plain rice and salted pork into the hospital. They also bring two different soups, which are thought to bring heat, the "yang," into her body, thereby removing the impurities from her system.

In traditional Chinese culture, good health means achieving a balance between yin and yang. The belief is that all body systems interact with each other and with the environment to produce a balanced state of wellness. In consultation with the mother, you are able to assess and understand why she is refusing to shower and eat the hospital food. With this increased understanding, you are able to mutually negotiate with the mother some alternatives for her care to accommodate her needs, without jeopardizing her care or causing her distress. You appropriately assess that rather than showering, the mother would prefer a basin of water and a cloth that she could use to clean herself. In terms of her dietary requests, you determined that she can eat the food from home as long as it does not interfere with or jeopardize her health status. As a result, your sensitivity and respect for the new mother's cultural beliefs enable her to relax and recover in a culturally appropriate manner. You were open to learning about the cultural beliefs of the new mother and then collaborating with her on decisions about care.

Application of Cultural Assessment Components to Aboriginal Peoples of Canada

Aboriginal peoples represent an important and growing group within Canada. In 2006, the number of people who identified themselves as Aboriginal (i.e., North American Indian [First Nations], Métis, and Inuit) surpassed one million (Statistics Canada, 2008a). Since the mid-1990s, the Aboriginal population has increased significantly. Between 1996 and 2006, it grew by 45%, nearly six times faster than the 8% rate of increase for the non-Aboriginal population (Statistics Canada, 2008a). In 2006, Aboriginal peoples accounted for almost 4% of the total population of Canada (Statistics Canada, 2008a). Of the three Aborginal groups in Canada, the Métis population increased the most. Aboriginal peoples in Canada also increasingly live in urban centres. In 2006, 54% lived in urban areas (including large cities or census metropolitan areas and smaller urban centres); this proportion increased from 50% in 1996 (Statistics Canada, 2008a). Furthermore, the Aboriginal population is, on average, younger than the non-Aboriginal population. Almost half (48%) of the Aboriginal population consists of children and youth aged 24 and younger, in comparison with 31% of the non-Aboriginal population (Statistics Canada, 2008a).

The three Aboriginal groups—First Nations, Métis, and Inuit—have their own unique languages, heritages, cultural practices, and spiritual beliefs. These groups contain many subgroups, each with its own unique culture. The term *Indian* describes all the Aboriginal peoples in Canada who are not Métis or Inuit. These include the nations or groups of people who were originally living in Canada before the European explorers began to arrive in the 1600s. Three legal definitions are used to describe Indians in Canada: Status, Non-Status, and Treaty Indians. Status Indians are registered under the *Indian Act* (Indian and Northern Affairs Canada, 2004), which regulates the management of reservations and sets out certain federal obligations. Non-Status Indians are not registered under the *Indian Act* (Indian and Northern Affairs Canada, 2004). A *Treaty Indian* is a Status Indian who belongs to a First Nation that signed a treaty with the United Kingdom (Indian and Northern Affairs Canada, 2004).

Many Aboriginal people find the term *Indian* offensive and outdated; in the 1970s, the term *First Nation* became preferred to *Treaty Indians*. In addition, many Indian people adopted the term *First Nation* to replace the word *band*, and also amended the term *First Nation* to the name of their community, such as the *Nuxalk First Nation* (Indian and Northern Affairs Canada, 2004; Wasekeesikaw, 2006). Some Aboriginal people prefer the more inclusive term *First Peoples* rather than the word *Nation* because in English, *Nation* does not fit with the Aboriginal social structure. The first European explorers to arrive in North America used the term *Indian* because they thought they had reached India (Canadian Health Network, 2004). First Nations peoples claim that the roots of the term *Indian* reflect a history of colonialism and that the term is, therefore, inappropriate (Wasekeesikaw, 2006).

The following sections describe the variations from the non-Aboriginal culture that exist among Canadian Aboriginal peoples. Bear in mind that these discussions are general in nature, and each client must be assessed as an individual.

Ethnohistory

"I am an Indian. I am proud to know who I am and where I originated. I am proud to be a unique creation of the Great Spirit. We are part of Mother Earth . . . .
We have survived, but survival by itself is not enough.
A people must also grow and flourish."
(Snow, Chief John. [1977]. *These mountains are our sacred places.* Toronto, ON: Samuel Stevens.)

An understanding of specific cultural Aboriginal groups in Canada is important in order to appreciate contemporary health issues affecting Aboriginal peoples. The First Nations of Canada are exceptionally diverse, culturally, linguistically, socially, economically, historically, and in other ways. As Waldram et al. (2006) emphasized, "the recognition and acceptance of such diversity is essential to an appreciation of developments in the health care field and to an appreciation of the myriad processes that have affected the health status of Aboriginal people in both the pre-contact and post-contact periods" (p. 23).

Pre-European contact refers to the history of Aboriginal people before exploration and settlement of the Americas by Europeans. During that period, Aboriginal people were composed of distinct cultures from the Arctic, Western Subarctic, Easter Subarctic, Northeastern Woodlands, Plains, Plateau, and Northwest Coast. Traditional health beliefs, shamans, herbalists, and folk medicine were aspects of how Aboriginal communities experienced healing and well-being. **European contact** began on Canada's east coast, where French explorers and fur traders settled and introduced diseases such as smallpox, tuberculosis, and measles, which killed thousands of Aboriginal people. Scarce resources diminished Aboriginal livelihoods, and malnutrition, starvation, and alcohol consumption made circumstances worse (Dickason, 2006). During **post-European contact,** Europeans established relationships with Aboriginal people, and colonization influenced Aboriginal systems of government, trade, and health care. Over the years, the Canadian government displaced Aboriginal people from their traditional lands and developed policies to isolate them, "civilize" them, and assimilate them into Canadian society, which resulted in the destruction of Aboriginal cultures. These oppressive and suppressive policies, and the acts that followed, had extensive negative effects on Aboriginal cultural identities and governances (Wasekeesikaw, 2006). The Indian residential school system, for instance, which no longer exists in Canada, left a multi-generational legacy of physical and psychological abuse that "lives on in the form of significant pain and suffering among residential school survivors and their families" (Barton et al., 2005b, p. 295).

Social Organization

Many First Nations peoples live on reserves and in communities in each of the Canadian provinces and territories, and many Inuit live in settlements throughout the territories. The reserves are easily accessible in the southern regions but remote and isolated in the northern regions. Métis live in communities across Canada and in settlements set aside for them in Alberta. For many Aboriginal people, the biological family is the traditional centre of social organization and includes all members of the extended family. The principles that guide family and community social organization by which they live their lives include the notion of wholeness, whereby "all things are interrelated, and everything in the universe is part of a signal whole. Everything is connected in some way to everything else, and it is only possible to understand something if one understands how it is connected to everything else" (Hunter et al., 2004, p. 274).

Socioeconomic Status

Cultural disorganization resulting from colonization underpins the culture of poverty, circumstances that are experienced by many Aboriginal people in contemporary Canadian society. Large proportions of the Aborginal population live in remote communities (Statistics Canada 2008a) and travel back and forth between rural and urban environments. In general, the Aboriginal population experiences both poorer health and reduced access to health services in comparison with most Canadians living in rural and urban locations. Along with other inequities and social injustices that contribute to their vulnerability, they are socially, economically, and politically marginalized from mainstream society. "Thus, there is a complex interplay between geographical context and the historical socio-economic and political context of Aboriginal people's health, and it has profoundly influenced the health and social status of Aboriginal Canadians" (Tarlier et al., 2007, p. 129).

Biocultural Ecology and Health Risks

Since the 1950s, dramatic changes in lifestyle have affected the social, environmental, and health status of Aboriginal people (Waldram et al., 2006). The disease patterns in many First Nations and Inuit communities continue to resemble those found in low-income countries, despite improvements since the 1990s (Health Canada, 2003). In addition, the prevalence of major chronic diseases, including diabetes, cardiovascular disease, cancer, arthritis, and rheumatitis, appears to be increasing in this population (Vollman et al., 2008). Rates of unintentional injuries, deaths from drowning, and other accidents are also high among children and families in Aborginal communities (Vollman et al., 2008).

Tuberculosis. Although the overall incidence of tuberculosis has dropped steadily since the 1960s, the incidence among First Nations and Inuit people is almost seven times higher than the national rate, according to 1998 statistics (Health Canada, 2008a). Factors contributing to such a high rate include overcrowding and unsafe or unreliable water supplies in these communities.

Hepatitis A. The rate of hepatitis A virus infection among First Nations and Inuit people tends to be significantly higher than the overall Canadian rate (Minuk & Uhanova, 2003). The major factors believed to contribute to these periodic outbreaks are poor housing, poor water supplies, and lack of sewage treatment.

Diabetes Mellitus. Diabetes is considered to be an epidemic in progress for Canadian Aboriginal peoples, with a prevalence of diabetes of three to five times higher, according to location, than that in non-Aboriginal communities (Health Canada, 2003). The factors contributing to this rate appear to be a combination of genetic susceptibility, a change from a physically active lifestyle to a sedentary lifestyle, and a diet high in sugar, fats, and salt. Type 2 diabetes is diagnosed with increasing frequency in Aboriginal children (Health Canada, 2003). Earlier onset of the disease leads to an earlier onset of complications, as well as excessive mortality rates among young and middle-aged adults. In Inuit communities, the rate of diabetes is still relatively low, but concerns have been raised that this may change if the Inuit alter their traditional eating patterns and lifestyle (Health Canada, 2003).

HIV and AIDS. Human immunodeficiency virus (HIV) infections and cases of acquired immune deficiency syndrome (AIDS) among Canadian Aboriginals have increased steadily since the 1990s, whereas the annual number of AIDS cases has levelled off in the rest of the population. The proportion of Aboriginal people who tested positive for HIV infection increased from 19% in 1998 to 24% in 2002. This number may be misleadingly low, however, inasmuch as ethnic identity is unknown for about 15% of clients with AIDS. Aboriginal clients with AIDS differ significantly from non-Aboriginal clients with AIDS. Among Aboriginal clients, for example, the proportion of female clients is much higher than that of male clients (25% in comparison with 9%), and the proportion of intravenous drug users is higher among non-Aboriginal clients (38% in comparison with 7%) (Waldram et al., 2006).

Alcohol and Substance Abuse. It is difficult to collect accurate data, but the abuse of alcohol and other substances is perceived to be common in some Aboriginal communities (Health Canada, 2008b). Alcohol and substance abuse can be viewed as part of a set of complex issues affecting the social and physical well-being of the client, the family, and the community. The National Native Alcohol and Drug Abuse Program was established to assist First Nations and Inuit community members in instituting and operating programs aimed at reducing the level of alcohol, drug, and solvent abuse among target groups on reserves. The program emphasizes prevention and treatment, as well as training, research, and development.

Suicide. The suicide rates in Inuit and First Nations communities are five to six times higher than the rates found in the non-Aboriginal population (Statistics Canada, 2008c). Possible factors contributing to the suicide rate include psychobiological factors (pre-existing mental illness, personality disorders, dysfunctional cognitive style), situational life history factors (early childhood trauma, family dysfunction, substance abuse, conflict with authority, absence of spirituality), socioeconomic factors (poverty, unemployment), and cultural stress (low self-esteem, lack of cultural heritage) (Waldram et al., 2006).

Language and Communication

Approximately 53 Aboriginal languages exist, with Algonquian being the largest and most widespread language family in Canada (Dickason, 2006). Many of these languages have identifiable dialects. Interpreters who can speak the various dialects within a language are invaluable, but locating them poses challenges to the health care system. Knowledgeable interpreters, however, not only understand and translate the clients' words but also interpret the culture and make relevant the concepts underlying it as well. For some Aboriginal Canadians, for instance, it is important to realize that reflection may lead to gaps, and thus long silences, in the conversaton (Watts & McDonald, 2007).

Religious and Spiritual Practices

The spiritual approaches of Aboriginal peoples incorporate a mind–body–spirit connection that is harmonious with nature. For some, the circle of life is often viewed as having four aspects or directions: spiritual, physical, mental, and emotional. The presence of all components together enables the person to heal the self and restore well-being. It is in the understanding of wholeness that the spiritual, physical, mental, emotional, and relational parts of the self are integrated. Transcending these dimensions, however, is the spiritual component, which assists the person in discovering his or her human potential (Hunter et al., 2004).

Caring Beliefs and Practices

Aboriginal peoples subscribe to a holistic concept of health but exemplify tremendous diversity of background and experience in terms of culture, language, and traditions (Wasekeesikaw, 2006). The caring beliefs and practices of various groups are linked to being alive and well, which may be understood as the interconnected relationship people create with the land and the plants and animals of nature. Aboriginal health and healing incorporates many aspects within the circle of life that includes, for instance, being human, stewarding the land, hunting wild animals, eating traditional foods, and practising herbal medicine. In a study that focused on the experience of diabetes among Aboriginal people living in a rural Canadian community (Barton et al., 2005a), the findings revealed cultural themes associated with Western and traditional medicines; dietary changes, exercise, and weight loss; culturally relevant communication; Aboriginal life choices and the responsibility to choose; and a belief in living day by day. Within this particular First Nations community, the researchers found that "(i) consultative meetings with community members; (ii) the use of a cultural awareness program for health professionals; and (iii) the involvement of Aboriginal people in the development of their own diet, exercise and prevention strategies would greatly enhance [diabetes] programs in the future. [Such initiatives] could contribute not only to the culturally safe management of diabetes, but also encourage its early detection now and in the future" (Barton et al., 2005a, p. 245).

Experience With Professional Health Care

Although cultural sensitivity frameworks will guide you in your relationships with clients, systematized and taxonomic descriptions of characteristics particular to a cultural group do not always "accommodate peoples' diet preferences, communication styles, family dynamics, and culturally-based responses to pain, child-birth, childrearing, etc." (Browne & Varcoe, 2006, p. 158). You need to ask yourself how you can think about notions of culture without stereotyping or thinking simplistically about Aboriginal people and without inciting hurtful and nonconstructive assumptions about cultural difference. In contemplating this question, Dion Stout and Downey (2006) described the conceptual links between nursing, Aboriginal peoples, and cultural safety. They contended that (1) "the caring spaces that are occupied by Indigenous people and nurses are also potentially the new arenas of struggle for both sides"; (2) "attention between the totality of self and the totality of one's environment is inherent in cultural safety affecting both nurses and Indigenous people"; and (3) "an overemphasis on culture as a health determinant can bring about an abdication of responsibility over all other health determinants by health determiners like Indigenous people and nurses" (p. 327).

Implications for Nursing Practice

The importance of cultural competency and safety for health care administrators, practitioners, and educators has been recognized by the National Aboriginal Health Organization (NAHO). NAHO's (2008) document describes the origins of cultural competency and cultural safety; a theoretical and methodological approach to cultural safety, an approach that originated with Aboriginal peoples; and the importance of its application to health care.

Increasingly, nurse scholars are researching the health challenges faced by Aboriginal peoples and discovering how to provide culturally competent care (Majumdar et al., 2004; Smith, 2003). Smith et al. (2006) focused on establishing safety and responsiveness as a mainstay of care for pregnant and parenting Aboriginal people. Their findings revealed "that safety and healthcare relationships and settings, and responsiveness to individuals' and families' experiences and capacities must be brought into the forefront of care. [These] results suggest that the intention of care must be situated in a broader view of colonizing relations to improve early access to, and relevance of, care during pregnancy and parenting for Aboriginal people" (p. E27).

One reason why people become nurses is a desire to "act in ways that are respectful, compassionate, and equitable and that leaves [nurses] feeling that [they] have somehow 'done good'" (Hartrick Doane & Varcoe, 2005, p. 16). A relational approach to nursing shapes the places of inquiry and practice that determine how to find your way through relationships, culture, safety, ethics, diversity, power, economics, communication, and history. A deep consideration of **relational practice** and nursing obligations offers you the means to understand experience and to imagine how you might incorporate reflexivity, intentionality, and openness into practice, education, and research.

In regard to practice, Hartrick Doane and Varcoe (2007) presented an example of a nurse recalling the interaction with an elderly woman in the emergency department who needed to be invited to reveal her "whole" experience. The woman's story "exemplifies the significance of a nurse–patient relationship and the profound difference it can make in promoting health and healing" (p. 195). In terms of education, Smith et al. (2007) described "community-based stakeholders' views of how safe and responsive care 'makes a difference' to health and well-being for pregnant and parenting Aboriginal people." Smith et al. concluded that "design and evaluation of care based upon community values and priorities and using a strengths-based approach can improve early access to a relevance of care during pregnancy and parenting for Aboriginal people" (p. 321). In considering research, Barton (2004) focused on a form of narrative inquiry as a relational method of critically analyzing its appropriateness as an innovative approach to researching Aboriginal people's experience of living with diabetes. By locating Aboriginal epistemology in a relational method such as narrative inquiry, "the ability to adapt a methodology for use in a cultural context, preserve the perspectives of Aboriginal peoples, maintain the holistic nature of social problems, and value co-participation in respectful ways are strengths of an inquiry partial to a responsive and embodied scholarship" (p. 519).

* KEY CONCEPTS

- Culture is the context for interpreting human experiences such as health and illness and provides direction for decisions and actions.
- Transcultural nursing is a comparative study and understanding of cultures to identify culture-specific and culture-universal caring constructs across ethnic groups.
- Culturally congruent care is meaningful, supportive, and facilitative because it conforms to valued life patterns of clients; it is achieved through cultural assessment.
- Culturally competent care requires knowledge, attitudes, and skills supportive of implementation of culturally congruent care.
- Cultural safety is an outcome of nursing education that enables safe service to be defined by clients who receive the service.
- Cultural assessment requires a comprehensive inquiry into the client's cultural values, beliefs, and practices; it may involve assessing ethnohistory, social organization, socioeconomic status, biocultural ecology and health risks, language and communication, religion and spirituality, caring beliefs and practices, and experiences with professional health care.
- Relational practice is the nursing obligation to examine relationships, ethics, and effective nursing practice, and the personal and contextual elements that continuously shape and influence nursing relationships.

* CRITICAL THINKING EXERCISES

1. You are about to begin giving an Arab Muslim man his morning care when he states, "I don't want a bath now." He becomes annoyed when you try to explain that you must give him a bath at this time. Before you leaqve the room, he asks you to leave a basin of water and towel by his bedside. He also asks you to get his prayer rug from his closet.
   a. How should you respond to the client?
   b. What may be the reasons for his refusal and annoyance?
2. A 50-year-old Chinese woman is hospitalized with a respiratory condition. She insists that you give her warm water and rub her back with Tiger balm liniment. When she receives her lunch, consisting of a turkey sandwich, tossed salad, and milk, she keeps the turkey sandwich and tossed salad but asks that you take the milk away.
   a. How should you respond to the client's requests?
   b. What is the significance of her requests?
   c. Why does she refuse her lunch?
3. You are assigned to a 60-year-old South Asian Hindu widow who is admitted with chest pain and shortness of breath. The client recently arrived from India to visit her son and pregnant daughter-in-law. She can speak only Gujarati and understands very little English. She is accompanied by her son.
   a. What areas should you include in your focused cultural assessment?
   b. How should you communicate with the client?
   c. Identify ways to preserve and accommodate the client's culture in her care.
   d. What aspects of the client's way of life may need repatterning?

* REVIEW QUESTIONS

1. Socialization into one's primary culture during childhood is known as
   1. Enculturation
   2. Acculturation
   3. Assimilation
   4. Multiculturalism
2. Multiculturalism results when a person
   1. Has an experience with a new or different culture that is extremely negative
   2. Maintains his or her culture and interacts peacefully with people of other cultures
   3. Gives up his or her ethnic identity in favour of the dominant culture
   4. Adapts to and adopts a new culture
3. Cultural awareness involves an in-depth self-examination of one's
   1. Background, recognizing biases and prejudices
   2. Social, cultural, and biophysical factors
   3. Engagement in culturally safe interactions
   4. Motivation and commitment to caring
4. Culturally competent care is the process of
   1. Learning about vast cultures
   2. Delivering care that is based on knowledge of the client's cultural heritage, beliefs, and attitudes
   3. Influencing treatment and care of clients
   4. Motivation and commitment to caring

5. Ethnocentrism is the root of
   1. Stereotypes, biases, and prejudices
   2. Meanings by which people make sense of their experiences
   3. Cultural beliefs
   4. Individualism and self-reliance in achieving and maintaining health
6. When a person acts on his or her prejudices,
   1. Discrimination occurs
   2. Sufficient comparative knowledge of diverse groups is obtained
   3. Delivery of culturally congruent care is ensured
   4. Effective intercultural and relational communication develops
7. The prevailing value orientation in Western society is
   1. Use of rituals symbolizing the supernatural
   2. Group reliance and interdependence
   3. Healing emphasizing naturalistic modalities
   4. Individualism and self-reliance in achieving and maintaining health
8. Disparities in health outcomes between rich and poor clients illustrate
   1. The attribution of illness to natural, impersonal, and biological forces
   2. Biological and sociocultural health risks
   3. Influence of socioeconomic factors in morbidity and mortality
   4. Combination of naturalistic, religious, and supernatural modalities
9. Culture strongly influences pain expression and need for pain medication. However, cultural pain
   1. May be suffered by a client whose valued way of life is disregarded by practitioners
   2. Is more intense, thus necessitating more medication
   3. Is not expressed verbally or physically
   4. Is expressed only to others of similar culture
10. The prevailing values in Western society on individual autonomy and self-determination
    1. Rarely have an effect on other cultures
    2. Do not have an effect on health care
    3. May hinder ability to get into hospice programs
    4. May be in direct conflict with the values of diverse groups

✻ RECOMMENDED WEB SITES

Canadian Ethnocultural Council: http://www.ethnocultural.ca/
This Web site explains the purposes of the Canadian Ethnocultural Council, which is a nonprofit, nonpartisan coalition of national ethnocultural organizations representing ethnocultural groups across Canada. Links to other related publications and sites related to ethnocultural groups are included.

Citizenship and Immigration Canada: Cultural Profiles Project: http://www.settlement.org/cp/
This Web site provides an overview of the life and customs of immigrants to Canada. Each profile includes a summary fact sheet and information about their culture, food, health, landscape, climate, arts, holidays, and literature.

Aboriginal Nurses Association of Canada: http://www.anac.on.ca/
This Web site offers a valuable resource of information regarding this association, founded by Jean Goodwill and Jocelyn Bruyere. Similar to provincial groups in existence, the association is available to provide support to Aboriginal nurses and Aboriginal student nurses, and it recognizes the need for increased numbers of Aboriginal nurses in Canada. It is also a valuable resource for students in nursing programs who do not self-identify as Aboriginal people.

11

Nursing Leadership, Management, and Collaborative Practice

Original chapter by Patricia A. Stockert, RN, BSN, MS, PhD

Canadian content written by Susan M. Duncan, RN, PhD

objectives

Mastery of content in this chapter will enable you to:

- Define the key terms listed.
- Describe entry-level staff nurse competencies related to leadership, management, and collaborative practice.
- Describe the relationships between nursing leadership and healthy practice environments, client safety, and quality client care outcomes.
- Discuss how a nurse leader can contribute to collaborative practice and best practices implementation.
- Discuss ways to apply skills of clinical care coordination in nursing practice.
- Discuss principles for the appropriate delegation of client care activities.
- Describe the purpose, elements, and models for quality practice environments and client safety.

key terms

Accountability, p. 138
Authority, p. 138
Autonomy, p. 138
Best practice guidelines, p. 137
Case management, p. 136
Collaborative practice, p. 133
Competencies for safe practice, p. 142
Continuity of care, p. 135
Decentralized management, p. 137
Delegation, p. 140
Functional nursing, p. 136
Healthy practice environment, p. 133
Interprofessional nursing teams, p. 136
Intraprofessional teams, p. 136
Leadership and management, p. 133
Nurse-sensitive outcome, p. 142
Outcomes, p. 133
Primary nursing, p. 136
Quality improvement (QI), p. 141
Responsibility, p. 138
Team nursing, p. 136
Total client care, p.136

media resources

evolve Web Site

- Audio Chapter Summaries
- Glossary
- Multiple-Choice Review Questions
- Student Learning Activities
- Weblinks

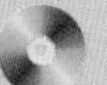
Companion CD

- Glossary
- Interactive Learning Activities
- Fluids and Electrolytes Tutorial
- Test-Taking Skills

All nurses must be leaders, and nurses assume positions of leadership in health care delivery much earlier in their careers today than in previous generations. As you develop the knowledge and skills to enter the nursing workforce, you also learn how to become a leader among colleagues for the delivery of care in many health care settings. It is therefore important that you develop an understanding of **leadership and management** roles in nursing early in your educational program because this is one of the competencies required of entry-level nurses. You can see from the list of competencies required of entry-level nurses in Box 11–1 that leadership begins with a strong professional identity and accountability. For optimal nursing care, managers and leaders are needed to ensure both the vision for quality care and the management skills required for best practices and quality care (Hibberd et al., 2006). Whereas *leadership* refers to a shared vision, values, organizational strategy, and relationships, *management* most often refers to the competencies required to ensure the day-to-day delivery of nursing care according to available resources and standards of professional practice. To be effective in promoting a healthy work environment, leaders and managers must demonstrate leadership practices that honour the importance of relationships, values, and culture (Cummings, 2004; Gifford et al., 2006). Figure 11–1 provides a conceptual model of transformational leadership practices that have been identified as contributing to health **outcomes.**

In the current context of health care in which qualified health care professionals are in short supply, competencies related to leadership in nursing relate to creating environments for healthy working relationships and teamwork. A healthy work environment is most likely to retain nurses in practice settings in which they are both satisfied and able to provide high-quality care. RNs must work collaboratively with other members of the nursing team, as well as with professionals from other disciplines and with clients and their families. The importance of such work is most often discussed as **collaborative practice**, defined as working together toward mutually identified goals while valuing different perspectives and accountabilities of individual team members (Gardner, 2005; RNAO, 2006b; Tschannen, 2004). This chapter therefore focuses on current thinking in nursing leadership and management, including definitions, roles and relationships, shifts to collaborative practice models, and the role of leaders in ensuring healthy practice environments and best practices. The ideas and examples included in this chapter apply to the different practice settings in which nurses work: in homes, in institutions, and in communities.

➤ BOX 11-1 Entry-Level Staff Nurse Competencies Related to Leadership and Management

- Is accountable and responsible for own actions and decisions, including personal safety.
- Demonstrates leadership in providing client care by promoting healthy and culturally safe work environments.
- Displays initiative, self-confidence, and self-awareness, and encourages collaborative interactions within the nursing and health care team.
- Organizes own workload and develops time-management skills for meeting responsibilities.
- Integrates quality improvement principles and activities into nursing practice.
- Uses relational knowledge and ethical principles when working with students and other health care team members to maximize collaborative client care.
- Participates in and contributes to nursing and health care team development.
- Supports professional efforts in the field of nursing to achieve a healthier society (e.g., lobbying, conducting health fairs, and promoting principles of the *Canada Health Act*).
- Demonstrates an awareness of healthy public policy and social justice.
- Develops support networks with registered nurse (RN) colleagues, health care team members, and community suppports.

Adapted from College of Registered Nurses of British Columbia (2006). *Competencies in the context of entry-level registered nurse practice in British Columbia. Leadership and management practices for healthy work environments.* Vancouver: Author.

Management and Leadership Roles for Nurses

Nurses assume a wide variety of management and leadership roles in health care organizations in order to ensure that clients receive safe and high quality care. Research has revealed that nurses must provide leadership to ensure that nursing care takes place in quality practice environments. (Aiken et al., 2002; Canadian Nursing Advisory Committee, 2002; Scott et al., 1999; Silas, 2007) and that these work environments are essential for health, high-quality client care, and client safety (Estabrooks et al., 2005). A high-quality practice environment is also a healthy work environment, defined as “a practice setting that maximizes the health and well-being of nurses, quality client outcomes, organizational performance and societal outcomes” (RNAO, 2006a, p. 13).

A **healthy practice environment** begins with the senior nurse leader in the organization, who most often holds the title of Chief Nurse Executive, Chief Nursing Officer, or Director or Vice President of Nursing or of Patient Care (Canadian Nurses Association [CNA], 2002). In 1999, the government of Canada instituted the first Office of Nursing Policy with Dr. Judith Shamian, RN, Executive Director, hired to provide leadership needed to ensure that attention was paid in government to the nursing perspective on programs and policies (Health Canada, n.d.). Since then, several provinces have followed suit, instituting provincial nursing policy offices led by nurses in executive positions. These positions are key to ensuring that nurses influence the policy directions that governments take to ensure high-quality nursing services for Canadians. In policy roles, nurses act as policy advocates, by which they have made a difference throughout history and continue to advocate today for progressive public policy in primary health care and population health (Spenceley et al., 2006; see Unit I in this text). As a student, you will learn the skills involved in nursing advocacy and assume the role of advocate in order to promote the health of people. Advocacy is key to nursing leadership at all levels. Nurses today “stand on the shoulders of giants”; the nurse leaders of the past held a powerful vision for the development of nursing as a profession and advocated tirelessly to bring this vision to fruition (“A century of progress,” 2005). One such leader was Ethel Johns, Director of the University of British Columbia's first nursing school. She inspired other nurses with her vision and challenged them to think for themselves (Boxes 11–2 and 11–3).

As in the past, a strong nurse executive unites the strategic direction of the organization with the values and goals of nursing. Nurse executives must also build teams of leaders who work across the organization to implement best practices and develop high-quality work environments in which nursing practice can flourish. Although it takes a strong senior nursing leader to inspire a healthy work

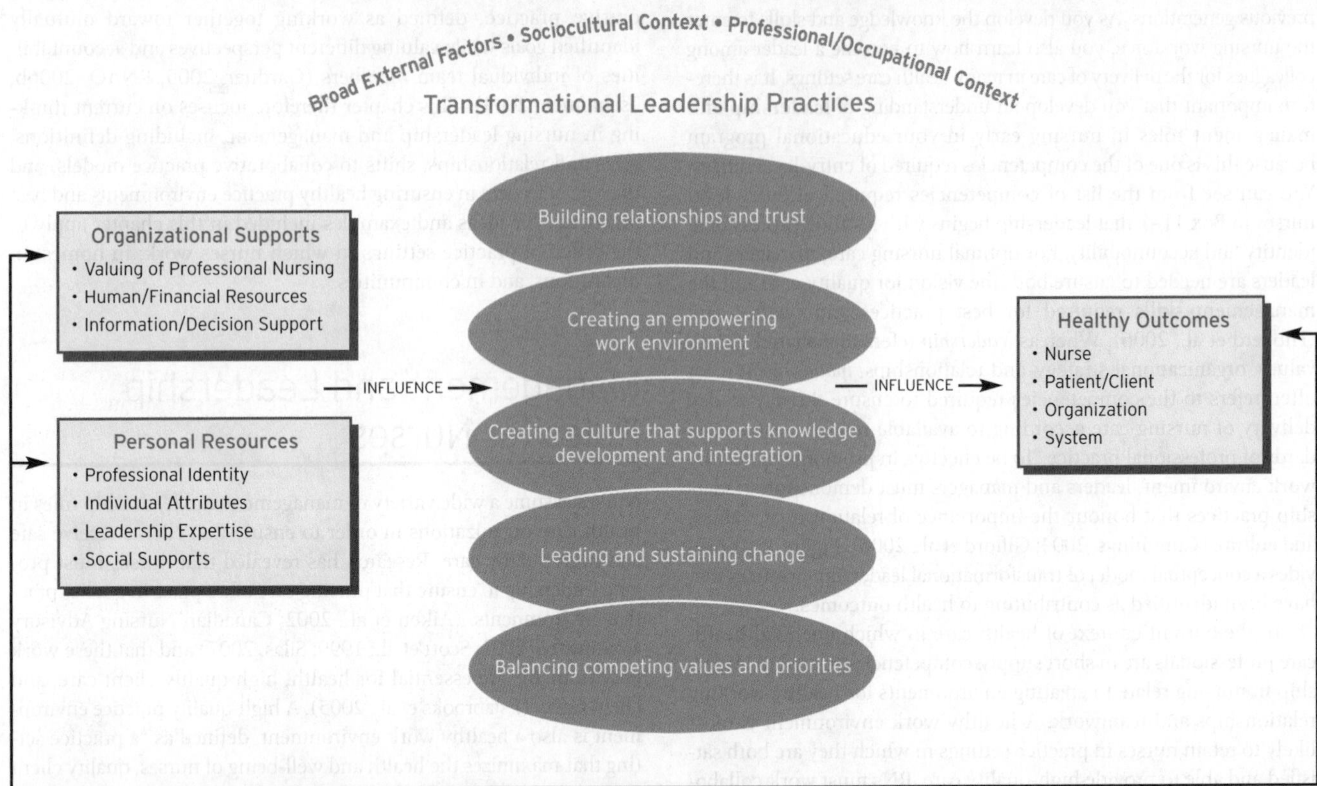

Figure 11-1 Conceptual model for developing and sustaining leadership. This model organizes and guides the discussion of the Registered Nurses Association of Ontario (RNAO) recommendations. It provides a framework for understanding the leadership practices needed to achieve healthy work environments and the organizational supports and personal resources that enable effective leadership practices. **Source:** From Registered Nurses Association of Ontario. (2006a). *Healthy work environments best practices guidelines: Developing and sustaining nursing leadership* (p. 22). Toronto, ON: Author.

BOX 11-2 Milestones in Canadian Nursing History

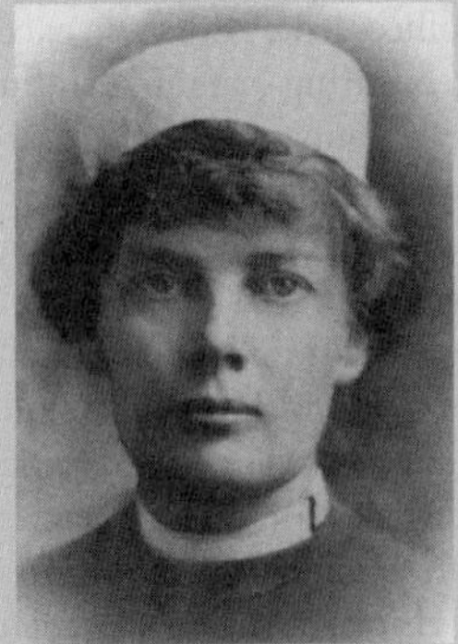

Ethel Johns, 1879–1968

A 1902 graduate of the Winnipeg General Hospital School of Nursing, Ethel Johns served as head nurse of several units at this hospital before becoming the first staff nurse to oversee its X-ray department. In 1907, she assumed editorship of its *Nurses Alumnae Journal* and began contributing to *Canadian Nurse.* Her literary talent, combined with her ability to challenge nurses to think independently, led to her nomination for membership in the Canadian Women's Press Club in 1911.

In 1913, Johns took a position as head surgical nurse at Good Samaritan Hospital in Los Angeles. After returning to Manitoba in 1915, she assumed the post of superintendent of the Children's Hospital of Winnipeg. She also worked tirelessly for the registration of nurses in Manitoba.

Johns held strong convictions about social issues and nursing, and she supported needed reforms. During the Winnipeg General Strike of 1919, her pro-labour views led her into conflict with the Children's Hospital board of directors, and she resigned.

Subsequently, Johns was appointed director of the Department of Nursing at the University of British Columbia, which offered the first Canadian university degree program in nursing. In 1929, she became director of nursing studies at New York Hospital–Cornell Medical College. She also worked on a landmark study of nursing education in the United States.

In 1933, Johns became editor of *Canadian Nurse,* which enabled her to communicate with a wide audience of nurses. Dr. Rae Chittick, president of the CNA during Johns's tenure as editor, praised Johns for bringing to the position "a world perspective on nursing, a hospitality of the mind from her rich experience . . . . She . . . reached out to challenge nurses to think for themselves and to create a body of nursing opinion on the changes essential to meet the health needs of a rapidly expanding nation." In 1947, Johns helped establish a new journal, *Just Plain Nursing,* which continued publication for the next 13 years. Also in 1947, Johns Hopkins Hospital asked her to write a history of its School of Nursing; this history was published in 1953. Later, she published the *Winnipeg General Hospital School of Nursing, 1887–1953.*

The CNA awarded Johns the Mary Agnes Snively Memorial Medal in 1940 and an honorary life membership in 1958 in recognition of her leadership in Canadian nursing.

Based on Street, M. M. (1973). *Watch-fires on the mountains: The life and writing of Ethel Johns.* Toronto, ON: University of Toronto Press.

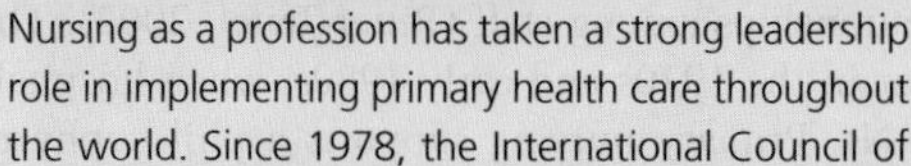

BOX 11-3 FOCUS ON PRIMARY HEALTH CARE

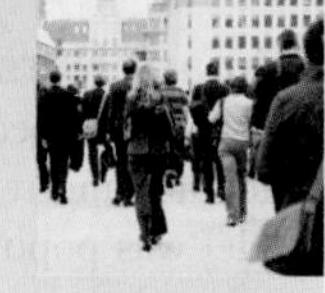

Nursing Leadership in Primary Health Care

Nursing as a profession has taken a strong leadership role in implementing primary health care throughout the world. Since 1978, the International Council of Nurses, the CNA, and other national, provincial, and territorial nursing associations have been instrumental in lobbying for inclusion of primary health care principles and programs in health care professional education, in service planning and delivery, and in research and evaluation. The CNA actively promotes initiatives to incorporate primary health care into nursing practice and policy. Primary health care principles enshrined in policy is the way to promote health for all people and is based on social justice model and values (Ogilvie & Reutter, 2003). Nursing advocacy for primary health care as the foundation of health care is required of leaders at all levels of practice and organizations.

Nurses continue to have a leadership role in primary health care. As Kaaren Neufeld, the president of the CNA, stated in an open letter in September 2008, "Nurses are leaders working to advance health for everyone. We are also system thinkers, advocating for an improved, publicly funded, not-for-profit system for all Canadians. . . . CNA believes that because nurses experience and participate in health system renewal every day, we have facts and insights that are relevant to the policy decisions that shape Canada's health system. We are well placed to give voice to the ideas and innovations that can improve health services or prevent illness in the first place."

Nurses provide primary health care at all levels and maintain links between individuals, families, communities, and the rest of the health care system. Working with other members of the health care team and other sectors or on their own, nurses explore new and better ways of staying well, improving health, and preventing disease and disability. Nurses improve equity and access to health care and add quality to the outcome of care.

From Canadian Nurses Association. (2003). *International Council of Nurses position statement: Nurses and primary health care; annual report*. Retrieved September 5, 2004, from http://www.icn.ch/psprimarycare.htm. Reprinted with permission from the Canadian Nurses Association.

environment, the role and responsibility of every nurse is to be a leader (CNA, 2002), displaying attributes such as articulating a vision, enabling others to act, encouraging others, and taking initiative. The leader and nursing staff must share a philosophy of care that integrates purpose, best practices, and concern for relationships, including how staff will work together and with clients and families (Box 11–4).

Nursing Care Delivery Models, Collaborative Practice, and Nursing Teams

Integral to the philosophy of care is the selection of a nursing care delivery model and a management structure that support professional nursing practice. Ideally, the vision for client care should drive the selection of a care delivery model (RNAO, 2006a). However, scarcity of resources and business initiatives from the health care organization influence this selection (Smith et al., 2006). The care delivery model must help nurses achieve desirable client outcomes. Key factors contributing to success are strong nursing leadership, decision-making authority for nurses who provide direct care, and effective respectful communications with colleagues, physicians, and other health care professionals (Canadian Nursing Advisory Committee, 2002; Canadian Patient Safety Institute, 2007; Hinshaw, 2008; Manojlovich et al., 2008).

Nursing care delivery models are designs that determine how nurses provide care. Historically, the choices of a nursing care delivery models have been influenced by the social and economic conditions, and this is the case today when care models are changing because of a shortage of nurses and other health care professionals (Manojlovich et al., 2008). **Continuity of care** is an extremely important concept in determining the choice of a nursing care delivery model. *Continuity of care* is defined as "a seamless continuous implementation of a plan of care that is reviewed and revised to meet the changing needs of the client" (RNAO, 2006b, p. 61). It refers to continuity of information or knowledge, continuity of relationships between a client and one or more health care professionals over time, and continuity of management of care across organizational boundaries (Smith et al., 2006). In the choice of nursing care delivery models, it is important to consider how nurses ensure that a client's plan of care is as consistent as possible. Functional, team, total client care and primary nursing, and case management models have been used. As change occurs in health care delivery and nursing practice, new care delivery models are evolving (Kimball et al., 2007). In the current context, a client care model known as the *collaborative practice model*, which includes nurses and others; it incorporates some of the features of earlier models.

Nursing care delivery models entail higher staff ratios of unregulated care providers (UCPs) in many settings of practice, including

BOX 11-4 Developing a Vision for a Nursing Unit

What Is the Nursing Unit's Purpose or Mission?

- Articulating why it exists
- Ensuring that nursing services are based on primary health care principles
- Knowing the background of health needs and perspectives of clients and population (internal and external)
- Knowing the background of its collaborative team members: their professional preparation, identity, and unique contributions
- Demonstrating how it accomplishes organizational goals or vision

How Will Staff Work With Clients and Families?

- By placing client's and family's needs first with a client-focused approach
- By involving clients and families as members of a collaborative practice team
- By making effective communication a priority

What Are the Standards of the Work Unit?

- Staff members adhere to professional accountability practice according to standards of practice and codes of ethics
- Staff members practise within a culture of safety
- The work unit integrates evidence-informed best practices
- Staff members work collaboratively with all members of the health care team

What Are the Key Values?

- Creating and maintaining a healthy practice environment
- Recognizing social justice issues
- Supporting relational practice
- Being self-aware, motivated, and accountable
- Supporting a learning environment

home care, institutional acute care, and residential long-term care, than do other models. The title of the UCP typifies the role of providing front-line personal and delegated care to increasing numbers of clients across different health care settings in Canada. UCP practice is not defined by qualifications or established standards. The title of the role differs from province to province, as does its requirement for training or educational programs. In British Columbia, for example, UCPs are referred to as *home support/resident care attendants* (HSRCAs), and they are required to take a preparatory six-month certification program offered in public and private post-secondary educational institutions. This is not the case in all provinces; for example, in Alberta, UCPs are not required to have educational prepartion, and they are referred to as *patient care attendants* (PCAs).

Functional Nursing. **Functional nursing** became popular during World War II in response to a nursing shortage. This model is task focused, not client focused. Tasks are divided; for example, one nurse may assume responsibility for hygiene and dressing changes, and another nurse may assume responsibility for medication administration. A lead nurse on a shift assigns tasks to staff members according to their qualifications, their abilities, and the tasks required. Nurses become highly competent with tasks that they perform repeatedly. The disadvantages of functional nursing are problems with continuity of care, absence of a holistic view of clients, and the possibility that care will become mechanical (Dadich, 2003). A task-focused approach does not ensure that clients' needs are met from shift to shift. Communication is not always clear, because one nurse is not responsible for the overall care of the client. The task-focused approach and ineffective communication lead to fragmented care and client dissatisfaction (Dadich, 2003).

Team Nursing. **Team nursing** developed in response to the nursing shortage after World War II (Marriner Tomey, 2004). It involves the delivery of nursing care by various staff members. An RN leads a team of other RNs, registered psychiatric nurses (RPNs), licensed practical nurses (LPNs), UCPs, or a combination of these professionals. The team leader, an experienced RN, develops client care plans, coordinates care delivered by the nursing team, and provides care that requires complex nursing skills. The team leader also performs problem solving with physicians and members of other disciplines and assists the team in evaluating the effectiveness of their care (Wywialowski, 2004). One of the limitations of the model is that the team leader does not spend a large amount of time with clients. Depending on the mix of staff members, this sometimes means that clients interact with any RN infrequently. Risks exist if an RN is unable to make necessary client assessments and cannot be involved in important clinical decision making. The task orientation of the model and the fact that nurses do not always interact with the same clients each day can result in a lack of continuity of care. An advantage of team nursing is the collaborative style that encourages each member of the team to help the other members. This model has a high level of autonomy for the team leader and is an example of decision making at a clinical level (Marriner Tomey, 2004).

Total Client Care. **Total client care** delivery was the original care model developed in the nineteenth century, during Florence Nightingale's time. It became popular in the 1970s and 1980s, when the numbers of RNs were increasing. In this model, an RN is responsible for all aspects of care for one or more clients. The RN may assign or delegate aspects of care to an RPN, an LPN, or a UCP but remains accountable for care of all assigned clients. The nurse works directly with the client, family, physician, and health care team members. The model typically has a shift-based focus. The same nurse does not necessarily care for the same client over time. Continuity of care from shift to shift or day to day is compromised if staff members do not clearly communicate the client's needs to one another.

Primary Nursing. The **primary nursing** model aimed to place RNs at clients' bedsides and improve nursing accountability for client outcomes and relationships among staff (Ritter-Teitel, 2002). The model was popular in the 1970s and early 1980s, when hospitals employed more RNs. Primary nursing supports a philosophy of strong nurse–client relationships. An RN assumes responsibility for a caseload of clients (Smith et al., 2006). Typically, the RN selects the clients and cares for the same clients during their stay in the health care setting. The RN assesses clients' needs, develops care plans, and ensures that appropriate nursing care is delivered. Primary nursing maintains continuity of care across shifts, days, or visits. It can be applied in any health care setting. When a primary nurse is off duty, associate nurses, including RPNs, LPNs, or other RNs, follow the care plan. If differences in opinion occur, associate and primary nurses collaborate to redefine the plan as necessary. Although primary nursing requires more RNs, the model is not necessarily more costly than others. The strengths of this model may be realized in case management and the collaborative practice model.

Case Management. The **case management** model coordinates health care services and links them to clients and their families while streamlining costs and maintaining quality (Dadich, 2003). The term *case managers* has been criticized because clients and families are not "cases" to be managed (Smith et al., 2006). In view of the importance of language and discourse in denoting the values of care, the term *case management* may, in the future, more appropriately refer to care or service coordination, or another descriptive label may communicate the value of client-centredness. Case management, as it has evolved, is "a collaborative process which assesses, plans, implements, coordinates, monitors, and evaluates the options and services required to meet an individual's health needs, using communications and available resources to promote quality, cost-effective outcomes" (Case Management Society of America, 2008). Clinicians, as individuals or in teams, care for clients with specific conditions and associated care needs (e.g., clients with complex nursing and medical problems) and are usually held accountable for quality and cost management. Many case managers use critical pathways, or "care maps," which are multidisciplinary treatment plans for clients with specific case types (see Chapter 13). The plans help in the delivery of timely, coordinated care.

Roles of case managers vary across health care settings, including long-term care, home care, community mental health, and acute care institutions, and these professionals increasingly coordinate and integrate care across these settings. Roles and responsibilities of case managers across settings include those of clinical experts, advocates, educators, facilitators, negotiators, managers, and researchers (Smith et al., 2006).

Collaborative Practice Model. The collaborative practice model is increasingly used by **intraprofessional nursing teams** (teams whose members provide nursing care) and by other health care professionals who are members of the **interprofessional team.** A call for interprofessional team and collaborative practice development has been sounded across Canada because this model is viewed as the way to ensure that all professionals and providers can practice to the full potential of their role and competencies. Collaborative practice is therefore also the best way to ensure that health human resources are used most effectively during a time of shortage. It is important for students in nursing and other professional health care programs to learn the competencies associated with collaborative practice during their educational programs. As a student, you are an integral member of both nursing and interprofessional teams that cross health care settings, including acute care, mental health care, community and home care, and public and population health care (RNAO, 2006b). One of first and most important responsibilities is to learn about the roles and responsibilities of other team members. Central to the collaborative practice model are the client, family, and population as full participants in care or service delivery. Nurse leaders in the Vancouver Coastal Health Authority (2007) launched an important initiative to support the shift in thinking required for collaborative practice among teams of nurses and health care professionals and across disciplines. This initiative provides opportunities for RNs, LPNs, UCPs, and members of other health care professions to learn from each other and to understand and respect their different roles and responsibilities. It also provides educational sessions in which team members learn about the competencies necessary in collaborative practice on a day-to-day basis in the work setting.

The RNAO (2006b) developed evidence-informed **best practice guidelines** for collaborative practice. These guidelines show how teamwork and collaborative practice can be supported at individual, team, organizational, and system levels of nursing practice. These guidelines are comprehensive and indicate the need for transformational leadership to support a culture of teamwork and collaboration. Thus, a collaborative practice model potentially incorporates the best of other care delivery models, including team, primary, and case management models previously discussed. It is important for students and entry-level nurses to acquire competencies that promote collaboration among teams as identified in Box 11–5.

> **BOX 11-5 RNAO Best Practice Guideline: Nursing Collaborative Practice**
>
> Guideline 1.4: Nursing teams establish clear processes and structures that promote collaboration and teamwork that leads to quality work environments and outcomes for clients by
>
> - Establishing processes for conflict resolution and problem solving
> - Establishing processes to develop, achieve, and evaluate team performance
> - Developing systems and processes to recognize and reward success
> - Incorporating nonhierarchical, democratic working practices to validate all contributions from team members
> - Incorporating processes that support continuity of care with clients to enhance staff satisfaction, staff self-worth, and client satisfaction
> - Developing and implementing processes that clarify their understanding of the unique and shared aspects of roles within the teams
> - Ensuring that the composition of the team is adequate to achieve their goals and meet their responsibilities to the needs of the client population
> - Establishing processes for decision making for a variety of circumstances such as
>   - Emergencies
>   - Day-to-day functioning
>   - Long-term planning
>   - Policy development
>   - Care planning
>
> From Registered Nurses Association of Ontario. (2006b, November). *Healthy work environments best practices guidelines: Collaborative practice among nursing teams* (p. 33). Toronto: Author.

Nurses are well situated to provide leadership for collaborative practice in many health care settings. One example may be found in the home care setting, in which nurses work closely with UCPs, who provide a large amount of the continuous day-to-day care for clients who have been discharged from hospitals after undergoing surgery or who have chronic illnesses and disabilities. UCPs must have opportunities to meet and communicate regularly with the nurses and other professionals involved in the care of the clients, to ensure that they understand the client situation and receive support for the challenges they face in providing care. Nurses can also aid UCPs by providing education and other supports so that they are able to contribute to best practices in important areas such as safety, emotional support, and wound healing. In this way, UCPs are recognized and valued for their role, and the continuity of care to a single client or family is supported by UCPs, nurses, and other health care professionals. Nurses who are employed in long-term or residential care settings may also provide leadership for collaborative practice by ensuring opportunities for communication and learning among professionals involved in teams or systems of care.

Home care delivery also often includes social workers, physicians, nutritionists, physiotherapists, and other health care professionals, as well as nurses and UCPs. At the centre of the collaborative practice model is the client and family; research is just beginning into how health care professionals and other caregivers include clients as part of the team or the social network of care (Cott et al., 2008). A nurse in home care or another practice setting is well situated to provide leadership for collaborative practice by providing opportunities for clients and families to meet with caregivers and and by ensuring that the client's voice is heard in his or her care planning.

Decentralized Decision Making

One of the most important recommendations to achieve healthy practice environments is that staff at all levels be involved in decision making about nursing practice. Of equal importance is that the most senior nurse in the organization be included in the executive decision-making level of the organizations and agencies, including those responsible for the delivery of home care, mental health care, public health care, or hospital care. The nurse executive supports managers and staff by creating a management structure that helps achieve organizational goals and provides support for democratic decision making and collaborative practice models. With a vision for nursing established, the manager helps staff realize that vision.

Decentralized management, in which decision making occurs at the staff level, is common in health care organizations. The advantage of this structure is that managers and staff are actively involved in shaping an organization's identity and determining success. Decentralized management requires workers to be empowered to accept greater responsibility for the quality of client care (Ellis & Hartley, 2005). A decentralized structure has the best potential to lead to positive outcomes, such as increased collaboration among staff, best practice implementation, and client satisfaction (Table 11–1).

The nurse manager is crucial for the successful functioning of nursing units and systems. Figure 11–2 illustrates the responsibilities and competencies of nurse managers, including supervising, planning, scheduling and staffing, as situated within a framework of leadership competencies.

For decentralized decision making to work, managers must enable decision making by the professionals who are most involved and must encourage inclusion rather than exclusion of staff (RNs, RPNs, LPNs, UCPs, unit administrators, and secretaries). Key elements in organizational decision making are responsibility, autonomy, authority, and accountability (Anders & Hawkins, 2006). CNA (2003b) outlined principles and criteria for decentralized decision making (Box 11–6).

TABLE 11-1 Examples of Management Structures

Structural Approach	Characteristics
Centralized management	A single administrator leads the organization, and directors oversee departments or programs. Decisions are made by the leader and directors, with little staff input. Managers have minimal responsibility or accountability for operation of nursing unit. Staff do not feel involved in care processes, and collaborative practice is not supported.
Decentralized management	Structure may be similar to that of centralized management. Often, the number of directors is lower. Staff members with the most knowledge about an issue make decisions. Managers often have 24-hour accountability and responsibility for staff, budget, and day-to-day management of work unit.
Matrix	Traditional units are reorganized into business units. Staff may report to multiple managers—such as one with responsibility for professional practice (e.g., nursing) and another with responsibility for a specific program (e.g., child and family health)—who may be from a variety of professional practice backgrounds.

Responsibility refers to the duties and activities that an individual is employed to perform. A professional nurse's responsibilities in a given role are outlined in a position description of the nurse's duties in client care and of participation as a member of the nursing team. Managers must be sure that staff members understand their responsibilities, particularly during change. For example, when hospitals restructure and client care delivery models change, the manager must clearly define the nurse's role within the new care delivery model. If decentralized decision making is in place, professional staff can help shape the new nurse role. All nurses are responsible for knowing their role.

Autonomy is the freedom of choice and responsibility for choices (Marriner Tomey, 2004). With autonomy, a nurse can make independent decisions about client care according the role and scope of practice. Innovation by nurses, increased productivity, higher employer retention of nurses, and greater client satisfaction are results of autonomy in nursing practice (Canadian Nursing Advisory Committee, 2002; Estabrooks et al., 2005; Hicks, 2003).

Authority to act is the right to act in areas in which a nurse has been given and accepts responsibility according to legislation, standards, and the code of ethics governing the professional practice of nursing. Nurses have authority to act and to question actions concerning the practice of other professionals in relation to this scope of responsibility. For example, a nurse who as a case manager finds that the nursing team did not follow a discharge teaching plan for an assigned client has the authority to consult with other nurses to learn why the plan was not followed. The nurse as case manager has accepted responsibility for the care of a group of clients and therefore has the final authority in selecting the best course of action for the client's care, while collaborating with others to ensure quality outcomes.

Accountability means being answerable for one's actions. It means that as a nurse, you accept the commitment to provide excellent client care and the responsibility for the outcomes of actions in providing that care (Anders & Hawkins, 2006). A nurse is accountable for clients' outcomes. In the example just described, the nurse as case manager is accountable for the client's health outcomes by ensuring a continuity of care across hospitalization and home care.

A successful decentralized nursing unit exercises the four elements of decision making: responsibility, autonomy, authority, and accountability. The staff must meet routinely to discuss how to maintain an

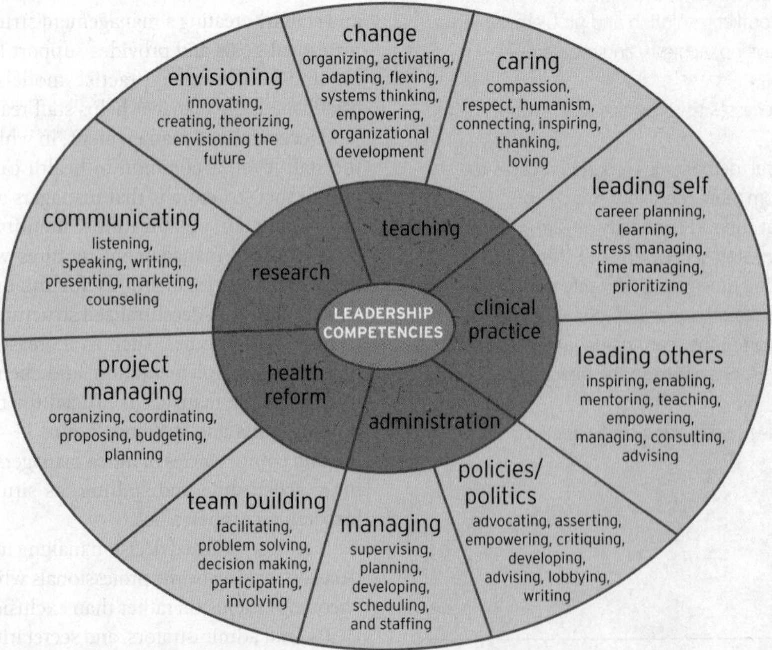

Figure 11-2 Management and leadership competencies. **Source:** From Canadian Nurses Association. (2005). *Nursing leadership development in Canada* (p. 28). Ottawa, ON: Author.

> **BOX 11-6 Principles of Decentralized Decision Making**
>
> - Decision making is based on having the appropriate number of positions and the competencies required to ensure safe, competent, and ethical care.
> - Nurse administrators and managers (including supervisors, middle managers, and senior managers) are responsible for ensuring the appropriate staff mix.
> - Legislative, professional, and organizational parameters are respected.
> - The safety of clients must never be compromised by substituting less qualified workers when the competencies of an RN are required.
> - The staffing decision-making process recognizes the unique and shared competencies of each health care professional group.
> - Responsibility and accountability of health care professionals are clear.
> - RNs at all levels in the organization are involved in decision making that affects nursing practice, client care, and the work environment.
> - Staffing decisions are evidence informed.
> - Organizations and other stakeholders, including RNs, ensure that the elements necessary for a high-quality professional practice environment are in place.
> - RNs are leaders in implementing collaborative practice and promoting effective communication among all members of the health care team.
>
> Adapted from Canadian Nurses Association. (2003b). *Staffing decisions for the delivery of safe nursing care—Position statement.* Ottawa, ON: Author.

equality and balance in these elements. Individuals should be comfortable in expressing differences in opinion and in challenging the status quo, while understanding their own responsibility, autonomy, authority, and accountability.

Supporting Staff Involvement. In decentralized decision-making structures, all staff members actively participate in unit or agency activities (Figure 11–3). Staff members benefit from the knowledge and skills of the entire team. If the staff members value knowledge and their colleagues' contributions, client care improves. The nursing manager supports staff involvement through the following approaches.

Establishment of Nursing Practice or Professional Shared Governance Councils. Chaired by senior clinical staff, these councils are empowered to maintain care standards for nursing practice (Gokenbach, 2007). The councils review and establish standards of care, develop policy and procedures, resolve client satisfaction issues, or develop new documentation tools. Mechanisms are established to empower all staff to contribute input on practice issues. Managers might not sit on the council, but they receive progress reports. The types of work in the nursing unit determines council membership. Professionals from other disciplines (e.g., pharmacy, respiratory therapy, social work, medicine, or clinical nutrition) might participate in these councils. Professional practice councils can advocate for resources and conditions necessary for healthy practice environments and safety.

Interprofessional Collaboration. As previously described, collaborative practice among professionals from different disciplines is essential to ensuring that health human resources are used in the best possible way. Whenever systems or programs are redesigned, interprofessional involvement is crucial because most health care processes involve more than one discipline (CNA, 2003a). Nurses must recognize the importance of prompt referrals and timely communication with other health care professionals. Inclusion of professionals from various disciplines in practice projects, in-service programs, conferences, and staff meetings fosters interprofessional collaboration.

Staff Communication. Communication with staff is one of the manager's greatest challenges, especially in a large work group in which change is constant. It is difficult to ensure that all staff members receive the correct messages. In the current health care environment, staff quickly become uneasy and distrusting if they fail to hear about planned changes in their work unit. A manager cannot be responsible for all communication but can use several approaches to communicate quickly and accurately with all staff: increasing presence on work units, circulating newsletters, posting minutes of committee meetings, and using list servers and e-mail. Of most importance is that staff members have the opportunity to meet and to discuss issues pertinent to their role and ability to provide care. Professional councils must be valued and invited to provide advice on emerging issues.

Developing a Learning Organization. Nurses must continually update their knowledge and incorporate best practices that are evidence informed (Cullum et al., 2008). Leaders and managers are challenged to develop the conditions for learning to flourish in what has been described as a *learning organization* (Senge, 2006). In learning organizations, many forms of knowledge are shared. Leadership strategies are needed to help nurses incorporate evidence-informed best practice guidelines into their nursing practice. These strategies include "support, role modelling commitment to best practices and reinforcing organizational policies and goals consistent with evidence based care" (Gifford et al., 2006, p. 73).

Leadership Skills for Nursing Students

Nursing students prepare for leadership roles. This does not mean you must quickly learn how to lead a nursing team; rather, you first learn to become an accountable and competent health care professional. Leadership development is ongoing throughout a career, and individual leadership styles are influenced from a variety of sources including theories, best practices, mentors, role models, and experiences. You learn leadership by making good clinical decisions, advocating for public health and quality care, learning from mistakes, seeking guidance, engaging in collaborative practice with nursing teams and other professionals, seeking mentors, and striving to improve during each client interaction. Your nursing education program provides you with the opportunity to develop leadership competencies: advocacy, conflict management, collaborative practice, client centredness, delegation, and evidence-informed decision making.

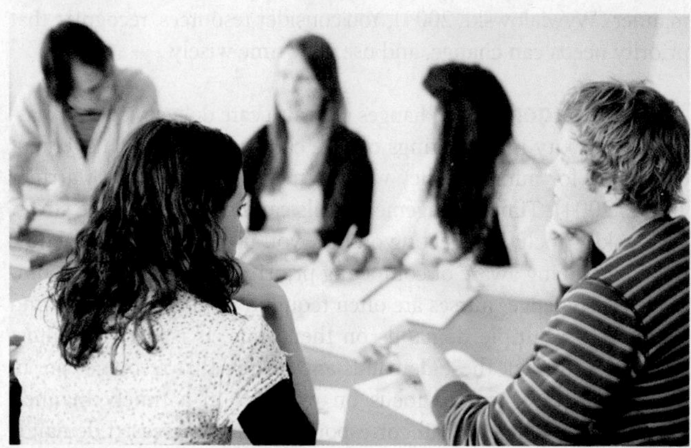

Figure 11-3 Students in nursing and other health care professional programs learning about their roles and contributions to collaborative practice. **Source:** © René Mansi, iStockPhoto.

Clinical Care Coordination

As a nursing student, you develop the skills necessary to ensure timely and effective client care. At first, you may have only one client, but eventually you will coordinate the care of groups of clients. Clinical care coordination includes decision making, priority setting, use of organizational skills and resources, time management, and evaluation.

Clinical Decisions. Leadership and decision-making skills are required as the nurse engages in the complex interactions—collaboration, negotiation, conflict resolution, and delegation—necessary to elicit the involvement of other people. You learn to value and practice client centredness in every interaction. You will adopt a critical thinking approach, applying understanding of clients' perspectives, your knowledge, evidence-informed best practice guidelines, and experience to the decision-making process (see Chapter 12).

Priority Setting. You must establish priorities of care as they relate to actions taken to meet clients' needs. This is particularly important in caring for groups of clients with health challenges involving immediate needs and actions to be taken. Hendry and Walker (2004) classified client problems in three priority levels on the basis of the time frame in which you must act:

- *High (first-order) priority:* An immediate threat to a client's survival or safety, such as a physiological episode of obstructed airway, loss of consciousness, injury, or an anxiety attack.
- *Intermediate (second-order) priority:* Nonemergency, non–life-threatening actual or potential needs that the client and family members are experiencing, such as anticipating teaching needs of clients with regard to a new drug, wound care, or measures to decrease falls among older adults.
- *Low (third-order) priority:* Actual or potential problems that may or may not be directly related to the acute phase of the client's health challenge. This means that they are not as time sensitive; however, they should be viewed as important to the health outcomes over the slightly longer term. Examples include promoting family members' understanding of a diabetic diet or other aspects of chronic illness management.

Many clients can have all three types of priorities, which requires you to use careful judgement in choosing a course of action. First-order priority needs require your immediate attention and, most often, immediate assistance in meeting these needs. Setting priorities also requires that you know the priority needs of each client, assessing each client's needs as soon as possible, including the client and family determination of priorities, and addressing needs in a timely manner (Wywialowski, 2004). You consider resources, recognize that priority needs can change, and use your time wisely.

Time Management. Changes in health care delivery and increasing complexity in all settings of care can create time management challenges for nurses as they work to meet clients' needs (Marriner Tomey, 2004). Time management skills can help you manage stress. These skills include reflecting on how you use time, planning effectively, and being aware of competing priorities. Because of the complexity of practice, nurses are often required to juggle priorities and respond to multiple demands on their time. It is therefore most important to track these demands and ensure that resources are in place that allow you to focus on priorites in a timely manner. Technology such as e-mail correspondence has increased demands on nurses' time, which often require immediate responses to issues. It is therefore important for you to to realize and reflect on the impact of technology and other forces and to acquire the ability to set limits and refuse demands that are unreasonable.

Evaluation. Evaluation is one of the most important aspects of clinical care coordination. Evaluation is an ongoing process that provides focus and direction for each phase of nursing care. Once you begin to provide care, you should also learn to immediately evaluate its effectiveness and the client's response. In the evaluation process, you compare expected client outcomes with actual outcomes. For example, a clinic nurse assesses a diabetic client's foot ulcer to determine whether healing is progressing and expected outcomes are met. Evaluation reveals the need to revise approaches to care and introduce new therapies. Focusing on evaluation of a client's progress and outcomes, rather than on tasks, lessens the chance of distraction. You learn to keep the client at the centre of the care by asking the client for his or her ideas and evaluation of how he or she is experiencing the care plan.

Delegation. Changes in staff mix have resulted in more UCPs delivering care to clients (CNA, 2005b; McGillis Hall, 2004). In the new working environment, a nurse must understand the evolving role of nursing and delegated care responsibilities in order to ensure the safety and quality of nursing care delivery. **Delegation** refers to the transferring of responsibility for the performance of an activity or task while retaining accountability for the outcome (College of Registered Nurses of British Columbia, 2005). Delegated tasks are those that are outside of the role description of the UCP. As a student, you will work with teams of nurses and UCPs during your practica in many health care settings, including home care, residential care, community health care, and acute care settings. As you develop in your role, it is important to learn about the roles and scopes of practice of UCPs in different practice settings. You will learn about how your role relates to that of the UCP and how the principles of delegation are applied in practice. Students and nurses also have access to valuable resources such as nursing practice consultants and practice guidelines to assist them in making complex decisions about delegation. The nurse may also assume responsibility for the education, supervision, and support of UCPs as they perform delegated nursing activities (Box 11–7).

Provincial regulations define the scope of an RN's practice, including activities that only RNs can perform (e.g., client assessment and planning care). Although most provinces identify the delegation and supervision of work as an RN's responsibility, each province addresses the specifics of delegation differently. In Ontario, British Columbia, and Alberta, for example, legislation that applies to all regulated health care professions identifies specific tasks or activities that can be performed by only certain professions. In British Columbia, these authorized tasks are known as *reserved acts;* in Ontario, they are called *controlled acts;* and in Alberta, they are known as *restricted activities.* UCPs are not allowed to perform actions authorized for RNs unless those actions have been properly delegated by an RN and only if they are within the UCP's job description and employer policy (Sorrentino, 2004).

An institution's policies, procedures, and job descriptions for UCPs provide specific guidelines regarding which tasks or activities can be delegated. The job description should specify any required education and the types of tasks UCPs can perform, either independently or under an RN's direct supervision. Institutional policy helps in defining the amount of training required of UCPs while they are employed. Procedures specify who is qualified to perform a given nursing procedure, whether supervision is necessary, and the type of reporting required. Job descriptions, policies, and procedures should comply with provincial laws and regulations. Nurses should have a means of accessing policies easily or have supervisory staff who can inform them about the UCP's job duties.

Effective delegation requires trust between the RN and UCPs. It also requires constant communication: sending clear messages and

> **BOX 11-7 The Five Rights of Delegation**
>
> **Right Task**
>
> The right task is one that can be delegated for a specific client, such as tasks that are repetitive, require little supervision, and are relatively non-invasive (bathing, toileting, feeding, some oral medication administration, positioning, and assisting with mobility).
>
> **Right Circumstances**
>
> The appropriate client setting, available resources, and other relevant factors are considered. In an acute care setting, clients' conditions can change quickly. Good clinical decision making is needed to determine what to delegate.
>
> **Right Person**
>
> The right person (e.g., the nurse) is delegating the right tasks to the right person (e.g., the UCP) to be performed on the right person (the correct client).
>
> **Right Direction or Communication**
>
> A clear, concise description of the task, including its objective, limits, and expectations, is given. Communication must be ongoing between RN and UCPs during a shift of care.
>
> **Right Supervision**
>
> Appropriate monitoring, evaluation, intervention as needed, and feedback are provided. UCPs should feel comfortable asking questions and seeking assistance.
>
> Modified from National Council of State Boards of Nursing. (1995). *Delegation: Concepts and decision-making process.* Chicago, IL: Author; National Council of State Boards of Nursing. (1997). *The five rights of delegation.* Chicago, IL: Author; and American Nurses Association (ANA) and National Council State Boards of Nursing. (2006). *Joint statement on delegation.* Retrieved April, 2008, from http://www.ncsbn.org/pdfs/joint_statement.pdf.

listening so that all participants understand expectations regarding client care. An RN should provide clear instructions when delegating tasks. These instructions may initially focus on the procedure itself, as well as on the unique needs of the client. As the RN becomes more familiar with a staff member's scope of practice, trust builds and fewer instructions may be needed, but clarification of clients' specific needs is always necessary.

A key step in delegation is evaluation of the staff member's performance and the client's outcomes. When UCPs do a good job, it is important to provide praise and recognition. If the staff member's performance is unsatisfactory, the RN must give constructive feedback, specifically discussing mistakes and how they could have been avoided. Giving feedback in private in a professional manner preserves the staff member's dignity. A UCP may fail to meet expectations because of inadequate training or assignment of too many tasks. The RN may need to review or demonstrate a procedure with staff or schedule additional training with the education department. The delegation of too many tasks might be a nursing practice issue. All staff should discuss delegation on their unit because UCPs may need help in learning how to prioritize and RNs may need to ensure that they are not overdelegating.

A few tips for nurses on appropriate delegation (College of Registered Nurses of British Columbia, 2006; Keeling et al., 2000) are as follows:

- *Assess the knowledge and skills of the delegate.* Nurses should determine what the UCP knows and what he or she can do by asking open-ended questions that will elicit conversation and details; for example, "Can you tell me what you would observe in Mr. S when you visit him today that would alert you to call me immediately?"
- *Match tasks to the delegate's skills.* Nurses need to know what skills are included in the UCP training program at their facility and to determine whether personnel have learned critical thinking skills, such as knowing the difference between normal clinical findings and changes to report.
- *Communicate clearly.* Nurses should provide unambiguous directions by describing a task, the desired outcome, and the time period for completion of the task. Rather than giving instructions through another staff member, nurses should make the delegate feel part of the team. For example, "I'd like you to help me by getting Mr. Floyd up to ambulate before lunch. Be sure to check his blood pressure before he stands and write your finding on the graphic sheet. OK?"
- *Listen attentively.* Nurses should listen to the UCP's responses as they give directions. Is the UCP comfortable asking questions or requesting clarification? Nurses need to be especially attentive if the UCP has a deadline assigned by another nurse and to help sort out priorities.
- *Provide feedback.* Nurses should give feedback about performance, regardless of outcome. They must tell the person about a job well done or, if an outcome is undesirable, find a private place to discuss what occurred, any miscommunication, and how to achieve a better outcome in the future.

Quality Care and Client Safety

As discussed throughout this chapter, safe and high-quality care is delivered when leadership, staffing models, and collaborative practice are in place to support it. Studies reveal that high-quality practice environments produce better client outcomes and more satisfied clients and staff (Aiken et al., 2001, 2002; CNA, 2005b; Tourangeau et al., 2002). Initiatives such as the College of Nurses of Ontario's (2004) *Quality Assurance Practice Consultation Program* and the Registered Nurses Association of British Columbia's (2003) *Quality Practice Environment Program* assess organizational attributes that enhance practice. The assessment is voluntary, but response by health care agencies is encouraging.

Organizational programs such as total quality management (TQM) and **continuous quality improvement (CQI)** were developed to encourage staff to reflect on how to improve work. In quality management, the client's or customer's definition of quality is recognized (Wendt & Vale, 2003). Most organizations have moved away from programs identified as TQM or CQI and focus instead on the more generic and pervasive concept of **quality improvement** (QI), defined by the Canadian Council on Health Services Accreditation (2003) as "an organizational philosophy that seeks to meet clients' needs and exceed their expectations by using a structured process that selectively identifies and improves all aspects of service" (p. 1). This council describes quality as responsiveness, system competency, client or community focus, and work life. QI focuses on improving organizational performance related to processes.

Quality in Nursing Practice

Quality Defined. Standards or guidelines define the meaning of quality. For example, to judge whether rehabilitation has been delayed, a standard of when rehabilitation should begin must exist. Quality of care in nursing practice is not arbitrarily defined. A definition of quality begins with the mission, vision, philosophy, and values of the nursing department. These statements define how all nurses within an organization are to perform and which services must be provided. Written values give direction for professional standards and care guidelines that lead to positive client outcomes.

Professional Standards. Professional standards are authoritative statements used by the profession in describing the responsibilities for which its practitioners are accountable (Peters, 1995). They include the policies and position descriptions that identify performance expectations within an organization. Standards are an organization's interpretation of the professional's competency. The adherence to professional standards is measured through professional outcomes.

Care and Best Practice Guidelines. Care guidelines encompass best practice guidelines, which are statements to assist in providing care according to the best evidence available (RNAO, 2003). Guidelines can be developed by single disciplines or can be multidisciplinary in focus. Examples of nursing practice guidelines are found on the RNAO Web site encompassing some of the examples referred to in this chapter, including wound care and prevention of falls. The effectiveness of nursing practice is measured through client outcomes and and the accumulation of evidence (Graham & Harrison, 2008).

Nurse-Sensitive Outcomes. Outcomes are conditions to be achieved as a result of care. It is important that the outcomes selected to measure the effectiveness of nursing care are related to the work that nurses do. A **nurse-sensitive outcome** reveals whether interventions are effective, whether clients progress, how well standards are being met, and whether changes are necessary. Examples of outcomes related to the implementation of best practice guidelines may include incidence of pressure sores, falls in elderly clients, and hypertension control measures.

To judge whether standards of care are met, processes and outcomes are measured. For example, a staff measures its success in implementing a new process of diabetes instruction and also measures the outcome: Can clients administer insulin correctly? When selecting quality indicators, teams should consider processes and related outcomes that are most likely to improve nursing practice. Processes to improve may include the following:

- A weak process that is causing problems (e.g., poor pain management for clients with cancer who are at home).
- A stable process that is adequate but can improve (e.g., access to education and support for people with diabetes in rural communities).
- A process linked to negative outcomes (e.g., care of intravenous access sites with the occurrence of phlebitis).

Building a Culture of Safety

Client safety has been recognized as a crucial component of health care delivery. The Canadian Patient Safety Institute (2007) defined client safety as "the reduction and mitigation of unsafe acts within the health care system, as well as through the use of best practices shown to lead to optimal patient safety." Issues such as staff shortages, new technology, and other demands on health care systems have prompted a re-examination of how errors and adverse events for clients can be prevented. Increasingly, the emphasis is on enabling health care professionals and providers to communicate effectively and to acknowledge and receive timely assistance for errors. This assistance includes the education of nursing and other health care professional students to view mistakes as learning, to know and prevent conditions that lead to unsafe practices, and to develop the **competencies for safe practice** (Canadian Association of Schools of Nursing, 2006; Davidson Dick et al., 2006). The Canadian Patient Safety Institute (2007) identified seven core domains of abilities for all health care professionals, including their contributions to developing a culture of client safety as a most important foundation (Box 11–8).

Coming Full Circle: Leadership for a High-Quality Work Life and High-Quality Health Care. Leaders and managers at all levels of health care organizations must do what they can to improve the quality of work life in health care in order to ensure client safety and quality health care; evidence and awareness of this need are growing. A forward thinking and exciting partnership of 10 leading health care organizations in Canada, including the CNA and the Canadian Council on Health Services Accreditation (now known as "Accreditation Canada"), have formed the Quality Worklife–Quality Healthcare Collaborative (QWQHC) with the mandate and a guiding conceptual framework to "improve the health of health workplaces." The foundational belief of the QWQHC is that "A fundamental way to better healthcare is through healthier health care workplaces; it is unaccceptable to work in, receive care in, govern, manage and fund unhealthy workplaces" (QWQHC, n.d.).

Transformational leadership, including the concepts and competencies discussed in this chapter, is needed to shift the current culture of health care to achieve the vision of health care professionals delivering high-quality health care, adopted by the collaborative. This means that nurses and other professionals working directly with clients and the midlevel managers have key roles to play in leading change. They must be inspired and supported through mentoring and by the implementation of leadership best practices guidelines and collaborative practice. Senior leaders must ensure adequate staffing and support for the culture of a healthy workplace. The way forward is to inspire lifelong learning at all levels of the organization and provide access and resources to education that enables staff to work with the client and the client's family at the centre of health care delivery and decision making.

Nurses working at all levels of organizations can contribute by making a commitment to this vision and being part of the change that is required to transform Canadian health care. Indeed, the CNA in its centenary year inspires the theme of leadership for a transformed

> **BOX 11-8 The Safety Competencies**
>
> **Domain 1: "Creating a Culture of Patient Safety" (http://www.patientsafetyinstitute.ca/education/safetycompetencies.html)**
>
> Health care professionals must be enabled to contribute to health care organizations, large or small, in ways that promote client safety in their structure and function. Content in this domain could include but is not limited to the following aspects:
>
> - Understanding of client safety concepts, epidemiology, and basic theories
> - Awareness of health care error
> - Promotion of a systems approach to care and safety
> - Promotion of staff empowerment to resolve unsafe situations
> - Role modelling and demonstration of a commitment to leadership in safe practice
> - Ensuring feedback on safety issues
> - Integration of safe practices into daily activities
> - Commitment to communication, teamwork, and quality
> - Reporting of adverse events
> - Commitment to a just, nonpunitive culture

Canadian health care system and calls for Canadian Nurses to "be the change" required to sustain quality health care for all. As a student and as as a qualified nurse, you have the opportunity and the challenge to effect positive change in nursing practice and Canadian health care (Box 11–9).

BOX 11-9 NURSING STORY

Leadership for Best Practices in Falls Prevention

Kaley Hart is a recently graduated RN working in a residential care facility. Ann Best, the nurse manager of the facility, is aware of Kaley's interest in leadership for best practices. As a fourth-year student, Kaley had completed a special project on falls prevention in the facility, using local statistics on falls and evidence-informed practice guidelines. Ann wishes to enroll the long-term care facility in the *National Collaborative on Falls in Long-Term Care* (RNAO, 2007a). This program requires the commitment of an improvement team consisting of five to seven staff members. Ann's vision is that the improvement team would be supported by the educational and research resources of this national program and by access to national experts in falls prevention. She sees this as an excellent opportunity for Kaley to be involved and to continue to develop her leadership skills in the areas of collaborative practice and best practices implementation.

At Ann's invitation, Kaley becomes involved with the quality improvement team, which also includes a nurse researcher from the university. Kaley begins her work by inspiring other nurses to become involved with the initiative, and she advocates for UCPs and other professionals to become members of the team in order to achieve a broad perspective on the changes required to prevent falls. She refers to the Canadian statistic that 50% of elderly residents in nursing homes fall every year (RNAO, 2007a), which results in a negative impact on their quality of life and increased costs to the health care system. Kaley inspires a vision of changes to be made in the interest of preventing falls and achieving the best possible health outcomes for the residents in the facility. She advocates for residents' and their families' involvement in the initiative and seeks input from all clients and professionals as to how the learning sessions should take place, in order to promote engagement as a learning community.

As a member of the team, Kaley contributes her knowledge of the RNAO (2007b) *Falls Prevention* Best Practices Guidelines and helps develop a practical approach to identifying residents who are at risk for falls. Drawing on her knowledge of collaborative practice, Kaley ensures that other team members, including the physiotherapist, UCP, recreation therapist, nutritionist, and housekeeping manager, are able to contribute their experiences and ideas about risk management and participate in the learning sessions. Kaley takes the opportunity to praise the contributions of diverse team members and to facilitate input and participation from the residents.

An evaluation of the quality improvement team reveals high levels of participation and interest within the facility. The experience of being involved in a national initiative has contributed to the capacity for best practices implementation and evidence-informed practice. Kaley has been inspired by the experience and has further developed her management and leadership competencies in the areas of inspiring a vision, leading change, facilitating collaborative practice, and developing respectful and supportive relationships among team members. She has worked with the nurse researcher at the local university to develop the plan for studying the impact of the changes on the incidence of falls, over time. Of most importance is that Kaley looks forward to the next opportunity to make a difference in the health outcomes of the residents through the exercise of progressive management and leadership initiatives.

* KEY CONCEPTS

- A leader must set a vision or philosophy for a work unit, ensure appropriate staffing, mobilize staff and institutional resources to achieve objectives, motivate staff members to carry out their work, set standards of performance, and make the right decisions to achieve objectives.
- Management and leadership are related processes; both are essential to nursing practice and health care delivery.
- Healthy practice environments are key to quality nurse and client care outcomes.
- Leadership plays a key role in ensuring healthy practice environments.
- An empowered nursing staff has decision-making authority to change how they practise.
- Nursing care delivery models vary by the responsibility of the RN in coordinating care delivery and the roles other staff members play in assisting with care.
- Continuity of nursing care can be compromised in total client care delivery, functional nursing practice, and team nursing.
- Best practice guidelines are evidence informed and contain recommendations for developing and sustaining collaborative practice models and leadership.
- For decentralized decision making to succeed, staff members must be aware that they have the responsibility, authority, autonomy, and accountability for the care they give and the decisions they make.
- A nurse manager can foster decentralized decision making by establishing nursing practice committees, supporting collaborative practice, implementing quality improvement plans, and maintaining timely staff communication.
- Clinical care coordination involves accurate clinical decision making, establishing priorities, efficient organizational skills, appropriate use of resources and time management skills, and an ongoing evaluation of care activities.
- To promote an enriching professional environment, each member of a nursing work team is responsible for open, professional communication.
- Delegation involves transferring responsibility for performing an activity while retaining accountability for the outcome.
- When accomplished correctly, delegation can improve job efficiency and job enrichment.
- An important responsibility for the nurse who delegates nursing care is evaluation of the staff member's performance and client outcomes.
- In a quality improvement-oriented environment, every staff member becomes involved in finding ways to improve or change work processes so as to promote client safety and quality care outcomes.
- The QWQHC was developed to transform Canadian health care delivery systems.

* CRITICAL THINKING EXERCISES

1. John, an RN, is working with Tammy, a UCP, to manage care for five clients. John has completed morning assessments and rounds on the assigned clients and is giving Tammy directions for what she needs to do in the next hour. John says to Tammy, "Why don't you go to Room 415 and see what Mr. Thomas needs, and go to Room 418 to check if Mrs. Landry is doing all right." Based on what you know about delegation, were these appropriate or inappropriate delegations to Tammy? Provide a rationale for your answer.

2. You are a recently graduated RN working in a home care setting. The manager of the nursing program asks you to assist with the implementation of a collaborative practice model. She asks you to help her set the agenda for the first meeting to discuss the concept and principles of collaborative practice. What ideas and resources would you contribute to the agenda?
3. You have just received morning shift reports on your clients. You have been assigned the following clients:
   - A 52-year-old man who was admitted yesterday with a diagnosis of angina. He is scheduled for a cardiac stress test at 0900.
   - A 60-year-old woman who was transferred out of intensive care at 0630 today. She underwent uncomplicated coronary bypass surgery yesterday.
   - A 45-year-old man who experienced a myocardial infarction three days ago and is complaining of chest pain, which he rates as 5 on a scale of 0 to 10.
   - A 76-year-old woman who had a permanent pacemaker inserted yesterday and is complaining of incision pain, which she rates as 7 on a scale of 0 to 10.

   Which one of these clients do you need to see first? Explain your answer.

* REVIEW QUESTIONS

1. The nursing model of client care in which specific tasks are divided (e.g., one nurse assumes responsibility for hygiene and dressing changes, and another nurse assumes responsibility for medication administration) is
   1. Team nursing
   2. Total client care
   3. Functional nursing
   4. Primary nursing
2. Collaborative practice models aim to
   1. Improve delegation between staff
   2. Improve communication between staff
   3. Place the client at the centre of care delivery
   4. Ensure that health care professionals can cover for one another
3. The type of care management approach that coordinates and links health care services to clients and their families while streamlining costs and maintaining quality is
   1. Case management
   2. Total client care
   3. Functional nursing
   4. Primary nursing
4. The type of management structure that has a potential for greater collaborative effort, increased competency of staff, and ultimately a greater sense of professional accomplishment and satisfaction is
   1. Case management
   2. Primary nursing
   3. Total client care
   4. Decentralized
5. While administering medications, the nurse realizes she has given the wrong dose of medication to a client. The nurse acts by completing an incident report and notifying the client's physician. The nurse is exercising
   1. Authority
   2. Responsibility
   3. Accountability
   4. Decision making
6. A manager who wishes to improve client safety in the health care organization should focus on
   1. Problem-solving committees
   2. Staffing models and ratios
   3. Systems for reporting mistakes
   4. Staff communication
7. A home care nurse is working with three UCPs who were recently hired and are new to their roles. For the first two weeks of their employment, the UCPs have been providing care for clients at home with complex wounds and caring for families in palliative care situations. The nurse believes in the principles of collaborative practice and wishes to support the UCPs in their development. An important first step would be to
   1. Provide an opportunity for the UCPs to talk about their experiences, questions, and roles
   2. Provide an educational session on palliative care
   3. Set up a mentoring system among the UCPs
   4. Discuss the role of the RN in home care
8. A client is experiencing an anxiety attack. This is which priority nursing need for this client?
   1. First-order priority
   2. Second-order priority
   3. Third-order priority
9. The nurse checks on a client who was admitted to the hospital with pneumonia. He has been coughing profusely and has required nasotracheal suctioning. He has an intravenous infusion of antibiotics. He is febrile. The client asks the nurse whether he can have a bath because he has been perspiring profusely. The nurse may delegate to the UCP working with her today the task of
   1. Assessing vital signs
   2. Changing intravenous dressing
   3. Nasotracheal suctioning
   4. Administering a bed bath
10. An example of a nurse-sensitive outcome based on best practice guidelines is
    1. Rates of emergency room readmission after postsurgical discharge
    2. Percentage of time it takes to count narcotics by nursing staff every shift
    3. Number of falls among residents in a long-term care setting
    4. Time it takes for a client to be transported from the emergency department to an inpatient nursing unit

* RECOMMENDED WEB SITES

Academy of Canadian Executive Nurses (ACEN): http//www.acen.ca

This is an association of nurses in leadership positions across the spectrum of health services. ACEN activities support leadership, advocacy and policy intitiatives, and mentorship for emerging nurse leaders and executives.

Accreditation Canada: http//www.cchsa.ca/default.aspx

Accreditation Canada, formerly known as the Canadian Council on Health Services Accreditation, is a national, nonprofit, independent organization whose role is to help health services organizations, across Canada and internationally, examine and improve the quality of care and service they provide to their clients.

Canadian Association of Schools of Nursing (CASN): http://www.casn.ca

The Canadian Association of Schools of Nursing (CASN) is the national voice for nursing education, research, and scholarship and represents baccalaureate and graduate nursing programs across Canada.

Canadian Health Services Research Foundation: http://www.chsrf.ca

The Web site of the Canadian Health Services Research Foundation contains research resources for policymakers and for health system leaders and managers pertaining to staffing models, high-quality health work life, and high-quality health care.

Canadian Nurses Association (CNA): http//www.cna-nurses.ca/cna

The CNA is a federation of 11 provincial and territorial nursing associations representing more than 120,000 RNs. The CNA's mission is to advance the quality of nursing in the interest of the public.

Canadian Nursing Students Association (CNSA): http//www.cnsa.ca/

The CNSA is the national voice of nursing students in Canada. For more than 30 years, the CNSA has represented the interests of nursing students to federal, provincial, and international governments and other nursing and health care organizations.

Canadian Patient Safety Institute: http://www.patientsafetyinstitute.ca/index.html

The Canadian Patient Safety Institute (CPSI) is an independent not-for-profit corporation, operating collaboratively with health professionals and organizations and with regulatory governments and bodies to build and advance a safer health care system for Canadians.

International Council of Nurses (ICN): http://www.icn.ch/

The ICN is a federation of national nurses' associations, representing nurses in more than 120 countries. Operated by nurses for nurses, ICN works to ensure quality nursing care for all clients, sound health policies globally, and the advancement of nursing knowledge.

Interprofessional Network of BC (In-BC): http:/www.in-bc.ca

The Interprofessional Network of BC promotes the development of interprofessional development and education for collaborative practice. Its Web site contains resources that include information about interprofessional competencies.

Interprofessional Rural Program of BC (IRPbc): http://www.bcahc.ca/irpbc/

The IRPbc offers a unique opportunity for students from various health care professional programs to experience life and work in a rural community in British Columbia and to participate in a number of interprofessional team activities. The Web site offers access to a 10-minute film, *Learning Together in Rural Communities,* which highlights the voices of the students about their experiences.

Registered Nurses Association of Ontario (RNAO): http://www.rnao.org

This Web site offers a complete and up-to-date inventory of best practice guidelines, including implementation and evaluation.

Quality Worklife-Quality Healthcare Collaborative (QWQHC): http://www2.cchsa.ca/qwqhc

This Web site describes the national interprofessional coalition of health care leaders who work together to develop an integrated action-oriented strategy to transform the quality of work life for Canada's health care professionals. According to the QWQHC, this strategy enables client safety and high-quality client care and system outcomes.

12

Critical Thinking in Nursing Practice

Original chapter by Patricia A. Potter, RN, MSN, PhD, GMAC, FAAN

Canadian content written by Donna M. Romyn, RN, PhD

objectives

Mastery of content in this chapter will enable you to:

- Define the key terms listed.
- Describe characteristics of a critical thinker.
- Describe the components of a critical thinking model for clinical decision making.
- Explain the relationship between clinical experience and critical thinking.
- Discuss critical thinking competencies used in nursing practice.
- Discuss the nurse's responsibility in making clinical decisions.
- Discuss the relationship of the nursing process to critical thinking.
- Discuss the critical thinking qualities used in clinical decision making.
- Explain how professional standards influence a nurse's clinical decisions.
- Describe how reflective journal writing promotes critical thinking.
- Discuss how concept maps can improve a nurse's ability to think critically.

key terms

Clinical decision-making process, p. 147
Clinical inference, p. 151
Concept map, p. 154
Critical thinking, p. 147
Decision making, p. 157
Diagnostic reasoning, p. 151
Evidence-informed knowledge, p. 147
Nursing process, p. 152
Problem solving, p 151
Reflection, p. 154
Reflective journal writing, p. 154
Scientific method, p. 150

media resources

evolve Web Site

- Audio Chapter Summaries
- Glossary
- Multiple-Choice Review Questions
- Student Learning Activities
- Weblinks

Companion CD

- Glossary
- Interactive Learning Activities
- Fluids and Electrolytes Tutorial
- Test-Taking Skills

As a nurse, you will face many complex situations involving clients, family members, and other health care workers. To deal with these experiences effectively, you need to develop sound **critical thinking** skills so that you can approach each new problem involving a client's care with open-mindedness, creativity, confidence, and wisdom. When a client develops a new set of symptoms, asks you to provide comfort, or requires a procedure, it is important to think critically and make prudent clinical judgements so that the client receives the best nursing care possible. Critical thinking is not a simple, step-by-step linear process that you can learn overnight. Your ability to think critically will increase as you gain experience and progress from novice to expert nurse (Benner, 1984). Critical thinking is central to professional nursing practice because it allows you to test and refine nursing approaches, learn from successes and failures, apply new knowledge (e.g., nursing research findings), and ensure holistic client-centred care.

Critical Thinking Defined

Most definitions of critical thinking emphasize the use of logic and reasoning (Di Vito-Thomas, 2005) to make accurate clinical judgements and decisions. Accordingly, nurses recognize that an issue (e.g., client problem or health-related concern) exists, analyze information about the issue (e.g., clinical data about the client), evaluate information (e.g., reviewing assumptions and evidence), and draw conclusions (Settersten & Lauver, 2004). In consultation with clients, nurses consider what is important in a situation, imagine and explore alternative solutions, consider ethical principles, and then make informed decisions about how to proceed. Consider the following case example:

Mr. Jacobs is a 58-year-old client who had a radical prostatectomy for prostate cancer yesterday. His nurse, Tonya, finds him lying supine in bed with his arms extended along his sides and his hands clenched. When Tonya checks his sugical wound and drainage device, she notes that he winces when she gently palpates over the incisional area. She asks Mr. Jacobs when he last turned onto his side, and he responds, "Not since sometime last night." Tonya asks Mr. Jacobs if he is having incisional pain and he nods, saying, "It hurts too much to move." Tonya considers her observations and the information she has learned from the client to determine that his pain is severe and his mobility is reduced because of it. Together, she and Mr. Jacobs decide to take action to relieve Mr. Jacob's pain so he can turn more frequently and begin to get out of bed to aid his recovery.

Critical thinking requires purposeful and reflective reasoning during which you examine ideas, assumptions and beliefs, principles, conclusions, and actions within the context of the situation (Brunt 2005a, 2005b). When you care for a client, you begin to think critically by asking questions such as "What do I know about the client's situation?" "How do I know it?" "What is the client's situation now? How might it change?" "What else do I need to know to understand this situation better or improve it? How can I obtain that information?" "In what way will a specific therapy affect the client?" "Are other options available?" By answering these questions, you are able to identify alternative solutions to resolve the client's health-related concerns.

As you gain experience in nursing, avoid letting your thinking become routine or standarized. Instead, learn to look beyond the obvious in any clinical situation, explore the client's unique responses to actual or potential health alterations, and recognize what actions are needed to benefit the client. Over time, your experience with many clients will help you recognize patterns of behaviour, see commonalities in signs and symptoms, and anticipate reactions to nursing interventions. Reflecting on your experiences will allow you to better anticipate clients' needs and recognize problems when they develop. It will also help you determine how the knowledge you gained working with one client may be applicable to another client's situation.

In Tonya's case, she knows that the client is likely to have pain because the surgery was extensive. Her review of her observations and the client's report of pain confirm that pain is a problem. Her options include giving Mr. Jacobs an analgesic and then waiting until it takes effect so that she can help him find a more comfortable position. Once his pain is less acute, Tonya might also ask Mr. Jacobs whether he would like to try some relaxation exercises and mobilization techniques she learned while caring for another postoperative client that may be effective in increasing his mobility.

You can begin to learn to think critically early in your practice. For example, as you learn about administering bed baths and other hygiene measures to your clients, take time to read this book and the nursing literature about the concept of comfort. What are the criteria for comfort? How do clients from other cultures perceive comfort? What are the many factors that promote comfort? Learning and thinking critically about the concept of comfort prepares you to better anticipate your clients' needs. You will also identify comfort problems more quickly and offer appropriate care. The use of **evidence-informed knowledge**—knowledge based on research or clinical expertise—makes you an informed critical thinker.

Critical thinking requires not only cognitive skills, such as interpretation, analysis, inference, evaluation, explanation, and self-regulation, but also a nurse's habit (disposition) to ask questions, to be well informed, to be honest in facing personal biases, and to always be willing to reconsider and think clearly about issues. Without these dispositions, sound critical thinking is unlikely to occur (Facione, 1990; Facione & Facione, 1996; Profetto-McGrath, 2003). When applied to nursing, these core critical thinking skills and critical thinking dispositions reveal the complex nature of the **clinical decision-making process** (Table 12–1). Being able to apply all of these skills and acquiring all of these critical thinking habits take time and practice. You also need to have a sound knowledge base and thoughtfully consider the knowledge you gain when caring for clients.

Nurses who apply critical thinking in their work consider all aspects of a situation and make well-reasoned judgements about a variety of possible alternative actions rather than hastily and carelessly implementing solutions (Kataoka-Yahiro & Saylor, 1994). For example, nurses who work in crisis situations such as child abuse and suicide prevention programs act quickly when client problems develop. These nurses must, however, exercise discipline in decision making to avoid premature and inappropriate decisions. Learning to think critically helps you to care for clients as their advocate and to make better informed choices about their care. Critical thinking is more than just problem solving; it is an attempt to continually improve how you apply knowledge when faced with problems in client care.

Levels of Critical Thinking in Nursing

Your ability to think critically grows as you gain new knowledge and experience in nursing practice. Kataoka-Yahiro and Saylor (1994) developed a critical thinking model that incorporates three levels of critical thinking in nursing: basic, complex, and commitment. As a beginning nursing student, you apply the critical thinking model at the basic level. As you advance in practice, you adopt complex critical thinking and commitment.

TABLE 12-1 Critical Thinking Skills and Dispositions

Elements of Decision-Making Process	Critical Thinking Behaviour
Skill	
Interpretation	Be orderly in data collection. Look for patterns to categorize data (e.g., formulate nursing diagnoses [see Chapter 13]). Clarify any data about which you are uncertain.
Analysis	Be open-minded as you look at information about a client. Do not make careless assumptions. Ask whether the data reveal what you believe is true or whether other scenarios are possible.
Inference	Examine meanings and relationships in the data. Form reasonable hypotheses and conclusions, on the basis of the patterns observed.
Evaluation	Assess all situations objectively. Use criteria (e.g., expected outcomes) to determine the effectiveness of nursing actions. Identify required changes. Reflect on your own behaviour.
Explanation	Support your findings and conclusions. Use knowledge and experience to select the strategies you use in the care of clients.
Self-regulation	Reflect on your experiences. Adhere to standards of practice. Apply ethical principles in your nursing practice. Identify in what way you can improve your own performance.
Dispositions or Habits	
Truth seeking	Learn what is actually happening in a situation. Be courageous about asking questions. Consider scientific principles and evidence, even if they do not support your preconceptions or personal beliefs.
Open-mindedness	Be receptive to new ideas and tolerant of other points of view. Respect the right of other people to hold different opinions. Be aware of your own prejudices.
Analyticity	Determine the significance of a situation. Interpret meaning. Anticipate possible results or consequences. Value reason. Use evidence-informed knowledge in your nursing practice.
Systematicity	Be organized and focused in data collection. Use an organized approach to problem solving and decision making.
Self-confidence	Trust your own reasoning processes. Seek confirmation from experts when uncertain.
Inquisitiveness	Actively seek new knowledge. Value learning for learning's sake.
Maturity	Accept that multiple solutions are possible. Reflect on your own judgements; be willing to consider other explanations. Use prudence in making, suspending, or revising judgements.

Modified from Facione, P. (1990). *Critical thinking: A statement of expert consensus for purposes of educational assessment and instruction. The Delphi report: Research findings and recommendations prepared for the American Philosophical Association* (ERIC Doc No. ED 315-423). Washington, DC: Educational Resources Information Center (ERIC).

Basic Critical Thinking

At the basic level of critical thinking, a learner trusts that experts have the right answers for every problem. Thinking is concrete and based on a set of rules or principles. For example, as a student nurse, you use a hospital's procedure manual to confirm how to insert a Foley catheter. In completing this procedure for the first time, you will probably follow the procedure step by step without adjusting the procedure to meet a client's unique needs (e.g., positioning to minimize the client's pain or mobility restrictions) because you do not have enough experience to know how to individualize the procedure. At this level, answers to complex problems are seen to be either right or wrong (e.g., the Foley catheter balloon contains too much or not enough air), and you may believe that one right answer exists for each problem. As you gain more experience in nursing, you will begin to explore the diverse opinions and values of experts (e.g., instructors and role models among staff nurses) and engage in more complex critical thinking.

Complex Critical Thinking

When you engage in complex critical thinking, you begin to separate your thinking processes from those of authorities and to analyze and examine choices more independently. Your thinking abilities and initiative to look beyond expert opinion begin to change, as you realize that alternative, and perhaps conflicting, solutions to a problem or issue exist.

Consider the following case study:

Mr. Rosen is a 36-year-old man who injured his back in a skiing accident. He suffers from chronic pain but is refusing to take a prescribed analgesic. While discussing the importance of rehabilitation with Mr. Rosen, the nurse, Edwin, learns that Mr. Rosen practises meditation at home. In complex critical thinking, Edwin recognizes that for pain relief, the client has options other than accepting analgesics. Edwin decides to discuss meditation and other nonpharmacological interventions with Mr. Rosen and his other health care professionals as pain control options.

In complex critical thinking, you are willing to consider other options in addition to routine procedures when complex situations develop. As a nurse, you learn to weigh the benefits and risks of each potential solution before making a final decision. Thinking becomes more creative and innovative as you explore a broad range of perspectives and alternative solutions.

Commitment

The third level of critical thinking is commitment. You anticipate the need to make choices without assistance from other professionals, and then you assume responsibility and accountability for those choices. As a nurse, you do more than just consider the complex alternative solutions that a problem poses. At the commitment level, you choose an action or belief on the basis of the alternative solutions available, and you stand by your choice. Sometimes an action is to not take action, or you may choose to delay an action until a later time as a result of your experience and knowledge. Because you take accountability for the decision, you give attention to the results of the decision and determine whether it was appropriate.

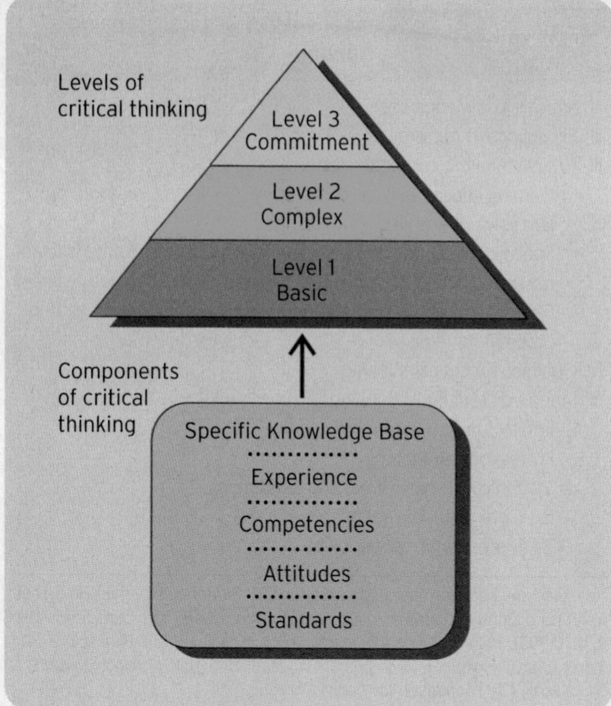

Figure 12-1 Critical thinking model for nursing judgement. **Source:** Redrawn from Kataoka-Yahiro, M., & Saylor, C. (1994). A critical thinking model for nursing judgment. *Journal of Nursing Education, 33*(8), 351. Adapted from Glaser, E. (1941). *An experiment in the development of critical thinking.* New York: Bureau of Publications, Teachers College, Columbia University; Miller, M., & Malcolm, N. (1990). Critical thinking in the nursing curriculum. *Nursing & Health Care, 11*, 67; Paul, R.W. (1993). The art of redesigning instruction. In Wilsen, J., Blinker, A.J.A. (Eds.). *Critical thinking: How to prepare students for a rapidly changing world.* Santa Rosa, California: Foundation for Critical Thinking; and Perry, W. (1979). *Forms of intellectual and ethical development in the college years: A scheme.* New York: Holt, Rinehart, & Winston.

A Critical Thinking Model for Clinical Decision Making

Thinking critically is becoming the benchmark or standard for professional nursing competence. To help you in the development of critical thinking, this text offers a model for critical thinking. Because critical thinking in nursing is complex, a model helps explain what is involved as you make clinical decisions and judgements about your clients. Kataoka-Yahiro and Saylor (1994) developed a model of critical thinking for nursing judgement based in part on previous work by Paul (1993), Glaser (1941), Perry (1979), and Miller and Malcolm (1990) (Figure 12–1). The model defines the outcome of critical thinking: nursing judgement that is relevant to nursing problems in a variety of settings. According to this model, critical thinking consists of five components: knowledge base, experience, competencies, qualities, and standards. The elements of the model combine to explain how nurses make clinical judgements that are necessary for safe, effective nursing care (Box 12–1).

Throughout this text, this model is used for applying critical thinking during the nursing process. Each clinical chapter of the text (Chapters 31 to 49) is organized by the steps of the nursing process and includes both scientific and nursing knowledge. It is your knowledge base (the first critical thinking component) that prepares you to make clinical judgements as a nurse. Figure 12–1 demonstrates how to apply elements of critical thinking in assessing clients, in planning the interventions you provide, and in evaluating your results. If you learn to apply each element of this model in the way you think about clients, you will be become a confident and effective professional.

Specific Knowledge Base

To think critically, establish accurate clinical judgements and decisions, and improve clinical practice (Di Vito-Thomas, 2005), nurses must possess a sound knowledge base. Your knowledge base includes information and theory from the basic sciences, humanities, behavioural sciences, and nursing. Nurses use their knowledge base in a different way than other health care professionals because they think holistically about client problems and health-related matters. For example, a nurse's broad knowledge base offers a physical, psychological, social, moral, ethical, and cultural view of clients and their health concerns. The depth and breadth of knowledge influences your ability to think critically about nursing problems. Consider this scenario:

Robert Perez previously earned a bachelor's degree in education and taught high school for one year. He has successfully completed the required courses in his nursing program in the sciences, health ethics, fundamental nursing concepts, and communication principles. His first clinical course focuses on health promotion with a clinical assignment in an outpatient primary care clinic. Although he is still new to nursing, his experiences as a teacher and his preparation and knowledge base in nursing will help him know how to begin to make clinical decisions about clients' health promotion practices.

Experience

Nursing is a practice discipline. Clinical nursing experiences are necessary for you to acquire clinical decision-making skills (Roche, 2002). In clinical situations, you learn from observing, sensing, talking with

> **BOX 12-1 Components of Critical Thinking in Nursing**
>
> I. Specific knowledge base
> II. Experience in nursing
> III. Critical thinking competencies
>   A. General critical thinking competencies (scientific method, problem solving, and decision making)
>   B. Specific critical thinking competencies in clinical situations (diagnostic reasoning, clinical inference, and clinical decision making)
>   C. Specific critical thinking competency in nursing (use of nursing process)
> IV. Qualities for critical thinking
> V. Standards for critical thinking
>   A. Intellectual standards
>   B. Professional standards
>   1. Ethical criteria for nursing judgement
>   2. Criteria for evaluation
>   3. Professional responsibility
>
> Adapted from Kataoka-Yahiro, M., & Saylor, C. (1994). A critical thinking model for nursing judgment. *Journal of Nursing Education, 33*(8), 351. Data from Paul, R. W. (1993). The art of redesigning instruction. In Willsen, J., & Blinker, A. J. A. (Eds.). *Critical thinking: How to prepare students for a rapidly changing world.* Santa Rosa, CA: Foundation for Critical Thinking.

clients and families, and then reflecting actively on your experiences. Clinical experience is the laboratory for testing nursing knowledge. You learn that "textbook" approaches form the basis for nursing practice, but you make safe adaptations or revisions in approaches to accommodate the setting, the unique qualities of the client, and the experience you gained from caring for previous clients. With experience, you begin to understand clinical situations, recognize cues of clients' health patterns, and interpret cues as relevant or irrelevant (Tanner, 2006). You also learn to seek new knowledge as needed, act quickly when events change, and make quality decisions that promote the client's well-being. It is important for you to admit to any limitations in your knowledge and skills. Critical thinkers admit what they do not know and try to acquire the knowledge needed to make proper decisions. A client's safety and welfare are at risk if you do not admit your inability to deal with a practice problem. You must rethink the situation, acquire additional knowledge, and then use new information to form opinions, draw conclusions, and take appropriate action. Perhaps the best lesson to be learned by a new nursing student is to value all client experiences, which enable you to build new knowledge and inspire innovative thinking.

During the previous summer, Robert worked as a nurse assistant in a long-term care facility. This experience provided him with valuable experience in interacting with older adults and in giving basic nursing care. Specifically, he has been able to develop good interviewing skills and understand the importance of the family in an individual's health, and he has learned how nurses advocate for clients. He has also learned that older adults require more time to perform activities such as eating, bathing, and grooming, and so he has adapted skill techniques for dealing with this requirement. His time in the physical assessment laboratory and the time he worked in the nursing home helped him begin to be a careful observer. As he reflects on his experiences, Robert also knows that much of what he learned can be applied in promoting health, wellness, and independence among the older clients who attend the outpatient clinic for routine follow-up visits.

Becoming familiar with practice standards developed by clinical experts also assists you in enhancing your knowledge base. For example, the *Nursing Best Practice Guidelines* developed by the Registered Nurses Association of Ontario (RNAO; n.d.) include standards for nursing care for a number of clinical conditions, such as asthma, chronic obstructive pulmonary disease, diabetes, and depression. Other standards focus on nursing practice issues such as embracing cultural diversity and fostering collaborative practice. Visit the RNAO's Web site (http://www.rnao.org/bestpractices/), as well as the Web site of the professional nursing association in the province or territory in which you reside, to learn more about the wide range of practice guidelines and to develop a sound knowledge base for your nursing practice.

Critical Thinking Competencies

Kataoka-Yahiro and Saylor (1994) described critical thinking competencies as the cognitive processes that a nurse uses to make judgements about the clinical care of clients. They include general critical thinking, specific critical thinking in clinical situations, and specific critical thinking in nursing. General critical thinking competencies are not unique to nursing. They include the scientific method, problem solving, and decision making. Specific critical thinking competencies in clinical situations include diagnostic reasoning, clinical inference, and clinical decision making. The specific critical thinking competency in nursing involves use of the nursing process.

General Critical Thinking Competencies

Scientific Method. The scientific method is a systematic, ordered approach to gathering data and solving problems that is used in nursing, medicine, and various other disciplines. Nurse researchers use the scientific method to verify that a set of facts is true when testing research questions in nursing practice situations. Research incorporating the scientific method contributes to evidence-informed nursing practice and the development of best practice guidelines.

The scientific method has five steps:

- Identification of the problem
- Collection of data
- Formulation of a research question or hypothesis
- Testing of the question or hypothesis
- Evaluation of the results of the test or study

Consider the following example of the scientific method in nursing practice:

A nurse caring for clients who receive large doses of chemotherapy for ovarian cancer detects a pattern whereby these clients develop severe inflammation of the mouth (mucositis) (identifies the problem). The nurse reads research articles (collects data) about mucositis and learns about evidence that cryotherapy, in which clients keep ice in their mouths during the chemotherapy infusion, reduces the severity of the mucositis after treatment. The nurse asks (forms research question), "Can ovarian cancer clients who receive chemotherapy have less severe mucositis when given cryotherapy instead of standard mouth rinse in the oral cavity?" The nurse then designs a study that compares the incidence and severity of mucositis in a group of clients who use cryotherapy with those in clients who use traditional mouth rinse (tests the question). The nurse hopes that the results from the study will give oncology nurses a better approach for reducing the frequency and severity of mucositis in cancer clients. A nurse in another oncology setting critically analyzes the study before implementing its recommendations for client care (evaluates the results of the study).

Problem Solving. Everyone faces problems every day. When a problem arises, people obtain information and then use the information, in addition to what they already know, to find a solution. Clients routinely present problems in nursing practice. For example, a home care nurse visits a client and learns that the client cannot describe what medications she has taken for the past three days. The nurse must solve the problem of why the client is not adhering to her medication schedule. The nurse knows the client was recently discharged from the hospital, and five medications were prescribed. When the nurse asks the client to show the medications that she takes in the morning, the nurse notices that the client has difficulty reading the medication labels. The client is able to tell the nurse the names of the medications she is to take but is uncertain about the times of administration. The nurse recommends having the client's pharmacy relabel the medications in larger lettering. In addition, the nurse shows the client examples of pill organizers that will help her sort her medications by time of day for a period of 7 days.

Effective **problem solving** also involves evaluating the solution over time to be sure that it is still effective. It becomes necessary to try different options if a problem recurs. As a continuation of the example just described, the nurse finds during a follow-up visit that the client has organized her medications correctly and is able to read the labels without difficulty. The nurse obtained information that correctly clarified the cause of the client's problem, and the nurse tested a solution that proved successful. Having solved a problem in one situation adds to the nurse's experience in practice and allows the nurse to apply that knowledge in future situations with clients.

Decision Making. When you face a problem or situation and need to choose a course of action from several options, you are making a decision. **Decision making** is a product of critical thinking that focuses on problem resolution. Following a set of criteria helps you make a well-reasoned decision. For example, decision making occurs when a person chooses a fitness consultant. To make a decision, the person has to recognize and define the problem (need for a physical activity), assess all options (consider recommended trainers or choose one on the basis of proximity to the person's home). The person has to weigh each option against a set of criteria (e.g., credentials, reputation, experience), test possible options (interview potential trainers; assess safety of equipment), consider the consequences of the decision (increased fitness; risk of injury), and then make a final decision. Although the criteria follow a sequence of steps, decision making involves moving back and forth between steps when all criteria are considered. Decision making leads to informed conclusions that are supported by evidence and reason. Examples of decision making include deciding on a choice of dressings for a client with a surgical wound or selecting the best approach for teaching a family how to assist a client who is returning home after a stroke. You learn to make sound decisions by approaching each clinical situation thoughtfully and by applying each component of the decision-making process described previously.

Specific Critical Thinking Competencies in Clinical Situations

Diagnostic Reasoning and Inference. As soon as you receive information about a client in a clinical situation, you begin **diagnostic reasoning**, a process of determining a client's health status after you make physical and behavioural observations and after you assign meaning to the behaviours, physical signs, and symptoms exhibited by the client. The information that you collect and analyze leads to a diagnosis of the client's condition. An expert nurse sees the context of a client situation (e.g., recognize that a client who is feeling lightheaded, has blurred vision, and has a history of diabetes is experiencing a problem with blood glucose levels), observes patterns and themes (e.g., symptoms including weakness, headache, hunger, and visual disturbances that suggest hypoglycemia), and chooses an appropriate intervention quickly (e.g., offers a food source containing glucose) (Ferrario, 2004). Considering the context of the situation enhances the nurse's analytic skills (Ironside, 2005) and results in a more accurate diagnosis.

Part of diagnostic reasoning is **clinical inference**: the process of drawing conclusions from related pieces of evidence (Smith Higuchi & Donald, 2002). An inference involves forming patterns of information from data before making a diagnosis. Seeing that a client has lost his appetite and experienced a loss of weight over the past month, the nurse infers that the client has a nutritional problem. An example of diagnostic reasoning is forming a nursing diagnosis such as *imbalanced nutrition, less than body requirements* (see Chapter 43).

Often you cannot make a precise nursing diagnosis during your first meeting with a client. You will sometimes sense that a problem or health concern exists, but you do not have sufficient data to make a specific diagnosis. Some clients' physical conditions limit their ability to tell you about symptoms. Other clients may choose not to share sensitive and important information during your initial assessment. Clients' behaviours and physical responses may become observable only under certain conditions not present during your initial assessment. When you are uncertain of a diagnosis, continue data collection, which may include consulting with expert nurses or other health care professionals. As a nurse, you have to critically analyze changing clinical situations until you are able to determine the client's unique situation. Diagnostic reasoning is a continuous behaviour in nursing practice.

In diagnostic reasoning, use client data that you gather to logically explain a clinical judgement. For example, after turning a client over in bed, you see an area of redness on his right hip. You palpate the area and note that it is warm to the touch, and the client complains of tenderness there. You push on the area with your finger, and, after you release pressure, the area does not blanch or turn white. You think about what you know about normal skin integrity and the effects of pressure. You form the conclusion the client has a pressure ulcer. As a new student, confirm your judgement with experienced nurses. At times, your clinical judgement may be incorrect; however, nurse experts will give you feedback to build on in future clinical situations.

Nurses do not make medical diagnoses, but they do assess and monitor clients closely and compare the client's signs and symptoms with those that are common to a medical diagnosis. This type of diagnostic reasoning helps nurses and other health care professionals pinpoint the nature of a problem more quickly and select proper interventions. Similarities and differences between medical and nursing diagnoses are described in more detail in Chapter 13.

Clinical Decision Making. Clinical decision making is a problem-solving activity that focuses on defining client problems and selecting appropriate treatments (Smith Higuchi & Donald, 2002). Nurses are responsible for making accurate and appropriate clinical decisions. Clinical decision making distinguishes professional nurses from technical personnel. It is the professional nurse, for example, who takes immediate action when a client's clinical condition deteriorates, decides whether a client is experiencing complications that call for notification of a physician, or decides whether a teaching plan for a client is ineffective and necessitates revision. Benner (1984) described clinical decision making as judgement that includes critical and reflective thinking and action and the application of scientific and practical knowledge.

Clinical judgement requires that you recognize the salient aspects of a clinical situation, interpret their meanings, and respond appropriately. It includes four components: noticing or grasping the situation; interpreting or developing a sufficient understanding of the situation to respond; responding or deciding on a course of action; and reflecting on or reviewing the actions taken and their outcomes. In making a clinical judgement, you consider the context of the situation and rely on analytic processes, intuition, and narrative thinking (i.e., thinking that occurs as a result of telling and interpreting stories). As you reflect on actions taken, you acquire clinical learning, which contributes to future clinical judgements (Tanner, 2006).

Most clients have health concerns for which no clear textbook solutions exist. Each client's problems are unique and products of many factors, including the client's physical health, lifestyle, culture, relationship with family and friends, living environment, and experiences. As a nurse, you do not always have a clear picture of the client's needs and the appropriate actions to take when you first meet a client. Instead, you must learn to question and explore different perspectives and interpretations in order to find a solution that benefits the client.

When you approach a clinical problem, such as a client who is experiencing difficulty walking, you make a decision that identifies the problem (e.g., right-sided weakness) and choose nursing interventions (e.g., teaching the use of appropriate assistive devices) for that client. Nurses constantly make clinical decisions to improve a client's health or maintain wellness. Clinical decision making requires careful reasoning so that you choose the options for the best client outcomes on the basis of the client's condition and the priority of the problem or health concern.

You improve your clinical decision making by knowing your clients. Nurse researchers found that expert nurses develop a level of knowing that leads to pattern recognition of client's symptoms and responses (White, 2003). For example, an expert nurse who has worked on a general surgery unit for many years is more likely to detect signs of internal hemorrhage (e.g., fall in blood pressure, rapid pulse, change in consciousness) than is a new nurse. Over time, a combination of knowledge, experience, time spent in a specific clinical area, and the quality of relationships formed with clients allow expert nurses to know clinical situations and quickly anticipate and select the right course of action (Tanner et al., 1993). Spending more time during initial client assessments to both observe client behaviour and measure physical findings is a way to improve knowing your clients. Also, consistently monitoring clients as problems occur helps you see how clinical changes develop over time. The selection of nursing actions is built on both clinical knowledge and client data, including the following:

- The identified status and situation of the client.
- Knowledge about the clinical variables (e.g., client's age, seriousness of the problem, pathological process of the problem, client's pre-existing disease conditions) involved in the situation and how the variables are linked together.
- Knowledge about the usual patterns of any diagnosed problem or prognosis and a judgement about the likely course of events and outcomes of the diagnosed problem, in view of any health risks the client also has.
- Any additional relevant information about requirements in the client's daily living situation, functional capacity, and social resources.
- Knowledge about the nursing interventions available and the way in which specific actions will predictably affect the client's situation.

Making an accurate clinical decision allows you to set priorities for nursing action (see Chapter 13). Because each situation involves different clients and different variables, a certain activity is sometimes more of a priority in one situation and less of a priority in another. For example, if a home care client is physically dependent, unable to eat, and incontinent of urine, skin integrity is of higher priority than if the client were immobile but continent of urine and able to eat a normal diet. Do not assume that certain health situations produce automatic priorities. For example, an adolescent who has embarked on a smoking cessation program is expected to experience some withdrawal symptoms, which often become a priority of care. However, if the client is experiencing anxiety about potential weight gain that decreases her ability to participate fully in the program, it becomes necessary for you to focus on ways to relieve the anxiety before the smoking cessation measures will be effective.

After determining a client's nursing care priorities, you select actions most likely to relieve each problem or to promote health, wellness, and quality of life. A wide range of choices is often available, from nurse-administered to client self-care strategies. You collaborate with the client and then select, test, and evaluate the chosen approaches.

Nurses make decisions about individual clients and about groups of clients. You use criteria such as the clinical condition of the clients, Maslow's hierarchy of needs, risks involved in treatment delays, and clients' expectations of care to determine which clients have the most urgent priorities for care. For example, a client in a community care centre who is experiencing a sudden drop in blood pressure along with a change in consciousness requires your attention immediately, as opposed to a small child who requires a routine immunization or a group of expectant parents attending a prenatal class. In order for you to manage the wide variety of problems associated with groups of clients, skillful, prioritized decision making is crucial (Box 12–2).

Nursing Process as a Critical Thinking Competency

Nurses apply the **nursing process** as a critical thinking competency when delivering client care (Kataoka-Yahiro & Saylor, 1994). The nursing process is a five-step clinical decision-making approach that

➤ BOX 12-2 Clinical Decision Making for Groups of Clients

- Identify the nursing diagnosis and collaborative problems of each client (see Chapter 13).
- Analyze clients' diagnoses or problems and decide which are most urgent on the bases of basic needs, the clients' changing or unstable status, and problem complexity (see Chapter 13).
- Consider the resources available for managing each problem, including unregulated care providers assigned to work with you, as well as clients' family members.
- Consider how to involve the clients as decision makers and participants in care.
- Decide how to combine activities to resolve more than one client problem at a time.
- Decide what, if any, nursing care procedures to delegate to unregulated care providers so that you are able to spend your time on activities requiring professional nursing knowledge.

consists of assessment, diagnosis, planning, implementation, and evaluation (see Chapters 13 to 15). The purpose of the nursing process is to assist nurses in identifying and treating clients' health concerns. Use of the nursing process allows nurses to help clients meet agreed-upon outcomes for better health (Figure 12–2). The nursing process incorporates general (e.g., scientific method, problem solving, and decision making) and specific critical thinking competencies (e.g., diagnostic reasoning, inference, and clinical decision making), described earlier in this chapter, in a manner that focuses on a particular client's unique needs. The format of the nursing process is unique to the discipline of nursing and provides a common language and process for nurses to "think through" clients' clinical problems (Kataoka-Yahiro & Saylor, 1994). Chapter 13 describes the nursing process in more detail.

The nursing process is often called a *blueprint* or *plan for care.* It allows flexibility for use in all clinical settings. When you use the nursing process, you identify a client's health-related concerns, clearly define a nursing diagnosis or collaborative problem, determine priorities of care, and set goals and expected outcomes of care. Then you develop and communicate a plan of care, perform nursing interventions, and evaluate the effects of your care. Involving your client in each step of the nursing process helps ensure that care is client centered. When you become more competent in using the nursing process, you are able to focus not merely on a single client problem or diagnosis but on multiple problems or diagnoses and to move back and forth between steps when considering all of the information available to you about a client's concerns. With each step, you apply critical thinking to provide the very best professional care to your clients.

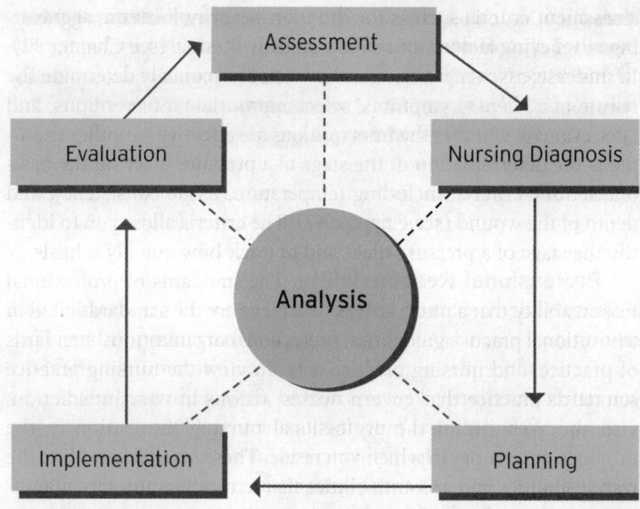

Figure 12-2 Five-step nursing process model.

Qualities for Critical Thinking

The fourth component of the critical thinking model is qualities. An important part of critical thinking is interpreting, evaluating, and making judgements about the adequacy of various arguments and available data. Qualities define how a successful critical thinker approaches a problem or a situation that necessitates decision making. For example, when a client complains of anxiety before undergoing a diagnostic procedure, the curious nurse explores possible reasons for the client's concerns. The nurse also exhibits discipline and perseverance in taking responsibility to complete a thorough assessment to find the sources of the client's anxiety. The quality of inquiry involves an ability to recognize that problems exist and that you need evidence in support of what you suppose to be true (Watson & Glaser, 1980). Knowing when you need more information, knowing when information is misleading, and recognizing your own knowledge limits and personal biases are examples of how critical thinking qualities play a key role in decision making.

Standards for Critical Thinking

The fifth component of the critical thinking model includes intellectual and professional standards (Kataoka-Yahiro & Saylor, 1994).

Intellectual Standards. An intellectual standard is a guideline or principle for rational thought. You apply such standards when you conduct the nursing process. When you consider a client problem, apply intellectual standards such as thoroughness, preciseness, accuracy, and consistency to make sure that all clinical decisions are sound. Efficacious use of the intellectual standards in clinical practice ensures that you do not perform critical thinking haphazardly.

Professional Standards. Professional standards for critical thinking refer to ethical criteria for nursing judgements, evidence-informed criteria used for evaluation, and criteria for professional responsibility. Professional standards promote the highest level of quality nursing care for individuals and groups in institutional and community-based settings.

Ethical Criteria for Nursing Judgement. Client care requires more than just the memorization and application of scientific knowledge (Ironside, 2005). Efficacious nursing practice reflects sound ethical principles. Being able to focus on a client's values and beliefs helps you make clinical decisions that are just, faithful to the client's choices, and beneficial to the client's health and well-being. The *Code of Ethics for Registered Nurses* (Canadian Nurses Association, 2008) is based on core values that serve as a guide to ethical decision making in nursing practice. Among these values and ethical responsibilities are providing safe, compassionate, competent, and ethical care; promoting health and well-being; promoting and respecting informed decision making; preserving dignity; maintaining privacy and confidentiality; promoting justice; and being accountable. Critical thinkers maintain a sense of self-awareness through conscious awareness of their own values, beliefs, and feelings and of the multiple perspectives of clients, family members, staff, and peers in clinical situations. Chapter 8 summarizes ethical standards to use when you are faced with ethical dilemmas or problems.

One of the clients in a community health clinic is a young man who has signs and symptoms of chlamydia, a sexually transmitted disease. The client has had the symptoms for more than 3 weeks and voices concern about what it will mean to have the disease. Richard, a nurse, examines the young man and finds that the client has redness and itching on his penis, with a yellowish discharge. Richard checks further and asks whether the client has pain on urination. He also assesses the client for fever. Richard has limited knowledge about chlamydia, and so he consults with the clinic nurse practitioner, who explains the nature of the infection, the risks it poses to the client, the usual course of treatment, and some of the legal and ethical guidelines that govern nurses' actions when working with clients with sexually transmitted diseases. Richard returns to the client and speaks confidently with him about chlamydia, the reason for his symptoms, the need to tell sex partners about the infection, and the importance of wearing a condom.

Criteria for Evaluation. Nurses routinely use evidence-informed criteria to assess clients' conditions and to determine the efficacy of nursing interventions. For example, accurate assessment of symptoms such as pain or shortness of breath requires use of assessment criteria such as the duration, severity, location, aggravating or relieving factors, and effects on daily lifestyle (see Chapter 42). In this case, assessment criteria allow you to accurately determine the nature of a client's symptoms, select appropriate interventions, and later evaluate whether the interventions are effective. Another example is the determination of the stage of a pressure ulcer on the basis of scientific criteria, including temperature, tissue consistency, and depth of the wound (see Chapter 47). The criteria allow you to identify the stage of a pressure ulcer and to track how quickly it heals.

Professional Responsibility. The standards of professional responsibility that a nurse strives to achieve are the standards cited in institutional practice guidelines, professional organizations' standards of practice, and nursing practice acts. To view the nursing practice standards practice that govern nurses' actions in your jurisdiction, visit the Web site of the professional nursing association in the province or territory in which you reside. These standards outline the responsibilities and accountabilities that a nurse assumes in guaranteeing high-quality health care to the public.

Developing Critical Thinking Skills

To develop critical thinking skills, it is important to learn how to connect knowledge and theory in practice (Box 12–3). Making sense of what you learn in the classroom, from reading, or from dialogue with other students and then applying it during client care are always challenging. Learning approaches will assist you in developing and improving your critical thinking skills.

Reflective Journal Writing

How often do you think back on a situation to consider why it occurred? How did you act? What could you have done differently? What knowledge could you have used? **Reflection** is the process of purposefully thinking back or recalling a situation to discover its purpose or meaning. Reflection is necessary for self-evaluation and improvement of nursing practice.

Reflective journal writing is a tool for developing critical thought and reflection through clarifying concepts (Bilinski, 2002). Reflective writing gives you the opportunity to define and express a clinical experience in your own words (Di Vito-Thomas, 2005). By keeping a reflective journal of each of your clinical experiences, you are able to explore personal perceptions or understanding of the experience and develop the ability to apply theory in practice. The use of a journal improves your observation and descriptive skills.

The "Circle of Meaning" model, which was adapted to nursing practice, encourages reflection, concept clarification, and a search for meaning in nursing practice (Bilinski, 2002). The model features a series of questions that enable nurses to journey through the clinical experience and find meaning and connections. The questions include the following:

- What experience or situation in your clinical practice seems confusing, difficult, or interesting?
- What is the meaning of the experience? What feelings did you have about it? What feelings did your client have? What influenced the experience?
- Do your responses to the preceding questions remind you of any experience from the past or present, or something that you think is desirable future experience? How does it relate? What are the implications or significance?
- What are the connections between what is being described and the things you have learned about nursing science, research, and theory? What are some possible solutions? What approach or solution would you choose, and why would you choose it? What is the effectiveness of this approach?

Keeping a journal of your client care experiences will help you become aware of how you use clinical decision making skills (Kessler & Lund, 2004). Begin by recording notes after a clinical experience. Telling a story and drawing a picture are two additional ways to identify the experience you wish to reflect on. Describe in detail what you felt, thought, and did. Analyze your experience by considering thoughts, feelings, and possible meanings for you and the client. Challenge any preconceived ideas you have when you look at actual clinical situations. Describe the significance of the experience. Refer to your journal often when you care for clients in similar circumstances. Reflecting on your experiences is an important component of monitoring your competence in nursing practice. It also promotes knowledge transfer by enabling you to identify how previously acquired knowledge can be applied in a current or future situation (Nielsen et al., 2007).

Concept Mapping

As a nurse, you care for clients who have multiple nursing diagnoses or collaborative problems. A **concept map** is a visual representation of client problems and interventions that depicts their relationships to one another (Schuster, 2003). The primary purpose of concept

BOX 12-3 RESEARCH HIGHLIGHT

How to "Think Like a Nurse"

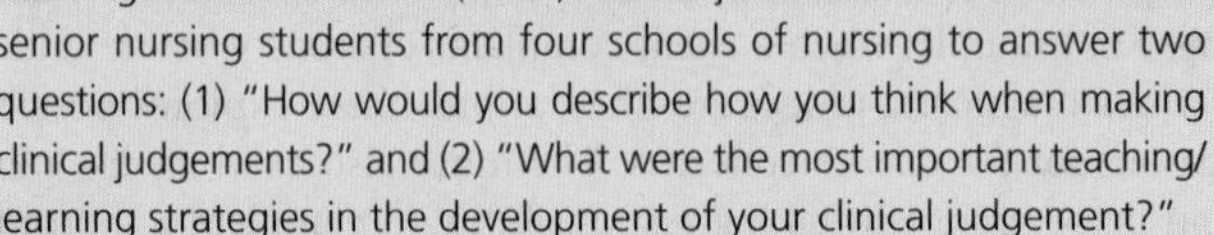

Research Focus

Faculty members use a variety of teaching and learning strategies to aid students in developing critical thinking. Di Vito-Thomas (2005) invited junior and senior nursing students from four schools of nursing to answer two questions: (1) "How would you describe how you think when making clinical judgements?" and (2) "What were the most important teaching/learning strategies in the development of your clinical judgement?"

Research Abstract

Students described their thinking as a process that developed through experience in practice. Education and practice are combined so that knowledge gained in the classroom becomes second nature in practice. Students noted that they learned to think through different options and then to weigh those options determine what to do first to improve client outcomes. Clinical experience was the most important strategy in developing clinical judgement. Concept maps showing the interrelatedness of all aspects of client care were also useful. Case studies allowed students to focus on, think critically about, and understand the relationships between those aspects.

Evidence-Informed Practice

Teaching and learning strategies that help develop clinical judgement include the following:

- Scrutinizing case studies displayed on concept maps
- Having in-depth discussion with instructors while observing clinical changes in clients
- Making joint decisions with peers and instructors on client care

References: Di Vito-Thomas, P. (2005). Nursing student stories on learning how to think like a nurse. *Nurse Education, 30*(3), 133.

mapping is to synthesize relevant data about a client, including assessment data, nursing diagnoses, health needs, nursing interventions, and evaluation measures (Hill, 2006). Through drawing a concept map, you learn to organize or link information in a unique way so that the diverse information you have about a client begins to connect to form meaningful patterns and concepts. When you see the relationship between the various client diagnoses and the data that support them, you gain a better understanding of a client's clinical situation. Over time, concept maps become more detailed, integrated, and comprehensive as you learn more about the care of a client and as you care for similar clients (Ferrario, 2004). You will see similarities and differences between clients, which helps you hone decision-making skills.

Concept maps take many visual forms. Several examples of concept maps are included in Chapters 31 to 49 of this textbook. Additional resources are also found in the reference list at the end of this chapter. Most students follow a model that makes the concept map a working document. As a student, you develop the map during your care for the client. You begin by obtaining client data from a variety of sources (e.g., the medical record, pertinent nursing literature, the client's history and physical examination, and other health care professionals). The client's major medical diagnosis and any comorbid conditions (unrelated medical conditions) usually form the center of the map. From there, you group patterns of assessment data along the edges of the map. As you identify the different nursing diagnoses, you draw dotted lines to connect the diagnoses that are related. The links must be accurate in order to show true clinical relationships. On the map, you also list the nursing interventions chosen for the client. Once again, you see how any one intervention applies to more than one nursing diagnosis. While caring for a client, you write down the client's responses to your interventions and any clinical impressions you may have.

The final map gives you a broader and more complex understanding of your client's health care needs. Save the concept maps you create and use them as a reference as you care for other clients with similar health concerns.

Critical Thinking Synthesis

Critical thinking is a reasoning process by which you reflect on and analyze your own thoughts, knowledge, and actions (Figure 12–3). To be think critically requires dedication and a desire to grow intellectually. For novice nurses, it is important to learn the steps of the nursing process and to incorporate the elements of the critical thinking model in your practice. The two processes are intertwined in making quality decisions about client care. The key components of critical thinking are integrated into Chapters 31 to 49 of this text to help you better understand its relationship to the nursing process and to making quality judgements and decisions about client care.

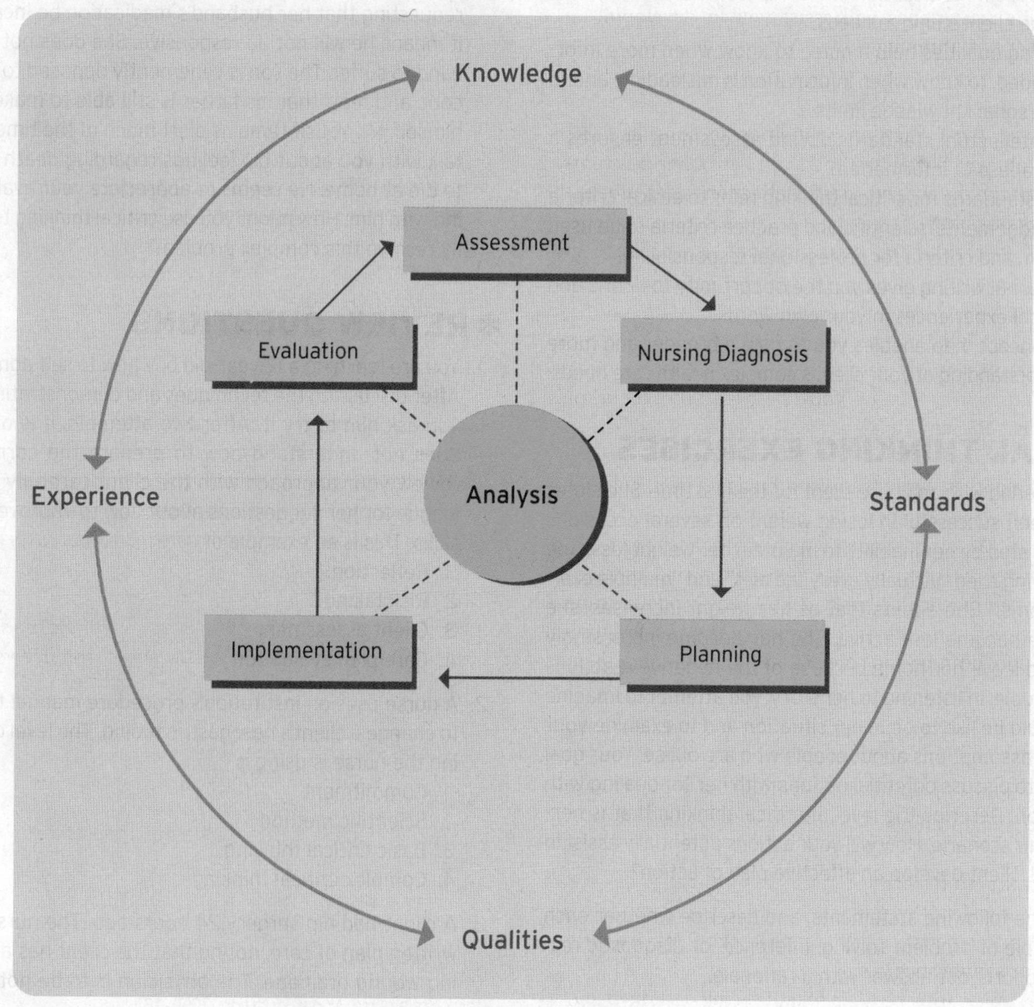

Figure 12–3 Synthesis of critical thinking with the nursing process competency.

* KEY CONCEPTS

- Critical thinking is a process acquired through experience and an active curiosity about learning.
- Nurses who apply critical thinking in their work focus on options for solving problems and making decisions, rather than rapidly and carelessly quickly adopting simple solutions.
- Following a procedure step by step without adjusting to a client's unique needs is an example of basic critical thinking.
- In complex critical thinking, a nurse learns that alternative, and perhaps conflicting, solutions to problems exist.
- The critical thinking model combines a nurse's knowledge base, experience, competence in nursing process, qualities, and standards to explain how nurses make clinical judgements that are necessary for safe, effective nursing care.
- In diagnostic reasoning, you collect client data and then logically develop a clinical judgement, such as a nursing diagnosis.
- When you face a clinical problem or situation and choose a course of action from several options, you are making a clinical decision.
- Clinical learning experiences are necessary for you to acquire clinical decision-making skills.
- You improve your clinical decision making by knowing your clients.
- Clinical decision making involves judgement that includes critical and reflective thinking and the action and application of scientific and practical knowledge.
- The nursing process is a blueprint for client care that involves both general and specific critical thinking competencies in a way that focuses on the client's unique needs.
- Critical thinking qualities help a nurse to know when more information is needed, to know when information is misleading, and to recognize personal knowledge limits.
- The use of intellectual standards during assessment ensures a complete database of information.
- Professional standards for critical thinking refer to ethical criteria for nursing judgements, scientific and practice criteria to be used for evaluation, and criteria for professional responsibility.
- Reflective journal writing gives you the opportunity to define and express clinical experiences in your own words.
- Drawing a concept map enables you to gain a broader and more complex understanding of your client's complex health care needs.

* CRITICAL THINKING EXERCISES

1. You are meeting with an obese client for the first time. She states that she been successful in losing weight on several occasions but is frustrated by her inability to maintain her weight loss. She reports having tried "virtually every fad diet" and "multiple exercise programs." She admits that as her weight increases, she tends to be become less active. She has become increasingly reluctant to leave her home because of the negative reactions of other people. In listening to her story, you attempt to imagine what it would be like to be in her situation and to examine your biases and assumptions about people who are obese. Your goal is to begin to discuss potential options with her for dealing with her situation. Describe the level of critical thinking that is necessary in this scenario. How will your actions potentially assist in helping this client develop an effective plan of action?
2. Consider the following statements, and describe whether each is an example of problem solving, inference, or diagnostic reasoning. Support your answer with a rationale.
   a. As the nurse enters a client's room, she observes that the intravenous line is not infusing at the ordered rate. The nurse checks the flow regulator on the tubing, looks to see whether the client is lying on the tubing, checks the connection between the tubing and the intravenous catheter, and then checks the condition of the site where the intravenous catheter enters the client's skin. She readjusts the flow rate, and the infusion begins at the correct rate.
   b. The nurse sits down to talk with her client, who lost her sister 2 weeks ago. The client reports that she is unable to sleep, feels very fatigued during the day, and is having trouble at work. The nurse asks her clarify the type of trouble, and the client explains that she cannot concentrate or even solve simple problems. The nurse records the results of her assessment, describing the client's problem as ineffective coping.
   c. In observing a new mother breastfeeding her baby, the public health nurse observes that the baby is fussy and is not sucking effectively. The nurse reviews the baby's record and finds that he has lost a considerable amount of weight since birth. The nurse conducts an assessment and notes that the baby has poor skin turgor. The mother reports that he urinates infrequently and sleeps only for very short periods of time between feedings. The nurse concludes that the baby is dehydrated and is at risk of becoming malnourished.
3. Mr. Yousif is a terminally ill client receiving home care. His wife and son are asking you about his pain control. Mrs. Yousif is requesting that her husband's medication be increased, even if it means he will not be responsive. She does not want her husband to suffer. The son is vehemently opposed to too much narcotic and feels that his father is still able to make decisions for himself. Mr. Yousif remains alert much of the time and is able to talk with you about his feelings regarding death and his desire to die at home. He seems to appreciate your availability in talking with him. How might you use critical thinking to help the family resolve this complex problem?

* REVIEW QUESTIONS

1. You are teaching a 12-year-old boy how to self-administer insulin. After discussing the techniques and demonstrating an injection, you ask him to try it. After two attempts, it is obvious that he does not understand how to prepare the correct dose. You review your approach with the client carefully and ask a colleague for her suggestions about how to improve your teaching skills. This is an example of
   1. Reflection
   2. Risk taking
   3. Client assessment
   4. Care plan evaluation
2. A nurse uses an institution's procedure manual to confirm how to change a client's nasogastric tubing. The level of critical thinking the nurse is using is
   1. Commitment
   2. Scientific method
   3. Basic critical thinking
   4. Complex critical thinking
3. A client had hip surgery 24 hours ago. The nurse refers to the written plan of care, noting that the client has a device collecting wound drainage. The physician is to be notified when the

accumulation in the device exceeds 100 mL for the day. When the nurse enters the room, the nurse looks at the device and carefully notes the amount of drainage currently in the device. This is an example of
1. Planning
2. Evaluation
3. Intervention
4. Assessment

4. The nurse asks a client how she feels about her impending surgery for breast cancer. Before the discussion, the nurse reviewed the description in his textbook of loss and grief in addition to therapeutic communication principles. The critical thinking component involved in the nurse's review of the literature is
   1. Experience
   2. Problem solving
   3. Knowledge application
   4. Clinical decision making

* RECOMMENDED WEB SITES

Canadian Nurses Association: http://www.cna-nurses.ca
A wide range of valuable resources, including the *Code of Ethics for Registered Nurses* (CNA, 2008), can be found on the Web site of the Canadian Nurses Association. This Web site also links to the Web sites of each of the provincial and territorial professional nursing associations in Canada. Visit these Web sites and become familiar with the kinds of resources that are available to you. The position papers and other documents found on these Web sites demonstrate how Canadian nurse leaders have used critical thinking to explore important issues in nursing and nursing practice.

IHMC CMap Tools: A Modelling Kit: http://cmap.ihmc.us
This Web site not only provides an example of a concept map but also provides instruction about how to create one. It illustrates components of a concept map and their relationship to each other.

Insight Assessment/California Academic Press: http://www.insightassessment.com/articles.html
A wide array of articles and case studies related to critical thinking, tools to measure your critical thinking skills, and other vauable resources can be found on this Web site. Many of these resources can be downloaded for free; others are available for purchase.

The Critical Thinking Community: http://www.criticalthinking.org
The section of this Web site titled "The Thinker's Guide Series" includes links to a number of short booklets that explore subjects such as critical thinking concepts and tools, improving your reading, writing and study skills, and ethical reasoning.

Critical Thinking on the Web: A Directory of Quality Online Resources: http://www.austhink.org/critical/index.htm
This Web site links to a wide range of articles in which critical thinking is examined from a variety of perspectives, including nursing. It also contains links to a variety of tutorials that you can use to improve your critical thinking skills.

Critical Thinking Strategies: Concept Mapping: http://cord.org/txcollabnursing/onsite_conceptmap.htm
This Web site provides examples of the use of concept maps in nursing practice.

Student Resources: Critical Thinking Skills: http://distance.uvic.ca/courses/critical/index.htm
This online tutorial assists students in exploring the importance of critical thinking in reading, writing, reasoning, and making judgements.

13

Nursing Assessment and Diagnosis

Original chapter by Patricia A. Potter, RN, MSN, PhD, GMAC, FAAN

Canadian content written by Marilynn J. Wood, RN, BSN, MPH, DrPH, and Janet C. Ross-Kerr, RN, BScN, MS, PhD

objectives

Mastery of content in this chapter will enable you to:

- Define the key terms listed.
- Discuss the steps of nursing assessment.
- Explain the relationship of critical thinking to assessment.
- Differentiate between subjective and objective data
- Discuss the purposes of a client interview.
- Discuss how the use of interview techniques helps clients describe their health histories.
- Describe the components of a nursing history.
- Describe the relationship between data collection and data analysis.
- Explain the relationship between data interpretation, validation, and clustering.
- Conduct a nursing assessment.
- Differentiate between a nursing diagnosis, medical diagnosis, and collaborative problem.
- Discuss the relationship of critical thinking to the nursing diagnostic process.
- Describe the steps of the nursing diagnostic process.
- Explain how defining characteristics and the etiological process individualize a nursing diagnosis.
- Explain the benefit of using the NANDA International nursing diagnoses in practice.
- Describe sources of diagnostic errors.
- Identify nursing diagnoses from a nursing assessment.

key terms

Actual nursing diagnosis, p. 170
Assessment, p. 159
Client-centred plan of care, p. 172
Clinical criteria, p. 169
Closed-ended questions, p. 164
Collaborative problem, p. 167
Cue, p. 160
Data analysis, p. 166
Database, p. 159
Defining characteristics, p. 169
Diagnosis, p. 159
Diagnostic label, p. 171
Etiology, p. 172
Evaluation, p. 159
Health-promotion nursing diagnosis, p. 171
Implementation, p. 159
Inference, p. 160
Interview, p. 163
Medical diagnosis, p. 167
NANDA International, p. 170
Nursing diagnosis, p. 167
Nursing health history, p. 161
Nursing process, p. 159
Objective data, p. 162
Open-ended questions, p. 164
Planning, p. 159
Related factor, p. 172
Review of systems, p. 161
Risk nursing diagnosis, p. 171
Standards, p. 160
Subjective data, p. 162
Validation, p. 165
Wellness nursing diagnosis, p. 171

media resources

evolve Web Site

- Audio Chapter Summaries
- Glossary
- Multiple-Choice Review Questions
- Student Learning Activities
- Weblinks

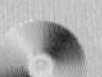
Companion CD

- Glossary
- Interactive Learning Activities
- Fluids and Electrolytes Tutorial
- Test-Taking Skills

The **nursing process** is a problem-solving approach to identifying, diagnosing, and treating the health issues of clients. It is fundamental to how nurses practice. As a nursing student, you will learn the five steps of the nursing process—assessment, diagnosis, planning, implementation, and evaluation—as if they were a linear process (Figure 13–1). However, the nursing process is, in fact, continuous, and in practice, you will learn to move back and forth between the various steps (Potter et al., 2005).

Consider the following scenario:

Lisa, a registered nurse on an orthopedic nursing unit, enters Ms. Devine's room for the first time at 0700 when her shift begins. Ms Devine is a 52-year-old woman who sustained an injury, a ruptured lumbar disc, in a fall 2 months ago. She is scheduled for a lumbar laminectomy this afternoon. When Lisa first observes Ms. Devine, she notes the client is moving in bed awkwardly and is grimacing when she turns. Ms. Devine looks up and states, "Oh, I am so glad you are here. [Sighs] The pain in my back seems worse, and I cannot get comfortable. I cannot sit at all, so I will stay in bed for now. I just dread having this surgery, I will be so glad when this is all over [looks away and avoids eye contact]." Lisa observes Ms. Devine's facial grimace and notes her sighing. She responds, "Ms. Devine, you obviously look uncomfortable and a bit upset. Let me ask you a few questions: Show me where the pain is. On a scale of 0 to 10, with 10 the worst pain ever and 0 no pain, how would you rate your pain? Does it become worse when you turn?" As Ms. Devine responds to the questions, Lisa analyzes the data and considers other relevant information, such as the client's medical diagnosis (ruptured lumbar disc) and knowledge of the alterations that the condition typically causes (e.g., sciatic pain and change in sensation of the lower extremities). Lisa decides that Ms. Devine has acute pain related to pressure on the spinal nerves. Lisa explains to Ms. Devine a plan to help relieve the discomfort. She then administers an ordered analgesic, repositions Ms. Devine, and discusses how Ms. Devine can practice relaxation exercises. Forty minutes later, Lisa returns to Ms. Devine's room to determine whether the pain is relieved and whether she wants to try the relaxation exercises.

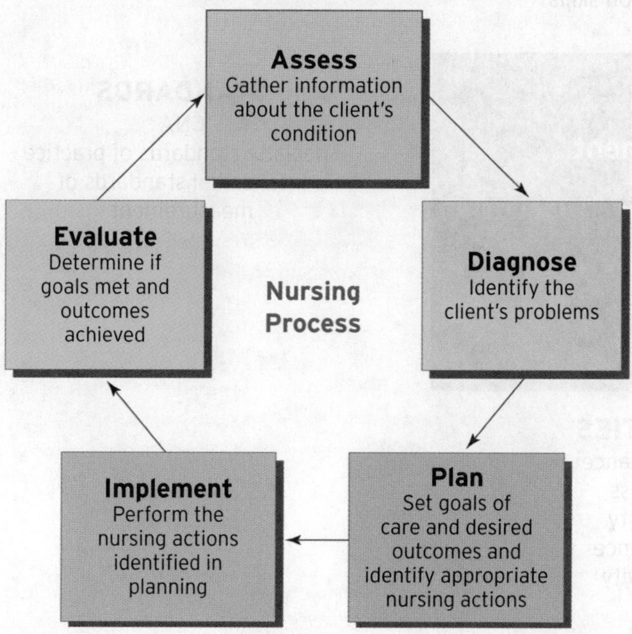

Figure 13–1 Five-step nursing process.

Lisa applied the nursing process while caring for Ms. Devine. Each time you meet a client, you will apply the nursing process to provide appropriate and effective nursing care. The process begins with the first step, **assessment**, the gathering and analysis of information about the client's health status. In the next step, **diagnosis**, you then make clinical judgements about the client's response to health problems in the form of nursing *diagnoses*. Once you establish appropriate nursing diagnoses, you create a plan of care. **Planning** includes interventions individualized to each of the client's nursing diagnoses. The next step, **implementation**, involves the actual performance of planned interventions. After administering interventions, you conduct an **evaluation** of the client's response and whether the interventions were effective. The nursing process is central to your ability to provide timely and appropriate care to your clients.

The nursing process is a variation of scientific reasoning that allows you to organize and systematize nursing practice. You learn to make inferences about the meaning of a client's response to a health problem or generalize about the client's functional state of health. A pattern begins to form. For example, if Ms. Devine is having acute back pain, the data allow Lisa to infer that the client's mobility is limited. Lisa gathers more information (e.g., noting how the client moves and whether the client is able to walk, stand, and sit normally) until the client's problem is classified accurately: for example, as the nursing diagnosis *impaired physical mobility related to acute back pain.* The clear definition of the client's problems provides the basis for planning and implementing nursing interventions and evaluating the outcomes of care.

Critical Thinking Approach to Assessment

Assessment is the deliberate and systematic collection of data to determine a client's current and past health status and functional status and to determine the client's present and past coping patterns (Carpenito-Moyet, 2005). Nursing assessment consists of two steps:

- Collection and verification of data from a primary source (the client) and secondary sources (e.g., family, health professionals, and patient record).
- The analysis of all data as a basis for developing nursing diagnoses, identifying collaborative problems, and developing a plan of individualized care.

The purpose of assessment is to establish a **database** about the client's perceived needs, health problems, and responses to these problems. In addition, the data reveal related experiences, health practices, goals, values, and expectations about the health care system.

When a plumber comes to your home to repair a problem you describe as a "leaking faucet," the plumber checks the faucet, its attachments to the water line, and the water pressure in the system to determine the actual malfunction. Similarly, you see clients who will present an initial health problem to you. You then proceed to observe each client's behaviour, ask questions about the nature of the problem, listen to the cues the client provides, and conduct a physical examination (see Chapter 32). Sometimes you also interview family members who are familiar with the client's health problem, and you review any existing medical record data. All of the data you collect form different sets or patterns of information that point to a diagnostic conclusion. Once a plumber knows the source of the faucet leak, he or she is able to repair the faucet. Similarly, once you know the nature and source of a client's health problems, you are able to provide interventions that will restore, maintain, or improve the client's health.

Critical thinking is important to good assessment (see Chapter 12). Critical thinking allows you to see the big picture when you form conclusions or make decisions about a client's health condition. While gathering data about a client, you synthesize relevant knowledge, recall prior clinical experiences, apply critical thinking **standards** and available evidence, and use standards of practice to direct your assessment in a meaningful and purposeful way (Figure 13–2). Your knowledge of the physical, biological, and social sciences enables you to ask relevant questions and collect history and physical assessment data relevant to the client's presenting health care needs. For example, by knowing that a client has a history of a ruptured lumbar disc, you know to ask whether the client has sciatic pain (characteristic pain that radiates or spreads from the buttocks down the leg) and to question how the discomfort affects the client's ability to walk or sit, inasmuch as these are common symptoms of disc disease. By using good communication skills and critical thinking intellectual standards, you can collect complete, accurate, and relevant data.

Prior clinical experience contributes to the skills of assessment. For example, if you have cared for a client with back pain, you know the pain is sometimes disabling and limits the client's normal motion. Thus, you thoroughly assess the extent to which the pain affects the current client's ability to walk normally and to perform daily living activities. By validating abnormal assessment findings and personally observing assessments performed by skilled professionals, you become competent in assessment. You also learn to apply standards of practice and accepted standards of "normal" for physical assessment data when assessing clients. Use of critical thinking qualities such as creativity, perseverance, and confidence ensure that you compile a comprehensive database.

Data Collection

As you begin a client assessment, think critically about what to assess. On the basis of your clinical knowledge and experience and your client's health history and responses, determine what questions or measurements are appropriate. When you first meet a client, make a quick observational overview or screening. Usually an overview is based on a treatment situation. For example, a community health nurse assesses the neighbourhood and the community of the client; an emergency room nurse uses the airway-breathing-circulation (ABC) approach; and an oncology nurse focuses on the client's symptoms from disease and from treatment and grief response. In the case of Ms. Devine, Lisa first focuses on the nature and severity of her client's pain, the risk of limited mobility, and the extent of the client's anxiety. She will later expand her assessment to determine whether Ms. Devine has been psychologically prepared for her upcoming surgery.

You learn to differentiate important data from the total data collected. A **cue** is information that you obtain through use of the senses. An **inference** is your judgement or interpretation of those cues. For example, a client's crying is a cue that possibly implies fear or sadness. You ask the client about any concerns and make known any nonverbal expressions you notice in an effort to direct the client to share his or her feelings. It is possible to miss important cues when you conduct an initial overview. However, always try to interpret cues from the client to know how in-depth to make your assessment. Remember that thinking is human and imperfect. You will acquire appropriate thinking processes in the conduct of assessment, but expect to make mistakes in missing important cues (Lunney, 2006).

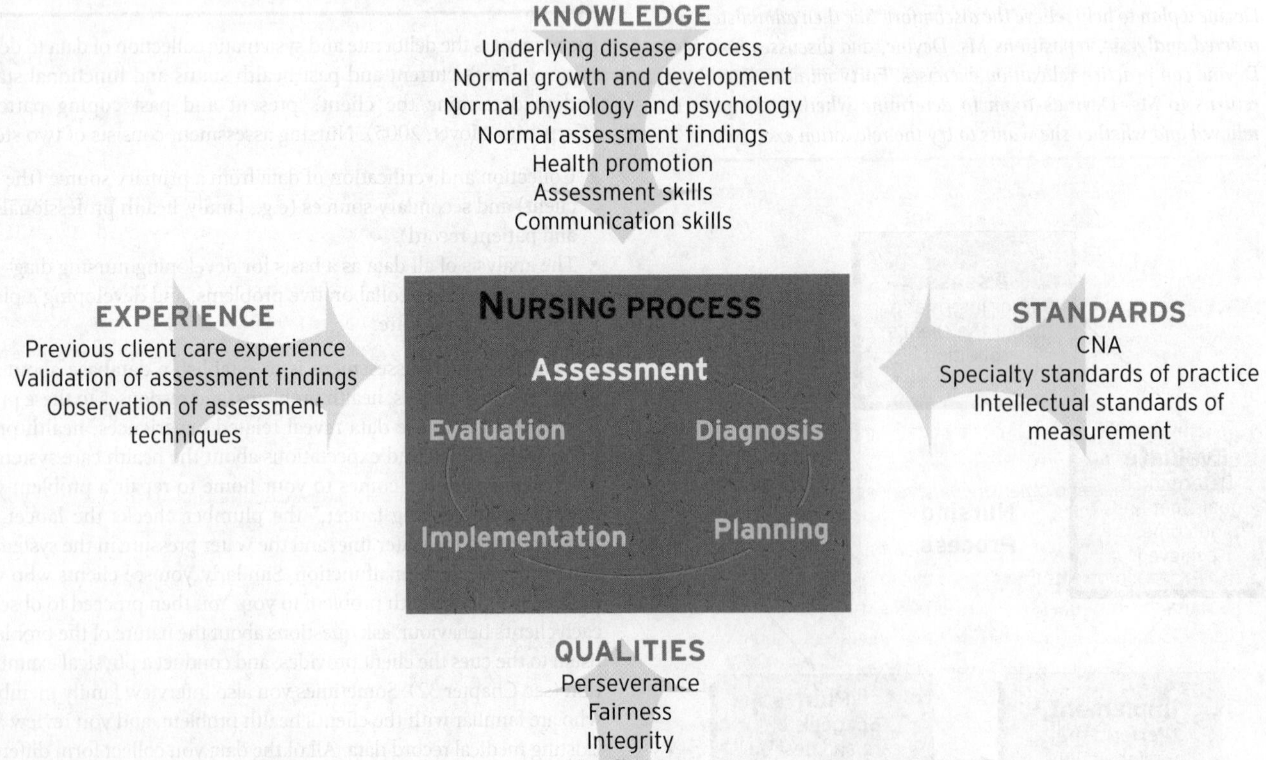

Figure 13-2 Critical thinking and the assessment process.

Assessment is dynamic and allows you to freely explore relevant client problems as you discover them.

Begin your assessment by documenting a comprehensive **nursing health history**, a detailed database that allows you to plan and carry out nursing care to meet the client's needs. Box 13–1 presents guidelines for documenting a comprehensive history. This approach encourages you to focus on your client's strengths and available supports, as well as on the presenting problem.

As you collect data, you begin to categorize cues, make inferences, and identify emerging patterns, potential problem areas, and

➤ BOX 13-1 Guidelines for Documenting a Comprehensive Nursing Health History

A. Identifying Data

Name, age, sex, date, and place of birth.

B. Reason for Health History Interview

Explain why you are interviewing the client at the present time (e.g., the client has just been admitted to an inpatient unit or clinic).

C. Current State of Health

General state of health and health goals. If an illness is present, gather data about the nature of the illness by conducting a symptom analysis (see Chapter 32).

D. Developmental Variables

- Marital status: single, married, separated, widowed, divorced.
- Number of children.
- Developmental stage (see Chapter 22).
- Current occupation.
- Significant life experiences (e.g., education, previous occupations, financial situations, retirement, coping or stress tolerance, and measures normally used to reduce stress).
- Safety hazards (e.g., biological, chemical, ergonomic, physical, psychosocial, reproductive).
- Housing, environmental hazards (e.g., type of housing, location, living arrangements; specific hazards in the home or community).
- Safety measures (e.g., use of seat belts, presence of smoke detectors and fire extinguishers, and other measures related to specific hazards of work, community, and home).

E. Psychological Variables

Mental processes, relationships, support systems, statements regarding client's feelings about self.

F. Spiritual Variables

Rituals, religious practices, beliefs about life, clients' source of guidance in acting on beliefs, and the relationship with family in exercising faith.

G. Sociocultural Variables

- Culture: beliefs and practices related to health and illness (see Chapter 10).
- Primary language and other languages spoken.
- Recreation (exercise, hobbies, socializing, use of leisure time).
- Family and significant others. Include family composition, relationships, special problems experienced by family, client's and family's response to stress, roles, and support systems. The family history provides information about family structure, interaction, and function that may be useful in planning care. For example, a cohesive, supportive family can help a client adjust to an illness or disability and should be incorporated into the plan of care. However, if the client's family members are not supportive, it may be better not to involve them in care. Outline a family tree (genogram; see Chapter 20) to determine whether the client is at risk for genetic illnesses and to identify areas of health promotion and illness prevention.

H. Physiological Variables (Body Structure and Function)

History of Past Illnesses and Injuries

Including dates.

Current Medications

Prescribed, over-the-counter, or illicit drugs. Include name, dosage, schedule, duration of and reason for use, and expected effects and side effects; if illicit drug, include type, amount, response, adverse reaction, drug-related accidents or arrests, attempts to quit.

Review of Systems

The **review of systems** is a systematic method for collecting data on all body systems. Not all questions in each system may be covered in every history. Nevertheless, some questions about each system are included, particularly when a client mentions a symptom or sign. The nurse begins with questions about the usual functioning of each body system and any noted changes and follows with specific questions such as the ones noted as follows for each system. Nurses also focus on measures taken by the client to promote and maintain health and those to prevent illness or injury. The following are included in the review of systems:

- *General manifestation of symptoms:* fever, chills, malaise, pain, sleep patterns and disturbances, fatigue, recent alterations in weight.
- *Integumentary:* itching, colour or texture change, lesions, dryness and use of creams or lotions, changes in hair or nails.
- *Ocular:* visual acuity, blurring, eye pain, recent change in vision, discharge, excessive tearing, date of last examination.
- *Auditory:* hearing loss, pain, discharge, dizziness, perception of ringing in ears, wax.
- *Upper respiratory:* nosebleeds, nasal discharge, nasal allergies, sinus problems, frequency of colds and usual method of treatment, sore throat and usual type of home remedy, hoarseness or voice changes.
- *Lower respiratory:* use of tobacco (amount and number of years of smoking; exposure to tobacco smoke; if smoker, attempts to stop smoking), exposure to airborne pollutants, cough, sputum, wheezing, shortness of breath, tuberculosis test and results, date of last chest X-ray examination.
- *Breasts and axillae:* rashes, lumps, discharge, pain, breast self-examination practices.
- *Lymphatic:* pain, swelling.
- *Cardiovascular:* chest pain or distress, precipitating causes, timing and duration, relieving factors, dyspnea, orthopnea, edema, hypertension, exercise tolerance, circulatory problems, varicose veins.
- *Gastrointestinal:* appetite, digestion, food intolerance, dysphagia, heartburn, abdominal pain, nausea or vomiting, bowel regularity, use of laxatives, change in stool colour or contents, constipation or diarrhea, flatulence, hemorrhoids, rectal examinations.
    a. Dietary pattern: calculate number of servings per day of each of the food groups, using *Canada's Food Guide to Healthy Eating* (http://www.nms.on.ca/Elementary/canada.htm) for serving size (see Chapter 43); restrictions to food choice; special diets; use of salt; calculate adequacy of fluid intake (should be 30 to 40 mL of fluid per kilogram of body weight); indicate sources of calcium and

Continued

BOX 13-1 Guidelines for a Comprehensive Nursing Health History *continued*

amounts per day, alcohol use (average number of ounces per week, recent changes in pattern of consumption).

- *Urinary:* painful urination; blood, stones, or pus in urine; bladder or kidney infections; difficulty stopping urinary stream; dribbling or hesitancy; sudden feeling of need to urinate; frequent urination; nocturia (having to get up to void during the night); incontinence (see Chapter 44).
- *Genital and reproductive:*
  a. Male: puberty onset, difficulty with erections, emissions, testicular pain, libido, infertility, urethral discharge, genital lesions, exposure to and history of sexually transmitted infections, testicular self-examinations, testicular lump or pain, hernias, sexual preference, birth control method, and safer sex practices used.
  b. Female: menses (onset, duration, regularity, flow, discomfort, date of most recent menstrual period), age at menopause (occurrence of hot flashes, night sweats, vaginal discharge), date of last Pap smear, pregnancies (number, miscarriages, abortions), exposure to and history of sexually transmitted infections, sexual preference, birth control method, and safer sex practices used.
- *Musculoskeletal:* pain, joint stiffness or swelling, restricted motion, muscle wasting, weakness, general mobility.
- *Neurological:* injury, headaches, dizziness, fainting, abnormalities of sensation or coordination, tremors, seizures.
- *Endocrine:* excessive sweating, thirst, hunger, or urination; intolerance of heat or cold; changes in distribution of facial hair; thyroid enlargement or tenderness; unexplained weight change; change in glove or shoe size.
- *Hematological:* anemia; bruise or bleed easily; transfusions.
- *Psychiatric:* depression, mood changes, difficulty concentrating, nervousness, anxiety, suicidal thoughts, irritability.
- *Immunological:* communicable diseases (indicate disease and age at or year of onset), immunization status (indicate year of most recent immunization), allergies (known allergens and reactions; MedicAlert identification worn).

Adapted from Skillen, D. L., & Day, R. A. (2004). *A syllabus for adult health assessment.* Edmonton, AB: University of Alberta, Faculty of Nursing.

solutions. To do this well, you critically anticipate patterns, problems, and solutions, which means you try to stay a step ahead of the assessment. Before you make an inference, remember to document cues that support the inference. Your inferences will direct you to further questions. Once you ask a question of a client or make an observation, the information "branches" to an additional series of questions or observations (Figure 13–3). If you do not anticipate assessment questions, your assessment may be incomplete, or you may fail to recognize cues and dismiss relevant problem areas. Knowing how to probe and frame questions is a skill that you hone with experience. You learn to decide which questions are relevant to a situation and to interpret the data accurately.

Types of Data

Data can be obtained from two primary sources: subjective and objective. **Subjective data** are your clients' verbal descriptions of their health problems. Only clients provide subjective data. For example, Ms. Devine's report of back pain and her expression of dread over anticipating surgery are subjective findings. Subjective data usually include feelings, perceptions, and self-report of symptoms. Although only clients provide subjective data relevant to their health condition, be aware that the data sometimes reflect physiological changes, which you further explore through objective data collection.

Objective data are observations or measurements of a client's health status. Inspection of the condition of a wound, a description of an observed behaviour, and the measurement of blood pressure are examples of objective data. The measurement of objective data is based on an accepted standard, such as the Fahrenheit or Celsius measure on a thermometer, centimetres on a measuring tape, or known characteristics of behaviours (e.g., anxiety or fear). When you collect objective data, apply critical thinking intellectual standards (e.g., whether the data are clear, precise, and consistent) so that you can correctly interpret your findings.

Sources of Data

As a nurse, you obtain data from a variety of sources. Each source of data provides information about the client's level of wellness, strengths, anticipated prognosis, risk factors, health practices and goals, and patterns of health and illness.

Client. A client is usually your best source of information. Clients who are conscious, alert, and able to answer questions correctly provide the most accurate information about their health care needs, lifestyle patterns, current and past illnesses, perception of symptoms, and changes in activities of daily living. Always consider the setting for your assessment. A client experiencing acute symptoms in an emergency department will not offer as much information as one who comes to an outpatient clinic for a routine checkup. Always be attentive, and show a caring presence with the client (see Chapter 19). Let the client know you are interested in what he or she has to say. Clients are less likely to reveal the nature of their health care problems fully when nurses show little interest or are easily distracted by activities around them.

Family and Significant Others. Family members and significant others are primary sources of information for infants or children, critically ill adults, and mentally handicapped, disoriented, or unconscious clients. In cases of severe illness or emergency situations, families are sometimes the only available sources of information for nurses and clients' health care professionals. The family and significant others are also important secondary sources of information. They confirm findings that a client provides (e.g., whether a client takes medications regularly at home or how well the client sleeps or eats). Include interviewing the family when appropriate. Remember also that a client does not always wish you to question the family.

Spouses or close friends often sit in during an assessment and provide their view of the client's health problems or needs. They not only supply information about the client's current health status but also are able to tell when changes in the client's status occurred. Family members are often very well informed because of their experiences living with the client and observing how health problems affect daily living activities. Family and friends make important observations about the client's needs that can affect the way care is delivered (e.g., how a client eats a meal or how a client makes choices).

Health Care Team. You frequently communicate with other health care team members in gathering information about clients. In the acute care setting, the change-of-shift report is the way for nurses from one shift to communicate information to nurses on the next

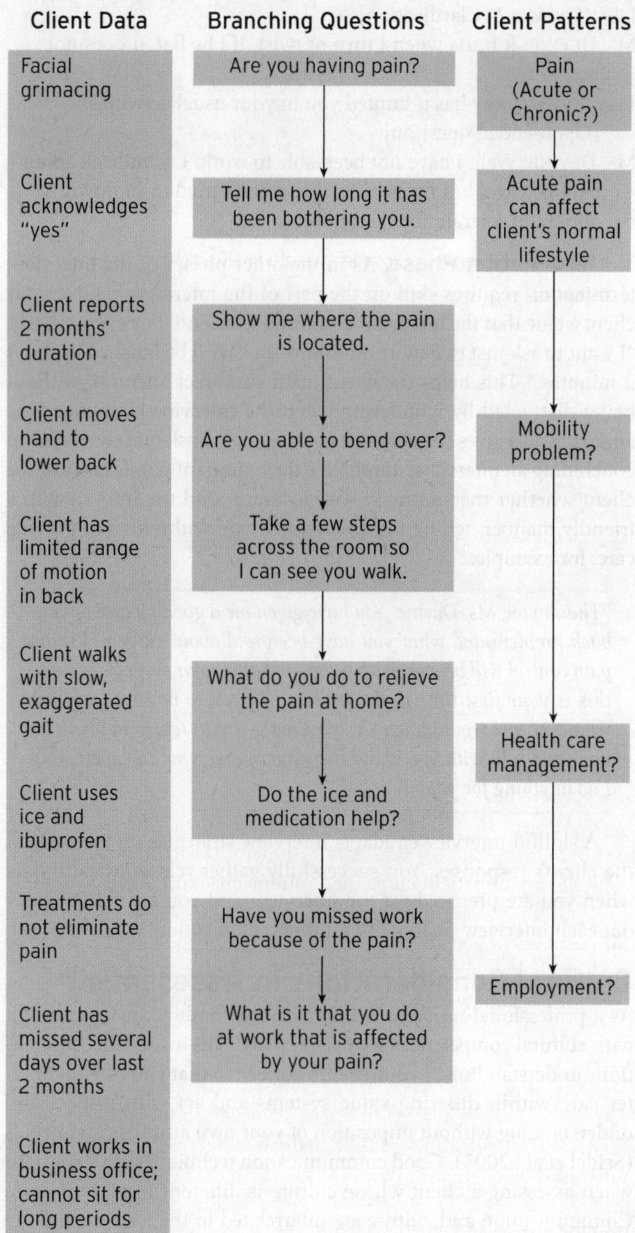

Figure 13-3 Example of branching logic for selecting assessment questions.

shift (see Chapter 16). When nurses, physicians, physical therapists, social workers, or other staff consult about a client's condition, they typically have information about the client. This information includes how the client is interacting within the health care environment, the client's physical or emotional reactions to treatment, the result of diagnostic procedures or therapies, and how the client responds to visitors. Every member of the team is a source of information for identifying and verifying information about the client.

Medical Records. The medical record is a source of the client's medical history, laboratory and diagnostic test results, current physical findings, and the medical treatment plan. Data in the records offer baseline and ongoing information about the client's response to illness and progress to date. Information in a client's record is confidential. The medical record is a valuable tool for checking the consistency and similarities of personal observations.

Literature. You complete your assessment database by reviewing nursing, medical, and pharmacological literature about a client's illness. This review increases your knowledge about the client's diagnosed problems, expected symptoms, treatment, prognosis, and established standards of therapeutic practice. A knowledgeable nurse obtains relevant, accurate, and complete information for the assessment database.

Nurse's Experience. Benner and Wrubel (1989) noted that through experience, a nurse learns to ask the right questions, choosing only the questions that will elicit the most useful information. A nurse's expertise develops after testing and refining propositions, questions, and principle- or standard-based expectations. For example, after Lisa has cared for Ms. Devine, she has learned some lessons. Lisa will more quickly recognize the behaviour the client showed while in acute pain when she cares for the next client with similar health problems. Lisa will also note how positioning techniques helped Ms. Devine relax and ameliorated her discomfort. Practical experience and the opportunity to make clinical decisions strengthen your critical thinking.

Methods of Data Collection

As a nurse, you use the client interview, nursing health history, physical examination findings, and results of laboratory and diagnostic tests to establish a client's assessment database.

Interview. The first step in establishing a database is to collect subjective information by interviewing the client. An **interview** is an organized conversation with the client. The initial formal interview involves obtaining the client's health history and information about the current illness. During the initial interview, you have the opportunity to do the following:

- Introduce yourself to the client, explain your role, and explain the role of other health care professionals during care.
- Establish a caring therapeutic relationship with the client.
- Obtain insight about the client's concerns and worries.
- Determine the client's goals and expectations of the health care system.
- Obtain cues about which parts of the data collection phase necessitate further in-depth investigation.

You and the client become partners during the interview, rather than your controlling the interview. An interview consists of three phases, similar to that of a therapeutic relationship: orientation, working, and termination.

A successful interview requires preparation. Collect any available information about the client, and then create a favourable environment for the interview. An environment in which the client is comfortable and relaxed helps you conduct a good interview. Some clients interviewed at home prefer that the interview take place in a bedroom, away from other family members, or in the living room, with a spouse present. Remember to let a client decide whether to involve the family. Finally, select a place private enough to allow the client to be comfortable when providing personal information.

Orientation Phase. During the orientation phase of the interview, you introduce yourself, describe your position, and explain the purpose of the interview. Explain to clients why you are collecting data (e.g., for a nursing history or for a focused assessment) and assure them that any information obtained will remain confidential and will be used only by health care professionals who provide their care.

After making Ms. Devine more comfortable, Lisa decides that it is time to get to know her client better. Lisa reviews the interview process and its objectives, confidentiality, and length. "I want to spend some time better understanding your back pain and then what you know about your surgery. If you are comfortable, I would like to spend about 10 minutes discussing this with you. Everything you share will be confidential." Lisa and Ms. Devine agree mutually on the interview time.

LISA: Now, I want to ask you some questions about your health so we can plan your care together. Before we get started, do you have any questions for me?

MS. DEVINE: Yes. I know they plan to remove the disc in my back. It has been hurting so bad. I can't even bend over. Is there a chance I could be paralyzed?

LISA: Tell me what your doctor has explained about surgery.

MS. DEVINE: She has told me that I have a, what was it called, a herniated disc. She said it is pinching nerves in my back. Well, if it pinches nerves, could I not become paralyzed? She did tell me that she has done this procedure many times before.

LISA: A herniated disc is serious. The disc is normally situated between two vertebrae, but in your case it is now pinching on your spinal nerves. That is why you have so much discomfort. Your surgery is aimed at removing pressure on your nerves. I would suggest you talk with your doctor about your concerns before going into surgery.

MS. DEVINE: Okay, that makes me feel a little better. I have some important things going on at my work. My husband and I own our own business. I just want this to be over.

LISA: Tell me more about your pain.

Working Phase. In the working phase of the interview, you gather information about the client's health status. Remember to stay focused, orderly, and unhurried. Use a variety of communication strategies such as active listening, paraphrasing, and summarizing to promote a clear interaction (see Chapter 18). The use of open-ended questions encourages clients to describe their health histories in detail.

During the working phase, obtain a nursing health history by exploring the client's current illness, health history, and expectations of care. The objective for collecting a health history is to identify patterns of health and illness, risk factors for physical and behavioural health problems, changes from normal function, and available resources for adaptation. The initial interview is normally the most extensive. Ongoing interviews, which occur each time you interact with your client, do not need to be as extensive; their purpose is to update the client's status and focus more on changes in previously identified ongoing and new problems. An example of Lisa's interview techniques is as follows:

LISA: Tell me, Ms. Devine, about your back pain. [Open-ended question]

MS. DEVINE: Sometimes it is really sharp, especially when I stand and try to walk.

LISA: On a scale of 0 to 10, with 0 being no pain and 10 being the worst imaginable, how would you rate your pain when it becomes sharp? [Close-ended question]

MS. DEVINE: Oh, it can be bad; I would rate it an 8 or 9.

LISA: Point to where you notice the pain. [Asking for specificity]

MS. DEVINE: [points to her lower sacral area] It hurts here, and I also get a deep burning pain in my right buttock.

LISA: Can you tell me if anything else aggravates the pain?

MS. DEVINE: This morning I sneezed and thought I was going to faint. Then I could feel the pain go down my right leg.

LISA: Does anything else worsen the pain? [Probes for completeness]

MS. DEVINE: Well, just about any way I move tends to make my back hurt.

LISA: Any way? [Clarification]

MS. DEVINE: It hurts when I turn or twist. If I lie flat, it does not bother me.

LISA: In what way has it limited you in your usual activities? [Open-ended question]

MS. DEVINE: Well, I have not been able to work. I went back about a month ago, but I was miserable when I tried to sit down. I could not tolerate the discomfort.

Termination Phase. As in the other phases of the interview, termination requires skill on the part of the interviewer. Give your client a clue that the interview is coming to an end. For example, say, "I want to ask just two more questions" or "We'll be finished in about 2 minutes." This helps the client maintain direct attention without being distracted by wondering when the interview will end. This approach also gives the client an opportunity to ask questions. When concluding an interview, summarize the important points and ask the client whether the summary was accurate. End the interview in a friendly manner, telling the client when you will return to provide care; for example:

"Thank you, Ms. Devine. You have given me a good picture of your back problem and what you have been told about surgery. I think pain control will be a priority before and after your surgery. Because this is your first time in the hospital, I want to be sure I explain whatever you would like to know. I am going to return in about an hour and talk with you about the surgery and what to expect. Can I do anything for you now?"

A skillful interviewer adapts interview strategies on the basis of the client's responses. You successfully gather relevant health data when you are prepared for the interview, and you are able to carry out each interview phase with minimal interruption.

Cultural Considerations in Assessment

As a professional nurse, it is important to conduct any assessment with cultural competence (see Chapter 10). This involves a conscientious understanding of your client's culture so that you can offer better care within differing value systems and act with respect and understanding without imposition of your own attitudes and beliefs (Seidel et al., 2003). Good communication techniques are important when assessing a client whose culture is different from your own. Communication and culture are interrelated in the way feelings are expressed verbally and nonverbally. If you can learn the variations in how people of different cultures communicate, you will probably be able to gather more accurate information from clients. For example, the Spanish and French use firm eye contact when speaking. However, this is considered rude or immodest by certain Asian or Middle Eastern cultures. North Americans often tend to let the eyes wander (Seidel et al., 2003). By using the right approach with eye contact, you show respect for your client, and the client is probably encouraged to share more information.

When you interact to assess any specific client, first know your own cultural self. You need to avoid forming a sense of the client on the basis of prior information about the client's culture. Instead, draw upon your knowledge and then ask questions in a constructive and probing way to allow you to truly understand the client.

Use **open-ended questions** whenever you are not sure what the answer will be and when you want description in the client's own words (Box 13–2). Remember that **closed-ended questions** can all be answered by "yes" or "no" (or a choice of answers that you provide), and limit these to issues in which you do not need additional information from the client.

> **BOX 13-2 Examples of Open- and Closed-Ended Questions**
>
> **Open-Ended Questions**
>
> Tell me how you are feeling.
> Your discomfort affects your ability to get around in what way?
> Describe how your wife has been helping you.
> Give me an example of how you get relief from your pain at home.
>
> **Closed-Ended Questions**
>
> Do you feel as if the medication is helping you?
> Who is the person who helps you at home?
> Do you understand why you are having the X-ray examination?
> Has the warm compress given you relief from your back pain?
> Are you having pain now?
> On a scale of 0 to 10, how would you rate your pain?

Nursing Health History

You document a nursing health history during either your initial contact or an early contact with a client. The history is a major component of assessment. Although many health history forms are structured, you learn to use the questions as starting points. A good assessor learns to refine and broaden questions as needed in order to correctly assess the client's unique needs. Time and client priorities determine how complete a history is. Identify patterns of information about a client's health and illness by collecting data about all health dimensions (see Box 13–1). Incorporating data from all dimensions allows you to develop a complete plan of care.

Family History

The purpose of documenting the family history is to obtain data about immediate and blood relatives. The objectives are to determine whether the client is at risk for illnesses of a genetic or familial nature and to identify areas of health promotion and illness prevention (see Chapter 21). The family history also provides information about family structure, interaction, and function that is often useful in planning care (see Chapter 20). For example, a close, supportive family will help a client adjust to an illness or disability, and so you incorporate information from the family into the plan of care. If the client's family is not supportive, however, it is better to not involve family members in care. Stressful family relationships are sometimes a significant barrier when you try to help clients with problems involving loss, self-concept, spiritual health, and personal relationships.

Documentation of History Findings

As you conduct the nursing health history, record your assessment in a clear, concise manner, using appropriate terminology. Standardized forms make it easy to enter data as the client responds to questions. In settings that have computerized documentation, entry of assessment data is very easy. A clear, concise record is necessary for use by other health care professionals (see Chapter 16). Regardless of the model used in a documentation system, you want a thorough database that provides historical and current information about the client's health. This information then becomes the baseline against which you evaluate any future changes.

Physical Examination

A physical examination is an investigation of the body to determine its state of health. A physical examination involves use of the techniques of inspection, palpation, percussion, auscultation, and smell (see Chapter 32). A complete examination includes measurements of a client's height, weight, and vital signs and a head-to-toe examination of all body systems. By performing actual hands-on physical assessment, you gather valuable objective information that helps in forming accurate diagnostic conclusions. Always conduct an examination with sensitivity and competence to prevent your client from becoming anxious.

Observation of Client Behaviour. Throughout an interview and physical examination, it is important for you to observe a client's verbal and nonverbal behaviours closely. The information enhances your objective database. You learn to determine whether data obtained by observation matches what the client verbally communicates. For example, if a client expresses no concern about an upcoming diagnostic test but shows poor eye contact, shakiness, and restlessness, all suggestive of anxiety, then verbal and nonverbal data conflict. Observations direct you to gather additional objective information to form accurate conclusions about the client's condition. An important aspect of observation includes a client's level of function: the physical, developmental, psychological, and social aspects of everyday living. Observation of the level of function differs from observations you make during an interview. Observation of level of function involves watching what a client does, such as eating or making a decision about preparing a medication, rather than what the client tells you he or she can do. Observation of function can occur in the home or in a health care setting during a return visit.

Diagnostic and Laboratory Data. The results of diagnostic and laboratory tests reveal or clarify alterations questioned or identified during the nursing health history and physical examination. For example, during the history documentation, the client reports having a bad cold for 6 days and at present has a productive cough with brown sputum and mild shortness of breath. On physical examination, you notice an elevated temperature, increased respirations, and decreased breath sounds in the right lower lobe. You review the results of a complete blood cell count and note that the white blood cell count is elevated (indicating an infection). In addition, the radiologist's report of a chest X-ray examination shows the presence of a right lower lobe infiltrate. Such findings combined are suggestive of the medical diagnosis of pneumonia and the associated nursing diagnosis of *impaired gas exchange.*

Some clients collect and monitor laboratory data in the home. For example, clients with diabetes mellitus often perform daily blood glucose monitoring. Ask clients about their routine results to determine their responses to illness and elicit information about the effects of treatment measures. Compare laboratory data with the established norms for a particular test result, age group, and gender.

Interpreting Assessment Data and Making Nursing Judgements. The successful analysis and interpretation of assessment data requires critical thinking. When you correctly analyze data, you recognize patterns that lead you to make necessary clinical decisions about your client's care. These decisions are in the form of either nursing diagnoses or collaborative problems that require treatment from several disciplines (Carpenito-Moyet, 2005). When you critically think about interpreting assessment information, you determine the presence of abnormal findings, what further observations you need to clarify information, and the client's health problems.

Data Validation. Before you begin analyzing and interpreting data, validate the collected information you have, in order to avoid making incorrect inferences (Carpenito-Moyet, 2005). **Validation** of assessment data is the comparison of data with another source to determine data accuracy. For example, you observe a client crying and logically infer it is related to hospitalization or a medical diagnosis. Making such an initial inference is not wrong, but problems result if you do not validate the inference with the client. Instead, say, "I notice that you have been crying. Can you tell me about it?" By questioning the client, you will discover the real reason for the crying behaviour. Ask your client to validate the information obtained during the interview and history. Validate findings from the physical examination and observation of client behaviour by comparing data in the medical record and by consulting with other nurses or health care team members. Often family or friends are able to validate your assessment information. Validation opens the door for gathering more assessment data because it involves clarifying vague or unclear data. On occasion, you need to reassess previously covered areas of the nursing history or gather further physical examination data. Continually analyze and think about a client's database to make concise, accurate, and meaningful interpretations. Critical thinking applied to assessment enables you to fully understand the client's problems, to judge the extent of the problems carefully, and to discover possible relationships between the problems.

Lisa gathered initial data about the character of Ms. Devine's back pain. She applied critical thinking in her assessment as she considered what she knew about ruptured lumbar discs and the anticipated type of symptoms that clients experience. As she assessed Ms. Devine, she applied intellectual standards, obtaining information that was precise (location of pain), consistent and accurate (use of pain rating scale), and complete (probing for factors that worsen pain). Lisa learned additional information about Ms. Devine's concerns about surgery. Ms. Devine tells Lisa, "I hope the surgery goes well. You know, I have a friend who had back surgery, and she took a long time to recover. I want to get back to work without a long absence. If this had just not happened—why did I have to fall?" Lisa could make several inferences from this information, but she applies the critical thinking attitude of discipline and stays focused to ensure her assessment is accurate and comprehensive. She validates her inferences with Ms. Devine, "You sound anxious about having surgery. You know of others who have had difficult outcomes after surgery. Do you think you are uncertain about what to expect?" Ms. Devine confirms Lisa's assessment, "Yes, I am worried. I have never been in a hospital, as you know, and I feel I do not know what that involves. I am a person who likes to have information, so I can make the right decisions and know what to do."

Analysis and Interpretation. After you collect extensive information about a client, you analyze and interpret the data. You begin analysis by organizing the information into meaningful and usable clusters, keeping in mind your client's response to illness. A data cluster is a set of signs or symptoms that you group together in a logical way. During data clustering, organize data and focus attention on client functions for which support or assistance for recovery is needed. **Data analysis** involves recognizing patterns or trends in the clustered data, comparing them with standards, and then establishing a reasoned conclusion about the client's responses to a health problem (Box 13–3). Patterns of meaning begin to form, enabling you to make inferences about client problems. Through reasoning and judgement, you decide what information explains the client's health status. At times, you need to gather additional information to clarify your interpretation. For example, Ms. Devine told Lisa that she had not been in a hospital and did not know what that involved. Lisa inferred or guessed that Ms. Devine had limited knowledge about the laminectomy and the associated nursing care. Instead of making that conclusion, Lisa sought further information by asking, "Tell me what your doctor has told you about your surgery." Ms. Devine related, "Well I know the doctor is going to remove something between my vertebrae. She said I will be in the hospital about 2 or 3 days." Lisa asked, "Has anyone talked with you about your care after surgery?" Ms. Devine replied, "No, not really. I have several questions I would like to ask about it." Lisa listened to the additional information provided by Ms. Devine. In looking for patterns of data, Lisa decided that Ms. Devine had a knowledge deficiency because of her limited preparation for the surgery but was interested in learning. If you are successful in clustering data well in your analysis, you will become proficient in identifying individualized nursing diagnoses and in identifying collaborative problems (see Figure 13–6).

During clustering, a cue or an individual sign, symptom, or finding will alert you more than others do. Such cues are especially helpful in identifying nursing diagnoses. In time, you will become experienced in recognizing clusters that indicate problems such as pain, anxiety, or immobility. Clustering also helps make documentation more concise and focused.

Data Documentation

Data documentation is the last part of a complete assessment. The timely, thorough, and accurate documentation of facts is necessary when client data are recorded. If you do not record an assessment finding or problem interpretation, that information is lost and unavailable to anyone else caring for the client. If specific information is lacking, the person reading the report is left with only general impressions. Observation and recording of client status is a legal and professional responsibility. Recording factual information is easy after it becomes a habit. The basic rule is to record all observations. When you record data, pay attention to facts, and make an effort to be as descriptive as possible. Anything heard, seen, felt, or smelled should be reported exactly. Record objective information in accurate terminology (e.g., "weighs 170 lbs," "abdomen is soft and nontender to palpation"). Record subjective information from a client in quotation marks. When entering data, do not generalize or form judgements through written communication. Conclusions about such data become nursing diagnoses and thus must be accurate. As you gain experience and become familiar with clusters and patterns of signs and symptoms, you will conclude the existence of the correct problem. (Review Chapter 16 for details on documentation.)

Concept Mapping. Most of the clients you care for have more than one health problem. A concept map is a visual representation that allows you to graphically show the connections between a client's many health problems. Hinck et al. (2006) showed that concept mapping is an effective learning strategy to understand the relationships that exist between client problems. Your first step in concept mapping is to organize the assessment data you collect for your client. Placing all of the cues together into clusters that form patterns will

➤ BOX 13-3 Steps of Data Analysis

1. Recognize a pattern or trend by cues:
   - Turns slowly
   - Is unable to bend over
   - Walks with hesitation
2. Compare with normal standards:
   - Has normal range of motion
   - Initiates movement without hesitation
3. Make a reasoned conclusion:
   - Has limited mobility
   - Has reduced activity level

lead you to the next step of the nursing process: nursing diagnosis. Through concept mapping, you obtain a holistic perspective of your client's health care needs, which ultimately leads you to make better clinical decisions (King & Shell, 2002). Figure 13–4 shows the first step in a concept map that Lisa will develop for Ms. Devine as a result of her nursing assessment.

Nursing Diagnosis

After you assess a client thoroughly to compile a database, the next step of the nursing process is to form diagnostic conclusions that determine the nursing care that a client receives (Figure 13–5). Some of the conclusions lead to nursing diagnoses, whereas others do not. Diagnostic conclusions include problems treated primarily by nurses (nursing diagnoses) and problems necessitating treatment by several disciplines (collaborative problems). Together, nursing diagnoses and collaborative problems represent the range of client conditions that necessitate nursing care (Carpenito-Moyet, 2005).

When physicians refer to commonly accepted medical diagnoses, such as myocardial infarction, diabetes mellitus, or osteoarthritis, they all know the meaning of the diagnoses and the standard approaches to treatment. A **medical diagnosis** is the identification of a disease condition on the basis of a specific evaluation of physical signs, symptoms, the client's medical history, and the results of diagnostic tests and procedures. Physicians are licensed to treat diseases or pathological processes described in medical diagnostic statements. Nurses have a similar diagnostic language. **Nursing diagnosis,** the second step of the nursing process, determines health problems within the domain of nursing. The process of diagnosing is the result of your analysis of data and your resultant identification of specific client responses to health care problems. The term *diagnose* means "distinguish" or "know." A nursing diagnosis is a clinical judgement about individual, family, or community responses to actual and potential health problems or life processes that is within the domain of nursing (NANDA International, 2007).

A **collaborative problem** is an actual or potential physiological complication that nurses monitor to detect the onset of changes in a client's status (Carpenito-Moyet, 2005). When collaborative problems develop, nurses intervene in collaboration with personnel from other health care disciplines. Nurses manage collaborative problems such as hemorrhage, infection, and cardiac arrhythmia by using both physician-prescribed and nursing-prescribed interventions to minimize complications. For example, a client who has a surgical wound is at risk for developing an infection, and so a physician prescribes antibiotics. The nurse monitors the client for fever and other signs of infection and implements appropriate wound care measures.

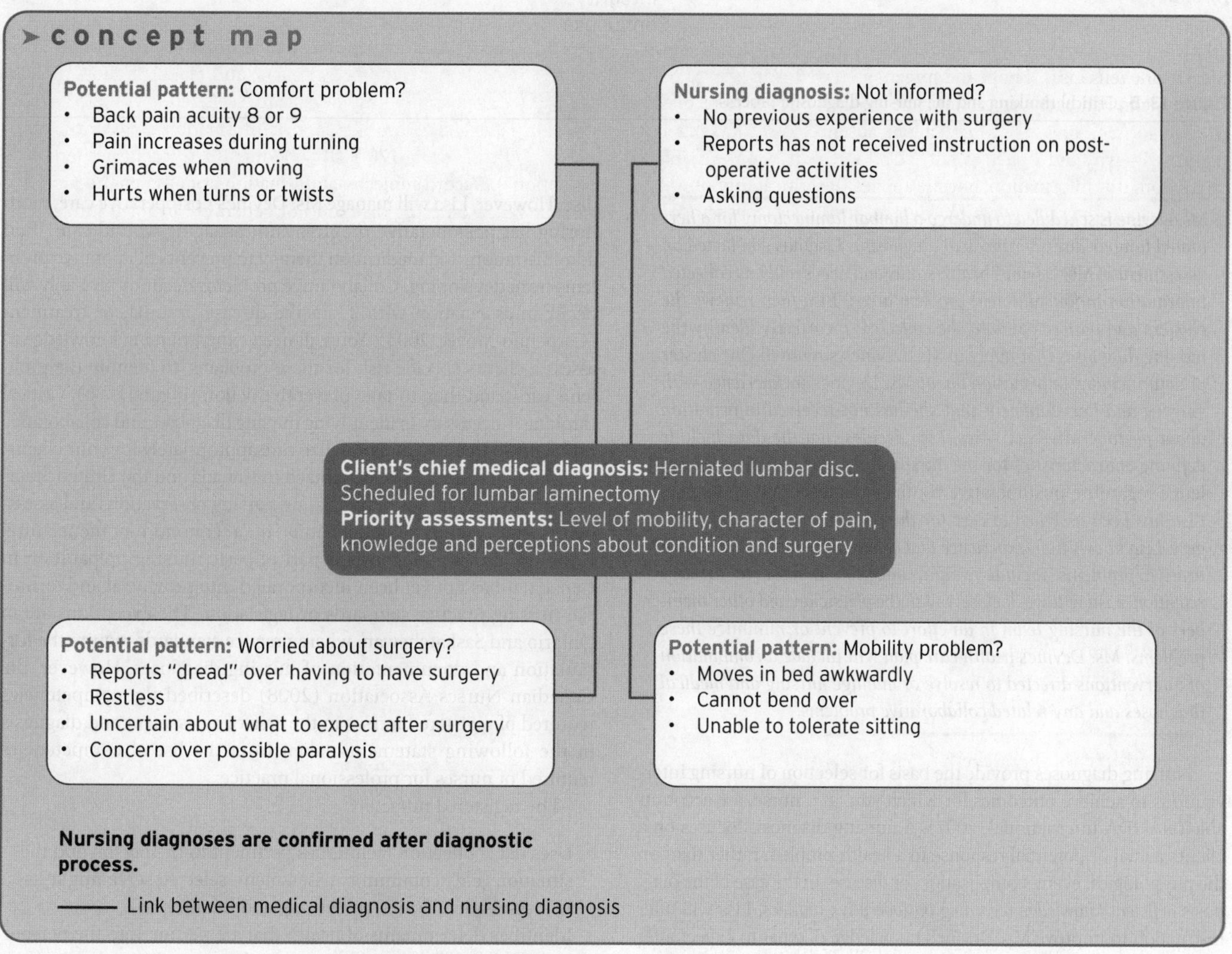

Figure 13–4 Concept map for Ms. Devine's nursing assessment findings.

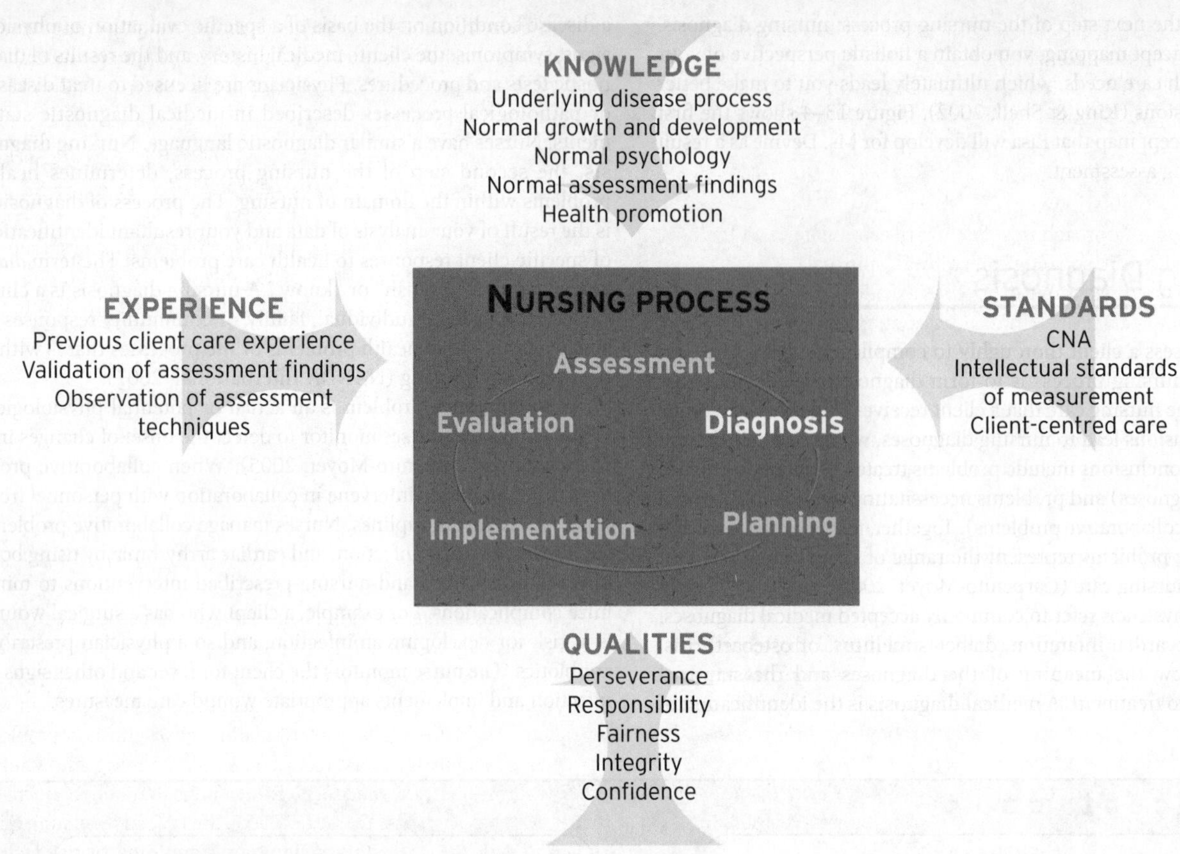

Figure 13-5 Critical thinking and the nursing diagnostic process.

Ms. Devine is scheduled to undergo a lumbar laminectomy for a herniated lumbar disc (her medical diagnosis). Lisa has conducted an assessment of Ms. Devine's health status and needs and has collected information in four different problem areas. Lisa then reviews the clusters and patterns of data she collected to correctly identify the nursing diagnoses that apply to Ms. Devine's situation. One cluster of data includes information about Ms. Devine's inexperience with surgery and her statement that she has not received information about postoperative activities. Lisa decides that the data include defining characteristics for the nursing diagnosis deficient knowledge regarding postoperative routines related to inexperience. *Lisa has been assigned to care for the client on the day after surgery. Lisa knows from experience that common postoperative collaborative problems include wound infection and acute urinary retention. Lisa will work closely with the physician and other members of the nursing team in an effort to prevent or minimize these problems. Ms. Devine's health care plan will include a combination of interventions directed to resolve or manage nursing and medical diagnoses and any related collaborative problems.*

Nursing diagnoses provide the basis for selection of nursing interventions to achieve outcomes for which you, as a nurse, are accountable (NANDA International, 2007). A nursing diagnosis focuses on a client's actual or potential response to a health problem rather than on the physiological event, complication, or disease. In the case of the diagnosis *deficient knowledge regarding postoperative routines,* Lisa will offer instruction to improve Ms. Devine's knowledge of what to expect after surgery and how she is able to participate in her postoperative care. A nurse cannot independently treat a medical diagnosis such as a herniated disc. However, Lisa will manage Ms. Devine's postoperative care, monitoring her postoperative progress and managing wound care, fluid administration, and medication therapy to prevent collaborative problems from developing. Collaborative problems occur or probably will occur in association with a specific disease, trauma, or treatment (Carpenito-Moyet, 2005). You will need expert nursing knowledge to assess a client's specific risk for these problems, to identify the problems early, and then to take preventive action (Figure 13–6). Critical thinking is necessary in identifying nursing diagnoses and collaborative problems so that you individualize care appropriately for your clients.

Nursing diagnosis is recognized in Canada and the United States as an innovative means of translating nursing observations and assessments into standard conclusions in a common nomenclature. Although nursing diagnosis is part of basic nursing preparation in Canada, it has not yet been incorporated into provincial and territorial nursing practice standards or legislation. The exceptions are in Ontario and Saskatchewan, where practice standards require the formulation and documentation of nursing diagnoses. However, the Canadian Nurses Association (2008) described the competencies required of registered nurses in the area of assessment and diagnosis in the following statements taken from the list of competencies required of nurses for professional practice:

The registered nurse:

- Uses data collection techniques pertinent to the person and the situation (e.g., community assessment, selected screening tests, risk assessment scales, measuring and monitoring).
- Identifies determinants of health that are pertinent to the person and the situation (e.g., income, social status, education, employment, work conditions).

- Identifies actual or potential health problems/risk factors (e.g., hypertension, diabetes, obesity).
- Identifies actual or potential safety risks to the person (e.g., incidents and accidents, environmental pollution, mechanical equipment).
- Identifies actual or potential risks of abuse (e.g., domestic violence, elder abuse, bullying).
- Uses a holistic approach in collecting relevant data (e.g., biological, psychological, sociological, cultural, spiritual).
- Collects data from a range of appropriate sources (e.g., the person, previous and current health records/nursing care plans/collaborative plans of care, family members/significant persons/substitute decision maker, census data, and epidemiological data, other health care providers).
- Uses appropriate assessment techniques for data collection (e.g., observation, inspection, auscultation, palpation, percussion, selected screening tests, interview, consultation, focus group, measuring and monitoring).
- Assesses psychological and psychosocial adaptation (e.g., recognizes depression and uses resources to assess depression).
- Individualizes the assessment to the person (e.g., growth and development stage, culture, physical and mental challenges).
- Validates data collected with the person and appropriate sources.
- Analyses data to establish relationships among the various data collected (e.g., determines relationship between health assessment and laboratory values).
- Integrates nursing knowledge with knowledge from the arts, humanities, and medical and social sciences to interpret data.
- Identifies actual and potential health problems or issues.

It is clear from these statements regarding nursing competencies that nursing diagnosis is intrinsic to professional practice in Canada. The use of standard formal nursing diagnostic statements (Box 13–4) serves several purposes:

1. They provide a precise definition that gives all members of the health care team a common language for understanding the client's needs.
2. They allow nurses to communicate their actions among themselves, to other health care professionals, and to the public.
3. They distinguish the nurse's role from that of the physician or other health care professionals.
4. They help nurses focus on the scope of nursing practice.
5. They foster the development of nursing knowledge.

Critical Thinking and the Nursing Diagnostic Process

Diagnostic reasoning is a process of using assessment data about a client to logically explain a clinical judgement: in this case, a nursing diagnosis. The diagnostic process flows from the assessment process and includes decision-making steps. These steps include data clustering, identifying client needs, and formulating the diagnosis or problem.

Clusters and patterns of data often contain **defining characteristics**, the clinical criteria or assessment findings that help confirm an actual nursing diagnosis. **Clinical criteria** are objective or subjective signs and symptoms, clusters of signs and symptoms, or risk factors

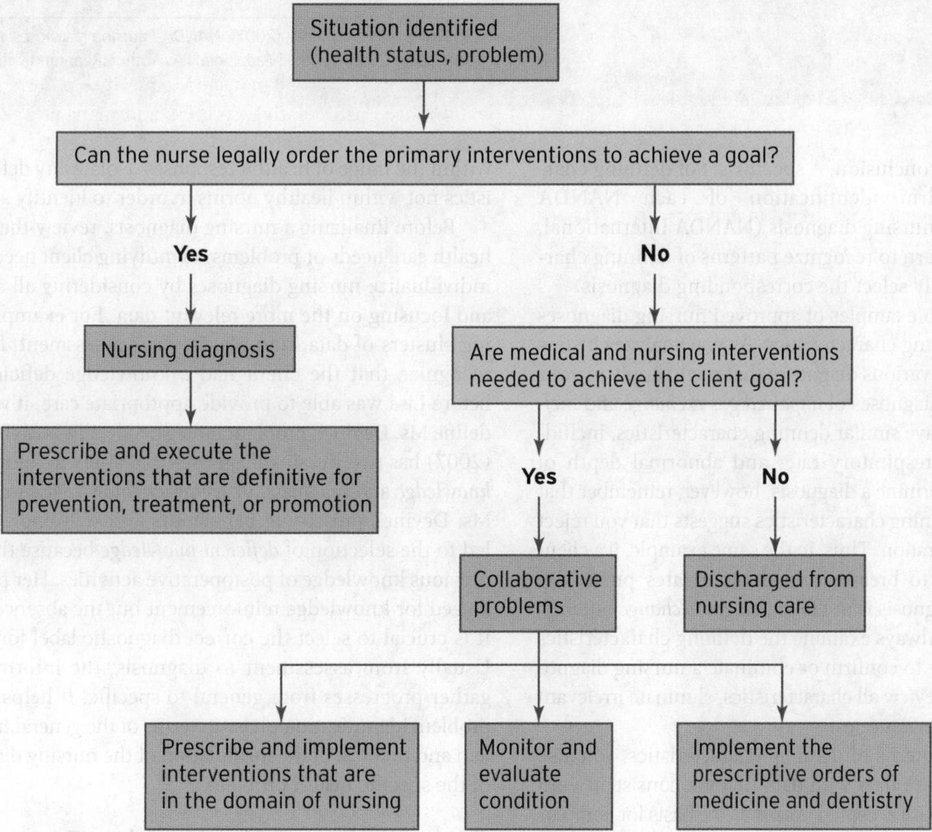

Figure 13-6 Differentiating nursing diagnoses from collaborative problems. **Source:** Copyright 1990, 1988, 1985 by Lynda Juall Carpenito. Redrawn from Carpenito, L. J. (1995). *Nursing diagnosis: Application to clinical practice* (6th ed.). Philadelphia, PA: J. B. Lippincott.

➤ BOX 13-4 Examples of NANDA International Nursing Diagnoses

Activity intolerance
Risk for *activity* intolerance
Ineffective *airway* clearance
Latex *allergy* response
Risk for latex *allergy* response
Anxiety
Death *anxiety*
Risk for *aspiration*
Risk for impaired parent–child *attachment*
Autonomic dysreflexia
Risk for *autonomic* dysreflexia
Risk-prone health *behaviour*
Disturbed *body* image
Risk for imbalanced *body* temperature
Bowel incontinence
Effective *breastfeeding*
Ineffective *breastfeeding*
Interrupted *breastfeeding*
Ineffective *breathing* pattern
Decreased *cardiac* output
Caregiver role strain
Risk for *caregiver* role strain
Readiness for enhanced *comfort*
Impaired verbal *communication*
Readiness for enhanced *communication*
Decisional *conflict*
Parental role *conflict*
Acute *confusion*
Chronic *confusion*
Risk for acute *confusion*
Constipation
Perceived *constipation*
Risk for *constipation*
Contamination
Risk for *contamination*
Compromised family *coping*
Defensive *coping*
Disabled family *coping*
Ineffective *coping*
Ineffective community *coping*
Readiness for enhanced *coping*
Readiness for enhanced community *coping*
Readiness for enhanced family *coping*
Risk for sudden infant *death* syndrome
Readiness for enhanced *decision making*
Ineffective *denial*
Impaired *dentition*
Risk for delayed *development*
Diarrhea
Risk for compromised human *dignity*
Moral *distress*
Risk for *disuse* syndrome
Deficient *diversional* activity
Disturbed *energy* field
Impaired *environmental* interpretation syndrome
Adult *failure* to thrive
Risk for *falls*
Dysfunctional *family* processes: alcoholism
Interrupted *family* processes

From NANDA International. (2007). *NANDA-I nursing diagnoses: Definitions and classification, 2007–2008*. Philadelphia, PA: Author. Reprinted with permission.

that lead to a diagnostic conclusion. A specific set of defining characteristics helps confirm identification of each **NANDA International**–approved nursing diagnosis (NANDA International, 2007). As a nurse, you learn to recognize patterns of defining characteristics and then readily select the corresponding diagnosis.

Table 13–1 shows two examples of approved nursing diagnoses and their associated defining characteristics. As you analyze clusters of data, begin to consider various diagnoses that might apply to your client. For example, the diagnoses of *impaired gas exchange* and *ineffective breathing pattern* have similar defining characteristics, including dyspnea, abnormal respiratory rate, and abnormal depth of breathing. When you determine a diagnosis, however, remember that the absence of certain defining characteristics suggests that you reject a diagnosis under consideration. Thus, in the same example, if a client uses accessory muscles to breathe and demonstrates pursed-lip breathing, the correct diagnosis is not *impaired gas exchange* but *ineffective breathing pattern*. Always examine the defining characteristics in your database carefully to confirm or eliminate a nursing diagnosis. To be more accurate, review all characteristics, eliminate irrelevant ones, and confirm the relevant ones.

While focusing on patterns of defining characteristics, you also compare a client's pattern of data with data that are consistent with normal, healthy patterns. Use accepted norms as the basis for comparison and judgement. These norms include laboratory and diagnostic test values, professional standards, and normal anatomical or physiological limits. When comparing patterns, judge whether the grouped signs and symptoms are normal for the client and whether they are within the range of healthy responses. Isolate any defining characteristics not within healthy norms in order to identify a problem.

Before finalizing a nursing diagnosis, review the client's general health care needs or problems. Identifying client needs allows you to individualize nursing diagnoses by considering all assessment data and focusing on the more relevant data. For example, after reviewing clusters of data from Ms. Devine's assessment, Lisa was able to recognize that the client had a knowledge deficiency. However, before Lisa was able to provide appropriate care, it was necessary to define Ms. Devine's problem more specifically. NANDA International (2007) has two nursing diagnoses that apply to knowledge: *deficient knowledge* and *readiness for enhanced knowledge*. A careful review of Ms. Devine's presenting behaviours and self-report of the problem led to the selection of *deficient knowledge* because the client had no previous knowledge of postoperative activities. Her problem was not a need for knowledge reinforcement but the absence of knowledge. It is crucial to select the correct diagnostic label for a client's need. Usually from assessment to diagnosis, the information that you gather progresses from general to specific. It helps to think of the problem identification phase in terms of the general health care problem and to think of the formulation of the nursing diagnosis in terms of the specific health problem.

Formulation of the Nursing Diagnosis

NANDA International (2007) identified four types of nursing diagnoses: actual diagnoses, risk diagnoses, health promotion diagnoses, and wellness diagnoses. An **actual nursing diagnosis**

➤ TABLE 13-1 Examples of NANDA International-Approved Nursing Diagnoses With Defining Characteristics

Diagnosis: Impaired Gas Exchange	Diagnosis: Ineffective Breathing Pattern
Defining Characteristics	
Dyspnea	Dyspnea
Abnormal rate, rhythm, depth of breathing	Bradypnea: in clients aged 14 years and older, ≤11 respirations/minute
Abnormal arterial pH	Decreased vital capacity
Abnormal skin colour (pale, dusky)	Orthopnea
Hypoxemia	Altered chest excursion
Hypercarbia	Use of accessory muscles to breathe
Hypoxia	Tachypnea: in clients aged 14 years and older, >24 respirations/minute
Confusion	Pursed-lip breathing
Related Factors	
Ventilation perfusion imbalance	Hyperventilation
Alveolar–capillary membrane changes	Pain
	Chest wall deformity
	Anxiety
	Musculoskeletal impairment
	Body position

Data from NANDA International. (2007). *NANDA-I nursing diagnoses: Definitions and classification, 2007–2008*. Philadelphia, PA: Author.

describes responses to health conditions or life processes that exist in an individual, family, or community. Defining characteristics (manifestations, signs, and symptoms) that cluster in patterns of related cues or inferences support this diagnostic judgement (NANDA International, 2007). The selection of an actual diagnosis indicates that sufficient assessment data are available to establish the nursing diagnosis. In the case of Ms. Devine, Lisa assessed the client to have back pain with a severity rated from 8 to 9 on a 10-point scale. The pain increased with movement. As a result of the pain, Ms. Devine has slept poorly. *Acute pain* is an actual nursing diagnosis.

A **risk nursing diagnosis** describes human responses to health conditions or life processes that will possibly develop in a vulnerable individual, family, or community (NANDA International, 2007). For example, after Ms. Devine undergoes the laminectomy, she has a surgical incision. The hospital environment poses a risk for infection. Thus, after Ms. Devine's surgery, Lisa chooses the nursing diagnosis *risk for infection*. The key assessment for this type of diagnosis is the presence of data that reveal risk factors (incision and hospital environment) that confirm Ms. Devine's vulnerability. Such data include physiological, psychosocial, familial, lifestyle, and environmental factors that increase the client's vulnerability to, or likelihood of developing, the condition.

A **health-promotion nursing diagnosis** is a clinical judgement of a person's, family's, or community's motivation and desire to increase well-being and actualize human health potential, as expressed in their readiness to enhance specific health behaviours, such as nutrition and exercise. Health-promotion diagnoses can be used in any health state; they do not reflect current levels of wellness (NANDA International, 2007).

A **wellness nursing diagnosis** describes levels of wellness in an individual, family, or community that can be enhanced (NANDA International, 2007). It is a clinical judgement about an individual, group, or community in transition from a specific level of wellness to a higher level of wellness. You select this type of diagnosis when the client wishes to or has achieved an optimal level of health. For example, *readiness for enhanced coping related to successful cancer treatment* is a wellness diagnosis, and the nurse and the family unit work together to adapt to the stressors associated with cancer survivorship. In doing so, the nurse incorporates the client's strengths and resources into a plan of care, with the outcome directed at improving the level of coping.

Components of a Nursing Diagnosis

The nursing diagnosis results from the assessment and diagnostic process. Throughout this text, nursing diagnoses are in a two-part format: the diagnostic label followed by a statement of a related factor (Table 13–2). It is this two-part format that provides a diagnosis meaning and relevance for a particular client. In addition, all NANDA International–approved diagnoses have a definition. Risk factors are a component of all risk nursing diagnoses.

Diagnostic Label. The **diagnostic label** is the name of the nursing diagnosis as approved by NANDA International (2007) (see Table 13–1). It describes the essence of a client's response to health conditions in as few words as possible. Diagnostic labels include

➤ TABLE 13-2 NANDA International (2007) Nursing Diagnosis Format

Diagnostic Statement	Related Factors
Acute pain	Biological, chemical, physical, or psychological injury agents (e.g., inflammation, edema, burn)
Anxiety	Stress Unmet needs Interpersonal transmission Situational or maturational crises
	Fluid retention Impaired skin integrity Excessive secretions Immobilizations Altered circulation

descriptors used to give additional meaning to the diagnosis. For example, the diagnosis *impaired physical mobility* includes the descriptor *impaired* to describe the nature or change in mobility that best describes the client's response. Examples of other descriptors are *compromised, decreased, deficient, delayed, effective, imbalanced, impaired,* and *increased.*

Related Factors. The **related factor** is a condition or **etiology** identified from the client's assessment data. It is associated with the client's actual or potential response to the health problem and can be changed through the use of nursing interventions. For example, in the case of Ms. Devine, Lisa assessed that Ms. Devine had not received instruction on postoperative activities and that Ms. Devine was asking questions. Lisa also learned that Ms. Devine had not undergone surgery before. The nursing diagnostic statement for Ms. Devine will include the diagnostic label (e.g., *deficient knowledge regarding postoperative routines*) and the related factor (e.g., *related to lack of exposure to instruction*) (Figure 13–7). Because of the related factor *lack of exposure to instruction,* Lisa will implement client instruction on postoperative activities. The "related to" phrase is not a cause-and-effect statement; rather, it indicates that the etiology contributes to or is associated with the client's diagnosis (Figure 13–8). The inclusion of the "related to" phrase requires you to use critical thinking skills to individualize the nursing diagnosis and then select nursing interventions (Table 13–3). The origin or cause of the nursing diagnosis is always within the domain of nursing practice and a condition that responds to nursing interventions.

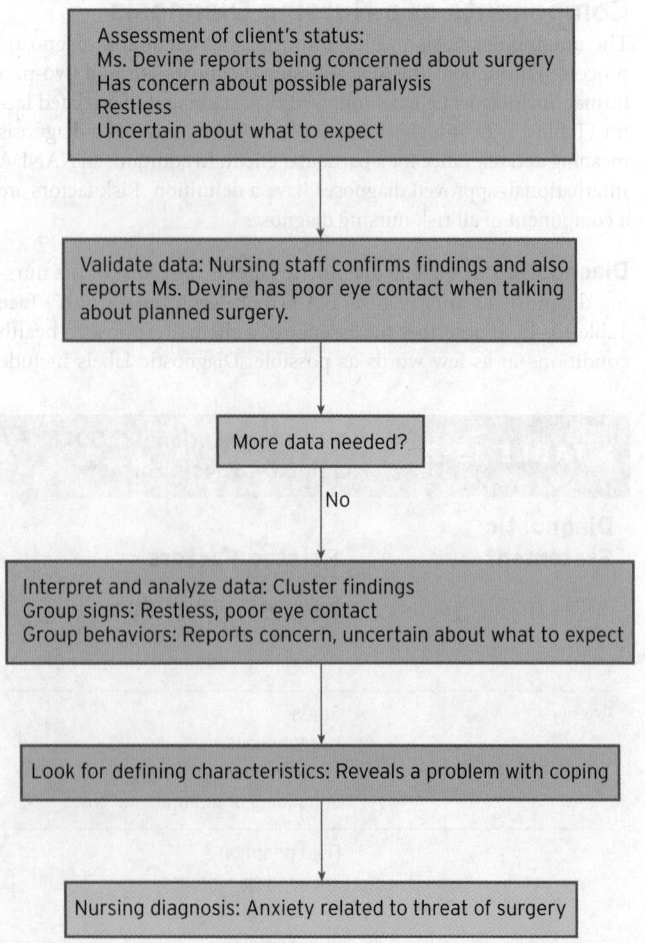

Figure 13-7 Diagnostic process for Ms. Devine.

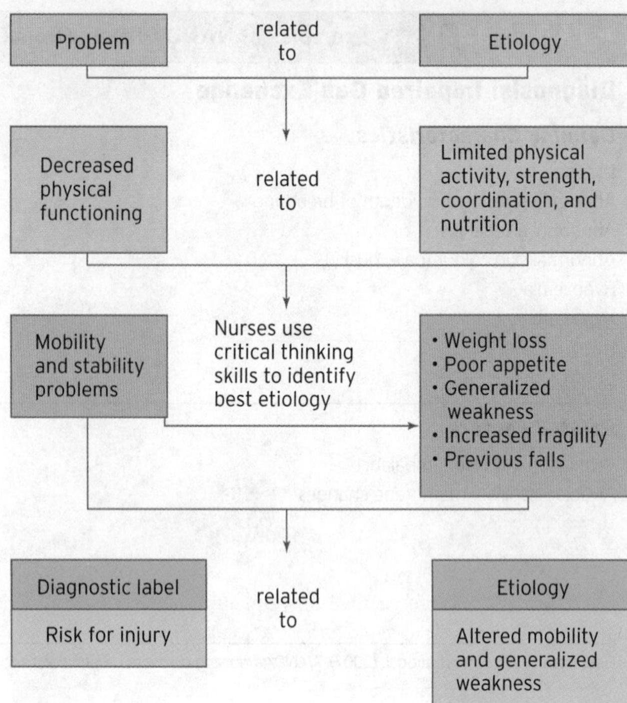

Figure 13-8 Relationship between a diagnostic label and an etiology (related factor). **Source:** Redrawn from Hickey, P. (1990). *Nursing process handbook.* St. Louis, MO: Mosby.

Sometimes health care professionals record medical diagnoses as the etiology in the nursing diagnosis. This is incorrect. Nursing interventions do not change a medical diagnosis. However, you direct nursing interventions at behaviours or conditions that you are able to treat or manage. For example, the nursing diagnosis *acute pain related to herniated disc* is incorrect; nursing actions do not affect the medical diagnosis of a herniated disc. Instead, a diagnosis of *acute pain related to pressure on spinal nerves* results in nursing interventions directed at reducing stress on the vertebrae, improving body alignment, and offering nonpharmacological comfort measures.

Table 13–4 demonstrates the association between a nurse's assessment of a client, the clustering of defining characteristics, and formulation of nursing diagnoses. The diagnostic process results in the formation of a total diagnostic label that enables a nurse to develop an appropriate, **client-centred plan of care.** The defining characteristics and relevant etiologies are from NANDA International (2007).

Definition. NANDA International (2007) approved a definition for each diagnosis that follows clinical use and testing. The definition describes the characteristics of the human response identified. For example, the definition of the diagnostic label *impaired physical mobility* is the "limitation in independent, purposeful physical movement of the body or of one or more extremities" (NANDA International, 2007). You will refer to definitions of nursing diagnoses to assist in identifying a client's correct diagnosis.

Risk Factors. Risk factors are environmental, physiological, psychological, genetic, or chemical elements that increase the vulnerability of an individual, family, or community to an unhealthful event (NANDA International, 2007). They are a component of all risk nursing diagnoses. The risk factors are cues to indicate that a risk nursing diagnosis is applicable to a client's condition. Examples of risk factors for the nursing diagnosis *risk for infection* include

➤ TABLE 13-3 Comparison of Interventions for Nursing Diagnoses with Different Etiologies

Nursing Diagnoses	Interventions
Client A	
Anxiety related to uncertainty over surgery	Provide detailed instructions about the surgical procedure, recovery process, and postoperative care activities Plan formal time for client to ask questions
Impaired physical mobility related to acute pain	Administer analgesics 30 minutes before planned exercise Instruct client in technique to splint painful site during activity
Client B	
Anxiety related to loss of job	Consult with social work to arrange for job consulting Encourage client to continue health promotion activities (e.g., exercise, routine social activities)
Impaired physical mobility related to musculoskeletal injury	Have client perform active range-of-motion exercises to affected extremity every 2 hours Instruct client on use of three-point crutch gait

invasive procedures, trauma, malnutrition, immunosuppression, and insufficient knowledge to avoid exposure to pathogens. The risk factors help you select the correct risk diagnosis, similar to the manner in which defining characteristics help you formulate actual nursing diagnoses. In addition, risk factors are valuable when you plan preventive nursing interventions.

Support of the Diagnostic Statement. Nursing assessment data must support the diagnostic label, and the related factors need must be included in these data. To collect complete, relevant, and correct assessment data, it helps to identify assessment activities that produce specific kinds of data. For example, asking the client about the quality and perception of pain elicits subjective data. However, if palpating an area elicits a facial grimace, that grimace is objective information. Likewise, asking a client to describe the perception of an irregular heartbeat elicits subjective information, and using auscultation to obtain a pulse elicits an objective measurement of heart rate and rhythm. When you review assessment data to look for clusters of defining characteristics, consider whether you have probed and assessed the client accurately and thoroughly to gather a complete database.

Concept Mapping for Nursing Diagnoses

When caring for a client or groups of clients, you need to think critically about client needs and how to prevent problems from developing. Your holistic view of a client heightens the challenge of thinking about all client needs and problems. Few clients have single problems. Nurses often care for clients with multiple nursing diagnoses. Therefore, a "picture" of each client usually consists of several interconnections between sets of data all associated with identified client problems (Mueller et al., 2002). Concept mapping is one way to graphically represent the connections between concepts and ideas that are related to a central subject (e.g., the client's health problems).

Hsu and Hsieh (2005) described a concept map as a scheme that displays visual knowledge in the form of a hierarchical graphic network. In a concept map, assessment data are depicted as the relationships of a client's problems to one another (Schuster, 2003). As you proceed in applying each step of the nursing process, your concept map expands with more detail about planned interventions. A concept map promotes critical thinking by causing you to identify,

➤ TABLE 13-4 Defining Characteristics and Etiologies to Confirm Nursing Diagnoses

Assessment Activities	Defining Characteristics (Clustering Cues)	Nursing Diagnoses	Etiologies ("Related to")
Ask client to rate severity of pain on a scale from 0 to 10 Observe client's positioning in bed	Client verbally reports pain at a level of 8 or 9 when it becomes sharp Client bends knees while on back to lessen pain	Acute pain	Physical pressure on spinal nerves
Ask whether client has difficulty falling asleep or awakens during night from pain Observe for any nonverbal signs of discomfort	Client reports feeling tired, awakens easily Client moans and sighs when attempting to find comfortable position in bed	Acute pain	Physical pressure on spinal nerves
Observe client's eye contact when client is talking Observe client's body language Ask client to describe feelings about surgery	Client has poor eye contact when discussing surgery Client is restless Client is uncertain about what to expect after surgery and the outcome of surgery	Anxiety	Threat to health status as a result of surgery
Give instruction in topic of interest, and return in 15 minutes to measure retention	Client forgets details of explanation	Anxiety	Threat to health status as a result of surgery

graphically display, and link key concepts by organizing and analyzing information (Hsu & Hsieh, 2005).

Figure 13–9 shows the development of Lisa's concept map for Ms. Devine. Lisa began during the assessment step of the nursing process to gather a database for Ms. Devine. Her assessment included Ms. Devine's perspective of her health problems, as well as the objective and subjective data Lisa collected through observation and examination. Lisa validated findings and added to the database as she learned new information. Data sources include physical, psychological, and sociocultural domains.

Lisa applies clinical reasoning and intuition that reflects her own basic nursing knowledge, her past experiences with clients, patterns that she observed in similar situations, and reference to institutional standards and procedures (e.g., pain management policies or postoperative teaching protocols) (Ferrario, 2004). As Lisa begins to observe patterns of defining characteristics, she places labels to identify the four nursing diagnoses that apply to Ms. Devine. She is also able to see the relationship between the diagnoses and connects them on the care map graphic. If Ms. Devine continues to be anxious, Lisa knows from her experience in caring for clients with pain that Ms. Devine's pain will increase. Likewise, increased pain will heighten anxiety. Anxiety also influences how well Ms. Devine will attend to any instructions, but until she understands what to expect, her anxiety will not diminish. Ms. Devine's pain, if unrelieved, will likely worsen her immobility.

Concept mapping organizes and links information to allow you to see new wholes and appreciate the complexity of client care (Ferrario, 2004). Lisa's next step on the care map will be to identify the nursing interventions appropriate for Ms. Devine's care.

The advantage of a concept map is its central focus on the client rather than on the client's disease or health alteration. This focus encourages students of nursing to concentrate on clients' specific health concerns and nursing diagnoses (Mueller et al., 2002). It also promotes client participation with the eventual plan of care.

Sources of Diagnostic Errors

Errors occur in the nursing diagnostic process during data collection, interpretation and analysis, clustering, and in statement of the diagnosis. As a nurse, you need to apply methodical critical thinking so that the nursing diagnostic process is accurate.

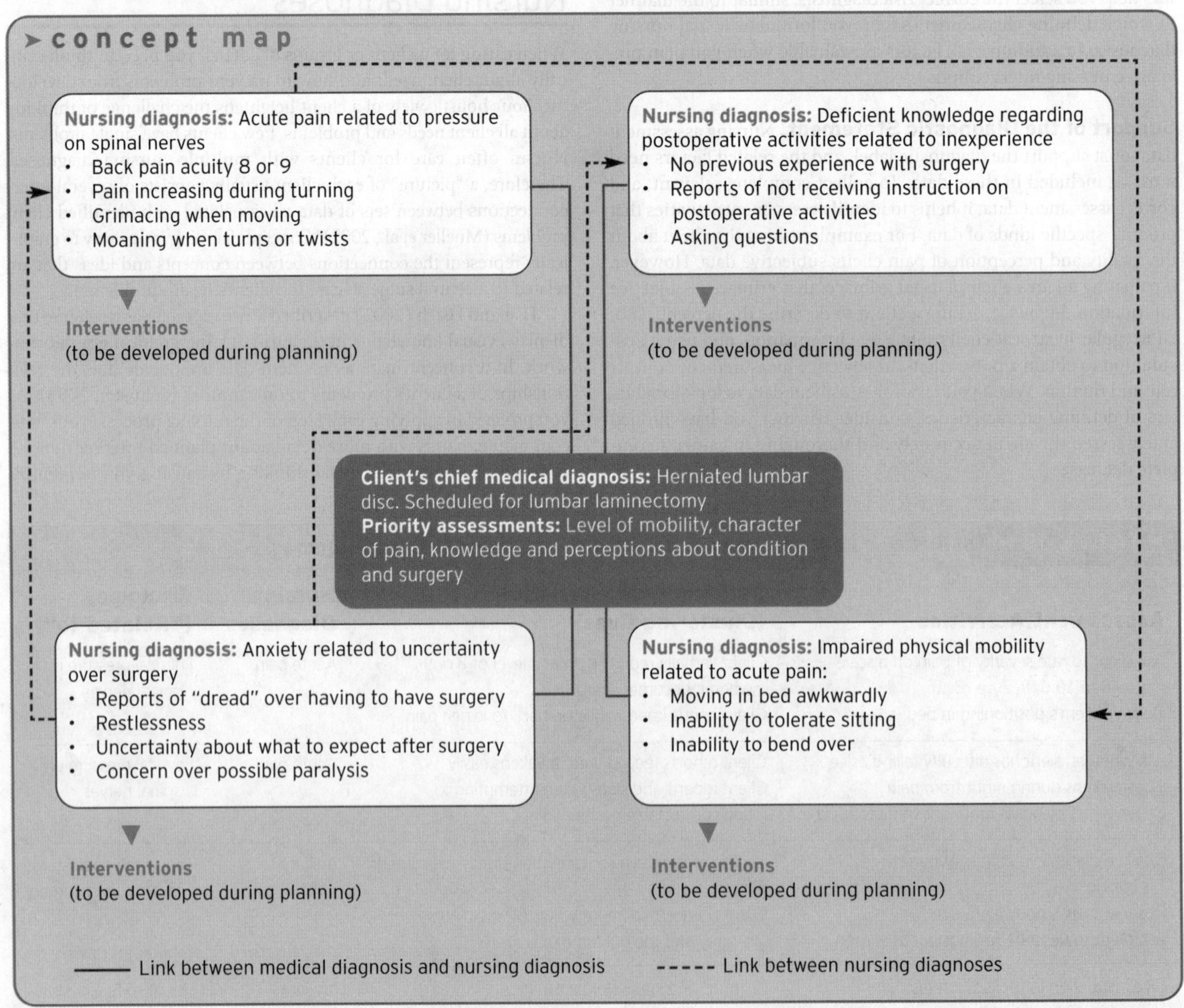

Figure 13-9 Concept map for Ms. Devine's nursing assessment findings.

Errors in Data Collection

To avoid errors in data collection, you should be knowledgeable and skilled in all assessment techniques (Box 13–5). Check for inaccurate or missing data, and collect data in an organized way. The following practice tips are essential to avoid data collection errors:

- Review your level of comfort and competence with interview and physical assessment skills before you begin data collection.
- Approach assessment in steps. Focus on completing a client interview before starting a physical examination. Perhaps focus on only one body system to learn how to gather a complete assessment. Then move to a more complex head-to-toe examination.
- Review your clinical assessments in clinical or classroom settings. They will provide you with a constructive learning opportunity to determine how to revise an assessment or to gather additional information.
- Determine the accuracy of your data. When you auscultate abnormal lung sounds for the first time, be sure of what you hear through the stethoscope. If assessment data are inaccurate, you will misinterpret data from clients, select inappropriate interventions, compromise the quality of care, and possibly endanger the client (Lunney, 1998). To minimize the risk of inaccuracy, have a more experienced coworker validate your findings or explain why they are incorrect.
- Be organized in any examination. Have the appropriate forms and examination equipment ready to use. Be sure the environment is private, quiet, and comfortable for the client.

Errors in Interpretation and Analysis of Data

After data collection, review your database to decide whether it is accurate and complete. Review data to confirm that measurable, objective physical findings support subjective data. For example, when a client reports "difficulty breathing," you should also listen to lung sounds, assess respiratory rate, and measure the client's chest excursion. When you are not able to validate data, the correspondence between clinical cues and the nursing diagnosis is inaccurate (Lunney, 1998). Begin interpretation by identifying and organizing relevant assessment patterns to confirm the presence of client problems. Be careful to consider any conflicting cues or to decide whether cues are insufficient for forming a diagnosis. Also, it is very important to consider a client's cultural background or developmental stage when you interpret the meaning of cues. For example, clients from the Middle East may express pain very differently than do Asian clients. Misinterpreting clients' expressions of pain will easily lead to an inaccurate diagnosis.

Errors in Data Clustering

Errors in data clustering occur when data are clustered prematurely or incorrectly or are not clustered at all. Premature closure of clustering occurs when you make the nursing diagnosis before grouping all data. For example, you learn that a client has had urinary incontinence and complains of urgency and nocturia. You cluster the available data and consider that *impaired urinary elimination* is a probable diagnosis. However, incorrect clustering occurs when you try to make the nursing diagnosis fit the signs and symptoms obtained. In this example, further assessment reveals the client has bladder distension and dribbling, and the condition is probably overflow incontinence. As a result of these findings, you are able to make a more accurate diagnosis: *urinary retention*. Always identify the nursing diagnosis from the data, not the reverse. An incorrect nursing diagnosis affects quality of client care.

➤ BOX 13-5 Sources of Diagnostic Error

Collecting

Lack of knowledge or skill
Inaccurate data
Missing data
Disorganization

Interpreting

Inaccurate interpretation of cues
Failure to consider conflicting cues
Using an insufficient number of cues
Using unreliable or invalid cues
Failure to consider cultural influences or developmental stage

Clustering

Insufficient clustering of cues
Premature or early closure of clustering
Incorrect clustering

Labelling

Wrong diagnostic label selected
Existence of evidence that another diagnosis is more likely
Condition incorrectly overlooked as a collaborative problem
Failure to validate nursing diagnosis with client
Failure to seek guidance

Errors in the Diagnostic Statement

The correct selection of a diagnostic statement is more likely to result in the selection of appropriate nursing interventions and outcomes (Dochterman & Jones, 2003). To reduce errors, word the diagnostic statement in appropriate, concise, and precise language. Use correct terminology reflecting the client's response to the illness or condition. Use of standardized nursing language from NANDA International (2007) helps ensure accuracy. A diagnostic statement such as "unhappy and worried about health" is not a scientifically based diagnosis, and it will lead to errors. The language needs to be more precise and appropriate, such as *ineffective coping related to fear of medical diagnosis*. Also, the problem and etiological portions of the diagnostic statement need to be within the scope of nursing in order to be diagnosed and treated.

Documentation

Once you identify a client's nursing diagnoses, list them on the written plan of care. In the clinical facility, list nursing diagnoses chronologically as you identify them. When you initiate the original care plan, always list the highest priority nursing diagnoses first.

Thereafter, add additional nursing diagnoses to the list. Date a nursing diagnosis at the time of entry. When you care for a client, always review the list and identify the nursing diagnoses with the highest priority, regardless of chronological order.

Nursing Diagnoses: Application to Care Planning

Nursing diagnosis is a mechanism for identifying the nursing care necessary for clients. Diagnoses provide direction for the planning process and the selection of nursing interventions to achieve desired outcomes for clients. Just as the medical diagnosis of diabetes guides a physician to prescribe a low-carbohydrate diet and medication for blood glucose control, the nursing diagnosis of *impaired skin integrity* directs a nurse to apply certain support surfaces to a client's bed and to initiate a turning schedule. In Chapter 14, you learn how unifying the language of NANDA International, along with the Nursing Interventions Classification (NIC), and Nursing Outcomes Classification (NOC), facilitate the process of matching nursing diagnoses with accurate and appropriate interventions and outcomes (Dochterman & Jones, 2003). The care plan is a map for nursing care and demonstrates your accountability for client care. By learning to make accurate nursing diagnoses, your subsequent care plan will assist in communicating to other professionals the client's health care problems and ensure that you select relevant and appropriate nursing interventions.

* KEY CONCEPTS

- The nursing process employs critical thinking to identify, diagnose, and treat clients' responses to health and illness.
- Nursing assessment involves the collection and verification of data and the analysis of all data to establish a database about a client's perceived needs, health problems, and responses to those problems.
- By interpreting the meaning of cues, you form an inference, which then enables you to identify meaningful clusters of information.
- To conduct a comprehensive assessment, you use a structured database format or a problem-oriented approach.
- The interview is an organized conversation with a client that begins by establishing a therapeutic relationship with the client and that aids in the investigation and discussion of the client's health care needs.
- Open-ended questions encourage clients to describe their health histories in detail, whereas closed-ended questions present a list of possible choices for the client.
- An interview includes three phases: orientation, working, and termination.
- Once a client provides subjective data, you consider exploring the findings further by collecting objective data.
- During assessment, you critically anticipate and use an appropriate branching set of questions or observations to collect data, and cues of assessment information are clustered to identify emerging patterns and problems.
- Written data statements are descriptive, to the point, and complete and do not include inferences or interpretative statements.
- Family members and friends sometimes offer observations about the client's needs; these observations will affect the way you deliver care.
- During assessment, you encourage clients to describe their histories of illnesses or health care problems.
- To form a nursing judgement, you critically assess a client, validate the data, interpret the information gathered, and look for diagnostic cues that will lead you to identify the client's problems.
- NANDA International has developed a common language that enables all members of the health care team to understand a client's needs.
- The analysis and interpretation of data requires you to validate data, recognize patterns or trends, compare data with healthful standards, and then form diagnostic conclusions.
- The absence of defining characteristics suggests that you reject a proposed diagnosis.
- Three types of nursing diagnoses exist: actual, at risk, and wellness diagnoses.
- A nursing diagnosis is written in a two-part format, including a diagnostic label and an etiologic or related factor.
- The "related to" factor of the diagnostic statement assists you in individualizing a client's nursing diagnoses and provides direction for your selection of appropriate interventions.
- Risk factors serve as cues to indicate that a risk nursing diagnosis applies to a client's condition.
- Concept mapping is a visual representation of a client's nursing diagnoses and their relationship with one another.
- Nursing diagnostic errors occur through errors in data collection, in interpretation and analysis of data, in clustering of data, or in the diagnostic statement.
- Nursing diagnoses improve communication between nurses and other health professionals.

* CRITICAL THINKING EXERCISES

1. Mrs. Lewis comes to the well-baby clinic for her infant's 1-month examination. She tells her nurse, Ethan, that the baby has not been sleeping well during the night. In addition, Mrs. Lewis has noted a rash on the baby's abdomen. Write three questions that Ethan might ask to assess the two potential problems Mrs. Lewis has presented. What assessment technique might the nurse apply to assess the rash that would not be used to assess the baby's sleep pattern?
2. Mrs. Spezio has a pressure ulcer over the coccyx that is 5 cm in diameter and approximately 1 cm deep. The tissue surrounding the ulcer is inflamed and tender to touch. Mrs. Spezio is transferring from a long-term care facility where she had resided for 6 months after a massive stroke. She is unable to move independently in bed and does not sense pressure or discomfort over her coccyx or hips. In view of this clinical situation, identify the defining characteristics and related factors for the nursing diagnosis *impaired skin integrity.*

* REVIEW QUESTIONS

1. The purpose of assessment is to
   1. Make a diagnostic conclusion
   2. Delegate nursing responsibility
   3. Teach the client about his or her health
   4. Establish a database concerning the client
2. Assessment data must be descriptive, concise, and complete. An assessment should *not* include
   1. Subjective data from the client
   2. A detailed physical examination
   3. The use of interpersonal and cognitive skills
   4. Inferences or interpretative statements not supported by data
3. During data clustering, a nurse
   1. Provides documentation of nursing care
   2. Reviews data with other health care professionals
   3. Makes inferences about patterns of information
   4. Organizes cues into patterns that enable the nurse to identify nursing diagnoses
4. You gather the following assessment data. Which of the following cues form a pattern? (Choose all that apply.)
   1. The client is restless.
   2. Fluid intake for 8 hours is 800 mL.
   3. The client complains of feeling short of breath.
   4. The client has drainage from surgical wound.
   5. Respirations are 24 per minute and irregular.
   6. Client reports loss of appetite for more than two weeks.

5. A nursing diagnosis is
   1. The diagnosis and treatment of human responses to health and illness
   2. The advancement of the development, testing, and refinement of a common nursing language
   3. A clinical judgement about individual, family, or community responses to actual and potential health problems or life processes
   4. The identification of a disease condition on the basis of a specific evaluation of physical signs, symptoms, the client's medical history, and the results of diagnostic tests
6. Lisa reviews data that she has collected regarding Ms. Devine's pain symptoms. She compares the defining characteristics for *acute pain* with those for *chronic pain*. In the end, she selects *acute pain* as the correct diagnosis. This is an example of how Lisa avoids an error in
   1. Data collection
   2. Data clustering
   3. Data interpretation
   4. Making a diagnostic statement
7. One of the purposes of the use of standard formal nursing diagnostic statements is to
   1. Evaluate nursing care
   2. Gather information on client data
   3. Help nurses to focus on the role of nursing in client care
   4. Facilitate understanding of client problems among health care professionals
8. The nursing diagnosis *readiness for enhanced communication* is an example of
   1. A risk nursing diagnosis
   2. An actual nursing diagnosis
   3. A potential nursing diagnosis
   4. A wellness nursing diagnosis
9. The nursing diagnosis *hypothermia* is an example of
   1. A risk nursing diagnosis
   2. An actual nursing diagnosis
   3. A potential nursing diagnosis
   4. A wellness nursing diagnosis
10. The word *impaired* in the diagnosis *impaired physical mobility* is an example of a
    1. Descriptor
    2. Risk factor
    3. Related factor
    4. Nursing diagnosis
11. In the following examples, which nurse is acting to avoid a data collection error?
    1. The nurse asks a colleague to chart his or her assessment data.
    2. The nurse considers conflicting cues in deciding the correct nursing diagnosis.
    3. The nurse assessing the edema in a client's lower leg is unsure of its severity and asks a coworker to check it with him or her.
    4. After performing an assessment, the nurse critically reviews his or her level of comfort and competence with interview and physical assessment skills.
12. Casey is reviewing a client's list of nursing diagnoses in the medical record. The most recent nursing diagnosis is *diarrhea related to intestinal colitis*. This is an incorrectly stated diagnostic statement, best described as
    1. Identifying the clinical sign instead of an etiology
    2. Identifying a diagnosis on the basis of prejudicial judgement
    3. Identifying the diagnostic study rather than a problem caused by the diagnostic study
    4. Identifying the medical diagnosis instead of the client's response to the diagnosis
13. Which of the following are defining characteristics for the nursing diagnosis *impaired urinary elimination?* (Choose all that apply.)
    1. Nocturia
    2. Frequency
    3. Urine retention
    4. Inadequate urinary output
    5. Treatment with intravenous fluids
    6. Sensation of bladder fullness

* RECOMMENDED WEB SITES

Center for Nursing Classification & Clinical Effectiveness: www.nursing.uiowa.edu/excellence/nursing_knowledge/clinical_effectiveness/index.htm
The University of Iowa's Center for Nursing Classification & Clinical Effectiveness was established to facilitate ongoing research of the Nursing Interventions Classification (NIC) and Nursing Outcomes Classification (NOC). This site provides an overview of the NIC and NOC and offers information about new classification material and publications.

NANDA International: http://www.nanda.org/
Through this Web site, NANDA International (formerly the North American Nursing Diagnosis Association) provides current information on nursing diagnosis research, publications, links, and Internet resources.

Registered Nurses Association of Ontario (RNAO): Nursing Best Practices Guidelines: http://www.rnao.org/bestpractices/
The RNAO has developed an extensive process to develop best practices guidelines in a variety of areas of clinical nursing. They have received federal as well as provincial funding for this process, and their work has been made available to all Canadian nurses through this Web site, which lists all current guidelines that have been developed.

14

Planning and Implementing Nursing Care

Original chapter by Patricia A. Potter, RN, MSN, PhD, GMAC, FAAN

Canadian content written by Janet C. Ross-Kerr RN, BScN, MS, PhD, and Marilynn J. Wood, RN, BSN, MPH, DrPH

objectives

Mastery of content in this chapter will enable you to:

- Define the key terms listed.
- Explain the relationship between planning and nursing assessment and diagnosis.
- Discuss the criteria used in priority setting.
- Describe goal setting.
- Discuss the difference between a goal and an expected outcome.
- List the seven guidelines for writing an outcome statement.
- Develop a plan of care from a nursing assessment.
- Discuss the differences between nurse-initiated, physician-initiated, and collaborative interventions.
- Discuss the process of selecting nursing interventions.
- Describe the purposes of a written nursing care plan.
- Describe the elements of a concept map.
- Describe the consultation process.
- Explain the relationship of implementation to the nursing diagnostic process.
- Discuss the differences between protocols and medical directives or standing orders.
- Describe the association between critical thinking and selecting nursing interventions.
- Identify preparatory activities to perform before implementation.
- Discuss steps taken to revise a plan of care before performing implementation.
- Define the three implementation skills.
- Describe and compare direct and indirect nursing interventions.
- Select appropriate interventions for an assigned client.

key terms

Activities of daily living, p. 194
Adverse reaction, p. 195
Client-centred goal, p. 180
Collaborative interventions, p. 183
Consultation, p. 190
Counselling, p. 195
Critical pathways, p. 187
Dependent nursing intervention, p. 183
Direct care, p. 190
Expected outcome, p. 180
Goal, p. 180
Independent nursing interventions, p. 183
Instrumental activities of daily living, p. 195
Kardex, p. 187
Lifesaving measure, p. 195
Long-term goal, p. 180
Medical directive, p. 192
Nursing care plan, p. 187
Nursing intervention, p. 190
Nursing-sensitive client outcome, p. 182
Planning, p. 179
Preventive nursing actions, p. 195
Priority setting, p. 179
Scientific rationale, p. 184
Short-term goal, p. 180
Standing order, p. 192

media resources

evolve Web Site

- Audio Chapter Summaries
- Glossary
- Multiple-Choice Review Questions
- Student Learning Activities
- Weblinks

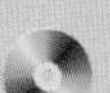

Companion CD

- Glossary
- Interactive Learning Activities
- Fluids and Electrolytes Tutorial
- Test-Taking Skills

Planning Nursing Care

Lisa is beginning to plan the nursing care for Ms. Devine. In the diagnostic step of the nursing process (see Chapter 13), Lisa identified four nursing diagnoses relevant to Ms. Devine's case: acute pain, anxiety, deficient knowledge, *and* impaired physical mobility. *Lisa is responsible for planning Ms. Devine's care from this morning until the time Ms. Devine leaves for surgery. Lisa will have left work on the unit by the time Ms. Devine returns from surgery, but as her primary nurse, Lisa will provide direction for the staff who assume Ms. Devine's care. Careful planning involves seeing a relationship between a client's problems, recognizing that certain problems take precedence over others, and proceeding with a safe and efficient approach to care. For each of the diagnoses, Lisa identifies the goals and expected outcomes that she and the client hope to achieve. The goals and outcomes direct Lisa in selecting appropriate therapeutic interventions. Ms. Devine is a client who will partner well with Lisa in selecting interventions suited to her own needs, strengths, and limitations. Lisa knows she needs to develop a plan quickly, because Ms. Devine is to go to the operating room by noontime.*

After you identify a client's nursing diagnoses and strengths, you begin planning nursing care. **Planning** is a category of nursing behaviour in which a nurse sets client-centred goals, outlines expected outcomes, plans nursing interventions, and selects interventions that will resolve the client's problems and achieve the goals and outcomes. Planning requires critical thinking, applied through deliberate decision making and problem solving. Another aspect of planning is to set priorities for a client. Many clients have multiple diagnoses and a number of health problems. Successful planning requires that you collaborate with the client and family, consult with other members of the health care team, and review related literature. This literature includes available evidence concerning the client's health care problems. A plan of care is dynamic and will change as you meet the client's needs or identify new needs.

Establishing Priorities

Priority setting is the ordering of nursing diagnoses or client problems, through the use of principles such as urgency or importance, to establish a preferential order for nursing actions (Hendry & Walker, 2004; Figure 14–1). By ranking nursing diagnoses in order of importance, you attend to the client's most important needs first. Priorities help you to anticipate and sequence nursing interventions for a client who has multiple nursing diagnoses and health problems. You and your clients select mutually agreed-on priorities on the bases of the urgency of the problems, safety, the nature of the treatment indicated, and the relationship among the diagnoses.

Establishing priorities is not merely a matter of numbering the nursing diagnoses on the basis of severity or physiological importance. Fontana (1993) suggested that nurses establish priorities in relation to importance and time. Nursing diagnoses of conditions that, if untreated, result in harm to the client or others have the highest priorities. For example, *risk for other-directed violence, impaired gas exchange,* and *decreased cardiac output* are typically high-priority nursing diagnoses that raise issues of safety, adequate oxygenation, and adequate circulation. High priorities are sometimes both physiological and psychological and may address other basic human needs. Consider Ms. Devine's case. Among Ms. Devine's nursing diagnoses,

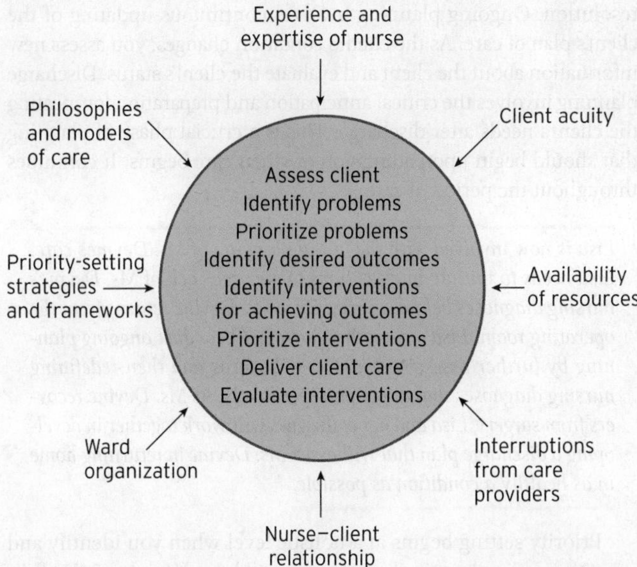

Figure 14-1 A model for priority setting. **Source:** Modified from Hendry, C., & Walker, A. (2004). Priority setting in clinical nursing practice. *Journal of Advanced Nursing, 47,* 427–436.

acute pain and *anxiety* are of the highest priority. Lisa knows that she needs to relieve Ms. Devine's acute pain and lessen the client's anxiety so that the client will approach surgery in less distress.

Intermediate priority nursing diagnoses involve the non-emergency, non–life-threatening needs of the client. In Ms. Devine's case, *deficient knowledge* is an intermediate diagnosis. It is very important that Lisa properly prepare Ms. Devine for surgery. Focused and individualized instruction will help Ms. Devine understand what to expect during her preoperative preparation and how to participate in postoperative care activities. Attending to the diagnosis of *deficient knowledge* will help minimize postoperative complications. Once Lisa addresses the higher priority nursing diagnoses of pain and anxiety, Ms. Devine will probably be more able to learn postoperative care. Also, greater understanding of the surgical procedure may help relieve Ms. Devine's anxiety.

Low-priority nursing diagnoses are not always directly related to a specific illness or prognosis but affect the client's future well-being. Many low-priority diagnoses focus on the client's long-term health care needs. In Ms. Devine's situation, *impaired physical mobility* is caused in part by her pain but also by her medical condition: a herniated disc. Lisa will monitor this diagnosis carefully, especially postoperatively. For now, Lisa will try to make Ms. Devine as comfortable as possible, which may improve Ms. Devine's ability to turn and position herself. After the surgery, Lisa will reassess her client. If *impaired physical mobility* remains a problem, the diagnosis is a higher priority because it is essential for Ms. Devine to achieve more normal mobility for a full recovery and to prevent postoperative complications.

The order of priorities changes as a client's condition changes, sometimes within a matter of minutes. Ongoing client assessment is crucial for determining the status of your client's nursing diagnoses.

In considering time as a factor in setting priorities, White (2003) explained that the planning of nursing care occurs in three phases: initial, ongoing, and discharge. Initial planning involves development of a preliminary plan of care after admission assessment and initial selection of nursing diagnoses. Because of progressively shorter lengths of hospitalization, initial planning is important in addressing nursing diagnoses and collaborative problems in order to hasten problem resolution. Ongoing planning involves continuous updating of the client's plan of care. As the client's condition changes, you assess new information about the client and evaluate the client's status. Discharge planning involves the critical anticipation and preparation for meeting the client's needs after discharge. This is a crucial phase of planning that should begin upon admission or when care begins. It continues throughout the period of care.

Lisa is now involved with the initial planning of Ms. Devine's care. Lisa needs to initiate interventions to manage each of Ms. Devine's nursing diagnoses before surgery. Once Ms. Devine returns from the operating room, Lisa, or another nurse, will conduct ongoing planning by further assessing Ms. Devine's status and then redefining nursing diagnoses that apply postoperatively. As Ms. Devine recovers from surgery, Lisa and her colleagues will work together in developing a discharge plan that will assist Ms. Devine in returning home in as healthy a condition as possible.

Priority setting begins at a holistic level when you identify and prioritize a client's main diagnoses or problems (Hendry & Walker, 2004). However, you also need to prioritize the specific interventions or strategies that you will use to help a client achieve desired goals and outcomes. For example, as Lisa considers the high-priority diagnosis of *acute pain* for Ms. Devine, she decides which intervention, among the interventions of administering an analgesic, repositioning, and teaching relaxation exercises, to perform first. Lisa knows that a certain degree of pain relief is necessary before a client can attend to relaxation exercises. She may decide to turn and reposition Ms. Devine and then give her an analgesic. However, if Ms. Devine is too uncomfortable to turn, Lisa will select administering the analgesic as her first priority. It is important to involve the client in priority setting whenever possible; in some situations, you and your client have different priorities.

Critical Thinking in Establishing Goals and Expected Outcomes

Once you identify a nursing diagnosis, you must identify the best approach to address and resolve the problem. What do you plan to achieve? **Goals** and **expected outcomes** are specific client behaviour or physiological responses that you set to achieve through nursing diagnosis or collaborative problem resolution. They provide a clear focus for the type of interventions necessary to care for your client.

For example, in the case of Ms. Devine, who has a diagnosis of *acute pain related to pressure on spinal nerves,* a goal of care includes "Client achieves improved pain control before surgery." To monitor Ms. Devine's progress, Lisa must use expected outcomes or measurable criteria to evaluate goal achievement. Measurable outcomes for the goal of pain relief include "Client's self-report of pain will be 3 or less on a scale of 0 to 10," and "Client will be able to turn without reported discomfort." The outcomes will reflect Lisa's success in selecting interventions for Ms. Devine's pain relief. After administering an analgesic and repositioning the client a few minutes later, Lisa will return to Ms. Devine's room in 30 minutes and ask the client to rate her pain and to report on her comfort level. If Ms. Devine rates her pain at a 3 or less and similarly reports minimal discomfort when turning, her goals will have been met. Lisa will follow her plan until Ms. Devine goes to the operating room. Goals and expected outcomes serve two purposes: to provide clear direction for the selection and use of nursing interventions and to provide focus for evaluating the effectiveness of the interventions.

Planning nursing care requires critical thinking (Figure 14–2). You need to carefully evaluate the identified nursing diagnoses, the urgency of the problems, and the resources of the client and the health care delivery system. You apply knowledge from the medical, sociobehavioural, and nursing sciences to plan client care. To select goals, expected outcomes, and interventions, you must consider your previous experience with similar client problems, as well as any established standards for clinical problem management. Goals and outcomes need to be relevant to client needs and to be specific, observable, measurable, and time-limited; they must also have the greatest likelihood of success.

For example, in choosing a plan for managing the client's acute pain, Lisa creatively selects a comfort measure that Ms. Devine practises at home. The diagram in Figure 14–3 graphically illustrates the relationships between nursing diagnoses, goals, expected outcomes, and nursing interventions.

Goals of Care

A **client-centred goal** is a specific and measurable behavioural response that reflects a client's highest possible level of wellness and independence in function. Examples are "Client will perform self-care hygiene independently" and "Client will remain free of infection." A goal is realistic and based on client needs and resources. A client-centred goal represents predicted resolution of a diagnosis or problem, evidence of progress toward resolution, progress toward improved health status, or continued maintenance of good health or function (Carpenito-Moyet, 2005). A goal involves only one behaviour or response. The example of "Client will administer a self-injection and demonstrate infection control measures" is incorrect because the statement includes two different behaviours: "administer" and "demonstrate." Instead, the goal should be worded as follows: "Client will administer a self-injection." The specific criteria you use to measure success of the goal are the expected outcomes: for example, "Client will prepare medication dose correctly" and "Client uses medical asepsis when preparing injection site." Each goal is time-limited so that the health care team has a common time frame for problem resolution. The time frame depends on the nature of the problem, etiology, overall condition of the client, and treatment setting.

A **short-term goal** is an objective behaviour or response that you expect a client to achieve in a short time, usually less than a week. In an acute care setting, you set goals for over a course of just a few hours. Such was the case when Lisa set for Ms. Devine the goal "Client's level of comfort will improve before surgery." A **long-term goal** is an objective behaviour or response that you expect a client to achieve over a longer period, usually over several days, weeks, or months: for example, "Client will be tobacco free within 60 days." Goal setting establishes the framework for the nursing care plan. Table 14–1 outlines the progression from nursing diagnoses to goals and expected outcomes, which Lisa individualizes to meet Ms. Devine's needs.

Role of the Client in Goal Setting. It is important to work closely with clients in setting goals. Mutual goal setting is an activity that includes clients and families in prioritizing goals of care and in developing plans for action (Bulechek et al., 2008). Clients need to be able to engage in problem solving and decision making in order to participate effectively in goal-setting. Unless you set goals mutually and make a clear plan for action, clients will not follow the care plan. For example, Lisa and Ms. Devine set the goal "Client will report greater comfort." They agreed that this would be demonstrated by pain acuity rated less than 3 on a scale of 0 to 10, a level that Ms. Devine reports is tolerable for her.

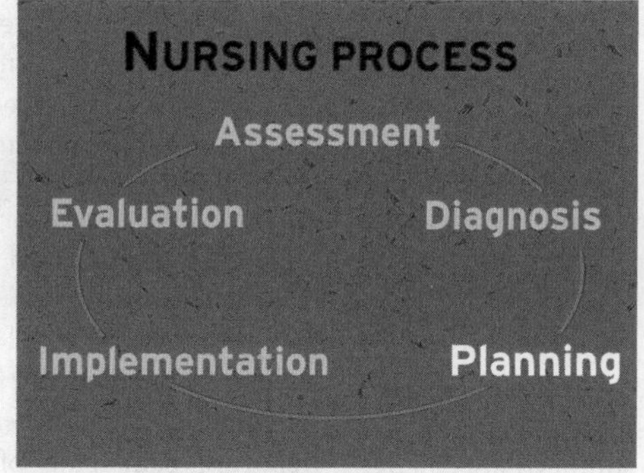

Figure 14-2 Critical thinking and the process of planning care. **Source:** CNA, Canadian Nurses Association. (2008). *Nursing practice: The practice of nursing.* Retrieved September 26, 2008, from http://www.cna-nurses.ca/CNA/practice/scope/default_e.aspx

Expected Outcomes

An expected outcome is a specific measurable change in a client's status that you expect in response to nursing care. Expected outcomes provide a focus or direction for nursing care because they are the desired physiological, psychological, social, developmental, or spiritual responses that indicate resolution of clients' health problems. Derived from both short- and long-term goals, outcomes determine when a specific client-centred goal has been met.

Usually you list several expected outcomes for each nursing diagnosis and goal. The reason for the multiple expected outcomes is that sometimes one nursing action is not enough to resolve a specific problem. In addition, the listing of the step-by-step expected outcomes assists in planning interventions. Write expected outcomes sequentially, specifying time frames for each (see Table 14–1). Time frames provide progressive steps to recovery and assist in ordering nursing interventions. In addition, time frames set limits for problem resolution. In the case of Ms. Devine, Lisa plans to relieve the client's pain enough so that she is able to turn comfortably in bed within the next two hours and to successfully reduce pain severity before surgery.

Write expected outcome statements in measurable terms. This enables you to note the specific behaviour or physiological response expected for resolution of the problem. For example, "Client will have less pain" is an inaccurate outcome statement because the phrase "less pain" is nonspecific. The statement "Client will report pain acuity of less than 3 on a scale of 0 to 10" is accurate.

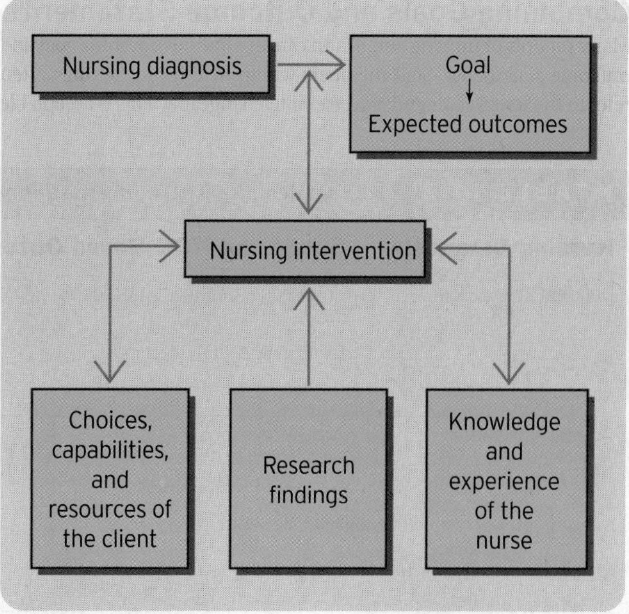

Figure 14-3 From diagnosis to outcome. **Source:** Revised and redrawn from Gordon, M. (1994). *Nursing diagnosis: Process and application* (3rd ed.). St. Louis, MO: Mosby.

➤ TABLE 14-1 Examples of Goal Setting with Expected Outcomes for Ms. Devine

Nursing Diagnoses	Goals	Expected Outcomes
Acute pain related to pressure on spinal nerves	Ms. Devine's level of comfort will improve before surgery	Client will be able to turn without reported discomfort in two hours Client's self-report of pain will be 3 or less on a scale of 0 to 10 by the time of scheduled surgery
Anxiety related to uncertainty over surgery	Ms. Devine will accept plan for surgical care before scheduled surgery	Client will express less uneasiness about surgical experience in next four hours
Deficient knowledge regarding postoperative activities related to inexperience	Ms. Devine will understand treatment procedures planned postoperatively within four hours	Client will exhibit less facial tension before scheduled surgery Client will describe purpose of postoperative exercises before scheduled surgery Client will demonstrate use of incentive spirometer and coughing before scheduled surgery Client will explain purpose of postoperative monitoring activities before scheduled surgery
Impaired physical mobility related to acute back pain	Ms. Devine will move independently in bed before surgery	Client will initiate turning without discomfort within 2 hours. Client will position self for care procedures within 2 hours

Nursing Outcomes Classification. The current health care environment pays considerable attention to measuring outcomes sensitive to nursing interventions. Many health care administrators focus on outcomes in determining staffing and other resources in health care settings. The Iowa Intervention Project published the Nursing Outcomes Classification (NOC) and has linked the outcomes to NANDA International (2007) nursing diagnoses (University of Iowa College of Nursing, 2008). The Iowa researchers defined a **nursing-sensitive client outcome** as an individual, family, or community state, behaviour, or perception that is measurable along a continuum in response to a nursing intervention. For any given NANDA International nursing diagnosis, multiple outcomes are suggested in NOC. These outcomes provide descriptions of the focus of nursing care and include indicators for measuring success with interventions (Table 14–2).

Combining Goals and Outcome Statements

Many schools of nursing and health care institutions combine goal and outcome statements. Staff members within health care settings often refer to the terms *goals* and *outcomes* interchangeably. This is acceptable as long as the criteria for writing goals and outcomes are met. For example, the statement "Client will achieve pain control as evidenced by reporting pain acuity of less than 3 on a scale of 0 to 10 within 24 hours" is an acceptable statement. The goal portion of the statement broadly describes the desired client status ("achieve pain control"), and the outcome portion of the statement contains the observable criterion ("3 on a [pain] scale") needed to measure success.

Guidelines for Writing Goals and Expected Outcomes

There are seven guidelines for writing goals and expected outcomes: client-centred, singular, observable, measurable, time-limited, mutual, and realistic.

Client-Centred Goal or Outcome. Outcomes and goals reflect client responses that are expected after nursing interventions. Write a goal to reflect client behaviour, not to reflect your goals or interventions. A correct outcome statement is "Client will ambulate in the hall three times a day." A common error is to write "Ambulate client in the hall three times a day."

➤ TABLE 14-2 Examples of NANDA International Nursing Diagnoses and Suggested NOC Linkages

Nursing Diagnosis	Suggested NOC-Based Outcomes (Examples)	Outcome Indicators (Examples)
Deficient knowledge	Knowledge: treatment procedures	Description of treatment procedure Description of steps in procedure
	Client satisfaction: teaching	Explanations provided in understandable terms Explanation of activity restrictions
Activity intolerance	Activity tolerance	Oxygen saturation with activity Pulse rate with activity Respiratory rate with activity
	Self-care status	Bathes self Dresses self Prepares food and fluid for eating

Source: Moorhead, S., Johnson, M., & Maas, M. (2008). *Nursing Outcomes Classification* (4th ed.). St. Louis, MO: Mosby.
NOC, Nursing Outcomes Classification.

Singular Goal or Outcome. Be precise in evaluating a client response to a nursing action. Each goal and outcome addresses only one behaviour or response.

Observable Goal or Outcome. You need to be able to observe whether change in a client's status occurs. Changes in physiological findings and in the client's knowledge, perceptions, and behaviour are observable. You observe outcomes by directly asking clients about their condition and by using assessment skills. For the outcome "Lungs will be clear on auscultation by 8/31," you auscultate the client's lungs routinely after therapy. The outcome statement "Client will appear less anxious" is not a correct statement because no specific behaviour for "will appear" is observable.

Measurable Goal or Outcome. You will learn to write goals and expected outcomes that set standards against which to measure the client's response to nursing care. Examples such as "Body temperature will remain 98.6°F" and "Apical pulse will remain between 60 and 100 beats per minute" enable you to objectively measure changes in the client's status.

Time-Limited Goal or Outcome. The time frame for each goal and expected outcome indicates when you expect the response to occur. Time frames assist in determining progress toward goals and outcomes.

Mutual Goal or Outcomes. Mutually set goals and expected outcomes ensure that client and nurse agree on the direction and time limits of care. Mutual goal setting increases clients' motivation and cooperation.

Realistic Goal or Outcome. Set goals and expected outcomes that are reachable. This provides clients with a sense of hope that increases motivation and cooperation. In order to establish realistic goals, you need to assess the resources of the health care facility, the family, and the client. You also need to be aware of the client's physiological, emotional, cognitive, and sociocultural potential and the economic cost and resources available to reach expected outcomes in a timely manner.

Types of Interventions

Nursing interventions belong to three categories: nurse-initiated, physician-initiated, and collaborative. Interventions are based on client needs. Some clients require all three categories of interventions, whereas others need only nurse- and physician-initiated interventions.

Nurse-initiated interventions are **independent nursing interventions.** These do not require direction or orders from other health care professionals. As a nurse, you act independently for clients. Nurse-initiated interventions are informed by the best available evidence. Examples include elevating an edematous extremity, instructing clients in side effects of medications, or directing a client to splint an incision during coughing.

Physician-initiated interventions are **dependent nursing interventions,** or actions that require orders or directions from physicians or other health professionals. The interventions are directed toward treating or managing a medical diagnosis. Nurse practitioners working under collaborative agreements with physicians or who are licensed through provincial or territorial nursing legislation are also able to provide such orders or directions for care. As the nurse, you intervene by carrying out these written or verbal orders. Administering a medication and changing a dressing are examples of physician-initiated interventions.

Each physician-initiated intervention requires specific nursing responsibilities that are based on nursing knowledge. For example, when administering medications, you are responsible for knowing the classification of the drug, its physiological action, the normal dosage, side effects, and nursing interventions related to its action or side effects (see Chapter 34).

Interdependent nursing interventions, or **collaborative interventions,** are therapies that require the combined knowledge, skill, and expertise of a number of health care professionals. Typically, when you plan care for a client, you review the necessary interventions and determine whether the collaboration is necessary. An interdisciplinary health care team conference about a client's care is useful in determining interdependent nursing interventions.

In the case study involving Lisa and Ms. Devine, Lisa will initiate independent interventions to help calm Ms. Devine's anxiety and to begin teaching her about postoperative care. In addition, Lisa independently positions Ms. Devine to minimize her discomfort and promote more normal mobility. Among the dependent interventions Lisa plans to implement are administering an analgesic and completing any necessary preoperative diagnostic tests. Lisa decides that consultation with the unit social worker is another way to help Ms. Devine with her anxiety over surgery.

Every nurse faces an inappropriate or incorrect order at some time (Table 14–3). The nurse with a strong knowledge base recognizes and questions errors. The ability to recognize incorrect therapies is particularly important in administering medications or implementing procedures. Errors may occur in writing or transcribing orders. Clarifying an order is competent nursing practice and protects clients from harm. When you carry out an incorrect or inappropriate intervention, you are responsible for an error in judgement and are legally responsible for any complications resulting from the error (see Chapter 9).

Selection of Interventions

Interventions are not selected randomly. Clients with the diagnosis of *anxiety,* for example, may require a variety of interventions. You treat anxiety related to the uncertainty of impending surgery very differently than anxiety related to a possible loss of family role function. When choosing interventions, consider six factors: (1) the nursing diagnosis, (2) goals and expected outcomes, (3) the evidence base (e.g., research or proven practice guidelines), (4) feasibility, (5) acceptability to the client, and (6) your own competence (Bulechek et al., 2008) (Box 14–1). During deliberation, review resources such as the nursing literature, standard protocols or guidelines, the Nursing Interventions Classification (NIC), critical pathways, policy or procedure manuals, and textbooks. As you select interventions, collaborate with other professionals, review your clients' needs and priorities, and review your previous experiences to select interventions that have the best potential for achieving the expected outcomes.

Nursing Interventions Classification

The Iowa Intervention Project (1993) developed a set of nursing interventions that provides a level of standardization, which enhances communication of nursing care across all health care settings and enables health care professionals to compare outcomes (Bulecheck et al., 2008; McCloskey & Bulechek, 2004). The NIC model includes three levels: domains, classes, and interventions for

TABLE 14-3 Frequent Errors in Writing Nursing Interventions

Type of Error	Incorrectly Stated Nursing Intervention	Correctly Stated Nursing Intervention
Failure to precisely or completely indicate nursing actions	Turn client every two hours	Turn client every two hours, using the following schedule: 8 A.M.: supine 10 A.M.: left side Noon: prone 2 P.M.: right side (repeat this routine beginning at 4 P.M. and midnight)
Failure to indicate frequency	Perform blood glucose measurements	Measure blood glucose before each meal: 7 A.M., 11 A.M., and 5 P.M.
Failure to indicate quantity	Irrigate wound once a shift: 6 A.M., 11 A.M., and 5 P.M.	Irrigate wound with 100 mL normal saline until clear: 6 A.M., 11 A.M., and 5 P.M.
Failure to indicate method	Change client's dressing once a shift: 6 A.M., 2 P.M., and 10 P.M.	Replace client's dressing with Neosporin ointment to wound and two dry 4×4 dressings secured with hypoallergenic tape, once a shift: 6 A.M., 2 P.M., and 10 P.M.

ease of use. The domains are the highest level (Level 1) of the model, worded in broad terms (e.g., "safety" and "physiological: basic") to organize the more specific classes and interventions (Table 14–4). The second level of the model includes 30 classes, which offer useful clinical categories for reference in selecting interventions. The third level of the model includes the 514 interventions, defined as any treatment based on clinical judgement and knowledge, that a nurse performs to enhance the condition of a client who presents an alteration within the class (Bulechek et al., 2008) (Box 14–2). Each intervention can be performed with a variety of nursing activities (Box 14–3). Nursing activities are those commonly used in a plan of care. NIC-based interventions are also linked with NANDA International (2007) nursing diagnoses for ease of use. For example, if a client has a nursing diagnosis of *acute pain*, 21 recommended interventions, including pain management, cutaneous stimulation, and anxiety reduction, may be used. A variety of nursing care activities are presented with each of the recommended interventions.

BOX 14-1 Choosing Nursing Interventions

Characteristics of the Nursing Diagnosis

Interventions should alter the etiological ("related to") factor or signs and symptoms associated with the diagnostic label.

- When an etiological factor cannot change, direct the interventions toward treating the signs and symptoms (e.g., NANDA International [2007] defining characteristics).
- For potential or high-risk diagnoses, direct interventions at altering or eliminating risk factors for the diagnosis.

Expected Outcomes

Because nurses state outcomes in terms used to evaluate the effect of an intervention, this language assists in selecting the intervention.

NIC is designed to show the link to NOC (University of Iowa College of Nursing, 2008).

Evidence Base

Research evidence in support of a nursing intervention indicates the effectiveness of the intervention in certain types of clients.

- Refer to the evidence (e.g., research articles or evidence-informed practice protocols that describe the use of the evidence in similar clinical situations and settings.
- When research is not available, use scientific principles (e.g., infection control) or consult a clinical expert about your client population.

Feasibility

A specific intervention has the potential for interacting with other interventions.

- Be knowledgeable about the total plan of care.
- Consider cost: Is the intervention clinically effective and cost efficient?
- Consider time: Are time and personnel resources available?

Acceptability to the Client

A treatment plan needs to be acceptable to the client and family and must match the client's goals, health care values, and culture.

- Promote informed choice; help a client know how to participate in and anticipate the effect of interventions.

Capability of the Nurse

The nurse needs to have up-to-date knowledge of the intervention, its scientific basis, and considerations for implementation.

- Be prepared to carry out the intervention.
- Know the **scientific rationale** for the intervention.
- Have the necessary psychosocial and psychomotor skills to complete the intervention.
- Be able to function within the specific setting and to use health care resources effectively and efficiently.

Modified from Dochterman, J. M., & Bulechek, G. M. (2004). *Nursing Interventions Classification (NIC)* (4th ed.). St. Louis, MO: Mosby.

TABLE 14-4 Nursing Interventions Classifications (NIC) Taxonomy

Domain 1	Domain 2	Domain 3	Domain 4	Domain 5	Domain 6	Domain 7
Level 1 Domains						
1. Physiological: Basic Care that supports physical functioning	2. Physiological: Complex Care that supports homeostatic regulation	3. Behavioural Care that supports psychosocial functioning and facilitates lifestyle changes	4. Safety Care that supports protection against harm	5. Family Care that supports the family	6. Health System Care that supports effective use of the health care delivery system	7. Community Care that supports the health of the community
Level 2 Classes						
A. *Activity and Exercise Management:* Interventions to organize or assist with physical activity and energy conservation and expenditure	G. *Electrolyte and Acid–Base Management:* Interventions to regulate electrolyte/acid–base balance and prevent complications	O. *Behaviour Therapy:* Interventions to reinforce or promote desirable behaviours or alter undesirable behaviours	U. *Crisis Management:* Interventions to provide immediate short-term help in both psychological and physiological crises	W. *Childbearing Care:* Interventions to assist in understanding and coping with the psychological and physiological changes during the childbearing period	Y. *Health System Mediation:* Interventions to facilitate the interface between patient/family and the health care system	c. *Community Health Promotion:* Interventions that promote the health of the whole community
B. *Elimination Management:* Interventions to establish and maintain regular bowel and urinary elimination patterns and manage complications due to altered patterns	H. *Drug Management:* Interventions to facilitate desired effects of pharmacological agents	P. *Cognitive Therapy* Interventions to reinforce or promote desirable cognitive functioning or alter undesirable cognitive functioning	V. *Risk Management:* Interventions to initiate risk-reduction activities and continue monitoring risks over time	Z. *Childrearing Care:* Interventions to assist in rearing children	a. *Health System Management:* Interventions to provide and enhance support services for the delivery of care	d. *Community Risk Management:* Interventions that assist in detecting or preventing health risks to the whole community
C. *Immobility Management:* Interventions to manage restricted body movement and the sequelae	I. *Neurologic Management:* Interventions to optimize neurologic functions	Q. *Communication Enhancement:* Interventions to facilitate delivering and receiving verbal and nonverbal messages		X. *Lifespan Care:* Interventions to facilitate family unit functioning and promote the health and welfare of family members throughout the lifespan	b. *Information Management:* Interventions to facilitate communication among health care providers	

Continued

TABLE 14-4 Nursing Interventions Classifications (NIC) Taxonomy *continued*

Domain 1	Domain 2	Domain 3	Domain 4	Domain 5	Domain 6	Domain 7
Level 2 Classes						
D. *Nutrition Support:* Interventions to modify or maintain nutritional status	J. *Perioperative Care:* Interventions to provide care before, during, and after surgery	R. *Coping Assistance:* Interventions to assist another to build on own strength, to adapt to a change in function, or to achieve a higher level of function				
E. *Physical Comfort Promotion:* Interventions to promote comfort using physical techniques	K. *Respiratory Management:* Interventions to provide care before, during, and immediately after surgery	S. *Patient Education:* Interventions to facilitate learning				
F. *Self-Care Facilitation:* Interventions to provide or assist with routine activities of daily living	L. *Skin/Wound Management:* Interventions to maintain or restore tissue integrity	T. *Psychological Comfort Promotion:* Interventions to promote comfort using psychological techniques				
	M. *Thermoregulation:* Interventions to maintain body temperature within a normal range					
	N. *Tissue Perfusion Management:* Interventions to optimize circulations of blood and fluids to the tissue					

From Bulechek, G. M., Butcher, H. K., & Dochterman, J. M. (2008). *Nursing Interventions Classification (NIC)* (5th ed.). St. Louis, MO: Mosby.

➤ BOX 14-2 **Example of Interventions for Physical Comfort Promotion**

Class: Physical Comfort Promotion

Interventions to promote comfort [by] using physical techniques

Interventions (Examples)

Acupressure
Aromatherapy
Cutaneous stimulation
Environmental management
Heat/cold application
Nausea management
Pain management
Progressive muscle relaxation
Simple massage

Examples of Linked Nursing Diagnoses

Acute pain
Chronic pain

From Dochterman, J. M., & Bulechek, G. M. (2004). *Nursing Interventions Classification (NIC)* (4th ed.). St. Louis, MO: Mosby.

➤ BOX 14-3 **Example of Interventions and Associated Nursing Activities**

Class: Physical Comfort Promotion
Intervention—Environmental Management

Examples of Activities

Create a safe environment for client
Provide a clean, comfortable bed and environment
Avoid unnecessary exposure, drafts, overheating, or chilling
Provide music of choice
Limit visitors
Manipulate lighting for therapeutic benefit
Bring familiar objects from home
Allow family/significant other to stay with client

From Dochterman, J. M., & Bulechek, G. M. (2004). *Nursing Interventions Classification (NIC)* (4th ed.). St. Louis, MO: Mosby.

Planning Nursing Care

In any health care setting, a nurse is responsible for developing a written plan of care for clients. The plan of care sometimes takes several forms (e.g., a nursing card-filing system, standardized care plans, and computerized plans). In general, a written **nursing care plan** includes nursing diagnoses; goals, expected outcomes, or both; and specific nursing interventions, so that any nurse is able to quickly identify a client's clinical needs and situation. In hospitals and community-based settings, the client often receives care from more than one nurse, physician, or allied health professional. A written nursing care plan makes possible continuity and coordination of nursing care and consultation by a number of health professionals.

Written care plans organize information exchanged by nurses in change-of-shift reports (see Chapter 16). You will learn to focus your reports on the nursing care, treatments, and expected outcomes documented in your care plans, and the end-of-shift report allows for discussion of care plans and the overall progress with the next caregiver. The nursing care plan (Box 14–4) on p. 188 provides an example of a care plan for Ms. Devine.

When developing an individualized care plan, involve the family and client. The family is a resource for helping the client meet health care goals. In addition, meeting some of the family's needs may improve the client's level of wellness.

Institutional Care Plans

Institutional care plans become part of a client's legal medical record. Many hospitals still use a written Kardex nursing care plan. The **Kardex** card-filing system allows quick reference to the needs of the client for certain aspects of nursing care (see Chapter 16). The care plan section of a Kardex system varies by agency and focuses on planned interventions to meet the needs of the client and family and to prepare the client for discharge from the hospital. The focus of a nursing care plan differs by setting and the evolving client situation. For example, nursing care plans developed for clients returning home are usually based solely on long-term health needs. Nursing care plans for same-day surgeries are usually focused on clients' short-term needs (e.g., immediate recovery from surgery and instructions for self-care at home). In a long-term care facility, plans of care focus on clients' long-term rehabilitation needs.

Computerized Care Plans. A majority of health care facilities now have some type of electronic health record (EHR) and documentation system (Moody et al., 2004). Software programs are available for nursing care plans. In many facilities, the format is for standardized plans that are based on nursing diagnoses or select problem areas, which nurses are able to individualize for a specific client. Even if a standardized care plan is generally appropriate for a client, you need to add or delete information on the standardized form to individualize it for a client's needs. For example, you select a nursing diagnosis and then individualize the standard care plan by making selections from menus. Each care plan lists generalized nursing diagnoses, goals, outcome criteria, and interventions for specific clients. Computerized and standardized nursing care plans organize and enhance care planning. Their design incorporates current evidence-informed practice guidelines to achieve the desired client outcomes for a specific group of clients.

Care Plans for Community-Based Settings. Planning care for clients in community-based settings—for example, clinics, community centres, or clients' homes—involves using the same principles of nursing practice. In these settings, however, you need to complete a more comprehensive community, home, and family assessment. Ultimately, the client or family unit must be able to provide the majority of health care independently.

Critical Pathways. Critical pathways are multidisciplinary treatment plans that outline treatments or interventions that clients may require for treatment of a condition. Most pathways are based on medical rather than nursing diagnoses, but they incorporate related nursing diagnoses and associated nursing interventions. A critical pathway maps out, day to day or even hour to hour, the recommended interventions and expected outcomes. For example, a pathway for a surgical procedure such as a bowel resection will recommend on a day-by-day basis the client's activities, procedures, and discharge planning activities. A critical pathway ensures better continuity of care because it clearly maps out the responsibility of each health discipline. Well-developed pathways incorporate current evidence in caring for clients with a specific condition. Nurses

BOX 14-4 NURSING CARE PLAN

Acute Pain

Assessment

Ms. Devine is a 52-year-old woman who was injured in a fall two months ago that caused rupture of a lumbar disc. She is scheduled for a lumbar laminectomy this afternoon. Ms. Devine is the office manager for a realty business she runs with her husband. She was not able to work regularly over the first month after the injury. She has sciatic pain that is sharp and burning, radiating down from her right hip to her right foot. The pain worsens when she sits. Her vital signs are as follows: temperature, 99.2°F; blood pressure, 138/82 mm Hg; pulse, 84 beats per minute; and respirations, 24 breaths per minute.

Assessment Activities	*Findings and Defining Characteristics**
Observe client's body movements	Client limps **slightly with right leg. Turns** in bed **slowly.**
Observe client's facial expression	Client **grimaces** when she attempts to sit down.
Ask client to rate pain at its worst	Client **rates pain on a scale of 0 to 10 at an 8 or 9 at its worst.**

*Defining characteristics are in boldface type.

Nursing Diagnosis: Acute pain related to pressure on spinal nerves

Planning

Goal (Nursing Outcomes Classification)†	*Expected Outcomes†*
Pain Control	**Knowledge of Treatment Procedures**
Client will achieve improved pain control before surgery.	Client's self-report of pain will be 3 or less on a scale of 0 to 10 Client's facial expressions reveal less discomfort when turning and repositioning.

†Outcomes classification labels from Moorhead S, Johnson, M., & Maas, M. (2008). *Nursing Outcomes Classification (NOC)* (3rd ed). St. Louis, MO: Mosby.

Interventions (Nursing Interventions Classification)‡	**Rationale**
Analgesic Administration	
Set positive expectations regarding effectiveness of analgesics.	Optimizes client's response to medication (Bulechek et al., 2008).
Give analgesic 30 minutes before turning or positioning client and before pain increases in severity.	Medication will exert peak effect when client attempts to increase movement.
Pain Management	
Reduce environmental factors in client's room (e.g., noise, lighting, temperature extremes).	Pleasurable sensory stimuli reduce pain perception.
Offer client information about any procedures and efforts at reducing discomfort.	Information satisfies client's interests and enables client to evaluate and communicate pain (McCaffery & Pasero, 1999).
Progressive Muscle Relaxation	
Direct client through progressive muscle relaxation exercise. Coach client through exercise.	Relaxation techniques enable self-control when pain develops, reversing the cognitive and affective–motivational component of pain perception.

‡Intervention classification labels from Bulechek, G. M., Butcher, H. K., & Dochterman, J. M. (2008). *Nursing Interventions Classification (NIC)* (4th ed.). St. Louis, MO: Mosby.

Evaluation

Nursing Actions	*Client Response and Finding*	*Achievement of Outcome*
Ask client to report severity of pain 30 minutes after analgesic administration.	Ms. Devine reports pain at a level of 5 on a scale of 0 to 10.	Pain is reduced, necessitates further nonpharmacological intervention to achieve outcome.
Observe client's facial expressions.	Ms. Devine is observed to have a relaxed facial expression.	Client's level of comfort is improving.

and other health care team members use these to monitor a client's progress. When critical pathways are used to plan care, some forms of documentation are eliminated (e.g., the nursing care plan, flow sheets, and nurses' notes) because all of the pertinent components are included in the pathway.

Concept Maps

Concept maps and their use in care planning are described in Chapter 13. Because you care for clients with multiple health problems and related nursing diagnoses, concept maps are useful in that they incorporate a visual representation of client problems and interventions and of their relationships to one another (Schuster, 2003). The concept map groups and categorizes nursing concepts to give you a holistic view of your client's health care needs and to help you make better clinical decisions in planning care (King & Shell, 2002). There are different approaches to writing concept maps. Schuster (2003) suggested some simple steps in preparing for concept mapping and in developing a clinical plan of care:

1. First, retrieve the clinical assessment database from the medical record, including health history, physical assessment data, laboratory and diagnostic data, medication history, and treatment plan.
2. Review all information concerning health problems, treatments, and medications in the literature, course textbooks, pharmacology texts, and other resources.
3. On the nursing unit, review standardized nursing care plans, critical pathways, clinical protocols, or client education materials.
4. Develop a preliminary diagram of the client's chief medical diagnosis and the patterns of assessment data that you have gathered. Write the client's major medical diagnoses in the middle of the map, and then add the assessment patterns like spokes on a wheel (see Chapter 13). Identify and group the related patterns of clinical assessment and medical history data. Remember that sometimes symptoms apply to more than one nursing diagnosis. Repeat symptoms under different categories when appropriate: for example, when pain is a symptom of both a problem with comfort and a problem with mobility.
5. Next, review your assessment patterns and attempt to identify the nursing diagnoses (see Chapter 13). Do not worry if you have difficulty developing nursing diagnoses at first. It is important to recognize the major nursing care focus for the client. Add diagnostic statements later if necessary.
6. Analyze relationships among nursing diagnoses, and draw dotted lines between them to indicate relationships (Figure 14–4). It is important for you to make meaningful associations between concepts because the links need to be accurate, meaningful, and complete. You need to be able to explain why nursing diagnoses are related. For example, in the case of Ms. Devine, anxiety and acute pain are interrelated, and pain is a cause of her reduced mobility.
7. List nursing interventions to attain the outcomes for each nursing diagnosis (see Figure 14–4). This step corresponds to the planning phase of the nursing process.
8. While caring for the client, use the map to write down the client's responses to each nursing activity. Also, note your clinical impressions and inferences about effectiveness of interventions and progress toward meeting expected outcomes.
9. Keep the concept map with you throughout the clinical day. As you revise the plan, take notes and add or delete nursing interventions. Use the information recorded on the map for your documentation of client care.

Concept maps help nurses link concepts such as nursing diagnoses and to identify relationships between them to organize and understand information.

Consulting Other Health Care Professionals

Planning involves **consultation** with members of the health team. Although consultation can occur at any step in the nursing process, it occurs most often during planning and implementation, when problems necessitating additional knowledge, skills, or resources arise. Consulting involves seeking the expertise of a specialist, such as a nursing instructor, registered nurse, or clinical nurse specialist to identify ways of approaching and managing the planning and implementation of therapies.

Nurse consultants frequently offer advice about difficult clinical problems. For example, a nursing student will consult with the registered nurse assigned to the same client about ways to individualize interventions, with a clinical specialist for wound care techniques, or with an educator for useful teaching resources. Nurses are consulted for their clinical expertise, client education skills, or staff education skills. Nurses also consult with other members of the health care team, such as physical therapists, nutritionists, and social workers.

Implementing Nursing Care

Lisa enters Ms. Devine's room to administer morphine sulphate ordered for her severe back pain. The client is probably not going to the operating room for another four to six hours, and so Lisa aims to reduce the client's discomfort before then. Lisa administers the medication, using physical care principles to promote safety and prevent infection. She communicates with Ms. Devine in a calm and reassuring manner to allay anxiety. Lisa explains that she will return to Ms. Devine's room in about 30 minutes to help her turn and become comfortable and to offer basic instruction about anticipated postoperative routines. Lisa's interventions are designed to prepare Ms. Devine for her upcoming surgery.

Implementation. With a care plan based on clear and relevant nursing diagnoses, you initiate interventions that are most likely to achieve goals and expected outcomes needed to support or improve the client's health status. A **nursing intervention** is any treatment, based on clinical judgement and knowledge, to enhance client outcomes (Bulechek et al., 2008). Ideally, interventions are evidence informed (see Chapter 7), providing the most current, up-to-date, and effective approaches addressing client problems and include both direct and indirect care measures.

Direct care interventions are treatments performed through interactions with clients. For example, a client receives direct intervention in the form of medication administration, insertion of an intravenous infusion, or counselling during a time of grief. Indirect care interventions are treatments performed away from the client but on behalf of the client or group of clients (Bulechek et al., 2008). For example, indirect care measures include actions for managing the

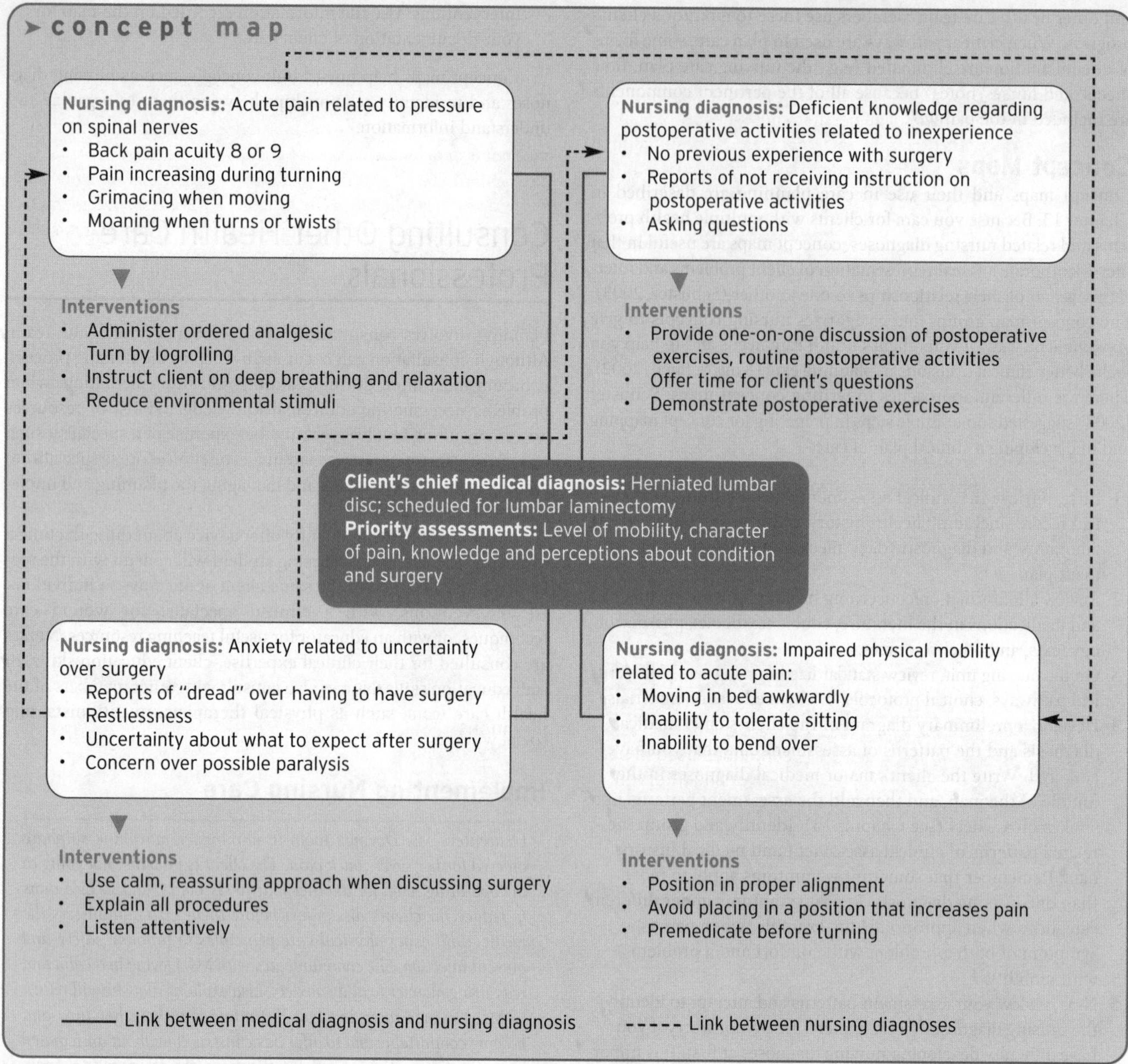

Figure 14-4 Concept map for planning Ms. Devine's nursing care.

client's environment (e.g., safety and infection control), documentation, and interdisciplinary collaboration. Both direct and indirect care measures can be nurse-initiated, physician-initiated, and collaborative interventions. For example, client teaching is a direct, nurse-initiated intervention. The indirect intervention of consultation is a collaborative intervention.

Nursing is both an art and a science. Each intervention is rendered within the context of a client's unique situation. As you learn to intervene for a client, consider the context of the clinical situation. What is the client's particular situation? Why do you need to intervene in the clinical situation? How does the client perceive your proposed interventions? How can you support the client as you intervene? The answers to these questions enable you to deliver care compassionately and effectively with the best outcomes for your clients.

Critical Thinking in Implementation

The selection of nursing interventions involves complex decision making and is based on critical thinking to ensure that an intervention is correct and appropriate for the clinical situation. Even though you have planned a set of interventions for a client, good judgement, decision making, and reassessment are needed before each intervention is actually performed, inasmuch as clients' conditions sometimes change rapidly. Some points to consider when you work with clients to meet their needs are as follows:

- Review the set of all possible nursing interventions for the client's problem (e.g., for Ms. Devine's pain, Lisa considers analgesic administration, positioning, relaxation, and other nonpharmacological approaches).

- Review all possible consequences associated with each possible nursing action (e.g., Lisa considers that the analgesic may relieve pain, may have little or insufficient effect, or may cause an adverse reaction).
- Determine the probability of all possible consequences (e.g., if Ms. Devine's pain has decreased with analgesia and positioning in the past, it is unlikely adverse reactions will occur, and the intervention will probably be successful; however, if the client continues to remain highly anxious, her pain may not be relieved).
- Determine the effect of the intervention on the client (e.g., if the administration of an analgesic is effective, Ms. Devine will become less anxious and will be more responsive to preoperative instruction).

The selection and performance of nursing interventions for a client is part of clinical decision making. The critical thinking model described in Chapter 12 provides a framework for making decisions about nursing care. As you proceed with an intervention, you should consider the purpose of the intervention, the steps in performing the intervention correctly, and the medical condition of the client (Figure 14–5). It is essential to know the clinical standards of practice of each agency because procedures and standards of practice vary considerably. The standards of practice are guidelines for selection of interventions, their frequency, and information about whether they can be delegated.

Standard Nursing Interventions

To facilitate good care planning, systems of standard nursing interventions are available to help you. These are based on common health care problems for which standard interventions can serve as a reference point in determining what is necessary. Of more importance, if the standards are informed by evidence, interventions are more likely to improve client outcomes (see Chapter 7). Standard interventions, both nurse initiated and physician initiated, are available in the form of clinical guidelines or protocols, preprinted medical directives or standing orders, and NIC-based interventions.

Clinical Practice Guidelines and Protocols

A clinical guideline or protocol is a document that guides decisions and interventions for specific health care problems. The guideline or protocol is developed on the basis of an authoritative examination of current scientific evidence and assists nurses, physicians, and other health care professionals in making decisions about appropriate health care for specific clinical circumstances. Clinicians within a health care agency sometimes choose to review the scientific literature and their own standard of practice to develop guidelines and protocols in an effort to improve their standard of care. For example, a hospital develops a rapid assessment protocol to improve the identification and early treatment of clients

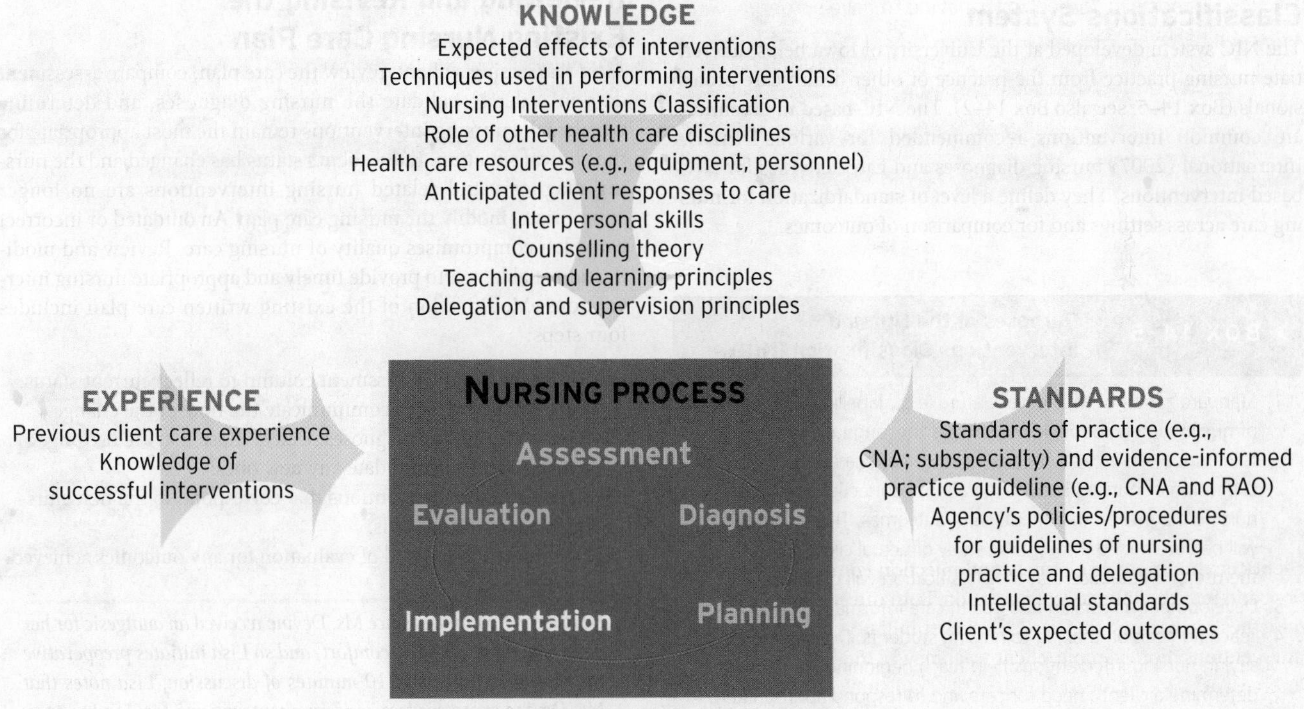

Figure 14-5 Critical thinking and the process of implementing care.

suspected of having a stroke. Clinical practice guidelines also assist you in providing the best possible care. The *Best Practice Guidelines* developed by the Registered Nurses Association of Ontario (2008) is an excellent example of these.

Medical Directives or Standing Orders

A **medical directive** or **standing order** is a statement of orders for the conduct of routine therapies, monitoring guidelines, or diagnostic procedures, or a combination of these, for specific clients with identified clinical problems. These statements direct client care in various clinical settings and must be approved and signed by the prescribing physician or health care professional. Medical directives or standing orders are common in critical care settings and other specialized practice settings in which clients' needs change rapidly and require immediate attention. Examples include those for preoperative blood tests, those for postoperative exercises and positioning, and those for certain medications (such as lidocaine or propranolol) for an irregular heart rhythm. When these statements are in place, the critical care nurse may administer the specified medication or conduct the specified action without first notifying the physician. Medical directives or standing orders are also common in community health settings in which physicians are not immediately available for contact. Medical directives, standing orders, and clinical protocols give the nurse legal protection to intervene appropriately in the client's best interest.

Nursing Intervention Classifications System

The NIC system developed at the University of Iowa helps differentiate nursing practice from the practice of other health care professionals (Box 14–5; see also Box 14–2). The NIC-based interventions are common interventions recommended for various NANDA International (2007) nursing diagnoses and care activities for NIC-based interventions. They define a level of standardization for nursing care across settings and for comparison of outcomes.

➤ BOX 14-5 Purposes of the Nursing Interventions Classification (NIC)

1. Standardization of the nomenclature (e.g., labelling, describing) of nursing interventions. Standardizes the language nurses use to describe sets of actions in delivering client care.
2. Expansion of nursing knowledge about connections between nursing diagnoses, treatments, and outcomes. These connections will be determined through the study of actual client care through the use of a database that the classification will generate.
3. Development of nursing and health care information systems.
4. Teaching decision making to nursing students. Defining and classifying nursing interventions help teach beginning nurses how to determine a client's need for care and to respond appropriately.
5. Determination of the cost of services provided by nurses.
6. Planning for resources needed in all types of nursing practice settings.
7. Language to communicate the unique functions of nursing.
8. Link with the classification systems of other health care professionals.

Modified from Dochterman, J. M., & Bulechek, G. M. (2004). *Nursing Interventions Classification (NIC)* (4th ed.). St. Louis, MO: Mosby.

Implementation Process

Preparation for implementation ensures efficient, safe, and effective nursing care. Preparatory activities include reassessing the client, reviewing and revising the existing nursing care plan, organizing resources and care delivery, anticipating and preventing complications, and implementing nursing interventions.

Reassessing the Client

Assessment is a continuous process that occurs each time you interact with a client. When you collect new data and identify a new client need, you modify the care plan. You also modify a plan when you resolve a client's health care need. During the initial phase of planning nursing care, assessment is partial and sometimes focuses on one dimension of the client, such as level of comfort, or on one system, such as the cardiovascular system. Reassessment helps you decide whether the proposed nursing action continues to be appropriate for the client's level of wellness. For example, Lisa plans to spend a few minutes talking further with Ms. Devine about her concerns relating to surgery. However, her reassessment reveals that Ms. Devine is still a bit uncomfortable and fatigued, and so Lisa must postpone her discussion. She decides to combine her discussion of Ms. Devine's concerns when she begins preoperative teaching in 30 minutes.

Reviewing and Revising the Existing Nursing Care Plan

After reassessing a client, review the care plan, compare assessment data in order to validate the nursing diagnoses, and determine whether the nursing interventions remain the most appropriate for the clinical situation. If the client's status has changed and the nursing diagnosis and related nursing interventions are no longer appropriate, modify the nursing care plan. An outdated or incorrect care plan compromises quality of nursing care. Review and modification enable you to provide timely and appropriate nursing interventions. Modification of the existing written care plan includes four steps:

1. Revise data in the assessment column to reflect current status. Date any new data to communicate the time of the change.
2. Revise the nursing diagnoses. Delete those that are no longer relevant, and add and date any new ones.
3. Revise specific interventions that correspond to the new nursing diagnoses and goals.
4. Determine the method of evaluation for any outcomes achieved.

It has been 45 minutes since Ms. Devine received an analgesic for her pain. She reports less discomfort, and so Lisa initiates preoperative instruction. After about 10 minutes of discussion, Lisa notes that Ms. Devine expresses less concern about surgery; Ms. Devine says, "I feel better now that I understand what surgery involves." Ms. Devine's movements are calmer and less restless. Lisa enters her new findings into the care plan. However, she decides not to delete the nursing diagnosis of anxiety just yet and adds an intervention to her plan: Encourage verbalization of client's remaining concerns about surgery *(see Figure 14–2). Seeing that Ms. Devine responded well to the analgesic, Lisa also adds more nonpharmacological interventions to her plan for pain management.*

Organizing Resources and Care Delivery

A facility's resources include equipment and skilled personnel. Organization of equipment and personnel makes timely, efficient, skilled client care possible. Preparation for giving care involves preparing the environment, as well as clients.

Equipment. Most nursing procedures require some equipment or supplies. Before you perform an intervention, you must identify which supplies are needed, determine whether they are available, and ensure that equipment is in working order to ensure safe use.

Personnel. You are responsible for determining whether to perform an intervention or to delegate it to another member of the nursing team. Your assessment of a client directs delegation decisions. For example, trained nursing assistants are able to competently measure a client's vital signs, but if you learned in the change-of-shift report that a particular client experienced cardiac irregularities during that shift, you must measure the client's vital signs yourself to evaluate cardiac status. Your judgement is important for determining health status and the need for intervention.

Environment. A care environment needs to be safe and conducive to the implementation of therapies. Client safety is your first concern. If the client has sensory deficits, a physical disability, or an alteration in level of consciousness, arrange the environment to prevent injury. Ensure privacy during procedures that may require some body exposure. Also, ensure that lighting is adequate for performing procedures correctly.

Client. Before you provide care, be sure the client is as physically and psychologically comfortable as possible. Ensure that clients are comfortable during interventions. Control environmental factors at the outset, taking care of physical needs (e.g., elimination), minimizing the potential for interruptions, and positioning the client correctly. Also, consider the client's strength and endurance, and plan only the level of activity that the client is able to tolerate comfortably. Awareness of the client's psychosocial needs helps you create a favourable emotional climate. Some clients feel reassured by having a significant other present for encouragement and moral support.

Anticipating and Preventing Complications

Risks to clients arise from both illness and treatment. Be alert for and recognize these risks, adapt your choice of interventions to the situation, evaluate the benefit of the treatment in relation to the risk, and, finally, initiate risk-prevention measures (Figure 14–6). Many conditions heighten the risk for complications. For example, the client with pre-existing left-sided paralysis that followed a stroke two years earlier is at risk for developing a pressure ulcer after orthopedic surgery because postoperative care entails traction and bed rest.

Your knowledge of pathophysiology and your experience with previous clients help you identify risk of complications. A thorough assessment reveals the level of the client's current risk. The **scientific rationale**, which concerns how certain interventions (e.g., pressure-relief devices, repositioning, or wound care) prevent or minimize complications, helps you select the most useful preventive measures. For example, if an obese client has uncontrolled postoperative pain, the risk for pressure ulcer development increases because the client may be unwilling or unable to change position frequently. The nurse anticipates when the client's pain will be aggravated, administers ordered analgesics, and then positions the client to remove pressure on the skin and underlying tissues. If the client continues to have difficulty turning or repositioning, the nurse may then select a pressure-relief device to place on the client's bed.

Identifying Areas of Assistance. Certain nursing situations require you to obtain assistance by seeking additional knowledge, nursing skills, unregulated care providers, or a combination of these. Before you begin care, review the plan to determine the need for assistance. Sometimes you need assistance in performing a procedure, comforting a client, or preparing the client for a diagnostic test. For example, when you care for an overweight, immobilized client, you may require additional personnel to help turn and position the client safely. Be sure to determine the number of additional personnel in advance. You can consult about this matter with other nurses or unregulated care providers.

You require additional knowledge and skills in situations with which you are less familiar or experienced. Because of the continual updating of health care technology, you may lack the skills to perform a procedure. In these situations, you need to prepare by seeking the necessary knowledge and requesting assistance from a more experienced nurse.

Implementation Skills

Nursing practice includes cognitive, interpersonal, and psychomotor (technical) skills. You need each type of skill to implement direct and indirect nursing interventions. You are responsible for knowing which skill is needed in a particular situation and for having the necessary knowledge and skill to perform each.

Cognitive Skills. Cognitive skills involve the application of critical thinking in the nursing process. To perform any intervention, always use good judgement and make sound clinical decisions. No nursing intervention is automatic or routine. You must continually think and anticipate so that you individualize care for clients. For example, Lisa knows the pathophysiological process of a ruptured disc, the anatomy of the spinal cord, and normal pain mechanisms. She considers each of these as she observes Ms. Devine, noting how the client's movement, posture, and position either aggravate or lessen her back pain. Lisa focuses on relieving Ms. Devine's acute pain with an analgesic but then considers the noninvasive interventions needed to minimize stress on the back so that the client will remain comfortable.

Interpersonal Skills. Interpersonal skills are essential for effective nursing action. The nurse develops a trusting relationship, expresses a caring attitude, and communicates clearly with the client and family (see Chapter 19). Good interpersonal communication is crucial for keeping clients informed, providing individualized client teaching, and effectively supporting clients with challenging emotional needs.

Psychomotor Skills. Psychomotor skills require the integration of cognitive and motor activities. For example, when giving an injection, you need to understand anatomy, physiology, and pharmacology (cognitive skills) and use good coordination and precision to administer the injection correctly (motor skills). You are responsible for acquiring necessary psychomotor skills, through your experience in the nursing laboratory, through the use of interactive instructional technology, or through actual hands-on care of clients. In the case of a new skill, always assess your level of competency and obtain the necessary resources to ensure that the client receives safe treatment.

> concept map

Nursing diagnosis: Acute pain related to pressure on spinal nerves
- Back pain acuity 8 or 9 when sharp
- Pain increasing during turning
- Reports of sleeping poorly since injury
- Moaning and sighing when turning

Interventions
- Administer ordered analgesic
- Turn by logrolling
- Reduce environmental stimuli
- Introduce client to deep breathing and relaxation
- Reduce number of care activities before surgery

Nursing diagnosis: Impaired physical mobility related to acute pain
- Client turns hesitantly
- Unable to tolerate sitting
- Slow, hesitant gait when walking

Interventions
- Position in proper alignment
- Avoid placing in a position that increases pain
- Premedicate before turning

Client's chief medical diagnosis: Herniated lumbar disc. Scheduled for lumbar laminectomy
Priority assessments: Level of mobility, character of pain, knowledge and perceptions about condition and surgery

Nursing diagnosis: Anxiety related to uncertainty over surgery
- Reports of being concerned about surgery
- Restlessness
- Uncertainty about what to expect after surgery
- Concern about possible paralysis

Interventions
- Use calm, reassuring approach when discussing surgery
- Explain all procedures
- Listen attentively
- Encourage verbalization of remaining concerns

Nursing diagnosis: Deficient knowledge regarding postoperative activities related to inexperience
- No previous experience with surgery
- Reports of not receiving instruction on postoperative activities
- Asking questions

Interventions
- Provide one-to-one discussion on postoperative exercises, routine postoperative activities
- Offer time for client's questions
- Demonstrate postoperative exercises

—— Link between medical diagnosis and nursing diagnosis   - - - - Link between nursing diagnoses

Figure 14-6 Concept map for planning Ms. Devine's postoperative nursing care.

Direct Care

Nurses provide a wide variety of direct care measures. How a nurse interacts affects the success of any direct care activity, and a caring approach is essential. You need to be sensitive at all times to a client's clinical condition, values and beliefs, expectations, and cultural views. All direct care measures require safe and competent practice.

Activities of Daily Living

Activities of daily living (ADLs) are activities usually performed in the course of a normal day, including ambulation, eating, dressing, bathing, brushing the teeth, and grooming (see Chapter 38). A client's need for assistance with ADLs is temporary, permanent, or rehabilitative. A client with impaired mobility because of bilateral arm casts has a temporary need for assistance. A client with an irreversible injury to the cervical spinal cord is paralyzed and thus has a permanent need for assistance. Occupational and physical therapists play key roles in rehabilitation to restore ADL function.

When your assessment reveals that a client is experiencing fatigue, a limitation in mobility, confusion, and pain, the client probably needs assistance with ADLs. For example, a client who experiences shortness of breath avoids eating because of the associated fatigue. Assist the client by setting up meals, offering to cut up food, and planning for small and frequent meals to maintain nutrition. Determine the client's preferences when you assist with ADLs, and let the client participate as much as possible. Involving the client in planning the timing and types of interventions enhances the client's self-esteem and willingness to assume more independence.

Instrumental Activities of Daily Living

Illness or disability sometimes alters a client's ability to be independent in society. **Instrumental activities of daily living** (IADLs) include such skills as shopping, preparing meals, writing checks, and taking medications. Nurses within the home care and community health care settings frequently assist clients in finding ways to accomplish IADLs. Often, family and friends are excellent resources for assisting clients. In acute care, it is important to anticipate how illness will affect the client's ability to perform IADLs and to involve other health professionals such as occupational therapists.

Physical Care Techniques

You routinely perform a variety of physical care techniques when caring for a client. Examples include turning and positioning, changing dressings, administering medications, and providing comfort measures. Considerations in providing physical care include protecting yourself and the client from injury, using proper infection control practices, staying organized, and following applicable practice guidelines. To carry out a procedure, you need to be knowledgeable about the procedure and how to perform it and about the expected outcomes.

Lifesaving Measures

A **lifesaving measure** is a physical care technique performed when a client's physiological or psychological state is threatened (see Chapter 39). The purpose of lifesaving measures is to restore physiological or psychological equilibrium. Such measures include administering emergency medications, instituting cardiopulmonary resuscitation, intervening to protect a confused or violent client, and obtaining immediate counselling from a crisis centre for an emotionally disturbed client. If an inexperienced nurse faces a situation necessitating emergency measures, the proper nursing action is to summon an experienced health professional.

Counselling

Counselling is a direct care method that helps the client use a problem-solving process to recognize and manage stress and to facilitate interpersonal relationships. Counselling involves emotional, intellectual, spiritual, and psychological support. A client and family who need nursing counselling may be upset or frustrated, but they are not necessarily disabled psychologically. Family caregivers need assistance in adjusting to the physical and emotional demands of caregiving. Likewise, the recipient of care also needs assistance in adjusting to the disability. Clients with psychiatric diagnoses require therapy provided by psychiatric nurses or by social workers, psychiatrists, or psychologists.

Many counselling techniques foster cognitive, behavioural, developmental, experiential, and emotional growth in clients. Most of the techniques listed in Box 14–3 require additional knowledge beyond the scope of this text. Counselling encourages individuals to examine available alternatives and decide which choices are useful and appropriate.

Teaching

Teaching is an important nursing responsibility and is related to counselling. Both involve using communication skills to create a change in the client. However, in counselling, the focus is on the development of new attitudes and feelings, whereas in teaching, the focus is on intellectual growth or the acquisition of new knowledge or psychomotor skills (Redman, 2005).

The purpose of health teaching is to help clients learn about their health status, ways of promoting health, and ways of caring for themselves. Some common examples of teaching by nurses are related to medication administration, activity restrictions, health promotion activities (e.g., diet and exercise), and knowledge about disease and related implications. Your role includes assessment of clients' learning needs and readiness to learn. It is important to know your client and to be aware of cultural and social factors that influence a client's willingness and ability to learn. It is also important to know the client's health literacy levels: that is, whether the client can read directions or make calculations that sometimes are necessary with self-care skills. The teaching–learning process is an interaction between you and the client in which you address specific learning objectives (see Chapter 21).

Controlling for Adverse Reactions

An **adverse reaction** is a harmful effect of a medication, diagnostic test, or therapeutic intervention. Because adverse reactions can follow any nursing intervention, it is important to know which ones might occur. Nursing actions that control for adverse reactions reduce or counteract the reaction. For example, when applying a moist heat compress, you must take steps to prevent burning the client's skin. First, assess the area where the compress is to be applied. Then, inspect the area every five minutes for any adverse reaction, such as excessive reddening of the skin from the heat or skin maceration from the moisture of the compress. When completing a physician-directed intervention, such as medication administration, you need to understand the known and potential side effects of the drug. After administration of the medication, you evaluate the client for any adverse effects. Also, be aware of drugs that counteract the side effects. For example, a client has a previously unknown hypersensitivity to penicillin, and hives develop after three doses. You record the reaction, stop further administration of the drug, and consult with the physician. You then administer an ordered dose of diphenhydramine (Benadryl), an antihistamine and antipruritic medication, to reduce the allergic response and to relieve the itching.

Preventive Measures

Preventive nursing actions promote health and prevent illness in order to avoid the need for acute or rehabilitative health care. Health promotion and illness prevention are very important. Prevention includes assessment and promotion of the client's health potential, carrying out prescribed measures (e.g., immunizations), health teaching, and identification of risk factors for illness, trauma, or both. Consider, for example, the case of Ms. Devine. Lisa learns that her client does not exercise regularly. Ms. Devine is 5 feet 6 inches tall and weighs 160 pounds. Because she is overweight and inactive, she is at risk when she performs activities that place stress on her back. If the client is able to lose some weight and start exercise therapy, she will be less likely to reinjure her back. Lisa plans to consult with the surgeon and physical therapist after surgery to design a plan to help Ms. Devine with weight loss and strengthening of back muscles.

Indirect Care

Indirect care measures are actions that support the effectiveness of direct care interventions (Bulechek et al., 2008). Many of the measures, such as emergency care maintenance and environmental and supply management, are managerial in nature (Box 14–6). Nurses spend a good amount of time in indirect and unit management activities. Communication of information about clients (e.g., change-of-shift report and consultation) is essential to ensure that direct care activities are planned, coordinated, and performed with the proper

➤ BOX 14-6 Examples of Indirect Care Activities

- Documentation
- Delegation of care activities to unregulated care providers
- Medical order transcription
- Infection control (e.g., proper handling and storage of supplies, use of protective isolation)
- Environmental safety management (e.g., make client rooms safe, strategically assigning clients in a geographic proximity to a single nurse)
- Computer data entry
- Telephone consultations with physicians and other health care professionals
- Change-of-shift report
- Collecting, labelling, and transporting laboratory specimens
- Transporting patients to procedural areas and other nursing units

Modified from Dochterman, J. M., & Bulechek, G. M. (2004). *Nursing Interventions Classification (NIC)* (4th ed.). St. Louis, MO: Mosby.

resources. Delegation of care to unregulated care providers is another indirect care activity.

Communicating Nursing Interventions

Any intervention you provide for a client will be communicated in a written or oral format, or both. Written interventions are part of both the nursing care plan and the permanent medical record. In many institutions, staff develop interdisciplinary care plans, which are plans that represent the contributions of all disciplines involved in caring for a client. For example, when Ms. Devine begins recovering from back surgery, her nursing diagnosis of *impaired physical mobility* will prompt interventions by nurses (e.g., nonpharmacological pain control and positioning), the surgeon (e.g., activity guidelines and pharmacological pain control), and the physical therapist (e.g., ambulation training and exercises).

After completing nursing interventions, you document the treatment and client's response in the appropriate record (see Chapter 16). The entry usually includes a brief description of pertinent assessment findings, the specific procedure, the time and details of the procedure, and the client's response. You also communicate nursing interventions verbally to other health care professionals. Unless communication is clear, concise, accurate, and timely, caregivers can be uninformed, interventions may be needlessly duplicated, procedures may be delayed, or tasks may be left undone.

Delegating, Supervising, and Evaluating the Work of Other Staff Members

Depending on the staffing system, not all of the nursing interventions may be performed by the nurse who develops the care plan. Some activities are delegated to other members of the health care team.. Interventions such as skin care, ambulation, grooming, measuring vital signs in stable clients, and hygiene measures are examples of care activities that you may assign to unregulated care providers and licensed practice nurses who are competent to carry out these activities. When a nurse delegates aspects of a client's care to another staff member, the nurse assigning tasks is responsible for ensuring that each task is appropriately assigned and completed.

Achieving Client-Centred Goals

You implement nursing care to meet client-centred goals and outcomes. In most clinical situations, multiple interventions are necessary to achieve selected outcomes. Because clients' conditions may change rapidly, it is important to apply principles of care coordination, such as good time management, organizational skills, and appropriate use of resources, to ensure that you deliver interventions effectively and that clients achieve desired outcomes. Priority setting is also crucial in successful implementation because it helps you to anticipate and sequence nursing interventions when a client has multiple nursing diagnoses and collaborative problems. Another way to achieve client-centred goals is to encourage and assist clients to follow their treatment plan.

Effective discharge planning and teaching for clients and families require individualized care that is consistent with culture and health beliefs. The process should be initiated at the outset of care. Adequate and timely discharge planning and education of the client and family are the first steps in promoting a smooth transition from one health care setting to another or to home. To be effective with discharge planning and education, you individualize your care and take into consideration the various factors that influence a client's health beliefs. For example, to help Ms. Devine adopt better exercise habits when she returns home, Lisa needs to determine what knowledge and psychosocial factors may influence Ms. Devine to exercise when she returns home. Reinforcing successes with the treatment plan encourages clients to follow their care plans.

* KEY CONCEPTS

- During planning, you determine client-centred goals, set priorities, develop expected outcomes of nursing care, and develop a nursing care plan.
- Priority setting helps you anticipate and sequence nursing interventions when a client has multiple nursing diagnoses and collaborative problems.
- Multiple factors in the nursing care environment influence your ability to set priorities.
- Goals and expected outcomes provide clear direction for the selection and use of nursing interventions and provide focus for evaluation of the effectiveness of the interventions.
- In setting goals, the time frame depends on the nature of the problem, etiology, overall condition of the client, and treatment setting.
- A client-centred goal is singular, observable, measurable, time limited, mutual, and realistic.
- An expected outcome is an objective criterion for goal achievement.
- Care plans and critical pathways increase communication among nurses and facilitate the continuity of care from one nurse to another and from one health care setting to another.
- A concept map provides a visually graphic way to understand the relationship between a client's nursing diagnoses and interventions.
- The NIC taxonomy provides a standardization to assist you in selecting suitable interventions for clients' problems.
- Correctly written nursing interventions include actions, frequency, quantity, and method, and they specify the person to perform them.

- Consultation increases your knowledge about a client's problem and helps you learn skills and obtain the resources needed to solve the problem.
- Implementation is the step of the nursing process in which you provide direct and indirect nursing care interventions to clients.
- Clinical guidelines or protocols are evidence-informed documents that guide decisions and interventions for specific health care problems.
- During the initial phase of implementation, you reassess the client to determine whether the proposed nursing action is still appropriate for the client's level of wellness.
- To anticipate and prevent complications, you identify risks to the client, adapt interventions to the situation, evaluate the benefit of a treatment in relation to the risk, and initiate risk-prevention measures.
- Successful implementation of nursing interventions requires you to use appropriate cognitive, interpersonal, and psychomotor skills.
- Counselling is a direct care method that helps clients use problem solving to recognize and manage stress and to facilitate interpersonal relationships.
- Preventive nursing actions include assessment and promotion of the client's health potential, application of prescribed measures (e.g., immunizations), health teaching, and identification of risk factors for illness, trauma, or both.

* CRITICAL THINKING EXERCISES

Shawn, a nurse, has two different clients. Mr. Gordon is a 52-year-old client who was admitted to the hospital after a motor vehicle accident. He suffered rib fractures and has a laceration along his right thigh. Shawn has identified the following nursing diagnoses: *ineffective breathing pattern related to chest pain, acute pain related to musculoskeletal trauma,* and *risk for infection related to open wound.* Shawn's second client, Ms. Lawrence, is a 63-year-old woman who had surgery yesterday evening for repair of a foot fracture. Her foot is in a cast. Ms. Lawrence's nursing diagnoses include *acute pain related to tissue swelling, impaired mobility related to restricted movement from cast,* and *deficient knowledge regarding cast care related to inexperience.* Ms. Lawrence will probably be discharged in the morning. She lives alone. Shawn begins to plan care by establishing goals and outcomes for the nursing diagnoses.

1. Between the two clients, which diagnoses are high priority and which are intermediate priority?
2. Of the two clients, which one has higher priority regarding pain management?
3. For the nursing diagnosis *deficient knowledge regarding cast care related to inexperience,* write one goal and two expected outcomes.

Sue is a nursing student. She is to care for Mr. Nelson, a 63-year-old client who was admitted to the hospital with congestive heart failure and pneumonia. He is receiving medications to improve his heart failure and intravenous antibiotics to treat his pneumonia. He reports becoming fatigued easily during care activities and states, "I feel short of breath if I try to do too much." Sue notes he has 3+ edema in his lower extremities. Sue has identified nursing diagnoses of *decreased cardiac output* and *activity intolerance.* Sue must still perform hygiene measures, change the client's intravenous dressing, get him up into a chair, and measure noontime vital signs.

4. Before she begins to intervene, how can Sue make Mr. Nelson more comfortable?
5. What type of intervention is vital sign measurement?
6. Because Sue thinks that Mr. Nelson may be at risk of falling, she decides to get assistance from a colleague before trying to get him into a chair. This is an example of what type of implementation skill?
7. When changing Mr. Nelson's intravenous dressing, Sue cleans the insertion site in accordance with clinical practice guidelines and checks the site for signs of phlebitis. These steps are examples of what type of direct care measure?

* REVIEW QUESTIONS

1. Sheila, a nurse, is assigned to a client who has returned from the recovery room after surgery for a colorectal tumour. After an initial assessment, Sheila anticipates the need to monitor the client's abdominal dressing, intravenous infusion, and function of drainage tubes. The client is in pain and will not be able to eat or drink until intestinal function returns. Sheila will have to establish priorities of care in which of the following situations? (Choose all that apply.)
   1. The family comes to visit the client.
   2. The client expresses concern about pain control.
   3. The client's vital signs change, showing a drop in blood pressure.
   4. The charge nurse approaches Sheila and requests a report at end of shift.
2. Sheila's client signals with her call light. Sheila enters the room and finds that the drainage tube is disconnected, the intravenous line has 100 mL of fluid remaining, and the client has asked to be turned. Which of the following should Sheila perform first?
   1. Reconnect the drainage tubing.
   2. Inspect the condition of the intravenous dressing.
   3. Improve client's comfort, and turn her onto her side.
   4. Go to the medication room, and obtain the next intravenous fluid bag.
3. In her nursing care plan, Sheila writes expected outcomes for her client. Which of the following expected outcomes are written correctly? (Choose all that apply.)
   1. Client will remain afebrile until discharge.
   2. Intravenous site will be without phlebitis by the third postoperative day.
   3. Provide incentive spirometer for deep breathing every 2 hours.
   4. Client will report pain and turn more freely by the first postoperative day.
4. The nurse writes an expected outcome statement in measurable terms. An example is:
   1. Client will be pain free
   2. Client will have less pain
   3. Client will take pain medication every 4 hours
   4. Client will report pain acuity less than 4 on a scale of 0 to 10

5. Collaborative interventions are therapies that require:
   1. Nurse and client intervention
   2. Physician and nurse intervention
   3. Client and physician intervention
   4. Multiple health care professionals
6. When does implementation begin in the nursing process?
   1. During the assessment phase
   2. Immediately, in some critical situations
   3. After the care plan has been developed
   4. After mutual goal setting by the nurse and client
7. Mr. Switzer is a 34-year-old client who underwent surgical repair of an abdominal hernia this morning. At noon, the nurse records Mr. Switzer's vital sign measurements on the recovery room flow sheet. The recording of vital sign measurements is an example of:
   1. Psychomotor skill
   2. Indirect care measure
   3. Physical care technique
   4. Anticipating complications
8. Environmental factors heavily affect a client's care. Your first concern for the client includes which of the following?
   1. Safety
   2. Nurse staffing
   3. Confidentiality
   4. Adequate pain relief
9. An out-of-date care plan:
   1. Means the client was discharged
   2. Compromises the quality of care
   3. Ensures that the nursing care was delivered
   4. Identifies that the client response was successful

* RECOMMENDED WEB SITES

Center for Nursing Classification & Clinical Effectiveness: http://www.nursing.uiowa.edu/excellence/nursing_knowledge/clinical_effectiveness/index.htm

The University of Iowa's Center for Nursing Classification and Clinical Effectiveness was established to facilitate ongoing research of the Nursing Interventions Classification (NIC) and Nursing Outcomes Classification (NOC). This Web site provides an overview of the NIC and NOC and offers information about new classification material and publications.

NANDA International: http://www.nanda.org/

Through this Web site, NANDA International provides current information on nursing diagnosis research, publications, and Internet resources.

Registered Nurses Association of Ontario: Best Practices Guidelines: http://www.rnao.org/bestpractices/

The Registered Nurses Association of Ontario has an extensive process for developing best practices guidelines in a variety of areas of clinical nursing. They have received federal and provincial funding for this process, and the results of their work have been made available to all Canadian nurses through this Web site, which lists all current guidelines that have been developed.

15

Evaluation of Nursing Care

Original chapter by Patricia A. Potter, RN, MSN, PhD, GMAC, FAAN

Canadian content written by Marilyn J. Wood, RN, BSN, MPH, DrPH, and Janet C. Ross-Kerr, RN, BScN, MS, PhD

objectives

Mastery of content in this chapter will enable you to:

- Define the key terms listed.
- Discuss the relationship between critical thinking and evaluation.
- Identify the five elements of the evaluation process.
- Explain the relationship between goals of care, expected outcomes, and evaluative measures in evaluating nursing care.
- Give examples of evaluation measures for determining a client's progress toward outcomes.
- Evaluate a set of nursing actions selected for a client.
- Describe how evaluation leads to discontinuation, revision, or modification of a plan of care.

key terms

Evaluation, p. 200
Evaluative measures, p. 202
Outcome, p. 202
Standard of care, p. 206

media resources

evolve Web Site

- Audio Chapter Summaries
- Glossary
- Multiple-Choice Review Questions
- Student Learning Activities
- Weblinks

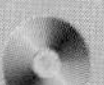 **Companion CD**

- Glossary
- Interactive Learning Activities
- Fluids and Electrolytes Tutorial
- Test-Taking Skills

When a plumber comes to a home to fix a leaking faucet, he or she turns on the faucet to determine the problem, changes or adjusts parts to the faucet, and then turns on the faucet once again to determine whether the leak is fixed. Similarly, after a client with a diagnosis of pneumonia completes a five-day dose pack of antibiotics, the physician often has the client return to the office to have a chest X-ray examination to determine whether the pneumonia has cleared. When a nurse delivers an intervention such as applying a warm compress to a wound, several steps are involved. The nurse assesses the appearance of the wound, determines the severity of the wound, applies the appropriate form of compress, and then returns to determine whether the condition of the wound has improved. These three scenarios depict what ultimately occurs during the process of **evaluation.** The plumber rechecks the faucet, the physician orders a chest X-ray film, and the nurse inspects the wound.

Evaluation involves two components: an examination of a condition or situation and then a judgement as to whether change has occurred. Ideally, after an intervention takes place, evaluation will reveal an improvement.

Chapters 13 and 14 describe how you use critical thinking skills to gather client data, form nursing diagnoses, develop a plan of care, and implement the care plan. Evaluation, the final step of the nursing process, is crucial for determining whether, after application of the nursing process, the client's condition or well-being improves. You apply all that you know about a client and the client's condition, as well as experience with previous clients, to evaluate whether nursing care was effective. *You conduct evaluative measures to determine whether expected outcomes were attained, not whether nursing interventions were completed.* The expected outcomes are the standards against which you judge whether goals have been met and if care is successful.

In the continuing case study, Lisa is now making final preparations to send Ms. Devine to the operating room. Lisa evaluates the interventions she has implemented for the goals of achieving pain control, reducing anxiety, improving mobility, and improving Ms. Devine's knowledge of postoperative activities. Lisa had returned to Ms. Devine's room 30 minutes after administering an analgesic. At that time, the client reported having pain at a level of 4 on a scale of 1 (none) to 10 (worst). Lisa had documented the expected outcome of reduction of pain to a level of 3. Lisa then implemented further nonpharmacological interventions. It is now two hours later, and Lisa finds Ms. Devine lying in bed with her eyes closed. The client awakens as Lisa enters and says, "I just had my eyes closed; I am ready to get this over." Lisa asks, "Tell me how you are feeling." Ms. Devine responds, "Okay, really okay; I feel better, and I am a little less worried than when I first got here." Lisa asks, "On a scale of 0 to 10, tell me how you would rate your pain now." Ms. Devine, "I would say about a 4; it is still there but not as sharp." Lisa continues, "You said you were feeling less worried." Ms. Devine replies, "Yes, I think you have helped me feel less anxious. You know, surgery is nothing anyone wants to have, but I feel better knowing what to expect." Lisa observes that Ms. Devine is relaxed and does not grimace when she turns slightly to her side. Lisa asks, "Can you take just a moment to go over with me what we discussed about your care after surgery?" Ms. Devine responds, "Sure, that would be fine."

Critical Thinking and Evaluation

Evaluation is an ongoing process whenever you have contact with a client. Once you perform an intervention, you gather subjective and objective data from the client, family, and health care team members. You also review knowledge regarding the client's current condition, treatment, resources available for recovery, and the expected outcomes. By referring to previous experiences caring for similar clients, you are in a better position to know how to evaluate your client's needs. Apply critical thinking qualities and standards to determine whether expected outcomes of care are achieved (Figure 15–1). If expected outcomes are achieved, the overall goals for the client also are met. Client behaviour and responses that you assessed before performing nursing interventions are compared with behaviour and responses that occur after you perform nursing care. Critical thinking directs you to analyze the findings from evaluation (Figure 15–2): Has the client's condition improved? Is the client able to improve, or do physical factors preventing recovery exist? To what degree does this client's motivation or willingness to pursue healthier behaviour influence response to therapies?

During evaluation, you make clinical decisions and continually redirect nursing care. For example, when Lisa evaluates Ms. Devine for a change in pain severity, she applies knowledge of the disease process, physiological responses to interventions (e.g., analgesics), and the correct procedure for pain severity measurement to interpret whether a change has occurred and whether the change is desirable. Lisa knows that the condition of the herniated disc will not change as a result of an analgesic, but the opioid medication she administered will alter the client's perception and reaction to pain (see Chapter 42). Use of the pain severity rating scale helps Lisa obtain an accurate measure of change in the client's pain perception. Evaluative findings determine Lisa's next course of action. In Ms. Devine's case, the pain score is a bit higher (4) than expected (3). However, the client is about to leave for surgery. Ms. Devine will probably receive a preoperative medication just before she goes to the preoperative holding area. The preoperative medication will include an analgesic, and so Lisa knows she cannot administer an additional analgesic at this time. She evaluates that Ms. Devine's pain has been reduced and decides to continue to use basic comfort measures to afford further pain relief.

Positive evaluations occur when you meet desired outcomes, and they lead you to conclude that the nursing intervention or interventions effectively met the client's goals. For example, in the case study, Lisa notes that Ms. Devine's pain rating fell from an 8 or 9 to a 4. With an expected outcome of a pain severity of 3, Lisa's interventions showed a successful reduction in pain severity, but

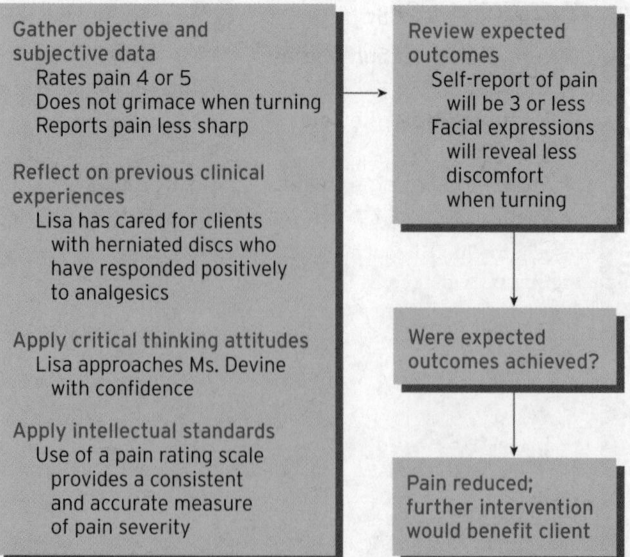

Figure 15-1 Critical thinking and the evaluation process.

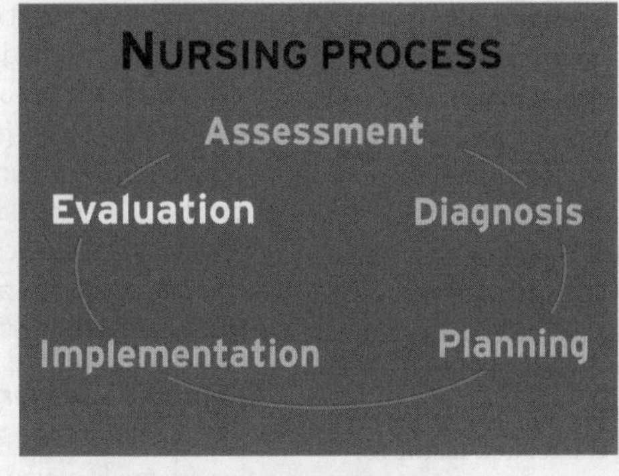

Figure 15-2 Critical thinking and evaluation.

continuing intervention is necessary. Unmet or undesirable outcomes, such as the continuation of severe pain, indicate that interventions are not effective in minimizing or resolving the actual problem or avoiding the risk of a problem. Outcomes need to be realistic and adjusted on the basis of the client's prognosis and nursing diagnoses. An unmet outcome reveals the client has not responded to interventions as planned. As a result, the nurse changes the plan of care by trying different therapies or changing the frequency or approach of existing therapies.

This sequence of critically evaluating and revising therapies continues until you and the client successfully and appropriately resolve the problems, as defined by nursing diagnoses. Remember that evaluation is dynamic and ever changing, depending on the client's nursing diagnoses and condition. As problems change, so will expectations of outcomes. A client whose health status continuously changes requires more frequent evaluation. In addition, you will evaluate high-priority diagnoses first. For example, Lisa evaluates Ms. Devine's diagnosis of *acute pain* before evaluating the status of the diagnosis of *deficient knowledge.*

The Evaluation Process

The purpose of nursing care is to assist the client in resolving actual health problems, preventing the occurrence of potential problems, and maintaining a healthy state. The evaluation process, which determines the effectiveness of nursing care, consists of five elements: (1) identifying evaluative criteria and standards; (2) collecting data to determine whether the criteria or standards are met; (3) interpreting and summarizing findings; (4) documenting findings and any clinical judgement; and (5) terminating, continuing, or revising the care plan.

Identifying Criteria and Standards

You evaluate nursing care by knowing what to look for. A client's goals and expected outcomes are the objective criteria by which to judge a client's response to care.

Goals. A goal is the expected behaviour or response that indicates resolution of a nursing diagnosis or maintenance of a healthy state. It is a summary statement of what will be accomplished when the client has met all expected outcomes. In the case of Ms. Devine, Chapter 14 described Lisa's plan of care for *acute pain.* Lisa selected the goal "Client achieves improved pain control before surgery." Successful achievement of this goal depends on the success of Lisa's interventions, chosen from the Nursing Interventions Classification (NIC; Bulechek et al., 2008), for analgesic administration, pain management, and progressive muscle relaxation. Goals are also often based on standards of care or guidelines established for minimal safe practice. When a nurse cares for a client with a peripheral intravenous line, the goal "The intravenous site will remain free of phlebitis" is established on the basis of sound practice standards. (The Registered Nurses Association of Ontario's [2008] *Best Practice Guidelines* contains specific recommendations for care of peripheral intravenous lines).

Expected Outcomes. Outcomes have been broadly defined in the health care literature. Donabedian (1980) defined outcomes as favourable or adverse changes in clients' health states caused by prior or concurrent care. When nurses apply the nursing process, expected outcomes are the expected favourable and measurable results of nursing care. A nursing-sensitive client outcome is a measurable client or family state, behaviour, or perception largely influenced by and sensitive to nursing interventions (Moorhead et al., 2008). Examples of nursing-sensitive outcomes include reductions in pain severity, in incidence of pressure ulcers, and in incidence of falls (Box 15–1). In comparison, outcomes influenced largely by medical interventions include client mortality, hospital readmissions, and length of stay. **Outcomes** are statements of progressive, step-by-step responses or behaviours that must be achieved in order to accomplish the goals of care. An outcome defines the effectiveness, efficiency, and measurement of the results of nursing interventions. When you achieve outcomes, the related factors for a nursing diagnosis usually no longer exist. In Ms. Devine's case, the expected outcomes for the goal of achieving improved pain control are "Client's self-report of pain will be 3 or less on a scale of 0 to 10" and "Client's facial expressions reveal less discomfort when turning and repositioning." When Lisa evaluates Ms. Devine's pain at a level of 4 and notes an absence of facial grimacing during turning, she knows the client's pain has been reduced but that further pain relief is needed. However, the related factor for Ms. Devine's diagnosis of *acute pain* is pressure on spinal nerves, which will not be totally relieved until surgery. The analgesics and noninvasive nursing interventions are designed to reduce the perception of pain from pressure on the nerves, as well as to minimize additional pressure on nerves. It is important to understand that evaluation is not a description of the achievement of an intervention. Evaluation of Ms. Devine does *not* involve observation of her ability to turn correctly; it *does* involve observation of the client's behaviour (facial expression) during turning. During the planning phase of the nursing process (see Chapter 14), it is important for you to select an observable client state, behaviour, or self-reported perception that will reflect goal achievement.

One valuable resource is the Nursing Outcomes Classification (NOC; Moorhead et al., 2008), which provides a classification system of nursing sensitive outcomes. NOC is designed to provide the language for the evaluation step of the nursing process. The purposes of NOC are (1) to identify, label, validate, and classify nursing-sensitive client outcomes; (2) to field test and validate the classification; and (3) to define and test measurement procedures for the outcomes and indicators using clinical data. The NOC project complements the work of NANDA International (2007) and the NIC project. The NOC system offers nursing-sensitive outcomes for NANDA International nursing diagnoses (Table 15–1). For each outcome, the NOC system specifies recommended evaluation indicators: the client behaviours or responses that are measures of outcome achievement.

Collecting Evaluative Data

Proper evaluation enables you to determine the client's response to nursing care and whether the therapy was effective in improving the client's physical or emotional health. It is important to evaluate whether each client reaches a level of wellness or recovery that the health care team and client established in the goals of care. In addition, you must determine whether you met the client's expectations of care. You will ask clients questions about their perceptions of care, such as "Did you receive the type of pain relief you expected?" and "Did you receive enough information to care for your baby at home?" This level of evaluation is important for determining the client's satisfaction with care and for strengthening the partnering between you and the client. Always select appropriate evaluative measures to evaluate client response and expectations. Evaluating a client's response to nursing care requires the use of **evaluative measures,** which are simply assessment skills and techniques (e.g., auscultation of lung sounds, observation of a client's skill performance, discussion of the client's feelings, and inspection of the skin) (Figure 15–3). In fact, evaluative measures are the same as assessment measures, but you perform them when you make decisions about the client's status and progress.

The intent of assessment is to identify any problems that exist. The intent of evaluation is to determine whether the known problems have remained the same, improved, worsened, or otherwise changed. In many clinical situations, it is important to collect evaluative measures over a period of time to determine whether a pattern of improvement or change exists. A one-time observation of a pressure ulcer is insufficient to determine that the ulcer is healing. It is important to note a consistency in change. For example, over a period of two days, you can observe whether the pressure ulcer is gradually decreasing in size, whether the amount of drainage is declining, and whether the redness of inflammation is resolving. Recognizing a pattern of improvement or deterioration allows you to reason and decide whether the client's problems are resolved. The primary source of data for evaluation is the client. However, you also use input from the family and other caregivers. For example, if a client is at home, you can ask a family member to report on the amount of food the client eats during a meal or how well a client prepares to take medications. You will sometimes consult with a colleague about how a hospitalized client responded to pain medication during another shift.

BOX 15-1 RESEARCH HIGHLIGHT

Nursing-Sensitive Outcomes

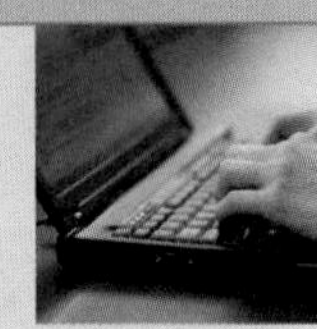

Evidence Summary

Although members of the general public recognize that oncology nurses aim to deliver high-quality care to people with cancer and to their families, nurses themselves struggle with ways to measure their influence on client outcomes. The Oncology Nursing Society (ONS) implemented a project to define and list nursing-sensitive patient outcomes (NSPOs) for the field of oncology. For each outcome, the ONS is working to provide references and links to best evidence in the literature, provide clinical guidelines, review existing knowledge, and discuss measurement of outcomes. Examples of NSPOs include control and management of symptoms (e.g., pain, fatigue, insomnia, nausea, constipation, breathlessness, diarrhea), functional status (activities of daily living, instrumental activities of daily living, role functioning, activity tolerance, nutritional status), psychological health status (anxiety, depression, spiritual distress, coping), and economic outcomes (home care visits, costs per day per episode of illness).

Application to Nursing Practice

- Establishing NSPOs for clients with cancer helps provide tools for you to use in measuring the impact of nursing care.
- Development of core measures linked to evidence-informed practice guidelines will improve nursing practice at the client's bedside.
- Use of NSPOs helps you clearly indicate to consumers the value nursing contributes to health care.

References: Given, B. A., & Sherwood, P. R. (2005). Nursing-sensitive patient outcomes—A white paper. *Oncology Nurses Forum, 32,* 773.

➤ TABLE 15-1 Linkages Between Nursing Outcomes Classification and Nursing Diagnoses

Nursing Diagnosis	Suggested Outcomes	Indicators (Examples)
Pain	Comfort level	Reported physical well-being Reported satisfaction with symptom control Expressed satisfaction with pain control
	Pain control	Recognition of pain onset Appropriate use of analgesics Control of reported pain
	Pain level	Reported pain severity Frequency of pain Muscle tension
Deficient knowledge	Knowledge: treatment procedures Knowledge: illness care	Description of treatment procedures Description of disease process Description of prescribed activity

Modified from Moorhead, S., Johnson, M., & Maas, M. (2008). *Nursing Outcomes Classification (NOC)* (4th ed.). St. Louis, MO: Mosby.

Interpreting and Summarizing Findings

During an acute illness, a client's clinical condition changes, often minute by minute. In contrast, chronic illness results in slow, subtle changes. When you evaluate the effect of interventions, you learn to recognize relevant evidence about a client's condition, even evidence that sometimes does not match clinical expectations. By applying your clinical knowledge and experience, you learn to recognize complications or adverse responses to illness and treatment in addition to expected outcomes. Using evidence, you make judgements about a client's condition. To develop clinical judgement, you learn to match the results of evaluative measures with expected outcomes to determine whether a client's status is improving. When interpreting findings, you compare the client's behavioural responses and the physiological signs and symptoms you expect to observe with those you actually observe in your evaluation. Comparing expected and actual findings allows you to interpret and judge the client's condition and whether predicted changes have occurred (Table 15–2).

To objectively evaluate the degree of success in achieving outcomes of care, use the following steps:

1. Examine the outcome criteria to identify the exact desired client behaviour or response.
2. Assess the client's actual behaviour or response.
3. Compare the established outcome criteria with the actual behaviour or response.
4. Judge the degree of agreement between outcome criteria and the actual behaviour or response.
5. If the outcome criteria are not in agreement or are in only partial agreement with the actual behaviour or response, what are the barriers to agreement? Why was agreement not complete?

Evaluation is easier to perform after you care for a client over a long period. You are then able to make subtle comparisons of client responses and behaviours. When you have not had the chance to care for a client over an extended time, you improve evaluation by referring to previous experiences or asking colleagues who are familiar with the client to confirm evaluation findings. The accuracy of any evaluation improves when you are familiar with the client's behaviour and physiological status or have cared for more than one client with a similar problem. Remember to evaluate whether each expected outcome was achieved and its place in the sequence of care. If you do not, it will be difficult to determine which expected outcome in the sequence was not achieved, and you cannot revise and redirect the plan of care at the most appropriate time. If the client

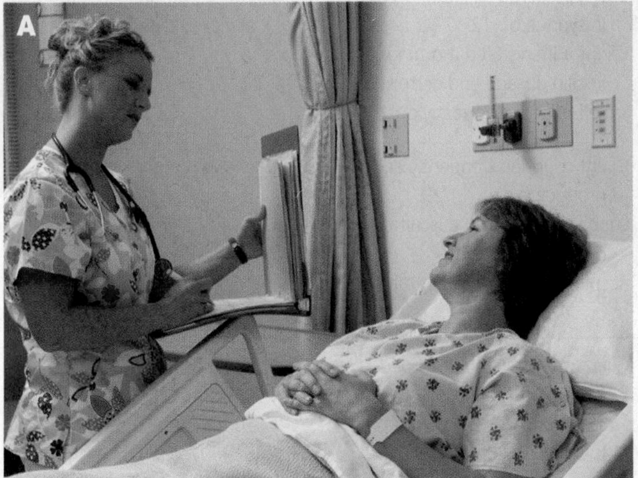

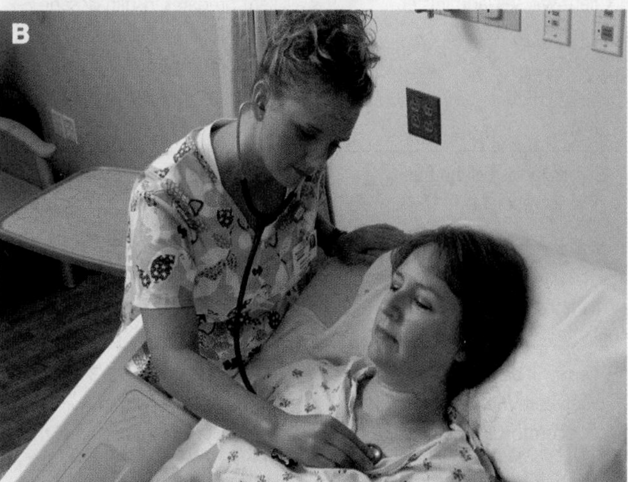

Figure 15-3 Evaluative measures. A, Nurse confirms client's medical history. B, Nurse evaluates client's lung sounds.

TABLE 15-2 Evaluative Measures to Determine the Success of Goals and Expected Outcomes

Goals	Evaluative Measures	Expected Outcomes
Client's pressure ulcer will heal within seven days	Inspect colour, condition, and location of pressure ulcer Measure diameter of ulcer daily Note odour and colour of drainage from ulcer	Erythema will be reduced in two days Diameter of ulcer will decrease in five days Ulcer will have no drainage in two days Skin overlying ulcer will be closed in seven days
Client will tolerate ambulation to end of hall by 11/20	Palpate client's radial pulse before exercise Palpate client's radial pulse 10 minutes after exercise Assess respiratory rate during exercise Observe client for dyspnea or breathlessness during exercise	Pulse will remain below 110 beats per minute during exercise Respiratory rate will remain within two breaths of client's baseline rate Client will deny feeling of breathlessness
Client will have improved grief resolution by 1/15	Ask client about frequency of periods of crying, sadness Review client's sleeping log Review client's dietary intake	Client reports decreased frequency of crying and sadness in two months Client has periods of six to seven hours of sleep without interruption within 10 days Client has no weight loss in one month

achieves the expected outcomes, you either continue the care plan to maintain a therapeutic status or discontinue interventions because the goal of care is met. If evaluation reveals that the expected outcomes were not achieved or were only partially achieved, you begin reassessment and revision of the care plan. Goals are achieved in different degrees. If the client's response matches or exceeds the outcome criteria, the goal is met. If the client's behaviour begins to show changes but does not yet meet criteria set, the goal is partially met. If progress is not made, the goal is not met (Table 15–3).

Documenting Findings

Documentation and reporting are an important part of evaluation. For you to make ongoing clinical decisions, a client's medical record must contain accurate information. When documenting the client's response to interventions, always describe the same evaluative measures. Your aim is to present a clear description, informed by the evaluative data, of a client's progress or lack of progress. Written nursing progress notes, assessment flow sheets, and information shared between nurses during change-of-shift reports (see Chapter 16) communicate a client's progress toward meeting expected outcomes and goals for the nursing plan of care.

Care Plan Revision

Evaluate expected outcomes, and determine whether the goals of care have been met. Then decide whether you need to adjust the plan of care. If you meet a goal successfully, discontinue that portion of the care plan. If goals are unmet or partially met, you must continue intervention. After you evaluate a client, you may want to modify or add nursing diagnoses with appropriate goals and expected outcomes, and establish interventions. You must also redefine priorities. This is an important step in critical thinking: knowing how the client is progressing and how problems either resolve or worsen.

TABLE 15-3 Examples of Objective Evaluation of Goal Achievement

Goals	Outcome Criteria	Client Response	Evaluation Findings
Client will self-administer insulin by 12/18	Client prepares insulin dosage in syringe by 12/17 Client demonstrates self-injection by 12/18	Client prepared accurate dosage in syringe on 12/17 Client administered morning insulin dosage and performed self-injection correctly on 12/18	Client has progressed and achieved desired behaviour
Client's lungs will be free of secretions by 11/30	Coughing will be nonproductive by 11/29 Lungs will be clear to auscultation by 11/30 Respirations will be 20 per minute by 11/30	Client coughed frequently and productively on 11/29 Lungs were clear to auscultation on 11/30 Respirations were 18 per minute on 11/29	Client will require continued therapy Condition is improving
Client will be able to perform self-care measures without discomfort in two days	Client will rate pain as 3 on a scale of 0–10 within two days Client will initiate bathing within two days	Client rates severe right-sided abdominal pain as 5 on a scale of 0–10 while attempting bathing on day 2	Client's condition still indicates a problem Client requires continued therapy with possibly new care measures

In the case of Ms. Devine, Lisa's initial evaluation at the beginning of this chapter revealed the following: The client reported feeling better, rated pain at a level of 4, was lying in bed relaxed, felt less worried, and did not grimace when turning over.

When matching these actual behaviours and responses to expected outcomes, Lisa determines that Ms. Devine's pain and anxiety have lessened. Because the pain is less acute, Ms. Devine's mobility is less restricted. However, Lisa knows that the cause of Ms. Devine's pain has not been corrected. The surgery is still pending, and thus the client's anxiety will possibly increase. Lisa decides to continue the plan of care but makes revisions by adding additional basic comfort measures. The comfort measures help control both the pain and anxiety and help maintain the client's mobility. Lisa next evaluates whether Ms. Devine remembers the postoperative activities that they discussed earlier: "Ms. Devine, we talked about several things that you will be asked to do after surgery. I want to know whether you understand what we discussed. Tell me what to expect about your pain control and activity." Ms. Devine responds, "You said that I would have a device that lets me control how much pain medication I receive. I should not be afraid to use it. I know the doctors will get me up early to move around. You said if I can get control of the pain, it will be easier to get up and walk. What I do not remember is something you said about breathing." Lisa says, "Good, the device is a PCA. As for breathing, let's practise the incentive spirometer I showed you one more time." Lisa recognizes that Ms. Devine has learned about select postoperative activities but requires further instruction on the incentive spirometer. Deficient knowledge now becomes Lisa's priority until Ms. Devine leaves for surgery.

Careful monitoring and early detection of problems are a client's first line of defence. Always make clinical judgements of your observations of what is occurring with a specific client and not merely of what happens to clients in general. Frequently, changes are not obvious. Evaluations are client specific: based on a close familiarity with each client's behaviour, physical status, and reaction to caregivers. Critical thinking skills promote accurate evaluation, which enables appropriate revision of ineffective care plans and discontinuation of therapy that has successfully resolved a problem.

Discontinuing a Care Plan

After you determine that expected outcomes and goals have been met, you confirm this finding with the client when possible. If you and the client agree, then you discontinue that portion of the care plan. Documentation of a discontinued plan ensures that other nurses will not unnecessarily continue interventions for that portion of the plan of care. Continuity of care ensures that care provided to clients is relevant and timely. If you do not communicate achieved goals, you will waste much time.

Modifying a Care Plan

When goals are not met, you identify the factors that interfere with goal achievement. Change in the client's condition, needs, or abilities usually necessitates alteration of the care plan. For example, when teaching self-administration of insulin, you discover that the client has developed a new problem, a tremor associated with a side effect of a medication. The client is unable to draw medication from a syringe or inject the needle safely. As a result, the original outcomes "Client will correctly prepare insulin in a syringe" and "Client will administer insulin injection independently" cannot be met. You introduce new interventions (instructing a family member in insulin preparation and administration) and revise outcomes to meet the goal of care.

At times a lack of goal achievement results from an error in nursing judgement or failure to follow each step of the nursing process. Clients often have multiple and complex problems. Always remember the possibility of overlooking or misjudging something. When a goal is not achieved, no matter what the reason, repeat the entire nursing process sequence for that nursing diagnosis to discover which changes in the plan are needed. You then reassess the client, determine accuracy of the nursing diagnosis, establish new goals and expected outcomes, and select new interventions.

A complete reassessment of all client factors relating to the nursing diagnosis and etiology is necessary when you modify a plan. Reassessment requires critical thinking as you compare new data about the client's condition with previously assessed information.

Knowledge from previous experiences helps you direct the reassessment process. Caring for clients and families who have had similar health problems gives you a strong background of knowledge to use for anticipating client needs and knowing what to assess. Reassessment ensures that the database is accurate and current. It also reveals "missing links" (i.e., critical pieces of new information that were overlooked, which thus interfered with goal achievement). You sort, validate, and cluster all new data to analyze and interpret differences from the original database. You also document reassessment data to alert other nursing staff to the client's status. After reassessment, determine what nursing diagnoses are accurate for the situation. Ask whether you selected the correct diagnosis and whether it and the etiological factor are current. Then revise the problem list to reflect the client's changed status.

Sometimes you make a new diagnosis. You base your nursing care on an accurate list of nursing diagnoses. Accuracy is more important than the number of diagnoses selected. As the client's condition changes, the diagnoses also change. For example, you identified the nursing diagnosis *deficient knowledge related to inexperience* for a client with newly diagnosed diabetes. The original plan was to instruct the client in how to self-administer insulin. After finding that the client has difficulty self-administering insulin because of reduced visual acuity, you reassess the situation and find that a family member is available as a resource. To develop a plan designed to educate a caregiver about the administration of insulin, you then establish a new diagnosis: *ineffective health maintenance related to impaired dexterity.*

Goals and Expected Outcomes

When you revise care plans, review the goals and expected outcomes for needed changes. You even need to examine the appropriateness of goals for unchanged nursing diagnoses, because a change in one problem sometimes affects other problems. Determining that each goal and expected outcome is realistic for the problem, etiology, and time frame is particularly important. Unrealistic expected outcomes and time frames hamper goal achievement. Clearly document goals and expected outcomes for new or revised nursing diagnoses so that all team members are aware of the revised care plan. When the goal is still appropriate but has not yet been met, try changing the evaluation data to allow more time. You may also decide at this time to change interventions. For example, when a client's pressure ulcer does not show signs of healing, you choose to use a different support surface or a different type of wound cleanser. All goals and expected outcomes are client centred, with realistic expectations for client achievement.

Interventions

The evaluation of interventions concerns two factors: the appropriateness of the interventions selected and the correct application of the intervention. The appropriateness of an intervention is based on the standard of care for a client's health problem. A **standard of care** is the minimum level of care acceptable to ensure high quality of care. Standards of care define the types of therapies typically administered to clients with defined problems or needs. If a client who is receiving chemotherapy for leukemia has a specific nursing diagnosis, such as *nausea related to pharyngeal irritation,* the standard of care established by a nursing department for this problem includes pain control measures for pharyngeal irritation, mouth care guidelines, and diet therapy. The nurse reviews the standard of care to determine whether the right interventions have been chosen or whether additional ones are required. Increasing or decreasing the frequency of interventions is another approach for ensuring appropriate application of an intervention. You adjust interventions on the basis of the client's actual response to therapy, as well as previous experience with similar clients. For example, if a client continues to have congested lung sounds, you increase the frequency of the client's coughing and deep breathing exercises to remove secretions.

During evaluation, you find that some planned interventions are designed for an inappropriate level of nursing care. If you need to change the level of care, substitute a different action verb, such as *assist* in place of *provide* or *demonstrate* in place of *instruct,* in the revised care plan. For example, to assist a client to walk, a nurse must be at the client's side during ambulation, whereas providing an assistive device helps the client ambulate more independently. Also, demonstrating requires you to show a client how a skill is performed rather than simply telling the client how to perform it. Sometimes the level of care is appropriate but the interventions are unsuitable because of a change in the expected outcome. In this case, discontinue the interventions and plan new ones. Make any changes in the plan of care according to the nature of the client's unfavourable response. Consult with other nurses to obtain suggestions for improving the approach to care delivery. Senior nurses are often excellent resources because of their experience. Simply changing the care plan is not enough. Implement the new plan, and re-evaluate the client's response to the nursing actions. *Evaluation is continuous.*

On occasion, you will discover unmet client needs during evaluation. This is normal. The nursing process is a systematic, problem-solving approach to individualized client care, but many factors affect each client with health care problems. Clients with the same health care problem are not treated the same way. As a result, you will sometimes make errors in judgement. The systematic use of evaluation provides a way for you to catch these errors. By consistently incorporating evaluation into practice, you will minimize errors and ensure that the client's plan of care is appropriate and relevant.

The evaluation of nursing care is a professional responsibility, and it is a crucial component of nursing care. Evaluation that focuses on a single client's plan of care enables you as a nurse to know the effectiveness of interventions and whether expected outcomes are met. At a system or institutional level, evaluation involves quality improvement and performance improvement activities that focus on the delivery of care provided by an agency or a specific nursing division within an agency. Through the continuous evaluation of care, nurses play a key role in the ongoing improvement of client care.

* KEY CONCEPTS

- Evaluation is a step of the nursing process that allows nurses to determine whether nursing interventions are successful in improving a client's condition or well-being.
- During evaluation, the appropriateness of the intervention should be assessed, as should the outcome.
- Evaluation involves two components: an examination of a condition or situation and a judgement as to whether change has occurred.
- During evaluation, apply critical thinking to make clinical decisions and redirect nursing care to best meet clients' needs.
- Evaluation findings are positive when you meet desired outcomes; this enables you to conclude that your interventions were effective.
- When the client's actual response (e.g., behaviours and physiological signs and symptoms) to nursing interventions are compared with expected outcomes established during planning, you determine whether goals of care are met. At this time, you should also determine whether the goals, outcomes, or both were realistic.
- Evaluative measures are assessment skills or techniques that you use to collect data for evaluation.
- It sometimes becomes necessary to collect evaluative measures over time to determine whether a pattern of change exists.
- To interpret evaluative findings, examine the outcome criteria, assess the client's actual behaviour or response, compare the outcome criteria with the actual behaviour or response, and judge the degree of agreement.
- Documentation of evaluative findings allows all members of the health care team to know whether a client is progressing.
- As a result of evaluation, a client's nursing diagnoses, priorities, and interventions sometimes change.

* CRITICAL THINKING EXERCISES

1. Mr. Jacko has recently received a diagnosis of asthma and is to be discharged tomorrow. His physician has ordered a metered-dose inhaler for Mr. Jacko to use daily. The client has not used an inhaler before. He asks the nurse, "What do I do at home if I have trouble using this thing?" The nursing diagnosis for Mr. Jacko is *deficient knowledge regarding use of a metered-dose inhaler related to inexperience.* Write a goal and expected outcome for this clinical scenario.
2. Mr. Vicar has been visiting the clinic for more than a month. He visits weekly for follow-up care for a chronic venous stasis ulcer of the left leg. The nurse's note at the time of his first visit contained the following information: "Ulcer with irregular margins, 4 cm wide by 5 cm long, approximately 0.5 cm deep, draining foul-smelling purulent yellowish drainage. Subcutaneous tissue visible. Skin around ulcer, brownish rust in colour. Zinc oxide and calamine gauze applied to ulcer; elastic wrap bandage applied to gauze. Client instructed to return in 1 week." The stated goal is "Wound will demonstrate healing within 4 weeks." As the nurse who is caring for the client on the follow-up visit, what expected outcomes would you anticipate for this goal? What evaluative measures would you use to determine whether the wound is healing?

* REVIEW QUESTIONS

1. A nurse caring for a client with pneumonia sits the client up in bed and suctions the client's airway. After suctioning, the client describes some discomfort in his abdomen. The nurse auscultates the client's lung sounds and provides a glass of water for the client. Which of the following is an evaluative measure used by the nurse?
    1. Suctioning the airway
    2. Sitting client up in bed
    3. Auscultating lung sounds
    4. Asking client to describe type of discomfort

2. A nurse caring for a client with pneumonia sits the client up in bed and suctions the client's airway. After the suctioning, the client describes some discomfort in his abdomen. The nurse auscultates the client's lung sounds and provides a glass of water to the client. Which of the following is an appropriate evaluative criterion used by the nurse? (Choose all that apply.)
   1. The client drinks the contents of the water glass.
   2. The client's lungs are clear to auscultation in bases.
   3. The client reports abdominal pain on scale of 0 to 10.
   4. The client's rate and depth of breathing are normal with the head of the bed elevated.
3. The evaluation process, which determines the effectiveness of nursing care, includes five elements, one being interpreting findings. Which of the following is an example of interpretation?
   1. Evaluating the client's response to selected nursing interventions
   2. Selecting an observable or measurable state or behaviour that will reflect goal achievement
   3. Reviewing the client's nursing diagnoses and establishing goals and outcome statements
   4. Matching the results of evaluative measures with expected outcomes to determine client's status
4. A goal specifies the expected behaviour or response that indicates
   1. The specific nursing action was completed
   2. The validation of the nurse's physical assessment
   3. The nurse has made the correct nursing diagnoses
   4. Resolution of a nursing diagnosis or maintenance of a healthy state
5. A client is recovering from surgery for removal of an ovarian tumour. It is one day after her surgery. Because she has an abdominal incision and dressing, the nurse has selected a nursing diagnosis of *risk for infection*. Which of the following is an appropriate goal statement for the diagnosis?
   1. The client will remain afebrile to the time of discharge.
   2. The client's wound will remain free of infection by discharge.
   3. The client will receive ordered antibiotic on time over next three days.
   4. The client's abdominal incision will remain covered with a sterile dressing for two days.
6. Unmet and partially met goals require the nurse to do which of the following? (Choose all that apply.)
   1. Redefine priorities
   2. Continue intervention
   3. Discontinue care plan
   4. Gather assessment data on a different nursing diagnosis
   5. Compare the client's response with that of another client

* RECOMMENDED WEB SITES

Center for Nursing Classification & Clinical Effectiveness: www.nursing.uiowa.edu/excellence/nursing_knowledge/clinical_effectiveness/index.htm
The University of Iowa's Center for Nursing Classification & Clinical Effectiveness was established to facilitate ongoing research of the Nursing Interventions Classification (NIC) and Nursing Outcomes Classification (NOC). This Web site provides an overview of the NIC and NOC and offers information about new classification material and publications.

NANDA International: http://www.nanda.org/
Through this Web site, NANDA International provides current information on nursing diagnosis research, publications, support resources, and Internet resources.

Registered Nurses Association of Ontario: Nursing Best Practice Guidelines: http://www.rnao.org
The Registered Nurses Association of Ontario has developed an extensive process for developing best practices guidelines in a variety of areas of clinical nursing. They have received federal and provincial funding for this process, and the results of their work have been made available to all Canadian nurses through this Web site, which lists all current guidelines that have been developed.

16

Documenting and Reporting

Original chapter by Barbara Maxwell, RN, BSN, MS, MSN, CNS

Canadian content written by Maureen A. Barry, RN, MScN

objectives

Mastery of content in this chapter will enable you to:

- Define the key terms listed.
- Describe multidisciplinary communication within the health care team.
- Identify purposes of a health care record.
- Discuss legal guidelines for documentation.
- Identify ways to maintain confidentiality of records and reports.
- Describe six quality guidelines for documentation and reporting.
- Describe the different methods used in record keeping.
- Discuss the advantages of standardized documentation forms.
- Identify elements to include when documenting a client's discharge plan.
- Describe the role of critical pathways in multidisciplinary documentation.
- Identify the important aspects of home care and long-term care documentation.
- Discuss the role of computerized charting and use of electronic health records in documentation.
- Describe the purpose and content of a change-of-shift report.
- Explain how to verify telephone orders.

key terms

Acuity records, p. 223
Care maps, 216
Case management, p. 216
Change-of-shift report, p. 229
Charting by exception (CBE), p. 216
Clinical decision support, p. 228
Computerized physician order entry (CPOE), p. 228
Consultations, p. 210
Critical pathways, p. 216
Data–action–response (DAR) notes, p. 214
Documentation, p. 209
Electronic health record (EHR), p. 228
Flow sheets, p. 223
Focus charting, p. 214
Incident reports, p. 231
Kardex, p. 223
Personal digital assistants, p. 225
Personal Information Protection and Electronic Documents Act (PIPEDA), p. 209
Point-of-care information systems, p. 227
Problem–intervention–evaluation (PIE), p. 214
Problem-oriented medical record, p. 214
Record, p. 209
Referrals, p. 210
Reports, p. 209
Residents, p. 227
Situation–background–assessment–recommendation (SBAR) technique, p. 228
Source record, p. 215
Standardized care plans, p. 223
Subjective–objective–assessment–plan (SOAP), p. 214
Subjective–objective–assessment–plan–intervention–evaluation) SOAPIE, p. 214
Transfer reports, p. 230
Variances, p. 216
Workload measurement systems, p. 223

media resources

evolve Web Site

- Audio Chapter Summaries
- Glossary
- Multiple-Choice Review Questions
- Student Learning Activities
- Weblinks

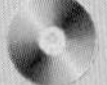

Companion CD

- Glossary
- Interactive Learning Activities
- Fluids and Electrolytes Tutorial
- Test-Taking Skills

Documentation is anything written or electronically generated that describes the status of a client or the care or service given to that client. Documentation within a client health care record is a vital aspect of nursing practice. Nursing documentation must be accurate, comprehensive, and flexible enough for members of the health care team to retrieve critical data, maintain continuity of care, and track client outcomes, and it must reflect current standards of nursing practice. Information in the client record provides a detailed account of the quality of care delivered to clients. Documentation ensures continuity and quality of care, furnishes legal evidence of care, provides evidence for quality assurance purposes, and constitutes a database for planning future health care (Cheevakasemsook et al., 2006).

Effective documentation can positively affect the quality of life and health outcomes for clients and minimize the risk of errors. Accrediting agencies such as Accreditation Canada (formerly the Canadian Council on Health Services Accreditation) offer guidelines for documentation. However, documentation and reporting practices differ among institutions and jurisdictions and are influenced by ethical, legal, medical, and agency guidelines.

As a member of the health care team, you need to communicate information about clients accurately and in a timely, effective manner. The quality of client care depends largely on caregivers' ability to communicate with one another. All health care professionals require accurate information about clients in order to devise an organized, comprehensive care plan. If the care plan is not communicated to all members of the health care team, care can be fragmented, tasks repeated, and therapies delayed or omitted. Data recorded, reported, or communicated to other health care professionals are confidential, and the confidentiality of these data must be protected.

The health care environment creates many challenges to accurately documenting and reporting client care. Because of the quality of care, the standards of regulatory agencies and nursing practice, and the legal guidelines for nursing practice, documentation and reporting are critical responsibilities of a nurse.

Confidentiality

Whether the transfer of client information occurs through verbal reports, written documents, or electronic transfer, nurses must follow certain principles to maintain confidentiality of information. You are legally and ethically obligated to keep information about clients confidential. You may not discuss a client's examination, observation, conversation, or treatment with other clients or with staff who are not involved in the client's care. Only staff directly involved in a specific client's care have legitimate access to the records. Many clients request copies of their health records, and they have the right to read their records. Each institution has policies for controlling the manner in which records are shared. In most situations, institutions are required to obtain written permission from clients to release medical information.

As a nurse, you are also responsible for protecting records from all unauthorized readers. When nurses and other health care professionals have a legitimate reason to use records for data gathering, research, or continuing education, they must obtain appropriate authorization according to agency policy. Nursing students and faculty may be required to present identification indicating they are authorized to access records. The health care agency stores the records after the treatment ends.

Before the beginning of clinical placements, students and instructors may be required to sign confidentiality agreements with the agencies in question. Students need to understand the practice standards and laws concerning confidentiality. A breach of confidentiality is often a careless rather than a deliberate act. Students need to make sure that client-identifiable information (e.g., files, stickers, information in notebooks, worksheets) is not taken home and is disposed of correctly in a secure bin for shredding. Examples of breaches of confidentiality include accessing information not related to your duties, discussing client information in an inappropriate area such as an elevator or on public transport, revealing to a caller confidential client or coworker details, emailing client information through a public network such as the Internet, and leaving confidential material in a public area. Even after you are no longer on placement at an agency, you are obligated to maintain the confidentiality of clients and coworkers at that agency.

Personal Information Protection and Electronic Documents Act (PIPEDA)

PIPEDA is federal legislation that protects personal information, including health information. *PIPEDA* delineates how private sector organizations may collect, use, or disclose personal information in the course of commercial activities. Individuals have the right to access and request correction of any personal information collected about them as well. *PIPEDA* applies to all organizations engaged in commercial activities unless the federal government exempts an organization or activity in a province with similar legislation. *PIPEDA* is discussed in more detail in Chapter 17.

Multidisciplinary Communication Within the Health Care Team

Client care requires effective communication among members of the health care team. Communication takes place through the client's record or chart and reports.

A client's **record**, or chart, is a confidential, permanent legal documentation of information relevant to a client's health care. Information about the client's health care is recorded after each contact with the client. The record is a continuing account of the client's health care status and is available to all members of the health care team. All health records contain the following information:

- Client identification and demographic data
- Informed consent for treatment and procedures
- Advance directives
- Admission nursing history
- Nursing diagnoses or problems and the nursing or multidisciplinary care plan
- Record of nursing care treatment and evaluation
- Medical history
- Medical diagnosis
- Therapeutic orders
- Progress notes for various health care professions
- Reports of physical examinations
- Reports of diagnostic studies
- Record of client and family education
- Summary of operative procedures
- Discharge plan and summary

Reports are oral, written, or audiotaped exchanges of information between caregivers. Reports commonly compiled by nurses include change-of-shift reports, telephone reports, transfer reports, and incident reports (see "Reporting" section on page 228). A physician or nurse practitioner may call a nursing unit to receive a verbal report on a client's condition and progress. A laboratory submits a written report about the results of diagnostic tests.

Team members communicate information through discussions or conferences (Figure 16–1).For example, a discharge planning conference often involves members of all disciplines (e.g., nursing, social work, dietary, medicine, and physiotherapy), who meet to discuss the client's progress toward established discharge goals. **Consultations** are another form of discussion whereby one professional caregiver gives formal advice about the care of a client to another caregiver. For example, a nurse caring for a client with a chronic wound may need a consultation with a wound care specialist. **Referrals** (an arrangement for services by another care provider), consultations, and conferences must be documented in a client's permanent record so that all caregivers can plan care accordingly.

Purposes of Records

A record is a valuable source of data that is used by all members of the health care team. Its purposes include communication and care planning, legal documentation, education, funding and resource management, research, and auditing–monitoring.

Communication and Care Planning

The record is a means by which health care team members communicate client needs and progress, individual therapies, content of conferences, client education, and discharge planning. The plan of care needs to be clear to everyone reading the chart. The record should be the most current and accurate source of information about a client's health care status.

In the record, always communicate the manner in which you conduct the nursing process with a client. The admitting nursing history and physical assessment are comprehensive and provide baseline data about the client's health status on admission to the facility. These data usually include biographical information (e.g., age and marital status), method of admission, reason for admission, a brief medical–surgical history (e.g., previous surgeries or illnesses), allergies, current medication (prescribed and over-the-counter), the client's perceptions about illness or hospitalization, and a review of health risk factors. Results of a physical assessment of all body systems are either documented in the nursing history or included on a separate form (see Chapter 32).

The medical progress notes should complement nursing process information. The notes detail the physician's or nurse practitioner's findings at the time of assessment. Nurses first refer to the client's health care record for relevant assessment findings so that they can anticipate the client's status and then conduct an individualized client assessment.

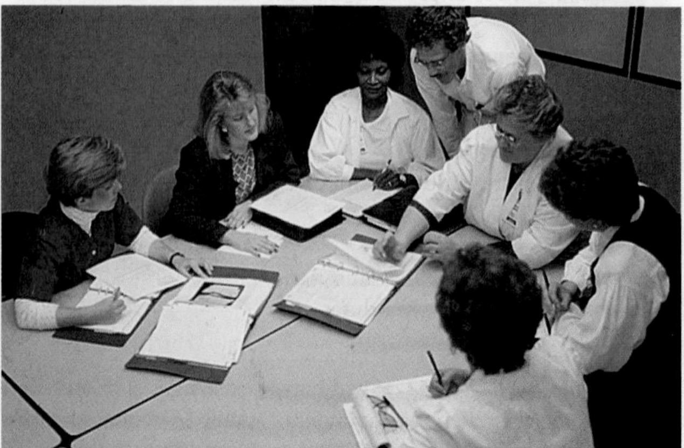

Figure 16-1 Staff communicate information about their clients during a change-of-shift report.

The record provides data that you use to identify and support nursing diagnoses, establish expected outcomes of care, and plan and evaluate interventions. Information from the record adds to your observations and assessment. You do not need to collect information that is already available. If you have reason to believe that the information is inaccurate, information should be verified and appropriate changes made to the client's record.

Legal Documentation

Accurate documentation is one of the best defences against legal claims associated with nursing care (see Chapter 9). From a legal perspective, the purpose of documentation is "always to accurately and completely record the care given to patients, as well as their response to that care" (Monarch, 2007, p. 58). To limit nursing liability, you must clearly document that individualized, goal-directed nursing care, based on the nursing assessment, was provided to a client. The record must describe exactly what happened to a client. Charting should be performed immediately after care is provided. Nursing care may have been excellent, but in a court of law, care not documented is care not provided (Graves Ferrell, 2007). In the health care record, you need to indicate all assessments, interventions, client responses, instructions, and referrals. It is important to complete all documentation on appropriate forms and to be sure that client-identifying information (client's name and identification number) is on every page of documentation.

The Nurses Service Organization (2008) (a medical malpractice, professional liability, and risk management company) identified eight common charting mistakes that can result in malpractice: (1) failing to record pertinent health or drug information, (2) failing to record nursing actions, (3) failing to record the administration of medications, (4) recording on the wrong chart, (5) failing to document a discontinued medication, (6) failing to record drug reactions or changes in the client's condition, (7) transcribing orders improperly or transcribing improper orders, and (8) writing illegible or incomplete orders. Table 16–1 provides guidelines for legally sound documentation.

Education

A client's record contains a variety of information, including diagnoses, signs and symptoms of disease, successful and unsuccessful therapies, diagnostic findings, and client behaviours. By reading the client care record, you can learn the nature of an illness and the client's response to the illness. No two clients have identical records, but patterns of information can be identified in records of clients with similar health problems. With this information, you can identify patterns for various health problems and begin to anticipate the type of care required for a client.

Funding and Resource Management

The client care record shows how health care agencies have used their financial resources. Various tools help monitor the timing and reasons for health team–client interactions. These data are then compared with documented entries on the chart to demonstrate the need for and efficacy of health care resources. In some workload assignment systems, health care interactions and tasks are assigned specified points in relation to time spent with each client.

Research

Statistical data relating to the frequency of clinical disorders, complications, use of specific medical and nursing therapies, recovery from illness, and deaths can be gathered from client records. For example,

➤ TABLE 16-1 Legal Guidelines for Recording

Guidelines	Rationale	Correct Action
Do not erase, apply correction fluid to, or scratch out errors made while recording.	Charting becomes illegible: It may appear as if you were attempting to hide information or deface record.	Draw single line through error; write "error," "mistaken entry," "delete," or "void" above it; and sign your name or initials and date. Then record note correctly.
Do not write retaliatory or critical comments about client or care by other health care professionals.	Statements can be used as evidence of non-professional behaviour or of poor quality of care.	Enter only objective descriptions of client's behaviour; direct quotes from client are preferred.
Correct all errors promptly.	Errors in recording can lead to errors in treatment or may imply an attempt to mislead or hide evidence.	Avoid rushing to complete charting; be sure that information is accurate.
Record all facts.	Record must be accurate, factual, and objective.	Be certain entry is factual and thorough; do not speculate or guess. A person reading the documentation should be able to determine that the client was adequately cared for.
Do not leave blank spaces in nurse's notes.	Another person can add incorrect information in spaces.	Chart consecutively, line by line; if space is left, draw line horizontally through it and sign your name at end.
Record all entries legibly and in black ink. Do not use felt-tip pens or erasable ink.	Illegible entries can be misinterpreted, thereby causing errors and lawsuits; felt-tip pen ink smudges or runs when wet and may destroy documentation; erasures are not permitted in client charting. Black ink is more legible when records are photocopied or transferred to microfilm.	Chart legibly in black ink; avoid the use of erasers, correction fluid, and pencils for documentation.
If an order is questioned, record that clarification was sought.	If you perform an order known to be incorrect, you are just as liable for prosecution as the prescriber is.	Do not record, "physician made error"; instead, chart that "Dr. Wong was called to clarify order for analgesic." Include the date and time of phone call, whom you spoke with, and the outcome.
Chart only your own actions.	You are accountable for information you enter into chart.	Never chart for someone else, except for the following situation: If caregiver has left unit for the day and calls with information that needs to be documented, include the date and time of entry, and reference the specific date and time you are referring to and the name of source of information in the entry, and include that the information was provided by telephone.
Avoid using generalized, empty phrases such as "status unchanged" or "had good day."	Such information is too generalized and has no meaning. Specific information about client's condition is missing.	Use complete, concise descriptions of care so that documentation is objective and factual.
Begin each entry with the date and time, and end with your signature and title.	This guideline ensures that correct sequence of events is recorded; signature indicates who is accountable for care delivered.	Do not wait until end of shift to record important changes that occurred several hours earlier; be sure to sign each entry (e.g., Mei Lin, RN).
Avoid "precharting" (documenting an entry before performing a treatment or an assessment or before giving a medication)	Precharting invites error and thus endangers the health and safety of the client; it is also illegal and can constitute falsification of health care records.	Document during or immediately after giving care or after administering a medication.
For computer documentation, keep your password to yourself.	This maintains security and confidentiality.	Once logged on to the computer, do not leave the computer screen unattended. Make sure the computer screen is not accessible for public viewing.

as part of a quality improvement program for clients receiving intravenous therapy, a nurse manager reviews clients' records to investigate the incidence of infection in clients with a specific type of intravenous catheter. This review reveals that the infection rate is increased, and the nurse manager and staff nurses design a new specific method for intravenous catheter care. Once this new intervention is implemented, the manager again reviews clients' records to determine whether the infection rate decreases.

A nurse may use clients' records during a clinical research study to investigate a new nursing intervention. For example, a nurse wants to compare a new method of pain control with a standard pain protocol, by using two groups of clients. The client records provide data on the two types of interventions: the new method and the standard pain control. The nurse researcher collects data from the clients' records that describe the types and doses of analgesic medications used, objective assessment data, and clients' subjective reports of pain relief. The researcher then compares the findings to determine whether the new method was more effective that the standard pain control protocol.

Some data collection activities may be part of the quality improvement practices at an agency, whereas other activities may be actual clinical research studies. Different types of permission must be secured before a researcher can review client records for any type of research study or data analysis. The researcher must be sure that the data collection and analysis adhere to provincial, territorial, and agency policies.

Auditing–Monitoring

A regular review of information in client records helps you evaluate the quality and appropriateness of care. This audit may be either a review of care received by discharged clients or an evaluation of care currently being given. Most Canadian health care agencies have continuous quality improvement programs and teams to monitor and improve the delivery of heath care services. These teams often contain members from across the organization, and they normally perform the self-assessment requirements of Accreditation Canada (see Chapter 11). Nurses or cross-discipline members of a committee monitor or review records throughout the year to determine the degree to which quality improvement standards are met. Deficiencies are explained to the nursing staff so that corrections in policy or practice can be made.

Guidelines for Quality Documentation and Reporting

High-quality documentation and reporting enhance efficient, individualized client care. High-quality documentation and reporting have six important characteristics: They are factual, accurate, complete, current, and organized, and they comply with standards set by Accreditation Canada and by provincial or territorial regulatory bodies.

Factual

A factual record contains descriptive, objective information about what a nurse sees, hears, feels, and smells. An objective description is the result of direct observation and measurement: for example, "BP 80/50, client diaphoretic, heart rate 102 and regular. L. Woo, RPN" (where "BP" stands for "blood pressure"). The use of inferences (e.g., "client appears to be in shock") without supporting factual data is not acceptable because inferences can be misunderstood.

The use of vague terms, such as *appears, seems,* or *apparently,* is not acceptable because these words reflect opinion. For example, the description "the client seems anxious" does not accurately communicate facts and does not inform another caregiver of the details regarding the behaviours exhibited by the client that led to the use of the word *anxious*. The phrase *seems anxious* is a conclusion without supported facts. Objective documentation includes the observations of the client's behaviours. For example, objective signs of anxiety can include increased pulse rate, increased respirations, and increased restlessness.

When recording subjective data, document the client's exact words within quotation marks whenever possible (e.g., "Client states, 'I feel very nervous and out of control'").

Accurate

The use of exact measurements establishes accuracy. For example, a description such as "Intake, 360 mL of water" is more accurate than "Client drank an adequate amount of fluid." These measurements can later be used as a means to determine whether a client's condition has changed. Charting that an abdominal wound is "5 cm in length without redness, drainage, or edema" is more descriptive than "large wound healing well."

Documentation of concise data should be clear and easy to understand. Avoid the use of unnecessary words and irrelevant detail. For example, the fact that the client is watching TV is relevant only when this activity has relevance to the client's status and plan of care.

Most health care institutions develop a list of standard abbreviations, symbols, and acronyms to be used by all members of the health care team in documenting or communicating client care and treatment. Approved abbreviations and acronyms vary, depending on the type of facility (i.e., long-term versus acute-care facility). Use of an institution's accepted abbreviations, symbols, and system of measures (e.g., metric) ensures that all staff members use the same language in their reports and records. Always use abbreviations carefully to avoid misinterpretation. For example, "od" (every day) can be misinterpreted to mean "O.D." (right eye). If abbreviations are confusing, then to minimize errors, you should spell them out in their entirety.

The Joint Commission on Accreditation of Healthcare Organizations (JCAHO) published a minimum list of dangerous abbreviations that should no longer be used in written medical documents (Karch, 2004). Suggestions include writing "unit" instead of "U"; always using a zero before a decimal point in a decimal fraction (e.g., "0.25 mg"); and not writing a zero alone after a decimal point (e.g., writing "5 mg," not "5.0 mg"). The Institute for Safe Medication Practices (2007) published a more extensive list of error-prone abbreviations, symbols, and dose designations that health care institutions also need to consider adding to their "Do Not Use" lists (see Chapter 34).

Correct spelling demonstrates a level of competency and attention to detail. Many terms can easily be misinterpreted (e.g., *dysphagia* and *dysphasia*). Some spelling errors can also result in serious treatment errors; for example, the names of certain medications, such as *digitoxin* and *digoxin* or *morphine* and *hydromorphone,* are similar and must be transcribed carefully to ensure that the client receives the correct medication.

Record entries must be dated, and a method for identifying the authors of entries must be in place. Therefore, each entry in a client's record ends with the caregiver's full name or initials and status, such as "Holly Lee, RPN." Each time initials are used, the full name and status must previously appear on the same page so that the individual entering initials can be readily identified. A nursing student enters full name, student nurse abbreviation (e.g., "SN" or "NS"), and educational institution: for example, "Henri Gauthier, SN 1 [student nurse, year one], U of S [University of Saskatchewan]."

Records must reflect accountability during the time frame of the entry. Accountability is best accomplished when you chart only your own observations and actions. Your signature holds you accountable for information recorded. If information was inadvertently omitted from the record, it is acceptable for you to ask colleagues to chart information on your behalf after you leave work. The entry needs to clearly show what was done and by whom (e.g., "At 1100 hrs, Sam Roustas, RN, called and reported that at 0800 hrs, morphine sulphate, 5 mg subcutaneous, was administered to client for abdominal pain. F. Khan, R.N.").

You should refer to agency policy before making late entries, correcting errors, or completing an omission. Late entries are often documented by writing the current date and time in the next available space as close to the late entry as possible and writing "late entry for [date and shift]." For adding information to an existing entry, using the current date and time in the next space and adding "addendum to note of [date and time of prior note]" is a good practice.

Complete

The information within a recorded entry or a report must be complete, containing appropriate and essential information. Criteria for thorough communication exist for certain health problems or nursing activities (Table 16–2). Your written entries in the client's health care record describe the nursing care you administer and the client's response. An example of a thorough nurse's note is as follows:

> *"1915: Client verbalizes sharp, throbbing pain localized along lateral side of right ankle, beginning approximately 15 minutes ago after twisting his foot on the stairs. Client rates pain as 8 on a scale of 0–10. Pain increased with movement, slightly relieved with elevation. Pedal pulses equal bilaterally. Right ankle circumference 1 cm larger than left. Capillary refill less than 3 seconds bilaterally; right foot warm to touch and pale pink; skin intact on right foot; responds to tactile stimulation on right foot. Ice applied. Percocet 2 tabs (PO) given for pain. Client states pain somewhat relieved with ice, rates pain as 6 on a scale of 0–10. Dr. P. Yoshida notified. Lee Turno, RN."*

Current

Timely entries are essential to the client's ongoing care. Documentation should occur during or as soon as possible after the incident or intervention, and events should be described chronologically to reflect a clear record of exactly what happened (College of Nurses of Ontario, 2005). To increase accuracy and decrease unnecessary duplication, many health care agencies use bedside records, which facilitate immediate documentation of information as it is collected from a client.

Flow sheets (described later in this chapter) are a means of entering current information quickly. Portable electronic work stations or secure wall cabinets in client rooms help ensure that client confidentiality is maintained. Nurses often keep notes on a worksheet when caring for several clients, making notes as the care occurs to ensure that entries recorded later in the record are accurate. The following activities and findings should be communicated at the time of occurrence:

- Vital signs
- Administration of medications and treatments
- Preparation for diagnostic tests or surgery
- Change in client's status and who was notified (e.g., nurse practitioner, physician, manager, client's family)
- Admission, transfer, discharge, or death of a client
- Treatment for a sudden change in client's status
- Client's response to treatment or intervention

Health care agencies use military time, a 24-hour system that avoids misinterpretation of "A.M." and "P.M." times (Figure 16–2). Instead of two 12-hour cycles in standard time, the military clock is one 24-hour time cycle. The military clock ends with midnight (2400) and begins with 1 minute after midnight (0001). For example, 10:22 A.M. is 1022 military time; 1:00 P.M. is 1300 military time.

TABLE 16-2 Examples of Criteria for Reporting and Recording

Topic	Criteria to Report or Record
Assessment	
Subjective data	Description of episode in quotation marks; for example, "I feel as if I have an elephant sitting on my chest, and I can't catch my breath." Onset, location, description of condition (severity, duration, frequency; precipitating, aggravating, and relieving factors); for example, "The pain in my left knee started last week after I knelt on the ground. Every time I bend my knee, I have a shooting pain on the inside of my knee."
Client behaviour (e.g., anxiety, confusion, hostility)	Onset, behaviours exhibited, precipitating factors, client's verbal response; for example, "Client observed pacing in her room, avoiding eye contact with nurse, and repeatedly stating, 'I have to go home now.'"
Objective data (e.g., rash, tenderness, breath sounds)	Onset, location, description of condition (see "Subjective data" above); for example, "1100 hrs: 2-cm raised pale red area noted on back of left hand."
Nursing Interventions and Evaluation	
Treatments (e.g., enema, bath, dressing change)	Time administered, equipment used (if appropriate), client's response (objective and subjective changes) in comparison with previous treatment; for example, "Client denied pain during abdominal dressing change" or "Client reported severe abdominal cramping during enema."
Medication administration	Immediately after administration, document time when medication is given, preliminary assessment (e.g., pain level, vital signs), client response or effect of medication; for example, "1500: Client reports a 'throbbing headache all over her head.' Rates pain as 6 (scale 0–10). Tylenol 650 mg given PO. 1530: Client reports pain level 2 (scale 0–10) and states 'the throbbing has stopped.'"
Client teaching	Information presented, method of instruction (e.g., discussion, demonstration, videotape, booklet), and client response, including questions and evidence of understanding such as demonstration of correct self-care or change in behaviour.
Discharge planning	Measurable client goals or expected outcomes, progress toward goals, need for referrals.

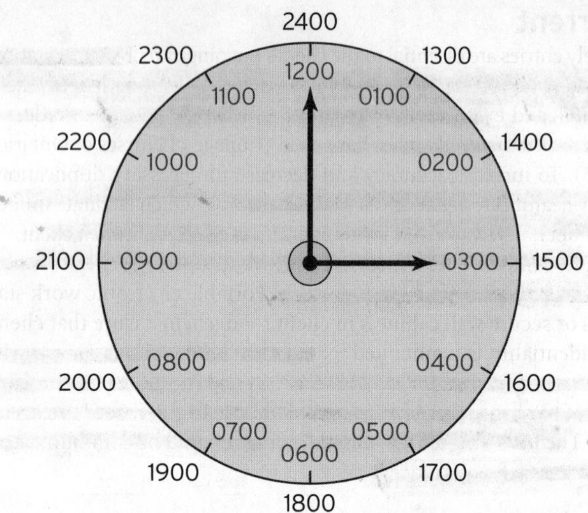

Figure 16-2 Military time clock.

Organized

As a nurse, you want to communicate information in a logical order. For example, an organized note describes the client's pain, the nurse's assessment and interventions, and the client's response. To write notes about complex situations in an organized manner, think about the situation and make notes of what is to be included before you begin to write in the permanent legal record.

Compliant With Standards

Documentation needs to follow standards set by Accreditation Canada and by provincial or territorial regulatory bodies to maintain institutional accreditation and to decrease the risk of liability. Current standards require that all clients who are admitted to a health care institution undergo physical, psychosocial, environmental, and self-care assessments; receive client education; and be provided discharge planning. In addition, criteria for standards stress the importance of evaluating client outcomes, including the client's response to treatments, teaching, or preventive care.

The nursing service department of each health care agency selects a method of documenting client care. The method reflects the philosophy of the nursing department and incorporates the standards of care. Because the nursing process shapes a nurse's approach and direction of care, effective documentation also reflects the nursing process.

Common Documentation Systems

Client data can be recorded in several documentation systems. Each nursing service selects a documentation system that reflects the philosophy of its department. The same documentation system is used throughout a specific agency and may also be used throughout a health care system.

Narrative Documentation

Narrative documentation is the traditional method for recording nursing care. It is simply the use of a story-like format to document information specific to client conditions and nursing care. Narrative charting, however, has many disadvantages, including the tendency to have repetitious information, to be time consuming to complete, and to require the reader to sort through much information to locate desired data.

Problem-Oriented Medical Records or Health Care Records

The **problem-oriented medical record** is a method of documentation that emphasizes the client's problems. Data are organized by problem or diagnosis. Ideally, each member of the health care team contributes to a single list of identified client problems. This assists in coordinating a common plan of care. The problem-oriented medical record has the following major sections: database, problem list, care plan, and progress notes.

Database. The database section contains all available assessment information pertaining to the client (e.g., history and physical examination findings, the nurse's admission history and ongoing assessment, the dietitian's assessment, laboratory reports, and radiological test results). The database is the foundation for identifying client problems and planning care. As new data become available, you revise the database. The database accompanies clients through successive hospitalizations or clinic visits.

Problem List. After analyzing data, health care team members identify problems and make a single problem list. The problems include the client's physiological, psychological, social, cultural, spiritual, developmental, and environmental needs. Team members list the problems in chronological order and file the list in the front of the client's record to serve as an organizing guide for the client's care. Add new problems as they are identified. When a problem has been resolved, record the date of resolution, and highlight the date or draw a line through the problem and its number.

Care Plan. A care plan is developed for each problem by the members of the health care team from each discipline involved in the client's care. Nurses document the plan of care in a variety of formats. In general, these plans of care include nursing diagnoses, expected outcomes, and interventions.

Progress Notes. Health care team members monitor and record the progress of a client's problems (Box 16–1). The information can be expressed in various formats. One method is the **subjective–objective–assessment–plan (SOAP)** charting, involving subjective data (verbalizations of the client), objective data (data that are measured and observed), assessment (diagnosis based on the data), and plan (what the caregiver plans to do). Some institutions add intervention (I) and evaluation (E) (i.e., **SOAPIE**). The logic for SOAP and SOAPIE notes is similar to that of the nursing process: to collect data about the client's problems, draw conclusions, and develop a plan of care. The nurse numbers each SOAP or SOAPIE note and titles it according to the problem on the list.

A second progress note method is the **problem–intervention–evaluation (PIE)** format (see Box 16–1). It is similar to SOAP charting in its problem-oriented nature. However, it differs from the SOAP method in that PIE charting originated in nursing practice, whereas SOAP charting originated from medical records. The PIE format simplifies documentation by unifying the care plan and progress notes. PIE notes differ from SOAP notes because the narrative does not include assessment information. A nurse's daily assessment data appear on flow sheets, preventing duplication of data. The narrative note includes the problem, the intervention, and the evaluation. The PIE notes are numbered or labelled according to the client's problems. Resolved problems are dropped from daily documentation after the nurse's review. Continuing problems are documented daily.

A third progress note format is **focus charting.** It involves use of **data–action–response (DAR) notes,** which include both subjective

> **BOX 16-1 Examples of Progress Notes Written in Different Formats**
>
> **Subjective-Objective-Assessment-Plan (SOAP)**
>
> 01/19/08 Knowledge deficit related to inexperience regarding surgery 1630 hrs
>
> **S:** "I'm worried about what it will be like after surgery."
>
> **O:** Client asking frequent questions about surgery.. Has had no previous experience with surgery. Wife present, acts as a support person.
>
> **A:** Knowledge deficit regarding surgery related to inexperience. Client also expressing anxiety.
>
> **P:** Explain routine preoperative preparation. Demonstrate and explain rationale for turning, coughing, and deep breathing (TCDB) exercises. Provide explanation and teaching booklet on postoperative nursing care. S. Lazarus, RPN
>
> **Problem-Intervention-Evaluation (PIE)**
>
> **P:** Knowledge deficit regarding surgery related to inexperience.
>
> **I:** Explained to client normal preoperative preparations for surgery. Demonstrated TCDB exercises. Provided booklet to client on postoperative nursing care.
>
> **E:** Client demonstrates TCDB exercises correctly. Needs review of postoperative nursing care. S. Lazarus, RPN
>
> **Focus Charting: Data-Action-Response (DAR)***
>
> **D:** Client stating, "I'm worried about what it will be like after surgery." Client asking frequent questions about surgery. Has had no previous experience with surgery. Wife present; acts as a support person.
>
> **A:** Explained to client normal preoperative preparations for surgery. Demonstrated TCDB exercises. Provided booklet to client on postoperative nursing care.
>
> **R:** Client demonstrates TCDB exercises correctly. Needs review of postoperative nursing care. Client states, "I feel better knowing a little bit of what to expect." S. Lazarus, RPN
>
> *Some agencies also add P (Plan) to make DARP.

and objective data, the action or nursing intervention, and the response of the client (i.e., evaluation of effectiveness). One distinction of focus charting is its movement away from charting only problems, which has a negative connotation. Instead, a DAR note addresses client concerns: a sign or symptom, a condition, a nursing diagnosis, a behaviour, a significant event, or a change in a client's condition. Documentation is written in accordance with the nursing process; nurses are encouraged to broaden their thinking to include any client concerns, not just problem areas; and critical thinking is encouraged. The benefits of focus charting are that it incorporates all aspects of the nursing process, highlights the client's concerns, and can be integrated into any clinical setting (*Mosby's Surefire Documentation*, 2006).

Source Records

In a **source record**, the client's chart is organized so that each discipline (e.g., nursing, medicine, social work, respiratory therapy) has a separate section in which to record data. One advantage of a source record is that caregivers can easily locate the proper section of the record in which to make entries. Table 16–3 lists the components of a source record.

TABLE 16-3 Organization of Traditional Source Record

Sections	Contents
Admission sheet	Specific demographic data about client: legal name, identification number, sex, age, birth date, marital status, occupation and employer, health card number, nearest relative to notify in an emergency, religious affiliation, name of attending physician, date and time of admission
Physician's order sheet	Record of physician's orders for treatment and medications, with date, time, and physician's signature
Nurse's admission assessment	Summary of nursing history and physical examination
Graphic sheet and flow sheet	Record of repeated observations and measurements such as vital signs, daily weights, and intake and output
Medical history and examination	Results of initial examination performed by physician, including findings, family history, confirmed diagnoses, and medical plan of care
Nurses' notes	Narrative record of nursing process: assessment, nursing diagnosis, planning, implementation, and evaluation of care
Medication administration record	Accurate documentation of all medications administered to client: date, time, dose, route, and nurse's signature
Progress notes	Ongoing record of client's progress and response to medical therapy and review of disease process completed by physician or nurse practitioner
Health care disciplines' records	Entries made into record by all health care–related disciplines: radiology, social work, laboratories, and so forth
Discharge summary	Summary of client's condition, progress, prognosis, rehabilitation, and teaching needs at time of dismissal from hospital or health care agency

A disadvantage of the source record is that details about a specific problem may be distributed throughout the record. For example, in the case of a client with bowel obstruction, the nurse describes in the nurses' notes the character of abdominal pain and the use of relaxation therapy and analgesic medication. In a separate section of the record, the physician's notes describe the progress of the client's condition and the plan for surgery. The findings of X-ray examinations that reveal the location of the bowel obstruction are in the test results section of the record.

The notes section is where nurses enter a narrative description of nursing care and the client's response (Box 16–2). It is also a section for documenting care that is provided by the physician or nurse practitioner in the nurse's presence. The nurse may record key diagnostic test results from other sections of the record in the nurses' notes if they are of major importance in the care of the client.

Charting by Exception

Charting by exception (CBE) focuses on documenting deviations from the established norm or abnormal findings. This approach reduces documentation time and highlights trends or changes in the client's condition (*Mosby's Surefire Documentation*, 2006). It is a shorthand method for documenting normal findings and routine care on the basis of clearly defined standards of practice and predetermined criteria for nursing assessments and interventions. Clearly defined standards of practice that specify nurses' responsibilities to clients provide the framework for routine care of all clients. With standards integrated into documentation forms, such as predefined normal assessment findings or predetermined interventions, a nurse needs only to document significant findings or exceptions to the predefined norms. In other words, the nurse writes a progress note only when the standardized statement on the form is not met. Assessments are standardized on flow sheets or other forms so that all caregivers evaluate and document findings consistently (Figure 16–3).

Because the standard assessments are located in the chart, client data are already present on the permanent record, and so nurses do not need to keep temporary notes for later transcription, and caregivers have easy access to current data. The assumption with CBE is that all standards are met unless otherwise documented. When nurses see entries in the chart, they know that something out of the ordinary has been observed or has occurred. For that reason, when changes in a client's condition have developed, it is easy to track them.

When clients' conditions change, it is essential to describe thoroughly and precisely what happens to clients and the actions taken. CBE can pose legal risks if nurses are not diligent in documenting exceptions. This charting method fails to provide a thorough picture of a client's developing condition and does not reflect communication among members of the health care team (*Mosby's Surefire Documentation*, 2006). If nurses rely too heavily on charting standard categories and do not enter exception notes, the client's situation will not be clear. CBE can also be problematic when related documentation forms do not have space allotted for documenting client and family perspectives.

> **➤ BOX 16-2 Sample Narrative Note**
>
> 04/03/08
>
> 1100 hrs: Client states, "I'm having a hard time catching my breath." Respirations [R], laboured at 32/min; P [pulse] 120; BP 112/70. Oxygen saturation 90% on room air. Client alert and oriented. Client using intercostal muscles during inhalation. Breath sounds auscultated, crackles and wheezes over both lower lobes. Chest excursion equal bilaterally. Elevated head of bed to Fowler's position. Obtained arterial blood gas (ABG) sample at 1045. O_2 started at 2 L/min per nasal prongs as ordered. Remained at bedside to calm client. P. Haske, RN
>
> 1130 hrs: Results of ABGs reported to Dr Stein are pH 7.34; PCO_2 [partial pressure of carbon dioxide] 44 mm Hg; PO_2 [partial pressure of oxygen] 80 mm Hg.
>
> Client states, "It is easier to breathe now." R 24/min; P 96; BP 110/72. Oxygen saturation 97% on O_2 at 2 L/min per nasal prongs, lips pale pink; capillary refill less than 3 seconds. Crackles and wheezing still audible on auscultation. Client remains in high Fowler's position. P. Haske, RN

Case Management Plan and Critical Pathways or Care Maps

The **case management** model of delivering care (see Chapter 11) incorporates a multidisciplinary approach to documenting client care. In many organizations, the standardized plan of care is summarized into critical pathways for a specific disease or condition. The **critical pathways** or **care maps** are multidisciplinary care plans that include client health concerns, key interventions, and expected outcomes within an established time frame (Figure 16–4). In a computerized charting system, professionals from many disciplines may access the chart, and this integration of information from the different disciplines can be accessed easily from every computer terminal in the institution at any time. The nurse and other team members such as physicians, nurse practitioners, dietitians, social workers, physiotherapists, and respiratory therapists use the same critical pathway to monitor the client's progress during each shift or, in the case of home care, during every visit.

Critical pathways eliminate the need for nurses' notes, flow sheets, and nursing care plans because the pathway document integrates all relevant information. Unexpected occurrences, unmet goals, and interventions not specified within the clinical pathway time frame are called **variances.** A variance is present when the activities on the clinical pathway are not completed as predicted or the client does not meet the expected outcomes. An example of a negative variance is when a client postoperatively develops pulmonary complications necessitating oxygen therapy and monitoring with pulse oximetry. An example of a positive variance is when a client progresses more rapidly than expected (e.g., use of a Foley catheter may be discontinued a day early). A variance analysis is necessary to review the data for trends and for developing and implementing an action plan to respond to the identified client problems (Box 16–3). In addition, variances may result from changes in the client's health or may occur as a result of other health complications not associated with the primary reason why the client requires care. Once a variance has been identified, the nurse modifies the client's care to meet the needs associated with the variance.

Consensus on the definition and impact of critical pathways is lacking. The pathways were developed to improve the efficiency of care in hospitals and as a cost containment measure to reduce length of hospital stay. According to Dy et al. (2005), critical pathways may be effective only under certain circumstances (e.g., first pathway implemented in a particular practice area or for lesser severity of illness).

Queensway Carleton Hospital

PATIENT CARE SERVICES
Interdisciplinary Systems Flowsheet

Key:	
Initials in Box	=Assessment findings meet standards and procedures. Interventions tolerated or care provided.
* & Initials in Box	=Significant finding(s) **abnormal or changed.** Document in progress notes.
→ & Initials in Box	=Significant finding(s) has **not changed.**
√	= Monitored on High Frequency Flow Sheet.

Initial all relevant items. Leave others blank. ***Document Clinical Pathway items on Clinical Pathway.***

CLINICAL PATHWAY NAME:											
Year______	DATE										
Month______	TIME 24 hr										
NEUROLOGICAL	Alert & oriented to person, place, time. Behaviour appropriate to situation. Follow simple commands. Verbalization clear and understandable. Pupils equal. Purposeful movement of all extremities and symmetry of strength. Sensation intact. Swallows without choking. **Post Op:** Mild to moderately sedated for first 24 hours. Easy to rouse.										
☐ See pre-existing condition Assessment											
SLEEP	Patient wakes feeling rested or sleep pattern within patient's norm.										
☐ See pre-existing condition Assessment											
CARDIOVASCULAR	Regular radial pulse 60 to 100 bpm. No edema, no chest pain, no diaphoresis. No calf tenderness. BP – Systolic 90 – 140, Diastolic 50 – 90 mmHg.										
☐ See pre-existing condition Assessment											
RESPIRATORY	Respirations quiet, regular, unlaboured, 10 – 20 per min. at rest. Sputum absent or clear. No pallor or cyanosis of nailbeds or mucous membranes. Oximetry as per patient standard. **Auscultation:** Breath sounds clear & audible both lung fields. **BiPAP:** 1=Mask off, 2=Mask on.										
☐ See pre-existing condition Assessment											
Assessment Auscultation											
BiPAP											
Chest Physio											
Tracheotomy Care											
Suctioning											
PERIPHERAL VASCULAR	Extremities pink, warm. Sensation present. Peripheral pulses palpable. No limb edema, no calf tenderness. Capillary refill < 3 seconds. **CSM**-Pulses 0=Absent 1+=Weak & Thready 2+=Normal 3+=Full and Bounding. Sensation/movement - (all limbs) Y-Yes N-No										
☐ See pre-existing condition Assessment											
CSM Location: Pulses											
CSM Location: Sensation/ Movement											

Page 1 of 2

INTERDISCIPLINARY SYSTEMS ASSESSMENT FLOWSHEET
Initial all relevant items. Leave others blank.
Document Clinical Pathway items on Clinical Pathway.

CLINICAL PATHWAY NAME:											
Year______	DATE										
Month______	TIME 24 hr										
GASTROINTESTINAL	No nausea, vomiting or pain. Bowel movements within patient's norm. Continent. Abdomen soft. Bowel sounds active in all 4 quadrants. **Post-op:** bowel sounds: Absent – sluggish – normal first 24 hrs. **Post-op:** nausea (scale 0-5). 0=none, 1-2=mild, 3-4=moderate, 5=severe. **Nasogastric drainage:** bile coloured fluid.										
☐ See pre-existing condition Assessment											
Bowel sounds: Hypoactive											
Bowel sounds: Absent											
Nausea Scale											
Skin Care Protocol											
Nasogastric Drainage (Colour)											
GENITOURINARY	**Genitalia:** No edema, bruising, lesions, abnormal discharge. **Vaginal Flow:** Scant to moderate, light pink to serosanguinous to brownish drainage. No foul odours or bright red bleeding. Few clots may be present. **Bladder:** Able to empty bladder. Output: >30 cc q 1 h. Not distended. Urine clear, yellow to amber, continent. No pain or burning on voiding. **Catheter:** Urinary drainage system patent. Cleansed q shift. Change as per protocol - Δ.										
☐ See pre-existing condition Assessment Genitalia											
Assessment Vaginal Flow											
☐ See pre-existing condition Assessment Bladder											
Catheter ☐ Indwelling ☐ Intermittent											
Sitz Bath											
MUSCULOSKELETAL/ ADL	No swelling, tenderness, weakness or muscle spasms. Functional ROM for all joints. **Mobility:** Able to ambulate; steady balance; purposeful gait. **Post op:** as ordered. **ADL**=Progressing to optimal level of functioning. **Mobility/ADL Levels:** 1-Total Assistance 2-Maximum Assistance 3-Moderate Assistance 4-Minimun Assistance 5-Supervision Only 6-Independent with Aide 7-Independent.										
☐ See pre-existing condition Assessment											
Mobility											
ADL											
Activity											
PSYCHOSOCIAL DISCHARGE PLANNING	**Psychosocial:** Has realistic perception of what is happening. Affect appropriate. No mood swings noted. **Discharge Planning:** Plans progressing according to Care Plan.										
Assessment: Psychosocial											
Discharge Planning											

Page 2 of 2

Figure 16-3 Example of a standardized form (in this case, a client care flow sheet) that can be used for charting by exception; predefined normal assessment findings are listed on the form, and the nurse notes when assessment findings are not normal or have changed. ADL, activities of daily living; AP, anteroposterior (film); BiPAP, bilevel positive airway pressure; CSM, circulation, sensation, and movement; ROM, range of motion; subcut, subcutaneous; TPN, total parenteral nutrition. **Source:** Courtesy Queensway-Carleton Hospital (2004), Nepean, Ontario.

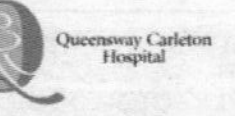

PATIENT CARE SERVICES
Interdisciplinary Care Flowsheet

Key: Initials in Box =Assessment findings meet standards and procedures. Interventions tolerated or care provided.
• **& Initials** in Box=Significant finding(s) **abnormal or changed.** Document in progress notes.
→ **& Initials** in Box=Significant finding(s) has **not changed.**
☐√ = Monitored on High Frequency Flow Sheet.

Initial all relevant items. Leave others blank. ***Document Clinical Pathway items on Clinical Pathway.***

CLINICAL PATHWAY NAME:	
Year______	DATE
Month______	TIME 24 hr
NUTRITION	Maintaining healthy body weight. Feeds self. No dehydration. **Oral Intake:** Consuming at least 3/4 of prescribed diet. **Swallowing:** No coughing/choking on liquids/solids. **Tube Feed/TPN:** Tolerating prescribed type, rate & amount of feeding. Flush entral tube and change dressing as per protocol. Δ=dressing change
☐ See pre-existing condition Assessment	
Assessment: Oral Intake	
Assessment: Swallowing	
Assessment: Tube Feeding/TPN	
INTEGUMENTARY	Skin warm, dry & intact; mucous membranes moist. Able to reposition self. Normal Braden Scale.
☐ See pre-existing condition Assessment	
Hygiene	
Reposition as per protocol	
Pressure support surface:______	
WOUND / ULCER / INCISION	**Site:** No redness, inflammation. Incision well approximated. Sutures, steristrips, staples intact. D/C=staples, sutures removed. **Stage:** I-red, non-blanchable, II-blister, broken epidermis, III-subcutaneous tissue visible, IV-muscle, bone or tendon exposed, X-black necrotic tissue on wound. **Dressing:** dry and intact. Δ=dressing change. **Drainage:** S=serous, SG=serosanguineous **Amount:** 1=nil, 2=small, 3=moderate, 4=copious.
Site 1:______ Assessment/Stage	
Dressing Type:______	
Drainage	
Site 2:______ Assessment	
Dressing Type:______	
Drainage	
Site 3:______ Assessment	
Dressing Type:______	
Drainage	

Page 1 of 2

INTERDISCIPLINARY CARE FLOWSHEET
Complete and initial all relevant items. Leave others blank.
Document Clinical Pathway items on Clinical Pathway.

CLINICAL PATHWAY NAME:	
Year______	DATE
Month______	TIME 24 hr
PAIN / COMFORT	Patient describes pain as nil, mild, or moderate & is satisfied with management. **Pain Scale:** 0-10 (none to excruciating)
Location # 1______ Pain Score	
Location # 2______ Pain Score	
Ice/heat	
SAFETY	Low risk for falls or wandering. Basic safety precautions in place. Low risk to harm self or others. Restrained as per protocol.
Assessment	
Restraint:______	
TEACHING / LEARNING	Verbalizing & understands treatment goals & care needs. Educational goals met as per teaching plan.
Assessment	
PERIPHERAL / CENTRAL LINES / SALINE LOCK	Absence of redness, swelling or tenderness at site. IV infusing at prescribed rate. IV site checked as per protocol. Saline lock patent. Flushed as per protocol. Δ=dressing change
Site Assessment ☐Lock ☐Peripheral ☐Central ☐Other ☐S/C line	
Site Assessment ☐Lock ☐Peripheral ☐Central ☐Other ☐S/C line	
Site Assessment ☐Lock ☐Peripheral ☐Central ☐Other ☐S/C line	
DRAINS	Patent & draining as expected. **Drainage:** S=serous, SS=sanguineous, SG=serosanguineous, P=purulent, B=bile, I=Irrigated **Amount:** 1=nil, 2=small, 3=moderate, 4=copious, SH=shortened D/C=discontinued.
Type:______ Location #1:______	
Type:______ Location #2:______	
Type:______ Location #3:______	
Type:______ Location #4:______	
TRANSURETHRAL PROCEDURES	**Urine:** C=Clear, P=pink, T=tea coloured, M=moderate sanguineous, SC=Sanguineous with clots, D/C=discontinued.
Bladder Irrigation – Continuous	
Bladder Irrigation – Intermittent	
Urine Drainage	
CHEST TUBE	Patent. Dressing dry and intact. Suction method as ordered. **Drainage:** S=serous,SS=sanguineous SG=serosanguineous, P=purulent.
Assessment	
Drainage	
CAST SITE	Cast dry and intact; nil-minimal drainage; sensation normal; swelling nil-minimal. Damp 24-48 hours.
Assessment	
Damp	

Page 2 of 2

Figure 16-3 Continued

The Ottawa Hospital | L'Hôpital d'Ottawa

CLINICAL PATHWAY – PLAN CLINIQUE

Hemi-Knee Arthroplasty
Hemi-genou arthroplastie

IN PATIENT 5 FLOW SHEET

☐ Civic ☐ Gen.-Gén.

Addressograph/Plaque

PAU — Unité pré-admission

Date: yyaa ______ mm ______ dj ______

Critical Path

- **Assessment & teaching per PAU standard of care and procedure specific education material**
- **Pre-operative diagnostic testing as per PAU Medical Directive for Pre-Admission Diagnostic Testing for Elective Surgery**

Tests
- CBC
- PTT, INR
- Type and screen

Additional Orders
- Social work consult if indicated
- X-ray:
  1) Standing AP of both knees
  2) Lateral and skyline patella view of operative knee

Discharge Planning
- Discuss expected length of stay (LOS)
- Discuss issues that could cause delay of discharge & discuss discharge preparation
- Provide patient with Hemi-Knee Arthroplasty education booklet

Patient Outcomes

Patient/Family Teaching
- Understands pre-op instructions and events
- Understands usual post-op course, plan for pain management, and usual self care measures to prevent post-op complications

Discharge Planning
- Understands usual LOS
- Appropriate discharge plan in place or if not suitable discharge plan in place – social work has been consulted

Patient progress corresponds with clinical pathway

Nursing:
☐ Yes ☐ No Signature: ______________
Time: ______ NTV – circle above, VC ______

Day of Surgery Pre-op — SDA/SDCU — Jour de la chirurgie pré-opératoire

Date: yyaa ______ mm ______ dj ______

Critical Path

- **Assessment and teaching per same day admission standard of care and procedure specific education material.**

Tests
- Glucose meter: for diabetic patient
- PTT/INR: for patient normally taking warfarin (Coumadin) – Unless normal result obtained after warfarin discontinued per pre-op instructions
- Electrolytes: for dialysis dependant patient unless acceptable post-dialysis results obtained within 24 h of surgery
- CBC if autologous blood donor

Additional Orders
- IV NS at 50 mL/h if IV medications to be given in SDA/SDCU

OR

If patient is insulin-dependent diabetic: IV D5W @ 100 mL/h

Antibiotics:
- If No history of allergy to penicillin or to other beta-lactam antibiotics;

or

- History of non-life threatening reaction to penicillin or other beta-lactam antibiotics (eg. rash, diarrhea, stomach upset)

IV Cefazolin *on chart for administration in OR:*
- 1 g if weight < 60 kg
- 2 g if weight ≥ 60 kg

Or

- If patient has a history of life threatening reaction (hypotension, bronchospasm, urticaria, angioedema) to penicillin or other beta-lactam antibiotics

IV Vancomycin:
- 1 g if weight < 90 kg (infuse over 60 minutes pre-op)
- 1.5 g if weight ≥ 90 kg (infuse over 90 minutes pre-op)

Patient Outcomes

Patient Teaching
- Adherence with pre-op instructions
- Understands usual events/expectations of operative day
- Understands usual post-op course, plan for pain management, and usual self care measures to prevent post-op complications

Patient progress corresponds with clinical pathway

Nursing:
☐ Yes ☐ No Signature: ______________
Time: ______ NTV – circle above, VC ______

Variance Codes (VC)

Code	Description	Code	Description
186	Activity variance	**510**	Not discharged by end of pathway – non-medical reason
653	Consult not sent by Day 3	**NTV**	Non-Tracked Variance
492	Not discharged by end of pathway – continued need for acute care	**OFF**	Ordered off clinical pathway

CP 22A (REV 01–2008) (12–2006) CHART – DOSSIER © THE OTTAWA HOSPITAL – L'HÔPITAL D'OTTAWA

Figure 16-4 Example of a critical pathway (care map) for a hemi-knee arthroplasty. ALC, alternate level of care; AP (anterior-posterior [film]); APS, acute pain service; CBC, complete blood cell count; CPM, continuous passive motion; D/C, discontinue; DVT, deep vein thrombosis; IHT, interhospital transfer; INR, international normalized ratio; IV D5W, intravenous 5% dextrose in water; IV NS, intravenous normal saline; NPO, nothing by mouth; NVS, neurovascular system; O_2, oxygen; PRN, as needed; PACU, postanaesthesia care unit; PTT, partial thromboplastin time; SDA, same-day admission; SDCU, surgical day care unit; SpO_2, pulse oximetry; VS, vital signs. **Source:** Courtesy The Ottawa Hospital (L'Hôpital d'Ottawa) (2008), Ottawa, Ontario.

Patient(e) ______________________ **Chart No. – Nº du dossier** ______________________

Day of Surgery Post-op / PACU Jour de la chirurgie / Post-opératoire / Unité de soins post-anesthésiques		Day of Surgery Post-op Ward Jour de la chirurgie / Post-opératoire / Unité regulière	
Date: yyaa ________ mm ______ dj ______		Date: yyaa ________ mm ______ dj ______	
Critical Path	**Patient Outcomes**	**Critical Path**	**Patient Outcomes**
• **SpO_2 monitoring and O_2 administration per PACU protocol** • **VS, assessment, treatment, and teaching per PACU standard of care** **Additional Orders** • Bedrest • NPO to Clear fluids prn	• Achieves PACU criteria for transfer to Ward	**Assessments/Treatments** • VS, NVS, pain q4h x 24 hrs, SpO_2 • Monitor Hemovac drainage • Monitor Dressing • Monitor Intake & Output • Pain management as per APS **Activity** • Up in chair x 1 ________ initial • Ambulate x 1 with assistance, if able ________ initial • CPM as ordered (when dressing removed) **Nutrition** • Diet as ordered **Elimination** • Catheter as ordered **Patient Teaching** • Reinforce: - Deep Breathing and Coughing (DB&C) - ankle pumping - positioning of the leg when on back and on side • Pain management • Ensure patient has Hemi-Knee Arthroplasty booklet **Discharge Planning** • Per Discharge Preparation indicators	**Pain Control** • Adequate pain control achieved: Pain ≤ 3 rest, ≤ 5 activity; pain not preventing movement; satisfied with pain control **Activity** • Demonstrates understanding of positioning **Prevention of DVT** • Performs ankle exercises **Prevention of Infection** • Verbalizes importance of adequate hydration • Performs DB&C **Patient Teaching** • Demonstrates: - DB&C - Positioning of leg - Ankle exercises
Patient progress corresponds with clinical pathway		**Patient progress corresponds with clinical pathway**	
Nursing: ☐ Yes ☐ No Signature: ________ Time: ________ NTV – circle above, VC ________		**Nursing:** **D** ☐ Yes ☐ No Signature: ________ Initials ________ Time: ________ NTV – circle above, VC ________ **E** ☐ Yes ☐ No Signature: ________ Initials ________ Time: ________ NTV – circle above, VC ________ **N** ☐ Yes ☐ No Signature: ________ Initials ________ Time: ________ NTV – circle above, VC ________	

D = 8-12 h day shift **E** = evening shift, if applicable **N** = 8-12 h night shift

Variance Codes (VC)

186	Activity variance	**510**	Not discharged by end of pathway – non-medical reason
653	Consult not sent by Day 3	**NTV**	Non-Tracked Variance
492	Not discharged by end of pathway – continued need for acute care	**OFF**	Ordered off clinical pathway

CP 22A (2 – 5) CHART – DOSSIER © THE OTTAWA HOSPITAL – L'HÔPITAL D'OTTAWA

Figure 16-4 Continued

Patient(e) ______________________ **Chart No. – Nº du dossier** ______________________

Post-op Day 1 — Jour 1 post-opératoire

Date: yyaa ________ **mm** ________ **dj** ________

Critical Path	Patient Outcomes
Consults ☐ Outpatient physio *or* ☐ Short Term Rehab **Assessments/Treatments** • VS, NVS, pain q4h → q shift, SpO_2 • Monitor Intake & Output • D/C Hemovac • D/C dressing & change to strip – If drainage notify MD • Pain management as per APS. Discontinue APS modality as per weaning guideline if patient meets criteria **Activity** • DB&C • Exercise program • Up in chair x 2 ________ initial, ________ initial • Ambulate x 2 with assistance: ________ initial, ________ initial • Assistive devices, specify: ________ • CPM as ordered **Nutrition** • Diet as ordered **Elimination** • Discontinue Foley catheter **Patient Teaching** • Reinforce exercise program • If patient on Low Molecular Weight Heparin – start self injection teaching • Pain Management **Discharge Planning** • Equipment needs addressed • Confirm out-patient physio if applicable • If patient is not expected to achieve discharge criteria by Post-op Day 2, and meets the criteria for rehab, consult service for transfer • Discharge plan confirmed with patient / family – If transferring to another facility: Specify facility ________ • Confirm (✓) arrangements re: ☐ Discharge Summary ☐ Doctor's letter ☐ IHT / Nurses letter ☐ Ambulance booked or transportation arranged *(see last page for rehab criteria)*	**Patient Teaching** • Verbalizes understanding of "Hemi-Knee Arthroplasty" instructions and exercise program • Understands the basics of self injection if applicable • Demonstrates: – Proper positioning – Understanding of mobility aids **Pain Control** • Adequate pain control achieved: Pain ≤ 3 rest, ≤ 5 activity; pain not preventing movement; satisfied with pain control **Activity** • Completes transfer with assistance • Performs exercises according to self directed program **Prevention of DVT** • Demonstrates appropriate exercises & positioning for prevention of DVT • Verbalizes understanding of anticoagulant therapy

Patient progress corresponds with clinical pathway

Physiotherapy:
☐ Yes ☐ No Signature: ________ Time: ________ NTV – circle above, VC ________

Nursing:
D ☐ Yes ☐ No Signature: ________, Initial ________ Time: ________ NTV – circle above, VC ________
E ☐ Yes ☐ No Signature: ________, Initial ________ Time: ________ NTV – circle above, VC ________
N ☐ Yes ☐ No Signature: ________, Initial ________ Time: ________ NTV – circle above, VC ________

D = 8-12 h day shift **E** = evening shift, if applicable **N** = 8-12 h night shift

Variance Codes (VC)

186	Activity variance	**510**	Not discharged by end of pathway – non-medical reason
653	Consult not sent by Day 3	**NTV**	Non-Tracked Variance
492	Not discharged by end of pathway – continued need for acute care	**OFF**	Ordered off clinical pathway

© THE OTTAWA HOSPITAL – L'HÔPITAL D'OTTAWA **CHART – DOSSIER** **CP 22A (3 – 5)**

Figure 16-4 Continued

Patient(e) ______ Chart No. – Nº du dossier ______

Post-op Day 2 / Discharge Day — Jour 2 post-opératoire / Jour de congé

Date: yyaa ______ mm ______ dj ______

Critical Path	Patient Outcomes
Assessments/Treatments • VS / NVS q shift, SpO_2 • Pain q4h • Wound care **Activity** • Continue exercise program • Ambulate x 2 • CPM as ordered • Assistive devices, specify: ______ • Gait training on stairs if required **Nutrition** • Diet as ordered **Elimination** • Assess for patient's normal bowel pattern **Patient Teaching** • Review physician specific discharge instructions and provide discharge instruction sheet • Assess patient for knowledge of discharge instructions / Hemi-Knee Arthroplasty precautions • Review anticoagulant therapy and self injection teaching if applicable • Review Question and Answer sheet in booklet • Review pain management plan **Discharge Planning** • Patient to be discharged unless otherwise indicated by physician • Discharge patient after seen by Physio in p.m., once discharge criteria met • If unable to discharge today: – Verify ALC status if discharge delayed and acute care no longer required – Document appropriate delay of discharge variance code – Discontinue pathway after Day 2	**Discharge Criteria** • Patient / family understand post-discharge care and follow-up plan • Adequate pain control • No clinical evidence of DVT • If patient on Low Molecular Weight Heparin – is able to give own injection • No clinical signs of infection • Adequate bowel function and understands bowel managment plan • Appropriate gait aides arranged • Ambulates independently with assistive devices • Safe on stairs (if needed) • Transfers independently with mobility devices • Appropriate place to go and support available as required post-discharge

Patient progress corresponds with clinical pathway

Physiotherapy:

☐ Yes ☐ No Signature: ______ Time: ______ NTV – circle above, VC ______

Nursing:

D ☐ Yes ☐ No Signature: ______, Initial ______ Time: ______ NTV – circle above, VC ______

E ☐ Yes ☐ No Signature: ______, Initial ______ Time: ______ NTV – circle above, VC ______

N ☐ Yes ☐ No Signature: ______, Initial ______ Time: ______ NTV – circle above, VC ______

D = 8-12 h day shift **E** = evening shift, if applicable **N** = 8-12 h night shift

Variance Codes (VC)

186 Activity variance
653 Consult not sent by Day 3
492 Not discharged by end of pathway – continued need for acute care
510 Not discharged by end of pathway – non-medical reason
NTV Non-Tracked Variance
OFF Ordered off clinical pathway

CP 22A (4 – 5) CHART – DOSSIER © THE OTTAWA HOSPITAL – L'HÔPITAL D'OTTAWA

Figure 16-4 Continued

Common Record-Keeping Forms

A variety of forms are specially designed for the type of information that nurses routinely document. The categories within a form are usually derived from institutional standards of practice or guidelines established by accrediting agencies.

Admission Nursing History Forms

A nursing history form is completed when a client is admitted to a nursing care unit. The history form guides the nurse through a complete assessment to identify relevant nursing diagnoses or problems (see Chapter 13). Data on history forms provide baselines that can be compared with changes in the client's condition.

Flow Sheets and Graphic Records

Flow sheets are forms in which nurses can quickly and easily enter assessment data about the client, including vital sign measurements and routine repetitive care actions, such as hygiene measures, ambulation, meals, weights, and safety and restraint checks (Box 16–4). The format of the flow sheet varies in accordance with the agency and the data being recorded. For example, some flow sheets may be used only to record vital sign measurements (often called *graphic records*); others may be more comprehensive (Figure 16–5; note that Figure 16–3 shows a flow sheet that is used for CBE). For flow sheets, a coding system is used for data entry. It is important to fill out all spaces on the flow sheet, even for items that are "not applicable" (for which you can write "N/A"). A blank space can raise doubts about whether an intervention was or was not performed. If an occurrence recorded on the flow sheet is unusual or changes significantly, a focus note is needed (see Box 16–3). For example, if a client's blood pressure becomes dangerously high, the nurse completes a focus assessment and records the findings, as well as action taken, in the progress notes. Flow sheets provide a quick, easy reference for the health care team members in assessing a client's status. Critical care and acute care units commonly use flow sheets for all types of physiological data.

Client Care Summary or Kardex

Many agencies now have computerized systems that provide basic, summative information in the form of a client care summary. This is printed out for each client during each shift. This summary is continually updated and provides the nurse with a current detailed list of orders, treatment, and diagnostic testing. In some settings, a **Kardex** system, a portable "flip-over" file or notebook, is kept at the nurses' station. Most Kardex forms have an activity and treatment section and a nursing care plan section that organize information for quick reference as nurses give change-of-shift reports or make walking rounds. An updated Kardex form eliminates the need for repeated referral to the chart for routine information throughout the day. In many institutions, entries on Kardex forms are made in pencil because of the need for frequent revisions as the client's needs change. In settings in which the Kardex form is a permanent part of the client's record, entries are made in ink. Information commonly found on the client care summary or Kardex form includes the following:

- Basic demographic data (e.g., age, sex, religious affiliation)
- Hospital identification number
- Physician's name
- Primary medical diagnosis
- Medical and surgical history
- Current physician's or nurse practitioner's treatment orders to be carried out by the nurse (e.g., dressing changes, ambulation, glucose monitoring)
- Nursing care plan
- Nursing orders (e.g., education sessions, symptom relief measures, counselling)
- Scheduled tests and procedures
- Safety precautions to be used in the client's care
- Factors related to activities of daily living
- Contact information about nearest relative or guardian or person to contact in an emergency
- Emergency code status
- Allergies

> **BOX 16-3 Example of Variance Documentation**
>
> A 56-year-old client is on a surgical unit one day after a bowel resection. His temperature is slightly elevated, his breath sounds are decreased bilaterally at the bases of both lobes of the lungs, and he is slightly confused. Ordinarily, one day postoperatively, a client should be afebrile with clear lungs. The following is an example of the variance documentation for this client.
>
> 9/23/05
> 1000 hrs: Breath sounds diminished bilaterally at the bases. T [temperature] 37.8°C; P 92; R 28/min; oxygen saturation 84%. Daughter states he is "confused" and did not recognize her when she arrived a few minutes ago. Oxygen started at 2 L/min via nasal prongs as per standing orders. Will monitor pulse oximetry and vital signs every 15 minutes. Dr. P. Yoshida notified of change in status. Daughter at bedside. R. Balliol, RN

> **BOX 16-4 Benefits of Using a Flow Sheet**
>
> - Information is accessible to all members of the health care team.
> - Time spent on writing a narrative note is decreased.
> - Information is current.
> - Errors resulting from transfer of information are decreased.
> - Team members can quickly see trends over time.

Acuity Records or Workload Measurement Systems

Acuity records (also known as **workload measurement systems**) provide a method of determining the hours of care and staff required for a given group of clients. A client's *acuity level* is based on the type and number of nursing interventions required for providing care in a 24-hour period. The acuity level determined by the nursing care allows clients to be rated in comparison with one another. For example, an acuity system might rate bathing clients from 1 to 5 (1 means client is totally dependent on others for bathing, 5 means client bathes independently). A client who has just undergone surgery and who requires frequent monitoring and extensive care may be listed with an acuity level of 1. On the same continuum, another client awaiting discharge after a successful recovery from surgery has an acuity level of 5. Accurate acuity ratings may also be used to justify overtime and the number and qualifications of staff needed to safely care for clients. The client-to-staff ratios established for a unit depend on a composite gathering of data for the 24-hour interventions that are necessary for each client receiving care.

Standardized Care Plans

Some institutions use **standardized care plans** to make documentation easier for nurses. The plans, based on the institution's standards of nursing practice, are preprinted, established guidelines that are used to care for clients who have similar health problems. After a nursing assessment is completed, the staff nurse identifies the standard care plans that are appropriate for the client. The care plans are

Ottawa–Carleton Hospital Post-Op Flow Sheet

Key to Amount		Key to Colour		Key to Urine Colour	
–	Nil	br	Bright Red	c	clear
S	Small	dr	Dark Red	tc	tea colour
M	Moderate	b	Brown	p	pink
L	Large	dg	Dark Green	br	bright red
Sc	Scant	lg	Light Green	dr	dark red
		y	yellow	rc	red with clots
		p	pink	b	brown

DATE	MONTH YEAR													
	TIME													
PAIN	– absent/comfortable													
	– relieved with meds													
	– meds not effective													
CHEST														
	– clear													
	– congested													
	– D B & C													
	– D B & C with encouragement													
ABDOMEN														
	– soft													
	– distended													
BOWEL SOUNDS														
	– absent													
	– sluggish													
	– normal													
	– passing flatus													
DRESSING														
	– dry, intact													
	– reinforced													
	– amount of drainage (key)													
	– colour of drainage (key)													
DIET														
	NPO													
	– sips/ice chips													
	– fluids													
	– diet tolerated													
	– diet not tolerated													

Ottawa–Carleton Hospital Post-Op Flow Sheet

Key to Amount		Key to Colour		Key to Urine Colour	
–	Nil	br	Bright Red	c	clear
S	Small	dr	Dark Red	tc	tea colour
M	Moderate	b	Brown	p	pink
L	Large	dg	Dark Green	br	bright red
Sc	Scant	lg	Light Green	dr	dark red
		y	yellow	rc	red with clots
		p	pink	b	brown

DATE	MONTH YEAR													
	TIME													
AMBULATION	– active exercise in bed													
	– dangles													
	– up as ordered													
	– up and about													
	– not tolerating activity													
URINE														
	– colour (key)													
P.V. LOSS														
	– colour (key)													
	– amount (key)													
CIRCULATION														
	– temp. satis.													
	– temp. unsatis.													
	– pulses – present													
	– absent													
	– edema – absent													
	– present													
	– cyanosis/pallor													
	– sensation – absent													
	– present													
DRAINAGE														
	– N.G. tube													
	– colour (key)													

Figure 16-5 Example of a client care flow sheet. D B & C, deep breathing and coughing; N.G., nasogastric; NPO, nothing by mouth. **Source:** Adapted from Ottawa-Carleton Hospital, 2000. Queensway-Carleton Campus. Nepean, ON: Author.

placed in the client's health care record. The standardized plans can be modified (and changes are noted in ink) to individualize the therapies. Most standardized care plans also allow the nurse to write in specific goals or desired outcomes of care and the dates by which these outcomes should be achieved.

One advantage of standardized care plans is establishment of clinically sound standards of care for similar groups of clients. These standards can be useful when quality improvement audits are conducted. These care plans can help nurses recognize the accepted requirements of care for clients and also improve continuity of care.

The use of standardized care plans is controversial. The major disadvantage is the risk that the standardized plans prevent nurses from providing unique, individualized therapies for clients. Standardized care plans cannot replace the nurse's professional judgement and decision making. In addition, care plans need to be updated on a regular basis to ensure that content is current and appropriate.

Discharge Summary Forms

It is important to prepare clients for an efficient, timely discharge from a health care facility. A client's discharge should also result in desirable outcomes. Multidisciplinary involvement in discharge planning helps ensure that a client leaves the hospital in a timely manner with the necessary resources in place (Box 16–5).

Ideally, discharge planning begins at admission. You need to revise the care plan as the client's condition changes. Remember to involve the client and family members in the discharge planning process so that they have the information needed to return the client home. Discharge information and instructions should include data such as the following:

- Instruction about potential food–drug interactions, nutrition intervention, and modified diets
- Rehabilitation techniques to support adaptation to, or functional independence in, the environment, or both
- Access to available community resources
- Circumstances in which clients should obtain further treatment or follow-up care
- Methods of obtaining follow-up care
- The client's and family's responsibilities in the client's care
- Medication instructions, including the times and reasons to take each medication, the dose, the route, precautions, possible adverse reactions, and information about when and how to get prescriptions refilled

Furthermore, a common standard in nursing practice is to educate clients about the nature of their disease process, its likely progress, and the signs and symptoms of complications.

When a client is discharged from inpatient care, a discharge summary that includes information from members of the health care team is prepared. The summary is given to the client or family or to the home care, rehabilitation, or long-term care agency. Discharge summary forms help make the summary concise and instructive (Figure 16–6). A summary form emphasizes previous learning by the client and family and care that should be continued in any restorative care setting. When given directly to clients, the form may be attached to pamphlets or teaching brochures.

Home Health Care Documentation

As a result of shorter hospitalizations and larger numbers of older adults who require home care services, home health care is expanding. Because clients are leaving acute care settings earlier, increasing numbers of home care clients are presenting in the community setting with more acuity (i.e., sicker). The focus in home health care is on family-centered care and forming a partnership or collaboration with the client and the family to help the client regain health, help the family take over the client's care, or to help accomplish both. Documentation in the home health care system has different implications than in other areas of nursing. Two primary differences are that the majority of the care is performed by the client and family and that the nurse is often teaching and helping the client and family achieve greater independence. Nurses must have astute assessment skills to gather the needed information about changes in the client's health care status. In addition, documentation systems need to provide the entire health care team with the information needed for them to work together effectively (Box 16–6).

In the home care setting, the client is the guardian of the health care record. A hard copy of the health care record is kept in the client's home, and the client is responsible for its safekeeping. Communication is crucial in home care because much of the interaction between health care professionals is conducted virtually by phone or fax over password-protected voice mail or secure fax lines. With the increasing availability of hand-held devices such as **personal digital assistants** and laptop computers or tablets, records can be available in multiple locations, which enables easier access to the multidisciplinary needs that are often associated with home care. Privacy remains a unique challenge in home health care, however, inasmuch as not all member of the health care team have access to secure electronic transmission of confidential material (e.g., as is the case in physicians' offices).

BOX 16-5 Discharge Summary Information

- Use clear, concise descriptions in client's own language.
- Provide step-by-step description of how to perform a procedure (e.g., home medication administration). Reinforce explanation with printed instructions.
- Identify precautions to follow when the client performs self-care or administers medications.
- Review signs and symptoms of complications that should be reported to the primary care practitioner.
- List names and phone numbers of health care professionals and community resources that the client can contact.
- Identify any unresolved problem, including plans for follow-up and continuous treatment.
- List actual time of discharge, mode of transportation, and who accompanied the client.

BOX 16-6 Home Care Forms for Documentation

The usual forms used to document home care include the following:

- Assessment forms
- Referral source information or intake form
- Discipline-specific care plans
- Physician's plan of treatment
- Professional order form (e.g., MD, speech language pathologist, specialty nurses)
- Medication administration record
- Clinical progress notes
- Miscellaneous (case conference notes, professional communication forms, private billing forms, insurance company forms)
- Discharge summary

Adapted from Iyer, P. W., & Camp, N. H. (1999). *Nursing documentation: A nursing process approach*. St. Louis: Mosby.

Ottawa–Carleton Hospital
Discharge Protocol

ADMITTING INFORMATION
(Completed by Nurse on Admission)

Admission Date:________ Doctor:________
Diagnosis:________

Support Systems: ☐ Spouse ☐ Children ☐ Friend/Neighbour ☐ None
☐ Other:________

Community Services: CCAC: ☐ Nursing ☐ OT ☐ PT ☐ Homemaking
☐ GAOT ☐ Helpline ☐ Day Hospital ☐ Meals on Wheels
☐ Seniors Support ☐ Other (describe):________

If not admitted from home, name of facility:________

DISCHARGE SUMMARY (Completed on Discharge)
Discharge Date:________ Time:________ Level:________ Quad:________

Discharge Destination: ☐ Home alone ☐ Home with other:________
☐ Facility:________ ☐ Informed of DC Date:________
☐ Transfer & Referral Form ☐ Transportation arranged:________

Accompanied By: ☐ Spouse ☐ Relative/friend ☐ Alone ☐ Other:________

Appliances/Aids: ☐ None ☐ Crutches ☐ Cane ☐ Walker ☐ Other:________

Community Referrals Arranged: CCAC: ☐ Nursing ☐ OT ☐ PT ☐ Homemaking
☐ GAOT ☐ Helpline ☐ Day Hospital ☐ Meals on Wheels
☐ Seniors Support ☐ Other (describe):________

Outpatient Follow-Up: ☐ None ☐ Clinic ☐ Physician's office ☐ Other:________
☐ Tests________

Discharge Medications: ☐ None Prescription ☐ Yes ☐ No Teaching ☐ Yes ☐ No

Discharge Teaching Completed: ☐ Yes ☐ No Comments:________

Incision Assessed: ☐ Yes ☐ No ☐ Not applicable Comments:________

Patient's Condition on Discharge:
Bladder Function: ☐ Good ☐ Fair ☐ Poor Independence: ☐ Good ☐ Fair ☐ Poor
Bowel Function: ☐ Good ☐ Fair ☐ Poor Nutrition: ☐ Good ☐ Fair ☐ Poor
Emotional Status: ☐ Good ☐ Fair ☐ Poor Skin: ☐ Good ☐ Fair ☐ Poor

Date:________ Nurse's Signature:________

KEY:
ADL = Activities of Daily Living
CNS = Clinical Nurse Specialist
GAOT = Geriatric Assessment Outreach Team
N/A = Not Applicable
RRT = Registered Respiratory Therapist
ARDU = Alzheimer & Related Disorder Unit
DC = Discharge
LTC = Long-Term Care
OT = Occupational Therapy
Rx = Treatment
CCAC = Community Care Access Centre
Dx = Diagnosis
MRSA = Methicillin-Resistant *Staphylococcus Aureus*
PT = Physiotherapy
SOB = Short of Breath

CLIENT PROBLEMS (Referral Criteria):
Multidisciplinary Team members to ✓ and date problems applicable to client.

MEDICAL HISTORY
☐ ____ Many chronic medical problems **Refer: Social Worker** **Refer: CNS** (if patient >75 yrs)
☐ ____ Many ER visits or hospital admissions **Refer: Social Worker**
☐ ____ Cancer, AIDS/HIV, or terminal illness & client/family needing support **Dr. to consider Palliative Care**
☐ ____ Behavioural or psychological problems **Dr. to consider Geriatrician, Psychogeriatric/Psychiatry, ARDU**
☐ ____ Other (describe)

HEALTH MANAGEMENT
☐ ____ Positive MRSA screen **Refer: Infection Control**
☐ ____ Needs stress management training **Refer: OT**

MEDICATIONS
☐ ____ Noncompliant or needs education
☐ ____ Uncertain of drug allergy reaction
☐ ____ DC medications differ from admission & is taking >6 schedule medications
☐ ____ Frequent medication changes or multiple generic brands, numerous herbal preparation **Refer: Pharmacist**
☐ ____ Taking multiple medications (>75 yr) **Refer: CNS**
☐ ____ Other (describe)

RESPIRATORY
☐ ____ O_2 titration, spirometry
☐ ____ Home O_2 or home O_2 candidate
☐ ____ Needs education: disease, devices
☐ ____ Candidate for Asthma Clinic **Refer: RRT**
☐ ____ Respiratory problem with mobility restrictions & safety issues
☐ ____ Respiratory deficiency, SOB, difficulty clearing secretions **Refer: PT**
☐ ____ Pneumonia **Refer: PT Refer: RRT**
☐ ____ Needs energy conservation, work simplication, & relaxation training **Refer: OT**
☐ ____ Other (describe)

SKIN
☐ ____ Delayed wound healing
☐ ____ Decubitus ulcer, exudating open wound, large burn, nutritional edema
☐ ____ Positioning & pressure relief **Refer: Dietitian Refer: CNS Refer: OT**
☐ ____ Limited mobility due to wound on joint **Refer: PT Refer: CNS**
☐ ____ Lymphedema, skin care problem **Refer: CNS**
☐ ____ Other (describe)

PAIN
☐ ____ Needs pain/symptom management **Dr. to consider Palliative Care**
☐ ____ Origin is musculoskeletal, articular, neural, gross edema
☐ ____ Palliative patient with pain **Refer: PT Refer: OT**

NUTRITION
☐ ____ Dysphagia **Refer: Speech Therapy Refer: Dietitian**
☐ ____ Malnutrition or weight loss
☐ ____ Inadequate food intake (prolonged)
☐ ____ Special diet
☐ ____ Enteral/parenteral nutrition
☐ ____ Needs diet intervention/teaching
☐ ____ Diabetic — new or uncontrolled
☐ ____ Candidate for Diabetes Info. Program
☐ ____ Candidate for Lipid Clinic **Refer: Dietitian**
☐ ____ Other (describe)

ELIMINATION
☐ ____ Stoma care problem (any age)
☐ ____ Altered bowel function
☐ ____ Altered urinary function **Refer: CNS**
☐ ____ Other (describe)

COGNITIVE & SENSORY
☐ ____ Cognitive impairment **Refer: OT Refer: CNS (if patient >75 yr)**
☐ ____ Motivational problems **Refer: CNS (if patient >75 yr) Refer: OT**

☐ ____ Communication difficulty (recent) **Refer: Speech Therapy**
☐ ____ Other (describe)

MOBILITY
☐ ____ Concern for ADL safety/independence
☐ ____ Need for wheelchair
☐ ____ Meal preparation **Refer: OT Refer: Dietitian**
☐ ____ Restricted/unsafe mobility
☐ ____ Severe general weakness/balance difficulties
☐ ____ Recent inability to do stairs at home
☐ ____ Problem moving in bed or transferring **Refer: PT Refer: CNS (if patient >75 yr)**
☐ ____ Other (describe)

PSYCHOSOCIAL
☐ ____ Lives alone and at risk
☐ ____ Unable to return to previous living situation
☐ ____ Financial concerns for living needs
☐ ____ Indications of abuse
☐ ____ Needs 24-h supervision
☐ ____ Anticipated DC to a facility
☐ ____ Sole caregiver for dependent person
☐ ____ Caregiver unable to manage **Refer: Social Worker Refer: CNS (if patient >75 yr) Refer: OT Refer: Geriatric Day Hospital**
☐ ____ Other (describe)

SPIRITUAL
☐ ____ Fear or anxiety related to Dx or Rx
☐ ____ Questioning meaning or purpose of life, self or situation, values & beliefs
☐ ____ Non-urgent sacramental care needed **Refer: Hospital Chaplain**
☐ ____ Acute fear or anxiety or grief
☐ ____ Urgent sacramental care needed **Notify on-call chaplain**
☐ ____ Other (describe)

Figure 16-6 Example of a discharge summary form. AIDS, acquired immune deficiency syndrome; HIV, human immunodeficiency virus. **Source:** Adapted from Ottawa-Carleton Hospital, 2000. Queensway-Carleton Campus. Nepean, ON: Author.

Long-Term Health Care Documentation

An increasing number of older adults require care in long-term care or residential facilities. Many individuals live in this setting for the rest of their lives and are therefore referred to as **residents** rather than as *clients*. In long-term care settings, nursing personnel face challenges much different from those in acute care settings. Residents' health is often stable, and so daily documentation can be completed on flow sheets. Assessments performed several times a day in acute care settings are required only weekly or monthly in long-term care settings.

Governmental agencies and provincial and territorial laws are instrumental in determining the standards and policies for documentation. Documentation is used to review the levels of care given to and needed by residents in long-term care facilities. Although most long-term care facilities have different documentation systems, these systems are based on the need for a concise, nonduplicating method of documentation and on the importance of nursing documentation in support of evidence-informed practice (Box 16–7).

> **BOX 16-7 Components of Documentation in Long-Term Care**
>
> **Section 1: The Health Care Record**
>
> The health care record includes the resident's name and medical number; date and time of admission; change in resident's condition; informed consent; note or discharge summary; incident reporting; monthly summary charting; and type of therapy and treatment time.
>
> **Section 2: Resident Assessments and Related Documents**
>
> This section consists of the admission record; preadmission assessment; admission assessment; assessment of risk for falls; skin assessment; bowel and bladder assessment; physical restraint assessment; record of self-administration of medication; nutrition assessment; and activities, recreation, or leisure interests.
>
> **Section 3: Other Records**
>
> Other records include drug therapy records, medication or treatment records, flow sheets or other graphic records, laboratory and special reports, consent forms, acknowledgements and notices, advance directives, and discharge or transfer records.

Computerized Documentation

Many hospitals are using computerized documentation systems or are in the process of transitioning to computerized charting. Current software programs enable nurses to quickly enter specific assessment data, fill in forms with typical entry choices, and enter narrative for unique situations; computer memory is also adequate for large amounts of data, and information can be automatically transferred to different reports. Computers can also help generate nursing care plans and document all facets of client care.

Hand-held devices such as personal digital assistants also have the potential to increase nursing productivity by providing access to clinical and reference material, providing a means for decreasing medication errors, and reducing documentation time (Scordo, Yeager, & Young, 2003). Nurses can document at the client's bedside—at the point of care. **Point-of-care information systems** consist of hand-held devices such as personal digital assistants or computers that nurses bring to the client's bedside.

Nursing Information Systems

A good information system supports the work you do. As a nurse, you need to be able to easily access a computer program, review the client's medical history and physician order, and then go to the client's bedside to conduct a comprehensive assessment. Once you have completed the assessment, you enter data into the computer terminal at the client's bedside and develop a plan of care from the information gathered. Periodically, you will return to the computer to check on laboratory test results and document the therapies you administer. The computer screens and optional pop-up windows make it easy to locate information, enter and compare data, and make changes.

Nursing information systems have two basic designs. The nursing process design is the most traditional. It organizes documentation within well-established formats, such as admission and postoperative assessment, problem lists, care plans, discharge planning instructions, and intervention lists or notes. The nursing process design also includes formats for the following tasks:

- Generation of a nursing worklist that indicates routine scheduled activities related to the care of each client.
- Documentation of routine aspects of client care, such as hygiene, positioning, fluid intake and output, wound care measures, and blood glucose measurements.
- Progress note entries with the use of narrative notes, CBE, and flow sheet charting.
- Documentation of medication administration.

The second design model for a nursing information system is the protocol, or critical pathway, design (Hebda et al., 2005). This design offers a multidisciplinary format to managing information. All health care professionals use a protocol system to document the care that they provide clients. Evidence-informed clinical protocols or critical pathways provide the formatting or design for the type of information that clinicians enter into the system. The information system allows a user to select one or more appropriate protocols for a client. An advanced system merges multiple protocols so that a master protocol, or path, is used to direct client care activities. The system identifies variances of the anticipated outcomes on the protocols as they are charted. This system provides all caregivers the ability to analyze variances and to obtain an accurate clinical picture of the client's progress.

Advantages of a Nursing Information System. Few formal well-designed studies have demonstrated the impact of computerized record systems on nursing practice or client outcomes. Anecdotal reports and descriptive studies suggest that nursing information systems do offer important advantages to nurses in practice. Hebda et al. (2005) outlined some specific advantages of nursing information systems:

- Increased time to spend with clients
- Bettter access to information
- Enhanced quality of documentation
- Reduced numbers of errors of omission
- Reduced hospital costs
- Increased nurse job satisfaction
- Enhanced compliance with accreditation standards
- Development of a common clinical database

Security Mechanisms. Computerized documentation has legal risks. Any given person could theoretically access a computer station within a health care agency and obtain information about almost any client. Protection of privacy of information in computer systems is a top priority. As described in Chapter 17, Canada has both provincial and national privacy legislation to protect personal health information in electronic or other form.

In most security mechanisms for information systems, a combination of logical and physical restrictions is used to protect information and computer systems. These measures include the installation of firewalls, antivirus software, and spyware-detection software. A firewall is a combination of hardware and software that protects private network resources (e.g., a hospital's information system) from outside hackers, network damage, and theft or misuse of information. An example of a logical restriction is an automatic sign-off, a mechanism that logs a user off the computer system after a specified period of inactivity on the computer (Hebda et al., 2005).

Physical security measures include the placement of computers or file servers in restricted areas. This form of security may have limited benefit, especially if an organization uses mobile wireless devices such as notebooks, tablet personal computers, or personal digital assistants. Such devices can be easily misplaced or lost, which allows them to be accessed by unauthorized persons. An organization may use motion detectors or alarms with devices to help prevent theft.

One method of authenticating access to automated records is the use of access codes and passwords. A password is a collection of alphanumeric characters that a user types into the computer before he or she can access a program. A user is usually required to enter a password after the entry and acceptance of an access code or user name. A password does not appear on the computer screen when it is typed, nor should it be known to anyone but the user and information systems administrators (Hebda et al., 2005). Efficacious passwords contain combinations of letters, numbers, and symbols that are not easily guessed. When using a health care agency computer system, you must not share your computer password, under any circumstances, with anyone. A secure system requires frequent and random changes in personal passwords to prevent unauthorized persons from tampering with records. In addition, most staff members have access to clients in their work area only. Select staff members (e.g., administrators or risk managers) may be given authority to access all client records.

Handling and Disposal of Information. It is important to keep medical records confidential, but it is equally important to safeguard the information that is printed from the record or extracted for report purposes. For example, you print a copy of a nursing activities worklist to use as a day planner while administering care to clients. You refer to information on the list and hand-write notes to enter later into the computer. Information on the list is considered to be personal health information and must be kept confidential and not left out for view by unauthorized persons. You must destroy anything that is printed when the printed information is no longer needed.

All papers containing personal health information (e.g., client's health care number, date of birth, age, name, or address) must be destroyed if they are not part of the client's health record. Most agencies have shredders or locked receptacles for shredding and later incineration. Be sure you familiarize yourself with the disposal policies for records in the institution where you work.

Clinical Information Systems

Any clinician, including nurses, physicians, pharmacists, social workers, and therapists, will use programs available on a clinical information system. These programs include monitoring systems; order entry systems; and laboratory, radiology, and pharmacy systems. A monitoring system includes devices that automatically monitor and record biometric measurements (e.g., vital signs, oxygen saturation, cardiac index, and stroke volume) in critical care areas and specialty areas. The devices electronically send measurements directly to the nursing documentation systems.

Order entry systems enable nurses to order supplies and services from another department. Such systems eliminate the need for written order forms and expedite the delivery of needed supplies to a nursing unit. The **computerized physician order entry (CPOE)** is one type of order entry system gaining popularity in many larger hospitals. CPOE is a process by which the physician or nurse practitioner directly enters orders for client care into the hospital information system. CPOE can eliminate the issues related to illegible handwriting and transcription errors, prevent duplication, and speed the implementation of ordered diagnostic tests and treatments. It can improve staff productivity and save money. Orders made through CPOE are integrated within the record and sent to the appropriate departments (e.g., pharmacy and radiology). In advanced systems, CPOE is linked to **clinical decision support**, which has a range of computerized tools such as built-in reminders and alerts that help the health care professional select the most appropriate medication or diagnostic test or remind the practitioner about drug interactions, allergies, and the need for subsequent orders. Medication errors and adverse drug-related events can potentially be reduced. Few studies have measured the effects of CPOE with clinical decision support on these variables, however, and more research (especially randomized controlled trials) in this area is needed (Wolfstadt et al., 2008).

The Electronic Health Record

The traditional paper health care record no longer meets the needs of today's health care industry. A paper record is episode oriented, with a separate record for each client visit to a health care agency (Hebda et al., 2005). Key information can be lost from one episode of care to the next, which can jeopardize a client's safety. An **electronic health record (EHR)** is a longitudinal record of client health information accessible online from many separate but interoperable automated systems within an electronic network (Health Canada, 2007; see Chapter 17). A unique feature of an EHR is its ability to integrate all pertinent client information into one record, regardless of the number of times a client enters a health care system.

The development and implementation of an EHR to support effective health care delivery for Canadians is in progress through Canada Health Infoway Inc. (Infoway; Health Canada, 2007). Infoway has set a target of 50% of Canadians to have EHRs by 2010 (Canada Health Infoway, 2007).

Reporting

Nurses communicate information about clients so that all team members can make appropriate decisions about the care of clients. Any verbal report must be timely, accurate, and relevant. Some Canadian hospitals having been using the **situation–background–assessment–recommendation (SBAR)** communication technique to provide "a common and predictable structure to communication" between members of the health care team about a client's care (Leonard et al., 2004, p. 86). The SBAR technique is an attempt to align ways of communicating important information that often necessitates immediate attention, and it fosters a culture of client safety.

Nurses commonly make four types of reports: change-of-shift reports, telephone reports, transfer reports, and incident reports. The SBAR technique (Box 16–8) can be incorporated into a variety of ways of reporting (e.g., a nurse's report to a physician about a critically ill client, change-of-shift reports about individual clients) and can be adapted for use with or by other health care professionals.

Change-of-Shift Reports

At the end of each shift, nurses report information about their assigned clients to the nurses working on the next shift. The purpose of the report is to provide continuity of care among nurses who are caring for a client.

Nurses give a **change-of-shift report** orally in person, by audiotape recording, by writing information on a summary report sheet, or during "walking–planning" rounds at each client's bedside. Oral reports can be given in conference rooms, with staff members from both shifts participating. Oral reports can also take the form of one-to-one reports: for example, a report given by the night nurse to the day nurse. An advantage of oral reports is that they allow staff members to ask questions or clarify explanations. When nurses make rounds, the client and family members also have the opportunity to participate in any decisions. The nurses can see the client together to perform needed assessments, evaluate progress, and discuss the interventions best suited to the client's needs. An audiotape report is given by the nurse who has completed care for the client; this type of report is left for the nurse on the next shift to review. Taped reports can improve efficiency by being recorded before the end of the shift when time is available and by avoiding social conversations between peers. However, it is essential to schedule an opportunity for the incoming nurses to ask questions for clarification after they listen to the taped report.

Because nurses have many responsibilities, it is important to compile a change-of-shift report quickly and efficiently (Table 16–4). An effective report describes clients' health status and tells staff on the next shift exactly what kind of care the clients require. A change-of-shift report should *not* simply be a reading of documented information. Instead, significant facts about clients are reviewed (e.g., condition of wounds, episodes of chest pain) to provide a baseline for comparison during the next shift. Data about clients need to be objective, current, and concise.

An organized report follows a logical sequence. To prepare for the report, the nurse gathers information from worksheets, the client's records, and the care plan. The following is an example of a change-of-shift report:

Background information: Cy Tolan in bed 4, a 32-year-old client of Dr. Lang, is scheduled for a colon resection this morning at 0800 hours. He has had ulcerative colitis for two years with recent bouts of frank bleeding in his stools. He was admitted at 0600 hours this morning with slight abdominal discomfort. This is his first experience with surgery. He knows he may require a colostomy. He has been NPO [had nothing by mouth] since midnight at home.

Assessment: Mr. Tolan mentioned that he was unable to sleep last night. He had many questions about surgery on admission this morning.

Nursing diagnosis: His chief nursing care problems are anxiety related to inexperience with surgery and risk for body image disturbance.

Teaching plan: I talked to him about postoperative routines and answered all his questions. He attended the preoperative admission clinic two weeks ago, but he did not have as many concerns at that time. He stated that he felt less anxious now that he knows what to expect.

Treatments: I started a intravenous infusion of normal saline in his left arm at 125 mL/hr at 0645 hrs.

Family information: His wife came with him this morning and will wait in the surgical waiting room till his surgery is complete.

Discharge plan: Mr. Tolan is a very active person and participates in strenuous sports such as swimming. Mrs. Tolan is concerned about how he might react to a colostomy. I suggest making a referral to the enterostomal therapist early, if the colostomy is performed.

Priority needs: Right now, Mr. Tolan is relaxing in his room. All preoperative procedures have been completed except for his preoperative antibiotic, due on call to the operating room.

A professional demeanour is essential when you give a report about clients or family members. It is often necessary to describe the interactions among clients, nurses, and family members in behavioural terms. Nurses must avoid using judgemental language such as *uncooperative*, *difficult*, or *bad* when describing such behaviours.

In many settings, unregulated care providers (UCPs) are involved in the change-of-shift report. UCPs are part of the health care team and can contribute more when they also know a client's condition and the nursing team's priorities in care. The nurse can use the report to emphasize to UCPs the tasks that need to be accomplished.

Telephone Reports

Nurses inform physicians of changes in a client's condition and communicate information to nurses on other units about client transfer. The laboratory staff or a radiologist may phone to report results of

➤ BOX 16-8 The Situation-Background-Assessment-Recommendation (SBAR) Technique

When calling the physician, follow the SBAR process as follows:

Situation: What is the situation you are calling about?

- Identify yourself, the unit, the client, and the room number
- Briefly state the problem: what it is, when it started, and the severity

Background: Provide background information related to the situation, including the following:

- The client's health care record
- The admitting diagnosis and date of admission
- A list of current medications, allergies, intravenous fluids, and laboratory tests
- The most recent vital signs
- Laboratory results, with the date and time each test was performed and results of previous tests for comparison
- Other clinical information
- Code status

Assessment: What is your assessment of the situation?

Recommendations: What is your recommendation, or what do you want?

Examples include the following:

- Client to be admitted
- Client to be seen now
- Order to be changed

Source: Joint Commission on Accreditation of Healthcare Organizations. (2005, February). The SBAR technique: Improves communication, enhances patient safety. *Joint Commission Perspectives on Patient Safety, 5*(2), 2.

TABLE 16-4 Change-of-Shift Reports: Dos and Don'ts

Dos	Don'ts
Do provide only essential background information about client (i.e., name, sex, age, physician's diagnosis, and medical history).	Don't review all routine care procedures or tasks (e.g., bathing, scheduled changes).
Do identify client's nursing diagnoses or health care problems and their related causes.	Don't review all biographical information already available in written form.
Do describe objective measurements or observations about client's condition and response to health problem, and emphasize recent changes.	Don't use critical comments about client's behaviour, such as "Mrs. Wills is so demanding."
Do share significant information about family members as it relates to client's problems.	Don't make assumptions about relationships between family members.
Do continuously review ongoing discharge plan (e.g., need for resources, client's level of preparation to go home).	Don't engage in idle gossip.
Do relay to staff significant changes in the way therapies are given (e.g., different position for pain relief, new medication).	Don't describe basic steps of a procedure.
Do describe instructions given in teaching plan and client's response.	Don't explain detailed content unless staff members ask for clarification.
Do evaluate results of nursing or medical care measures (e.g., effect of back rub or analgesic administration), and describe results specifically.	Don't simply describe results as "good" or "poor."
Do be clear about priorities to which incoming staff must attend.	Don't force incoming staff to guess what to do first.

diagnostic tests. Telephone reports should provide clear, accurate, and concise information. Information in a telephone report is documented when significant events or changes in a client's condition have occurred. In documenting a phone call, the nurse includes information about when the call was made, who made it (if other than the writer of the information), who was called, to whom information was given, what information was given, and what information was received. An example is as follows: "At 1005 hrs called Dr. Morgan's office; S. Thomas, RN, was informed that Mr. Rush's stat potassium level drawn at 0800 hrs was 3.2. C. Skala, RN."

Telephone or Verbal Orders

A telephone order (often written "TO") involves a physician stating a prescribed therapy over the phone to a registered nurse. A verbal order (often written "VO") may be accepted when the physician has no opportunity to write the order, as in emergency situations. Clarifying for accuracy is important when you accept a physician's orders over the telephone or verbally. You need to verify the order by repeating it clearly and precisely. You are responsible for writing the order on the physician's order sheet in the client's permanent record and signing it. An example is as follows: "1/16/2008, 1920 hrs: acetaminophen 325 mg PO [orally] 2 tabs now and q4h [every four hours] prn [as needed]. TO Dr. Reiss/Carol Skala, RN." The physician later verifies the telephone order legally by signing it within a set time period (e.g., 24 hours). Many telephone orders are given at night or during an emergency and need to be used only when absolutely necessary. In some situations, it may be prudent to have a second person listen to telephone orders. Box 16–9 provides guidelines that can be used to prevent errors when receiving telephone orders and verbal orders.

Transfer Reports

Clients may transfer from one unit to another to receive different levels of care. For example, clients transfer from an intensive care unit or the recovery room to general nursing units when they no longer require intense monitoring. To promote continuity of care, you may give **transfer reports** by phone or in person. When giving a transfer report, you need to include the following information:

- Client's name, age, name of primary physician, and medical diagnosis
- Summary of progress up to the time of transfer
- Client's current health status (physical and psychosocial)
- Client's allergies
- Client's emergency code status
- Client's family support (e.g., spouse or partner, children, parents)

BOX 16-9 Guidelines for Telephone Orders and Verbal Orders

- Clearly determine the client's name, room number, and diagnosis.
- Repeat any orders back to the prescribing physician.
- Ask for clarification to avoid misunderstandings.
- Write telephone order ("TO") or verbal order ("VO"), including date and time, name of client, and the complete order, and sign the names of the physician and nurse.
- Follow agency policies; some institutions require telephone (and verbal) orders to be reviewed and signed by two nurses.
- The physician must co-sign the order within the time frame required by the institution (usually 24 hours).

- Client's current nursing diagnoses or problem and care plan
- Any critical assessments or interventions to be completed shortly after transfer (helps receiving nurse to establish priorities of care)
- Need for any special equipment, such as isolation equipment, suction equipment, or traction

After completion of the transfer report, the receiving nurse needs an opportunity to ask questions about the client's status. In some cases, written documentation must include a record of information reported.

Incident Reports

An incident is any event that is not consistent with the routine operation of a health care unit or routine care of a client. Examples of incidents include client falls, needle-stick injuries, a visit by someone who has symptoms of illness, medication administration errors, accidental omission of ordered therapies, and circumstances that led to injury or risk for client injury. Analysis of **incident reports** (also known as *adverse occurrence reports*) helps with the identification of trends in systems and unit operations that justify changes in policies and procedures or the scheduling of in-service seminars. Incident reports are an important part of a unit's quality improvement program and should not be used for punitive purposes (see Chapter 11).

✻ KEY CONCEPTS

- The health care record is a legal document and requires information describing the care that is delivered to a client.
- All information pertaining to a client's health care management that is gathered by examination, observation, or conversation or as a result of treatment is confidential.
- Multidisciplinary communication is essential within the health care team.
- Accurate record keeping requires an objective interpretation of data with precise measurements, correct spelling, and proper use of abbreviations.
- A nurse's signature on an entry in a record designates that particular nurse's accountability for the contents of that entry.
- Any change in a client's condition warrants immediate documentation to keep a record accurate.
- Problem-oriented health care records are organized by the client's health care problems.
- The intent of SOAP, SOAPIE, PIE, and DAR charting is to organize entries in the progress notes according to the nursing process.
- Critical pathways or care maps provide members of the health care team with a way to document their contributions to the client's total plan of care.
- Home care documentation is accessible to a variety of caregivers in the home.
- Long-term care documentation is multidisciplinary. Assessments performed several times a day in the acute care setting are required only weekly or monthly in long-term care.
- Computerized information systems contain information about clients that is organized and easily accessible.
- Protection of the confidentiality of client health information and the security of computer systems should be a top priority.
- The major purpose of the change-of-shift report is to maintain continuity of care.
- When information pertinent to care is communicated by telephone or verbally, the information needs to be verified.
- Incident reports objectively describe any event that is not consistent with the routine care of a client.

✻ CRITICAL THINKING EXERCISES

1. Joseph Vojnovic is an 80-year-old man admitted with a diagnosis of possible pneumonia. He complains of general malaise and a frequent productive cough, worse at night. Vital sign measurements are as follows: blood pressure, 150/90 mm Hg; pulse rate, 92 beats per minute; respiration rate, 22 breaths per minute; and temperature, 38.5°C. During your initial assessment, he coughs violently for 40 to 45 seconds without expectorating. He exhibits wheezes and coarse crackles at both bases of the lungs. He states, "It hurts in my chest when I cough." Differentiate between objective and subjective data in this case example.

2. The nurse positions Mr. Vojnovic in a semi-Fowler's position, encourages him to increase his fluid intake, and gives him acetaminophen (Tylenol), 650 mg PO, as ordered for fever. One hour later, the client is resting in bed. Vital sign measurements are as follows: blood pressure, 130/86 mm Hg; pulse, 86 beats per minute; respiration rate, 22 breaths per minute; and temperature, 37.7°C. He states that he has been able to sleep. His fluid intake over the past hour has been 200 mL of water. Use the given information to write a nurse's progress note in the PIE format.

3. Near the end of your shift, you have identified *fluid volume deficit* as a nursing diagnosis for Mr. Vojnovic. Since his admission, he has had fluid intake of about 600 mL, and his urine output was 300 mL of dark, concentrated urine. His temperature is back up to 38.4°C, his mucous membranes are dry, and he states that he feels very weak. List what should be included in the change-of-shift report.

4. Several days later, after treatment with intravenous antibiotics, Mr. Vojnovic is feeling much better, and preparations are being made for discharge. He is to take cephalexin (Keflex) 500 mg every six hours, for the next 10 days; continue to drink extra fluids; and get extra rest. He lives alone. Although he is generally cooperative, he does not like drinking water or taking pills. He is to make an appointment with his physician for one week from today and should call the physician if symptoms recur. Write a discharge summary that is concise and instructive.

✻ REVIEW QUESTIONS

1. A fellow nursing student is a client in the hospital where you have your clinical placement. You became aware of his admission when you transferred your own client to his unit today. What should you do?
   1. Keep the information to yourself.
   2. Advise a few of his friends so that they can visit him.
   3. Visit him on his unit during your lunch break.
   4. Access his EHR to see if he is well enough for you to visit.

2. A manager is reviewing the nurses' notes in a community client's health care record. She finds the following entry, "Client is difficult to care for, refuses advice for improving appetite." Which of the following suggestions should the manager give to the community health nurse who entered the note?
   1. Avoid rushing when charting an entry.
   2. Use correction fluid to remove the entry.
   3. Draw a single line through the statement and initial it.
   4. Enter only objective and factual information about the client.

3. A client tells the nurse, "I have stomach cramps and feel nauseated." This is an example of which type of data?
   1. Objective
   2. Historical
   3. Subjective
   4. Assessment
4. During your visit to a client's home, your client says, "I do not know what is going on; I cannot get an explanation from my doctor about the results of my test. I want something done about this." Which of the following is the most appropriate documentation of the client's emotional status?
   1. The client has a defiant attitude.
   2. The client appears to be upset with his physician.
   3. The client is demanding and complains frequently.
   4. The client stated he felt frustrated by the lack of information he has received regarding test results.
5. Clients frequently request copies of their health care records. Which of the following statements is true regarding client access to health care records?
   1. Clients have the right to read those records.
   2. Clients are not allowed to read those records.
   3. Only the health care workers have access to the records.
   4. Only the families may read the records.
6. Accurate entries are an important characteristic of good documentation. Which of the following charting entries is most accurately written?
   1. Client ambulated in hall with assistance, exercise well tolerated.
   2. Client ambulated 15 m (50 feet) up and down hall, exercise well tolerated.
   3. Client ambulated 15 m (50 feet) up and down hall with assistance from nurse.
   4. Client ambulated 15 m (50 feet) with assistance from nurse. HR 88 before exercise and HR 94 after exercise.
7. What is the purpose of acuity records?
   1. To guide all nursing care
   2. To document the client admission
   3. To determine hours of care needed
   4. To establish guidelines for client care
8. Match the correct numbered entry with the appropriate SOAP category.

S	1. Repositioned client on right side. Encouraged client to use patient-controlled analgesia.
O	2. "The pain increases every time I try to turn on my left side."
A	3. Acute pain related to tissue injury from surgical incision.
P	4. Left lower abdominal surgical incision, 3 inches in length, closed, sutures intact, no drainage. Pain noted on mild palpation.

* RECOMMENDED WEB SITES

Accreditation Canada: http://www.cchsa.ca

Accreditation Canada (formerly the Canadian Council on Health Services Accreditation) is a national, nonprofit, independent organization whose role is to help health and social service organizations, across Canada and internationally, examine and improve the quality of care and service they provide to their clients through a voluntary external peer review.

Canada Health Infoway: http://www.infoway-inforoute.ca

Canada Health Infoway (Infoway) is a federally funded, independent, not-for-profit organization. Members include the 14 federal, provincial and territorial Deputy Ministers of Health. Infoway has a mandate to accelerate the use of electronic health information systems and EHRs across Canada.

Canadian Nurses Association: Provincial/Territorial Organizations: http://www.cna-aiic.ca/CNA/about/members/provincial/default_e.aspx

This part of the Web site of the Canadian Nurses Association provides links to each provincial and territorial nursing association. Most associations provide information about documentation standards and requirements in their province or territory.

Canadian Nursing Informatics Association: http://cnia.ca/

The Canadian Nursing Informatics Association (CNIA) is affiliated with the Canadian Nurses Association and has been established as the voice for health informatics in Canada. *Nursing informatics* refers to the integration of nursing science, computer science, and information science to document and communicate data and knowledge in nursing practice.

17

Nursing Informatics and Canadian Nursing Practice

Written by Kathryn J. Hannah, RN, PhD,
and Margaret Ann Kennedy, RN, PhD

objectives

Mastery of content in this chapter will enable you to:

- Define the key terms listed.
- Differentiate how nursing informatics differs from routine use of technologies in nursing practice.
- Identify key issues and challenges in managing nursing data in Canada.
- Identify and compare strategies in Canada for identifying and documenting key nursing data.
- Discuss how health information data standards influence nursing practice in Canada.
- Discuss why using the standardized nursing data is important for acknowledging the professional contributions of nursing to health outcomes of Canadians.
- Develop a beginning understanding of the scope of nursing informatics concepts and the ways in which nurses can be involved in nursing informatics.
- Discuss the relationship of national privacy legislation to nursing practice in a digital practice environment.
- Discuss how the national *E-Nursing Strategy* influences current and future nursing practice.

key terms

American Medical Informatics Association (AMIA), p. 243
Canada Health Infoway Inc. (Infoway), p. 236
Canadian Institute for Health Information (CIHI), p. 234
Canadian Nursing Informatics Association (CNIA), p. 243
Canadian Organization for Advancement of Computers in Health (COACH), p. 234
Electronic health record (EHR), p. 234
Health Information: Nursing Components (HI:NC), p. 238
Health Outcomes for Better Information and Care (HOBIC) project, p. 242
International Classification for Nursing Practice® (ICNP®), p. 239
International Council of Nurses (ICN), p. 239
International Health Terminology Standards Development Organisation (IHTSDO®), p. 236
International Medical Informatics Association (IMIA), p. 243
International Medical Informatics Association–Special Interest Group in Nursing Informatics (IMIA-SIGNI), p. 243
Nursing informatics, p. 234
Personal Information Protection and Electronic Documents Act (*PIPEDA*), p. 241
Standards, p. 236
Systematized NOmenclature of MEDicine—Clinical Terms (SNOMED CT®), p. 236

media resources

evolve Web Site

- Audio Chapter Summaries
- Glossary
- Multiple-Choice Review Questions
- Student Learning Activities
- Weblinks

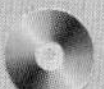 **Companion CD**

- Glossary
- Interactive Learning Activities
- Fluids and Electrolytes Tutorial
- Test-Taking Skills

As health care systems respond to an increasingly complex technological environment, long-standing routines and tools are being superseded by strategic, evidence-informed practices that mandate high-quality, timely health information. In an era when complex health care is provided by dynamic multidisciplinary teams, effective nursing documentation is crucial for supporting clinical decision making, as well as for supporting aggregation with documentation from other nurses and clinical disciplines, in enabling optimal client outcomes. Current information needs in health care challenge nurses to identify the elements of their practice that are most critical for consideration in decision making. **Nursing informatics**, a specialty area of nursing practice dedicated to optimal use of technology to support professional practice and enable optimal client outcomes, has responded to this challenge and continues to support the progression of effective nursing practice and documentation.

Hannah et al. (2006) tracked the evolution of technology in health care, noting that since its introduction in the health care sector, nurses have recognized the value of technology to inform effective practice and have fostered technological development in support of client care. Current technological applications include client scheduling and transfer, billing and financial management, diagnostic imaging, laboratory results reporting, order entry applications, pharmacy, client documentation systems, clinical support tools, and resource management applications. Developers of health care software offer integrated suites of applications that incorporate multiple tools for health care facilities or regions, and many health care institutions customize software to meet specific needs. Efforts are under way in every Canadian province and territory to develop a jurisdictional **electronic health record (EHR)**—a longitudinal record of an individual's health status (including diagnosed morbid conditions), diagnostic tests, treatments, and results—that will be interoperable with a pan-Canadian EHR. This movement toward provincial and national EHRs requires that developers or vendors incorporate into their information systems the capacity for interoperability with other vendors' systems so that client information can be communicated to caregivers as clients move across all sectors of the regional, provincial, or national health care delivery system.

However, despite of the vast array of technologies available in current health care, nurses must continue to contextualize technology within the scope of their professional practice. For example, Hannah (2005, p. 48) noted that "the issues for nurses are no longer computers or management information systems, but rather information and information management. The computer and its associated software are merely tools to support nurses as they practise their profession."

Nursing Informatics and the Canadian Health Care System

As the use of technology in health care settings burgeoned, pioneers in nursing informatics recognized that nurses needed to adopt strategically those information technologies that support professional practice. Furthermore, nursing informatics pioneers realized that there was also a need to consider the impact on nurses and nursing workflow of the demands related to using information technology. The term *nursing informatics* was introduced initially by Dr. Marion Ball at the 1983 International Medical Informatics Association (IMIA) Conference in Amsterdam (IMIA, 2004). In the 1980s, nursing informatics emerged as a new nursing specialty in health care information management. Since the 1984 publication of the first text devoted to nursing informatics, by Ball and Hannah, relevant journals and texts have proliferated across Canada and internationally. Hannah et al. (2006) noted that, despite the escalation of technology in health care and the recognition of the importance of nursing informatics, methods for defining and coding nursing contributions to health care outcomes have not been universally accepted, and the persistent absence of such methods is a significant obstacle to the collection of nursing data.

Defining Nursing Informatics

As research, education, and practice continue to inform nursing informatics, and as nursing informatics continues to evolve, definitions have correspondingly evolved. Early definitions of nursing informatics focused on technology and its effective use in practice, whereas current definitions focus more on the role of information management and the role of the nurse as an information manager. Table 17–1 is an overview summary of definitions that reflect the evolving understanding of nursing informatics (Staggers & Bagley Thompson, 2002).

Evolution of Informatics in the Canadian Health Care System

Health informatics encompasses all health care disciplines, and unique informatics knowledge and skills reflect specialties such as medical informatics and nursing informatics. The **Canadian Organization for Advancement of Computers in Health (COACH)**, Canada's Health Informatics Association, defines health informatics as the "intersection of clinical, IM/IT [Information Management/Information Technology] and management practices to achieve better health" (COACH, 2007, p. 7). The importance of informatics was recognized over many years and as the result of dedicated efforts of many professionals. Although other types of informatics practices exist, the focus of this chapter is on nursing informatics.

From the mid-1980s onward, Canada's health information infrastructure experienced numerous evolutions and reconfigurations, all of which had significant implications for nursing. The 1989 Canadian merger of the National Hospital Productivity Improvement Program and the Management Information System Project, which resulted in the Management Information System (MIS) Group, was an important event in Canadian health care information management (Hannah et al., 2006). The MIS Group, according to Hannah et al. (2006), developed guidelines on the collection of data for demographic, statistical, and resource use and consumption purposes. The problem with the MIS data is that, like hospital discharge summaries, this health information was restricted to physician-driven data and contained no clinical nursing data elements. Hannah et al. (2006, p. 89) made the point that "noteworthy, again, is the *total absence* of clinical nursing data."

The *Wilk Report* (National Task Force on Health Information, 1991) had a significant effect on health information in Canada, triggering the 1993 merger of the MIS Group, Hospital Medical Records Institute (HMRI), portions of Statistics Canada, and Health and Welfare Canada to create the **Canadian Institute for Health Information (CIHI)** (Alvarez, 1993; Hannah, 2005). CIHI is the national, independent, and not-for-profit body that records, analyzes, and disseminates essential data and analyses on Canada's health system and the health of Canadians (CIHI, 2007). Although not initially attentive to nursing data, this institution later became more important to several issues directly influencing nursing, including issues related to nursing workforce recruitment and retention.

In response to recommendations issued by the National Forum on Health for a pan-Canadian EHR, the federal government committed an initial $500 million to the development of e-health, which included the EHR, telehealth, and Internet-based health information (Canadian Nurses Association [CNA], 2006a; Hannah, 2005).

➤ TABLE 17-1 Evolution of Nursing Informatics Definitions

Focus of Definition	Date	Author	Definition
Information technology	1984; 1994	Ball & Hannah (p. 181); Hannah, Ball, & Edwards (p. 5)	"any use of information technologies by nurses in relation to the care of their patients, the administration of health care facilities, or the educational preparation of individuals to practise the discipline is considered nursing informatics"
	1986	Saba & McCormick (p. 116)	"systems that use computers to process nursing data into information to support all types of nursing activities"
	1990	Zielstorff, Abraham, Werley, Saba, & Schwirian	Central role of technology
	1996	Saba & McCormick (p. 226)	"use of technology and/or a computer system to collect, store, process, display, retrieve, and communicate timely data and information in and across health care facilities that administer nursing services and resources, manage the delivery of patient and nursing care, link research resources and findings to nursing practice, and apply educational resources to nursing education"
	1998	International Medical Informatics Association (IMIA; http://www.imia.org/working_groups/WG_Profile.lasso?-Search=Action&-Table=CGI&-MaxRecords=1&-SkipRecords=15&-Database=organizations&-KeyField=Org_ID&-SortField=workgroup_sig&-)	The integration of nursing, its information, and information management with information processing and communication technology, to support the health of people worldwide
	2000	Ball, Hannah, Newbold, & Douglas (p. 10)	"all aspects of nursing—clinical practice, administration, research and education—just as computing holds the power to integrate all four aspects"
	2001b	Canadian Nurses Association (http:www.cnia.ca/documents/OHIHfinalappendixA.doc)	"the application of computer science and information science to nursing. NI promotes the generation, management and processing of relevant data in order to use information and develop knowledge that supports nursing in all practice domains"
Conceptual	1986	Schwirian (p. 134)	"solid foundation of nursing informatics knowledge [that] should have focus, direction, and cumulative properties"
	1989	Graves & Corcoran (p. 227)	"A combination of computer science, information science, and nursing science designed to assist in the management and processing of nursing data, information, and knowledge to support the practice of nursing and the delivery of nursing care"
	1996	Turley	Development of a NI model which included cognitive science, information science, and computer science
Role centred	1992	American Nurses Association (ANA) Council on Computer Applications in Nursing (p. 1)	"specialty that integrates nursing science, computer science, and information science in identifying, collecting, processing, and managing data and information to support nursing practice, administration, education, and research and to expand nursing knowledge. The purpose of nursing informatics is to analyze information requirements; design, implement and evaluate information systems and data structures that support nursing; and identify and apply computer technologies for nursing"
	1994	ANA (p. 1)	"specialty that integrates nursing science, computer science, and information science in identifying, collecting, processing, and managing data and information to support nursing practice, administration, education, research, and expansion of nursing knowledge. It supports the practice of all nursing specialties, in all sites and settings, whether at the basic or advanced level. The practice includes the development of applications, tools, processes, and structures that assist nurses with the management of data in taking care of patients or in supporting their practice of nursing"

Continued

TABLE 17-1 Evolution of Nursing Informatics Definitions *continued*

2002	Staggers & Bagley Thompson (p. 260)	Nursing informatics is a specialty that integrates nursing science, computer science, and information science to manage and communicate data, information, and knowledge in nursing practice. Nursing informatics facilitates the integration of data, information, and knowledge to support patients, nurses, and other providers in their decision making in all roles and settings. This support is accomplished through the use of information structures, information processes, and information technology

NI, nursing informatics.

From American Nurses Association. (1994). *The scope of practice for nursing informatics.* Washington, DC: Author.

Canada Health Infoway Inc. (Infoway), incorporated in 2001, was a key outcome of the federal, provincial, and territorial partnership (CNA, 2006b). Infoway is a national body with a national mandate to generate consensus on health information standards, to drive forward the national agenda of creating an EHR, and to act as the liaison to international standards development organizations (Canada Health Infoway, 2007). Infoway has experienced significant growth since its inception; by 2008, Infoway had spent approximately $1 billion on electronic health systems in Canada (Canada Health Infoway, 2008a). In 2006, Infoway launched the Standards Collaborative, which is a "Canada-wide coordination function created to support and sustain health information standards in Canada" (Canada Health Infoway, 2008b, p. 4). The global mandate for the Standards Collaborative was endorsed by the federal, provincial, and territorial Ministries of Health to coordinate support for (1) development and implementation, (2) education for general and specific users groups (e.g., information management specialists, programmers, change management and adoption specialists, clinicians), (3) conformance (testing and evaluation), and (4) maintenance of EHR standards developed by Infoway and its jurisdictional partners.

The Standards Collaborative also incorporates nine Standards Collaborative Working Groups (SCWGs), in which clinicians, information technology experts, academics, researchers, and policymakers collaborate to address standards development for health information and systems in Canada. Membership in these groups is voluntary and open to any individual with an interest in contributing to the development of a specific aspect of the EHR. Box 17–1 illustrates the nine SCWGs and their respective focus of attention.

By March 31, 2007, Infoway had approved more than $1 billion, or 85% of its total funding, across all its program areas (Canada Health Infoway, 2008a). At the time of its publication, Infoway had committed more than $33 million to various provincial and territorial initiatives; as a result, in more than 20 projects have been completed or are nearing completion (Canada Health Infoway, 2008b). For example, one implementation project is the Picture Archiving & Communication Systems (PACS) initiative in Nova Scotia, through which diagnostic images are transmitted by computers to local and remote physicians, which enables a much faster response time between assessment and treatment. Projects in various stages of planning, implementation, or completion are recorded in every province in Canada.

The technological advances since the 1970s have directed national attention to the need for timely, secure, and appropriate health information access. Multiple health care and standards development organizations operate to coordinate broad documentation of health information and to monitor the Canadian health care system. You must have both an awareness and understanding of the roles and relevance of each of these entities in relation to your nursing practice.

Standards in Health Informatics

Standards Development in Canada

Standards for health care data are the established and formally endorsed coding protocols for all health information, including coding types of care provided, location of care provision, pharmaceutical ordering and dispensing, and coding for billing messages. A broader meaning for the term *standards* is the standardization of forms of technology, information, or business processes (Canada Health Infoway, 2004). Canada Health Infoway (2008b) noted that standards ensure interoperability by supporting information exchange and identified standards as a critical foundation for the interoperable electronic health record. Additional benefits of standards for various stakeholder groups are identified in Table 17–2.

Standards play a role in shaping health care data in a number of ways. Standards such as the **Systematized NOmenclature of MEDicine—Clinical Terms (SNOMED CT®)**, client registry standards, provider registry standards, diagnostic imaging standards, drug standards, and laboratory messaging and nomenclature standards all influence how nurses document clinical practice and access health data. For example, SNOMED CT (originally developed by the College of American Pathologists, enhanced over time by collaboration with other health care professionals, and currently managed by the **International Health Terminology Standards Development Organisation** [**IHTSDO®**] in Copenhagen, Denmark) contains clinical terminology used to describe multidisciplinary clinical practice. In addition, standards operate in the background to support consistent packaging or coding of data. These standards include security and consent standards, interoperable EHR technical standards, and interoperable EHR clinical messaging standards.

In Canada, Infoway uses a consistent process to bring standards forward from initiation to conformance, implementation, and maintenance. Two types of needs can trigger the development of a standard. *Technical needs* are generated from gaps in information management; to address these needs, a consistent manner of communicating health data is needed among providers or between institutions or jurisdictions. *Business needs* are identified from analysis of the actual clinical work processes; for example, a particular condition or clinical situation may not be described consistently. Infoway has a three-option process of standards development, in decreasing order of preference: (1) *adopt* an existing standard; (2) *adapt* an existing standard; and (3) *develop* a new standard (Canada Health Infoway, 2008b). Upon adoption, adaptation, or development of a standard, Infoway issues a "Stable for Use" designation to indicate that the standard is ready for limited implementation and testing. Before formal approval, the proposed standard must undergo rigorous evaluation, and testing, as well as demonstrate a

BOX 17-1 Standards Collaborative Working Groups

Standards Collaborative Working Groups (SCWGs)	Scope
SCWG 1: Population Health (Delivery of Care)	Immunization Communicable disease management • Public health case • Public health outbreak • Public health investigations

SCWG 2: Individual Care (Delivery of Care)	Electronic health records (EHRs)
	Shared health record
	• Adverse event
	• Allergy
	• Clinical observations
	• Discharge care summary
	• Health conditions
	  • Care compositions (e.g., encounters and episodes)
	  • Professional services
	  • Referral and referral note
	Health summary records
	Chronic disease management

SCWG 3: Managing the Health System	Claims Client administrative Wait times Secondary use Research Clinical data warehouse
SCWG 4: Medication Management	Prescribing Dispensing Client (drug) queries Drug queries Contraindications
SCWG 5: Labs & Diagnostics	Human laboratory Nonhuman laboratory Diagnostic imaging Diagnostic investigations
SCWG 6: Infostructure & Architecture	Data types Common message element types Message wrappers Common message patterns Broadcast EHR record retrieval Event tracking Queue management (polling) Retract OIDs
SCWG 7: Non-Clinical Registries	Client registry and identification management Provider registry and identification management Location registry and identification management Organization registry and identification management
SCWG 8: IT Privacy & Security Services	Security Privacy Consent User registries (Access & Authentication) *Note: This SCWG does not address privacy and security policy, regulatory issues, or legislation.*
SCWG 9: Terminology Representation & Services	Terminology services HL7 Common terminology servers Terminology models HL7 Vocabulary worksheet

From Canada Health Infoway. (2008b). *Standards Collaborative: Enabling solutions, enhancing health outcomes . . . together* (p. 11). Toronto, ON: Author.
HL7, Health Level 7 Standards; OIDS, object identifiers.

consensus among users (balloting). Various international standards form the foundation of pan-Canadian standards:

- Health Level 7 (HL7)
- SNOMED CT®
- Logical Observation Identifier Names and Codes (LOINC®)
- *The Canadian Enhancement of ICD-10 [International Statistical Classification of Diseases and Related Health Problems, 10th Revision]* (ICD-10-CA) (CIHI, 2001)
- Canadian Classification of Health Interventions (CCI)
- Integrating the Healthcare Enterprise (IHE)
- Digital Imaging and Communication in Medicine (DICOM)
- Unified Codes for Units of Measure (UCUM)
- Health Canada Drug Product Database (DPD)

Standardizing Nursing Language

A widely held perception among many nurses is that nursing, as a professional practice, is generally considered invisible in regard to formal and tangible recognition (CNA, 2000; Clark, 1999; Clark & Lang, 1992; Hannah et al., 2006; Marck, 1994; Norwood, 2001; Powers, 2001; Weyrauch, 2002). Clark (1999, p. 42) observed that despite its being the largest group of health care clinicians, nursing was invisible in health policy decisions, in descriptions of health care, and in contracts and service specifications.

Clark and Lang (1992, p. 109), in their assessment of the invisibility of nursing, noted that nurses cannot control what cannot be named, stating that "if we cannot name it, we cannot control it, finance it, teach it, research it, or put it into public policy." According to the stance of Clark and Lang (1992) and other scholars (such as Graves & Corcoran, 1989; Werley, 1988), giving nursing visibility requires a standardized language to reflect what nursing is and what nursing does. Clark (1999, p. 42) advocated for a standardized nursing language, using the argument that ". . . without a language to express our concepts we cannot know whether our understanding of their meaning is the same, so we cannot communicate them with any precision to other people." More recently, the argument has shifted from the issue of visibility to the value and necessity of client safety and professionals' accountability, along with accurate data for system and clinical evaluation. Adopting a standardized nursing language is urgent, as the pan-Canadian interoperable EHR moves forward and information management further enables evidence-informed practice.

Health Information: Nursing Components

Before a standard nursing language is adopted, the most important data elements required for effective nursing decision making and evaluation must be identified. The minimum number of essential nursing data elements are referred to as a *minimum nursing data set*. In Canada, the process of capturing nursing data was led by the Alberta Association of Registered Nurses (AARN) in 1992. This provincial nursing body, in conjunction with the CNA, hosted a national conference focused on generating and validating a Canadian nursing minimum data set (NMDS) (Giovannetti et al., 1999). The Canadian version of an NMDS is known as **Health Information: Nursing Components (HI:NC)**. The CNA (2000, p. 5)

TABLE 17-2 Benefits of Standards for Stakeholder Groups

Stakeholder Group	Benefits of Standards in Health Care Data
Clients	• Reduced repetition of health information • Accessible personal health history • Improved coordination of care • Reduced duplication of tests and procedures • Improved health outcomes
Providers	• Timely access to health data • Availability of more reliable health information • Reduced duplication of efforts • Shorter response time between assessment and treatment • Improved quality and consistency of care resulting from enhanced information access • Enhanced client outcomes
Service delivery organizations	• Reuse of solutions, benefiting from lessons learned and change management strategies • Greater breadth of data to use for evaluating outcomes • Enhanced ability to work collaboratively with other organizations or jurisdictions • Increased confidence in products when suitability for use is determined
Educators	• Support for curriculum design that is aligned with accreditation process • Increased value of data for educational purposes • Enabling of educators and students to understand the health informatics environment at early stages of education • Enhanced ability to extract data, such as best practice guidelines, from published sources
Researchers	• Availability of higher quality data • Reduced time to prepare data for use • Comprehensive data sets • Improved ability to monitor and assess health outcomes and determinants

Adapted from Hannah, K. J. (2005). Health informatics and nursing in Canada. *Healthcare Information Management and Communications, 19*(3), 45–51. Reprinted by permission of Healthcare Computing and Communications Canada, Inc.

described HI:NC as the "most important pieces of data about the nursing care provided to the client during a health care episode." Since 1992, the majority of Canadian nurses have agreed that HI:NC is composed of five categories of elements: client status, nursing interventions, client outcomes, nursing resource intensity, and primary nurse identifier (AARN, 1994; CNA, 2000, 2001a). Table 17–3 presents the HI:NC definitions.

Chapter 16 provides an overview of computerized nursing documentation. Many clinical information systems incorporate the HI:NC into the architecture or design of the nursing system. This enables capture of the most significant nursing data. Computerized nursing documentation systems continue to evolve, and their design relies on an underlying philosophy of documentation. For example, many systems do not encourage narrative documentation; instead, they provide checklists of common activities and encourage exception charting. This issue is further discussed in Chapter 16.

International Classification for Nursing Practice®

In 2001, the CNA endorsed the **International Classification for Nursing Practice (ICNP®)** "for use in Canada as a foundational classification system for nursing practice in Canada" (CNA, 2001b, p. 1). This endorsement was renewed in 2006 (CNA, 2006a). The **International Council of Nurses (ICN)**—an international federation of countries representing national nursing organizations that advances professional nursing practice, advocates for effective health policy, and enhances health globally—developed the ICNP in response to concerns regarding the visibility of nursing contributions in health care and calls for standardization of nursing data for comparability and analysis, as well as for evidence-informed practice. ICN proposed the use of a single unified nomenclature to represent nursing practice; ICNP is the only unified international terminology for recording nursing practice. The goals were to capture nursing practice across practice settings, cultures, languages, and geographical settings, as well as to ensure that professionals who used this new terminology could communicate electronically with the numerous nursing terminologies already in use in information systems and software. Initially endorsed in 1989 by resolution at the ICN's nineteenth quadrennial conference (ICN, 2005), the Alpha version of the ICNP® was released in 1995. Version 1.0 was released in 2005 and is substantively different from previous iterations (Alpha, Beta, Beta 2): To unify all previous ICNP® axes, it comprises seven axes with associated terms for describing nursing practice (Figure 17–1).

ICNP® is used to generate statements of nursing diagnoses, nursing actions, and nursing outcomes, in which terms arranged in a hierarchical order are used (Figure 17–2), and in catalogues (or subsets) of previously combined terms. Catalogues comprise nursing data subsets of diagnoses, actions, and outcomes specific to various practice areas or specialties (such as wound care) and continue to be developed. To begin catalogue development, nurses select a health care topic on the basis of the needs of clients. The organization of the catalogue content would be determined by the nurses as ICNP® diagnoses, outcomes, and interventions are identified. ICN (2005) suggested that catalogues can fill a practical need in building health information systems with all the benefits of being part of a unified nursing language.

As stated earlier, the Canadian Nurses' Association endorsed ICNP® as the terminology of choice for documenting professional nursing practice in Canada (CNA, 2001b, 2006a). Although Canada Health Infoway, in consultation with various stakeholder groups, adopted SNOMED CT® as the terminology of choice for the pan-Canadian EHR, ICNP® remains the preferred terminology for nursing. ICN, which holds the intellectual property rights to ICNP®, is in discussions with SNOMED CT® to identify means of linking the two standardized clinical terminologies to ensure that nursing practice is accurately documented.

As illustrated in Figure 17–1, Version 1.0 of ICNP® is constructed with seven axes: Focus, Judgement, Means, Action, Time, Location, and Client. Table 17–4 lists definitions for each axis and examples of terms. According to ICNP® requirements, both nursing diagnoses and nursing outcomes *must* contain a term from the Focus axis and the Judgement axis and may include terms from additional axes as needed to fully describe the phenomenon of attention. Nursing

TABLE 17-3 Health Information: Nursing Components

Nursing Component	Definition
Client status	A label for the set of indicators that reflect the phenomena for which nurses provide care, relative to the health status of clients (McGee, 1993). Although client status is similar to nursing diagnosis, the term *client status* is preferred because it represents a broader spectrum of health and illness. The common label *client status* is inclusive of input from all disciplines. The summative statements referring to the phenomena for which nurses provide care (i.e., nursing diagnosis) are merely one aspect of client status at a point in time, in the same way as medical diagnosis.
Nursing interventions	Purposeful and deliberate health-affecting interventions (direct and indirect), based on assessment of client status, which are designed to bring about results which benefit clients (Alberta Association of Registered Nurses [AARN], 1994).
Client outcome	A "client's status at a defined point(s) following health care [affecting] intervention" (Marek & Lang, 1993). It is influenced to varying degrees by the interventions of all care providers.
Nursing intensity	"Refers to the amount and type of nursing resource used to [provide] care" (O'Brien-Pallas & Giovannetti, 1993).
Primary nurse identifier	A single unique, lifetime identification number for each individual nurse. This identifier is independent of geographic location (province or territory), practice sector (e.g., acute care, community care, public health), or employer.

From Hannah, K. J. (2005). Health informatics and nursing in Canada. *Healthcare Information Management and Communications, 19*(3), 49.

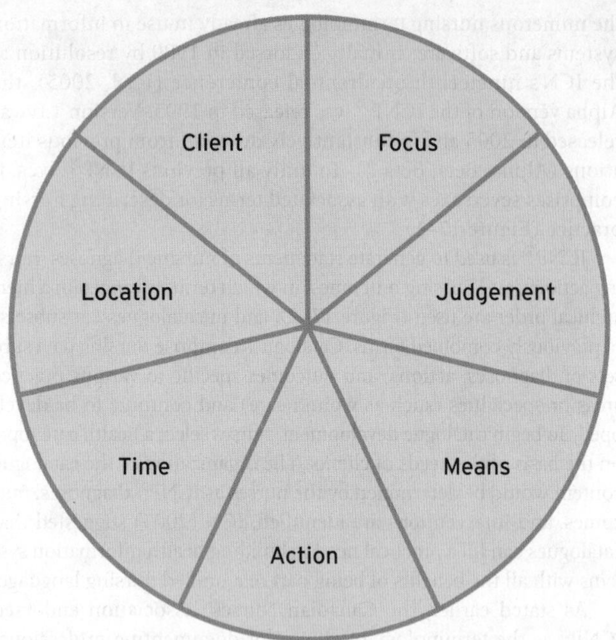

Figure 17-1 7-Axes model of the International Classification for Nursing Practice (ICNP®), Version 1.0. **Source:** From International Council of Nurses. (2005). *International Classification for Nursing Practice®, Version 1.0.* (p. 29). Geneva, Switzerland: Author. Reproduced with permission of the International Council of Nurses © 2005.

Interventions *must* include a term from the Action axis and the Target axis, and may include additional terms from other axes as necessary. ICN (2005) described a "Target term" as a term originating in any axis except the Judgement axis.

The format of these nursing diagnosis statements may not correspond with those identified in previous chapters. These statements may not be used literally in daily verbal communication among nurses; they will be used for nursing documentation in the EHR to enable aggregation. The following examples reflect the core details for coding key nursing data in the EHR:

Nursing diagnosis: *Decreasing level of pain in right knee joint*

- *Pain* is from the Focus axis.
- *Decreasing level* is from the Judgement axis.
- Both *right* and *knee joint* are from the Location axis.

Nursing intervention: Analgesic injected

- *Injected* and *injecting* are from the Action axis.
- *Analgesic* is from the Means axis.

Nursing outcome: Sputum decreased

- *Sputum* is from the Focus axis.
- *Decreased* is from the Judgement axis.

As with all languages, development of ICNP® is continuous, and research is under way in many countries (Boxes 17–2 and 17–3). Version 1.0 is subjected to ongoing evaluation to refine and enhance terms, catalogues, and translations.

Canadian Privacy Legislation

Although both provincial standards of practice and the CNA (2008a) *Code of Ethics* address confidentiality, you also need to be aware of Canadian privacy legislation that also affects nursing practice and the protection of client data. Even as you fulfill the standards of practice, it is possible to violate privacy legislation. Canadians recognize this risk of privacy violation, and "two thirds of Canadian citizens believe that personal health information is one of the most important areas in need of protection under privacy laws" (Roch, 2008, p. 8). Although privacy legislation varies between provinces, you must develop a working knowledge of the relevant legislation, both provincial and national.

Two federal legislative acts address the privacy of personal information. These include the *Privacy Act* (Government of Canada,

Figure 17-2 Hierarchical structure of the International Classification for Nursing Practice (ICNP®), Version 1.0. **Source:** From Hierarchical structure of International Council of Nurses Version 1.0. Reproduced with permission of the International Council of Nurses © 2005.

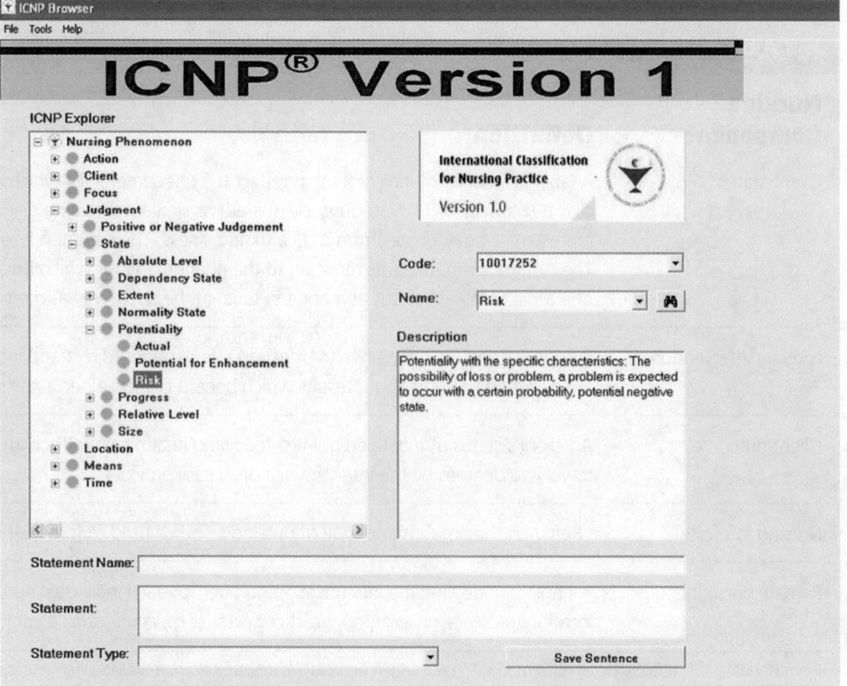

TABLE 17-4 Definitions and Examples of Terms in ICNP® Version 1

Axis	Definition	Sample Terms
Focus	The area of attention relevant to nursing	*Elder abuse, sputum, air, child labour law*
Judgement	Clinical opinion or determination related to the focus of nursing practice	*High, enhanced, partial, risk*
Means	A manner or method of accomplishing an intervention	*Wound drainage bag, nebulizer, bed rail, cardiac monitor*
Action	An intentional process applied to or performed by a client	*Violence prevention, explaining, listening, resuscitating*
Time	The point, period, interval, or duration of an occurrence	*Rarely, chronic, discharge, intermittent*
Location	Anatomical or spatial orientation of a diagnosis or intervention	*Chest wall, distal, residential building, supine, intravenous route*
Client	Subject to which a diagnosis refers and who is the recipient of an intervention	*Extended family, community, adolescent, older adult, infant*

Adapted from International Council of Nurses. (2005). *International Classification for Nursing Practice®, Version 1.0* (p. 29). Geneva, Switzerland: Author. Reproduced with permission of the International Council of Nurses © 2005.

1983) and the ***Personal Information Protection and Electronic Documents Act (PIPEDA)*** (Government of Canada, 2004). Both acts identify specific limitations to the disclosure of personal information, whether in electronic or other forms. Regardless of the practice setting or mode, you are professionally and ethically obligated to protect all personal information of clients in your care. Knowledge of these two pieces of federal privacy legislation can help you uphold the standards of practice and *Code of Ethics*.

According to the *Privacy Act*, Section 8.1, "Personal information under the control of a government institution shall not, without the consent of the individual to whom it relates, be disclosed by the institution . . . ." (Government of Canada, 1983). The *PIPEDA* is federal legislation governing the disclosure of personal health information in any electronic environment. This act extends the *Privacy Act* by addressing specific risks associated with electronic data collection, storage, retrieval, and communication. *PIPEDA* addresses personal health information specifically and identifies *personal health information*, with regard to any individual, whether living or deceased, as having any of the following meanings (Government of Canada, 2004, Section 1.2):

1. Information concerning the physical or mental health of the individual
2. Information concerning any health care service provided to the individual
3. Information concerning the donation by the individual of any body part or any bodily substance of the individual or information derived from the testing or examination of a body part or bodily substance of the individual
4. Information that is collected in the course of providing health care services to the individual
5. Information that is collected incidentally to the provision of health care services to the individual

Furthermore, *PIPEDA* restricts the disclosure of personal information to only the most stringent of conditions, such as law enforcement requirements (Government of Canada, 2004, Division 1, Section 7.3). You must exercise diligence in examining and adhering to these pieces of legislation in your professional nursing practice. Chapter 16 explores how *PIPEDA* applies to specific nursing documentation.

BOX 17-2 RESEARCH HIGHLIGHT

Evaluating Standardized Nursing Terminology

Nursing data have not been included in national data repositories for a variety of reasons, including the lack of a single nursing terminology to describe nursing practice. Consequently, health care decisions have been made in the absence of valuable nursing data. The need for a standardized nursing language stimulated the development of the ICNP®. Testing was necessary to evaluate the representational capacity of this terminology for Canadian nursing practice. Kennedy (2005) examined the effectiveness of the ICNP® in representing the contributions of nursing care to health care outcomes in Canada. The ICNP® was used to code retrospective nursing data extracted from client records originating in acute care, in-patient mental health, home health care, and long-term care practice settings. In spite of a wide variation in documentation practices, ICNP® achieved matches with a significant majority of nursing data, thereby confirming the utility of ICNP® for documenting nursing practice in Canada.

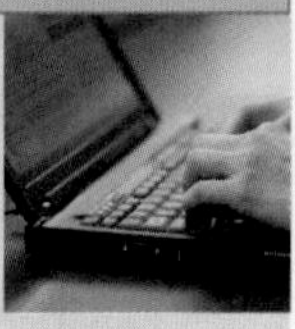

Representing Nursing Practice

ICNP® represents Canadian nursing practice with high accuracy. Variations and gaps in nursing documentation practices are further evidence of the need for standardized terminology to ensure that at least minimum nursing data are recorded.

References: Kennedy, M. A. (2005). *Packaging nursing as politically potent: A critical reflexive cultural studies approach to nursing informatics.* Unpublished doctoral dissertation, University of South Australia, Adelaide, Australia; Kennedy, M. A., & Hannah, K. J. (2007). Representing nursing practice: Evaluating the effectiveness of a nursing classification system. *Canadian Journal of Nursing Research, 39*(7), 58–79.

> BOX 17-3 **Creating Canadian Nursing History**

The C-HOBIC Initiative

The CNA launched a multiprovince project in 2007, in collaboration with the provinces of Ontario, Saskatchewan, Manitoba, and Prince Edward Island, with financial contribution from Canada Health Infoway. This project focused on collecting information reflecting evidence-informed, nursing-sensitive client outcomes (CNA, 2008b). Drawing on the work of the original **Health Outcomes for Better Information and Care (HOBIC) project**, the Canadian Health Outcomes for Better Information and Care (C-HOBIC) project (http://www.cna-aiic.ca/c-hobic/about/default_e.aspx) implements a standardized nursing documentation approach for capturing, analyzing, and reporting nursing-sensitive outcomes for acute care, complex continuing care, long-term care, and home care.

The C-HOBIC project addresses gaps in health information related to the contribution of nursing care to client outcomes and also addresses the need for standardized nursing data to be included in client admission and discharge summaries. The C-HOBIC project is a systematic approach to gathering nursing content that is documented with a standardized clinical terminology, ICNP®, and coded in a format suitable for inclusion in the EHRs being developed or implemented by the participating provinces. C-HOBIC provides an opportunity for Canadian nurses to make substantive contributions to the ongoing development of ICNP® through research that adds new terms or concepts to ICNP®. One particular component of the C-HOBIC project was the mapping of outcomes concepts to the ICNP® Version 1.0.

Mapping challenges provided an immediate opportunity for Canadian nurses to contribute to the iterative development of ICNP® by proposing multiple new terms and a catalogue of precombined terms for inclusion in ICNP® that are uniquely Canadian and reflect C-HOBIC concepts. The mapping was validated at a national forum (Kennedy, 2008; Kennedy et al., 2008) that included C-HOBIC partners, nursing informatics experts, nurse educators, nurse researchers, representatives from government ministries, policy institutions and practice environments, and two international ICNP® experts.

In total, 96 concepts were addressed in the mapping aspect of the C-HOBIC project: 58 HOBIC concepts were matched and validated as C-HOBIC terms; 13 HOBIC concepts were partially mapped to ICNP®, and a new term was required in ICNP® in order to fully communicate the original concept in C-HOBIC; 24 concepts did not match and new C-HOBIC terms were proposed for inclusion in ICNP®; and only one HOBIC concept ("Activity did not occur") could not be mapped to ICNP®. In addition, two HOBIC ordinal scales (for pain scale and for the number of falls) were retained for use in C-HOBIC. Consensus by the group was achieved for all concepts, terms and issues. Critical next steps include the creation of the C-HOBIC catalogue by ICNP® and the establishment of a Nursing Terminology Working Group.

National E-Nursing Strategy

The CNA (2006b) released the *E-Nursing Strategy for Canada* to direct the coordinated integration of technology into Canadian nursing practice. The strategy addresses both medium- and long-term targets, with the overall goal of improving both nursing practice and outcomes for clients. This strategy is intended to completely integrate information and communication technologies (ICT) in such a way that the "e" in *e-nursing* is no longer required; ICT will simply be another tool that nurses use in their practice (CNA, 2006b). The CNA (2006b, p. 4) identified seven key outcomes that are projected to emerge from the *E-Nursing Strategy.* These include:

1. Nurses will integrate ICT into their practice to achieve desirable client outcomes.
2. Nurses will have the required information and knowledge to support their practice.
3. Human resources planning will be facilitated.
4. New models of nursing practice and health services delivery will be supported.
5. Nursing groups will be well connected.
6. ICT will improve the quality of nurses' work environments.
7. Canadian nurses will contribute to the global community of nursing.

Three fundamental directions for CNA's *E-Nursing Strategy* were developed among working groups and from national feedback: access, competencies, and participation. *Access* to quality ICT in the practice environment is imperative if Canadian nurses are to realize the full benefits of technology in their practices. The CNA (2006b) noted that health care organizations have a responsibility to ensure that nurses have connectivity—tools such as computers, mobile technology (e.g., laptops, personal digital assistants wireless technology), as well as resource databases and Internet resources—that will support professional practice.

The CNA (2006b) encouraged nurses to develop *Competencies* in the application of ICT and recommended that such competencies be part of both undergraduate and graduate level nursing programs. Just as you have a responsibility to develop competencies in performing a variety of client care tasks, such as assessments and treatments, it is also your responsibility to develop and maintain competencies in technological applications that support information management in professional practice.

Many examples of innovative nursing practice incorporating ICT are evident in Canada. Two such examples are the mobile wound assessment program used by the Victorian Order of Nurses and the standardized assessment approaches currently being integrated in the Local Health Integration Network in Ontario. Goodwin et al. (2008) combined telemedicine and telemonitoring with client education and peer supports in assisting chronically ill clients to stay at home in rural Ontario. Without this program, these clients would have had to travel for care provision and would have potentially experienced more frequent hospitalizations, loss of independence, and significantly less self-care. Tracey (2008) described how a standardized assessment approach is in pilot testing at two sites. This pilot format will ultimately replace six different assessment forms; therefore, data collection will be more systematic and the capacity for data aggregation and analysis will be greater.

The CNA (2006b, p. 12) identified *Participation* as including strategic partnerships with nurses in clinical practice; with employers and administrators; with federal, provincial, and territorial ministries; with nursing organizations (professional associations, regulatory bodies, educational groups, and unions); and with educators and researchers. The concept of partnership has far-reaching consequences: With effective partnerships, you can contribute to the selection and design of information technology applications, as well as to educational programs. For example, many health care institutions and agencies have clinical committees that collaborate with information technology experts in the design and selection of electronic documentation systems. Especially as a novice nurse, you have both the knowledge and the opportunity to contribute insights into which information management systems are user friendly or present unexpected challenges. It is also helpful to have this type of clinician involvement when the system requires revision or adaptation. Even small changes can sometimes have significant impact on the capture of appropriate nursing data and on how other nurses view the system. Without partnerships, however, you, and all nurses, risk being excluded from decision making and risk being required to use systems that are selected without valuable clinician contributions.

The Canadian Nurses Portal is a key component of the *E-Nursing Strategy.* The portal was initially funded from a grant from the First Nations and Inuit Health Branch (FNIHB) of Health Canada (CNA, 2006c). The nursing portal, now known as NurseONE, enables you to register, create a personal profile, and customize use of the site's tools and resources. NurseONE provides such services as the following:

- Professional links (resources with clinical or professional orientation)
- Professional development (including resources for continuing competence, online and continuing education, and career development)
- Library (access to numerous articles and publications)
- NurseConnect (use of the portal to create discussion groups among individual subscribers)

Resources available to subscribers include activities for conducting self-assessments, creating individualized learning plans, and developing an online professional portfolio. You can also track current news and nursing information, receive updates and alerts on items of interest, access educational opportunities, and search for practice support on the NurseONE site. This site will continue to develop over time and provides a centralized professional nursing forum for Canadian nurses. You should sign up today!

Clinician Engagement and Informatics Communities

Many Canadian and international health informatics communities offer exciting opportunities for participation: support, educational programs, and networking opportunities. Of most importance, these communities always welcome new members who are interested in advancing informatics. As noted throughout this chapter, involving clinicians in the selection, design, and revision of technology is crucial. As a professional, you have both an obligation and a right to be involved in issues that affect your professional practice and your work environment.

Many informatics organizations have specific strategies to foster clinician engagement or encourage clinicians to become involved; however, literature on the topic of clinician engagement is scarce. Mercer (2008) promoted involvement through five questions (the "5 Ws"): (1) What is it? (2) Who should be involved? (3) Why is it important? (4) Where does it fit? (5) When should clinicians get involved? Mercer advocated immediate involvement and in any clinical environment.

The CNA is the national professional body representing Canadian nurses. The CNA's mandate of supporting professional nursing practice also includes supporting the integration of nursing informatics in Canada. The CNA has issued many position statements and professional guidelines to support all nurses as technology has become increasingly integrated into Canadian practice environments. The CNA provides an excellent starting point from which you can explore nursing informatics in Canada.

The **Canadian Nursing Informatics Association** (CNIA) is the national special interest group dedicated to the advancement of nursing informatics in Canada. CNIA is designated as a group affiliated with the CNA. Also affiliated with COACH, CNIA is the Canadian nursing representative to the **International Medical Informatics Association–Special Interest Group in Nursing Informatics (IMIA-SIGNI).** Originally functioning as a special interest group within COACH, this group disbanded in 2000 and resumed as the CNIA (CNIA, 2000). This group was agreed to include the following mandates (CNIA, 2000):

- To provide nursing leadership for the development of nursing and health informatics in Canada
- To establish national networking opportunities for nurse informaticians
- To facilitate informatics educational opportunities for all nurses in Canada
- To engage in international nursing informatics initiatives
- To act as a nursing advisory group in matters of nursing and health informatics

Since being founded, the CNIA has hosted successful national nursing informatics conferences, launched a national online journal (*Canadian Journal of Nursing Informatics*), provided educational offerings, and advocated for the advancement of nursing informatics in Canada.

As noted earlier in this chapter, COACH is another organization dedicated to promoting health informatics within the Canadian health system through education, information, networking, and communication. COACH was formed in 1975 by software developers and health care clinicians (COACH, 2008). Their original focus was to support effective use information technology and systems among Canadian health institutions by sharing ideas and efforts. This focus has expanded to include the effective use of health information for decision making.

COACH's multidisciplinary membership encompasses more than 1300 individuals, including health care executives, physicians, nurses and allied health care professionals, researchers and educators, chief information officers, information managers, technical experts, consultants, and information technology vendors (COACH, 2008). Member organizations include health care service delivery agencies, government and nongovernment agencies, consulting firms, commercial providers of information and telecommunications technologies, and educational institutions.

In addition to the previous groups, you can also contribute your clinician perspective to the various SCWGs sponsored by Infoway. These groups, as noted previously in this chapter, are open and voluntary in nature, which means that you need only express your interest; you do not need to be nominated or elected as a member. You will be welcomed to any SCWG or multiple groups. Participating in these SCWGs not only supports your professional practice but also offers you an opportunity for professional development and mentoring. Many experienced nurses are currently involved in advisory groups of the Standards Collaborative, but the SCWGs consistently need and solicit clinician engagement.

Many international informatics organizations exist, in which you can be involved. These include the **American Medical Informatics Association (AMIA)**, the **International Medical Informatics Association (IMIA)**, and the Health Informatics Society of Australia (HISA), all of which host special interest groups in nursing informatics. You can be involved at every level of information management in health care. Your challenge and your opportunity are to decide how your interest and energy can be best used.

In addition to the formal organizations that you may consider joining, numerous informal communities are devoted to nursing informatics and creating dialogue among nurses. You may decide to explore a variety of informal communities or social entities, including the following:

- Blogs: These are online diaries generally sponsored by individuals, which are occasionally interactive but typically present only the thoughts or opinions of the blog's sponsor.
- Wikis: These are Web pages that are interactive and allow subscribers to modify or contribute to the content. Subscribers are able to use any Web browser. Wikis also allows users to incorporate hyperlinks and use a simplified language to create new pages and linkages rapidly.
- Listserv and discussion groups: These are e-mail distributions lists. Many nursing informatics sites allow and encourage you to subscribe to the listserv or discussion groups so that you can receive regular contact and updates in regard to content, activities, or networking opportunities. These tools also allow you to ask questions, post messages, and network with colleagues.
- Social networks: Communities such as MySpace and Facebook allow subscribers to join groups of individuals who are interested in shared interests and activities. These Web-based communities include a variety of ways in which subscribers may communicate, including chat, messaging, e-mail, blogs, video, voice chat, file sharing, discussion groups, and message boards.

The value of interest in informal networking cannot be underestimated; however, you should not depend on these types of forums for consistent, professional, and credible health informatics information. Some sites may offer highly professional informatics advice or information; unfortunately, no standard exists with regard to either content or process. Many sites offer only personal or anecdotal commentary and may provide misleading information, which can create liability if used in your professional practice. Consequently, you must critically evaluate the content of these informal sites and groups to determine the validity of the content, the credibility of the organization or group, and the intent of the networking tool. The most effective way to obtain reliable and authoritative information is through formalized organizations that are committed to the professional advancement of informatics.

✻ CRITICAL THINKING EXERCISES

1. You are making a presentation to a group of nursing peers. Your task is to lead the selection of an electronic documentation tool. How do you prepare your peers for evaluation discussions preceding the selection decision? What factors do you consider when determining what are the most important pieces of nursing documentation to record?
2. During the course of documenting an admission assessment, you note that your client has in the past been admitted to a psychiatric unit. One of your colleagues is a neighbour of the client and asks you to share whether this client has a psychiatric history. Your colleague is not providing care to the client today or tomorrow. How do you respond to this inquiry? What pieces of legislation do you consider in making a decision?

✻ REVIEW QUESTIONS

1. What changes that occurred in the health care system since the 1950s have led to the recognition of nursing informatics?
2. What factors are behind the need for standardized nursing documentation?
3. How is standardized nursing terminology being used in Canada?
4. How does privacy legislation influence nursing practice in Canada?
5. How can nurses implement the *E-Nursing Strategy?*
6. What nursing or health informatics communities are available to nurses?

✻ RECOMMENDED WEB SITES

American Medical Informatics Association (AMIA): http://www.amia.org/

AMIA is a national association in the United States and is dedicated to the adoption and advancement of technology in health care.

American Medical Informatics Association–Nursing Informatics: http://www.amia.org/mbrcenter/wg/ni/

The American Medical Informatics Association–Nursing Informatics is a special interest group within the American Medical Informatics Association. This group is focused on the advancement of informatics as it relates specifically to American professional nursing practice.

Canada Health Infoway: http://www.infoway-inforoute.ca/

Canada Health Infoway is Canada's national not-for-profit body that generates consensus on health information standards, drives forward the national agenda of creating an EHR, and acts as the liaison to international standards development organizations.

Canadian Nursing Informatics Association (CNIA): http://cnia.ca/intro.htm

The Canadian Nursing Informatics Association is Canada's national body with a mission to advance nursing informatics in Canada. CNIA is also the publisher of the *Canadian Journal of Nursing Informatics*.

Canadian Organization for Advancement of Computers in Health (COACH): http://www.coachorg.com/

COACH is a Canadian not-for-profit association that is dedicated to the effective integration of technology in health care. This association is one of the largest informatics associations in Canada and includes members from all health care disciplines.

Health Informatics Society of Australia (HISA): http://www.hisa.org.au/

HISA is the national not-for-profit association for advancing informatics in Australia.

Health Informatics Society of Australia–Nursing Informatics: http://www.hisa.org.au/nursing

The Health Informatics Society of Australia–Nursing Informatics is a special interest group within the Health Informatics Society of Australia. This group is focused on the advancement of informatics as it relates specifically to professional nursing practice in Australia.

International Medical Informatics Association (IMIA): http://www.imia.org/

IMIA is an international not-for-profit association and is dedicated to the adoption and advancement of technology in health care.

International Medical Informatics Association–Nursing Informatics: http://www.imia.org/working_groups/WG_Profile.lasso?-Search=Action&-Table=CGI&-MaxRecords=1&-SkipRecords=15&-Database=organizations&-KeyField=Org_ID&-SortField=workgroup_sig&-SortOrder=ascending&type=wgsig

The International Medical Informatics Association–Nursing Informatics is a special interest group within the International Medical Informatics Association. This group is focused on the advancement of nursing informatics with international implications.

NurseONE: http://www.nurseone.ca/

The NurseONE site is one of the outcomes of the Canadian Nurses Association's *E-Nursing Strategy.* This site offers nurses a diverse array of educational tools, professional practice supports, and networking opportunities.

18

Communication

Original chapter by Jeri Burger, RN, PhD

Canadian content written by Nancy C. Goddard, RN, BScN, MN, PhD

objectives

Mastery of content in this chapter will enable you to:

- Define the key terms listed.
- Describe aspects of critical thinking that are important to the communication process.
- Describe the five levels of communication and their uses in nursing.
- Describe the basic elements of the communication process.
- Identify significant features and therapeutic outcomes of nurse–client helping relationships.
- List nursing focus areas within the four phases of a nurse–client helping relationship.
- Identify significant features and desired outcomes of nurse–health care team member relationships.
- Describe qualities, behaviours, and communication techniques that affect professional communication.
- Discuss effective communication techniques for clients at various developmental levels.
- Identify client health states that contribute to impaired communication.
- Discuss nursing care measures for clients with special communication needs.

key terms

Active listening, p. 257
Assertive, p. 254
Autonomy, p. 254
Channels, p. 249
Communication, p. 246
Empathy, p. 257
Environment, p. 249
Feedback, p. 249
Interpersonal communication, p. 248
Interpersonal variables, p. 249
Intrapersonal communication, p. 248
Message, p. 249
Metacommunication, p. 251
Nonverbal communication, p. 250
Perception, p. 247
Perceptual biases, p. 247
Public communication, p. 248
Receiver, p. 248
Referent, p. 248
Sender, p. 248
Small-group communication, p. 248
Symbolic communication, p. 251
Sympathy, p. 260
Therapeutic communication techniques, p. 256
Transpersonal communication, p. 248
Verbal communication, p. 249

media resources

evolve Web Site

- Audio Chapter Summaries
- Glossary
- Multiple-Choice Review Questions
- Student Learning Activities
- Weblinks

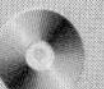

Companion CD

- Glossary
- Interactive Learning Activities
- Fluids and Electrolytes Tutorial
- Test-Taking Skills

Communication is a lifelong learning process for the nurse. Nurses are intimately involved with clients and their families from birth to death. It is important to build therapeutic communications for this journey. Nurses must communicate effectively with people under stress. They must function as client advocates and as members of interdisciplinary teams, other members of which often have different priorities for client care. Nurses must also be able to communicate their own needs to avoid burnout and to continue providing effective care within a high-stress environment (Balzer Riley, 2004). Despite the competing demands on nurses' time and despite current technological complexity, it is the intimate nurse–client connection that makes the difference in the quality of care and in the meaning of the illness experience for both (Balzer Riley, 2004). Therefore, nurses must be competent in a variety of communication techniques in order to develop and maintain therapeutic relationships. Effective communication promotes collaboration and interdisciplinary teamwork, helps ensure that ethical and legal responsibilities and professional practice standards are met, and contributes to positive client outcomes. It is an essential element of professional nursing practice (Apker et al., 2006). Ineffective communication may lead to poor client outcomes, increases in adverse incidents, and decreases in professional credibility. The Conference Board of Canada considers communication and interpersonal relationship skills to be crucial for successful employment and the establishment of healthy work environments (Devito et al., 2005).

The qualities, behaviours, and therapeutic communication techniques described in this chapter characterize professionalism in helping relationships. Although the term *client* is often used, the same principles can be applied in communicating with any person, in any nursing situation.

Communication and Interpersonal Relationships

At the core of nursing care are therapeutic interpersonal relationships based on caring, mutual respect, and dignity. Communication is the means to establish these helping–healing relationships. Because all behaviour communicates, and all communication influences behaviour, nurses must become experts in communication if they are to provide effective care.

The nurse's ability to relate to other people—to take initiative in establishing and maintaining a relationship, to be authentic, and to respond appropriately to the other person—is a crucial aspect of interpersonal communication. Effective interpersonal communication also requires a sense of mutuality, a belief that the nurse–client relationship is a partnership and that both partners are equal participants. Mutuality requires that both participants respect each other's autonomy and value system and are committed to the client's well-being (Arnold & Boggs, 2007). Nurses honour the fact that people are complex and ambiguous beings. Often, more is communicated than is at first apparent, and client responses are not always what you might expect. It is helpful for nurses to purposefully focus on shared problem solving and on positive client outcomes and to develop a mutual vision of hope and shared responsibility for health care outcomes (Grover, 2005).

According to one perspective of human relationships, energy fields permeate and connect all beings. Although the use of energy to heal is relatively new concept in Western cultures, it has long existed in Eastern cultures. Healers in early cultures treated their clients holistically and often focused on the concept of balancing energy within each human being to maintain health (McCaffrey & Fowler, 2003). Therefore, it is not surprising that nurses often perceive a strong sense of connection to other people within a helping relationship. Most nurses embrace the profession's view of people as holistic beings and have experienced synergy in human interactions. When clients and nurses work together, they accomplish much more.

Therapeutic communication occurs within a healing environment between a nurse and a client (Arnold & Boggs, 2007). Nurses know that attitudes and emotions are easily transmitted and can be communicated intentionally or unintentionally. Every nuance of posture, every small expression and gesture, every word chosen, every attitude held—all have the potential to hurt or heal. Because thought patterns (positive or negative), intention, and behaviour directly influence human energy fields and therefore health, nurses have a tremendous ethical responsibility to do no harm to people entrusted to their care. Communication must be respected for its potential power and not carelessly misused to hurt, manipulate, or coerce clients. Good communication empowers clients and enables them to know themselves and make their own choices, which is an essential aspect of the healing process. Nurses have the opportunity to create positive outcomes for themselves, their clients, and their colleagues through therapeutic communication.

Developing Communication Skills

Gaining expertise in communication, as in any aspect of nursing, requires both an understanding of the communication process and reflection about your personal communication experiences. Developing good critical thinking skills enables the most effective communication. You can draw on theoretical knowledge about communication and integrate this knowledge with previously learned knowledge gained through personal experience. You can interpret messages received from other people, analyze their content, make inferences about their meaning, evaluate their effect, explain the rationale for communication techniques used, and self-examine personal communication skills (Balzer Riley, 2004).

Other qualities of good critical thinking are also important to the communication process. Curiosity, perseverance, creativity, self-confidence, independence, fairness, integrity, and humility are useful in approaching a problem. Curiosity motivates you to learn more about a person, and clients are more likely to communicate with nurses who express an interest in them. Perseverance and creativity are necessary for identifying innovative solutions. Self-confidence enables you to more readily establish interpersonal helping-trust relationships and conveys competence in the professional role. A sense of independence enables you to take the risk of communicating ideas about nursing interventions even though colleagues may question your suggestions. An attitude of fairness enables you to listen to both sides in any discussion: You are able to recognize when your opinions conflict with those of the client, to review positions objectively, and to decide how to communicate to reach mutually beneficial decisions. Integrity prompts you to communicate responsibly and ask for help if you are uncertain or uncomfortable with any aspects of client care. Humility is necessary for you to recognize and communicate the need for more information before a decision can be made (Paul & Elder, 2001). In summary, critical thinking that is based on established nursing practice standards and a professional code of ethics promotes effective communication and facilitates high-quality client care.

Interpersonal communication may be challenging because it is based on an individual's perception of received information and is therefore subject to misinterpretation. **Perception** is based on information acquired through the five senses of sight, hearing, taste, touch, and smell (Stuart & Laraia, 2005). It is a process of mentally organizing and interpreting sensory information to arrive at a meaningful conclusion. An individual's culture, education, and personal background also influence perception. Critical thinking can help nurses overcome **perceptual biases**, which are human tendencies that interfere with accurately perceiving and interpreting messages from other people. People often assume that others would think, feel, act, react, and behave as they themselves would in similar circumstances. People tend to distort or ignore information that goes against their expectations, preconceptions, or stereotypes (Beebe et al., 2004). By thinking critically about personal communication habits, you will learn to control these tendencies and become more effective in interpersonal relationships.

As communication skills develop, competence in the nursing care process also grows. You need to integrate communication skills throughout the nursing care process as you collaborate with clients and members of the health care team to achieve goals (Box 18–1). Communication skills are used to gather, analyze, and transmit information and to accomplish the work of each step of the process. Assessment, diagnosis, planning, implementation, and evaluation all depend on effective communication among nurse, client, family, and other members of the health care team. Although the nursing care process is a reliable framework for client care, it does not work well unless you master the art of effective interpersonal communication.

The nature of the communication process requires nurses to constantly make decisions about what, when, where, why, and how to convey messages to other people. Decision making is always contextual: The unique features of any situation influence the nature of the decisions made. For example, the importance of following a prescribed diet will be explained differently to a client with a newly diagnosed medical condition than to a client who has repeatedly chosen not to follow diet restrictions. Effective communication techniques are easy to learn, but their application is more difficult. Deciding which techniques best fit each unique nursing situation is challenging. Communication about specific diagnoses such as cancer or end-of-life conditions and dealing with client and family emotions can be challenging, and some nurses struggle to cope with their own reactions and emotions (Sheldon et al., 2006).

Throughout this chapter, brief clinical examples guide you in the use of effective communication techniques. Situations that challenge nurses' decision-making and communication skills and call for careful consideration of therapeutic techniques often involve the styles of individuals described in Box 18–2. Because the best way to acquire skill is through practice, it is useful for you to discuss and role-play these scenarios before experiencing them in the clinical setting. Consider that clients, family, nurse colleagues, unregulated care providers, physicians, or other members of the health care team might be involved, and decide which communication techniques might be most effective.

➤ BOX 18-1 Communication Throughout the Nursing Care Process

Assessment

Verbal interviewing and history taking
Visual and intuitive observation of nonverbal behaviour
Documentation of visual, tactile, and auditory data during physical examination
Written medical records, diagnostic test results, and literature review

Nursing Diagnosis

Intrapersonal analysis of assessment findings
Validation of health care needs and priorities through verbal discussion with client
Handwritten or electronic documentation of nursing diagnosis

Planning

Interpersonal or small-group planning sessions with health care team
Interpersonal collaboration with client and family to determine implementation methods
Written documentation of expected outcomes
Written or verbal referral to members of the health care team

Implementation

Delegation and verbal discussion with health care team
Verbal, visual, auditory, and tactile health teaching activities
Provision of support through therapeutic communication techniques
Contact with other health care resources
Written documentation of client's progress in medical record

Evaluation

Acquisition of verbal and nonverbal feedback
Comparison of actual and expected outcomes
Identification of factors affecting outcomes
Modification and update of care plan
Verbal or written explanation, or both, of revisions of care plan to client

Levels of Communication

Nurses use different levels of communication in their professional role. The nurse's communication skills need to include techniques that reflect competence in each level.

➤ BOX 18-2 Challenging Communication Styles of Clients

- Silent, withdrawn; do not express any feelings or needs
- Sad, depressed; have slow mental and motor responses
- Angry, hostile; do not listen to explanations
- Uncooperative; resent being asked to do something
- Talkative, lonely; want someone with them all the time
- Demanding; want someone to wait on them or meet their requests
- Ranting and raving; blame nursing staff unfairly for their misfortunes or difficulties
- Sensory impaired; cannot hear or see well
- Verbally impaired; cannot articulate needs or desires
- Gossiping; violate confidentiality and cause friction
- Mentally handicapped; are frightened and distrustful
- Confused, disoriented; are bewildered and uncooperative
- Foreign-born; speak very little of the dominant culture's language
- Anxious, nervous; cannot cope with what is happening
- Grieving, crying; have sustained a major loss
- Screaming, kicking (toddlers); want their parents
- Flirtatious, sexually inappropriate
- Loud, obscene; cause disturbances or violate rules

Intrapersonal Communication

Intrapersonal communication, also known as *self-talk* or *inner thought*, is a powerful form of communication that occurs within an individual. It is exemplified in one's thinking (Beebe et al., 2004). People's thoughts strongly influence perceptions, feelings, behaviour, and self-concept; thus, it is important for you to be aware of the nature and content of your thinking. Nurses and clients use intrapersonal communication to develop self-awareness and a positive self-concept that can facilitate self-expression and improve health and self-esteem by replacing negative thoughts with positive assertions. Another type of intrapersonal communication, self-instruction, can provide a mental rehearsal for difficult tasks or situations.

Interpersonal Communication

Interpersonal communication is one-to-one interaction between the nurse and another person that often occurs face to face. It is the level most frequently used in nursing situations and is the crux of nursing practice. It takes place within a social context and includes all the symbols and cues used to give and receive meaning.

Sometimes messages are received differently than the messenger intended. Nurses work with people who have different opinions, experiences, values, and belief systems; therefore, meaning must be validated or mutually negotiated between participants. Meaningful interpersonal communication results in exchange of ideas, problem solving, expression of feelings, decision making, goal accomplishment, team building, and personal growth.

Transpersonal Communication

Transpersonal communication is interaction that occurs within a person's spiritual domain. Interest in the influence of religion and spirituality has increased dramatically since the 1980s and much has been written to promote nurses' understanding of the role spirituality plays in facilitating health care and coping ability (Burkhardt & Nagai-Jacobson, 2002; Taylor, 2002). Many people use prayer, meditation, guided reflection, religious rituals, or other means to communicate with their "higher power." Nurses who value the importance of human spirituality often use this form of communication with clients and for themselves. Nurses have a moral and ethical responsibility to assess clients' spiritual needs and to intervene to meet those needs.

Small-Group Communication

Small-group communication is interaction that occurs when a small number of people meet together and share a common purpose. This type of communication is usually goal directed and requires an understanding of group dynamics. When nurses work on committees, lead client support groups, form research teams, or participate in client care conferences, they are using a small-group communication process. For small groups to function effectively, members must feel accepted, comfortable in sharing ideas and thoughts openly and honestly, able to actively listen to other group members and consider possible alternative viewpoints (Sully & Dallas, 2005).

Public Communication

Public communication is interaction with an audience. Nurses have opportunities to speak with groups of consumers about health-related topics, present scholarly work to colleagues at conferences, or lead classroom discussions with peers or students. Public communication requires special adaptations in eye contact, gestures, and voice inflection and the use of media materials to communicate messages effectively. Effective public communication increases audience knowledge about health-related topics, health care issues, and other issues important to the nursing profession.

Basic Elements of the Communication Process

Communication is an ongoing, dynamic, and multidimensional process. Its basic elements are illustrated in Figure 18–1 and described in the following paragraphs. This simple model represents a very complex process, but it helps identify its essential components. Nursing situations have many unique aspects that influence the nature of communication and interpersonal relationships. In the professional role, you use critical thinking to focus on each aspect of communication so that interactions can be purposeful and effective.

Referent

The **referent** motivates one person to communicate with another. In a health care setting, sights, sounds, odours, time schedules, messages, objects, emotions, sensations, perceptions, ideas, and other cues trigger communication. The nurse who knows the stimulus that triggered communication is able to develop and organize messages more efficiently and better perceive meaning in another person's message. For example, a client's request for help prompted by difficulty breathing triggers a different nursing response than does a request prompted by boredom.

Sender and Receiver

The **sender** is the person who encodes and delivers the message, and the **receiver** is the person who receives and decodes the message. The sender puts ideas or feelings into a form that can be transmitted and is responsible for accuracy and emotional tone. The sender's message acts as a referent for the receiver, who is responsible for attending to, decoding, and responding to the sender's message. Sender and receiver roles are fluid and change back and forth as people interact; sometimes sending and receiving even occur simultaneously. The more the sender and receiver have in common and the closer their

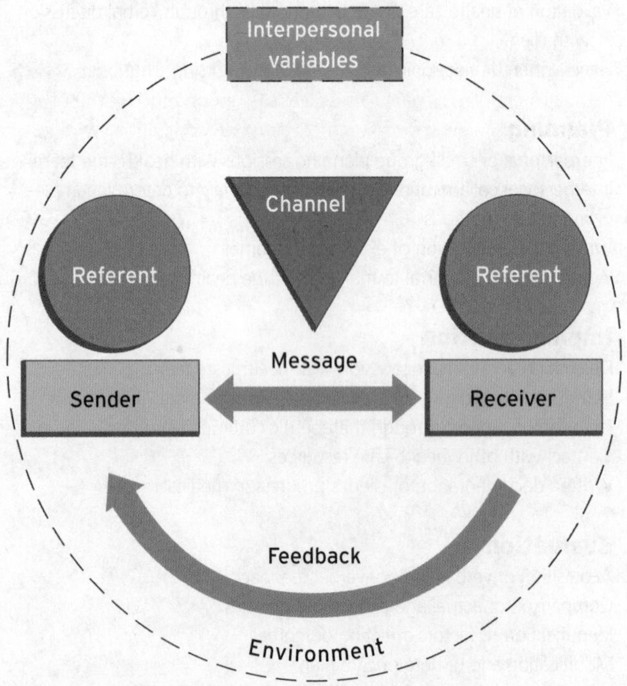

Figure 18-1 Communication is an active process between sender and receiver.

relationship is, the more likely they will accurately perceive one another's meaning and respond accordingly.

Messages

The **message** is the content of the communication. It contains verbal, nonverbal, and symbolic expressions of thoughts or feelings that are transmitted from the sender to the receiver (Arnold & Boggs, 2007). Personal perceptions sometimes distort the receiver's interpretation of the message. Two nurses can provide the same information and yet convey very different messages according to their personal communication styles. One nurse can send the same message to two people and be understood differently by each. You can send effective messages by expressing yourself clearly, directly, and in a manner familiar to the receiver. By watching the listener for nonverbal cues that suggest confusion or misunderstanding, you can determine whether the message needs to be clarified. Communication can be difficult when participants have different levels of education and experience. "Your incision is well approximated without purulent drainage," means the same as "Your wound edges are together, and you have no signs of infection," but the latter is easier to understand. You must be sure clients are able to read before you send messages in writing.

Channels

Channels are means of conveying and receiving messages through visual, auditory, and tactile senses. Facial expressions send visual messages, spoken words travel through auditory channels, and touch traverses tactile channels. The more channels the sender uses to convey a message, the more clearly the message is usually understood. For example, when teaching about insulin self-injection, the nurse talks about and demonstrates the technique, gives the client printed information, and encourages hands-on practice with the vial and syringe. Nurses use verbal, nonverbal, and mediated (technological) communication channels. They send and receive information in person, by informal or formal writing, over the telephone or pager, by audiotape and videotape, through fax and electronic mail, and through electronic online interactive and information sites.

Feedback

Feedback is the message returned by the receiver. It indicates whether the meaning of the sender's message was understood by the receiver. Senders need to seek verbal and nonverbal feedback to ensure that good communication has occurred. To be effective, the sender and receiver must be sensitive and open to each other's messages, clarify the messages, and modify behaviour accordingly. In a social relationship, both participants assume equal responsibility for seeking openness and clarification, but in the nurse–client relationship, this responsibility is primarily the nurse's.

Interpersonal Variables

Interpersonal variables are characteristics within both the sender and receiver that influence communication. Perception is one such variable that provides a uniquely personal view of reality that is informed by the person's expectations and experiences. People sense, interpret, and understand events differently. A nurse might say, "You have been very quiet since your family left. Is something on your mind?" One client might perceive the nurse's question as showing caring and concern; another might perceive the nurse as being intrusive. Other interpersonal variables include educational and developmental levels, sociocultural backgrounds, values and beliefs, emotions, gender, physical health status, and roles and relationships. Variables associated with illness, such as pain, anxiety, and medication effects, can also affect nurse–client communication (Feldman-Stewart et al., 2005).

Environment

The **environment** is the setting for sender–receiver interaction. For effective communication, the environment should meet participants' needs for physical and emotional comfort and safety. Noise, temperature extremes, distractions, and lack of privacy or space create confusion, tension, and discomfort. Environmental distractions are common in health care settings and interfere with messages sent between people; therefore, nurses must try to control the environment as much as possible to create favourable conditions for effective communication.

Forms of Communication

Messages are conveyed verbally, nonverbally, concretely, and symbolically. As people communicate, they express themselves through words, movements, voice inflection, facial expressions, and use of space. These elements work in harmony to enhance a message, or they conflict with one another to contradict and garble the message.

Verbal Communication

Verbal communication entails the use of spoken or written words. Verbal language is a code that conveys specific meaning through a combination of words. The most important aspects of verbal communication are discussed as follows.

Vocabulary. Communication is unsuccessful if senders and receivers cannot decode each other's words and phrases. When a nurse cares for a client who speaks another language, the services of an interpreter may be necessary. Even those who speak the same language use subcultural variations of certain words: *dinner* may mean a noon meal to one person and the last meal of the day to another. Medical jargon (technical terminology used by health care professionals) may sound like a foreign language to clients and should be used only with other members of the health care team. Children have more limited vocabularies than do adults and may use special words to describe bodily functions or a favourite blanket or toy. Teenagers often use words in unique ways that are unfamiliar to adults.

Denotative and Connotative Meaning. A single word can have several meanings. Individuals who use a common language share the denotative meaning: *Baseball* has the same meaning for everyone who speaks English, but *code* denotes cardiac arrest primarily to health care professionals. The connotative meaning is the shade or interpretation of a word's meaning influenced by the thoughts, feelings, or ideas that people have about the word. Families who are told that a loved one is "in serious condition" may believe that death is near, but to nurses *serious* may simply describe the nature of the condition. You need to select words carefully, avoiding terms that can be easily misinterpreted, especially when explaining a client's medical condition or therapy. Even a much-used phrase such as "I'm going to take your vital signs" can be unfamiliar to an adult or frightening to a child.

Pacing. Messages are conveyed more successfully when sent at an appropriate speed or pace. Speak slowly enough to enunciate clearly. Talking rapidly, using awkward pauses, or speaking slowly and deliberately can convey an unintended message. Long pauses and rapid shifts to another topic may give the impression that you are hiding the truth. Pacing is improved by thinking before speaking and by developing awareness of the cadence of your speech.

Intonation. Tone of voice dramatically affects the meaning of a message. Depending on intonation, even a simple question or statement can express enthusiasm, anger, concern, or indifference. To avoid sending unintended messages, be aware of your tone of voice. For example, clients may interpret a nurse's tone of voice as condescending, and further communication may be inhibited. A client's voice tone often provides information about his or her emotional state or energy level.

Clarity and Brevity. Effective communication is simple, brief, and direct. Fewer words result in less confusion. You achieve clarity by speaking slowly, enunciating clearly, and using examples to make explanations easier to understand. Repeating important parts of a message also clarifies communication. Phrases such as "you know" or "OK?" at the end of every sentence detract from clarity. Brevity is achieved by using short sentences and words that express an idea simply and directly. "Where is your pain?" is much better than "I would like you to describe for me the location of your discomfort."

Timing and Relevance. Timing is critical in communication. Even though a message is clear, poor timing can limit its effectiveness. For example, you should not begin routine teaching when a client is in severe pain, is in emotional distress, or is distracted by pressing matters. Often the best time for interaction is when a client expresses an interest in communicating. If messages are relevant or important to the situation at hand, they are more effective. When a client is facing emergency surgery, discussing the risks of smoking is less relevant than explaining preoperative procedures.

Nonverbal Communication

Nonverbal communication makes use of all five senses and refers to transmission of messages that do not involve the spoken or written word. Researchers have estimated that approximately 7% of meaning is transmitted by words, 38% is transmitted by vocal cues, and 55% is transmitted by body cues. Nonverbal communication serves to accent, complement, contradict, regulate, repeat, or substitute for verbal messages (Devito et al., 2005). Nonverbal communication is unconsciously motivated and therefore reflects a person's intended meaning more accurately than do spoken words (Stuart & Laraia, 2005). When verbal and nonverbal communication are incongruous, the receiver usually "hears" the nonverbal message as the true message.

All kinds of nonverbal communication are important, but interpreting them is often difficult. Sociocultural background is a major influence on the meaning of nonverbal behaviour. Nonverbal messages between people of different cultures are easily misinterpreted. Because the interpretation of nonverbal behaviour is subjective, it is important to check its perceived meaning (Adler et al., 2004). Assessing nonverbal messages is an important nursing skill (Grover, 2005).

Personal Appearance. Personal appearance includes physical characteristics, facial expression, manner of dress and grooming, and adornments. These factors help communicate physical well-being, personality, social status, occupation, religion, culture, and self-concept. First impressions are largely based on appearance. Nurses learn to develop a general impression of client health and emotional status through appearance, and clients develop a general impression of the nurse's professionalism and caring in the same way.

Posture and Gait. Posture and gait are forms of self-expression. The ways that people sit, stand, and move reflect attitudes, emotions, self-concept, and health status. For example, an erect posture and a quick, purposeful gait communicate a sense of well-being and confidence. Leaning forward conveys attention. A slumped posture and a slow, shuffling gait may be indicative of depression, illness, discomfort, or fatigue.

Facial Expression. The face is the most expressive part of the body. Facial expressions convey emotions such as surprise, fear, anger, happiness, and sadness. Some people have an expressionless face, or flat affect, which reveals little about what they are thinking or feeling. An inappropriate affect is a facial expression that does not match the content of a verbal message: for example, smiling when describing a sad situation. People are sometimes unaware of the messages their expressions convey. For example, a nurse may frown in concentration while doing a procedure and the client may interpret this as anger or disapproval. Clients closely observe nurses. Consider the impact a nurse's facial expression might have on a person who asks, "Am I going to die?" The slightest change in the eyes, lips, or facial muscles will reveal the nurse's feelings. Although it is hard to control all facial expression, try to avoid showing shock, disgust, dismay, or other distressing reactions in the client's presence.

Eye Contact. People signal readiness to communicate through eye contact. In European and American cultures, maintaining eye contact during conversation shows respect and willingness to listen. Eye contact also allows people to closely observe one another. Lack of eye contact may indicate anxiety, defensiveness, discomfort, or lack of confidence in communicating. However, people from some Asian and Aboriginal cultures consider eye contact intrusive, threatening, or harmful, and they minimize or avoid its use. Eye movements can also communicate feelings and emotions. Standing above a person (looking downward) conveys authority, whereas interacting at the same eye level indicates equality in the relationship. Rising to the same eye level as an angry person communicates self-assertion.

Gestures. Gestures emphasize, punctuate, and clarify the spoken word. Gestures alone carry specific meanings, or they create messages with other communication cues. A finger pointed toward a person may communicate several meanings, but when accompanied by a frown and stern voice, the gesture conveys an accusation or a threat. Pointing to an area of pain may be more accurate than verbally describing the location.

Sounds. Sounds such as sighs, moans, groans, or sobs also communicate feelings and thoughts. When combined with other nonverbal communication, sounds help send clear messages. Sounds can be interpreted in several ways: sighing often suggests boredom or anxiety, moaning may convey pleasure or suffering, and crying may communicate happiness, sadness, or anger. You need to validate such nonverbal messages with the client in order to interpret them accurately.

Territoriality and Personal Space. Territoriality is the need to gain, maintain, and defend one's right to space. Territory is important because it provides people with a sense of identity, security, and control. Territory can be distinguished and made visible to other people, as with a fence around a yard or a curtain around a bed in a hospital room. Personal space, however, is invisible and individual, and it travels with the person. During interpersonal interaction, people maintain varying distances between each other, depending on their culture, the nature of their relationship, and the situation. When personal space becomes threatened, people respond defensively and communicate less effectively. Specific situations dictate whether the interpersonal distance between nurse and client is appropriate. Nurses often must move into clients' territory and personal space because of the nature of caregiving. Before entering into a client's personal space, it is essential that you prepare both your client and the environment. By explaining to your client what you will do and preparing the environment for particular nursing interventions, your client will recognize a shift toward the establishment of a therapeutic interaction. You need to convey confidence, gentleness, and respect for privacy, especially when your actions will require intimate contacts or involve a client's vulnerable zone. Box 18–3 provides examples of nursing actions within zones of personal space (Stuart & Laraia, 2005) and zones of touch.

> **BOX 18-3 Zones of Personal Space and Touch**
>
> **Zones of Personal Space**
>
> ***Intimate Zone (0 to 45 cm)***
> Holding a crying infant
> Performing physical assessment
> Bathing, grooming, dressing, feeding, and toileting a client
> Changing a client's dressing
>
> ***Personal Zone (45 cm to 1 m)***
> Sitting at a client's bedside
> Taking the client's nursing history
> Teaching an individual client
> Exchanging information with health care staff at change of shift
>
> ***Social Zone (1 to 4 m)***
> Participating in client care rounds
> Sitting at the head of a conference table
> Teaching a class for clients with a specific disease
> Conducting a family support group session
>
> ***Public Zone (4 m and greater)***
> Speaking at a community forum
> Testifying at a legislative hearing
> Lecturing to a class of students
>
> **Zones of Touch**
>
> ***Social Zone (permission not needed)***
> Hands, arms, shoulders, back
>
> ***Consent Zone (permission needed)***
> Mouth, wrists, feet
>
> ***Vulnerable Zone (special care needed)***
> Face, neck, front of body
>
> ***Intimate Zone (great sensitivity needed)***
> Genitalia, rectum

Symbolic Communication

Good communication requires awareness of **symbolic communication**, the verbal and nonverbal symbolism used to convey meaning. Art and music are forms of symbolic communication that nurses use to enhance understanding and promote healing. Lane (2006) found that creative expressions such as art, music, and dance have a healing effect on clients. Clients reported decreased pain and greater joy and hope.

Metacommunication

Metacommunication is a broad term that refers to all factors that influence how a message is perceived by other people (Arnold & Boggs, 2007). It is communication *about* communication (Devito et al., 2005) that reflects the relational aspects of messages (Adler et al., 2004) and helps people better understand what has been communicated. For example, a nurse observes a young client holding his body rigidly erect, and his voice is sharp as he says, "Going to surgery is no big deal." The nurse replies, "You say having surgery doesn't bother you, but you look and sound tense. I'd like to help." Awareness of the tone of the verbal response and the nonverbal behaviour may result in further exploration of the client's feelings and concerns.

Professional Nursing Relationships

The nurse's application of knowledge, understanding of human behaviour and communication, and commitment to ethical behaviour all contribute to the formation of professional relationships. Having a philosophy based on caring and respect for other people will help you be more successful in establishing professional relationships.

Nurse–Client Helping Relationships

Helping relationships are the foundation of clinical nursing practice. In such relationships, the nurse assumes the role of professional helper and comes to know the client as an individual who has unique health care needs, human responses, and patterns of living. The relationship is therapeutic, promoting a psychological climate that facilitates positive change and growth. Therapeutic communication allows clients to achieve their health care–related goals and attain optimal personal growth (Arnold & Boggs, 2007). It includes an explicit time frame and a goal-directed approach, and confidentiality is an expected feature. The nurse establishes, directs, and takes responsibility for the interaction, and the client's needs take priority over the nurse's needs. The relationship is also characterized by the nurse's nonjudgemental acceptance of the client. Acceptance conveys a willingness to hear a message or to acknowledge feelings. It does not mean you always agree with the client or approve of the client's decisions or actions. A helping relationship between nurse and client does not just happen; you create it through care, skill, and the development of trust.

The nurse–client helping relationship is characterized by a natural progression of four goal-directed phases: preinteraction, orientation, working, and termination phases (Box 18–4). These phases often begin before the nurse meets the client and continue until the caregiving relationship ends. Even a brief interaction is characterized by an abbreviated version of these four phases. For example, the student nurse gathers client information to prepare in advance for caregiving, meets the client and establishes trust, accomplishes health care–related goals through use of the nursing care process, and says goodbye at the end of the shift or when the client leaves the unit.

Socializing is an important initial component of interpersonal communication. It helps people get to know one another and relax. It is easy, superficial, and not deeply personal, whereas therapeutic interactions are often more difficult, intense, and uncomfortable. A nurse often uses social conversation to lay a foundation for a closer relationship: "Hi, Mr. Simpson. I hear it's your birthday today. Happy birthday!" A friendly, informal, and warm communication style helps establish trust, but nurses must get beyond social conversation to talk about issues or concerns affecting the client's health. During social conversation, clients may ask personal questions about the nurse's family, place of residence, and so forth. Students often wonder whether it is appropriate to reveal such information. The skillful nurse uses judgement about what to share and provides minimal information or deflects such questions with gentle humour and refocuses conversation back to the client.

BOX 18-4 Phases of the Helping Relationship

Pre-interaction Phase

Before meeting the client, the nurse accomplishes the following tasks:

- Reviews available data, including the medical and nursing history
- Talks to other caregivers who may have information about the client
- Anticipates health care concerns or issues that may arise
- Identifies a location and setting that will foster comfortable, private interaction with the client
- Plans enough time for the initial interaction

Orientation Phase

When the nurse and client meet and get to know one another, the nurse accomplishes the following tasks:

- Sets the tone for the relationship by adopting a warm, empathetic, caring manner
- Recognizes that the initial relationship may be superficial, uncertain, and tentative
- Expects the client to test the nurse's competence and commitment
- Closely observes the client and expects to be closely observed by the client
- Begins to make inferences and form judgements about client messages and behaviours
- Assesses the client's health status
- Prioritizes the client's problems and identifies the client's goals
- Clarifies the client's and nurse's roles
- Negotiates a contract with the client that specifies who will do what
- Lets the client know when to expect the relationship to be terminated

Working Phase

When the nurse and client work together to solve problems and achieve goals, the nurse accomplishes the following tasks:

- Encourages and helps the client to express feelings about his or her health
- Encourages and helps the client to explore own feelings and thoughts
- Provides information that the client needs to understand and change behaviour
- Encourages and helps the client to set goals
- Takes actions to meet the goals set with the client
- Uses therapeutic communication skills to facilitate successful interactions
- Uses appropriate self-disclosure and confrontation

Termination Phase

During the ending of the relationship, the nurse accomplishes the following tasks:

- Reminds the client that relationship termination is near
- Evaluates goal achievement with the client
- Reminisces about the relationship with the client
- Separates from the client by relinquishing responsibility for his or her care
- Facilitates a smooth transition for the client to other caregivers as needed

Creating a therapeutic environment depends on the your ability to communicate, comfort, and help clients meet their needs. Comfort is crucial in the practice of nursing. Therapeutic interactions increase feelings of personal control by helping clients feel secure, informed, and valued. Optimizing personal control facilitates emotional comfort, which minimizes physical discomfort and promotes recovery (Williams & Irurita, 2006) (Box 18–5).

In a therapeutic relationship, nurses often encourage clients to share personal stories, which are called *narrative interactions.* Through narrative interactions, such as reminiscing with clients, you begin to understand the context of clients' lives and learn what is meaningful to the clients from their perspective (Shattell & Hogan, 2005). For example, a nurse asked a client to tell about a time in his life when he had to make a hard decision. The client related the following story:

"When I was a young man, I worked on the family farm. An uncle died and left me some money. All of a sudden, I could afford to go to college, but Dad didn't want me to go because he needed me there. I had to decide whether to stay or go, and it was real hard because at first I just wanted to get away. I talked to our preacher, and he said it was up to me, to pray about it and do what my heart told me to. So I stayed. Oh, I've thought from time to time what I might have made of myself, but I never regretted it. I had a good life in farming."

From this brief story, the nurse understood that it was important to the client to put his family's needs above his personal desires and that seeking spiritual guidance was an important component of his decision making. This same information may not have been

BOX 18-5 EVIDENCE-INFORMED PRACTICE GUIDELINE

Emotional Comfort

Evidence Summary

In a study by Williams and Irurita (2006), recently hospitalized clients described emotional comfort as a pleasant positive feeling and state of relaxation that resulted from therapeutic interactions. Clients described emotional discomfort as unpleasant negative feelings and tension. Personal control over the situation contributed to emotional comfort. Therapeutic interactions helped the client achieve control and were associated with emotional comfort. Clients perceived a positive link between emotional comfort and recovery.

Application to Nursing Practice

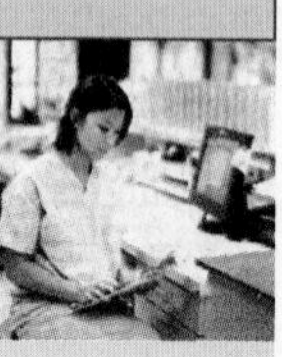

- Clients perceive a connection between the mind and body.
- Increased emotional comfort increases physical comfort and enhances recovery.
- Nurse–client therapeutic interactions improve the client's emotional and physical comfort.
- By using therapeutic communication to increase the client's perceived control of the situation and the environment, nurses increase the client's comfort.

References: Williams, A. M., & Irurita, V. F. (2006). Emotional comfort: The patient's perspective of a therapeutic context. *International Journal of Nursing Studies, 43*(4), 405–415.

revealed had the nurse used a standard history that usually elicits only short answers.

Collaboration between nurses and clients builds relationships and is based on principles of mutual gain and respect. It reflects a desire to satisfy the needs of both parties (Dubrin & Geerinck, 2006). Collaborative communication promotes personal responsibility, enables self-expression, and strengthens the client's problem-solving ability.

Nurse-Family Relationships

Many nursing situations, especially those in community care and home care settings, require the nurse to form helping relationships with entire families. The same principles that guide one-to-one helping relationships also apply when the client is a family unit; however, communication within families requires additional understanding of the complexities of family dynamics, needs, and relationships (see Chapter 20).

Nurse-Health Care Team Relationships

Nurses function in roles that require interaction with multiple members of the health care team. Many elements of the nurse–client helping relationship also apply to collegial relationships, which focus on accomplishing the work and goals of the clinical setting. Communication in such relationships may be geared toward team building, facilitating group process, collaboration, consultation, delegation, supervision, leadership, and management (see Chapter 11). You need a variety of communication skills, including presentational speaking, persuasion, group problem solving, providing performance reviews, and writing business reports.

Social and therapeutic interactions are needed between the nurse and members of the health care team to build morale and strengthen relationships within the work setting. Everyone has interpersonal needs for acceptance, inclusion, identity, privacy, power and control, and affection (Stewart & Logan, 2005). Nurses need friendship, support, guidance, and encouragement from one another to cope with the many stressors imposed by the nursing role and must extend the same caring communication used with clients to build positive relationships with colleagues and coworkers.

Nurse-Community Relationships

Many nurses form relationships with community groups by participating in local organizations, volunteering for community service, or becoming politically active. In a community-based practice, you must be able to establish relationships with their community to be an effective agent for change (see Chapter 4). Understanding the importance of community-oriented, population-focused nursing practice and developing the skills to practise it are crucial in attaining a leadership role in health care, regardless of the practice setting (Stanhope & Lancaster, 2004). Through neighbourhood newsletters, public bulletin boards, newspapers, radio, television, and electronic information sites, you can share information and discuss issues important to community health care.

Elements of Professional Communication

Professional appearance, demeanour, and behaviour are important in establishing your trustworthiness and competence. They communicate the impression that you have assumed the professional helping role, are clinically skilled, and are focused on the client. Nothing harms the professional image of nurses as much as an individual nurse's inappropriate appearance or behaviour.

A health care professional is expected to be clean, neat, well-groomed, conservatively dressed, and free of scent and odour. Visible tattoos and body piercings other than ear piercings are not acceptable in the professional setting. Professional behaviour should reflect warmth, friendliness, confidence, and competence. Professionals speak in a clear well-modulated voice, use good grammar, listen to other people, help and support colleagues, and communicate effectively. Being punctual, organized, well-prepared, and equipped for the responsibilities of the nursing role also communicate professionalism.

Courtesy

Common courtesy is part of professional communication. To practise courtesy, say hello and goodbye to clients, knock on doors before entering, and use self-introduction. A courteous nurse will also state his or her purpose, address people by name, say "please" and "thank you" to members of the health care team, and apologize for inadvertently causing distress. When a nurse is discourteous, he or she is perceived as rude or insensitive. Such behaviour sets up barriers between nurse and client and causes friction among members of the health care team.

Use of Names

Self-introduction is important. Failure to give a name, indicate status (e.g., student nurse, registered nurse, or licensed practical nurse), or acknowledge the client creates uncertainty about the interaction and conveys a lack of commitment or caring. Making eye contact and smiling at other people communicates recognition. Addressing other people by name conveys respect for human dignity and uniqueness. Because using last names is respectful in most cultures, nurses usually use the client's last name in the initial interaction, but they may use the first name in subsequent interactions at the client's request. It is important to ask other people how they would like to be addressed and to honour their preferences. Using first names is appropriate for infants, young children, confused or unconscious clients, and close colleagues. Terms of endearment such as "honey," "dear," "Grandma," or "sweetheart" are not appropriate; they may be perceived as disrespectful. The use of plural pronouns such as "we" when referring to clients implies a loss of independence and may be interpreted as condescending (Williams et al., 2004). Referring to a client by diagnosis, room number, or another attribute is demeaning and implies that you do not care enough to know the client as an individual.

Trustworthiness

Trust entails relying on someone without doubt or question. Being trustworthy means helping other people without hesitation. To foster trust, you need to communicate warmth and demonstrate consistency, reliability, honesty, integrity, competence, and respect. Sometimes it is not easy for a client to ask for help. Trusting another person involves risk and vulnerability, but it also fosters open, therapeutic communication and enhances the expression of feelings, thoughts, and needs. Without trust, a nurse–client relationship rarely progresses beyond social interaction and superficial care. Avoid dishonesty. Knowingly withholding key information, lying, or distorting the truth violates both legal and ethical standards of practice. Maintaining confidentiality and protecting a client's privacy are also important aspects of professional behaviour. Sharing personal information or gossiping about other people communicates the message that you cannot be trusted and damages interpersonal relationships.

Autonomy and Responsibility

Autonomy is the ability to be self-directed and independent in accomplishing goals and advocating for other people. Professional nurses make choices and accept responsibility for the outcomes of their actions (Townsend, 2005). They take initiative in solving problems and communicate in a manner that reflects the importance and purpose of the therapeutic interaction (Arnold & Boggs, 2007). It is also important to recognize the client's autonomy because people who seek health care are often concerned about losing control of decisions regarding how they live.

Assertiveness

Assertive communication allows individuals to act in their own best interests without infringing on or denying the rights of other people (Devito et al., 2005). Assertiveness conveys self-assurance and respect for other people (Stuart & Laraia, 2005).

Nurses teach assertiveness skills to other people as a means of promoting personal health. Assertive people express feelings and emotions confidently, spontaneously, and honestly. They make decisions and control their lives more effectively than do nonassertive individuals. They can deal with criticism and manipulation by other people and learn to say "no," set limits, and resist other people's efforts to impose guilt.

Assertive responses are characterized by feelings of security, competence, power, optimism, and professionalism. They are good tools for dealing with criticism, change, negative conditions in personal or professional life, and conflict or stress in relationships. Assertive responses often contain "I" messages, such as "I want," "I need," "I think," and "I feel."

> **BOX 18-6 Contextual Factors That Influence Communication**
>
> **Psychophysiological Context**
>
> This refers to the internal factors that influence communication:
> - Physiological status (e.g., pain, hunger, weakness, dyspnea)
> - Emotional status (e.g., anxiety, anger, hopelessness, euphoria)
> - Growth and development status (e.g., age, developmental tasks)
> - Unmet needs (e.g., safety or security; love or belonging)
> - Attitudes, values, and beliefs (e.g., meaning of illness experience)
> - Perceptions and personality (e.g., optimistic or pessimistic, introverted or extroverted)
> - Self-concept and self-esteem (e.g., positive or negative)
>
> **Relational Context**
>
> This refers to the nature of the relationship between the participants:
> - Social, helping, or working relationship
> - Level of trust between participants
> - Level of caring expressed
> - Level of self-disclosure between participants
> - Shared history of participants
> - Balance of power and control
>
> **Situational Context**
>
> This refers to the reason for the communication:
> - Information exchange
> - Goal achievement
> - Problem resolution
> - Expression of feelings
>
> **Environmental Context**
>
> This refers to the physical surroundings in which communication takes place:
> - Privacy level
> - Noise level
> - Comfort and safety level
> - Distraction level
>
> **Cultural Context**
>
> This refers to the sociocultural elements that affect the interaction:
> - Educational level of participants
> - Language and self-expression patterns
> - Customs and expectations
> - Media influences

Communication Within the Nursing Care Process

In the following sections, the focus of the nursing care process is on providing care for clients who need special assistance with communication. However, the section on implementation contains examples of therapeutic communication techniques that are appropriate strategies for use in any interpersonal nursing situation.

❖Assessment

Assessment of a client's ability to communicate includes gathering data about the many contextual factors that influence communication. The word *context* refers to all the parts of a situation that help determine its meaning. A context includes all the environmental factors that influence the nature of communication and interpersonal relationships. This includes the participants' internal factors and characteristics, the nature of their relationship, the situation prompting communication, the environment, and the sociocultural elements present (Beebe et al., 2004). Box 18–6 lists the contextual factors that influence communication. Understanding these contextual factors helps you make sound decisions during the communication process.

Physical and Emotional Factors

Assessing the psychophysiological factors that influence communication is especially important. Many altered health states and human responses limit communication. People with hearing or visual impairments have fewer channels through which to receive messages (see Chapter 48). Facial trauma, laryngeal cancer, tracheostomy, or endotracheal intubation often prevents movement of air past vocal cords or mobility of the tongue, which results in inability to articulate words. An extremely breathless person must use oxygen to breathe rather than speak. People with aphasia after a stroke or in late-stage Alzheimer's disease often cannot understand or form words. People with delirium cannot focus attentively, and those with dementia often cannot make sense of what is being said. Certain mental illnesses such as psychoses or depression cause clients to demonstrate flight of ideas (words do not keep up to rapidly changing thoughts), constant verbalization of the same words or phrases, a loose association of ideas, or slowed speech pattern. People who are highly anxious are sometimes unable to perceive environmental stimuli or hear explanations. Unresponsive or heavily sedated people cannot send or respond to verbal messages.

Review of the client's medical record helps provide relevant information about the client's ability to communicate. Through the health history and physical examination, you document physical barriers to speech, neurological deficits, and pathophysiological conditions that affect hearing or vision. Reviewing the client's medication record is also important. For example, opiates, antidepressants, neuroleptics, hypnotics, or sedatives may cause a client to slur words or use incomplete sentences. The nursing progress notes may reveal other factors that contribute to communication difficulties, such as the absence of family members who could provide more information about a confused client.

Assessment should include communicating directly with clients to provide information about their ability to attend to, interpret, and respond to stimuli. If clients have difficulty communicating, it is important to assess the effects of the problem. Clients who cannot communicate effectively will often have difficulty expressing their needs and responding appropriately to the environment. A client who is unable to speak is at risk for injury unless the nurse identifies an alternative communication method. If barriers make it difficult to communicate directly with the client, then family or friends become important sources of information about the client's communication patterns and abilities.

Developmental Factors

Aspects of a client's growth and development also influence nurse–client interactions. For example, an infant's self-expression is limited to crying, body movement, and facial expression, whereas most older children express their needs more directly, through speech and specific actions such as pointing. Nurses adapt communication techniques to the special needs of infants and children. Communication with children and their parents requires special considerations. It is important to include the parents, child, or both as sources of information about the child's health, depending on the child's age. If a young child is given toys or other distractions, parents can give you their full attention. Children are especially responsive to nonverbal messages, and sudden movements, loud noises, or threatening gestures can be frightening. Children often prefer to initiate interpersonal contacts and, like adults, do not like adults to stare or look down at them. A child who has received little environmental stimulation may have delayed language development, which makes communication more challenging.

Age also influences communication. Age alone does not determine an adult's capacity for communication. However, approximately 12% of Canadians aged 65 and older have speech or hearing disorders that limit self-expression or their ability to understand other people (Canadian Association of Speech–Language Pathologists and Audiologists, n.d.). Although many older adults have some form of communication barrier, you need to communicate with them on an adult level to avoid being perceived as patronizing or condescending (Williams et al., 2004). Box 18–7 highlights tips for communicating with older adults who have communication needs and barriers. These tips can be applied to all clients with communication problems.

Sociocultural Factors

Culture is a blueprint for thinking, feeling, behaving, and communicating. Nurses need to be aware of the typical patterns of interaction that characterize various cultures. For example, most Inuit and First Nations peoples value privacy, respect, and silence. Whereas Canadians of European descent are more open and willing to discuss private family matters, Aboriginal Canadians may be reluctant to reveal personal or family information to strangers. Personal information is often conveyed indirectly through storytelling. For example, Hutterite colonies, which form a large portion of the rural Canadian population, have a hierarchical social order, and elders make decisions that affect all community members. For the Hutterites, taking individual responsibility for health care–related choices would not be consistent with communalism and their culture (Fahrenwald et al., 2001). Awareness of such cultural values will facilitate communication between you and your clients (see Chapter 10).

Foreign-born people may not speak or understand English or French. Those who speak a second language often experience difficulty with self-expression or language comprehension. To practise cultural sensitivity in communication, you must understand that people of different cultures use different degrees of eye contact, personal space, gestures, voice modulation, pace of speech, touch, silence, and meaning of language. Make a conscious effort to avoid interpreting messages from your own cultural perspective and to consider communication within the context of the client's background. Do not stereotype, patronize, or make fun of other cultures. Lack of knowledge by both nurses and clients about each other's cultural background and expectations frequently leads to feelings of anxiety, doubt, embarrassment, anger, and frustration (Spence, 2001). Language and cultural barriers prevent effective communication and not only are frustrating but also may lead to delayed or inappropriate care. Developing cultural competence increases understanding between clients and health care professionals and promotes positive client outcomes.

Gender

Gender is another factor that influences how people think, act, feel, and communicate. Male and female communication patterns tend to differ, which can sometimes create barriers to effective communication (Beebe et al., 2004). Boys and men tend to use less verbal communication but are more likely to initiate conversations and address issues directly. Girls and women tend to disclose more personal information, use more active listening, and respond in ways that encourage continued conversation. A male nurse might say to his colleague, "Help me turn Jeremy." A female nurse might say, "Jeremy needs to be turned," expecting her colleague to understand the implied request for help.

To practise gender sensitivity in communication, recognize the differences in male and female communication patterns to avoid misinterpreting messages sent by someone of the opposite gender. Avoid conversations with sexual overtones, gender-denigrating jokes, and male–female stereotyping.

BOX 18-7 FOCUS ON OLDER ADULTS

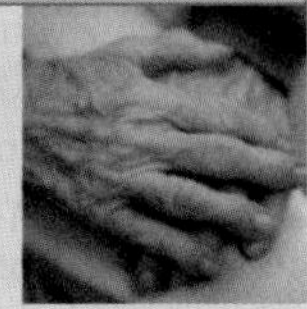

Tips for Improved Communication With Older Adults Who Have Communication Needs or Barriers

- Capture the client's attention before speaking.
- Check for hearing aids and glasses.
- Introduce yourself.
- Choose a quiet, well-lit environment, and minimize visual and auditory distractions.
- Face the client, and use facial expressions and gestures as needed.
- Amplify your voice if necessary, but do not shout because it distorts sound and your facial expression could be misinterpreted. Speak clearly at a moderate rate.
- Allow time for the client to respond. Do not assume the client is being uncooperative if the client makes no response or a delayed response.
- Give clients time to ask questions and clarify responses.
- Whenever possible, ask a family member or caregiver to join you and the client in the room. Such people are usually most familiar with the client's communication patterns and can assist in the communication process.

❖Nursing Diagnosis

Most individuals experience difficulty with some aspect of communication. People who are free of illness or disability may lack skills in attending, listening, responding, and self-expression. Often, you will direct your care toward individuals who experience more serious communication impairments.

The primary nursing diagnostic label used to describe the client with limited or no ability to communicate verbally is *impaired verbal communication*. This is the state in which the ability to receive, process, transmit, and use symbols is decreased or absent (Doenges et al., 2005). Defining characteristics include the inability to articulate words, inappropriate verbalization, difficulty forming words, and difficulty in comprehending, which the nurse clusters together to form the diagnosis. This diagnosis is useful for a wide variety of clients with special problems and needs related to communication, such as impaired perception, reception, and articulation. Although a client's primary problem may be impaired verbal communication, the associated difficulty in self-expression or altered communication patterns may also contribute to other nursing diagnoses:

- Anxiety
- Social isolation
- Ineffective coping
- Compromised family coping
- Powerlessness
- Impaired social interaction

The related (contributing) factors for a nursing diagnosis focus on the causes of the communication disorder. In the case of impaired verbal communication, these are physiological, mechanical, anatomical, psychological, cultural, or developmental in nature. Accuracy in the identification of related factors is necessary so that you can select interventions that can effectively resolve the diagnostic problem. For example, the diagnosis of *impaired verbal communication related to cultural difference* (Ukrainian heritage) would be managed very differently than the diagnosis of *impaired verbal communication related to deafness*.

❖Planning

Once you have identified the nature of the client's communication dysfunction, you must consider several factors as you design the nursing care plan. Motivation is a factor in improving communication, and clients often must be encouraged to try different approaches. It is especially important to involve the client and family in decisions about the plan of nursing care to determine whether suggested methods are acceptable. Make sure that basic comfort and safety needs are met before you introduce new communication methods and techniques, and allow plenty of time for practice. Participants must be patient with themselves and with each other when learning new skills if communication is to be effective. When the focus is on practising communication, it is best to arrange for a quiet, private place that is free of distractions such as television or visitors. Communication aids, such as a writing board for a client with a tracheostomy or a special call system for a paralyzed client, enhance communication.

Goals and Outcomes

The primary goal of nursing interventions is to facilitate the development of trust between the client and members of the health care team. It is important to identify expected outcomes for all clients, particularly when impaired communication is a concern. Outcomes are specific and measurable and provide the means to determine whether the broader goal is met. For example, outcomes for the client might be as follows:

- The client initiates conversation about diagnosis or health care problem.
- The client is able to attend to appropriate stimuli.
- The client conveys clear and understandable messages with family members and members of the health care team.
- The client expresses increased satisfaction with the communication process.

At times, you will care for well clients whose difficulty in sending, receiving, and interpreting messages interferes with healthy interpersonal relationships. In this case, impaired communication may be contributing to other nursing diagnoses such as *impaired social interaction* or *ineffective coping*. In such cases, you need to plan interventions to help your clients improve their communication skills. For example, you could model effective communication techniques and provide feedback regarding the client's communication. Role-play helps clients rehearse situations in which they have difficulty communicating. Expected outcomes for a client in this situation might include demonstrating the ability to appropriately express needs, feelings, and concerns; communicating thoughts and feelings more clearly; engaging in appropriate social conversation with peers and staff; and increasing feelings of autonomy and assertiveness.

Setting of Priorities

It is essential for the nurse to always be available for communication so that the client is able to express any pressing needs or problems. This may involve an intervention as simple as keeping a call light within reach for a client restricted to bed or providing a communication augmentative device for the client to use (e.g., message board, Braille keyboard). When you plan to have lengthy interactions with a client, it is important to address physical care priorities (i.e., pain or elimination needs) first, so that the client is comfortable and the discussion is not interrupted.

Continuity of Care

To ensure an effective care plan, you may need to collaborate with other members of the health care team who have expertise in communication strategies. Speech therapists help clients with aphasia, interpreters are often needed for clients who speak a foreign language, and psychiatric nurse specialists help angry or highly anxious clients communicate more effectively.

❖Implementation

In carrying out any care plan, nurses use communication techniques that are appropriate for the client's individual needs. Before learning how to adapt communication methods to help clients with serious communication impairments, it is necessary to learn the communication techniques that serve as the foundation for professional communication. It is also important to understand techniques that create barriers to effective interaction.

Therapeutic Communication Techniques

Therapeutic communication techniques are specific responses that encourage the expression of feelings and ideas and convey acceptance and respect. By learning these techniques, you develop awareness of the variety of nursing responses available for use in different situations. Although some of the techniques seem artificial at first, skill and comfort in using them increase with practice. Tremendous satisfaction will result from the development of therapeutic relationships and achievement of desired client outcomes.

Active Listening. **Active listening** means to be attentive to what the client is saying both verbally and nonverbally. Active listening enhances trust and facilitates client communication because it demonstrates acceptance and respect for the client. Several nonverbal skills facilitate attentive listening. They can be identified by the acronym *SOLER* (Townsend, 2005):

S: *Sit* facing the client. This posture indicates that you are there to listen and are interested in what the client is saying.
O: Keep an *open* posture (i.e., keep arms and legs uncrossed). This posture suggests that you are receptive ("open") to what the client has to say. A "closed" position may convey a defensive attitude, possibly invoking a similar response in the client.
L: *Lean* toward the client. This posture indicates that you are involved and interested in the interaction.
E: Establish and maintain intermittent *eye contact*. This behaviour conveys your involvement in and willingness to listen to what the client is saying. Absence of eye contact or shifting of the eyes indicates that you are not interested in what the client is saying.
R: *Relax*. It is important to communicate a sense of being relaxed and comfortable with the client. Restlessness communicates a lack of interest and also conveys a sense of discomfort that may extend to the client.

Sharing Observations. Nurses make observations by commenting on how the client looks, sounds, or acts. Stating observations often helps the client communicate without the need for extensive questioning, focusing, or clarification. This technique helps start a conversation with quiet or withdrawn people. Do not state observations that might anger, embarrass, or upset the client, such as telling someone "You look a mess!" Even if such an observation is made with humour, the client can become resentful.

Sharing observations differs from making assumptions, which means drawing unwarranted conclusions about the client without validating them. Making assumptions puts the client in the position of having to contradict the nurse. Examples might include the nurse interpreting fatigue as depression or assuming that untouched food indicates lack of interest in meeting nutritional goals. Making observations is a gentler and safer technique: "You look tired," "You seem different today," or "I see you haven't eaten anything."

Sharing Empathy. **Empathy** is the ability to emotionally and intellectually understand another person's reality, to accurately perceive unspoken feelings, and to communicate this understanding to the other person (Devito et al., 2005). Empathy is expressed when you reflect understanding of the other person's feelings. Cultivating an ability to empathize requires patience, a sense of curiosity, and a willingness to understand a client's viewpoint (Larson & Yao, 2005). Such empathic understanding requires you to be both sensitive and imaginative, especially if you have not had similar experiences. Although nurses are not always empathic, it is an important goal to work toward, a key to unlocking concern and communicating support for other people. Statements reflecting empathy are highly effective because they indicate that you heard the emotional content, as well as the factual content, of the communication. Empathy statements are neutral and nonjudgemental and help establish trust in difficult situations. For example, to an angry client who has limited mobility after a stroke, you might say, "It must be very frustrating to know what you want to do and not be able to do it."

Sharing Hope. You must recognize that hope is essential for healing, and you must learn to communicate a "sense of possibility" to other people. Appropriate encouragement and positive feedback are important in fostering hope and self-confidence and for helping people achieve their potential and reach their goals. You can instill hope by commenting on the positive aspects of the other person's behaviour, performance, or response. Sharing a vision of the future and reminding clients of their internal resources and coping abilities also strengthens hope. You can reassure clients that many kinds of hope exist and that meaning and personal growth can arise from illness experiences. For example, you might say to a client discouraged about a poor prognosis: "I believe you will find a way to face your situation, because I have seen your courage and creativity in the past."

Sharing Humour. Humour is an important but underused resource in nursing interactions. Research suggests that a sense of humour is a useful coping strategy for clients, health care professionals, and families (Wanzer et al., 2005) and an essential communication tool for nurses (Dziegielewski et al., 2004). Humour has been shown to have positive effects on both a person's psyche and physiology. Laughter signifies positive events to people and contributes to feelings of togetherness, closeness, and friendliness (Balzer Riley, 2004). Shulman and Haugo (2003) noted that humour positively influences the immune system by decreasing levels of stress-related hormones that suppress immune function and by increasing numbers of defensive immune cells. Humour fosters feelings of power and security, creates nurturing environments, provides a means for expressing empathy, and facilitates social bonding, intimacy, and conflict resolution. Chauvet and Hofmeyer (2006) found that humour also promoted health and well-being, strengthened social connections, enhanced communication, and fostered resilience and coping abilities. Humour is a social lubricant that facilitates therapeutic communication and interpersonal interactions. It reduces tension, increases trust, promotes social bonding, improves self-esteem, stimulates creativity, and broadens one's perspectives, thereby permitting cognitive reframing of difficult situations (Dziegielewski et al., 2004.

Today it is common for nurses to care for clients from different cultures. When nurses interact with clients who do not have a full grasp of the language, it is important to realize that their clients may misunderstand or misinterpret jokes and statements that are meant to be humorous. It is also important to recognize that when either a nurse or a client tries to speak in another language, mistakes can sometimes occur.

Health care professionals sometimes use negative humour after difficult or traumatic situations as a way to deal with extreme tension and stress. This coping humour has a high potential for misinterpretation as lack of caring by people not involved in the situation. For example, student nurses are sometimes offended and wonder how staff can laugh and joke after unsuccessful resuscitation efforts. When nurses use coping humour within earshot of clients or their loved ones, great emotional distress can result.

Sharing Feelings. Emotions are subjective feelings that result from thoughts and perceptions. Feelings are not right, wrong, good, or bad, although they may be pleasant or unpleasant. If individuals do not express their feelings, stress and illness may worsen. You can help clients express their emotions by making observations, acknowledging feelings, encouraging communication, giving them permission to express "negative" feelings, and modelling healthy emotional self-expression. At times, clients direct anger or frustration prompted by their illness toward nurses, who should not take such expressions personally. Acknowledging clients' feelings demonstrates empathy and communicates that you listened to and understood the emotional aspects of their illness situation.

When you care for clients, you must be aware of your own emotions because feelings are difficult to hide. Students may wonder whether it is helpful for nurses to share their feelings with clients. Sharing emotion makes nurses seem more human and often brings people closer. It is appropriate to share feelings of caring, or even cry with other people, as long as you are in control of the expression of those feelings and do so in a way that does not burden the client or break confidentiality. Clients are perceptive and can sense a nurse's emotions. It is usually inappropriate to discuss negative personal emotions such as anger or sadness with clients. A social support system of colleagues is helpful, and employee assistance programs, peer group meetings, and the use of interdisciplinary teams such as social work and pastoral care provide other means for nurses to safely express feelings away from clients.

Using Touch. In today's fast-paced technical environments, nurses are required more than ever to bring the sense of caring and human connection to their clients (see Chapter 19). Touch is one of the nurse's most potent forms of communication. Touch conveys many messages, such as affection, emotional support, encouragement, tenderness, and personal attention. Comfort touch, such as holding a hand, is especially important for vulnerable clients who are experiencing severe illness with its accompanying physical and emotional losses. Nurses often use touch with older people to provide comfort and reassurance (Gleeson & Timmins, 2004), to convey caring and consolation, to add emphasis to explanations, and to convey empathy in situations when speaking might break a mood (Arnold & Boggs, 2007). It is important for nurses to abide by cultural norms when interacting with clients from other cultures (Figure 18–2).

Students may initially find giving intimate care stressful, especially when caring for clients of the opposite gender. Students learn to cope with intimate contact by changing their perception of the situation. Because much of what nurses do involves touching, you must learn to be sensitive to other people's reactions to touch and use it wisely. Touch should be as gentle or as firm as needed and delivered in a comforting, nonthreatening manner. In certain situations, you must withhold touch, for example, when interacting with highly suspicious or angry people who may respond negatively or even violently when touched.

Using Silence. It takes time and experience to become comfortable with silence. Most people have a natural tendency to fill silences with words, but sometimes silences serve the need for time for the nurse and client to observe one another, sort out their feelings, think about how to say things, and consider what has been communicated. Silence prompts some people to talk. Silence allows clients to think and gain insight into their situations. In general, you should allow the client to break the silence, particularly when the client has initiated it (Stuart & Laraia, 2005).

Silence is particularly useful when people are confronted with decisions that require much thought. For example, silence may help a client gain confidence needed to share the decision to refuse medical treatment. Silence also allows the nurse to pay particular attention to nonverbal messages such as worried expressions or loss of eye contact. Remaining silent demonstrates the nurse's patience and willingness to wait for a response when the other person is unable to reply quickly. Silence may be especially therapeutic during times of profound sadness or grief (Box 18–8).

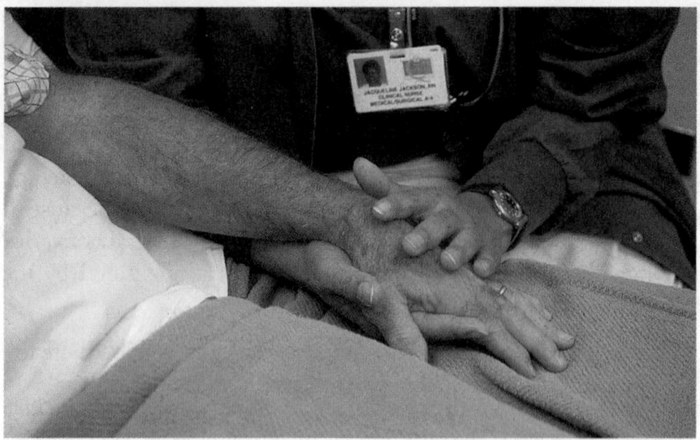

Figure 18-2 The nurse uses touch to communicate.

Providing Information. Providing relevant information that the client needs or wants to know empowers the client to make informed decisions, experience less anxiety, and feel safe and secure. It is also an integral aspect of health teaching. Hiding information from clients is not usually helpful, particularly when they are seeking it. If a physician withholds information, you need to clarify the reason with the physician. Clients have a right to know about their health status and what is happening in their environment. Information of a distressing nature needs to be communicated with sensitivity, at a pace appropriate to what the client can absorb, and in general terms at first: "John, your heart sounds have changed from earlier today, and so has your blood pressure. I'll let your doctor know." It is important to provide information that enables clients to understand what is happening and what to expect: "Ms. Evans, John is getting an echocardiogram right now. This test uses painless sound waves to create a moving picture of his heart structures and valves and should tell us what is causing his murmur."

BOX 18-8 NURSING STORY

Communication With a Dying Client

A young third-year nursing student who was assigned to care for a dying client came to me, as her nursing instructor, to discuss her assignment. The student nurse appeared to be anxious and distraught and was tearful. She requested a change of assignment and, when asked why she felt she needed to be moved, she stated: "I just don't know what I'm supposed to be *doing* with her. She is asking for her family, but they aren't here. She's dying and I just don't know what to do to *help* her." I asked the student what she was doing while she was in the room and she said: "I'm just sitting there holding her hand and listening to her when she's awake. She really isn't talking much, and she drifts off to sleep a lot, but she's afraid of being left alone, so I'm just holding her hand and letting her know I'm there, even when she's sleeping; that way she'll know she's not alone whenever she wakes up. I make sure she's comfortable but I don't know what else she needs. I'm just not *doing* anything." As I looked into her tear-filled eyes, I simply asked her: "So, what makes you think you aren't doing anything?" Communication involves so much more than dialogue. In this case, communication involved very little verbal interaction; it involved active listening, shared empathy, comfort care, gentle touch, silence, presence, and "being with," as the student compassionately accompanied the client through her final stage of life and assisted with her transition into death.

Clarifying. To check whether understanding is accurate, restate an unclear or ambiguous message to clarify the sender's meaning or ask the other person to rephrase it, explain further, or give an example of what he or she means. Without clarification, you may make invalid assumptions and miss valuable information. Despite efforts at paraphrasing, you sometimes will still not understand the client's message and should let the client know that this is the case: "I'm not sure I understand what you mean by 'sicker than usual.' What is different now?"

Focusing. Focusing centres on key elements or concepts of a message. If conversation is vague or rambling or if clients begin to repeat themselves, focusing is a useful technique. Do not use focusing if it interrupts clients while they are discussing an important issue. Rather, use focusing to guide the direction of conversation to important areas: "We've talked a lot about your medications, but let's look more closely at the trouble you're having in taking them on time."

Paraphrasing. Paraphrasing is restating another person's message more briefly in your own words. Through paraphrasing, you let the client know you are actively involved in the search for understanding. Practice is required to paraphrase accurately. If the meaning of a message is changed or distorted through paraphrasing, communication becomes ineffective. For example, a client may say, "I've been overweight all my life and never had any problems. I can't understand why I need to be on a diet." Paraphrasing this statement by saying, "You don't care if you're overweight or not," is incorrect. It would be more accurate to say, "You're not convinced you need a diet because you've stayed healthy."

Asking Relevant Questions. Nurses ask relevant questions to seek information needed for decision making. You should ask only one question at a time and fully explore one topic before moving to another area. During client assessment, questions should follow a logical sequence and proceed from general to more specific. Open-ended questions allow the client to take the conversational lead and introduce pertinent information about a topic. For example, "What's your biggest concern at the moment?" Focused questions are used when more specific information is needed in an area: "How has your pain affected your life at home?" Allow clients to fully respond to an open-ended question before asking more focused questions. Closed-ended questions elicit "yes," "no," or one-word responses: "How many times a day are you taking pain medication?" Although they are helpful during assessment, they are generally less useful during therapeutic exchanges.

Asking too many questions is sometimes dehumanizing. Seeking primarily factual information does not allow you or your client to establish a meaningful relationship or deal with important emotional issues. It is a way to ignore uncomfortable areas in favour of more comfortable, neutral topics. A useful exercise is to try conversing without asking the other person a single question. By giving general leads ("Tell me about it."), making observations, paraphrasing, focusing, providing information, and so forth, you may discover important information that would have remained hidden if communication were limited primarily to questions.

Summarizing. Summarizing is a concise review of key aspects of an interaction. Summarizing brings a sense of satisfaction and closure to an individual conversation and is especially helpful during the termination phase of a nurse–client relationship. By reviewing a conversation, participants focus on key issues and add additional relevant information as needed. Beginning a new interaction by summarizing a previous one helps the client recall topics discussed and shows the client that you have analyzed the communication. Summarizing also clarifies expectations, as in this example of a nurse manager who has been working with a dissatisfied employee: "You've told me a lot of reasons about why you don't like this job and how unhappy you've been. We've also come up with some possible ways to make the situation better, and you've agreed to try some and let me know if any of them help."

Self-Disclosure. Self-disclosures are subjectively true, personal experiences about the self that are intentionally revealed to another person. This is not therapy for the nurse; rather, it shows clients that you understand and that their experiences are not unique. You may choose to share experiences or feelings that are similar to those of the client and emphasize both the similarities and differences. This kind of self-disclosure is indicative of the closeness of the nurse–client relationship and involves a particular kind of respect for the client. It is offered as an expression of genuineness and honesty and is an aspect of empathy (Stuart & Laraia, 2005). Self-disclosure should be relevant and appropriate and made to benefit the client. Self-disclosure should be used sparingly so that the client remains the focus of the interaction: "That happened to me once, too. I was devastated . . . . I went for counselling, and it really helped. What are your thoughts about seeing a counsellor?"

Confrontation. To confront someone in a therapeutic way, you help the other person become more aware of inconsistencies in his or her feelings, attitudes, beliefs, and behaviours (Stuart & Laraia, 2005). This technique improves client self-awareness and helps the client recognize growth and deal with important issues. Confrontation should be used only after you have established a trusting relationship with the client, and it requires gentleness and sensitivity: "You say you've already decided what to do, but you're still talking a lot about your options."

Nontherapeutic Communication Techniques

Certain communication techniques hinder or damage professional relationships. These specific techniques are referred to as *nontherapeutic* or *blocking* and will often cause recipients to activate defences to avoid being hurt or negatively affected. Nontherapeutic techniques tend to discourage further expression of feelings and ideas and may engender negative responses or behaviours in other people.

Asking Personal Questions. Asking personal questions that are not relevant to the situation but simply to satisfy your curiosity (e.g., "Why don't you and John get married?") is not appropriate professional communication. Such questions are invasive and unnecessary. If clients wish to share private information, they will. To learn more about the client's interpersonal roles and relationships, ask a question such as "How would you describe your relationship with John?"

Giving Personal Opinions. When you provide a personal opinion (e.g., "If I were you, I'd put your mother in a long-term care facility"), it takes decision making away from the client. It inhibits spontaneity, stalls problem solving, and creates doubt. Personal opinions differ from professional advice. At times, clients need suggestions and help to make choices. Suggestions should be presented to clients as options because the final decision rests with the client. Remember that the problem and its solution belong to the client. A much better response is "Let's talk about what options are available for your mother's care."

Changing the Subject. When another person is trying to communicate something important, changing the subject (e.g., "Let's not talk about your problems with the insurance company. It's time for your walk") is rude and shows a lack of empathy. It tends to block further communication, and the sender then withholds important messages or fails to openly express feelings. Thoughts and spontaneity are interrupted, ideas become tangled, and information provided may be inadequate. In some instances, changing the subject serves as a face-saving manoeuvre. If this happens, reassure the client that you will return to his or her concerns: "After your walk, let's talk some more about what's going on with your insurance company."

Automatic Responses. Stereotypes (e.g., "Older adults are always confused" or "Administration doesn't care about the staff") are generalized beliefs held about people. Making stereotyping remarks about other people reflects poor nursing judgement and can threaten nurse–client or nurse–team relationships. A cliché is a generalizing comment such as "You can't win them all" that tends to belittle the other person's feelings and minimize the importance of his or her message. These automatic phrases communicate that you are not taking concerns seriously or responding thoughtfully. Another kind of automatic response is parroting, repeating what the other person has said, word for word. Parroting is easily overused and is not as effective as paraphrasing. If the client says something that takes you by surprise, responding simply "Oh?" will give you time to think.

A nurse who is excessively task oriented automatically makes the task or procedure the entire focus of interaction with clients, missing opportunities to communicate with them as individuals and meet their needs. Task-oriented nurses are often perceived as cold, uncaring, and unapproachable. When you first perform technical tasks, you may have difficulty integrating therapeutic communication because of your need to focus on the procedure. In time, you will learn to integrate communication with high-visibility tasks and accomplish several goals simultaneously.

False Reassurance. When a client is seriously ill or distressed, you may be tempted to offer hope to the client with statements such as "Don't worry, everything will be all right"; "You'll be fine"; or "You have nothing to worry about." When a client is reaching for understanding, false reassurance discourages open communication. Offering reassurance not supported by facts or based in reality does more harm than good. Although you may be attempting to be kind, such reassurance has the secondary effect of helping you avoid the client's distress, tends to block conversation, and discourages further expression of feelings. A more facilitative nursing response is "It must be difficult not to know what the surgeon will find. What might be helpful to you at this time?"

Sympathy. Sympathy is concern, sorrow, sadness, or pity felt for the client generated by personal identification with the client's needs (Grover, 2005). Sympathy is a subjective vision of another person's viewpoint that prevents a clear perspective of the issues confronting that person. If you over-identify with the client (e.g., "I'm so sorry about your mastectomy; it must be terrible to lose a breast"), you will lose objectivity and be unable to effectively help the client work through his or her situation (Arnold & Boggs, 2007). Although sympathy is a compassionate response to another's situation, it is not as therapeutic as empathy. Your own emotional issues may prevent effective problem solving and impair your judgement. A more empathetic approach is "The loss of a breast is a major change. How do you think it will affect your life?"

Asking for Explanations. You may be tempted to ask your client to explain why he or she believes, feels, or has acted in a certain way (e.g., "Why are you so anxious?"). Clients frequently interpret "why" questions as accusations or think you already know the reason and are simply testing them. "Why" questions tend to interrupt clients' descriptions of their feelings and experience and cause them to refocus their energy into intellectual or defensive responses (Shattell & Hogan, 2005). Regardless of your motivation, "why" questions can cause resentment, insecurity, and mistrust. If you require additional information, it is best to phrase your questions to avoid using the word "why": "You seem upset. What's on your mind?" is more likely to help the anxious client to communicate.

Approval or Disapproval. Do not impose your personal attitudes, values, beliefs, and moral standards on other people while in the professional helping role (e.g., "You shouldn't even think about assisted suicide; it's not right"). Other people have the right to speak their minds and make their own decisions. Judgemental responses often contain terms such as *should, ought, good, bad, right,* and *wrong.* Agreeing or disagreeing conveys the subtle message that you are making value judgements about the client's decisions. Approving implies that the behaviour being praised is the only acceptable one. Often the client shares a decision not in an effort to seek approval but to provide a means to discuss feelings. On the other hand, disapproving implies that the client needs to meet your expectations or standards. Instead, help clients explore their own beliefs and decisions. The nursing response "I'm surprised you're considering assisted suicide; tell me more" gives the client a chance to express ideas or feelings without fear of being judged.

Defensive Responses. Becoming defensive in response to criticism (e.g., "No one here would intentionally lie to you") implies that the other person has no right to an opinion. The sender's concerns are ignored when you focus on the need for self-defence, defence of the health care team, or defence of other people. When clients express criticism, it is important to listen to what they have to say. Listening does not imply agreement. To discover reasons for the client's anger or dissatisfaction, you must listen uncritically. By avoiding defensiveness, you can defuse anger and uncover deeper concerns: "It sounds as if you believe people have been dishonest with you. That must make it difficult for you to trust anyone."

Passive or Aggressive Responses. Passive responses (e.g., "Things are bad, and I can't do anything about it") serve to avoid conflict or sidestep issues. They reflect feelings of sadness, depression, anxiety, powerlessness, and hopelessness. Aggressive responses (e.g., "Things are bad, and it's all your fault") provoke confrontation at the other person's expense and reflect feelings of anger, frustration, resentment, and stress. When nurses lack assertiveness skills, they may also use triangulation, complaining to a third party rather than confronting the problem or expressing concerns directly to the source. This lowers team morale and draws other people into the conflict situation. Assertive communication is a far more professional approach to take.

Arguing. Challenging or arguing against perceptions (e.g., "How can you say you didn't sleep a wink, when I heard you snoring all night long?") denies that they are real and valid to the other person. They imply that the other person is lying, misinformed, or uneducated. Skillful nurses give information or present reality in a way that avoids argument: "You feel as if you didn't get any rest at all last night, even though I thought you slept well because you seemed peaceful when I checked your room during the night."

Adapting Communication Techniques for the Client With Special Needs

With Canada's steadily aging population, increasing numbers of clients have visual, hearing, and speech impairments or other difficulties communicating. Interacting effectively with clients who have conditions that impair communication requires special thought and sensitivity. Such clients benefit greatly when you adapt communication techniques to their unique circumstances or developmental level. For example, if you are caring for a client with impaired verbal communication related to cultural differences, you can provide a table of simple words in the client's language. You and the client can use the table to help communicate about basic needs such as food, water, toileting, pain relief, sleep, and so forth. Similar techniques can be used with clients suffering with aphasia or some dementias (Goldfarb & Santo Pietro, 2004). Research findings suggest that many of the difficulties in communicating with clients with severe communication impairment arise from the lack of an understandable nurse–client communication system.

Clients who are deaf or hard of hearing have the greatest risk for miscommunication with health care professionals (Meador & Zazove, 2005). For some people, being deaf may seem worse than being blind because being blind isolates people from things but being deaf isolates people from other people. In a study of people who were deaf or hard of hearing, findings suggested that one of the most important actions of the nurse was to ask the client how best to communicate with him or her (Iezzoni et al., 2004).

You need to direct nursing actions toward meeting the goals and expected outcomes identified in the plan of care, addressing both the communication impairment and its contributing factors. Box 18–9 lists many methods available to encourage, enhance, restore, or substitute

➤ BOX 18-9 Communicating With Clients Who Have Special Needs

Clients Who Cannot Speak Clearly (Aphasia, Dysarthria, Muteness)

Listen attentively, be patient, and do not interrupt.
Ask simple questions that require "yes" or "no" answers.
Allow time for understanding and response.
Use visual cues (e.g., words, pictures, and objects) when possible.
Allow only one person to speak at a time.
Do not shout or speak too loudly.
Encourage the client to converse.
If you have not understood the client, let him or her know.
Collaborate with a speech therapist as needed.
Use communication aids:

- Pad and felt-tipped pen or Magic Slate
- Communication board with commonly used words, letters, or pictures denoting basic needs
- Call bells or alarms
- Sign language
- Use of eye blinks or movement of fingers for simple responses ("yes" or "no")

Clients Who Are Cognitively Impaired

Reduce environmental distractions while conversing.
Capture client's attention before you speak.
Use simple sentences, and avoid long explanations.
Ask one question at a time.
Allow time for the client to respond.
Be an attentive listener.
Include family and friends in conversations, especially in topics known to the client.

Clients Who Are Hearing Impaired

Check for the presence of hearing aids and glasses.
Reduce environmental noise.
Get the client's attention before you speak.
Face the client so that your mouth is visible.
Do not chew gum.
Speak at normal volume; do not shout.
Rephrase rather than repeat, if your message is misunderstood.
Provide a sign language interpreter if this is indicated.

Clients Who Are Visually Impaired

Check for use of glasses or contact lenses.
Identify yourself when you enter room, and notify client when you leave room.
Speak in a normal tone of voice.
Do not rely on gestures or nonverbal communication to convey messages.
Use indirect lighting, avoiding glare.
Use at least 14-point print.

Clients Who Are Unresponsive

Call the client by name during interactions.
Communicate both verbally and by touch.
Speak to the client as though he or she can hear.
Explain all procedures and expected sensations.
Provide orientation to person, place, and time.
Avoid talking about client to other people in his or her presence.
Avoid saying things that the client should not hear (e.g., gossip or speculations about client's condition).
Always assume that clients can hear and understand everything said at their bedside.

Clients Who Do Not Speak English

Speak to the client in a normal tone of voice (shouting may be interpreted as anger).
Establish a method for the client to signal a desire to communicate (call light or bell).
Provide an interpreter (translator) as needed.
Avoid using family members, especially children, as interpreters.
Develop communication board, pictures, or cards.
Translate words from the English list into the client's native language for the client to make basic requests.
Ensure that a dictionary (English–French, English–Cree, and so forth) is available if client can read.

for verbal communication. You must be sure that the client is physically able to use the chosen method and that it does not cause frustration by being too complicated or difficult.

Because nursing care of the older adult is ideally provided through an interdisciplinary model, your primary goal is to establish a reliable communication system that is easily understood by all members of the health care team. Effective communication involves adapting to any special needs resulting from sensory, motor, or cognitive impairments that are present. You can also encourage older adults to share life stories and reminisce about the past, which has a therapeutic effect and increases their sense of well-being. Avoid sudden shifts from topic to topic. It is helpful to include the client's family and friends and to become familiar with the client's favourite topics for conversation.

❖Evaluation

To determine whether the plan of care has been successful, both the nurse and the client evaluate the client's communication outcomes. You need to evaluate nursing interventions to determine what strategies or interventions were effective and what changes in the client's situation resulted because of the interventions. For example, if using a pen and paper proves frustrating for a nonverbal client whose handwriting is shaky, you need to revise the care plan to include use of a picture board instead. If expected outcomes are not met or progress is not satisfactory, you need to determine what factors influenced the outcomes and then modify the plan of care.

You can evaluate the effectiveness of your own communication by videotaping practice sessions with peers, making process recordings, and analyzing written records of your verbal and nonverbal interactions with clients. Process recording analysis reveals faults in personal communication techniques, so that you can improve their effectiveness. Box 18–10 contains a sample communication analysis of such a record. Analyzing a process recording enables you to evaluate the following:

- Determine whether the nurse encouraged openness and allowed the client to "tell his or her story," expressing both thoughts and feelings.
- Identify any missed verbal or nonverbal cues or conversational themes.
- Examine whether nursing responses blocked or facilitated the client's efforts to communicate.
- Determine whether nursing responses were positive and supportive or superficial and judgemental.
- Examine the type and number of questions that were asked.
- Determine the type and number of therapeutic communication techniques used.
- Discover any missed opportunities to use humour, silence, or touch.

Evaluation of the communication process helps you gain confidence and competence in interpersonal skills. Becoming an effective communicator greatly increases your professional satisfaction and success. No skill is more basic, and no tool more powerful, than communication.

➤ BOX 18-10 Sample Communication Analysis

NURSE: Good morning, Mr. Simpson. [*Smiles and approaches bed, holding clipboard*]
- Acknowledging by name, social greeting to begin conversation

CLIENT: What's good about it? [*Arms crossed over chest, frowning, with a direct stare*]
- Nonverbal signs of anger

NURSE: You sound unhappy. [*Pulls up chair and sits at bedside*]
- Sharing observation, nonverbal communication of availability

CLIENT: You'd be unhappy, too, if nobody would answer your questions. [*Angry tone of voice, challenging expression*]
- Further expression of feelings, facilitated by nurse's accurate observation

NURSE: This hospital has a fine staff, Mr. Simpson. I'm sure no one would intentionally keep information from you.
- Feeling threatened and being defensive: a nontherapeutic technique

CLIENT: All right, then: Why wouldn't that girl tell me what my blood sugar was?

NURSE: I'm not sure. If I were you, I'd forget about it and get a fresh start.
- Giving advice and using cliché, which is nontherapeutic; would have been better to acknowledge that client had a right to know the information

NURSE: I'm going to test your blood sugar levels in a minute, and I'll tell you the results. [*Performs test*] Your blood sugar level was 20.
- Providing information, demonstrating trustworthiness

CLIENT: That's up pretty high, isn't it? [*Worried facial expression*]
- Feeling very concerned about test results

NURSE: [*Nods; long pause*]
- Nonverbal affirmation, use of silence to allow client time to absorb information and gather thoughts

CLIENT: I'm so afraid complications will set in because my blood sugar is high. [*Stares out window*]
- Feeling free to express deeper concerns, which are hard to face

NURSE: What kinds of things are you worried about?
- Open-ended question to elicit information

CLIENT: I could lose a leg, as my mother did. Or go blind. Or have to live hooked up to a kidney machine for the rest of my life.

NURSE: You've been thinking about all kinds of things that could go wrong, and it adds to your worry not to be told what your blood sugar is.
- Summarizing to let client "hear" what he has communicated

CLIENT: I always think the worst. [*Shakes head in exasperation*]
- Expressing insight into his "inner dialogue"

NURSE: I'll pass along to the technician that it's OK to tell you your blood sugar levels. And later this afternoon, I'd like us to talk more about some things you can do to help avoid these complications and set some goals for controlling your blood sugar. [*Stands up, keeps looking at client*]
- Providing information, encouraging collaboration and goal setting; giving nonverbal cue that conversation is nearing end

CLIENT: OK, I'll see you later.

✻ KEY CONCEPTS

- Communication is a powerful therapeutic tool and an essential nursing skill used to influence other people and achieve positive health care outcomes.
- Communication involves the entire human being: body, mind, emotions, and spirit.
- Critical thinking facilitates communication through creative inquiry, focused self-awareness and awareness of other people, purposeful analysis, and control of perceptual biases.
- Nurses consider many contexts and factors influencing communication when making decisions about what, when, where, how, why, and with whom to communicate.
- Nurses use intrapersonal, interpersonal, transpersonal, small-group, and public interaction to achieve positive change and health goals.
- Communication is most effective when the receiver and sender accurately perceive the meaning of each other's messages.
- Message transmission is influenced by the sender's and receiver's physical and developmental status, perceptions, values, emotions, knowledge, sociocultural background, roles, and environment.
- Effective verbal communication requires appropriate vocabulary, intonation, clear and concise phrasing, proper pacing of statements, and proper timing and relevance of a message.
- Nonverbal communication often conveys the true meaning of a message more accurately than verbal communication.
- Helping relationships are strengthened when the nurse demonstrates caring by establishing trust, empathy, autonomy, confidentiality, and professional competence.
- Effective communication techniques are facilitative and tend to encourage the other person to openly express ideas, feelings, or concerns.
- Ineffective communication techniques are inhibitive and tend to block the other person's willingness to openly express ideas, feelings, or concerns.
- The nurse must blend social and informational interactions with therapeutic communication techniques so that other people can explore feelings and manage health issues.
- Older adult clients with sensory, motor, or cognitive impairments require the adaptation of communication techniques to compensate for their loss of function and special needs.
- Clients with impaired verbal communication require special consideration and alterations in communication techniques to facilitate the sending, receiving, and interpreting of messages.
- Desired outcomes for clients with impaired verbal communication include increased satisfaction with interpersonal interactions, the ability to send and receive clear messages, and attending to and accurately interpreting verbal and nonverbal cues.

✻ CRITICAL THINKING EXERCISES

1. Ms. Mary Goodrunning, an Aboriginal Canadian of Chipewyan descent, must learn how to manage her diabetes mellitus and self-administer insulin injections. What communication techniques could you use to help her?

2. Jan, a nurse colleague of Mary Ellen, is having difficulty interacting assertively with Dr. Fielding, a physician who has an abrupt, intimidating communication style. Jan frequently complains of tension headaches, pent-up anger, and crying easily. What can Mary Ellen do to help Jan?

3. Mr. Hess, a client with Parkinson's disease living at a long-term care facility, has a stiff, expressionless face as a result of his disease. He sits slumped in a recliner chair all day and seems lost in his own world, rarely looking at or interacting with anyone. When he does talk, he mumbles in a soft voice, and his words are difficult to understand. What nursing interventions could you use to establish a helping-healing relationship with Mr. Hess?

4. Ms. Velma Eberhard, a member of a Hutterite colony in western Canada, is considering whether she should have her two young children immunized before they begin attending school. What communication techniques could you use to help her decide, and what traps must you avoid in such a situation?

5. Ms. Esther Simons, a client who is receiving palliative care, confides in you that she feels overwhelmed with the number of issues she must attend to, now that she's facing the possibility of death. She says, "My thoughts are all over the place. I don't know where to start." What communication techniques, based on the critical thinking model, can you use to help her at this point?

✻ REVIEW QUESTIONS

1. Communication is not about the message that was intended but rather the message that was received. The statement that best helps explain this is as follows:
   1. Clear communication can ensure the client will receive the message intended.
   2. Sincerity in communication is the responsibility of the sender and the receiver.
   3. Attention to personal space can minimize misinterpretation of communication.
   4. Contextual factors, such as attitudes, values, beliefs, and self-concept, influence communication.

2. As a nurse, you would demonstrates active listening by
   1. Agreeing with the client
   2. Repeating everything the client says to clarify
   3. Assuming a relaxed posture, establishing eye contact, and leaning toward the client
   4. Smiling and nodding continuously throughout the interview

3. During the orientation phase of the helping relationship, you might
   1. Discuss the cards and flowers in the room
   2. Work together with the client to establish goals
   3. Review the client's history to identify possible health concerns
   4. Use therapeutic communication to manage the client's confusion

4. If you are working with a client who has expressive aphasia, it would be most helpful for you to
   1. Ask open-ended questions
   2. Speak loudly and use simple sentences
   3. Allow extra time for the client to respond
   4. Encourage a family member to answer for the client

5. The statement that best explains the role of collaboration with other members of the health care team for the client's plan of care is that the professional nurse
   1. Collaborates with colleagues and the client's family to provide combined expertise in planning care
   2. Consults the physician for direction in establishing goals for clients
   3. Depends on the latest literature to complete an excellent plan of care for clients
   4. Works independently to plan and deliver care and does not depend on other staff for assistance
6. "I'm not sure I understand what you mean by 'sicker than usual.' What is different now?" This statement reflects the therapeutic technique of
   1. Paraphrasing
   2. Providing information
   3. Clarifying
   4. Focusing
7. "We've talked a lot about your medications, but let's look more closely at the trouble you're having in taking them on time." In this situation, you would be using the therapeutic technique of
   1. Paraphrasing
   2. Providing information
   3. Clarifying
   4. Focusing
8. As a nursing student, you give yourself positive messages regarding your ability to do well on a test. This type of communication is
   1. Public
   2. Intrapersonal
   3. Interpersonal
   4. Transpersonal
9. When working with an older adult, you should remember to avoid
   1. Touching the client
   2. Shifting from subject to subject
   3. Allowing the client to reminisce
   4. Asking the client how he or she feels
10. You should consider zones of personal space and touch when caring for clients. If you are taking the client's nursing history, you should be
    1. 0 to 45 cm from the client
    2. 45 cm to 1 m from the client
    3. 1 to 4 m from the client
    4. 4 m or farther from the client

* RECOMMENDED WEB SITES

American Sign Language Browser: http://www.commtechlab.msu.edu/sites/aslweb/browser.htm
This Web site provides an English and manual alphabet and dictionary, a brief history of sign language, and links to other relevant Web sites.

Communicative Disorders Assistant Association of Canada: http://www.cdaac.ca/links.htm
This Web site provides links to various Canadian and international resources for people with conditions that affect communication.

Hutterites and Peaceful Societies: http://www.hutterites.org/organizationStructure.htm; http://www.peacefulsocieties.org/Society/Hutter.HTML
Both of these Web sites provide links to articles and resources about Hutterite culture and social organization.

Jest for the Health of It!: http://www.jesthealth.com
This Web site provides links to articles and resources about using therapeutic humour in nursing practice.

Medscape: http://www.medscape.com/px/urlinfo
Medscape is a resource for physicians and nurses that requires a one-time registration (free of charge) and offers links to current literature on numerous health care topics. Enter "Communication" in the search frame, and the site will list current articles on communication in health care.

National Institute on Deafness and Other Communication Disorders: http://www.nidcd.nih.gov/
Part of the National Institutes of Health (NIH) in the United States, the National Institute on Deafness and Other Communication Disorders (NIDCD) is mandated to conduct and support biomedical and behavioural research and research training in the normal and disordered processes of hearing, balance, smell, taste, voice, speech, and language.

19

Caring in Nursing Practice

Original chapter by Anne G. Perry, RN, EdD, FAAN

Canadian content written by Cheryl Sams, RN, BScN, MSN

objectives

Mastery of content in this chapter will enable you to:

- Define the key terms listed.
- Discuss the role that caring plays in building a nurse–client relationship.
- Compare and contrast theories on the concept of caring.
- Discuss the potential implications when nurses' perceptions of caring differ from the clients' perceptions of caring.
- Explain how an ethic of care influences nurses' decision making.
- Describe ways to express caring through presence and touch.
- Describe the therapeutic benefit of listening to clients.
- Explain the relationship between knowing a client and clinical decision making.

key terms

Caring, p. 266
Comfort, p. 271
Cultural aspects of care, p. 267
Ethic of care, p. 270
Presence, p. 271
Transcultural, p. 266
Transformative, p. 267

media resources

evolve Web Site

- Audio Chapter Summaries
- Glossary
- Multiple-Choice Review Questions
- Student Learning Activities
- Weblinks

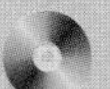
Companion CD

- Glossary
- Interactive Learning Activities
- Fluids and Electrolytes Tutorial
- Test-Taking Skills

Caring is central to nursing practice, and it is of great importance because of today's hectic health care environment. The demands, pressure, and time constraints in the health care environment leave little room for caring practice; as a result, nurses and other health care professionals may become cold and indifferent to clients' needs (Watson 2006a). Cara (2003) believed that the current health care climate, with its emphasis on restructuring, threatens to dehumanize client care. She stressed that the nursing profession must ensure that caring continues to be a strong force within all areas of nursing: in the clinical, administrative, educational, and research fields. Increasing use of technological advances for rapid diagnosis and treatment often causes nurses and other health care professionals to perceive their relationship with the client as relatively unimportant. Technological advances become dangerous without a context of skillful and compassionate care. Caring practices and expert knowledge that are at the heart of competent nursing practice must be valued and embraced (Benner & Wrubel, 1989; Lesniak, 2005). When you engage clients in a caring and compassionate manner, you learn that the therapeutic gains in the health and well-being of your clients are enormous.

Think about your own experiences of being ill or having a problem that necessitated health care intervention. Then consider the following two scenarios, and select the situation that you believe most successfully demonstrates a sense of caring.

A nurse enters a client's room, greets the client warmly while touching the client lightly on the shoulder, makes eye contact, sits down for a few minutes, and asks about the client's thoughts and concerns. The nurse listens to the client's story, looks at the intravenous solution being administered, briefly examines the client, and then checks the vital sign summary on the bedside computer screen before departing the room.

A second nurse enters the client's room, looks at the intravenous solution being administered, checks the vital sign summary sheet on the bedside computer screen, and acknowledges the client but never sits down or touches the client. The nurse makes eye contact from above while the client is in the vulnerable horizontal position. The nurse asks a few brief questions about the client's symptoms and then leaves.

The first scenario depicts the nurse in specific acts of caring. The nurse's calm presence, parallel eye contact, attention to the client's concerns, and physical closeness all express a client-centred, comforting approach. In contrast, the second scenario is task-oriented and expresses a sense of indifference to the client's concerns. During times of illness or when a person seeks the professional guidance of a nurse, caring is essential in helping the individual reach positive outcomes.

Theoretical Views on Caring

Caring is a universal phenomenon influencing the ways in which people think, feel, and behave in relation to one another. Since the time of Florence Nightingale, nurses have studied caring from a variety of philosophical and ethical perspectives. A number of nursing scholars developed theories about caring because of its importance to the practice of nursing. This chapter does not detail all of the theoretical positions on caring, but it helps you understand why caring is at the heart of your ability to work with all clients in a respectful and therapeutic way.

Caring Is Primary

Benner (1984) and Benner and Wrubel (1989) offered nurses a rich, holistic understanding of nursing practice and caring through the interpretation of expert nurses' stories. After listening to nurses' stories and analyzing their meaning, Benner described caring as the essence of professional nursing practice. The stories revealed the nurses' behaviour and decisions that expressed caring. *Caring* means concern about a person, events, projects, and things (Benner & Wrubel, 1989). It is a word for being connected.

Caring reflects what matters to a person; it describes a wide range of involvements, from parental love to friendship, from caring for one's work to caring for one's pet, to caring for and about one's clients. Benner and Wrubel (1989, p. 1) noted, "Caring creates possibility." Personal concern for another person, an event, or a thing provides motivation and direction for people to care. Caring as a framework has practical implications for transforming nursing practice (Boykin et al., 2003). Caring is an inherent feature of nursing practice whereby nurses help clients recover from illness, give meaning to that illness, and maintain or re-establish connection with other people. Caring helps nurses identify successful interventions, and this concern then guides future caregiving.

Each individual client has a unique background of experiences, values, and cultural perspectives. As you acquire more experience, you learn that caring helps you focus on the clients for whom you are caring. Caring facilitates your ability to understand a client, which enables you to recognize a client's problems and to find and implement individualized solutions.

In addition to their work in understanding caring, Benner and Wrubel (1989) described the relationship between health, illness, and disease. Health is not the absence of illness, nor is illness identical to disease (see Chapter 1 for further information). Health is a state of being that people define in relation to their own values, personality, and lifestyle. Health exists along a continuum. Illness is the experience of loss or dysfunction, whereas disease is the manifestation of an abnormality at the cellular, tissue, or organ level. Some clients have a disease (e.g., arthritis or diabetes) but do not experience the sense of being ill or a decrease in function. Some individuals do not seek health care until they experience a disruption, loss, or concern. For example, a client who has had diabetes for a number of years may not sense being ill until the disease causes serious visual impairment, which threatens the ability to work. Illness therefore has meaning only within the context of the person's life.

Because illness is the human experience of loss or dysfunction, any treatment or intervention given without consideration of its meaning to an individual is likely to be worthless. Expert nurses understand the difference between health, illness, and disease. Through caring relationships, you learn to listen to clients' stories about their illness so that you obtain an understanding of the meaning of illness to them. With this understanding, you provide therapeutic, client-centred care.

The Essence of Nursing and Health

From a **transcultural** perspective, Leininger (1978) described the concept of care as the essence and the central, unifying, and dominant domain that distinguishes nursing from other health disciplines. Care is an essential human need, necessary to the health and survival of all individuals. Care, unlike cure, assists an individual or group in improving a human condition. Acts of caring are the nurturant and skillful activities, processes, and decisions to assist people in ways that are empathetic, compassionate, and supportive. An act of caring is dependent on the needs, problems, and values of the client. Leininger's studies of numerous world cultures have revealed that care helps protect, develop, and nurture people and enable them to survive. Care is vital to recovery from illness and to the maintenance of healthy life practices in all cultures.

Leininger (1988) stressed the importance of understanding cultural caring behaviours and other **cultural aspects of care**. Event though caring is a universal phenomenon, the expressions, processes, and patterns of caring vary among cultures (Box 19–1). Caring is very personal, and thus expressions of caring differ for each client. For caring to be effective and meaningful to clients, you need to learn culturally specific behaviours and words that reflect human caring in different cultures. Refer to Chapter 10 for more information on culture and ethnicity.

Transpersonal Caring

Clients and their families should receive high-quality human interaction with nurses. Unfortunately, many of the conversations occurring between clients and their nurses are brief and disconnected. According to Watson's (1979, 1988, 2008) theory of caring (a holistic nursing model), a conscious intention to care promotes healing and wholeness (Hoover, 2002). This intention is complementary to conventional science and modern nursing practices. The theory integrates human caring processes with healing environments, incorporating the life-generating and life-receiving processes of human caring and healing for both nurses and their clients (Watson, 2006b). The theory describes a consciousness that allows nurses to raise new questions about what it means to be a nurse, what it means for a client to be ill, and how caring and healing should take place. Transpersonal caring theory rejects the disease orientation of health care and stresses care as more important than cure (Watson, 1988). Instead of focusing on the client's disease and its treatment by conventional means, transpersonal caring explores inner sources of healing to protect, enhance, and preserve a person's dignity, humanity, wholeness, and inner harmony.

In Watson's (2006b) view, caring is almost spiritual. Caring preserves human dignity in the technological, cure-dominated health care system. The emphasis is on the nurse–client relationship, as well as the caring relationship. During a single caring moment between the nurse and client, the nurse and client may communicate to each other on a level deeper than simple verbal exchange. There may be a sense of connection between the one cared for and the one caring. Caring on a deep, interpersonal level can promote healing (Watson 2006b). Application of Watson's caring model may enhance your caring practices. The model is **transformative** because the relationship influences both the nurse and the client, for better or for worse (Hoover, 2002). Watson further developed her caring science theory, described in her 2008 book. Her carative factors are now called *carative processes* and are outlined in Table 19–1. Evidence-informed material that enhances caring is described in Box 19–2.

BOX 19-1 CULTURAL ASPECTS OF CARE

Nurse Caring Behaviours

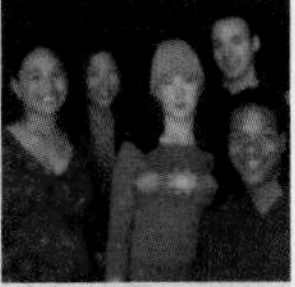

As a nurse, you must provide caring behaviours that are based on clients' cultural values and beliefs. Although the need for human caring is universal, its application is based on cultural norms. For example, providing time for family presence is often more valuable to traditional Asian families than is nursing presence. Using touch to convey caring sometimes crosses cultural norms. Sometimes gender-congruent caregivers or the client's family need to provide caring touch. In some cultures, maintaining eye contact while listening to the client is considered disrespectful.

Implications for Practice

- Know the client's cultural norms for caring practices.
- Know the client's cultural practices regarding end-of-life care. In some cultures, it is considered insensitive to tell the client that he or she is dying.
- Determine whether a member of the client's family or cultural group is the most appropriate resource for presence or touching.
- Determine the need for gender-congruent caregivers.
- Avoid the use of idioms because they can often create misunderstanding between the caregiver and the client or family.
- Know the client's cultural practices regarding the removal of life support.

Data from Galanti, G. A. (2004). *Caring for patients from different cultures* (3rd ed.). Philadelphia, PA: University of Pennsylvania Press; and Watson, J. (2006). Caring theory as an ethical guide to administrative and clinical practices. *Nursing Administration Quarterly, 30*(1), 48–55.

Swanson's Theory of Caring

In an effort to develop a theory of caring applicable for nursing practice, Swanson (1991) studied clients and professional caregivers. Three different groups were interviewed: women who miscarried, parents and health care professionals in a neonatal intensive care unit, and socially at-risk mothers who had received long-term, public health intervention. All groups were interviewed before, during, or after labour and delivery of a child and had experienced the phenomenon of caring. Researchers asked each subject questions regarding how they experienced caring in their situation. After analyzing the stories and descriptions of the three research groups, Swanson developed a theory of caring, whereby caring consists of five categories or processes: knowing, "being with," "doing for," enabling, and maintaining belief (Table 19–2).

Swanson's (1991) contributions are valuable in providing direction for how to develop useful and effective caring strategies. Each of the caring processes are crucial in making positive differences in clients' health and well-being outcomes. Thus, research findings used to develop the theory are useful in guiding clinical nursing practice. For example, Swanson (1999) tested the effects of caring-based counselling on women's emotional well-being in the first year after the miscarriage. Caring-based counselling was significant in reducing women's depression and anger, particularly during the first four months after the miscarriage.

The Human Act of Caring

Roach (1997) also focused on the integration of caring and spirituality in her "human act of caring" theory. She was requested by the Canadian Nurses Association (CNA) in 1977 to develop the first Canadian code of ethics for Canadian nurses. This first code was based on her caring theory, which comprised five concepts: compassion, competence, confidence, conscience, and commitment (Table 19–3). This foundational work set the stage for a value-based code that has been updated over time but continues to retain Roach's caring principles as the framework (Storch, 2007). The CNA (1997) *Code of Ethics* was revised and published in the summer of 2008.

Pusari (1998) applied Roach's theory in work with people with life-threatening illnesses. She proposed that Roach's caring elements be extended to include the concepts of courage, culture, and communication; thus, the theory would be more holistic. These eight concepts incorporate physical, psychological, emotional, spiritual, and cultural components to guide nurses as they provide comprehensive and individualistic care.

TABLE 19-1 Watson's Carative Processes

Carative Factors or Caritas Processes	Description
Humanistic–altruistic values	Practising loving-kindness and equanimity for self and others
Instilling or enabling faith and help	Being authentically present: enabling, sustaining, and honouring deep belief system and subjective world of self and others
Cultivating sensitivity to oneself and others	Cultivating one's own spiritual practices; deepening self-awareness, going beyond "ego-self"
Developing a helping–trusting, human caring relationship	Promoting and supporting a relationship that is characterized by trust, authenticity, helping and caring
Promoting and accepting expression of positive and negative feelings	Being present to and supportive of the expression of positive and negative feelings, recognizing both as important to a deep, interpersonal connection between self and person being cared for
Systematic use of scientific (creative) problem-solving process	Creatively using self and all ways of knowing, being, and doing as part of the caring process (engaging in artistry of caring–healing practices)
Providing for a supportive, protective, or corrective mental, social, spiritual environment	Creating healing environment at all levels: physical and nonphysical, whereby wholeness, beauty, comfort, dignity, and peace are potential (being or becoming the environment)
Assisting with the gratification of human needs	Reverentially and respectfully assisting with basic needs; holding an intentional, caring consciousness of touching and working with the embodied spirit of another; honouring a sense of unity within oneself; allowing for spirit-filled connection
Allowing for existential–phenomenological dimensions	Being open-minded and attending to spiritual, mysterious, unknown existential dimension of life, death, and suffering: "allowing for a miracle"

Adapted from Watson, J. (2008). *Nursing: The philosophy and science of caring* (rev. ed., p. 31). Boulder, CO: University Press of Colorado. Reprinted by permission of University Press of Colorado.

The Moral and Ethical Bases of Responsive Nurse-Client Relationships

Tarlier (2004), a Canadian author, presented another perspective on the principle of caring as a foundational nursing concept: that the concept of caring has not been well defined and that the nursing ethic of caring must be empirically shown to make a difference in client outcomes. For the nursing profession, it is important to provide evidence that caring is tied to a broader ethical knowledge base.

A personal moral sense that is shared by other people needs to be agreed on as a principle and integrated specifically into the

BOX 19-2 EVIDENCE-INFORMED PRACTICE GUIDELINE

Enhancing Caring

Evidence Summary

Caring facilitates healing and improves client satisfaction with nursing care. However, does the instructional process influence human caring? Do nurse educators present instructional methods that improve students' caring practices? In Hoover's (2002) study, undergraduate nursing students attended a 15-week educational module on nursing as human caring. The purpose of the module was to improve students' understanding of caring practice and to thus make them more caring practitioners. Researchers interviewed the students before and after completing the module to understand the effect of this module on their caring practices. For example, they asked students about factors that facilitate and impede their caring practices. The students reported an increase in self-awareness in regard to (1) connecting in relationships with self and others, (2) finding purpose and meaning in life, and (3) clarifying values. Several students spoke of becoming more tolerant of others, recognizing each person's uniqueness, and appreciating a person's perspectives. By recognizing themselves as caring persons, the students gained meaning in their lives. Many were able to report a great deal of satisfaction in recognizing that they were caring persons and how nursing allowed them to express that characteristic. Students worked through the emotional issues and practical constraints, which allowed them to grow spiritually and connect with clients at a deeper level. Finally, students also expressed an enhanced appreciation of what they valued.

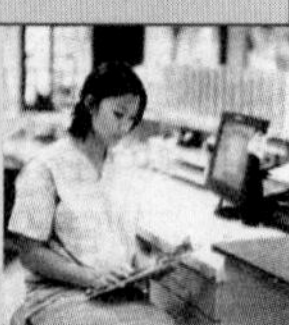

Application to Nursing Practice

- Increasing knowledge and understanding of caring helps nurses begin to understand clients' worlds and to change their approach to nursing care.
- The use of caring in nursing practice encourages a more holistic approach to nursing care.
- As nurses use caring, they get to know their clients and therefore better meet their needs.
- The caring model involves closeness, commitment, and involvement in the nurse–client relationship.

From Hoover, J. (2002). The personal and professional impact of undertaking an educational module on human caring. *Journal of Advanced Nursing, 37*(1), 79–86.

➤ TABLE 19-2 Swanson's Theory of Caring

Caring Process	Definitions	Subdimensions
Knowing	Striving to understand an event as it has meaning in the life of the other person	Avoiding assumptions about the life of the other person Centring on the one cared for Seeking cues
"Being with"	Being emotionally present for the other person	Engaging the self or both the self and the other person "Being there" Conveying ability Sharing feelings
"Doing for"	Doing for (assisting) the other person with actions that he or she would do for himself or herself if it were at all possible	Not burdening Comforting Anticipating Performing skillfully Protecting
Enabling	Facilitating the other person's passage through life transitions (e.g., birth, death) and unfamiliar events	Preserving dignity Informing and explaining Supporting and allowing Focusing Generating alternatives
Maintaining belief	Sustaining faith in the other person's capacity to get through an event or transition and face a future with meaning	Validating and giving feedback Believing in and holding in esteem Maintaining a hope-filled attitude Offering realistic optimism Spending extra effort to help the other person

From Swanson, K. M. (1991). Empirical development of a middle-range theory of caring. *Nursing Research, 40*(3), 161–166.

discipline of nursing and the nursing ethical knowledge base. Tarlier (2004) put forward the idea of responsive nurse–client relationships that are conceptualized in the nursing literature. Responsive relationships are based on respect, trust, and mutuality. These relationships can tie together theory, ethical knowledge, and clinical outcomes and strengthen the nursing ethical knowledge base.

Summary of Theoretical Views

Nursing caring theories have common themes. Caring is highly relational. Caring relationships open up possibilities (e.g., for comfort, touch, and solace) or close them down (Benner, 2004). The nurse and the client enter into a relationship that is much more than one person simply "doing tasks for" another. A mutual give-and-take

➤ TABLE 19-3 The Human Act of Caring

Compassion	• Way of living born out of an awareness of one's relationship to all living creatures • Engendering a response of participation in the experience of another • A sensitivity to the pain and brokenness of the other; a quality of presence that allows one to share with and make room for the other
Competence	• State of having the knowledge, judgement, skills, energy, experience, and motivation required to respond adequately to the demands of one's professional responsibilities
Confidence	• Quality that fosters trusting relationships • Goals of service rendered within an environment and under conditions of mutual trust and respect
Conscience	• State of moral awareness • Compass directing one's behaviour according to the moral fitness of things
Commitment	• Complex affective response characterized by a convergence between one's desires and one's obligations and by a deliberate choice to act in accordance with them

From Roach, S. (1992). *The human act of caring. A blueprint for the health professions.* Ottawa, ON: Canadian Hospital Association.

develops as nurse and client begin to know and care for one another. In his own experience with cancer, sociologist Arthur Frank (1998) noted that what he wanted when he was ill was a mutual relationship with persons who were also clinicians and clients. It was important for Frank to be seen as one of two fellow human beings, not the dependent client being cared for by the expert technical clinician.

Caring seems highly invisible at times when a nurse and client enter a relationship of respect, concern, and support. The nurse's empathy and compassion become a natural part of every client encounter. The absence of caring, however, is very obvious. For example, if the nurse shows lack of interest or chooses to avoid a client's request for help, the nurse's inaction quickly conveys an uncaring attitude. Benner and Wrubel (1989, p. 14) related the story of a clinical nurse specialist who learned from a client what caring is all about: "I felt that I was teaching him a lot, but actually he taught me. One day he said to me (probably after I had delivered some well-meaning technical information about his disease), 'You are doing an OK job, but I can tell that every time you walk in that door you are walking out.'" In this nurse's story, the client perceived that the nurse was simply going through the motion of teaching and showed little caring toward the client. Clients quickly sense nurses' failure to empathize with them.

As a nurse is being caring, the client senses commitment on the part of the nurse and is willing to allow the nurse to gain an understanding of the client's experience of illness. In a study of oncology clients' descriptions of their nursing care, Radwin et al. (2005, p. 166) found that clients characterized a caring nurse as one who would "quietly try to care for every need I had" and "be there when you need them" versus "treat[ing] you like a number or a case rather than a person." Thus, you become a coach and partner rather than a detached provider of care.

Imagine the situation in which a nurse is working with a client who recently received a diagnosis of diabetes mellitus and who must learn to administer daily insulin injections. In this scenario, the nurse's caring behaviour might be enabling. When a nurse practises enabling, the client and nurse work together to identify treatment alternatives and resources. The nurse enables the client to understand diabetes management, and the nurse supports the client in progressing through self-care activities.

Another common theme in caring is to understand the context of the client's life and illness. It is difficult to demonstrate caring without gaining an understanding of who the other person is and that person's perception of his or her illness. By exploring the following questions with the client, you can begin understanding the client's perception of illness: "How was your illness first recognized?" "How do you feel about the illness?" "How does the illness affect your daily life practices?" Knowing the context of a client's illness helps you choose and individualize interventions that will actually help the client. This approach is more successful than simply selecting interventions on the basis of the client's symptoms or the disease process.

Client's Perceptions of Caring

Swanson's (1991) theory of caring is a foundation for understanding the behaviours and processes that characterize caring. Other researchers have also studied caring from clients' perceptions (Table 19–4). Identifying nurse behaviours that clients perceive as caring helps nurses understand what clients expect of them as caregivers. Clients continue to value nurses' effectiveness in performing tasks; however, clients clearly also value the affective dimension of nursing care (Williams, 1997): establishing a reassuring presence, recognizing an individual as unique, and being attentive to the client. Each client has a unique background of experiences, values, and cultural perspectives; however, understanding common behaviours that clients associate with caring helps you learn to express caring in practice.

The study of clients' perceptions is important because health care emphasizes client satisfaction. What clients experience in their interactions with institutional services and health care professionals, and what they think of that experience, determines how clients use the health care system and how they can benefit from it (Gerteis et al., 1993; Mayer, 1986). When clients believe that health care professionals are sensitive, sympathetic, compassionate, and interested in them as people, they usually become active partners in the plan of care (Attree, 2001). Williams (1997) studied the relationship between clients' perceptions of four dimensions of caring and their satisfaction with nursing care. Clients in the study indicated that they were more satisfied when they perceived nurses to be caring. Radwin (2000) found that oncology clients associated excellent nursing care with attentiveness, partnership, individualization, rapport, and caring. As institutions look to improve client satisfaction, creating a caring environment is a necessary and worthwhile goal. Client's satisfaction with nursing care is an important factor in their decision to return to a hospital.

As a new clinical practitioner, you must account for how clients perceive caring and the best approaches to providing care. To start, consider behaviours associated with caring and consider an individual client's perceptions and unique expectations. Clients and nurses frequently differ in their perceptions of caring (Mayer, 1987; Wolf et al., 2003). For example, consider the situation in which your client is fearful of having an intravenous catheter inserted, and you are still a novice at catheter insertion. Instead of giving a lengthy description of the procedure to relieve the client's anxiety, you decide the client will benefit more if you obtain assistance from a skilled staff member. Understanding clients' perceptions helps you select caring approaches that are most appropriate to the clients' needs.

Ethic of Care

Caring is a moral imperative. Through caring for others, human dignity is ultimately protected, enhanced, and preserved. Watson (1988) suggested that caring, as a moral ideal, provides the stance from which a nurse intervenes. This stance ensures the practice of ethical standards for good conduct, character, and motives. Chapter 8 explores the importance of ethics in professional nursing. The term *ethic* refers to the ideals of right and wrong behaviour. In any client encounter, a nurse needs to know what behaviour is ethically appropriate. An **ethic of care** ensures that nurses do not make decisions solely on the basis of intellectual or analytical principles. Instead, an ethic of care places caring at the centre of decision making. For example, consider whether placing a disabled relative in a long-term care facility is truly caring.

An ethic of care is concerned with relationships between people and with a nurse's character and attitude toward others. Nurses who function according to an ethic of care are sensitive to unequal relationships that can lead to an abuse of one person's power over another, intentional or otherwise. In health care settings, clients and families are often on unequal footing with professionals because of the client's illness, lack of information, regression caused by pain and suffering, and unfamiliar circumstances. According to an ethic of care, the nurse is the client's advocate, solving ethical dilemmas by attending to relationships and by recognizing each client's uniqueness as a human being.

TABLE 19-4 Comparison of Research Studies Exploring Clients' Perceptions of Nurse Caring Behaviour

Wolf et al. (2003) Clients With Cardiac Conditions	Wolf et al. (2003) Male Clients	Attree (2001): General Medical Clients and Families	Chang et al. (2005): Clients With Cancer
Managing equipment skillfully	Being physically present so that client feels valued	Checking up on client	Being accessible to client and family
Being perceptive and compassionate	Returning voluntarily without being called	Being compassionate and patient	Providing comfort
Being physically present	Making client feel comfortable, relaxed, and secure	Demonstrating sensitivity and sympathy	Being trustworthy
Using a soft, gentle voice	Attending to comfort and needs of client before performing tasks	Using a calm, gentle, and kind approach	Anticipating client and family needs
Returning to client voluntarily without being asked	Using a kind, soft, pleasant, gentle voice and attitude		
Providing comfort and security			
Helping reduce pain			

Caring in Nursing Practice

It is impossible to prescribe ways that will guarantee whether or when a nurse becomes a caring professional. Experts disagree as to whether caring is teachable or fundamentally a way of being. Cook and Cullen (2003) wrote about the importance of teaching caring as an integral part of a nursing curriculum. In order for the value of caring to be internalized by the student nurse, caring behaviours must be demonstrated, and clinical opportunities to practise these behaviours must be built into the program. Caring models are essential to help in the development of a student's capacity to care (Roach, 1992). For example, Watson's nursing model has been adopted by many nursing programs in which the concept of caring is integrated throughout the curriculum.

For people who view caring as a normal part of their lives, caring is a product of their cultures, values, experiences, and relationships with other people. Persons who do not experience care in their lives often find it difficult to act in caring ways. As nurses deal with health and illness in their practice, their ability to care grows. Nursing behaviours that show caring include providing presence, a caring touch, and listening in each encounter with clients.

Providing Presence

Providing **presence** is to have a person-to-person encounter that conveys closeness and a sense of caring. Fredriksson (1999) explained that presence involves "being there" and "being with." "Being there" is not only physical presence but also communication and understanding. The interpersonal relationship of "being there" seems to depend on the fact that a nurse is attentive to the client (Cohen et al., 1994). You offer this type of presence to the client with the purpose of achieving some goal, such as support, comfort, or encouragement, to diminish the intensity of unwanted feelings or for reassurance (Fareed, 1996; Pederson, 1993).

"Being with" is also interpersonal. It means being available and at your clients' disposal (Pederson, 1993). If clients accept the nurse, they will invite the nurse to see and share their vulnerability and suffering. One person's human presence never leaves another person unaffected (Watson, 2003). The nurse then enables the client to articulate his or her feelings and to understand himself or herself in a way that leads to identifying solutions, seeing new directions, and making choices (Gilje, 1997).

By establishing presence—through eye contact, body language, voice tone, listening, and having a positive and encouraging attitude—you create openness and understanding. The message conveyed this way is that the client's experience matters to you (Swanson, 1991). Establishing presence with a client enhances your ability to learn from the client, which enhances nursing care.

It is especially important to establish presence when clients are experiencing stressful events or situations. Awaiting a physician's report of test results, preparing for an unfamiliar procedure, and planning to return home after serious illness are just a few examples of events in the course of a person's illness that can create unpredictability and dependency on health care professionals. Your presence can help calm a client's anxiety and fear in such situations. Giving reassurance and thorough explanations about a procedure, remaining at the client's side, and coaching the client through the experience all convey caring, which is invaluable to the client's well-being.

Touch

Clients face situations that can be embarrassing, frightening, and painful. Whatever the feeling or symptom, clients look to nurses for **comfort**. Touch is one comforting approach in which the nurse communicates concern and support.

Touch is relational and leads to a connection between nurse and client. Touch involves contact (physical) and noncontact touch. Contact touch involves obvious skin-to-skin contact, whereas noncontact touch refers to eye contact. It is difficult to separate the two. Both are described within three categories: task-orientated touch, caring touch, and protective touch (Fredriksson, 1999).

Nurses use task-orientated touch when performing a task or procedure. The skillful and gentle performance of a nursing procedure conveys security and a sense of competence. An expert nurse learns that any procedure is more effective when administered carefully and with consideration for any client concern. For example, if a client is anxious about a procedure such as an insertion of a nasogastric tube, the nurse provides comfort through full explanation of the procedure and what the client will feel. The nurse then assures the client that the procedure will be performed safely, skillfully, and successfully. This assurance is conveyed in the way that supplies are prepared, the client is positioned, and the nasogastric tube is gently manipulated and inserted. Throughout the procedure, the nurse talks quietly with the client to provide reassurance and support.

Caring touch is a form of nonverbal communication that successfully influences a client's comfort and security, enhances self-esteem, and improves reality orientation (Boyek & Watson, 1994). The nurse can express this caring touch by holding a client's hand, by giving the client a back massage, by gently positioning a client, or by participating in a conversation. When using a caring touch, the nurse is making a connection with showing acceptance of the client (Tommasini, 1990).

Protective touch is a form of touch that protects the nurse, the client, or both. The client views it either positively or negatively. The most obvious form of protective touch is in preventing an accident, such as holding and bracing the client to avoid a fall. This protects the client. Sometimes a nurse withdraws from a client or distances himself or herself when he or she is unable to tolerate suffering or needs to escape from a tense situation. This protects the nurse but elicits negative feelings in a client (Fredriksson, 1999).

Because touch conveys many messages, it must be used with discretion. Touch itself is a concern when crossing cultural boundaries of either the client or the nurse (Benner, 2004). Clients generally permit task-orientated touch because most individuals give nurses and doctors authority to enter their personal space to provide care. However, exceptions can exist because of clients' cultural backgrounds. You should understand whether clients are accepting of touch and how they interpret your intentions.

Listening

Caring involves an interpersonal interaction that is much more than two people simply talking back and forth. In a caring relationship, the nurse establishes trust, opens lines of communication, and listens to the client (Figure 19–1). Listening is key because it conveys the nurse's full attention and interest. Listening includes "taking in" what a client says, as well as interpreting and understanding what is the client is saying and conveying that understanding to the person talking (Kemper, 1992). Listening to the meaning of what a client says helps create a mutual relationship. True listening leads to truly knowing and responding to what really matters to the client and family (Boykin et al., 2003).

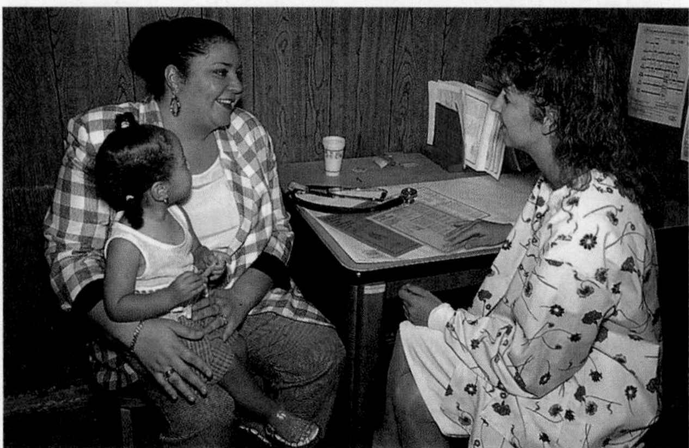

Figure 19-1 Nurse listening to a client.

When an individual becomes ill, he or she usually has a story to tell about the meaning of the illness. Any critical or chronic illness affects all of a client's life choices and decisions and sometimes the individual's identity. Being able to tell that story helps the client deal with the distress of illness. Thus, a story needs a listener. Frank (1998) described his own feelings during his experience with cancer, saying that he needed a health care professional's gift of listening in order to make his suffering a relationship between them instead of an iron cage around him. He needed to be able to express what he needed when he was ill. The personal concerns that are part of a client's illness story are what is at stake for the client. Caring through listening enables the nurse to be a participant in the client's life.

To listen effectively, listeners need to silence themselves (Fredriksson, 1999). Fredriksson described silencing one's mouth and also one's mind: that is, to silence one's own thoughts that might distract from fully listening to a client. It is important to remain intentionally silent and to concentrate on what the client has to say. You need to be able to give clients your full, focused attention as they tell their stories.

When an ill person chooses to tell his or her story, it involves reaching out to others. Telling the story implies a relationship that can develop only if the clinician exchanges his or her stories as well. Frank (1998) argued that professionals do not routinely take seriously their own need to be known as part of a clinical relationship. Yet, unless the professional acknowledges this need, the relationship is not reciprocal; it is only an interaction (Campo, 1997). The clinician is pressured to know as much as possible about the client, but this pressure isolates the clinician from the client. In contrast, in knowing and being known, each supports the other (Frank, 1998).

Through active listening, you begin to truly know the client and what is important to him or her (Bernick, 2004). Learning to listen to a client is sometimes difficult. It is easy to become distracted by tasks at hand, colleagues shouting instructions, or other clients waiting to have their needs met. However, the time you take to listen is worthwhile both in the information gained and in the strengthening of the nurse–client relationship. Listening involves paying attention to the individual's words and tone of voice and understanding his or her perspective. Chapter 18 provides more detailed information on the art of communication. By observing the expressions and body language of the client, you will find cues to help assist the client in exploring ways to achieve a greater sense of peace and well-being.

Knowing the Client

One of the five caring processes described by Swanson (1991) is knowing the client. This concept comprises both your understanding of a specific client's situation and your subsequent selection of interventions (Radwin, 1995). Knowing develops over time as you learn the clinical conditions within a specialty and the behaviours and physiological responses of clients. Intimate knowing helps you respond to what really matters to the client (Bulfin, 2005). To know a client means that you avoid assumptions, focus on the client, and engage in a caring relationship with the client so that you can detect information and cues that facilitate critical thinking and clinical judgements (see Chapter 8 for further details on nursing values and ethics). Knowing that the client is at the core of the process, you use this process to make clinical decisions. By establishing a caring relationship, you develop the understanding that helps you better know the client as a unique individual and choose the most appropriate and helpful nursing therapies.

The caring relationships that you develop over time, coupled with your growing knowledge and experience, enable you to detect changes in a client's clinical status. Expert nurses develop this ability to detect such changes almost effortlessly. Clinical decision making, perhaps the most important nursing responsibility, involves various aspects of knowing the client: responses to therapies, routines, and habits; coping resources; physical capacities and endurance; and body typology and characteristics (Tanner et al., 1993). The experienced nurse knows additional facts about his or her clients, such as their experiences, behaviours, feelings, and perceptions (Radwin, 1995). When you make clinical decisions accurately in the context of knowing a client well, client outcomes are improved. Swanson (1999b) noted that when nurses base care on knowing the client, the clients perceived care as personalized, comforting, supportive, and healing.

The most important thing for a beginning nurse to recognize is that knowing a client is more than simply gathering data about the client's clinical signs and condition. Success in knowing the client depends on the relationship you establish. To know a client is to enter into a caring, social process that results in "bonding," whereby the client comes to feel known by the nurse (Lamb & Stempel, 1994). The bonding then enables the relationship to evolve into "working" and "changing" phases so that you can help the client become involved in his or her care and accept help when needed (Bulfin, 2005).

Spiritual Caring

Spiritual health occurs when a person finds a balance between his or her own life values, goals, and belief systems and those of others (see Chapter 28 for more information on spiritual health). Human beings have physical, emotional, spiritual, and psychological dimensions. An individual's beliefs and expectations do have effects on his or her physical well-being.

Establishing a caring relationship with a client involves an interconnectedness between the nurse and the client. This interconnectedness is why Watson (1979, 2006a, 2006b, 2008) described the caring relationship in a spiritual sense. Spirituality offers a sense of connection intrapersonally (connected with oneself), interpersonally (connected with others and the environment), and transpersonally (connected with an unseen higher power). In a caring relationship, the client and the nurse come to know one another so that the relationship becomes one of healing through the following actions:

- Mobilizing hope for the client and for the nurse
- Finding an interpretation or understanding of illness, symptoms, or emotions that is acceptable to the client
- Assisting the client in using social, emotional, or spiritual resources

Family Care

Each individual experiences life through relationships with others. Thus, caring for an individual does not occur in isolation from that person's family. It is important for you as a nurse to know the family almost as thoroughly as they know the client (Figure 19–2). The family is an important resource. Success with nursing interventions often depends on the family's willingness to share information about the client, their acceptance and understanding of therapies, whether the interventions fit with the family's acceptance and understanding of therapies, whether the interventions fit with the family's daily practices, and whether the family supports and provides the therapies recommended.

Many nurse caring behaviours are perceived as most helpful by families of clients with cancer (Box 19–3). Ensuring the client's well-being and helping the family become active participants in the client's care are critical for family members. These behaviours, although specific to families of clients with cancer, are useful for developing a caring relationship with all families. Begins a relationship by learning who makes up the client's family and what family members' roles are in the client's life. Showing the family care and concern for the client creates an openness that then enables a relationship to form with the family. Caring for the family takes into consideration the context of the client's illness and the stress it imposes on all members. Chapter 20 contains more material on family nursing.

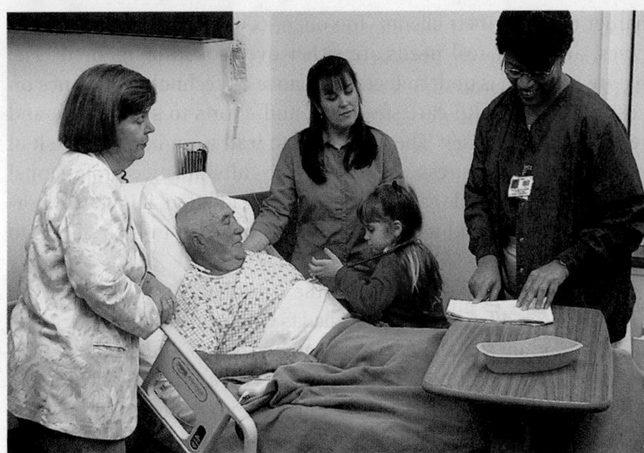

Figure 19-2 The nurse discusses the client's health care needs with the family.

The Challenge of Caring

Assisting individuals during a time of need is the reason that many people enter the field of nursing. When nurses are able to affirm themselves as caring individuals, they reinforce a meaning and purpose to their lives (Benner, 2004; Hoover, 2002). Caring is a motivating force for people to become nurses, and it becomes the source of satisfaction when nurses know they have made a difference in their clients' lives.

It is becoming more of a challenge to care in today's health care system. Being a part of the helping professions is difficult and demanding. Nurses are torn between the human caring model and the task-oriented biomedical model and institutional demands that consume their practice (Watson & Foster, 2003). The time that nurses can spend with clients is diminishing, which makes it much

➤ BOX 19-3 Nurse Behaviours Perceived by Families as Caring

- Being honest
- Giving clear explanations
- Keeping family members informed
- Trying to make the client comfortable
- Showing interest in answering questions
- Providing necessary emergency care
- Assuring the client that nursing services will be available
- Answering family members' questions honestly, openly, and willingly
- Allowing the client to do as much for himself or herself as possible
- Teaching the family how to keep the client physically comfortable

Data from Brown, C. L., Holcomb, L., Maloney, J., Naranjo, J., Gibson, C., & Russell, P. (2005). Caring in action: The patient care facilitator role. *International Association for Human Caring Journal, 9*(3), 51–58; Mayer, D. K. (1986). Cancer patients' and families' perceptions of nurse caring behaviors. *Topics in Clinical Nursing, 8*(2), 63–69; and Radwin, L. (2000). Oncology patients' perceptions of quality nursing care. *Research in Nursing & Health, 23*(3), 179–190.

harder to know their clients. Too often, clients are perceived as just cases, and their real needs are either overlooked or ignored. The nature of caring is undermined by reliance on technology, reliance on cost-effective health care strategies, and efforts to standardize and refine work processes. These factors can lead to an increased risk of burnout from the stress and inability to fully practice professional standards that include caring behaviours. In addition, it is very important that student and novice nurses are supported in their efforts to be client focused.

The CNA has partnered with the Canadian Council on Health Services Accreditation, Health Canada's Office of Nursing Policy, and other important stakeholders to research, develop, and promote quality of worklife indicators (CNA, 2002). These fundamental indicators are designed to help organizations improve the health of their work environments. Healthy work environments are important for implementing client-focused care, preventing burnout, and preserving the practice of caring. Providing safe, compassionate, competent, and ethical care is a hallmark of the new CNA (2008) *Code of Ethics*.

The Registered Nurses Association of Ontario (2006) developed a guideline for nursing best practices that is informed by evidence about how to provide client-centred care. This guideline includes practice, education, organization, and policy recommendations that can help the individual nurse, educational organizations, and health care organizations implement client-centred care and integrate the ethic of caring into practice.

If health care is to make a positive difference in their lives, human beings cannot be treated like machines or robots. Instead, health care must become more humanized. Nurses play an important role in making caring behaviours an integral part of the health care delivery. First, nurses must make caring a part of the philosophy and environment in the workplace. By incorporating care concepts into standards of nursing care, nurses establish the guidelines for professional conduct. Finally, during day-to-day practice with clients and families, nurses need to be committed to caring and be willing to establish the relationships necessary for personal, competent, compassionate, and meaningful nursing care.

* KEY CONCEPTS

- Caring is at the heart of a nurse's ability to work with people in a respectful and therapeutic way.
- Caring is always specific and relational for each nurse-client encounter.
- For caring to be effective and meaningful to clients, nurses must learn culturally specific behaviours and words that reflect human caring in different cultures.
- Because illness is the human experience of loss or dysfunction, any treatment or intervention given without consideration of its meaning to the individual is likely to be worthless.
- Swanson's theory of caring includes five caring processes: knowing, "being with," "doing for," enabling, and maintaining belief.
- Roach's caring theory comprises five concepts: compassion, competence, confidence, conscience, and commitment.
- Caring involves a mutual give-and-take that develops as nurse and client begin to know and care for one another.
- It is difficult to demonstrate caring to clients without gaining an understanding of who they are and their perception of their illness.
- Presence involves a person-to-person encounter that conveys closeness and a sense of caring that involves "being there" and "being with" clients.
- Research has shown that touch, both contact and noncontact, includes task-orientated touch, caring touch, and protective touch.
- The skillful and gentle performance of a nursing procedure conveys security and a sense of competence in the nurse.
- Listening includes interpreting and understanding what is said.
- Knowing the client is at the core of the process by which nurses make clinical decisions.
- A nurse demonstrates caring by helping family members become active participants in a client's care.

* CRITICAL THINKING EXERCISES

1. Mrs. Lowe is a 52-year-old client being treated for lymphoma (cancer of the lymph nodes) that occurred 6 years after lung transplantation. Mrs. Lowe is discouraged about her current health status and a lot of what she describes as muscle pain. The unit where Mrs. Lowe is receiving care has a number of very sick clients and is short-staffed.
   a. You enter her room to perform a morning assessment and find Mrs. Lowe crying. How are you going to use caring practices to help Mrs. Lowe, knowing that you have only begun your tasks for the day?
   b. When you listened to Mrs. Lowe, she explained that her muscle pain was very bothersome and it was worse particularly when she was alone. Both you and Mrs. Lowe determine that an injection for her pain would be beneficial. In what way are you caring when you administer the injection to Mrs. Lowe?
   c. Mrs. Lowe seems more comfortable and is crying less. What else can you do for Mrs. Lowe?
2. During your next clinical practicum, select a client to talk with for at least 15 to 20 minutes. Ask the client to tell you about his or her illness:
   a. What do you believe the client was trying to tell you about his or her illness?
   b. Why was it important for the client to share his or her story?
   c. What did you do that made it easy or difficult for the client to talk with you? What did you do well? What could you have done better?
   d. Would you rate yourself a good listener? How can you listen better?

* REVIEW QUESTIONS

1. A nurse hears a colleague tell a student nurse that she never touches the clients unless she is performing a procedure or doing an assessment. The nurse tells the colleague that
   1. She does not touch the clients either
   2. Touch is a type of verbal communication
   3. Using touch is never a problem
   4. Touch forms a connection between nurse and client
2. Of the five caring processes, "knowing" the client is best described as
   1. Anticipating the client's cultural preference
   2. Determining the client's physician preferences
   3. Gathering task-oriented information during assessment
   4. Establishing an enhanced understanding of the client's needs
3. Helping a new mother through the birthing experience demonstrates which of the five caring behaviours?
   1. Knowing
   2. Enabling
   3. "Doing for"
   4. "Being with"
   5. Maintaining belief

4. Mr. Kline is fearful of upcoming surgery and a possible cancer diagnosis. He discussed his love for the Bible with Jada, his nurse, and she recommends a favourite Bible verse. Another nurse tells Jada that spiritual caring has no place in nursing. Jada replies:
    1. "Spiritual care should be left to a professional."
    2. "You are correct; expressions of spirituality are a personal decision."
    3. "Nurses should not force their spiritual beliefs on clients."
    4. "Healing can be promoted by assisting the client in using spiritual resources."

5. A number of strategies have potential for creating work environments that enable nurses to demonstrate more caring behaviours. Some of these include
    1. Increases in working hours
    2. Increases in monetary gain
    3. Flexibility, autonomy, and improvements in staffing
    4. Increases in physicians' input concerning nursing functions

6. A nurse demonstrates caring by helping family members
    1. Become active participants in care
    2. Provide activities of daily living
    3. Remove themselves from personal care
    4. Make health care decisions for the client

7. Listening is not only "taking in" what a client says; it also includes
    1. Incorporating the views of the physician
    2. Correcting any errors in the client's understanding
    3. Injecting the nurse's personal views and statements
    4. Interpreting and understanding what the client means

8. Presence involves a person-to-person encounter that
    1. Enables clients to care for themselves
    2. Provides personal care to a client
    3. Conveys a closeness and sense of caring
    4. Describes being in close contact with a client

9. By considering the clients' perceptions of caring, nurses are better able to
    1. Understand what clients expect of them as caregivers
    2. Be more efficient in performing tasks
    3. Provide continuity of care
    4. Establish nursing priorities

* RECOMMENDED WEB SITES

International Association for Human Caring: http://www.humancaring.org

The focus of this Web site is to advance nursing and other related disciplines in the knowledge of caring and caring theory. This site provides access to the *International Journal for Human Caring*, a well-recognized journal that details research on caring.

Nursing as Caring: http://www.nursingascaring.com/index.html

This Web site describes current research, development, practice, and education projects related to the theory of "nursing as caring." It also lists a bibliography of publications on the subject of caring.

20

Family Nursing

Written by Lorraine M. Wright, RN, PhD, Maureen Leahey, RN, PhD, and Francis Loos, RN, MN, CNCC(C)

Based on the original chapter by Anne G. Perry, RN, EdD, FAAN

objectives

Mastery of content in this chapter will enable you to:

- Define the key terms listed.
- Discuss how the term *family* can be defined.
- Examine current trends in the Canadian family.
- Discuss how family members influence one another's health.
- Compare family as context with family as client and explain how these perspectives influence nursing practice.
- State the three major categories of the Calgary Family Assessment Model (CFAM) and understand subcategories important to consider in a family assessment.
- Describe key concepts of the Calgary Family Intervention Model (CFIM).
- Ask assessment questions to learn relevant information about family functioning in the context of health or illness.
- Discuss family nursing skills needed to conduct a family interview.

key terms

Alliances and coalitions, p. 286
Beliefs, p. 285
Calgary Family Assessment Model (CFAM), p. 280
Calgary Family Intervention Model (CFIM), p. 286
Circular communication, p. 284
Circular questions, p. 286
Commendation, p. 286
Ecomap, p. 283
Emotional communication, p. 284
Family, p. 277
Family forms, p. 277
Family nursing, p. 277
Genogram, p. 283
Hardiness, p. 279
Illness narrative, p. 287
Influence, p. 285
Linear questions, p. 286
Nonverbal communication, p. 284
Problem solving, p. 285
Reciprocity, p. 288
Resiliency, p. 280
Roles, p. 285
Verbal communication, p. 284

media resources

evolve Web Site

- Audio Chapter Summaries
- Glossary
- Multiple-Choice Review Questions
- Student Learning Activities
- Weblinks

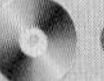
Companion CD

- Glossary
- Interactive Learning Activities
- Fluids and Electrolytes Tutorial
- Test-Taking Skills

The family continues to be a central institution in Canadian society. The role of the family in health care has been evolving. In the early twentieth century, visiting public health nurses and private duty nurses worked closely with family members while providing nursing care in the client's home. After World War II and the implementation of Medicare, most nursing services were provided in hospitals rather than in homes. As a result, families were generally excluded from their relatives' nursing care, and physicians and nurses were considered to be the final authorities to determine what was best for the client (Canadian Nurses Association [CNA], 1997). Since the 1970s, however, families and health care professionals have been forging more collaborative relationships, in which families' needs and contributions are taken into consideration.

Today, nurses strive to provide *family-centred care,* also known as *family nursing.* **Family nursing** is based on the assumption that every person, regardless of age, is a member of some type of family form and that individuals are best understood within the context of the family. A change in one family member, such as an illness or health condition, affects the other family members. Family nursing promotes, supports, and provides for the well-being and health of the family and individual family members (Astedt-Kurki et al., 2002). Nurses are responsible for first understanding the makeup (configuration), structure, and coping capacity of the family and then building on the family's relative strengths and resources (Feeley & Gottlieb, 2000). Studies have shown that when nurses and families establish meaningful relationships, families are better able to manage the illness, and nurses gain greater clinical confidence and job satisfaction (Leahey et al., 1995). The goal of family nursing is to help the family and its individual members achieve and maintain optimal health throughout and beyond the illness experience. Family nursing is the focus of the future across all practice settings and is emphasized in all health care environments.

What Is a Family?

Defining *family* may initially appear to be a simple undertaking. However, different definitions have resulted in heated debates among social scientists and legislators. The family can be defined as a biological entity, as a legal entity, or as a social network with personally constructed ties and ideologies. To some clients, family may include only people who are related by marriage, birth, or adoption. Other clients consider aunts, uncles, close friends, cohabiting people, and even pets as family. Families are as diverse as the individuals that compose them, and clients may have deeply ingrained values about their families that must be respected. Thus, **family** is defined as a set of relationships that each client identifies as family or as a network of individuals who influence each other's lives, regardless of whether actual biological or legal ties exist. In other words, each person has an individual definition of who or what constitutes family (Baumann, 2006).

Your personal beliefs do not have to coincide with those of the client. To provide individualized care, you must understand that families have many forms and have diverse cultural and ethnic orientations. In addition, no two families are alike; each has its own strengths, weaknesses, resources, and challenges (Bell et al., 2001). However, some general characteristics of a family include future obligations and caregiving functions, such as protection, nourishment, and socialization of its members (Stuart, 1991).

Current Trends in the Canadian Family

Although the institution of the family remains strong, the family itself is changing. You should be aware of current trends and social factors that affect the structure and function of the family. The following information about current family trends is based on data from Statistics Canada's 2001 and 2006 censuses (Statistics Canada, 2002, 2003a, 2003b, 2004, 2007a, 2007b, 2007c, 2007d, 2007e).

Family Forms

Family forms are patterns of people considered by family members to be included in the family (Box 20–1). Although all families have some common characteristics, each family form has unique problems and strengths. You need to keep an open mind about what constitutes a family so that potential resources and concerns are not overlooked.

The proportion of "traditional" families (married parents and their biological children) has been declining since about 1980, whereas the proportions of common-law and lone-parent families have been increasing (Figure 20–1). The number of couples without children at home is also increasing: In 1981, 32% of married and common-law

➤ BOX 20-1 Family Forms

Traditional Nuclear Family
Consists of a mother and father (married or common-law) and their children

Extended Family
Includes the nuclear family and other relatives (perhaps grandparents, aunts, uncles, cousins)

Step-Family
Formed when at least one child in a household is from a previous relationship of one of the parents

Blended Family
Formed when both parents bring children from previous relationships into a new, joint living situation or when children from the current union and children from previous unions are living together

Lone-Parent Family
Consists of one parent (either father or mother) and one or more children. The lone-parent family is formed when one parent leaves the nuclear family because of death, divorce, or desertion or when a single person decides to have or adopt a child.

Other Family Forms
These relationships include married and common-law couples without children, "skip-generation" families (grandparents caring for grandchildren), "nonfamilies" (adults living alone), and same-sex couples (with or without children).

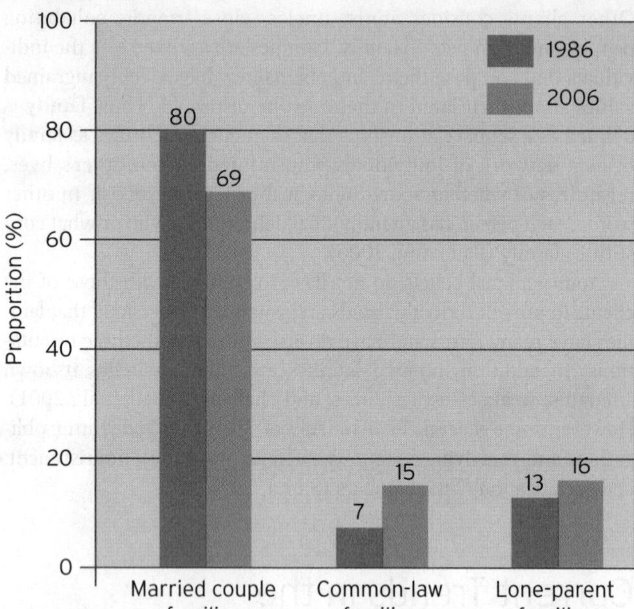

Figure 20-1 Proportion of married, common-law, and lone-parent families, 1986 and 2006. **Source:** Adapted from Statistics Canada. (2007, September 12). *2006 Census: Families, marital status, households, and dwelling characteristics.* Retrieved October 20, 2008, from www.statcan.ca/Daily/English/070912/d070912a.htm

couples had no children living at home; by 2001, this number had risen to 37%. This increase is partly a result of lower fertility rates, couples' delay in having children, and increased life expectancy, which is resulting in greater numbers of older couples with independent adult children (Statistics Canada, 2002).

Divorce rates have increased dramatically since the 1950s, and although the rate seems to be dropping, it is now estimated that 38% of Canadian marriages will end in divorce (Statistics Canada, 2004). Most divorced people eventually remarry, which results in blended families with complex sets of relationships among step-parents, stepchildren, half-brothers and half-sisters, and extended family members. When transitioning to a blended family, parents must deal with sometimes hostile or upset reactions of the children, the extended families, and an ex-spouse. Parents also must address the new family organization, including roles and relationships.

Same-sex couples define their relationships in family terms. According to the 2006 census, same-sex couples accounted for 0.6% of all couples, and 16.5% of these couples were married. Some families of same-sex couples include children, through adoption, through artificial insemination, or from prior relationships. About 16% of female couples and 3% of male couples have children (Statistics Canada, 2007b).

Grandparents are also increasingly taking responsibility for raising their grandchildren. In 2001, about 1% of all grandparents were living with their grandchildren without either of the children's parents involved (Statistics Canada, 2003a). This parenting responsibility is most often a consequence of legal intervention when parents are deemed unfit or renounce their parental obligations.

The proportion of teenagers who give birth has declined steadily since 1980, probably as a result of increased sex education, the availability of contraceptives, and the use of abortion (Dryburgh, 2000). Nevertheless, adolescents who give birth are now more likely to raise their children themselves than to place the children for adoption (The Vanier Institute of the Family, 2000). A teenage pregnancy tends to have health and social consequences for the baby and mother and often severely strains family relationships and resources. In addition, these families are at increased risk for continued poverty. Child-bearing often interrupts the mother's education, thereby limiting her employment opportunities. Many adolescent parents—already struggling with the normal tasks of development and identity—must also accept a responsibility for which they may not be ready physically, emotionally, socially, or financially.

Marital Roles

Marital roles are also more complex as families increasingly comprise two wage earners. The majority of mothers—both wives and lone mothers—work outside the home; more than 75% of mothers with children older than 6 years are in the workforce (The Vanier Institute of the Family, 2000). Balancing employment and family life creates a variety of challenges in terms of child care and household work. Concerns that maternal employment is detrimental for children are unsubstantiated (Harvey, 1999). However, finding high-quality substitute child care is a major issue for parents. Managing household tasks can also be a major challenge. Both the management of household tasks and parenting responsibilities can vary substantially from family to family. Fathers are now expected to participate more fully in day-to-day parenting responsibilities.

Economic Status

In 2000, the median annual income of Canadian families was about $67,600. The median annual income for lone-parent households is $30,000 (Statistics Canada, 2007e). In fact, in 2000, about 13% of all families had low annual income, and almost half (46%) of all lone-parent families with children younger than 18 years had low annual incomes (Statistics Canada, 2003b). Distribution of wealth greatly affects the capacity to maintain health. Low educational preparation, poverty, and decreased amounts of support magnify each other's impact on sickness in the family and increase the amount of sickness in the family.

Aboriginal Families

Aboriginal families are the fastest growing group with children younger than 24 years. They are undergoing substantial changes while trying to maintain their traditional structure and function. Aboriginal families, in their multigenerational form, consist of a network of grandparents, parents, children, aunts, uncles and cousins. Each member has obligations to the family. Children are held in high esteem and are expected to be treated gently and protected from harm (Castellano, 2002).

Aboriginal peoples include First Nations, Métis, and Inuit. The number of individuals of Aboriginal origin increased 54% (and at six times the growth rate of other groups) between 1996 and 2006 (Statistics Canada, 2007c). Half of the Aboriginal population lives in urban areas, in comparison with 80% of the non-Aboriginal population. In the non-Aboriginal population, the median age is 40 years; in contrast, the median age of Aboriginal people is 27 years. Therefore, approximately half (48%) of Aboriginal people are younger than 24 years, in comparison with 31% of non-Aboriginal people. In addition, life expectancy is shorter and fertility rates are higher among Aboriginal peoples (Statistics Canada, 2007d).

Aboriginal families thus tend to be larger, be younger, and contain more diverse family members than do non-Aboriginal families. Their needs must be considered on an individual basis as more Aboriginal peoples move to urban centres and fewer remain in traditional living arrangements. Each group of Aboriginal peoples has its own traditions, relationships, and functions. The Calgary Family Assessment Model is well suited for evaluating these individual situations.

Family Caregivers

The fastest growing age group in Canada is 80 years of age and older. One per seven Canadians is a senior citizen. The growth in this group is projected to accelerate in 2011 as baby boomers turn 65 years old. Life expectancy is 82.5 years for women and 77.7 years for men (Statistics Canada, 2007a). This aging of the population has affected family life cycle, especially the middle generation. Often, family members serve as informal caregivers for older adults and other persons with disabilities. The majority of these caregivers are women, and they frequently provide 10 hours or more of unpaid assistance per week (The Vanier Institute of the Family, 2000). Family caregiving involves the routine provision of services and personal care activities for a family member by spouses, siblings, or children. Caregiving activities might include personal care (bathing, feeding, or grooming), monitoring for complications or side effects of medications, instrumental activities of daily living (shopping or housekeeping), and ongoing emotional support.

Whenever an individual becomes dependent on another family member for care and assistance, both the caregiver and the care recipient are under significant stress. The caregiver must continue to meet the demands of his or her normal lifestyle (e.g., raising children, working full time, or dealing with personal problems or illness). In many cases, older adult children care for their parents or older relatives. Although family caregivers often find that providing care has many rewards, they usually also have to balance caregiving with career and other family responsibilities. This group frequently must make major adjustments to integrate the challenges and time commitments of caring for a family member with their own lives (Hunt, 2003). Caregivers' physical and emotional health may suffer, as may their careers and family relationships (The Vanier Institute of the Family, 2000). Box 20–2 provides a list of family nursing gerontological concerns.

BOX 20-2 FOCUS ON OLDER ADULTS

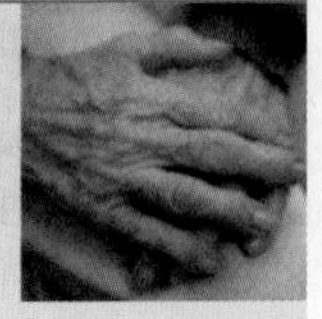

- The nurse must consider caregiver strain; caregivers are usually either spouses, who may also be older adults and whose own physical stamina may be declining, or middle-age children, who often have other responsibilities.
- Older families have a different social network than do younger families because friends and same-generation family members may have died or have been ill themselves. The nurse may need to look for social support within the community and within the client's religious affiliation.
- Greater physical health impairment increases the risk of depression in older adults.
- As in the other stages of life, members of older families need to work on developmental tasks (see Chapter 25).
- Abuse of older adults in families occurs across all social classes. Family members and family caregivers are the most frequent abusers. Unexplained bruises and skin trauma should not be ignored by health care professionals.

The Family and Health

The family is the primary social context in which health promotion and disease prevention take place (Box 20–3). The health of the family is influenced by many factors (e.g., its relative position in society, economic resources, and geographical boundaries). The family's beliefs, values, and practices also strongly influence health-promoting behaviours of its members (Hartrick, 2000). In turn, the health status of each individual influences how the family unit functions and its ability to achieve goals. When the family functions satisfactorily to meet its goals, its members tend to feel positive about themselves and their family. Conversely, when they do not meet goals, families view themselves as ineffective.

Good health may not be highly valued in some families; in fact, detrimental practices may be accepted. In some cases, a family member may provide mixed messages about health. For example, a parent may continue to smoke while telling children that smoking is "bad" for them. Family environment is crucial because health behaviour reinforced in early life has a strong influence on later health practices. In addition, the family environment can be a crucial factor in an individual's adjustment to a crisis. Although illness can strain relationships, research indicates that family members have the potential to be a primary force for coping.

Attributes of Healthy Families

In his classic work, Hill (1958/2003) noted that it is possible to explain the reactions of crisis-proof and crisis-prone families. A crisis-proof, or effective, family is able to integrate the need for stability with the need for growth and change. This type of family has a flexible structure that allows adaptable performance of tasks and acceptance of help from outside the family system. The structure is flexible enough to allow adaptability but not so flexible that the family lacks cohesiveness and a sense of stability. An effective family has control over the environment and exerts influence on the immediate environment of home, neighbourhood, and school. A crisis-prone, or ineffective, family may lack or believe it lacks control over these environments.

Health promotion researchers have focused on the stress-moderating effect of hardiness and resiliency as factors that contribute to long-term health. Family **hardiness** has been defined as the internal strengths and durability of the family unit and is characterized by a

BOX 20-3 FOCUS ON PRIMARY HEALTH CARE

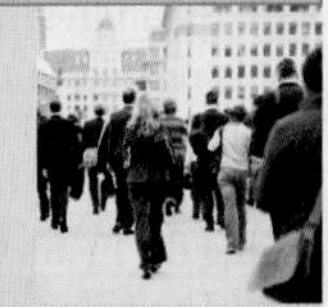

Community health nurses meet families in a wide variety of settings and have many opportunities to use holistic family nursing practices. Nursing duties in health promotion include neonatal assessments, bereavement visits, school health care, occupational health care, substance abuse programs, palliative care, infusion clinics, home care, and numerous other clinical encounters.

When family nursing care is implemented, health promotion interventions are needed to improve or maintain the physical, social, emotional, and spiritual well-being of the family and its members (Ford-Gilboe, 2002). Individual members and the total family are encouraged to reach their optimal levels of wellness. Identifying attributes that contribute to health and resilience in families has been a focus of ongoing research since at least the 1970s. "Strong" families that adapt to expected transitions and unexpected crises and change tend to be characterized by clear communication among members, good problem-solving skills, a commitment to each other and to the family unit, and a sense of cohesiveness and spirituality (Svavarsdottir et al., 2000; also see Chapter 28). Health promotion programs aimed at enhancing these attributes are available for families and children in many communities. You must be aware of family-oriented community offerings so that families can be referred as needed. Health promotion behaviours that you need to encourage are often tied to the developmental stage of the family, such as programs for the child-bearing family about adequate prenatal care.

sense of control over the outcome of life, a view of change as beneficial and growth producing, and an active rather than passive orientation in adapting to stressful events (McCubbin et al., 1996). A hardy family can transcend long periods and inevitable lifestyle changes. Family **resiliency** is the ability to cope with expected and unexpected stressors: role changes, developmental milestones, and crises. The goal of the family is not only to survive the challenge but also to thrive and grow as a result of the newly gained knowledge. Resources and techniques that a family or individuals within the family use to maintain health can demonstrate a family's level of resiliency (Black & Lobo, 2008; Svavarsdottir et al., 2000).

Family Nursing Care

Nursing practice is enhanced by a family-centred approach. Nurses should examine family patterns, relationships, and interactions when they consider how a health problem or illness affects a family and how a family affects a health problem or illness. A nurse's relationship with the family has a significant influence on client and family functioning (Leahey & Harper-Jaques, 1996). A positive collaborative relationship with family members must be based on mutual respect and trust (Figure 20–2).

To begin working with families, you must have a scientific knowledge base in family theory and an adequate knowledge base in family nursing. Although health care systems in the past tended to emphasize the individual, a family focus is now needed in order to be able to safely discharge clients to the care of the family or community settings. The current emphasis on home nursing care provides another opportunity for family nursing care.

Family nursing care can be described as focusing either on family as context or on family as client. The choice of approach used depends on the situation and the abilities of the nurse.

Family as Context

When considering the family as context, you focus either on the individual client within the context of his or her family or on the family with the individual as context (CNA, 1997). The approach that you use is related to the clinical setting, the clinical problem, and realistic and practical considerations. An example of the first approach is the situation in which a nurse interviews a man with heart disease, asking the man's wife about the family's diet and possible family stressors. The wife's abilities to support her husband's efforts at changing eating patterns and use of stress management techniques are also assessed. The main focus is on the health of the client within the environment of the family. An example of the second approach is the situation in which a community health nurse interviews the adult daughter of a woman with multiple sclerosis, discussing how the daughter is coping with her mother at home. Family members may need direct interventions themselves.

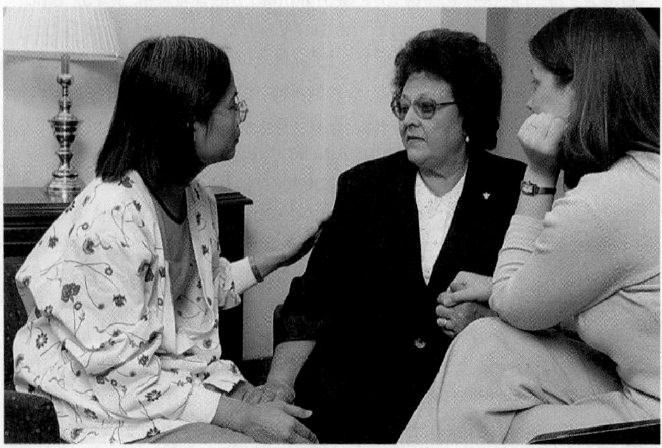

Figure 20-2 Nurse (*left*) and family members.

With both approaches, you assess the extent to which the family provides the individual's basic needs. Family members should be considered valuable resources. They can provide you with information about how they have been helping the client maintain health and manage health problems. When clients are unable to communicate, families can provide important information about the client and indicate the client's wishes. All nurses should be competent at considering the family as context. Even if you do not have an opportunity to involve the family directly, you should still consider the client as a member of a family.

Family as Client

When the family as client is the approach, you focus on the entire family: its processes and relationships (e.g., parenting or family caregiving). The focus of nursing assessment is usually on family patterns and interactions among family members rather than on individual characteristics. The nursing process concentrates on the extent to which these patterns and processes are consistent with achieving and maintaining family and individual health. Nursing practice that focuses on family as client is also known as *family systems nursing*, and it usually requires an in-depth knowledge of family dynamics and family systems theory. Therefore, nurses who specialize in family systems nursing usually have extensive clinical practice skills and a postgraduate degree. Dealing with complex family system problems often requires an interdisciplinary approach. You must always be aware of the limits of nursing practice and make referrals when appropriate. When you view the family as the client, you aim to support communication among all family members. This support ensures that the family remains informed of the nurse's intent and progress in providing health care. Often you must support conflict resolution between family members so that each member can confront and resolve problems in a healthy way. You also help family members use the external and internal resources that are necessary. Ultimately, your aim is to help the family achieve optimal function.

Assessing the Needs of the Family: The Calgary Family Assessment Model

Family assessment is essential in providing adequate family care and support. To help families adjust to acute and chronic illness, nurses need to understand the family unit, what the illness means to the family members, what the illness means to family functioning, how the family has been affected by the illness, and the support that the family requires (Neabel et al., 2000). Box 20–4 lists the particular features of families who should be considered for a family assessment. During an assessment, the nurse, client, and family collaboratively engage in conversation to systematically collect information and reflect on issues important to the client's well-being at this particular time.

The **Calgary Family Assessment Model (CFAM)** can be used by nurses to perform a thorough family assessment (Wright & Leahey, 2005). It has received wide recognition, and faculties and schools of nursing around the world have adopted it. The International Council of Nurses recognizes it as one of the four leading family assessment models in the world (Schober & Affara, 2001). The CFAM focuses on

> **BOX 20-4 Features of Families Who Should Be Considered for a Family Assessment**
>
> Families who may benefit most from a family assessment include those who
>
> - Are experiencing emotional, physical, or spiritual suffering or disruption caused by a family crisis (e.g., acute illness, injury, or death)
> - Are experiencing emotional, physical, or spiritual suffering or disruption caused by a developmental milestone (e.g., birth, marriage, or child leaving home)
> - Define a problem as a family issue (e.g., the impact of chronic illness on the family)
> - Have a child or adolescent whom they identify as having difficulties (e.g., school phobia or fear of cancer treatment)
> - Are experiencing issues that are serious enough to jeopardize family relationships (e.g., terminal illness or abuse)
> - Have a family member who is about to be admitted to the hospital for psychiatric treatment
> - Have a child who is about to be admitted to the hospital
>
> From Wright, L. M., & Leahey, M. (2000). *Nurses and families: A guide to family assessment and intervention* (3rd ed., p. 17). Philadelphia: F. A. Davis.

three major categories of family life: the structural dimension, the developmental dimension, and the functional dimension. Each category has several subcategories; however, not all subcategories are relevant to all families (Figure 20–3). You must decide, on a family-by-family basis, which subcategories are relevant at each time. Using too many subcategories may result in an overwhelming amount of data; using too few may yield insufficient data, which can distort a family's strengths, problems, or both. The model can be consulted during discussions about family issues.

Structural Assessment

The structural dimension of the family includes the following:

- Internal structure: the people who are included in the family and how they are connected to each other
- External structure: the relationships the family has with people and institutions outside the family
- Context: the whole situation or background relevant to the family

Internal Structure. The internal structure of the family—its composition and connections among family members—can be further divided into six subcategories: family composition, gender, sexual orientation, rank order, subsystems, and boundaries.

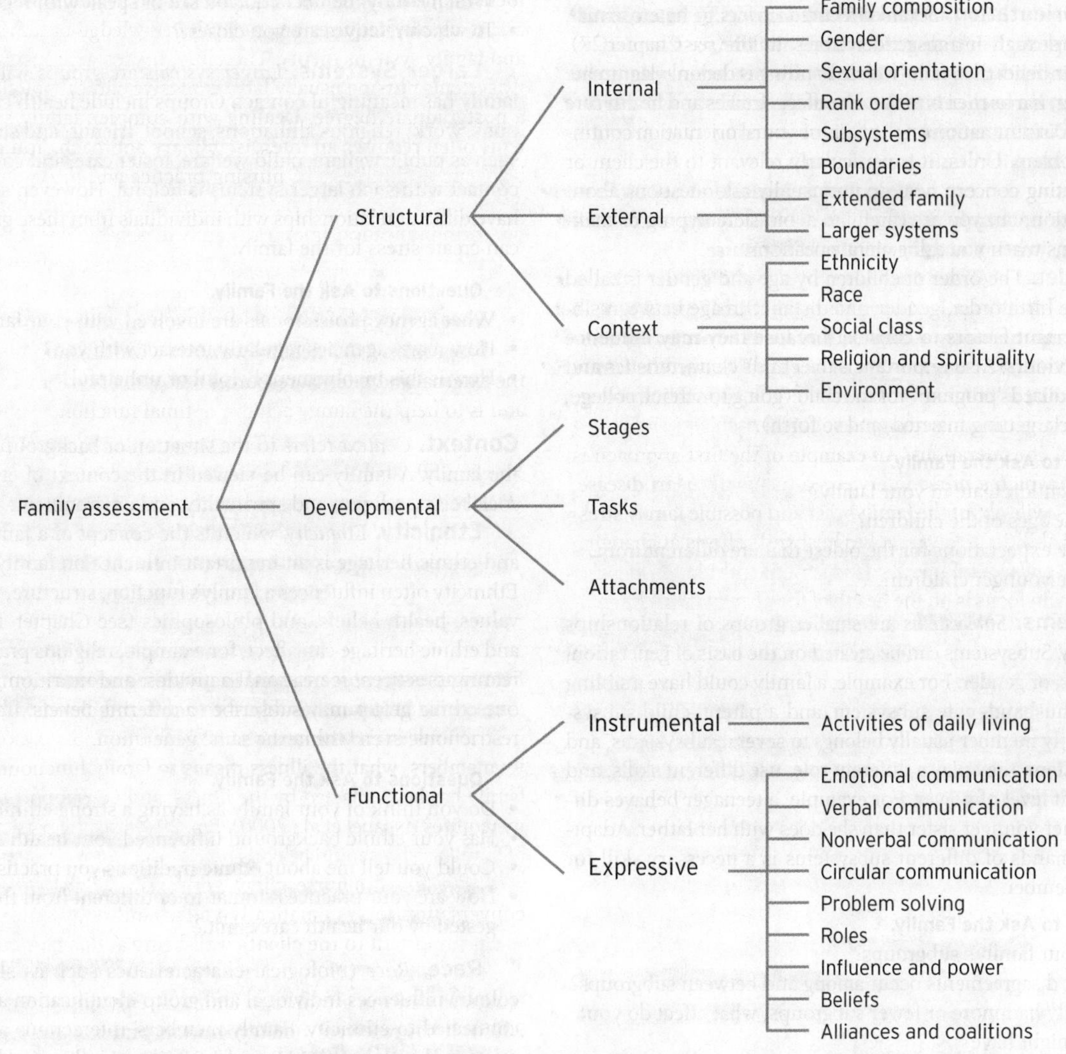

Figure 20-3 Branching diagram of the Calgary Family Assessment Model (CFAM). **Source:** From Wright, L. M., & Leahey, M. (2005). *Nurses and families: A guide to family assessment and intervention* (4th ed., p. 68, Fig. 3-1). Philadelphia: F. A. Davis.

Family Composition. *Family composition* refers to the individual members who form the family. The family composition is not limited to the traditional, nuclear family; it may include any of the various family forms discussed earlier (see Box 20–1). It is important to note whether any recent additions or losses in the family composition have occurred.

Questions to Ask the Family.
- Who is in your family?
- Does anyone else live with you: for example, grandparents, boarders?
- Has anyone recently moved out, married, or died?
- Can you think of anyone else who is like a family member but is not biologically related?

Gender. *Gender* is the set of beliefs about or expectations of masculine and feminine behaviours and experiences. These beliefs are fundamental to male and female relationships and are influenced by culture, religion, and family. It is useful to understand how male and female members of a particular family may view the world differently.

Questions to Ask the Family.
- How have your parents' ideas about masculinity and femininity affected your own?
- Do you have expectations of your children on the basis of their gender?
- Is the division of labour in your family based on gender roles?

Sexual Orientation. *Sexual orientation* refers to heterosexual, homosexual, bisexual, or transgendered orientation (see Chapter 27). Heterosexism, a belief that male–female bonding is the only legitimate type of bonding, is a form of bias that can affect families and health care professionals. Discrimination on the basis of sexual orientation continues to be a problem. Unless it is particularly relevant to the client or family's presenting concern, you do not usually ask questions about sexual orientation, but you are careful to avoid stereotyping or making assumptions when you ask general questions.

Rank Order. The order of children by age and gender is called *rank order.* The birth order, gender, and distance in age between siblings are important factors to consider because they may influence roles and behaviours. Also important is the child's characteristics and the family's idealized "program" for the child (going to school, college, university, work, getting married, and so forth).

Questions to Ask the Family.
- How many children are in your family?
- What are the ages of the children?
- Do you have expectations for the oldest that are different from those for the younger children?

Subsystems. *Subsystems* are smaller groups of relationships within a family. Subsystems can be created on the basis of generation, interests, skills, or gender. For example, a family could have a sibling subsystem, a husband–wife subsystem, and a parent–child subsystem. Each family member usually belongs to several subsystems, and in each subsystem, they play a different role, use different skills, and have a different level of power. For example, a teenager behaves differently with her younger sister than she does with her father. Adapting to the demands of different subsystems is a necessary skill for each family member.

Questions to Ask the Family.
- What are your family's subgroups?
- Do frequent disagreements occur among and between subgroups?
- If your family had more or fewer subgroups, what effect do you think that might have?

Boundaries. *Boundaries* define family subsystems and distinguish one subsystem from another. They influence how members participate in each subsystem. For example, a child in a parent–child subsystem may be given certain responsibilities and power but is not be expected to be involved with family decision making. Boundaries can be weak, rigid, or flexible, and they change over time as family members age or are gained or lost.

Questions to Ask the Family.
- Whom do you talk with when you feel happy?
- Whom do you talk with when you feel sad?
- Does the family have any "unwritten" rules about topics that are never to be discussed with someone outside of the family?

External Structure. *External structure* refers to the connections that family members have to persons outside the family. Two subcategories of external structure exist: extended family and larger systems.

Extended Family. *Extended family* includes the family of origin, the current generation, and steprelatives. How each member sees himself or herself as an individual, yet also as part of the family, should be critically assessed. You should note whether family members make many references to the extended family during the interview.

Questions to Ask the Family.
- Where do your parents live?
- How often do you have contact with them and your brothers and sisters?
- Which family members do you see or speak with regularly?
- To which relatives are you closest?

Larger Systems. *Larger systems* are groups with whom the family has meaningful contact. Groups include health care organizations, work, religious affiliations, school, friends, and social agencies such as public welfare, child welfare, foster care, and courts. Usually, contact with such larger systems is helpful. However, some families have difficult relationships with individuals from these groups, which can create stress for the family.

Questions to Ask the Family.
- What agency professionals are involved with your family?
- How many agencies regularly interact with you?
- How is this involvement helpful or unhelpful?

Context. *Context* refers to the situation or background relevant to the family. A family can be viewed in the context of ethnicity, race, social class, religion and spirituality, and environment.

Ethnicity. *Ethnicity,* which is the concept of a family's cultural and ethnic heritage is an important influence on family interaction. Ethnicity often influences a family's function, structure, perspectives, values, health beliefs, and philosophies (see Chapter 10). Cultural and ethnic heritage can affect, for example, religious practices, child-rearing practices, recreational activities, and nutrition. Members of one ethnic group may subscribe to differing beliefs, traditions, and restrictions, even within the same generation.

Questions to Ask the Family.
- Do you think of your family as having a strong ethnic identity?
- Has your ethnic background influenced your health care?
- Could you tell me about ethnic traditions you practise?
- How are your practices similar to or different from those suggested by our health care clinic?

Race. *Race* (biological characteristics such as skin and hair colour) influences individual and group identification and is closely connected to ethnicity. Family members' interactions among themselves and with health care professionals are influenced by racial attitudes, stereotypes, and discrimination. If ignored, these influences can harm the nurse and family's relationship.

Questions to Ask the Family.

- If you and I were of the same race, would our conversation be different?
- If so, how?

Social Class. *Social class* is shaped by education, income, and occupation. Each class has its own values, lifestyles, and behaviours that influence family interaction and health care practices.

Questions to Ask the Family.

- What is your job, and how many hours a week do you work?
- Does anyone in the family work shifts?
- How does that influence your family functioning?
- What level of education have you completed?
- Does your family have economic problems at this time?

Religion and Spirituality. Family members' spiritual or religious beliefs, rituals, and practices can influence their ability to cope with or manage an illness or health concern (Wright, 2004). Spirituality is often an underused resource in family work (see Chapter 28).

Questions to Ask the Family.

- Are you involved in a church, temple, mosque, or synagogue?
- Would you discuss a family problem with anyone from your place of worship?
- Do you consider your spiritual beliefs a resource?

Environment. The family *environment* refers to the larger community, neighbourhood, and home. Environmental factors that may affect family functioning include availability or lack of adequate space and of access to schools, day care, recreation, and public transportation.

Questions to Ask the Family.

- What are the advantages and disadvantages of living in your neighbourhood?
- What community services does your family use?
- What community services would you like to learn about?

Structural Assessment Tools.

The CFAM encourages you to create genograms and ecomaps to help document and understand the structure of a family and its contact with outside individuals and organizations. A **genogram** is a sketch of the family structure and relevant information about family members (Figure 20–4). Some agencies have genogram forms, but genograms can also be sketched on other forms, such as admission forms or Kardex cards. The genogram becomes part of the documentation about the client and family. In some facilities, the information is collected on admission and then hung at the client's bedside, serving as a visual reminder to all health care professionals involved with the client to think about the family. An **ecomap** is a sketch of the family's contact with persons outside the family (Figure 20–5). The family members who share the household are depicted in the centre of the ecomap, and various important extended family members or larger systems are sketched in to show their relationship to the family.

You should draw genograms and ecomaps for families with whom you will be involved for more than one day. Information for brief genograms and ecograms can be gleaned from family members during the structural assessment. The most essential information for genograms includes data about ages, occupation or school grade, religion, ethnicity, and current health status of each family member. For a brief genogram, you focus only on information that is relevant to the family and the health problem.

Developmental Assessment

Families, like individuals, change and grow over time. Although each family is unique, all families tend to go through certain stages that require family members to adjust, adapt, and change roles. Each developmental stage presents challenges and includes tasks that need to be completed before the family can successfully move on to the next stage. Family development is more than the concurrent development of children and adults. It is the interaction between an individual's development and the phase of the family developmental life cycle that can be significant for family functioning. Therefore, in addition to understanding family structure, you should understand the developmental life cycle of each family.

In their model of family life stages, McGoldrick and Carter (1982; Carter & McGoldrick, 1999) described the emotional aspects of lifestyle transition and the changes and tasks necessary for the family to proceed developmentally (Table 20–1). You can use this model to promote behaviours to achieve essential tasks and help families prepare for transitions. The model presented in Table 20–1, however, does not address diverse family forms, such as blended families, lone-parent families, families without children, or common-law partners.

Functional Assessment

A *functional assessment* focuses mainly on how family members interact and behave toward each other. You assess how family members function by closely observing their interactions. Family functioning consists of two subcategories: instrumental and expressive functioning.

Instrumental Functioning. *Instrumental functioning* refers to the normal activities of daily living such as preparing meals, eating, sleeping, and attending to health needs. For families with health problems, these activities often become a challenge. Roles may change as family members cope with a relative's illness and disability.

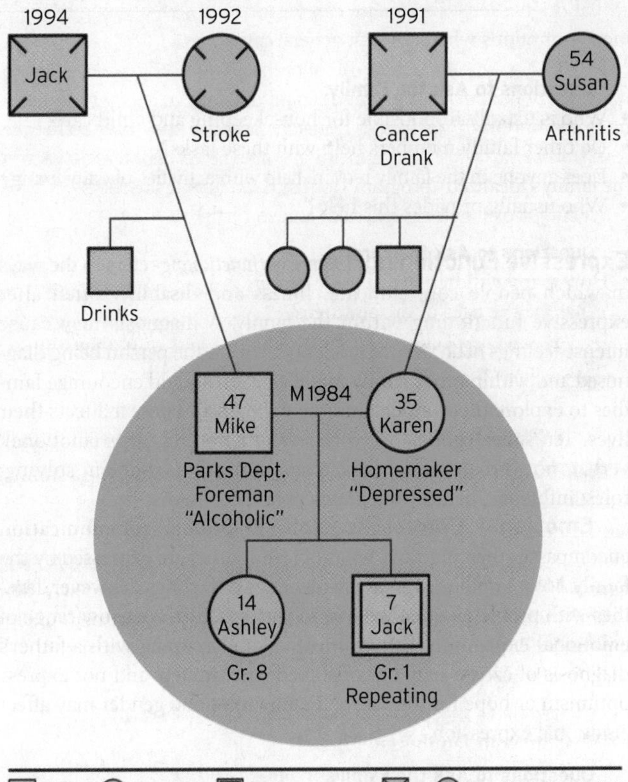

Figure 20-4 Sample family genogram. **Source:** Adapted from Wright, L. M., & Leahey, M. (2000). *Nurses and families: A guide to family assessment and intervention* (3rd ed., p. 90, Fig. 3-9). Philadelphia: F. A. Davis.

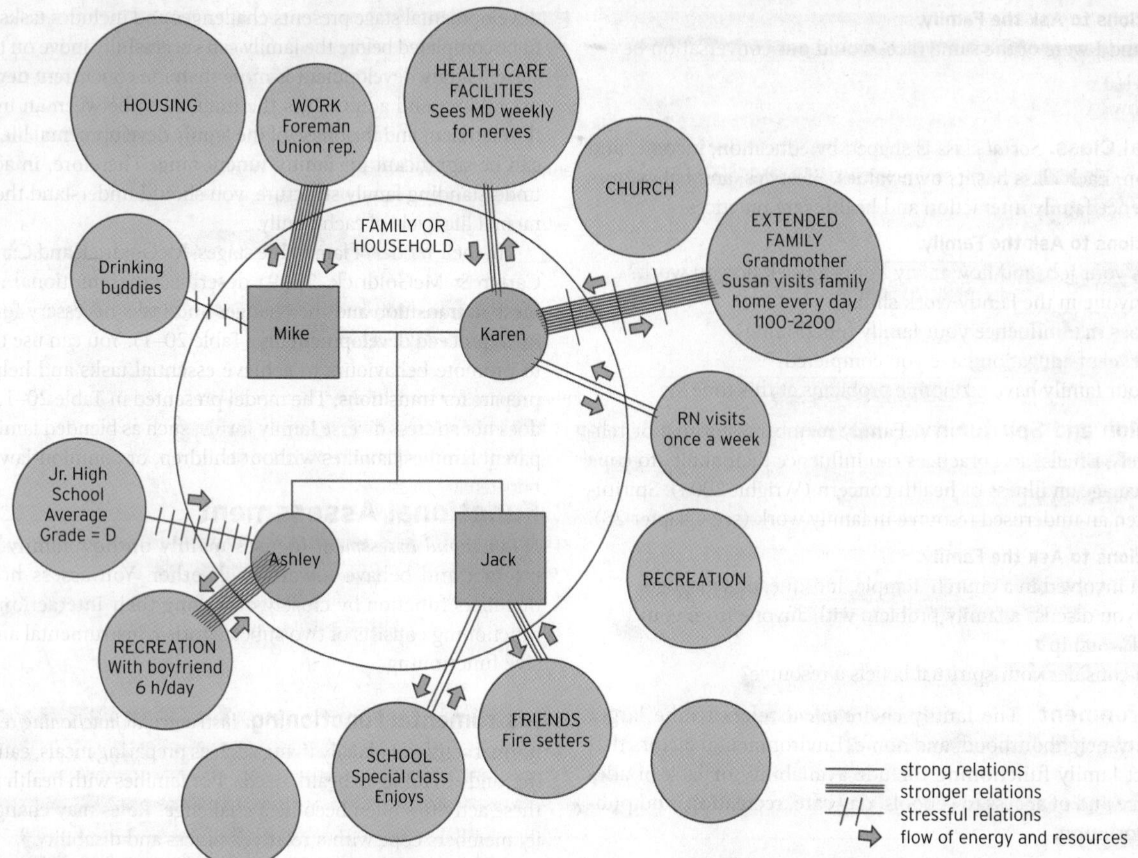

Figure 20-5 A sample family ecomap. RN, registered nurse. **Source:** Adapted from Wright, L. M., & Leahey, M. (2000). *Nurses and families: A guide to family assessment and intervention* (3rd ed., p. 96). Philadelphia: F. A. Davis.

Questions to Ask the Family.

- Who is usually responsible for housekeeping and child care?
- Do other family members help with these tasks?
- Does anyone in the family require help with activities of daily living?
- Who usually provides this help?

Expressive Functioning. *Expressive functioning* refers to the ways in which people communicate. Illness and disability often alter expressive functioning within the family. A diagnosis may cause intense feelings of anxiety or grief, both within the person being diagnosed and within other family members. You should encourage families to explore their understanding of illness and how it affects their lives. Ten subcategories of expressive functioning exist: emotional, verbal, nonverbal, and circular communication; problem solving; roles; influence; beliefs; and alliances and coalitions.

Emotional Communication. **Emotional communication** encompasses the range and types of feelings that are expressed by the family. Most families express a wide range of feelings. However, families with problems often have rigid patterns with a narrow range of emotional expression. For example, a family coping with a father's diagnosis of cancer may be consumed with anxiety and not express optimism or hope for the future. Family roles and gender may affect emotional expression.

Questions to Ask the Family.

- How can you tell when each member of your family is happy, sad, or under stress?
- How do you express happiness, sadness, or stress?

Verbal Communication. You should observe a family's verbal **communication**, focusing on the meaning of the words in terms of the relationship. Is communication among family members clear and direct, or is it vague and indirect? You should also ask family members their opinions about how well the family communicates.

Questions to Ask the Family.

- Which family member communicates most clearly?
- How might your family members communicate with each other more effectively?

Nonverbal Communication. Nonverbal communication consists of messages conveyed without words, including body language, eye contact, gesturing, crying, and tone of voice.

Questions to Ask the Family.

- How do you think your daughter feels when your son rolls his eyes while she's talking?
- Who shows the most distress when talking about your dad's drinking?

Circular Communication. **Circular communication** refers to communication between family members that is reciprocal; that is, each person influences the behaviour of the other. Circular communication can be adaptive or maladaptive. For example, an adaptive communication pattern occurs when a parent comforts a child because the child cries. Because the parent responds to the child, the child feels safe and secure. An example of a maladaptive communication pattern is when a parent criticizes a teenager for not phoning home. The teenager is angry for being criticized and avoids the

TABLE 20-1 Stages of the Family Life Cycle

Family Life Cycle Stage	Emotional Process of Transition: Key Principles	Changes in Family Status Required to Proceed Developmentally
Between families: unattached young adult	Accepting parent–offspring separation	Differentiation of self in relation to family of origin Development of intimate peer relationships Establishment of self in work
Joining of families through marriage: newly married couple	Commitment to new system	Formation of marital system Realignment of relationships with extended families and friends to include spouse
Family with young children	Accepting new generation of members into system	Adjusting marital system to make space for children Taking on parental roles Realignment of relationships with extended family to include parenting and grandparenting roles
Family with adolescents	Increasing flexibility of family boundaries to include children's independence	Shifting of parent–child relationships to permit adolescents to move into and out of system Refocus on midlife material and career issues Beginning shift toward concerns for older generation
Launching children* and moving on	Accepting multitude of exits from and entries into family system	Renegotiation of marital system as dyad Development of adult-to-adult relationships between grown children and their parents Realignment of relationships to include in-laws and grandchildren Dealing with disabilities and death of parents (grandparents)
Family in later life	Accepting shifting of generational roles	Maintaining own or couple functioning and interests in the face of physiological decline; exploration of new familial and social role options Support for more central role for middle generation Making room in system for older adults' wisdom and experience Supporting older generations without overfunctioning for them Dealing with loss of spouse, siblings, and other peers, and preparation for own death; life review and integration

From McGoldrick, M., & Carter, E. (1982). The stages of the family life cycle. In Walsh, F. (Ed.), *Normal family processes* (pp. 375–398). New York: Guilford Press.

*Enabling children to move out of the family home.

parent. Because the teenager avoids the parent, the parent becomes angrier and criticizes more.

Questions to Ask the Family.

- You mentioned that your teenager does not phone home. What do you do then?
- How do you think that affects her?

Problem Solving. **Problem solving** refers to how a family thinks about actions to take to resolve difficult situations.

Questions to Ask the Family.

- Who first notices problems?
- How does your family tend to deal with problems?
- Is one member more proactive than others about solving problems?

Roles. **Roles** are established patterns of behaviour for family members, often developed through interactions with others. Formal roles include those of mother, husband, friend, and so forth. Informal roles can include, for example, those of "the softy," "the angel," or "the scapegoat."

Questions to Ask the Family.

- Who is the "good listener" in your family?
- Who is "the angel"?

Influence. **Influence** refers to methods of affecting or controlling another person's behaviour. Influence may be instrumental (the use of privileges as reward for behaviour; e.g., the promise of candy, computer time), psychological (the use of communication to influence behaviour; e.g., praise, admonishment), or corporal (the use of body contact; e.g., hugging, hitting).

Questions to Ask the Family.

- What method does your mom use to get you to go to bed at the right time?
- How does your grandma get your brother to attend school when he refuses?

Beliefs. **Beliefs** are individual- and family-held fundamental ideas, values, opinions, and assumptions (Wright et al., 1996). Beliefs influence behaviour and how the family adapts to illness. For example, if a family believes that vaccinations may cause long-term disabilities, the parents may decline vaccinating an infant.

Questions to Ask the Family

- What do you believe is the cause of your husband's depression?
- What do you believe would be the effect on your chronic pain if you choose to participate in that treatment?

Alliances and Coalitions. Alliances and coalitions involve the directionality, balance, and intensity of relationships among family members or between families and nurses.

Questions to Ask the Family.

- If the children are playing well together, who would be most likely to get them to start fighting?
- Who would stop them from fighting?

Family Intervention: The Calgary Family Intervention Model

After the assessment, you need to intervene to help families meet their needs. A range of family nursing interventions can be offered to families. Some, such as parent education and caregiver support, are general; others are specific and require therapeutic communication and family interviewing skills. The ultimate goal is to help family members discover solutions that reduce or alleviate emotional, physical, and spiritual suffering. Whether caring for a client with the family as context or directing care to the family as client, nursing interventions aim to increase family members' abilities in certain areas, to remove barriers to health care, and to perform actions that the family cannot perform for itself. You guide the family in problem solving, provide practical services, and convey a sense of acceptance and caring by listening carefully to family members' concerns and suggestions.

You must tailor your interventions to each family and the chosen domain of family functioning. You must remember that each family is unique. In addition, you can only offer interventions to the family; you should not instruct or insist on a particular kind of change or way of family functioning.

The **Calgary Family Intervention Model (CFIM)** is a companion to the CFAM and can be used as a guide for family interventions (Wright & Leahey, 2005). The CFIM focuses on promoting and improving family functioning in three domains: cognitive (thinking), affective (feeling), and behavioural (doing). Interventions may affect functioning in any or all of the three domains. For example, when a clinic nurse informs a wife that her husband, who has amyotrophic lateral sclerosis, is still capable of large gross motor movement, the nurse can suggest that he help with chores in the house, such as bringing the laundry upstairs. This intervention challenges the wife's thinking that her husband was incapable of work, influences the wife to feel less depressed over her husband's declining physical capacity, and leads the wife to change her behaviour by including her husband when performing other household chores.

The CFIM recommends many nursing practices that promote family functioning, including asking interventive questions, offering commendations, providing information, validating emotional responses, encouraging illness narratives, supporting family caregivers, and encouraging respite.

Asking Interventive Questions

One of the simplest but most effective ways that nurses can help families is by engaging in conversations with families and asking them questions. Questions lead the family to reflect on their situation, clarify their opinions and ideas, and understand how they are affected by their family member's illness or condition. By hearing their own responses to questions, family members can better understand themselves and each other and perhaps discover new solutions. Interventive questions also elicit information important to the nurse.

Interventive questions are of two types: linear and circular (Tomm, 1987, 1988). **Linear questions** elicit information about a client or family. They explore a family member's descriptions or perceptions of a problem. For example, when exploring a couple's perceptions of their daughter's anorexia nervosa, you could begin with linear questions: "When did you notice that your daughter had changed her eating habits?" "Has she been hospitalized in the past for this problem?" These questions inform you of the daughter's eating patterns and illuminate family perceptions or beliefs about eating patterns.

Circular questions help determine changes that could be made in a client's or family's life. They help explain a problem. For example, with the same family, you could ask, "Who is most worried about Cheyenne's anorexia?" or "How does Mother show that she's worrying the most?" Circular questions help you understand relationships between individuals, beliefs, and events, and they elicit valuable information to help create change. In this way, circular questions often help clients make new cognitive connections, paving the way for changes in family behaviours. Whereas linear questions may imply that you knows what is best for the family, circular questions facilitate change by inviting the family to discover their own answers. Linear questions tend to target specific "yes" or "no" answers, thereby limiting the options for the family: for example, "Have you tried time out to discipline your three-year-old?" An alternative circular question might be "Which type of discipline seems to work best for your three-year-old?" Several types of circular questions exist, and each can affect the cognitive, affective, and behavioural domains. These types include difference questions, behavioural effect questions, hypothetical or future-oriented questions, and triadic questions (Wright & Leahey, 2005; Table 20–2).

Offering Commendations

Families do not always view their own system as one that has inherently positive components. You can help the family become aware of its own unique strengths, thereby increasing its potential and capabilities. A **commendation** is a statement that emphasizes the strengths or abilities of the family. While spending time with the family, you may observe many instances in which the family displays positive attributes. It is important to acknowledge these to the family so that they can appreciate their own strengths. By commending a family's strengths and competencies, you can offer family members a new view of themselves. You should look for patterns of behaviour to commend, rather than a single occurrence. For example, you may say, "Your family is showing much courage in living with your wife's cancer for five years" or "I'm very impressed with how the family worked together during the crisis." Families coping with chronic, life-threatening, or psychosocial problems frequently feel hopeless in their efforts to overcome or live with the illness. Therefore, you should offer as many truthful commendations as possible. In a study of families experiencing chronic illness, families reported that the nursing team's commendations were "an extremely important facet of the process" (Robinson, 1998).

Family strengths include clear communication, adaptability, healthy child-rearing practices, support and nurturing among family members, and the use of crisis for growth. You can help the family focus on these strengths instead of on its problems and weaknesses.

Providing Information

Families need information from health care professionals about developmental issues, health promotion, and illness management, especially if the illness is complex (Levac et al., 2002; Robinson, 1998). Accurate and timely information is essential for the family to make decisions and cope with difficult situations. One of the roles

TABLE 20-2 Types of Circular Questions

Purpose of Question	Examples to Elicit Change: Cognitive Domain	Affective Domain	Behavioural Domain
Difference Question Explores differences between people, relationships, time, ideas, or beliefs	What is the best advice given you about supporting your son with AIDS? What is the worst advice?	Who in the family is most worried about how AIDS is transmitted?	Which family member is best at getting your son to take his medication on time?
Behavioural Effect Question Explores connections between how one family member's behaviour affects other members	What do you know about the effect of life-threatening illness on children?	How does your son show that he is afraid of dying?	What could you do to show your son that you understand his fears?
Hypothetical/Future-Oriented Question Explores family options and alternative actions or meanings in the future	What do you think will happen if these skin grafts continue to be painful for your son?	If your son's skin grafts are not successful, what do you think his mood will be? Angry? Resigned?	When will your son engage in treatment for his contractures?
Triadic Question Question posed to a third person about the relationship between two other people	If your father were not drinking daily, what would your mother think about his receiving treatment for alcoholism?	What does your father do that makes your mother less anxious about his condition?	If your father were willing to talk with your mother about solutions to his addiction, what do you think he might say?

Adapted from Wright, L. M., & Leahey, M. (2000). *Nurses and families: A guide to family assessment and intervention* (3rd ed., pp. 162–163). Philadelphia: F. A. Davis.
AIDS, acquired immunodeficiency syndrome.

you will need to adopt is that of an educator. Health education is a process by which information is exchanged between nurse and client. Family and client needs for information may be elicited through direct questioning, but they are generally far more subtle. You may recognize, for example, that a new father is fearful of cleaning his newborn's umbilical cord stump or that an older woman is not using her cane safely. Respectful communication is required. Often, you can express your need for information subtly: "I notice you are trying to not touch the umbilical cord stump; I see that a lot with other new parents" or "You use the cane the way I did before I was shown a way to keep from falling or tripping over it; do you mind if I show you?" When you assume a humble position instead of coming across as an authority on the subject, this attitude often decreases the client's defences and invites the client to listen without feeling embarrassed.

Validating or Normalizing Emotional Responses

Validation of intense emotions can alleviate a family's feelings of isolation and loneliness and help family members make the connection between a family member's illness and their own emotional response. For example, after a diagnosis of a life-shortening illness, families frequently feel powerless or frightened. It is important for you to validate these strong emotions as normal and to reassure families that they will adjust and learn new ways to cope.

Encouraging Illness Narratives

Too often, clients and family members are encouraged to talk only about medical aspects of their illness rather than emotional aspects. An **illness narrative** is the person's story of how the illness affects his or her whole being, including emotional, intellectual, social, and spiritual dimensions. Hearing the person's illness narrative helps you understand the person's strengths and challenges. This information enables you to offer commendations of the client's abilities. Many people also find that the telling of their story helps them better understand themselves, their experience, and their family's experience.

The need to communicate what it is like to live with individual, separate experiences, particularly the experience of illness, is powerful in human relationships (Nichols, 1995; Wright, 2004). Frequently, nurses believe that listening entails an obligation to "fix" whatever concerns or problems are raised. However, showing compassion and offering commendations are usually more therapeutic or helpful than is offering solutions to problems (Bohn et al., 2003; Hougher Limacher, 2003; Hougher Limacher & Wright, 2003; Moules, 2002).

Encouraging Family Support

You can enhance family functioning by encouraging and assisting family members to listen to each other's concerns and feelings. This assistance can be particularly useful if a family member is embracing some constraining beliefs when a loved one is dying or has died (Wright & Nagy, 1993). For example, a family may believe that talking with the ill person about death and dying would hasten the person's death.

Supporting Family Caregivers

Family members are often afraid of becoming involved in the care of an ill member without a nurse's support. One way you can best provide family care is through supporting family caregivers. Without adequate preparation or support, caregiving can be stressful, causing a decline in the health of the caregiver and the care receiver or even the development of abusive relationships.

Despite its demands, caregiving can be a positive and rewarding experience (Picot et al., 1997). Whether it is one spouse caring for the other or a child caring for a parent, caregiving is an interactional process. The interpersonal dynamics between family members influence the ultimate quality of caregiving. Thus, you can play a key role in helping family members develop better communication and problem-solving skills needed for successful caregiving.

Researchers have identified variables, such as caregiver and care recipient expectations of one another, that influence caregiving quality. Carruth (1996) studied the concept of **reciprocity**, in which care recipients acknowledge the importance of the caregiver's help, which contributes to a caregiver's perception of self-worth. When the caregiver knows that the care recipient appreciates his or her efforts and values the assistance provided, the caregiving relationship is healthier and more satisfying. When caregiver and client solve problems together, overprotection or oversolicitous behaviour can be avoided. Clients feel in control of their care and responsible for care decisions. The caregiver also feels very positive and enjoys the caregiving experience (Isaksen et al., 2003).

Encouraging Respite

Nurses should encourage respite for caregivers, who may feel guilty about needing or wanting to withdraw, even temporarily, from the caregiving role. Caregivers may not recognize their needs for respite. Sometimes an ill person may be encouraged to accept another person's temporary assistance so that family members can take a break. Whatever the situation, you should remember that each family's need for respite varies.

Providing care and support for family caregivers often involves using available family and community resources for respite. A caregiving schedule is useful when all family members participate, when extended family members share any financial burdens posed by caregiving, and when distant relatives send cards and letters communicating their support. However, it is imperative for you to understand the relationship between potential caregivers and care recipients. If the relationship is not a supportive one, community services may be a resource for both the client and family.

Use of community resources might include locating a service required by the family or providing respite care so that the family caregiver has time away from the care recipient. Services that may be beneficial to families include caregiver support groups, housing and transportation services, food and nutrition services, housecleaning, legal and financial services, home care, hospice, and mental health resources. Before referring a family to a community resource, it is crucial that you understand the family's dynamics and know whether support is desired or welcomed. Often a family caregiver resists help, feeling obligated to be the sole source of support to the care recipient. You must be sensitive to family relationships and help caregivers understand the normality of caregiving demands.

Interviewing the Family

Once you have a clear conceptual framework for assessment and intervention, you can begin to learn the competencies and skills needed to conduct family interviews. Family interviews follow the same basic principles as any client interview (see Chapter 13). However, family interviews can be more complex because more people are involved. You must develop keen perceptual, conceptual, and executive skills. *Perceptual skills* refer to the ability to make relevant observations. In family interviewing, the nurse must observe multiple interactions and relationships simultaneously. *Conceptual skills* constitute the ability to formulate observations of the entire family and give meaning to those observations. Remember, however, that observations and subsequent judgements are subjective and not conclusive. Executive skills are the actual therapeutic interventions that you carry out in an interview. These therapeutic interventions elicit responses from family members and are the basis for further observations and conceptualizations. During an interview, you monitor responses from a client and family to form opinions and concepts about therapeutic interventions. The type of therapeutic intervention that you provide depends on your clinical expertise and experience in working with families.

Table 20–3 lists four stages of a family interview and the executive skills that might be used during each stage. By using the skills presented in Table 20–3, you can engage a family to assess, explore, and identify strengths and problems. You can also decide to intervene or refer the family to another health professional. These skills should not necessarily be applied to all families. You should tailor the interview to each family's individual context.

It is important to realize that not all family interviews are formal, lengthy processes. Even if you do not have the time to organize a formal family interview, you can still engage the family in productive, therapeutic conversation. Every conversation between you and client or family members improves communication and understanding, and no conversation is trivial. Therapeutic conversations can be as short as one sentence or as long as time allows. All conversations, regardless of time, have the potential to unite the family (Hougher Limacher & Wright, 2003; McLeod, 2003). Even brief interviews, or conversations, have tremendous healing potential because they offer families the opportunity to acknowledge and affirm their problems and seek solutions (Hougher Limacher, 2003; Moules, 2002; Tapp, 2001).

The integration of task-oriented client care with interactive, purposeful conversation distinguishes a time-effective interview (taking less than 15 minutes; Box 20–5). Providing information and involving the family in decision making are integral parts of the process. You should search for opportunities to engage in purposeful conversations with families, which may include the following:

- Routinely inviting families to accompany the client to the unit, clinic, or hospital
- Routinely including families' participation in the admission procedure
- Routinely inviting families to ask questions
- Acknowledging the client and family's expertise in managing the health problem at home
- Routinely consulting clients and families about their ideas regarding treatment and discharge

TABLE 20-3 Family Interviewing Skills for Nurses Using the CFAM and CFIM

Perceptual and Conceptual Skills You understand the following:	Executive Skills You might do the following:
Stage 1: Engagement	
1. An individual family member is best understood in the context of the family.	1. Invite to the first interview all family members who are concerned about or involved in the problem.
2. Involvement of partners, parents, or both helps you obtain a broad view of the family and increase engagement among its members.	2. Try to involve partners, parents, or both in initial sessions.
3. Providing structure to the interview reduces anxiety and increases engagement, especially during times of crisis.	3. Explain the purpose, length, and structure of the interview to family members, and ask whether they have any questions about the interview.
4. Family members are most comfortable talking about the structural aspects of the family.	4. Introduce yourself, and ask family members to share their names, ages, work or school information, number of years married, and so forth.
Stage 2: Assessment	
1. The CFAM can be used to understand family dynamics.	1. Explore the components of the structural, developmental, and functional aspects of the CFAM to assess strengths and problem areas. Not all components of the CFAM need to be explored if they are not relevant to the situation.
2. A detailed description and history of the presenting problem are important.	2. Ask family members, including children, to explain their understanding of the presenting problem: "How do you see the problem?"
3. The presenting problem is often related to other concerns in the family. For example, a child's outbursts may be related to a family conflict.	3. Explore with the family whether other problems or concerns connected to the presenting problem exist.
4. Noting differences generates more specific information: • Clarifying *differences between individuals* reveals information about family functioning. • Clarifying *differences between relationships* reveals information about family structure. • Clarifying *differences between family members or in relationships* at various times reveals information about family development.	4. Inquire about differences between individuals, relationships, and points in time. For example: • Ask the child, "Who is better at getting you to do those things in the evening, your mother or father?" • "Do your father and Ingo fight more or less than your father and Hannah do?" • "Do you worry more, less, or the same about your husband's health since his heart attack?"
5. The information obtained from the family assessment is used to create a list of strengths and problems. Strengths and problems may be present in the structural, functional, or developmental dimensions of family life. For example: • Structural: adjusting to lone parenthood • Developmental: adjusting to children's leaving home • Functional: reacting to a family-held belief, such as "Father would be displeased with us for still crying about his death"	5. State to the family your understanding of its strengths and problems, and ask whether you are correct. After verifying them with the family, record your conclusions. For example: • "I've identified your being a newly single parent and also having to cope with your children's leaving home as your two major concerns. Have I understood this correctly?"
6. Some problems are beyond the scope of the nurse's competence. Referral is necessary when medical symptoms have not been fully assessed or when longstanding emotional or behavioural problems exist.	6. Tell the family members whether you will continue to work with them on problems or will refer them to another professional. (If you refer them, proceed to Stage 4, Termination.) For example: • "Now that I have a more complete understanding of your concerns, I think it is necessary to have your son examined by a pediatrician."
7. An extensive inquiry into the most pressing problems is necessary before you intervene.	7. Ask the family members which issue they think is most important, and then explore it in depth. If the family members cannot agree, discuss the lack of consensus. For example: • "About which of the problems we have discussed today are you most concerned?"
8. Assessment is complete when you have obtained sufficient information to clearly understand the presenting problem.	8. State your understanding of the problem or problems to the family members, and obtain their commitment to work on a specific problem.

Continued

➤ TABLE 20-3 Family Interviewing Skills for Nurses Using the CFAM and CFIM *continued*

Perceptual and Conceptual Skills You understand the following:	**Executive Skills** You might do the following:
Stage 3: Intervention	
1. Families have problem-solving abilities. Families not only possess the capability to change but also the capability to identify and implement solutions.	1. Encourage family members to explore possible solutions to problems. For example: • "You've mentioned that your mother is critical of herself. What do you think she could do to feel more positive?"
2. Interventions are focused on the cognitive, affective, and behavioural domains of functioning, as described in the CFIM. It is not always necessary to design interventions for all domains simultaneously.	2. Plan interventions to influence one or all of the domains of functioning described in the CFIM. For example: • Cognitive: invite the family to think differently. • Affective: encourage different affective expressions. • Behavioural: ask the family to perform new tasks.
3. Lack of information can inhibit the family's problem-solving abilities. With additional information, many families can provide their own creative and unique solutions to problems.	3. Provide information to the family that will support further problem solving. For example: • Ask the family members whether they would like to hear about some typical reactions a three-year-old has to a new baby. This intervention targets cognitive functioning.
4. Persistent, intense emotions can block the family's problem-solving abilities. • Families who experience predominantly negative emotions such as sadness or anger are often unable to deal with problems until the emotional constraint is removed.	4. When appropriate, validate family members' emotional responses. For example: • A son who is suppressing grief may need confirmation that the grieving process is normal. This intervention targets the affective functioning.
5. Suggestions of specific tasks often provide new ways for family members to behave in relation to one another.	5. Assign tasks aimed at improving family functioning. For example: • Suggest that the mother and daughter spend one evening a week together in a common activity. This intervention influences behavioural functioning.
Stage 4: Termination	
A. If Consultation or Referral Is Necessary	
1. Families appreciate additional professional resources when problems are complex.	1. Refer individuals, family members, or both for consultation or ongoing treatment. For example: • "I think that your family needs professional input beyond what I can offer. Therefore, I would like to refer you to the learning centre."
B. If Family Interviewing With the Nurse Continues	
1. Evaluating the family interviews at regular intervals is important.	1. Collaborate with family members about the current status of problems, and initiate termination when sufficient progress is made.
2. Interviews over a prolonged period can foster excessive dependency. The nurse must be careful to not inadvertently encourage dependency.	2. If necessary, mobilize other supports for the family, and begin to initiate termination by decreasing the frequency of sessions. You can inadvertently provide "paid friendship" unless other supports, such as partner, friends, or relatives, are available.
3. Recognizing family members' constructive efforts to solve problems is helpful.	3. Commend family members' positive efforts to resolve problems, regardless of whether you think significant improvement has occurred. For example: • "Your family has made tremendous efforts to find ways to care for your aging father at home and still attend to your children's needs."
4. Individuals and families appreciate backup support in times of stress.	4. If appropriate, extend an invitation for further meetings if problems recur or if the family wants consultation.

CFAM, Calgary Family Assessment Model; CFIM, Calgary Family Intervention Model.

Adapted from Wright, L. M., & Leahey, M. (2000). *Nurses and families: A guide to family assessment and intervention* (3rd ed., pp. 195–202). Philadelphia: F. A. Davis.

BOX 20-5 NURSING STORY

Using Family Interviewing Strategies to Introduce Information, Commend Family Strengths, and Identify Family Needs

Mr. S., 82 years old, was re-admitted today with a diagnosis of severe congestive heart failure. He had suffered a myocardial infarction three months ago. He is accompanied by his daughter Jean, who lives nearby. Jean tells you that other family members are on their way from three hours out of town. Jean tells you that her sister, her brother, and their spouses and children do not really understand how sick her father is. Because the physician can offer Mr. S. only medical management of his congestive heart failure, Jean recognizes that her father's condition is terminal. Jean has also expressed some concern about the level of understanding and acceptance of this situation by other family members. The nurse plans to meet with the whole family when they arrive.

During the nurse's admission assessment of Mr. S., he indicated that he did not want any heroic measures taken to maintain his life and that both his doctor and Jean knew about his wishes. Mr. S. is severely short of breath, receiving high-flow oxygen, and requires diuretics three times daily and doses of morphine as needed to remain even slightly comfortable. He is also taking antiarrhythmic, antihypertensive, and beta-blocking medications to maintain a heart rate of 50 to 70 bpm, and his blood pressure is about 90/60 mm Hg. Despite the antiarrhythmic medications, he has bouts of atrial fibrillation with pounding in his chest. His heart rate can speed up to 150 to 180 bpm, and he turns ashen in colour. The heart rate drops back to 50 to 70 bpm after a few minutes, although he says these episodes are becoming more frequent. His physician has written "do not resuscitate" orders, which include no intubation, no defibrillation, and only comfort measures.

Mr. S.'s other children Mark and Sue, their spouses, and four preteenage children join Jean to meet with the nurse. The nurse engages the family by drawing a genogram to determine who is in the family and their relationships to one another. Then the nurse uses questioning strategies to determine what the family knew previously about Mr. S.'s condition. In response to the question "Who best understands Mr. S.'s condition?" both Mark and Sue indicate that Jean was most knowledgeable. The nurse then asks Mark, "If I asked Sue what she knew about Mr S.'s condition, what would she say?" Mark believes that because Sue talks to her father weekly, she can describe how he is doing and what is wrong with him. The nurse asks Jean what she understands about her father's illness. Jean explains that her father has had heart failure. She indicats that the drugs do not seem to be working very well, her dad is "getting worse," and he does not want "anything else done." On the last visit with the physician at his office, Mr. S. had told the physician that if his condition deteriorated, he did not want to receive further lifesaving treatment.

The nurse then asks Mark and Sue to explain what they understand about congestive heart failure. Both seem to have an adequate understanding of the condition. When asked who best understands what Mr. S. meant by "not wanting anything more done," Mark replies that when they were working on the farm together, his father expressed on a number of occasions that he did not want to be kept alive by artificial means and that unless he was feeling good, he would "rather be dead." Sue indicates that she had talked to her dad a couple of times about his wishes regarding terminal care. The nurse commends the family for their closeness and their knowledge of Mr. S.'s condition. The nurse indicates that the family appears to understand the situation very well.

The nurse asks the family, "Who is having the most difficulty accepting the situation?" The family responds that Mark is, inasmuch as he seems to have been in the least contact with Mr. S. Mark responds that "although it's hard, I'll be O.K." because he knows that "this is the way my dad wants it."

The nurse includes the children in the discussion by asking, "Who is most concerned that Grandpa may not get well?" The two older children indicate that their parents had explained that Grandpa might not get well and that this might be their last chance to see him. The nurse asks the two younger children, "Who will have the most difficult time visiting Grandpa?" and "What would you need to know to feel better about visiting Grandpa?" The responses to the questions indicate that the two younger children would have the most trouble visiting, and they need to know how their grandfather looks and whether he will recognize them. The nurse responds to both questions with information about Mr. S.'s appearance and cognitive state.

The nurse continues exploring the need for support over the next while and whether the family can do other things for each other. The brief interview with the family provides Jean with information about the knowledge and acceptance levels of other members of the family. The family acknowledges Jean's burden in taking Mr. S. to appointments and helping him because she lives close by. The family demonstrates that they can support each other and would need little additional support. The family believes that if they need anything, they would feel comfortable asking the nursing staff. The nursing staff continues to explore the family's response to Mr. S.'s situation and helps prepare them for the time ahead.

Additional interviews are used to explore the family's understanding of the dying process, to provide information, and to promote support for the children.

* KEY CONCEPTS

- Family members influence one another's health beliefs, practices, and status.
- The concept of family is highly individual; thus, you should base care on the client's definition of family rather than on an inflexible definition of family.
- Family nursing care requires that nurses continually examine the current trends in the Canadian family and its health care implications.
- A healthy, resilient family is able to integrate the need for stability with the need for growth and change. The family can be viewed as context, in which you focus either on the individual client within the context of his or her family or on the family with the individual as context, or the family can be viewed as client (family systems nursing), in which you focus on family interactions.
- The CFAM is a conceptual framework that guides you in assessing the structural, developmental, and functional aspects of the family.
- Genograms and ecomaps are structural assessment tools that provide you with a pictorial image of the family's structure and relation to outside influences.
- Family members as caregivers are often spouses who may be either older adults themselves or adult children trying to work full time, care for aging parents, and enable children to move out of the home (launch children) successfully.
- Illness and disability often alter expressive functioning and communication within the family.
- The CFIM is a companion to the CFAM that guides you in implementing family interventions; it is focused on improving family functioning in three domains: cognitive (thinking), affective (feeling), and behavioural (doing).
- One of the simplest and most effective ways that you can help families is by asking them interventive questions.
- Offering commendations is important because they encourage the family to recognize their strengths and competencies.
- Other nursing interventions to help the family include providing information, validating emotional responses, encouraging clients to provide illness narratives, supporting family caregivers, and encouraging respite for family caregivers.
- Family caregiving is an interactional process that occurs within the context of the relationships among its members.
- Family interviews require you to have perceptual, conceptual, and executive skills; interviews may be formal and lengthy or casual and brief.

* CRITICAL THINKING EXERCISES

1. Kathy is a palliative care nurse working with a family of four: Wai-Ling, a 45-year-old single mother; her adolescent sons, Chun and Wang; and Heng, her 76-year-old mother, who is in the last stages of terminal breast cancer. The family has lived together for 10 years, ever since they immigrated to Canada from Hong Kong. Heng helped Wai-Ling parent Chun and Wang and supported Wai-Ling when her husband died five years ago. Wai-Ling has decided to care for her mother in the family's home until Heng dies. Kathy will assist this family in achieving their goal. Kathy has just had in-service training in using CFAM.
   a. What parts of the CFAM should Kathy use when assessing the family's needs?
   b. How can Kathy help the family achieve their goal of caring for their aging family member at home?
   c. How can Kathy determine this family's strengths, suffering, and resources?
   d. What cultural aspects are important to consider for a family who has immigrated to Canada and is now facing the death of a loved one?
2. Dan and Kim divorced seven years ago, and neither has remarried. They have three daughters, aged 10, 12, and 14. At the time of the divorce, Dan was HIV-positive, and has remained so for five years. Kim has had repeated tests and remains HIV-negative. Dan is responding to therapy slowly. Kim and Dan share parenting responsibilities and have a friendly relationship. They have decided it would be easier for the family to live together again so that Dan can actively participate in his children's lives without placing caregiver demands on Kim when the extended family visits overnight. Kim also wants to care for her former husband.
   a. What family development tasks are important to assess for this family as the members attempt to reunite?
   b. How should the nurse determine what support services the family needs?
   c. What assessment questions would be useful to ask in order to assess how the illness is affecting this family? Do family members have any signs of emotional, physical, or spiritual suffering?
3. Mr. and Mrs. Baillargeron, both in their early 50s, are the youngest members of large families. They work full-time and have two teenage children. Both sets of their parents are in their 80s and have chronic health problems. All of their siblings live farther away.
   a. How can the nurse help Mr. and Mrs. Baillargeron access resources to aid in caring for their parents and maintain the responsibilities of their own family unit?
   b. What developmental tasks does this family have?
   c. What kinds of questions can you ask to assess the family's emotional and verbal communication (found in CFAM's functional assessment category)?

* REVIEW QUESTIONS

1. The nurse must think of family as
   1. Parents and their children
   2. People related by marriage, birth, or adoption
   3. The nuclear family and aunts, uncles, grandparents, and cousins
   4. A set of relationships that the client identifies as family
2. The client is remarried, and her two children from a previous marriage live in the same household. Her husband's children visit on the weekend. This is an example of
   1. A nuclear family
   2. A blended family
   3. An extended family
   4. An alternative family

3. Which of the following is *not* a current trend?
   1. The proportion of couples without children at home is increasing.
   2. The proportion of "traditional" families is declining.
   3. The proportions of common-law and lone-parent families are increasing.
   4. The proportion of teenagers giving birth has increased steadily.
4. The primary social context in which health promotion and disease prevention take place is
   1. At educational institutions
   2. From friends and colleagues
   3. From physicians and nurses
   4. In the family
5. Two factors that contribute to the long-term health of a family are
   1. Structure and function
   2. Caregiving and reciprocity
   3. Hardiness and resiliency
   4. Context and system
6. When nurses view the family as client, their primary focus is on the
   1. Health and development of an individual member existing within a specific environment
   2. Family process and relationships
   3. Family relational and transactional concepts
   4. Family within a system
7. Asking a client "Who is in your family?" helps you assess
   1. Internal structure
   2. External structure
   3. Context
   4. Instrumental functioning
8. According to the CFAM, emotional communication is a subcategory of
   1. Instrumental functioning
   2. Development
   3. Internal structure
   4. Expressive functioning
9. "What do you think when your husband won't visit your son in the hospital?" is an example of a circular question. Asking the family circular questions is an effective way to
   1. Facilitate change by inviting the family to discover their own answers
   2. Encourage family members to be caregivers
   3. Validate their emotional responses
   4. Target specific "yes" or "no" answers
10. During a family interview, the nurse can
    1. Educate the family
    2. Enforce change
    3. Engage a family to assess, explore, and identify strengths and problems
    4. Establish roles

* RECOMMENDED WEB SITES

The Vanier Institute of the Family: http://www.vifamily.ca

The Vanier Institute of the Family was established in 1965 under the patronage of Governor General Georges P. Vanier and Madame Pauline Vanier. It is a national voluntary organization dedicated to promoting the well-being of Canadian families through research, publications, education, and advocacy. This Web site provides links to numerous publications related to important trends and issues affecting Canadian families, including a link to an online publication of *Profiling Canada's Families*.

21

Client Education

Original chapter by Amy M. Hall, RN, BSN, MS, PhD

Canadian content written by Nancy A. Edgecombe, RN-NP, BN, MN, PhD

objectives

Mastery of content in this chapter will enable you to:

- Define the key terms listed.
- Identify appropriate topics for a client's health education.
- Identify the role of the nurse in client education.
- Identify the purposes of client education.
- Use communication principles when providing client education.
- Describe the domains of learning.
- Identify basic learning needs.
- Differentiate factors that determine readiness to learn from those that determine the ability to learn.
- Compare and contrast the nursing and teaching processes.
- Write learning objectives for a teaching plan.
- Establish an environment that promotes learning.
- Include client teaching while performing routine nursing care.
- Use appropriate methods to evaluating learning.

key terms

Affective learning, p. 298
Analogies, p. 307
Cognitive learning, p. 297
Learning, p. 296
Learning objectives, p. 301
Motivation, p. 299
Psychomotor learning, p. 298
Reinforcement, p. 306
Return demonstration, p. 306
Social learning theory, p. 300
Teaching, p. 296

media resources

evolve Web Site

- Audio Chapter Summaries
- Glossary
- Multiple-Choice Review Questions
- Student Learning Activities
- Weblinks

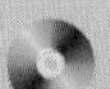
Companion CD

- Glossary
- Interactive Learning Activities
- Fluids and Electrolytes Tutorial
- Test-Taking Skills

Client education is one of the most important roles for nurses in any health care setting. Clients and family members have the right to health education so that they can make informed decisions about their health care and lifestyle. Shorter hospital stays, increased demands on nurses' time, increase in numbers of clients with acute conditions, the severity of these acute conditions, and the increase in numbers of chronically ill clients emphasize the importance of high-quality client education. Initial client education often takes place in the hospital while clients are in the highly stressful acute stage of their illness and may not be completed at the time of discharge. Hospitals need to have clear guidelines to provide for follow-up. Client education helps ensure continuity of care as clients move from one health care setting to another. Nurses often clarify information provided by physicians and other health care professionals and may become the primary source of information for people adjusting to health problems (Falvo, 2004). In primary health care settings, nurses are often the main source of information about health promotion and illness prevention (Box 21–1).

The general public has become more assertive in seeking knowledge, understanding health, and finding resources available within the health care system. Nurses need to assist clients in navigating the vast amount of information available to them, through all forms of media. The Internet and other forms of technology (telehealth, e-health) provide nurses and clients with vast amounts of information, some reliable and some not. Clients need guidance regarding the selection of current and reliable resources. Nurses must be able to discuss with clients the criteria for evaluating sources for validity and reliability. The teaching material provided by nurses must honour copyright rules and must reference both written information and illustrations that are used to support client learning.

You need to be mindful of the increasing emphasis on "scientific" evidence and the diminished focus on other kinds of evidence of the efficacy or effectiveness of therapeutic interventions. You need to have a broad perspective of what constitutes meaningful evidence to support the significance of testimonials, lived experiences, and other ways of knowing. Because critical thinking is essential in nursing care, you need to be mindful that knowledge is limited, beliefs change, and conclusions are temporary. A well-designed, comprehensive teaching plan that meets a learner's needs can reduce health care costs, improve quality of care, help clients gain optimal wellness, and increase independence (Bastable, 2006).

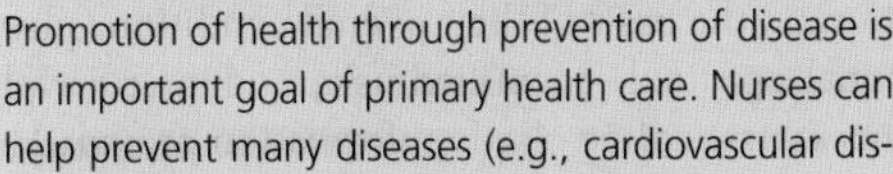

BOX 21-1 FOCUS ON PRIMARY HEALTH CARE

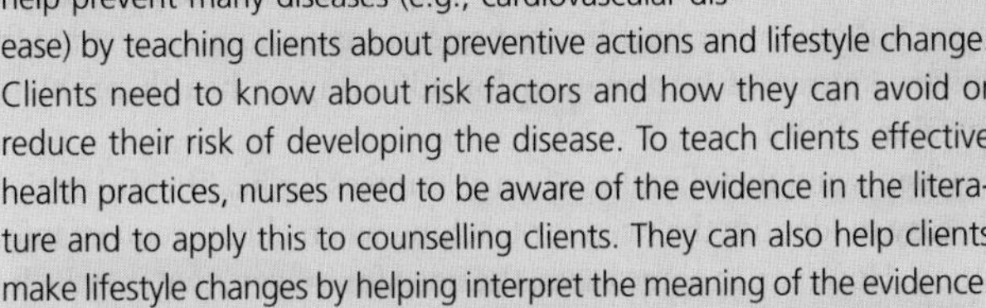

Educating Clients in Order to Promote Health and Prevent Disease

Promotion of health through prevention of disease is an important goal of primary health care. Nurses can help prevent many diseases (e.g., cardiovascular disease) by teaching clients about preventive actions and lifestyle change. Clients need to know about risk factors and how they can avoid or reduce their risk of developing the disease. To teach clients effective health practices, nurses need to be aware of the evidence in the literature and to apply this to counselling clients. They can also help clients make lifestyle changes by helping interpret the meaning of the evidence.

In order to communicate information successfully, nurses need to use simple, clear, and nontechnical language that clients can understand and develop a rapport with clients so that clients are able to receive and act on the information. Characteristics of a positive relationship with the client include empathic understanding, genuineness, intimacy and reciprocity, respect for the client's right to control lifestyle, and mutual trust.

Because clients may face serious barriers to making lifestyle changes, nurses need to carry out an assessment to determine the readiness for behaviour change and the feasibility of carrying out the change. To determine whether meaningful lifestyle change is possible for clients, nurses must understand principles of learning and behavioural change theories.

Clients need to develop an awareness of their own behaviour, a process that can be enhanced by self-monitoring. When clients can identify areas of difficulty and determine how these can be addressed, goals can be set collaboratively to ensure that clients are able to change their behaviour. Breaking down long-term goals into shorter term goals tends to enhance self-efficacy and client satisfaction. Focusing on behaviour change rather than physiological outcomes is recommended because the former is within the control of the client. Once the client identifies a goal, feedback is given to support the client in the process of achieving the goal. Social support from family or friends can be a positive influence in helping clients achieve their goals.

From Burke, L. E., & Fair, J. (2003). Promoting prevention: Skill sets and attributes of health care providers who deliver behavioural interventions. *Journal of Cardiovascular Nursing, 18*(4), 256–266.

Goals of Client Education

The goal of client education is to assist individuals, families, or communities in achieving optimal health (Edelman & Mandle, 2006). Education is a main tool of primary health care; it helps individuals, families, and communities maintain and improve their health, reduces hardship, helps contains health care costs, and enables people to take control of their own health (Canadian Nurses Association, 2003). Client education has three main goals (Box 21–2):

- Maintaining and promoting health and preventing illness
- Restoring health
- Optimizing quality of life with impaired functioning

Maintaining and Promoting Health and Preventing Illness

In the home, clinic, or other community health care setting, you provide information and skills that people need to maintain and improve their health (see Box 21–2). For example, in prenatal classes, nurses teach expectant parents about fetal development and physical and psychological changes during pregnancy. They also teach about the importance of healthy food choices, exercise, and avoiding substances that might harm the fetus. Greater knowledge can result in better health. When clients become more health conscious, they are more likely to seek early diagnosis of health problems (Redman, 2007).

Restoring Health

Many clients seek information and skills that will help them regain or maintain their health (see Box 21–2). However, clients who find it difficult to adapt to illness may be more passive. You learn to identify barriers to learning, to recognize clients' willingness to learn, and to help motivate interest in learning (Redman, 2007).

The family can be a vital part of a client's return to health and may need to know as much as the client. If you exclude the family from a teaching plan, conflicts may arise. For example, if the family does not understand a client's need to regain independent function, their efforts may encourage dependency and slow recovery. You should assess the client–family relationship before involving the family in a teaching plan (see Chapter 20).

> BOX 21-2 Topics for Health Education

Health Maintenance and Promotion and Illness Prevention

Educate clients about:

- First aid
- Avoidance of risk factors (e.g., smoking, alcoholism)
- Stress management
- Typical growth and development patterns
- Proper hygiene
- Required immunizations
- Prenatal care and normal child-bearing
- Nutrition
- Exercise
- Safety (in home and health care setting)
- Screening for common conditions (e.g., blood pressure, poor vision, cholesterol level)
- Behaviour modification to change risky behaviours (e.g., quitting smoking, treatment for substance abuse)

Restoration of Health

Educate clients about:

- Client's disease or condition
- Anatomy and physiology of body system affected by disease or condition
- Cause of disease
- Origin of symptoms
- Expected effects on other body systems
- Prognosis
- Limitations on function
- Rationale for treatment
- Medications
- Tests and therapies
- Nursing measures
- Surgical intervention
- Expected duration of care
- Hospital or clinic environment
- Hospital or clinic staff
- Long-term care implications
- Methods for client's participation in care
- Limitations imposed by disease or surgery

Optimizing Quality of Life When Functions Are Impaired

Educate clients about:

- Home care
- Medications
- Intravenous therapy
- Diet
- Activity
- Self-help devices
- Rehabilitation of remaining function
- Physiotherapy
- Occupational therapy
- Speech therapy
- Prevention of complications
- Knowledge of risk factors
- Implications of noncompliance with therapy
- Environmental alterations
- Self-help and support groups

Coping With Impaired Functioning

Some clients must learn to cope with permanent health alterations. For example, a client who loses the ability to speak after surgery of the larynx must learn new ways to communicate. A client with severe heart disease must learn to modify risk factors that might cause further heart damage. After the client's needs are identified and the family has displayed willingness to help, you teach family members to assist the client with health care management (e.g., giving medications through gastric tubes and performing passive range-of-motion exercises).

Teaching and Learning

Teaching is an interactive process that promotes learning. Teaching and learning generally begin when a person identifies a need for knowing or acquiring an ability to do something. A nurse-teacher provides information that prompts the client to engage in activities that lead to a desired change (Box 21–3). Teaching is most effective when it addresses the learner's needs, learning style, and capacity. The teacher assesses these needs by asking questions, observing the client, and determining the client's interests. With successful teaching, clients can learn new skills or change existing attitudes (Redman, 2007).

Role of the Nurse in Teaching and Learning

Nurses have an ethical responsibility to teach their clients about health enhancement (Redman, 2005, 2007). The Canadian Nurses Association's (2008) *Code of Ethics* indicates that clients have the right to make informed decisions about their care. The information that clients need to make such decisions must be accurate, complete, and relevant to their needs. You should anticipate clients' needs for information on the basis of their overall condition (physical, mental, emotional, spiritual), identified risks, and interdisciplinary treatment plans. Nurses often clarify information provided by physicians and other health care professionals and may become the primary source of information for adjusting to health problems (Bastable, 2006).

Clients and their families often ask nurses for health information. It is easy to identify the need for teaching when clients request information. However, in some cases, the need for information may be less apparent. You must observe and listen carefully to determine clients' needs for information and learning. When you value education and ensure that your clients learn necessary information, clients are better prepared to assume health care responsibilities. To be an effective educator, you must do more than just pass on facts; you must determine what clients need to know, find time when they are ready to learn, and evaluate the impact of client education on client outcomes (Bastable, 2003, 2006; Redman, 2007).

Teaching as Communication

Effective teaching depends on effective communication (see Chapter 18). To be a good teacher, you must listen empathetically, observe astutely, and speak clearly. Many intrapersonal variables—including attitudes, values, culture, emotions, and knowledge—influence both the nurse's and client's styles and approaches. Both you and the client and are also affected by the client's motivation and ability to learn, which depend on physical and psychological health, education, developmental stage, and previous knowledge.

Domains of Learning

Learning occurs in three domains: cognitive (understanding), affective (attitudes), and psychomotor (motor skills); (Bloom, 1956). Any topic to be learned may involve one domain, all domains, or any combination of the three. For example, clients with diabetes must

BOX 21-3 RESEARCH HIGHLIGHT

The Effectiveness of Nurse-Directed Client Education

Research Focus

Clients living with heart failure need education about their diagnosis and related care to prevent multiple hospitalizations and promote optimal functioning.

Research Abstract

Kutzleb and Reiner (2006) wanted to know whether clients who participated in a nurse-directed client education program (the treatment group) had fewer admissions to the hospital, were more knowledgable about self-management, and had better quality of life and functional ability than did clients who did not participate (the control group). Clients in the treatment group were evaluated by a medical physician with a subspecialty in cardiology. The cardiac clinical nurse specialists performed physical assessments and taught the clients the importance of weighing themselves daily and recording the weights. An educational booklet outlining behaviours for successfully managing heart failure was provided to the clients and their families. The clinical nurse specialists also provided individualized counselling and telephone follow-up between monthly clinic visits. The clients in the control group saw a cardiologist every three months in a cardiology clinic and received standardized care. Both groups completed a quality-of-life survey and a walking test to measure functional status. The results of this study revealed no actual difference in functional capacity between the two groups. However, the group that received nurse-directed client education program reported greater quality of life and a positive correlation between quality of life and functional capacity.

Research Highlights

- Nurse-directed client education about lifestyle choices and exercise enhanced quality of life in clients with heart failure.
- Cardiac clinical nurse specialists who collaborated with physicians successfully managed clients with heart failure in the outpatient setting.
- Improving quality of life enhanced the perception of functional capacity in clients with heart failure.
- Clients who receive nurse-directed client education improved their ability to manage their diet and medication.

References: Kutzleb, J., & Reiner, D. (2006). The impact of nurse-directed patient education on quality of life and functional capacity in people with heart failure. *Journal of the American Academy of Nurse Practitioners, 18*(3), 116–123.

learn how diabetes affects the body and how to control blood glucose levels for better health (cognitive domain). They must also learn to accept the chronic nature of diabetes by learning positive coping mechanisms (affective domain). Finally, many clients with diabetes must learn to test their blood glucose levels at home. This requires learning how to use a glucose meter (psychomotor domain). By understanding each learning domain, you can select appropriate teaching methods (Box 21–4).

Cognitive Learning

Cognitive learning includes all intellectual behaviours and requires thinking (Bastable, 2003). In the hierarchy of cognitive behaviours, the simplest behaviour is acquiring knowledge, whereas the most complex is evaluation. Cognitive learning includes the folowing:

- Knowledge: the learning of new facts or information and the ability to recall them

BOX 21-4 Appropriate Teaching Methods Based on Domains of Learning

Cognitive

Discussion (One-on-One or Group)

May involve nurse and one client or nurse with several clients
Promotes active participation and focuses on topics of interest to client
Facilitates peer support
Enhances application and analysis of new information

Lecture

Is more formal method of instruction because it is teacher controlled
Helps learner acquire new knowledge and gain comprehension

Question-and-Answer Session

Is designed specifically to address client's concerns
Assists client in applying knowledge

Role Play and Discovery

Encourages client to actively apply knowledge in controlled situation
Promotes synthesis of information and problem solving

Independent Projects (e.g., Computer-Assisted Instruction) and Field Experience

Assists client to assume responsibility for learning at own pace
Promotes analysis, synthesis, and evaluation of new information and skills

Affective

Role Play

Encourages expression of values, feelings, and attitudes

Discussion (Group)

Enables client to acquire support from other people in group
Encourages client to learn from other people's experiences
Promotes responding, valuing, and organizing

Discussion (One-on-One)

Facilitates discussion of personal, sensitive topics of interest or concern

Psychomotor

Demonstration

Provides presentation of procedures or skills by nurse
Encourages client to model nurse's behaviour
Allows nurse to control questioning during demonstration

Practice

Enables client to perform skills by using equipment in a controlled setting
Allows repetition

Return Demonstrations

Enables client to perform skill as nurse observes
Provides excellent source of feedback and reinforcement

Independent Projects and Games

Require teaching method that promotes adaptation and initiation of psychomotor learning
Enable learner to use new skills

- Comprehension: the ability to understand the meaning of learned material
- Application: the use of abstract, newly learned ideas in a practical situation
- Analysis: the breaking down of information into organized parts
- Synthesis: the ability to apply knowledge and skills to produce a new whole
- Evaluation: a judgement of the worth of information given for a specific purpose

Affective Learning

Affective learning concerns expressions of feelings and acceptance of attitudes, opinions, or values. Values clarification (see Chapter 8) is an example of affective learning. The simplest behaviour in the affective learning hierarchy is receiving, and the most complex is characterizing (Krathwohl et al., 1964).

- Receiving: the willingness to attend to another person's words
- Responding: active participation through listening and reacting verbally and nonverbally
- Valuing: attachment of worth to an object, concept, or behaviour, demonstrated by the learner's actions
- Organizing: development of a value system by identifying and organizing values and resolving conflicts
- Characterizing: action and response with a consistent value system

Psychomotor Learning

Psychomotor learning involves acquiring skills that require the integration of mental and muscular activity, such as the ability to walk or to use an eating utensil. The simplest behaviour in the hierarchy is perception and the most complex is origination (Rankin & Stallings, 2005; Redman, 2007).

- Perception: awareness of objects or qualities through the use of sense organs.
- Set: a readiness (mental, physical, or emotional) to take a particular action.
- Guided response: the performance of an act under the guidance of an instructor, involving imitation of a demonstrated act
- Mechanism: a higher level of behaviour by which a person gains confidence and skill in performing a behaviour that is more complex or involves several more steps than does a guided response
- Complex overt response: the smooth and accurate performance of a motor skill that requires a complex movement pattern
- Adaptation: the ability to change motor response when unexpected problems occur
- Origination: use of existing psychomotor skills and abilities to perform a highly complex motor act that involves creating new movement patterns

Basic Learning Principles

Before nurses can teach, they must understand how people learn. Learning depends on the learning environment and on the individual's ability to learn, learning style, and motivation to learn. Learning takes place both in formal learning sessions, which involve planned learning activities, and in teachable moments, which allow you to spontaneously take advantage of teaching opportunities as they occur in the day-to-day contact with the client.

Learning Environment

Client education takes place in a variety of settings: the client's home, community centres, classrooms, and hospital rooms. The ideal environment for learning is a well-lit, well-ventilated room with appropriate furniture and a comfortable temperature. A quiet setting with few distractions and interruptions helps concentration. You can provide privacy even in a busy hospital by closing cubicle curtains or taking the client to a quiet spot. In the home, a bedroom might separate the client from household activities. If the client desires, family members or significant others may share in discussions. However, some clients may be reluctant to discuss their illness when other people, even close family members, are in the room. An ideal environment is not always achievable, however, and rather than miss a teachable moment, you can adapt the environment as much as possible to provide privacy and minimize distractions.

Ability to Learn

The ability to learn depends on emotional, intellectual, and physical capabilities and on developmental stage. If a client's learning ability is impaired, you should modify or postpone teaching activities.

Emotional Capability. Emotions can aid or prevent learning. Mild anxiety may help a person focus. However, stronger levels of anxiety can be incapacitating, creating an inability to attend to anything other than to relieve the anxiety. The prospect of change makes many people anxious. Seriously ill people, who are faced with multiple losses, may be extremely anxious and distressed. Nurses must be sensitive to a client's level of anxiety. If a person is incapacitated by anxiety, you need to find a way to alleviate the anxiety. This may mean teaching relaxation techniques before attempting to teach a task or a procedure.

Intellectual Capability. Clients have different levels of intellectual ability. You must assess the client's knowledge and intellectual level before beginning a teaching plan. For example, measuring liquid or solid food portions requires the ability to perform mathematical calculations. Reading a medication label or discharge instructions requires reading and comprehension skills. Following directions when performing self-care in accordance with limitations requires comprehension and application skills.

Physical Capability. The ability to learn often depends on physical health. To learn psychomotor skills, a client must possess the necessary strength, coordination, and sensory acuity. You should not overestimate the client's physical ability. The following physical attributes are necessary for learning psychomotor skills:

- Size (height and weight adequate for performing the task or using the equipment, such as crutch walking)
- Strength (ability of the client to follow a strenuous exercise program)
- Coordination (dexterity needed for complicated motor skills, such as using utensils, changing a bandage, or opening a medication container)
- Sensory acuity (visual, auditory, tactile, gustatory, and olfactory resources needed to receive and respond to messages taught)

Any physical condition (e.g., pain, fatigue, or hunger) that depletes energy also impairs the ability to learn. For example, a client in a weakened state who has just spent hours undergoing diagnostic tests is likely to be too fatigued to learn. Nurses must assess the client's energy level by noting the client's willingness to communicate, the degree of activity initiated, and the client's responsiveness to questions. You may halt teaching if the client needs rest.

Developmental Stage. Age and stage of development affect the ability to learn (Box 21–5). Without proper biological, motor, language, and personal–social development, many types of learning cannot take place.

> **BOX 21-5 Teaching Methods Based on Client's Developmental Capacity**
>
> **Infant**
>
> Maintain consistent routines (e.g., feeding, bathing).
>
> Hold infant firmly while smiling and speaking softly, to convey sense of trust.
>
> Have infant touch different textures (e.g., soft fabric, hard plastic).
>
> **Toddler**
>
> Use play to teach procedure or activity (e.g., handling examination equipment, applying bandage to doll).
>
> Offer picture books that describe a story of children in a hospital or clinic.
>
> Use simple words such as "cut" instead of "laceration," to promote understanding.
>
> **Preschooler**
>
> Use role-playing, imitation, and play to make learning fun.
>
> Encourage questions and offer explanations; use simple explanations and demonstrations.
>
> Encourage several children to learn together through pictures and short stories about how to perform hygiene.
>
> **School-Age Child**
>
> Teach necessary psychomotor skills. (Complicated skills, such as learning to use a syringe, may take considerable practice.)
>
> Offer opportunities to discuss health problems and answer questions.
>
> **Adolescent**
>
> Help adolescent learn about feelings and need for self-expression.
>
> Collaborate with adolescent on teaching activities.
>
> Let adolescent make decisions about health and health promotion (safety, sex education, substance abuse).
>
> Use problem solving to help adolescent make choices.
>
> **Young or Middle-Aged Adult**
>
> Encourage participation in teaching plan by setting mutual goals.
>
> Encourage independent learning.
>
> Offer information so that adult can understand effects of health problem.
>
> **Older Adult**
>
> Teach when client is alert and rested.
>
> Involve adult in discussion or activity.
>
> Focus on wellness and the person's strength.
>
> Use approaches that enhance sensorially impaired client's reception of stimuli (see Chapter 48).
>
> Keep teaching sessions short.

Learning in Children. As a child matures, intellectual growth progresses from concrete to abstract. Therefore, information should be understandable, and the expected outcomes should be realistic and based on the child's developmental stage. Developmentally appropriate teaching aids should also be used (Figure 21–1).

Adult Learning. Many adults are independent, self-directed learners. However, they may become dependent in new learning situations. Adults typically learn more successfully when they are encouraged to use past experiences to solve problems. Adult clients and nurses should collaborate on educational topics and goals. Needs or issues that are important to the adult should be addressed early in the teaching–learning process. Ultimately, adults must accept responsibility for changing their own behaviours. Assessing what the adult client currently knows, teaching what the client wants to know, and setting mutual goals will improve the outcomes of care and education (Bastable, 2003).

Learning Style and Preference

People have different learning styles. Everyone processes information differently by seeing and hearing, reflecting and acting, reasoning logically and intuitively, and analyzing and visualizing. Some people are visual learners; they learn best by watching. Audiovisual presentations and visual demonstrations often work best for this type of learner. Other people are kinesthetic learners; they learn best when they are able to manipulate tools and find out how they work. Some people learn by taking detailed notes; others prefer to only listen. Some people need to be engaged in activities and discussion in order to learn effectively. Others may be too shy to enjoy this type of learning and prefer to learn from an orderly, structured presentation.

Environmental, social, emotional, psychological, and physical stimuli affect people differently. Some people prefer complete silence in the learning environment, whereas others prefer background sounds. Some prefer to learn in a group; others, on their own. Different people prefer different times of the day for learning experiences.

When developing teaching plans, you should assess the favoured learning style and preferences of the client. With groups, it may not be possible to address every client's preferences. However, including a combination of approaches to meet multiple learning styles can ensure that most people's learning preferences are met (Bastable, 2006). When the client is having difficulty with learning, you should consider a change to accommodate a different learning style.

Motivation to Learn

Motivation is a person's desire or willingness to learn, and it influences a person's behaviour (Redman, 2007; Box 21–6). If a person is not ready or does not want to learn, learning is unlikely to occur. The stimuli for motivation vary between individuals and may be social, task mastery, or physical in nature. *Social motives* reflect a need for connection, social approval, or self-esteem. For example, the motivation to exercise may be linked to the social aspects of the exercise activities (Heading, 2008). *Task mastery motives* are driven by desire for achievement. For example, a high school student with diabetes begins to test blood glucose levels and determine insulin dosages before leaving home and establishing independence. The

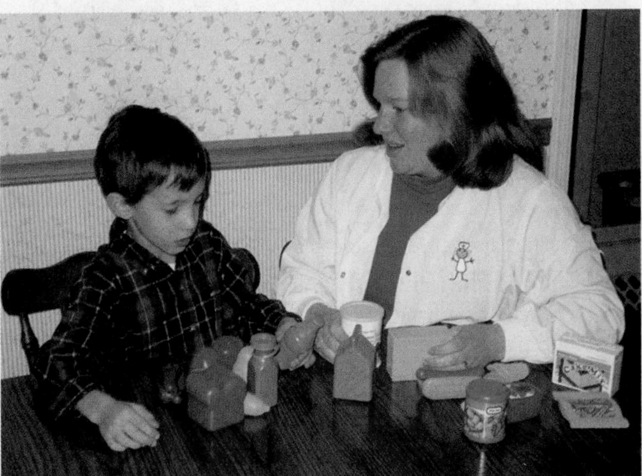

Figure 21-1 The nurse uses developmentally appropriate food models to teach healthy eating behaviours to the school-aged child.

desire to live independently and manage the disease provides the motivation to master the task or skill. After succeeding at a task, a person is usually motivated to achieve more. *Physical motives* come from a desire to maintain and improve health. Clients motivated by the need to survive or overcome hardship are often more motivated than those who wish merely to improve their health (Rankin & Stallings, 2005). For example, a client who has undergone a leg amputation may be extremely motivated to learn to use assistive devices, whereas a client who is overweight but otherwise healthy may not be motivated to exercise.

BOX 21-6 NURSING STORY

"To Take or Not to Take"

In preparation for a trip to Vietnam and Cambodia, Mr. and Mrs. Bennet visited a travel clinic, which recommended that they update their immunization (diphtheria-pertussis-tetanus, hepatitis A, typhoid) and take antimalarial drugs for the Cambodia portion of the trip (atovaquone/proguanil [Malarone], one pill daily starting one day before stay and continuing during stay and one week after). When they came in for their immunizations, they expressed some concerns about taking the antimalarial drugs. They had been talking to friends who told them these antimalarial drugs had severe side effects and caused hallucinations. They had investigated several Internet sites that their friends had recommended; these sites indicated that antimalarial drugs were not required for where they were going. Mrs. Bennet e-mailed the Cambodian Consulate in Canada and was told that malaria was not a concern where they were going.

Assessment

- Concerned about health but received mixed messages about the need for antimalarial drugs.
- Concerned about serious side effects of drugs.
- Motivated to learn.

Plan

- Discussed with Mr. and Mrs. Bennet criteria for evaluating Web sites for health information (author, age, conflict of interest, whether evidence informed rather than opinion based)
- Provided list of known travel health sites (Health Canada; World Health Organization; US Centers for Disease Control and Prevention)
- Identified other measures to reduce risk of contracting malaria (using mosquito repellent, limiting time outside at night, staying in air-conditioned rooms or mosquito nets, wearing protective clothing)
- Discussed various drugs used for malaria and the incidence and types of side effects
- Explored the risk of not taking medication and implications of contracting malaria
- Identified other resources of information (travel agents, pharmacists)

Outcome

Mr. and Mrs. Bennet visited several reliable sources on the Internet and talked to their pharmacist. They identified several strategies to minimize exposure to mosquitoes on their travels. Mr. Bennet learned that the risk of side effects from the Malarone was minimal and decided to take the drug. Mrs. Bennet also recognized that the risk for side effects was minimal; however, because of her concern about those side effects, she decided not to take the Malarone. She was more comfortable taking the risk because she understood that if she developed a high fever and flu-like illness at any time up to a year after the trip, she had to seek immediate medical attention.

Many people do not adopt new health behaviours or change unhealthy behaviours unless they perceive a disease as a threat, overcome barriers to changing health practices, and see the benefits of such changes (Pender et al., 2006). Thus, a client with lung disease may continue to smoke. An obese client may worsen a heart condition by refusing to follow a low-fat diet.

Motivation and Social Learning Theory. Health education often involves changing people's attitudes and values. Change can occur only when education plans and interventions are based on sound learning theories. A number of theories address the complex client education process (Bastable, 2003; Redman, 2007). One of these is **social learning theory**, which helps educators understand learners and develop interventions that enhance motivation and learning (Bandura, 2001; Bastable, 2003; Saarmann et al., 2002).

When people believe that they can execute a particular behaviour, they are more likely to perform the behaviour consistently and correctly (Bandura, 1997). *Self-efficacy*, a social learning theory concept, is a person's perceived ability to successfully complete a task. Beliefs about self-efficacy arise from four sources: verbal persuasion, vicarious experiences, enactive mastery experiences, and physiological and affective states (Bandura, 1997). Understanding these sources lets nurses develop appropriate interventions. For example, a nurse teaching a boy with asthma to use an inhaler expresses positive reinforcement (verbal persuasion). The nurse then demonstrates how to use the inhaler (vicarious experience). The boy uses the inhaler (enactive mastery experience). As the boy's wheezing and anxiety decrease from using the inhaler, the nurse gives him positive feedback, which further enhances his confidence to use the inhaler (physiological and affective states). Interventions such as these enhance perceived self-efficacy, which in turn improves the achievement of desired outcomes.

Motivation and Transtheoretical Model of Change. Health education may involve changes in behaviour. Behavioural change is often challenging and difficult. It involves a process that occurs over time through a series of stages. By identifying the client's stage of change and focusing learning activities to match the client's stage, you faciliate the learner's motivation to change and his or her transition from one stage to the next. Five stages have been identified and used in smoking cessation activities (DiClemente et al., 1991; Prochaska & DiClemente, 1992):

- Precontemplation: is unaware of need for change and has no intention of changing behaviour
- Contemplation: is aware of need for change and intends to change behaviour sometime in the future
- Preparation: alters behaviour in minor ways with the intention to make substantive changes in the immediate future
- Action: modifies behaviour and experiences in order to make sustainable change
- Maintenance: focuses on not reverting to previous behaviour and on solidifying new behaviours

Integrating the Nursing and Teaching Processes

The nursing and teaching processes are related (Redman, 2007) and usually take place concurrently. Like the nursing process, the teaching process requires assessment, nursing diagnosis, planning, implementation, and evaluation. However, the processes are not exactly the same: The nursing process is broader. For example, determining a client's health needs requires assessing all data sources. The teaching process is focused on data sources that reveal the client's learning needs, willingness and ability to learn, and available teaching resources. Table 21–1 compares the teaching and nursing processes.

The teaching process requires assessment. The client's ability to learn, motivation, and needs should be assessed and analyzed. A diagnostic statement specifies the information or skills that the client requires. You set specific **learning objectives** (i.e., what the learner will be able to do after successful instruction) and implement the teaching plan by using teaching and learning principles to ensure that the client acquires knowledge and skills. Finally, the teaching process requires an evaluation of learning; this evaluation is based on learning objectives.

❖Assessment

During assessment, you determine the client's health care needs (see Chapter 13). The client may reveal a need for health care information, or you may identify a need for education. Learning needs identified by both the client and the nurse determine the content to be learned. By performing an effective assessment, you can individualize instruction for each client (Wingard, 2005). Ask specific questions to assess a client's unique learning needs (Box 21–7).

Learning Needs

Most clients can identify at least some of their own learning needs. Effective questioning and assessment tools help you determine a client's perceived learning needs. By listening carefully and using open-ended and closed-ended questions (see Chapter 18), nurses can often find out what a client's needs are. Because a client's health status is dynamic, assessment is an onging activity. Assess the following:

- Information or skills needed by the client to perform self-care and to understand the implications of a health problem. (Health care team members anticipate learning needs related to specific health problems. For example, you teach an adolescent boy to perform testicular self-examination.)
- Client's experiences that influence the need to learn.
- Information that the family members or significant others require to support the client's needs. (The amount of information needed depends on the exent of the family's role in helping the client.)

Ability to Learn

The ability to learn can be impaired by many factors, including body temperature, electrolyte levels, oxygenation status, and blood glucose level. Several factors may influence a client at one time. You assess the client's ability to learn by considering the following:

- Physical strength, movement, dexterity, and coordination (you determine the client's ability to perform skills)
- Sensory deficits that may affect the ability to understand or follow instruction (see Chapter 48)
- Reading level (reading level can be difficult to assess because functional illiteracy is often easy to conceal; one way to assess a client's reading level and level of understanding is to ask the client to read instructions from a teaching brochure and then explain its meaning)
- Developmental level (developmental level influences teaching approaches [see Box 21–5])
- Cognitive function (cognitive function includes memory, knowledge, association, and judgement)

Motivation to Learn

You ask questions that identify a client's motivation level, which help you determine whether the client is prepared and willing to learn. You assesses the client's motivation by studying the following:

- Behaviour (e.g., attention span, tendency to ask questions, memory, and ability to concentrate during the teaching session)
- Health beliefs and perception of a health problem and the benefits and barriers to treatment (e.g., you ask a client with coronary

➤TABLE 21-1 Comparison of the Nursing and Teaching Processes

Basic Steps	Nursing Process	Teaching Process
Assessment	Collect data about client's physical, psychological, social, cultural, developmental, and spiritual needs from client, family, diagnostic tests, medical record, health history, learning style, and literature.	Gather data about client's learning needs, motivation, ability to learn, and teaching resources from client, family, learning environment, medical record, health history, and literature.
Nursing diagnosis	Identify appropriate nursing diagnoses based on assessment findings, including deficits.	Identify client's learning needs on basis of three domains of learning.
Planning	Develop individualized care plan. Set diagnosis priorities on the basis of client's immediate needs. Collaborate with client on care plan.	Establish learning objectives, stated in behavioural terms. Identify priorities regarding learning needs. Collaborate with client on teaching plan. Identify type of teaching method to use.
Implementation	Perform nursing care therapies. Include client as active participant in care. Involve family or significant other in care as appropriate.	Implement teaching methods. Actively involve client in learning activities. Include family or significant other in participation as appropriate.
Evaluation	Identify success in meeting desired outcomes and goals of nursing care. Alter interventions as indicated when goals are not met.	Determine outcomes of teaching–learning process. Measure client's ability to achieve learning objectives. Reinforce information as needed .

> **BOX 21-7 Nursing Assessment Questions**
>
> **Ask Clients**
>
> What do you want to know?
>
> What do you know about your illness and your treatment plan?
>
> How does (or will) your illness affect your current lifestyle?
>
> What barriers currently exist that are preventing you from managing your illness the way you would like to manage it?
>
> What cultural or spiritual beliefs do you have regarding your illness and the prescribed treatment?
>
> What experiences have you had that are similar to what you are experiencing now?
>
> Together we can choose the best way for you to learn about your disease. How can I best help you?
>
> What role do you believe your health care professional should take in helping you manage your illness or maintain health?
>
> When you learn new information, do you prefer to have the information given to you in pictures or written down in words?
>
> When you give someone directions to your house, do you tell the person how to get there, write out the instructions, or draw a map?
>
> How involved do you want your family to be in the management of your illness?
>
> **Ask Family Members**
>
> When are you available to help, and how do you plan to help your loved ones?
>
> Your spouse needs some help. How do you feel about learning how to assist him [her]?

artery disease, "Explain how heart disease will affect you over time. What is the value of eating a low-fat diet?")

- Perceived ability to complete a required healthy behaviour
- Desire to learn
- Attitudes about health care professionals (e.g., role of client and nurse in making decisions, such as your asking, "In what way can I best help you?")
- Knowledge of information to be learned (the client must play an active role in seeking health-related information)
- Pain, fatigue, anxiety, or other physical symptoms that can interfere with the ability to maintain attention and participate (in acute care settings, a client's physical condition can easily detract from learning)
- Sociocultural background (a client's beliefs and values about health and various therapies may be influenced by sociocultural norms or tradition [see Chapter 10]; educational efforts can be especially challenging when clients and educators do not speak the same language)
- Learning style preference (clients who learn better by seeing and hearing may benefit from a video; clients who learn best by reasoning logically and intuitively may learn better if presented with written material that they can analyze and discuss with others)

Teaching Environment

You assess the following factors when choosing a teaching environment:

- Distractions or persistent noise (a quiet area should be set aside for teaching)
- Comfort of the room, including ventilation, temperature, lighting, and furniture
- Room facilities and available equipment

Resources for Learning

Assessment of resources includes a review of available teaching tools. If a client requires family support, you evaluate the readiness and ability of family and friends to learn to care for the client, and you review resources in the home. You assess the following:

- Client's willingness to have family members involved in the teaching plan and care (information about the client's health care is confidential unless the client chooses to share it)
- Family members' perceptions and understanding of the client's illness and its implications (family members and clients' perceptions should match; otherwise, conflicts may arise in the teaching plan)
- Family's willingness and ability to participate in care (family members must be responsible, willing, and able to assist in care activities, such as bathing or administering medications)
- Resources in the home (these resources include health care equipment and a suitable rearrangement of rooms)
- Teaching tools, including brochures, audiovisual materials, or posters. Printed material should present current and easy-to-understand information that matches the client's reading level.

❖Nursing Diagnosis

After assessing the client's ability and need to learn, you interpret data to form an accurate diagnosis. This diagnosis ensures that teaching will be goal directed and individualized. If a client has several learning needs, the nursing diagnoses guide priority setting. By classifying diagnoses according to the three learning domains, you can focus on subject matter and teaching methods. Examples of nursing diagnoses that indicate a need for education include the following:

- *Ineffective health maintenance*
- *Health-seeking behaviours*
- *Impaired home maintenance*
- *Deficient knowledge*
- *Ineffective therapeutic regimen management*
- *Ineffective community therapeutic regimen management*
- *Ineffective family therapeutic regimen management*

When health care problems can be managed through education, the diagnostic statement is *deficient knowledge*. For example, an older adult may be unable to manage a medication regimen because of the number of medications that must be taken at different times of the day. Education may improve the client's ability to schedule and take the medications.

Some nursing diagnoses also indicate that teaching is inappropriate. You may identify conditions that hinder learning (e.g., nursing diagnosis of pain or activity intolerance). In these cases, you should delay teaching until the nursing diagnosis is resolved or the health problem is controlled.

❖Planning

After identifying a client's learning needs and making a nursing diagnosis, you develop a teaching plan, set goals and expected outcomes, and work with the client to select a teaching method (Box 21–8). Expected outcomes or learning objectives determine which teaching strategies and approaches are appropriate. Client participation is essential.

BOX 21-8 NURSING CARE PLAN

Learning Needs

Assessment

Connie, a nurse in a surgeon's office, is preparing Mr. Holland for a colon resection, which is scheduled in one week. Mr. Holland, aged 75, has recently received a diagnosis of colorectal cancer. Connie's assessment focuses on Mr. Holland's readiness to learn and factors that might affect his ability to understand the procedure and related postoperative care.

Assessment Activities	***Findings and Defining Characteristics***
Assess Mr. Holland's readiness to learn, and ask what the surgeon has already told him about the surgery.	Mr. Holland responds, "I can't remember what the doctor told me at my last appointment. My surgery is scheduled for next week."
Ask Mr. Holland to explain postoperative care, including performing a return demonstration of deep breathing and coughing.	Mr. Holland is unable to describe postoperative care or provide a return demonstration of deep breathing and coughing.
Assess Mr. Holland's visual acuity.	Mr. Holland says he has difficulty reading small print.

Nursing Diagnosis: Deficient knowledge related to lack of recall and exposure to information

Planning

Goal (Nursing Outcomes Classification)*	***Expected Outcomes****
	Knowledge of Treatment Procedures
Mr. Holland will describe preoperative and postoperative care to nurse before surgery.	Mr. Holland will verbalize understanding of surgical procedure and related care on the day of surgery.
Mr. Holland will participate in postoperative care during hospitalization.	Mr. Holland will demonstrate deep breathing and coughing; he will advance his level of activity after his surgery.

*Outcome labels from Moorhead, S., Johnson, M., & Maas, M. L. (Eds.). (2004). *Nursing Outcomes Classification (NOC)* (3rd ed.). St. Louis, MO: Mosby.

Interventions (Nursing Interventions Classification)†	**Rationale**
Learning Readiness Enhancement	
Determine readiness to learn and what the client perceives as important to know.	Adult clients' learning is enhanced when they are ready to learn and the information is perceived as important (Bastable, 2003).
Learning Facilitation	
Give client large-print brochure describing preoperative and postoperative care during educational session.	Providing clients with educational methods that use multiple senses is effective in educating older adults. Large fonts with contrasting colours are easier for older adults to visualize (Wendell et al., 2003).
Explain postoperative care, demonstrate deep breathing and coughing, and have client perform return demonstration.	Improving self-efficacy by using role modelling and by having the client perform behaviours enhances the successful adoption of healthy behaviours (Bandura, 1997).

†Intervention classification labels from Dochterman, J. M., & Bulechek, G. M. (Eds.). (2004). *Nursing Interventions Classification (NIC)* (4th ed.). St. Louis, MO: Mosby.

Evaluation

Nursing Actions	***Client Response and Finding***	***Achievement of Outcome***
Ask Mr. Holland what he can expect before and after surgery.	Mr. Holland is able to state understanding of preoperative and postoperative care.	Mr. Holland's anxiety level has decreased, and he reports that he is ready for surgery.
Observe client as he demonstrates deep breathing and coughing and advances his activity postoperatively.	Mr. Holland is able to cough and breathe deeply postoperatively, but he is hesitant to advance his activity level after surgery.	Outcome of advancing activity postoperatively has not been totally achieved. Address and manage barriers inhibiting attainment of this outcome (e.g., pain), and continue to encourage and educate client.

Developing Learning Objectives

Learning objectives identify the expected outcome of instruction and establish learning priorities. Objectives help you manage time and resources.

Objectives are either for a short term or a long term. Short-term objectives meet the client's immediate learning needs, such as needing knowledge about an upcoming test. Long-term objectives, which are often broader, help a client adapt to a long-term challenge. Learning objectives, which will guide the teaching plan, include the same criteria as outcomes in a nursing care plan:

- Singular behaviours
- Observable or measurable content
- Timing or conditions under which the objective is measured
- Goals mutually set by the nurse and client

Each objective focuses on a single behaviour that will determine the client's ability to meet health care outcomes. A behavioural objective contains an active verb, describing what the learner will do after the objective is met (e.g., "*will administer* an injection." Behavioural objectives are measurable and observable and indicate how learning will be evidenced (e.g., "will perform *three-point crutch gait*"). The objective describes precise behaviours and content. Nurses should avoid vague or nonspecific objectives that do not explain what the learner is to do.

An objective is more precise when it describes the conditions or timing under which the behaviour occurs. Conditions and time frames should be realistic and designed for the learner's needs (e.g., "will identify the side effects of medication by discharge"). It also helps to consider conditions under which the client or family will perform the behaviour (e.g., "will walk from bedroom to bathroom, using crutches"). You set criteria for acceptable performance on the basis of the desired level of accuracy, success, or satisfaction. For example, "a client undergoing therapy for a fractured leg will walk on crutches to the end of the hall within 3 days." Criteria are more acceptable when the teacher and learner establish them mutually. However, you serve as a resource in setting the minimum criteria for success.

After formulating objectives, you and the client establish a teaching plan. You integrate basic teaching principles and develop a well-timed, organized teaching plan.

Setting Priorities

The teaching plan is prioritized according to the client's immediate needs, nursing diagnoses, learning objectives, main concerns, anxiety level, and the time available to teach.

Timing

When is the right time to teach? Before a client is hospitalized? When a client enters a clinic or a long-term care facility? At discharge? At home? All of these times are correct because clients continue to have learning needs and opportunities as long as they stay in the health care system. You should plan to teach when a client is most attentive, receptive, and alert. However, timing can be difficult, particularly in an acute care setting, because the focus is on an early discharge. By the time the client is ready to learn, discharge may already be scheduled. Therefore, you need to anticipate a client's educational needs.

The length of teaching sessions also influences learning. Concentration decreases with prolonged sessions. You should assess a client's level of concentration by observing nonverbal cues such as poor eye contact or slumped posture. Teaching sessions should be held often enough to document the client's learning progress. The frequency of sessions depends on the learner's abilities and the complexity of the material. For example, a child in whom diabetes has been newly diagnosed will require more visits to an outpatient centre than will an older adult who has been managing diabetes for 15 years. Intervals between teaching sessions should not be so long that the client might forget information.

Organizing Teaching Material

An outline helps organize information into a logical sequence. Material should progress from simple to complex. A person must learn simple facts and concepts before learning associations or complex concepts.

Essential content should be taught first because people are more likely to remember information that is taught early. Repetition reinforces learning. Summarizing key points helps the learner remember important information (Bastable, 2003).

Maintaining Attention and Promoting Participation

Active participation is key to learning. People learn better when more than one of the body's senses is stimulated. Nurses should engage the clients' interest by changing the tone and intensity of their voice, making eye contact, using gestures, asking questions, and encouraging participation with activities such as role-playing.

Building on Existing Knowledge

An effective teacher presents information that builds on a learner's existing knowledge. For example, a client who has had multiple sclerosis must begin a new medication that is given subcutaneously. On assessment, you ask the client about experience with injections. The client explains that she gave her father insulin injections for many years. You then individualize the teaching plan by building on the client's previous knowledge and experience with insulin injections.

Selecting Teaching Methods

A teaching method is the way that the teacher delivers information. It is based on the client's learning needs. More than one method may be used for instruction. For example, a client who learns best in the psychomotor domain will benefit from demonstrations and supervised practice. The client masters skills by manipulating equipment and practising manual skills. Discussions, question-and-answer sessions, and formal lectures can all be effective methods, depending on the client's needs and learning style. When choosing appropriate teaching methods, you should encourage the client to offer suggestions (Box 21–9).

Selecting Resources

You are responsible for ensuring that clients' educational needs are met. Sometimes clients' needs are highly complex. In these cases, you identify appropriate health education resources within the health care system or the community. Examples of resources for client education include diabetes education clinics, cardiac rehabilitation programs, prenatal classes, and support groups. You obtain a referral if necessary, encourage clients to attend these sessions, and reinforce information taught.

Writing Teaching Plans

In all health care settings, nurses develop written teaching plans for use by colleagues. The nurse responsible for developing the teaching plan incorporates all pertinent information into the plan, including topics for instruction, resources (e.g., equipment, teaching booklets, and referrals to education programs), recommendations for involving family, and objectives of the teaching plan. A plan may be detailed or in outline form.

In an acute care setting, plans are concise and focused on the primary learning needs of the client because time for teaching is limited. A home care teaching plan or outpatient clinic plan may be more comprehensive because nurses may have more time to instruct clients, and clients are often less anxious in outpatient settings.

A plan should provide continuity of instruction, particularly when several nurses are involved in a client's care. The more specific the plan is, the easier it is to follow.

❖Implementation

Implementing a teaching plan depends on your ability to analyze assessment data when identifying learning needs and developing the teaching plan (see Box 21–8). You evaluate the learning objectives

BOX 21-9 CLIENT TEACHING

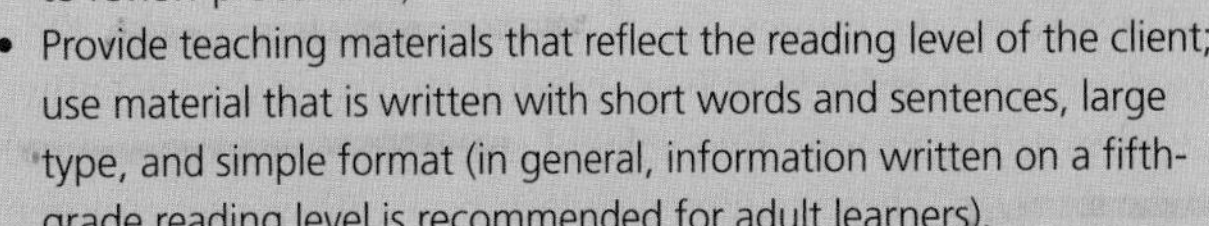

Teaching Strategies

- Establish trust with the client before beginning the teaching–learning session.
- Limit teaching objectives.
- Use simple terminology to enhance the client's understanding.
- Avoid medical jargon. If necessary, explain medical terms by using basic one- or two-syllable words.
- Schedule short teaching sessions at frequent intervals; minimize distractions during teaching sessions.
- Begin and end each teaching session with the most important information.
- Present information slowly; pacing to provide ample time for the client to understand the material.
- Repeat important information.
- Provide many examples that have meaning to the client; for example, relate new material to a previous life experience.
- Build on existing knowledge.
- Use visual cues and simple analogies when appropriate.
- Ask the client for frequent feedback to determine whether the client comprehends information.
- Demonstrate procedures such as measuring dosages; ask for return demonstrations (which provide opportunities to clarify instructions and time to review procedures).
- Provide teaching materials that reflect the reading level of the client; use material that is written with short words and sentences, large type, and simple format (in general, information written on a fifth-grade reading level is recommended for adult learners).
- Model appropriate behaviour and use role-playing to help client learn how to ask questions and ask for help effectively.
- Pace the delivery of material so that clients can progress at their own speed.
- Include family members or other caregivers in the education process.

Data from Bastable, S. (2003). *Nurse as educator: Principles of teaching and learning for nursing practice.* Sudbury, MA: Jones & Bartlett; Cutilli, C. C. (2006). Do your patients understand? How to write effective health care information. *Orthopaedic Nursing, 25*(1), 39–50; and Mennies, J. (2001). Teaching adult patients with learning disabilities. *Nursing Spectrum, 14*(21), 20.

and determine the best teaching and learning methods to help the client to meet expected goals and outcomes. You use a diversified approach to create an active learning environment (Box 21–10).

Teaching Approaches

A teaching approach is different from a method. Because a learner's needs and motives can change over time, you must be ready to modify teaching approaches.

Telling. The telling approach is useful when limited information must be taught (e.g., preparing a client for an emergency diagnostic procedure). You outline the task to be done by the client and give instructions. This method provides no opportunity for feedback.

Selling. The selling approach entails two-way communication. You pace instruction according to the client's response. Specific feedback is given to the client who learns successfully. For example, the client learns a step-by-step procedure for changing a dressing.

Participating. Participating involves setting objectives and becoming involved in the learning process together. The client helps decide content, and you guide and counsel the client with pertinent information. Opportunities are provided for discussion, feedback, mutual goal setting, and revision of the teaching plan.

Entrusting. The entrusting approach provides the client with the opportunity to manage self-care. You observe the client's progress and remain available to assist without introducing more new information.

BOX 21-10 Example of Nursing Interventions Based on Client's Learning Needs

Assessment Data

Mr. Kennedy, aged 67, has a 15-year history of type 2 diabetes. He is in the hospital because of an infected foot ulcer that necessitates frequent dressing changes. Mr. Kennedy used to take oral hypoglycemic agents to control his blood glucose levels. However, he now needs to start home insulin injections because of the infection and wound. He must also learn how to change his dressings. Mr. Kennedy is anxious about his discharge and requests information about a local diabetes support group. The case manager indicates that Mr. Kennedy will be discharged soon.

Cognitive Interventions

- Ask Mr. Kennedy about what he believes he needs to know before his discharge.
- Encourage Mr. Kennedy to help establish learning outcomes and goals.
- Provide Mr. Kennedy with teaching materials regarding insulin preparation, administration, and how to recognize and manage hypoglycemia and hyperglycemia.
- During teaching sessions, give Mr. Kennedy examples of what problems he might experience at home and ask him how he would respond to the situations (e.g., "If the wound's drainage increases and becomes purulent, what would you do?").

Affective Interventions

- Encourage Mr. Kennedy to attend a support group meeting if possible to facilitate learning from others' experiences.
- Encourage Mr. Kennedy to verbalize his feelings and fears about this change in his health status.
- Have Mr. Kennedy role-play how he will respond to his friends when they ask him about his health status.
- As he acquires new skills and behaviours, provide Mr. Kennedy with feedback and positive reinforcement.

Psychomotor Interventions

- Demonstrate insulin preparation and injection techniques.
- Demonstrate use of blood glucose meter and recording of blood glucose measurements.
- Demonstrate dressing changes.
- Ask Mr. Kennedy to perform return demonstrations of insulin preparation and injection, blood glucose testing, and dressing changes.

Reinforcing. **Reinforcement** is the use of a stimulus that increases the probability of a response. A person who receives positive reinforcement before or after learning a desired behaviour is likely to repeat the behaviour. People usually respond better to positive reinforcement (Bastable, 2003). The effects of negative reinforcement, such as criticizing, can decrease an undesired response but are less predictable and often undesirable. Feedback is a common form of reinforcement.

Three types of reinforcers are social, material, and activity. Most nurses use social reinforcers (e.g., encouraging words) to acknowledge a learned behaviour. Examples of material reinforcers are food, toys, and music. These reinforcers work best with young children. Activity reinforcers are based on the principle that people are motivated to engage in an activity if after its completion they are able to engage in a more desirable activity. For example, clients with dementia may be more willing to bathe if they can go for a walk with you afterward. Activity reinforces work when a client is self-motivated. Choosing an appropriate reinforcer requires attention to individual preferences. Observing behaviour often helps reveal the best reinforcer to use. Reinforcers should never be used as threats and are not effective with every client.

Incorporating Teaching Into Nursing Care

Many nurses teach effectively while delivering nursing care. This activity becomes easier as you gain confidence in clinical skills. For example, while hanging a blood bag, you explain why the blood is needed, and you describe the symptoms of transfusion reactions that should be reported immediately. When you follow a teaching plan informally, the client feels less pressure to perform, and learning becomes more of a shared activity. Teaching during routine care is efficient and cost effective (Figure 21–2).

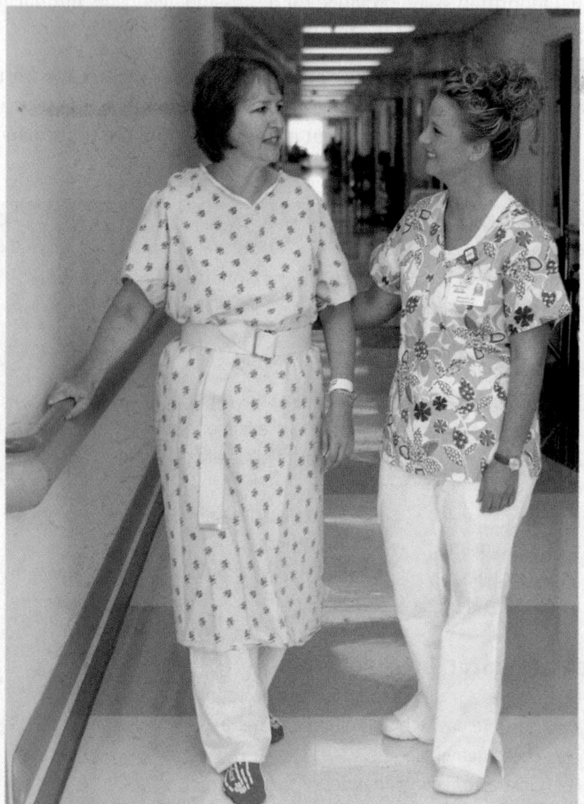

Figure 21-2 Teaching postoperative care while walking with the client is an effective use of time.

Implementing Teaching Methods

Your choice of teaching methods depends on the client's learning needs, the time available for teaching, the environment, the resources, and the nurse's own comfort level with teaching. Skilled teachers are flexible in altering teaching methods according to the learner's responses and in using teaching tools that work best with a particular method. Various teaching tools are detailed in Table 21–2.

One-on-One Discussion. In one-on-one discussion, you present information informally, providing the client with the opportunity to ask questions or share concerns. During the discussion, you can use various teaching aids such as models or diagrams, depending on the client's learning needs.

Group Instruction. Groups are an economical way to teach several clients at once. Clients interact and learn from others' experiences. Groups can also foster positive attitudes that help clients meet learning objectives (Rankin & Stallings, 2005).

Group instruction often involves both lecture and discussion. Lectures are highly structured and help clients learn standard content. However, they do not encourage active thinking; thus, discussion and practice sessions are essential (Rankin & Stallings, 2005).

Preparatory Instruction. Clients are often anxious about unfamiliar tests or procedures. By providing information about procedures, you help clients anticipate what will happen. Guidelines for giving preparatory explanations are as follows:

- Describe physical sensations during the procedure, but do not evaluate them. For example, when you draw a blood specimen, explain that the client will feel a sticking sensation as the needle punctures the skin.
- Describe the cause of the sensation to prevent misinterpretation of the experience. For example, explain that a needle stick burns because the alcohol used to cleanse the skin enters the puncture site.
- Prepare clients only for aspects of the experience that are common to other clients. For example, explain that it is normal for a tight tourniquet to cause a person's hand to tingle and feel numb.

Demonstrations. Demonstrations help teach psychomotor skills such as preparing a syringe, bathing an infant, walking with a crutch, or measuring a pulse. Clients are able to observe a skill before practising it. Demonstrations are most effective when clients first observe you and then perform a **return demonstration** to practise the skill. A demonstration should be combined with discussion to clarify concepts and feelings. An effective demonstration requires advanced planning:

- Position the client to provide a clear view of the demonstration.
- Review the rationale and steps of the procedure.
- Assemble and organize equipment. Make sure it works.
- Perform each step in sequence while analyzing the knowledge and skills involved.
- Determine when to give explanations, considering the client's learning needs.
- Adjust speed and timing of the demonstration according to the client's abilities and anxiety level.

You demonstrate the steps of a procedure in the same order in which the client will perform them. The demonstration involves the following:

- Performing each step slowly and accurately
- Encouraging the client to ask questions so that each step is understood

- Explaining the rationale for each step
- Allowing the client to observe each step
- Providing the client with the opportunity to handle equipment and practise the procedure under supervision

The client demonstrates the procedure to ensure that learning has occurred. The demonstration should occur under the same conditions that will be experienced at home or in the place where the procedure is to be performed. For example, for a client learning to walk with crutches, you simulate the home environment. If short, narrow steps lead to the client's bedroom, the client should learn to climb similar stairs in the hospital.

Analogies. Learning occurs when a teacher translates complex language or ideas into words or concepts that the client understands. Analogies aid learning by supplementing verbal instruction with familiar images that make complex information simpler and understandable. For example, to explain arterial blood pressure, an analogy is the flow of water through a hose. To use analogies, follow these general principles:

- Be familiar with the concept.
- Know the client's background, experience, and culture.
- Keep the analogy simple and clear.

Role-Playing. Role-playing helps teach new ideas and attitudes. During role-playing, clients play themselves or someone else and rehearse a desired behaviour. For example, you can teach a parent to respond to a child's behaviour by pretending to be a child having a temper tantrum. This role-playing provides the parent with the opportunity to practise responding in this situation. You evaluate the parent's response and determine whether an alternative approach would be more appropriate. Role-playing helps clients learn skills and feel confident in their ability to perform them independently.

TABLE 21-2 Teaching Tools for Instruction

Description of Tool	Implications for Learning
Printed Material	
Written teaching tools such as pamphlets, booklets, and brochures	Material must be easily readable for learner. Information must be accurate and current. Method is ideal for understanding complex concepts and relationships.
Programmed Instruction	
Written sequential presentation of learning steps requiring that learners answer questions and that teachers tell them whether their answers are right or wrong	Instruction is primarily verbal, but teacher may use pictures or diagrams. Method requires active learning, giving immediate feedback, correcting wrong answers, and reinforcing right answers. Learner works at own pace.
Computer Instruction	
Programmed instruction format in which computers store response patterns for learners and select further lessons on basis of these patterns (programs can be individualized)	Method requires reading comprehension, psychomotor skills, and familiarity with computer.
Audiovisual Materials	
Diagrams	
Illustrations that show interrelationships by means of lines and symbols	Method demonstrates key ideas and summarizes and clarifies key concept.
Graphs (Bar, Circle, or Line)	
Visual presentations of numerical data	Graphs help learner to grasp information quickly about single concept.
Charts	
Highly condensed visual summaries of ideas and facts that may highlight series of ideas, steps, or events	Charts demonstrate relationship of several ideas or concepts. Method helps learners know what to do.
Pictures	
Photographs or drawings used to teach concepts in which the third dimension of shape and space is not important	Photographs are more desirable than diagrams because they more accurately portray the details of the real item. Drawings are pertinent for removing the superfluous detail present in real objects.
Physical Objects	
Use of actual equipment, objects, or models to teach concepts or skills	Models are useful when real objects are too small, large, or complicated or are unavailable. Learners can manipulate objects that are to be used later in skill.
Other Audiovisual Materials	
Slides, audiotapes, television, and videotapes used with printed material or discussion	Materials are useful for clients with reading comprehension problems and visual deficits.

Simulation. Simulation helps teach problem solving, application, and independent thinking. During individual or group discussion, a nurse poses a problem or situation for clients to solve. For example, clients with heart disease are asked to plan a low-fat meal. You ask the clients to present their diet, providing an opportunity to identify mistakes and reinforce correct information.

Paying Attention to Learning Barriers. Many situations or conditions present a barrier to learning. For example, the client may have a low reading level (functionally illiterate), a learning disability, a sensory alteration, or depression; may be suffering the effects of prescribed medications or adjusting to life changes or transitions; or may have a poor memory. Clients understand fewer medical words than health care professionals predict. Unfortunately, health care professionals often use medical terminology and jargon, which prevents clients from understanding the written health information they are given (Sand-Jecklin, 2007). Professionals should pay special attention to the learning needs of clients who have reading problems, learning disabilities, and sensory alterations and of those whose first language is not English or French.

Illiteracy and Learning Disabilities. A 2005 survey on literacy rates in Canada (Statistics Canada & Organisation for Economic Co-operation and Development, 2005) revealed that about 15% of Canadian adults fall within the lowest level of literacy. These people have only rudimentary reading and writing skills; for example, they are not able to read and understand a label on a medicine container. An additional 27% of Canadians can read only material that is simple and familiar. Therefore, almost half of Canadians have problems with reading materials encountered in everyday life. To compound this problem, the readability of printed material ranges from elementary school level to college level. Researchers have found that printed educational material is consistently written above most clients' reading level (Cutilli, 2005; Demir et al., 2008). Health care professionals need to screen materials for readability and clarity.

Some people have learning disabilities, which are disorders that may impair ability to acquire, organize, remember, understand, or apply information (Learning Disabilities Association of Canada, 2002). The ability to learn or use oral or written language, mathematics, or both may be poor. Teaching strategies need to be adapted to accommodate their learning needs. For example, clients with attention deficit–hyperactivity disorder may have difficulty recalling information and staying focused during educational sessions; they may also have a low threshold of frustration (Mennies, 2001). Teaching activities should be kept short in an environment with minimal competing stimuli.

Sensory Alteration and Other Barriers. Some clients, including many older adults, have sensory deficits (see Chapter 48). Sensory changes such as visual and hearing deficits necessitate teaching methods that enhance functioning. For example, you face a client with hearing problems and speak in a low tone of voice during discussions (lower tones are easier to hear than are higher tones). Clearly, written materials should be provided. Clients with visual problems can benefit from large-print materials. Clients with slower cognitive function and reduced short-term memory (such as some older adults and clients who have had strokes) learn and remember effectively if the learning is paced properly and the material is relevant to the learner's needs and abilities.

Language

The diverse backgrounds of Canadians can challenge you to provide culturally sensitive care (see Chapter 10). Clients may not understand instructions that are not in their native language (see Chapter 18). You need to ascertain a client's fluency in English or French before you choose teaching methods or tools.

Cultural Diversity

You need to have knowledge of clients' cultural background, values, and beliefs (see Chapter 10), as well as the client's ability to understand both verbal and written material (Cutilli, 2006). When educating clients of cultural groups different from your own, you need to be aware of the distinctive aspects of their cultures and develop teaching strategies that are respectful of cultural beliefs, values, and behaviours.

Needs of Clients With Severe Illness

Adapting to serious illness or disability is difficult for most people. They need to grieve. The grieving process gives them time to adapt psychologically to the emotional and physical implications of illness. People experience the stages of grieving as theorized by Kübler-Ross (1969; see Chapter 29) at different rates and sequences, depending on their self-concept before illness, the severity of the illness, and the changes and losses caused by the illness. Not everyone experiences every stage. Sensitivity is required to educate clients while they are grieving and adjusting to their illness.

Readiness to learn is related to the grieving stage (Table 21–3). Clients cannot learn when they are unwilling or unable to accept the reality of illness. However, properly timed teaching can help a client to adjust to illness or disability. You must identify the client's stage of grieving on the basis of the client's behaviours. When the client enters the stage of acceptance, the stage compatible with learning, you can introduce a teaching plan. Continuous assessment of the client's behaviours determines the stages of grieving.

❖Evaluation

Client education is not complete until you evaluate outcomes of the teaching–learning process (see Box 21–8). You must determine whether clients have learned the material. Evaluation reinforces correct behaviour, helps learners realize how they should change incorrect behaviour, and helps you determine the adequacy of the teaching (Redman, 2007). Success depends on the client's ability to meet the established outcome and goals by which you can evaluate success. The following checklist helps evaluate client education (Rankin & Stallings, 2005):

- Were the objectives clearly stated in a way that allowed client behaviours to be observed?
- Were the client's goals or outcomes realistic?
- Were the learner's needs assessed thoroughly?
- Did the client perceive the education as important, and did the client state a willingness to change behaviour?
- What obstacles or problems were encountered that provided barriers to change?
- Were educational goals set mutually between the nurse and the client?

➤ TABLE 21-3 **Relationship Between Learning and Psychosocial Adaptation to Illness**

Stage	Client's Behaviour	Nursing Activities	Rationale
Denial or disbelief	Client avoids discussion of illness ("Nothing is wrong with me"), withdraws from others, and disregards physical restrictions. Client suppresses and distorts information that has not been presented clearly.	Provide support, empathy, and careful explanations of all procedures while they are being done. Let client know you are available for conversation. Explain situation to family or significant other if appropriate. Teach in present tense (e.g., explain what client needs to know to be discharged).	Client is not prepared to deal with problem; attempts to teach client will result in further anger or withdrawal. Provide only information that client. pursues or requires.
Anger	Client blames, complains, and often directs anger toward nurse or others.	Do not argue with client, but listen to concerns. Teach in present tense. Reassure family of the normality of client's behaviour.	Client needs opportunity to express feelings and anger. Client is still not prepared to face future.
Bargaining	Client offers to live better life in exchange for promise of better health (e.g., "If God lets me live, I promise to manage my disease better").	Continue to introduce only reality and teaching in present tense.	Client is still unwilling to accept limitations.
Resolution	Client begins to express emotions openly, realizes that illness has created changes, and begins to ask questions.	Encourage expression of feelings. Begin to share information needed for future, and set aside formal times for discussion.	Client begins to perceive need for assistance and is ready to accept responsibility for learning.
Acceptance	Client recognizes reality of condition, actively pursues information, and strives for independence.	Focus on future skills and knowledge required. Continue to teach in present tense. Involve family in planning and teaching for discharge.	Client is more easily motivated to learn. Acceptance of illness reflects willingness to deal with its implications.

- Were the interventions individualized to help the client meet the learning objectives?
- Was the client's behavioural change measured and documented accurately?
- Does the client continue to have a skill deficiency? If so, what changes in interventions should be made to enhance skill attainment?
- Does any follow-up or reassessment need to be performed?

Measurement Methods

Under direct observation, the client should demonstrate the behaviours described in the learning objectives. If the evaluation process indicates a deficit in knowledge or skill, you must repeat or modify the teaching plan. By watching clients demonstrate behaviours, you can see whether correct techniques are used. However, a client may behave differently later. Therefore, observation works best in real-life situations.

Oral and written questioning are other useful evaluation methods. Questions are best used for behaviours that are not easily demonstrated. You should phrase questions to ensure that the learner understands them and that objectives are truly measured.

Another form of evaluation includes self-reports (oral and written) and self-monitoring (written). An example is a client's written log of the foods eaten in a specific time period, in comparison with a new diet. You rely on the client's honesty and memory in self-reporting.

Client Expectations

Evaluations of nursing care and teaching sessions help determine whether a client's needs and expectations have been met. At the end of the session, you ask the client whether he or she has questions; in this way, you can identify information that was missing and should have been covered. Clients may also fill out written evaluations of a teaching session or course. Anonymous written evaluations may be more truthful than are face-to-face evaluations.

Evaluation may reveal new learning needs or new factors that are interfering with learning, in which case you should try alternative teaching methods. When a client has difficulty in an acute care setting, you may make a referral to resources, such as home care or an outpatient clinic, for further education and evaluation.

Documentation

Because client teaching often occurs informally, it is difficult to document it consistently. You are legally responsible for providing accurate, timely information that promotes continuity of care; therefore, it is essential to document the outcomes of teaching. Rankin and Stallings (2005) suggested documenting the following with regard to client education:

- *Assessment data and reassessment of learning needs.* Such data and evaluation provide important information needed when the teaching plan is developed.

- *Nursing diagnoses, client needs, and educational priorities.* These provide support for goals and outcomes that are established.
- *Interventions planned.* A specific plan, including the methods to be used in instruction, enhances continuity of care. When viewing the planned interventions, you can determine what information needs to be provided to the client.
- *Interventions provided.* Specifically describing the subject matter enables other nurses to follow up and reinforce teaching (e.g., "Explained side effects of Inderal" or "Demonstrated umbilical cord care"). Note the date, time, and specific client or clients taught. Avoid generalizations (e.g., "medications taught"). Resources used, such as pamphlets or audiovisual materials, are documented in the client's record.
- *Client's response and outcomes of care.* In documenting evidence of learning (e.g., a return demonstration or the ability to verbalize the purpose and side effects of a medication), you inform staff about the client's progress and determine information that must still be taught.
- *Ability of client, family, or both to manage needs after discharge.* An evaluation of remaining educational needs on discharge helps identify the need for outpatient or home health care follow-up. If referrals are appropriate, the client, family, or both are often able to meet their needs.

* KEY CONCEPTS

- The nurse ensures that clients, families, and communities receive information needed to maintain optimal health.
- Health education is aimed at the promotion, restoration, and maintenance of health.
- Teaching is most effective when it is responsive to the learner's needs.
- Teaching is a form of interpersonal communication, with the teacher and student actively involved in a process that increases the student's knowledge and skills.
- The ability to learn depends on a person's physical and cognitive attributes.
- The ability to attend to the learning process depends on physical comfort and anxiety levels and on the presence of environmental distraction.
- A person's health beliefs influence the willingness to gain knowledge and skills necessary to maintain health.
- Teaching must be timed to coincide with the client's readiness to learn.
- Clients of different age groups require different teaching strategies as a result of developmental capabilities.
- The client should be an active participant in a teaching plan: agreeing to the plan, helping choose instructional methods, and recommending times for instruction.
- Learning objectives describe what a person is to learn in behavioural terms.
- A combination of teaching methods improves the learner's attentiveness and involvement.
- A teacher is more effective when presenting information that builds on a learner's existing knowledge.
- Nurses should assess which learning materials, methods, and approaches will be most effective for each client, on the basis of each client's individual abilities and challenges.
- A nurse evaluates a client's learning by observing performance of expected learning behaviours under desired conditions.
- Effective documentation describes the entire process of client education, promotes continuity of care, and demonstrates that educational standards have been met.

* CRITICAL THINKING EXERCISES

1. Mrs. S. has a 10-year history of hypertension and a 5-year history of diabetes. Recently, her hypertension has worsened and she has received a diagnosis of depression. Her medications, which have recently been changed, include 25 mg of captopril (Capoten) three times a day; 240 mg of diltiazem (Cardizem CD) every morning; 1500 mg of metformin (Glucophage XR) before the evening meal; and 100 mg of sertraline (Zoloft) by mouth at bed time. You identify the priority nursing diagnosis as *deficient knowledge related to change in medications.* You want to develop a plan of care in which the three domains of learning are used. What are the client's teaching priorities? Which learning needs would necessitate a cognitive method? Which needs would be more appropriate to satisfy through affective or psychomotor methods?
2. You are caring for a client who is being discharged after an appendectomy. He takes medication to treat attention deficit-hyperactivity disorder. Which teaching strategies should you use when providing discharge information to this client?
3. A 23-year-old man has recently sustained a spinal cord injury after being involved in a diving accident that has left him paralyzed from the waist down. He verbally abuses the staff and expresses anger toward his family and friends when they come to visit. He needs to begin learning transfer techniques. Which stage of grieving is this client experiencing? What approach should you take in planning education for this client?
4. A 65-year-old woman is taking her 72-year-old husband home after surgery. Which strategies should you use in helping this couple make the transition to home smoothly?

* REVIEW QUESTIONS

1. A client must learn to use a walker. Acquisition of this skill will require learning in which domain?
   1. Cognitive
   2. Affective
   3. Psychomotor
   4. Attentional
2. You should plan to teach a client about the importance of exercise
   1. When visitors are in the room
   2. When the client's pain medications are effectively managing pain
   3. Just before lunch, when the client is most awake and alert
   4. When the client is talking about current stressors in his or her life
3. A client with newly diagnosed cervical cancer is going home. The client is avoiding discussion of her illness and postoperative orders. In teaching the client about discharge instructions, you should
   1. Teach the client's spouse
   2. Focus on knowledge the client will need in a few weeks
   3. Provide only the information the client needs to go home
   4. Convince the client that learning about her health is necessary

4. A community health nurse is about to teach a Grade 12 health class about nutrition. To achieve the best learning outcomes, you should
   1. Provide information by using a lecture
   2. Use simple words to promote understanding
   3. Complete an extensive literature search focusing on eating disorders
   4. Develop topics for discussion that necessitate problem solving
5. You are going to teach a client how to perform a breast self-examination. The behavioural objective that would best measure the client's ability to perform the examination is as follows:
   1. The client will verbalize the steps involved in breast self-examination within 1 week.
   2. You will explain the importance of performing breast self-examination once a month.
   3. The client will perform breast self-examination correctly before the end of the teaching session.
   4. You will demonstrate breast self-examination on a breast model provided by the Canadian Cancer Society.
6. A client who is having chest pain is about to undergo an emergency cardiac catheterization. Which of the following is the most appropriate teaching approach in this situation?
   1. Telling
   2. Selling
   3. Entrusting
   4. Participating
7. You are teaching a parenting class to a group of pregnant adolescents and have given the adolescents baby dolls to bathe and talk to. This is an example of
   1. Discovery
   2. An analogy
   3. Role-playing
   4. A demonstration
8. A client with a learning disability is starting to take a new antihypertensive medication. In teaching the client about the medication, you should
   1. Demonstrate measuring dosages and ask for return demonstration
   2. Provide only written material
   3. Present the information once
   4. Expect the client to understand the information quickly
9. A client must learn how to administer a subcutaneous injection. You know the client is ready to learn when the client
   1. Has been given written instructions
   2. Expresses the importance of learning the skill
   3. Can see and understand the markings on the syringe
   4. Has the dexterity needed to prepare and inject the medication
10. A client who is hospitalized has just received a diagnossis of diabetes. He needs to learn how to give himself injections. The best teaching method would be
    1. Demonstration
    2. Group instruction
    3. One-on-one discussion
    4. Simulation

* RECOMMENDED WEB SITES

Public Health Agency of Canada: http://www.phac-aspc.gc.ca/chn-rcs/index-eng.php

This Web site provides information and resources on a variety of public health issues and topics, including health promotion, healthy living, diseases, and injury prevention.

Health Canada: http://www.hc-sc.gc.ca/

This Web site provides many resources on a variety of health issues and topics to assist in client education:

- TeleHealth: http://www.hc-sc.gc.ca/fnih-spni/services/ehealth-esante/tele/index_e.html
- E-health: http://www.hc-sc.gc.ca/hcs-sss/ehealth-esante/index_e.html
- Travel health: http://www.hc-sc.gc.ca/hl-vs/travel-voyage/index_e.html

Canadian Public Health Association: http://www.cpha.ca/en/default.aspx

This Web site provides both national and international information and resources on public health issues and services.

National Institutes of Health: http://health.nih.gov/

This Web site provides a great many resources for client education, prepared by the National Institutes of Health in the United States.

22

Developmental Theories

Original chapter by Karen Balakas, RN, PhD, CNE

Canadian content written by Nicole Letourneau, RN, PhD

objectives

Mastery of content in this chapter will enable you to:

- Define the key terms listed.
- Identify basic principles of growth and development.
- Discuss factors influencing growth and development.
- Identify five major traditions that underlie modern developmental theories.
- Name and describe the major developmental theories associated with each tradition.
- Describe and compare the mechanisms that underlie the major developmental theories.
- Discuss nursing implications associated with the application of developmental principles to client care.

media resources

evolve Web Site

- Audio Chapter Summaries
- Glossary
- Multiple-Choice Review Questions
- Student Learning Activities
- Weblinks

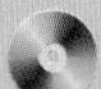

Companion CD

- Glossary
- Interactive Learning Activities
- Fluids and Electrolytes Tutorial
- Test-Taking Skills

key terms

Accommodation, p. 316
Assimilation, p. 316
Attachment, p. 320
Autonomous stage, p. 316
Biophysical developmental theories, p. 313
Bowlby's attachment and separation theory, p. 320
Bronfenbrenner's bioecological theory, p. 324
Cognitive developmental theories, p. 316
Contextual tradition, p. 324
Conventional stage, p. 316
Developmental health, p. 325
Dialectic tradition, p. 325
Differentiation, p. 315
Dynamic maturational model of attachment, p. 320
Ego, p. 318
Epigenesis, p. 320
Erikson's theory of eight stages of life, p. 319
Exosystem, p. 325
Freud's psychoanalytic model of personality development, p. 318
Gould's development themes, p. 323
Havighurst's developmental tasks, p. 323
Id, p. 318
Individuation, p. 318
Kohlberg's theory of moral development, p. 317
Libido, p. 318
Macrosystem, p. 325
Maturation, p. 315
Mechanisms of development, p. 313
Mechanistic tradition, p. 323
Mesosystem, p. 325
Microsystem, p. 324
Moral developmental theories, p. 316
Organicism, p. 313
Piaget's theory of cognitive development, p. 316
Piaget's theory of moral development, p. 316
Population health approach, p. 325
Premoral stage, p. 316
Protective processes, p. 326
Psychoanalytic and psychosocial tradition, p. 318
Resilience, p. 326
Separation, p. 318
Superego, p. 318
Temperament, p. 315
Vulnerability processes, p. 326
Zone of proximal development, p. 325

All people progress through phases of growth and development, from the simple to the complex, at a highly individualized rate. Understanding typical growth and development helps nurses to predict, prevent, and detect any changes from clients' expected patterns and to develop approaches and programs that can further enhance the developmental well-being of individuals (Berk, 2006; Bukatko & Daehler, 2004). Understanding the impact of early experience on development in adulthood provides the foundation for nurses to advocate for appropriate developmental care for vulnerable children and families (McCain et al., 2007). Developmental theories also help nurses to assess and treat a client's response to an illness. Understanding the process of human development helps caregivers to plan appropriate individualized care for clients (Berk, 2008; Edelman & Mandle, 2006).

For many years, human growth and development have been described as orderly, predictable processes beginning with conception and continuing until death. This view is increasingly being recognized as overlooking differences in gender, culture, and sexuality. Today, it is no longer assumed that all people progress through universal linear phases of growth and development. Human growth and development are now seen as processes in which sociocultural, biological, and psychological forces interact with the individual over time (Berk, 2008). As a result, theorists have changed focus from describing growth and development to explaining it. How do humans develop? What are the mechanisms, or explanatory components, that underlie human growth and development?

In this chapter, five broad traditions of human development are introduced, and the mechanisms of development espoused by key theorists are outlined. Examples of implications for the nursing process that follow from the mechanisms are offered. Detailed descriptions of human development appear in Chapters 23, 24, and 25.

Growth and Development

Growth and development are synchronous processes that are interdependent in the healthy individual. Growth and development depend on a sequence of endocrine, genetic, constitutional, environmental, and nutritional influences (Edelman & Mandle, 2006).

Physical Growth

Growth is the quantitative, or measurable, aspect of an individual's increase in physical measurements. Measurable growth indicators include changes in height, weight, teeth, skeletal structures, and sexual characteristics. For example, children generally double their birth weight by 5 months of age and their birth height by 36 months. Physical growth is not only genetic but is also affected by other contextual factors such as socioeconomic status.

Development

Development is a progressive and continuous process of change leading to increased skill and capacity to function. Development is the result of complex interactions between biological and environmental influences (Salkind, 2004). These changes are qualitative in nature and difficult to measure in exact units. Developmental changes have certain predictable characteristics: They proceed from simple to complex, from general to specific, from head to toe (cephalocaudal), and from the trunk to the extremities (proximodistal). For example, a child's progressions from rolling over to crawling to walking are developmental changes.

Factors Influencing Growth and Development

Three major categories of factors influence human growth and development: (1) genetic or natural forces within the person, (2) the environment in which the person lives, and (3) the interaction that takes place between these two factors (Table 22–1). You apply knowledge of these factors when selecting approaches to promote typical growth and developmental progression. It is important, for example, that as part of planning for a client's pregnancy, you consider the client's genetic endowment, age, socioeconomic status, culture (Box 22–1), available support system, and preconceived state of health.

Traditions of Developmental Theories

A theory is an organized, often observable, logical set of statements about a subject. Human developmental theories are models intended to account for how and why people develop as they do (Thomas, 1997). All of the theories of development discussed in this chapter make different contributions to our understanding of the developmental process.

To help you understand the number of developmental theories, this chapter has been grouped into five traditions of (or ways of thinking about) theory development: organicism, psychoanalytic and psychosocial, mechanistic, contextualism, and dialecticism. The areas of learning and spiritual development are covered in Chapters 21 and 28, respectively.

Each tradition of developmental theory emphasizes different underlying developmental mechanisms. **Mechanisms of development** are the explanatory components of each theory, or the means by which the developmental tasks are achieved. They are the processes or factors that underlie the developmental process within each theory, and they enable developmental progression. These underlying mechanisms are proposed to be universal and to function across the lifespan, not just in childhood. Although developmental theories are often presented within a framework of stagelike progressions, what the stages actually represent are the outcomes produced by these mechanisms at each specific age.

Organicism

Organicism refers to a theoretical focus on the organism itself. According to theories in this tradition, development is a result of biologically driven behaviour and the person's adaptation to the environment. Biophysical and cognitive–moral theories of development are included in this tradition.

Biophysical Developmental Theories

Biophysical developmental theories describe and explain how the physical body grows and changes. The changes that occur as a newborn grows into adulthood can be quantified and compared against established norms; however, regional and cultural differences may exist, as may differences related to the availability of resources in the environment for adequate growth.

How does the physical body age? What are the triggers that change the body's physical characteristics from childhood through adolescence to adulthood? Biological influences on development include many factors such as genetics and exposure to teratogens

TABLE 22-1 Major Factors That Influence Growth and Development

Categories	Implications
Genetic or Natural Factors	
Heredity	Genetic endowment determines sex, skin, hair and eye colour, physical growth, stature, and, to some extent, psychological uniqueness.
Temperament	Temperament is the characteristic psychological mood with which the child is born; it influences interactions between an individual and the environment.
Environmental Factors	
Family	Family purposes are to protect, teach, and nurture its members. Family functions include means for survival, security, assistance with emotional and social development, assistance with maintenance of relationships, instruction about society and world, and assistance in learning roles and behaviours. Family influences through its values, beliefs, customs, and specific patterns of interaction and communication.
Peer group	Peer group provides a new and different learning environment. Peer group provides different patterns and structures of interaction and communication, necessitating a different style of behaviour. Functions of peer group include allowing individual to learn about success and failure; to validate and challenge thoughts, feelings, and concepts; to receive acceptance, support, and rejection as a unique person apart from family; and to achieve group purposes by meeting demands, pressures, and expectations.
Health environment	Level of health affects an individual's responsiveness to environment and responsiveness of others to the individual. It determines availability and accessibility of resources to support health.
Nutrition	Growth is regulated by dietary factors. Adequacy of nutrients influences whether and how physiological needs, as well as subsequent growth and development needs, are met. The availability of quality nutrients also affects growth.
Rest, sleep, and exercise	Balance between rest, sleep, and exercise is essential for rejuvenating the body. Disturbances diminish growth, whereas equilibrium reinforces physiological and psychological health.
Living environment	Factors affecting growth and development include season, climate, community life, socioeconomic status, and quality of the physical environment (air, water, land). An embryo may be exposed to teratogenic substances (e.g., alcohol, chemicals, or radiation) that cause abnormal development.
Political and policy environment	Municipal, provincial, and federal policies directly affect the health and well-being of individuals, families, and communities.
Interacting Factors	
Life experiences	Individuals develop by applying what has been learned through experience to their current situation. Experiences emerge from both biological and environmental sources. The individual deduces meaning from these experiences and bases further actions on them.
Prenatal health	Biological and maturational factors (genetics; maternal age; medical problems) and environmental factors (maternal health; nutrition; use of tobacco, drugs, and alcohol; use of prenatal services) together affect fetal growth and development.
State of health	Health is a product of both intrinsic (biology) and extrinsic (quality of environment, availability of resources for health) factors. Changes to health status such as illness or injury may cause inability to cope with and respond to underlying processes and demands of development.

(e.g., maternal diseases, drugs, X-rays, or other hazardous substances that interfere with the normal development of the fetus). All biophysical developmental theories give some credence to the roles of nature (genetics) and nurture (caregiving environment and resources). However, the theories differ sharply on how much influence individual and environmental forces have on development (Berk, 2006).

Gesell's Theory of Maturational Development. Arnold Gesell (1880–1961) was a psychologist who obtained his medical degree to help him explain the physiological processes he observed in the behaviour of children. Through extensive observations in the 1940s, he developed behavioural norms that serve as a primary source of information for childhood development today.

Fundamental to Gesell's theory of development is the notion that the pattern of growth and development is directed by the activity of the genes, although at that time, the genetic mechanism was unknown to him. He believed that environmental factors can support, change, and modify the pattern but that they do not generate the progressions of development (Gesell, 1948). Gesell proposed that the pattern of maturation follows a fixed developmental sequence in all

BOX 22-1 CULTURAL ASPECTS OF CARE

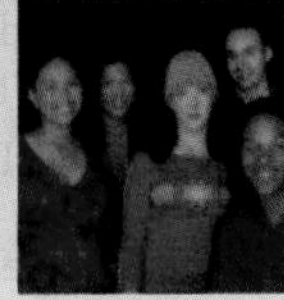

You need to assess the cultural background of each client and be prepared to change your practice so that it is congruent with the client's beliefs and values concerning growth and development. For example, within many Aboriginal cultures, the concept of a circle or cycle is a fundamental theme (Smylie, 2001) and can be applied to human development. Human states and concepts are considered to be part of the life cycle of the earth, which also includes plants, animals, and seasons (Smylie, 2000). For people, this life cycle may be described as a continuum of age-related roles and qualities of being, including physical, mental, emotional, and spiritual well-being. All aspects of human development are viewed as being in harmony with the cycle of life in nature. As in nature, each part of the cycle needs to be balanced with the other parts. Roles and expectations related to developmental age reflect traditional values of respect, honour, balance, and harmony. Figure 22–1 represents the circle of life, or the medicine wheel, as applied to the human life cycle.

humans and that critical periods exist in which the presence or absence of particular experiences makes a biological system functional or nonfunctional (Keating & Hertzman, 1999). For example, if a child's visual defect is not identified until the start of school, usual message pathways in the brain may not become fully developed, and long-term vision may be impaired (Cynader & Frost, 1999).

Sequential development is seen in fetuses, in which the order of development of the various organ systems is specific (Crain, 2005). After birth, children grow according to their genetic blueprint and gain skills in an orderly manner, but at each individual's own pace. For example, most children learn first how to hold a cup with digital grasp at about 15 months of age and later how to lift, drink from, and replace the cup at 21 months of age. Gesell clarified that not every child develops those skills at exactly the same ages. He pointed out that the environment does play a part in the development of the child but that it does not have any part in the sequence of development. Gesell believed that children could not be pushed to develop faster than their own unique timetables permitted. He also proposed that the biological body determines behavioural development. Researchers continue to use Gesell's theories today, probing for gene–environment interactions in human development (Cicchetti & Nurcombe, 2007).

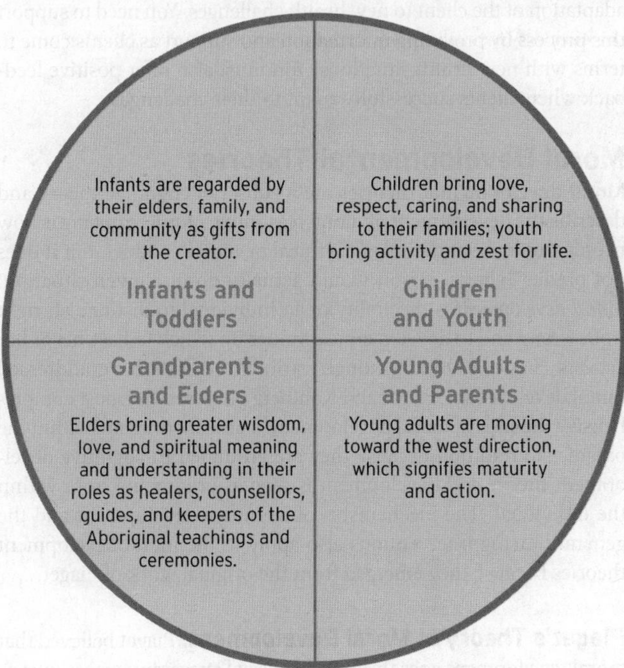

Figure 22-1 An Aboriginal perspective on human development: the circle of life, or the medicine wheel, as applied to the human life cycle. **Source:** Redrawn from Smylie, J. (2001, January). A guide for health professionals working with Aboriginal peoples: Health issues affecting Aboriginal peoples. *Journal SOGC, 100*, 55.

Mechanisms of Maturational Development. **Maturation** is the biological internal regulatory mechanism that governs the emergence of all new skills and abilities that appear with advancing age (Nelson et al., 2006). Maturation involves an individual's biological ability, physiological condition, and desire to learn more mature behaviour. To mature, the individual may have to relinquish previous behaviour and learning, integrate new patterns into existing behaviour, or both. Maturation influences the sequence and timing of the changes associated with growth and development. For example, the child relinquishes crawling for walking because walking permits greater investigation of the environment and more learning. However, the child cannot walk until the biological ability and structures to perform the action (i.e., increased muscle cells and tone) have developed.

Differentiation is the process by which cells and structures become modified and refine their characteristics. Development of activities and functions progresses from simple to complex. Embryonic cells begin as vague and undifferentiated and develop into complex, highly diversified cells, tissues, and organs.

Nursing Implications of Maturational Development. As a nurse, you consider maturational development in your care planning when you help mothers sequence play activities appropriate for learning of sitting, rolling, creeping, crawling, and walking. You consider sequential development of fetuses and critical periods when you counsel expectant mothers about environmental teratogens during the first trimester of pregnancy. You also support development during critical periods when you develop early intervention programs for parents.

Chess and Thomas's Theory of Temperament Development. **Temperament** is a physical and emotional response style that affects a child's interactions with others (Hockenberry & Wilson, 2007). It is the way a person adjusts to life experiences, and it is thought to originate within the person's genetic makeup. A child's temperament influences how others respond to the child and to his or her needs. Knowledge of temperament helps parents to have a clearer perspective of their child and enables health care professionals to guide them appropriately (Hockenberry & Wilson, 2007).

Psychiatrists Stella Chess (1914–2007) and Alexander Thomas (1915–2003) conducted a landmark 20-year longitudinal study of development that included children from a range of populations, including children of middle-income parents and intellectually disabled children of lower-income parents. The breadth of the data allowed them to look at the behaviour of people from childhood to early adulthood as they interacted with their environment. Their work defined the concept of temperament (Chess & Thomas, 1995), and they proposed that temperament is biologically derived.

Chess and Thomas (1995) described three common categories of temperament, but individual variation meant that approximately 30% of children cannot be classified in any of these groups:

- The *easy child* is easygoing and even-tempered, regular and predictable in his or her habits, and open-minded and adaptable to change. Mood expressions are mild to moderately intense and typically positive.

- The *difficult child* is highly active, irritable, and irregular in habits. Negative withdrawal from other people is typical, and the child requires a highly structured environment. He or she adapts slowly to new routines, new people, or new situations. Mood expressions are usually intense and primarily negative.
- The *slow-to-warm-up child* typically reacts negatively and with mild intensity to new stimuli. He or she adapts slowly with repeated contact unless pressured and responds with mild but passive resistance to novelty or changes in routine.

Mechanisms of Temperament Development. According to temperament theory, biologically derived temperament characteristics drive children's interaction with the environment. Chess and Thomas (1995) proposed that it is through "goodness of fit" between the individual and the immediate environment that human development is modulated. This proposal places significant responsibility for child development outcomes within the family. For instance, the difficult child who has trouble making the transition from one activity or environment to a new one functions best in a family that maintains routine and has a slow, easy attitude toward the introduction of change. The same child in a family that has few routines has much more difficulty moving from one activity (such as play) to the next activity (such as sleep). The first scenario is an example of "goodness of fit" between the temperament of the child and the family environment.

Nursing Implications of Temperament Development. Nurses can help families identify the unique characteristics of their infants and children. For instance, an approach called "Keys to Caregiving" (Sumner, 1995) assists nurses in helping new parents identify their infants' usual behaviour and communication styles. Keys to Caregiving teaches new parents about infant cues and behaviours that signify needs (e.g., hunger or desire for playful attention), infant states and how to modulate infant states (e.g., helping soothe and comfort a fussy baby), and optimal parenting practices that promote sensitive, nurturant relationships between caregivers and infants. This information helps families adapt their habits and routines to match their children's temperaments. You can also consider temperament styles when working with adults and families in teaching or support situations.

Cognitive Developmental Theories

Cognitive developmental theories focus on reasoning and thinking processes, including the changes in how people perform intellectual operations. These operations are related to the ways people learn to understand the world in which they live. Mental processes, including perceiving, reasoning, remembering, and believing, affect certain types of emotional behaviour. For example, a child will have a different emotional reaction to the death of a grandparent than to the death of an older sibling or a parent.

Unlike biophysical developmental theories, cognitive developmental theories emphasize that although the developmental process originates with the person, it is greatly influenced by interactions between the person and the environment. Therefore, theories of cognitive development emphasize the active role that the individual plays in the developmental process. Cognitive theories are considered to be within the organicism tradition because development is still viewed as originating within the organism.

Piaget's Theory of Cognitive Development. Jean Piaget (1896–1980), a Swiss biologist and philosopher, studied how people come to know their world. **Piaget's theory of cognitive development** addresses the development of children's intellectual organization and how they think, reason, perceive, and make meaning of the physical world. His theory includes four periods, each of which subsumes a number of stages (Table 22–2). He recognized that people move through these specific periods at different rates but in the same sequence or order (Berk, 2006; Crain, 2005). Piaget also theorized that this would be true in all cultures. He acknowledged that biological maturation plays a role in this developmental theory but believed that rates of development depend on the intellectual stimulation and challenge in the environment of the person. Piaget found that children acquire knowledge through acting on the environment. In other words, the individual plays an active role in his or her development.

Mechanisms of Cognitive Development. Although it is helpful to be aware of the stages, the importance of Piaget's theory is that development is considered a spontaneous process in which individuals play an active role in their own development. Environmental challenges are internalized through the mechanisms of assimilation and accommodation. **Assimilation** is the process of making sense of new information in comparison with what is already known. **Accommodation** is the process of adapting ways of thinking to a new experience or new information. Together, these processes reflect adaptation to new information or experience. In a health care situation, a person who has a headache can evaluate it as an everyday or usual experience. In this process, the person is assimilating it to what he or she knows already as the experience of his or her body; that is, the person occasionally has headaches. When headaches become extreme or constant, then the person needs to understand the headache pain differently in the experience of his or her body. For instance, the person may learn to see himself or herself as a person who has migraines or as a person with a brain tumour who requires surgery.

The mechanisms of cognitive development apply across the lifespan and to all client situations. As such, they also apply to the moral theories and theories of adult development that are described in the following sections.

Nursing Implications of Cognitive Development. Most clients need to know about new ways of adjusting or behaving with regard to their health. Assimilation and accommodation represent adaptation of the client to new health challenges. You need to support this process by providing information and support as clients come to terms with new health situations. You must also offer positive feedback when clients successfully adapt to their challenges.

Moral Developmental Theories

Moral developmental theories are a subset of cognitive theory and describe the development of moral reasoning. *Moral reasoning* is how people think about the rules of ethical or moral conduct, but it does not predict what a person would actually do in a given situation. *Moral development* is the ability of an individual to distinguish right from wrong and to develop ethical values on which to base his or her actions (Berk, 2006). Although various theorists have addressed moral development, Piaget and Kohlberg proposed the most comprehensive theories of moral development. These theories are within the organicism tradition because they are grounded in cognitive development theory and development is seen as originating from within the individual. The mechanisms of cognitive development and the general nursing interventions also apply to the moral development theories because they emerged from the original work of Piaget.

Piaget's Theory of Moral Development. Piaget believed that moral development goes through a series of successive stages, just as cognition and learning do. **Piaget's theory of moral development** presents three stages of morality: the **premoral stage**, the **conventional stage**, and the **autonomous stage**. In the premoral stage, the child feels no obligation to follow rules. In the conventional stage, children follow the rules set up by people in authority, such as their

TABLE 22-2 Piaget's Theory of Cognitive Development

Stage	Description	Nursing Implications
Period 1: Sensorimotor (birth to 2 years of age)	The infant develops the schema or action pattern for dealing with the environment (Berk, 2006; Singer & Revenson, 1996). These schemas may include hitting, looking, grasping, or kicking (Figure 22–2). Schemas become self-initiated activities; for example, the infant who learns that sucking achieves a pleasing result generalizes the action to suck fingers, blanket, or clothing. Successful achievement leads to greater exploration. In the second year, children are able to form primitive mental images as they acquire object permanence. Before this, they do not realize that objects out of sight exist. When a 6-month-old is shown a toy before it is hidden, he or she will not search for it. At 18 months, the child can understand that even if it cannot be seen, it still exists and will search for it.	Educate parents about the need to promote infants' exploration of the environment. Such education supports development of action patterns that help the children achieve motor and cognitive skills.
Period 2: Preoperational (2 to 7 years of age)	Children learn to think with the use of symbols and mental images. Still egocentric, the child sees objects and people from only one point of view: the child's own. Play is the initial method of nonlanguage use of symbols. This is a time of parallel play. Parallel play can be observed as children engage in activities side by side without a common goal. Imitation and make-believe play are ways to represent experience (Berk, 2006; Singer & Revenson, 1996). Later, language develops and broadens possibilities for thinking about the past or the future. Children can now communicate about events with others. As the language fits into a logical form, it mirrors the thinking process at the time.	Recognize the use of play as the way the child understands the events taking place. Parents can be assisted in the use of play materials such as toy thermometers and stethoscopes to encourage children to communicate feelings about health care procedures.
Period 3: Concrete operations (7 to 11 years of age)	Children achieve the ability to perform mental operations. For example, the child can think about an action that before was performed physically. At the earlier stage, the child could count to 10, but at this stage, he or she can count and understand what each number represents. Children can describe a process without actually performing it. At this stage, they are able to coordinate two perspectives. In other words, they can appreciate the difference between their perspective and that of a friend. Reversibility is the primary characteristic of concrete operational thought. Children can mentally reverse the direction of their thoughts. Children can mentally classify objects according to their quantitative dimensions, known as seriation. Another major accomplishment of this stage is conservation, or the ability to see objects or quantities as remaining the same despite a change in their physical appearance (Berk, 2006; Singer & Revenson, 1996). Children can begin to cooperate and share with new information about the acts they perform.	Encourage parents to guide the child to perform helpful activities within the home, such as doing chores in exchange for privileges (TV time, play with friends).
Period 4: Formal operations (11 years to adulthood)	The individual's thinking moves to abstract and theoretical subjects. Thinking can venture into such subjects as achieving world peace, finding justice, and seeking meaning in life. Adolescents can organize their thoughts in their minds. They have the capacity to reason with regard to possibilities. New cognitive powers allow the adolescent to achieve more far-reaching problem solving. This thinking matures, and the depth of understanding increases with experience.	Include the adolescent in decision making about his or her own health care that is based on his or her ability to think abstractly.

parents, teachers, clergy, or police. When a person reaches the stage of autonomous morality, moral judgements are based on mutual respect for the rules. A person also considers the consequences of a moral decision. In making moral judgements that involve others, the person at this stage starts to consider information related to the subjective intent (Berk, 2006).

Piaget believed that children initially follow the rules without understanding them. Children see these rules as fixed and handed down by adults or by God and therefore think they cannot change them. Young children base their moral decisions on the extent of the consequences to the action, not necessarily on the action itself. For example, a young child will not eat a cookie before supper, not because the mother said not to but because the child is afraid of the punishment that would result if he or she did. Around 10 or 11 years of age, children's cognitive ability matures and the rules they follow are understood within the context of community life. Children understand that the rules can be modified "by legal channels" if everyone agrees to change the rules (Singer & Revenson, 1996). Moral maturity is the internalization of the principles: that is, the desire to weigh all of the relationships and circumstances before making a decision.

Kohlberg's Theory of Moral Development. Lawrence Kohlberg (1927–1987) expanded on Piaget's moral developmental theory. From a series of moral dilemmas presented to boys aged 10, 13, and 16 years, he identified six stages of moral development occurring at three levels (Kohlberg, 1981; Table 22–3). Kohlberg found a link between moral development and Piaget's cognitive development theory. He theorized that a child's moral development does not advance if the child's cognitive development does not also mature. In this way, **Kohlberg's theory of moral development** follows Piaget's

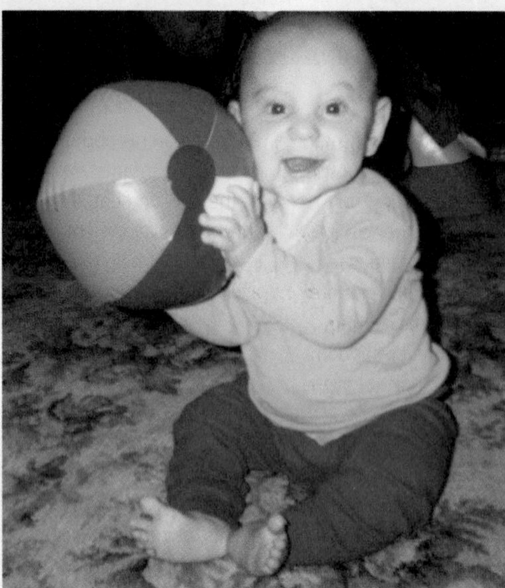

Figure 22-2 Successfully achieving action patterns, such as grasping, leads to learning and more exploration.

cognitive developmental theory. According to Kohlberg, levels and stages do not occur at specific ages, and people attain different levels of moral development.

Kohlberg's Critics. Although Kohlberg is recognized as a leader in moral developmental theory, critics have questioned the applicability of his study beyond the study population of male adolescents of the Western philosophical tradition. Research attempting to support Kohlberg's (1981) theory with people raised in the Eastern philosophies found that those study participants never proceeded beyond stages 3 or 4 of Kohlberg's model. Does that mean that they have not reached as high a level of moral development as most of the adults raised in the Western traditions? Or is it that Kohlberg's research design did not allow a way to measure moral development in people raised within a different culture?

Kohlberg's (1981) study has also been criticized for age and gender biases. Gilligan (1982), an associate, concentrated on the differences in Kohlberg's findings that could have been related to gender. According to Gilligan, all developmental theories are subject to gender bias, and only since the 1990s have scholars researched and recognized the differences between men and women in the way they think and how they have been raised to make decisions (Kail, 2002).

Gilligan's Theory. Carol Gilligan (1936–present) proposed that Kohlberg's (1981) theory is biased in favour of men. She believed that men and women develop in parallel ways, with one not being superior to the other. Gilligan's argument is basically that the developmental difference between women and men is in relationships and issues of dependency (Berk, 2006; Crain, 2005; Gilligan, 1982). Separation and individuation are critically tied to male development. **Separation** refers to the boy's recognition of biological distinctness and is based on his emergence from a dependent relationship with his mother. This separation from the mother is essential for the boy in his development of masculinity. Girls do not need to separate from their mothers to achieve feminine identity; it is through this attachment to their mother that their identity is formed. In most developmental theories, the achievement of increasing separation is a developmental norm. When women are measured against this norm as it relates to their need to maintain relationships, they are seen as failures or as less evolved developmentally. **Individuation** is based on the child's awareness of differences in will, viewpoint, and needs. This process enables the individual to gradually assume a more independent role and identity.

Male moral development may focus on logic, justice, and social organization, whereas female moral development focuses on interpersonal relationships. Of interest is that in studies whose research design is based on Gilligan's critique, findings have been inconclusive. As a result, Gilligan's position remains controversial (Cavanaugh & Blanchard-Fields, 2006).

Psychoanalytic and Psychosocial Tradition

Theories in the **psychoanalytic and psychosocial tradition** describe the development of personality, thinking, behaviour, and emotions. This development is thought to occur with varying degrees of influence from internal biological forces and external societal and cultural forces.

Sigmund Freud

The first scholar to provide a formal, structured theory of personality development was Sigmund Freud (1856–1939). His goal was to promote successful participation in society through the development of balance between pleasure-seeking drives and societal pressures. In **Freud's psychoanalytic model of personality development**, he asserted that mature adults should have a strong sense of conscience that allows for the experience of pleasure within the boundaries of society. He believed that two internal biological forces essentially drive psychological change in the child: sexual (**libido**) and aggressive energies. Motivation for behaviour is to achieve pleasure and avoid pain created by these forces. These forces come into conflict with the reality of the world as maturational changes occur.

Freud's theory accounts for five psychosexual developmental stages, each associated with different pleasurable zones that serve as the foci for gratification and bodily pleasure (Berk, 2006; Kliegman et al., 2007; Table 22–4). Freud's theory has been soundly criticized for gender and cultural biases. Some of Freud's critics contend that people are more influenced by their life experiences than by their sexual energies. Despite these criticisms, it is clear that Freud gave other theorists a basis for observation of emotion and behaviour. According to many other psychoanalytic theories, development is an ongoing process of resolving conflict between issues of biological maturation and societal expectations.

Mechanisms of Freud's Theory. Components of personality emerge through Freud's developmental stages. The mechanisms of Freud's personality development theory are the id, the ego, and the superego. Freud believed that the functions of these mechanisms regulate behaviour. The **id**—basic instinctual impulses and drives to achieve pleasure—is the most primitive part of the personality and originates in the infant. The **ego** represents the reality mechanism mediating conflicts between the environment and the forces of the id. The ego helps us judge reality accurately, regulate impulses, and make good decisions. The third mechanism, the **superego**, performs regulating, restraining, and prohibiting actions. Often referred to as the *conscience*, the superego is influenced by the standards of outside social forces (parent, teacher).

Nursing Implications of Freud's Theory. The functions of the id, ego, and superego form the historical basis of many, if not all, subsequent theories of personality and social emotional development. You need to remember that according to Freudian theory, mature human personality is the product of conflict between instinctual drives to achieve pleasure and the restraints of adaptive human society. When activities associated with basic pleasure (e.g., eating, sexual activity, and elimination) are altered by illness or disability, knowledgeable and empathetic nursing care is required.

Erikson's Theory of Eight Stages of Life

Erik Erikson (1902–1994) expanded Freud's psychoanalytic stages into a psychosocial model that covered the whole lifespan, not just childhood and adolescence (Erikson, 1993, 1997; Kliegman et al., 2007). He broadened the factors responsible for influencing development to include socialization.

According to **Erikson's theory of eight stages of life**, each person goes through eight stages of development (Table 22–5). In each stage, the person needs to accomplish a particular task before moving on to the next stage. Each task is framed with opposing conflicts that the person must balance. For example, an adolescent needs to develop a sense of personal identity despite many conflicting societal choices (stage 5, identity versus role confusion). Each stage builds upon the successful resolution of the previous developmental conflict. Readiness for the task is necessary for success. Once mastered, tasks are challenged and tested during new situations or at times of conflict (Hockenberry & Wilson, 2007). For example, the infant's trust is built through consistent, reliable caregiving, and

TABLE 22-3 Kohlberg's Moral Development Theory

Level and Stage	Description	Nursing Implications
Level I: Preconventional level	The person reflects on moral reasoning based on personal gain. The person's moral reason for acting, the "why," relates to the consequences that the person believes will occur. These consequences can occur in the form of punishment or reward. Therefore, children may view illness as a punishment for fighting with their siblings or disobeying their parents.	As a nurse, you should be aware of this thinking and reinforce teaching that the child cannot become ill because of wrongdoing.
Stage 1: Punishment and obedience orientation	Response to a moral dilemma is in terms of absolute obedience to authority and rules. Avoidance of punishment or the unquestioning deference to authority is characteristic behaviour. The child will do something because an authority figure tells him or her to do it.	
Stage 2: Instrumental relativist orientation	The person recognizes that more than one view may be correct. The decision to do something morally correct is based on satisfying one's own needs and occasionally the needs of others.	
Level II: Conventional level	The person sees moral reasoning based on his or her own personal internalization of societal and others' expectations. A person wants to fulfill the expectations of the family, group, or nation, develop loyalty to the dominant order, and actively maintain, support, and justify the order. Moral decision making at this level moves from "What's in it for me?" to "How will it affect my relationships with others?"	You may observe this level of moral development when family members make end-of-life decisions for their loved ones. Grief support will involve an understanding of the level of moral decision making of each family member (see Chapter 29).
Stage 3: Good boy–nice girl orientation	The individual wants to please others and win approval by "being nice," which means having good motives, showing concern for others, and keeping mutual relationships through trust, loyalty, respect, and gratitude.	
Stage 4: Society-maintaining orientation	Focus expands from relationships with others to societal concerns. Correct behaviour is doing one's duty, showing respect for authority, and maintaining the social order. Adolescents in this stage may choose not to attend a party at which drugs will be used, not because they are afraid of getting caught but because they know that using drugs is not healthy.	
Level III: Postconventional level	The person finds a balance between basic human rights and obligations and societal rules and regulations. Individuals reject moral decisions based on authority or conformity to groups in favour of defining their own moral values and principles. Individuals at this stage start to envision an ideal society.	You focus not only on your individual practice but also on social determinants that affect the well-being of a community, such as poverty and homelessness.
Stage 5: Social contract orientation	An individual follows the laws but recognizes the possibility of changing the law to improve society. The individual also recognizes that different social groups may have different values but believe in basic rights, such as liberty and life.	
Stage 6: Universal ethical principle orientation	"Right" is defined by the decision of conscience in accord with self-chosen ethical principles. These principles, such as the Golden Rule, are abstract and appeal to logical comprehensiveness, universality, and consistency (Kohlberg, 1981). Whereas stage 5 emphasizes the basic rights and the democratic process, stage 6 defines the principles by which agreements will be most just.	

TABLE 22-4 Freud's Five Stages of Psychosexual Development

Stage	Description	Nursing Implications
Stage 1: Oral (birth to age 12–18 months)	Initially, sucking and oral satisfaction is not only necessary for living but also extremely pleasurable in its own right. Late in this stage, the infant begins to realize that the mother or parent is something separate from self. Disruption in the physical or emotional availability of the parent (e.g., inadequate bonding or chronic illness) could have an impact on the infant's development.	For an infant, feeding and sucking produces pleasure and comfort. Teach parents that feedings should be offered whenever the infant requires them.
Stage 2: Anal (ages 12–18 months to 3 years)	The focus of pleasure changes to the anal zone. Children become increasingly aware of the pleasurable sensations of this body region with interest in the products of their effort. Through the toilet-training process, the child is asked to delay gratification in order to meet parental and societal expectations.	Teach the parents that toilet training should be as positive an experience as possible. Praise helps the child achieve a sense of control.
Stage 3: Phallic or Oedipal (ages 3–6 years)	The genital organs become the focus of pleasure. The boy becomes interested in the penis; the girl becomes aware of the absence of the penis, known as *penis envy*. This is the time of exploration and imagination as the child fantasizes about the parent of the opposite sex as his or her first love interest, known as the *Oedipal complex* (in boys) or *Electra complex* (in girls). By the end of this stage, the child attempts to reduce this conflict by identifying with the parent of the same sex in a way to win recognition and acceptance.	Assure parents that a child's identifying with the parent of the same sex is a normal developmental phase.
Stage 4: Latency (ages 6–12 years)	Sexual urges from the earlier Oedipal stage are repressed and channelled into productive activities that are socially acceptable. Within the educational and social worlds of the child, much is to be learned and accomplished. The child places energy and effort into these worlds.	Encourage the child to pursue physical and intellectual challenges.
Stage 5: Genital (puberty through adulthood)	This is a time of turbulence when earlier sexual urges reawaken and are directed toward an individual outside the family circle. Unresolved prior conflicts surface during adolescence. Once conflicts are resolved, the individual is then capable of having a mature adult sexual relationship.	Educate parents that the child needs to be encouraged to be independent and make his or her own decisions, within safe limits.

the concept of trust is tested when an infant is hospitalized or after the birth of a new sibling.

Mechanisms of Erikson's Theory. *Maturation* and *ego* activity are the primary mechanisms of development in Erikson's theory of eight stages of life. The ego mediates the conflicts between the biological needs and societal norms, and maturation establishes the timeline of this mediation. The developmental result of these mechanisms is described as an **epigenesis** (successive gradual change). If the process is adaptive, then a person has successive positive outcomes.

Nursing Implications of Erikson's Theory. The theory of the eight stages of life implies that the quality of early developmental work is important. For instance, children who live in environments in which violence is common and trust has not been attained are at greater risk of experiencing poor intimate relationships. The mechanism of epigenesis implies that the original required trust elements cannot be retrieved; at best, such a person can learn only to live with the fear and anger associated with this mistrust. You therefore need to practise within the health promotion model to build the familial, community, and societal supports necessary for growing, vulnerable children to achieve successful transitions at each stage (e.g. trust, autonomy, and initiative).

John Bowlby

John Bowlby (1907–1990) was a child psychiatrist interested in children's mental health. According to **Bowlby's attachment and separation theory**, the conflict between attachment and separation needs to be resolved in order to produce healthy social and emotional developmental outcomes across the lifespan. **Attachment** means a bond or tie between an individual and another person, such as a parent or caregiver. A basic premise of the theory is that the quality of attachment relationships stems from interactions between infants and their caregivers. These interactions reflect the degree to which infants can rely on their caregivers to provide proximity and companionship, a safe haven in the presence of threat or anxiety, and a secure base from which to explore. Failure to achieve secure attachment results in an inability throughout the lifespan to separate from caregivers and reconnect to new relationships (including work, friendship, and intimate relationships) in a healthy way.

Mechanisms of Bowlby's Theory. Early in life, two complementary behavioural systems, attachment and caregiving, combine into a self-regulating system that supports people in their healthy attachments to and separations from others. The child's experiences within this self-regulating system cause the child to develop a cognitive working model (or "map") of self, other, and the relationship between them. The ability to regulate emotion and behaviour (Box 22–2) are influenced by this working model at each developmental stage throughout life.

Patricia Crittenden

Psychologist Patricia Crittenden (1945–present) was heavily influenced by the work of attachment theorists Bowlby and Ainsworth (1979) in developing her **dynamic maturational model of attachment** (Crittenden & Claussen, 2003; Crittenden, 2008). In this

TABLE 22-5 Erikson's Theory of Eight Stages of Life

Stage	Description	Nursing Implications
1. Trust versus mistrust (infancy: birth to age 1 year)	The infant learns to trust others. Trust is achieved when the infant will let the caregiver out of sight without undo distress. Key to this stage is consistent caregiving. The question answered at this stage is "Can I trust the world?"	The parent's struggle with building competence can be assisted by your use of anticipatory guidance and other educative interventions. The parent may need guidance to understand the importance of a safe, nurturing environment when meeting the child's needs.
2. Autonomy versus sense of shame and doubt (toddler years: ages 1–3 years)	The toddler learns to be independent and develops self-confidence. Not learning independence creates feelings of shame and self-doubt. Independence is accomplished through self-care activities, including walking, feeding, and toileting. Toddlers also develop autonomy by making choices. The question answered at this stage is "Can I control my own behaviour?"	You can use empathetic guidance to offer support for and understanding of the challenges of this stage. Harsh punishment and never offering choices are not appropriate.
3. Initiative versus guilt (preschool years: ages 3–6 years)	The child learns to initiate his or her activities. Accomplishing this task teaches the child to seek challenges in later life. Children use fantasy and imagination to explore their environment. Conflicts often arise between the child's desire to explore and the limits placed on his or her behaviour. These conflicts may lead to feelings of frustration and guilt. The questioned answered during this stage is "Can I become independent of my parents and explore my limits?"	Teaching impulse control and cooperative behaviours to the child are necessary at this stage.
4. Industry versus inferiority (middle childhood: ages 6–11 years)	The child develops a sense of competence in physical, cognitive, and social areas. Not learning new skills may lead to a sense of inadequacy and inferiority. Successfully achieving this task leads to positive attitudes toward work in adulthood (Erikson, 1993). The question answered at this stage is "Can I master the skills necessary to survive and adapt?"	You can encourage parents to offer the child many opportunities to pursue new interests and challenges.
5. Identity versus role confusion (adolescence: ages 12–18 years)	The task of adolescence is to try out several roles and form a unique identity. Dramatic physiological changes associated with sexual maturation also mark this stage. Acquiring a sense of identity is essential for making later adult decisions such as vocation or marriage partner. New social demands, opportunities, and conflicts arise in relation to the emergent identity and separation from family. The question answered at this stage is "Who am I, and what are my beliefs, feelings, and attitudes?"	You can provide education and anticipatory guidance for the parent about the changes in and challenges to the adolescent. You can also assist hospitalized adolescents in dealing with their illness by giving them enough information to allow them to make decisions about their treatment plan.
6. Intimacy versus isolation (young adulthood: ages 18–35 years)	The primary task of young adulthood is to form close, personal relationships. This is the time to become fully active in the community. If young adults have not achieved a sense of personal identity, they may be unable to form meaningful attachments, and they experience feelings of isolation. The question answered during this stage is "Can I give of myself fully to another?"	Understand that during hospitalization, young adults may benefit from the support of their partners or significant others because this support helps fulfill their need for intimacy.
7. Generativity versus self-absorption and stagnation (middle adulthood: ages 35–65 years)	The task of middle adulthood is to help younger people. The ability to expand one's personal and social involvement is crucial for this stage of development. Middle-aged adults should be able to see beyond their needs and accomplishments and view the needs of society. Dissatisfaction with one's achievements often leads to self-absorption and stagnation. The question answered during this stage is "What can I offer succeeding generations?"	You can assist adults in choosing creative ways to foster social development. Middle-aged people may find a sense of fulfillment from volunteering some time in a local school, hospital, or place of worship.

Continued

TABLE 22-5 Erikson's Theory of Eight Stages of Life *continued*

Stage	Description	Nursing Implications
8. Integrity versus despair (old age: age 65 years and older)	Older adults reflect on their life and feel satisfaction or disappointment. By suffering physical and social losses, such as those through retirement or illness, the adult may also suffer loss of status and function. The person may also have internal struggles, such as the search for meaning in life. Meeting these challenges creates the potential for growth and wisdom (Figure 22–3). The question answered during this stage is "Has my life been worthwhile?"	You can contribute to the valuing of people at all ages and stages in their communities. For example, by promoting older adults' involvement in volunteer activities, such as youth mentoring, that you display value for the skills and experience of older people, and such mentoring helps the younger generation feel important.

Adapted from Salkind, N. (2004). *An introduction to theories of human development.* Thousand Oaks, CA: Sage.

model, behavioural and psychiatric developmental disorders are considered within the context of family attachment relationships. Unlike the previous work of attachment theorists, the model considers the impact of intimate relationships on development over the lifespan.

Mechanisms of the Dynamic Maturational Model. The interaction between brain development and experiences with caregivers is central in the development of self-protective strategies that individuals use over their lifespan. Attachment strategies are employed to promote safety and security in relationships. Patterns of attachment are dominated by "cognitive" and "affective" strategies and may be categorized as types A and C, respectively. People with type A patterns tend to minimize awareness of negative feelings, compulsively perform what they expect will be reinforced, and avoid doing what will be punished. People with type C patterns rely on feelings as guides to behaviour because they lack confidence in what will happen next. When familial relationships fail to protect the child (or adult parent), type A and type C coping strategies become more extreme. For example, a child reared by an unresponsive caregiver may learn that "acting out" elicits a needed response from the caregiver. As the child grows and becomes an adult, he or she may seek attention by extreme emotional outbursts, acting coercively or aggressively in other adult relationship (type C). Another pattern, type B, is characterized by a tendency to use a balance of type A and type C strategies.

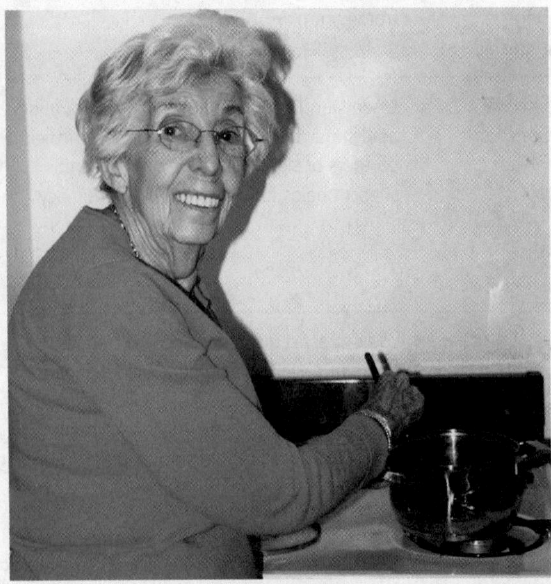

Figure 22-3 Maintaining independence is important to a person's self-esteem.

BOX 22-2 NURSING STORY

Stress and Child Development

Jonathan is 5 years old. His mother has brought him to the pediatrician at the advice of his kindergarten teacher. You are the clinic nurse, charged with taking Jonathan's history. His mother works to organize and seat her three other children (two older, one younger than Jonathan) in the office. She removes their warm winter coats and collects their mittens and hats. She takes a few minutes and, chattering away to each child, locates toys, crayons, paper, crackers, and juice boxes for her children, who each settle in to their activity. However, Jonathan does not settle for long. As you begin your assessment, you observe Jonny, as she calls him, spend a minute or two on one toy before moving on to the next one that intrigues him more. Most of the time, the one that intrigues him is in the hands of a brother or sister. You watch him walk over and remove his newest object of interest (mostly without a fight) from his older or younger sibling. Jonny's siblings appear to be used to his behaviour, and his mother makes no move to correct him. Jonny smiles at you and seems to get along well with his siblings in spite of his rampaging through their toys. He has no interest in the crayons and paper, preferring instead the cars and moving toys. He seems content to chaotically move about in the company of his siblings.

As you proceed through your assessment, you learn that Jonny accomplished typical milestones (walking, talking, toilet training) on time and had a few ear infections but no other physical health problems. His weight and height are normal. He gets along well with the other kids, except for the occasional skirmish over a toy. His mother notes that he does not sit still for very long, except when she has time to read to him alone or when he is watching TV or playing computer games. She has given up on trying to make him sit still in church, leaving him instead in a supervised playroom. But, she says, Jonny loves to be read to and can easily curl up for half an hour easily during storytime. The mother tells you that since her military husband was deployed 3 months ago, she rarely has individual time for each child. She adds that the kids miss their dad but that the older ones grew accustomed to his absences over time. As she begins to talk about Jonny's dad, Jonny climbs into his mother's lap and starts playing a shooting game with a car on the counter. As you switch subjects to talk about kindergarten, Jonny slides to the floor but returns with a book held out to his mother. She says, "Sorry, not now, Jonny," and tells you the teacher's concern about his activity level, inability to hold a pencil properly, and failure to pay attention to learning tasks in class. The mother relays the teacher's concern that he may have attention deficit–hyperactivity disorder. You wonder whether Jonny's activity level has anything to do with his father's deployment and the increased demands on his mother's time. The mother wonders whether medication would help Jonny have an easier time in kindergarten, and she asks you for your opinion.

Nursing Implications of the Dynamic Maturational Model. You need to design approaches that address both the quality of the attachment system and the caregiving system. Crittenden and Claussen (2003) asserted that recognizing clients' attachment strategies is crucial for providing helpful treatments and reducing the risk of inappropriate treatment. For instance, in the situation in which a young child is hospitalized, you would need to consider the security of the child and to provide high-quality substitute care, including making developmentally appropriate efforts to keep the child attached to his or her primary caregiver (e.g., using pictures, phone calls, liberal visiting hours, parent sleepovers). If you are working in mental health care, you need to recognize that clients' apparently maladaptive coping strategies (e.g., obsessive–compulsive disorder, anxiety) may be strategies developed to cope with adverse relationships with attachment figures. Alternatively, in working with parents in impoverished environments, you need to support the caregivers through provision of material, social, and educational resource that will promote safety and security of their children. You need to advocate for appropriate support resources for families in which caregiving may be compromised as a result of stress associated with parental poverty, mental illness, or lack of education (Middlebrooks & Audage, 2008; Mustard, 2006).

Havighurst's Developmental Tasks

Robert Havighurst (1900–1991) was influenced by Erikson's work and observations of the developmental tasks crucial for healthy development. Havighurst defined a series of age-specific essential tasks, such as learning to walk, getting ready to read, learning social and gender roles, developing independence, selecting a mate, rearing children, and, finally, adjusting to decreasing physical strength and health. The essential tasks arise from predictable internal and external pressures, such as increasing physical maturity, cultural pressure of society, and the individual's personal goals and aspirations.

According to **Havighurst's developmental tasks**, several sources of pressure may be present at the same time. Increasing physical maturity is associated with the development of skills such as walking, talking, or eating. Cultural pressure creates the conditions necessary to learn social behaviours and ethical norms. An adolescent girl may be physically able to bear a child, but the preparation and timing for the onset of parenthood can also be considered from a perspective of pressure from both the youth and adult cultures.

Havighurst believed that at certain critical periods, the individual is most receptive to the learning necessary to achieve success in performing these tasks. Effective learning and achievement of tasks during one period lead to happiness and success with later tasks. Failure leads to unhappiness, disapproval by society, and difficulty with later tasks. An example is the struggle that adolescents might experience in preparing for a work career after having failed to develop fundamental skills in reading and math.

Havighurst's theory is limited in its cultural application, according to critics who believe that it describes developmental milestones from the perspective of middle-class norms within the United States. It would be difficult to fit all cultural or ethnic mores within this theoretical framework.

Mechanisms and Nursing Implications of Havighurst's Theory. Havighurst's work built on that of Freud and Erikson. Therefore, the mechanisms and nursing implications from Freud and Erikson also apply to Havighurst's developmental tasks.

Roger Gould

Psychiatrist Roger Gould (ca. 1935–present) reviewed the work of other theorists and found a lack of understanding of how the adult years contributed to the maturing and changing of personality (Gould, 1972). (The major themes of the three most prominent theorists of adulthood personality are compared in Table 22–6.) Gould conducted extensive research that supported a set of development themes within stages of adult development. Gould found that over the adult years, people dismantle the protective thinking developed during childhood. Over a period of years, beliefs are shed, which marks a shift from childhood into adult consciousness.

Gould's development themes start when individuals are in their twenties with the theme "I have to get away from my parents." This theme is challenged in minor ways before the end of high school but culminates as young people begin to live away from home. The move away from parental influence is gradual as young adults establish themselves as adults.

The second theme occurs when individuals reach their early thirties and ask, "Is what I am the only way for me to be?" This question occurs when young adults experience the consequences of the decisions of their independence. Everything does not work out magically as might have been expected. Failures must be overcome. Acceptance for who they are is essential. So, too, is acceptance of their own growing children as being unique and separate.

The third theme occurs when individuals reach their middle to late thirties: "Have I done the right thing? Do I have time to change?" These questions recognize the complexities of adult decisions. The impact of a growing family and aging parents influences this theme. Individuals begin to have a sense of how much time is left to meet desired goals.

The fourth theme, identified in individuals in their forties, "The die is cast," is indicative of resignation and the belief that possibilities are limited. The personality is believed to be set. Changes in career are believed to be less likely to be successful. Parents are blamed for their lack of choices. Mistakes made in raising children are regretted.

During the period when individuals are in their fifties, a decrease in negativism occurs. Gould (1972) found that people at this age generally recognize their mortality and are concerned for their state of health. They have less responsibility for the welfare of the children and experience more attachment to the spouse, as might be expected.

Gould (1972) believed that his research described a sequential process that takes place between the internal life (personality) of adults and their outer world (culture, lifestyle). For example, Gould studied the timing and sequencing of an event, as well as the individual's adjustment and transition into a particular stage. It seemed clear to Gould that events of adulthood may be similar in adults; however, the timing and sequencing affects the adjustment and consequences in different individuals. Marriage, for example, may occur before or after pregnancy, the time interval between the birth of the first and second children may differ, and retirement may occur in one's fifties or sixties.

Mechanisms and Nursing Implications of Gould's Theory. As with Havighurst, Gould's (1972) work built on that of Freud and Erikson. Therefore, the mechanisms and nursing implications from Freud and Erikson also apply to Gould's theory of development.

Mechanistic Tradition

According to the **mechanistic tradition**, the organism is similar to a machine. Development depends on the level of stimulation, the kind of stimulation, and the history of stimulation from the environment. The environment is considered to activate human development (Bornstein & Lamb, 1999), and behaviour is seen as responsive to environmental forces rather than driven only by internal causes such as maturation. Social learning theory follows from this tradition and is presented in Chapter 21.

TABLE 22-6 Developmental Theorists for Adult Stages

Adult Stages	Erikson's Description	Havighurst's Description	Gould's Description
Early-early adult (ages 16–22 years)	Intimacy versus isolation	Early adulthood stage	Theme: "I have to get away from my parents."
Middle-early adult (ages 22–28 years)	Ability to form intimate relationships	Selecting a mate Learning to live with a marriage partner Starting a family Rearing children Getting started in an occupation Taking on civic responsibilities Finding a congenial social group	Gradually establishing control of self as an adult
Late-early adult (ages 28–35 years)			Theme: "Is what I am the only way for me to be?" Demonstrating independent competence while overcoming failures
Early-middle adult (ages 35–45 years)	Generativity versus self-absorption and stagnation Ability to expand personal and social involvement	Middle age Assisting teenage children to become responsible adults Achieving adult social and civic responsibility Reaching and maintaining satisfactory performance in one's occupation Developing adult leisure-time activities Relating to one's spouse as a person Accepting and adjusting to the physiological changes of middle age Adjusting to aging of parents	Themes: "Have I done the right thing?" "Do I have time to change?" Learning to live with ambivalence without need to prove self Beginning sense of limited time to effect desired results
Middle-middle adult (continued) (ages 40–50 years)			Theme: "The die is cast." Believing that possibilities are limited Seeing time as having an end point
Late-middle adult (continued) (50–65 years)			Decreased negativism Increased feelings of self-satisfaction Recognizing own mortality and concern for health
Late adult–old age (age 65 years and older)	Integrity versus despair, disgust Ability to adapt to changes in lifestyle, functional level, and family structure	Later maturity Adjusting to decreasing physical strength and health Adjusting to retirement and reduced income Adjusting to death of a spouse Establishing an affiliation with one's age group Adopting and adapting social roles in a flexible way Satisfactory physical living space	

Contextualism

The way that human development is described and explained is increasingly tied to the understanding of environment and context. Developmental theories within the **contextual tradition** focus on the relationship between the individual and his or her social context. Within this tradition, the individual and the environment are viewed as mutually influential, acting on one another in dynamic interaction (Bornstein & Lamb, 1999). Human development is the process of continuously adapting to changing environments.

Bioecological Theory

Urie Bronfenbrenner (1917–2005), a developmental psychologist at Cornell University, developed a theory that stresses the importance of the interaction between the developing individual and his or her surrounding social environments. **Bronfenbrenner's bioecological theory** involves considering multiple "layers" of the environment:

- The **microsystem** consists of the immediate settings, activities, and personal relationships of the individual. Examples include family, classroom, workplace, and recreation group.

- The **mesosystem** is made up of the relationships between the different settings in which the person spends time. Examples include relationships between families and schools, between workplaces and schools, and between families and spiritual organizations (church parish, mosque, temple), and spiritual organizations and schools.
- The **exosystem** is a set of specific social structures that do not directly contain the individual but exert direct and indirect influence on individual development. Examples include the health care system, the education system, the justice system, and religious institutions.
- The **macrosystem** consists of all of the elements contained in the individual's microsystem, mesosystem, and exosystem, as well as the general underlying philosophy, cultural orientation, and values by which the person lives (Salkind, 2004). Examples include overarching dimensions such as political orientation, economic model, and cultural values.

Mechanisms of the Bioecological Theory. Lev Semenovich Vygotsky (1896–1934) introduced a concept called the **zone of proximal development**, which is the key developmental mechanism of ecological theories. This zone is the space between the individual's potential and his or her actual developmental status. For instance, a toddler may have a 10-word vocabulary but potentially could have a repertoire of hundreds of words. Activity that links those two states promotes development. For instance, parents who use joint referencing (looking at things that their toddlers are looking at and naming them) promote toddler vocabulary development within the zone of proximal development.

Bronfenbrenner's modern conception of developmental processes expands upon Vygotsky's idea of the zone of proximal development. In language acquisition, developmental support processes occur in all levels of the system. At the macrosystem level, a process that would support language development in young children would be the adoption of a national child care policy to support working parents. Such a policy would inform regulations concerning issues such as education level of child care workers, ratio of children to worker in child care centres, and space requirements per child.

Nursing Implications of the Bioecological Theory. An appropriate goal of nursing practice is to influence wellness by promoting health in all layers of the bioecological system. The ecological model applies to nursing practice beyond the individual level of health promotion to higher levels of the social context. Therefore, Bronfenbrenner's theory fits well with current emphasis on primary health care (Box 22–3).

Dialecticism

In the **dialectic tradition**, all developmental theories are considered mutually interactive. Developmental theorists are increasingly proposing that change or development can occur within the framework of multiple theories. A key element of the dialectic tradition is the ability to incorporate multiple contexts. An example of a dialectic approach from the biomedical sciences is the theory of gene expression. The theory of gene expression links genetics, the environment, and their influences on human behaviour and disease. In the human development disciplines, examples of dialectical thinking include the growing awareness of the effect of the economic environment on human development at the population level. Resilience theory is an approach in which the interaction between two processes, previously studied separately, is examined.

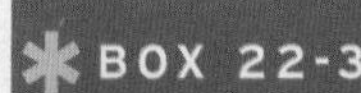

BOX 22-3 FOCUS ON PRIMARY HEALTH CARE

Bronfenbrenner's Ecological Theory and Primary Health Care

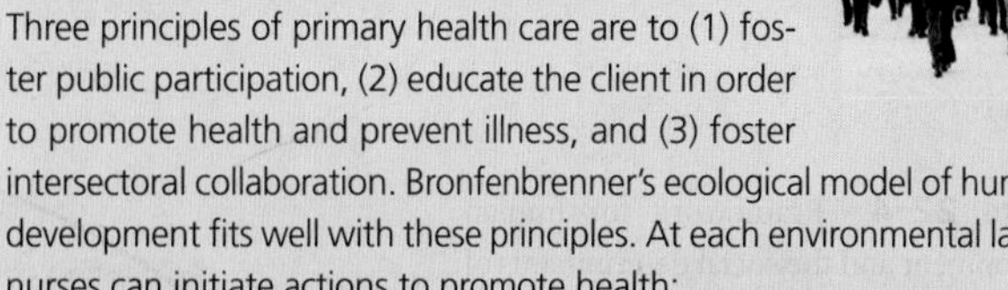

Three principles of primary health care are to (1) foster public participation, (2) educate the client in order to promote health and prevent illness, and (3) foster intersectoral collaboration. Bronfenbrenner's ecological model of human development fits well with these principles. At each environmental layer, nurses can initiate actions to promote health:

- *Microsystem,* which includes the individual and his or her immediate setting (e.g., family, school, workplace, neighbourhood). You can help the individual develop personal skills, healthy lifestyles and activities, and supportive environments. For example, you can help teach family members caring for an elderly parent how to balance family care and self-care to keep themselves healthy.
- *Mesosystem,* which consists of relations among the individual's various immediate settings. To strengthen the mesosystem, you can work toward strengthening community action. You can link the family to community supports such as adult respite services and older adults' activities groups.
- *Exosystem,* which comprises relations among structures, sectors, services, and policies. The exosystem is strengthened when nurses promote healthy public policy. You are practising at this level when you help develop links between typically separate services such as the health care system and the social service system. For example, you can volunteer to be on planning committees and other decision-making bodies.
- *Macrosystem,* which consists of societal values. To promote optimum health at the macrosystem level, the nurse can be an advocate for social change. For example, if you believe that more value should be placed on older adults in society, you may advocate for higher standards and staff-to-resident ratios in long-term care facilities. Such advocacy might include writing letters to the editor, joining community or national advocacy groups, and lobbying politicians.

Keating and Hertzman's Population Health Theory

Human development has historically been considered an individual characteristic. According to Daniel P. Keating (1949–present) and Clyde Hertzman's (1953–present) (1999) **population health approach,** human development is a population phenomenon. These Canadian developmental theorists referred to the strong association between the health of a population, developmental outcomes, and the social and economic forces affecting the larger society. They based their developmental theory on epidemiological evidence that improved literacy (one marker of human development) is related to improvements in family economic status, in school community economic status, and in national economic status.

Keating and Hertzman (1999) proposed that health, behaviour, and cognitive functions are largely set in early life and are then influenced further by succeeding events in the socioeconomic environment. **Developmental health** is defined as the physical and mental health, well-being, coping, and competence of human populations. Developmental health is primarily a function of the overall quality of the social environment, including the national socioeconomic environment, civil society, and social network. Keating and Hertzman's population approach to human development is outlined in Figure 22–4.

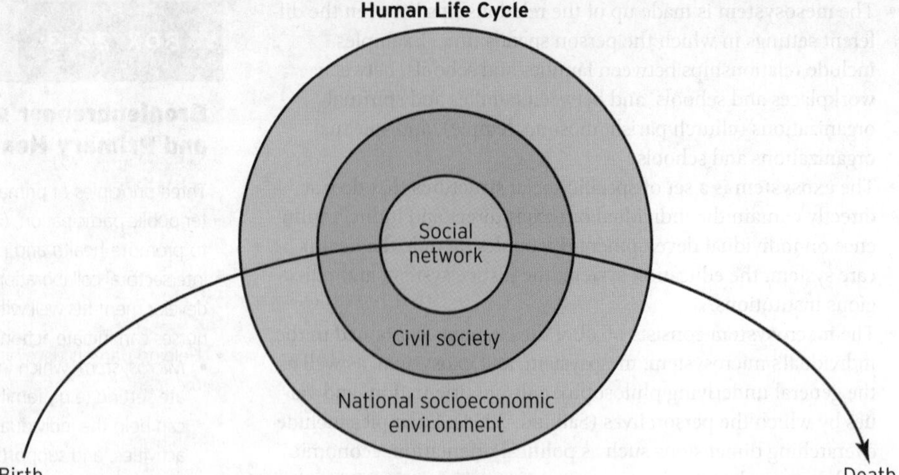

Figure 22-4 Framework for human development and the social determinants of health. **Source:** Redrawn from Keating, D. P., & Hertzman, C. (Eds.). (1999). *Developmental health and the wealth of nations: Social, biological and educational dynamics* (p. 30). New York: Guilford Press.

Mechanisms of the Population Health Theory. Keating and Hertzman (1999) proposed three interrelated regulatory systems as the mechanisms for human population development: emotional regulation, attention regulation, and social regulation. Each regulatory system develops in interaction between the individual's biological processes and his or her multiple socioeconomic environments. *Emotional regulation,* which involves the modulation of emotional reactions, plays an important role in competent social functioning. *Attention regulation,* which involves regulation of arousal and reactivity of the brain, contributes to the ability to pursue goals and respond to challenges to those goals. *Social regulation* involves regulation of social interactions, including aspects such as mutual affection and warmth, particularly in nurturing relationships. Together, these three regulatory systems are thought to influence later competence as individuals interact reciprocally with their socioeconomic environments.

Nursing Implications of the Population Health Theory. Nurses have typically focused on the health and well-being of clients. To promote well-being, health professionals need to implement practices that take into account the impact of the socioeconomic context on the health of the individuals in society. The ecological levels of health promotion activities are directly applicable to the population health approach (see Box 22–2). A population health approach helps identify these socioeconomic factors and provides direction for designing nursing interventions that address them.

Resilience Theory

Resilience is defined as the maintenance of positive adjustment under challenging life conditions (Cicchetti & Curtis, 2007). This approach arose in the field of child psychiatry when clinicians observed that some children and adolescents were able to thrive in severely adverse conditions (e.g., poverty, maternal depression, and paternal criminality), whereas others faltered.

Mechanisms of Resilience. Resilience theory focuses on the interaction between protective processes and vulnerability processes. **Vulnerability processes** (physical illness, psychological stresses, social risk) and **protective processes** (self-efficacy, good parenting and problem solving, social support acquisition and maintenance) are examined together to understand and explain human growth and development. Individual factors found to promote resilience include self-efficacy, positive attitude, literacy, social competence, and a history of success. Family-level processes that protect from adversity include coherent response to crisis, social supports, stability, flexibility, effective parenting, and responsibilities outside the home (Drummond et al., 1996–1997). Community-level processes that promote resilience include control over policy, collaborative and cooperative organization, widespread citizen participation in community, and volunteerism.

Resilience and family adaptation theory has been used to design interventions to support children and families at risk, focusing on protective processes within the context of key risk situations, usually defined by factors such as poverty, chronic illness, and civil conflict. This emphasis is a progression from the previous emphasis on only pathological processes, but the challenge is to design research that enables scholars to study both protective processes and vulnerability processes as they occur together.

Nursing Implications of Resilience. The focus of nursing practice is directly on the individual, family, and community factors that promote health. Nursing practice is usually used in situations that are stressful and challenging for individuals and families, such as illness and loss. Resilience theorists acknowledge the complexity of these moments and ask what nurses can use from these challenging situations that help the family succeed (Box 22–4). For example, a young single woman dealing with the birth of her first child will benefit from nursing interventions that focus both on protective processes (linking to support group, learning parenting skills) and on vulnerability processes (ensuring adequate health care, arranging for financial support).

Developmental Theories and Nursing

The diverse set of theories included in this chapter suggest that human behaviour is truly complex. No single theory successfully describes human growth and development in all of its complexity. Theorists demonstrate their own values and beliefs in their focus and the subjects chosen for their work, and they work within cultural and historical perspectives. The theories described in this chapter are meant to provide the basis for meaningful thought and observation of an individual's pattern of growth and development and the role of

BOX 22-4 RESEARCH HIGHLIGHT

Supporting Parents: Can Intervention Improve Parent–Child Relationships?

Research Focus

Healthy child development has been identified as one of the key determinants of health and resiliency in adulthood. In two studies reported by Letourneau et al. (2001), researchers examined interventions aimed at improving the parent–child relationship and enhancing resiliency among children considered to be at risk because of poverty or parents' young age, inexperience, or lack of education.

Research Abstract

These two pilot studies were randomized control trials designed to test the effects of two support interventions. In the first intervention, Keys to Caregiving, a family-centred approach, was used to provide parents with tools necessary for high-quality interactions with their infants. A post-test experimental design was used to study 16 adolescent mothers and their infants. The second intervention, Natural Teaching Strategies, focused on developing mutually satisfying methods for parents to communicate with their preschoolers. A pretest–post-test design was used to study 29 families of children enrolled in Head Start programs. In both groups, parent–child interactions were enhanced in the treatment groups. Results of both interventions revealed the potential effect of supportive intervention on parent–child interactions over time.

Evidence-Informed Practice

- Helping parents develop realistic expectations of their child's development and improving the quality of parent–child relationships are important support mechanisms for families at risk.
- Parent training and support has the potential to positively alter the style of interactions between parents and children.

References: Letourneau, N., Drummond, J., Fleming, D., Kysela, G., McDonald, L., & Stewart, M. (2001). Supporting parents: Can intervention improve parent–child relationships? *Journal of Family Nursing, 7*(2), 159–187.

environments in it. This observation and reflection provide you with a framework within which you can predict human responses to health and illness and recognize deviations from the norm.

Patterns of growth and development help determine future patterns of adjustment to life (Edelman & Mandle, 2006). A clear understanding of these patterns and of the contexts within which they occur assists you in planning questions for health screening and health history and in health teaching for clients of all ages. You need to consider an individual's development within the context of his or her families, social relationships, communities, and the larger society.

Developmental theories help you use critical thinking skills when you consider how and why people respond as they do. Your assessment of a client requires a thorough analysis and interpretation of data to form accurate conclusions about a client's developmental needs. To accurately identify clients' needs, you need the ability to consider developmental theory in data analysis. Typical developmental behaviours are compared with those projected by the developmental theory.

KEY CONCEPTS

- Nurses provide care for individuals and families throughout their lives. Developmental theories provide a basis for nurses to assess, interpret, and understand the responses seen in their clients.
- Development continues throughout life.
- Individuals have unique patterns of growth and development within broad limits.
- Development is not just a series of distinct linear tasks; it is also a process that varies across and within individuals (Hartup, 2002).
- Three major categories of factors influence human growth and development: (1) genetic or natural forces within the person, (2) the environment in which the person lives, and (3) the interaction that takes place between these two.
- Theories within the organic tradition explore how individuals develop when mostly biological components are believed to stimulate developmental progress.
- Theories in the psychoanalytic and psychosocial tradition describe development of the human personality with regard to conflict resolution between the internal biological forces and the external societal and cultural forces.
- According to the mechanistic approach, human development and behaviour are responses to environmental forces rather than driven by internal causes such as maturation.
- Within the contextual tradition, the individual and the environment are viewed as mutually influential, acting on one another in dynamic interaction.
- In the dialectical tradition, the complete complexity of development is acknowledged. Theorists who work in this tradition strive to combine divergent ways of viewing human development.

CRITICAL THINKING EXERCISES

1. A 50-year-old woman is anxious because her children, 20 and 23 years of age, are no longer living at home. Her husband is still working full time but planning to retire in two years. She is concerned that she is not needed, and she is bored with her life. Identify the developmental task of Erickson's theory that best fits this woman's situation. How will you assist this client in changing her lifestyle while understanding her developmental tasks?
2. A public health nurse conducting a routine assessment of an 18-month-old is concerned about the child's being underweight for his age. Upon further discussion, the father reveals that he is not working at present and the family is having financial troubles. Using your knowledge of Bronfenbrenner's bioecological theory, what approach and subsequent strategies would be helpful for these parents?
3. Two 11-year-old girls are spending the day together at the mall. They exit one store, and one of the girls shows her friend a small purse that she stole from the store. Her friend is upset and wonders how she should respond. Use moral development theory to discuss this issue.
4. A women visits her nurse practitioner at her local health clinic. The women is struggling with depression and seeking to increase her medication dosage. She also reveals that she is struggling to cope with her 8-year-old son's problem behaviours, such as refusing to do homework and having tantrums when he fails to get his way. Using the dynamic maturational model of attachment, discuss how her mental health state could be influencing her child's behaviour.

✻ REVIEW QUESTIONS

1. Children generally double their birth weight by 5 months of age. This is an example of
   1. Development
   2. Heredity
   3. State of health
   4. Physical growth

2. ________ development is the ability of an individual to distinguish right from wrong and to develop ethical values on which to base his or her actions.
   1. Moral
   2. Cognitive
   3. Psychosocial
   4. Psychoanalytic

3. Theories in the ________ tradition hold that development is a result of biology and adaptation.
   1. Organicism
   2. Psychoanalytic and psychosocial
   3. Contexualism
   4. Dialecticism

4. Which of the following factors is considered an environmental factor that affects human development:
   1. Family
   2. Heredity
   3. State of health
   4. Genetics

5. The developmental theorist who believed his research described a sequential process that resolved conflict between the internal life (personality) of adults and their outer world (culture) was
   1. Erickson
   2. Crittenden
   3. Freud
   4. Gould

6. "The die is cast" is consistent with Gould's theme for the
   1. Thirties
   2. Forties
   3. Fifties
   4. Seventies

7. According to Piaget's theory of cognitive development, during what stage does the individual's moral thinking move to abstract and theoretical subjects, such as achieving world peace, finding justice, and seeking meaning in life?
   1. Formal operations
   2. Concrete operations
   3. Sensorimotor
   4. Preoperational

8. The nurse who is working with a school committee to develop playground safety guidelines is focusing on which level of the bioecological model?
   1. Mesosystem
   2. Microsystem
   3. Exosystem
   4. Macrosystem

9. Which of the following nursing interventions is representative of a population health approach?
   1. Parent teaching
   2. Developing a clinical practice guideline
   3. Participating in a community coalition to improve community housing
   4. Assisting an individual in obtaining funding support for home care

10. A resilient individual is able to experience positive development despite challenging life circumstances. For a young single mother with two young children, access to high-quality day care represents the following:
    1. A vulnerability process
    2. A critical period
    3. Attachment
    4. A protective process

✻ RECOMMENDED WEB SITES

Canadian Institute of Child Health: http://www.cich.ca

The Canadian Institute of Child Health (CICH) is dedicated to improving the health of children and youth in Canada. Activities range from research and policy recommendations to community development and resource building. CICH focuses on four key areas of activity: supporting healthy pregnancy and childbirth, fostering healthy child development, ensuring that the environment is safe for children, and monitoring the state of children's health.

Centre of Excellence for Early Childhood Development: http://www.excellence-jeunesenfants.ca/home.asp?lang=EN

The mandate of the Centre of Excellence for Early Childhood Development (CEECD) is to foster the dissemination of scientific knowledge about the social and emotional development of young children and about the policies and services that influence this development. The CEECD also formulates recommendations for the services needed to ensure optimum early childhood development. This page of the CEECD Web site lists a variety of issues and behaviours common to children younger than 5 years, with links to articles on the subjects written by leading researchers in the field.

Centre for Health Promotion (CHP): http://www.phac-aspc.gc.ca/chhd-sdsh/index-eng.php

The CHP uses a life stages approach and is responsible for implementing policies and programs that enhance the conditions conducive to healthy development. The CHP addresses the determinants of health and facilitates successful movement through the life stages. The CHP acts through programs addressing healthy child development, families, aging and lifestyles, public information, and education (Canadian Health Network), as well as on issues related to rural health and support of the voluntary sector.

Nursing Child Assessment Satellite Training (NCAST): http://www.ncast.org/

Based in the University of Washington, this organization aims to give professionals, parents, and other caregivers the knowledge and skills to provide nurturing environments for young children. NCAST disseminates and develops research-informed products and training programs for practitioners and researchers in many disciplines and settings, which can be used with typically developing children, with those at risk for developmental delays, and with those in whom special health care needs have been identified.

23

Conception Through Adolescence

Original chapter by Karen Balakas, RN, PhD, CNE

Canadian content written by Shirley M. Solberg, RN, PhD

objectives

Mastery of content in this chapter will enable you to:

- Define the key terms listed.
- Discuss physiological and psychosocial health concerns during the transition of the child from intrauterine to extrauterine life.
- Describe characteristics of physical growth of the fetus and of the child from birth to adolescence.
- Describe cognitive and psychosocial development from birth to adolescence.
- Describe the interactions that occur between parent and child.
- Explain the role of play in the development of the child.
- Identify factors that contribute to self-esteem in youth.
- Describe the influence of the school environment on the development of the child.
- Plan culturally appropriate health promotion activities for children of all backgrounds.
- Discuss ways in which you can help parents meet their children's developmental needs.

key terms

Adolescence, p. 353
Animism, p. 346
Apgar score, p. 331
Artificialism, p. 346
Blastocyst, p. 330
Bonding, p. 331
Classification, p. 350
Concrete operations, p. 350
Differentiation, p. 331
Embryo, p. 330
Estrogen, p. 354
Fertilization, p. 330
Fetus, p. 331
Fontanels, p. 333
Formal operations, p. 356
Hyperbilirubinemia, p. 335
Immanent justice, p. 346
Implantation, p. 330
Inborn errors of metabolism, p. 335
Infancy, p. 335
Lanugo, p. 331
Menarche, p. 356
Molding, p. 333
Morula, p. 330
Nagele's rule, p. 330
Neonatal period, p. 330
Object permanence, p. 343
Organogenesis, p. 331
Placenta, p. 330
Prematurity, p. 334
Preoperational thought, p. 343
Preschool period, p. 346
Preterm labour, p. 332
Puberty, p. 349
Quickening, p. 331
School-age, p. 347
Sensorimotor period, p. 335
Sexually transmitted infections (STIs), p. 359
Teratogens, p. 332
Testosterone, p. 354
Toddlerhood, p. 340
Vernix caseosa, p. 331
Zygote, p. 330

media resources

evolve Web Site

- Audio Chapter Summaries
- Glossary
- Multiple-Choice Review Questions
- Student Learning Activities
- Weblinks

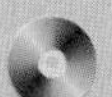

Companion CD

- Glossary
- Interactive Learning Activities
- Fluids and Electrolytes Tutorial
- Test-Taking Skills

Human growth and development are continuous, intricate, complex processes that are divided into stages organized by age groups. This arbitrary, chronological division is used because it coincides with the timing and sequence of maturational changes that allows children to progress through a series of developmental stages and associated tasks (Box 23–1). This chapter focuses on the various physical, psychosocial, and cognitive changes. It also focuses on health risks and concerns during the various stages of growth and development. Major developmental theories are discussed in Chapter 22.

Selecting a Developmental Framework for Nursing

Providing developmentally appropriate nursing care is easier when the care plan is based on a theoretical framework (see Chapter 22). An organized, systematic approach ensures that children's needs are assessed and met by the care plan. In a developmental approach, organized care is directed at an individual child's current level of functioning to motivate self-direction and health promotion; for example, you might instruct parents to encourage toddlers to feed themselves in order to advance their developing independence and thus promote their sense of autonomy. Understanding an adolescent's need to be independent should prompt you to negotiate with the adolescent to establish a contract about the care plan and its implementation. All care must be planned so that it is culturally safe (see Chapter 10), ethical and legal (see Chapters 8 and 9), and informed by the best evidence available (see Chapter 7).

Conception

From the moment of conception, human growth proceeds at a predictable and rapid rate. During the prenatal period, the embryo grows from a single cell to a complex, physiological being. All major organ systems develop in utero, and most function before birth.

Intrauterine Life

Intrauterine life that reaches full term usually lasts approximately 9 calendar months, or 40 weeks. The length of pregnancy is computed according to **Nagele's rule**, in which you count back 3 months from the first day of the pregnant woman's last menstrual period and then add 7 days. **Fertilization** occurs when a sperm penetrates the ovum and the material from both cell nuclei unites. The newly formed organism, known as a **zygote**, has its full genetic complement (1 pair of sex chromosomes and 22 pairs of autosomal chromosomes). The ovum and the sperm each contribute one chromosome to each pair. Through this mechanism. genetically determined characteristics (such as eye colour) are transmitted from parent to child and genetic conditions (such as Down's syndrome) can result.

The zygote moves through the fallopian tube to the uterus within 3 to 4 days. During this time, the zygote continues to divide. Within 3 days, a solid ball of cells, the **morula**, has formed. The morula continues to develop and forms a central cavity, or **blastocyst**. Even at this early stage of development, cells begin to differentiate in structure and function. Cells at one end of the blastocyst develop into the **embryo**, and those at the opposite end form the **placenta**. Between days 6 and 10, some of the cells secrete enzymes that allow the blastocyst to burrow into the endometrium and become completely covered; this process is known as **implantation**. Chorionic villi—fingerlike projections that emerge from the outer sac surrounding the embryo—obtain oxygen and nutrition from the maternal blood supply and dispose of carbon dioxide and waste products.

➤ BOX 23-1 Developmental Age Periods

Prenatal Period: Conception to Birth

Germinal: Conception to approximately 2 weeks
Embryonic: 2 to 8 weeks
Fetal: 8 to 40 weeks (birth)

Because of rapid growth rate and total dependency, this is one of the most mutable and vulnerable periods in the developmental process. The relationship between maternal health and certain manifestations of normalities and abnormalities in the newborn emphasizes the importance of adequate prenatal care to the health and well-being of the infant.

Infancy Period: Birth to Approximately 12 to 18 Months

Neonatal: Birth to 28 days
Infancy: 1 to approximately 12 to 18 months

The infancy period is one of rapid motor, cognitive, and social development. Through bonding with the parent or other caregiver, the infant establishes a basic trust in the world and the foundation for future interpersonal relationships. The critical first month of life, termed the **neonatal period,** although part of infancy, is often differentiated from the remainder of infancy because it is characterized by major physical adjustments to extrauterine existence and by the psychosocial adjustment of the parents to their new roles.

Early Childhood: 1 to 6 Years

Toddler: 1 to 3 years
Preschooler: 3 to 6 years

This period, which extends from the time children begin walking until school entry, is characterized by intense activity and discovery. It is a time of marked physical and psychosocial development. Motor development advances steadily. Children at this age acquire language and wider social relationships, learn role standards, gain self-control and skill mastery, develop increasing awareness of dependence and independence, and begin to develop a self-concept.

Middle Childhood: 6 to 12 Years

Frequently referred to as the *school age,* this period of development is one in which children expand relationships outside the family group and activities revolve around peer relationships. Physical, cognitive, and psychosocial development advance steadily, with emphasis on developing skill competencies. Social cooperation and early moral development take on more importance, with relevance for later life stages. This is a critical period in the development of a self-concept.

Adolescence: 12 to Approximately 19 Years

The period of rapid maturation and change known as adolescence is considered to be a transitional period that begins at the onset of puberty and extends to the point of entry into the adult world—in Canada, usually high school graduation. Biological and psychological maturation are accompanied by physical changes and emotional turmoil, and the self-concept is redefined. In the late adolescent period, children begin to internalize all previously learned values and to focus on an individual, rather than a group, identity.

Adapted from Hockenberry, M. J., & Wilson, D. (2007). *Wong's nursing care of infants and children* (8th ed.). St. Louis, MO: Mosby.

The placenta produces essential hormones that maintain the pregnancy. It also provides nutrients to the developing fetus and removes wastes. Because the placenta is porous, noxious materials such as viruses and drugs can pass from mother to child. The effect of noxious agents on the fetus depends on the developmental stage in which exposure takes place; the embryonic stage (2 to 8 weeks after conception) is critical because the organ systems and the main external features are developing. The period of gestation is divided equally into three periods called *trimesters*.

First Trimester. During the first trimester, the first 3 calendar months, fetal cells continue to differentiate and develop into essential organ systems. As cellular change (**differentiation**) and rapid organ growth (**organogenesis**) occur, each organ is vulnerable to conditions in the environment. Interference with growth can cause the congenital absence of an organ system or extensive structural or functional alterations. Because several organ systems develop at the same time, disruption of one system often occurs with disruption of others. Toward the end of the first trimester, it is possible to detect fetal heart tones by fetoscopy or ultrasonography.

Second Trimester. During the second trimester, from the end of the third month to the end of the sixth month, the height of the mother's uterus above the symphysis pubis is an indicator of fetal growth and approximate gestational age. Between 16 and 20 weeks, the mother begins to feel fetal movement. This feeling of life is referred to as **quickening**.

By the end of the sixth month, most of the fetal organ systems are complete and can function. The **fetus** is therefore considered viable, or capable of life outside the uterus, if given intensive environmental support. Fingers and toes are differentiated, rudimentary kidneys function, and the genitalia are defined. The fetus is covered with **vernix caseosa**, a cheeselike substance coating the skin. **Lanugo**, or fine hair, covers most of the body. These substances protect the thin, fragile skin and decrease in amount as the pregnancy nears its completion; thus, infants born before 38 weeks' gestation have more of these protective coverings than do full-term infants.

Third Trimester. During the last 3 months of gestation, the fetus grows to approximately 50 cm in length. Subcutaneous fat is stored, and weight increases to between 3.2 and 3.4 kg. The skin thickens, lanugo begins to disappear, and the fetal body becomes rounder and fuller.

A tremendous spurt in brain growth begins during this trimester and lasts well into the first few years of life. The central nervous system has established its total number of neurons and connections between neurons, and myelination of nerve fibres progresses at a rapid rate.

At the end of the third trimester, the normal fetus is physically able to make the transition from intrauterine to extrauterine life. The circulatory system, which bypasses the right side of the heart (which, in turn, supplies the lungs with oxygen), can change its circulation to include the lungs. The lungs are capable of maintaining the inflated state for gas exchange. The primitive temperature maintenance systems, reflexes, and sensory organs are ready for use.

Health Promotion

You can address many topics with a pregnant client in order to protect her health and that of the fetus. Topics may vary, depending on the stage of pregnancy. Box 23–2 lists some of the many topics that you can address with pregnant women and their partners. You can make a significant difference in supporting the functions of young families. After an assessment of the couple's strengths and weaknesses, you can direct parents to available services to enhance their coping skills (Petch & Halford, 2008).

Transition from Intrauterine to Extrauterine Life

The transition from intrauterine to extrauterine life requires rapid changes in the newborn. You need to assess the newborn's ability to make these changes, and you should begin to plan before the birth for appropriate nursing interventions (Murray & McKinney, 2006). Circulatory, pulmonary, and thermal changes all contribute to the infant's adaptation to neonatal life. Gestational age and development, exposure to depressant drugs before or during labour, and the newborn's own behavioural style also influence the adjustment to the external environment. Therefore, initial assessment encompasses a variety of physical and psychosocial elements. You can also provide early opportunities for the parents and infant to develop close emotional bonds.

Physical Changes

The most extreme physiological change occurs when the newborn leaves the in utero circulation and assumes independent respiratory functioning. Nursing care is directed at maintaining an open airway, stabilizing and maintaining body temperature, and protecting the newborn from infection. The most widely used assessment tool is the **Apgar score**, in which heart rate, respiratory effort, muscle tone, reflex irritability, and colour are rated in order to determine overall status. The Apgar assessment is generally conducted at 1 and 5 minutes after birth and may be repeated until the newborn's condition stabilizes. Table 23–1 outlines the scoring criteria of physiological functioning. A total score of 0 to 3 signifies severe distress, a score of 4 to 6 represents moderate difficulty, and a score of 7 to 10 indicates little difficulty in adjusting to extrauterine life. You can use the Apgar score to determine areas requiring further assessment and careful observation. In addition, you need to monitor and record the newborn's early elimination patterns (i.e., voiding and passage of meconium), as well as body temperature and other vital signs.

Psychosocial Changes

After conducting a physical evaluation and applying identification bracelets, promote the parents' and newborn's need for close physical contact. Early parent–child interaction encourages parent–child attachment or bonding. Physical factors (e.g., fatigue, hunger, and health) and emotional factors (e.g., needs for affection and for touch) are assessed.

Merely placing the family together does not promote closeness. The parents and newborn must be willing and able to respond to each other. Most healthy newborns are awake and alert for the first half-hour after birth. This is a good time for parent–child interaction to begin. Close body contact, often including skin-to-skin contact and breastfeeding, is a satisfying way for most families to start. If immediate contact is not possible, incorporate it into the care plan as early as possible, which may mean bringing the newborn to an ill parent or bringing the parents to an ill or premature child.

Bonding occurs when parents and newborn elicit reciprocal and complementary behaviour. Parental bonding behaviours include attentiveness and physical contact. Newborn bonding behaviour involves maintenance of physical contact with the parent. Preterm newborns, ill newborns, and ill mothers may have difficulty forming this bond if separation is prolonged; they need to be carefully assessed for any problems with attachment. The bonding process is further complicated if parents are unable to care for the infant. You should give the parents support throughout the early bonding process, particularly if the newborn or mother is ill or if the newborn is separated from the parents.

BOX 23-2 FOCUS ON PRIMARY HEALTH CARE

Health Promotion Topics for the Pregnant Client

First Trimester Health Concerns

Nutrition

Mothers with good nutritional practices have fewer complications of pregnancy and childbirth and bear healthier babies than do mothers with poor nutritional intake (Murray & McKinney, 2006). Inadequate prenatal nutrition has been associated with lower birth weight (Health Canada, 1999), and infants with low birth weight have an increased risk for learning disorders, temperament problems, neurological and motor impairment, and developmental delays. Folic acid (vitamin B_9) intake must be adequate before and during pregnancy; the recommended daily dose is 0.4 mg. Mothers should eat foods rich in folic acid, such as green leafy vegetables, liver, kidney, and asparagus. Folic acid intake is believed to be responsible for decreasing the incidence of neural tube defects (Health Canada, 2001). See Chapter 43 for a fuller description of the nutritional needs of the pregnant woman.

Teratogens

Agents capable of producing functional or structural damage to the developing fetus are called **teratogens.** You need to educate the mother about avoiding exposure to teratogenic agents. One such teratogen is the rubella virus, which can cause stillbirth or congenital anomalies, primarily when exposure occurs in the first trimester. Many drugs are teratogenic during the first trimester. You should assess the mother's past and current use of home remedies, medications (prescription and over-the-counter), and illegal drugs. The benefits of any drug needed to maintain the mother's health must be weighed against potential harm to the fetus.

Cigarette smoke and alcohol are also teratogens. Smoking during pregnancy has been shown to reduce birth weight and increase the incidences of premature birth, fetal death, and neonatal death (Murray & McKinney, 2006). It is also considered a risk factor for impaired growth and development among young children (Santock, 2007). Alcohol consumed during pregnancy is known to cause fetal alcohol syndrome, fetal alcohol effect, and alcohol-related birth defects. Pregnant women must be educated about the risks of cigarette smoke and alcohol on the fetus.

Second Trimester Health Concerns

Preterm Labour

Preterm labour is labour that begins before the 37th week of pregnancy. With technological advances, it is possible for 500-g babies of 24 to 26 weeks' gestation to survive; however, the risk of morbidity and disability is significant. Causes of preterm labour are poorly understood and may be the result of maternal or fetal problems. Maternal risk factors include physiological stresses such as renal and cardiovascular disease, diabetes mellitus, and uterine and cervical abnormalities. Urinary tract infections greatly increase the risk of preterm labour. Because of dramatic changes occurring in the maternal renal system, it is possible for a mother to have an asymptomatic urinary tract infection. Voiding habits should be discussed with the mother during this time. Mothers living in poverty, smokers, and mothers receiving poor prenatal care are at higher risk for preterm labour (Behrman et al., 2008). The presence of multiple fetuses and fetal infections are two of the potential fetal factors for preterm labour. Interventions to prevent preterm labour include medications, intravenous fluids, and bed rest.

Third Trimester Health Concerns

Choices of Birth Setting

In Canada, childbirth was gradually moved into hospital settings, starting in the early 1920s, and by 1950, approximately 76% of births occurred in hospitals (Mitchinson, 2002) because emergency backup was available in case of birth complications. Many hospitals have taken a family-centred approach to childbirth.

In some areas of the country, birthing centres are available for mothers who prefer a more homelike setting. Women delivering in this setting are required to attend childbirth classes, and the pregnancy must be considered low risk. Physicians and midwives with hospital privileges may attend births in these facilities. Mothers must understand that they may be transferred to a hospital if the conditions warrant.

A growing number of mothers choose to deliver at home when professional midwifery services are available. Control over the birth process and the desire for a more natural birth are common reasons why some mothers choose home births. Another reason is so that the entire family or other people close to the family can be part of the birth. You can support the mother by offering information and resources to help her choose the birth setting.

Health Risks

The removal of nasopharyngeal and oropharyngeal secretions with suction or a bulb syringe ensures airway patency. Newborns are susceptible to heat loss and cold stress (Behrman et al., 2008). Because hypothermia increases oxygen needs, the newborn's body temperature must be stabilized and maintained. The newborn may be placed directly on the mother's abdomen and covered in warm blankets; dried and wrapped in warm blankets, with the head well covered; or placed unclothed in an infant warmer with a temperature probe in place. For newborns unable to sustain adequate body temperature, isolettes and incubators, which supply radiant heat, are preferred.

Prevention of infection is a major concern in the care of the newborn, whose immune system is immature. Good hand-washing technique is the most important factor in protecting the newborn and yourself from infection. Once the blood and amniotic fluid have been removed from the infant's skin, you do not need to wear cover gowns while you provide care for the healthy newborn (Hockenberry & Wilson, 2007). Other precautions include wearing gloves when touching mucous membranes or skin that is not intact (e.g., as a result of surgery or injury) and when drawing blood (e.g., heel stick).

The most commonly used prophylactic treatment against ophthalmic conjunctivitis is erythromycin (0.5%) because it prevents infections with *Neisseria gonorrhoeae* and other organisms, which can be transmitted during passage through an infected vaginal canal. This treatment should be applied during the newborn's initial assessment.

Vitamin K is administered in a single intramuscular injection shortly after birth. Vitamin K is important for the synthesis of prothrombin necessary for clotting. Normally, the intestinal flora synthesizes vitamin K, and by about the third day, the infant should have enough intestinal flora to start to synthesize its vitamin K.

The stump of the moist umbilical cord is an excellent medium for bacterial growth. The cord should be cleansed with soap and water and dried at each diaper change. Until the stump dries and falls off, the diaper should be folded below the umbilicus to prevent accumulation of moisture.

TABLE 23-1 Apgar Scoring

Sign	Score 0	Score 1	Score 2
Heart rate	Absent	Slow, <100 bpm	>100 bpm
Respiratory effort	Absent	Irregular, slow, weak cry	Strong cry
Muscle tone	Limp	Some flexion of extremities	Strong flexion of extremities
Reflex irritability	No response	Grimace	Cry, sneeze
Colour	Blue, pale	Body pink, extremities blue	Completely pink

Adapted from Hockenberry, M. J., & Wilson, D. (2007). *Wong's nursing care of infants and children* (8th ed., p. 261). St. Louis, MO: Mosby.

Newborn

The neonatal period is the first month of life. During this stage, the newborn's physical functioning is mostly reflexive, and stabilization of major organ systems is the body's primary task. Behaviour greatly influences interaction between the newborn and the environment and caregivers. For example, the average 2-week-old newborn may smile and is able to regard the mother's face. The effect of these reflexive behaviours is generally a surge of feelings of love that prompt the mother to cuddle the baby.

You can apply your knowledge of this stage of growth and development to promote neonatal and parental health. If you understand, for example, that the newborn's cry is usually a response to an unmet need (such as hunger), you can assist parents in identifying ways to meet those needs, such as counselling the parents to feed their baby on demand rather than on a rigid schedule.

Physical Changes

A comprehensive nursing assessment is usually performed as soon as the newborn's physiological functioning is stable, generally within a few hours after birth. Measure the infant's height, weight, head circumference, temperature, pulse, and respirations, and observe general appearance, body functions, sensory capabilities, reflexes, and responsiveness.

The average newborn weighs 3400 g, is 50 cm in length, and has a head circumference of 35 cm. Up to 10% of birth weight is lost in the first few days after birth, primarily through fluid losses by respiration, urination, defecation, and low fluid intake. Birth weight is usually regained by the second week after birth, and a gradual pattern of increase in weight, height, and head circumference is evident. During the first month, weekly increases average 226 to 455 g in weight, 0.6 to 2.5 cm in length, and 2 cm in head circumference.

The newborn's heart rate ranges from 120 to 160 beats per minute. The average blood pressure is 85/54 mm Hg. The newborn's respiratory movements are primarily abdominal and vary in rate and rhythm, with an average rate of 30 to 60 breaths per minute. The axillary temperature ranges from 36°C to 37.5°C and generally stabilizes within 24 hours after birth.

Normal physical characteristics include the continued presence of lanugo on the skin of the back; cyanosis of the hands and feet for the first 24 hours; and a soft, protuberant abdomen. Skin colour varies according to racial and genetic heritage and gradually changes during infancy. **Molding**, or overlapping of the soft skull bones, allows the fetal head to adjust to various diameters of the maternal pelvis and is a common occurrence with vaginal births. The bones readjust within a few days, producing a rounded appearance. The sutures and **fontanels** are usually palpable at birth. The diamond shape of the anterior fontanel and the triangular shape of the posterior fontanel between the unfused bones of the skull are shown in Figure 23–1.

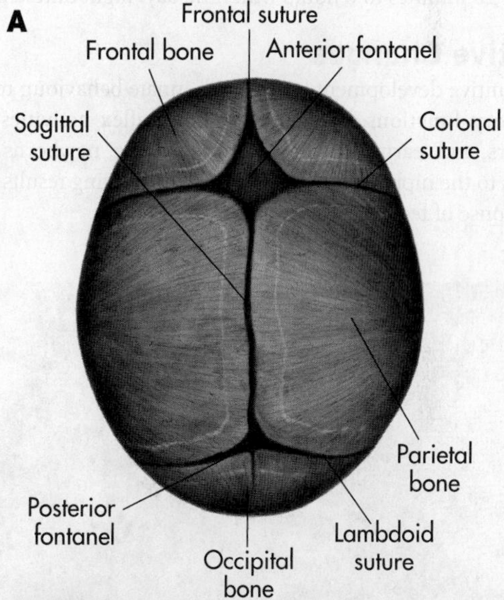

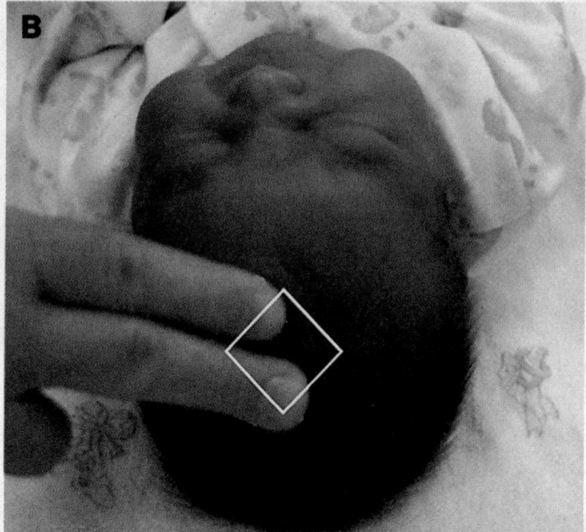

Figure 23-1 Fontanels and suture lines. **Source:** Adapted from Hockenberry, M. J., & Wilson, D. (2007). *Wong's nursing care of infants and children* (8th ed., p. 275, Fig. 8-7). St. Louis, MO: Mosby.

To assess neurological function, observe the newborn's level of activity, alertness, irritability, responsiveness to stimuli, and reflexes. Normal reflexes include sucking, rooting, grasping, yawning, coughing, sneezing, hiccuping, blinking in response to bright lights, and startling (pulling arms and legs inward) in response to sudden, loud noises. An absence of any of these or other reflexes indicates **prematurity**, possible trauma, or central nervous system complications. Because the newborn depends largely on reflexes for survival and in response to its environment, it is necessary to assess them. Figure 23–2 shows the tonic neck reflex: When newborns are lying supine, they reflexively turn the head to one side, extend the arm and leg on that side, and flex the opposite arm and leg.

Normal newborn behaviours include periods of sucking, crying, sleeping, and wakefulness. Movements are generally sporadic, but they are symmetrical and involve all four extremities. The relatively flexed fetal position of intrauterine life continues as the newborn attempts to maintain an enclosed, secure feeling. Newborns respond to sensory stimuli, particularly the primary caregiver's face, voice, and touch.

Except for the first hour after birth, when they are in a quietly alert state, newborns sleep almost continuously for the first 2 to 3 days to recover from the exhausting birth process. Thereafter, sleep periods vary from 20 minutes to 6 hours with little day–night differentiation.

Cognitive Changes

Early cognitive development begins with innate behaviour, reflexes, and sensory functions. Newborns initiate reflex activities, learn behaviours, and learn their desires. For example, newborns reflexively turn to the nipple (rooting) and learn that crying results in parents' response of feeding, diapering, and cuddling.

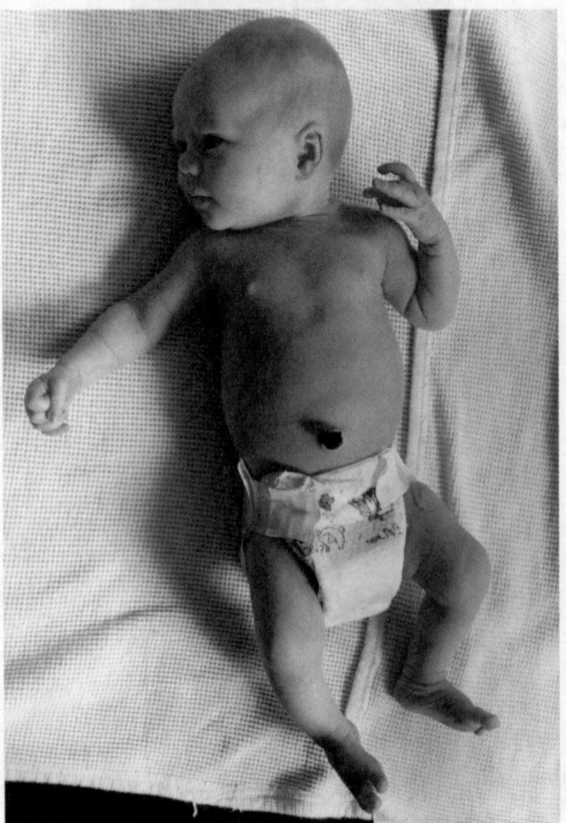

Figure 23-2 Tonic neck reflex. **Source:** Courtesy Paul Vincent Kuntz, Texas Children's Hospital.

Sensory functions contribute to cognitive development in the newborn. At birth, children can fixate on moving objects about 20 to 25 cm from their faces (Hockenberry & Wilson, 2007). A preference for the human face is apparent. Auditory and vestibular (i.e., equilibrium) systems function from birth. These sensory capabilities allow newborns to elicit stimuli rather than simply receive them. Parents should be taught the importance of providing sensory stimulation, such as talking to their newborns and holding them to see their faces. This allows infants to seek or take in stimuli, thereby enhancing learning and promoting cognitive development.

Psychosocial Changes

During the first month of life, parents and newborns normally develop a strong bond that grows into a deep attachment. Interactions during routine care enhance or detract from the attachment process. The processes of feeding, changing, bathing, and comforting an infant promote interaction and provide a foundation for deep attachments. Early on, older siblings should have the opportunity to be involved with the newborn. Family involvement helps support growth and development and promotes nurturing (Figure 23–3).

If parents or newborns experience health complications after birth, bonding may be compromised. Infants' behavioural cues may be weak or absent, and caregiving may be less mutually satisfying. Tired, ill parents have difficulty interpreting and responding to their infants' cues. Children who have congenital anomalies are often too weak to be responsive to parental cues and require special supportive nursing care. For example, infants born with heart defects may tire easily during feedings. They may rest frequently after several bursts of sucking. They may awaken frequently, crying because they are hungry again. Mothers may think that they are inadequate as mothers or that the infants are being fussy. Both infants and mothers may feel frustrated. In this case, bonding is not enhanced and may even be reduced unless nursing intervention breaks the sequence of events.

For newborns, crying is a means of communication and provides cues to parents (Santock, 2007). Although it can be a sign of distress, such as from pain, crying is an adaptive response to extrauterine life. Babies may cry because their diapers are wet, they are hungry, they want to be held, or they need a change in position or activity. Their crying may frustrate the parents if no cause is apparent. With help, parents can learn to recognize infants' cry patterns and take appropriate action when necessary (Herman & Le, 2007).

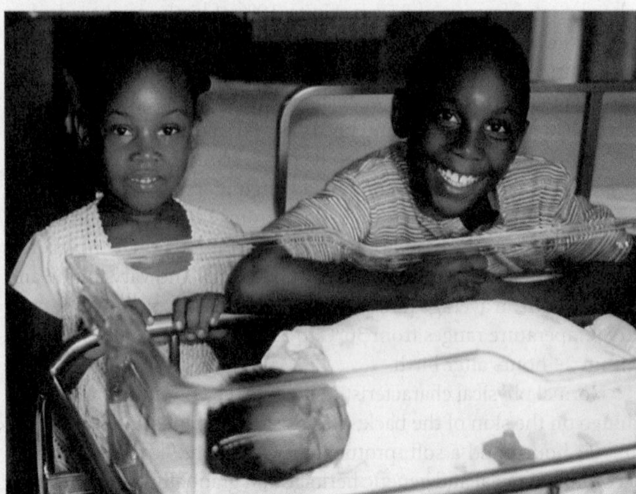

Figure 23-3 Siblings should be encouraged to visit with the newborn as soon as possible. **Source:** Courtesy Elaine Polan, RNC, BSN, MS.

Health Risks

Hyperbilirubinemia is a condition in which an excessive amount of bilirubin accumulates in the blood, and it is characterized by a yellowish colouring of the skin, or jaundice. The accumulation occurs when the infant's immature liver is unable to balance the destruction of red blood cells with the use or excretion of by-products. The balance can be further upset by prematurity, inadequate intake during breastfeeding, excess production of bilirubin, certain disease states, or a disturbance in the liver. Bilirubin at high levels is highly toxic to neurons, and affected newborns are at risk for brain injury. Phototherapy is used to help break down the bilirubin for easier excretion. During phototherapy, the infant's eyes must be shielded because they can be damaged by the light. Because excretion of the extra bilirubin can cause watery stools, adequate fluid balance in the infant must be maintained.

Health Concerns

Screening. Coordinate screening tests and other laboratory tests as needed. Blood tests can determine **inborn errors of metabolism.** This term applies to genetic disorders caused by the absence or deficiency of a substance, usually an enzyme, essential to cellular metabolism that results in abnormal protein, carbohydrate, or fat metabolism. Although inborn errors of metabolism are rare, they account for a significant proportion of health problems in children. Neonatal screening can detect phenylketonuria (PKU), hypothyroidism, and galactosemia and thus allow appropriate treatment that can prevent permanent intellectual disability and other health problems. Routine screening of newborns for PKU is recommended (Behrman et al., 2008). Other screening (e.g., for cystic fibrosis or hemophilia) may be necessary depending on the family history.

Circumcision. Circumcision is controversial in this country and is not recommended as a routine procedure by the Canadian Paediatric Society (1996). The controversy surrounds the risks and benefits, especially with regard to pain control. Risks have been identified as hemorrhage, infection, adhesions, and meatal stenosis. Benefits include prevention of penile cancer, prevention of urinary tract infections, and preservation of male body image to be consistent with that of peers when circumcision is part of the culture (Hockenberry & Wilson, 2007). Parents must give informed consent before the procedure. Care of the circumcized site depends on the type of method used for the procedure. Circumcized newborns should be checked frequently for evidence of swelling or oozing and the ability to void.

Infant

Infancy, the period from 1 month to 1 year of age, is characterized by dramatic physical growth and change. Psychosocial development advances, and interaction between infants and the environment is greater and more meaningful. Infants who giggle and roll over in response to tickling are interacting more with their social environments than when they merely smile in response to a hug.

Physical Changes

Steady and proportional growth of the infant is more important than absolute growth values. The infant's growth can be compared with charts of normal age- and gender-related growth measurements. Using growth charts, you can also evaluate an infant's growth patterns by recording weight, length, and head circumference at selected intervals. Measurements recorded over time are the best way to monitor growth and identify problems. An infant with a growth problem may have measurements generally below the expected norms at all intervals or may experience an acute, brief interference with growth. An infant with a feeding problem or a genetic condition such as cystic fibrosis may have a weight below the expected norm.

Size increases rapidly during the first year; birth weight doubles in approximately 5 months and triples by 12 months. On average, weight gain is 680 g during the first 5 months and 340 g for months 7 to 12. Height increases an average of 2.5 cm during each of the first 6 months and 3.8 cm for the next 6 months. This 50% increase in birth height occurs primarily in the trunk, with the chest diameter approximating that of the head by the first birthday (Hockenberry & Wilson, 2007). The fontanels become smaller; the posterior fontanel closes at about 2 months.

Physiological functioning stabilizes, and by the end of the first year, the heart rate is 90 to 140 beats per minute, the blood pressure averages 95/65 mm Hg, and the respiratory rate is 30 to 35 breaths per minute. Patterns of body function also stabilize, as evidenced by predictable sleep, elimination, and feeding routines. Motor development proceeds steadily in a cephalocaudal direction (from the head toward the feet).

Cognitive Changes

The infant learns by experiencing and manipulating the environment. Developing motor skills and increasing mobility expand an infant's environment and, with developing visual and auditory skills, enhance cognitive development. For these reasons, Piaget (1952) named his first stage of cognitive development, which extends until around the third birthday, the **sensorimotor period** (see Chapter 22). Before the acquisition of language, the extraordinary development of the mind occurs through children's developing senses and motor abilities. Improved visual acuity and eye–hand coordination allow grasping and exploration of objects. In addition, rudimentary colour vision begins by 2 months and improves throughout the first year, making the environment more interesting to see and explore. Infants' hearing also improves, allowing localization and discrimination of sounds.

Infants need opportunities to develop and use their senses. Evaluate the appropriateness and adequacy of these opportunities. For example, ill or hospitalized infants may lack the energy to interact with their environments, and thus their cognitive development may be slowed. Infants need to be stimulated according to their temperament, energy, and age. Use stimulation strategies that maximize the development of infants while conserving their energy and orientation. An example of this approach is talking to an infant and encouraging him or her to suck on a pacifier while administering a tube feeding.

Language. Speech is an important aspect of cognition that develops during the first year. Infants proceed from crying, cooing, and laughing to imitating sounds, comprehending the meaning of simple commands, and repeating words with knowledge of their meaning. By age 1 year, children recognize their own names and have two- or three-word vocabularies, usually including "Da-Da," "Ma-Ma," and "no." You can promote language development by encouraging mothers to name objects on which their infants' attention is focused.

Psychosocial Changes

Separation. During their first year, infants begin to differentiate themselves from other people, understanding that they are separate beings capable of acting on their own. Initially, infants are unaware of the boundaries of self, but through repeated experiences with the environment, they learn where the self ends and the external world begins. As infants determine their physical boundaries, they begin to respond to others.

At 2 or 3 months of age, infants begin to smile responsively rather than reflexively. Similarly, they can recognize differences in people when their sensory and cognitive capabilities improve. By 8 months, most infants can differentiate a stranger from a familiar person and respond differently to the two. Close attachment to the primary caregivers, most often parents, is usually established by this age. Infants seek out these people for support and comfort during times of stress. The ability to distinguish self from others allows children to interact and socialize within their environments. By 9 months, for example, children play simple social games such as patty-cake and peekaboo. More complex interactive games such as hide-and-seek involving objects are possible by the age of 1 year. Erikson (1963) described the psychosocial developmental crisis for the infant as trust versus mistrust. If the infant's physical and emotional needs are met, then the infant begins to develop a sense of security (see Chapter 22).

Assess the availability and appropriateness of experiences contributing to psychosocial development. Hospitalized infants may have difficulty establishing physical boundaries because of repeated bodily intrusions and painful sensations. Limiting these negative experiences and providing pleasurable sensations are interventions that support early psychosocial development. Extended separations from parents complicate the bonding process and increase the number of caregivers with whom the infant must interact. Ideally, the parents should provide the majority of care during hospitalization. When parents are not present, an attempt should be made to limit the number of caregivers who have contact with the infant and to follow the parents' directions for care. These interventions will foster the infant's continuing development of trust.

Play. Play is a meaningful set of activities through which individuals interact with their environment and relate to others. Play provides opportunities for the infant to develop many motor skills. Much of infant play is exploratory, inasmuch as infants use their senses to observe and examine their own bodies and objects of interest in their surroundings. For example, placing their toes in their mouths provides infants with pleasure and information about their own body and helps form their early self-concept. Play becomes manipulative as children learn control of the hands. Adults can facilitate infant learning by planning activities that promote the development of milestones and by providing toys that are safe for infants to explore with the mouth and manipulate with the hands, such as rattles, blocks, stacking rings, and washable stuffed animals. Infants most frequently engage in solitary (one-sided) play but do enjoy watching others, particularly siblings. Infants need to be played with and stimulated through interactions with others.

Health Risks

Sudden Infant Death Syndrome. Sudden infant death syndrome (SIDS) is the sudden and unexpected death of an apparently healthy infant. SIDS is rare before 1 month of age, but its incidence peaks among infants between 2 and 4 months of age, and it can occur in infants up to a year old. Three babies die of SIDS every week in Canada (Public Health Agency of Canada, 2002). The cause of SIDS is not understood, but the Public Health Agency of Canada recommends the following precautions:

- Infants should sleep on their backs on a firm, flat surface.
- A smoke-free environment should be provided before and after birth.
- A baby's crib must be free of such clutter as pillows, pillowlike items, comforters, and duvets.
- The infant should be dressed and covered lightly to avoid overheating.
- Mothers should breastfeed if possible.

Accidental Injury. Injury is a major cause of death in children 6 to 12 months old. An understanding of the major developmental accomplishments during this time period helps you plan for injury prevention. Box 23–3 lists the main types of injuries occurring in this age group and possible prevention strategies.

Child Maltreatment. You need to be aware that child maltreatment can occur during any stage of a child's life, beginning in infancy. *Child maltreatment* refers to violence, emotional or sexual mistreatment, or neglect of a child or adolescent. More children suffer from neglect than from any other type of maltreatment. Many suffer from more than one type of maltreatment. The approximate numbers of reported cases for every 1000 children of categories of maltreatment of children in Canada except Quebec were six cases of neglect, five cases of physical maltreatment, three cases of emotional maltreatment, and one case of sexual maltreatment (Trocmé et al., 2005). Protection of children from maltreatment comes under the jurisdiction of a province or territory. If you suspect any type of maltreatment of children, you are legally required to report it. Box 23–4 includes possible signs and symptoms of child maltreatment. These indications are relevant for children from infancy through adolescence.

A combination of signs and symptoms or a pattern of injury should arouse suspicion. It is important for you to be aware of certain birthmarks (e.g., mongolian spots, which are flat, dark birthmarks that may look like bruises) and cultural practices (e.g., coining, in which the skin is rubbed or scratched with a coin to improve circulation or restore balance) that may mimic signs of maltreatment.

Health Concerns

Nutrition. The quality and quantity of nutrition influence the infant's growth and development. Help parents select a nutritionally adequate diet for their infant. Nutrition is influenced by many variables (e.g., culture, food preferences, slow eating, or food allergies), and no diet is effective for all children or for one age group.

Feeding Alternatives. Supplying essential nutrients to the infant is an important goal. Support the parents' choice of feeding methods and facilitate a successful feeding process (Box 23–5). Breastfeeding is considered the most complete nutritional source until the infant is about 6 months of age. Breast milk contains protein, fats, and carbohydrates, as well as immunoglobulins that bolster the infant's ability to resist infection. Breastfeeding has been associated with a decreased frequency of gastroenteritis, otitis media, and food allergies (Health Canada, 2004; Hockenberry & Wilson, 2007).

If breastfeeding is not possible or not desired by the parent, an acceptable alternative is commercially prepared formula that is fortified with iron. Formulas are convenient, contain standard ingredients, and are also fortified with vitamins and minerals. Cow's milk and imitation milks are not recommended in the first year because infants are not able to properly digest the contained fat. Cow's milk also contains more sodium and protein and less iron than does formula (Hockenberry & Wilson, 2007). Because cow's milk has low levels of iron and high levels of calcium and phosphorus, absorption of iron may be decreased, causing anemia.

The average 1-month-old infant takes approximately 540 to 630 mL of breast milk or formula per day. This amount increases slightly during the first 6 months and decreases when solid foods are introduced. The amount of formula per feeding and the number of feedings vary among infants.

➤ BOX 23-3 Injury Prevention During Infancy

Age: Birth to 4 Months

Major Developmental Accomplishments

Involuntary reflexes, such as the crawling reflex, may propel infant forward or backward, and the startle reflex may cause the body to jerk.
The infant may roll over.
Eye–hand coordination improves, and the voluntary grasp reflex increases.

Injury Prevention

Aspiration

Aspiration is not as great a danger in this age group as in others, but you should begin to practise safeguarding early (see "Age: 5 to 7 Months" section).
Never shake baby powder directly on the infant; place powder in your hand and then on infant's skin. Store container closed and out of the infant's reach.
Hold the infant for bottle feeding; do not prop the bottle.
Know emergency procedures for choking.
Use pacifiers with one-piece construction and loop handle.

Suffocation and Drowning

Keep all plastic bags stored out of the infant's reach; discard large plastic garment bags after tying them in a knot.
Do not cover the infant's mattress with plastic.
Use a firm mattress and loose blankets; use no pillows.
Make sure crib design follows federal regulations and mattress fits snugly; crib slats should be no farther than 6 cm apart.
Position the crib away from other furniture and away from radiators.
Do not tie a pacifier on a string around the infant's neck.
Remove bibs at bedtime.
Never leave the infant alone in a bath.
If the infant is younger than 12 months, do not leave him or her alone on an adult- or youth-sized mattress or on "beanbag"-type pillows.

Falls

Always raise crib rails.
Never leave the infant on a raised, unguarded surface.
When in doubt as to where to place the child, use the floor.
Restrain the child in an infant seat, and never leave him or her unattended while the seat is resting on a raised surface.
Avoid using a high chair until the child can sit well with support.

Poisoning

Poisoning is not as great a danger in this age group as in others, but you should begin to practise safeguards early (see "Age: 5 to 7 Months" section).

Burns

Install smoke detectors in the home.
Use caution when warming formula in a microwave oven; always shake the bottle and check temperature of liquid before feeding.
Check bath water temperature.
Do not pour hot liquids when the infant is close by (e.g., sitting on your lap).
Do not leave infant in the sun for more than a few minutes; keep exposed areas covered.
Wash flame-retardant clothes according to label directions.
Use cool-mist (rather than hot-mist) vaporizers.
Do not leave the child in a parked car.
Check the surface heat of the car restraint before placing the child in it.

Motor Vehicles

Transport the infant in a federally approved, rear-facing infant seat, in the back seat* (Figure 23–4).
Never place an infant seat in the front passenger seat with an air bag.*
Do not place the child in a carriage or stroller behind a parked car.

Bodily Damage

Avoid sharp, jagged objects.
Keep diaper pins closed and away from the infant.
Never shake a baby (which can cause shaken baby syndrome); advise caregivers to seek help if they feel irritated or overwhelmed by a baby's crying.

Age: 5 to 7 Months

Major Developmental Accomplishments

The infant rolls over.
The infant sits momentarily.
The infant grasps and manipulates small objects.
The infant picks up a dropped object.
The infant has well-developed eye–hand coordination.
The infant can focus on and locate very small objects.
The infant's tendency to put objects in his or her mouth is very prominent.
The infant can push up on hands and knees.
The infant crawls backward.

Injury Prevention

Aspiration

Keep buttons, beads, syringe caps, and other small objects out of the infant's reach.
Keep the floor free of any small objects.
Do not feed the infant hard candy, nuts, food with pits or seeds, or whole or circular pieces of hot dog.
Exercise caution when giving the infant teething biscuits, because large chunks may be broken off and aspirated.
Do not feed the infant while he or she is lying down.
Inspect toys for removable parts.

Suffocation

Keep all latex balloons out of the child's reach.
Remove all crib toys that are strung across the crib or playpen when the child begins to push up on hands or knees or is 5 months old.
Keep baby powder and baby oil, if used, out of the child's reach.

Falls

Restrain the child in a high chair.
Keep crib rails raised to their full height.
Do not use baby walkers (baby walkers are no longer sold in or imported to Canada because of the high rate of injuries that they cause).

Poisoning

Make sure that paint for furniture or toys does not contain lead.
Hang plants, or place them on high surfaces rather than on the floor.
Store any toxic substances, such as cleaning fluid, paints, and pesticides, out of the reach of babies on a high shelf or in a locked cabinet.
Discard used containers of poisonous substances.
Do not store toxic substances in food containers.
Know the telephone number of the local poison control centre (usually listed in the beginning of telephone directories)
Keep faucets out of reach.
Place hot objects (candles, incense) on high surfaces.
Limit the child's exposure to sun; apply sunscreen.

Continued

BOX 23-3 Injury Prevention During Infancy *continued*

Motor Vehicles

See "Age: Birth to 4 Months" section

Bodily Damage

Give the child toys that are smooth and rounded, preferably made of natural wood or plastic.
Avoid long, pointed objects as toys.
Avoid toys that are excessively loud.
Keep sharp objects out of the infant's reach.
See also the "Age: Birth to 4 Months" section.

Age: 8 to 12 Months

Major Developmental Accomplishments

The child crawls and creeps.
The child stands, holding on to furniture.
The child stands alone.
The child cruises around furniture.
The child walks.
The child climbs.
The child pulls on objects.
The child throws objects.
The child is able to pick up small objects and has pincer grasp.
The child explores objects by putting them in his or her mouth.
The child dislikes being restrained.
The child explores away from parents.
The child's understanding of simple commands and phrases increases.

Injury Prevention

Aspiration

Keep small objects out of the reach of children.
Feed very small pieces solid table food.
Do not use beanbag toys or allow the child to play with dried beans.
See also the "Age: 5 to 7 Months" section.

Suffocation and Drowning

Keep doors of appliances (ovens, dishwashers, refrigerators, coolers, and front-loading clothes washers and dryers) closed at all times.
If you are storing an unused appliance, such as a refrigerator, remove the door.
Supervise contact with inflated balloons; immediately discard popped balloons, and keep uninflated balloons out of children's reach.
Fence in swimming pools.
Always supervise the child when near any source of water, such as baths, cleaning buckets, drainage areas, and toilets.
Keep bathroom doors closed.
Eliminate unnecessary pools of water.
Keep one hand on the child at all times when he or she is in the tub.

Falls

Fence stairways at the top and bottom if the child has access to either end.
Dress the child in safe shoes (soles that do not "catch" on the floor, tied shoelaces) and clothing (pant legs that do not touch the floor).
Ensure that furniture is sturdy enough for the child to hold while pulling himself or herself to a standing position and cruising.

Poisoning

Never call medications "candy."
Do not administer medications unless they are prescribed by a practitioner.
Put away medications and poisons immediately after use; put child-protector caps on properly.

Burns

Place guards in front of or around any heating appliance, fireplace, or furnace.
Keep electrical wires hidden or out of the child's reach.
Place plastic guards over electrical outlets; place furniture in front of outlets.
Keep hanging tablecloths out of reach (the child may pull down hot liquids or heavy or sharp objects).

*Further information available from Transport Canada (2006) and Health Canada (2006).

Adapted from Hockenberry, M. J., & Wilson, D. (2007). *Wong's nursing care of infants and children* (8th ed., pp. 553–554). St. Louis, MO: Mosby.

Developmentally, infants are not ready for solid food until 6 months of age. Before 6 months, the infant's gastrointestinal tract cannot handle the complex nutrients in solid food, and the extrusion reflex causes food to be pushed out of the mouth. Also, early introduction to solid foods may cause food allergies.

Cereals and well-cooked and pureed fruits, vegetables, and meats eaten during the second 6 months of life provide iron and additional sources of vitamins. These nutrients become especially important when infants stop consuming breast milk or formula and begin drinking whole cow's milk after the first birthday. Because the amount and frequency of feedings vary among infants, discuss differing feeding patterns with parents.

Honey has been used to sweeten water and coat pacifiers. However, honey should not be given to infants younger than 1 year because of the potential for infant botulism poisoning (Behrman et al., 2008).

Supplementation. The need for dietary vitamin and mineral supplements depends on the infant's diet. Full-term infants are born with some iron stores. The breastfed infant absorbs adequate iron from breast milk during the first 4 to 6 months of life. After age 6 months, iron-fortified cereal is generally considered an adequate

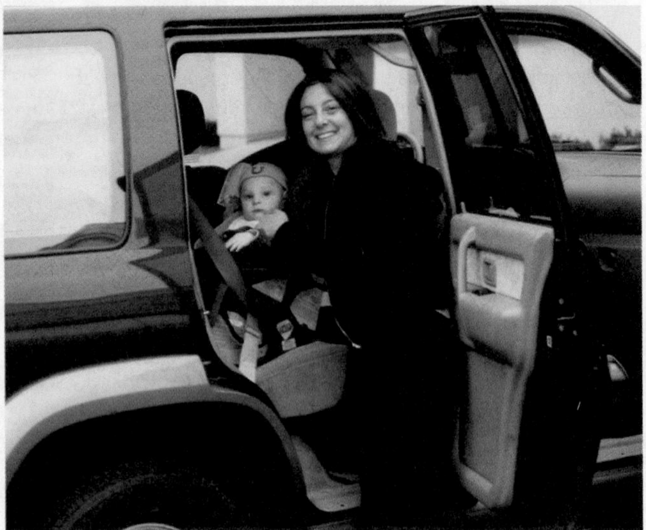

Figure 23-4 Federally approved infant car restraint. Note that the seat is rear facing in the back seat. **Source:** Courtesy Elaine Polan, RNC, BSN, MS.

supplemental source. Because iron in formula is less readily absorbed than that in breast milk, formula-fed infants should receive iron-fortified formula throughout the first year. Infants who are breastfed, especially those in more northerly areas with less sunlight in winter months, need to receive a vitamin D supplement to prevent rickets (Ward et al., 2007).

Adequate concentrations of fluoride to protect against dental caries are not available in human milk, and therefore fluoridated water or supplemental fluoride is generally recommended. The presence of fluoride in formula depends on the type of formula and the source of water used in preparing the concentrated forms. Fluoride supplementation may be necessary.

Overfeeding and Infant Obesity. The association between overfeeding, infant obesity, and later adult obesity is still controversial. However, early feeding experiences can influence later eating habits. You should therefore emphasize balanced nutrition and good

> **BOX 23-4 Clinical Manifestations of Potential Child Maltreatment**

Physical Neglect

Suggestive Physical Findings

Failure to thrive (infants), signs of malnutrition (e.g., unhealthy looking skin and hair, sunken eyes or cheeks), evidence of poor health care
Poor personal hygiene, especially of teeth; unclean or inappropriate dress
Frequent injuries resulting from lack of supervision

Suggestive Behaviours

Dull and inactive (infants)
Self-stimulatory behaviours, such as finger sucking or rocking
Begging or stealing food, vandalism, or shoplifting
Absenteeism from school
Drug or alcohol addiction

Emotional Maltreatment and Neglect

Suggestive Physical Findings

Failure to thrive
Feeding disorders, such as rumination
Enuresis (bed wetting after toilet training has been established)
Sleep disorders

Suggestive Behaviours

Self-stimulatory behaviours such as biting, rocking, sucking
Stranger anxiety and lack of social smile (infants)
Withdrawal and unusual fearfulness
Antisocial behaviour, such as destructiveness, stealing, cruelty
Extremes of behaviour, such as overcompliance, passivity, aggressiveness, or being demanding
Lags in emotional and intellectual development, especially language
Suicide attempts

Physical Maltreatment

Suggestive Physical Findings

Bruises and welts on face, lips, mouth, back, buttocks, thighs, or areas of torso
Regular patterns on skin that are descriptive of certain objects, such as belt buckle; hand; wire hanger; chain; wooden spoon; squeeze or pinch marks; round cigar or cigarette burns; burns in the shape of an iron, radiator, or electric stove burner
Burns, injuries, fractures, lacerations, or bruises in various stages of healing on soles of feet, palms of hands, back, or buttocks
Presence of symmetrical burns in the absence of "splash" marks
Unusual symptoms, such as abdominal swelling, pain, and vomiting from punching
Marks such as those resembling human bites, or pulling out of hair
Unexplained repeated poisoning or unexplained sudden illness

Suggestive Behaviours

Wariness of physical contact with adults
Apparent fear of parents or of going home
Lying very still while surveying environment, lack of reaction to frightening events
Inappropriate reaction to injury, such as failure to cry from pain
Apprehensiveness when hearing other children cry
Indiscriminate friendliness and displays of affection, superficial relationships
Acting-out behaviour, attention-seeking behaviours
Withdrawn behaviour

Sexual Maltreatment

Suggestive Physical Findings

Bruises, bleeding, lacerations, or irritation of external genitalia, anus, mouth, or throat
Torn, stained, or bloody underclothing
Pain on urination or pain, swelling, and itching of genital area; penile discharge; unusual odour in the genital area
Sexually transmitted infection, nonspecific vaginitis, venereal warts, or presence of sperm
Difficulty in walking or sitting
Recurrent urinary tract infections
Pregnancy in a young adolescent

Suggestive Behaviours

Sudden emergence of sexually related problems, including excessive or public masturbation, age-inappropriate sexual play, promiscuity, or overtly seductive behaviour
Withdrawn behaviour, excessive daydreaming, preoccupation with fantasies, especially in play
Poor relationships with peers
Sudden changes, such as anxiety, loss or gain of weight, clinging behaviour
In incestuous relationships, a child's excessive anger at one parent for not protecting the child from the other parent
Regressive behaviour, such as bed-wetting or thumb-sucking
Sudden onset of phobias or fears, particularly fears of the dark, men, strangers, or particular settings or situations (e.g., undue fear of leaving the house, of staying at the day care centre, or of staying at the babysitter's house)
Running away from home
Substance abuse, particularly of alcohol or mood-elevating drugs
Profound and rapid personality changes, especially extreme depression, hostility, and aggression (often accompanied by social withdrawal)
Rapidly declining school performance
Suicidal attempts or ideation about suicide

Adapted from Hockenberry, M. J., & Wilson, D. (2007). *Wong's nursing care of infants and children* (8th ed., p. 701). St. Louis, MO: Mosby.

BOX 23-5 RESEARCH HIGHLIGHT

Breastfeeding

Research Focus

Success in breastfeeding largely depends on the woman's self-confidence in her ability to breastfeed. You can play an important role in assisting new mothers to feel more confident in their ability to breastfeed by being aware of some of the factors that promote successful breastfeeding.

Research Abstract

Kingston et al. (2007) explored some of the factors that enhanced women's self-efficacy in breastfeeding 48 hours and 4 weeks after the birth of their babies. Kingston et al. examined such influences as previous successful breastfeeding experiences, professional assistance with breastfeeding, watching other mothers breastfeed, watching videos of other women breastfeeding, giving positive feedback and consistent advice, receiving praise from family members and friends, encouraging mothers to continue breastfeeding, and encouraging mothers to think positively about the breastfeeding experience, as well as physiological influences on breastfeeding such as pain, fatigue, and feeling overwhelmed. Self-efficacy was measured by the Breastfeeding Self-Efficacy Scale–Short Form. The study was performed with a small sample of mothers ($N = 65$) in a hospital in central Canada. The researchers found that self-efficacy was significantly higher in women who had seen videotapes of women breastfeeding as part of their breastfeeding education or had received praise from their partners or own mothers. Women who reported pain or received help with breastfeeding from professionals had significantly lower scores. Women receiving more help would have a greater need for assistance, and this might affect self-efficacy.

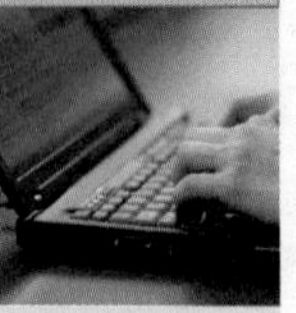

Evidence-Informed Practice

- Assess the breastfeeding self-efficacy of new mothers.
- Examine the educational material used with clients, and show clients videos of successful breastfeeding.
- Consider the physiological condition of the mother, and address issues such as pain.
- Include the mother's partner and, if possible, the woman's own mother in supporting and offering praise to the breastfeeding mother.
- Examine other factors that increase or decrease the mother's self-confidence in her ability to breastfeed.

References: Kingston, D., Dennis, C.-L., & Sword, W. (2007). Exploring breast-feeding self-efficacy. *Journal of Perinatal and Neonatal Nursing, 21*, 207–215.

dietary habits through feeding experiences mutually satisfying for the parents and infant. Eating habits are frequently affected by the family's sociocultural background. Because some cultures consider a fat baby to be a sign of good mothering, any suggestion to limit intake or slow weight gain may be seen as a threat. It is important for you to develop an understanding of the cultural influences to develop effective nursing interventions.

Dentition. The average age at which the first tooth erupts is 7 months, but considerable variation exists among infants because of their genetic endowment. An occasional infant is born with a tooth, whereas others remain toothless at 1 year. The order of tooth eruption is fairly predictable: The lower central incisors are first to appear, closely followed by the upper central incisors. Most 1-year-olds have six teeth.

Teething may result in considerable discomfort for some infants and little or none for others. The inflammation of the gums before the tooth emerges may result in a low-grade fever and irritability. Some infants exhibit increased drooling, biting, or finger sucking. Biting on a frozen teething ring or ice cube wrapped in a washcloth may be soothing. Over-the-counter teething medications to rub on the inflamed gums and appropriate doses of acetaminophen are helpful when the infant is irritable and has difficulty eating or sleeping.

Most dentists recommend that parents cleanse their infant's teeth after each feeding. The parent can place a clean, wet washcloth or piece of gauze over a finger and use it to wipe the infant's teeth. Because of the risk of developing dental caries, discourage prolonged breast- or bottle-feeding, especially just before the infant goes to sleep because the infant is likely to leave milk in the mouth and around the teeth. The infant should never go to bed with a bottle of juice or milk (Behrman et al., 2008).

Immunizations. The widespread use of immunizations has resulted in the dramatic decline of infectious diseases since the 1950s and is therefore a most important factor in health promotion during childhood. Although most immunizations can be given to people of any age, the Public Health Agency of Canada (2006) recommended that the administration of the primary series begin soon after birth and be completed during early childhood (Table 23–2). Minor side effects may occur, but serious reactions are rare. Parents must receive instructions regarding the potential side effects of immunizations. High fever and extreme irritability should be reported to their health care professional.

As a result of complacency and fear regarding the side effects of certain vaccines, especially diphtheria and tetanus toxoids and pertussis vaccine (DTP), not all children receive appropriate immunizations (Leitch, 2007). An important role for you is to discuss the importance of vaccination for infants and children, provide up-to-date information to parents, and encourage them to make an informed decision for their children. General contraindications to vaccination include moderate illness, allergic response to a previous dose of a particular vaccine, immunosuppression, and taking high doses of corticosteroids.

Sleep. Sleep patterns vary among infants; many having their days and nights "mixed up" until 3 to 4 months of age. By that age, most infants sleep between 9 and 11 hours a night. Total daily sleep averages 15 hours. Most infants take one or two naps a day by the end of the first year. Sleep disturbances with a physiological basis are rare, with the possible exception of colic. Common sleep disturbances are described in Table 23–3.

Toddler

Toddlerhood ranges from 12 to 36 months. Toddlers have increasing independence, physical mobility, and cognitive abilities. Toddlers become aware of their abilities to control their environments and are pleased with successful efforts. This success leads them to continue attempting to control their environments. Unsuccessful attempts at control may result in the toddler refusing to do something, saying "no" frequently, or engaging in temper tantrums.

➤ TABLE 23-2 Canadian Routine Immunization Schedule for Infants and Children

Age at Vaccination	DTaP-IPV	Hib	MMR	Var	HB	Pneu-C-7	Men-C	Tdap	Inf
Birth					Infancy: 3 doses				
2 months	✪	✦			★	◆	⊙		
4 months	✪	✦				◆	(⊙)		
6 months	✪	✦				◆	⊙ or		6–23 months
12 months			■	●	or	◆ 12–15 months	⊙ if not yet given		○
18 months	✪	✦	■ or						1–2 doses
4–6 years	✪		■						
14–16 years					Preteen/teen: 2–3 doses		⊙ if not yet given	▲	

Legend

- ( ) Symbols with brackets around them imply that these doses may not be required, depending upon the age of the child or adult. Refer to the relevant chapter [in Public Health Agency of Canada, 2006] for that vaccine for further details.
- ✪ Diphtheria, tetanus, acellular pertussis, and inactivated polio virus vaccine (DTaP-IPV): DTaP-IPV(± Hib) vaccine is the preferred vaccine for all doses in the vaccination series, including completion of the series in children who have received one or more doses of DPT (whole cell) vaccine (e.g., recent immigrants). Year dose can be omitted if the fourth dose was given after the fourth birthday.
- ✦ Haemophilus influenzae type b conjugate vaccine (Hib): The Hib schedule shown is for the Haemophilus b capsular polysaccharide–polyribosylribitol phosphate (PRP) conjugated to tetanus toxoid (PRP-T). For catching up, the number of doses depends on the age at which the schedule is begun (see Public Health Agency of Canada, 2006, "Haemophilus Vaccine" chapter). Not usually required past age 5 years.
- ■ Measles, mumps, and rubella (MMR) vaccine: A second dose of MMR vaccine is recommended for children at least 1 month after the first dose for the purpose of better measles protection. For convenience, options include giving it with the next scheduled vaccination at 18 months of age or at school entry (4–6 years) (depending on the provincial or territorial policy) or at any intervening age that is practical.
- ● Varicella vaccine (Var): children aged 12 months to 12 years should receive one dose of varicella vaccine. Susceptible individuals 13 years of age should receive two doses at least 28 days apart.
- ★ Hepatitis B vaccine (HB): hepatitis B vaccine can be routinely given to infants or preadolescents, depending on the provincial or territorial policy. For infants born to chronic carrier mothers, the first dose should be given at birth (with hepatitis B immunoglobulin); otherwise, the first dose can be given at 2 months of age to fit more conveniently with other routine infant immunization visits. The second dose should be administered at least 1 month after the first dose, and the third at least 2 months after the second dose, but these may fit more conveniently into the 4- and 60-month immunization visits. A two-dose schedule for adolescents is an option (see Public Health Agency of Canada, 2006, "Hepatitis B Vaccine" chapter).
- ◆ Pneumococcal conjugate vaccine–7-valent (Pneu–C-7): Recommended for all children under 2 years of age. The recommended schedule depends on the age of the child when vaccination is begun (see Public Health Agency of Canada, 2006, "Pneumococcal Vaccine" chapter).
- □ Pneumococcal polysaccharide–23-valent (Pneu–P-23): Recommended for all adults 65 years of age (see Public Health Agency of Canada, 2006, "Pneumococcal Vaccine" chapter).
- ⊙ Meningococcal C conjugate vaccine (Men-C): Recommended for children under 5 years of age, adolescents, and young adults. The recommended schedule depends on the age of the individual (see Public Health Agency of Canada, 2006, "Meningococcal Vaccine" chapter) and the conjugate vaccine used. At least one dose in the primary infant series should be given after 5 months of age. If the provincial or territorial policy is to give Men-C to persons 12 months of age, one dose is sufficient.
- ▲ Diphtheria, tetanus, acellular pertussis vaccine–adult or adolescent formulation (Tdap): A combined adsorbed "adult type" preparation for use in people 7 years of age; contains less diphtheria toxoid and pertussis antigens than preparations given to younger children and is less likely to cause reactions in older people.

Continued

➤ TABLE 23-2 Canadian Routine Immunization Schedule for Infants and Children *continued*

❖ Diphtheria, tetanus vaccine (Td): A combined adsorbed "adult type" preparation for use in people 7 years of age; contains less diphtheria toxoid antigen than preparations given to younger children and is less likely to cause reactions in older people. It is given to adults not immunized in childhood as the second and third doses of their primary series and subsequent booster doses; Tdap is given only once under these circumstances, as it is assumed that previously unimmunized adults will have encountered *Bordetella pertussis* and have some pre-existing immunity.

o Influenza vaccine (Inf): Recommended for all children 6–23 months of age and all persons 65 years of age. Previously unvaccinated children <9 years of age require two doses of the current season's vaccine with an interval of at least 4 weeks. The second dose within the same season is not required if the child received one or more doses of Influenza vaccine during the previous Influenza season (see Public Health Agency of Canada, 2006, "Influenza Vaccine" chapter).

\+ Inacivated polio virus (IPV).

From Public Health Agency of Canada. (2006). *Canadian immunization guide: Seventh edition—2006.* Retrieved October 30, 2008, from http://www.phac-aspc.gc.ca/publicat/cig-gci/index-eng.php. Reproduced with permission of the Minister of Public Works and Government Services Canada, 2008.

➤ TABLE 23-3 Selected Sleep Disturbances During Infancy and Early Childhood

Disorder and Description	Management
Nighttime Feeding	
Colic, irritability Prolonged need for bottle or breastfeeding at night Going to sleep at the breast or with a bottle Irregular sleep patterns Returning to sleep after feeding; other comfort measures (e.g., rocking or holding) are usually ineffective	Soothe, rock for brief periods, offer pacifier. Gradually increase daytime feeding intervals to 4 hours or more. Offer last feeding as late as possible at night. Gradually increase amount of fluid during day. Offer no bottles in bed. Put child to bed when awake. When child is crying, check at progressively longer intervals each night; reassure child but do not hold, rock, take to parent's bed, or give bottle or pacifier.
Developmental Night Crying	
Child aged 6–12 months with undisturbed nighttime sleep now awakes abruptly; awakening may be accompanied by nightmares	Be assured that this phase is temporary. Enter room immediately to check on child, but keep reassurances brief. Avoid feeding, rocking, taking to parent's bed, or any other routine that may initiate trained nighttime crying.
Trained Night Crying (Inappropriate Sleep Associations)	
Child typically falls asleep in a place other than own bed (e.g., rocking chair or parent's bed) and is brought to own bed while asleep; on awakening, cries until usual routine is instituted (e.g., rocking)	Put child in own bed when child is awake. If possible, arrange sleeping area separate from other family members. Check crying child at progressively longer intervals each night; reassure child but do not resume usual routine.
Refusal to Go to Sleep	
Child resists bedtime and comes out of room repeatedly Nighttime sleep may be continuous, but frequent awakenings and refusal to return to sleep may occur and become a problem if parent allows child to deviate from usual sleep pattern	Evaluate whether bedtime is too early (child may resist sleep if not tired). Adapt consistent bedtime routine. If child persists in leaving bedroom, close door for progressively longer periods. Reinforce positive behaviour.
Nighttime Fears	
Child resists going to bed or wakes during the night because of fears Child seeks parent's physical presence and falls asleep easily with parent nearby	Evaluate whether bedtime is too early (child may fantasize when he or she has nothing to do but think in a dark room). Calmly reassure the frightened child; keeping a night light on may be helpful. Use reward system with child to provide motivation to deal with fears. Avoid patterns that can lead to additional problems (e.g., sleeping with child or taking child to parent's room).
Overwhelming fears	If child's fear is overwhelming, consider desensitization (e.g., progressively spending longer periods of time alone); obtain professional help for protracted fears. Distinguish between nightmares and sleep terrors (confused partial arousals).

Physical Changes

The rapid development of motor skills allows toddlers to participate in self-care activities such as feeding, dressing, and toileting. Initially, toddlers walk with a broad stance and gait, protuberant abdomen, and arms out to the sides for balance. Soon they begin to navigate stairs, using a rail or the wall to maintain balance. Locomotion skills eventually include running, jumping, standing on one foot for several seconds, and kicking a ball. Most toddlers can ride tricycles, climb ladders, and run well by their third birthday.

Fine motor capabilities move from scribbling spontaneously to drawing circles and crosses accurately. By age 3 years, children draw simple stick people and can usually stack a tower of small blocks. Increased locomotion skills, the ability to undress, and development of sphincter control allow toilet training if a toddler has developed the necessary language and cognitive abilities. Parents often consult nurses for an assessment of readiness for toilet training. A child's recognition of the urge to urinate and defecate is a crucial component in the child's mental readiness. At this stage, children usually show a willingness to please parents and take pride in their accomplishments (Santock, 2007). You must remind parents that patience, consistency, and a nonjudgemental attitude, in addition to the child's readiness, are essential for successful toilet training.

The cardiopulmonary system becomes stable in the toddler years. The heart and respiratory rates slow to an average of 110 beats and 25 breaths per minute, respectively, and the blood pressure varies slightly from infancy. The average blood pressure in toddlers is 90/50 mm Hg.

The anterior fontanel closes between 12 and 18 months of age, ending the period of the most rapid growth of the skull and brain. However, head circumference should be measured routinely until a toddler is 3 years of age.

The rate of increase in a toddler's weight and length slows. By age 2.5 years, children's weights are four times the birth weight. Height during the toddler years increases by approximately 7.5 cm a year, mainly as a result of increases in leg length. The average height of 2-year-olds is 85 cm. Slowed growth rates are accompanied by decreased caloric need, and smaller food intake leads some parents to worry about the adequacy of dietary intake. Parents need encouragement to offer appropriate servings of food from *Eating Well With Canada's Food Guide* (Health Canada, 2007) and to avoid force-feeding or allowing children to fill up on foods that have high levels of fat and sugar. You can reassure parents that a child's nutrition is adequate by demonstrating the child's satisfactory status on a growth chart.

Cognitive Changes

Toddlers' completion of the development of **object permanence**, their ability to remember events, and their beginning ability to put thoughts into words at about 2 years of age, signal their transition to Piaget's (1952) **preoperational** stage of cognitive development (see Chapter 22). Toddlers recognize that they are separate beings from their mothers, but they are unable to assume another person's point of view. They use symbols to represent objects, places, and people. This function is demonstrated when children imitate the behaviour of another person that they viewed earlier (e.g., pretend to shave like daddy), pretend one object is another (e.g., pretend that a doll is a baby), and use language to stand for absent objects (e.g., request a bottle).

Language. An 18-month-old child uses approximately 50 words (Santock, 2007). A 24-month-old child has a vocabulary of up to 200 words and is generally able to speak in two-word sentences. "Who's that?" and "What's that?" typify questions asked during this period. First-person expressions such as "me do it" and "that's mine" demonstrate 2-year-old children's use of pronouns and desire for independence and control. Despite the expanded vocabulary of older toddlers, the word they use most often is "no" until well into the third year. Offering choices to toddlers helps reduce their sense of frustration and builds their sense of independence (Santock, 2007).

Because children's moral development is closely associated with their cognitive abilities, the moral development of toddlers is only beginning and is also egocentric. Toddlers do not understand concepts of right and wrong. However, they understand that some behaviours bring pleasant results and others elicit unpleasant results. Therefore, until toddlers achieve a higher level of cognitive function, they behave simply to avoid the unpleasant and seek out the pleasant (Hockenberry & Wilson, 2007).

Psychosocial Changes

According to Erikson (1963), a sense of autonomy emerges during the toddler years (see Chapter 22). Children strive for independence by using their developing muscles to do everything for themselves and control their bodily functions. Their strong wills are frequently exhibited in negative behaviour when caregivers attempt to direct their actions; for example, temper tantrums may result when toddlers are frustrated by parental restrictions. Parents need to provide toddlers with graded independence, allowing them to do things that do not result in harm to themselves or others. This strategy prevents them from doubting their abilities or feeling a sense of shame for what they have done. Firm consistent limits, patience, and support allow toddlers to develop socially acceptable behaviour and cope with the frustration of learning self-control (Santock, 2007).

Socially, toddlers remain strongly attached to their parents and fear separation from them. In their parents' presence, toddlers feel safe, and their curiosity is evident in their exploration of the environment. Children continue to engage in solitary play during toddlerhood but also begin to participate in parallel play, which is playing beside rather than with another child. Toddlers who are just learning what belongs to them are often possessive of their toys. They learn the joy of sharing when they offer parents or caregivers toys to hold and the parents or caregivers express pleasure.

Health Risks

Their newly developed locomotion abilities and insatiable curiosity put toddlers at risk for injury. Toddlers need close supervision at all times, particularly when in environments that have not been childproofed (Figure 23–5). Creating a safe, childproof environment in the home is essential for preventing accidental injuries.

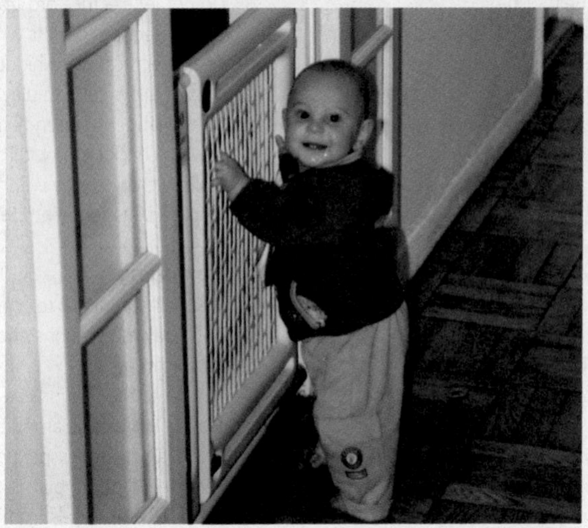

Figure 23-5 Safety precautions should be provided for toddlers.
Source: Courtesy Elaine Polan, RNC, BSN, MS.

Poisonings occur frequently in children nearing 2 years of age because they are interested in placing any object or substance in their mouths to learn about it. Parents must remove or lock up all possible poisons, including plants, cleaning materials, and medications. Lead poisoning can pose a health hazard for younger children (Leitch, 2007). Health care professionals need to educate families living in older homes about the risks, screening, and treatment of lead poisoning. Because of toddlers' lack of awareness regarding the danger of water and their newly developed walking skills, drowning is a major cause of accidental death in this age group. Toddlers can easily become separated from a parent because they often wander away. It is important to closely supervise toddlers, especially if they are in an open public space. Setting limits is extremely important for toddlers' safety. In automobiles, toddlers must remain in car seats (Transport Canada, 2006). Children often learn to release the car restraints, and parents must be firm in their resolve not to drive unless the children are securely restrained. Toddlers depend completely on their parents for physical safety. Health care professionals must educate parents on the proper use of child passenger restraint use. Table 23–4 identifies developmental abilities acquired during this age period and injury prevention strategies.

TABLE 23-4 Injury Prevention for Toddlers and Preschoolers

Developmental Abilities Related to Risk of Injury	Injury Prevention
Walks, runs, and climbs Is able to open doors and gates Can ride tricycle Can throw ball and other objects	***Motor Vehicles*** Continue to use federally approved car restraint. A toddler weighing 10 to 18 kg should be placed in a forward-facing child seat that is anchored to the vehicle frame with a tether strap. A child weighing 18 to 36 kg should be seated in a booster seat. Supervise child while he or she is playing outside, to prevent child from entering street. Do not allow child to play on curb or behind a parked car. Do not permit child to play in pile of leaves, snow, or anywhere that he or she is not visible. Supervise tricycle riding. Supervise child playing outside. Teach children to obey pedestrian safety rules. Supervise child when near traffic.
Has great curiosity Is helpless in water, unaware of its danger at any depth	***Drowning*** Supervise closely when child is near any source of water, including buckets. Keep bathroom doors and lid on toilet closed. Have fence around swimming pool, and lock gate. Teach the child swimming and water safety (and continue to protect him or her from injury).
Is able to reach heights by climbing, stretching, standing on toes, and using objects as a ladder Pulls objects Explores any holes or openings Can open drawers and closets Is unaware of potential sources of heat or fire Plays with mechanical objects	***Burns*** Turn pot handles toward back of stove. Place electric appliances, such as coffeemaker or frying pan, toward back of counter. Place guard rails in front of radiators, fireplaces, and heating appliances. Store matches and cigarette lighters in locked or inaccessible area; discard carefully. Place burning candles, incense, hot foods, ashes, embers, and cigarettes out of reach. Do not let tablecloth hang within child's reach. Do not let electric cord from iron or other appliance hang within child's reach. Cover electrical outlets with protective devices. Keep electrical wires hidden or out of reach. Do not allow child to play with electrical appliance, wires, or lighters. Stress danger of open flames; teach child what "hot" means. Always check bath water temperature; adjust hot-water heater temperature to 49°C or lower; do not allow child to play with faucets. Apply a sunscreen with SPF 15 or higher when child is exposed to sunlight.
Explores by putting objects in mouth Can open drawers, closets, and most containers Climbs Cannot understand warning labels	***Poisoning*** Place all potentially toxic agents (including plants) in a locked cabinet or out of reach. Put away medications and poisonous substances immediately after use; positon (and tighten) child-resistant caps properly. Refer to medications as "drugs," not as "candy." Do not store large amounts of toxic agents. Promptly discard empty poison containers; never reuse such containers to store a food item or other poison. Teach child not to play in trash containers. Never remove labels from containers of toxic substances. Know number and location of nearest poison control centre (usually listed at beginning of telephone directories).

TABLE 23-4 Injury Prevention for Toddlers and Preschoolers *continued*

Developmental Abilities	Injury Prevention
Is able to open doors and some windows Goes up and down stairs Has unrefined depth perception	***Falls*** Keep screen in window, nail securely, and install guard rail. Place gates at top and bottom of stairs. Keep doors locked or use child-resistant doorknob covers at entry to stairs, high porch, or other elevated area, such as laundry chute. Remove unsecured or scatter rugs. Apply nonskid mat in bathtub or shower. Keep crib rails fully raised and mattress at lowest level. Place carpeting under crib and in bathroom. Keep large toys and bumper pads out of crib or playpen (child can use these as "stairs" to climb out). Move child to youth bed when he or she is able to climb out of crib. Dress child in safe clothing (soles that do not "catch" on floor, tied shoelaces, pant legs that do not hang on floor). Never leave child unattended in shopping cart or stroller. Supervise child at playgrounds; select play areas with soft ground cover and safe equipment.
Puts things in mouth May swallow hard or nonedible pieces of food	***Choking and Suffocation*** Do not give child large, round chunks of meat, such as whole hot dogs (instead, slice into thin pieces). Do not give child fruit with pits, fish with bones, dried beans, hard candy, chewing gum, nuts, popcorn, grapes, or marshmallows. Choose large, sturdy toys without sharp edges or small removable parts. Discard unused refrigerators, unused ovens, and other unused appliances; if storing old appliance, remove doors. Keep automatic garage door opener in inaccessible place. Select safe toy boxes or chests without heavy, hinged lids. Keep window blind strings out of child's reach. Remove drawstrings from clothing.
Is still clumsy in many activities Is easily distracted from tasks Is unaware of potential danger from strangers or other people	***Bodily Damage*** Avoid giving child sharp or pointed objects—such as knives, scissors, or toothpicks—especially when child is walking or running. Do not allow lollipops or similar objects in the child's mouth when he or she is walking or running. Teach safety precautions (e.g., to hold fork or scissors with pointed end away from face). Store all dangerous tools, garden equipment, and firearms in locked cabinet. Be alert to danger of animals, including household pets. Use safety glass and decals on large glass areas, such as sliding glass doors. Teach personal safety. Teach child his or her name, address, and phone number, and teach child to ask for help from appropriate people (cashier, security guard, police officer) if lost; have identification on child (sewn in clothes, inside shoe). Avoid dressing child in personalized clothing in public places. Teach child to never go anywhere with a stranger. Teach child to tell parents if anyone makes child feel uncomfortable in any way. Always listen to child's concerns regarding others' behaviour. Teach child to say "no" when confronted with uncomfortable situations.

Adapted from Hockenberry, M. J., & Wilson, D. (2007). *Wong's nursing care of infants and children* (8th ed., pp. 631–632). St. Louis, MO: Mosby.

Health Concerns

Nutrition. Most toddlers stop drinking breast milk or formula and begin drinking cow's milk. Nutritional requirements are increasingly met by solid foods. Because the consumption of more than 1 L of milk per day usually decreases children's appetite for these essential solid foods and results in inadequate iron intake, you should advise parents to limit milk intake to between 500 and 750 mL (two to three servings) per day. Children should not drink low-fat or skim milk until 2 years of age because they need the fat in whole milk for physical and intellectual growth. Healthy toddlers require a balanced daily intake of bread and grains, vegetables, fruit, dairy products, and proteins (see Chapter 43). Because parents frequently overestimate the size of a normal serving for their child, you should discuss normal serving sizes with parents.

Special dietary considerations are required for children who are ill, are undergoing surgery, or have conditions involving ingestion, absorption, or use of nutrients. Alterations in the type of foods and caloric requirements may be necessary. Strict vegetarian diets for children also require careful planning to ensure adequate, balanced protein intake. Regardless of children's health status, several basic principles of nutrition apply. Mealtime has psychosocial and physical significance. If the parents struggle to control toddlers' dietary intake, problematic behaviour and conflicts may result. Toddlers often develop "food jags," or the desire to eat one food repeatedly. Rather than becoming disturbed by this behaviour, parents should be encouraged to offer a variety of nutritious foods at meals and to provide only nutritious snacks between meals. Serving finger foods to toddlers allows them to eat by themselves and to satisfy their need for independence and control. Small, reasonable servings allow toddlers to eat all of their meals.

Preschooler

The **preschool period** encompasses the years between 3 and 5 years of age. Children refine the mastery of their bodies and often are eager to begin school. Many people consider these the most intriguing years of parenting because children exhibit positive emotions and can more effectively share their thoughts, interact, and communicate. Physical development occurs at a slower pace than does cognitive and psychosocial development.

Physical Changes

Physical development continues in the preschool years. Heart and respiratory rates range from 60 to 100 beats and 23 to 25 breaths per minute, respectively. Blood pressure rises slightly to an average of 92/56 mm Hg. Children gain about 2.27 kg per year; the average weight is 14.5 kg at 3 years, 16.8 kg at 4 years, and about 18.6 kg at 5 years. Preschoolers grow 6 to 7.5 cm per year, double their birth length at about 4 years of age, and stand an average of 1 m tall by their fifth birthday. The elongation of the legs results in a more slender appearance. Little difference exists between the sexes, although boys are slightly larger with more muscle and less fatty tissue.

Large and fine muscle coordination improves. Preschoolers run well, walk up and down steps with ease, and learn to hop. By age 5 years, they can usually skip on alternate feet, can jump rope, and begin to skate and swim. Improvements in fine motor skills allow intricate manipulations. Children learn to copy crosses and squares. Triangles and diamonds are usually mastered between ages 5 and 6 years. Scribbling and drawing help children develop fine muscle skills and eye–hand coordination needed for the printing of letters and numbers.

Children need opportunities to learn and practise new physical skills. Early intervention programs are helpful in developing these skills, especially among disadvantaged children. Nursing care of healthy and ill children includes an assessment of the availability of these opportunities. Although children with acute illnesses benefit from rest and exclusion from usual daily activities, children who have chronic conditions or who have been hospitalized for long periods need ongoing exposure to developmental opportunities. With the parents, weave these opportunities into the children's daily experiences, depending on their abilities, needs, and energy level.

Cognitive Changes

Preschoolers continue to master the preoperational stage of cognition. The first phase of this period, known as *preconceptual thought* (2 to 4 years), is characterized by perception-bound thinking, in that children judge people, objects, and events by their outward appearance or what seems to be true (Piaget, 1952). For example, a child may think that a 240-mL glass full of fluid contains more than a 300-mL glass that also contains 240 mL of fluid because the smaller glass appears fuller. Even if they watch the fluid from the smaller glass being poured into the larger glass and the smaller glass refilled, they still assert that the full, smaller glass contains more.

Children's thinking is hindered by their limited attention and attending skills. **Artificialism**, the misconception that everything in the world has been created by humanity, may result in children's asking questions such as "Who built the mountains?" Another misconception of preschool thinking, **animism**, the attribution of animal life to inanimate objects, often results in statements such as "Trees cry when their branches are broken." A third misconception is a type of reasoning called **immanent justice**, the notion that if a built-in code of law and order is broken, punishment will occur immediately (Santock, 2007). For example, a child might think that he became sick because he lied to his mother.

At about the age of 4 years, the intuitive phase of preoperational thought develops. Children's ability to think more complexly is demonstrated by their ability to classify objects according to size or colour and by questions such as "Why do they call it the 31st day of the month instead of the 30 last?" Egocentricity persists, but during these 3 years, it begins to be replaced with social interaction; for example, a 5-year-old child offers a bandage to a child with a cut finger. Children become aware of cause-and-effect relationships, as illustrated by the statement, "The sun sets because people want to go to bed." Early causal thinking is also evident in preschoolers' transductive thoughts (reasoning occurs from one particular to another). If two events are related in time or space, children link them in a causal manner. A hospitalized child, for example, may reason, "I cried last night, and that's why the nurse gave me the shot." As children near the age of 5 years, they begin to use or can be taught to use rules to understand causation. They then begin to reason from the general to the particular. This development forms the basis for more formal logical thought. The hospitalized child now reasons, "I get a shot twice a day, and that's why I got one last night."

Preschoolers' knowledge of the world remains closely linked to concrete (perceived by the senses) experiences. Even their rich fantasy life is grounded in the perception of reality. The mixing of the two aspects can lead to many childhood fears, and adults may misinterpret children's stories as lying when children are actually presenting reality from their perspective.

The greatest fear of this age group appears to be that of bodily harm, and it can be seen in children's fear of the dark, thunderstorms, and medical personnel. This fear often makes children unwilling to allow nursing interventions such as measurement of vital signs. Preschoolers may cooperate if they are allowed to help you measure the blood pressure of a doll or teddy bear or if they are allowed to handle the equipment you will use.

Preschoolers' moral development expands to include a beginning understanding of behaviours considered socially right or wrong. Children continue to be motivated, however, by the wish to avoid punishment and the desire to obtain a reward. The primary difference between this stage of moral development and that of toddlers is that preschoolers are better able to identify behaviours that elicit rewards or punishment and begin to label these behaviours as "right" or "wrong."

Language. Preschoolers' vocabularies continue to increase rapidly, and by the age of 5 years, children know more than 2100 words and can construct sentences containing 5 to 6 words (Hockenberry & Wilson, 2007). Language is more social, and questions expand to "Why?" and "How come?" Phonetically similar words such as "die" and "dye" or "wood" and "would" might cause confusion in preschool children. Avoid such words when you prepare children for procedures, and assess their comprehension of explanations.

Psychosocial Changes

The world of preschoolers expands beyond the family into the neighbourhood, where children meet other children and adults. Their curiosity and developing initiative lead to the active exploration of the environment, the development of new skills, and the making of new friends. Preschoolers have much energy, which enables them to plan and attempt many activities that may be beyond their capabilities, such as pouring milk into their cereal bowls. Guilt arises within children when they overstep the limits of their abilities and feel they have not behaved correctly. Children who in anger have wished their sibling were dead experience guilt if that sibling becomes ill. Children need to be taught that "wishing" for something to happen does not make it occur. Parents should allow preschoolers to perform tasks on their own but must set firm limits and provide guidance.

During times of stress or illness, preschoolers may revert to bedwetting or thumb-sucking and want the parents to feed, dress, and hold them. These dependent behaviours are often confusing and embarrassing to parents, who can benefit from your reassurance that they are the children's normal coping behaviours. You should provide experiences that these children can master. Such successes help children return to their prior level of independent functioning. As language skills develop, children should be encouraged to talk about their feelings. Play is also an excellent way for preschoolers to vent frustration or anger and is a socially acceptable way to deal with stress.

Play. Children become more social after their third birthday as they shift from parallel to associative play. Children playing together engage in similar if not identical activity; however, no division of labour or rigid organization or rules exist. Most 3-year-old children are able to play with one other child in a cooperative manner in which they make something or play designated roles such as mother and baby. By the age of 4 years, children play in groups of two or three, and by 5 years, the group has a temporary leader for each activity.

In many play activities, preschoolers display awareness of social context. Sex role identification is strengthening, and children most often assume roles of people of their own sex. Children frequently mimic or repeat social experiences. This tendency is especially significant in hospitalized children. Through play, children may express questions, fears, anger, and misunderstanding about their illnesses and care. Be alert to such clues, and ensure that children can play within energy limits. Play can provide a healthy outlet for frustration, especially when children have been subjected to painful or restrictive experiences against their will.

Imaginary play depends on children's memory of things they have seen or heard. This sociodramatic play involving other children occupies about a third of 5-year-old children's playtime. Pretending allows children to learn to understand others' points of view, develop skills in solving social problems, and become more creative. Some children have imaginary playmates, which are a sign of creativity and healthy development.

Health Risks

As fine and gross motor skills develop, children become more coordinated with better balance; nevertheless, falls and other accidents remain a leading cause of injury. Guidelines for injury prevention in toddlers also apply to preschoolers (see Table 23–4). You should alert parents of children in this age group to the risks of poisoning and pedestrian–motor vehicle accidents. The leading cause of death in Canadian children is unintentional injury. All of these injuries are preventable. Children should be taught about safety in the home, and this teaching should be reinforced early in elementary school.

Health Concerns

Nutrition. Nutrition requirements for preschoolers vary little from those for toddlers. The average daily intake is 1800 calories. Parents may nonetheless worry about the amount of food their child is consuming. In most situations, however, the quality of the food is more important than quantity. Preschoolers consume about half of the average adult portions. Finicky eating habits are characteristic of 4-year-olds; in contrast, 5-year-olds are more interested in trying new foods. It is important to monitor children's food intake because obesity may be evident first in preschool years (Leitch, 2007).

Sleep. Preschoolers average 12 hours of sleep a night and take infrequent naps. Sleep disturbances are common during these years. Disturbances may range from trouble getting to sleep to nightmares to prolonging bedtime with extensive rituals. Many preschoolers have had an overabundance of activity and stimulation during the day. Having children follow a set routine before bedtime helps them prepare for sleep.

Vision. Preschoolers should routinely be screened for vision problems. One of the common problems in the preschool period is amblyopia (blindness from disuse of an eye if a child has untreated strabismus). Early detection and treatment can improve vision for most children (Hockenberry & Wilson, 2007).

School-Age Children and Adolescents

School-age children and adolescents lead demanding, challenging lives. The changes that occur between 6 and 19 years of age are diverse and span all areas of growth and development. Physical, psychosocial, cognitive, and moral skills are developed, expanded, refined, and synchronized. The environment in which the individual develops skills also expands and diversifies. Instead of only family and close friends, the environment now may include the school, community, and religious institution. Because of expectations for development, increasing skill and knowledge base, and environmental expansion, the individual experiences new difficulties and dilemmas. With age-specific assessment, review the appropriate developmental expectations for each age group. For example, before assessing risk-taking behaviours, recognize that adolescents normally strive to achieve a sense of identity while developing a moral code compatible with society.

Direct school-age children and adolescents toward normal developmental behaviours, assisting them in improving their abilities and using them to cope. Table 23–5 provides an overview of developmental behaviours typical of school-age children and adolescents. You must also increasingly involve children or adolescents in charting a developmental course. Not only can they describe their feelings about the changes but also they can think through these changes. Problem solving becomes more purposeful and sophisticated and results in the achievement of the outcomes that they desire. This paced, active participation may initiate a style of involvement in lifelong self-care.

School-age children and adolescents must cope with many changes, and these changes can be a source of stress for children. For example, 6-year-old children beginning school are confronted with new authority figures, teachers, and new rules and restrictions. They need to work and play cooperatively with a large group of children of various cultural backgrounds. School-age children must meet the challenge of developing cognitive skills that enhance their reasoning and allow them to learn to read, write, and manipulate numbers. Because of the stress of these changes, children may develop physical and psychosocial health problems (e.g., increased susceptibility to upper respiratory infections, inadequate peer relationships, or poor performance in school). Design health promotion interventions that are based on an individual child's developmental stage.

TABLE 23-5 Developmental Behaviours of School-Age Children and Adolescents

School-Age Children	Adolescents
Relationships With Parents	
Children gradually learn that parents are less than perfect; children can become disillusioned with parents and wish that friends' parents were their own. They still rely on parents for unconditional love, security, guidance, and nurturing.	Adolescents desire increasing independence and autonomy and yet continue needing some dependence and limit setting by parents; this conflict places strain on the parent–child relationship. Effective communication and democratic parenting are the best tools for meeting this challenge.
Relationships With Siblings	
Siblings seem to be at odds with one another at home, and yet they tend to be each other's best defenders away from home. Younger children often idolize older siblings, and this frequently leads to competition. Older children may envy attention that younger siblings require and can be quite bossy and somewhat abusive.	Younger siblings rarely understand their adolescent siblings' need for privacy. Adolescents often enjoy interacting with and guiding younger brothers and sisters when timing is convenient for them and they can remain in control.
Relationships With Peers	
During primary grades (6–7 years), children of both sexes play together, depending on who is available and interested. Around age 8, social groupings of same-sex peers form. These groups allow children to declare their independence from parental rules and establish their own rules of membership and behaviour. Preadolescent (ages 10–12 years) friendships are characterized by having a best friend of the same sex. These relationships may be transient, but they are intense and allow discussion of all areas of life. Childhood "crushes" are common.	Peer group is of critical influence on adolescents, who increasingly need recognition and acceptance. Companionship offered by peer groups provides a secure environment for individuals to try out new ideas and share similar feelings and attitudes. Adolescents often form cliques with peers with similar interests from the same socioeconomic group. Cliques, which are highly exclusive, help their members develop their identities.
Self-Concept	
Children's feelings of competence regarding mastery of tasks are key elements in forming self-esteem. Children need to receive positive feedback regarding their efforts. It is important for children to develop skills in at least one area such as reading, music, or swimming.	Formal and informal peer groups are a primary force in shaping self-concept of group members. Popularity and recognition within the peer group enhance self-esteem and reinforce self-concept. Total immersion in the peer group may make it appear that adolescents have no original thoughts and are incapable of making decisions. Adolescents who withdraw from peers into isolation struggle with developing identity.
Fears	
Fears related to body safety decline. Fears of supernatural beings such as ghosts and witches persist and decline slowly. New fears related to school and family occur. Children fear ridicule from teachers and friends and disapproval and rejection of parents. They also become frightened about death and events that they hear on the news, such as war and destruction of the environment.	Fears in this age group centre on peer group acceptance, body changes, loss of self-control, and emerging sexual urges. Adolescents constantly examine their bodies for changes and signs of imperfection. Any defect, real or imagined, is a cause of endless worry.
Coping Patterns	
To deal with stress, school-age children use problem solving and defence mechanisms such as denial and aggression. Several categories of coping behaviours of hospitalized school-aged children include inactivity (total silence, lack of activity, and apathy), orientation or precoping (looking and listening, walking around and exploring, and asking questions), cooperation (compliance with care), resistance (attempt to get away from the situation by turning away or making physical or verbal attacks), and controlling (assuming responsibility for self-care and suggesting how things could be done).	Coping behaviours expand with experiences adolescents have gained from life and from developing cognitive maturity. By age 15, most adolescents use a full range of defence mechanisms, including rationalization and intellectualization. Adolescents' problem-solving abilities have matured, and they can reason through philosophical discussions and complex situations that require abstract thinking and proposition of hypotheses. Some adolescents use avoidance coping strategies in which a problem is denied or repressed and an attempt is made to reduce tension by engaging in substance abuse or avoiding people.
Morals	
Children learn rules from parents, but their understanding of rules or reasons for them is limited until about age 10 years. Before that, they are concerned with their own needs first and may cheat to win games. After 10 years of age, they advocate justice and believe that punishment should fit the crime (e.g., if children break something, they should pay to have it fixed).	According to Kohlberg (1964), as youths approach adolescence, they reach conventional level, where internalization of expectations of their family and society begins. Initially, youths exhibit considerable conformity to rules to win praise or approval from others and to avoid social disapproval or rejection; later, they seek to avoid criticism from people of authority in institutions.

➤ TABLE 23-5 Developmental Behaviours of School-Age Children and Adolescents *continued*	
Diversional Activities	
School-age children play cooperatively in group activities such as sports and jumping rope. Play becomes competitive, and children often have difficulty learning to accept losing. Teasing, insults, dares, superstitions, and increased sensitivity are characteristics of this age.	Many teenagers develop special interests in certain sports and concentrate on developing maximal skills therein. Recreational activities are often determined by what is popular with peers and what can provide independence from parents (e.g., computers, cars).
Nutrition	
Children have definite likes and dislikes. Few nutritional deficiencies occur in this age group. Children have voracious appetites after school and need quality snacks such as fruit and sandwiches to avoid empty-calorie foods such as chips and candy.	Total nutritional needs become greater during adolescence. Girls' caloric needs decrease, and their need for protein increases slightly. Adolescents need to increase their consumption of iron-rich foods, and growth spurts increase calcium demand.

School-Age Child

During these "middle years" of childhood, the foundation for adult roles in work, recreation, and social interaction is laid. In industrialized countries, this period begins when children start formal schooling at about the age of 6 years. **Puberty**, which occurs at about 12 years of age, signals the end of middle childhood. Great developmental strides are made during these years as children develop competencies in physical, cognitive, and psychosocial skills.

The school or educational experience expands children's world and is a transition from a life of relatively free play to a life of structured play, learning, and work. The school and home influence growth and development, necessitating adjustment by parents and children. Children must learn to cope with rules and expectations presented by the school and peers. Parents must learn to allow their children to make decisions, accept responsibility, and learn from life's experiences.

Physical Changes

The rate of growth during these early school years is slower than at any time since birth but continues steadily. A particular child may not follow the pattern precisely. School-age children appear slimmer than preschoolers as a result of changes in fat distribution and thickness (Edelman & Mandle, 2006). Growth accelerates at different times for different children. The average increase in height is 5 cm per year, and weight, which is more variable, increases by 1.8 to 3.2 kg per year. An average 6-year-old is 112.5-cm tall and weighs 20.9 kg; the average 12-year-old is 147.5-cm tall and weighs 40 kg. Many children double their weight during these middle childhood years (Hockenberry & Wilson, 2007).

School provides children with the opportunity to compare themselves with children of the same age. The physical examination is an excellent opportunity to discuss with a child and parents the influences of genetic endowment, nutrition, and exercise on height and weight. Annual measurement of height and weight may reveal alterations in growth that are symptoms of the onset of a variety of childhood diseases.

Boys are slightly taller and heavier than girls during these early school years. Approximately 2 years before puberty, children experience a rapid acceleration in skeletal growth. Girls, who generally reach puberty first, begin to surpass boys in height and weight, which causes embarrassment to both sexes. In North America, puberty occurs between the ages of 9 and 13 years in girls and between the ages of 11 and 14 years in boys.

Cardiovascular functioning is refined and stabilized during the school years. The heart rate averages 75 to 100 beats per minute, the blood pressure normalizes to approximately 110/65 mm Hg, and the respiratory rate stabilizes to 20 to 30 breaths per minute. Lung growth is minimal, and respirations become slower, deeper, and more regular. However, by the end of this period, the heart is six times the size it was at birth and has generally reached its adult size.

School-age children become more graceful during the school years because their large-muscle coordination improves and their strength doubles. Most children practise the basic gross motor skills of running, jumping, balancing, throwing, and catching during play, which results in refinement of neuromuscular function and skills. Fine motor skills improve and as control is gained over fingers and wrists, children become proficient in a wide range of activities, although much individual difference exists in the rate and degree of proficiency.

Most 6-year-olds can hold a pencil adeptly and print letters and words. By age 12 years, children can make detailed drawings and write sentences in script. Activities such as painting, drawing, playing computer games, and making models allow children to practise and improve newly refined skills. Parents should encourage children to pursue these activities. Table 23–6 describes specific gross motor and fine motor skills and their use in self-care activities.

The improved fine motor capabilities of school-age children allow them to become very independent in bathing, dressing, and taking care of other personal needs. They develop strong personal preferences in the way these needs are met. Illness and hospitalization threaten children's control in these areas; therefore, it is important to allow them to participate in care and maintain as much independence as possible. For example, children whose care mandates restriction of fluids cannot be allowed to decide the amount of fluids they will drink in 24 hours, but they can help decide the type of fluids and can help keep a record of intake.

Assessment of neurological development is often based on fine motor coordination. This assessment may include penmanship, stacking ability, and performance of sequential, rapid, alternating movements such as touching the finger to the nose and then to the examiner's finger (smooth movement without tremors is the normal response). Fine motor coordination is crucial for academic success because children must be able to hold pencils and crayons, use scissors and rulers, and develop computer skills. The opportunity to practise these skills through schoolwork and play is essential for the acquisition of coordinated, complex behaviours.

Other physical changes take place during the school years. Steady skeletal growth in the trunk and extremities occurs, and small- and long-bone ossification is present but not complete by age 12 years. Dental growth is prominent during the school years. The first permanent or secondary teeth begin to erupt at approximately 6 years of age. Development of the permanent teeth has, however, been occurring for some time before eruption. The root of a primary tooth is absorbed, leaving the crown, which causes the tooth to become loose

TABLE 23-6 Average Motor Development in School-Age Children

Ages 6–7 Years	Ages 8–10 Years	Ages 11–12 Years
Fine Motor Skills		
Uses knife to butter bread and learns to cut tender meat	Uses knife and fork simultaneously	Learns to peel apples and potatoes
Cuts, folds, and pastes paper	Learns to thread needle and tie knot	Sews simple garments on machine
Prints with pencil	Uses hammer, saw, and screwdriver	Builds simple objects like birdhouse
Draws person with 12–16 details	Becomes proficient at cursive writing	Enjoys writing in decorative script
Copies triangle at age 6 years and diamond by age 7 years	Uses symbols in drawing (e.g., bird, star)	Begins to use creative and artistic talents
Colours within lines of picture	Builds simple models of cars and planes and does simple handicrafts	Builds complex models of cars and planes and does complex handicrafts
Needs assistance to clean teeth thoroughly	Can learn to floss teeth effectively and be independent in tooth care	Learns to play musical instrument
		Becomes proficient in caring for teeth with braces and other appliances
Gross Motor Skills		
Remains in constant motion when awake	Catches, throws, and hits a baseball	Can perform standing broad jump of 1.5 m
Moves more cautiously at age 7 years than at age 6 years	Engages in alternate rhythmic hopping	Can perform standing high jump of 1 m
Hops and jumps into small squares	Engages in complex styles of skipping rope while reciting verbal jingles	Engages in sports involving simultaneous use of two or more complex motor skills, such as ice skating, skateboarding, or playing hockey
Learns to roller skate, skip rope, ride a bicycle, and swim		
Self-Care		
Takes bath without supervision	Learns to clean bathroom after bath	Dusts, vacuums, and straightens own room
Often returns to finger feeding	Enjoys fixing own snacks and sack lunch	Learns to cook simply prepared foods
Learns to brush and comb hair in acceptable manner without help	Learns to part hair and insert barrettes	Washes, dries, and fixes own hair
Puts on most clothes but may need assistance with final adjustments	Dresses self completely and can help younger siblings with clothes	Learns to sort, wash, dry, and press own clothing
	Can make own bed	Learns to care for fingernails and toenails

and fall out, making room for the permanent tooth. Eruption of secondary teeth usually begins with the 6-year molars, and the others follow the same order as with the primary teeth. By 12 years, all primary teeth have been shed, and the majority of permanent teeth have erupted. Infrequent or inadequate dental care remains a persistent problem for many children.

As skeletal growth progresses, body appearance and posture change. Earlier posture, which was characterized by a stoop-shouldered, slight lordosis and prominent abdomen, changes to a more erect posture. It is essential that children, especially girls after the age of 12 years, be evaluated for scoliosis, the lateral curvature of the spine.

Eye shape alters because of skeletal growth. This improves visual acuity, and normal adult 20/20 vision is achievable. Screening for vision and hearing problems is easier, and results are more reliable because school-age children can more fully understand and cooperate with the test directions. The public health nurse typically assesses the dental, visual, and auditory status of school-age children and refers those with possible deviations to their family practitioner or pediatrician.

Cognitive Changes

Cognitive changes provide school-age children with the ability to think in a logical manner and to understand the relationship between things and ideas (Hockenberry & Wilson, 2007). The thoughts of school-age children are no longer dominated by their perceptions, and thus their ability to understand the world greatly expands. At about 7 years of age, children enter Piaget's (1952) third stage of cognitive development, known as **concrete operations**, in which they are able to use symbols to carry out operations (mental activities) in thought rather than in action. They begin to use logical thought processes with concrete materials (people, events, and objects they can touch and see).

Children in the concrete operational stage are considerably less egocentric than are younger children and develop the ability to concentrate on more than one aspect of a situation. School-age children now have the ability to recognize that the amount or quantity of a substance remains the same even when its shape or appearance changes. For instance, they can understand that two balls of clay of equal size retain the same amount of clay even when one is flattened and the other remains in ball shape.

The mental process of **classification** becomes more complex during the school years. Younger children can separate objects into groups according to shape or colour, whereas school-age children understand that the same element can exist in two classes at the same time. School-age children are becoming "thinkers" and are more capable of understanding another person's views and feelings (Santock, 2007).

In middle childhood, youngsters can use their newly developed cognitive skills to solve problems. Some individuals are better than others at problem solving because of intelligence level, education, and experience, but all children can improve these skills. Children who are good problem solvers demonstrate the following characteristics: a positive attitude that the problem can be solved with persistence, a concern for accuracy, the ability to divide the problem into parts for study, and the ability to avoid guessing while searching for facts. Adults can help children improve their problem-solving strategies by helping them define the problem, plan a solution, and then evaluate their solution. You can use these strategies to help hospitalized school-age children understand their illness and assume responsibility for their general health.

Language Development. Language growth is so rapid during middle childhood that these ages cannot be matched with language achievements. Children improve their use of language and expand their structural knowledge. They become more aware of the rules for linking words into phrases and sentences. They can also identify generalizations and exceptions to rules. They accept language as a means for representing the world in a subjective manner and realize that words have arbitrary, rather than absolute, meanings. They can use different words for the same object or concept, and they understand that a single word may have many meanings. Like younger children, school-age children watch parents and other adults to obtain clues about how to understand events (Santock, 2007). Many school-age children use "bad language" to gain peer status and to shock adults. It often begins with bathroom language and progresses to sexual or genital words. Children begin to think about language, which enables them to appreciate jokes and riddles. Language acquisition is nurtured by social interactions with their parents and caretakers.

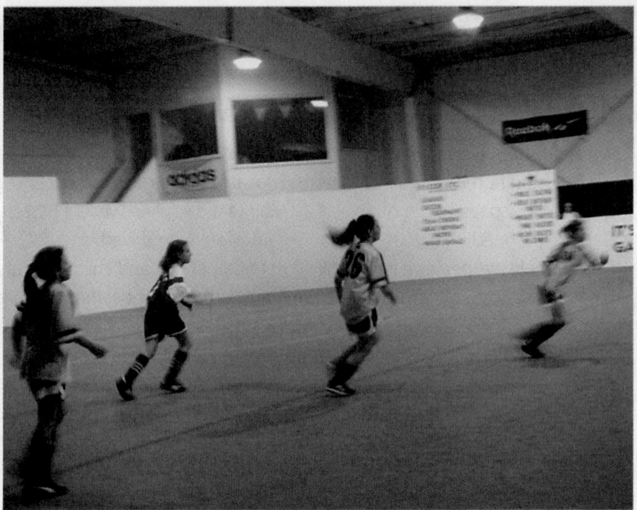

Figure 23-6 School-age children gain a sense of achievement by working and playing with peers. **Source:** Courtesy Elaine Polan, RNC, BSN, MS.

Psychosocial Changes

Erikson (1963) identified the developmental task for school-age children as industry versus inferiority (see Chapter 22). During this time, children strive to acquire competence and skills necessary for them to function as adults. School-age children who are positively recognized for success feel a sense of worth. Those faced with failure can feel a sense of unworthiness, which may result in withdrawal from school activities and peers.

Moral Development. The need for a moral code and social rules becomes more evident as school-age children's cognitive abilities and social experiences increase. For example, 12-year-old children are able to consider what society would be like without rules because of their ability to reason logically and their experiences with group play. They view rules as necessary principles of life, not just dictates from authorities. In the early school years, children strictly interpret and adhere to rules. As they grow older, their judgements become more flexible and they can evaluate rules for applicability to a given situation. School-age children consider motivations and behaviour when making judgements about the way their behaviours affect themselves and others. The abilities to be flexible when applying rules and to take the perspective of other people are essential in developing moral judgements. These abilities are present at times in earlier years but are more consistently displayed in later school years.

Peer Relationships. Group and personal achievements are important to school-age children. Success is important in physical and cognitive activities. Play involves peers and the pursuit of group goals. Although solitary activities are not eliminated, they are overshadowed by group play. Learning to contribute, collaborate, and work cooperatively toward a common goal becomes a measure of success (Figure 23–6).

School-age children prefer same-sex peers to opposite-sex peers. In general, girls and boys view the opposite sex negatively. Peer influence becomes diverse during this stage of development. Conformity is evidenced in mannerisms, clothing styles, and speech patterns, which are reinforced and influenced by contact with peers. During this period, clubs and peer groups become prominent. Group identity increases as school-age children approach adolescence.

Sexual Identity. Sigmund Freud described middle childhood as the *latency period* because he believed that children of this age had little interest in their sexuality. Today, many researchers believe that school-age children have a great deal of curiosity about their sexuality. Some may experiment, but this play is usually temporary. Children's curiosity about adult magazines or meanings of sexually explicit words is also an example of their sexual interest. This is the time for children to have exposure to sex education, including information on sexual maturation, reproduction, and relationships (Edelman & Mandle, 2006).

Health Risks

Accidents and injuries are major health problems affecting school-aged children. Motor vehicle accidents and accidents related to recreational activities or equipment are the leading causes of death or injury from the age of 1 year to adulthood (Edelman & Mandle, 2006). Unintentional injuries account for nearly half of all childhood deaths (Table 23–7).

Although falls account for a major portion of pediatric hospital admissions, they account for less than 5% of pediatric deaths resulting from injury. However, even though an accident may not result in death, it still can be a major cause of disability in children. More children die from automobile accidents than from all major preventable childhood diseases. The rates of injury and death decreased since the institution of automobile child restraint laws.

School-age children are also significantly affected by respiratory illnesses, especially asthma, cancer, and heart disease (Hockenberry & Wilson, 2007). In this age group, these problems have a relatively low mortality rate but a high morbidity rate in comparison with accidents. Cancers are the second leading cause of death in children 5 to 14 years of age (Hockenberry & Wilson, 2007). Leukemia is the most frequent type, and brain tumours and lymphoma are second and third, respectively.

Infections account for the majority of all childhood illnesses; respiratory infections are the most prevalent. The common cold remains the chief illness of childhood. Children living in poverty are more prone to disease and disability. Intellectual disabilities, learning disorders, sensory impairments, and malnutrition are far more prevalent among children living in poverty (Campaign 2000, 2007).

Poverty and the prevalence of illness are highly correlated, probably because access to health promotion and preventive health care activities are minimal for children living in poverty. Poor nutrition and access to early intervention programs continue to be major health concerns for impoverished families. Education, social and health care reform, and environmental change are necessary to positively influence the health of children. Children's developing cognitive and psychomotor skills make it possible for them to become more involved in health promotion and the management of chronic illness.

TABLE 23-7 Injury Prevention for School-Age Children

Developmental Abilities Related to Risk of Injury	Injury Prevention
	Motor Vehicles
Is increasingly involved in activities away from home Is excited by speed and motion Can be reasoned with Does not always perceive injury risk Is easily distracted by environment	Educate child regarding proper use of seat belts while a passenger in a vehicle. Maintain discipline while a passenger in a vehicle (e.g., keep arms inside, do not lean against doors, do not interfere with driver). Remind parents and children that no one should ride in the bed of a pickup truck. Emphasize safe pedestrian behaviour. Insist that child wears safety apparel (e.g., helmet) when applicable, such as when riding a bicycle or using a skateboard, all-terrain vehicle, or snow machine.
	Drowning
Is apt to overdo activities May work hard to perfect a skill Is cautious but not fearful	Teach child to swim. Teach basic rules of water safety. Select safe and supervised places to swim. Check sufficient water depth for diving. Insist that child swims with a companion. Use an approved flotation device in water or boat. Learn cardiopulmonary resuscitation (CPR).
	Burns
Demonstrates increasing independence Enjoys trying new things	Make sure smoke detectors are in homes. et hot water temperatures (49°C–54°C) to avoid scald burns. Instruct child in behaviour in areas involving contact with potential burn hazards (e.g., gasoline, matches, bonfires or barbecues, lighter fluid, firecrackers, cigarette lighters, cooking utensils, chemistry sets). Instruct child to avoid climbing or flying kites around high-tension wires. Instruct child in proper behaviour in the event of fire (e.g., fire drills at home and school). Teach child safe cooking (use low heat; avoid frying; be careful of steam burns, scalds, or exploding foods, especially in microwave ovens). Teach children about the danger of fire, and instruct them that if their clothing is on fire, they should "stop," "drop," and "roll."
	Substance Abuse and Poisoning
May be easily influenced by peers Has strong allegiance to friends	Educate child regarding hazards of taking nonprescription drugs and chemicals, including tobacco and alcohol. Teach child to say "no" if he or she is offered illegal or dangerous drugs or alcohol. Keep potentially dangerous products in properly labeled receptacles, preferably locked and out of child's reach.
	Bodily Damage
Demonstrates increased physical skills Needs strenuous physical activity Is interested in acquiring new skills and perfecting attained skills Is daring and adventurous, especially with peers Frequently plays in hazardous places Confidence often exceeds physical capacity Desires group loyalty and has strong need for friends' approval Attempts hazardous feats Delights in physical activity Is likely to overdo activity Has growth in height that exceeds muscular growth and coordination	Help provide facilities for supervised activities. Encourage playing in safe places. Keep firearms safely locked up. Teach proper care of, use of, and respect for devices with potential danger (e.g., power tools). Teach children not to tease or surprise dogs, invade their territory, take dogs' toys, or interfere with dogs' feeding. Teach safety regarding use of corrective devices (glasses); if child wears contact lenses, monitor duration of wear to prevent corneal damage. Stress careful selection, use, and maintenance of sports and recreation equipment such as skateboards and in-line skates. Emphasize proper conditioning, safe practices, and use of safety equipment for sports or recreational activities. Caution against engaging in hazardous sports, such as those involving trampolines. Use safety glass and decals on large glassed areas, such as sliding glass doors. Use window guards to prevent falls. Teach stranger safety. Avoid personalized clothing in public places. Caution child to never go anywhere with a stranger. Have child tell parents if anyone makes child feel uncomfortable in any way. Always listen to child's concerns regarding others' behaviour. Teach child to say "no" when confronted with uncomfortable situations. Help child avoid carrying more than 10%–15% of body weight in a backpack, and teach child to always put backback on to evenly distribute weight; a light-weight backpack with wide shoulder straps, a waist strap, a padded back, and multiple compartments should be used.

Adapted from Hockenberry, M. J., & Wilson, D. (2007). *Wong's nursing care of infants and children* (8th ed., p. 733). St. Louis, MO: Mosby; and from KidsHealth. (2007). *Backpack safety.* Retrieved October 30, 2008, from http://kidshealth.org/parent/positive/learning/backpack.html

Health Concerns

During the school years, identity and self-concept become stronger and more individualized. School-age children are aware of their bodies and are sensitive about being exposed. Provide for privacy and offer explanations of common procedures. This approach helps foster children's self-esteem and lessens their fear of pain and intrusion (Hockenberry & Wilson, 2007).

Health Education. The school years are crucial for the acquisition of behaviours and health practices for a healthy adult life. Because cognition is advancing during the period, effective health education must be developmentally appropriate. Promotion of good health practices is a nursing responsibility. A comprehensive school health approach includes programs, activities, and services that take place in schools and their surrounding communities in order to enable children and youth to improve their health and develop to their fullest potential (*Canadian Consensus Statement,* 2007; Box 23–6).

School-age children should receive age-appropriate sexual health education that begins before the onset of sexual activity (Behrman et al., 2008). Other topic areas for elementary health education curricula include the promotion of adequate nutrition, oral hygiene, and regular health supervision. School-age children should also be educated about prevention of tobacco, drug, and alcohol use (Public Health Agency of Canada, 1999b).

Instruct parents regarding health promotion appropriate for school-age children. Parents need to recognize the importance of annual checkups for immunizations, screenings, and dental care. When school-age children reach 10 years of age, their parents need to talk with the children about upcoming pubertal changes. Topics should include introductory information regarding menstruation, sexual intercourse, and reproduction. Provide age-appropriate written materials to aid parents in their efforts. The settings in which health promotion activities can occur are varied: the classroom, a school-based clinic, a community-based clinic, or community settings such as a public library or community centre.

Table 23–8 presents a list of possible health promotion topics for school-age children.

➤ BOX 23-6 Critical Functions of Comprehensive School Health

A comprehensive approach to promoting health in schools includes the following:

- Promote healthy habits and illness prevention measures, with attention to multicultural, linguistic, physical, cognitive, and emotional factors.
- Intervene to assist children and youth who are in need or at risk.
- Help support children who are already experiencing poor health.
- Foster parental education on health issues.
- Identify learning disabilities early, and begin appropriate interventions to foster learning and self-esteem.
- Facilitate growth and self-actualization.
- Emphasize positive health attitudes.
- Foster positive life skills that enhance successful coping.
- Encourage physical activity.
- Encourage involvement of individuals, families, and communities as active partners in the health care of school-age children.

Adapted from Communities and Schools Promoting Health. *Canadian consensus statement (Revised 2007): Comprehensive school health.* Retrieved December 21, 2008, from http://www.safehealthyschools.org/CSH_Consensus_Statement2007.pdf

Safety. Because accidents are the leading cause of death and injury in school-age children, safety is a priority health teaching consideration. You can contribute to the general health of children by educating them about safety measures to prevent accidents. At this age, children should be encouraged to take responsibility for their own safety.

Nutrition. You can contribute to the promotion of healthy lifestyle habits, including nutrition. School-age children should participate in educational programs that enable them to plan, select, and prepare healthy meals and snacks. These foods should be consistent with the recommendations in *Canada's Food Guide* (Health Canada, 2007), which include limiting intake of fats and increasing intake of complex carbohydrates, fruits, and vegetables. Box 23–7 outlines several learning activities appropriate for this age group. In addition, encourage daily physical activity for all children.

Growth may slow down during the school years in comparison with infancy and adolescence. Obesity is the most common nutritional problem during childhood. Obesity is believed to begin during infancy and childhood (Edelman & Mandle, 2006). Obesity increases the risk for hypertension, diabetes, and coronary heart disease, but its emotional effects are less clear (Wardle & Cooke, 2005); some children with obesity are extremely dissatisfied with their bodies and have low self-esteem. Obesity may occur because children often rush into the home after school or play and eat the most easily obtainable and appealing foods. Unfortunately, these foods are often high in calories and low in nutrition. Providing nutritious snacks is often the best way for a parent to ensure good nutritional intake. Caregivers should provide ready access to fresh fruit, raw vegetables, cheese, popcorn, and high-protein snacks such as skim-milk pudding and hot chocolate. Consider cultural, economic, and social issues when planning successful eating interventions (Edelman & Mandle, 2006).

Help families and children prevent obesity through proper nutrition and exercise. Many families often eat in fast-food restaurants in which the food is high in fat, calories, and salt. Encourage healthy food choices in these situations. Selections should include meats that are not breaded and are broiled, shakes that are made with low-fat yogurt or skim milk, and fruits and vegetables that are fresh or prepared in a low-calorie manner.

Adolescent

Adolescence is the period of development between childhood and adulthood, usually between 12 and 19 years of age. The term *adolescent* usually refers to psychological maturation of the individual, whereas *puberty* is to the point at which reproduction becomes possible. The hormonal changes of puberty result in changes in the appearance of the young person: the primary sexual characteristic changes (maturation of the reproductive organs) and the secondary sexual characteristic changes (such as the development of pubic hair and female breasts). Mental development during puberty results in the ability to hypothesize and deal with abstractions. In addition, adolescents become much more social, and their behavioural patterns become much less predictable. Adjustments and adaptations are needed to cope with these simultaneous changes and the attempt to establish a mature sense of identity. Many people refer to adolescence as a stormy and stressful period filled with inner turmoil, but it is recognized that most teenagers successfully meet the challenges of this period. These challenges may cause adolescents to be moody and difficult. Within adolescence, three subphases exist: early adolescence, including puberty (ages 12 to 14 years), middle adolescence (ages 14

TABLE 23-8 Health Promotion for School-Age Children

School-Age Health Concerns	Health Promotion Interventions
Nutrition	Provide nutrition education that promotes healthy lifestyle: for example, limiting fat intake to 30% of calories, limiting saturated fat to 10% of calories, avoiding overeating.
Oral hygiene	Provide examples of low cariogenic snacks. Review mechanics of dental hygiene: brushing, flossing. Stress importance of biannual dental checkups.
Infections	Provide immunization information and follow-up. Teach infection prevention practices (handwashing, care of minor skin injuries). Teach concepts of viral and bacterial illness. Promote handwashing and regular bathing.
Tobacco, alcohol, and drug use	Provide programs in preventing tobacco use. Provide information regarding the hazards of alcohol and drug use.
Human sexuality	Provide information about sexual maturation and reproduction in age-appropriate manner. Encourage parents to view their children's sexual curiosity as part of the developmental process. Discuss with parents the learning needs of their children regarding sexuality. Provide age-appropriate sexual health education.

to 17 years), and late adolescence (ages 17 to 19 years). Opportunities, challenges, changes, skills, pressures, and physical, cognitive, and psychosocial development vary widely among the subphases (Table 23–9).

Your understanding of development provides a unique perspective for helping teenagers and parents anticipate and cope with the stresses of adolescence. Primary health care activities, particularly education, can promote healthy development. These activities occur in a variety of settings and can be directed at adolescents, parents, or both. For example, you can conduct seminars in a high school to provide practical suggestions for solving problems of concern to a large group of students, such as treating acne or making responsible decisions about drugs or alcohol use. Similarly, a group education program for parents about how to cope with teenagers would promote parental understanding of adolescent development. These programs can be held in the school, clinic, private office, or community centre. To learn more about specific topics or problems, you need to identify teenagers' needs and desires. Involvement produces more active, interested learners.

Physical Changes

Physical changes occur rapidly in adolescence. Sexual maturation occurs with the development of primary and secondary sexual characteristics. Four main focuses of the physical changes are as follows:

- Increased growth rate of skeleton, muscle, and viscera
- Sex-specific changes, such as changes in shoulder and hip width
- Alteration in distribution of muscle and fat
- Development of the reproductive system and secondary sex characteristics

The timing of physical changes associated with puberty varies widely between sexes and within the same sex. Girls tend to begin their physical changes earlier than boys. Variations are more pronounced in boys (Behrman et al., 2008). The sequence of pubertal growth changes is the same in most individuals (Table 23–10).

Changes are created by hormonal fluctuations within the body when the hypothalamus begins to produce gonadotropin-releasing hormones. This change sends the pituitary gland a signal to secrete gonadotropic hormones. Gonadotropic hormones stimulate ovarian cells to produce **estrogen** and testicular cells to produce **testosterone**. These hormones contribute to the development of secondary sex characteristics such as hair growth and voice changes and play an essential role in reproduction. The changing concentrations of these hormones are also linked to acne and body odour. Understanding these hormonal changes enables you to reassure adolescents and educate them about body care needs.

Boys who mature early have been shown by some researchers to be more poised, relaxed, good-natured, skilled in athletic activities, and more likely to be school leaders than are boys who mature late. In contrast, girls who mature early have been found to be less sociable and more shy and introverted, perhaps as a result of feeling so conspicuous (Edelman & Mandle, 2006). Such girls are more conscious of body development, such as breast development, and thus stand out from many of their peers.

Being like their peers is extremely important for adolescents. You need to stress that normal sexual changes are quite variable. As with

BOX 23-7 Interventions to Promote Education About Nutrition

- Include healthy eating as part of the education programs at school.
- Make healthy foods available in school vending machines and at school sporting or other events.
- Encourage nutritious and nonfood items for school fund-raising projects.
- Use positive messages to reinforce healthy eating and physical activity.
- Have teachers and school personnel model healthy eating habits.
- Limit access to unhealthy foods and beverages.
- Provide positive reinforcement for healthy food choices.
- Create a pleasant environment for eating.
- Promote safe food handling practices.
- Involve parents and the community in promoting healthy eating in schools.

Adapted from Knowledge Network. (n.d.). *Making it happen: Healthy eating at school.* Burnaby, BC: Author. Retrieved October 29, 2008, from http://www.knowledgenetwork.ca/news/2005/feb2005/Making%20It%20Happen.pdf

TABLE 23-9 Growth and Development During Adolescence

Early Adolescence (11–14 Years)	Middle Adolescence (14–17 Years)	Late Adolescence (17–20 Years)
Growth		
Rapidly accelerating growth reaches peak velocity. Secondary sex characteristics appear.	Growth decelerates in girls. Stature reaches 95% of adult height. Secondary sex characteristics are well advanced.	The body is physically mature. Structural and reproductive growth are almost complete.
Cognition		
The person explores newfound ability for limited abstract thought. The person experiences uncertainty when confronted with new values. One's "normality" is compared with that of peers of same sex.	Capacity for abstract thinking develops. Intellectual powers, often in idealistic terms, are increased. Concerns with philosophic, political, and social problems arise.	Abstract thought is established. The person can perceive and act on long-range operations. The person is able to view problems comprehensively. Intellectual and functional identity are established.
Identity		
The person is preoccupied with rapid body changes. The person tries out various roles. Attractiveness is measured by acceptance or rejection by peers. Conformity to group norms is typical.	Body image is modified. Person is very self-centred; narcissism is increased. Tendency toward inner experience and self-discovery develops. Fantasy life is rich. The person becomes idealistic. The person is able to perceive future implications. of current behaviour and decisions; variable. application.	Body image and gender role definition is nearly secured. Sexual identity is mature. Identity is consolidated. Self-esteem stabilizes. The person is comfortable with physical growth. Social roles are defined and articulated.
Relationships With Parents		
Independence–dependence boundaries are defined. The person has a strong desire to remain dependent on parents while trying to detach from them. No major conflicts over parental control occur.	Major conflicts over independence and control occur. This is the low point in parent–child relationship. The person makes the greatest push for emancipation and disengagement. Emotional detachment from parents is final and irreversible; mourning occurs.	Emotional and physical separation from parents are completed. Independence is achieved from family with less conflict. Emancipation is nearly secured.
Relationships With Peers		
The person seeks peer affiliations to counter instability generated by rapid change. The person experiences upsurge of close, idealized friendships with members of the same sex. Struggle for mastery takes place within peer group.	The person has a strong need for identity to affirm self-image. Behavioural standards are set by peer group. Acceptance by peers is extremely important; rejection is feared. The person explores ability to attract the opposite sex.	Peer group recedes in importance in favour of individual friendship. Male–female relationships are tested against possibility of permanent alliance. Relationships are characterized by giving and sharing.
Sexuality		
Self-exploration and evaluation occur. Dating is limited; the person usually socializes with a group. Intimacy is limited.	Multiple plural relationships are characteristic. The person decisively turns toward hetero-sexuality or homosexuality. "Self-appeal" is explored. Feeling of "being in love" is common. Relationships are tentatively established.	The person forms stable relationships and attachment to another person. Capacity for mutuality and reciprocity grows. Dating is common. Intimacy involves commitment rather than exploration and romanticism.
Psychological Health		
Wide mood swings occur. Intense daydreaming is characteristic. Anger is outwardly expressed with moodiness, temper outbursts, verbal insults, and name-calling.	Tendency toward inner experiences is exhibited; person becomes more introspective. The person tends to withdraw when upset or when feelings are hurt. Emotions vacillate in time and range. Feelings of inadequacy are common; asking for help is difficult.	The person experiences more constancy of emotion. Anger is more apt to be concealed.

Adapted from Hockenberry, M. J., & Wilson, D. (2007). *Wong's nursing care of infants and children* (8th ed., p. 813). St. Louis, MO: Mosby.

TABLE 23-10 Average Sequences of Physiological Changes in Adolescence

Characteristics	Age Range (Years) Girls	Boys
Beginning of skeletal growth spurt	8–14.5 (peak: 12)	10.5–16 (peak: 14)
Beginning of breast development	8–13	—
Enlargement of testes and scrotal sac	—	10–13.5
Appearance of straight, pigmented pubic hair, which gradually becomes curly	8–14	10–15
Early voice changes (cracks)	—	11–14.5
Enlargement of penis and prostate gland	—	11–14.5
Menarche	10–18 (average: 12.25)	—
Spermatogenesis (ejaculation of sperm)	—	11–17 (average: 13.5)
Ovulation and completion of breast development	14–18 (average: 15.52)	—
Appearance of downy facial hair	—	12–17
Appearance of axillary (underarm) hair and increased output of oil and sweat-producing glands, which may lead to acne	10–16	12–17
Widening and deepening of female pelvis, with deposition of subcutaneous fat that gives rounded appearance to body	10–18	—
Increase in shoulder width	—	11–21
Deepening of male voice, with appearance of coarse and pigmented facial hair and appearance of chest and axillary hair as well as other body hair becoming more prominent, such as that on forearms and legs	—	16–21

increases in height and weight, the pattern of sexual changes is more significant than their time of onset. Large deviations from normal patterns necessitate investigation.

Any deviation in the timing of the physical changes can be extremely difficult for adolescents to accept. Provide emotional support for those undergoing early or delayed puberty. Even adolescents whose physical changes are occurring at the normal times may seek reassurance about their normality.

Height and weight usually increase during the prepubertal growth spurt. The growth spurt for girls generally begins between 8 and 14 years of age. Height increases 5 to 20 cm, and weight increases by 7 to 25 kg. The growth spurt in boys usually occurs between 10 and 16 years of age. Height increases approximately 10 to 30 cm, and weight increases by 7 to 30 kg. In both sexes, the final 20% to 25% of adult height and 50% of adult weight are attained during this time (Hockenberry & Wilson, 2007).

Girls attain 90% to 95% of their adult height by **menarche** (the onset of menstruation) and reach their full height by 16 to 17 years of age, whereas boys continue to grow taller until 18 to 20 years of age. Fat is redistributed into adult proportions as height and weight increase, and gradually the adolescent torso takes on an adult appearance. Despite individual and sex differences, growth follows a similar pattern for both sexes. Growth in the length of the extremities occurs earliest, making the hands and feet appear very large and the legs very long; the individual often appears awkward and clumsy. At the same time, the lower jaw and nose become longer and the forehead higher and wider as the baby face of childhood disappears. Next, the thighs widen; then the shoulders broaden, and growth of the trunk proceeds. The female hips widen and the male shoulders broaden throughout adolescence.

Personal growth curves help you assess physical development. The individual's sustained progression along the curve, however, is more important than a comparison of measurements with the norm. To evaluate changes, you should chart growth measurements during routine health assessments.

Adolescents are sensitive about physical changes that make them different from peers. For this reason, they are generally interested in the normal pattern of growth and in their personal growth curves. Therefore, you should share this information to reassure adolescents that their own patterns are normal.

Cognitive Changes

According to Piaget (1952), the changes that occur within the mind and the widening social environment of adolescents result in the highest level of intellectual development, known as **formal operations** (see Chapter 22). However, without an appropriate educational environment, some people may not attain this stage. Those who are guided toward rational thinking may reach this stage early.

Adolescents develop the ability to determine possibilities, rank possibilities, solve problems, and make decisions through logical operations. The teenager can deal effectively with hypothetical problems. When confronted with a problem, the teenager is able to consider an infinite variety of causes and solutions. Adolescents can move beyond the physical or concrete properties of a situation and use reasoning powers to understand the abstract. School-age children think about what is, whereas adolescents can imagine what might be. These newly developed abilities allow the individual to have more insight and skill in playing video games, computer games, and board games that necessitate abstract thinking and deductive reasoning about many possible strategies. A teenager can solve problems by simultaneously manipulating several abstract concepts.

Development of this ability to reason abstractly is important in the pursuit of an identity. For example, newly acquired cognitive skills enable the teenager to define appropriate, effective, and comfortable sex role behaviours and to consider their impact on peers, family, and society. The ability to think logically about these behaviours and their outcomes encourages adolescents to develop personal thoughts and means of expressing sexual identity. In addition, because their level of cognitive functioning is higher, adolescents are receptive to more detailed and diverse information about sexuality and sexual behaviours. For example, sex education can include an explanation of physiological sexual changes and birth control measures.

By middle adolescence, an introspective quality emerges. At this time, adolescents believe that they are unique. They also may believe, because of their new physical skills, that they are invulnerable, and so they engage in risk-taking behaviours: Many state that they "can drive fast and not get into an accident." Other typical adolescent behaviours include self-consciousness and the desire for privacy.

The complex development of thought during this period leads adolescents to question society and its values. Although adolescents have the capability to think as logically as adults, they do not yet have experiences from which gain perspective. It is common for teenagers to consider their parents too narrow-minded or too materialistic. This perception can result in conflicts between teenagers and their parents. Cognitive abilities and performance vary greatly among adolescents. In fact, an adolescent may perform at different levels in different situations on the basis of past experiences, formal education, and motivation in the use of logic and effective deductive reasoning.

Language Skills. Language development is fairly complete by adolescence, although vocabulary continues to expand. The primary focus becomes communication skills that can be used effectively in various situations. Adolescents need to communicate thoughts, feelings, and facts to others. The skills used in communication situations are varied. Adolescents must select the person with whom to communicate, decide on the message, and choose the way to transmit the message. For example, the way teenagers tell parents about failing grades is not the same as the way that they tell friends. Adolescents develop different skills and styles of communication and learn how and when to use them most effectively. These diverse communication skills are used and refined throughout life (Santock, 2007). Good communication skills are crucial for overcoming peer pressure and unhealthy behaviours. The following are some hints for communicating with adolescents:

- Do not avoid discussing sensitive issues. Asking questions about sex, drugs, and school demonstrates your interest in their well-being and may open the channels for further discussion.
- Ask open-ended questions.
- Try to discern the meaning behind their words or actions.
- Be alert to clues to their emotional state.
- Involve other individuals and resources when necessary.

Psychosocial Changes

The search for personal identity is the major characteristic of adolescent psychosocial development. Teenagers must establish close peer relationships or risk remaining socially isolated. Erikson (1963) viewed identity (or role) confusion as the prime danger of this stage and suggested that the cliquishness and intolerance of differences seen in adolescent behaviour are defences against identity confusion (Erikson, 1968). Adolescents work at becoming emotionally independent from their parents, while retaining family ties. In addition, they need to develop their own ethical systems that are based on personal values. Choices about vocation, future education, and lifestyle must be made. The various components of identity evolve from these stages and compose a total adult personal identity that is unique to the individual. Indecisiveness and the inability to make an occupational choice are behaviours indicating the lack of resolution to certain developmental tasks.

Gender Identity. Achievement of gender identity is enhanced by the physical changes of puberty. According to Freud, these physiological changes of puberty stimulate the libido, the energy source that fuels the sex drive (see Chapter 22). This change is evidenced by teenagers' interest in romantic relationships, as well as by their practice of masturbation. The physical evidence of maturity encourages the development of masculine and feminine behaviours. If these physical changes involve deviations, the person has more difficulty developing a comfortable sexual identity. Adolescents depend on these physical clues because they want assurance of maleness or femaleness and because they do not wish to be different from peers.

Other influences on gender identity are cultural attitudes and expectations of sex role behaviour and available role models. The masculine and feminine behaviours that teenagers see affect the way that they express sexuality.

Group Identity. Adolescents seek a group identity because they need esteem and acceptance (Figure 23–7). Similarity in dress, speech, or both is common in teenage groups. Popularity is a major concern for teenagers. Peer groups provide adolescents with a sense of belonging, approval, and the opportunity to learn acceptable behaviour. Popularity with both opposite-sex and same-sex peers is important. The strong need for group identity seems to conflict at times with the search for personal identity. It is as though adolescents require close bonds with peers so that they can later achieve a sense of individuality.

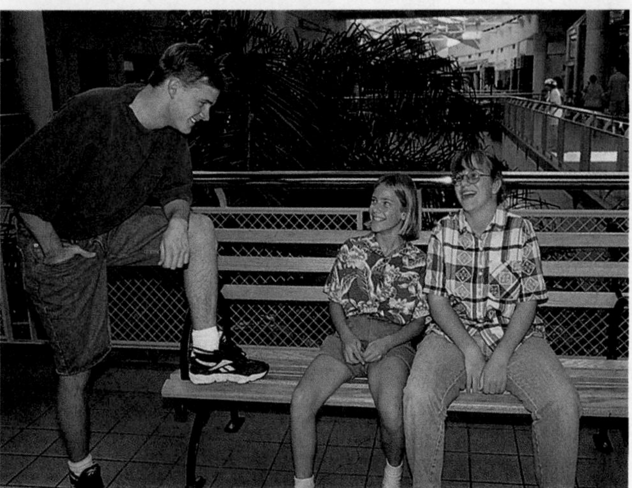

Figure 23-7 Social interactions strengthen a teenager's group identity.
Source: Courtesy Elaine Polan, RNC, BSN, MS.

Family Identity. The movement toward stronger peer relationships contrasts with adolescents' movements away from parents. Although financial independence for adolescents is not the norm in Canadian society, many adolescents work part-time, using their income to bolster independence. When adolescents cannot have a part-time job because of studies, school-related activities, and other factors, parents can provide allowances for clothing and incidentals, which encourage adolescents to develop decision-making and budgeting skills.

Some adolescents and families have more difficulty during these years than others. Adolescents need to make choices, act independently, and experience the consequences of actions. This testing, however, is best done against the background of firm family support. The family needs to allow independence while providing a haven in which adolescents can contemplate actions. Families unable to provide this support complicate movement toward identity formation. Health care support of a family and an adolescent may be essential to their success.

Assist families in considering ways that are appropriate for them to foster the independence of their adolescent while maintaining family structure. Many of these discussions involve curfews, jobs, and participation in family chores. Emancipation from the immediate family is most successful when accomplished gradually and results in a balance between independence and family ties.

Vocational Identity. Selecting an occupation or a vocational direction in life is a goal for adolescents. Because of society's changing needs, adolescents must be future oriented when making these choices. However, adolescents do not know which jobs will be available and rewarding 10 or 20 years in the future, and selecting a career is thus a complicated task. You need to be supportive to the family during this process and help adolescents select courses of action that promote self-satisfaction, identity, and continued opportunity for growth.

Moral Identity. The development of moral judgement depends heavily on cognitive and communication skills and peer interaction. Although moral development begins in early childhood, it is consolidated in adolescence because of the presence of certain skills. Adolescents learn that rules are cooperative agreements that can be modified to fit the situation, rather than absolute. Adolescents learn to use their own judgement rather than to use the rules to avoid punishment as in earlier years. Kohlberg (1964) explained moral development in terms of stages (see Chapter 22). At the highest level, morality is derived from individual principles of conscience. Adolescents judge themselves by internalized ideals, which often leads to conflict between personal and group values. Group values become less significant in later adolescence.

Not all adolescents attain the same level of moral development; however, they generally advance through the stages of moral development, and the sequence of the stages is similar for all individuals, even though the time at achievement varies. Kohlberg's (1964) moral development theory focuses on justice based on reciprocity and equal respect. Adolescent girls have been found to be more likely to give caring responses to moral problems, whereas adolescent boys have been found to give more justice-oriented responses (Gilligan, 1982).

Health Identity. Healthy adolescents evaluate their own health according to feelings of well-being, ability to function normally, and absence of symptoms (Hockenberry & Wilson, 2007).

Interventions to improve health perception might, therefore, concentrate on the adolescent period. The rapid changes during this period make primary health care programs especially crucial. Adolescents try new roles, begin to stabilize their identity, and acquire values and behaviours from which their adult lifestyle will evolve.

Health Risks

Injuries. Injuries, including self-inflicted injuries and injuries caused by motor vehicle accidents and poisoning, are the leading causes of death in adolescents (Pan et al., 2007). Feelings of being indestructible lead to risk-taking behaviour. Many injuries are preceded by the use of alcohol (Pickett et al., 2005). Youths continue to be both the victims and perpetrators of violence.

Suicide. Suicide is increasing as a cause of death in adolescents between 15 and 19 years of age. Depression and social isolation commonly precede a suicide attempt, but suicidal thoughts probably result from a combination of several factors (Box 23–8).

You must be able to identify the factors associated with adolescent suicide risk and precipitating events. In addition, you should be alert

> **BOX 23-8 Suicide Risk Assessment**
>
> **History**
>
> Previous suicide attempt
> Suicide attempt by family member or friend
> History of child maltreatment
> Past psychiatric hospitalization
> Death of a parent when child was young
>
> **Individual Factors**
>
> Hopelessness
> Marked, persistent depression
> Alcohol or drug abuse
> Impulsiveness
> Difficulty tolerating frustration
> Feelings of self-hatred, excessive guilt, or humiliation
> Thinking disorder (wishes to join a deceased person, hears voices telling to kill self)
> Physical problems or problems with body image (delayed puberty, chronic illness, disability, attention deficit–hyperactivity disorder, learning disorders)
> Gender identity concerns; being gay or lesbian in an unsupportive environment
> Seeing self as totally helpless: a victim of fate
> Needing to do things perfectly
>
> **Family Factors**
>
> Difficult home situation: long, bitter parent–child conflict
> Hostile parents
> Overt rejection by one or both parents
> Divorce or separation of parents
> Recent or impending move
> Family breakup or loss of parent
> Stress of unrealistically high parental expectations
> Parental indifference with very low expectations
>
> **Social and Environmental Factors**
>
> Firearms in the home
> Incarceration
> Lack of effective social support system
> Isolation
> Suicide of someone known
> Few social, vocational, educational opportunities
>
> Adapted from Hockenberry, M. J., & Wilson, D. (2007). *Wong's nursing care of infants and children* (8th ed., p. 912). St. Louis, MO: Mosby.

to the following warning signs, which often occur for at least a month before suicide is attempted:

- Deterioration in school performance
- Social withdrawal
- Loss of initiative
- Loneliness, sadness, and crying
- Appetite and sleep disturbances
- Verbalization of suicidal thought

Immediate referrals to mental health professionals are needed when assessment findings suggest that adolescents may be considering suicide. Guidance can help them focus on the positive aspects of life and strengthen coping abilities.

Substance Abuse. Adolescents may believe that mood-altering substances create a sense of well-being or improve level of performance. All adolescents are at risk for experimental or recreational substance use, but those who have dysfunctional families are more at risk for chronic use and physical dependency. Some adolescents believe that substance use makes them more mature. They further believe that they will look and feel better with drug usage. Alcohol is the substance most commonly used, followed by cannabis. Other substances frequently abused by teenagers include steroids, which are used to enhance their athletic performances. It is believed that the use of these products may increase the likelihood of using other illicit drugs (Canadian Centre on Substance Abuse, 2007). Tobacco use, although decreasing, continues to be a problem among adolescents.

Eating Disorders. The number of eating disorders is on the rise in adolescents, particularly girls, and knowledge of growth progression may be a way to discourage radical weight reduction activities. If an adolescent's growth deviates radically from the usual pattern, further assessment is necessary to identify the cause. Areas to include in the assessment are past and present diet history, food records, eating habits, attitudes, health beliefs, and socioeconomic and psychosocial factors (Hockenberry & Wilson, 2007). Weight extremes resulting from excessive or inadequate caloric intake are common during the adolescent years. Allowing an adolescent to see when and how the weight curve changed can be a first step in identifying the problem and implementing dietary changes.

Although anorexia nervosa and bulimia are classified as separate eating disorders, manifestations of the two significantly overlap (Health Canada, 2002). Anorexia nervosa is considered a clinical syndrome with both physical and psychosocial components. The majority of clients are adolescents and young women. Attending a highly competitive high school and being from a professional, upper-middle-class family increase the risk for this disorder. People with anorexia nervosa have an intense fear of gaining weight and refuse to maintain body weight at the normal minimum for their age and height.

Bulimia nervosa is most identified with binge eating and behaviours to prevent weight gain, including self-induced vomiting, misuse of laxatives and other medications, and excessive exercise (Hockenberry & Wilson, 2007). Because adolescents rarely volunteer information about behaviours to prevent weight gain, it is important to take a thorough dietary history. Society's expectations for thinness may have a strong influence on the development of these eating disorders. Eating disorders are thought to be more common among girls, but it is important to note that boys may suffer from these disorders as well. Causes of eating disorders are the same for both girls and boys.

Obesity and Physical Inactivity. Overweight and obesity, together with a decrease in physical activity, are becoming serious public health problems in Canada. In adolescents aged 12 to 17 years, rates of overweight have doubled and rates of obesity have tripled since the 1990s (Leitch, 2007). A contributing factor is a lack of physical activity; children and adolescents spend more time watching television and using computers, especially engaging in playing computer games. Parents and other people working with adolescents must encourage greater physical activity among this age group, must monitor computer use, and must promote healthy nutrition.

Sexual Experimentation. Sexual experimentation is common among adolescents. Peer pressure, physiological and emotional changes, and societal expectations contribute to early heterosexual and homosexual relations. Two prominent consequences of adolescent sexual activity are sexually transmitted infections and pregnancy (Sex Facts in Canada, 2006).

Sexually Transmitted Infections. The incidence of **sexually transmitted infections (STIs)** reported is increasing in adolescents (Sex Facts in Canada, 2006). Therefore, sexually active adolescents must be screened for STIs, even when they have no symptoms, because STIs can be asymptomatic. The annual physical examination of a sexually active adolescent should include a thorough sexual and genitourinary history and a careful examination of the genitalia so that genital warts, herpes, and other STIs are not missed. Recommended tests for women include Papanicolaou (Pap) smears, cervical cultures for gonorrhea and *Chlamydia* species, and syphilis tests; for men, urethral cultures for gonorrhea and *Chlamydia* species and syphilis tests are recommended. If men have participated in homosexual activities, rectal and pharyngeal cultures also need to be taken to check for gonorrhea. Because the human papillomavirus is a common STI, in some provinces adolescent girls are given a vaccine that is effective against some human papillomaviruses associated with cervical cancer (Public Health Agency of Canada, 2007). The health care professional can be proactive by using the client interview process to identify risk factors in adolescents. Once identified, the risk factors should lead to strategies for prevention.

The human immunodeficiency virus (HIV), which causes acquired immune deficiency syndrome (AIDS), is transmitted through unprotected sexual intercourse, the use of shared needles, and infected blood products (see Chapter 27). Therefore, the risk-taking behaviours of sexual activity and drug use make adolescents vulnerable to the threat of AIDS and other STIs. Adolescents who have placed themselves at risk for AIDS should be tested for HIV infection. All adolescents need improved knowledge about HIV and AIDS.

Pregnancy. Adolescent pregnancy occurs across socioeconomic classes, in public and private schools, among all ethnic and religious backgrounds, and in all parts of the country. Adolescent pregnancy with early prenatal supervision is considered less physically harmful to both mother and child than earlier believed. Pregnant teenagers need special education about nutrition, as well as health supervision and psychological support.

Health Concerns

Adolescents must form healthy habits of daily living. You need to emphasize the importance of exercise, sleep, nutrition, and stress reduction and to identify ways to adapt them to each adolescent. To do this, you must assess the individual's positive and negative habits and attitudes about health. Extensive and long-term follow-up is required if individualized interventions are to succeed. You must be aware of the prevalence of health problems and make assessments accordingly.

Health Education. Community and school-based health programs for adolescents focus on health promotion and illness prevention. You can become involved in community health through screening and teaching programs (Table 23–11).

➤ TABLE 23-11 Health Promotion for Adolescents	
Adolescent Health Concerns	**Health Promotion Intervention**
Unintentional injuries	Advise adolescent to take a driver's education course and to wear seat belts. Inform the adolescent of risk associated with drinking and driving and with use of drugs. Promote helmet use by adolescents who use bicycles, motorcycles, all-terrain vehicles, and snow machines. Ensure adolescent receives proper orientation in the use of all sports equipment. Encourage adolescent to swim with a "buddy."
Firearm use and violence	Teach conflict resolution skills.
Tobacco, alcohol, and drug use	Screen for tobacco (including smokeless), alcohol, and drug use, and inform adolescent of the risks of use.
Suicide	Offer suicide prevention information. Teach methods of dealing with a suicidal peer. Promote suicide alternatives.
Sexually transmitted infections	Provide adolescent with information regarding disease, mode of transmission, and related symptoms. Encourage safer sexual practices, including abstinence from sexual activity or the use of condoms. Provide accurate information about the consequences of sexual activity.

Through primary health care efforts in the school and community, you can contribute to improvements in the health of adolescents. Discussions with adolescents must be private and confidential. Adolescents must first feel comfortable and respected as individuals to reveal intimate information about their risk-taking behaviours. Developing and implementing programs to respond to adolescents' needs are important strategies. Helping adolescents make decisions about their health care strengthens their autonomy and promotes healthy behaviours.

You can play an important role in preventing injuries and accidental deaths. Important activities include injury prevention activities; support of organizations that promote responsible behaviour, including Mothers Against Drunk Driving (MADD) and Drug Abuse Resistance Education (DARE); and encouragement of students to participate in organizations such as Students Against Drunk Driving (SADD). By stimulating adolescents to discuss alternatives to driving when under the influence of drugs or alcohol, you prepare them to consider alternatives when such an occasion arises. You need to identify adolescents at risk for substance abuse, provide education to prevent accidents related to substance abuse, and provide counselling to clients in rehabilitation programs.

You can play a strategic role in an antismoking movement. Smoking prevention programs can be initiated in schools. Communities can also play a role in creating tobacco control policies at the local level (Greaves et al., 2006).

You need to provide sex education and counselling. You can play a key role in counselling teenagers on ways to avoid pregnancies. You can also assist adolescents in making decisions about pregnancies that do occur (e.g., becoming a parent, adoption, or abortion). Some schools have instituted day care programs so that adolescent mothers can continue their schooling after their babies are born. Whatever choice an adolescent makes, it is important that she receive appropriate health care, including counselling.

Extensive educational efforts to prevent the spread of AIDS and other STIs in this age group are a nursing responsibility. Formal or informal education, in a one-on-one or group setting, may be provided in the school or community. Speakers and organizations can be used to help in the educational process.

Adolescents in Rural Communities. Approximately 20% of Canadians live in rural areas and small towns; however, this percentage varies by province and territory. Although adolescents living in these areas have many of the same health needs as their urban counterparts, they also have some unique risks. For example, those living on farms are at increased risks for accidents because of exposure to heavy equipment, huge vehicles, and large animals (Safe Kids Canada, n.d.). Other concerns for adolescents living in rural areas and small towns are limited availability of recreational facilities and limited access to specialized services.

You can play an important role in improving the health of adolescents who live in rural areas. You can address decreasing barriers to care, health promotion education, development of coping strategies, and assessment of health beliefs.

Minority Adolescents. By the next century, it is expected that minorities as a group will become the majority. Minority adolescents have been identified as experiencing a greater percentage of health problems and barriers to health care.

Issues of concern for minority adolescents living in a high-risk environment include learning or emotional difficulties, death related to violence, unintentional injuries, and increased rates of adolescent pregnancy and STIs, including AIDS. Poverty has a major negative effect on the lives of minority adolescents. Access to culturally appropriate health services is commonly limited. You can make a significant contribution to improving access to appropriate health care for adolescents. Health promotion initiatives must be based on topics of concern for these adolescents.

It is important when working in the community that you adopt culturally sensitive interventions to meet the needs of minority adolescents and their families (Hockenberry & Wilson, 2007). You must be able to communicate in another language by speaking it or using an interpreter's services. Educational materials need to be written in the appropriate language. Information regarding health beliefs and healing practices must be assessed. With knowledge about various cultures and the means to care for minority adolescents, you act as an advocate to ensure accessibility of appropriate services.

Aboriginal Adolescents. Health status and factors affecting it are generally worse for Canadian Aboriginal adolescents (i.e., First Nations, Inuit, and Métis) than any other adolescent populations (Leitch, 2007). Suicide rates are higher among Aboriginal youth than among other youth in Canada, especially among boys (MacNeil, 2008). Aboriginal adolescents are more likely to have crowded living conditions and to live in communities in which alcohol abuse and substance abuse are high. Likewise, the incidence of unemployment and reported sexual and physical abuse is higher than in non-Aboriginal communities (Public Health Agency of Canada, 1999b). Some problems persist for Aboriginal peoples, such as overcrowded living conditions and high rates of unemployment, when they live in urban areas of Canada.

When working with Aboriginal adolescents, you need to be aware of the unique factors that may affect these young people's health. First, you need to be aware that health beliefs and practices, as well as health problems, vary among Aboriginal populations and communities. You need to be sensitive to culturally appropriate interventions. Many Aboriginal communities take responsibility for their own health and well-being, develop their own health services, and include traditional methods of healing to improve well-being.

Lesbian, Gay, and Bisexual Adolescents. Although research on lesbian, gay, and bisexual youth is limited, special consideration must be given to the developmental and health challenges that may result from sexual orientation and societal attitudes to those orientations (Hockenberry & Wilson, 2007). It may be difficult for adolescents to discuss some of these challenges because of the stigma associated with being lesbian, gay, or bisexual. As a consequence, lesbian, gay, or bisexual adolescents could be at greater risk for emotional distress, depression, and suicide, as well as for alcohol or other drug abuse. Lesbian, gay, and bisexual youth need assistance with disclosing their sexual orientation and, before they disclose this information, a plan for dealing with negative and sometimes violent reactions. It is important to respond to these individuals in a sensitive and nonjudgemental way.

✻ KEY CONCEPTS

- A developmental perspective helps you understand commonalities and variations in each stage and the impact they have on the client's health.
- During the intrauterine period, while embryo and fetus grow and develop, genetic factors and environmental factors (teratogens) may cause impairments in any body system.
- Physiological, cognitive, and psychosocial development continue from conception through adolescence, and you must be familiar with normal parameters to determine potential problems and promote normal development.
- Physical growth during the school years is slow and steady until the skeletal growth spurt just before puberty.
- The major psychosocial developmental task of school-age children is the development of a sense of competence.
- Cognitively, young school-age children develop the ability to think in a logical manner.
- The prepubertal growth spurt usually occurs 2 years earlier in girls than in boys.
- Adolescents move forward to the last stage of cognitive development, formal operations, in which they begin to think in an abstract manner, reflect on thought processes, and plan for the future.
- Adolescence begins with puberty, when the primary sexual characteristic changes (maturation of the reproductive organs) and the secondary sexual characteristic changes (such as the development of pubic hair and female breasts) begin.
- Adolescents are able to solve complex mental problems by using deductive reasoning.
- Adolescents' rapid change in physical appearance heightens self-consciousness and concerns regarding body image.
- Accidents are the major cause of death in all age groups.
- Motor vehicle accidents are the major cause of accidental death in adolescence.
- Adolescents begin the long process of emancipation from their parents and need parental support to accomplish this in a timely manner.

✻ CRITICAL THINKING EXERCISES

1. Ms. Yeigh, who is in her first trimester of pregnancy, is attending the antepartum clinic for the first visit. What are the main health promotion topics you need to explore with her at this stage in her pregnancy?

2. The parents of 2-year-old Mark are concerned because his language does not seem to be at the same level as that of their neighbour's 2-year-old daughter. How would you reassure these parents and help them with language development?

3. Eight-year old Lisa sometimes says to her parents that she feels "like a failure." According to Erickson's task for this stage of development, what measures can her parents and teacher use to help negate these feelings and help her meet this stage of development?

4. Twelve-year-old Maya is brought to the pediatric clinic for a physical examination. She is concerned about her lack of physical development in comparison with her peers. Discuss ways to educate Maya about puberty and the variations that occur.

5. Fifteen-year-old Ricardo wants very much to belong and be accepted by his peers. He expresses concern when his peers begin to plan a party with alcohol and drugs. What should be discussed to help support his feelings and need to belong?

✻ REVIEW QUESTIONS

1. Maternal risk factors associated with preterm labour include
   1. Physiological stresses, such as renal disease
   2. Ethnicity
   3. Fetal infections
   4. Nutrition

2. A newborn lying supine, with head turned to one side, arm and leg extended on that side, and the opposite arm and leg flexed, is exhibiting a
   1. Startle reflex
   2. Moro reflex
   3. Tonic neck reflex
   4. Perez reflex

3. The recommended age for beginning immunization for diphtheria and tetanus toxoids and acellular pertussis vaccine (DTaP) in healthy children is
   1. 18 months
   2. 2 months
   3. 12 months
   4. 4 months
4. A toddler pretends to shave after watching his father shave. This is an example of Piaget's
   1. Sensorimotor stage
   2. Intuitive phase of preoperational thought stage
   3. Autonomy stage
   4. Preoperational thought stage
5. The type of play characteristic of the early preschool years is
   1. Selfish
   2. Onlooker
   3. Associative
   4. Parallel
6. Preschoolers sleep an average of
   1. 8 hours a night and take frequent naps
   2. 12 hours a night and take infrequent naps
   3. 10 hours a night and take frequent naps
   4. 6 hours a night and take frequent naps
7. You can counsel a parent that her child can floss his teeth effectively and be independent in tooth care by the age of
   1. 8 to 10 years
   2. 6 to 7 years
   3. 11 to 12 years
   4. 7 to 8 years
8. The most common nutritional disturbance of childhood is
   1. Obesity
   2. Anorexia nervosa
   3. Type 2 diabetes
   4. Bulimia
9. When you are communicating with adolescents, it is best to
   1. Avoid discussing sensitive issues, such as asking questions about sex and drugs
   2. Ask closed-ended questions to get straight answers
   3. Be alert to clues to their emotional state
   4. Avoid looking for meaning behind adolescents' words or actions
10. The leading cause of death in adolescence is
    1. Homicide
    2. Substance abuse
    3. Injuries
    4. Eating disorders

✻ RECOMMENDED WEB SITES

Campaign 2000: http://www.campaign2000.ca
Campaign 2000 is a nonpartisan, cross-Canada coalition of more than 120 national, provincial, and community organizations committed to working together to end child and family poverty in Canada.

Canadian Institute of Child Health: http://www.cich.ca/
The Canadian Institute of Child Health (CICH) is a national charitable organization dedicated to promoting the health of children and youth in Canada. The CICH works with government and industry to address children's safety and health care issues and develop appropriate policies. This Web site offers evidence-based resources of interest to health care professionals, teachers, and parents.

Canadian Paediatric Society: Position Statements: http://www.cps.ca/English/publications/StatementsIndex.htm
This Web site includes the Canadian Paediatric Society's position statements on a variety of child health issues. It has updates as they are developed.

24

Young to Middle Adulthood

Original chapter by Patsy Ruchala, RN, DNSc

Canadian content written by Marion Clauson, RN, MSN, PNC(C)

objectives

Mastery of content in this chapter will enable you to:

- Define the key terms listed.
- Discuss major life events and developmental tasks of young and middle-aged adults.
- Discuss the significance of family in the life of the adult.
- Describe normal physiological changes in young and middle adulthood and in pregnancy.
- Discuss cognitive and psychosocial changes that occur during the adult years.
- Describe health concerns of young and middle-aged adults.
- Apply clinical decision making to administer care to young and middle-aged adults.

key terms

Braxton-Hicks contractions, p. 368
Breastfeeding, p. 365
Doula, p. 365
Infertility, p. 367
Menopause, p. 372
Nesting, p. 368
Perimenopause, p. 372
Prenatal care, p. 368
Puerperium, p. 368
Sandwich generation, p. 372

media resources

evolve Web Site

- Audio Chapter Summaries
- Glossary
- Multiple-Choice Review Questions
- Student Learning Activities
- Weblinks

Companion CD

- Glossary
- Interactive Learning Activities
- Fluids and Electrolytes Tutorial
- Test-Taking Skills

Young to middle adulthood is a period of challenges, rewards, and crises. Challenges may include the demands of working and raising families; rewards may include career, family, and personal successes; and crises may include job loss and caring for aging parents.

Adult developmental changes are based on earlier characteristics that help shape subsequent behaviour and characteristics. Each person's development, however, is a unique process (Fortinash & Holoday Worret, 2004). Young adulthood is the period between the late teens and the mid- to late thirties (Edelman & Mandle, 2002). Young adults constituted approximately 24% of the Canadian population in 2007 (Statistics Canada, 2008b). During young adulthood, individuals move away from their families of origin, establish career goals, and decide whether to marry and begin families or to remain single. Young adults must adapt to new experiences and newly acquired independence.

Middle age is the period between the mid- to late thirties and the mid-sixties, when people become aware of changes in reproductive and physical abilities. This is a time when individuals may reassess life goals. In 2007, about 43% of the Canadian population were middle-aged adults (Statistics Canada, 2008b). The population aged 45 to 64 years increased by 36% between 1991 and 2001 and is expected to increase an additional 30% by 2011.

Developmental theories provide you with a basis for understanding the life events and developmental tasks of young and middle-aged adults. Developmental theorists Erikson (1963, 1982), Gould (1972), Havighurst (1972), and Gilligan (1993) described the phases of adulthood and related developmental tasks (see Chapter 22).

You may be a young or middle-aged adult yourself, coping with the demands of your respective developmental period. You must be careful to recognize the needs of your clients even if you are not experiencing the same challenges and events. You can help young and middle-aged adult clients achieve their potential by offering support and providing information and appropriate referrals.

Young Adulthood

Physical Changes

Most young adults have completed physical growth by the age of 20 years. Young adults are usually quite active, experience fewer severe illnesses than do older age groups, tend to ignore physical symptoms of illness, and often postpone seeking health care. Physical characteristics of young adults begin to change as middle age approaches.

Clients in this developmental stage may benefit from a personal lifestyle assessment to identify habits that increase the risk for cardiac, malignant, pulmonary, renal, or other chronic diseases. A personal lifestyle assessment of the young adult includes assessment of general life satisfaction; hobbies and interests; habits such as diet, sleeping, exercise, sexual practices, and use of caffeine, alcohol, and illicit drugs; home conditions, including housing and finances; and occupational environment, including type of work, exposure to hazardous substances, and physical or mental strain.

Cognitive Changes

Cognitive changes are variations in reasoning and thinking. Critical thinking habits increase steadily through the young and middle adult years. Formal and informal education, life experiences, and work opportunities increase the individual's conceptual and problem-solving skills. Because young adults are continually evolving and adjusting to changes in the home, workplace, and personal lives, those with flexible decision-making processes cope more effectively.

Choosing an occupation is a major task of young adults and involves knowing their skills, talents, and personality characteristics. Many young adults, however, lack the resources or the support systems to pursue higher education or develop work skills. As a result, some young adults may have limited occupational choices.

By understanding how adults learn, you can develop teaching plans (see Chapter 21). Adults enter the learning situation with a background of unique life experiences, including illness. Therefore, you should always view each adult as an individual. When determining what amount of information the individual needs to make decisions about the prescribed course of therapy, you should consider factors that may affect the individual's compliance with the regimen, including educational level, socioeconomic factors, motivation, and desire to learn.

Psychosocial Changes

The emotional health of the young adult is related to the individual's ability to address and resolve personal and social tasks. The young adult often wants to prolong adolescence and yet assume adult commitments. Between the ages of 23 and 28 years, people usually refine self-perception and capability for intimacy. From ages 29 to 34 years, people usually focus on achieving personal and occupational goals and improving their socioeconomic status. For many young adults, a dual-income family is needed to achieve and maintain middle-class status. Career and personal counselling can help individuals identify career choices and set realistic goals.

Ethnicity and gender issues influence an adult's life and can pose challenges for nursing care. Each person holds culture-bound definitions of health and illness. An understanding of ethnicity, race, and gender differences enables you to provide individualized care (see Chapter 10). The traditional gender roles of men and women have changed. In many cultures, the man traditionally assumed familial authority. However, since the 1970s, women have been entering the workforce and pursuing careers in high numbers. About 58% of Canadian women aged 15 years and older are in the labour force (Statistics Canada, 2008c). Women contribute significantly to their families' incomes. As a result, many women deal with the stresses of being wife, mother, and employee. Likewise, men are assuming more parental and household responsibilities (Fortinash & Holoday Worret, 2004). Some men choose to put careers on hold to be stay-at-home fathers.

Career. Young men and women hope to have fulfilling careers. They may formulate short- and long-term career goals. Successful employment ensures economic security and promotes friendships, social activities, support, and self-respect.

The number of two-career marriages is increasing. When both partners are working, they experience many benefits (e.g., improved finances) but also many potential stressors (e.g., child care demands; household needs; increased physical, mental, or emotional demands). To reduce stress in a two-career family, neither partner should assume all household responsibilities. For some families, a solution is to hire a housekeeper. Others may set up an equal division of household and child care duties.

Sexuality. Young adults usually have the emotional maturity necessary to develop fulfilling sexual relationships and establish intimacy. Young adults who have failed to achieve the developmental tasks of adolescence may develop relationships that are superficial (Fortinash & Holoday Worret, 2004).

For most young adults, the emotional aspect of sexual activity is as important as its type or frequency. Adults should be encouraged to explore various aspects of their sexuality and be aware that their sexual needs and concerns evolve (see Chapter 27).

Singlehood. Social pressure to get married is not as great as it once was. In Canada, the average ages for first marriage are 29 years for women and 31 years for men (Statistics Canada, 2008b). For young adults who remain single, parents and siblings become the nucleus of a family, although the single young adult usually maintains independence. Close friends and associates of the single young adult may also be viewed as the individual's "family." Some singles choose to become parents, either biologically or through adoption.

The single population is increasing partly because women have greater career opportunities than before and partly because single individuals often choose to live together rather than marry. In addition, many adults become single again after a marriage ends.

Marriage. Every married couple's relationship is unique. Although no rules guarantee a successful marriage, some guidelines are useful for building a happy marriage. Before marriage, the couple ideally should (1) ensure that their emotions are based on love rather than physical attraction, (2) explore their motivations for marriage, (3) develop clear communication, (4) accept that behaviour and habits are unlikely to change after marriage, and (5) determine their compatibility in important beliefs and values.

When establishing a household and family, the married couple must work as a team. Individuals require maturity and self-esteem to accomplish the following major tasks of marriage: establishing an intimate relationship; deciding on and working toward mutual goals; establishing guidelines for decision-making issues; setting standards for social interactions; and choosing morals, values, and ideologies acceptable to both. Accomplishing these tasks provides the foundation for a stable relationship.

Marriage also requires the couple to learn patterns of sexual expression, establish roles, and practise effective conflict resolution and decision-making skills. Each partner may experience a sense of loss of individuality in the transition from being single to being married.

Child-Bearing Cycle. Conception, pregnancy, birth, and the puerperium (postpartum period) are phases of the child-bearing cycle. The changes during these phases are complex (Box 24–1). Childbirth education classes can prepare the pregnant woman, her partner, and other supportive people to participate in the birthing process. Social support has a positive impact on pregnant women and their families (Box 24–2). A current trend is to have a lay **doula**, or support person, in addition to the woman's partner, present during labour to offer physical, emotional, and informational support (Campbell et al., 2006). Professional midwives offer choices regarding home or hospital birth.

Breastfeeding offers many advantages to both the new mother and baby (see Chapter 43). However, for the inexperienced mother, breastfeeding may cause anxiety and frustration. Women who have had no contact with newborns and other mothers who breastfeed may require assistance to breastfeed successfully. You must be alert for signs that the mother needs information and assistance. By observing the mother while she breastfeeds, you may catch problems such as improper positioning or ineffective sucking by the infant (Registered Nurses Association of Ontario, 2003).

The personal and social changes occurring in the lives of a couple after the birth of a baby cannot be underestimated (Figure 24–1). The nursing assessment of the couple's response to the birthing experience and parent–child attachment are discussed later in this chapter.

Parenthood. Contraception allows couples to decide when and whether to start a family. One factor influencing this decision is the reason for wanting a child. Social pressures may encourage a couple to have a child or may influence them to limit the number of children they have. Economic considerations frequently enter into the decision because raising children is expensive. Because couples are getting married later and are postponing pregnancies, general health status and age are also factors in whether a couple decides to have children.

Parenting roles must be defined and practised. Nurturing and socialization needs of the children can put pressure on the couple's intimate relationship. In addition, parents' images of the "perfect parent" may conflict with reality.

Alternative Family Structures and Parenting. The norms and values about family life in Canada continuously evolve, as demonstrated by judicial rulings on same-sex marriage since 2000. Greater numbers of infants are born to cohabiting (common-law) couples (see Chapter 20). Parents may also be single or same-sex couples. Families may be combined from previous relationships. Many parents from alternative family structures feel a lack of support and bias from the health care system (McManus et al., 2006). The needs of same-sex parents and their children may include support for the adoption of children and for the parenting role.

Hallmarks of Emotional Health

Most young adults have the physical and emotional resources and support systems to meet their many challenges, tasks, and responsibilities. During psychosocial assessment of young adults, you can assess for 10 hallmarks of emotional health that indicate successful maturation in this developmental stage (Box 24–3). If one or more of these hallmarks are not attained, further assessment and action may be required.

BOX 24-1 FOCUS ON PRIMARY HEALTH CARE

Preparation for Parenthood

Preparing for child-bearing and parenthood involves many decisions and choices for the child-bearing family. These include the decision to have a baby and the choices of health care professional, place of birth, how to obtain information and prepare for childbirth, and how to feed and care for the newborn.

In a hospital or community prenatal clinic, you have many opportunities to assist the child-bearing family by providing information that aids decision making. You may help families to seek preconceptional counselling for known or suspected health risks that might affect the mother or fetus during pregnancy. You may also refer families to other health care professionals for unique concerns. By providing a list of questions that could be asked of a health care professional on a first visit, you may encourage expectant parents to select a health care professional with whom they will be comfortable and who will meet their needs.

Prenatal education programs offered by hospital and community nurses and by midwives provide information about coping strategies and support during pregnancy, labour, and the early postpartum period. Classes specifically about preparation for Caesarean birth or for siblings and grandparents may also be available. Prenatal education programs should be structured to meet the unique needs, goals, and learning styles of the expectant family.

Adapted from Olds, S. B., London, M. L., Ladewig, P. A., & Davidson, M. R. (Eds.). (2004). *Maternal–newborn nursing and women's health care* (7th ed., pp. 285–293). Upper Saddle River, NJ: Pearson Prentice Hall.

BOX 24-2 RESEARCH HIGHLIGHT

Culture and Social Support During Pregnancy

Research Focus

Although Mexican Americans have poorer prenatal care and lower socioeconomic status than do other North Americans, they have relatively the same or better infant mortality rates and favourable birth-weight distributions. Domian (2001) studied the reasons why, and the conclusions about the value of social support during pregnancy can also apply to Canadian settings.

Research Abstract

The purpose of Domian's study was to describe the role of social supports of American Hispanic families during pregnancy. Hispanic mothers, Hispanic family members, and Hispanic health care professionals were interviewed, and regional data and demographics were analyzed. Findings indicated that pregnancy outcomes were positive because of a socialization process that helped pregnant Hispanic women and family members adapt and change to support the pregnancy. The aspects of mutual adaptation helped reinforce the family structure, integrate cultural beliefs, define roles for both mother and family members, define the nature of mother–child and family–child relationships, and facilitate a positive process through a supportive orientation.

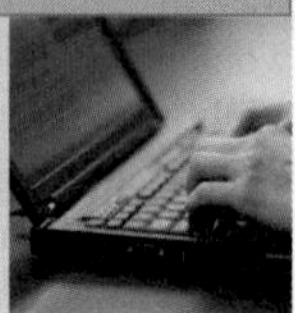

Evidence-Informed Practice

- Recognizing the importance of cultural and social contexts in which pregnancies occur is an important aspect of nursing care and intervention.
- Family support of pregnant women is a major factor in the well-being of pregnant women and their unborn children.
- Health care practices and policy focused on increasing social support of pregnant women could improve birth outcomes.

References: Domian, E. (2001). Cultural practices and social support of pregnant women in a northern New Mexico community. *Journal of Nursing Scholarship, 33*(4), 331–336.

Health Risks

Health risk factors for a young adult originate in the environment and occupation, lifestyle patterns, and family history.

Lifestyle. Lifestyle habits such as poor food choices, smoking, stress, substance abuse, and inactivity increase the risk of illness. For example, prolonged stress can cause ulcers, emotional disorders, and infections (see Chapter 30). Smoking and second-hand smoke can cause lung cancer and pulmonary, cardiac, and vascular diseases. Your role in health promotion is to identify lifestyle risk factors and provide education and support to reduce unhealthy behaviours.

Family History. A family history of a disease may put a young adult at risk for developing that disease in the middle or older adult years. For example, a family history of certain cancers or cardiovascular, renal, endocrine, or neoplastic disease increases the family member's risk of developing the disease.

Accidental Death and Injury. Accidents are the leading causes of injury and death in young adults (Lemone & Burke, 2004). Death and injury can result from motor vehicle or other accidents, physical assaults, and suicide attempts. Motor vehicle accidents are the primary cause of death in 15- to 19-year-olds and the second leading cause of death in 20- to 24-year-olds (Statistics Canada, 2008a). They also may cause permanent disability.

Physical assault and violence also may cause injury or death. Factors that may predispose to violence include poverty, breakdown of family relations, child abuse and neglect, and access to firearms. To detect personal and environmental risk factors for violence, it is important that you perform a thorough psychosocial assessment, including such factors as behaviour patterns, history of physical abuse and substance abuse, education, work history, and social support systems.

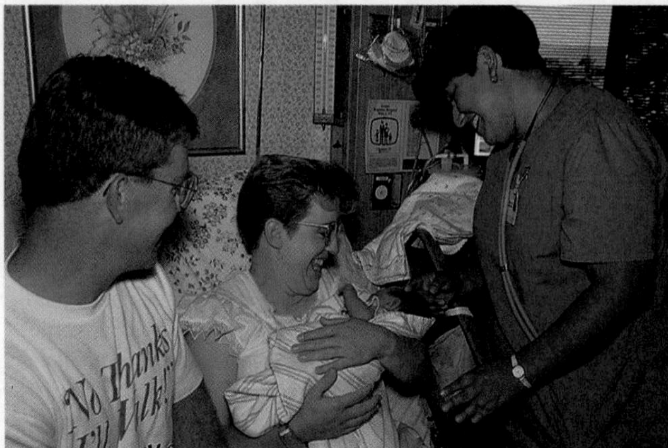

Figure 24-1 The birth of a newborn causes many personal and social changes in the parents' lives. **Source:** From Stanhope, M., & Lancaster, J. (2004). *Community and public health nursing* (6th ed.). St. Louis, MO: Mosby.

Substance Abuse. Substance abuse directly or indirectly contributes to mortality and morbidity in young adults. Regular heavy drinking (five or more drinks on one occasion) is most common among youth aged 20 to 24 (Statistics Canada, 2008a). Intoxication is often a factor in motor vehicle accidents.

Dependence on stimulant or depressant drugs can result in death. Overdose of a stimulant drug ("upper") can stress the cardiovascular and nervous systems and lead to death. The use of depressants ("downers") can lead to an accidental or intentional overdose and death. You can provide counselling and support for clients seeking treatment for substance abuse.

Substance abuse cannot always be diagnosed, particularly in its early stages. Nonjudgemental questions about use of legal drugs (prescribed drugs, over-the-counter drugs, tobacco, and alcohol),

BOX 24-3 Ten Hallmarks of Emotional Health

- A sense of meaning and direction in life
- Successful negotiation through transitions
- Absence of feelings of being cheated or disappointed by life
- Attainment of several long-term goals
- Satisfaction with personal growth and development
- When married, feelings of love for partner; when single, satisfaction with social interactions
- Satisfaction with friendships
- Generally cheerful attitude
- Acceptance of constructive criticism
- No unrealistic fears

so-called soft drugs (marijuana), and illegal drugs (cocaine or heroin) should be a routine part of any physical assessment. Important information may be obtained by making specific inquiries about past medical problems, changes in food intake or sleep patterns, or problems of emotional lability. Reports of arrests because of driving while intoxicated, because of domestic or child abuse, or because of disorderly conduct should alert you to the possibility of drug abuse.

Unplanned Pregnancies. Unplanned pregnancies, although more common among adolescents, also occur in young and middle-adult Canadian women. Unplanned pregnancies are a source of stress that can result in adverse health outcomes for the mother, infant, and family. Many young adults have educational and career goals that take precedence over family development. Interference with these goals can affect future relationships and later parent–child relationships.

Determining situational factors that may affect the outcome of an unplanned pregnancy is important. When assessing the woman with an unplanned pregnancy, it is important for you to explore issues such as family support systems; potential parenting disorders; depression; coping mechanisms; and possible financial, career, or housing problems.

Sexually Transmitted Infections. Sexually transmitted infections (STIs) are a major health problem in young adults (Public Health Agency of Canada, 2007; Society of Obstetricians and Gynaecologists of Canada, 2006). STIs include syphilis, chlamydia, gonorrhea, genital herpes, human papilloma virus (HPV) infection, and acquired immune deficiency syndrome (AIDS) (see Chapter 27). STIs have immediate physical effects such as discharge and discomfort. STIs also can lead to chronic disorders (from genital herpes), infertility (from gonorrhea), or death (from AIDS). Many people have an STI without experiencing symptoms. Young adults need information about transmission, prevention, symptoms, and management of STIs.

Many young adults have misconceptions regarding transmission and treatment of STIs. Partners are encouraged to know one another's sexual history and sexual practices. You should be alert for STIs when clients come to clinics with complaints of urological or gynecological problems (see Chapter 32). Young adults should be assessed for their knowledge and use of safer sex practices and genital self-examinations.

Environmental or Occupational Factors. A common environmental or occupational risk factor is exposure to work-related hazards or agents, which may cause diseases and cancer (Table 24–1). Such diseases include silicosis from inhalation of talcum and silicon dust, emphysema from inhalation of smoke, and hearing loss from noise exposure. Cancers resulting from occupational exposures may involve the lungs, liver, brain, blood, or skin. Environmental exposures with leisure activities include outdoor exposure to mosquitoes (which may transmit West Nile virus) and ticks (which may transmit Lyme disease). Questions regarding environmental and occupational exposures should be a routine part of your assessment.

Health Concerns

Infertility. Infertility refers to a prolonged time to conceive, usually more than 1 full year. An estimated 17% of reproductive couples are infertile, and many are young adults (University of Toronto, 2007). However, about half the couples evaluated and treated in infertility clinics become pregnant. In about 20% of affected couples, the cause of infertility is unknown. Female factors, such as ovulatory dysfunction or a pelvic factor, and male factors, such as sperm and semen abnormalities, are responsible for about 80% of cases of infertility (Breslin & Lucas, 2003). Couples who delay conception until their mid-thirties may also experience fertility problems. For some infertile couples, you may be the first resource contacted. Nursing assessment of infertile couples should include comprehensive histories of both the male and female partners to determine factors that may have affected fertility, as well as pertinent physical findings (Lowdermilk & Perry, 2003).

Exercise. Exercise patterns can affect health status. Exercise three times a week that produces a sustained increase in the pulse rate for 15 to 20 minutes improves cardiopulmonary function by decreasing blood pressure and heart rate. In addition, exercise decreases fatigue, insomnia, tension, and irritability. You should conduct a thorough

TABLE 24-1 Occupational Hazards or Exposures Associated With Diseases and Cancers

Job Category	Occupational Hazard or Exposure	Work-Related Condition
Agricultural workers	Pesticides, infectious agents, gases, sunlight	Pesticide poisoning, "farmer's lung," skin cancer
Automobile workers	Asbestos, plastics, lead, solvents	Asbestosis, dermatitis
Carpenters	Wood dust, wood preservatives, adhesives	Nasopharyngeal cancer, dermatitis
Cement workers	Cement dust, metals	Dermatitis, bronchitis
Dry cleaners	Solvents	Liver disease, dermatitis
Glass workers	Heat, solvents, metal powders	Cataracts
Hospital workers	Infectious agents, cleansers, latex gloves, radiation	Infections, latex allergies, unintentional injuries, back injuries
Insulators	Asbestos, fibrous glass	Asbestosis, lung cancer, mesothelioma
Office computer workers	Repetitive wrist motion on computers and eye strain	Tendonitis, carpal tunnel syndrome, tenosynovitis

From Stanhope, M., & Lancaster, J. (2004). *Community and public health nursing* (6th ed., p. 1074, Tab. 44-1). St. Louis, MO: Mosby.

musculoskeletal assessment, including evaluations of joint mobility and muscle tone, and a psychosocial assessment for improved tolerance of stress to determine the effects of exercise.

Routine Health Screening. Routine screening examinations lower the risk for severe illnesses because they enable early detection. Clients should be encouraged to perform monthly skin, breast, or male genital self-examination (see Chapter 32). In Canada, lung cancer is the leading cause of death, followed by colorectal cancer (Canadian Cancer Society, 2008). Thirty percent of new cancer cases and 18% of cancer deaths occur in young and middle-aged adults (Canadian Cancer Society, 2008). The incidence of breast cancer is steadily increasing. Therefore, your role is extremely important in educating female clients about breast self-examination and the current breast screening recommendations, and you must provide male clients with information about testicular self-examination. In adolescence and early adulthood, prolonged exposure to ultraviolet rays of the sun or in tanning salons can increase the risk for development of skin cancer later in life. You should encourage clients to undergo routine assessment of the skin for recent changes in colour or presence of lesions and changes in their appearance.

Job Stress. Job stress can occur every day or from time to time. Most young adults are able to handle day-to-day crises (Figure 24–2). Situational job stress may occur when a new boss enters the workplace, a deadline is approaching, or the worker is given new responsibilities. Corporate downsizing and mergers, which may lead to layoffs and increased responsibilities for remaining employees, are major sources of stress. Job stress also occurs when a person becomes dissatisfied with a job. Because individuals perceive jobs differently, the types of job stressors vary from person to person. Your assessment of the young adult should include a description of the adult's work, including conditions and hours, duration of employment, changes in sleep or eating habits, and evidence of increased irritability or nervousness.

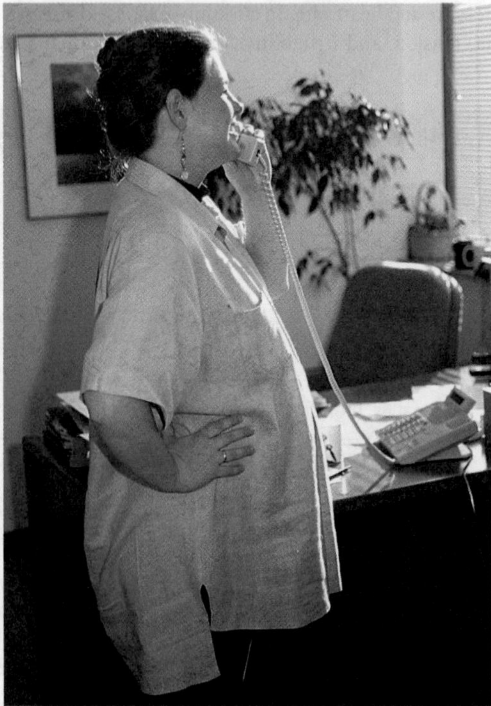

Figure 24-2 The ability to handle day-to-day challenges at work minimizes stress.

Family Stress. Family stressors can occur at any time in family life. Family life has peaks, when everyone in the family works together, and valleys, when everyone appears to pull apart. Situational stressors occur during events such as births, deaths, illnesses, marriages, and job losses. Because of changing relationships and structures in the emerging young adult family, stress levels are frequently high. Stress may be related to a number of variables and may lead to dysfunction in the young adult family. Stress and the possible resulting family dysfunction may account for the high divorce rate during the first 3 to 5 years of marriage for young adults younger than 30 years of age. When a client seeks health care and exhibits stress-related symptoms, you should ask whether the person has recently experienced a life-changing event.

Each family has certain predictable roles or jobs for members. These roles enable the family to function and be an effective part of society. One necessary role is the family leader. In most families, one parent is the leader or both parents act as co-leaders. In lone-parent families, the parent or, on occasion, a member of the extended family is the family leader. When this role changes as a result of illness, a situational crisis may occur. You should assess environmental and familial factors, including support systems and coping mechanisms commonly used by family members.

Pregnancy. Although the physiological changes of pregnancy and childbirth occur only in women, cognitive and psychosocial changes and health concerns affect the entire child-bearing family (Somers-Smith, 1999). The entire family, therefore, needs education about pregnancy, labour, delivery, breastfeeding, and integration of the newborn into the family structure.

Women who are anticipating pregnancy benefit from good health practices before conception, including eating a balanced diet, exercising, attending regular dental checkups, and avoiding alcohol, drugs, and smoking. Women trying to become pregnant should not follow weight-reduction diets.

Prenatal Care. **Prenatal care** includes routine assessment of the pregnant woman by a nurse, family physician, obstetrician, nurse practitioner, or midwife. Health promotion interventions are important during the prenatal period and can improve the well-being of the woman and fetus (Box 24–4). Prenatal care includes a thorough physical assessment of the pregnant woman during regularly scheduled intervals; provision of information regarding STIs, vaginal infections, and urinary infections that could adversely affect the fetus; and counselling about exercise patterns, diet, and child care. Regular prenatal care can address health concerns that arise during the pregnancy.

Physiological Changes. The physiological changes and needs of the pregnant woman vary with each trimester (Table 24–2). Temporary changes in visual and hearing acuity, taste, and smell also occur. You must be familiar with these physiological changes, their causes, and helpful interventions. All women experience some physiological changes in the first trimester, but some changes affect only certain women. During the second trimester, growth of the uterus and fetus results in some of the physical signs of pregnancy, and the woman will be able to see her growing abdomen and feel the fetal movements. During the third trimester, irregular, short contractions (**Braxton-Hicks contractions**), fatigue, and urinary frequency may occur. Close to the onset of labour, the woman may experience a burst of energy during which she prepares for the baby's arrival, a period called **nesting**.

The **puerperium** is a period of approximately 6 weeks after delivery. During this time, the woman's body reverts to its prepregnant physical status. You should assess the woman's knowledge of and ability to care for both herself and her newborn. Assistance with infant

TABLE 24-2 Major Physiological Changes During Pregnancy

Signs and Symptoms	Causes
First Trimester	
Amenorrhea	Fertilization and implantation of egg Increases in hormone levels
"Morning sickness" (nausea, sometimes vomiting)	Increased serum hormone levels
Breast changes: enlargement, tenderness, darkened and enlarged nipples	Increased estrogen levels
Urinary frequency	Pressure of uterus on bladder
Fatigue	Increased nutritional demands Decreased nutritional intake resulting from morning sickness
Second Trimester	
Integumentary changes: pigment changes in nipple and breast, hyperpigmentation of abdominal line (linea nigra), mottling of cheeks or forehead (chloasma, or "mask of pregnancy"), localized or generalized pruritis	Increased levels of melanocyte-stimulating hormone
Hypertrophy of gums, causing gingival swelling and bleeding	Proliferation of interdental papillary blood vessels, caused by increased estrogen levels
Increasing height of uterine fundus	Growth of fetus
Sensation of movement or of abdominal gas (quickening)	Fetal movement
Third Trimester	
Braxton-Hicks contractions	Expansion and preparation of uterus for labour
Increased colostrum	Hormonal influence; preparation of breasts for lactation
Increased urinary frequency	Pressure on bladder from enlarged fetus
Shortness of breath	Pressure on diaphragm from enlarged uterus
Supine hypertension	Uterine pressure on inferior vena cava
Heartburn	Slower gastric emptying and esophageal reflux

Data from Lowdermilk, D., & Perry, S. (2003). *Maternity nursing* (6th ed.). St. Louis, MO: Mosby.

feeding and care and assessment of parenting skills and mother–infant interactions are particularly important (Dunn et al., 2006).

Psychosocial Changes. Like the physiological changes of pregnancy, psychosocial changes may occur at various times during the 9 months of pregnancy and in the puerperium. Table 24–3 summarizes the major categories of psychosocial changes and the implications for nursing intervention.

Acute Care. The young adult years are generally a time of good physical and emotional health. Potential health hazards may be related to lifestyle. Acute care for young adults is frequently related to accidents, substance abuse, exposure to environmental and occupational hazards, stress-related illnesses, respiratory infections, gastroenteritis, influenza, urinary tract infections, and minor surgery.

Approximately 10,000 cancers are diagnosed in young adults every year in Canada, and cancer is diagnosed in more women are than men because of the frequency of breast and reproductive system cancers (Cancer Care Ontario, 2006).

An acute, minor illness can cause a disruption in the life activities of the young adult and increase stress in an already hectic lifestyle. Dependency and limitations posed by treatment regimens can also increase frustration for the young adult. To give young adults control of their health care choices, it is important for you to keep them informed about their health status and involve them in health care decisions.

Restorative and Continuing Care. Chronic conditions in young adulthood, although not common, do occur. Chronic illnesses such as hypertension, coronary artery disease, and diabetes may have their onset in young adulthood without being known to the young adult until later in life. Causes of chronic illness and disability in a young adult can include accidents, multiple sclerosis, rheumatoid arthritis, AIDS, and cancer. Chronic illness and disability can affect the accomplishment of important developmental tasks in young adulthood. They can reduce a young adult's independence and require the person to change personal, family, and career goals. A young adult with chronic illness or disability may experience developmental problems related to sense of identity. The person needs support in the establishment of independence, reorganization of intimate relationships and family structure, and launching of a chosen career (Lemone & Burke, 2004).

Middle Adulthood

The middle adult years begin around the early to mid-thirties and last through the mid-sixties. Personal and career achievements have often already been experienced. Many middle-aged adults enjoy assisting their children and other young people to become productive and responsible adults. Middle-aged adults may also begin to

TABLE 24-3 Major Psychosocial Changes During Pregnancy

Type of Change	Implications for Nursing Intervention
Body image	Morning sickness and fatigue may contribute to poor body image. Increase in breast size may make the woman feel more feminine and sexually appealing but may also be uncomfortable. The woman begins to "show" during the second trimester. The woman may experience a general feeling of well-being; she can feel the baby move and hear the baby's heartbeat.
Role changes	Both partners think about impending role changes and can have feelings of uncertainty about them. Both partners may have feelings of ambivalence about becoming parents and concern about ability to be parents.
Sexuality	Partners need reassurance that sexual activity will not harm the fetus. Desire for sexual activity may be influenced by body image. Partners may desire cuddling and holding rather than sexual intercourse.
Coping mechanisms	Partners need reassurance that childbirth and child rearing are natural and positive experiences but can also be stressful. Partners should be provided guidance in preparation for childbirth and encouraged to participate in childbirth classes.
Stresses during puerperium	Partners may return home from hospital fatigued and unfamiliar with infant care. Partners may experience physical discomfort or feelings of anxiety. The woman may have to return to work soon after delivery, with subsequent feelings of guilt, anxiety, or, possibly, sense of freedom or relief.
Postpartum blues and depression	Postpartum blues symptoms include transient emotional or mood disturbances such as weepiness, insomnia, anxiety, and poor concentration about 3 to 6 days after birth. Postpartum depression symptoms include extreme anxiety, sense of failure, feelings of guilt, sleep disturbances, appetite disorders, excessive concerns about the baby, and suicide ideation. Interventions include medication, therapy, counselling and support.

help aging parents. Technology has an increasing impact on work, pleasure, and play for middle-aged adults. Using leisure time in satisfying and creative ways is a challenge that, if met satisfactorily, enables middle-aged adults to prepare for retirement.

Although most middle-aged adults have achieved socioeconomic stability, trends in corporate downsizing have left many middle-aged adults either jobless or forced to accept lower paying jobs.

Men and women must adjust to inevitable biological changes. Middle-aged adults adapt self-concept and body image to physiological realities and changes in physical appearance. Exercising, eating well, getting enough sleep, and practising good hygiene promote good health and a positive attitude toward physiological changes.

Physical Changes

Major physiological changes occur between the ages of 40 and 65 years. Table 24–4 summarizes the normal developmental changes that you consider when conducting a physical examination. The most visible changes are greying of the hair, wrinkling of the skin, and thickening of the waist. Decreases in hearing and visual acuity are often noted during this period. Often these physiological changes have an

BOX 24-4 NURSING STORY

Support During Pregnancy

Melinda was a 24-year-old woman who was pregnant with her first child. She has had a healthy pregnancy, and the fetus appearred to be growing well. She signed up to attend childbirth education classes beginning in her sixth month of pregnancy. The classes were taught by a community health nurse who also worked in Melinda's community. The nurse noticed that Melinda's boyfriend, Troy, accompanied her to the first class but did not attend after that. During the second class, the nurse observed that Melinda was by herself and appeared a bit withdrawn. Concerned about whether Melinda would have adequate support during labour and birth, the nurse asked Melinda whether Troy was going to be coming back. Melinda replied that Troy had gone up north to work, as his job had ended at home, and that he would be gone for at least 3 months. She said she was missing him already and was worried that he might miss the birth. The camp where he was working very remote, and because only a few flights out each week were available, Melinda was not sure that he would be able to leave when she went into labour. The nurse asked Melinda about other family members who might be able to support her. Melinda said that she is estranged from her mother, who lives in another province, but her 19-year-old sister might be able to be with her for the birth, depending on when it occurs and if she can take time off work. The nurse suggested that Melinda consider arranging to have a doula who could be present during labour to offer physical, emotional, and informational support. The doula would meet with Melinda sometime before her due date to talk with her about what would be most helpful to her during labour and would be at her side through the birth. The nurse provided several names of doulas and encouraged Melinda to consider this as an additional support person in case her boyfriend or sister could not make it in time. During the next class, Melinda said that she had contacted a doula and made arrangements to meet with her. She stated that she was relieved to know that she would have labour support if Troy could not attend the birth. She was very appreciative of the nurse's help. Several months later, Melinda phoned the nurse to say that Troy had caught a flight in time to be with her and that both he and the doula had really helped her during the birth. They were thrilled to have given birth to a healthy baby boy.

impact on self-concept and body image. For women, the most significant physiological change during middle age is menopause. Men may also notice several sexual changes as androgen levels decrease, such as less firm erections and less frequent ejaculation (see Chapter 27). However, many middle-aged men are still capable of producing fertile sperm and fathering a child.

TABLE 24-4 Physical Assessment Findings in the Middle-Aged Adult

Body System	Expected Findings
Integument	Intact condition Appropriate distribution of pigmentation Slow, progressive decrease in skin turgor Greying and loss of hair (baldness patterns in men are established by age 55; hair loss after this time might have other causes)
Head and neck	Symmetry of scalp, skull, and face
Eyes	Normal accessory organs of vision Visual acuity (according to Snellen chart) that is less than 20/50 Normal pupillary reaction to light and accommodation Normal visual fields and extraocular movements Normal retinal structures
Ears	Normal auditory structures and acuity
Nose, sinuses, and throat	Patent nares and intact sinuses, mouth, and pharynx Location of trachea at midline Nonpalpable lateral thyroid lobes
Thorax and lungs	Increased anteroposterior diameter Respiratory rate: 12–20 breaths per minute and regular Ratio of respiratory rate to heart rate: 1:4 Normal tactile fremitus, resonance, and breath sounds
Heart and vascular system	Normal heart sounds Systole: first heart sound loudest at apex Diastole: first heart sound loudest at base Point of maximal impulse: at fifth intercostal space in midclavicular line and 2 cm or less in diameter Temperature: 36.1°C–37.6°C Pulse: 60–100 bpm (in conditioned athlete, 50 bpm) Blood pressure: 130 mm Hg systolic, 85 mm Hg diastolic All pulses palpable
Breasts	Decreased size resulting from decreased muscle mass Normal nipples
Abdomen	No tenderness or organomegaly Decreased strength of abdominal muscles
Female reproductive system	Change in menstrual cycle and in duration and quality of menstrual flow to cessation of menses "Hot flashes"
Male reproductive system	Normal penis and scrotum Prostatic enlargement in some individuals
Musculoskeletal system	Decreased muscle mass Decreased range of joint motion
Neurological system	Appropriate affect, appearance, and behaviour Lucidity and appropriate level of cognitive ability Intact cranial nerves Adequate motor responses Responsive sensory system

Perimenopause and Menopause. Menstruation and ovulation occur in a cyclical rhythm in women from adolescence into middle adulthood. **Perimenopause** is the period during which ovarian function declines, which results in a diminishing number of ova and irregular menstrual cycles. During this perimenopause time, however, women can still become pregnant. **Menopause** is the permanent cessation of menstruation. It occurs primarily because the ovaries stop producing the hormones estrogen and progesterone. Menopause typically occurs between the ages of 45 and 60 years. Approximately 10% of women have no symptoms of menopause other than cessation of menstruation, 70% to 80% are aware of other changes but have no problems, and approximately 10% experience changes severe enough to interfere with activities of daily living, such as hot flashes and insomnia (Condon, 2004).

Cognitive Changes

Changes in the cognitive function of middle-aged adults are rare except with illness or trauma. The middle-aged adult can learn new skills and information. Some middle-aged adults enter educational or vocational programs to prepare themselves for entering the job market or changing jobs.

Psychosocial Changes

The psychosocial changes in middle-aged adults may involve expected events, such as children moving away from home, or unexpected events, such as a marital separation or the death of a loved one. Many middle-aged adults may find themselves in the so-called **sandwich generation**, simultaneously having the responsibilities of raising their own children and caring for aging parents. These changes may result in stress that can affect middle-aged adults' overall health. During middle age, the person examines life goals and relationships. Often a "midlife crisis" results, in which the person feels turmoil or anxiety about the course of his or her life and desires change. As a result, the person may change relationships, lifestyle, or occupation.

You should assess the major life changes occurring in the middle-aged adult and the impact that the changes have on that person's state of health. Your assessment should also include individual psychosocial factors such as coping mechanisms and sources of social support.

In the middle adult years, as children depart from the household, the family enters the postparental family stage. Time and financial demands on the parents decrease, and the couple faces the task of redefining their relationship. If grandchildren are born, grandparenting styles must be chosen. Many middle-aged adults begin to adopt a healthier lifestyle. Health promotion needs for the middle-aged adult include adequate rest, leisure activities, regular exercise, good nutrition, reduction or cessation in the use of tobacco or alcohol, and regular screening examinations. A middle-aged adult's social environment is also important, including relationship concerns; communication and relationships with children, grandchildren, and aging parents; and caregiver concerns with their own aging or disabled parents.

According to Erikson's (1968, 1982) developmental theory, the primary developmental task of the middle adult years is to achieve generativity (see Chapter 22). *Generativity* is the willingness to care for and guide others. Middle-aged adults can achieve generativity with their own children or other younger people (Figure 24–3). If middle-aged adults fail to achieve generativity, stagnation occurs. This state is manifested by excessive concern with themselves or destructive behaviour toward their children and the community.

Career Transition. Career changes may occur by choice or as a result of changes in the workplace or society. Middle-aged adults more often change occupations for a variety of reasons, including limited upward mobility, decreasing availability of jobs, and seeking an occupation that is more challenging. In some cases, technological advances or other changes force middle-aged adults to seek new jobs. Some middle-aged adults choose not to retire and continue to work as long as they are able to work. Such changes, particularly when unanticipated, may result in stress that can affect health, family relationships, self-concept, and other dimensions.

Sexuality. After the departure of their last child from the home, many couples rejuvenate their relationships and find increased marital and sexual satisfaction during middle age. The onset of menopause can affect the sexual health of the middle-aged woman. A woman may desire increased sexual activity because pregnancy is no longer possible. Menopausal women may also experience vaginal dryness and dyspareunia or pain during sexual intercourse (see Chapter 27). During middle age, a man may notice changes in the strength of his erection and a decrease in his ability to experience repeated orgasm. Other factors influencing sexuality during this period include work stress; diminished health of one or both partners; and the use of prescription medications with side effects that may influence sexual desire or functioning (e.g., antihypertensive agents). Both partners may experience stresses related to sexual changes or a conflict between their sexual needs and self-perceptions and social attitudes or expectations.

Family Types. Psychosocial factors involving the family may include the stresses of singlehood, marital changes, transition of the family as children leave home, and the care of aging parents.

Singlehood. Many adults older than 35 years have never been married. Many of them have chosen to delay marriage and parenthood. Some single middle-aged adults, however, have chosen to become parents, either biologically or through adoption. Many single middle-aged adults may have no relatives but share a family type of relationship with close friends or work associates. Consequently, some single middle-aged adults may feel isolated during traditional "family" holidays. In times of illness, single adults may have to rely on relatives or friends. Your assessment of single middle-aged adults should include a thorough assessment of psychosocial factors, including the individual's definition of family and available support systems.

Marital Changes. Marital changes that may occur during middle age include death of a spouse, separation, divorce, and the choice of remarrying or remaining single. A widowed, separated, or divorced

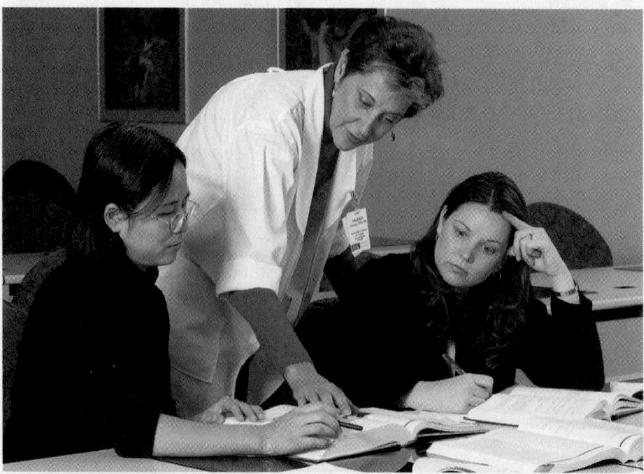

Figure 24-3 Mentoring younger people is important to many middle-aged adults.

client goes through a period of grief and loss in which it is necessary to adapt to the change in marital status. Normal grieving progresses through a series of phases, and resolution of grief may take a year or more. You should assess middle-aged adults' coping with the grief and loss associated with certain life changes (Chapter 29).

If a single middle-aged adult decides to marry, the stressors of marriage are similar to those for the young adult.

Family Transitions. The departure of the last child from the home may be a stressor. Many parents welcome freedom from child-rearing responsibilities, whereas others feel lonely or without direction because of this change (known as "empty-nest" syndrome). Eventually parents must reassess their marriage, resolve conflicts, and plan for the future. On occasion, this readjustment phase may lead to marital conflicts, separation, and divorce.

Care of Aging Parents. Increasing lifespans have led to increased numbers of older adults in the population. Therefore, greater numbers of middle-aged adults must address the personal and social issues confronting their aging parents. Many become caregivers for their older parents.

Housing, employment, health, and economic realities have changed the traditional social expectations between generations in families. The middle-aged adult and the older adult parent may have conflicting priorities concerning their relationship while the older adult strives to remain independent. Negotiations and compromises help in defining and resolving problems. You may encounter middle and older adults in the community, in long-term care facilities, and in hospitals. You can help identify the health needs of both groups and can assist the multigenerational family in determining the health and community resources available to them as they make decisions and plans. You should also assess family relationships to determine family members' perceptions of responsibility and loyalty in relation to caring for older adult members. It is also important to assess environmental resources (e.g., number of rooms in the house, stair rails, or handrails in bathrooms) needed for adults to care for their older parents.

Health Concerns

Physiological concerns for middle-aged adults include stress, level of wellness, obesity, and the formation of positive health habits. When adults seek health care, your focus on the goal of wellness can guide clients to evaluate health behaviours, lifestyle, and environment. Clients' health can be undermined by such alterable factors as stress, obesity, use of tobacco, excessive alcohol consumption, poor nutrition, and unsafe sexual practices. Attention to these risk factors can increase the quality of life and add years to it.

Stress and Stress Reduction. Middle-aged adults' perceptions of health and health behaviours are often important factors in maintaining health. Individuals are prone to stress-related illnesses such as heart attacks, hypertension, migraine headaches, ulcers, colitis, autoimmune disease, backache, arthritis, and cancer. Stress levels may also increase as the middle-aged adult tries to balance responsibilities related to employment, family life, care of children, and care of aging parents.

Throughout life, people are exposed to many stressors (see Chapter 30). After these stressors are identified, you and the client can work together to intervene and modify the stress response. Stress can be reduced in three ways. First, the frequency of stress-producing situations can be minimized. Together, you and the client identify approaches to prevent stressful situations, such as habituation, change avoidance, time blocking, time management, and environmental modification. Second, stress resistance can be increased by psychophysiological preparation, such as increasing self-esteem, improving assertiveness, redirecting goal alternatives, and reorienting cognitive appraisal. Third, the physiological response to stress can be avoided. You can teach the client relaxation techniques, imagery, and biofeedback to recondition the client's response to stress. Chapter 35 explains these general interventions in greater detail.

Levels of Wellness. You must be able to assess the health status of the middle-aged client. Such assessment offers direction for planning nursing care and is useful in evaluating the effectiveness of nursing interventions. You can consult Table 24–4, which shows the expected physical assessment findings of the middle-aged adult, and use standard assessment techniques as guides for physical assessment (see Chapter 32).

Obesity. Obesity, defined as having a body mass index of 30 or more, is a health concern for many middle-aged adults. Among Canadian adults, 13% of women and 14% of men are classified as obese (Canadian Institute for Health Information, 2004). Health consequences of obesity include such conditions as high blood pressure, high blood cholesterol levels, type 2 (non–insulin-dependent) diabetes mellitus, coronary heart disease, osteoarthritis, and obstructive sleep apnea. Continued focus on the goal of wellness can assist clients in evaluating health behaviours and lifestyle that contribute to obesity during the middle adult years. Counselling related to physical activity and nutrition is an important component of the plan of care for overweight and obese clients.

Forming Positive Health Habits. A habit is a person's usual practice or manner of behaviour. This behaviour pattern is reinforced by frequent repetition until it becomes the individual's customary way of behaving. Some habits support health, such as exercise, eating a balanced diet, participating in routine screening and diagnostic tests (e.g., laboratory work for cholesterol, mammography), reducing stress, and daily brushing and flossing of teeth. Other habits involve behaviours harmful to health, such as smoking, consuming excessive alcohol, using illegal drugs, or eating foods with little or no nutritional value.

During assessment, you frequently obtain data about clients' positive and negative health behaviours. In the planning, implementation, and evaluation phases, you help the client maintain habits that protect health and offer healthier alternatives to poor habits.

Health teaching and health counselling are often directed at improving health habits (Box 24–5). The more fully you understand the dynamics of behaviour and habits, the more likely your interventions are to help the client to achieve or reinforce health-promoting behaviours.

To help clients form positive health habits, you become a teacher and facilitator. By providing information about how the body functions and how habits are formed and changed, you raise clients' understanding of the impact of behaviour on health. You cannot change clients' habits. Clients have control of and are responsible for their own behaviours. You can explain psychological principles of changing habits and offer information about health risks. Ultimately, however, the client decides which behaviours will become habits of daily living. Barriers to change exist (Box 24–6). Unless these barriers are minimized or eliminated, it is futile to encourage the client to take actions that are going to be blocked.

As with adolescents and young adults, you continue educating middle-aged adults about STIs, substance abuse, and accident prevention.

BOX 24-5 CLIENT TEACHING

Encouraging Positive Health Habits

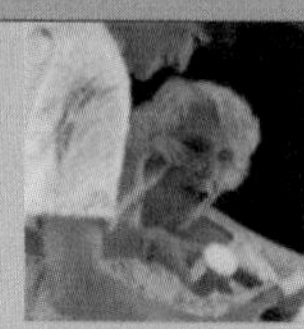

Objective

- Client will increase exercise patterns to include three 2-km walks per week to assist in weight loss and to improve cardiopulmonary functions.

Teaching Strategies

- Review with client the daily work schedule and identify potential times for exercise.
- Inform client about the effect of exercise on weight control and improved cardiac function.
- Demonstrate how to calculate target heart rate and assess pulse correctly.
- Provide warm-up and cool-down exercises, and demonstrate how to do them.
- Instruct client about the importance of support shoes for walking exercises.

Evaluation

- Have client keep log of exercise periods.
- Have client demonstrate pulse measurement.
- Have client demonstrate warm-up and cool-down exercises.
- Inspect client's feet for blisters or sores.

Anxiety. Anxiety is a common response to change, conflict, and perceived control of the environment (Fortinash & Holoday Worret, 2004). Adults often experience anxiety in response to the physiological and psychosocial changes of middle age. Such anxiety can motivate the adult to rethink life goals and can stimulate productivity. For some adults, however, this anxiety precipitates psychosomatic illness and preoccupation with death. Such middle-aged adults view life as being half or more over and think in terms of the time left to live.

Clearly, a life-threatening illness, marital transition, or job stressor increases the anxiety of the client and family. You may need to use crisis intervention or stress management techniques to help the client adapt to the changes of the middle adult years (see Chapter 30).

Depression. Depression is a mood disorder that manifests itself in many ways. Although its onset occurs most frequently between the ages of 25 and 44 years, it is common among adults in the middle years and may have many causes (Fortinash & Holoday Worret, 2004). The risk factors for depression include being female; disappointments or losses at work, school, or in family relationships; departure of the last child from the home; and family history. The incidence of depression in women is twice that in men.

People experiencing mild depression describe feeling sad, "blue," downcast, "down in the dumps," and tearful. Other symptoms include difficulty in sleeping (insomnia) or sleeping too much (hypersomnia), irritability, feelings of social disinterest, and decreased alertness. Physical changes such as weight loss or weight gain, headaches, or feelings of fatigue regardless of the amount of rest may also be depressive symptoms. Depression that occurs during the middle years is commonly characterized by moderate to high anxiety and physical complaints. Mood changes and depression are common phenomena during menopause. Depression may be worsened by the abuse of alcohol or other substances. Your assessment of a depressed middle-aged adult includes focused data collection regarding individual and family history of depression, mood changes, cognitive changes, behavioural and social changes, and physical changes. Assessment data should be collected from both the client and the client's family. Family data may be particularly important, depending on the level of depression being experienced by the middle-aged adult.

BOX 24-6 Barriers to Changing Negative Health Habits

External Barriers	Internal Barriers
Lack of facilities	Lack of knowledge
Lack of materials	Lack of motivation
Lack of social supports	Insufficient skills to effect change in health habits
	Undefined short- and long-term goals

Primary Health Care Programs. Primary health care programs for young and middle-aged adults are designed to prevent illness, promote health, and detect disease in the early stages. You can make valuable contributions to the community's health by taking an active part in the planning of screening programs, teaching programs, and support groups for young and middle-aged adults.

Family planning, birthing, and parenting skills are program topics in which adults might be interested. Health screening for diabetes, hypertension, eye disease, and cancer is a good opportunity for you to perform assessment and provide health teaching and health counselling.

Health education programs can promote changes in behaviour and lifestyle. As a health teacher, you offer information that enables the client to make decisions about health practices. You must be sure that educational programs are culturally appropriate (Box 24–7). Encouraging young to middle adults to adopt more positive health practices during young and middle adulthood may lead to fewer or less complicated health problems during older adulthood. During

BOX 24-7 CULTURAL ASPECTS OF CARE

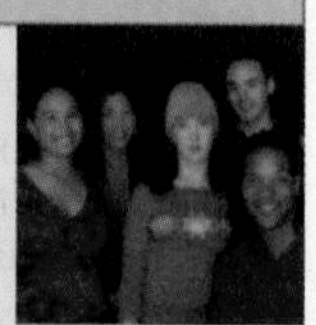

All women experience menopause, but the experience itself of menopause is unique for every woman. The culture in which women participate, beginning in early childhood, contributes to how women learn to respond. The experience of menopause for Korean women in Canada has been studied. Elliott et al.'s (2002) findings revealed that although menopause symptoms required management, Korean women considered menopause to be a natural process. They used herbs and maintained healthy diets, as well as used Western medicine, to deal with menopause symptoms.

Implications for Practice

- Be aware of cultural influences that may affect the experience of menopause, and how women seek assistance from health care professionals.
- Educational materials that combine Western remedies with traditional approaches may be more easily accepted and utilized.
- Cultural norms and taboos may influence women's willingness to discuss personal issues such as menopause. Information sessions on the topic, or more broadly related to women and aging, should be held in community settings where women might gather and feel comfortable.

From Elliott, J., Berman, H., & Kim, S. (2002). A critical ethnography of Korean Canadian women's menopause experience. *Health Care for Women International, 23*(4), 377–388.

health counselling, you and the client should design a plan of action that addresses the client's health and well-being. Through objective problem solving, you help the client grow and change.

Acute Care. Acute illnesses and conditions experienced in middle adulthood may be similar to those in young adulthood. Injuries and acute illnesses in middle adulthood, however, may take a longer recovery period because of the slowing of recuperative processes. In addition, acute illnesses and injuries experienced in middle adulthood are more likely to become chronic conditions.

Restorative and Continuing Care. Chronic illnesses such as diabetes mellitus, hypertension, rheumatoid arthritis, chronic obstructive pulmonary disease, or multiple sclerosis may affect the roles and responsibilities assumed by the middle-aged adult. Strained family relationships, modifications in family activities, increased health care tasks, increased financial stress, the need for housing adaptation, social isolation, medical concerns, and grieving may all result from chronic illness. The degree of disability and the client's perception of both the illness and the disability determine the extent to which lifestyle changes will occur. A few examples of the problems experienced by clients who develop debilitating chronic illness during adulthood include role reversal, changes in sexual behaviour, and alterations in self-image. Along with the current health status of the chronically ill middle-aged adult, you must assess the knowledge base of both the client and family. This assessment should include the medical course of the illness and the prognosis for the client. In addition, you determine the coping mechanisms of the client and family, their adherence to treatment and rehabilitation regimens, and the need for community and social services, along with appropriate referrals.

* KEY CONCEPTS

- Adult development involves orderly and sequential changes that adults experience over time.
- Young adults are generally in a stable period of physical development, except for changes related to pregnancy.
- Cognitive development continues throughout the young and middle adult years.
- Emotional health of young adults is correlated with the ability to address and resolve personal and social problems.
- Young adults must choose a career and decide whether to remain single or marry and begin a family.
- Pregnant women need to understand physiological changes occurring during each trimester.
- Psychosocial changes and health concerns during pregnancy and the puerperium period affect the mother and the rest of the family.
- Health promotion interventions are important during the prenatal period and can improve the well-being of the woman and fetus.
- Midlife transition begins when a person becomes aware that physiological and psychosocial changes signify passage to another stage in life.
- Two significant physiological changes of the middle years are menopause in women and changes in sexual response in men.
- Cognitive changes are rare in middle age except in cases of illness or physical trauma.
- Psychosocial changes for middle-aged adults may be related to career transition, sexuality, marital changes, family transition, and care of aging parents.
- Health goals of middle-aged adults commonly involve preventing stress-related illnesses, participating in health assessments, and adopting positive health habits.

* CRITICAL THINKING EXERCISES

1. Katya is a 24-year-old woman who smokes two packs of cigarettes per day. She began smoking when she was 14 years old. Katya complains to you at the clinic, "I just can't seem to kick the habit no matter how hard I try." What information do you need to know to assist Katya in quitting smoking?
2. Rohan, 48 years old, married, and the father of 13- and 16-year-old sons, has recently had to assume the responsibility of caring for his 78-year-old mother after she suffered a stroke. Describe your role in assisting Rohan to care for his mother.

* REVIEW QUESTIONS

1. Most young adults have completed physical growth by the age of
   1. 18 years
   2. 20 years
   3. 25 years
   4. 30 years
2. Young adults usually have good health. However, it is important to direct health care education in this population toward activities related to
   1. Health promotion
   2. Primary prevention
   3. Secondary prevention
   4. Tertiary prevention
3. When determining what amount of information the individual needs to make decisions about the prescribed course of therapy, you should consider factors that may affect the individual's compliance with the regimen, including educational level, socioeconomic factors, and
   1. Sexuality
   2. Lifestyle
   3. Gender
   4. Motivation and desire to learn
4. A common physiological change in the second trimester of pregnancy is
   1. Morning sickness
   2. Amenorrhea
   3. Increased colostrum
   4. Quickening
5. The most common cause of death in young adults is
   1. Suicide
   2. Accidents
   3. Substance use
   4. Cancer
6. Close friends and associates of the single young adult may also be viewed as the individual's
   1. Siblings
   2. Family
   3. Alternative family structure
   4. Substitute parents
7. A young man's father and paternal grandfather had myocardial infarctions (heart attacks) in their 50s. Therefore, he is at risk for a future myocardial infarction. The young man faces what type of health risk?
   1. Lifestyle
   2. Poor personal hygiene
   3. Family history
   4. Hereditary disease

8. In the middle adult years, the family enters which stage?
   1. Generative stage
   2. Independence stage
   3. Postparental family stage
   4. Family orientation stage
9. To improve an adult's health habits, you often use health counselling and
   1. Medications
   2. Referrals
   3. Health teaching
   4. Stress management techniques
10. To help recondition the client's response to stress, you can use biofeedback, imagery, and
    1. Medication
    2. Time management strategies
    3. Relaxation techniques
    4. Assertiveness training

* RECOMMENDED WEB SITES

Breastfeeding Committee for Canada: http://www.breastfeedingcanada.ca

The Breastfeeding Committee for Canada was established in 1991 as a Health Canada initiative. This Web site addresses Canadian breastfeeding issues.

Canadian Cancer Society: http://www.cancer.ca

This site provides information on specific cancers, clinical trials, support services, and ways to get involved.

Canadian Women's Health Network: http://www.cwhn.ca

The goal of the Canadian Women's Health Network is to share information, resources, and strategies to improve women's health.

Health Canada, Population and Public Health Branch: http://www.gov.pe.ca/infopei/index.php3?number=53989

This Web site has links to topics concerning health issues of Canadian adults, including information on chronic diseases, infectious diseases, and healthy living.

La Leche League Canada: http://www.lllc.ca

This Web site encourages, promotes, and provides mother-to-mother breastfeeding support and educational opportunities as an important contribution to the health of children, families, and society.

25

Older Adulthood

Written by Wendy Duggleby, RN, PhD, AOCN

Based on the original chapter by Annette Lueckenotte, RN, MS, BC, GNP, GCNS

objectives

Mastery of content in this chapter will enable you to:

- Define the key terms listed.
- Discuss demographic trends related to older adults in Canada.
- Identify common myths and stereotypes about older adults.
- List the types of community-based and institutional health care services available to older adults.
- Identify selected biological and psychosocial theories of aging.
- Discuss common developmental tasks of older adults.
- Describe common physiological changes associated with aging.
- Differentiate among delirium, dementia, and depression.
- Discuss issues related to psychosocial changes connected with aging.
- Describe selected health concerns of older adults.
- Identify nursing interventions related to the physiological, cognitive, and psychosocial changes of aging.

key terms

Abuse, p. 388
Ageism, p. 379
Alzheimer's disease, p. 386
Cognitive stimulation, p. 394
Delirium, p. 386
Dementia, p. 386
Depression, p. 387
Geriatrics, p. 378
Gerontic nursing, p. 379
Gerontological nursing, p. 378
Gerontology, p. 378
Nonstochastic theories, p. 380
Personal care home, p. 381
Polypharmacy, p. 393
Reminiscence, p. 394
Stochastic theories, p. 380

media resources

evolve Web Site

- Audio Chapter Summaries
- Glossary
- Multiple-Choice Review Questions
- Student Learning Activities
- Weblinks

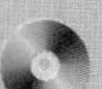
Companion CD

- Glossary
- Interactive Learning Activities
- Fluids and Electrolytes Tutorial
- Test-Taking Skills

The identification of 65 years of age as the start of older adulthood dates back to social reform in Germany in the nineteenth century. The age of 65 years continues to be used as the lower boundary for "old age" in demographics and social policy, although many older adults consider themselves to be "middle-aged" well into their 70s (Statistics Canada, 2008). Chronological age may have little relation to the reality of aging for an older adult. Each person ages in his or her own ways according to his or her own schedules and life histories. Even though generalizations are made in this chapter about the aging process and its effect on individuals, every older adult is unique and must be treated as a unique individual by nurses.

The number of older adults in Canada is growing, both absolutely and as a proportion of the total population. In 2005, 4.2 million adults were older than 65 years in Canada; they represented 13.2% of the population (Statistics Canada, 2008). This number represented an increase of 4.2 % since 1997. Geographic variations in the aging population exist across Canada; the proportion of older adults is lowest in Nunavut (2.6%) and highest in Saskatchewan (14.8%; Statistics Canada, 2008). The number of older adults is expected to increase to 9.8 million (24.5% of the population) by 2036 (Statistics Canada, 2008). Part of that increase is a result of the extension of the average lifespan. Since 2001, life expectancy has increased. On average, a 65-year-old woman could expect to live another 20.8 years, and a 65-year-old man, another 17.4 years. In 2002 the average life expectancy at birth for Canadians was 79.7 years: 77.2 years for men and 82.1 years for women (Statistics Canada, 2008).

Two other factors contribute to the projected increase in the number of older adults: the aging of the baby boom generation and the growth of the population segment older than 85 years. The baby boomers are the large cohort of adults born between 1946 and 1964. The oldest baby boomers will reach the age of 65 years in 2011. As baby boomers age, social and health care programs will need to expand to meet their needs, as well as the needs of the fastest-growing group of adults: those aged 85 years and older. The numbers in this group have doubled since 1981 to 430,000 in 2001 and are expected to grow to 2.5 million by 2021 (5.8% of the population; Statistics Canada, 2008).

The diversity of the population older than 65 years is also projected to increase. Approximately 26.2% of Canadian older adults were born outside of Canada. Most immigrated when they were young. Between 1995 and 2004, 2% to 4% of immigrants arriving each year were older adults. This number is expected to increase as immigration patterns change. Of all immigrant older adults, 96% can speak one or both of Canada's official languages. Of the population older than 65 years, more women than men are unable to speak either French or English. In 2001, 5.0% of older women and 3.2% of older men were unable to speak either official language. Currently, older adults make up a small proportion (4%) of Canada's Aboriginal population (Statistics Canada, 2008). However, the number of older Aboriginal people is expected to triple by 2016 as their population ages and lives longer. As they care for older adults from these groups, nurses must account for the diversity in cultures, values, and languages. Examples of culturally safe nursing approaches to older adults include respect for preferences in food, music, and religion; attentive listening; use of physical assessment norms appropriate for diverse groups; and asking about personal health practices, family customs, lifestyle preferences, and spiritual resources (Ebersole et al., 2008). Chapter 10 provides further information on culturally safe care.

Variability Among Older Adults

The nursing care of older adults poses special challenges because of great variation in their physiological, cognitive, and psychosocial health. Levels of functional ability also vary widely among older adults. The majority of older adults are active and involved members of their communities. A smaller number have lost the ability to care for themselves, are confused or withdrawn, are unable to make decisions concerning their needs, or have a combination of these factors. Most older adults live in noninstitutional settings, either with family members or alone (28.9% of older adults live alone). Only 7.4% of all older adults reside in institutions such as long-term care facilities (National Advisory Council on Aging [NACA], 2006). Age influences living arrangements: The proportion of older adults living with a spouse decreases with age, the proportion living alone increases with age, and the proportion living in an institution increases with age.

Aging does not inevitably lead to disability and dependence. Most older people remain functionally independent despite the increasing prevalence of chronic disease. Nursing assessment, a complex and challenging process, can provide valuable clues to the effect of a disease or illness on a client's functional status. Chronic conditions add to the complexity of assessment and care of the older adult. Approximately 91% of older adults report one or more chronic conditions; arthritis, hypertension, heart disease, vision impairment, and diabetes mellitus are the most common conditions in noninstitutionalized older adults (NACA, 2006). These chronic conditions impose limitations on activities: Slightly more than 22% of adults 65 to 74 years of age and nearly 50% of adults aged 85 years or older report some limitations in activities (NACA, 2006).

The physical, cognitive, and psychosocial aspects of aging are closely related. For the older person, a reduced ability to respond to stress, the experience of multiple losses, and the physical changes associated with normal aging may combine to increase the risk for illness and functional deterioration. Although the interaction of these physical and psychosocial factors can be serious, you should not assume that all older adults have signs, symptoms, or behaviours representing disease and decline or that these are the only items to be assessed. An older adult's strengths and abilities must also be identified during the assessment.

Terminology

As the number of older adults increases, the specialty of gerontological nursing is gaining in importance. Several terms are used, at times interchangeably, to describe this specialty (Meiner & Lueckenotte, 2006):

- **Geriatrics** is the branch of medicine that deals with the physiological and psychological aspects of aging and with the diagnosis and treatment of diseases affecting older adults.
- **Gerontology** is the study of all aspects of the aging process and its consequences.
- **Gerontological nursing** is concerned with assessment of the health and functional status of older adults; diagnosis, planning, and implementing health care and services to meet the identified needs; and evaluating the effectiveness of such care. This is the term most often used by nurses specializing in this field.

- **Gerontic nursing**, a seldom-used term that is gaining popularity, is the art and practice of nurturing, caring, and comforting older clients, rather than merely the treatment of disease.

Myths and Stereotypes

Despite ongoing research in the field of gerontology, false beliefs and myths about older adults persist. These stereotypes include beliefs about the physical and psychosocial characteristics and the lifestyles of older adults. Younger and older adults may believe in stereotypes, both positive and negative, but this does not automatically imply age-based prejudice (Chasteen et al., 2002). However, negative stereotypes may adversely affect the quality of the care provided to older clients. Nurses, although personally susceptible to the myths and stereotypes held by society, have the responsibility to dispel the myths and replace the stereotypes with accurate information.

Older adults are sometimes stereotyped as ill and disabled. However, although many experience chronic conditions or have at least one disability that limits their performance of activities of daily living (ADLs), only 23% of older adults describe their health as poor or fair (Statistics Canada, 2008). Other common misconceptions are that older adults are generally not interested in sex and that any interest in sexual activities is abnormal and should be discouraged. However, many older adults report continued enjoyment of sexual relationships.

Some people believe that older adults are forgetful, confused, rigid, bored, and unfriendly and that they are unable to understand and learn new information. However, centenarians, the oldest of the old, are described as having an optimistic outlook on life, good memories, broad social contacts and interests, and tolerance for others (Ebersole et al., 2008). Although the process of learning may be affected by age-related changes in vision or hearing or by reduced energy and endurance, older adults are lifelong learners. You should use teaching techniques that compensate for sensory changes, provide additional time for remembering and responding, and present concrete rather than abstract material to facilitate learning by older adults. Other effective teaching techniques draw from older adults' past experiences and correspond to their identified interests rather than to the content areas believed important by the health care professional. Box 25–1 presents additional teaching strategies that you can use to address the learning needs of older adults.

Stereotypes about lifestyles include mistaken notions about living arrangements and finances. As mentioned previously, most older adults live in noninstitutional settings, either with family members or alone. Misconceptions about the financial status of older adults range from beliefs that many are affluent to beliefs that many are poor. In 2004, about 5.6% of noninstitutionalized Canadian older adults were living in low-income households (NACA, 2006). Rates of poverty among older adults in Canada are among the lowest such rates in industrialized countries. However, unattached older adults, particularly women, are more likely to have low incomes. This statistic is expected to change because of women's increased workforce participation. In a society that values attractiveness, energy, and youth, these myths and stereotypes lead to the undervaluing of older adults. Some people believe that older adults are unattractive and become worthless to society after they leave the workforce. Others consider the knowledge and experience of older adults to be too old-fashioned to have any current value. These notions underlie the concept of **ageism**, which is discrimination against people because of increasing age, just as racism and sexism are discrimination based on skin colour and gender, respectively. Ageism has the potential to undermine the self-confidence of older adults, limit their access to care, and distort caregivers' understanding of the uniqueness of each older adult (Hess, 2006).

Today, discrimination on the grounds of age is illegal. The economic and political power of older adults also acts against ageism. Older adults are a significant proportion of the consumer economy. As voters and activists in various issues, they influence the formation of public policy. Their participation adds a unique perspective to social, economic, and technological issues because they have experienced so much change. In the past 100 years, transportation has progressed from horse-drawn carriages to space shuttle flights. Gaslights and steam power have given way to electricity and nuclear power. Typewriters and carbon paper have been replaced by computers and copier machines. Many older adults have lived through the Great Depression and two world wars; all have lived through the Korean War and the Afghanistan conflict. Health care has changed as the era of the family doctor gave way to the age of specialization. After witnessing the government initiatives that established the Old Age Security Program, Canada Pension Plan, and National Health Insurance System (Medicare), older adults are currently living with

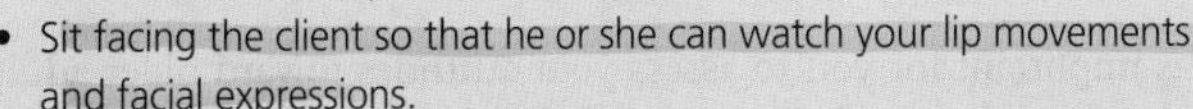

BOX 25-1 FOCUS ON OLDER ADULTS

Older Adult Clients' Learning Needs

Teaching Strategies

- Make sure the client is ready to learn before you try to teach him or her. Watch for clues that would indicate that the client is preoccupied or too anxious to comprehend the material.
- Sit facing the client so that he or she can watch your lip movements and facial expressions.
- Speak slowly.
- Keep your tone of voice low; older adults can hear low-frequency sounds better than high-frequency sounds.
- Give the client enough time in which to respond because older adults' reaction times may be longer than those of younger people.
- To help the client concentrate, focus on a single topic.
- Keep environmental distractions to a minimum.
- With permission of the client, invite another member of the household to join the discussion.
- Use auditory, visual, and tactile cues to enhance learning and help the client remember information.
- Ask for feedback to ensure that the information has been understood.
- Refer to the client's past experience; connect new learning to that already learned.
- Compensate for physical discomfort and sensory alterations if necessary.
- Support a positive self-image in the learner.
- Use creative teaching strategies.
- Respond to identified interests of learners.
- Emphasize and integrate emotional and personal values in the acquisition of skills and ideas.

Adapted from Ebersole, P. & Hess, P. (2008). *Geriatric nursing and healthy aging* (p. 552). St. Louis, MO: Mosby; and SPRY Foundation. (2000). *Senior citizens can learn quite well, thank you.* Retrieved November 5, 2008, from http://www.rwjf.org/pr/product.jsp?id=17930

the changes imposed by health care reform. Having lived through all of these events and changes, older adults have stories and examples of coping with change to share with other people.

Nurses' Attitudes Toward Older Adults

It is important for you to assess your attitudes toward older adults, your own aging, and the aging of your family, friends, and clients. Your attitudes toward older adults result partly from personal experiences with older adults, education, employment experiences, attitudes of coworkers and employers, and your own age. Cultivation of positive attitudes toward older adults and specialized knowledge about aging and the health care needs of older adults are priorities for nurses.

Positive attitudes are based in part on a realistic portrayal of the characteristics and health care needs of older adults. In the past, negative attitudes about aging and older adults have contributed to the persistence of stereotypes of older adults as dependent and less attractive than younger clients. Health care professionals, under the influence of these attitudes, often lacked respect for older clients and ignored the opportunity to actively involve them in care decisions and activities. At times, hospitals and long-term care facilities have treated older adults as objects to be acted upon rather than as independent, dignified adults. The time has come for all nurses to recognize and address ageism by questioning prevailing negative attitudes and sterotypes and advocating for older adults in all care settings.

Theories of Aging

Various theorists have attempted to describe the complex biopsychosocial process of aging. Although many theories have been developed, no single universally accepted theory predicts and explains the complexities of the aging process. You must be aware of the scientific attempts to explain the aging process and the concepts included in the theories. Although the theories are in various stages of development and have limitations, you can use them to increase your understanding of the phenomena affecting the health and well-being of older adults.

The biological theories of aging are categorized as either stochastic theories or nonstochastic theories. **Stochastic theories** view aging as the result of random cellular damage that occurs over time. The accumulated damage leads to the physical changes characteristic of the aging process. According to the **nonstochastic theories**, genetically programmed physiological mechanisms within the body control the process of aging.

The psychosocial theories of aging attempt to explain changes in behaviour, roles, and relationships that come with aging. As with biological theories of aging, no single psychosocial theory is universally accepted. The psychosocial theories also reflect the values held by the theorist and society at the time the theory was first articulated. The three classic psychosocial theories of aging are disengagement theory, activity theory, and continuity theory. According to disengagement theory, the oldest psychosocial theory, aging individuals withdraw from customary roles and engage in more introspective, self-focused activities as society disengages from them (Cummings & Henry, 1961). In the activity theory, unlike the disengagement theory, the continuation of activities performed during middle age is considered necessary for successful aging (Lemon et al., 1972). According to continuity theory or developmental theory (Neugarten, 1964), personality remains the same and behaviour becomes more predictable as people age. The personality and behaviour patterns developed during a lifetime determine the degree of engagement and activity in older adulthood.

Critics suggest, however, that all three psychosocial theories either fail in some measure to consider the many factors that affect an individual's response to the aging process or address those factors in a simplistic manner. Biologically, psychosocially, and spiritually, each individual ages in a unique way.

Developmental Tasks for Older Adults

Theories of aging are closely linked to the concept of developmental tasks appropriate for distinct stages of life. Although no two individuals age in the same way, either biologically or psychosocially, frameworks outlining developmentally appropriate tasks for older adult have been developed. Seven developmental tasks of the older adult are listed in Box 25–2.

These developmental tasks are common to many older adults and are associated with varying degrees of change and loss. The more common losses involve health, significant others, a sense of being useful, socialization, income, and independent living. The ways that older adults adjust to the changes of aging are highly individualized. For some, adaptation and adjustment are relatively easy. For others, coping with the changes caused by aging may require the assistance of family, friends, and health care professionals. You must be sensitive to the effect of such losses on older adults and their families and be prepared to offer support.

Older adults must adjust to the physical changes that accompany aging. The extent and timing of these changes vary from individual to individual, but as body systems age, changes occur in appearance and functioning. These changes are not associated with a disease but are normal changes. The presence of disease may alter the timing of the changes or their impact on daily life. Structural and functional changes associated with aging are described in the "Physiological Changes" section.

The great majority of Canadian older adults are retired; 6% of them are employed outside the home (NACA, 2006). A large number (85%) of employed older adults work on a part-time basis. Many return to paid work after initial retirement; in 2002, 22% of Canadian retirees reported they had returned to paid work. Older adults retired from employment outside the home are challenged to cope with the loss of that work role. Older adults who worked at home and the spouses of those who worked outside the home also face role changes as they retire.

➤ BOX 25-2 Developmental Tasks for the Older Adult

- Adjusting to decreasing health and physical strength
- Adjusting to retirement and reduced or fixed income
- Adjusting to the death of a spouse
- Accepting one's self as an aging person
- Maintaining satisfactory living arrangements
- Redefining relationships with adult children
- Finding ways to maintain quality of life

Adapted from Erikson, E. H., Erikson, J. M., & Kivnick, H. Q. (1986). *Vital involvement in old age: The experience of old age in our time.* New York: W. W. Norton.

Because retirement is usually anticipated, people can plan for financial changes and replacement activities. Many older adults welcome retirement as a time to pursue new interests and hobbies, to participate in volunteer activities, to continue their education, or to start a new business career. Retirement plans for some older adults include changes of residence, such as moving to a different city or province or moving to a different type of housing.

Reasons other than retirement may also lead to changes of residence. For example, physical impairments may necessitate relocation to a smaller, single-level home. Because of health problems, an older adult may need to live with relatives or friends or move to an assisted-living or long-term care facility. A change in living arrangements for an older adult may require an extended period of adjustment, during which assistance and support from health care professionals, friends, and family members are needed. However, although they may change residence, the majority of Canadian older adults report that they enjoy good housing (NACA, 2006).

The majority of older adults are faced with the death of a spouse. In 2001, 28% of all older women were widows, and 12.7% of older men were widowers (Statistics Canada, 2008). Some older adults must cope with the death of adult children and grandchildren. All experience the deaths of friends. These deaths represent both losses and reminders of personal mortality. Coming to terms with these deaths is often difficult. By assisting older adults through the grieving process, you can help them resolve the issues posed by these deaths.

The redefining of relationships with children that occurs as the children of older adults grow up and leave home, continues as older adults experience the challenges of aging. A variety of issues may arise, such as role reversal, control of decision making, dependence, conflict, guilt, and loss. How these issues surface in situations and how they are resolved depends in part on the past relationship between the older adult and the adult children. All of the involved parties are influenced by past experiences and powerful emotions. When adult children assist the older adults of their family, they must find ways to balance the demands of their own children and their careers. Adult children also determine how much assistance to provide and how much decision-making authority to assume. As adult children and aging parents negotiate the parameters of the changed roles, you may act as a counsellor to both the parents and the children. You can assist adult children by listening and by helping them distinguish between changes and behaviours related to illness, normal aging changes, and their parents' lifelong preferences and patterns of behaviour.

Faced with the changes that come with aging, older adults must find ways to maintain their quality of life. The definition of quality of life varies from person to person. You must listen to what an older adult considers to be most important rather than making assumptions about that individual's priorities. Together, you and the client may set objectives for maintaining quality of life, whether quality of life is defined as maintenance of social relationships, continuing to live alone, or continuing activities such as driving or gardening.

Community-Based and Institutional Health Care Services

You may encounter older adult clients in a wide variety of community-based and institutional health care settings. Outside of the acute care hospital setting, you and other nurses may care for older adults in private homes and apartments, adult day care centres, assisted-living facilities (also known as *supportive housing*), and long-term care facilities. Long-term care facilities provide accommodations, 24-hour nursing care, and support services for people who cannot care for themselves at home but do not need hospital care. Assisted-living facilities are designed for residents who need only minimal to moderate care. Residents live independently in their own apartments and are provided with support services such as homemaking or personal care. Some assisted-living facilities are small group homes where residents share common eating and living areas. In some provinces, personal care homes are offered as a type of assisted-living facility. A **personal care home** is a private business that provides accommodation, meals, and supervision or assistance with personal care in a family-like atmosphere. Nursing services are not usually included in assisted-living facilities.

You can also assist older adults and their families by providing information and answering questions as they make choices among care options. During the decision-making period, the actual move from a private home to an assisted-living or long-term care facility, and the time after the move, your role is to support the older adult and the family. You can provide information about the selection of a good assisted-living or long-term care facility (Box 25–3). The best way to evaluate quality is to visit that facility and inspect it personally (Rantz et al., 2001).

Assessing the Needs of Older Adults

Gerontological nursing offers creative approaches for maximizing the potential of older adults. The standards of practice of the Canadian Gerontological Nursing Association (1996) were developed to define the uniqueness and scope of gerontological nursing practice, which includes functions such as assessment. With comprehensive assessment information regarding an older client's strengths, resources, and

BOX 25-3 FOCUS ON OLDER ADULTS

Selecting a Personal Care Home

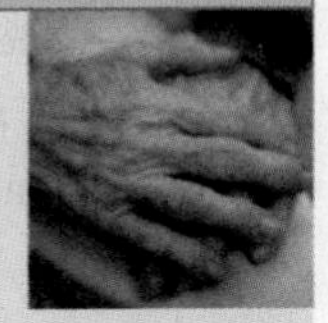

A personal care home, like all assisted-living facilities, is designed for adults who need minimal to moderate assistance. It provides an adult with accommodation, meals, and supervision or assistance with personal care. Advise clients that an important step in the selection process is to visit the facility. Clients should select a home that offers the features that are most important to them. Suggest to clients that they do the following when visiting a personal care home:

- Notice the atmosphere. The facility should feel like a home. Residents should be able to personalize their rooms and have privacy. Space should be adequate to meet residents' requirements.
- Ask to see the facility's license.
- Talk to the staff and residents about the care services provided, recreation activities, and transportation.
- Ask about the experience and training of staff.
- Ask whether residents are encouraged to do things they like to do around the home, such as tidying their room.
- Talk about how much money you will pay to live in the home and what you will receive in return.
- Ask to see the menu plan.
- Ask to see a copy of the residents' rights and privileges.
- Ask about the rules of the home.

Adapted from Saskatchewan Health. (2008). *Selecting a personal care home.* Retrieved November 6, 2008, from http://www.health.gov.sk.ca/rr_selecting_prsnl_care.HTML

limitations, you and the client can identify needs and problems and select interventions that maintain the client's physical abilities and create an environment for psychosocial and spiritual well-being. A thorough assessment requires you to actively engage older adults and provide them with enough time to share important information about their health. You should assess for changes in physiology, cognition, and psychosocial behaviour.

Nursing assessment must take into account five key points to ensure an age-specific approach: (1) the interrelation between physical and psychosocial aspects of aging, (2) the effects of disease and disability on functional status, (3) the decreased efficiency of homeostatic mechanisms, (4) the lack of standards for health and illness norms, and (5) altered manifestations of and responses to specific disease (Meiner & Lueckenotte, 2006). Obtaining a comprehensive assessment of an older adult often takes more time than does an assessment of a younger adult because of the longer life and medical history and the potential complexity of that history. By planning to spend extra time with the assessment, you and an older adult are less likely to feel rushed. During the physical examination, you may find it necessary to allow rest periods or to conduct the assessment in several sessions because of the reduced energy and limited endurance experienced by some frail older adults.

Sensory changes may also affect data gathering. Your choice of communication techniques is influenced by any visual or hearing impairments experienced by the client. If older adults are unable to understand your visual or auditory cues, assessment data may be inaccurate or misleading. For example, if a client has difficulty hearing your questions, his or her responses may be inappropriate, and you may wrongly believe that the client is confused. You can use the following communication techniques with an older adult who has a visual impairment:

- Sit or stand in front of the client, in full view.
- Face the client while speaking; do not cover your mouth.
- Provide diffuse, bright, nonglare lighting.
- Encourage clients with assistive devices such as glasses or magnifiers to use them.

You can use the following techniques with an older adult who has a hearing impairment:

- Speak directly to the client; do not cover your mouth.
- Speak in clear, low-pitched tones at a moderate rate and volume.
- Reduce background noises; move to a quiet, private room.
- Ask whether the client has a "good ear," and speak toward that ear.
- Encourage clients with assistive devices such as hearing aids or "microphone plus earphones" to use them.
- Make sure the hearing aid is working properly (check the battery, check that the hearing aid is turned on, adjust volume controls).
- Check the ear canal for cerumen impaction.

Memory deficits, if present, will affect the accuracy and completeness of the data collected. Information contributed by a family member or other caregiver, such as a history of allergies and documentation of immunizations, may be necessary to supplement the client's recollection of past medical events and information. You must use tact when involving another person in the assessment interview with an older adult. The additional person supplements the answers of the client with the client's consent, but the client remains the focus of the interview.

Interpreters must be present when an older adult does not speak your language. The spoken word must be interpreted within the context of the client's culture. To ensure culturally safe means of communication during assessment, (1) identify how the client wishes to be addressed (use culturally appropriate titles); (2) assess the health-related beliefs and practices of the client; and (3) know the beliefs and practices of the older client's culture group with regard to spatial requirements, eye contact, and touch, and use them to establish rapport.

In older clients, signs and symptoms of diseases and laboratory values may be different from those in younger clients; the classic signs and symptoms of diseases may be absent, blunted, or atypical in older adults (Meiner & Lueckenotte, 2006). These differences may result from age-related changes in organ systems and homeostatic mechanisms, from progressive loss of physiological and functional reserves, or from coexisting acute or chronic conditions. As a result, for example, an older adult with a urinary tract infection may present with confusion, loss of appetite, weakness, dizziness, or fatigue instead of fever, dysuria, frequency, or urgency; an older adult with pneumonia may have tachycardia, tachypnea, and confusion without the more common symptoms of fever and productive cough; and instead of substernal chest pain and diaphoresis, an older adult with a myocardial infarction may experience epigastric discomfort, restlessness, hypotension, confusion, or referred or no pain. Variations from the usual norms for laboratory values may result from age-related changes in cardiac, pulmonary, renal, and metabolic function (Beers & Berkow, 2000). Examples of laboratory values that may be increased by these changes include, but are not limited to, levels of alkaline phosphatase, serum cholesterol, triglycerides, serum glucose (postprandial), and serum uric acid. Examples of laboratory values that may be decreased by the aging process include, but are not limited to, levels of serum calcium, and serum creatine kinase, as well as creatinine clearance.

It is important to recognize the early indicators of acute illness in older adults: change in mental status, falls, dehydration, decrease in appetite, loss of function, dizziness, and incontinence (Amella, 2004). Two key principles of providing age-appropriate nursing care are timely detection of these cardinal signs of illness and a focus on finding underlying causes so that treatment can begin (Box 25–4). As a result of mistaken assumptions about what normal aging is, attention is often not paid to underlying causes (King, 2005). Many health challenges can coexist, which adds to the difficulty in isolating the causes of symptoms. Mental status commonly changes as a result of disease and psychological issues, but more often in relation to drug toxicity or adverse drug events. A fall is a complex event, and careful investigation is necessary to find out whether it has environmental causes or is the symptom of a new-onset illness; such illnesses include cardiac, respiratory, msuculoskeletal, neurological, urological, and sensory disorders. Dehydration is common in older adults because the thirst response is reduced, which results in less water intake, and because less free water is available as a consequence of decreased muscle mass. Vomiting and diarrhea can accompany the onset of an acute illness, and older adults are then at risk for further dehydration. Decrease in appetite is a common symptom with the onset of pneumonia, heart failure, and urinary tract infection. Loss of functional ability occurs either in a subtle manner over a period of time or suddenly, depending on the underlying cause. Thyroid disease, infection, cardiac or pulmonary conditions, metabolic disturbances, and anemia are common causes of functional decline, and so you need to identify them early and notify health care professionals so that proper treatment can be initiated. Dizziness is a common sign of various acute illnesses, including anemia, arrhythmia, infection, myocardial infarction, stroke, and brain tumour. New-onset urinary incontinence in an older adult is often associated with a urinary tract infection, but it can also be a symptom of an electrolyte abnormality or an adverse drug event.

> BOX 25-4 **Examples of Indicators of Acute Illness in Different Settings**

Hospital

- Confusion is not inevitable. Look for neurological events, new medication, or the presence of risk factors for delirium.
- Many hospitalized older adults suffer from chronic dehydration accelerated by acute illness.
- Not all older adults have fevers with infection. Symptoms instead may include increased respiratory rate, falls, incontinence, or confusion.

Nursing Home

- Health care professionals often undertreat pain in older adults, especially those with dementia. Look for nonverbal cues such as grimacing or resistance to care.
- Decline in functional ability (even a minor one, such as the inability to sit upright in a chair) is a signal of new illness.
- Residents with less muscle mass—both frail and obese persons—are at heightened risk for toxicity from protein-binding drugs such as phenytoin (Dilantin) and warfarin (Coumadin).
- Urinary or fecal incontinence is often a sign of the onset of a new illness.

Ambulatory Care

- Complaints of fatigue or decreased ability to perform usual activities are signs of anemia, thyroid problems, depression, or neurological or cardiac problems.
- Severe gastrointestinal problems in older adults do not always manifest with the same acute symptoms seen in younger clients. Ask about constipation, cramping sensations, and changes in bowel habits.
- Older adults reporting increased dyspnea and confusion, especially those with a cardiac history, need to go to the emergency department; these are the most common manifestations of myocardial infarction in this population.
- Depression is common among older adults with chronic illnesses. Watch for lack of interest in formerly pleasurable activities, and be alert to significant personal losses or changes in role or home life.

Home Care

- Investigate all falls, focusing on balance, gait, and neurological issues.
- Monitor older adults with late-stage heart disease for loss of appetite, which is an early symptom of impending heart failure.
- Monitor for drug–drug interactions in older clients who are seeing more than one health care professional and taking multiple medications.

Adapted from Amella, E. J. (2004). Presentation of illness in older adults. *American Journal of Nursing, 104*(10), 40–51.

Physiological Changes

Perception of well-being can define quality of life. Understanding a client's perceptions about health status is essential for accurate assessment and development of clinically relevant interventions. Older adults' concepts of health generally depend on personal perceptions of functional ability. Therefore, older adults engaged in ADLs usually consider themselves healthy, whereas those whose activities are limited by physical, emotional, or social impairments may perceive themselves as ill.

Many observed physiological changes in older adults are called "normal." Finding such changes during an assessment is not unexpected. These physiological changes are not always pathological processes, but they may make older adults more vulnerable to some common clinical conditions and diseases. Some older adults experience all of these physiological changes, and others experience only a few. The body changes continuously with age, and specific effects on particular older adults depend on health, lifestyle, stressors, and environmental conditions. You should know about these commonly experienced changes in order to provide appropriate care for older adults and to assist with adaptation to the changes. Common physiological changes are summarized in Table 25–1.

General Survey. The general survey occurs during your initial encounter with an older adult and includes a quick, but careful, head-to-toe scan of the client, which you should document in a concise description. An initial inspection of an older adult might reveal whether eye contact and facial expression are appropriate to the situation, as well as common aging changes such as facial wrinkles, grey hair, loss of body mass in the extremities, and an increase of body mass in the trunk.

Integumentary System. With aging, the skin loses resilience and moisture. The epithelial layer thins, and elastic collagen fibres shrink and become rigid. Wrinkles of the face and neck reflect lifelong patterns of muscle activity and facial expressions, the pull of gravity on tissue, and diminished elasticity.

Spots and lesions may also be present on the skin. Smooth, brown, irregularly shaped spots ("age spots," or senile lentigo) initially appear on the backs of the hands and on forearms. Small, round, red or brown cherry angiomas may be found on the trunk. Seborrheic lesions or keratoses may appear as irregular, round or oval, brown, watery lesions. Years of sun exposure contribute to the aging of the skin and may lead to premalignant and malignant lesions. In examining skin lesions, you must rule out three malignancies related to sun exposure: melanoma, basal cell carcinoma, and squamous cell carcinoma (see Chapter 32).

Head and Neck. The facial features of older adults become more pronounced as a result of loss of subcutaneous fat and skin elasticity. Facial features may appear asymmetrical because of missing teeth or improperly fitting dentures. In addition, common vocal changes include a rise in pitch and a loss of power and range.

Visual acuity declines with age. This decline may be the result of retinal damage, reduced pupil size, development of opacities in the lens, or loss of lens elasticity. Presbyopia (the gradual decline in the ability to focus on close objects) is common in older adults. The ability to see in darkness is reduced, and adaptation to abrupt changes from dark areas to light areas (and the reverse) is slower. Ambient lighting (soft, indirect light that usually illuminates the entire room) is generally the best type of lighting for older adults. However, older adults also have increased sensitivity to the effects of glare, and interventions to increase ambient light should not increase glare. Changes in colour vision and discoloration of the lens make it difficult to distinguish between blues and greens and among pastel shades.

Auditory changes are often subtle. The earliest losses of hearing acuity may be ignored until friends and family members comment on it. Presbycusis, a common age-related change in auditory acuity, is a decrease in the ability to hear high-pitched sounds and sibilant consonants such as "s," "sh," and "ch." Before you assume that presbycusis is present, you must inspect the client's external auditory canal for the presence of cerumen (earwax). Impacted cerumen is an easily treated cause of diminished hearing acuity.

Taste buds atrophy and lose sensitivity. Older adults are less able to discern among salty, sweet, sour, and bitter tastes. The sense of smell is also decreased, which further reduces the sense of taste. Salivary secretion is reduced as well.

Thorax and Lungs. Because of changes in the musculoskeletal system, the configuration of the thorax sometimes changes. After the age of 55 years, respiratory muscle strength begins to decrease (Beers & Berkow, 2000). The anteroposterior diameter of the thorax increases. The incidence of osteoporosis is increased in older adults; vertebral changes caused by osteoporosis lead to dorsal kyphosis, the curvature of the thoracic spine sometimes called "dowager's hump." Calcification of the costal cartilage can cause decreased mobility of the ribs. The chest wall gradually becomes stiffer. Lung expansion decreases. If kyphosis or chronic obstructive lung disease is present, breath sounds are distant.

Heart and Vascular System. Decreased contractile strength of the myocardium results in decreased cardiac output. The decrease is significant when an older adult experiences stress from anxiety,

TABLE 25-1 Common Physiological Changes With Aging

Anatomical Part	Common Changes	Anatomical Part	Common Changes
System		***Sensory***	
Integument	Loss of skin elasticity (resulting in wrinkles, sagging, dryness, easily tears) Pigmentation changes, glandular atrophy (oil, moisture, sweat glands) Thinning hair (facial hair: decreased in men, increased in women) Slower nail growth, atrophy of epidermal arterioles	Eyes	Decreased ability to focus on near objects (presbyopia) Difficulty adjusting to changes from light to dark Yellowing of the lens Altered perception of colours Increased sensitivity to glare Smaller pupils
Respiratory	Decreased cough reflex Decreased removal of mucus, dust, irritants from airways (decreased cilia) Decreased vital capacity (increased anterior-posterior chest diameter) Increased chest wall rigidity Fewer alveoli, increased airway resistance Increased risk of respiratory infections	Ears	Loss of ability to hear high-frequency tones (presbycusis) Thickening of tympanic membrane Sclerosis of inner ear Possible buildup of cerumen (earwax)
		Taste	Often diminished; possibly fewer taste buds
		Smell	Often diminished
Cardiovascular	Thickening of blood vessel walls Narrowing of vessel lumen Loss of vessel elasticity Lower cardiac output Decreased number of heart muscle fibres Decreased elasticity and calcification of heart valves Decreased baroreceptor sensitivity Decreased efficiency of venous valves Increased pulmonary vascular tension Increased systolic blood pressure Decreased peripheral circulation	Touch	Decreased skin receptors
		Proprioception	Decreased awareness of body positioning in space
		Genitourinary	Fewer nephrons Decreased renal blood flow Decreased bladder capacity Men: enlargement of prostate Women: reduced sphincter tone
		Reproductive	
		Female	Decreased estrogen production Degeneration of ovaries Atrophy of vagina, uterus, breasts
Gastrointestinal	Periodontal disease Loss of teeth Decrease in saliva, gastric secretions, and pancreatic enzymes Changes in smooth muscle, with decreased esophageal peristalsis and small intestinal motility	Male	Diminished sperm count Smaller testes Less firm and slower erections
		Endocrine	
		General	Alteration in hormone production with decreased ability to respond to stress
Musculoskeletal	Decreased muscle mass and strength Decalcification of bones Degenerative joint changes Dehydration of intervertebral disks (decreased height)	Thyroid	Decreased secretion
		Thymus	Involution of thymus gland
		Cortisols, glucocorticoids	Increased levels of anti-inflammatory hormones
Neurological	Degeneration of nerve cells Decrease in neurotransmitters Decrease in rate of conduction of impulses	Pancreas	Increased fibrosis, decreased secretion of enzymes and hormones

Adapted from Ebersole, P., & Hess, P. (2008). *Geriatric nursing and healthy aging.* St. Louis, MO: Mosby.

excitement, illness, or strenuous activity. The body tries to compensate for decreased cardiac output by increasing the heart rate during exercise. However, after exercise, it takes longer for an older adult's rate to return to baseline.

Systolic or diastolic blood pressure, or both, may be abnormally elevated. More than 50% of older adults have systolic hypertension (systolic pressure >140 mm Hg) or diastolic hypertension (diastolic pressure >90 mm Hg; Beers & Berkow, 2000). Although it is a common chronic condition, hypertension is not a normal aging change; it predisposes older adults to heart failure, stroke, renal failure, coronary heart disease, and peripheral vascular disease.

Peripheral pulses become frequently weaker in the lower extremities, although they are still palpable. Older adults may report that their lower extremities are cold, particularly at night. Changes in the peripheral pulses in the upper extremities are less common.

Breasts. In older women, the breasts sag as a result of decreased muscle mass, tone, and elasticity. Atrophy of glandular tissue, coupled with more fat deposits, cause breasts to become slightly smaller, less dense, and less nodular. Gynecomastia (enlarged breasts in men) may be caused by medication side effects, hormonal changes, or obesity. Both older men and women are at risk for breast cancer.

Gastrointestinal System and Abdomen. Aging leads to an increase in the amount of fatty tissue in the trunk. As a result, the abdomen increases in size. Because muscle tone and elasticity decrease, the abdomen also becomes more protuberant. Gastrointestinal function changes include a slowing of peristalsis and alterations in secretions. Older adults may experience these changes as the development of intolerance to certain foods and as discomfort caused by delayed gastric emptying. Alterations in the lower gastrointestinal tract may lead to constipation, flatulence, or diarrhea.

Reproductive System. Changes in the structure and function of the reproductive system occur as the result of hormonal alterations. Menopause is related to a reduced responsiveness of the ovaries to pituitary hormones and a resultant decrease in estrogen and progesterone levels. In men, fertility does not cease in association with aging. Spermatogenesis begins to decline during the fourth decade but continues into the ninth. The changes in reproductive structure and function, however, do not affect libido. Sexual activity can become less frequent as a result of illness, death of a sexual partner, decreased socialization, or loss of sexual interest.

Urinary System. Hypertrophy of the prostate gland may develop in older men. The gland enlarges, and pressure is displaced to the neck of the bladder. As a result, urinary retention, frequency, incontinence, and urinary tract infections may occur. In addition, prostatic hypertrophy can result in difficulty initiating voiding and maintaining a urinary stream. Benign prostatic hypertrophy must be distinguished from cancer of the prostate. Cancer of the prostate is the malignancy most frequently diagnosed in men older than 70 years, and it results in the death of 1 per 27 men in whom it is diagnosed (Canadian Cancer Society, 2008).

Urinary incontinence is an abnormal condition, although it is experienced by 50% of women older than 45 years (Canadian Continence Foundation, 2007). The prevalence of incontinence increases with age. Older women, particularly those who have borne children, can experience stress incontinence, which is an involuntary release of urine that occurs when they cough, sneeze, or lift an object. This type of incontinence results from a weakening of the perineal and bladder muscles. Other types of urinary incontinence are transient, urge, overflow, functional, reflex, and mixed incontinence (see Chapter 44). The Registered Nurses Association of Ontario [RNAO] (2002b) recommended assessing risk factors for urinary incontinence, which include individual factors (fluid intake, medications, functional ability, and medical history) and environmental factors.

Musculoskeletal System. With aging, muscle fibres are reduced in size. Muscle strength diminishes in proportion to the decline in muscle mass. Bone mass also declines. Older adults who exercise regularly do not lose as much bone and muscle mass or muscle tone as do those who are inactive. Of Canadian women older than 50 years, 25% have osteoporosis (Osteoporosis Canada, 2008). Women who maintain calcium intake throughout life and into menopause have less bone demineralization than do women with low calcium intake. Older men with poor nutrition and decreased mobility are also at risk for bone demineralization. One per eight men in Canada has osteoporosis.

Neurological System. The decrease in the number of neurons in the nervous system that begins in the middle of the second decade can lead to changes such as the sensory disturbances described earlier. In addition, older adults may experience a decreased sense of balance or uncoordinated motor responses. Older adults frequently report alterations in the quality and the quantity of sleep, including difficulty falling asleep, difficulty staying asleep, difficulty falling asleep again after waking during the night, waking too early in the morning, and excessive daytime napping (see Chapter 39).

Functional Changes

Declines in physical, psychological, cognitive, and social function that can occur with aging are usually linked to illness or disease and its degree of chronicity. However, the complex relationship among all of these areas ultimately influences an older adult's functional abilities and overall well-being. Keep in mind that it is difficult for older adults to accept the changes that occur in all the areas of their lives, which in turn have a profound effect on function. Some older adults may deny the changes and continue to expect the same performance from themselves regardless of age. Conversely, some overemphasize these changes and then prematurely limit their activities and involvement in life. Also, the fear of becoming dependent is overwhelming for an older adult who is experiencing functional decline as a result of aging. You should educate older adults to promote understanding of age-related changes, appropriate lifestyle adjustments, and effective coping. Factors that promote the highest level of function in all the areas include a healthy, well-balanced diet; paced and appropriate activity; regularly scheduled visits with a health care professional; regular participation in meaningful activities; use of stress management techniques; and avoidance of alcohol, tobacco, and illicit drugs. *Functional status* in older adults ordinarily refers to the capacity and safe performance of ADLs, and it is a sensitive indicator of health or illness in older adults. ADLs are essential to independent living; therefore, you must carefully assess whether an older adult has changed the way in which he or she completes these tasks. In fact, a sudden change in function, as evidenced by a decline or change in an older adult's ability to perform any one or combination of ADLs, is often a sign of the onset of an acute illness or worsening of a chronic problem (Kresevic & Mezey, 2003). Pneumonia, urinary tract infection, dehydration, electrolyte disturbances, and delirium are examples of acute illnesses that may manifest as a change in function. Worsening of chronic conditions such as diabetes, cardiovascular disease, and chronic lung disease can also manifest as a change in function.

Various health care professionals in a range of different settings are able to perform functional assessment. Several standardized functional assessment tools are widely available; an online collection of tools is available at www.geronurseonline.org. When you identify a decline in function, focus nursing interventions on maintaining, restoring, and maximizing the client's functional status so that he or she can maintain independence while preserving dignity.

Cognitive Changes

A common misconception about aging is that cognitive impairments are widespread among older adults. Forgetfulness is not an expected consequence of aging. Older adults often fear that they are, or soon will be, cognitively impaired. Younger adults often assume that older adults are confused and no longer able to handle their affairs. Structural and physiological changes within the brain—such as reduction in the number of cells, deposition of lipofuscin and amyloid in cells, and change in neurotransmitter levels—are normal with aging and are observed in older adults whether they do or do not have cognitive impairment. Symptoms of cognitive impairment such as disorientation, loss of language skills, loss of the ability to calculate, and poor judgement are not normal aging changes. When you identify these changes during the assessment, you must further investigate the underlying causes.

The three common conditions affecting cognition are delirium, dementia, and depression (Table 25–2). You may find that distinguishing among these three conditions is challenging but essential for selecting appropriate nursing interventions. The RNAO (2003) published best practice guidelines to screen for delirium, dementia, and depression in older adults. Appropriate nursing interventions specifically address the cause of the cognitive impairment.

Delirium. **Delirium**, or acute confusional state, is a potentially reversible cognitive impairment that often has a physiological cause. Physiological causes of delirium include, but are not limited to, electrolyte imbalances, cerebral anoxia, hypoglycemia, medications, drug effects, tumours, subdural hematomas, pain, infection, and cerebrovascular infection, infarction, or hemorrhage. Delirium in older adults sometimes accompanies systemic infections and may be the presenting symptom for pneumonia or urinary tract infection. Delirium may also have environmental causes, such as sensory deprivation or unfamiliarity with surroundings, or psychosocial causes, such as emotional distress or pain. Although delirium may occur in any setting, an older adult in the acute care setting is especially at risk because of predisposing factors (physiological, psychosocial, and environmental) in combination with the medical condition that led to the hospital admission.

Delirium is characterized by fluctuations in cognition, mood, attention, arousal, and self-awareness. Other signs may be hallucinations, occasional incoherent speech, disturbed sleep–wake cycle, and disorientation. The onset of delirium is typically sudden, and symptoms and severity fluctuate rapidly. The presence of delirium necessitates prompt assessment and intervention. The cognitive impairment secondary to delirium is usually reversed once the cause of delirium is identified and treatment is started, unless permanent brain injury has occurred. The story in Box 25–5 is a true one and exemplifies the importance of finding and treating the cause of delirium.

Treatment of delirium is focused on determining causative factors; however, prevention of delirium is also important. To prevent delirium and maintain a client's functioning, you must address the causative factors, which may be multidimensional. A strategy for delirium prevention and treatment that targets risk factors is the implementation of a delirium protocol. An example of such a protocol was described by Gillis and MacDonald (2006). In this protocol, you would assess the client's cognition on a regular basis, using an assessment tool such as the Confusion Assessment Method (Waszynski, 2007). A medication profile and therapeutic environmental modification are also aspects of this protocol.

Dementia. **Dementia** is a syndrome consisting of a number of symptoms that include loss of memory, judgement, and reasoning and changes in mood, behaviour, and communication abilities. The deterioration of cognitive function leads to a decline in the ability to perform basic and instrumental ADLs. Unlike delirium, dementia is characterized by a gradual, progressive, irreversible cerebral dysfunction. Because of the close resemblance of delirium to dementia, the presence of delirium must be ruled out whenever dementia is suspected. The Alzheimer Society of Canada (2008) classifies five major types of dementia: Alzheimer's disease, diffuse Lewy body disease, frontotemporal dementia, Creutzfeldt-Jacob dementia, and vascular dementia. The most common form of dementia is Alzheimer's disease. In Canada, approximately 34.5% of adults older than 85 years have dementia, in comparison with 2.4% of those aged 65 to 74 years (Alzheimer Society of Canada, 2008).

The cause of **Alzheimer's disease** is not known, and although several theories are being studied, none is definitive. Cholinesterase-inhibiting medications—memantine (Exiba), donepezil (Aricept), rivastagmine (Exelon), and galantamine (Reminyl)—are currently prescribed to slow the progression of symptoms. These medications prevent the breakdown of the neurotransmitter acetylcholine by the

TABLE 25-2 A Comparison of the Clinical Features of Delirium, Dementia, and Depression

Clinical Feature	Delirium	Dementia	Depression
Onset	Acute or subacute, depending on cause; often occurs at twilight or in darkness	Chronic and generally insidious, depending on cause	Chronic and generally insidious, depending on cause
Course	Short episodes; diurnal fluctuations in symptoms; worse at night, in darkness, and on awakening	Long episodes; no diurnal effects; symptoms progressive and yet relatively stable over time	Diurnal effects; typically worse in the morning; fluctuations situational but less so than those of delirium
Progression	Abrupt	Slow but uneven	Variable, rapid, or slow but even
Duration	Hours to less than 1 month; seldom longer	Months to years	At least 6 weeks; can last several months to years

Adapted from Rapp, C. G., Mentes, J. C., & Titler, M. G. (2001). Acute confusion/delirium protocol. *Journal of Gerontological Nursing, 27*(4), 21–33.

BOX 25-5 NURSING STORY

Pain and Delirium

Mr. D. R. was a 75-year-old man who underwent an elective right hip arthoplasty and was given patient-controlled anesthesia (PCA) for 48 hours. During that time, he did not use any additional dosages of morphine and was drowsy but alert and moving well. Approximately 10 hours after the PCA had been discontinued, he started to have episodes of confusion, in which he would not remember where he was. His wife, who was visiting him, came to the nurses station, concerned about his confusion. The nurse measured his vital signs, which appeared to be normal with a slightly elevated pulse, but he had no fever. The nurse asked Mr. D. R. whether he was having pain; he responded, "Not really, just not feeling right." Throughout the night, he became increasingly confused. The nurse on the night shift applied her knowledge of postoperative delirium: In looking back at the medical record, she realized that Mr. D. R. had not had anything to control pain since the PCA had been discontinued. She also asked him whether he had pain, and he again said, "Not really." She used the Faces Pain Scale to assess Mr. D. R.'s pain, as recommended by the Hartford Foundation for Geriatric Nursing (Flaherty, 2007); his rating suggested that he was indeed having pain. The nurse gave him his oral pain medication on a regular basis, and by morning, he was alert.

enzyme cholinesterase (Conn, 2001). It is hypothesized that by increasing the amount of acetylcholine available to transmit impulses among neurons, cognition in some older adults with Alzheimer's disease will improve. The characteristic progressive symptoms of Alzheimer's disease are loss of memory (amnesia), loss of the ability to recognize objects and people (agnosia), loss of the ability to perform familiar tasks (apraxia), and loss of language skills (aphasia). As Alzheimer's disease progresses, the affected adult becomes more dependent on caregivers for assistance with ADLs. Safety issues must be addressed as the disease progresses and the ability to judge risks diminishes.

Like Alzheimer's disease, diffuse Lewy body disease is progressive. The features of diffuse Lewy body disease include dementia, fluctuating cognition, visual or auditory hallucinations (or both), and the motor features of Parkinsonism.

Frontotemporal dementia has an insidious onset and progresses slowly. Early symptoms include poor hygiene, lack of social tact, hyperorality, and sexual disinhibition. Incontinence is also an early symptom in frontotemporal dementia, whereas it is a late symptom in the more common Alzheimer's disease. Repetitive behaviours (wandering, clapping, singing, picking up objects) are frequently observed. Safety and behaviour managements are major concerns for caregivers.

A sudden onset of memory loss, behaviour changes, or difficulties with speech and movement occur with Creutzfeldt-Jakob disease (CJD). CJD is a rare, rapid, and fatal form of dementia caused by infectious agents called *prions.* Two types of CJD exist: *Classical CJD* (also called *sporadic CJD*) occurs at random. *Variant CJD* (vCJD) is a disease linked to eating beef products from cattle with bovine spongiform encephalopathy, also called "mad cow disease." The infectious agent attacks the central nervous system, and the infection is fatal if illness develops. Both types of CJD typically cause memory loss and behavioural changes (Alzheimer Society of Canada, 2008).

The cause of vascular dementia is interruption of blood supply to areas of the brain by thromboembolism, hemorrhage, or ischemia (Bolla et al., 2000). Symptoms of vascular dementia vary according to the areas of the brain affected. Progression of vascular dementia may be either stepwise, with repeated episodes of damage to the brain over time, or steadily progressive. Management of vascular dementia parallels the recommendations for cerebrovascular disease (i.e., reduction of risk factors by treatment of hypertension, hyperlipidemia, carotid disease, arrhythmias, diabetes mellitus, and polycythemia vera). Because the use of nicotine has been linked with vascular disease, older adults with vascular dementia should stop or reduce their use of tobacco products. If an older adult has a cardiac arrhythmia such as atrial fibrillation, anticoagulant therapy may be indicated to reduce the risk of thromboembolism.

In the nursing management of older adults with any form of dementia, you must consider the needs of the client with dementia and the needs of the family. Those needs change because the progressive nature of dementia leads to increased cognitive deterioration. In addition to the client's physical needs, his or her safety needs and psychosocial needs must be considered. The client's family needs information and support. Nursing care objectives are the promotion of the use of remaining functional abilities and behavioural interventions to decrease the incidence of disruptive behaviours. The Alzheimer Society of Canada (2008) has compiled suggestions for care of persons with dementia. The most challenging behaviours are those that include verbal and physical aggression. You should be calm and reassuring, look for an immediate cause, try distracting the client, and, if safety is an issue, leave the situation and get assistance. Restraints cause physical harm and are not an efficacious alternative. Minimal restraint (policy of least restraint) for the shortest period of time should be used only as the last resort when safety is an issue.

Depression. Late-life **depression** may be experienced by 15% to 20% of older adults who live in the community (RNAO, 2003). Depression reduces happiness and well-being, contributes to physical and social limitations, complicates the treatment of concomitant medical conditions, and increases the risk of suicide. The manifestation of depression in older adults differs from that in younger adults. Older adults are more likely to talk about being "blue" or "down in the dumps" and may express feelings of diminished life satisfaction (Miller, in press). The mental health of seniors is a major issue facing older Canadians. It is estimated (Canadian Coalition for Seniors' Mental Health, 2008) that 20% of Canadians older than 65 years are living with mental illness. Best practice guidelines for mental health treatment have been developed by the Canadian Coalition for Seniors' Mental Health (2008).

Delirium and depression, both reversible disorders, are often mistaken for irreversible dementia in older adults because cerebral dysfunction and cognitive impairment occur with these conditions, as well as with dementia. Careful and thorough assessment of older adults with cognitive impairment is essential in order to distinguish among delirium, dementia, and depression. As a beginning nurse, you may choose to consult with a clinical nurse specialist in gerontology. Accurate assessment is necessary in order to select appropriate nursing interventions.

Psychosocial Changes

The psychosocial changes that occur with aging involve changes in roles and relationships. Roles and relationships within the family change as parents become grandparents, as adult children become caregivers for aging parents, or as spouses become widows or widowers. Group membership roles and relationships change as older adults retire from work, move from a familiar neighbourhood, or stop attending social activities because of declining health status.

You should assess both the nature of the psychosocial changes facing an older adult and the adaptation of that person to those changes. In the assessment, ask how the client feels about himself or herself, about himself or herself in relation to others, and about himself or herself as aging. Areas to be addressed during the assessment include the family, intimate relationships, past and current occupation, finances, housing, social networks, activities, and spirituality. Specific topics related to these areas include retirement, housing and environment, social isolation, abuse, sexuality, and death.

Retirement. Retirement is often mistakenly associated with passivity and seclusion. In actuality, it is a stage of life characterized by transitions and role changes. The psychosocial stresses of retirement may be related to role changes within the marital relationship or within the family and to loss of role. Problems may arise in relation to social isolation and finances. Retirement, which may be mandatory or voluntary, occurs at a variety of ages. Regardless of the age at retirement, it is one of the major turning points in life.

Planning for retirement is an important, advisable task for middle-aged individuals. People who plan in advance for retirement generally have a smoother transition into that stage of life. Financial planning for retirement, although important, is only one aspect of retirement planning. Planning begins with consideration of the "style" of retirement desired and includes an inventory of interests, current skills, and general health. Meaningful retirement planning is critical because retirement can last for 30 years or more.

Retirement has an impact on other individuals besides the retired person. Spouses, adult children, and grandchildren are all affected. When the spouse is still working, the retired person faces time alone. For example, the working spouse may have new ideas about the amount of participation in housework expected of the retired person. Friction may develop when the plans of the retired person conflict with the work responsibilities of the working spouse. The working spouse's expectations of the retired person must be clarified. For couples, the adjustment to retirement is affected by the quality of their communication with each other, their process of decision making about issues such as money or activities, their adherence to either traditional or shared role orientations, and their level of affection and intimacy (Ebersole et al., 2008). Adult children may expect the retired person to become an automatic babysitter for the grandchildren.

Loss of the work role has a major impact on some retired people. When so much of life has revolved around work and the personal relationships at work, the loss of the work role may be devastating. Personal identity may be rooted in the work role, and with retirement, a new identity must be constructed. The structure imposed on daily life by a work schedule is also lost with retirement, as are the social exchanges and interpersonal support that occur in the workplace. In the adjustment to retirement, older adults are challenged to develop a personally meaningful schedule and a supportive social network.

The most powerful factors that influence the retired person's satisfaction with life are health status, the option to continue working, and sufficient income (Ebersole et al., 2008). Positive expectations also contribute to satisfaction in retirement. You can help an older adult and the family prepare for retirement by discussing with them several key areas, including relationships with spouse and children, meaningful activities to replace the work role, adjusting or rebuilding social networks, issues related to the promotion and maintenance of income and health, and long-range planning, including wills and advance directives.

Social Isolation. Social isolation and loneliness are significant issues for older adults regardless of gender and geographic location (Havens et al., 2004). Social isolation is the lack of contacts with other people. Loneliness is the dissatisfaction with the level of social contact. Isolation exists in two forms: It may be a choice to not interact with others, or it may be a response to conditions that inhibit the ability or the opportunity to interact with others (Ebersole et al., 2008). For example, geographic dispersion of families leads to decreased opportunities for interaction among family members. Regardless of whether isolation is a choice for older adults, they are vulnerable to its consequences.

Living alone and having multiple chronic illnesses are factors contributing to social isolation and loneliness (Havens et al., 2004). Some older adults see themselves as unattractive and rejected because of changes in their personal appearance as a result of normal aging or because of body image changes caused by illness or surgery (Ebersole et al., 2008). Older adults who are confused or incontinent, who are unable to communicate, who are institutionalized, or who are poor or homeless may feel isolated.

You can assist lonely older adults to rebuild social networks and reverse patterns of isolation (Ebersole et al., 2008). Many communities have outreach programs designed to make contact with isolated older adults. Outreach programs, such as Meals on Wheels, may help meet nutritional needs; daily telephone calls by volunteers may help meet socialization needs; and outings may help meet needs for activities. Social service agencies in most communities welcome older adults as volunteers and provide them with the opportunity to serve and to be served. Other organizations within communities such as religious institutions, colleges, and libraries offer a variety of programs for older adults that increase the opportunity to meet people with similar activities, interests, and needs.

Abuse. Elder **abuse** is the mistreatment of an older person by other people who are in a position of trust or power or who are responsible for the person's care. Neglect is commonly associated with abuse. For example, elder abuse includes not performing an action (inaction) that a caretaker has a duty to perform, such as not providing medications to an older adult who needs them (Canadian Network for the Prevention of Elder Abuse, 2008). Types of abuse are as follows:

- Physical abuse: use of physical force that may result in bodily injury, physical pain, or impairment
- Sexual abuse: nonconsensual sexual contact of any kind, which includes sexual contact with any person incapable of giving consent
- Psychological or emotional abuse: infliction of anguish, emotional pain, or distress through verbal or nonverbal acts
- Material abuse (financial abuse): illegal or improper exploitation of an older person's funds, property, or assets
- Neglect: the intentional or unintentional harmful behaviour on the part of an informal or formal caregiver in whom the older person has placed his or her trust
- Self-neglect: behaviour by an older adult that threatens his or her own health and safety

In most provinces in Canada, elder abuse must be reported. As a nurse, you play an important role in assessment, recognition, and reporting of elder abuse, as well as its prevention, through education and resources for families (Box 25–6).

Sexuality. Sexuality is increasingly recognized as an important factor in the lives of older adults. All older adults, whether healthy or frail, need to express sexual feelings. Sexuality involves love, warmth, sharing, and touching, not just the act of intercourse. Sexuality is linked with identity and validates the belief that people can give of themselves to others and have the gift appreciated.

Maintaining sexual health requires integration of somatic, emotional, intellectual, and social aspects of the sexual being. To help an older adult achieve or maintain sexual health, you should understand the physical changes in sexual response (see Chapter 27). You should provide privacy for any discussion of sexuality and should maintain a nonjudgemental attitude. Open-ended questions inviting the client to explain sexual activities or concerns may elicit more information than do closed-ended questions about specific activities or symptoms. Older adults may appreciate information about the typical age-related changes in sexuality. Information about the prevention of sexually transmitted infections should be included when appropriate.

The libido does not decrease in older adults, although frequency of sexual activity may decline. An older woman who does not understand physical changes affecting sexual activity may be concerned that her sex life is nearly over. The older man may feel the same when he discovers a change in the firmness of his erection, a decreased need for ejaculation with each orgasm, or a longer recovery period between episodes of intercourse.

In addition to the physical changes that affect sexual functioning, many older adults use prescription medications that depress libido, such as antihypertensives, antidepressants, sedatives, and hypnotics. Some drugs increase libido in older adults. For example, phenothiazines increase sexual desire in women, and levodopa has a similar effect in men.

While considering an older adult's need for sexual expression, you must not ignore the important need to touch and be touched. Touch is an overt expression with many meanings and is an important part of sexuality in some cultures. Touch can complement traditional sexual methods or serve as an alternative sexual expression when physical intercourse is not desired or possible, and thus it can serve as an important method of achieving intimacy (Atkinson, 2006). Before using touch, you should respect the fact that it may not be appropriate for some older persons because of culturally associated meanings. Experience in caring for older adults, in combination with the ability to establish therapeutic connection, enables you to learn how to explore clients' sexual concerns. Knowing an older adult's sexual needs allows you to incorporate this information into the nursing care plan.

The sexual preferences of older adults are as diverse as those of younger adults. Not all older adults are heterosexual. Little information regarding older homosexual adults and their health care needs is available. To be effective caregivers for older homosexual clients, you need to be aware of their own beliefs about sexuality and the potential impact of those beliefs on their ability to provide care.

> **BOX 25-6 Elder Abuse: Signs and Action Required**
>
> **Signs**
>
> Physical signs of abuse
> Isolation from others
> Withdrawal
> Feeling of the victim, that he or she is to blame
> Verbalized threats against the victim
>
> **Action Required**
>
> Assess the presence of physical danger
> Take legal action
> Support the victim's decision to leave the situation or to stay in it
> Develop a workable safety plan
> Provide specific information about places of safety
>
> Adapted from Ebersole, P., Hess, P., Touhy, T., Jett, K., & Luggen, A. (2008). *Toward healthy aging: Human needs and nursing response* (7th ed.). St. Louis, MO: Mosby.

Improving communication and creating open and supportive environments of care are necessary to promote successful, healthy sexual expression.

You may find that you are called on to advise older adults and help other health care professionals understand the sexual needs of older adults. You may feel uncomfortable counselling older adults about sexual health and need not feel obligated to do so. But you should be prepared to refer older adults to appropriate professional counsellors.

Housing and Environment. Housing choices are strongly determined by an older adult's ability to live independently. Changes in social roles, family responsibilities, and health status influence this ability. Some older adults choose to live with family members. Others prefer their own homes or apartments near their families. Leisure or retirement communities provide older people with living and social opportunities in a one-generation setting. Federally subsidized housing, where available, offers apartments with communal, social, and, in some cases, food service arrangements.

When assisting older adults with housing needs, you should assess their activity level, their financial status, the availability of access to public transportation and community activities, environmental hazards, and their support systems. Housing choices should also account for anticipated future needs of the clients. A housing unit with only one floor and without exterior steps may be a prudent choice for an older adult with severe arthritis who has already had some lower extremity joint replacement surgeries and anticipates the need for future surgeries.

Housing and environment have a major impact on the health of older adults. The environment can support or hinder physical and social functioning, can enhance or drain energy, and can complement or tax existing physical changes such as vision and hearing. For example, older adults can most easily see the colours red, orange, and yellow; in contrast, they have difficulty distinguishing between green and blue and among pastel shades. To help older adults in health care settings find their rooms, pictures or other decorations near their doors can be used as landmarks. To improve perception of the boundaries of halls and rooms, door frames and baseboards should be painted in a colour that contrasts with the colour of the wall. Glare from highly polished floors, metallic fixtures, and windows is poorly tolerated.

Furniture should be comfortable and designed for the musculoskeletal changes of older adults. Older adults should examine furniture carefully for size, comfort, and function before purchasing it. Furniture should be easy to get into and out of and should provide back support. Dining room chairs should be tested for comfort during meals and for height in relation to the table. Older adults may prefer transferring out of a wheelchair to another chair for meals because some styles of wheelchairs prevent sitting close enough to the table to eat comfortably. Raising the table to clear the wheelchair arms may bring the table closer to the person but may make it too high for comfortable use. To make getting out of bed easier and safer, the height of the bed should allow the person's feet to be flat on the floor when the person is sitting on the side of the bed.

The goal of nursing assessment of the environment is the promotion of independence and functional ability. Assessment of safety, a major component of an older adult's environment, includes determining risks within the environment and the person's ability to recognize and respond to the risks (see Chapter 30). Risks include factors leading to injury within the home (such as water heaters set at excessively hot temperatures or throw rugs that could cause a fall) and factors outside of the home (such as deteriorating sidewalks and steps or a high incidence of street crime).

Death. Part of the life history of an older adult is the experience of the death of family members and friends (see Chapter 29). This experience includes the loss of the older generations of their families and sometimes the loss of a child or grandchild. As adults age, friends gradually die. Despite these experiences, it would be wrong to assume that older adults are comfortable with the idea of death. A key role for nurses is supporting older adults in coping with these losses and facilitating adjustment to the life changes imposed by them.

Older people have a wide variety of attitudes and beliefs about death. To support a client at the end of life, you can use the dignity-conserving model of care (Chochinov, 2007). In this model, you use your attitudes, behaviours, compassion, and dialogue acknowledging the individual's attitudes and beliefs about death to ensure his or her dignity at the end of life. Another model of care that you can use is a Living with Hope program (Duggleby et al., 2007) to foster his or her hope and improve quality of life (Box 25–7). Such strategies to improve end-of-life care can be easily incorporated into everyday nursing practice. You will often be the person to whom the client and family members or friends turn for assistance in coping with death and loss. It is critical that you understand the grieving process, have excellent communication skills, understand the legal issues, are familiar with community resources, and are aware of your own feelings, limitations, and strengths as they relate to care of clients confronting death.

Addressing the Health Concerns of Older Adults

The two most common causes of death in Canadian older adults are cancer and heart disease, Other frequently reported causes of death are respiratory diseases, stroke, accidents or falls, diabetes, kidney disease, and liver disease (Statistics Canada, 2008). For all these causes of death, preventive measures exist, and these measures could potentially reduce the frequency of these conditions and delay disability, death, or both.

Health Canada's NACA (2006) identified the following areas in which action to improve the health of older adults is necessary:

- Improving chronic disease management (e.g., self-management and community supports to adopt healthier lifestyles)
- Improving personal health practices (e.g., physical activity and healthy eating)
- Strengthening programs for preventing falls and injuries
- Reducing suicide rates among men aged 85 years and older
- Increasing affordable housing options
- Improving accessibility of transportation for all older persons
- Improving instituational standards of care

You may participate in activities such as health screenings and fairs, in which you can identify older adults at risk and advise them about disease prevention and health promotion measures (Davidhizar et al., 2002). Many communities offer wellness programs (Box 25–8) in which older adults can access information about health promotion and disease prevention (Resnick, 2003). In acute-care and long-term care settings, you must also assess the health status of older adults, intervene in acute situations, and, with the clients, plan strategies to reduce risk and manage chronic conditions. Each contact with an older adult, regardless of setting, offers opportunities to teach and counsel. To be most effective, use an individualized approach to health promotion activities with each client (Resnick, 2003).

Nursing interventions for older adults are directed toward improving or maintaining their health needs and concerns. Although various interventions cross all three levels of care—health promotion, acute care, and restorative care—approaches to each level are unique. When you plan interventions, it is important to incorporate a client's routines or rituals when possible because clients feel more secure when routines are continued. In general, the interventions are aimed at promoting independence and supporting self-care abilities.

Health Promotion and Maintenance: Physiological Health Concerns

Older adults, like persons of any age, vary in their desire to participate in health promotion activities; therefore, you should use an individualized approach, taking into account the person's beliefs about the importance of staying healthy and fit and remaining independent. Researchers have not fully identified the factors that lead to good health in advanced age, but four factors seem to be important: genetics, luck, good health habits, and preventive measures. You cannot alter an older adult's genetic heritage or luck, but you can promote health habits by establishing health maintenance programs, and you can recommend preventive measures. Health maintenance programs have been found to have a positive impact on the physical, mental, and social health of older adults (Buijs et al., 2003). Community centres, houses of worship, schools, shopping malls, libraries, and hospital lobbies can be used as settings to conduct screening tests and

✱ BOX 25-7 EVIDENCE-INFORMED PRACTICE GUIDELINE

Living With Hope Program for Older Adults at the End of Life

Evidence Summary

Clients who are terminally ill with cancer endure and cope with their psychosocial pain by maintaining hope. The overall purpose of a study by Duggleby et al. (2007) was to evaluate the effectiveness of the Living with Hope program in increasing hope and quality of life for older adults who were living in the community and terminally ill with cancer. The program consisted of viewing a film about hope and choosing from one of three activities to work on for a week. The activities were (1) to start a "hope collection," (2) to write a letter to someone or to have someone help the client write a letter, and (3) to start an "about me" collection. Subjects enrolled in the Living with Hope program had statistically hope scores ($df = 3$, $F = 30.087$, $p = .000$) and quality-of-life scores ($df = 3$, $F = 9.022$, $p = .000$) at the second visit that were significantly higher than the scores of subjects in the control group. Qualitative data confirmed this finding: The majority of subjects in the treatment group (61.5%) reported that the program increased their hope.

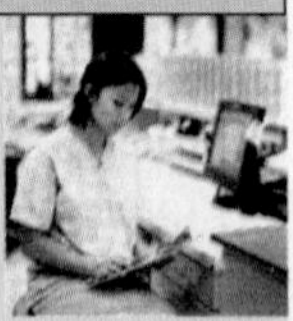

Application to Nursing Practice

- Hope is situational; therefore, it can be changed.
- By increasing hope, quality of life is also improved.
- The Living with Hope program may be effective in increasing hope in seniors with terminal illness.

Based on Duggleby, W., Degner, L., Williams, A., Wright, K, Cooper, D., Popkin, D., et al. (2007). Living with hope: Initial evaluation of a psychosocial hope intervention for older palliative home care patients. *Journal of Pain and Symptom Management, 33*(3), 247–257.

BOX 25-8 FOCUS ON PRIMARY HEALTH CARE

Older Adult Wellness Programs

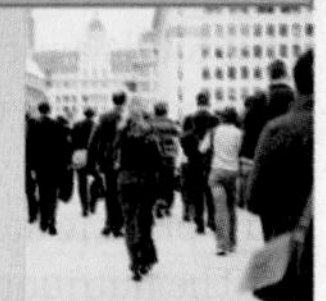

Focusing on self-care abilities and practices that foster health during the aging process are important nursing interventions (Pender et al., 2002). Factors that have been reported to affect older adults' willingness to engage in health promotion activities include socioeconomic factors, beliefs and attitudes, encouragement by a health care professional, availability of access to resources, age, number of chronic illnesses, and mental and physical health (Resnick, 2003). In general, older adults seem to be less interested in engaging in health promotion activities for the purpose of lengthening their lives, but they may have greater interest in these activities if they improve quality of life (Resnick, 2003).

In order to help older adults maintain function and improve quality of life, the Saskatoon Health Region (2006), in conjunction with several other community agencies, established an Older Adult Wellness Program. The program goals are as follows:

1. Encourage older adults to adopt lifestyle choices and practices that preserve their health.
2. Promote the concept of mutual aide and social support among older adults in the community (capacity building).
3. Alter or adapt social, economic, or physical surroundings to preserve and enhance the health of older adults.

The program is housed in a public health centre. As part of this program, the nurses provide educational programs about promoting older adults' health to the community, health care professionals, and older adults themselves. The nurses also organize and provide a program ("Steady as You Go" [SAYGO]; Robson et al., 2003) to increase physical activity and decrease falls. Preventive services such as health screening and immunizations are also offered to older adults. A community resource directory has been published and is used by older adults and the nurses to access services for program participants.

From Saskatoon Health Region. (2006). *Older Adult Wellness Program: Annual report* (pp. 1–25). Saskatoon, SK: Author.

present information on health topics. Using creative approaches, you can include health promotion activities for older adults in all health care settings.

Approximately 80% of older adults living at home have at least one chronic health condition. The most common conditions are arthritis, high blood pressure, back problems, chronic heart problems, cataracts, and diabetes (Statistics Canada, 2008). The effect of chronic conditions on the lives of older adults varies widely, but, in general, chronic conditions diminish well-being and threaten the independence of older adults. Nursing interventions are often directed at the management of these conditions, but interventions can also focus on prevention. You can recommend the following general preventive measures:

- Regular exercise
- Weight reduction if the client is overweight
- Management of hypertension
- Smoking cessation
- Immunization for influenza, pneumococcal pneumonia, and tetanus

Approximately 70,000 to 75,000 hospitalizations and 6700 deaths each year in Canada are attributed to influenza (Menec et al., 2003). Annual immunization against influenza is strongly recommended for all older adults, especially residents of long-term care facilities, and for clients of any age with chronic cardiovascular, pulmonary, and metabolic disorders (Gomolin & Kathpalia, 2002). Vaccination against pneumococcal pneumonia is recommended for all adults older than 65 years. Influenza vaccine is needed every year, whereas pneumococcal pneumonia vaccine is given only once (although some authorities recommend revaccination 6 to 8 years after the initial vaccination; Beers & Berkow, 2000). For tetanus immunization, booster injections every 10 years are recommended for adults who have received the primary series for tetanus immunization. However, not all older adults are up to date with their booster injections, and some have never received the primary series of injections. You should ask an older adult client about the current status of all three types of immunizations, provide information about the immunizations, and make arrangements for the client to receive the immunizations as needed. You should also refer older adults for screening for the early detection of cancer and depression.

Most older adults are interested in their health and are capable of taking charge of their lives. They want to remain independent and to prevent disability (Figure 25–1). Initial screenings establish baseline data that can be used to determine wellness, identify health needs, and design health maintenance programs. After initial screening sessions, you can share information on nutrition, exercise, medications, and safety precautions with older adults. You may also provide information about specific conditions, such as hypertension or arthritis, or about self-care procedures, such as foot and skin care. By providing information about health promotion and self-care, you can significantly improve the health and well-being of older adults.

Cancer. Malignant neoplasms are the most common cause of death among older adults (Statistics Canada, 2008). You may participate in programs to educate older adults about early detection, treatment, and risk factors. Examples include smoking cessation programs, teaching breast self-examination (see Chapter 5), and encouraging all older adults to have annual screening for fecal occult blood. It is also important to educate older adults about the signs of cancer and encourage prompt reporting of nonhealing skin lesions, unexpected bleeding, change in bowel habits, and unexplained weight loss. Detection is complicated when cancer symptoms are mistakenly identified by clients and health care professionals as part of the normal aging process, and you must carefully distinguish between normal aging and pathological conditions.

Heart Disease. Heart disease is the second leading cause of death in older adults. Common cardiovascular disorders are hypertension and coronary artery disease. Hypertension is diagnosed when repeated diastolic blood pressure measurements are 90 mm Hg or

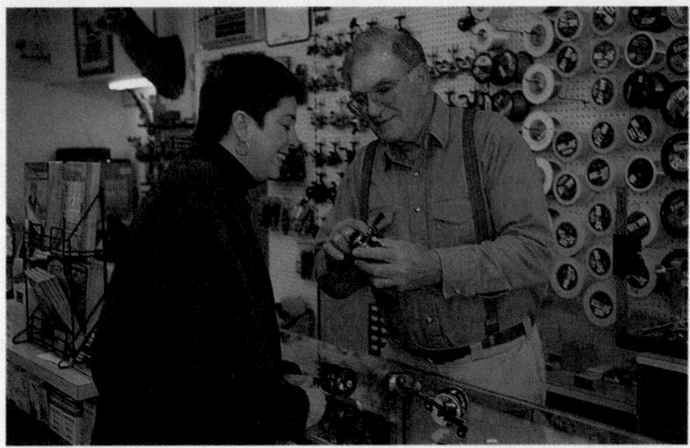

Figure 25-1 This older adult works part-time at a sporting goods store.

greater and systolic measurements are 140 mm Hg or greater. Although over 45% of Canadians have elevated diastolic or systolic pressures, or both (NACA, 2006), the fact that hypertension is common does not mean it is normal or harmless. Systolic pressures higher than 160 mm Hg are associated with increased risk of stroke, increased risk of cardiovascular mortality, and increased risk of overall mortality (Beers & Berkow, 2000). In coronary artery disease, partial or complete blockage of one or more coronary arteries leads to myocardial ischemia and myocardial infarction. The risk factors for both hypertension and coronary artery disease include smoking, obesity, lack of exercise, and stress. Additional risk factors for coronary artery disease include hypertension, hyperlipidemia, and diabetes mellitus. Nursing interventions for hypertension and coronary artery disease address weight reduction, exercise, dietary changes to limit salt and fat, stress management, and smoking cessation. Client education includes information about medications, blood pressure monitoring, nutrition, stress reduction techniques, and the symptoms that indicate the need for emergency care.

Smoking. Cigarette smoking has been recognized as the major preventable cause of death and disease in Canada (Canadian Council on Social Development for the Division of Aging and Seniors, Public Health Agency of Canada, 2004). Smoking cessation is a health promotion strategy as much for older adults as for younger adults. Older smokers can benefit from smoking cessation (Flaherty et al., 2003). In addition to reducing risk, smoking cessation may help stabilize existing conditions such as chronic obstructive pulmonary disease. Smoking cessation may even contribute to the extension of life or of independent functioning.

You can use four sequential approaches, referred to as the "Four A's" (Flaherty et al., 2003), to encourage smoking cessation. First, *ask* the older client about the type of tobacco product used, the frequency of smoking, and the number of years he or she has smoked. Then *advise* quitting. It is useful at this time for you to provide information about the ill effects of smoking and the benefits of quitting. Next, *assist* the client with quitting by helping him or her develop a plan (e.g., discuss the use of nicotine gum or nicotine patches, and ask family members to reduce smoking). Also consider referral to a local smoking cessation program. Last, *arrange* with the client a date to quit; offer encouragement and assistance in modifying the plan as necessary. Although some people mistakenly believe that older adults do not want to quit smoking or are unable to quit, some older adults do quit smoking successfully.

Alcohol Abuse. It is estimated that up to 12% of older adults consume 14 or more drinks a week (Statistics Canada, 2008). Studies of alcohol abuse in older adults have revealed two patterns: a lifelong pattern of frequent heavy drinking and a late-onset pattern in which heavy drinking begins late in life. Frequently cited causes of excessive alcohol use are depression, loneliness, and lack of social support.

Abuse of alcohol may be underidentified in older adults (Ebersole et al., 2008). Signs of alcohol abuse are subtle, and the assessment may be complicated by coexisting dementia or depression. Alcohol abuse should be suspected when the client has a history of repeated falls and accidents, exhibits a change in behaviour or personality, is socially isolated, has recurring episodes of memory loss and confusion, has a history of skipping meals or medications, and has difficulty managing household tasks and finances. When abuse of alcohol is suspected, treatment includes age-specific approaches in which you acknowledge the stresses experienced by the client and encourage involvement in activities that match the client's interests and boost feelings of self-worth. The identification and treatment of coexisting depression is also important.

Nutrition. Lifelong eating habits and situational factors influence how older adults meet their needs for good nutrition. Lifelong eating habits based in tradition, ethnicity, and religion influence choices of what foods are eaten and how those foods are prepared. Situational factors affecting nutrition include availability of access to food stores, finances, the physical and cognitive capability for food preparation, and a place to store food and prepare meals.

The nutritional needs of older adults are affected by their levels of activity and by clinical conditions. Level of activity has implications for the total amount of calories: More sedentary older adults usually need fewer calories than do more active older adults. However, caloric requirements are not determined solely by activity. Additional calories may be required in clinical situations such as recovery from surgery, whereas calories may be restricted when the client is diabetic or overweight. Beyond caloric requirements, therapeutic diets may restrict fat, sodium, or simple sugars or may increase fibre or foods with high levels of calcium, iron, vitamin A, or vitamin C.

Good nutrition for older adults includes appropriate caloric intake and limited intake of fat, salt, refined sugars, and alcohol. Although the nutritional guidelines displayed in Canada's Food Guide (Health Canada, 2007) are the basic recommendations for nutrition in older adults (see Chapter 43), some older adults do not follow these guidelines. Protein intake may be lower than recommended if clients have reduced financial resources or limited access to grocery stores. Difficulty chewing meat may also limit protein intake. Fat intake may be higher than recommended because fast-food restaurant meals may be substituted for meals prepared at home or because methods of cooking may feature fried foods and sauces made with butter and cream. Extra salt and sugar may be used in cooking or at the table to compensate for a diminished sense of taste. Vitamin intake may be reduced if the person has difficulty shopping for fresh fruits and vegetables.

Older adults with dementia have special nutritional needs. As their memory and their functional skills decline, they lose the ability to remember when to eat, how to prepare food, and, eventually, how to feed themselves. At the same time, their caloric needs may increase because of the energy expended in pacing and wandering activities. You and other caregivers of older adults with dementia should routinely monitor weight and food intake, serve food that is easy to eat, provide assistance with eating, and offer food supplements as needed to maintain weight (Amella, 2004). Mealtime interventions for older adults with dementia also provide opportunities for socialization and practice with functional skills.

Dental Problems. Dental problems are common in older adults and include conditions involving natural teeth and dentures. Dental caries, gingivitis, broken or missing teeth, and ill-fitting or missing dentures may affect nutritional adequacy, cause pain, and lead to infection. You can help prevent dental and gum disease through education about routine dental care (see Chapter 38). You can also help older adults find dental services that offer reduced rates and that are accessible to clients with impaired mobility.

Exercise. Older adults should be encouraged to maintain physical exercise and activity. The primary benefits of exercise include maintaining and strengthening functional ability and promoting a sense of enhanced well-being. An exercise such as walking builds endurance, increases muscle tone, improves joint flexibility, strengthens bones, reduces stress, and contributes to weight loss. Other benefits of an exercise program include improvement of cardiovascular function, improved plasma lipoprotein profiles, increased metabolic rate, increased gastrointestinal transit time, and improved quality of sleep. Frail older adults who exercise may experience improvements in mobility, gait, and balance, as well as less difficulty getting up from a chair or climbing stairs. Exercise also substantially delays the onset of functional impairment and loss of independence.

An exercise program should meet physical needs while allowing for physical impairments, and you should encourage the client to persevere with the exercise program. Willingness to participate in and persevere with an exercise program is influenced by general beliefs about exercise, specific benefits from exercise, past experiences with exercise, personal goals, personality, and any unpleasant sensations associated with exercise. Walking is the preferred exercise of many older adults (Figure 25–2). Walking and other low-impact exercises such as riding an exercise (stationary) bicycle or exercises in a swimming pool protect the musculoskeletal system and joints. Other exercises can be incorporated into an older adult's ADLs. For example, the person can perform arm and leg circles while watching television. However, before beginning an exercise program, the client should have a physical examination. Exercise programs for sedentary older adults who have not been exercising regularly should begin conservatively and progress slowly. Safety considerations include wearing shoes and clothing appropriate for the exercise, drinking water before and after exercising, avoiding outdoor exercise when the weather is very warm or very cold, and exercising with one or more partners. You should instruct the client to stop exercising and seek help if he or she experiences a sensation of tightness or pain in the chest, shortness of breath, dizziness or lightheadedness, or palpitations during exercise.

Arthritis. Arthritis is a common condition in older adults, especially in women. The degree to which the mobility of older adults is impaired depends on the extent of the disease and which joints are affected. The changes in joint range of motion and stability, combined with the amount of pain experienced, affect quality of life. Arthritis has no cure, but pharmacological agents can decrease pain and swelling and therefore increase joint motion. Nursing interventions are aimed at promoting comfort, functional ability, and safety. Education about self-care techniques, joint protection, and exercises for flexibility and strength is also important.

Falls. Falls are a safety concern and one of the most common causes of functional dependence in seniors. Falls may lead to fear of additional falls, withdrawal from usual activities, and loss of independence (see Chapter 37). Hospitalization and placement in a long-term care facility may be required. Falls account for 87% of unintentional injuries that result in hospitalization for adults aged 71 years and older and for 75% of the deaths from injury in this age group (NACA, 2006). A fracture is sustained in 5% of falls in this age group. Falls are more frequent and have more serious consequences among adults older than 85 years.

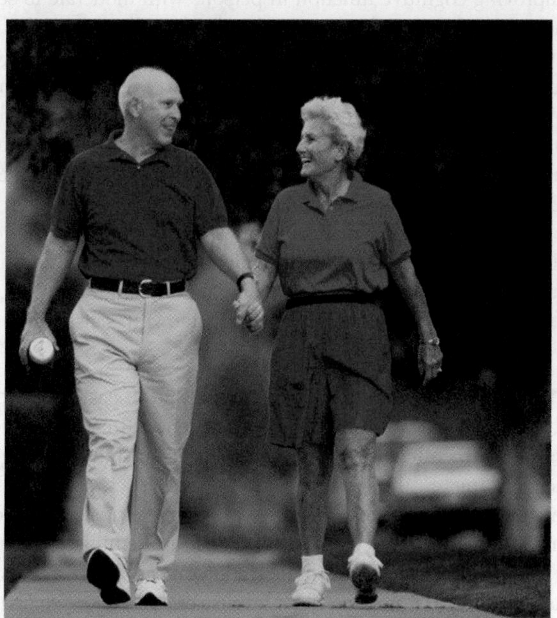

Figure 25-2 This couple enjoys walking together.

Falls are caused by a combination of individual and environmental factors (RNAO, 2002a). Individual factors include impaired vision; cardiovascular conditions, such as postural hypotension or syncope; conditions affecting mobility, such as arthritis, muscle weakness, and foot problems; conditions affecting balance; alterations in bladder function, such as frequency or incontinence; cognitive impairment; and adverse medication reactions. Environmental factors include, but are not limited to, poor lighting, slippery or wet floors, stairs or sidewalks in poor repair, shoes in poor repair or with slippery soles, and household items that could be tripped over, such as throw rugs, foot stools, and electric extension cords.

Multifactoral falls-prevention programs such as "Stand-Up" have been found to significantly reduce falls in community-dwelling older people (Filiatrault et al., 2007). This program includes exercises to increase balance and strength, adoption of active lifestyles and safe behaviours, and actions to reduce hazards in the home environment. You can encourage older adults to perform exercises aimed at increasing leg strength and balance, which also reduce the risk of falls. Simple interventions in the home, such as rearranging furniture to provide a clear pathway to the bathroom and providing a night light in the bathroom, can reduce falls related to nighttime trips to the toilet. Removing throw rugs and other items on the floor helps reduce slipping and tripping. You can also instruct older adults in the safe use of assistive devices such as canes, walkers, and wheelchairs. Older adults taking medications that may have adverse effects, such as postural hypotension, dizziness, or sedation, can be instructed to be aware of these potential effects and to take precautions such as changing position slowly or holding on to sturdy furniture if they are unsteady. Other health conditions such as ear infections can also contribute to falls.

Sensory Impairments. Most older adults have changes in vision, hearing, taste, and smell as a result of normal aging. Chapter 48 describes in detail the nursing interventions used to maintain and improve sensory function.

Pain. At least 50% of older persons suffer pain at any one time, and pain is undertreated (Hadjistavropoulos & Fine, 2006). The causes of pain in older adults include acute and chronic conditions (e.g., trauma, infection, and neuropathies). The consequences of persistent pain include depression, sleep difficulties, changes in gait and mobility, and decreased socialization. Many factors influence the management of pain, including cultural influences on the meaning and expression of pain in older adults, fears related to the use of analgesic medications, and the problem of pain assessment with cognitively impaired older adults. In caring for older adults, you must advocate for appropriate and effective pain management and for the use of standardized pain tools in assessing pain (see Chapter 42). The goal of nursing management of chronic pain in older adults is to maximize function and improve quality of life.

Medication Use. Older adults take more prescription and over-the-counter drugs than do people of any other age group. Older adults account for 12% of the population but use as much as 40% of prescription medications (NACA, 2006). In 2003, 92% of Canadian older adults reported using medications in the previous month (NACA, 2006). The medications most commonly used are cardiovascular drugs, antihypertensives, analgesics, sedatives, tranquilizers, laxatives, and antacids. **Polypharmacy** (the concurrent use of many medications) increases the risk for adverse reactions. Although polypharmacy may reflect inappropriate prescribing, the concurrent use of multiple medications may be necessary if the client has multiple acute and chronic conditions. However, a periodic and thorough review of all medications being used is important in helping the client use the fewest necessary medications. Your role with an older adult undergoing drug therapy is to ensure the greatest therapeutic benefit with the least amount of harm. A good resource to help you is *Medication Matters* (Division of Aging and Seniors, Public Health Agency of Canada, 2008).

Older adults are at risk for adverse reactions because of age-related changes in the absorption, distribution, metabolism, and excretion of drugs (see Chapter 34). Medications may interact with one another; one drug may augment or negate the effect of another. Medications may also cause confusion; affect balance and mobility; cause dizziness, nausea, and vomiting; or lead to constipation, urinary frequency, or incontinence. Because of these effects, some older adults are unwilling to take medications, and others do not adhere to the prescribed dosing schedule.

Managing medications is a very important component of maintaining and promoting good health in old age. For some older adults taking large numbers of medications, safely managing medications can be a complex activity that can easily become overwhelming. You can provide valuable assistance to these clients as they carry out this important self-care activity.

You should work collaboratively with an older adult to ensure safe and appropriate use of prescribed and over-the-counter medications. The client should be taught the names of all drugs being taken, when and how to take them, and the desirable and undesirable effects of the drugs. You should also teach how to avoid adverse effects and interactions of drugs and how to establish and follow an appropriate self-administration pattern. To reduce the risk for an adverse medication reaction in an older adult, you should review the medications with the client at each visit; examine for potential interactions with food or other drugs; simplify and individualize the drug regimen; take every opportunity to inform the client and family about all aspects of medication use; and encourage the client to question the physician, advanced practice nurse, pharmacist, or all three about all prescribed and over-the-counter drugs.

When drugs are used in the management of confusion, special care is necessary. The sedatives and tranquilizers sometimes prescribed for acutely confused older adults may themselves cause or exacerbate confusion. These drugs should be carefully administered; age-related changes in body systems can affect the pharmacokinetic activity. When confusion has a physiological cause (such as an infection), the cause, rather than the confused behaviour, should be specifically treated. When confusion varies by time of day or is related to environmental factors, you can use creative, nonpharmacological measures such as changing the environment to include things that are familiar to the client, providing adequate light, encouraging use of assistive devices (glasses, hearing aids), or even encouraging the client to make telephone calls to friends or family members to hear reassuring voices.

Health Promotion and Maintenance: Psychosocial Health Concerns

Interventions supporting the psychosocial health of older adults resemble those for other age groups. However, some interventions are more crucial for older adults experiencing social isolation, cognitive impairment, or stresses related to retirement, relocation, or approaching death. These interventions include therapeutic communication, touch, cognitive stimulation, reminiscence, and interventions to improve body image.

Therapeutic Communication. With therapeutic communication, you perceive and respect the client's uniqueness and meet his or her expectations. Older adults expect you to be attentive, caring, and knowledgeable. Being attentive means that you provide care in a timely manner, meeting client's expressed or unexpressed needs. As a caring nurse, you convey concern, kindness, and compassion. To show that you are knowledgeable, you not only demonstrate procedural competence but also are adept at recognizing needs and relaying information. Older adult clients also expect you to respect their individuality. When you meet these expectations and communicate effectively, clients accept you as someone who has a genuine concern for their welfare. However, you cannot simply enter an older adult's environment and immediately establish a therapeutic relationship; you must first be knowledgeable and skilled in communication techniques (see Chapter 18).

Touch. Throughout life, touch tells people about their environment and the people around them. Gentle touch conveys affection and friendliness. A firm hand clasp may convey security. Touch is a therapeutic tool that you can use to help comfort older adults. Hawranick et al. (2008) found that agitation levels of older adults with dementia were significantly lower when they received a touch intervention (Box 25–9). Touch can provide sensory stimulation, induce relaxation, provide physical and emotional comfort, orient the person to reality, convey warmth, and communicate interest. It is a powerful physical expression of a relationship.

Older adults may be deprived of touching when separated from family or friends. An older adult who is isolated, dependent, or ill; who fears death; or who lacks self-esteem has a greater need for touch. You may recognize touch deprivation by behaviours as simple as a client's reaching for your hand or standing close to you. When you use touch, you must be aware of cultural variations and individual preferences (see Chapter 10). Touch should convey respect and sensitivity. Touch should not be used in a condescending way, such as patting a client on the head.

Cognitive Simulation. Cognitive stimulation, in which persons engage in cognitive activities such as games, appears to show promise in improving cognitive function in persons with moderate to severe dementia (Forbes, 2004). It is considered more effective and less confrontational than reality orientation techniques, although it does include some aspects of reality orientation. An example of cognitive stimulation is the use of a reality orientation board with personal and oreitnation information combined with sessions of cognitive exercises involving memory, problem solving, and conversation (Spector et al., 2003). Some clients may benefit more from cognitive stimulation than do others, but this still remains unknown. Until more information is available, you should be sensitive to individuals responses. You should always be respectful, patient, and calm, and in communicating, you should answer questions simply, honestly, and with sensitivity.

Reminiscence. Reminiscence is recalling the past. Many older adults find enjoyment in sharing past experiences. In reminiscence as therapy, the recollection of the past is used to find meaning and understanding of the present and to resolve current conflicts. Remembering positive resolutions to problems reminds older adults of previous coping strategies used successfully. Reminiscing is also a way to express personal identity. Reflection on past achievements supports self-esteem. For some older adults, the process of remembering past events uncovers new meanings for those events and fosters hope (Duggleby & Wright, 2005).

BOX 25-9 EVIDENCE-INFORMED PRACTICE GUIDELINE

Therapeutic Touch and Agitation in Individuals With Alzheimer's Disease

Evidence Summary

Very few strategies to alleviate or treat disruptive behaviour are effective in people with Alzheimer's disease. The purpose of a 2008 study by Hawranik et al. was to compare the effectiveness of therapeutic touch (identifying and correcting energy imbalances by passing hands several inches above the client's body), simulated therapeutic touch (moving hands over the client's body without energy transfer), and usual care on the disruptive behaviour of 51 subjects with Alzheimer's disease who were receiving long-term care. Disruptive behaviour was classified into three categories: physical aggression, physical nonaggression, and verbal agitation. Physical nonaggressive behaviours decreased significantly in subjects who received therapeutic touch, in comparison with those who received the simulated version and usual care. All categories of disruptive behaviours decreased over time in both the subjects receiving therapeutic touch and those receiving simulated therapeutic touch.

Application to Nursing Practice

- Therapeutic touch and simulated therapeutic touch are effective in reducing disruptive behaviours in clients with Alzheimer's diaease.
- These touch techniques can be taught to family members, staff, and volunteers.
- These techniques can help calm the agitated person and enhance communication during visits.

Based on Hawranik, P., Johnston, P., & Deatrich, J. (2008). Therapeutic touch and agitation in individuals with Alzheimer's disease. *Western Journal of Nursing Research, 30*(4), 417–434.

During the assessment process, you may use reminiscence to assess self-esteem, cognitive function, emotional stability, unresolved conflicts, coping ability, and expectations for the future. Reminiscence also occurs during direct care activities. Taking time to ask the client questions about his or her experiences and listening attentively conveys to an older adult your attitude of respect and concern.

Although reminiscence is often useful in a one-on-one situation with the older adult, reminiscence can also be useful in group therapy for cognitively impaired or depressed older adults. You can organize the group and selects strategies to start a conversation. For example, you might ask the group to discuss families or childhood memories. The group's size, structure, process, goals, and activities are adapted to meet its members' needs.

Body-Image Interventions. The way that older adults present themselves influences body image and feelings of isolation. Some physical characteristics of older adulthood, such as distinguished-looking grey hair, may be socially desirable. Other features, such as a lined face that displays character or wrinkled hands that convey a lifetime of hard work, may also be impressive. Consequences of illness and aging that threaten the older adult's body image include invasive diagnostic procedures, pain, surgery, loss of sensation in a body part, skin changes, loss of scalp hair, and incontinence. Body image is also affected by the use of devices such as dentures, hearing aids, artificial limbs, in-dwelling catheters, ostomy devices, and enteral feeding tubes.

The importance to the older adult of presenting a socially acceptable image must be considered. When older adults have acute or chronic illnesses, the related physical dependence makes it difficult for them to maintain body image. You can influence the older adult's appearance by assisting with grooming and hygiene, such as combing hair, cleaning dentures, shaving, or changing clothing. You should also be sensitive to odours in the environment. Odours may be created by urine and some illnesses. By controlling odours, you may encourage visitors to stay longer or visit more often.

Older Adults and the Acute Care Setting

Older adults in the acute care setting need special attention to help them adjust to the acute care environment and to meet their basic needs for comfort, safety, nutrition, hydration, and skin integrity. The acute care setting poses increased risk for adverse events such as delirium, dehydration, malnutrition, nosocomial infections, urinary incontinence, and falls.

The risk for delirium is increased when hospitalized older adults experience immobilization, infection, dehydration, pain, and hypoxia. Multiple medications and multiple medical diagnoses are also risk factors for delirium (Flaherty et al., 2003). Nonmedical causes of delirium include placement in unfamiliar surroundings, separation from supportive family members, and stress. Impaired vision or hearing contributes to confusion and interferes with nurses' attempts to reorient the client. When the prevention of delirium fails, the basis of nursing management is identification and treatment of the cause of delirium. Supportive interventions include encouraging family visits, providing memory cues (clocks, calendars, name tags), and compensating for sensory deficits. Reality orientation techniques may be useful.

Older adults are at greater risk for dehydration and malnutrition during hospitalization because of standard procedures such as limiting food and fluids in preparation for diagnostic tests. The risk for dehydration and malnutrition is also increased when older adults are unable to reach beverages or to feed themselves while in bed or connected to medical equipment. Interventions include getting the client out of bed, providing beverages and snacks frequently, and including favourite foods and beverages in the diet plan.

The risk for nosocomial infections in older adults is increased by age-related reductions in immune system response. Of all health care agency–acquired infections, 65% occur in hospitalized clients older than 60 years: urinary catheter-related bacteriuria in older adults is the most common infection (Beers & Barklow, 2000). Other nosocomial infections include surgical site infection, pneumonia, and blood stream infections. Prevention begins with hand hygiene and measures to minimize the risk of infection from procedures (see Chapter 33). Prevention also includes measures to increase the older adult's resistance to infection.

Older adults in acute care settings are also at risk for acquiring urinary incontinence (transient incontinence). Causes of transient urinary incontinence include delirium, untreated urinary tract infection, excessive urine production, medications, restricted mobility, and constipation or impaction (Dowling-Castronovo & Bradway, 2003). Interventions for transient urinary incontinence should be geared to correcting contributing factors. The interventions may include an individualized plan to provide voiding opportunities and modification of the environment to improve access to the toilet. In-dwelling urinary catheters should be avoided if possible. Skin breakdown should be prevented.

The risk for skin breakdown and the development of pressure ulcers is increased by changes in aging skin and situations that arise in the acute care setting, such as immobility, incontinence, and malnutrition. To prevent skin breakdown in older clients, you must avoid pressure on the skin, reduce shear forces and friction, provide skin care and moisture management, and provide nutritional support (see Chapter 43).

Older adults in the acute care setting are at risk for falling and sustaining injuries. Many of the falls occur as they get out of bed without assistance. Sedating medications may increase unsteadiness. Medications causing orthostatic hypotension may also increase the risk for falls because the blood pressure drops when the client arises from a bed or chair. Diuretics increase the risk for falling because the person must get out of bed often to void. Attempts to get out of bed when physically restrained may lead to injury if the client becomes entangled in the restraint. Equipment such as wires from monitors, intravenous tubing, urinary catheters, and other medical devices become obstacles to safe ambulation. Impaired vision may prevent the client from seeing tripping hazards such as garbage cans. Confused older adults who may try to get out of bed although weak, unsteady, or drowsy may benefit from the presence of family members and friends. Interventions to reduce the risk for falling include assistance with ambulation, strengthening exercises, medication monitoring, assistance with toileting, and removal of tripping hazards (see Chapter 37). Falls may be reduced by minimizing fall risk factors; through staff, client, and family education; and through individualized fall-reduction interventions. The goal is to minimize the risk of falling without compromising mobility and functional independence.

Older Adults and Restorative Care

Restorative care consists of two types of ongoing care: (1) continuing the convalescence from acute illness or surgery that began in the acute care setting and (2) addressing chronic conditions that affect day-to-day functioning. Both types of restorative care take place in private homes and in long-term care settings.

Interventions during convalescence from acute illness or surgery are directed toward regaining or improving the prior level of independence in ADLs. Interventions that began in the acute care setting should be continued and later modified as convalescence progresses. To achieve this continuation, the acute care setting's discharge information should describe the ongoing interventions (e.g., exercise routines, wound care routines, medication schedules, vital sign monitoring, and blood glucose monitoring). To ensure that all the client's needs are addressed, a team approach to discharge planning is important. Interventions should also address the restoration of interpersonal relationships and activities either at their previous level or at the level desired by the client.

When restorative care addresses chronic conditions, the goals of care include stabilizing the chronic condition, promoting health, and promoting independence in ADLs. Interventions to stabilize the chronic condition may focus on regulation or prevention. An example of a regulatory intervention is the monitoring of blood glucose levels in diabetes. An example of promoting health is a smoking cessation program for the older adult with chronic obstructive pulmonary disease.

Health promotion interventions for older adults, as addressed in this chapter, should occur in all health care settings. For example, nurse-directed programs in long-term care settings improve ambulation, reverse urinary incontinence, and reduce confusion.

Interventions to promote independence in ADLs address physical ability, cognitive ability, and safety. The physical ability to perform ADLs requires strength, flexibility, and balance. Impairments of vision, hearing, and touch must be accommodated. The cognitive ability to perform ADLs requires the ability to recognize, judge, and remember. Cognitive impairments, such as Alzheimer's disease, may interfere with the safe performance of ADLs, although the affected client is still physically capable of the activities. Interventions to promote independence in ADLs adapt these requirements to the needs and lifestyle of the older adult. Safety is always an important consideration. An older adult should be able to perform the ADLs with the least amount of risk.

Beyond the basic ADLs, the older adult's ability to perform instrumental ADLs must be assessed and appropriate interventions implemented. Instrumental ADLs are tasks such as using a telephone, preparing meals, shopping, doing laundry, cleaning the home, and driving an automobile. To remain independent at home or in assisted-living residences, older adults must be able to perform instrumental ADLs, be able to purchase services by outside workers, or have a supportive network of family and friends who assist with these tasks.

Restorative care measures focus on activities to prevent, improve, reduce, or eliminate problems. Priorities of care are established, client goals and expected outcomes are determined, and appropriate interventions are selected. These are done with the client's participation so that the interventions are understood and conflicts in approaches or priorities can be avoided. An older adult's lifetime experiences, values, and sociocultural background are the bases for planning individual care. When deterioration of the client's cognitive status prevents participation in health care decisions, the family or significant others must be consulted. Family and friends are rich sources of data because they knew the client before the impairment. Frequently, they can provide explanations for the older adult's behaviours and suggest methods of management. Thoughtful assessment and planning involve consideration of the influence of normal aging changes, facilitate an optimal level of comfort and coping, and promote independence in self-care activities.

* KEY CONCEPTS

- The number of older adults, especially the number of older adults older than 85 years, is increasing.
- Because your attitudes toward older adults influence the quality of care, those attitudes should be based on accurate information about older adults, rather than on myths and stereotypes.
- Biological and psychosocial theories of aging offer possible explanations for the changes seen in aging, but every older adult is a unique individual who ages in a unique way.
- The physical changes that accompany aging are considered normal, not pathological, although they may predispose the older adult to disease.
- Cognitive impairment is not normal in older adults, and necessitates assessment and intervention.
- Cognitive impairment includes acute, potentially reversible disorders and chronic, irreversible, progressive disorders.
- Areas affected by psychosocial changes of aging include retirement, social isolation, change in housing, death, and sexuality.
- Nursing interventions for psychosocial concerns include therapeutic communication, touch, cognitive stimulation, reminiscence, and interventions to improve body image.
- The leading causes of death in the older population are cancer, heart disease, stroke, lung disease, accidents and falls, diabetes, kidney disease, and liver disease.

- Health promotion recommendations for older adults include good nutrition, regular exercise, smoking cessation, measures to reduce the risk for falls, and measures to reduce adverse medication reactions.
- Acute care settings increase older adults' risk for delirium, dehydration, malnutrition, nosocomial infections, urinary incontinence, and falls.
- Restorative nursing interventions, whether accomplished in the older adult's home or in long-term care institutions, stabilize chronic conditions, promote health, and promote independence in basic and instrumental ADLs.

✻ CRITICAL THINKING EXERCISES

1. Mr. Brown, 73 years old, has come to the clinic for a routine check of his blood pressure. It is normal (130/80 mm Hg). He tells you that he wants to do everything he can to stay healthy. What advice can you give him on health promotion and disease prevention?
2. Mrs. Shephard's daughter has come with her to the clinic. She is concerned about her mother's memory. She tells you that her mother's memory has been excellent but has suddenly become poor. Two days ago, Mrs. Shephard phoned her daughter six times in 2 hours, asking where her husband (the late Mr. Shephard) was, and, when told of his death 4 years ago, Mrs. Shephard denied this fact. When her daughter arrived at her house to check on her, she found that Mrs. Shephard had emptied the contents of all the closets onto the floor and accused her daughter of theft. Her daughter brought Mrs. Shephard to her own home that night because of concern about Mrs. Shephard's safety. From Mrs. Shephard's daughter's report, you suspect delirium (acute confusional state). What questions should you ask, and what areas should you assess to identify the possible causes of Mrs. Shephard's confusion?
3. A nursing colleague tells you that she does not know very much about assessing older adults, and she asks for some pointers on how to perform a thorough assessment. What advice can you give her about the process of geriatric assessment?

✻ REVIEW QUESTIONS

1. Two factors contribute to the projected increase in the number of older adults:
   1. Financial success and improved environment
   2. Fewer medical problems associated with aging
   3. Improved medication plan and increase in federal health care funding
   4. The aging of the "baby boom" generation and the growth of the population segment older than 85 years
2. Which of the following is true about the theories of aging?
   1. Genetic changes are solely responsible.
   2. Environment is the main factor.
   3. No single theory explains aging.
   4. Disease causes a decline in function.
3. The three common conditions affecting cognition in older adults are
   1. Stroke, heart attack, and cancer of the brain
   2. Cancer, Alzheimer's disease, and stroke
   3. Delirium, depression, and dementia
   4. Blindness, hearing loss, and stroke
4. Sexuality is recognized as a factor in the lives of older adults; thus,
   1. Any expression of sexuality should be discouraged
   2. All older adults, whether healthy or frail, need to express sexual feelings
   3. An older adult's need for sexual expression decreases
   4. The need to touch and be touched is decreased
5. The libido does not decrease in older adults; however,
   1. Frequency of sexual activity may decline
   2. Physical changes do not usually affect sexual functioning
   3. The need to touch and be touched is decreased
   4. The sexual preferences of older adults are not as diverse
6. Visual acuity declines with age. Presbyopia is a progressive decline in
   1. Distinguishing between blues and greens and among pastel shades
   2. The ability to see in darkness
   3. The ability to focus on near objects
   4. Adaptation to abrupt changes from darkness to light
7. A common age-related change in auditory acuity is called
   1. Presbycusis
   2. Presbyopia
   3. Calcification
   4. Hypertrophy
8. Taste buds atrophy and lose sensitivity. Older adults are less able to discern
   1. Salty, sweet, sour, and bitter tastes
   2. Hot and cold temperatures
   3. Moistness and dryness
   4. Spicy and bland tastes
9. Changes in the musculoskeletal system lead to changes in the configuration of the thorax. This is known as
   1. Hypertrophy
   2. Calcification
   3. Presbycusis
   4. Kyphosis
10. Frontotemporal dementia has an insidious onset and progresses slowly. Early symptoms include
    1. Poor hygiene, lack of social tact, and sexual disinhibition
    2. More involvement in surroundings and social situations
    3. Fluctuating cognition and visual or auditory hallucinations (or both)
    4. Motor features of parkinsonism

✻ RECOMMENDED WEB SITES

Alzheimer Society of Canada: http://www.alzheimer.ca
The Alzheimer Society of Canada provides current information about Alzheimer's disease, related dementias, caregiving, support, research, treatment, and programs and services.

Canadian Gerontological Nursing Association: http://www.cgna.net
This Web site provides information about gerontological nursing practice in Canada, including current standards of practice.

Public Health Agency of Canada, Division of Aging and Seniors: http://www.phac-aspc.gc.ca/seniors-aines
This federal Web site provides links to new services, publications, and news releases on issues relevant to aging.

26

Self-Concept

Original chapter by Victoria N. Folse, APRN, BC, LCPC, PhD
Canadian content written by Judee E. Onyskiw, RN, BScN, MN, PhD

objectives

Mastery of content in this chapter will enable you to:

- Define the key terms listed.
- Discuss factors that influence the following components of self-concept: identity, body image, and role performance.
- Identify stressors that affect self-concept and self-esteem.
- Describe the components of self-concept as related to psychosocial and cognitive developmental stages.
- Explore ways in which a nurse's self-concept and nursing actions can affect a client's self-concept and self-esteem.
- Incorporate research findings to promote evidence-informed practice for identity confusion, disturbed body image, low self-esteem, and role conflict.
- Examine cultural considerations that affect self-concept.
- Apply the nursing process to promote a client's self-concept.

key terms

media resources

evolve Web Site

- Audio Chapter Summaries
- Glossary
- Multiple-Choice Review Questions
- Student Learning Activities
- Weblinks

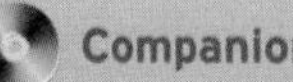

Companion CD

- Glossary
- Interactive Learning Activities
- Fluids and Electrolytes Tutorial
- Test-Taking Skills

Self-concept is described as how a person thinks about himself or herself. It is a subjective sense of the self and a complex mixture of conscious and unconscious thoughts, attitudes, and perceptions. Self-concept comprises several domains: social, emotional, physical, academic, and nonacademic. Self-concept affects how a person manages situations and relationships. Self-concept also affects self-esteem, or how a person feels about himself or herself. Although the terms *self-concept* and *self-esteem* are often used interchangeably, it is important to understand the distinction. Self-esteem stems from self-concept, and self-esteem influences self-concept. *Self-concept* is a descriptive term, whereas *self-esteem* is an evaluative term. By using these terms appropriately, health care professionals facilitate communication and ensure that the nursing care plan is individualized to meet each client's needs.

Nurses care for clients with a variety of health problems that can threaten their self-concept and self-esteem. The loss of a bodily function, a decline in activity tolerance, and difficulty managing a chronic illness are all situations that can potentially affect a client's self-concept. Nurses play a key role in helping clients adjust to alterations in self-concept and in supporting components of self-concept that enable clients to cope with difficulties.

Scientific Knowledge Base

The development and maintenance of self-concept and self-esteem begin at a young age and continue across the lifespan. Parents and other primary caregivers, as well as culture and environment, influence the development of a child's self-concept and self-esteem. In general, young children tend to rate themselves higher on measures of self-esteem than they rate other children, which is perhaps a reflection of their egocentric view of the world. Self-concept becomes more clearly differentiated during the transition into puberty and during adolescence. Adolescence is a particularly critical time, when many factors affect self-concept and self-esteem (Figure 26–1). The adolescent experience appears to adversely affect self-esteem, more so for girls than for boys (Birndorf et al., 2005). Maturational changes are generally regarded as positive for boys: No sudden physical change indicates puberty. For girls, adolescence brings menarche, its associated symptoms, the development of breasts, and a gain in body fat. As a result, adolescent girls may be more sensitive to their appearance and how others view them (Park, 2003).

In adulthood, men tend to report higher levels of self-esteem than do women. However, the exact magnitude of this gender difference

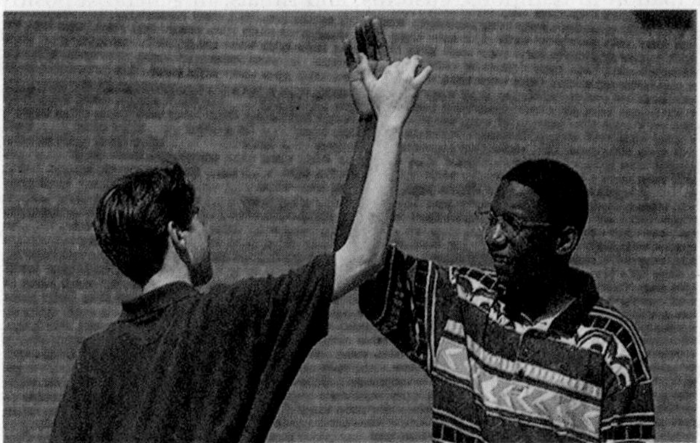

Figure 26-1 Participating in group activities can foster adolescents' self-esteem. **Source:** From Birchenall, J., & Streight, E. (2003). *Mosby's textbook for the home care aide* (2nd ed.). St. Louis, MO: Mosby.

and the way it varies across the lifespan remain unclear. Job satisfaction and job performance are linked to self-esteem. When individuals lose a job, they lose their position-related identity, and their self-perceptions may be altered or diminished. They may not be motivated to be active socially or may even become depressed. A developmental goal of adulthood is to establish a sense of self that is stable and transcends relationships and situations.

In older adults, the sense of self may be negatively affected by emotional and physical changes associated with aging (Robins et al., 2002). When older adults lose a partner or develop health problems, for example, they may experience negative changes in independence or social interaction. These changes may alter their self-concept and self-esteem.

Ethnic and cultural differences in self-concept and self-esteem have also been demonstrated across the lifespan, and research findings suggest that differences in the development of self-concept may exist (Twenge & Crocker, 2002). To ensure an individualized approach to health care, nurses must be sensitive to factors that affect self-concept and self-esteem in diverse cultures.

Individuals' perceptions of themselves and of their health are closely related. Clients' beliefs about their personal health can enhance their self-concept. Statements such as "I can get through anything" or "I've never been sick a day in my life" indicate that a person's thoughts about personal health are positive. Self-concept is also affected by illness, hospitalization, and surgery. Chronic illness may affect the ability to provide financial support, thereby affecting an individual's self-esteem and perceived roles within the family. Negative perceptions regarding health status may be reflected in such statements as "It's not worth it anymore" or "I'm a burden to my family." Chronic illness can affect identity and body image. This is reflected in statements such as "I'll never get any better" or "I can't stand to look at my body this way."

What individuals think and how they feel about themselves affect the way they care for themselves physically and emotionally and the way they care for others. How a person behaves is generally consistent with both self-concept and self-esteem. Individuals who have poor self-concepts often do not feel in control of situations and may not feel worthy of care, which can influence decisions regarding health care. Knowledge of variables that affect self-concept and self-esteem is crucial for providing effective treatment.

Nursing Knowledge Base

Knowledge developed from medical and social sciences, humanities, and psychology, as well as knowledge from nursing research and clinical practice, is used to provide clients with evidence-informed practice. This broad knowledge base allows nurses to have a holistic view of clients, which promotes quality client care that best meets the self-concept needs of each client and family.

Development of Self-Concept

The development of self-concept is a complex lifelong process that involves many factors. In his psychosocial theory of development, Erikson (1963) described key tasks that individuals face at various stages of development. Each stage builds on the tasks of the previous stage, and successful mastery of each stage leads to a positive sense of self (Box 26–1).

Nurses learn to recognize an individual's failure to achieve an age-appropriate developmental stage or an individual's regression to an earlier stage in a period of crisis. This understanding enables nurses to individualize care and determine appropriate nursing interventions. Self-concept is always changing and is based on the following:

- Sense of competency
- Perceived reactions of other people to own body
- Ongoing perceptions and interpretations of other people's thoughts and feelings
- Personal and professional relationships
- Racial identity

➤ BOX 26-1 Self-Concept: Erikson's Developmental Tasks

Trust Versus Mistrust (Birth to Age 1 Year)
Develops trust from consistency in caregiving and nurturing interactions of parents and others
Distinguishes self from environment

Autonomy Versus Shame and Doubt (Ages 1 to 3 Years)
Begins to communicate likes and dislikes
Is increasingly autonomous in thoughts and actions
Appreciates body appearance and function
Develops self through modelling, imitation, and socialization

Initiative Versus Guilt (Ages 3 to 6 Years)
Takes initiative
Identifies with a gender
Gains enhanced self-awareness
Increases language skills, including identification of feelings
Is sensitive to family feedback

Industry Versus Inferiority (Ages 6 to 12 Years)
Incorporates feedback from peers and teachers
Increases self-esteem with new skill mastery (e.g., reading, math, sports, music)
Experiences strengthening of sexual identity
Is aware of strengths and limitations

Identity Versus Role Confusion (Ages 12 to 20 Years)
Accepts body changes and maturation
Examines attitudes, values, and beliefs; establishes goals for the future
Feels positive about expanded sense of self
Interacts with people whom he or she finds sexually attractive or intellectually stimulating

Intimacy Versus Isolation (Ages Mid-20s to Mid-40s)
Has intimate relationships with family and significant others
Has stable, positive feelings about self
Experiences successful role transitions and increased responsibilities

Generativity Versus Self-Absorption (Mid-40s to Mid-60s)
Accepts changes in appearance and physical endurance
Reassesses life goals
Shows contentment with aging

Ego Integrity Versus Despair (Ages Late 60s and Older)
Feels positive about own life and its meaning
Is interested in providing a legacy for the next generation

- Sexual identity
- Academic and employment-related identity
- Spiritual identity
- Personality structure
- Perceptions of events that have an impact on the self
- Mastery of prior and new experiences
- Current feelings about the physical, emotional, and social self
- Self-expectations

Components and Interrelated Terms of Self-Concept

A positive self-concept provides a sense of meaning, wholeness, and consistency. A healthy self-concept has a high degree of stability and generates positive feelings toward the self. The components of self-concept frequently considered by nurses are identity, body image, and role performance. Self-esteem is traditionally viewed as a closely related concept.

Identity. Identity involves the internal sense of individuality, wholeness, and consistency of a person over time and in various circumstances. Identity implies being distinct and separate from others. Identity develops over time and ends in being a "unique" person. The core of identity is being "oneself." A child learns culturally and socially accepted values, behaviours, and roles through observing other people and modelling their behaviour. Identity is often gained from self-observation and from what individuals are told about themselves (Stuart & Laraia, 2005). A child first identifies with parental figures and later with teachers, peers, and role models. To form an identity, a child must be able to integrate learned behaviours and expectations into a coherent, consistent, and unique whole (Erikson, 1963).

Identity is expressed in relationships with others. Sexuality is a part of one's identity. Gender identity is a person's sense of self as a man or as a woman and includes a person's sexual orientation. This image and its meaning depends on culturally determined values that are affected by socialization (see Chapter 23).

Religious faith also may foster identity formation through participation in traditions and rituals (Good & Willoughby, 2007; Sinclair & Milner, 2005; Smith, 2003a, 2003b). Association with religious friends and mentors provide strong identity experiences that influence an individual's sense of self.

Racial or cultural identity develops from identification and socialization within an established group, as well as through the experience of integrating the response of individuals outside the cultural or racial group into a person's sense of self. Differences in ethnic identity (e.g., Vietnamese Canadian, Polish Canadian) exist through participation in traditions, customs, and rituals. In general, a positive relationship exists between identification with social groups and personal self-esteem. Self-esteem tends to be high when racial identity is central to self-concept and is positive (Twenge & Crocker, 2002). People who experience discrimination, prejudice, or environmental stressors such as poverty or living in high-crime neighbourhoods may conceptualize themselves differently than those who have not experienced the same stressors (Ruiz et al., 2002). Furthermore, the opinion or approval of others may not constitute the basis for self-esteem in the same way for all racial and cultural groups. Cultural differences in self-concept exist and may also demonstrate some age-specific trends (Box 26–2).

Body Image. Body image involves attitudes related to the body, including physical appearance, structure, or function. Feelings about body image include those related to sexuality, femininity and masculinity, youthfulness, health, and vitality. These mental images are

BOX 26-2 CULTURAL ASPECTS OF CARE

Racial and Cultural Background

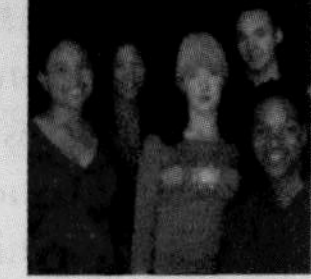

Racial and cultural identity are important components of a person's self-concept. Early in growth and development, an individual develops a racial and cultural identity within the family context. As the individual grows, the cultural aspects of their self-concept may be reinforced through family, social, or cultural experiences. An individual's self-concept may be strengthened or challenged through political, social, or cultural influences experienced in school or work environments. Positive or negative cultural role modelling and past experiences also influence self-concept.

Implications for Practice

- To improve a client's self-concept, develop an open, nonrestrictive attitude when assessing for and encouraging cultural practices.
- Ask clients what they think is important to help them feel better or gain a stronger sense of self.
- Encourage cultural identity by individualizing hygiene practices, dietary choices, and clothing to meet each client's self-concept needs.

Data from Birndorf, S., Ryan, S., Auinger, P., & Aten, M. (2005). High self-esteem among adolescents: Longitudinal trends, sex differences, and protective factors. *Journal of Adolescent Health, 37,* 194–201; Biro, F. M., Streigel-Moore, R. H., Franco, D. L., Padgett, J., & Bean, J. A. (2006). Self-esteem in adolescents females. *Journal of Adolescent Health, 39,* 501–507; Robins, R. W., Trzesniewski, K. H., Tracy, J. L., Gosling, S. D., & Potter, J. (2002). Global self-esteem across the life span. *Psychology and Aging, 17*(3), 423; Ruiz, S. Y., Roosa, M. W., & Gonzales, N. A. (2002). Predictors of self-esteem for Mexican American and European American youths: A reexamination of the influence of parenting. *Journal of Family Psychology, 16*(1), 70; and Twenge, J. M., & Crocker, J. (2002). Race and self-esteem: Meta-analyses comparing Whites, Blacks, Hispanics, Asians, and American Indians. *Psychology Bulletin, 128*(3), 371–408.

not always consistent with a person's actual physical structure or appearance. Some body image distortions have deep psychological origins, such as those that occur in an eating disorder (e.g., anorexia nervosa). Other alterations occur as a result of situational events such as an amputation of a limb as a result of trauma.

The majority of men and women experience some degree of body dissatisfaction, which can affect body image and overall self-concept. Disturbances in body image can be exaggerated when a change in health status occurs. The way other people view a person's body and the feedback offered are also influential. For example, a controlling, violent husband might tell his wife that she is ugly and that no one else would want her. Over time, with repeated humiliation and degradation, she may incorporate this devalued image into her self-concept.

Body image is affected by cognitive growth and physical development. Normal developmental changes such as puberty, menopause, and aging have an effect on body image. Body image is influenced by hormonal changes during adolescence. The development of secondary sex characteristics and changes in body fat distribution affect an adolescent's self-concept. In the older adult, changes associated with aging (e.g., decreasing visual acuity, hearing, and mobility) can also affect body image.

Cultural and societal attitudes and values also influence body image. Culture and society dictate accepted norms for body image that can influence a person's attitudes (Figure 26–2). Values such as ideal body weight and shape, as well as attitudes toward body markings, piercing, and tattoos, are culturally based. In North American culture, people have been socialized to dread the normal aging process. Youth, beauty, and wholeness are emphasized, as apparent in television programs, movies, and advertisements. The media play an important role in creating and perpetuating a cultural standard for unrealistic thinness, youth, and beauty that is difficult for individuals to attain (Strahan et al., 2008). Exposure to societal messages that reflect the sociocultural norm have a negative impact on women. Although these media images target mostly women, men also have been shown to be influenced by idealized media images (Strahan et al., 2006).

Body image depends only partly on the reality of the body. When physical changes occur, individuals may or may not incorporate these changes into their body image. For example, people who have experienced significant weight loss may not perceive themselves as thin and thus may have a distorted body image. Body image issues are often associated with impaired self-concept and self-esteem.

Role Performance. Role performance is the way in which individuals perceive their ability to carry out significant roles. Common roles include those of parent, child, spouse, employee, and student. An individual's perception of competency in a role may or may not match other people's evaluation. Roles that individuals follow in given situations involve socialization to expectations or standards of behaviour. Patterns are stable and change only minimally during adulthood. Individuals learn behaviours that are approved by society through the following processes:

- *Reinforcement–extinction:* Certain behaviours become common or are avoided, depending on whether they are approved and reinforced or are discouraged and punished.
- *Inhibition:* An individual learns to refrain from certain behaviours, even when tempted to engage in them.
- *Substitution:* An individual replaces one behaviour with another, which provides the same personal gratification.
- *Imitation:* An individual acquires skills or behaviours by observing and then imitating the skills and behaviours of other members of the family or other social or cultural groups.
- *Identification:* An individual internalizes the beliefs, behaviour, and values of role models into a personal, unique expression of self.

Ideal societal role behaviours are often hard to achieve in real life. Individuals have multiple roles and personal needs that often conflict. For example, an individual may be a mother of three children, a child of elderly parents, a student, and an employee. Each role involves meeting certain expectations. To function effectively in multiple roles, a person must know the expected behaviour and values, desire to conform to them, and be able to meet the role requirements. Successful adults

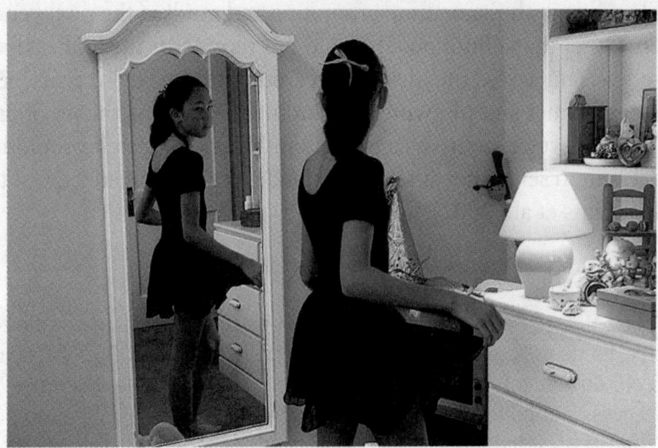

Figure 26-2 An individual's appearance influences self-concept. **Source:** From Sorrentino, S. A. (2004). *Mosby's textbook for nursing assistants* (6th ed.). St. Louis, MO: Mosby.

learn to distinguish between ideal role expectations and realistic possibilities. Fulfillment of these expectations leads to an enhanced sense of self. Difficulty or failure in meeting role expectations leads to deficits in the sense of self and often contributes to decreased self-esteem or altered self-concept.

Self-Esteem. Self-esteem is described as an individual's overall sense of self-worth or the emotional appraisal of self-concept. It represents the overall judgement of personal worth or value. Self-esteem is positive when a person feels capable, worthwhile, and competent (Rosenberg, 1965). Self-esteem is shaped by the individual's appraisals of how he or she is perceived by significant others.

According to Erikson (1963), young children begin to develop a sense of usefulness or industry by learning to act on their own initiative. Children's self-esteem is related to their evaluation of their effectiveness at school, within the family, and in social settings. The evaluation of other people such as parents, teachers, and peers has a profound influence on children's self-esteem.

Global self-esteem levels tend to be highest in childhood, possibly because children's sense of self is inflated by a variety of positive sources (Robins et al., 2002). Self-esteem tends to decline in adolescence. This may be partially understood in the context of maturational changes associated with puberty and increased expectations associated with the transition from primary to secondary school. This decline may also be associated with a shift to more realistic information about the self. Some gender differences exist in the adolescent years; for example, boys report greater self-esteem than do girls (Birndorf et al., 2005).

Several factors have been shown to be positively associated with self-esteem in adolescents: for example, parental support and social and emotional support from other adult role models in early adolescence (Gomez & McLaren, 2006; Park, 2003). Adults may foster self-esteem in adolescents by providing positive communication through supportive and caring relationships (Birndorf et al., 2005; Park, 2003). Other factors related to greater self-esteem include family income above the poverty level, safe and nurturing environments, and religious community. Participating in physical activity that is developmentally appropriate and enjoyable can lead to positive self-esteem in boys (Strong et al., 2005) and in girls (Schmatz et al., 2007).

Self-esteem levels rise gradually during adulthood and decline sharply in old age (Robins et al., 2002). In general, this pattern holds true across gender, socioeconomic status, and ethnicity. Erikson's (1963) emphasis on the generativity stage (see Chapter 22) may explain the rise in self-esteem and self-concept in adulthood. The individual is focused on being increasingly productive and creative at work, while at the same time promoting and guiding the next generation. Other than childhood, the mid-60s represents the highest level of self-esteem across the lifespan. At around the age of 70 years, self-esteem declines sharply, which, according to Erikson's theory of psychosocial development, reflects a diminished need for self-promotion and a shift in self-concept to a more modest and balanced view of the self (Robins et al., 2002).

safety alert Lower levels of self-esteem may increase adolescents' tendency to engage in risky behaviours (Biro et al., 2006; Wild et al., 2004). Adolescents are more likely than people of other ages to engage in practices harmful to their health. A decline in self-esteem in adolescence is often associated with an increased need for attention. This need for attention may be demonstrated in unsafe behaviours, such as premature sexual activity, unprotected sex, or substance abuse. In addition, adolescents may take more risks when they begin to drive. These risks threaten adolescents' health and have implications for health care interventions.

To better understand self-esteem, consider the relationship between a person's self-concept and his or her ideal self. The *ideal self* consists of the aspirations, goals, values, and standards of behaviour that a person considers ideal and strives to attain. The ideal self originates in the preschool years and develops throughout life. It is influenced by societal norms and by the expectations and demands of parents and significant others. In general, a person whose self-concept comes close to matching the ideal self has high self-esteem, whereas a person whose self-concept varies widely from the ideal self suffers from low self-esteem. A child who excels in school and who is liked by peers is more likely to have higher self-esteem than is a child who has difficulty in school and is not liked by peers.

Self-evaluation is an ongoing mental process. A positive sense of self-esteem is an important variable in determining how an individual functions in the world. A person's ability to contribute to society in a meaningful way often affects self-concept and self-esteem. Once established, basic feelings about the self tend to be constant, although they may fluctuate somewhat. A situational crisis may temporarily affect one's self-esteem. Individuals who are sick and unable to be involved in society may feel worthless. Accepting a client as an individual with worth and dignity can help maintain and improve the client's self-esteem.

Stressors Affecting Self-Concept

A self-concept stressor is any real or perceived change that threatens identity, body image, or role performance (Figure 26–3). A stressor challenges a person's adaptive capacities. The most important factor in determining an individual's response is the individual's perception of the stressor. The ability to re-establish balance is related to numerous factors, including the number of stressors, duration of the stressors, and health status (see Chapter 30). The normal process of maturation and development itself is a stressor. Changes that occur in physical, spiritual, emotional, sexual, familial, and sociocultural health can affect self-concept. Being able to adapt to stressors is likely to lead to a positive sense of self, whereas failure to adapt often leads to a negative sense of self.

Any change in health can be a stressor that potentially affects self-concept. A physical change in the body can alter body image, thereby affecting identity and self-esteem. Chronic illnesses often alter role performance, which may affect identity and self-esteem. Loss of a partner can lead to loss of identity and lower self-esteem (Van Baarsen, 2002). An essential process in adjusting to loss is the development of a new self-concept. The following case study illustrates the interrelationships among the components of self-concept.

Amil, a 48-year-old man, has a sudden, unexpected stroke. He had not even been aware that he was hypertensive. Amil awakens in the hospital to find that he cannot move his right hand. He cannot care for himself and is unable to turn himself for days. With the nurses' and physiotherapists' constant encouragement, he is finally able to pull himself out of bed and into a chair. He wonders what lies ahead for him. Amil's body image has dramatically changed from that of a physically strong man to a helpless individual. He worries about his family's future. His older child is away at college, and his younger child is still in high school. Amil and his wife, Meredith, are scared. Although Meredith works, they are not able to meet their monthly expenses or to educate their children without his wages. Amil's role as primary financial provider for the family may be drastically changed if his condition does not improve.

Amil's self-esteem diminishes as his recovery and rehabilitation progress slowly. His self-concept has changed from a person who is self-sufficient to someone who must rely on others. Although he returns home and is in the rehabilitation process, Amil is not able to

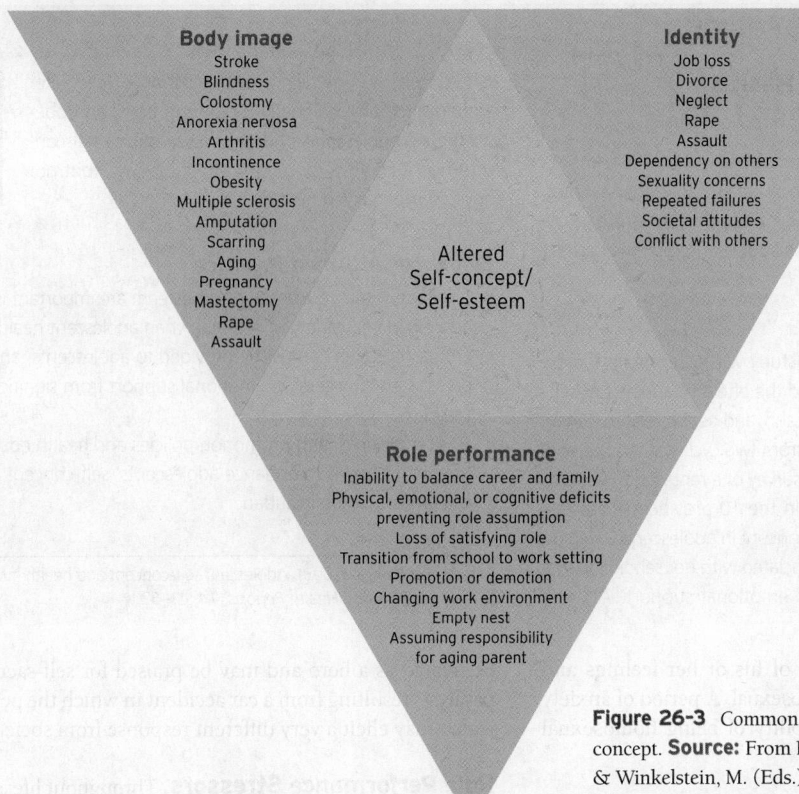

Figure 26-3 Common stressors that influence self-concept. **Source:** From Hockenberry, M., Wilson, D., & Winkelstein, M. (Eds.). (2003). *Wong's nursing care of infants and children* (7th ed.). St. Louis, MO: Mosby.

perform tasks for his family and must wait until his wife and younger child get home to help him with activities that require strength. Amil's adaptation capabilities are stretched to the maximum, although his physician tells him that he is very fortunate to be alive. Amil's identity is not clear to him anymore. He has no clear role within the family, his body image has been drastically altered, and his self-esteem is spiralling lower.

Amil continues in outpatient physiotherapy. He requires significant time and energy even for simple tasks. Nevertheless, he slowly begins to gain some strength. After several months of rehabilitative therapy and support from an interdisciplinary team of health care professionals, he is able to return to work, with a few modifications to ensure his safety. He has some diminished mental agility and muscle weakening, but he is able to perform most aspects of his job. His self-esteem improves, and his body image is enhanced. Although he still feels somewhat altered, his physical capabilities closely resemble those he had before the stroke.

Crisis occurs when a person cannot overcome obstacles with his or her usual methods of problem solving and adaptation. Any crisis potentially threatens self-concept and self-esteem. Some crises, such as the one described in the preceding case study, directly affect all components of self-concept. Self-esteem has been shown to be negatively affected by stroke, and this development is strongly associated with depressive mood (Vickery et al., 2008). The stressors created by a crisis—identity confusion, disturbed body image, low self-esteem, role conflict, role strain, role ambiguity, and role overload—may result in illness. For example, a diagnosis of cancer places additional demands on a person's established living pattern. It changes the person's appraisal of and satisfaction with the current level of physical, emotional, and social functioning. Learned resourcefulness, social support, and, in particular, self-esteem are predictive of health-related quality of life for long-term survivors of cancer (Pedro, 2001). Health-related quality of life may increase with interventions such as nurse-led support groups aimed at supporting and improving self-esteem. During self-concept crises, supportive and educative resources can help a person learn new ways of coping and responding to the stressful event or situation in order to maintain or enhance self-concept.

Identity Stressors. Developmental markers such as puberty, menopause, retirement, and decreasing physical abilities may affect identity. Identity, like body image, is closely related to appearance and abilities. An individual's identity is affected by stressors throughout life, but it is particularly vulnerable during adolescence, a time characterized by physical, emotional, and mental changes of increasing maturity, which can result in insecurity and anxiety. It is also a time when adolescents are developing psychosocial competence, including coping strategies (see Chapter 30). A positive self-concept in adolescence enhances psychological and physical health in young adulthood (Box 26–3).

Adults generally have a more stable identity and thus a more firmly developed self-concept than do younger people. Cultural and social stressors, rather than personal stressors, may have more effect on an adult's identity. For example, an adult may have to balance career and family or make choices regarding religious or cultural traditions. Retirement may mean the loss of an important means of achievement and continued success. People at retirement may begin to re-evaluate their identities and accomplishments. Loss of a significant other can lead the surviving individual to re-examine aspects of his or her identity.

Identity confusion results when people do not maintain a clear, consistent, and continuous consciousness of personal identity. It may occur at any stage of life if a person is unable to adapt to identity stressors. Under extreme stress, an individual may experience disturbed personal identity, a state in which the differences between the self and others cannot be determined. One example of identity confusion is

BOX 26-3 RESEARCH HIGHLIGHT

Adolescent Self-Concept and Health

Research Focus

The literature on adolescent self-concept is considerable, but little is known about the long-term effect of self-concept on health. By understanding the role of self-concept in adolescent health, you can develop strategies to promote adolescent health and design health education programs to meet the needs of this population.

Research Abstract

The purpose of Park's (2003) longitudinal study was to examine factors associated with adolescent self-concept and the effect of adolescent self-concept on psychological health, physical health, and health-related behaviour in later adulthood. Park analyzed data from two cycles of the National Population Health Survey, a general health survey of a representative sample of Canadians aged 12 years or older in the 10 provinces. The data revealed that girls tend to have lower self-concept in adolescence than do boys of the same age. Self-concept was associated with household income and with adolescents' perceived level of emotional support. A weak self-concept was predictive of depression 6 years later among girls, physical inactivity among boys, and obesity among adolescents of both sexes. A strong self-concept had a positive long-term effect on girls' (but not boys') self-perceived health.

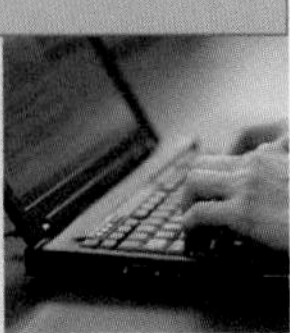

Evidence-Informed Practice

- Adolescent self-concept and self-esteem are important issues to be addressed in a variety of settings when adolescent health is promoted.
- Emotional support must be provided to adolescents, and they must be assisted in accessing emotional support from significant others in their lives.
- To strengthen health promotion policies and health education programs, strategies to enhance adolescents' self-concept and self-esteem should be included.

References: Park, J. (2003). Adolescent self-concept and health into adulthood [Catalogue 82-003]. *Health Reports, 14,* 41–52.

when an adolescent realizes that some of his or her feelings and behaviours could be understood as homosexual. A period of anxiety and confusion begins, when the possibility of being homosexual clashes with a heterosexual self-image.

Body Image Stressors. Changes in the appearance, structure, or function of a body part requires an adjustment in body image. An individual's perception of the change and the relative importance placed on body image affects the significance of the loss of function or change in appearance. For example, if a woman's body image incorporates reproductive functions as the ideal, a hysterectomy performed to combat uterine cancer may be a significant alteration and may result in a perceived loss of femininity or wholeness. Changes in body appearance, such as an amputation, facial disfigurement, or scars from burns, are physically obvious stressors affecting body image. Mastectomy and colostomy are surgical procedures that alter body appearance and function; although these changes are usually undetected by other people, they nonetheless have a significant effect on the individual. Even some elective changes such as breast augmentation or reduction can affect body image. Chronic illnesses such as heart and renal disease affect body image because the body no longer functions at an optimal level. Anticipated body changes resulting from developmental processes can also affect body image. In addition, the effects of pregnancy, significant weight gain or loss, pharmacological management of illness, or radiation therapy change body image. Negative body image can lead to adverse health outcomes.

Many people associate success with a specific body part or function. For example, athletes may consider their bodies and physical activities to be the focus of personal success. Adaptation and rehabilitation may be affected if they can never again participate in athletics because of an accident or injury. To a surgeon, an amputation of a finger would significantly alter his or her ability to perform surgery. This change may affect the surgeon's perception of his or her worth as an individual. Body image changes necessitate the revision of long-accepted self-perceptions, as well as alterations in lifestyle. To regain a positive self-concept and self-esteem, each person must adapt to his or her body image stressors.

Society's response to an individual's physical changes may be affected by the conditions surrounding the alteration. For example, in response to paralysis resulting from an act of war, an individual may be treated as a hero and may be praised for self-sacrifice. However, paralysis resulting from a car accident in which the person was intoxicated may elicit a very different response from society.

Role Performance Stressors. Throughout life, a person undergoes numerous role changes. Normal changes associated with growth and maturation result in developmental transitions. Situational transitions occur when parents, spouses, children, or close friends die or when people move, marry, divorce, or change jobs. A health–illness transition is changing from a state of health or well-being to one of illness. A shift along the continuum from illness to wellness is as stressful as a shift from wellness to illness. Any of these transitions may lead to role conflict, role ambiguity, role strain, or role overload.

Role conflict results when a person simultaneously assumes two or more roles that are inconsistent, contradictory, or mutually exclusive. For example, when a middle-age woman with teenage children assumes responsibility for caring for her older parents, conflicts may arise in relation to being both the adult child and the caregiver of her parents. Negotiating a balance of time and energy between her children and parents may also create role conflicts. The perceived importance of each conflicting role influences the degree of conflict experienced. The **sick role** involves the expectations of other people and society about how a person should behave when sick. Role conflict may occur when general societal expectations ("take care of yourself and you will get better") and the expectations of coworkers ("we need to get the job done") collide. The conflict of taking care of oneself while getting everything done can be a major challenge.

Role ambiguity involves unclear role expectations. When expectations are unclear, people may be unsure about what to do or how to behave. Such situations are often stressful and confusing. Role ambiguity is common in adolescence. Adolescents are pressured by parents, peers, and the media to assume adult-like roles, but many adolescents lack the resources to move beyond the role of dependent children. Role ambiguity is also common in employment situations. In complex, rapidly changing, or highly specialized organizations, employees often become unsure about job expectations.

Role strain is the stress or strain experienced by an individual when behaviours, expectations, or obligations associated with a single social role are incompatible. Role strain may be experienced by individuals who feel inadequate or unsuited for a new social role. For example, individuals who marry someone with children often feel unprepared to assume the parental role. Role strain is also associated with gender role stereotypes (Stuart & Laraia, 2005). Some people perceive women in positions traditionally held by men as less competent, less objective, or less knowledgeable than their male counterparts. Women may feel that they must work harder and perform better in order to compete. Men in traditionally female roles may also encounter gender bias; for example, male nurses frequently report gender stereotyping by clients and other health care professionals (Meadus & Twomey, 2007). One such stereotype suggests that male nurses are viewed as less caring than are female nurses.

Role overload involves having more roles or responsibilities within a role than are manageable. It is frequently reflected in unsuccessful attempts to meet the demands of work and family while still having some personal time. During periods of illness or change, the people involved, either as the person who is ill or as a significant other, often find themselves in role overload.

Self-Esteem Stressors. Individuals with high self-esteem are generally more resilient and are better able to cope with demands and stressors than are those with low self-esteem. High self-esteem is associated with more optimal mental and physical health, greater control over circumstances, and greater adaptation and productivity as an adult (Trzesniewski et al., 2006). Low self-worth can contribute to feeling unfulfilled and isolated from others and can result in depression and unremitting uneasiness or anxiety. Illness, surgery, or accidents that change life patterns can also influence feelings of self-worth. Chronic illnesses such as diabetes, arthritis, and cardiac dysfunction necessitate changes in accepted and long-assumed behavioural patterns. The more the chronic illness interferes with the ability to engage in activities contributing to feelings of worth or success, the more it affects self-esteem.

Self-esteem stressors vary with developmental stages. Perceived inability to meet parental expectations, harsh criticism, inconsistent discipline, and unresolved sibling rivalry may reduce children's sense of self-worth. Ineffective parenting also is associated with low self-esteem in children. Low self-esteem takes a toll on children. Children with low self-esteem and self-worth are more likely to bully other children and are more likely to be bullied (Christie-Mizell, 2003; Box 26–4). Low self-esteem in adolescence is one of the strongest predictors of depression (MacPhee & Andrews, 2006) and is related to thoughts about suicide (Wilburn & Smith, 2005). A developmental milestone such as pregnancy also introduces unique self-concept stressors and has significant implications for health care. Low self-esteem is one of the strongest predictors of postpartum depression (Beck, 2008). In older adults, self-concept stressors include health problems, reduced functional ability, declining socioeconomic status, spousal loss or bereavement, loss of social support, and decline in achievement experiences after retirement (Box 26–5).

The Family's Effect on Development of Self-Concept

The family plays a key role in creating and maintaining each family member's self-concept. Children develop a basic sense of who they are from their caregivers. Bowlby's (1982) attachment theory suggests that the quality of the attachment that children develop with their caregivers influences the development of a set of expectations about the self, their interpretations of the actions of other people, and ideas about how to respond to them. Attachment theory suggests that children who experience sensitive and supportive caring will develop expectations that they are worthy of other people's love and that other people are supportive. The quality of parenting interactions also influences children's development. Parents who respond in a firm, consistent, and warm manner promote positive self-esteem in their children (Ruiz et al., 2002). Parents who are harsh, behave inconsistently, or have low self-esteem themselves may foster negative self-concepts in their children. Even well-meaning parents can cultivate negative self-concepts in children. To assist clients in developing a positive self-concept, it is important to assess the family's style of relating (see Chapter 20).

BOX 26-4 RESEARCH HIGHLIGHT

Bullying and Self-Concept

Research Focus

Bullying is defined as physical, psychological, or verbal intimidation or attack, or a combination of these, that is meant to cause distress, harm, or both to an intended victim. In Canada, approximately 15% of school-aged children report being bullied in the classroom, schoolyard, or playground. Some studies however, indicate that bullying behaviour among children is increasing and is committed by younger children than in the past. Bullying is a serious problem both for the victims and the children who bully others.

One of the explanations for why children bully other children focuses on self-concept. Studies have shown that children with a positive self-concept are less likely to bully other children, engage in delinquent behaviour, or be instigators of peer conflict (Coloroso, 2002). In addition, children with a positive self-concept are less likely to be bullied. The family environment and, in particular, parenting behaviours influence children's self-concept.

Research Abstract

The objective of Christie-Mizell's (2003) study was to examine how the quality of the parental relationships (specifically, conflict between the parents) affects children's self-concept and participation in bullying behaviour. The researcher analyzed data from children aged 8 to 14 years who participated in the National Longitudinal Survey of Youth, a national survey of children in the United States. The data revealed that participation in bullying behaviour is significantly tied to a child's self-concept. Lower self-concept was associated with an increase in bullying behaviour. In addition, the effect of parental conflict on children's bullying behaviour was mediated by the child's self-concept.

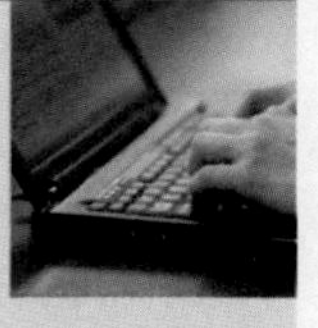

Evidence-Informed Practice

- Building children's self-concept is an important strategy to prevent bullying behaviour in children and to prevent victimization by a bully.
- Parents must be helped to understand how children are affected by parental conflict and the family environment.
- It is important to involve the entire family system in the intervention process when children are identified as victims or bullies.
- Referral to other health care professionals may be necessary to assist vulnerable children and families.

References: Christie-Mizell, C. A. (2003). Bullying: The consequences of interparental discord and child's self-concept. *Family Process, 42*(2), 237–251.

BOX 26-5 FOCUS ON OLDER ADULTS

- Promoting a positive self-concept in all older adults is essential, but it is especially important for those experiencing disability, frailty, or reduced functional capacity (Vickery et al., 2008).
- Conducting a life review or participating in a reminiscence group, recording an oral history, or arranging a photo scrapbook of meaningful life events are examples of activities to help older adults feel a sense of self-worth about their lives while providing a legacy for younger family members (Eliopoulos, 2005).
- Potential threats to the self-esteem of older adults may arise from the institutional environments where they receive care. These threats can include dependence, devaluation, depersonalization, functional impairments, and lack of control over one's environment. Nursing interventions directed toward reducing or eliminating these threats result in improved quality of life for the older adult.
- Self-concept may be negatively affected in older adulthood by a number of life changes, including health problems, declining socioeconomic status, spousal loss or bereavement, loss of social support, and decline in achievement experiences after retirement (Stuart & Laraia, 2005).
- Health care professionals should be alert to older adults' preoccupation with physical complaints; they should conduct a comprehensive assessment and encourage clients to verbalize needs, feelings, and emotions such as fear, insecurity, and loneliness (Robins et al., 2002).
- By actively listening and accepting the person's feelings, being respectful, praising health-seeking behaviours, and recognizing, acknowledging, and praising accomplishments, health care professionals convey respect for the older adult's worth.

The Nurse's Effect on the Client's Self-Concept

Your acceptance of a client with an altered self-concept helps promote positive change. When a client's physical appearance has changed, likely both the client and the family will observe your verbal and nonverbal responses and reactions. You need to be aware of your own feelings, ideas, values, expectations, and judgements. Self-awareness is critical in initially understanding and accepting others. Nurses who are secure in their own identities more readily accept and thus reinforce clients' identities. It is important to assess and clarify the following self-concept issues:

- Thoughts and feelings about lifestyle, health, and illness
- Awareness of how nonverbal communication may affect clients and families
- Personal values and expectations and how they affect clients
- Ability to convey a nonjudgemental attitude toward clients
- Preconceived attitudes toward cultural differences in self-concept and self-esteem

Some clients with a change in body appearance or function are very sensitive to health care professionals' verbal and nonverbal responses. A positive and matter-of-fact approach to care can provide a model for the client and family to follow. You can have a positive effect by conveying genuine interest and acceptance. By recognizing and including self-concept issues in planning and delivering care, you can positively influence client outcomes. By building a trusting nurse–client relationship and appropriately involving the client and family in decision making, you can enhance self-concept. An individualized approach may highlight a client's unique needs, including incorporating alternative health care practices or methods of spiritual expression.

You also can significantly influence a client's body image. For example, for a woman who has undergone a mastectomy, you can affect her body image in a positive way by showing acceptance of the mastectomy scar. Clients closely watch other people's reactions to their wounds and scars. A facial expression of shock or disgust can lead to development of a negative body image. It is important to monitor your responses toward clients. Statements such as "This wound is healing nicely" or "The tissue looks healthy" are very affirming for a client. Nonverbal behaviours help to convey caring for a client and can affect self-esteem (Figure 26–4). For example, the self-concept of an incontinent client can be threatened by the perception that the caregivers find the situation unpleasant. Anticipate personal reactions, acknowledge them, and focus on the client instead of on the unpleasant task or situation. Imagining yourself in the client's position will help you find strategies and measures to ease your client's embarrassment, frustration, and anger.

Preventive measures, early identification, and appropriate treatment can minimize the intensity of self-esteem stressors and the potential effects on the client and family. Learn to design specific self-concept interventions to fit a client's profile of risk factors. It is essential to assess the client's perception of a problem and to work collaboratively with the client to resolve self-concept issues (Box 26–6). It may also be necessary to work with other members of the health care team to resolve issues related to self-concept.

Critical Thinking

Self-concept profoundly influences a person's response to illness. A critical thinking approach to care is essential. This approach requires synthesis of knowledge, experience, information gathered from clients and families, critical thinking qualities, and intellectual and professional standards. Solid clinical judgement requires anticipating the required information, collecting and analyzing the data, and making appropriate decisions regarding client care.

In the case of self-concept, it is essential to integrate knowledge from nursing and other disciplines, including self-concept theory and communication principles, and to consider cultural and developmental factors. Previous experience in caring for clients with alterations in self-concept assists you in individualizing care for each client. The nursing process continues until the client's self-concept is improved, restored, or maintained.

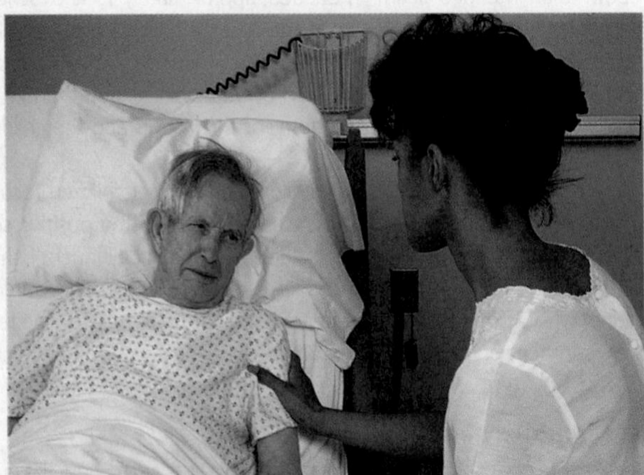

Figure 26-4 Nurses can use touch and eye contact to enhance a client's self-esteem.

BOX 26-6 RESEARCH HIGHLIGHT

Promoting a Healthy Body Image

Research Focus

In North American society, sociocultural norms for appearance suggest to girls and women that their value is determined by their appearance. The media typically plays an important role in depicting women as thin, youthful, and beautiful. Women for whom this standard is unrealistic feel self-conscious and dissatisfied with their bodies. The extent to which women internalize society's standards for thinness is associated with body dissatisfaction and represents a risk factor for eating disorders.

Research Abstract

Strahan et al. (2008) tested whether sociocultural norms for ideal appearance leads women to base their self-worth more strongly on appearance. In the first study, the researchers presented images reflecting norms of thinness (e.g., one commercial featuring models wearing Victoria's Secret bras) to female university students; then they measured whether these images had a direct effect on the students' body satisfaction and concern with others' perceptions and whether appearance-contingent self-worth accounted for these effects. Results showed that exposure to images conveying the sociocultural norm for beauty influenced the students' perceptions of satisfaction with their bodies. The second study was conducted with students in public schools. Students received an intervention that challenged the legitimacy of sociocultural norms for ideal appearance. Results of the second study showed that in comparison with control subjects, students receiving the intervention were less accepting of sociocultural norms for appearance, based their self-worth less strongly on appearance, and in turn were less concerned with others' perceptions and were more satisfied with their bodies.

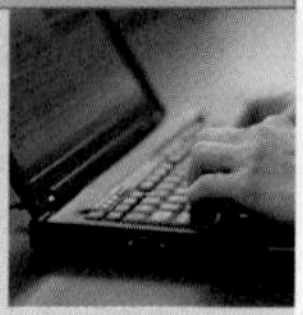

Evidence-Informed Practice

- Promoting empowerment, building self-esteem, and developing positive self-concept in girls and women are important health promotion strategies.
- Body weight concerns and coping strategies are important issues for nurses to address with girls and women.
- Nurses should increase clients' awareness of the role of the media and popular culture in promoting unrealistic and unhealthy standards.

References: Strahan, E. J., Lafrance, A., Wilson, A. E., Ethier, N., Spencer, S. J., & Zanna, M. P. (2008). Victoria's dirty little secret: How sociocultural norms influence adolescent girls and women. *Personality and Social Psychology Bulletin, 34*(2), 288–301.

Self-Concept and the Nursing Process

❖Assessment

In assessing self-concept and self-esteem, you must focus on the various components of self-concept (identity, body image, and role performance). Assessment should also include observing behaviours suggestive of an altered self-concept (Box 26–7), actual and potential self-concept stressors (see the earlier case study), and coping patterns. An awareness of cultural differences is crucial because some behaviours suggestive of an altered self-concept for someone in one cultural group may be quite normal for individuals in other cultures. For example, in many First Nations and Asian cultures, eye contact is a sign of disrespect. In order to gather comprehensive assessment, information from multiple sources must be synthesized critically (Figure 26–5).

➤BOX 26-7 Behaviours Suggestive of Altered Self-Concept

- Avoidance of eye contact
- Slumped posture
- Unkempt appearance
- Being overly apologetic
- Hesitant speech
- Being overly critical or angry
- Frequent or inappropriate crying
- Negative self-evaluation
- Being excessively dependent
- Hesitancy in expressing views or opinions
- Lack of interest in what is happening
- Passive attitude
- Difficulty in making decisions

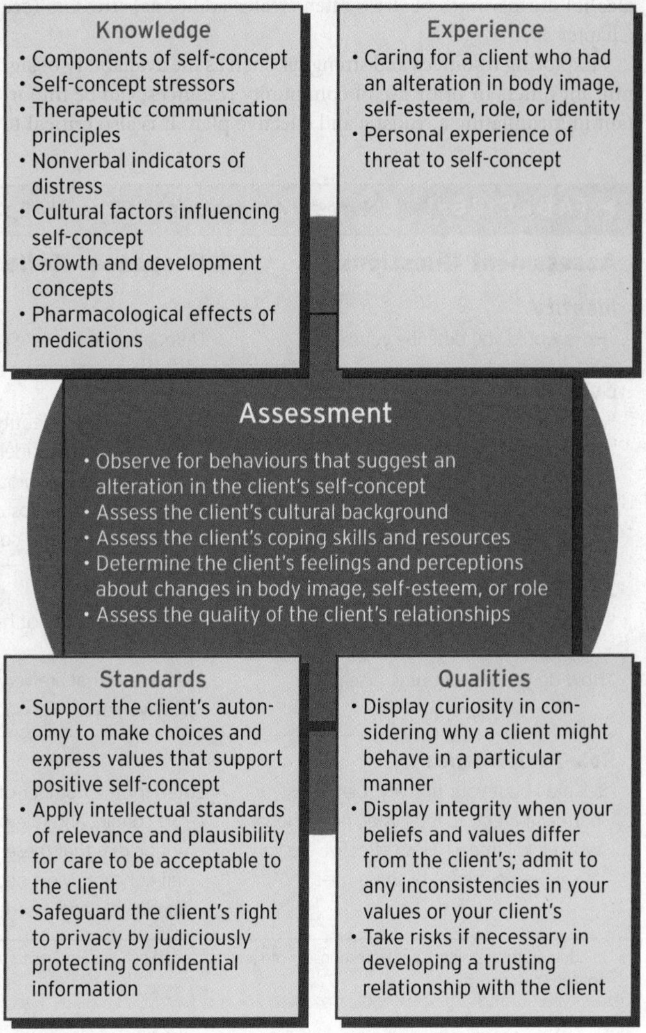

Knowledge
- Components of self-concept
- Self-concept stressors
- Therapeutic communication principles
- Nonverbal indicators of distress
- Cultural factors influencing self-concept
- Growth and development concepts
- Pharmacological effects of medications

Experience
- Caring for a client who had an alteration in body image, self-esteem, role, or identity
- Personal experience of threat to self-concept

Assessment
- Observe for behaviours that suggest an alteration in the client's self-concept
- Assess the client's cultural background
- Assess the client's coping skills and resources
- Determine the client's feelings and perceptions about changes in body image, self-esteem, or role
- Assess the quality of the client's relationships

Standards
- Support the client's autonomy to make choices and express values that support positive self-concept
- Apply intellectual standards of relevance and plausibility for care to be acceptable to the client
- Safeguard the client's right to privacy by judiciously protecting confidential information

Qualities
- Display curiosity in considering why a client might behave in a particular manner
- Display integrity when your beliefs and values differ from the client's; admit to any inconsistencies in your values or your client's
- Take risks if necessary in developing a trusting relationship with the client

Figure 26-5 Critical thinking model for self-concept assessment.

You can gather much of the data regarding self-concept by observing the client's nonverbal behaviour and by paying attention to the client's conversation, in addition to direct questioning. Take note of the manner in which clients talk about significant people in their lives. This can provide clues to both stressful and supportive relationships, as well as to key roles that the client assumes. Using knowledge of developmental stages to determine what areas are likely to be important to the client, inquire about these aspects of the person's life. For example, ask an older client about his or her life and what has been important to him or her. At this stage of development, individuals are examining their lives and considering the effects they have had in the world. The individual's conversation will probably provide data relating to role performance, identity, self-esteem, stressors, and coping patterns. At appropriate times, it may be useful to ask specific questions (Table 26–1).

Coping Behaviours

The nursing assessment should also include consideration of previous coping behaviours; the nature, number, and intensity of the stressors; and the client's internal and external resources. Knowledge of how a client has handled past stressors can enable insight into the client's style of coping. People do not address all issues in the same way, but they often use a familiar coping pattern for newly encountered stressors. As previous coping patterns are identified, it is useful to determine whether these patterns have contributed to healthy functioning or created more problems. For example, the use of drugs or alcohol during times of stress often creates additional stressors (see Chapter 30).

Exploring resources and strengths, such as the availability of significant others or prior use of community resources, can be important in formulating a realistic and effective plan. It is also critical to understand how a client views a situation. For example, older women may be more accustomed to changes in their health status because of the aging process in general, and experiencing heart disease may be one more aspect of growing older. On the other hand, a cardiac event occurring in middle age may be less expected and more problematic for women in terms of family and career responsibilities and may thus elicit a dramatic increase in anxiety.

Significant Others

Significant others can help identify changes in a client's behaviour that may be suggestive of alterations in self-concept. These individuals may have insights into the client's way of dealing with stressors or knowledge about what is important to the client's self-concept. The way a significant other talks about the client and the significant other's nonverbal behaviours may provide information about what kind of support is available for the client.

Clients' Expectations

Another important factor in assessing self-concept is the person's expectations. Asking a client what he or she thinks you can do to help is important. You need to collaborate with clients so that interventions are acceptable to them. Asking a client how he or she thinks the interventions will make a difference elicits useful information regarding the client's expectations. It also provides an opportunity to discuss the client's goals. For example, while working with a client who is experiencing anxiety related to an upcoming diagnostic test, you might ask about the relaxation exercise that the client has been practising. The client's response provides valuable information about his or her beliefs and attitudes regarding the efficacy of the intervention, as well as the potential need to modify the nursing approach.

➤TABLE 26-1 Nursing Assessment of Client's Self-Concept

Assessment Questions*	Responses Reflecting Difficulties With Self-Concept
Identity	
"How would you describe yourself?"	Derogatory answers (e.g., "I don't know; not too much is worth mentioning") should raise concern.
Body Image	
"What aspects of your appearance do you like?" "Would you like to change any aspects of your appearance? If yes, describe the changes you would make."	Most people can identify something about their appearance that they like (e.g., "I have nice eyes"). If a person cannot identify any positive characteristic, this may suggest a negative body image and poor self-esteem. Most people have something that they would like to change (e.g., "My nose is too big" or "My hips are too large"), but a long list of problem areas may be suggestive of difficulties with self-concept.
Self-Esteem	
"Tell me about the things you do that make you feel good about yourself."	Statements about not having any strengths or being able to do anything well should raise concern.
"How do you feel about yourself?"	Statements that are very negative about themselves should raise concern (e.g., "I am hopeless" or "I have never felt good about myself").
Role Performance	
"Tell me about your primary roles (e.g., partner, parent, friend, sister, professional worker, volunteer). How effective are you at carrying out each of these roles?"	Listen for the number of primary roles identified. A large number of primary roles increase the risk for role conflict and role overload. As with previous questions, if the client indicates that he or she does not believe that these roles are adequately covered, the client may be experiencing alterations in self-concept. Most people carry out several roles and often feel as though some of them are not adequately addressed; listen for the client's perception about his or her overall role competency.

*In addition to the client's verbal response, note any nonverbal behaviours. Hesitant speech, lack of interest in what is happening, and slumped posture are suggestive of negative self-concept.

❖Nursing Diagnosis

Carefully consider the assessment data to identify a client's actual or potential problem areas. Rely on knowledge and experience, apply appropriate professional standards, and look for clusters of defining characteristics that indicate a nursing diagnosis. Although multiple nursing diagnostic labels exist for altered self-concept, the following list provides examples of self-concept–related nursing diagnoses:

- *Impaired adjustment*
- *Anxiety*
- *Disturbed body image*
- *Caregiver role strain*
- *Decisional conflict*
- *Ineffective coping*
- *Ineffective denial*
- *Fearful*
- *Hopelessness*
- *Disturbed personal identity*
- *Risk for loneliness*
- *Ineffective role performance*
- *Chronic low self-esteem*
- *Situational low self-esteem*
- *Ineffective sexuality patterns*
- *Impaired social interaction*
- *Spiritual distress*
- *Risk for self-directed violence*

Making nursing diagnoses about self-concept is complex. Often, isolated data could be the defining characteristics for more than one nursing diagnosis (Box 26–8). For example, a client might express feelings of uncertainty and inadequacy. These are defining characteristics for both anxiety and situational low self-esteem. If you are aware that the client is demonstrating defining characteristics for more than one nursing diagnosis, gather specific data to validate and differentiate the underlying problem. To further assess the possibility of anxiety as the nursing diagnosis, you might consider whether the client has any of the following defining characteristics: Is the person experiencing increased muscle tension, shakiness, a sense of being "rattled," or restlessness? These symptoms are more suggestive of anxiety than of low self-esteem. On the other hand, if the person expresses a predominantly negative self-appraisal, including inability to handle situations or events and difficulty making decisions, then situational low self-esteem may be the more appropriate nursing diagnosis. To further aid in differentiating between the two diagnoses, information regarding recent events in the person's life and how the person has viewed himself or herself in the past provides insight into the most appropriate nursing diagnosis. As additional data are gathered, usually the priority nursing diagnosis becomes evident.

To validate critical thinking regarding a nursing diagnosis, it is important to share observations with the client and allow the client to provide input and verify perceptions. This approach often encourages the client to provide additional data, which further clarifies the situation. In the example in Box 26–8, if you said, "I notice you haven't eaten much lunch today," the response to this statement, coupled with the client's nonverbal communication, could facilitate further discussion. An alternative approach may be to state, "I notice you jumped when I came up behind you. Are you feeling uneasy today?" This statement allows the client to verify whether he or she is in fact anxious and to discuss any concerns.

❖Planning

During planning, synthesize knowledge, experience, critical thinking qualities, and standards (Figure 26–6). Critical thinking ensures that the client's care plan integrates all that you know about the individual, as well as key critical thinking elements (Box 26–9). Professional standards are especially important to consider when you develop a plan of care. These standards often establish ethical or evidence-informed practice guidelines for selecting effective nursing interventions.

A concept map is another method to assist in planning nursing care. The concept map illustrated in Figure 26–7 shows the relationship between a medical diagnosis, postoperative reconstruction of severe facial scars, and the four nursing diagnoses. The concept map also links the nursing diagnoses and shows how they are interrelated. In this example, disturbed body image is related to situational low self-esteem. As the client's facial scars improve, she should begin to feel better about her appearance.

Goals and Outcomes

In collaboration with the client, an individualized plan of care for each nursing diagnosis is developed. Together, you and the client set realistic expectations for care. Goals should be individualized and realistic with measurable outcomes. In establishing goals, it is important to consult with the client about whether the goals are perceived as realistic. By consulting with significant others, mental health clinicians, and community resources, you can design a more comprehensive and workable plan. Once a goal has been formulated, consider how the data that illustrated the problem would change if the problem were diminished. These changes should be reflected in the outcome criteria. For example, a client receives a diagnosis of *situational low self-esteem related to a recent job layoff.* You and the client establish a goal:

➤BOX 26-8 NURSING DIAGNOSTIC PROCESS

Assessment Activities	***Defining Characteristics***	***Nursing Diagnosis***
Observe client's behaviour during conversation.	Client demonstrates restlessness, inability to maintain eye contact, facial tension, increased perspiration, and self-preoccupation.	*Anxiety related to accidental injury, pain, uncertainty of outcome of upcoming surgery*
Empathically communicate, "Tell me how you are coping" or "Let's talk about what you are thinking and feeling about tomorrow's procedure."	Client replies, "I'm scared. They may amputate my leg tomorrow. I just don't know how I'll manage. I couldn't sleep last night. On top of the pain, I just kept thinking about everything."	

Knowledge
- Principles of caring to establish trust
- Nursing interventions to promote self-awareness and facilitate change in self-concept
- Family dynamics
- Available services offered by health care professionals and community agencies

Experience
- Establishing rapport with diverse clients
- Previous client responses to planned nursing interventions to enhance or support a client's self-concept

Planning
- Select therapies that strengthen or maintain the client's coping skills
- Involve the client to ensure that realistic therapies are chosen
- Refer to community services as appropriate
- Minimize stressors affecting the client's self-concept

Standards
- Maintain the client's dignity and identity
- Demonstrate the ethics of care

Qualities
- Think independently; explore various approaches to address the issue or problem
- Be creative; be willing to try unique interventions
- Exhibit perseverance because changes in self-concept often happen slowly; continue to support the vision that change is possible

Figure 26-6 Critical thinking model for self-concept planning.

"Client's self-esteem and self-concept should begin to improve in 2 weeks." Examples of expected outcomes directed toward that goal include the following:

- The client will discuss a minimum of three areas of his or her life in which he or she is functioning well.
- The client will be able to voice the recognition that losing the job is not reflective of his or her worth as a person.
- The client attends a support group for out-of-work individuals.

Setting Priorities

The care plan lists the goals, expected outcomes, and interventions for a client with an alteration in self-concept. Interventions focus on helping the client adapt to the stressors that led to the disturbance in self-concept and on supporting successful coping. A client may perceive a situation as overwhelming and may feel hopeless about returning to the previous level of functioning. The client may need time to adapt to physical changes.

Establishing priorities may include therapeutic communication to address self-concept issues to ensure that the client's ability to address physical needs is maximized. Look for strengths in both the client and the family, and provide resources and education to assist the client in changing limitations into strengths. Client teaching creates understanding of the normality of certain situations (e.g., the nature of a chronic disease, change in a relationship, or the effect of a loss). Often, once this is understood, the sense of hopelessness and helplessness decreases.

Continuity of Care

The perceptions of significant others must be incorporated into the plan of care. Clients who have experienced deficits in self-concept before the current episode of treatment may have established a system of support that includes mental health clinicians, clergy, and other community resources. Before involving the family, consider the client's desires for the family's involvement and cultural norms regarding who most frequently makes decisions in the family.

➤ BOX 26-9 NURSING CARE PLAN

Disturbed Body Image

Assessment

You have been assigned to care for Ms. Johnson, a 45-year-old married woman who underwent a unilateral radical mastectomy because of malignancy. Ms. Johnson's physical assessment has been completed, and she has received adequate medication for pain. You sit down to discuss how the mastectomy has affected Ms. Johnson's self-concept.

Assessment Activities	*Findings and Defining Characteristics*
Assess identity concerns (e.g., sexual role, femininity).	Ms. Johnson looks away, shakes her head, and states, "I don't feel feminine. My husband says it doesn't affect how he feels about me, but I feel it does"
Ask Ms. Johnson how the mastectomy is affecting her sense of self.	Intermittent eye contact, frequent crying when alone, pulling hospital gown tightly across chest
Observe Ms. Johnson's mood and interactions with others, including family members.	Has superficial conversations with staff and family members
Determine Ms. Johnson's participation in self-care activities.	Avoids looking in mirror and touching or looking at the dressing; refuses to bathe, comb hair, or brush her teeth

Nursing Diagnosis: Disturbed body image related to negative thoughts and feelings to actual change in body

➤ BOX 26-9 NURSING CARE PLAN *continued*

Planning

*Goal (Nursing Outcomes Classification)**	*Expected Outcomes*
Ms. Johnson will identify and express feelings verbally and nonverbally.	**Body Image** Ms. Johnson will discuss disturbed body image with staff members and significant others within 3 days. Ms. Johnson will consider exploring support groups by the time of discharge.
Ms. Johnson will participate in self-care related to mastectomy.	**Acceptance and Health Status** Ms. Johnson will look at tissue surrounding surgical site within 2 days. Ms. Johnson will begin to attend to basic hygiene needs within 2 days.
Ms. Johnson will identify and use resources outside the hospital.	**Social Involvement** Ms. Johnson will verbalize commitment to participating in community resources (e.g., mastectomy support group) by the time of discharge. By postoperative visit, Ms. Johnson will determine whether she wishes to attend support group.

*Outcome classification labels from Moorhead, S., Johnson, M., & Maas, M. (Eds.). (2004). *Nursing Outcomes Classification (NOC)* (3rd ed.). St. Louis, MO: Mosby.

Interventions (Nursing Interventions Classification)†	Rationale
Initially assign the same staff members to work with Ms. Johnson.	Continuity in care will facilitate the establishment of a therapeutic relationship; familiarity and trust will enhance communication.
Approach Ms. Johnson and initiate conversation; use silence and active listening to promote communication.	Ms. Johnson's ability to initially find the words for what she is experiencing may be limited.
Remain aware of your own feelings regarding Ms. Johnson's bodily changes and physical appearance.	Inadvertently communicating your own discomfort or negativity will interfere with Ms. Johnson's ability to openly communicate her feelings.
Have Ms. Johnson spend time alone and with supportive family members for crying, recording in her journal, reflection, or prayer.	This use of time encourages expression of thoughts and feelings, including depression, grief, resentment, and fear of rejection.
Facilitate evaluation of overall self-concept.	The effect on body image may influence other aspects of self-concept and self-esteem, including perception of identity and role performance.
Involve Ms. Johnson's husband in discussion of uncomfortable issues, such as sexual concerns.	Family involvement is an essential element of comprehensive care. Sexuality is a basic need and concern for both men and women, and yet it can be one of the most difficult discussions for clients to initiate.
Assist Ms. Johnson in identifying and using appropriate support systems outside the hospital, including home health care.	Support can assist the client in feeling normal again and in integrating a new body image into her self-concept.

†Intervention classification labels from Dochterman, J. M., & Bulechek, G. M. (Eds.). (2004). *Nursing Interventions Classification (NIC)* (4th ed.). St. Louis, MO: Mosby.

Evaluation

Nursing Actions	*Client Response and Finding*	*Achievement of Outcome*
Ask Ms. Johnson how effective she feels in her ability to identify and express feelings verbally and nonverbally.	Ms. Johnson responds, "It's hard for me to talk about myself, but I have really made an effort to talk about what the loss of my breast means to me."	Ms. Johnson reports improvement in communication skills and success with discussing disturbed body image with primary nurse and husband.
Observe Ms. Johnson's participation in self-care related to mastectomy.	Ms. Johnson assumes responsibility for basic hygiene immediately after establishing the goal and has used a mirror to examine her mastectomy scar.	Ms. Johnson has increased her independence and has begun to integrate body image change into her self-concept.
Assist Ms. Johnson in identifying resources outside the hospital; secure a commitment to use resources.	Ms. Johnson verbalizes commitment to participating in community resources (e.g., mastectomy support group).	Outcome has not been completely achieved; Ms. Johnson has expressed hesitancy in attending a support group but is receptive to home care. Home care nurse will ensure that goal is re-evaluated and addressed as appropriate.

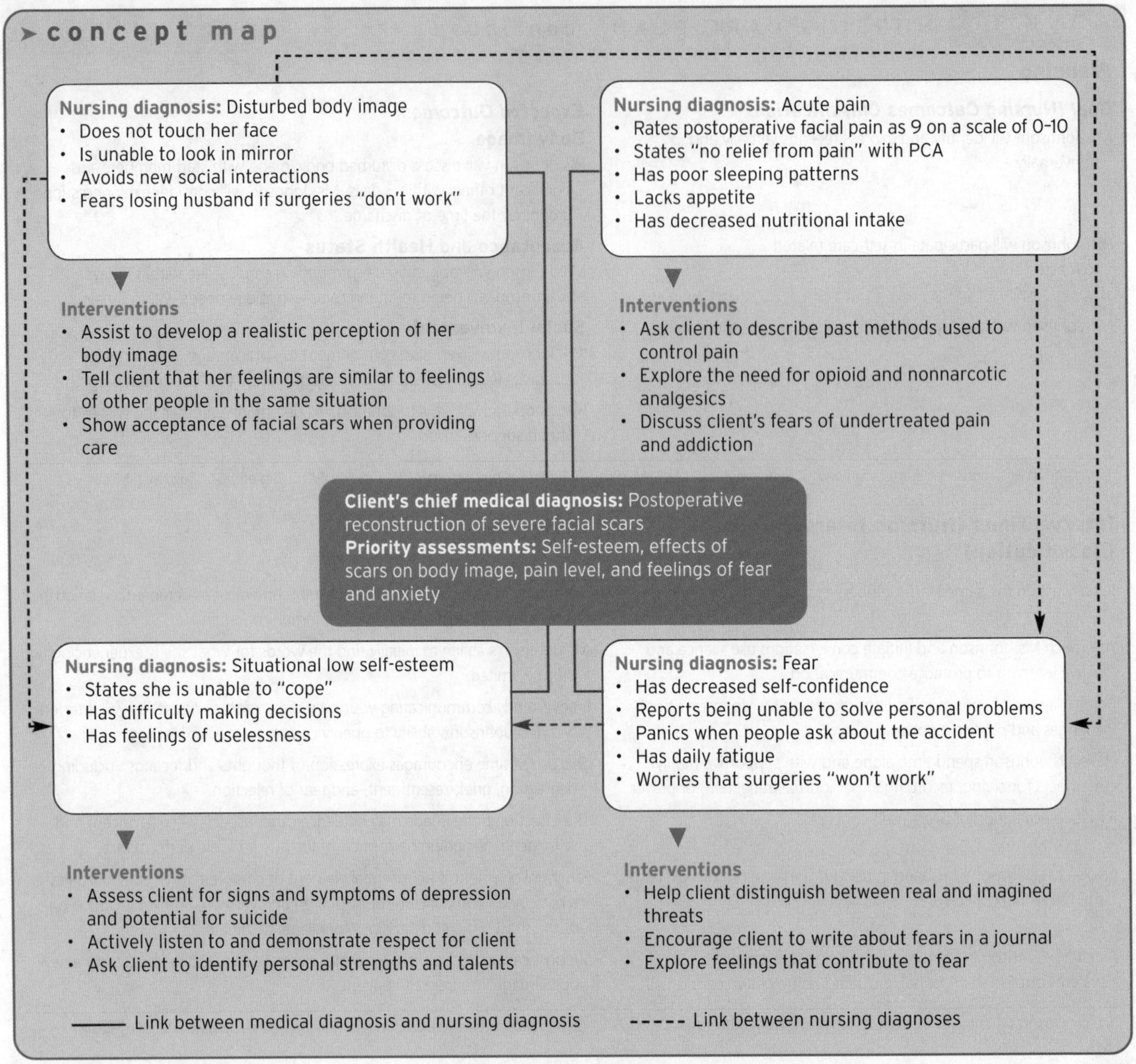

concept map

Nursing diagnosis: Disturbed body image
- Does not touch her face
- Is unable to look in mirror
- Avoids new social interactions
- Fears losing husband if surgeries "don't work"

Interventions
- Assist to develop a realistic perception of her body image
- Tell client that her feelings are similar to feelings of other people in the same situation
- Show acceptance of facial scars when providing care

Nursing diagnosis: Acute pain
- Rates postoperative facial pain as 9 on a scale of 0–10
- States "no relief from pain" with PCA
- Has poor sleeping patterns
- Lacks appetite
- Has decreased nutritional intake

Interventions
- Ask client to describe past methods used to control pain
- Explore the need for opioid and nonnarcotic analgesics
- Discuss client's fears of undertreated pain and addiction

Client's chief medical diagnosis: Postoperative reconstruction of severe facial scars
Priority assessments: Self-esteem, effects of scars on body image, pain level, and feelings of fear and anxiety

Nursing diagnosis: Situational low self-esteem
- States she is unable to "cope"
- Has difficulty making decisions
- Has feelings of uselessness

Interventions
- Assess client for signs and symptoms of depression and potential for suicide
- Actively listen to and demonstrate respect for client
- Ask client to identify personal strengths and talents

Nursing diagnosis: Fear
- Has decreased self-confidence
- Reports being unable to solve personal problems
- Panics when people ask about the accident
- Has daily fatigue
- Worries that surgeries "won't work"

Interventions
- Help client distinguish between real and imagined threats
- Encourage client to write about fears in a journal
- Explore feelings that contribute to fear

—— Link between medical diagnosis and nursing diagnosis

- - - - Link between nursing diagnoses

Figure 26-7 Concept map for client after surgical reconstruction of severe facial scars. PCA, patient-controlled analgesia.

❖Implementation

As with all the steps of the nursing process, a therapeutic nurse–client relationship is central to the implementation phase. Once the goals and outcome criteria have been developed, consider nursing interventions to promote a healthy self-concept and help the client move toward achieving the goals. To develop effective nursing interventions, consider the nursing diagnosis and broad interventions that address the diagnosis. These broad, standard interventions should be tailored to the individual client. Regardless of the health care setting, it is important to work with clients and their families or significant others to promote a healthy self-concept. For example, nursing interventions may include strategies to help clients regain or restore the elements that contribute to a strong and secure sense of self. The approaches that you choose will vary according to the level of care required.

Health Promotion

Work with clients to help them develop healthy lifestyle behaviours that contribute to a positive self-concept (Box 26–10).

Acute Care

In the acute care setting, some clients experience potential threats to their self-concept because of the nature of the treatment and diagnostic procedures. Threats to a person's self-concept can result in anxiety or fear. Numerous stressors, including unknown diagnoses, the need to make changes in lifestyle, and change in functioning, may be present and need to be addressed. In the acute care setting, more than one stressor is often present, which increases the overall stress level for the client and family.

Nurses in the acute care setting also encounter clients who are faced with the need to adapt to an altered body image as a result of surgery or other physical change. Often a visit to the client by someone

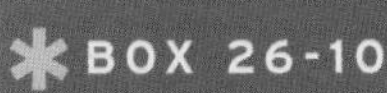

BOX 26-10 FOCUS ON PRIMARY HEALTH CARE

Promoting Client's Self-Concept

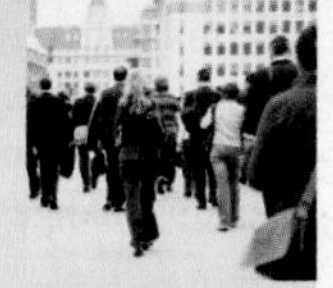

The focus of primary health care is to promote health and prevent illness by stressing client education and self-care. Measures that contribute to a healthy self-concept and therefore promote health and well-being include those that support adaptation to stress, such as proper nutrition and regular exercise within the client's capabilities; those that facilitate adequate sleep and rest; and those that reduce stress.

Nurses are in a unique position to identify lifestyle practices that put a client's self-concept at risk or are suggestive of an altered self-concept. For example, a young adult visits a clinic with complaints of being unable to sleep and experiencing anxiety attacks. In gathering the nursing health history, you may learn of lifestyle practices such as excessive use of alcohol or nonprescription drugs, too little rest, or a large number of life changes occurring simultaneously. These data, when taken together, may suggest actual or potential self-concept disturbances. In this situation, you determine how the client views the various lifestyle elements so that you can facilitate the client's insight into behaviours. If necessary, you provide needed health teaching or make appropriate referrals to other community services. Clients who are experiencing threats to or alterations in self-concept often benefit from mental health and community resources to promote increased awareness. Knowledge of available community resources enables you to make appropriate referrals.

who has experienced similar changes and adapted to them (e.g., someone who has undergone a laryngectomy) may be helpful. The timing of such a visit is important. Because addressing these needs may be difficult while the client is in an acute care setting, appropriate follow-up and referrals, including home care, are essential. Remain sensitive to the client's level of acceptance of the change. Forcing confrontation with the change before the client is ready could delay the client's acceptance. Signs that a client may be receptive to such a visit include the client's asking questions related to how to manage a particular aspect of what has happened or looking at the changed area. As the client expresses readiness to integrate the body change into his or her self-concept, let the client know about groups that are available, and make the initial contact.

Restorative Care

Often, in a long-term nurse–client relationship in a home care environment, nurses have the opportunity to work with clients to attain a more positive self-concept (Box 26–11). Interventions designed to help clients attain a positive self-concept are based on the premise that the client first develops insight and self-awareness concerning problems and stressors and then acts to solve the problems and cope with the stressors. This approach, outlined by Stuart and Laraia (2005), can be incorporated into client teaching for alterations in self-concept, including situational low self-esteem, which might manifest in the home care setting.

Increasing the client's self-awareness is achieved through establishing a trusting nurse–client relationship that allows the client to openly explore thoughts and feelings. A priority nursing intervention is the expert use of communication skills to clarify client and family expectations. Open exploration can make the situation less threatening for the client and encourages behaviours that expand self-awareness. You encourage the client's self-exploration by accepting the client's thoughts and feelings, by helping the client clarify interactions with others, and by being empathetic. Encourage self-expression, and

BOX 26-11 CLIENT TEACHING

Alterations in Self-Concept

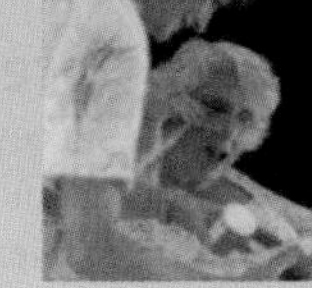

Objective

- Risks for situational low self-esteem will be reduced in the home care setting.

Teaching Strategies

- Reinforce the client's expression of thoughts and feelings; clarify meaning of verbal and nonverbal communication.
- Encourage opportunities for self-care.
- Elicit the client's perceptions of strengths and weaknesses.
- Convey verbally and behaviourally that the client is responsible for his or her own behaviour.
- Identify relevant stressors with the client, and ask for the client's appraisal of these stressors.
- Explore the client's adaptive and maladaptive coping responses to problems.
- Collaboratively identify alternative solutions; encourage the client to use alternatives not previously tried.
- Continue to reinforce the client's strengths and successes.

Evaluation

- Confirm the client's perception of and actual use of improved communication skills.
- Observe the client's level of participation in decisions that affect care.
- Confirm with the client and family that the increase in activities and tasks has been a positive experience.
- Observe the client's establishment of a simple routine.
- Observe the client take necessary action to change maladaptive coping responses and maintain adaptive responses.
- Confirm with the client and family how new coping resources can be applied to continued change.

Modified from Stuart, G. W., & Laraia, M. T. (2005). *Principles and practice of psychiatric nursing* (8th ed.). St. Louis, MO: Mosby.

stress the client's self-responsibility. To promote the client's self-evaluation, help the client to define problems clearly, and identify positive and negative coping mechanisms. Work closely with the client to help analyze adaptive and maladaptive responses; contrast different alternative responses, and discuss outcomes.

Collaborating with the client in establishing realistic goals involves helping the client identify alternative solutions and develop realistic goals based on them. This collaboration facilitates real change and encourages further goal-setting behaviours. Design opportunities that result in success, reinforce the client's skills and strengths, and assist the client in getting needed assistance. To assist the client in becoming committed to decisions and actions to achieve goals, teach the client to stop using ineffective coping mechanisms and develop successful coping strategies. Supporting attempts that are health promoting is essential, because with each success, another attempt can be made. Supporting adaptive, flexible coping is crucial in helping a client with alterations in self-concept.

Establishing a therapeutic environment and a therapeutic relationship (see Chapter 18) and increasing self-awareness are also crucial in successfully helping clients who have alterations in self-concept, whether care is focused on health promotion, dealing with an acute process, or addressing restorative care. To support a client in developing a positive self-concept, you must convey genuine caring (see Chapter 19). You can then establish a partnership with the client to address underlying problems.

❖Evaluation

Client Care

Evaluating success in meeting each client's goal and the established expected outcomes requires critical thinking (Figure 26–8). Frequent evaluation of client progress is recommended so that changes can be instituted if necessary. You use knowledge of behaviours and characteristics of a healthy self-concept when you review the client's behaviours. This method determines whether outcomes have been met.

Expected outcomes for a client with a self-concept disturbance may include nonverbal behaviours indicating a positive self-concept, statements of self-acceptance, and acceptance of change in appearance or function. Nonverbal behaviours can be key indicators of clients' self-concept. For example, a client who has had difficulty making eye contact may demonstrate a more positive self-concept by making more frequent eye contact. Social interaction, adequate self-care, acceptance of the use of prosthetic devices, and statements indicating understanding of teaching all indicate progress. A positive attitude toward rehabilitation and increased movement toward independence facilitate a return to pre-existing roles at work or at home. Patterns of interacting can also reflect changes in self-concept. For example, a client who has been hesitant to express his or her views may more readily offer opinions and ideas as self-esteem increases. The goals of care may be unrealistic or inappropriate as the client's condition changes. The plan may need to be revised, to reflect on successful experiences with other clients. Client adaptation to major changes may take a year or longer, but such length is not suggestive of problems with adaptation. Look for signs that the client has reduced some stressors and that some behaviours have become more adaptive. Changes in self-concept also take time. For some clients, the sense of hopelessness and helplessness may persist. Referral to other mental health specialists may be necessary for some clients with a poor self-concept.

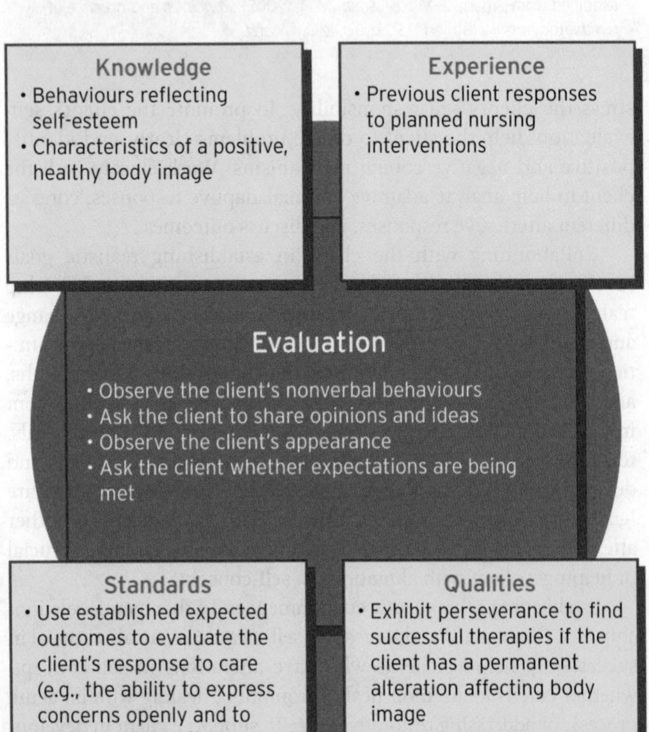

Figure 26-8 Critical thinking model for self-concept evaluation.

Client Expectations

If you have a good rapport with the client, the client may be able to share how things are going from his or her perspective. You may be able to facilitate this sharing by initiating a review of what has happened over time. This offers the opportunity to share perceptions and encourages clients to consider and voice how they have conceptualized any changes.

✻ KEY CONCEPTS

- Self-concept is an integrated set of conscious and unconscious attitudes and perceptions about the self.
- Components of self-concept are identity, body image, and role performance.
- Each developmental stage involves factors that are important to developing a healthy, positive self-concept.
- Identity is particularly vulnerable during adolescence.
- Body image is the mental picture of a person's own body and is not necessarily consistent with a person's actual body structure or appearance.
- Body image stressors include changes in physical appearance, structure, or functioning that are caused by normal developmental changes or illness.
- Self-esteem is the emotional appraisal of self-concept and reflects the overall sense of being capable, worthwhile, and competent.
- Self-esteem stressors include developmental and relationship changes, illness (particularly chronic illness involving changes in what were normal activities), surgery, accidents, and the responses of other individuals to changes resulting from these events.
- Role stressors, including role conflict, role ambiguity, and role strain, may originate in unclear or conflicting role expectations and may be aggravated by illness.
- Your self-concept and nursing actions can have an effect on a client's self-concept.
- Planning and implementing nursing interventions for self-concept disturbance involve increasing the client's self-awareness, encouraging self-exploration, aiding in self-evaluation, helping formulate goals for adaptation, and assisting the client in achieving those goals.

✻ CRITICAL THINKING EXERCISES

1. You are assigned to care for a 23-year-old Chinese Canadian client who sustained multiple fractures to his face and femur 4 days ago in a motor vehicle accident. He had surgery the evening of admission to repair his femur but was admitted to wait for surgery to his face. The client lives with his girlfriend and their 7-month-old daughter and works as a janitor in the local university. He left China with his mother when he was a young child and has grown up in Canada. You have been with him for most of the morning. He was in moderate pain, which was treated with an analgesic. His pain rating decreased from 6 to 3 on a scale of 0 to 10, but the morphine left him drowsy. During the morning, he shared with you some of his concerns about when he will be able to return to work. You are in the room when the surgeon tells him about his upcoming surgery. A temporary tracheotomy is planned because of the extensive surgery needed in the nasal and throat area. After the surgeon leaves, the client tells you that he does not want the tracheotomy. He indicates that he is unclear about what it actually entails, even though the surgeon explained it in fairly simple terms. He states, "I just want to get back to normal." How would you address his comment regarding "get back to normal" and his lack of understanding regarding the tracheotomy?

2. A 16-year-old girl is preparing for discharge from the hospital after giving birth 2 days earlier. She is unmarried, is uninvolved with the baby's father, and has minimal support from her family to assist her in caring for her newborn. Before admission, she arranged to give the baby up for adoption. She reaffirms this as a good decision because she will be able to return to school immediately and still graduate with her peers. The client confides in you that her biggest concerns right now are how she feels about herself and how she looks. Taking into account the developmental needs of this adolescent, how will you collaborate with her to establish priority interventions to address her self-concept difficulties?
3. As a part of your community health experience, you are assigned to visit a 75-year-old woman who has gone to live with her daughter after being hospitalized for agitation and aggression secondary to Alzheimer's disease. When you go to their home, you find the 55-year-old daughter tearful. She says, "I just don't know if I can do this. She is so confused. She calls me two or three times a night to sit with her; sometimes she doesn't even recognize me. I've been missing a lot of work. Even when I'm there, I'm not as productive as I was before she came to live with us." What additional assessment data would be important to gather? What provisional nursing diagnosis could be made for the daughter?

✻ REVIEW QUESTIONS

1. When a nurse is caring for a client after mastectomy, interventions to promote physiological stability and pain control are necessary. In addition, the nurse also needs to design nursing interventions directed toward improving the client's
   1. Mobility
   2. Self-concept
   3. Activity tolerance
   4. Self-care activities
2. Developing self through modelling, imitation, and socialization is a self-concept developmental task during the ages of
   1. 0 to 1 year
   2. 1 to 3 years
   3. 3 to 6 years
   4. 6 to 12 years
3. Which of the following involves the internal sense of individuality, wholeness, and consistency of a person over time and in various circumstances?
   1. Body image
   2. Self-concept
   3. Role performance
   4. Identity
4. Adolescents are at risk for body image disturbance. An accurate statement about body image is that
   1. Body image is not influenced by the opinions of others
   2. Body image refers to the external features of a person
   3. Body image includes actual and perceived perceptions of one's body
   4. Physical changes during adolescence are quickly incorporated into the person's body image
5. Certain behaviours become common or are avoided, depending on whether they are approved and reinforced or are discouraged and punished. This process is called
   1. Reinforcement-extinction
   2. Inhibition
   3. Substitution
   4. Identification
6. When an individual internalizes the beliefs, behaviour, and values of role models into a personal, unique expression of self, the process is called
   1. Reinforcement-extinction
   2. Inhibition
   3. Substitution
   4. Identification
7. An individual's identity is affected by stressors throughout life, but the age group that is particularly vulnerable to stressors because that age is a time of great change is
   1. Infants
   2. Children
   3. Adolescents
   4. Adults
8. When a person does not maintain a clear, consistent, and continuous consciousness of personal identity, it results in
   1. Identify confusion
   2. Low self-esteem
   3. Low self-concept
   4. Body image difficulties
9. The nurse asks the client, "How do you feel about yourself?" The nurse is assessing the client's
   1. Identity
   2. Body image
   3. Self-esteem
   4. Role performance
10. Increasing a client's self-awareness is achieved
    1. By establishing a trusting nurse–client relationship that allows the client to explore his or her thoughts and feelings
    2. By accepting the client's thoughts and feelings
    3. By helping the client to define his or her problems clearly
    4. Through having the client identify his or her positive and negative coping mechanisms

✻ RECOMMENDED WEB SITES

Canadian Mental Health Association: Children and Self-Esteem: http://www.cmha.ca/bins/content_page.asp?cid=2-29-68
This Web page offers advice about how to promote positive self-esteem in children.

Statistics Canada: Adolescent Self-Concept and Health into Adulthood: http://www.statcan.ca/Daily/English/031119/d031119b.htm
In this report, published in 2003, factors associated with adolescent self-concept are examined, and the effect of adolescent self-concept on later health and health-related behaviour in young adulthood is described.

Status of Women Canada: Mental Health Promotion Among Newcomer Female Youth: Post-Migration Experiences and Self-Esteem, Chapter 5: http://www.swc-cfc.gc.ca/index_e.html
This Web site presents the findings of a research project on newcomer Canadian adolescent girls; mental health promotion issues for this group are examined, and recommendations are offered. Enter the search term "self-esteem" after going to the home page.

The Canadian Women's Health Network: Body Image and the Media: http://www.cwhn.ca/resources/faq/biMedia.html
This site contains a discussion of the impact of the media on body image, and it provides advice to help young women have a healthy body image.

27

Sexuality

Original chapter by Amy M. Hall, RN, BSN, MS, PhD

Canadian content written by Anne Katz, RN, PhD

objectives

Mastery of content in this chapter will enable you to:

- Define the key terms listed.
- Discuss the nurse's role in maintaining or enhancing a client's sexual health.
- Discuss the complexities of sexual identity, gender identity, and sexual orientation.
- Describe key concepts of sexual development across the lifespan.
- Describe the sexual response cycle.
- Identify high-risk and safer sex behaviours.
- Identify common sexually transmitted infections (STIs).
- Identify major types of sexual dysfunction and potential causes.
- Assess a client's sexuality.
- Define appropriate nursing diagnoses for clients with alterations in sexuality.
- Identify and describe nursing interventions to promote sexual health.
- Evaluate a client's sexual health.
- Identify potential referral resources for clients' sexual concerns outside the nurse's level of expertise.
- Use critical thinking skills to assist clients in meeting their sexual needs.

key terms

Bisexuality, p. 417
Contraception, p. 422
Dyspareunia, p. 418
Gender identity, p. 417
Heterosexuality, p. 417
Homophobia, p. 417
Homosexuality, p. 417
Infertility, p. 424
Safer sex, p. 420
Sexual dysfunction, p. 425
Sexual health, p. 417
Sexual identity, p. 417
Sexual orientation, p. 417
Sexual response cycle, p. 419
Sexuality, p. 417
Sexually transmitted infections (STIs), p. 417
Transsexuality, p. 417
Vasocongestion, p. 419

media resources

evolve Web Site

- Audio Chapter Summaries
- Glossary
- Multiple-Choice Review Questions
- Student Learning Activities
- Weblinks

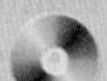 **Companion CD**

- Glossary
- Interactive Learning Activities
- Fluids and Electrolytes Tutorial
- Test-Taking Skills

Sexuality and its expression are vital elements to the wholeness we feel as human beings. Sexuality is seen as "a central aspect of being human throughout life and encompasses sex, gender, identities and roles, sexual orientation, eroticism, pleasure, intimacy, and reproduction" (Wagner et al., 2005). People's view of themselves and others as sexual beings is influenced by their cultural, ethnic, and religious beliefs and practices. Sexuality also concerns people's sexual relationships with others and how they are perceived by others (van der Riet, 1998). Sexual functioning is seen as what people *do* as sexual beings; it is thought to consist of the four phases of the sexual response cycle as conceived by Masters and Johnson (1966; Barton et al., 2004). Sexual functioning, according to this definition, is the same as sexual behaviour; sexual dysfunction is thought to occur when behaviour does not follow some predetermined path and is seen as wrong or abnormal or necessitating intervention.

The World Health Organization (2004) defined **sexual health** as "a state of physical, emotional, mental and social well-being related to sexuality; it is not merely the absence of disease, dysfunction or infirmity. Sexual health requires a positive and respectful approach to sexuality and sexual relationships, as well as to the possibility of having pleasurable and safe sexual experiences, free of coercion, discrimination and violence. For sexual health to be attained and maintained, the sexual rights of all persons must be respected, protected and fulfilled."

Nurses have a role in the promotion of positive, healthful sexuality for youth, adolescents, young and middle-aged adults, and older adults. Nurses can also educate clients to help prevent adverse outcomes such as unwanted pregnancy, **sexually transmitted infections (STIs)**, or sexual dysfunction (Health Canada, 2008).

Religious teachings, culturally prescribed gender roles, beliefs about sexual orientation, and social and environmental climates influence both the client's and the health care professional's value systems. You need to explore your own beliefs and prejudices and strive to develop a nonjudgemental and caring approach that integrates sexual health care into everyday practice.

Scientific Knowledge Base

To assist clients in meeting their sexual needs, you must have a sound scientific knowledge base about sexual and gender identity, sexual orientation, sexual development, the sexual response cycle, high-risk and safer sex behaviours, STIs, contraception, and abortion.

Sexual and Gender Identity

Sexual identity is the objective labelling of a person as male or female. Most people would probably say that two sexes exist and that sexual identification is fairly straightforward. Conventional wisdom is that a person's genitalia determines whether the person is male or female (Vilain, 2004). According to the XY sex-determination system, the two sex chromosomes are the same in female humans (XX), and different in male humans (XY). However, people do not always fit neatly within these systems of sexual identification. Variations in genitalia, gonads, chromosomes, or hormones occur in an estimated 17 of 1000 births in Canada (Johnson, 2004). For example, some people are born with ambiguous genitalia, which makes determining the sex of the infant difficult. Several genetic conditions can disrupt the development of the fetus in such a way that the baby is neither fully male nor fully female (Liao, 2003). A child with an androgen disorder may have male-appearing genitalia and might genetically be a girl; another child might have male hormones and may have the external appearance of a girl.

Gender identity is the degree to which a person identifies as male, female, or some combination. It begins in early childhood as the child becomes aware of the differences of the sexes and perceives that he or she is male or female. Gender identity is usually consistent with physical sex at birth; however, this is not always the case. For example, in **transsexuality**, the physical body is incongruous with the gender identity. A transsexual person may have a female body but feel like a man or may have a male body but feel like a woman (Johnson, 2004). Current research findings indicate that gender identity disorder is caused by hormonal fluctuations at a crucial time in fetal development (Society for Human Sexuality, 2004). Many transsexual people choose to undergo sex reassignment so that their physical sex is congruent with their gender identity; this process involves surgery and the administration of hormones.

Sexual Orientation

Sexual orientation describes the predominant gender preference of a person's sexual attraction over time. **Heterosexuality** is sexual preference for members of the opposite sex; **homosexuality** is sexual preference for members of the same sex. **Bisexuality** is an equal or almost equal preference for both sexes. In a recent Statistics Canada (2004) survey, 1% of the respondents identified themselves as homosexual (gay men and lesbians), and about 0.7% of respondents identified themselves as bisexual. As a nurse, you must not assume that you know your clients' gender identity or sexual orientation. Anyone could be lesbian, gay, bisexual, transsexual, or heterosexual. If you learn a client's sexual orientation, you should not assume that you may tell anyone else or include it in the medical record without the client's knowledge. Some people might want to keep their sexual orientation confidential.

Earlier thinking about sexual orientation led many to believe that heterosexuality was normal and mentally healthy and that all other orientations were abnormal or signs of a psychological disorder. Today, this theory is summarily rejected; scientists agree that homosexuality, transsexuality, and bisexuality are not disorders and are not associated with mental illness or abnormal psychological functioning. Nevertheless, **homophobia**—the prejudicial treatment of or negative attitudes about lesbian, gay, bisexual, or transsexual people and those who are perceived to have these gender or sexual identities—still exists. Homophobia can include a range of emotions and behaviour from discomfort, fear, and disgust to hatred and violence. If you are nonjudgemental and equipped with an appropriate knowledge base, you can help address the problems of homophobia and provide nursing care that does not discriminate against the client's sexual orientation.

Sexual Development

As a person grows and develops, so does his or her sexuality. Each stage of development brings changes in sexual functioning and in the role of sexuality in relationships.

Infancy and Childhood. The awareness of one's sexual identity and sexual development begins in infancy, when the attitudes about the physical body are communicated by the caregivers (Haroian, 2000). From birth on, children are treated differently according to their gender. The differential treatment shapes the behaviour of the child. During the school years, children expand their horizons from parents and family. Parents, teachers, and the child's peer group serve as role models and teach about how men and women act and relate with each other. School-aged children generally have questions regarding the physical and emotional aspects of sex (Finan, 1997). They need accurate information from home and school about physical and emotional changes during this period and what to expect as they move into puberty. This knowledge may help decrease anxieties as these changes begin to happen. An uninformed child may be frightened by menstruation or nocturnal emission and view them as evidence of a dreadful disease.

Puberty and Adolescence. Puberty is characterized by the development of secondary sex characteristics; in girls, these changes generally begin between the ages of 8 and 11 years. The first signs are usually the development of breast buds and, later, growth of pubic hair. The labia begin to enlarge, as do the internal reproductive organs. Sometime after the tenth year, the girl may experience her first menstrual period, and her body shape takes on a more womanly form. By the time she has her period, the breasts are usually fully developed, and pubic hair and axillary (underarm) hair are present. Over time, the menstrual cycle ordinarily becomes regular.

In boys, the changes usually occur about a year later. In some boys, starting at about age 9 years, the testicles begin to enlarge, and the skin of the scrotum becomes darker and coarser. Pubic hair appears and the boy grows taller and more muscular. Genital growth continues over the next 2 years, and the boy begins to look like a male adult, with broad shoulders and narrow hips. When the larynx enlarges, the voice begins to deepen. Fine facial hair and axillary hair also begin to grow. Over time, pubic hair becomes coarser, and penile growth starts to slow down; the testicles continue to grow until they reach full size. Many boys between the ages of 15 and 19 years experience ejaculation, either spontaneously at night (nocturnal emission) or as a result of masturbation. By the end of puberty, the young man is close to his adult height, but further growth can occur into the third decade.

This is a developmental period in which social and emotional changes are also significant. Peer group attachments are strong; sexual attraction to other people is common (Figure 27–1). These emotional and social changes do not always keep up with the physical changes; as a result, an adolescent may look like an adult but still acts and thinks like a child. Perception of body image is important through this stage. Many adolescents are very unhappy with the way they look. They may constantly compare themselves with their peers or with images in the media, and they may consequently experience great dissatisfaction. Self-esteem may be affected negatively; low self-esteem may result in dangerous social and sexual behaviours. Cognitive changes that occur during adolescence are the ability to think in an abstract manner and to anticipate potential consequences (Duncan et al., 2003). These changes are useful in view of the physical and emotional changes.

It is the norm for youth, rather than the exception, to experiment sexually and often with multiple partners (Beitz, 1998); thus, it is essential that youth have access to sexual health services, including information on topics such as body changes, sexual health promotion, STIs, contraception, and pregnancy. Such services are designed to promote sexual health and to encourage responsible decision making with regard to sexual behaviour.

Public health care professionals have been alarmed by the trend toward greater sexual activity at increasingly younger ages, particularly because of the adverse consequences. In 1998 in Canada, 21,000 girls between 15 and 19 years of age had elective abortions, and almost 20,000 girls of that age group gave birth; these statistics translate into a rate of 19.8 births for every 1000 girls (Canadian Institute of Health Information, 2004). After teenage pregnancy, mothers and their children often experience health, financial, and social problems (Jewell et al., 2000). Similarly, exposure to STIs and unwanted sexual activity can lead to psychological disturbances, impairments in the development of healthy social and interpersonal relationships, and long-term physical health problems.

You may be most effective in your goals to support teenagers by helping parents develop confidence in educating their children about sexuality. Factual information regarding sexuality and sexual activity is important, but equally or perhaps more important is guidance in establishing a personal value or belief system to use as a framework for decision making. In healthy family networks, much of this guidance is conveyed in the course of child rearing. Parents need to understand the importance of providing information, sharing their values, and promoting sound decision-making skills. Parents and significant others need to be counselled that even with the best guidance and information, adolescents will make their own decisions and must be held accountable for those decisions.

Adolescence is often a time when individuals explore their primary sexual orientation. Some teenagers may recognize their preference as distinctly homosexual, which can be frightening and confusing. Support for the adolescent's sexual identity is important during this time and can come from a variety of sources, such as school counsellors, clergy, family, and health care professionals.

Adulthood. Adults have matured physically but continue to explore and define emotional maturation in relationships. Intimacy and sexuality are issues for all adults of all sexual orientations, whether they are in a sexual relationship, choose to abstain from sex, are single, are widowed, are divorced—whatever circumstances arise. People can be sexually healthy in numerous ways.

As sexually active adults develop intimate relationships, they need to learn techniques of stimulation that are satisfying to both themselves and their sexual partners. Some adults may need confirmation that alternative ways of sexual expression other than penile–vaginal intercourse are normal. Other individuals may require significant education or therapy to achieve mutually satisfying sexual relationships.

Through middle adulthood, physical changes can affect sexual functioning. Decreasing levels of estrogen in perimenopausal women (during the years leading up to menopause) and menopausal women (after menstruation has ceased) may result in diminished vaginal lubrication and decreased vaginal elasticity. Both of these changes may lead to **dyspareunia**, which is painful intercourse. Declining levels of testosterone result in decreased desire for sexual activity. Suggestions such as using vaginal lubrication and creating time for caressing and tenderness can help clients adjust to normal changes related to aging.

As men age, they are likely to experience an increase in the post-ejaculatory refractory period, delayed ejaculation, and erectile dysfunction. Advising clients of these normal changes related to aging can ease concerns regarding functioning. Aging adults may also need

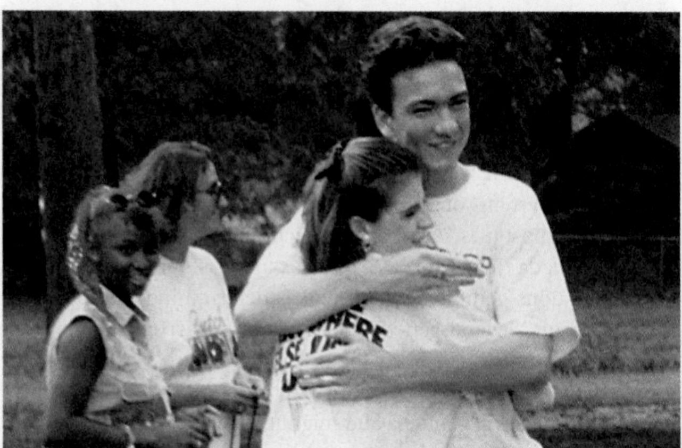

Figure 27-1 Adolescents function within a powerful network of peers as they explore their sexual and gender identity.

to adjust to the effects of chronic illness, medications, aches, pains, and other health concerns that affect sexuality.

Older Adulthood. As people age, some shift their priority from genital sex to other ways of expressing sexual desire. Activities that promote affection, romance, intimacy, and companionship may be enough to satisfy the sexual needs of some older adults (Figure 27–2). However, not all older adults experience a decline in interest in sex. The majority of people have the capacity to stay sexually active into very late life and regard sexual activity as important to their overall well-being and quality of life (Gott, 2001). Aging does, however, affect sexual functioning (Box 27–1). The accompanying psychological and physical transitions require flexibility in thinking and adjustment to the changes; people who successfully manage the transition are poised for emotional and sexual satisfaction (Palacios et al., 2002).

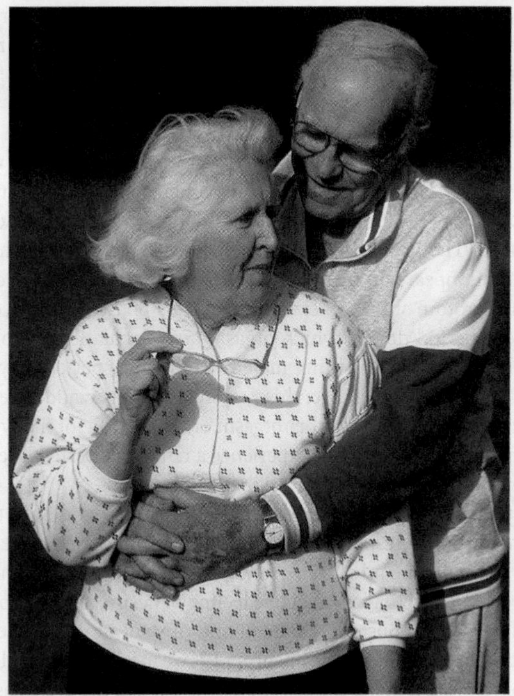

Figure 27-2 Intimacy and affection are important to older adults. **Source:** From Sorrentino, S. A. (2004). *Mosby's Canadian textbook for the support worker* (p. 166). Toronto: Elsevier.

Sexual Response Cycle

Masters and Johnson (1966) developed a four-stage model explaining the human **sexual response cycle**. The model suggested that major similarities exist between men and women. The four stages of the model are excitement, plateau, orgasm, and resolution, and they represent episodes of **vasocongestion** (swelling of tissues) and muscle contractions.

In the *excitement* stage, the heart rate and blood pressure increase, and blood flows into the sexual organs. In women, the breasts enlarge in size, and a reddish flush may be seen over the upper torso. The nipples become more erect. Increased blood flow to the genitalia results in enlargement of the clitoris; engorgement of the labia majora, which flatten and spread outward; and swelling of the labia minora. The upper two thirds of the vagina enlarge, and the vaginal walls thicken. The vaginal walls also secrete a fluid that allows for penile penetration. In men, the penis becomes erect as blood flows into the spongy tissues. The skin of the scrotum thickens, and the testicles swell; the scrotum elevates, and the testicles move in toward the body.

The *plateau* phase is a state of advanced arousal. Blood pressure and heart rate continue to increase, and breathing may become rapid. In women, the lower third of the vagina (at the entry to the vagina) swells. The upper vagina continues to expand, and the uterus moves into an upright position. The labia minora become more engorged with blood and become a darker colour. The clitoris shortens and withdraws below the clitoral hood. The breasts continue to increase in size. In men, the testicles continue to enlarge. The head or glans of the penis changes to a deeper colour.

Orgasm is the phase of significant muscular contractions. During this phase, respiration and heart rates peak, and subjective feelings of intense pleasure radiate through the body. Most of the major muscles in the body contract and may go into spasm. In women, the pelvic muscles contract between 3 and 15 times. The muscles of the anal sphincter and the uterus itself contract. Orgasm in the male occurs in two stages; in the first phase, seminal fluid is forced into the bulb of the penis by contractions of the vas deferens, the two seminal vesicles, the ejaculatory ducts, and the prostate gland. The bladder neck closes off to prevent urine from mixing with the semen. The second stage of

BOX 27-1 RESEARCH HIGHLIGHT

Erectile Dysfunction and Relationships: Viewpoints of Men With Erectile Dysfunction and Their Partners

Research Focus

The viewpoints of the partners of men with erectile dysfunction have not been considered in much of the research on this topic.

Research Abstract

McCabe and Matic's (2008) study was designed to evaluate the effect that erectile dysfunction has on the man, his partner, their sexual and general relationship, and their functioning. The participants were 40 heterosexual men and their female partners. All completed a questionnaire that measured their reaction to the man's erectile dysfunction, their past and current sexual activity, their sexual and relationship satisfaction, their levels of self-esteem, and their perceptions of their quality of life. The results showed that sexual acitivity had been reduced since the occurrence of erectile dysfunction and that couples were interested in solving this. Men with erectile dysfunction had lower levels of self-esteem, poorer quality of life, and poorer sexual satisfaction than did their female partners, but levels of relationship satisfaction were not different.

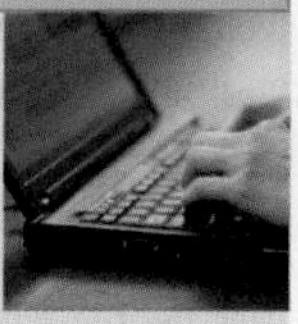

Evidence-Informed Practice

- Erectile dysfunction has a significant impact on self-esteem, quality of life, and sexual satisfaction for affected men.
- The female partner is also affected by the man's erectile dysfunction and must adapt to his difficulties.
- When the health care professional assesses or intervenes for sexual problems, it is important to consult the client's partner.
- Medical treatments for erectile dysfunction do not address the psychological and relationship factors that often accompany erectile dysfunction.

References: McCabe, M. P., & Matic, H. (2008). Erectile dysfunction and relationships: Views of men with erectile dysfunction and their partners. *Sexual and Relationship Therapy, 23*(1), 51–60.

orgasm for the man occurs when the muscles around the urethra contract and fluid is propelled along the urethra and out of the urethral meatus. These contractions are accompanied by subjective feelings of intense pleasure.

In the *resolution* phase, vasocongestion diminishes, and the rest of the body returns to its normal state: Muscle tension is reduced within minutes, and heart rate, blood pressure, and respiration rate return to normal. During this phase in women, blood flow to the pelvic organs is reduced. The breasts return to their normal size, and flushing of the skin disappears. In men, the penis loses its rigidity, and the testicles and scrotum shrink in size. In men, this phase is followed by a refractory period during which orgasm and ejaculation are physiologically impossible. In young men, the refractory period may last a few minutes, but as men age, this period lasts longer, and older men may not be able to have another orgasm or ejaculation for many hours or even days. Women do not experience a refractory period; they may have multiple orgasms with continued stimulation.

Kaplan (1979) introduced the idea of desire in her description of the human sexual response cycle. Her model comprised three parts: desire, excitement, and orgasm. In Kaplan's model, emotion and cognition, which lead to the subjective feeling of desire, are an important part of sexual response. Excitement and orgasm in this model is as described in Masters and Johnson's (1966) model. Kaplan did not include resolution in her model; she suggested that the cycle has three independent phases. Also, according to this model, it is possible to experience excitement without having experienced desire first.

Basson (2005) more recently described an alternative model of the female sexual response cycle. It relied heavily on psychoemotional processes, as opposed to the more physiological basis of Masters and Johnson's (1966) and Kaplan's (1979) models. In her model, desire (or *libido*) is thought to occur at a variety of points in the sexual response cycle. The female sexual response cycle is conceptualized as a circular rather than linear process, as described in the two previous models. Basson suggested that women rely on different reasons to be receptive to or instigators of sexual activity; rewards such as emotional intimacy, feelings of well-being, and lack of negative feelings resulting from avoiding sex are all factors that may cause a woman to feel desire. With varied motivations for sexual activity, women respond to sexual stimuli from a partner. When the woman receives these stimuli, they are processed psychologically and physically; this may then lead to subjective feelings of arousal and a responsive feeling of desire. Sexual satisfaction is thought to further increase motivation and willingness to be receptive at a future time. Basson reasoned that satisfaction does not necessarily mean orgasm; she suggested that for many women, feelings of closeness and intimacy and the partner's satisfaction may be enough to cause satisfaction for the woman.

Sexual Behaviour

Sexual behaviour typically comprises the broad array of sexual activities people participate in, such as masturbation, hugging, kissing, manual stimulation of a partner, vaginal or anal penetration, oral–genital stimulation, oral–anal stimulation, sexual excitement while looking at erotica, and telephone or "cyber" sex (Bernhard, 2002; Engender Health, 2004). It is difficult to define "normal" and "abnormal" because wide variation exists between cultures and at different times in society. An inclusive attitude is that whatever people find pleasurable is "normal" as long as it occurs between consenting adults who engage in sexual behaviour by choice, in a safe environment where rules and boundaries are negotiated and respected.

High-Risk Sexual Behaviour. Because body fluids can be transferred between partners, unprotected sex can result in pregnancy or the transmission of STIs. **Safer sex** refers to sexual activities that present minimal or reduced risk for disease transmission or unintended pregnancy. Unsafe sex refers to activities through which risk for infection, unintended pregnancy, or injury is decreased. Unsafe sex includes anal–penile or vaginal–penile intercourse without a condom (Society for Human Sexuality, 2004). Without the use of barriers such as condoms or latex dental dams, penile–anal intercourse is probably the riskiest activity, followed by penile–vaginal intercourse, oral–anal sex, and oral–genital sex.

The dynamics of sexual risk taking are not fully understood, but numerous studies have revealed that drug and alcohol use are highly correlated with sexual abuse and unsafe sex (Keller et al., 1996; Kenney et al., 1998). Adolescents, especially, tend to have a sense of being invincible, believing that unwanted pregnancy, STIs, and other negative outcomes of sexual behaviour are not likely to happen to them (Ross et al., 2000).

Sexually Transmitted Infections

A number of STIs are of concern to public health officials and health care professionals. In Canada, health officials report increases in all of the infections that, by law, must be reported, including chlamydia, gonorrhea, and syphilis (Public Health Agency of Canada, 2004).

A major problem in dealing with STIs is finding and treating the people who have them. Because symptoms may be absent or go unnoticed, some people may not even know that they are infected. Sexual behaviour may include the whole body rather than just the genitalia; therefore, many parts of the body are potential sites for an STI. The mouth, tongue, and throat are commonly used for sexual pleasure. The vagina, perineum, anus, and rectum are also frequently included in sexual activity. Furthermore, any contact with another person's body fluids near an open lesion on the skin, anus, or genitalia can result in transmission of an STI.

Sometimes people do not seek treatment because they are embarrassed to discuss sexual symptoms or concerns. They may also hesitate to talk about their sexual behaviour if they believe that it is not "normal." This hesitation to seek help often hinders the detection of an STI.

Syphilis. Syphilis, a bacterial infection, can be transmitted through oral, vaginal–penile, or anal sex with an infected person. A pregnant woman with syphilis can pass it on to her baby, which can lead to birth defects or death in the baby. Syphilis also can be transmitted through injection drug use or through broken skin or sores, although transmission by these routes is not common. Syphilis can be diagnosed with a simple blood test and is easily treated with antibiotics. If it is not treated, syphilis can affect the brain, blood vessels, heart, and bones. It can also cause death. Males older than 30 years account for the majority of syphilis cases in Canada (Public Health Agency of Canada, 2004), and local outbreaks are reported periodically across the country.

Chlamydia. The most common of all bacterial STIs, chlamydial infection may cause an abnormal genital discharge and burning with urination; however, it is often asymptomatic. It is treated by an antibiotic.

Chlamydia produces many serious complications in women. If undetected and thus untreated, it can progress to pelvic inflammatory disease in women, a very painful and sometimes debilitating disease

safety alert Increasingly, adolescents engage in oral sex, thinking that this entails less risk for acquiring STIs. However, herpes can be transmitted from genitals to mouth or from mouth to genitals during unprotected oral sex, and it is possible to acquire gonorrhea, syphilis, or chlamydia from oral sex. Consistent use of condoms or latex dental dams can decrease the risk of infection.

that is linked to infertility. An untreated chlamydial infection may cause scarring of the uterine tubes, which increases the risk for ectopic pregnancy and infertility. Research findings suggest that chlamydial infection is also a risk factor for the transmission of the human immunodeficiency virus (HIV), and it could be a risk factor for cervical cancer (Anttila et al., 2001). It is estimated that fewer than 10% of chlamydial infections are diagnosed and treated (Public Health Agency of Canada, 2004). Women, particularly those younger than 30 years, are most affected; women account for two thirds of all reported chlamydia cases in Canada (Public Health Agency of Canada, 2004).

Gonorrhea. Gonorrhea is easily transmitted during vaginal–penile intercourse, anal–penile intercourse, and oral sex (Birley et al., 2002). It can affect the penis, cervix, rectum or anus, throat, and eyes. Pain during sex or during urination, or unusual discharge, may be indications of a gonorrheal infection. Gonorrhea must be treated with antibiotics. If left untreated, it may cause serious health problems, including infertility. It can also cause blood, joint, and eye infections in a baby born to an infected woman (Planned Parenthood Federation of America, 2008b). Gonorrhea is the second most commonly reported bacterial STI in Canada, and its prevalence is also increasing. Men aged 20 to 29 years are the most affected age group in Canada. Of the cases among women, 70% occur in those aged 15 to 24 years. Antibiotic-resistant strains of the bacterium are becoming a problem in some regions of Canada (Public Health Agency of Canada, 2004).

Human Papillomavirus. Human papillomavirus (HPV) is not required to be reported, although it is a very serious STI. It is strongly linked with cervical cancer (Division of STD Prevention and Control, 2000). It may be manifested as external genital warts that can occur on the penis, scrotum, perineum, vulva, and perianal area; they usually appear as small, hard, painless bumps. These warts can also occur in the vagina, on the cervix, inside the urethra, and inside the anus (Beutner et al., 1998). If untreated, they may grow and develop a fleshy, cauliflower-like appearance. Because they are caused by a virus, genital warts cannot be cured. They are treated with a topical drug (applied to the skin), by freezing, or, if they recur, with injections of medication. If the warts are very large, they can be removed surgically. A preventive vaccine for HPV has been approved; it offers protection against against four HPV types, which together cause 70% of cervical cancers and 90% of genital warts (Centers for Disease Control and Prevention, 2008). The recommendation is that girls and women between the ages of 9 and 26 be offered this vaccine; it is important that the vaccine be given before the initiation of sexual activity. Women who are sexually active may receive the vaccine but, because they may have already been exposed to some of the strains of HPV, are less likely to benefit.

Genital Herpes. Genital herpes, caused by the herpes simplex virus, is the most common manifestation of genital ulceration and is often transmitted by people who have no visible or symptomatic lesions (Public Health Agency of Canada, 2004). Genital herpes can cause extensive ulceration (painful blisters or open sores), with severe pain. Without treatment, episodes can last for 3 or more weeks, and many people with herpes have recurrent episodes. At present, the viral infection is incurable; antiviral drugs can only control the symptoms and suppress transmission.

Human Immunodeficiency Virus Infection. HIV is the virus that causes acquired immune deficiency syndrome (AIDS). Essentially, HIV destroys the body's ability to defend against infection. Many people do not have symptoms when they first are infected with HIV, although some may have a flulike illness within 1 to 2 months after exposure. More persistent or severe symptoms may not appear for 10 years or more after infection. During the asymptomatic period, however, the virus is actively multiplying, infecting, and killing cells of the immune system. As the immune system weakens, various complications occur (National Institute of Allergy and Infectious Diseases, 2003).

AIDS represents the most advanced stages of HIV infection. The syndrome can result in many infections that do not usually affect healthy people. In people with AIDS, these infections are often severe and sometimes fatal. People with AIDS are particularly prone to developing cancers, especially those caused by viruses (such as Kaposi's sarcoma or cervical cancer) and those of the immune system (such as lymphomas).

In an infected person, HIV is present in the majority of body fluids. For transmission to occur, therefore, some exchange of body fluid, particularly blood, must occur. Primary routes of transmission include contaminated intravenous needles, unprotected sexual activity (anal intercourse, vaginal intercourse, and oral–genital sex), and transfusion of blood and blood products. HIV can also be spread from infected mothers to their babies during pregnancy, at birth, or during breastfeeding. HIV has not been proved to be transmitted through sweat, tears, saliva, or urine.

In Canada, by the end of 2004, it was estimated that 57,674 positive results of HIV tests were confirmed and reported to the Public Health Agency of Canada. Rates of infection are highest in men who have sex with men, in Aboriginal people, in injection drug users, and in immigrants from countries where HIV is endemic (Centre for Infectious Disease Prevention and Control, 2003). Women account for 25% of all HIV infections in Canada (Public Health Agency of Canada, 2004). Many Canadians who are currently infected with HIV do not know that they are.

Although medications enable individuals with HIV to stay healthy longer, and although they help prevent the transmission of HIV from a pregnant woman to her newborn, medications cannot cure the disease (McIlhaney, 2000).

Prevention of Sexually Transmitted Infections. People most likely to be infected with an STI are those who have unprotected sex. Exposure to multiple partners or to a sexual partner who has many partners increases the risk of acquiring an STI. Injection drug users are also a high-risk group. Primary prevention of STIs starts with changing the sexual behaviour that heightens the risk for infection. Health promotion must be targeted toward high-risk groups and must emphasize education and counselling regarding safer sexual behaviour. STIs often occur together, and screening is usually performed for all STIs at the same time.

Safer Sex. *Safer sex* refers to the sexual practices and behaviour that reduce the risk of contracting and transmitting STIs, especially HIV. When a partner is infected or when the infection status of a partner is not known, it is crucial to practise safer sex. For vaginal–penile and penile–anal intercourse, partners should use condoms. Safer sex practices are also necessary for oral sex; if one of the partners is a woman, a thin piece of rubber, a latex dental dam, a female condom, or an unlubricated male condom cut open to form a flat piece of latex should be placed between the other partner's mouth and the woman's vulva before any oral contact is made. Male partners should cover their penis with an unlubricated condom before any oral contact is made (Engender Health, 2004).

Using Condoms. Condoms were originally sold to promote birth control. However, when used correctly, they also provide protection against STIs. A condom acts as a barrier to keep blood, semen, and vaginal fluids from passing from one person to another. In Canada, condoms are free at many public health clinics and are readily available from drugstores and supermarkets. The condom can be made from latex, polyurethane, or natural membranes such as sheepskin or lambskin. Latex and polyurethane condoms reduce the risk of most STIs (including HIV) and help protect against pregnancy. Natural membrane condoms do not protect against STIs because some bacteria and viruses can pass through the small pores in the material (Centre for Infectious Disease Prevention and Control, 2002).

A female condom is a strong, soft, clear sheath made of polyurethane with two rings at either end. It is placed inside the vagina before sex and protects against pregnancy and STIs (including HIV). When placed correctly, one end covers the cervix and the other end covers part of the external genitalia (Planned Parenthood Federation of America, 2008a).

Contraception

Contraception is a crucial facet of sexual health to avoid unwanted pregnancies. Some forms of contraception require a health care professional's intervention: hormonal contraceptives (e.g., birth control pills or patch, injectable contraceptives), intrauterine devices (IUDs), the diaphragm, the vaginal contraceptive ring, and the cervical cap. Surgical procedures that provide permanent contraception are also available to men (vasectomy) and women (tubal ligation). Other forms of contraception do not require a prescription or intervention from a health care professional: condoms, contraceptive sponges, vaginal spermicides, and fertility awareness methods (i.e., timing of intercourse in relation to the menstrual cycle). Table 27–1 summarizes some of the contraceptive choices available.

Effective contraception involves factors relating to the sexually active couple, the method of contraception, the couple's understanding of the contraceptive method, the consistency of contraceptive use, and the compliance with the requirements of the chosen method. Personal characteristics that have been identified as positively influencing contraceptive use include motivation to avoid unplanned pregnancy, ability to plan, comfort with sexuality, and previous contraceptive use (Running & Berndt, 2003). Cultural and religious background may permit certain practices and prohibit others. For example, the teachings of the Roman Catholic Church prohibit the use of contraception except for the fertility awareness method.

Emergency Contraception. Emergency contraception pills (ECPs, or "morning after" pills) can prevent a woman from becoming pregnant after unprotected vaginal–penile sex. ECPs are most effective up to 72 hours after intercourse, and the sooner they are taken, the more effective they are (Public Health Agency of Canada, 2006. They are recommended to women when contraception was not used, when a condom broke, when a diaphragm slipped, when a birth control injection was given over 1 week late, when two or more birth control pills were missed, or in cases of rape. When hormonal ECPs are taken within 72 hours (3 days) after unprotected sex, the risk of getting pregnant is reduced by approximately 75%. ECPs have been shown to be effective up to 5 days after intercourse.

Women can obtain ECPs from family physicians, nurse practitioners and midwives, hospital emergency rooms, or walk-in clinics. As of 2005, Canadian pharmacists may dispense ECPs without a physician's prescription; however, pharmacists have the right to refuse to do so if it conflicts with their personal beliefs. ECPs are available for free or at minimum cost at many university health services, sexual health clinics, birth control clinics, Planned Parenthood clinics, and women's health clinics. Adolescent girls do not require parental consent to obtain ECPs, and no medical examination is required.

Abortion

Since 1988, Canada has been one of the few countries without any legal restrictions on abortion. Canada has no requirements for waiting periods, parental or spousal consent, gestational limits, or restrictions on types of elective abortion. Abortion is also a safe procedure, especially if performed within the first trimester of pregnancy. Some provinces fully fund all elective abortions; others fund only those performed in hospitals. However, access to abortion services is often a problem for women living outside major cities. Two thirds of abortions are performed in hospitals; the remainder are performed in abortion clinics and health centres. However, only 18% of hospitals across the nation provide abortions (Canadian Abortion Rights Action League, 2003). In Prince Edward Island and Nunavut, no hospitals provide abortions.

Abortion continues to be a hotly debated issue. Women and their partners who are faced with an unwanted pregnancy may consider an elective abortion. As a nurse, you can provide an environment in which the issue of abortion can be discussed openly and various options with an unwanted pregnancy can be explored. You should discuss religious, social, and personal issues in a nonjudgemental manner with clients. Reasons for choosing an elective abortion vary and may include terminating an unwanted pregnancy or aborting a fetus known to have abnormalities. When abortion is chosen as a way of dealing with an unwanted pregnancy, the woman, and often her partner, may experience a sense of loss, grief, or guilt, or a combination of these. Guilt may surface immediately, or it may be more covert and manifest as sexual dysfunction.

Health care professionals must reflect on their own personal values related to abortion. The health care professional is entitled to personal views and should not be forced to participate in counselling or procedures contrary to beliefs and values. Nurses should choose specialties or places of employment in which their personal values are not compromised and the health care that a client needs is not jeopardized.

Nursing Knowledge Base

In planning to help clients address their sexual needs, you should use critical thinking skills and basic nursing knowledge. You may draw from the following areas of nursing knowledge: sociocultural dimensions of sexuality; how to discuss sexual issues; alterations in sexual health (infertility, sexual abuse, sexual dysfunction); and conditions that create sexual health concerns (pregnancy, surgery, illness, and disability).

Sociocultural Dimensions of Sexuality

Sexuality is influenced by cultural rules and norms that determine which behaviour is acceptable within the culture. Society plays a powerful role in shaping sexual values and attitudes and in supporting specific expression of sexuality in its members. Each cultural and social group has its own set of rules and norms that guide the behaviour of its members. These rules become an integral part of an individual's thinking and underlie sexual behaviour; they include, for example, how people find partners, their choices of partners, how they relate to one another, how often they have sex, and what they do when they have sex.

It is widely suggested that nurses include information about sexual health and the implications for sexuality when they care for clients. Nurses should also routinely ask clients whether they have any sexual concerns related to their condition or treatments (Albaugh

TABLE 27-1 Available Contraceptives

Type	Effectiveness	Description
Male condom	86%–97%	A thin, skin-tight sheath placed on an erect penis to stop sperm from entering a partner's body. Water-based lubricants can make them more comfortable, increase sensation, and reduce the risk of breakage.
Female condom	79%–85%	A lubricated pouch that is placed in the vagina before penile insertion; it stops sperm from entering the woman's body. It may break or slip, and some women may have difficulty placing it correctly.
Birth control pills	98%–99%	Pills taken every day that contain a low dose of hormones (estrogen and progestin or progestin alone). The ovaries are prevented from releasing an egg for fertilization, eggs are prevented from implanting, and the mucus around the cervix is thickened, which makes entry of the sperm more difficult. They are available only by prescription.
Cervical cap	80%–91%	A small, flexible cup that is inserted into the vagina before penile insertion. It covers the cervix and prevents sperm from entering the uterus. The caps are available in different sizes; proper fitting by a trained health care professional is required.
Intrauterine device (IUD)	99%	A small piece of plastic or copper that is inserted into the uterus by a physician. Sperm is prevented from fertilizing an egg, or, if an egg is fertilized, the egg is prevented from implanting in the uterus. Some IUDs also release hormones to prevent pregnancy. IUDs can stay in place for 1–8 years.
Birth control patch	99.2%–99.4%	A thin, 2-cm • 2-cm patch that can be worn on the lower abdomen, buttock, upper arm, or upper torso. The patch is applied once a week for 3 consecutive weeks; the fourth week is patch free. The mechanism of action is the same as that of oral contraceptives.
Injectable contraceptive	99.7%	Progestin is injected into a woman's arm or buttocks once every 12 weeks. The hormone prevents the ovaries from releasing eggs. A physician or nurse administers the injections.
Vaginal contraceptive ring	98.3%–99.4%	A soft, flexible, transparent ring that is self-inserted into the vagina and delivers hormones over 3 weeks, after which time the ring is removed for 1 week. A new ring is then inserted.
Contraceptive sponge	80%–91%	A soft sponge that is filled with spermicide and placed in the vagina before vaginal–penile intercourse. It is effective for 24 hours after placement. The sponge must be kept in place for 6 hours after intercourse.
Vaginal spermicides	78%–90%	Gels, films, and suppositories, which contain a spermicidal agent, that are inserted into the vagina before vaginal–penile intercourse. The agent kills sperm and acts as a physical barrier to prevent any surviving sperm cells from entering the cervix. This approach may be used by women who are at low risk for STIs and whose partners are at low risk.
Fertility awareness method	90%–98%	A woman can monitor her fertility patterns and know, on the basis of daily observations of body temperature and cervical mucus, when she is most likely and least likely to conceive. She must abstain from vaginal–penile intercourse when she is most likely to conceive. This method can also be used to achieve pregnancy.
Tubal ligation	99.5%	A surgical procedure in which a woman's uterine tubes are tied into a loop and then cut. This procedure is performed with the woman under general anaesthesia, and its effects should be considered permanent.
Vasectomy	99.9%	A minor surgical procedure for men in which the vas deferens that carry the sperm are cut, "tied," cauterized, or otherwise interrupted. The semen no longer contains sperm after the tubes are cut, and conception cannot occur. The procedure can be performed in a physician's office with a local anaesthetic. The results of this procedure should be considered permanent.

Adapted from Planned Parenthood Federation of Canada. (2004). *Contraception.* Retrieved June 25, 2004, from http://www.ppfc.ca/ppfc/content.asp?articleid=248; and from Pettinato, A., & Emans, S. J. (2003). New contraceptive methods: Update 2003. *Current Opinion in Pediatrics, 15,* 362–369.

& Kellog-Spadt, 2003). However, this question is frequently omitted, and a valuable opportunity to be proactive and holistic in the care provided is thus missed (Haboubi & Lincoln, 2003). You may feel that asking about sexuality is an invasion of clients' privacy (Bartlik et al., 2005), or you may think that gender is a barrier (Burd et al., 2006). Nurses appear to be more likely to wait for the client to initiate the discussion than to assess this routinely (Guthrie, 1999). You may think that the client does not expect you to ask questions about this (Magnan et al., 2005), or you may believe that it is the physician's responsibility (Herson et al., 1999). As a result, sexual problems may not be recognized and thus may be ignored. Some nurses may presume that because of the seriousness of the client's disease or because of the client's stage of life, sexuality is not an important issue (Huang, 1999); this presumption can have consequences such as lack of education for the client.

Discussing Sexual Issues

Sexuality is a significant part of each person's being; however, sexual assessment and interventions are not always included in health care. The area of sexuality can be emotionally charged for nurses as well as for clients. Discomfort with talking about sexual issues, lack of information, and differences between a client's values and the nurse's values may prevent the nurse from discussing issues of sexuality with clients. The most valuable tool that you can develop for providing care in areas of sexuality is effective, nonjudgemental communication. If you have difficulty discussing topics related to sexuality, you should understand why, and you should develop a plan for addressing your discomfort.

Discussing matters of a sexual nature can also be embarrassing for clients. Often, clients do not mention sexual health issues; they may worry about looking stupid, using incorrect words, or being offensive, or they may simply have no way of describing their concerns. It is crucial that you be comfortable in asking questions about sexuality and in responding to issues that arise from such questioning. By using a perceptive and educated approach to talking about sexuality, you can offer the support that many clients require.

Effective communication about sexuality requires caring, sensitivity, tact, compassion, the use of appropriate language, and nondiscriminatory attitudes. When talking with clients about sexuality, it is important not to have preconceived notions about their sexual identity or activity. Homosexual and bisexual people may not receive adequate health care if health care professionals assume heterosexual sexual orientation and fail to obtain complete sexual histories. Older adults' sexual health may also be overlooked if health care professionals stereotype these clients as asexual.

Alterations in Sexual Health

Infertility. Infertility is the inability of a couple to conceive after 1 year of unprotected intercourse. A couple who wants to conceive and cannot may experience a sense of failure and may feel that their bodies are somehow defective. Infertility may become an emotionally draining facet of their lives, and the treatments also affect their sexual lives and relationship. With advances in reproductive technology, infertile couples face many choices, some of which involve challenges to their religious and ethical values and may cause financial strain.

Choices for the infertile couple include medical assistance with fertilization, adoption, or exploring the possibility of remaining childless. Infertility support groups can provide such couples with emotional and educational help. For example, the Infertility Awareness Association of Canada, a national support group for couples with infertility, can be helpful in offering educational resources and assistance for a couple.

Sexual Abuse. Sexual abuse is a widespread health problem. Abuse crosses all gender, socioeconomic, age, and ethnic groups. Most often, this abuse is perpetrated by a former intimate partner or by a family member. Sexual abuse has far-ranging effects on physical and psychological functioning (Dickinson et al., 1999). Increasingly, sexual abuse is occurring through the Internet: Sexual predators recruit victims on social networking sites and then arrange to meet the victims, after which the abuse begins.

Evidence of sexual abuse in children may be uncovered during history taking or physical examination (see Chapter 32). Symptoms that should raise suspicion of sexual abuse include a child showing an early, exaggerated awareness of sex or exhibiting seductive behaviour toward adults; swelling or bruising of the external genitalia, anus, breasts, or buttocks; lacerations of or a foreign substance in the vagina or anus; and an STI in a child younger than 15 years. In Canada, nurses are required by law to report suspected child abuse to child protection authorities. Signs and symptoms of sexual abuse in adults are listed in Box 27–2.

When sexual abuse is recognized, support needs to be mobilized for the victim and the family. All family members may require therapy in situations of incest to promote healthy interactions and relationships. Rape victims may need to come to terms with the crisis before feeling comfortable with intimate expressions of affection. The victim's partner may need support in understanding this process and ways to assist the victim. Children who have been sexually abused need to understand that they are not at fault for the incident. The parents must understand that their response is critical to how the child reacts and adapts. You may come in contact with clients confronting these stressors. You are in an ideal position to assess occurrences of sexual violence and to educate individuals about

➤ BOX 27-2 Signs and Symptoms That May Indicate Current or Previous Sexual Abuse

- Irritation or injury (such as cuts and bruises or scarring) of the thighs, perineum, or breasts
- Trauma to mouth and throat, including petechiae of the oral cavity
- Oral STIs
- Intense fear of bathing or perineal care
- Vaginal discharge, genital odour, and painful urination
- Difficulty walking or sitting
- Avoidance of casual touching
- Sleep pattern disturbances
- Nightmares
- Depression
- Anxiety
- Decreased self-esteem
- Difficulties with intimate relationships
- Substance abuse
- Frequent visits to health care professionals
- Headaches
- Gastrointestinal problems
- Eating disorders
- Abdominal pain
- Vaginal pain
- Dysmenorrhea

Adapted from Bohn, D., & Holz, K. (1996). Sequelae of abuse: Health effects of childhood sexual abuse, domestic battering, and rape. *Journal of Nurse-Midwifery, 41*(6), 442.

community services. You should be aware of resources for referral and support in the community.

Sexual Dysfunction. Sexual dysfunction is a common, complex problem that arises because of biological, psychological, and interpersonal factors (Table 27–2). Sexual problems and dysfunction are often associated with health problems such as heart disease, diabetes, cancer, and mental illness. It is not known how many people experience sexual dysfunction, and it is most probably a minority who seek help. Researchers estimate that between 10% and 52% of men and 25% and 63% of women have sexual problems, although the prevalence of sexual dysfunctions that meet the diagnostic criteria of the fifth edition of the *Diagnostic and Statistical Manual of Mental Disorders* (American Psychiatric Association, in press) is lower (Heiman, 2002). For most people, sexual dysfunction is perplexing and emotionally disturbing, and it adversely affects their primary relationship.

Sexual dysfunction can usually be treated with either medical interventions (mostly pharmacological) or psychological interventions (e.g., cognitive and behavioural methods). The aim is typically to achieve changes in physical (genital response, orgasms) or subjective (greater desire, ease of orgasm) responses (Heiman, 2002).

Sexual Dysfunction in Women. Loss of sexual desire is the most common reason that women seek help for sexual dysfunction (Butcher, 1999a). Despite considerable research, sexual desire is poorly understood. Some medical conditions (including depression), stress, and fatigue affect sexual desire. Painful intercourse is another common sexual dysfunction in women. Recurring sexual pain can produce a cycle in which trepidation because of previous pain leads to avoidance of the sexual activity that produced it, which in turn leads to lack of arousal, failure to achieve orgasm, and loss of sexual desire (Butcher, 1999b). This cycle can evolve to avoidance of sexual activity altogether.

Sexual Dysfunction in Men. One of the most common types of sexual dysfunction for men is erectile dysfunction. It is estimated that about 27% of sexually active Canadian men experience erectile dysfunction, which is the repeated inability to achieve or maintain an erection (Auld & Brock, 2002). Erectile dysfunction can be caused by any health problem, including heart disease, hypertension (or its treatment), diseases of the prostate, diabetes mellitus, multiple sclerosis, and depression. Indeed, erectile dysfunction might be a warning sign of undiagnosed cardiovascular disease.

Clients With Particular Sexual Health Concerns

Pregnant and Postpartum Women. Female sexual interest tends to fluctuate during pregnancy; it increases during the second trimester and often decreases during the first and third trimesters. The decrease in libido during the first trimester may be caused by nausea, fatigue, and breast tenderness. During the second trimester,

TABLE 27-2 Types of Sexual Dysfunction

Category	Type*	Definition
Sexual desire disorders	Hypoactive sexual desire disorder	Persistent or recurrent deficiency or absence of sexual fantasies and desire for sexual activity
	Sexual aversion disorder	Persistent or recurrent extreme aversion to, and avoidance of, all or almost all genital sexual contact with a sexual partner
Sexual arousal disorders	Female sexual arousal disorder	Failure in a woman to attain or maintain the lubrication-swelling response or to experience a subjective sense of sexual excitement and pleasure during sexual activity
	Male erectile dysfunction	Persistent or recurrent inability to attain an adequate erection or to maintain an adequate erection until completion of the sexual activity
Orgasmic disorders	Female orgasmic disorder (anorgasmia)	The recurrent and persistent inhibition of the female orgasm, as manifested by the absence or delay of orgasm after a period of sexual excitement the clinician judges adequate in intensity and duration to produce such a response
	Male orgasmic disorder (retarded ejaculation)	Persistent or recurrent delay in, or absence of, orgasm after a normal sexual excitement phase during sexual activity that the clinician, taking into account the man's age, judges to be adequate in focus, intensity, and duration
	Male orgasmic disorder (premature ejaculation)	Persistent or recurrent ejaculation with minimal sexual stimulation before, upon, or shortly after penetration and before the man wishes it
Sexual pain disorders	Dyspareunia	Recurrent or persistent genital pain in either a man or a woman before, during, or after sexual intercourse that is not associated with vaginismus or with lack of lubrication
	Vaginismus	An involuntary constriction of the outer third of the vagina that prevents penile insertion and intercourse
Sexual dysfunction resulting from drug use or diseases		Sexual dysfunction judged to be caused by the direct physiological effects of a general medical condition or use of a substance

*According to American Psychiatric Association. (in press). *Diagnostic and statistical manual of mental disorders* (5th ed.). Washington, DC: Author.

blood flow to the pelvic area is increased to supply the placenta, and sexual enjoyment and libido accordingly increase. During the third trimester, increased abdominal size may make finding a comfortable position difficult.

The most prevalent sexual problem during pregnancy is fear of harming the fetus. However, pregnancy and birth complications are not associated with sexual intercourse (von Sydow, 1999). If women have a history of miscarriages or premature labour, they may be advised to avoid sexual intercourse during the later months of pregnancy. Other restrictions such as no orgasms or no sexual arousal may be necessary to protect high-risk pregnancies (Mayo Foundation for Medical Education and Research, 2004).

Clients Recovering From Surgery. Surgeries that result in disfigurement, especially of the face, breasts, genitalia, and reproductive organs, frequently have harmful effects on a client's self-image and sexuality (de Marquiegui & Huish, 1999). The effects of surgery, whether temporary or permanent, are often not fully anticipated and may not be fully manifested until after discharge from the hospital. Clients' partners might also have adjustments to make and may find it difficult to resume sexual activity. Coping with anxiety, fear, or depression about the surgery is essential. You need to support clients to discuss their concerns, especially sexual anxieties, because problems can become deep-rooted, complicated, and more difficult to resolve over time (de Marquiegui & Huish, 1999). Clients who have had ileostomies, colostomies, or urostomies are particularly concerned about possible loss of control, unpleasant smells or sounds, seepage or broken bags, and their partners' responses (see Chapter 45). Perioperative counselling and support are essential for these clients.

Clients With Illness or Disabilities. Illness and disability often affect sexual health. During periods of illness, individuals may experience major physical changes, the effects of drugs or treatments, the emotional stress of a prognosis, concern about future functioning, and separation from significant others. Situational stressors could include a heart attack (myocardial infarction); cancer diagnosis and treatment; or chronic disease such as diabetes, multiple sclerosis, or Parkinson's disease. You should not assume, because of a client's age or severity of prognosis, that sexual functioning is not a concern. In some instances, clients may wrongly believe that their condition prohibits sexual activity, or they may need some guidance to promote satisfactory sexual functioning (Nusbaum et al., 2003).

Many myths are prevalent about people with a disability, including the idea that they are asexual or somehow different. Without doubt, long-term disability can have profound effects on a person's sense of sexuality and sexual function. Congenital or birth impairments commonly affect sexual development; for example, the resulting lack of privacy and independence may mean that people with disabilities miss out on typical sexual experiences (Glass & Soni, 1999). Acquired disabilities may have different implications: Impairments sustained in youth may bring about low social and sexual confidence, and people who sustain disabilities as adults may be far more aware of what they have lost. It is important that health care professionals validate a disabled person's sexuality. You can do this by sensitively initiating conversations about sexual function and safer sex practices.

Critical Thinking

Successful critical thinking requires synthesis of knowledge, experience, information gathered from clients, critical thinking qualities, and intellectual and professional standards. Clinical judgement requires you to anticipate the information necessary, analyze the data, and make appropriate decisions regarding client care. Figure 27–3 depicts numerous critical thinking elements, as well as client assessment data, that contribute to appropriate nursing diagnoses.

In the case of sexuality, you integrate knowledge from nursing and other disciplines. You must have a good understanding, for example, of the human sexual response cycle, safer sex practices, and the taxonomy of sexual problems, as well as solutions to these, to anticipate how to assess a client and then how to interpret findings. Previous experience in caring for clients whose sexuality becomes threatened helps you approach the next client in a more reflective and helpful way. Clients may have customs and values different from yours. Professional standards call for you to respect each client as an individual.

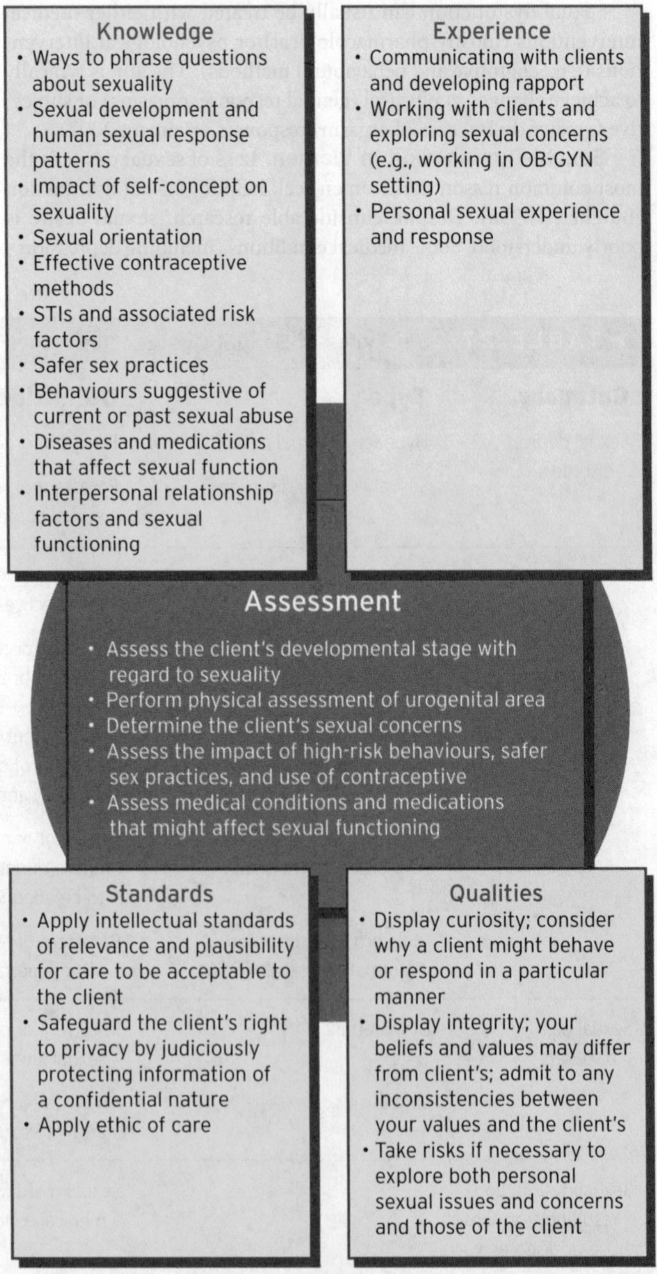

Knowledge
- Ways to phrase questions about sexuality
- Sexual development and human sexual response patterns
- Impact of self-concept on sexuality
- Sexual orientation
- Effective contraceptive methods
- STIs and associated risk factors
- Safer sex practices
- Behaviours suggestive of current or past sexual abuse
- Diseases and medications that affect sexual function
- Interpersonal relationship factors and sexual functioning

Experience
- Communicating with clients and developing rapport
- Working with clients and exploring sexual concerns (e.g., working in OB-GYN setting)
- Personal sexual experience and response

Assessment
- Assess the client's developmental stage with regard to sexuality
- Perform physical assessment of urogenital area
- Determine the client's sexual concerns
- Assess the impact of high-risk behaviours, safer sex practices, and use of contraceptive
- Assess medical conditions and medications that might affect sexual functioning

Standards
- Apply intellectual standards of relevance and plausibility for care to be acceptable to the client
- Safeguard the client's right to privacy by judiciously protecting information of a confidential nature
- Apply ethic of care

Qualities
- Display curiosity; consider why a client might behave or respond in a particular manner
- Display integrity; your beliefs and values may differ from client's; admit to any inconsistencies between your values and the client's
- Take risks if necessary to explore both personal sexual issues and concerns and those of the client

Figure 27-3 Critical thinking model for sexuality assessment. OB-GYN, obstetrical–gynecological; STIs, sexually transmitted infections.

Sexuality and the Nursing Process

A person's sexuality has physical, psychological, social, and cultural elements. You must assess all relevant elements to determine a client's sexual well-being. You should build a sound knowledge base and be willing to explore personal issues regarding sexuality. The nursing role in addressing sexual concerns can range from ongoing assessment to providing information to counselling to referral.

❖Assessment

Factors Affecting Sexuality

In gathering a sexual history, you should consider physical, functional, relationship, lifestyle, and self-esteem factors that may influence sexual functioning.

Sexual Health History

When taking a health history, you should include a few questions related to sexual functioning to determine whether the client has any sexual concerns. You can incorporate these questions in the review of systems and address them in a routine, matter-of-fact manner. It is important to ask these questions once you have established rapport with the client, and the sexual history is usually taken at the end of the general history. You need to understand the reasons for the questions and be able to provide these reasons to the client on request. An opening statement such as "Sex is an important part of life and can be affected by our health status. To better understand your health, it is useful to know . . ." is a possible introduction to these questions. Other questions for adults might include the following:

- How do you feel about the sexual aspects of your life?
- Have you noticed any changes in the way you feel about yourself (as a man, woman, husband, or wife)?
- How has your illness, medication, or surgery affected your sex life?
- It is not unusual for people with your condition to be experiencing some sexual changes. Have you noticed any changes, or do you have any concerns?

Conducting a sexual assessment of children and adolescents provides special challenges for health care professionals. Common challenges include issues of language, of promoting normal development while not minimizing problems, and of screening for sexual concerns while not unduly alarming children. In addition, the sexual counselling of minors raises ethical and legal issues regarding the client's rights to health care and education, on the one hand, and the parents' or guardian's right to supervise information, on the other. Use of an open, positive, interested disposition when introducing sexual questions is helpful. It is also helpful to inform that parents that you are going to be discussing this in private with their child or teenager and that this is a normal part of the nursing assessment.

When caring for older adults, nurses may adjust their assessment approach. When gathering a sexual history from an older adult, it is important to keep in mind that the older adult may have difficulty discussing intimate details with health care professionals because of cultural and social norms for their age group. You have the responsibility to help maintain healthy sexuality of older adults by offering the opportunity to discuss any concerns or to seek information. Often, asking questions on the topic of sexuality in a comfortable, relaxed manner facilitates older adults' discussion of their sexual needs.

Because of the prevalence of domestic violence and sexual abuse, questions relating to abusive relationships can be important. Questions that address domestic violence or abuse should be addressed to the client in private. A question such as "Are you in a relationship in which someone is hurting you?" may encourage a client to reveal current or previous abuse. An additional question such as "Has anyone ever forced you to have sex that you did not wish to participate in?" may more specifically encourage the client to discuss concerns. Recognizing both subjective and objective signs and symptoms of abuse can aid in recognition of this too-common problem (see Box 27–2). If a person identifies sex abuse as a current or past problem, appropriate referrals need to be made with the client's permission.

While you document the sexual history of a client, it is also helpful to explore the client's use of contraceptives and safer sex practices as appropriate. Adolescents may respond to a comment that reassures them that having questions related to sexuality is normal. A lead-in could be "Many teenagers have questions about whether their bodies are developing at the right rate. Do you have any questions about sex or your body?"

Some individuals are too embarrassed or do not know how to ask questions about sexuality. If a client makes a sexual joke or expresses concern about relations with his or her partner, he or she may have questions. Observing for and listening to concerns about sexuality takes practice. With experience, you develop skill in clarifying and paraphrasing to help clients express sexual concerns. By including sexuality in the health history, you acknowledge that sexuality is an important part of health and create an opportunity for the client to discuss sexual concerns.

Physical Assessment

The physical examination is important in evaluating the cause of sexual concerns or problems; however, this is beyond the scope of the generalist nurse and more appropriate for the advanced practice nurse or physician. Talking about sexuality at the time of the genital examination is not appropriate and can be miscontrued by the client, in addition to making him or her feel uncomfortable. Discussions about sexuality are best held when the client is fully clothed and sitting comfortably in a private room.

Client Expectations

As in the case of any client assessment, it is important to understand the client's expectations regarding his or her care. Questions such as "What would you like to have happen in regard to [expressed concern]?" and "What initial steps might you take?" can help the person identify desired outcomes. It is important for the nurse to set aside personal views and not assume what a client's expectations might be.

❖Nursing Diagnosis

After completing an assessment and applying critical thought to the diagnostic process (Box 27–3), you select diagnoses applicable to the client's needs. Possible nursing diagnoses related to sexual functioning (NANDA International, 2007) are listed as follows:

- *Anxiety*
- *Ineffective coping*
- *Interrupted family processes*
- *Deficient knowledge (about contraception or STIs or both)*
- *Sexual dysfunction*
- *Ineffective sexuality patterns*
- *Social isolation*
- *Risk for other-directed violence*
- *Risk for self-directed violence*

BOX 27-3 NURSING DIAGNOSTIC PROCESS

Assessment Activities	Defining Characteristics	Nursing Diagnosis
Observe readiness to discuss sexual concerns through verbalization (e.g., "When can I return to life as normal?" or "There goes my love life") or behaviour (e.g., exhibitionism).	Client verbalizes concern that sexual activity may cause another myocardial infarction or death.	*Ineffective sexuality patterns related to fear of recurrent myocardial infarction or death during intercourse.*
Ask client and spouse about previous level and method of sexual expression (e.g., frequency, initiator).		
Observe for affectionate behaviour (e.g., touching, hand holding, kissing).	Client's spouse exhibits reluctance to touch client.	
In privacy, ask spouse about perceptions of client's recovery and return to full functioning.	Spouse verbalizes concern that client will need continuous care, attention, and protection.	
Observe for anxiety (e.g., hand wringing).	Client maintains eye contact, shifts position frequently.	

Clues that may signal risk or an actual nursing diagnosis related to sexuality include a history of surgery involving the reproductive organs, changes in appearance, past or current physical or sexual abuse, chronic illness, and developmental milestones such as puberty or menopause. Before making nursing diagnoses related to sexual dysfunction, you must first assess anatomical, physiological, sociocultural, and situational issues thoroughly.

When making a nursing diagnosis in regard to sexuality, you must clarify with the client that the defining characteristics do in fact exist and that the client perceives a problem with regard to sexuality. Determining the etiological or contributing factors is important in order to focus effective planning and to select appropriate nursing interventions. For example, the nursing interventions appropriate for the nursing diagnosis *chronic low self-esteem* would be different from those appropriate for other etiological factors. For *self-esteem disturbance related to chronic, recurring herpes infection,* the appropriate interventions include counselling and education on how to maintain safer sexual practices. In contrast, *self-esteem disturbance related to sexual abuse* would necessitate counselling and referral to community resources (e.g., crisis services or sexual abuse support group).

❖Planning

Goals and Outcomes

During planning, you again synthesize information from multiple resources (Figure 27–4). You use critical thinking skills to integrate professional standards and knowledge about the client's sexuality into the care plan. It is especially important to maintain a client's dignity and identity when you develop the care plan. For example, convey respect for a gay client by including the help of a gay partner in the plan to the degree that the partner can assist the client in maintaining his or her identity and dignity.

You develop an individualized care plan for each nursing diagnosis (Box 27– 4). Together, you and the client set realistic goals for care. Expected outcomes must be individualized and realistic. For example, for a client with a nursing diagnosis of *sexual dysfunction related to dyspareunia,* you and the client develop a goal to be free from pain or discomfort during sexual intercourse. Expected outcomes for this goal may be as follows:

- The client will report decreased anxiety and greater satisfaction with sexual activity.
- The client will consistently use a water-soluble lubricant with sexual intercourse.
- The client will avoid the use of feminine hygiene products that destroy the natural flora and secretions of the vaginal walls.

A concept map is useful for organizing client care (Figure 27–5). A concept map shows the relationship of a medical diagnosis (e.g., decreased libido and depression) with the four nursing diagnoses identified from the client assessment data. The map also shows the links and relationship with the nursing diagnosis. For example, ineffective coping affects and contributes to social isolation; as long as the client has ineffective coping, the social isolation continues or perhaps worsens.

Setting Priorities

A framework useful in guiding planning is the "PLISSIT" model developed by Annon (1976). In this model, levels of intervention are progressively more involved. *P* stands for "permission giving." During assessment, you can bring up the topic of sexuality and give the individual permission to talk about sexual concerns. *LI* stands for "limited information," which is basic information regarding sexuality and sexual functioning. An example is discussing nocturnal emissions with a prepubescent boy to minimize fear that might develop if the boy did not know this was a normal part of development. *SS* stands for "specific suggestions": in this case, specific suggestions regarding a sexual concern or issue. For example, a postmenopausal woman might be concerned about her lack of vaginal lubrication, and you might suggest use of a water-based lubricant during sexual intercourse. If you are not equipped to address a particular concern, you should refer the client to another qualified health care professional. *IT* stands for "intensive therapy." At this level of intervention, your role is to refer the client to a qualified practitioner, such as a social worker or sexuality counsellor, for individualized therapy. The level

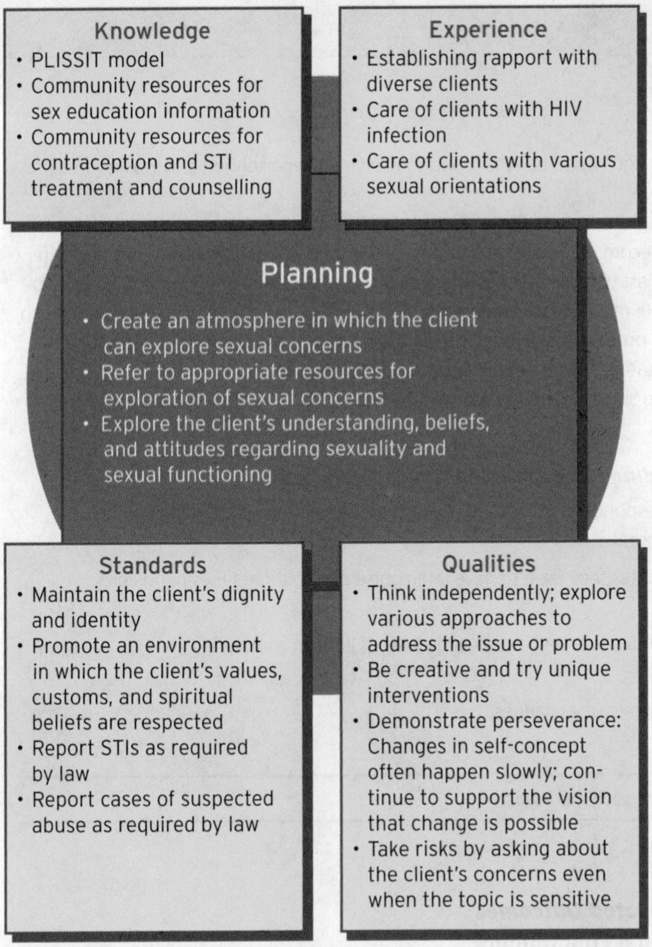

Knowledge
- PLISSIT model
- Community resources for sex education information
- Community resources for contraception and STI treatment and counselling

Experience
- Establishing rapport with diverse clients
- Care of clients with HIV infection
- Care of clients with various sexual orientations

Planning
- Create an atmosphere in which the client can explore sexual concerns
- Refer to appropriate resources for exploration of sexual concerns
- Explore the client's understanding, beliefs, and attitudes regarding sexuality and sexual functioning

Standards
- Maintain the client's dignity and identity
- Promote an environment in which the client's values, customs, and spiritual beliefs are respected
- Report STIs as required by law
- Report cases of suspected abuse as required by law

Qualities
- Think independently; explore various approaches to address the issue or problem
- Be creative and try unique interventions
- Demonstrate perseverance: Changes in self-concept often happen slowly; continue to support the vision that change is possible
- Take risks by asking about the client's concerns even when the topic is sensitive

Figure 27-4 Critical thinking model for sexuality planning. HIV, human immunodeficiency virus; PLISSIT, permission giving, limited information, specific suggestions, and intensive therapy; STI, sexually transmitted infection.

of intervention that you plan depends in part on your own experience and knowledge. When a client requires specific suggestions or intensive therapy, you may recommend referral to a specialist.

Continuity of Care

Planning in the area of sexuality may include referrals to community resources (Box 27–5). Sexual conflicts in marriage or trauma related to sexual abuse or incest may necessitate intensive treatment with a mental health care professional or a certified sex therapist. For women in abusive relationships, most communities have battered women's shelters that provide counselling and serve as a safe haven for them while they plan for their future.

❖Implementation

Health Promotion

Because of their education, clinical expertise, and wellness orientation, nurses are among the professionals best situated to develop and implement sexual health initiatives. You can promote sexual health by identifying clients at increased risk, providing appropriate information, helping individuals gain insight into their problems, and exploring methods to deal with problems effectively. A health promotion perspective ought to guide nurses in designing a number of programs: informal educational opportunities, continuing education, peer learning activities for adolescents, community and political initiatives, and health care professional education (Beitz, 1998). Topics for education vary, depending on the nursing diagnosis (Box 27–6).

Acute Care

In general, nursing interventions that address alterations in sexuality are aimed at raising awareness, assisting in clarification of issues or concerns, providing information, or performing a combination of these. Nurses who have pursued specialized education in sexual functioning and counselling may provide more intensive sex therapy. You should recognize when an individual's needs exceed your expertise, in which case you should provide appropriate referral.

In the initial intervention, you often explore current sexual practices of the client. The client should be encouraged to investigate and acknowledge social and ethical values and consider the role of sexuality in his or her self-concept. When significant discrepancy exists between values and past or current practices, the client may need referral for more intensive counselling.

Major developmental milestones (e.g., puberty or menopause) should prompt education about potential effects on sexuality. Situational crises such as a life change with pregnancy, illness, extreme financial stress, placement of a spouse in a long-term care facility, or loss and grief affect sexuality. Effects may last for days, months, or years and can generate performance anxieties that lead to continued sexual dysfunction. If an individual is prepared for possible changes in sexual functioning, performance anxieties may be minimized.

When concerns are assessed and identified, they can be addressed in the context of the client's value system. In response to identified concerns, you may initiate discussion in pertinent areas. It may be appropriate to discuss sexual practices such as oral–genital sex or mutual masturbation as methods of expressing intimate affection when vaginal–penile intercourse is contraindicated. A partner experiencing musculoskeletal problems that cause joint pain, muscle spasms, stiffness, or problems with flexibility or mobility may appreciate a discussion of various positions for intercourse. Pillows placed about the body or under joints may reduce pain during sexual activity. Additional relief may be obtained by taking a warm shower or bath before sexual activity or using a waterbed to minimize pressure on painful joints (Nusbaum et al., 2003). Use of fantasy or a sense of playfulness may add new romance or stimulation to a long-term relationship. A couple may need confirmation or assurance that the acting out of nonharmful fantasy is normal and healthy.

Restorative Care

In the client's home, you can help create an environment that is comfortable for sexual activity. This may involve recommending ways to arrange the bedroom to accommodate an individual's limitations. For example, a client in a wheelchair may prefer to move the chair close to the side of the bed at an angle that allows for more ease in touching and caressing. Suggestions regarding how to accommodate barriers such as Foley catheters or drainage tubes can contribute to enhanced sexual activity.

In the long-term care setting, facilities should make proper arrangements for privacy during clients' sexual experiences (Lueckenotte, 2000). The ideal situation is to set up a pleasant room that can be used for a variety of activities but may also be reserved for private visits with a spouse or partner. If this is not feasible, you can make arrangements for the roommate of a client to go to another place, in order to allow a client and his or her partner time alone.

BOX 27-4 NURSING CARE PLAN

Sexual Dysfunction

Assessment

Mr. Clements is a 46-year-old client who was last seen in the office 2 months ago, when he was found to have mild hypertension and was given a prescription for propranolol (Inderal). His blood pressure today is 122/82 mm Hg.

Jack, a nursing student, talks with Mr. Clements after reading his records, which include the recent diagnosis of mild hypertension, the order for propranolol, and the current blood pressure reading of 122/82 mm Hg. The record also indicates that Mr. Clements is married and living with his wife.

Jack tells Mr. Clements of the improvement in his blood pressure since his last visit. He inquires whether Mr. Clements is taking his medication regularly. Mr. Clements reports that he has been taking his medication regularly. He relates that it scared him when his blood pressure was up because both his parents had died of strokes. Jack then inquires whether Mr. Clements has noted any side effects from the medicine. Mr. Clements says that he has not, except that he may be a little more tired than he used to be. Jack then states, "Some people find that certain blood pressure medications affect their sexual performance. Have you noticed any changes in sexual functioning since you began your medication?" Mr. Clements replies that he has had some problems achieving an erection since starting the medication.

Assessment Activities	*Findings and Defining Characteristics*
Ascertain when Mr. Clements began noticing his inability to have an erection.	He responds that it was at about the same time he started taking propranolol.
Ask Mr. Clements about his sexual relationship with his wife before taking propranolol.	He states they used to have intercourse one to three times per week.
Ask Mr. Clements whether he has noticed any changes in his desire for sex.	He states that he has the same level of interest as before.
Ask Mr. Clements whether he has made any changes to his lifestyle since the first of the year.	He denies any changes.

Nursing Diagnosis: Erectile dysfunction related to side effects of antihypertensive medication

Planning

*Goal (Nursing Outcomes Classification)**	*Expected Outcomes*
Client will find resolution for this problem.	**Sexual Functioning** Client will talk to his physician about this problem, and a change of medication may be warranted.

*Outcome classification label from Moorhead, S., Johnson, M., & Maas, M. (Eds.). *Nursing Outcomes Classification (NOC)* (3rd ed.). St. Louis, MO: Mosby.

Interventions (Nursing Interventions Classification)†	**Rationale**
Sexual Counselling	
Establish trust and respect with client. Offer privacy during conversations.	Conveys sense of caring, increasing likelihood of client's ability to express concerns fully (Ross et al., 2000)
Discuss possible effects of antihypertensive on sexual functioning, and encourage client to discuss sexual concerns with physician.	Helps client understand possible cause for sexual difficulties and gives client important option to review with physician (Riley, 1999)
Encourage client to discuss concerns with his wife. Role-play so that client can practise ways to approach concerns.	Many of the sexual problems in relationships involve poor communication (Finan, 1997)
Anxiety Reduction	
Assure client that other blood pressure medications are available to can maintain blood pressure control and that do not negatively affect sexual function.	Knowing that options exist and that blood pressure can continue to be safely managed gives client sense of control (Running & Berndt, 2003)

†Intervention classification labels from Dochterman, J. M., & Bulechek, G. M. (2004). *Nursing Interventions Classification (NIC)* (4th ed.). St. Louis, MO: Mosby.

Evaluation

Nursing Actions	*Client Response and Finding*	*Achievement of Outcome*
At his next visit, ask Mr. Clements whether his problems have been resolved.	He responds that since he has been on new medication, he has had no trouble having an erection.	Mr. Clements reports sexual function with the new medication.

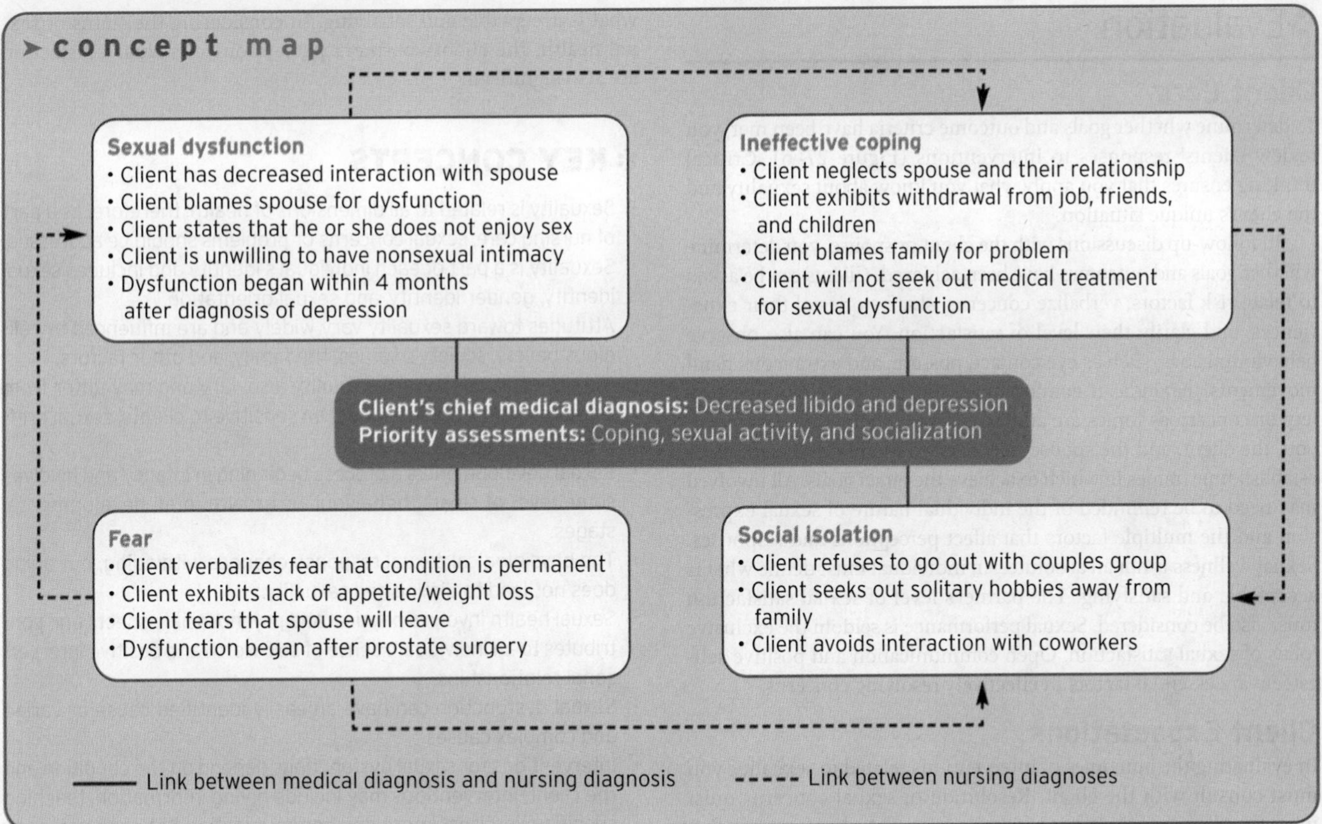

Figure 27-5 Concept map for client with decreased libido and depression.

BOX 27-5 Community Resources Relating to Sexuality

Planned Parenthood
Sex therapists
Clinical psychologists
Social workers
Health department (often for both family planning and treatment of STIs)

Groups that provide education and services for those with particular conditions include the following:

- Canadian Diabetes Association
- Heart and Stroke Foundation of Canada
- Muscular Dystrophy Canada

- Sexual abuse support groups
- Women's shelters (for those who have been physically abused, sexually abused, or both)
- Hotlines for help (which have lists of community support resources)

BOX 27-6 FOCUS ON PRIMARY HEALTH CARE

Sexual Health Education Topics

- Guidelines for normal development: For example, you might talk to a toddler's mother about preparing the toddler for a new baby, to a school-aged child about the appearance of pubic hair, or to a 60-year-old man about erectile difficulties. Details of physiological changes should be described as a part of general health care. Providing client education gives permission for a client to raise questions or concerns regarding personal functioning.
- Contraception, when talking with a client of child-bearing age: The discussion should include such topics as the desire for children, usual sexual practices, acceptable methods of contraception, frequency of sexual activity, comfort with genital touching, comfort with sharing contraceptive responsibility with the partner, and comfort with interruption of sexual acts. You might ask, "Are you using contraceptives with your partner now?" and then follow up, on the basis of the client's answer. For a client who does not have a regular contraceptive method, does not have a reliable contraceptive method, or is not satisfied with the current method, the various methods of contraception should be reviewed to provide necessary information for an informed choice. The best method is the one that the client will use consistently.

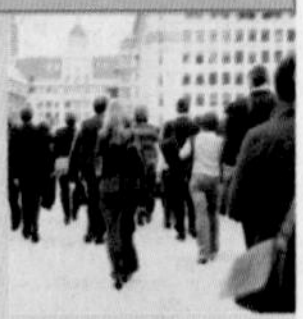

- Safer sex practices, when talking with a sexually active adolescent, with a client who has more than one sex partner, or with a client whose partner has multiple sexual partners: You should provide information regarding STI symptoms and transmission, use of condoms, and risky sexual activities (e.g., trauma from penile–anal sex). A topic to consider in discussing sexual relating is the emotional risks within a relationship. Role-play can be a useful educational tool in helping a person learn to say no or negotiate with a partner to use a condom.
- The need for regular physical examinations: Regular health examinations are important for maintaining sexual health. The annual health examination also provides an easy opportunity to discuss contraception and safer sex practices. Regular clinical breast examinations, mammography, and Papanicolaou (Pap) smears are important for women, as are testicular self-examinations for men.

❖Evaluation

Client Care

To determine whether goals and outcome criteria have been met, you review clients' responses to interventions (Figure 27–6). Critical thinking ensures that you apply what you know about sexuality and the client's unique situation.

In follow-up discussions with the client or spouse, you determine whether goals and outcomes have been achieved. Clients can be asked to relate risk factors, verbalize concerns, share stories of their experiences, and clarify their level of satisfaction. You can also observe behavioural cues, such as eye contact, posture, and extraneous hand movements, that indicate comfort or are suggestive of continued anxiety or concern as topics are addressed. As outcomes are evaluated, you, the client, and the spouse may need to modify expectations or establish time frames in which to achieve the target goals. All involved may need to be reminded of the individual nature of sexual expression and the multiple factors that affect perceptions and responses. Sexual wellness is not an absolute. An individual must define what is acceptable and satisfying. The partner's level of sexual satisfaction must also be considered. Sexual performance is seldom the exclusive focus of sexual satisfaction. Open communication and positive self-esteem are essential factors in effectively resolving concerns.

Client Expectations

In evaluating the outcomes of interventions related to sexuality, you must consult with the client. Resolution of sexual concerns must meet the client's perceptions of improvement. A client must define what is acceptable and satisfying. In considering the status of sexual health, the client's partner's perceptions of sexual satisfaction are also significant.

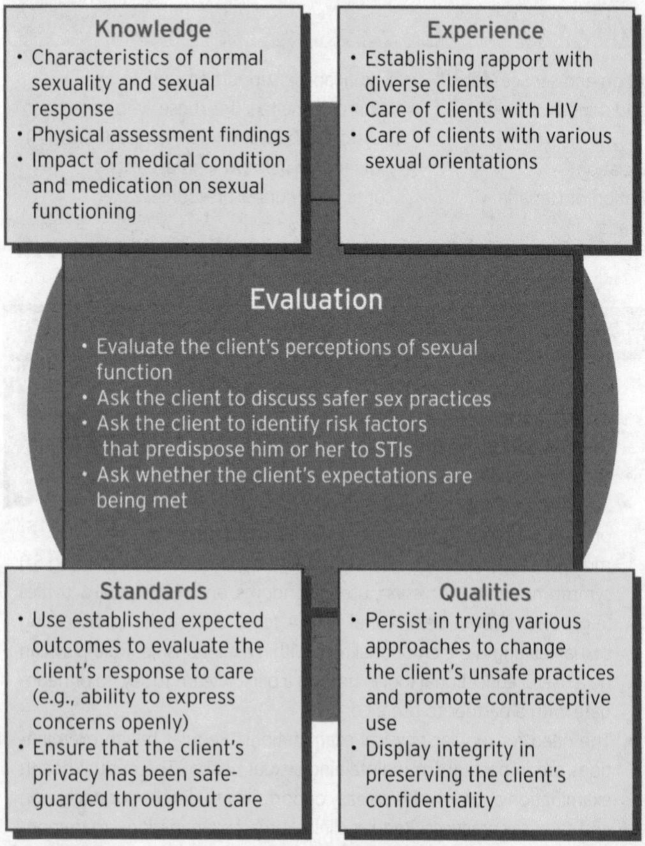

Knowledge
- Characteristics of normal sexuality and sexual response
- Physical assessment findings
- Impact of medical condition and medication on sexual functioning

Experience
- Establishing rapport with diverse clients
- Care of clients with HIV
- Care of clients with various sexual orientations

Evaluation
- Evaluate the client's perceptions of sexual function
- Ask the client to discuss safer sex practices
- Ask the client to identify risk factors that predispose him or her to STIs
- Ask whether the client's expectations are being met

Standards
- Use established expected outcomes to evaluate the client's response to care (e.g., ability to express concerns openly)
- Ensure that the client's privacy has been safeguarded throughout care

Qualities
- Persist in trying various approaches to change the client's unsafe practices and promote contraceptive use
- Display integrity in preserving the client's confidentiality

Figure 27-6 Critical thinking model for sexuality evaluation. HIV, human immunodeficiency virus; STI, sexually transmitted infection.

✻ KEY CONCEPTS

- Sexuality is related to all dimensions of health; therefore, as a part of nursing care, sexual concerns or problems should be addressed.
- Sexuality is a part of each individual's identity and includes sexual identity, gender identity, and sexual orientation.
- Attitudes toward sexuality vary widely and are influenced by religious beliefs, society's values, the family, and other factors.
- Nurses' attitudes toward sexuality also vary and may differ from those of clients; nurses should be sensitive to clients' sexual preferences and needs.
- Sexual development is a process beginning in infancy and involves some level of sexual behaviour or growth in all developmental stages.
- The physiological sexual response changes with aging, but aging does not lead to diminished sexuality.
- Sexual health involves physical and psychosocial aspects and contributes to an individual's sense of self-worth and positive interpersonal relationships.
- Sexual dysfunction can have an easily identified cause or varied and complex causes.
- Interventions for sexual dysfunctions depend on the condition and the client; interventions may include giving information, teaching specific exercises, improving communication between partners, and referral to a knowledgeable professional.
- Choice and use of contraceptive methods are affected by desire for children, usual sexual practices, acceptable methods of contraception, frequency of sexual activity, comfort with genital touching, comfort with sharing contraceptive responsibility with the partner, and comfort with interruption of sexual acts.
- A brief review of sexuality should be included in every nursing assessment of a client's level of wellness.
- Most nursing interventions to enhance a client's sexual health involve providing information and education.

✻ CRITICAL THINKING EXERCISES

1. Your current clinical experience is in a community health care setting. You are conducting the initial interview with a 48-year-old man who started taking antihypertensive medications 2 weeks ago. You take his blood pressure and find it to be 136/74 mm Hg. You ask him how he has been doing since his last visit. He looks down at the floor and says, "Oh, OK, I guess. Seems like I'm just getting old now." What kind of follow-up would be indicated on the basis of this information?

2. You are assigned to care for a 15-year-old girl who was admitted after a motor vehicle accident. Yesterday she underwent internal fixation of a fractured ankle. In gathering her nursing history, you explore sexuality and learn that she has just recently become sexually active with her boyfriend of 3 months. When you ask about safer sex and the use of birth control, she tells you that she knows she does not have to worry about STIs with him because he is just not one of those kinds of boys. In regard to birth control, she says that her boyfriend has reassured her that because he is pulling out before ejaculation, she does not risk becoming pregnant. How would you proceed?

3. You are working on a rehabilitation unit and caring for a 67-year-old man who had a stroke 3 weeks ago. He shares a room with another man who is recovering from a stroke. Your client has been progressing in his self-care skills and is now able to get around with a cane, feed himself, and perform most of his bathing. His wife is in fairly good health, and the plan is for him to return home within the next 1 to 2 weeks. As you work with him one morning, he says to you, "You know, one of the things that is hardest about being here is not being able to sleep in the same bed as Greta. I miss her so much. Even though she visits every day, it is just not the same." How would you explore his comment, and what planning would you consider?

* REVIEW QUESTIONS

1. Gender identity is the individual's
   1. Sexual behaviour
   2. Sexual orientation
   3. Sense of being male, female, or some combination
   4. Sense of preferring one sex over the other

2. Sexual health refers to
   1. Having no STIs
   2. Awareness of and positive attitudes toward sexual functioning
   3. Using contraception consistently
   4. Sexual activity with multiple partners

3. Inability or difficulty in sexual functioning caused by numerous factors is called
   1. Sexual behaviour
   2. Sexual response
   3. Sexual orientation
   4. Sexual dysfunction

4. A major problem in dealing with STIs is that
   1. Symptoms are often absent or go unnoticed
   2. Most STIs cannot be treated with antibiotics
   3. Little is known about how they are transmitted
   4. Little can be done to help

5. The most common bacterial STI is
   1. Syphilis
   2. Genital chlamydia
   3. Gonorrhea
   4. HIV infection and AIDS

6. Of the following methods of contraception, which *two* require a health care professional's intervention?
   1. Diaphragm and intrauterine device (IUD)
   2. Condoms and hormones
   3. Cervical caps and condoms
   4. Sterilization and vaginal spermicidals

7. Which of the following is the most effective contraception method for women?
   1. Female condom
   2. Birth control pill
   3. Contraceptive sponge
   4. Vaginal spermicide

8. The most valuable tool that you can use when providing sexual health care is
   1. Knowledge of right and wrong sexual behaviours
   2. Effective, nonjudgemental communication
   3. Nursing diagnoses
   4. Firm personal convictions about what constitutes normal sexual behaviour

9. When you are gathering a sexual history from an older adult, you must keep in mind that
   1. Older adults do not usually participate in sexual activity
   2. Older men always lose fertility
   3. Older adults may have difficulty discussing intimate matters
   4. Both older men and women are sexually dysfunctional

10. A useful framework for the nurse to guide planning and set priorities about sexual activity for a client is
    1. The PLISSIT model
    2. The NANDA International guidelines
    3. The *Nursing Interventions Classification* (NIC) and *Nursing Outcomes Classification* (NOC) guidelines
    4. Your own theory of sexual behaviour

* RECOMMENDED WEB SITES

Public Health Agency of Canada: *Canadian Guidelines for Sexual Health Education:* http://www.phac-aspc.gc.ca/publicat/cgshe-ldnemss/
This publication, developed by Health Canada in collaboration with sexual health experts, provides information for health care professionals and others to develop and improve sexual health education policies and programs that address the diverse needs of Canadians.

Public Health Agency of Canada: Sexual Health and Sexually Transmitted Infections: http://www.phac-aspc.gc.ca/std-mts/
The Public Health Agency of Canada works with provinces, nongovernmental organizations, and health care professionals to improve and maintain the sexual health and well-being of Canadians. This Web site offers links to sexual health and STI information, publications, and resources.

Sunnybrook and Women's College Health Sciences Centre: http://www.womenshealthmatters.ca/centres/sex/index.html
Developed by Sunnybrook and Women's College Health Sciences Centre and the Centre for Research in Women's Health, this Web site provides information about women's sexual matters, including sexual expression, how female bodies work, pregnancy, birth control, abortion, and safer sex.

28

Spiritual Health

Original chapter by Amy M. Hall, RN, BSN, MS, PhD

Canadian content written by Sonya Grypma, RN, PhD, and Barb Pesut, RN, PhD

objectives

Mastery of content in this chapter will enable you to:

- Define the key terms listed.
- Discuss research findings that suggest a relationship between spiritual practices and clients' health status.
- Describe the relationship between faith, hope, and spiritual well-being.
- Discuss theoretical foundations for spiritual care.
- Compare and contrast the concepts of religion and spirituality.
- Perform an assessment of a client's spiritual needs and resources.
- Explain how a nurse's caring relationship with clients affects clients' ability to gain spiritual insight.
- Discuss ethics related to spiritual nursing care.
- Discuss nursing interventions designed to promote spiritual well-being.

key terms

Agnostic, p. 437
Atheist, p. 437
Culture, p. 438
Faith, p. 437
Holistic, p. 447
Hope, p. 438
Religion, p. 438
Spiritual care, p. 437
Spiritual well-being, p. 437
Spirituality, p. 435
Transcendence, p. 437

media resources

evolve Web Site

- Audio Chapter Summaries
- Glossary
- Multiple-Choice Review Questions
- Student Learning Activities
- Weblinks

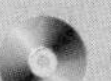 **Companion CD**

- Glossary
- Interactive Learning Activities
- Fluids and Electrolytes Tutorial
- Test-Taking Skills

The word **spirituality** is derived from the Latin word *spiritus*, which refers to breath or wind. The spirit gives life to, or animates, a person. It signifies whatever is at the centre of all aspects of a person's life, whatever gives that person ultimate meaning (Sessanna et al., 2007). Spirituality is often described as being connected to oneself, to others, to nature, and to God. A person's health depends on a balance of physical, psychological, sociological, cultural, developmental, and spiritual factors. Spirituality can be the important factor that helps individuals achieve the balance needed to maintain health and well-being and to cope with illness.

Spirituality is a highly personal matter. Caring for a client's spiritual needs means caring for the whole person, accepting his or her beliefs and experiences, and helping with issues concerning meaning and hope. Being able to determine the importance spirituality holds for clients depends on your ability to develop a caring relationship (see Chapter 19).

In your nursing practice, you must recognize spirituality in clients and be aware of your own spirituality to provide appropriate spiritual care. Expert nurses help clients use their spiritual resources as they identify what is meaningful in their lives and cope with the effects of illness and life stressors.

Scientific Knowledge Base

Research findings have revealed an association between spirituality and health. Health outcomes may be beneficial when individuals engage their beliefs in a higher power and sense a source of strength or support. For example, Spurlock (2005) found that caregivers who reported higher levels of spiritual well-being experienced less caregiver burden (feeling overloaded or overwhelmed) when providing care to family members. Holstad et al. (2006) found that clients with human immunodeficiency virus (HIV) or acquired immunodeficiency syndrome (AIDS) who found meaning and hope in their lives were more likely to follow their prescribed antiretroviral therapy. Many people use prayer as a method of coping because it is effective in minimizing physical stressors. Attending religious services and praying often positively affects health and the decision to participate in health promotion practices (Aaron et al., 2003; Banks-Wallace & Parks, 2004). The increased interest in studying the relationship between spirituality and health has greatly contributed to nursing science (Gray, 2006; Smith, 2006).

Mind, body, and spirit are linked; however, the relationship is not clearly understood. Nevertheless, studies show that an individual's beliefs and expectations have effects on the person's physical well-being. For example, Canadian studies showed that spirituality influences health for Orthodox Jewish women during child-bearing years (Semenic et al., 2004), for Punjabi Sikh living in Canada (Labun & Emblen, 2007), and for informal caregivers of older and disabled clients (Sawatzky & Fowler-Kerry, 2003). You will be more successful in helping clients achieve desirable health outcomes after learning to support clients and families spiritually, as well as mentally and physically.

Nursing Knowledge Base

Historical Perspectives

Nursing has a rich spiritual heritage. Spirituality was at the core of early nursing philosophies and practice until the nineteenth century (McSherry, 2001). Organized nursing originated from religious orders, in which nuns were primarily responsible for providing nursing care. In Canada, the earliest nurses belonged to Roman Catholic orders devoted to care of the sick: most notably, the Sisters of Charity of Montreal (Grey Nuns), an order founded by Marie Marguerite d'Youville in 1737 (Paul, 2000). This noncloistered order was responsible for bringing a Judeo-Christian model of nursing care to the most remote areas of western and northern Canada. Religion provided a lens through which to acknowledge spiritual needs, express spiritual care, and pursue spiritual health.

Florence Nightingale's ideas of modern nursing were first taught in London in 1860. Her model of Western nursing, rooted in Christianity, was spread around the world during the colonial era (Paul, 2000). Canadian missionary nurses were among those who brought modern nursing methods to China, India, Japan, and Korea in the first half of the of the twentieth century (Grypma, 2008). For many people, the concepts of spirituality and religion were linked, and until the 1970s, nurses used the terms interchangeably (Taylor, 2002).

In the twentieth century, confidence in religion was replaced by confidence in medical science. By the 1970s, nursing had evolved from a religious vocation to an increasingly secular profession. Religious aspects of care became less visible. Over time, the general public became dissatisfied with a purely medical approach to care, partly because people realized that scientific research could not answer all the existential questions raised by clients (McSherry, 2001). Nurses felt a spiritual gap in the profession and began to find ways to articulate and incorporate spirituality into practice and research. Spirituality was conceptualized as broader and more encompassing than any particular religion or culture. Between 1980 and 2000, renewed interest in spirituality was reflected by an increase in related subjects in nursing literature, as well as a growing interest in parish nursing as a way for faith communities in Canada to reclaim their healing mission (Olson et al., 1998). Clients and caregivers relied on nurses as leaders in spiritual care because of the unique spiritual heritage of the field of nursing and its continual leading role in health care delivery (McSherry, 2001).

Canadian nursing scholarship has shifted away from the notion of spirituality as a discrete concept, emphasizing instead the relationship between spirituality, religion, health, and culture (Browne & Fiske, 2001; Kulig et al., 2004; Labun & Emblen, 2007). For example, in their study of spirituality and health in Punjabi Sikh living in British Columbia, Labun and Emblen stated that an understanding of the interplay of spirituality, religion, and health informs culturally competent care. Just as Canadian nurses must understand cultural influences in health, illness, and caring patterns (see Chapter 10), they must also recognize the need for sensitive, safe, and ethical nursing care in which clients' spiritual needs and resources are recognized and supported. Because Canada is a pluralistic society in which diversity is valued, Canadian nurses must recognize how individual world views influence the way clients (and nurses) view the spiritual world and their place in the world (Pesut, 2006).

Although nurses have long integrated understandings of spirituality into their care, the development of systematic approaches to spiritual care is relatively recent. In the 1980s, the North American Nursing Diagnosis Association (NANDA) created an American and Canadian task force to determine nursing diagnoses for nurses to use as part of the nursing process. Although three nursing diagnoses related to spirituality are currently accepted by NANDA International (2007)—*readiness for spiritual well-being, spiritual distress,* and *risk for spiritual distress*—their use in nursing practice is debated. Some scholars are challenging what is perceived as the problematization of spirituality. For example, Pesut (2008) urged nurses to "resist the notion that there is some idealized spiritual state that the absence of which necessarily dictates some pathological process" (p. 172). If nurses accept the idea that spirituality is somewhat unique and individualized, they need to be cautious about creating normative criteria, particularly those based on positive emotions (Pesut & Sawatzky, 2006). Although the nursing process is still considered a helpful method of thinking about care, the use of nursing diagnoses has lost some of its earlier appeal. The transcendent nature and experience of spirituality must not be limited by being reduced to problems or nursing diagnoses.

Theoretical Perspectives

Many nursing theorists describe clients as biological–psychological–social–spiritual beings, and most advocate holistic care (Barnum, 2003; Taylor, 2002). The concept that humans are multidimensional beings is still used as a basis for nursing models today (Figure 28–1). Theorists who advocate for holistic care typically identify spirituality as an aspect of nursing care. Others view spiritual care as a "way of being" with patients that pervades all aspects of care.

Several theoretical nursing models have identified spirituality as an aspect of nursing practice (Taylor, 2002):

- Henderson (1966) identified three nursing abilities that are related to spirituality: ability to express feelings and thoughts, ability to play and re-create, and ability to learn and satisfy curiosity. *Spiritual care could entail assisting clients to worship or pursue recreational activities.*
- Travelbee (1966) portrayed nursing as an interpersonal process involving preventing, alleviating, or helping individuals, families, and communities find meaning in illness or suffering. By witnessing or assisting clients through experiences such as illness, nurses receive opportunities to create meaning. *Spiritual care could entail instilling meaning and hope through verbal communication.*
- Neuman (1982) maintained that each person or group constitutes a system of physiological, psychological, sociological, cultural, developmental, and spiritual variables that exist along a developmental continuum. The spiritual continuum can range from lack of awareness, or denial, to a highly developed spiritual consciousness. *Spiritual care could entail assisting clients to identify goals, increase spiritual awareness, and access spiritual resources.*
- Watson (1979) recognized a societal need for the universal, mysterious, and powerful forces of love and care. Human caring is an ethical and spiritual act that connects practitioners and patients within a unitary field of consciousness. This forms the basis for a healing relationship in which the sacredness and interconnectedness of all of life are recognized. *Spiritual care could entail authentic presence, consciousness and intentionality to create a healing environment.*

Nursing theories are broad and encompassing and are meant to be adapted for use in a variety of areas of nursing practice. *Nursing frameworks* are more specific, describing ways in which spirituality can be incorporated into care of culturally diverse clients (Andrews & Boyle, 2007). *Nursing models* may be expressly geared to spiritual caregiving, providing guidelines to a particular group of nurses (such as Christian or parish nurses; Mosgrove, 2007; Van Dover & Bacon-Pfeiffer, 2007)

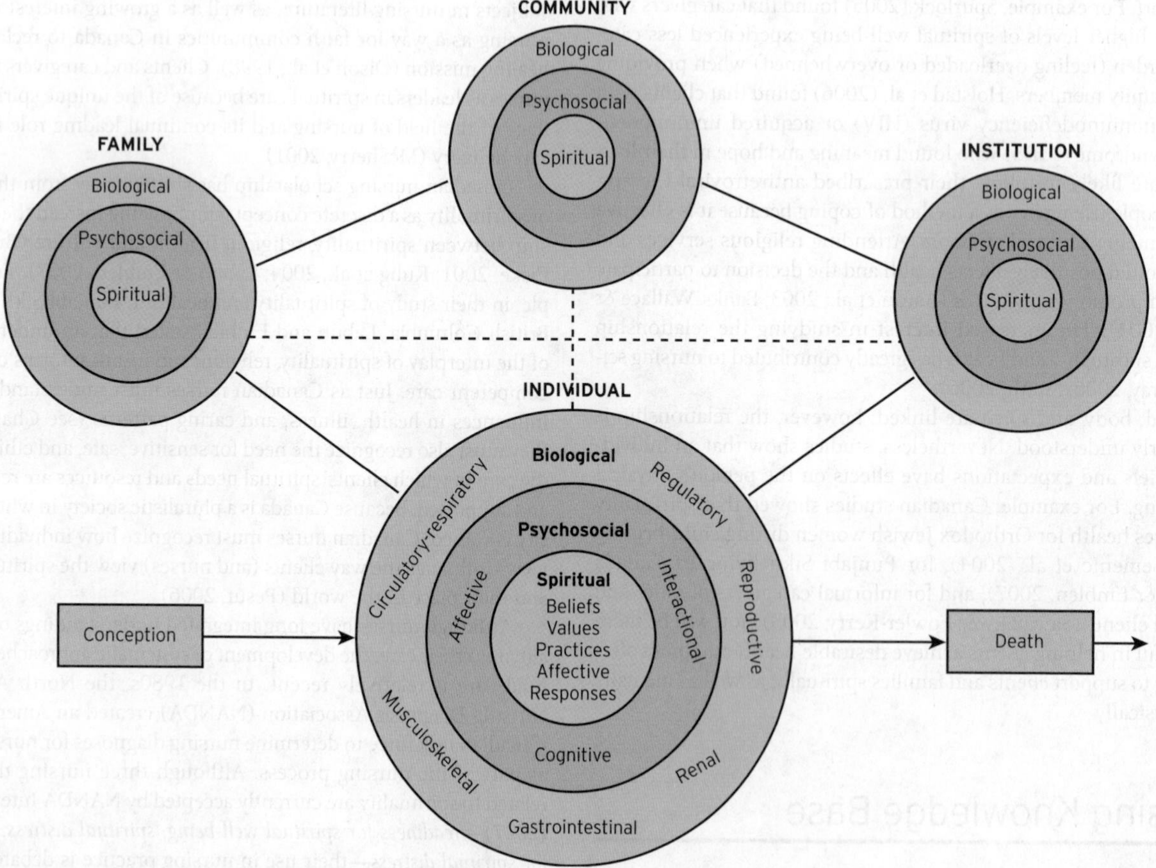

Figure 28-1 Model of spiritual relationships. **Source:** Adapted from Artinian, B. M., & Conger, M. M. (Eds.) (1997). *The intersystem model: Integrating theory and practice* (p. 5). Thousand Oaks, CA: Sage.

or a particular practice setting (such as a faith community; Clark & Olson, 2000; O'Brien, 2003). Nursing theories are not meant to address practical specifics about spiritual caregiving; rather, they serve to establish a system of assumptions and principles that nurses can use to guide their practice. You may draw from more than one theory to develop effective approaches to client care (Taylor, 2002).

Traditional Concepts Associated With Spiritual Health

Various concepts are used to describe spiritual health. To provide meaningful and supportive spiritual care, you must understand the concepts of spirituality, faith, religion, and hope. Each concept offers direction in understanding individuals' views of life and its value.

Spirituality. Spirituality is a concept that is unique to each individual and dependent on a person's culture, development, life experiences, beliefs, and ideas about life. Spirituality enables a person to love, have faith and hope, seek meaning in life, and nurture relationships with others. Spirituality offers a sense of being connected intrapersonally (connected within oneself), interpersonally (connected with others and the environment), and transpersonally (connected with the unseen, God, or a higher power; Delgado, 2005). The notion of "relationship" is central to the concept of spirituality in nursing.

Spiritual well-being is a state of wholeness or health. Spiritual health is enhanced when people find a balance between their life values, goals, and belief systems and their relationship within themselves and with others. **Spiritual care** involves nursing practices that support patients in their connectedness to self, others, and the sacred (Como, 2007). To enage in spiritual care, you must first be aware of the transcendent dimension and be comfortable with hearing about clients' spirituality. Spiritual care is an altruistic, relational, intuitive, and integrative process by which you seek to understand and reflect the client's spiritual values, beliefs, and experiences (Figure 28–2; Satwatzky & Pesut, 2005).

Spirituality begins as children learn about themselves and their relationships with others. Children's ideas of a higher power or supreme being are often based on what is presented to them in their homes or religious community. Adolescents may reconsider their childhood concept of a spiritual power and, in the search for an identity, may question values and practices. Many Canadian teenagers and young adults who have been reared in a religious tradition "drop out" of their religious system as they search for a personalized belief system and seek a clearer meaning of life (Bibby, 2002).

Many adults experience spiritual growth by entering into lifelong relationships. An ability to care meaningfully for others and the self is evidence of a healthy spirituality. Older adults often turn to important relationships and the giving of themselves to others as spiritual tasks. As people mature, they often turn inward to enduring values and to a concept of a supreme being or a higher meaning that has been sustaining and meaningful. A healthy spirituality in older adults is one that gives peace and acceptance of the self and that is often based on a lifelong relationship with a supreme being. A positive relationship to a higher power may help to protect older adults from the negative effects of loss and changing identity that occur with aging (Griffith et al., 2007). Illness and loss can threaten and challenge the spiritual developmental process or can precipitate a spiritual crisis. You can help clients cope with the spiritual health concerns triggered by critical events (Meyerhoff et al., 2002). It is thus important for you to understand the nature and status of a client's belief system and spiritual health.

Many individuals either do not believe in the existence of God (**atheist**) or believe that any ultimate reality is unknown (**agnostic**). Agnostics believe that the existence of a God or higher power cannot be proved or disproved. This does not mean that spirituality is not an important concept for the atheist or agnostic. Atheists may search for meaning in life through their work and their relationships with other individuals (Burnard, 1988). However, of importance is that the term *spirituality,* because of its long association with religion, may not be one that atheists or agnostics would use in reference to themselves (Paley, 2008). An important part of respect in nursing is using the language that is familiar or acceptable to clients.

Faith. Spirituality enables a person to love, have faith and hope, seek meaning in life, and nurture relationships. The concept of **faith** is described in the literature in two ways: First, faith is defined as a cultural or institutional religion, such as Judaism, Buddhism, Islam, or Christianity; second, faith is defined as a relationship with a divinity, a higher power, an authority, or a spirit that incorporates a reasoning faith (belief) and a trusting faith (action) (Benner, 1985). *Reasoning faith* is an individual's belief and confidence in something for which no scientific proof exists. Sometimes that faith involves a belief in a higher power, a spirit guide, God, or Allah (Mauk & Schmidt, 2004). However, faith also might be the manner in which a person chooses to live life. Faith in this sense enables action. For example, a person might believe that having a positive outlook on life is the best way to achieve life's goals.

The belief that comes with faith involves **transcendence**: an awareness of something that a person cannot see or know in ordinary physical ways (Perry, 2004). It gives purpose and meaning to an individual's life, allowing for action. For example, in clients with advanced cancer, faith may provide significant strength and resources to cope with their illness (Lin & Bauer-Wu, 2003).

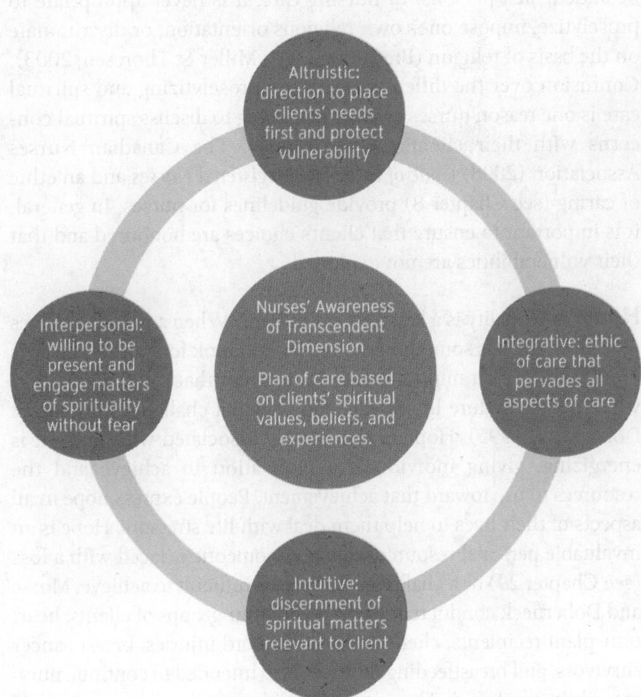

Figure 28-2 Attributes of spiritual care in nursing practice. **Source:** Adapted from Sawatzky, R., & Pesut, B. (2005). Attributes of spiritual care in nursing practice. *Journal of Holistic Nursing, 23,* 19–33. Copyright © 2005. Reprinted by permission of SAGE Publications.

Religion. Many people use the terms *religion* and *spirituality* interchangeably. Although closely associated, these terms are not synonymous. **Religion** is an organized system of beliefs concerning the cause, nature, and purpose of the universe, especially belief in or the worship of God or gods (Andrews & Boyle, 2007). It is a structured search for the spiritual and an outward expression of spirituality (Emblen, 1992). Religious practice encompasses spirituality, but spirituality need not include religious practice. Whereas the aim of religious care is to help clients maintain their belief systems and worship practices, the aim of spiritual care is to facilitate spiritual health (Taylor, 2002).

Spirituality is informed by, and expressed through, both culture and religion. **Culture** represents a way of perceiving, behaving, and evaluating the world. It provides a blueprint or guide for determining values, beliefs, and practices (Andrews & Boyle, 2007). A person's spiritual nature may be expressed in religious and philosophical beliefs and practices, and these may differ widely, depending on the person's race, gender, social status, religion, ethnicity, and experience (Taylor, 2002).

Thus, although nurses may make an intellectual distinction between spirituality and religion or culture, the boundaries are much less distinct in actual experience (Macrae, 2001). For many patients, the term *spirituality* may still be closely related to religion, and many individuals' spiritual practices are drawn from a variety of religious traditions (Pesut et al., 2008). Indeed, 53% of Canadians still describe spirituality in traditional terms such as *prayer, religion*, and *a power beyond* (Bibby, 2006). Organized religion can provide a framework for understanding the meaning of existence and a structure for worship. Considerable religious and cultural diversity exist in Canada, and many geographic regions provide health care to users of many faiths. Pluralism and respect for diversity is highly valued. Canadians generally disapprove of religious groups' aggressive attempts to convert others, particularly vulnerable people such as children, immigrants, and older adults (Bibby, 2002), and, it could be added, sick persons. In nursing care, it is never appropriate to proselytize, impose one's own religious orientation, or discriminate on the basis of religion (Bradshaw, 1994; Miller & Thoresen, 2003). Confusion over the difference between proselytizing and spiritual care is one reason nurses give for hesitating to discuss spiritual concerns with their clients (Vance, 2001). The Canadian Nurses Association (2008) *Code of Ethics for Registered Nurses* and an ethic of caring (see Chapter 8) provide guidelines for nurses. In general, it is important to ensure that client's choices are honoured and that their vulnerabilities are not exploited.

Hope. Spirituality is a key element in hope. When a person believes that he or she has something to live for and look forward to, **hope** is present. Hope is a multidimensional concept that provides comfort while people endure life threats and personal challenges (Morse & Doberneck, 1995). Hope is also closely associated with faith. It is energizing, giving individuals a motivation to achieve and the resources to use toward that achievement. People express hope in all aspects of their lives to help them deal with life stressors. Hope is an invaluable personal resource whenever someone is faced with a loss (see Chapter 29) or a challenge that seems difficult to achieve. Morse and Doberneck conducted research with four groups of clients: heart transplant recipients, clients with spinal cord injuries, breast cancer survivors, and breastfeeding mothers who intended to continue nursing while employed. The researchers identified seven concepts of hope: initially assessing threat, envisioning of options and setting goals, preparing for negative outcomes, assessing of resources, seeking out supportive relationships, evaluating signs that reinforce goals, and determining to endure. Thus, hope can be a complex and unique concept for each individual.

Spiritual Challenges

When illness, loss, grief, or a major life change affects a person, either spiritual resources help a person recover or spiritual needs and concerns develop. A catastrophic illness, for example, can upset a person's spiritual health sufficiently to cause doubt and loss of faith. The person may feel alone or even abandoned. Individuals may question their spiritual values, raising questions about their way of life and purpose for living. Spiritual concerns also arise when a person's beliefs conflict with prescribed treatment or when the person is unable to practise rituals.

Acute Illness. Sudden, unexpected illness can create significant spiritual concerns. For example, both a 50-year-old man who has a heart attack and a 20-year-old victim of a motor vehicle accident face crises that may threaten their spiritual health. The illness or injury creates an unanticipated scramble to integrate and cope with new realities (e.g., disability). People look for ways to remain faithful to their beliefs and value systems. They may pray, attend religious services, or reflect on the positive aspects of their lives. Conflicts often develop with regard to a person's beliefs and the meaning of life. Anger is not uncommon, and clients may express anger toward God, their families, themselves, or you. Spiritual dimensions of the illness experience may include reconsidering beliefs about life; maintaining spiritual or religious practices; connecting with God and significant others; and finding balance, courage, and growth (van Leeuwen et al., 2007).

Chronic Illness. People with chronic illness often suffer debilitating symptoms that change their lifestyles. A symptom is more than a signal for a persistent health problem or a clue for diagnosing a disease. A symptom can prompt permission to a person to take needed rest, can be a sign of impending disruption, or can even raise feelings about the person's self-worth and strength (Benner &Wrubel, 1989). Symptoms are meaningful to the individual, and that meaning is shaped by the person's history and the current context of the illness.

With chronic illness, independence can be threatened, causing fear, anxiety, and dispiritedness. Dependence on other people can create a feeling of powerlessness. A person may feel a loss of a sense of purpose in life, which affects the inner strength needed to deal with alterations in functioning. A person's spirituality can influence how he or she adapts to changes resulting from chronic illness. Successful adaptation can strengthen a person spiritually. A client may re-evaluate his or her life. Clients who have a sense of spiritual health, who feel connected with a higher power and other people, and who are able to find meaning and purpose in life are better able to cope with chronic illness; better coping helps them achieve their potential and enhances quality of life (Figure 28–3; Adegbola, 2006; Narayanasamy, 2004).

Terminal Illness. Terminal illness commonly causes fears of physical pain, isolation, losing control, and dying, as well as uncertainty about the future, both for oneself and for one's family. Individuals experiencing a terminal illness examine their life and question its meaning. Common questions include "Why is this happening to me?" or "What have I done to deserve this?" Family and friends can be affected just as much as the client. Terminal illness causes family members to ask important questions about its meaning and how it will affect their relationship with the client (see Chapter 29). However, spirituality may facilitate coping with terminal illness. Tanyi and Werner (2008) interviewed 16 women with end-stage renal disease and found that spirituality helped them accept illness and mortality, find strength and understanding amidst the experience, and counter negative emotions such as anger, fear, and depression.

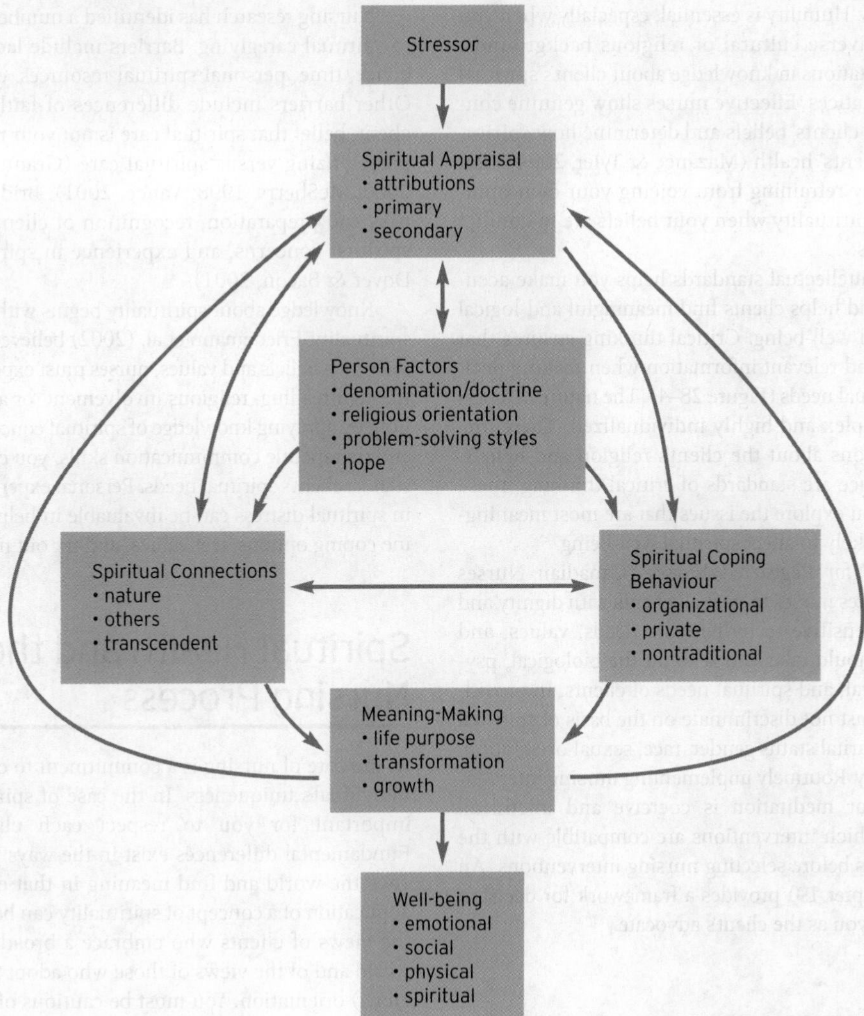

Figure 28-3 The spiritual framework of coping (an adaptation and application of the transactional model). **Source:** From Gall, T. L., Charbonneau, C., Clarke, N. H., Grant, K., Joseph, A., & Shouldice, L. (2005). Understanding the nature and role of spirituality in relation to coping and health: A conceptual framework. *Canadian Psychology, 46*(2), 88–104. Copyright 2005, Canadian Psychological Association. Permission granted for use of material.

Critical Thinking

The helping role is important in nursing practice (Benner, 1984). Clients rely on nurses for a different kind of help than that sought from other health care professionals. Expert nurses can anticipate the personal issues affecting clients' abilities to receive and seek help, including their spiritual well-being. Critical thinking knowledge and skills help you to enhance clients' spiritual well-being and health. While using the nursing process, you apply knowledge, experience, qualities, and standards in providing appropriate spiritual care.

Nurses who are comfortable with their own spirituality are more likely to care for their clients' spiritual needs than are other nurses (Miner-Williams, 2006). Nurses who foster their own personal, emotional, and spiritual health become resources for their clients and use their own spirituality as a tool when caring for themselves and their clients (Gray, 2006; Jackson, 2004).

Taking a faith history reveals client's beliefs about life, health, and a supreme being. Knowing the client's cultural preferences provides additional insight into the client's spiritual practices. Applying knowledge of spiritual concepts, principles of caring (see Chapter 19), and therapeutic communication skills (see Chapter 18) will help you recognize and understand your clients' spiritual beliefs.

A sound understanding of ethics and values (Chapter 8) is essential when you provide spiritual care. A person's values or beliefs about a given idea, attitude, or custom are linked to the individual's spiritual well-being. Application of ethical principles ensures respect for client's spiritual and religious convictions.

Personal experience in caring for clients in experiencing distress, anger, or confusion is valuable for helping clients select coping options. You need to determine whether your own spirituality is beneficial in assisting clients. Nurses who sense a personal faith and hope regarding life are usually better able to help their clients than are other nurses (Jackson, 2004). As a result of previous personal and professional experiences with dying clients, clients with chronic disease, or clients who have experienced significant losses, you can help clients face difficult challenges and offer support to family and friends (Wright, 2005).

Because each person has a unique spirituality, you need to know your own beliefs so that you are able to care for each client without bias. Use critical thinking when you assess each client's reaction to illness and loss and when you determine whether spiritual intervention is necessary. Humility is essential, especially when you care for clients from diverse cultural or religious backgrounds. Recognize personal limitations in knowledge about client's spiritual beliefs and religious practices. Effective nurses show genuine concern as they assess their clients' beliefs and determine how spirituality influences their clients' health (Mazanec & Tyler, 2004). You demonstrate integrity by refraining from voicing your own opinions about religion or spirituality when your beliefs are in conflict with your client's beliefs.

The application of intellectual standards helps you make accurate clinical decisions and helps clients find meaningful and logical ways to pursue spiritual well-being. Critical thinking ensures that you obtain significant and relevant information when making decisions about client's spiritual needs (Figure 28–4). The nature of a person's spirituality is complex and highly individualized. Therefore, avoid making assumptions about the client's religion and beliefs. Significance and relevance are standards of critical thinking; these standards ensure that you explore the issues that are most meaningful to clients and most likely to affect spiritual well-being.

The *Code of Ethics for Registered Nurses* (Canadian Nurses Association, 2008) requires nurses to treat all clients with dignity and respect. You must be sensitive to individual's needs, values, and choices. Nursing care should take into account the biological, psychological, social, cultural, and spiritual needs of clients. In providing nursing care, you must not discriminate on the basis of spiritual beliefs, age, ethnicity, marital status gender, race, sexual orientation, health status, or disability. Routinely implementing nursing interventions such as prayer or meditation is coercive and unethical. Therefore, determine which interventions are compatible with the client's beliefs and values before selecting nursing interventions. An ethic of caring (see Chapter 19) provides a framework for decision making and establishes you as the client's advocate.

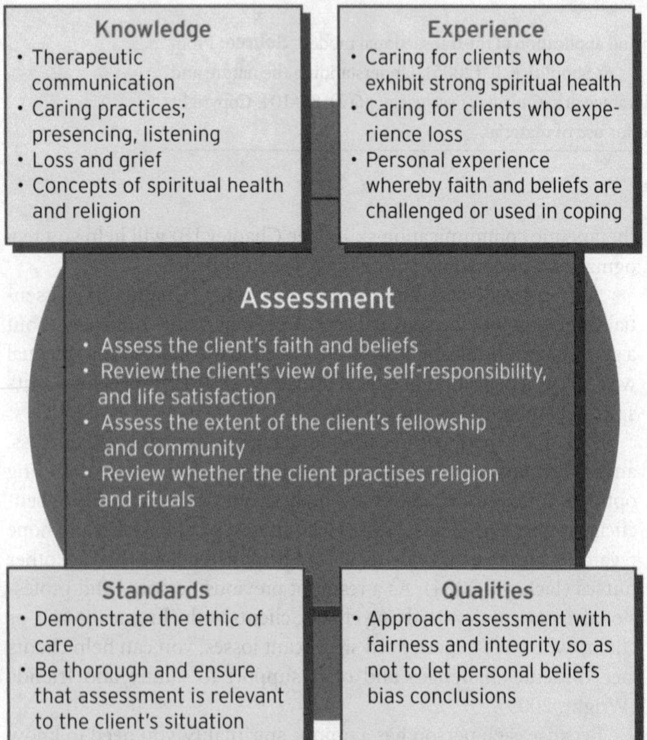

Knowledge
- Therapeutic communication
- Caring practices; presencing, listening
- Loss and grief
- Concepts of spiritual health and religion

Experience
- Caring for clients who exhibit strong spiritual health
- Caring for clients who experience loss
- Personal experience whereby faith and beliefs are challenged or used in coping

Assessment
- Assess the client's faith and beliefs
- Review the client's view of life, self-responsibility, and life satisfaction
- Assess the extent of the client's fellowship and community
- Review whether the client practises religion and rituals

Standards
- Demonstrate the ethic of care
- Be thorough and ensure that assessment is relevant to the client's situation

Qualities
- Approach assessment with fairness and integrity so as not to let personal beliefs bias conclusions

Figure 28-4 Critical thinking model for spiritual health assessment.

Nursing research has identified a number of barriers and bridges to spiritual caregiving. Barriers include lack of knowledge, confidence, time, personal spiritual resources, or institutional support. Other barriers include differences of faith between you and the client, belief that spiritual care is not your role, and confusion over proselytizing versus spiritual care (Grant, 2004; Louis & Alpert, 2000; McSherry, 1998; Vance, 2001). Bridges include your readiness and preparation, recognition of clients' and families' cues of spiritual concerns, and experience in spiritual intervention (Van Dover & Bacon, 2001).

Knowledge about spirituality begins with insight about your own spirituality. Friedemann et al. (2002) believed in order to understand their own beliefs and values, nurses must experience a self-exploration through reading, religious involvement, or activities such as meditation. By applying knowledge of spiritual concepts, principles of caring, and therapeutic communication skills, you can recognize and understand a client's spiritual needs. Personal experience in caring for clients in spiritual distress can be invaluable in helping each client to examine coping options, test values, and try out new behaviours.

Spiritual Health and the Nursing Process

At the core of nursing is a commitment to caring and respect for an individual's uniqueness. In the case of spirituality, it is even more important for you to respect each client's personal beliefs. Fundamental differences exist in the ways in which people experience the world and find meaning in that experience. Any blanket application of a concept of spirituality can be equally disrespectful of the views of clients who embrace a broadly religious view of the world and of the views of those who adopt a more secular (nonreligious) orientation. You must be cautious of personal biases or misconceptions and be willing to share and discover a client's meaning and purpose in life, sickness, and health. It is important for you to sort out value judgements about other people's belief systems. Working through values clarification exercises can be helpful (see Chapter 8). If you are a "believer," do you judge harshly the "unbeliever"? If you are agnostic or atheist, do you dismiss the believer? You must accept and acknowledge other people's beliefs and not try to convert them. Look beyond a personal view when establishing a client relationship. This approach means identifying the common values that make people human and respecting the commitments and values that make humans unique. Love, trust, hope, forgiveness, meaning, and community are spiritual needs of all people. Learning to respond appropriately to these needs helps you find a way to give clients spiritual care and support.

Application of the nursing process to a client's spirituality must be done with caution. The nursing process helps you learn how to provide care, but you should be cautious when using this problem-solving process for the delivery of spiritual care (Pesut & Sawatzky, 2006). Spiritual care is different from the physical aspects of care. Spirituality contains an element of mystery that cannot be assessed and treated in the same way that you might treat a physical problem, such as a pressure ulcer. Diagnosing and intervening in a client's spirituality may be considered disrespectful and intrusive. Instead, the nursing process should be be thought of as a tool to explore what is meaningful to clients and to support individualized spiritual health. Above all, the caregiving process should be grounded in an understanding of compassion and community (Heliker, 1992). The term *compassion* comes from the Latin words *pati* and *cum*, meaning "to suffer with." *Community* is derived from the Latin word *communio,* meaning "fellowship." To be compassionate is to "enter into places of pain, to share in brokenness with other human beings" (Heliker, 1992). To practise compassion as a nurse requires awareness of the very human tie between clients and a healing community. This kind of work generally consists of quiet conversations, effective listening, and communication through presence and touch (Draper & McSherry, 2002).

BOX 28-1 NURSING STORY

Encountering Spiritual Torment

In a phenomenological study of the lived experience of cross-cultural nurses (Grypma, 2001), participants described meaningful instances of deep human connection that were at once intuitive (expected) and startling (unexpected). Some participants described disturbing experiences of being with patients suffering from intense spiritual pain. To Vicki, a Canadian missionary nurse who has worked for almost 40 years in various remote and underdeveloped regions of the world, some of her most profound experiences involved what she described as encountering spiritual torment. Vicki recalled the following incident in Bolivia:

> From our home above the clinic, [my husband and I] could hear the patient crying out, calling out, panic-stricken. My husband [a physician] could find no medical explanation for her choking. But we kept her overnight anyway. By morning she had left the clinic with friends. Two days later we found out she had died. The people said a curse had been put on her . . . and that she was frightened to death.

Although it had been more than two decades since the experience, Vicki began to weep as she relived it:

> She literally had no physical symptoms, but we didn't know enough about cross-cultural caring at that point to be able to discern what was wrong with her *[voice falters, cries]*, and as Christians, we weren't even sensitive enough to pray for her, and pray for her healing, or pray for her protection . . . and she left.

Neither her Canadian nursing education nor her missionary orientation had exposed Vicki to the spiritual causes of physical illness. Vicki still does not completely understand the cause of death of this woman and presumes she died because of the curse itself (spiritual cause) or because she believed so strongly in the existence of a curse (psychological cause).

A few years after leaving Bolivia, Vicki and her husband cared for a patient in Zaire who had a bowel disease necessitating surgery. The patient refused treatment despite his deteriorating condition. It was the Zairian chaplain who identified the patient's problem as a spiritual one:

> The chaplain recommended that this patient go home to find out who caused his bowel problem—who may have placed a curse on him. After ten days back in his village, the patient returned to the clinic, at peace, and ready now for surgery.

Vicki learned to recognize spiritual needs, to realize that spiritual pain exists in ways that she cannot really comprehend, and to accept the judgement and intervention of local community members when they identify spiritual causes of physical symptoms. About the Zairian patient, she concluded:

> He was refusing his surgery for some reason . . . . It was such a powerful lesson of being able to listen without him necessarily saying anything to us, but listening, I guess, to our own spirit, to our own sensitivities that something was not right.

❖Assessment

Because spirituality is deeply subjective, it means different things to different people (McSherry & Ross, 2002). The ability to understand a client's spirituality is compromised when you have limited contact with the client or when you fail to build a therapeutic relationship. Once you establish a trusting relationship with a client and you reach a point of learning together, spiritual caring occurs (Taylor, 2003a). Focus the nursing assessment on aspects of spirituality that will probably be influenced by current health or illness experiences. Conducting an assessment is therapeutic because it expresses a level of caring and support.

Spiritual assessment is a fundamental part of the nursing assessment. Because nurses often have limited time to spend with their clients, it is often difficult to obtain an in-depth spiritual assessment. However, it is critical that you obtain information about religious and spiritual beliefs and practices when clients enter a health care facility. Inability to observe those practices can cause significant distress for clients (Box 28–1). Table 28–1 lists health beliefs and nursing implications for some Canadian religious groups. However, it is important to remember that clients have varying degrees of adherence to their religious traditions, and many clients choose their practices from a number of different traditions, and so it is important to discern what is relevant to the client.

A key to success is to conduct an ongoing assessment over the course of the client's stay in the health care setting. Establish trust and rapport, and make the opportunity to conduct meaningful conversations with clients a priority. One way to understand a client's spirituality is to ask direct questions (Box 28–2). This approach requires you to feel comfortable asking clients about spirituality and to be able to discern which questions might be appropriate, depending on a client's circumstances. For example, asking questions about life satisfaction and meaning may not be appropriate during the acute phase of an illness. You must also be sensitive about whether clients would consider such questions inappropriate or intrusive from health care professionals.

Many spiritual assessment tools are available to help nurses clarify values and assess spirituality (Elkins & Cavendish, 2004). The BELIEF assessment tool helps pediatric nurses evaluate the child and family's spiritual and religious needs (McEvoy, 2003). The acronym stands for the following:

B: belief system
E: ethics or values
L: lifestyle
I: involvement in a spiritual community
E: education
F: future events

The Spiritual Well-Being Scale has 20 items that assess the individual's view of life and relationship with a higher power (Gray, 2006). The Spiritual Perspective Scale is a 10-item tool that was developed by a nurse. It measures connectedness to a higher power, others, and self (Gray, 2006). The JAREL Spiritual Well-Being Scale also provides nurses and other health care professionals with a simple tool for assessing a client's spiritual well-being (Hungelmann et al., 1996). Items in the JAREL tool reflect three key dimensions: faith and belief, life and self-responsibility, and life satisfaction and self-actualization. Spiritual tools such as the BELIEF tool and the Spiritual Well-Being Scale are easy to use and help nurses remember important areas to assess. Responses to assessment tools often reveal areas that need further investigation. For example, if after using an assessment tool you find that a client is involved in a spiritual community, you must spend

➤ TABLE 28-1 Religious Beliefs About Health

Religious or Cultural Background	Possible Health Care Beliefs and Practices	Nursing Implications
Hinduism	Modern medical science is accepted. Illness is caused by past sins. Holy Days are celebrated with fasting, prayer, and feasting.	Privacy is needed for prayer and meditation. Modesty in clothing is important, and hospital gowns may be considered indecent; same-sex caregivers are preferred. Important sacraments are associated with birth, naming, puberty, and death. Religious symbols should not be removed.
Sikhism	Modern medical science is accepted. Baptized and nonbaptized Sikhs have different religious requirements.	Prayers are said twice a day; privacy is preferred. Modesty in clothing is important, and hospital gowns may be considered indecent; same-sex caregivers are preferred. Religious symbols include uncut hair, comb, steel bracelet, symbolic dagger, undershorts, and turban; these should not be removed. Cleanliness during eating and prayers is important.
Buddhism	Modern medical science is accepted. Understanding, rather than belief, is emphasized. Dharma, the law of nature, teaches that life is impermanent and all people have to age and die. Death is usually accepted as the last stage of life, and withdrawal of life support may be permitted. Buddhists may believe in rebirth after death.	Treatment may be refused on Holy Days. Prayers usually occur five times daily. Privacy is needed for meditation. The client may want a Buddhist monk in attendance for spiritual support.
Islam	Muslims must be able to practise the Five Pillars of Islam. Muslims may have a fatalistic view of health. Faith healing is used. Withdrawal of life support may be permitted. Autopsies are generally forbidden.	Prayers are said five times per day, facing toward Mecca. Privacy is important. Fasting may occur on Holy Days. Modesty in clothing is important, and hospital gowns are considered indecent; same-sex caregivers are required.
Judaism	Jews believe in the sanctity of life. God and medicine must have a balance. Observance of the Sabbath is important.	Prayers are said three times per day; men may wear prayer shawl and skull cap. Treatment may be refused on the Sabbath.
Christianity	Modern medical science is accepted. Many Christians follow complementary alternative medicine (see Chapter 35). Prayer and faith healing are used; some Christians use laying on of hands.	Times of prayer vary between individuals; privacy is preferred. Sacraments of Holy Communion and the Anointing of the Sick may be practised. Religious symbols may include cross and prayer beads.
Hutterites	Modern science is accepted. About 80% of Hutterites seek alternative therapies. All things are shared communally. Hutterites live on colonies to help avoid earthly distractions that impede spiritual practice and devotion. Praying for good health is not appropriate; rather, prayers may be for wisdom to live a healthy life or bear suffering without complaint. Created order is God over man, man above woman, elder adult above younger adult, and parent over child.	Education about health is appreciated. Straightforward discussions are preferred. Health professionals are respected. Families expect to be involved in health care discussions. Decision-making processes about what health concerns are important for the colony are made by the leaders. Individual decisions regarding medical treatment may be made in consultation with other members of the colony.
Ojibway (Anishinabe)	Central value is that everything belongs to everyone in extended family. Health is a spiritual experience. Disease and illness may be caused by soul loss or spiritual intrusion.	Families generally want to be involved in health care decisions and may wish to stay with the ill individual. They desire to get to know the nurse before sharing problems. They may use Western medicine blended with traditional healing practices (Davidhizar & Giger, 1998; Griffith, 1996).

> **BOX 28-2 Nursing Assessment Questions**
>
> **Spirituality and Spiritual Health**
> - Is spirituality important to you?
> - What aspects of your spirituality have been most helpful to you?
> - What aspects of your spirituality would you like to discuss?
>
> **Faith, Belief, Fellowship, and Community**
> - To what or to whom do you look as a source of strength, hope, or faith in times of difficulty?
> - How does your faith help you cope?
> - Do you use prayer?
> - What can I do to support your religious beliefs or faith commitment?
> - What gives your life meaning?
>
> **Life and Self-Responsibility**
> - How do you feel about the changes this illness has caused?
> - How do these changes affect what you now need to do?
>
> **Life Satisfaction**
> - How happy or satisfied are you with your life?
> - What accomplishments help you feel satisfied with your life?
>
> **Connectedness**
> - What feelings do you have after you pray?
> - Who do you feel is the most important person to you?
>
> **Vocation**
> - How has your illness affected the way you live your life spiritually, at home, or where you work?
> - In what way has your illness affected your ability to express what is important in life to you?

time understanding whether and how the client would like the spiritual community to be involved in the plan of care. Regardless of whether you use an assessment tool or direct an assessment with questions that are based on principles of spirituality, it is important not to impose personal value systems on the client. This is particularly true when the client's values and beliefs are similar to yours because it then becomes easy to make false assumptions. When you understand the overall approach to spiritual assessment, you are able to enter into thoughtful discussion with clients, gain a greater awareness of personal resources that clients bring to a situation, and incorporate the resources into an effective plan of care.

Faith and Belief

Assess the source of authority and guidance that a client uses in life to choose and act on his or her beliefs. Determine whether the client has a religious source of guidance that conflicts with medical treatment plans. This may affect the options that nurses and other health care professionals are able to offer clients. For example, if a client is a Jehovah's Witness, blood products are not an acceptable form of treatment. Christian Scientists often refuse any medical intervention, believing that their faith will heal them. It is also important to understand a client's religious philosophy of life (Semenic et al., 2004; see Box 28–2). Assessment data reveal the basis of the client's belief system with regard to meaning and purpose in life and the client's spiritual focus. This information often reflects the effect that illness, loss, or diability has on the person's life. For example, a client who believes that all circumstances are determined by God might experience illness quite differently than someone who believes that circumstances are random or based on "luck." Religious diversity is considerable in Canada. A client's religious faith and practices, views about health, and the response to illness often influence how nurses provide support (see Table 28–1).

Life and Self-Responsibility

Spiritual well-being includes response to life changes and self-responsibility. Individuals who accept change in life, make decisions about their lives, and are able to forgive others in times of difficulty may have high levels of spiritual well-being. During illness, many clients struggle with accepting limitations or not knowing how to regain a functional and meaningful life. In these situations, clients may use their spirituality as a resource as they adapt to changes and seek solutions to deal with limitations. Assess the extent to which a client understands the limitations or threats posed by an illness and the manner in which the client chooses to adjust to them.

Connectedness

People who are connected to themselves, others, nature, and God or another supreme being may have enhanced capacity to cope with the stress brought on by crisis and chronic illness (Narayanasamy, 2004). Clients remain connected with God, Allah, or another higher being by praying. Prayer is personal communication with one's god. In many cases, it provides a sense of hope, strength, and security, and it is a part of faith (Cavendish et al., 2004). Help clients become or remain connected by respecting each client's unique sense of spirituality.

Life Satisfaction

Spiritual well-being is tied to a person's satisfaction with life and what he or she has accomplished (Krebs, 2003). In assessing a client's satisfaction with life, you may obtain insight into appropriate nursing care. When people are satisfied with life, they have more energy to deal with new difficulties and to resolve problems. Closely tied to life satisfaction is a sense of purpose. For many individuals, spirituality provides a sense of purpose that endures despite circumstances of illness and loss.

Culture

Spirituality is a personal experience within a cultural context (Pincharoen & Congdon, 2003). It is important to know a client's culture of origin and to assess a client's values. Remaining connected with their cultural heritage often helps clients define their place in the world and express their spirituality. Asking clients about their faith and belief systems is a good beginning for understanding the relationship between culture and spirituality (Box 28–3).

Fellowship and Community

Fellowship is a type of relationship an individual has with other persons (e.g., family, close friends, fellow members of a religious community, or neighbours). Explore the extent and nature of the client's support networks. It is unwise to assume that a given network offers the kind of support a client desires. For example, calling the client's

BOX 28-3 RESEARCH HIGHLIGHT

Spiritual and Cultural Dimensions of Childbirth for Canadian Orthodox Jewish Women

Research Focus

Giving birth is a pivotal and life-changing event. A woman's perception of her childbirth experience is influenced by culture. Religious faith or spiritual belief lends perspective to the meaning of significant life experiences. Little is known about the spiritual and cultural meanings of giving birth.

Research Abstract

The purpose of Semenic et al.'s (2004) study was to understand the meaning of the childbirth experience to Canadian Orthodox Jewish women. Interviews were conducted with 30 Orthodox Jewish women who had given birth within the preceding 2 weeks to healthy full-term newborns at a Montreal Jewish hospital. Five themes reflecting spiritual and cultural dimensions of childbirth were identified: (1) birth as a significant life event, (2) birth as a bittersweet paradox, (3) the spiritual dimensions of giving birth, (4) the importance of obedience to rabbinical law, and (5) a sense of support and affirmation.

When speaking of their childbirth experiences, these women spoke of awe, reverence, purpose in the creation of a new life, and the meaning of birth as an integral part of the spiritual dimension of their lives. Meaning was created as women obeyed rabbinical law when bearing a child. Obedience to the laws of purity and modesty were foundational to family life. It was important to observe the Sabbath and other religious holidays even while hospitalized, and to maintain the ancient rituals of naming and circumcision.

Evidence-Informed Practice

- Appreciate the central role of motherhood to an Orthodox Jewish woman.
- Within the framework of rabbinical law, spirituality is infused into every aspect of daily lives.
- Women may request head covering or extra gowns to preserve modesty.
- A visit from extended family is considered a *mitzvah,* or good deed.
- One of the ways to allow mothers to observe the Sabbath might be for the nurse to diaper or bathe newborns.
- An amulet or prayer card might be used to keep the newborn safe from harm.
- Commercial cow milk-based formula is not kosher; ensure availability of soy formula if the mother chooses not to breastfeed.
- A newborn boy will be circumcised in an important religious ceremony on the eighth day after birth.
- Family may be reluctant to reveal the newborn's intended name (e.g., for the birth certificate) until after the naming ceremony.

References: Semenic, S. E., Callister, L. C., & Feldman, P. (2004). Giving birth: The voices of Orthodox Jewish women living in Canada. *Journal of Obstetric, Gynecologic, and Neonatal Nursing, 33*(1), 80–87.

religious advisor to request a visit is inappropriate if the client finds little fellowship with that person.

Ritual and Practice

By assessing the use of rituals and practices, you can understand a client's spirituality (Box 28–4). Rituals include participation in worship, prayer, participation in sacraments (e.g., baptism or communion), fasting, singing, meditating, reading religious works (e.g., the Torah, Quran, or New Testament), and making offerings or sacrifices. Different religions have different rituals for life events. For example, Buddhists practise baptism later in life and find burial or cremation acceptable at death. Muslims wash the body of a dead family member and wrap it in white cloth with the head turned toward the right shoulder. Orthodox and Conservative Jews circumcise their newborn sons 8 days after birth. Determine whether illness or hospitalization has interrupted a client's usual rituals or practices. A ritual often provides the client with structure and support during difficult times. If rituals are important to the client, account for them as part of nursing intervention.

Vocation

Individuals express their spirituality on a daily basis in life's routines, work, play, and relationships. Spirituality is often part of a person's identity and vocation in life (Skalla & McCoy, 2006). Determine whether illness or hospitalization alters the ability to express some aspect of spirituality as it relates to the person's work or daily activities. Expression of spirituality is highly individual and includes showing an appreciation for life in the variety of things people do, living in the moment and not worrying excessively about the future, appreciating nature, expressing love toward others, and being productive (McSherry et al., 2004). When illness or loss prevents clients from

BOX 28-4 CULTURAL ASPECTS OF CARE

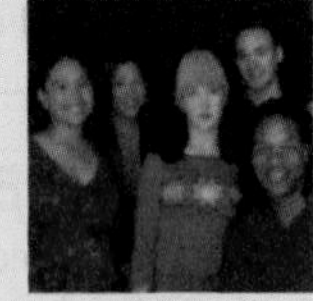

Spirituality should not be limited to a client's religious perspective; instead, it should include all of life. In caring for clients from different cultures, you must determine what is important in their lives and what provides them with inner strength and meaning. Clients are usually attempting to find meaning in the changing circumstances of their health and illness. Often spirituality and health are closely associated. For example, Chiu (2001) found that Chinese immigrant women with breast cancer used the following as spiritual resources: family; traditional Chinese values; art, prose, and literature; alternative therapy; Chinese support groups; and religion. Pincharoen and Congdon (2003) investigated how spirituality helped older Thai adults maintain health and found that finding harmony through a healthy mind and body was critical.

Implications for Practice

- Explore spirituality of clients from different cultures by assessing the meaning of health and how clients achieve balance, stability, peace, or comfort in their lives.
- Offer a universal and holistic approach to assessing clients' needs by demonstrating caring and using therapeutic communication techniques.
- Promote an environment during assessment in which human rights, values, customs, and spiritual beliefs are respected.
- Include appropriate spiritual care providers in the assessment process.
- Avoid use of language that alienates clients or discriminates between different religions (e.g., asking whether the client wants someone from his or her "faith community" to visit, rather than "temple," "church," or "synagogue").

expressing their spirituality in these ways, you need to understand the psychological, social, and spiritual implications and to provide the appropriate guidance and support.

Client Expectations

It is important to include in any client assessment a review of the clients' expectations for their health care. You and your client explore what the client expects of caregivers and what he or she hopes to gain. You should not anticipate a client's expectations. Your assumptions about a client's needs may have nothing to do with what the client actually expects or wants. Assessing client expectations requires you to ask questions such as "What do you hope we will be able to do for you?" or "Your expectations are important to us; how can we make your care most satisfactory?" During times of loss or crisis, the client might simply desire a trusting and open relationship with you. It might also be important that the client perceive caregivers to be accepting of his or her religious rituals. By asking clients what they expect of caregivers and then meeting those expectations, you can help establish a strong relationship.

❖Planning

During the planning step of the nursing process, you develop a plan of care for each of the concerns identified in the assessment. When selecting the most appropriate nursing interventions, you must reflect on previous experience and apply knowledge and critical thinking (Figure 28–5). Prior experience in selecting interventions that support clients' spiritual well-being is invaluable when you consider the best options for clients with similar types of situations or problems. To develop an individualized plan of care, you also integrate the knowledge gathered from assessment and knowledge of resources and therapies available for spiritual care (Box 28–5). You match the client's needs with interventions that are supported and recommended in the clinical and research literature.

Confidence becomes an important critical thinking quality as you attempt to build a caring relationship with the client. Confidence works to build trust, enabling you and your client to enter into a healing relationship together. Attempting to meet or support clients' spiritual needs is not simple, and many new nurses must accept the fact that additional resources may be needed. Your skills in helping clients interpret and understand the meaning of illness and loss, for example, may be limited. Because spiritual care is so personal, standards of autonomy and self-determination are critical in supporting the client's decisions about the plan of care.

Goals and Outcomes

A care plan usually includes realistic and individualized goals along with relevant outcomes. With spiritual care, however, devising a care plan is challenging. Human experience is complex, and it is unrealistic to set plans and time frames around goals such as finding acceptance, peace, meaning, or connections. These are often lifelong pursuits that extend beyond the time-limited nature of the nurse–client relationship. It is more appropriate to set limited, short-term goals that are based on the client's expressed desires. To set these goals, you need to know the client well. For example, a client may be estranged from a family member and express a desire for reconciliation or forgiveness. An appropriate goal would be to achieve contact with the family member, but it may be unrealistic to set a goal of harmonious connection, even though that would be the ultimate hope. This is an example of a situation in which the phenomenology of human experience is not easily adapted to a problem-solving process. Setting unrealistic, time-limited goals could be experienced as coercive in the context of spiritual care.

Setting Priorities

Spiritual health is closely tied to physical and psychological well-being. When a client is in acute distress, you focus your care on the relief of symptoms to provide the client with a sense of control. Then you support the client's efforts to express the emotional and intellectual aspects of his or her spirituality. When a client has a chronic or terminal condition, your priorities may shift to helping the client deal with unresolved losses and to connect with the spiritual resources available. You need to reinforce the everyday life patterns that the client uses to maintain coherence and practise individuation.

Continuity of Care

Significant others, such as spouses, siblings, parents, and friends, need to be involved in the client's care, as appropriate. You learn from the assessment which individuals or groups have formed a relationship with the client. These individuals may become involved in all levels of your plan. The client's support network may assist in giving physical care, providing emotional comfort, and sharing spiritual support.

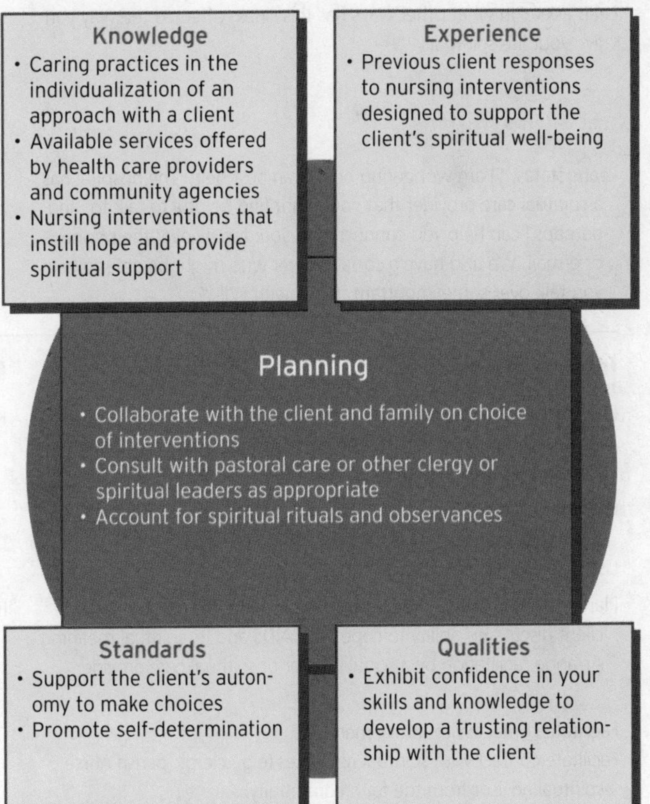

Figure 28-5 Critical thinking model for spiritual health planning.

In a hospital setting, one of the best resources to use in planning a client's spiritual care is the hospital's spiritual care department. A spiritual care provider in a health care setting has special expertise in dealing with the spiritual problems confronted by clients. These professionals should be part of the health care team, lending insight about how and when to best support clients and families.

➤ BOX 28-5 NURSING CARE PLAN

Spiritual Distress

Assessment

James, a 24-year-old, has recently received a diagnosis of AIDS and has been hospitalized. The nurse, Leah, has been talking with James and has discovered that spirituality is important to him. During that time, James has expressed a fear of dying. His partner, Will, visits James much less often now than he did before the diagnosis. Leah now talks with James in a private area with the purpose of gaining a deeper understanding of how his illness is affecting his spirituality.

Assessment Activities	***Findings and Defining Characteristics***
Leah asks James, "How has your illness affected your own source of strength or hope?"	James responds, "I don't believe this is happening to me. How can God do this to me? I have moments when I just feel so angry. What is going to happen to me?"
Leah responds, "This is obviously a very difficult time. Who in your life provides you the greatest source of support?"	James begins to cry and admits, "I feel so alone. Will has just not been there when I need him. My family wants to help, but they live out of town."
Leah clarifies, "You sound as though it would help to have someone to talk to."	James responds, "It would, but it is so hard to find someone I can trust and who will listen."
Leah questions, "You mentioned you could not understand why God has done this to you. How has this experience affected your faith and beliefs?"	James responds, "It has been hard. I have never been a religious person. My church does not accept homosexuality, but I always have had a faith in God. Will and I have attended a new ecumenical service at the local college. I have not been attending lately, and I miss that."
Leah asks, "In what other ways has this illness affected the way you live your life spiritually?"	James responds, "Well I have always been active in an HIV support group trying to help others with their illness. It provides a real sense of purpose for me, but I can't do that while I'm in here. This whole diagnosis has really shaken me up. I used to be able to pray, but now it just feels like talking to the wall."
Leahs states, "I am wondering how I can best help. The hospital has a spiritual care provider that you might find helpful to talk to, and perhaps I can help you connect with your family over the phone or e-mail. We also have a social worker who might be able to help you talk over some important things with Will."	James responds, "I would really appreciate that. But, can you do one more thing for me right now? Can you pray for me?"

Interventions	**Rationale**
Plan instructional session to discuss typical course of AIDS, emphasizing the typical pattern of remissions with drug therapy. Review therapies available for treatment.	Knowledge about disease will help client think as a person living with AIDS rather than dying with AIDS (Hall, 1998). Understanding how to manage disease course will help instill hope.
Encourage client's expression of loneliness through establishing a caring presence. Listen to client's feelings and concerns.	"Presencing" reflects being in tune with the client and displays caring. It is an effective technique that makes a topic of discussion more approachable (Benner & Wrubel, 1989).
Plan discussion session with client that includes his partner. Have client discuss his ability to cope with AIDS and its spiritual meaning. Arrange facilitation by a social worker or spiritual care provider.	People question and become amenable to discovering their unique spiritual meaning after a crisis that threatens health (Hall, 1998). It is important to ensure referral to a health care professional who has expertise in spiritual counselling.
Facilitate contact with family members. Facilitate contact with spiritual resources (e.g., clergy, parish nurse, spiritual advisor from the faith community).	Connections with a support system can enable client to find meaning in illness and can offer sources of hope.
Consider praying with or for James.	Prayer may be an appropriate intervention if specifically requested by the client. It is important for the nurse to be authentic (Taylor, 2003b). If the nurse does not believe in prayer, it may be more appropriate to offer to be present and listen while James prays.

If the client participates in a formal religion, members of the clergy, parish nurses, or members of the church, temple, mosque, or synagogue may need to be involved in the plan of care. Depending on the client's health status and needs, part of the plan will involve a continuation of appropriate religious rituals. You must make sure that any icons or religious materials, such as scriptures or a prayer book, are made available.

❖Implementation

To provide spiritual care, you must be able to establish a caring relationship with a client. Spiritual care interventions need not be time-consuming. Partnering with clients helps you determine the most appropriate and effective interventions, which may include touch, rest, nature, reminiscence, imagery, and humour (Meyerhoff et al., 2002). You and the client discover together the meaning that illness or loss poses for the client and the effect that it has on the meaning and purpose of life. Achieving this level of understanding with a client enables you to provide care in a sensitive, creative, and appropriate manner (Box 28–6).

Health Promotion

Spiritual care should be a central theme in promoting an individual's overall well-being. In settings where health promotion activities occur, clients are often in need of information, counselling, and guidance to make the necessary choices to remain healthy. Nurses providing primary health care can contribute to clients' spiritual well-being partly by establishing a positive presence (Box 28–7). They can also support a healing relationship through a variety of methods.

Supporting a Healing Relationship. A nurse looks beyond health problems and recognizes a client's broader needs. For example, you do not just treat a client's back pain; you also consider how the pain influences ability to function and achieve goals. A **holistic** view enables you to establish a helping role and a healing relationship. Three factors are evident when a healing relationship develops between nurse and client:

- Mobilizing hope for you, as well as for the client.
- Finding an interpretation or understanding of the illness, pain, anxiety, or other stressful emotion that is acceptable to the client.
- Assisting the client in using social, emotional, and spiritual resources (Benner, 1984).

Hope motivates people with strategies to face challenges in life. You can help a client find things to hope for. For example, a client with newly diagnosed diabetes might hope to learn how to manage the disease so as to continue a productive and satisfying way of life. Hope helps a client work toward recovery. To help clients achieve hope, you and the client work together to find an explanation of the situation. Then you help the client realistically exercise hope. This help might include supporting a client's positive attitude toward life or a desire to be informed and to make decisions.

To further support a healing relationship, you must remain aware of the client's spiritual resources and needs. It is always important for clients to express their beliefs and find spiritual comfort. When life stressors or illness create confusion or uncertainty for the client, you must recognize the possible effect on a client's health. How can spiritual resources be used and strengthened? You may begin by encouraging a client to discuss the effect that illness has had on personal beliefs and faith. This discussion gives you the chance to clarify any misconceptions or inaccuracies in information about their illness. A clear sense of how illness may affect an individual's life helps the person apply all resources toward recovery.

Acute Care. Within acute care settings, clients experience multiple stressors that threaten their sense of control. Support and enhancement of a client's spiritual well-being can be a challenge when

BOX 28-6 CASE STUDY

Spiritual Nursing Interventions

Case Study Focus

In this case study, Meyerhoff et al. (2002) described spiritual health interventions used by Canadian public health nurses to help a family confronted with a loss of meaning precipitated by the diagnosis of a child's chronic condition. These health interventions continued through the boy's childhood and adolescence.

The Perez Family

After their son Michael's lack of language development, unpredictability, erratic behaviour, and repetitive rocking movements prompted a diagnosis of autism, Marie and Edwin felt overwhelmed by emotional stress. They struggled to find meaning in their lives and in the life of their son, while experiencing a loss of hopes and dreams for a "normal" son.

Spiritual Interventions

Communication. When Michael's diagnosis was confirmed, the public health nurse focused on establishing a relationship with the family. Communication facilitated the processing of feelings and responses to the loss of hopes and dreams as the family struggled to find meaning in the presence of unwelcome challenges. Marie needed to express how tired she felt and occasionally questioned why this burden had been imposed on her family. Edwin needed solitude to cope with intense feelings, but this made Marie feel that he was withdrawing. The nurse suggested Edwin write down his feelings in a journal, which he found helpful.

Connectedness. The nurse helped the family identify and nurture significant relationships. The family identified significant family members, close friends, and members of their faith community, and asked them to meet as a group. At the first meeting, Marie and Edwin asked whether the group would be willing to provide support and counselling. Everyone agreed, and the group met weekly for 15 years. Marie and Edwin also nurtured connectedness with God by attending spiritual retreats, practising prayer, and partnering with a spiritual director.

Bibliotherapy. Bibliotherapy is the use of book reading to provide healing, enhance the expression of feelings, and gain insight. Through reading, the Perez family gained new information about families who cope with illness. The nurse encouraged Edwin, Marie, and Michael's sister, Mary, to compare their situation with those in the books and to write a new ending for one of the experiences. This exercise allowed the Perez family to reflect on changes they could make living with a child with a developmental disability a more positive experience.

Music Therapy. The healing power of music has long been established, even though music therapy as a spiritual intervention is new in the field of nursing. The nurse suggested a referral to a music therapist, who used and taught a variety of music styles to engage and calm Michael. Edwin and Marie also listened to tranquil music to relieve their own spiritual distress.

Prayer. Marie and Edwin prayed for their son's health and for strength for themselves. Other family and friends prayed for ongoing support. The Perez family said they could "feel" the prayers of others. They felt that God heard their prayers of petition, and they trusted God with Michael's future.

From Meyerhoff, H., Van Hofwegen, L., Harwood, C., Drury, M. & Emblen, J. (2002). Spiritual nursing interventions. *Canadian Nurse, 98*(3), 21–24.

BOX 28-7 FOCUS ON PRIMARY HEALTH CARE

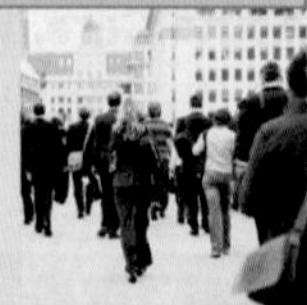

Establishing Presence

Clients have reported that the presence of nurses and their caregiving activities contribute to a sense of well-being and provide hope for recovery (Clark et al., 1991). Behaviours that establish the nurse's presence include giving attention, answering questions, listening, and having a positive and encouraging (but realistic) attitude. The ability to establish presence is part of the art of nursing. Establishing presence is not simply about being in the same room with a client while performing procedures or sharing information. Being present (or "presencing") involves "being with" a client, as opposed to "doing for" a client (Benner, 1984). It also involves offering a closeness with the client: physically, psychologically, and spiritually.

When health promotion is the focus of care, your presence becomes important in instilling confidence in clients' abilities to take the steps necessary to remain healthy. Research findings have shown that the best way to convey a caring presence is to listen to the client (Emblen & Halstead, 1993). Other ways include involving family in discussions about clients' health, displaying self-confidence when providing health instruction, and supporting clients' confidence in the choices they make. The client who seeks health care may be fearful of experiencing an illness that would threaten loss of control and looks for someone to offer competent direction. Your encouraging words of support and your calm and decisive approach establish a presence that builds trust and well-being (see Chapter 19).

the focus of health care seems to be one of treatment and cure rather than care. You work closely with clients and their support networks in finding ways to make spiritual resources part of the plan of care.

Support Systems. Use of support systems is important in any health care setting. Support systems provide clients with the greatest sense of well-being during hospitalization and serve as a human link connecting the client, you, and the client's pre-illness lifestyle (Clark et al., 1991). Part of the client's caregiving environment is the regular presence of supportive family and friends. You plan care with the client and the client's support network to promote the interpersonal bonding that is needed for recovery. The support system is a source of faith and hope, and it can be an important resource in conducting the religious rituals on which some clients rely.

When it is known that clients depend on family and friends for support, you encourage them to visit the client regularly. Often, illness and the treatment environment intimidate family members and friends. You help family members feel welcome and encourage them to act naturally during visits. Their support and presence can be used to promote healing. Encouraging the family to bring meaningful religious symbols to the client's bedside can offer significant spiritual support.

Another important resource to clients is spiritual advisors and members of the clergy. Many hospitals have spiritual care departments that assist in notifying community clergy of their congregants' admission or who can provide trained clergy for support. In addition, some congregations have parish nurses who provide hospitalized congregants with spiritual support. *Parish nurses* are registered nurses with specialized knowledge who are "called to ministry and affirmed by a faith community to promote health, healing and wholeness" (Canadian Association for Parish Nursing Ministry, 2008). Spiritual care providers, including parish nurses, are expert at giving attention to how an illness influences a person's beliefs and how beliefs can influence illness and recovery. You should ask whether clients desire to have a member of the clergy or a parish nurse visit during their hospitalization. All spiritual care providers should be made welcome on nursing units. A client or family may request that you keep pastoral care providers informed of any physical, psychosocial, or spiritual concerns affecting the client. You show respect for clients' spiritual values and needs by willingly cooperating with people who give spiritual care and by facilitating the administration of sacraments, rites, and rituals.

Providing privacy for the client, family, and spiritual care providers is a thoughtful and sensitive gesture. You determine the proper routine in a client's religion by asking the clergy, family, or client. Often a client within the hospital may want to discuss spiritual concerns in the evening or late at night, when support services such as clergy and social services are unavailable. You can help meet the client's needs through careful, skilled, and active listening.

Diet Therapies. Food and nutrition are important aspects of client care and often an important component of some religious observances (Table 28–2). Food and the rituals surrounding the preparation and serving of food can be important to a person's spirituality. You can consult with a dietitian to integrate the client's dietary preferences into daily care. In the event that an agency cannot prepare food in the preferred way, the family may be asked to bring meals that accommodate dietary restrictions.

Supporting Rituals. Nurses provide spiritual care by supporting clients' participation in spiritual rituals and activities. This support is especially important for older adults, who typically perceive themselves as highly spiritual (Isaia et al., 1999; Box 28–8). Personal care of the client should be planned to allow time for religious readings, visits by spiritual advisors, or attendance at religious services. Some churches and synagogues offer audiotapes of their services for those members who cannot attend in person. Family members can plan a prayer session or an organized reading of religious material on a regular basis. Arrangements may need to be made with spiritual care staff for the client and family to receive the sacraments. Clergy will routinely offer to make home visits for people unable to attend religious services. Taped meditations, classical or religious music, and televised religious services are other options. You should be respectful of icons, medals, prayer rugs, or crosses that clients bring to a health setting; be sure that they are not accidentally lost, damaged, or misplaced.

Restorative and Continuing Care.

For clients who are recovering from a long-term illness or disability or who suffer chronic or terminal disease, spiritual care becomes especially important. Many of the nursing interventions applicable in health promotion and acute care are applicable to this level of health care as well.

Prayer. The act of prayer gives an individual the opportunity to renew personal faith and belief in a higher being in a specific, focused way that may be highly ritualized and formal or quite spontaneous and informal. Prayer may be an effective coping resource for physical and psychological symptoms. Clients may pray in private or pursue opportunities for group prayer with family, friends, or clergy. You can be supportive of prayer by giving the client privacy if desired, by learning whether the client wishes to have you participate, and by suggesting prayer when it is known to be a coping resource for the client. If prayer is not suitable for a client, an alternative may be to read from a book (e.g., the Bible or the Quran) selected by the client or from poetry or other inspirational texts.

Supporting Grief Work. Clients who experience terminal illness or who have been recently disabled by disease or injury require your support in grieving over and coping with their loss (see Chapter 29). Supporting a client during times of grief can be enhanced by a spiritual relationship with the client.

➤ TABLE 28-2 Religious Dietary Regulations Affecting Health Care

Religion	Dietary Practices
Hinduism	Some sects are vegetarians. These sects believe in not killing any living creature.
Buddhism	Some Buddhists are vegetarians, and many do not use alcohol or tobacco and may hesitate to use medications. Many fast on Holy Days.
Islam	Islam prohibits consumption of pork and alcohol. Fasting takes place during the month of Ramadan.
Judaism	Some Jews observe the kosher dietary restrictions of avoiding pork, avoiding shellfish, and not preparing and eating milk and meat at the same time.
Christianity	Some Baptists, Evangelicals, and Pentecostals discourage the use of alcohol, caffeine, and tobacco. Some Roman Catholics may fast during Lent, Ash Wednesday, Good Friday, and 1 hour before receiving Communion.
Jehovah's Witnesses	Members may avoid food prepared with or containing blood.
Mormonism	Members abstain from alcohol, caffeine, and tobacco.
Russian Orthodox Church	Followers must observe fast days as well as a "no meat" rule on Wednesdays and Fridays. During Lent, all animal products, including dairy products and butter, are forbidden.
First Nations	Food practices are influenced by individual nations' beliefs.

BOX 28-8 FOCUS ON OLDER ADULTS

- An older adult's spirituality is associated with ability to adjust or cope with illness (Ebersole et al., 2004).
- Religious activities and spiritual experiences are common among older adults. Those who experience spiritual well-being have strong social support, better emotional health, and, to some extent, improved physical health (Koenig et al., 2004).
- Respecting privacy and dignity is an essential part of nursing care, especially in meeting the spiritual needs of the older adult (Narayanasamy et al., 2004).
- Older adults use a variety of strategies such as spiritual rituals, exercise, and complementary medicine to cope with pain and chronic illness, including religious activities and meditation. These activities positively enhance coping and feelings of peace (Barry et al., 2004; Lindberg, 2005).
- Feelings of connectedness are important for older adults. Enhance connectedness by helping older clients find meaning and purpose in life, by listening actively to their concerns, and by being present (Narayanasamy et al., 2004).
- Beliefs in the afterlife increase as adults grow older. Enable visits from clergy, social workers, lawyers, and financial advisors so that clients feel as though they can complete all unfinished business. Leaving a legacy to loved ones prepares older adults to leave the world with a sense of meaning (Ebersole et al., 2004). Legacies include oral histories, works of art, publications, photographs, or other objects of significance.
- Older adult caregivers, such as those caring for a person with Alzheimer's dementia, often use their spirituality and spiritual behaviours or practices to help them deal with crisis and conflict (Spurlock, 2005).
- Spiritual beliefs and practices may also help caregivers cope and find a sense of peace (Sawatzky & Fowler-Kerry, 2003).

❖Evaluation

The evaluation of a client's spiritual care requires you to think critically about spiritual health outcomes. You must consider spiritual concepts and stress and adaptation theory (see Chapter 30) in evaluating whether the client has been able to adjust to factors that threaten spiritual health. However, spiritual health outcomes are not easily evaluated, particularly in the short term. In addition, an ethic of caring ensures that you evaluate any ethical concerns that may arise in the course of the client's spiritual care and support. Your evaluation includes a review of the client's response to care and determining whether the client's expectations were achieved.

Client Care

Attainment of spiritual health is a lifelong goal. Clients experience the need to clarify values, reshape philosophies, strengthen relationships, and live experiences that help to shape their purpose in life. You provide spiritual care with an understanding that many interventions may not easily be evaluated. Relying on the patient's subjective evaluation is a central part of care. For example, if in your assessment you find that the client is losing hope, the follow-up evaluation involves a discussion with the client to determine whether the client has regained a purpose for living. Family and friends can also be a useful source of evaluative information. Successful outcomes may include an increased or restored sense of connectedness with significant others, family, or the faith community, or a combination of these;

maintaining, renewing, or reforming a sense of purpose in life; and, for some, establishing or renewing a confidence and trust in God, a supreme being, or a higher power.

For clients with a serious or terminal illness, evaluation may focus on the goal of helping the client retain faith and hope or openly express life's uncertainties. You evaluate how clients are accepting their illness and whether hope has enabled them to recognize their mortality and focus on living for each day. Fryback (1993) found that the terminally ill clients in their study, regardless of whether they followed a formal religion, held a belief in a higher power, which gave them a sense that God was with them and they were not alone. You must not assume that all clients have such faith. However, your aim is to help clients accept their destiny and to be at peace.

Client Expectations

You must evaluate whether client expectations were met. In regard to spiritual care, this involves evaluating whether the client's spiritual practices were respected and whether the nurse–client relationship was one of caring and support. Both the client and family should be able to relate whether opportunities were offered for religious rituals. With regard to the nurse–client relationship, does the client express trust and confidence in you? Is the client able to discuss important issues or topics? Is the client comfortable in expressing spiritual needs with you? Ask the client to reflect on the quality of the nurse–client relationship. The response to the question "Do you feel your expectations of me in supporting your spiritual needs were met?" helps you determine whether an effective healing relationship was developed.

* KEY CONCEPTS

- Nurses must develop a caring relationship to understand clients' spirituality.
- Spirituality may have beneficial health outcomes.
- Canadian nursing practice has a rich spiritual heritage that has influenced contemporary practice.
- Nursing theories can guide nurses in providing spiritual care.
- Spirituality is highly personal and unique to each individual.
- Faith is a relationship with God or a higher power or authority that enables action and gives purpose and meaning to an individual's life.
- Religion is a system of organized beliefs and worship that a person practises to express spirituality outwardly.
- Hope provides comfort and a motivation to achieve when a person is faced with a loss.
- When clients experience acute or chronic illness or a terminal disease, either spiritual resources help a person recover or spiritual concerns develop.
- Common religious rituals include private worship, prayer, singing, use of a rosary, and reading religious texts.
- A spiritual assessment is most successful when you apply knowledge that pertains to therapeutic communication, principles of loss and grief, and knowledge of caring practices.
- The personal nature of spirituality requires open communication and the establishment of trust between nurse and client.
- If a client's religious beliefs conflict with medical treatment, nurses' and other health care professionals' options can be limited.
- An important part of spiritual assessment is learning which of the client's friends or family share a community of faith.
- A hospital's spiritual care department is a valuable resource to use in planning a client's spiritual care.
- Central to a healing relationship is mobilizing the client's hope.
- Part of a client's caregiving environment can be the regular presence of family, friends, parish nurses, or spiritual advisors.
- Depending on a client's religion, certain foods may be forbidden.
- Prayer may be an effective coping resource for physical and psychological symptoms.
- When evaluating spiritual care, successful outcomes may include an increased or restored sense of connectedness with significant others and maintaining, renewing, or reforming a sense of purpose in life.

* CRITICAL THINKING EXERCISES

1. Mr. Gadacz is a 40-year-old businessman with more than 100 employees. A 12-hour workday is not unusual for him. He is married, has four teenaged children, and is solely responsible for providing financially for the family. Last evening, he was admitted to the cardiac care unit with severe chest pain resulting from a myocardial infarction (heart attack). He is now stabilized but frequently asks about his diagnostic tests and what he needs to do to be able to go home. He tells his nurse, "My doctor tells me I will need surgery once I am more stable. I hope he can do that soon. I just can't believe this is happening. I worry about what will happen to my business while I am gone and to my family if I can't keep my business going." He asks you, "Could I die from this?" You notice that Mr Gadacz has devotional literature at his bedside. How might you go about conducting a spiritual health assessment for Mr. Gadacz?
2. Tejal is a new graduate nurse caring for Ms. Rosenbaum for the first time. Ms. Rosenbaum is 27 years old and has recently received a diagnosis of uterine cancer. She is scheduled for an abdominal hysterectomy. Tejal notices from the patient chart that Ms. Rosenbaum has identified herself as Jewish. What factors might be important to consider in relation to Ms. Rosenbaum's spirituality or religion for the plan of care? How might Tejal determine which factors are relevant for Ms. Rosenbaum?
3. Critical thinking is an ongoing process. When you learn that you are assigned to care for Fangzhou Lin, you note that the Kardex information includes his religion (Buddhist) and his place of birth (Hong Kong). A colleague tells you he can speak some English. The client is 80 years old and reportedly has a hearing deficit. What knowledge might you wish to reflect on critically before beginning a spiritual assessment of this client?

* REVIEW QUESTIONS

1. Caring for a client's spiritual needs means
   1. You must have the same beliefs as the client
   2. Praying for the client
   3. Accepting the client's beliefs and experiences
   4. Calling for a religious leader if you determine a need
2. An individual who does not believe in the existence of God is an
   1. Agnostic
   2. Atheist
   3. Anarchist
   4. Agenic

3. Hope is a concept related to spirituality that can be best described as
   1. Satisfaction with someone or something
   2. Having a bond with another person for ongoing support
   3. Having confidence in something for which no proof exists
   4. Having something to live for and look forward to

4. Canadian Hutterites believe that suffering
   1. May be prevented through prayer
   2. May be caused by soul loss
   3. Is a public matter
   4. Is a burden to be borne without complaint

5. Clients' rituals and practice
   1. Have no place in modern medicine
   2. Have no place in the hospital
   3. Can get in the way of nursing care
   4. Provide structure and support for the client

6. Establishing presence is not simply being in the same room with a client; it also involves
   1. Offering a closeness with the client: physically, psychologically, and spiritually
   2. Performing procedures
   3. Sharing technical information with the client
   4. All team members

7. For Hindus, it is important to consider that
   1. Some sects are vegetarian
   2. Followers must observe fast days
   3. Many individuals avoid meats containing blood
   4. Members abstain from alcohol and caffeine

8. Jehovah's Witnesses may avoid
   1. Caffeine and chocolate
   2. Pork and shellfish
   3. Dairy products and caffeine
   4. Food prepared with or containing blood

9. Members of the Mormon faith
   1. Avoid pork and shellfish
   2. Avoid alcohol, caffeine, and tobacco
   3. Practise vegetarianism
   4. Do not eat milk and meat at the same time

10. Clients who experience terminal illness or who have suffered a recent disability because of a disease or injury can benefit from
    1. Grief work
    2. Diet therapy
    3. Acupuncture
    4. Values clarification

* RECOMMENDED WEB SITES

Canadian Association for Parish Nursing Ministry: http://www.capnm.ca
The Canadian Association for Parish Nursing Ministry is committed to the development of parish nursing as a health and ministry resource within Canada.

Center for Spirituality and Healing: http://www.csh.umn.edu
Established in 1995 at the University of Minnesota in the United States, the Center for Spirituality and Healing provides education about integrative medicine, combining biomedical, complementary, cross-cultural, and spiritual care.

Center for Spirituality, Theology and Health: http://www.dukespiritualityandhealth.org
The purpose of this center, which is part of Duke University in the United States, is to conduct research on the effects of spirituality on physical and mental health.

Nurses Christian Fellowship: http://ncf-jcn.org/ncfindex.html
Nurses Christian Fellowship, a US institution, is a Christian organization with the goal of integrating Christianity into nursing care. This Web site contains information about the scope and trend of research related to spiritual care. The Canadian chapter of Nurses Christian Fellowship can be found at http://www.ncfcanada.ca/

29

The Experience of Loss, Death, and Grief

Original chapter by Valerie Yancey, RN, PhD

Canadian content written by Jim Hunter, RN, BSN, MSN

objectives

Mastery of content in this chapter will enable you to:

- Define the key terms listed.
- Identify your role in assisting clients who have experienced loss, death, and grief.
- Describe and compare the phases of grieving from Kübler-Ross (1969), Bowlby (1980), and Worden (1991).
- List and discuss the five categories of loss.
- Describe the types of grief.
- Describe the characteristics of a person experiencing grief.
- Discuss variables that influence a person's response to grief.
- Develop a nursing care plan for a client or family experiencing loss and grief.
- Explain reasons for the need for improved end-of-life care for clients.
- Discuss principles of palliative care.
- Describe how to involve family members in palliative care.
- Describe the procedure for care of the body after death.
- Discuss your own loss experience when caring for dying clients.

key terms

Acceptance, p. 454
Actual loss, p. 453
Anger, p. 454
Anticipatory grief, p. 455
Bargaining, p. 454
Bereavement, p. 454
Denial, p. 454
Depression, p. 454
Disorganization and despair, p. 455
Grief, p. 454
Hope, p. 457
Hospice, p. 471
Maturational loss, p. 453
Necessary losses, p. 453
Numbing, p. 454
Palliative care, p. 467
Perceived loss, p. 453
Post-mortem care, p. 472
Reorganization, p. 455
Situational loss, p. 453
Yearning and searching, p. 454

media resources

evolve Web Site

- Audio Chapter Summaries
- Glossary
- Multiple-Choice Review Questions
- Student Learning Activities
- Weblinks

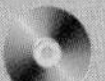

Companion CD

- Glossary
- Interactive Learning Activities
- Fluids and Electrolytes Tutorial
- Test-Taking Skills

Loss and grief are experiences that affect not only clients and their families, but the nurses who care for them as well. In Canada and other Western societies, palliative and end-of-life care has played a secondary role in health care because in the more dominant medical model, the focus is on cure (Allan et al., 2005). As a result, Canadians often deny death, as well as the need to express grief and to feel the pain associated with a loss, both of which are beneficial to healing. Grief affects survivors physically, psychologically, socially, and spiritually as a result of very real concrete and perceived losses. Death of a client, for example, leaves family, friends, and caregivers feeling powerless. Most nurses enter the profession with the intent of helping clients recover from illness, adjust to illness-related changes in lifestyle, and move toward health restoration. It is often frightening to learn that knowledge, skill, and technology do not always result in cure.

Your role in facilitating the grief process includes assisting survivors to feel the loss, express the loss, and complete the stages of the grief process. To be effective, you must have a thorough understanding of a client's loss, its significance and meaning to the client and family, and how it affects the client and family's ability to carry on. Providing care for clients in crisis from loss or during the end of life requires knowledge, caring, and compassion to help bring comfort to clients and families, even when a hope for cure is gone. Helping clients to a peaceful, dignified death is an important aspect of your nursing care. Although working with dying clients can be challenging, many nurses also find it to be a rewarding and often life-changing experience, both professionally and personally (Chochinov, 2006).

Scientific Knowledge Base

Loss

Throughout their lives, people form attachments and suffer losses. They develop independence from their parents, start and leave school, change friends, begin careers, and form relationships. The growing-up process is natural and positive, and yet as peoples' lives unfold, they suffer necessary losses (Hasler, 1996). **Necessary losses** are an integral part of each person's life. People expect their losses to be recovered and replaced by something different or better, but other losses cause an unbearable change in their sense of safety and security (Hasler, 1996). Losses such as death of a loved one, divorce, or loss of independence are significant and can have long-term effects on physical and psychological health.

Loss comes in many forms, depending on the values and priorities learned within a person's sphere of influence, which includes family, friends, society, and culture. A person experiences loss in the absence of an object, person, body part or function, emotion, or idea that was formerly present (Table 29–1). Losses may be actual or perceived. An **actual loss** is any loss of a person or object that can no longer be felt, heard, known, or experienced by the individual. Examples could include the loss of a body part, a child, a relationship, or a role at work. Lost objects that have been valued by a client include any possession that is worn out, misplaced, stolen, or ruined. For example, a child may grieve over the loss of a favourite toy. A **perceived loss** is any loss that is defined uniquely by the grieving client. It may be less obvious to others. An example is the loss of confidence or prestige. Perceived losses are easily overlooked or misunderstood, and yet the process of grief follows the same sequence and progression as that for actual losses. Individual interpretation makes a difference in how the perceived loss is uniquely valued and the response that a person will have during grieving.

Losses may also be maturational, situational, or both. A **maturational loss** includes any change in the developmental process that is normally expected during a lifetime. One example would be a parent's feeling of loss as a child goes to school for the first time. Events associated with maturational loss are part of normal life transitions, but the feelings of loss persist as grieving helps a person cope with the change. **Situational loss** includes any sudden, unpredictable external event. Often this type of loss includes multiple losses rather than a single loss; for example, an automobile accident may leave a driver paralyzed, unable to return to work, and grieving over the death of a passenger in the accident.

The type of loss and the perception of the loss influence the depth and duration of grief that a person experiences. Each individual responds to loss differently. It is incorrect to assume that the loss of an object does not generate the same level of grieving as loss of a loved one. The value an individual places on the lost object (e.g., a family heirloom) determines the emotional response to the loss. You

TABLE 29-1 Types of Loss

Definition	Implications of Loss
Loss of external objects (e.g., loss, misplacement, deterioration, theft, destruction by natural causes)	Extent of grieving depends on object's value, sentiment attached to it, and its usefulness.
Loss of known environment (e.g., moving from a neighbourhood, hospitalization, leaving or losing a job, moving out of intensive care unit)	Loss occurs through maturational or situational events and through injury or illness. Loneliness or newness of an unfamiliar setting threatens self-esteem and makes grieving difficult.
Loss of a significant other (e.g., through being promoted, moving, or running away; loss of a family member, friend, trusted nurse, acquaintance, or animal companion)	Significant other typically fulfills another person's need for psychological safety, love and belonging, and self-esteem.
Loss of an aspect of self (e.g., body part, psychological function, or physiological function)	Illness, injury, and developmental changes result in loss of aspect of self that causes grief and permanent changes in body image and self-concept.
Loss of life (e.g., death of family members, friend, or acquaintance; own death)	Loss of life creates grief for the survivors. The person facing death often fears pain, loss of control, and dependency on others.

must assess the special meaning that a loss has for a client and validate its effect on the client's health and well-being.

Hospitalization, chronic illness, and disability are special circumstances that are associated with multiple losses. When clients enter a hospital, they lose their privacy, control over their daily routines, and any illusions that they may have about their personal indestructibility. In addition, modesty and control over bodily functions may be compromised. A chronic illness or disability often engenders concern over financial security. Furthermore, long-term illness may necessitate a job change, threaten independence, and force alterations in lifestyle. Even a brief illness or hospitalization necessitates temporary shifts in family role functioning. Chronic or debilitating illness may pose a major threat to the stability of relationships.

Death is the ultimate loss. Although death is part of the continuum of life and a universal and inevitable part of being human, it is also a mystical event that generates anxiety and fear. Death ends relationships and separates people. Even with a strong spiritual grounding, facing death is often difficult for the dying person, as well as for the person's family, friends, and caregivers. A person's terminal illness reminds close friends and associates of their own mortality. A person with an advanced, progressive, ultimately fatal illness, such as chronic renal failure, end-stage heart failure, amyotrophic lateral sclerosis, or metastatic cancer, faces many—often progressive—levels of suffering. It is difficult to be sick, and many people dislike seeking help from others; however, nearly all want companionship and want to strengthen relationships with significant others when death is imminent (Chochinov, 2006).

When faced with death, feelings of guilt, anger, and fear arise. It may cause family members and caregivers to withdraw at a time when the dying person needs a trusted, unhurried companion, acting with gentle advocacy and humility. Clients faced with death are increasingly choosing to die at home (Allan et al., 2005); as a result, family members are becoming more involved in the care of their loved one. The way a person approaches dying is influenced by personal fundamental beliefs and values, past experiences with death, culture, spirituality, and the quality of the human emotional support available.

Grief

Grief is the emotional response to a loss or a death (Waldrop, 2007). Each individual responds to loss differently and therefore grieves differently (Perry, 2005). These differences are based on past experience and coping strategies, cultural expectations, and spiritual beliefs (Verosky, 2006; see Chapters 10 and 28). Coping with grief after a loss involves the process of mourning and the process of adapting to a loss (Waldrop, 2007). It involves working through the grief until an individual accepts and adapts to his or her expectations to go on in life without that which was lost.

Bereavement includes grief and mourning; it is the state of having lost a significant other to death (Waldrop, 2007). Survivors go through a bereavement period that is not linear. It does not proceed in sequential stages that can be precisely predicted, which may imply passivity on the part of the bereaved person. Rather, a survivor will move back and forth through a series of stages, tasks, or both many times, possibly over a period of several years, before the process is completed. Although no one really "gets over" a loss, the individual can heal and adapt to the loss. A useful analogy is to think of a new ring on a finger. Initially, the wearer is always aware that it is there, but over time, it will be less noticeable and yet still present. Several theorists have formulated stages of the grieving process and a series of tasks for survivors to work through their bereavement and adapt to life with a loss.

Theories of Grief

Kübler-Ross's Stages of Dying. The framework for Kübler-Ross's (1969) theory is behaviour oriented and includes five stages (Table 29–2). During **denial**, an individual acts as though nothing has happened and may refuse to believe or understand that a loss has occurred. In the **anger** stage, the individual resists the loss and may strike out at everyone and everything. During **bargaining**, the individual postpones awareness of the reality of the loss and may try to deal in a subtle or overt way as though the loss can be prevented. A person finally realizes the full impact and significance of the loss during the stage of **depression**, when the individual may feel overwhelmingly lonely and withdraw from interpersonal interaction. Finally, during the **acceptance** stage, the individual accepts the loss and begins to look to the future.

Bowlby's Phases of Mourning. Bowlby's (1980) attachment theory is the foundation for his theory on mourning. Attachment is described as an instinctive behaviour that leads to the development of affectionate bonds between children and their primary caregiver. These bonds are present and active throughout the life cycle. Later, the bonds are generalized to other people with whom individuals form close relationships. Attachment behaviour ensures human survival because it keeps people in close contact with other people who can offer protection and support.

Bowlby (1980) described four phases of mourning (see Table 29–2). As in the case of the other grief theories, a person can move back and forth between any two of the phases while responding to the loss. The **numbing** phase may last from a few hours to a week or more and may be interrupted by periods of extremely intense emotion. It is the briefest phase of mourning. The grieving person may describe this phase as feeling "stunned" or "unreal." Numbing may serve to protect the body from the onslaught or consequence of the loss. The second phase of **yearning and searching** arouses emotional outbursts of tearful sobbing and acute distress in most people. This phase is painful but must be endured (Hasler, 1996). Parkes (1972) explained that it is necessary for the bereaved person to experience the pain of grief in order to finish the work of grief. Therefore, anything that continually allows the person to avoid or suppress the pain can be expected to prolong the course of mourning. Common physical symptoms include

TABLE 29-2 The Grief Process

Kübler-Ross's (1969) Five Stages of Dying	Bowlby's (1980) Four Phases of Mourning	Worden's (1991) Four Tasks of Mourning
Denial	Numbing	Accepting the reality of loss
Anger	Yearning and searching	Working through the pain of grief
Bargaining	Disorganization and despair	Adjusting to the environment without the deceased
Depression	Reorganization	Emotionally relocating the deceased and moving on with life
Acceptance		

tightness in the chest and throat, a shortness of breath, feelings of weakness and lethargy, insomnia, and loss of appetite. A person may also experience an intense yearning for the object or individual who is lost. This phase may last for months or years. During the phase of **disorganization and despair**, an individual may constantly examine how and why the loss occurred. It is common for the person to express anger at anyone who might be responsible. This examination gradually gives way to an acceptance that the loss is permanent. During the final phase of **reorganization**, which may require as much as a year or more, the person begins to accept unaccustomed roles, acquire new skills, and build new relationships. People experiencing this phase must be encouraged to untie themselves from their old relationship, without devaluing it or feeling that in so doing they are lessening its importance (Hasler, 1996).

Worden's Four Tasks of Mourning. Worden's (1991) four tasks of mourning imply that people who mourn can be actively involved in helping themselves and can be assisted by outside intervention. Although time varies greatly among individuals, working through the tasks typically requires a minimum of a full year.

- *Task 1: To accept the reality of the loss.* Even when a death has been expected, some period of disbelief and surprise that the event has really happened always occurs. This task involves the processes required to accept that the person or object is gone and will not return.
- *Task 2: To work through the pain of grief.* Even though people respond to loss differently, it is impossible to experience a loss and work through grief without emotional pain. Individuals who deny or shut off the pain prolong their grief.
- *Task 3: To adjust to the environment in which the deceased is missing.* According to Worden (1991), a person does not realize the full impact of a loss for at least 3 months. At this point, many friends and associates make less frequent contact, and the person is left to ponder the full impact of loneliness. People completing this task must take on roles formerly filled by the deceased, including some tasks that they never fully appreciated.
- *Task 4: To emotionally relocate the deceased and move on with life.* The goal of this task is not to forget the deceased or give up the relationship with the deceased but to have the deceased take a new, less prominent place in a person's emotional life. This is often the most difficult task to complete because people fear that if they make other attachments, they will forget their loved one or be disloyal. A person completes this stage after realizing that it is possible to love other people without loving the deceased person less.

Types of Grief. Knowledge of types of grief, which are based on characteristics or signs and symptoms of grief, enables you to implement appropriate bereavement therapies.

Normal Grief. Normal or uncomplicated grief consists of the normal feelings, behaviours, and reactions to a loss, including resentment, sorrow, anger, crying, loneliness, and temporary withdrawal from activities. Often the "healthy" grief response to a loss can prove positive, helping an individual mature and develop as a person as he or she comes to terms with the changes that have occurred in his or her life and works to rearrange and reorganize internal models (Grassi, 2007). This results in the development of adaptive coping strategies on which the person can rely in the future.

Anticipatory Grief. The process of disengaging, or "letting go," that occurs before an actual loss or death has occurred is called **anticipatory grief.** For example, once a person or family receives a terminal diagnosis, they begin the process of saying goodbye and completing life affairs. The process becomes more stressful when the client is unable to make decisions as a result of the progression of illness. Unless guided by a client's explicit decisions regarding end-of-life care, the family, in consultation with health care professionals, assumes the responsibility of deciding whether to continue life-sustaining measures. The family must weigh factors such as the client's known values and choices, the medical facts, opinions and probabilities, the burden of treatment, the expected future quality of life for the client, and the limitations of their own emotional resources (Tilden et al., 2001).

When dying takes a long time, the client's loved ones may exhibit few symptoms of grief once the death occurs. This seeming absence of grief symptoms may result because the family has engaged in the grief process over time. By the time the moment of death arrives, much of the shock, denial, and tearfulness have already been experienced.

Anticipatory grieving entails some risks. Family members may withdraw emotionally from the client too soon, leaving the client with no emotional support as death approaches. Complications may also arise if a person who was thought to be near death survives. Family members may then have difficulty reconnecting and may even be resentful that the person has lived past life expectancy.

Complicated Grief. When a person has difficulty progressing through the normal (generally accepted) phases or stages of grieving, bereavement becomes complicated. In these cases, bereavement appears to "go wrong" and loss has not been adequately dealt with. This can threaten a person's relationships with others. Complicated grief includes four types:

- *Chronic grief:* active acute mourning that is characterized by normal grief reactions that do not subside and continue over very long periods of time (Egan & Arnold, 2003). Affected people verbalize an inability to "get past" the grief.
- *Delayed grief:* characterized by normal grief reactions that are suppressed or postponed and by the survivor's conscious or unconscious avoidance of the pain of the loss (Egan & Arnold, 2003). Active grieving is held back, only to resurface later, usually in response to a trivial loss or upset. For example, a wife may appear to grieve for only a few weeks after the death of her spouse, but then she may become distraught and sad a year later when she attends a family gathering. The extreme sadness is a delayed response to the death of her husband.
- *Exaggerated grief:* grief that overwhelms people to the point that they cannot function. This may be reflected in the form of severe phobias or self-destructive behaviour such as alcoholism, substance abuse, or suicide.
- *Masked grief:* Lack of awareness by survivors that behaviours that interfere with normal functioning are a result of their loss (Egan & Arnold, 2003). For example, a person who is grieving may develop alterations in eating or sleeping patterns.

Disenfranchised Grief. People experience grief when a loss is experienced and cannot always be openly acknowledged, socially sanctioned, or publicly shared (Egan & Arnold, 2003). Examples include the loss of a partner from acquired immunodeficiency syndrome (AIDS) or the loss of a child in utero or at birth.

Application of Grief Theory to Other Types of Loss. Although grief theories apply mainly to the way that individuals cope with the death of a loved one, they also apply to other losses. The theories are relevant to the way people respond to a loss of body function, as in the case of organ transplantation or heart attack, and to disability, such as amputation of a limb or paralysis. Grief theory applies to individuals who progress through stages of mourning for lost independence, body integrity, and a change in body image. These individuals experience genuine emotional pain as they progress through the stages of grieving.

Nursing Knowledge Base

Nursing knowledge has traditionally focused on the acute care setting, in which losses are more physical in nature. As you enter home and community settings, the definitions of loss are more comprehensive and in many ways different. You must develop interventions for each unique client situation.

Factors Influencing Loss and Grief

The way that an individual perceives a loss and responds to it during bereavement is influenced by many factors.

Human Development. People of differing ages and stages of development display different and unique symptoms of grief. For example, toddlers are unable to understand loss or death, but they feel great anxiety over loss of objects and separation from parents. School-aged children experience grief over the loss of a body part or function. They often associate misdeeds with causing death. Middle-aged adults usually begin to re-examine life and are sensitive to their own physical changes. Older adults often experience anticipatory grief because of aging and the possible loss of self-care abilities. Aging is frequently associated with losses such as physical changes, loss of employment, loss of social respect, loss of relationships, and threats to a sense of fulfillment and contributions made in life. However, Lund (1989) found that older adults are often resilient in responding to grief, despite its being a highly stressful process (Box 29–1).

Psychosocial Perspectives of Loss and Grief. Loss and death are life experiences that each person faces. Death is an overwhelming experience that affects everyone involved in the loss situation or in the death of the individual. Culture can have a significant influence on people's views of death and how the dying should be cared for. In each culture is a set of beliefs and values that are the result of positive and negative experiences, cultural influences, and spiritual beliefs (Verosky, 2006). You are part of that same psychosocial environment and share many of the biases or perspectives gained during sociological development. Norms for psychosocial patterns of loss and grief are reflected in caregivers as well as in clients. You need to be aware of your own personal perspectives that may influence your approach and attitudes in caring for dying clients and their families (Verosky, 2006).

BOX 29-1 FOCUS ON OLDER ADULTS

- Bereavement adjustments are multidimensional in that nearly every aspect of a person's life can be affected by a loss.
- The overall effect of bereavement on the physical and mental health of many older spouses is not as devastating as expected.
- Older bereaved spouses commonly experience both positive and negative feelings simultaneously.
- Loneliness and problems associated with completing the tasks of daily living are two of the most common and difficult adjustments for older bereaved spouses.
- Older bereaved adults adjust to the deaths of spouses in diverse ways.

Data from Lund, D. A. (1989). Conclusions about bereavement in later life and implications for interventions and future research. In D. A. Lund (Ed.), *Older bereaved spouses: Research with practical application*. New York: Hemisphere.

An individual's expression of grief evolves as the person matures. Personal experiences shape the coping mechanisms that the individual uses to deal with stressors. As psychologists explain, the coping mechanisms that were effective in the past are repeated as a first response to the pain of a loss. When older coping strategies are unsuccessful, new coping mechanisms are attempted (see Chapter 30). When faced with a loss, a client learns what is needed for his or her own coping through repetition that is based on the successes and failures of different coping mechanisms. Sometimes the number or depths of losses become overwhelming, and familiar coping styles are not successful. For example, in the case of disenfranchised grief, society has different expectations than the person who experiences the loss, and routine coping strategies become ineffective, unavailable, or maladaptive. Professional assistance is often required to help the client and family understand and deal realistically with losses.

Socioeconomic Status. Socioeconomic status influences a person's ability to obtain options and use support mechanisms when coping with loss. In general, people feel greater burden from a loss when financial, educational, or occupational resources are lacking. For example, a client with limited finances may not be able to replace a home lost in a fire or may not be able to purchase necessary medications to manage a newly diagnosed disease. These clients require referral to community social service and support agencies that can provide needed resources.

Personal Relationships. When loss involves a loved one, the quality and meaning of the relationship are critical in understanding a survivor's grief experience. It has been said that to lose parents is to lose the past, to lose a spouse is to lose the present, and to lose a child is to lose the future. When a relationship between two individuals has been very close, the one left behind can have great difficulty coping. Support from family and friends is based in part on the person's relationships with members of a social network and the manner and circumstances of the loss. People who do not receive support and compassion from others may have difficulty grieving.

Nature of the Loss. The ability to manage grief depends on the meaning of the loss and the situation surrounding the loss. A bereaved person's ability to accept help from others influences whether he or she will be able to cope. The visibility of a loss influences the support a person receives. For example, the loss of one's home from a fire prompts support from the community, whereas a private loss of an important possession may prompt less support from others. Some losses are not highly visible, such as reproductive loss (e.g., miscarriage, stillbirth, abortion, giving up a child for adoption, infertility). The Centre for Reproductive Loss was founded in Montreal to help people who have suffered such a loss so that they can acknowledge and deal with their unspoken grief (Gray & Lassance, 2003).

The suddenness of a loss can delay resolution from grief. For example, a sudden and unexpected death is generally more difficult for a family to accept than death after a long-term chronic illness.

Culture and Ethnicity. A person's cultural background strongly influences attitudes toward life-sustaining treatments during terminal illness (Verosky, 2006). Cultural background and family practices also influence people's interpretation of a loss and the expression of grief (Box 29–2). Culture affects how clients and their support systems or families respond to loss (see Chapter 10). For example, in the Western hemisphere, the grieving process is usually personal and private; individuals show restrained emotion. However, the ceremonies surrounding a person's death offer time for grief resolution and reminiscing. In Eastern hemisphere nations, such as the Philippines or China, respect for the dead is shown by wailing and physically demonstrating grief for a specified period of time. Despite these trends, members of the same ethnocultural background may respond to loss and death differently. You must acquire an understanding and appreciation of each client's cultural values as they apply to the experience of loss, death, and grieving.

Canada is a multicultural society, and as a nurse, you can anticipate many cultural contexts and responses to loss, death, and bereavement. You must be able to support and guide clients and families through the end-of-life process in a culturally informed and acceptable manner. Culturally sensitive practices are needed to guide the development of effective nursing interventions. When individuals lose control over aspects of their life because of illness, you must provide respectful and appropriate culturally safe care to individual clients. This is best achieved through asking specific questions of the client or the family (Verosky, 2006).

BOX 29-2 CULTURAL ASPECTS OF CARE

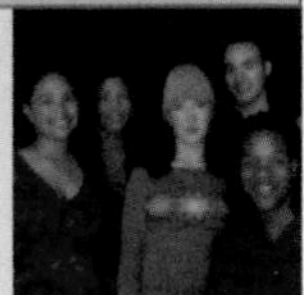

At the end of life, rituals, mourning practices, and specific expressions of grief are necessary for participants of all cultures, in order to have a sense of acceptance and inner peace. Whether appropriate care at the end of life achieves a "good death" or an "acceptable death" for clients is controversial. Do clients achieve a sense of comfort and peace during the death experience? Most hospital policies and procedures support an "acceptable death"—nontheatrical, disciplined, and with minimal exchange of emotions—for the client who is dying. This means providing basic standard levels of care and support, which may or may not take into account a client's cultural beliefs and practices. A "good death" or "acceptable death" is also known as a "meaningful death" and can be defined as a dying process "during which the patient is physically, psychologically, spiritually and emotionally supported by his or her family, friends, and caregivers" (Chochinov, 2006, p. 85). In contrast, Kagawa-Singer (1998) described a "good death" as one that allows social adjustments and personal preparations for the transition that will occur. A "good death" allows time for the family and client to make both the private and public preparations that are needed to help the family begin the adjustment to a world without their loved one and for the client to complete unfinished tasks. The disengagement that occurs between the person who is dying and loved ones takes many forms because of cultural differences:

- Hindus envision a circular pattern of life and death with multiple deaths and rebirths.
- Christians believe in a more linear trajectory, as expressed in the construct of a heaven, in which all good people will gather after death, and a hell to which lost souls will go for eternity.
- Some Aboriginal cultures envision the land of the dead as a parallel world, where the spirits of the dead can directly affect the lives of the living.
- In some cultures, disengagement can be abrupt and final, even to the point of sanctions against speaking names of the deceased, to avoid keeping them from leaving earth and obtaining peace.

Implications for Practice

- Your nursing concept of social support must be broadened to include greater variation in the timing, form, and mode of support provided to grieving clients and families.
- Cultural beliefs influence who makes up a client's support network and what support is acceptable to both give and receive during death.
- Care provided at the end of life within the client's and family's cultural context draws from the resources of their whole lives.

Data from Kagawa-Singer, M. (1998). The cultural context of death rituals and mourning practices. *Oncology Nursing Forum, 25*(10), 1752.

Spiritual Beliefs. Individuals' spirituality significantly influences their ability to cope with loss. Some of the spiritual resources on which clients may depend during a loss include faith in a higher power or influence, their community of fellowship with friends, their sources of hope and meaning in life, and their use of religious rituals and practices. Loss can sometimes cause internal conflicts about spiritual values and the meaning of life. Clients who have a strong interconnectedness with a higher power or others are often very resilient and able to face death with relatively minimal discomfort (see Chapter 28). Alternatively, clients faced with a life-threatening or terminal illness may begin to question their faith and wonder why this would be allowed to happen to them.

Coping With Grief and Loss

In order to support clients and families during loss, you must understand how people normally cope with grief and loss. Nursing interventions involve reinforcing the client's successful coping mechanisms and introducing new coping approaches. Chapter 30 summarizes the nursing care principles for assisting clients in coping with stressful situations.

Hope. Hope is the anticipation of a continued good or of an improvement in, or lessening of, something unpleasant. It is a multidimensional concept that is energizing and provides comfort while a person endures life threats and personal challenges (Smith & Kautz, 2007). Hope enhances coping skills by building on a client's control. A person often reveals hope through an expression of expectations for life, the present, and the future. Many clients with terminal illness focus hope on milestones or something other than a prognosis (Chochinov, 2006). Spiritual distress is often based on the person's definition of hope or lack of hope. People may view hope as encouragement to work toward recovery. Other people may view hope more negatively by not being able to envision any future favourable outcomes.

Hope has purpose and direction and, in a palliative client, can contribute to enhancing control, maintaining dignity, and sustaining relationships (Smith & Kautz, 2007). The existence and maintenance of hope depend on a person's having strong relationships and a sense of emotional connectedness to others. Nurses and other health care professionals may provide that personal connectedness essential to hope. Hope is often the basis from which clients find meaning in their illness. Hopefulness enables people to see life as enduring or having sustained meaning or purpose (Chochinov, 2006). Nurses have reported that they believe they make the greatest difference in clients' lives by helping them keep hope alive; by increasing a client's awareness of what is possible, nurses can, in addition, maintain a renewed sense of purpose through hope (Smith & Kautz, 2007). Chapter 28 discusses the conceptual components of hope and related nursing care implications.

Critical Thinking

When you care for clients who have experienced losses, successful critical thinking requires a synthesis of knowledge, previous experience with loss and grief, and information gathered from clients and families. To provide appropriate and responsive nursing care, you must apply both critical thinking qualities and intellectual and professional standards.

During assessment, you must analyze all sources of information in order to select appropriate nursing diagnoses (Figure 29–1). To understand the process of grief and its effect on the client and family, you integrate knowledge from nursing and other disciplines and from previous experiences in caring for clients suffering loss. Knowledge of the stages of grief, for example, enables you to better empathize with a client and family and to understand the client's behaviours. Through identification of the stages of grief, you are able to direct assessment questions. Critical thinking qualities and standards then help you apply this information in a relevant and therapeutic way for the client's benefit. For example, you need the critical thinking quality of perseverance so that you can learn as much as possible about the type of grief a client is experiencing, in order to ultimately select the most appropriate nursing interventions. The use of intellectual standards such as significance and relevance helps ensure that the information gathered is pertinent to the client's unique situation. Guiding standards include those of bioethics, the dying person's bill of rights (Box 29–3), clinical standards such as guidelines for managing cancer pain, the Canadian Nurses Association (CNA; 2008) *Code of Ethics for Registered Nurses*, and provincial regulatory bodies' professional standards and practice standards. All provide evidence-informed guidelines for a thorough assessment and humane, compassionate nursing care.

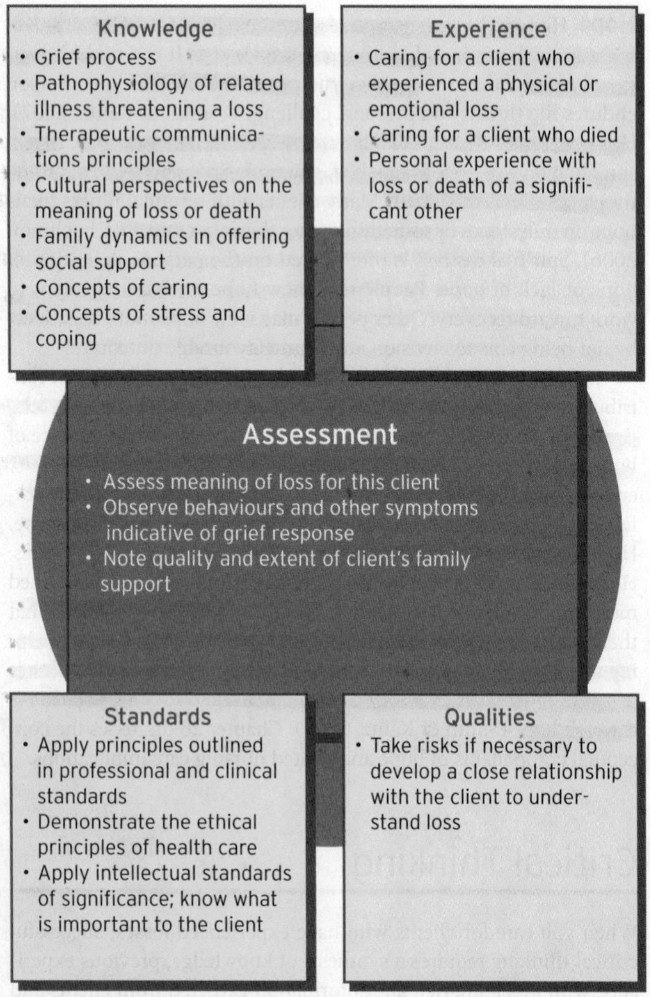

Knowledge
- Grief process
- Pathophysiology of related illness threatening a loss
- Therapeutic communications principles
- Cultural perspectives on the meaning of loss or death
- Family dynamics in offering social support
- Concepts of caring
- Concepts of stress and coping

Experience
- Caring for a client who experienced a physical or emotional loss
- Caring for a client who died
- Personal experience with loss or death of a significant other

Assessment
- Assess meaning of loss for this client
- Observe behaviours and other symptoms indicative of grief response
- Note quality and extent of client's family support

Standards
- Apply principles outlined in professional and clinical standards
- Demonstrate the ethical principles of health care
- Apply intellectual standards of significance; know what is important to the client

Qualities
- Take risks if necessary to develop a close relationship with the client to understand loss

Figure 29-1 Critical thinking model for loss, death, and grieving assessment.

BOX 29-3 A Dying Person's Bill of Rights

I have the right to be in control.
I have the right to be treated as a living human being until I die.
I have the right to have a sense of purpose.
I have the right to be cared for by those who can maintain a sense of hopefulness.
I have the right to express my feelings and emotions about my approaching death in my own way.
I have the right to have a respected spirituality.
I have the right to participate in decisions about my care.
I have the right to expect continuing medical and nursing attention even though "cure" goals must be changed to "comfort" goals.
I have the right not to die alone.
I have the right to be comfortable.
I have the right to have my questions answered honestly.
I have the right not to be deceived.
I have the right to have help from and for my family in accepting my death.
I have the right to die in peace and dignity.
I have the right to laugh and to be angry and sad.
I have the right to retain my individuality and not be judged for my decisions that may be contrary to beliefs of others.
I have the right to be cared for by caring, sensitive, knowledgeable people who will try to understand my needs and will be able to gain some satisfaction in helping me face my death.

Adapted from Barbus, A. J. (1975). The dying person's bill of rights. *American Journal of Nursing, 75,* 99; and from Hospice RN. (2003). *Patient's bill of rights.* Retrieved November 21, 2008, from http://www.geocities.com/HotSprings/5120/bill.htm

The Nursing Process and Grief

❖Assessment

When you care for a client who has experienced or is facing a loss, assessment includes the client, family, significant others, and the context. Grief assessment is ongoing throughout the course of an illness for the client and family and for the bereavement period after the death for the survivors (Verosky, 2006). You should not assume how or whether the client or family experiences grief. You should also avoid assuming that a particular behaviour indicates grief; rather, you should allow clients to share what is happening in their own way. An effective nurse encourages clients to tell their stories. This requires you to establish trust with clients and to evoke a caring presence. It is helpful to have clients and families find a time and place to express their grief and describe their experiences (Figure 29–2). During an assessment, you interview clients and families separately unless a client requests having family members present. A thorough and comprehensive approach to the assessment of grief will result in a well-designed plan of care that will facilitate clients' and families' abilities to work through grief.

You begin by interviewing the client and then the family, using honest and open communication. Listening carefully and observing the client's responses and behaviours are important. You assume a neutral perspective and remain alert for nonverbal cues such as affect, facial expressions, voice tones, and topics that are avoided. While gathering data, you summarize and validate any impressions formed with the client and family so that appropriate nursing diagnoses can be made. Information from other health care workers, such as physicians, social workers, and providers of pastoral care will contribute to the database.

Type and Stage of Grief

It is important for you to assess how a client *is reacting* rather than how the client should be reacting. The sequencing of stages or behaviours of grief may occur in order, they may be skipped, or they may recur. A single behaviour can be representative of any number of types of grief. Therefore, the identification of the type and stage of grief should be used only to guide your assessment and not to judge the outcomes of the grieving process. By understanding a theorist's phase of grief, you can accurately assess a situation. For example, if a client is complaining of loneliness and difficulty falling asleep, you consider all factors surrounding the loss. When did the loss occur? What type of loss occurred? The client may be experiencing a normal grief reaction, or, if the loss occurred 2 years previously, the client may be experiencing chronic grief.

Ask clients to describe their loss and how it has affected them: "Tell me how your diagnosis of heart disease makes you feel." You can anticipate characteristics or responses during a phase of grieving, but you should allow clients to describe their feelings as thoroughly as possible: "How has this change in your life affected you today?" "Tell me more." Then probe and validate feelings expressed in the client's emotions: "You seem angry; tell me more . . . ," "You seem sad; tell me . . . ," "What are your feelings about . . . ?" Avoid premature assumptions about the phase of grief that a client might be experiencing, so that you do not terminate the assessment too early.

Grief Reactions

You will use psychological and physical assessment skills to compile a complete database about the client, family, or both. Although no two people grieve exactly the same way, most people who grieve have at least some outward signs and symptoms (Box 29–4). Clinical reasoning is needed to analyze the data cues and to determine the appropriate related cause. For example, a client who is experiencing dysfunctional grieving may have a changing affect, lowered activity level, somatic complaints such as headache or upset stomach, and alterations in sleep patterns, memory, and concentration. You might associate these symptoms with any number of problems such as anxiety, gastrointestinal disturbances, or even impaired memory. However, the focus is to assess the client's symptoms in context. What are the meaning and significance of the loss, and how are they affecting the client in physical and psychological ways? With what does the client associate the symptoms? In what way are the symptoms related to one another when they occur? What symptoms are observed when the client openly expresses grief? Over what time period have the symptoms been present: before the loss or during the loss? Careful analysis refines your ability to make judgements about the client's condition.

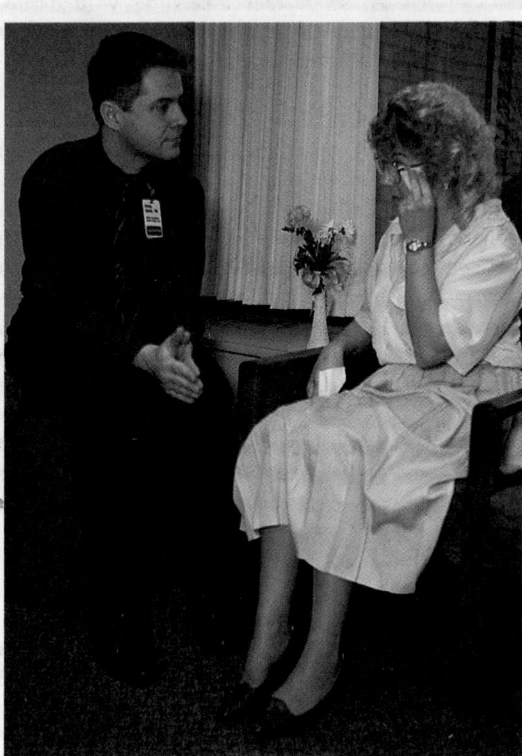

Figure 29-2 Nurses find a private place to listen to clients express their grief.

➤ BOX 29-4 Symptoms of Normal Grief

Feelings
Sadness
Anger
Guilt or self-reproach
Anxiety
Loneliness
Fatigue
Helplessness
Shock or numbness (lack of feeling)
Yearning
Feeling of emancipation or relief

Cognitions (Thought Patterns)
Disbelief
Confusion
Preoccupation about the deceased
Sense of the presence of the deceased
Auditory hallucinations
Perceptual disturbances
Hopelessness ("I'll never be OK again")

Physical Sensations
Hollowness in the stomach
Tightness in the chest
Tightness in the throat
Oversensitivity to noise
Depersonalization ("Nothing seems real")
Shortness of breath
Muscle weakness
Lack of energy
Dry mouth
Headache
Abdominal pain

Behaviours
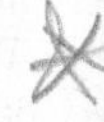
Sleep pattern changes
Appetite disturbances
Absent-minded behaviour
Dreams about the deceased
Sighing
Emotional lability
Carrying objects that belonged to the deceased

A loss takes place in a social context. When the primary provider in a family has a terminal illness, the family begins to reorganize itself as soon as the client is no longer able to fulfill the same number and types of roles. When a person is disabled, the client and family undergo similar reorganization, realigning roles and responsibilities to meet the demands. During this time, clients and families can experience a variety of physical and psychological symptoms. You assess the entire family's response to loss, recognizing that family members may be dealing with aspects of grief different from those of the client. Good interviewing and physical assessment skills guide you as caregiver and as an advocate of the client in planning appropriate nursing care. It is important that you assess for any changes in family relationships or interactions during a client's illness. Terminal illness may bring distant family members together, which can result in additional stressors on families. An awareness of this potential allows you to identify strategies for adaptive family coping if they are required.

Factors That Affect Grief

Because a number of factors influence loss and the grief response, it helps to discuss the meaning of loss to the client and family. This discussion usually elicits information that allows you to explore a number of topics in detail, such as personal characteristics of the person experiencing loss, the nature of family relationships, support systems, and cultural and spiritual beliefs (Table 29–3). You must then apply assessment skills from appropriate specialty areas (e.g., family or spiritual assessment; see Chapters 20 and 28, respectively) to acquire a thorough understanding of the client's loss.

End-of-Life Decisions

Although living wills or advance directives may not be recognized legally in all provinces, the CNA (1994), along with other national health organizations, developed the *Joint Statement on Advance Directives*. In this document, the CNA stated that "all persons have the right to make decisions regarding their health care and treatment, including the right to request or refuse life-sustaining treatment" (p. 1). An advance directive documents a person's preferences regarding life-sustaining treatment and communicates these preferences if the person becomes incapable of doing so for himself or herself (CNA, 1998). You must be aware of the legal status of advance directives in your province or territory and the laws regarding a person's competence to consent to treatment, as well as legislation regarding the selection and responsibilities of substitute decision makers (see Chapter 9).

When a person has a terminal illness, family members must face end-of-life decisions that have ethical, legal, and practical implications. Families may experience higher levels of stress, discomfort, or even guilt when deciding whether to initiate or withdraw life-sustaining treatments. Some treatments may offer symptom relief but simultaneously prolong life, which creates conflict or dilemmas for both families and caregivers. Although some clients may have advance directives, it is important for family members to know in advance a client's wishes in regard to life-sustaining measures.

The *Code of Ethics for Registered Nurses* (CNA, 2008) identifies three values that are pertinent to nurses assisting individuals in end-of-life decision making:

1. Health and well-being: Nurses must ensure that an individual's wishes as stated in an advance directive are respected and that continuing care and support are provided.
2. Choice: Nurses must respect and promote the autonomy of individuals, help clients express their needs and values, and help clients obtain appropriate care.
3. Dignity: Nurses must advocate on the client's behalf and examine biological, psychological, social, cultural, and spiritual factors that affect end-of-life treatment decisions (CNA, 1998).

Responsibility statements associated with each value in the code give more direction to nurses in upholding the values. For example, the value "health and well-being" includes the responsibility statement: "When a person receiving care is terminally ill or dying, nurses foster comfort, alleviate suffering, advocate for adequate relief of discomfort and pain and support a dignified and peaceful death" (CNA, 2008, p. 14).

Benner et al. (2003) articulated a set of core nursing principles regarding end-of-life care, in which "attending to death as a human passage" is central. You must assess the client's and family's wishes for end-of-life care, including the preferred place for death, the use and extent of life-sustaining measures, and expectations regarding pain control and symptom management (Box 29–5). Does the client want to try all available treatments? Does the family or client insist on use of a feeding tube for continued nutritional support after the client stops eating? When life support requires use of a mechanical ventilator, is this something the client wants? Does the family feel comfortable in administering analgesics? You must give the client and family time to discuss their preferences. Often it is necessary to return to a conversation on a subsequent day or visit. If you feel uncomfortable in assessing a client's wishes, it is important to find a health care professional who is experienced with discussing end-of-life issues and can assist in communicating a client's preferences to the health care team. For example, physicians may be helpful when discussing issues related to probability or futility, or a social worker may be able to help with decision making with regard to family roles, responsibilities, and relationships.

End-of-life care is one of the more significant topics you will discuss with clients (Box 29–6). Good interdisciplinary teamwork is essential to provide quality end-of-life care. Thus, you must communicate what is known about client preferences and decisions in change-of-shift reports, health team conferences, written care plans, documentation in the client's record, and ongoing consultation with physicians and other health team members.

Nurses' Experience With Grief

When caring for grieving clients, you must assess your own emotional well-being. Self-reflection, which is a part of critical thinking, is a valuable tool in assessing whether a person's sadness is related to the client, to unresolved personal experiences from the past, or to a combination of both. It is normal to have personal feelings and emotions about certain illnesses and death. However, it is inappropriate to emphasize your personal family situations and values over those of the client. Talking with friends and professional colleagues may help you to resolve conflicts about caring for dying clients. Some nurses choose to work in a specialty area in which deaths are unusual. Part of being a professional involves knowing yourself and when to move away from a situation. Nurses who choose to work in palliative care settings obtain support from their peers, as well as from interdisciplinary team debriefings.

Client Expectations

You must assess the client's and family's expectations for nursing care. The client's perceptions and expectations can influence how you prioritize nursing diagnoses. For example, if clients perceive that their pain and discomfort are severe, they will be less attentive to your attempts to discuss the significance and meaning of their loss. Before you can begin meaningful discussion or counselling, the client must be comfortable. On occasion, clients are hesitant to accept, and families reluctant to administer, narcotic analgesics because of fears of addiction.

TABLE 29-3 Assessment of Factors That Influence Grieving

Factor	Areas, Suggestions, and Questions to Explore
Nature of relationships	Functions of the family, community, and society *Examples:* "How long have you known your friend?" "What role has your mother played in your family?" "What is your relationship? Will it change?" "How will family relationships change as a result of the loss?"
Social support system	Availability of family, friends, health care professionals *Examples:* Who is present? Absent? Supportive? Nonsupportive? What do family and friends do that is most meaningful? Are family and friends available when needed? Are health care professionals accepting and exploring ways to preserve the client's dignity and lifestyle?
Nature of loss	Actual versus perceived; death issues; impact on roles *Examples:* "Tell me what the loss means to you." "What factors help you to grieve?" "What factors interfere with grieving?" "What past experiences or outcomes have you had with loss?"
Cultural and spiritual beliefs	Values, cultural norms, spirituality, customs, attitudes *Examples:* "What is your belief about death? About the meaning of life?" "What customs do you value at the time of death?" "How is this loss viewed by other people of your culture or religious group?" "Do medical treatments interfere with religious practices?" "Who has the right to say 'yes' or 'no' to life-sustaining measures?"
Loss of personal life goals	Actual or perceived individual losses affecting future decisions and options *Examples:* "What is your goal in life for . . . ?" "How has this goal changed as a result of your diagnosis?" "How will your role change your personal goals?" "What planning have you and your family made for your own life?"
Family's grief	Relationships, involvement with the dying process *Examples:* Observe client and family's level of grief, patterns of behaviour, rank of leadership or power. What has helped family members deal with problems in the past? What was not helpful? What are the family's strengths and weaknesses?
Survivor risk factors	High risk, such as sudden death, violent death, loss of a child *Examples:* "Describe your feelings at this time." "Let's talk about why you think you could have prevented this. Are you feeling guilty because . . . ?" "What are unresolved issues or perceptions toward others?"
Hope	Goals, worth, adaptation to future changes *Examples:* "Tell me what you think about your treatment plan." "What do you expect will happen to you?" "How does this illness affect your goals in life?' "What are you hoping for after your surgery?"

BOX 29-5 RESEARCH HIGHLIGHT

Family Perception of End-of-Life Care

Research Focus

Family members are often involved in providing care during a dying person's last month of life, regardless of the setting (home, hospice, or hospital). Their perspectives of how the person's last days of life are spent provide valuable insight into the quality of end-of-life care.

Research Abstract

Tolle et al. (2000) conducted a retrospective study of decedents and their families. Data about family views of health services and clinicians' care during the last month of life were collected. Using a 58-item questionaire, the researchers also conducted telephone surveys of family members. The survey obtained information about family members' perceptions of end-of-life care.

Findings suggested that the rate of advance planning and clinicians' respect for client–family preferences were high. Aggressive, life-sustaining treatments were not used extensively, and decisions to forgo aggressive treatments were more frequent than decisions to discontinue them once started. All clients who died at home preferred that location. However, almost half of clients who received care in a hospital preferred that setting. One third of the families indicated that their family member experienced moderate to severe pain in the final week of life. Families had more complaints about the management of pain for decedents who died at home, even though they did not report higher levels of pain. In general, families were highly satisfied with clinicians' efforts to manage pain.

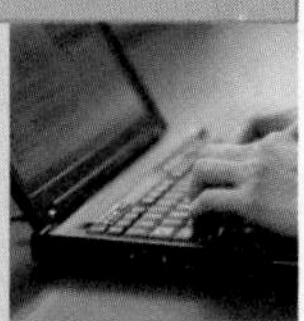

Evidence-Informed Practice

- It is important to learn directly from clients and families their wishes regarding preferred location of the client's death.
- Families of dying clients may have low expectations of pain management; nevertheless, aggressive therapies are needed to help comfort dying clients.
- You should recognize that family members are more aware of pain management problems and bear more responsibility for direct care of such needs.
- You should provide guidance and support to help families administer necessary pain therapies.
- Pain management in palliative care is complex and involves a variety of interventions and medications. Nurses require sound pharmacological knowledge in this area.

References: Tolle, S., Tilden, V. P., Rosenfeld, A. G., & Hickman, S. E. (2000). Family reports of barriers to optimal care of the dying. *Nursing Research, 49*(6), 310–317.

Significant medication teaching may be required in these situations. Once the client is assessed as comfortable and the client considers pain level acceptable or under control, you should assess the client's expectations within the context of the loss by asking questions such as "How can we help you cope with your loss?" "What do you feel is necessary from us for you to be able to manage the grief you feel?" "What is most important that we do for you while you are under our care?"

It is important to give family members the chance to explain how they perceive your role, explain what they think are the goals of the health care team, and ask any questions they may have. This helps you clarify any misunderstandings that might exist. For example, the family may have unrealistic expectations regarding the treatment available to the client and the anticipated effects, or different family members may have conflicting opinions.

BOX 29-6 NURSING STORY

Nursing Roles With Loss, Grief, and End-of-Life Issues: John's Story

Nurses from many areas and disciplines are involved in the experiences of loss, death, and grief. John is an 81-year-old with recurrent small-cell lung cancer and is considered eligible for palliative care. Several years ago, he received a diagnosis of limited-stage small-cell lung cancer. A course of chemotherapy and radiotherapy resulted in a remission of several years' duration. Subsequent follow-up revealed that the cancer had returned, and John's condition was considered terminal. Throughout John's experience with his illness, he has interacted with many nurses with varying roles and responsibilities. Although these nurses all had different roles, functions, and work areas, they were all involved and sharing with John and his family's sense of loss, grief, celebrations, and eventual preparation for death.

Initially, John interacted with the clinic nurse at his family physician's office. Although not involved directly in his care, this nurse was able to provide support, reassurance, and encouragement each time John visited the office. While John was receiving his treatments at the cancer centre, he relied on the chemotherapy clinic nurses to check how he was feeling, and he counted on them to be caring but not gloomy, to keep his spirits up, and to encourage him to keep "fighting" while it was beneficial. One nurse in particular had frequent contact with John, and he looked forward to seeing her. She was a clinical trials research nurse, and John had enrolled in a medication trial. This advanced practice nurse was, to John, like his own private nurse, someone who wanted to see him regularly, took a genuine interest in him, and provided tremendous support to him and his family.

Home care nurses also played an important role in John's experience. The initial home assessment, enrolment in a community palliative care program, and discussion of "do not recusitate" protocols were managed in a caring and compassionate manner. John's health is now relatively stable and appears to have reached a plateau in the disease course. Each time the home care nurse visits and performs her assessment and documentation, John sees this as a "social" visit but finds the support to be very important. Being a reserved person, John finds it easier to discuss some of his issues with a professional. John has not decided yet whether he wishes to die at home or in a hospital; however, caring and compassionate palliative care nurses will at that point became key components of John's and his family's experience.

John's story is not unique, and most nurses are involved in the experience of loss, death, and grief, regardless of the area of practice. Having a sound understanding of these concepts will enable you to provide supportive, understanding, and compassionate care to your clients, anywhere along the continuum of life, loss, grief, and eventually death.

❖Nursing Diagnosis

From data collected during assessment, you identify a nursing diagnosis that accurately reflects the needs of the client or family experiencing the loss. Critical thinking skills are the tools used to apply concepts of assessment, clustering of cues, and drawing a conclusion of the actual or perceived needs of the client. You cluster defining characteristics and identify the nursing diagnosis applicable to the client's situation (Box 29–7). Clustering of client or family behaviours, actual or potential losses, the client's attempts at coping, and data involving the nature and meaning of the loss will lead to individualized nursing diagnoses, such as the following:

- *Anticipatory grieving*
- *Anxiety*
- *Caregiver role strain*
- *Compromised family coping*
- *Dysfunctional grieving*
- *Fear*
- *Hopelessness*
- *Ineffective coping*
- *Ineffective denial*
- *Powerlessness*
- *Readiness for enhanced spiritual well-being*
- *Social isolation*
- *Spiritual distress*

The presence of one or two defining characteristics is usually insufficient to make an accurate diagnosis. You must carefully review the data to consider whether competing diagnoses exist. For example, if a dying person cries, displays anger, and reports nightmares, this could signal several possible nursing diagnoses, in as much as these characteristics are common to more than one diagnosis. Possibilities include *pain, ineffective coping,* and *spiritual distress*. You examine all available data, and you inquire about and observe for the presence of other behaviours and symptoms until you can identify an accurate diagnosis.

Part of the diagnostic process is to identify the appropriate related factor for each diagnosis. For example, *dysfunctional grieving related to the loss of the ability to walk from paralysis* necessitates different interventions than does *dysfunctional grieving related to the loss of a job*.

In order to promote a holistic approach to care, wellness-oriented diagnoses need to be included, such as *readiness for enhanced spiritual well-being*. These diagnoses allow for recognizing and drawing from client strengths. In addition, the nursing diagnostic process is continual because the client situation will change.

When identifying nursing diagnoses for the dying client, other problems are identified separately according to specific standards of care. Other nursing diagnoses can include *disturbed body image, impaired physical mobility,* or *ineffective role performance*. More physical nursing diagnoses are identified when the client begins to experience the physical changes accompanying the progression of illness, including *impaired urinary elimination and/or bowel incontinence, acute pain, nausea, disturbed sensory perception,* and *ineffective breathing pattern*. The comfort of dying clients, including specialized pain control and the acceptance of the dying process by the family, is a realistic expectation. With terminal illness, physical assessment of the dying process is ongoing so that you can adapt or validate the actual nursing diagnoses with the changing condition of the client.

❖Planning

Grieving is the natural response to loss and thus has a therapeutic value. The focus in planning nursing care is to support the client physically, emotionally, developmentally, and spiritually in the expression of grief. Figure 29–3 illustrates the interrelatedness of critical thinking factors during the planning phase of the nursing process. Through critical thinking, you ensure a well-designed plan in which you support the client's personhood, self-esteem, and autonomy by including the client in making decisions about the plan of care. When caring for the dying client, it is important to devise a plan that helps a client die with dignity and offers family members the assurance that their loved one is cared for compassionately (Box 29–8). The care planning process is highly individual to the client and family, and when possible, both must be included as active participants in your planning, goal setting, and development of realistic interventions and timelines.

Goals and Outcomes

You establish realistic goals and expected outcomes on the basis of the client's nursing diagnoses. Client resources such as physical energy and activity tolerance, supportive family members, spiritual faith, and methods for coping are integrated into the plan of care. For example, if a client with a life-threatening illness has the diagnosis *powerlessness related to planned cancer therapy,* a goal of "Client will be able to discuss expected course of disease" is realistic if the client is able to remain attentive and participate in educational discussions without becoming fatigued. In contrast, the expected outcome

BOX 29-7 NURSING DIAGNOSTIC PROCESS

Assessment Activities	Defining Characteristics	Nursing Diagnosis
Ask client to discuss future goals and plans.	Client sighs and says, "I have no future."	*Hopelessness related to failing physical condition*
Observe client's nonverbal behaviour.	Client becomes passive with little affect and turns away from speaker.	*Ineffective individual coping related to low mood, and inability to manage loss*
Offer client choices and observe responses.	Client shrugs and says, "What does it matter?"	*Powerlessness related to precieved poor outcomes*
Assess activity level.	Client refuses to eat. Client sleeps all the time, keeping blinds closed and lights out. Client refuses to participate in care.	*Self-care deficit related to inability to perform activities of daily living* *Social islolation related to inability to cope with loss*

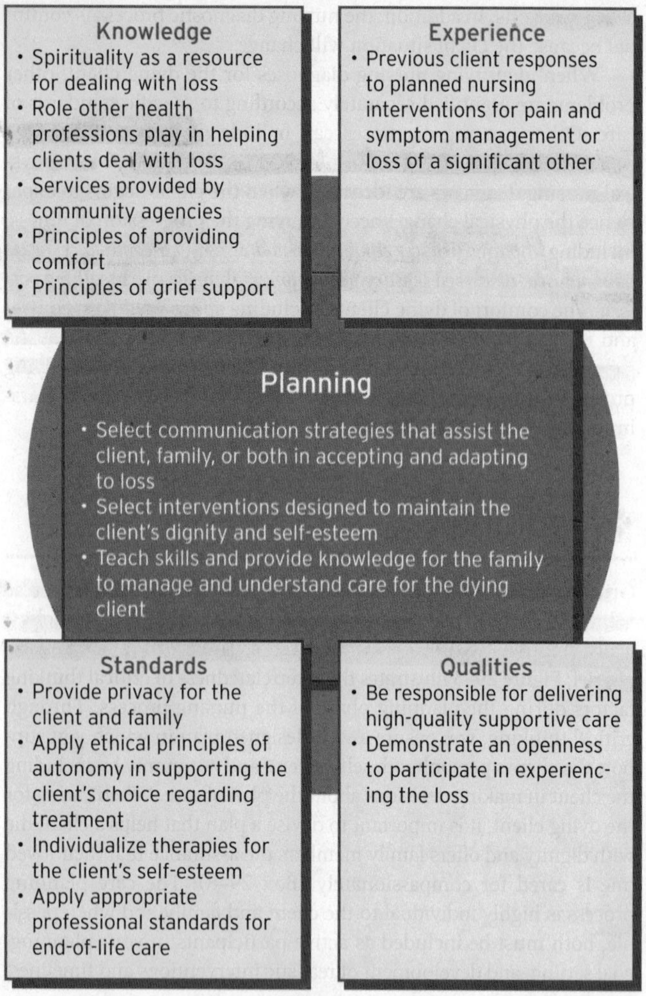

Knowledge
- Spirituality as a resource for dealing with loss
- Role other health professions play in helping clients deal with loss
- Services provided by community agencies
- Principles of providing comfort
- Principles of grief support

Experience
- Previous client responses to planned nursing interventions for pain and symptom management or loss of a significant other

Planning
- Select communication strategies that assist the client, family, or both in accepting and adapting to loss
- Select interventions designed to maintain the client's dignity and self-esteem
- Teach skills and provide knowledge for the family to manage and understand care for the dying client

Standards
- Provide privacy for the client and family
- Apply ethical principles of autonomy in supporting the client's choice regarding treatment
- Individualize therapies for the client's self-esteem
- Apply appropriate professional standards for end-of-life care

Qualities
- Be responsible for delivering high-quality supportive care
- Demonstrate an openness to participate in experiencing the loss

Figure 29-3 Critical thinking model for loss, death, and grieving planning.

"Client will participate in series of short planned teaching discussions about disease" accounts for the client's need for teaching sessions to be short so as to avoid exhaustion.

Goals of care for a client dealing with loss might be long or short term, depending on the nature of the loss and the client's phase of grieving, and the nature of the illness. Many terminally ill clients experience plateaus (periods or relatively stable health) interspersed with periods of exacerbation of symptoms. Because a client may move back and forth between phases of grief, you may need to revise goals and outcomes to ensure that they remain relevant. Help from the client's partner in deciding which goals are relevant is important. General nursing care goals for clients with a loss include accommodating grief, accepting the reality of a loss, and renewing regular relationships. When a client has a terminal illness, controlling pain and symptoms, maintaining autonomy, and achieving spiritual comfort are important goals. For the goal "achieving a sense of dignity," expected outcomes might include the following:

- Client will be able to continue parental responsibilities in care of toddler.
- Client will express hopefulness that cancer treatment will control symptoms.
- Client will engage in playing chess with friends on a weekly basis.

Setting Priorities

When a client has multiple nursing diagnoses, the problems cannot be addressed simultaneously. At any given time, two or three problems dominate your attention. Figure 29–4 is a concept map developed for a client with a medical diagnosis of depression after the death of his wife 6 months previously. As a result of the client's medical condition, associated health problems include the nursing diagnoses *dysfunctional grieving, disturbed sleep pattern,* and *imbalanced nutrition: less than body requirements.* You must determine which of the three diagnoses necessitates greater attention. The continuing grief experienced by the client might be the focus. Until the client is able to accept his loss and begin resolving his grief, he may be unable to attend to interventions that will improve his nutritional intake and sleep status.

BOX 29-8 NURSING CARE PLAN

Ineffective Coping

Assessment

Jan Runyon is the nurse who admits Mr. Miller, a 48-year-old man, from the emergency department to the intensive care unit (ICU) after traumatic brain injury incurred in a motor vehicle accident. Mr. Miller is a successful business executive who has a wife and two sons. The physician has explained to the family that Mr. Miller's prognosis is poor. Tests are under way to determine the extent of brain injury. Mrs. Miller and the children are in the ICU waiting area, waiting on word about Mr. Miller.

Assessment Activities	*Findings and Defining Characteristics*
Jan asks Mrs. Miller, "Tell me how you are feeling about your discussion with the physician."	"I know they are doing everything they can. He is going to be OK, I just know he is. He has never been sick a day in his life."
Jan observes Mrs. Miller's interaction with her children.	Mrs. Miller has difficulty problem solving. The family has posed several questions to her as to what she plans to say to the insurance company and Mr. Miller's employees. Mrs. Miller is unable to decide what to say at this time.
Jan overhears Mrs. Miller on the phone in the waiting area.	Mrs. Miller states over the phone, "Don't worry, he's having some tests right now. I know Bill: he will be back in the office before you know it. Tell the staff everything will be OK."
Jan accompanies the transplant coordinator, who asks Mrs. Miller if the family has ever discussed organ donation.	Mrs. Miller responds, "Bill will be fine. That's not important right now!"

Nursing Diagnosis: Ineffective coping related to husband's traumatic brain injury and poor prognosis

➤ BOX 29-8 NURSING CARE PLAN *continued*

Planning

*Goal (Nursing Outcomes Classification)**	*Expected Outcomes**
	Grief Resolution
Wife will accept the fact that the client will probably die within 48 hours.	Wife will verbalize to caregiver within the next 6 hours that husband's death is actually imminent. Wife will inform children within 24 hours of their father's likely death. Wife will make a decision about organ donation within the next 12 hours. Wife will discuss immediate lifestyle changes that will occur as a result of husband's death over next 48 hours.
Wife will demonstrate effective expression of grief within next 48 hours.	Wife will discuss with children their concerns about what they need to do as a family to prepare for father's impending death within next 48 hours. Wife will discuss effects loss has on her personally with caregiver within next 48 hours.

*Outcome classification label from Moorhead, S., Johnson, M., & Maas, M. L. (2004). *Nursing Outcomes Classification (NOC)* (3rd ed.). St. Louis, MO: Mosby.

Interventions (Nursing Interventions Classification)†	**Rationale**
Presence	
Display interest in wife's situation and accept her behaviours of denial.	Recognizing denial (based on Kübler-Ross's [1969] theory) gives the staff direction for planning unique interventions based on grief theory (Verosky, 2006).
Establish trust and a positive regard by creating an atmosphere of sharing. Offer privacy and security.	Privacy offers a place of security to exhibit personal needs and to work through feelings (Chochinov, 2006). Anxiety about losing dignity when expressing grief will hinder an honest expression of feelings.
Grief Work Facilitation	
Offer wife encouragement to explore and verbalize feelings of grief.	Encouragement refocuses on current needs and assists in initiating grief process.
Identify personal coping strategies used in the past; assess their effectiveness, and promote them when appropriate.	Previously successful coping strategies are the first to be used when a person is under stress (Grassi, 2007). Discouraging maladaptive behaviours helps minimize dysfunctional grieving.
Determine wife's acceptance of available community resources and initiate as appropriate: significant other (business partner), children, clergy, or other health care professionals.	Professionals can use their expertise to direct the grieving process (Verosky, 2006). Trust in relationships already formed will speed the therapeutic communication process

†Intervention classification labels from Dochterman, J. M., & Bulechek, G. M. (2004). *Nursing Interventions Classification (NIC)* (4th ed.). St. Louis, MO: Mosby.

Evaluation

Nursing Actions	*Client Response and Finding*	*Achievement of Outcome*
Say to client's wife, "This has been a difficult time. Your husband's injury has been so sudden."	Wife responds, "I still cannot believe it. The doctors do not believe he will live through the night."	Wife begins to acknowledge client's impending death.
Ask, "Tell me how you are feeling now."	Wife explains, "I am worried about my kids. Both boys are close to their dad. I feel this unbelievable sadness."	Wife is able to express normal grieving behaviours.
Observe wife's behaviour when with children.	Wife discusses decisions that must be made because of impending death of husband. She allows the children to express their sadness.	Wife is able to express grief with family; maintains role as supportive mother.

Clients' conditions always change. In the ongoing assessment of a client's condition, you can quickly discover a new problem. You must always consider which of the client's most urgent physical or psychological needs require immediate intervention. You consider the client's expectations and preferences in regard to the priorities of care. If a terminally ill client's priorities include controlling pain and maintaining self-esteem, pain control is the priority when analgesics become ineffective and the client experiences acute distress. If the client is progressing as desired, you may refocus priorities to address unmet needs. For example, the client suffering depression caused by his wife's death

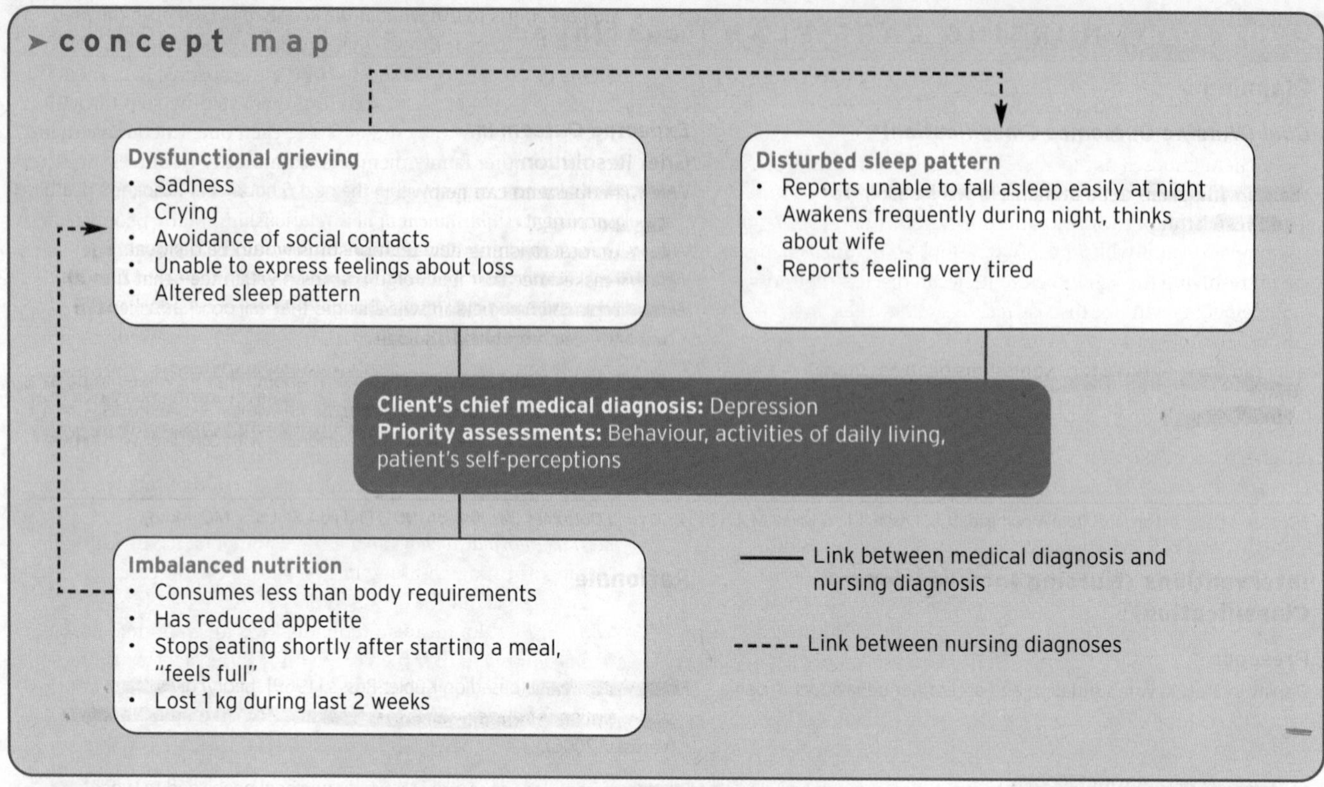

Figure 29-4 Concept map for a client with depression after the death of his wife.

also has problems of imbalanced nutrition and a disturbed sleep pattern. If the client reports an improved appetite and has shown weight stabilization since the last clinic visit, you can focus more attention on the sleep pattern disturbance. You must remember that the client's expectations, clinical condition, and preferences influence priorities. If a terminally ill client places more emphasis on spiritual support than on other priorities such learning about planned treatments, you must attend to the client's priorities. Meeting client priorities may allow you to then address other needs more effectively with less effort.

Continuity of Care

Interdisciplinary teams help identify and meet the needs of people who experience losses. Dietitians, clergy, physicians, social workers, physiotherapists, psychologists, chaplains, and other specialty health care professionals can assist a client and family in their grief. A coordinated team approach to managing a client's needs results in a well-managed care plan. When a client dies, the loss that you and your colleagues experience can be shared within the interprofessional group. Support is needed to promote healing for all who worked with the dying client and the family. Conflicts and differences can be discussed openly and solutions found in a healthy manner with the client as the primary focus. For example, ethical conflicts may have arisen related to proposed or performed medical treatments or interventions. Through working together, the sharing of experiences, feelings, alternatives, and solutions becomes the basis for dealing with future losses.

Many terminally ill clients return home and require continued intensive nursing care. Home care nurses collaborate closely with family members to meet the client's ongoing needs. Important interventions to include in planning a return home are arranging for main-floor access, arranging appropriate medical equipment, and providing sufficient family respite. When it is realistic for the client to remain independent, therapeutic strategies should bolster the client's sense of autonomy and the ability to function as independently as possible (Smith & Kautz, 2007). For example, judicious application of orthotic devices, along with physiotherapy and occupational therapy, can often bolster a client's functional capacity. In the home, safety issues related to the environment may exist, and clients often benefit from nurse-initiated referrals to community occupational therapists.

❖Implementation

Health Promotion

Although a return to full function is not an expected outcome for a terminally ill client or even for a client who has significant disability, optimal physical and emotional functioning is a realistic goal. The goal of nursing care is to help clients and families cope with the stressors in their lives and to achieve healthy grief resolution. You help clients and families in dealing with loss, making decisions about the client's health care, and adjusting to any disappointment, frustration, and anxiety created by their loss.

Therapeutic Communication. Nursing care of the grieving client and family begins with establishing a caring presence and determining the significance of their loss. This is difficult if the client is unwilling or unable to express feelings or is experiencing numbing or denial. You must use therapeutic communication strategies that enable clients to discuss their loss and find ways to work through it. Your presence, attentive listening, and use of open-ended questions enable clients to freely share their thoughts and concerns. Closed-ended questions often reflect only what you presume is the problem. For example, in response to the question "Does knowing you have cancer make you fearful?" a client will probably not reveal as much as to "Tell me how your diagnosis of cancer is making you feel." You should acknowledge the client's grief and show support by demonstrating caring behaviours throughout the discussion (see Chapter 19). You will gain the client's trust by showing a desire to enter into a caring, therapeutic relationship with the client. Listening attentively to the client can be very therapeutic for the client, and you may discover details that help you plan effective care.

If a client chooses not to share feelings or concerns, you should convey a willingness to be available when needed. If you are reassuring and respectful of the client's need for dignity and privacy, a therapeutic relationship will probably develop. Sometimes clients need to begin resolving their grief before they can discuss their loss.

Some clients will not discuss feelings about their loss, or sometimes a client does not want to discuss loss, symptoms, or impending death. You must observe for expressions of anger, denial, depression, or guilt. You must also know your own feelings before encouraging clients to express their anger. Individuals may express anger toward family, staff, or physicians. Clients can also become demanding and accusing. You must remain supportive by letting clients and family members know that feelings such as anger are normal. For example, you might say, "You are obviously upset. I just want you to know I am here to talk with you if you want." You must avoid barriers to communication such as denying the client's grief, providing false reassurance, or avoiding discussion of sensitive issues (see Chapter 18).

No topic that a dying client wishes to discuss should be avoided. When the client wants to talk, it is important for you to find time to do so. This can be challenging for a nurse with limited experience with dying clients or who works in a busy acute care setting. You should respond to questions openly and honestly and provide information that helps clients and their families to understand their condition, the trajectory or future course of their disease, the benefits and burdens of treatment, and values and goals (Verosky, 2006). In some cases, you may recognize the need for pastoral care or counselling services, and you can initiate a referral for the client to consult with such professionals.

Promoting Hope. Hope can be an energizing resource for clients experiencing loss. For each dimension of hope, nursing strategies that promote hope exist.

- *Affective dimension:* Show empathic understanding of the client's strengths. Reinforce expressions of courage, positive thinking, and realistic goal setting. Encourage expression of both positive and negative feelings.
- *Cognitive dimension:* Offer information about the illness and treatments, and correct any misunderstanding or misinformation. Clarify or modify the client's perceptions.
- *Behavioural dimension:* Assist the client in using personal resources and making use of external supports to balance the need for independence with healthy interdependence and dependence.
- *Affiliative dimension:* Encourage clients to foster supportive relationships with others.
- *Temporal dimension:* Focus on short-term goals as life expectancy diminishes.
- *Contextual dimension:* Encourage development of achievable goals. Allow time to reminisce about achievements or positive moments.

Facilitating Mourning. Nursing care strategies can help clients move through uncomplicated grief (Worden, 1991). The following guidelines are helpful for people who are mourning a death, facing death, and grieving over an actual loss:

- *Help the client accept that loss is real.* Discuss how the loss or illness occurred or was discovered, when, under what circumstances, who told the client about it, and other similar topics to help make the event real and to place it in perspective.
- *Support efforts to live without the deceased person or in the presence of disability.* A problem-solving approach is often helpful. Have clients or the family make a list of their problems, help them prioritize the problems, and then lead them step-by-step through a discussion of how they might tackle each one. Encourage them to rely on other family members, community resources, or other people who can help.
- *Encourage establishment of new relationships.* Many people fear that establishing new relationships would be disloyal. They need reassurance that new relationships do not mean that they are replacing the person who has died. Encourage the client to become involved in social relationships that are nonthreatening (e.g., religious gatherings or volunteer activities).
- *Allow time to grieve.* It is common to have "anniversary reactions" around the time of the loss in subsequent years. Some people worry that they are mentally or emotionally unstable when sadness or other signs of grief recur after a period of relative calm. Encourage the client to reminisce.
- *Interpret "normal" behaviour.* Being distractible, having difficulty sleeping or eating, thinking one has heard the deceased's voice, or dreaming about the deceased are common after loss. These symptoms do not mean an individual has an emotional problem or is becoming ill in some way. Reinforce the fact that these occurrences are normal and will resolve over time.
- *Provide continuing support.* Clients and their families may need to talk and may look to you for support for many months or years after a loss. If you have occasion to see the client or family after an extended time, it is appropriate to ask about how they are coping or adjusting. This gives them the opportunity to talk if they need to.
- *Be alert for signs of ineffective coping.* Be aware of coping mechanisms that may be maladaptive, such as increased alcohol or substance abuse, which can include excessive use of over-the-counter pain medications or sleep aids.

Acute Care

Palliative Care. For people who face life-threatening illnesses, many medical and technological advances are available to reverse the course of the disease or to prolong life. For clients with serious life-limiting illness, it becomes important for health care professionals to find ways to help clients approach their end of life. The aim of **palliative care** is to relieve suffering and improve the quality of living and dying (Chochinov, 2006). More than 220,000 Canadians die each year; approximately 160,000 need palliative care. However, only an estimated 5% of dying Canadians and their families receive palliative care services (Senate of Canada, 2000).

Palliative care is for any age, any diagnosis, at any time, and not just during the last few months of life. Chochinov (2006) explained that when the preservation of dignity becomes the goal of palliation, care options encompass the physical, psychological, social, spiritual, and existential aspects of the client's illness. Palliative care thus allows clients to make more informed choices, to better alleviate symptoms, and to have more opportunity to manage unfinished business. Ferris et al. (2002) designed the *Model to Guide Patient and Family Care,* which provides a comprehensive approach for palliative caregiving with nationally accepted principles and norms of practice.

According to the World Health Organization (2008), when health care professionals provide palliative care, they do the following:

- Provide relief from pain and other distressing symptoms
- Affirm life and regard dying as a normal process
- Neither hasten nor postpone death
- Integrate psychological and spiritual aspects of client care

- Offer a support system to help clients live as actively as possible until death.
- Offer a support system to help families cope during the client's illness and their own bereavement
- Enhance the quality of life

Chochinov (2006) added that palliative care also helps clients and families "combine the best of modern medicine and symptom management techniques [and] provides an opportunity to achieve dignity-conserving end of life care" (p. 84) and "encompasses the psychosocial, existential and spiritual aspects of the patient's experience" (p. 84).

Palliative care is a philosophy of total care. A palliative care approach ensures that a client experiences a "meaningful death," free of avoidable pain and suffering, in accordance with the client's and family's wishes, and "is the difference between technically competent symptom management [and] a holistic approach to end of life care" (Chochinov, 2006, p. 84). Palliative care is highly dependent on an interdisciplinary team–based approach, in which each team member has individual expertise and makes an individual commitment to common goals. The team includes physicians, nurses, social workers, pastoral care providers, physiotherapists, occupational therapists, and pharmacists. Massage therapists, music therapists, or art therapists—who provide alternative therapies—might also be a part of the team (see Chapter 35). Volunteers are also part of the team and can provide additional psychosocial support and simple comfort measures.

The Canadian Hospice Palliative Care Association Nursing Standards Committee (2002) has developed nursing standards of practice for hospice palliative care. These nursing standards reflect the six dimensions of the supportive care model: valuing, connecting, empowering, doing for, finding meaning, and preserving integrity (Davies & Oberle, 1990).

Palliative care is compassionate and supportive of dying people and their families. Nurses play a key role in providing care to the dying and are "often the most intimate contact and constant presence" (CNA, 2000). Thus, one of the most important skills you provide in palliative care is establishing a caring relationship with both client and family. It also becomes very important for you to provide appropriate symptom-control measures for maintaining the client's dignity and self-esteem, to prevent feelings of abandonment or isolation, and to provide a comfortable and peaceful environment at the time of death.

Symptom Control. Comfort for a dying client requires management of symptoms of disease and therapies. For many clients, symptom distress is characteristic of the dying experience (Chochinov, 2006). *Symptom distress* is the experience of discomfort or anguish related to the progression of a disease. Clients experience anguish from not knowing or being unaware of aspects of their health status or treatment. Worry and fear are common among clients and may heighten their perception of discomfort. You assess the character of the client's symptoms carefully in order to select appropriate therapies. Chapter 42 details the assessment of pain. By providing information about treatment options or the anticipated course of an illness, you help preserve the dignity of clients and families (Kirk et al., 2004). Complementary therapies are sometimes used for symptom management: for example, therapeutic touch, massage, aromatherapy, music therapy, biofeedback, homeopathy, acupuncture, and relaxation therapy. On occasion, clients may inquire about culture-specific complementary therapies.

One symptom common among terminally ill clients is dyspnea (air hunger). The sense of suffocation can cause anxiety or panic in the client and significant stress in the caregiver (Kouch, 2006). As the client's anxiety increases when he or she is unable to breathe adequately, the dyspnea worsens. Family who are in attendance may likely become more anxious. Kirk et al. (2004) interviewed terminally ill clients and caregivers and found that collaborative decision making, including the client's views, helps the client maintain a sense of control. For example, a client may choose to switch oxygen devices, even though they deliver the same concentration of oxygen. However, if the client believes that a different device makes a difference, the switch might be enough to relieve the dyspnea at least briefly. A client who is breathing by mouth may receive more benefit from a mask than from a nasal cannula; however, a mask can also increase anxiety, which results in worsening dyspnea. When options in respiratory therapy exist, it helps to give the client a choice.

Management of air hunger also involves the judicious administration of morphine and antianxiolytics for relief of respiratory distress. Table 29–4 summarizes nursing care measures for additional symptoms of terminal disease. Because therapies and clinical practice standards are constantly evolving, you must keep your knowledge current.

Maintaining Dignity and Self-Esteem. The notion of dignity varies from client to client and between one circumstance and the next, and it is an overarching value or goal inherent in palliative care (Chochinov, 2006). Personal dignity may revolve around a person's positive sense of self-regard, is individualistic, and is closely linked with the client's personal goals and social contexts (Chochinov, 2006). Dignity may also revolve around the extent to which clients feel valued and how they are treated by caregivers.

You can promote a client's self-esteem and dignity by conveying respect for the client as a whole person with feelings, accomplishments, and passions independent of the illness experience (Chochinov, 2006). Giving importance to autonomy, acceptance, resilience, and maintaining hope acknowledges individual personhood; it also strengthens the empathic, therapeutic communication between the client, the client's family, and yourself. Providing time for clients to share their life experiences, particularly about what has been meaningful, enables you to know clients better. Knowing clients then facilitates choice of therapies that promote client decision making and autonomy.

For many clients, receiving spiritual comfort helps preserve dignity and self-esteem. Facilitating connections to a spiritual practice or community and supporting the expression of culturally held beliefs is very important. Clients may also benefit by being assured that some aspect of their lives may transcend death. In other words, the client gains comfort from knowing that something of his or her life will continue after death. Participating in a life project such as making an audiotape or videotape for the family, writing letters, or keeping a journal can offer clients the comfort of knowing that something of their essence will survive (Chochinov, 2006). Chapter 28 further discusses some of the spiritual practices and religious rituals that can support people in need of spiritual comfort.

Basic to promoting self-esteem and dignity is attending to the client's appearance and surroundings. Cleanliness, absence of body odours, attractive clothing, and personal grooming all contribute to a sense of worth. When helping a client tend to bodily functions, you always show respect, even when the client becomes dependent. It is important to keep the client's immediate surroundings pleasant by opening curtains and letting light change from the bright of day to the dark of night. The quick removal of liquid stool or vomitus will help avoid unpleasant odours.

Disabilities experienced by the client may threaten dignity, especially when caregivers take control of the client's life. You allow the client to participate in nursing care decisions (e.g., how and when to administer personal hygiene, diet preferences, and timing of nursing therapies). You keep the client and family well informed about planned therapies, their purpose, and anticipated effects. It is also

TABLE 29-4 Promoting Comfort in Terminally Ill Clients

Symptoms	Characteristics or Causes	Nursing Implications
Discomfort	Any source of physical irritation may worsen pain.	Provide thorough skin care—including daily baths, lubrication of skin, and dry, clean bed linens—to reduce irritants. Assess for appropriateness of special mattresses.
	As client approaches death, mouth remains open, tongue becomes dry and edematous, and lips become dry and cracked.	Provide oral care at least every 2 to 4 hours. Use foam or premoistened swabs for frequent mouth care. Apply a light film of water-soluble lubricant to lips and tongue (see Chapter 38).
	Blinking reflexes diminish near death, which causes drying of the cornea.	Remove crusts from eyelid margins. Administer artificial tears to reduce corneal drying.
Fatigue	Metabolic demands of a cancerous tumour cause weakness and fatigue.	Help client identify values or desired tasks; then help client conserve energy for only those tasks. Promote frequent rest periods in a quiet environment.
	Exhaustion phase of the general adaptation syndrome causes energy depletion.	Time and pace nursing care activities (ensure periods of rest between blocks of care). Encourage use of energy-saving devices such as mobility aids.
Nausea	Nausea may occur as a side effect of medications and as a result of severe pain, as a symptom of certain illnesses, or as a result of palliative chemotherapy or radiation therapy.	Administer antiemetics: provide oral care at least every 2 to 4 hours; offer clear liquid diet and ice chips; avoid liquids that increase stomach acidity, such as coffee, milk, and citric acid juices. Encourage high-calorie nutritional supplements (e.g., Ensure, Boost).
Constipation	Narcotic medications and immobility slow peristalsis.	Provide preventive care, which is most effective: increase fluid intake; include bran, whole grain products, and fresh vegetables in diet; encourage exercise (Chapter 43).
	Lack of bulk in diet or reduced fluid intake may occur with appetite changes.	Administer prophylactic stool softeners on a regular basis.
	Constipation can add to discomfort.	Administer laxatives as necessary.
Diarrhea	Diarrhea results from disease process (e.g., colon cancer), from complications of treatment or medications, or from fecal impaction caused by constipation.	Assess for fecal impaction (if sudden liquid stool occurs) and treat if required. Provide thorough perineal care if required. Administer antidiarrheals as needed. Confer with physician to change medication if possible. Provide low-residue diet.
Urinary incontinence	Incontinence results from progressive disease (e.g., involvement of spinal cord, reduced level of consciousness).	Protect skin from irritation or breakdown. Implement use of barrier creams to help protect skin integrity. Use disposable incontinence briefs if appropriate. Use indwelling urinary catheter or condom catheters if appropriate (Chapter 44).
Inadequate nutrition	Nausea and vomiting can decrease appetite.	Serve smaller portions and bland foods, which may be more palatable. Encourage intake of nutritional supplements.
	Depression from grieving may cause anorexia.	Allow home-cooked meals, which may be preferred by client and gives the family a chance to participate in care.
Dehydration	As disease progresses, client is less willing or able to maintain oral fluid intake.	Remove factors causing decreased intake; give antiemetics, and apply topical analgesics to oral lesions. Reduce discomfort from dehydration; provide mouth care at least every 4 hours; offer ice chips or moist cloth to lips.
Ineffective breathing patterns (e.g., dyspnea, shortness of breath)	Disease progression that involves lung tissue (e.g., progression of cancer, pneumonia, pulmonary edema) may affect breathing.	Treat or control underlying cause. For example, in some cases of pulmonary edema, a diuretic may be appropriate and may temporarily relieve symptoms. Provide reassurance and comfort measures to the client. Place client in semi-Fowler's position, which will help.
	Anemia reduces oxygen-carrying capacity.	Maximize client's oxygenation (e.g., place the client in semi-Fowler's position or upright; provide supplemental oxygen; maintain a patent airway; reduce anxiety or fever).
	Anxiety increases oxygen demand.	Administer medications such as bronchodilators, inhaled steroids, or narcotics and antianxiolytics to suppress cough, ease breathing, and alleviate apprehension.
	Fever increases oxygen demand.	Administer antipyretics as needed. Promote comfort through measures such as removing some clothing and bedding.
Confusion, disorientation, and restlessness	These manifestations may be caused by hypoxia, metabolic changes, brain metastases, or medication side effects.	Ensure safe environment. Monitor client frequently. Reorient the client as needed. Administer medications as prescribed and as needed.

important to provide the client with privacy during nursing care procedures and when the client and family need time together.

Preventing Abandonment and Isolation. Many terminally ill clients are fearful of dying alone. Therefore, it is important for you to answer the call light quickly and to explain when staff will be giving care and performing assessments throughout the day and night. You should establish presence and use appropriate touch when performing care measures. You must be available to answer questions, even if data are not needed, no further decisions are left to make, or no further curative interventions are available (Kirk et al., 2004). Clients may feel a sense of involvement when sharing a room and interacting with staff. Clients can share conversation and companionship with roommates and visitors. The choice of private or shared room should be discussed with the client and family whenever possible.

Family is always considered as the unit of care in palliative care. If family members have difficulty accepting the client's impending death, they may avoid visitation, exhibit denial, or express unrealistic expectations. When family members do visit, it is important for you to talk with them and keep them informed of the client's progress. It may be useful to give family members helpful hints about what to discuss with clients. For example, you can help improve the family member's communication skills by role modelling attentive listening and offering reassurance. You should encourage the family to discuss activities other family members are involved in, to reminisce about enjoyable times, and to inquire about the client's concerns. It is important for you to advocate for the client to ensure that the client does not become exhausted by visits. A useful strategy is to establish a schedule for family to be in attendance or to suggest family or friends visit two at a time. It is also helpful to find simple and appropriate care activities for the family to perform, such as feeding the client, washing the client's face, combing hair, and filling out the client's menu. Older adults often become particularly lonely at night and may feel more secure if a family member stays at the bedside during the night. You should allow visitors to remain with dying clients at any time if the client wants them. Also, you must know how to contact family members at any time if the client requests a visit or if the client's condition worsens.

Providing a Comfortable and Peaceful Environment. You keep a client comfortable through frequent and regular repositioning, keeping bed linens dry, and controlling extraneous environmental noise. Pictures, cherished objects, cards or letters from family members and friends, and plants and flowers create an environment that is more familiar and comforting. You offer the client frequent back, lower leg, and foot massage, or guided imagery exercises, and allow the client time to listen to preferred types of music. A comfortable, pleasant environment helps clients to relax, which promotes their ability to sleep and minimizes severity of symptoms.

Fear of Dying and Death. People are afraid of dying and death for many different reasons: the process of dying, with its associated pain and loss of dignity; not knowing what will happen after death; and dying before fulfilling dreams and goals. The intensity of the fear varies with each person and his or her circumstances, including age, culture, sex, personal experiences, family situation, social supports, and religious beliefs. Kirk et al. (2004) pointed out that nurses need to help clients realistically appraise these fears. Nurses also need to listen and understand as clients express their emotions.

Support for the Grieving Family. The family may be the primary caregivers when the client chooses to die at home. Family members need your support, and they benefit from being taught ways to care for their loved one (Box 29–9). Caring for a family member can be emotionally stressful and physically exhausting for the family caregiver. Not all families can manage care on their own. In the home setting, you provide the opportunity for the family to be temporarily relieved of their duties so that they can rest. Such respite care is a resource available through hospice programs, in which respite workers can come into the home, or a client can go to a facility for a respite stay.

Families also need to be informed of home care, hospice, and community service options so that they can choose among the resources available. The Saint Elizabeth Health Care Foundation in Canada has sponsored a free-of-charge publication called *Family Hospice Care: Pre-planning and Care Guide*. This is a practical and informative resource written to help families meet the needs of their terminally ill loved ones (van Bommel, 2006). Each province and health region has varying resources; therefore, you are required to know what is available to them in the individual family's jurisdiction. In some cases, families may need assistance and support in making the decision about placement in a health care facility.

You must keep the family informed so that they can anticipate the type of symptoms the client will probably experience and the implications for care. You encourage family members to express their grief openly with the client and to give the client the opportunity to discuss any remaining concerns or requests. The family also needs personal time to share their concerns with you and to ask questions about treatment options, the course of the client's disease, and the meaning of the client's behaviours. It is wise for you to communicate news of the client's impending death when the family is together, if possible. Family members can provide support for one another. Convey the news in a private area, and be willing to remain with the family as needed. In some situations in which families are large or cannot all be together, it may be beneficial to have a designated family spokesperson or representative through whom information can be relayed.

BOX 29-9 CLIENT TEACHING

Preparing the Dying Client's Family

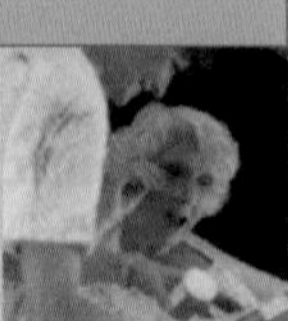

Objectives

- Improve the family's ability to provide appropriate physical care for the dying client in the home.
- Improve the family's ability to provide appropriate psychological support to the dying client.

Teaching Strategies

- Describe and demonstrate feeding techniques and selection of foods to facilitate the client's ease of chewing and swallowing.
- Demonstrate bathing, mouth care, and other hygiene measures, and allow the family to perform return demonstration.
- Show the family a video on simple transfer techniques to prevent injury to themselves and the client; help the family practise these techniques.
- Instruct the family on the need to take rest periods.
- Teach the family to recognize signs and symptoms to expect as the client's condition worsens, and provide information on whom to call in an emergency.
- Discuss ways to support the dying client, and listen to needs and fears.
- Solicit questions from the family, and provide information as needed.

Evaluation

- Ask the family members to demonstrate physical care techniques (e.g., turning, feeding, mouth care).
- Ask the family members to describe how they vary approaches to care when the client has symptoms such as pain or fatigue.
- Ask the family to discuss how they feel about their ability to support the client.

It is important for you to educate the family regarding the signs of impending death. Tissue perfusion becomes impaired, which results in cool and clammy skin. Alterations in heart rate or rhythms, hypotension, and pooling of blood in dependent areas may occur. The extremities often have a mottled appearance. Breathing patterns may be impaired. Clients may exhibit shortness of breath or increased secretions. Later signs include increasingly longer and more frequent periods of apnea, alternating with hyperpnea; this pattern is known as Cheyne-Stokes respirations. Clients may exhibit alterations in level of consiousness and changes in behaviour; for example, disorientation and restlessness may occur. Urine output decreases, and incontinence may occur. In addition, periods of sleep increase, and eventually some clients may become unconscious as death nears.

In the hospital setting, you assist in planning a visitation schedule for family members, to prevent the client and family from excessive fatigue. Young children should visit dying parents. During the final moments of a client's life, you help the family to stay in communication with the client through frequent visits, caring silence, attentive listening, touch, and telling the client of their love. After the client's death, you need to encourage the family to remain with the deceased as long as as long as they feel they need to. You are required to provide support and to assist the family with decision making, such as notification of a funeral home or mortician, transportation of additional family members, and collection of the client's belongings.

Hospice Care. Hospice care is an alternative care delivery model for terminally ill clients. It is one phase of palliative care. **Hospice** is not necessarily a facility but a concept for family-centred care designed to assist the client in being comfortable and maintaining a satisfactory lifestyle until death. Hospice services are available in the home, hospital, stand-alone facilities, and long-term care settings. Availability and accessibility vary across Canada. Hospice care programs include the following components:

- Client and family as the unit of care
- Coordinated home care with access to beds in available inpatient and long-term care facilities
- Control of symptoms (physical, sociological, psychological, and spiritual)
- Physician-directed services
- Provision of an interdisciplinary care team of physicians, nurses, spiritual advisors, social worker, and counsellors
- Availability of medical and nursing services at all times
- Bereavement follow-up after a client's death
- Use of trained volunteers for frequent visitation and respite support

Canada's first hospice was established in Toronto in 1979. Casey House in Toronto and the John Gordon home in London, Ontario, provide hospice care for people dying from AIDS. Canuck Place, in Vancouver, is the only children's hospice in North America and provides a continuum of care that comprises three components: respite, palliative, and bereavement (Davies et al., 2003). In general, clients accepted into a hospice program are believed to have less than 6 months to live, although this criterion is being challenged across Canada.

Your role in hospice care is to meet the primary wishes of the dying client and to be amenable to individual desires of each client. You support a client's choice in maintaining comfort and dignity. Whether the client ultimately dies at home or in a health care facility, the client's wishes are followed with the understanding that whatever his or her choice, it is made "for the good of all who are involved." When options are complicated by family needs, hospice professionals will try to work with the clients' wishes. A hospice program emphasizes palliative care with the client and family as active participants. Client care goals are mutually set, and all participants fully understand the options and desires of the client. Efforts by the hospice team are made to meet the client's desires and to encourage the family to stay within those guidelines. One or more bereavement visits are often made by the staff of the hospice team to the family even after the death of the client to help the family move through the grieving process successfully.

Many clients prefer to die at home in a familiar setting, whereas others, not wishing to burden their families, choose to die in a hospital or long-term care facility. Alternatively, some families are ill-prepared or unable to care for a client at home. It is important that the hospice team know the client's preference. Many clients suffer physical ailments that prevent them from being cared for at home despite the willingness of family and friends to care for the client. The health and welfare issues are viewed from a broader perspective than just the client's desires. The concern for family needs is also taken into consideration by the hospice team.

A client receiving hospice care may be hospitalized because of a change in condition or exacerbation of symptoms, and the health care team coordinates care between the home and inpatient setting. An effort is always made to keep clients at home for as long as possible. The family provides basic supportive care. However, if the family cannot meet all of the client's needs, a nurse is available to coordinate and administer symptom management therapies. The goal of the interdisciplinary team is 24-hour accessibility as needed. As a client's death becomes imminent, members of the hospice team are available to give support to the client and family.

Care After Death. When a client dies in a hospital setting, you provide **post-mortem care**. It is important to care for the client's body with dignity and sensitivity and in a manner consistent with the client's religious or cultural beliefs. After death, the body undergoes many physical changes. For that reason, care must be provided as soon as possible to prevent tissue damage or disfigurement of body parts.

Hospitals are required to formulate policies and procedures that are based on current provincial and territorial laws to validate death, identify potential organ or tissue donors, and provide post-mortem care. For transplantation of organs, the client must be maintained in an intensive care unit on ventilatory and circulatory support until vital organs are harvested. The family must clearly understand that the client is "brain dead" and that the equipment (i.e., ventilator and vasopressor medications) is not keeping the client alive but keeping the physical body in a state so that the organs will not be damaged before being harvested.

Family support is crucial at the time of the client's death. If family members are not present at that time, the assigned nurse (or another staff member who knows the family) makes contact with the family. If you are the assigned nurse, you inform the family of the death and respond to any immediate questions from the family. It is important that you find out from the family whether they will come to the facility to view the deceased and to collect any personal belongings. Make note of which family members will come and when. In some situations, family members may be too distraught to safely drive themselves and need to be encouraged to have someone else drive or to take alternative transportation.

Once the family has arrived to view the deceased, it is beneficial, before they view the body, for you to explain to the family what they may expect to see. Typically, a deceased person has a peaceful expression (as facial muscles have relaxed); however, the body feels cool to touch and appears grayish-white. This appearance may be difficult for some family members to observe.

You can be very helpful in supporting families through the organ and tissue request process. It is important to provide a private area in which to discuss all issues with the family. The staff member designated to make a request, such as a formal transplant coordinator, a social worker, chaplain, or you, must offer the family clarification of what defines brain death because support systems must remain in place even after the client is pronounced "dead" for vital organ retrieval (i.e., heart, lungs, kidneys, and liver). You reinforce explanations throughout the organ retrieval process. The family must know who legally can give final consent, the options for organ or tissue donation, any associated costs, and how donation will affect burial or cremation. Nonvital tissues such as corneas, skin, long bones, and middle ear bones can be harvested when the client is proclaimed dead without artificially maintaining vital functions. If the client did not make specific documented requests before death, the family must agree on organ and tissue donation. You should review the organ retrieval laws in the family's province or territory, as well as your institution's policy and procedure regarding the formal consent process.

Another topic that creates tension or anxiety is autopsy. The physician usually asks for permission for an autopsy, but nurses are often the professionals who answer questions and support the family's choices. It is very difficult to approach a grieving family with such a request; ideally, the topics of autopsy and donation are discussed before the client's death. The value of an autopsy is that it may improve knowledge in the field of medicine or bring answers or clarification for the family. To help the living, the autopsy can lead to new therapies or new understanding of diseases. The more reasons you can think of to support organ donation, tissue donation, or autopsy, the more the family will be helped to realize the good that can be accomplished by either donation or research autopsy.

Clients' and families' cultural beliefs are very important in postmortem care (see Chapter 10). Maintaining the integrity of rituals and mourning practices helps families accept the client's death and achieve an inner peace. The ethical decisions that surround a client's death are based on the values of a culture. Health care professionals must determine the makeup of a family network and which members should be involved about decisions such as organ donation and end-of-life care.

You are responsible for coordination of all aspects of care surrounding a client's death. Box 29–10 summarizes the nurse's and physician's responsibilities for care of the body after death. It is important for you to be familiar with institutional policies and procedures

➤ BOX 29-10 Procedural Guidelines

Care of the Body After Death

Delegation Considerations: Care of the body after death can be delegated to unregulated care providers except in cases of organ or tissue donation. Check agency policy for which staff member is authorized to remove any invasive tubes or catheters.

Equipment: Bath towels, washcloths, wash basin, scissors, shroud kit with name tags, bed linen, room deodorizer, documentation forms.

Procedure

1. Physicians must complete the death certificate: cause of death, time when death was pronounced, therapy used, and actions taken. In some provinces such as British Columbia, nurses may pronounce the death but may not complete the death certificate. (This may not be the policy in all agencies. Follow your agency's policy.)
2. Physicians may request an autopsy, especially for deaths under unusual circumstances.
3. Trained staff members offer survivors the option of donating the organs or tissue of the deceased; personal, religious, and cultural needs should be included during this process.
4. Nurses work with sensitivity to preserve the client's and family's dignity.
   A. Check orders for any specimens or special orders needed by the physician.
   B. Make arrangements for staff, spiritual advisor, or others to stay with the family while the body is prepared for viewing; find out whether survivors have special requests for viewing (e.g., shaving, a special gown, Bible in hand, rosary at the bedside).
   C. Before shaving of male client: Determine whether the family wishes the client to remain unshaven if it was his custom to wear a beard. Determine whether client's religion or culture has a preference regarding facial hair.
   D. Remove all equipment, tubes, supplies, and dirty linens according to agency protocol. Exceptions to this process include organ donation (leave support systems in place), and sudden or unexpected deaths that necessitate coroner involvement or investigation (leave tubings and lines in situ, but cut them near the body and clamp them).
   E. Cleanse the body thoroughly, apply clean sheets, and remove all trash from the room.
   F. Brush and comb the client's hair. Apply any personal hairpiece.
   G. Position according to protocol: The eyes should be closed by gently holding the client's eyelids closed for a few minutes; dentures should be in the client's mouth to maintain facial alignment.
   H. Cover the body with a clean sheet up to the chin with arms outside covers if possible.
   I. Lower the lighting, and spray a deodorizer if possible to remove unpleasant odours.
   J. Give the family the option to view or not to view the dead body; clarify that either option is acceptable.
   K. If family members choose to view the dead body, go with them.
   L. Encourage the family to say goodbye through both touch and talk.
   M. Do not rush the goodbye process. Once the family is more comfortable, ask if they would like to be left alone. Remind them that they can call you if they need to.
   N. Clarify which personal belongings should stay with the body and who will take personal items; documentation requires both a descriptor of the objects (i.e., rings, jewelry, electronics) and the name of each person who received them, with the time and date.
   O. Do not discard items found after the family is gone; call the family and tell them what was found and ask who might pick it up. Descriptions of the articles help the client's family make decisions accordingly.
   P. Apply name tags according to protocol, such as on the wrist, on the right big toe, or outside a shroud.
   Q. Complete documentation in the nursing notes. Documents vary, depending on the agency (see Box 29–11).
   R. Remain sensitive to other hospitalized clients or visitors when transporting the body, such as covering the body with a clean sheet, temporarily and gently closing doors to clients' rooms, and watching to avoid visitors when moving the body to another part of the hospital or to the exit for the funeral home.
   S. Follow all protocol and policies to meet all legal requirements in caring for the body.

that are established for post-mortem care. Many of these practices also depend on the individuals' unique experiences and preferences.

The family becomes the primary client when the actual death has occurred, and the shift of concern moves from the deceased client to the living family. At this time, it is important to appropriately use the resources that are available. For example, pastoral care staff can be a helpful resource to assist the family even before the actual death, if no bereavement team is available. However, it is important to know whether the family chooses to have spiritual counsellors present. Some families prefer to grieve alone, whereas others may desire the support of other people. Social workers and counsellors can also offer assistance. If the family's expectations for support are unknown, any professional who assists the family can ask the simple questions and make suggestions for assistance.

Documentation of all of the events surrounding a client's death is important for avoiding misunderstandings and for clarifying final events in a client's life. Each facility's policies and procedures support legal guidelines that must be followed and accurately documented. Box 29–11 lists the content to be documented about end-of-life care. Documentation validates the success of meeting the goals identified for the client or provides a justification for the failure to meet any goals. Complete and accurate documentation offers a summary of activities that can become the focus for risk management or legal investigations.

A physician or coroner must sign some of the medical forms, but the registered nurse must record most of the forms. Gathering of information for the forms may be delegated to unregulated care providers, but you must chart the data in the nurse's notes. A licensed professional should witness the signing of forms.

In cases of legal matters, the family expects a clear, concise description of what occurred in the care of the client at the time of death. Opinions must be avoided, and facts are stated in a nonjudgemental, objective manner. Provincial and territorial guidelines direct what type of information is charted and when it is to be charted. Clients have the right to access their health records. Copies of parts of the chart can be given to family members upon written request and the approval of the physician and hospital (see your agency's guidelines). You must understand and uphold the legal guidelines of documentation at all times (see Chapter 16).

The Grieving Nurse. When you have cared for a client for a period of time, it is possible to have deep personal feelings of loss and sadness when the client dies. It is common for nurses to want to hold the hand of the client who is dying. By being present at the time of the client's death, you are able to "let go."

You can attempt in many ways to cope with the loss of a dying client. Attending the viewing at the mortuary or funeral is one way to say goodbye. Writing a letter of sympathy to the family can prove helpful. Some agencies routinely send out sympathy cards from the interdisciplinary team, in which you can write an individual note. It is natural for you to go through the grieving process. When you work in an area in which multiple losses occur, it is easy for bereavement overload to develop unless you have ways to process grief. You might feel frustration, anger, guilt, sadness, or anxiety. Often nurses seek out other nurses or health care professionals to discuss their own grief (Figure 29–5). It is important for you to develop your own support systems that allow time away from the care setting and provide opportunities to share personal feelings. Stress management techniques (see Chapter 30) can help restore a nurse's energy and continued enjoyment in caring for clients. Your self-care is crucial for your survival and recovery from loss, not only for your sake but also for the sake of future clients. Interdisciplinary team debriefings regarding complex or ethical issues are valuable in helping you cope with loss.

➤ BOX 29-11 Documentation of End-of-Life Care

The following items must be documented at the end of a client's life:

- Time of death and actions taken to prevent death, or cardiac arrest record if applicable
- The name of the person who pronounced the client's death
- Any special preparation and type of donation, including time, staff, and company
- The name of the family memeber or friend who was called and who came to the hospital: donor organization, morgue, funeral home, chaplain, and individual family members making any decisions
- Personal articles left on the body and taped to skin, or tubes left in
- Personal items given to the family: specific names and descriptors of items
- Time of discharge and destination of the body
- Location of name tags on the body
- Special requests made by the family
- Any other statements that might be needed to clarify the situation

❖Evaluation

Client Care

You care for clients and families at every phase of the grief process. This requires you to remain aware of signs and symptoms of grief, even when clients are not specifically seeking care directly related to a loss. These signs and symptoms help you evaluate whether a client is able to deal with a loss and progress through the grief process. Critical thinking ensures that the evaluation process is thorough and relevant to the client's situation (Figure 29–6).

To determine the effectiveness of nursing interventions, you must refer to the goals and expected outcomes established in the plan of care. By comparing actual client behaviours with expected outcomes, you evaluate the client's health status and whether the plan of care needs to be revised. For example, if the goal is to have the client communicate a sense of hope with family members, you evaluate the verbal and nonverbal communication process for cues related to hope. The client's responses indicate whether new therapies are needed or whether existing therapies should be revised. You continue to evaluate the progress of the client, the effectiveness of the interventions,

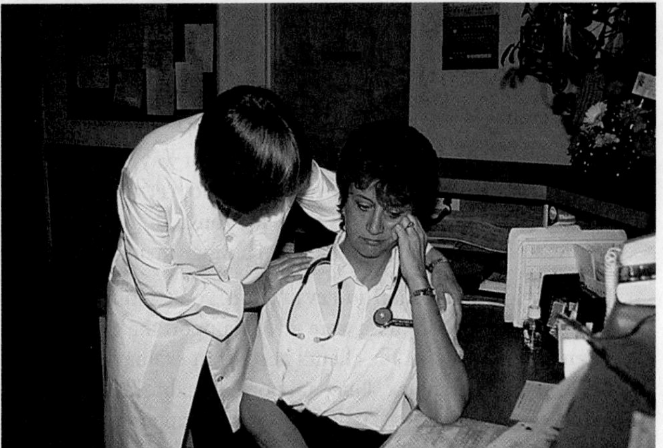

Figure 29-5 Nurses benefit from support of colleagues during their time of loss.

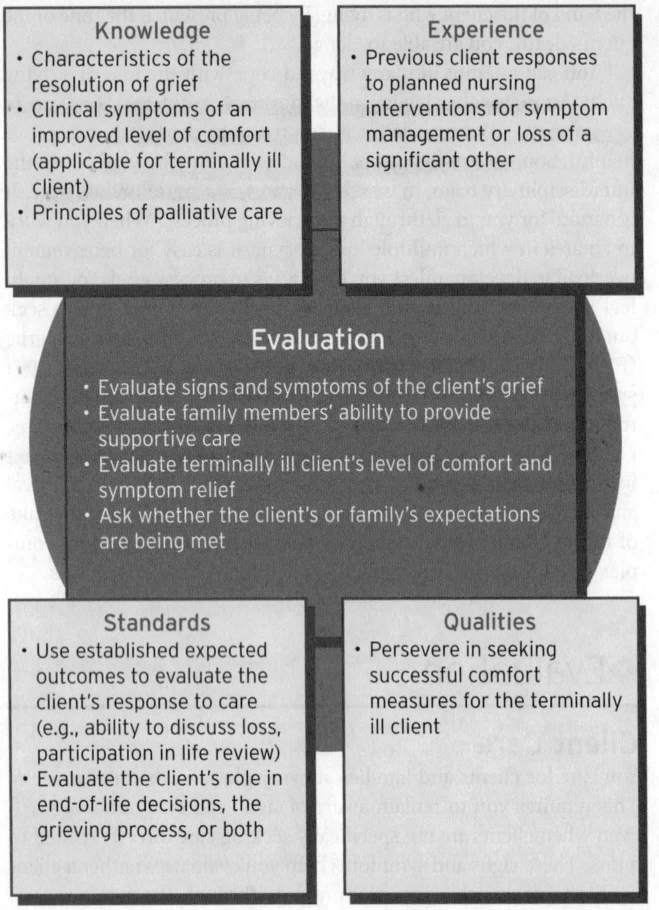

Knowledge
- Characteristics of the resolution of grief
- Clinical symptoms of an improved level of comfort (applicable for terminally ill client)
- Principles of palliative care

Experience
- Previous client responses to planned nursing interventions for symptom management or loss of a significant other

Evaluation
- Evaluate signs and symptoms of the client's grief
- Evaluate family members' ability to provide supportive care
- Evaluate terminally ill client's level of comfort and symptom relief
- Ask whether the client's or family's expectations are being met

Standards
- Use established expected outcomes to evaluate the client's response to care (e.g., ability to discuss loss, participation in life review)
- Evaluate the client's role in end-of-life decisions, the grieving process, or both

Qualities
- Persevere in seeking successful comfort measures for the terminally ill client

Figure 29-6 Critical thinking model for loss, death, and grieving evaluation.

and the interactions between the family and client. It is important for the client and family to share experiences and be active participants in the evaluation process.

Client Expectations

The client expects individualized care, including relief of symptoms, preservation of dignity, and support of the family to maximize quality of life. The success of the evaluation depends partially on the bond that you form with the client. If the client does not trust you, he or she is not likely to share personal expectations or desires with you. It becomes important for you to take the time to talk with the client and learn whether expectations are being met. The following are examples of questions that will validate whether client expectations have been achieved:

- "Am I helping you in the way you have hoped?"
- "Would you like me to assist you in a different way?"
- "Do you have a specific request that I have not yet met?"
- "What is most important for us to do for you at this time?"
- "Are we dealing with your problems in a timely manner?"

Through communication and evaluation, you continue to determine whether outcome criteria were met to support the goals of care. It is often easy to evaluate the client's needs, but evaluating the family's needs is more complex. Once rapport is established, you must be vigilant to avoid problems that threaten that rapport.

* KEY CONCEPTS

- When caring for clients who have experienced a loss, you facilitate the grief process by assisting survivors in feeling the loss, expressing the loss, and moving through the tasks of the grief process.
- Loss comes in many forms, depending on the values and priorities learned within a person's sphere of influence, which includes family, friends, society, and culture.
- The type of loss and the perception of the loss influence the degree of grief a person experiences.
- Death is difficult for the dying person, as well as for the person's family, friends, and caregivers.
- Survivors go through a bereavement period that is not linear; rather, a grieving individual will move back and forth through a series of stages, tasks, or both many times, possibly over a period of several years.
- Several theorists have formulated stages of the grieving process and a series of tasks for survivors to successfully complete their bereavement and adapt to life with a loss.
- Your knowledge of the types of grief enables you to implement appropriate bereavement therapies.
- The way an individual perceives and responds to a loss is influenced by development, psychosocial perspectives, socioeconomic status, personal relationships, the nature of the loss, culture, and spiritual beliefs.
- Nursing interventions involve reinforcing clients' successful coping mechanisms and introducing new coping approaches, such as the promotion of hope.
- When assessing clients in grief, you do not assume how or whether clients experience grief or whether a particular behaviour indicates grief; rather, you allow clients to share in their own way what is happening.
- You must assess the terminally ill client's and family's wishes for end-of-life care, including the preferred place for death, the level of life-sustaining measures to use, and expectations regarding pain and symptom management.
- You develop a plan of care by integrating clients' resources such as physical energy and activity tolerance, supportive family members, spiritual faith, and methods for coping.
- You establish a caring presence and use therapeutic communication strategies that enable clients to discuss their loss and find ways to manage it.
- Palliative care enables clients to make more informed choices, better alleviate symptoms, and have more opportunity to manage unfinished business.
- You can promote a client's self-esteem and dignity by conveying respect for the client as a whole person.
- Hospice is not a facility but a concept for family-centred care designed to assist the client in being comfortable and maintaining a satisfactory lifestyle until death.

* CRITICAL THINKING EXERCISES

1. Mr. Singh visits the community health clinic and tells you, "I don't know what's wrong with me. I lost my wife 6 months ago and I still get angry that God let her die. I still miss her so much. I have been going out with friends, but I just don't enjoy it that much. Sometimes I wake up at night and I think my wife is still here. What is wrong with me? I thought I would be feeling better by now." How could you respond to Mr. Singh?

2. You are assigned to care for Mrs. Nester. She has bone cancer and has experienced ongoing deep pain in her back and hips, with some discomfort also in her lower extremities. Discuss the management of pain for Mrs. Nester.

3. A nursing colleague is discussing her client with you. She says, "My client is a 48-year-old man with a degenerative neurological disease. The disease is progressive. He is having trouble walking and taking care of his daily needs. The only thing I can do is assist him with bathing, feeding, and walking. He really is not a candidate yet for palliative care." What would be your response to your colleague?

* REVIEW QUESTIONS

1. A child is grieving over the loss of a pet. This is an example of
   1. An actual loss
   2. A perceived loss
   3. A situational loss
   4. A maturational loss
2. A middle-aged man comes to a community clinic for his annual flu shot. In the discussion, you learn that he still works at a local law firm. However, he has recently lost two important cases, and his boss has been pressuring him "to turn it around." The client may be experiencing
   1. An actual loss
   2. A perceived loss
   3. A situational loss
   4. A maturational loss
3. The community health nurse's job is to provide grief counselling for the residents of a community in which a major flood has occurred. The loss associated with flooding is best described as
   1. An actual loss
   2. A perceived loss
   3. A situational loss
   4. A maturational loss
4. A client has received a diagnosis of terminal brain cancer. When you visit him during rounds, he asks you whether the cancer could have been caused by something he ate or by exposure to some chemical toxin. The client is probably experiencing
   1. Bowlby's phase of numbing
   2. Kübler-Ross's stage of acceptance
   3. Worden's tasks of emotionally relocating
   4. Bowlby's phase of disorganization and despair
5. According to Kübler-Ross's stages of dying, a client may feel overwhelmingly lonely and withdraw from interpersonal interaction during this phase:
   1. Denial
   2. Anger
   3. Bargaining
   4. Depression
6. Since the death of his wife, the client has assumed full responsibility for the care of his children. He has noticed over the past few weeks that friends are calling less often. He is most likely in which of the following phases of mourning?
   1. Anticipatory grieving
   2. Worden's task 3 of mourning
   3. Kübler-Ross's phase of bargaining
   4. Bowlby's phase of disorganization and despair
7. Which of the following is one of the most common and difficult issues faced by older bereaved spouses?
   1. Adjusting to physical problems
   2. Overcoming mental health problems
   3. Completing the tasks of daily living
   4. Managing finances
8. "Client will express hopefulness that cancer treatment will control symptoms" is an example of
   1. A goal
   2. An intervention
   3. A plan
   4. An expected outcome
9. A 16-year-old client has been admitted to the intensive care unit after suffering a closed-head injury. The client is soon declared brain dead. The physician and nurse are preparing to approach the family to consider donation of the client's heart and lungs. When working with families in this situation, it is important to explain that
   1. The ventilator is being used to prevent brain death
   2. The ventilator maintains organ perfusion until time for harvesting
   3. Tissues such as corneas can be harvested only if the client remains ventilated
   4. Organ donation can occur only if the client has made a request to donate organs in the past
10. Which of the following types of care allows clients to make more informed choices, achieve better alleviation of symptoms, and have more opportunity to manage unfinished business?
    1. Acute care
    2. Mourning care
    3. Palliative care
    4. Terminal care

* RECOMMENDED WEB SITES

Bereaved Families of Ontario: http://www.bereavedfamilies.net

This Web site provides support programs and resources for people of all ages who have lost a family member.

Canadian Hospice Palliative Care Association: http://www.chpca.net/home.htm

The Canadian Hospice Palliative Care Association (CHPCA) is a national organization that promotes excellence in care for people approaching death. One of its goals is to advocate for improved hospice palliative care policy, resource allocation, and supports for caregivers.

Regional Palliative Care Program in Edmonton, Alberta: http://www.palliative.org

The objective of this program is to provide information to health care professionals that will help them to reflect on their practice with the terminally ill. This Web site offers palliative care tips, nursing notes, a caregiver guide, and links to publications and other resources.

30

Stress and Adaptation

Written by Marjorie Baier, RN, PhD, and

Kathy Hegadoren, RN, BScN, MSc, PhD

objectives

Mastery of content in this chapter will enable you to:

- Define the key terms listed.
- Describe how stress is conceptualized.
- Define the key biological systems involved in stress responses.
- Describe how overwhelming stress or chronic stress can affect health.
- Differentiate acute stress disorder and post-traumatic stress disorder.
- Discuss the integration of stress theory with nursing theories.
- Formulate nursing diagnoses from assessment data.
- Describe stress management techniques beneficial for coping with stress.
- Discuss the process of crisis intervention.
- Develop a care plan for clients experiencing stress.
- Discuss how stress in the workplace can affect health care professionals.

key terms

Acute stress disorder, p. 480
Adaptation, p. 477
Alarm reaction, p. 477
Appraisal, p. 477
Burnout, p. 487
Coping, p. 477
Crisis, p. 477
Crisis intervention, p. 489
Developmental crises, p. 477
Distress, p. 480
Endorphins, p. 479
Eustress, p. 480
Exhaustion stage, p. 477
Fight-or-flight response, p. 477
Flashbacks, p. 480
General adaptation syndrome, p. 477
Homeostasis, p. 477
Post-traumatic stress disorder (PTSD), p. 480
Primary appraisal, p. 477
Resistance stage, p. 477
Secondary appraisal, p. 477
Situational crises, p. 477
Stress, p. 477
Stressors, p. 477
Trauma, p. 480

media resources

evolve Web Site

- Audio Chapter Summaries
- Glossary
- Multiple-Choice Review Questions
- Student Learning Activities
- Weblinks

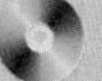

Companion CD

- Glossary
- Interactive Learning Activities
- Fluids and Electrolytes Tutorial
- Test-Taking Skills

Stress: Everyone has experienced it, but the term **stress** is difficult to define and is often loosely used. It has been used to describe a stimulus, a process, a response, and a state, which leads to confusion and ambiguity (Le Moal, 2007). In this chapter, the term **stressors** is used to describe events that activate stress response systems: that is, act as stimuli. This activation of multiple biological systems and psychological schemas have a collective goal of maintaining a state of dynamic equilibrium. Stressors can arise in the external environment and range from motivational prompts, such as taking a school examination, to devastating personal events, such as a life-threatening illness, a motor vehicle crash, a sexual assault, or a natural disaster (e.g., an earthquake or a tornado). Internal stressors, such as hunger or infection, can also activate stress response systems. Behavioural responses to stressors presumably reflect the activation of numerous stress hormone systems. Behavioural responses can change over time, inasmuch as previous stressful experiences and individual contextual factors can produce **adaptation** in stress response systems. Among animals, biological systems help alert the animal to some type of threat in the environment and prepare it to mount a defense. These systems also turn off when the threat is past. For humans, in addition to acute threats to body integrity, psychological well-being and sense of self-worth can be threatened. Physical and psychological health can be severely affected by serious stressors, and these effects can be long-standing and pervasive. It is important for health care professionals to understand conceptual frameworks that have been developed to understand the relationship between stress (overwhelming or chronic) and health.

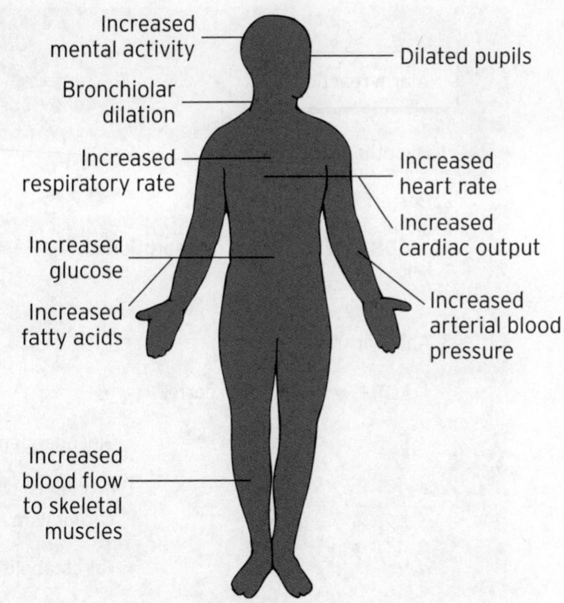

Figure 30-1 Fight-or-flight response.

Conceptualizations of Stress

Physiological Conceptualizations

Walter Cannon was one of the pioneers of the early twentieth century who laid the groundwork for regulatory physiology and concepts of adaptation. He demonstrated that the sympathetic–adrenal–medullary (SAM) system acted to maintain homeostasis of the internal environment. He first coined the term **fight-or-flight response**, in 1915, to describe an animal's response to threats through the activation of the SAM system (Figure 30–1; Le Moal, 2007). Hans Selye, another pioneer, focused on maladaptation and the pathology of stress. He demonstrated the existence of a biological stress syndrome, which he called the **general adaptation syndrome** (Selye, 1974; Figure 30–2). This three-stage syndrome occurs in response to serious stressors. The first stage is the **alarm reaction**, analogous to Cannon's fight-or-flight response to stress. In this stage, complex physiological changes help the organism mobilize energy and react to the stressor. The second stage of the general adaptation syndrome is the **resistance stage**. During resistance, the organism maintains arousal while the body works to defend against and adapt to the stressor and maintain homeostasis. Should the stressors continue for an extended period, organisms use up their finite ability to adapt, and they enter a third stage of the adaptation syndrome, called the **exhaustion stage.** This is a pathological state in which organisms start showing diverse health consequences, which may eventually result in death. Selye was also the first to emphasize the role of the pituitary–adrenal axis in the pathological processes of stress.

At this point, two systems for stress were proposed: (1) the SAM system for behavioural fight-or-flight responses to stress and immediate adaptation and (2) the pituitary–adrenal axis for maintaining homeostasis. The concept of the pituitary–adrenal axis was expanded to the hypothalamic–pituitary–adrenal (HPA) axis; this axis is thought to mediate a bidirectional brain–body communication during physiological and psychological stress and is activated to promote homeostasis and to adapt to threatening or stressful situations (Engelmann & Ludwig, 2004). Bruce McEwan (2007), elaborating on the concept of **homeostasis** (the return of systems to a stable set point), used the term *allostasis* to describe how serious stressors can change physiological set points through adaptation. In this way, organisms are readied to respond and adapt to stressors, but maintaining this state of readiness has an energy cost. This cost is called *allostatic load.* When this load becomes too great, the stress response changes from adaptation to health problems and stress-related disorders.

Psychological Conceptualizations

In addition to physiological models of stress and stress responses, cognitive approaches to stress were also studied. The general adaptation syndrome and fight-or-flight responses to stress did not explicitly take into account perceptions and appraisals of stress in humans. Researchers began to look at the relationship between the person and the environment. The roles of perception and appraisal in the stress response is integral in the framework of stress proposed by Richard Lazarus. Lazarus (1999) maintained that a person is under stress only if the person evaluates the event or circumstance as personally significant. **Appraisal** of an event or circumstance is an ongoing perceptual process (Aguilera, 1998). Evaluating an event for its personal meaning is called **primary appraisal.** If as a result of primary appraisal the person identifies the event or circumstance as a harm, loss, threat, or challenge, the person experiences stress. If stress is present, **secondary appraisal** focuses on possible coping strategies. **Coping** is the active process of managing taxing circumstances, expending effort to solve personal and interpersonal problems, and seeking to master, minimize, reduce, or tolerate stress or conflict. Balancing factors contribute to restoring equilibrium.

If previous ways of coping are not effective, a **crisis** may occur, in which the person faces a turning point in life and the person must change. Caplan (1981) distinguished two types of crises: those associated with changing developmental levels, or **developmental crises,** and **situational crises.** The frame of reference for a crisis is the viewpoint of the person experiencing the crisis. According to Aguilera's (1998) crisis theory, the vital questions for a person in crisis are "What does this mean to you?" and "How is it going to affect your life?" A

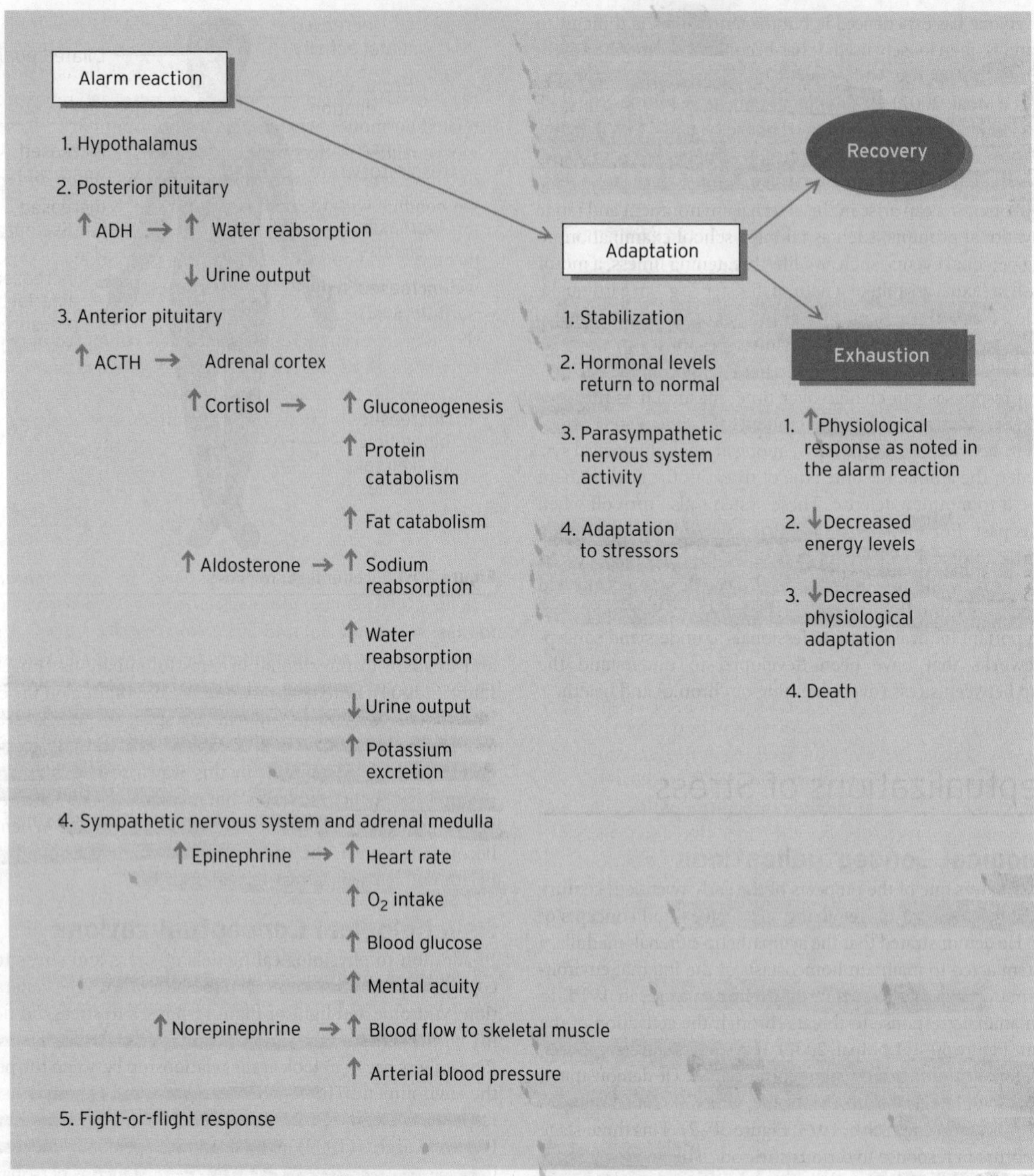

Figure 30-2 General adaptation syndrome. ACTH, adrenocorticotropic hormone; ADH, antidiuretic hormone.

basic assumption of crisis theory is that a person can either advance or regress as a result of a crisis, depending on how the crisis is managed. Feedback cues lead to ongoing reappraisals of original perceptions. Therefore, coping behaviours constantly change as new information is perceived.

Later work in the important role of appraisal and perception focused on the contribution of gender to responses to stressful events. Gender differences may be conceptualized as an interaction between biologically based sex differences and an individual's social context (Desbonnet et al., 2008; Kimerling et al., 2000). Women and men may perceive a stressor differently and thus may have different responses and reactions to that same stressor (Davis et al., 1999).

In summary, individual differences in response to stressors can be affected by previous vulnerabilities and experiences, coexisting health problems, gender, allostatic load, and coping resources. Psychological and biological conceptualizations are not mutually exclusive. Indeed, the integration of the various frameworks help explain the complexity of the relationship between stress and health.

Stress Response Systems

Sympathetic-Adrenal-Medullary System

Activation of the SAM system results in increased heart rate, diversion of blood from the intestines to the brain and skeletal muscles, increased blood pressure, bronchodilation and increased respiratory rate, and increases in blood glucose levels (Chrousos et al., 1988; Selye,

1991). All these changes are meant to prepare for fight-or-flight responses. A stressor activates specific cells in the brain stem that release norepinephrine into the bloodstream. Norepinephrine stimulates the adrenal medulla to release epinephrine. Epinephrine produces the cardiovascular, respiratory, and metabolic changes and the heightened awareness or alertness. Chronic stimulation brings about a chronic arousal state, with sleep disturbance, edginess and irritability, gastrointestinal upset, and increased startle responses. Brain areas that are involved in this stress response system include the following:

- *Reticular formation:* This is a small, integrative cluster of neurons in the brain stem and spinal cord that continuously monitors the physiological status of the body through connections with sensory and motor tracts. For example, certain cells within the reticular formation can cause a sleeping person to regain consciousness or increase the level of consciousness when a need arises.
- *Limbic system:* This is another integrative cluster of neurons that interconnect several parts of the brain that is involved in processing strong emotional experiences. Stress will cause increased activity within this system.
- *Midbrain and pons:* The midbrain joins the lower part of the brain stem and the spinal cord with the higher part of the brain and acts as a reflex centre for certain auditory, visual, and postural stimuli. The pons mainly relays impulses to and from the medulla oblongata to other parts of the brain and the peripheral nervous system, and it also controls the rate and depth of breathing.
- *Medulla oblongata:* This controls vital functions necessary for survival, including heart rate, blood pressure, and respiration. Impulses travelling to and from the medulla oblongata can increase or decrease these vital functions. For example, the heartbeat is regulated by sympathetic or parasympathetic nervous system impulses travelling from the medulla oblongata to the heart. The heart rate increases in response to pulses from sympathetic fibres and decreases with impulses from parasympathetic fibres.

Hypothalamic-Pituitary-Adrenal Axis

Activation of the HPA axis results in the release of a cascade of hormones (Dunn, 1989). A stressor activates the hypothalamus to release corticotropin-releasing hormone. This hormone activates receptors in the anterior pituitary, which signals the release of adrenocorticotropic hormone (ACTH) into the bloodstream. ACTH interacts with its receptors in the adrenal cortex to release glucocorticoids. In humans, the major glucocorticoid is cortisol. Cortisol has effects similar to those of epinephrine, contributing to the increase in heart rate and blood pressure, causing shunting of blood to skeletal muscles, and increasing the availability of glucose in the bloodstream. This stress response system is tightly controlled by negative feedback, whereby rising cortisol levels activate receptors in the hypothalamus and the pituitary gland, shutting off further release of corticotropin-releasing hormone and ACTH (Brunello et al., 2001).

This part of the endocrine system interacts with other parts that regulate sex hormone levels, thyroid hormones, electrolyte and fluid balance, and insulin release. Therefore, overwhelming or chronic stressors can have diverse and compex impacts on health. The following brain areas are involved in this stress response system:

- *Hypothalamus:* This region of the brain is involved with many basic phsyiological processes, including appetite, sexual drive, sleeping, motor activity, and mood states (all of which are affected by stress). The hypothalamus is highly interconnected with multiple other areas of the brain. Dysregulation of the hypothalamus is thought to be involved in depression.
- *Pituitary gland:* This small gland, attached to the hypothalamus, produces and releases hormones that control vital functions. It is divided into the anterior and posterior portions. The anterior pituitary releases stress-, thyroid-, growth-, and reproduction-related hormones, whereas the posterior pituitary releases hormones related to electrolyte and water balance, as well as oxytocin, which is involved in uterine contraction and in maternal bonding with the newborn. Both the pituitary gland and the hypothalamus can produce endorphins. **Endorphins**, such as morphine and opiates, are hormones that produce a sense of well-being and reducing pain (Lazarus, 1999).
- *Adrenal glands:* One of these glands rests atop each kidney, and they are key to stress responses. Each is composed of two very different regions. The outer region, or cortex, is where glucocorticoids such as cortisol are produced, and the inner region, or medulla, is where epinephrine is produced and released.

Stress and the Immune System

Physiological responses to stress also include immunological responses, although the mechanisms through which stress affects the immune system are not fully understood (Aldwin, 2000; Box 30–1). The immune system differentiates between self and non-self material, so that, under normal conditions, one's own cells are not treated as threats in the way that bacteria, viruses, parasites, or toxins are treated. An antigen on the surface of the bacteria cells identifies the bacteria as invaders. After being exposed to a particular antigen, the immune system remembers how to respond to that antigen and is prepared to respond with antibodies when the same antigen appears at a later time. Problems occur when the immune system misinterprets antigens and responds too vigorously, which leads to an autoimmune illness. Glucocorticoids are also powerful anti-inflammatory agents and play a role in the cascade of homeostatic immune responses that are activiated by infection or inflammation. Dysregulation or chronic activation of the SAM system and the HPA axis may increase the risk of cardiovascular disease, insulin resistance, metabolic syndromes, and autoimmune illnesses.

➤ BOX 30-1 Factors Influencing the Response to Stressors

Aspects of a Stressor That Influence the Stress Response

Intensity
Scope
Duration
Number and nature of other stressors
Past exposure to serious stressors
Predictability

Characteristics of the Individual That Influence the Stress Response

Gender
Perception of personal control or inescapability
Availability of social supports
Feelings of competence
Cognitive appraisal

The Relationship Between Type of Stressor and Health

Selye (1974) identified two types of stress: **distress**, or damaging stress, and **eustress**, or stress that protects health. Eustress is motivating energy, such as happiness, hopefulness, and purposeful movement (Varcarolis, 2002). Eustress is a positive, healthy adaptation to stressors in daily life. In reference to this concept, Selye (1974) wrote his book *Stress Without Distress*. However, Aldwin (2000) wrote that the idea of healthy stress is controversial because it is difficult to tell whether a person has benefited from stress or is coping by denying the stress in some way.

Distress can be categorized in many ways, including work stressors, family stressors, chronic stressors, acute stressors, daily hassles, trauma, and crisis: "Work and family stress interact, family being the background for work stress, and work the background for family stress" (Lazarus, 1999). Chronic stress arises in stable conditions and from stressful roles. Another example of chronic stress is living with a long-term illness. Conversely, acute stress is provoked by time-limited events that are threatening for a relatively brief period. Further complicating chronic or acute stress are daily hassles that are recurrent, such as commuting to work, maintaining a home, dealing with difficult people, and managing money. **Trauma** can refer to any physical damage to the body or in mental health terms can refer to witnessing or experiencing an emotionally painful, distressful, or shocking event(s). Severe stressors such as natural disasters or interpersonal events such as family violence or childhood abuse are often considered traumatic events; however, as in other types of stressors, perception plays a major role in the individual's response to such events. Indeed, for some people, trauma can have positive effects, leading to greater self-knowledge, improved coping skills, stronger social ties, and positive changes in values and perspectives (Hyer & Sohnle, 2001).

Stress-Related Disorders

Prolonged exposure to a serious stressor or an acute stressor that overwhelms the ability to cope can lead to stress-related disorders (Box 30–2). However, even if an individual's stress-related symptoms do not meet full criteria for a stress disorder, it is important to recognize that those symptoms may have a significant effect on the individual's life. If interventions are not implemented, these symptoms can decrease quality of life and increase the risk of developing the full disorder. Early emerging stress-related symptoms include poor sleep, tension and jitteriness, and inability to concentrate, to a degree that day-to-day activities are affected.

Although stress-related psychiatric disturbances are usually considered to be acute stress disorder and PTSD, these are only two potential health outcomes. It is important to recognize the diversity of health effects from serious stressors. Indeed, clinical depression, chronic pain syndromes, somatization disorder, and irritable bowel syndrome have all been linked to chronic stress (Blackburn-Munro & Blackburn-Munro, 2001; Matthews et al., 2001). Health professionals need to perform thorough, multifaceted assessments to identify the full range of health effects.

Acute Stress Disorder. **Acute stress disorder** is a time-limited reaction to experiencing, witnessing, or being confronted with a traumatic event; the reaction is one of intense fear, helplessness, or horror (American Psychiatric Association, 2000). Other criteria of acute stress disorder are as follows: (1) The client displays at least three acute dissociative symptoms; (2) the client has at least one recurring symptom (intense memories, **flashbacks** [recurring, intensely vivid mental images of a past traumatic experience], or distressing dreams); (3) the client displays marked avoidance of stimuli that arouse memories of the trauma; (4) the client shows marked hyperarousal; and (5) these symptoms emerge between 2 days and 4 weeks after the traumatic event (Hyer & Sohnle, 2001). These symptoms must have

BOX 30-2 RESEARCH HIGHLIGHT

Understanding Risks for Developing Psychological Distress

Research Focus

When caring for clients who have experienced trauma such as motor vehicle crashes, assaults, and industrial accidents, nurses focus first on life-threatening effects of the trauma. However, other consequences of trauma, such as psychological distress, may not be evident. You need to be aware of risk factors for anxiety, depression, acute stress disorder, and post-traumatic stress disorder after trauma.

Research Abstract

The purpose of Joy et al.'s (2000) study was to describe the pretrauma characteristics of people who experienced significant psychological distress shortly after physical injury. Individuals who had received treatment in the emergency department were contacted and asked to complete three questionnaires: the Posttraumatic Stress Disorder Scale, the Impact of Event Scale (IES), and the Hospital Anxiety and Depression Scale. A fourth questionnaire, the Abbreviated Injury Scale, was completed by the researchers on the basis of a medical record review. Significant psychological distress was documented in 152 people (87 women and 65 men) of all of the people receiving emergency treatment. Overall, the people identified with distress reported very little functional impairment and a high level of contentment before the traumatic event. Most of their injuries were relatively minor and not life-threatening. However, 141 (93%) of the subjects met the diagnostic criteria for **post-traumatic stress disorder (PTSD).** The IES revealed that the subjects were experiencing high levels of trauma-related distress. The researchers examined the relationship between pretrauma variables and the total score on the IES. The pretrauma factors of being unemployed and having experienced previous trauma were shown to be important contibutors to the total IES score. The researchers concluded that (1) trauma perceived as mild by medical personnel can nonetheless result in severe stress, anxiety, and depression for the client; (2) high functioning before a traumatic event does not protect the client from developing PTSD; and (3) pretrauma unemployment can contribute to psychological distress after a traumatic injury.

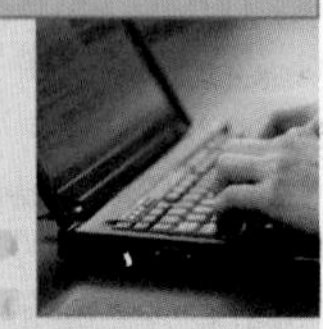

Evidence-Informed Practice

- Regardless of the severity of trauma or previous level of functioning, clients who have experienced a traumatic injury are at risk for developing PTSD.
- Nurses must monitor the client's perception of the meaning and impact of a traumatic injury, regardless of the apparent severity of the trauma.
- Two risk factors for developing PTSD after a traumatic injury are unemployment before the trauma and previous trauma.

References: Joy, D., Probert, R., Bisson J. I., & Shephard, J. P. (2000). Post-traumatic stress reactions after injury. *Journal of Trauma, 48*(3), 490–494.

a significant effect on the individual's occupational, social, or personal functioning to meet full criteria for acute stress disorder. Examples of traumatic events that lead to acute stress disorder are motor vehicle crashes, natural disasters, violent personal assault, emergency service work experiences, and military combat. Nurses are also not immune to acute stress disorder. Treatment usually focuses on symptoms: to aid in sleeping and to relieve the jitteriness and irritability.

Post-Traumatic Stress Disorder. Symptoms of PTSD are more persistent, having endured for at least 1 month. They may emerge immediately after a traumatic event, or their onset may be delayed (American Psychiatric Assocation, 2000). The symptom clusters are similar to those of acute stress disorder, with less emphasis on dissociative symptoms (Breslau & Kessler, 2001). The diagnosis of PTSD was formulated from work with men returning from the Vietnam war and was first thought to be quite rare. Ongoing community-based studies showed it to be more prevalent, with lifetime prevalence rates of 6.8% (Brunello et al., 2001). Treatment guidelines for PTSD have been published and include multimodal interventions with drug therapy and targeted psychotherapy (Adshead, 2000; Shalev et al., 1996).

Nursing Knowledge Base

Nurses have proposed theories related to stress and coping. Because stress plays a role in vulnerability to disease, symptoms of stress often necessitate nursing intervention.

Nursing Theory and the Role of Stress

Neuman's (1995) systems model is based on the concepts of stress and reaction to stress. Nurses are viewed as being responsible for developing interventions to prevent or reduce stressors on the client or to make them more bearable for the client (Neuman, 1995). Because Neuman's model is a systems model, it is applied not only to understand clients' individual responses to stressors but also to understand families' and communities' responses. All systems experience multiple stressors, each of which has a differing potential to disturb the person's, family's, or community's dynamic balance. Every person has developed a set of responses to stress that constitute the "normal line of defence" (Neuman, 1995). This line of defence helps maintain health and wellness. However, when "physiological, psychological, sociocultural, developmental, or spiritual influences" are unable to buffer stress, the normal line of defence is broken, and disease can result. Neuman's systems model coincides with Selye's (1974) general adaptation syndrome and McEwan's (2007) concept of allostatic load.

Neuman's (1995) systems model stresses the importance of accuracy in assessment and interventions that promote optimal wellness through the use of primary, secondary, and tertiary prevention strategies. According to Neuman's theory, the goal of primary prevention is to promote client wellness by stress prevention and reduction of risk factors. Secondary prevention occurs after symptoms appear. You help the client determine the meaning of the illness and stress, and you find resources available to handle them. Tertiary prevention begins when the client system is becoming more stable and recovering. At the tertiary level of prevention, you support rehabilitation processes involved in healing, moving the client back to wellness, and the primary level of disease prevention.

In their health promotion model, Pender et al. (2003) proposed that health promotion is directed toward increasing the level of well-being of an individual or group. Conversely, primary, secondary, and tertiary prevention (health protection) focus on avoiding negative events. Pender et al. considered stress reduction strategies important to reduce threats to well-being, to help people fulfill their potential, and to shape and maintain health behaviours. To change behaviour, the client must initiate the change and behave differently in interactions. On the basis of core assumptions regarding the capability and desire of people to be healthy, Pender et al. suggested strategies for prevention and health promotion related to stress management.

Situational, Maturational, and Sociocultural Factors

Multiple factors affect the types of potential stressors and coping mechanisms. Age is one; for example, adolescence, adulthood, and old age bring different stressors (Andersen & Teicher, 2008). Appraisal of stressors, amount and type of social support, and coping strategies are other factors that affect appraisal of stressors, as are previous life experiences (Aguilera, 1998).

Situational Factors. Situational stress can arise from the person's current circumstances, such as moving, changing jobs (stressful job changes can include promotions, transfers, downsizing, restructuring, changes in supervisors, and changes in responsibilities), and adjusting to a chronic illness or condition. Common diseases and conditions that can be exacerbated by stress are obesity, hypertension, diabetes, depression, asthma, and coronary artery disease. Being a family caregiver may also cause situational stress, although the source of stress may be not necessarily the caregiving but other factors in the caregiver's life, such as work, finances, or lack of respite (Chiriboga 1992). Spouses and other family members also experience stress when a loved one is ill (Box 30–3).

Maturational Factors. Stressors vary with life stage and are not necessarily related to negative events. Important individual and family developmental milestones can be anticipated with excitement but can nonetheless be stressful. Preadolescents may experience stress related to self-esteem issues, changes in family structure as a result of divorce or death of a parent, or hospitalizations. As adolescents search for their identity with peer groups and separate from their families, they undergo stress. In addition, they must make decisions about using mind-altering substances, peer pressure, sexuality, jobs, school, and career choices; the decision-making process causes stress. Stress for adults can arise from major changes in individual and family life circumstances (Aguilera, 1998). These changes include the many milestones of beginning a family and a career, losing parents, helping children leave home, and accepting physical aging. In old age, stressors include the loss of autonomy and mastery, as a result of general frailty or health problems that limit stamina and strength, and the loss of spouse, close friends, and family that provided social support over the years (Box 30–4).

Sociocultural Factors. Low socioeconomic status is not necessarily associated with more stress than better financial status is. You must not make assumptions about the sources of stress for an individual or family. However, some circumstances create higher risk of experiencing serious stressors or trauma. For example, living under conditions of continuing violence, living in disintegrated neighbourhoods, and homelessness can be damaging, especially for young people (Pender et al., 2002).

A person's cultural background also greatly influences the perception of and reaction to stress (Aldwin, 2000). Cultural context must be integrated into any assessment. Differences are observed from culturally distinct groups within the general population, such as

BOX 30-3 RESEARCH HIGHLIGHT

Spousal Support for Psychological Distress

Research Focus

Holistic nursing care includes the client's family. Family members, especially the spouse, influence the client's recovery from cardiac disease and surgery. More information is needed about stress experienced by spouses of clients in cardiac rehabilitation and interventions to help spouses cope with stress.

Research Abstract

The purposes of O'Farrell et al.'s (2000) study were (1) to describe the distress experienced by 213 spouses of men in cardiac rehabilitation, (2) to identify the most common heart disease stressors experienced by the women, (3) to compare distressed and nondistressed spouses in terms of demographic variables and coping strategies, and (4) to identify specific intervention needs for spouses of clients undergoing cardiac rehabilitation. Spouses were recruited by telephone at the time of the client's admission to the cardiac rehabilitation program. Subjects agreed to participate in five spousal support group sessions and to complete five questionnaires to assess psychological distress, coping, marital intimacy, family functioning, and heart disease–related stressors. The Brief Symptom Inventory was a measure of psychological distress. On the basis of responses to this scale, 66 subjects were categorized as being psychologically distressed. Symptoms of distress were feeling tense, having trouble falling asleep, and feeling easily hurt. The spouses who were distressed were, on average, significantly younger than those who were not distressed. The distressed spouses coped with the stress by disengagement strategies, such as avoidance, wishful thinking, self-criticism, and withdrawal. The Heart Disease Hassles Scale has 75 items to identify common heart disease–related stressors. The five stressors ranked highest by spouses in this study were (1) worries about treatment, recovery, and prognosis; (2) moodiness of the client; (3) worries about the client returning to work and about money; (4) sexual concerns; and (5) helplessness or apathy of the client and increased responsibilities of the spouse.

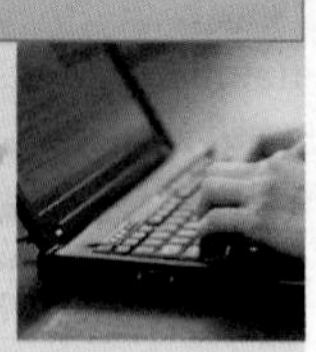

Evidence-Informed Practice

- Spouses of clients in cardiac rehabilitation could benefit from the following interventions:
  - Stress-management techniques, such as relaxation training, assertiveness training, and self-care techniques
  - Training in problem-solving and cognition-based coping strategies
  - Support groups for spouses
- Younger women especially need to be offered supportive interventions when their husbands are in cardiac rehabilitation.

References: O'Farrell, P., Murray, J., & Hotz, S. B. (2000). Psychologic distress among spouses of patients undergoing cardiac rehabilitation. *Heart & Lung, 29*(2), 97–104.

Aboriginal cultures, as well as from immigrant populations. It is important to recognize that Aboriginal culture is not singular. Indeed, potential stressors vary by geographic region (e.g., whether clients live in urban centres, rural areas, or remote parts of Canada); by historical events, such as residential schooling; and by the financial status of a specific Aboriginal group. Although stresssors related to immigration have been well described, ongoing stressors also may influence the health of families for generations. Initial stressors can include career and financial issues related to underemployment, loss of extended family supports, language barriers, and unfamiliarity regarding accessing health services (Mollica et al., 2001; Shen & Takeuchi, 2001). Later stressors can be related to raising children in a dual context (between cultural norms of the country of origin and the current environment; Guendelman et al., 2001). An example of how cultural background may influence health is behavioural responses to pain (Box 30–5).

BOX 30-4 FOCUS ON OLDER ADULTS

- Older adults are incorrectly presumed to be more vulnerable to the psychosocial effect of stressors (Kasl, 1992). However, HPA axis activity does change with age; higher evening levels of cortisol have been observed (Magri et al., 2006). As a result, memory may be impaired (Lupien et al., 2005) and immune system functioning may be blunted (Graham et al., 2006). These changes can lead to increasing physical and mental frailty (Butcher & Lord, 2004).
- A study of stress and coping in old-old clients (aged 75 to 91 years) revealed that such clients, in comparison with clients of other ages, were less likely to view their lives as having problems, and they expended less effort in coping (Aldwin et al., 1996). This may be because the life experiences and perspectives of older adults may make most problems seem insignificant, because older adults have acquired appropriate stress management techniques, or both.
- The timing of stress-inducing events can significantly influence older adults' ability to cope. Many older adults experience several stressful events (e.g., loss of a spouse and new medical diagnosis) within a brief time frame, which may result in reduced coping ability.
- Older adults with strong spiritual beliefs effectively use religious coping in response to medical illness and disasters (Foster, 1997).
- Depression and anxiety disorders are the most prevalent mental health disorders in later life (Chapman & Perry, 2008; Skultety & Rodriguez, 2008).

Critical Thinking

When caring for a client who is experiencing stress, you integrate knowledge from nursing and other disciplines, previous experiences, and information gathered from clients to understand stress and its effect on the client and family. You must know the neurophysiological changes that occur in response to overwhelming or chronic stress. You must also be able to determine the client's perception of the situation and help the client identify and use coping strategies that have helped in the past. If the client's usual coping skills are unsuccessful or support systems are inadequate, you must implement crisis intervention counselling (see "Crisis Intervention" section).

You should be confident in the belief that you can help the client manage the current situation effectively. Clients who are overwhelmed and perceive events as being beyond their capacity to cope rely on you as an expert and may require short-term intervention or guidance. Through a nurse's expert advice and counsel, many clients gain confidence in their ability to move past the stressful event or illness. Standards of practice can help you make an accurate assessment of a client's stress, coping mechanisms, and support system before you intervene.

BOX 30-5 CULTURAL ASPECTS OF CARE

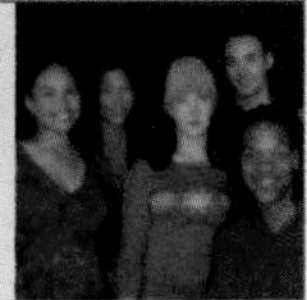

Cultural context shapes the types of environmental stimuli that produce stress. For example, diverse cultures address developmental transitions and life's turning points differently. How a person leaves the parental home, experiences health crises or chronic illness, cares for the family, or becomes disabled or dependent are all culturally bound. Furthermore, how a person appraises stress is also dependent on the person's culture. Coping strategies are also influenced by culture. According to Aldwin (1992), cultures vary in their emotion-focused and problem-focused coping strategies. According to some cultures, emotions should be controlled; according to others, they should be expressed. *Problem-focused coping* refers to controlling or managing stress. In addition, cultures provide different institutions for coping with stress. These include the legal system for conflict resolution, advice givers or support groups, and rituals.

Implications for Practice

- Realize that stressors and coping styles vary with different cultures.
- Use introspection to examine your own perceptions of stress and coping in a cultural context.
- Assess the influence of culture on a client's appraisal of stress.
- Determine the available resources within a client's culture that may facilitate coping.

From Aldwin, C. M. (2000). *Stress, coping and development: An integrative perspective* (pp. 30–22). New York: Guilford Press.

Nursing Process

❖Assessment

When assessing a client's stress level and coping resources, you must ask the client to share personal and sensitive information. Therefore, you must first establish a trusting nurse–client relationship. By asking open-ended questions, listening carefully, observing the client's nonverbal behaviour, and observing the client's environment, you learn about the client's stress. You use critical thinking skills to synthesize and analyze information (Figure 30–3). Often clients have difficulty expressing what is troubling them until they have the opportunity to talk with someone who has time to listen.

Subjective Findings

When assessing a client's level of stress and coping resources, you arrange a nonthreatening physical environment, without a desk as a barrier, for the interaction (Varcarolis, 2002). You assume the same height as the client, arranging the interview environment so that eye contact can be comfortably maintained or avoided. By placing chairs at a 90-degree angle or side by side, you can reduce the intensity of the interaction (Varcarolis, 2002). You use the interview to determine the client's view of the stress, past successful coping resources, any possible maladaptive coping, and adherence to prescribed medical recommendations, such as medication or diet (Monat & Lazarus, 1991; Table 30–1). If the client is using denial as a coping mechanism, you must be alert to whether he or she is overlooking necessary information. Other clients may state that they feel overwhelmed and unable to cope, but with help, they can reduce their multiple interacting stressors to manageable pieces. As in all interactions with the client, you must respect the confidentiality and sensitivity of the information shared.

safety alert Medical conditions such as sleep apnea and thyroid dysfunction that are common in older adults can initially cause symptoms that mimic stress-related symptoms. For this reason, a thorough physical assessment of an older adult who appears stressed or anxious is necessary to rule out potentially serious medical disorders. In addition, in older adults, signs of stress and crisis must be differentiated from emerging dementia and also from acute confusion, a condition that can be life-threatening.

Objective Findings

You obtain further findings about stress and coping by observing the client's appearance and nonverbal behaviour during the interview, including grooming and hygiene, handshake and gait, body language, speech quality, eye contact, and attitude. Before or at the end of the interview, depending on the client's anxiety level, you take basic vital signs to assess for physiological signs of stress, such as elevated blood pressure, heart rate, or respiratory rate (Figure 30–4).

Client Expectations

It is crucial that you understand the meaning the client attaches to the precipitating event and how stress is affecting the client's life. You must allow the client time to express priorities for coping. For example, if a woman has just been told that a breast mass was identified on a routine mammogram, you must discern what the client wants and needs most from you. Some clients identify an immediate need for information about biopsy or mastectomy; others need guidance and support on how to share the news with family members. In some cases, when nothing can be done to change or improve the situation, allowing the client to use denial as a coping mechanism can be

Figure 30-3 Critical thinking model for stress and coping assessment.

TABLE 30-1 Focused Assessment Interview

Factors to Assess	Questions and Approaches	Physical Assessment Strategies
Perception of stressor	Ask the client what is of most concern at this time. Ask the client about problems sleeping, eating, working, and concentrating. Ask whether the client has had accidents in the home, in the car, or on the job. Ask about previous stressors that are influencing current appraisals.	Observe nonverbal behaviour and expressions of feelings that indicate anxiety, fear, anger, irritability, or tension.
Available coping resources	Ask the client about current friendships and contacts with family members. Ask what the client has done in the past to cope with similar problems or stress. Ask how the client spends leisure time. Ask the client to describe any specific stress management techniques.	Observe whether the client is alone or with others. Observe grooming and hygiene. Observe the client's communication skills. Determine whether the client is able to ask for help. Observe developmental level and sociocultural circumstances.
Maladaptive coping used	Assess current and past patterns of use of tobacco, prescription or over-the-counter drugs, and caffeine.	Observe for effects of heavy use of tobacco, alcohol, illegal drugs, and caffeine.
Adherence to healthy practices	Ask whether the client visits a physician or nurse practitioner regularly for checkups. Ask about nutritional habits, exercise, use of seat belts, helmets (if applicable), and safer sexual practices.	Monitor pulse, blood pressure, weight. Observe nonverbal behaviour.

helpful. However, once you understand client expectations, you must not exclude important aspects of care simply because a client does not identify them as needs.

❖Nursing Diagnosis

You cluster data that indicate a potential or actual stressor and the client's response. Keeping in mind previous knowledge and experiences with clients under stress, you then make individualized nursing diagnoses (Box 30–6).

Nursing diagnoses for people experiencing stress generally focus on coping. Major defining characteristics of *ineffective coping* include verbalization of both an inability to cope and an inability to ask for help. You identify defining characteristics by asking clients what currently concerns them most and allowing them sufficient time to answer. You observe for nonverbal signs of anxiety, fear, anger, irritability, and tension. Other defining characteristics include the presence of life stressors, an inability to meet role expectations and basic needs, alteration in societal participation, self-destructive behaviour, change in usual communication patterns, high rate of accidents, excessive food intake, drinking, smoking, and sleep disturbances. Stress can result in multiple nursing diagnoses, such as the following:

- *Anxiety*
- *Caregiver role strain*
- *Chronic pain*
- *Post-traumatic stress disorder*
- *Powerlessness*

Crises differ from stressors in the degree of severity, although stressors and crises have many similarities. A client who perceives a situation as stressful, who is unable to cope in ways that have worked before, and who has insufficient support is experiencing a crisis. A crisis can be devastating and requires you to help mobilize all resources available (Aguilera, 1998).

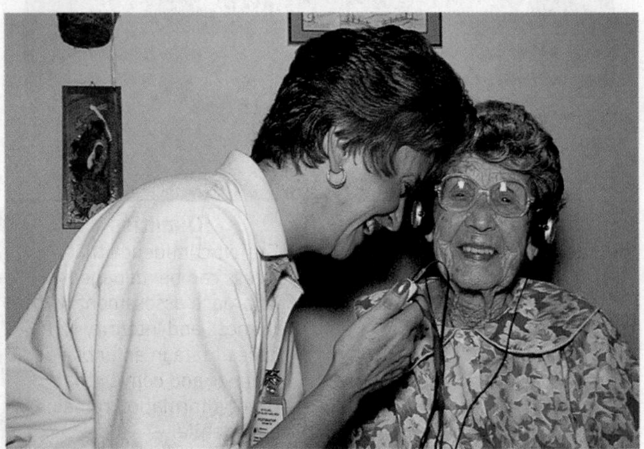

Figure 30-4 Sharing a joke or laughing with clients can reduce stress and support a therapeutic relationship.

❖Planning

Goals and Outcomes

Desirable outcomes for people experiencing stress are (1) effective coping, (2) coping by their family, (3) emotional health of the caregiver, and (4) psychosocial adjustment to life changes (Moorhead et al., 2004). You may select interventions for stress and improved coping such as coping enhancement or crisis intervention, which are in the *Nursing Interventions Classification (NIC)* (Dochterman & Bulechek, 2004). In addition, you select individualized interventions after you consider the nursing diagnosis, the resources available to the client, and the goals identified by the client and nurse (Figure 30–5).

BOX 30-6 NURSING DIAGNOSTIC PROCESS

Assessment Activities	*Defining Characteristics*	*Nursing Diagnosis*
Ask client about change in sleeping patterns.	Sleep disturbance; difficulty falling asleep at night or staying asleep Nightmares or disturbing dreams Sighing	*Anxiety*
Ask client to complete a sleep diary for 2 weeks.	Excessive sleeping	
Observe client's behaviour and response to questions during assessment.	Fatigue Inability to concentrate Inaccurate response to questions Inappropriate laughing or crying	
Observe client's appearance.	Poor grooming Self-harm	
Ask client about changes in eating patterns.	Weight gain or loss Lack of interest in food	

Nursing interventions may be designed within the framework of primary, secondary, and tertiary prevention. At the primary level of prevention, individuals and populations who may be at risk for stress are identified (Stuart & Wright, 1995). At the secondary level, nursing actions are directed at symptoms, such as protecting the client from self-harm. At the tertiary level, nursing interventions assist the client in readapting and might include relaxation training and time management training (Box 30–7). Another method of planning care involves using a concept map (Figure 30–6). You create the map after identifying relevant nursing diagnoses from the assessment database. In this example, the nursing diagnoses are linked to the client's medical diagnosis of PTSD. The concept map shows the relationships with the nursing diagnoses: *post-traumatic stress disorder* (PTSD), *ineffective coping, anxiety,* and *risk for other-directed violence.* In this approach, you use critical thinking skills to organize client data and plan for client-centred care.

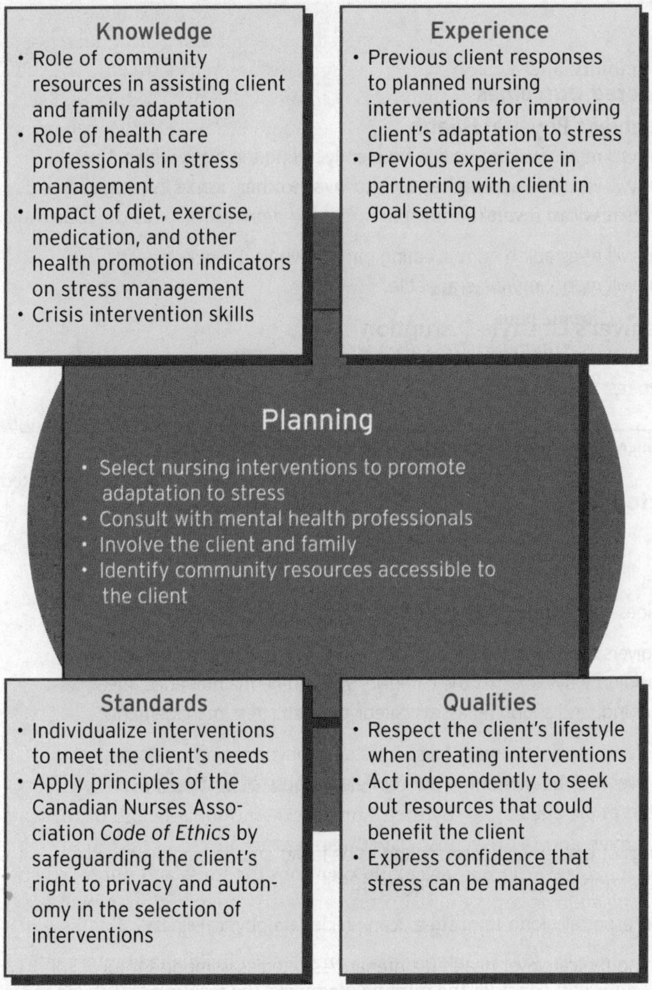

Just as the nursing assessment of stress and coping depends on the client's perception of the problem and coping resources, the interventions focus on a partnership of the nurse with the client and support system, usually the family. In the case of a family or community stressor and impaired family or community coping, the view of the situation and resources is broader.

Knowledge
- Role of community resources in assisting client and family adaptation
- Role of health care professionals in stress management
- Impact of diet, exercise, medication, and other health promotion indicators on stress management
- Crisis intervention skills

Experience
- Previous client responses to planned nursing interventions for improving client's adaptation to stress
- Previous experience in partnering with client in goal setting

Planning
- Select nursing interventions to promote adaptation to stress
- Consult with mental health professionals
- Involve the client and family
- Identify community resources accessible to the client

Standards
- Individualize interventions to meet the client's needs
- Apply principles of the Canadian Nurses Association *Code of Ethics* by safeguarding the client's right to privacy and autonomy in the selection of interventions

Qualities
- Respect the client's lifestyle when creating interventions
- Act independently to seek out resources that could benefit the client
- Express confidence that stress can be managed

Figure 30-5 Critical thinking model for stress and coping planning.

Setting Priorities

When you prioritize needs for a person experiencing stress or a crisis, the first question to be answered is "What is happening in your life that you needed to come today?" or "What happened in your life that is *different*?" This question requires the client to focus. You should then assess the client's perception of the event, situational supports, and what the client usually does when faced with a problem (Aguilera, 1998). As in all areas of nursing, safety of the client and family is the first priority.

safety alert Direct questions help to determine whether the person is suicidal or homicidal. You might ask, "Have you thought that life is not worth living? Are those thoughts with you most of the day?" "Have you thought your problems would be solved if that other person were not around any more?" If so, you should calmly determine whether the client has a plan and determine how lethal the means are. If suicide or homicide is not an issue, you should consider other threats to the safety of people who are under the client's care and provide for their temporary care or supervision if necessary. When immediate assessment is completed and safety is ensured, the problem-solving process should begin (Aguilera, 1998).

BOX 30-7 NURSING CARE PLAN

Caregiver Role Strain

Assessment

When the professional nurse first goes to Carl's house, she finds the home to be in slight disarray. The lawn is overgrown, dirty dishes are in the sink, and an empty can of soup is sitting on the kitchen counter. Carl is standing in the living room, folding clothes from a laundry basket, and Evelyn, Carl's wife, is sitting in a chair watching TV. Evelyn recently received a diagnosis of Alzheimer's disease.

Assessment Activities	***Findings and Defining Characteristics***
Ask Carl about his recent stressors and coping strategies.	He continues to fold clothes during the visit, stating, "There's so much to do that I don't even know where to begin." Carl describes being awakened three to four times per night to find Evelyn wandering in the house. He states that he has no outside activities and his children live in other provinces. He does have several close friends who live nearby, but he does not know of community resources.
Observe Carl's grooming and hygiene.	Carl is unshaven and appears dishevelled.
Ask Carl about his sleep and nutrition patterns.	Carl states that he has lost 9 kg in the past 6 months and that his appetite has been poor.
Assess Carl's mood and affect by asking how he is feeling.	Carl states, "I feel very tired. Everything feels overwhelming."
Assess Carl's suicide potential.	Carl denies being suicidal.
Assess health status and health care status.	Carl has not seen a nurse practitioner or physician for his own health in over a year.

Nursing Diagnosis: Caregiver role strain related to recent diagnosis of wife's Alzheimer's disease

Planning

Goal (Nursing Outcomes Classification)*	***Expected Outcomes***
	Caregiver's Physical Health
Client will appear rested in 1 month.	Client will report waking up less frequently during the night within 1 week. Client will verbalize approaches used to involve other people in caregiving activities within 2 weeks.
Client will maintain a stable weight over next 4 weeks.	Client will re-establish normal eating pattern within 1 week. Client will report improved appetite.
	Caregiver's Lifestyle Disruption
Client will state that he has resumed one outside activity within 1 month.	Client will report within 1 week a balanced routine that incorporates time for own rest or relaxation.

*Outcome classification labels from Moorhead, S., Johnson, M., & Maas, M. (Eds.). (2004). *Nursing Outcomes Classification (NOC)* (3rd ed.). St. Louis, MO: Mosby.

Interventions (Nursing Interventions Classification)†	**Rationale**
Caregiver Support	
Assist client in establishing a consistent care routine.	Routines can help tasks be simplified and more time efficient.
Discuss ways that client agrees will simplify care routine, such as hiring a teenage neighbour to mow the lawn, buying frozen meals, having groceries delivered, and having a cleaning service twice a month.	Caregivers experience stress outside of their caregiving roles. Frequently, providing ways to assist the caregiver with home maintenance, meal planning, and shopping assists caregivers with stress management.
Identify sources of respite care by encouraging client to identify available friends who can assist with caregiving.	Caregiving cannot normally be successful if it involves only one caregiver. Caregiver may be hesitant to ask for help because of past family conflict (Etters et al., 2008).
Explore community resources such as home care, adult day care, and Meals on Wheels with client.	Feelings of burden have been found to be lower among caregivers with social supports (Solomon & Draine, 1995).
Teach client stress-management techniques.	Stress, especially long-term stress, can precipitate physical illness.
Set up monthly health checks for client that include vital sign and weight measurements.	Teaching the caregiver health maintenance strategies is important for sustaining his own physical and mental health (Dochterman & Bulechek, 2004).

†Intervention classification labels from Dochterman, J. M., & Bulechek, G. M. (Eds.). (2004). *Nursing Interventions Classification (NIC)* (4th ed.). St. Louis, MO: Mosby.

➤ BOX 30-7 NURSING CARE PLAN *continued*

Evaluation

Nursing Actions	*Client Response and Finding*	*Achievement of Outcome*
Observe for signs of fatigue.	Carl states he feels more rested and less depressed.	Carl is able to sleep for 6 hours during night and takes a 30-minute nap in the afternoon.
Review new care routines. Ask client what other modifications may need to be made.	Carl buys frozen meals to use when he is busy with other caregiving responsibilities.	Carl has reduced his personal expectation that he must cook every meal himself.
Ask client about how community and additional family support is helping to relieve stress.	Meals on Wheels delivers lunch 5 days per week. A neighbour mows the lawn for Carl.	Carl is mobilizing community resources.
Ask client to compare past and current energy levels.	Carl reports having more energy and smiles spontaneously.	Carl has improved balance between Evelyn's and his own routines.
Weigh client regularly.	Carl reports gaining 2 kg in 1 month.	Carl has resumed a normal eating pattern.
Ask client about recent food intake.	Carl reports having eaten lunch with Evelyn on the day of the visit.	Carl has been able to sustain reasonable food intake recently.

Continuity of Care

Sometimes the scope of nursing practice is insufficient to meet all of the client's needs. For clients experiencing stress from medical conditions or psychiatric disorders, you must consult with advanced practice mental health nurses, psychiatrists, psychologists, psychiatric social workers, or other mental health experts. Such a multidisciplinary approach to care is often most effective in addressing the holistic needs of the client and should be included in the planning of care. Your role is to recognize the need for collaboration and consultation, inform the client about potential resources, and make arrangements for interventions, such as consultations, group sessions, or therapy as needed.

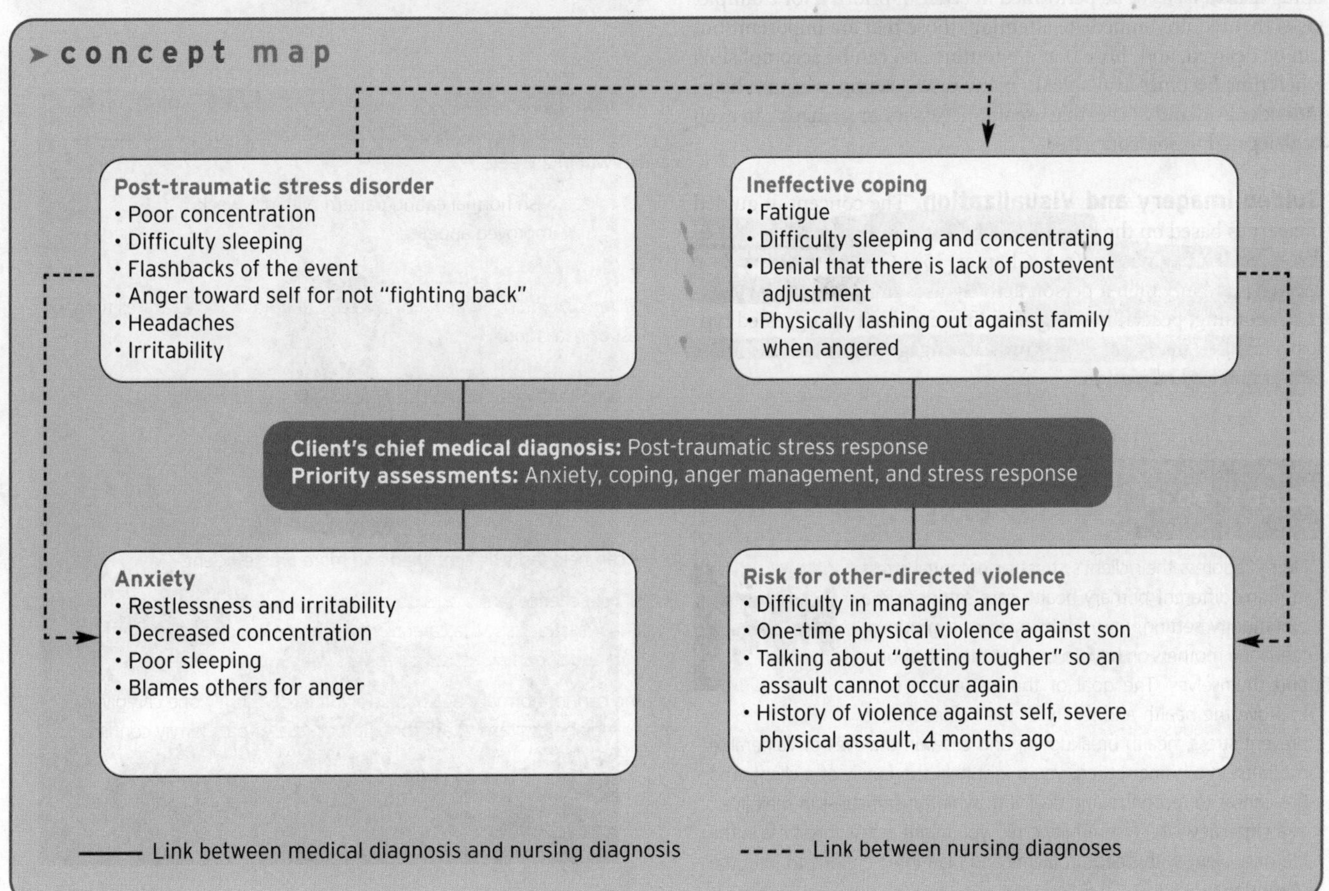

Figure 30-6 Concept map for client with PTSD after experiencing a severe phsyical assault 4 months ago.

❖Implementation

Health Promotion

Three primary modes of intervention for stress are to decrease stress-producing situations, increase resistance to stress, and learn skills that reduce physiological response to stress (Pender et al., 2002). You are in a position to educate clients and families about the importance of health promotion (Boxes 30–8 and 30–9). Several strategies help increase resistance to stress and reduce response to stress.

Regular Exercise. A regular exercise program improves muscle tone and posture, controls weight, reduces tension, and promotes relaxation. In addition, exercise reduces the risk of cardiovascular disease and improves cardiopulmonary functioning. Clients who have a history of a chronic illness, who are at risk for developing an illness, or who are older than 35 years should begin a physical exercise program only after discussing the plan with a physician. In general, for a fitness program to have positive physical effects, a person should exercise daily for an hour (Figure 30–7).

Support Systems. A support system of family, friends, and colleagues who listen, offer advice, and provide emotional support benefits clients experiencing stress. Many support groups are available to individuals, such as those sponsored by the Heart and Stroke Foundation of Canada, the Canadian Cancer Society, local hospitals and churches, and mental health organizations.

Time Management. Time management techniques include developing lists of tasks to be performed in order of priority: for example, tasks that require immediate attention, those that are important but can be delayed, and those that are routine and can be accomplished when time becomes available. In many cases, setting priorities helps individuals identify tasks that are not necessary or perhaps can even be delegated to someone else.

Guided Imagery and Visualization. The concept of guided imagery is based on the belief that a person can significantly reduce stress with imagination (see Chapter 35). Guided imagery is a relaxed state in which a person actively uses imagination to visualize a soothing, peaceful setting. The image created or suggested typically evokes many sensory words to engage the mind and offer distraction and relaxation.

✱ BOX 30-8 FOCUS ON PRIMARY HEALTH CARE

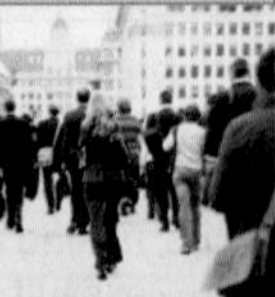

Nurses address their client's stress or potential stress in many different primary health care settings. In a community setting, you might instruct a group of teenaged mothers on how to care for their newborns and themselves. The goal of the instruction is to improve the health and safety of the babies and to prevent stress, health breakdown, and crises in the lives of vulnerable mothers. In a home setting, you might help the family of a client who has cancer to recognize and deal with symptoms of stress in their lives. In an interview at a community clinic, you might assess the stress in the life of a client with sleep problems and plan interventions to help the client sleep.

✱ BOX 30-9 CLIENT TEACHING

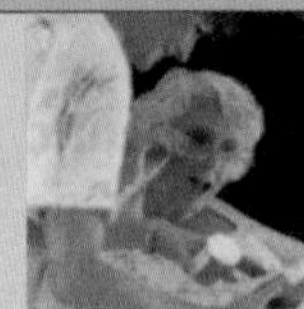

Stress Management Strategies

Objective

- Improved coping with daily hassles in the workplace

Teaching Strategies

- Teach the client how to break down hassles into specific aspects in order to begin coping with them.
- Instruct the client to avoid impulsive changes in lifestyle when stressed.
- Instruct the client in time management skills to become more organized and set priorities.
- Assist the client in examining lifestyle issues that may serve as stress relievers, such as walking during the lunch hour and other recreatonal activities.
- Assist the client in examining dietary sources of increased tension, such as excessive caffeine intake (e.g., coffee, tea, chocolate).
- Assist the client in building a network of social support.
- Train the client in progressive muscle relaxation or other relaxation techniques.

Evaluation

- Observe the client for signs of active coping strategies.
- Ask the client to keep a record of hours of sleep.
- Ask the client to list activities that are soothing or enjoyable.

Data from Pender, N. J., Murdaugh, C., & Parsons, M. A. (2002). *Health promotion in nursing practice* (4th ed.). Upper Saddle River, NJ: Haworth Press.

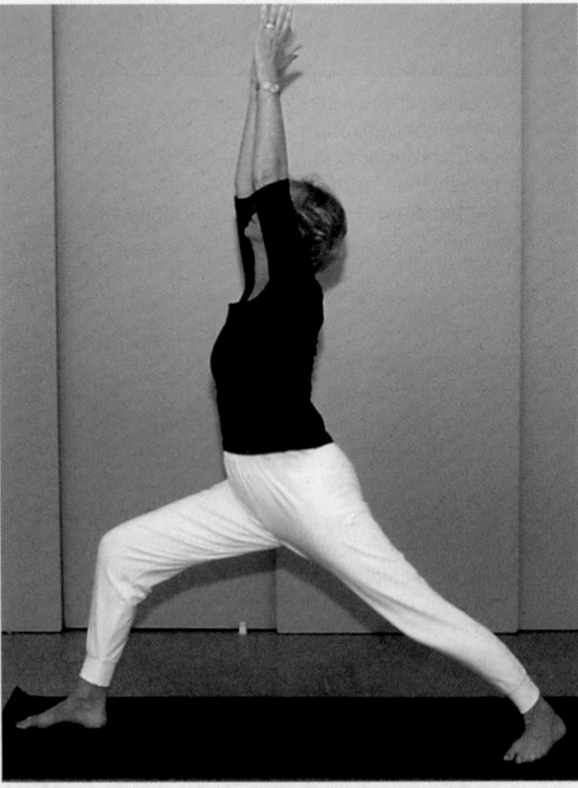

Figure 30-7 Regular exercise assists in coping with stress.

Progressive Muscle Relaxation. In the presence of anxiety-provoking thoughts and events, a common physiological symptom is muscle tension. Physiological tension is diminished through a systematic approach to releasing tension in major muscle groups. A relaxed state is achieved typically through deep chest breathing, and then the client is directed to alternately tighten and relax muscles in specific groupings (see Chapter 35).

Assertiveness Training. Assertiveness comprises skills that help individuals communicate their needs and desires effectively. The ability to resolve conflict through assertiveness training is important for reducing stress. When assertiveness is taught in a group setting, benefits of the experience are increased.

Journal Writing. For many people, keeping a private, personal journal provides a therapeutic outlet for stress, and it is well within the realm of nursing to suggest journal keeping to clients experiencing difficult situations. In a private journal, clients can express a full range of emotion and vent their feelings honestly without hurting anyone's feelings and without concern for how they might appear to others.

Stress Management in Your Workplace. Rapid changes in health care technology, diversity in the workforce, organizational restructuring, and changing work systems can place stress on nurses (Bauman et al., 2001; Manning et al., 1999). Additional causes of job stress include particular job assignments (Box 30–10), difficult schedules that include more than two different work shifts in short periods of time, working predominantly night shifts, fear of failure, and inadequate support services (Manning et al., 1999). **Burnout** occurs as a result of chronic stress. Burnout is "a syndrome of emotional exhaustion, depersonalization of others, and perceptions of reduced personal accomplishment, resulting from intense involvement with people in a care-giving environment" (Aguilera, 1998). This can be reflected in high rates of sick leave, irritability with coworkers, increased risk of errors at work, and increased home stress. Nurses are not immune to maladaptive coping, such as use of alcohol, in response to chronic stress or burnout.

Primary prevention is key to addressing risk for burnout and is important for all health professionals. Personal stress management strategies need to be a part of professional practice; they can include working on crafts, scheduled social outings with friends, participation in a team sport or an individual recreational or physical activity, limiting amount of overtime worked, taking an art class, or simply reading for pleasure. If nurses recognize feelings of burnout, they can engage in some of the same strategies that help clients: increase their own self-reflections regarding potential sources of stress, use daily journal writing to increase recognition of contextual factors, seek a colleague or mentor to help with their reflections, create an inventory of available personal and support resources, and devise a plan for addressing the various stressors in a manageable and positive manner. An important step is identifying the limits and scope of responsibilities at work (Aguilera, 1998). It is essential that you recognize the areas over which you have control and can change and those for which you do not have responsibility.

Acute Care

Crisis Intervention. When stress overwhelms a person's usual coping mechanisms and all available resources must be mobilized, the situation becomes a crisis (Aguilera, 1998). A crisis creates a turning point in a person's life because it changes the direction of a person's life in some way. According to Aguilera (1998), the precipitating event usually occurs 1 to 2 weeks before the individual seeks help, but it may have occurred within the past 24 hours. In general, a crisis is resolved in some way within approximately 6 weeks. The aim of crisis intervention is to return the person to a precrisis level of functioning and to promote growth (Figure 30–8). The use of unfamiliar strategies can result either in a heightened awareness of previously unrecognized strengths and resources or in deterioration in functioning. Thus, a crisis is often referred to as a situation of both danger and opportunity. Some people or families emerge from a crisis state functioning more effectively, whereas others are weakened, and still others are rendered completely dysfunctional.

Crisis intervention is a specific type of brief psychotherapy with prescribed steps (Aguilera, 1998). Crisis intervention is more directive than traditional psychotherapy or counselling and can be used by any member of the health care team who has been trained in its techniques. The basic approach is problem solving, and the focus is on only the problem presented by the crisis.

When using a crisis intervention approach, you help the client make the mental connection between the stressful event and the client's reaction to it. This is crucial because the client may be unable to envision the whole situation clearly. You also help the client become aware of current feelings, such as anger, grief, or guilt, in order to

BOX 30-10 NURSING STORY

Missing What Is Important

I was so keen! I wanted to be such a good nurse. Thus, in the second year of my nursing program, I began my first day on an assessment unit within our provincial psychiatric hospital with eager anticipation of testing my newly learned communication techniques, mixed with some curiosity and admitted anxiety about how I would react to clients. As it turned out, what I was stressed about was so far off the mark! I was so concerned about how I would react to clients that I did not consider how clients would react to me! We were to complete verbatim reports regarding our interactions with our clients. However, my assigned client was a middle-aged man with paranoid schizophrenia, who apparently was suspicious of new people. It was suggested that I "hang around" the unit for a few days, so that my client could get used to seeing me before I actually approached him. But what about those verbatim reports? How could I initiate the first conversation? Maybe discreet observations could fill in for the time being. I was caught up in my role as an unobtrusive casual staff member. On the second day, the client abruptly approached me and in an angry tone stated, "You have been following me and watching me for 2 days!" So much for my discretion. In focusing only on my perceptions and needs, I had thought little about how perception, like communication, can be different for the participants. My spontaneous response was "You're right, I have. I just didn't know how to approach you." His anger dissolved into a laugh at my awkwardness. That clear, honest response was the start of a very rewarding nurse–client relationship that spanned the entire 2-month rotation. He taught me so much about mental health nursing: how perceptions about potential stressors affected our interactions, how spontaneity could be powerful in interactions, and how my self-perceptions needed to be checked against the perceptions of my clients, regardless of diagnosis. I subsequently enjoyed mental health, which spanned more than 30 years. I worked with many different clinical populations over the years, but I still remember my stress and distress over my first client and how it made me blind to what was really going on.

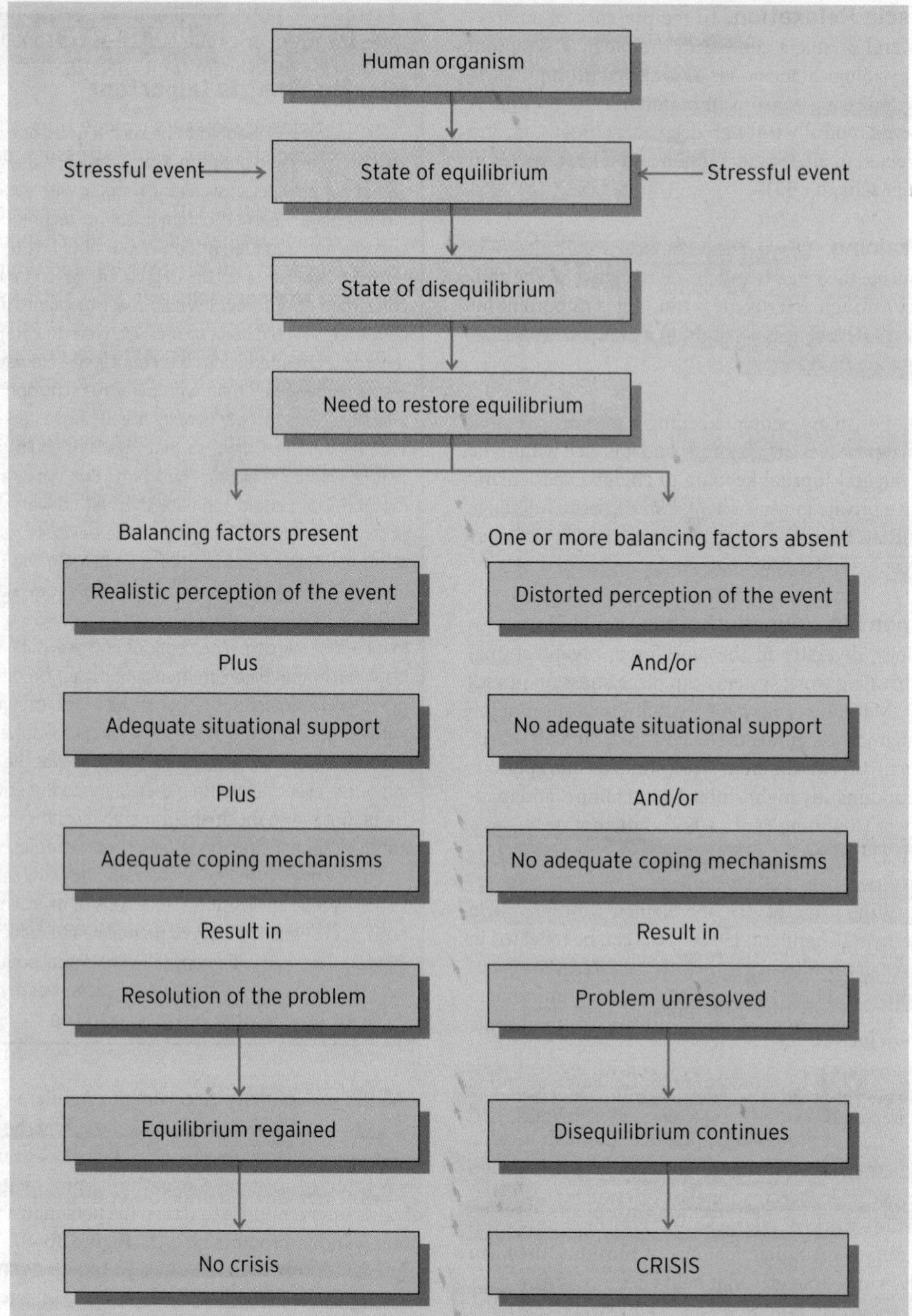

Figure 30-8 Crisis intervention model. **Source:** Redrawn from Aguilera, D. C. (1998). *Crisis intervention: Theory and methodology* (8th ed.). St. Louis, MO: Mosby.

reduce tension. In addition, you help the client explore coping mechanisms, perhaps identifying ways of coping that the client had not thought of. Finally, you may help increase the client's social contacts if the client has been internally focused and isolated (Aguilera, 1998).

Restorative and Continuing Care

A person under stress recovers when the stress is removed or coping strategies are successful; however, a person who has experienced a crisis has changed, and the effects may last for years or for the rest of the person's life (Shontz, 1975). The final stage of adapting to a crisis is acknowledgement of the long-term implications of the crisis (Shontz, 1975).

❖Evaluation

Client Care

By evaluating the goals and expected outcomes of care, you know whether the nursing interventions were effective and whether the client is coping with the identified stress. You review the measurable goals and assess whether the client has met the criteria for success as stated in the outcomes. If the nursing interventions have not been effective in helping the client achieve targeted goals, you must re-evaluate the strategies implemented and revise the care plan in light of the client's current health status (Figure 30–9).

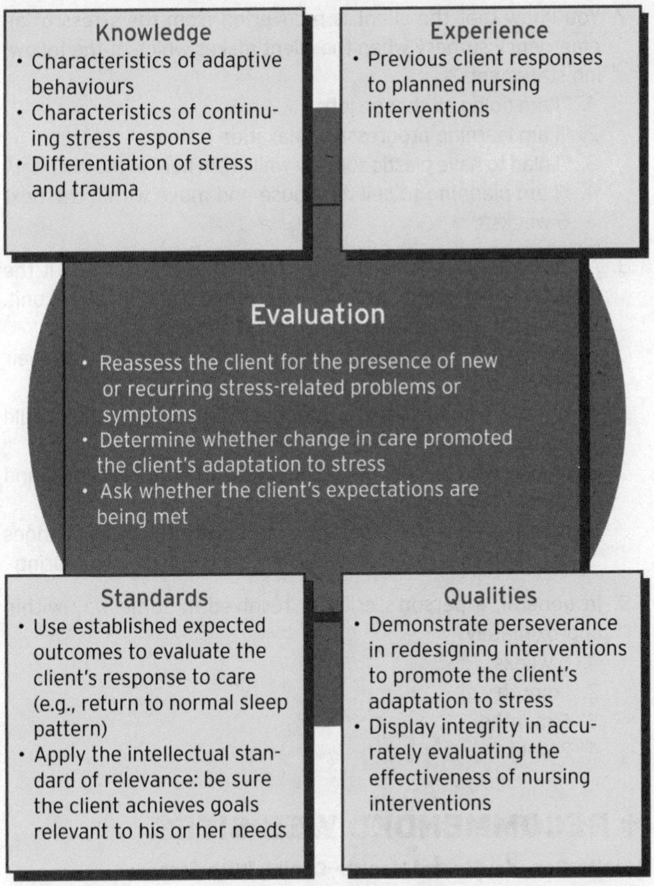

Knowledge
- Characteristics of adaptive behaviours
- Characteristics of continuing stress response
- Differentiation of stress and trauma

Experience
- Previous client responses to planned nursing interventions

Evaluation
- Reassess the client for the presence of new or recurring stress-related problems or symptoms
- Determine whether change in care promoted the client's adaptation to stress
- Ask whether the client's expectations are being met

Standards
- Use established expected outcomes to evaluate the client's response to care (e.g., return to normal sleep pattern)
- Apply the intellectual standard of relevance: be sure the client achieves goals relevant to his or her needs

Qualities
- Demonstrate perseverance in redesigning interventions to promote the client's adaptation to stress
- Display integrity in accurately evaluating the effectiveness of nursing interventions

Figure 30-9 Critical thinking model for stress and coping evaluation.

To evaluate whether goals and outcomes of care have been achieved, you observe client behaviours and interactions between the client and family, if appropriate. If your contact with a client ends before goals have been achieved, the client should be referred to appropriate resources so that progress is not delayed or interrupted.

Client Expectations

It is crucial to maintain ongoing communication with clients in regard to the care plan. Clients under severe stress or trauma often feel powerless and vulnerable. You can help reduce these feelings by actively involving clients and families in assessment, prioritizing, goal setting, and evaluation. Being involved enables clients to direct their energy positively and encourages them to take responsibility for their health. It also facilitates open communication, which makes it easier for the client to report on interventions that are successful and helps you better understand why some interventions fail to meet their goals.

* KEY CONCEPTS

- Physiological and psychological frameworks have been developed to describe how stress affects biological systems and psychological well-being.
- Overwhelming or chronic stress can increase the risks of (1) serious and long-standing health problems; (2) choosing coping strategies that are unhealthy, such as isolating oneself, not getting enough rest or a proper diet, or using tobacco, alcohol, or caffeine; (3) ignoring warning signs of illness; and (4) neglecting to take prescribed medicines or treatments.
- A person is under psychological stress only if the person evaluates the event or circumstance as personally significant. Such an evaluation of an event for its personal meaning is called *primary appraisal*.
- Several types of stressors include work stressors, family stressors, chronic stressors, acute stressors, daily hassles, trauma, and crisis.
- Rapid changes in health care technology, diversity in the workforce, organizational redesign, and changing work systems can place nurses at risk for stress-related symptoms and burnout.
- Potential stressors and coping mechanisms vary across the lifespan: from childhood through adolescence, adulthood, and old age.
- Coping is a means of managing psychological stress and reflects a dynamic process in response to the current situation, past experiences, and available resources.
- Three primary modes for stress intervention are to decrease stress-producing situations, increase resistance to stress, and learn skills that reduce physiological response to stress.
- If stress is so severe that the client is unable to cope in any ways that have worked before, the client is experiencing a crisis.
- A crisis is a turning point in life and can be developmental or situational.
- In general, a crisis is resolved in some way within approximately 6 weeks. Crisis intervention aims to return the person to a precrisis level of functioning and to promote growth.

* CRITICAL THINKING EXERCISES

1. You are caring for a 30-year-old woman who has recently received a diagnosis of metastatic breast cancer. She is the lone parent and sole provider for three young children (all younger than 7 years). Discuss the various stressors that must be considered when you write an appropriate discharge plan.
2. A client comes to the emergency department with complaints of dizziness, which are not related to any physical finding on examination. During the health history, the client reports that her life is very stressful and she is barely coping. She finalized her divorce 3 months ago, is working 32 hours per week, and is attending college. Her ex-husband recently lost his job and can no longer pay child support. She tearfully confesses that she thinks she might be pregnant but does not want her ex-husband to know. Develop nursing diagnoses related to this situation.
3. An older woman is admitted to the hospital with a fractured hip. Before her injury, she lived with her husband, who has advancing Alzheimer's disease. While she is hospitalized, he is staying with a niece who lives 50 km away, but this cannot be a permanent situation because her niece is also in frail health. The client has no children who can help her when she returns home. She is concerned not only about who will care for her after she is discharged but also about her husband's care. What approach would be the best to take in establishing goals for treatment?

* REVIEW QUESTIONS

1. The vital functions necessary for survival, which include heart rate, blood pressure, and respiration, are controlled by the
   1. Medulla oblongata
   2. Reticular formation
   3. Pituitary gland
   4. Limbic system

2. While assessing a person for effects of the general adaptation syndrome, you should be aware that
   1. Heart rate increases in the adaptation state
   2. Blood volume increases in the exhaustion stage
   3. Vital signs return to normal in the exhaustion stage
   4. Blood glucose level increases during the alarm reaction stage
3. When performing an assessment of a young woman who was in an automobile accident 6 months before, you learn that the woman has vivid images of the crash whenever she hears a loud, sudden noise. You recognize that these reactions are flashbacks, which are symptoms of
   1. Social phobia
   2. Acute anxiety
   3. Post-traumatic stress disorder
   4. Borderline personality disorder
4. A man is adjusting to a chronic illness; the chronic illness can be considered
   1. A sociocultural stressor
   2. A maturational stressor
   3. A situational stressor
   4. An environmental stressor
5. A child who has been in a house fire comes to the emergency department with her parents. The child and parents are upset and tearful. During your first assessment for stress, what should you say?
   1. "Tell me whom I can call to help you."
   2. "Tell me what upsets you the most about this experience."
   3. "I will contact someone who can help get you temporary housing."
   4. "I will sit with you until other family members can come help you get settled."
6. You are evaluating the coping strategies of a client experiencing stress from receiving a new diagnosis of multiple sclerosis and psychomotor impairment. You realized that the client is coping successfully when the client makes which of the following statements?
   1. "I am going to learn to drive a car so I can be more independent."
   2. "My sister says she feels better when she goes shopping, so I will go shopping."
   3. "I have always felt better when I go for a long walk. I will do that when I get home."
   4. "I am going to attend a support group to learn more about multiple sclerosis and what I will be able to do."
7. You know that the client is recovering from the stress of an emergency surgery when the client makes which of the following statements?
   1. "I am going to change jobs."
   2. "I am learning progressive relaxation training."
   3. "I plan to have plastic surgery while I am here in the hospital."
   4. "I am planning to sell my house and move within the next 6 weeks."
8. A staff nurse is talking with her nursing supervisor about the stress she feels from having transferred to a new inpatient unit. The supervising nurse recognizes that
   1. Nurses who feel stress usually pass the stress along to their clients
   2. A nurse who feels stress is ineffective as a nurse and should not be working
   3. Nurses who talk about feeling stress are unprofessional and should calm down
   4. Nurses frequently experience stress with the rapid changes in health care technology and organizational restructuring
9. In general, a person's crisis is resolved in some way within approximately
   1. 6 weeks
   2. 1 month
   3. 6 months
   4. 2 weeks

* RECOMMENDED WEB SITES

Health Canada: Mental Health—Coping With Stress: http://www.hc-sc.gc.ca/hl-vs/iyh-vsv/life-vie/stress-eng.php

This Web page provides links to taking care of your mental health by identifying symptoms of stress and strategies to decrease its effect on health.

Heart & Stroke Foundation Reduce Your Stress: http://www.heartandstroke.ab.ca/site/c.lqIRL1PJJtH/b.3650923/

This Web page provides information and resources related to coping with stress.

Yahoo! Health: Stress Management: http://health.yahoo.com/stress-overview/stress-management/healthwise-rlxsk.html

This Web site provides information on identification of stress-related symptoms and some strategies for managing stressors.

31

Vital Signs

Original chapter by Susan J. Fetzer, RN, PA, BSN, MSN, MBA, PhD

Canadian content written by Phyllis Castelein, RN, MN

objectives

Mastery of content in this chapter will enable you to:

- Define the key terms listed.
- Explain the principles and mechanisms of thermoregulation.
- Describe nursing measures that promote heat loss and heat conservation.
- Discuss physiological changes associated with fever.
- Accurately assess tympanic, oral, rectal, and axillary temperatures.
- Accurately assess pulse, respirations, oxygen saturation, and blood pressure.
- Explain the physiology of normal regulation of blood pressure, pulse, oxygen saturation, and respirations.
- Describe factors that cause variations in body temperature, pulse, oxygen saturation, respirations, and blood pressure.
- Describe ethnic variations in blood pressure.
- Identify ranges of acceptable vital sign values for an infant, a child, and an adult.
- Explain variations in technique used to assess an infant's, a child's, and an adult's vital signs.
- Describe the benefits and precautions involving self-measurement of blood pressure.
- Identify when vital signs should be measured.
- Accurately record and report vital sign measurements.
- Appropriately delegate vital sign measurement to unregulated care providers.

key terms

Afebrile, p. 497
Antipyretics, p. 508
Auscultatory gap, p. 533
Basal metabolic rate (BMR), p. 495
Blood pressure, p. 523
Bradycardia, p. 516
Cardiac output, p. 509
Celsius, p. 503
Conduction, p. 496
Convection, p. 496
Core temperature, p. 494
Diaphoresis, p. 496
Diastolic, p. 523
Diffusion, p. 516
Dysrhythmia, p. 516
Eupnea, p. 517
Evaporation, p. 496
Fahrenheit, p. 503
Febrile, p. 497
Fever, p. 497
Fever of unknown origin, p. 497
Frostbite, p. 498
Heat exhaustion, p. 498
Heatstroke, p. 498
Hematocrit, p. 524
Hypertension, p. 524
Hyperthermia, p. 498
Hypotension, p. 525
Hypothalamus, p. 495
Hypothermia, p. 498
Hypoxemia, p. 516
Malignant hyperthermia, p. 498
Masked hypertension, p. 525
Nonshivering thermogenesis, p. 495
Orthostatic hypotension, p. 526
Perfusion, p. 516
Postural hypotension, p. 526
Pulse deficit, p. 516
Pulse pressure, p. 523
Pyrexia, p. 497
Pyrogens, p. 497
Radial pulse, p. 510
Radiation, p. 495
Shivering, p. 495
Sphygmomanometer, p. 526
Stroke volume, p. 509
Systolic, p. 523
Tachycardia, p. 516
Thermoregulation, p. 495
Tidal volume, p. 517
Ventilation, p. 516
Vital signs (VS), p. 494
White coat hypertension, p. 525

media resources

evolve Web Site

- Audio Chapter Summaries
- Glossary
- Multiple-Choice Review Questions
- Student Learning Activities
- Weblinks

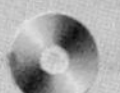

Companion CD

- Glossary
- Interactive Learning Activities
- Fluids and Electrolytes Tutorial
- Test-Taking Skills

The most frequent measurements obtained by health care professionals are those of temperature, pulse, blood pressure, respiratory rate, and oxygen saturation. These measurements indicate the effectiveness of circulatory, respiratory, neural, and endocrine body functions. Because of their importance, they are referred to as **vital signs (VS)**. Many factors—such as pain, environmental temperature, physical state or activities, or illness—cause vital signs to change, sometimes to values outside an acceptable range.

Vital signs provide data to determine the usual state of health (baseline data). A change in vital signs indicates a change in physiological function, which may signal the need for medical or nursing intervention. Measuring vital signs is a quick and efficient way of monitoring a client's condition, identifying problems, or evaluating the response to intervention. With knowledge of the physiological variables influencing vital signs, and recognition of the relationship of vital signs changes to other physical assessment findings, precise determinations of health are made. Inspection, palpation, and auscultation are used to determine vital signs. These simple skills should not be taken for granted. Careful measurement techniques ensure accurate findings. Vital signs and other physiological measurements are the basis for clinical problem solving.

Guidelines for Measuring Vital Signs

Vital signs are a part of the assessment database. You obtain them during a complete physical assessment (see Chapter 32) or as needed to assess a client's condition. Vital sign measurements during a routine physical examination provide a baseline for future assessments. The client's needs and condition determine when, where, how, and by whom vital signs are measured. You must measure them correctly or delegate their measurement appropriately. Values must be understood and interpreted, findings communicated appropriately, and interventions begun as needed. Box 31–1 lists acceptable adult values.

Use the following guidelines to incorporate vital sign measurement into your nursing practice:

- Unregulated care providers may measure selected vital signs (i.e., in stable clients), and then the nurse responsible for the client may interpret and act upon these measurements.
- Use equipment that is functional and appropriate for the size and age of the client to ensure accurate findings (e.g., an oral thermometer is not appropriate for use in an infant).
- Select equipment on the basis of the client's condition and characteristics (e.g., an adult-size blood pressure cuff should not be used for a child).
- Minimize environmental factors that may affect vital signs (e.g., assessing the client's temperature in a warm, humid room may yield a value that is not a true indicator of the client's condition).
- Use an organized, step-by-step approach to ensure accuracy.
- Approach the client in a calm, caring manner while demonstrating proficiency in handling supplies needed for vital sign measurement. The manner of approach can alter vital signs.
- Follow guidelines cited in Box 31–2 to decide frequency of vital sign assessment. Increase the frequency of vital sign assessment if the client's condition warrants it (i.e., frequency of vital signs ordered by the prescribing health care professional is the *minimum* number of times that they should be checked).
- Use vital sign measurements to determine indications for prescribed medication administration (e.g., certain cardiac drugs are given only if pulse or blood pressure values are in a certain range, and antipyretics are administered only when temperature is elevated outside the acceptable range for the client).
- Analyze the results of vital sign measurement by using knowledge of the client's usual values, medical history, therapies, and prescribed medications. A client's usual values may differ from the acceptable range for that age or physical state. Some illnesses or treatments cause predictable changes in vital signs. Some medications affect one or more vital signs. You are often in the best position to assess all clinical findings about a client. You must know related physical signs or symptoms and be aware of the client's ongoing health status.
- Baseline measurements allow the identification of changes in vital signs. When vital signs appear abnormal, it may help to have another nurse repeat the measurement. Verify, document, and communicate significant changes in vital signs to the prescribing health care professional or nurse in charge.
- Develop a teaching plan to instruct client or caregiver in vital sign assessment and the significance of findings.

➤ BOX 31-1 Vital Signs: Acceptable Ranges for Adults

Temperature Range: 36°C to 38°C
Average oral/tympanic: 37°C
Average rectal: 37.5°C
Average axillary: 36.5°C

Pulse
60 to 100 beats per minute

Respirations
12 to 20 breaths per minute

Blood Pressure
Average: 120/80 mm Hg
Pulse pressure: 30 to 50 mm Hg

Body Temperature

Physiology

The body temperature is the difference between the amount of heat produced by body processes and the amount of heat lost to the external environment. Despite extremes in environmental conditions and physical activity, temperature-control mechanisms keep the body's **core temperature** (temperature of the deep tissues) relatively constant (Figure 31–1). Surface temperature fluctuates, depending on blood flow to the skin and the amount of heat lost to the external environment. Because of these surface temperature fluctuations, acceptable body temperature ranges from 36°C to 38°C, a narrow range in which the body's tissues and cells function best.

The site of temperature measurement (oral, rectal, axillary, tympanic membrane, temporal artery, esophageal, pulmonary artery, or even urinary bladder) is one factor that determines the measurement of the client's temperature. For healthy young adults, the average oral temperature is 37°C. In clinical practice, nurses learn the temperature range of individual clients, inasmuch as no single temperature is normal for all people.

The measurement of body temperature is aimed at obtaining a representative average temperature of core body tissues. Sites reflecting core temperatures are more reliable indicators of body temperature

> **BOX 31-2 When to Measure Vital Signs**
>
> Upon admission to a health care facility
> During a home care visit
> According to the prescribing health care professional's order or the health facility's standards of practice
> Before and after a surgical procedure or an invasive diagnostic procedure
> Before, during, and after the administration of blood products
> Before, during, and after administration of medications that affect cardiovascular, respiratory, and temperature-control function
> When client's general physical condition changes (e.g., loss of consciousness or increased pain)
> Before and after nursing interventions that affect a vital sign (e.g., before a client previously on bed rest ambulates or before a client performs range-of-motion exercises)
> When a client reports nonspecific symptoms of physical distress (e.g., feeling "funny" or "different")

than are sites reflecting surface temperatures (Box 31–3). In addition, the temperature value obtained may differ between one measurement site and another.

Regulation. The balance between heat lost and heat produced, or **thermoregulation**, is precisely regulated by physiological and behavioural mechanisms. For body temperature to stay constant and within an acceptable range, the relationship between heat production and heat loss must be maintained. This relationship is regulated by neurological and cardiovascular mechanisms. To regulate clients' temperatures, you apply knowledge of temperature-control mechanisms.

Neural and Vascular Control. The **hypothalamus**, located between the cerebral hemispheres, controls body temperature the same way that a thermostat works in a building. A comfortable temperature is the *set point* at which a heating system operates. In the building, a decrease in environmental temperature activates the furnace, whereas a rise in temperature shuts the system down. The hypothalamus is like the building's furnace; it senses minor changes in body temperature. The anterior hypothalamus controls heat loss, and the posterior hypothalamus controls heat production.

When nerve cells in the anterior hypothalamus become heated above the set point, impulses are sent to reduce body temperature. Mechanisms of heat loss include sweating, vasodilation (widening) of blood vessels, and inhibition of heat production. Blood is redistributed to surface vessels to promote heat loss. If the posterior hypothalamus senses that the body's temperature is lower than the set point, heat conservation mechanisms are instituted: Vasoconstriction (narrowing) of blood vessels reduces blood flow to the skin and extremities.

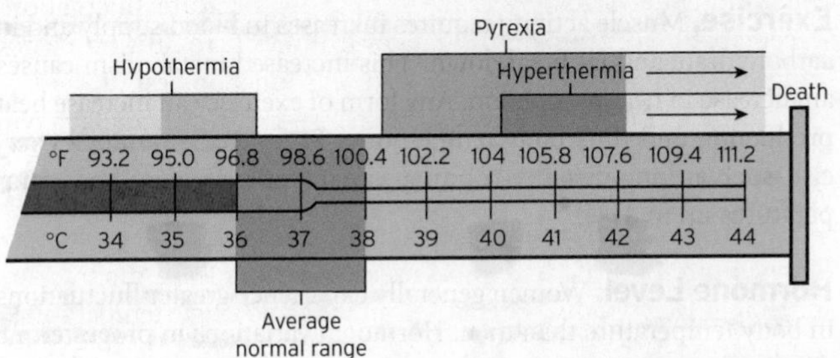

Figure 31-1 Ranges of normal temperature values and physiological consequences of abnormal body temperature.

Compensatory heat is produced through voluntary muscle contraction and muscle shivering. When vasoconstriction is ineffective in preventing additional heat loss, shivering begins. Disease or trauma to the hypothalamus or to the spinal cord, which carries hypothalamic messages, can cause serious alterations in temperature control.

Heat Production. Thermoregulation depends on the normal function of heat production processes. Heat is produced in the body as a by-product of metabolism, the chemical reaction in all body cells. Food is the primary fuel source for metabolism. Activities requiring additional chemical reactions increase metabolic rate. As metabolism increases, additional heat is produced. When metabolism decreases, less heat is produced. Heat production occurs during rest, voluntary movements, involuntary shivering, and nonshivering thermogenesis.

Basal metabolism accounts for the heat produced by the body at absolute rest. The average **basal metabolic rate (BMR)** depends on the body surface area. Thyroid hormones also affect the BMR. By promoting the breakdown of body glucose and fat, thyroid hormones increase the rate of chemical reactions in almost all cells of the body. When large amounts of thyroid hormones are secreted, the BMR can increase 100% above normal. Absence of thyroid hormones can cut the BMR in half, causing a decrease in heat production. The male sex hormone testosterone increases BMR. Men have a higher BMR than do women.Voluntary movements such as muscular activity during exercise require additional energy. Metabolic rate can increase up to 2000 times normal during exercise. Heat production can increase up to 50 times normal.

Shivering is an involuntary body response to temperature differences in the body. The skeletal muscle movement during shivering requires significant energy. In vulnerable clients, shivering can seriously deplete energy sources, which results in further physiological deterioration. Shivering can increase heat production four to five times greater than normal. The heat produced assists in equalizing body temperature, and shivering ceases.

Nonshivering thermogenesis occurs primarily in newborns. Until they are approximately 2 weeks old, newborns cannot shiver, so they rely on vasoconstriction through an increase in norepinephrine. In addition, a limited amount of vascular brown tissue (fat) is metabolized for heat production.

Heat Loss. Heat loss and heat production occur simultaneously. The skin's structure and exposure to the environment result in constant, normal heat loss through radiation, conduction, convection, and evaporation.

Radiation is the transfer of heat from the surface of one object to the surface of another without direct contact between the two. Up to 85% of the human body's surface area radiates heat to the environment.

> **BOX 31-3 Sites of Measurement of Core and Surface Temperature**
>
> **Core Temperature**
> Rectum
> Tympanic membrane
> Temporal artery
> Esophagus
> Pulmonary artery
> Urinary bladder
>
> **Surface Temperature**
> Skin
> Mouth
> Axillae

Peripheral vasodilation increases blood flow from internal organs to the skin to increase radiant heat loss. Peripheral vasoconstriction minimizes radiant heat loss. Radiation increases as the temperature difference between the objects increases. If the environment is warmer than the skin, the body absorbs heat through radiation.

Heat loss is increased through radiation by removing clothing or blankets. The client's position enhances radiation heat loss (e.g., standing exposes a greater radiating surface area, and lying in a fetal position minimizes heat radiation). Covering the body with dark, closely woven clothing also reduces the amount of heat lost from radiation.

Conduction is the transfer of heat from one object to another with direct contact. Heat conducts through contact with solids, liquids, and gases. When the warm skin touches a cooler object, heat is lost. Conduction normally accounts for a small amount of heat loss. Interventions such as applying a cool cloth increase conductive heat loss. Applying several layers of clothing reduces conductive loss. The body gains heat by conduction when contact is made with materials warmer than skin temperature (e.g., application of an aquathermia pad).

Convection is the transfer of heat away by air movement. A fan promotes heat loss through convection. Convective heat loss increases when moistened skin comes into contact with slightly moving air.

Evaporation is the transfer of heat energy when a liquid is changed to a gas. The body continuously loses heat by evaporation. About 600 to 900 mL per day evaporates from the skin and lungs, which results in water and heat loss. By regulating perspiration (sweating), the body promotes additional evaporative heat loss. Millions of sweat glands located in the dermis of the skin secrete sweat through tiny ducts on the skin's surface. When body temperature rises, the anterior hypothalamus signals the sweat glands to release sweat. Sweat evaporates from the skin surface, which results in heat loss. During exercise and emotional or mental stress, sweating is one way to lose excessive heat produced by the increased metabolic rate.

Diaphoresis is visible perspiration, which occurs primarily on the forehead and upper thorax, although it can also be seen elsewhere on the body. Excessive evaporation can cause skin scaling and itching, as well as drying of the nares and pharynx. A lowered body temperature inhibits sweat gland secretion. People who have a congenital absence of sweat glands or a serious skin disease that impairs sweating are unable to tolerate warm temperatures because they cannot cool themselves adequately.

Skin in Temperature Regulation. The skin regulates temperature through insulation of the body, vasoconstriction (which affects the amount of blood flow and heat loss to the skin), and temperature sensation. The skin, subcutaneous tissue, and fat keep heat inside the body. When blood flow between skin layers is reduced, the skin alone is an excellent insulator. People with more body fat have more natural insulation than do slim and muscular people.

In the human body, the internal organs produce heat. During exercise or increased sympathetic stimulation, the amount of heat produced is greater than the usual core temperature. Blood flows from the internal organs, carrying heat to the body surface. The skin is well supplied with blood vessels, especially the areas of the hands, feet, and ears. Blood flow through these vascular areas of skin may vary from minimal flow to as much as 30% of the blood ejected from the heart. Heat transfers from the blood through vessel walls to the skin's surface and is lost to the environment through the heat-loss mechanisms. The body's core temperature remains within safe limits.

The degree of vasoconstriction determines the amount of blood flow and heat loss to the skin. If the core temperature is too high, the hypothalamus inhibits vasoconstriction. As a result, blood vessels dilate, and more blood reaches the skin's surface. On a hot, humid day, the blood vessels in the hands are dilated and easily visible. In contrast, if the core temperature becomes too low, the hypothalamus initiates vasoconstriction and blood flow to the skin lessens, thus conserving body heat.

Behavioural Control. Healthy individuals voluntarily act to maintain a comfortable body temperature when exposed to temperature extremes. A person's ability to control body temperature depends on (1) the degree of temperature extreme, (2) the person's ability to sense feeling comfortable or uncomfortable, (3) thought processes or emotions, and (4) the person's mobility or ability to remove or add clothes. Body temperature control is difficult if any of these abilities is absent. Infants can sense uncomfortably warm conditions but cannot change their environment. Older adults may need help in detecting cold environments and minimizing heat loss. Illness, a decreased level of consciousness, or impaired thought processes result in an inability to recognize the need to change behaviour for temperature control. When temperatures become extremely hot or cold, health-promoting behaviours, such as removing or adding clothing, have a limited effect on controlling temperature. Assess for factors that place clients at high risk for ineffective thermoregulation.

Factors Affecting Body Temperature

Many factors affect body temperature. Changes in body temperature within an acceptable range occur when the relationship between heat production and heat loss is altered by physiological or behavioural variables. Be aware of these factors when assessing temperature variations and evaluating deviations from normal.

Age. At birth, the newborn leaves a warm, relatively constant environment and enters one in which temperatures fluctuate widely. Temperature-control mechanisms are immature. An infant's temperature may respond drastically to changes in the environment. Extra care is needed to protect the newborn from environmental temperatures. Clothing must be adequate, and exposure to temperature extremes must be avoided. A newborn loses up to 30% of body heat through the head and therefore needs to wear a cap to prevent heat loss. When protected from environmental extremes, the newborn's body temperature is normally maintained between 35.5°C and 37.5°C.

Temperature regulation is unstable until children reach puberty. The normal temperature range gradually drops as individuals approach older adulthood. Older adults have a lower and narrower range of body temperatures than do younger adults. An oral temperature of 35°C is not unusual for older adults in cold weather. However, the average body temperature of older adults is approximately 36°C. Older adults are particularly sensitive to temperature extremes because of deterioration in control mechanisms, particularly poor vasomotor control (control of vasoconstriction and vasodilation), reduced amounts of subcutaneous tissue, reduced sweat gland activity, and reduced metabolism.

Exercise. Muscle activity requires increases in blood supply and in carbohydrate and fat breakdown. This increased metabolism causes an increase in heat production. Any form of exercise can increase heat production and thus body temperature. Prolonged strenuous exercise, such as long-distance running, can temporarily raise body temperatures up to 41°C.

Hormone Level. Women generally experience greater fluctuations in body temperature than men. Hormonal variations in progesterone during the menstrual cycle cause body temperature fluctuations. When progesterone levels are low, the body temperature is a few tenths of a degree below the baseline level. The lower temperature persists until ovulation occurs. During ovulation, greater amounts of progesterone enter the circulatory system and raise the body temperature to previous baseline levels or higher. These temperature variations can be used to predict a woman's most fertile time to achieve pregnancy.

Body temperature changes also occur during menopause (cessation of menstruation). Menopausal women may experience times of intense body heat and sweating that last from 30 seconds to 5 minutes. Skin temperature may increase intermittently up to 4°C during these times, called *hot flashes*. These increases result from the instability of the vasomotor controls for vasodilation and vasoconstriction.

Circadian Rhythm. Body temperature normally changes 0.5°C to 1°C during a 24-hour period. In persons who are awake during the day and sleep during the night, the temperature is usually lowest between 0100 and 0400 hours (Figure 31–2). During the day, body temperature rises steadily, until a maximum temperature value at about 1800 hours, and then declines to early morning levels. It takes 1 to 3 weeks for temperature patterns to reverse in people who work at night and sleep during the day. In general, the circadian temperature rhythm does not change with age.

Stress. Physical and emotional stress increase body temperature through hormonal and neural stimulation. These physiological changes increase metabolism, which increases heat production. The client who is anxious about entering a hospital may register a higher normal temperature (see Chapter 30).

Environment. Environment influences body temperature. If body temperature is measured in a very warm room, a client may be unable to regulate body temperature by heat-loss mechanisms, and the body temperature is elevated. If the client has just been outside in the cold without warm clothing, body temperature may be low because of extensive radiant and conductive heat loss. Infants and older adults are most likely to be affected by environmental temperatures because their temperature-regulating mechanisms are less efficient.

Temperature Alterations. Body temperatures outside the usual range affect the hypothalamic set point. Such changes can be related to excess heat production, excessive heat loss, minimal heat production, minimal heat loss, or any combination of these alterations. The nature of the change affects the type of clinical problems experienced.

Fever. Pyrexia, or fever, occurs because heat-loss mechanisms are unable to keep pace with excess heat production; as a result, body temperature rises to an abnormal level. A fever is usually not harmful if it stays below 39°C, and a single temperature reading may not indicate a fever. In addition to physical signs and symptoms of infection, determination of fever is based on several temperature readings at different times of the day that are compared with the usual value for that person at those times.

A true fever results from an alteration in the hypothalamic set point. **Pyrogens** such as bacteria and viruses cause a rise in body temperature. Pyrogens act as antigens, triggering immune system responses. The hypothalamus reacts to raise the set point, and the body responds by producing and conserving heat. Several hours may pass before the body temperature reaches the new set point. During this period, the person experiences chills, shivers, and feels cold, even though the body temperature is rising (Figure 31–3). The chill phase resolves when the new set point, a higher temperature, is achieved. During the next phase, the plateau, the chills subside, and the person feels warm and dry. If the new set point is "overshot" or the pyrogens are removed (e.g., destruction of bacteria by antibiotics), the third phase of a febrile episode occurs. The hypothalamus set point drops, initiating heat loss responses. The skin becomes warm and flushed because of vasodilation. Diaphoresis assists in evaporative heat loss. When the fever "breaks," the person becomes **afebrile**.

Fever is an important defence mechanism. Temperature elevations up to 38°C enhance the body's immune system. During a **febrile** episode, white blood cell production is stimulated. Increased temperature reduces the concentration of iron in the blood plasma, suppressing the growth of bacteria. Fever also fights viral infections by stimulating production of interferon, the body's natural virus-fighting substance.

By analyzing a fever pattern, health care professionals can make diagnoses. Fever patterns differ, depending on the causative pyrogen. The increase or decrease in pyrogen activity results in fever spikes and declines at different times of the day. The duration and degree of fever depend on the pyrogen's strength and the ability of the individual to respond. The term **fever of unknown origin** refers to a fever that does not have a determined cause.

During a fever, cellular metabolism increases and oxygen consumption rises. The body's metabolism increases 10% for every degree Celsius of temperature elevation (Henker & Carlson, 2007). Heart and respiratory rates increase to meet the metabolic needs of the body for nutrients. The increased metabolism entails the use of energy that produces additional heat. If the client has a cardiac or respiratory problem, the stress of a fever can be great. A prolonged fever can weaken a person by exhausting energy stores. Increased metabolism

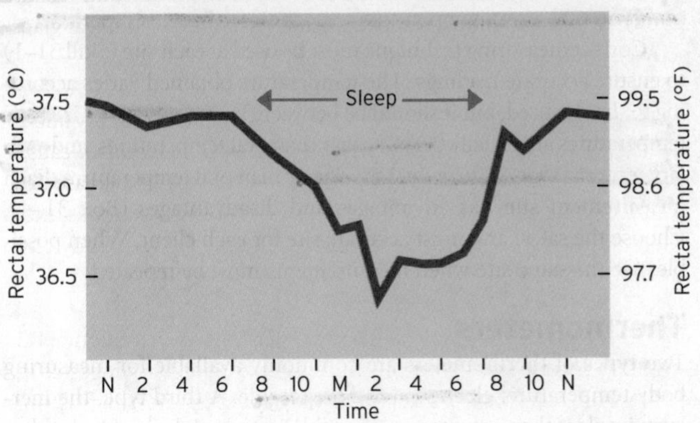

Figure 31-2 Temperature cycle for 24 hours.

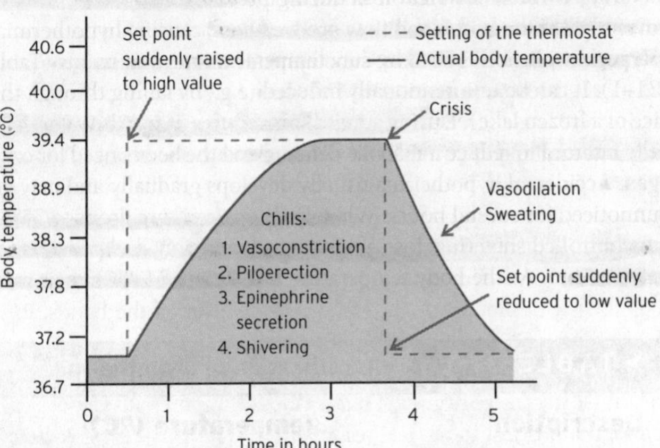

Figure 31-3 Effect of changing the set point of the hypothalamic temperature control during a fever. **Source:** Adapted from Guyton, A. C., & Hall, J. E. (2005). *Textbook of medical physiology* (10th ed., p. 899). Philadelphia, PA: W. B. Saunders.

requires additional oxygen. If the demand for additional oxygen cannot be met, cellular hypoxia (inadequate oxygenation) occurs. Myocardial hypoxia produces angina (chest pain); cerebral hypoxia produces confusion. Interventions during a fever may include oxygen therapy. Water loss through increased respiration and diaphoresis can be excessive, placing a client at risk for fluid volume deficit. Dehydration is a serious problem for older adults and for children with low body weight. Maintaining optimum fluid volume status is an important nursing intervention (see Chapter 40).

Hyperthermia. **Hyperthermia** is body temperature that is elevated as a result of the body's inability to promote heat loss or reduce heat production. Whereas fever is an upward shift in the set point, hyperthermia results from an overload of the body's thermoregulatory mechanisms. Any disease or trauma to the hypothalamus can impair heat-loss mechanisms. **Malignant hyperthermia** is a hereditary condition of uncontrolled heat production, occurring when susceptible people receive certain anaesthetic drugs.

Heatstroke. Prolonged exposure to the sun or high environmental temperatures can overwhelm the body's heat-loss mechanisms. Heat also depresses hypothalamic function. These conditions cause **heatstroke,** a dangerous heat emergency with a high mortality rate. Clients at risk include those who are very young, those who are very old, and those who have cardiovascular disease, hypothyroidism, diabetes, or alcoholism. Also at risk are clients who take medications that decrease the body's ability to lose heat (e.g., phenothiazines, anticholinergics, diuretics, amphetamines, and β-adrenergic receptor antagonists) and those who exercise or engage in strenuous physical labor (e.g., athletes, construction workers, and farmers).

Signs and symptoms of heatstroke include confusion, delirium, excess thirst, nausea, muscle cramps, visual disturbances, giddiness, and incontinence. The most important sign is hot, dry skin. Clients with heatstroke do not sweat because of severe electrolyte loss and hypothalamic malfunction. Vital signs reveal a body temperature sometimes as high as 45°C, with an increase in heart rate and lowering of blood pressure. If the condition progresses, the person becomes unconscious with fixed, unreactive pupils. Permanent neurological damage occurs unless cooling measures are rapidly started.

Heat Exhaustion. **Heat exhaustion** occurs when profuse diaphoresis results in excess water and electrolyte loss. The client exhibits signs and symptoms of fluid volume deficit (see Chapter 40). First aid includes transporting the client to a cooler environment and restoring fluid and electrolyte balance.

Hypothermia. Heat loss during prolonged exposure to cold overwhelms the body's ability to produce heat, causing hypothermia. **Hypothermia** is classified by core temperature measurements (Table 31–1). It can be unintentionally induced (e.g., by falling through the ice of a frozen lake). During surgical procedures, it may be intentionally induced to reduce metabolic demand and the body's need for oxygen. Accidental hypothermia usually develops gradually and may go unnoticed for several hours. When body temperature drops to 35°C, uncontrolled shivering, loss of memory, depression, and poor judgement occur. As the body temperature falls below 34.4°C, heart rate, respiratory rate, and blood pressure fall. The skin becomes cyanotic. If hypothermia progresses, a person exhibits cardiac dysrhythmia, loss of consciousness, and unresponsiveness to painful stimuli. In cases of severe hypothermia, a person may demonstrate clinical signs similar to death (e.g., lack of response to stimuli and extremely slow respirations and pulse). The assessment of core temperature is critical when hypothermia is suspected. A special thermometer that displays low readings may be required because standard devices do not register below 35°C.

TABLE 31-1 Classification of Hypothermia

Description	Temperature (°C)
Mild	34–36
Moderate	30–34
Severe	<30

Frostbite occurs when the body is exposed to subnormal temperatures. Ice crystals forming inside cells can result in permanent circulatory and tissue damage. Areas particularly susceptible to frostbite are the earlobes, tip of the nose, fingers, and toes. The injured area becomes white, waxy, and firm to the touch. The client loses sensation in the affected area. Intervention includes gradual warming measures, analgesia, and protection of the injured tissue.

Nursing Process and Thermoregulation

Knowledge of the physiology of body temperature regulation is essential for assessing and evaluating the client's response to temperature alterations and for intervening safely. Independent measures can be implemented to increase or minimize heat loss, promote heat conservation, and increase comfort. These measures complement the effects of medically ordered therapies. Many measures can be taught to family members, parents of children, and other caregivers.

❖Assessment

Sites

Core and surface body temperature may be measured at several sites. The core temperatures of the pulmonary artery, esophagus, and urinary bladder are measured in intensive care settings. These measurements require the use of continuous invasive devices placed in body cavities or organs and continually display readings on an electronic monitor.

Intermittent temperature measurements are obtained invasively from the sites of the mouth, rectum, and tympanic membrane or noninvasively from the axilla and temporal artery sites. Chemically prepared thermometer patches can also be applied to the skin. In order to measure oral, rectal, axillary, and skin temperature, blood circulation at the measurement site must be effective. The heat of the blood is conducted to the thermometer probe. Tympanic temperature relies on the radiation of body heat to an infrared sensor. Temporal artery measurements detect cutaneous blood flow temperature. Because they share the same arterial blood supply as the hypothalamus, tympanic and temporal artery temperature are considered core temperatures.

Correct measuring technique must be used at each site (Skill 31–1) to ensure accurate readings. The temperature obtained varies according to the site used, but it should be between 36.0°C and 38.0°C. Rectal temperatures are usually 0.5°C higher than oral temperatures, and axillary temperatures are usually 0.5°C lower than oral temperatures. Each measurement site has advantages and disadvantages (Box 31–4). Choose the safest and most accurate site for each client. When possible, use the same site when measurements must be repeated.

Thermometers

Two types of thermometers are commonly available for measuring body temperature: electronic and disposable. A third type, the mercury-in-glass thermometer, was once the standard device for the clinical setting. Most municipalities have now prohibited the sale or use of mercury-containing medical devices because of potential hazards.

➤ SKILL 31-1 Measuring Body Temperature

video

Delegation Considerations

The task of measuring temperature can be delegated to unregulated care providers (UCPs). The nurse is responsible for assessing the impact of changes in body temperature; therefore, when the task of measuring temperature is delegated, it is important to *inform the unregulated care provider* about the following:

- The appropriate route and device to measure temperature
- Client-specific factors that can falsely raise or lower temperature
- Appropriate precautions when positioning the client
- Frequency of temperature measurement for the client
- Usual values for client
- Abnormalities that should be reported to the health care professional

Equipment

- Appropriate thermometer
- Soft tissue or wipe
- Lubricant (for rectal measurements only)
- Pen and either vital sign flow sheet or record form
- Disposable gloves
- Plastic thermometer sleeve or disposable probe cover

Procedure

STEPS	RATIONALE
1. Assess for signs and symptoms of temperature alterations and for factors that influence body temperature.	• Physical signs and symptoms may indicate abnormal temperature. You can accurately assess the nature of variations.
2. Determine any previous activity that would interfere with accuracy of temperature measurement. Wait before measuring oral temperature in the following situations: 2 minutes after client has smoked, 5 minutes after client has chewed gum, and 20 minutes after client has ingested hot or cold liquids or foods.	• Smoking, mouth breathing, and oral intake of food or fluids can cause false oral temperature readings (Henker & Carlson, 2007).
3. Determine appropriate temperature site and device for client.	• This choice is based on advantages and disadvantages of each site (see Box 31–4). Use a disposable, single-use thermometer for a client who has isolation precautions.
4. Explain to client the route by which temperature will be measured and the importance of maintaining proper position until the reading is complete.	• Clients are often curious about measurements and should be cautioned against prematurely removing the thermometer to read results.
5. Perform hand hygiene.	• Hand hygiene reduces transmission of microorganisms between the client and the nurse.
6. Obtain temperature reading.	
A. **Oral temperature measurement with electronic thermometer**	
(1) Put on disposable gloves (optional).	• Use of oral probe cover, removed without physical contact, minimizes need to wear gloves.
(2) Remove thermometer pack from charging unit. Attach oral probe (blue tip) to thermometer unit. Grasp top of probe stem, being careful not to press the ejection button.	• Charging provides battery power. Removal of handheld unit from base prepares it to measure temperature. Pressing ejection button releases plastic probe cover from tip.
(3) Slide disposable plastic probe cover over thermometer probe until cover locks in place (see Step 6A[3] illustration).	• Soft plastic cover will not break in client's mouth, and it prevents transmission of microorganisms between clients.

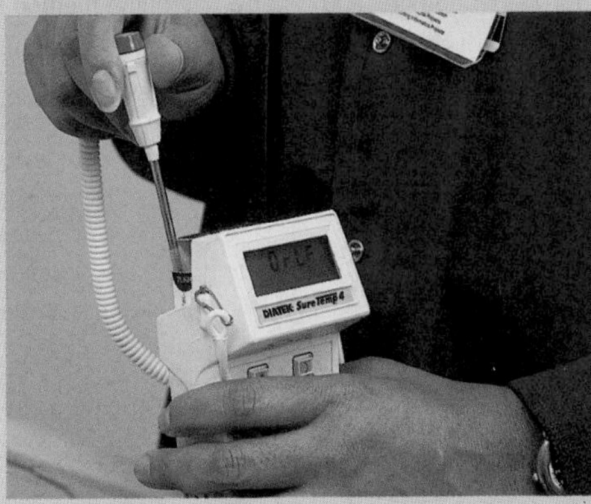

Step 6A(3) Inserting thermometer stem into plastic probe cover.

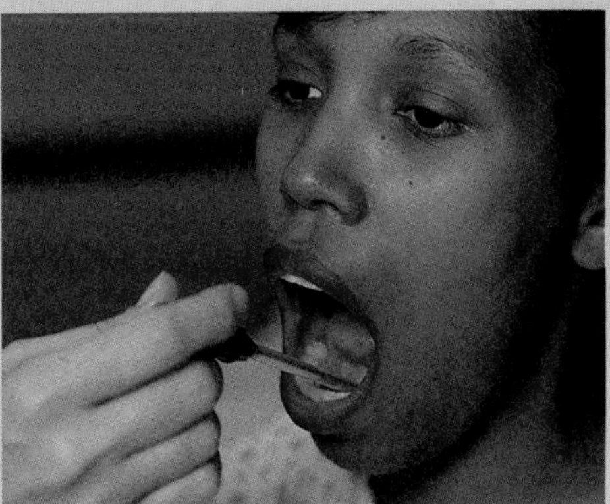

Step 6A(4) Probe under tongue in posterior sublingual pocket.

STEPS	RATIONALE
(4) Have client sit or lie in bed. Ask client to open mouth; gently place thermometer probe under client's tongue in posterior sublingual pocket lateral to centre of lower jaw (see Step 6A[4] illustration).	• Heat from superficial blood vessels in sublingual pocket produces temperature reading. Temperatures in right and left posterior sublingual pockets are significantly higher than in area under front of tongue.

Continued

➤ SKILL 31-1 Measuring Body Temperature *continued*

STEPS	RATIONALE
(5) Ask client to hold thermometer probe with lips closed.	• Holding the probe this way helps maintain proper position of thermometer during recording.
(6) Leave thermometer probe in place until audible signal occurs and client's temperature appears on digital display; remove thermometer probe from under client's tongue.	• Probe must stay in place until signal occurs, to ensure accurate reading.
(7) Push ejection button on thermometer stem to discard plastic probe cover into appropriate receptacle.	• Discarding probe cover reduces transmission of microorganisms between clients.
(8) Return thermometer stem to storage well of recording unit.	• Proper storage protects probe from damage. Returning probe automatically causes digital reading to disappear.
(9) If gloves were worn, remove and dispose in appropriate receptacle. Perform hand hygiene.	• Glove disposal and hand hygiene reduce transmission of microorganisms between clients.
(10) Return thermometer to charger.	• Charging provides battery power.
B. Rectal temperature measurement with electronic thermometer	
(1) Prepare client for procedure. (a) Draw curtain around client's bed or close room door, or do both. (b) Assist client to Sims' position with upper leg flexed. (c) Move aside bed linen to expose only anal area. Keep client's upper body and lower extremities covered with sheet or blanket. (d) Remind client to remain in Sims' position until procedure is complete.	• These actions maintain client's privacy, minimize embarrassment, and promote comfort. Anal area is exposed for correct thermometer placement.
(2) Put on disposable gloves.	• Gloves help you maintain standard precautions and routine practices during exposure to items soiled with body fluids (e.g., feces).
(3) Remove thermometer pack from charging unit. Attach rectal probe (red tip) to thermometer unit. Grasp top of probe stem, being careful not to press the ejection button.	• Charging provides battery power. Removal of handheld unit from base prepares it to measure temperature. Pressing the ejection button releases plastic probe cover from tip.
(4) Slide disposable plastic probe cover over thermometer probe until cover locks in place.	• Probe cover prevents transmission of microorganisms between clients.
(5) Squeeze liberal portion of lubricant on tissue. Dip thermometer's blunt end into lubricant, covering 2.5 to 3.5 cm for adult client.	• Lubrication minimizes trauma to rectal mucosa during thermometer insertion. Tissue avoids contamination of remaining lubricant in container.
(6) With nondominant hand, separate client's buttocks to expose anus. Ask client to breathe slowly and relax.	• Separating buttocks fully exposes anus for thermometer insertion. Relaxing anal sphincter facilitates thermometer insertion.
(7) Gently insert thermometer into client's anus in direction of umbilicus, 3.5 cm for adult client. Do not force thermometer.	• Insertion in this direction ensures adequate exposure against blood vessels in rectal wall.
(8) If resistance is felt during insertion, withdraw thermometer immediately. Never force thermometer.	• This action prevents trauma to mucosa.

Critical Decision Point: If thermometer cannot be adequately inserted into rectum, remove thermometer and consider alternative method for obtaining temperature.

STEPS	RATIONALE
(9) Once positioned, thermometer probe should be left in place (see Step 6B[9] illustration) until audible signal occurs and client's temperature appears on digital display; remove thermometer probe from anus.	• Probe must stay in place until signal occurs, to ensure accurate reading.

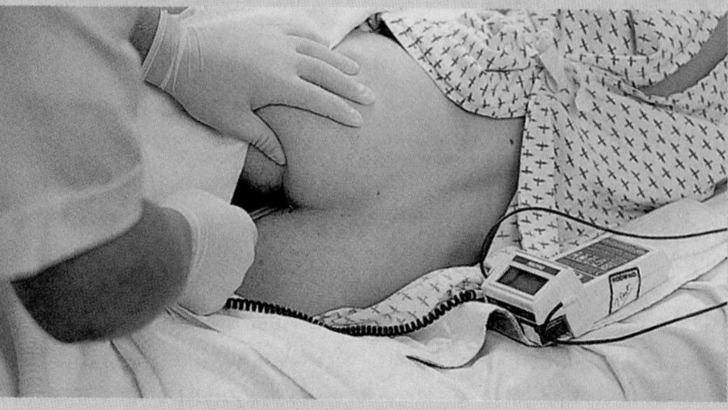

Step 6B(9) Probe positioned in anus.

➤ SKILL 31-1 Measuring Body Temperature *continued*

STEPS	RATIONALE
(10) Push ejection button on thermometer stem to discard plastic probe cover into appropriate receptacle. Wipe probe with alcohol swab, paying particular attention to ridges where probe cover connected to probe.	• Discarding probe cover reduces transmission of microorganisms between clients.
(11) Return thermometer stem to storage well of recording unit.	• Proper storage protects probe from damage. Returning probe automatically causes digital reading to disappear.
(12) Wipe client's anal area with soft tissue to remove lubricant or feces, and discard tissue. Assist client to assume a comfortable position and sufficiently covered with linens.	• These actions provide for comfort and hygiene.
(13) Remove and dispose of gloves in appropriate receptacle. Perform hand hygiene.	• Glove disposal and hand hygiene reduce transmission of microorganisms between the client and the nurse.
(14) Return thermometer unit to charger. Verify that charger and probes are wiped with alcohol daily (in isolation areas, they are wiped whenever they are removed from the room).	• Charging provides battery power. Wiping with alcohol reduces transmission of microorganisms between the client and the nurse.
C. **Axillary temperature measurement with electronic thermometer**	
(1) Prepare client for procedure.	
(a) Draw curtain around client's bed or close room door, or do both.	• These actions maintain client's privacy, minimize embarrassment, and promote comfort.
(b) Assist client to a supine or sitting position.	• These positions enable easy access to axilla.
(c) Move clothing or gown away from client's shoulder and arm.	• This action exposes axilla for correct thermometer probe placement.
(2) Remove thermometer pack from charging unit. Be sure oral probe (blue tip) is attached to thermometer unit. Grasp top of probe stem, being careful not to press the ejection button.	• Charging provides battery power. Removal of handheld unit from base prepares it to measure temperature. Pressing ejection button releases plastic cover from probe.
(3) Slide disposable plastic probe cover over thermometer probe until cover locks in place.	• Soft plastic cover prevents transmission of microorganisms between clients.
(4) Raise client's arm away from torso; inspect for skin lesions and excessive perspiration. Insert probe into centre of client's axilla, lower client's arm over probe, and place arm across client's chest (see Step 6C[4] illustration).	• Maintains proper position of probe against blood vessels in axilla.

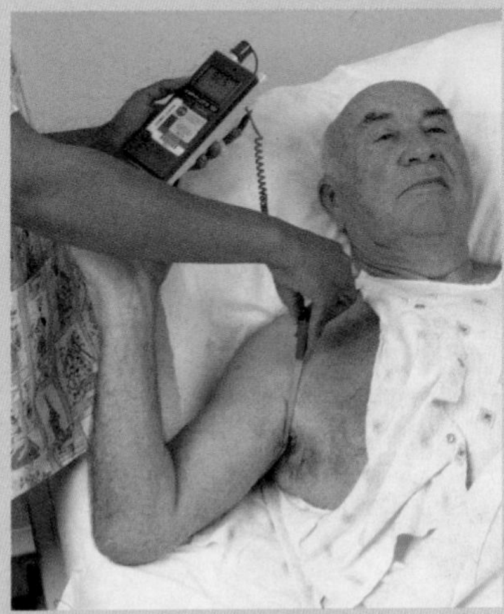

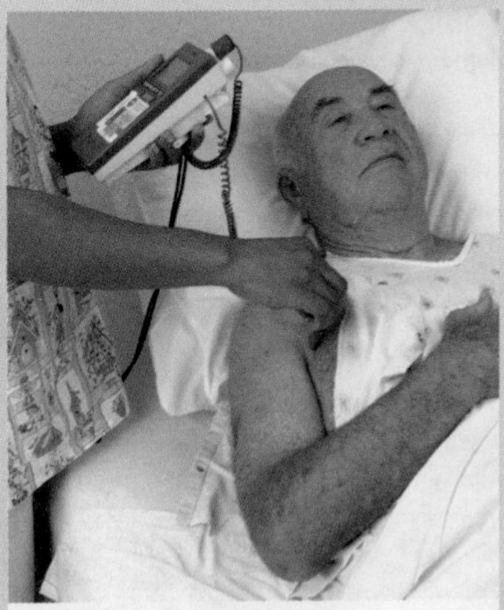

Step 6C(4) Thermometer tip in axilla.

Critical Decision Point: Do not use axilla if skin lesions are present because local temperature may be altered and area may be painful to touch. Wipe off excessive perspiration.

(5) Hold probe in place until audible signal occurs and temperature appears on digital display.	• Probe must stay in place until signal occurs, to ensure accurate reading.
(6) Remove probe from client's axilla.	
(7) Push ejection button on thermometer stem to discard plastic probe cover into appropriate receptacle.	• Discarding probe cover reduces transmission of microorganisms between the client and the nurse.

Continued

➤ SKILL 31-1 Measuring Body Temperature *continued*

STEPS	RATIONALE
(8) Return thermometer stem to storage well of recording unit.	• Proper storage protects probe from damage. Returning probe automatically causes digital reading to disappear.
(9) Assist client to assume a comfortable position, and move linen or gown back over client's shoulder.	• Restores comfort and promotes privacy.
(10) Perform hand hygiene.	• Hand hygiene reduces transmission of microorganisms between the client and the nurse.
(11) Return thermometer to charger.	• Charging provides battery power.
D. Tympanic membrane temperature measurement with electronic thermometer	
(1) Assist client in assuming comfortable position with head turned toward to side, away from nurse. Right-handed caregivers should obtain temperature from client's right ear. Left-handed caregivers should obtain temperature from client's left ear.	• This positioning ensures comfort and exposes auditory canal for accurate temperature measurement. The less acute the angle of approach is, the better the probe seal is.
(2) Check for the presence of obvious cerumen in the client's ear canal.	• To ensure clear optical pathway, lens cover of speculum must not be impeded by cerumen. Switch to other ear or select alternative measurement site if necessary.
(3) Remove thermometer handheld unit from charging base, being careful not to press the ejection button.	• Charging provides battery power. Removal of handheld unit from base prepares it to measure temperature. Pressing ejection button releases plastic probe cover from tip.
(4) Slide clean disposable speculum cover over otoscope-like lens tip until it locks into place; be careful not to touch lens cover.	• Lens cover must be clear of dust, fingerprints, and cerumen to ensure clear optical pathway.
(5) Insert speculum into client's ear canal in accordance with manufacturer's instructions for tympanic probe positioning:	• Correct positioning of the probe with regard to ear canal ensures accurate readings. Operator errors cause false readings.
(a) For adults, pull client's pinna backward, up, and out. For children younger than 2 years, point covered speculum tip toward midpoint between eyebrow and sideburn.	• Ear tug straightens the external auditory canal, allowing maximum exposure of the tympanic membrane (Hockenberry & Wilson, 2007).
(b) Move thermometer in a figure-eight pattern.	• Some manufacturers recommend movement of the speculum tip in a figure-eight pattern, which allows the sensor to detect maximum tympanic membrane heat radiation.
(c) Fit otoscope probe snugly into canal and do not move (see Step 6D[5][c] illustration).	• Gentle pressure seals ear canal from ambient temperature, which can alter readings as much as 2.8°C.
(d) Point speculum tip toward client's nose.	

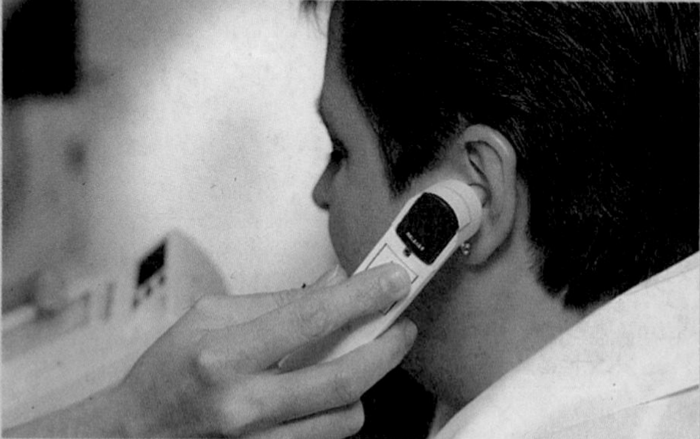

Step 6D(5)(c) Tympanic thermometer with probe cover inserted into auditory canal.

STEPS	RATIONALE
(6) When probe is in place, press scan button on handheld unit. Leave thermometer probe in place until audible signal occurs and client's temperature appears on digital display.	• When scan button is pressed, probe detects infrared energy. Otoscope tip must stay in place until signal occurs, to ensure accurate reading.
(7) Carefully remove speculum from auditory meatus.	• Careful removal prevents rubbing of sensitive outer ear lining.
(8) Push ejection button on handheld unit to discard plastic probe cover into appropriate receptacle.	• Discarding probe cover reduces transmission of microorganisms between the client and the nurse and automatically causes digital reading to disappear.

➤ SKILL 31-1 Measuring Body Temperature *continued*

STEPS	RATIONALE
(9) If a second reading is necessary, replace probe lens cover and wait 2 to 3 minutes before inserting probe tip.	• Lens cover must be free of cerumen to maintain optical path. Time allows ear canal to regain usual temperature.
(10) Return handheld unit to charging base.	• Proper storage protects probe from damage.
(11) Assist client to assume a comfortable position.	• This action restores comfort and sense of well-being.
(12) Perform hand hygiene.	• Hand hygiene reduces transmission of microorganisms between the client and the nurse.
7. Discuss findings with client as needed.	• Such discussion promotes client's participation in care and understanding of health status.
8. If client's temperature is being assessed for the first time and is within normal range, document temperature as baseline.	• Baseline is used to compare future temperature measurements.
9. Compare current temperature reading with client's previous baseline and with acceptable temperature range for client's age group.	• Normal body temperature fluctuates within narrow range; comparison helps reveal presence of abnormality. Improper placement or movement of thermometer causes inaccuracies. Second measurement confirms initial findings of abnormal body temperature.

Unexpected Outcomes and Related Interventions

Temperature 1°C Above Usual Range

- Assess possible sites (e.g., central line catheter, wounds) for localized infection and for related data suggestive of a systemic infection.
- Implement appropriate nursing measures (see Box 31–10).

Persistent Fever

- Notify prescribing health care professional, and administer antipyretic and antibiotics as ordered.

Temperature 1°C Below Usual Range

- Remove any drafts, wet clothing, or damp linens.
- Apply extra blankets, and, unless contraindicated, offer warm liquids.

Recording and Reporting

- Record temperature on vital sign flow sheet. Document temperature after administration of specific therapies in nurses' narrative notes.
- Report abnormal findings to nurse in charge or to prescribing health care professional.

Home Care Considerations

- Assess temperature and ventilation of client's environment to determine existence of any environmental condition that may influence outcome of client's temperature.
- In the home, clients may continue to use mercury-in-glass thermometers (see Box 31–6). Assess whether the storage of these thermometers is adequate to protect them from breakage and to prevent mercury spills. Educate client and caregiver about mercury hazards.

Each device measures temperature according to the **Celsius** or **Fahrenheit** scale. Electronic thermometers allow conversion to alternative scales by activating a switch. When it is necessary to convert temperature readings, the following formulas can be used:

- To convert a Fahrenheit reading to Celsius, subtract 32 from the Fahrenheit reading and multiply the result by 5/9 (e.g., 40°C = [104°F – 32] × 5/9)
- To convert a Celsius reading to Fahrenheit, multiply the Celsius reading by 9/5 and add 32 to the product (e.g., 104°F = [40°C × 9/5] + 32)

Electronic Thermometer. The electronic thermometer consists of a rechargeable battery-powered display unit, a thin wire cord, and a temperature-processing probe covered by a disposable plastic cover (Figure 31–4). Separate unbreakable probes are available for oral and rectal use. The oral probe can also be used for axillary temperature measurement. Electronic thermometers provide two modes of operation: a 4-second predictive temperature and a 3-minute standard temperature. When the first mode is used, a reading appears on the display unit within 20 to 50 seconds of insertion. A signal is sounded when the peak temperature reading has been measured.

Another form of electronic thermometer is used exclusively for tympanic temperature. An otoscope-like speculum with an infrared sensor tip detects heat radiated from the tympanic membrane. Within 2 to 5 seconds after the speculum is placed in the auditory canal, a reading appears on the display unit. A signal is sounded when the peak temperature reading has been measured.

Another type of electronic thermometer measures the temperature of the superficial temporal artery. A handheld scanner with an infrared sensor tip detects the temperature of cutaneous blood flow: The sensor is swept across the forehead and just behind the ear (Figure 31–5). Once scanning is complete, a reading appears on the display. Temporal artery temperature is a reliable noninvasive measure of core temperature (Box 31–5).

The greatest advantages of electronic thermometers are that they can be inserted immediately and read easily within seconds. The plastic sheath is unbreakable, and so these devices are ideal for use in children. Their expense is a major disadvantage. Maintaining cleanliness of the probes is an important consideration. If a rectal probe is not properly cleaned between clients, contamination of the rectal probe by gastrointestinal disease organisms can be a vector of disease transmission. The thermometer must be wiped daily with alcohol, and the thermometer probe must be wiped with an alcohol swab after each use. Particular attention must be paid to the probe hub, which has ridges, where the probe cover is secured to the probe.

Chemical Dot Thermometers. Single-use or reusable chemical dot thermometers are thin strips of plastic with a temperature sensor at one end. The sensor consists of chemically impregnated dots that change colour at different temperatures in increments of 0.1°C between 35.5°C and 40.4°C (Figure 31–6). Most of these devices are intended for single use, but the dots on reusable ones return to their original colour in seconds. The devices are used for measuring oral or axillary temperatures, particularly in children, and may be used rectally

BOX 31-4 Advantages and Disadvantages of Select Temperature Measurement Sites

Tympanic Membrane

Advantages

This site is easily accessible; minimal client repositioning is required.

The temperature reading can be obtained without disturbing or waking client.

The device provides core reading, inasmuch as the eardrum is close to the hypothalamus.

Measurement is very rapid (2 to 5 seconds).

Measurement is unaffected by oral intake of food of fluids or by smoking.

This device can be used for tachypneic clients without affecting breathing.

This device can be used in newborns to reduce handling of infants and heat loss.

Disadvantages

Measurement is more variable with this device than with other core temperature devices.

Hearing aids must be removed before measurement.

This site cannot be used in clients who have had surgery of the ear or tympanic membrane.

Readings are altered by cerumen impaction and otitis media.

Disposable probe cover comes in only one size.

The device does not accurately measure core temperature changes during and after exercise.

Positioning the device correctly in newborns, infants, and children younger than 3 years is challenging because of the anatomy of the ear canal (Holtzclaw, 2003).

Inaccuracies result from incorrect positioning of unit (Maxton et al., 2004).

Obtaining continuous measurement is not possible.

Temperature readings are affected by ambient temperature devices such as incubators, radiant warmers, and fans.

Rectum

Advantages

This site is argued to be more reliable when oral temperature cannot be obtained.

Disadvantages

Measurement at this site lags behind those at sites of core temperature during rapid temperature changes (Maxton et al., 2004).

This site should not be used in clients with diarrhea, rectal surgery, a rectal disorder, or bleeding tendencies.

This site should not be used for routine measurement of vital signs in newborns.

Measurement at this site requires special positioning, which may be a source of client embarrassment and anxiety.

Impacted stool alters readings (Maxton et al., 2004).

Measurement at this site carries risk of exposure to body fluids.

Lubrication is required.

Mouth

Advantages

This site is accessible, and no position change is required.

Measurement at this site is comfortable for clients.

Measurement at this site provides accurate reading of surface temperature.

Measurement at this site reflects rapid change in core temperature.

Disadvantages

Temperature readings are affected by ingestion of fluids or foods, by smoking, and by oxygen delivery.

Measurement at this site is not suitable for clients who have had oral surgery, have suffered trauma, have a history of epilepsy, or have shaking chills.

Temperature should not be measured at this site in infants, in small children, or in confused, unconscious, or uncooperative clients.

Measurement at this site carries risk of exposure to body fluids.

Axilla

Advantages

Measurement at this site is safe and noninvasive.

Temperature can be measured at this site in newborns and in uncooperative or unconscious clients.

Disadvantages

The measurement time is long.

Measurement at this site necessitates continuous positioning by nurse.

Measurement at this site lags behind those at sites of core temperature during rapid temperature changes.

This measure requires exposure of thorax, which can result in temperature loss, especially in newborns.

Readings are affected by exposure to environment during device placement (Maxton et al., 2004).

Measurement at this site is not recommended for detecting fever in infants and young children.

Skin

Advantages

Continuous reading can be obtained at this site.

Measurement at this site is safe and noninvasive.

Measurement at this site does not require disturbing client.

Temperature can be measured at this site in newborns.

Disadvantages

Measurement at this site lags behind those at other sites during temperature changes, especially during hyperthermia.

Adhesion of the thermometer can be impaired by diaphoresis or sweat.

Measurement at this site can be affected by environmental temperature.

Measurement cannot be measured at this site in clients who have allergy to adhesive.

Temporal Artery

Advantages

Measurement is rapid.

Measurement at this site reflects rapid change in core temperature.

This site is easy to access without changing the client's position.

Measurement at this site is comfortable and eliminates need to remove clothing.

Measurement at this site is useful in premature infants, newborns, and children.

Disadvantages

Measurement at this site is not effective through head covering or hair.

Results are affected by diaphoresis or sweating.

Continuous measurement is not possible.

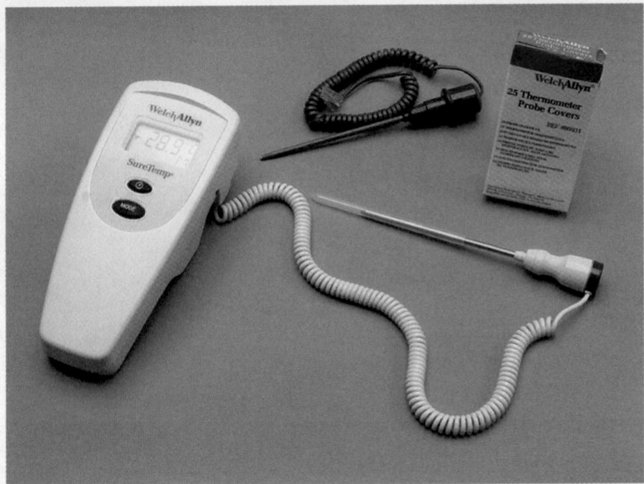

Figure 31-4 Electronic thermometer. The blue probe is for oral or axillary use. The red probe is for rectal use.

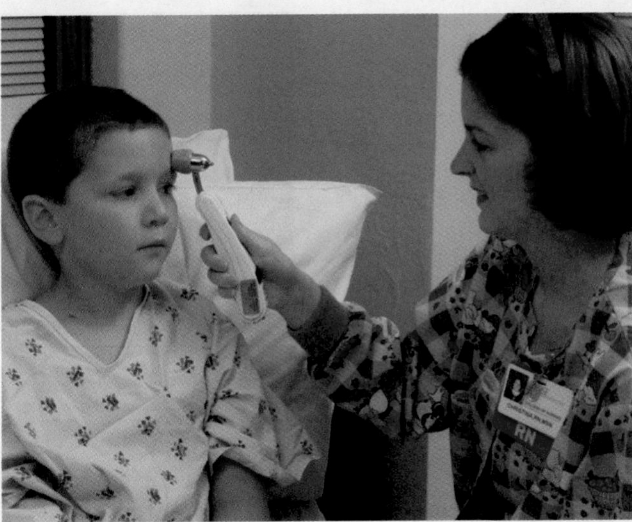

Figure 31-5 Temporal artery thermometer scanning the child's forehead.

in a special sheath. The thermometer is removed after 60 seconds and read after another wait of 10 seconds to ensure that the temperature reading has stabilized. Research has shown that disposable single-use thermometers tend to overestimate or underestimate true temperature readings. The device is recommended only for screening purposes. When an abnormal temperature is suspected, the temperature should be confirmed with an electronic thermometer. The chemical dot thermometers are useful in caring for clients with isolation precautions (see Chapter 33), to avoid the need to take electronic instruments into these clients' rooms. Research has shown them to be effective with intubated clients.

Another type of disposable thermometer is a temperature-sensitive patch or tape. Applied to the forehead or abdomen, the patch changes colour at different temperatures. These thermometers are also useful for screening clients, especially infants, for altered temperature. If an abnormal temperature is suspected, the temperature must be confirmed with an electronic temperature device. Disposable thermometers are not appropriate for monitoring temperature therapies.

Glass Thermometers. The mercury-in-glass thermometer is a glass tube sealed at one end and with a mercury-filled bulb at the other. Exposure of the bulb to heat causes the mercury to expand and rise in the enclosed tube. The length of the thermometer is marked with Centigrade (Celcius) calibrations. Obtaining a temperature with a mercury-in-glass thermometer requires careful preparation of the device (Box 31–6). In addition to proper positioning of the thermometer at the oral, rectal, or axillary site, this position must be maintained for the appropriate length of time to obtain an accurate reading. In addition to the time delay, the mercury-in-glass device is easily breakable and, when broken, releases hazardous mercury. Although health care agencies no longer use glass thermometers, clients may have mercury-in-glass thermometers in their homes. If such a thermometer is broken or a mercury spill is suspected, take immediate action (Box 31–7). It is important to teach clients and their families what to do in the event of breakage of a mercury-in-glass thermometer.

➤ BOX 31-5 Procedural Guidelines

Measurement of Temporal Artery Temperature

Delegation Considerations: The measurement of temporal artery temperature can be delegated to unregulated care providers. The nurse is responsible for assessing changes in pulse; therefore, when measurement of temporal artery temperature is delegated, it is important to *inform the unregulated care provider* about the following:

- Frequency of temperature measurement
- Factors that falsely raise or lower temperature readings
- Reporting abnormalities to the nurse for further assessment

Equipment: Temporal artery thermometer, alcohol wipes or probe cover (optional).

Procedure

1. Perform hand hygiene.
2. Ensure that the client's forehead is dry; wipe it with towel if it is moist.
3. Place the probe flush on the client's forehead to avoid measuring ambient temperature.
4. Press the red scan button with your thumb. Scanning for the highest temperature will be continuous until you release the scan button.
5. Slowly slide the thermometer straight across the client's forehead while keeping the probe flush on the client's skin.
6. Keeping scan button pressed, lift the probe from the client's forehead, and touch the probe to the client's neck just behind the earlobe (the area where perfume is typically applied).
7. While the probe is scanning, a clicking sound occurs; this sound stops when peak temperature is scanned.
8. Release the scan button; read and record the temperature. Reading remains on for 15 seconds after you release the button.
9. Clean the probe with an alcohol wipe, or, if a probe cover was used, remove and dispose of the probe cover.

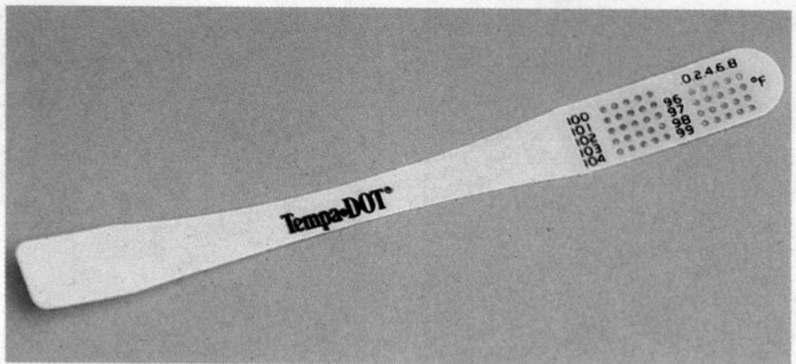

Figure 31-6 Disposable, single-use thermometer strip.

> **BOX 31-6 Procedural Guidelines**

Use of a Mercury-in-Glass Thermometer

Delegation Considerations: Client, family, or unregulated care provider will safely perform temperature measurement.

Equipment: Mercury-in-glass thermometer (rectal or oral), plastic sleeve, lubricating jelly (rectal only), disposable gloves.

Procedure

1. Perform hand hygiene. Apply disposable gloves to avoid contact with body fluids (e.g., saliva, stool).
2. Hold the nonbulb end of the glass thermometer (if colour-coded, tip will be blue or red) with your fingertips to reduce contamination of the bulb.
3. Read the mercury level while gently rotating the thermometer at eye level. If the mercury is above the desired level, grasp the tip of the thermometer securely, stand away from solid objects, and sharply flick your wrist downward. Brisk shaking lowers the mercury level in the glass tube. Continue shaking the thermometer until the mercury reading is below 35.6°C. The thermometer reading must be lower than the client's actual temperature before the thermometer is used.
4. Insert the thermometer into a plastic sleeve cover to protect it from body secretions (e.g., saliva, stool). Apply lubricant to cover 2.5 cm to 3.5 cm of a rectal thermometer.
5. Place the thermometer according to the technique appropriate for the oral, rectal, or axillary site (see Skill 31–1).
6. Leave the thermometer in place 3 minutes for oral or rectal temperature, 5 minutes for axillary temperature, or according to agency policy.
7. Remove the thermometer. Carefully discard the plastic sleeve. Wipe off secretions with a clean tissue, moving toward the bulb.
8. Read the thermometer at eye level. Record the findings. Store the thermometer in its storage container. Remove your gloves, and perform hand hygiene.

> **BOX 31-7 Steps to Take in the Event of a Mercury Spill**

1. *Do not touch* spilled mercury droplets. If skin contact has occurred, immediately flush area with water for 15 minutes.
2. If possible, remove client from immediate contaminated environment, and shut door to contaminated area.
3. *Using rubber gloves,* remove any clothing, linen, or shoes contaminated with mercury, and place these items in a plastic trash bag.
4. *Using rubber gloves,* contain visible mercury beads with moistened rags or paper towel. Turn off heating or air conditioning systems that could circulate air from spill site to other areas. Turn down thermostat.
5. Follow procedures for mércury removal outlined by local health authority. Notify environmental services department or occupational health services to obtain a mercury spill kit or instructions.
6. Spills are removed using *special* absorbent materials, filtered vacuum equipment, and protective clothing. Everything is sealed in plastic to be discarded or cleaned according to Health Canada (2007) guidelines.
7. Keep area well ventilated for 24 hours.
8. Complete incident report as directed by institution procedure.

Adapted from Environment Canada. (2004). *Cleaning up small mercury spills: Mercury and the environment*. Retrieved December 4, 2008, from http://www.ec.gc.ca/mercury/en/cu.cfm

❖Nursing Diagnosis

Identify assessment findings and cluster defining characteristics to form a nursing diagnosis. Nursing diagnoses for clients with body temperature alterations include the following:

- *Risk for imbalanced body temperature*
- *Hyperthermia*
- *Hypothermia*
- *Ineffective thermoregulation*

For example, an increase in body temperature, flushed skin, skin warm to touch, and tachycardia are indicative of the diagnosis *hyperthermia*. The nursing diagnosis is stated as either an at-risk or an actual temperature alteration. If the client has risk factors for temperature alterations, minimize or eliminate them.

Once the diagnosis is established, accurately determine the related factor or cause (Box 31–8). The related factor directs the selection of appropriate nursing interventions. In the example of hyperthermia, a related factor of vigorous activity will result in interventions much different from those for a related factor of decreased ability to perspire.

BOX 31-8 NURSING DIAGNOSTIC PROCESS

Assessment Activities	Defining Characteristics	Nursing Diagnosis
Measure vital signs, including temperature, pulse, respirations, and pulse oximetry (SpO_2).	Increased body temperature above usual range Tachycardia Tachypnea Hypoxemia	*Ineffective thermoregulation related to aging and inability to adapt to environmental temperature*
Palpate skin.	Warm, dry skin	
Observe client's appearance and behaviour while talking and resting.	Restlessness Confusion Flushed appearance	
Review medical history.	Location (e.g., found in unventilated apartment during heat wave) and other client characteristics (e.g., 85 years old with history of dementia)	

❖Planning

During planning, integrate knowledge gathered from assessment and client history to develop an individualized care plan (Box 31–9). Match client's needs with interventions that are supported and recommended in the clinical research literature.

Goals and Outcomes

The care plan for a client with alteration in temperature must include realistic and individualized goals along with relevant outcomes. Collaborate closely with the client in setting goals and outcomes and choosing nursing interventions. Expected outcomes are established to gauge progress toward returning the body temperature to an acceptable range. Goals may be short term, such as regaining normal range of body temperature in 24 hours, or long term, such as helping the client modify the environment, (e.g., obtaining appropriate clothing to wear in cold weather). Outcomes must be related to what is learned about the client.

Setting Priorities

The severity of temperature alteration and its effects, together with the client's general health status, influence care priorities. Safety is a top priority. In many cases, other medical problems complicate the care plan. For instance, alterations in body temperature affect the body's requirements for fluids. Clients with cardiac disease may have difficulty tolerating required fluid replacement therapy.

Continuity of Care

Clients at high risk for alterations in body temperature require an individualized care plan directed at maintaining normothermia (normal body temperature) and reducing risk factors. For example, the outcome of care may be that the client can explain actions to take during a heat wave. Teach the client and caregiver the importance of thermoregulation and actions to take during very hot weather. Education is particularly important for parents who need to know how to take action at home when an infant or child develops temperature alteration.

❖Implementation

Health Promotion

Health promotion for clients at risk for altered body temperature is directed toward promoting balance between heat production and heat loss. Client activity, temperature of the environment, and clothing are all considered. Teach clients to avoid strenuous exercise in hot, humid weather; to drink fluids such as water or clear fruit juices before, during, and after exercise; to wear light, loose-fitting, light-coloured clothes; to avoid exercising in areas with poor ventilation; to wear a protective covering over the head when outdoors; and, when entering hot climates, to expose themselves to the heat gradually.

Prevention is key for clients at risk for hypothermia. Prevention involves educating clients, family members, and friends. Clients most at risk include very young persons, very old persons, and people debilitated by trauma, stroke, diabetes, drug or alcohol intoxication, sepsis, and Raynaud's disease. Mentally ill and disabled clients may acquire hypothermia because they are unaware of the dangers of cold conditions. People without adequate home heating, shelter, diet, or clothing are also at risk. Fatigue, skin colour (Black clients are more susceptible), malnutrition, hypoxemia, and body piercing also contribute to the risk of frostbite.

Acute Care

Fever. When body temperature is elevated, initiate interventions to treat fever. The objective of therapy is to increase heat loss, reduce heat production, and prevent complications.

The procedures used to intervene and treat the temperature depend on the cause, any adverse effects, and the strength, intensity, and duration of the elevation. You play a key role in assessing and implementing temperature-reducing strategies (Box 31–10). The prescribing health care professional may try to determine the cause of the elevated temperature by isolating the causative pyrogen. You may need to obtain necessary culture specimens for laboratory analysis, such as urine, blood, sputum, and tissue from wound sites (see Chapter 33). After the cultures have been obtained, the prescribing health care professional orders administration of antibiotic medications to destroy pyrogenic bacteria and eliminate the cause of the elevated temperature.

Most fevers in children are caused by viruses, last only briefly, and have limited effects. Children still have immature temperature-control mechanisms, and so temperatures can rise rapidly. Dehydration and febrile seizures can occur while temperatures are rising in children between 6 months and 3 years of age. Febrile seizures are unusual in children older than 5 years. The actual temperature, often exceeding 38.8°C, seems to be more important than the rapidity of the temperature increase. Children are at particular risk for fluid volume deficit because they can quickly lose large

BOX 31-9 NURSING CARE PLAN

Hyperthermia

Assessment

Mr. Coburn is a 45-year-old teacher who arrives at the outpatient clinic complaining of malaise. His medical history includes a past urinary tract infection. Several of his students have had colds lately. He has been feeling unwell for the past 3 days.

Assessment Activities	***Findings and Defining Characteristics***
Palpate skin.	Skin *warm and dry* to touch
Observe client's behaviour when talking and resting.	Breathing appears laboured; face is *flushed*
Measure vital signs.	Blood pressure: right arm, 116/62 mm Hg; left arm, 114/64 mm Hg Right radial pulse, *128 per minute,* regular and bounding Respiratory rate regular at *26 breaths per minute* SpO_2, 98% on room air Oral temperature, *39.2°C*
Review medical history.	Smokes one pack of cigarettes per day and recently began expectorating *yellow-green sputum* *Tired* for past 3 days and dizzy upon rising in the morning

Nursing Diagnosis: Hyperthermia related to infectious process

Planning

Goal (Nursing Outcomes Classification)*	***Expected Outcomes***
	Thermoregulation
Client will regain normal range of body temperature within next 24 hours.	Body temperature will decline at least 1°C within next 8 hours.
Client will attain sense of comfort and rest within next 48 hours.	Client will verbalize increased satisfaction with rest and sleep pattern. Client will report increase in energy level within next 3 days.

*Outcome classification label from Moorhead, S., Johnson, M., & Maas, M. L. (2004). *Nursing Outcomes Classification (NOC)* (3rd ed.). St. Louis, MO: Mosby.

Interventions (Nursing Interventions Classification)†	**Rationale**
Fever Treatment	
Instruct client to reduce external coverings and keep clothing and bed linen dry.	Heat loss is promoted through conduction and convection.
Instruct client to monitor temperature at home and take acetaminophen every 4 hours as ordered for temperature higher than 38°C.	Antipyretics reduce set point.
Instruct client to limit physical activity and increase frequency of rest periods over next 2 days.	Activity and stress increase metabolic rate, contributing to heat production.

†Intervention classification label from Dochterman, J. M., & Bulechek, G. M. (Eds.). (2004). *Nursing Interventions Classification (NIC)* (4th ed.). St. Louis, MO: Mosby.

Evaluation

Nursing Actions	***Client Response and Finding***	***Achievement of Outcome***
Obtain body temperature measurement.	Body temperature, 37.8°C	Body temperature is within normal limits.
Ask Mr. Coburn whether his energy level has changed since the last visit.	He responds, "I am sleeping much better and have returned to work with a lot more energy."	Rest and sleep pattern have improved, and energy level has increased.

amounts of fluids in proportion to their body weight. Maintain accurate intake and output records, and encourage fluid consumption.

A fever may be a hypersensitivity response to a drug. Drug fevers can be accompanied by other symptoms of allergy, such as rash or pruritus (itching). Treatment involves withdrawing the particular medication.

Antipyretics are drugs that reduce fever. Nonsteroidal drugs such as acetaminophen, salicylates, indomethacin, and ketorolac reduce fever by increasing heat loss. Corticosteroids reduce heat production by interfering with the immune system and can mask signs of infection. Corticosteroids are not used to treat a fever. However, be aware of their effect on suppressing the client's ability to develop a fever in response to a pyrogen.

Nonpharmacological therapy for fever involves methods that increase heat loss by evaporation, conduction, convection, or radiation. Blankets cooled by circulating water delivered by motorized units increase conductive heat loss. Manufacturer's instructions for applying these hypothermia blankets must be followed because of risk for skin breakdown and "freeze burns." Placing a bath blanket between the client and the hypothermia blanket and wrapping distal extremities (fingers, toes, and genitalia) are recommended to reduce the risk of injury to the skin and tissue from hypothermia therapy. Traditional methods such as tepid sponge baths, bathing with alcohol water solutions, applying ice packs to axillae and groin areas, and cooling fans should be used cautiously because they lead to shivering.

> **BOX 31-10 Nursing Measures for Clients with a Fever**
>
> **Assessment**
>
> - Obtain core temperature during each phase of a febrile episode.
> - Assess for contributing factors such as dehydration, infection, and environmental temperature.
> - Identify physiological response to temperature.
> - Measure all vital signs.
> - Observe skin colour.
> - Assess skin temperature.
> - Observe for shivering and diaphoresis.
> - Assess the client's comfort and well-being.
> - Determine phase of fever: chill, plateau, or fever break.
>
> **Interventions (Unless Contraindicated)**
>
> - Obtain blood cultures when ordered: Blood specimens are obtained to coincide with temperature spikes when the antigen-producing organism is most pervasive.
> - Minimize heat production: Reduce frequency of activities that increase oxygen demand, such as excessive turning in bed; allow rest periods; limit physical activity.
> - Maximize heat loss: Reduce external covering on client's body to promote heat loss through radiation and conduction without inducing shivering; keep clothing and bed linen dry to increase heat loss through conduction and convection.
> - Meet requirements for increased metabolic rate: Provide oxygen as ordered to improve oxygen delivery to body cells; provide measures to stimulate appetite; offer well-balanced meals; provide fluids (3 L per day for client with normal cardiac and renal function) to replace fluids lost through insensible water loss and sweating.
> - Promote client comfort: Encourage the client to practise oral hygiene for dry oral mucous membranes; control environmental temperature without inducing shivering (between 21°C and 27°C).
> - Identify febrile episode phases: Examine previous temperature measurements to identify trends.
> - Initiate health teaching as indicated.

These methods have no demonstrated advantage over antipyretic medications. Nursing measures to enhance body cooling must avoid stimulating shivering. Shivering is counterproductive and increases energy expenditure up to 400%. Wrapping the client's extremities has been recommended to reduce the incidence and intensity of shivering.

Heatstroke. Heatstroke is an emergency. First aid treatment for heatstroke includes moving client to a cooler environment, reducing clothing covering body, placing cool, wet towels over skin, and using oscillating fans to increase convective heat loss. Emergency medical treatment may include intravenous fluids, irrigation of the stomach and lower bowel with cool solutions, and hypothermia blankets.

Hypothermia. The priority of treatment for hypothermia is to prevent a further decrease in body temperature. Removing wet clothes, replacing them with dry clothes, and wrapping the client in blankets are key nursing interventions. Away from a health care setting, the client should be laid under blankets next to a warm person. A conscious client should drink hot liquids (e.g., soup) and avoid alcohol and caffeine. Keep the client's head covered, place the client near a fire or in a warm room, or place heating pads next to areas of the client's body (head and neck) that lose heat most rapidly.

Restorative and Continuing Care

Educate the client who has been febrile about the importance of taking and continuing antibiotics as directed until the course of treatment is completed. Children and older adults are at risk for fluid volume deficit because they can quickly lose large amounts of fluids in proportion to their body weight. Encourage intake of preferred fluids.

❖Evaluation

All nursing interventions are evaluated by comparing the client's actual response with the expected outcomes of the care plan. This evaluation reveals whether goals of care have been met or whether the plan must be revised. After any intervention, measure the client's temperature to evaluate for change. Use other evaluative measures such as palpation of the skin and assessment of pulse and respirations. If therapies are effective, body temperature will return to an acceptable range, other vital sign measurements will stabilize, and the client will report a sense of comfort.

Pulse

The pulse is the bounding of blood flow that is palpable at various points on the body. Blood flows through the body in a continuous circuit. The pulse is an indicator of circulatory status.

Physiology and Regulation

Electrical impulses originating from the sinoatrial node travel through heart muscle to stimulate cardiac contraction. Approximately 60 to 70 mL of blood enters the aorta with each ventricular contraction (**stroke volume**). With each stroke volume ejection (blood pushed out of the heart), the walls of the aorta distend, creating a pulse wave that travels rapidly toward the distal ends of the arteries. When a pulse wave reaches a peripheral artery, it can be felt by palpating the artery lightly against underlying bone or muscle. The number of pulsing sensations occurring in 1 minute is the *pulse rate*.

The volume of blood pumped by the heart during 1 minute is the **cardiac output**: the product of heart rate and ventricular stroke volume. In an adult, the heart pumps about 5000 mL of blood per minute (e.g., if heart rate is 70 beats per minute and stroke volume is 70 mL, the cardiac output is 4900 mL per minute). A change in heart rate or stroke volume does not always change the heart's output or the amount of blood in the arteries. Mechanical, neural, and chemical factors regulate the strength of heart contractions and its stroke volume. When these factors are unable to alter stroke volume, a change in heart rate results in a change in blood pressure (BP). As heart rate increases, the heart has less time to fill. Without a change in stroke volume, blood pressure decreases. As the heart rate slows, filling time is increased, and blood pressure increases. The inability of blood pressure to respond to increases or decreases in heart rate may indicate a health deviation and must be reported to the prescribing health care professional. An abnormally slow, rapid, or irregular pulse alters cardiac output. Assess the ability of the client's heart to meet the demands of the body's tissue for nutrients by palpating a peripheral pulse or by using a stethoscope to listen to heart sounds (apical rate).

Assessment of Pulse

Any artery can be assessed for pulse rate, but the radial artery is commonly used because it is easily palpated. When a client's condition suddenly worsens, the carotid artery is the recommended site for quickly finding a pulse. The heart will continue delivering blood through the carotid artery to the brain as long as possible. When cardiac output declines significantly, peripheral pulses weaken and are difficult to palpate. Nurses most commonly assess the radial and apical pulses, but people who are learning to monitor their own heart rates use the radial or carotid pulse (e.g., athletes, clients taking medications for cardiac disease, and clients starting a prescribed exercise regimen). If the radial pulse at the wrist is abnormal or intermittent, or if it is inaccessible because of a dressing or cast, assess the apical pulse. When a client takes medication that affects the heart rate, the apical pulse provides a more accurate assessment of cardiac function. In infants or young children, it is best to assess the brachial or apical pulse because other peripheral pulses are deep and difficult to palpate accurately.

Assessment of other peripheral pulse sites, such as the popliteal or femoral artery, is unnecessary in routine measurement of vital signs. Other peripheral pulses are assessed during a complete physical examination, when surgery or treatment has impaired blood flow to a body part, or when a client has clinical indications of impaired peripheral blood flow (see Chapter 32). Table 31–2 summarizes pulse sites and criteria for measurement. Skill 31–2 outlines pulse rate assessment. Table 31–3 lists acceptable pulse rate ranges.

Use of a Stethoscope. Use a stethoscope to assess the apical rate (Figure 31–7). The five major parts of the stethoscope are the earpieces, binaurals, tubing, bell chestpiece, and diaphragm chestpiece.

The plastic or rubber earpieces fit snugly and comfortably in your ears. The binaurals are angled and strong enough so that the earpieces stay firmly in the ears without causing discomfort. To ensure the best reception of sound, the earpieces follow the contour of the ear canal, pointing toward the face when the stethoscope is in place. Stethoscopes can have single or dual tubes. The tubing has thick walls and is flexible and yet moderately rigid to eliminate transmission of environmental noise and to prevent the tubing from kinking, which distorts sound wave transmission. Tubing that is longer than 30 to 40 cm decreases the transmission of sound waves.

The chestpiece consists of a bell and a diaphragm that are rotated into position. The diaphragm or bell must be in proper position to hear sounds through the stethoscope. Test the position of the chestpiece by tapping lightly on the diaphragm to determine which side is functioning. The diaphragm is the circular, flat portion of the chestpiece and is covered by a thin plastic disk. It transmits high-pitched sounds created by the high-velocity movement of air and blood. You auscultate bowel, lung, and heart sounds by using the diaphragm. Position the diaphragm to make a tight seal against the client's skin (Figure 31–8). Exert enough pressure to leave a temporary red ring on the client's skin when the diaphragm is removed.

The bell is the bowl-shaped chestpiece usually surrounded by a rubber ring. The ring avoids chilling the client with cold metal when the chestpiece is placed on the skin. The bell transmits low-pitched sounds created by the low-velocity movement of blood. Heart and vascular sounds are auscultated through the bell. Apply the bell lightly, resting the chestpiece on the client's skin (Figure 31–9). Compressing the bell against the skin reduces low-pitched sound amplification and creates a "diaphragm of skin." Some stethoscopes have one chestpiece that combines the features of the bell and diaphragm. With the use of light pressure, the chestpiece acts as a bell; with more pressure, it acts as a diaphragm.

The stethoscope is a delicate instrument and requires proper care for optimal function. The earpieces should be removed regularly and cleaned according to the manufacturer's instructions (to remove cerumen). The bell and diaphragm are cleaned (to remove dust, lint, and body oils). The tubing is cleaned with mild soap and water. Nurses are encouraged to have their own stethoscope. If several nurses use the same stethoscope, the earpieces should be cleansed with an antiseptic before each use.

➤ TABLE 31-2 Pulse Sites

Site (Artery)	Location	Use and Assessment Criteria
Temporal	Over temporal bone of head, above and lateral to eye	To assess pulse in children
Carotid	Along medial edge of sternocleidomastoid muscle in neck	During physiological shock or cardiac arrest, when other sites are not palpable
Apical	Fourth to fifth intercostal space at left midclavicular line	To auscultate for apical pulse
Brachial	Groove between biceps and triceps muscles at antecubital fossa	To assess status of circulation to lower arm; to ausculate blood pressure
Radial	Radial or thumb side of forearm at wrist	To assess character of pulse peripherally and assess status of circulation to hand
Ulnar	Ulnar side of forearm at wrist	To assess status of circulation to hand; also to perform Allen's test (test for patency of radial artery)
Femoral	Below inguinal ligament, midway between symphysis pubis and anterior superior iliac spine	To assess character of pulse during physiological shock or cardiac arrest when other pulses are not palpable; to assess status of circulation to leg
Popliteal	Behind knee in popliteal fossa	To assess status of circulation to lower leg
Posterior tibial	Inner side of ankle, below medial malleolus	To assess status of circulation to foot
Dorsalis pedis	Along top of foot, between extension tendons of the great toe and the toe next to it	To assess status of circulation to foot

➤ SKILL 31-2 Assessing the Radial and Apical Pulses

video

Delegation Considerations

The task of pulse measurement can be delegated to unregulated care providers (UCPs). The nurse is responsible for assessing changes in pulse; therefore, when the task of pulse measurement is delegated, it is important to *inform the unregulated care provider* about the following:

- Client's history or risk for irregular pulse
- Frequency of pulse measurement in client
- Client's usual pulse values
- Abnormalities that should be reported to the health care professional

Equipment

- Stethoscope (to measure apical pulse only)
- Watch or clock with second hand or digital display
- Pen and either vital sign flow sheet or record form
- Alcohol swab

Procedure

STEPS	RATIONALE
1. Determine need to assess radial or apical pulse.	• You use clinical judgement to determine need for assessment.
A. Note risk factors for alterations in apical pulse.	• Certain conditions heighten risk for pulse alterations. These conditions include cardiac disease, cardiac dysrhythmias, sudden chest pain or acute pain from any site, invasive cardiovascular diagnostic tests, surgery, sudden infusion of large volume of intravenous fluid, hemorrhage, and administration of medications that alter cardiac function.
B. Assess for signs and symptoms of altered stroke volume and cardiac output, such as dyspnea, fatigue, chest pain, orthopnea, syncope, palpitations (unpleasant awareness of heartbeat), jugular venous distension, edema of dependent body parts, and cyanosis or pallor of skin.	• Physical signs and symptoms may indicate alteration in cardiac function.
2. Assess for factors that normally influence pulse rate and rhythm: age, exercise, position changes, fluid balance, medications, temperature, sympathetic stimulation.	• These assessments enable you to accurately evaluate the presence and significance of pulse alterations. Acceptable range of pulse rate changes with age (see Table 31–3).
3. Determine previous baseline apical rate (if available) from client's record. Otherwise, note baseline radial rate.	• By comparing rates, you can assess for change in client's condition and evaluate future apical pulse measurements.
4. Explain to client that pulse or heart rate is to be assessed. If client was active, wait 5–10 minutes before taking his or her pulse. Encourage client to relax and not to speak.	• Activity and anxiety elevate heart rate. Client's voice interferes with your ability to hear sound when you measure apical pulse. Measuring pulse rates at rest allows for objective comparison of values.
5. Perform hand hygiene.	• Hand hygiene reduces transmission of microorganisms between the client and the nurse.
6. If necessary, draw curtain around client's bed or close room door, or do both.	• These actions maintain client's privacy, minimize embarrassment, and promote comfort.
7. Obtain pulse measurement.	
A. **Radial pulse**	
(1) Assist client to assume a supine or sitting position.	• These positions enable easy access to pulse sites.
(2) If client is supine, place client's forearm straight alongside body, across lower chest, or across upper abdomen with wrist extended straight (see Step 7A[2] illustration). If client is sitting, bend client's elbow 90 degrees and support lower arm on chair or on your arm. Slightly flex client's wrist with palm down (see Step 7A[2] illustration).	• Relaxed position of lower arm and slight flexion of wrist promotes exposure of artery to palpation without restriction.
(3) Place tips of your first two or middle three fingers over groove along radial or thumb side of client's inner wrist (see Step 7A[3] illustration).	• Fingertips are the most sensitive parts of the hand to palpate arterial pulsation. Your thumb has pulsation that may interfere with accuracy.

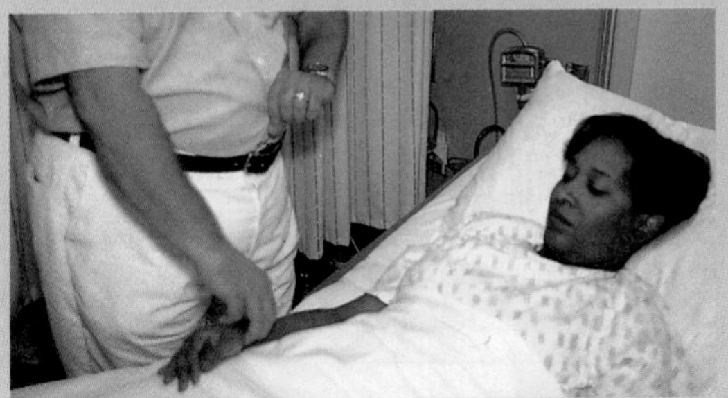

Step 7A(2) Pulse check with client's forearm at side with wrist extended.

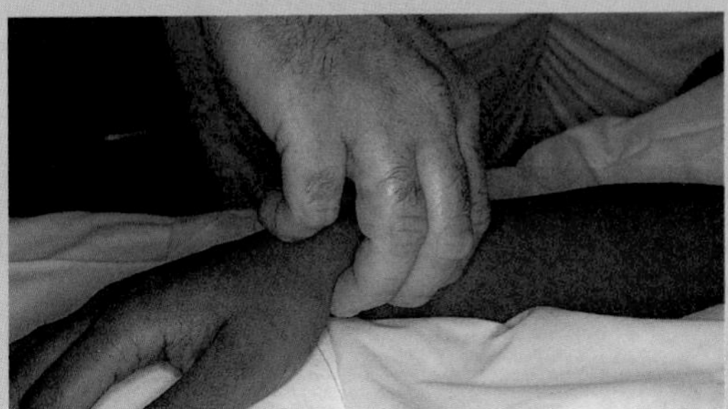

Step 7A(3) Hand placement for pulse checking radial pulse.

Continued

➤ SKILL 31-2 Assessing the Radial and Apical Pulses *continued*

STEPS	RATIONALE
(4) Lightly compress your fingertips against client's radius, obliterate pulse initially, and then relax pressure so that pulse becomes easily palpable.	• Pulse is more accurately assessed with moderate pressure. Too much pressure occludes pulse and impairs blood flow.
(5) Determine strength of pulse. Note whether thrust of vessel against your fingertips is bounding (+4), strong (+3), weak (+2), thready (+1), or absent (0).	• Strength reflects volume of blood ejected against arterial wall with each heart contraction. Accurate description of strength improves communication among health care professionals.
(6) After you can feel a regular pulse, look at watch and begin to count pulse rate when second hand reaches a number on watch dial; start counting pulse with "one," then "two," and so on.	• You can determine pulse rate accurately only after you can palpate the pulse. Count of "one" is the first beat palpated after you begin timing.
(7) If pulse is regular, count rate for 30 seconds and multiply total by 2.	• A 30-second count is accurate for rapid, slow, or regular pulse rates.
(8) If pulse is irregular, count rate for 1 minute (60 seconds). Assess frequency and pattern of irregularity. Compare bilateral radial pulses.	• Inefficient contraction of heart fails to transmit pulse wave, interfering with cardiac output, resulting in irregular pulse. Longer time ensures accurate count.

Critical Decision Point: If pulse is irregular, assess apical or radial pulse to detect a pulse deficit. Count apical pulse rate while a colleague counts radial pulse rate. Begin apical pulse count out loud to simultaneously assess pulses. If pulse count differs by more than two, a pulse deficit exists; this can indicate altered cardiac output.

STEPS	RATIONALE
B. Apical pulse	
(1) Perform hand hygiene; clean earpieces and diaphragm of stethoscope with alcohol swab.	• These actions reduce transmission of microorganisms between clients.
(2) Draw curtain around client's bed or close room door, or do both.	• These actions maintain client's privacy, minimize embarrassment, and promote comfort.
(3) Assist client to supine or sitting position. Move aside bed linen and gown to expose sternum and left side of chest.	• Expose portion of client's chest wall to select auscultatory site.
(4) Locate anatomical landmarks to identify the *point of maximal impulse* (PMI), also called the *apical impulse* (see Steps 7B[4][a] to 7B[4][d] illustrations). Heart is located behind and to left of sternum with base at top and apex at bottom. Find angle of Louis just below suprasternal notch between sternal body and manubrium; it can be palpated as a bony prominence (see Step 7B[4][a] illustration). Slip fingers down each side of angle to find second intercostal space (ICS; see Step 7B[4][b] illustration). Carefully move fingers down left side of sternum to fifth ICS (see Step 7B[4][c] illustration) and laterally to the left midclavicular line (MCL; see Step 7B[4][d] illustration). A light tap felt in an area within 1 to 2 cm of the PMI is reflected from the apex of the heart.	• Use of anatomical landmarks allows correct placement of stethoscope over apex of heart, enhancing ability to hear heart sounds clearly. In a client with large breasts, ask the client to move the breast aside so that you can access the PMI site. If you are unable to palpate the PMI, reposition client on left side. In the presence of severe cardiac disease, the PMI may be located to the left of the MCL or at the sixth ICS.

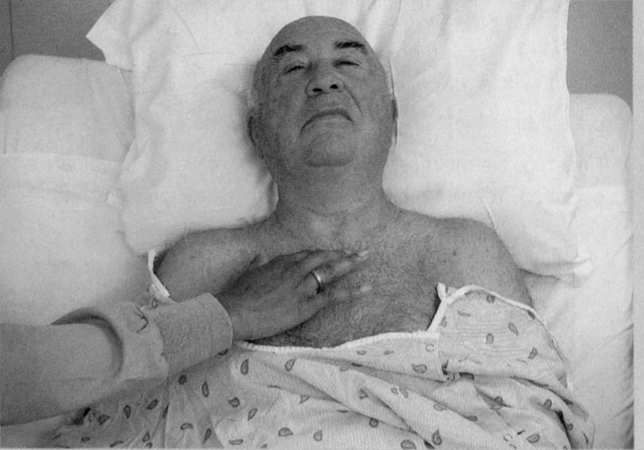

Step 7B(4)(a) Locating the angle of Louis.

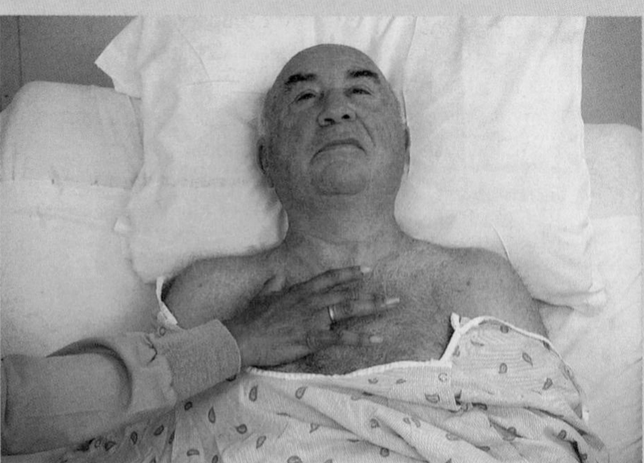

Step 7B(4)(b) Locating the second intercostal space.

➤ SKILL 31-2 Assessing the Radial and Apical Pulses *continued*

STEPS	RATIONALE
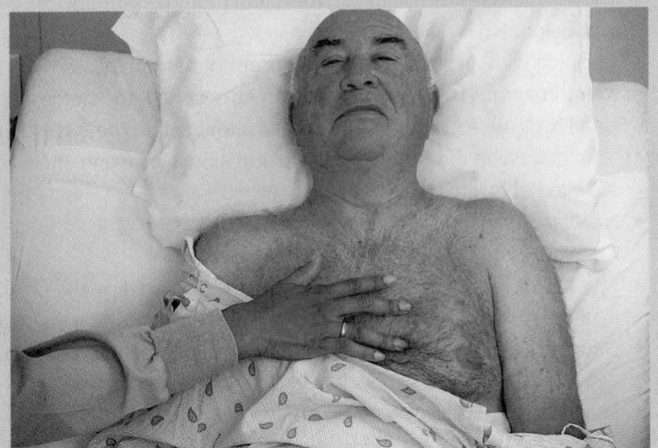 Step 7B(4)(c) Locating the fifth intercostal space.	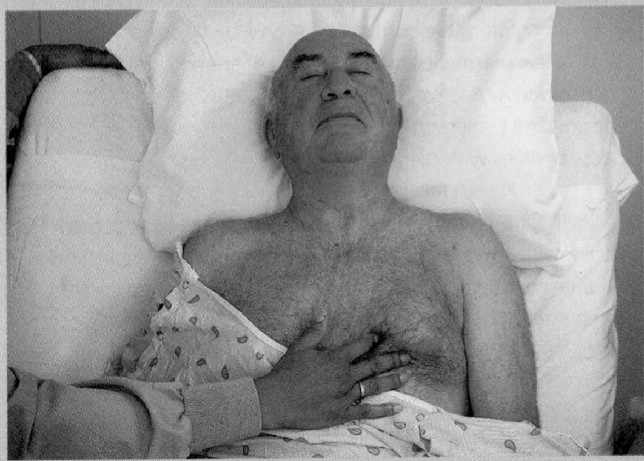 Step 7B(4)(d) Identifying the midclavicular line.
(5) Place diaphragm of stethoscope in palm of your hand for 5 to 10 seconds.	• By warming metal or plastic diaphragm, you avoid startling client and promote client's comfort.
(6) Place diaphragm of stethoscope over PMI at the fifth ICS, at left MCL, and auscultate for normal S_1 and S_2 heart sounds (heard as "lub-dub"; see Step 7B[6] illustrations).	• Allow stethoscope tubing to extend straight without kinks that would distort sound transmission. Normally, S_1 and S_2 heart sounds are high-pitched and best heard with the diaphragm.

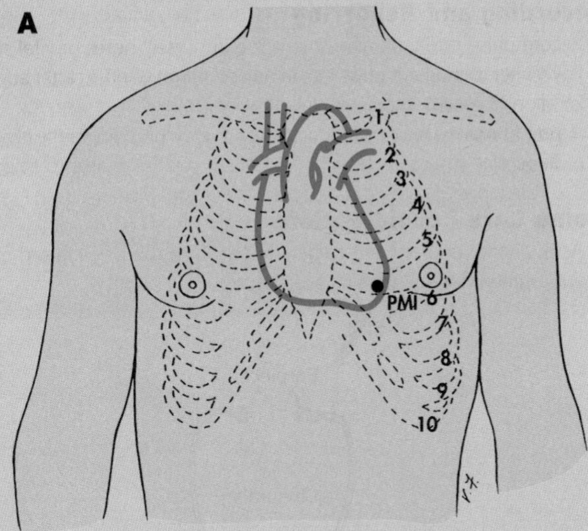

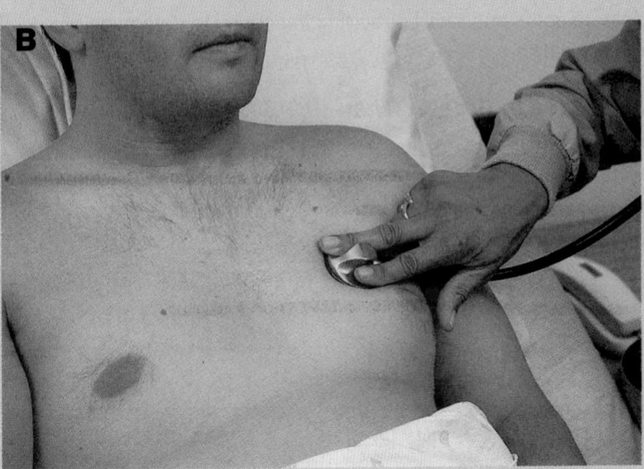

Step 7B(6) **A,** Location of point of maximal impulse (PMI) in adult. **B,** Stethoscope placement over PMI.

STEPS	RATIONALE
(7) When S_1 and S_2 are heard with regularity, look at watch and begin to count rate: When second hand reaches a number on watch dial, start counting with "one," then "two," and so on.	• You can accurately determine apical rate only after you can auscultate sounds clearly. Count of "one" is first sound auscultated after timing begins.
(8) If apical rate is regular, count for 30 seconds and multiply by 2.	• Regular apical rate can be assessed within 30 seconds.

Critical Decision Point: If heart rate is irregular or if client is receiving cardiovascular medication, count for 1 minute (60 seconds). An irregular rate is more accurately assessed when measured over a longer interval.

STEPS	RATIONALE
(9) If heart rate is irregular, or client is receiving cardiovascular medication, count for a full 1 minute (60 seconds), describe pattern of irregularity (S_1 and S_2 occurring early or later after previous sequence of sounds; e.g., every third or every fourth beat is skipped).	• Regular occurrence of dysrhythmia within 1 minute may indicate inefficient contraction of heart and alteration in cardiac output.

Continued

SKILL 31-2 Assessing the Radial and Apical Pulses *continued*

STEPS	RATIONALE
(10) Move back client's gown and bed linen; assist client to return to comfortable position.	• These actions restore client's comfort and promote sense of well-being.
(11) Clean earpieces and diaphragm of stethoscope with alcohol swab as necessary.	• Cleaning with an alcohol swab helps control transmission of microorganisms between clients when nurses share the stethoscope.
8. Perform hand hygiene.	• Hand hygiene reduces transmission of microorganisms between clients.
9. Discuss findings with client as needed.	• Such discussion promotes client's participation in care and understanding of health status.
10. Compare current readings with previous baseline measurement or acceptable range of heart rate for client's age (see Table 31–3).	• Evaluate for change in condition and alterations.
11. Compare peripheral pulse rate with apical rate, and note any discrepancy.	• Differences between measurements indicate pulse deficit and possibly cardiovascular compromise. Abnormalities may necessitate therapy.
12. Compare radial pulse equality, and note any discrepancy.	• Differences between radial arteries indicate compromised peripheral vascular system.
13. Correlate pulse rate with data obtained from blood pressure and related signs and symptoms (palpitations, dizziness).	• Pulse rate and blood pressure are interrelated.

Unexpected Outcomes and Related Interventions

Radial Pulse Is Weak or Thready

- Assess both radial pulses and compare findings. Local obstruction to one extremity (e.g., clot, edema) may decrease peripheral blood flow.
- Perform complete assessment of all pulses (see Chapter 32).
- Observe for symptoms associated with decreased tissue perfusion, such as pallor and cool skin temperature of tissue distal to the weak pulse.
- Measure apical and radial pulse simultaneously to determine presence of pulse deficit.

Apical Pulse Is Greater Than 100 Beats per Minute (Tachycardia)

- Assess for presence of fever, anxiety, pain, recent exercise, hypotension, decreased oxygenation, or dehydration, all of which can elevate pulse.
- Measure all vital signs.
- Assess for factors associated with decreased cardiac output, such as chest pain, dizziness, cyanosis, fatigue, and orthopnea.

Apical Pulse Is Less Than 60 Beats per Minute (Bradycardia)

- Assess for the presence of factors that may alter heart rate, such as digoxin or other cardiac medications. It may be necessary to withhold prescribed medications until the prescribing health care professional can evaluate the need to adjust dosage.
- Assess for factors associated with decreased cardiac output.

Recording and Reporting

- Record pulse rate with assessment site in nurses' notes or vital signs flow sheet. Document pulse rate in nurses' narrative notes after administration of specific therapies.
- *Report abnormal findings* to nurse in charge or prescribing health care professional.

Home Care Considerations

- Assess home environment to determine which room will afford quiet environment for auscultating apical rate.

TABLE 31-3 Acceptable Ranges of Heart Rate

Age	Heart Rate (Beats per Minute)
Infant	120–160
Toddler	90–140
Preschooler	80–110
School-age child	75–100
Adolescent	60–90
Adult	60–100

Data from Kinney, M. R., Dunbar, S. B., Brooks-Brunn, J., Molter, N., & Vitello-Cicciu, J. M. (1998). *AACN's clinical reference for critical care nursing* (4th ed.). St. Louis, MO: Mosby.

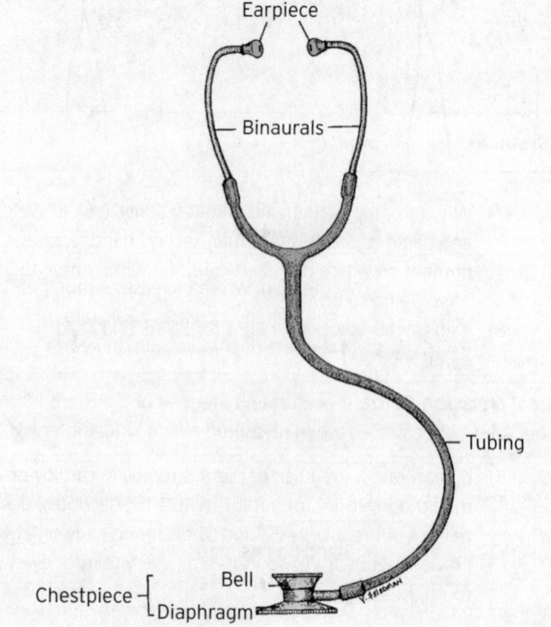

Figure 31-7 Parts of a stethoscope.

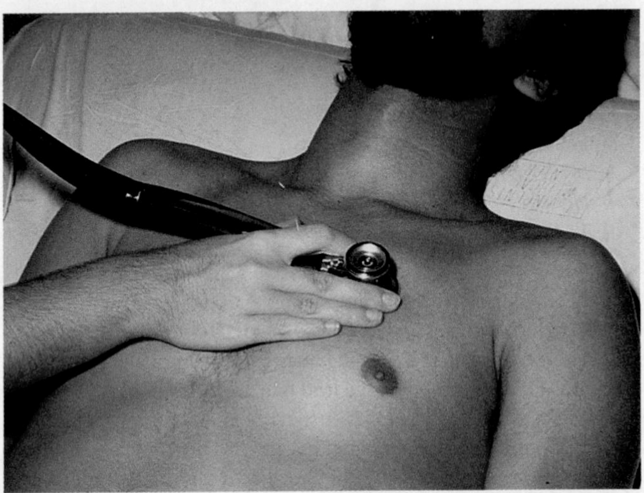

Figure 31-8 Positioning the diaphragm of the stethoscope firmly and securely when high-pitched heart sounds are auscultated.

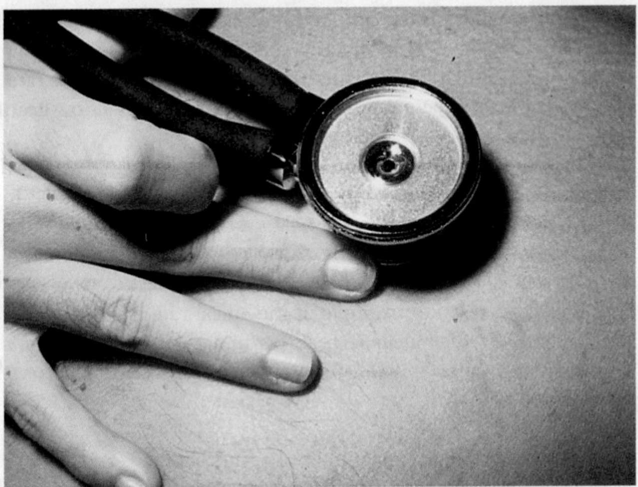

Figure 31-9 Positioning the bell of the stethoscope lightly on the skin to hear low-pitched heart sounds.

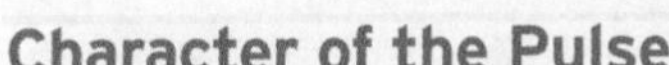

Character of the Pulse

Assessment of the radial pulse includes measurement of the rate, rhythm, strength, and bilateral equality. When auscultating an apical pulse, assess rate and rhythm only.

Rate. Before measuring a pulse, review the client's baseline rate for comparison (see Table 31–3). Some practitioners make baseline measurements of the pulse rate with the client sitting, standing, and lying. Changes in posture cause changes in pulse rate because of alterations in blood volume and sympathetic nervous system activity. The heart rate temporarily increases when a person changes from a lying to a sitting or standing position.

Always consider the variety of factors influencing the pulse rate (Table 31–4). A single factor or a combination of factors can cause significant changes. If you detect an abnormal rate while you palpate a peripheral pulse, the next step is to assess the apical rate. This requires auscultation of heart sounds, which provides a more accurate assessment of cardiac contraction (see Chapter 32).

Identify the first and second heart sounds (S_1 and S_2). At normal slow rates, S_1 is low-pitched and dull, sounding like a "lub." S_2 is higher pitched and shorter, creating the sound "dub." Each set of "lub-dub" is counted as one heartbeat. Using the diaphragm or bell of the stethoscope, count the number of "lub-dubs" occurring in 1 minute.

➤ TABLE 31-4 Factors Influencing Pulse Rates

Factor	Increases Pulse Rate	Decreases Pulse Rate
Exercise	Short-term exercise	Long-term exercise, which conditions the heart and results in a lower resting pulse and a quicker return to resting level after exercise
Temperature	Fever and heat	Hypothermia
Emotions	Anxiety increases sympathetic stimulation, affecting heart rate	Relaxation
Pain	Acute pain, which increases sympathetic stimulation and thereby increases heart rate The effect of chronic pain on heart rate varies	Unrelieved severe pain, which increases parasympathetic stimulation and thereby affects heart rate
Drugs	Positive chronotropic drugs such as epinephrine	Negative chronotropic drugs such as digitalis, β-adrenergic blockers, and calcium channel blockers
Hemorrhage	Loss of blood increases sympathetic stimulation	
Postural changes	Standing or sitting	Lying down
Pulmonary conditions	Diseases causing poor oxygenation, such as asthma and chronic obstructive pulmonary disease (COPD)	

Peripheral and apical pulse rate assessment may reveal variations in heart rate. Two common abnormalities in pulse rate are tachycardia and bradycardia. **Tachycardia** is an abnormally fast heart rate, more than 100 beats per minute in adults. **Bradycardia** is a slow heart rate, less than 60 beats per minute in adults.

An inefficient contraction of the heart that fails to transmit a pulse wave to the peripheral pulse site creates a pulse deficit. To detect a **pulse deficit**, you assess either radial or apical rate, and a colleague simultaneously assesses the other rate; then you compare the two rates. The difference between the apical and radial pulse rates is the pulse deficit. For example, if the apical rate is 92 beats per minute and the radial rate is 78 beats per minute, the pulse deficit is 14 beats per minute. Pulse deficits are frequently associated with abnormal rhythms.

Rhythm. Normally, a regular interval occurs between each pulse or heartbeat. An interval interrupted by an early or late beat or a missed beat indicates an abnormal rhythm, or **dysrhythmia**. Dysrhythmia threatens the heart's ability to provide adequate cardiac output, particularly if it occurs repetitively. You identify dysrhythmia by palpating an interruption in successive pulse waves or auscultating an interruption between heart sounds. If dysrhythmia is present, assess the regularity of its occurrence and auscultate the apical rate (see Chapter 32). Dysrhythmias are described as "regularly irregular" or "irregularly irregular."

To document a dysrhythmia, a prescribing health care professional may order electrocardiography, Holter monitoring, or telemetry. In electrocardiography, the electrical activity of the heart is recorded for a 12-second interval. The Holter monitor records 24 hours of electrical activity in a small tape recorder that the client wears. Access to the information recorded is not available until after the 24 hours have passed and the data are printed for review. In cardiac telemetry, the heart's electrical activity is monitored continuously, and the data are transmitted to a stationary monitor. Telemetry enables observation of heart rhythm during all the client's daily activities and thus allows for immediate treatment if the rhythm becomes erratic or unstable. Many children have a sinus dysrhythmia, which is an irregular heartbeat that speeds up with inspiration and slows down with expiration. This is a normal finding.

Strength. The strength of a pulse reflects both the volume of blood ejected against the arterial wall with each heart contraction and the condition of the arterial vascular system leading to the pulse site. Normally, the pulse strength remains the same with each heartbeat. Pulse strength may be graded or described as bounding, strong, weak, thready, or absent. It is included during assessment of the vascular system (see Chapter 32).

Equality. Pulses on both sides of the peripheral vascular system should be assessed, in order to compare their characteristics. A pulse in one extremity may be unequal to the pulse in the other extremity in strength, or it may be absent in many disease states (e.g., thrombus [clot] formation). All symmetrical pulses can be assessed simultaneously except for the carotid pulses, which should never be measured simultaneously because excessive pressure may occlude blood supply to the brain or trigger carotid reflexes that may result in altered cardiac output.

Nursing Process and Pulse Determination

Pulse assessment helps you determine the general state of cardiovascular health and the body's response to other system imbalances. Tachycardia, bradycardia, and dysrhythmia are defining characteristics of many nursing diagnoses, including the following:

- *Activity intolerance*
- *Anxiety*
- *Decreased cardiac output*
- *Deficient/excess fluid volume*
- Impaired gas exchange
- *Hyperthermia*
- *Hypothermia*
- *Acute pain*
- *Ineffective tissue perfusion*

The nursing care plan includes interventions specific for the nursing diagnosis identified and its related factors. For example, the defining characteristics of an abnormal heart rate, exertional dyspnea, and a client's verbal report of fatigue lead to a diagnosis of *activity intolerance*. When the related factor is "inactivity after a prolonged illness," interventions focus on increasing the client's daily exercises. Evaluate client outcomes by assessing the pulse rate, rhythm, strength, and equality after each intervention.

Respiration

Human survival depends on the ability of oxygen (O_2) to reach body cells and of carbon dioxide (CO_2) to be removed from the cells. Respiration is the mechanism that the body uses to exchange gases between the atmosphere and the blood and between the blood and the cells. Respiration involves **ventilation** (the movement of gases in and out of the lungs), **diffusion** (the movement of oxygen and carbon dioxide between the alveoli and the red blood cells), and **perfusion** (the distribution of red blood cells to and from the pulmonary capillaries). To analyze respiratory efficiency, you must integrate assessment data from all three processes. You assess ventilation by determining respiratory rate, respiratory depth, and respiratory rhythm. You assess diffusion and perfusion by determining oxygen saturation.

Physiological Control

Breathing is generally a passive process; a person thinks little about it. The respiratory centre in the brain stem regulates the involuntary control of respirations. Adults normally breathe in a smooth, uninterrupted pattern, 12 to 20 times a minute.

Ventilation is regulated by levels of carbon dioxide, oxygen, and hydrogen ion concentration (pH) in the arterial blood. The most important factor is the level of CO_2 in the arterial blood. An elevation in the CO_2 level causes the respiratory control system in the brain to increase the rate and depth of breathing. The increased ventilatory effort removes excess CO_2 (which is the state of hypercarbia) by increasing exhalation. However, clients with chronic lung disease have ongoing hypercarbia. For them, chemoreceptors in the carotid artery and aorta become sensitive to **hypoxemia**, or low levels of arterial O_2. If arterial O_2 levels fall, these receptors signal the brain to increase the rate and depth of ventilation. Hypoxemia helps control ventilation in clients with chronic lung disease. Because low levels of arterial O_2 provide the stimulus that allows the client to breathe, administration of high oxygen levels can be dangerous for these clients.

Mechanics of Breathing

Although breathing is normally passive, muscular work is involved in moving the lungs and chest wall. Inspiration is an active process. During inspiration, the respiratory centre sends impulses along the phrenic nerve, causing the diaphragm to contract. Abdominal organs move downward and forward, increasing the length of the chest cavity to move air into the lungs. The diaphragm moves approximately 1 cm, and the ribs retract upward from the body's midline approximately 1.2 to 2.5 cm. During a normal, relaxed breath, a person inhales 500 mL of air. This amount is referred to as the **tidal volume.** During expiration, the diaphragm relaxes and the abdominal organs return to their original positions. The lung and chest wall return to a relaxed position (Figure 31–10). Expiration is a passive process. The normal rate and depth of ventilation, **eupnea**, is interrupted by sighing. The sigh, a prolonged deeper breath, is a protective physiological mechanism for expanding small airways and alveoli not ventilated during a normal breath.

The accurate assessment of respiration depends on the recognition of normal thoracic and abdominal movements. During quiet breathing, the chest wall gently rises and falls. Contraction of the accessory muscles of breathing (i.e., the intercostal muscles between the ribs and the muscles in the neck and shoulders) is not visible. During normal quiet breathing, diaphragmatic movement causes the abdominal cavity to rise and fall slowly.

Assessment of Ventilation

Special equipment is not needed to measure respirations, but measurement must not be haphazard. You must not estimate respirations. Accurate measurement requires observation and palpation of chest wall movement.

A sudden change in the character of respirations is important. Because respiration is tied to the function of numerous body systems, consider all variables when changes occur (Box 31–11). For example, abdominal trauma may injure the phrenic nerve, which is responsible for diaphragmatic contraction. The extent of the injury and the implications for the respiratory system are important to understand.

Do not let a client know that you are assessing his or her respiration. A client aware of your intentions may consciously alter the rate and depth of breathing. The best time to measure respiration is immediately after you measure pulse rate, with your hand still on the client's wrist as it rests over the chest or abdomen. When assessing, keep in mind the client's usual ventilatory rate and pattern, the influence any disease or illness has on respiratory function, the relationship between respiratory and cardiovascular function, and the influence of therapies on respiration. The objective measurements in assessing respiratory status include the rate and depth of breathing and the rhythm of ventilatory movements (Skill 31–3).

Respiratory Rate. Observe both inspiration and expiration when you count ventilation or respiration rate. The respiratory rate varies with age (Table 31–5) and usually decreases with age.

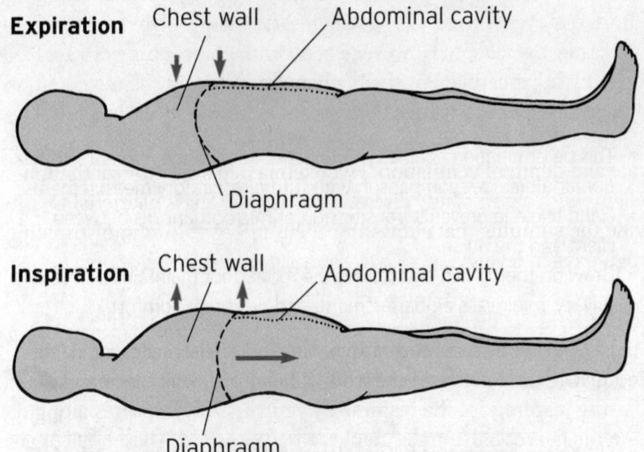

Figure 31-10 Illustration of diaphragmatic and chest wall movement during inspiration and expiration.

BOX 31-11 Factors Influencing Character of Respiration

Exercise

Exercise increases respiratory rate and depth to meet body's need for additional O_2 and to rid body of CO_2.

Acute Pain

Pain alters rate and rhythm of respiration; breathing becomes shallow.

Client inhibits or splints chest wall movement when pain is in area of chest or abdomen.

Anxiety

Anxiety increases respiratory rate and depth as a result of sympathetic stimulation.

Smoking

Chronic smoking changes pulmonary airways, resulting in increased rate of respirations at rest when the person is not smoking.

Body Position

A straight, erect posture promotes full chest expansion.

A stooped or slumped position impairs ventilatory movement.

Lying flat prevents full chest expansion.

Medications

Narcotic analgesics, general anaesthetics, and sedative hypnotics depress respiratory rate and depth.

Amphetamines and cocaine may increase respiratory rate and depth.

Bronchodilators slow respiratory rate by causing airway dilation.

Neurological Injury

Injury to the brain stem impairs the respiratory centre and inhibits respiratory rate and rhythm.

Hemoglobin Function

In the state of anemia, decreased hemoglobin levels reduce O_2-carrying capacity of the blood, which results in increases in respiratory rate.

Increased altitude lowers the amount of saturated hemoglobin, which increases respiratory rate and depth.

Abnormalities in blood cell function (e.g., sickle cell disease) reduce ability of red blood cells to carry oxygen, which results in increases in respiratory rate and depth.

An apnea monitor is a respiratory monitoring device that aids in respiratory assessment. Leads that sense movement are attached to the client's chest wall. Absence of chest wall movement triggers the apnea alarm. Apnea monitoring is used frequently with infants in hospitals and at home to observe for prolonged apneic events.

Ventilatory Depth. You assess the depth of respiration by observing the degree of excursion or movement in the client's chest wall. Describe ventilatory movements as "deep," "normal," or "shallow." A deep respiration involves a full expansion of the lungs with full exhalation. Respirations are shallow when only a small quantity of air passes through the lungs and ventilatory movement is difficult to see. Objective techniques are used if chest excursion is unusually shallow (see Chapter 32). Table 31–6 summarizes alterations in breathing pattern.

SKILL 31-3 Assessing Respirations video

Delegation Considerations

The task of measuring respiration can be delegated to unregulated care providers (UCPs). The nurse is responsible for assessing for change in respiration rate, rhythm, and depth; therefore, when the task of measuring respiration is delegated, it is important to *inform the unregulated care provider* about the following:

- The client's history or risk for abnormal respiratory status
- The frequency of respiration measurement for a specific client
- Abnormalities that should be reported to the health care professional

Equipment

- Watch with second hand or digital display
- Pen and either vital sign flow sheet or record form

Procedure

STEPS	RATIONALE
1. Determine need to assess client's respiration:	
A. Note presence of risk factors for respiratory alterations.	• You use clinical judgement to determine need for assessment. • Conditions that heighten risk for alterations in ventilation—detected by changes in respiratory rate, depth, and rhythm—include fever, pain, anxiety, diseases of chest muscles, constrictive chest or abdominal dressings, gastric distension, chronic pulmonary diseases, traumatic chest injury, presence of a chest tube, respiratory infection, pulmonary edema and emboli, anemia, and head injury with damage to brain stem.
B. Assess for signs and symptoms of respiratory alterations, such as bluish (cyanotic) appearance of nail beds, lips, mucous membranes, and skin; restlessness, irritability, confusion, and reduced level of consciousness; pain during inspiration; laboured or difficult breathing; adventitious breath sounds (see Chapter 32), inability to breathe spontaneously; thick, frothy, blood-tinged, or copious sputum produced on coughing.	• Physical signs and symptoms indicate alterations in respiratory status related to ventilation.
2. Assess pertinent laboratory values.	
A. **Arterial blood gases** (normal values may vary slightly between institutions): *pH:* 7.35–7.45 mm Hg *$PaCO_2$:* 35–45 mm Hg *PaO_2:* 80–100 mm Hg *SaO_2:* 95%–100%	• Arterial blood gases measure arterial blood pH, partial pressure of O_2 (PaO_2) and CO_2 ($PaCO_2$), and arterial O_2 saturation (SaO_2), which reflects client's oxygenation status.
B. **Pulse oximetry (SpO_2):** Normal levels are 90%–100%; 85%–89% may be acceptable for certain chronic disease conditions; less than 85% is abnormal (see Skill 31–4).	• Although 95% is considered normal, 90% is an acceptable value in clients with sleep disorders. SpO_2 less than 85% is often accompanied by changes in respiratory rate, depth, and rhythm.
C. **Specific tests of the complete blood cell count (CBC):** (normal values for adults may vary between institutions and references consulted): *Hemoglobin:* 132–173 g/L in male clients; 117 to 155 g/L in female clients *Hematocrit:* 0.43 to 0.49 in male clients; 0.38 to 0.44 in female clients *Red blood cell count:* 4.7 to 5.74 × 10^{12}/L in male clients; 4.2 to 4.87 × 10^{12}/L in female clients	• Hemoglobin, hematocrit, and red blood cell count (three of several CBC tests), measure the concentration of hemoglobin volume of red blood cells, and red blood cell count, all of which reflect client's capacity to carry O_2.
3. Determine previous baseline respiratory rate (if available) from client's record.	• This determination enables you to assess for change in client's condition and provides comparison with future respiratory measurements.
4. Perform hand hygiene.	• Hand hygiene prevents transmission of microorganisms between the client and the nurse.
5. Draw curtain around client's bed or close room door, or do both.	• Drawing the curtain and closing the room door maintains client's privacy, minimizes embarrassment, and promotes comfort.

Critical Decision Point: Clients with difficulty breathing (dyspnea), such as those with congestive heart failure, with abdominal ascites, or in late stages of pregnancy, should be assessed in the position of greatest comfort. Repositioning may increase the work of breathing, which increases respiratory rate.

STEPS	RATIONALE
6. Be sure client is in comfortable position, preferably sitting or lying with the head of the bed elevated 45 to 60 degrees. Move bed linen or gown to be sure client's chest is visible.	• Sitting erect promotes full ventilatory movement. A clear view of the chest wall and abdominal movements is needed for assessment.

➤ SKILL 31-5 Assessing Respirations *continued*

STEPS	RATIONALE
7. Place client's arm in relaxed position across his or her abdomen or lower chest, or place your hand directly over client's upper abdomen (see Step 7 illustration).	• A similar position used during pulse assessment allows you to assess respiratory rate inconspicuously. Client's hand or your hand rises and falls during respiratory cycle.

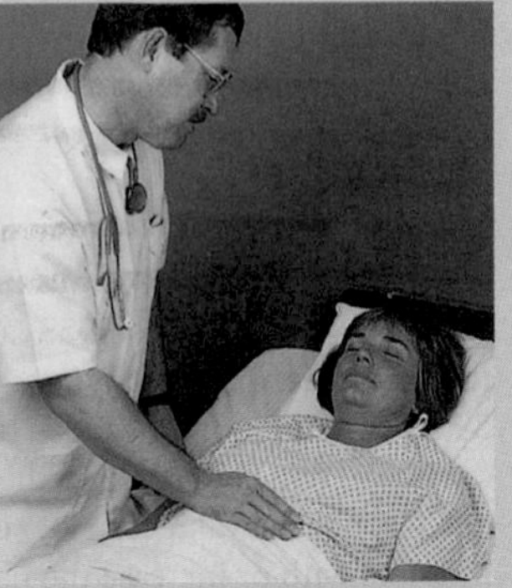

Step 7 Nurse's hand over client's abdomen to check respiration.

STEPS	RATIONALE
8. Observe complete respiratory cycle (one inspiration and one expiration).	• You can determine rate accurately only after you have viewed client's respiratory cycle.
9. After observing cycle, look at watch's second hand. When second hand reaches a number on watch dial, begin counting respiratory cycles, starting with "one" for the first full cycle, then "two," and so on.	• Timing begins with count of one. Respirations occur more slowly than pulse.
10. If rhythm is regular, count number of respiratory cycles in 30 seconds and multiply by 2. If rhythm is irregular, slower than 12 per minute, or faster than 20 per minute, count for 1 full minute.	• Respiratory rate is equivalent to number of respiratory cycles per minute. Suspected irregularities necessitate assessment for at least 1 minute.
11. Note depth of respirations, which you subjectively assess by observing degree of chest wall movement while counting respiratory rate. You can also objectively assess respiratory depth by palpating client's chest wall excursion or auscultating the posterior thorax after respiratory rate has been counted (see Chapter 32). Depth is described as "shallow," "normal," or "deep."	• Character of ventilatory movement may reveal specific disease state restricting volume of air from moving into and out of the lungs.
12. Note rhythm of ventilatory cycle. Normal breathing is regular and uninterrupted. Sighing should not be confused with abnormal rhythm.	• Character of ventilations can reveal specific types of alterations. Without being aware of it, people periodically take single deep breaths or sighs to expand small airways prone to collapse.

Critical Decision Point: Any irregular respiratory pattern or period of apnea (the cessation of respiration for several seconds) in an adult is a symptom of underlying disease and must be reported to the prescribing health care professional or nurse in charge. Further assessment may be required (see Chapter 32), and immediate intervention may be needed. An irregular respiratory rate and short apneic spells are normal only in newborns.

STEPS	RATIONALE
13. Move back bed linen and client's gown.	• This action restores client's comfort and promotes sense of well-being.
14. Perform hand hygiene.	• Hand hygiene reduces transmission of microorganisms between clients.
15. Discuss findings with client as needed.	• Such discussion promotes client's participation in care and understanding of health status.
16. If client's respiration is assessed for the first time, document rate, rhythm, and depth as baseline values if they are within normal ranges.	• These data are used for comparing data from future respiratory assessments.
17. Compare respiration data with client's previous baseline values and with normal values for rate, rhythm, and depth.	• These data allow you to assess for changes in client's condition and for presence of respiratory alterations.

Unexpected Outcomes and Related Interventions

Client's Respiratory Rate Is Less Than 12 (Bradypnea) or More than 20 (Tachypnea) Breaths per Minute, Depth Is Increased or Decreased, Rhythm Is Irregular, or Client Feels "Short of Breath"

- Observe for related factors, including obstructed airway, abnormal breath sounds, productive cough, restlessness, irritability, anxiety, and confusion.
- Position client in a supported sitting position (semi-Fowler's or high Fowler's), unless contraindicated.
- Provide oxygen as ordered.
- When possible, remove respiratory irritants from the environment, such as second-hand smoke and perfumes.

Recording and Reporting

- Record respiratory rate and character in nurses' notes or vital sign flow sheet. Indicate type and amount of oxygen therapy if it was used by the client during assessment. Document respiratory rate in nurses' narrative notes after administration of specific therapies.
- Report abnormal findings to nurse in charge or to prescribing health care professional.

Home Care Considerations

- Assess for environmental factors in the home that may influence client's respiration, such as second-hand smoke, poor ventilation, or gas fumes.

➤ TABLE 31-5 Acceptable Ranges of Respiratory Rates by Age

Age	Rate (Breaths per Minute)
Newborn	30–60
Infant (6 months)	30–50
Toddler (2 years)	25–32
Child and preadolescent (3–12 years)	20–30
Adolescent (13–18 years)	16–19
Adult (older than 18 years)	12–20

Ventilatory Rhythm. Breathing pattern can be determined by observing the chest or the abdomen. Diaphragmatic breathing results from the contraction and relaxation of the diaphragm and is best observed by watching abdominal movements. Healthy men and children usually demonstrate diaphragmatic breathing. Women tend to use thoracic muscles to breathe; movements are observed in the upper chest. Laboured respirations involve the accessory muscles of respiration visible in the neck. When something such as a foreign body interferes with the movement of air in and out of the lungs, the intercostal spaces retract during inspiration. A longer expiration phase is evident when the outward flow of air is obstructed (e.g., as in asthma).

With normal breathing, a regular interval occurs after each respiratory cycle. Infants tend to breathe less regularly. The young child may breathe slowly for a few seconds and then suddenly breathe more rapidly. Estimate the time interval after each respiratory cycle. Respiration is regular or irregular in rhythm.

Assessment of Diffusion and Perfusion

To evaluate the respiratory processes of diffusion and perfusion, measure the oxygen saturation of the blood. Blood flow through the pulmonary capillaries contains red blood cells for oxygen attachment. After oxygen diffuses from the alveoli into the pulmonary blood, most of it attaches to hemoglobin molecules in red blood cells; these cells carry the oxygenated hemoglobin molecules through the left side of the heart and out to the peripheral capillaries, where the oxygen detaches, depending on the needs of the tissues.

The percentage of hemoglobin that is bound with oxygen in the arteries is the percentage of saturation of hemoglobin (SaO_2). This value is usually between 95% and 100%. SaO_2 is affected by factors that interfere with ventilation, perfusion, or diffusion (see Chapter 39). The saturation of venous blood (SvO_2) is lower because the tissues have removed some of the oxygen from the hemoglobin molecules. A normal value for SvO_2 is 70%. SvO_2 is affected by factors that interfere with or increase the tissue's need for oxygen.

Measurement of Arterial Oxygen Saturation. A pulse oximeter permits the indirect measurement of oxygen saturation (Skill 31–4). It is a probe with a light-emitting diode (LED) and photo detector connected by cable to an oximeter (Figure 31–11). The LED emits light wavelengths that are absorbed differently by the oxygenated and deoxygenated hemoglobin molecules. The photo detector detects the amount of oxygen bound to hemoglobin molecules, and the oximeter calculates the pulse saturation (SpO_2).

The photo detector is in the oximeter probe. Select the appropriate probe to reduce measurement error. Digit probes are spring-loaded and conform to various sizes. Earlobe probes have greater accuracy at lower saturations and are least affected by peripheral vasoconstriction. Disposable sensor pads can be applied to a variety of sites, even the bridge of an adult's nose or the sole of an infant's foot. Factors that affect light transmission or peripheral arterial pulsations also affect the ability of the photo detector to measure SpO_2

➤ TABLE 31-6 Alterations in Breathing Pattern

Alteration	Description
Bradypnea	Rate of breathing is regular but abnormally slow (<12 breaths per minute).
Tachypnea	Rate of breathing is regular but abnormally rapid (>20 breaths per minute).
Hyperpnea	Respirations are laboured, increased in depth, and increased in rate (>20 breaths per minute). This occurs normally during exercise.
Apnea	Respirations cease for several seconds. Persistent cessation results in respiratory arrest.
Hyperventilation	Rate and depth of respirations increase. Hypocarbia may occur.
Hypoventilation	Respiratory rate is abnormally low, and depth of ventilation may be depressed. Hypercarbia may occur.
Cheyne-Stokes respiration	Respiratory rate and depth are irregular, characterized by alternating periods of apnea and hyperventilation. Respiratory cycle begins with slow, shallow breaths that gradually increase to abnormal rate and depth. The pattern reverses, breathing slows and becomes shallow, climaxing in apnea before respiration resumes.
Kussmaul's respiration	Respirations are abnormally deep, regular, and increased in rate.
Biot's respiration	Respirations are abnormally shallow for two to three breaths, followed by irregular period of apnea.

➤ SKILL 31-4 Measuring Oxygen Saturation (Pulse Oximetry)

Delegation Considerations

The task of measuring oxygen saturation can be delegated to unregulated care providers (UCPs). The nurse is responsible for assessing the effect of changes in oxygen saturation; therefore, when the task of measuring oxygen saturation is delegated, it is important to *inform the unregulated care provider* about the following:

- The importance of notifying the nurse immediately of any reading lower than SpO_2 of 90%
- How to select appropriate sensor site and probe for measurement of oxygen saturation.
- The frequency of oxygen saturation measurements for the client.
- Factors that can falsely lower SpO_2 (see Box 31–12).

Equipment

- Oximeter
- Oximeter probe appropriate for client and recommended by manufacturer
- Acetone or nail polish remover, if needed
- Pen and either vital sign flow sheet or record form

Procedure

STEPS	RATIONALE
1. Determine need to measure client's oxygen saturation:	• You use clinical judgement to determine need for assessment.
A. Note risk factors, including acute or chronic compromised respiratory function; recovery from general anaesthesia or conscious sedation; traumatic injury to chest; ventilator dependence; activity intolerance; and changes in supplemental oxygen therapy.	• Certain conditions heighten risk for decreased oxygen saturation.
B. Assess for signs and symptoms such as altered respiratory rate, depth, or rhythm; adventitious breath sounds (see Chapter 32); cyanotic appearance of nail beds, lips, mucous membranes, and skin; restlessness, irritability, or confusion; reduced level of consciousness; and laboured or difficult breathing.	• Physical signs and symptoms may be indicative of abnormal oxygen saturation.
2. Assess for factors that normally influence measurement of SpO_2 (see Box 31–12), such as oxygen therapy, hemoglobin level, temperature, and medications (e.g., bronchodilators).	• This assessment enables you to accurately assess oxygen saturation variations. Peripheral vasoconstriction related to hypothermia can interfere with SpO_2 determination.
3. Review client's medical record for order, or consult agency policy or procedure manual for standard of care.	• Medical order may be needed to assess oxygen saturation.
4. Determine site most appropriate for sensor probe placement (e.g., digit, earlobe) by assessing capillary refill (see Chapter 32) and skin condition. If capillary refill is less than 3 seconds, choose another site. A. Site needs to have adequate circulation and be free of moisture. B. If peripheral digit is used, it must be free of polish or artificial nail. C. If tremors are present, use earlobe as site. D. If client is obese, clip-on probe may not fit; obtain a single-use tape-on probe.	• Sensor requires pulsating vascular bed to identify hemoglobin molecules that absorb emitted light. Changes in SpO_2 are reflected in the circulation of the finger capillary bed within 30 seconds and the capillary bed of earlobe within 5–10 seconds. Moisture prevents the sensor from detecting SpO_2 levels. Artificial nails and nail polish colors alter readings. Motion artifact is the most common cause of a false reading.
5. Determine previous baseline SpO_2 (if available) from client's record.	• Baseline information provides basis for comparison and assists in assessment of current status and evaluation of interventions.
6. Explain purpose of procedure to client and how oxygen saturation will be measured.	• Explaining procedures promotes client's cooperation and increases compliance.
7. Perform hand hygiene.	• Hand hygiene reduces transmission of microorganisms between the client and the nurse.
8. Position client comfortably. If finger is chosen as monitoring site, support client's lower arm.	• This positioning enables probe positioning and decreases motion artifact that interferes with SpO_2 determination.
9. Instruct client to breathe normally.	• Normal breathing prevents large fluctuations in respiratory rate and depth and prevents possible errors in SpO_2 reading.
10. If finger is to be used, remove any fingernail polish with acetone from digit to be assessed.	• Nail polish interferes with accuracy of readings. Opaque coatings decrease light transmission; nail polish containing blue pigment can absorb light emissions and falsely alter saturation measurement.
11. Attach sensor probe to monitoring site. Inform client that clip-on probe feels like a clothespin on the finger but will not hurt.	• To avoid startling client, prepare client to feel pressure of sensor probe's spring tension on a peripheral digit or earlobe.

Critical Decision Point: Do not attach probe to finger, ear, or bridge of nose if area is edematous or skin integrity is compromised. Do not attach probe to hypothermic fingers. Select ear or bridge of nose if adult client has history of peripheral vascular disease. Do not use sensors on earlobe and bridge of nose in infants and toddlers because of skin fragility. Do not use disposable adhesive probes if client has latex allergy. Do not place probe on same extremity as electronic blood pressure cuff because blood flow to finger is temporarily interrupted when cuff inflates; this results in inaccurate readings that trigger alarms.

Continued

➤ SKILL 31-4 Measuring Oxygen Saturation (Pulse Oximetry) *continued*

STEPS	RATIONALE
12. Once sensor is in place, turn on oximeter. Observe pulse waveform and intensity display, and listen for audible beep. Correlate oximeter pulse rate with client's radial pulse. Oximeter pulse rate and client's radial pulse should be the same. If differences are present, re-evaluate oximeter probe placement, and reassess pulse rates.	• Pulse waveform and intensity display enables detection of valid pulse or presence of interfering signal. Pitch of audible beep is proportional to SpO_2 value. Double-checking pulse rate ensures oximeter accuracy.
13. Leave probe in place until oximeter readout reaches constant value and pulse display reaches full strength during each cardiac cycle. Inform client that oximeter will sound alarm if probe falls off or if client moves probe. Read SpO_2 on digital display.	• Reading takes 10 to 30 seconds, depending on site selected.
14. If SpO_2 monitoring is to be continuous, verify SpO_2 alarm limits and alarm volume, which are preset by the manufacturer at a minimum of 85% and a maximum of 100%. Determine limits for SpO_2 and pulse rate alarms on the basis of each client's condition. Verify that alarms are functional. Assess skin integrity under sensor probe every 2 hours. Relocate sensor probe at least every 4 hours and more frequently if skin integrity is altered or tissue perfusion compromised.	• Alarms must be set at appropriate limits and volumes to avoid frightening clients and visitors. Spring tension of sensor probe or sensitivity to disposable sensor probe adhesive can cause skin irritation and lead to disruption of skin integrity.
15. Assist client to return to comfortable position.	• This action restores client's comfort and promotes sense of well-being.
16. Perform hand hygiene.	• Hand hygiene reduces transmission of microorganisms between the client and the nurse.
17. Discuss findings with client as needed.	• Such discussion promotes client's participation in care and understanding of health status.
18. If SpO_2 measurements are intermittent or spot-checked, remove probe and turn oximeter power off between measurements. Store probe in appropriate location.	• Batteries will be depleted if oximeter is left on. Sensor probes are expensive and vulnerable to damage.
19. Compare SpO_2 readings with client's baseline and acceptable values.	• Comparison reveals presence of abnormality.
20. Correlate SpO_2 with SaO_2 obtained from arterial blood gas measurements (see Chapter 40) if available.	• Reliability of noninvasive assessments is documented.
21. Correlate SpO_2 reading with data obtained from assessment of respiratory rate, depth, and rhythm (see Skill 31–3).	• Measurements of ventilation, perfusion, and diffusion are interrelated.

Unexpected Outcomes and Related Interventions

SpO_2 Is Less Than 90%

- Verify that oximeter probe is intact and that outside light transmission does not influence measurement.
- Observe for signs associated with decreased oxygenation (e.g., anxiety, restlessness, tachycardia, cyanosis).
- Verify that supplemental oxygen delivery system is delivered as ordered and is functioning properly.
- Minimize factors that alter SpO_2 (e.g., lung secretions, increased activity, hyperthermia).
- Position client to promote optimal ventilation (e.g., high Fowler's position for obese client).

Pulse Rate Indicated on Oximeter Is Lower Than Client's Radial or Apical Pulse

- Reposition sensor probe to alternative site with increased blood flow.
- Assess client for signs of altered cardiac output (e.g., decreased blood pressure, cool skin, confusion).

Recording and Reporting

- Record SpO_2 value on nurses' notes or vital sign flow sheet, indicating type and amount of oxygen therapy used by client during assessment. Record any signs and symptoms of oxygen desaturation in nurses' narrative notes. Report abnormal findings to nurse in charge or prescribing health care professional.
- Document SpO_2 in nurses' narrative notes after administration of specific therapies.
- Record in nurses' notes client's use of continuous or intermittent pulse oximetry.

Home Care Considerations

- Pulse oximetry is used in home care to noninvasively monitor oxygen therapy or changes in oxygen therapy.
- Instruct caregivers to examine oximeter site before applying sensor.
- Instruct caregivers on procedure to implement when oxygen saturation not within acceptable values.

(see Box 31–12). Control of these factors allows accurate interpretation of abnormal SpO_2 measurements.

Nursing Process and Respiratory Vital Signs

Measurements of respiratory rate, pattern, and depth, along with SpO_2, enable you to assess ventilation, diffusion, and perfusion. Other assessments also involve respiratory status (see Chapter 32). Each measurement provides clues in determining the nature of a client's problem. Respiratory assessment data are defining characteristics of many nursing diagnoses, including the following:

- *Activity intolerance*
- *Ineffective airway clearance*
- *Anxiety*
- *Ineffective breathing pattern*
- *Impaired gas exchange*

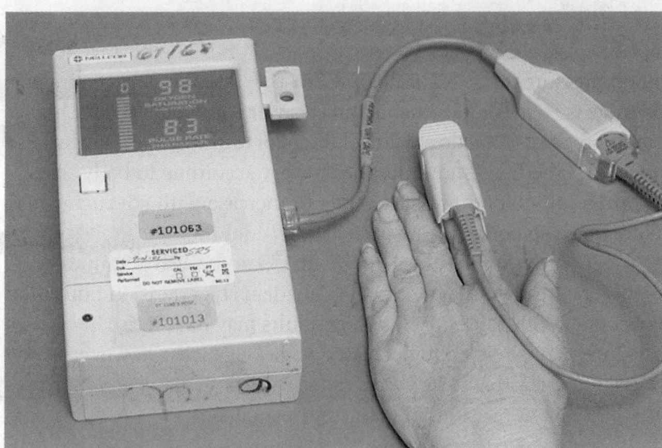

Figure 31-11 Portable pulse oximeter with digit probe.

- *Acute pain*
- *Ineffective tissue perfusion*
- *Dysfunctional ventilatory weaning response*

The nursing care plan includes interventions specific for the nursing diagnosis identified and the related factors. For example, the defining characteristics of tachypnea, changes in depth of respirations, use of accessory muscles, cyanosis, and a decline in SpO_2 lead to a diagnosis of *impaired gas exchange*. Related factors may include lung surgery, a history of chronic obstructive lung disease, and history of heavy smoking. Evaluate client outcomes by assessing the respiratory rate, ventilatory depth, rhythm, and SpO_2 after each intervention.

> **BOX 31-12 Factors Affecting Determination of Pulse Oxygen Saturation (SpO_2)**
>
> **Interference With Light Transmission**
>
> Outside light sources interfere with oximeter's ability to process reflected light.
> Carbon monoxide (caused by smoke inhalation or poisoning) artificially elevates SpO_2 by absorbing light in a similar way than oxygen does.
> Client motion interferes with oximeter's ability to process reflected light.
> Jaundice interferes with oximeter's ability to process reflected light.
> Intravascular dyes (e.g., methylene blue) absorb light in a similar way that deoxyhemoglobin does and artificially lower saturation.
> Nail polish, artificial nails, and metal studs in nails interfere with light absorption and the ability of the oximeter to process reflected light.
> Dark skin pigment sometimes results in signal loss or overestimation of saturation.
>
> **Reduction of Arterial Pulsations**
>
> Peripheral vascular disease (atherosclerosis) reduces pulse volume.
> Hypothermia at assessment site decreases peripheral blood flow.
> Pharmacological vasoconstrictors (epinephrine, dopamine) decrease peripheral pulse volume.
> Low cardiac output and hypotension decrease blood flow to peripheral arteries.
> Peripheral edema obscures arterial pulsation.
> Tight probe records venous pulsations in the finger that compete with arterial pulsations.

Blood Pressure

Blood pressure is the force exerted on the walls of an artery by the pulsing blood under pressure from the heart. Blood flows throughout the circulatory system because of pressure changes. It moves from an area of high pressure to an area of low pressure. Systemic or arterial blood pressure (the blood pressure in the system of arteries in the body) is a good indicator of cardiovascular health. The heart's contraction forces blood under high pressure into the aorta. The peak of maximum pressure when ejection occurs is the **systolic** blood pressure. When the ventricles relax, the blood remaining in the arteries exerts **diastolic** blood pressure, which is the minimal pressure exerted against the arterial walls at any time.

The standard unit for measuring blood pressure is millimetres of mercury (mm Hg). The measurement indicates the height to which the blood pressure can raise a column of mercury. It is recorded as the systolic reading over the diastolic reading (e.g., 120/80). The difference between systolic and diastolic pressure is the **pulse pressure.** For a blood pressure of 120/80, the pulse pressure is 40.

Physiology of Arterial Blood Pressure

Blood pressure reflects the interrelationships of cardiac output, peripheral vascular resistance, blood volume, blood viscosity, and artery elasticity. Knowledge of these hemodynamic variables helps in the assessment of blood pressure alterations.

Cardiac Output. Blood pressure depends on cardiac output. When volume increases in an enclosed space, such as a blood vessel, the pressure in that space rises. Thus, as cardiac output increases, more blood is pumped against arterial walls, causing the blood pressure to rise. Cardiac output increases as a result of an increase in heart rate, greater heart muscle contractility, or an increase in blood volume. Changes in heart rate can occur faster than changes in heart muscle contractility or blood volume. A rapid or significant increase in heart rate decreases the heart's filling time. As a result, blood pressure decreases.

Peripheral Resistance. Blood pressure depends on peripheral vascular resistance. Blood circulates through a network of arteries, arterioles, capillaries, venules, and veins. Arteries and arterioles are surrounded by smooth muscle that contracts or relaxes to change the size of the lumen. The size of arteries and arterioles changes to adjust blood flow to the needs of local tissues. For example, when more blood is needed by a major organ, the peripheral arteries constrict, decreasing their supply of blood. More blood becomes available to the major organ because of the resistance change in the periphery. Normally, arteries and arterioles remain partially constricted to maintain a constant flow of blood. Peripheral vascular resistance is the resistance to blood flow determined by the tone of vascular musculature and diameter of blood vessels. The smaller the lumen of a vessel is, the greater the peripheral vascular resistance to blood flow. As resistance rises, arterial blood pressure rises. As vessels dilate and resistance falls, blood pressure drops.

Blood Volume. The volume of blood circulating within the vascular system affects blood pressure. Most adults have a circulating blood volume of 5000 mL. Normally, the blood volume remains constant. However, if volume increases, more pressure is exerted against arterial walls. For example, the rapid, uncontrolled infusion of intravenous fluids elevates blood pressure. When circulating blood volume falls, as in the case of hemorrhage or dehydration, blood pressure falls.

Viscosity. The thickness or viscosity of blood affects the ease with which blood flows through small vessels. The **hematocrit,** or percentage of red blood cells in the blood, determines blood viscosity. When the hematocrit rises and blood flow slows, arterial blood pressure increases. The heart must contract more forcefully to move the viscous blood through the circulatory system.

Elasticity. Normally, the walls of an artery are elastic and easily distensible. As pressure within the arteries increases, the diameter of vessel walls increases to accommodate the pressure change. Arterial distensibility prevents wide fluctuations in blood pressure. However, in certain diseases, such as arteriosclerosis, the vessel walls lose their elasticity and are replaced by fibrous tissue that cannot stretch well. With reduced elasticity, resistance to blood flow is greater. As a result, when the left ventricle ejects its stroke volume, the vessels no longer yield to pressure. Instead, a given volume of blood is forced through the rigid arterial walls, and the systemic pressure rises. Systolic pressure is more significantly elevated than diastolic pressure as a result of reduced arterial elasticity.

Each hemodynamic factor significantly affects the others. For example, as arterial elasticity declines, peripheral vascular resistance increases. The complex control of the cardiovascular system normally prevents any single factor from permanently changing the blood pressure. For example, if the blood volume falls, the body compensates with increased vascular resistance.

Factors Influencing Blood Pressure

Blood pressure is not constant; it is continually influenced by many factors. One measurement cannot adequately reflect a client's blood pressure. Blood pressure changes from heartbeat to heartbeat. Blood pressure trends, not individual measurements, guide nursing interventions. By understanding these factors, you can more accurately interpret blood pressure readings.

Age. Normal blood pressure levels vary throughout life (Table 31–7). Blood pressure increases during childhood. The level of a child's or adolescent's blood pressure is assessed with regard to body size and age. An infant's systolic blood pressure ranges from 65 to 115 systolic, and the diastolic pressure ranges from 42 to 80. The normal systolic blood pressure for a 7-year-old is 87 to 117, and the normal diastolic pressure is 48 to 64. Larger children (heavier and/or taller) have higher blood pressures than do smaller children of the same age. During adolescence, blood pressure continues to vary according to body size.

An adult's blood pressure tends to increase with advancing age. The optimal blood pressure for a healthy, middle-aged adult is lower than 120/80. Systolic values of 130 to 139 and diastolic values of 85 to 89 are considered high normal (Canadian Hypertension Education Program, 2008; Table 31–8). Older adults may have a rise in systolic pressure that is related to decreased vessel elasticity; however, blood pressure higher than 140/90 is defined as hypertension and increases an older adult's risk for hypertension-related illness.

➤ TABLE 31-7 Average Optimal Blood Pressure for Age

Age	Blood Pressure (mm Hg)
Newborn (average, 3000 g)	40 (mean)
1 month	85/54
1 year	95/65
6 years*	105/65
10–13 years*	110/65
14–17 years*	120/75
>18	<120/80

*In children and adolescents, hypertension is defined as blood pressure that is, on repeated measurement, at the 95th percentile or higher, adjusted for age, height, and gender (Chobanian et al., 2003).

From Chobanian, A. V., Bakris, G. L., Black, H. R., Cushman, W. C., Green, L. A., Izzo, J. L., Jr., et al. (2003). The seventh report of the Joint National Committee on Detection, Evaluation, and Treatment of High Blood Pressure: The JNC 7 report. *Journal of the American Medical Association, 289,* 2560.

Stress. Anxiety, fear, pain, and emotional stress result in stimulation of the sympathetic nervous system, which increases heart rate, cardiac output, and peripheral vascular resistance. These alterations, in turn, increase blood pressure. Anxiety raises blood pressure by as much as 30 mm Hg.

Ethnicity. The incidence of hypertension is higher among ethnic groups such as South Asian, Aboriginal, and Black Canadians. Genetic and environmental factors are believed to be contributing factors.

Gender. Boys and girls do not have clinically significant differences in blood pressure levels. After puberty, boys tend to have higher blood pressure readings. After menopause, women tend to have higher levels of blood pressure than do men of similar ages.

Daily Variation. Blood pressure varies over the course of a day. In people who are active during the day, it is typically lowest during sleep between midnight and 0300 hours (Jones et al., 2006). Between 0300 and 0600 hours, blood pressure rises steadily. When the client awakens, blood pressure surges (Redon, 2004). Blood pressure is highest between 1000 and 1800 hours (Redon, 2004). No two people have the same pattern or degree of variation.

Medications. Some medications directly or indirectly affect blood pressure. During blood pressure assessment, ask whether the client is receiving antihypertensive or other cardiac medications, which lower blood pressure (Table 31–9). Another class of medications affecting blood pressure is opioid analgesics, which can lower blood pressure. Vasoconstrictors and an excess of intravenous fluids increase blood pressure.

Activity, Weight, and Smoking. Blood pressure can be reduced for several hours after a period of exercise. Older adults often experience a 5- to 10-mm Hg fall in blood pressure about 1 hour after eating. Increase in oxygen demand by the body during activity leads to increases in blood pressure. Inadequate exercise contributes to weight gain; obesity is a factor in hypertension. Smoking results in vasoconstriction. Blood pressure rises when a person is smoking, and it returns to baseline 15 minutes after smoking ceases.

Hypertension

The most common alteration in blood pressure is **hypertension.** Hypertension is often asymptomatic. The diagnosis of high normal blood pressure in adults is made when, on at least two visits to a health care professional after an initial high reading, an average of three or more diastolic readings is between 85 and 89 mm Hg or when the average of multiple systolic blood pressures on two or more subsequent visits is between 130 and 139 mm Hg. Hypertension is

TABLE 31-8 Classification of Blood Pressure for Adults Aged 18 and Older

Category	Systolic Pressure (mm Hg)	Diastolic Pressure (mm Hg)
Optimal	<120	<80
Normal	<130	<85
High normal	130–139	85–89
Grade 1 hypertension	140–159	90–99
Grade 2 hypertension	160–179	100–109
Grade 3 hypertension	≥180	≥110
Isolated systolic hypertension)	>140	<90

Adapted from Canadian Hypertension Education Program. (2008). *Recommendations for the management of hypertension. Part 1: Hypertension as a public health risk.* Retrieved April 1, 2008, from http://www.hypertension.ca/chep/educational-resources/slides (Introduction Slide 5).

noted with diastolic readings higher than 90 mm Hg and systolic readings higher than 140 mm Hg (Canadian Hypertension Education Program, 2008). Categories of hypertension have been developed and are used to determine medical intervention (see Table 31–8). One elevated blood pressure measurement does not qualify as a diagnosis of hypertension. However, if a high reading (e.g., 150/90 mm Hg) is obtained during the first blood pressure measurement, the client is encouraged to return for another checkup within 2 months. Home measurement of blood pressure is an important facet in the diagnosis of white coat hypertension and masked hypertension (Canadian Hypertension Education Program, 2008). In **white coat hypertension**, blood pressure is elevated during a visit to a health care professional. Affected clients are more likely to develop true hypertension over time. In **masked hypertension**, the blood pressure reading is normal while the client is with a health care professional but becomes elevated at home (Canadian Hypertension Education Program, 2008). Box 31–13 describes a nursing example.

Hypertension is associated with the thickening and loss of elasticity in the arterial walls. Peripheral vascular resistance increases within thick and inelastic vessels. The heart must continually pump against greater resistance. As a result, blood flow to vital organs such as the heart, brain, and kidney decreases.

People with a family history of hypertension are at significant risk. Modifiable risk factors linked to hypertension include obesity, cigarette smoking, heavy alcohol consumption, high sodium (salt) intake, sedentary lifestyle, and continued exposure to stress. The incidence of hypertension is higher among people with diabetes, among older adults, and in some ethnic groups. It is a major factor underlying deaths from strokes and is a factor contributing to myocardial infarctions (heart attacks). When hypertension is diagnosed, educate the client about blood pressure values, long-term follow-up care and therapy, the usual lack of symptoms (the fact that it may not be "felt"), the ability of therapy to control but not cure hypertension, and the importance of consistently following a treatment plan to ensure a relatively normal lifestyle (Canadian Hypertension Education Program, 2008).

Hypotension

Hypotension is considered present when the systolic blood pressure falls to 90 mm Hg or lower. Some adults have a low blood pressure normally; however, for the majority of people, low blood pressure is an abnormal finding associated with illness.

Hypotension occurs because of the dilation of the arteries in the vascular bed, the loss of a substantial amount of blood volume (e.g., as in hemorrhage), or the failure of the heart muscle to pump adequately (e.g., as in myocardial infarction). Hypotension associated with pallor, skin mottling, clamminess, confusion, increased heart rate, or decreased urine output is life-threatening and should be reported to a prescribing health care professional immediately.

TABLE 31-9 Antihypertension Medications

Medication Type	Names	Action
Diuretics	Furosemide (Lasix), spironolactone (Aldactone), metolazone, polythiazide, triamterene (Dyazide)	These lower blood pressure by reducing kidneys' reabsorption of sodium and water, thus lowering circulating fluid volume.
β-Adrenergic blockers	Atenolol (Tenormin), nadolol (Corgard), timolol maleate (Blocadren), propranolol (Inderal)	These combine with β-adrenergic receptors in the heart, arteries, and arterioles to block response to sympathetic nerve impulses; they reduce heart rate and thus cardiac output.
Vasodilators	Hydralazine hydrochloride (Apresoline), minoxidil (Loniten)	These act on arteriolar smooth muscle to cause relaxation and reduce peripheral vascular resistance.
Calcium channel blockers	Diltiazem (Cardizem, Dilacor XR), verapamil hydrochloride (Calan SR), nifedipine (Procardia)	These reduce peripheral vascular resistance by systemic vasodilation.
Angiotensin-converting enzyme (ACE) inhibitors	Ramipril (Altace), captopril (Capoten), enalapril (Vasotec), lisinopril (Prinivil, Zestril), benazepril (Lotensin)	These lower blood pressure by blocking the conversion of angiotensin I to angiotensin II, thereby preventing vasoconstriction; they also reduce aldosterone production and fluid retention, thereby lowering circulating fluid volume.
Angiotensin-II receptor blockers	Losartan (Cozaar), olmesartan (Benicar)	These lower blood pressure by blocking the binding of angiotensin-II, which prevents vasoconstriction.

BOX 31-13 NURSING STORY

White Coat Hypertension

Between the ages of 45 and 49, my neighbour, M. J., had a blood pressure reading of approximately 140/85 during her annual checkups. After each visit, I informed her that she may have white coat hypertension and recommended that she monitor her blood pressure at home because individuals who have white coat hypertension are at risk of developing true hypertension. I advised her to reduce her sodium dietary intake and to exercise regularly; she did not drink alcohol. I monitored her blood pressure at home; results were all below 135/85. At her annual checkup after her fiftieth birthday, her blood pressure was 140/86; at a follow-up visit 2 months later, it was 142/88. During that time, her blood pressure at home ranged between 136 and 140 (systolic) and 82 and 86 (diastolic). She went to the hypertension clinic to have a 24-hour blood pressure monitor applied. I informed her that this test would provide the physician with information to make treatment decisions. Because of high readings during the test, Dyazide [triamterene], 25 mg daily, was prescribed. I continued to monitor her blood pressure at home, but because her results remained in the hypertensive range, enalapril (Vasotec), 2.5 mg, was added to her blood pressure drug regimen at her next visit 4 months later. Since then, all of her blood pressure readings, both at home and in the physician's office, have been below 126 (systolic) and 82 (diastolic). Four years later, M. J.'s blood pressure continues to be controlled.

Orthostatic hypotension, also referred to as **postural hypotension**, occurs when a normotensive person (a person with normal blood pressure) develops symptoms of low blood pressure when rising to an upright position. When a healthy individual changes from lying down to a sitting or standing position, the peripheral blood vessels in the legs constrict. Vasoconstriction in the lower extremities during standing prevents the pooling of blood in the legs caused by gravity. Thus, no symptoms are normally felt in standing. In contrast, when clients have a decreased blood volume, their blood vessels are already constricted. When a volume-depleted client stands, blood pressure drops significantly, and heart rate increases to compensate for the drop in cardiac output. Clients who are dehydrated, are anemic, or have experienced prolonged bed rest or recent blood loss are at risk for orthostatic hypotension. Some medications can cause orthostatic hypotension if misused, especially in older adults or young clients. Blood pressure should always be measured before such medications are administered.

Assess for orthostatic hypotension during vital sign measurements by obtaining blood pressure and pulse with the client supine, sitting, and standing. The readings are obtained 1 to 3 minutes after the client changes position. In most cases, orthostatic hypotension is detected within a minute of standing up. If it occurs, assist the client to a lying position and notify the prescribing health care professional or nurse in charge. While obtaining orthostatic measurements, observe for other symptoms of hypotension such as fainting, weakness, or light-headedness. When recording orthostatic blood pressure measurements, record the client's position, in addition to the blood pressure measurement: for example: "140/80 supine, 132/72 sitting, 108/60 standing." Because the skill of orthostatic measurements requires critical thinking and ongoing nursing judgement, *do not delegate this procedure* to unregulated care providers.

Measurement of Blood Pressure

Arterial blood pressure may be measured either directly (invasively) or indirectly (noninvasively). The direct method requires the insertion of a thin catheter into an artery. Tubing connects the catheter to electronic monitoring equipment. The monitor displays a constant arterial pressure waveform and reading. Because of the risk of sudden blood loss from an artery, invasive blood pressure monitoring is used only in intensive care settings. The more common noninvasive method requires use of the sphygmomanometer and stethoscope. Measure blood pressure indirectly by auscultation or palpation. Auscultation is the most widely used technique (Skill 31–5).

Blood Pressure Equipment. Before assessing blood pressure, make sure that you know how to use a sphygmomanometer and stethoscope. A **sphygmomanometer** includes a pressure manometer, an occlusive cloth or vinyl cuff that encloses an inflatable rubber bladder, and a pressure bulb with a release valve that inflates the bladder. Manometers are of two types: aneroid (Figure 31–12) and mercury. Aneroid manometers have the advantages of being safe, lightweight, portable, and compact. The aneroid manometer has a glass-enclosed circular gauge containing a needle that registers millimetre calibrations. Before you use the aneroid model, make sure that the needle is pointing to zero and that the manometer is correctly calibrated. Aneroid sphygmomanometers require biomedical calibration every 6 months in order to verify accuracy (Jones et al., 2003).

Mercury manometers, once the "gold standard," are less common because they contain mercury, a hazardous substance. Most municipalities have prohibited the sale or use of mercury-containing devices because of potential hazards. However, some agencies or specific units (e.g., operating rooms or intensive care units) still use them. Pressure created by the inflation of the compression cuff moves the column of mercury upward against the force of gravity. Millimetre calibrations mark the height of the mercury column. To ensure accurate readings, the mercury column should fall freely as pressure is released and should always be at zero when the cuff is deflated. Obtain accurate readings by looking at meniscus of the mercury at eye level; looking up or down results in distorted readings.

Cloth or disposable vinyl compression cuffs contain an inflatable bladder and come in several sizes. The size selected is proportional to the circumference of the limb being assessed (Figure 31–13). Ideally, the width of the cuff should be 40% of the circumference (or 20% wider than the diameter) of the midpoint of the limb on which the cuff is used. The bladder, enclosed by the cuff, should encircle at least 80% of the arm of an adult and the entire arm of a child. Place the lower edge of the cuff above the client's antecubital fossa, allowing room for placement of the stethoscope bell or diaphragm. Many adults require a large cuff. Using the forearm when a large cuff is not available is not recommended (Box 31–14). Blood pressure measurements are not accurate unless the correct size blood pressure cuff is applied appropriately (Table 31–10).

The release valve of the aneroid or mercury sphygmomanometer should be clean and freely moveable in either direction. The valve, when closed, holds the pressure constant. A sticky valve makes pressure cuff deflation hard to regulate. The pressure bulb should be free of leaks.

Auscultation. The best environment for blood pressure measurement by auscultation is a quiet room at a comfortable temperature. Although the client may lie or stand, sitting is the preferred position. In most clients, blood pressure readings obtained in the supine, sitting, and standing positions are similar.

The client's position during routine blood pressure determination should be the same during each measurement to enable a meaningful comparison of values. Before measuring blood pressure, attempt to control factors responsible for artificially high readings, such as pain, anxiety, or exertion. The client's perceptions that the physical or interpersonal environment is stressful affects blood pressure measurement.

➤ SKILL 31-5 Measuring Blood Pressure

video

Delegation Considerations

In most provinces and territories, the task of measuring blood pressure can be delegated to unregulated care providers (UCPs). The nurse is responsible for assessing changes in blood pressure; therefore, when the task of measuring blood pressure is delegated, it is important to *inform the unregulated care provider* about the following:

- Selection of appropriate limb for blood pressure measurement
- Selection of appropriate-size blood pressure cuff for designated extremity
- Frequency of blood pressure measurement for client
- Client's usual values
- Abnormalities that should be reported to the health care professional

Equipment

- Aneroid sphygmomanometer
- Cloth or disposable vinyl pressure cuff of appropriate size for client's extremity
- Stethoscope
- Alcohol swab
- Pen and either vital sign flow sheet or record form

Procedure

STEPS	RATIONALE
1. Determine need to assess client's blood pressure:	• You use clinical judgement to determine need for assessment.
A. Note risk factors for alteration in blood pressure, including cardiovascular disease, renal disease, diabetes, circulatory shock, acute or chronic pain, rapid intravenous infusion of fluids or blood products, increased intracranial pressure, postoperative conditions, and toxemia of pregnancy.	• Certain conditions heighten risk for blood pressure alteration.
B. Observe for signs and symptoms of blood pressure alterations. (1) High blood pressure (hypertension): headache (usually occipital), flushing of face, nosebleed, and fatigue in older adults; high blood pressure is often asymptomatic until pressure is very high (2) Low blood pressure (hypotension): dizziness, mental confusion; restlessness; pale, dusky, or cyanotic skin and mucous membranes; and cool, mottled skin over extremities	• Physical signs and symptoms may indicate alterations in blood pressure.
2. Determine best site for blood pressure assessment. Avoid applying cuff to extremity when intravenous fluids are infusing; when an arteriovenous shunt or fistula is present; when breast or axillary surgery has been performed on that side; and when extremity has been traumatized, is diseased, or requires a cast or bulky bandage. Use lower extremities when the brachial arteries are inaccessible.	• Inappropriate site selection results in poor amplification of sounds, causing inaccurate readings. Application of pressure from inflated cuff bladder temporarily impairs blood flow and can exacerbate existing impairment of circulation in extremity.
3. Determine previous baseline blood pressure (if available) from client's record.	• Baseline measurement enables you to assess for change in client's condition and provides comparison with future blood pressure measurements.
4. Identify factors likely to interfere with accuracy of blood pressure measurement: exercise, caffeine, and smoking. Encourage client to avoid exercise and smoking for 15–30 minutes and ingestion of caffeine for 60 minutes before blood pressure is assessed (Canadian Hypertension Education Program, 2008).	• Exercise and smoking cause false elevations in blood pressure. Smoking increases blood pressure immediately, and this effect lasts up to 15 minutes. Caffeine (e.g., in coffee) increases blood pressure for up to 3 hours.
5. Explain to client that blood pressure is to be assessed, and have client rest at least 5 minutes before blood pressure is measured in sitting or lying position; wait 1 minute if client is standing. Ask client not to speak when blood pressure is being measured.	• These preparations allow client to relax and helps avoid falsely elevated readings. Blood pressure readings taken at different times can be objectively compared with readings taken with client at rest. Talking to a client when the blood pressure is being assessed may increase readings (Canadian Hypertension Education Program, 2008).
6. Select appropriate cuff size.	• Improper cuff size results in inaccurate readings. If cuff is too small, it comes loose when inflated or results in false high readings. A cuff that is too large may produce false low readings.
7. Perform hand hygiene.	• Hand hygiene reduces transmission of microorganisms between the client and the nurse.
8. Have client assume sitting or lying position. Be sure room is warm, quiet, and relaxing.	• These actions maintain client's comfort during measurement. The client's perceptions that the physical or interpersonal environment is stressful affect the blood pressure measurement.

Continued

➤ SKILL 31-5 Measuring Blood Pressure *continued*

STEPS	RATIONALE
9. With client sitting or lying, position client's forearm at heart level; position client's thigh flat (provide support as needed). To measure at client's arm, turn palm up (see Step 9 illustration); to measure at client's thigh, position with knee slightly flexed. If client is sitting, instruct client to sit with feet touching floor without crossing legs (Canadian Hypertension Education Program, 2008).	• If extremity is unsupported, client may perform isometric exercise that increases diastolic blood pressure. Leg crossing falsely elevates blood pressure.
10. Expose client's extremity (arm or leg) fully by removing constricting clothing.	• Exposure ensures proper cuff application.

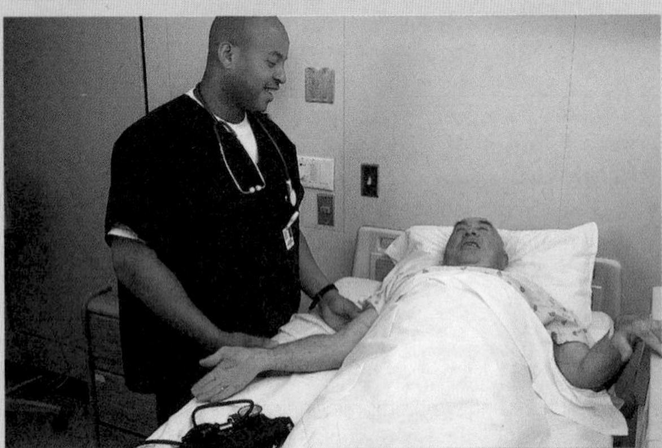

Step 9 Client's forearm supported in bed.

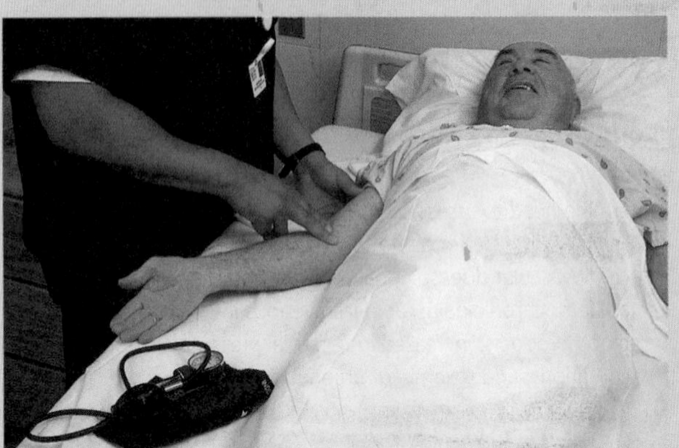

Step 10 Palpating client's brachial artery.

STEPS	RATIONALE
11. Palpate client's brachial artery (arm; see Step 10 illustration) or popliteal artery (leg). With cuff fully deflated, apply bladder of cuff above artery by centring cuff over artery. If no centre arrows appear on the cuff, estimate the centre of the bladder and place this centre over artery. Position cuff 2.5 cm above site of pulsation (antecubital or popliteal space). Wrap cuff evenly and snugly around extremity (see Step 11 illustrations). Do not place blood pressure cuff over clothing.	• Inflating bladder directly over artery ensures that proper pressure is applied during inflation. Loose-fitting cuff causes false high readings.

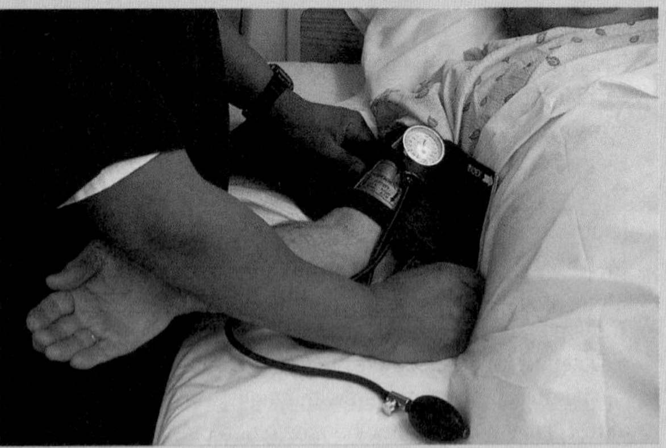

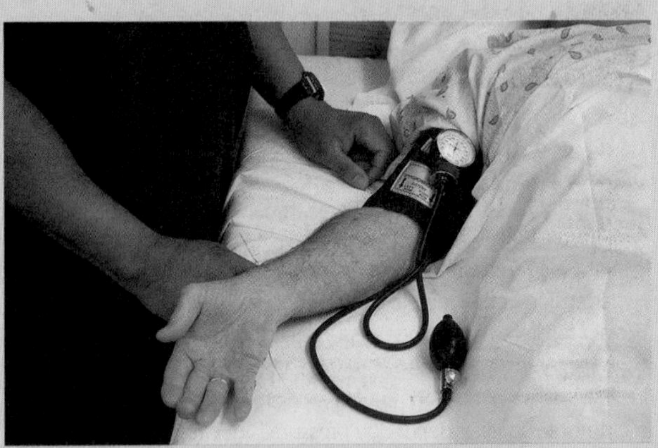

Step 11 **Left,** Bladder of cuff centred above artery. **Right,** Blood pressure cuff wrapped around upper arm.

STEPS	RATIONALE
12. Position aneroid needle no further than 1 metre away.	• Aneroid needle indicates correct readings.
13. Measure blood pressure.	
A. **Two-step method**	
(1) Relocate client's brachial pulse. Palpate the artery distal to the cuff with fingertips of nondominant hand while inflating cuff rapidly to pressure 30 mm Hg above point at which pulse disappears. Slowly deflate cuff, and note reading when pulse reappears. Deflate cuff fully and wait 30 seconds.	• Relocating prevents false low readings. Maximal inflation point for accurate reading can be determined by palpation. If you are unable to palpate artery because of weakened pulse, you can use an ultrasonic stethoscope (see Chapter 32). Completely deflating cuff prevents venous congestion and false high readings.

➤ SKILL 31-5 Measuring Blood Pressure *continued*

STEPS	RATIONALE
(2) Place stethoscope earpieces in your ears, and be sure sounds are clear, not muffled.	• Each earpiece should follow angle of ear canal to facilitate hearing.
(3) Relocate client's brachial or popliteal artery and place bell or diaphragm chestpiece of stethoscope over it. Do not allow chestpiece to touch cuff or clothing (see Steps 13A[3] illustration).	• Proper stethoscope placement ensures optimal sound reception. Stethoscope improperly positioned causes muffled sounds that often result in false low systolic readings and false high diastolic readings.

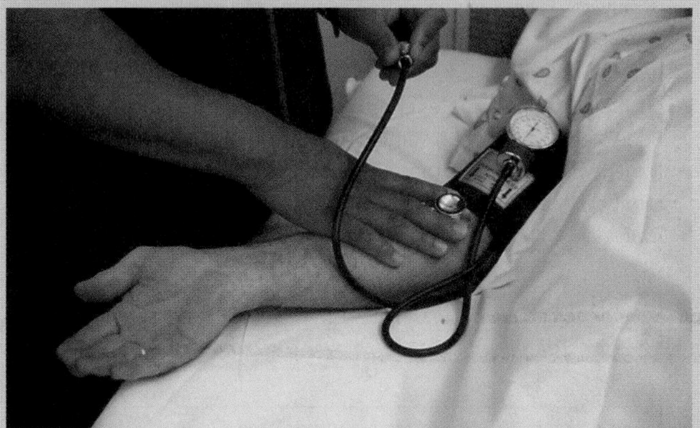

Step 13A(3) Stethoscope over brachial artery to measure blood pressure.

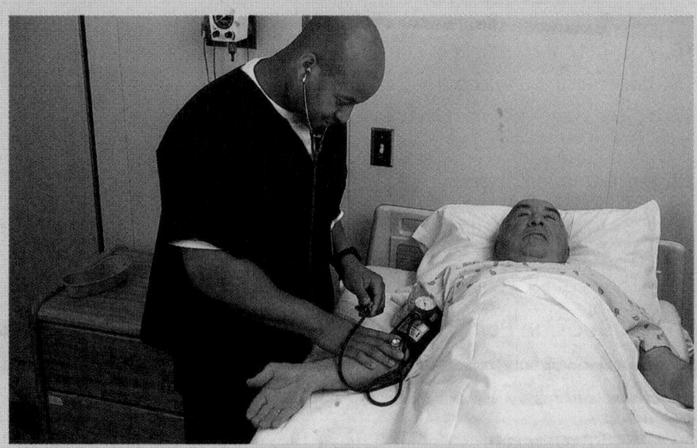

Step 13A(5) Inflating blood pressure cuff.

STEPS	RATIONALE
(4) Close valve of pressure bulb clockwise until it is tight.	• Tightening of valve prevents air leak during inflation.
(5) Quickly inflate cuff to 30 mm Hg above palpated systolic pressure (client's estimated systolic pressure; see Step 13A[5] illustration).	• Rapid inflation ensures accurate measurement of systolic pressure.
(6) Slowly release pressure bulb valve, and allow needle of manometer gauge to fall at rate of 2 to 3 mm Hg/second. Make sure no extraneous sounds are audible.	• Too rapid or slow a decline in pressure can cause inaccurate readings. Noise interferes with precise determination of Korotkoff phases.
(7) Note point on manometer when first clear sound is heard. The sound will slowly increase in intensity.	• First Korotkoff sound indicates systolic pressure.
(8) Continue to deflate cuff, noting point at which sound becomes muffled or dampened.	• Fourth Korotkoff sound is distinctly muffled and is indication of diastolic pressure in children.
(9) Continue to deflate cuff gradually, noting point at which sound disappears in adults. Listen for 10 to 20 mm Hg after the last sound, and then allow remaining air to escape quickly.	• Beginning of the fifth Korotkoff sound is indication of diastolic pressure in adults. Cuff is deflated as soon as possible because continuous cuff inflation causes arterial occlusion, resulting in numbness and tingling sensation in client's arm.
B. One-step method	
(1) Place stethoscope earpieces in your ears, and be sure sounds are clear, not muffled.	• Each earpiece should follow angle of ear canal to facilitate hearing.
(2) Relocate client's brachial or popliteal artery, and place bell or diaphragm chestpiece of stethoscope over it. Do not allow chestpiece to touch cuff or clothing.	• Proper stethoscope placement ensures optimal sound reception. Stethoscope improperly positioned causes muffled sounds that often result in false low systolic readings and false high diastolic readings.
(3) Close valve of pressure bulb clockwise until tight. Quickly inflate cuff to 30 mm Hg above palpated systolic pressure.	• Tightening of valve prevents air leak during inflation. Inflation above systolic level ensures accurate measurement of systolic pressure.
(4) Slowly release pressure bulb valve, and allow needle of manometer gauge to fall at rate of 2 to 3 mm Hg/second.	• Too rapid or slow a decline in pressure can cause inaccurate readings.
(5) Note point on manometer when first clear sound is heard. The sound will slowly increase in intensity.	• First Korotkoff sound indicates systolic pressure.
(6) Continue to deflate cuff, noting point at which sound becomes muffled or dampened.	• Fourth Korotkoff sound is distinctly muffled and indicates diastolic pressure in children.
(7) Continue to deflate cuff gradually, noting point at which sound disappears in adults. Listen for 10 to 20 mm Hg after the last sound, and then allow remaining air to escape quickly.	• Beginning of the fifth Korotkoff sound is indication of diastolic pressure in adults. Cuff is deflated as soon as possible because continuous cuff inflation causes arterial occlusion, resulting in numbness and tingling sensation in client's arm.

Continued

SKILL 31-5 Measuring Blood Pressure *continued*

STEPS	RATIONALE
14. Canadian Hypertension Education Program (2008) recommended that two readings separated by 2 minutes should be taken. If readings are different by more than 5 mm Hg, additional readings are necessary.	• Two sets of blood pressure measurements help prevent false-positive readings resulting from a client's sympathetic nerve response (alert reaction). Averaging minimizes the effects of anxiety, which often causes a first reading to be higher than subsequent measurements (Canadian Hypertension Education Program, 2008).
15. Remove cuff from extremity unless measurement must be repeated. If client's blood pressure is being assessed for the first time, repeat blood pressure assessment on other extremity.	• By comparing blood pressure in both extremities, you can detect circulation problems. (Difference of 5 to 10 mm Hg between extremities is normal.)
16. Assist client to return to comfortable position, and cover client's upper arm if it was previously clothed.	• These actions restore client's comfort and promote sense of well-being.
17. Discuss findings with client as needed.	• Such discussion promotes client's participation in care and understanding of health status.
18. Perform hand hygiene.	• Hand hygiene reduces transmission of microorganisms between the client and the nurse.
19. Compare reading with previous baseline value, acceptable value of blood pressure for client's age, or both.	• Evaluate for change in condition and alterations.

Critical Decision Point: In some situations (e.g., critically ill clients or those with peripheral vascular disease), it is often necessary to compare blood pressure readings in both arms, both legs, or all four extremities. If using upper extremities, use the arm with the higher pressure for subsequent assessments, unless this is contraindicated.

20. Correlate blood pressure with data obtained from pulse assessment and related cardiovascular signs and symptoms.	• Blood pressure and heart rate are interrelated.

Unexpected Outcomes and Related Interventions

Blood Pressure Reading Cannot Be Obtained

- Determine whether any immediate crisis is present by measuring pulse and respiratory rate.
- Assess for signs of decreased cardiac output (e.g., weak or thready pulse, confusion, pallor, or cyanosis). If any sign is present, notify nurse in charge or prescribing health care professional immediately.
- Use alternative sites or procedures to obtain blood pressure. Auscultate blood pressure in lower extremity, or use a Doppler ultrasonic instrument or a palpation method to obtain systolic measurement.
- Repeat blood pressure measurement with sphygmomanometer. Electronic blood pressure devices are less accurate in conditions of low blood flow.

Blood Pressure Is Not Sufficient for Adequate Perfusion and Oxygenation of Tissues

- Compare blood pressure value with baseline value. A systolic reading of 90 mm Hg is an acceptable value for some clients.
- Position client in supine position to enhance circulation, and restrict activity if it is causing blood pressure to decrease.
- Assess for signs of decreased cardiac output (e.g., weak or thready pulse, confusion, pallor, or cyanosis). If any sign present, notify nurse in charge or prescribing health care professional immediately.
- Increase rate of intravenous infusion, or administer vasoconstrictor drugs if ordered.

Blood Pressure Is Elevated Above Acceptable Range

- Repeat measurement in client's other arm, and compare findings. Verify correct selection and placement of cuff.
- Ask colleague to repeat measurement in 1 to 2 minutes.
- Observe for related symptoms (e.g., headache, confusion), although symptoms are sometimes not apparent until blood pressure is extremely elevated.
- Report elevated blood pressure to nurse in charge or prescribing health care professional immediately.
- Administer antihypertensive medications as ordered.

Recording and Reporting

- Inform client of value and need for periodic reassessment of blood pressure.
- Record blood pressure in nurses' notes or vital sign flow sheet. Document blood pressure in nurses' narrative notes after administration of specific therapies.
- Report abnormal findings to nurse in charge or prescribing health care professional.

Home Care Considerations

- Assess home noise level to determine which room will provide the quietest environment for assessing blood pressure.
- Consider using electronic blood pressure cuff in the home if client has hearing difficulties, adequate financial resources, and adequate dexterity.

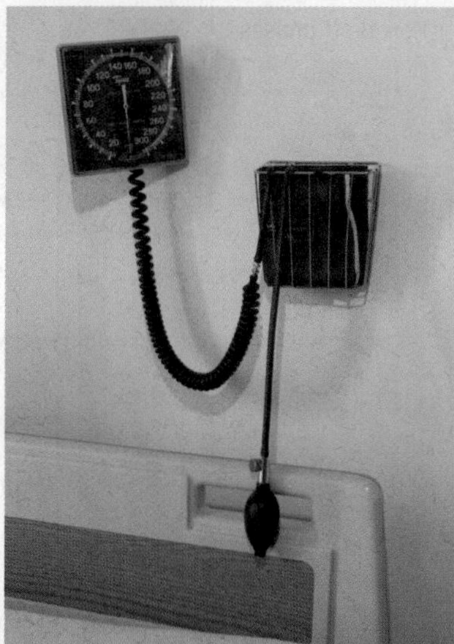

Figure 31-12 Wall-mounted aneroid sphygmomanometer.

During the initial assessment, measure and record the blood pressure in both arms. Normally, pressures in the arms differ by 5 to 10 mm Hg. In subsequent assessments, measure the blood pressure in the arm with the higher pressure. Pressure differences greater than 10 mm Hg indicate vascular problems and are reported to the prescribing health care professional or nurse in charge.

Ask the client to state his or her usual blood pressure. If the client does not know, inform the client after measuring and recording the blood pressure. Educate the client about optimal values of blood pressure, the risk factors for developing hypertension, and the dangers of hypertension.

Indirect measurement of arterial blood pressure works on a basic principle of pressure: Blood flows freely through an artery until an inflated cuff applies pressure to tissues and causes the artery to collapse. After the cuff pressure is released, the point at which blood flow returns and sound appears through auscultation is the systolic pressure.

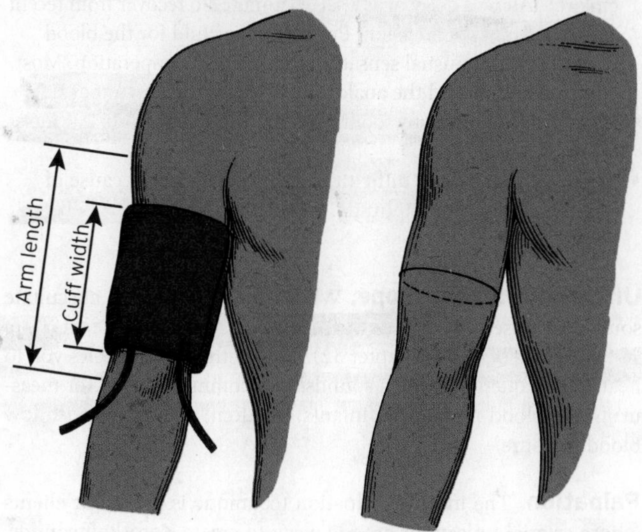

Figure 31-13 Guidelines for proper blood pressure cuff size. Cuff width should be 20% more than upper arm diameter, or 40% of circumference and two-thirds of arm length.

BOX 30-14 EVIDENCE-INFORMED PRACTICE GUIDELINE

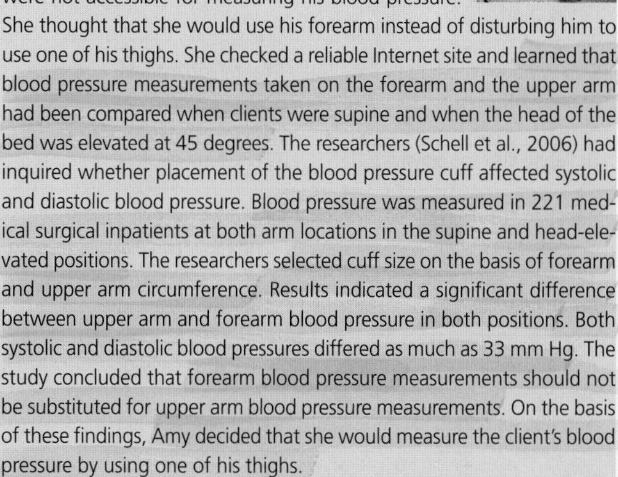

Forearm Versus Upper Arm Blood Pressure Measurements

Amy, a registered nurse, had a client whose upper arms were not accessible for measuring his blood pressure. She thought that she would use his forearm instead of disturbing him to use one of his thighs. She checked a reliable Internet site and learned that blood pressure measurements taken on the forearm and the upper arm had been compared when clients were supine and when the head of the bed was elevated at 45 degrees. The researchers (Schell et al., 2006) had inquired whether placement of the blood pressure cuff affected systolic and diastolic blood pressure. Blood pressure was measured in 221 medical surgical inpatients at both arm locations in the supine and head-elevated positions. The researchers selected cuff size on the basis of forearm and upper arm circumference. Results indicated a significant difference between upper arm and forearm blood pressure in both positions. Both systolic and diastolic blood pressures differed as much as 33 mm Hg. The study concluded that forearm blood pressure measurements should not be substituted for upper arm blood pressure measurements. On the basis of these findings, Amy decided that she would measure the client's blood pressure by using one of his thighs.

Application to Nursing Practice

Forearm blood pressure measurements should not be substituted for upper arm blood pressure measurements.

References: Schell, K., Lyons, D., Bradley, E., Bucher, L., Seckel, M., Wakai, S., et al. (2006). Clinical comparison of automatic noninvasive measurements of blood pressure in the forearm and upper arm with the client supine or with the head of the bed raised 45 degrees: A follow-up study. *American Journal of Critical Care, 15,* 196–205.

In 1905, Nikolai Korotkoff, a Russian surgeon, first described the sounds heard over an artery distal to the blood pressure cuff. The first Korotkoff sound is a clear rhythmical tapping that corresponds to the pulse rate and gradually increases in intensity. *Onset of the sound corresponds to the systolic pressure.* A blowing or swishing sound occurs as the cuff continues to deflate; this is the second Korotkoff sound. As the artery distends, blood flow becomes turbulent. The third Korotkoff sound is a crisper and more intense tapping. The fourth Korotkoff sound is muffled and low-pitched as the cuff is further deflated. At this point, the cuff pressure has fallen below the pressure within the vessel walls; *this sound is the diastolic pressure in infants and children.* The fifth Korotkoff "sound" is actually the disappearance of sound. *In adolescents and adults, the fifth sound corresponds to the diastolic pressure* (Figure 31–14). In some clients, the sounds are clear and distinct. In other clients, only the beginning and ending sounds are clear.

The Canadian Hypertension Education Program (2008) recommended recording two numbers for a blood pressure measurement: the point on the manometer when the first sound is heard, for the systolic reading, and the point on the manometer when the fifth sound is heard, for the diastolic reading. Some institutions recommend recording the point when the fourth sound is heard as well, especially for clients with hypertension. Divide the numbers by

TABLE 31-10 Common Mistakes in Blood Pressure Assessment

Error	Effect
Bladder or cuff too wide	False low reading
Bladder or cuff too narrow or too short	False high reading
Cuff wrapped too loosely or unevenly	False high reading
Deflating cuff too slowly	False high diastolic reading
Deflating cuff too quickly	False low systolic reading and false high diastolic reading
Arm below heart level	False high reading
Arm above heart level	False low reading
Arm not supported	False high reading
Stethoscope that fits poorly or impairment of the examiner's hearing, causing sounds to be muffled	False low systolic reading and false high diastolic reading
Stethoscope applied too firmly against antecubital fossa	False low diastolic reading
Cuff inflating too slowly	False high diastolic reading
Repeating assessments too quickly	False high systolic reading
Inadequate inflation level	False low systolic reading
Multiple examiners using different Korotkoff sounds for diastolic readings	False high systolic reading and low diastolic reading

slashed lines (e.g., "120/80" or "120/100/80"). Note the arm used to measure the blood pressure (e.g., "right arm [RA] 130/70"), and the client's position (e.g., "sitting").

Blood pressure findings prompt many medical decisions and nursing interventions concerning a client's health care. Obtaining an accurate blood pressure measurement is essential. Error can arise from several sources (see Table 31–10). When you are unsure of a reading, ask a colleague to reassess the blood pressure.

Assessment in Children. All children 3 years of age through adolescence should have blood pressure checked at least yearly. Blood pressure in children changes with growth and development. Help parents understand the importance of this routine screening in children who may be at risk for hypertension. The measurement of blood pressure in infants and children is difficult for several reasons:

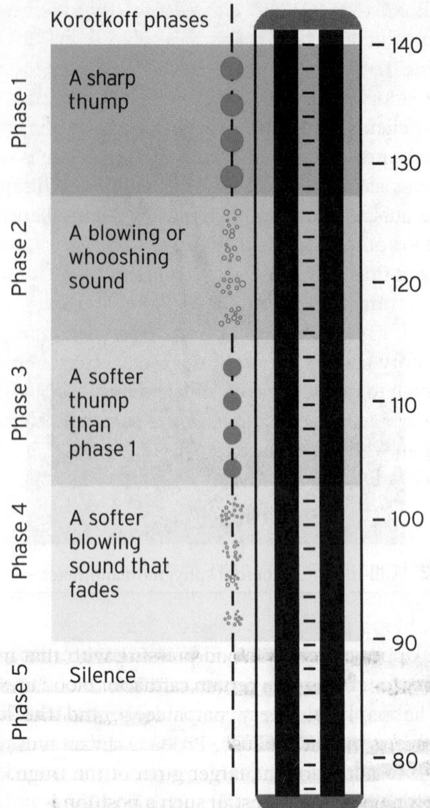

Figure 31-14 The sounds auscultated during blood pressure measurement can be differentiated into five Korotkoff phases. In this example, blood pressure is 140/90.

- Different arm sizes necessitate careful selection of appropriate cuff size. Do not choose a cuff on the basis of the name of the cuff; for example, an "infant" cuff may be too small for some infants.
- Readings are difficult to obtain in restless or anxious infants and children. Allow a delay of at least 15 minutes to recover from recent activities and apprehension. Preparing the child for the blood pressure cuff's unusual sensation can increase cooperation. Most children understand the analogy of a "tight hug on your arm."
- Placing the stethoscope too firmly on the antecubital fossa causes errors in auscultation.
- Korotkoff sounds are difficult to hear in children because of low frequency and amplitude. A pediatric stethoscope bell can be helpful.

Ultrasonic Stethoscope. When you are unable to auscultate sounds because of a weakened arterial pulse, you can use an ultrasonic stethoscope (see Chapter 32). This stethoscope enables you to hear low-frequency systolic sounds. It is commonly used for measuring the blood pressure of infants, children, and adults with low blood pressure.

Palpation. The indirect palpation technique is useful for clients whose arterial pulsations are too weak to create Korotkoff sounds. Severe blood loss and decreased heart contractility are examples of conditions that result in blood pressure too low to auscultate accurately. In these cases, the systolic blood pressure can be assessed by palpation; the diastolic pressure, however, is difficult to assess by palpation (Box 31–15). When using the palpation technique, record the systolic value and how it was measured (e.g., "RA 90/—, palpated, supine").

The palpation technique can be used with auscultation. In some hypertensive clients, the sounds usually heard over the brachial artery when the cuff pressure is high disappear as pressure is reduced, and then they reappear at a lower level. This temporary disappearance of sound is the **auscultatory gap.** It typically occurs between the first and second Korotkoff sounds. The gap in sound may cover a range of 40 mm Hg and thus may cause you to underestimate the systolic pressure or overestimate the diastolic pressure. You must be certain to inflate the cuff high enough to hear the true systolic pressure before the auscultatory gap. Palpation of the radial artery helps you determine how high to inflate the cuff. Inflate the cuff to 30 mm Hg above the pressure at which the radial pulse was palpated. Record the range of pressures in which the auscultatory gap occurs (e.g., "blood pressure RA 180/94 with an auscultatory gap from 180 to 160, sitting").

Lower Extremity Blood Pressure. Dressings, casts, intravenous catheters, or arteriovenous fistulas or shunts can render the upper extremities inaccessible for blood pressure measurement. In such cases, blood pressure is measured in the lower extremities. Comparing upper extremity blood pressure with that in the legs is also necessary for clients with certain cardiac or blood pressure abnormalities. The popliteal artery, palpable behind the knee in the popliteal space, is the site for auscultation. The cuff must be wide and long enough to allow for the larger girth of the thigh. Placing the client in a prone position is best. If such a position is impossible, ask the client to flex the knee slightly for easier access to the artery. Position the cuff 2.5 cm above the client's popliteal artery with the bladder over the posterior aspect of the midthigh (Figure 31–15). The procedure is identical to that for brachial artery auscultation. Systolic pressure in the legs is usually higher by 10 to 40 mm Hg than in the brachial artery, but the diastolic pressure is the same.

> **BOX 31-15** Procedural Guidelines
>
> ### Palpating the Systolic Blood Pressure
>
> **Delegation Considerations:** The skill of palpation of blood pressure *may not be delegated* to unregulated care providers.
>
> **Equipment:** Sphygmomanometer.
>
> **Procedure**
>
> 1. Perform hand hygiene.
> 2. Apply the blood pressure cuff to the client's extremity selected for measurement.
> 3. Continually palpate the pulse of the client's brachial, radial, or popliteal artery with fingertips of one of your hands.
> 4. Inflate the blood pressure cuff 30 mm Hg above the point at which the client's pulse cannot be palpated.
> 5. Slowly release the valve and deflate the cuff; if you are using a mercury manometer, allow the mercury in the manometer needle to fall 2 mm Hg per second.
> 6. Note the manometer reading when the pulse is again palpable; this is the systolic blood pressure.
> 7. Deflate the cuff rapidly and completely. Remove the cuff from the client's extremity unless repeat measuremennt is needed.
> 8. Perform hand hygiene. Record pressure as "[systolic]/—" and palpated (e.g., "blood pressure 108/—, palpated").

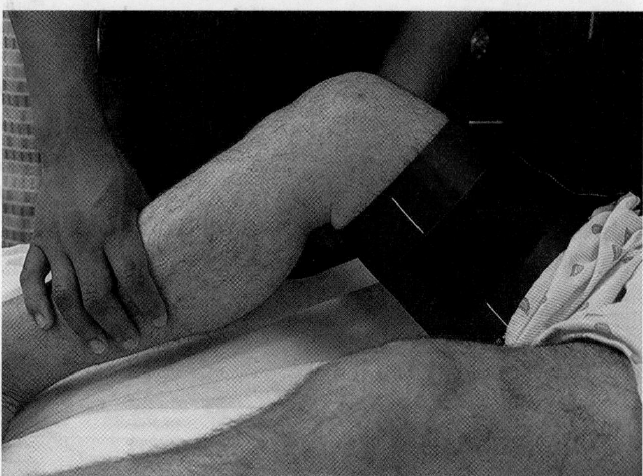

Figure 31-15 Lower extremity blood pressure cuff positioned above the popliteal artery at midthigh with knee flexed. **Source:** Courtesy St. Mary's Health Center. St. Louis, MO.

Automatic Blood Pressure Devices. Many styles of electronic devices are available to determine blood pressure automatically (Figure 31–16). For example, some devices rely on an electronic sensor to detect the vibrations caused by the rush of blood through an artery. When the cuff deflates, the sensor determines the initial burst of vibrations and translates the information into a systolic pressure reading. When the vibrations are lowest, just before they stop, the diastolic pressure is determined. Use electronic blood pressure machines when frequent blood pressure assessment is required, as in

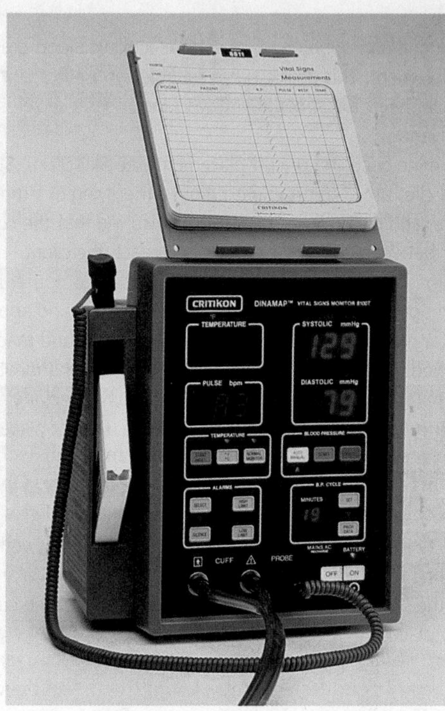

Figure 31-16 Automatic blood pressure monitor. **Source:** Dinamap Vital Signs Monitor is a trademark of Critikon, Inc. Photo courtesy Critikon, Inc., Tampa, FL.

critically ill or potentially unstable clients; during or after invasive procedures; or when therapies necessitate frequent monitoring (e.g., intravenous medications for cardiac and blood pressure conditions; Box 31–16). For some client conditions, the use of automatic blood pressure devices is not appropriate (Box 31–17).

Automatic devices are easy to use and efficient when measurements must be repeated or frequent. The ability to use a stethoscope is not required. However, automatic devices are more sensitive to outside interference, and their readings are susceptible to error. Most automatic blood pressure devices cannot process sounds or vibrations of low blood pressure. The range of device sophistication also can make blood pressure measurement comparisons difficult. The use of automatic blood pressure devices enables assessment of blood pressure during interpersonal interactions. However, avoid speaking to the client for at least a minute before you initiate a blood pressure recording. Talking to a client when the blood pressure is being assessed can increase readings 10% to 40% .

➤ BOX 31-16 Procedural Guidelines

Electronic Blood Pressure Measurement

Delegation Considerations: The task of obtaining an electronic blood pressure measurement can be delegated to an unregulated care provider unless the client is considered unstable or needs close monitoring. The nurse is responsible for assessing the impact of changes in blood pressure; therefore, when the task of obtaining an electronic blood pressure measurement is delegated, it is important to *ensure that the unregulated care provider* performs the following tasks:

- Selects appropriate limb for measurement.
- Selects appropriate-size cuff for designated limb.
- Selects blood pressure cuff recommended by manufacturer.
- Obtains blood pressure measurement for client with ordered frequency.
- Reports abnormalities.

Equipment: Electronic blood pressure machine and blood pressure cuff of appropriate size as recommended by manufacturer.

Procedure

1. Determine appropriateness of using electronic blood pressure measurement. This device is not suitable for use in clients with irregular heart rates, peripheral vascular disease, seizures, tremors, or shivering.
2. Determine best site for cuff placement (see Skill 31–5, Step 2).
3. Assist client to comfortable position, either lying or sitting. Plug in device, and place device near client, ensuring that the connector hose, between cuff and machine, will reach the client.
4. Turn machine on to enable device to self-test computer systems.
5. Select appropriate cuff size for client's extremity and appropriate cuff for machine. Electronic blood pressure cuff and machine are matched by the manufacturer and are not interchangeable.
6. Expose client's extremity for measurement by removing restrictive clothing, to ensure proper cuff application. Do not place blood pressure cuff over clothing.
7. Prepare blood pressure cuff by manually squeezing all air out of the cuff and connecting cuff to connector hose.
8. Wrap flattened cuff snugly around client's extremity, verifying that only one finger fits between cuff and client's skin. Make sure the "artery" arrow marked on the outside of the cuff is correctly placed.
9. Verify that connector hose between cuff and machine is not kinked. Kinking prevents proper inflation and deflation of cuff.
10. In accordance with manufacturer's directions, set frequency control to automatic or manual, and then press "start" button. The first blood pressure measurement will pump the cuff to a pressure of about 180 mm Hg. After this pressure is reached, the machine begins a deflation sequence that helps measure the blood pressure. The first reading is the peak pressure inflation for additional measurements.
11. When deflation is complete, digital display provides most recent values and flashes time (in minutes) that has elapsed since measurement occurred.
12. Set frequency of blood pressure measurements and upper and lower alarm limits for systolic, diastolic, and mean blood pressure readings. Intervals between blood pressure measurements are set from 1 to 90 minutes. Determine measurement frequency and alarm limits on the basis of client's acceptable range of blood pressure, your nursing judgement, and health care professional's order.
13. Obtain additional readings at any time by pressing the start button. (Sometimes you need these readings for unstable clients.) Pressing the "cancel" button immediately deflates the cuff.
14. If blood pressure determinations must be frequent, leave the cuff in place. Remove cuff at least every 2 hours to assess underlying skin integrity, and, if possible, alternate blood pressure sites. Clients with abnormal bleeding tendencies are at risk for microvascular rupture from repeated inflations. When electronic blood pressure machine is no longer needed, clean cuff according to facility policy to reduce transmission of microorganisms between clients.
15. Compare electronic blood pressure readings with auscultatory blood pressure measurements to verify accuracy of the electronic blood pressure device.
16. Record blood pressure and site assessed on vital sign flow sheet or in nurses' notes. Record associated signs of blood pressure alterations in nurses' narrative notes. Report abnormal findings to nurse in charge or health care professional.

➤ BOX 31-17 Client Conditions Not Appropriate for Electronic Blood Pressure Measurement

- Irregular heart rate
- Peripheral vascular obstruction (e.g., clots, narrowed vessels)
- Shivering
- Seizures
- Excessive tremors
- Inability of client to cooperate
- Systolic blood pressure of less than 90 mm Hg

You should obtain a baseline blood pressure measurement by using the auscultatory method before you apply automatic devices. A comparison assists in evaluation of a client's status and allows proper programming of the device. Once the blood pressure cuff is applied, program the device to obtain and record blood pressure readings at preset intervals. Alarm limits can be programmed to alert you if the blood pressure measurement is outside desired parameters.

Self-Measurement of Blood Pressure. More people measure their own blood pressure because of improved technology in home monitoring devices and a greater interest in health promotion. Portable home devices include aneroid sphygmomanometers and electronic digital readout devices that do not require use of a stethoscope. The electronic devices inflate and deflate cuffs with the push of a button. The electronic devices are easier to manipulate but require recalibration more than once a year. Because of their sensitivity, improper cuff placement or movement of the arm causes electronic devices to give incorrect readings.

Stationary automatic blood pressure devices can be found in public places such as grocery stores, drug stores, fitness clubs, airports, and worksites. Users simply rest their arms within the machine's inflatable cuff, which contains a pressure sensor. The cuff fits over clothing. A visual display tells users their blood pressure within 60 to 90 seconds. The reliability of the stationary machines is limited. Blood pressure values (both systolic and diastolic) may vary by 5 to 10 mm Hg or more in comparison with values measured by a manual sphygmomanometer.

Self-measurement of blood pressure has several benefits. Elevated blood pressure may be detected in people previously unaware of a problem. People with high normal blood pressure can provide information about the pattern of blood pressure values. Clients with hypertension can benefit from participating actively in their treatment through self-monitoring, which may enhance compliance with treatment. The disadvantages of self-measurement include improper use of the device and inaccurate readings. A client may be needlessly alarmed by one elevated reading. Clients with hypertension may become overly conscious of their blood pressure and inappropriately adjust medication intake.

Clients can learn to use self-measurement devices if they have the information needed to perform the procedure correctly and if they know when to seek medical attention. Advise clients that because of possible inaccuracies in the blood pressure devices, they must not adjust their medication regimens without consulting the health care professional. Help them understand the meaning and implications of readings, and teach them proper measurement techniques.

Nursing Process and Blood Pressure Determination

In assessing blood pressure and pulse, you evaluate the client's general state of cardiovascular health and responses to other system imbalances. Hypotension, hypertension, orthostatic hypotension, and narrow (small difference) or wide (large difference) pulse pressures are defining characteristics of certain nursing diagnoses, including the following:

- *Activity intolerance*
- *Anxiety*
- *Decreased cardiac output*
- *Deficient/excess fluid volume*
- *Risk for injury*
- *Acute pain*
- *Ineffective tissue perfusion*

The nursing care plan includes interventions specific for the nursing diagnosis identified and the related factors. For example, the defining characteristics of hypotension, dizziness, pulse deficit, and dysrhythmia lead to a diagnosis of *decreased cardiac output*. Related factors may include poor oral intake, excessive heat exposure, and a history of valvular heart disease. The related factor guides the choice of nursing interventions. Evaluate client outcomes by assessing the blood pressure after each intervention.

Health Promotion and Vital Signs

The emphasis on health promotion and health maintenance, as well as early discharge from hospital settings, has resulted in an increase in the need for clients and their families to monitor vital signs in the home. Teaching considerations affect all vital sign measurements. Incorporate them within the client's plan of care (Box 31–18).

Recording Vital Signs

Measurements of vital signs can be recorded on special graphic flow sheets (Figure 31–17). Identify your institution's procedure for documenting on the graphic or vital sign flow sheet. In addition to the actual vital sign values, record in the nurses' notes any accompanying or precipitating symptoms, such as chest pain and dizziness with abnormal blood pressure, shortness of breath with abnormal respiration, cyanosis with hypoxemia, or flushing and diaphoresis with elevated temperature. Document any interventions initiated as a result of abnormal vital sign measurements, such as administration of oxygen therapy or an antihypertensive medication.

For clients for whom critical paths or care maps are used, vital sign values may be listed as outcomes (see Chapter 13). If a vital sign value is higher or lower than the anticipated outcomes, write a variance note to explain the nature of the variance and your course of action. For example, a care map for a client who has undergone a thoracotomy may list a postoperative outcome of "afebrile." If the client has a fever, the nurse's variance note addresses possible sources of fever (e.g., retained pulmonary secretions) and nursing interventions (e.g., increased suctioning, postural drainage, or hydration).

BOX 31-18 FOCUS ON PRIMARY HEALTH CARE

Health Promotion and Vital Signs

Temperature

- Identify client's ability to initiate preventive health care and recognize alteration in body temperature. Educate client and caregiver about ways to prevent body temperature alterations.
- Teach clients risk factors for hypothermia and frostbite: fatigue; malnutrition; hypoxemia; cold, wet clothing; and alcohol intoxication.
- Teach clients risk factors for heat stroke: strenuous exercise in hot, humid weather; sudden exposure to hot climates; insufficient fluid intake before, during, and after exercise.
- Teach clients importance of taking and continuing to take antibiotics as directed until course of treatment is completed (e.g., to decrease chance of resurgence of infection or the development of antibiotic-resistant organisms).

Pulse Rate

- Clients taking certain cardiac medications need to learn to assess their own pulse rates to detect side effects.
- Clients undergoing cardiac rehabilitation need to learn to assess their own pulse rates to determine their response to exercise.

Blood Pressure

- Clients with family history of hypertension are at significant risk for hypertension. Teach risk factors for hypertension: obesity, cigarette smoking, heavy alcohol consumption, high blood cholesterol and triglyceride levels, and continued exposure to stress.
- Clients with hypertension need to learn about their blood pressure values, long-term follow-up care and therapy, the usual lack of symptoms, ability of therapy to control but not cure hypertension, and benefits of consistently following treatment plan.
- Teach client importance of appropriate-size blood pressure cuff for home use.
- Instruct client or primary caregiver to measure blood pressure at same time each day and after client has had a brief rest. Clients should measure blood pressure while sitting or lying down, and they should use the same position and arm each time they measure pressure.
- Instruct client or primary caregiver that if it is difficult to hear the pressure, the cuff may be too loose, not big enough, or too narrow; the stethoscope is not over arterial pulse; the cuff was deflated too quickly or too slowly; or the cuff was not pumped high enough for systolic readings.

Respirations

- Clients who demonstrate decreased ventilation benefit from learning deep breathing and coughing exercises (see Chapter 49).
- Instruct caregiver to contact home care nurse or prescribing health care professional if unusual fluctuations in respiratory rate occur.
- Teach client signs and symptoms of hypoxemia: headache, somnolence, confusion, dusky colour of skin and mucous membranes, shortness of breath, and dyspnea.
- Teach client effect of high-risk behaviours, such as cigarette smoking, on oxygen saturation.

When you consider how to teach clients and their families about vital sign measurements and their importance and significance, the client's age is an important factor. Because of the increase in the population of older adults, caregivers must be more aware of changes that are unique to older adults. Box 31–19 identifies some of these variations.

BOX 31-16 FOCUS ON OLDER ADULTS

Vital Signs

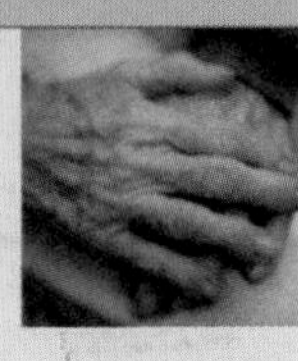

Temperature

- Normal body temperature ranges from 36°C to 36.8°C orally and 36.6°C to 37.2°C rectally. Temperatures considered to be within normal range sometimes reflect a fever in an older adult.
- Older adults are very sensitive to slight changes in environmental temperature because their thermoregulatory systems are not as efficient as they once were (Ebersole et al., 2004).

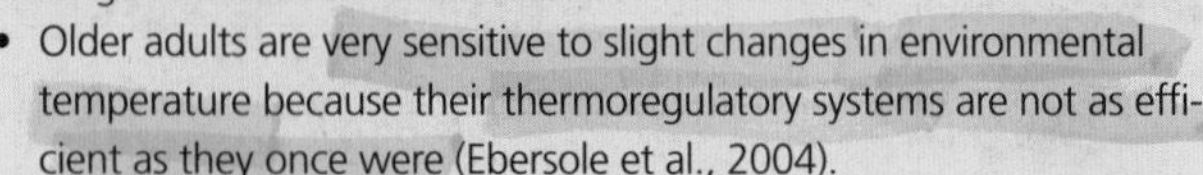

- Sweat gland reactivity decreases in older adults; as a result, sweating may not occur until temperatures are very high, and this leads to hyperthermia and heatstroke.
- For older adults, be especially attentive to subtle temperature changes and other manifestations of fever, such as tachypnea, anorexia, falls, delirium, and decline in overall function.
- Loss of subcutaneous fat reduces the insulating capacity of the skin; older men are especially at high risk for hypothermia.

Pulse Rate

- If it is difficult to palpate the pulse of an older adult or an obese client, a Doppler device provides a more accurate reading.
- Older adults have a decreased heart rate at rest (Ebersole et al., 2004).
- In older adults, it takes longer for the pulse rate to rise to meet sudden increased demands that result from stress, illness, or excitement. Once elevated, the pulse rate of an older adult takes longer to return to normal resting rate (Ebersole et al., 2004).
- Heart sounds are sometimes muffled or difficult to hear in older adults because of an increase in air space in the lungs.

Blood Pressure

- In older adults with decreased upper arm mass, blood pressure cuff size must be selected especially carefully.
- The normal range for blood pressure is the same in older adults as in younger adults. An older adult's blood pressure may elevate with age. Such elevations should not be considered a normal aspect of aging; minor elevations in older adults must be monitored (Chobanian et al., 2003).
- Older adults may have an increase in systolic pressure in relation to decreased vessel elasticity. The diastolic pressure remains the same, which results in a wider pulse pressure.
- Instruct older adults to change position slowly and wait after each change before beginning activity, to avoid orthostatic hypotension and prevent injuries.

Respirations

- Aging causes ossification of costal cartilage and causes the ribs to slant downward, which result in more rigidity of the rib cage, which in turn reduces chest wall expansion. Kyphosis and scoliosis that can occur in older adults restrict chest expansion and decrease tidal volume.
- Older adults depend more on accessory abdominal muscles during respiration than on weaker thoracic muscles.
- The respiratory system matures by the time a person reaches the age of 20 and begins to decline in healthy people after the age of 25. Despite this decline, older adults are able to breathe effortlessly as long as they are healthy. Sudden events that increase demand for oxygen (eg., stress, exercise, illness) lead to shortness of breath in the older adult (Ebersole et al, 2004).
- Identifying an acceptable site for the pulse oximeter probe may be difficult in older adults because of the likelihood of peripheral vascular disease, decreased cardiac output, cold-induced vasoconstriction, and anemia.

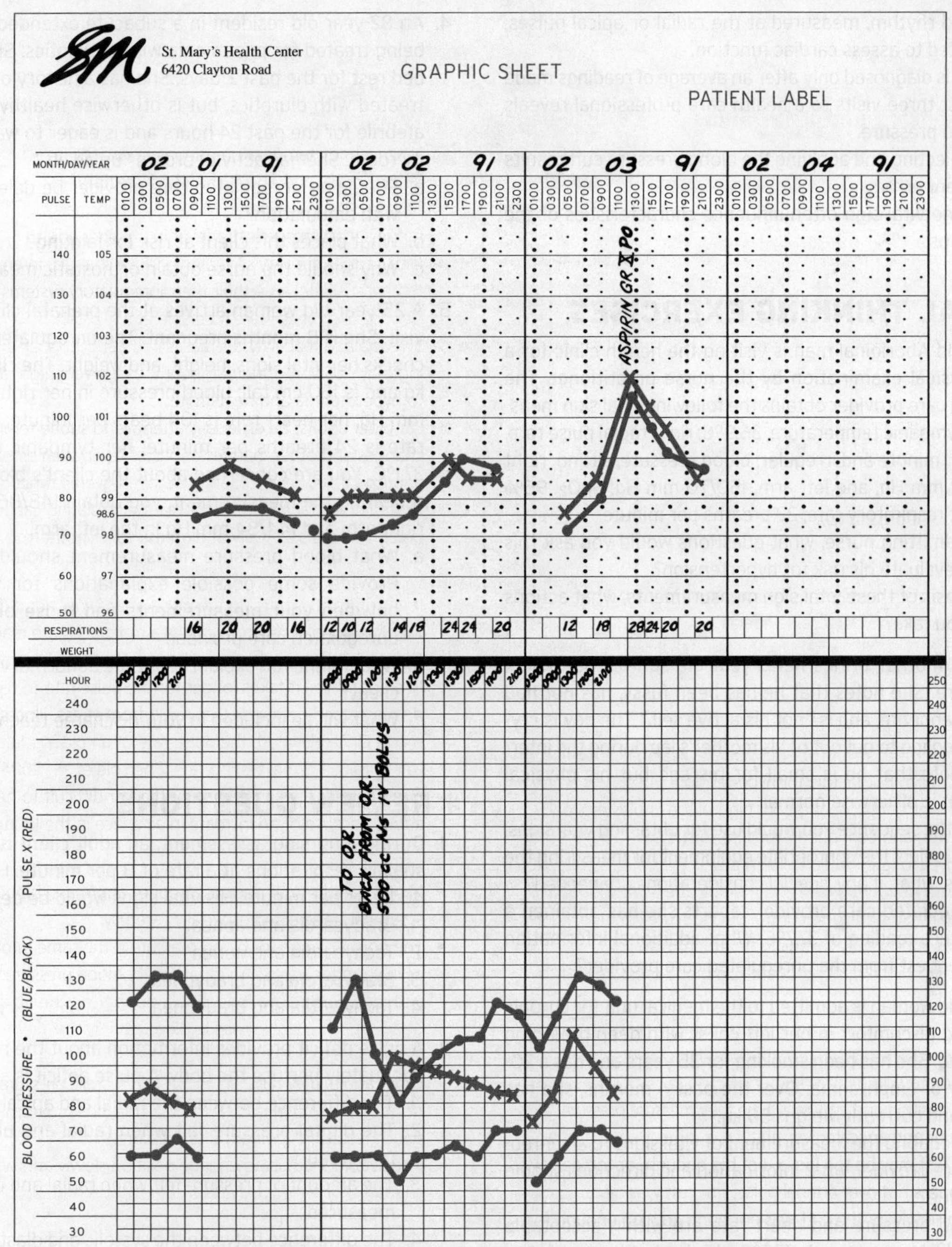

Figure 31-17 Vital signs graphic flow sheet. **Source:** Courtesy St. Mary's Health Center. St. Louis, MO.

✻ KEY CONCEPTS

- Vital sign measurement includes the physiological measurement of temperature, pulse, blood pressure, respiration, and oxygen saturation.
- Vital signs are measured as part of either a complete physical examination or a review of a client's condition.
- Changes in vital signs are evaluated with other physical assessment findings; clinical judgement is used to determine frequency of measurement.
- Knowledge of the factors influencing vital signs assists in determining and evaluating abnormal values.
- Vital signs provide a basis for evaluating response to nursing interventions.
- Vital signs should be measured when the client is inactive and the environment is controlled for comfort.
- Clients should be assisted in maintaining body temperature by interventions that promote heat loss, production, or conservation.
- A fever is one of the body's normal defence mechanisms.
- Measurement of temperature with the temporal artery is the least invasive, most accurate method of obtaining core temperature.
- Respiratory assessment includes determining the effectiveness of ventilation, perfusion, and diffusion.
- Assessment of respiration involves observing ventilatory movements through the respiratory cycle.
- Variables affecting ventilation, perfusion, and diffusion influence oxygen saturation.

- Pulse rate and rhythm, measured at the radial or apical pulses, are documented to assess cardiac function.
- Hypertension is diagnosed only after an average of readings made during at least three visits to a health care professional reveals elevated blood pressure.
- Improperly selecting and applying the blood pressure cuff results in measurement errors.
- Changes in one vital sign often influence characteristics of the other vital signs.

* CRITICAL THINKING EXERCISES

1. A 47-year-old Aboriginal man is visiting the health clinic for a routine physical examination by the nurse practitioner. The unregulated care provider obtains the following vital sign measurements: tympanic temperature, 36.9°C; right radial pulse rate, 96 beats per minute and irregular; blood pressure, sitting, right arm, 162/82 mm Hg, and left arm, 150/70 mm Hg; SpO_2, 95% on room air; respiratory rate, 22 breaths per minute.
   a. As the admitting nurse, what questions would you ask this client to evaluate his risk for hypertension?
   b. On the basis of these vital sign measurements, what actions should you take?
2. A teenaged mother brings her 3-year-old son to the walk-in health centre. She notes that he has been fussy, has not had much of an appetite, and is "not his active self." The boy is crying and struggling to get out of his mother's lap during the interview. You note that he is small for his age but his physical development is otherwise normal.
   a. Describe the sequence you would use for obtaining vital signs.
   b. When you select the appropriate equipment for measuring the vital signs, what, if any, special considerations are needed?
   c. The unregulated care provider reports she has obtained a temperature reading of 37.7°C. What additional information do you request from the unregulated care provider?
3. A 52-year-old woman is admitted to the medical unit for chronic dyspnea and discomfort in her left chest with deep breathing and coughing. She has been smoking for 35 years and has a 20-year history of emphysema. Over the past 4 months, she has lost 4.5 kg and currently weighs 50 kg.
   a. When delegating the measurement of vital signs to an unregulated care provider, what information and directions should you provide?
   b. The blood pressure and heart rate are within acceptable ranges. The temperature is 37.5°C, obtained with an oral electronic thermometer; the respiratory rate 32 breaths per minute and shallow; and the SpO_2 is 89%. On the basis of these results, list your actions in priority order.
4. An 82-year-old resident in a subacute extended care facility is being treated for pneumonia with antibiotics. She has been on bed rest for the past 2 days. She has a history of hypertension, treated with diuretics, but is otherwise healthy. She has been afebrile for the past 24 hours and is eager to walk to the activity room. She has activity orders "up ad lib."
   a. Should an unregulated care provider be delegated to assist with ambulation?
   b. What places this client at risk for fainting?
   c. Why should the nurse obtain orthostatic measurements?
5. A 25-year-old woman arrives at the prenatal clinic for her first visit. She is 8 months pregnant. The unregulated care provider checks her vital signs, height, and weight. The client weighs 104 kg and is 160 cm tall; blood pressure in her right arm is 210/92 mm Hg; her heart rate is 104 beats per minute; her respiratory rate is 24 breaths per minute; her tympanic temperature is 37.1°C. You are concerned about the client's blood pressure. In repeating the measurement, you obtain 148/86 mm Hg in the right arm and 144/84 mm Hg in the left arm.
   a. What blood pressure measurement should be recorded? Provide some possible explanations for the difference between your measurements and those obtained by the unregulated care provider.
   b. What might you explain about the abnormal vital signs to the client?
   c. What will be included in your discharge teaching?

* REVIEW QUESTIONS

1. During a nursing assessment, an adult client is noted to have shallow respirations at a rate of 8 per minute. His heart rate is 46 beats per minute. His vital signs would be described as
   1. Bradycardia and apnea
   2. Tachycardia and apnea
   3. Bradycardia and bradypnea
   4. Tachycardia and bradypnea
2. A pulse deficit provides information about the heart's ability to adequately perfuse the body. A pulse deficit is
   1. The difference between the radial and apical pulse rates
   2. The digital pressure felt when radial and ulnar pulses are measured
   3. The amount of pressure felt when radial and ulnar pulses are measured
   4. The difference between the systolic and diastolic blood pressure readings

3. As individuals approach older adulthood, body temperature tends to
   1. Gradually drop
   2. Gradually rise
   3. Fluctuate
   4. Remain the same

4. If a blood pressure cuff is too small, the blood pressure reading is
   1. Falsely low
   2. Falsely high
   3. Difficult to hear because sounds are muffled
   4. Dependent on the examiner's hearing acuity

5. Clients with apnea experience
   1. Difficult respiration that requires more effort
   2. Slowness of breathing, followed by rapid breathing
   3. Cessation of breathing that may be temporary
   4. Lack of oxygen to body tissues and organs

6. An older adult recently on bed rest is assisted out of bed. The nurse measures his blood pressure as the client changes position, and the results are as follows: 140/80 supine, 132/72 sitting, 108/60 standing. The client also mentions that he feels light-headed. The nurse should immediately
   1. Assist the client to return to a supine position
   2. Obtain a blood pressure measurement in the other arm
   3. Report the findings to the nurse in charge
   4. Help the client walk

7. A nurse is measuring a client's vital signs. The nurse notes that the radial pulse is initially strong, diminishes in intensity, and has an interruption in rhythm about every four to six beats. The nurse should immediately
   1. Report the findings to a health care professional
   2. Measure the apical pulse for 60 seconds
   3. Connect the client to a cardiac monitor
   4. Measure apical and radial pulse rates simultaneously for 60 seconds

8. Nursing interventions such as applying cool cloths act to decrease body temperature through
   1. Conduction
   2. Convection
   3. Evaporation
   4. Radiation

9. Poor oxygenation of the blood ordinarily affects the pulse rate, causing it to become
   1. Bounding
   2. Irregular
   3. Faster than normal
   4. Slower than normal

10. Which of these basic techniques are used to determine vital signs?
    1. Inspection, palpation, and auscultation
    2. Inspection, blood work, and radiography
    3. Rhythm and rate measurements and open communication
    4. Psychology, physiology, and nursing skills

* RECOMMENDED WEB SITES

Canadian Hypertension Society: http://www.hypertension.ca/
This Web site has links to three key organizations dealing with hypertension in Canada: (1) the Canadian Hypertension Society (CHS), (2) the Canadian Hypertension Education Program (CHEP), and (3) Blood Pressure Canada (BPC). The site offers information on hypertension to health professionals and the public. It also includes valuable links to related topics (e.g., Heart and Stroke Canada). The mission of CHS is to promote the prevention and control of hypertension through research and education. CHEP is the volunteer, non-profit hypertension education program that provides annually updated, relevant, evidence-informed hypertension guidance. BPC is committed to providing high-quality educational material and sources for clients. All sites provide educational tools.

Centre for Chronic Disease Prevention and Control: Cardiovascular Disease: http://www.phac-aspc.gc.ca/ccdpc-cpcmc/cvd-mcv/links_e.html
This Web page, part of the Web site of the Public Health Agency of Canada, provides links to a variety of Canadian resources on cardiovascular health, including the Heart and Stroke Foundation of Canada and the Canadian Stroke Network.

British Columbia Ministry of Health Services, Guidelines and Protocols Advisory Committee (GPAC): Hypertension–Detection, Diagnosis and Treatment of Hypertension: http://www.bcguidelines.ca/gpac/submenu_cardi.html
Part of the British Columbia Ministry of Health Services, the Guidelines and Protocols Advisory Committee developed several documents to recommend proper blood pressure management, including, in Appendix A, recommended technique for measuring blood pressure. Other topics include home blood pressure monitoring, dietary approaches, and a patient guide.

Heart & Stroke Foundation of Alberta, Northwest Territories, and Nunavut: Blood Pressure Action Plan: http://www.heartandstroke.ab.ca/site/c.lqIRL1PJJtH/b.3945715/k.8AB3/Blood_Pressure_Action_Plant.htm
Sponsored by the Public Health Agency of Canada (Health Canada) and the Heart and Stroke Foundation of Canada, this Web site provides information on several issues related to cardiovascular health, including high blood pressure and heart disease.

32

Health Assessment and Physical Examination

Written by D. Lynn Skillen, RN, PhD
Marjorie C. Anderson, RN, PhD
Rene A. Day, RN, PhD and
Tracey C. Stephen, MN RN

objectives

Mastery of content in this chapter will enable you to:

- Define the key terms listed.
- Conduct a symptom/sign analysis as the basis for a focused physical examination.
- List basic physical examination techniques.
- Describe the preparation of the nurse, client, and environment for the physical examination.
- Describe the essential techniques used in the physical examination of body systems and regions.
- Explain the rationale for the techniques and procedures of physical examination.
- List the specific characteristics to be assessed during the physical examination of body systems and regions.
- Describe the findings expected from the physical examination of adults.
- List age-related changes expected to be identified in the physical examination of adults.
- Integrate data from preventive screening examinations and client self-examinations with those from the physical examination.
- Identify the focus for client health promotion.
- Document physical examination findings using the standard format, appropriate terminology, physical examination criteria, and principles of recording.

key terms

Adventitious sounds, p. 590
Anatomical position, p. 551
Apical impulse, p. 592
Audible sounds, p. 546
Auscultation, p. 541
Benign, p. 578
Borborygmi, p. 602
Bruit, p. 580
CAGE questions, p. 544
Capillary refill, p. 614
Capillary return, p. 566
Cultural sensitivity, p. 541
Cyanosis, p. 562
Delirium, p. 558
Direct lighting, p. 544
Distension, p. 601
Edema, p. 564
Fasciculations, p. 614
General survey, p. 624
Health history, p. 541
Hernias, p. 600
Induration, p. 563
Inflammation, p. 562
Inspection, p. 541
Integument, p. 561
Intertriginous, p. 562
Jaundice, p. 563
Lesions, p. 561
Melanoma, p. 562
Mental status, p. 557
Metastasize, p. 595
Objective data, p. 541
Oblique (tangential) lighting, p. 544
Palpation, p. 541
Papanicolaou (Pap) smear, p. 607
Patency, p. 576
Percussion, p. 541
Peristalsis, p. 600
Petechiae, p. 562
Physical assessment, p. 541
Precordium, p. 592
Primary prevention, p. 541
Routine practices and additional precautions, p. 557
Screening, p. 557
Secondary prevention, p. 541
Sign, p. 542
Sternal angle, p. 587
Subjective data, p. 541
Symptom/sign analysis, p. 541
Symptoms, p. 542
Syncope, p. 580
Tactile fremitus, p. 590
Turgor, p. 563
Vital signs, p. 542

media resources

evolve Web Site

- Animations
- Audio Chapter Summaries
- Glossary
- Multiple-Choice Review Questions
- Student Learning Activities
- Weblinks

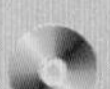 **Companion CD**

- Glossary
- Interactive Learning Activities
- Fluids and Electrolytes Tutorial
- Test-Taking Skills

Whether employed in urban, rural, remote, or international health care settings, as a Canadian nurse, you must have a firm foundation in the knowledge and skills required for physical examination. You will use four basic examination modes—**inspection**, **palpation**, **percussion**, and **auscultation**—to perform the following tasks:

- Obtain baseline client data for comparison with future assessment findings.
- Refute, confirm, or supplement an existing client database.
- Obtain information to be used for symptom/sign analysis, which helps determine the focus of the physical examination.
- Identify client response to treatment and changes in client condition or function.
- Detect treatable client conditions early.
- Determine learning needs and opportunities for clients.
- Identify high-risk clients through screening.
- Interpret patterns in examination findings and make clinical nursing judgements.
- Determine whether more comprehensive examinations, including diagnostic tests, are required.
- Individualize client care.
- Practise **primary**, **secondary**, and tertiary **prevention**.
- Document physical examination findings to inform other members of the interdisciplinary health care team.

Purposes of Physical Examination

Subjective data are collected while taking the **health history** (see Chapter 13) and conducting a symptom/sign analysis, and **objective data** are collected during the physical examination. By obtaining the client history first, you initiate a relationship with the client, which promotes trust and sharing of key information. Clients' subjective data determine the areas of focus in the physical examination. Similarly, the **symptom/sign analysis** helps you to plan a focused physical examination and address clients' presenting concerns. You conduct a focused physical examination when constraints of time, personnel, and health care settings exist, or when clients' conditions or responses warrant the shortest, most relevant examination, guided by the symptom/sign analysis. Acutely ill clients, for example, require nursing assessments that are efficient and focused only on the affected body systems or regions.

Subjective information helps you understand the life context of your clients, discuss health needs with them, and focus on their main concerns. Objective information enables you to make clinical judgements, identify teaching opportunities, and document the health status of clients using standardized assessment techniques. The level of accuracy of your assessments will influence the management of clients' health problems.

Comprehensive examinations, the preferred method for collecting baseline data, facilitate identification of clients' strengths and resources; promotion of wellness behaviours; early detection of potential and actual health problems; eligibility determination for health insurance, military service, and new employment; and recommendations for admission to a health care facility.

Integrate focused, context-based **physical assessment** into your daily routine. While providing a bed bath to a client, you can assess the condition of the integumentary system. You observe ambulatory clients to assess their gait, balance, and range of motion. When performing oral hygiene on debilitated clients, you observe the structures of the oral cavity. By integrating assessment skills into all your encounters with clients, you make efficient use of the available time.

Physical assessment should become an automatic practice whenever you interact with your clients. The same skill that you use to assess a client's condition (e.g., palpating a pulse) is the one you use to evaluate your nursing care (e.g., evaluating tolerance to an exercise plan). Your measurements and observations help determine whether expected outcomes of care are being met and whether the client's status is stable, improving, or deteriorating (Box 32–1).

Cultural Sensitivity and Responsiveness

In Canada's multicultural society, clients and nurses often bring many cultural differences to their interactions (Box 32–2). As a nurse, you demonstrate **cultural sensitivity** when you respect and respond sensitively to differences (see Chapter 10) and take into consideration clients' health beliefs, use of alternative therapies, nutritional habits, family and community relationships, and level of comfort with physical closeness and examination.

Never stereotype clients on the basis of their gender or racial background. Education, experience, and sensitivity help you distinguish between cultural characteristics and physical characteristics of clients. Learn about the genetic disorders that are commonly found in the ethnic populations in your service area. Be aware of biological variations that can be observed during physical examination. For example, clients of European descent commonly have RH-negative

BOX 32-1 Purposes of Physical Examination by Nurses

- Gathering baseline data on clients' health status
- Supplementing, confirming, or refuting data obtained during history taking
- Providing clients with learning opportunities for self-examinations or understanding of body changes
- Identifying potential and actual health problems
- Determining or confirming nursing diagnoses
- Monitoring clients' response to nursing interventions
- Making clinical judgements about clients' changing health status and management of care
- Determining eligibility for employment, insurance, or admission to a health care facility
- Evaluating the physiological outcomes of care

BOX 32-2 CULTURAL ASPECTS OF CARE

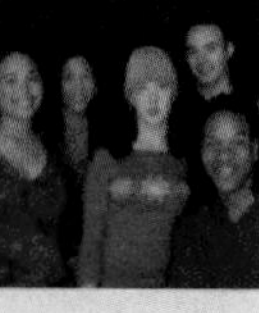

Culture influences the following aspects of health care:

- Interpretation of symptoms by health care professionals
- Client's decision to consult with family or community members
- Client's willingness to seek professional health care
- Client's preference for alternative medicine
- Client's willingness to assume responsibility for health
- Expectations of health care professionals
- Client's gender preference for health care professionals
- Client's response to health care professionals' assessments

blood types, in contrast to individuals of African and Asian backgrounds, who present as RH negative less often, and Inuit clients, who show no evidence of RH-negative blood. Acceptance of ethnic diversity enables you to respect the uniqueness of each client, consider alternative explanations for presenting concerns, make accurate observations about health status, and provide culturally safe care.

Mobility

Many Canadians are highly mobile and travel for work, study, family occasions, or pleasure; they are at risk for environment-related or infectious diseases (Box 32–3). Therefore, inquire about travel when you take a health history, and consider possible travel-related reasons for observations made during the physical examination of symptomatic clients.

Analyzing Signs and Symptoms

Collect data on clients' signs and symptoms in order to make a thorough assessment. A substantial database is the foundation for accurate diagnosis, treatment, intervention, referral, and education.

A **sign** is an observeable action or physical manifestation. In the health care context, it may be a physical finding, expression, or bodily movement that is observed using visual, olfactory, tactile, and auditory senses. Because signs can be seen, measured, felt, heard, or smelled, they are considered objective data. Measurements of blood pressure, height, weight, visual acuity, and temperature are examples of objective data. Other objective data include diagnostic test results (e.g., X-rays) and laboratory findings (e.g., blood work). Because objective data are observable, they can help validate subjective reports. For example, your client reports having an itchy patch of skin, and you see an area of dryness; your objective data thus validate the client's subjective information.

Symptoms are sensations or emotions reported by a client, unobservable by others and not always verifiable (e.g., nausea, numbness, and tingling). Subjective data therefore come from the client and may be collected at any time in the course of history taking and physical examination. Some essential data can only be collected through client reports. Using *symptom/sign analysis,* a systematic way of collecting more information about a sensation, emotion, or physical manifestation, helps the client describe the symptom or sign as completely and accurately as possible (Table 32–1). Accuracy of the information depends on two major factors: client reliability and your interpretation of the findings. Other factors to keep in mind when analyzing symptoms and signs are cultural response to the situation, underlying disease or dysfunction, language barriers, socioeconomic factors, and ethical or legal issues.

Analysis of a client concern (e.g., headache, bruising) provides comprehensive information about the symptom or sign. The analysis includes descriptions of 10 characteristics of a symptom or sign (see Table 32–1), all of which contribute to a substantive database containing important information. First, ask the client a broad question, for example, "Can you describe your headache?" After the client provides as much information as possible, use direct questioning about all 10 important characteristics.

➤ BOX 32-3 Examples of Diseases Acquired by Canadians During Travel

Ascariasis	Japanese encephalitis
Chagas' disease	Malaria
Cholera	Rabies
Cryptosporidiasis	Salmonellosis
Dengue fever	SARS (sudden acute respiratory syndrome)
Filariasis	Shigellosis
Giardiasis	Schistosomiasis
Hepatitis (A–E)	STIs (sexually transmitted infections)
HIV/AIDS (human immunodeficiency virus/acquired immune deficiency syndrome)	Tetanus
Hookworm infestation	Yellow fever

Physical Examination Modes

Physical examination techniques incorporate the basic examination modes of inspection, palpation, percussion, and auscultation.

Inspection

Inspection is always used first to avoid missing any significant signs.

General Inspection. General inspection precedes local inspection. Use your visual, auditory, and olfactory senses during inspection from the first moment of your encounter with a client. Even when the client is behind a screen or curtain, you could be using your senses of hearing and smell (Table 32–2).

During general inspection of a client, you must know which client characteristics to scrutinize (Table 32–3) and integrate the information obtained into the global picture of the client. By carefully planning your general inspection, you minimize the risk of discounting or failing to detect significant signs. Take the time to be thorough, and pay attention to detail. *General inspection is perhaps the examination mode by which you will detect the majority of physical signs.* With experience, you will gain the skills to make several observations almost simultaneously, recognize the range of expected findings, and detect early warnings of alterations in client health status.

In this chapter, findings are described as *expected* and *unexpected.* Consider clients' age, developmental stage, gender, biological variations, ethnicity, and occupation when interpreting findings as expected or unexpected. This terminology emphasizes the range of findings to be encountered and the need to be precise; it also takes into account the risk that what one health care professional describes as "normal" may be in the "normal" range for the individual who reads the record at a different point.

Vital Signs. General inspection includes measuring clients' vital signs and height and weight. **Vital signs** are indicators of clients' circulatory, respiratory, endocrine, and neural functions, and any changes in them indicate alterations in physiological functioning. Vital signs include blood pressure, heart rate and rhythm, respirations, oxygen saturation, and temperature. Pain is considered the fifth vital sign (Jackson, 2002). Conduct a complete symptom analysis for reported pain, and observe for its signs (see Chapter 42). In older adults, another vital sign to be measured is functional ability.

Know when and how to measure vital signs, what range of results to expect, why you use certain techniques, how to record findings accurately, and when to report findings to the nurse in charge, nurse practitioner, or physician (see Chapter 31). Assess changes in light of

➤ TABLE 32-1 Characteristics of Symptoms and Signs

Characteristic	Explanation	Sample Questions
1. Location	The specific anatomical area that is affected	"Describe where your pain is." (symptom) "Where is your rash?" (sign)
• Localization	Occurs in one specific area of the body	"Is your pain in one spot?" (symptom) "Is the rash only on your left elbow?" (sign)
• Generalization	Occurs over larger area of the body, or over whole body	"Is the rash only on your chest and back, or does it cover other areas, too?" (sign)
• Radiation	Moves to or from another area	"Does the tingling move from your back down your legs?" (symptom) "Is the redness moving along your arm?" (sign)
2. Quality	The nature or feature of a symptom or sign	"Describe what the sputum looks like." (sign) "What colour is the rash?" (sign)
	Refers to colour, consistency (thick, thin, hard, soft), and type (crushing, throbbing, aching, burning, cutting, stabbing) of a symptom or sign	"Is it itchy?" (symptom) "Has the mole changed colour?" (sign)
3. Timing		
• Onset (slow or fast)	When the symptom or sign began and the speed of onset	"When did you first notice the pain?" (symptom)
• Duration	The length of time the symptom or sign occurs	"How long does the pain usually last?" (symptom)
• Constancy	Whether the symptom or sign is constant or intermittent	"Is the rash itchy always or only sometimes?" (symptom)
• Time of day/month/year		"Does the rash appear all through the year, or mainly in the winter?" (sign)
4. Intensity/severity	Quantity of a symptom or sign	"On a scale of 0 to 10 (0 = no pain, 10 = worst pain), how would you rate your pain?" (symptom) "How many towels did you use to soak up the blood?" (sign)
5. Aggravating factors	Activities or exposures that worsen the symptom or sign	"What makes the pain worse?" (symptom) "What makes the rash worse?" (sign)
6. Alleviating factors	Activities or exposures that reduce the symptom or sign	"What lessens the pain?" (symptom) "What reduces the rash?" (sign)
7. Associated symptoms or signs	Other symptoms that may be related	"Are you experiencing any other symptoms like nausea or dizziness?"
8. Environmental factors	Anything in the client's surroundings that may be related to the symptom or sign	"What is going on in your life, at home, or at work that might be causing this?" "Are any renovations going on at home or at work?" "Did you travel anywhere recently?" "Have you made any major changes in your life that might be affecting how you are feeling?" "Is anyone else sick at home?"
9. Significance to client	The impact of the symptom or sign on the client's lifestyle and well-being	"How does this affect your lifestyle? Your work?"
10. Client perspective	What the client thinks is happening	"What do you think is causing your pain?" (symptom) "What do you think caused your rash?" (sign)

Adapted from Stephen, T. C. (1997). "Symptom Analysis." In *Adult Health Assessment Series* [CD-ROM]. Edmonton, AB: DataStar Education Systems & Services.

TABLE 32-2 Assessment of Characteristic Odours During General Inspection

Odour	Site or Source	Potential Causes
Alcohol	Oral cavity	Ingestion of alcohol
Ammonia	Urine	Urinary tract infection
Body odour	Skin	Excessive or foul-smelling perspiration
	Axillae, under breasts, groins	Inadequate hygiene; yeast infection
	Clothing	Vomiting
	Wound	Abscess
Feces	Rectal area	Incontinence
		Obstruction
	Clothing	Malabsorption syndrome
Halitosis	Oral cavity	Poor dental hygiene
		Dental abscess
		Gum disease
	Stomach	Nervousness or anxiety
Sweet, fruity odour	Oral cavity	Diabetic acidosis (ketones)
	Breath	Ingestion or inhalation of solvent
Stale urine	Skin	Uremic acidosis
	Clothing	Incontinence
Thick odour (sweet, heavy)	Wound drainage	Bacterial infection
	Vagina	Poor hygiene
Mustiness	Cast area	Infection
Fetid and sweet	Mucous secretions	Bacterial infection
	Tracheostomy	Bacterial infection

other physical findings, using your clinical judgement to determine the frequency of measurement.

Height, Weight, and Waist Circumference. Height and weight are routinely measured during screenings, visits to primary care providers, and admissions to health care facilities. Weight is the basis for determining drug dosages, limitations on caregiver lifting, or care plans for position changes. The health history would suggest possible causes for weight changes (Table 32–4).

Measure weight and height to monitor growth, development, relationship to nutrition and fluid intake, and change over time. Use a standing scale (which must be calibrated at each use) to measure ambulatory clients or an electronic scale (which automatically adjusts to display the weight within seconds). Compare your observations with standardized tables, while taking into account age-related changes. Compare data with a weight classification system devised for adults 18 years of age and older, except in the case of pregnant and lactating women (Health Canada, 2003; see www.hc-sc.gc.ca/ hpfb-dgpsa/onpp-bppn/cg_bwc_introduction_e.html). The Canadian system (Tables 32–5A and 32–5B) is based on a body weight–height calculation using a nomogram, the body mass index (BMI), and the amount of abdominal fat measured using waist circumference. The BMI divides weight in kilograms by height in metres squared (kg/m^2). For example, to calculate the BMI for a 66-year-old woman who weighs 65 kilograms and has a height of 160 cm, divide 65 by 1.6 squared (2.56) to obtain a BMI of 25.4.

Local Inspection. Local inspection *follows* general inspection. Select an anatomical region or body part, and focus your attention on specific characteristics. The observations you make at this stage build on those made during general inspection. If you notice clinical indications of abuse (Box 32–4), you need to be aware that clients may feel further victimized (stressed, anxious) by your scrutiny.

Recognize red flags for possible substance abuse (Box 32–5). Approach the client in a caring and nonjudgemental way, as substance abuse usually involves both emotional and lifestyle issues. Ask the following **CAGE questions**: Have you ever felt the need to *Cut down* on your drinking or drug use? Have people *Annoyed* you by criticizing your drinking or drug use? Have you ever felt bad or *Guilty* about your drinking or drug use? Have you ever used or had a drink first thing in the morning as an *Eye-opener* to steady your nerves or feel normal? If two or more answers are positive, suspect abuse, and consider how you can motivate the client to seek treatment (Stuart & Laraia, 2003).

During local inspection (Table 32–6), be aware of client's physical exposure and the lighting in the examination room. Avoid unnecessary exposure for the client's comfort, but ensure sufficient exposure for accurate assessment. Diffused natural lighting is preferable, but artificial lighting is usually adequate. Nurses commonly use a penlight for inspection. Use **direct** (perpendicular) **lighting** to detect the colour of the skin and mucous membranes and to examine the characteristics of skin lesions (type, configuration, distribution, colour). Use **oblique (tangential) lighting**, by shining the penlight at an angle, to clearly detect movement, pulsations, and contour in the body region you are examining.

Palpation

Palpation, the second basic examination mode, uses the sense of touch. It is based on tactile, temperature, kinesthetic, and vibratory sensations and is a technique that can be mastered with experience and education. The different anatomical areas of the hand vary in their receptiveness to sensations, and distinguishing these sensations depends on the appropriate use of your hands (Table 32–7).

Palpation Techniques. During palpation, vary the pressure, movement, and position of your hand(s) depending on the type of data required. Bones, tendons, muscles, superficial arteries, salivary ducts, abdominal viscera, and structures accessible through body orifices are all palpable. Using data from the history and inspection, select key areas for palpation, and determine the amount of pressure to exert. Two types of pressure are used during palpation: light and deep (Figure 32–1). Light palpation detects characteristics of skin surfaces or structures located close to the surface to a depth of about 1 cm. Deep palpation detects structures that are 3 to 4 cm from the skin surface. Generally, you would use light palpation throughout a physical examination and deep palpation according to your discretion.

When you begin palpation, ensure that your hands are warm, and use light pressure, which will promote clients' confidence, relaxation, and cooperation. As clients can initially perceive deep palpation as

safety alert The risk for further abuse is high after a victim has reported abuse or tries to leave an abusive situation. Provide the person with counselling options.

TABLE 32-3 Client Characteristics to Be Assessed During General Inspection

Client Characteristic	Focus of Assessment
Gender	Body type, sexual development, type of clothing
Genetic background	Integument, body type
Body type	Shape, muscularity, obesity, thinness
Apparent age	Face, posture, motor activity, gait, type of clothing
Level of consciousness	Eyes, verbal response, motor response (see Glasgow Coma Scale, Table 32–16)
Orientation	Personal identity (name), place, time
Signs of distress	Anxiety, difficulty breathing, perspiration, pallor, restlessness, dilated pupils, agitation, consciousness Indicators of pain (see Chapter 42)
Outstanding anatomical malformations	Head, neck, torso, limbs
Appearance of health	Physical, mental, emotional
Posture	Vertical alignment (coronal and median planes)
Affect and mood	Congruence of verbal and nonverbal communication Facial expression, voice, demeanour, emotion
Motor activity and gait	Coordination, balance, arm and head movement, mobility Purposeful movements, tremors
Signs of abuse	All socioeconomic levels (see Box 32–4 for clinical indicators in adults)
Signs of substance abuse	All socioeconomic levels Men and women Childhood, adolescence, adulthood Alcohol, medications, illegal drugs (see Box 32–5 for clinical indicators)
Clothing	Amount, appropriateness for weather and temperature, fastened correctly, right side out, context
Facial expression at rest and during interaction	Symmetry, congruence with nonverbal communication
Odours	Physical activity, body and oral hygiene, disease (see Table 32–2 for causes)
Personal grooming and hygiene	Cleanliness of hair, skin, nails, clothing Use of cosmetics
Cognitive functions	Orientation, short- and long-term memory, attention, learning ability
Insight and judgement	Awareness of normality Comparison and evaluation of alternatives for action
Sexual development	Age, gender, type of clothing (see Chapter 27)
Speech and language	Clarity, pace, inflection, tone, fluency
Thought processes and content	Logic, coherence, relevance, insight, judgement Patterns (e.g., compulsions, obsessions, phobias, anxieties, delusions)

➤ TABLE 32-4 Health History for Weight Assessment

Assessment Category	Rationale
Ask about total weight lost or gained; compare with usual weight, note period of loss (e.g., gradual, sudden) and type of loss (e.g., desired, undesired).	Determines severity of problem and may reveal relationship to any disease process, change in eating pattern, or pregnancy.
In case of desired weight loss, ask about eating pattern, diet plan followed, usual daily calorie intake, and appetite.	Helps determine appropriateness of diet plan.
In case of undesired weight loss, find out about anorexia, vomiting, diarrhea, thirst, frequent urination, and change in lifestyle or activity.	Focuses on problems that may cause weight loss.
Assess whether client has noticed any changes in social aspects of eating: more meals in restaurants, rushing to eat meals, eating poorly due to stress at work, or skipping meals.	Determines lifestyle contributions to weight changes.
Find out whether client is on chemotherapy, diuretics, insulin, psychotropics, steroids, nonprescription diet pills, or laxatives.	Weight gain or loss can be side effects.

roughness, light palpation always precedes deep palpation. Light palpation involves exerting gentle pressure with fingers together and extended. Keep your fingernails short. Performing light palpation first may help you discover tender areas. Clients who experience tenderness to palpation might increase muscular resistance, which would inhibit your detection of important findings, so palpate the tender areas last.

Deep palpation always involves firm but discontinuous pressure, as continuous pressure on the nerve endings of finger pads or fingertips reduces their tactile sensitivity. To maintain sensitivity, apply firm hand pressure with fingers together and extended, and release the pressure. You may use both hands (bimanual) to achieve firm pressure for deep palpation of the abdominal structures. Your top hand exerts the pressure, while the bottom hand stays relaxed and sensitive to tactile sensations.

Movements of Palpation. The type of data collected through light and deep palpation depends on the position and movement of the hand(s) (Table 32–8). Palpation may detect feces in the colon, a bladder distended with urine, a pregnant uterus, a mobile right kidney, or bulkiness in the right lower quadrant (cecum) and left lower quadrant (descending colon).

Percussion

Sounds produced when body tissues are percussed assist you to interpret the size of body organs and the density of underlying tissues (Figure 32–2).

Characteristics of Sound. Audible sounds have *pitch* (high, low), *intensity* (loud, soft), *duration* (short, long), and *quality* or *nature* (varied). Pitch refers to the *frequency* of sound pressure waves. Frequency is a measure of the number of wave cycles per second (cps) and is expressed in Hertz (Hz).

The intensity (loudness) of sound is measured in decibels (dbs) on the "A" scale of a sound pressure level meter. Intensity may be measured objectively and independently of frequency (pitch).

➤ TABLE 32-5A Health Risk Classification According to Body Mass Index (BMI)*

Classification	BMI Category (kg/m^2)	Risk of Developing Health Problems
Underweight	<18.5	Increased
Normal weight	18.5–24.9	Least
Overweight	25.0–29.9	Increased
Obese		
• Class I	30.0–34.9	High
• Class II	35.0–39.9	Very high
• Class III	≥40.0	Extremely high

*For use in adults age 18 years and older. Not for use in pregnant and lactating women. *Note:* For people 65 years and older, the "normal" weight range may begin slightly above BMI 18.5 and extend into the overweight weight range.

Adapted from World Health Organization. (2000). *Obesity: Preventing and managing the global epidemic: Report of a WHO consultation on obesity* (p. 9). Geneva, Switzerland: Author.

➤ TABLE 32-5B Health Risk Classification According to Waist Circumference (WC)*

WC Cut-off Points		Health Risk (Relative to WC Below Cut-off Point)
Men	≥102 cm	Increased risk of developing health problems†
Women	≥88 cm	Increased risk of developing health problems

For BMIs in the 18.5 to 34.9 range, use WC as an additional indicator of health risk. For BMIs ≥35, WC measurement does not provide additional information on level of risk.

*For use in adults age 18 years and older. Not for use in pregnant and lactating women.

†Risk for type 2 diabetes, coronary heart disease, hypertension.

World Health Organization. (2000). *Obesity: Preventing and managing the global epidemic: Report of a WHO consultation on obesity* (p. 9). Geneva, Switzerland: Author.

➤ BOX 32-4 Clinical Indicators of Abuse in Adults

Physical Findings	Behavioural Findings
Domestic Abuse	
Injuries, fractures, or trauma inconsistent with reported cause Multiple injuries involving head, face, neck, breasts, abdomen, and genitalia (e.g., black eyes, orbital fractures, broken nose, fractured skull, lip lacerations, broken teeth, strangulation marks) X-ray films show old and new fractures at different stages of healing Abrasions, lacerations, bruises, or welts Burns Human bite marks	Attempted suicide Eating or sleeping disorders Anxiety Panic attacks Pattern of substance abuse (follows physical abuse) Low self-esteem Depression Sense of helplessness Guilt Increased forgetfulness Stress-related complaints (headache, anxiety)
Elder Abuse	
Injuries and trauma inconsistent with reported cause (cigarette burns, scratches, bruises, or bite marks) Hematomas Bruises at various stages of resolution Bruises, chafing, excoriations on wrists and legs (restraints) Burns Fractures inconsistent with cause described Dried blood	Dependent on caregiver Physically or cognitively impaired Combative Wandering Verbally belligerent Minimal social support Prolonged interval between injury and medical treatment Diminished capacity for self-care

Data from Gerard, M. (2000). "Domestic Violence: How to Screen and Intervene," *RN, 63*(12), pp. 52–56; Hoban, S., & Kearney, K. (2000). "Elder Abuse and Neglect," *American Journal of Nursing, 100*(11), pp. 49–50; and Kramer, A. (2002). "Domestic Violence: How to Ask and How to Listen," *Nursing Clinics of North America, 37*, pp. 189–210.

➤ BOX 32-5 Red Flags for Possible Substance Abuse

- Frequently missed appointments
- Frequent requests for written excuses from work
- Chief complaints of insomnia, "bad nerves," and pain that do not fit a particular pattern
- Frequent reports of lost prescriptions (e.g., tranquilizers or pain medications) or frequent requests for refills
- Frequent emergency department visits
- History of changing doctors or bringing in medication bottles prescribed by several health care professionals
- History of gastrointestinal bleeds, peptic ulcers, pancreatitis, cellulitis, or frequent pulmonary infections
- Frequent STIs, complicated pregnancies, multiple abortions, or sexual dysfunction
- Complaints of chest pains or palpitations or history of admissions to rule out myocardial infarctions
- History of activities that place the client at risk for HIV infections (multiple sexual partners, multiple rapes)
- Family history of addiction; history of childhood sexual, physical, or emotional abuse; or social, financial, or marital problems

Adapted from Master, S., & Terpstra, J. K. (1992). "Recognition and Diagnosis," In Schnoll, S. H., Horvatich, P. K., & Terpstra, J. K. (Eds.). *Prescribing drugs with abuse liability* (p. 18), Richmond, VA: DSAM, MCV-VCU; and Friedman, L., et al. (1996). *Source book of substance abuse and addiction.* Baltimore: Williams & Wilkins.

➤ TABLE 32-6 Characteristics Assessed During Local Inspection

Alignment	Depressions	Lesion characteristics	Pigmentation	Secretions
Closure	Development	Lustre	Pulsations	Shape
Colour	Elevations	Mass	Range of motion	Size
Contour	Hair characteristics	Mobility	Reaction to light	Sounds
Coordination	Hygiene	Moisture	Reflections	Spacing
Contraction	Integrity	Movements	Reflexes	Symmetry
Curvatures	Inversion	Parasites	Rhythm	Vascularity

Adapted from Skillen, D. L. (2004). *A primer on physical examination techniques* [WebCT]. Edmonton, AB: Faculty of Nursing, University of Alberta.

TABLE 32-7 Sensory Properties of the Hand for Specific Characteristics

Anatomical Area of Hand	Specific Characteristics to Be Assessed	Rationale
Finger pads	Consistency, contour, moisture, position, and texture	Sensory nerve fibres are abundant in the finger pads and facilitate tactile discriminations.
Finger tips	Elasticity, fluid content of tissues, mobility, pulsatility, thickness, tissue turgor, and vascularity	Sensory nerve fibres are particularly abundant in the fingertips and facilitate fine tactile discriminations.
Dorsal surface (back of hand)	Temperature	Skin on dorsal surfaces is thinner, which increases sensitivity to temperature.
Ball of hand, palmar surface	Vibrations	Metacarpophalangeal joints (ball of hand) on skin surface are sensitive to vibrations.
Ulnar edge (side of hand that includes little finger)	Temperature and vibrations	Skin on ulnar edge is thinner, which facilitates sensitivity to temperature and vibrations.

Adapted from Skillen, D. L. (2004). *A primer on physical examination techniques* [WebCT]. Edmonton, AB: Faculty of Nursing, University of Alberta.

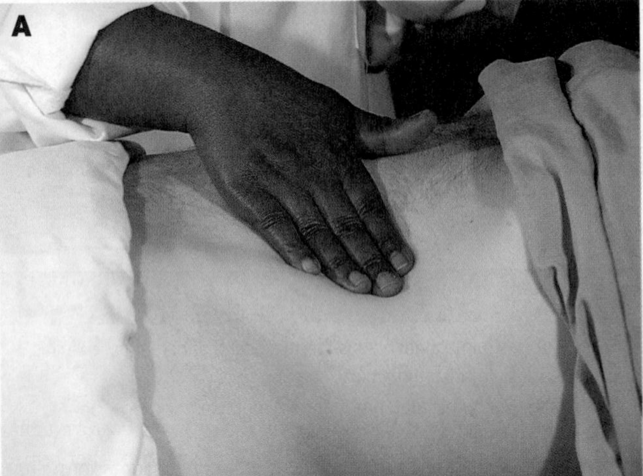

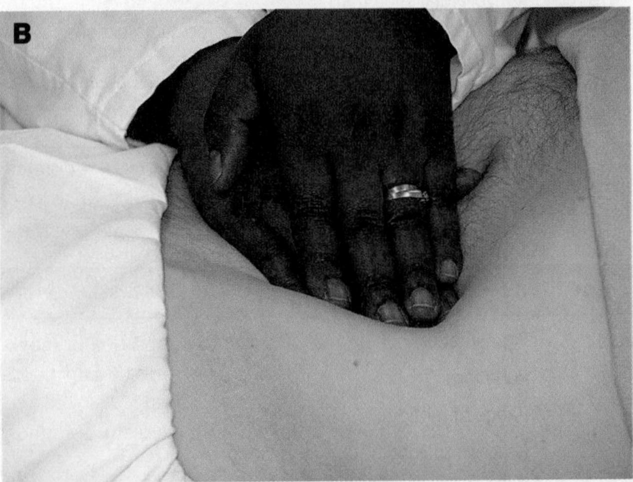

Figure 32-1 A, Light palpation. B, Deep palpation. **Source:** From Skillen, D. L., Day, R. A., Anderson, M. C., Stephen, T. C., Gilbert, J. A., & Day, L. W. (2004). *Physical examination images* [CD-ROM]. Edmonton, AB: Faculty of Nursing, University of Alberta.

Intensity is dependent on the amplitude of the vibrations or sound waves produced by stimulating the source. Loudness refers to human physiological perception of intensity. Striking a drum produces a relatively loud sound because of the drum's capacity to vibrate freely. In contrast, tapping on the tissues of the human forearm produces a sound that is always of low intensity, as relatively dense tissues do not vibrate freely. The force used to increase vibration may affect the intensity but not the frequency (high, medium, or low pitch). The duration of sound is the length of time in seconds, minutes, or hours that a sound is heard. Tapping on soft tissue (muscle, adipose tissue) may shorten the duration of sound. The quality (nature, timbre) of sound pertains to its musical nature or its blowing, gurgling, or clicking quality.

Use a tuning fork of 1024 or 512 Hz to test hearing, and a tuning fork of 128 or 256 Hz to test vibration. A 1024 Hz tuning fork produces a sound that is higher pitched, more musical, of longer duration, and *within the range of human hearing*. A 256-Hz tuning fork produces a buzzing noise that is lower pitched, of shorter duration, and possibly outside the human hearing range.

Sound Transmission in the Body. Gases are poor transmitters of sound; fluids are better transmitters, and solids are the best. Knowing the sound transmission capabilities of these media enables you to detect alterations in body tissues (e.g., breath sounds are altered by lung and other tissue changes). Audible sound is a pressure wave that moves more quickly through the solids and fluids than through the gases in the body. Sounds detected during percussion and auscultation depend on tissue density and elasticity. Elasticity permits vibration of body structures, which in turn creates sound waves that are transmitted to the exterior of the body and perceived as sound by the examiner. All the sounds detected during percussion or auscultation are interpreted in terms of the characteristics of pitch, intensity, quality, and duration. In the case of dense tissue, sounds have a higher pitch, softer intensity, and shorter duration and

safety alert To prevent any injury to clients, nursing students are supervised when they perform deep palpation.

TABLE 32-8 Movements of the Hand for Palpation of Specific Characteristics

Palpation Movement	Techniques and Rationale
Gliding	Slide finger pads over skin surface in both horizontal and vertical planes to detect subtle differences. *Assesses moisture, surface contour, tenderness, and texture.*
Circular movements	Roll surface tissue over underlying structures with finger pads to accentuate the characteristics of structures or masses. *Assesses consistency, contour, discreteness of a mass, mobility, shape, size, and tenderness.*
Grasping	Grasp skin surfaces with the finger pads (pincer action) to obtain data about structures immediately below the skin surface. *Assesses amplitude, association with respiratory movements, consistency, elasticity, mobility, position, pulsations, shape, size, tenderness, tissue turgor, and thickness.*
Direct perpendicular pressure	Apply direct pressure with fingertips, pads, ulnar surfaces, or palmar surfaces to detect blanching, fluid content, tenderness, guarding, pulsations, resistance, or an association with respiration. *Assesses blood vessels, excursion, fremitus, masses, muscle, pulsations, rate, rhythm, skin lesions, and subcutaneous tissue.*
Dipping	Use finger pads during palpation of the abdomen while visualizing the underlying structures to guide documentation and interpretation of findings. *Assesses consistency, contour, elasticity, guarding, masses, mobility of underlying structure, resistance, shape, size, status of underlying viscera, and tenderness.*

Adapted from Skillen, D. L. (2004). *A primer on physical examination techniques* [WebCT]. Edmonton, AB: Faculty of Nursing, University of Alberta.

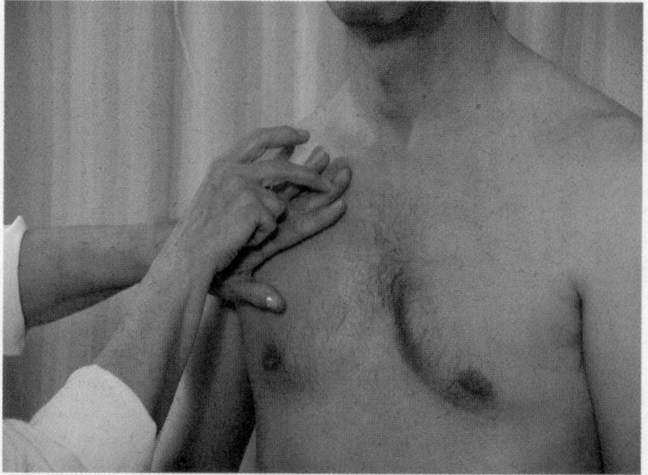

Figure 32-2 Indirect percussion. **Source:** From Skillen, D. L., Day, R. A., Anderson, M. C., Stephen, T. C., Gilbert, J. A., & Day, L. W. (2004). *Physical examination images* [CD-ROM]. Edmonton, AB: Faculty of Nursing, University of Alberta.

are less musical in quality. In the case of less dense tissue, sounds have a lower pitch, louder intensity, and longer duration and more musical quality.

Percussion Notes. Sounds produced as a result of percussion are described as flat, dull, resonant, hyper-resonant, and tympanic. Percussion notes have pitch, intensity, duration, and quality (Table 32–9).

Simulating Sounds. To familiarize yourself with sounds, tap your puffed-out cheek to simulate tympany. Percuss the scapula of another adult to produce a flat percussion note. Percuss your own chest just inferior to the clavicle to hear resonance and your anterior thigh to hear dullness. Percuss hyper-resonance on a thin child's chest.

Percussion Techniques. Density influences sound, so you can map the size and location of underlying organs by paying attention to the percussion notes produced. Percussion also elicits tissue tenderness, if present, and stimulates reflex action of a partially stretched deep tendon. Two types of percussion are used: indirect (mediated) and direct (nonmediated). Indirect percussion is the most commonly used (Skill 32–1; see Figure 32–2). Indirect percussion can be achieved by striking the dorsum of one hand with the ulnar edge of the fist of the other hand (e.g., fist percussion of the kidney in the costovertebral angle) to detect underlying tenderness. Direct percussion is performed with the plexor finger directly on body surfaces (e.g., percussion over the clavicle to detect resonance of apical lung tissue).

Practise percussion techniques often until you learn to elicit a clear percussion note. When comparing symmetrical areas, use the technique consistently to ensure accuracy and avoid misinterpretations. Results of percussion vary according to the technique used. To perceive differences among the five percussion notes most accurately (see Table 32–9), percuss from areas of lesser density to areas of greater density. It is easier to detect the change from a resonant note to a dull note than from dullness to resonance or hyper-resonance.

Auscultation

Use a stethoscope to auscultate sounds created by vibration or movement of underlying tissues. Binaural stethoscopes are the most popular; they have right and left earpieces, single tubing, and bell and diaphragm chestpieces. A poor-quality stethoscope distorts sounds, compromising the quality of findings.

Use the chestpieces to detect the pitch, duration, intensity, and quality of body sounds. The bell chestpiece has an outer rim bordered by rubber material and a hollow centre. If a chestpiece has a flat surface joining its outer rim, it is a diaphragm. The bell accentuates low-frequency sounds, filtering out high-pitched sounds. As it is an open

TABLE 32-9 Characteristics of Percussion Notes

Percussion Note	Pitch	Intensity	Duration	Quality	Tissue Density	Example
Flat	High	Soft	Short	Flat noise	Dense	Thigh muscle, scapula
Dull	Medium	Medium	Moderate	Thud-like noise	Dense	Heart, liver, distended urinary bladder
Resonant	Low	Loud	Long	Hollow noise	Less dense	Air-filled lung
Hyper-resonant	High	Loud	Longer than resonant	Pronounced hollow noise	Less dense	Hyperinflated lung, child's thin chest
Tympanic	High	Loud	Moderate	Musical, drum-like	Less dense	Gas in bowel, gastric air bubble, cheek puffed out

system, it requires a complete seal with the skin but only light pressure. A complete seal prevents sound leaks and distortion of sound by environmental noise. If the bell is applied with firm pressure, the skin functions like a diaphragm and accentuates high-pitched sounds.

The diaphragm chestpiece picks up high-frequency sounds (think "di-hi") and filters out low-pitched sounds. It does not require a complete seal with the skin surface because it is a closed system. For accuracy and hygiene, use only your own stethoscope. See Box 32–6 for care of the stethoscope. If you must use a shared stethoscope, clean the earpieces with alcohol first. To block outside noise, earpieces should fit snugly in the external opening of your ear. A too-small earpiece may enter too far into your auditory canal and obstruct sound transmission. Insert earpieces facing forward, medially toward your nose, and pointing somewhat inferiorly so that they fit the natural curvature of your ear canals. Earpieces must fit comfortably. Composition of earpieces (rubber or plastic) affects comfort and fit. For effective sound conduction, you need short, flexible, thick-walled tubing of about 3 mm diameter. The preferred length of the tubing is about 30 cm. An electronic stethoscope is useful to amplify sound.

SKILL 32-1 Critical Components of Indirect Percussion Techniques

Equipment

- None

Procedure

STEPS	RATIONALE
1. Trim your fingernail short on the plexor finger.	• Perpendicular blows to pleximeter will not draw blood and will cause less soreness.
2. Place pleximeter finger (finger being struck) on the skin surface over the area to be percussed.	• Contact with skin surface permits blow to pleximeter, which makes underlying body structures vibrate, producing a percussion note.
3. Place pleximeter firmly.	• Body structures will not vibrate fully if finger is not firmly placed.
4. Do not move pleximeter.	• Movement reduces and diffuses underlying vibrations.
5. Limit contact of pleximeter to one small area on the skin; preferably only the distal interphalangeal (DIP) joint touches the skin surface.	• Limiting the area of contact produces a clearer percussion note.
6. Strike a sharp, perpendicular blow to the DIP joint of the pleximeter with the plexor (striking) finger.	• Striking sharply produces a clearer percussion note.
7. Perform brisk arc-like wrist action with relaxed wrist.	• Produces sharp perpendicular blow.
8. Restrict movement to wrist action; avoid movement at elbow.	• Produces sharp perpendicular blow.
9. Limit percussion to one or two sharp blows.	• Detects percussion note more accurately.
10. Select the appropriate force of blow to achieve a clear percussion note.	• Clarity facilitates interpretation of percussion note.
11. Use the lightest blow possible to achieve a clear percussion note.	• Note elicited is restricted to a small body area. Examiners adjust the force of the blow according to body build of clients, using a more forceful blow with a heavily muscled or obese client, and a less forceful blow if client is emaciated or very thin.
12. Use consistent technique when comparing symmetrical areas.	• Promotes accuracy of interpretation.
13. Percuss from an area of lesser density to an area of greater density.	• Facilitates detection of changes.

Adapted from Skillen, D. L. (2004). *A primer on physical examination techniques* [WebCT]. Edmonton, AB: Faculty of Nursing, University of Alberta.

> **BOX 32-6 Care of the Stethoscope**
>
> Remove regularly the earwax that accumulates on earpieces. Keep the bell and diaphragm free of dust, lint, and body oils (avoid draping the stethoscope around your neck next to your skin). Clean the entire stethoscope (diaphragm, tubing, etc.) with alcohol or soapy water.

Auscultation Techniques. To maximize sound volume, apply the diaphragm chestpiece with enough pressure so that it can move in synchrony with body movements caused by breathing and to avoid creation of frictional noise. Close your eyes to shut out environmental stimuli and focus better on a particular sound. Avoid sliding or moving your fingers on the chestpiece, rubbing the tubing, moving the chestpiece on the skin, or breathing on the tubing, as all of these contribute to extraneous noise that obscures detection of significant sounds. Place the stethoscope on the client's bare skin, as clothing obscures sound. Movement of the stethoscope on the coarse hair on the skin of a hirsute individual can create frictional noise. To prevent this, wet the hair so that it lies closer to the skin. Tap the chestpiece first to verify that it is turned on.

During auscultation, concentrate on one sound at a time. Consider the area you are auscultating and the causes for the sounds you detect. For example, closure of the mitral valve causes the first heart sound "lub." Learn well the types of sounds arising from each body structure and where to hear them best. The location, timing, rate, and rhythm of the sounds you hear vary with the body system you auscultate.

Anatomical Terms

Anatomical Position

By international convention, nurses use the **anatomical position** for standardized verbal and written documentation (Box 32–7). This practice promotes accurate, safe, and clear communication and protects clients' best interests. When clients are in the prone, supine, standing, or side position, you visualize the anatomical position in order to describe your findings (Figure 32–3A). The client record is a legal document. Clearly communicated findings using the anatomical position facilitate accurate comparison of change in client condition over time, even if examiners change.

Anatomical Planes

For precise descriptions, use four major and imaginary planes to divide the body (see Figure 32–3B). Start by visualizing the client in the anatomical position, then consider the four imaginary planes (Table 32–10):

- Median
- Coronal (frontal)
- Sagittal
- Horizontal (transverse)

> **BOX 32-7 Standardized Anatomical Position**
>
> Visualize the client in the following position:
> - Upright (erect)
> - Head, eyes, and toes facing forward (anteriorly)
> - Heels and great toes touching
> - Arms hanging by the sides and palms facing forward (anteriorly)

Anatomical Surfaces

Anatomical planes are reference points for anatomical surfaces (Table 32–11) that are used to describe body structures in relation to one other. Always visualize clients in the anatomical position. Describe your observations in relation to anatomical surfaces and use a combination of terms to indicate location. For example, you record that you changed a wound dressing on the medial surface of the right forearm. You may also indicate direction in relation to anatomical surfaces. For example, the diameter from the front of the chest to the back (anteroposterior diameter of the thorax) is less than the lateral diameter. When assessing the shape of the thorax, you compare the two directions in length. Also, the "position of function" indicates whether a surface is ventral or dorsal when you describe the foot, hand, penis, and tongue.

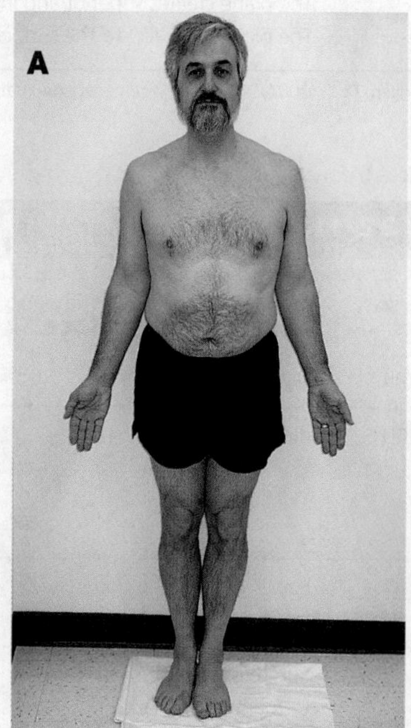

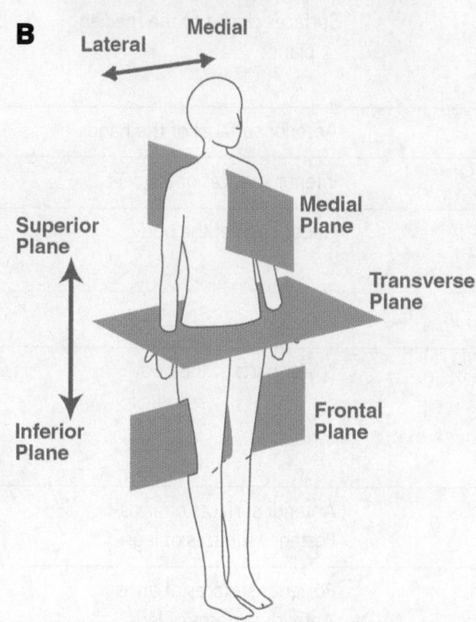

Figure 32-3 A, Anatomical position. B, Anatomical planes. **Source:** From Skillen, D. L., Day, R. A., Anderson, M. C., Stephen, T. C., Gilbert, J. A., & Day, L. W. (2004). *Physical examination images* [CD-ROM]. Edmonton, AB: Faculty of Nursing, University of Alberta.

TABLE 32-10 Imaginary Anatomical Planes

Name of Plane	Location and Outcome of Plane
Median	The plane passes vertically through the body from back to front, creating right and left symmetrical halves.
Coronal (Frontal)	Beginning at the coronal suture of the skull, the plane passes vertically through the body at right angles to the median plane and posteriorly through the ankles and feet, creating anterior and posterior regions.
Sagittal	The plane passes vertically through the body, parallel to the median plane, creating sections of right and left symmetrical halves.
Midsagittal	The plane passes vertically through the median plane, separating the sections of right and left symmetrical halves.
Horizontal (Transverse)	The plane passes through the body at right angles to the sagittal, median, and coronal planes through the umbilicus anteriorly and the intervertebral disc between third lumbar vertebra (L3) and fourth lumbar vertebra (L4). The plane creates superior and inferior regions. The plane is parallel to the surface on which the individual stands.

Adapted from Skillen, D. L. (2004). *A primer on physical examination techniques* [WebCT]. Edmonton, AB: Faculty of Nursing, University of Alberta.

TABLE 32-11 Anatomical Surfaces

Name of Surface	Location of Surface	Additional Information
Anterior (ventral)	Front of the body	In neuroanatomy and embryology, the term used is *ventral*.
Dorsal (posterior)	Back of the body	It is helpful to think of the dorsal fin of a fish. The term *dorsal* can be confusing. For example: • The superior surface of the foot or tongue is the dorsal surface or dorsum. • The anterior part of the flaccid (non-erect) penis is also referred to as the dorsum.
Inferior	Lower parts of the body	Observations are closer to the client's feet than to the head. For example: • The knee is inferior to the hip.
Lateral	Surfaces farthest away from the median plane	In the anatomical position, • The little toe is lateral to the great toe.
Medial	Surfaces closest to the median plane	In the anatomical position, • The little finger is medial to the thumb. • The surfaces of the arms and legs closest to the torso are medial surfaces.
Palmar	Anterior surfaces of the hands	Palmar surfaces of the fingers.
Plantar	Inferior surfaces of the feet	Includes soles of the toes.
Superior	Upper parts of the body	Includes torso above umbilicus and intervertebral disc between L3 and L4, arms, and the head and neck. Structures may be described as superior to another structure. For example, • Shoulders are superior to the elbows.
Inferior	Lower parts of the body	Includes torso below the umbilicus and the intervertebral disc between L3 and L4, the legs, and feet. Structures may be described as inferior to another structure. For example: • The ankle is inferior to the knee.
Flexor	Anterior surfaces of arms Posterior surfaces of legs	Surfaces that come closer to one another with flexion (bending).
Extensor	Posterior surfaces of arms Anterior surfaces of legs	Surfaces that move farther away from one another with extension (straightening).

Adapted from Skillen, D. L. (2004). *A primer on physical examination techniques* [WebCT]. Edmonton, AB: Faculty of Nursing, University of Alberta.

Anatomical Quadrants and Regions

Anatomical Quadrants. Quadrants are created by imaginary intersecting vertical and horizontal lines in the median and horizontal planes (Figure 32–4). The abdomen and breasts are commonly described in terms of their quadrants. Labels for breast quadrants (Figure 32–5) are different from those for the abdominal quadrants. Also, each breast has an area that is labelled the tail of Spence.

Anatomical Regions. To describe your findings more precisely, you may also divide the abdomen systematically into nine regions (Figure 32–6). Two imaginary vertical lines (parallel to the median plane) and two imaginary horizontal lines (parallel to the horizontal plane) create the nine regions.

Anatomical Terms of Comparison

When using terms of comparison, draw upon your knowledge of the anatomical positions, planes, surfaces, quadrants, and regions to describe the position of a structure with respect to another (Table 32–12). When making comparisons, avoid using such words as *on, over, above,* and *under* to describe location. For example, if you describe a mass as lying "under" the umbilicus, it will not be clear to the reader whether it is located inferior, posterior, or deep to the umbilicus. Precision of descriptions is important for client safety.

Anatomical Terms of Movement

Describe movements at the articulations of bones and range of motion (ROM) in relation to anatomical planes (Table 32–13). The median and coronal planes are the most common planes of reference for movements. The median plane creates imaginary right and left body halves; the coronal plane creates imaginary anterior and posterior body halves. As a nurse, you will be guided by standardized anatomical terms of movement, position, and plane when systematically inspecting body structures for the type and range of movements. You will frequently compare movements made by symmetrical areas of the body, such as the arms and legs, and describe ROM relative to a neutral position, often the midline.

Common terms of movement are described in Table 32–13. Some less common terms of movement are *opposition, protraction, retraction, elevation, depression,* and *circumduction.*

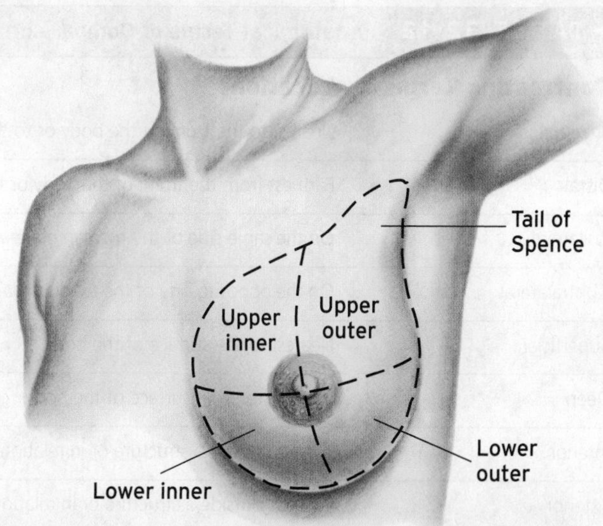

Figure 32-5 Quadrants of the breast. **Source:** From From Seidel, H. M., Ball, J. W., Dains, J. E., Benedict, G. W. (2006). *Mosby's guide to physical examination* (6th ed., p. 493, Figure 16–2). St. Louis, MO: Mosby.

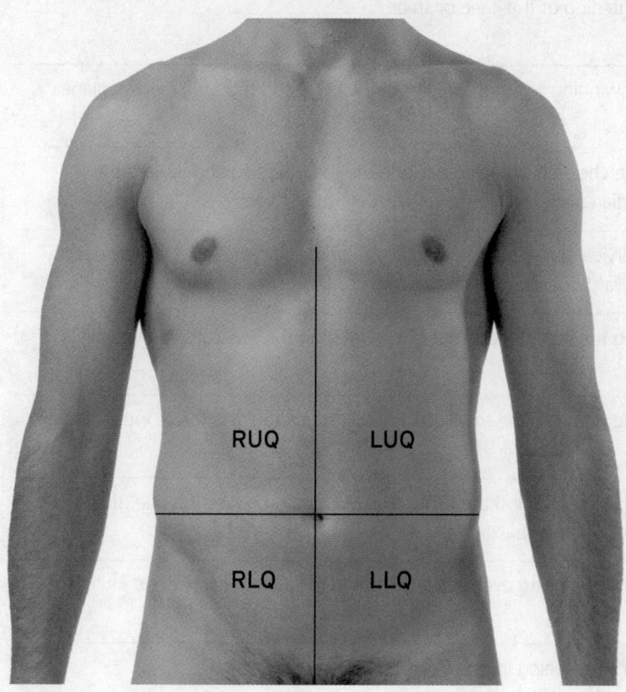

Figure 32-4 Quadrants of the abdomen. RUQ, right upper quadrant; LUQ, left upper quadrant; RLQ, right lower quadrant; LLQ, left lower quadrant. **Source:** From Seidel, H. M., Ball, J. W., Dains, J. E., & Benedict, G. W. (2006). *Mosby's guide to physical examination* (6th ed., p. 532, Figure 17–4). St. Louis, MO: Mosby.

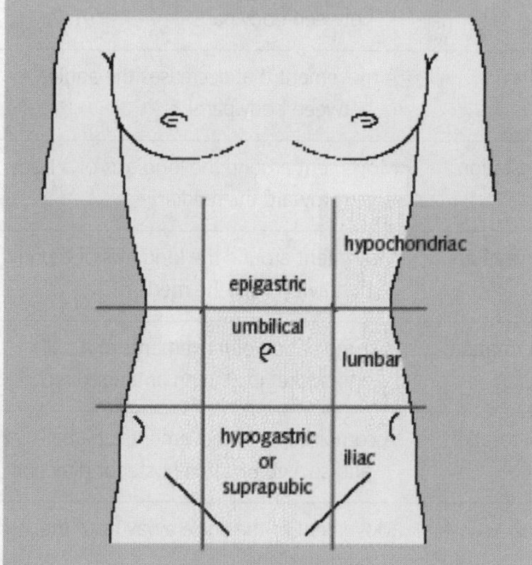

Figure 32-6 Nine abdominal regions. **Source:** From Skillen, D. L., Day, R. A., Anderson, M. C., Stephen, T. C., Gilbert, J. A., & Day, L. W. (2004). *Physical examination images* [CD-ROM]. Edmonton, AB: Faculty of Nursing, University of Alberta.

➤ TABLE 32-12 Anatomical Terms of Comparison

Contrasting Terms	Location
Proximal	Nearest to the trunk of the body or to the origin of a structure.
Distal	Farthest from the trunk of the body or from the origin of a structure.
Ipsilateral	On the same side of the median plane as another structure observed. *A term used in neurological assessments.*
Contralateral	On the opposite side of the median plane from another structure observed. *A term used in neurological assessments.*
Superficial	Nearest to the surface of the body.
Deep	Distant from the surface of the body.
Interior	Located within a structure or in relation to the body core.
Exterior	Located outside a structure or in relation to the body surface.

Adapted from Skillen, D. L. (2004). *A primer on physical examination techniques* [WebCT]. Edmonton, AB: Faculty of Nursing, University of Alberta.

➤ TABLE 32-13 Common Terms of Movement

Movement	Description	Examples
Flexion	A bending movement that reduces the angle between body parts	Plantar flexion—posterior movement toward the floor in the coronal plane ("plant" the foot down). Dorsiflexion—anterior movement (upward) of the foot at the ankle. Lateral flexion—sideways movement away from the midline position in the coronal plane.
Extension	A movement that increases the angle between body parts	Straightening of the knee or spine.
Abduction	A movement that increases the angle between body parts	Arms swinging out and away from the body and from the median plane.
Adduction	A movement that decreases the angle between body parts	Outstretched leg swinging back beside the other leg and toward the median plane.
Medial rotation	Movement around the long axis of a body part toward the median	The cervical spine rotating medially when turning the head to look directly forward or anteriorly.
Lateral rotation	Movement around the long axis of a body part away from the median	Turning the head to look back, thus rotating the cervical spine laterally.
Internal rotation	A combination of movements of a ball-and-socket joint in an anterior direction	Moving hands to the small of the back, thus shoulders rotate internally.
External rotation	A combination of movements of a ball-and-socket joint in a posterior direction	Placing hands behind the head, elbows pointing out to the side, thus shoulders rotate externally
Eversion	Movement at the ankle away from the median plane	Soles of feet being everted when turned away from each other.
Inversion	Movement at the ankle toward the median plane	Soles of feet being inverted when facing each other.
Supination	Lateral rotation of a structure around the long axis of the radius	The elbow being flexed at a right angle, causing lateral rotation of the radius around its long axis, and the palm of the hand turning upward.
Pronation	Medial rotation around the long axis of the radius	The pronated palm of the hand facing downward (e.g., with this movement, a bowl of soup would be dropped because it would be upside down).

Adapted from Skillen, D. L. (2004). *A primer on physical examination techniques* [WebCT]. Edmonton, AB: Faculty of Nursing, University of Alberta.

Preparation for Physical Examination

Preparation of the client, environment, and yourself ensures a smooth examination with few interruptions. An unorganized approach reduces client confidence in you, creates client discomfort or embarrassment, and causes you to make errors or miss observations. Pay careful attention to both the physical and psychological preparation of your client to ensure a successful assessment. See Table 32–14 for client positions that facilitate physical examination.

Client safety during physical examination is paramount. Be sure that clients are not at risk of losing their balance, falling, or being hurt by equipment. Do not leave a confused, weak, combative, or uncooperative client alone. Be aware that seriously ill or older clients are easily chilled.

TABLE 32-14 Positions for Examination

Position	Areas Assessed	Rationale	Limitations
Sitting	Head and neck, back, posterior thorax and lungs, anterior thorax and lungs, breasts, axillae, heart, and upper extremities; to measure vital signs	Sitting upright facilitates full expansion of lungs and better visualization of symmetry of upper body parts.	A physically weakened client may be unable to sit. The examiner would place the client in the supine position, with the head of the bed elevated.
Supine	Head and neck, anterior thorax and lungs, breasts, axillae, heart, abdomen, extremities; to measure pulses	This is the most normally relaxed position. It facilitates easy access to pulse sites.	If the client easily becomes short of breath, the examiner may need to raise head of the bed.
Dorsal recumbent	Head and neck, anterior thorax and lungs, breasts, axillae, heart, abdomen	This position is used for abdominal assessment because it promotes relaxation of abdominal muscles.	Clients with painful disorders are more comfortable with knees flexed.
Lithotomy*	Female genitalia and genital tract	This position provides maximal exposure of the genitalia and facilitates insertion of the vaginal speculum.	The lithotomy position is embarrassing and uncomfortable for most clients; therefore, the examiner minimizes time that the client is in it, and the client is kept well draped.
Sims'	Rectum and vagina	Flexion of hip and knee provides better exposure of rectal area.	Joint deformities may hinder the client's ability to bend the hip and knee.
Prone	Musculoskeletal system	This position is used only to assess extension of the hip joint.	This position is poorly tolerated in clients with respiratory difficulties.
Lateral recumbent	Heart	This position aids in detecting murmurs.	This position is poorly tolerated in clients with respiratory difficulties.
Knee–chest*	Rectum	This position provides maximal exposure of rectal area.	This position is embarrassing and uncomfortable for most clients.

*Clients with arthritis or other joint deformities may be unable to assume this position.

The physical environment for client examination can vary greatly. The Canadian Nurses Association's *Code of Ethics for Registered Nurses* (2008) mandates that nurses provide initial assessment and emergency care wherever needed. Regardless of the setting, be mindful of the client's dignity and ensure privacy to the extent possible (e.g., use room curtains, or sheets or blankets held up by assistants).

You must know how to conduct a complete physical examination to be able to attend to the needs and circumstances of every client. After mastering the techniques and skills, your challenge is to focus your examinations and interpret findings in light of the client's age, developmental stage, gender, genetic background, and occupation. Nurses who are dedicated to client health promotion and illness prevention include specific screening examinations according to age groups considered at risk (Table 32–15). The Registered Nurses Association of Ontario (RNAO) is one example of a Canadian professional nursing association that has introduced guidelines for nursing best practice developed from evidence-informed nursing research (see http://www.rnao.org/bestpractices/).

➤ TABLE 32-15 Recommended Preventive Screenings

Disease or Condition	Age Group in Years	Screening Measures
Breast cancer	20–39	• Client familiarity with how breasts look and feel through regular breast self-examination • Client ability to recognize monthly breast changes • Annual physical examination by physician, nurse practitioner, or other health care professional • Awareness of risk factors for breast cancer and early detection guidelines for all age groups
	40–49	• Clinical breast examination by a trained health care professional at least every 2 years • Regular breast self-examination • Client discussion with physician about risk for breast cancer and the risks and benefits of mammography
	50–69	• Mammography every 2 years between the ages of 50 and 69 (women) • Clinical breast examination by a trained health care professional at least every 2 years • Regular breast self-examination and report of any changes to physician
	70 and over	• Client discussion with physician about a screening program • Clinical breast examination by a trained professional at least every 2 years • Regular breast self-examination and report of any changes to physician
Colorectal cancer	50 and over	• Fecal occult blood test (FOBT) at least every 2 years (FOBT blood testing helps identify polyps early before they become cancerous.) • Client discussion with physician about individual plan of surveillance, if in the high-risk group
Ear disorders	All ages Over age 65	• Periodic hearing checkups, as needed • Regular hearing checkups
Eye disorders	40 and under 40–64 65 and up	• Complete eye examination every 3 to 5 years (more if positive history) • Complete eye examination every 2 years • Complete eye examination every year
Heart and vascular disorders	Men 45–65 Women 45–65	• Regular measurement of total blood cholesterol levels and triglycerides; blood pressure screenings
Obesity	All ages	• Periodic height, weight, and waist measurements • Calculation of BMI
Oral cavity and cancer of pharynx	All ages	• Regular dental examinations every 6 months
Ovarian cancer	18 and over, or on becoming sexually active	• Annual pelvic examination by health care professional
Prostate cancer	40 and over	• Client discussion about prostate-specific antigen (PSA) test with physician if family history of prostate cancer or African background (The PSA test measures the level of a protein [prostate-specific antigen] in the blood. PSA levels vary with age.)
	50 and over	• Client discussion about annual digital rectal examination (DRE) with physician/nurse practitioner (DRE is a physical examination in which the examiner palpates the prostate by inserting a finger in the rectum.) • Client discussion about the PSA test with physician/nurse practitioner for measuring the level of prostate-specific antigen in the blood and comparing it with age range

Continued

TABLE 32-15 Recommended Preventive Screenings *continued*

Skin cancer	All ages	• Client learning about what to look for and checking skin regularly, as most skin cancers can be cured if caught early enough • Client making sure to check or have checked "hard-to-get-at" places such as the back, back of neck and ears, and backs of legs
Testicular cancer	15 and over	• Regular testicular self-examination (TSE), which informs what is usual for testicles and detects any changes
Uterine cancer	18 and up, or on becoming sexually active	• Annual pelvic examination by health care professional plus an annual Pap test
Cervical cancer	All women on becoming sexually active; to continue even on cessation of sexual activities	• Pap test and pelvic examination every 1 to 3 years, depending on provincial screening guidelines
Endometrial cancer	18 and up, or on becoming sexually active	• Endometrial biopsy at age 35 in high-risk clients • Information to women at menopause at average and high risk about high risks and the signs and symptoms to report

From Canadian Cancer Society (CCS). (2008). *Get to know your breasts.* Retrieved November 15, 2008, from http://www.cancer.ca; Canadian Cancer Society. (2007). *Canadian cancer statistics 2007*. Toronto, ON: Author; Canadian Cancer Society. (2006). *Canadian Cancer Encyclopedia*. Retrieved November 15, 2008, from http://www.cancer.ca/Canada-wide/About%20cancer/Cancer%20encyclopedia.aspx?sc_lang=en; Canadian Task Force on Preventive Health Care. (2005). *New reviews (2001–2005 Publications).* Retrieved June 9, 2008, from http://www.ctfphc.org/Whats%20New/whats_new.htm; Public Health Agency of Canada. (2004). *Progress report on cancer control in Canada.* Retrieved April 27, 2008, from http://www.phac-aspc.gc.ca/publicat/prccc-relccc/index.html; and American Cancer Society. (2008). *Cancer prevention and early detection facts and figures 2008.* Retrieved April 27, 2008, from http://www.cancer.org/docroot/STT/content/STT_1x_Cancer_Prevention_ _Early_ Detection_Facts_ _Figures_2008.asp

Nurses conduct **screening** (shortened assessments to detect deviations) of clients according to age groups and known risk factors (see Table 32–15).

Infection Control Practices

For reasons of safety and comfort, be aware of the biological, chemical, ergonomic, physical, and psychosocial hazards to which you and your clients may be exposed during physical examinations (Rogers, 2003). Provincial regulations exist for Canadian nurses for their protection and that of their clients and for the promotion of health, safety, and wellness. For example, **routine practices and additional precautions** must be followed for the protection of both nurses and clients against contact with blood, body fluids, and body substances that transmit infectious agents. Routine practices include hand hygiene, use of disposable gloves, and use of appropriate barriers against spray or splash exposures. Additional precautions may be the use of dedicated equipment or facilities, airborne precautions, droplet precautions, and contact precautions (Health Canada, 1999). Depending on the situation, masks and safety glasses may be needed in addition to gloves and gown (see Chapter 33).

Both Health Canada and the Public Health Agency of Canada routinely use their Web sites (www.hc-sc-gc.ca and www.phac-aspc.gc.ca) to provide guidelines, a biweekly journal on communicable diseases, recommendations, reports of outbreaks, or summaries for health professionals.

safety alert Perform hand hygiene before preparing equipment, and before and after examinations. Use disposable gloves if you or the client has nonintact skin or if exposure to blood and body fluids is possible.

Assessing Mental and Emotional Status

Much can be learned about the client's mental capacity and emotional state from interaction during the history. Ask questions throughout the examination, and observe the appropriateness of the client's affective response and ideas. Special assessment tools are available to screen a client's current **mental status**. Kahn and Goldfarb's Mental Status Questionnaire (MSQ; 1960) is a widely used 10-item instrument (Kahn et al., 1960). Folstein, Folstein, and McHugh (1975) developed the Mini-Mental State Examination (MMSE) to assess orientation and cognitive function in older adults. Box 32–8 presents sample questions from this examination. A maximum score on the MMSE is 30. A score of 25 or less is suggestive of delirium, dementia, or possible depression, and the client requires further evaluation (Kennedy-Malone, Fletcher, & Plank, 2000).

To ensure objective assessment, take into account the client's values, beliefs, cultural and educational background, and previous experiences, as they influence the client's responses to questions. Alterations in mental or emotional status may reflect a disturbance in cerebral functioning, inasmuch as the cerebral cortex controls and

> **BOX 32-8 Mini-Mental State Examination Sample Questions**

Orientation to time

"What is the date?"

Registration

"Listen carefully. I am going to say three words. You say them back after I stop.

Ready? Here they are . . .

HOUSE (pause), CAR (pause), LAKE (pause). Now repeat those words back to me."

[Repeat up to 5 times, but score only the first trial.]

Naming

"What is this?" [Point to a pencil or pen.]

Reading

"Please read this and do what it says." [Show examinee the words on the stimulus form.]

CLOSE YOUR EYES

From Folstein, M., Folstein, S., & McHugh, P. (2001). *Mini-mental state examination (MMSE)*. Psychological Assessment Resources, Inc. Copyright 1975, 1998, 2001 by Mini-Mental, LLC, Inc. Reproduced by special permission of the Publisher, Psychological Assessment Resources, Inc., 16204 North Florida Avenue, Lutz, Florida 33549. Further reproduction is prohibited without permission of PAR, Inc. The MMSE can be purchased from PAR, Inc. by calling (800) 331-8378 or (813) 968-3003.

> **BOX 32-9 Clinical Criteria for Delirium**

Definition

Delirium is an acute disturbance of consciousness accompanied by a change in cognition. Cannot be accounted for by pre-existing or evolving dementia. Develops over a short period of time, usually hours to days, and tends to fluctuate during the course of the day. Is usually a direct physiological consequence of a general medical condition. A reduced clarity of awareness of the environment.

Delirium is also characterized by the impaired ability to focus, sustain, or shift attention (questions must be repeated). Easy distraction by irrelevant stimuli. A change in cognition (memory impairment, disorientation, or language disturbance). Recent memory most commonly affected. Disorientation usually shown, with client disoriented regarding time or place. Language disturbance involving impaired ability to name objects or ability to write; speech may ramble. Perceptual disturbances, which include misinterpretation, illusions, or hallucinations.

Adapted from American Psychiatric Association. (2000). *Diagnostic and statistical manual of mental disorders* (4th ed. Rev.). Washington, DC: Author; and Stuart, G., & Laraia, M. (2003). *Principles and practice of psychiatric nursing* (8th ed.). St. Louis, MO: Mosby.

integrates emotional and intellectual functioning. Primary brain disorders, medication, and metabolic changes are factors that may change cerebral function.

A common mental disorder affecting older adults is **delirium**, an acute confusional disorder characterized by changing levels of disorientation, consciousness, and sleep–wake cycle. Delirium is often caused by infection, dehydration, surgical procedure, or adverse effects of medication and is amenable to treatment. This acute condition is often misdiagnosed as a form of dementia such as Alzheimer's disease. In the client who already has a dementia (organic loss of intellectual function), symptoms of delirium may go untreated if attributed to the dementia. When delirium occurs in an older adult, you risk dismissing it as expected behaviour in a person of that age. Fortunately, when correctly assessed, the condition can be reversed with treatment of the underlying cause—central nervous system (CNS), metabolic, and cardiopulmonary disorders; systemic illnesses; and sensory deprivation or overload (Stuart & Laraia, 2003). To recognize delirium early, be sure that you know the criteria for delirium, and obtain a full history of the client's behaviour (Box 32–9).

Level of Consciousness

Level of consciousness exists along a continuum from full awakening, alertness, and cooperation to lack of response to any form of external stimuli. A fully conscious client responds to questions spontaneously. As consciousness decreases, a client may show irritability, shorter attention span, or unwillingness to cooperate. To avoid ambiguity when assessing the level of consciousness, the Glasgow Coma Scale (GCS) measures consciousness by an objective numerical scale in three domains: spontaneity of eye opening, best verbal response, and best motor response (Table 32–16). Take extra care when using the scale with clients who have sensory losses (e.g., vision or hearing) or motor paralysis. As consciousness deteriorates, clients become disoriented to name, time, and place. Ask short, to-the-point questions about things that the client knows (e.g., "What is your name?" "What is the name of this place?" and "What day is this?"). The client's ability to understand and answer questions affects your ability to complete an examination. Rouse the client to full alertness before you take a history.

A client may be unable to follow simple commands such as "Squeeze my finger" or "Move your toes." As the level of consciousness declines, the client may respond only to painful stimuli. Apply firm pressure with your thumb on the root of the fingernail. Expect a client to withdraw that hand from the painful stimulus. Serious neurological damage causes clients to respond to pain with unusual posturing. A flaccid response indicates absent muscle tone in the extremities and severe injury to brain tissue.

> **TABLE 32-16 Glasgow Coma Scale**

Action	Response	Score
Eyes open	Spontaneously	4
	To speech	3
	To pain	2
	None	1
Best verbal response	Oriented	5
	Confused	4
	Inappropriate words	3
	Incomprehensible sounds	2
	None	1
Best motor response	Obeys commands	6
	Localized pain	5
	Flexion withdrawal	4
	Unexpected flexion	3
	Unexpected extension	2
	Flaccid	1
Total score		15

The GCS allows you to evaluate a client's neurological status over time. The oriented client who responds to commands would score a full 15 points. A client with a score of 8 points or less is in a coma. A client who fails to respond to pain, open eyes, or move in any way to stimulation would score 3 points.

Behaviour and Appearance

A client's behaviour, moods, hygiene, grooming, and choice of dress provide relevant information about his or her mental status. Be aware of mannerisms and actions during the entire assessment, noting both nonverbal and verbal behaviours. Does the client respond appropriately to directions? Does the client's mood vary for no apparent cause? Does the client show concern about appearance? Is the client's hair clean and neatly groomed, and are the nails trimmed and clean? Expect the client to be alert. Remember that making eye contact and expressing feelings related to the situation are culturally bound. Choice and appropriateness of clothing may reflect socioeconomic status or personal taste rather than deficient self-concept or self-care. Focus also on the appropriateness of clothing for the weather. Older adults may neglect their appearance because of a lack of energy, finances, or reduced vision.

Language

Individuals' ability to understand spoken or written words and to express themselves through writing, speaking, or gesturing is a function of the cerebral cortex. Assess voice inflection, tone, and manner of speech. The voice should have inflections, be clear and strong, and have appropriate variations in volume. Speech should be fluent, and the rate of speech, content, and use of words should be appropriate to the situation. Allow extra time for older adults to respond, as information processing may be slowed in them. When communication is clearly ineffective (e.g., omission or addition of letters and words, wrong use of words, or hesitations), assess for aphasia that may have been caused by an injury to the cerebral cortex. Aphasia is the loss of ability to understand or formulate speech. Language capabilities can be assessed by simple techniques:

- Point to a familiar object, and ask the client to name it (naming).
- Ask the client to respond to simple verbal and written commands, such as "Stand up" or "Sit down" (word comprehension).
- Ask the client to read simple sentences out loud (reading comprehension)

Intellectual Function

Intellectual function includes memory (recent, immediate, and past), knowledge, abstract thinking, association, and judgement. Test each aspect of intellectual function with a specific technique. Culture and education influence a client's ability to respond to test questions. Do not ask questions related to concepts or ideas unfamiliar to the client. Before testing the client, ask his or her permission to do it.

Memory. Assess immediate recall as well as recent and remote memory. Often, a problem with memory becomes apparent when taking the health history. To assess immediate recall, have the client repeat a series of numbers (e.g., *7, 4, 1*) in the order presented or in reverse order. Gradually increase the number of digits (e.g., *7, 4, 1, 8, 6*) until the client fails to repeat the digits correctly. Expect digit span to be five to eight digits forward and four to six digits backward.

To test recent memory, say clearly and slowly the names of three unrelated objects (MMSE; see Box 32–8) and ask the client to repeat each. Continue this until the client is successful. Later in the assessment, ask the client to repeat the three words, and the client should be able to do this. Asking the client to recall earlier events of the day (e.g., what was eaten for breakfast) is another test. You may need to ask a family member to validate the information provided by the client.

To assess past memory, ask open-ended questions, for example, about the client's mother's maiden name, a birthday, or a special date in history, and expect immediate recall of such information. With older adults, determine if the client suffers from any hearing loss before attributing his or her failure to recall to confusion.

Knowledge. Assess the client's knowledge by asking questions about the illnesses or the reason for seeking health care. You thus determine client ability to learn or understand. If an opportunity to teach exists, you can evaluate understanding by asking for feedback during a follow-up visit. Older adults can learn new tasks, but they need more time to do so.

Abstract Thinking. Interpreting abstract ideas or concepts reflects one's capacity for abstract thinking. A higher level of intellectual functioning is required for individuals to explain idioms and sayings, such as "A stitch in time saves nine" or "Don't count your chickens before they're hatched." Note whether the client's explanations are relevant and concrete. The client with altered mentation will likely interpret the phrase literally or merely rephrase the words. Older adults should be able to perform this task successfully.

Association. Another higher level of intellectual functioning involves identifying similarities or associations between concepts: for example, a dog is to a Beagle as a cat is to a Siamese. Alternatively, you can ask the client how an apple and a pear are similar, expecting a response such as "They are both fruits." Questions should be appropriate to clients' level of intelligence and cultural background. It is sufficient to use simple concepts. Older adults are expected to successfully perform this task.

Judgement. Judgement requires comparison and evaluation of facts and ideas to understand their relationships and to form appropriate conclusions. Attempt to measure the client's ability to make logical decisions. By assessing judgement, you also measure the ability to organize thought processes. You may choose to ask clients why they decided to seek health care or how they plan to adjust to limitations after returning home. A simpler test would involve asking what clients would do if locked out of their homes or if they suddenly became ill when alone at home. Expect logical and realistic answers. If clients do not provide such answers, their safety may be an issue. Cognitively intact adults of all ages should be able to do this.

Assessing Cranial Nerve Function

The peripheral nervous system contains 12 paired cranial nerves, and their function can be assessed when examining the peripheral nervous system or when assessing structures in the head and neck. You may test a single cranial nerve, assess a related group of cranial nerves, or examine all 12 cranial nerves at one time. For example, a test of the oculomotor nerve measures pupillary response to light; integrity of the gag reflex confirms vagus and glossopharyngeal nerve function. Dysfunction reflects an alteration at some point along the nerve distribution. Use the following mnemonic (memory aid), "On old Olympus' towering tops, a Finn and German viewed some hops," to remember the order of the 12 paired nerves. The first letter of each word in the phrase is the same as the first letter of the names of the cranial nerves (Table 32–17). Eight cranial nerves have either sensory or motor functions, and four have both functions.

TABLE 32-17 Cranial Nerve Function and Assessment

Number	Name	Type	Function	Method
I	Olfactory	Sensory	Sense of smell	Ask the client to identify different nonirritating aromas, such as that from coffee or vanilla.
II	Optic	Sensory	Visual acuity	Use the Snellen chart, or ask the client to wear his or her glasses and read printed material.
III	Oculomotor	Motor	Extraocular eye movement Pupil constriction and dilation	Assess directions of gaze. Measure pupillary reaction to light reflex and accommodation.
IV	Trochlear	Motor	Upward and downward movement of eyeball	Assess directions of gaze.
V	Trigeminal	Sensory and motor	Sensory nerve to skin of face Motor nerve to muscles of jaw	Lightly touch cornea with wisp of cotton to assess corneal reflex. Measure sensation of light pain and touch across skin of face. Palpate temples as client clenches teeth.
VI	Abducens	Motor	Lateral movement of eyeballs	Assess directions of gaze.
VII	Facial	Sensory and motor	Facial expression Taste	Look for asymmetry as the client smiles, frowns, puffs out cheeks, and raises and lowers eyebrows. Have the client identify taste by placing salty or sweet things on the front of the tongue.
VIII	Auditory	Sensory	Hearing	Assess ability to hear the spoken word.
IX	Glossopharyngeal	Sensory and motor	Taste Ability to swallow	Ask the client to identify taste by placing sour or sweet things on the back of the tongue. Use the tongue blade to elicit the gag reflex.
X	Vagus	Sensory and motor	Sensation of pharynx Movement of vocal chords	Ask the client to say "ah." Observe the movement of the palate and pharynx. Assess speech for hoarseness.
XI	Spinal accessory	Motor	Movement of head and shoulders	Ask the client to shrug the shoulders and turn the head against passive resistance.
XII	Hypoglossal	Motor	Position of tongue	Ask the client to stick out the tongue to the midline and to move the tongue from side to side.

Assessing Sensory and Motor Functions

Sensory Function

Be sure that you know the sensory and motor functions of the CNS before examining the head and neck, torso, or extremities. Sensory pathways of the CNS conduct sensations of pain, temperature, position, vibration, crude touch, and fine touch. Different nerve pathways relay the sensations. Most peripheral nerves have sensory as well as motor fibres. For most clients, screening of sensory function is sufficient unless the client reports symptoms of reduced sensation, motor impairment, or paralysis.

safety alert Impaired sensation creates the risk of skin breakdown. Do a complete integuement assessment of the area affected by the sensory loss. Teach clients to avoid pressure, thermal, or chemical trauma to the affected area.

Most clients exhibit sensory responses to all stimuli. Usually, sensations on body surfaces are felt equally on both sides of the head, torso, and extremities. To assess the major sensory nerves, you need to know the sensory dermatomes (see Figure 32–30, page 622). Skin areas are innervated by specific dorsal root cutaneous nerves.

Demonstrate to the client what you are using for the test. During all sensory testing, the client must keep the eyes closed so that no clues are provided. Apply stimuli in a random, unpredictable order to maintain the client's attention and to avoid anticipation. Ask the client to indicate when and where each stimulus is felt, and what it is. Compare results for symmetrical areas.

Motor Function

Motor pathways of the CNS consist of upper and lower motor neurons and their synapses. The higher motor neurons affect movement through the lower motor neurons. Three primary motor pathways mediate muscle tone, posture, muscular activity, reflex activity, balance, coordination, gait, and equilibrium. These pathways are the cerebellar system, corticospinal tract, and basal ganglia system.

Assessment of central and peripheral nervous system motor functions is done primarily during examination of the extremities and, to a lesser extent, during examination of the head and neck or torso.

Assessing the Integumentary System

Use inspection and palpation to assess the function and integrity of the **integument** (i.e, skin, hair, scalp, nails, sebaceous glands, and sweat glands).

Skin

Assessment of the skin reveals a variety of conditions, including changes in circulation, hydration, integrity of tissues, nutrition, and oxygenation. The skin (epidermis, dermis, and subcutaneous tissues) provides the body's external protection, regulates body temperature, synthesizes vitamin D, excretes some metabolic wastes (e.g., sugars, uric acid, urea), absorbs certain chemicals, and acts as a sensory organ for pain, temperature, pressure, and touch.

The thin, avascular epidermis of the skin is divided into the basal cell layer (where melanin and keratin are formed) and the outer horny cell layer (where dead keratinized cells are shed). The underlying dermis supplies nutrition to the epidermis. Connective and elastic tissues predominate in the dermis, where blood vessels, nerves, lymphatics, hair follicles, sebaceous glands, and sweat glands are located. With the exception of the skin on the palms and soles, all skin has sebaceous glands. Widely distributed in the skin, eccrine sweat glands open directly onto skin surfaces to help maintain body temperature. Apocrine sweat glands, which mainly open into hair follicles in the axillae and genital area, are stimulated by stress, and sweating in these areas produces body odour. The subcutaneous layer is composed of adipose tissue, which contributes to skin mobility.

During history taking (see Chapter 13), use open-ended questions to inquire about the skin (e.g., colour, pigmentation, rashes, **lesions**, itching, bruising, dryness, moisture), hair (e.g., loss, dryness, oiliness), nails (e.g., brittleness, colour, shape), changes in known lesions, workplace and lifestyle exposures to chemicals, and previous history of skin disease (including familial predisposition, allergies). Table 32–18 provides the approach to history taking for skin assessment.

TABLE 32-18 Health History for Skin, Hair, Scalp, and Nail Assessment

Assessment Category	Rationale for Assessment
Skin	
Question the client about his or her knowledge of risk factors for skin cancer and the presence of any of those risk factors.	Knowledge of risk factors, such as skin tones, sun exposure, exposure to hazardous toxins, and sunburns early in life, can increase the client's level of self-care and reduce risk of skin cancer, for example, by reducing the time spent outdoors and in tanning booths.
Inquire about the number and nature of skin lesions, moles, and freckles.	Presence of more than 40 moles increases the risk of skin cancer.
Ask the client about changes in skin condition and when the last self-assessment and clinical assessment of the skin were conducted.	Regular self-assessment and clinical examination of the skin ensures proper care of skin.
Inquire about the use of lotions and creams on skin surfaces and about regular hygiene practices.	Regular hygiene and use of appropriate lotions can ensure proper skin care.
Ask the client about the presence of any allergies.	Skin rashes are commonly allergic responses.
Question the client on the use of hats, sunglasses, protective lotions, and long-sleeved clothing during exposures to the sun.	Protecting skin surfaces is the best way to prevent skin cancer.
Inquire about skin exposure to chemical substances during work, study, hobbies, or recreation.	Skin absorption of toxic chemicals contributes to organic or systemic conditions and malignancies.
Hair and Scalp	
Inquire about usual hygiene routine for hair and scalp.	Hygiene practices contribute to the health of hair and scalp.
Ask about any changes in the hair or scalp.	Changes in nutrition can affect the condition of hair. Chemicals and heat can cause dryness and brittlenesss. Changes are noticed by the client during self-care.
Inquire about current disease conditions, treatments, or medications that may affect the integrity of the hair and scalp.	Chemotherapy destroys cells that multiply rapidly (e.g., hair cells, tumour cells). Vasodilators may cause excessive hair growth.
Nails	
Inquire about usual nail care practices.	Frequent manicures or exposure to chemicals may damage nails.
Inquire about recent changes in nails and changes over time.	Systemic conditions may affect colour, growth, or shape; local trauma may affect shape and growth.
Determine risks for nail problems.	Diseases such as diabetes as well as trauma can affect the vascularity of the peripheral tissues, including nails. Poor vision, inability to bend, or lack of coordination may make it difficult to practise regular nail care.

safety alert Skin can absorb certain chemicals, which creates risks for those who are exposed to chemicals during work, study, hobby, or recreation. Inquire about such exposures during history taking. The protective functions of the skin become impaired with compromised mobility, circulation, nutrition, and hydration. Friction and moisture increase the risk of skin breakdown in bedridden clients.

Counsel clients about protecting their skin and avoiding harmful exposures. The Slip! Slap! Slop! Message, which originated in Australia (http://www.asebp.ab.ca/slip_slap_slop.html), can be used for this purpose. Broaden your health promotion focus to include the integument (Box 32–10). Use your knowledge of teaching and learning principles to ensure that clients are fully informed about skin self-examination (Box 32–11). Cutaneous malignancies are the most commonly identified neoplasms. Approximately 4600 new cases of **melanoma**, an aggressive form of skin cancer, and 69,000 new cases of the highly curable nonmelanoma (basal cell and squamous cell) cancers were expected in 2007 (Canadian Cancer Society, 2007). Basal cell carcinomas frequently occur in sun-damaged skin.

Trauma to the skin during bedside care, exposure to pressure during immobilization, or reaction to treatment medications lead to risks for skin lesions. Individuals most at risk are chronically ill, neurologically impaired, orthopedic clients, or clients with diminished mental status, poor tissue oxygenation, low cardiac output, or inadequate nutrition. In long-term care facilities, clients may be at risk for similar problems in relation to their level of mobility and multiple chronic illnesses.

Routinely assess clients' skin for early indications of change or development of lesions. *Primary lesions* can quickly deteriorate to become *secondary lesions* that require more extensive nursing care. The development of a pressure ulcer, for example, can lengthen hospital stay unless it is prevented or discovered early and treated properly (see Chapter 47). The condition of the client's skin is a good indication of the need for nursing care. Assessment findings determine the hygiene measures, nutrition, and hydration required to maintain the integrity of the integument (see Chapters 38 and 43).

Inspection of Skin. Inspect colour, hygiene (including odours), and lesions. During physical examination you observe each part of the body, but ensure that you make a brief but careful visual sweep of the entire body. This informs you of the distribution and extent of any lesions, as well as the overall symmetry of skin colour. Because you inspect all skin surfaces, clients will need to assume several positions.

Colour. For accurate inspection of skin colour and for identification of the type, colour, configuration, and distribution of skin lesions, adequate lighting is necessary. Sunlight is best for detecting skin changes in dark-skinned clients (Talbot & Curtis, 1996). Despite individual variations among clients, skin colour is usually uniform over the body, although ambient temperature may affect findings. A warm environment may cause superficial vasodilation, increasing redness of the skin. A cool environment may cause sensitive clients to develop **cyanosis** (bluish discoloration) around the lips and nail beds (Talbot & Curtis, 1996). Skin pigmentation ranges in tone from ivory or light pink to ruddy pink in light skin and from light to deep brown or olive in dark skin. Pigmentation from melanin is more pronounced in sun-exposed areas. While inspecting the skin, be aware that cosmetics or tanning agents may mask the true colour. Table 32–19 lists colour variations, underlying causes, and the assessment focus.

It is more difficult to note changes such as pallor or cyanosis in dark-skinned clients. Usually, hues are best seen in the palms, soles, lips, tongue, hard palate, earlobes, and nail beds where pigmentation is reduced. Skin creases and folds are darker than the rest of the body in dark-skinned clients. Look for loss of the underlying red tones in dark skin, and remember that melanin in the lips may be mistaken for cyanosis. In dark-skinned clients, use palpation after inspection to detect heat and warmth from erythema (e.g., presence of skin **inflammation**; Talbot & Curtis, 1996).

Odours. Using your sense of smell, inspect for generalized, localized, or **intertriginous** (skin fold) body odour in areas such as the axillae, groins, and breasts (see Table 32–2).

Lesions. Expect to see skin pigmentation as freckles, moles, and birthmarks during inspection, noting their distribution. You may also see primary and secondary skin lesions that require further examination during palpation (Box 32–12). For example, **petechiae** are pinpoint, red or purple spots on the skin caused by small hemorrhages in the skin layers. They may indicate serious blood-clotting disorders, drug reactions, or liver disease. Inspect any lesion for colour, location, size, shape, type, grouping (e.g., clustered, linear, circular), and distribution (localized or generalized). Using a small, clear, flexible ruler, measure length, width, and depth of lesions. Assess exudate for amount, colour, odour, and consistency, and document tattoos and body piercings.

During skin inspection, you might detect indications of substance abuse in skin colour, lesions, and perspiration (Box 32–13). Clients who have repeatedly and recently injected illegal drugs intravenously may have edematous, reddened, and warm areas along the arms and legs. Old injection sites are shiny, scarred, or hyperpigmented. Do not confuse clients who donate blood regularly with those who abuse drugs.

BOX 32-10 FOCUS ON PRIMARY HEALTH CARE

Integument

- Basic hygiene
- Prevention of head lice in at-risk clients
- Skin self-examination (asymmetry, borders, colour, diameter, elevation of lesions)
- Protection of integument (skin, hair, scalp, and nails)
- Adequate vitamin D intake
- Prevention of work-related skin problems

BOX 32-11 Skin Self-Examination

Advise clients to perform skin self-examination in appropriate light and to be aware of the locations and appearance of moles and birthmarks.

Instruct clients to examine hard-to-see areas of the body using full-length and hand-held mirrors in a systematic manner; they require a head-to-toe approach, concentrating especially on the shoulders and back, where dysplastic nevi most commonly occur, and on areas where ordinary moles are rarely found—scalp, breast, and buttocks. Clients should also be instructed to check the soles of their feet and between the toes.

Suggest that clients take photographs of moles and compare them with the appearance of the moles during self-examination. Teach them to monitor change in size by measuring the moles with a small ruler.

Urge clients to consult their physician promptly if any pigmented skin spots look like melanoma, if new moles appear, or if existing moles change.

Adapted from Seidel, H. M., Ball, J. W., Dains, J. E., & Benedict, G. W. (2006). *Mosby's guide to physical examination* (6th ed., p. 174, Box 8–1). St. Louis, MO: Mosby.

➤ TABLE 32-19 Inspection of Skin Colour

Colour	Underlying Cause	Focus of Assessment
Bluish (cyanosis)	Increased amount of deoxygenated hemoglobin, which is associated with hypoxia (e.g., congenital heart disease, advanced lung disease, abnormal hemoglobins) Cold environment, anxiety	Lips, oral mucosa, sclera, palpebral conjunctiva, tongue, nails, palms, soles, dorsum of hands and feet Nails, hands, feet
Black	Necrosis of tissue	
White (pallor)	Decreased amount of oxyhemoglobin, which is associated with anemia, decreased blood flow (prolonged elevation, immobilization, or edema) Fainting, shock, arterial insufficiency or occlusion Lack of pigmentation due to congenital condition (e.g., albinism) or loss of pigmentation due to autoimmune condition (e.g., vitiligo)	Fingernails, lips, mucous membranes of mouth and palpebral conjunctivae, ear lobes, face, palms, soles Eyes, skin Head, neck, torso, arms, legs
Yellow-orange (**jaundice**)	Increased deposit of bilirubin in tissues, associated with liver disease or excessive destruction of red blood cells High levels of carotene in diet	Palpebral conjunctivae, lips, hard palate, undersurface of tongue, tympanic membrane, skin Face, palms, soles
Red (erythema)	Increased visibility of oxyhemoglobin associated with dilation or increased blood flow, fever, direct trauma, pressure, blushing, or alcohol intake	Face, sacrum, shoulders, elbows, hips, buttocks, knees, scrotum, heels, area of trauma
Tan-brown (pigmentation)	Increased melanin in skin; examples: • Suntan, artificial tanning • Pregnancy • Age-related change	Areas exposed to sun or tanning agent: face, neck, arms, legs, torso Face, areolae, nipples Dorsum of hands

Palpation of Skin. During palpation, assess moisture, temperature, texture, thickness, mobility, turgor, and lesions. Use disposable gloves if open, moist, or draining lesions are present. Use fingertips to palpate skin surfaces for moisture (wetness and oiliness). Hydration of the skin and mucous membranes reveals body fluid imbalances, changes in the environment, and regulation of body temperature. Expect minimal perspiration or oiliness, except for the intertriginous areas (e.g., axillae, inguinal regions). Increased perspiration may be associated with rigorous activity, warm environments, obesity, postmenopausal hot flashes, anxiety, or excitement. Dry skin may result from low humidity, exposure to sun, stress, smoking, excessive perspiration, and dehydration (Hardy, 1996). Excessive dryness can aggravate existing inflammatory conditions such as eczema and dermatitis. Both flaking and scaling indicate extreme dryness (Hardy, 1996). Flakes resembling dandruff appear when the skin surface is lightly rubbed. Fish-like scales rub off the skin surface easily.

Skin temperature depends on the amount of blood circulating through the dermis. Increased or decreased skin temperature indicates an increase or decrease in blood flow. If an examination room is cold, the client's skin temperature and colour may be affected. Assess temperature by palpating the skin with the dorsum (back) of the hand and comparing symmetrical body parts; the skin temperature should be warm. Localized erythema or redness is often accompanied by an increase in the temperature of the skin. A stage I pressure ulcer can be identified early by detecting warmth and erythema of a skin area (see Chapter 47). Always assess skin temperature in clients at risk for impaired circulation (e.g., after a cast application).

Texture is a characteristic of the surface and deeper portions of the skin. Stroke the skin lightly with your fingertips and finger pads to assess smoothness, thickness, and firmness. Skin on the palms and soles tends to be thicker. Local changes may be a result of trauma, surgical wounds, or lesions. Irregularities in texture, such as scars or **induration** (hardening), may be an indication of recent injury. Deeper palpation may reveal tenderness or localized induration often caused by repeated intramuscular or subcutaneous injections into specific areas. Palpate those areas last in diabetic clients or clients receiving vitamin B_{12} or iron injections.

Assess elasticity of the skin by using fingertips and pads to grasp a fold of skin in the area under the clavicle (Figure 32–7) or on the back of the forearm, and then release it. Note the degree of ease with which the skin moves and how quickly it returns to place. Usually, skin lifts easily into a fold (mobility) and falls back immediately into place (**turgor**). If the skin fold remains pinched, evaluate the client's hydration, and take further action, as needed. Clients with reduced skin turgor do not have resilience to the usual wear and tear on the skin and are predisposed to skin breakdown.

Skin circulation affects the appearance of superficial blood vessels. After a client has been lying or sitting in one position for a considerable amount of time, localized pressure areas appear as pale, pink, or reddened (see Chapter 47). Assess these areas for blanching to pressure.

Fluid buildup makes areas of the skin become swollen or edematous. Direct trauma and impaired venous return are two common causes of edema. First, inspect swollen or edematous areas for location, colour, and shape. In clients with dependent edema caused by poor

BOX 32-12 Types of Skin Lesions

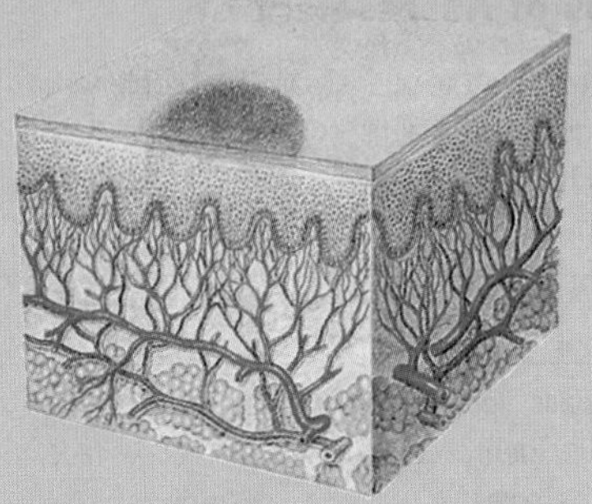

Macule: A flat, circumscribed area that is a change in the colour of the skin; less than 1 cm in diameter (e.g., freckle, petechiae)

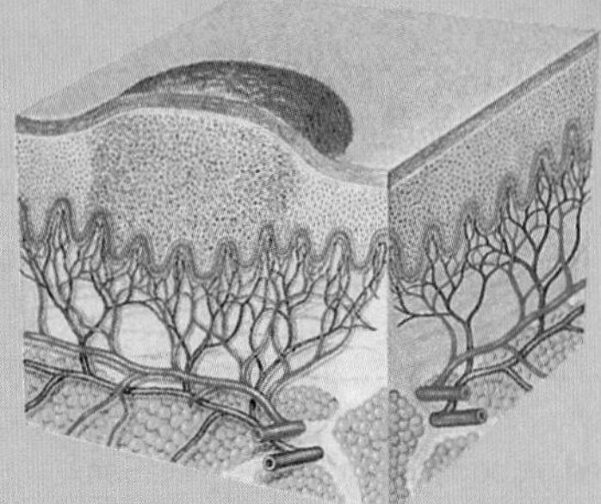

Papule: An elevated, firm circumscribed area; less than 1 cm in diameter (e.g., wart, elevated mole)

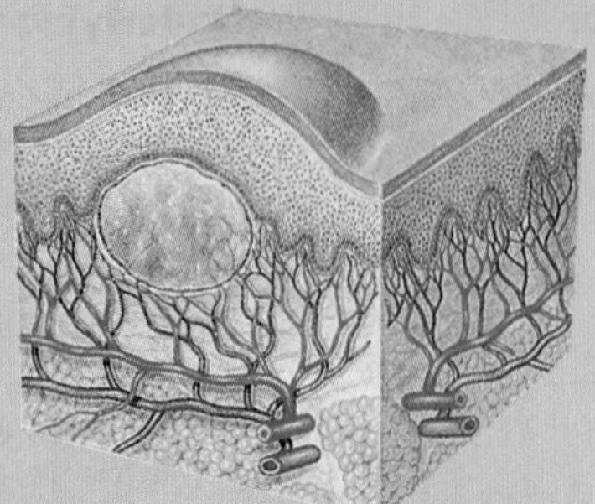

Nodule: Elevated, firm, circumscribed lesion; deeper in the dermis than a papule; 1 to 2 cm in diameter (e.g., lipoma)

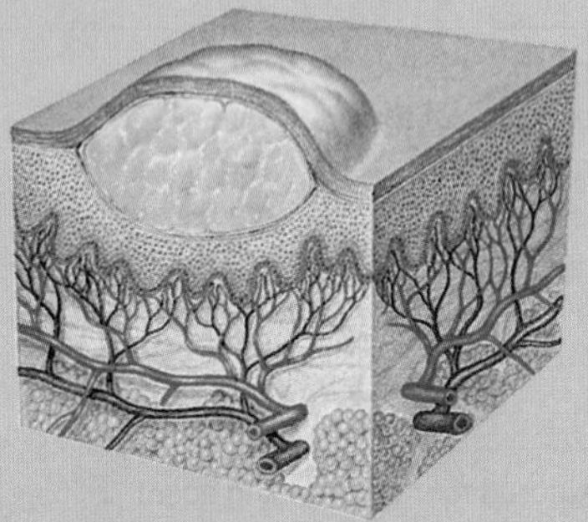

Tumour: Elevated, solid lesion; may or may not be clearly demarcated; deeper in the dermis; greater than 2 cm in diameter (e.g., neoplasm)

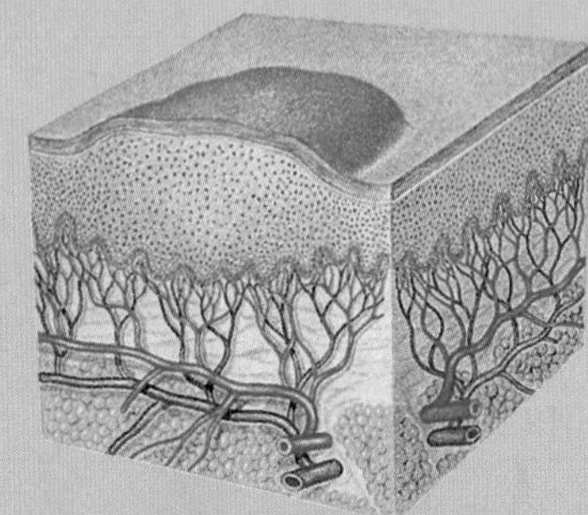

Wheal: Elevated, irregular-shaped area of cutaneous edema; solid, transient, variable diameter (e.g., allergic reaction)

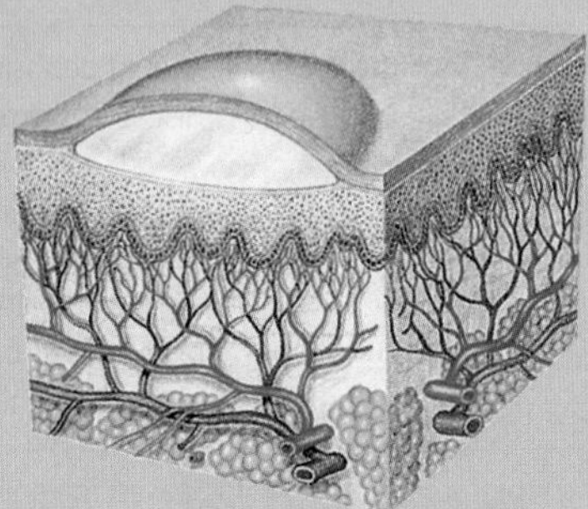

Vesicle: Elevated, circumscribed, superficial lesion, not into the dermis; filled with serous fluid; less than 1 cm in diameter (e.g., herpes zoster)

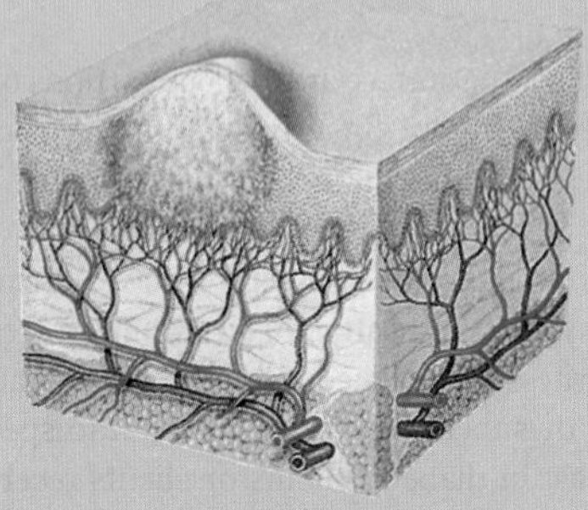

Pustule: Elevated, superficial lesion; similar to a vesicle but filled with purulent fluid (e.g., acne)

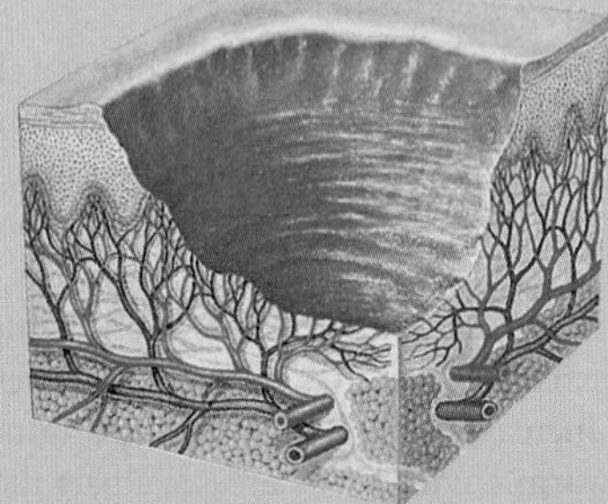

Ulcer: Loss of epidermis and dermis; concave lesion; varies in size (e.g., decubitus ulcer)

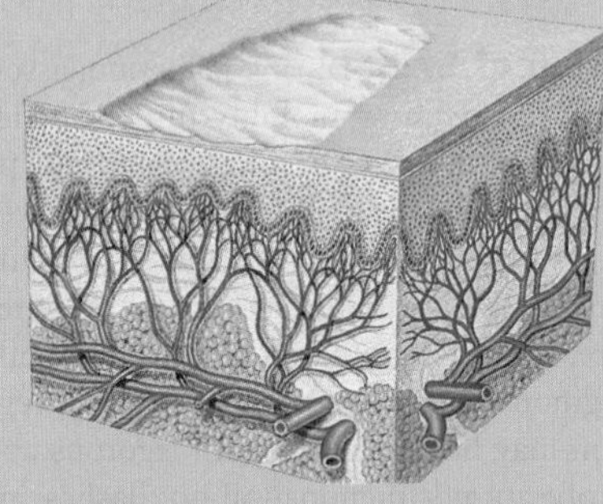

Atrophy: Thinning of skin surface and loss of skin markings; skin translucent and paper-like (e.g., aged skin)

From Seidel, H. M., Ball, J. W., Dains, J. E., & Benedict, G. W. (2006). *Mosby's guide to physical examination* (6th ed., pp. 183–188). St. Louis, MO: Mosby.

venous return, typical locations are the feet, ankles, and sacrum. **Edema** separates the skin surface from the pigmented and vascular layers, masking true skin colour. Edematous skin looks stretched and shiny. Palpate areas of edema to determine skin mobility, consistency, tenderness, and extent. When pressure from the your thumb leaves an indentation in the edematous area, it is called **pitting edema** (Figure 32–8). To assess the degree of pitting edema, press the edematous area firmly with your thumb for 5 seconds, and release. The depth of pitting, recorded in millimetres, determines the degree of edema (Figure 32–8; Seidel et al., 2006). For example, 1 degree of edema equals a 2-mm depth, 2 degrees equals a 4-mm depth, and so on.

Palpation determines the lesion's mobility, contour (flat, raised, or depressed), and consistency (soft or indurated). Classification of lesions as primary or secondary includes descriptions of size and elevation (see Box 32–12). Primary lesions occur as initial spontaneous manifestations of a pathological process (e.g., wheal caused by an insect bite); secondary lesions are alterations in primary lesions (e.g., a pressure ulcer).

Age-Related Changes in Skin. In older adults, skin pigmentation increases unevenly, causing discoloured areas. Skin becomes wrinkled because of decrease in collagen, subcutaneous fat, and sweat

➤ BOX 32-13 Physical Findings of the Skin Indicative of Substance Abuse

Physical Finding	Commonly Associated Drug
Diaphoresis	Sedative hypnotic (including alcohol)
Spider angiomas	Alcohol, stimulants
Burns (especially fingers)	Alcohol
Needle marks	Opioids
Contusion, abrasions, cuts, scars	Alcohol, other sedative hypnotics
"Homemade" tattoos (prevents detection of injection sites)	Cocaine, intravenous opioids
Increased vascularity of face	Alcohol
Red, dry skin	Phencyclidine (PCP)

Adapted from Caulker-Burnett, I. (1994). Primary care screening for substance abuse. *The Nurse Practitioner, 19*(6), 42–48; and Friedman, L., Fleming, N. F., Roberts, D. H., & Hyman, S. E. (1996). *Source book of substance abuse and addiction*. Baltimore, MD: Williams & Wilkins.

glands. Very dry skin is common in older adults. Capillaries are more fragile, and skin loses elasticity. Skin lesions may appear as skin tags, thickenings (senile keratosis), ruby red papules (cherry angiomas), and atrophic warts.

Documentation. Record your findings from inspection and palpation of the skin (Table 32–20).

Hair and Scalp

The two types of hair on the body are terminal and vellus. Terminal hair is long, coarse, thick, and visible on the scalp, in the eyebrows or beards, and in the axillae and pubic areas. Clients with Aboriginal and Asian backgrounds have less terminal hair and are assessed using relevant norms. Vellus hair is short, soft, inconspicuous, and lightly pigmented, covering the entire body except for the palms and soles. Assess the type and distribution of body hair. Discuss diet and hygiene to promote hair and scalp health.

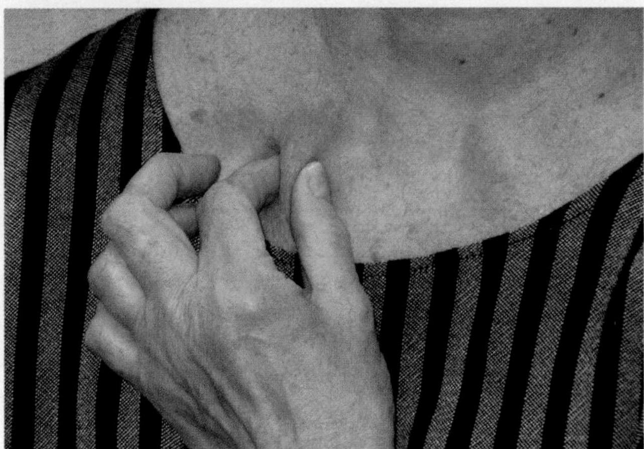

Figure 32-7 Assessment of skin turgor in the subclavicular area. **Source:** From Skillen, D. L., Day, R. A., Anderson, M. C., Stephen, T. C., Gilbert, J. A., & Day, L. W. (2004). *Physical examination images* [CD-ROM]. Edmonton, AB: Faculty of Nursing, University of Alberta.

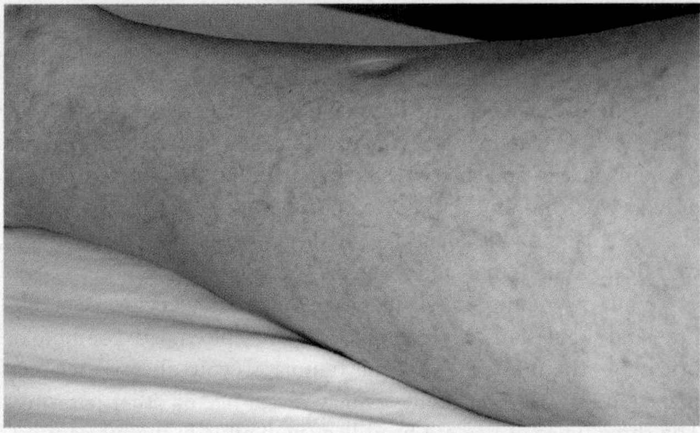

Figure 32-8 Pitting edema in leg. **Source:** From Skillen, D. L., Day, R. A., Anderson, M. C., Stephen, T. C., Gilbert, J. A., & Day, L. W. (2004). *Physical examination images* [CD-ROM]. Edmonton, AB: Faculty of Nursing, University of Alberta.

Inspection of Hair and Scalp. Clients are sensitive about their personal appearance . Before inspection, explain the need to examine the scalp, and use gloves from the beginning as you may encounter lesions or lice. During inspection, examine the colour, distribution, and quantity of body hair. Wide variations in hair colour may be

➤ TABLE 32-20 Examples of Documentation for Integumentary System

Specific Characteristic	Expected Findings
Skin	
Colour	Uniformly olive
Odour	Free of odour
Lesions	Occasional nevus on extremities and torso
Moisture	Minimally moist bilaterally
Temperature	Warm bilaterally
Texture	Smooth bilaterally
Turgor	Skin is mobile; skin fold returns to place quickly
Vascularity	Occasional red papules noted on torso
Edema	Edema not present bilaterally at ankles
Hair and Scalp	
Colour	Brown
Texture	Coarse and curly
Moisture	Dry
Distribution	Evenly distributed over skull
Quantity	Uniformly thick
Scalp	Uniformly pinkish white
Nails	
Nail plate	Smooth and trimmed right, left
Nail bed	Pink bilaterally Capillary return <2 seconds
Nail base	Firm bilaterally
Nail folds	Smooth, colour of surrounding skin, nontender right, left
Nail angle	160 degrees with nail base right, left

Adapted from Chambers, J., Bazin, M., Nutting, L., & Stephen, T. (2008). *Year I lab guide* (pp. 45, 49). Edmonton, AB: Faculty of Nursing, University of Alberta.

present because of the use of rinses or dyes. Expect age-related and genetically based variations in distribution and quantity. Unexpected changes may be the result of inadequate nutrition, hormonal or endocrine disturbances, or excessive use of chemical agents. For example, hirsutism in women manifests as hair growth on the upper lip, chin, cheeks, and coarser vellus hair over the body. In thyroid disorders, hair thinning or loss (alopecia) occurs. Recognize that a change in hair growth can negatively affect body image and emotional well-being in both men and women.

While examining scalp hair, make note of colour, evidence of dryness, and skin lesions. Moles on the scalp may bleed with combing or brushing. Inquire about recent trauma if you observe lesions. Inspection of scalp hair follicles may reveal lice or other parasites. The three types of lice are head lice (pediculus humanus capitis), body lice (pediculus humanus corporis), and crab lice (pediculus pubis). They attach their waxy, yellowish eggs firmly to the hair and are not easily detected. Head and body lice have very small greyish-white bodies, and crab lice have red legs. Bites or pustular eruptions in the hair follicles and skin irritations behind the ears and in the warm intertriginous areas indicate their presence. In a nonjudgemental and calm manner, teach clients about treating the infestation and about using a medicated shampoo.

Palpation of Hair and Scalp. During palpation, examine scalp hair for thickness, texture, and lubrication. The hair may be coarse, fine, curly, or straight. Expect hair to be shiny, smooth, pliant, and evenly distributed. Hair is lubricated by the sebaceous glands. Excessive oiliness is associated with androgen hormone overstimulation; extreme dryness may be a result of a thyroid condition or poor self-care practices.

Age-Related Changes in Hair. In older adults, hair is drier and more brittle and loses pigment, becoming dull grey, white, or yellow. The amount of scalp hairs decreases in a generalized pattern, and the hair diameter becomes smaller. Hairline recession starts as a result of genetics, beginning at the temples and proceeding to the vertex. In women, the pattern of hair loss is similar but less severe. Older men experience reduction in facial hair growth, but older women may develop hair on the chin and upper lip. Age-related hair loss occurs on the torso, axillae, pubic area, and legs as well.

Documentation. Record your findings from the inspection and palpation of the hair and scalp (see Table 32–20).

Nails

The condition of the nails reflects a person's general state of health, nutritional status, occupation, and level of self-care. The client's psychological state may be indicated by evidence of nail biting or picking. Nails usually grow at a constant rate, but direct injury or generalized disease can impair growth. The most visible portion of the nails is the plate of keratin that covers the nail bed. Vascularity of the underlying epithelial cells in the nail bed and the state of the circulating blood give the nail its colour. The semilunar, opaque white area at the base of the nail bed is called lunula, from which the nail plate develops. Nail folds overlap the lateral and proximal borders of the nail plate. The cuticle protects the nail matrix, where new keratin cells develop. Before assessing the nails, take a brief history from the client (see Table 32–18).

Inspection of Nails. Inspect the nail bed for colour, cleanliness, and length; the nail plate for contour and surface; the angle between the nail and the nail bed in degrees; and the lateral and proximal nail folds for colour, shape, and integrity. Expect nails to be smooth, pink, transparent, well rounded, and convex; cuticles are smooth, intact, and clear. In dark-skinned clients, longitudinal bands of brown or black pigment may be seen. Bands in nail beds can be caused by changes in nutrient and electrolyte levels. Splinter hemorrhages may indicate trauma or chronic conditions.

The nail bed angle is about 160 degrees, although the angle in clients with chronic oxygenation problems from heart or lung conditions may increase. For example, in clubbing, the distal phalanx is rounded and bulbous, the angle of the nail bed is 180 degrees or greater, and the nail plate is convex.

If nails are ragged, dirty, and poorly kept, consider the client's reported frequency of nail care, ability to perform care, and type of employment. Work such as farming, mining, or mechanics (e.g., oil and gas industry) may cause dirty nails despite excellent nail care. Jagged, bitten, or broken nail edges or cuticles can predispose a person to infection and risks from exposure to substances and infectious agents in the workplace. Inspection of the skin around the nails may reveal thickenings of the epidermis, such as calluses or corns, caused by friction or pressure from shoes, tools, and instruments.

Palpation of Nails. Palpate the nail base for firmness, and the nail plate for thickness, texture, smoothness, and capillary return. When you note an angle of 180 degrees or more during inspection, you will detect a base that feels spongy or floating. You can check **capillary return** by pressing firmly, quickly, and gently on the nail plate. With pressure, the nail bed blanches; on release of pressure, the pink colour returns within 1 or 2 seconds, unless circulatory insufficiency delays it. Reduced amounts of oxyhemoglobin is the cause for continual pallor of the nail beds; increased amounts of deoxygenated hemoglobin will create a bluish colour. During inspection and palpation of the nails, take advantage of the opportunity to promote nail health by discussing diet, hygiene, and protective measures.

safety alert Clients with impaired circulation are at greater risk for localized infection. Observe the condition of the nails on their hands and feet to identify early signs of infection.

Age-Related Changes to Nails. With aging, nails become harder and thicker, and nail growth slows down. Nails are more brittle, dull, and opaque and develop longitudinal striations. If calcium uptake or intake is insufficient, nails may turn yellow. Cuticles become thinner and narrower.

Documentation. Record your findings from inspection and palpation of the nails (see Table 32–20).

Assessing the Head and Neck

Assessment of the head and neck requires inspection and palpation in close sequence as well as auscultation.

Head

Inspection. History taking includes screening for intracranial injuries and local or congenital deformities (Table 32–21). Begin by inspecting the client's head position and all facial features, expecting the head to be held upright and still. A slight asymmetry of features is a common finding. Note whether all features on one side of the face are affected or whether only part of the face is. Note the size, shape, and contour of the skull, which is generally round with prominences in the frontal and occipital areas.

➤ TABLE 32-21 Health History for Head Assessment

Assessment Category	Rationale for Assessment
Ask whether the client has a history of headache or any trauma to the head; document results of a symptom analysis.	Characteristics of a headache can help determine causative factors, and the nature of trauma will guide examination.
Inquire about the client's occupational history, especially use of safety helmets.	Certain occupations have risks for head injury.
Question the client about participation in sporting events and use of protective equipment.	Many sporting activities have the potential for head injuries when proper protective equipment is not used.

Palpation. Local skull deformities are typically caused by trauma. Palpate the skull for nodules, masses, and tenderness. Gently rotate your fingertips over the skull for irregularities. Note the pulse characteristics of the temporal arteries bilaterally; then assess movement in the temporomandibular joint (TMJ) space, which should be smooth, although it is not unusual to hear or feel a click or snap. At this time, the motor and sensory branches of cranial nerve V (trigeminal) and the motor function of cranial nerve VII (facial) may also be tested (Skill 32–2).

Eyes

Assessment of the eyes includes visual acuity, visual fields, extraocular movements, and external and internal eye structures. If you detect visual alterations, assess the level of assistance that the client requires when ambulating or performing self-care activities. The client may need special aids for reading instructions, such as those on medication labels. Table 32–22 contains the health history that guides the eye examination. Box 32–14 highlights the focus of health promotion for the eyes.

➤ SKILL 32-2 Assessing the Face

Equipment

- Splintered tongue blade
- Cotton ball

Procedure

EXAMINATION SKILL AND FOCUS	TECHNIQUES AND RATIONALE
Inspection: Skin, face, lips	1. Inspect skin, face, and lips.
Palpation:	
Temporal arteries	1. Palpate temporal arteries with fingertips or pads. *Fine tactile discrimination is required.*
Temporomandibular joint	1. Position your index fingertips in front of each tragus. *Fingertips will slip into joint space when the client opens the mouth.* 2. Instruct the client to open and close the mouth, while you keep your fingertips in position in front of the tragus.
Cranial nerve (CN) V (trigeminal) motor function	1. Instruct the client to clench the teeth during palpation. *Assesses motor function of paired CN V.* 2. Palpate temporal and masseter muscles with fingertips or pads. 3. Note strength and symmetry of contraction. *Detects differences.*
Sensory function	1. Demonstrate how sharp, dull, or light touch feels before beginning tests. *Client knows what to expect and report.* 2. Instruct the client to close the eyes and indicate when he or she feels your touch. *Ensures that sensation, not vision, is being tested.* 3. Test side to side, varying rhythm, touching ophthalmic, maxillary, and mandibular regions lightly with cotton ball. *Prevents client's anticipation of being touched and tests all three sensory branches of the nerve.* 4. Repeat with splintered tongue blade. Use the dull touch to check the reliability of the client's response at least once. *Validates client is sensing pain, not pressure.* 5. Compare sides for differences.
CN VII (facial) motor function	1. Instruct client to: A. Show upper and lower teeth. B. Puff out cheeks. C. Smile. 2. Test functions of paired CN VII: A. Observe for symmetry. B. Instruct client to: (1) Frown. (2) Raise eyebrows. C. Attempt to open the client's closed eyes by exerting pressure on the bony orbit, avoiding pressure on the eye. D. Observe for symmetry and strength of motion.

From Stephen, T. C., Day, R. A., & Skillen, D. L. (Eds.). (2008). *A syllabus for adult health assessment* (pp. 33–34). Edmonton, AB: Faculty of Nursing, University of Alberta.

TABLE 32-22 Health History for Eye Assessment

Assessment Category	Rationale for Assessment
Ask whether the client has a history of eye disease, eye trauma, diabetes, hypertension, or eye surgery.	Some disease conditions create risk for partial or complete vision loss.
Inquire about family history of eye disorders.	Some eye disorders are hereditary.
Question client about use of protective eyewear for occupational or recreational activities as well as protection for sun exposure.	Some occupations and recreational events create risk for eye injuries. Sun exposure can damage the eyes or surrounding tissues.
Ask the client about use of glasses or contact lenses.	Vision is tested with glasses; use of contact lens necessitates questions regarding lens hygiene.
Inquire whether the client undergoes regular examinations by an eye specialist.	Regular eye examinations indicate preventive care taken by client.
Ask the client about use of medications for eye problems.	Certain eye medications may cause visual disturbances.

Visual Acuity. Assessment of visual acuity (ability to see small details) includes tests for central vision. Ask clients to read printed material in adequate lighting. Clients who wear glasses for distance vision should wear them during the test. Find out the first language of the client and whether he or she can read.

Assessment of distant vision requires a well-illuminated Snellen chart (paper chart or projection screen), which has standardized numbers at the end of each line. The numerator is the number 20 (6.1 m) (the distance the client stands away from the chart). The denominator is the distance from which the client can read the line of the chart. Vision is expected to be 20/20 (6.1/6.1). The larger the denominator, the poorer is the client's visual acuity. A value of 20/40, for example, means that the client has to stand 20 feet away to read a line that a person with unaffected vision can read from 40 feet away.

Test vision without corrective lenses first, but have your client leave contact lenses in place. The client sits or stands 20 feet (6.1 m) away from the chart and tries to read all letters out loud, beginning at any line, with one eye at a time (opposite eye covered with index card or eye cover) and then with both eyes. The client should avoid applying pressure to the covered eye. Note the lowest line for which the client can read more than half the letters correctly, and record the visual acuity for that line (Bickley & Szilagyi, 2007). Repeat the test with the client wearing corrective lenses. Do the test rapidly enough that the client does not memorize the chart (Seidel et al., 2006), or have the client do part of the test by starting to read the letters from right to left. Observe for signs of straining (head turning, squinting, frowning) while clients read the chart. Record visual acuity without correction or with correction.

If clients cannot see even the largest letters or figures on the Snellen chart, test their ability to count your upraised fingers or their ability to distinguish light. Holding your hand 30 cm (1 ft) in front of the client's face, instruct the client to count your upraised fingers. For light perception, shine a penlight into the client's eye and then turn the light off. If clients are able to tell when the light is turned on or off, light perception is intact. If clients are unable to read, use an E chart or one with pictures of familiar objects. Ask the client to mimic the direction in which each E is pointing or name the object. Score visual acuity for each eye separately and for both eyes.

Assess near vision by asking the client to read from a hand-held card containing a vision screening chart. Ask the client to hold the card at a comfortable distance (about 30 cm) and read the smallest line possible.

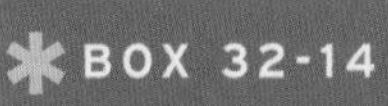

BOX 32-14 FOCUS ON PRIMARY HEALTH CARE

Eyes

- Regular eye examinations
- Protective eyeware
- Precautions for older adults

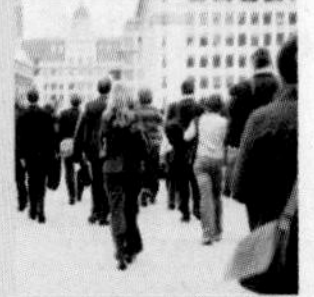

Inspection of External Eye Structures

Position and Alignment. Stand directly in front of the client at eye level, and ask the client to look at your face. Inspect the external structures, position, and alignment (Skill 32–3) of the client's eyes. Expect the eyes to be parallel to each other and without bulging or protrusion. Bulging (*exophthalmos*) of both eyes is usually caused by hyperthyroidism. If only one eye protrudes, suspect tumours or inflammation of the orbit. Crossed eyes (*strabismus*) may be caused by neuromuscular injury or may be genetic.

Eyebrows. Inspect the eyebrows for symmetry, size, distribution, alignment, movement, and hair texture. Loss or absence of hair may indicate a hormonal disturbance or may be the result of waxing or plucking. The client is expected to be able to raise and lower the eyebrows symmetrically. Facial nerve paralysis prevents eyebrow movement.

Eyelids. Inspect the eyelids for position, colour, and the condition of the lid surface and eyelashes. Assess the client's ability to open, close, and blink eyelids. Eyelids lie close to the eyeball and close symmetrically. Eyelashes are distributed evenly and curve outward away from the eye. Edema caused by allergies or heart or kidney failure may prevent the eyelids from closing. Inspect any lesions present for specific characteristics, and wear gloves if drainage is present. Failure of the eyelids to close creates the risk of drying of corneas, a common condition in unconscious clients or clients with facial nerve paralysis. Usually, a person blinks involuntarily and bilaterally up to 20 times a minute, which helps lubricate the cornea. Continuous and long periods of computer use can also reduce the frequency of eye blinking and cause drying of the cornea.

Lacrimal Apparatus. The anterior surface of the eye is made up of the sensitive cornea and conjunctivae and is lubricated by tears secreted from the lacrimal gland, which lies in the upper outer wall of each anterior orbit. Tears from the gland flow across the eye surface to the lacrimal duct in the nasal corner (inner canthus) of the eye. Inspect the lacrimal gland area for edema and redness. The flow of tears may be blocked if the nasolacrimal duct becomes obstructed. If the client reports excessive tearing, look for the presence of edema in the inner canthus.

Palpation. Although the lacrimal gland is not usually felt, palpate the area gently to detect tenderness. Mild palpation of the duct at the lower eyelid just inside the lower orbital rim (not on the nose) may cause regurgitation of tears.

Conjunctivae and Sclerae. Bulbar conjunctivae cover the exposed surface of the eyeballs up to the outer edge of the cornea; palpebral conjunctivae are the delicate membranes lining the eyelids. Usually, conjunctivae are transparent, and allow you to view the tiny underlying blood vessels that give the conjunctivae their light pink colour. Sclerae are seen under the bulbar conjunctivae and are the colour of white porcelain in individuals of European origin, light yellow in those of African origin. Sclerae may become pigmented and appear yellow or green if liver disease is present. Conjunctivae are inspected for colour, texture, edema, and lesions. Localized bright red blood surrounded by clear conjunctivae usually

➤ SKILL 32-3 Inspecting the External Structures of the Eyes

Equipment

- Penlight
- Cotton ball

Procedure

EXAMINATION SKILL AND FOCUS	TECHNIQUES AND RATIONALE
Inspection: Eyebrows, lids, lashes	1. Inspect eyebrows, lids, lashes.
Cornea	1. Use tangential lighting, with penlight, to inspect cornea. *Tangential lighting shows contour better than direct lighting can.*
Lens, iris, pupils	1. Inspect: • The lens from the anterior view. • The iris of each eye. • The size, shape, and equality of pupils in natural lighting.
Sclera, conjunctiva	Find out whether the client wears contact lenses. *Contact lenses might come out during the inspection of the sclera and conjunctiva.* 1. Instruct the client to look up while gently retracting the lower lid to inspect the sclera and conjunctiva. *Ensures adequate exposure of the conjunctivae.* 2. Instruct the client to look down and from side to side while gently retracting the upper lid to view the sclera and possibly the lacrimal gland.
Lacrimal sacs/glands	1. Inspect the lacrimal sac puncta/gland regions bilaterally.
Pupillary reaction CN II, III (optic, oculomotor)	Test each eye separately. *Prevents a false reflex from accommodation.* 1. Instruct the client to look past you.
Pupillary reaction to light; direct, consensual reactions	2. Shine a bright light from the temporal region on each pupil in turn. *Tangential lighting prevents a false reflex from accommodation.* 3. Inspect for direct and consensual reactions. *The afferent nerve synapses with both sides of the brain.*
Near reaction (accommodation)	Test each eye separately.
Dilatation	1. Instruct the client to look into the distance with one eye at a time. 2. Observe the pupil for dilatation.
Constriction	3. Instruct the client to look at your finger held 10 cm from client's eye. *Pupils dilate for distance and constrict to see near objects.* 4. Observe for pupillary constriction while the client focuses on your finger. 5. Repeat the test for the other eye.
Convergence CN III, IV (oculomotor, trochlear)	1. Instruct the client to follow the movement of your finger.
Convergence	2. From directly in front of client, move your finger to within 5 to 8 cm from the bridge of the client's nose. *Convergence occurs in this range.* 3. Observe convergence.
Corneal reflex	Test each eye separately.
CN V, VII (trigeminal, facial)	1. Ask the client about use of contact lenses. *Contact lenses obstruct the cornea, which then cannot be tested. Long-term contact lens wearers may have a diminished corneal reflex.* 2. Instruct the client to look up and away from you. 3. Position yourself on the client's side. 4. With fine wisp of cotton, touch the cornea, avoiding the eyelashes and sclera.
Bilateral blink	5. Observe for bilateral blink. *CN V, VII integrity can be observed.*

From Stephen, T. C., Day, R. A., & Skillen, D. L. (Eds.). (2008). *A syllabus for adult health assessment* (pp. 29–31). Edmonton, AB: Faculty of Nursing, University of Alberta.

indicates subconjunctival hemorrhage. Expose the bulbar conjunctivae by retracting the eyelids, avoiding pressure on the eyeball. While you are doing this, clients tend to blink. Conjunctivae should be free of erythema, which can indicate allergic or infectious conjunctivitis.

Palpation. Pale conjunctivae result from anemia; inflammation creates a fiery red appearance and indicates an infection that is highly contagious. Crusty drainage on eyelid margins can be carried from one eye to the other. Perform hand hygiene before and after palpation; wear gloves for palpation.

Corneas. The cornea is the transparent, colourless cover of the pupil and iris. Laterally, it looks like the crystal in a wristwatch. Ask the client to look straight ahead, and examine the cornea for clarity, shine, transparency, and smooth contour. Any irregularity in the surface may indicate an abrasion or tear that warrants immediate examination by a physician. Assess corneal reflex using the bilateral blink test. Expect to observe a brisk, bilateral blink when touching each cornea with a wisp of cotton (test of fifth and seventh cranial nerves).

Pupils and Irises. Observe the pupils for size, shape, equality, accommodation (near reaction), and reaction to light. Pupils are expected to be black, round, regular, and equal in size (3 to 7 mm in diameter; Figure 32–9). The iris should be clearly visible and intact. A thin white ring along the corneal margin (arcus senilis) is not expected in anyone under age 40.

Cloudy pupils are an indication of cataracts. Dilated pupils can result from glaucoma, trauma, neurological disorders, eye medications (e.g., atropine), or withdrawal from opioids. Constricted pupils may be caused by inflammation of the iris or use of certain drugs (e.g., pilocarpine, morphine, or cocaine). Pinpoint pupils are a common sign of opioid intoxication. When a beam of light is shone through the pupil onto the retina, the third cranial nerve is stimulated and innervates the muscles of the iris to constrict. Any irregularity along the nerve pathways from the retina to the iris alters pupillary ability to react to light. Changes in intracranial pressure, locally applied ophthalmic medications, lesions along nerve pathways, and direct trauma to the eye may alter pupillary reaction.

Pupillary reflexes are easier to observe when the test is conducted in a dimly lit room. A directly illuminated pupil constricts, and the pupil in the other eye also constricts consensually. Observe the speed and equality of responses.

When testing for accommodation (near reaction), expect equal pupillary responses. The pupils converge and accommodate by constricting when looking at close objects. To remember this response, think of "constrict" with "close" and "dilate" with "distance."

Visual Fields. Assess visual fields to confirm peripheral vision (Skill 32–4). When looking straight ahead, a client is expected to be able to see all objects in the periphery. The visual field of each eye covers 180 degrees. Clients who are unable to see all objects surrounding them may be at risk for injury.

Extraocular Movement. Six small muscles move the eyes in parallel directions in each of the six directions of gaze (see Skill 32–4). Assess parallel eye movement, position of the upper eyelid in relation to the iris, and any unexpected movements during conjugate movement. As the eyes move in each direction, the upper eyelids cover the iris only slightly. Stop the movement of your finger periodically in order to assess nystagmus, which is an involuntary, rhythmical oscillation of the eyes. Local injury to the eye muscles or supporting structures and any disorders of the cranial nerves that innervate muscles can be detected by doing this. You can also assess the extraocular muscles of the eyes by using the corneal light reflex test (see Skill 32–4). A weakness or imbalance of the extraocular muscles may cause misalignment. Expect the light to reflect off the cornea in the same spot on both eyes. The cover test is an alternative for the corneal light reflection test.

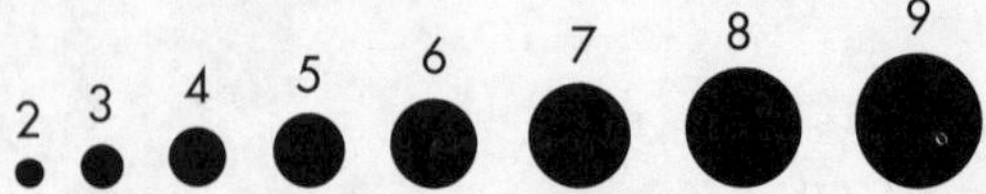

Figure 32-9 Chart depicting pupillary size in millimetres.

Inspection and Internal Eye Structures

Funduscopic Examination. Examine the internal eye with the ophthalmoscope to inspect the fundus (retina, choroid, optic nerve disc, macula, fovea centralis, and retinal vessels). The ophthalmoscope has a battery tube light source, two dials or discs, and a keyhole viewer. The dial at the top of the battery tube changes the light image. Five lenses are available, but only the small white light is used for general examination. To adjust the focus, rotate clockwise the dial at the top of the viewer.

Practise holding the ophthalmoscope in each hand, using the index finger to rotate the lens dial (putting the "digit on the widget"). Turn the white light on, rotate the lens dial to *0*, look through the keyhole, and focus on near objects, for example, the palm of your hand. Reading a newspaper through the ophthalmoscope is useful practice. Keep both eyes open when looking through the keyhole.

During the assessment, dim the room lighting. You and the client should stand or sit in comfortable positions facing each other with your eyes at the same level. The client removes his or her eyeglasses but can leave contact lenses in place; you may decide to keep your own eyeglasses on if the correction in diopters is high. Hold the ophthalmoscope against your face (Skill 32–5). A bright orange glow, called the red reflex, is usually seen in the client's pupil. Light from the ophthalmoscope causes the pupil to constrict. Moving slowly toward the pupil while keeping the light focused on the red reflex, you begin to see the structures of the fundus. By rotating the lens dial, you can bring the internal structures into focus. Inspect for size, colour, and disc clarity; integrity of the vessels; presence of retinal lesions; and the appearance of the macula and fovea (Figure 32–10). Expect to see the following:

- Clear, yellow optic nerve disc
- Reddish-pink retina (White client) or darkened retina (Black client) (Figure 32–10)
- Light red arterioles and dark red veins
- A 3:2 vein-to-artery ratio in size
- Avascular macula

Do not illuminate the fundus for extended periods. The bright light of the ophthalmoscope can be very irritating to the eye and can cause discomfort and tearing.

Age-Related Changes. Aging causes loss of the lateral third of the eyebrows. Often, lid margins turn out (ectropion) or in (entropion). An entropion permits lashes to irritate the cornea and conjunctiva, increasing the risk of infection. Elastic tissues around the eyes atrophy, creating wrinkles (crow's feet). Orbital fat decreases, and eyes appear sunken. Decreased tear production, loss of lustre in the cornea, and fading of the iris occur. A thin white ring along the margin of the cornea (arcus senilis) is seen commonly in older adults. Visual acuity gradually declines after 50 years of age, necessitating visual aids. Changes in the lens reduce peripheral vision and alter accommodation.

Documentation. Record your findings from inspection and palpation of the eyes (see Table 32–26, page 584).

➤ SKILL 32-4 Assessing Visual Fields and Extraocular Movements

Equipment

- Penlight
- Splintered tongue blade
- Cotton ball

Procedure

EXAMINATION SKILL AND FOCUS	TECHNIQUES AND RATIONALE
Visual fields by confrontation CN II (optic) Visual fields	**1.** Position yourself 60 cm away from the client at eye level. *Ensures comfortable distance for focus.* **2.** Instruct the client to cover one eye and to look at your eye directly opposite. *Tests each eye separately.* **3.** Cover your own eye opposite to client's covered eye. *Allows comparison to examiner's field of vision.* **4.** Instruct the client to indicate when your wiggling finger can be seen. **5.** Test the client's temporal, inferotemporal, and superotemporal fields of vision by placing your wiggling finger somewhat behind the client and slowly bringing it within the client's visual field. *Assesses all fields for each eye.* **6.** Test the client's nasal, superior, and inferior fields of vision in turn by keeping your wiggling finger equidistant between the client and yourself. Test eight different positions for each eye. **7.** Slowly bring your wiggling finger within the client's visual fields. **8.** Compare the client's visual field against your own.
Extraocular muscles and movements CN III, IV, VI (oculomotor, trochlear, abducens)	**1.** Inspect extraocular muscle function by performing: A. Cardinal directions test **AND** B. Cover test **OR** C. Corneal reflection test
Cardinal directions (extraocular movements)	**1.** Find out whether the client wears contact lenses. *Contact lenses may be dislodged by lateral and medial movements of the eyes.* **2.** Position yourself so that the client can focus. **3.** Instruct the client to follow the movement of your finger or a pen (take client's age into consideration) with the eyes, without moving the head. *Ensures movement of eyes is assessed, not movement of head.* **4.** Move your finger slowly (avoid straight up-and-down midline position) to client's right in line with shoulder, upward to right of midline, downward to right of midline, then to client's left in line with shoulder, upward to left of midline, and downward to left of midline. *Assesses all directions.*

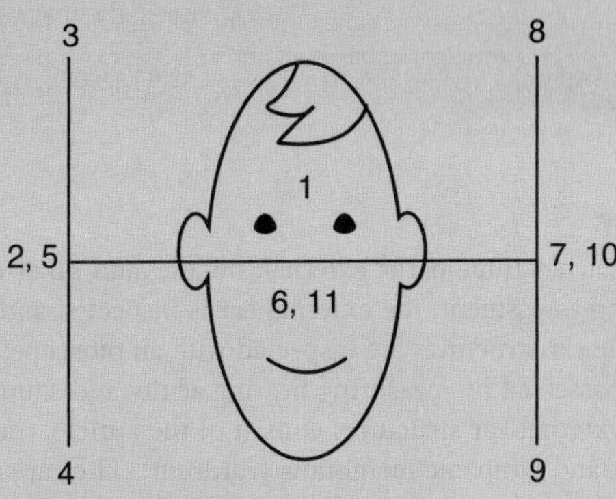

EXAMINATION SKILL AND FOCUS	TECHNIQUES AND RATIONALE
Parallel tracking, nystagmus, lid lag	**5.** Avoid asking the client to fix vision on extreme lateral points. *This is uncomfortable for the client.* **6.** Observe for parallel tracking (conjugate movements), nystagmus, and lid lag.
Cover test	**1.** Keep your eyes level with those of client. **2.** Instruct the client to look at yourself. **3.** Hold an opaque cover over one eye of the client for 5 to 10 seconds before removing it quickly, without warning and without touching the client. *Gives time for eye to deviate before cover is removed.* **4.** Observe the eye that was covered. *Eye movement after uncovering indicates movement while covered.* **5.** Repeat the test with the other eye.
Corneal reflections	**1.** Stand at least 0.6 m away from client. **2.** Shine a penlight from your midline directly onto bridge of client's nose; ask the client to look directly at the light. **3.** Observe the site on each cornea from which light is reflected. *Observe symmetry to assess alignment.*

From Stephen, T. C., Day, R. A., & Skillen, D. L. (Eds.). (2008). *A syllabus for adult health assessment* (pp. 30–32). Edmonton, AB: Faculty of Nursing, University of Alberta.

➤ SKILL 32-5 Assessing the Internal Structures of the Eyes

Equipment

- Ophthalmoscope

Procedure

EXAMINATION SKILL AND FOCUS	TECHNIQUES AND RATIONALE
Fundus	Both eyes
Inspection with ophthalmoscope	**1.** Instruct the client to look slightly up and over your shoulder at a specific point on a wall. *Helps dilate the pupil.*
	2. Turn the lens disc of the ophthalmoscope to 0 diopters. *Neutral starting point.*
	3. Maintain your index finger on the lens disc for refocusing during examination. *Ensures that refocusing can be done easily.*
	4. Use your right hand and your right eye for assessing the client's right eye. *Avoids uncomfortable positioning of client and examiner.*
	5. Use your left hand and left eye to assess the client's left eye.
	6. Shine a *small* light beam on the client's pupil from about 40 cm away from client and 15 degrees lateral to the client's midline. *A small light beam reduces the amount of pupil constriction. The angle helps see the optic disc better.*
	7. Place your hand, with thumb extended, on the client's forehead above the eye being examined. *Stabilizes the ophthalmoscope; ensures correct distance from eye.*
Red reflex	**8.** Observe for red reflex.
	9. Move toward client while maintaining focus on the pupil, until the client's eyelashes almost touch the ophthalmoscope.
Disc, cups, arterioles	**10.** Inspect the disc, cup, arterioles, veins, and crossings, adjusting lens disc if necessary. *Adjusts lens until structures are in focus and not a red blur.*
Veins, crossings	**11.** Move your head and the ophthalmoscope as one unit and follow vessels peripherally in four directions. *Ensures proper visualization of structures.*
Macula	**12.** Instruct the client to briefly look at the light directly. *Helps better visualize the macula and fovea (central vision).*
	13. Inspect the macula and fovea.

From Stephen, T. C., Day, R. A., & Skillen, D. L. (Eds.). (2008). *A syllabus for adult health assessment* (p. 32). Edmonton, AB: Faculty of Nursing, University of Alberta.

Ears

The ear has three parts: external, middle, and inner ear structures. During assessment, the external ear is inspected and palpated; the middle ear structures are inspected with an otoscope; and the inner ear is assessed by measuring hearing acuity and sound conduction. The external ear structures consist of the auricle, tragus, outer ear canal, and tympanic membrane (eardrum). The ear canal is usually curved and about 2.54 cm long in an adult. It is lined with skin containing fine hairs, nerve endings, and glands secreting cerumen (earwax). The middle ear is an air-filled cavity that contains three bony ossicles (malleus, incus, and stapes). The eustachian tube connects the middle ear to the nasopharynx and helps balance the pressure between the outer atmosphere and the middle ear. The inner ear contains the cochlea, vestibule, and semicircular canals. Assess the integrity of the ear structures and the acuity of hearing.

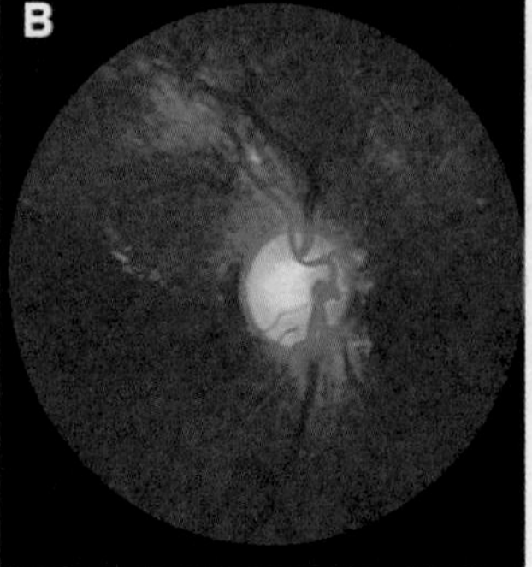

Figure 32-10 Fundus of White client (A) and Black client (B). **Source:** Courtesy MEDCOM. Cypress, CA.

Health history data (Table 32–23; Box 32–15) help identify risks for hearing disorders, and understanding the mechanisms for sound transmission helps identify the nature of hearing disorders. Sound travels through the ear by air and bone conduction in the following sequence:

1. Sound waves in the air enter the external ear, passing through the outer ear canal.
2. Sound waves reach the tympanic membrane, causing it to vibrate.
3. Vibrations are transmitted through the middle ear by the bony ossicular chain to the oval window at the opening of the inner ear.
4. The cochlea receives the sound vibration.
5. Nerve impulses from the cochlea travel to the auditory (eighth cranial) nerve and cerebral cortex.

Ear disorders result from mechanical dysfunction (blockage by cerumen or foreign body), trauma (foreign bodies or noise exposure), neurological disorders (auditory nerve damage), acute illnesses (viral infection), and toxic effects of medications.

External Ear Structures

Auricles and Tragus. Inspect the auricle size, shape, symmetry, landmarks, position, and colour (Skill 32–6). Expect the auricles to be at the same level. The upper point of attachment is in a straight line

TABLE 32-23 Health History for Ear Assessment

Assessment Category	Rationale for Assessment
Document behaviours that suggest hearing loss, such as failure to respond when spoken to, requests to repeat instructions, leaning forward to hear, or seeming inattentiveness.	Clients with hearing loss may compensate by responding to certain behavioural cues.
Ask whether the client is experiencing any hearing difficulties or illnesses related to his or her ears, and conduct a symptom analysis.	Different symptoms reveal the causes of different ear problems, for example, pain indicating an ear infection.
Find out about excessive accumulation of cerumen in ear canals.	Excessive cerumen can interfere with the client's ability to hear well.
Question the client about the presence of any risks for hearing impairment, such as head trauma or excessive occupational or recreational noise, and about the client's use of protective ear equipment.	Prolonged exposure to loud noises alters hearing temporarily or permanently.
Ask the client about medication use, such as large doses of aspirin or other ototoxic drugs.	Ringing in the ears or hearing loss may be a side effect of some medications.
Ask whether the client uses a hearing aid.	This alerts you to adjust your tone of voice and to face the client while speaking.
Inquire about regularity of hearing tests.	Date of last hearing test will indicate preventative care of ears.

BOX 32-15 FOCUS ON PRIMARY HEALTH CARE

Ears

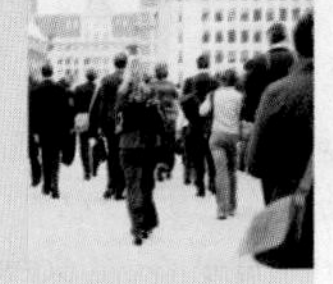

- Cleaning technique
- Hearing protection
- Hearing tests
- Age-related changes

with the lateral canthus (corner of the eye). The auricle should also be almost vertical. Ears that are at an unusual angle or low set may indicate a chromosomal abnormality (e.g., Down syndrome). The colour of the auricle is the same as that of the face, without moles, cysts, deformities, or nodules. Any redness is a sign of inflammation or fever; extreme pallor can indicate frostbite.

Palpate the auricles for texture, tenderness, and skin lesions. If the auricle or tragus is tender when palpated, an auditory canal infection is likely (see Skill 32–6). If palpation of the auricle and tragus does not elicit or change the level of reported pain, the client could have a middle ear infection. Tenderness in the mastoid area can indicate an infection (mastoiditis).

Hearing Acuity. Often, you detect hearing loss in a client from the manner in which he or she responds during a conversation. Three types of hearing loss occur: conductive, sensorineural, and mixed. A conduction loss interrupts sound waves travelling from the outer ear to the cochlea of the inner ear, preventing transmission through the outer and middle ear structures. Swelling of the auditory canal and

SKILL 32-6 Inspecting and Palpating the Ears

Equipment

- None

Procedure

EXAMINATION SKILL AND FOCUS	TECHNIQUES AND RATIONALE
Inspection:	Ears fully exposed
Auricle, mastoid surface	1. Inspect the auricle and mastoid bilaterally, moving the client's hair away, as needed, for clear vision.
Alignment	1. Inspect the alignment of the ears from anterior and lateral views (angle of attachment, horizontal, vertical). *Allows comparison between ears and alignment with eyes.*
Palpation:	1. Inquire about tenderness during palpation. *Tenderness may indicate an inflammatory or infectious process.*
Mastoid surface	2. Palpate both mastoid surfaces of the temporal bones with the pads of your fingers.
Auricle	3. Pull each auricle up.
Tragus	4. Press on each tragus with your fingertip.

From Stephen, T. C., Day, R. A., & Skillen, D. L. (Eds.). (2008). *A syllabus for adult health assessment* (p. 28). Edmonton, AB: Faculty of Nursing, University of Alberta.

perforations in the tympanic membrane can cause conduction loss. A sensorineural loss involves the inner ear, auditory nerve, or hearing centre of the brain. Sound is still conducted through the outer and middle ear structures, but the transmission of sound becomes interrupted at some point beyond the bony ossicles. A mixed loss involves both conduction and sensorineural losses. Clients who work or live in the middle of loud noises are at risk for permanent hearing loss.

Gross Hearing. During the assessment, the client should remove any hearing aid worn. Note the client's response to your questions. If you suspect hearing loss, check the client's response to whispered questions (Skill 32–7). Clients usually hear numbers clearly even when whispered, responding correctly at least 50% of the time (Seidel et al., 2006).

Weber Test. To assess hearing acuity, tests are performed using a tuning fork or audiometer. The Weber test assesses for lateralization of sound (see Skill 32–7). With the Weber test, clients with unimpaired hearing are expected to hear sound equally in both ears. If clients have conduction deafness, they hear the sound best in the impaired ear. If they have sensorineural hearing loss, they identify the sound only in the unimpaired ear.

Rinné Test. The Rinné test compares air and bone conduction (see Skill 32–7). Air-conducted sound is heard twice as long as bone-conducted sound. Clients with conduction deafness are able to hear bone-conducted sound longer. In sensorineural loss, sound is reduced and heard for a short time through air and bone.

Otoscopic Examination

External Ear Canals and Eardrums. Inspect the opening of the ear canal for size and presence of any discharge; in some cases, discharge may have an odour. Yellow or green, foul-smelling discharge indicate possible infection or presence of a foreign body. The meatus should not be swollen or occluded. Cerumen, a yellow, waxy substance, is often present.

Using an otoscope, observe the deeper structures of the external and middle ear (Skill 32–8). Specula come in different sizes. For best visualization, use the largest speculum that fits comfortably into the client's ear canal. Before insertion, check for foreign bodies in the opening of the auditory canal. The client must keep the head still to avoid the occurrence of any damage to the canal and tympanic membrane during the examination. Hold the handle of the otoscope in the

➤ SKILL 32-7 Assessing Hearing Acuity

Equipment

- Tuning fork (512 Hz or 1024 Hz)

Procedure

EXAMINATION SKILL AND FOCUS	TECHNIQUES AND RATIONALE
CN VIII (acoustic)	Assess each ear separately.
Test hearing	**1.** Block the hearing in one ear by moving a fingertip in the client's auditory canal. *Ensures that the ear being tested can hear without help from the other ear.*
Gross hearing	**2.** Stand 30 to 60 cm from the client (ensuring that client does not lip-read).
Cranial nerve VIII	**3.** Exhale fully, and then whisper directly toward the ear being tested.
	4. Start with three low-whispered, two-syllable, equally accented numbers or words. *Only if* the client does not identify the first numbers or words in low whispers, gradually increase the intensity of whispering (while saying different numbers or words) and go up to the spoken voice.
Weber test	**1.** Select a tuning fork of 512 or 1024 Hz. *Assesses sound within human speech range.*
	2. Activate the tuning fork using: A. Thumb and finger **OR** B. Reflex hammer **OR** C. Another part of your hand. *Creates a sound for testing.*
	3. Hold the base of the vibrating tuning fork.
	4. Press the end of the base of the vibrating tuning fork firmly on: A. The midline of the skull **OR** B. The midline of the forehead.
	5. Ask the client, "Where do you hear the sound?" *Assesses for lateralization of sound (heard in one ear only).*
Rinné test	**1.** Select a tuning fork of 512 or 1024 Hz.
	2. Activate the tuning fork using: A. Thumb and finger **OR** B. Reflex hammer **OR** C. Another part of your hand.
	3. Hold the base of the vibrating tuning fork, and place the end on the mastoid surface, level with the ear canal.
	4. Request the client to indicate when the sound is no longer heard.
	5. Based on client response, place the vibrating tuning fork about 2.54 cm from the auditory meatus of the same ear with the "U" of the tuning fork facing forward (anteriorly). *Assesses bone conduction of sound.*
	6. Ask the client whether the sound can be heard. *Assesses whether air conduction is longer than bone conduction.*

From Stephen, T. C., Day, R. A., & Skillen, D. L. (Eds.). (2008). *A syllabus for adult health assessment* (pp. 28–29). Edmonton, AB: Faculty of Nursing, University of Alberta.

➤ SKILL 32-8 Otoscopy

Equipment

- Otoscope

Procedure

EXAMINATION SKILL AND FOCUS	TECHNIQUES AND RATIONALE
Inspection by otoscopy:	*Otoscopic examination* (each ear, tender ear last)
	1. Select the largest ear speculum that fits in the canal.
	2. Brace your hand against the client's head when holding the otoscope. *Stabilizes the otoscope and prevents injury to the client.*
	3. Lift the auricle upward, backward, and slightly out from the client's head *before inserting* the speculum. *Helps straighten the ear canal of an adult for better visualization.*
	4. Insert the speculum gently and not deeply in a downward and forward direction.
Auditory canal	**5.** Inspect the auditory canal.
Tympanic membrane, cone of light, umbo, handle of the malleus, short process	**6.** Inspect the tympanic membrane, handle of malleus, umbo, cone of light, short process (structures and vascularity).
	7. Adjust the position of the speculum in order to visualize the ear drum in its entirety.
	8. Remove the speculum before releasing the auricle. *Prevents any trauma to the ear canal.*

From Stephen, T. C., Day, R. A., & Skillen, D. L. (Eds.). (2008). *A syllabus for adult health assessment* (p. 29). Edmonton, AB: Faculty of Nursing, University of Alberta.

space between your thumb and index finger, supporting the instrument on the middle finger. This leaves the ulnar side of your hand to brace against the client's head, stabilizing the otoscope as you insert it into the canal (Seidel et al., 2006).

You may use one of two types of grip on the otoscope: (1) holding the battery tube along the length of the client's face with fingers against the face or neck or (2) lightly bracing the inverted otoscope against the side of the client's head or cheek. This grip, used with children and any adult who might move unexpectedly, prevents accidental insertion of the otoscope deeper into the ear canal. You can straighten the ear canal in adults by pulling the auricle upward, backward, and slightly out (Figure 32–11). Insert the speculum slightly down and forward 1.0 to 1.5 cm into the ear canal, avoiding contact with the sensitive lining of the ear canal (the skin of the lining has little subcutaneous fat between it and the underlying bone). The canal usually has some cerumen and is uniformly pink, with tiny hairs in its outer third. Observe for colour, discharge, scaling, lesions, foreign bodies, and cerumen. The cerumen is expected to be dry (light brown to grey and flaky) or moist (dark yellow or brown) and sticky. Dry cerumen occurs in clients of Asian or Aboriginal origin about 85% of the time (Seidel et al., 2006). In others, accumulated cerumen is common and can cause a mild hearing loss. A reddened canal with discharge is a sign of inflammation or infection.

The light from the otoscope facilitates visualization of the tympanic membrane (Figure 32–12). Moving the otoscope slowly enables you to see the entire tympanic membrane and its periphery. Because the tympanic membrane is angled toward you, the light reflected from the otoscope appears as a cone. A ring of fibrous cartilage surrounds the oval membrane. The umbo is near the centre of the membrane, and the attachment of the malleus is behind it. A knoblike structure at the top of the tympanic membrane is created by the underlying short process of the malleus. Check carefully to make sure that the membrane has no tears or breaks. The tympanic membrane is translucent, shiny, and pearly grey. It is taut, except for the small triangular pars flaccida near the top. A pink or red bulging membrane indicates inflammation. A white colour indicates pus behind the tympanic membrane.

Figure 32-11 Otoscopic examination. **Source:** From Skillen, D. L., Day, R. A., Anderson, M. C., Stephen, T. C., Gilbert, J. A., & Day, L. W. (2004). *Physical examination images* [CD-ROM]. Edmonton, AB: Faculty of Nursing, University of Alberta.

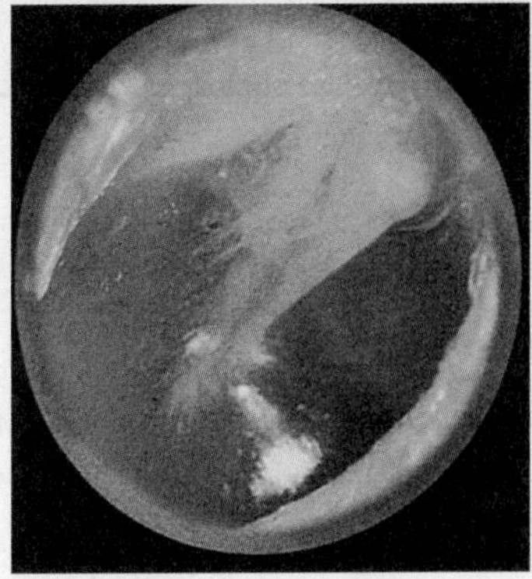

Figure 32-12 Healthy right tympanic membrane. **Source:** Courtesy Dr. Richard A. Buckingham. Abraham Lincoln School of Medicine, University of Illinois, Chicago, IL.

Age-Related Changes. The ability to hear high-frequency sounds and consonants (e.g., *s, z, t,* and *g*) is gradually reduced due to the deterioration of the cochlea and the thickening of the tympanic membrane. In older adults, the tympanic membranes may be whiter and duller than in younger adults. High-maintenance doses of antibiotics (e.g., the aminoglycosides) may create the risk for hearing loss due to ototoxicity (injury to auditory nerve). Coarse hairs appear at the canal opening, and the earlobes become pendulous and have linear creases.

Documentation. Record your findings from the inspection and palpation of the ears (see Table 32–26, page 584).

Nose

The nose consists of bone, cartilage, nares, and septum, all of which can be examined while the client is in the sitting position. Expect the healthy nose to be smooth, symmetrical, located in the centre of the face, and the same skin colour as of the face. Air usually passes freely through both nostrils as a person breathes. The nasal septum is highly sensitive to touch, so you must take care to avoid any direct contact with it. The health history guides your examination of the nose and paranasal sinuses (Table 32–24).

Data collection during health history taking provides you with opportunities for health promotion related to the nose and paranasal sinuses (Box 32–16).

Inspection. Inspect the nose from two perspectives for size, shape, skin characteristics, midline alignment, and any deformities. Assess **patency** (open, no obstruction) of the nares by listening to breathing sounds during full respirations. Assess the client's ability to smell (function of cranial nerve I, the olfactory nerve) by using pungent odours (e.g., coffee, spices, alcohol). In a healthy client, you can expect quiet breathing and the ability to identify odours.

Palpation. Palpate the nose to detect any tenderness, masses, or underlying deviations. Nasal structures are usually firm, stable, and nontender.

Inspection With a Nasal Speculum. Using a nasal speculum, inspect the vestibule, septum, and inferior and middle turbinates, keeping in mind that the septum is very sensitive. While illuminating the anterior nares (vestibule), inspect the mucosa for colour, lesions, discharge, swelling, and evidence of bleeding. Expect the mucosa to be pink and moist, with clear mucus and no lesions. In a client with an allergy, the mucosa may be pale pink and boggy. Inspect the septum for alignment, perforation, or bleeding. Expect the septum to be intact and aligned along the midline. Hair and red mucous membranes line the vestibule. Inspect the mucosa and inferior turbinates for colour, dryness, bleeding, and irritation.

Paranasal Sinuses

Assess paired sinuses in the frontal and maxillary facial areas by inspection and palpation (Figure 32–13; Skill 32–9). The skin over the sinuses is usually the same colour as the surrounding skin of the face; neither sinus area is expected to be tender to palpation. After inspecting the skin over the frontal and maxillary sinuses, assess for tenderness by palpating both areas. Gentle pressure elicits tenderness if sinus irritation is present and indicates the severity of sinus irritation. Avoid pressure near the eyes.

Mouth and Pharynx

After taking the health history for the mouth and pharynx (see Table 32–24), assess for the overall health of the mouth and pharynx and the status of oral hygiene (Skill 32–10). These data provide guidance for health promotion (Box 32–17).

Inspection of the Mouth

Lips. Before inspecting the lips for colour, texture, hydration, contour, and lesions, ask the client to keep the mouth closed, and in female clients, ensure that lipstick has been removed. Expect lips to be moist, smooth, and symmetrical at rest.

Buccal Mucosa, Gums, and Teeth. You can easily determine the quality of dental hygiene by inspecting the teeth; at this time, you will also note the position and alignment of the teeth. When examining the posterior surface of the teeth, ask the clients to keep the

TABLE 32-24 Health History for Nose, Sinus, Mouth, and Pharynx Assessment

Assessment Category	Rationale for Assessment
Nose and Sinuses	
Ask the client about any history of nasal trauma.	Past trauma may create tissue alteration, leading to impaired air entry.
Inquire about history of nosebleeds, postnasal drip, allergies, and nasal discharge.	History helps determine the nature of a nasal condition.
Question the client about the use of nasal sprays, medications, or illicit drugs.	Overuse of over-the-counter nasal sprays can cause damage to the nasal mucosa and recurring (rebound) symptoms. Cocaine, when inhaled, damages the septum.
Ask whether the client snores at night or experiences any breathing difficulties when sleeping.	Snoring or breathing difficulties may be caused by obstructions in the nostrils.
Mouth and Pharynx	
Ask whether the client wears dentures or other dental appliances and whether they are comfortable.	Poorly fitting dental appliances irritate the gums and mucosa, causing open sores.
Inquire about tobacco use (smoking, chewing).	Tobacco use increases the risks for mouth and throat cancers.
Question the client about usual dental hygiene practices, including dental checkups, cleaning, use of fluoride toothpaste, and frequency of brushing and flossing.	Regular hygiene and dental care indicates preventive self-care practices. You can assess the need for further education.
Question the client about appetite or recent changes in appetite.	Mouth disease affects appetite and nutritional intake.

BOX 32-16 FOCUS ON PRIMARY HEALTH CARE

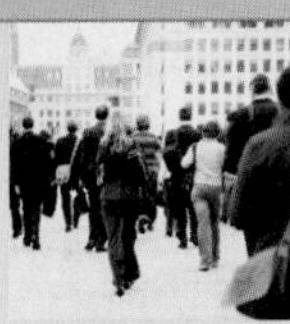

Nose and Sinuses

- Safe use of over-the-counter nasal sprays.
- Safety precautions in older adults who experience loss of smell (olfaction).

mouth open and the lips relaxed. You may need a tongue depressor to retract the lips and cheeks, especially when viewing the molars. Healthy teeth are smooth, white, and shiny. To view the mucosa and gums, ask the client to remove any dentures. View the inner oral mucosa by having the client open and relax the mouth slightly, gently retracting the client's lower lip away from the teeth. Repeat this process with the upper lip. With a penlight, inspect the mucosa for colour, hydration, texture, and such lesions as ulcers, abrasions, or cysts. The healthy mucous membrane is pinkish-red, smooth, and moist. If lesions are present, palpate them with a gloved hand to assess tenderness, size, and consistency. Palpate the cheek with one finger inside the mouth and the thumb on the cheek to check for lesions or thickening. Inspect the gums for colour, edema, retraction, or bleeding. Inspect gums around the back molars, an area that is difficult to reach when cleaning teeth. Healthy gums are pink, smooth, moist, tight around each tooth, and nontender.

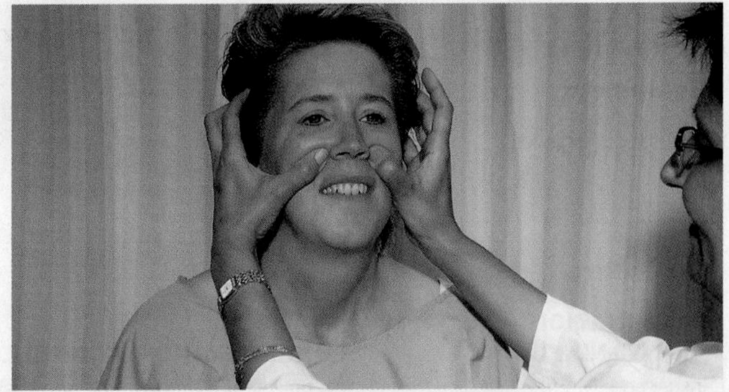

Figure 32-13 Palpation of maxillary sinuses. **Source:** From Skillen, D. L., Day, R. A., Anderson, M. C., Stephen, T. C., Gilbert, J. A., & Day, L. W. (2004). *Physical examination images* [CD-ROM]. Edmonton, AB: Faculty of Nursing, University of Alberta.

SKILL 32-9 Assessing the Nose and Paranasal Sinuses

Equipment

- Penlight
- Nasal speculum

Procedure

EXAMINATION SKILL AND FOCUS	TECHNIQUES AND RATIONALE
Inspection: Nose	1. Inspect the nose from the anterior and lateral views. *Ensures full inspection.*
Frontal and maxillary sinuses	2. Inspect the frontal and maxillary sinus regions.
Palpation: Nose	1. Palpate the entire length of the nose with your finger pads. *Alterations might only be detectable by palpation.*
	2. Ask the client about any tenderness.
Frontal, maxillary sinuses	3. Palpate the maxillary sinuses simultaneously by pressing upward on the maxillae with your thumbs, and ask the client about any tenderness. *Congested or irritated sinuses create tenderness.*
	4. Palpate the frontal sinuses by pressing upward, inferior to the supraorbital ridge, from the medial border of the eyebrow to the mid-eyebrow, using your thumbs, and ask the client about any tenderness.
Test for patency	1. Occlude each nostril in turn. *Focuses on one nostril at a time.*
	2. Instruct the client to breathe with the mouth closed. *Detects nasal alterations.*
	3. Listen to a complete inspiration for each nostril. *Obstructed breathing may only occur in one phase of respiration.*
Test of smell (cranial nerve)	1. Instruct the client to close the eyes. *Client is prevented from identifying the pungent odour by seeing its source.*
	2. Occlude one nostril (naris).
CN I	3. Hold the object with the pungent odour near the opposite nostril. Ask the client to identify the odour. *The sensation of smell is affected by abnormalities in cranial nerve I.*
	4. Change over to another object with a different pungent odour, and repeat on other side.
Inspection with nasal speculum:	Both nostrils
Nose	1. Instruct the client to tilt the head back slightly.
	2. Insert the nasal speculum posteriorly in the horizontal plane into the vestibule of the nares.
	3. Stabilize the speculum (with your index finger on the client's nose or on the cheek). *Avoids causing injury if the client moves.*
	4. Avoid touching the septum. *The nasal septum is highly sensitive.*
Mucous membrane, septum, inferior and middle turbinates	5. Inspect the mucous membrane, septum, and inferior turbinates by moving the speculum slowly upward. *The middle turbinates become visible.*
	6. Inspect the middle turbinates and mucous membranes.
	7. Offer the client a tissue, if needed.

From Stephen, T. C., Day, R. A., & Skillen, D. L. (Eds.). (2008). *A syllabus for adult health assessment* (pp. 32–33). Edmonton, AB: Faculty of Nursing, University of Alberta.

➤ SKILL 32-10 Assessing the Mouth and Pharynx

Equipment

- Disposable gloves
- Penlight
- Tongue blade

Procedure

EXAMINATION SKILL AND FOCUS	TECHNIQUES AND RATIONALE
Inspection: Mouth	1. Ask the client to remove the dentures. *Permits full inspection of the gums.*
	2. Instruct the client to sip some water.
	3. Use the penlight and tongue blade to inspect:
	• The buccal mucosa bilaterally
Gums	• The upper and lower gums
Teeth	• The upper and lower teeth
Tongue	• The dorsal and ventral surfaces and sides of the tongue
Floor of mouth	• The floor of the mouth
Uvula, palates	• The uvula and the soft and hard palates
Tonsils, tonsillar pillars	• The tonsils and the tonsillar pillars
Posterior pharynx	• The posterior pharyngeal wall
	4. If any lesion is present, palpate it with a gloved hand. *Gloves prevent transmission of microorganisms.*
Cranial nerve (CN) IX, X (glossopharyngeal, vagus)	1. Depress the client's tongue with a tongue blade, and instruct the client to say "ah."
Motor and sensory	2. Watch the uvula and soft palate rise while the client makes the "ah" sound.
Uvula, soft palate, gag reflex	3. Touch each side of the posterior pharyngeal wall to elicit the gag reflex (the ability to swallow is tested during examination of the thyroid). *Cranial nerves are in pairs.*
CN XII (hypoglossal)	1. Observe the tongue at rest on the floor of the client's mouth.
Motor function	2. Instruct the client to protrude the tongue, and take a close look at it.
Symmetry and strength	3. Instruct the client to:
	A. Wag the tongue laterally.
	B. Stick the tongue into each cheek.
	4. Palpate each cheek to assess strength.

From Stephen, T. C., Day, R. A., & Skillen, D. L. (Eds.). (2008). *A syllabus for adult health assessment* (pp. 34–36). Edmonton, AB: Faculty of Nursing, University of Alberta.

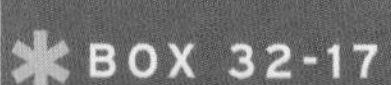

BOX 32-17 FOCUS ON PRIMARY HEALTH CARE

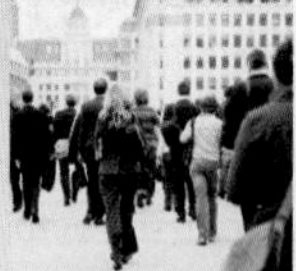

Mouth and Pharynx

- Oral hygiene
- Regular dental examinations
- Age-related changes

Tongue and Floor of Mouth. Using a penlight, examine the ventral and dorsal surfaces of the tongue for colour, size, position, texture, coating, or lesions, and the side surfaces for any lesions. The healthy tongue is medium or dull red in colour, moist, slightly rough on the dorsal surface, and smooth along the margins. The ventral surface is highly vascular. Inspect the floor of the mouth for nodules, ulcerations, or white patches, and palpate for lesions or indurations with a gloved hand. To determine cranial nerve XII (hypoglossal) functioning, look for symmetry, purposeful movements, and stillness at rest of the tongue.

safety alert The risk of oral cancer is high in clients who chew tobacco or smoke cigarettes, cigars, or pipes. They may have leukoplakia or other lesions anywhere in the oral cavity at an early age.

Palates. Inspect the hard and soft palates for colour, shape, symmetry, texture, and lesions. The healthy hard palate (roof of the mouth) is dome-shaped, whitish pink in colour, and located superiorly. A **benign** enlargement (torus palatinus) may be present in the midline of clients of Aboriginal or Asian origin (Overfield, 1995). The soft palate is light pink in colour, smooth, and located posteriorly. The uvula is in the midline position, pink in colour, and rises with the soft palate. The soft palate and uvula are innervated by cranial nerve X (vagus) and rise along the midline as the client says "ah."

Pharynx. Inspect the arch formed by the anterior and posterior pillars, soft palate, and uvula. Tonsils, if present, are seen in the cavities between the anterior and posterior pillars and are oval in shape, with a rough surface or crypts. Grade tonsils on a 4-point scale (1 = visible, 4 = touching; Figure 32–14). The posterior pharynx lies behind the pillars and tonsils. Expect healthy pharyngeal tissues to be pink in colour and smooth. Test the gag reflex on the posterior pharyngeal wall bilaterally (cranial nerves IX and X).

Age-Related Changes. Loose or missing teeth are common due to increased bone resorption. In older adults, teeth often feel rough as the tooth enamel calcifies. Yellow or darkened teeth are also commonly seen in older adults due to general wear and tear exposing the darker, underlying dentin. The oral mucosa become drier with

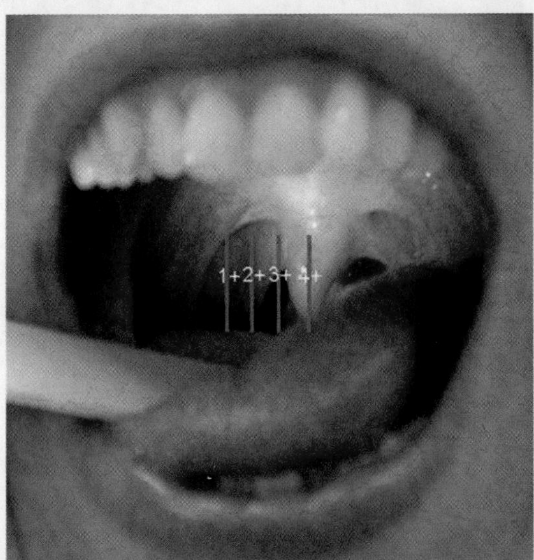

Figure 32-14 How to grade tonsil size in relation to the uvula. **Source:** From Skillen, D. L., Day, R. A., Anderson, M. C., Stephen, T. C., Gilbert, J. A., & Day, L. W. (2004). *Physical examination images* [CD-ROM]. Edmonton, AB: Faculty of Nursing, University of Alberta.

decreased salivation, and the gums often appear pale. Tonsillar tissue is not usually seen. The bony ridges of the jaw that surround each tooth gradually are resorbed, especially in the lower jaw.

Documentation. Record your findings from the inspection and palpation of the nose, sinuses, mouth, and pharynx (see Table 32–26, page 584).

Neck

Muscles, lymph nodes, carotid arteries, jugular veins, thyroid gland, and trachea are located within the neck. Each structure can be examined as part of the assessment of the neck or during a systems approach. For example, examination of the jugular veins and carotid arteries (Figure 32–15) can be part of a cardiovascular assessment or part of a regional assessment of the head and neck.

The sternomastoid and the trapezius muscles are the two major neck muscles. The sternomastoid muscles begin at the sternum and the medial aspect of the clavicle, lie diagonally across the neck, and end at the mastoid process behind the ears. The two trapezius muscles begin at the occipital bone and the vertebrae and end at the scapula and the distal end of the clavicle. The sternomastoid and trapezius muscles are useful landmarks for identifying and describing neck structures, functions, and findings. The neck is divided into two imaginary triangles by the sternomastoids (Figure 32–16). The anterior triangle lies in front of the sternomastoid muscle and contains the trachea, thyroid gland, carotid artery, and the anterior cervical lymph nodes. The posterior triangle lies between the trapezius muscles (at the back), the sternomastoid muscle (in the front), and the clavicle (at the bottom). The posterior lymph nodes are located in the posterior triangle. Figure 32–17 presents the lymph nodes of the head and neck.

Table 32–25 contains the health history for the examination of the neck. Box 32–18 presents the focus of health promotion during the neck assessment. The examination of the neck is best performed with the client in the sitting position, the neck fully exposed. You will mainly use your inspection and palpation skills, along with auscultation of the carotid arteries.

Inspection. Inspect the neck from two perspectives, noting the client's position. The head may be observed to be directly over the neck, slightly backward (extension) or forward (flexion); this information may be useful in health teaching. Examine the structures of the neck (muscles, arteries, veins, thyroid cartilage, cricoid cartilage, thyroid) for symmetry, alignment, and integrity. Inspect the skin of the neck for lesions and the carotid arteries and jugular veins for pulsations.

Carotid Arteries. When the left ventricle of the heart pumps blood into the aorta, pressure waves are transmitted through the arterial system. These pressure waves are manifested as pulses that are palpable in the arteries close to the skin or lying over bones. Assess

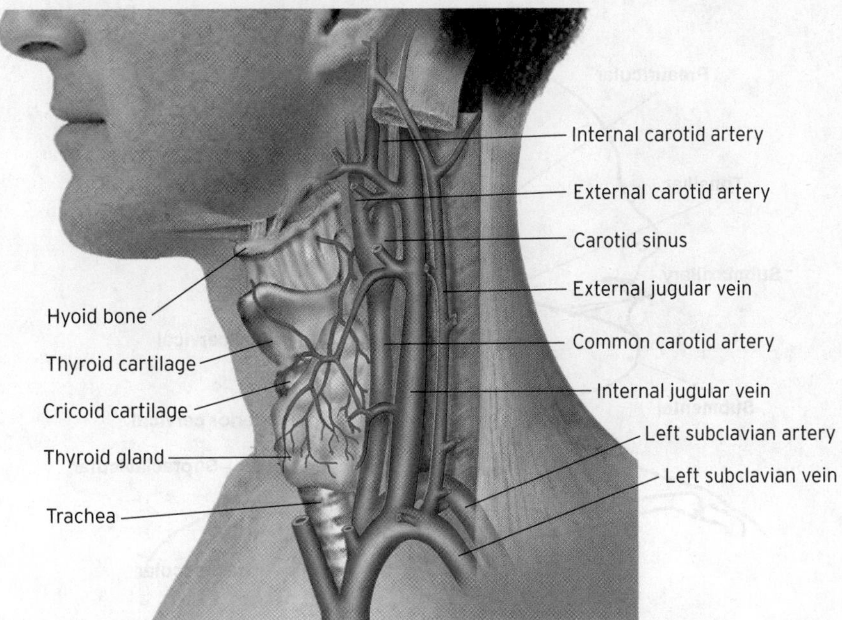

Figure 32-15 Arteries and veins of neck. **Source:** From Seidel, H. M., Ball, J. W., Dains, J. E., & Benedict, G. W. (2006). *Mosby's guide to physical examination* (6th ed., p. 256, Figure 10–3b). St. Louis, MO: Mosby.

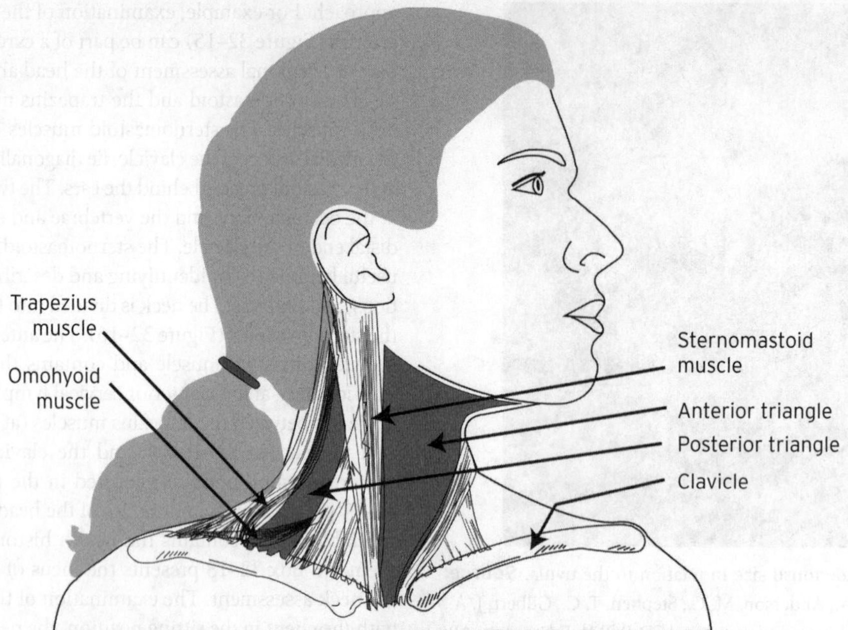

Figure 32-16 Neck muscles, anterior triangle, and posterior triangle. **Source:** From Skillen, D. L., Day, R. A., Anderson, M. C., Stephen, T. C., Gilbert, J. A., & Day, L. W. (2004). *Physical examination images* [CD-ROM]. Edmonton, AB: Faculty of Nursing, University of Alberta.

the carotid arteries to obtain information about heart function and any pathological changes in the aortic valve.

The carotid arteries supply oxygenated blood to the head and neck (see Figure 32–15) and are protected by the overlying sternomastoid muscle. The carotid sinus is located in the upper third of the neck, level with the superior border of the thyroid cartilage. The sinus sends impulses along the vagus nerve. Stimulation of the carotid sinus by such activities as palpation, massage, or a quick turning of the head can cause a reflex drop in heart rate and blood pressure, causing **syncope** (fainting) or circulatory arrest. This effect can be a particular problem in older adults.

Inspection. To examine the carotid arteries, have the client sit or lie supine, with the head of the bed elevated 30 degrees. With the client's head turned slightly away from the artery being examined, inspect first for obvious pulsation of each artery (Skill 32–11).

Auscultation. The carotid artery is the artery most commonly auscultated for bruits. Others include the renal and abdominal arteries. Blood flow is disturbed as blood passes through a narrowed section, which creates a turbulence that causes a blowing or swishing sound. The sound is called a **bruit** (pronounced "brew-ee"). Auscultation is an especially important consideration in middle-aged and older clients if a thrill is present or in clients suspected of having

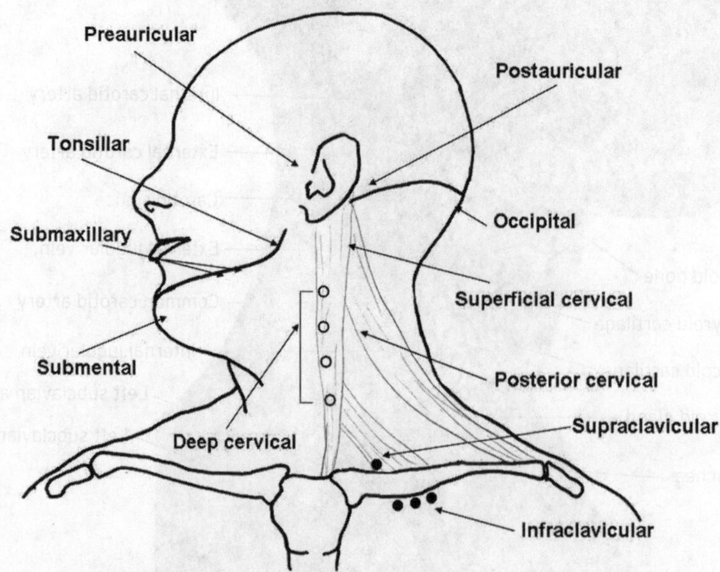

Figure 32-17 Lymph nodes of the head and neck. **Source:** From Skillen, D. L., Day, R. A., Anderson, M. C., Stephen, T. C., Gilbert, J. A., & Day, L. W. (2004). *Physical examination images* [CD-ROM]. Edmonton, AB: Faculty of Nursing, University of Alberta.

TABLE 32-25 Health History for Neck Assessment

Assessment Category	Rationale for Assessment
Ask the client about any history of recent cold, infection, or trauma to neck.	Colds and infections can cause lymph node swelling.
Ask the client about any pain or restriction with neck movement.	Muscle strain or trauma to the neck may result in painful or restricted movement.
Inquire about any history of thyroid problems or thyroid treatments.	Diseases or medications may influence tissue growth of the gland.
Ask the client about any current symptoms of thyroid problems, such as a change in temperature preference; swelling in the neck; change in the texture of hair, skin, and nails; and emotional instability.	These symptoms may indicate the presence of thyroid disease.
Inquire about any enlarged lymph nodes, and document the results of a symptom analysis, as necessary.	Specific signs and symptoms guide the examination.

BOX 32-18 FOCUS ON PRIMARY HEALTH CARE

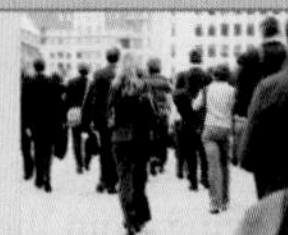

Neck

- Thyroid health

SKILL 32-11 Assessing Neck Veins and Arteries and Range of Motion

Equipment

- Stethoscope
- Light source

Procedure

EXAMINATION SKILL AND FOCUS	TECHNIQUES AND RATIONALE
Inspection: Neck, carotid arteries, jugular veins	Neck fully exposed. Client in the sitting position or supine at 30-degree angle. *Ensures visibility.* 1. Use tangential lighting on the neck. *Casting shadows improves visualization of pulsations.* 2. Inspect the neck. *Pulsations of the carotid arteries and the level of pulsations of the external and internal jugular veins become visible.* 3. Inspect the carotid arteries and jugular veins.
Palpation: Carotid arteries	1. Palpate each carotid artery *separately* (at the level of the cricoid cartilage), using your thumb or index and middle fingers. *Avoids decreasing blood flow to the brain.* 2. Assess the amplitude, contour, and presence of thrills (humming vibrations). 3. Avoid the carotid sinus. *Pressure on the carotid sinus (level with top border of thyroid cartilage) can cause syncope.*
Auscultation: Carotid arteries	1. Instruct the client to hold the breath while you also hold your own breath. *Alerts you to when client needs to breathe again.* 2. Use the bell of the stethoscope to auscultate over each carotid artery. *Stethoscopes amplify a bruit.*
Inspection: Jugular veins	Neck and upper thorax exposed. *Ensures visibility.* Client in the supine position with the head on a pillow and elevated 45 degrees. *Avoids hyperextension or flexion of the neck and thus prevents kinking or stretching of veins. Uses a standardized position for inspecting jugular venous distention.* 1. Use tangential lighting on the neck. *Facilitates better visibility of pulsations.* 2. Locate the external jugular vein first and then the internal jugular vein. *The external jugular vein is easier to find.* 3. Repeat on the other side.
Inspection: Range of motion of neck	Client is in the sitting or standing position. 1. Inspect the range of motion of the cervical vertebrae by instructing the client to: A. Touch the chin to the chest (flexion). B. Look up at the ceiling (extension). C. Touch the ear to the shoulder bilaterally (lateral flexion) while you restrict the client's shoulder movement. D. Turn the head to each side, looking over the shoulder (rotation). *The client demonstrates active range of motion (four movements), and any restrictions are noted.*

From Stephen, T. C., Day, R. A., & Skillen, D. L. (Eds.). (2008). *A syllabus for adult health assessment* (p. 35). Edmonton, AB: Faculty of Nursing, University of Alberta.

cerebrovascular disease manifested by carotid artery obstruction. During carotid auscultation, place the diaphragm of the stethoscope over the artery (Figure 32–18). Ask the client to hold the breath for a moment so that breath sounds do not obscure a bruit. No bruit is usually heard during carotid auscultation.

safety alert If both arteries are occluded during palpation, the client can lose consciousness as a result of inadequate blood circulation to the brain. Avoid vigorous palpation or massage of the carotids. If a bruit is heard in a carotid artery, do not proceed to palpate of the artery.

Palpation. The carotid arteries should always be palpated one at a time (Figure 32–19). For palpation of the carotid pulse, ask the client to turn the head slightly toward the side being examined, as this position relaxes the neck muscles. To avoid the carotid sinus, palpate the carotid pulse in the lower third of the neck, level with the cricoid cartilage. Slide your index and middle fingers or thumb around the medial edge of the sternomastoid muscle. Gentle palpation helps avoid occlusion of circulation. In the past, the use of the thumb to assess major pulses was discouraged. It is now acceptable practice to use the thumb to palpate large arteries such as the carotids (Bickley & Szilagyi, 2007). During palpation, you may feel vibrations or a thrill like a cat's purr. The carotid pulse is strong, with a thrusting quality. The pulsation does not change with breathing or with moving from the sitting position to the supine position. The carotid arteries should exhibit equal pulse rate, rhythm, and strength. Unequal or diminished carotid pulsations can indicate atherosclerosis or aortic arch disease.

Jugular Veins. The most accessible veins are the internal and external jugular veins in the neck. Both drain bilaterally from the head and neck into the superior vena cava. The external jugular vein lies superficially and is seen just above the clavicle. The internal jugular vein lies deeper, along the carotid artery (see Figure 32–15), and only its pulsations are visible.

Inspect the jugular veins to assess venous pressures. Usually, when a client lies supine, the external jugular vein distends and becomes easily visible. In contrast, the jugular veins usually become flattened when the client is sitting. Clients with heart disease, however, may have distended jugular veins even while in the sitting position. Factors that create greater blood volume in the venous system cause elevated venous pressure.

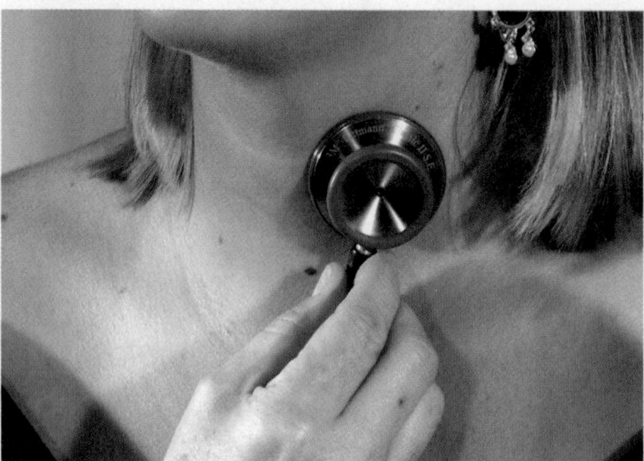

Figure 32-18 Auscultation of the carotid artery. **Source:** From Skillen, D. L., Day, R. A., Anderson, M. C., Stephen, T. C., Gilbert, J. A., & Day, L. W. (2004). *Physical examination images* [CD-ROM]. Edmonton, AB: Faculty of Nursing, University of Alberta.

Range of Motion of the Neck

Inspection. Inspect for symmetry of the neck muscles and range of motion (ROM) of cervical vertebrae and neck muscles during flexion, extension, lateral flexion, and rotation (Skill 32–12). Flexion, lateral flexion, and rotation test the function of the sternomastoid muscles; extension and rotation test the trapezius muscles. The neck should move freely without causing discomfort or dizziness. Test muscle strength and function of the neck during assessment of the musculoskeletal system.

Age-Related Changes. The cervical concave curvature of the neck increases, and the head and jaw move forward. Older adults are more likely to experience dizziness when turning the head.

Documentation. Record your findings from the inspection, palpation, and auscultation of the vascular structures of the neck; record the findings from the inspection of ROM as well (Table 32–26).

Lymph Nodes. The lymphatic system consists of vessels and lymph nodes and is separate from the cardiovascular system. Lymph, a clear watery liquid, moves from tissue spaces into the lymphatic system. Lymph nodes are clusters of lymphatic tissue that occur at intervals and look like beads on a string. They filter the lymph, trap foreign organisms and damaged cells, and provide a partial barrier to

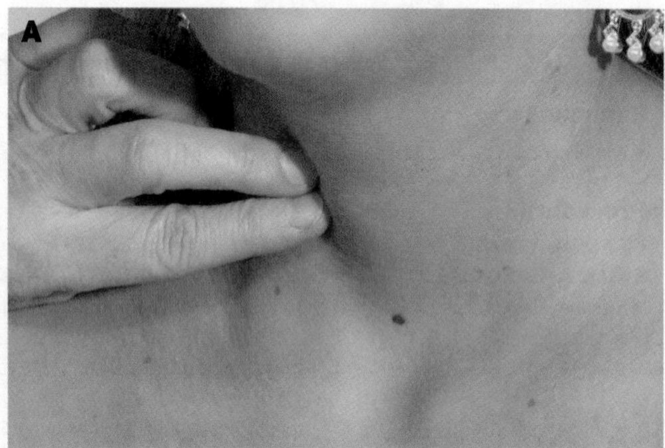

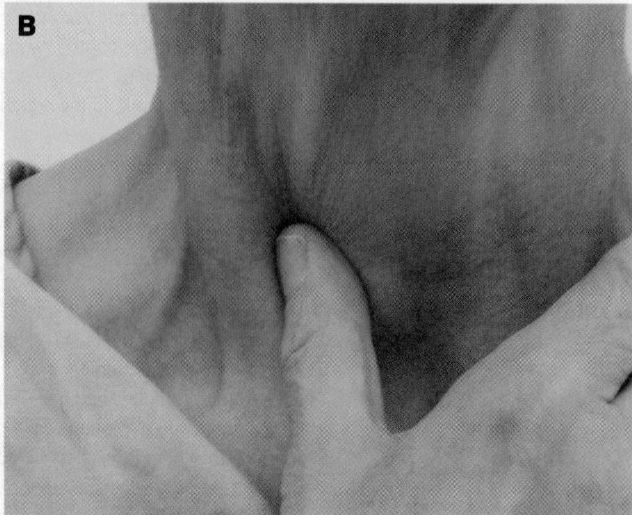

Figure 32-19 A, Palpation of carotid artery with finger pads. B, Palpation of carotid artery with thumb. **Source:** From Skillen, D. L., Day, R. A., Anderson, M. C., Stephen, T. C., Gilbert, J. A., & Day, L. W. (2004). *Physical examination images* [CD-ROM]. Edmonton, AB: Faculty of Nursing, University of Alberta.

➤ SKILL 32-12 Assessing Lymph Nodes of the Neck, Trachea, and Thyroid Gland

Equipment

- Stethoscope
- Glass of water

Procedure

EXAMINATION SKILL AND FOCUS	TECHNIQUES AND RATIONALE
Inspection: Lymph nodes	1. Inspect the area of each set of lymph nodes. *Assesses swelling and changes in skin.*
Palpation: Lymph nodes	Client in the sitting position, while you stand in front of the client. 1. Palpate the lymph nodes (bilaterally) using your finger pads in a circular (rotary) motion to move the skin over the underlying structure. *Finger pads are useful in assessing the characteristics of nodes.* You may palpate the following areas simultaneously: • Preauricular • Postauricular • Occipital • Tonsillar • Submaxillary • Submental (brace top of client's head with one hand) • Superficial cervical • Deep cervical • Posterior cervical • Supraclavicular
Palpation: Trachea	Client in the sitting or supine position. 1. Locate the trachea above the suprasternal notch with your index finger, and compare the spacing from the sternomastoid on each side. *Assesses for deviation from the midline.*
Inspection: Cricoid cartilage and below thyroid	Client in the sitting position, while you stand in front of the client. 1. Instruct the client to extend the head slightly. *Tightens skin to improve visualization.* 2. Direct tangential lighting from the tip of the client's chin toward the thyroid region. *Assists in seeing movement and masses.* 3. Inspect the region below the cricoid cartilage at rest. *Inspects at level of thyroid isthmus.* 4. Ask the client to hold some water in the mouth. *Water helps the client swallow and accentuates the swallow.* 5. Instruct the client to extend the head slightly again. *Extension makes muscles and skin more taut for better visibility.*
Inspection: Thyroid gland movement Cranial nerve (CN) IX, X	6. Inspect for thyroid gland movement when the client is swallowing. *The isthmus and the thyroid gland rise with swallowing. The motor function of CN IX and X is intact if the client can swallow.*
Palpation: Thyroid	1. From the front, palpate down midline to identify each structure. *Ensures you are aware of the location of structures before examining the client from behind.* 2. From behind the client, place your index fingers just below the cricoid cartilage on the client's neck. 3. Instruct the client to flex the head *slightly* toward the side being examined. 4. Instruct the client to swallow some water while you are palpating for the thyroid isthmus. 5. Displace the trachea to one side. 6. Palpate to locate the thyroid lobe between the displaced trachea and sternomastoid. 7. Displace the trachea to other side. 8. Palpate to locate the other thyroid lobe between the displaced trachea and sternomastoid.
Auscultation: Thyroid gland	1. Place the bell of the stethoscope lightly over the thyroid lobe. 2. Ask the client to hold the breath while you also hold own breath. *Alerts you to when client needs to breathe again. Increased blood flow in an enlarged thyroid can be heard better if the client holds the breath.* 3. Listen for bruit. 4. Ask the client to breathe and then hold the breath again. 5. Repeat auscultation on the other side.
Test motor function of CN XI (spinal accessory)	Client in the sitting position. 1. Observe the client shrug shoulders. *Assesses active movement.* 2. Instruct the client to shrug the shoulders while you apply resistance with your hands on client's shoulders. *Assesses muscle strength.* 3. Instruct the client to look straight ahead. 4. Place your hand on the side of the client's face, then instruct the client to turn the head to the same side against resistance. Observe opposite sternomastoid contraction and force against your hand. *Assesses muscle strength.* 5. Repeat on the other side.

From Stephen, T. C., Day, R. A., & Skillen, D. L. (Eds.). (2008). *A syllabus for adult health assessment* (pp. 35–36). Edmonton, AB: Faculty of Nursing, University of Alberta.

➤ TABLE 32-26 Examples of Documentation for Assessment of the Head and Neck

Focus of Assessment	Expected Findings
Head	Head held upright and still, face symmetrical, intact, round skull, full, smooth and nontender temporomandibular joint (TMJ) movements.
Eyes	
Eyebrows, lids, lashes	Full, lying close to eye, colour consistent with complexion, complete closure over sclera; no scaling, edema, lesions, or lid lag; symmetrical palpebral folds; curling outward, equal hair distribution
Cornea, lens	Clear, transparent, shiny
Corneal reflex	Brisk bilateral blinking
Iris	Blue, green, brown; circular, equal size, shape, and colour; flat when viewed from side
Conjunctiva, sclera	Pink, white, clear
Lacrimal sacs, glands	No swelling or redness
Pupils (cranial nerves II and III)	Equal and round at 3 mm
Pupillary reaction to light	PERRLA (pupils equal, round, reactive to light, and accommodation)
Near reaction (accommodation)	Pupils dilate with distant gaze and constrict with near gaze
Convergence	Present to 5 cm
Confrontation	Full visual fields bilaterally
Extraocular muscles	Parallel movement in six positions of gaze; no nystagmus or lid lag; gaze maintained in cover test; corneal light reflected symmetrically
Funduscopy (lens)	Clear, full red reflex bilaterally
Funduscopy (vessels)	Arterioles two-thirds the size of veins, smooth crossings; arterioles have bright light reflections
Funduscopy (disc)	Round, margins well-defined, yellowish pink in colour
Ears	
Auricle	Pink, smooth, intact, complete bilaterally
Mastoid	Smooth, hard, nontender right and left
Gross hearing test (cranial nerve VIII)	Correctly identifies three numbers bilaterally at a distance of 50 cm
Weber test	Hearing in right and left equally
Rinné test	AC > BC bilaterally; 2:1 ratio
Otoscope (canal)	Pink, smooth, clear bilaterally
Otoscope (cerumen)	Soft, light amber bilaterally
Otoscope (tympanic membrane)	Intact, shiny, pearly grey bilaterally
Otoscope (landmarks)	Cone of light shiny bilaterally; right at 5 o'clock and left at 7 o'clock; well-defined handle of malleus, umbo, and annulus right and left
Nose	Air entry easy and effortless right and left Nose smooth, symmetrical, and located at centre of face Nasal structures firm, stable, without tenderness Nasal mucosa pink, moist, with clear mucus bilaterally Frontal and maxillary sinuses nontender right and left Accurate identification of pungent odours right and left
Mouth	
Lips	Pink, moist, symmetrical, smooth
Oral cavity	Oral mucosa glistening, pink, soft, moist, and smooth Gums pink, smooth, moist, with tight margins around each tooth Tongue medium or dull red in colour, moist, slightly rough on dorsal surface, smooth along lateral margins, and highly vascular on ventral surface Gag reflex present bilaterally Uvula and soft palate rise centrally when saying "ah"
Neck	Symmetrical, smooth, no fullness over thyroid
Carotid arteries	Smooth contour, 2+ strength bilaterally, no bruits heard over right or left arteries
Jugular veins	At a 45-degree angle, no distension bilaterally
Range of motion (ROM) of neck	Full ROM bilaterally without discomfort or dizziness
Lymph nodes	Bilaterally nonpalpable
Tracheal position	Midline, posterior to suprasternal notch
Thyroid	Isthmus smooth, lobes nonpalpable, lobes and isthmus move upward with swallowing
Cranial nerves IX, X	Motor function of both nerves intact
Cranial nerve XI	Motor function intact right and left Muscle strength strong right and left

Adapted from Chambers, J., Bazin, M., Nutting, L., & Stephen, T. (2008). *Year I lab guide* (pp. 93–94). Edmonton, AB: Faculty of Nursing, University of Alberta.

the growth of cancerous (malignant) cells within the body. The superficial lymph nodes are the only component of the lymphatic system that is accessible for examination. They are located in the head, neck, axillae, arms, and inguinal regions. You need to assess lymph nodes competently, particularly when caring for clients with severe infections, suspected cancer, and reduced immunity evidenced by the presence of allergies, autoimmune diseases (e.g., lupus erythematosus), or human immunodeficiency virus (HIV) infection.

The head and neck are well supplied with lymph nodes (see Figure 32–22, page 590). They are known by different names, so one commonly used system of nomenclature is provided here. The fact that the names refer to nearby structures aids in memorizing the location of the nodes. To avoid overlooking any single node or chain of nodes, use a systematic approach of inspection and palpation to examine lymph nodes, and evaluate each node or chain for the following:

- Location
- Enlargement
- Size
- Shape (round, regular, irregular)
- Consistency (soft, firm, hard)
- Delineation (borders clearly defined or not)
- Mobility
- Surface characteristics
- Tenderness
- Skin warmth over the nodes

For inspection and palpation of lymph nodes, ask the client to flex the neck slightly forward (see Skill 32–12), which relaxes tissues and muscles. Lymph nodes are not usually visible; if they can be visualized, examine them for swelling, erythema, or red streaks. During palpation, face or stand to the side of the client to easily access all the nodes. It is important to press underlying tissue in each area and not simply move your fingers over the skin; however, if you apply too much pressure, you may miss the small nodes and obliterate the palpable nodes. Nodes can be examined in sets of three. The preauricular, postauricular, and occipital nodes comprise one set. Another set consists of the tonsillar, submaxillary, and submental lymph nodes. The third set includes the superficial, deep, and posterior cervical nodes. Usually, lymph nodes are not palpable, but small, mobile, nontender nodes are commonly encountered during the examination and are mostly benign. Lymph nodes that are large, fixed in position, inflamed, or tender indicate a health problem, such as a systemic disease, a local infection, or a neoplasm or cancer (Seidel et al., 2006). When you find enlarged nodes, explore adjacent areas drained by the nodes for signs of infection or malignancy. To locate the site of an infection, note which nodes are enlarged. For example, ear infections usually drain to the deep cervical or preauricular nodes. A serious infection may leave a node permanently enlarged, and nontender. Malignancy is usually associated with nontender, hard, fixed nodes with irregular borders.

Trachea. The trachea is located in the midline of the neck, above the suprasternal notch. Masses in the neck or mediastinum and pulmonary alterations can cause the trachea to deviate laterally (see Skill 32–12). Assess the tracheal position using gentle pressure to avoid causing the coughing reflex in the client.

Thyroid Gland. The thyroid gland lies in the middle and front of the neck and is fixed to the trachea. It consists of two irregular, cone-shaped lobes that lie behind the sternomastoid muscles. The lobes are connected by a bridge of tissue (thyroid isthmus) that is located over the second and third tracheal rings. Assess the thyroid gland using inspection, palpation, and auscultation (see Skill 32–12).

Inspection. Stand in front of the client to inspect the area of the lower neck overlying the thyroid gland for visible masses, symmetry, and any fullness. Usually, a hollow area or a groove is seen on each side of the neck between the trachea and the sternomastoid. At the level of the thyroid isthmus, observe for fullness and the disappearance of the natural grooves. When the client swallows, look for upward movement of the isthmus and any bulging of the thyroid gland. The thyroid gland is not usually visible.

Palpation. Begin palpation by identifying the midline structures from the front. For the posterior approach, have the client sit so that the neck is more accessible. With both your hands placed around the client's neck, rest two fingers of each hand on the sides of the trachea just below the cricoid cartilage. This permits you to assess enlargement and movement of the thyroid isthmus while the client swallows. Move your fingers between the sternomastoid and trachea to gently palpate each thyroid lobe separately for any enlargement, masses, or nodules. The lobes are usually small, smooth, and free of nodules, but you may be able to palpate them more easily in extremely thin individuals. Enlargement indicates thyroid dysfunction. Masses or nodules may indicate malignancy, but not all nodules are malignant.

Auscultation. When you find the gland enlarged, place the bell of the stethoscope over the thyroid. Enlargement causes blood flow through the thyroid arteries to increase, which causes a fine vibration. During auscultation, the vibration is heard as a soft, rushing sound (bruit).

Cranial Nerves. Assess the motor function of cranial nerves IX (glossopharyngeal) and X (vagus) by observing the client swallowing water as part of the thyroid examination or as part of the neurological examination. Assess cranial nerve XI (spinal accessory) by observing the client shrug the shoulders (movement) and by testing muscle strength of shoulders and neck.

Age-Related Changes. The submandibular (submaxillary) salivary gland may prolapse and be incorrectly identified as a tumour in older adults. The prolapse occurs bilaterally, and the glands feel soft (Jarvis, 2004).

Documentation. Record your findings from the inspection and palpation of the lymph nodes, trachea, and thyroid gland (see Table 32–26).

Assessing the Torso

Inspection, palpation, percussion, and auscultation are used in the assessment of the torso (spine, thorax, lungs, heart, breasts, abdomen, female and male genitalia, inguinal regions, anus, rectum, and prostate).

Assessing the Spine

The vertebral column has four curvatures—cervical, thoracic, lumbar, and sacral—which ease the impact of active movements and distribute weight from the upper body to the lower body. Muscles are attached at the transverse and spinous processes. The trapezius and latissimus dorsi are large muscles attached to each side of the spine. Coordination of the 24 vertebrae, vertebral discs, muscles, and interconnecting ligaments contributes to the healthy mechanics of the spine. After taking the health history, you will use inspection and palpation to examine the spine.

Inspection. Conduct the inspection with the client standing and draped (Skill 32–13). The standing posture is an upright stance with parallel alignment of shoulders and hips. When viewing the client from the side, expect to see a slight convex curve in the thoracic region and a concave curve in the lumbar area. A pronounced lordosis (exaggerated concave curvature in the lumbar spine; Figure 32–20A) or a kyphosis (exaggerated convex curvature of the thoracic spine; Figure 32–20B) are not expected. A lateral curvature of the spine viewed from the back is called scoliosis and is an important deviation that is detected early in youth (Figure 32–20C). After examining the spinal curvatures, assess the spine for vertical alignment. Look for symmetrical horizontal alignment of landmarks (shoulders, spinous processes, paravertebral muscles, scapulae, iliac crests, and posterior superior iliac spines).

Range of Motion. By inspecting the range of motion (ROM) of the spine (see Skill 32–13), you assess flexibility, ease of movement, symmetry, and curvatures in the back. Expect clients to demonstrate full flexion (the hands should almost touch the toes) and extension (backward lean from hips), as well as symmetrical lateral bending (the hand at the side almost reaches the knee) and rotation of the spine.

Palpation. Palpation of the spinous processes and paravertebral muscles begins when you track two fingers down the client's spine assessing vertical alignment of the spinous processes. Obvious protrusions of the vertebral discs or processes are not expected findings. Using circular motions with finger pads or thumbs on both sides of the spine, expect to find nontenderness and similar muscle bulk bilaterally.

Age-Related Changes. Changes in the musculoskeletal system become increasingly evident in the posture and gait of persons 80 years or older. Height is gradually lost due to thinning intervertebral discs and collapsed vertebral bodies as a result of osteoporosis. Knee and hip flexion contributes to loss of height. Collapse of vertebral bodies makes a significant contribution to kyphosis. The head may tilt backward due to the kyphosis or bend forward due to the collapsed cervical vertebral bodies. Flexion at the knees and hips and the limbs (especially arms) appearing longer in proportion to the trunk create a stooped posture.

➤ SKILL 32-13 Assessing the Spine

Equipment

- None

Procedure

EXAMINATION SKILL AND FOCUS	TECHNIQUES AND RATIONALE
Spine	Client in standing position, loosely draped, feet together. Pants resting just below sacroiliac joints. *Adequate exposure ensures that the spinal curves are visible.*
Inspection:	
Curvatures	1. Inspect from the side (profile). *Permits assessment of thoracic and lumbar curvatures.*
Vertical alignment	2. Inspect from the back in the midline position.
Horizontal alignment	1. Look for symmetry of shoulders, scapulae, iliac crests, sacroiliac joints, and gluteal folds. *Comparison facilitates identification of horizontal alignment.*
Palpation:	2. Palpate structures to confirm symmetry.
Inspection:	1. Instruct the client to touch the toes (flexion).
Range of motion	2. Place your hand on the client's posterior superior iliac spine, fingers pointing toward the midline.
	3. Instruct the client to bend backward as far as possible (extension).
	Urgent: During extension and lateral bending, you should protect the client from injury by stabilizing the client at the hips.
	4. Place your hands on the client's hips.
	5. Instruct the client to bend sideways as far as possible (lateral bending).
	6. Repeat on the other side.
	7. Place one hand on the client's hip and the other on the opposite shoulder.
	8. Rotate the client's trunk by pulling the shoulder and then the hip (rotation). *Flexion, extension, lateral bending, and rotation are movements that are possible if the spine and musculature are intact.*
	9. Repeat on the other side.
Palpation:	Client in standing position.
Spinous processes	1. Palpate the spinous processes from C1 to L5. *Spinous processes are landmarks for the 24 vertebrae of the vertebral column.*
	2. Move your finger pads or thumbs in rotary motion. *Motion detects deviations or tenderness. Thumbs and finger pads are sensitive to characteristics to be assessed.*
	3. Inquire about any tenderness.
	4. Assess alignment by running two fingers down the client's spine from C1 to L5. *Palpation emphasizes vertical alignment.*
Paravertebral muscles	1. Palpate the paravertebral muscles bilaterally from the level of C1 to L5. *Paravertebral muscles attach to all spinous processes.*
	2. Use your finger pads or thumbs.
	3. Inquire about any tenderness.

From Stephen, T. C., Day, R. A., & Skillen, D. L. (Eds.). (2008). *A syllabus for adult health assessment* (pp. 36–37). Edmonton, AB: Faculty of Nursing, University of Alberta.

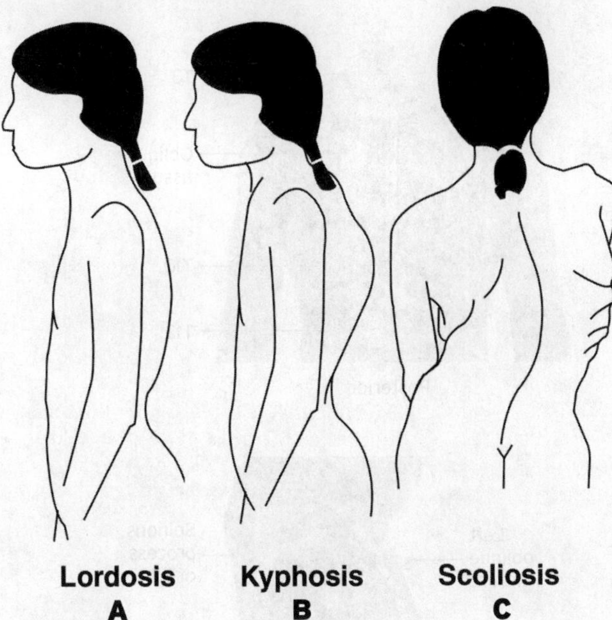

Figure 32-20 Abnormalities of the spine. A, Lordosis. B, Kyphosis. C, Scoliosis. **Source:** From Skillen, D. L., Day, R. A., Anderson, M. C., Stephen, T. C., Gilbert, J. A., & Day, L. W. (2004). *Physical examination images* [CD-ROM]. Edmonton, AB: Faculty of Nursing, University of Alberta.

Documentation. Record your findings from the inspection and palpation of the spine (see Table 32–33, page 605).

Assessing the Thorax and Lungs

Accurate physical assessment of the thorax and lungs requires knowledge of anatomical terms, landmarks, underlying structures, and ventilatory and respiratory functions of the lungs. Assess the thorax and lungs posteriorly, anteriorly, and laterally (both sides). Be alert to changes in certain body systems possibly caused by alterations in the respiratory system. For example, reduced oxygenation of the blood can change the client's mental alertness due to the reaction of the brain to lowered oxygen levels. Similarly, alterations in other body systems can cause respiratory alterations. Inspection, palpation, percussion, and auscultation are used during this assessment.

Thorax. The thorax is a bony structure created by the sternum, clavicle, ribs, thoracic spine, scapulae, and vertebrae. The nonpalpable costochondral junctions connect the ribs with the costal cartilages. Anteriorly, important midline structures are the manubrium, body of the sternum, and xiphoid process.

The suprasternal notch on the superior border of the manubrium guides identification of the **sternal angle** (angle of Louis), a bony prominence or ridge where the manubrium joins the body of the sternum. The left and right second ribs articulate with this prominence. Anteriorly, count the ribs and intercostal spaces (spaces between ribs) starting from the sternal angle and the second rib. The number of each intercostal space corresponds to the rib just above it. To describe findings on the anterior thorax, use the sternal angle, midsternal line, numbered ribs, interspaces between ribs, and costal margins.

Posteriorly, the inferior margin of the scapula lies at the level of the seventh rib, which helps locate the seventh thoracic vertebra. Use the ribs, interspaces, inferior tip of the scapula, spinous processes, and costal margin to describe your findings. The vertebral line posteriorly and the midsternal line anteriorly are very precise. Less precise but useful vertical lines are: scapular, midclavicular, anterior and posterior axillary, and midaxillary. To describe your findings, use the anatomical terms *supraclavicular, infraclavicular, interscapular, infrascapular, bases, apices, and upper, middle,* and *lower lung fields*.

Lungs. Oblique and horizontal fissures divide the right lung into the right upper lobe (RUL), right middle lobe (RML), and right lower lobe (RLL; Figure 32–21). In the anterior thorax, the apex of the RUL and the left upper lobe (LUL) rises 2 to 4 cm above the medial clavicles. The lower lung borders cross the eighth ribs in the midaxillary lines and the sixth ribs in the midclavicular lines (MCLs). Posteriorly, the lower border of the lungs is at approximately the tenth thoracic (T10) spinous process and descends to the T12 spinous process with deep inspiration (Swartz, 2005). Anteriorly, the trachea bifurcates at the level of the sternal angle into right and left main bronchi and posteriorly at the level of the fourth thoracic (T4) spinous process. The right main bronchus is somewhat straighter than the left one.

Lungs are covered by serous membranes, called visceral pleura. Parietal pleura line the rib cage and the superior surface of the diaphragm. Between the pleura is a potential space. Pleural fluid permits surfaces to move without friction during respiration.

Respiration depends on an intact brainstem and the muscles of respiration. During inspiration, the diaphragm contracts and descends, increasing the vertical dimension of the thoracic cavity and compressing abdominal contents. To increase the anterior or posterior diameter of the thorax, the external intercostal muscles elevate the ribs and the sternum. The intrathoracic pressure falls, causing air to flow through the trachea, bronchi, and bronchioles into the alveoli (air sacs). In the expanded state of the lungs at the alveolar–capillary interface, oxygen diffuses into the blood, and carbon dioxide diffuses out. During expiration, which is a primarily passive activity, the diaphragm and external intercostals relax, the intrathoracic pressure increases, air in the alveoli and tracheobronchial tree flows in the opposite direction, and the thoracic cage returns to its former position.

The act of breathing is usually quiet, effortless, and automatic. Respiratory rates in healthy adults vary from 12 to 20 respirations per minute. When respiration requires effort due to exercise or disease, breathing becomes audible, and effort is visible. Accessory muscles assist the respiratory effort. The sternomastoid and scalene muscles in the neck lift the sternum and first two ribs to enlarge the upper thoracic cavity during inspiration. During forced expiration, the abdominal muscles and internal intercostals contract to decrease the vertical and anteroposterior diameters.

Before initiating respiratory assessment, conduct a health history interview (Table 32–27). Use the data from the interview to determine the focus of the assessment and to plan health promotion (Box 32–19).

Posterior Thorax and Lung Fields. When assessing the thorax and lungs, it is essential to inspect, palpate, percuss, and auscultate on symmetrical areas of the thorax and compare the sides (Skill 32–14). While examining posteriorly, drape a female client's anterior chest. Bedridden clients may be allowed to remain supine and be assisted onto their side, but ambulatory clients are best examined posteriorly in the sitting position.

Inspection. In the midline position, examine the posterior thorax for shape, skin condition, and movement, during both rest and respiration. Expect the scapulae to be symmetrical and closey attached to the thoracic wall. You will routinely inspect rate, rhythm, depth, and effort of breathing. Always look for any indication of respiratory difficulty, including colour (lips, nails), displacement of the trachea from the midline, audible sounds of breathing, and client

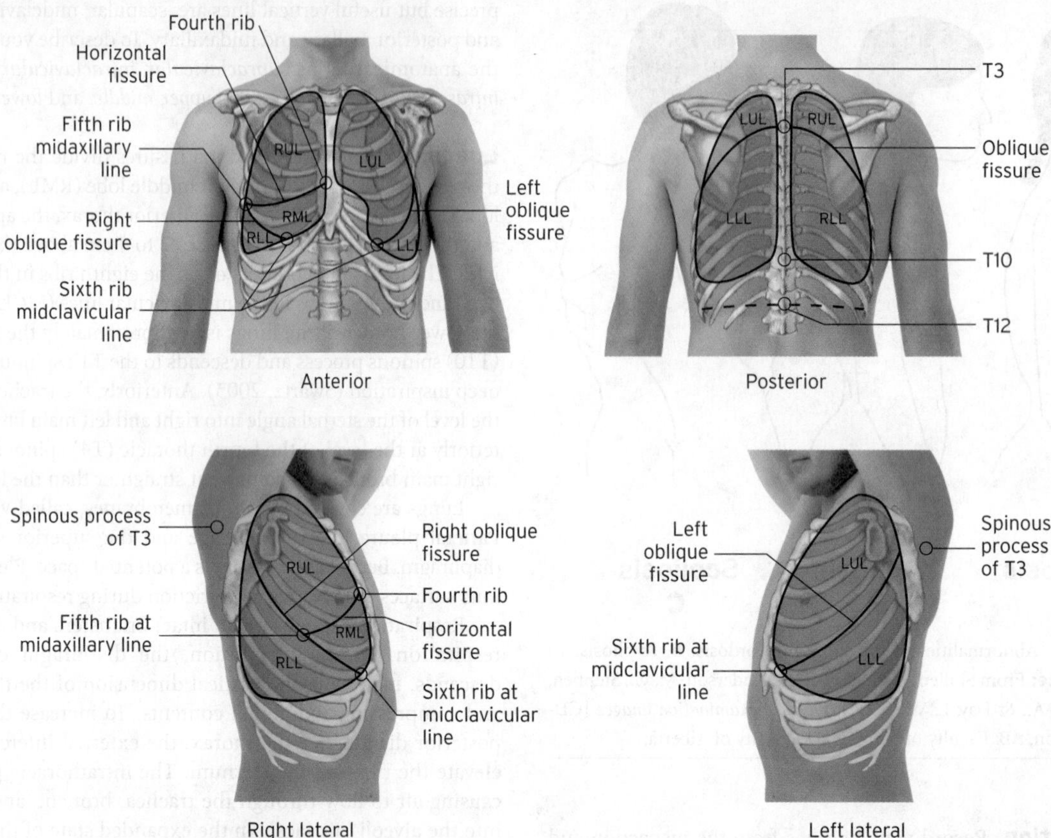

Figure 32-21 Visualizing the lungs from the surface. **Source:** From Seidel, H. M., Ball, J. W., Dains, J. E., & Benedict, G. W. (2006). *Mosby's guide to physical examination* (6th ed., p. 365, Box 13–1). St. Louis, MO: Mosby.

TABLE 32-27 Health History for Lung Assessment

Assessment Category	Rationale for Assessment
Ask the client about any tobacco use, including duration, amount, frequency of use in pack-years,* age at initiation of smoking, type of tobacco, and efforts to quit.	Smoking is a risk factor for lung cancer, other lung diseases, and heart disease.
Inquire about cough, sputum, chest pain, activity tolerance, shortness of breath, recurrent infections.	Symptoms may help localize objective data.
Question the client about workplace environmental pollutants (e.g., asbestos, coal dust, secondhand smoke, chemicals).	These exposures increase risk for lung disease.
Inquire about history of substance abuse, HIV infection, low income, residential living, or recent immigration.	These are risk factors for tuberculosis.
Ask the client about persistent cough, fatigue, hemoptysis, unexplained weight loss, night sweats, or fever.	These signs and symptoms are associated with tuberculosis and HIV infection.
Ask about any hoarseness of voice.	This may indicate a laryngeal disorder or a lifestyle-related issue (substance abuse).
Inquire about family history of cancer, tuberculosis, allergies, or chronic obstructive pulmonary disease.	These factors increase the client's risk for lung disease.
Ask about allergies to pollutants, dust, or other airborne irritants, and to foods, drugs, or chemical irritants.	Allergic responses can cause signs and symptoms such as dyspnea and wheezes.

*Pack-years = number of years smoked x number of packs per day.

BOX 32-19 FOCUS ON PRIMARY HEALTH CARE

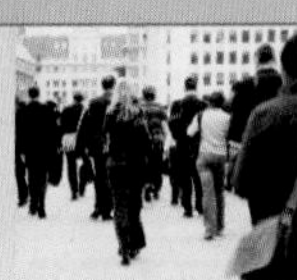

Lungs

- Influenza vaccination
- Tobacco cessation
- Warning signs for lung disease
- Respiratory protection in the workplace

SKILL 32-14 Examination of the Posterior Thorax and Lungs

Equipment

- Stethoscope

Procedure

EXAMINATION SKILL AND FOCUS	TECHNIQUES AND RATIONALE
Thorax inspection: Anteroposterior (AP) and lateral	Client in sitting position, disrobed to waist. *Ensures chest is fully visible.* **1.** Inspect from the side (profile). *Assesses anteroposterior diameter in relation to lateral diameter.* **2.** Inspect the posterior thorax from the midline. **3.** Compare the ratios.
Posterior lung fields Palpation: Chest expansion	**1.** Place your thumbs at the level of and parallel to the tenth ribs. **2.** Wrap your hands *loosely* around lateral rib cage. *Loosely wrapped hands permit unrestricted movement of the thorax.* **3.** Slide your hands medially to raise the client's skinfolds between your thumb and the client's spine. **4.** Instruct the client to inhale deeply and then exhale. *As client inhales, a flattened skinfold indicates symmetrical movement of the thorax.* **5.** Observe the distance between your thumbs during inspiration. **6.** Observe and feel for the range and symmetry of expansion during inhalation and exhalation. **7.** Compare the sides.
Tactile fremitus	**1.** Instruct the client to "round" the shoulders by folding the arms across chest and placing each hand on the opposite shoulder. *As shoulders are rounded, the scapulae separate, increasing access to posterior lung fields.* **2.** Palpate and compare symmetrical areas: • Upper (apices and interscapular) • Lower • Lateral (in midaxillary line) *Ensures that all the posterior lung fields, including the lateral lung fields, are fully palpated.* **3.** Ask the client to say the number "99" **OR** the words "blue moon" in a deep voice. *A deep voice produces vibrations that carry more effectively to the periphery.* **4.** Use the ball of your hand (the palm at the base of the fingers) **OR** the ulnar aspect of the hand. *The ulnar surface and ball of the hand are equally sensitive to vibrations.* **5.** Use one **OR** both hands to assess fremitus in symmetrical areas (upper, lower, and lateral).
Percussion: Posterior chest	**1.** Instruct the client to continue "rounding" the shoulders. *As the shoulders are rounded, the scapulae separate, increasing access to posterior lung fields.* **2.** Percuss and compare symmetrical areas at 5-cm intervals: • Upper (apices and interscapular) • Lower • Lateral (in midaxillary line) *Ensures that all posterior lung fields are fully percussed.* **3.** Press the distal phalanx and the joint of the middle (pleximeter) finger *firmly* over the intercostal space (avoiding contact with other fingers). *Contact on the thorax from fingers other than the pleximeter finger dampens percussion notes. Avoids percussing over bone.* **4.** Aim at the distal phalanx or interphalangeal joint. **5.** Strike the pleximeter with a sharp perpendicular blow with the tip of your middle (plexor) finger (you may support the plexor finger with the thumb). *Consistent, quick, sharp blows are most effective in eliciting percussion notes. No more than one or two blows per site are needed to facilitate identification of the percussion note.* **6.** Use wrist action only.
Auscultation: Posterior lung fields	**1.** Instruct the client to continue rounding the shoulders. *Ensures access to posterior lung fields.* **2.** Auscultate with the diaphragm of stethoscope. **3.** Instruct the client to breathe with mouth open, more deeply than usual, and to let you know if he or she feels dizzy. *Dizziness alerts you to hyperventilation and need for rest.* **4.** Listen to at least ONE full breath in each area. *Assesses both inspiratory and expiratory breath sounds. Timing in respiratory cycle assists with interpretation of findings.* **5.** Listen to and compare symmetrical areas. *Comparison aids detection of alterations.* • Upper (apices and interscapular) • Lower • Lateral (in midaxillary line) *Ensures all posterior lung fields are fully ausculated.*

From Stephen, T. C., Day, R. A., & Skillen, D. L. (Eds.). (2008). *A syllabus for adult health assessment* (pp. 37–39). Edmonton, AB: Faculty of Nursing, University of Alberta.

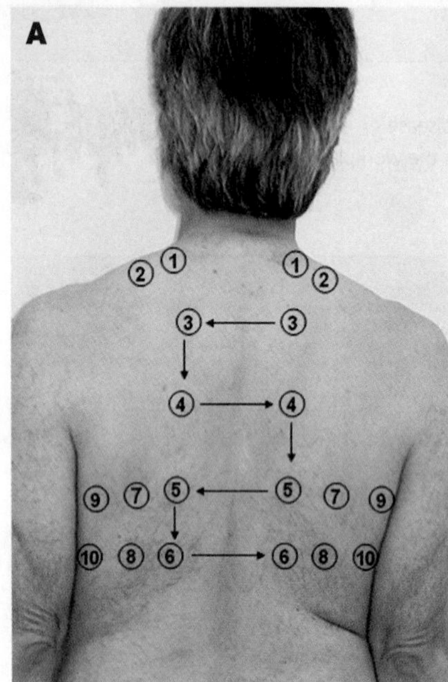

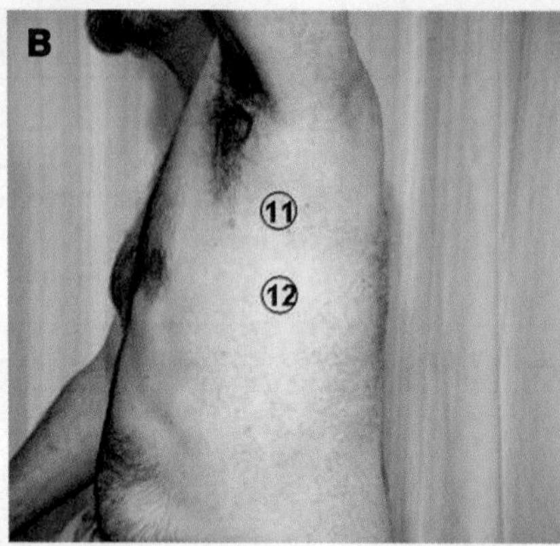

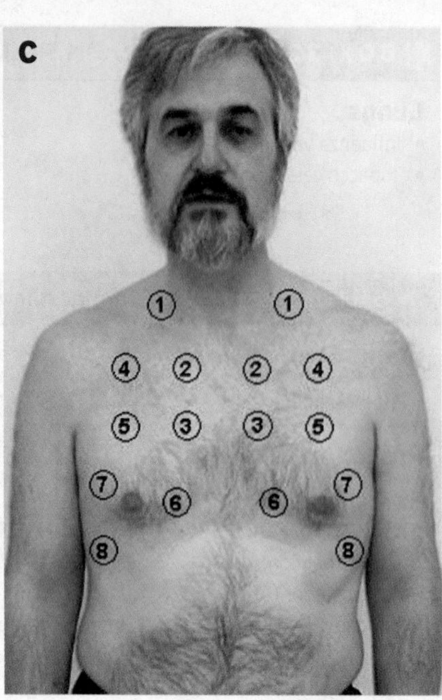

Figure 32-22 A, Sites on posterior thorax to be compared. **B**, Sites on lateral thorax to be compared. C, Sites on anterior thorax to be compared. **Source:** From Skillen, D. L., Day, R. A., Anderson, M. C., Stephen, T. C., Gilbert, J. A., & Day, L. W. (2004). *Physical examination images* [CD-ROM]. Edmonton, AB: Faculty of Nursing, University of Alberta.

position that aids breathing. Look for a lateral diameter (Lat) wider than the anteroposterior diameter (AP), and estimate their ratio when recording findings. The AP:Lat ratio ranges from 1:2 to 5:7. Deformities, asymmetry of movement, or use of accessory respiratory muscles are unexpected findings.

Clients who lean forward, supporting their arms against a chair, pillow, their knees, or something else, may be doing so because they are having difficulty breathing. This position aids expiration and is commonly seen in clients with chronic obstructive pulmonary disease (COPD). Watch for pursed lips during expiration, or splinting or holding of the chest wall to minimize localized pain aggravated by respirations. This causes clients to bend toward the affected side and impairs ventilatory movement.

Palpation. Examine skin lesions noted during inspection, and palpate the chest for tenderness, masses, and skin temperature. The thoracic muscles and skeleton are expected to be nontender. While examining respiratory expansion, assess symmetry of chest expansion, which may be limited by pain, postural deformity, or fatigue. Evaluate symmetry of chest vibrations by assessing **tactile fremitus**, a palpable vibration generated when the client repeats certain sounds (as instructed by you) during thoracic palpation. If fremitus is faint, ask the client to speak in a louder or deeper voice. You can detect the vibrations of sound waves with either the ball of your hand or the ulnar edge. Use one hand, or both hands simultaneously unless one is more sensitive to vibrations than the other. Compare the thoracic regions systematically as you palpate from the apices to the bases (Figure 32–22). Palpable vibrations are present bilaterally and are equal; the intensity is greater over the apices and interscapular areas and reduced over the lung bases. Lung lesions, collapsed lungs, or mucus accumulations all decrease the intensity.

Percussion. Percussion over the intercostal spaces identifies underlying tissues as air-filled, fluid-filled, or solid. Percuss the posterior thorax in all areas used for palpation and auscultation (see Figure 32–22), comparing the sides. As lungs are filled with air, resonance is expected for all thoracic regions. Percussion over the scapulae, ribs, or spine produces a dull percussion note. Adults with hyperinflated lungs (e.g., in asthma or emphysema) will have hyperresonance. When lung tissue is consolidated or contains fluid, the percussion note is dull. A lung mass causes a flat sound. A dull or flat sound may suggest atelectasis, pleural effusion, or hemothorax.

Auscultation. By recognizing sounds created by airflow during inspiration and expiration (Table 32–28), you are able to detect the sounds caused by open, narrowed, or obstructed airways. Listen to an entire inspiration and expiration with the diaphragm chestpiece of your stethoscope at each indicated position. If the sounds are faint, as may occur in an obese client, ask the client to breathe deeper. Always move the stethoscope systematically from the right to the left and back (see Figure 32–22A) to compare sounds in one region with those of the same region on the other side. Similarly, compare symmetrical regions to detect unexpected **adventitious sounds**, which may be superimposed over the expected sounds. Four common types of adventitious sounds are crackles, rhonchi, wheezes, and pleural friction rub (Table 32–29).

Anterior and Lateral Thorax and Lung Fields

Anterior Thorax. Inspect, palpate, percuss, and auscultate the anterior thorax for most of the same features as with the posterior thorax. Nurses commonly assess the respiratory rate, rhythm, and effort in the anterior thorax. The right middle lobe (RML) is best assessed while examining the right anterior lung field. Clients may be sitting or supine. The supine position facilitates displacement of the breasts for the examination of the female client. The costal angle (between the right and left costal margins) is usually more than 90 degrees. Men may have diaphragmatic respirations; women usually have thoracic or costal respirations.

Avoid palpating over the heart and, in women, over the breasts when assessing tactile fremitus. Gently retract the breasts, or have the client lift them up. You will feel the fremitus best next to the sternum at the second intercostal space, at the level of the bronchial bifurcation.

Percussion of the anterior thorax follows a systematic pattern. Begin above the clavicles, moving side to side, and end at the lower thorax. In women, move the breasts away, as needed. Proceeding downward, you will detect heart and liver dullness and the tympanic gastric air bubble.

Auscultation of the anterior thorax follows the same pattern as that for percussion. Vesicular sounds are heard in the apices, below the clavicles, and over the peripheral lung fields. Bronchovesicular sounds are heard below the clavicles. Bronchial sounds heard over the trachea are loud, high pitched, and hollow. Pay special attention to the lower lobes, where fluids commonly collect in adult clients with illness.

➤ TABLE 32-28 Description of Expected Breath Sounds

Type of Breath Sound	Location	Origin
Vesicular sounds are soft, breezy, and low pitched. The inspiratory phase is three times longer than the expiratory phase.	Best heard over the peripheral lung fields (except over the scapula)	Created by air moving through the smaller airways
Bronchovesicular sounds are blowing sounds that are medium pitched and of medium intensity. The inspiratory phase is equal to the expiratory phase.	Best heard posteriorly between the scapulae and anteriorly over the bronchioles lateral to the sternum at the first and second intercostal spaces	Created by air moving through the large airways
Bronchial sounds are loud and high pitched and have a hollow quality. Expiration lasts longer than inspiration (3:2 ratio).	Best heard over the trachea	Created by air moving through the trachea close to the chest wall

➤ TABLE 32-29 Description of Adventitious Breath Sounds

Fine crackles: high-pitched, discrete, discontinuous crackling sounds heard during the end of inspiration; not cleared by a cough

Medium crackles: lower, more moist sounds heard during the midstage of inspiration; not cleared by a cough

Coarse crackles: loud, bubbly noise heard during inspiration; not cleared by a cough

Rhonchi (sonorous wheeze): loud, low, rumbling coarse sounds, like a snore, most often heard continuously during inspiration or expiration; coughing may clear the sound (usually means mucus accumulation in the trachea or the large bronchi)

Wheeze (sibilant wheeze): musical noise that sounds like a squeak; most often heard continuously during inspiration or expiration; usually louder during expiration

Pleural friction rub: dry, rubbing, or grating sound, usually caused by inflammation of pleural surfaces; heard during inspiration or expiration; loudest over lower lateral anterior surface

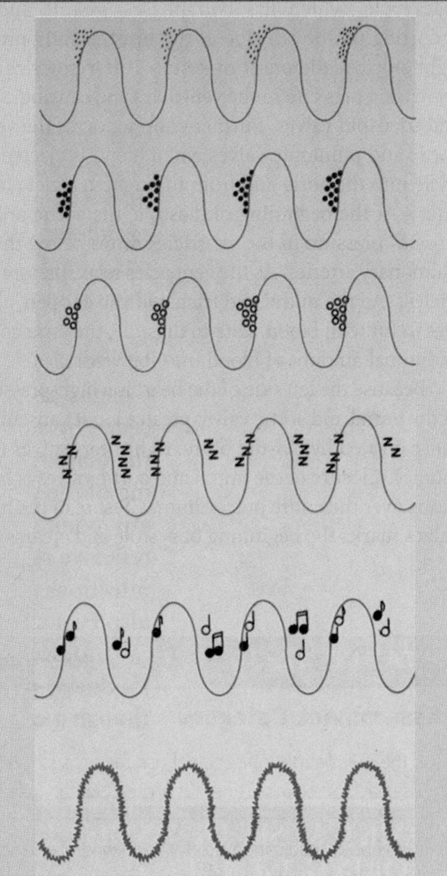

Data from Seidel, H. M., Ball, J. W., Dains, J. E., & Benedict, G. W. (2006). *Mosby's guide to physical examination* (6th ed., p. 387). St. Louis, MO: Mosby.

Lateral Thorax. Using the same systematic pattern, inspect, palpate, percuss, and auscultate the lateral lung fields on both sides (see Figure 32–22B). This is usually done as an extension of the assessment of the posterior thorax when you ask the client to lift the arms away from the chest. In the healthy client, percussion notes are expected to be resonant and breath sounds vesicular.

Age-Related Changes. The mobility of the thorax diminishes as costal cartilages become increasingly calcified. Muscles of respiration lose strength. Elastic properties of the lung tissue become diminished, affecting extensibility and recoil. The small airways are more likely to close early, reducing the amount of air that can be expelled during expiration and increasing the amount of residual air in the lungs. At the alveolar level, the surface area for oxygen and carbon dioxide exchange is reduced. Ventilation of the lung bases decreases. Skeletal changes increase the anteroposterior diameter and emphasize the thoracic curvature; they have little effect on function in healthy older adults but make the chest more of a barrel shape.

Documentation. Record your findings from the inspection, palpation, percussion, and auscultation of the thorax and lungs (see Table 32–33 on page 605).

Assessing the Heart

Assess cardiac function anteriorly. Visualize the location of the heart chambers and valves and the direction in which the great vessels arise from the heart in relation to the sternum and ribs. The adult heart lies posterior to the **precordium** (area of the thorax that lies over the heart), is rotated so that the right ventricle forms most of its anterior surface, and extends almost to the xiphoid process where it rests on the diaphragm. A small part of the right atrium extends to the right of the sternum. The superior border of the heart that is formed mostly by the great vessels—called the "base" of the heart—is located at about the right and left second interspaces close to the sternum. The left ventricle lies posterior to the right ventricle, its left lateral border extending beyond the right ventricle. The left ventricle forms the left lateral border and the bottom tip or "apex" of the heart. The apex lies just medial to the left MCL at about the fifth intercostal space. Contraction of the left ventricle produces the **apical impulse**.

To understand the significance of your cardiac assessment findings, you must have a clear understanding of the dynamics of the cardiac cycle, which has two phases: systole and diastole. Events occurring on the left side of the heart slightly precede those on the right side. At the onset of systole, the ventricles begin to contract, increasing pressure in the ventricles and causing closure of the mitral and tricuspid valves. Further contraction of the ventricles opens the aortic and pulmonic valves when blood is ejected from the left ventricle into the aorta and from the right ventricle into the pulmonary artery. At the beginning of diastole, the aortic and pulmonic valves close as pressure in the ventricles drops below that in the aorta and pulmonary arteries. As the ventricles relax, pressure drops in the ventricles, and the mitral and tricuspid valves open, allowing the ventricles to fill with blood. Late in diastole, the atria contract, pushing an additional amount of blood into the ventricles.

Because the left side of the heart is a high-pressure system, closure of the mitral and aortic valves creates louder auscultatory sounds than those created by closure of the right heart valves (tricuspid and pulmonic). Closure of the mitral and aortic valves is heard with a stethoscope over the entire precordium. Closure of the mitral and tricuspid valves marks the beginning of systole and creates S_1 ("lub"), usually loudest at the apex (mitral area). At the beginning of diastole, the aortic and pulmonic valves close together, creating the second heart sound, S_2 ("dub"). Because sound is carried in the direction of blood flow, S_2 is usually loudest at the base of the heart in the second right interspace (aortic area) and second left interspace (pulmonic area). As systole is usually shorter than diastole, S_1 is followed by S_2 ("lub-dub"), then by a slightly longer interval before S_1 is heard again.

As the ventricular pressures fall below the atrial pressures, the mitral and tricuspid valves open, allowing the ventricles to fill. The rapid filling of the left ventricle may create a third heart sound (S_3), more often in children and young adults. In a person older than 40 years, an S_3 is considered pathological, likely associated with congestive heart failure or regurgitant valves. Near the end of diastole, when the atria contract to enhance ventricular filling, a fourth heart sound (S_4) may be heard in some healthy older adults and trained athletes. More commonly, it is pathological, caused by hypertensive heart disease, in which the left ventricular wall stiffens, increasing resistance to ventricular filling following atrial contraction. A useful way to remember the timing of S_3 and S_4 heart sounds is given below (Swartz, 2005):

SLOSH' –	ing in	a STIFF' wall
S_1	S_2 S_3	S_4 S_1 S_2

Events on the left side of the heart usually occur slightly earlier than those on the right side; however, following a deep inspiration, S_2 may split, making closure of the aortic valve (A_2) heard first, and then the pulmonic valve (P_2) closure becomes audible in the left second and third interspaces close to the sternum. Current understanding of this physiological splitting of the second heart sound is as follows: deep inspiration increases the capacity of the pulmonary vasculature, prolongs right ventricular contraction, and delays closure of the pulmonic valve. The left ventricle contracts comparatively earlier, followed by aortic valve closure (Bickley & Szilagyi, 2007; Seidel et al., 2006).

The health history interview (Table 32–30) provides guidance for the assessment, which, in turn, provides opportunities for client health promotion (Box 32–20).

TABLE 32-30 Health History for Heart Assessment

Assessment Category	Rationale for Assessment
Ask the client about presence of risk factors such as smoking, alcohol or drug use, lack of exercise, high fat and salt dietary patterns, and high stress levels.	These factors are related to heart disease.
Inquire about medication use for cardiovascular function and whether the client has a clear understanding of dosage, purpose, and side effects.	You can assess client knowledge and plan teaching, as needed.
Ask the client about any history of chest pain, palpitations, fatigue, cough, dyspnea, leg pains or cramps, edema of extremities, fainting, and orthopnea. Inquire whether these happen at rest or during activity, and conduct a symptom analysis.	These can be symptoms of heart disease.
Question the client about family history of cardiac problems.	Family history of heart disease increases the risk for heart disease.
Inquire about the presence of conditions such as diabetes, lung disease, obesity, or hypertension.	These disorders can affect heart function.
Question the client about any habit of ingesting caffeine-containing drinks (coffee, tea, soft drinks) or chocolate.	Caffeine can cause cardiac arrhythmia.

BOX 32-20 FOCUS ON PRIMARY HEALTH CARE

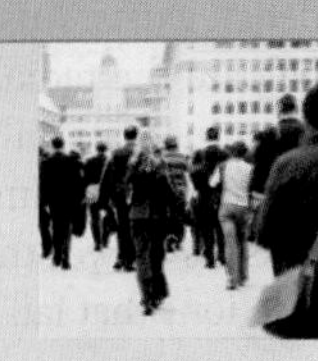

Heart

- Risk factors for heart disease
- Regular examinations
- Dietary intake
- Physical activity
- Stress management

Before assessing the heart, ensure that the client is relaxed, comfortable, in the supine position, with the upper body elevated 30 degrees, and in a quiet environment with good lighting. To relieve any anxiety, provide the client with ongoing explanations of procedures. The client should not be allowed to talk during auscultation.

Inspection. Using tangential lighting, inspect the entire precordium for pulsations or lifts. Begin at the base of the heart near the second right and left interspaces, and progress downward to the apex; or begin at the apex and progress upward to the base. Inspect the epigastric region. Absence of pulsations over the precordium and epigastric region is expected. In thin clients, you may see pulsations at the apex (apical impulse) or in the epigastric area (aortic pulsations). If you observe pulsation or lifts at other locations usually they indicate cardiac pathology.

Palpation. Six anatomical landmarks on the precordium are important for palpation and auscultation (Figure 32–23). Using fingertips, first locate the angle of Louis (sternal angle). Then glide your fingers across the angle to feel the attached second ribs on each side and just below the right and left second intercostal spaces. Mark the left second interspace with a felt pen as a reference point.

Skill 32–15 provides the sequence and techniques for palpation of the precordium and epigastric area. Each time that you ask a client to exhale and briefly hold the breath during palpation, hold your own breath to determine when the client needs to breathe again. Palpate for pulsations, lifts, or thrills while the client holds the breath. The presence of pulsations may indicate cardiac pathology. For example, an impulse against the palpating fingertip in the epigastric area suggests enlargement of the right ventricle.

Assess the apical impulse for location, diameter, amplitude, and duration (Figure 32–24A). Expect apical pulsations to be palpable in about the fifth interspace, medial to the left MCL; to be less than 2.5 cm (one interspace) in diameter; to feel like a brisk tap against your fingers; and to be brief in duration (first two thirds of systole). To assess duration, identify systole by listening to the heart sounds. If the apical impulse is lateral to the left MCL, is larger than 2.5 cm, and lasts most of systole, suspect an enlarged left ventricle.

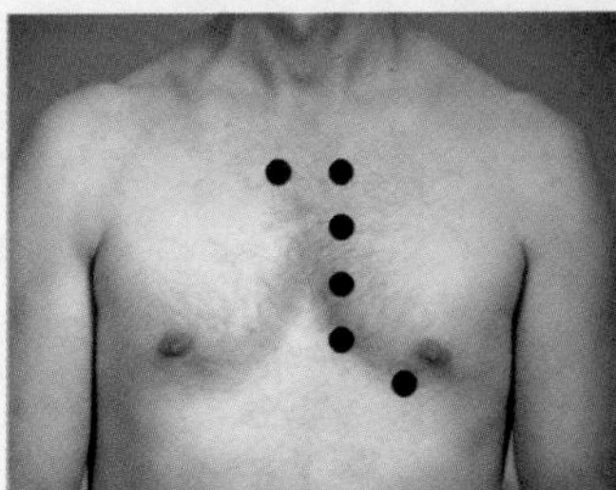

Figure 32-23 Landmarks on the precordium. **Source:** From Skillen, D. L., Day, R. A., Anderson, M. C., Stephen, T. C., Gilbert, J. A., & Day, L. W. (2004). *Physical examination images* [CD-ROM]. Edmonton, AB: Faculty of Nursing, University of Alberta.

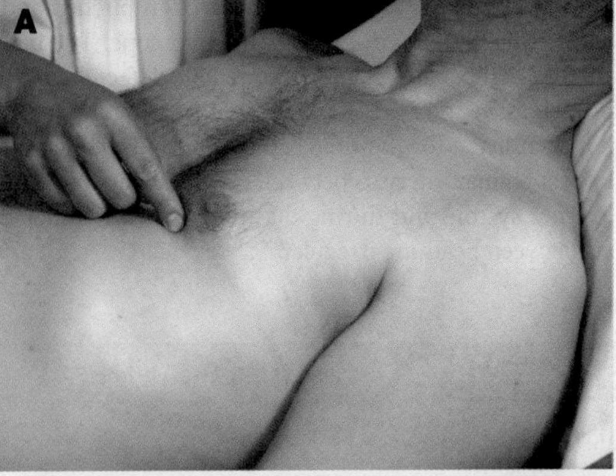

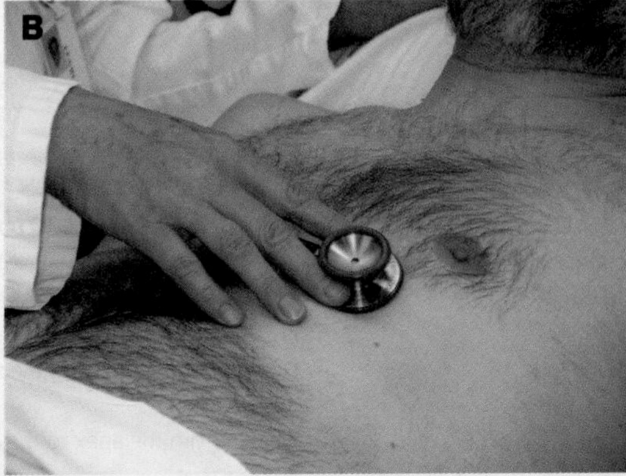

Figure 32-24 A, Palpation of the apical impulse. B, Auscultation of the apex. **Source:** From Skillen, D. L., Day, R. A., Anderson, M. C., Stephen, T. C., Gilbert, J. A., & Day, L. W. (2004). *Physical examination images* [CD-ROM]. Edmonton, AB: Faculty of Nursing, University of Alberta.

If the apical impulse is not initially palpable, ask the client to exhale fully and hold the breath before you palpate again. If it still cannot be found, ask the client to roll onto the left side (left lateral recumbent position), support the client's back with your left hand flat on the table, and encourage the client to lean back on your left arm. This manoeuvre brings the heart closer to the chest wall for palpation but may increase the diameter of the apical impulse. Palpation of the apical impulse may be difficult if the anteroposterior diameter is enlarged or if the client is very muscular or overweight.

Auscultation. Auscultation of the heart detects expected heart sounds, extra heart sounds, and murmurs. You will first become skilled at hearing and interpreting expected heart sounds (Skill 32–15). At each location, you identify the "lub-dub" sound created primarily by closure of the mitral valves (S_1) and then the aortic valves (S_2). Each combination of S_1 and S_2, or the "lub-dub", counts as one heartbeat.

Systole is the period between the "lub" and "dub" and is usually shorter than diastole. If the heart rate is rapid, systole and diastole may be similar in length, making it difficult to distinguish one from the other. To deal with this, palpate the carotid pulse as you auscultate. This pulse occurs during early systole. At the apex, assess heart rate and rhythm with the diaphragm of the stethoscope (see Figure 32–24B).

During auscultation, carefully assess the character of the heartbeats. Listen for S_1 to be louder at the apex and S_2 to be louder at the base of the heart. These are both relatively high pitched and heard best with the diaphragm ('di-hi') of the stethoscope. The bell chestpiece of the stethoscope is better suited to detect lower-pitched sounds, such as S_3 and S_4. Listen for the interval between S_1 and S_2 (systole); then listen for the time between S_2 and the next S_1 (diastole). Expect regular intervals between each beat and a distinct silent pause during systole and during diastole. A dysrhythmia exists if intervals between beats are irregular.

When you find that the heart rhythm is irregular, compare the apical and radial pulse rates simultaneously to determine if a pulse deficit exists. Auscultate the apical pulse first, and then immediately palpate the radial pulse (one-examiner technique). When another examiner is available, both of you can assess the apical and radial pulses at the same time. A pulse deficit is present when the radial pulse is slower than the apical pulse. It is caused by ineffective contractions that fail to send pulse waves to the periphery.

➤ SKILL 32-15 Assessing the Heart

Equipment

- Penlight
- Stethoscope
- Felt pen

Procedure

EXAMINATION SKILL AND FOCUS	TECHNIQUES AND RATIONALE
Inspection: Precordium	Client in the supine position, with head elevated 30 degrees; anterior thorax and epigastric area exposed; you at the client's right side. *Provides best access to precordium.*
	1. Inspect the precordium shining the penlight tangentially. *Enhances the visibility of pulsations.*
Palpation:	1. Locate a landmark using the sternal angle. *Assists in locating accurate site for palpation and auscultation.*
	2. Palpate from the apex to the base **OR** from the base to the apex. *Either direction is acceptable as long as it is consistent.*
Apical area	1. Use your finger pads to palpate the fifth interspace medial to the left midclavicular line (MCL).
	2. Ask the client to exhale and hold the breath if you are unable to locate the apical area. *Exhalation brings the left ventricle closer to the chest wall, facilitating palpation.*
	3. Analyze the impulses in the apical area using your fingertips and then one finger. *Assesses location, size, amplitude, and duration.*
Right ventricular area	1. Place the tips of your curved fingers in the left third, fourth, and fifth interspaces close to the sternum.
	2. Ask the client to exhale and hold the breath. *Exhalation brings the chest wall closer to the right ventricle and the palpating fingers.*
Epigastric area (subxiphoid)	1. Press the index finger of your flattened hand under the left costal margin and up toward the client's left shoulder.
	2. Ask the client to inhale and hold the breath. *Inhalation brings the right ventricle closer to the palpating finger and also moves your hand away from the aorta.*
Left second interspace (pulmonic area)	1. Place your index finger pad in the second left interspace close to the sternum.
	2. Ask the client to exhale and hold the breath, and palpate firmly. *Exhalation brings the chest wall closer to the heart and the pulmonary artery.*
Right second interspace (aortic area)	1. Place your index finger pad in the second right interspace.
	2. Ask the client to exhale and hold the breath, and palpate firmly. *Exhalation brings the chest wall closer to the heart and the aorta.*
Auscultation:	1. Use the diaphragm and bell of the stethoscope to listen to all six areas. *The diaphragm picks up higher-pitched sounds (S_1 and S_2). The bell picks up lower-pitched sounds (S_3 and S_4).*
	2. Place the bell of the stethoscope lightly on the chest wall. *Placing the bell lightly, with just enough pressure to ensure a full seal with the skin, prevents stretching the underlying skin and creating a diaphragm.*
	3. Auscultate from the apex to the base **OR** from the the base to apex.
	4. Listen for 5 seconds in each area with the diaphragm and bell of the stethoscope. *Five seconds allows enough time for careful assessment of the heart sounds.*
	5. Auscultate the following:
Right second interspace	• Right second interspace close to sternum
Left second interspace	• Left second interspace close to sternum
Third interspace	• Left third interspace close to sternum
Fourth interspace	• Left fourth interspace close to sternum
Fifth interspace	• Left fifth interspace close to sternum
Apex	• Apex
Apical rate	6. Listen for 1 minute at the apex for rate, using the diaphragm of the stethoscope.

From Stephen, T. C., Day, R. A., & Skillen, D. L. (Eds.). (2008). *A syllabus for adult health assessment* (pp. 40–41). Edmonton, AB: Faculty of Nursing, University of Alberta.

When you are able to identify S_1 from S_2 and diastole from systole, listen for sounds that occur during diastole and systole. During diastole, listen for an S_3 or S_4 (either is an extra heart sound) with the bell chestpiece of the stethoscope placed at the apex. Also, assess for physiological splitting, by listening for the two components of S_2: aortic closure (A_2) followed by pulmonic closure (P_2). A physiological split may or may not be present. Finally, assess for a murmur, which is a sustained swishing or blowing sound heard at the beginning, middle, or end of the systolic or diastolic phase. Murmurs are created by turbulent blood flow over a stenosed or incompetent heart valve. The intensity of a murmur varies from barely audible to a sound that can be heard without the aid of a stethoscope.

Age-Related Changes. Differentiating between age-related and disease-related cardiac changes is difficult, as both are influenced by lifestyle and environment. Some authorities believe that age-related changes in the myocardium include slight hypertrophy of the left ventricle, which develops gradually over the years in response to increased peripheral vascular resistance and elevated systolic blood pressure from stiffening of the arteries. Over the long term, circulatory efficiency may be impaired. In addition, thickening of the atrioventricular and aortic valves is common in older adults. In the aortic valve, thickening is often accompanied by calcification, which is called *aortic sclerosis*. In at least one third of people over 60 years of age, aortic sclerosis results in a mild aortic systolic murmur heard best with the diaphragm of the stethoscope in the right second interspace. If the sclerosis worsens, aortic stenosis (pathological) may develop. Degenerative changes in the sinus node and myocardial pacemaker cells result in more frequent ectopic beats (Miller, 2009).

Documentation. Record your findings from the inspection, palpation, and auscultation of the heart (see Table 32–33, page 605).

Assessing the Breasts

Inspection and palpation of the breasts needs to be carried out in both female and male clients. Glandular tissue is the potential site for the growth of cancer cells; men have a small amount and women have a large amount of glandular tissue.

Female Breasts. The breasts are located anterior to the pectoralis major and serratus anterior muscles and usually extend from the sternum to the midaxillary line, and from the clavicle and second rib to the sixth rib. The nipple, which is round in shape, is situated slightly below the centre of the breast. It is usually protuberant, and its surface may be smooth or wrinkled. The areola surrounds the nipple and is round or oval in shape. Areolae are almost equal bilaterally, and their colour ranges from pink to brown. In light-skinned women, the areola turns brown during pregnancy and remains dark. In dark-skinned women, the areola is brown even before pregnancy (Seidel et al., 2006). To describe the locations of your findings, use imaginary lines drawn through the nipple, which will divide the breast into quadrants and the tail of Spence (Figure 32–25).

Breasts consist of glandular tissue, fibrous supportive ligaments, and adipose (fat) tissue. The proportion of the three types varies according to age, pregnancy, lactation, nutritional status, and time in the menstrual cycle (Jarvis, 2004). Glandular tissue is organized into lobes that end in ducts that open on the nipple surface. The largest portion of glandular tissue is in the upper outer quadrant and tail of the breast. Fibrous suspensory ligaments connect to skin and fascia underlying the breast to support it and maintain its upright position. Fatty tissue is located superficially and to the sides of the breast.

Lymphatics. A large portion of lymph from the breasts drains into axillary lymph nodes, which are commonly involved when cancerous lesions **metastasize** (spread) (see Figure 32–25). The central nodes are located along the chest wall and high up in the axillae. The other three sets of axillary nodes (pectoral, subscapular, and lateral) drain lymph into the central nodes. Pectoral nodes are located at the edge of the pectoralis major muscle along the anterior axillary line. Lymph from the anterior chest wall and much of the breast drains into these nodes. Subscapular nodes are found along the lateral border of the scapula, deep in the posterior axillary fold. Lymph from the posterior chest wall and part of the arm drains into these nodes. Lateral nodes are located along the upper part of the humerus and drain lymph from much of the arm. Lymph collected in the central nodes then drains to infraclavicular nodes and supraclavicular nodes. Some lymph drains directly into the infraclavicular nodes and deep into the chest, which is why a tumour in one breast may spread to the nodes on the opposite side as well as to those on the same side.

Breast Cancer. The Canadian Cancer Society (2008a, 2008b) estimated that over 22,000 women would be diagnosed with breast cancer in 2008, and 5300 would die of it. It is only second to lung cancer as the cause of death from cancer in women. However, current mortality rates for breast cancer are at the lowest point in Canada since 1950; a decline has also been reported in Australia, the United States, and the United Kingdom. The density of breast tissue is now recognized as a significant risk factor. It accounts for up to 30% of breast cancers, while family history and known genes account for a lower percentage (Boyd et al., 2007). One in nine women is expected to develop breast cancer and 1 in 28 to die from it (Canadian Cancer Society, 2008a, 2008b). Mortality rates for First Nation women, both on and off reserves, in Canada are lower than those for all other Canadian women (Health Canada, 2007).

Early detection is the key to cure. While most breast lumps are found by the client herself by accident (not from breast self-examination [BSE]) (Kearney & Murray, 2006), you have the responsibility to offer to teach techniques of BSE to willing clients, using your knowledge of teaching and learning principles. No consensus has been reached in North America regarding the criteria for BSE, and studies suggest that only a minority of women actually perform BSE. The Canadian Breast Cancer Foundation (2006) recommends the following guidelines for the early detection of breast cancer:

- BSE performed monthly (Box 32–21).
- Examination by a health care provider annually.
- Mammograms every 2 years for women 50 to 69 years of age (every province and territory in Canada, except Nunavut, has followed this practice since 2003).
- Women's knowledge of what their breasts look and feel like (BSE done monthly is one way to accomplish this).

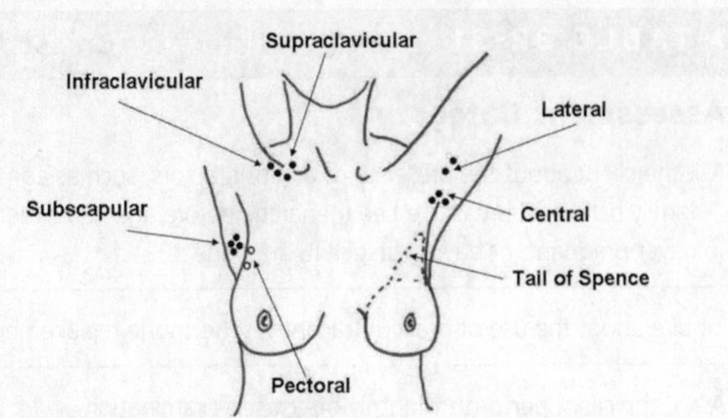

Figure 32-25 Lymph nodes of axillae and thorax. **Source:** From Skillen, D. L., Day, R. A., Anderson, M. C., Stephen, T. C., Gilbert, J. A., & Day, L. W. (2004). *Physical examination images* [CD-ROM]. Edmonton, AB: Faculty of Nursing, University of Alberta.

BOX 32-21 Breast Self-Examination

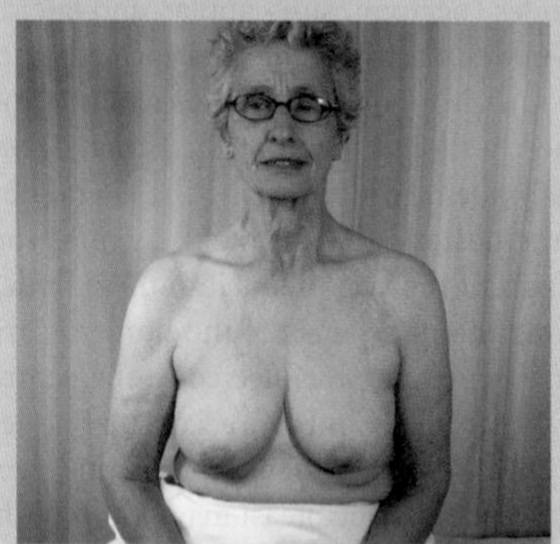
Arms at sides.

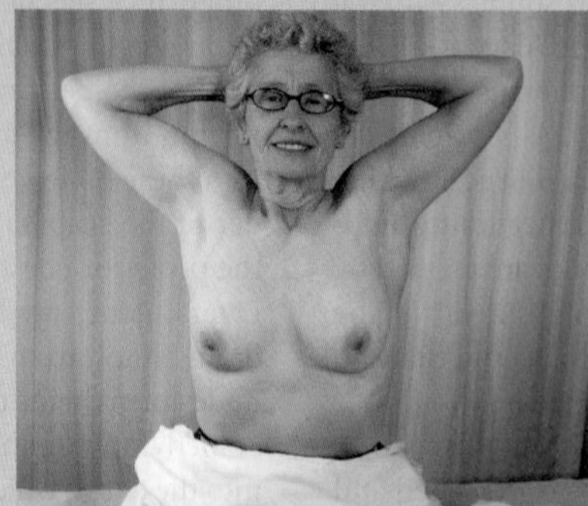
Arms above head.

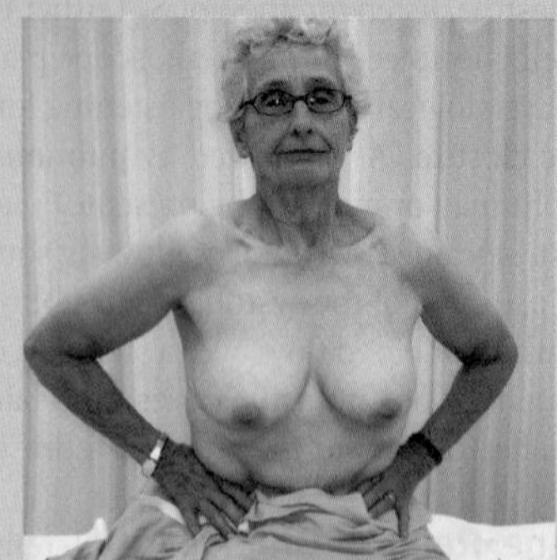
Pressing on hips.

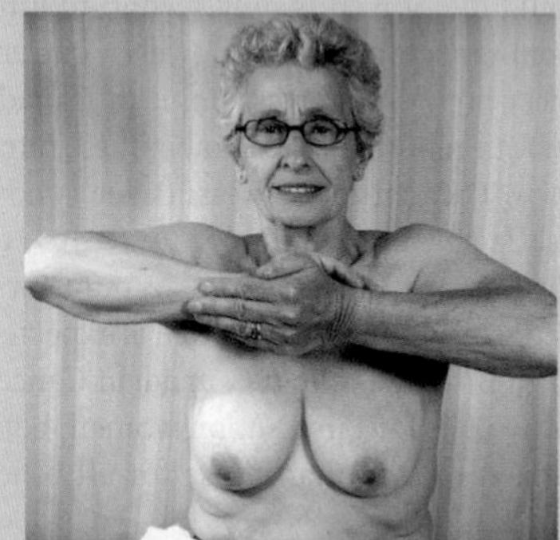
Pressing in front, below, or above breasts.

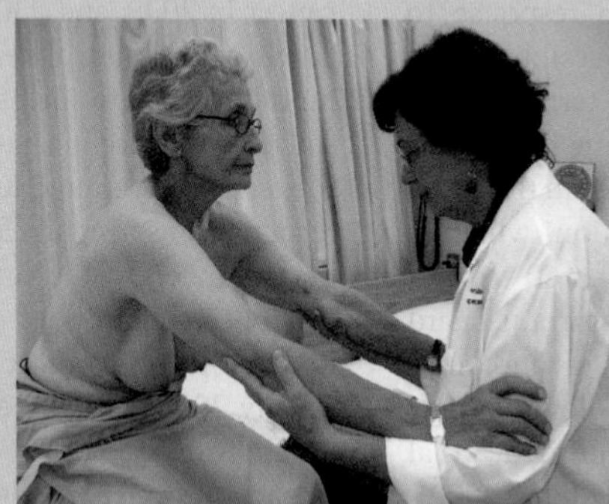
Arms forward and leaning forward.

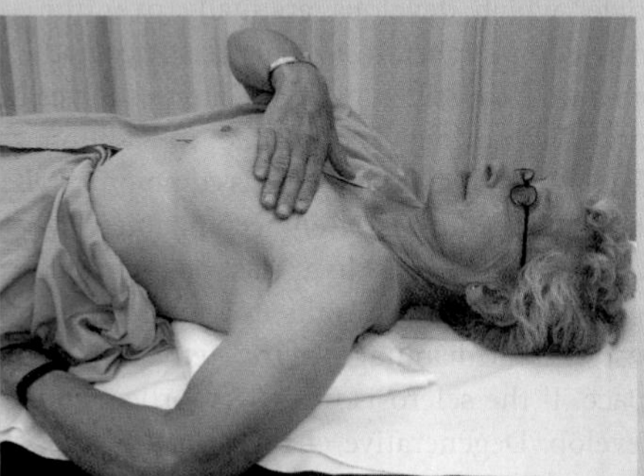
Lying position.

Photos from Skillen, D. L., Day, R. A., Anderson, M. C., Stephen, T. C., Gilbert, J. A., & Day, L. W. (2004). *Physical examination images* [CD-ROM]. Edmonton, AB: Faculty of Nursing, University of Alberta.

Examination of Breasts. The client's history (Table 32–31) should alert you to any signs of breast disease and expected developmental changes. Because of its glandular structure, the breast undergoes changes throughout a woman's life. Knowledge of these changes helps you complete an accurate assessment that includes health promotion (Box 32–22).

While assessing the client's breasts, you use many of the same techniques that the client can learn to use herself. It may be difficult for the client to learn to palpate for lymph nodes. Lying down with the arm abducted makes the area more accessible. Instruct the client to use her left hand to examine the right axillary and clavicular areas and then her right hand to palpate the nodes on the left side. You can hold her fingerpads and move them in the correct circular fashion. The best time for BSE is 7 days from the start of the menstrual period when the breasts of premenopausal women are no longer swollen or tender from hormone elevations. Women need to continue to check their breasts monthly, even during pregnancy. It is important for postmenopausal women to check the breasts at the same time each month

TABLE 32-31 Health History for Breast Assessment

Assessment Category	Rationale for Assessment
Ask the client about the presence of any risk factors, such as age over 40, personal or family history of breast cancer, menarche before age 12 or menopause after age 50, never pregnant, or having first child after age 30.	These are risk factors for breast cancer.
Inquire about the use of oral contraceptives, hormone replacement, steroids, or caffeine.	These can affect breast tissue.
Ask if the client performs monthly breast self-examination.	This facilitates early detection of breast changes.
Question the client about discovery of any lumps, thickening of tissue, pain, discharge or tissue distortion, nipple retraction, or changes in the breast generally. Conduct a symptom analysis, as necessary.	These are potential signs and symptoms of breast disease, and conducting a symptom analysis will help determine the nature of the problem.

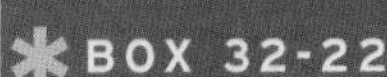

BOX 32-22 FOCUS ON PRIMARY HEALTH CARE

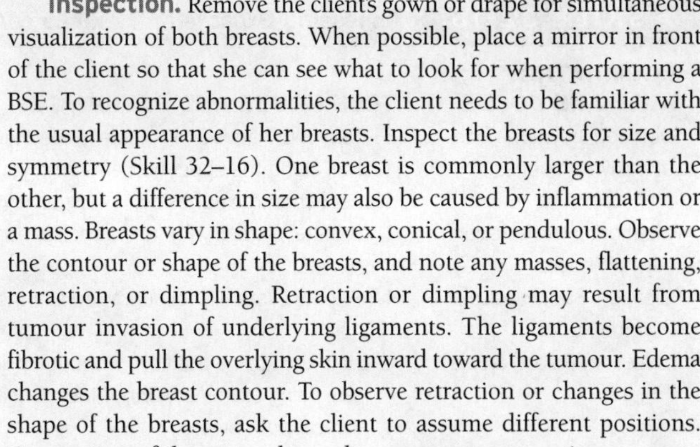

Breasts

- Breast size and support
- Breast self-examination
- Clinical breast examinations
- Mammography and magnetic resonance imaging
- Risk factors for breast cancer and benign disorders
- Signs and symptoms of breast cancer and fibrocystic disease

and pay special attention to regular BSE. Some may ignore changes in their breasts, assuming they are age-related. Some may not be aware that cancer of the breast can occur in older women and may avoid breast examinations or mammograms. Musculoskeletal changes, reduced eyesight, changes in the ROM of joints, and diminished peripheral sensation may limit their ability to inspect and palpate during BSE.

Inspection. Remove the client's gown or drape for simultaneous visualization of both breasts. When possible, place a mirror in front of the client so that she can see what to look for when performing a BSE. To recognize abnormalities, the client needs to be familiar with the usual appearance of her breasts. Inspect the breasts for size and symmetry (Skill 32–16). One breast is commonly larger than the other, but a difference in size may also be caused by inflammation or a mass. Breasts vary in shape: convex, conical, or pendulous. Observe the contour or shape of the breasts, and note any masses, flattening, retraction, or dimpling. Retraction or dimpling may result from tumour invasion of underlying ligaments. The ligaments become fibrotic and pull the overlying skin inward toward the tumour. Edema changes the breast contour. To observe retraction or changes in the shape of the breasts, ask the client to assume different positions. Contraction of the pectoral muscles accentuates retraction.

Carefully inspect the overlying skin for colour and venous pattern. You can see venous patterns more easily in thin women and in pregnant women. Note the presence of lesions, inflammation, or edema. Ask the client to lift each breast while you examine its lower and lateral aspects for changes in colour and texture. The breasts are

➤ SKILL 32-16 Assessing Breasts and Axillae

Equipment

- Small pillow or towel
- Disposable gloves (if signs of infection or discharge are present)

Procedure

EXAMINATION SKILL AND FOCUS	TECHNIQUES AND RATIONALE
Inspection: Breast, areola, nipple	Client in sitting position and disrobed to waist. *Both breasts need to be visible.* 1. Inspect the breast, areola, and nipple bilaterally in anterior and lateral views. *Different positions may allow changes in contour of breasts to be visible.* Client should sit: • With the arms at the sides. • With the arms raised over the head. • With the hands pressed against the hips **OR** pressed together, not obstructing the view of the breasts. *Contraction of pectoral muscles may make masses or skin changes more visible.* 2. Inspect the breasts, with the client leaning forward and then with the breasts lifted. *Masses are seen more easily in this position. Skin underneath the breasts is checked for rashes.*
Palpation: Large breasts	1. With the client leaning forward, palpate the breast tissue between your hands. *Brings the breast tissue away from the chest wall and allows you to feel the masses that may not be accessible when the client is in the supine position.*
Inspection: Axillae	1. Inspect the skin of the axillae, with the client raising the arms overhead. *Permits examination of total skin surface of axillae.* 2. *Only* if signs of infection are present, put on gloves for palpation. *Gloves are important to prevent transmission of microorganisms.*
Palpation: Axillary lymph nodes	1. Assist the client to dry the axillae. 2. Support the client's left hand and wrist with your left hand to examine the left axilla; and support the client's right hand and wrist with your right hand for the right axilla. 3. Instruct the client to relax the arm. *Keeps the client's arm close to the side to reduce tension on the axilla.*
Central lymph nodes	4. Cup your fingers together. 5. Reach as high as possible into the apex of the left axilla. 6. Press your fingers against the client's chest wall. *Nodes may be felt when the tissue is pressed against the chest wall.* 7. Bring your finger pads down over the client's ribs and palpate for the central nodes (Figure 32–26A).
Pectoral lymph nodes	8. Slide your fingers under the client's anterior axillary fold, palpating the chest wall with the finger pads for pectoral nodes. 9. Grasp the anterior axillary folds (pectoral) and palpate with your finger pads, using the thumbs as an anchor and palpating over the ribs (Figure 32–26B and C). 10. Slide your fingers under the posterior axillary fold, palpating the chest wall with the finger pads for subscapular nodes.

Continued

➤ SKILL 32-16 Assessing Breasts and Axillae *continued*

EXAMINATION SKILL AND FOCUS	TECHNIQUES AND RATIONALE
Subscapular lymph nodes	11. Turn your hands and palpate inside the posterior axillary folds with the finger pads (subscapular) (Figure 32–26D).
Lateral lymph nodes	12. Feel along the upper humerus with your finger pads (lateral) (Figure 32–26E).
	13. Repeat on the right side.
Palpation: Infraclavicular lymph nodes	1. Palpate bilaterally for infraclavicular nodes below the clavicle in the first interspace with your finger pads.
Palpation: Supraclavicular lymph nodes	1. Palpate bilaterally for supraclavicular nodes above the clavicle with your finger pads.
Inspection: Breast, areola, nipple	Client in the supine position, without a pillow under the head. Place a small pillow under the client's shoulder on the side being examined, *only if the client's breasts are large. The pillow shifts the breast tissue medially.* 1. Inspect both breasts.
Palpation: Breast, areola, nipple, tail of Spence	Ask the client to move the arm away from the chest on the side being examined. 1. Palpate each breast. 2. Use the flat of your second, third, and fourth fingers in a rotating motion to compress the breast tissue. 3. Flex, from your wrist, not from the fingers. *Allows your fingers to stay flat, in contact with the client's skin.* 4. Apply moderate pressure, keeping constant contact with the client's skin. 5. Move your fingers back and forth across the breast in straight lines, making constant small circles. 6. Slide your hand down one finger width for each pass. 7. Cover the full area from below the clavicle to 3 cm below the breast, from the midaxillary line to the midsternal line: • Glandular tissue • Areolar area • Nipple • Tail of Spence

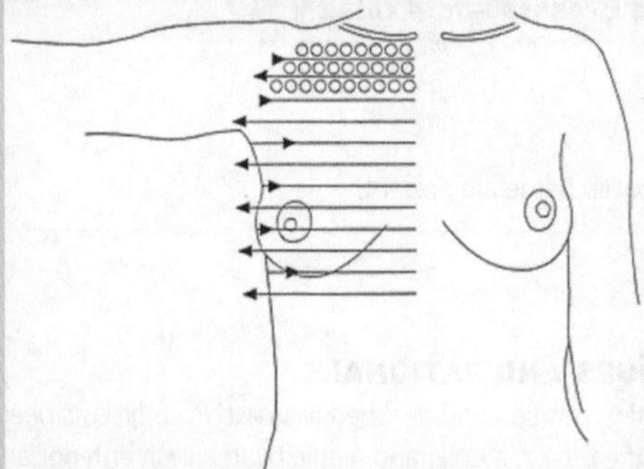

Illustration of direction of strokes in breast examination adapted from Canadian Cancer Society Alberta, NWT Division. (2002). *Breast self-examination: What you can do* [Brochure]. Calgary, AB: Author.

From Stephen, T. C., Day, R. A., & Skillen, D. L. (Eds.). (2008). *A syllabus for adult health assessment* (pp. 41–43). Edmonton, AB: Faculty of Nursing, University of Alberta.

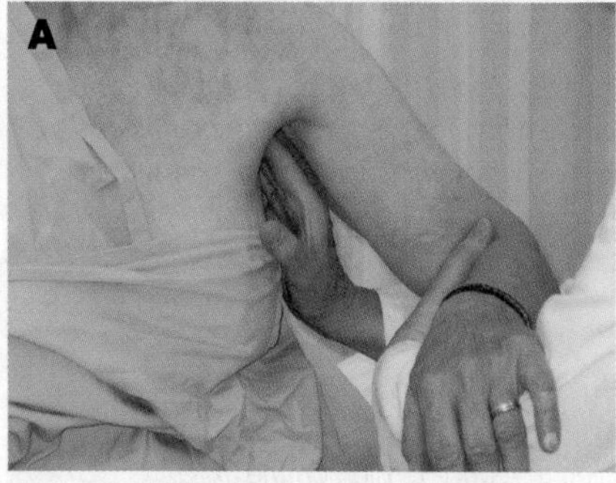

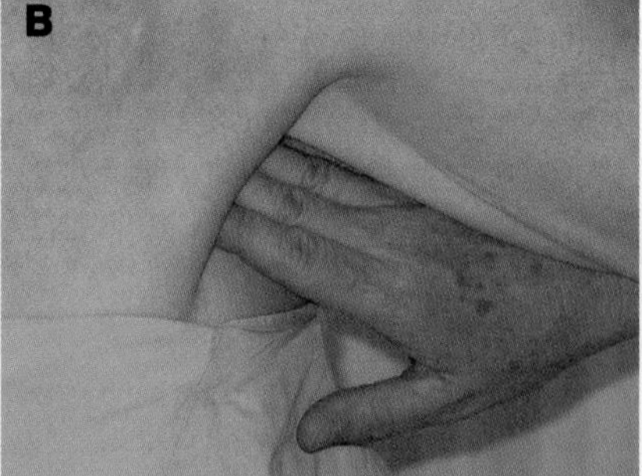

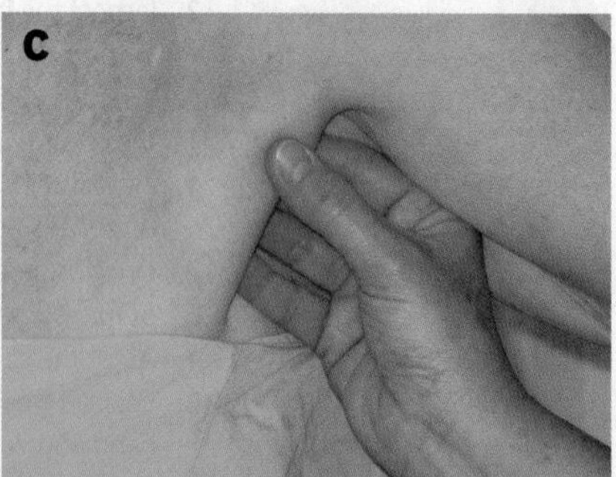

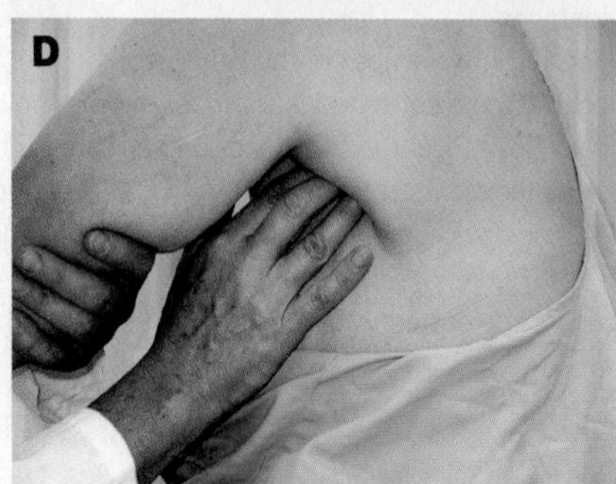

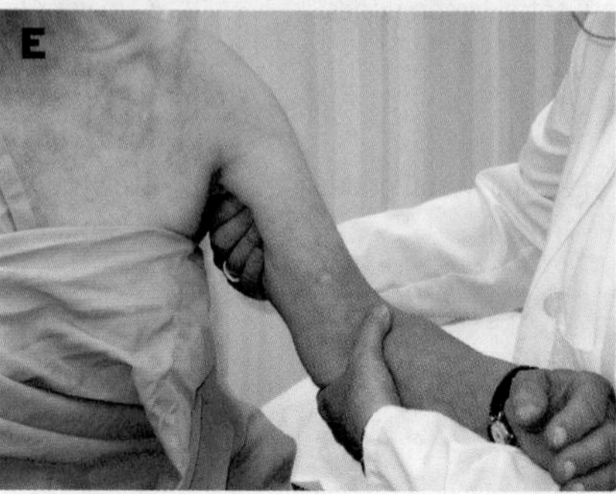

Figure 32-26 A, Palpation of the central lymph nodes. B and C, Palpation of the pectoral lymph nodes (two techniques). D, Palpation of the subscapular lymph nodes. E, Palpation of the lateral lymph nodes. **Source:** From Skillen, D. L., Day, R. A., Anderson, M. C., Stephen, T. C., Gilbert, J. A., & Day, L. W. (2004). *Physical examination images* [CD-ROM]. Edmonton, AB: Faculty of Nursing, University of Alberta.

the colour of neighbouring skin, and venous patterns are the same bilaterally. Inspect the skin of the axillae for any signs of a rash, an infection, or increased pigmentation. In women with large breasts, examine the undersurface, a common site for redness and excoriation caused by rubbing of skin surfaces.

Inspect the nipple and areola for size, colour, shape, discharge, and the direction of the nipples. The nipples point in symmetrical directions, are everted, and have no drainage. If the nipples are inverted, ask the client if this has always existed. A recent inversion or inward turning of the nipple may indicate an underlying growth. Note ulcerations and rashes on the breasts or nipples. It is not recommended that you squeeze the nipples to test for discharge. A clear yellow discharge that occurs 2 days after childbirth is expected. Bleeding or discharge from the nipple is a concern, particularly if it occurs persistently and only on one side. While inspecting the breasts, describe to the client the observed characteristics and the significance of any unusual signs and symptoms. If the breasts are large and pendulous, use a bimanual technique for palpation, with the client still in the sitting position for inspection (see Skill 32–16).

Palpation. Use palpation to determine the condition of the underlying breast tissue and lymph nodes. The lymph nodes are best palpated with the client in the sitting position, but she may also be in the supine position. Easy access to the axillary nodes is gained with the client's arms at her sides and the muscles relaxed. The lymph nodes are not usually palpable, but when they are, the central nodes are the most likely to be felt (see Figure 32–26A). Assess the axillary areas carefully to avoid missing enlarged nodes (see Figure 32–26A–E). Assess the infraclavicular and supraclavicular nodes. You may find one or two small, soft, nontender nodes. A palpable node is like a small mass and may be hard, tender, and fixed. Note the number, size, consistency, and mobility of the nodes.

Palpation of the breast is best performed with the client in the supine position, without a pillow under the head and with one arm out from the side (alternating positions for each breast). Breast tissue flattens evenly over the chest wall in the supine position. If the breasts are large, place a small pillow or towel under the client's shoulder blade to further spread breast tissue.

Using the pads of four fingers, make constant small circles to compress breast tissue gently against the chest wall, noting tissue consistency (see Skill 32–16). The approach recommended by the Canadian Cancer Society/Alberta/NWT Division (2002) is to palpate the breast in horizontal lines back and forth, systematically covering the area from below the clavicle to 3 cm below the breast and from the midsternal line to the midaxillary line. Palpating along the vertical lines (American Cancer Society, 2008) is the most validated method (Barton, et al., 1999). It is essential to examine the entire breast and the tail of Spence, focusing on any areas of tenderness. During palpation, note the consistency of the breast tissue. The breast tissue feels dense, firm, and elastic. With menopause, breast tissue shrinks and becomes softer. Glandular tissue usually feels lobular. The lower edge of each breast (inframammary ridge) may feel firm and hard; it should not be interpreted as a tumour. Point out any tissue variations to the client.

If the client presents with a breast mass, examine the opposite breast first to determine if a mass is present in the other breast in the symmetrical position and to ensure an objective comparison of breast tissue.

Palpate masses to determine the following:

- Location in relation to quadrants
- Diameter in centimetres
- Shape
- Consistency (soft, firm, or hard)
- Tenderness
- Mobility
- Discreteness (whether boundaries of mass are clear or not).

Cancerous lesions tend to be hard, fixed, irregular in shape, and usually, but not always, painless. A common benign (noncancerous) condition of the breast is fibrocystic breast disease (lumpy, painful breasts and sometimes nipple discharge). Symptoms of this condition are more apparent during menstruation. Located in both breasts, cysts (lumps) are soft, well-defined, and mobile. Fibroadenoma, a round, very mobile, firm, and circumscribed mass, is also noncancerous and occurs mainly in young women.

After you complete your examination, ask the client to demonstrate BSE. Observe the client's technique and stress the importance of a systematic approach, as needed. Urge the client to report any unusual masses discovered during BSE.

Male Breasts. Examine the male breast with the client in the supine or sitting position. Inspect the nipple and areola for nodules, edema, and ulceration. An enlarged male breast may be a result of obesity or glandular enlargement. When palpated, fatty tissue feels soft; glandular tissue feels firm. Gynecomastia, a temporary, unilateral enlargement of undeveloped breast tissue, feels smooth, firm, and mobile and usually occurs in puberty. Breast enlargement in young males may indicate steroid use. Palpate any masses for the same characteristics as in the female breast. Breast cancer in men is relatively rare; approximately 170 cases and 50 deaths were reported in 2007 (CCS, 2007).

safety alert All men, especially men who have a first-degree relative (e.g., mother or sister) with breast cancer, are at risk for breast cancer and should examine their breasts at regular intervals. Men should also be scheduled for routine mammograms.

Documentation. Record your findings from the inspection and palpation of the breasts and axillae (see Table 32–33, page 605).

Assessing the Abdomen

Examination of the abdomen can be complex because of the organs located within and near the abdominal cavity. A thorough health history (Table 32–32) helps you interpret physical signs and plan for health promotion (Box 32–23). The examination includes assessment of the liver, stomach, spleen, kidneys, bladder, and structures of the lower gastrointestinal (GI) tract. Abdominal pain is a common symptom that clients report when seeking medical care. An accurate assessment requires that client history data be matched with a careful assessment of the location of physical symptoms.

Certain landmarks help map out the abdominal region. The xiphoid process marks the upper boundary of the abdominal region; the symphysis pubis delineates the lower boundary. Use the costal margins as a landmark for the liver and stomach, and the costovertebral angle for kidney percussion (see "Thorax" section).

The abdomen is divided into four imaginary quadrants (see Figure 32–4, page 553). You can record your assessment findings in relation to each quadrant. For example, you may determine that a client is experiencing tenderness over the left lower quadrant (LLQ) and that expected bowel sounds are present. The system of dividing the abdomen into nine regions (see Figure 32–6, page 553) is not used as often, but some terms from that approach remain in common use, for example, hypogastric, epigastric, umbilical, and suprapubic (Jarvis, 2004).

It is important to visualize the location of the abdominal organs during the examination of the abdomen. For example, the liver is in the right upper quadrant (RUQ), with the lower border of the liver extending just below the costal margin. This knowledge is essential for percussion and palpation of the liver. The stomach and the spleen are located in the left upper quadrant (LUQ). Posteriorly, the kidneys

TABLE 32-32 Health History for Abdominal Assessment

Assessment Category	Rationale for Assessment
Ask the client about usual dietary habits, bowel routine, characteristics of the stool, and any use of laxatives.	Information about usual habits helps identify irregularities, if present.
Question the client about any recent weight changes or intolerance to any food (e.g., nausea, vomiting, cramping, especially in the last 24 hours).	Data may indicate alterations in the upper GI tract (stomach or gallbladder) or lower colon.
Ask the client about medication use, including anti-inflammatory medications or antibiotics.	Some medications irritate the gastric mucosal lining, causing pain, nausea, or vomiting.
Inquire about the presence of any problems such as flatulence, belching, swallowing, heartburn, diarrhea, or constipation.	These signs and symptoms may indicate changes within the GI tract.
Ask the client if she is pregnant, writing down the date of last menstrual period.	Pregnancy affects the shape and contour of the abdomen.
Find out about family or personal history of hypertension, alcoholism, kidney or heart disease, abdominal trauma, or surgeries.	These data may reveal identifiable alterations during physical examination.
Carefully observe the client's movements and positions, such as lying still with knees drawn up, restlessness, and lying on the side during history taking; conduct a symptom analysis, as necessary.	Positions assumed by client may reveal the nature and source of pain.
Ask the client about knowledge and presence of the following risk factors: health care occupation, hemodialysis, IV drug use, household or sexual contact with a hepatitis B virus (HBV) carrier, international travel in area of high HBV infection rate, multiple heterosexual partners in the last 6 months, active male homosexuality or bisexuality.	These are risk factors for HBV infection.

are between the T12 and L3 vertebrae and are protected by the lower ribs and back muscles.

Tightened abdominal muscles hinder accuracy of palpation and auscultation. To promote relaxation, ask the client to void before the examination, and ensure that your hands, the room, and the stethoscope are warm. To distract the client from the discomfort of the examination, maintain a conversation, except during auscultation. The client lies supine, with the arms at the sides and the knees slightly bent. If the client places the arms under the head, the abdominal muscles will tighten. Expose the abdomen from just above the xiphoid process to the symphysis pubis, and drape the client's upper chest and legs. Ask the client to report any pain or tender areas before beginning the assessment; then proceed calmly and slowly, observing the client's face closely and checking regularly for any signs of discomfort. Always examine the tender areas last.

The sequence of steps in the abdominal examination differs from that of other assessments in that *auscultation immediately follows inspection*.

Inspection. Inspect the entire abdomen for skin characteristics, contour, symmetry, pulsations, and peristalsis (Skill 32–17). Skin characteristics to assess include colour, scars, venous patterns, lesions, and striae (stretch marks). The skin is subject to the same colour variations as on the rest of the body. Venous patterns are usually faint, except in thin clients. Striae result from stretching of tissue due to obesity or pregnancy. An artificial opening may indicate a drainage site resulting from surgery or an ostomy. Scars indicate past trauma or surgery that may have created permanent changes in the anatomy of underlying organs. Bruises may indicate accidental injury, physical abuse, or a bleeding disorder. Ask about the history of any marks. Ask if the client self-administers injections (e.g., heparin or insulin). Colour changes (as in jaundice or cyanosis) and glistening, taut skin (ascites) are unexpected findings.

Note the position, shape, and colour of the umbilicus, as well as any signs of inflammation, discharge, or protruding masses (Box 32–24). The umbilicus is usually a flat or concave hemisphere positioned in the midline midway between the xiphoid process and the symphysis pubis. Its colour is the same as that of the surrounding skin. Underlying masses can cause displacement. An everted (pouched-out) umbilicus usually indicates abdominal distension. **Hernias** (anterior protrusions of abdominal organs through the muscle) cause umbilical protrusion. Discharge in the umbilical area is not an expected finding.

Inspect for abdominal contour, symmetry, and surface motion, noting masses, bulging, or distension. Expect the abdomen to be flat or rounded. The contour is smooth and symmetrical at rest, and with a deep breath. Suspect pathology if a mass or asymmetry is present.

Intestinal gas, a tumour, or fluid in the abdominal cavity may cause **distension** (swelling). When distension is generalized, the entire abdomen appears protuberant. The skin often appears taut, as if stretched tightly over the abdomen. Ask the client if the abdomen

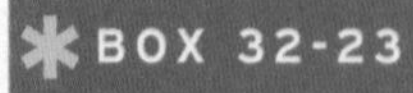

FOCUS ON PRIMARY HEALTH CARE

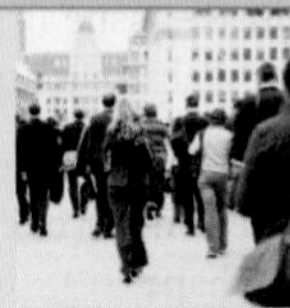

Abdomen

- Digestive health
- Hepatitis A and B immunization
- Screening for colon cancer
- Alcohol and substance abuse

➤ SKILL 32-17 Inspecting and Auscultating the Abdomen

Equipment

- Stethoscope

Procedure

EXAMINATION SKILL AND FOCUS	TECHNIQUES AND RATIONALE
Inspection: Abdomen	Abdomen fully exposed; bladder empty; client draped. *Ensures client comfort and complete visibility of the abdomen.*
	Client in the supine position, with arms at the sides **OR** folded across the chest. *Relaxes abdominal muscles.*
	1. Inspect tangentially from the right side and from the foot of the table. *Aids assessment of contour and movements.*
	2. Inspect across the abdomen.
	3. Ask the client to inhale deeply and hold the breath. *Aids assessment of symmetry.*
	4. Inspect for symmetry.
Auscultation: Bowel sounds	1. Inquire about any abdominal tenderness, and ask the client to point to the area. *Tender areas are assessed last.*
	2. Auscultate before percussion and palpation. *Percussion and palpation may change the frequency of bowel sounds.*
	3. Place the diaphragm of the stethoscope gently on the client's abdomen.
	4. Listen in all four quadrants. *Ensures no sounds are missed.*
Auscultation:	1. Press the diaphragm of the stethoscope *gently* against the client's abdomen.
Aorta	2. Listen slightly to the left of the midline in the epigastric region (aorta).
Renal arteries	3. Listen to the left and right of the midline just superior to the umbilicus (renal).
Iliac arteries	4. Listen just above the inguinal ligament, midway between the anterior superior iliac spine and the symphysis pubis (iliac).

From Stephen, T. C., Day, R. A., & Skillen, D. L. (Eds.). (2008). *A syllabus for adult health assessment* (pp. 43–44). Edmonton, AB: Faculty of Nursing, University of Alberta.

feels unusually tight. Measure abdominal girth with a tape measure around the abdomen at the level of the umbilicus. Use a felt pen to mark where the tape measure is applied. Consecutive measurements show any increase or decrease in distension. Do not confuse distension with obesity. In obesity, the abdomen is large, rolls of adipose tissue are often present along the flanks, and the client does not complain of tightness in the abdomen.

Remember that men tend to breathe abdominally and women costally. If clients have severe pain, respiratory movement is diminished; to guard against the pain, they tighten their abdominal muscles. By looking closely across the abdomen from the side, you may detect peristaltic movements and aortic pulsations. It may take several minutes to see a peristaltic wave. In contrast, aortic pulsations occur with each beat of systole and appear in the midline above the umbilicus (epigastric area).

Auscultation. In abdominal assessment, auscultation always precedes percussion and palpation (Skill 32–18). Auscultation is easier and more accurate if the client is not talking. **Peristalsis** (intestinal motility) is a function of the small and large intestines. Bowel sounds

BOX 32-24 NURSING STORY

A Surprise Ending

At 0130 hours one Saturday night, the on-call registered nurse (Skillen) for the Health Centre in a remote northern Alberta community was awakened by the ringing of the phone. Jimmy Coutreille identified himself and said, "Nurse, I have appendicitis." The nurse instructed him to go to the Health Centre right away where she would meet him. She dressed quickly and started thinking about the logistics of requesting a medivac, if needed.

Upon arrival at the door of the Health Centre, the nurse saw Jimmy, the 22-year-old man, being held up by two friends, his jeans dropped to his ankles, and clutching the left side of his abdomen. While assisting Jimmy into the emergency room of the Health Centre, the nurse took a brief history and noted a strong smell of alcohol. As she helped him lie down on the examination table, she started her symptom analysis. The nurse then draped Jimmy for a complete abdominal assessment, exposing the abdomen from the xiphoid process to the margins of the pubic hair. First, she inspected the abdomen tangentially from Jimmy's right side and from the foot of the table. Next, she inspected across the abdomen, and asked him to inhale deeply and hold his breath while she inspected for symmetry. It looked as if he had a lop-sided pregnancy! What she observed was a highly distended bladder that deviated to the left, filling the left lower quadrant and reaching into the left upper quadrant. She then asked Jimmy when he had last urinated, and he could not remember. When he said that he thought he could urinate, she walked with him to the washroom. Jimmy voided a very large amount of urine and reported to the nurse that he had emptied his bladder. He then hugged the nurse and thanked her profusely because his pain was gone now. He agreed to return for follow-up the next day at the nurse's clinic and left, walking by himself, with his two buddies.

The nurse knew that she would be able to obtain more accurate information after he had slept off the alcohol he had consumed. She planned to take a more detailed history, especially with respect to his nutritional and fluid intakes, use of alcohol and other substances, immunizations, sexual history, and psychosocial needs. She would focus on a review of his gastrointestinal and genitourinary systems and would conduct a complete abdominal assessment that would include tests of urine and any urethral discharge. For health promotion, she planned to address safer sex practices, genital and testicular self-examination, prevention of STIs, and drinking practices. She hoped that by helping him when he was in pain, she had initiated a relationship of trust with him.

occur due to the audible passage of air and fluid created by peristalsis. Air and fluid move through the intestines, creating soft gurgling or clicking sounds that occur irregularly 5 to 35 times per minute (Seidel et al., 2006). Sounds may last 0.5 seconds to several seconds. It usually takes 5 to 20 seconds to hear a bowel sound. The best time to auscultate is between meals, as bowel sounds tend to be increased right after a meal and if a meal is overdue. Bowel sounds are generally described as absent, audible, hyperactive, or hypoactive. Absence of sounds indicates cessation of GI motility that may result from late-stage bowel obstruction, paralytic ileus, or peritonitis. Absent sounds are expected postoperatively following general anaesthesia. Listen for 5 minutes before concluding that bowel sounds are absent (Seidel et al., 2006). Loud, growling hyperactive sounds (**borborygmi**) indicate increased motility of the GI tract. Altered motility results from anxiety, diarrhea, bleeding, bowel inflammation, excessive ingestion of laxatives, and reaction to certain foods.

The presence of bruits can reveal aneurysms or stenosed blood vessels in the abdomen. With the diaphragm of the stethoscope, auscultate over the aorta and over the renal and iliac arteries (see Skill 32–17; Figure 32–27). No vascular sounds are expected to be heard. Any bruit over the arteries should be considered an unexpected finding and be reported immediately to a physician or nurse practitioner.

Percussion. Percussion of the abdomen helps map out the underlying organs, bone, and masses and reveals the presence of air in the GI system (see Skill 32–18). Always percuss potentially painful areas last. Tympany usually predominates because of the presence of air in the stomach and intestines. The sounds are dull over the liver, the spleen, the pancreas, the kidneys, a pregnant uterus, a distended bladder, or a tumour.

Percussion allows you to identify the borders of the liver to detect organ enlargement. The note changes from tympany to dullness at the lower border of the liver near the right costal margin and changes from resonance to dullness at the upper border of the liver (usually in the fifth, sixth, or seventh intercostal space). The liver span (distance) between the upper and lower borders is 6 to 12 cm in the right

➤ SKILL 32-18 Percussing the Abdomen

Equipment

- Felt pen
- Tape measure

Procedure

EXAMINATION SKILL AND FOCUS	TECHNIQUES AND RATIONALE
Percussion: Abdomen	1. Place the distal phalanx and the joint of the middle (pleximeter) finger on the abdominal wall (avoiding contact with other fingers). *Ensures best percussion note achieved.* 2. Aim at the distal phalanx or the interphalangeal joint. 3. Strike the pleximeter with a sharp, light blow with tip of your middle (plexor) finger. 4. Percuss lightly over the entire abdomen. *Percussion notes vary from tympany to dullness.* 5. Inquire about areas of tenderness. 6. Observe the client's facial expressions during percussion. *Facial expressions may be the only indications of tenderness.*
Percussion: Liver	1. Percuss along the right midclavicular line from lung resonance to liver dullness (upper border); mark the level. 2. Start at a level below the umbilicus along the right midclavicular line, and percuss upward to liver dullness (lower border); mark the level. *Identifies upper and lower borders for measurement.* 3. Measure the vertical span of liver dullness in centimetres. 4. Ask the client to inhale deeply. 5. Percuss upward toward the lower border. *Identifies the lowest border of the liver when the diaphragm descends during inhalation, pushing the liver downward.* 6. Identify the new level of dullness; mark the level.
Splenic percussion sign	1. Percuss the lowest interspace along the left anterior axillary line. 2. Instruct the client to take a deep breath, and repeat the percussion in lowest interspace of the left anterior axillary line. *If the note changes to dullness, splenic enlargement may be present.* 3. Note any change in percussion.
Percussion: Bladder	1. Percuss downward along the midline from the umbilicus to the pelvic brim. *Tympany changes to dullness over a distended bladder.*
Percussion: Kidney	Client in sitting or standing position. Inform the client about the procedure. 1. Inquire about any kidney tenderness. *If the area is tender, percussion should not be done over it.* 2. If the client reports tenderness, press in each costovertebral angle with your fingertips. 3. Inquire about any tenderness. 4. If tenderness is present, place the palm (fingers not touching the client) of your nondominate hand over each costovertebral angle. *The palm of your hand is positioned over the lower pole of the kidney.* 5. Strike the dorsum of your hand with the ulnar surface of your fist. *Blunt, indirect percussion is used to elicit kidney tenderness.* 6. Inquire about any tenderness.

From Stephen, T. C., Day, R. A., & Skillen, D. L. (Eds.). (2008). *A syllabus for adult health assessment* (p. 44). Edmonton, AB: Faculty of Nursing, University of Alberta.

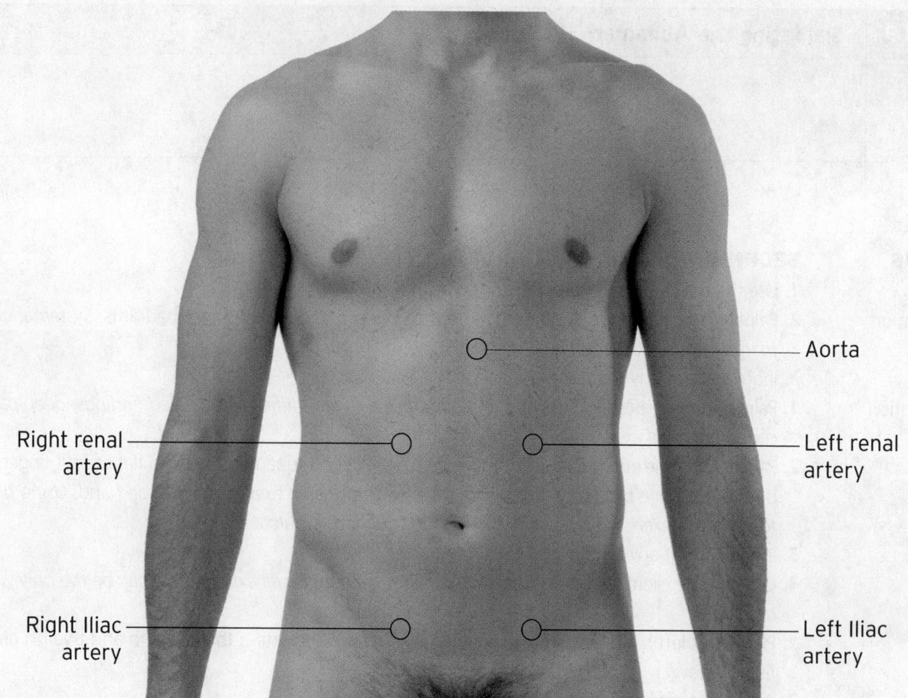

Figure 32-27 Sites to auscultate for bruits: renal arteries, iliac arteries, and the aorta. **Source:** Adapted from Thompson, J., & Wilson, S. (1996). *Health assessment for nursing practice* (p. 451, Figure 17–8). St. Louis, MO: Mosby.

MCL. Liver enlargement occurs in diseases such as cirrhosis, cancer, and hepatitis.

Alert the client, in the sitting or standing position, before performing direct or indirect percussion to assess for kidney inflammation (see Skill 32–18). If the kidneys are inflamed, the client will report tenderness to percussion, sometimes exquisite tenderness. When assessing the spleen (see Skill 32–18), expect to hear a tympanic note that remains tympanic even after the client takes a deep breath. Change to a dull note with a deep breath is an unexpected finding that suggests splenic enlargement.

Palpation. With palpation, you are primarily concerned with detecting areas of abdominal tenderness, unexpected distension, or masses (Skill 32–19). As you gain more skill, you will palpate for specific organs such as the liver, and use deep palpation as well as light palpation (see Figure 32–1, page 548). Palpate lightly, using smooth coordinated movements and avoiding quick jabs. The pads of your fingers should depress approximately 1.3 cm in a gentle dipping motion during light palpation. Leave palpation of painful areas to the last. Palpation assesses for muscular resistance, distension, tenderness, and superficial organs or masses. Observe the client's face for any signs of discomfort. Expect the abdomen to be smooth, soft, nontender, and without masses. If you palpate a sensitive area, guarding or muscle tenseness may occur. A distended bladder is detected easily with light palpation; the client is more comfortable if it is detected with percussion. Assess masses for size, location, shape, consistency, tenderness, pulsation, and mobility.

safety alert Never use deep palpation over a surgical incision or over extremely tender organs. Do not use deep palpation on unexpected masses. Deep pressure over the cecum, sigmoid colon, aorta, and the midline near the xiphoid process may cause tenderness in the healthy client (Seidel et al., 2006).

With experience, you can perform deep palpation to delineate the abdominal organs and to detect less obvious masses. You need to keep your fingernails short. It is important for the client to be relaxed as you press your hands approximately 2.5 to 7.5 cm into the client's abdomen. The liver lies in the right upper quadrant under the rib cage. Use deep palpation to locate the lower edge of the liver and any liver enlargement (see Skill 32–19; Figure 32–28). The liver is often not palpable; when palpable, it is found to be nontender, with a firm, regular, and sharp edge. An irregular edge or a boggy or tender liver is not an expected finding.

Lymphatics. Most lymphatics from the lower extremities, external genitalia, and abdominal wall drain into the inguinal lymph nodes, but lymphatics from the testes drain into the abdomen where you cannot access enlarged lymph nodes. The inguinal area lies between the anterior superior iliac spine and the symphysis pubis. The inguinal ligament runs between them; the inguinal canal lies about parallel to the ligament and is the conduit for the vas deferens through the abdominal muscles. Assess the horizontal and vertical chains of the inguinal lymph nodes for tenderness and inflammation (see Skill 32–19). You may find nontender, mobile, and horizontal or vertical nodes less than 1 cm in size. If nodes are larger than 1 cm, tender, and fixed (not mobile), suspect local, systemic, or malignant disease.

Age-Related Changes. In older adults, adipose tissue tends to increase on the abdomen and hips. Reduced abdominal tone makes it easier to palpate the underlying organs and to visualize pulsations and peristalsis. The incidence of constipation and gallstones increases, although age-related changes should not cause adverse effects in fecal movement in the large intestine. Most liver functions do not change with aging (Jarvis, 2004).

Documentation. Record your findings from the inspection, auscultation, percussion, and palpation of the abdomen (Table 32–33).

➤ SKILL 32-19 Palpating the Abdomen

Equipment

- None

Procedure

EXAMINATION SKILL AND FOCUS	TECHNIQUES AND RATIONALE
Palpation	1. Use the flat of four fingers held together, in a light, dipping motion.
Light abdominal palpation	2. Palpate over the entire abdomen, more than once in each of the four quadrants. *Systematic palpation ensures that the entire abdomen is palpated.* 3. Inquire about any tenderness.
Deep abdominal palpation	1. Palpate deeply *after* light palpation. *If light palpation identifies unexpected findings, deep palpation may be contraindicated.* 2. Palpate over the entire abdomen, more than once in each quadrant. Use the flat of four fingers of one hand OR use both hands, one placed on top of the other, with pressure exerted by the top hand. *Using both hands allows the top hand to exert the pressure and the bottom hand to palpate.* 3. Inquire about any tenderness. 4. Observe the client's facial expressions during palpation. *Facial expressions may be the only way client indicates discomfort.*
Palpation: Liver	1. Place your left hand behind the client parallel to and supporting the eleventh and twelfth ribs and the soft tissue below. 2. Press your left hand forward while the client relaxes. 3. Place your right hand on the client's abdomen: • Below the lower border of liver dullness percussed upon deep inspiration. *Percussed level of liver indicates how low to start palpation.* • Lateral to the rectus muscle with your hand held parallel or obliquely to the midline of the client's body **OR** parallel to the costal margin. 4. Palpate deeply with the flat of four fingers. 5. Instruct the client to take a deep breath, and try to feel the liver edge as it comes down to meet your fingertips **OR** the lateral edge of your index finger. *When the client inhales, the diaphragm descends, pushing the liver down toward your hand.* 6. If the liver is not palpable: • Inch your hand closer to the right costal margin, and repeat the procedure. • Exert more pressure inward while the client exhales, and repeat the procedure.
Inguinal nodes: Horizontal	1. Palpate inferior to the inguinal ligament from the symphysis pubis to the anterosuperior iliac spine. *Lymph nodes are found to be linked, as in a chain, in this area.*
Vertical	2. Palpate medial to the femoral canal from the superior ramus to an area 5 cm distally. *Ensures that both chains of nodes are palpated.*

From Stephen, T. C., Day, R. A., & Skillen, D. L. (Eds.). (2008). *A syllabus for adult health assessment* (p. 45). Edmonton, AB: Faculty of Nursing, University of Alberta.

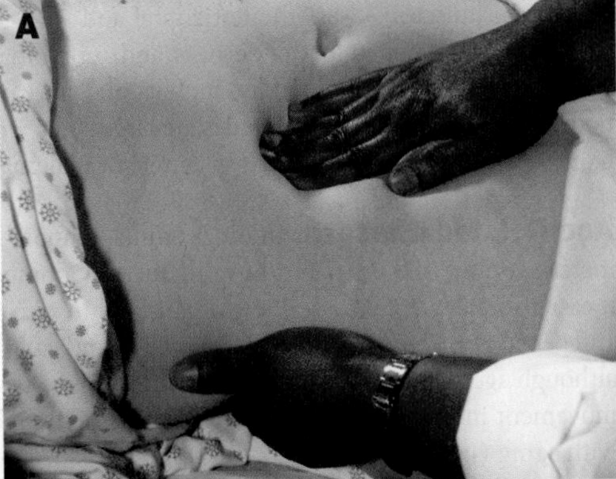

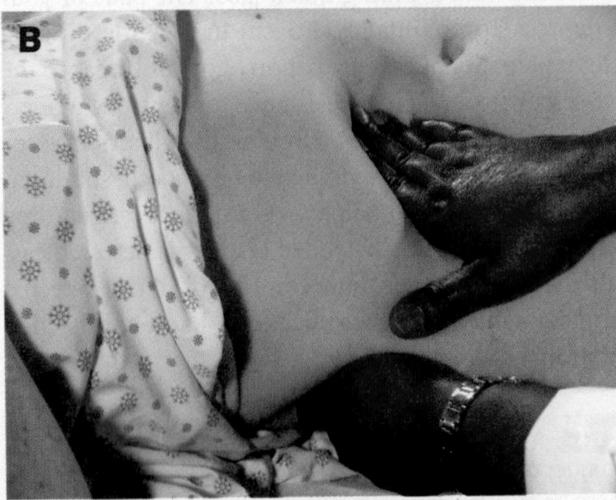

Figure 32-28 Liver palpation. A, The hand is parallel to the rectus abdominus muscle. B, The hand is oblique to the rectus abdominus muscle. **Source:** From Skillen, D. L., Day, R. A., Anderson, M. C., Stephen, T. C., Gilbert, J. A., & Day, L. W. (2004). *Physical examination images* [CD-ROM]. Edmonton, AB: Faculty of Nursing, University of Alberta.

➤ TABLE 32-33 Examples of Documentation of Assessments of the Spine, Posterior Thorax, Lungs, Heart, Breasts, Axillae, and Abdomen

Focus of Assessment	Expected Findings
Spine	
Spinal curvatures	Thoracic curve convex; lumbar curve concave. Vertebrae vertically aligned.
Symmetry	Shoulders, scapulae, iliac crests, sacroiliac joints, and gluteal folds horizontally aligned.
Range of motion (ROM)	Touches right and left toes in flexion, full ROM in extension, lateral bending and rotation. Lateral bending and rotation symmetrical.
Spinous processes	Nontender to palpation from C1 to L5. No protrusions evident.
Paravertebral muscles	Nontender bilaterally from C1 to L5, without spasm; equal muscle bulk.
Thorax	
Shape	Elliptical; AP:Lat ratio is 1:2.
Symmetry	Shoulders, scapulae, iliac crests, and posterior superior iliac spines aligned horizontally; muscle development symmetrical; nontender bilaterally.
Skin	Intact; pink; smooth; warm; scattered freckles over shoulders and upper thorax.
Respiratory expansion	Symmetrical upward and outward movement on inspiration; equal movement during expiration.
Lungs	
Tactile fremitus	Vibrations equally palpable and intense over apices and interscapular areas; less intense over right and left lower lung fields.
Percussion	Resonant throughout right and left lung fields.
Breath sounds	Vesicular sounds over right and left lung fields; bronchovesicular breath sounds over right interscapular area; no adventitious sounds heard.
Heart	
Inspection	No pulsations evident in right or left second intercostal space (ICS), along left sternal border, or epigastric region. Pulsations evident in fifth ICS, medial to left midclavicular line (MCL).
Palpation	No palpable pulsations or lifts in aortic or pulmonic areas, along left sternal border, or epigastric region. Point of maximal impulse (PMI) palpable in fifth ICS, medial to left MCL.
Apical impulse	PMI palpable in fifth ICS, medial to left MCL as light tap, 2 cm in diameter; spans first half systole.
Auscultation	S_1 louder than S_2 at apex, S_2 louder than S_1 at second right interspace, splitting of S_2 evident in second left interspace following deep inspiration, no extra heart sounds or murmurs heard.
Rate/rhythm	76 beats per minute (bpm), regular rhythm.
Axillae	Skin smooth, intact; no palpable lymph nodes bilaterally; no tenderness.
Breasts	
Nipples	Colour darker than breast; no rashes or discharge bilaterally; everted bilaterally; point in symmetrical directions.
Areola	Symmetrical; round; colour darker than breast.
Breast tissue	Breasts lobular; right slightly larger than left; colour similar to body. Firm and smooth. No masses, lesions, edema, dimpling, retraction or peau d'orange (orange peel) skin noted bilaterally.
Abdomen	
Skin	Pink; smooth; intact; striae present
Umbilicus	Pink; flat; round
Contour and symmetry	Rounded; symmetrical
Movement or pulsations	Pulsations visible in aortic region less than 1 cm diameter
Bowel sounds	Bowel sounds present in all four quadrants
Vascular sounds	No vascular sounds auscultated in aortic, iliac, or renal areas
Percussion	Dullness in RUQ; tympany in LUQ, LLQ, and RLQ
Liver size	Liver span 8 cm at midclavicular line
Kidney tenderness	No report of tenderness on direct percussion
Splenic percussion note	Percussion note tympanic before and after inhalation
Palpation	Soft; nontender
Liver	Not palpable
Inguinal nodes	Not palpable

Adapted from Chambers, J., Bazin, M., Nutting, L., & Stephen, T. (2008). *Year I lab guide* (pp. 56, 83, 89, 101). Edmonton, AB: Faculty of Nursing, University of Alberta.

Assessing the Female Genitalia and Reproductive Tract

External Genitalia. The external genitalia comprise the mons pubis, labia majora, labia minora, clitoris, urethral meatus, and vaginal orifice. The mons pubis is a pad of fatty tissue lying anterior to the symphysis pubis. Hair growth forms a triangle over the adult perineum and along the medial thighs. Labia majora are folds of fatty tissue spanning an area from the mons pubis to the perineum (area between vaginal orifice and anus). The inner surfaces of the labia majora appear dark pink and moist. Labia majora may be gaping or closed. After childbirth, the labia majora are more separated and prominent. Labia minora are smaller folds joined anteriorly at the clitoris, forming a hood or prepuce, and posteriorly by the frenulum. The clitoris is erectile tissue 0.5 cm wide that varies in length from 2 cm to less.

The labial structures form the vestibule, which has several openings. The urethral meatus is anterior to the vaginal orifice, pink, and at times difficult to locate. It may appear as a pinhole opening or a small slit 2.5 cm below the clitoris, just above the vaginal canal. After several vaginal childbirths, the opening to the vaginal canal often extends upward, interfering with the view of the meatus. Small glands (Skene's) surround the urethral meatus. The vaginal orifice (introitus) is a thin vertical slit or a large orifice with moist tissue. The hymen is just inside the introitus. In virgins, the hymen can narrow the vaginal opening. Remnants of the hymen remain after initiation of sexual activity. During sexual intercourse, secretions from Bartholin's glands (located on either side of the vaginal orifice) provide lubrication.

Internal Genitalia. The internal genitalia consist of the vagina, cervix, uterus, fallopian tubes, and ovaries. The vagina begins at the vaginal orifice and extends back into the pelvis. Secretions are usually thin, clear or cloudy, and odourless. The vaginal walls are pink and moist, with folds of tissue (rugae) that allow the canal to expand during childbirth. The cervix extends into the end of the vagina. It is pink, smooth, glistening, and round, with a diameter of 2.5 to 3 cm in young women. An opening in the cervix (cervical os) increases in size after childbirth. At the os, the surface of the cervix is lined with layers of vaginal squamous cells that meet the columnar cells. Columnar cells secrete mucus and line the passageway that leads up into the central cavity of the uterus. Squamous cells protect the cervix; columnar cells help sperm to enter the uterus for fertilization. The space around the cervix is called the anterior fornix and posterior fornix. A pear-shaped uterus measures 5.5 to 8 cm long by 3.5 to 4 cm wide and 2 to 2.5 cm thick (Jarvis, 2004, p. 767). The fallopian tubes extend out from the fundus of the uterus and curve down toward the ovaries, which lie on each side of the uterus in line with the anterosuperior iliac spine.

The history you collect from female clients about the genitalia and reproductive tract (Table 32–34) determines the focus for health promotion (Box 32–25).

Examination of the genitalia can be embarrassing for many women, but you can make it less embarrassing by using a calm, relaxed approach. The gynecological examination can be one of the most difficult experiences for adolescents. Cultural background also contributes to apprehension. You need to provide thorough explanations in advance about procedures so that clients are mentally prepared for them. The lithotomy position required for the examination

TABLE 32-34 Health History for Female Genitalia and Reproductive Tract Assessment

Assessment Category	Rationale for Assessment
Ask the client about any history of illness, surgery, or sexually transmitted infections (STIs) involving reproductive organs.	Illness or surgery can influence the appearance and position of the organs being examined.
Inquire about client's menstrual history, including age at menarche, frequency, duration, characteristics of menstrual flow; dysmenorrhea (painful menstruation); pelvic pain; and premenstrual symptoms.	All this information provides a good indication of reproductive health.
Ask the client about obstetrical history, including number of pregnancies, abortions, or miscarriages.	Observed physical findings will vary, depending on the client's obstetric history.
Inquire about the client's contraceptive and safer sex practices.	Use of certain types of contraceptives may influence reproductive health (e.g., sensitivity to spermicidal jelly). This information helps determine reproductive risks. Sexual history reveals risk for and understanding of STIs.
Ask the client about any history of genitourinary problems, including burning during urination, frequency, urgency, nocturia, hematuria, or incontinence.	Urinary problems may be associated with gynecological disorders.
Determine if the client is postmenopausal, obese, or infertile; had early menarche (before the age of 12 years); had late menopause (after age 50); has a history of hypertension, diabetes, or liver disease; or has a family history of endometrial, breast, or colon cancer.	These are risk factors for endometrial cancer.
Ask the client about the presence of vaginal discharge, painful or swollen tissues, or genital lesions.	These signs and symptoms may indicate STIs or yeast infection (candidiasis).

BOX 32-25 FOCUS ON PRIMARY HEALTH CARE

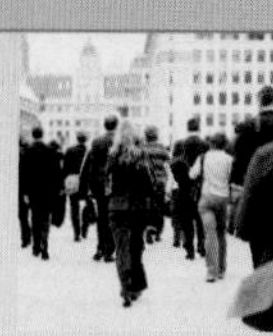

Female Genitalia

- Safer sex practices
- Regular gynecological examinations
- Self-examination by at-risk clients
- Immunization (females 9 to 26 years of age) to prevent cancer of the cervix and genital warts
- Prevention of STIs

is an added source of embarrassment. Client comfort can be achieved by correct positioning and draping of the client. Adolescents may choose to have a parent or guardian present during the examination.

The client may require a complete examination of the reproductive organs, which includes assessment of the external genitalia and a vaginal examination. You can examine the rectum and anus also when the client is in the lithotomy position. You will often examine external genitalia during routine hygiene measures or urinary catheter care; you may perform parts of the vaginal examination in obstetric clinics, family planning clinics, or sexually transmitted infection (STI) clinics. More complete examinations are performed by nurse practitioners and midwives. You need to have a clear understanding of all the procedures because you will often assist at those complete examinations.

The examination of the reproductive system is part of each woman's preventive health care, as uterine cancers have a high incidence rate (about 5500 cases and over 1100 deaths in 2007) and ovarian cancer causes more deaths (1700 deaths and 2500 cases in 2007) than any other cancer of the female reproductive system (CCS, 2007). Young adults and adolescents are routinely examined because of the increasing incidence of STIs. On average, menarche occurs at an earlier age now than in the 1950s, and the majority of teenagers (male and female) are sexually active by the age of 19 years (Hockenberry et al., 2007). Clients at risk for STIs should learn to perform a genital self-examination using a mirror to detect any signs (e.g., sores, blisters, or warts). Many women do not realize they have an STI, so some STIs remain undetected for years. During history taking (see Table 32–34), assess the client's anxiety level and previous experiences of vaginal examinations.

Examination of External Genitalia

Preparation of the Client. Before beginning the examination (Skill 32–20), assemble all the necessary equipment, and ask the client to empty her bladder. Assist the client into the lithotomy position on a bed or an examination table. Help her feet into stirrups if a speculum examination is to be performed (see Table 32–14, page 555). Place your hands at the edge of the table, and instruct the client to slide her buttocks down the examination table until they touch your hands. Ensure that the client's arms are at her sides or folded across her chest and not under her head. Women with joint pain or deformity may be unable to assume the lithotomy position. They can instead lie on their left side, with the right thigh and knee drawn up to the chest, or they can abduct only one leg. Ensure that your client is adequately draped. Only when beginning the examination should you lift the drape to expose the perineum. Male nurses should always have a female colleague present during the examination. A female nurse may examine the client alone but may have another female present if the client is particularly anxious.

Inspection and Palpation. Ensure that the perineal area is well illuminated. Wear gloves on both hands to prevent the transmission of microorganisms. The perineum is extremely sensitive and tender and should not be touched without warning the client. Touch the thigh first before proceeding to the perineum. Skill 32–20 presents the sequence and techniques for examining the external genitalia.

Inspect the labia majora for edema, inflammation, lesions, or lacerations. Gently retract the labia minora outward, using a firm hold to avoid retracting sensitive tissues repeatedly. Look for atrophy, inflammation, or adhesions of the remaining external structures. An inflamed clitoris is bright red in colour; in young women, it is a common site for syphilitic chancres (small open ulcers with serous discharge). Older women may have malignant changes such as dry, scaly, nodular lesions. Examine the urethral orifice for colour and position; note any polyps, discharge, or fistulas. With the labia still retracted, examine Skene's and Bartholin's glands for tenderness and any discharge.

Assess the adequacy of muscle support. If it is lacking, the vaginal walls bulge and block the introitus. Ask the client to tighten or try to close the vaginal orifice; with your hand gloved, insert your index and middle fingers into the vaginal orifice, palpate for tension in the muscles. Women who have undergone vaginal childbirth have reduced muscle tone. You may also inspect the anus at this time, looking for lesions and hemorrhoids (see Skill 32–22, page 613). Discard the gloves, and provide perineal hygiene care to the client.

Examination of Internal Genitalia

Speculum Examination. When assisting an examiner with the internal examination, ensure that the client's feet are comfortably positioned in the stirrups. The examiner uses a plastic or metal speculum and selects the appropriate size of speculum (small, medium, or large) for the client. The smallest is used for a virgin. If a woman is sexually active, a medium-sized speculum is best. For women who have had vaginal deliveries, a medium or large speculum is used. The speculum, which consists of two blades and an adjustable thumbscrew, is inserted into the vagina to examine the internal genitalia for cancerous lesions and other abnormalities.

Papanicolaou (Pap) Smear. During the examination, the examiner collects a specimen to test for cancer. A **Papanicolaou (Pap) smear** is a simple, painless screening test for cervical cancer and has no side effects. Smears are taken from the endocervix and ectocervix. The test is performed annually during the pelvic examination of women who are, or have been, sexually active. After three or more consecutive annual examinations with expected findings, the test may be done less frequently (e.g., every 2 or 3 years), based on provincial screening guidelines and the discretion of the health care provider. Women at high risk for cervical cancer and those over 40 years should have annual smears.

After the speculum has been withdrawn, assist the client to the sitting position; allow her to perform hygiene and to dress. In a hospital, the client may need assistance with performing perineal hygiene.

Age-Related Changes. Pubic hair diminishes and becomes grey in older adults. At menopause (often between the ages of 46 and 55 years), the labia majora become thinner; with advancing age, they atrophy. Sex organs such as the clitoris also atrophy. The cervical diameter becomes narrower. Vaginal secretions become reduced, sometimes causing pain during sexual intercourse. Urinary infections tend to occur with thinning of tissues.

Documentation. Record your findings from the inspection and palpation of external female genitalia (Table 32–35).

➤ SKILL 32-20 Assessing the External Female Genitalia

Equipment

- Examination table with stirrups
- Adjustable light source
- Sink
- Disposable gloves
- Cotton-tipped applicators
- Culture media

Procedure

EXAMINATION SKILL AND FOCUS	TECHNIQUES AND RATIONALE
Inspection: Pubic hair	Client in lithotomy position, with feet in stirrups; draped with pubis and genitalia exposed; your hands gloved; and light coming over your shoulders. *This position allows for best visibility and access to structures. Gloves prevent transmission of microorganisms. Good lighting is essential for visibility.* 1. Inspect the hair, hair distribution, and skin of the pubis.
Labia majora	1. Inspect the labia majora. 2. Place the thumb and index finger of your nondominant hand, inside labia minora and gently but firmly retract the tissues forward. *This position provides better visibility.* 3. Inspect the labia minora. *Repeated repositioning of sensitive tissues can damage them.*
Palpation: Labia minora	1. With your other hand, palpate the labia minora between your thumb and index finger on one side. 2. Repeat on the other side.
Inspection: Clitoris	1. Inspect the clitoris.
Urethral meatus	1. Identify the urethral meatus above the vaginal canal. 2. Inspect the meatus. *Correct identification of the meatus is essential for procedures such as inserting a urinary catheter.*
Vaginal orifice (introitus)	1. With the labia minora still retracted, inspect the introitus. 2. With the labia minora still retracted and using your dominant hand, first dip the index finger into a basin of warm water for lubrication. *Water should be the only lubricant used when specimens are collected.* 3. With the palm facing upward, insert your index finger as far as the proximal interphalangeal joint (second finger joint) into the vagina.
Palpation: Skene's glands	4. Exert upward pressure by moving your fingers outward (milking action) on either side of the urethra and directly over the urethra. *Milking helps elicit discharges.* 5. Inquire about any tenderness. 6. Arrange to culture any discharge obtained. 7. Remove your retracting hand. 8. Insert your index finger into the posterior vaginal opening toward the left side, and palpate the posterior labia majora between the index finger and the thumb. 9. Repeat on the other side. 10. Arrange to culture any discharge obtained. 11. Change your gloves. *This prevents contamination.*
Bartholin's glands	Performed by experienced nurses. See specialized texts.
Perineum, vaginal orifice	1. Insert first two fingers into the client's vagina and instruct the client to tense the vaginal wall so that she can squeeze your fingers. *Assesses vaginal tone (important for sexual satisfaction and prevention of urinary incontinence).* 2. Instruct the client to strain downward as if voiding. Determine if any structures touch your examining fingers. *Bulging of vaginal walls may indicate prolapse of the bladder (cystocele) or the rectum (rectocele).* 3. Remove your fingers from the cleint's vagina; then, using the first two fingers of both hands, separate the vaginal orifice. 4. Instruct the client to bear down. 5. Inspect the vaginal orifice.
Inspection: Anus	See Skill 32–22, page 613.

From Day, R. A. (2008). Female external and internal genital examination. In T. C., Stephen, R. A., Day, & D. L. Skillen (Eds.), *A syllabus for adult health assessment* (pp. 93–94). Edmonton, AB: Faculty of Nursing, University of Alberta.

➤ TABLE 32-35 Examples of Documentation of Assessment of External Female Genitalia

Focus of Assessment	Expected Findings
Pubic hair	Uniform and thick; triangular distribution of coarse, curly hair over pubis and medial thighs; free of parasites.
External genitalia	No swelling, lesions, or discharge noted. No urethral swelling or discharge.

Adapted from Day, R. A. (2004). Documentation. In Faculty of Nursing, University of Alberta. (Ed.), *Health assessment self-test modules* (WebCT Vista). Edmonton, AB: Author.

Assessing Male Genitalia

Examination of the external male genitalia includes inspection, palpation, and occasional auscultation of the penis, scrotum, external inguinal ring, and inguinal canal. Internal genital structures that are assessed are the testis, epididymis, and vas deferens.

The shaft of the penis contains the urethra and columns of erectile tissue: corpus cavernosum (two) and corpus spongiosum (one). The urethra is located ventrally in the shaft and opens into the urethral meatus, somewhat ventrally on the cone-shaped glans penis. The dorsal vein is usually easily identifiable. At the base of the glans is the corona. In uncircumcised men, the prepuce (foreskin) covers the glans, so secretions may collect under the prepuce. The scrotum, which has a wrinkled surface, has two compartments, each containing a testis (testicle). Testes are ovoid and somewhat rubbery, range in length from 3.5 to 5.5 cm, and produce testosterone and spermatozoa. The left testis commonly lies at a lower level in the scrotum. On the superior margin of each testis, the epididymis is located posteriorly and laterally and is comma shaped. The vas deferens (cord-like structure) transmits the sperm from the testes and epididymis via a circuitous route to the urethra, along with secretions from the seminal vesicles, prostate, and the vas deferens. The spermatic cord contains the vas deferens, blood vessels, nerves, and muscle fibres.

Lymphatics from the penis and scrotal sac drain into the inguinal lymph nodes but drain directly from the testes into the abdomen, where they are not accessible. The inguinal area lies between the anterosuperior iliac spine and the symphysis pubis. The inguinal ligament runs between them. The inguinal canal lies parallel to the ligament and carries the vas deferens through the abdominal muscles. The external inguinal ring lies superolateral to the pubic tubercle and is accessible to the examining finger.

When you take a health history (Table 32–36), ensure that the subsequent examination is complete. Box 32–26 presents health promotion topics that you may discuss during the assessment of male genitalia.

Use a calm, gentle approach to lessen client anxiety about inspection and palpation of the genitalia and inguinal regions. Respect the client's modesty and strive to preserve the client's dignity. Men, especially adolescents, may worry about their genitals not being "normal." Adolescent and adult males often fear that they may have an erection while being examined. Gentle manipulation of the genitalia and not discussing the client's sex life during the examination helps avoid causing an erection. Do not joke, and avoid displaying any facial expressions that may convey concern or worry. Delay client education until the examination has been completed. Male clients need to know how to perform genital self-examination as part of routine self-care. Use your knowledge of teaching and learning principles to instruct them how to examine themselves. As the incidence of STIs in adolescents and young adults is increasing, assessment of genitalia should be a routine part of physical examination in this age group.

Penis

Inspection. Follow standard practice and use disposable gloves from the start of the examination to prevent transmission of infections from any unexpected discharge or skin lesions (Skill 32–21). Assess the sexual maturity of the client, noting the size and shape of the penis and testes, the colour and texture of the scrotal skin, and the

➤ TABLE 32-36 Health History for the Assessment of Male Genitalia

Assessment Category	Rationale
Ask the client about urinary elimination patterns, including frequency of voiding, nocturia, urine characteristics, burning, urgency, hematuria, difficulty starting stream, and daily fluid intake.	Problems in the urinary and genitourinary systems can be related due to the anatomical proximity of the two systems.
Inquire about the client's sexual history, safer sex practices, and sexual orientation.	Sexual history and practices reveal the level of risk for STIs, including HIV/AIDS.
Ask the client about history of surgery or illness involving urinary or reproductive organs, including STIs.	Alterations in the involved organs may underlie reported symptoms or changes.
Inquire about the presence of penile swelling, genital lesions, urethral discharge, or pain in the testicles or scrotum.	These signs and symptoms are associated with STIs.
Inquire about irregular or painless lumps or painless enlargement of testes, a feeling of heaviness in the scrotum, or a dull ache in the abdomen.	These are signs and symptoms of testicular cancer.
Inquire about any history of undescended testes in childhood and about frequency of testicular self-examination.	Risk for testicular cancer increases in men who had undescended testes in early childhood. Frequency of self-examination is an indication for potentially early detection.
Ask the client about any enlargements noticed in the inguinal area, duration, and association with lifting, coughing, or straining.	These signs and symptoms are associated with hernias.
Ask the client about current medication use (e.g., antihypertensives, sedatives, diuretics, or tranquilizers) and alcohol intake. Also, inquire about satisfaction with sex life and any difficulty achieving erection or ejaculating.	Medications or alcohol may affect sexual performance.

BOX 32-26 FOCUS ON PRIMARY HEALTH CARE

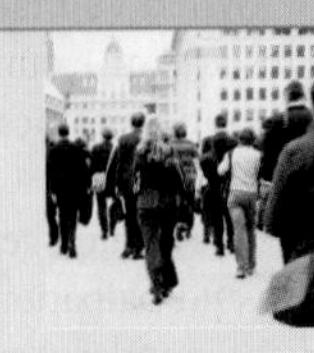

Male Genitalia

- Safer sex practices
- Genital self-examination
- Testicular self-examination
- Prevention of STIs
- Prevention of hernias

character and distribution of pubic hair. In adults, the length of the penis reaches down to the bottom of the scrotum, the testicles are fully grown, and the scrotal skin is darker and rugated. Coarse, curly pubic hair extends from the base of the penis over the pubic area and medial thighs and toward the umbilicus.

Inspect the skin in the genital area for evidence of rashes, lesions, lice, or excoriations. Inspection for inflammation and swelling of the shaft, corona, prepuce, glans, and urethral meatus of the penis follows. Note if the client is circumcised. It is common to see venereal lesions

SKILL 32-21 Assessing Male Genitalia and Inguinal Regions

Equipment

- Disposable gloves
- Glass slide
- Culture media

Procedure

EXAMINATION SKILL AND FOCUS	TECHNIQUES AND RATIONALE
Inspection:	Client in standing or supine position; pubis and genitalia exposed; you are gloved. *Clear visibility of the area to be examined is essential. Gloves prevent the transmission of microorganisms.*
Pubic hair	1. Inspect the hair and skin of the pubis.
Penis	1. Inspect the shaft of the penis.
Skin prepuce	2. Ask the client to retract the prepuce (foreskin), if present. *Visibility of the penis is essential for assessment in an uncircumcised male.*
Glans, corona	3. Inspect the glans and the corona.
Urethral meatus	4. Inspect the location of the meatus. *Congenital displacements may be present.*
	5. Compress the glans gently. *Compression exposes the meatus for full inspection.*
	6. Inspect the meatus. *Culture any discharge and obtain glass smear.*
	7. Replace the prepuce, if retracted. *Retracted prepuce creates the risk for impeded arterial circulation (constriction).*
Palpation:	1. Palpate the shaft between the thumb and the first two fingers. *Induration (hardened plaque) is palpable.*
Shaft	2. Inquire about any tenderness.
Inspection:	1. Inspect the anterior and lateral surfaces. *Visibility is essential for detection of changes.*
Scrotum	2. Lift the scrotum gently to inspect the posterior surface.
Palpation:	1. Use the thumb and first two fingers of your examining hand. *This captures the mobile structures for examination.*
	2. Palpate each side in sequence: A. Testis B. Epididymis C. Spermatic cord (and vas deferens). *Sequence permits structures to be located easily.*
	3. Repeat on the other side. *Comparison permits detection of differences.*
Inspection:	Client in standing position. *This position facilitates visibility of any hernia, full effects of gravity, and increased intra-abdominal pressure with bearing down.*
Inguinal region	1. Inspect the left and right inguinal regions.
Pubic tubercle to antero-superior iliac spine (inguinal canal)	2. Instruct the client to strain or bear down. 3. Inspect the regions using tangential lighting. *Increases detection of contours, bulges, enlarged nodes.* 4. Compare the regions. *Comparison detects alterations.*
Femoral canal	1. Inspect the left and right femoral regions.
	2. Use tangential lighting. *Expansile impulses and bulges are more readily detected.*
	3. Instruct the client to cough or strain down on the right and left sides. *Hernias may be bilateral.*
Palpation:	1. Place your finger pads on the anterior thigh in the region of the femoral canal. *The finger pads will feel the pressure of a hernia.*
	2. Instruct the client to cough and to strain down.
	3. Assess for any bulge or impulse felt against your fingers.
	4. Observe the relationship to the pubic tubercle.
	5. Repeat on the opposite thigh. *Hernias may be bilateral.*
Inguinal lymph nodes	See Skill 32–20, page 608.

From Skillen, D. L. (2008). Male genitalia examination. In T. C. Stephen, R. A. Day, & D. L. Skillen (Eds.), *A syllabus for adult health assessment* (pp. 90–91). Edmonton, AB: Faculty of Nursing, University of Alberta.

between the foreskin and the glans; you may retract the prepuce for inspection, or ask the client to do so. Foreskins retract easily.

Inspect any lesions for size, shape, location, colour, type, and discharge. A small amount of thick, white secretion between the glans and foreskin is expected. If any discharge is present, take a specimen for culture. The urethral meatus is slitlike and is situated on the ventral surface only millimetres from the tip of the glans. In some congenital conditions, the meatus is displaced along the ventral penile shaft. The meatal opening is expected to be glistening, pink, and without discharge; however, the meatus should be inspected for lesions, edema, and inflammation. When inspection of the penis is completed, ensure that the foreskin is returned to its original position. Never leave it retracted.

Palpation. Palpate the shaft between your thumb and first two fingers to detect any localized areas of hardness (induration) and tenderness on the dorsal or lateral surfaces. These indicate a risk in older males for fibrotic plaques associated with painful erections.

Scrotum

Inspection. Be particularly cautious when examining the scrotum because of the sensitivity of structures in the scrotal sac. Inspect the size, shape, and symmetry of the scrotum, and observe for lesions or edema. The scrotal skin is coarse, rugated, loose, and usually more deeply pigmented than the body skin. Look for excoriated skin in bedridden clients who are susceptible to friction or moisture in the scrotal area. Tightening of the skin may indicate edema. The scrotum size usually changes with temperature, as the dartos muscle contracts in cold and relaxes in warm temperatures. Obtain the occupational history (e.g., exposure to heat, if the client is a baker) to assess its effects on scrotal contents. Remember that testicular cancer, a solid tumour, is a known risk among young men ages 18 to 34 years or more. For early detection, clients must learn to perform testicular self-examination and be aware of its importance (see Box 32–27).

Palpation. Gently palpate the testicles and epididymis between your thumb and first two fingers. Scrotal structures are sensitive to even gentle compression. They feel smooth, rubbery, and free of nodules. The most common signs of testicular cancer are a painless enlargement of one testis, and a palpable, small, pea-sized, hard lump on the anterior or lateral testicle. Note the size, shape, consistency, and tenderness of the scrotal organs. Palpate the vas deferens separately, to look for nodules or swelling. Expect it to be smooth and discrete. The external inguinal ring provides the opening for the spermatic cord to pass into the inguinal canal.

Inguinal Region

Inspection. Inspect with the client in the standing position. Ask the client to strain or bear down. This causes an expansile impulse, enlargement, or bulge to become more obvious. When a portion of abdominal tissue or intestine protrudes through the inguinal or femoral canal, it creates a hernia. Intestinal loops can even enter the scrotum, and bowel sounds can be heard in that area on auscultation.

Palpation. Complete your examination by palpating for the inguinal lymph nodes (see Skill 32–19). You may find a nontender, mobile, and horizontal or vertical node less than 1 cm in size. Tender, nonmobile nodes over 1 cm in size require further examination. With experience, you would palpate the external inguinal ring, medial inguinal canal, and femoral canals to rule out a hernia. If you detect an expansile impulse or bulge, note its relationship to the pubic tubercle. This helps distinguish an inguinal hernia from a femoral hernia.

Age-Related Changes. Pubic hair diminishes and turns grey in older adults. The penis decreases in size. The testicles are less firm to palpation and may be reduced in size during a prolonged illness. Production of spermatozoa and testosterone declines. Muscle tone of the dartos muscles in the scrotum decreases, and the scrotal sac becomes more pendulous, causing the scrotal contents to hang lower. Sexual function remains, but sexual response becomes less intense. Erections are slower and less firm; ejaculation occurs more quickly and is less forceful. The refractory period between orgasm and the next erection lengthens.

Documentation. Record your findings from the inspection and palpation of the male genitalia and inguinal region (Table 32–37).

➤ BOX 32-27 Male Genital Self-Examination

All men aged 15 years and older should perform regular self-examination of genitalia. A warm bath or shower allows the scrotal sac to relax. Clients should inspect for any bumps, sores, warts, or blisters on the penis. They should scrutinize the skin under the pubic hair for the presence of excoriations or crab lice. Using a mirror, they should check for any swelling or lumps in the scrotal skin. By gently rolling the testicle between the index and middle fingers, they should palpate for lumps, thickening, or hardening. Impress upon clients the importance of consulting with a physician if they find small, pea-sized lumps on the anterior or lateral surfaces of the testicle.

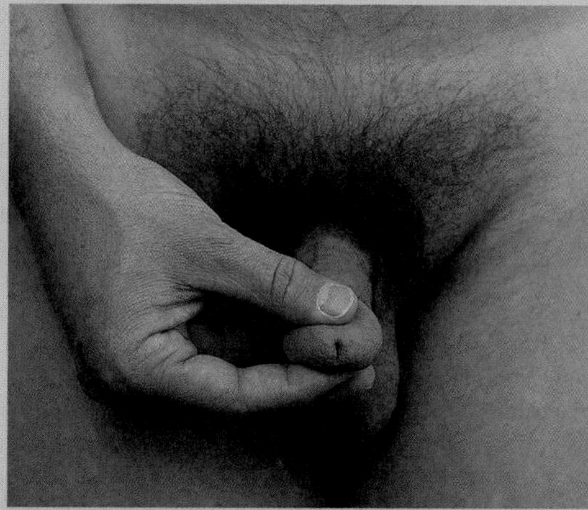

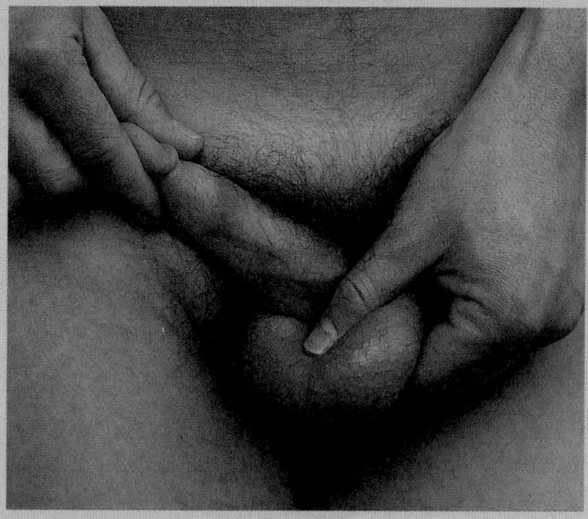

Illustrations from Seidel, H. M., Ball, J. W., Dains, J. E., & Benedict, G. W. (2006). *Mosby's guide to physical examination* (6th ed., p. 651). St. Louis, MO: Mosby.

Assessing the Anus, Rectum, and Prostate

Anus and Rectum. A good time to perform the rectal examination in both men and women is after the genital examination. Inspection and palpation are used for the assessment. The anus is a tightly closed, hairless, moist, visible structure, which is the external opening of the anal canal and the termination of the GI tract. The anal canal is surrounded by the internal sphincter muscle (under involuntary control) and the external sphincter muscle (under voluntary control). The canal is 3.8 cm long and extends in a line toward the umbilicus before turning into the mucus-lined rectum. *Somatic sensory nerves in the anal canal are very sensitive to a poorly directed examining finger or instrument.* At the anorectal junction, the rectum dilates and turns posteriorly into the hollow of the coccyx and sacrum. The rectum is about 12 cm long and joins the sigmoid colon at the distal end of the GI tract. The rectum contains three transverse valves of Houston; the inferior valve (fold) may be palpable. The upper portion of the rectum is covered by the peritoneum, which is only accessible to the examining finger on the anterior rectal surface. This permits you to assess for peritoneal inflammation through the rectum (e.g., in suspected appendicitis). In men, the peritoneum reflects on itself to form the rectovesical pouch; in women, the reflection forms the rectouterine pouch. Examination of the rectum can detect colorectal cancer at an early stage. In men, the rectal examination can also detect prostate tumours.

Use a calm, slow-paced, gentle approach when you explain the rectal examination to the client. Inform the client that a sensation as if the bowels will move may occur but bowel movement will not happen. This helps the client who has concerns about discomfort or embarrassment to relax. When examined by male nurses, men may be asked to bend forward with hips flexed and the upper body resting across an examination table; however, when examined by female nurses, they will be asked to assume the left lateral side-lying (Sims') position. Examine the female client immediately after the examination of the genitalia while the client is still in the dorsal recumbent position; otherwise the client should assume Sims' position. A non-ambulatory client should be in Sims' position for this examination.

Collect a thorough history (Table 32–38) to identify the client's learning needs and risk for bowel, rectal, or prostate disease. Box 32–28 provides the focus for health promotion.

Anus

Inspection. Inspect the perianal and sacrococcygeal areas to see if the skin is smooth and intact (Skill 32–22). Anal tissues are expected to be intact and usually moist and hairless compared with perianal skin; the tissue is coarser and more darkly pigmented. Look for lesions, rashes, inflammation, excoriation, linear splits (fissures), scars, and skin or mucous protrusions. A tuft of hair or dimple at the midline near the coccyx may indicate a pilonidal cyst. Protrusions from the anus may be hemorrhoids; external hemorrhoids are dilated or thrombosed veins that appear as bluish protrusions; internal hemorrhoids are reddish.

Rectum

Palpation. Some agencies may not permit you to perform digital examinations. As mandated in some regions, nursing students may require supervision during the first examination. Explain to both male and female clients that they may feel the urge to pass urine when they are palpated but that it will not happen. Ensure that your finger nails are kept trimmed to ensure client comfort.

The tone of the anal sphincter is tight. Weakness may indicate a neurological problem or may be the result of practising anal intercourse. Assess the anal canal and the lower rectum for smooth, nontender surfaces. Digital insertion should never be rough. Palpate the entire rectal wall for tenderness, irregularities, polyps, masses, or nodules. When the client bears down, lesions situated high in the rectum

TABLE 32-37 Examples of Documentation of Assessment of Male Genitalia

Focus of Assessment	Expected Findings
Pubic hair	Uniform and thick distribution of coarse, curly, red hair over the pubis, medial thighs, and midway to umbilicus; free of parasites
Penis	Circumcised (or uncircumcised); free of lesions; reaches to the bottom of the scrotum; meatus slit-like, pink, glistening; corona smooth and pink
Scrotum	Skin darker, rugated, and free of excoriations
Testicle	Palpated bilaterally; firm; 4 cm long bilaterally
Epididymis	Smooth; comma-shaped; nontender; situated on posterolateral testicular surface bilaterally
Spermatic cord	Smooth; nontender on the right and left
Inguinal canal	No bulge on straining bilaterally
Femoral canal	No impulse or bulge on cough bilaterally
Inguinal lymph nodes	Nonpalpable horizontal and vertical nodes bilaterally

Adapted from Skillen, D. L. (2004). Documentation. In Faculty of Nursing, University of Alberta. (Ed.), *Health assessment self-test modules* (WebCT Vista). Edmonton, AB: Author.

➤ TABLE 32-38 Health History for Assessment of the Anus, Rectum, and Prostate

Assessment Category	Rationale for Assessment
Question the client about dietary intake of fat and fibre.	High fat or low fibre intake may be linked to bowel cancer and the characteristics of stool.
Ask the client about any history of rectal bleeding, black or tarry stools, rectal pain, or change in bowel habits.	These are warning signs of colorectal cancer and other gastrointestinal disorders.
Inquire about family or personal history of colorectal cancer, polyps, or inflammatory bowel disease; find out if the client is over 40 years of age.	These are risk factors for colorectal cancer.
Question the client about medication use, including laxatives or cathartic medications, iron supplements, and codeine.	These medications affect the characteristics of the stool and bowel habits.
Inquire about previous screening for colorectal cancer.	This will help determine the client's health-promoting behaviours.
Ask a male client about weak or interrupted urine flow, inability to urinate, difficulty in starting or stopping the flow; ask both male and female clients about presence of polyuria, nocturia, hematuria, dysuria, and any pain in the lower back, pelvis, or upper thighs.	These are warning signs of prostate cancer, prostate enlargement, and urinary infection.

✱ BOX 32-28 FOCUS ON PRIMARY HEALTH CARE

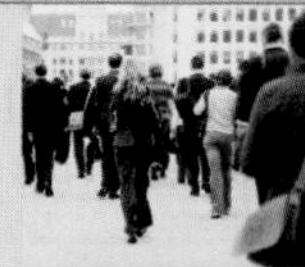

Anus, Rectum, and Prostate

- Regular digital rectal examinations, as appropriate for age
- Warning signs and symptoms for colorectal and prostate cancer
- Dietary fibre intake
- Screening for occult blood

➤ SKILL 32-22 Assessing the Anus and Rectum

Equipment

- Disposable gloves
- Lubricant
- Culture media
- Occult blood test

Procedure

EXAMINATION SKILL AND FOCUS	TECHNIQUES AND RATIONALE
Inspection: Anus	Client in the forward-bending or side-lying (Sims') position. *This position permits directing of the index finger toward the umbilicus, promotes client comfort, and protects the client's modesty.* Anal area exposed. *Exposure permits inspection.* Your hand gloved. *Gloves prevent transmission of microorganisms.*
Palpation	1. Spread the client's buttocks apart. *This exposes the perianal and sacrococcygeal regions.* 2. Inspect the perianal and sacrococcygeal regions. 3. Lubricate the index finger of your dominant hand by applying lubricant on the gloved finger. *Lubrication facilitates insertion of the finger.* 4. Place your finger pad across the client's anus. 5. Instruct the client to bear down. *This helps the external sphincter relax to facilitate easy insertion of the examining finger.* 6. Assess the tone of the anal sphincter. *This detects any neurological problems or lifestyle-related practice.*
Palpation: Rectum	1. Flex your fingertip and insert the finger gently into the client's anal canal. *Somatic nerve fibres supply anal canal.* 2. Insert your finger in the direction of the umbilicus. *Using a natural angle reduces discomfort.* 3. Offer the client tissues to perform personal hygiene. *The client removes the lubricant before dressing self.*

Adapted from Skillen, D. L. (2008). Anus, rectum, and prostate examination. In T. C. Stephen, R. A. Day, & D. L. Skillen (Eds.), *A syllabus for adult health assessment* (p. 97). Edmonton, AB: Faculty of Nursing, University of Alberta.

descend against the fingertip. Acute rectal pain may be associated with irritation, fissures, inflamed or thrombosed hemorrhoids, or rock-hard stools in constipation.

Anterior Rectal Surface. In female clients, on the anterior surface of the rectum, you can assess the posterior region of the cervix, which will feel like a small round mass. Do not mistake a retroverted uterus or a tampon in the vagina for a tumour. In male clients, with experience, you will be able to palpate the prostate through the anterior rectal surface.

Prostate

Palpation. The prostate gland is palpable anteriorly as a rounded, heart-shaped structure, about 2.5 to 4 cm in diameter, protruding less than 1 cm into the rectum. A small median groove separates the gland into two lateral lobes. The surface is smooth, elastic or rubbery, and nontender. With experience, you will be able to palpate to determine the size, shape, and consistency. The gland usually is firm and without nodules, bogginess, or tenderness. Hardness or nodules may indicate the presence of a cancerous lesion. Prostate enlargement is classified based on the extent of projection into the rectum: grade I is 1 to 2 cm protrusion; grade II, 2 to 3 cm; grade III, 3 to 4 cm; grade IV, more than 4 cm (Seidel et al., 2006).

Age-Related Changes. Usually, the prostate starts to enlarge in middle life. If the person is straining down, the perianal musculature may relax, causing less control of the external sphincter muscle.

Documentation. Record your findings from the inspection and palpation of the anus and rectum (Table 32–39).

Assessing the Extremities

To assess the extremities, you need to examine four body systems: integumentary, neurological, peripheral vascular, and musculoskeletal. Inspection and palpation of the integument and pulses of the extremities, as well as measurement of blood pressure, form part of the assessment of the integumentary and vascular systems. Examination of musculoskeletal function includes assessment of the joints and surrounding tissues, in addition to range of motion. Assessment of the neurological system includes examination of the cranial nerves, sensation, coordination, muscle tone, muscle strength, and reflexes. You will integrate aspects of the musculoskeletal and neurological examinations when observing the client's gait, movements in bed, and other activities that require coordination. You will routinely test cranial nerve function when examining the head and neck. Table 32–40 contains the health history for the assessment of the vascular, musculoskeletal, and neurological systems in the upper and lower extremities. Box 32–29 presents the focus for health promotion for the extremities.

➤ TABLE 32-39 Examples of Documentation of the Assessment of the Anus and Rectum

Focus of Assessment	Expected Findings
Perianal and sacrococcygeal area	Skin smooth and uniform; no lesions
Anus	Pigmented; tightly closed; no lesions Anal canal smooth and nontender
Rectum	All surfaces smooth and uniform; stool on glove is brown

Adapted from Skillen, D. L. (2004). Documentation. In Faculty of Nursing, University of Alberta. (Ed.), *Health assessment self-test modules* (WebCT Vista). Edmonton, AB: Author.

Assessing the Upper Extremities

Inspection

Integument and Muscle Mass. Roll up the sleeves of the client's gown to fully expose the arms and part of the shoulders. Inspect the integument and muscle mass of the hands, arms, and shoulders, critically comparing findings from both sides (Skill 32–23). Expect to find symmetrical muscle development and no wasting or **fasciculations** (localized twitching of muscle cells innervated by a single motor neuron). Inspect for signs of skin inflammation (swelling and redness), and note any lesions, including scars, nevi, freckles, and petechiae, or changes in skin colour due to sun or chemical exposure. Depending on the client's work, you may observe calluses and thickened epidermis on the palmar surfaces of the hands as a result of pressure and friction. Assess the nails for surface integrity and colour. Nail beds may be cyanosed (indicating hypoxia) or pale (indicating anemia).

Range of Motion. Inspect the arms for active ROM when the client voluntarily and without assistance moves the limb against gravity (see Skill 32–23). It helps if you demonstrate the required ROM. In healthy adults, expect bilaterally symmetrical and full ROM. Document any restrictions to ROM. If the client is unable to perform active ROM, attempt to move the supported joint through a passive ROM without client assistance. If you achieve passive ROM, you can determine that the client lacks the muscle strength to move the joint. If you cannot achieve passive ROM, you can determine that the problem lies within the joint.

safety alert Never force a joint through ROM if pain or muscle spasm is present.

Palpation. Use the dorsum of your hand to palpate the integument for temperature, expecting uniform warmth and slight moisture bilaterally (Skill 32–24). The client's hands may be cooler than the upper arms if the ambient air temperature is cool. In a warm environment, or when the client is anxious, the palms, axillae, and skin may be noticeably moist. Expect the skin to be mobile (you can pinch a fold of skin easily; see Figure 32–7). If turgor (elasticity) is intact, the skin immediately returns to the original position when released. In dehydration, decreased skin turgor causes the skin to stay "tented" even when released. Nail plates are firm and uniformly thick. Assess **capillary refill**, to test blood circulation to the fingers, by pressing firmly, quickly, and gently on the nail plate. Pressure on the nail bed causes blanching; when pressure is released, the natural pink colour returns almost instantly (in 1 to 2 seconds).

Joints. Palpate the joints, noting size, shape, tenderness, and temperature. Warm, swollen, tender, or boggy joints may indicate inflammation and the presence of fluid in the joint. To assess the shoulder joint (see Skill 32–24), you must know the surface landmarks created by the bony structure of the shoulder girdle: the sternoclavicular

➤ TABLE 32-40 Health History for the Vascular, Musculoskeletal, and Neurological Assessment of the Extremities

Assessment Category	Rationale for Assessment
Vascular System	
Ask if the client experiences legs cramps, numbness or tingling in the extremities, cold hands or feet, leg pains, or swelling or cyanosis of the feet, ankles, or hands. Conduct a symptom analysis, as required.	These signs and symptoms indicate vascular disease.
Ask the client about use of tight-fitting hosiery or long-term sitting or lying with crossed legs.	These can impair venous return.
Inquire about any history of heart disease, hypertension, diabetes, or varicose veins and any related treatments.	These guide the focus or your assessment and interpretation of findings.
Musculoskeletal System	
Inquire about activity patterns, including type of exercise usually performed, and any alterations in usual habits; inquire about the effect of the alterations on activities of daily living, including bathing, feeding, dressing, toileting, ambulating, and recreational and sexual activities.	Provides baseline assessment to determine further investigation related to need for assistance.
Conduct a symptom analysis if pain or disability is reported.	Helps to determine the nature of the alteration.
Question the client about any involvement in sports, including contact or competitive sports.	These are risk factors for sports-related injuries.
Inquire about history of heavy alcohol use; smoking; constant dieting; calcium intake less than 500 mg daily; thin and light body frame; nulliparous status; menopause before age 45; family history of osteoporosis; menopause status; Caucasian, Asian, or northern European ancestry.	These are risk factors for osteoporosis.
Neurological System	
Ask the client about use of medications, including analgesics, antipsychotics, antidepressants, nervous system stimulants, alcohol, sedative-hypnotics, or recreational drugs.	These medications can alter the level of consciousness or cause behavioural changes.
Ask about any history of seizures or convulsions, and conduct a symptom analysis, as necessary.	Characteristics of seizures help determine the cause of the seizures.
Inquire about the presence of headaches, tremors, dizziness, vertigo, numbness or tingling in a body part, visual changes, weakness, pain, changes in speech, hearing, vision, taste, smell, or touch.	These signs and symptoms may indicate a pathological condition.
Ask the client or family members about any recent changes in behaviour, including mood changes, irritability, or memory loss, or any change in activity level.	May indicate pathology. Client may not notice changes immediately.
Inquire about past history of head or spinal cord injury, hypertension, or psychiatric disorders.	May provide information to guide assessment.
If an older adult displays sudden onset of confusion (delirium; see Box 32–9), review medications, gather information about possible serious infections, metabolic disturbances, heart failure, or severe anemia.	These conditions are potentially reversible.

(SC) joint, acromion, clavicle, and acromioclavicular (AC) joint. Detect the AC joint by asking the client to rotate the arm externally. Expect the joints to be nontender, to move smoothly, and to be free of crepitations (grating sensations) that result from roughened articular cartilage and suggest osteoarthritis. Locate the greater tubercle of the humerus by palpating over the lateral border of the acromion process, which forms the crest of the shoulder. Medial to the greater tubercle is the bicipital groove where the long head of the biceps tendon lies. Asking the client to externally rotate the arm makes the groove and the lesser tubercle more accessible. Gently palpate the biceps tendon; it rolls beneath the finger pads during external rotation of the arm and is nontender.

Muscle Tone. Muscle tone is the slight muscular tension retained in a voluntarily relaxed muscle. Assess tone before assessing strength. The state of the muscle tone guides your interpretation of your findings from strength testing (Skill 32–25). The client relaxes the arm, and you support and move it smoothly through ROM. Expect mild and even resistance. Range of motion may be difficult if the client has arm pain. Increased or decreased muscle tone signals a possible neurological deficit and alterations during strength testing. Hypertonicity means that your passive stretch of a muscle is met with considerable resistance, but continued movement eventually causes the muscle to relax. Hypotonic muscle feels flabby or flaccid, and the arm may hang loosely.

✱ BOX 32-29 FOCUS ON PRIMARY HEALTH CARE

Extremities

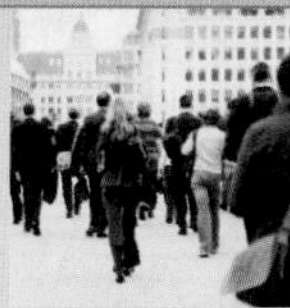

- Warning signs and symptoms for vascular conditions
- Prevention of osteoporosis
- Physical activity
- Safety measures for clients with sensory or motor impairments
- Skin self-assessment in at-risk clients
- Avoidance of exposure to neurotoxins in the workplace

Muscle Strength. Assess the strength of muscle groups (see Skill 32–25). Ask the client to either extend or flex the muscles around a joint and then apply an opposing force. For example, when testing the strength of wrist extension, ask the client to extend the wrist and then resist as you attempt to flex the wrist. When possible, test the muscle strength of both limbs at the same time, as this

➤ SKILL 32-23 Inspecting the Upper Extremities

Equipment

- Reflex hammer
- Splintered tongue blade or cotton-tip applicator
- Tuning fork (128 Hz)
- Cotton ball

Procedure

EXAMINATION SKILL AND FOCUS	TECHNIQUES AND RATIONALE
Skin, nails, hair, symmetry	**1.** Fully expose the hands and arms of the sitting or supine client. **2.** Inspect the skin, nails, and symmetry of both arms and hands.
Range of motion (ROM)	Inspect ROM. Full ROM includes: • Flexion and extension of the distal and proximal interphalangeal joints. • Flexion, extension, abduction, and adduction of the metacarpophalangeal joints. • Flexion, extension, abduction, adduction, and opposition of the thumbs. • Flexion, extension, and ulnar and radial deviation of the wrists. • Flexion, extension, supination, and pronation of the elbows. • Flexion, extension, adduction, abduction, external rotation, and internal rotation of the shoulders. Each arm is inspected, either separately or simultaneously and the findings compared. *Comparison detects alterations.* Only if the client is unable to perform active ROM should you attempt passive ROM.
Thumbs	Instruct the client to: **1.** Supinate the hands. **2.** Touch the base of the fifth finger with the thumb (flexion). **3.** Move the thumb back and forth away from the fingers (extension). **4.** Move the thumb anteriorly away from palm (abduction). **5.** Move the thumb back down (adduction). **6.** Touch the tip of the thumb to each fingertip (opposition).
Fingers	Instruct the client to: **1.** Make a fist (flexion), with the thumb across the knuckles. **2.** Straighten the fingers (extension). **3.** Spread the extended fingers (abduction). **4.** Close the extended fingers together (adduction).
Wrists	Inspect each wrist separately. Instruct the client to: **1.** Flex the wrist. **2.** Extend the wrist. **3.** With your help, stabilize the forearm and hand in supination. **4.** Move the hand medially (radial deviation). **5.** Move the hand laterally (ulnar deviation).
Elbows	Instruct the client to: **1.** Bend the elbows (flexion). **2.** Straighten the elbows (extension). **3.** Hold the flexed elbows close to the sides and turn the palms upward (supination). *Ensures that only the ROM of elbow (not shoulder) is tested.* **4.** Turn the palms downward (pronation).
Shoulders	Instruct the client to: **1.** Extend the arms forward (flexion). **2.** Extend the straightened arms as far back as possible (extension). **3.** Bring the straightened arms across the anterior midline (adduction). **4.** Lift the arms laterally in an arc, starting from the sides and ending with both arms extended above the head, palms facing (abduction). **5.** Place the hands behind the neck (external rotation). **6.** Place hands behind small of back (internal rotation).

From Stephen, T. C., Day, R. A., & Skillen, D. L. (Eds.). (2008). *A syllabus for adult health assessment* (pp. 45–47). Edmonton, AB: Faculty of Nursing, University of Alberta.

➤ SKILL 32-24 Palpating Temperature and Joints of the Upper Extremities

Equipment

- None

Procedure

EXAMINATION SKILL AND FOCUS	TECHNIQUES AND RATIONALE
Palpation: Temperature	1. Use the dorsum of your hands or fingers to compare the temperature of each hand with that of the forearm and upper arm above it. *Dorsal skin is thin and sensitive to temperature.* 2. Compare both sides. *Comparison detects alterations.*
Palpation: Joints	Instruct the client to indicate whether any tenderness is experienced during joint palpation. Palpate both limbs separately, and compare the findings. *One or more joints may become swollen and inflamed due to trauma or chronic conditions.*
Fingers: interphalangeal (IP) joints	1. Palpate with the thumb and index finger of one hand all of the distal and proximal IP joints of the fingers and thumb of both hands at the medial and lateral aspects of each joint. *Palpation detects tenderness and bogginess.*
Fingers: metacarpophalangeal (MCP) joints	1. Palpate with the thumbs of both your hands the MCP joints of the client's hands just distal to and on each side of the knuckle.
Wrists	1. Palpate the medial and lateral surfaces of each wrist (distal radius and ulna). 2. Palpate each wrist dorsally with your thumbs and ventrally with your fingers.
Elbows	1. Support the slightly flexed left arm of the client with your left hand and forearm. *Palpation detects the presence of nodules around the elbow.* 2. Palpate: A. The olecranon process. B. The groove on either side of the olecranon process. C. The lateral and medial epicondyles. 3. Inquire about any tenderness. 4. Repeat on the right side.
Shoulders	1. Cup a hand over each of the client's exposed shoulders. *Crepitus in the shoulder may be felt (and sometimes heard) when the client is performing ROM.* 2. Feel for crepitus during adduction, abduction, and external and internal rotations. 3. Palpate the acromioclavicular (AC) and the sternoclavicular (SC) joints. *Palpation of the SC and AC joints and the biceps tendon detects tenderness.* 4. Palpate the biceps groove for the long head of the biceps tendon. 5. Inquire about any tenderness during steps 3 and 4.

From Stephen, T. C., Day, R. A., & Skillen, D. L. (Eds.). (2008). *A syllabus for adult health assessment* (pp. 46–48). Edmonton, AB: Faculty of Nursing, University of Alberta.

facilitates the best comparison. Expect the client to demonstrate strength commensurate with the muscle mass present. Compared with women, men exhibit greater strength because of their greater muscle mass. The client should demonstrate sustained and bilaterally equal strength and resistance. Grade muscle strength from 0 (no active movement) to 5+ (strong active sustained resistance). See Table 32–41 for a grading scheme. If you identify any weakness, compare the size of the muscle with its counterpart on the other side by measuring the circumference of the muscle with a tape. Arophied muscle feels soft and contracts with less force (muscle weakness).

Peripheral Pulses. Palpate the peripheral pulses with your finger pads or thumbs, as both are sensitive to arterial pulsations. You get better access to the arteries if the client slightly flexes the arm at the elbow and wrist. Apply firm pressure, but avoid occluding the pulse. Arterial walls are elastic and easily palpable. When a pulse is difficult to find, vary the pressure, and feel all around the area. A hard, inelastic artery suggests arteriosclerosis. Assess the pulses for rate, rhythm, amplitude, and equality (see Chapter 31). Grade the amplitude (force at which blood is ejected against the arterial wall) on a scale of 0 (absent) to 4+ (bounding; Table 32–42). The expected amplitude is 2+. Pulse amplitude should be consistent between pulsations. Variability in amplitude suggests pathology.

Assess all peripheral pulses for equality and symmetry, and compare findings from both arms (Skill 32–26). Pulse inequality may indicate a local obstruction. You can palpate the brachial artery at two locations (Figure 32–29). If brachial circulation is blocked, the hands do not receive adequate blood flow. If circulation is impaired in the radial or ulnar arteries, the hand still receives adequate perfusion because an interconnection between the two arteries guards against arterial occlusion.

Epitrochlear Nodes. Epitrochlear nodes are located between the biceps and triceps muscles about 3 cm above the medial epicondyle on the inner aspect of the forearm. They drain the medial aspect of forearms and hands. Do not expect to find a palpable epitrochlear node (see Skill 32–26).

Coordination. Coordination is achieved through the integrated function of four components of the nervous system: (1) the motor system provides strength; (2) the sensory system contributes to position sense; (3) the vestibular system contributes to balance by integrating eye, head, and body movements; and (4) the cerebellar system manages rhythmic movements and upright posture. Use two rapid alternating tests and one point-to-point test to assess the coordination of the upper extremities. It helps to demonstrate each and provide verbal instructions to the client (Skill 32–27). Expect the alternating

➤ SKILL 32-25 Assessing Muscle Tone and Strength of the Upper Extremities

Equipment

- None

Procedure

EXAMINATION SKILL AND FOCUS	TECHNIQUES AND RATIONALE
Palpation: Muscle tone	1. Support the client's relaxed arm at the hand and elbow. *Tone is the residual tension.*
	2. Move each arm of the client (fingers, wrist, elbow, shoulder) through a modified passive range of motion (ROM).
	3. Note the resistance.
	4. Test muscle tone before testing muscle strength. *Results of strength testing may be misinterpreted without knowledge of the residual tension.*
Muscle strength Fingers	1. Place your two crossed fingers in each hand of the client. *Avoids injury to you during grip testing.*
	2. Instruct the client to squeeze your fingers firmly (grip). *Tests the integrity of C7, C8, T1.*
	3. Compare findings from both sides; you may assess both sides simultaneously.
	4. Try, against resistance, to force the client's outspread fingers of each hand together (abduction). *Tests the integrity of C8, T1, and the ulnar nerve.*
	5. Instruct the client to touch the thumb to the tip of the little finger.
	6. Ask the client to resist the pull of your thumb against his or her thumb (opposition). *Tests the integrity of C8, T1, and the median nerve.*
	7. Compare findings from both sides; you may assess both sides simultaneously. *Comparison helps detect alterations.*
Wrists	1. Instruct the client to hold the flexed elbows close to the sides with the forearm in pronation. *Isolates movement at the wrist.*
	2. Instruct the client to make a fist and flex the wrists.
	3. Try to pull the client's fist up against resistance (flexion). *Tests integrity of C6 to C8, and the radial nerve.*
	4. Instruct the client to make a fist and extend the wrist.
	5. Try to pull the client's fist down against resistance (extension).
	6. Compare findings from both sides; you may assess both sides simultaneously.
Elbows	1. Instruct the client to flex the arm at the elbow.
	2. Try, against resistance, to extend the client's flexed elbows (biceps). *Tests strenth of biceps (C5, C6) and triceps (C6 to C8) muscles.*
	3. Instruct the client to flex the arm at the elbow.
	4. Try, against resistance, to further flex the client's elbows (triceps).
	5. Compare findings from both sides; you may assess both sides simultaneously.
Shoulders	1. Instruct the client to raise both extended arms above the head. *Tests strength of shoulder girdle, primarily the abductor muscles (deltoid and supraspinatus, C5, C6).*
	2. Try, against resistance, to force the client's arms to the sides.
	3. Compare findings from both sides; you may assess both sides simultaneously.

From Stephen, T. C., Day, R. A., & Skillen, D. L. (Eds.). (2008). *A syllabus for adult health assessment* (pp. 48–49). Edmonton, AB: Faculty of Nursing, University of Alberta.

➤ TABLE 32-41 Muscle Strength Grading Scheme

	Scales		
Muscle Function Level	**Grade**	**% Normal**	**Lovett Scale**
No evidence of contractility	0	0	0 (zero)
Slight contractility, no movement	1	10	T (trace)
Full range of motion, gravity eliminated*	2	25	P (poor)
Full range of motion with gravity	3	50	F (fair)
Full range of motion against gravity, some resistance	4	75	G (good)
Full range of motion against gravity, full resistance	5	100	N (normal)

*Passive movement.

Adapted from Barkauskas, V. H., Baumann, L. C., & Darling-Fisher, C. S. (2002). *Health and physical assessment* (3rd ed., p. 433). St. Louis, MO: Mosby.

TABLE 32-42 Grading of Peripheral Pulses

Description of Amplitude	Grade
Absent, not palpable	0
Pulse diminished, barely palpable	1+
Easily palpable, brisk, expected	2+
Full pulse, increased	3+
Strong, bounding pulse, cannot be obliterated	4+

movements with either hand to be smooth, rapid, and rhythmic. The dominant hand often exhibits slightly more dexterity. Point-to-point testing should demonstrate movements that are smooth, accurate, and without tremor. Deviations suggest pathology (cerebellar or motor systems). If the client's movements are accurate with eyes open but not with eyes closed, position sense may be impaired.

Sensory System. Assess the integrity of the sensory nerve tracts within the spinal column, medulla, and sensory cortex (Skill 32–28). Pain and temperature sensations are carried in the spinothalamic tracts; if the pain sensation is intact, temperature is usually not tested. Position and vibration sensations are carried in the posterior columns. Touch sensation is carried in both spinal tracts: crude-touch fibres are carried in the spinothalamic tracts; fine-touch fibres are carried in the posterior columns. Perception of sensory stimuli should be equal on both sides of the client's body. Assess major sensory nerves using your knowledge of the sensory dermatome zones (Figure 32–30), which are innervated by specific dorsal root cutaneous nerves. The client must keep the eyes closed during all sensory testing so he or she cannot see what stimulus you use.

Pain and Light Touch. Systematically assess the dermatomes of the shoulder (C4), upper arm (C6 and T1), forearm (C5 and T1), and hand (C6–C8; see Skill 32–28; see Figure 32–30) to assess perception of pain and light touch. Use a splintered tongue blade or cotton-tipped applicator as the pain stimulus. Vary the rhythm or pace of dermatome testing to ensure that the client responds to an actual touch sensation rather than an anticipated touch. Compare the sensations of pain and light touch in both arms by applying the stimulus first on

SKILL 32-26 Palpating Pulses and Epitrochlear Nodes in the Upper Extremities

Equipment

- None

Procedure

EXAMINATION SKILL AND FOCUS	TECHNIQUES AND RATIONALE
Palpation:	1. Palpate the brachial artery with your finger pads or thumbs at the antecubital crease (fossa) **OR** above the elbow in the groove between the biceps and triceps muscles.
Brachial pulse	2. Compare findings from both sides. *Comparison helps detect alterations.*
Radial pulse	1. Palpate the radial artery with your finger pads on the lateral flexor surface of the client's wrist. *Slight flexion at the wrist may provide better access to the radial artery.*
	2. Compare findings from both sides.
Palpation: Epitrochlear nodes	1. Support the client's right forearm with your right hand as the client flexes the elbow about 90 degrees. *Provides better access to nodes.*
	2. Palpate for the epitrochlear node in the groove between the biceps and triceps muscles with the finger pads of your left hand medially and approximately 3 cm above the medial epicondyle.
	3. Reverse the hand position to examine the client's left arm.

From Stephen, T. C., Day, R. A., & Skillen, D. L. (Eds.). (2008). *A syllabus for adult health assessment* (p. 49–50). Edmonton, AB: Faculty of Nursing, University of Alberta.

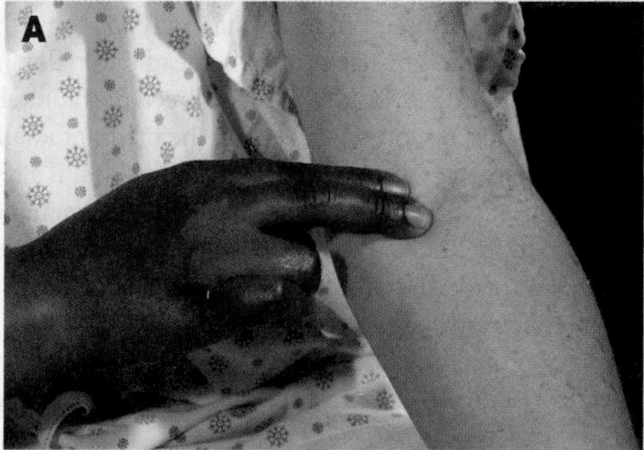

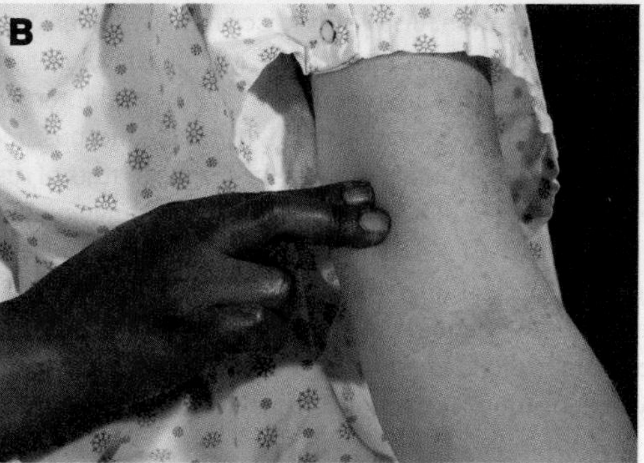

Figure 32-29 A, Brachial palpation in the antecubital fossa. B, Brachial palpation between the biceps and triceps muscles.
Source: From Skillen, D. L., Day, R. A., Anderson, M. C., Stephen, T. C., Gilbert, J. A., & Day, L. W. (2004). *Physical examination images* [CD-ROM]. Edmonton, AB: Faculty of Nursing, University of Alberta.

➤ SKILL 32-27 Inspecting Coordination in the Upper Extremities

Equipment

- None

Procedure

EXAMINATION SKILL AND FOCUS	TECHNIQUES AND RATIONALE
Coordination	Test each hand separately. *Testing separately ensures that coordination in one hand is not affected by the other.*
Rapid alternating testing	1. Instruct the client to pat the thigh as rapidly as possible with the palm and the dorsum of hand alternately. 2. Compare findings from both sides. 3. Instruct the client to touch the distal joint of the thumb with the index fingertip repeatedly, as rapidly as possible. 4. Compare findings from both sides. *Comparison helps detect alterations.*
Point-to-point testing	Instruct the client to: 1. Extend the arm. 2. Alternately touch the nose, then your finger with fully extended arm. 3. Alter the finger position. 4. Hold the finger in one place. 5. Raise the extended arm over the head and then lower it to touch the finger. 6. Repeat the above with eyes closed. *Tests position sense.* 7. Repeat steps 5 and 6 with other arm.

From Stephen, T. C., Day, R. A., & Skillen, D. L. (Eds.). (2008). *A syllabus for adult health assessment* (p. 49). Edmonton, AB: Faculty of Nursing, University of Alberta.

one arm and then on the symmetrical dermatome on the other arm. Expect pain and light touch sensations to be intact bilaterally over dermatomes C4–C8 and T1. If the sensations are unequal, map out the area of sensory loss (hyposensitivity) or hypersensitivity by testing from the area of decreased sensitivity and moving proximally until the client reports a change in sensory perception.

Vibration Sense. Testing the sensation of vibration assesses the integrity of the posterior columns of the sensory system (see Skill 32–28). The client must keep the eyes closed during the testing. Grasp the stem of the 128-Hz tuning fork, tap the tines of the fork on the heel of your hand, and place on the distal interphalangeal (DIP) joint. Expect the client to report a buzz-like sensation at the DIP joint and to correctly indicate when the vibration stops. If the client does not feel the vibration, continue testing by progressing upward through the proximal interphalangeal (PIP) joint, metacarpophalangeal (MCP) joint, wrist, and elbow until vibrations are felt by the client.

Position Sense. Testing position sense also assesses the integrity of the posterior columns of the sensory system. Focus on one digit separated from the others (see Skill 32–28). Always return the digit to the neutral position before testing again. Ask the client to identify, with eyes closed, if digit is "up" or "down."

Discriminative Sensation. Assessing discriminative sensation involves three tests of fine touch that require a higher level of sensory cortex function, as clients are required to analyze and interpret a stimulus with eyes closed. Sensations of light touch and position sense must be intact or nearly intact for positive results in tests of discriminative sensation (see Skill 32–28). Unexpected findings suggest pathology in the sensory cortex and posterior columns. Test for stereognosis, extinction, and graphesthesia (Figure 32–31; see Skill 32–28). In the test for extinction, the client is expected to report that two places were touched and identify the areas touched. If the client identifies only one location, extinction is considered impaired.

Reflexes. The neurological system has defence mechanisms (reflexes) that facilitate quick reactions to potentially harmful stimuli and contribute to the maintenance of muscle tone and balance. Reflexes range from monosynaptic to polysynaptic. The monosynaptic reflex arc pathway is shown in Figure 32–32. Each muscle contains a small sensory unit (spindle) that detects changes in the length of the muscle fibre. If the tendon of a partially stretched muscle is tapped with the reflex hammer, muscle spindles lengthen. The spindle sends impulses along afferent nerve pathways to the dorsal horn of the spinal cord segment. In milliseconds, impulses reach the spinal cord to synapse with the efferent motor neuron. A motor nerve sends impulses back to the muscle, causing the monosynaptic reflex response.

Two types of reflexes are tested: deep tendon and cutaneous. In the upper extremities, test deep tendon reflexes in the biceps (Figure 32–33A), triceps (Figure 32–33B), and brachioradialis (supinator). The correct technique involves consistently holding the reflex hammer somewhat loosely between your thumb and fingers and swinging the head of the hammer in an arc using a rapid wrist action (not elbow action).

Use only the required force to elicit an expected response, and apply the same amount of force bilaterally for comparison purposes. Either the pointed or flat end of the head of a reflex hammer is useful for this purpose, as long as it is directed accurately. The flat end causes less discomfort when testing the brachioradialis reflex.

Compare the reflex responses on both sides. If a reflex is *symmetrically* absent or diminished, use a reinforcement technique. Just before striking the tendon, ask the client to clench the teeth or press firmly on the thigh with the free hand. This increases the likelihood of the reflex arc being completed.

As your technique can affect the reflex, practise it to ensure consistency (Skill 32–29). Expect a reflex response at all sites. Grade

➤ SKILL 32-28 Assessing Sensation in the Upper Extremities

Equipment

- Tongue blade
- Cotton ball
- 128 Hz tuning fork
- Familiar small objects

EXAMINATION SKILL AND FOCUS	TECHNIQUES AND RATIONALE
Inspection and palpation:	Both arms are tested.
Sensation	Demonstrate how sharp, dull, and light touches feel before beginning tests. *The client learns what to expect and report.*
Superficial pain	**1.** Instruct the client to close the eyes and describe each touch as "sharp" or "dull." *Ensures vision does not influence perception.*
	2. Touch the client's arms lightly and alternately in corresponding areas with the sharp end of a splintered tongue blade (occasionally using the blunt end), covering the C4 to C8 and T1 dermatomes in the upper arms, forearms, and hands. *The blunt (dull) end validates client perception of pressure, not pain, and assesses the reliability of client responses. Further testing with the sharp end assesses client perception of pain in the area.*
	3. Compare findings from both sides. *Comparison helps detect asymmetry.*
Light touch	**1.** Instruct the client to close the eyes and report each time the touch of a cotton wisp is perceived.
	2. Touch the client's arms lightly, avoiding pressure and alternately in corresponding areas, with a cotton wisp, testing the C4 to C8 and T1 dermatomes in the upper arms, forearms, and hands. *The touch must be light, as touch is being tested, not pressure.*
	3. Vary the intervals between touches. *By varying the rhythm of the touches, you can be more certain that the client is responding to the touch.*
	4. Compare findings from both sides.
Vibration	**1.** Instruct the client to close the eyes and describe the sensation felt.
	2. Place a vibrating 128-Hz tuning fork firmly over the distal interphalangeal (DIP) joint of one finger and proceed proximally to the proximal interphalangeal (PIP) and metacarpophalangeal (MCP) joints, and so on, until vibrations are felt and reported. *Vibrations from the 128-Hz tuning fork can be felt through bone. Asking the client to report cessation of the vibrations validates its perception.*
	3. Compare findings from both sides.
Position sense	**1.** Demonstrate the "up" and "down" positions of a finger. *Identifying the test finger ensures that adjacent digits do not influence the sensation felt.*
	2. Instruct the client to close the eyes and identify the position of the finger.
	3. Grasp the distal phalanx by the medial and lateral aspects and move it "up" or "down." Ensure that adjacent digits are not involved.
	4. Compare findings from both sides.
Inspection and palpation: Tactile discrimination	Both sides are tested.
Stereognosis	**1.** Instruct the client to close the eyes and identify the object placed in the palm.
	2. Place a small, familiar object in each palm, one at a time. The object can only be manipulated by the hand being tested. *Coins, safety pins, and keys are examples of familiar objects.*
	3. Compare findings from both sides.
Graphesthesia	**1.** Instruct the client to close the eyes and identify the number being drawn on the skin. *Ensures that you draw the number in one connected movement while facing the client.*
	2. Draw a number with a blunt object on the palm of the client's hand positioned facing toward the client.
	3. Compare findings from both sides.
Extinction	**1.** Instruct the client to close the eyes and identify the area that is touched.
	2. Touch the client in corresponding areas on both arms simultaneously. *Corresponding areas must be touched simultaneously to accurately assess extinction.*
	3. Ask the client to identify the areas touched.

From Stephen, T. C., Day, R. A., & Skillen, D. L. (Eds.). (2008). *A syllabus for adult health assessment* (p. 50–51). Edmonton, AB: Faculty of Nursing, University of Alberta.

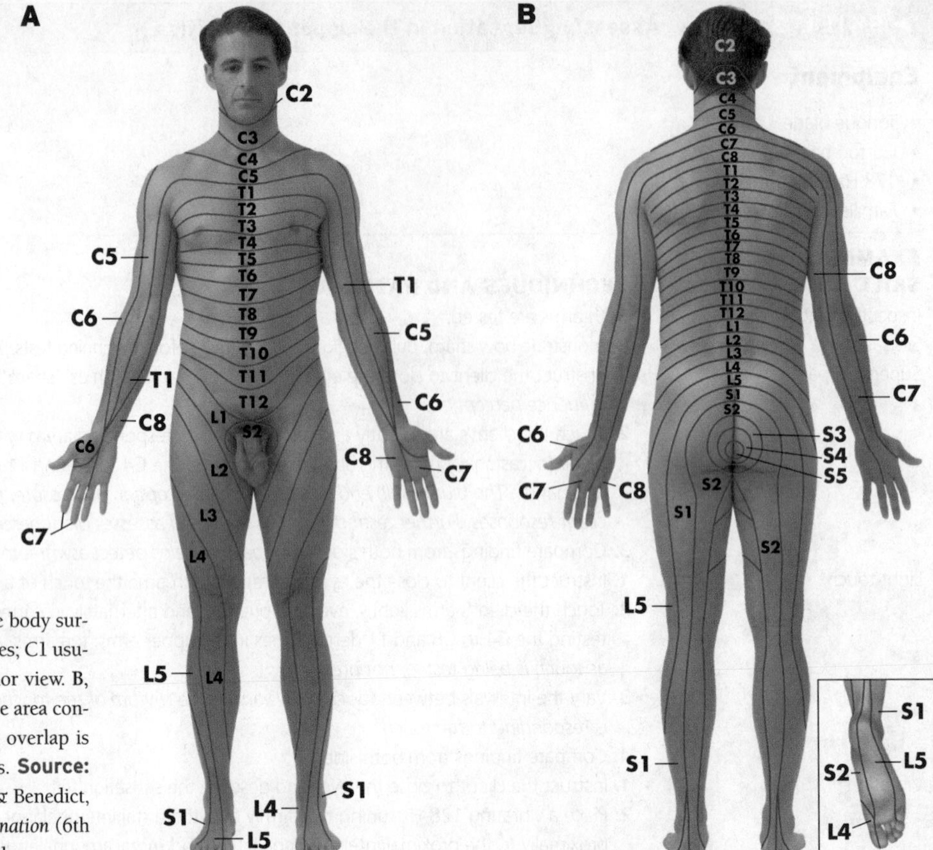

Figure 32-30 Dermatomes of the body, the body surface areas innervated by particular spinal nerves; C1 usually has no cutaneous distribution. A, Anterior view. B, Posterior view. A distinct separation of surface area controlled by each dermatome is apparent, but overlap is almost always present between spinal nerves. **Source:** From Seidel, H. M., Ball, J. W., Dains, J. E., & Benedict, G. W. (2006). *Mosby's guide to physical examination* (6th ed., p. 768, Figure 22–8). St. Louis, MO: Mosby.

responses on a scale of 0 (no response) to 4+ (hyperactive). Table 32–43 contains the grading scale. An average response is graded as 2+. A hyperactive response, accompanied by clonus (rapidly alternating involuntary contraction and relaxation of the skeletal muscle), or an absent response may signal a neuromuscular deviation. Some individuals may exhibit symmetrically diminished or even absent deep tendon reflexes in spite of not having any pathology.

Documentation. Record your findings from the inspection and palpation of the upper extremities (Table 32–44).

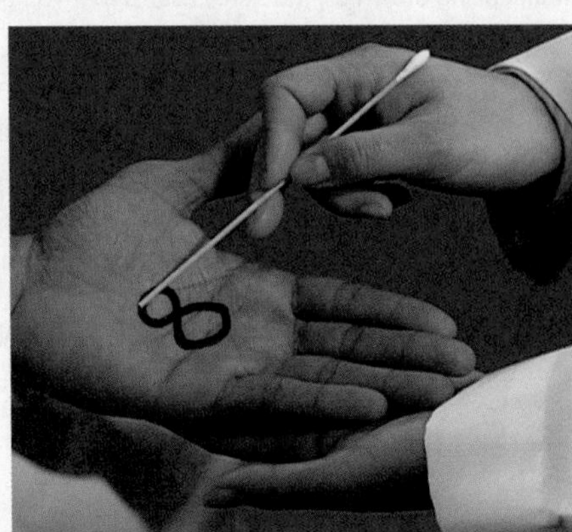

Figure 32-31 Graphesthesia. **Source:** From Seidel, H. M., Ball, J. W., Dains, J. E., & Benedict, G. W. (2006). *Mosby's guide to physical examination* (6th ed., p. 787, Figure 22–25c). St. Louis, MO: Mosby.

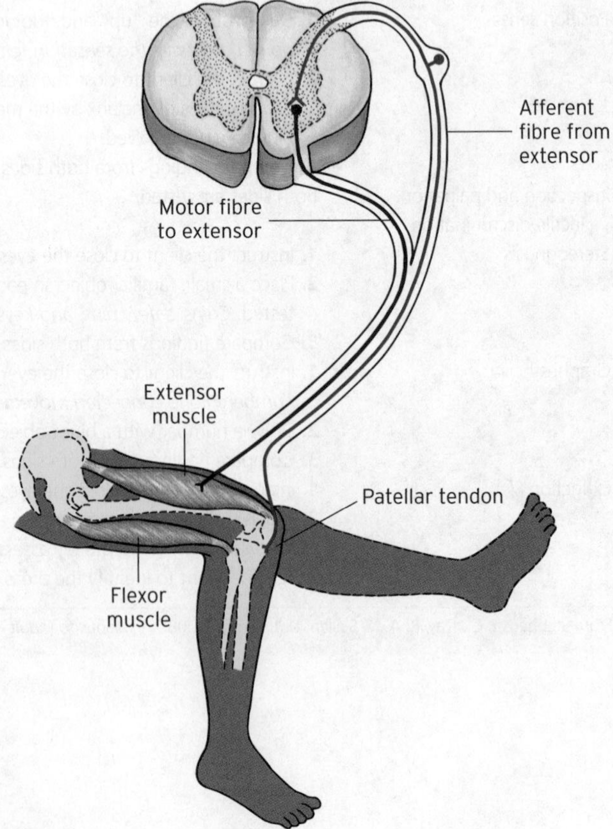

Figure 32-32 Pathway of the reflex arc.

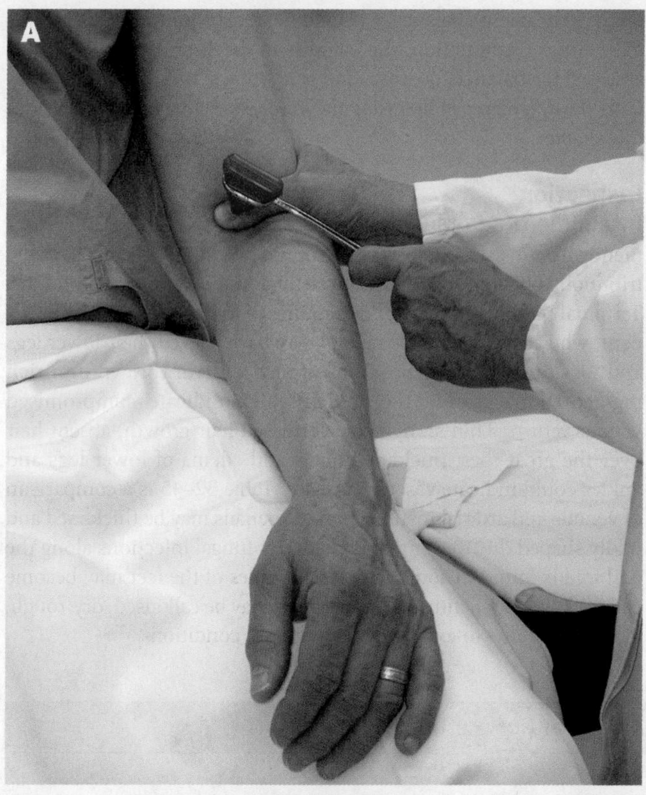

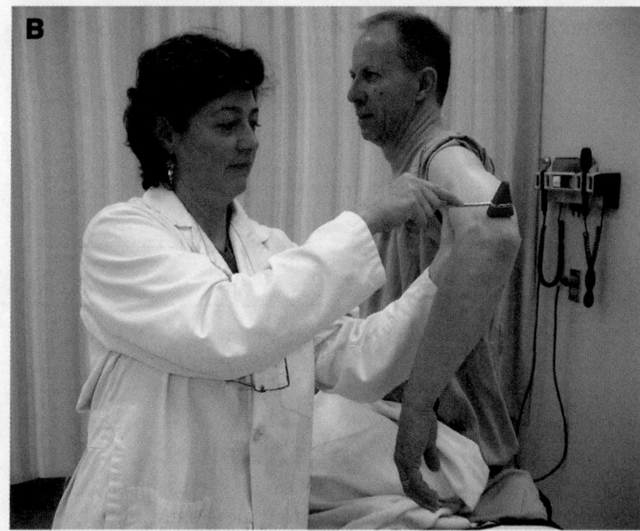

Figure 32-33 A, Biceps reflex. B, Triceps reflex. **Source:** From Skillen, D. L., Day, R. A., Anderson, M. C., Stephen, T. C., Gilbert, J. A., & Day, L. W. (2004). *Physical examination images* [CD-ROM]. Edmonton, AB: Faculty of Nursing, University of Alberta.

➤ SKILL 32-29 Assessing Deep Tendon Reflexes of the Upper Extremities

Equipment

- Percussion hammer

Procedure

EXAMINATION SKILL AND FOCUS	TECHNIQUES AND RATIONALE
Inspection and percussion: Deep tendon reflexes	Both sides are tested and findings compared. *Only if* responses are symmetrically diminished or absent should you use reinforcement (augmentation). *Failure to ensure that reflexes are symmetrically diminished before using reinforcement could mask unequal reflexes.* Strike the slightly stretched tendon briskly with the reflex hammer held loosely between your thumb and fingers and the head of the hammer swung freely in an arc using a rapid wrist action. *A consistent force ensures accurate results.*
Biceps reflex	1. Position the client with the arm supported and relaxed, the elbow flexed, and the palm placed downward on the thigh (in a seated client) or the abdomen (in a supine client). *A relaxed arm ensures a valid response.* 2. Use the hammer to tap your own thumb placed over the client's biceps tendon at the antecubital fossa (crease). *The pressure of the thumb provides a slight stretch.* 3. Compare the flexion of the forearm on each side. *Forearm flexion implies intact reflex arc at C5 to C6.*
Triceps reflex	1. Position the client with the arm supported and relaxed and the elbow flexed **OR** abducted and flexed at the right angle, in the "hang-to-dry" position. 2. Use the hammer to tap the triceps tendon 2 to 5 cm above the elbow. 3. Compare the extension of the forearm on each side. *Forearm extension suggests intact reflex arc at C6 to C7.*
Brachioradialis reflex	1. Position the client with the arm resting on the lap (in a sitting client) or the abdomen (in a supine client), palm down, and forearm slightly pronated. 2. Use the hammer to tap the brachioradialis tendon 2 to 5 cm above the wrist. *The tap generates the needed slight stretch of the tendon.* 3. Compare the flexion and supination of the hand on each side. *Flexion and supination of the hand suggests intact reflex arc at C5 to C6.*

From Stephen, T. C., Day, R. A., & Skillen, D. L. (Eds.). (2008). *A syllabus for adult health assessment* (p. 51). Edmonton, AB: Faculty of Nursing, University of Alberta.

TABLE 32-43 Grading of Reflexes

Description of Response	Grade
No response (absent)	0
Somewhat diminished with slight muscle contraction	1+
Average, as expected, visible muscle twitch with movement of arm or leg	2+
Brisker than expected; exaggerated but acceptable	3+
Very brisk, with clonus; often associated with spinal cord disorders	4+

Assessing the Lower Extremities

Assess the integumentary, peripheral vascular, musculoskeletal, and neurological systems in the lower extremities. Many procedures are identical to those for the assessment of the upper extremities, but some are different. For example, during the **general survey**, you observe the client's balance, gait, and posture. For much of the lower extremities examination, the client is in the supine position but is assessed for balance, posture, and gait when standing and walking. *Only the differences in assessing the lower extremities are presented in this chapter.*

Inspection

Integument and Muscles. Expect symmetrical muscle development without fasciculations or wasting (Skill 32–30). Vellus hair distribution is bilaterally uniform over the toes, lower legs, and thighs. Terminal hair over the lower extremities of males is usually fully evident, whereas some female clients may have shaved their lower legs and toes. Inspect for depositions of hemosiderin (brown iron-rich pigmentation) around the ankles which indicate compromised venous return. Thin shiny skin, decreased hair growth, absent hair over the great toes, thickened nails, and edema of lower legs and ankles could indicate vascular disease. Table 32–45 is a comparison of venous and arterial insufficiencies. Toenails may be thickened and oddly shaped due to trauma. Evidence of fungal infections along the nail fold is found in some individuals. Soles of the feet may become callused due to repetitive pressure; heels may be calloused, dry, rough, and cracked due to exposure to harsh, dry conditions.

TABLE 32-44 Examples of Documentation of the Assessment of the Upper Extremities

Focus of Assessment	Expected Findings
Skin	Pink tone; moist; elastic; scattered nevi bilaterally. No other lesions visible. Fine, evenly distributed light-coloured hair over both arms and proximal and distal phalanges. Skin temperature uniformly warm over arms and hands. Turgor and mobility intact.
Muscles	Muscle mass symmetrical in size and contour, without atrophy or fasciculations—in hands, forearms, upper arm, and shoulder girdle.
Nails	Short; rounded; manicured, without polish. Nail bed firm. No lesions around cuticles.
Range of motion (ROM)	Full ROM—in thumbs, fingers, wrists, elbows, and shoulders. No discomfort reported with ROM.
Joints	Distal interphalangeal (DIP), proximal interphalangeal (PIP), and metacarpophalangeal (MCP) joints without tenderness, swelling, or bogginess to palpation bilaterally. Wrists, elbows, and shoulder girdle without tenderness or swelling to palpation bilaterally. Same temperature as surrounding skin in all joints.
Muscle tone	Slight tension felt to passive movements bilaterally.
Muscle strength	Strong, sustained (5+) bilaterally—in fingers, wrists, elbows, and shoulders.
Coordination	Performance of rapid alternating movements rapidly, smoothly, with even rhythm, dominant right side slightly faster than left. Point-to-point testing smooth and accurate bilaterally, with eyes open or closed.
Pulses	Radial and brachial pulses 2+ bilaterally. Rhythm regular.
Epitrochlear nodes	Nonpalpable bilaterally.
Sensation	Superficial pain and light touch intact bilaterally over dermatomes C4 to C8 and T1; vibration and position senses intact bilaterally at fingers.
Tactile discrimination	Stereognosis, graphesthesia, and extinction intact bilaterally.
Reflexes	Biceps, triceps, and brachioradialis reflexes 2+ bilaterally.

From Anderson, M. C. (2004). Documentation. In Faculty of Nursing, University of Alberta. (Ed.), *Health assessment self-test modules* (WebCT Vista). Edmonton, AB: Author.

➤ SKILL 32-30 Inspecting the Lower Extremities, Including Range of Motion

Equipment

- None

Procedure

EXAMINATION SKILL AND FOCUS	TECHNIQUES AND RATIONALE
Skin, nails, hair, symmetry	**1.** Fully expose the legs and feet of the supine client. *Symmetry of skin condition and hair distribution provides clues to vascular perfusion.* **2.** Inspect the skin, nails, muscle mass, and symmetry of both legs and feet. **3.** Inspect the knee for expected depressions on either side of the patella.
Range of motion	Test each leg either separately or simultaneously, and compare the findings. Only if the client is unable to perform active ROM would you attempt passive ROM. Full ROM includes: • Dorsiflexion, plantar flexion, inversion, and eversion of ankles. • Flexion and extension of knees. • Flexion, extension, adduction, abduction, and internal and external rotation of hips.
Toes	Instruct the client to: **1.** Bend the toes downward (flexion). **2.** Straighten the toes and point upward (extension).
Ankles	Instruct client to: **1.** Bring foot upward toward the shin (dorsiflexion). **2.** Bend foot downward away from the shin (plantar flexion). **3.** Tilt foot inward with sole toward midline (inversion), while you stabilize the ankle and hold the heel. **4.** Tilt foot outward with sole facing laterally (eversion), while you stabilize the ankle and hold the heel. Repeat on the other foot.
Hips and knees	**1.** Place your hand under the client's lumbar spine. *This stabilizes the pelvis; further flexion originates at the hip.* **2.** Instruct the client to bring each knee, by turns, up toward the chest and press it firmly on the abdomen (flexion at hip and knee). **3.** Note when the client's back touches your hand. **4.** Ensure that the client's opposite thigh remains flat on the table. **5.** Instruct the client to straighten the leg (extension).
Hips	**1.** Stabilize the pelvis by pressing on one anterosuperior iliac crest with your left hand. **2.** Grasp the opposite leg at the ankle with your right hand, and move that leg over the other leg (adduction). **3.** Repeat on the other side. **4.** Stabilize the pelvis by pressing on one anterosuperior iliac crest with your left hand. *At the end of the range for either abduction or adduction, the pelvis begins to move and is felt by your left hand on the anterosuperior iliac crest.* **5.** Grasp the opposite leg at the ankle, and abduct the leg until the iliac spine moves (abduction). **6.** Repeat on the other side. **7.** Flex the leg at the hip and knee to 90 degrees. **8.** Support the thigh with your left hand and the ankle with your right hand. **9.** Turn the lower leg medially (external rotation) and then laterally (internal rotation). **10.** Repeat on the other side.

From Stephen, T. C., Day, R. A., & Skillen, D. L. (Eds.). (2008). *A syllabus for adult health assessment* (pp. 51–53). Edmonton, AB: Faculty of Nursing, University of Alberta.

➤ TABLE 32-45 Signs of Venous and Arterial Insufficiency

Assessment Criterion	Venous	Arterial
Colour	Expected or cyanotic	Pale; worsened by elevation of extremity; dusky red when extremity lowered
Temperature	Expected	Cool (blood flow blocked to extremity)
Pulse	Expected	Decreased or absent
Edema	Often marked	Absent or mild
Skin changes	Brown pigmentation around ankles	Thin, shiny skin; decreased hair growth; thickened nails

Range of Motion. Assess for active ROM by focusing on the hip, knee, ankle, and toe joints (see Skill 32–30). In well adults, expect full ROM at the toes, ankles, knees, and hips. Figure 32–34 shows four expected movements at the hip: abduction, adduction, internal rotation, and external rotation.

Palpation

Temperature. Expect the skin to be uniformly warm (Skill 32–31). If the ambient air temperature is cool, both feet may feel cooler than shins and thighs. If one leg is cooler than the other, ensure that you look for additional indications of arterial insufficiency, such as absent hair on toes and thin, shiny skin over shins (see Table 32–45).

Peripheral Edema. Assess the dorsum of the foot, ankle, and lower leg for edema (see Figure 32–8; see Skill 32–31). In a client who must remain standing during working hours, slight edema (1+) is not unusual at the end of a work day. Table 32–46 provides a useful grading system based on depth and duration of pitting edema.

Joints. Palpate each joint separately for temperature, warmth, tenderness, and swelling or bogginess (sensation that fluid is present) (see Skill 32–31).

The knee joint is subject to wear and injury, making it a frequent site for degenerative changes such as osteoarthritis. Feel for crepitations and crackling or grating sounds produced by roughened bony surfaces rubbing together. Expect the patella to glide smoothly over the trochlear groove of the femur.

The tibiofemoral joint of the knee is lined with a synovial capsule. The suprapatellar pouch lies under the quadriceps muscle and patella and extends posteriorly to the popliteal fossa and laterally to fill the joint space. When inflamed, the synovial capsule produces fluid, causing bulging of the capsule that is evident on inspection and palpation. Access the tibiofemoral joint space by asking the client to flex the knee to about 90 degrees and keep the foot on the examining surface (Figure 32–35). The patellar tendon inserts on the tibial tuberosity on the anterior surface of the tibia. Slightly superior are the lateral and medial condyles of the tibia. Palpate the joint spaces created by the medial femoral epicondyle and the tibial condyle and by the lateral femoral epicondyle and the tibial condyle. Assess for warmth, tenderness, swelling, and bogginess. Expect joint margins to be smooth, nontender, and without swelling.

Muscle Tone. Although slightly more difficult to test because the leg is naturally longer and heavier than the arm, the muscle tone of the leg is also assessed (Skill 32–32). Pain in any joint of the legs may make the manoeuvre difficult to perform.

Muscle Strength. Beginning at the feet and moving proximally to the hips, assess the strength of the muscle groups in the legs (see Skill 32–32). Expect the client to demonstrate sustained strength

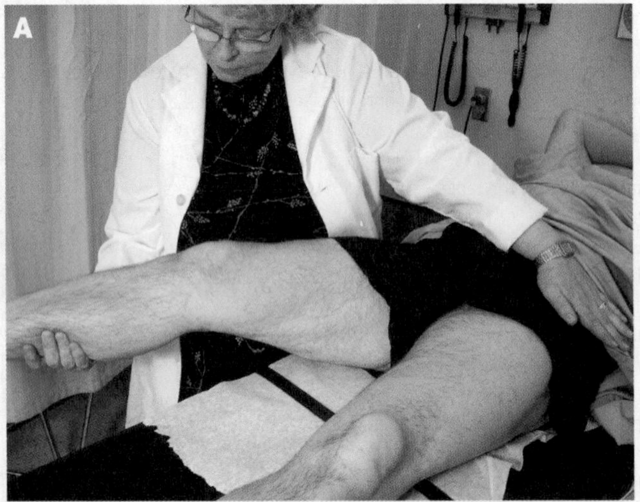

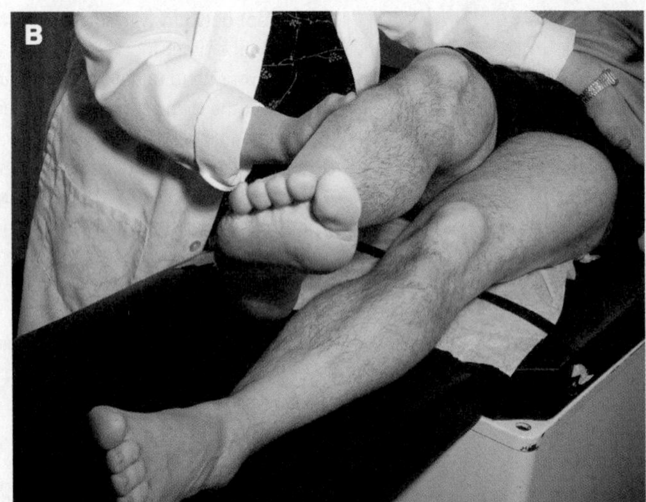

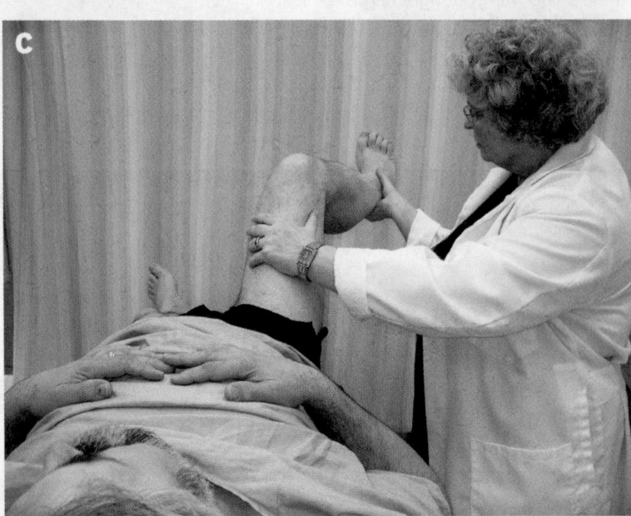

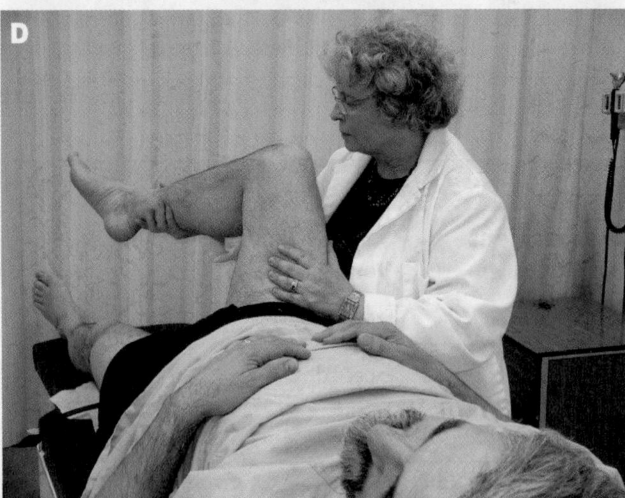

Figure 32-34 A, Hip abduction. B, Hip adduction. C, Hip internal rotation. D, Hip external rotation. **Source:** From Skillen, D. L., Day, R. A., Anderson, M. C., Stephen, T. C., Gilbert, J. A., & and Day, L. W. (2004). *Physical examination images* [CD-ROM]. Edmonton, AB: Faculty of Nursing, University of Alberta.

➤ SKILL 32-31 Palpating Joints and Skin Surface for Temperature and Edema

Equipment

- None

Procedure

EXAMINATION SKILL AND FOCUS	TECHNIQUES AND RATIONALE
Temperature	1. Use the dorsum of your hands or fingers to compare temperature of each foot with that of the lower leg and thigh above it. *Thin dorsal skin increases sensitivity to temperature.*
	2. Compare findings from both sides.
Edema	1. Press firmly and gently with your thumb for 5 seconds over the dorsum of each foot or medial malleolus. *Fluid in tissues disperses under pressure, leaving a depression that can be graded.*
	2. Assess for the extent of depression in the skin.
	3. Press firmly and gently with your thumb for 5 seconds over each shin.
	4. Assess for the extent and duration of depression in the skin.
Feet	
Interphalangeal (IP) joints	1. Palpate with the thumb and index finger of one hand all of the distal and proximal IP joints of the toes. *One or more joints may be swollen and inflamed due to trauma or chronic conditions.*
Metatarsophalangeal (MTP) joints	2. Compress each forefoot just proximal to the MTP joints with your thumb and fingers placed on the medial and lateral surfaces.
Heels	3. Palpate each heel.
Ankles	1. Place your thumbs dorsally and your fingers ventrally.
Ankle joint	2. Palpate the anterior aspect of each ankle joint.
Achilles tendon	3. Palpate along each Achilles tendon with your thumb and fingers.
Knees	1. Instruct the client to bend the knees (flexion).
	2. Cup your hands over each knee, by turns, as the client moves the leg back to the resting position (extension). *Crepitations may be felt and even heard.*
Suprapatellar pouch	3. Note any crepitations.
	4. Palpate each side of the quadriceps in progressive steps, from 10 cm above the superior border of the patella to the patellar pouch. *An inflamed synovial capsule produces fluid, distending the capsule.*
Patella	5. Continue palpating along the sides of the patella. *Distension is evident because the hollows on either side of the patella bulge and feel boggy on palpation.*
Tibiofemoral joint	6. Instruct the client to slightly flex the knee.
	7. Palpate the tibiofemoral joints (inferior, medial, and lateral to patella).

From Stephen, T. C., Day, R. A., & Skillen, D. L. (Eds.). (2008). *A syllabus for adult health assessment* (pp. 53–54). Edmonton, AB: Faculty of Nursing, University of Alberta.

commensurate with the muscle mass present. For example, Figure 32–36A demonstrates assessment of knee flexion strength; Figure 32–36B demonstrates assessment of knee extension strength. Expect equal strength and resistance. Grade muscle strength from 0 to 5+ (see Table 32–41). If you identify weakness, compare the size of the muscle in that leg with its counterpart in the other leg.

Peripheral Pulses. Assess the peripheral pulses for rate, rhythm, amplitude, and equality (Skill 32–33). An interconnection between the posterior tibial and the dorsalis pedis arteries guards against local arterial occlusion. The popliteal pulse is located behind the knee in the popliteal fossa and may be difficult to palpate. Expect the popliteal pulse to feel diffuse. The posterior tibial pulse is located behind and below the medial malleoli and is palpated with the finger pads, but it may be obscured by edema or fat. The dorsalis pedis pulse is located on the dorsum of the foot lateral to the extensor tendon of the great toe, but it may be congenitally absent. You may palpate these pulses simultaneously with your finger pads (Figure 32–37). Expect the amplitude of the pulses to attain a grade of 2+ bilaterally, but 1+ is acceptable in the feet. Asymmetrical pulses may indicate local obstruction.

Coordination. When assessing coordination in the lower extremities, one rapid alternating test and one point-to-point test are used (Skill 32–34). Test each leg separately, as the dexterity in one leg can affect the dexterity in the other. Expect rapid alternating movements (rhythmic patting of the foot against your hand) to be smooth and rhythmic, but not as rapid or dextrous as those in the same test for

➤ TABLE 32-46 Description and Grading of Dependent Edema

Description	Depression	Grade
Slight pitting, disappears rapidly	2 mm	1+
Deeper pitting, disappears in 10 to 15 seconds	4 mm	2+
Visibly swollen; dependent extremity; pitting takes more than 60 seconds to disappear	6 mm	3+
Grossly swollen and distorted dependent extremity; pitting may take 3 minutes to disappear	8 mm	4+

Adapted from Dillon, P. M. (2007). *Nursing health assessment: Clinical pocket guide* (p. 170). Philadelphia: F. A. Davis.

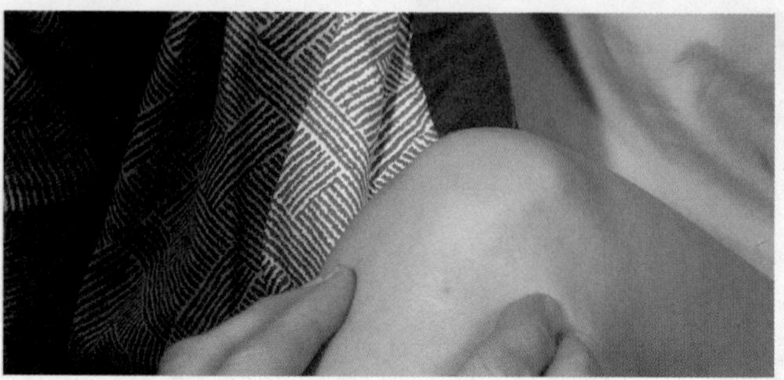

Figure 32-35 Palpation of the tibiofemoral joint. **Source:** From Skillen, D. L., Day, R. A., Anderson, M. C., Stephen, T. C., Gilbert, J. A., & Day, L. W. (2004). *Physical examination images* [CD-ROM]. Edmonton, AB: Faculty of Nursing, University of Alberta.

the hands. In contrast, the client's performance of the point-to-point test is expected to be smooth, accurate, and without tremor. Deviations suggest pathology within the cerebellar or motor system or both. If point-to-point test is performed by the client accurately with eyes open but not with eyes closed, a deviation in position sense is possible.

Sensory System. Assess the integrity of the sensory system in the lower extremities in a similar sequence and with the same techniques that you use when examining the upper extremities. The client is in the supine position and must keep the eyes closed during all sensory testing to avoid seeing the stimulus. Assess pain and light touch as you did when assessing the upper extremities. Expect the sensations of pain and light touch to be intact bilaterally from L2 to S1. For assessing vibration sense, apply the vibrating tuning fork to the DIP joint on the great toe. Use the great toe to also assess position sense. In the lower extremities, the only test of discriminative sensation is extinction.

➤ SKILL 32-32 Assessing Muscle Tone and Muscle Strength of the Lower Extremities

Equipment

- None

Procedure

EXAMINATION SKILL AND FOCUS	TECHNIQUES AND RATIONALE
Muscle tone Legs	1. Support the leg at the foot and lower thigh. 2. Move each leg (ankle, knee, hip) through a modified ROM. 3. Assess the resistance offered. 4. Test muscle tone before testing muscle strength. *Assessment of tone permits you to interpret muscle strength results accurately.*
Muscle strength Feet	1. You may test both sides separately or simultaneously. 2. Place your hands on the soles of the client's feet. 3. Ask the client to plantar-flex the foot against the resistance offered. *Tests strength of plantar flexion (L4 to L5)* 4. Compare findings from both sides. *Comparison helps detect asymmetry.* 5. Place your hands on the dorsum of the client's feet. 6. Ask the client to dorsiflex the feet against resistance offered. *Tests dorsiflexion (S1) at the ankle.* 7. Compare findings from both sides.
Legs	1. Instruct the client to flex the knee. *Flexion tests strength of hamstring muscles (L4 to L5, S1 to S2), and extension tests strength of quadriceps muscles (L2 to L4).* 2. Place your left hand at the knee, and grasp the client's ankle with your right hand. 3. Instruct the client to keep the foot in contact with the table as you attempt to straighten the client's leg (flexion at knee). 4. Compare findings from both sides. 5. Instruct the client to flex the knee. 6. Support the client's flexed knee with your left hand and push against the lower shin with your right hand as the client attempts to straighten the leg (extension at the knee). 7. Compare findings from both sides.
Hip	1. Place both your hands on the client's thigh. 2. Try to force the thigh downward as the client raises the leg against your hand (flexion). *Tests strength of iliopsoas muscle (L2 to L4).* 3. Place your hand under the client's thigh. 4. Instruct the client to force the thigh downward on your hand (extension). *Tests strength of the gluteus maximus muscle (S1).* 5. Compare findings from both sides. 6. Place both your hands firmly on the surface between the client's knees. 7. Instruct the client to bring the legs together (adduction). *Tests strength of the adductors (L2 to L4).* 8. Place your hands firmly on the surface at lateral aspect of client's knees. 9. Instruct the client to spread the legs (abduction). *Tests strength of the gluteus medium and minimus muscles (L4 to L5, S1) of the hip.* 10. Compare findings from both sides.

From Stephen, T. C., Day, R. A., & Skillen, D. L. (Eds.). (2008). *A syllabus for adult health assessment* (p. 54). Edmonton, AB: Faculty of Nursing, University of Alberta.

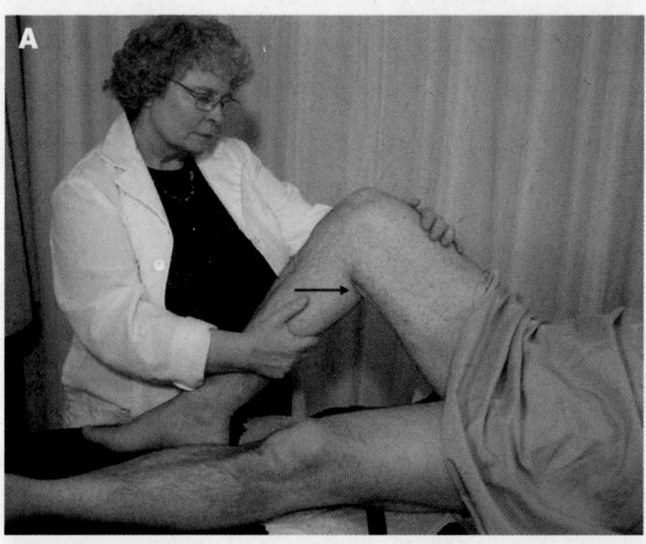

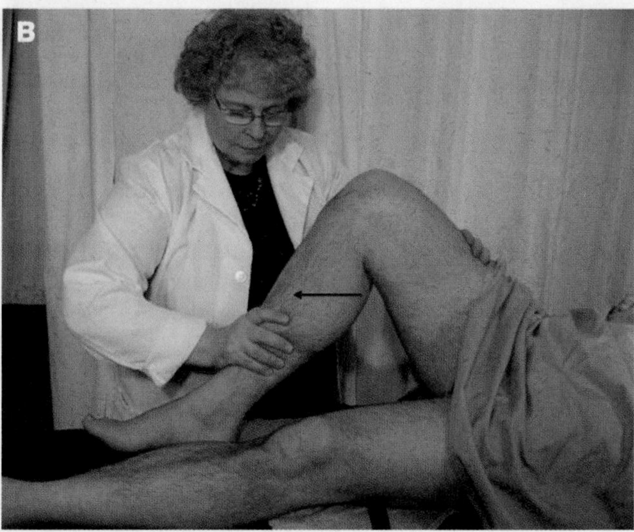

Figure 32-36 A, Assessment of knee flexion strength. B, Assessment of knee extension strength. **Source:** From Skillen, D. L., Day, R. A., Anderson, M. C., Stephen, T. C., Gilbert, J. A., & Day, L. W. (2004). *Physical examination images* [CD-ROM]. Edmonton, AB: Faculty of Nursing, University of Alberta.

➤ SKILL 32-33 Assessing Pulses in the Lower Extremities

Equipment

- None

Procedure

EXAMINATION SKILL AND FOCUS	TECHNIQUES AND RATIONALE
Popliteal pulses	1. Instruct the client to flex the leg slightly and relax the muscles. 2. Palpate the popliteal artery with the fingertips of both hands at the midline in the popliteal fossa, pressing deeply. *The popliteal artery is more deeply situated than are other peripheral pulses.* 3. Compare findings from both sides. 4. If you are unable to palpate the popliteal artery, ask the client to lie prone on the examination surface with the legs flexed at the knee and then try to palpate.
Posterior tibial pulses	1. Palpate the posterior tibial artery behind and below the medial malleolus with your finger pads. 2. Compare findings from both sides. You may palpate both sides simultaneously.
Dorsalis pedis pulses	1. Palpate the dorsalis pedis artery with your finger pads on the dorsum of the foot just lateral to the extensor tendon of the great toe. 2. Compare findings from both sides. You may palpate both sides simultaneously.

From Stephen, T. C., Day, R. A., & Skillen, D. L. (Eds.). (2008). *A syllabus for adult health assessment* (pp. 54–55). Edmonton, AB: Faculty of Nursing, University of Alberta.

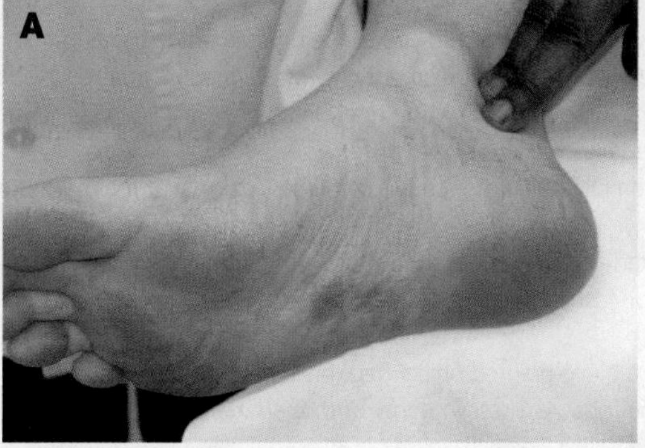

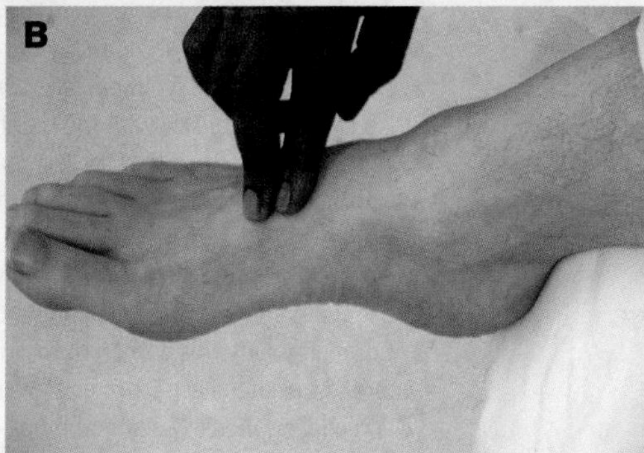

Figure 32-37 A, Palpation of the posterior tibial artery. B, Palpation of the dorsalis pedis artery. **Source:** From Skillen, D. L., Day, R. A., Anderson, M. C., Stephen, T. C., Gilbert, J. A., & Day, L. W. (2004). *Physical examination images* [CD-ROM]. Edmonton, AB: Faculty of Nursing, University of Alberta.

➤ SKILL 32-34 Assessing Coordination of the Lower Extremities

Equipment

- None

Procedure

EXAMINATION SKILL AND FOCUS	TECHNIQUES AND RATIONALE
Coordination	Test each leg separately.
Rapid alternating movements	1. Instruct the client to pat the foot against your hand as rapidly as possible (rhythmic patting).
Point-to-point test	2. Instruct the client to place the heel on the opposite knee and run the heel down the shin and off the great toe on each side, with eyes open.
Position sense	3. Repeat on both sides with eyes closed. *Testing with eyes open and then closed assesses both coordination and position sense.*
	4. Compare findings from both sides.

From Stephen, T. C., Day, R. A., & Skillen, D. L. (Eds.). (2008). *A syllabus for adult health assessment* (p. 54). Edmonton, AB: Faculty of Nursing, University of Alberta.

Reflexes. Assess the patellar and ankle deep tendon reflexes and the plantar superficial reflex (Skill 32–35; Figure 32–38). Encourage the client to relax the leg. Only if a reflex is symmetrically absent or diminished would you use a reinforcement technique (augmentation), that is, asking the client to lock the fingers together and then pull them apart hard without breaking the grasp. Just before striking the tendon, tell the client to perform this manoeuvre. Expect a response at all sites. See Table 32–43 for the grading scheme. Some individuals may consistently exhibit diminished or even absent deep tendon reflexes in the legs. Test the plantar superficial reflex by using a continuous firm stroke on the sole of the foot with a blunt object, such as the end of the handle of the reflex hammer. Expect the toes to flex bilaterally.

Ask the client to stand so that you can complete the examination of the lower extremities.

Inspection and Palpation of a Standing Client. Assess the symmetry of muscle development, evidence of distended saphenous veins (varicose veins), and integrity of the arches and popliteal fossa (Skill 32–36). Assess the popliteal fossa for swelling or bogginess; none should be present. As with the upper extremities, expect muscle development to be symmetrical, and no wasting should be apparent. Although the veins in the legs may become more evident with the client in the standing position, they should not appear distended and tortuous, which suggests the presence of varicose veins.

Coordination. With the client in the standing position, assess the client's cerebellar function, position sense, muscle strength, posture, balance, and gait (see Skill 32–36). The Romberg test performed with client's eyes open assesses cerebellar function; with client's eyes closed, it assesses position sense. Test muscle strength and coordination by asking the client to perform tandem walking, shallow knee

➤ SKILL 32-35 Assessing Deep Tendon and Superficial Reflexes of the Lower Extremities

Equipment

- Reflex hammer

Procedure

EXAMINATION SKILL AND FOCUS	TECHNIQUES AND RATIONALE
Deep tendon reflexes	Both sides are tested.
	Only if responses are symmetrically diminished or absent would you use reinforcement (augmentation). *Failure to ensure reflexes are symmetrically diminished before reinforcement may mask unequal reflexes.*
	Strike the tendon briskly with the hammer held loosely and swung freely in an arc.
Patellar reflex	1. Position the client so that the leg is relaxed and the knee is flexed.
	2. Use the hammer to tap the patellar tendon just below the patella. *Assesses integrity of the reflex arc at L2 to L4.*
	3. Compare extension on both sides.
Ankle reflex	1. Position the client so that the knee is flexed and the foot is supported in the dorsiflexed position by you.
Superficial reflex	2. Use the hammer to tap the Achilles tendon just above the heel. *Assesses integrity of the reflex arc primarily at S1.*
	3. Compare plantar flexion on both sides.
Plantar reflex	1. Stroke the lateral aspect of the sole with a blunt-pointed object beginning at the heel, laterally along the sole, and curving medially across the ball of the foot. *Assesses integrity of the reflex arc at L5 and S1.*
	2. Compare the toe movement on both sides.

From Stephen, T. C., Day, R. A., & Skillen, D. L. (Eds.). (2008). *A syllabus for adult health assessment* (p. 56). Edmonton, AB: Faculty of Nursing, University of Alberta.

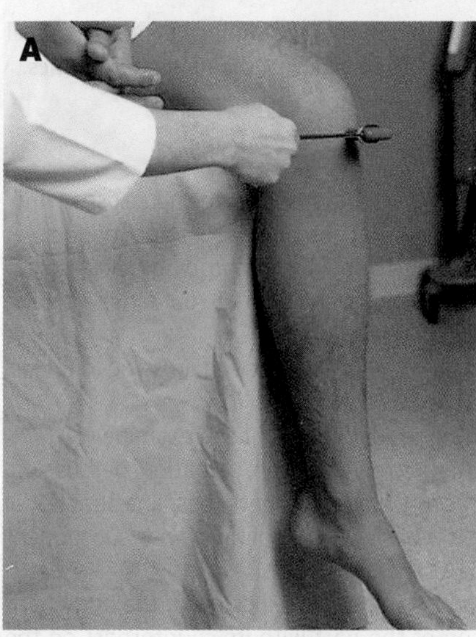

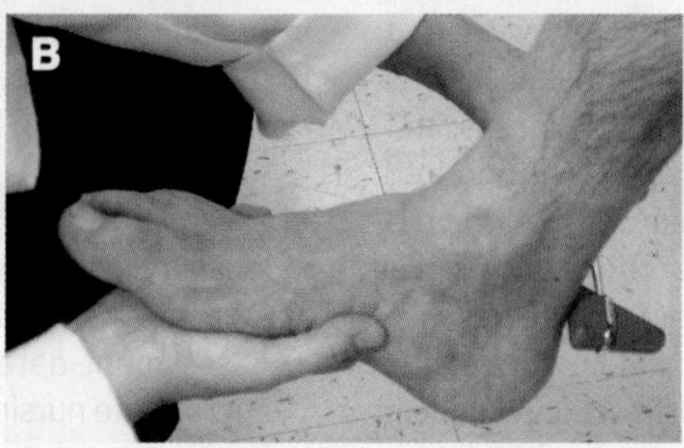

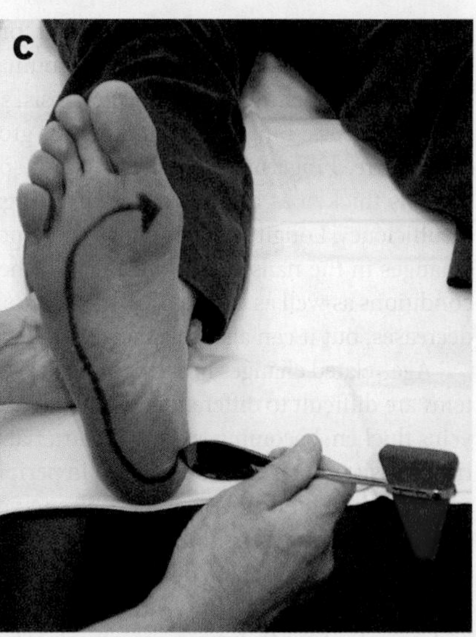

Figure 32-38 A, Position for eliciting the patellar deep tendon reflex. B, Achilles deep tendon reflex. C, Plantar superficial reflex. **Source:** Photos B and C from Skillen, D. L., Day, R. A., Anderson, M. C., Stephen, T. C., Gilbert, J. A., & Day, L. W. (2004). *Physical examination images* [CD-ROM]. Edmonton, AB: Faculty of Nursing, University of Alberta.

bends, hopping in one place, heel walking, and toe walking. Expect the client to perform these tests without difficulty, showing strength and coordinated movement. To assess balance, posture, and gait, ask the client to walk. The client is expected to walk unassisted, at an even pace, with the heel striking first followed by a push off with the toe, with arms swinging easily in the opposite direction to the leg movements, and the head leading on the turn.

Age-Related Changes for Extremities. With aging, the epidermis, dermis, and subcutaneous skin layers thin, and vascularity decreases. The skin, especially over the dorsal surface of the hands, forearms, and lower legs becomes more transparent, thin, fragile, and loose. Skin mobility increases, and turgor decreases. The rate of epidermal proliferation slows down, which delays wound healing. Skin on the extremities is often dry (xerosis), flaky, and itchy because

➤ SKILL 32-36 Inspecting the Legs and Assessing Coordination With the Client in the Standing Position

Equipment

- None

Procedure

EXAMINATION SKILL AND FOCUS	TECHNIQUES AND RATIONALE
Legs and feet	1. Inspect both legs with the client in the standing position, noting symmetry, veins, arches, and popliteal fossae. *Effects of gravity are maximized for assessing integrity of venous return, arches of the feet, and popliteal fossae.*
Symmetry, veins, arches, and popliteal fossae	2. Palpate the popliteal fossae.
Cerebellar tests, position sense	1. Instruct the client to stand without support, arms at the sides and feet together, first with eyes open, then with eyes closed for 20 seconds (Romberg test). *The Romberg test, with client's eyes open, assesses cerebellar function; with client's eyes closed, assesses position sense.*
	2. Protect the client from risk of falling.
	Urgent: The client must be protected from falling because some sway is expected, especially when the client has the eyes closed.
	3. Instruct the client to walk in a straight line by placing heel of foot directly before toes of other foot (tandem walking). *The tandem walk and the heel–toe walk test coordination (balance) and motor strength.*
Muscle strength	4. Instruct the client to hop in place, first on one foot and then on the other. *Hopping and shallow knee bends demonstrate strength and coordination of legs.*
Shallow knee bend	5. Instruct the client to stand on one foot and do a shallow knee bend, first on one leg and then on the other.
	6. Support the client's elbow if the client has a risk of falling.
Heel walk	7. Instruct the client to walk on the heels.
Toe walk	8. Instruct the client to walk on the toes.
Gait, balance, and posture	1. Instruct the client to walk away and then back toward you.
	2. When the client is walking, observe posture, gait (stance and swing), balance, arm swing, leg movement, and position of head on turning. *Critical observation of gait assesses the integrity of the motor and cerebellar components of the nervous and musculoskeletal systems.*

From Stephen, T. C., Day, R. A., & Skillen, D. L. (Eds.). (2008). *A syllabus for adult health assessment* (pp. 56–57). Edmonton, AB: Faculty of Nursing, University of Alberta.

eccrine sweat glands decrease in number, producing less sweat, and the sebaceous glands produce less sebum. Common skin lesions include actinic lentigines, actinic keratosis, seborrheic keratosis, and actinic purpura. Fingernails and toenails grow more slowly and lose their lustre. Fingernails usually thin and split more easily, whereas toenails thicken as a result of trauma, fungal infection, or vascular insufficiency. Longitudinal ridging is commonly seen in all the nails. Changes in the nails reflect the effects of health and environmental conditions as well as aging. Growth of hair on the lower legs and feet decreases, but it can also be an adverse effect of vascular disease.

Age-related changes in the peripheral vascular and lymphatic systems are difficult to differentiate from disease processes. Arteries and veins thicken, becoming less elastic. Arterial thickening is called arteriosclerosis, which causes increases in peripheral vascular resistance and systolic blood pressure. Less elastic veins dilate more readily, which increases susceptibility to venous stasis and varicose veins.

Skeletal muscle mass decreases due to the deterioration of muscle fibres, resulting in loss of strength and endurance. Whereas bones and muscles benefit from exercise, joints and articular surfaces are adversely affected by years of use. Articular surfaces thin and are subject to fraying and cracking. Elastic fibres degenerate and contribute to loss of tensile strength in the ligaments and tendons. The result is loss of joint stability, decreased ROM, and pain. Osteoarthritis occurs at the joint surface.

Hands reflect age-related musculoskeletal changes quite graphically. Many older adults develop enlarged IP joints called Heberden's nodes at the distal joints and Bouchard's nodes at the proximal joints. Hands appear bony because of loss of subcutaneous fat and muscle mass between the metacarpals. Muscle mass is lost in the base of the thumb (thenar eminence on the palm).

Pain sensation remains intact, but pressure, vibration, and position senses may be diminished due to a decline in density of cutaneous nerve endings (Miller, 2009). Ability to do tandem walking, walking on heels or toes, and deep knee bends may diminish, in part due to loss of muscle strength but also due to difficulty in maintaining balance. Swaying may occur during the Romberg test, especially when the client has the eyes closed, due to changes in vision and position sense. Gait is usually slower, with a shorter stride, decreased steppage height, and decreased arm swing.

Documentation. Record your findings from the inspection and palpation of the lower extremities Table 32–47 provides examples of documentation for the assessment of the standing client. Findings for the examination of the lower extremities in the supine client are parallel to the expected findings in the assessment of the upper extremities.

* KEY CONCEPTS

- When a client presents with a symptom or sign, the nurse uses symptom or sign analysis to gather data about the symptom or sign.
- Assessment data are used to make nursing diagnoses, select appropriate nursing interventions, and evaluate outcomes of nursing care.
- Physical assessment of different age groups requires you to understand age-related changes.
- Health promotion is integrated throughout the examination.
- Physical examination modes of inspection, palpation, percussion, and auscultation are used to assess clients' baseline functional abilities and to serve as a basis for comparison with subsequent assessments.
- Inspection requires good lighting, full exposure of the body part, and careful comparison of the part with its counterpart on the opposite side of the body.
- Palpation involves the use of parts of your hand to detect different types of physical characteristics.
- Percussion is the detection of differences in the density of underlying tissues by listening to audible sounds produced while striking the client's body surface.
- Auscultation with a stethoscope facilitates assessment of the character of sounds created in various organs.
- Physical examination is performed only after proper preparation of the client (both physically and psychologically), the environment, and the equipment.
- Throughout the examination, you need to ensure that the client is safe, warm, comfortable, and informed of each step of the process.
- You always use a systematic approach when conducting a physical assessment and learn to integrate the assessments of different body systems simultaneously.
- During assessments of the skin, breast, and genitalia, you take the opportunity to explain to the client the techniques for self-examination.
- You always assess clients' cognitive function (mental status and intellectual function) continually throughout the examination.
- At the end of the examination, you would provide for the client's comfort, review your findings, facilitate closure, and document the assessment findings.

TABLE 32-47 Examples of Documentation of the Assessment of the Lower Extremities, Client Standing

Focus of Assessment	Expected Findings
Skin	Brownish hair over proximal and distal phalanges. Skin pink; moist; elastic. Skin temperature uniformly warm over thighs; cooler over shins and feet.
Muscle development	Muscle mass symmetrical in size and contour; without atrophy or fasciculations in the legs. Standing: arches high bilaterally; popliteal fossae without swelling.
Nails	Nails short; firm; uniformly thick; cut straight across. No evidence of lesions around cuticles.
Posture, gait, balance	Gait coordinated, heel strike with push-off at toe, arm swing opposite to leg, head leads on turn.
Cerebellar and muscle strength	Minimal sway during the Romberg test, client with eyes open and closed; tandem walking smooth, coordinated; standing on one foot, followed by shallow knee bend without assistance bilaterally; coordinated walking on heels and toes.

From Anderson, M. C. (2004). Documentation. In Faculty of Nursing, University of Alberta. (Ed.), *Health assessment self-test modules* (WebCT Vista). Edmonton, AB: Author.

* CRITICAL THINKING EXERCISES

1. Examine the image of the eyes.

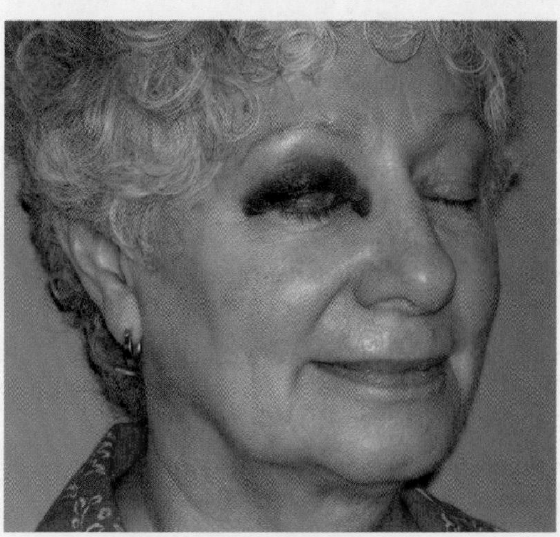

Source: From Skillen, D. L., Day, R. A., Anderson, M. C., Stephen, T. C., Gilbert, J. A., & Day, L. W. (2004). *Physical examination images* [CD-ROM]. Edmonton, AB: Faculty of Nursing, University of Alberta.

   a. What questions will you ask the client to complete a symptom and sign analysis?
   b. If you suspect physical abuse, what questions would you ask the client?
   c. If you suspect a fall related to substance abuse, what questions would you ask the client?
   d. What techniques will you use to examine the right eye?
   e. What age-related change might influence the sign observed in this client?
   f. What is your documentation for inspection?

2. Examine the image of the right breast.

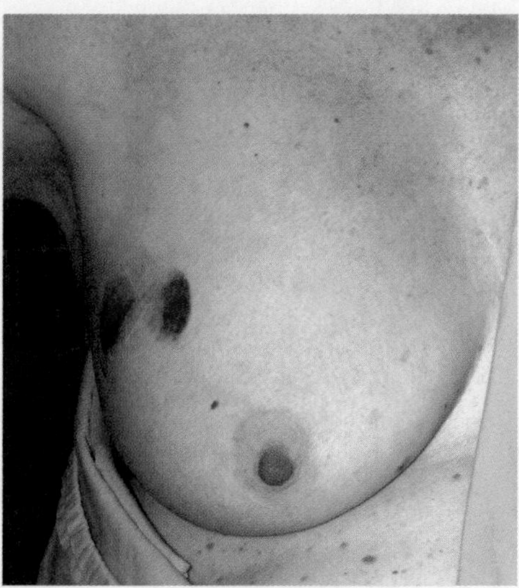

Source: From Skillen, D. L., Day, R. A., Anderson, M. C., Stephen, T. C., Gilbert, J. A., & Day, L. W. (2004). *Physical examination images* [CD-ROM]. Edmonton, AB: Faculty of Nursing, University of Alberta.

   a. What questions will you ask the client when taking a health history?
   b. What specific characteristics will you assess in the breast?
   c. What examination mode(s) will you use with this client?
   d. What do you expect to find when you examine the breast?
   e. What is your documentation for inspection?

3. Examine the image of the left leg in a female client.

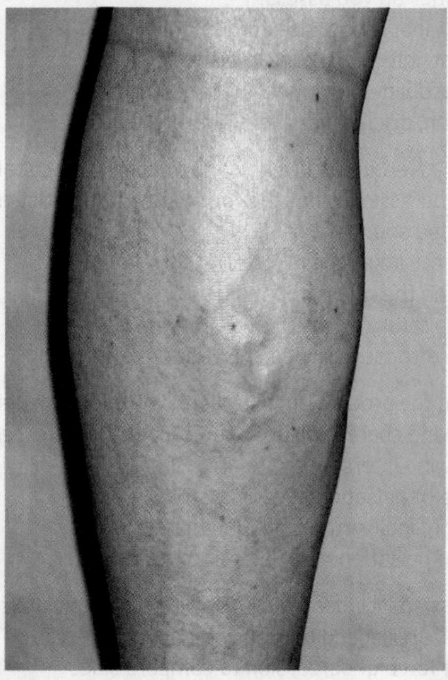

Source: From Skillen, D. L., Day, R. A., Anderson, M. C., Stephen, T. C., Gilbert, J. A., & Day, L. W. (2004). *Physical examination images* [CD-ROM]. Edmonton, AB: Faculty of Nursing, University of Alberta.

   a. What questions will you ask the client when taking the health history?
   b. What anatomical structures are accessible to examination?
   c. What system(s) will you examine?
   d. What health promotion activities will you integrate in your assessment?
   e. What specific characteristics are you going to assess during your examination?
   f. What aspects of your assessment would change if this were a male client?

* REVIEW QUESTIONS

1. Your analysis of a symptom includes a focus on all of the following characteristics, *except:*
   1. Quality or nature
   2. Intensity or severity
   3. Location and radiation
   4. Diagnosis or hypothesis

2. Recent memory is measured by asking the client to recall events that occurred:
   1. One week ago
   2. One month ago
   3. Three minutes ago
   4. Within the past 24 hours

3. To ensure a thorough inspection of the tympanic membrane, you do all of the following, *except:*
   1. Straighten the ear canal
   2. Instruct the client to tilt the head slightly towards you
   3. Use the largest ear speculum that the client's ear canal will accommodate
   4. Move the otoscope slowly to see as much of the tympanic membrane as possible

4. When palpating the lymph nodes of the neck, which of the following characteristics do you assess?
   1. Congruency, induration, size, turgor
   2. Enlargement, integrity, shape, moisture
   3. Consistency, delineation, mobility, tenderness
   4. Configuration, discreteness, temperature, colour
5. If you identify adventitious breath sounds during auscultation of the lungs, you assess all of the following characteristics of those unexpected sounds, *except*:
   1. Location in the lung fields
   2. Timing during the respiratory phases
   3. Ratio of inspiratory phase to expiratory phase
   4. Persistence after several deep inspirations and coughs
6. When palpating the precordium of a client, you expect to detect all of the following characteristics of apical pulsations, *except:*
   1. Isolation to one interspace
   2. Prominence of pulsation in early systole
   3. Brisk tapping against the palpating finger
   4. Detection of pulsation 4 cm lateral to the left MCL
7. Indirect percussion includes all the following techniques, *except:*
   1. Use of brisk, arclike and relaxed wrist action
   2. Variation of force of percussion to compare sides
   3. Application of pleximeter finger firmly to skin surface
   4. Use of the lightest blow to achieve clear percussion notes
8. Inspection of the spine includes assessment of all of the following characteristics, *except*:
   1. Bilateral lateral bending
   2. Curvatures and prominences
   3. Attachments of paravertebral muscles
   4. Alignment of shoulders and iliac crests
9. When examining the external genitalia of an elderly male client, you expect to detect all of the following age-related changes, *except*:
   1. Sparse pubic hair
   2. Pendulous scrotal sac
   3. Smooth, rubbery testicles
   4. Small, uncircumcised penis
10. When conducting a point-to-point test of the upper extremities, you observe that the client performs the test accurately with eyes open, but inaccurately with eyes closed. This finding suggests a:
    1. Vestibular anomaly
    2. Position sense deficit
    3. Cerebellar dysfunction
    4. Discriminatory sensory loss

* RECOMMENDED WEB SITES

Canadian Breast Cancer Foundation: http://www.cbcf.org
Provides information about breast cancer research programs.

Canadian Cancer Society: http://www.cancer.ca/
Provides access to current cancer statistics and information about screening and early detection.

Canadian Nurses Association: http://www.cna-aiic.ca
Provides access to the national code of ethics for nurses.

Canadian Nurses Protective Society: http://www.cnps.ca
Provides access to legal information related to documentation of examinations by nurses.

Canadian Task Force on Preventive Health Care: http://www.ctfphc.org
Offers recommendations from review of publications related to preventive health care.

Public Health Agency of Canada: http://www.phac-aspc.gc.ca/
Provides information about chronic diseases, emergency preparedness, health promotion, immunization, infectious diseases, injury prevention, travel health, documentation, and surveillance.

33

Infection Control

Original chapter by Katherine West, BSN, MSEd, CIC

Canadian content written by Colleen M. Astle, RN, MN, CNeph (C)

and Deborah Hobbs, RN, BScN, CIC

objectives

Mastery of content in this chapter will enable you to:

- Define the key terms listed.
- Explain the relationship between the chain of infection and the transmission of infection.
- Identify the body's normal defences against infection.
- Discuss the events in the inflammatory response.
- Describe the signs and symptoms of a localized and a systemic infection.
- Identify clients most at risk for infection.
- Explain conditions that promote the transmission of health care–associated infection.
- Explain the difference between medical and surgical asepsis.
- Give an example for preventing infection for each element of the infection chain.
- Perform proper procedures for hand hygiene.
- Explain the rationale and practices for standard precautions or routine practices.
- Explain the rationale and practices for transmission-based (isolation) precautions.
- Explain how infection-control measures in the home may differ from those the hospital.
- Properly don a surgical mask, sterile gown, and sterile gloves.

key terms

Aerobic, p. 637
Anaerobic, p. 637
Asepsis, p. 649
Broad-spectrum antibiotics, p. 640
Carriers, p. 636
Colonizing, p. 636
Communicable, p. 636
Disinfection, p. 650
Edema, p. 641
Endogenous infection, p. 641
Epidemiology, p. 662
Exogenous infection, p. 641
Exudates, p. 641
Hand hygiene, p. 651
Handwashing, p. 651
Iatrogenic infection, p. 641
Immune response, p. 639
Immunocompromised, p. 636
Inflammatory response, p. 641
Invasive, p. 636
Isolation precautions, p. 657
Leukocytosis, p. 641
Localized, p. 639
Medical asepsis, p. 649
Microorganisms, p. 636
Necrotic, p. 640
Normal flora, p. 639
Nosocomial infection, p. 641
Pathogens, p. 636
Pathogenicity, p. 639
Phagocytosis, p. 641
Purulent, p. 641
Routine practices, p. 649
Sanguineous, p. 641
Serosanguineous, p. 641
Serous, p. 641
Standard precautions, p. 649
Sterile field, p. 665
Sterilization, p. 650
Superinfection, p. 640
Surgical asepsis, p. 662
Susceptibility, p. 639
Systemic, p. 639
Virulence, p. 636

media resources

evolve Web Site

- Animations
- Audio Chapter Summaries
- Glossary
- Multiple-Choice Review Questions
- Skills Performance Checklists
- Student Learning Activities
- Video Clips
- Weblinks

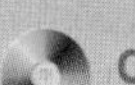

Companion CD

- Glossary
- Interactive Learning Activities
- Fluids and Electrolytes Tutorial
- Test-Taking Skills

Good health depends in part on a safe environment. Practices or techniques that control or prevent transmission of infection help to create an environment that protects clients and health care workers from disease. Clients in all health care settings are at risk for acquiring infections because they often have lower resistance to infectious **microorganisms** and increased exposure to numbers and types of disease-causing microorganisms, and they sometimes undergo **invasive** procedures wherein a body cavity or organ is entered by either puncture or incision. Microorganisms can only be seen with the aid of a microscope and are typically a single cell. They include bacteria, protozoans, certain types of algae, and fungi. In acute care or ambulatory care facilities, clients can be exposed to pathogens, some of which may be resistant to most antibiotics. By practising infection-prevention and -control techniques, you can avoid spreading microorganisms to clients.

In all settings, clients and their families must be able to recognize sources of infections and be able to institute protective measures. Client teaching should include information concerning infections, modes of transmission, and methods of prevention.

Health care workers can protect themselves from contact with infectious materials or exposure to communicable diseases by having knowledge of the infectious process and appropriate barrier protections. The spread of diseases such as hepatitis B and C, acquired immune deficiency syndrome (AIDS), sudden acute respiratory syndrome (SARS), and tuberculosis have resulted in a greater emphasis on infection-control techniques. Infection control has two purposes: (1) protecting clients from acquiring infections and (2) protecting health care workers from becoming infected. Many of the techniques used to protect clients also provide effective protection for nurses. You must remain constantly vigilant to prevent the spread of infection while providing care.

Scientific Knowledge Base

Microorganisms live and grow on inanimate objects and in air, water, food, soil, plants, and animals. They also live and grow in and on persons. Most microorganisms are nonpathogens, meaning that they do not cause a person to be ill; however, some are **pathogens**, meaning that they are capable of causing disease. An infection is a disease state resulting from the entry and multiplication of a pathogen in the tissues of a host causing the body to manifest clinical signs and symptoms. If the infection can be transmitted from one person to another, it is a **communicable** (infectious, contagious) disease.

Chain of Infection

The presence of a pathogen does not mean that an infection will begin. The development of an infection occurs in a cycle that depends on the presence of all the following elements:

- An infectious agent (pathogen)
- A reservoir (source for pathogen growth)
- A portal of exit from the reservoir
- A mode of transmission
- A portal of entry to a host
- A susceptible host

An infection develops if this chain remains intact (Figure 33–1). You will follow infection-prevention and -control practices to break the chain so that infections do not develop.

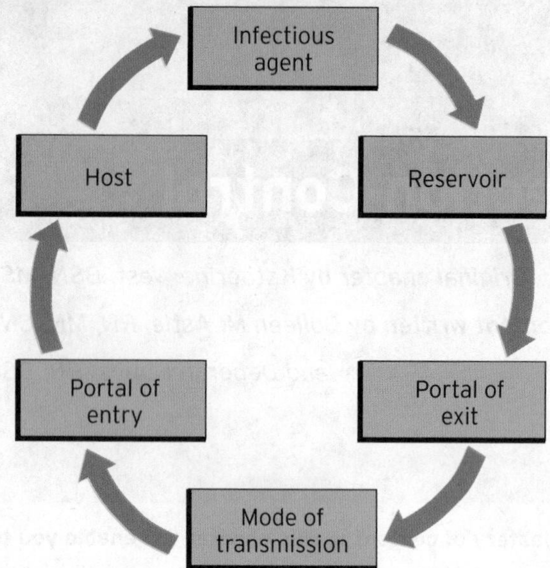

Figure 33-1 Chain of infection.

Infectious Agents. Microorganisms include bacteria, viruses, fungi, and protozoa (Table 33–1). Microorganisms on the skin are called *resident* or *transient flora.* Resident organisms are considered permanent residents of the skin, where they survive and multiply without causing harm. They are not easily removed by handwashing with plain soaps unless considerable friction is used. Resident microorganisms in deep skin layers are usually killed only by performing hand hygiene with products containing antimicrobial ingredients.

Transient microorganisms attach to the skin when a person has contact with another person or object. For example, when you touch a bedpan or a contaminated dressing, transient bacteria adhere to your skin. The organisms attach loosely to the skin in dirt and grease and under fingernails. These organisms may be readily transmitted unless removed by handwashing (Larson, 1996).

The potential for microorganisms to cause disease depends on the following factors:

- A sufficient number of organisms
- **Virulence**, or the ability to produce disease
- The ability to enter and survive in the host
- The susceptibility of the host

Resident skin microorganisms are usually nonpathogenic. However, they can cause serious infection when surgery or other invasive procedures allow them to enter deep tissues or when a client is severely **immunocompromised** (has an impaired immune system).

Reservoir. A reservoir is a place where a pathogen can survive but may or may not multiply. For example, hepatitis A virus survives in shellfish but does not multiply; *Pseudomonas* organisms can survive and multiply in nebulizer reservoirs used in the care of clients with respiratory problems. The most common reservoir is the human body. A variety of microorganisms live on the skin and within body cavities, fluids, and discharges. When a pathogen is present on or in the body but does not cause harm, the pathogen is **colonizing** the site. **Carriers** are animals or persons who show no symptoms of illness but who have pathogens on or in their bodies that can be transferred to others. For example, a person can be a carrier of hepatitis B virus without having any signs or symptoms of infection. Animals, food, water, insects, and even inanimate objects can also be reservoirs for infectious organisms. For example, the bacterium *Legionella pneumophila*, which causes legionnaires' disease,

TABLE 33-1 Common Pathogens and Resulting Major Infections

Organism	Major Reservoir(s)	Major Infections
Bacteria		
Clostridium difficile	Colon	Colitis, diarrhea
Escherichia coli	Colon	Gastroenteritis, urinary tract infection
Staphylococcus aureus	Skin, hair, anterior nares	Wound infection, pneumonia, food poisoning, cellulitis, bacteremia
Streptococcus (β-hemolytic group A) organisms	Oropharynx, skin, perianal area	"Strep throat," rheumatic fever, scarlet fever, impetigo, wound infection
Streptococcus (β-hemolytic group B) organisms	Adult genitalia	Urinary tract infection, wound infection, postpartum sepsis, neonatal sepsis
Mycobacterium tuberculosis	Droplet nuclei from lungs	Tuberculosis
Neisseria gonorrhoeae	Genitourinary tract, rectum, mouth	Gonorrhea, pelvic inflammatory disease, infectious arthritis, conjunctivitis
Rickettsia rickettsii	Wood tick	Rocky Mountain spotted fever
Staphylococcus epidermidis	Skin	Wound infection, bacteremia
Viruses		
Hepatitis A virus	Feces	Hepatitis A
Hepatitis B virus	Blood and body fluids	Hepatitis B
Hepatitis C virus	Blood	Hepatitis C
Herpes simplex virus (type 1)	Lesions of mouth or skin, saliva, genitalia	Cold sores, aseptic meningitis, genital herpes, herpetic whitlow
Human immunodeficiency virus	Blood, semen, vaginal secretions, breast milk (has also been isolated in saliva, tears, and urine, but these have not proved to be sources of transmission)	Acquired immune deficiency syndrome
Fungi		
Aspergillus organisms	Soil, dust, construction dust, decaying or organic matter	Sinusitis or skin, lung, wound, or central nervous system infection (Wilson, 2006)
Candida albicans	Mouth, skin, colon, genital tract	Candidiasis, pneumonia, sepsis
Protozoan		
Plasmodium falciparum	Blood	Malaria

lives in contaminated water and water systems. To thrive, pathogens require a reservoir that provides food, oxygen (or no oxygen, depending on the pathogen), water, an appropriate temperature and pH, and minimal light.

Food. Microorganisms require nourishment. Some—such as *Clostridium perfringens*, the microbe that causes gas gangrene—thrive on organic matter. Others, such as *Escherichia coli*, consume undigested food in the bowel. Carbon dioxide and inorganic materials such as soil provide nourishment for other organisms.

Oxygen. **Aerobic** bacteria require oxygen to survive and to multiply sufficiently to cause disease. Aerobic organisms cause more infections than do **anaerobic** organisms (i.e., organisms that can only survive in the absence of oxygen). Examples of aerobic organisms are *Staphylococcus aureus* and strains of *Streptococcus* organisms.

The gastrointestinal tract is colonized by large numbers of anaerobic bacteria that can cause infections if the bowel is damaged. Infections deep within the pleural cavity, in a joint, or in a deep sinus tract are typically caused by anaerobes. Bacteria that cause tetanus, gas gangrene, and botulism are anaerobes.

Water. Most organisms require water or moisture for survival. For example, microorganisms thrive in the moist drainage from a surgical wound. However, some bacteria assume a form called a *spore*. Spores remain viable even when deprived of water and are resistant to drying. Spore-forming bacteria, such as those that cause anthrax, botulism, and tetanus, can live without water.

Temperature. Microorganisms can live only in certain temperature ranges. The ideal temperature for most pathogens in humans is 35°C (Keroack & Rosen-Kotilainen, 1996); however, some can survive temperature extremes that would be fatal to humans. Cold temperatures tend to prevent the growth and reproduction of bacteria.

pH. The acidity of an environment determines the viability of microorganisms. Most microorganisms prefer an environment within a pH range of 5 to 8. Bacteria, in particular, thrive in urine with an alkaline pH. Most organisms cannot survive the acidic environment of the stomach. In clients receiving acid-reducing medications (e.g., antacids and histamine$_2$ blockers), these can cause an overgrowth of gastrointestinal organisms, which can contribute to nosocomial pneumonia (Centers for Disease Control and Prevention [CDC], 2004).

Minimal Light. Microorganisms thrive in dark environments such as those under dressings and within body cavities. Ultraviolet light may be effective in killing certain forms of bacteria (e.g., *Mycobacterium tuberculosis*).

Portal of Exit. After microorganisms find a site in which to grow and multiply, they must find a portal of exit if they are to enter another host and cause disease. A *portal of exit* is the path by which the pathogen leaves the reservoir (Sorrentino, 2004). Exits in the human body include body openings (mouth, nose, and rectal, vaginal, and urethral openings; and artificial openings such as those resulting from ostomies), breaks in the skin (a scrape, cut, or other wound), and breaks in the mucous membranes (the skin in the mouth, eyes, nose, vagina, and rectum). Pathogens are carried through portals of exit by blood, body fluids, excretions, and secretions (e.g., urine, stool, vomitus, saliva, mucus, pus, vaginal discharge, semen, wound drainage, bile, and sputum). For example, pathogens that infect the respiratory tract, such as *M. tuberculosis,* can be released from the body through the mouth and nose when an infected person sneezes, coughs, talks, or even breathes. In clients with artificial airways such as tracheostomy or endotracheal tubes (see Chapter 39), organisms easily exit the respiratory tract through these devices. Similarly, when a client has a urinary tract infection, microorganisms exit during urination or through urinary diversions such as ileal conduits, urostomies, and suprapubic drains (see Chapter 44).

Modes of Transmission. Microorganisms can be transmitted from the reservoir to the host in many ways. Certain infectious diseases tend to be transmitted more commonly by specific modes (Table 33–2). However, a microorganism may be transmitted by more than one mode. For example, human herpesvirus 3 (varicella-zoster) may be spread by the airborne route or through direct contact.

Indirect contact is a major mode of transmission in health care facilities. The health care worker's hands can easily pick up microbes from one person, place, or thing and then transmit them to other persons, places, or things. However, almost any object within the environment (e.g., a stethoscope or thermometer) can be a mode of indirect transmission of pathogens. Some organisms, such as *Clostridium difficile,* which can produce spores, can live in hospital environments for months. *C. difficile* can be spread by direct or indirect contact. All health care workers providing direct care (e.g., nurses, physiotherapists, and physicians) or performing diagnostic and support services (e.g., laboratory technicians, respiratory therapists, and dietary workers) must follow practices to minimize the spread of infection. Each group follows procedures for handling equipment and supplies used by a client. For example, respiratory therapists perform hand hygiene before working with each client and dispose of contaminated therapy equipment in a

TABLE 33-2 Modes of Transmission

Mode of Transmission	Examples of Organisms
Contact Transmission	
The transfer of microbes by physical touch; may be by direct contact, indirect contact, or droplet	Direct: Hepatitis A, B; herpes simplex virus; methicillin-resistant *Staphylococcus aureus* (MRSA); vancomycin-resistant enterococci (VRE) Indirect: Hepatitis A, B, C; MRSA;, VRE; *Pseudomonas;* multidrug–resistant *Acintobacter* Droplet: Influenza virus, rubella virus, sudden acute respiratory syndrome
Direct Contact	
Physical skin-to-skin contact between an infected or colonized individual and a susceptible host (e.g., via touching client)	Hepatitis A virus, *Shigella, Staphylococcus,* herpes simplex virus, MRSA, VRE, multidrug-resistant *Acinetobacter*
Indirect Contact	
Contact between a susceptible host and a contaminated intermediate object (e.g., via touching soiled linen, equipment, or dressings; transferring pathogens to a client via hands that are not washed between handling clients)	Hepatitis A, B, and C viruses, *Staphylococcus,* respiratory syncytial virus, *Pseudomonas,* MRSA, VRE, multidrug-resistant *Acinetobacter*
Droplet Transmission	
Large particles (droplets) from the respiratory system of an infected source propelled up to 1 m through the air and deposited onto a susceptible host (e.g., droplets produced via coughing, sneezing, or talking)	Influenza virus, rubella virus, sudden acute respiratory syndrome virus
Airborne Transmission	
Small airborne particles (droplet nuclei) containing microbes remain suspended in the air for long periods of time (e.g., droplets and aerosolized airborne particles produced via coughing and sneezing); air currents transmit these particles long distances (>1 m); susceptible host inhales them	*Mycobacterium tuberculosis* (causes tuberculosis), human herpesvirus 3 (varicella-zoster virus; causes chickenpox), *Aspergillus,* measles virus
Vehicle Transmission	
A single contaminated source (e.g., water, drugs, blood, food, equipment) transmits infection to multiple hosts, possibly resulting in an outbreak	*Pseudomonas* (via water, drugs), *Escherichia coli* (via food, water), hepatitis B and C viruses (via blood), human immunodeficiency virus (via blood), *Salmonella* (via food)
Vectorborne Transmission	
Insects (fleas, mites, ticks, mosquitoes) or pests (e.g., mice) transmit microbes to humans	*Vibrio cholerae, Plasmodium falciparum* (causes malaria), West Nile virus

Adapted from Health Canada. (1999). Infection control guidelines: Routine practices and additional precautions for preventing the transmission of infection in health care. *Canada Communicable Disease Report, 25*(Suppl. 4), 83–111.

prescribed manner. Certain medical devices and diagnostic procedures provide avenues for the spread of pathogens. Invasive procedures such as cystoscopy (the use of an endoscope to visualize the bladder) facilitate the diagnosis of problems but also increase the risk of infection transmission. Because so many factors can promote the spread of infection to a client, all health care workers must be conscientious about using infection-control practices, such as proper handwashing and ensuring that equipment has been adequately disinfected or sterilized.

Portal of Entry. Organisms can enter the body through the same routes they use to exit (i.e., body openings and breaks in the skin or mucous membranes). For example, organisms enter the body when a needle pierces the skin. As long as the device is in place, more organisms are able to enter the body. In clients with a urinary catheter, any obstruction to the flow of urine allows organisms to travel up the urethra. Factors that reduce the body's defences enhance the chances of pathogens entering the body.

Susceptible Host. Whether a person acquires an infection is related to his or her susceptibility to an infectious agent—**susceptibility** depends on the individual's degree of resistance to a pathogen. Although everyone is constantly in contact with large numbers of microorganisms, an infection does not develop until an individual becomes susceptible to the strength and numbers of microorganisms capable of producing infection. The more virulent an organism is, the greater the likelihood is that a person will be susceptible to it. Organisms with resistance to antibiotics are becoming more common in acute care settings—this is believed to be associated with the frequent and sometimes inappropriate use of antibiotics. A person's resistance to an infectious agent may be enhanced by receiving an appropriate vaccine or actually contracting the disease.

➤ BOX 33-1 Course of Infection, by Stage

Incubation Period

- Interval between the entrance of pathogen into body and the appearance of first symptoms (e.g., in chickenpox, 2 to 3 weeks; in the common cold, 1 to 2 days; in influenza, 1 to 3 days; in mumps, 15 to 18 days).

Prodromal Stage

- Interval from the onset of nonspecific signs and symptoms (malaise, low-grade fever, and fatigue) to more specific symptoms (during this time, microorganisms grow and multiply and the client may be more capable of spreading disease to others).

Illness Stage

- Interval when the client manifests signs and symptoms specific to type of infection (e.g., the common cold is manifested by a sore throat, sinus congestion, and rhinitis; mumps is manifested by an earache, a high fever, and parotid and salivary gland swelling).

Convalescence

- Interval when the acute symptoms of infection disappear and the body tries to replenish its resources and return to a state of homeostasis; the length of recovery depends on the severity of the infection and the client's general state of health (may take several days to months).

Infectious Process

By understanding the chain of infection, you can intervene to prevent infections from developing. If a client is at risk for acquiring an infection, you should observe for signs and symptoms of infection and take appropriate actions to prevent its spread. Infections follow a progressive course (Box 33–1). The severity of a client's illness depends on the extent of the infection, the ability of the microorganism to cause disease (**pathogenicity** of the microorganisms), and the susceptibility of the host (client).

If infection is **localized** (e.g., a wound infection), proper care controls the spread and minimizes the illness. The client may experience localized symptoms such as pain and tenderness at the wound site. An infection that affects the entire body instead of just a single organ or part is **systemic** and can be fatal.

The course of an infection influences the level of nursing care provided. You are responsible for properly administering antibiotics and monitoring the response to drug therapy (see Chapter 34). Supportive therapy includes providing adequate nutrition and rest to bolster the client's defences against the infectious process. The complexity of care depends on body systems affected by the infection.

Regardless of whether an infection is localized or systemic, you play a critical role in minimizing its spread. For example, an organism causing a simple wound infection can spread to involve an intravenous needle–insertion site if you use an improper technique when changing a dressing at this site. Nurses who have breaks in their own skin can also acquire infections from clients if their techniques for controlling infection transmission are inadequate.

Defences Against Infection

The body has several mechanisms that protect it against infection. Normal body flora that reside inside and outside the body protect a person from several pathogens. Each organ system has defence mechanisms that fight infectious microorganisms. The **immune response** is a protective reaction that neutralizes pathogens and repairs body cells. The immune system is composed of cells and molecules that help the body resist disease; certain responses of the immune system are nonspecific and protect against microorganisms regardless of prior exposure (e.g., normal flora, body system defences, and inflammation), whereas others are specific defences against particular pathogens. If any of the body's defences fail, an infection can quickly progress to a serious health problem.

Normal Flora. The body normally contains microorganisms that reside on the surface and in deep layers of skin, in the saliva and oral mucosa, and in the gastrointestinal and genitourinary tracts. A person normally excretes trillions of microbes daily through the intestines. The skin also has a large population of resident flora—these **normal flora** do not typically cause disease when residing in their usual area of the body but, instead, participate in maintaining health.

Normal flora of the large intestine exist in great numbers without causing injury. They also secrete antibacterial substances within the intestine's walls. The skin's normal flora exert a protective action by inhibiting the multiplication of organisms landing on the skin. The mouth and pharynx are also protected by flora that impair the growth of invading microbes. The mass of normal flora maintains a sensitive balance with other microorganisms to prevent infection. Any factor that disrupts this balance places a person at increased risk for acquiring an infectious disease. For example, according to studies, when a client acquires microorganisms within the hospital, the person's resident flora changes, which may lead to an infection (Green, 1996; Health Canada, 1999).

In addition, the use of **broad-spectrum antibiotics** for the treatment of infection can lead to a **superinfection**, which develops when broad-spectrum antibiotics eliminate a wide range of microorganisms, not just those causing infection. Normal bacterial flora are eliminated, reducing the body's defences and, thus, allowing disease-producing microorganisms to multiply (Siegel et al., 2007).

Body System Defences. A number of the body's organ systems have unique defences against infection (Table 33–3). The skin, respiratory tract, and gastrointestinal tract are easily accessible to microorganisms: pathogenic organisms easily adhere to the skin's surface, are inhaled into the lungs, or are ingested with food. Each organ system has defence mechanisms physiologically suited to its structure and function. For example, the lungs cannot completely control the entrance of microorganisms; however, the airways are lined with hairlike projections (cilia) that rhythmically beat to move a blanket of mucus and adherent or trapped organisms up to the pharynx to be removed. Conditions that impair an organ's specialized defences increase the person's susceptibility to infection.

Inflammation. Inflammation is the body's cellular response to injury or infection. Inflammation is a protective vascular reaction that delivers fluid, blood products, and nutrients to interstitial tissues in an area of injury. The process neutralizes and eliminates pathogens or **necrotic** (dead) tissues and establishes a means of repairing body cells and tissues. Signs of localized inflammation are swelling, redness, heat, pain or tenderness, and loss of function in the affected body part. When infection becomes systemic, other signs and symptoms develop, including fever, leukocytosis, malaise, anorexia, nausea, vomiting, and lymph node enlargement.

TABLE 33-3 Normal Defence Mechanisms Against Infection

Defence Mechanisms	Action	Factors That May Alter Defence
Skin		
Intact multilayered surface (body's first line of defence against infection)	Provides barrier to microorganisms and antibacterial activity	Cuts, abrasions, wounds, areas of maceration (softening of the skin due to moisture)
Shedding of outer layer of skin cells	Removes organisms that adhere to skin's outer layers	Failure to bathe regularly
Sebum	Contains fatty acid that kills some bacteria	Excessive bathing
Mouth		
Intact multilayered mucosa	Provides mechanical barrier to microorganisms	Lacerations, trauma, extracted teeth
Saliva	Washes away particles containing microorganisms, contains microbial inhibitors (e.g., lysozyme)	Poor oral hygiene, dehydration
Eye		
Tearing and blinking	Blinking prevents entry of particles containing pathogens, and tearing helps to wash particles away	Injury
Respiratory Tract		
Cilia lining upper airway, coated with mucus	Trap inhaled microbes and sweep them outward in mucus to be expectorated or swallowed	Smoking, high concentration of oxygen and carbon dioxide, decreased humidity, cold air
Macrophages	Engulf and destroy microorganisms that reach the lung's alveoli	Smoking
Urinary Tract		
Flushing action of urine flow	Washes away microorganisms on lining of bladder and urethra	Obstruction to normal flow by urinary catheter placement, obstruction from growth or tumour, delayed micturition
Intact multilayered epithelium	Provides barrier to microorganisms	Introduction of urinary catheter, continual movement of catheter in urethra
Gastrointestinal Tract		
Acidity of gastric secretions	Acids destroy some microorganisms	Administration of antacids to neutralize acids
Increased peristalsis in small intestine	Prevents retention of bacterial contents	Delayed motility resulting from impaction of fecal contents in large bowel or mechanical obstruction by masses
Vagina		
At puberty, normal flora causing vaginal secretions to achieve low pH	Inhibit growth of many microorganisms	Use of antibiotics or oral contraceptives, which disrupt normal flora

The **inflammatory response** may be triggered by physical agents, chemical agents, or microorganisms. Mechanical trauma, temperature extremes, and radiation are examples of physical agents. Chemical agents include external and internal irritants such as harsh poisons or gastric acid.

After tissues are injured, the inflammatory response, a series of well-coordinated events, occurs:

- Vascular and cellular responses
- The formation of inflammatory **exudates** (fluid and cells that are discharged from cells or blood vessels, e.g., pus or serum)
- Tissue repair

Vascular and Cellular Responses. Acute inflammation is an immediate response to cellular injury. Arterioles supplying the infected or injured area dilate, allowing more blood into the local circulation. The increase in local blood flow causes the characteristic redness of inflammation. The symptom of localized warmth results from a greater volume of blood at the inflammatory site. Local vasodilation enables blood and white blood cells (WBCs) to travel to the injured tissues.

Injury causes tissue necrosis, and, as a result, the body releases histamine, bradykinin, prostaglandin, and serotonin. These chemical mediators increase the permeability of small blood vessels, allowing fluid, protein, and cells to enter interstitial spaces. Accumulated fluid appears as localized swelling (**edema**).

Another symptom of inflammation is pain—the swelling of inflamed tissues increases the pressure on nerve endings, causing pain. Chemical substances such as histamine stimulate nerve endings. As a result of physiological changes occurring with inflammation, the involved body part usually undergoes a temporary loss of function. For example, a localized infection of the hand causes the fingers to become swollen, painful, and discoloured. Joints may become stiff as a result of the swelling, but the function of the fingers returns when inflammation subsides.

The cellular response of inflammation involves WBCs arriving at the site. These cells pass through the blood vessels and into the tissues. Through the process of **phagocytosis**, specialized WBCs, called *neutrophils* and *monocytes*, ingest and destroy microorganisms and other small particles. As inflammation becomes systemic, other signs and symptoms develop. **Leukocytosis**, or an increase in the number of circulating WBCs, is the body's response to WBCs leaving blood vessels. A serum WBC count is normally 5000/mm^3 to 10,000/mm^3 but may rise to 15,000/mm^3 or even higher during inflammation. Fever is caused by the phagocytic release of pyrogens from bacterial cells that cause a rise in the hypothalamic set point (see Chapter 31).

Inflammatory Exudates. The accumulation of fluid, dead tissue cells, and WBCs forms an exudate at the site of inflammation (see Chapter 47). The exudate may be **serous** (clear, watery plasma), **sanguineous** (bloody drainage), **serosanguineous** (thin, watery drainage that is blood tinged), or **purulent** (thick drainage that contains pus). Eventually, the exudate is cleared away through lymphatic drainage. Platelets and plasma proteins such as fibrinogen form a meshlike matrix at the site of inflammation to prevent the spread of infection.

Tissue Repair. When tissues are injured, healing involves the inflammation, proliferation, and remodelling stages (see Chapter 47). Damaged cells are eventually replaced with healthy new ones, which undergo a gradual maturation until they take on the same structural characteristics and appearance as the previous cells. However, unless a wound is minor, the healed wound does not usually have the tensile strength of the tissue it replaces and scarring may occur.

Health Care-Acquired Infections

Clients in health care settings have an increased risk of acquiring infections. A health care–acquired infection (HAI), also known as **nosocomial infection or iatrogenic infection**, is an infection acquired after admission to a health care facility that was not present or incubating at the time of admission. Clients in hospitals are at risk for infections because they may have a high acuity of illness and frequently undergo aggressive treatments, many of which compromise immunity (Health Canada, 1999). Transmission of antibiotic-resistant organisms also can occur in health care facilities because a large population of susceptible people who frequently receive antibiotics are in close proximity to each other.

Health care–acquired infections can result from a diagnostic or therapeutic procedure, such as a urinary tract infection that develops after catheter insertion. The incidence of nosocomial infections can be reduced if you use critical thinking when practising aseptic techniques. You should always consider the client's risks for infection and anticipate how the approach to care may increase or decrease the chances of infection transmission (Box 33–2).

HAIs may be exogenous or endogenous. An **exogenous infection** arises from microorganisms external to the individual that do not exist as normal flora; examples are *Salmonella* organisms and *Clostridium tetani*. An **endogenous infection** can occur when some of the client's flora become altered and overgrowth results. Examples are infections caused by enterococci, yeasts, and streptococci. When sufficient numbers of microorganisms normally found in one body cavity or lining are transferred to another body site, an endogenous infection develops. For example, the transmission of enterococci, normally found in fecal material, from the hands to the skin is a common cause of wound infections. The number of microorganisms needed to cause an infection depends on the virulence of the organism, the host's susceptibility, and the site affected.

A client's risk of infection is influenced by the number of health care workers having direct contact with the client, the type and number of invasive procedures, the therapy received, and the length of hospitalization. Major sites for HAI include surgical and traumatic wounds, urinary and respiratory tracts, and the bloodstream (Box 33–3).

Older adults have an increased susceptibility to HAIs because they are more likely to have a chronic disease and because of the effects of the aging process itself (Box 33–4). Extended stays in health care institutions, increased disability, and prolonged recovery times are all potential outcomes of HAIs. HAIs decrease the client's quality of life and increase costs to the health care system. Therefore, their prevention is an important part of managed care.

Serous - clear watery
Sanguinous - bloody drainage
serosanguinous - both
purulent - thick, pus drainage

BOX 33-2 NURSING CARE PLAN

The Perils of Central Venous Catheters

Assessment

Susan Serious is a 48-year-old woman in end-stage renal failure secondary to focal segmental glomerulosclerosis, diagnosed 2 months previously. She is dialysis dependent, which required the insertion of a central venous catheter. Susan was admitted to the nephrology service on Friday evening from the emergency department with complaints of chills, nausea, vomiting, headache, and fatigue. She stated that she had felt well until the end of her dialysis treatment that day.

Susan related that she is allergic to co-trimoxazole (Bactrim). Her medication list is composed of amlodipine (Norvasc), ramipril (Altace), furosemide (Lasix), prednisone, calcium carbonate, multivitamins (Replavite), iron dextran, and darbepoetin alpha (Aranesp).

Assessment Activities	*Findings and Defining Characteristics*
Review signs and symptoms of localized and systemic infections.	Signs of localized infection include swelling, redness, heat, pain, or tenderness and loss of function in the affected body part. Signs and symptoms of systemic infection include fever, leukocytosis, malaise, anorexia, nausea, vomiting, and lymph node enlargement.
Research susceptibility to infection in clients with end-stage renal failure.	The literature shows that infections are a significant cause of morbidity and mortality in clients with end-stage renal failure as a result of the clinical setting where treatment is received and the use of immunosuppressive medications (Parker, 1998). Susan has been taking prednisone 30 mg daily.
Review effects of medications.	Prednisone suppresses the body's response to infection.

Nursing Diagnosis: Risk for infection related to disease, immunosuppressive medications, and the use of a central venous catheter.

Planning

Goals	*Expected Outcomes*
Susan will be treated for infection and will remain free of future infections.	Follow up results of chest radiographs, complete blood count with differential, and blood cultures with attending nephrologist to diagnose and treat existing infection. Initiate IV antibiotics, as ordered, to treat existing infection. Arrange to have the tunnelled central venous catheter removed, for 48 hours while receiving antibiotics as ordered, to eliminate the source of infection. After 48 hours the catheter may be reinserted using sterile techique. Susan will recover from existing infection and will not develop signs or symptoms of new infections.
Susan will become knowledgeable of infection risks.	Susan will self-monitor for signs and symptoms of infection, report these to health care professionals, and will observe for good aseptic technique during catheter care by the health care professionals. Review the use and dosage of prednisone with Susan to increase her understanding of immunosuppressive medications.

Interventions

Prevention and Early Detection	*Rationale*
Monitor Susan's temperature, vital signs, and inspect the central venous catheter exit site for evidence of infection.	Interventions are designed to prevent and ensure early detection of infection.
Practise hand hygiene before and after catheter care.	Handwashing reduces bacterial counts on hands (Boyce & Pittet, 2002).
Teach Susan to perform hand hygiene.	
Teach Susan about her catheter: aseptic technique, infection rates, care, and indications of infection.	Increased knowledge will aid in the early detection of infection.
Teach Susan about her medications, indications, side effects, and dosages.	Increased knowledge will increase adherence to the medication regimen and reporting of any related issues.

Evaluation

Nursing Actions	*Client Response and Finding*	*Achievement of Outcome*
Compare Susan's temperature, vital signs, and physical findings with baseline data.	Susan remains afebrile, free of signs and symptoms of infection.	Susan has no active infection at this time.
Ask Susan to review knowledge of catheter-related infections.	Susan is able to identify signs and symptoms of catheter-related infections.	Susan has demonstrated a good knowledge base of catheter-related infections.
Ask Susan to explain the importance of hand hygiene related to catheter care.	Susan is able to relate that hand hygiene eliminates microorganisms that may contribute to infections.	Susan understands the principles and rationale of hand hygiene.
Ask Susan to discuss central venous catheters and the use of aseptic technique during care of the catheters.	Susan is able to describe aseptic technique during catheter care.	Susan has demonstrated knowledge of catheter care.
Ask Susan to review the medications she is currently using.	Susan is able to list and explain the use of her current medications.	Susan has demonstrated an understanding of her medications, regarding their use, effects, and potential concerns.

> **BOX 33-3 Sites for and Causes of Health Care-Acquired Infections**
>
> **Surgical and Traumatic Wounds**
> Improper skin preparation (shaving and bathing) before surgery
> Failure to cleanse skin surface properly
> Failure to use aseptic technique during dressing changes
> The use of contaminated antiseptic solutions
> Improper hand hygiene
>
> **Urinary Tract**
> Inappropriate and unsterile catheterization techniques
> Inadequate monitoring of in-dwelling urinary catheters
> Obstruction or blockages in tubing
> An improper specimen-collection technique
> Urine in the catheter or drainage tube being allowed to re-enter bladder (reflux)
> Improper hand hygiene
>
> **Respiratory Tract**
> Contaminated respiratory therapy equipment
> Failure to use aseptic technique while suctioning airway
> Improper disposal of secretions
> Improper hand hygiene
>
> **Bloodstream**
> Contamination of intravenous fluids by tubing or needle changes
> The insertion of drug additives to intravenous fluid
> The addition of a connecting tube or stopcocks to an intravenous system
> Improper care of a needle-insertion site
> Improper insertion technique
> Contaminated needles or catheters
> Failure to change the intravenous access site when inflammation first appears
> Improper technique during the administration of multiple blood products
> Improper care of peritoneal or hemodialysis catheters
> Improper hand hygiene

> **BOX 33-4 FOCUS ON OLDER ADULTS**
>
> - An age-related decline in immune system function, termed *immune senescence,* increases the body's susceptibility to infection and lessens the strength of the overall immune response (Eliopoulos, 2001).
> - Chronic disease, prevalent among older adults, allows infectious agents to readily invade; hospitalization and institutionalization as a result of chronic disease also increases older adults' exposure to pathogens (Eliopoulos, 2001).
> - Risks associated with the development of infections in older clients include poor nutrition, unintentional weight loss, and low serum albumin levels (Lueckenotte, 2000).
> - Age-related changes in immunity contribute to the increased risk for acquiring pneumonia and influenza in older adulthood, both of which have significant age-related increases in mortality rates (Miller, 1999).
>
> Data from Eliopoulos, C. (2001). *Gerontologic nursing* (5th ed.). Philadelphia, PA: Lippincott; Lueckenotte, A. G. (2000). *Gerontologic nursing* (2nd ed.). St. Louis, MO: Mosby; and Miller, C. A. (1999). *Nursing care of older adults: Theory and practice* (3rd ed.). Philadelphia, PA: Lippincott.

Nursing Process in Infection Control

❖Assessment

When considering infection prevention, you must assess a client's defence mechanisms, susceptibility, and knowledge of infections. A review of disease history with the client and family may reveal an exposure to a communicable disease. A thorough review of the client's clinical condition may allow you to detect signs and symptoms of an infection or a risk for infection. Information about the client's defences against infection can be determined by an analysis of laboratory findings. By knowing the factors that increase susceptibility or risk for infection, you are better able to plan preventive therapy that includes aseptic techniques. Recognizing early signs and symptoms of infection allows you to alert others on the health care team to the potential need for therapy and to initiate supportive nursing measures.

Status of Defence Mechanisms

You can determine the status of the client's normal defence mechanisms against infection through a review of the physical assessment findings and the client's medical condition. For example, any break in the skin or mucosa is a potential site for infection. Similarly, a chronic smoker is at greater risk for acquiring a respiratory tract infection after general surgery because the cilia of the lung are less likely to propel retained mucus from the lung's airways. Any reduction in the body's primary or secondary defences against infection places a client at risk (Box 33–5).

Client Susceptibility

Many factors influence susceptibility to infection. You will gather information about each factor through the client's and family's history.

Age. Throughout the lifespan, susceptibility to infection changes. An infant has immature defences against infection. Born with only the antibodies provided by the mother, the infant's immune system is incapable of producing the necessary immunoglobulins and WBCs to adequately fight some infections. However, breast-fed infants have greater immunity than do bottle-fed infants because they receive the mother's antibodies through the breast milk. As the child grows, the immune system matures; however, the child is still susceptible to organisms that cause the common cold, intestinal

> **BOX 33-5 Risk Factors for Infection**
>
> **Inadequate Primary Defences**
> Broken skin or mucosa
> Traumatized tissue
> Decreased ciliary action
> Obstructed urine outflow
> Altered peristalsis
> A change in the pH of secretions
> Decreased mobility
>
> **Inadequate Secondary Defences**
> A reduced hemoglobin level
> The suppression of WBCs (drug or disease related)
> A suppressed inflammatory response (drug or disease related)
> A low WBC count (leukopenia)

infections, and, if the child is not vaccinated, infectious diseases such as mumps and measles.

The young or middle-aged adult has refined defences against infection. Normal flora, body system defences, inflammation, and the immune response provide protection against invading microorganisms. Viruses are the most common cause of infectious illness in young and middle-aged adults.

Defences against infection change with aging (Gantz et al., 2000). The immune response, particularly cell-mediated immunity, declines. Older adults also undergo alterations in the structure and function of the skin, urinary tract, and lungs. For example, the skin loses its turgor and the epithelium thins; as a result, the skin is more easily abraded or torn. This increases the potential for invasion by pathogens (Table 33–4).

Nutritional Status. When protein intake is inadequate as a result of poor diet or debilitating disease, the rate of protein breakdown exceeds that of tissue synthesis (see Chapter 43). A reduction in the intake of protein and other nutrients such as carbohydrates and fats reduces the body's defences against infection and impairs wound healing (see Chapter 43). Clients with illnesses or problems that increase protein requirements are at further risk. These problems include traumatic injury, extensive burns, and conditions causing fever. Clients who have had surgery also require increased protein.

You need to assess clients' dietary intake and ability to tolerate solid foods. Clients who have difficulty with swallowing, who experience alterations in digestion, or who are too confused or weak to feed themselves are at risk for inadequate dietary intake. A dietitian may be called in to assess the nutritional adequacy of a client's diet.

TABLE 33-4 Assessing the Risk of Infection in Older Adults

Component	Possible Changes With Age	Possible Outcomes
Skin	Thinner dermal and epidermal layers, decreased collagen strength, decreased skin elasticity, decreased sweating	Pressure ulcers
Peripheral nerves	Reduced sensitivity, particularly in clients with a history of alcohol abuse, vitamin B_{12} deficiency, and diabetes mellitus	Pressure ulcers, clients unaware of trauma to skin, leading to infection
Circulation	Congestive heart failure, calcified mitral and aortic valves	Pneumonia, bacterial endocarditis
Peripheral circulation	Loss of elasticity of veins (prone to distension), less effective venous valves, blood pooling in lower extremities	Venous stasis ulcers
Mouth	Dehydration, reduction in saliva production, functional inability to maintain oral hygiene	Parotid gland infection, periodontal disease, localized abscess, bacteremia (i.e., bacteria in the blood)
Gastrointestinal tract	Loss of ability to secrete stomach acid in 30% of persons older than 70 years	*Salmonella* diarrhea
Pulmonary system	Increased colonization of oropharynx, impaired mucociliary clearance, decreased macrophage function, decreased cough reflex	Viral and bacterial pneumonia
Genitourinary tract	Prostatic hypertrophy or hyperplasia, urethral strictures, age-related hormonal changes in vaginal wall, pelvic floor relaxation, ureterocele or cystocele, degeneration of nerves leading to neurogenic bladder, use of tricyclic antidepressants result in urinary retention, dehydration	Asymptomatic bacteriuria (i.e., bacteria in the urine), cystitis, pyelonephritis
Nutrition	Malnutrition, vitamin deficiency (vitamin A, vitamin C, pyridoxine, and riboflavin), protein and caloric deficiencies	Impaired immune response to infection
Drug therapy	Corticosteroid and cytotoxic drugs	Impaired immune response to infection in patients already at risk for decline in immune system function
Long-term care residency	Exposure to nosocomial infections including influenza, *Proteus* and *Providencia* organisms with an in-dwelling catheter, tuberculosis, and wound infections (incidence of bacteremia after admission is 50%)	Frequent serious infection, increased risk of pneumonia

Data from Gantz, N. M., Tkatch, L. S., & Makris, A. T. (2000). Geriatric infections. In J. A. Pfeiffer (Ed.), *APIC text of infection control and epidemiology* (pp. 35.1–35.13). Washington, DC: Association for Professionals in Infection Control and Epidemiology.

When preparing a client for discharge, you should evaluate the client's and family's understanding of nutritional needs.

Stress. The general adaptation syndrome is the body's response to emotional or physical stress (see Chapter 30). During the alarm stage, the basal metabolic rate increases as the body uses energy stores. Adrenocorticotropic hormone acts to increase serum glucose levels and decrease unnecessary anti-inflammatory responses through the release of cortisone. If stress continues or becomes intense, elevated cortisone levels result in a decreased resistance to infection. Continued stress leads to exhaustion, wherein energy stores are depleted and the body has no resistance to invading organisms. The same conditions that increase nutritional requirements, such as surgery or trauma, also increase physiological stress.

Disease Process. Clients with diseases of the immune system are at particular risk for infection. Leukemia, AIDS, lymphoma, and aplastic anemia are conditions that compromise a host by weakening defences against infectious organisms. Clients with leukemia, for example, are unable to produce normal WBCs to effectively ward off infection.

Clients with chronic diseases such as diabetes mellitus and multiple sclerosis are also more susceptible to infection because of general debilitation and nutritional impairment. Cancer (which alters the immune response), peripheral vascular disease (which reduces blood flow to injured tissues), and diseases that impair body system defences, such as emphysema and bronchitis (which impair ciliary action and thicken mucus), increase susceptibility to infection. Clients with burns have a very high susceptibility to infection because of the damage to skin surfaces. The greater the depth and extent of the burns are, the higher the risk for infection is.

Medical Therapy. Some drugs and medical therapies compromise immunity to infection. You will need to assess your clients' history to determine whether they take medications at home that increase infection susceptibility. A review of therapies received within the health care setting may further reveal risks. Adrenal corticosteroids, prescribed for several conditions, are anti-inflammatory drugs that cause protein breakdown and impair the inflammatory response against bacteria and other pathogens. Cytotoxic or antineoplastic drugs attack cancer cells but cause side effects including depression of bone marrow activity and normal cell toxicity. When bone marrow activity is depressed, the body is unable to produce lymphocytes and sufficient WBCs. When normal cells become altered by antineoplastic agents, cellular defences against infection fail. Cyclosporine and other immunosuppressant drugs, which decrease the body's immune response, are commonly taken by organ transplant recipients. The immunosuppressants prevent organ and tissue rejection, but they also increase the recipients' susceptibility to infection.

Clients with cancer who are receiving radiotherapy are at risk for infection. The massive doses of radiation that destroy cancerous cells can also depress bone marrow activity and destroy normal cells.

Clinical Appearance

The signs and symptoms of infection may be local or systemic. Localized infections are most common in areas of skin or mucous membrane breakdown, such as surgical and traumatic wounds, pressure ulcers, and mouth lesions. Infections also develop locally in cavities beneath the skin; an example is an abscess.

To assess an area for localized infection, you should first inspect the area for redness and swelling caused by inflammation. Because drainage from open lesions or wounds may occur, you must wear disposable gloves. Infected drainage may be yellow, green, or brown, depending on the pathogen. Ask the client about pain or tenderness around the site. The client may complain of tightness and pain caused by edema. If the infected area is large enough, movement of a body part may be restricted. Gentle palpation of an infected area usually results in some degree of tenderness.

Systemic infections cause more generalized symptoms than do local infections. Systemic infections usually result in fever, fatigue, and malaise. Lymph nodes that drain the area of infection often become enlarged, swollen, and tender during palpation. For example, an abscess in the peritoneal cavity may cause the enlargement of the lymph nodes in the groin. An infection of the upper respiratory tract may cause cervical lymph node enlargement. If an infection is serious and widespread, all major lymph nodes may enlarge. Systemic infections commonly cause a loss of appetite, nausea, and vomiting.

Systemic infections may develop after treatment for a localized infection has failed. You should be alert for changes in a client's level of activity and responsiveness. As systemic infections develop, the client may become lethargic and complain of a loss of energy. An elevation in body temperature may lead to episodes of increased heart and respiratory rates and low blood pressure. The involvement of major body systems may produce specific signs. For example, a pulmonary infection may result in a productive cough with purulent sputum. A urinary tract infection may result in cloudy, foul-smelling urine.

In older adults, infection may not present with typical signs and symptoms. Fever, pain, and swelling are often absent in older adults because they tend to have lower body temperatures, decreased pain sensation, and less immune response to infection. As a result, in older adults, infection is often advanced before it is identified. Atypical symptoms such as a change in behaviour (e.g., new or increased confusion, incontinence, or agitation) may be the only symptoms of an infectious illness (Gantz et al., 2000). For example, as many as 20% of older adults with pneumonia do not have the typical signs and symptoms of fever, shaking, chills, and "rusty" productive sputum. The only symptoms present may be an increased heart rate with no apparent reason, confusion, or generalized fatigue.

Laboratory Data

A review of laboratory test results may confirm infection (Table 33–5). However, laboratory values alone are not sufficient to detect infection; other clinical signs must be assessed. Factors other than infection may alter test values. For example, trauma and physical stress can cause an elevation in the number of neutrophils. A culture may show the growth of an organism in the absence of overt signs of infection.

Clients With Infection

A client with infection may have a variety of health problems. You need to assess ways that the infection affects the client's and family's needs—these may be physical, psychological, social, or economic. For example, a client with a chronic disease such as AIDS may experience serious psychological problems as a result of self-imposed isolation or rejection by family and friends. Using a case-management approach, you can determine the client's and family's ability to adjust to the disease and the resources available to help them manage health care challenges (Grimes & Grimes, 1994).

TABLE 33-5 Laboratory Tests to Screen for Infection

Laboratory Value	Normal (Adult) Values	Indication of Infection
White blood cell (WBC) count	4–11 × 10^9/L	Increased in acute infection, decreased in certain viral or overwhelming infections
Erythrocyte sedimentation rate	Up to 15 mm/hour for men and 20 mm/hour for women	Elevated in presence of inflammatory process
Iron level	60–90 g/100 mL	Decreased in chronic infection
C-reactive protein	30–35 mg/dL	Elevated in the presence of acute inflammatory process
Cultures of urine and blood	Normally sterile, without microorganism growth	Presence of infectious microorganism growth
Cultures and Gram stain of wound, sputum, and throat	No WBCs on Gram stain, possible normal flora	Presence of infectious microorganism growth and WBCs on Gram stain
WBC	**Differential Count (Percentage of Each Type of WBC)**	**Indication of Infection**
Neutrophils	55%–70%	Increased in acute suppurative infection, decreased in overwhelming bacterial infection (older adult)
Lymphocytes	20%–40%	Increased in chronic bacterial and viral infection, decreased in sepsis
Monocytes	2%–8%	Increased in protozoal, rickettsial, and tuberculosis infections
Eosinophils	1%–4%	Increased in parasitic infection
Basophils	0.5%–1%	Normal during infection

❖Nursing Diagnosis

During assessment, you gather objective findings, such as an open incision or a reduced caloric intake, and subjective data, such as a client's complaint of tenderness over a surgical wound site (Box 33–6). You then interpret the data carefully, looking for clusters of defining characteristics or risk factors that create a pattern suggesting a specific nursing diagnosis. The following are examples of nursing diagnoses that may apply:

- *Disturbed body image*
- *Risk for infection*
- *Risk for injury*
- *Imbalanced nutrition—less than body requirements*
- *Impaired oral mucous membrane*
- *Risk for impaired skin integrity*
- *Social isolation*
- *Impaired tissue integrity*

It may be necessary for you to validate data (e.g., by inspecting the integrity of a wound more carefully). Likewise, additional data such as laboratory findings may be helpful. The proper selection of appropriate nursing diagnoses depends on the correct analysis and organization of data.

The diagnosis must have the correct etiological factor for you to establish an appropriate and well-thought-out plan. For example, minimizing the risk for infection related to broken skin requires

BOX 33-6 NURSING DIAGNOSTIC PROCESS

Assessment Activities	*Defining Characteristics*	*Nursing Diagnosis*
Check results of laboratory tests.	WBC count 3.9 × 10^9/L	*Risk for infection related to neutropenia.*
Review current medications.	Client receiving azathioprine (Imuran), an immunosuppressant	
Identify potential sites of infection.	Intravenous catheter in right forearm in place for 3 days	
	Foley catheter draining amber-coloured urine	

good hygiene measures and wound care; minimizing the risk for infection related to malnutrition requires good nutritional support and fluid balance.

You may diagnose a risk for infection or make diagnoses that result from the effects of infection on the client's health status. Your success in planning appropriate nursing interventions depends on the accuracy of the diagnosis and your ability to meet the client's needs.

❖Planning

Goals and Outcomes

The client's care plan is based on each nursing diagnosis and related factors (Box 33–7). You develop a plan that sets attainable outcomes so that interventions are purposeful and directed. If you are caring for a client with the nursing diagnosis *risk for infection related to broken skin,* you must implement skin and wound care measures to promote healing. The expected outcomes "reduction in wound size by 1 cm" and "absence of drainage" represent targets for measuring the client's improvement. Once outcomes are met, the goal of "skin intact and without drainage" can be reached. Interventions are selected in collaboration with the client, the family, and others on the health care team. You direct the care in the acute care setting; care may also involve other professionals in assisting with instructions on postdischarge procedures. Common goals of care relating to infection include the following:

- Preventing exposure to infectious organisms
- Controlling or reducing the extent of the infection
- Maintaining resistance to infection
- Educating the client and family about infection-control techniques

Setting Priorities

In collaboration with the client, you establish priorities for the goals of care. For example, for a client who has an open wound and cancer and cannot tolerate solid foods, the priority of administering therapies that promote wound healing exceeds the goal of educating the client to assume self-care therapies at home. When the client's condition improves, the priorities will change, and client education will become an essential intervention.

Continuity of Care

The development of a care plan includes infection-prevention practices. You may initiate appropriate referrals, such as to a dietitian, infection-control professional, or home care nurse, to collaborate in a client's care. When care is being administered in the home, you should ensure that the environment supports good infection-control practices. For example, if a client does not have running water, you need to bring a waterless antimicrobial solution during visits to ensure adequate hand hygiene. Educating clients and families is also an important aspect of prevention.

➤BOX 33-7 NURSING CARE PLAN

Risk for Infection

Assessment

Mrs. Spicer was admitted to the medical nursing unit 3 days ago with a diagnosis of lymphoma. She received her first dose of multiagent chemotherapy yesterday. Jess Ralston is the student nurse caring for Mrs. Spicer. He begins his shift by conducting a focused assessment.

Assessment Activities	*Findings and Defining Characteristics*
Review client's chart for laboratory data reflecting immune function.	Data show a reduction in number of WBCs (leukopenia).
Ask client to describe appetite and review food intake for past 24 hours. Weigh client. Measure height.	Mrs. Spicer reports she has not had an interest in eating for a couple of weeks. She has lost approximately 2.5 kg. Her current weight is 57 kg, and her height is 170 cm. Her food intake yesterday consisted of a small cup of applesauce, a half-bowl of soup, some crackers, and two glasses of juice. Mrs. Spicer states, "I get full easily and lose interest in food."
Palpate client's cervical and clavicular lymph nodes.	Lymph nodes are enlarged and painless.
Review effects of chemotherapy in drug reference.	Multiagent chemotherapy causes drug-induced pancytopenia.

Nursing Diagnosis: Risk for infection related to immunosuppression and reduced food intake

Planning

*Goals (Nursing Outcomes Classification)**	*Expected Outcomes*
	Risk Detection
Client will remain free of infection.	Client will remain afebrile. Client will develop no signs or symptoms of local infection (e.g., will remain free of cough, cloudy or foul-smelling urine, and purulent drainage from open wound or normal body opening).
	Knowledge: Infection Control
Client will become knowledgeable of infection risks.	Client will identify routines to follow in the home that reduce the transmission of microorganisms. Client will identify signs and symptoms indicating infection to report to her health care professional.

*Outcome classification labels from Moorhead, S., Johnson, M., & Maas, M. (Eds.). (2004). *Nursing Outcomes Classification (NOC)* (3rd ed.). St. Louis, MO: Mosby.

Continued

BOX 33-7 NURSING CARE PLAN *continued*

Interventions (Nursing Intervention Classification)†	Rationale
Prevention and Early Detection	
Monitor client's body temperature routinely, inspect oral cavity for lesions, inspect urethral and vaginal orifices for drainage or discharge, inspect intravenous access site for drainage, and observe client for evidence of cough.	Interventions are designed to prevent and ensure early detection of infection in a client at risk (Dochterman & Bulechek, 2004).
Practise hand hygiene routinely before caring for a client, between clients, and before any invasive procedures.	Rigorous hand hygiene reduces bacterial counts on the hands (Boyce & Pittet, 2002).
Teach client how to perform hand hygiene correctly.	Client can easily come in contact with infectious agents that can cause infection.
Consult with dietitian about providing a high-calorie, high-protein, low-bacteria diet. Minimize the intake of salads, undercooked meat, pepper, paprika, and raw fruits and vegetables. Offer small, frequent meals.	Maintaining calorie and protein intake will prevent weight loss. Foods high in bacteria should be avoided because they increase the risk for gastrointestinal infection (Ignatavicius & Workman, 2002).
Infection Control	
Instruct client to report the following to the physician: temperature >38°C, persistent cough with or without sputum, pus or foul-smelling drainage from the body site, the presence of an abscess, urine that is cloudy or foul smelling, or burning on urination.	Signs and symptoms are indicative of local or systemic infection.
Teach client to follow these activities at home: • Avoid crowds and large gatherings of persons. • Bathe daily. • Do not share personal hygiene items with family members (e.g., toothbrush, washcloth, and deodorant stick). • Take your temperature twice daily. • Do not drink water that has been standing for >15 minutes. • Do not reuse cups or glasses without washing.	These measures are designed to prevent infection in clients with impaired immune function (Ignatavicius & Workman, 2002).

†Intervention classification labels from Dochterman, J. M., & Bulechek, G. M. (Eds.). (2004). *Nursing Interventions Classification (NIC)* (4th ed.). St. Louis, MO: Mosby.

Evaluation

Nursing Actions	*Client Response and Finding*	*Achievement of Outcome*
Compare client's body temperature and other physical findings with baseline data.	Mrs. Spicer remains afebrile and denies having cough or burning on urination. No signs of drainage or discharge from body site are evident.	Mrs. Spicer has no active infection at this time.
Ask client to describe signs and symptoms to report to health care professional.	Mrs. Spicer is able to identify the temperature range to report. She is able to describe cough. She is unable to identify signs of urinary infection or local discharge.	Mrs. Spicer has a partial understanding of signs and symptoms to report. I will require additional instruction and information sheet.
Ask client to explain the measures to take at home to reduce exposure to infectious agents.	Mrs. Spicer is able to discuss need to avoid sharing personal hygiene articles. She has asked for a list of other precautions and requested that her husband be included in discussion.	Mrs. Spicer has a partial understanding of restrictions. I will obtain printed guidelines and include her husband in discussion this evening.

❖Implementation

By recognizing and assessing a client's risk factors and implementing appropriate measures, you can reduce the risk of infection.

Health Promotion

You may prevent an infection from developing or spreading by minimizing the numbers and kinds of organisms transmitted to potential infection sites. Eliminating reservoirs of infection, controlling portals of exit and entry, and avoiding actions that transmit microorganisms prevent pathogens from finding a new site in which to grow. The proper use of sterile supplies, barrier protection, and proper hand hygiene are examples of methods that nurses use to control the spread of microorganisms. A further preventive measure is to strengthen a potential host's defences against infection. Nutritional support, rest, maintenance of physiological protective mechanisms, and receipt of recommended immunizations (Box 33–8) protect a client from invasion by pathogens.

BOX 33-8 FOCUS ON PRIMARY HEALTH CARE

Immunizations

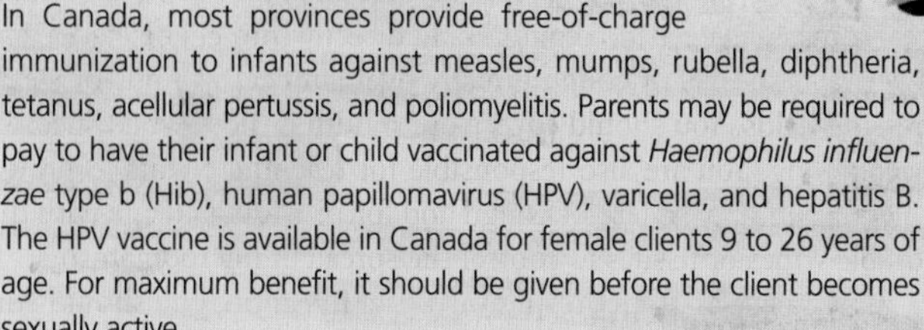

Immunizations are an essential component of disease prevention. You should encourage proper immunization of infants, children, those at risk, and older adults. In Canada, most provinces provide free-of-charge immunization to infants against measles, mumps, rubella, diphtheria, tetanus, acellular pertussis, and poliomyelitis. Parents may be required to pay to have their infant or child vaccinated against *Haemophilus influenzae* type b (Hib), human papillomavirus (HPV), varicella, and hepatitis B. The HPV vaccine is available in Canada for female clients 9 to 26 years of age. For maximum benefit, it should be given before the client becomes sexually active.

Older adults and those who have underlying medical conditions are at risk for influenza and pneumonia and are therefore offered influenza vaccines each year and pneumococcal vaccines as per the recommended schedule, which varies according to the recipient's age. You should remind clients of the importance of having a tetanus–diphtheria booster vaccination every 10 years. Health care workers who care for persons at high risk for complications from influenza should be immunized for influenza yearly as well.

In most provinces and territories, public health nurses or community nurses hold free immunization clinics for clients at risk during an outbreak of a potentially deadly infection such as bacterial meningitis.

From Health Canada. (2006). *Canadian immunization guide* (7th ed.). Ottawa, ON: Public Health Agency of Canada. Retrieved December 19, 2008, from http://www.naci.gc.ca

Being vigilant about infection control helps you to apply good medical–surgical aseptic practices at the right time and in the right clinical situation. When a client develops an infection, you need to continue preventive care so that health care personnel and other clients are not exposed to the infection. Isolation precautions may be necessary for clients with communicable diseases; the environment is controlled by barriers against the transmission of infection (see "Isolation Guidelines" section).

Acute Care Measures

Treatment of an infectious process includes eliminating the infectious organisms and supporting the client's defences. To identify the causative organism, you may collect specimens of body fluids or drainage from infected body sites for cultures. When the disease process or causative organism has been identified, the physician prescribes the treatment that is most effective for the situation. You properly administer antibiotics and other treatments, watch for adverse reactions, and assess the progress of the infection.

Systemic infections necessitate measures to prevent complications of fever (see Chapter 33). Maintaining the client's intake of fluids prevents dehydration resulting from diaphoresis. Because of the client's increased metabolic rate, adequate nutritional intake must be ensured. Rest preserves energy for the healing process.

Localized infections often necessitate measures to remove debris to promote healing. You will need to apply the principles of wound care to remove any infected drainage from the wound site and support the integrity of healing wounds. Special dressings can be applied to facilitate the removal of infectious drainage and promote healing of wound margins. Drainage tubes may be inserted to remove infected drainage from body cavities. You must use medical and surgical aseptic techniques to manage wounds and ensure correct handling of all drainage or body fluids (see Chapter 47).

During the course of infection, you can support the client's body defence mechanisms. For example, if a client has infectious diarrhea, you must maintain skin integrity to prevent breakdown and the entrance of microorganisms. Other routine hygiene measures such as bathing and oral care protect the skin and mucous membranes from invasion and overgrowth of microorganisms.

Asepsis

Your efforts to minimize the onset and spread of infection are based on the principles of aseptic technique. **Asepsis** is the absence of pathogenic (disease-producing) microorganisms. *Aseptic technique* refers to practices that keep a client as free from pathogens as possible. The two types of aseptic technique are medical asepsis and surgical asepsis.

Medical asepsis, or clean technique, includes procedures used to reduce and prevent the spread of microorganisms. Hand hygiene, using clean gloves (i.e., disposable gloves) to prevent direct contact with blood or body fluids, and cleaning the environment routinely are examples of medical asepsis. The principles of medical asepsis are commonly followed in the home, as in washing hands before preparing food.

After an object becomes unsterile or unclean, it is considered *contaminated*. In medical asepsis, an area or object is considered contaminated if it contains or is suspected of containing pathogens. For example, a used bedpan, the floor, and a used dressing are contaminated.

You need to follow certain principles and procedures, including **standard precautions** (also known as **routine practices**), to prevent infection and control its spread (see "Isolation Guidelines" section). During your daily routine care, use basic medical aseptic techniques to break the infection chain. Because infections are readily transmitted between clients and caregivers, it may become necessary for you to follow isolation precautions as appropriate (see "Isolation Guidelines" section).

You are responsible for providing the client with a safe environment. The effectiveness of infection-control practices depends on you and your colleagues' conscientiousness and consistency in using effective aseptic technique. It is easy to forget key procedural steps or, in a hurry, to take shortcuts that break aseptic procedures. However, your failure to be meticulous places the client at risk for an infection that can seriously impair recovery or lead to death.

Control or Elimination of Infectious Agents. Proper cleaning, disinfection, and sterilization of contaminated objects significantly reduce and often eliminate microorganisms. In health care centres, a sterile processing department disinfects and sterilizes reusable supplies. However, you also may be required to perform these functions. Many principles of cleaning and disinfection also apply to the home.

Cleaning. Cleaning is the physical removal of foreign material (e.g., dust, soil, and organic material such as blood, secretions, excretions, and microorganisms) from objects and surfaces (Health Canada, 1998). In general, cleaning involves the use of water and mechanical action with detergents or enzymatic products. When an object comes in contact with infectious or potentially infectious material, the object is contaminated. Reusable objects must be cleaned thoroughly before reuse and then either disinfected or sterilized according to the manufacturer's recommendations.

When cleaning equipment that is soiled by organic material such as blood, fecal matter, mucus, or pus, you should take appropriate measures to protect yourself against contamination. These may include wearing a mask and protective eyewear (or a face shield) and waterproof gloves. These barriers provide protection from infectious organisms. A brush and detergent or soap are needed for cleaning.

The following steps ensure that an object is clean:

1. Rinse a contaminated object or article with cold running water to remove organic material. Hot water causes the protein in organic material to coagulate and stick to objects, making removal difficult.
2. After rinsing, wash the object with soap and warm water. Soap or detergent reduces the surface tension of water and emulsifies the dirt or remaining material. Rinse the object thoroughly to remove the emulsified dirt.
3. Use a brush to remove dirt or material in grooves or seams. Friction dislodges the contaminated material for easy removal. Open any hinged items for cleaning.
4. Rinse the object in warm water.
5. Dry the object and prepare it for disinfection or sterilization if indicated by the intended use of the item.
6. The brush, gloves, and sink in which the equipment is cleaned should be considered contaminated and should be cleaned and dried.

Disinfection and Sterilization. Disinfection is the elimination of all pathogens except bacterial spores (Health Canada, 1998). Disinfectants are used on inanimate objects; antiseptics are used on living tissue. Disinfection usually involves chemicals, heat, or ultraviolet light. An item must be thoroughly cleaned before it is disinfected. Examples of disinfectants are alcohols, chlorines, glutaraldehydes, phenols, and quaternary ammonium compounds. These chemicals can be caustic and toxic to tissues. Some disinfectants are indicated only for use on noncritical items; you should read the label and follow the manufacturer's recommendations for use.

Sterilization is the destruction of all microorganisms, including spores. Steam under pressure, ethylene oxide gas, hydrogen peroxide plasma, and chemicals are the most common sterilizing agents. Items must be cleaned thoroughly before they can be sterilized.

Whether an item is to be simply cleaned, or cleaned and disinfected or sterilized, depends on the intended use of the item. Devices are classified in three categories (Box 33–9). You should be familiar with your agency's policy and procedures for cleaning, handling, and delivering care items for eventual disinfection and sterilization. Workers especially trained in disinfection and sterilization should perform most of the procedures. Efficacy of the disinfecting or sterilizing method is influenced by the following factors:

- *Concentration of solution and duration of contact.* A weakened concentration or shortened exposure time may lessen effectiveness.
- *Type and number of pathogens.* Certain organisms are killed more easily than others by disruption. Higher numbers of pathogens on an object necessitate longer disinfecting time.
- *Surface areas to treat.* All dirty surfaces and areas must be fully exposed to disinfecting and sterilizing agents.
- *Temperature of the environment.* Disinfectants tend to work best at room temperature.
- *Presence of soap.* Soap may cause certain disinfectants to be ineffective. Thorough rinsing of an object is necessary before disinfecting.
- *Presence of organic materials.* Disinfectants can become inactivated unless blood, saliva, pus, or body excretions are already washed off.

Table 33–6 lists processes for disinfection and sterilization and their characteristics. Selection of the method for disinfecting or sterilizing an item depends on the intended use and nature of the item (e.g., some delicate instruments cannot tolerate steam and must be sterilized with gas or plasma).

Control or Elimination of Reservoirs. To control or eliminate reservoir sites for infection, you need to eliminate or control sources of body fluids, drainage, or solutions that might harbour microorganisms. You must also carefully discard articles that become contaminated with infectious material (Box 33–10). All health care institutions must have guidelines for the disposal of infectious waste according to provincial or territorial laws.

Control of Portals of Exit. You will need to follow several measures to minimize or prevent infectious organisms from exiting the body. To control organisms exiting via the respiratory tract, you should wear a mask as needed, avoid talking directly into clients' faces, and never talk, sneeze, or cough directly over surgical wounds or sterile dressing fields. You should cover your mouth or nose when sneezing or coughing. You are also responsible for teaching clients to protect others when they sneeze or cough and for providing clients with disposable wipes or tissues to control the spread of microorganisms.

If you have an upper respiratory tract infection, you should consider not working; you may be required to remain at home. If you continue to work with clients, you should wear a mask when working closely with a client and pay special attention to hand hygiene. You should not be caring for clients who are highly susceptible to infection (e.g., an immunosuppressed client or a neonate).

Another way of controlling the exit of microorganisms is through the careful handling of blood, body fluids, secretions, or excretions (e.g., urine, feces, vomitus, and exudate). Contaminated fluids can

➤ BOX 33-9 Categories for Sterilization, Disinfection, and Cleaning

Critical Items

Critical items are instruments and devices that enter sterile tissue or the vascular system. They present a high risk of infection if the items are contaminated with microorganisms, including bacterial spores. Critical items must be thoroughly cleaned and sterilized. Examples of these items include the following:

- Surgical instruments
- Intravascular catheters
- Urinary catheters
- Needles

Semicritical Items

Semicritical items are devices that come in contact with mucous membranes or nonintact skin but do not penetrate them. These items also present a risk of infection and must be free of all microorganisms (except bacterial spores). Semicritical items must be thoroughly cleaned and disinfected. The following are examples of these items:

- Electronic thermometers
- Respiratory therapy equipment
- Endotracheal tubes
- Gastrointestinal endoscopes
- Vaginal and nasal specula

Noncritical Items

Noncritical items are items that either touch only intact skin but not mucous membranes or do not directly touch the client. Noncritical items must be cleaned or cleaned and disinfected. Examples of these items include the following:

- Bedpans, urinals, and commodes
- Blood pressure cuffs
- Linens
- Stethoscopes
- Some eating utensils

TABLE 33-6 Examples of Disinfection and Sterilization Processes

Characteristics	Examples of Use
Moist Heat	
Steam is moist heat under pressure. When exposed to high pressure, water vapour can attain a temperature above boiling point to kill pathogens and spores.	An autoclave is used to sterilize surgical instruments and dressings.
Chemicals	
A number of chemical disinfectants are used in health care, including alcohols, chlorines, formaldehyde, glutaraldehydes, hydrogen peroxide, iodophors, phenolics, and quaternary ammonium compounds. Each product performs in a unique manner and is used for a specific purpose.	Chemicals are used for the disinfection of instruments and equipment such as thermometers and endoscopes. Use the appropriate facility-approved disinfectant in a safe manner (e.g., with gloves, proper ventilation) for the approved purpose.
Ethylene Oxide Gas	
Ethylene oxide gas destroys spores and microorganisms by altering cells' metabolic processes. Fumes are released within an autoclave-like chamber. This gas is toxic to humans, and aeration time varies with products.	This gas sterilizes some rubber and plastic items.
Boiling Water	
Boiling is the least expensive method of sterilization for use in the home. Bacterial spores and some viruses resist boiling. It is not used in hospitals.	The items (e.g., glass baby bottles) should be boiled for at least 15 minutes.

BOX 33-10 Infection Control to Reduce Reservoir Sites

Bathing

Use soap and water to remove drainage, dried secretions, or excess perspiration.

Dressing Changes

Change dressings that become wet or soiled (see Chapter 47).

Contaminated Articles

Place tissues, soiled dressings, and soiled linen in moisture-resistant bags for proper disposal.

Contaminated Needles

Engage the safety features of all sharp devices and dispose of them in a puncture-proof container. Place syringes, uncapped hypodermic needles, and intravenous needles in puncture-proof containers, which should be located in client rooms or treatment areas so that exposed, contaminated equipment need not be carried a distance (see Chapter 34). *Do not recap needles* or attempt to break them.

Bedside Unit

Keep table surfaces clean and dry.

Bottled Solutions

Do not leave bottled solutions open for prolonged periods. Keep solutions tightly capped. Date bottles when opened and discard according to your facility's policy.

Surgical Wounds

Keep drainage tubes and collection bags patent to prevent the accumulation of serous fluid under the skin surface.

Drainage Bottles and Bags

Empty and dispose of drainage suction bottles according to your health agency's policy. Empty all drainage systems on each shift unless otherwise ordered by a physician. Never raise a drainage system (e.g., urinary drainage bag) above the level of the site being drained unless the drainage system is clamped off.

easily splash while being discarded or cleaned up. You should always wear disposable gloves when handling blood, body fluids, secretions, or excretions. Masks, gowns, and protective eyewear should be worn if splashing or contact with any fluids is possible. You should appropriately dispose of disposable soiled items in impervious plastic bags. Laboratory specimens from all clients are handled as if they were infectious.

Control of Transmission. Effective control of infection requires you to remain aware of the modes of transmission and ways to control them. In the hospital, home, or long-term care facility, a client should have a personal set of care items. The sharing of bedpans, urinals, bath basins, and eating utensils can easily lead to transmission of infection. Thermometers, even when individually used, warrant special care. Because the client's own mucus can become a source of microorganism growth, the electronic thermometer is used with a disposable sheath over the probe; the sheath is discarded after each use. Single-use chemical strip thermometers present less risk of infection than do other thermometers. Use of electronic thermometers for rectal temperatures has been associated with nosocomial diarrhea (Jernigan et al., 1998). The organism *C. difficile* is able to survive on inanimate surfaces such as a thermometer probe for weeks to months. In institutions where nosocomial diarrhea occurs, electronic thermometers are not recommended for rectal temperatures.

To prevent transmission of microorganisms through indirect contact, soiled items and equipment must not touch your clothing. A common error is to carry dirty linen in the arms against the uniform. Fluid-resistant linen bags should be used, or soiled linen should be carried with hands held out from the body. Laundry hampers should be replaced before they are overflowing.

Hand Hygiene. **Hand hygiene** is the most important and most basic technique in preventing the transmission of infections. Hand hygiene includes using an instant alcohol hand antiseptic before and after providing client care, handwashing with soap and water when hands are visibly soiled, and performing a surgical scrub when necessary. The components of good **handwashing** include using an adequate amount of soap, rubbing the hands together to lather the soap and create friction, and rinsing under a stream of water (Health Canada, 1998). The purpose is to remove soil and transient organisms from the hands and to reduce total microbial counts over time.

Contaminated hands are a prime cause of cross-infection. For example, imagine you are caring for a client who has excessive pulmonary secretions, and you assist the client in expectorating mucus and disposing of the tissues in a bedside container. The client's roommate asks you to open containers of food on the meal tray. You then leave the client's room to pour a dose of medication that is to be taken in 5 minutes. If you fail to perform hand hygiene before opening the containers of food or pouring the medication, organisms from the first client's mucus can easily be transmitted to the roommate's food and to the medication container. Decreased nosocomial infection rates have been reported with improved handwashing compliance (Pittet et al., 2000).

The decision regarding when and what type of hand hygiene should occur depends on the following: the intensity of contact with clients or contaminated objects, the degree or amount of contamination that could occur with that contact, the susceptibility of the client or the health care worker to infection, and the procedure or activity to be performed (Larson, 1996). For example, after prolonged and direct contact with a client's wound drainage, you must perform thorough hand hygiene.

Washing times of at least 15 seconds are needed to remove most transient microorganisms from the skin (CDC, 2002). If the hands are visibly soiled, more time may be needed. Routine handwashing may be performed with plain soap. Plain soap with water can physically remove a certain level of microbes, but antiseptic agents are necessary to kill or inhibit microorganisms and reduce the level still further (CDC, 2002). Skill 33–1 lists the steps for hand hygiene.

➤ SKILL 33-1 Hand Hygiene

video

Delegation Considerations

- Monitor an unregulated care provider (UCP) to ensure that he or she is using the proper method of hand hygiene.
- Instruct the UCP to report any skin irritation from soaps or antimicrobials.

Equipment

- Easy-to-reach sink with warm running water
- Antimicrobial or regular soap
- Alcohol-based waterless antiseptic
- Paper towels or air dryer
- Clean orangewood stick (optional)

Procedure

STEPS	RATIONALE
1. Inspect surface of hands for breaks or cuts in skin or cuticles. Report and cover lesions before providing client care.	• Open cuts or wounds can harbour high concentrations of microorganisms. Agency policy may prevent you from caring for high-risk clients. If dermatitis occurs, additional interventions may be needed.
2. Inspect hands for visible soiling.	• Lengthier handwashing is needed if soiling is heavy.
3. Inspect nails for length and presence of artificial acrylics or chipped nail polish.	• Nails should be short and filed because most microbes on hands come from beneath the fingernails. Nails should be free of artificial applications and chipped or old nail polish (CDC, 2002; Gruendeman & Mangum, 2001; Health Canada, 1998). (See Box 33–11.)
4. Assess client's risk for, or extent of, infection (e.g., WBC count, extent of open wounds, known medical diagnosis).	• Use of alcohol-based waterless antiseptic is encouraged if you will be working with clients who are immunosuppressed (CDC, 2002; Health Canada, 1998).
5. Push wristwatch and long uniform sleeves above wrists. Avoid wearing rings. If worn, remove during procedure.	• Provide complete access to fingers, hands, and wrists. Wearing of rings increases number of microorganisms on hands (Garner, 1996).
6. If hands are visibly dirty or contaminated with protein-containing material, use water and plain soap or antimicrobial soap for handwashing:	
A. Stand in front of sink, keeping hands and uniform away from sink surface. (If hands touch sink during handwashing, repeat procedure.)	• Inside of sink is a contaminated area. Reaching over the sink increases the risk of touching the edge, which is contaminated.
B. Turn on water. Turn faucet on or push knee pedals laterally or press pedals with foot to regulate flow and temperature (see Step 6B illustration).	
C. Avoid splashing water against uniform.	• Microorganisms travel and grow in moisture.
D. Regulate flow of water so that temperature is warm.	• Warm water removes less of the protective oils than does hot water.
E. Wet hands and wrists thoroughly under running water. Keep hands and forearms lower than elbows during washing.	• Hands are the most contaminated parts to be washed. Water flows from least to most contaminated area, rinsing microorganisms into the sink.
F. Apply a small amount of soap, lathering thoroughly (see Step 6F illustration). Soap granules and leaflet preparations may be used.	• Antimicrobial soaps used exclusively can be drying to hands and can cause skin irritations. The decision of whether to use an antimicrobial soap or alcohol-based hand antiseptic should depend on the procedure to be performed and the client's immune status.

➤ SKILL 33-1 Hand Hygiene *continued*

G. Wash hands using plenty of lather and friction for at least 10 to 15 seconds. Interlace fingers and rub palms and back of hands with circular motion at least five times each. Keep fingertips down to facilitate removal of microorganisms. Rub knuckles of one hand into the palm of the other; repeat with other hand (see Step 6G illustration).	• Soap cleanses by emulsifying fat and oil and lowering the surface tension of water. Friction and rubbing mechanically loosen and remove dirt and transient bacteria. Interlacing fingers and thumbs and rubbing knuckles ensures that all surfaces are cleansed.
H. Rub thumb on one hand with the palm of the other hand; repeat with other hand (see Step 6H illustration).	• Thumbs are frequently missed areas.
I. Work the fingertips on one hand into the palm of the other. Massage soap into nail spaces; repeat with other hand (see Step 6I illustration).	• Fingertips are frequently missed areas.
J. Areas under fingernails are often soiled. Clean them with orange-wood stick or fingernails of other hand and additional soap.	• Areas under nails can be highly contaminated, which increases the risk of infection.

Critical Decision Point: Do not tear or cut skin under or around nail.

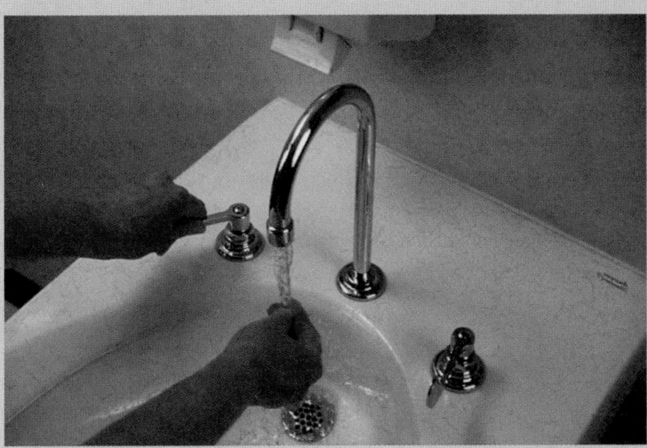

Step 6B Turn on water.

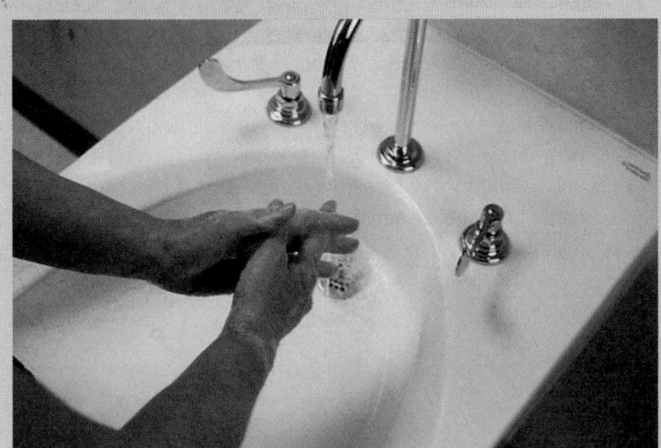

Step 6F Lather hands thoroughly.

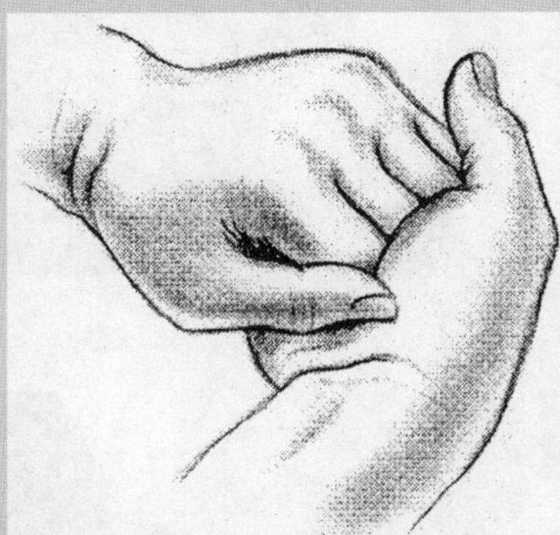

Step 6G Rub the knuckles of one hand into the palm of the other. **Source:** From MacMillan, S. (1996). *Demonstration of a proper medical handwash* [Brochure]. Toronto, ON: St. Michael's Hospital. Reprinted with permission.

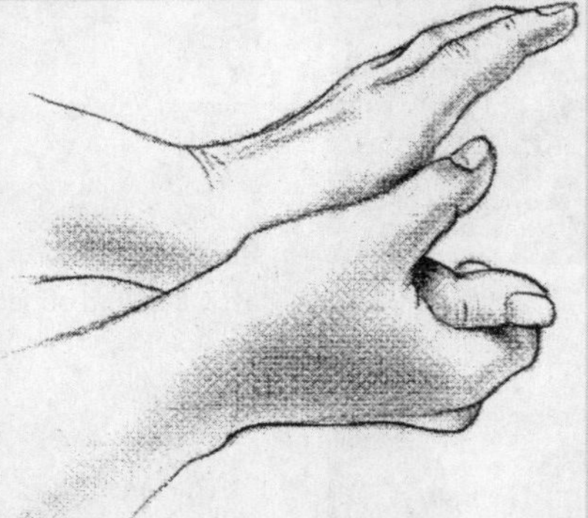

Step 6H Rub the thumb into the palm of the other hand. **Source:** From MacMillan, S. (1996). *Demonstration of a proper medical handwash* [Brochure]. Toronto, ON: St. Michael's Hospital. Reprinted with permission.

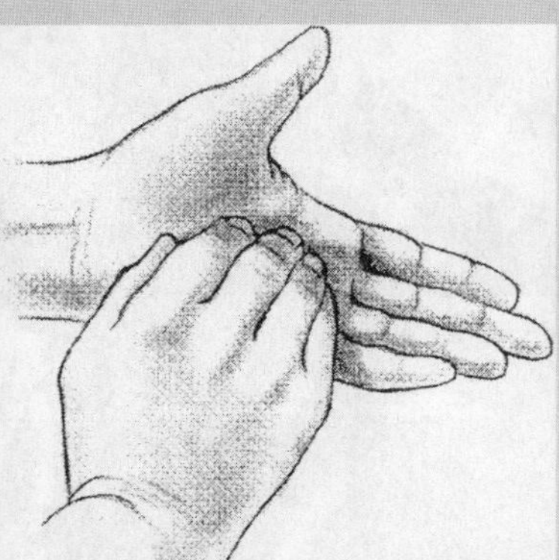

Step 6I Work the fingertips into the palm of the other hand. **Source:** From MacMillan, S. (1996). *Demonstration of a proper medical handwash* [Brochure]. Toronto, ON: St. Michael's Hospital. Reprinted with permission.

Continued

➤ SKILL 33-1 Hand Hygiene *continued*

Steps	Rationale
K. Rinse hands and wrists thoroughly, keeping hands down and elbows up (see Step 6K illustration).	• Rinsing mechanically washes away dirt and microorganisms.
L. Optional: Repeat steps A through J and extend period of washing if hands are heavily soiled.	
M. Dry hands thoroughly from fingers to wrists and forearms with paper towel, single-use cloth, or warm air dryer.	• Drying from cleanest (fingertips) to least clean (forearms) area avoids contamination. Drying hands prevents chapping and roughened skin.
N. If paper towel is used, discard it in proper receptacle.	• Prevents transfer of microorganisms.
O. Turn off water with foot or knee pedals. To turn off hand faucet, use clean, dry paper towel; avoid touching handles with hands (see Step 6O illustration).	• Faucets are contaminated. Using paper towels to touch faucet prevents contamination of hands.
P. If hands are dry or chapped, a small amount of lotion or barrier cream can be applied.	• Use agency-provided container of lotion because many lotions may interfere with antimicrobial action or disintegrate gloves.
Q. Inspect surfaces of hands for obvious signs of soil or other contaminants.	• Determine whether handwashing is adequate.
R. Inspect hands for dermatitis or cracked skin.	• The presence of these conditions indicates complications from excessive handwashing.
7. If hands are not visibly soiled, use an alcohol-based waterless antiseptic for routine decontamination of hands in all clinical situations.	
A. Apply an ample amount of product to palm of one hand (see Step 7A illustration).	• Enough product is needed to thoroughly cover the hands.
B. Rub hands together, covering all surfaces of hands and fingers with antiseptic (see Step 7B illustration).	• Complete coverage of the hands and fingers by using friction ensures antimicrobial effect
C. Rub hands together for several seconds until alcohol is dry. Allow hands to dry before applying gloves.	• Drying ensures full antiseptic effect (Health Canada, 1998).
D. If hands are dry or chapped, a small amount of lotion or barrier cream can be applied.	• Use the agency-provided container of lotion because many lotions may interfere with antimicrobial action or disintegrate gloves.

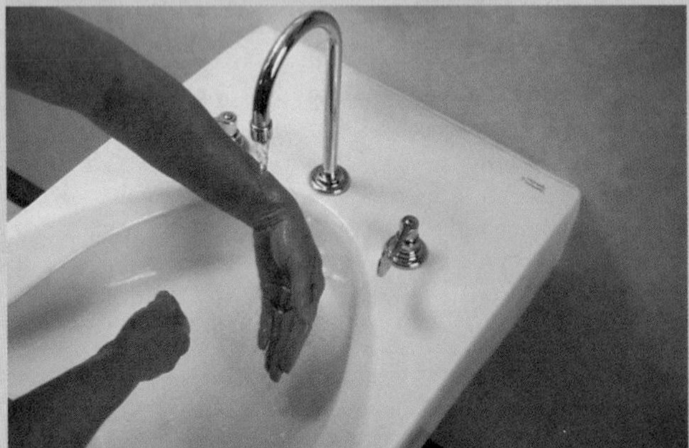

Step 6K Rinse hands.

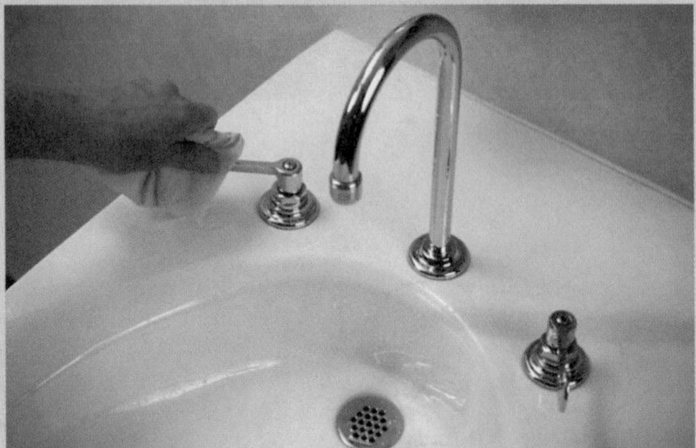

Step 6O Turn off faucet.

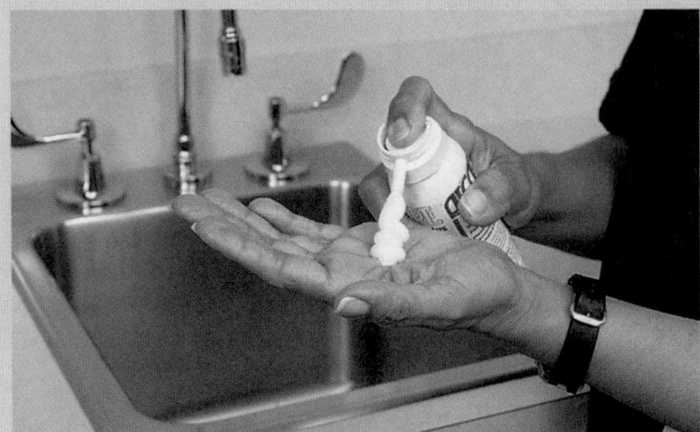

Step 7A Apply waterless antiseptic to palm of hand.

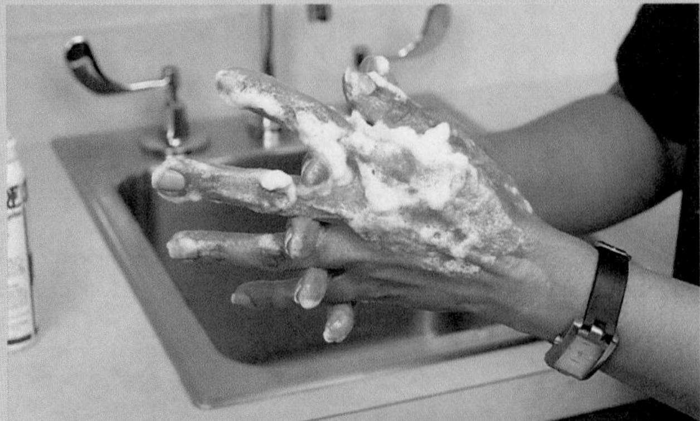

Step 7B Rub hands thoroughly.

➤ SKILL 33-1 Hand Hygiene *continued*

Recording and Reporting

- It is not necessary to record or report this procedure.
- Report any dermatitis to employee health or infection control per agency policy.

Home Care Considerations

- Evaluate the handwashing facilities in the home to determine the possibility of contamination, the proximity of the facilities to the client, and available supplies in the area.
- Evaluate the availability of warm running water and soap when conducting home visits, and anticipate the need for alternative handwashing products such as alcohol-based hand rubs and detergent-containing towels.
- Instruct the client and primary caregiver in the proper techniques and situations for handwashing.

The use of alcohol-based waterless antiseptics is recommended by the CDC (2002) to improve hand hygiene practices, protect health care workers' hands, and reduce the transmission of pathogens to clients and personnel in health care settings. Alcohols have excellent germicidal activity and are more effective than either plain soap or antimicrobial soap and water. Emollients are added to alcohol-based antiseptics to prevent drying of the skin. Researchers have found that these antiseptics may be more effective than water because they are used quickly and are available at the bedside (Girou et al., 2002; Parienti et al., 2002).

The CDC (2002) recommended that hands be washed with plain soap or with antimicrobial soap and water when hands are visibly soiled. If your hands are not visibly soiled, use an alcohol-based waterless antiseptic agent for routine decontamination of hands in all other clinical situations:

- Before direct contact with each client (e.g., taking a pulse or blood pressure, lifting a client)
- After direct contact with each client
- Before donning sterile gloves
- After removing gloves (i.e., after removing sterile gloves or clean, nonsterile gloves)
- After contact with body fluids or excretions, mucous membranes, nonintact skin, or wound dressings, as long as hands are not visibly soiled (if visibly soiled, wash with soap and water)
- When moving from a contaminated body site to a clean body site during client care
- After contact with inanimate objects (including medical equipment) in the immediate vicinity of the client

Alternatively, if antiseptic agents are not available, you may wash hands in all clinical situations (CDC, 2002). Also, health care workers are advised to wash their hands with soap and water if client exposure to *C. difficile* is suspected or proven. The physical action of washing and rinsing hands under such circumstances is recommended because antiseptic agents have poor activity against spores (Louie & Meddings, 2004).

You need to instruct clients and visitors about the proper technique and times for hand hygiene. Ensure that clients and visitors understand the importance of cleaning under their nails and that artificial nails should not be worn because they harbour increased numbers of pathogens (Box 33–11). Teaching hand hygiene is particularly important if health care is to continue at home. Clients should wash their hands before eating or handling food; after handling contaminated

✱ BOX 33-11 RESEARCH HIGHLIGHT

Pathogens and Artificial Fingernails

Research Focus

Some health care workers have artificial or manicured nails. Researchers posed the question as to whether bacteria can reside in higher-than-normal numbers on artificial nail material.

Research Abstract

Hedderwick et al. (2000) and McNeil et al. (2001) conducted two separate studies comparing the identity and quantity of microbial flora from health care workers wearing artificial nails with those from health care workers with natural nails. In both studies, nail surfaces were swabbed and subungual (area under nails) debris was collected to obtain material for culture. In the first study, 12 health care workers who did not normally wear artificial nails wore polished artificial nails on their nondominant hand for 15 days. The identity and quantity of microflora were compared between the artificial nails and the polished natural nails of the other hand. Potential pathogens were isolated from more samples obtained from the artificial nails than from the natural nails. Also, the colonization in artificial nails increased over time. More organisms were found on the surface of the artificial nails than on natural nails.

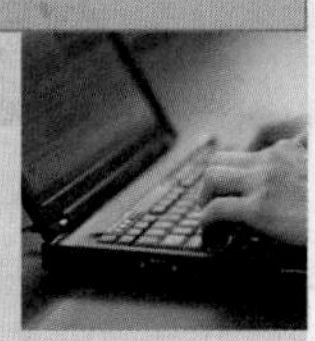

In the second study, the flora of the nails of 30 health care workers who wore permanent acrylic artificial nails were compared with those of the natural nails of health care workers. In health care workers wearing artificial nails, pathogens were more likely to be isolated than in those with natural nails.

In this study, artificial nails were more likely to harbour pathogens, especially Gram-negative bacilli and yeasts, than were natural nails. The longer the artificial nails were worn, the more likely it was that a pathogen was isolated.

Evidence-Informed Practice

- You should not wear artificial nails when performing client care.

References: Hedderwick, S. A., McNeil, S. A., Lyons, M. J., & Kauffman, C. A. (2000). Pathogenic organisms associated with artificial fingernails worn by health-care workers. *Infection Control and Hospital Epidemiology, 21*, 505–509.
McNeil, S. A., Foster C. L., Hedderwick, S., & Kauffman, C. A. (2001). Effect of hand cleansing with antimicrobial soap or alcohol-based gel on microbial colonization of artificial fingernails worn by health care workers. *Clinical Infectious Disease, 32*, 367–372.

equipment, linen, or organic material; and after elimination. Visitors are encouraged to wash their hands before eating or handling food, after coming in contact with infected clients, and after handling contaminated equipment or organic material.

Control of Portals of Entry. Many measures that control the exit of microorganisms likewise control their entrance. Maintaining the integrity of skin and mucous membranes reduces the chances of microorganisms reaching a host. The client's skin should be kept well lubricated by using lotion as appropriate. Immobilized and debilitated clients are particularly susceptible to skin breakdown. Clients should not be positioned on tubes or objects that might cause breaks in the skin. Dry, wrinkle-free linen also reduces the chances of skin breakdown. Frequent turning and positioning are needed before a client's skin becomes reddened. Frequent oral hygiene prevents the drying of mucous membranes. A water-soluble ointment keeps the client's lips well lubricated.

After elimination, a woman should clean the rectum and perineum by wiping from the urinary meatus toward the rectum. Cleansing in a direction from the least to the most contaminated area helps reduce genitourinary infections. Meticulous and frequent perineal care is especially important in women who wear incontinence pads.

Clients, health care workers, and even housekeepers are at risk for acquiring infections from accidental needle sticks. After administering an injection or inserting an intravenous catheter, you should engage any safety device and carefully dispose of needles in a puncture-resistant box (see Chapter 34). A stray needle lying in the bed linen or carelessly thrown into a wastebasket is a prime source of exposure to bloodborne pathogens. Hepatitis B and C are the infections most commonly transmitted by contaminated needles. A needle stick should be reported immediately. Health care agencies require the victim of a needle stick to complete an injury report and seek appropriate treatment. The Canadian Needle Stick Surveillance Network (2003) has the mandate to monitor health care workers exposed to needle sticks and the subsequent outcomes of these exposures.

Another cause of microorganism entrance into a host is improper handling and management of urinary catheters and drainage sets (see Chapter 44). The point of connection between a catheter and drainage tube should remain closed and intact. As long as such systems are closed, their contents are considered sterile. Outflow spigots on drainage bags should also remain closed to prevent the entrance of bacteria. Movement of the catheter at the urethra should be minimized by stabilizing the catheter with tape to reduce chances of microorganisms ascending the urethra into the bladder. Urine-measuring containers should not be shared between clients.

You may care for clients with closed drainage systems that collect wound drainage, bile, or other body fluids. In each example, the site from which a drainage tube exits should remain clear of excess moisture and accumulated drainage. All tubing should remain connected throughout use. Drainage receptacles should only be opened when it is necessary to discard or measure the volume of drainage.

At times, you will obtain specimens from drainage tubes or intravenous tubing ports. First, you must perform hand hygiene; then disinfect tubes and ports by wiping the surface outward with alcohol, iodine, or a chlorhexidine alcohol solution before entering the system. Temporarily placing squares of sterile gauze around the ends of an open drainage tube, such as a urinary catheter, adds further protection against bacteria. However, keeping drainage tubes closed and secure is the best practice.

A final method for reducing the entrance of microorganisms is the technique for cleansing wounds (see Chapter 47). A surgical wound is considered to be sterile. To prevent the entrance of microorganisms into the wound, you should clean outward from a wound site. When applying an antiseptic or cleaning with soap and water, wipe around the wound edge first and then clean outward away from the wound. Clean gauze should be used for each revolution around the wound's circumference.

Protection of the Susceptible Host. Clients' resistance to infection improves as you protect their normal body defences against infection. You can intervene to maintain the body's normal reparative processes (Box 33–12). You must also protect yourself and others by following your agency's isolation guidelines.

Isolation Guidelines. The risk of transmitting a nosocomial infection or infectious disease among clients is high. When a client has a suspected or known infection, health care workers are alerted and follow infection-control practices. However, sometimes health care workers are not aware that clients have infections. The majority of organisms causing nosocomial infections are found in the colonized body substances of clients regardless of whether a culture has confirmed infection and a diagnosis has been made (Garner, 1996). Body substances such as feces, saliva, mucus, and wound drainage always contain potentially infectious organisms.

The CDC issued isolation guidelines in 1996 that contain a two-tiered approach (Garner, 1996). These guidelines were updated and expanded upon in 2007 and have been adopted by most health care agencies. Some health care agencies have adopted Health Canada's isolation guidelines (1999), which contain a similar two-tiered approach. The Health Canada guidelines were written to accommodate acute, long-term, home, and ambulatory care settings, whereas the CDC guidelines were written specifically for acute care settings. Nevertheless, the CDC guidelines and Health Canada's guidelines are essentially interchangeable.

The first tier of the isolation guidelines contains precautions designed to care for all clients in any setting, regardless of their diagnosis or presumed infectiousness. In the CDC's guidelines, this tier is called *standard precautions* (Table 33–7); in Health Canada's guidelines, it is called *routine practices*. Standard precautions or routine

➤ BOX 33-12 Infection Control: Protecting the Susceptible Host

Protecting Normal Defence Mechanisms

Regular bathing removes transient microorganisms from the skin's surface. Lubrication helps keep the skin hydrated and intact.

Regular oral hygiene removes proteins in the saliva that attract microorganisms. Flossing removes tartar and plaque that can cause infection.

Maintenance of adequate fluid intake promotes normal urine formation and a resultant outflow of urine to flush the bladder and urethral lining of microorganisms.

For physically dependent or immobilized clients, you should encourage routine coughing and deep breathing to keep clients' lower airways clear of mucus.

You should encourage proper immunization of children and adult clients (see Box 33–8).

Maintaining Healing Processes

Promote the intake of adequate fluids and a well-balanced diet containing essential proteins, vitamins, carbohydrates, and fats. You should also use measures to increase the client's appetite.

Promote a client's comfort and sleep so that energy stores are replenished daily.

You can assist a client in learning techniques to reduce stress.

practices apply when a health care worker is or potentially may be exposed to (1) blood; (2) all body fluids, secretions, and excretions except sweat; (3) nonintact skin; or (4) mucous membranes. Standard precautions or routine practices include the appropriate use of gowns, gloves, masks, eyewear, and other protective devices or clothing. Barrier protection is indicated for use with all clients because every client has the potential to transmit infection via blood and body fluids and the risk for infection transmission can be unknown. Standard precautions or routine practices also include rules on appropriate handwashing, cleaning of equipment, and disposal of contaminated linen and sharps.

The second tier of the isolation guidelines is *transmission-based precautions.* (In the Health Canada guidelines, the second tier is called *additional precautions.*) These precautions are designed to contain pathogens in one area, usually the client's room; therefore, they are often called **isolation precautions.** Only clients infected or colonized with certain highly transmissible or epidemiologically significant pathogens are placed under isolation precautions. These precautions

➤ TABLE 33-7 Centers for Disease Control and Prevention Isolation Guidelines

Standard Precautions (Tier One)

Standard precautions apply to blood, all body fluids, secretions, excretions (except sweat), nonintact skin, and mucous membranes.

Hands are washed between client contacts; after contact with blood, body fluids, secretions, and excretions and after contact with equipment or articles contaminated by them; and immediately after gloves are removed. (Refer to your agency's policy for use of alcohol-based waterless antiseptics.)

Gloves are worn when touching blood, body fluids, secretions, excretions, nonintact skin, mucous membranes, or contaminated items. Gloves should be removed and hand hygiene performed between care of clients. Gloves should also be changed between procedures on the same client and after contact with material that may be highly contaminated.

Masks, eye protection, or face shields are worn if client care activities may generate splashes or sprays of blood or body fluid.

Gowns are worn if soiling of clothing is likely from blood or body fluid. Remove used gowns as soon as possible. Perform hand hygiene after removing your gown.

Client care equipment is properly cleaned and reprocessed, and single-use items are discarded.

Contaminated linen is placed in a leak-proof bag and handled in a manner that prevents skin and mucous membrane exposure.

All sharp instruments and needles are discarded in a puncture-resistant container. Safety devices must be enabled after use to prevent injury. Never recap a used needle.

A private room is unnecessary unless a client's hygiene is unacceptable. Check with an infection-control professional.

Transmission-Based (Isolation) Precautions (Tier Two)

Category	*Description and Disease*	*Barrier Protection*
Airborne precautions	For known or suspected infections caused by microbes transmitted by airborne droplets; examples: measles, chickenpox (varicella), disseminated zoster, tuberculosis	Private room (room door kept closed), negative-pressure airflow of at least six exchanges per hour, respiratory protection device (e.g., N95 respirator) must be worn when the client has tuberculosis or when the client has varicella, disseminated zoster, or measles and the worker is not immune
Droplet precautions	For known or suspected infections caused by microbes transmitted by droplets produced by coughing, sneezing, or talking; examples: diphtheria (pharyngeal), rubella, influenza, pertussis, mumps, mycoplasmal pneumonia, meningococcal pneumonia, or sepsis	Private room or cohort clients (room door closed unless bed is more than 1 m from the door), mask is worn when within 1 m of the client
Contact precautions	For known or suspected infections caused by direct or indirect contact; examples: colonization or infection with multidrug-resistant organism; *C. difficile*; major wound infections; gastrointestinal, respiratory, or skin infections	Private room or cohort clients (door can be open); gloves and gown upon entry into isolation room; limiting patient movement outside of isolation room to necessary medical treatments or procedures; cleaning and disinfecting or discarding items before removal from isolation room

Adapted from Garner, J. S. (1996). Guideline for isolation precautions in hospitals. The Hospital Infection Control Practices Advisory Committee. *Infection Control and Hospital Epidemiology, 17*(1), 54–80.

are followed in addition to standard precautions or routine practices. Isolation precautions are categorized in three ways: airborne, droplet, and contact precautions (see Table 33–7). The precautions used depend on how the pathogen is spread. For example, a client diagnosed with (or suspected of having) active tuberculosis would require the use of airborne precautions, using a special mask and ventilated room, in conjunction with standard precautions or routine practices.

Regardless of the category of isolation precaution (Box 33–13), you must observe the following basic principles:

- Observe thorough hand hygiene before entering and leaving the room of a client in isolation.
- Dispose of contaminated supplies and equipment in a manner that prevents the spread of microorganisms to other persons as indicated by the mode of transmission of the organism.
- Apply knowledge of a disease process and the mode of infection transmission when using protective barriers.
- Ensure that all persons who might be exposed during transport of a client outside the isolation room are protected.

Psychological Implications of Isolation Precautions. A client required to be in isolation in a private room may become lonely because normal social relationships are disrupted. This situation can be psychologically harmful, especially for children (Box 33–14).

Clients' body image may be altered as a result of the infectious process. Clients may feel unclean, rejected, lonely, or guilty. Infection-prevention and -control practices further intensify these feelings of difference or undesirability. Isolation in a private room limits sensory contact. Unless you act to minimize feelings of psychological and physical isolation, your clients' emotional state can interfere with their recovery.

Before isolation measures are instituted, a client and family must understand the nature of the disease or condition, purposes of isolation, and steps for carrying out specific precautions. If they are able to participate in maintaining infection prevention, the chances of reducing the spread of infection are increased. The client and family should be taught to perform hand hygiene and use barrier protection if appropriate. Each procedure should be demonstrated, and the client and family should be given an opportunity to practise it. It is also important to explain how infectious organisms can be transmitted so that the client understands the difference between contaminated and clean objects.

You should take measures to improve the client's sensory stimulation during isolation. The room environment should be clean and pleasant. Drapes or shades should be opened, and excess supplies and equipment removed. You must listen to the client's concerns or interests. If you hurry through care or show a lack of interest, the client will feel rejected and even more isolated. Mealtime is a particularly good opportunity for conversation. Providing comfort measures such as repositioning, a back massage, or a tepid sponge bath increases physical stimulation. If appropriate for the client's condition, you should encourage the client to walk and sit up in a chair. Recreational activities such as board games or cards may be an option to keep the client mentally stimulated.

You must explain to the family the client's risk for depression or loneliness. Visiting family members should be taught the principles of isolation and encouraged to avoid expressions or actions that convey revulsion, fear, or disgust. Discuss ways to provide meaningful stimulation.

Protective Environment. Private rooms used for isolation may have negative-pressure airflow to prevent infectious particles from flowing out of the room. Special rooms with positive-pressure airflow are used for highly susceptible clients, such as organ transplant recipients. On the door or wall outside the room, post a card listing the precautions for the isolation category according to your agency's policy. The card is a handy reference for health care workers and visitors, and it alerts anyone who might enter the room that special precautions must be followed.

The isolation room or an adjoining anteroom should contain hand hygiene, bathing, and toilet facilities. Soap and antiseptic solutions must be made available. Personnel and visitors perform hand hygiene before approaching the client's bedside and again before leaving the room. If toilet facilities are unavailable, special procedures for handling portable commodes, bedpans, or urinals must be followed. Personal protective equipment should be stored in an anteroom between the room and hallway or in a convenient location close to the point of use.

All client care rooms, including those used for isolation, contain an impervious bag for soiled or contaminated linen as well as a waste receptacle with plastic liners. Impervious receptacles stop the transmission of microorganisms by preventing seepage and soiling of the outside surface. A disposable rigid container should be available in the room for discarding of used needles, syringes, and sharp objects.

You should remain aware of infection-prevention and -control techniques while working with clients in protected environments. Depending on the microorganism and the mode of transmission, you must evaluate what articles or equipment may be taken into an isolation room. For example, Health Canada (1997) recommends the dedicated use of articles such as stethoscopes, sphygmomanometers, and rectal thermometers in the isolation room of a client infected or colonized with vanomycin-resistant enterococci (VRE). These devices should not be used on other clients unless the devices are first adequately cleaned and disinfected. If you bring an article into the room, expose the article to infected material, and then touch or remove the article, you increase the risk of transmitting infection to other clients or personnel.

Personal Protective Equipment. Personal protective equipment (gowns, masks, protective eyewear, and gloves) should be readily available. The primary reason for gowning is to prevent the contamination of clothes during contact with the client. Gowns and cover-ups protect health care workers and visitors from coming in contact with infected material, blood, or body fluid. Gowns may also be required for contact precautions, depending on the expected amount of exposure to infectious material. Gowns used for barrier protection are made of a fluid-resistant material and should be changed immediately if damaged or heavily contaminated.

Isolation gowns usually open at the back and have ties or snaps at the neck and waist to keep the gown closed and secure. They should be long enough to cover all outer garments. Long sleeves with tight-fitting cuffs provide added protection. No special technique is required for applying clean gowns as long as they are fastened securely. However, you must be careful when removing a gown to minimize the contamination of your hands and uniform. Isolation gowns are disposable or reusable, depending on your agency's policy.

Full face protection (with eyes, nose, and mouth covered) should be worn when splashing or spraying of blood or body fluid into the face is possible. Masks should also be worn when working with a client placed on droplet precautions; they protect you from inhaling microorganisms from a client's respiratory tract and prevent the transmission of pathogens from your respiratory tract to the client. Surgical masks protect a wearer from inhaling large-particle aerosols that travel short distances (1 m). At times, a client who is susceptible to infection wears a mask to prevent inhalation of pathogens. Clients on droplet or airborne precautions who are transported outside of their rooms should wear masks to protect other clients and personnel. According to the CDC (Garner, 1996), masks may prevent the transmission of infection through direct contact with mucous membranes. In addition,

➤ BOX 33-13 Procedural Guidelines

Caring for a Client on Isolation Precautions

Delegation Considerations: Care of a client in isolation can be delegated to an unregulated care provider (UCP) when necessary procedures are within the UCP's competence.

Equipment:
- Barrier protection determined by type of isolation
- Supplies necessary for procedures performed in room

Procedure
1. Assess isolation indications (e.g., current laboratory test results or the client's history of exposure).
2. Review agency policies and precautions necessary for the specific isolation category, and consider care measures to be performed while in the client's room.
3. Review nurses' notes or confer with colleagues regarding the client's emotional state and adjustment to isolation.
4. Perform hand hygiene and prepare all equipment to be taken into the client's room.
5. Prepare for entrance into isolation room:
   A. Perform hand hygiene.
   B. Apply gown (when needed), making sure it covers you from neck to knees. Pull sleeves down to wrist. Tie securely at neck and waist (see Step 5B illustration).
   C. Apply either surgical mask or respirator around mouth and nose when needed. (Type will depend on type of isolation and facility policy.)
   D. Apply eyewear or goggles snugly and adjust to fit around face and eyes (when needed).
   E. Apply disposable nonsterile gloves for isolation. (Note: Unpowdered, latex-free gloves should be worn if the client or the health care worker has a latex allergy.) If gloves are worn with a gown, bring the glove cuffs over edge of the gown sleeves.
6. Enter the client's room. Arrange supplies and equipment. (If equipment will be removed from room for reuse, place it on a clean paper towel.)
7. Explain purpose of isolation and necessary precautions to the client and family. Offer an opportunity to ask questions. Assess for evidence of emotional problems that may be caused by being in isolation.
8. Assess vital signs:
   A. If client is infected or colonized with a resistant organism (e.g., vancomycin-resistant enterococci [VRE] or methicillin-resistant *Staphylococcus aureus* [MRSA]), the equipment remains in room. Proceed to assess vital signs. Avoid contact of stethoscope or blood pressure cuff with infectious material.
   B. If stethoscope is to be reused, the entire stethoscope must be thoroughly cleaned after leaving the room. You may use a few alcohol swabs to clean and disinfect the stethoscope. (Ideally, equipment is dedicated for the use of the patient with an antibiotic-resistant organism and remains in the room.) Clean diaphragm or bell with alcohol. Set aside on clean surface.
   C. Individual or disposable thermometers should be used.
9. Administer medications:
   A. Give oral medication in wrapper or cup.
   B. Dispose of wrapper or cup in plastic-lined receptacle.
   C. Administer injection.
   D. Discard syringe and uncapped needle or sheathed needle into special container.
   E. If gloves are not worn and hands contact contaminated article or body fluids, wash hands immediately.
10. Administer hygiene measures, encouraging the client to discuss questions or concerns about isolation. Informal teaching can be used at this time:
    A. Prevent the gown from becoming wet.
    B. Remove linen from the bed; avoid contact with the gown. Place linen in an impervious bag.
    C. Change gloves and wash your hands if they become excessively soiled and further care is necessary.
11. Collect specimens:
    A. Place specimen containers on a clean paper towel in the client's bathroom.
    B. Follow procedure for collecting specimen of body fluids.
    C. Transfer specimen to the container without soiling the outside of the container. Place the container in a plastic bag, and place a label on the outside of the bag or as per agency policy.
12. Dispose of linen and garbage bags as they become full:
    A. Use sturdy, moisture-resistant single bags to contain soiled articles.
    B. Tie bags securely at the top in a knot (see Step 12B illustration).

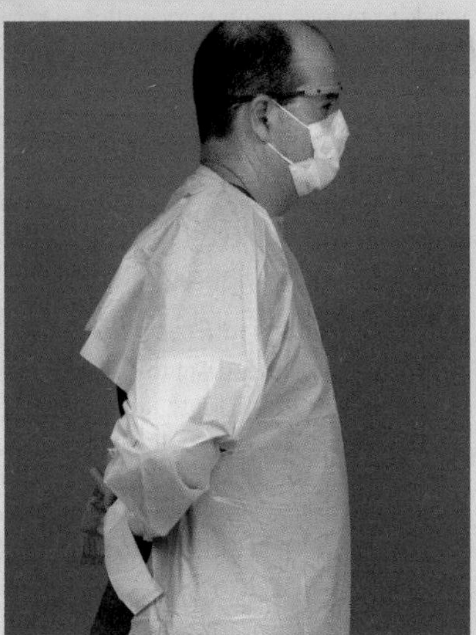

Step 5B Tie gown at waist.

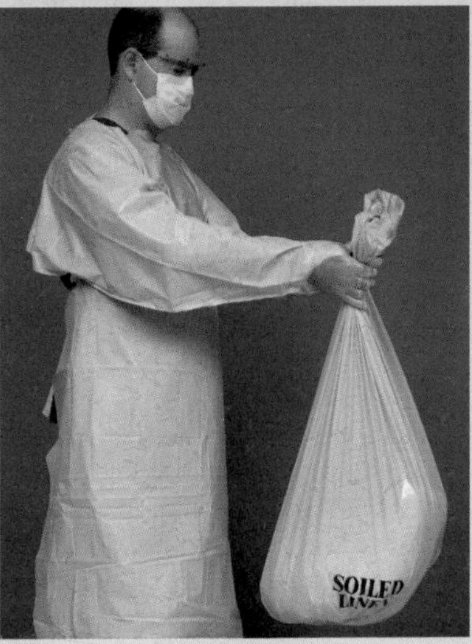

Step 12B Tie linen securely.

Continued

➤BOX 33-13 Procedural Guidelines *continued*

13. Resupply room as needed.
14. When leaving isolation room, remove personal protective equipment, except for N95 respirator, inside doorway or in anteroom. Remove N95 respirator after leaving the client's room and closing the door.
    A. Remove gloves. Remove one glove by grasping the cuff and pulling the glove inside out over the hand. Discard the glove. With the ungloved hand, tuck a finger inside the cuff of the remaining glove and pull it off, inside out.
    B. Perform hand hygiene.
    C. Untie waist and neck strings of the gown. Allow the gown to fall from your shoulders. Remove hands from sleeves without touching the outside of the gown (see Step 14C illustration). Hold the gown inside at shoulder seams and fold inside out; discard in laundry bag.
    D. Perform hand hygiene.
    E. Untie first top mask string and then bottom strings; pull the mask away from your face, and drop the mask into a waste receptacle (see Step 14E illustration). (Do not touch outer surface of mask.)
    F. Remove eyewear or goggles.
    G. Perform hand hygiene.
    H. Explain to the client when you plan to return to the room. Ask whether the client requires any personal care items, books, or magazines.
    I. Leave the room and close the door, if necessary. (Door should be closed if airborne precautions are being used.)
    J. All contaminated supplies and equipment should be disposed of in a manner that prevents the spread of microorganisms to other persons (see your agency's policy).

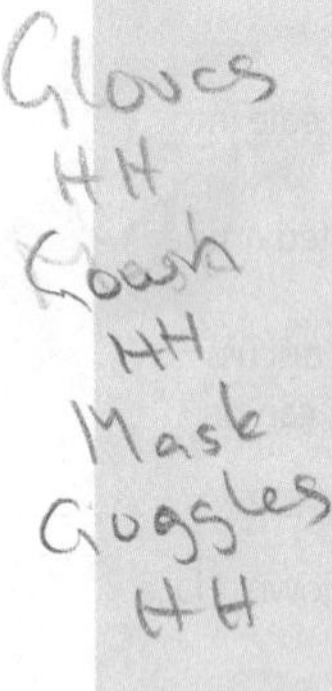

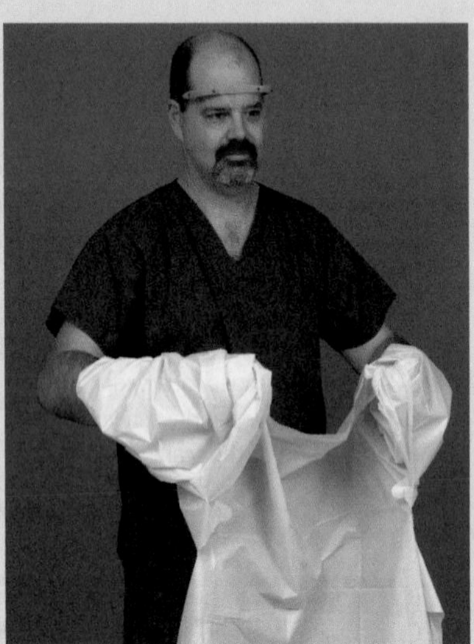

Step 14C Remove mask away from face.

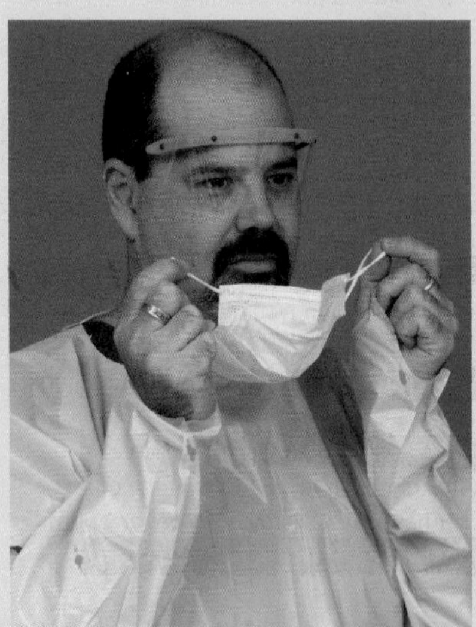

Step 14E Remove hands from sleeves without touching outside of the gown.

masks discourage the wearer from touching the eyes, nose, or mouth.

A properly applied mask fits snugly over the mouth and nose so that pathogens and body fluids cannot enter or escape through the sides (Box 33–15). If a person wears glasses, the top edge of the mask fits below the glasses so that the glasses do not cloud over as the person exhales. Talking should be kept to a minimum while wearing a mask to reduce respiratory airflow—a mask that has become moist may not provide a barrier to microorganisms and should be discarded.

✱BOX 33-14 RESEARCH HIGHLIGHT

Adverse Effects of Isolation

Research Focus

Stelfox et al. (2003) studied whether clients who are isolated in single rooms experience adverse effects as a result of the isolation.

Research Abstract

A Canadian and an American hospital were included in a study to examine the likelihood of adverse events. Clients who were cared for in isolation because they were infected with MRSA were compared with those who were not isolated. The research found that (1) isolated clients were more likely to complain about care than were nonisolated clients (8% versus 1%); (2) vital signs were not recorded on charts as ordered as often for isolated clients as for nonisolated clients (51% versus 31%); (3) nurses were less likely to record nursing notes for isolated clients (14% versus 10%); and (d) clients in isolation were eight times more likely to experience falls, pressure ulcers, and fluid or electrolyte disorders.

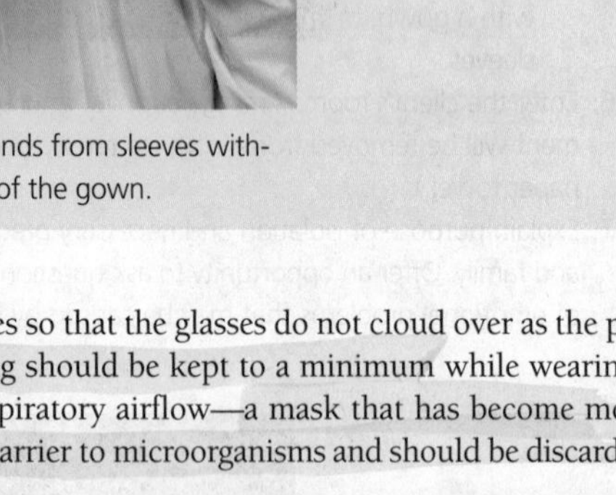

Evidence-Informed Practice

- You must be extra vigilant to ensure the standard of care is similar for all clients, including those on isolation precautions.
- You should ensure that both physical and psychological factors are addressed when planning and carrying out care for isolated clients.
- You must ensure that you record observations and complete nursing notes for all clients including those in isolation.

References: Stelfox, H. T., Bates, D. W., & Redelmeir, D. A. (2003). Safety of patients isolated for infection control. *Journal of the American Medical Association, 290,* 1899–1905.

➤ BOX 33-15 **Procedural Guidelines**

Donning a Surgical-Type Mask

Procedure

1. Find top edge of the mask (usually has a thin metal strip). The pliable metal fits snugly against bridge of nose.
2. Hold the mask by top two strings or loops. Tie the two top ties at the top of back of the head (see Step 2 illustration), with ties above ears (alternative: slip loops over each ear).
3. Tie the two lower ties snugly around the neck, with mask well under chin (see Step 3 illustration).
4. Gently pinch upper metal band around bridge of nose.

Note: Mask should be changed if it becomes wet, moist, or contaminated.

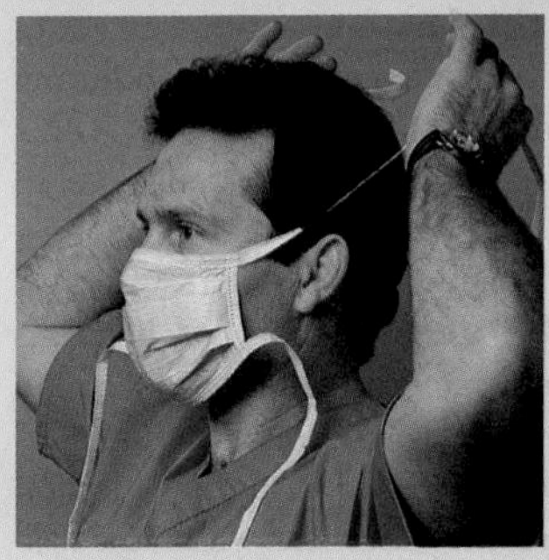

Step 2 Tie two top ties at top of back of head.

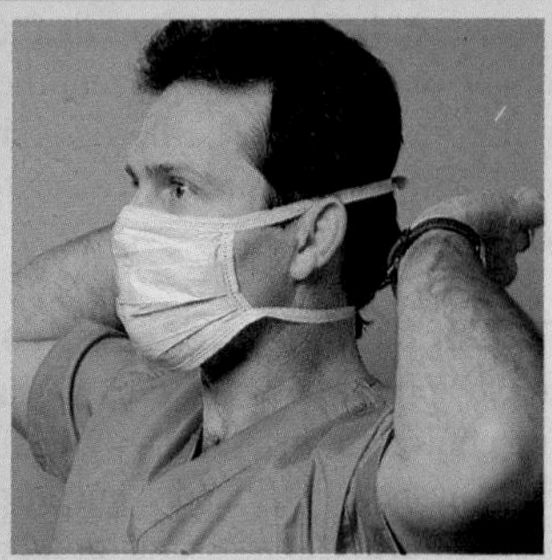

Step 3 Tie two lower ties snugly around the neck.

A mask should never be reused. Clients and family members should be warned that a mask can cause a sensation of smothering. If family members become uncomfortable wearing a mask, they should leave the room and discard the mask.

Specially fitted respiratory protective devices or masks are required when you care for a client with known or suspected tuberculosis or when the client has varicella, disseminated zoster, or measles and the worker is not immune. The mask must have a higher filtration rating than the regular surgical mask and be fitted snugly to the wearer's face to prevent leakage around the sides. You should be aware of your agency's policy regarding the type of respiratory protective device required.

Gloves help to prevent the transmission of pathogens by direct and indirect contact. Clean, nonsterile gloves (also called disposable gloves) should be worn when contact with blood, body fluid, secretions, excretions, or contaminated items is possible. Clean gloves should be donned just before you touch mucous membranes and nonintact skin. Gloves should be changed between tasks and procedures on the same client after contact with material that may contain a high concentration of microorganisms. Gloves should be removed promptly after use, before touching noncontaminated items and environmental surfaces, and before going to another client. Hand hygiene should be performed immediately after removing the gloves to avoid the transfer of microorganisms to other clients and environments. Facilities provide nonlatex gloves for health care staff who are allergic or sensitive to latex. When full protective apparel is needed, you must first perform hand hygiene, apply a mask and eyewear or goggles (as needed), apply a gown, and then put on gloves. Disposable gloves are easily applied and are designed to fit either hand. The glove cuffs should be pulled up over the wrists or over the cuffs of the gown. The gloves' thin rubber can be easily torn; if a break or tear is detected in a glove while providing care, you should change gloves if care is not completed. If you do not plan to have more contact with the client, reapplying gloves is unnecessary.

Family members visiting clients who are in isolation that necessitates the use of gloves must know when and how to apply gloves properly. You need to demonstrate the application of gloves to family members and explain the reason for glove use. Emphasize the importance of hand hygiene after the removal of gloves.

When participating in a procedure that may create droplets or splashing or spraying of blood or other body fluids, you must wear protective eyewear and a mask or a face shield (Garner, 1996). Examples of such procedures include the irrigation of a large abdominal wound or the insertion of an arterial catheter in which you assist a physician. Eyewear may be available in the form of plastic glasses or goggles. They should fit snugly around the face so that fluids cannot enter between the face and the glasses.

Specimen Collection. Often, many laboratory studies are required when a client is suspected of having an infectious disease. Body fluids and secretions suspected of containing infectious organisms are collected for culture and sensitivity tests. The specimen is placed in a medium that promotes the growth of organisms. A laboratory technologist then identifies the microorganisms growing in the culture. Additional test results indicate antibiotics to which the organisms are resistant or sensitive, and sensitivity reports determine the antibiotics to be used in treatment.

You need to obtain all culture specimens using disposable gloves and sterile equipment. Collecting fresh material from the site of the infection, such as wound drainage, ensures that the specimen is not contaminated by neighbouring microbes. All specimen containers should be sealed tightly to prevent spillage and contamination of the outside of the container. Box 33–16 describes the techniques for collecting specimens from a client with a suspected infection.

Bagging Waste or Linen. You should use special bagging procedures when removing contaminated items from a client's environment. Bagging contaminated items and ensuring the outside of the bag is not contaminated prevents accidental exposure of personnel and contamination of the surrounding environment.

Health Canada (1999) recommends using a single bag for discarding items if the bag is impervious and sturdy and if the article can be placed in the bag without contaminating the outside of the bag. Soiled linen should be placed in an impervious laundry bag in the client's room. Health Canada (1999) recommends double bagging *only* if it is impossible to prevent the contamination of the bag's outer surface. Studies have shown that double bagging is otherwise not necessary to control infection (Maki et al., 1986; Weinstein et al., 1989). The use of one standard-sized linen bag that is not overfilled, is tied securely, and is intact is adequate to prevent infection transmission. The same rule applies to garbage bags.

Transporting Clients. Before transferring clients to wheelchairs or stretchers, give them clean gowns to serve as robes. Clients infected with organisms transmitted by the airborne route should leave their rooms only for essential purposes, such as diagnostic procedures or surgery. These clients must also wear masks. Personnel transporting these clients should also wear barrier protection as needed.

At times, a client being transported may drain body fluids onto a stretcher or wheelchair. When this occurs, you must be sure to have the equipment cleaned and, if necessary, disinfected after the client returns to the room. An extra layer of sheets may be used to cover the stretcher or seat of the wheelchair.

Personnel in diagnostic or procedural areas or the operating room should be notified that the client is on isolation precautions. Record the type of isolation on the client's chart. Explain to the client ways that he or she can help prevent the transmission of infection during transport. A client on airborne or droplet isolation is provided with a mask and given tissues and a bag to allow for the proper disposal of secretions.

Role of the Infection-Control Professional. Many hospitals employ professionals who are specially trained in infection prevention and control; most of these professionals are nurses. These individuals are responsible for advising hospital personnel regarding infection prevention and control and for monitoring infections within the hospital. The Community and Hospital Infection Control Association of Canada (CHICA–Canada) is a voluntary multidisciplinary association of infection-control professionals. Its mission is to promote excellence in the practice of infection prevention and control (CHICA–Canada, 2004). The duties of an infection-control professional include the following:

- Provide staff with education on infection prevention and control
- Develop and review infection-prevention and -control policies and procedures
- Recommend appropriate isolation procedures
- Screen client records for community-acquired infections that may be reportable to the public health department
- Consult with employee health departments concerning recommendations to prevent and control the spread of infection among personnel, such as tuberculosis testing
- Gather statistics regarding the **epidemiology** (cause and effect) of HAIs
- Notify the public health department of incidences of communicable diseases within the facility
- Confer with all hospital departments to investigate unusual events or clusters of infection
- Recommend education for clients and families
- Identify infection-control problems regarding equipment
- Monitor antibiotic-resistant organisms in the institution
- Monitor construction sites in hospitals to ensure that appropriate dust containment measures are used

An infection-control professional can be a valuable resource for nurses in controlling nosocomial infections.

Infection Prevention and Control for Hospital Personnel. Health care workers are continually at risk of exposure to infectious microorganisms. Each agency has protocols in place to advise staff and to monitor infection protocols. Hospitals offer regularly scheduled staff education programs. Each province and territory has rules and procedures to ensure that health care workers are not unnecessarily exposed to pathogens.

Client Education. Often clients must learn to use infection-control practices at home (Box 33–17). Preventive technique will become almost second nature to you if practised daily, but your clients will be less aware of factors that promote the spread of infection and ways to prevent its transmission. The home environment does not always lend itself to infection prevention—often you must help clients adapt according to the resources available to maintain hygienic techniques. However, clients in a home care setting generally have a lower risk of infection than do clients in a hospital because they have less exposure to resistant organisms and undergo fewer invasive procedures.

Surgical Asepsis. **Surgical asepsis**, or sterile technique, requires precautions different from those of medical asepsis. Surgical asepsis includes procedures used to eliminate all microorganisms, including pathogens and spores, from an object or area. In surgical asepsis, an area or object is considered contaminated if touched by any object that is not sterile. While you are working with a sterile field or with sterile equipment, you must understand that the slightest break in technique results in contamination. Surgical asepsis should be used in the following situations:

- During procedures that require the intentional perforation of the client's skin (e.g., the insertion of intravenous catheters or administration of injections)
- When the skin's integrity is broken as a result of trauma, surgical incision, or burns
- During procedures that involve the insertion of catheters or surgical instruments into sterile body cavities

➤ BOX 33-16 Specimen Collection Techniques*

Wound Specimen

Clean the site with sterile water or saline before wound specimen collection. Wear gloves and use a cotton-tipped swab or a syringe to collect as much drainage as possible. Set a clean test tube or culture tube on a clean paper towel close by. After swabbing the centre of wound site, grasp the collection tube by holding it with a paper towel. Carefully insert the swab without touching the outside of the tube. After securing the tube's top, transfer the tube into a bag for transport and then perform hand hygiene.

Blood Specimen

Wearing gloves, use a syringe and culture media bottles to collect up to 10 mL of blood per culture bottle (check your agency's policy about exact amounts required). After prepping the client, perform a venipuncture at two different sites to decrease the likelihood of both specimens being contaminated with skin flora. Place the blood culture bottles on the bedside table or another surface; swab off the bottle tops with alcohol. Inject the appropriate amount of blood into each bottle. Remove your gloves and transfer the specimen into a clean, labelled bag for transport. Perform hand hygiene.

Stool Specimen

Wearing gloves, use a clean cup with sealing top (it does not need to be sterile) and a tongue blade to collect a small amount of stool, approximately the size of a walnut: place the cup on a clean paper towel in the client's bathroom; using the tongue blade, collect the needed amount of feces from the client's bedpan; transfer the feces to the cup without touching the cup's outside surface. Dispose of the tongue blade, and place the seal on the cup. Transfer the specimen into a clean bag for transport. Remove your gloves and perform hand hygiene.

Urine Specimen

Wearing gloves, use a syringe and sterile cup or tube to collect 1 to 5 mL of urine. Place the cup or tube on a clean towel in the client's bathroom. If client has a urinary catheter, use the syringe to collect specimen. If the client is not catheterized, have the client follow the procedure to obtain a clean voided specimen (see Chapter 40). Transfer the urine into a sterile container by injecting urine from the syringe or by pouring it from the used collection cup. Secure the top of the container and transfer the specimen into a clean, labelled bag for transport. Remove your gloves and perform hand hygiene.

*Agency policies may differ on the type of containers and amount of specimen material required.

Adapted from Pagana, K. D., & Pagana, T. J. (1998). *Diagnostic testing and nursing implications: A case study approach* (5th ed.). St. Louis, MO: Mosby.

Although surgical asepsis is commonly practised in the operating room, labour and delivery area, and major diagnostic areas, you may also use surgical aseptic techniques at the client's bedside, for example, when inserting intravenous or urinary catheters, suctioning the tracheobronchial airway, or reapplying sterile dressings. In an operating room, you must follow a series of steps to maintain sterile technique, including applying a mask, protective eyewear, and a cap; performing a surgical hand scrub; and applying a sterile gown and gloves. In contrast, when performing a dressing change at a client's bedside, you may only perform hand hygiene and apply sterile gloves (see "Principles of Surgical Asepsis" section).

BOX 33-17 CLIENT TEACHING

Infection Control

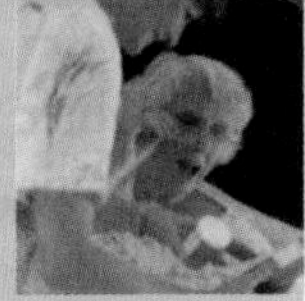

Objective

- Client will perform self-care using proper infection-control techniques.

Teaching Strategies

- Instruct the client about cleaning equipment using soap and water and disinfecting it with an appropriate disinfectant.
- Demonstrate proper hand hygiene, explaining that it should be done before and after all treatments and when infected body fluids are contacted.
- Instruct the client about the signs and symptoms of wound infection.
- For clients who receive tube feedings at home, explain the importance of preparing enough formula for only 8 hours (in the case of commercially prepared foods) or 4 hours (in the case of home prepared foods). Tell the client that contaminated enteral feedings can cause infections. Teach the client to rinse the feeding bag and tubing with mild soap and water daily and to dry them.
- Instruct the client to place contaminated dressings and other disposable items containing infectious body fluids in impervious plastic bags and to place needles in a puncture-proof and leak-proof container, such as an empty bleach bottle with the opening taped shut or a coffee can with the lid taped closed. Glass containers should not be used. Ensure that the client knows to contact the local municipality or public health department before disposing of contaminated items (Health Canada, 1998).
- Instruct the client (or family) to separate noticeably soiled linen from other laundry, wash it in water that is as hot as the fabric will tolerate, add 250 mL of bleach to detergent, and set the dryer temperature as high as the fabric will allow.

Evaluation

- Ask the client or family member to describe techniques used to reduce the transmission of infection.
- Ask the client demonstrate select techniques.
- Ask the client to explain the risks for infection based on the condition.

After clients are at home, you need to educate them about infection and techniques to prevent or control its spread, and you need to determine their compliance with infection-control practices. Family members caring for clients must be involved in the teaching plan—teach clients and family members a common-sense approach to controlling and preventing infection. Topics to address in a teaching session include the following:

- The client's susceptibility to infection
- The chain of infection, with specific reference to the means of transmission
- Hygienic practices that minimize organism growth and spread; emphasize handwashing
- Preventive health care (e.g., proper diet, immunizations, and exercise)
- The proper methods for handling and storage of food
- An awareness of family members who are at risk for acquiring infection

Client Preparation. Because surgical asepsis necessitates exact techniques, you must have the client's cooperation. Therefore, you must prepare the client before any procedure. Some clients may fear moving or touching objects during a sterile procedure, but others may try to assist. You need to explain how a procedure is to be performed and what the client can do to avoid contaminating sterile items, including the following:

- Avoid sudden movements of body parts covered by sterile drapes
- Refrain from touching sterile supplies, drapes, or the nurse's gloves and gown
- Avoid coughing, sneezing, or talking over a sterile area

Certain sterile procedures may take an extended period of time. You should assess the client's needs and anticipate factors that may disrupt a procedure. If a client is in pain, try to administer analgesics no more than half an hour before a sterile procedure begins. Give the client the opportunity to void. Often clients must assume uncomfortable positions during sterile procedures. Help the client to assume the most comfortable position possible. Finally, the client's condition may result in actions or events that contaminate a sterile field. For example, a client with a respiratory infection transmits organisms by coughing or breathing; you need to anticipate such a problem and offer the client a mask.

Principles of Surgical Asepsis. When beginning a surgically aseptic procedure, you must follow certain principles to ensure the maintenance of asepsis. Failure to follow these principles places clients at risk for infection. The following principles are important:

1. *A sterile object remains sterile only when touched by another sterile object.* This principle guides you in the placement of sterile objects and how to handle them.
   A. Sterile objects that touch sterile objects remain sterile; for example, sterile gloves are worn or sterile forceps are used to handle objects on a sterile field.
   B. Sterile objects that touch clean objects become contaminated; for example, if the tip of a syringe or other sterile object touches the surface of a clean disposable glove, the object is contaminated.
   C. Sterile objects that touch contaminated objects become contaminated; for example, when you touch a sterile object with an ungloved hand, the object is contaminated.
   D. Sterile objects that touch questionable objects are considered contaminated; for example, when a tear or break in the covering or packaging of a sterile object is found, the object is discarded regardless of whether the object itself appears untouched.
2. *Only sterile objects may be placed on a sterile field.* All items are properly sterilized before use. Sterile objects are kept in clean, dry storage areas. The package or container holding a sterile object must be intact and dry—a package that is torn, punctured, wet, or open is considered to be contaminated.
3. *A sterile object or field out of the range of vision or an object held below a person's waist is contaminated.* You must never turn your back on a sterile tray or leave it unattended. Contamination can occur accidentally by a dangling piece of clothing, falling hair, or an unknowing client touching a sterile object. Any object held below waist level is considered contaminated because it cannot be viewed at all times. Sterile objects should be kept in front of you with your hands as close together as possible.

4. *A sterile object or field becomes contaminated by prolonged exposure to air.* You need to avoid activities that may create air currents, such as excessive movements or rearranging linen after a sterile object or field becomes exposed. When sterile packages are being opened, it is important to minimize the number of persons walking into the area. Microorganisms travel by droplet through the air; therefore, no one should talk, laugh, sneeze, or cough over a sterile field or when gathering and using sterile equipment. Microorganisms travelling through the air can fall on sterile items or fields if you reach over the work area. When opening sterile packages, hold the item or piece of equipment as close as possible to the sterile field without touching the sterile surface. Keeping the movement or rearranging of sterile items to a minimum also reduces contamination by air transmission.
5. *When a sterile surface comes in contact with a wet, contaminated surface, the sterile object or field becomes contaminated by capillary action.* If moisture seeps through a sterile package's protective covering, microorganisms travel to the sterile object. When stored sterile packages become wet, you must discard the objects immediately or send the equipment for resterilization. When working with a sterile field or tray, you may have to pour sterile solutions. Any spill can be a source of contamination unless the object or field rests on a sterile surface that cannot be penetrated by moisture. Urinary catheterization trays contain sterile supplies that rest in a sterile, plastic container. In this example, sterile solutions spilled within the container will not contaminate the catheter or other objects. In contrast, if you place a piece of sterile gauze in its wrapper on a client's bedside table and the table surface is wet, the gauze is considered contaminated.
6. *Fluid flows in the direction of gravity.* A sterile object becomes contaminated if gravity causes a contaminated liquid to flow over the object's surface. To avoid contamination during a surgical hand scrub, hold your hands above the elbows. This allows water to flow downward without contaminating your hands and fingers. This is also the reason for drying from the fingers to elbows with hands held up, after the scrub.
7. *The edges of a sterile field or container are considered to be contaminated.* Frequently, sterile objects are placed on a sterile towel or drape (Figure 33–2). Because the edge of the drape touches an unsterile surface, such as a table or bed linen, a 2.5-cm border around the drape is considered contaminated. Objects placed on the sterile field must be inside this border. The edges of sterile containers become exposed to air after they are open and are thus contaminated. After a sterile needle is removed from its protective cap or after forceps are removed from a container, the objects must not touch the container's edge. The lip of an opened bottle of solution also becomes contaminated after it is exposed to air. When pouring a sterile liquid, first pour a small amount of solution to wash away microorganisms on the bottle lip. This small amount of solution is then discarded; pour a second time on the same side to fill a container with the desired amount of solution.

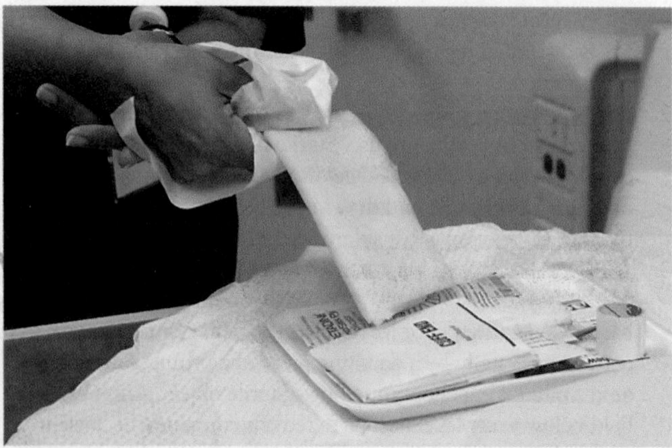
Figure 33-2 Placing sterile item on a sterile field.

Performing Sterile Procedures. All necessary equipment should be assembled before a procedure so that you avoid having to leave a sterile area to obtain equipment. A few extra supplies should be available in case objects accidentally become contaminated. Before the sterile procedure, each step should be explained so that the client can cooperate fully. If an object becomes contaminated during the procedure, you should discard it immediately.

Donning and Removing Caps, Masks, and Eyewear. For sterile procedures on a general nursing division, you may wear a surgical mask and eyewear without a cap. Eyewear is worn as a part of standard precautions or routine practices if fluid or blood could splash into your eyes. For sterile surgical procedures, you must first apply a clean cap that covers all the hair and then put on the surgical mask and eyewear. The mask must fit snugly around the face and nose to prevent contamination by droplet nuclei. After a mask is worn for several hours, the area over the mouth and nose often becomes moist. Because moisture promotes the spread of microorganisms, the mask should be changed if it becomes moist.

Protective glasses or goggles should fit snugly around the forehead and face to fully protect the eyes. Eyewear needs to be worn only for procedures that create the risk of body fluids splashing into the eyes.

Before removing a mask, eyewear, and cap, remove the gloves to prevent contamination of the hair, neck, and facial area. After untying the mask, hold it by the ties and discard it with the cap. Masks should not be worn hanging from the neck after removal from the face. Eyewear is removed and cleaned later for reuse. After removing all protective wear, perform hand hygiene thoroughly.

Opening Sterile Packages. Sterile items such as syringes, gauze dressings, and catheters are packaged in paper or plastic containers that are impervious to microorganisms as long as they are dry and intact. Some institutions wrap reusable supplies in a double thickness of paper, linen, or muslin. These packages are permeable to steam and thus allow for steam autoclaving. Sterile items are kept in clean, enclosed storage cabinets and are separated from nonsterile equipment.

Sterile supplies carry chemical tapes indicating that a sterilization process has taken place. The tapes change colour during the sterilization process; if the tapes do not changed colour, the item is not sterile. A sterile item should never be used if the integrity of the packaging is compromised. Health care facilities may apply the date processed and a lot number to the item after processing ("event-related expiration"), or they may apply an expiration date ("date-related expiration") to the item. With either system, it is important for you to check the integrity of the packaging before using an item.

Before opening a sterile item, perform thorough hand hygiene. Inspect the supplies for package integrity and sterility and assemble the supplies in the work area, such as the bedside table or treatment room, before opening the packages. A bedside table or countertop provides a large, clean working area for opening items. The work area should be above waist level. Sterile supplies should not be opened in a confined space where a dirty object might fall on or strike them.

Opening a Sterile Item on a Flat Surface. Sterile packaged items must be opened without contaminating the contents. Commercially packaged items are usually designed so that you only have to tear away or separate the paper or plastic cover. The item is held in one hand while the wrapper is pulled away with the other (Figure 33–3). Take care to keep the inner contents sterile before use. When opening items processed by the facility and packed in paper or linen, observe the following steps:

1. Place the item flat in the centre of the work surface.
2. Remove the sterilization tape or seal.
3. Grasp the outer surface of the tip of the outermost flap.
4. Open the outer flap away from the body, keeping the arm outstretched and away from the sterile field (Figure 33–4A).
5. Grasp the outside surface of the first side flap.
6. Open the side flap, allowing it to lie flat on the table surface. Keep your arm to the side and not over the sterile surface (Figure 33–4B). Do not allow the flaps to spring back over the sterile contents.
7. Grasp the outside surface of the second side flap and allow it to lie flat on the table surface (Figure 33–4C).
8. Grasp the outside surface of the last and innermost flap.
9. Stand away from the sterile package and pull the flap back, allowing it to fall flat on the surface (Figure 33–4D).
10. Use the inner surface of the package (except for the 2.5-cm border around the edges) as a sterile field to add additional sterile items. The 2.5-cm border can be grasped to manoeuvre the field on the table surface.

If the sterile supplies are not for immediate use, you can close the sterile package. In this case, touch only the wrapper's outside surface. To close a package, the order of unwrapping is reversed, and you should not touch the inside contents or reach over the field.

Opening a Sterile Item While Holding It. To open a small, sterile item, hold the package in your nondominant hand. Using the dominant hand, carefully open the side and top flaps away from the enclosed sterile item in the order previously mentioned. Open the item in a hand so that the item can be handed to a person wearing sterile gloves or transferred to a sterile field.

Preparing a Sterile Field. When performing sterile procedures, you need a sterile work area that provides room for the handling and placing of sterile items. A **sterile field** is an area free of microorganisms and prepared to receive sterile items. The field may be prepared by using the inner surface of a sterile wrapper as the work surface or by using a sterile drape or dressing tray. Skill 33–2 describes preparation of a sterile field. After the surface for the field is created, add sterile items by carefully placing them directly on the field or by transferring them with a sterile forceps. A sterile object that comes in contact with the 2.5-cm border must be discarded.

You may choose to wear sterile gloves while preparing items on the field. If this is done, you can touch the entire drape, but sterile items must be handed over by an assistant. Your gloves cannot touch the wrappers of sterile items.

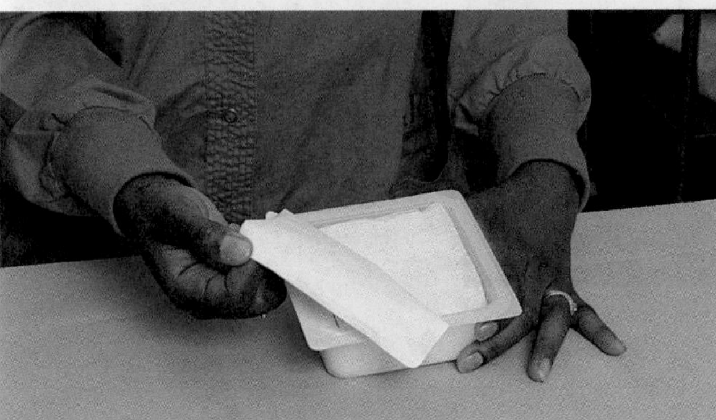

Figure 33-3 Opening a sterile package on a work area above waist level.

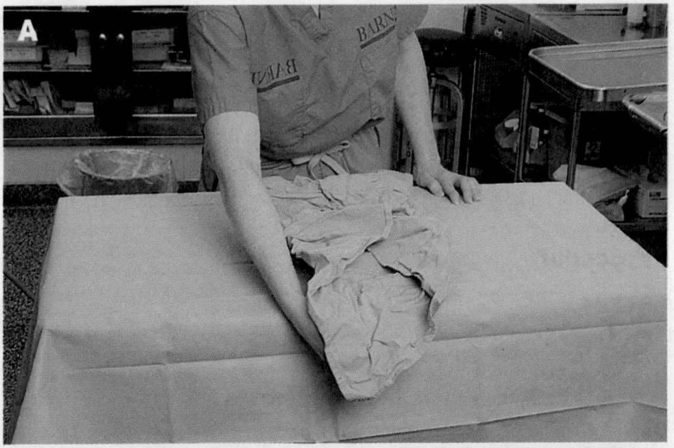

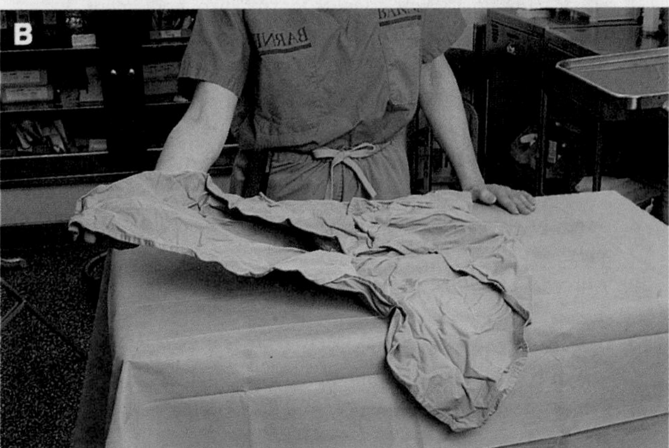

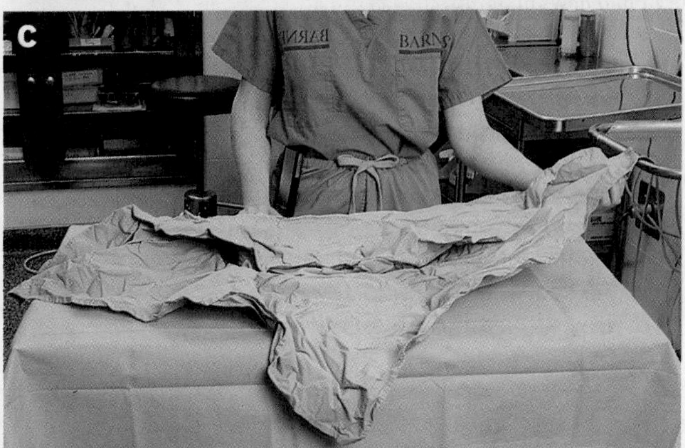

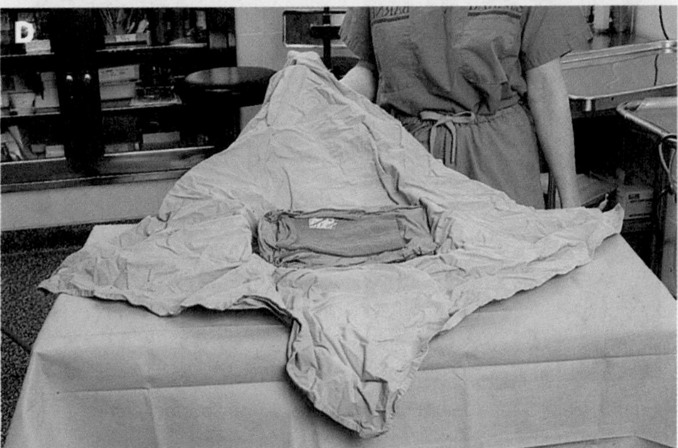

Figure 33-4 Opening sterile packaged items on a flat surface. **A**, Open the top flap away from the body. **B**, Keep your arm away from the sterile field while opening the side flap. **C**, Open the second side flap. **D**, Open the back flap.

SKILL 33-2 Preparation of a Sterile Field

Delegation Considerations

Delegation of the preparation of a sterile field is inappropriate unless you are delegating to an unregulated care provider (UCP) who has received specialized training. Operating room technicians are usually trained for this skill.

Equipment

- Sterile drape
- Assorted sterile supplies

Procedure

STEPS	RATIONALE
1. Prepare sterile field just before planned procedure. Supplies are to be used immediately.	• Prevents exposure of sterile field and supplies to air and contamination.
2. Select clean work surface above waist level.	• A once-sterile object held below waist is considered contaminated.
3. Assemble necessary equipment.	• Preparation of equipment in advance prevents a break in the technique.
4. Check dates or labels on supplies for sterility of equipment.	• Equipment stored beyond expiration date is considered unsterile.
5. Perform hand hygiene thoroughly. *Option:* Procedure may be performed with gloves on.	• Reduces microbial counts on skin.
6. Place pack containing sterile drape on work surface and open as described in Figure 33–4.	• Ensures sterility of packaged drape.
7. With fingertips of one hand, pick up folded top edge of sterile drape.	• The 2.5-cm border around drape is unsterile and may be touched with fingers or clean gloves.
8. Gently lift drape up from its outer cover and let it unfold by itself without touching any object. Discard outer cover with your other hand.	• If sterile object touches any nonsterile object, it becomes contaminated.
9. With your other hand, grasp adjacent corner of drape and hold it straight up and away from your body (see Step 9 illustration).	• Drape can now be properly placed while using two hands. Drape must be held away from unsterile surfaces.
10. Holding drape, first position and lay bottom half over intended work surface (see Step 10 illustration).	• Prevents you from reaching over sterile field.
11. Allow top half of drape to be placed over work surface last (see Step 11 illustration).	• Creates flat, sterile work surface.
12. Grasp 2.5-cm border around edge to position as needed.	• Assists in differentiating and organizing the sterile surface.
Adding Sterile Item	
13. Open sterile item (according to package directions) while holding outside wrapper in nondominant hand.	• Frees dominant hand for unwrapping outer wrapper.
14. Carefully peel wrapper onto nondominant hand.	• Item remains sterile.
15. Being sure wrapper does not fall down on sterile field, place item onto field at angle. Do not hold arm over sterile field (see Step 15 illustration).	• Prevents reaching over field and contaminating its surface.
16. Dispose of outer wrapper.	• Prevents accidental contamination of sterile field.
17. Perform procedure using sterile technique.	• Prevents transmission of infection to client.

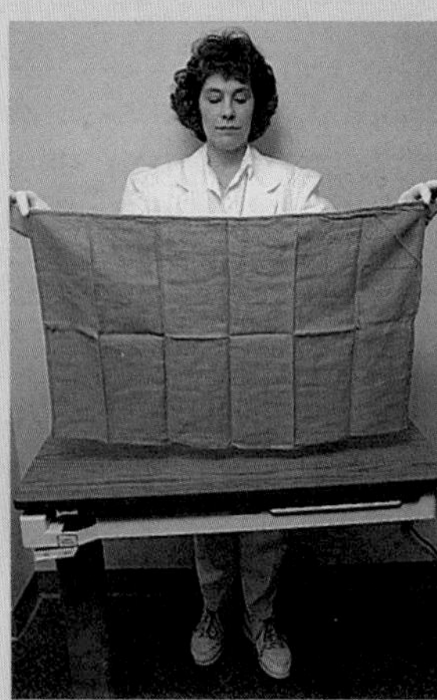
Step 9 Hold drape straight up and away from body.

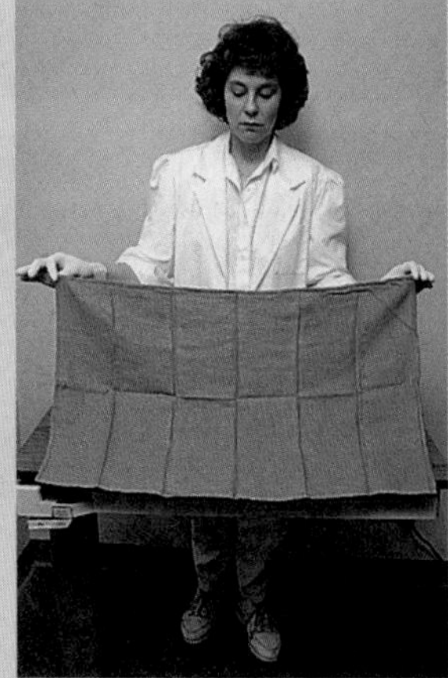
Step 10 Lay bottom half of drape over work surface.

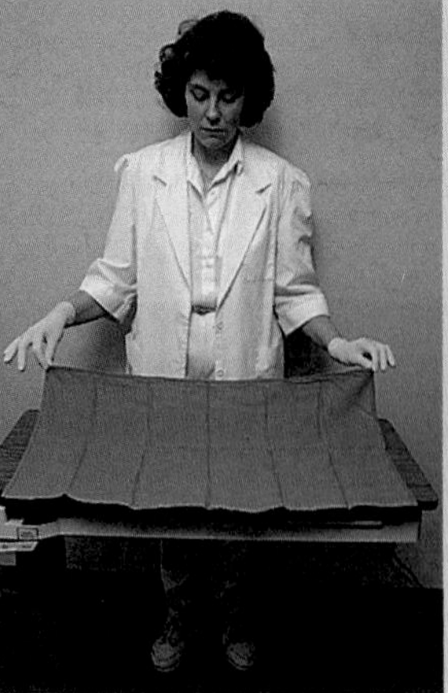
Step 11 Place top half of drape over work surface.

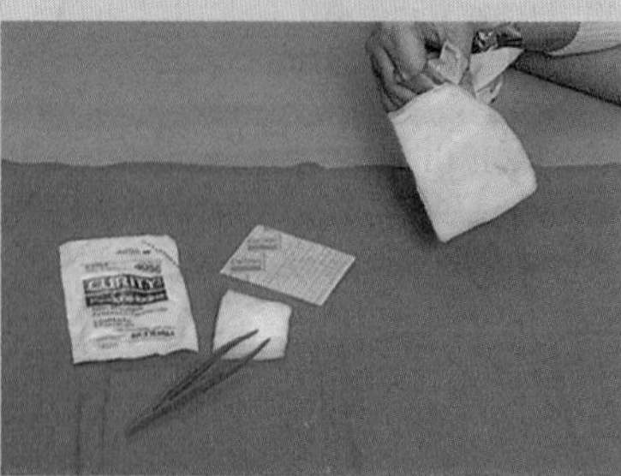
Step 15 Adding item to sterile field.

Recording and Reporting

- It is not necessary to record or report this procedure.

Pouring Sterile Solutions. Often you must pour sterile solutions into sterile containers. A bottle containing a sterile solution is sterile on the inside and contaminated on the outside; the outside neck of the bottle is also contaminated, but the inside of the bottle cap is considered sterile. After the cap or lid is removed, it is held in the hand or placed sterile side (inside) up on a clean surface. This means that the inside of the lid can be seen as it rests on the table surface. A bottle cap or lid should never rest on a sterile surface, even though the inside of the cap is sterile. The outer edge of the cap is unsterile and would contaminate the sterile surface. Likewise, placing a sterile cap down on an unsterile surface increases the chances of the inside of the cap becoming contaminated.

You need to check the label of the bottle to ensure it is the correct solution. Then hold the bottle with its label in the palm of the hand to prevent the possibility of the solution wetting and fading the label. Before pouring the solution into the container, pour a small amount (1 to 2 mL) into a disposable cap or plastic-lined waste receptacle. The discarded solution cleans the lip of the bottle. The edge of the bottle is kept away from the edge or inside of the receiving container. Pour the solution slowly to avoid splashing the underlying drape or field. The bottle should never be held so high above the container that even slow pouring will cause splashing. The bottle should be held outside the edge of the sterile field.

Surgical Scrub. Clients undergoing operative procedures are at an increased risk for infection. When working in operating rooms, you must perform surgical hand antisepsis to decrease and suppress the growth of skin microorganisms, in case your glove tears (Operating Room Nurses Association of Canada [ORNAC], 2003).

During surgical hand antisepsis before an operation, scrub from your fingertips to your elbows with an antiseptic soap. The optimum duration of the surgical hand scrub is unclear, although research indicates that it may be dependent on the type of antimicrobial product. The usual scrub time for both the initial and subsequent scrubs is 5 minutes (Meeker & Rothrock, 1999). Larson (1996) recommends that at least 2 minutes of friction be used for presurgery handwashing. You should follow your agency's policy for length of scrub time. For many years, preoperative handwashing protocols required nurses to scrub with a brush. However, this practice may damage the skin and can result in increased shedding of bacteria from the hands. Scrubbing with a disposable sponge or combination sponge–brush has been shown to reduce bacterial counts on the hands as effectively as scrubbing with a brush (Hsieh, et al, 2006). However, the study by Gupta et al. (2007) suggested that neither a brush nor a sponge is necessary to reduce bacterial counts on the hands, especially when an alcohol-based product is used.

For maximum elimination of bacteria, all jewellery should be removed and the nails should be kept clean and short (ORNAC, 2003). Artificial nails should not be worn because they may harbour a greater number of bacteria. Similarly, nail polish should be avoided because it conceals soil under the nails and because chipped nail polish may increase the bacterial load (Health Canada, 1998). Freshly applied polish (not chipped or worn for more than 4 days) may be acceptable, if permitted by your facility's policy (Gruendeman & Mangum, 2001). If you have active skin infections, open lesions or cuts, or respiratory infections, you should be excluded from the surgical team. Skill 33–3 describes the steps for surgical hand hygiene.

Applying Sterile Gloves. Sterile gloves are an additional barrier to bacterial transfer. If you work on general nursing divisions, use *open gloving* before procedures such as dressing changes and urinary catheter insertions. *Closed gloving*, which is performed after you apply sterile gowns, is practised in operating rooms and special treatment areas. Skills 33–4 and 33–5 review the steps of each sterile gloving technique. The proper glove size should be selected; the glove should not stretch so tightly that it can easily tear, yet it should be tight enough that objects can be picked up easily.

➤ SKILL 33-3 Surgical Hand Hygiene

Preparing for Gowning

Delegation Considerations

The role of the scrub nurse can be delegated to a surgical technologist or licensed practical nurse. UCPs can help the registered nurse in the circulating nurse role by opening sterile supplies, setting up sterile fields, and running errands under the direction of the registered nurse.

Equipment

- Deep sink with foot or knee controls for dispensing water and soap (faucets should be high enough for hands and forearms to fit comfortably)
- Antimicrobial detergent or alcohol-based waterless antiseptic, according to agency policy (product should be nonirritating, broad spectrum, fast acting, and effective in reducing skin microorganisms and have a residual effect) (Association of Perioperative Registered Nurses [AORN], 2004; ORNAC, 2003)
- Surgical scrub sponge with plastic nail pick
- Paper mask and cap or hood
- Sterile towel
- Proper scrub attire
- Protective eyewear (glasses or goggles)

Procedure

STEPS	RATIONALE
1. Consult your agency's policy regarding required length of scrub time and antiseptic to use for hand antisepsis.	• Guidelines vary regarding ideal time needed and antiseptic to use for surgical scrub.
2. Be sure fingernails are short, clean, and healthy. Artificial nails should be removed. Natural nails should be less than 0.5 cm long.	• Long nails and chipped or old polish increase number of bacteria residing on nails. Long fingernails can puncture gloves, causing contamination. Artificial nails are known to harbour Gram-negative microorganisms and fungus (Hedderwick et al., 2000).

Critical Decision Point: Remove nail polish if chipped or worn longer than 4 days because it may harbour microorganisms (AORN, 2004; ORNAC, 2003).

Continued

➤ SKILL 33-3 Surgical Hand Hygiene *continued*

STEPS	RATIONALE
3. Inspect hands for presence of abrasions, cuts, or open lesions.	• These conditions increase the likelihood of microorganisms residing on skin surfaces.
4. Apply surgical shoe covers, cap or hood, face mask, and protective eyewear.	• Mask prevents escape into air of microorganisms that can contaminate hands. Other protective wear prevents exposure to blood and body fluid splashes during the procedure.
5. Surgical handwashing:	
A. Turn on water using knee or foot controls.	
B. Wet hands and arms under running water and lather with detergent to 5 cm above elbows. (Hands need to be above elbows at all times.)	• Water runs by gravity from fingertips to elbows, flowing from least to most contaminated areas. Hands become cleanest part of upper extremity. Washing a wide area reduces risk of contaminating overlying gown that you later apply.
C. Rinse hands and arms thoroughly under running water. **Remember to keep hands above elbows.**	• Rinsing removes transient bacteria from fingers, hands, and forearms.
D. Under running water, clean under nails of both hands with nail pick. Discard after use (see Step 5D illustration).	• Removes dirt and organic material that harbour large numbers of microorganisms.
E. Wet clean sponge and apply antimicrobial detergent. Scrub nails of one hand with 15 strokes. Holding sponge perpendicular, scrub palm, each side of thumb and fingers, and posterior side of hand with 10 strokes each. The arm is mentally divided into thirds, and each third is scrubbed 10 times (see Step 5E illustrations). The duration of scrub is determined by the manufacturer's recommendations for the scrub agent used, which is usually 2 to 6 minutes (ORNAC, 2003). Rinse sponge and repeat sequence for other arm. A two-sponge method may be substituted. Check your agency's policy.	• Friction loosens resident bacteria that adhere to skin surfaces. Technique ensures coverage of all surfaces. Scrubbing is performed from cleanest area (hands) to marginal area (upper arms).
F. Discard sponge and rinse hands and arms thoroughly (see Step 5F illustration). Turn off water with foot or knee control and back into room entrance with hands elevated in front of and away from the body.	• After touching skin, the sponge is considered contaminated. Rinsing removes resident bacteria. Using foot or knee tap control and backing into room prevents accidental contamination.
G. Walk up to sterile tray and lean forward slightly to pick up a sterile towel (see Step 5G illustration). Dry one hand thoroughly, moving from fingers to elbow. Dry in a rotating motion. Dry from cleanest to least clean area (see Step 5G illustration).	• Drying prevents chapping and facilitates donning of gloves. Leaning forward prevents accidental contact of arms with scrub attire.
H. Repeat drying method for other hand by carefully reversing towel or using a new sterile towel.	• Prevents accidental contamination.
I. Discard towel.	• Prevents accidental contamination.
J. Proceed with sterile gowning (see Skill 33–4).	
6. Alternative method of surgical hand hygiene using alcohol-based antiseptic:	
A. Wash hands with soap and water for at least 15 seconds to remove soil.	• Removes dirt and organic material that harbour large numbers of microorganisms.
B. Under running water, clean under nails of both hands with nail pick. Discard after use and dry hands with paper towel.	

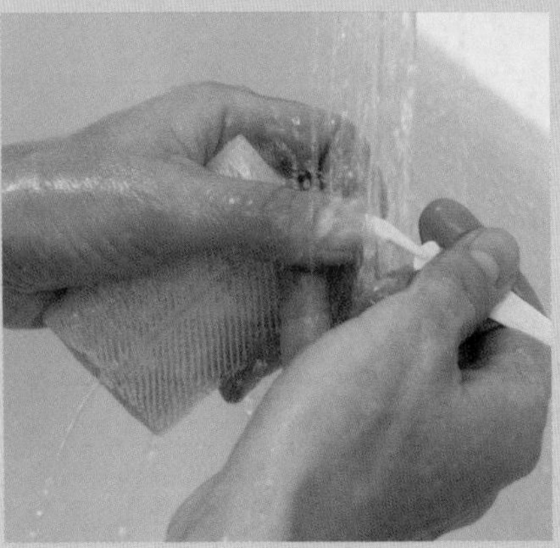

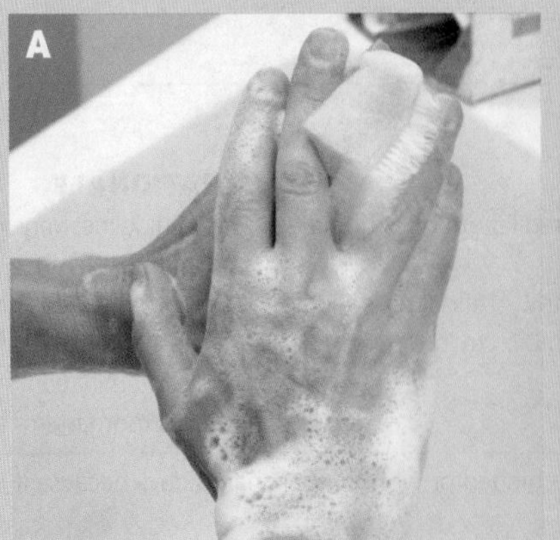

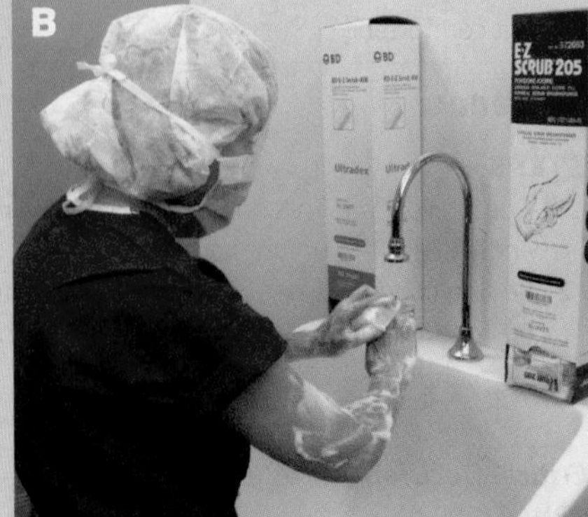

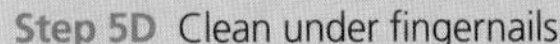
Step 5D Clean under fingernails.

Step 5E **A,** Scrub side of fingers. **B,** Scrub forearms.

➤ SKILL 33-3 Surgical Hand Hygiene *continued*

STEPS	RATIONALE
C. Apply enough alcohol-based waterless antiseptic to one palm to cover both hands thoroughly (see Step 6C illustration). Spread the antiseptic over all surfaces of the hands and fingernails. Follow product instructions for length of time to rub over hand surfaces. Allow to air-dry.	• Ensures coverage of all surfaces. Air-drying ensures complete antisepsis is achieved.
D. Repeat the process and allow hands to air-dry before applying sterile gloves.	

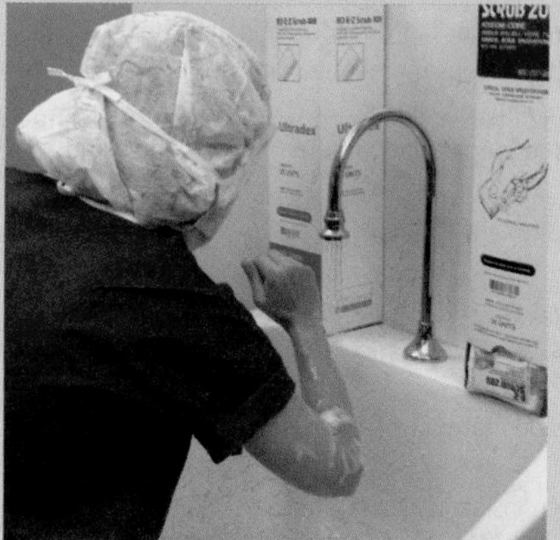

Step 5F Rinse arms.

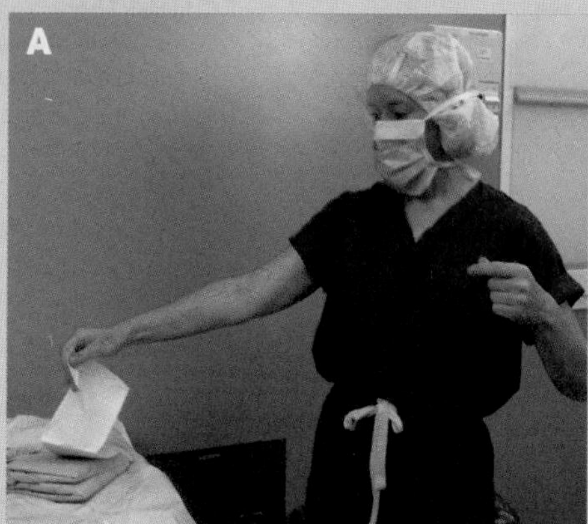

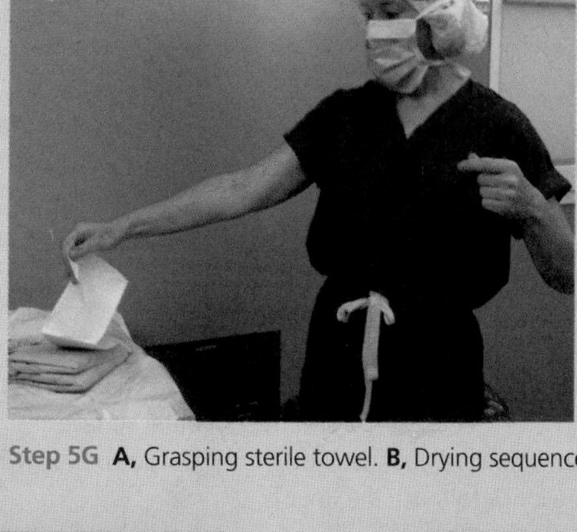

Step 5G **A,** Grasping sterile towel. **B,** Drying sequence.

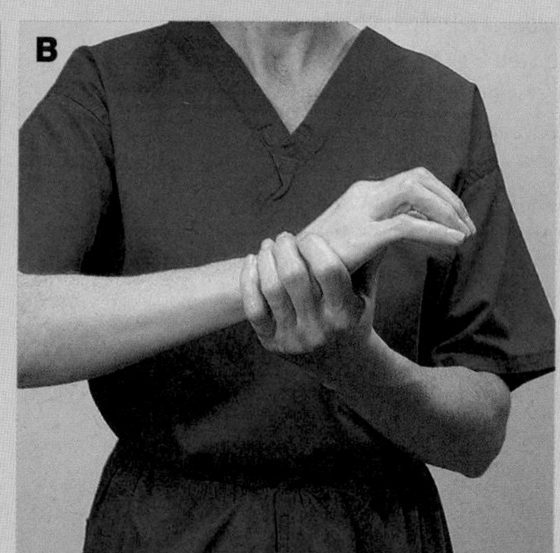

Step 6C Application of antimicrobial agent for brushless hand scrub. This nurse is using 3M Avagard.
Source: Photo courtesy of 3M Health Care.

Recording and Reporting

- It is not necessary to record or report this procedure.
- Report any dermatitis to employee health or infection control per your agency's policy.

Donning a Sterile Gown. You must wear a sterile gown when assisting at the sterile field in an operating room, delivery room, or special treatment areas so that sterile objects can be comfortably handled with less risk of contamination. If you are the circulating nurse, you do not usually wear a sterile gown. The sterile gown acts as a barrier to decrease the shedding of microorganisms from skin surfaces into the air, thus preventing wound contamination. You may also wear a sterile gown if you are caring for a client with a large open wound or assisting a physician during a major invasive procedure (e.g., inserting an arterial catheter).

After you have applied a mask and surgical cap and performed surgical handwashing, you apply a sterile gown. Pick up the gown from a sterile pack, or ask an assistant to hand the gown to you. Only a certain portion of the gown—the area from the anterior waist to, but not including, the collar and the anterior surface of the sleeves—is considered sterile. The back of the gown, the area under the arms, the collar, the area below the waist, and the underside of the sleeves are not sterile because you cannot keep these areas in constant view and ensure their sterility. Skill 33–4 reviews the steps for applying a sterile gown and closed gloving, and Skill 33–5 reviews the method of open gloving.

➤ SKILL 33-4 Applying a Sterile Gown and Performing Closed Gloving

Delegation Considerations

The role of the scrub nurse can be delegated to a surgical technician.

Equipment

- Surgical cap
- Surgical mask
- Eyewear
- Foot covers
- Sterile gown (prepared by circulating nurse)

Procedure

STEPS	RATIONALE
1. Before entering operating room or treatment area, apply cap, face mask, and eyewear. Foot covers are also required in operating room.	• Prevent hair and air droplet nuclei from contaminating sterile work areas. Eyewear protects mucous membranes of eye. Foot covers are paper or cloth and fit over work shoes.
2. Perform thorough surgical hand hygiene (see Skill 33–3).	• Remove transient and resident bacteria from fingers, hands, and forearms.
3. Ask circulating nurse to assist by opening sterile pack containing sterile gown (folded inside out).	• Gown's outer surface remains sterile.
4. Have circulating nurse prepare glove package by peeling outer wrapper open while keeping inner contents sterile. Inner glove package is then placed on sterile field created by sterile outer wrapper.	• This action keeps gloves sterile and allows nurse who has scrubbed to handle sterile items.
5. Reach down to sterile gown package; lift folded gown directly upward and step back away from table.	• This action provides wide margin of safety, avoiding contamination of gown.
6. Holding folded gown, locate neckband. With both hands, grasp inside front of gown just below neckband.	• Clean hands may touch inside of gown without contaminating outer surface.
7. Allow gown to unfold, keeping inside of gown toward body. Do not touch outside of gown with bare hands or allow it to touch the floor.	• Outside of gown will remain sterile surface.
8. With hands at shoulder level, slip both arms into armholes simultaneously (see Step 8 illustration). Ask circulating nurse to bring gown over shoulders by reaching inside to arm seams and pulling gown on, leaving sleeves covering hands.	• Careful application prevents contamination. Gown covers hands to prepare for closed gloving.
9. Have circulating nurse securely tie back of gown at neck and waist (see Step 9 illustration). (If gown is a wraparound style, sterile flap to cover gown is not touched until you have gloved.)	• Gown must completely enclose underlying garments.

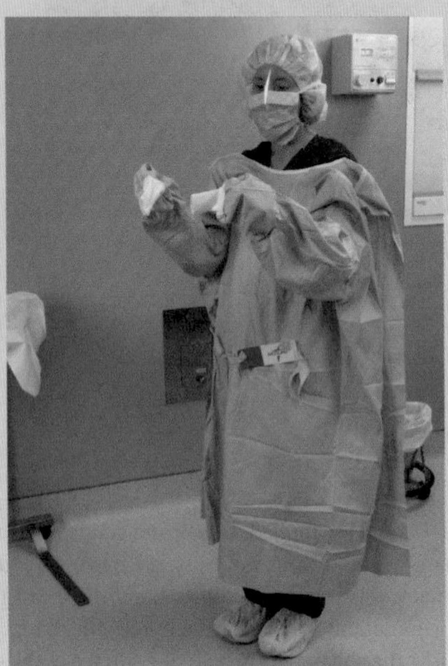

Step 8 Place arms in sleeves.

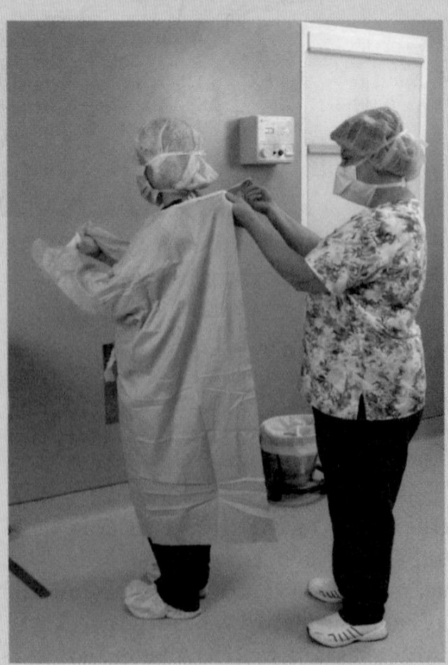

Step 9 Circulating nurse ties scrub gown.

➤ SKILL 33-4 Applying a Sterile Gown and Performing Closed Gloving *continued*

STEPS	RATIONALE
10. Closed gloving:	
A. With hands covered by gown sleeves, open inner sterile glove package (see Step 10A illustration).	• Hands remain clean. Sterile gown cuff will touch sterile glove surface.
B. With dominant hand inside gown cuff, pick up glove for non-dominant hand by grasping folded cuff.	• Sterile gown touches sterile glove.
C. Extend nondominant forearm with palm up and place palm of glove against palm of nondominant hand. Glove fingers will point toward elbow.	• Position glove for application over cuffed hand, keeping glove sterile.
D. Grasp back of glove cuff with covered dominant hand and turn glove cuff over end of nondominant hand and gown cuff (see Step 10D illustration).	• Seal that is created by glove cuff over gown prevents exit of microorganisms over operative sterile field.
E. Grasp top of glove and underlying gown sleeve with covered dominant hand. Carefully extend fingers into glove, being sure glove's cuff covers gown's cuff.	
F. Glove dominant hand in same manner, reversing hands (see Step 10F illustration). Use gloved nondominant hand to pull on glove. Keep hand inside sleeve (see Step 10F illustration).	• Sterile object touches sterile object and therefore stays sterile. Touching the sterile sleeve with the sterile gloved hand allows the gloved hands to remain sterile.
G. Be sure fingers are fully extended into both gloves.	• Ensure that you have full dexterity while using gloved hand.
11. For wraparound sterile gowns, take gloved hand and release fastener or ties in front of gown.	• Front of gown is sterile.
12. Hand tie to sterile team member, who stands still (see Step 12 illustration). Allowing margin of safety, turn around to the left, covering back with extended gown flap. Take back tie from team member and secure tie to gown.	• Contact with team member could contaminate gown and gloves. Gown must enclose undergarments.

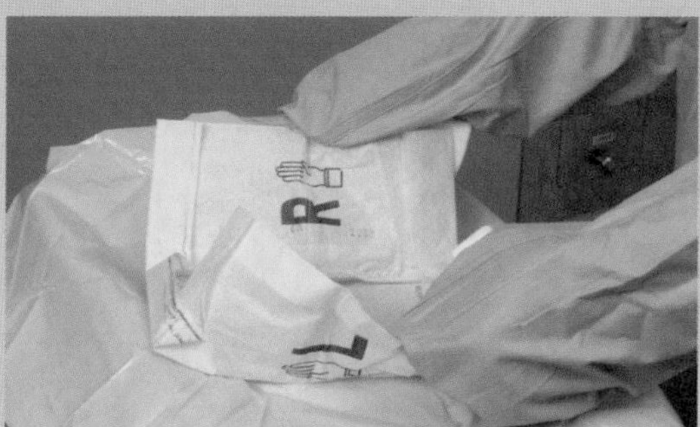

Step 10A Open glove package.

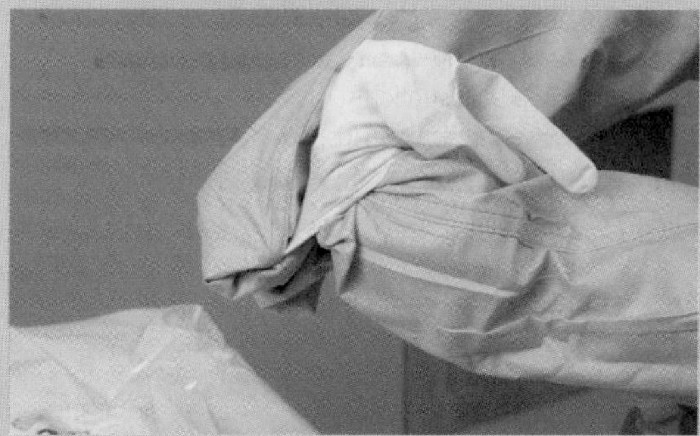
Step 10D Apply glove to left hand keeping right hand inside cuff.

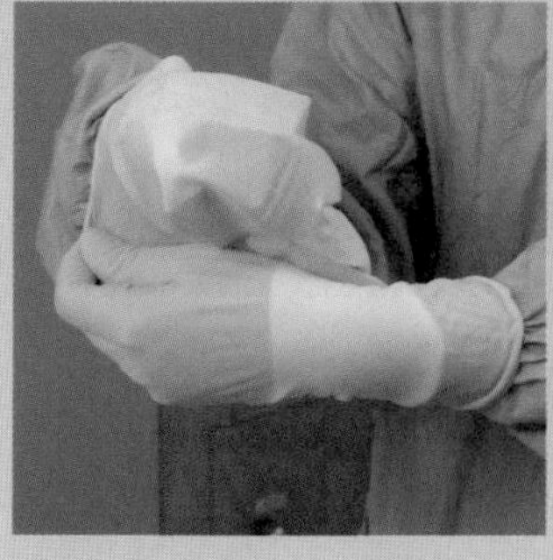
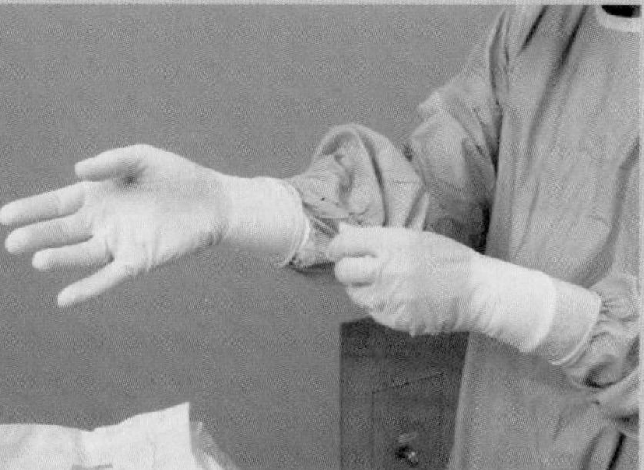
Step 10F Apply second glove.

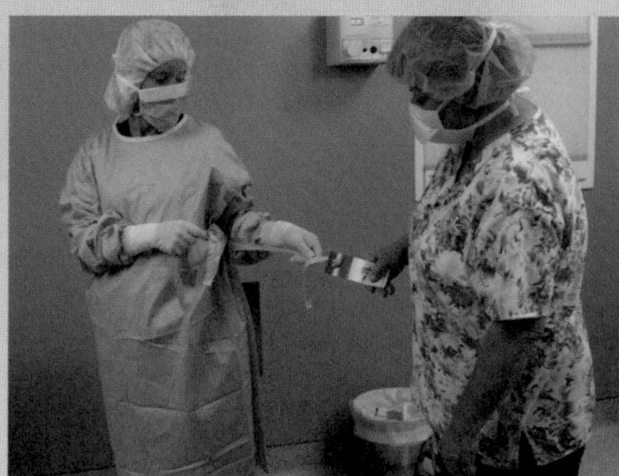
Step 12 Hand tie to sterile team member.

Recording and Reporting

- It is not necessary to record or report this procedure.

➤ SKILL 33-5 Open Gloving

Delegation Considerations

Delegation of open gloving depends on whether a UCP has received special training and is competent to perform the sterile procedure.

Equipment

- Sterile gloves (proper size)

Procedure

STEPS	RATIONALE
1. Perform thorough hand hygiene.	• Removes bacteria from skin surfaces and reduces risk of transmitting infection.
2. Remove outer glove package wrapper by carefully separating and peeling apart sides.	• Prevents inner glove package from accidentally opening and touching contaminated objects.
3. Grasp inner package and lay it on clean, dry flat surface just above waist level. Open package, keeping gloves on wrapper's inside surface (see Step 3 illustration).	• Sterile object held below waist is contaminated. Inner surface of glove package is sterile
4. If gloves are not prepowdered, take packet of powder and apply lightly to hands over sink or wastebasket.	• Powder allows gloves to slip on easily. (Some staff members do not use powder for fear of promoting growth of microorganisms.)
5. Identify right and left gloves. Each glove has cuff approximately 5 cm wide. Glove dominant hand first.	• Proper identification of gloves prevents contamination by improper fit. Gloving of dominant hand first improves dexterity.
6. With thumb and first two fingers of nondominant hand, grasp edge of cuff of glove for dominant hand. Touch only glove's inside surface.	• Inner edge of cuff will lie against skin and is thus not sterile.
7. Carefully pull glove over dominant hand, being sure cuff does not roll up wrist. Be sure thumb and fingers are in proper spaces (see Step 7 illustration).	• If glove's outer surface touches hand or wrist, then it is contaminated.
8. With gloved dominant hand, slip fingers underneath second glove's cuff (see Step 8 illustration).	• Cuff protects gloved fingers. Sterile surface touching sterile surface prevents glove contamination.
9. Carefully pull second glove over nondominant hand. Do not allow fingers and thumb of gloved dominant hand to touch any part of exposed nondominant hand. Keep thumb of dominant hand abducted back (see Step 9 illustration).	• Contact of gloved hand with exposed hand results in contamination.
10. After second glove is on, interlock hands. The cuffs usually fall down after application. Be sure to touch only sterile sides (see Step 10 illustration).	• Ensure smooth fit over fingers.

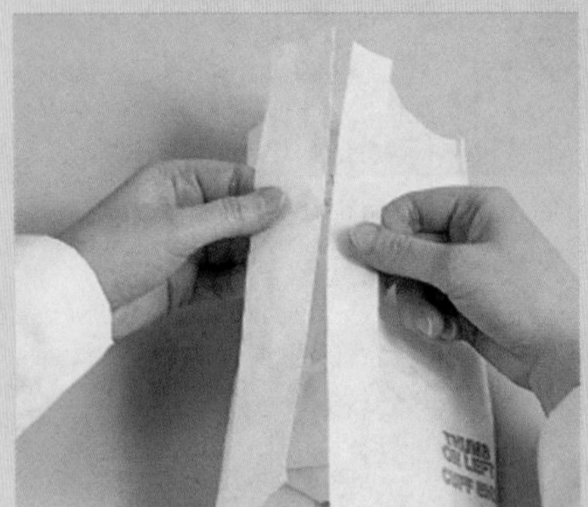
Step 3 Open package.

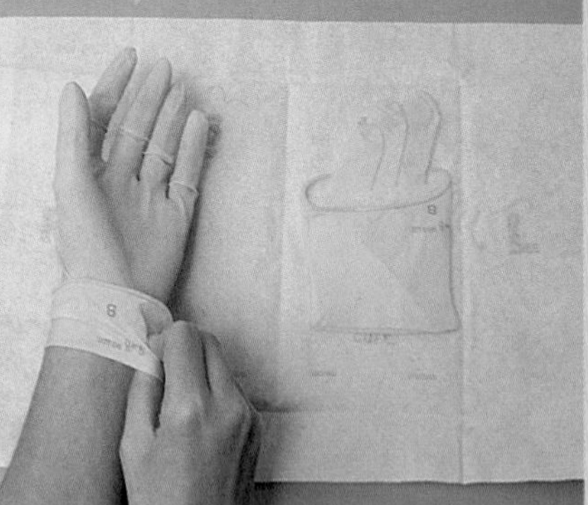
Step 7 Pull glove over dominant hand.

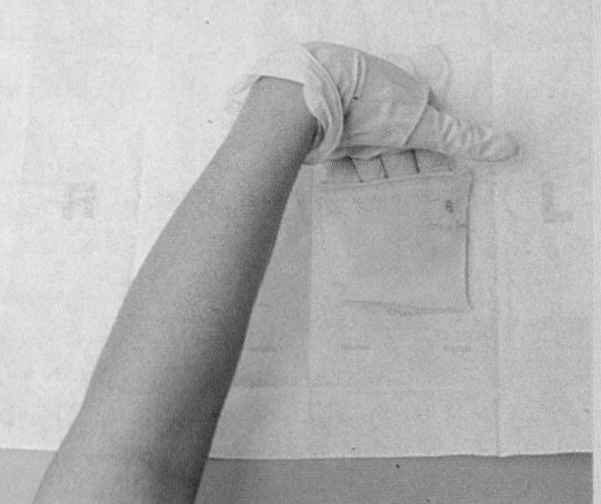
Step 8 Slip fingers underneath second glove's cuff.

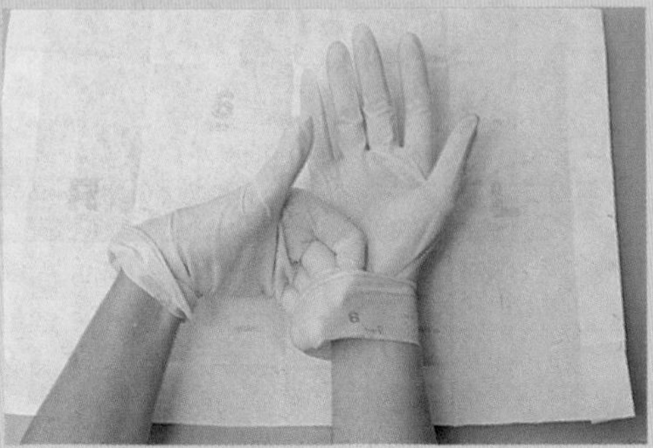
Step 9 Pull second glove over nondominant hand.

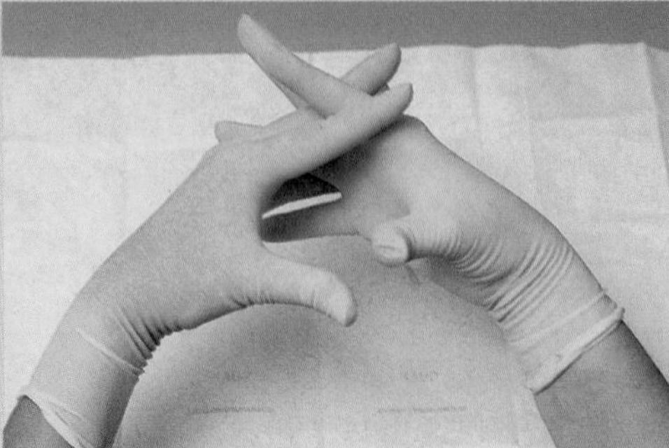
Step 10 Interlock hands.

➤ SKILL 33-5 Open Gloving *continued*

STEPS	RATIONALE
Glove Disposal	
11. Grasp outside of one cuff with other gloved hand; avoid touching wrist.	• Minimize contamination of underlying skin.
12. Pull glove off, turning it inside out. Discard in receptacle.	• Outside of glove does not touch skin surface.
13. Take fingers of bare hand and tuck inside remaining glove cuff. Peel glove off, inside out. Discard in receptacle. Perform hand hygiene.	

Recording and Reporting

- It is not necessary to record or report this procedure.

❖Evaluation

Your success when practising infection-control techniques is measured by determining whether the goals for reducing or preventing infection are achieved. By comparing the client's response, such as the absence of fever or development of wound drainage, with expected outcomes, you determine the success of nursing interventions. Similarly, you determine whether interventions should be revised or eliminated. Correctly assessing wounds for healing and conducting a physical assessment of body systems (see Chapter 32) are important skills in evaluation. You need to closely monitor clients, especially those at risk, for signs and symptoms of infection. For example, a client who has undergone a surgical procedure is at risk for infection at the surgical site, as well as at sites of invasive procedures such as a venipuncture or central line insertion. In addition, the client is at risk for a respiratory tract infection as a result of decreased mobility and for a urinary tract infection if an in-dwelling catheter is present. You must closely monitor all invasive and surgical sites for swelling, erythema, and purulent drainage. Breath sounds are monitored for changes, and sputum character is checked for purulence. Laboratory test results are reviewed for leukocytes in the urine, which may indicate a urinary tract infection. The absence of signs or symptoms of infection is the expected outcome of infection-prevention and -monitoring activities.

The client at risk for infection must understand the measures needed to reduce or prevent microorganism growth and spread. Providing clients or family members with the opportunity to discuss infection-control measures and to demonstrate procedures will increase their ability to comply with therapy. You may determine that clients require new information or that previously instructed information needs reinforcement.

You need to document the client's response to therapies for infection control. A clear description of any signs and symptoms of systemic or local infection is necessary to give all nurses a baseline for comparative evaluation. The efficacy of any intervention in reducing infection must be reported.

✻ KEY CONCEPTS

- Hand hygiene is the most important technique to use in preventing and controlling the transmission of infection.
- The potential for microorganisms to cause disease depends on the number of organisms, their virulence, their ability to enter and survive in a host, and the susceptibility of the host.
- Normal body flora help to resist infection by releasing antibacterial substances and inhibiting the multiplication of pathogenic microorganisms.
- The signs of local inflammation and infection are identical.
- An infection can develop as long as the six elements comprising the chain of infection are uninterrupted.
- Microorganisms are transmitted by direct and indirect contact, droplets, airborne particles, and contaminated vehicles and vectors.
- Advancing age, poor nutrition, stress, diseases of the immune system, chronic disease, and treatments or conditions that compromise the immune response increase a person's susceptibility to infection.
- The major sites for HAI include the urinary and respiratory tracts, the bloodstream, and surgical or traumatic wounds.
- The CDC now recommends the use of alcohol-based waterless antiseptics as an alternative to handwashing to more effectively reduce the transmission of pathogens.
- Invasive procedures, medical therapies, long hospitalization, and contact with health care personnel increase a hospitalized client's risk for acquiring an HAI.
- Isolation practices may prevent personnel and clients from acquiring infections and may prevent the transmission of microorganisms.
- Standard precautions or routine practices entail the use of generic barrier techniques in the care of all clients.
- Transmission-based (isolation) precautions are used for clients with specific, highly transmissible infections.
- Proper cleansing necessitates the mechanical removal of soil from an object or area.
- A client in isolation is subject to sensory deprivation because of the restricted environment.
- An infection-control professional monitors the incidence of infection within an institution and provides educational and consultative services to maintain infection prevention.
- Surgical asepsis necessitates more stringent techniques than does medical asepsis and is directed at eliminating all microorganisms.
- Surgical aseptic practices are followed if the skin is broken or if you perform an invasive procedure in a body cavity that is normally free of microorganisms.

✻ CRITICAL THINKING EXERCISES

1. Mrs. Jaycock had an in-dwelling urethral catheter for 1 week. The catheter has now been out for 24 hours. She complains of frequency of and pain on urination. Mrs. Jaycock suggests that the catheter be re-inserted so that she does not need to get up frequently. What can frequency of or pain on urination indicate? Should the catheter be re-inserted? Why or why not? Describe at least one appropriate assessment measure and independent nursing action for Mrs. Jaycock.

2. You are caring for Mr. Huang, who has a large, open, draining abdominal wound. You notice another health care worker changing Mr. Huang's dressing without wearing gloves or using sterile supplies or sterile technique. When you question the health care worker regarding this practice, the person says, "Don't worry, the wound is already infected, and the antibiotics and draining will take care of any contaminants." How would you respond to this comment? What would your next steps be in following up on this incident?
3. Mrs. Niles is 83 years of age and lives alone. She has difficulty walking and relies on a church volunteer group to deliver lunches during the week. Her fixed income limits her ability to buy food. Last week, Mrs. Niles's 79-year-old sister died. The two sisters had been very close. Explain the factors that might increase Mrs. Niles's risk for infection.
4. Mr. Vargas is admitted to your facility with a history of recent weight loss, a cough that has persisted for 2 months, and hemoptysis. His chest X-ray film shows a cavity in one lung, and his physician suspects tuberculosis. What type of isolation precautions would you use for Mr. Vargas? What protection would you use when providing care? What education would you provide for the client and his family?

* REVIEW QUESTIONS

1. If an infection can be transmitted from one person to another, it is a
   1. Communicable disease
   2. Portal of entry to a host
   3. Portal of exit from a reservoir
   4. Susceptible host
2. The mode of transmission for hepatitis A is
   1. Direct and indirect contact
   2. Droplet transmission
   3. Airborne transmission
   4. Vectorborne transmission
3. The interval when a client manifests signs and symptoms specific to a type of infection is the
   1. Incubation period
   2. Convalescence stage
   3. Prodromal stage
   4. Illness stage
4. The most important and basic way to break the chain of infection is by
   1. Wearing gloves
   2. Practising hand hygiene
   3. Placing clients in isolation
   4. Providing private rooms for clients
5. The minimum handwashing time necessary to remove most transient microorganisms is
   1. 1.5 seconds
   2. 15 seconds
   3. 60 seconds
   4. 3 minutes
6. A client is on isolation precautions for pulmonary tuberculosis. You note that the client seems to be angry, but you know this is a normal response to isolation. Your best intervention is to
   1. Provide a dark, quiet room to calm the client
   2. Explain the isolation procedures and provide meaningful stimulation
   3. Reduce the level of precautions to keep the client from becoming angry
   4. Limit family and other caregiver visits to reduce the risk of spreading the infection
7. A gown should be worn when
   1. The client's hygiene is poor
   2. The client has AIDS or hepatitis
   3. You are assisting with medication administration
   4. Blood or body fluids may get on your clothing from a task you plans to perform
8. You have dressed a client's wound and now plan to administer a medication (which is currently in the room) to the client. It is important to
   1. Remove your gloves and perform hand hygiene before leaving the room
   2. Remove your gloves and perform hand hygiene before administering the medication
   3. Leave your gloves on to administer the medication
   4. Leave the medication on the bedside table to avoid having to remove your gloves before leaving the client's room
9. A patient on your unit developes diarrhea, which is confirmed to be caused by *C. difficile*. What type of isolation should this patient be placed on?
   1. Airborne isolation
   2. Contact precautions
   3. Standard precautions or routine practices
   4. Droplet precautions
10. When performing surgical hand hygiene, your hands must be kept
    1. Above your elbows
    2. Below your elbows
    3. At a 45-degree angle
    4. In a comfortable position

* RECOMMENDED WEB SITES

Community and Hospital Infection Control Association of Canada: http://www.chica.org/

Community and Hospital Infection Control Association of Canada (CHICA-Canada) is a national, multidisciplinary, voluntary association of infection-control professionals committed to improving infection prevention and control.

Public Health Agency of Canada: http://www.phac-aspc.gc.ca/index-eng.php

This federal government site provides links to documents related to infection-control practices, including the *Canada Communicable Disease Report*.

34

Medication Administration

Written by Jill E. Vihos, RN, BScN, MN, PhD(c)

Based on the original chapter by Sheryl Buckner, RN-BC, MS, CNE

objectives

Mastery of content in this chapter will enable you to:

- Define the key terms listed.
- Examine the nurse's role and responsibilities regarding medication administration.
- Describe the physiological mechanisms of medication action, including absorption, distribution, metabolism, and excretion of medications.
- Differentiate among different types of medication actions.
- Discuss developmental factors that influence pharmacokinetics.
- Discuss factors that influence medication actions.
- Discuss methods of educating a client about prescribed medications.
- Compare and contrast the roles of the prescriber, the pharmacist, and the nurse in medication administration.
- Implement nursing actions to prevent medication errors.
- Describe factors to consider when choosing routes of medication administration.
- Calculate a prescribed medication dose.
- Discuss factors to use when assessing a client's needs for and response to medication therapy.
- Explain the seven rights of medication administration.
- Prepare and administer subcutaneous, intramuscular, and intradermal injections; intravenous medications; hypodermoclysis infusions; oral and topical skin preparations; eye, ear, and nose drops; vaginal instillations; rectal suppositories; and inhalants.
- Describe the importance of safe medication techniques.
- Describe the importance of establishing and adhering to agency policies and procedures when administering medications.
- Identify and describe how principles of primary health care are applied to medication administration in nursing practice.

key terms

Absorption, p. 678
Adverse effects, p. 680
Anaphylactic reactions, p. 680
Biotransformation, p. 679
Buccal, p. 683
Concentration, p. 681
Controlled substances, p. 678
Culture of safety, p. 691
Detoxify, p. 679
Hypodermoclysis, p. 748
Idiosyncratic reaction, p. 680
Infusions, p. 681
Inhalation, p. 684
Injection, p. 679
Instillation, p. 684
Intra-articular, p. 683
Intracardiac, p. 683
Intradermal (ID), p. 683
Intramuscular (IM), p. 683
Intraocular, p. 684
Intravenous (IV), p. 683
Irrigations, p. 684
Medication allergy, p. 680
Medication error, p. 690
Medication interaction, p. 680
Medication reconciliation, p. 691
Metered-dose inhalers (MDIs), p. 716
Metric system, p. 684
Narcotics, p. 678
Ophthalmic, p. 708
Parenteral administration, p. 683
Peak concentration, p. 681
Pharmacokinetics, p. 678
Polypharmacy, p. 701
Prescription, p. 687
Serum half-life, p. 681
Side effects, p. 680
Solution, p. 684
Subcutaneous, p. 683
Sublingual, p. 683
Synergistic effect, p. 680
Therapeutic effect, p. 680
Toxic effects, p. 680
Transdermal disc, p. 684
Verbal order, p. 687
Z-track method, p. 738

media resources

Web Site

- Animations
- Audio Chapter Summaries
- Glossary
- Multiple-Choice Review Questions
- Student Performance Checklists
- Student Learning Activities
- Video Clips
- Weblinks

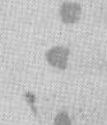
Companion CD

- Glossary
- Interactive Learning Activities
- Fluids and Electrolytes Tutorial
- Test-Taking Skills

Clients who have acute or chronic diseases or conditions use a variety of strategies to restore or maintain their health. A medication is a substance used in the prevention, diagnosis, relief, treatment, or cure of health alterations. Medications are the primary treatment that clients associate with restoration of health. No matter where clients receive their health care—in hospitals, at clinics, or at home—nurses play an essential role in preparing and administering medications, teaching clients about medications, and evaluating clients' responses to medications.

In the primary health care setting, clients often self-administer their medications. As a nurse, you are responsible for evaluating the effects of the medications on the client's health status, teaching clients about their medications and their side effects, ensuring client compliance with the medication regimen, and evaluating the client's technique for all routes of medication delivery. Additionally, you must assess the relationship between a client's medication regime and socioenvironmental influences, including accessibility to resources (e.g., financial and geographical). Consistent with principles of primary health care, nurses can implement interventions to address barriers to effective medication management.

In both acute and restorative health care settings, nurses spend a great deal of time administering medications to clients and ensuring that clients are adequately prepared to self-administer medications when they are discharged. If clients cannot administer their own medications when they are at home, family members or support persons can take responsibility for this task. As a nurse, you assess the effect of the medications in restoring or maintaining health and continue to educate the client, the client's family, and home care personnel about the medication's purpose, regimen, and side effects.

Scientific Knowledge Base

Medications are administered to clients to prevent, diagnose, or treat disease and health conditions. Because medication administration and evaluation are essential to nursing practice, you need to understand the actions and effects of the medications your clients take. To safely and accurately administer medications, you must have an understanding of pharmacology, pharmacokinetics (the study of how medications enter, affect, and exit the body), human growth and development, human anatomy, pathophysiology, psychology, nutrition, and mathematics. You need to apply your cumulative nursing knowledge when administering medications. The nursing process provides the framework for you to organize your thoughts and actions, and it is the foundation for medication administration.

Pharmacological Concepts

Drug Names. A medication may have as many as three different names. A medication's chemical name provides an exact description of the medication's composition and molecular structure. Chemical names are rarely used in clinical practice. For example, the chemical name N-acetyl-para-aminophenol is commonly known as Tylenol. The generic, or nonproprietary, name is given by the manufacturer that first develops the medication. Acetaminophen is the generic name for Tylenol. The generic name becomes the official name under which the medication is listed in official publications, such as the *Compendium of Pharmaceuticals and Specialties (CPS)*, the *Canadian Formulary (CF)*, or the *United States Pharmacopeia (USP)*. In addition to the drug name, all drug products approved for distribution in Canada have an eight-digit number, which is assigned by the Health Protection Branch of the federal government. This Drug Identification Number (DIN) is used by various groups and agencies to track drug information across Canada.

The trade name, brand name, or proprietary name is the name under which a manufacturer markets a medication. The trade name is followed by the symbol ™, which indicates that the manufacturer has trademarked the medication's name (e.g., Tempra™, Motrin™). Manufacturers choose trade names that are easy to pronounce, spell, and remember so that laypersons will remember the medication names. A medication may be produced by many different companies, and similarities in their trade names can be confusing. Because similarities in drug names are a common cause of medical errors, the Joint Commission (2007) in the United States publishes on its Web site a list of drugs whose names look like or sound like other drug names as well as recommendations for nurses, prescribers, other health care professionals, and health care organizations to prevent drug errors related to look-alike and sound-alike names of medications. Medications are available under a variety of different nomenclatures, or names, and you must be careful to obtain the exact name and spelling for the particular medications you administer.

Classification. Medication classification indicates the effect of the medication on a body system, the symptoms the medication relieves, or the medication's desired effect. For example, clients who have type 2 diabetes often take medications to control their blood glucose level. *Sulfonylureas* are one classification of medications often used by these clients. At least seven different medications are included in the sulfonylurea classification (McKenry et al., 2006). A prescriber chooses a particular medication on the basis of the client's characteristics; the medication's cost, efficacy, and dosing frequency; and the prescriber's experience with the medication. Some medications belong to more than one class. For example, aspirin is an analgesic, an antipyretic, and an anti-inflammatory medication.

Medication Forms. Medications are available in a variety of forms, or preparations (Figure 34–1). The form of the medication determines its route of administration. The composition of a medication is designed to enhance its absorption and metabolism. Many medications are made in several forms, such as tablets, capsules, elixirs, and suppositories. When administering a medication, you must be certain to use the proper form (Table 34–1).

Medication Legislation and Standards

Canadian Drug Legislation. Regulation of drug standards began in Canada in 1884, when the *Adulteration Act* set the conditions under

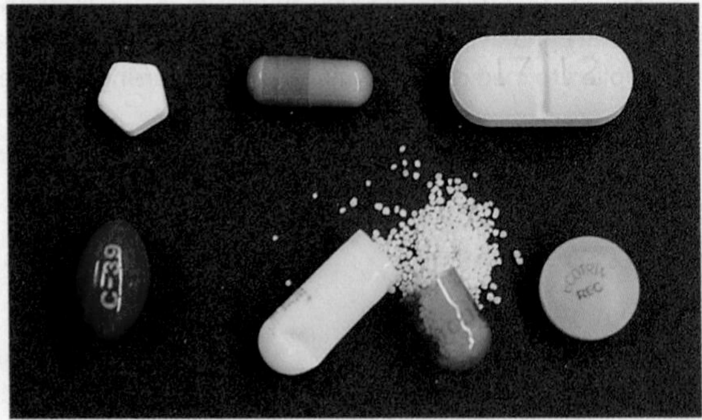

Figure 34-1 Forms of oral medications. Top row: Uniquely shaped tablet, capsule, scored tablet. Bottom row: Gelatin-coated liquid, extended-release capsule, enteric-coated tablet.

which a drug could be adulterated. The *Food and Drugs Act* of 1920 replaced this Act and, with amendments in 1950, gave the federal government control of the manufacture and sale of all drugs (except narcotics), all food, all cosmetics, and certain medical devices.

The federal government first attempted to control narcotic substances in 1908 through the *Opium Act*. Cocaine and morphine came under the jurisdiction of this Act in 1911. In 1961, the *Narcotic Control Act*, which controls the manufacture, distribution, and sale of narcotic drugs, was enacted. This Act was repealed in 1996 and replaced by the *Controlled Drugs and Substances Act*. The federal government has also passed legislation that regulates the manufacture and sale of herbs and other natural health products. This legislation addresses the content of these products as well as the products' packaging, labelling, distribution, and storage.

Drug Standards. Official publications, such as the *British Pharmacopoeia* (BP) and the *Canadian Formulary*, set standards for drug strength, quality, purity, packaging, safety, labelling, and dosage form. Physicians, nurses, and pharmacists depend on these standards to ensure that clients receive pure drugs in safe and effective dosages.

TABLE 34-1 Forms of Medication

Form	Description
Medication Forms Commonly Prepared for Administration by Oral Route	
Solid Forms	
Caplet	Shaped like a capsule and coated for ease of swallowing.
Capsule	Medication encased in a gelatin shell.
Tablet	Powdered medication compressed into a hard disc or cylinder; in addition to primary medication, contains binders (adhesives that allow the powder to stick together), disintegrators (to promote tablet dissolution), lubricants (for ease of manufacturing), and fillers (to make a convenient size for swallowing).
Enteric-coated tablet	Coated tablet that does not dissolve in stomach; coatings dissolve in intestine, where medication is absorbed.
Pill	Contains one or more medications; shaped into globules, ovoids, or oblongs; rarely used because most pills have been replaced by tablets.
Liquid Forms	
Elixir	Clear fluid containing medication and either water or alcohol, or both; often sweetened.
Extract	Syrup or dried form of pharmacologically active medication, usually made by evaporating the solution.
Aqueous solution	Medication dissolved in water.
Aqueous suspension	Finely divided drug particles dispersed in a liquid medium; when the suspension is left standing, particles settle to the bottom of the container.
Syrup	Medication dissolved in a concentrated sugar solution.
Tincture	Medicinal alcoholic extract from a plant or vegetable.
Other Oral Forms and Terms Associated With Oral Preparations	
Troche (lozenge)	Flat, round tablet that dissolves in the mouth to release medication; not intended for ingestion.
Aerosol	Aqueous medication sprayed and absorbed in the mouth and upper airway; not intended for ingestion.
Sustained release	Tablet or capsule that contains small particles of a medication coated with material that requires time to dissolve.
Medication Forms Commonly Prepared for Administration by Topical Route	
Ointment (salve or cream)	Semisolid, externally applied preparation, usually containing one or more medications.
Liniment	Preparation that usually contains medication and alcohol, oil, or soapy emollient; applied to the skin.
Lotion	Liquid suspension that usually protects, cools, or cleanses skin and can contain medication.
Paste	Thick ointment; absorbed through the skin more slowly than ointment; often used for skin protection.
Transdermal disc or patch	A disc or patch from which medication is absorbed through the skin slowly over a long period of time (e.g., 24 hours, 1 week).
Medication Forms Commonly Prepared for Administration by Parenteral Route	
Solution	Sterile preparation that contains water with one or more dissolved medicinal compounds.
Powder	Sterile particles of medication that are dissolved in a sterile liquid (e.g., water or normal saline) before administration.
Medication Forms Commonly Prepared for Instillation Into Body Cavities	
Solution	Medication dissolved in water or other liquid.
Intraocular disc	Small, flexible oval (similar to a contact lens) consisting of two soft, outer layers and a middle layer containing medication; slowly releases medication when moistened by ocular fluid.
Suppository	Solid medicine dosage mixed with gelatin and shaped into a pellet for insertion into a body cavity (rectum or vagina); melts at body temperature to release medication.

Accepted standards must be met in the following areas:

- *Purity:* Manufacturers must meet purity standards for the type and concentration of substances allowed in drug products.
- *Potency:* The concentration of the active drug in the preparation affects its strength, or potency.
- *Bioavailability:* The ability of a drug to be released from its dosage form and to be dissolved, absorbed, and transported by the body to the drug's site of action.
- *Efficacy:* Detailed laboratory studies help determine a drug's effectiveness.
- *Safety:* All drugs need to be continually evaluated to determine their side effects.

Control. Administration of the *Food and Drugs Act* and the *Controlled Drugs and Substances Act* is carried out by the Health Protection Branch (HPB) of the federal government. Before a new drug can be marketed in Canada, an application for approval must be made to the HPB. After intensive testing to ensure the drug's effectiveness and safety in humans, the HPB reviews the application. The HPB issues a Drug Identification Number and Notification of Compliance, which allow the drug to be sold in Canada. Stringent controls are applied to this new drug until sufficient information has been accumulated to ensure its safety and efficacy. Only then is the drug released for general use. Monitoring of the drug is ongoing to report adverse effects, safety concerns, or changes in the indications for a particular drug's use.

Provincial, Territorial, and Local Regulation of Medication. The provincial and territorial governments do not directly regulate the manufacture or sale of drugs. However, because the provincial and territorial governments have most of the legislative responsibility for health care, provincial and territorial legislation indirectly affects the use and sale of drugs within provincial and territorial boundaries. In addition, each province and territory has legislation regarding medical, dental, pharmacy, and nursing practice that dictates each health care professional's role in the ordering, dispensing, and administration of drugs. In particular, some provincial and territorial pharmacy legislation includes schedules that indicate the drugs that can be sold without prescription, behind the counter, and by prescription only. The National Association of Pharmacy Regulatory Authorities facilitates the activities of the regulatory authorities of all provinces and Yukon and promotes the harmonization of the practice of drug sales across the country.

Health care institutions establish policies that conform to federal and provincial regulations. The size of an institution, the types of services it provides, and the types of professional personnel it employs influence an institution's policies for drug control, distribution, and administration. Because an institution is primarily concerned with preventing health problems resulting from drug use, institutional policies are often more restrictive than government controls. For example, a common institutional policy is the automatic discontinuation of antibiotic therapy after a predetermined number of days. Although a prescriber may reorder an antibiotic, this policy helps to control unnecessarily prolonged drug therapy, which may lead to drug sensitivity or toxic reactions.

Medication Regulation and Nursing Practice. In Canada, you must be familiar with both the federal and provincial or territorial regulations affecting drug administration in your practice areas. If you move from one province or territory to another, you may discover significant differences in the laws governing drug administration. For example, laws vary concerning the prescription and administration of drugs. In the past, only physicians could prescribe medications. Today, most provinces have amended their nursing practice acts to include the prescription of medications by nurses in advanced practice. In most cases, this privilege is limited to nurse practitioners, clinical nurse specialists, and nurse midwives.

You are responsible for following legal provisions when administering **controlled substances** (drugs that affect the mind or behaviour), which can be dispensed only with a prescription. Violations of the *Narcotic Control Act* are punishable by fines, imprisonment, and loss of your nursing licence or your nursing registration. Hospitals and other health care institutions have policies for the proper storage and distribution of controlled substances, including **narcotics** (Box 34–1).

Pharmacokinetics as the Basis of Medication Actions

For medications to be therapeutic, they must be taken into a client's body, where they are absorbed and distributed to cells, tissues, or a specific organ, and they must alter physiological functions. **Pharmacokinetics** is the study of how medications enter the body, reach their site of action, metabolize, and exit the body. Use your knowledge of pharmacokinetics when timing medication administration, selecting the route of administration, considering the client's risk for alterations in medication action, and evaluating the client's response.

Absorption. **Absorption** refers to the passage of medication molecules into the blood from the medication's site of administration. Medication absorption is affected by the route of administration, the ability of the medication to dissolve, blood flow to the site of administration, the client's body surface area, and lipid solubility (maximum concentration of a chemical that will dissolve in fatty substances) of medication.

Route of Administration. Each route of medication administration has a different rate of absorption. When medications are applied to the skin, absorption is slow due to the physical makeup of the skin. Medications placed on the mucous membranes and respiratory airways are quickly absorbed because these tissues are highly vascular. Because orally administered medications must pass through the gastrointestinal (GI) tract to be absorbed, the overall rate of absorption

➤ BOX 34-1 Guidelines for Safe Narcotic Administration and Control

- Store all narcotics in a locked, secure cabinet or container. (Cabinets with computer-controlled locking devices are preferred.)
- Count narcotics frequently. Count and record inventories on a continuous basis, especially when narcotic drawers are opened and when nursing shifts change.
- Report discrepancies in narcotic counts immediately.
- Use a special inventory record each time a narcotic is dispensed. Records are often kept electronically and provide an accurate ongoing count of narcotics used, narcotics remaining, and information about narcotics that are wasted.
- After dispensing a narcotic, use the record to document the client's name, the date and time of medication administration, the name of the medication, the dose, and your signature.
- If you dispense only part of a premeasured dose of a controlled substance, a second nurse must witness disposal of the unused portion. If paper records are kept, both you and the nurse who witnesses the wastage are required to sign the form. Computerized systems record the nurses' names electronically. Do not place wasted portions in the sharps containers. Instead, flush wasted portions of tablets down a toilet and wash wasted liquids down a sink.

is usually slow. Intravenous (IV) **injection** produces the most rapid absorption because this route provides immediate access to systemic circulation.

Ability of the Medication to Dissolve. The ability of an oral medication to dissolve depends on its form or preparation. Solutions and suspensions in a liquid state are absorbed more readily than tablets or capsules. Acidic medications pass through the gastric mucosa rapidly. Medications that have a base pH are not absorbed before reaching the small intestine.

Blood Flow to the Site of Administration. When the site of administration contains a rich blood supply, the body absorbs medications more rapidly. As blood comes in contact with the site of administration, the medication is absorbed. Therefore, areas that have more blood supply will experience enhanced absorption, facilitating the passage of the medication into the bloodstream.

Body Surface Area. When a medication is in contact with a large surface area, the medication will be absorbed at a faster rate. This characteristic explains why most medications are absorbed in the small intestine, not in the stomach.

Lipid Solubility of a Medication. Because the cell membrane has a lipid layer, highly lipid-soluable medications easily cross the cell membrane and are absorbed quickly. The absorption of medication is also affected by the presence of food in the stomach. Some oral medications are absorbed more easily when administered between meals or on an empty stomach because food can change the structure of a medication and impair its absorption. When you administer medications, you should be aware of potential medication–medication interactions listed in the *CPS*, in drug manuals, and on drug packaging. If medications that interact are ordered at the same time, notify the prescriber immediately to revise medication administration times.

Safe medication administration requires knowledge of factors that may alter or impair the absorption of the prescribed medications. This information is based on an understanding of the medication's pharmacokinetics, the client's history, the physical examination of the client, and knowledge gained through daily interactions with clients. Use this knowledge to ensure that you administer all prescribed medications at the correct time. Consult and collaborate with the client's prescribers to ensure the client achieves the therapeutic effect of all medications. Before administering any medication, check pharmacology books or drug references, package inserts, or consult with pharmacists to identify medication–medication interactions or medication–nutrient interactions. Furthermore, because the safe delivery of many medications (e.g., blood pressure–lowering agents, blood glucose–lowering medications, and antiarrhythmics) are dependent on nursing assessments, ensure that physical assessment data are collected and interpreted before administering medications.

Distribution. After a medication is absorbed by the body, it is distributed to tissues and organs and to its specific site of action. The rate and extent of distribution depend on the physical and chemical properties of the medications and the physiology of the person taking the medication.

Circulation. After a medication enters the bloodstream, it is carried throughout the body's tissues and organs. The speed at which it reaches the site depends on the vascular content of the tissues and organs. Conditions that limit blood flow or blood perfusion inhibit the distribution of a medications. For example, clients who have experienced congestive heart failure have impaired circulation, which also impairs medication delivery to the intended site of action. Therefore, the efficacy of medications in congestive heart failure clients can be delayed or altered.

Membrane Permeability. For a medication to be distributed to an organ, it must pass through all the organ's tissues and biological membranes. Some membranes serve as barriers to the passage of medications. For example, the blood–brain barrier allows only fat-soluble medications to pass into the brain and cerebral spinal fluid. Therefore, central nervous system infections require treatment with antibiotics that selectively cross the blood–brain barrier. This change in the permeability of the blood–brain barrier can lead to confusion and other adverse effects in some older clients. The placental membrane also has a nonselective barrier to medications. Fat-soluble and non–fat-soluble agents can cross the placenta and result in fetal deformities, respiratory depression, and, when combined with narcotic use, withdrawal symptoms.

Protein Binding. Most medications bind to proteins to some extent. The degree to which medications bind to serum proteins, such as albumin, affects the medication's distribution. Medications bound to albumin cannot exert pharmacological activity. The unbound, or free, medication is the active form of the medication. Older adults have a decrease in albumin in their bloodstream, which is probably the result of a change in their liver function. The same is true for clients who have liver disease or malnutrition, who, along with older adults, have the potential for more medication being unbound, and thus may be at risk for an increase in medication activity or toxicity, or both.

Metabolism. After a medication reaches its site of action, it metabolizes into a less active or inactive form that is more easily excreted. **Biotransformation** occurs when enzymes **detoxify**, degrade (break down), and remove the biologically active chemicals. Most biotransformation occurs within the liver, although the lungs, kidneys, blood, and intestines also metabolize medications. The liver is especially important because its specialized structure oxidizes and transforms many toxic substances. The liver degrades many harmful chemicals before they are distributed to the tissues. If a decrease in liver function occurs, a medication is usually eliminated more slowly and results in an accumulation of the medication. If the organs that metabolize medications are altered, clients are at risk for medication toxicity. For example, a small sedative dose of a barbiturate may cause a client with liver disease to lapse into a hepatic coma.

Excretion. After medications are metabolized, they exit the body through the kidneys, liver, bowel, lungs, or exocrine glands. The chemical makeup of a medication determines the organ of excretion. Gaseous and volatile compounds, such as nitrous oxide and alcohol, exit through the lungs. Deep breathing and coughing (see Chapter 39) help the postoperative client to eliminate anaesthetic gases more rapidly. The exocrine glands excrete lipid-soluble medications. When medications exit through the sweat glands, the skin often becomes irritated. You can assist the client in good hygiene practices (see Chapter 38) to promote cleanliness and skin integrity. If a medication is excreted through the mammary glands, a nursing infant is at risk of ingesting the chemicals. You will need to check on the safety of any medication used by breastfeeding women.

The GI tract is another route for medication excretion. Many medications enter the hepatic circulation where they are broken down by the liver and excreted into the bile. After chemicals enter the intestines through the biliary tract, they may be reabsorbed by the intestines. Factors that increase peristalsis (e.g., laxatives and enemas) accelerate medication excretion through the feces, whereas factors that slow peristalsis (e.g., inactivity and improper diet) may prolong a medication's effects.

The kidneys are the main organs for medication excretion. Some medications escape extensive metabolism and exit unchanged in the urine. Other medications must undergo biotransformation in the liver before being excreted by the kidneys. If renal function declines, a client is at risk for medication toxicity. If the kidneys cannot adequately excrete a medication, the dose may need to be reduced. Maintenance of an adequate fluid intake (50 mL/kg/day) promotes proper elimination of medications for the average adult.

Types of Medication Action

Medications vary considerably in the way they act and in their types of action. Factors other than characteristics of the medication also influence medication actions. A client does not always respond in the same way to each successive dose of a medication. Sometimes, the same medication causes very different responses in different clients. Therefore, you need to understand all the effects that medications can have on clients.

Therapeutic Effects. The **therapeutic effect** is the expected or predictable physiological response that a medication causes. Each medication has a desired therapeutic effect, which is the reason it is prescribed. For example, nitroglycerine reduces the body's cardiac workload and increases myocardial oxygen supply. A single medication may have more than one therapeutic effect. For example, aspirin reduces platelet aggregation (clumping) and is an analgesic, an antipyretic, and an anti-inflammatory drug. Knowing the desired therapeutic effect for each medication allows you to provide client education to accurately evaluate the medication's desired effect.

Side Effects. **Side effects** are the unintended, secondary effects that a medication predictably will cause. Side effects may be harmless or injurious. If the side effects are serious enough to negate a medication's intended beneficial effects, the prescriber may decide to discontinue the medication. Clients often stop taking medications because of side effects.

Adverse Effects. **Adverse effects** are severe, negative responses to medication. For example, a client may become comatose after injesting a drug. When adverse responses to medications occur, the prescriber immediately discontinues the medication. Some adverse effects are unexpected effects that were not discovered during drug testing. When this situation occurs, health care professionals should report the adverse effect to the Health Protection Branch of the federal government (http://www.hc-sc.gc.ca/english/protection/drugs.html). This reporting system is voluntary.

Toxic Effects. **Toxic effects** develop after prolonged intake of a medication or after a medication accumulates in the blood because of impaired metabolism or impaired excretion. Excess amounts of a medication within the body may have lethal effects, depending on the medication's action. For example, toxic levels of morphine, which is an opioid, may cause severe respiratory depression and death. Antidotes are available to treat specific types of medication toxicity. For example, Narcan is used to reverse the effects of opioid toxicity.

Idiosyncratic Reactions. Medications sometimes cause unpredictable effects, such as an **idiosyncratic reaction**, which occurs when a client overreacts or underreacts to a medication or has a reaction different from the normal reaction. For example, a child receiving an antihistamine (Benadryl) may become extremely agitated or excited instead of becoming drowsy. It is not always possible to predict whether a client might have an idiosyncratic response to a medication.

Allergic Reactions. Allergic reactions are unpredictable responses to a medication. Some clients become immunologically sensitized to the initial dose of a medication. After repeated administration of the medication, the client develops an allergic response to the medication, its chemical preservatives, or a metabolite. The medication or chemical acts as an antigen, triggering the release of the body's antibodies. A client's **medication allergy** symptoms may vary, depending on the individual and the medication (Table 34–2). Among the different classes of medications, antibiotics cause a high incidence of allergic reactions.

Anaphylactic reactions are severe reactions that are life-threatening and are characterized by sudden constriction of bronchial muscles, edema of the pharynx and larynx, severe wheezing, shortness of breath, and circulatory collapse. Immediate use of antihistamines, epinephrine, or bronchodilators is required to treat anaphylactic reactions. Emergency resuscitation measures are sometimes required. A client with a known history of an allergy to a medication needs to avoid exposure to that medication and must wear a bracelet or medal engraved with emergency medical information, including medication allergies (e.g., a MedicAlert bracelet Figure 34–2). These bracelets and medals alert health care workers to the client's medical information, including allergies, if the client is unable to communicate this information when receiving medical care. Additionally, some clients with allergies leading to anaphylactic reactions carry their own epinephrine pens.

Medication Interactions

When one medication modifies the action of another medication, a **medication interaction** occurs. Medication interactions are common in clients who take several medications. Some medications increase or diminish the action of other medications or may alter the way another medication is absorbed, metabolized, or eliminated from the body. When two medications have a **synergistic effect**, the combined effect of the two medications is greater than the effect of the medications when given separately. For example, alcohol acts as a depressant on the central nervous system and has a synergistic effect on antihistamines, antidepressants, barbiturates, and narcotic analgesics.

Sometimes a medication interaction is desired. Prescribers combine medications to create an interaction that will have a beneficial effect on the client's condition. For example, a client with high blood pressure may be prescribed several medications, such as diuretics and vasodilators, which act together to control blood pressure when one medication alone is not effective.

Medication Dose Responses

After administration, a medication undergoes absorption, distribution, metabolism, and excretion. Except when administered intravenously, medications take time to enter the bloodstream. The quantity and distribution of a medication in different body compartments change constantly. When a medication is prescribed, the goal

➤TABLE 34-2 Mild Allergic Reactions

Symptom	Description
Urticaria	Raised, irregularly shaped skin eruptions with varying sizes and shapes; eruptions have reddened margins and pale centre.
Rash	Small, raised vesicles that are usually reddened; often distributed over entire body.
Pruritus	Itching of skin; accompanies most rashes.
Rhinitis	Inflammation of mucous membranes lining nose; causes swelling and clear, watery discharge.

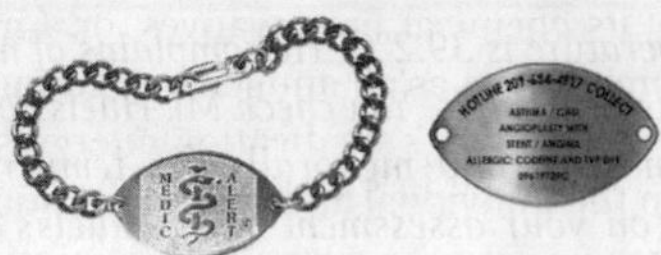

Figure 34-2 A MedicAlert bracelet is engraved with a person's emergency medical information, including drug allergies.

is to achieve a constant blood level of the medication within a safe therapeutic range. Repeated doses are required to achieve a constant therapeutic **concentration** of a medication because a portion of a drug is always being excreted. The highest serum concentration (**peak concentration**) of a medication usually occurs just before the body absorbs the last of the medication (McKenry et al., 2006). After peaking, the serum medication concentration falls progressively. After intravenous (IV) **infusions**, the peak concentration occurs quickly, but the serum level also begins to fall immediately (Figure 34–3). The point at which the lowest amount of drug is detected in the serum is called the trough concentration. Some medications doses (e.g., vancomycin) are based on peak and trough serum levels. The trough level is generally drawn 30 minutes before the drug is administered, and the peak level is drawn whenever the drug is expected to reach its peak concentration. The time a drug takes to reach its peak concentration varies depending on the medication's pharmacokinetics.

All medications have a **serum half-life**, which is the time it takes for the excretion processes to lower the serum medication concentration by half. To maintain a therapeutic plateau, the client needs to receive regular fixed doses. For example, current evidence indicates that pain medications are most effective when they are given "around the clock" to maintain an almost constant level of pain medication rather than being given when the client intermittently complains of pain. After an initial medication dose, the client receives each successive dose when the previous dose reaches its half-life.

Together with the client, you need to follow regular dosage schedules and adhere to prescribed doses and dosage intervals (Table 34–3). Some agencies set schedules for medication administration. However, nurses are able to alter this schedule on the basis of knowledge about a medication. For example, at some agencies, medications prescribed to be taken once a day are given at 9:00 A.M. However, if a medication works best when given before bedtime, administer the medication before the client goes to sleep.

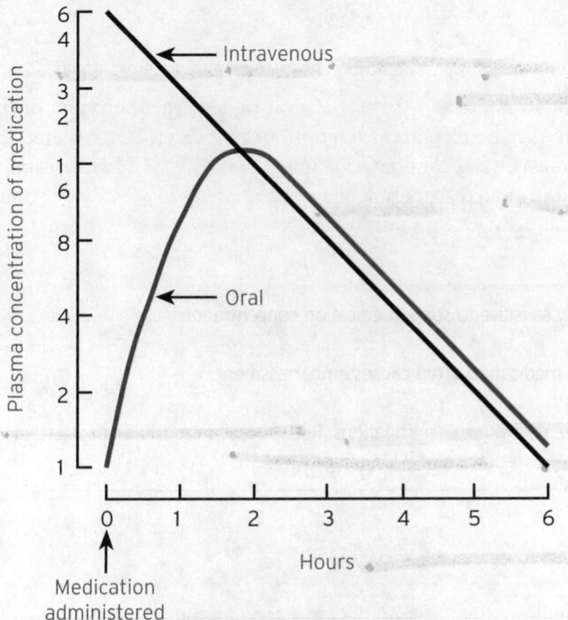

Figure 34-3 Curve showing therapeutic blood levels of medication. **Source:** From Clark, J. F., Queener, S. F., & Karb, V. B. (1998). *Pharmacological basis of nursing practice* (6th ed.). St. Louis, MO: Mosby.

When teaching clients about dosage schedules, use language that is familiar to the client. For example, when teaching a client about medication dosing twice a day, instruct the client to take a medication in the morning and again in the evening. Use knowledge about the time intervals of medications to anticipate a medication's effect and to educate the client about when to expect a response. Table 34–4 lists common terms associated with medication actions.

TABLE 34-3 Common Dosage Administration Schedules

Dosage Schedule	Abbreviation or Notation*
Before meals	AC, ac
As desired	ad lib
Twice a day	[Do not abbreviate]
Hour	h, hr
At bedtime	[Do not abbreviate; write out "nightly or at bedtime"]
After meals	PC, pc
Whenever there is a need	prn
Every morning, every *A.M.*	qam
Every day, daily	[Do not abbreviate]
Every hour	qh
Every 2 hours	q2h
Every 4 hours	q4h
Every 6 hours	q6h
Every 8 hours	q8h
Four times a day	[Do not abbreviate]
Every other day	[Do not abbreviate]
Give immediately	STAT
Three times a day	[Do not abbreviate]

*For some terms, it is safer to write out the term than to abbreviate it (see Table 34–7). Follow your agency's policy regarding the use of abbreviations.

TABLE 34-4 Terms Associated With Medication Actions

Term	Meaning
Onset	The time it takes for a medication to produce a response after it has been administered.
Peak	The time it takes for a medication to reach its highest effective concentration.
Trough	Minimum blood serum concentration of medication, typically reached just before the next scheduled dose.
Duration	The time during which a medication is present in sufficient concentration to produce a response.
Plateau	Blood serum concentration of a medication has been reached and is maintained after repeated fixed doses.

Routes of Administration

The route prescribed for administering a medication depends on the medication's properties, the medication's desired effect, and the client's physical and mental condition (Table 34–5). Collaborate with the prescriber to determine the best route for a client's medication, as in the following hypothetical situation:

Mr. Huels's temperature is 39.2°C. He complains of nausea and is unable to tolerate oral fluids. You check Mr. Huels's orders, which read, "Acetaminophen 650 mg orally for temperature above 38.5°C." Based on your assessment of Mr Huels's nausea, you determine that he will not be able to tolerate acetaminophen orally. You consult the prescriber and receive an order for acetaminophen

TABLE 34-5 Factors Indicating Choice of Administration Routes

Advantages	Disadvantages or Contraindications
Oral, Buccal, Sublingual Routes	
Convenient and comfortable for client	Avoid when client has alterations in gastrointestinal function (e.g., nausea, vomiting), reduced motility (after general anaesthesia or bowel inflammation), or surgical resection of a portion of the gastrointestinal tract.
Economical	Gastric secretions destroy some medications. Oral administration is contraindicated in clients who are unable to swallow (e.g., clients with neuromuscular disorders, esophageal strictures, mouth lesions).
Easy to administer	Oral medications may irritate the lining of the gastrointestinal tract, discolour teeth, or leave an unpleasant taste.
Medications may produce local or systemic effects.	An unconscious or confused client may be unable or unwilling to swallow or hold medication under the tongue.
Rarely cause anxiety for client	Oral medications cannot be given when the client has gastric suction. Oral medications are contraindicated in clients before some medical tests and surgeries.
Subcutaneous, Intramuscular (IM), Intravenous (IV), Intradermal (ID) Routes	
An alternative means of administration when oral medications are contraindicated	Risk of introducing infection. Some medications are expensive. Some clients experience pain from repeated needle sticks. Subcutaneous, IM, and ID routes are avoided in clients who have bleeding tendencies.
More rapid absorption than with topical or oral routes	Risk of tissue damage with subcutaneous injections
IV infusion provides medication delivery when client is critically ill or when long-term therapy is required. If peripheral perfusion is poor, IV route is preferred over injections.	IM and IV routes have higher absorption rates, which places the client at higher risk for reactions. Anxiety is caused in many clients, especially children.
Dermal Route	
Topical Medications	
Primarily provide local effects	Clients with skin abrasions are at risk for rapid medication absorption and systemic effects.
Painless	Medications slowly absorb through the skin.
Limited side effects	
Transdermal Medications	
Prolonged systemic effects with limited side effects	Leaves oily or pasty substance on skin and may soil clothing
Mucous Membranes*	
Therapeutic effects are provided by local application to the affected sites.	Mucous membranes are highly sensitive to some medication concentrations.
Aqueous solutions are readily absorbed and capable of causing systemic effects.	Insertion of rectal and vaginal medication often causes embarrassment.
An alternative means of administration when oral medications are contraindicated	Clients with ruptured eardrums cannot receive irrigations. Rectal suppositories are contraindicated if client has had rectal surgery or if active rectal bleeding is present.
Inhalation Routes	
Provides rapid relief for local respiratory problems	Some local inhalants can cause serious health effects.
Used for introduction of general anaesthetic gases	

*Includes eyes, ears, nose, vagina, rectum, and ostomy.

per rectum. By using a rectal suppository, you are able to administer the acetaminophen without increasing the client's symptoms of nausea.

Oral Routes. The oral route is the easiest and the most commonly used route of administering medication. Medications are given by mouth and swallowed with fluid. Oral medications have a slower onset of action and a more prolonged effect than parenteral medications. In general, clients prefer taking medication orally.

Sublingual Administration. Some medications are designed to be readily absorbed after being placed under the tongue to dissolve (Figure 34–4). A medication given by the **sublingual** route should not be swallowed because the medication will not have the desired effect. Nitroglycerine is commonly given sublingually. After giving a sublingual medication, avoid giving liquids; instruct the client not to drink anything until the medication is completely dissolved.

Buccal Administration. Administration of a medication by the **buccal** route involves placing solid medication in the mouth and against the mucous membranes of the cheek until the medication dissolves (Figure 34–5). To avoid mucosal irritation, teach clients to alternate cheeks with each subsequent dose. Advise clients not to chew or swallow the medication or to take any liquids with it. A buccal medication acts locally on the mucosa or systemically when it is dissolved in a person's saliva.

Parenteral Routes. Parenteral administration involves injecting a medication into body tissues. The following are the four major sites of injection:

Intradermal (ID): Injection into the dermis just under the epidermis
Subcutaneous: Injection into tissues just below the dermis
Intramuscular (IM): Injection into a muscle
Intravenous (IV): Injection into a vein

Some medications are administered into body cavities other than the four sites listed above. These routes of medication administration include epidural, intrathecal, intraosseous, intraperitoneal, intrapleural, and intra-arterial routes. Depending on agency policy, additional education or certification may be required for you to administer medications through some routes. Whether you actually administer the medication by these routes, you remain responsible for monitoring the integrity of medication delivery systems, understanding the therapeutic value of the medication, and evaluating the client's response to the therapy.

Epidural Route. Epidural medications are administered in the epidural space via a catheter, which is put in place by an anaesthesiologist.

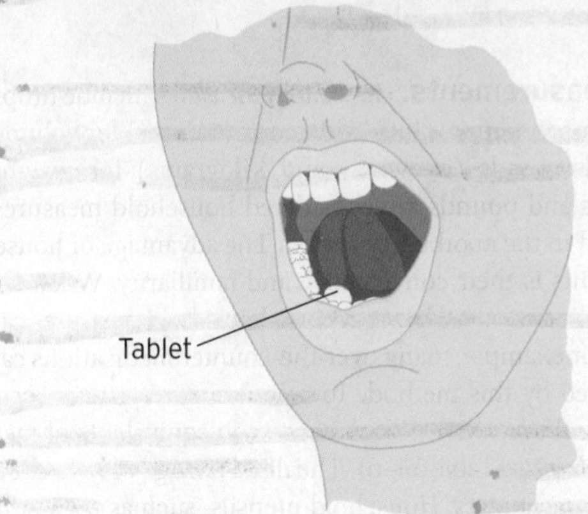

Figure 34-4 Sublingual administration of a tablet.

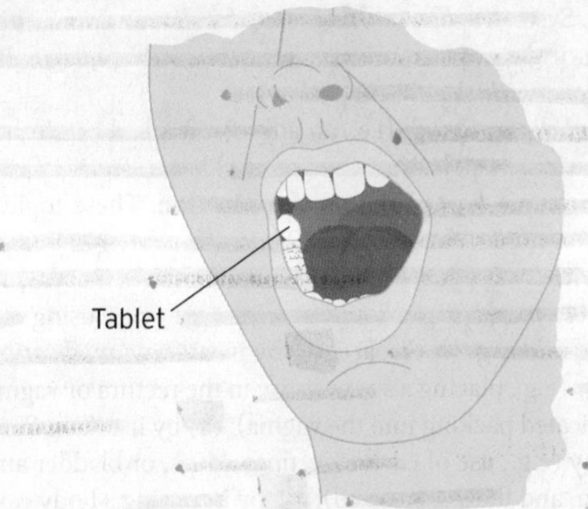

Figure 34-5 Buccal administration of a tablet.

This route is often used for the administration of analgesia both intraoperatively and postoperatively (see Chapter 42). If you have received extra education in the epidural route, you will be able to administer medications in bolus form or by continuous infusion. Be aware of agency policies regarding a client's physical assessment following epidural medication administration.

Intrathecal Route. Intrathecal medications are administered through a catheter that has been placed into the subarachnoid space or into one of the ventricles of the brain. Intrathecal administration is often associated with long-term medication administration through surgically implanted catheters.

Intraosseous Route. This method of medication administration involves the infusion of medication directly into the bone marrow. Intraosseous routes are most commonly used in infants and toddlers because their intravascular space is difficult to access. This method is most often used when an emergency arises and IV access is impossible. The physician inserts an intraosseous infusion needle into the bone, usually the tibia, for the administration of medication by the nurse.

Intraperitoneal Route. Medications are administered into the peritoneal cavity, where they are absorbed into the circulation system. Intraperitoneal routes are used to administer chemotherapeutic agents, insulin, and antibiotics.

Intrapleural Route. An injection or a chest tube is used to administer intrapleural medications directly into the pleural space. Chemotherapeutic agents are the most common medications administered by this method.

Intra-arterial Route. Intra-arterial medications are administered directly into the arteries and are commonly used to deliver tissue plasminogen activators in clients who have arterial clots. Often, intra-arterial medications are delivered through in-dwelling catheters. You are responsible for monitoring the integrity of infusions systems and evaluating clients for adverse responses to these medications, including systemic and gastrointestinal bleeding. Ensure that you are familiar with agency protocols, policies, and procedures for client assessment.

Other methods of medication administration that are usually limited to administration by a physician are **intracardiac** routes, in which medication is injected directly into cardiac tissue, and **intra-articular** routes, in which medication is injected into a joint.

Topical Administration. Medications applied to the skin and to mucous membranes usually result in local effects. Administer topical medications by painting or spreading the medication over the skin, applying moist dressings, soaking body parts in a solution, or giving medicated baths. Systemic effects often occur if a client's skin is thin or broken down, if the medication concentration is high, or if the medication's contact with the skin is prolonged.

A **transdermal disc** or patch (i.e., an adhesive-backed patch that releases nitroglycerine, scopolamine, or estrogens) has systemic effects. The disc secures the medicated ointment to the skin. These topical applications may be applied for as few as 12 hours or as long as 7 days.

Medications can be applied to mucous membranes in a variety of ways: (1) by directly applying a liquid or ointment (e.g., using eye drops, gargling, swabbing the throat); (2) by inserting a medication into a body cavity (e.g., placing a suppository in the rectum or vagina or inserting medicated packing into the vagina); (3) by instilling fluid into a body cavity (e.g., use of ear drops, nose drops, or bladder and rectal **instillation**, and fluid is retained); (4) by irrigating a body cavity (e.g., flushing with medicated fluid the eye, ear, vagina, bladder, or rectum, and fluid is not retained); and (5) by spraying (e.g., instillation into the nose or throat).

Inhalation Route. The deeper passages of the respiratory tract provide a large surface area for medication absorption. Medications can be administered through the nasal passages, the oral passage, or endotracheal or tracheostomy tubes. Endotracheal tubes are inserted into the client's mouth and extend to the trachea (Figure 34–6), whereas tracheostomy tubes directly enter the trachea through an incision in the client's neck. Medications that are administered by the **inhalation** route are readily absorbed and work rapidly because of the rich vascular alveolar–capillary network present in the pulmonary tissue. Inhaled medications may have either local or systemic effects.

Intraocular Route. In **intraocular** medication delivery, a medication in a form similar to a contact lens is inserted directly into the client's eye. The eye medication disc has two soft outer layers that enclose the medication. The disc can remain in the client's eye for up to 1 week. Pilocarpine, a medication used to treat glaucoma, is the most common medication delivered through the intraocular route.

Systems of Medication Measurement

The proper administration of a medication depends on your ability to compute medication doses accurately and to measure medications correctly. Mistakes can lead to a fatal errors. You are responsible for checking the accuracy of the dose before you give a medication.

The metric, apothecary, and household systems of measurement are used in medication therapy. Most nations, including Canada, use the metric system as their standard of measurement. Household measurements are used by health care professionals when they write prescriptions to be self-administered by clients.

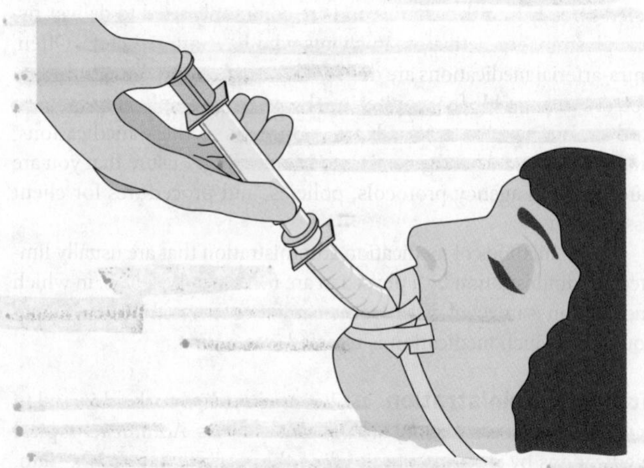

Figure 34-6 Medication being instilled through an endotracheal tube.

Metric System. Because it is a decimal system, the **metric system** (Système Internationale d'Unités [SI]) is the most logically organized system of measurement. Metric units can easily be converted and computed through simple arithmetic, such as multiplication and division. Each basic unit of measurement is organized into units of 10. Secondary units are formed by multiplying or dividing by 10. In multiplication, the decimal point moves to the right; in division, the decimal moves to the left. For example:

10 mg × 10 = 100 mg
10 mg/10 = 1 mg

When designating a metric dosage, *do not write a zero* alone after a decimal point (e.g., write 5 mg; not 5.0 mg) and always include a zero before the decimal point (e.g., 0.1 mg) to comply with current guidelines (Institute for Safe Medication Practices, 2006a; The Joint Commission, 2007).

The basic units of measurement in the metric system are the metre (length), the litre (volume), and the gram (weight). For medication calculations, use only the measurements for volume and weight. In the metric system, the basic units are designated by the use of lowercase or uppercase letters:

Gram = g or Gm
Litre = L or l

Lower-case letters are used for abbreviations for other units:

Milligram = mg
Millilitre = mL

A system of Latin prefixes designates a subdivision of the basic units: *deci-* (1/10 or 0.1), *centi-* (1/100 or 0.01), and *milli-* (1/1000 or 0.001). Greek prefixes designate multiples of the basic units: *deka-* (10), *hecto-* (100), and *kilo-* (1000). When medication doses are written in metric units, prescribers and nurses use either divisions or multiples of a unit. Convert any fractions to the decimal form.

500 mg or 0.5 g, *not* 1/2 g
10 mL or 0.01 L, *not* 1/100 L

Solutions. Solutions of various concentrations are used for injections, **irrigations**, and infusions. A **solution** is a given mass of solid substance dissolved in a known volume of fluid or a given volume of liquid dissolved in a known volume of another fluid. When a solid is dissolved in a fluid, the concentration is expressed in units of mass per units of volume (e.g., g/mL, g/L, mg/mL). A concentration of a solution may also be expressed as a percentage. A 10% solution, for example, is 10 g of solid dissolved in 100 mL of solution. A proportion also expresses concentrations. A 1/1000 solution represents a solution containing 1 g of solid in 1000 mL of liquid or 1 mL of liquid mixed with 1000 mL of another liquid.

Household Measurements. Household measures include drops, teaspoons, tablespoons, cups, pints, and quarts (or litres) for volume, and ounces and pounds (or grams and kilograms) for weight. Although ounces and pounds are considered household measures, they are also used in the apothecary system. The advantage of household measurements is their convenience and familiarity. When the accuracy of a medication dose is not critical, household measures can be safely used. For example, many over-the-counter medications can safely be measured by this method. To calculate medications accurately, you need to be familiar with the common equivalents of metric and household units (Table 34–6). The disadvantage of household measures is their inaccuracy. Household utensils, such as teaspoons and cups, often vary in size. The scales used to measure pints or quarts are often not well calibrated.

➤ TABLE 34-6 Equivalents of Measurement

Metric Measurement	Household Measurement
1 mL	15 drops (gtt)
4–5 mL	1 teaspoon (tsp)
15 mL	1 tablespoon (tbsp)
30 mL	2 tablespoons (tbsp)
250 mL	1 cup (c)
480 mL (approximately 500 mL)	1 pint (pt)
960 mL (approximately 1 L)	1 quart (qt)
3840 mL (approximately 5 L)	1 gallon (gal)

Nursing Knowledge Base

The Institute of Medicine (IOM) (2003) published the book *To Err Is Human: Building a Safer Health System.* According to this book, in any given year, an estimated 98,000 people die from medical errors that occur in hospitals; more people die from medical errors than from motor vehicle accidents, breast cancer, and workplace injuries; and medication-related errors for hospitalized clients cost approximately $2 billion annually.

Nurses play an important role in client safety, especially in the area of medication administration. To safely administer medications, ensure that you know how to calculate medication doses accurately, strictly adhere to agency policy and procedure, and report any medication errors that occur. Be aware of the different roles that members of the health care team play in prescribing and administering medications. Remember to apply your previous learning to medication administration. The nursing process provides the framework for organizing your thoughts and actions, and it is the foundation for medication administration (Box 34–2).

✱ BOX 34-2 EVIDENCE-INFORMED PRACTICE GUIDELINE

Reducing Distractions During Medication Administration

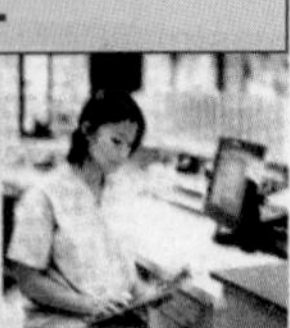

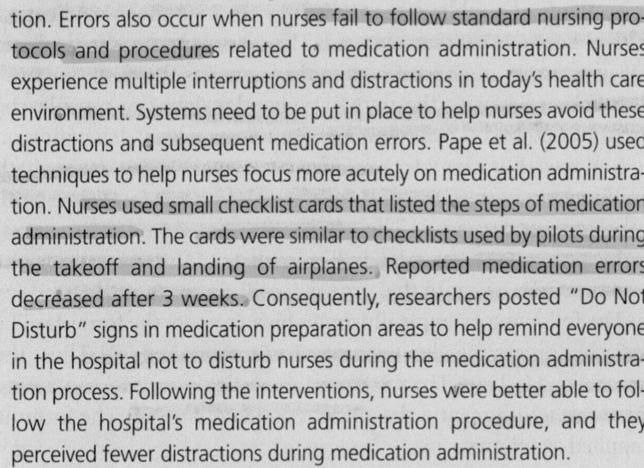

Evidence Summary

Many medication errors occur when nurses become distracted or lose focus during medication administration. Errors also occur when nurses fail to follow standard nursing protocols and procedures related to medication administration. Nurses experience multiple interruptions and distractions in today's health care environment. Systems need to be put in place to help nurses avoid these distractions and subsequent medication errors. Pape et al. (2005) used techniques to help nurses focus more acutely on medication administration. Nurses used small checklist cards that listed the steps of medication administration. The cards were similar to checklists used by pilots during the takeoff and landing of airplanes. Reported medication errors decreased after 3 weeks. Consequently, researchers posted "Do Not Disturb" signs in medication preparation areas to help remind everyone in the hospital not to disturb nurses during the medication administration process. Following the interventions, nurses were better able to follow the hospital's medication administration procedure, and they perceived fewer distractions during medication administration.

Application to Nursing Practice

- Consistently following nursing protocols for medication administration decreases medication errors.
- Nurses who experience fewer distractions during medication administration experience fewer medication errors.
- Placing "Do Not Disturb" signs in medication preparation areas helps reduce distractions and errors.
- Nurses need to investigate strategies that will decrease distractions, enhance their ability to follow nursing protocols, and improve their focus during medication administration.

From Pape, T. M, Guerra, D. M., Muzquiz, M., Bryant, J. B., Ingram, M., Schranner, B., et al. (2005). Innovative approaches to reducing nurses' distractions during medication administration. *Journal of Continuing Nursing Education, 36,* 108–116.

Clinical Calculations

To administer medications safely, you need an understanding of basic arithmetic to calculate medication doses, mix solutions, and perform a variety of other activities. This skill is important because medications are not always dispensed in the unit of measure in which they are ordered (Box 34–3). This discrepancy occurs because medication companies package and bottle certain standard dosages. For example, the prescriber may order 20 mg of a medication that is available only in 40-mg vials. You frequently need to convert available units of volume and weight to the prescribed doses. Therefore, be aware of approximate equivalents in all major measurement systems.

Conversions Within One System. To convert units of measurement in the metric system, divide or multiply. To change milligrams to grams, divide by 1000, moving the decimal three places to the left.

$$1000 \text{ mg} = 1 \text{ g}$$
$$350 \text{ mg} = 0.35 \text{ g}$$

To convert litres to millilitres, multiply by 1000 or move the decimal three places to the right.

$$1 \text{ L} = 1000 \text{ mL}$$
$$0.25 \text{ L} = 250 \text{ mL}$$

To convert units of measurement within the apothecary system or the household system, consult an equivalence table. For example, when converting fluid ounces to quarts, recall that 32 ounces is the equivalent of 1 quart. To convert 8 ounces to a quart measurement, divide 8 by 32 to get the equivalent, which is 0.25 quart.

Conversion Between Systems. Determine the proper dose of a medication by converting weights or volumes from one system of measurement to another. Before making a conversion, compare the measurement system available with the measurement system ordered. For example, the prescriber orders Robitussin 30 mL, but the client only has tablespoons at home. To provide proper instruction to the client, convert 30 millilitres to tablespoons, which requires knowing the equivalent; alternatively, you can refer to a table such as Table 34–6. Tables of equivalent measurements are available in all health care institutions.

➤ BOX 34-3 Common Reasons for Measurement Conversions

- Needing to convert fluid ounces to millilitres for measurement of intake and output
- Needing to convert body weight from pounds to kilograms and vice versa
- Needing to convert volume equivalents to calculate intravenous flow rates and to prepare wound irrigation solutions, enemas, or bladder irrigations

Dose Calculations. Many formulas can be used to calculate medication doses. Apply the following basic formula when preparing solid or liquid doses of a medication:

Dose ordered/Dose on hand × Amount on hand =
Amount to administer

The dose ordered is the amount of medication prescribed. The dose on hand is the dose of medication supplied by the pharmacy (e.g., milligrams, units) and is expressed on the medication label as the contents of a tablet or capsule or as the amount of medication dissolved per unit volume of liquid. The amount on hand is the basic unit or quantity of the medication that contains the dose on hand. For solid medications, the amount on hand may be one capsule; the amount of liquid on hand may be a millilitre or litre, depending on the container. For example, a liquid medication comes in the strength of 125 mg per 5 mL. Thus, 125 mg is the dose on hand, whereas 5 mL is the amount on hand. The amount to administer is the actual amount of medication you will administer. Always express the amount to administer in the same unit as the amount on hand.

The following example illustrates how to apply the formula. The prescriber orders the client to receive morphine 2 mg IV. Thus, the dose ordered is 2 mg. The medication is available in a vial containing 10 mg per millilitre, and the amount on hand is 1 mL. The formula is applied as follows:

2 mg/10 mg × 1 mL = Amount in millilitres to administer

To simplify the 2/10 fraction to decimal form, divide numerator and denominator by 2:

1/5 × 1 mL = 1/5 mL or 0.2 mL to administer

Syringes are calibrated only in decimals. After converting the fraction 1/5 to 0.2 mL, prepare the correct dose.

The following is an example of how the formula applies when calculating solid dose forms. The prescriber orders 0.125 mg orally (PO) of digoxin. The medication is available in tablets containing 0.25 mg of digoxin.

0.125 mg/0.250 mg × 1 tablet = Number of tablets to administer

The fraction 0.125/0.250 equals 1/2 or 0.5. Therefore,

0.5 × 1 tablet = 0.5 or 1/2 tablet to be administered

Many tablets are manufactured with scores, or indentations, across the centre of the tablet (Figure 34–7). A scored tablet is easy to break in half for divided doses. Do not cut unscored tablets because the potential for an incorrect dose is high.

Often, liquid medications are manufactured in volumes greater than 1 mL. In applying the formula, be careful to use the correct concentration to avoid a medication error. For example, a medication order is for "erythromycin suspension 250 mg PO." The pharmacy delivers 100-mL bottles with the label stating, "5 mL contains 125 mg of erythromycin." Thus, to obtain the correct dose of medication, the appropriate concentration is 125 mg in 5 mL.

250 mg/125 mg × 5 mL = Volume to administer

The fraction 250/125 equals 2. Therefore,

2 × 5 mL = 10 mL to administer

Some agencies require a nurse to double-check calculations with another nurse before administering the medication, especially when the risk of administering the wrong medication dose is high (e.g., heparin or insulin). Always double-check your calculations or confer with another nurse or health care professional if an answer to your calculation seems unreasonable.

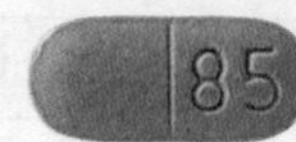

Figure 34-7 Scored medication tablet. **Source:** Courtesy *Mosby's GenRx 1999: The complete reference for generic and brand drugs* (9th ed.). (1999). St. Louis, MO: Mosby–Year Book.

Pediatric Doses. Use caution when calculating children's medication doses. Children metabolize medications at different rates than adults. For example, premature and newborn infants are especially vulnerable to adverse effects of medications because their livers and kidneys have not matured to full functioning levels. After the newborn period, the liver metabolizes some drugs more quickly, which may require that the child receive either larger doses or more frequent doses (Hockenberry & Wilson, 2007). Medication dosages for children are also affected by difficulty in evaluating whether the medication has the desired effect and the hydration status of the child. In most cases, the prescriber will calculate the dose for a child before ordering the medication. However, you are responsible for the safe dose range for any medication administered to a child. Be aware of the formulas used to calculate pediatric doses and recheck all doses before administration. Drug package inserts or medication references often list the normal ranges for pediatric doses.

Various formulas are used to determine the appropriate medication dosages for children. These formulas are often calculated on the basis of the child's age, weight, body surface area, and the medication amount. The most accurate method of calculating pediatric doses is based on a child's body surface area (Hockenberry & Wilson, 2007). Use Mosteller's formula or the standard nomogram (e.g. the West nomogram) to estimate a child's body surface area (Figure 34–8).

Use the following formula to calculate a pediatric dose. The formula is a ratio of the child's body surface area compared with the body surface area of an average adult, which is 1.7 square metres, or 1.7 m^2.

Child's dose = Surface area of child/1.7 m^2 × Normal adult dose

For example, a prescriber orders ampicillin for a child weighing 12 kg. The normal adult dose for ampicillin is 250 mg. According to the West nomogram (see Figure 34–8), a child weighing 12 kg has a surface area of 0.54 m^2. Using this information, calculate the appropriate child's dose:

Child's dose = 0.54 m^2/1.7 m^2 × 250 mg

The m^2 units are cancelled out.

Child's dose = 0.54/1.7 × 250 mg
0.54/1.7 = 0.3
Child's dose = 0.3 × 250 mg = 75 mg

An alternative method to determine medication doses for children involves basing the amount of medication to administer (usually in milligrams) on the weight of the child (usually in kilograms). For example, a prescriber orders 5 mg/kg to be given to a child weighing 14 kg. Using this information, calculate the appropriate dosage based on the following calculation:

Child's dose = 5 mg/kg × 14 kg = 70 mg to be delivered.

Collectively, the prescriber (i.e., the physician, nurse practitioner, or pharmacist) and the pharmacist help to ensure the right medication is delivered to the right client. When you administer medications, you

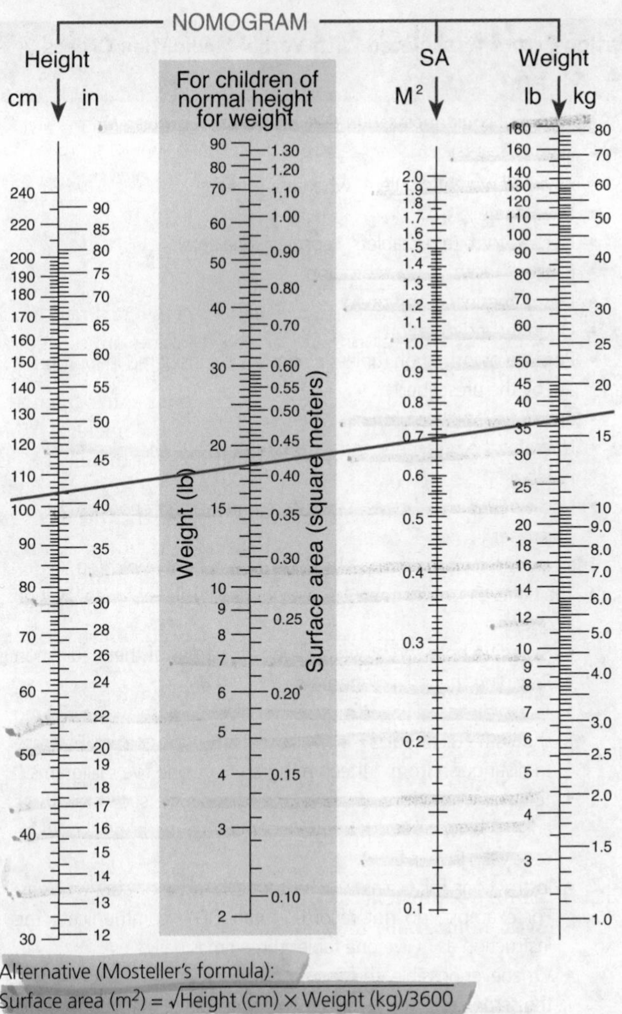

Figure 34-8 West nomogram used to estimate the body surface area of children. A straight line is drawn between a child's height and weight. The point where the line crosses the surface area column is the child's estimated body surface area. **Source:** From Behrman, R. E., Kliegman, R., & Jenson, H. B. (2004). *Nelson textbook of pediatrics* (17th ed.). Philadelphia: Saunders.

are accountable for knowing which medications are prescribed, their therapeutic and nontherapeutic effects, and any nursing implications associated with the medications. You are responsible for performing a physical assessment of the client (e.g., monitoring and interpreting blood pressure before administering an antihypertensive medication) and, on the basis of data from the physical assessment, for determining whether a medication is safe to administer. You should also know why the client needs the medication and be able to determine whether the client needs supervision when taking the medication or education about the medication and its effects. Always monitor the effect of the drug after it is administered and report any reactions to the prescriber.

Prescriber's Role

The physician, nurse practitioner, or pharmacist prescribes the client's medication by writing a medication order (**prescription**) on a form in the client's medical record, in an order book, or on a legal prescription pad; by transmitting the information on a paper form through a facsimile (fax) machine; or by sending the information through a computer terminal. For each medication ordered, prescribers must document the client's diagnosis, condition, or indication for use.

A prescriber may also order a medication by talking directly to the nurse or by telephone. A medication or medical treatment ordered in this way is called a **verbal order**. When you receive a verbal order, read it back and receive confirmation from the prescriber to ensure accuracy (Box 34–4). Immediately enter the order into the client's medical record and record the time and the name of the prescriber who gave the order (The Joint Commission, 2007). Lastly, sign the record. Most institutions require a prescriber's signature within 24 hours after the order is made. Institutional policies vary regarding the personnel who are authorized to receive verbal or telephone orders. Nursing students cannot receive these types of medication orders. Nursing students give newly ordered medications only after the order has been written and verified by a registered nurse.

Common abbreviations are used when writing orders. Abbreviations indicate dosage frequencies or times, routes of administration, and special information for administering the medication (see Table 34–3). Caution must be exercised when you use abbreviations because some shortened forms can lead to confusion and the potential for medication errors (Table 34–7). It is important to know your agency's policies on abbreviations. Do not use error-prone abbreviations when documenting medication orders or other information about medications (Institute for Safe Medication Practices, 2006a; National Coordinating Council for Medication Error Reporting and Prevention [NCCMERP], 2006; The Joint Commission, 2007).

Types of Orders

Five types of medication orders are common in acute care settings: routine, "prn," single (one-time), "STAT," and "now" orders. Medication orders are based on the frequency and the urgency of medication administration. Some conditions change the status of a client's medication orders. For example, in some agencies, the client's preoperative medications are automatically discontinued after surgery, and the health care professional needs to write new medication orders (see Chapter 49). The prescriber should review the medications and write new orders when a client is transferred to another health care agency, relocated to a different service within a hospital, or discharged.

Routine Medication Orders. A routine order is carried out until the prescriber cancels it by writing a new order or until a prescribed number of days have elapsed. A routine order may indicate a final date or the total number of treatments or doses. Many institutions have policies for automatically discontinuing routine orders. The following are examples of routine orders: "tetracycline 500 mg PO q6h" and "Decadron 10 mg daily ×5 days."

As-Needed ("prn") Orders. According to a "prn" order, a medication is to be given only when a client requires it. Use your skills in objective and subjective assessment and discretion when determining whether the client needs the medication. Often, the prescriber sets minimum intervals for the time of administration, which requires the medication not be given more often than a prescribed period of time. An example is "morphine sulphate 5 mg subcutaneously q3–4 h prn for incisional pain." This order indicates that the client needs to wait at least 3 hours between doses. When administering medications, document the assessment made and the time of medication administration. Make frequent evaluation of the effectiveness of the medication and record your findings in the appropriate record.

Single (One-Time) Orders. A prescriber will often order a medication to be given only once at a specified time. This order is common for preoperative medications or medications given before diagnostic examinations: for example, "Versed 25 mg IM on call to OR" and "Valium 10 mg PO at 0900."

STAT Orders. A STAT order signifies that a single dose of a medication is to be given immediately and only once. STAT orders are

➤ BOX 34-4 Recommendations Designed to Reduce Medication Errors Associated With Verbal Medication Orders and Prescriptions

Council Recommendations to Reduce Medication Errors Associated With Verbal Medication Orders and Prescriptions

Adopted February 20, 2001
Revised February 24, 2006

Preamble

Confusion over the similarity of drug names accounts for approximately 25% of all reports to the *USP* Medication Errors Reporting (MER) Program. To reduce confusion pertaining to verbal orders and to further support the Council's mission to minimize medication errors, the following recommendations have been developed.

In these recommendations, verbal orders are prescriptions or medication orders that are communicated as oral, spoken communications between senders and receivers face to face, by telephone, or by other auditory device.

Recommendations

1. Verbal communication of prescription or medication orders should be limited to urgent situations where immediate written or electronic communication is not feasible.
2. Health care organizations* should establish policies and procedures that:
   - Describe limitations or prohibitions on use of verbal orders
   - Provide a mechanism to ensure validity/authenticity of the prescriber
   - List the elements required for inclusion in a complete verbal order
   - Describe situations in which verbal orders may be used
   - List and define the individuals who may send and receive verbal orders
   - Provide guidelines for clear and effective communication of verbal orders.
3. Leaders of health care organizations should promote a culture in which it is acceptable, and strongly encouraged, for staff to question prescribers when there are any questions or disagreements about verbal orders. Questions about verbal orders should be resolved before the preparation, or dispensing, or administration of the medication.
4. Verbal orders for antineoplastic agents should *not* be permitted under any circumstances. These medications are not administered in emergency or urgent situations, and they have a narrow margin of safety.
5. Elements that should be included in a verbal order include:
   - Name of client
   - Age and weight of client, when appropriate
   - Drug name
   - Dosage form (e.g., tablets, capsules, inhalants)
   - Exact strength or concentration
   - Dose, frequency, and route
   - Quantity and duration
   - Purpose or indication (unless disclosure is considered inappropriate by the prescriber)
   - Specific instructions for use
   - Name of the prescriber and, when appropriate, the telephone number
   - Name of individual transmitting the order, if different from the prescriber
6. The content of verbal orders should be clearly communicated:
   - The name of the drug should be confirmed by any of the following:
     - Spelling
     - Providing both the brand and generic names of the medication
     - Providing the indication for use
     - To avoid confusion with spoken numbers, a dose such as 50 mg should be dictated as "fifty milligrams . . . five zero milligrams" to distinguish from "fifteen milligrams . . . one five milligrams."
     - To avoid confusion with drug name modifiers, such as prefixes and suffixes, additional spelling-assistance methods should be used (i.e., S as in Sam).
     - Instructions for use should be provided without abbreviations. For example, do not record "1 tab TID"; communicate the instruction as "Give one tablet three times daily."
     - Whenever possible, the receiver of the order should *write* down the complete order to enter it into a computer, then *read* it back, and receive confirmation from the individual who gave the order or test result.
7. All verbal orders should be committed immediately to writing and the written record should be signed by the individual receiving the order.
8. Verbal orders should be documented in the client's medical record, reviewed, and countersigned by the prescriber as soon as possible.

*Health care organizations include community pharmacies, physicians' offices, hospitals, nursing homes, home care agencies, and so on.

Copyright 1998–2007, National Coordinating Council for Medication Error Reporting and Prevention. All rights reserved.

often written for emergencies when the client's condition changes suddenly: for example, "Give Apresoline 10 mg IV STAT."

Now Orders. A "now" order is more specific than a one-time order; it is used only once, when a client needs medication quickly but not immediately, as in a STAT order. When you receive a "now" order, you have up to 90 minutes to administer the medication. An example of a "now" order is "Give Vancomycin 1 g IV piggyback now."

Prescriptions. The prescriber writes prescriptions for clients who are to be administered medications outside of the hospital setting. The prescription includes more detailed information than a regular order because the client must understand how to take the medication and when to refill the prescription if a refill is necessary. The parts of a prescription are illustrated in Figure 34–9. You need to assess the client's accessibility to pharmacies and other health care resources to determine whether the client needs additional support in the community.

Pharmacist's Role

The pharmacist prepares and distributes prescribed medications. Pharmacists work with nurses, physicians, and other health care professionals to evaluate the efficacy of clients' medication. The pharmacist is responsible for filling prescriptions accurately and for ensuring the prescriptions are valid. The pharmacist in a health care agency rarely needs to mix compounds or solutions, except in the case of intravenous solutions. Most medication companies deliver medications in a form that is ready for use. The pharmacist's main

➤ TABLE 34-7 Abbreviations, Symbols, and Dose Designations With Potential for Errors in Medication Administration

Intended Abbreviation	Meaning	Misinterpretation	Correction
U or u	Unit	Can be mistaken for the number 0 or 4, causing a 10-fold overdose or greater (e.g., "4U" can be misread as "40," or "4u" can be misread as "44"); can be mistaken for "cc," causing the dose to be administered in volume instead of in units (e.g., "4u" can be misread as "4cc")	Write out "unit"
IU	International unit	Can be mistaken for "IV" (intravenous) or "10" (ten)	Write out "international unit"
Q.D., q.d., QD, or qd	Every day	Can be mistaken for "q.i.d.," especially if the period after the letter "q" or the tail of the letter "q" is misunderstood as the letter "I"	Write out "daily"
Q.O.D., q.o.d., QOD, or qod	Every other day	Can be mistaken for "q.d." (daily) or "q.i.d." (four times daily) if the letter "o" is poorly written	Write out "every other day"
MS, MSO_4	Morphine sulfate	Can be mistaken for magnesium sulfate	Write out the complete drug name
$MgSO_4$	Magnesium sulfate	Can be mistaken for morphine sulfate	Write out the complete drug name
µg	Microgram	Can be mistaken for "mg" (milligram)	Write the abbreviation "mcg"
hs	At bedtime, hours of sleep (*hora somna*)	Can be mistaken for "half-strength"	Write out "bedtime" or "half-strength"
T.I.W. or tiw	3 times a week	Can be mistaken for 3 times a day or twice in a week	Write out "three times weekly"
S.C., S.Q., SC, and SQ	Subcutaneous	SC can be mistaken for S.L. (sublingual); SQ can be mistaken for the words "5 every": the letter "q" in "sub q" can be mistaken for the word "every" (e.g., a heparin dose ordered "sub q 2 hours before surgery" can be misunderstood as being required every 2 hours before surgery)	Write the abbreviation "subcut" or the term "subcutaneously"
D/C	Discharge or discontinue	When "discharge" is intended, can be mistaken for premature "discontinuation of medications," especially when followed by a list of discharge medications	Write out "discharge" and "discontinue"
cc	Cubic centimeters	Can be mistaken for the letter "u" (units)	Use the abbreviation "mL"

Adapted from The Joint Commission for Accreditation of Health Care. (2004). *2004 National patient safety goals: FAQs*. Retrieved January 8, 2009, from http://www.premierinc.com/safety/safety-share/10-03-downloads/01-2004-JCAHO-no7-NPSG.doc

task is dispensing the correct medication in the proper dosage and amount and labelling the medication accurately. The pharmacist also provides information about medication side effects, toxicity, interactions, and incompatibilities.

Distribution Systems

Systems for storing and distributing medications vary. Pharmacists provide the medications, but nurses distribute the medications to clients. Institutions that provide nursing care reserve a special area for stocking and dispensing medications. Examples of medication storage areas are special medication rooms, portable locked carts, medication cabinets with computer-controlled locking devices, and individual storage units next to clients' rooms. Ensure that all medications are in locked containers in a room (e.g., a medication room) or are under constant surveillance.

Stock Supply System. In a stock system, medications are available in quantity, in large, multidose containers. The stock system is time-consuming and costly because a nurse must dispense each medication separately for each client. This type of medication delivery has been associated with a high rate of medication errors and is not commonly used today.

Unit-Dose System. The unit-dose system uses portable carts containing a drawer with a 24-hour supply of medications for each client. Each drawer is labelled with the name of a client. The unit dose is the ordered dose of medication the client receives at one time. Each tablet or capsule is wrapped in a foil or paper container. At a designated time each day, the pharmacist or a pharmacy technician refills the drawers in the cart with a fresh supply. The cart also contains limited amounts of "prn" and stock medications. Controlled substances

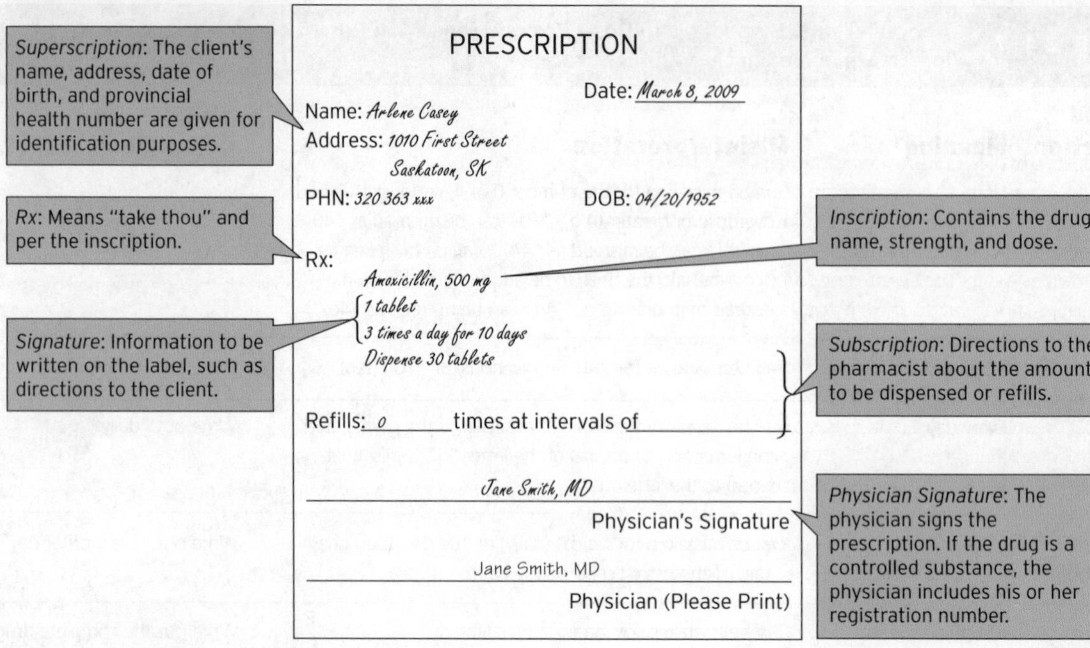

Figure 34-9. Sample medication prescription.

are not kept in the individual client drawers; they are kept in a larger locked drawer. The unit-dose system is designed to reduce the number of medication errors and to save the steps required when dispensing medications.

Automated Dispensing Systems. Automated medication dispensing systems (AMDS) are used successfully throughout Canada (Figure 34–10). These systems use computerized controls to dispense narcotics and unit-dose medication. Each nurse accesses the system by entering a security code. All procedures connected to an AMDS are controlled electronically via a client's profile. The client's name and drug profile must be accessed before the AMDS will dispense a medication. The nurse enters the client's identification number into the computer and selects the desired medication, the correct dose, and the route from a display on the computer screen. The system opens the drawer containing the medication and records the transaction. Nurses may also scan bar codes to identify the client, medication (name, dose, route), and the nurse administering the medication. This information is then automatically recorded in a computerized database.

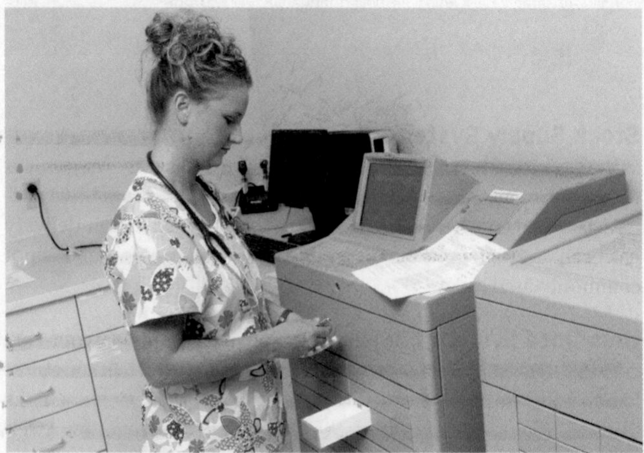

Figure 34-10 Nurse using automated medication dispensing system.

Nurse's Role

Administering medications to clients requires knowledge and skills that are unique to nurses. You must first determine that the medication ordered is the correct medication. Do not assume that all medications in the client's drawer or pill box are to be given to the client. Collect and interpret physical assessment data to determine whether a client should receive a medication at a given time, administer medications correctly, and monitor the effects of prescribed medications. Assess the client's ability to self-administer medications. An integral part of your role is educating the client and the client's family about proper medication administration and monitoring. Do not delegate any part of the medication administration process to unregulated care providers, and use the nursing process to integrate medication therapy into nursing care.

Medication Errors. A medication error is any event that could cause or lead to a client either receiving inappropriate medication therapy or failing to receive appropriate medication therapy. Most errors made by nurses are medication errors. A medication error can cause or lead to inappropriate medication use or client harm. A medication error can occur when you neglect routine procedures, such as checking dose calculations; administer unfamiliar medications; neglect to administer an ordered medication; fail to comply with the seven rights of medication administration; and fail to perform necessary assessments before medication administration (e.g., monitoring the client's blood glucose levels or blood pressure). Additional system issues that can lead to medication errors include distraction, illegible orders, transcription errors, and inappropriate use of abbreviations. Hospital medication delivery systems should be designed so that a system of checks and balances help reduce medication errors.

To demonstrate accountability and acting responsibly in professional practice, you need to acknowledge your errors when they occur. Because nurses play an essential role in the preparation and administration of medications, you need to be vigilant in preventing medication errors (Box 34–5) and advocate for work environments that are conducive to safe medication administration (Box 34–6).

Medication errors can also result from the design of health care products or from procedures and systems, such as product labelling and distribution. When an error occurs, the client's safety and well-being is top priority. Assess the client's condition and notify the physician or prescriber of the medication error as soon as possible. You may need to take measures to counteract the error. After the client's condition has stabilized, report the incident to the appropriate person in the institution (e.g., a manager or supervisor).

When a medication error occurs, you are responsible for preparing a written occurrence or incident report, which usually needs to be filed within 24 hours of the error. The report includes the client identification information; the location and time of the incident; an accurate, factual description of the error that occurred and measures taken to address the error; and your signature. The occurrence report is not a permanent part of the client's medical record and is not referred to in the record (see Chapters 9 and 18), which legally protects the health care professional and the institution. Institutions use occurrence reports to track incident patterns and to address quality improvement and risk-management issues. Many institutions have procedures in place for disclosing incidents to clients or their family members.

Report all medication errors, including errors that do not cause obvious or immediate harm and near misses. It is important for you to feel comfortable in reporting an error and not fear repercussions from managerial staff. Even when a client suffers no harm from a medication error, the institution can still learn why the mistake occurred and what steps can be taken to avoid similar errors in the future. Creating a culture of safety through strategies such as "Good Catch" or "Near Miss" reporting is becoming a popular method for addressing medication safety. Table 34–8 outlines error-prone conditions that lead to student nurse–related errors and specific strategies for avoiding these errors.

Medication errors often occur when a client is transferred to a different unit within a hospital or to another health care agency. Therefore, reconciling the list of client's medications during the transfer process is an important part of ensuring safe client care (The Joint Commission, 2007). Nurses play an essential role in medication reconcilliation (Box 34–7).

When admitting a client to any health care setting, compare the medications the client took in the previous setting (e.g., at home or in another nursing unit) with the client's current medication orders (Ptasinski, 2007). When a client is discharged, review the client's current medications with the health care professionals in the new setting. This action, **medication reconciliation**, may be time-consuming, but it is an essential step in ensuring medication safety. When reconciling medications, consult with the client, the client's caregivers and family members, the physician or advanced practice nurse, and the pharmacist.

➤ BOX 34-5 Steps to Take to Prevent Medication Errors

- Follow the seven rights of medication administration.
- Be sure to read labels at least three times (comparing medication administration record with label) before, during, and after administering the medication.
- Use at least two client identifiers whenever administering a medication.
- Do not allow any other activity to interrupt administration of medication to a client.
- Double-check all calculations, and verify with another nurse.
- Do not interpret illegible handwriting; clarify with prescriber.
- Question unusually large or small doses.
- Document all medications as soon as they are given.
- When you have made an error, reflect on what went wrong and ask how you could have prevented the error.
- Evaluate the context or situation in which a medication error occurred. This helps to determine whether you have the necessary resources for safe medication administration.
- When repeated medication errors occur within a work area, identify and analyze the factors that may have caused the errors and take corrective actions.
- Attend in-service programs that focus on the medications commonly administered.

Reprinted with permission of the National Coordinating Council for Medication Error Reporting and Prevention. © 2006. All rights reserved.

➤ BOX 34-6 Informatics and Medication Safety

Many medication errors occur when the nurse incorrectly administers medications at the client's bedside. The following innovations and advances in technology help to reduce the number of medication errors in nursing practice:

- Networked computers allow all the client's health care professionals to see a current list of ordered and discontinued medications.
- Internet and intranet access allow nurses and other health care professionals to access current information about medications (e.g., indications, desired effects, adverse effects) and specific agency policies that address medication administration (e.g., how fast to administer an intravenous [IV] push medication, how to administer medications through a nasogastric tube).
- In some agencies, prescribers enter medication orders directly into a networked computer system or a personal handheld computer.
- Automated medication dispensing systems and electronic medication administration records help with medication reconciliation, administration, and documentation (Manno, 2006; Paoletti et al., 2007).
- Bar-coding technology requires nurses to scan the medication, the client's identification bracelet, and the nurse's identification badge before administering the medication. This process helps to ensure compliance with the seven rights of medication administration (Mills et al., 2006; Paoletti et al, 2007; Skibinski et al., 2007).

Application to Nursing Practice

- Actively participate in the selection and evaluation of advanced technologies and the creation of nursing policies and protocols used for medication administration.
- Always follow agency policies when administering medications.
- Implement agency policies for when the technology cannot be used (e.g., during computer down time or power outages).
- Follow the manufacturer's guidelines for care of electronic equipment and report problems with technology immediately.

➤ TABLE 34-8 Error-Prone Conditions Leading to Student Nurse-Related Errors

Condition	Description	Strategies to Prevent Error
Preparing drugs for multiple clients	Preparing medications for multiple clients increases the risk of administering medications to the wrong client.	Organize the medication process by preparing medications for one client at a time. When preparing medications for multiple clients, apply client labels to medication cups, removable needle caps of syringes, and IV bags. Use two unique identifiers to verify the correct client before administering medications.
Nonstandard times	Medications scheduled for administration during nonstandard or less commonly used times are prone to dose omissions.	Develop a proactive plan with staff nurses to clarify the responsibility for administration of each ordered medication and how new medication orders received during the shift will be handled. Instructors and staff nurses should monitor the client's MARs and review potential omissions with the student nurses.
Documentation	When both staff nurses and student nurses are assigned to the same clients, neglecting to document or review previously administered medications can lead to dose omissions or extra doses.	Both student nurses and staff nurses should use the same MAR. The client's MAR should be taken to the client's bedside and the drug administration should be documented immediately after the client has been administered the medications. Review all sources of documented drug administration, especially for clients who are transferred from a different unit. Be involved in all verbal reports about the clients you are caring for.
MARs unavailable or not referenced	Neglecting to take the MAR to the client's bedside when administering medications can lead to errors.	Always use MARs when preparing and administering medications; *worksheets should not be used.* Prepare medications in accordance only with the original MAR, and take the MAR to the client's bedside for verification before administering medications. Always use two unique identifiers to verify the correct clients before administering medications.
Partial drug administration	Depending on the year of study, student nurses may not be involved in administering all of the prescribed medications to clients, such as IV medications.	For each unit that hosts student nurses, nursing instructors should provide a daily report that indicates the types of medications that the student nurses will and will not be administering. At the beginning of your shift, confirm with the staff nurse responsible for your client assignment the types of medications you will and will not be administering. Report medications that are not given when due.
Held or discontinued medications	Drugs that have been placed on hold or have been discontinued may be mistakenly administered when student nurses are unfamiliar with an agency's processes for holding and discontinuing medications.	Agencies should annually review their procedures for holding medications and make necessary revisions to ensure that the process is clear and reliable. Consult with nursing instructors and staff nurses regarding processes for holding or discontinuing medications.
Monitoring issues	Errors occur when nurses are unaware of medications that require vital signs monitoring or lab values assessment before medication administration.	Ensure you know how to access the most recent lab values. Ensure you know which medications require vital signs monitoring (e.g., antihypertensive medications) and lab values assessment (e.g., warfarin) before being administered.
Nonspecific doses dispensed	Excessive doses have been administered when student nurses expect the drug is provided in a client-specific dose, but the pharmacy has dispensed the drug in a larger dose or quantity.	The pharmacy should dispense medications in ready-to-use, client-specific doses whenever possible; otherwise, provide further instructions on the MAR and the dose itself. On MARs, list the client-specific dose first, as in the following example: "Lopressor 25 mg," followed by "25 mg = 1/2 of a 50-mg tab."
Oral liquids in parenternal syringes	Preparation of oral or enteral solutions in parenteral syringes can lead to nursing students incorrectly administering these products by the IV route.	Pharmacists should dispense all oral liquid products in oral syringes. Medication areas should be stocked with oral syringes. Use only oral syringes to prepare oral medications.

MAR = medical administration record.

Adapted from Institute for Safe Medication Practices. (2007). *Error-prone conditions that lead to student nurse-related errors.* Retrieved June 1, 2008, from http://www.ismp.org/Newsletters/acutecare/articles/20071018.asp?ptr=y

> **BOX 34-7 Process for Medication Reconciliation**
>
> 1. Verify: Obtain a current list of the client's medications.
> 2. Clarify: Ensure the accuracy of the medications, dosages, and frequencies; clarify the content of the list with as many people as necessary (e.g., the client, caregivers, health care professionals, pharmacists).
> 3. Reconcile: Compare new medication orders against the current list; investigate any discrepancies by contacting the client's health care professional.
> 4. Transmit: Communicate the updated and verified list to caregivers and the client as appropriate.
>
> Adapted from Ptasinski, C. (2007). Develop a medication reconciliation process. *Nurse Manager, 38*, 18.

Critical Thinking

Knowledge

To understand why a particular medication has been prescribed for a client and how the medication will alter the client's physiology and have a therapeutic effect, use knowledge you have acquired from many disciplines. For example, from physiology, you learn that potassium is a major intracellular ion. When clients do not have enough potassium in their body (hypokalemia), they experience signs and symptoms such as muscle fatigue or weakness. In some cases, severe hypokalemia is fatal because of the dysrhythmias that may occur as a result. To restore the client's potassium level to normal, medications may be prescribed, which will also relieve the client's signs and symptoms of hypokalemia.

Nurses administer a wide variety of medications, and new medications are constantly being approved for dispensation. As a result, you may not always have knowledge about the medications you are asked to administer. Responsible nurses admit what they do not know and acquire the knowledge needed to safely administer unfamiliar medications by consulting a medication book, electronic computer manuals, the prescriber, or a pharmacist.

Experience

Nursing students often have limited experience with medication administration as it applies to professional practice. Clinical experiences provide nursing students with the opportunity to apply the nursing process to medication administration. As you gain experiences in medication administration, your psychomotor skills (the steps you take to complete the task) become more refined; however, psychomotor skills represent only a small part of medication administration. The client's attitudes, knowledge, physical and mental status, and responses can make medication administration a complex experience.

Cognitive and Behavioural Attributes

Every step of safe medication administration requires a disciplined attitude and a comprehensive, systematic approach. To be consistent with professional, ethical, and legal nursing standards, you must always accept full responsibility for all your actions related to medication administration. When administering a medication to a client, ensure that your nursing actions do not harm the client in any way. Do not assume that the medication ordered for the client is the correct medication or the correct dose. You can be held accountable for administering an ordered medication that is knowingly inappropriate for the client. Thus, for all medications that you administer, you need to be familiar with the therapeutic effect, usual dosage, laboratory interferences, and side effects. Before administering medications, you must conduct a comprehensive physical assessment of the client and critically analyze the assessment data. You are also responsible for ensuring that clients who will self-administer medications have been properly informed about all aspects of self-administration.

Institutional policy may limit your ability to administer medications in certain units in acute care settings. You may be limited by certain medication routes or by certain dosages. In most institutions, nursing procedure manuals list the institution's policies that define the classes of medications that nurses may and may not administer. The types and doses of medications that nurses may deliver can also vary from unit to unit within the same facility. For example, Dilantin, a powerful medication that is prescribed to treat seizures, may be administered by mouth or by IV push. In large doses, Dilantin can affect the rhythm of the heart. Therefore, when a nursing unit does not have the ability to monitor the client's heart rate and rhythm, some institutions limit the amount of Dilantin that can be given to a client. To ensure safe medication administration, you must adhere to evidence-informed practice guidelines and agency policy and procedure. Not all prescribers are aware of the limitations of all health care institutions and may prescribe medications that cannot be given in a particular health care setting. You must recognize this possibility and ensure that the prescriber is informed of any limitations.

Standards

Standards are actions that ensure safe nursing practice. In Canada, the activity of medication administration by registered nurses is governed by the Canadian Nurses Association's Code of Ethics and professional practice standards set by provincial and territorial nursing associations. Nurses are legally and ethically responsible to acquire the knowledge needed to administer medications and to uphold the client's rights, dignity, and uniqueness in the process. To ensure safe nursing practice, each time you administer a medication, you must be aware of the seven rights of medication administration. All medication errors can be linked, in some way, to an inconsistency in adhering to the following seven rights of medication administration:

1. The right medication
2. The right dose
3. The right client
4. The right route
5. The right time
6. The right documentation
7. The right reason

Right Medication. A medication order is required for every medication you administer to a client. When medications are first ordered, compare the medication administration record or computer order with the prescriber's written order. Always verify new medication information when new orders are written or when clients transfer from one nursing unit or health care facility to another (The Joint Commission, 2007). When administering medications, compare the label of the medication container with the medication form. Check the label against the medication form three times: (1) before removing the container from the drawer or shelf; (2) when the amount of medication ordered is removed from the container; and (3) before returning the container to storage. Never prepare medications from unmarked containers or from containers with illegible labels (The Joint Commission, 2007). When you are using unit-dose prepackaged medications, check the label against the medication administration record when taking medications out of the medication dispensing system. After you determine that the information on the client's medication administration record is accurate, the record is used to prepare and administer the medications. Verify all medications against the medication administration record at the client's bedside before opening the medication packages and delivering the medications to the client.

Administer only the medications that you prepare. If an error occurs, the nurse who administers the medication is responsible. If a client questions the medication, do not ignore the client's concerns. An alert client will know whether a medication is different from one previously received. In most cases, the client's medication order has been changed; however, the client's questions might reveal an error. If an error does occur, withhold the medication and recheck it against the prescriber's orders.

Clients who self-administer medications should keep the medications in their original labelled containers, separate from other medications, to avoid confusion. Many hospitals request that all medication in the hospital setting be administered by nurses, rather than allowing clients to self-administer; this process ensures that clients do not receive double doses of medication. If a client refuses a medication, you should discard it; do not return it to the original container. Unit-dose packaged medications can be saved if they are unopened. However, because of infection control, some agencies require medication to be discarded if it has been taken into a client's room. If a client refuses narcotics, follow the proper hospital procedure of having another nurse witness the wastage of the medication.

Right Dose. The unit-dose system is designed to minimize errors. The chance of error increases when a medication must be prepared from a larger volume or strength than needed or when the prescriber, in ordering a medication, uses a system of measurement different from what the pharmacist supplies. When you perform a medication calculation or conversion, ensure that another nurse verifies the calculated dose.

After confirming the calculated dose, prepare the medication by using standard measurement devices. Use graduated cups, syringes, and scaled droppers to measure medications accurately. At home, clients should use measuring spoons and cups, not household spoons and cups, which vary in volume.

Only tablets that are scored by the manufacturer should be broken. When you need to break a scored tablet, ensure the break is even. You may cut a tablet in half by using a knife or a pill-cutting device. Discard tablets that do not break evenly. Some agencies allow nurses to save the unadministered portion of the scored medication tablet for subsequent doses if the remaining tablet is repackaged and labelled. Verify with agency policy before administering a tablet that has been opened, cut, and repackaged. In the home care setting, pill splitting is particularly problematic. The Institute of Safe Medication Practices (2006b) has developed suggestions to help with this process. Determine whether the client has both the motor dexterity and visual acuity needed to split tablets. If possible, prescribers need to avoid ordering medications that require splitting.

Often a nurse prepares a tablet by crushing it so that it can be mixed in food. The crushing device should always be cleaned completely before the tablet is crushed. Remnants of previously crushed medications may increase a medication's concentration or result in the client receiving a portion of an unprescribed medication. Crushed medications should be mixed with very small amounts of food or liquid. Do not mix crushed medications with the client's favourite foods or liquids because a medication may alter the taste of the food or liquid, and thereby decrease the client's desire for them. Pay particular attention to this concern when administering crushed medications to pediatric clients.

safety alert Not all medications can be crushed. Some medications, such as time-released or extended-release capsules, are coated with special material to prevent the medication from being absorbed too quickly. Before crushing a medication, refer to a medication manual or another medication reference to ensure that the medication can be safely crushed.

Right Client. Medication errors often occur because one client receives a medication intended for another client. An important step in administering medications safely is to ensure medications are given to the right client. Remembering every client's name and face is difficult. To identify a client correctly, check the medication administration record against the client's identification bracelet and ask the client to state his or her name to ensure that the client's identification bracelet has the correct information (Figure 34–11).

If an identification bracelet is missing or the text is smudged or illegible, acquire a new bracelet for the client. When asking the client's name, you should not merely speak the name and assume that the client's response indicates that he or she is the right person. Instead, ask the client to state his or her full name. To avoid making the client feel uneasy, simply explain that the question is routine for giving a medication.

Right Route. If a prescriber's order does not designate a route of administration, or if the specified route is not the recommended route, always consult with the prescriber.

When administering injections, take precautions to ensure that the medications are given correctly. Prepare injections only from preparations designed for parenteral use. The injection of a liquid designed for oral use can produce local complications, such as a sterile abscess, or fatal systemic effects. Medication companies label parenteral medications "for injectable use only."

Right Time. Nurses must know why a medication is ordered for certain times of the day and whether the time schedule can be altered. For example, two medications are ordered: one q8h (every 8 hours) and the other three times a day. Both medications are scheduled three times within a 24-hour period. The prescriber intends the

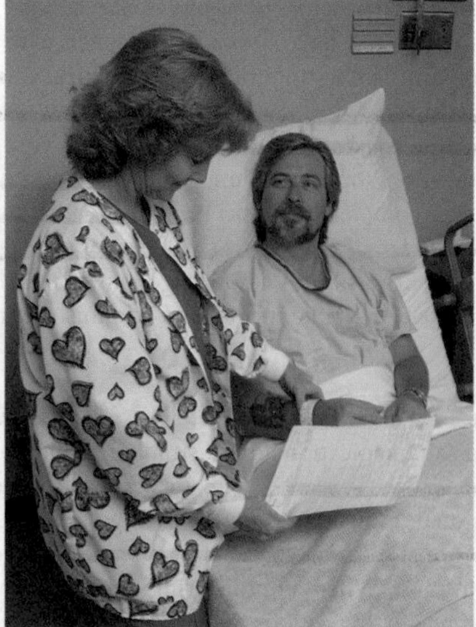

Figure 34-11 Before administering any medications, the nurse checks the client's identification bracelet. **Source:** From deWit, S. (2005). *Fundamental concepts and skills for nursing* (2nd ed.). Philadelphia, PA: W.B. Saunders.

q8h medication to be given around the clock to maintain therapeutic blood levels of the medication. In contrast, you need to give the three-times-a-day medication during the waking hours. Each institution has a recommended time schedule for medications ordered at frequent intervals. You may alter these recommended times if necessary or appropriate.

The prescriber often gives specific instructions for the timing of administration of a medication. For example, when a preoperative medication is to be given "on call," you need to administer the medication when the operating room notifies the nursing unit that the client can be transferred for surgery. A medication ordered pc (after meals) is to be given within half an hour after a meal, when the client has a full stomach. A "STAT" medication is to be given immediately.

Give priority to medications that must act at certain times. For example, insulin should be administered at a precise interval before a meal. Antibiotics should be administered on time around the clock to maintain therapeutic blood levels. All routinely ordered medications should be given within 60 minutes of the times for which they are ordered (i.e., 30 minutes before or after the prescribed time).

Some medications require you to use your clinical judgement to determine the proper time for administration. A "prn" sleeping medication should be administered when the client is prepared for bed or at another time appropriate for maximum benefit. Use your judgement when administering "prn" analgesics. For example, you may need to obtain a STAT order from the prescriber if the client requires a medication before the "prn" interval has elapsed. Always document your calls to the client's prescriber that were made to obtain a change in the medication order.

Before a client is discharged from the hospital setting, evaluate the client's need for home care, especially if the client was admitted to the hospital as the result of a problem with medication self-administration. Clients often leave the hospital with a basic knowledge of their medications but are unable to retreive and implement this knowledge after they return home. Before discharge, evaluate whether medications are adequate or are prescribed at therapeutic levels for the client. At home, a client may need to take several medications throughout the day. Help clients to plan their schedules on the basis of preferred medication intervals, the medications' pharmacokinetics, and the clients' own daily schedule. For clients who have difficulty remembering when to take medications, make a chart that lists the times when each medication is to be taken or prepare a special container to hold each timed dose.

Right Documentation. Nurses and other health care professionals use accurate documentation to communicate with each other. Correct documentation is essential to ensure safe medication administration. Because medication errors may result from inaccurate documentation, ensure that the documentation is appropriate before giving the medications. Appropriate documentation includes the client's name; the name of the ordered medication written out in full (no medication name abbreviations); the time the medication was administered; and the medication's dose, route, and frequency. Common problems with medication orders are incomplete information, inaccurate dose form or strength, illegible orders or signatures, incorrect placement of decimals leading to the wrong dosage, and nonstandard terminology (Hughes & Oritz, 2005). If any pieces of information are missing, contact the prescriber to verify the order. The prescribing health care professional is responsible for providing accurate, complete, and understandable medication orders.

After you administer a medication, complete the medication administration record according to agency policy to verify that the medication was administered as ordered. You are also responsible for documenting any preassessment data regarding the administration of certain medications (e.g., antihypertensive medications, blood glucose–lowering agents, and medications for pain management). Innaccurate documentation of medications, such as failing to document an administered medication, or documenting an incorrect dose, can lead to errors in subsequent decisions about the client's care. For example, errors in documentation about insulin often result in negative client outcomes. Consider the following situation: A client receives insulin at breakfast, but the nurse who gave the insulin neglected to document it. The nurse goes home, and a new nurse is assigned to care for the client. The new nurse notices that the previous nurse did not document the insulin and assumes that the ordered insulin was not given. Therefore, the new nurse gives the client another dose of insulin. Two hours later, the client experiences a low blood glucose level that causes the client to experience seizures. Timely and accurate documentation would have prevented this situation.

Right Reason. Nurses are professionally responsible for obtaining the rationale for prescribed medications. If you are unaware of a new medication, you have the professional responsibility to research the medication by using the following sources: the *Compendum of Pharmaceuticals and Specialties (CPS)*, drug manuals, or electronic drug information databases. When retrieving information about a medication, be attentive to nursing implications, including routes of administration, preadministration physical assessments, expected onset of action, contraindications, and follow-up nursing assessments and evaluation for both adverse effects and desired responses. You are professionally obligated to contact the prescriber for verification in any of the following situations: a prescriber orders a drug that you identify as contraindicated on the basis of either the client's medical history or the client's current condition, the ordered dose exceeds the recommended limits, or the ordered route is contraindicated for the client. Being vigilant in critically assessing a client's medication regimes is essential to maintain client safety.

Risk Management: Agency Policy and Procedure. Most institutions have nursing policy and procedure manuals to guide nursing practice. These manuals are updated annually based on current evidence-informed practice literature. Policy and procedure manuals contain vital information for medication administration, including the types of medications nurses are permitted to administer, the preparation of medications, the administration of medications, and guidelines for evaluating client's response to medications. For example, some agencies require nurses to complete specialized training to qualify them to safely administer intravenous chemotherapeutic agents. Furthermore, the administration of certain medications (e.g., intravenous inotropic medications for regulating a client's blood pressure) are prohibited on general medicine and surgery units and permitted only in critical care areas where the client is continuously monitored for responses to medication therapy.

Maintaining Clients' Rights. Because of the potential risks related to medication administration, clients have the right to the following:

- To be informed of the medication's name, purpose, action, and potential undesired effects
- To refuse a medication regardless of the consequences
- To have qualified nurses or physicians assess their medication history, including allergies and use of herbal therapies (Box 34–8)
- To be properly advised of the experimental nature of medication therapy and to give written consent for its use
- To receive labelled medications safely without discomfort in accordance with the seven rights of medication administration

> **BOX 34-8 Nursing Assessment Questions**
>
> - What prescription and nonprescription medications do you take, when do you take them, and how do you take them? Do you have a list of medications from your pharmacy or your health care professional?
> - What are your medications for?
> - What side effects have you experienced?
> - Have you ever stopped taking your medications? If so, why did you stop taking them?
> - How do you help yourself to remember to take your medications?
> - Do you have any allergies to medications or foods? If so, describe what happens when you take the medication or eat the food.
> - Describe your normal eating patterns. What foods do you eat, and at what times do you normally eat?
> - How do your religious or cultural beliefs influence your beliefs about your medications?
> - How do you pay for your medications? Do you have additional insurance through your employer or pension plan to help cover the costs of your medication? Do you live close to a pharmacy? How do you access prescription medications in your community?
> - What questions do you have about your medications?

- To receive appropriate supportive therapy in relation to medication therapy
- To not receive unnecessary medications
- To be informed whether medications are part of a research study

Be aware of these rights and handle all inquiries by clients and their families courteously and professionally. If a client refuses medication therapy, do not become defensive. Recognize that every person of consenting age has the autonomous right to refuse a medication.

Nursing Process and Medication Administration

❖Assessment

To determine the need for and potential response to medication therapy, nurses assess many factors. To ensure safe medication administration, perform thorough physical assessments of all clients before administering medications.

History

Before administering medications, you need to obtain or review the client's medical history. A client's medical history provides indications or contraindications for medication therapy. A client who has disease or illness is at risk for adverse medication effects. For example, if a client has a gastric ulcer, compounds containing aspirin will increase the likelihood of bleeding. If a client has a long-term health condition, such as diabetes or arthritis, the client requires medications to treat these conditions. A client's surgical history may also indicate the use of medications. For example, after a thyroidectomy, a client may require hormone replacement.

History of Allergies

If the client has a history of contact allergies or allergies to medication or food, inform the other members of the health care team. Food allergies should be carefully documented because many medications include ingredients also found in food sources. For example, a client who is allergic to shellfish may also be sensitive to any product containing iodine, such as Betadine or dyes used in radiological testing. To ensure client safety, when clients are admitted to a hospital, they are issued an identification band that lists the medications they are allergic to. Ensure that all allergies are noted on the nurse's admission notes, the medication records, and the physician's documentation of the client's history.

Medication Data

Assess information about each medication that the client takes, including length of time the medication has been taken, the current dosage, and whether the client has experienced any adverse effects. Review the medication data, including the action, purpose, normal dosages, routes, side effects, and nursing implications for administration and monitoring. Common questions to ask include the following: Is the smallest possible dose ordered? (a question pertinent for medications ordered for older adults) Can a certain medication interact with other medications the client is taking? Are special instructions required for administering the medication? Often, several resources must be consulted to gather the information you need. Some valuable resources are pharmacology textbooks, nursing journals, the *Compendium of Pharmaceuticals and Specialties* (*CPS*), online medication manuals, medication package inserts, nursing journals, and the pharmacist. You are responsible for knowing as much as possible about each medication you administer. Many nursing students prepare or purchase cards containing medication data to use as a quick resource.

Diet History

A diet history reveals the client's normal eating patterns and food preferences. Nurses can then plan the dosage schedule more effectively and advise clients to avoid foods that may interact with their medications. Be aware of clients' cultural preferences for food, and if these foods interact with medications, provide the clients and their families with comprehensive, respectful explanations.

Client's Perceptual or Coordination Problems

For a client with limited perceptual, fine motor, or coordination skills, self-administration of medication may be difficult. For example, a client with arthritis who takes insulin to manage blood glucose levels may have difficulty manipulating a syringe. Always assess the client's ability to prepare doses and take medications correctly. If the client is unable to self-administer medications, determine whether a family member or friend will be available to assist the client, or collaborate with the interdisciplinary team to refer the client to a home care service that can assist in medication administration.

Client's Current Condition

The physical or mental status of a client may affect whether a medication is given or how it is administered. Carefully assess a client before giving any medication. For example, check the client's blood pressure before giving an antihypertensive medication. A client who is nauseated may be unable to swallow a tablet. Assessment findings also serve as a baseline in evaluating the effects of medication therapy.

Client's Attitude Toward Medication Use

The client's attitude about medications may reveal the client's level of medication dependence or drug avoidance. Clients may not express their feelings about taking a particular medication, particularly if they have become dependent on it. Observe the client's behaviour for evidence of medication dependence or avoidance. Also be aware that the client's cultural beliefs about Western medicine could interfere with medication compliance (Box 34–9, and see Chapter 10).

Client's Knowledge and Understanding of Medication Therapy

The client's knowledge and understanding of medication therapy influence the willingness or ability to follow a medication regimen. Compliance is unlikely unless a client understands the medication's purpose, the importance of regular dosage schedules and proper administration methods, and the medication's possible side effects. When assessing a client's knowledge of a medication, ask, "What is it for? How is it taken? When is it taken? What side effects have you experienced? Have you ever stopped taking doses? Is there anything else you do not understand about the medication but would like to know?" When the client has a history of poor compliance, review resources available for the purchase of medications.

Client's Learning Needs

Determine the need for instruction by assessing the client's level of knowledge about a medication and the resources available to help the client to take medications regularly. You may need to explain the action and purpose of the medication, the expected side effects, the correct administration techniques, and steps the client can take to remember the medication regimen. If a client has a newly prescribed medication, your instruction will need to be more involved.

BOX 34-9 CULTURAL ASPECTS OF CARE

Influences on Medication Administration

Health beliefs vary by culture and often influence how clients manage and respond to drug therapy. Differences in values, beliefs, and attitudes affect a client's compliance with drug therapy. For example, cultures attach different symbolic meanings to medications and drug therapy.

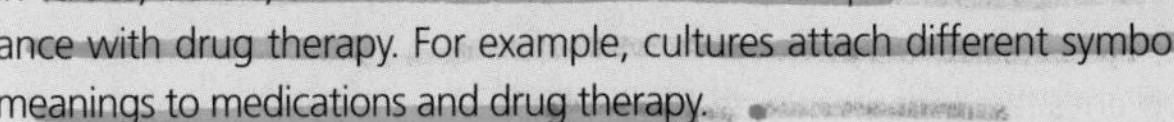

Herbal remedies and alternative therapies are common in some cultures and ethnic groups and can interfere with prescribed medications. In addition, differences between the health beliefs of health care professionals and their clients can affect a client's compliance with medical therapy.

Demographic changes in both age and race can affect the nursing practice in medication administration. In addition to the psychosocial aspect of medication therapy, pharmacological research has shown that some ethnic and racial groups experience differences in drug response, metabolism, and side effects.

Implications for Practice

- Assess a client's cultural beliefs, attitudes, and values when administering medications and teach clients about their medications.
- Resolve conflicts between medications and cultural beliefs to achieve optimal client outcomes.
- Ask whether the client practises any alternative therapies or takes any herbal preparations.
- If a client is not responding to drug therapy as expected, consider whether cultural influences affect the drug response, the rate at which it is metabolized, and side effects. Bear in mind that a change in the client's medication is sometimes necessary.
- Always exercise awareness of your personal beliefs and distinguish between your values and the clients'.

Data from Andrews, M. M., & Boyle J. S. (2007). *Transcultural concepts in nursing care* (5th ed.). Philadelphia, PA: Lippincott; and from McKenry, L. M., Tessier, E., & Hogan, M. A. (2006). *Mosby's pharmacology in nursing* (22nd ed.): St. Louis, MO: Mosby.

❖Nursing Diagnosis

Assessment of the client provides data about the client's condition, the ability to self-administer medications, medication management (e.g., diabetic management), and medication use patterns, which can be used to determine actual or potential problems with medication therapy. Certain data are defining characteristics; when clustered together, they reveal nursing diagnoses. For example, noncompliance related to a medication regimen may be indicated when a client admits that he or she is not taking prescribed medications correctly, or when evidence shows that a medication has not reversed symptoms as expected. The following nursing diagnoses may be observed during the administration of medications:

- *Anxiety*
- *Ineffective health maintenance*
- *Health-seeking behaviours*
- *Deficient knowledge of medications*
- *Noncompliance with prescribed medications*
- *Disturbed visual sensory perception*
- *Impaired swallowing*
- *Effective therapeutic regimen management*
- *Ineffective therapeutic regimen management*

After the client's diagnosis has been selected, identify the related factors, which guide the selection of nursing interventions. For example, the related factors of inadequate resources and lack of knowledge require different interventions. If the client's noncompliance is related to inadequate finances, collaborate with the client's family members, social workers, or community agencies to ensure the client receives the necessary medications. If the related factor is lack of knowledge, initiate referrals to ensure home care nurses follow up with the client and that they implement an extensive teaching plan.

❖Planning

Organize care activities to ensure the safe administration of medications. Hurrying to give clients medications can lead to errors. When preparing and administering medications, it is important to minimize distractions and interruptions (Pape et al., 2005).

Goals and Outcomes

Setting goals and related outcomes will help you to use your time wisely during medication administration. For example, establish the following goal and related outcomes for a client with newly diagnosed type 2 diabetes:

Goal: The client will safely administer all ordered medications before discharge.

Outcomes:

- The client will express an understanding of the desired effects and the adverse effects of medications.
- The client will state the signs, symptoms, and treatment of hypoglycemia.
- The client will be able to monitor and interpret blood glucose levels to determine medication management or treatment for hypoglycemia.

- The client will establish a daily routine that will coordinate timing of medication with mealtimes.

Setting Priorities

Prioritize care when administering medications. Use information gathered from your assessment of the client to determine whether the administration of medications is appropriate and, if it is, which medication should be given first. For example, if a client is in pain, provide pain medication as soon as possible. If the client is experiencing an elevated blood pressure, antihypertensive medications should be administered before other medications. Establish priorities when providing client education about medications. Provide the most important information about the medications first. For example, because hypoglycemia is a serious side effect of insulin, the client must be able to identify and treat hypoglycemia before learning how to administer an insulin injection.

Collaborative Care

Nurses collaborate with a variety of health care professionals when administering medications. It is also important when giving instruction to collaborate with the client's family or friends, who can reinforce the importance of medication regimens in the client's home setting. Interdisciplinary collaboration with the prescriber, the pharmacist, and the home care case manager helps to ensure the client receives medications safely. Ensure that clients are able to read both medication labels and printed teaching sheets. Collaborate with community resources (e.g., the home care nurse, social workers) if clients have difficulty in understanding medication management, adhering to medication routines due to functional ability, or accessing resources because of physical or financial restrictions.

When clients are hospitalized, do not postpone their medication and discharge instructions until the day of discharge. In order for the client to understand medications and self-administration guidelines, you must allow sufficient time for questions and discussion. Early planning is critical. Whether a client attempts self-administration or a nurse assumes responsibility for administering medications, the following goals and expected outcomes must be met: (a) the client and the client's family understand the medication therapy; (b) the client gains the therapeutic effect of the prescribed medications without discomfort or complications; (c) the client experiences no complications related to the route of administration; and (d) the client can safely self-administer the prescribed medications.

❖Implementation

Health Promotion

When working with clients to promote and maintain their health, you need to identify factors that may improve or diminish their well-being. Beliefs about health, personal motivations, socioeconomic factors, and habits (e.g., smoking) can influence the client's compliance with the medication regimen.

Teaching the client and the client's family about the benefit of a medication and the knowledge needed to take it correctly is an essential component of primary health care and can promote adherence to the medication regimen (Box 34–10). Integrating the client's health beliefs and cultural practices into the treatment plan can assist in establishing a schedule or routine with the client. You may make referrals to community resources if the client cannot afford to purchase the necessary medications, or if the client cannot arrange transportation to obtain the necessary medications. You should teach all clients the basic guidelines for medication safety. These guidelines ensure the proper use and storage of medications in the home (Box 34–11).

Acute Care

Clients are often hospitalized to receive expert nursing observation and documentation of their responses to medications. When receiving a medication order, several nursing interventions are essential for safe and effective medication administration.

Receiving Medication Orders. A medication order is required for any medication to be administered by a nurse. Before any other interventions, ensure the medication order contains all of the elements in Box 34–12. If the medication order is not complete,

> **BOX 34-10 FOCUS ON PRIMARY HEALTH CARE**
>
> ### Improving Drug Compliance
>
> When a client is discharged from hospital or sent home from a visit to a clinic, the ongoing treatment may include regularly taking medications at home. In cases of chronic illness, the success of the treatment may depend on the client's compliance with drug therapy. Nurses can play an important role in assisting clients to comply with their medication regimen.
>
> The following suggestions may improve client compliance:
>
> - Ensure that the client and the client's family understand the reason for the medication, proper administration of the medication, and the possible consequences of noncompliance.
> - Ensure that the client and the client's family and friends are able to recognize symptoms of medication side effects or toxicity, such as physiological changes and alterations in behaviour. Because the client's family members and friends are often the first people to recognize such effects in the client, they are an important resource for ensuring client compliance.
> - Teach proper self-administration of medications to clients for all routes. For example, demonstrate how to accurately measure a liquid medication. Show the client how to prepare and administer an injection correctly by using aseptic technique. Assess the client's ability to self-administer injections. If a client cannot independently self-administer injections, family members or friends can be taught to administer the injections. Alternatively, collaborate with community and home care services to administer injections when clients are discharged to their home. Provide specially designed equipment as necessary, such as syringes with enlarged calibrated scales for easier reading or Braille-labelled medication vials.
> - Help the client to address any economic issues that might affect compliance.
> - Explore with the client any factors that will influence his or her ability to comply; for some clients, keeping a daily medication log may be helpful.
> - Provide a written schedule that includes the name of the medication, the dose, and a description or picture of the medication.
> - Encourage clients to take their medication in conjunction with an activity they do every day, such as brushing their teeth or having breakfast.
> - Help clients to organize their pills into a box with daily dividers. If compliance is a major concern, home care nurses or family members can check the box and refill it on a weekly basis.
> - Work with the client's pharmacist to ensure the pharmacy calls to remind the client when a refill is required.

inform the prescriber and ensure completeness before carrying out the medication order.

Correct Transcription and Communication of Orders. Nurses or a designated unit secretary sometimes write the prescriber's complete order on the appropriate medication form, the medication administration record. The transcribed order includes the client's name, identification number, room, bed number, allergies, and the medication name, dose, frequency, and route of administration. Each time a medication dose is prepared, refer to the medication form. When the unit-dose system is used, only one transcription is necessary, which limits the opportunity for errors. When transcribing orders, ensure that names, doses, and symbols are legible. Rewrite any smudged or illegible transcriptions.

Some institutions have prescribed order entry. The prescriber enters an order directly into the computer, which avoids the need for the transcription of orders. Computer interfaces transfer the order to the medication administration record, the pharmacy record, and the automated dispensing system. The computer printout may be used as the medication administration record (Figure 34–12).

Always check all transcribed orders against the original order for accuracy and thoroughness. If an order is incorrect or inappropriate, consult the prescriber. If you give the wrong medication or an incorrect dose, you are legally responsible for the error. Other health care professionals involved in the error are also legally responsible.

BOX 34-11 CLIENT TEACHING

Safe Insulin Administration

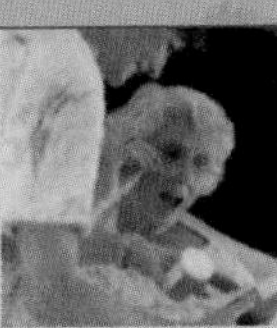

Objective

- The client will correctly administer subcutaneous insulin.

Teaching Strategies

- Instruct the client how to determine that insulin is not out of date.
- Instruct the client to keep insulin in its original labelled container.
- Instruct the client to keep insulin refrigerated if necessary.
- Assess the client's visual acuity to ensure that the client is able to prepare the appropriate amount of insulin.
- Demonstrate how to rotate the location of insulin injection sites.
- Help the client to determine the amount of insulin required based on the results of home capillary glucose monitoring, as ordered by the client's health care professional.
- Observe the client's ability to correctly assess the results of capillary blood glucose monitoring.
- Demonstrate to the client how to prepare a single insulin preparation.
- Demonstrate to the client how to administer a subcutaneous insulin injection.
- Show the client how to keep a daily log book to record insulin injections, including results of home capillary glucose monitoring, type and amount of insulin given, expiration date on insulin vial, time of insulin injection, and injection site used.

Evaluation

- Ask the client to describe the signs and symptoms of hypoglycemia and the associated interventions.
- Ask the client to describe the procedure used at home for determining the correct dose of insulin needed and the injection site.
- Observe the client preparing an insulin dose on the basis of the results of capillary glucose monitoring.
- Observe the client selecting the injection site and self-administering the insulin injection.
- Review the information recorded in the client's log book for completeness.

BOX 34-12 Components of Medication Orders

A complete medication order includes all the following information:

- Client's full name: The client's full name distinguishes the client from other persons with the same last name. In an acute care setting, clients may also be assigned a special identification number (e.g., a medical record number) to help differentiate clients with the same names. This number may be included on the order form.
- Date and time the order is written: The day, month, year, and time must be listed. Designating the time that an order is written helps to clarify when certain orders are to stop automatically. If an incident occurs involving a medication error, documentation is easier when this information is available.
- Medication name: The prescriber will order a medication by its generic or trade name. Correct spelling is essential to prevent confusion with medications with similar spelling.
- Dose: The amount or strength of the medication is included.
- Route of administration: The prescriber uses accepted abbreviations to indicate the medication routes. Accuracy is important because some medications can be administered by more than one route.
- Time and frequency of administration: Nurses need to know when to initiate medication therapy. Orders for multiple doses establish a routine schedule for medication administration.
- Signature of prescriber: The prescriber's signature makes the order a legal request.

Accurate Dose Calculation and Measurement. When measuring liquid medications, use a standard measuring container to reduce the chance of error. Calculate each dose when preparing the medication, pay close attention to the process of calculation, and avoid interruption from other nursing activities (Pape et al., 2005). Consult with other nurses when calculating a new or unusual dose.

Correct Administration. To help ensure safe administration, use aseptic techniques and proper procedures when handling and giving medications. Verify the client's identity by using at least two client identifiers (The Joint Commission, 2007) and perform the necessary assessments (e.g., assessing heart rate before giving antidysrhythmic medications). Carefully monitor the client's response to medication, especially when administering the first dose of a new medication. Document the client's response on the appropriate record forms.

Recording Medication Administration. After administering a medication, record it immediately on the appropriate record form (see Figure 34–12). Never chart a medication before administering it. Recording the medication immediately after its administration prevents errors.

The recording of a medication includes writing the name of the medication, the dose, the route, and the exact time of administration. Record assessment parameters (e.g., blood glucose level, blood pressure, pain score) and the site of any injections, in accordance with agency policy.

If a client refuses a medication or undergoes tests or procedures that result in a missed dose, the reason why the medication was not given must be recorded in both the medication administration record and nurse's notes.

Room: 3700-03

Patient: PDM, Pharmacy
Birth: 11/30/79 Admit: 01/03/09
MRN: 2000403 Acct: 900015
A Doctor: Jim Smith

Age: 29 y Ht: 1 m 57 cm Wt: 56.79 kg

MEDICATION ADMINISTRATION RECORD

Date: 01/18/09 – 01/19/09

ADEs/Nondrug allergies: Latex – Zosyn – Amoxicillin – Insulins – Darvocet – Lugols soln. – Antihi +

Medication	0800	0900	1000	1100	1200	1300	1400	1500	1600	1700	1800	1900	2000	2100	2200	2300	2400	0100	0200	0300	0400	0500	0600	0700
P00014 Bacitracin ointment AKA: Bacitracin ointment Dose: Apply STRGH: 30 gm/tube TID Topical: Right lower leg For external use only Testing			RL 10																					
P00029 Insulin/human regular AKA: Humulin R Dose: 15 units Strgh: 1 ml = 100 units AC Sub-Q	RL 0730																							
P00030 Fexofenadine 60 mg/pseudo 120 mg AKA: Allegra–D Sr Tab Dose: 1 tab STRGH: 60/120/tab BID Oral Auto Sub: 1 Allegra–D Tab bid For Claritin–D 12 hr and 24 hr Per P&T Comm			RL 10																					
P00036 Aspirin AKA: Aspirin 325 mg Tab Dose: 2 tab 650 mg STRGH: 325 mg/tab Q3–4h Oral Testing						RL 1315																		
P00039 Haloperidol tablet AKA: Haldol 0.5 mg tab Dose: 1 mg STRGH: 1 mg/tab QHS Oral																								
P00035 Zolpidem AKA: Ambien 5 mg tab Dose: 5 mg STRGH: 5/tab QHS PRN Oral MR × 1 Testing																								

Circle = Dose not given
Initials = Dose given
Deltoid = R.D., L.D.
Vastus Lateralis = R.V.L., L.V.L.
Lower Abdominal = R.L.A., L.L.A.
Anterior Gluteal = R.A.G., L.A.G.
Posterior Gluteal = R.P.G., L.P.G.

Page: 01 (continued)

Initials and signature	Initials and signature	Initials and signature
Rita Lassater RL		
Initials and signature	Initials and signature	Initials and signature
Initials and signature	Initials and signature	Initials and signature

Figure 34-12 Example of a medication administration record.

Restorative Care

Medication administration activities vary among the numerous types of restorative care settings. Clients with functional limitations may require you to fully administer all medications. In the home setting, clients usually administer their own medications. Regardless of the type of medication activity, you are responsible for instructing clients and their families in medication action, administration, and side effects. Additionally, you need to monitor the client's compliance with medication and determine the effectiveness of medications that have been prescribed.

Special Considerations for Administering Medications to Specific Age Groups

A client's developmental level affects the way that nurses administer medications. Your knowledge of a client's developmental needs helps you to anticipate responses to medication therapy.

Infants and Children. Children vary in age, weight, body surface area, and their ability to absorb, metabolize, and excrete medications. Children's medication doses are lower than doses for adults; therefore, special caution is needed when preparing medications for children. Medications are usually not prepared and packaged in standardized dose ranges for children. Preparing an ordered dose from an available amount of medication requires careful calculation.

All children require special psychological preparation before receiving medications. The child's parents are valuable resources for learning the best way to administer medications to their child. Sometimes the child will experience less trauma if a parent administers the medication and you supervise.

Supportive care is needed if a child is expected to cooperate. Explain the procedure to the child, using short words and simple language appropriate to the child's level of comprehension. Long explanations may increase the child's anxiety, especially for painful procedures such as an injection. You need to administer medications to children even when they refuse to cooperate or resist consistently despite explanation and encouragement. If the child is uncooperative, administer the medication to the child quickly and carefully (Hockenberry & Wilson, 2007). If you are able to involve the child, you may have greater success giving a medication. For example, when you say, "It's time to take your tablet now. Do you want it with water or juice?" you are allowing the child to make a choice. Do not give the child the option of not taking a medication. After a medication is given, praise the child; you may even offer a simple reward such as a star or a token. Tips for administering medications to children are listed in Box 34–13.

Older Adults. Older adults also require special consideration during medication administration (Box 34–14). In addition to physiological changes of aging (Figure 34–13), behavioural and economic factors influence an older person's use of medications.

Polypharmacy. **Polypharmacy** occurs when the client takes two or more medications to treat the same illness, when the client takes two or more medications from the same chemical class, when the client uses two or more medications with the same or similar actions to treat several disorders simultaneously, or when a client mixes nutritional supplements or herbal products with medications (Brager & Soland, 2005; Ebersole et al., 2004). Older adults also often experience polypharmacy when they self-medicate to seek relief from a variety of symptoms (e.g., pain, constipation, insomnia, and indigestion) by using over-the-counter (OTC) preparations, traditional folk medicines, or herbal remedies. Over-the-counter medications contain many different ingredients; when used inappropriately, they can cause indesirable side effects and adverse reactions, or they may be contraindicated by the client's condition.

➤ BOX 34-13 Tips for Administering Medications to Children

Oral Medications

- Use liquid forms when available. They are safer for children to swallow and they help to avoid aspiration.
- Use droppers to administer liquids to infants.
- If older childen have difficulty swallowing pills, suggest that they put the pill in their mouth and then sip liquid through a straw. The suction action pulls the liquid up the straw and makes it easier to swallow the pill.
- Offer juice, a soft drink, or a frozen juice bar after a medication is swallowed.
- To reduce nausea, pour carbonated beverages over finely crushed ice.
- When medications are mixed with palatable flavourings, such as syrup or applesauce, use only a small amount. Avoid mixing a medication with foods or liquids that the child enjoys because the child may in turn refuse them.
- A plastic, disposable syringe is the most accurate device for preparing liquid doses, especially doses of less than 10 mL (cups, spoons, and droppers are inaccurate.)
- When administering liquid medications, use a spoon, a plastic cup, or an oral syringe (without needle).

Injections

- Use caution when selecting IM injection sites for infants and small children. The deltoid muscle, which can be used for adults and older children, is underdeveloped and should not be used in infants and small children.
- Children can be unpredictable and uncooperative. Ensure that someone (preferably another nurse) is available to restrain a child if physical control is needed. The parent should act as a comforter, not a restrainer.
- Always awaken a sleeping child before giving him or her an injection.
- Distracting the child with conversation, a ringing bell, or a toy may reduce the child's perception of pain.
- Give the injection quickly and do not argue with the child.
- If time allows, use a eutectic mixture of local anaesthetics (EMLA) cream.

✱ BOX 34-14 FOCUS ON OLDER ADULTS

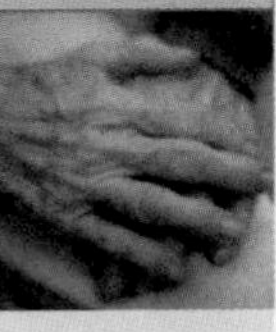

- Simplify the drug therapy plan whenever possible (McKenry et al., 2006).
- Keep instructions clear and simple and provide written material in large print (Ebersole et al., 2004).
- Assess the client's functional status to determine whether the client requires assistance in taking medications (McKenry et al., 2006).
- Have the client drink a little fluid before taking oral medications to ease swallowing. Encourage the client to drink at least 150–180 mL of fluid after taking medications (Ebersole et al., 2004).
- Older adults may have a greater sensitivity to drugs, especially drugs that act on the central nervous system. Therefore, you need to carefully monitor clients' responses to medications and anticipate dosage adjustments as needed (Meiner & Lueckenotte, 2006).
- If the client has difficulty swallowing a capsule or tablet:
  - Ask the physician to substitute a liquid medication if possible (Ebersole et al., 2004).
  - Ask the client to sit up straight and to tuck in the chin to decrease risk of aspiration (McKenry et al., 2006).
- Teach alternatives to medications, such as proper diet in place of vitamins and exercise in place of laxatives (Ebersole et al., 2004).
- On a frequent basis, review the client's medication history, including over-the-counter medications (Meiner & Luekenotte, 2006).

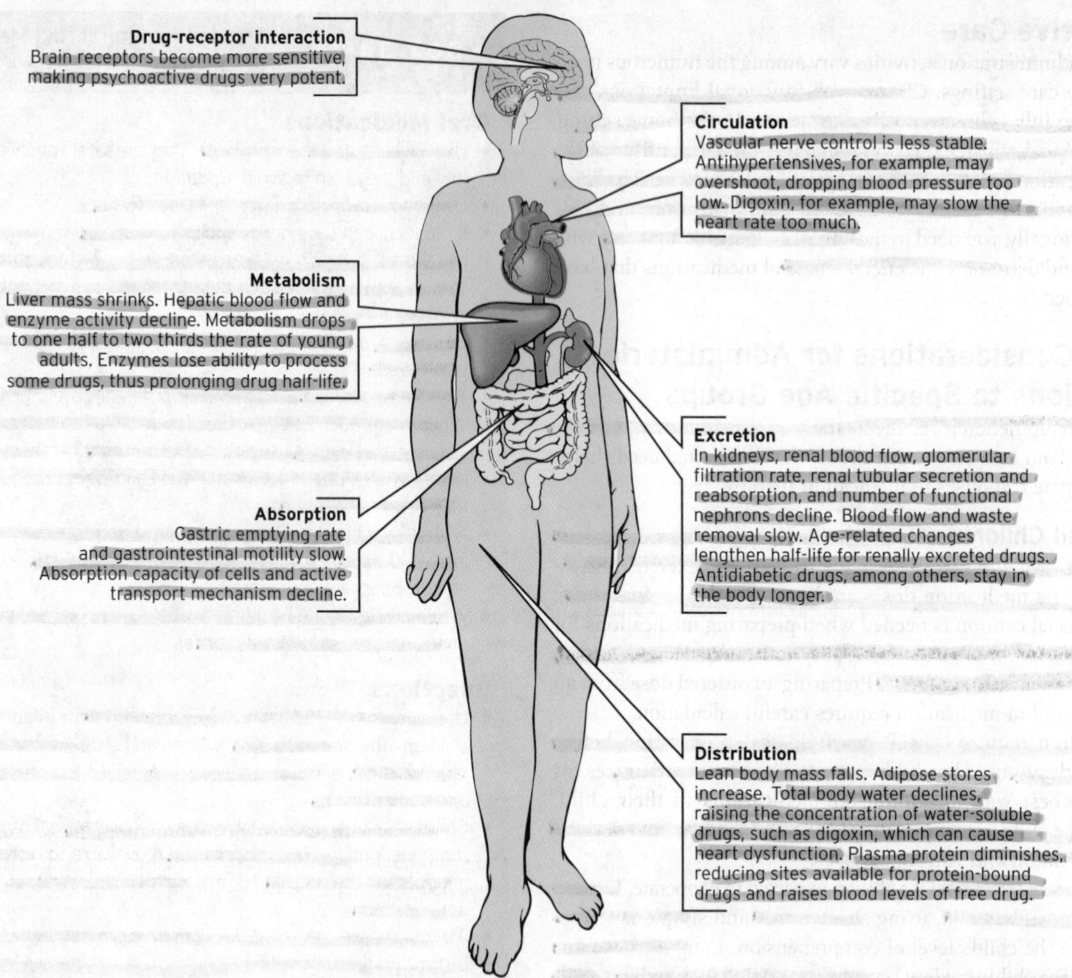

Figure 34-13 The aging body and drug use. **Source:** From Lewis, S. M., Heitkemper, M. M., & Dirksen, S. R. (2004). *Medical–surgical nursing* (6th ed.). St. Louis, MO: Mosby.

Because many older adults suffer chronic health problems, polypharmacy is common. The client who experiences polypharmacy is at an increased risk of adverse reactions and medication interactions with other medications and food.

Polypharmacy can be divided into two types: rational polypharmacy and irrational polypharmacy. Rational polypharmacy occurs when clients need to take several medications to treat their health conditions, which is often the case for older adults. For example, many older adults take multiple medications to lower their blood pressure. Irrational polypharmacy occurs when the client takes more medications than needed. Irrational polypharmacy results from several causes. For example, some older adults need to see more than one health care professional to treat their different health conditions. When health care professionals fail to take an accurate medication history or do not communicate with each other, the result can be clients taking many different medications, which increases their risk of polypharmacy (Brager & Soland, 2005).

Noncompliance. Noncompliance is defined as a deliberate misuse of medication, such as not taking a prescribed medication or altering the dose of a medication. In general, noncompliance occurs either because of drug ineffectiveness, uncomfortable side effects, or the prohibitive cost of the medicine.

❖Evaluation

Nurses monitor client responses to medications on an ongoing basis. For each medication, you require knowledge of the desired effect, the therapeutic action, and the common side effects. A change in a client's condition can be physiologically related to health status, medications, or both. Be alert for reactions in a client who takes several medications. To achieve the goal of safe and effective medication administration, a careful evaluation of both the client's response to therapy and the client's ability to assume responsibility for self-care is required.

To evaluate the effectiveness of nursing interventions in meeting established goals of care, use evaluative measures to identify whether client outcomes were met. Apply various evaluation measures in the context of medication administration, including direct observation of the client's behaviour or response, rating scales and checklists, and oral questioning. Physiological measurement is the most common method of evaluation. Examples of physiological measures are blood pressure, heart rate, and visual acuity. Client statements can also be used as evaluative measures. Table 34–9 gives examples of goals, expected outcomes, and corresponding evaluative measures.

TABLE 34-9 Example Evaluation for Client Goals

Goals	Expected Outcomes	Evaluative Measure With Example
The client and the client's family understand the client's medication therapy.	The client and the client's family describe information about the medication, its dosage, schedule, purpose, and adverse effects.	Written measurement: Ask the client to write out the medication schedule for a 24-hour period.
		Oral questioning: Ask the client to describe the purpose, dosage, and adverse effects of each prescribed medication.
	The client and the client's family identify situations that require medical intervention.	Oral questioning: Ask the client's family to describe what to do if the client has adverse effects from a medication.
	The client and the client's family demonstrate the appropriate administration technique.	Direct observation: Ask the client to demonstrate the filling of an insulin syringe and self-injection.
The client safely self-administers medications.	The client follows a prescribed treatment regimen.	Anecdotal notes: Have the client's family keep a log of the client's compliance with therapy for 1 week.
	The client performs administration techniques correctly.	Direct observation: Observe while the client instills eye drops.
	The client identifies available resources for obtaining the necessary medication.	Oral questioning: Ask the client's family to identify how to contact the local pharmacy or community clinic to obtain the client's medications.

Medication Administration

Medication administration is an essential part of nursing practice and requires a sound knowledge base in anatomy, physiology, pathophysiology, pharmacology, psychology, and research. The following sections illustrate the steps involved in administering medications through various routes.

Oral Administration

The easiest and most desirable way to administer medications is by mouth (Skill 34-1). Clients usually are able to ingest or self-administer oral medications with few problems. Most tablets and capsules should be administered and swallowed with approximately 60 to 100 mL of fluid (as allowed). Some situations contraindicate administering medications by mouth.

The primary contraindications to giving oral medications include the presence of gastrointestinal (GI) alterations, the inability of the client to swallow food or fluids, and the use of gastric suction. An important precaution to take when administering any oral preparation is to protect clients from aspiration. Aspiration occurs when food, fluid, or medication intended for GI administration is inadvertently administered into the respiratory tract. Protect the client from aspiration by assessing the client's ability to manage oral medications. Box 34–15 describes techniques you can use to protect the client from aspirating. Properly positioning the client is also essential in preventing aspiration. Position the client in a seated position when administering oral medications, if such a position is not contraindicated by the client's condition. Having the client slightly flex the head in a chin-down position usually reduces aspiration (Metheny, 2006). Use a multidisciplinary approach (e.g., consult with a speech therapist, a dietitian, and an occupational therapist) with clients who have difficulty swallowing (Morris, 2006).

For clients with nasogastric feeding tubes, liquid medications are preferred, but some tablets can be crushed and some capsules can be opened to mix in a solution for administration (Box 34–16).

Topical Medication Applications

Topical medications are medications that are applied locally, most often to intact skin but also to mucous membranes. They are prepared in many forms, including lotions, pastes, and ointments (see Table 34–1).

Skin Applications. Because many locally applied medications, such as lotions, pastes, and ointments, cause both systemic and local effects, apply these medications with the use of gloves and applicators. Use sterile techniques if the client has an open wound.

Skin encrustation and dead tissues harbour microorganisms and block contact of the medications from the tissues to be treated. Before applying medications, clean the area to be treated thoroughly by washing the skin gently with soap and water, soaking an involved site, or locally debriding tissue (see Chapter 47).

Apply each type of topical medication according to the directions to ensure proper penetration and absorption. When applying ointments or pastes, spread the medication evenly over the involved surface and cover the area well without applying an overly thick layer. Prescribers may order a gauze dressing to be applied over the medication to prevent soiling of clothes and wiping away of the medication. Lightly spread lotions and creams onto the skin's surface; rubbing often causes irritation. Apply a liniment by rubbing it gently but firmly into the skin. After that, dust a powder lightly to cover the affected area with a thin layer. During any application, assess the skin thoroughly. When you record the administration, note the area where the medication was applied, the name of the medication, and the condition of the skin.

➤ SKILL 34-1 Administering Oral Medications

video

Delegation Considerations

The administration of oral medications cannot be delegated to unregulated care providers (UCPs). Instruct UCPs to report the occurrence of medication side effects immediately.

Equipment

- Medication cart or tray
- Disposable medication cups
- Client identification labels
- Glass of water, juice, or preferred liquid
- Drinking straw
- Pill-crushing device (optional)
- Medication administration record or computer printout

STEPS	RATIONALE
1. Check the accuracy and completeness of each medication administration record (MAR) or computer printout against the prescriber's original medication order. Check the client's name and the medication name, dosage, route, and time for administration. Copy or rewrite any portion of the MAR that is difficult to read.	• The order sheet is the most reliable source and only legal record of medications the client is to receive. Adherence to the order ensures the client receives the correct medications. Illegible MARs are a source of medication errors.
2. Assess the client for any contraindications to receiving oral medication: Is the client experiencing nausea or vomiting? Has the client received a diagnosis of bowel inflammation or reduced peristalsis? Has client undergone recent gastrointestinal (GI) surgery? Does client have gastric suction? Is the client restricted to nothing by mouth (NPO)? Check the client's reflexes for swallowing, coughing, and gagging.	• Alterations in GI function interfere with a medication's ability to be distributed, absorbed, and excreted. Clients with GI suction might not receive benefit from medications because they are suctioned from the GI tract before they can be absorbed. Clients with impaired swallowing are at risk for aspiration (Metheny, 2006).
3. Assess the client's medical history, history of allergies, medication history, and diet history. List the client's food and drug allergies on each page of the MAR and prominently display the allergies on the client's medical record. This information may also be added to an identification bracelet.	• The information reflects the client's need for medications and the potential responses to medications. Communication of the client's potential food and drug interactions and allergies is essential for safe, effective care.
4. Gather information from the client's physical examination and laboratory data that may influence medication administration (e.g., vital signs, blood glucose levels, electrolyte levels, laboratory findings related to blood clotting times and to renal and liver function).	• Physical examination or laboratory data may contraindicate medication administration. Poor liver and kidney functions affect the metabolism and excretion of medications (McKenry et al., 2006).

Critical Decision Point: If the client has any contraindications for receiving oral medications, or if you are in doubt of the client's ability to swallow oral medications, temporarily withhold medication and inform the prescriber.

STEPS	RATIONALE
5. Assess the client's knowledge regarding health and medication use.	• This assessment helps to determine the client's need for medication education and whether the client adheres to medication therapy at home. The assessment may reveal difficulties with medication use problems, such as medication intolerance, noncompliance, abuse, addiction, or dependence.
6. Assess the client's preferences for fluids. Maintain fluid restriction when applicable.	• Offering fluids during medication administration increases the client's fluid intake. Fluids ease swallowing and facilitate absorption from the GI tract. Fluid restrictions must be maintained when applicable.
7. Prepare medications:	
A. Perform hand hygiene.	• Proper hygiene reduces the transfer of microorganisms.
B. If a medication cart is used, move it to a location outside the client's room.	• Organization of equipment saves time and reduces the chance for error.
C. Unlock the medicine drawer or cart or log on to the automated medication dispensing system.	• Medications are safeguarded when locked in cabinet or cart. Storage in a locked area prevents preparation error.
D. Prepare medication for one client at a time. If you are using paper copies of the MAR, keep all pages for one client together. If you are using the client's medication administration on the computer, view only one computer screen at a time.	• Preventing distractions limits preparation errors (Pape et al., 2005).
E. Select the correct medication from a stock supply or a unit-dose drawer. Compare the label on the medication with the MAR (see Step 7E illustration) or the computer screen. Check the expiration date on all medication labels.	• Comparing the labels on the medication with the transcribed orders reduces the chance for error. *This is the first accuracy check.*
F. Calculate the medication dose as necessary. Double-check all calculations, and verify your calculations with another nurse.	• Double-checking reduces the risk of error.

➤ SKILL 34-1 Administering Oral Medications ***continued***

STEPS	RATIONALE
G. If you are preparing a controlled substance, check the client's MAR or computer record to determine the last time the medication was administered. Check the record for the previous medication count and compare the current count with the supply available.	• Checking the medication count reduces the risk of double-dosing if the client is receiving controlled substances on a "prn" schedule. • Controlled substance laws require nurses to carefully monitor and count any dispensed narcotics.
H. To prepare tablets or capsules from a floor stock bottle, pour the required number into the bottle cap and transfer the medication to a medication cap. Do not touch the medication with your fingers. Return extra tablets or capsules to the bottle. Break prescored medications. If necessary, use a gloved hand or a clean pillating device. Identify prescored tablets by looking for a line that dividesthe tablet in half.	• A clean technique is required of medication administration. Cleaning the pillating (or pill-cutting) device ensures prior medications are cleaned out of the device and cannot contaminate this tablet. To ensure that you give the accurate dose to client, split only those tablets that are prescored.
I. To prepare unit-dose tablets or capsules, place the packaged tablet or capsule directly into a medicine cup. Do not remove the wrapper (see Step 7I illustration.)	• Wrappers maintain the cleanliness of medications and allow the nurse to identify the medication name and dose at the client's bedside.

Critical Decision Point: If you are preparing narcotics, check the narcotic record for the previous drug count and compare it against the supply available. You are responsible for being aware of and upholding laws regarding the use of controlled substance.

STEPS	RATIONALE
J. Place all tablets or capsules to be given to client in one medicine cup, with the client's identification label attached, except for those medications that require preadministration assessments (e.g., pulse rate or blood pressure); keep medications in their wrappers. After medication administration, remove the client's identification label and discard the label in the appropriate confidential waste disposal receptacle.	• Labelling the client's medication cup reduces the risk of administering medications to the incorrect client. • Keeping medications that require preadministration assessments separate from other medications makes it easier for the nurse to withhold medications as necessary. • Disposing of the client's label in confidential waste receptacles is necessary to protect client confidentiality.

Critical Decision Point: Not all medications can be crushed (e.g., capsules and enteric-coated drugs). When in doubt whether a medication can be crushed, consult with your pharmacist. When pills are crushed, the client is more likely to experience choking or aspiration of particles of medication or soft food.

STEPS	RATIONALE
K. If the client has difficulty swallowing, and liquid medications are not an option, use a pill-crushing device, such as a mortar and pestle to grind the pills (see Step 7K illustration). Before using a mortar and pestle, clean them. If a pill-crushing device is not available, place the tablet inside a medication cup, place another medication cup on top of it, and press on the top cup with a blunt instrument until the pill is crushed. Mix the ground tablet in small amount of soft food (custard or applesauce).	• Large tablets can be difficult to swallow. A ground tablet mixed with palatable soft food is usually easier to swallow. Cleaning pill-crushing devices ensures that contamination of medications does not occur.

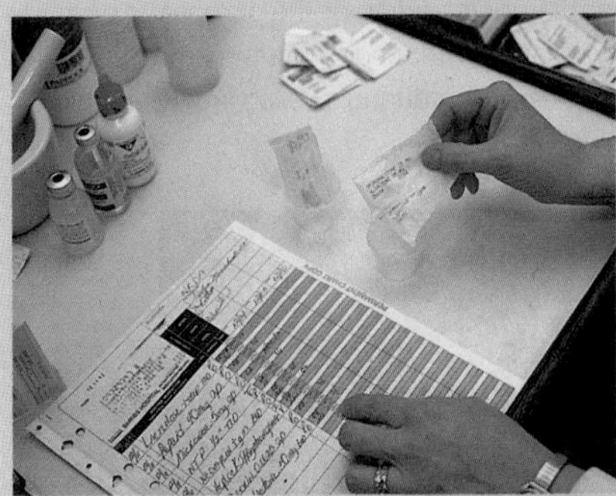

Step 7E The nurse verifies each medication with the MAR.

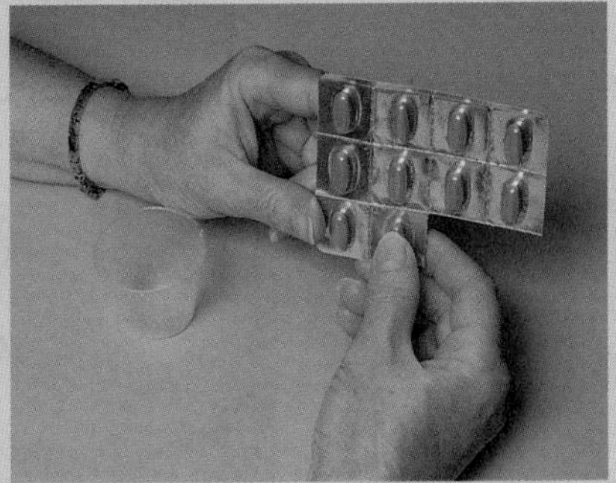

Step 7I Place tablet into medicine cup without removing wrapper.

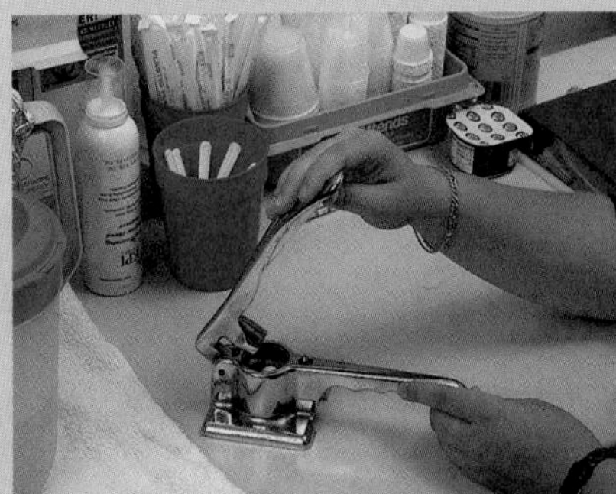

Step 7K Pill-crushing device used to crush pills when necessary.

➤ SKILL 34-1 Administering Oral Medications ***continued***

STEPS	RATIONALE
L. To prepare liquids:	
(1) Gently shake the container. If the medication is in a unit-dose container with the correct amount to administer, no further preparation is needed. If the medication is in a multidose bottle, remove the bottle cap from the container and place the cap so that the inside of the cap is not exposed.	• Shaking the container ensures the medication is mixed before administration. Correct placement of the cap of the bottle avoids contamination.
(2) Hold a multidose bottle with the label against the palm of your hand while pouring.	• Hold the bottle so that any spilled liquid will not soil or fade the label.
(3) Hold the medication cup at eye level and fill to the desired level on the scale (see Step 7L(3) illustration). The scale should be even with the fluid level at its surface or the base of the meniscus, not at its edges. Draw up volumes of less than 10 mL in a syringe without a needle (see Step 7L(3) illustration).	• Filling medication properly ensures accuracy of measurement. The use of a syringe enables greater accuracy for small doses of medication.
(4) Discard any excess liquid into a sink. Wipe the lip and neck of the multidose bottle with a paper towel.	• These steps prevent contamination of the bottle's contents and prevent the bottle cap from sticking to the counter. • Avoids unnecessary manipulation of the dose.
M. Compare the MAR, computer printout, or computer screen with the prepared medication and container.	• Reading labels a second time reduces the chance for error. *This is the second accuracy check.*
N. Return stock containers or unused unit-dose medications to the storage shelf or drawer and read the labels again.	• The *third accuracy check* of medication labels in multiple-dose containers further reduces administration errors.
O. Do not leave medications unattended.	• Nurses are responsible for the safekeeping of drugs.
8. Administering medications:	
A. Take medications to the client at the correct time.	• Medications are administered within 30 minutes before or after the prescribed time to ensure the intended therapeutic effect. Give STAT medications immediately or single-order medications at the time they are ordered.
B. Identify the client by using at least two client identifiers. Compare the client's name and one other identifier (e.g., the hospital identification number) on the MAR, computer printout, or computer screen with information on the client's identification bracelet. Ask the client to state his or her name if possible, for a third identifier.	• These steps comply with The Joint Commission's (2007) requirements and improve medication safety. In most acute care settings, the client's name and identification number on an armband and the MAR is used to identify clients. Identification bracelets are made at time of client's admission and are the most reliable source of identification. The client's room number is not an acceptable identifier.

Critical Decision Point: Replace client identification bracelets that are missing, illegible, or faded.

STEPS	RATIONALE
C. Compare labels of the medications with the MAR at the client's bedside.	• Perform a final check of medication labels against the MAR at the client's bedside to reduce medication administration errors.
D. Explain to the client the purpose of each medication and its action. Encourage the client to ask any questions about the drugs.	• The client has the right to be informed; questions often indicate the need for teaching, reveal noncompliance with therapy, or potential medication errors. A client's understanding of the purpose of each medication improves compliance with medication therapy.
E. Assist the client to a sitting position (or side-lying position if sitting is contraindicated).	• A sitting position prevents aspiration during swallowing (Metheny, 2006).

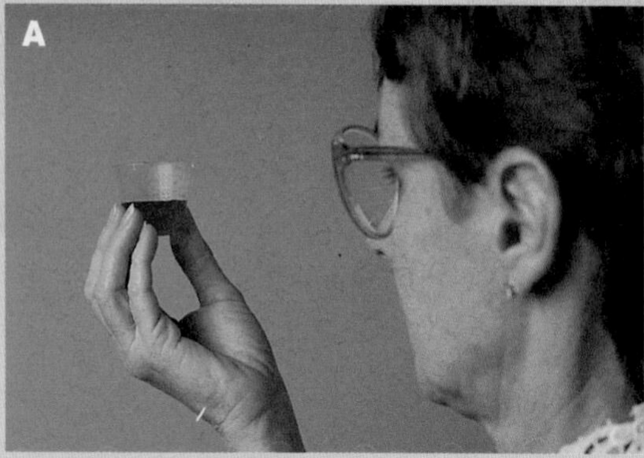

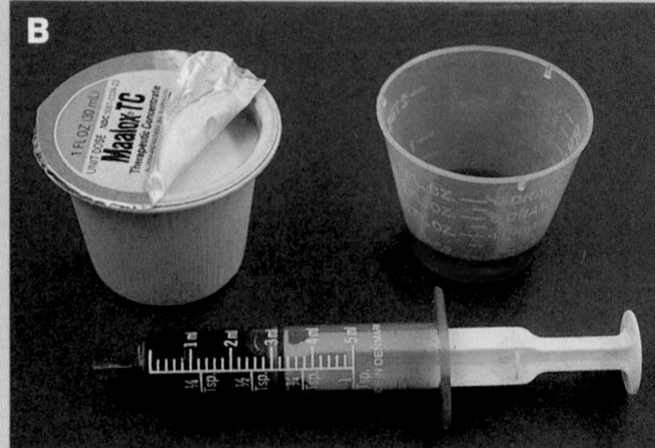

Step 7L(3) A, Pour the desired volume of liquid so that the base of the meniscus is level with the line on the scale. **B,** Use a needleless syringe to draw up volumes of less than 10 mL.

➤ SKILL 34-1 Administering Oral Medications *continued*

STEPS	RATIONALE
F. Administer medications:	
(1) *For tablets:* The client may wish to hold solid medications in the hand or in a cup before placing them in the mouth.	• The client can become familiar with medications by seeing each drug.
(2) Offer water or juice to help the client swallow the medications. Give cold carbonated water if it is available and not contraindicated.	• Offering a choice of fluids promotes the client's comfort and can improve fluid intake. Carbonated water helps passage of the tablet through the esophagus.
(3) *For sublingual-administered medications:* Have the client place the medication under the tongue and allow it to dissolve completely (see Figure 34–4). Caution the client against swallowing the tablet.	• Medication is absorbed through the blood vessels of the undersurface of the tongue. If medication is swallowed, it is destroyed by gastric juices or detoxified by the liver so rapidly that therapeutic blood levels are not attained.
(4) *For buccal medications:* Have the client place the medication in the mouth against the mucous membranes of the cheek until it dissolves (see Figure 34–5). Avoid administering liquids until the buccal medication has dissolved.	• Buccal medications act locally on mucosa or systemically as they are swallowed in saliva.
(5) *For powdered medications:* Mix with liquids at bedside and give to the client to drink.	• When prepared in advance, powdered medications may thicken and even harden, which makes swallowing difficult.
(6) Caution the client against chewing or swallowing lozenges.	• Medication acts through slow absorption through oral mucosa, not gastric mucosa.
(7) Give effervescent powders and tablets immediately after they have dissolved.	• Effervescence improves the unpleasant taste of the medication and often relieves GI problems.
G. If the client is unable to hold medications in the hand or in a cup, place the medication cup to the client's lips and gently introduce each drug into the mouth, one at a time. Do not rush.	• Administering a single tablet or capsule eases swallowing and decreases the risk of aspiration.
H. If a tablet or capsule falls to the floor, discard it and repeat the preparation.	• Medication is contaminated when it touches floor.
I. Stay at the bedside until the client has completely swallowed each medication. If you are uncertain whether the medication was swallowed, ask the client to open the mouth.	• You are responsible for ensuring the client receives the ordered dose. If left unattended, the client may not take the dose or may save medications, which could cause a risk to health.
J. For highly acidic medications (e.g., aspirin), offer the client a nonfat snack (e.g., crackers) if it is not contraindicated by the client's condition.	• A nonfat snack reduces the possible gastric irritation from highly acidic medication.
K. Assist the client in returning to a comfortable position.	• The client's comfort is maintained.
L. Dispose of soiled supplies and perform hand hygiene.	• Proper disposal reduces the transmission of microorganisms.
M. Replenish the stock, such as cups and straws. If a medication cart was used, return the cart to the medication room. Clean the work area.	• A clean and organized work space helps other staff to complete their duties efficiently.
9. Evaluate the client's response to medications at times that correlate with the medication's onset, peak, and duration.	• You can evaluate the medication's therapeutic benefit and detect the onset of side effects or allergic reactions.
10. Ask the client or the client's family member to identify the medication name and explain the purpose, action, dosage schedule, and potential side effects of the drug.	• You can determines the level of knowledge gained by the client and the client's family.

Unexpected Outcomes and Related Interventions

Adverse Effects (e.g., Side Effects, Toxic Effects, Allergic Reactions)

- Symptoms such as urticaria, rash, pruritus, rhinitis, and wheezing may indicate an allergic reaction.
- Withhold further doses, and add allergy information to the client's medical record.
- Always notify the prescriber and the pharmacy when the client exhibits adverse effects.

Client Refuses Medication

- Explore reasons why the client does not want the medication.
- If misunderstandings of the medication therapy are apparent, address the misconceptions by educating the client.
- Do not force the client to take the medication; clients have the right to refuse treatment.
- If the client continues to refuse medication despite your attempts to educate, record on client's chart why the drug was withheld and notify the prescriber.

Continued

➤ SKILL 34-1 Administering Oral Medications *continued*

Recording and Reporting

- Record the administration of oral medications on the computerized or paper copy of the medication administration record immediately after administering the medications. If you are using a paper copy of the medication administration record, include your initials or signature.
- Record the reason any drug was withheld and follow the agency's policy for proper recording.
- Record and report your evaluation of the medication's effect to the prescriber if required (e.g., report urine output following administration of a diuretic if ordered by the prescriber).

Home Care Considerations

- To ensure safe medication administration at home, instruct clients on all aspects of medication administration, including dosage, desired effect, when to take the medications, proper storage of the medications, anticipated side effects, and whether to take medication with or without food.
- Evaluate the client's ability to safely self-administer medications. If the client needs assistance in self-administration, introduce nursing interventions, such as a chart or pillbox. If interventions fail and the client still is unable to safely administer medications, notify the prescriber.

Some topical medications are applied in the form of a transdermal patch that remains in place for an extended period of time (e.g., 12 hours or 7 days). Many patches are clear, which makes them difficult to see. Nurses and clients may inadvertently leave old transdermal patches in place, which results in the client receiving an overdose ot the medication. Therefore, carefully assess the client's skin and ensure that you remove the existing patch before applying a new patch. The following guidelines are used to ensure safe administration of transdermal or topical medications (Institute for Safe Medication Practices, 2007):

1. Document on the medication administration record or computer record the area where the medication was applied.
2. When applying a transdermal patch, ask the client whether he or she has an existing patch.
3. Do not assume that a patch has fallen off or has been already been removed. Assess the skin thoroughly before administering the medication.
4. When taking a medication history or reconciling medications, specifically ask the client whether he or she takes any medications in the forms of patches, topical creams, or any route other than the oral route.
5. If the dressing or patch is difficult to see (e.g., it is clear), apply a noticeable label to the patch.
6. Document removal of the patch or medication on the medication administration record or computer record.

➤ BOX 34-15 Protecting the Client From Aspiration

- Determine the client's ability to swallow.
- Assess the client's cough.
- Determine the presence of a gag reflex.
- Prepare oral medications in the form that is easiest for the client to swallow.
- Allow the client to self-administer medications if possible.
- If the client has unilateral weakness, place the medication in the stronger side of the mouth.
- Administer pills one at a time, ensuring that each pill is properly swallowed before the next one is introduced.
- Thicken regular liquids or offer fruit nectars if the client cannot tolerate thin liquids.
- Have the client hold and drink from a cup if possible.
- When possible, medications should be timed to coincide with mealtimes or when the client is well rested and awake.
- Administer medications through another route if risk of aspiration is severe.

Nasal Instillation. Clients with nasal sinus alterations may receive medications by spray, drops, or tampons (Box 34–17). The most commonly administered form of nasal instillation is a decongestant spray or drops, which are used to relieve symptoms of sinus congestion and colds. Caution clients to avoid abuse of medications because overuse can lead to a rebound effect in which the nasal congestion worsens. When excess decongestant solution is swallowed, serious systemic effects can develop, especially in children. Saline drops are safer as a decongestant for children than nasal preparations that contain sympathomimetics (e.g., Afrin or Neo-Synephrine).

Self-administering sprays is easier because the client can control the spray and inhale as it enters the nasal passages. For clients who use nasal sprays repeatedly, check the nares for irritation. Position clients to permit the medication to reach the affected sinus.

Eye Instillation. Common eye medications used by clients are eye drops and ointments, including over-the-counter preparations, such as artificial tears and vasoconstrictors (e.g., Visine and Murine). Many clients receive prescribed **ophthalmic** medications for eye conditions, such as glaucoma, and after cataract extraction. In older adults, the ease with which eye medications can be self-administered can be affected by gerontological changes, including poor vision, hand tremors, and difficulty grasping or manipulating containers. Instruct clients and their family members about the proper techniques for administering eye medications (Skill 34–2). Determine the ability of the client and the client's family members to administer the eye medication by demonstrating the procedure. Showing clients each step of the procedure for instilling eye drops can improve their compliance. Follow these principles when administering eye medications:

- The cornea of the eye is richly supplied with pain fibres and thus is very sensitive to anything applied to it. Avoid instilling any form of eye medication directly onto the cornea.
- The risk of transmitting infection from one eye to the other is high. Avoid touching the eyelids or other eye structures with eyedroppers or ointment tubes.
- Use eye medication only for the client's affected eye.
- Never allow a client to use another client's eye medications.

Intraocular Administration. Some medications are administered intraocularly (see Skill 34–2). **Intraocular** medications resemble a contact lens. Place the medication into the conjunctival sac, where it remains in place for up to 1 week. Medications such as pilocarpine are administered this way. You will need to teach the client about monitoring for adverse reactions to the disc. Clients will also need to be taught how to insert and remove the disc.

Ear Instillation. Internal ear structures are very sensitive to temperature extremes. Failure to instill ear drops or irrigating fluid at room temperature may cause vertigo (severe dizziness) or nausea. Although the structures of the outer ear are not sterile, sterile drops and solutions are used in case the eardrum is ruptured. The entrance of nonsterile solutions into middle ear structures can result in infection. If the client has ear drainage, assess the ear to ensure the client does not have a ruptured eardrum. Never occlude the ear canal with the dropper or an irrigating syringe. Forcing medication into an occluded ear canal creates pressure that will injure the eardrum. Box 34–18 provides guidelines for administering ear drops and ear irrigations and describes the differences in straightening the ear canal for children and adults.

The external ear structures of children differ from those of adults. When instilling drops or irrigating solutions, you must first straighten the ear canal. In infants and young children, straighten the cartilaginous canal by grasping the auricle of the ear and pulling it gently down and backward. In adults, the ear canal is longer and composed of underlying bone. The adult ear canal is straightened by pulling the auricle upward and outward. Failure to straighten the canal properly may prevent medicinal solutions from reaching the deeper external ear structures.

➤ BOX 34-16 Procedural Guidelines

Giving Medications Through a Nasogastric Tube, Intestinal Tube, Gastrostomy Tube, or Small-Bore Feeding Tube

Delegation Considerations: The administration of medications through a nasogastric tube, intestinal tube, gastrostomy tube, or small-bore feeding tube cannot be delegated. Instruct unregulated care providers to report the occurrence of side effects immediately.

Equipment:
- 60-mL syringe (catheter tip for large-bore tubes, Luer-Lok tip for small-bore tubes)
- Gastric pH test strips (scale of 0.0 to 11.0 or 14.0 preferred)
- Graduated container
- Water
- Medication to be administered
- Pill crusher, if medication is in tablet form
- Medication administration record
- Clean gloves

Procedure
1. Check the accuracy and completeness of each medication administration record against the prescriber's written medication order. Check the client's name, the drug name and dosage, and the route and time of administration.
2. Investigate and, if possible, use alternative routes of medication administration (e.g., intravenous, transdermal, rectal).
3. Avoid complicated medication regimens that frequently interrupt enteral feedings.
4. Prepare medication (see Skill 34–1, Steps 7A–G and M–O). Check the label of the medication with the medication administration record three times.
5. Avoid giving elixirs or medications that have a pH of less than 4.
6. Verify the medication is compatible with enteral feeding. If the medication is incompatible with the feeding, stop the feeding 1 to 2 hours before giving medication, and restart the feeding 1 to 2 hours after the medication is given. Never add medications directly to a feeding tube. Before administering a medication, determine if it needs to be given on an emply stomach or if it is compatible with the enteral feeding. The amount of time the enteral feeding needs to be held before administration varies with the medication. Verify the amount of the time that you hold a feeding with agency policy or with a pharmacist.
7. Verify tube placement before administering medications (see Chapter 43).
8. Administer medications in a liquid form (suspension, elixir, or solution) when possible to prevent tube obstruction.
9. Before crushing tablets, ensure they are crushable. Buccal, sublingual, enteric-coated, or sustained-release medications cannot be crushed. Read medication labels carefully before crushing a tablet or opening a capsule.
10. Take medications to the client at the correct time and perform hand hygiene.
11. Identify the client by using at least two client identifiers. Compare the client's name and one other identifier (e.g., the hospital identification number) on the identification bracelet with the medication administration record. Ask the client to state his or her name if possible, for a third identifier.
12. Compare the labels on the medications against the medication administration record one more time at the client's bedside.
13. Explain the procedure and the medications to the client.
14. Dissolve crushed tablets, gelatin capsules, and powders in 15–30 mL of warm water. Dissolve each medication separately.
15. Do not give whole or undissolved medications through the feeding tube.
16. Put on clean, disposable gloves.
17. Verify the placement of any tube that enters the mouth or nose by using pH testing (see Chapter 43).
18. Assess gastric residual (see Chapter 43).
19. Draw up medication in syringe. Do not mix medications together.
20. Connect the syringe with medication to a nasogastric tube, G-tube, J-tube, or small-bore feeding tube. Do not use the pigtail vent for irrigation or instillation of fluid.
21. Administer medication either by pushing the medication through the tube by depressing the plunger of the syringe or by allowing the medication to flow into the body freely by using gravity. Administer each medication separately.
22. Flush the tube with 15–30 mL of warm water between each medication. Unless contraindicated, the total amount of liquid volume administered to the client is approximately 60 mL.
23. After giving all the medications, flush the tube once more with 30–60 mL of warm water.
24. Remove gloves and perform hand hygiene.
25. Document administration of medications on the medication administration record.
26. Continually evaluate the client's response to medication therapy. If the desired effect is not achieved, a different medication or a different route of administration may be indicated because of problems with the drug bioavailability when given by the enteral route.

Adapted from Jordan, S., Griffiths, H., & Griffin, R. (2003). Administration of medicines. II. Pharmacology. *Nursing Standard, 18*(3), 45–55.

➤ BOX 34-17 **Procedural Guidelines**

Administering Nasal Instillations

Delegation Considerations: The administration of nasal drops and ointments cannot be delegated. Instruct unregulated care providers to report the occurrence of medication side effects immediately.

Equipment:

- Prepared medication with a clean dropper or spray container
- Facial tissue
- Small pillow (optional)
- Washcloth (optional)
- Clean, disposable gloves (if client has extensive nasal drainage)
- Medication administration record
- Penlight (to inspect nares; if ointment is to be applied to a specific lesion inside the nares)

Procedure

1. Check the accuracy and completeness of each medication administration record (MAR) or computer printout against the prescriber's original medication order. Check the client's name and the medication name, dosage, route, and time for administration. Copy or rewrite any portion of the MAR that is difficult to read.
2. If nasal drops are to be administered, refer to the medical record to determine which sinus is affected, so that you can position the client appropriately for drug instillation.
3. Assess the client's medical history (e.g., cardiovascular disease, hyperthyroidism). Medical conditions can contraindicate the use of decongestants that stimulate the central nervous system. Side effects may occur, such as transient hypertension, tachycardia, palpitations, and headache.
4. List the client's food and drug allergies on each page of the MAR and prominently display the allergies on the client's medical record as per agency policy. Determine whether the client has any allergies to medications delivered via nasal instillation.
5. Review the physician's order, including the client's name and the medication name, dosage, route, time of administration, and indication.
6. Take the medication to the client at the correct time and perform hand hygiene. Using a penlight, inspect the condition of the nose and sinuses. Palpate sinuses for tenderness.
7. Assess the client's knowledge regarding the use of nasal instillations and the technique for instillation, and determine whether the client is willing to learn self-administration.
8. Prepare the medication (see Skill 34–1, Steps 7A–G, M–O). Ensure you compare the label of the medication against the MAR at least two times while preparing the medications.
9. Identify the client by using at least two identifiers. Compare the client's name and one other identifier (e.g., the hospital identification number) on the MAR, computer printout, or computer screen with information on the client's identification bracelet. Ask the client to state his or her name if possible, for a third identifier.
10. Compare the MAR with the medication labels at the client's bedside.
11. Explain the procedure to the client regarding the positioning and the sensations to expect, such as a burning or stinging of the mucosa, or a choking sensation as the medication trickles into the throat.
12. Arrange the supplies and medications at the bedside. Put on gloves if the client has nasal drainage.
13. Gently roll or shake the medication container.
14. Instruct the client to clear or blow the nose gently unless contraindicated (e.g., risk of increased intracranial pressure or nosebleeds). Clearing the nose helps to remove mucus and secretions that can block medication distribution.
15. Administer nasal drops:
    A. Assist the client to a supine position and position the head properly to facilitate access to the nasal passages.
        (1) To access the posterior pharynx, tilt the client's head backward.
        (2) To access the ethmoid and sphenoid sinuses, tilt the head back over the edge of the bed or place a small pillow under the client's shoulder and tilt the head back (see Step 15A(2) illustration).
        (3) To access the frontal and maxillary sinuses, tilt the head back over the edge of the bed or pillow with the head turned toward the side to be treated (see Step 15A(3) illustration). This position will allow the medication to drain into the affected sinus.
    B. Support the client's head with your nondominant hand to prevent the straining of neck muscles.
    C. Instruct the client to breathe through the mouth, which reduces the chance of aspirating nasal drops into the trachea and lungs.
    D. Hold the dropper 1 cm above the nares to avoid contamination of the dropper. Instill the prescribed number of drops toward midline of the ethmoid bone to facilitate distribution of medication over the nasal mucosa.
    E. Have the client remain in a supine position for 5 minutes to prevent premature loss of medication through the nares.
    F. Offer a facial tissue to blot a runny nose, but caution the client against blowing the nose for several minutes.

➤ BOX 34-17 **Procedural Guidelines** ***continued***

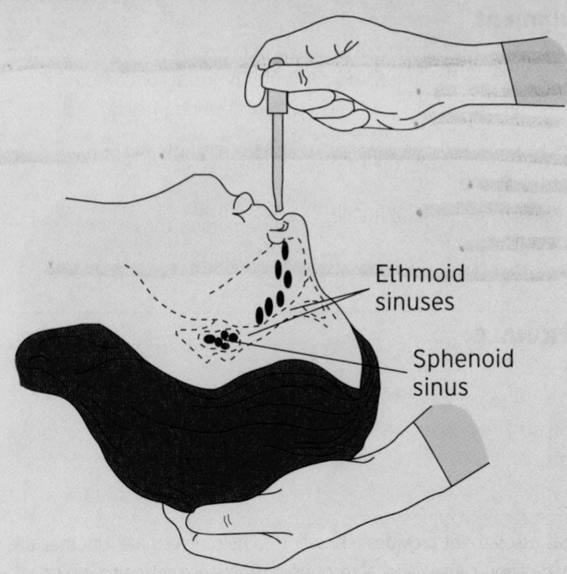

Step 15A(2) Position for instilling nose drops into the ethmoid and sphenoid sinuses.

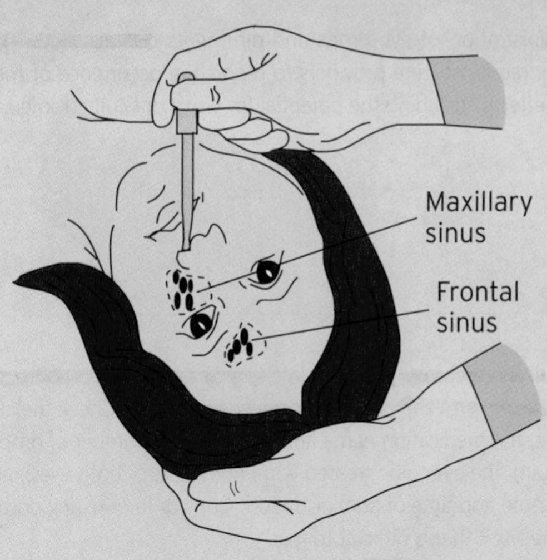

Step 15A(3) Position for instilling nose drops into the frontal and maxillary sinuses.

16. Assist the client to a comfortable position after the medication is absorbed.
17. Administering nasal spray:
    A. Assist the client to comfortable high Fowler's position or a sitting position.
    B. Administer the nasal spray with the client's head upright. Tipping the opening of the nasal spray container downward will cause the medication to be administered in a stream, not a spray, and will deliver more medication than the prescribed order.
    C. Offer a facial tissue to blot a runny nose, but caution the client against blowing the nose for several minutes.
18. Dispose of soiled supplies in the proper container and perform hand hygiene.
19. Document administration of medication on the MAR or in the computer.
20. Observe the client for the onset of side effects 15–30 minutes after administration. Drugs absorbed through mucosa can cause a systemic reaction.
21. Ask whether the client is able to breathe through the nose after decongestant administration to determine the drug's effectiveness. Sometimes the client will need to occlude one nostril at a time and breathe deeply.
22. Evaluate the client's response to the medications at times that correlate with the medication's onset, peak, and duration. Evaluate the client for both desired effects and adverse effects. Reinspect the condition of the nasal passages between the instillations.
23. Ask the client to review the risks of overuse of decongestants and methods for administration.
24. Have the client demonstrate self-medication.

➤ SKILL 34-2 Administering Ophthalmic Medications

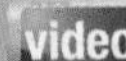

Delegation Considerations

The administration of eye drops and ointments cannot be delegated. Instruct unregulated care providers to report the occurrence of medication side effects, including the potential for visual difficulty, immediately.

Equipment

- Medication bottle with sterile eyedropper, ointment tube, or medicated intraocular disc
- Cotton ball or tissue
- Washbasin filled with warm water and washcloth if eyes have crust or need drainage
- Eye patch and tape (optional)
- Clean gloves
- Medication administration record (MAR) or computer printout

STEPS	RATIONALE
1. Check the accuracy and completeness of each MAR or computer printout against the prescriber's medication order. Check the client's name, the medication name and dosage (e.g., number of drops, if a liquid), the eye to be treated (e.g., right, left, or both eyes), and the route and time of administration. Copy or rewrite any portion of the MAR that is difficult to read.	
2. Assess the condition of the client's external eye structures. (This may also be assessed just before drug instillation.)	• This assessment provides a baseline to help determine whether the medication causes a local response. The assessment also indicates the need to clean the eye before medication application.
3. Determine whether the client has any known allergies to eye medications. Also ask whether the client has an allergy to latex.	
4. Determine whether the client has any symptoms of visual alterations.	• Certain eye medications act to either decrease or increase these symptoms. Determining the client's visual alteration status ensures that you are able to recognize a change in client's condition after the medication is administered.
5. Assess the client's level of consciousness and ability to follow directions.	• A client who becomes restless or combative during the procedure is at a greater risk of accidental eye injury.
6. Assess the client's knowledge regarding medication therapy and the desire to self-administer medication.	
7. Assess the client's ability to manipulate and hold an eye dropper.	
8. Prepare medication (see Skill 34–1, Steps 7A–G and M–O): Ensure that you check the label of the medication against the MAR at least two times while preparing the medication.	
9. Take the medication to the client at the correct time and perform hand hygiene.	
10. Identify the client by using at least two client identifiers. Compare the client's name and one other identifier (e.g., the hospital identification number) on the MAR, computer printout, or computer screen with information on client's identification bracelet. Ask the client to state his or her name if possible, for a third identifier.	
11. Compare labels of medications with the MAR or computer printout at the client's bedside.	
12. Arrange the medication supplies at the bedside and put on clean gloves. If eye drops are stored in the refrigerator, allow them to reach room temperature before instilling them.	• The use of gloves reduces the transmission of microorganisms and follows standards to prevent accidental exposure to body fluids. Warming the eye drops reduces irritation to the eye.
13. Gently roll the container.	• Rolling the container ensures the medication is mixed before administration. Shaking the bottle causes bubbles, which makes medication administration difficult.
14. Explain the procedure to the client, including the positioning and sensations to expect, such as burning or stinging.	
15. Ask the client to lie supine or to sit back in a chair with the head slightly hyperextended.	• This position provides easy access to the eye for medication instillation and minimizes drainage of medication through the tear duct.

Critical Decision Point: Do not hyperextend the neck of a client who has a cervical spine injury.

➤ SKILL 34-2 Administering Ophthalmic Medications *continued*

STEPS	RATIONALE
16. If crusts or drainage are present along the eyelid margins or the inner canthus, gently wash them away. Soak any crusts that are dried and difficult to remove by applying a damp washcloth or cotton ball over the eye for a few minutes. Always wipe from the inner canthus to the outer canthus.	• Crusts or drainage harbours microorganisms. Soaking allows easy removal of the crusts and prevents pressure from being applied directly over the eye. Cleansing from the inner canthus to the outer canthus avoids entrance of microorganisms into the lacrimal duct.
17. Hold a cotton ball or clean tissue in your nondominant hand on the client's cheekbone just below the lower eyelid.	• Cotton or tissue absorbs the medication that escapes the eye.
18. With the tissue or cotton resting below the lower lid, gently press downward with your thumb or forefinger against the bony orbit.	• This technique exposes the lower conjunctival sac. Retraction against the bony orbit prevents pressure and trauma to the eyeball and prevents your fingers from touching the eye.
19. Ask the client to look at the ceiling and explain the steps to the client.	• When the client looks toward the ceiling, this action retracts the sensitive cornea up and away from the conjunctival sac and reduces stimulation of the blink reflex.
A. Instill the eye drops:	
(1) With your dominant hand resting on the client's forehead, hold the filled medication eyedropper or the ophthalmic solution approximately 1–2 cm above the conjunctival sac (see Step 19A(1) illustration).	• This technique helps to prevent accidental contact of the eyedropper with eye structures, thus reducing risk of both injury to the eye and transfer of infection to dropper. Ophthalmic medications are sterile.
(2) Instill the prescribed number of medication drops into the conjunctival sac.	• The conjunctival sac normally holds 1 or 2 drops, which provides even distribution of medication across the eye.
(3) If the client blinks or closes the eye, or if the drops land on the outer lid margins, repeat the procedure.	• The client obtains the therapeutic effect of the drug only when the eyedrops enter the conjunctival sac.
(4) After instilling the drops, ask the client to close the eye gently.	• Closing the eye helps to distribute the medication. Squinting or squeezing of eyelids forces medication from the conjunctival sac (VisionRx, 2005).
(5) When administering medications that cause systemic effects, apply gentle pressure with your finger and a clean tissue on the client's nasolacrimal duct for 30–60 seconds.	• This action prevents both the overflow of medication into the nasal and pharyngeal passages and the absorption of the medication into the systemic circulation.
B. Instill eye ointment:	
(1) Ask the client to look at the ceiling.	• This action retracts the sensitive cornea up and away from the conjunctival sac and reduces stimulation of the blink reflex.
(2) Hold the ointment applicator above the lower lid margin, apply a thin stream of ointment evenly along the inner edge of the lower eyelid on the conjunctiva (see Step 19B(2) illustration) from the inner canthus to outer canthus.	• This technique distributes the medication evenly across the eye and lid margin.
(3) Have the client close the eye and use a cotton ball to rub the lid lightly in a circular motion, if rubbing is not contraindicated.	• This action further distributes the medication without traumatizing the eye.

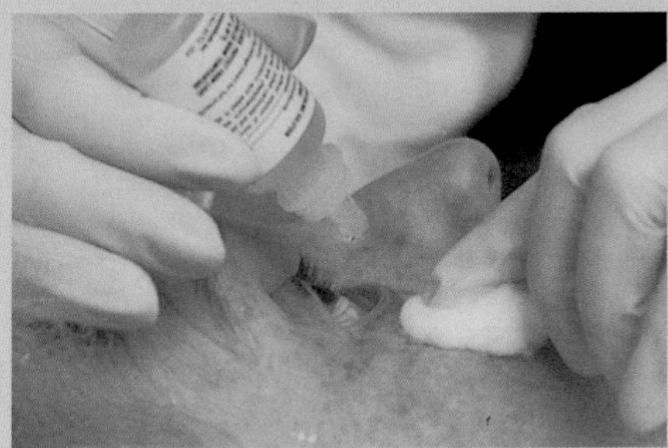

Step 19A(1) Hold the eyedropper above the conjunctival sac.

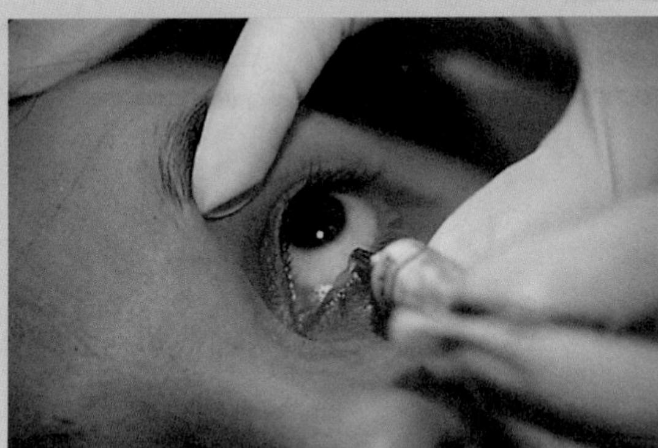

Step 19B(2) Apply ointment along the lower eyelid.

Continued

➤ SKILL 34-2 Administering Ophthalmic Medications *continued*

STEPS	RATIONALE
C. Intraocular disc	
(1) Application:	
(a) Open the package containing the disc. Gently press your fingertip against the disk so that it adheres to your finger. Position the convex side of the disc on your fingertip (see Step 19C(1)(a) illustration).	• These actions allow you to inspect the disc for damage or deformity.
(b) With your other hand, gently pull the client's lower eyelid away from the eye. Ask the client to look up.	• This action prepares the conjunctival sac for receiving the medicated disc.
(c) Place the disc in the conjunctival sac, so that it floats on the sclera between the iris and the lower eyelid (see Step 19C(1)(c) illustration).	• This placement ensures delivery of the medication.
(d) Pull the client's lower eyelid out and over the disc (see Step 19C(1)(d) illustration).	• This action ensures accurate medication delivery.

Critical Decision Point: You should not be able to see the disc at this time. If you can see the disc, repeat step 19C(1)d.

STEPS	RATIONALE
(2) Removal:	
(a) Perform hand hygiene and put on gloves.	
(b) Explain the procedure to the client.	
(c) Gently pull on the client's lower eyelid to expose the intraocular disc.	
(d) Using your forefinger and thumb of the opposite hand, pinch the disc and lift it out of the client's eye (see Step 19C(2)(d) illustration).	
20. If excess medication is on the eyelid, gently wipe it from the inner canthus to outer canthus.	• Wiping away of excess medication promotes the client's comfort and prevents trauma to eye (Vision Rx, 2005).
21. If the client wears an eye patch, apply a clean patch by placing it over the affected eye so that the entire eye is covered. Tape securely without applying pressure to eye.	• A clean eye patch reduces the chance of infection.

Critical Decision Point: If the client receives more than one eye medication to the same eye at the same time, wait at least 5 minutes before administering the next medication to avoid interaction between medications (Vision Rx, 2005).

STEPS	RATIONALE
22. If the client receives eye medication to both eyes at the same time, use a different tissue or cotton ball for each eye.	• The use of separate tissues or cotton balls prevents cross-contamination between eyes.
23. Remove gloves, dispose of soiled supplies in proper receptacle, and perform hand hygiene.	
24. Note the client's response to instillation; ask whether the client felt any discomfort.	• The client's response determines whether the procedure was performed correctly and safely and whether the client is experiencing adverse effects of the medication.
25. Observe the client's response to the medication by assessing any visual changes and noting any side effects.	
26. Ask the client to discuss the medication's purpose, action, side effects, and the technique of administration.	
27. Have the client demonstrate self-administration of the next dose.	

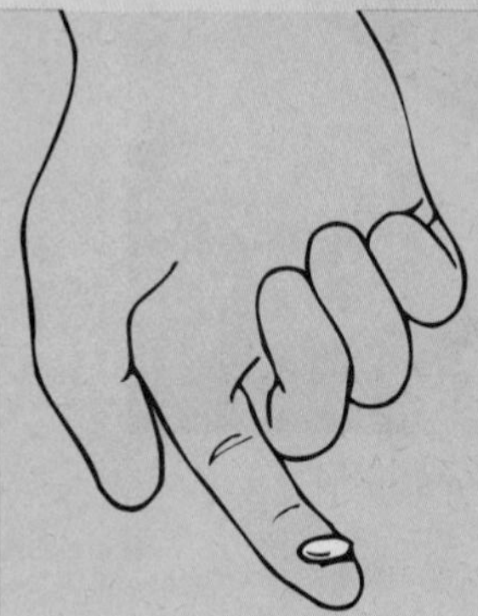

Step 19C(1)(a) Gently position the convex side of the disc against your fingertips.

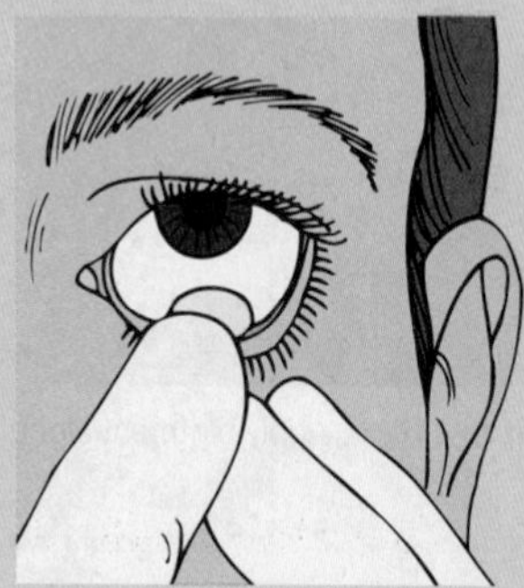

Step 19C(1)(c) Place the disc in the conjunctival sac between the iris and the lower eyelid.

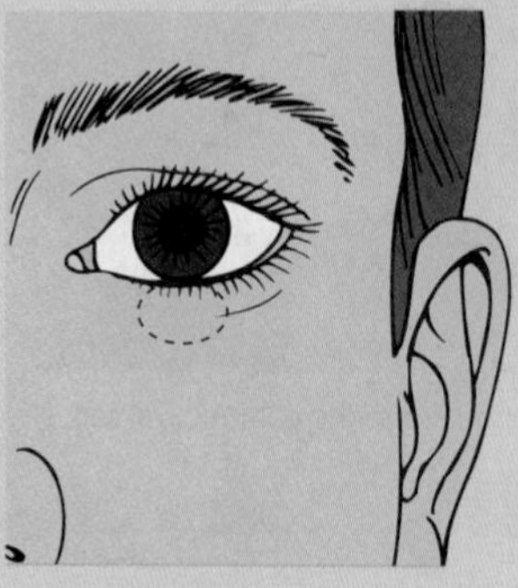

Step 19C(1)(d) Gently pull the lower eyelid over the disc.

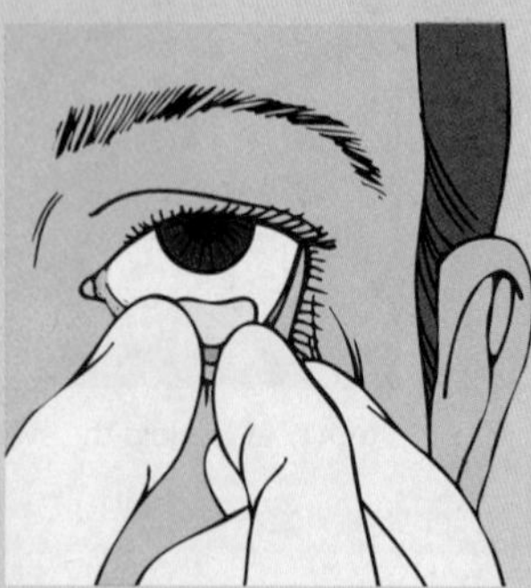

Step 19C(2)(d) Carefully pinch the disc to remove it from the client's eye.

➤ SKILL 34-2 **Administering Ophthalmic Medications** *continued*

Unexpected Outcomes and Related Interventions

Inability of Client to Instill Drops Without Supervision

- Reinforce your teaching and allow the client to self-administer drops as often as possible to enhance confidence.
- If the client cannot self-administer drops, teach others, such as family members, to instill drops into the client's eye.

Signs of Reaction to Medication, Such as Allergic Reaction (e.g., Tearing, Reddened Sclera) or Systemic Response (e.g., Bradycardia)

- Follow the institutional policy or guidelines for the reporting of adverse or allergic reaction to medications.
- Notify the client's health care professional immediately, and withhold further administration of the medication.
- Add information about the allergy to the client's medical record, according to agency policy.

Recording and Reporting

- Document on the MAR or the computer record the medication, concentration, number of drops, time of administration, and the eye (left, right, or both) that received medication.
- Record the appearance of the eye in the nurses' notes.

Home Care Considerations

- Clients with chronic health care problems should consult with their health care professional before they use over-the-counter eye medication.
- When they use eye drops at home, clients should not share medications with other family members because the risk of infection transmission is high.

➤ BOX 34-18 **Procedural Guidelines**

Administering Ear Medications

Delegation Considerations: The administration of ear medications cannot be delegated. Instruct unregulated care providers about the potential side effects of ear medications and the need to report their occurrence immediately.

Equipment:

- Medication administration record (MAR)
- Clean gloves if client has drainage from the ear
- Medication bottle with dropper, cotton-tipped applicator, and cotton ball (optional) if ear drops are being administered
- Irrigating syringe, kidney-shaped basin, and towel if ear is to be irrigated

Procedure

1. Check the accuracy and completeness of each MAR or computer printout against the prescriber's original medication order. Check the client's name and the medication name, dosage, route, and time for administration. Copy or rewrite any portion of the MAR that is difficult to read.
2. Prepare the medication. Ensure that you compare the label of the medication against the MAR at least two times during the medication preparation.
3. Take the medication to the client at the correct time and perform hand hygiene. Put on gloves if drainage is present.
4. Identify the client by using at least two client identifiers. Compare the client's name and one other identifier (e.g., the hospital identification number) on the MAR, computer printout, or computer screen with information on the client's identification bracelet. Ask the client to state his or her name if possible, for a third identifier.
5. Compare the label on the medication with the MAR one more time at the client's bedside. *This is the third accuracy check.*
6. Explain the procedure to the client regarding positioning and the sensations to expect, such as hearing bubbling or feeling water in the ear as medication trickles into the ear.
7. Teach the client about the medication.
8. Administer the ear drops:
   A. Have the client assume a side-lying position (if this position is not contraindicated by client's condition) with the ear to be treated facing up. Alternatively, the client may sit in a chair or at the bedside.
   B. Perform hand hygiene. Put on gloves if drainage is present.
   C. Straighten the ear canal by pulling the auricle down and back (for children under 3 years of age) or upward and outward (for adults).
   D. Hold the dropper 1 cm above the ear canal and instill the prescribed drops (see Step 8D illustration).

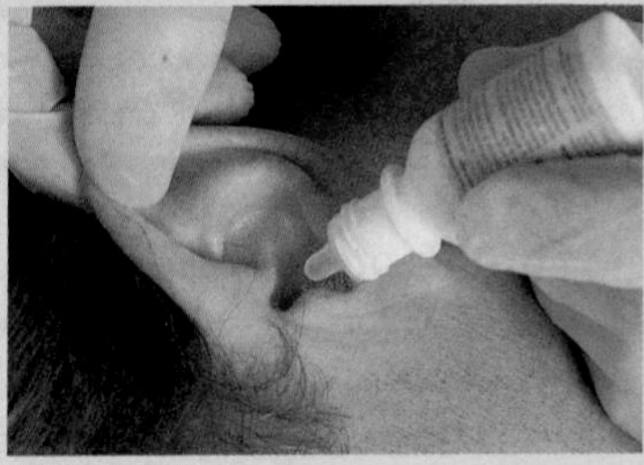

Step 8D Placing ear drop in ear.

   E. Ask the client to remain in a side-lying position for 2–3 minutes. Apply gentle massage or pressure to the tragus of the ear with your finger unless contraindicated due to pain.
   F. If a cotton ball is needed, place the cotton ball into the outermost part of the ear canal. Do not press cotton deep into the canal. Remove cotton after 15 minutes.
9. Administer ear irrigations:
   A. Assess the tympanic membrane or review the medical record for a history of eardrum perforation, which would contraindicate ear irrigation.
   B. Assist the client in assuming a sitting or lying position with the head tilted or turned toward the affected ear. Place a towel under the client's head and shoulder and have the client hold a kidney-shaped basin under the affected ear.
   C. Perform hand hygiene. Put on gloves if drainage is present.
   D. Fill the irrigating syringe with approximately 50 mL of the solution.
   E. Gently grasp the auricle and straighten the ear canal by pulling it down and back (for children under 3 years of age) or upward and outward (for children 4 years of age and older and adults).
   F. Slowly instill the irrigating solution by holding the tip of the syringe 1 cm above the opening of the ear canal. Allow the fluid to drain out during instillation. Continue until the canal is clean or until all solution is used.
10. Clean the work area and put the medication supplies away.
11. Remove gloves and perform hand hygiene.
12. Document medication administration on the MAR or computer record.
13. Evaluate the client's response to the medication.

Vaginal Instillation. Vaginal medications are available as suppositories, foam, jellies, and creams. Suppositories are individually packaged in foil wrappers and are sometimes stored in a refrigerator to prevent the solid, oval-shaped suppositories from melting. After a suppository is inserted into the vaginal cavity, body temperature causes it to melt and be distributed and absorbed. Foam, jellies, and creams are administered with an applicator inserter (Box 34–19). Give a suppository with a gloved hand in accordance with standard precautions and routine practices (see Chapter 33). Clients often prefer administering their own vaginal medications, which requires privacy. After instillation of the medication, a client may wish to wear a perineal pad to collect the drainage. Because vaginal medications are often given to treat infection, the discharge may be foul smelling. Follow aseptic techniques and offer the client frequent opportunities to maintain her perineal hygiene (see Chapter 38).

Rectal Instillation. Rectal suppositories are thinner and more bullet-shaped than vaginal suppositories. The rounded end prevents anal trauma during insertion. Rectal suppositories contain medications that exert local effects, such as promoting defecation, or systemic effects, such as reducing nausea. Rectal suppositories are usually stored in the refrigerator until administered.

During administration, place the suppository past the internal anal sphincter and against the rectal mucosa (Box 34–20). Otherwise, the suppository may be expelled before it can dissolve and be absorbed into the mucosa. With practice, you learn to recognize the sensation of the sphincter relaxing around the finger. Do not force the suppository into a mass of fecal material. If necessary, clear the rectum with a small cleansing enema before inserting a suppository.

Administering Medications by Inhalation

Medications administered by handheld inhalers are dispersed through an aerosol spray, mist, or powder that penetrates the lung airways. The alveolocapillary network absorbs medications rapidly. **Metered-dose inhalers (MDIs)**, dry powder inhalers (DPIs), and slow-stream inhaler devices usually produce local effects, such as bronchodilatation; however, some medications can lead to serious systemic side effects.

Clients who receive medications by inhalation frequently have chronic respiratory disease, such as chronic asthma, emphysema, or bronchitis. Medications given by inhalation provide these clients with control of their airway obstruction. Inhaled medications are often described as "rescue" or "maintenance" medications. Rescue medications are short-acting medications that are taken for immediate relief of acute respiratory distress. Maintenance inhalers are used on a daily scheduled basis to prevent acute respiratory distress. The effects of maintenance inhalers start within hours of administration and last for a longer period of time than rescue inhalers. Because these clients depend on these medications for disease control, they must learn about the inhalers and how to administer them safely (Skill 34–3). If a client uses more than one type of inhaler, the bronchodilator is given first.

A metered-dose inhaler (MDI) delivers a measured dose of medication with each push of the canister. Chemical propellants (e.g., hydrofluorocarbons) push the medication out of the MDI. MDIs are either squeeze-and-breathe inhalers or are inhalers activated by the client's breath. The squeeze-and-breathe MDI requires the application of approximately 2 to 5 kg of pressure to the top of the canister to administer the medication. To use this type of MDI, the client must have hand strength, which often diminishes as a result of aging or the effects of chronic respiratory disease. Lack of sufficient hand strength can restrict the client's ability to self-administer medication via MDIs. Breath-activated MDIs release the medication when the client inhales. Release of the medication is dependent on the strength of the client's breath on inspiration (Capriotti, 2005). The MDI can be used with a spacer to allow the particles of medication to slow down and break into smaller pieces, which improves the drug's absorption in the client's airway. Spacers are equipped with a facemask when they are used by infants and children younger than 4 years of age. Spacers are especially helpful for clients who have difficulty coordinating the steps involved in self-administering inhaled medications. When clients do not use their inhalers and spacers correctly, they do not receive the full effect of the medication. Therefore, client education is essential.

Dry powder inhalers (DPIs) hold dry, powdered medication and create an aerosol when the client inhales through a reservoir that contains a dose of the medication. DPIs require less manual dexterity than MDIs, and because the device is activated by the client's breath, the client does not need to coordinate puffs with inhalation, as required when an MDI is used. DPIs do not require use of a spacer; however, the medication inside the DPI may clump if the DPI is used in a humid climate, and some clients cannot inspire at the speed needed to administer the entire dose of the medication.

One important aspect of client teaching is to help the client determine when the MDI or DPI is empty and needs to be replaced. Floating the MDI to determine the amount of medication remaining is no longer recommended because extra propellant may cause buoyancy even if no medication remains in the inhaler. Furthermore, MDIs with hydrofluoroalkanes (HFA) should never be immersed (Capriotti, 2005). Some DPIs have mechanisms that indicate the number of doses remaining; however, these mechanisms are not always accurate. To calculate how long the medication in an MDI or DPI will last, divide the capacity of the canister by the number of doses the client takes per day. For example, a client is to take albuterol, a β-adrenergic agonist bronchodilator. The ordered dose is 2 puffs 4 times a day. The canister has a total of 200 puffs. Complete the following calculations to determine how long the MDI will last:

$$2 \text{ puffs} \times 4 \text{ times a day} = 8 \text{ puffs per day}$$
$$200 \text{ puffs} \div 8 \text{ puffs per day} = 25 \text{ days}$$

The canister in this example will last 25 days. To ensure the client does not run out of medication, teach the client to refill the medication prescription at least 7 to 10 days before it is expected to run out (MayoClinic.com, 2007).

Administering Medications by Irrigations

Some medications irrigate or wash out a body cavity and are delivered through a stream of solution. Irrigations most commonly use sterile water, saline, or antiseptic solutions to irrigate the eye, ear, throat, vagina, or urinary tract. Use aseptic technique if the client has a break in the skin or mucosa. When the cavity to be irrigated is not sterile, as in the case of the ear canal (see Box 34–18) or vagina, use a clean technique. In health care settings, sterile solutions are usually used. Irrigations are used to clean an area, instill a medication, or apply heat or cold to injured tissue.

Administering Parenteral Medications

Parenteral administration of medications is the administration of medications by injection. Parenteral administration is an invasive procedure that must be performed with aseptic techniques (Box 34–21). After a needle pierces the skin, the client is at risk of infection. Each type of injection requires the application of specific skills to ensure the medication reaches the proper location. The effects of a parenterally administered medication develop rapidly, depending on the rate of medication absorption. Always closely observe the client's response.

➤ BOX 34-19 **Procedural Guidelines**

Administering Vaginal Medications

Delegation Considerations: The administration of medications by the vaginal route cannot be delegated. Instruct unregulated care providers to report new or increased vaginal discharge or bleeding and occurrence of potential side effects of the medications immediately.

Equipment:

- Vaginal cream, foam, jelly, or suppository, or irrigating solution with applicator (if required)
- Clean, disposable gloves
- Towels, or a washcloth, or both
- Paper towels
- Perineal pad
- Drape or sheet
- Water-soluble lubricating jelly
- Medication administration record (MAR) or computer printout

Procedure

1. Check the accuracy and completeness of each MAR or computer printout against the prescriber's original medication order. Check the client's name and the medication name, form (cream, foam, jelly, or suppository), route, dosage, time of administration, and drug indication.
2. Review the client's history of allergies, including allergies to latex. Prepare the medication (see Skill 34–1, Steps 7A–G and M–O). Compare the label of the medication with the MAR two times while preparing the medication.
3. Take the medication to the client at the correct time and perform hand hygiene.
4. Identify the client by using at least two client identifiers. Compare the client's name and one other identifier (e.g., the hospital identification number) on the MAR, computer printout, or computer screen with information on the client's identification bracelet. Ask the client to state his or her name if possible, for a third identifier.
5. Allow the client to empty or attempt to empty her bladder before administration of vaginal medication. To facilitate adequate absorption, the client needs to lie quietly for at least 10 minutes.
6. Compare the label on the medication with the MAR one more time at the client's bedsidse.
7. Teach the client about the medication. Explain to the client the procedure for positioning and the sensations she can expect, such as feelings of moisture or wetness in the vaginal area. Assess the client's ability to manipulate the applicator or suppository and to position herself to insert the medication. Explain the procedure to the client. If the client plans to self-administer the medication, be specific in your explanation.
8. Close the room curtain or door and arrange the supplies at the bedside.
9. Assist the client to lie in a dorsal recumbent position. This position provides full exposure and easy access to the vaginal canal and allows the suppository to dissolve without escaping through an orifice.
10. Put on clean, disposable gloves.
11. Keep the abdomen and lower extremities draped.
12. Ensure the lighting is adequate to visualize the vaginal opening. Inspect the condition of external genetalia and the vaginal canal, noting the appearance of any discharge. Clean the area with a towel or washcloth if necessary.
13. Insert the vaginal suppository:
    A. Remove the suppository from its foil wrapper. Apply a liberal amount of sterile water-based lubricating jelly to the smooth or rounded end of the suppository. Lubricate the gloved index finger of your dominant hand.
    B. With your nondominant gloved hand, expose the vaginal orifice by gently retracting the labial folds.
    C. With your dominant gloved hand, gently insert the rounded end of the suppository along the posterior wall of the vaginal canal for the entire length of your finger (7.5–10 cm) to ensure equal distribution of the medication along the walls of the vaginal cavity (see Step 13C illustration).
    D. Withdraw your finger and wipe any remaining lubricant from around the orifice and labia.
14. Administer the cream or foam:
    A. Fill the cream or foam applicator, as described on the package directions.
    B. With your nondominant gloved hand, expose the vaginal orifice by gently retracting the labial folds.
    C. With your dominant gloved hand, insert the applicator approximately 5–7.5 cm. Push the applicator plunger to deposit the medication into the vagina to allow equal distribution of medication (see Step 14C illustration).
    D. Withdraw the applicator and place it on a paper towel. Wipe residual cream from the labia or vaginal orifice.
15. Dispose of supplies, remove gloves, and perform hand hygiene.
16. Instruct the client to remain on her back for at least 10 minutes.
17. Document the medication administration on the MAR or computer record.
18. If the applicator was used, wear gloves to wash it with soap and warm water, rinse, and store for future use.
19. Offer the client a perineal pad when she resumes ambulation to prevent vaginal discharge from spreading to clothing.
20. Inspect the appearance of discharge from the vaginal canal and the condition of external genitalia between applications to evaluate the medication's effectiveness.

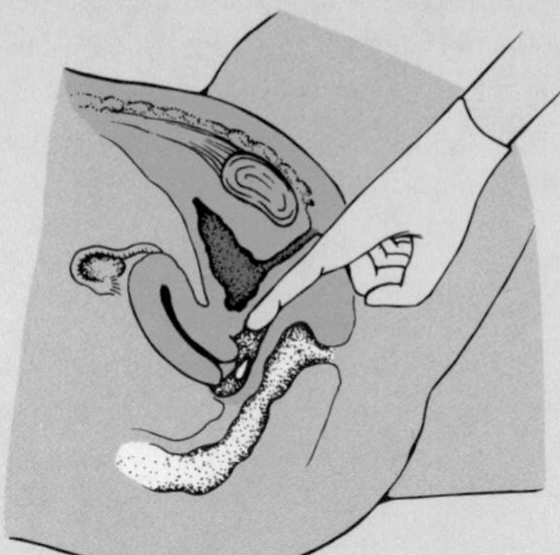

Step 13C Insertion of a suppository into the vaginal canal.

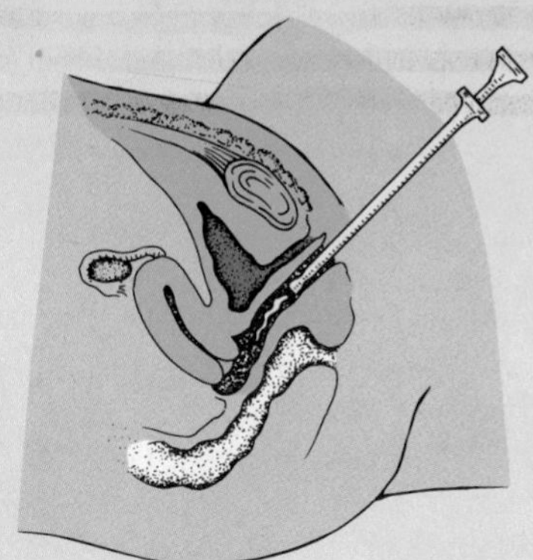

Step 14C Instillation of medication in the vaginal canal.

➤ BOX 34-20 **Procedural Guidelines** 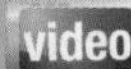

Administering Rectal Suppositories

Delegation Considerations: The administration of medications by the rectal route cannot be delegated. Instruct unregulated care providers to expect and report fecal discharge or a bowel movement and to report the occurrence of potential side effects or medications immediately.

Equipment:

- Rectal suppository
- Water-soluble lubricating jelly
- Clean gloves (two pair)
- Drape or sheet
- Tissue
- Medication administration record (MAR) or computer printout

Procedure

1. Check the accuracy and completeness of each MAR or computer printout against the prescriber's original medication order. Check the client's name and the medication name, route, dosage, and time of administration. Copy or rewrite any portion of the MAR that is difficult to read.
2. Review the medical record for information on rectal surgery, bleeding, and for a history of allergies.
3. Prepare medication (see Skill 34–1, Steps 7A–G and M–O). Ensure that you compare the label of the medication with the MAR two times during medication preparation.
4. Take the medication to the client at the correct time and perform hand hygeine.
5. Identify the client by using at least two client identifiers. Compare the client's name and one other identifier (e.g., the hospital identification number) on the MAR, computer printout, or computer screen with information on the client's identification bracelet. Ask the client to state his or her name if possible, for a third identifier.
6. Compare the label of the medication with the MAR or computer printout one more time at the client's bedside.
7. Teach the client about the medication. Explain the procedure to the client regarding the positioning and the sensations to expect, such as feelings of needing to defecate. Ensure that the client understands the procedure and he or she can self-administer the medication.
8. Close the room curtain or door and arrange supplies at the bedside.
9. Put on clean gloves.
10. Assist the client in assuming Sims' position to expose the anus and facilitate relaxation of the external anal sphincter. Keep the client draped with only the anal area exposed.
11. Ensure the lighting is adequate to visualize the anus. Check for evidence of active rectal bleeding. Examine the condition of the anus externally and palpate the rectal walls to assess for presence of feces, which may interfere with the suppository placement (see Chapter 32). Dispose of gloves in proper receptacle if they are soiled.
12. Put on a new pair of disposable gloves (if previous gloves were discarded).
13. Remove the suppository from its wrapper and lubricate the rounded end (see Step 13 illustration) with a sterile water-soluble lubricating jelly to reduce the friction when the suppository enters the rectal canal. Lubricate the index finger of your dominant hand with a water-soluble lubricant.

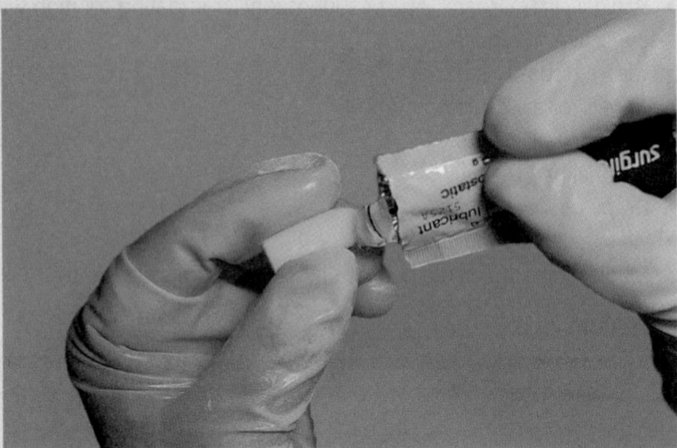

Step 13 Remove the suppository from its wrapper.

14. Ask the client to take slow deep breaths through the mouth and relax the anal sphincter.
15. Retract the buttocks with your nondominant hand. Insert the suppository gently through the anus, past the internal sphincter and against the rectal wall, 10 cm in adults, 5 cm in children and infants. Apply gentle pressure to hold the buttocks together momentarily if necessary to keep medication in place and to facilitate medication distribution and absorption.
16. Withdraw your finger and wipe the anal area with tissue.
17. Remove gloves and dispose of medication supplies in the appropriate receptacle and perform hand hygiene.
18. Ask the client to remain flat or on the side for 5 minutes to prevent expulsion of the suppository.
19. If the suppository contains a laxative or fecal softener, place a call light within the client's reach.
20. Document medication administration on the MAR or computer record.
21. Evaluate the effectiveness of the medication by observing the client for a response to the suppository (e.g., bowel movement, relief of nausea) at times that correlate with the medication's onset, peak, and duration.

➤ SKILL 34-3 Using Metered-Dose or Dry Powder Inhalers

Delegation Considerations

The administration of a metered-dose inhaler (MDI) or dry powder inhaler (DPI) and the supervision of clients who self-administer these medications cannot be delegated to unregulated care providers (UCPs). Instruct UCPs to report changes in the client's respiratory status, increased coughing, or the occurrence of potential side effects immediately.

Equipment

- MDI or DPI
- Spacer (optional with MDI)
- Facial tissues (optional)
- Washbasin or sink with warm water
- Paper towel
- Medication administration record (MAR) or computer printout

STEPS	RATIONALE
1. Check the accuracy and completeness of each MAR or computer printout against the prescriber's original medication order. Check the client's name and the medication name, route, dosage, and time of administration. Copy or rewrite any portion of the MAR that is difficult to read.	
2. Assess the client's respiratory pattern, auscultate the client's breath sounds.	• Assessment of the client's respiratory pattern establishes the baseline of airway status for comparison during and after treatment.
3. If the client has been previously instructed in self-administration, assess the client's technique in using the inhaler.	
4. Assess the client's ability to hold, manipulate, and depress the canister. Assess the client's strength of inhalation.	• Any impairment in the ability to grasp, to breathe, or to coordinate movements interferes with the client's ability to use the MDI or DPI correctly.
5. Assess the client's readiness to learn: for example, whether the client asks questions about the medication, disease, or complications; requests education in use of inhaler; is mentally alert; participates in self-care.	• The client's readiness to learn affects the ability to understand explanations and actively participate in the learning process (Bastable, 2003).
6. Assess the client's ability to learn: the client should not be fatigued, in pain, or in respiratory distress; assess the client's level of understanding of technical terms.	• The client's mental or physical limitations affect the ability to learn and the methods you can use for instruction (Bastable, 2003).
7. Assess the client's knowledge and understanding of the disease and the purpose and action of the prescribed medications.	• Knowledge of disease is essential for the client to understand the proper use of the inhaler.
8. Determine the medication schedule and the number of inhalations prescribed for each dose.	• The medication schedule influences the explanations you provide for use of inhaler.
9. Prepare the medication (see Skill 34–1, Steps 7A–G and M–O). Ensure that you compare the label of the medication with the MAR two times during medication preparation.	
10. Identify the client by using at least two client identifiers. Compare the client's name and one other identifier (e.g., the hospital identification number) on the MAR, computer printout, or computer screen with information on the client's identification bracelet. Ask the client to state his or her name if possible, for a third identifier.	
11. Compare the label on medications with the MAR one more time at the client's bedside.	
12. Instruct the client in a comfortable environment by sitting in a chair in the hospital room or by sitting at a kitchen table in the client's home.	• The client will be more likely to remain receptive to education if he or she is in a comfortable environment (Bastable, 2003).
13. Provide adequate time for the teaching session.	
14. Perform hand hygiene and arrange the equipment needed.	
15. Allow the client an opportunity to manipulate the inhaler, the canister, and the spacer device. Explain and demonstrate how the canister fits into the inhaler.	• Manipulating the various items facilitates the client's familiarity with the equipment.

Critical Decision Point: If the client is using an MDI with or without a spacer and the inhaler is new or has not been used for several days, push a "test spray" into the air (MayoClinic.com, 2007). A test spray is not needed for a DPI.

STEPS	RATIONALE
16. Explain to the client what a metered dose is and warn the client about overuse of the inhaler, including medication side effects.	• The client must not arbitrarily administer excessive inhalations because of the risk of serious side effects. If medication is given in recommended doses, side effects are uncommon.

Continued

➤ SKILL 34-3 Using Metered-Dose or Dry Powder Inhalers *continued*

STEPS	RATIONALE
17. Explain the steps for administering squeeze-and-breathe inhaled dose of medication of MDI (demonstrate steps when possible):	• Use of simple, step-by-step explanations allows the client to ask questions at any point during the procedure.
A. Insert the MDI canister into the holder.	
B. Remove the mouthpiece cover from the inhaler.	
C. Shake the inhaler vigorously five or six times.	• Shaking the inhaler ensures that fine particles are aerosolized.
D. Have the client take a deep breath and exhale.	• A deep breath followed by an exhalation empties the lungs and prepares the client's airway to receive the medication.
E. Instruct the client to position the inhaler in one of two ways.	
(1) Close the mouth around the MDI with the opening toward the back of the throat (see Step 17E(1) illustration).	
(2) Position the device 2–4 cm in front of the mouth (see Step 17E(2) illustration).	• This position directs the aerosol spray toward the airway. Positioning the mouthpiece in front of mouth is considered the best way to deliver the medication.
F. With the inhaler properly positioned, have client hold the inhaler with thumb at the mouthpiece and the index finger and middle finger at the top. This arrangement is called a three-point or lateral hand position.	• MDIs work best when clients use a three-point or lateral hand position to activate the canister.
G. Instruct the client to tilt the head back slightly and inhale slowly and deeply through the mouth for 3–5 seconds while depressing the canister fully.	• Medication is distributed to airways during inhalation. Inhalation through the mouth rather than than nose draws medication more effectively into airways.
H. Instruct the client to hold the breath for approximately 10 seconds.	• Holding the breath allows tiny drops of aerosol spray to reach the deeper branches of the airways.
I. Instruct the client to remove the MDI from the mouth and to exhale through pursed lips.	• Using pursed lips keeps the small airways open during exhalation.
18. Explain the steps to administer MDI by using a spacer, such as an AeroChamber (demonstrate when possible):	
A. Remove the mouthpiece cover from the MDI and the mouthpiece of the spacer. Inspect the spacer for foreign objects. If the spacer has a valve, ensure the valve is intact.	
B. Insert the MDI into the end of the spacer.	• The spacer traps medication released from the MDI; the client then inhales the drug from the device. These devices break up and slow down the medication particles, enhancing the amount of medication received by the client (Vella and Grech, 2005).
C. Shake the inhaler vigorously five or six times.	• Shaking the enhaler ensures the fine particles are aerosolized.
D. Have the client exhale completely before closing the mouth around the mouthpiece of the spacer. Avoid covering small exhalation slots with the lips (see Step 18D illustration).	• An exhalation empties the lungs and prepares them for the medication.
E. Have the client depress the medication canister, spraying one puff into the spacer.	• The spacer emits a spray that allows finer particles to be inhaled. Large droplets are retained in the spacer.
F. Instruct the client to inhale deeply and slowly through the mouth for 3–5 seconds.	• Deep inhalations maximize the amount of medication that enters the lungs.
G. Instruct the client to hold the breath for 10 seconds.	• Holding the breath ensures full medication distribution.
H. Instruct the client to remove the MDI and spacer before exhaling.	• Removing the MDI and spacer allows the client to exhale normally.

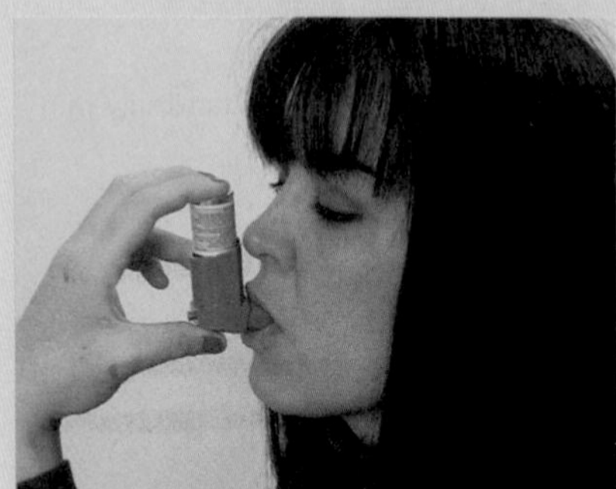

Step 17E(1) The client opens lips and places inhaler in mouth with opening toward back of throat.

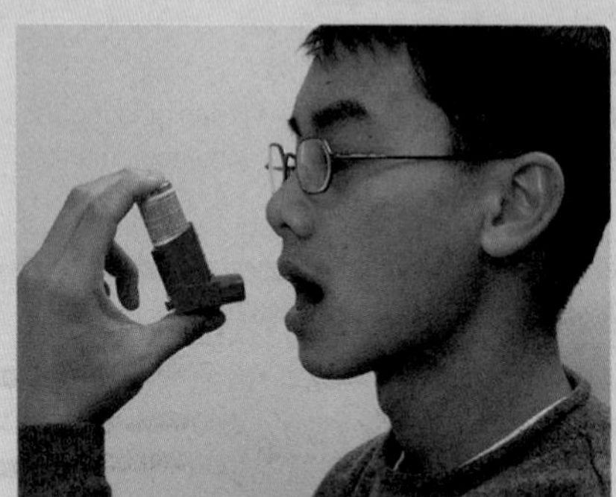

Step 17E(2) The client positions the mouthpiece 2 to 4 cm away from the mouth. This placement is considered the best way to deliver the medication.

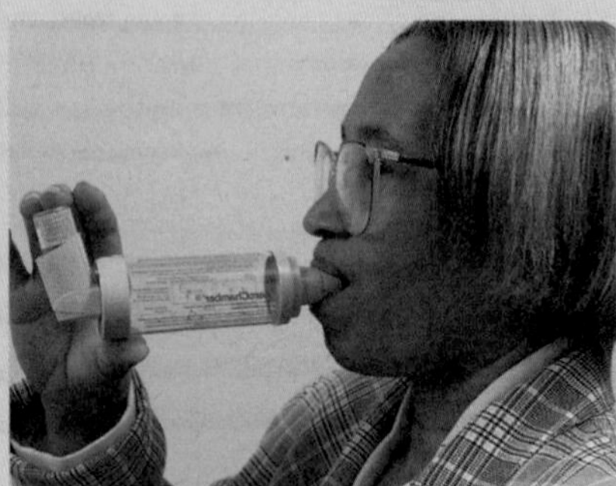

Step 18D Have the client place the mouthpiece in the mouth and close the lips, being careful to keep the exhalation slots exposed.

➤ SKILL 34-3 Using Metered-Dose or Dry Powder Inhalers *continued*

STEPS	RATIONALE
19. Explain the steps to administer DPI or breath-activated MDI (demonstrate when possible):	
A. Remove the cover from the mouthpiece. Do not shake the inhaler.	
B. Prepare the medication as directed by the manufacturer (e.g., hold the inhaler upright and turn the wheel to the right and then to the left until a click is heard, load the medication pellet, etc.).	• Preparing the medication properly primes the inhaler to ensure the medication will be delivered to the client (Capriotti, 2005).
C. Instruct the client to exhale away from the inhaler before inhalation.	• Exhaling before using the inhaler prevents loss of powder.
D. Position the mouthpiece between the client's lips.	• Properly positioning the mouthpiece prevents the medication from escaping through the mouth.
E. Instruct the client to inhale deeply and forcefully through the mouth.	• Deep inhalations create aerosol.
F. Instruct the client to hold the breath for 5–10 seconds.	• Holding the breath ensures full medication distribution.
20. Instruct the client to wait at least 20–30 seconds between inhalations of medications.	• Medications must be inhaled sequentially. The first inhalation opens the airways and reduces inflammation. The second or third inhalation penetrates the deeper airways.

Critical Decision Point: If two medications are to be administered, give the bronchodilator first.

STEPS	RATIONALE
21. Instruct the client against repeating inhalations before the next scheduled dose.	• Medications are prescribed at intervals during the day to provide constant drug levels and minimize side effects. β-Adrenergic MDIs are used either on an "as needed" basis or regularly every 4–6 hours.
22. Explain that the client may feel a gagging sensation in the throat caused by droplets of medication on the pharynx or tongue.	• The client should be aware of the results when the inhalant is sprayed incorrectly and inhaled incorrectly.

Critical Decision Point: If the client uses a corticosteroid, have the client rinse the mouth with water or salt water, or brush teeth after inhalation to reduce risk of fungal infection. Teach the client to inspect the oral cavity daily for redness, sores, or white patches. Report abnormal assessment findings to the client's health care professional (Capriotti, 2005).

STEPS	RATIONALE
23. Instruct the client in cleaning the inhaler:	
A. Once a day, the inhaler and its cap should be rinsed in warm running water. The inhaler must be completely dry before use.	• Accumulation of spray around the mouthpiece can interfere with proper distribution during use.
B. Twice a week, the L-shaped plastic mouthpiece should be washed with mild dishwashing soap and warm water. Rinse and dry well before placing the canister back inside the mouthpiece (Canadian Lung Association, n.d.).	• Regular cleaning removes residual medication. Do not place inhalers holding cromolyn, nedocromil, or HFA (hydrofluoroalkane) in water.
24. Ask whether the client has any questions.	• The client has an opportunity to clarify misconceptions or misunderstandings.
25. Have the client explain and demonstrate the steps in the use of an inhaler.	• A return demonstration provides feedback for measuring the client's learning.
26. Ask the client to explain the medication schedule, side effects, and when to call health care professionals.	• Reviewing the medication requirements improves the likelihood of compliance with the therapy.
27. Ask the client to calculate how many days the inhaler will last.	• This calculation helps the client to determine when to reorder a prescription.
28. After the medication has been taken, assess the client's respiratory status, including the ease of respirations, auscultation of lungs, and the use of pulse oximetry to assess the client's oxygenation status.	• Assessment of the respiratory status determines the status of the client's breathing pattern and adequacy of ventilation.

Unexpected Outcomes and Related Interventions

Need for a Bronchodilator More Frequently Than Every 4 Hours

- Respiratory problems are indicated. The type of medication and delivery methods need to be reassessed. Notify the health care professional if respiratory status does not improve.

Cardiac Dysrhythmias, Especially in Client Receiving β-Adrenergics

- If the client experiences symptoms with the dysrhythmias (e.g., lightheadedness, syncope), withhold all further doses of medication and notify the prescriber.

Inability of Client to Self-Administer Medication Properly

- Explore alternative delivery routes or alternative methods of medication administration.

Paroxysms of Coughing

- Aerosolized particles irritate the posterior pharynx. Notify the prescriber; reassess the type of medication or the delivery method.

Recording and Reporting

- Document the skills that you taught the client and the client's ability to perform these skills.
- Document on the MAR or computer record the medication, time of administration, and number of puffs.
- Report any undesirable effects from the medication.

Home Care Considerations

- Remind clients to carry their prescribed inhalers to use immediately in case of an acute asthma attack.

➤ BOX 34-21 Preventing Infection During an Injection

- To prevent contamination of the solution, draw the medication from the ampule quickly. Do not allow it to stand open.
- To prevent needle contamination, avoid letting the needle touch a contaminated surface (e.g., the outer edges of the ampule or vial, the outer surface of the needle cap, your hands, a countertop, a table surface).
- To prevent syringe contamination, avoid touching the length of the plunger or the inner part of the barrel. Keep the tip of the syringe covered with a cap or needle.
- To prepare the skin, wash skin soiled with dirt, drainage, or feces with soap and water and then dry. Use friction and a circular motion to clean the skin with an antiseptic swab. Swab from centre of site and move outward in a 5-cm radius.

Equipment. A variety of syringes and needles are available, each designed to deliver a precise volume of medication to a specific type of tissue. Use your nursing judgement when determining the syringe or needle that will be most effective.

Syringes. Syringes consist of a a close-fitting plunger and a cylindrical barrel with a tip designed to fit the hub of a hypodermic needle. Syringes, in general, are classified as being Luer-Lok or non–Luer-Lok. This nomenclature is based on the design of the syringe's tip. Luer-Lok syringes (Figure 34–14A) require special needles, which are twisted onto the tip and lock in place. This design prevents the inadvertent removal of the needle. Non–Luer-Lok syringes (Figure 34–14B–D) require needles that slip onto the tip. In clinical settings, all syringes now have safety devices to prevent needle-stick injuries.

Fill the syringe by aspiration, by pulling the plunger outward while the needle tip remains immersed in the prepared solution. You may handle the outside of the syringe barrel and the handle of the plunger. To maintain sterility, avoid letting any unsterile object touch the tip or the inside of the barrel, the hub, the shaft of the plunger, or the needle (Figure 34–15).

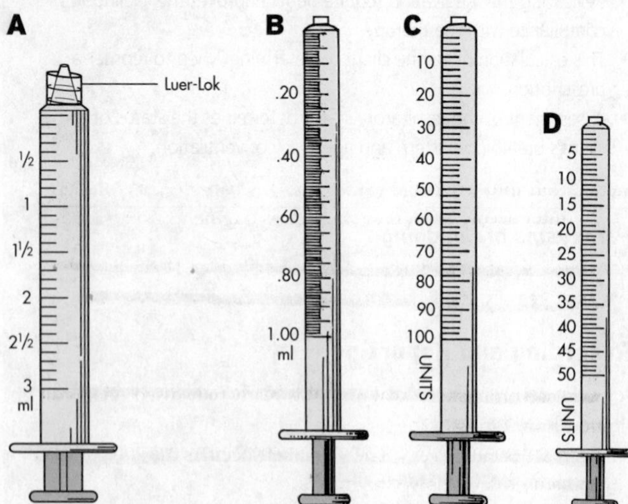

Figure 34-14 Types of syringes. A, Luer-Lok syringe marked in 0.1 (tenths). B, Tuberculin syringe marked in 0.01 (hundredths) for doses of less than 1 mL. C, Insulin syringe marked in units (100). D, Insulin syringe marked in units (50).

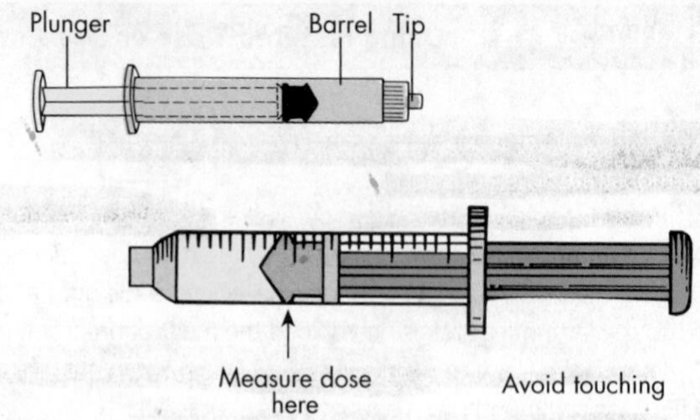

Figure 34-15 Parts of a syringe.

Syringes come in numerous sizes, from 0.5 mL to 60 mL. A 1- to 3-mL syringe is usually adequate for a subcutaneous or intramuscular injection. The use of a syringe larger than 5 mL is unusual for an injection. The larger volume creates discomfort. Instead, use larger syringes to administer certain intravenous medications, to add medications to intravenous solutions, and to irrigate wounds or drainage tubes. Syringes may be prepackaged with a needle attached; however, you may change the needle size depending on the route of administration and the size of the client.

Insulin syringes (see Figure 34–14C and D) are available in sizes from 0.3 mL to 1 mL and are calibrated in units. Insulin syringes that hold 0.3 mL are known as low-dose syringes (30 units per 0.3 mL). Most insulin syringes are known as U-100s and are designed to be used with insulin that has a strength of U-100. Each millilitre of U-100 insulin contains 100 units of insulin.

The tuberculin syringe (see Figure 34–14B) has a long, thin barrel with a preattached thin needle. The syringe is calibrated in sixteenths of a minim and in hundredths of a millilitre and has a capacity of 1 mL. Use a tuberculin syringe to prepare small amounts of medications (e.g., intradermal or subcutaneous injections). A tuberculin syringe is also useful when preparing small, precise doses for infants or young children.

Needles. Needles are packaged in individual sheaths to allow flexibility in choosing the right needle for a client. Some needles are preattached to standard-sized syringes. Most needles are made of stainless steel and are disposable.

The needle has three parts: the hub, which fits onto the tip of a syringe; the shaft, which connects to the hub; and the bevel, or slanted tip (Figure 34–16). The tip of a needle, or the bevel, is always slanted. The bevel creates a narrow slit when it is injected into tissue. When the needle is removed, the slit quickly closes to prevent leakage of medication, blood, or serum. Long bevelled tips are sharper and narrower to minimize discomfort to the client when entering tissue used for subcutaneous or intramuscular (IM) injections.

Needles vary in length from 0.6 to 7.6 cm (Figure 34–17). Choose the needle length according to the client's size and weight and the type of tissue into which the medication is to be injected. In general, a child or slender adult requires a shorter needle. Use longer needles (2.5 to 3.8 cm) for intramuscular injections and use a shorter needle (1 to 1.6 cm) for subcutaneous injections.

Needle diameter is measured by gauge. As the gauge becomes smaller, the needle diameter becomes larger (see Figure 34–17). Gauge selection depends on the viscosity of fluid to be injected or infused. An intramuscular injection usually requires an 18- to 27-gauge needle, depending on the viscosity of the medication. Subcutaneous injections require small-diameter needles, such as a 25-gauge needle. A 26-gauge needle is used for an intradermal injection.

Bevel
Gauge number
25
Shaft
Hub

Figure 34-16 Parts of the needle.

Disposable Injection Units. Disposable, single-dose, prefilled syringes are available for some medications. Ensure that you check the medication and concentration because all prefilled syringes look very similar. When using these syringes, you do not have to prepare medication doses, except perhaps to expel portions of unneeded medications.

The Tubex and Carpuject injection systems include reusable plastic mechanisms that hold prefilled, disposable, sterile cartridge-needle units (Figure 34–18). To prepare these systems, slip the cartridge into the syringe, secure it (by following the package directions), and check for air bubbles in the syringe. Advance the plunger to expel excess medication as you would with a regular syringe. A new type of injection system involves screwing a plunger-like device into the end of a prefilled vial that contains a needle. After the medication is given, safely dispose of the entire unit in a puncture-proof and leak-proof receptacle. The design of these injection systems reduces the risk of needle-stick injuries.

Preparing an Injection From an Ampule. Ampules contain single doses of medication in a liquid. Ampules are available in several sizes, from 1 mL to 10 mL or more (Figure 34–19A). An ampule is made of glass with a constricted neck that must be snapped off to access the medication. A coloured ring around the neck indicates where the ampule is prescored to be broken easily. Aspiration of the medication into a syringe (Skill 34–4) is sometimes completed by using a filter needle to prevent small glass fragments from entering the syringe (Stein, 2006). Change the filter needle to an appropriate-sized needle for the actual injection.

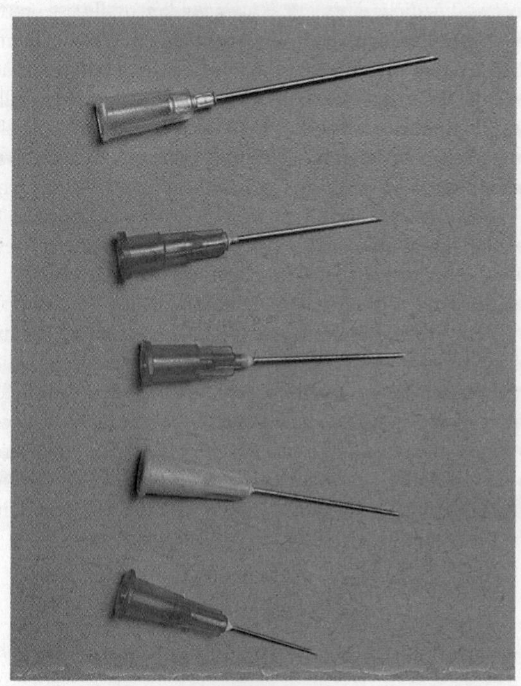

Figure 34-17 Needles. Top to bottom: 19 gauge, 3.8-cm length; 20 gauge, 2.5-cm length; 21 gauge, 2.5-cm length; 23 gauge, 2.5-cm length; and 25 gauge, 1.6-cm length.

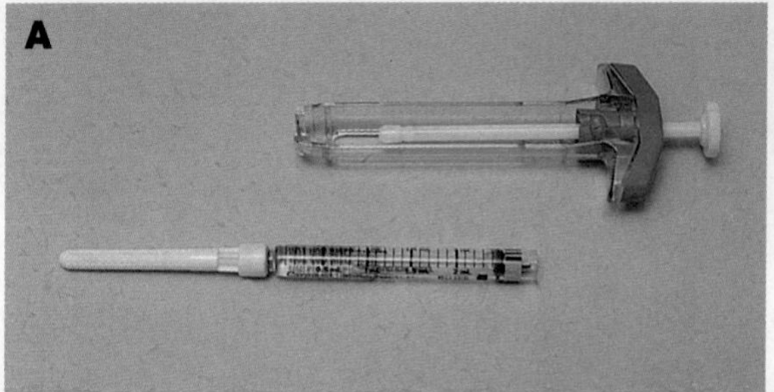

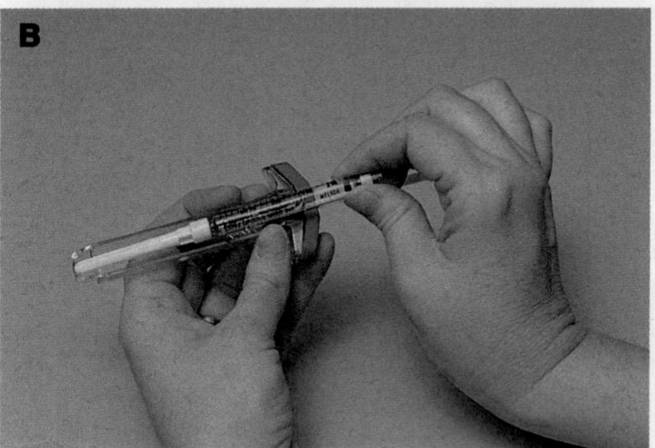

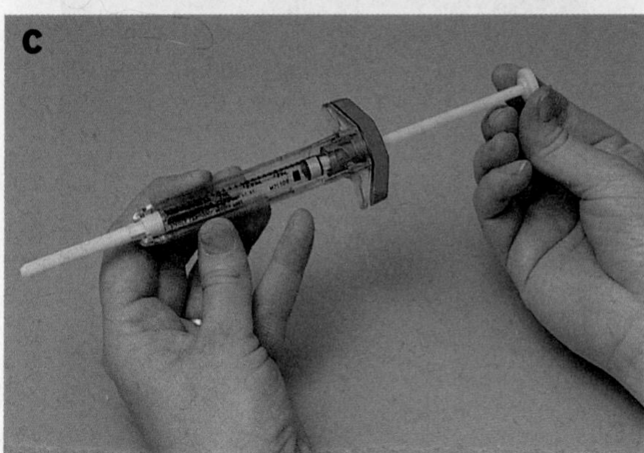

Figure 34-18 Disposable injection unit. **A**, Carpuject syringe and prefilled sterile cartridge with needle. **B**, Assembling the Carpuject system. **C**, Cartridge locks at needle end; plunger screws into opposite end.

Preparing an Injection From a Vial. A vial is a single-dose or multidose container with a rubber seal at the top (see Figure 34–19B). A metal cap protects the seal until it is ready to be used. Vials contain liquid or dry forms of medications. Medications that are unstable in solution are packaged dry. The vial label specifies the solvent or diluent to be used to dissolve the medication and the amount of diluent needed to prepare a desired medication concentration. Normal saline and sterile distilled water are solutions commonly used to dissolve medications.

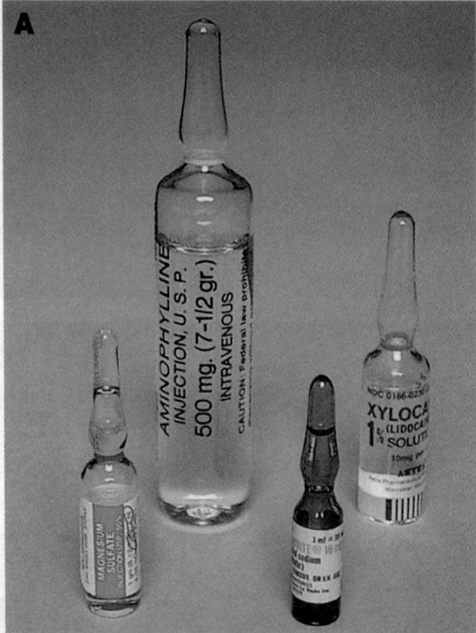

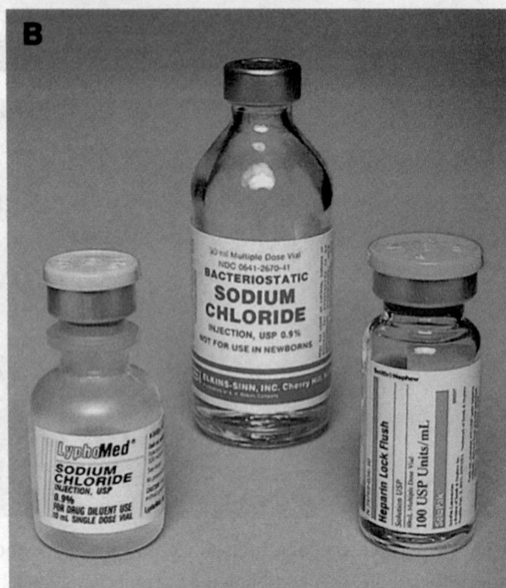

Figure 34-19 A, Medication in ampules. B, Medication in vials.

Unlike the ampule, the vial is a closed system, and air must be injected into the vial to permit easy withdrawal of the solution. Failure to inject air creates a vacuum within the vial that makes withdrawal difficult (see Skill 34–4). If you are concerned about drawing up parts of the rubber stopper or other particles into the syringe, use a filter needle when preparing medications from vials (Nicoll & Hesby, 2002).

To prepare a powdered medication, draw up the amount of diluent or solvent recommended on the vial's label. Inject the diluent into the vial in the same manner used for injecting air into the vial. Most powdered medications dissolve easily, but you may need to withdraw the needle to mix the contents thoroughly. If this step is needed, remove the needle and gently roll the vial between your hands to dissolve the powdered medication, then reinsert the needle to draw up the dissolved medication. After mixing multidose vials, make a label that records the date and time of the mixing and indicates the concentration of medication per millilitre. Multidose vials may require refrigeration after the contents are reconstituted.

Mixing Medications. If two medications are compatible, they can be mixed in one injection if the total dose is within accepted limits. When two or medications are mixed, the client will not have to receive more than one injection at a time. Most nursing units keep charts that list common compatible medications. If you have any uncertainty about medication compatibilities, consult a pharmacist.

Mixing Medications From Two Vials. Apply the following principles when mixing medications from two vials:

1. Do not contaminate one medication with another.
2. Ensure the final dose is accurate.
3. Maintain an aseptic technique.

To mix medications from two vials, use only one syringe with a needle or use a syringe with a needleless access device attached (Figure 34–20). Aspirate a volume of air equivalent to the first medication's dose (vial A). Inject the air into vial A, ensuring the needle does not touch the solution. Withdraw the needle and aspirate a volume of air equivalent to the second medication's dose (vial B). Inject the air into vial B. Immediately withdraw the medication from vial B into the syringe, then insert the needle back into vial A, being careful not to push the plunger and expel the medication in the syringe into the vial. Withdraw the desired amount of medication from vial A into the syringe. After withdrawing the necessary amount, withdraw the needle from the syringe. Insert into the syringe a new needle or a needleless access device suitable for injection.

Mixing Medications From One Vial and One Ampule. When mixing medication from a vial and an ampule, prepare medication from the vial first and then use the same syringe and filter needle to withdraw medication from the ampule. Prepare the medication combination in this order because you do not need to add air to withdraw medication from an ampule.

Insulin Preparation. Insulin is the hormone used to treat diabetes in some clients. Although inhaled insulin has recently been approved for use, insulin is most commonly administered by injection. Because insulin is a protein, if it were taken orally, it would break down and be destroyed in the gastrointestinal tract. Most clients who have diabetes that requires them to take insulin learn to self-administer the injections. In Canada, health care professionals usually prescribe insulin in concentrations of 100 units per millilitre of solution, which is called U-100 insulin. Insulin is also commercially available in concentrations of 500 units per milliliter of solution, which is called U-500 insulin. U-500 insulin is five times as strong as U-100 insulin and is used only in rare cases when clients are very resistant to insulin (American Diabetes Association [ADA], 2004).

Use the correct syringe when preparing insulin. For example, use a 100-unit insulin syringe to prepare U-100 insulin. Because no syringe is currently designed to prepare U-500 insulin, medication errors can result when preparing U-500 insulin. The Institute for Safe Medication Practices (2002) recommends that prescribers specify the units and volume (e.g., 150 units, 0.3 mL of U-500 insulin) and that nurses use tuberculin syringes to draw up doses of U-500 insulin. When U-500 insulin is ordered, the following medication calculation must be performed to correctly prepare the insulin:

Dose ordered/Dose on hand × Amount on hand =
Amount to administer

Example: Mr. Dobbs is ordered 250 units of U-500 insulin.

250 units ordered/500 units of insulin on hand × 1 mL =
0.5 mL to administer

Therefore, you need to prepare and administer 0.5 mL of U-500 insulin in a tuberculin syringe.

➤ SKILL 34-4 Preparing Injections

Delegation Considerations

The preparation of injections cannot be delegated to unregulated care providers (UCPs).

Equipment

- Medication administration record (MAR) or computer printout
- Medication in an ampule
  - Syringe, needle, and filter needle
  - Small gauze pad or unopened alcohol swab
- Medication in a vial
  - Syringe
    - Needles:
      - Blunt-tip vial access cannula (if a needleless system used)
      - Filter needle (if indicated)
      - Needle for drawing up medication (if needed) and needle for injection
  - Small gauze pad or alcohol swab
  - Diluent (e.g., normal saline or sterile water) (if indicated)

STEPS	RATIONALE
1. Check the accuracy and completeness of each MAR or computer printout against the prescriber's original medication order. Check the client's name and the medication name, route, dosage, and time of administration. Copy or rewrite any portion of the MAR that is difficult to read.	
2. Review the pertinent information related to the medication, including its action, purpose, side effects, and nursing implications.	
3. Assess the client's body build, muscle size, and weight.	• The client's body type determines the type and size of the syringe and the needles for injection.
4. Perform hand hygiene and assemble the medication supplies.	
5. Check the date of expiration on the medication vial or ampule.	• Medication potency may increase or decrease when medications are expired.
6. Prepare medication (see Skill 34–1, Steps 7A–G and M–O): Ensure that you compare the label of the medication with the MAR at least two times while preparing the medication.	
A. Ampule preparation	
(1) Tap the top of the ampule lightly and quickly with your finger until the fluid moves from the neck of the ampule (see Step 6A(1) illustration).	• Tapping the ampule dislodges any fluid that collects above the neck of the ampule. All solution moves into the lower chamber of the ampule.
(2) Place a small gauze pad or an unopened alcohol swab around the neck of the ampule (see Step 6A(2) illustration).	• Placing a pad around the neck of the ampule protects your fingers from injury when the glass tip is broken off.
(3) Snap the neck of the ampule quickly and firmly away from the hands (see Step 6A(3) illustration).	• Snapping the neck quickly and firmly protects your fingers and face from the shattering glass.
(4) Draw up the medication quickly, using a filter needle long enough to reach the bottom of the ampule.	• The injection system is vulnerable to airborne contaminants. The needle must be long enough to access the medication for preparation. Filter needles are used to sift out any fragments of glass (Stein, 2006).
(5) Hold the ampule upside down, or set it on a flat surface. Insert the filter needle into the centre of the ampule opening. Do not allow the needle tip or shaft to touch the rim of the ampule.	• The broken rim of the ampule is considered contaminated. When the ampule is inverted, the solution dribbles out if the needle tip or shaft touches the rim of the ampule.

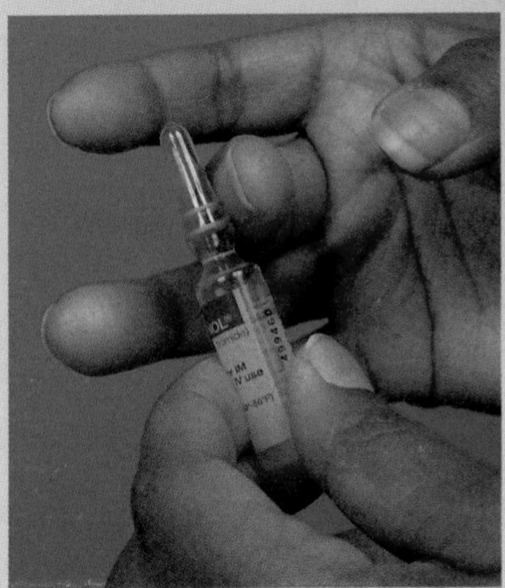

Step 6A(1) Tapping the ampule moves the fluid down the neck of the ampule.

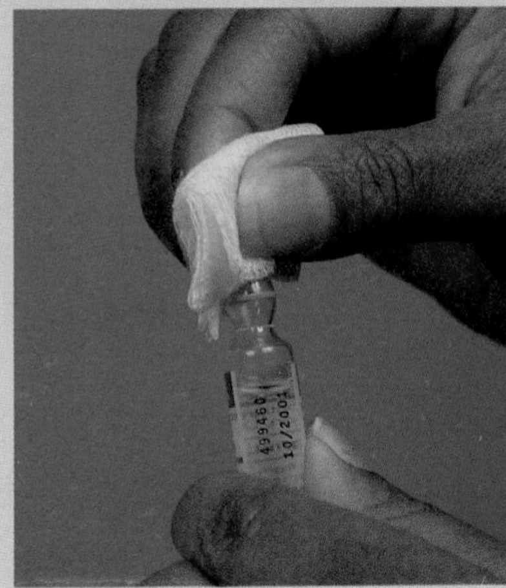

Step 6A(2) Gauze pad placed around the neck of the ampule.

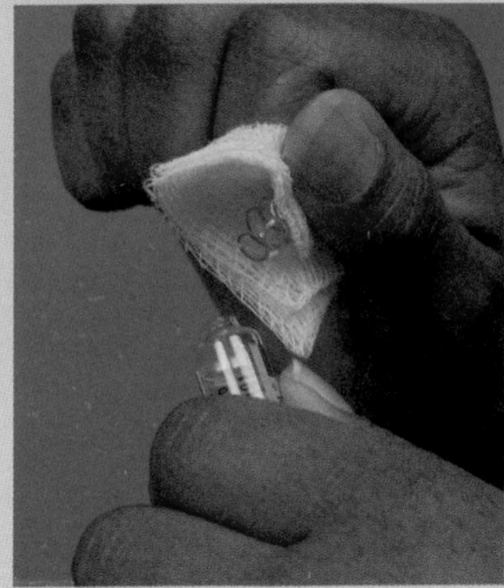

Step 6A(3) Snapping the neck of the ampule away from the hands.

Continued

➤ SKILL 34-4 Preparing Injections *continued*

STEPS	RATIONALE
(6) Aspirate the medication into the syringe by gently pulling back on the plunger (see Step 6A(6) illustrations).	• Withdrawal of the plunger creates negative pressure within the syringe barrel, which pulls the fluid into the syringe.
(7) Keep the needle tip under the surface of the liquid. Tip the ampule to bring all fluid within reach of the needle.	• Keeping the needle tip under the surface of the liquid prevents the aspiration of air bubbles.
(8) If air bubbles are aspirated, do not expel the air into the ampule.	• Expelling air into the ampule may force fluid out of the ampule, which could lead to loss of the medication.
(9) To expel excess air bubbles, remove the needle from the ampule. Hold the syringe with the needle pointing up. Tap the side of the syringe to cause the bubbles to rise toward the needle. Draw back slightly on the plunger, then push the plunger upward to eject the air. Do not eject any fluid.	• Withdrawing the plunger too far will remove it from the barrel. Holding the syringe vertically allows fluid to settle in the bottom of the barrel. Pulling back on the plunger allows the fluid within the needle to enter the barrel so that fluid is not expelled. Air at the top of the barrel and within the needle is then expelled.
(10) If the syringe contains excess fluid, dispose of it in a sink. Hold the syringe vertically with the needle tip up and slanted slightly toward the sink. Slowly eject the excess fluid into the sink. Recheck the fluid level in the syringe by holding it vertically.	• Medication is safely dispersed into the sink. The position of the needle allows the medication to be expelled without flowing down the needle shaft. Rechecking the fluid level ensures the proper dose.
(11) Cover the needle with its safety sheath or cap. Replace the filter needle with a needle or a needleless access device for injection.	• Covering the needle prevents contamination of the needle and minimizes needle-stick injuries. Filter needles cannot be used for injection.
B. Vial containing a solution	
(1) Remove the cap covering the top of the unused vial to expose the sterile rubber seal. If a multidose vial has been previously used, the cap has already been removed. Firmly and briskly wipe the surface of the rubber seal with an alcohol swab and allow it to dry.	• The vial comes packaged with a seal that cannot be replaced after the cap has been removed. Not all drug manufacturers guarantee that caps of unused vials are sterile. Therefore, seals must be swabbed with alcohol before preparing the medication. Allowing the alcohol to dry prevents the needle from being coated with alcohol, which could mix with the medication.
(2) Pick up the syringe and remove the needle cap or the cap covering the needleless vial access device (see Step 6B(2) illustration). Pull back on the plunger to draw an amount of air into the syringe equivalent to the volume of medication to be aspirated from the vial.	• Inject air into the vial to prevent the buildup of negative pressure in the vial when aspirating medication.

Critical Decision Point: Some medications require that a filter needle be used when preparing medications from a vial. The same policy is required by some institutions. Check the agency policy to determine whether the use of a filter needle is indicated (Nicoll & Hesby, 2002). If using a filter needle to aspirate the medication, use an appropriately sized needle to administer the medication.

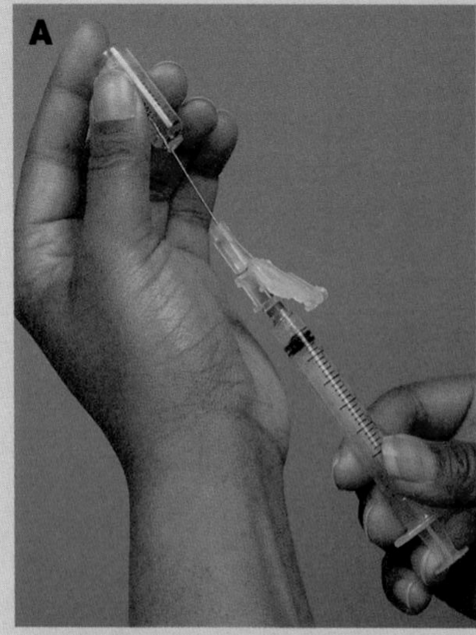

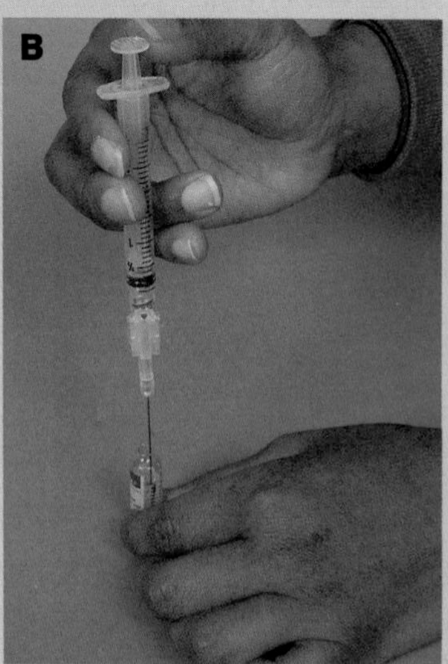

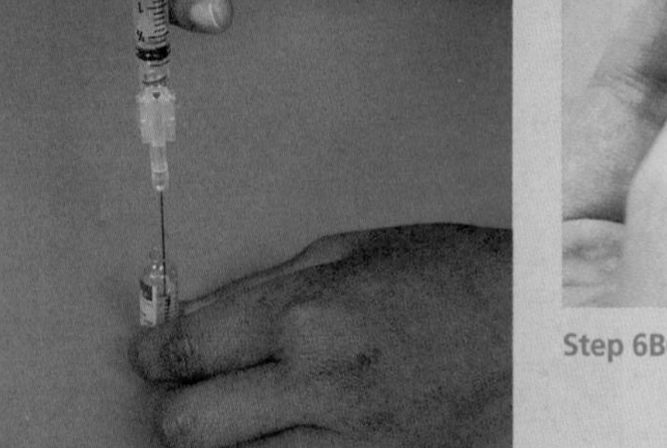

Step 6A(6) A, Medication aspirated with the ampule inverted. **B,** Medication aspirated with the ampule on a flat surface.

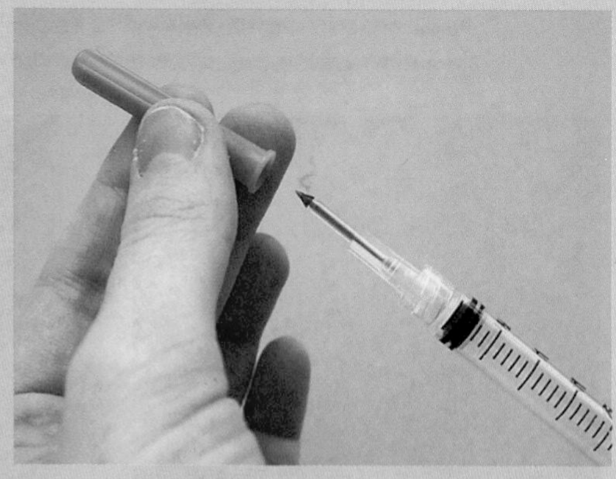

Step 6B(2) Syringe with needleless adapter.

➤ SKILL 34-4 Preparing Injections *continued*

STEPS	RATIONALE
(3) With the vial on a flat surface, insert the tip of the needle. Ensure the bevelled tip enters first, through the centre of the rubber seal (see Step 6B(3) illustration). Apply pressure to the tip of the needle during insertion.	• The centre of the seal is thinner and easier to penetrate than the sides of the seal. Injecting the bevelled tip of the needle first and using firm pressure prevents coring of the rubber seal, which could enter the vial or needle.
(4) Inject air into the vial's airspace, holding on to the plunger. Hold the plunger with firm pressure; the plunger may be forced backward by air pressure within the vial.	• Injecting air before aspirating the fluid creates a vacuum that is needed to allow the medication to flow into the syringe. Injecting air into the vial's airspace prevents the formation of bubbles, which can lead to an inaccurate dose.
(5) Invert the vial while keeping a firm hold on the syringe and plunger (see Step 6B(5) illustration). Hold the vial between your thumb and the middle fingers of your nondominant hand. Grasp the end of the syringe barrel and plunger with the thumb and forefinger of your dominant hand to counteract pressure in the vial.	• Inverting the vial allows the fluid to settle in the lower half of the container. Correct positioning of your hands prevents forceful movement of the plunger and permits easy manipulation of the syringe.
(6) Keep the tip of the needle below the fluid level.	• Keeping the needle tip under the surface of the liquid prevents the aspiration of air.
(7) Allow air pressure from the vial to fill the syringe gradually with medication. If necessary, pull back slightly on the plunger to obtain the correct amount of solution.	• Positive pressure within the vial forces the fluid into the syringe (unless the vial has been used several times).
(8) When the desired volume of solution is obtained, position the needle into the vial's airspace; tap the side of the syringe barrel carefully to dislodge any air bubbles. Eject any air remaining at the top of the syringe into the vial.	• Forcefully striking the barrel while the needle is inserted in the vial may bend the needle. The accumulation of air displaces the medication and can lead to dose errors.
(9) Remove the needle from the vial by pulling back on the barrel of the syringe.	• Accidentally pulling the plunger instead of the barrel can cause the plunger to separate from the barrel, which can result in the loss of medication.
(10) Hold the syringe at eye level, at a 90-degree angle, to ensure the correct volume has been obtained and no air bubbles are present. Remove any remaining air by tapping the barrel to dislodge the air bubbles (see Step 6B(10) illustration). Draw back slightly on the plunger; then push the plunger upward to eject the air. Do not eject the fluid. Recheck the volume of the medication.	• Holding the syringe vertically allows fluid to settle in the bottom of barrel. Pulling back on the plunger allows the fluid within the needle to enter the barrel so that fluid is not expelled. Air at the top of the barrel and within the needle is then expelled.
(11) If medication is to be injected into a client's tissue, change the needle to one of the appropriate gauge and length according to the route of medication and the client's size and weight.	• Inserting a needle through a rubber stopper may dull the bevelled tip. New needles are sharper. Because no fluid remains along the shaft, the needle will not track medication through the tissues.

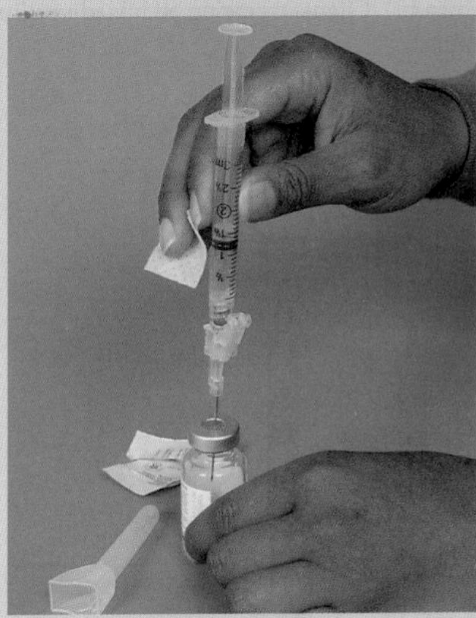

Step 6B(3) Insert the tip of the needle through the centre of the vial diaphragm (with the vial flat on the table).

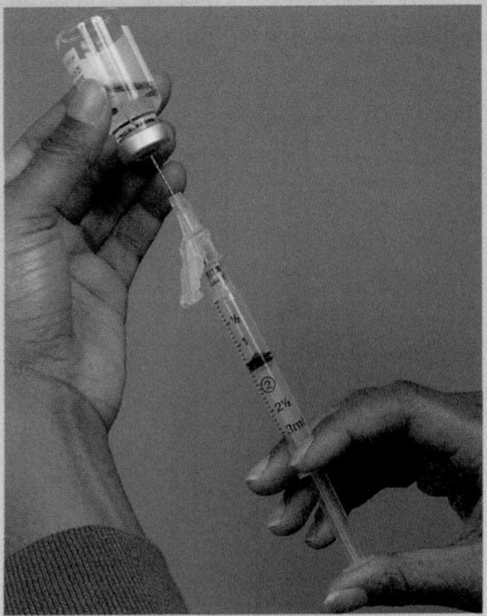

Step 6B(5) Withdraw fluid with the vial inverted.

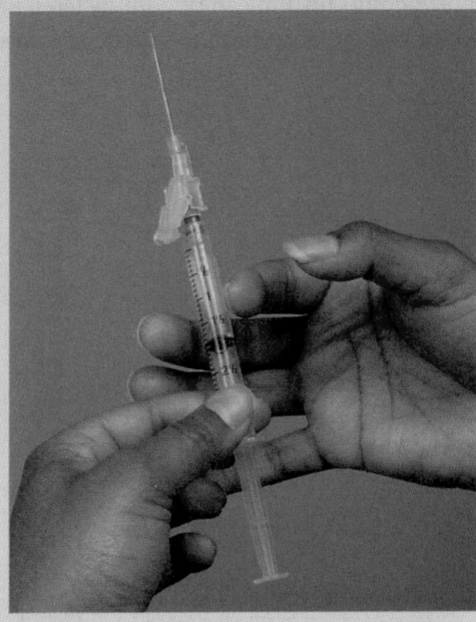

Step 6B(10) Hold the syringe upright and tap the barrel to dislodge air bubbles.

Continued

➤ SKILL 34-4 Preparing Injections *continued*

STEPS	RATIONALE
(12) For a multidose vial, make a label that includes the date of mixing, the concentration of the medication per millilitre, and your initials.	• Labelling ensures that future doses will be prepared correctly. Some medications must be discarded after a certain number of days have elapsed since the mixing of the vial.
C. Vial containing a powder (reconstituting medications)	
(1) Remove the cap covering the vial of powdered medication and the cap covering the vial of proper diluent. Firmly wipe both seals with the alcohol swab and allow to dry.	• Not all drug manufacturers guarantee that caps of unused vials are sterile. Therefore, seals must be swabbed with alcohol before preparing the medication. Allowing the alcohol to dry prevents the needle from being coated with alcohol, which could mix with the medication.
(2) Draw up diluent into the syringe following the Steps 6B(2) through 6B(10).	• Drawing up the diluent prepares the diluent for injection into a vial containing powdered medication.
(3) Insert the tip of the needle through the centre of the rubber seal on the vial of powdered medication. Inject the diluent into the vial. Remove the needle.	• The diluent begins to dissolve and reconstitute medication.
(4) Mix the medication thoroughly. Roll the vial in your palms. Do not shake.	• Rolling ensures proper dispersal of medication throughout the solution. Shaking produces bubbles.
(5) Reconstituted medication in the vial is ready to be drawn into a new syringe. Read the label carefully to determine the dose after reconstitution.	• After the diluent has been added, the concentration of medication (mg/mL) determines the dose to be given.
(6) Prepare medication in syringe following Steps 6B(2) through 6B(12).	

Critical Decision Point: Some institutions may require prepared parenteral medications to be verified for accuracy by another nurse. Check the agency policy before administering medication.

7. Dispose of all soiled supplies. Place broken ampule vials, used vials, and used needles in a puncture-proof and leak-proof container. Clean the medication work area and perform hand hygiene.	• Proper disposal of glass and needle prevents accidental injury to staff and controls the transmission of infection.

Unexpected Outcomes and Related Interventions

Air Bubbles Remaining in Syringe

- Expel air from the syringe and add medication to the syringe until the correct dose is prepared.

Incorrect Dose Prepared

- Discard the prepared dose and prepare the corrected new dose.

Insulin is classified by its rate of action: rapid-acting, short-acting, intermediate-acting, or long-acting. Each type has a different onset, peak, and duration of action (Table 34–10). Only regular (short-acting) insulin can be administered intravenously. Orders for insulin injections attempt to imitate the normal pattern of a client's insulin release from the pancreas. Some insulins come in a stable premixed solution (e.g., "70/30 insulin" comprises 70% NPH [neutral protamine Hagedorn], or intermediate-acting, insulin and 30% regular, or short-acting, insulin). Clients receiving premixed insulins do not need to mix insulins.

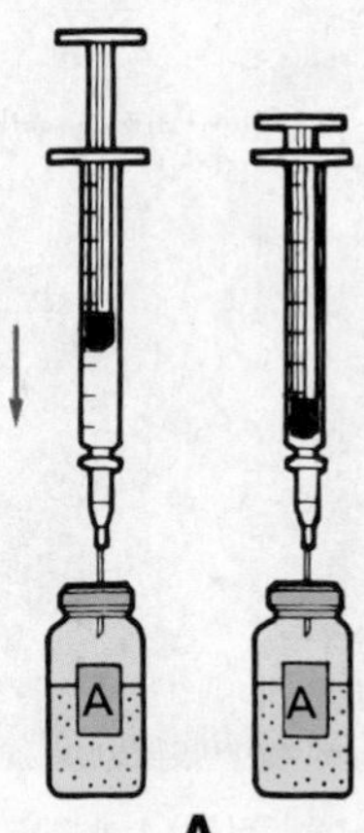

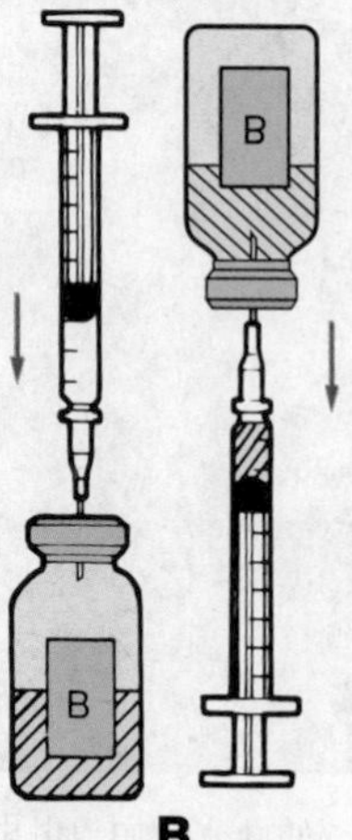

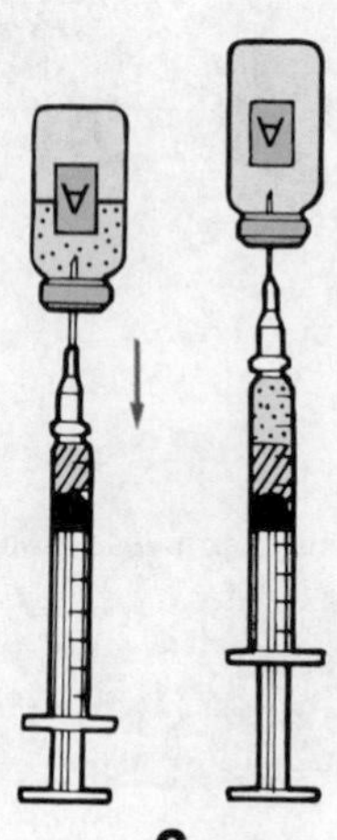

Figure 34-20 Mixing medications from two vials. A, Injecting air into vial A. B, Injecting air into vial B and withdrawing the dose. C, Withdrawing medication from vial A; the two medications are now mixed.

TABLE 34-10 A Comparison of Insulin Preparations

Type of Insulin	Onset	Peak	Duration
Rapid-Acting and Short-Acting			
Insulin glulisine (Apidra)	15 minutes	1 hour	2–3 hours
Insulin lispro (Humalog)	15 minutes	1 hour	4 hours
Insulin aspart (NovoLog)	30 minutes	1–3 hours	3–5 hours
Regular insulin*	30 minutes–1 hour	2–4 hours	5–7 hours
Intermediate-Acting			
Isophane insulin suspension (NPH insulin, Humulin N insulin)	3–4 hours	6–12 hours	18–28 hours
Insulin zinc suspension (Lente insulin)	1–3 hours	8–12 hours	36 hours
Long-Acting			
Extended insulin zinc suspension (Ultralente insulin)	4–6 hours	18–24 hours	36 hours
Insulin glargine (Lantus) †	1–5 hours	Plateau	24 hours
Insulin detemir (Levemir) †	3–4 hours	"Peakless"	24 hours
Combinations			
Isophane human insulin (50%) and regular human insulin (50%) (Humulin 50/50)	30 minutes	3 hours	22–24 hours
Isophane human insulin (70%) and regular human insulin (30%) (Humulin 70/30, Novolin 70/30)	30 minutes	4–8 hours	24 hours
Insulin lispro protamine (75%) and insulin lispro (25%) (Humalog Mix 75/25)	15 minutes	30 minutes–6 hours	24 hours
Insulin aspart protamine (70%) and insulin aspart (30%) (NovoLog Mix 70/30)	15 minutes	1–4 hours	24 hours

*Regular insulin is the only insulin for intravenous use; when administered intravenously, the onset of action is within 10–30 minutes and the peak effect is within 20–30 minutes.

†Cannot be mixed with other insulins.

Adapted from McKenry, L. M., Tessier, E., & Hogan, M. A. (2006). *Mosby's pharmacology in nursing* (22nd ed.). St. Louis, MO: Mosby; and from Novo Nordisk. (2007). *Levemir* [product description]. Retrieved January 24, 2009, from http://www.levemir-us.com/about-levemir-what-is.asp?DC_Options_Paid_MSN_Levemire_Product_Brand_09112008

A client with diabetes may require more than one type of insulin. For example, by receiving both a short-acting insulin and an intermediate-acting insulin, a client receives a more sustained control of blood glucose levels over 24 hours.

Insulin is ordered either by a specific dose at select times or by a sliding scale. A sliding scale dictates a certain dose on the basis of the client's blood glucose level (Box 34–22). Usually, rapid-acting or short-acting insulins are used for sliding scales. Before drawing up the insulin doses, gently roll all cloudy insulin preparations between the palms of the hands (or rotate the vial for at least 1 minute) to resuspend the insulin. Do not shake insulin vials; shaking causes the formation of bubbles, which take up space in the syringe and thereby alter the dose. If more than one type of insulin is required to manage the client's diabetes, you can mix two different types of insulin in one syringe if they are compatible (Box 34–23), by following the steps demonstrated in Figure 34–20. When two types of insulin are mixed, the single injection minimizes the client's discomfort that is associated with multiple injections. In hospitals, when you need to take capillary blood samples for blood glucose monitoring, always swab the client's anticipated sample site (e.g., the fingertip) with an alcohol swab before taking the sample. Use of an aseptic technique prevents the introduction of microorganisms and protects clients from infection while in the hospital. Although diabetic clients are commonly educated not to use alcohol swabs in the home care setting, their use is essential to maintain asepsis and infection control standards in hospital settings. Always consult with agency protocol for special care required when treating diabetic clients.

Administering Injections

Each injection route differs depending on the type of tissues the medication enters. The characteristics of the tissues influence the rate of medication absorption and thus the onset of medication action. Before injecting a medication, know the volume of the medication to administer, the medication's characteristics and viscosity, and the location of anatomical structures underlying the injection sites (Skill 34–5).

If you do not administer injections correctly, negative client outcomes can result. Failure to select an injection site in relation to anatomical landmarks can result in nerve or bone damage during needle insertion. An inability to maintain stability of the needle and syringe unit can result in pain for the client and possible tissue damage. If you fail to aspirate the syringe before injecting an intramuscular medication, the medication may accidentally be injected directly into an artery or vein. Injecting too large a volume of medication for the site selected causes the client extreme pain and may result in local tissue damage.

BOX 34-22 Example of a Sliding Scale Insulin Order

Give regular insulin subcutaneously:

2 units for glucose 11.1–13.3 mmol/L
4 units for glucose 13.4–13.8 mmol/L
6 units for glucose 13.9–16.7 mmol/L
For glucose greater than 16.8 mmol/L, call physician

Many clients, particularly children, fear injections. Clients with serious or chronic illness often are given several injections daily. You may be able to minimize the client's discomfort in the following ways:

- Use a sharp-bevelled needle in the smallest suitable length and gauge.
- Position the client as comfortably as possible to reduce muscular tension.
- Select the proper injection site, by using anatomical landmarks.
- Divert the client's attention from the injection by asking open-ended questions.
- Insert the needle quickly and smoothly to minimize tissue pulling.
- Hold the syringe steady while the needle remains in the tissues.
- Inject the medication slowly and steadily.

Subcutaneous Injections. Subcutaneous injections involve administering medications into the loose connective tissue under the dermis (see Skill 34–6, page 741). Because subcutaneous tissue is not as richly supplied with blood as the muscles, medication given by subcutaneous injection is absorbed slower than medication given by intramuscular (IM) injections; however, medications injected subcutaneously are absorbed completely if the client's circulatory status is normal. Because subcutaneous tissue contains pain receptors, the client may experience some discomfort.

The best subcutaneous injection sites are the outer posterior aspect of the upper arms, the abdomen from below the costal margins to the iliac crests, and the anterior aspects of the thighs (Figure 34–21). The site most frequently recommended for heparin injections is the abdomen (Figure 34–22). Other recommended sites are the scapular areas of the upper back and the upper ventral or dorsal gluteal areas. The injection site chosen should be free of skin lesions, bony prominences, and large underlying muscles or nerves.

The administration of low-molecular-weight heparin (LMWH) (e.g., enoxaparin) requires special considerations. The injection site is the right or left side of the abdomen at least 5 cm from the umbilicus. Do not pinch the injection site. Administer LMWH in its pre-filled syringe with the attached needle; do not expel the air bubble in the syringe before giving the medication (Sanofi-Aventis, 2006).

When giving U-100 insulin, use U-100 insulin syringes with preattached 26- to 31-gauge needles; when giving U-500 insulin, use 1-mL tuberculin syringes (Institute for Safe Medication Practices, 2002). Recommended sites for insulin injections include the upper arm and the anterior and lateral portions of the thigh, buttocks, and abdomen. Clients with diabetes who inject insulin should practise intrasite rotation (rotating injection sites within the same body part) to provide greater consistency in the absorption of insulin. For example, if the morning insulin is injected into the client's arm, then a subsequent injection should also be given in the arm but at least 2.5 cm away from the previous site. No injection site should be used again for

➤ BOX 34-23 Procedural Guidelines

Mixing Two Kinds of Insulin in One Syringe

Delegation Considerations: The mixing of two kinds of insulin in one syringe cannot be delegated.

Equipment:

- Insulin vials
- Insulin syringe
- Alcohol swabs
- Medication administration report (MAR) or computer printout

Procedure

1. Check the accuracy and completeness of each MAR or computer printout against the prescriber's original medication order. Check the client's name and the medication name, dosage, route, and time for administration. Copy or rewrite any portion of the MAR that is difficult to read.
2. Carefully verify the insulin labels; compare the medication labels against the MAR before preparing the dose to ensure the correct type of insulin is prepared.
3. Perform hand hygiene.
4. If the insulin is cloudy, roll the bottle of insulin between your hands to resuspend the insulin preparation.
5. Wipe the tops of both insulin vials with the alcohol swabs.
6. Verify the insulin dosage against the MAR a second time.
7. If mixing rapid- or short-acting insulin with intermediate- or long-acting insulin, take the insulin syringe and aspirate a volume of air equivalent to the dose of insulin to be withdrawn from the intermediate- or long-acting insulin first. If two intermediate- or long-acting insulins are mixed, either vial can be prepared first.
8. Insert the needle and inject air into the vial of the intermediate- or long- acting insulin. Do not let the tip of the needle touch the insulin.
9. Remove the syringe from the vial of intermediate- or long-acting insulin without aspirating the insulin.
10. With the same syringe, inject a volume of air that is equivalent to the dose of insulin to be withdrawn into the vial of the rapid- or short-acting insulin. Withdraw the correct dose into the syringe.
11. Remove the syringe from the rapid- or short-acting insulin vial after carefully removing air bubbles in the syringe to ensure the correct dose.
12. After verifying the insulin dosage with the MAR a third time, show the insulin preparation in the syringe to another nurse to verify the correct dose of insulin was prepared. Determine which point on the syringe scale represents the total of the combined units of insulin by adding the number of units of both insulins together (e.g., 3 units regular insulin + 10 units NPH insulin = 13 units total insulin).
13. Place the needle of the syringe back into the vial of the intermediate- or long-acting insulin. Be careful not to push the plunger, which would inject the insulin in the syringe into the vial.
14. Invert the vial, and carefully withdraw the desired amount of insulin into the syringe.
15. Withdraw the needle and check the fluid level in the syringe. Keep the needle of the prepared syringe sheathed or capped until you are ready to administer the medication. Show the syringe to another nurse to verify the correct dose was prepared.
16. Dispose of soiled medication supplies in the proper receptacle and perform hand hygiene.
17. Because rapid- or short-acting insulin binds with intermediate- or long-acting insulin, which reduces the action of the faster-acting insulin, administer the mixture within 5 minutes of preparing it.

Adapted from the Canadian Diabetes Association. (n.d.). *Insulin: Things you should know.* Retrieved June 8, 2008 from http://www.diabetes.ca/files/Insulin.pdf; and American Diabetes Association. (2004). Insulin administration: Position statement, *Diabetes Care, 27*(1S), S106–S109.

➤ SKILL 34-5 Administering Injections

Delegation Considerations

The administration of injections cannot be delegated to an unregulated care provider (UCP). Instruct UCPs to report the occurrence of potential medication side effects or any changes in the client's vital signs or level of consciousness (e.g., sedation) immediately.

Equipment

- Proper size syringe and needle:
  - *Subcutaneous:* Syringe (1–3 mL) and needle (25–27 gauge, 1–1.6 cm)
  - *Subcutaneous U-100 insulin*: Insulin syringe (0.3, 0.5, or 1 mL) with preattached needle (28–31 gauge)
  - *IM:* Syringe 2–3 mL for adult, 0.5–1 mL for infants and small children
- Needle, with length corresponding to the site of injection and the age of the client according to the following guidelines (Nicoll & Hesby, 2002):
  - *Any site (children):* 1.6–3.2 cm (depending on the size of the child)
  - *Vastus lateralis (adults):* 2.5–3.8 cm
  - *Deltoid (adults):* 2.5–3.8 cm
  - *Ventrogluteal (adults):* 3.8 cm
  - *Intradermal and subcutaneous U-500 insulin:* 1-mL tuberculin syringe with preattached 26- or 27-gauge needle
- Small gauze pad, or alcohol swab, or both
- Vial or ampule of medication or skin test solution
- Clean gloves
- Medication administration record (MAR) or computer printout

STEPS	RATIONALE
For All Injections	
1. Check the accuracy and completeness of each MAR or computer printout against the prescriber's original medication order. Check the client's name and the medication name, route, dosage, and time of administration. Copy or rewrite any portion of the MAR that is difficult to read.	• The order sheet is the most reliable source and only legal record of the medications that clients are to receive. Consistency between the MAR and the original medication order ensures the client recives the correct medications. Illegible MARs are a source of medication errors.
2. Assess the client's medical history, medication history, and history of allergies. Determine whether the client is allergic to any substances and the normal allergic reaction experienced.	• Certain substances have similar compositions; never administer a substance to which a client has a known allergy.
3. Check the date of expiration for the medication.	• Drug potency may increase or decrease when medications are expired.
4. Observe the client's verbal and nonverbal responses to receiving the injection.	• Injections can be painful. Some clients have anxiety, which can increase their experience of pain.
5. Assess the client for contraindications.	
A. For subcutaneous injections: Assess the client for factors such as circulatory shock and reduced local tissue perfusion. Assess the adequacy of the client's adipose tissue.	• Reduced tissue perfusion interferes with medication absorption and distribution. Physiological changes of aging and the client's health may affect the amount of the client's subcutaneous tissue. The amount of subcutaneous tissue influences the methods chosen for administering injections.
B. For intramuscular injections: Assess the client for muscle atrophy, reduced blood flow, and circulatory shock.	• Atrophied muscles absorb medication poorly. Factors that interfere with blood flow to muscles will impair the medication's absorption.

Critical Decision Point: Because of documented adverse effects to intramuscular injections, other routes of medication administration are safer. Verify that an intramuscular injection is necessary and explore alternative medication routes if possible (Nicoll & Hesby, 2002; World Health Organization [WHO], 2005).

STEPS	RATIONALE
6. Aseptically prepare the correct medication dose from an ampule or vial (see Skill 34–3). Ensure all air is expelled from the syringe. Check the label of medication against the MAR two times while preparing the medication. Create a removable label that shows the client's name, the name of the drug, and the dosage. Apply the label to the removable needle cap.	• Aseptic preparation ensures that the medication is sterile. Preparation techniques differ for ampules and vials. Checking the label against the MAR ensures the right medication is prepared for the right client.
7. Take the medication to the client at the right time and perform hand hygiene.	• Taking the medication according to schedule ensures the client receives the effect of the medication at the right time. Hand hygiene reduces the transfer of microorganisms.
8. Close the room curtain or door.	• Closing the curtain or door provides privacy and avoids distractions.
9. Identify the client using at least two client identifiers. Compare the client's name and one other identifier (e.g., the hospital identification number) on the MAR, computer printout, or computer screen against information on the client's identification bracelet. Ask the client to state his or her name if possible, for a third identifier.	• This process complies with The Joint Commission's (2007) requirements and improves medication safety. In most acute care settings, the name and identification number on the client's armband and the MAR are used to identify clients. Identification bracelets are made at the time of the client's admission and are the most reliable source of information. The client's room number is *not* an acceptable identifier.
10. Compare the label on the medication with the MAR one more time at the client's bedside.	• The final check of medication labels against the MAR at the client's bedside reduces medication administration errors.

Continued

➤ SKILL 34-5 Administering Injections *continued*

STEPS	RATIONALE
11. Describe the steps of procedure and inform the client that the injection will cause a slight burning or stinging sensation.	• Describing the process to the client helps to minimize the client's anxiety.
12. Perform hand hygiene; put on disposable gloves.	• Hand hygiene and the wearing of gloves reduces the transfer of microorganisms.
13. Keep a sheet or gown draped over the client's body parts that do not need to be exposed.	• Use of a sheet or gown respects the dignity of the client while only the area to be injected is exposed.
14. Select an appropriate injection site. Inspect the skin surface over the injection site for bruises, inflammation, and edema.	• Injection sites should be free of abnormalities that may interfere with medication absorption. Injection sites that are used repeatedly can become hardened from lipohypertrophy (increased growth in fatty tissue). Do not inject an area that is bruised or shows signs associated with infection.
A. *Subcutaneous injection:* Palpate the injection site for masses or tenderness. Avoid these areas. For clients who require daily insulin, rotate the injection site daily. Ensure the needle is the correct size by grasping a skinfold at the injection site with your thumb and forefinger. Measure the fold from top to bottom. The needle should be one-half the length of the skinfold.	• Subcutaneous injections can be inadvertently given in the muscle, especially when the injection site is in the abdomen or thigh (Annersten & Willman, 2005). Use of the appropriate size of needle ensures that medication will be injected in the subcutaneous tissue.
B. *Intramuscular injection:* Note the integrity and size of the muscle and palpate for tenderness or hardness. Avoid these areas. If injections are given frequently, rotate the injection sites. Use the ventrogluteal site if possible.	• Unless contraindications exist for this site, the ventrogluteal site is the preferred injection site for adults and children, including infants (Cook & Murtagh, 2006; Hockenberry & Wilson, 2007; Nicoll & Hesby, 2002; Small, 2004).
C. *Intradermal injection:* Note any lesions or discolourations of the client's forearm. Select an injection site three to four fingerwidths below the antecubital space and a handwidth above the wrist. If the forearm cannot be used, inspect the client's upper back. If necessary, sites for subcutaneous injections may be used.	• An intradermal site should be free from lesions or discolourations so that results of skin test can be seen and interpreted correctly.
15. Assist the client to a comfortable position:	
A. *Subcutaneous injection:* Have the client relax the arm, leg, or abdomen, depending on the site chosen for injection.	• Relaxation of the injection site minimizes the client's discomfort.
B. *Intramuscular injection:* Position the client depending on the site chosen (e.g., have the client sit, lie flat, lie on one side, or lie prone).	• The position of the client can reduce strain on the client's muscle and minimize the discomfort of the injection.
C. *Intradermal injection:* Have the client extend the elbow and support the elbow and forearm on a flat surface.	• The position of the client stabilizes the injection site for easy accessibility.
D. Speak with the client about a subject of interest. Ask open-ended questions.	• Distraction reduces anxiety.

Critical Decision Point: Ensure the client's position is not contraindicated by a medical condition.

STEPS	RATIONALE
16. Relocate the injection site using anatomical landmarks.	• Injection into the correct anatomical site prevents injury to nerves, bones, and blood vessels.
17. Clean the injection site with an antiseptic swab. Touch the swab to the centre of the site and rotate outward in a circular direction for about 5 cm (see Step 17 illustration).	• The mechanical action of the swab removes secretions containing microorganisms.

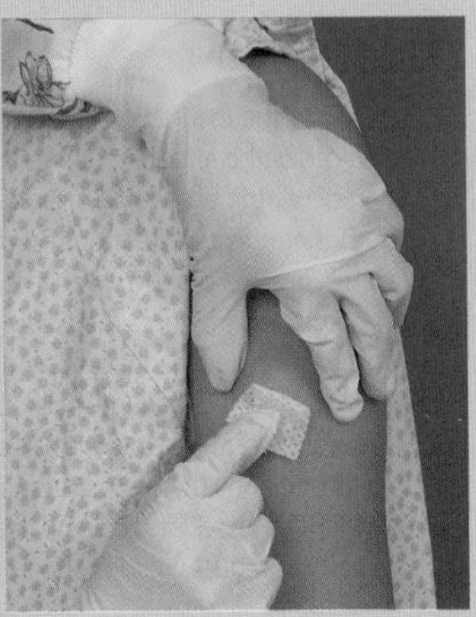

Step 17 Clean the injection site by using a circular motion.

➤ SKILL 34-5 Administering Injections *continued*

STEPS	RATIONALE
18. Hold the swab or gauze between the third and fourth fingers of your nondominant hand.	• The gauze or swab is readily accessible when the needle is withdrawn.
19. Remove the needle cap or sheath from the needle by pulling it straight off.	• Preventing the needle from touching the sides of the cap avoids the risk of contamination.
20. Hold the syringe between the thumb and forefinger of your dominant hand	
A. *Subcutaneous injection:* Hold the syringe as if you were holding a dart, palm down; or hold the syringe across the tops of your fingertips (see Step 20A illustration).	• Quick, smooth injection requires proper manipulation of the syringe parts.
B. *Intramuscular injection:* Hold the syringe as if you were holding a dart, palm down.	
C. *Intradermal injection:* Hold the bevel of the needle pointing up.	• With the bevel pointing up, the medication is less likely to be deposited into tissues below dermis.
21. Administer the injection:	
A. Subcutaneous injection	
(1) For an average-sized client, spread the skin tightly across the injection site or pinch the skin with your nondominant hand.	• The needle penetrates tight skin easier than loose skin. Pinching the skin elevates the subcutaneous tissue and may desensitize the area.
(2) Inject the needle quickly and firmly at a 45- to 90-degree angle. Then release the skin, if pinched.	• Quick, firm insertion minimizes the client's discomfort. (Injecting medication into compressed tissue irritates the nerve fibres). Injecting at the correct angle prevents accidental injection into the muscle.
(3) For an obese client, pinch the skin at the injection site and inject the needle at a 90-degree angle below the tissue fold.	• Obese clients have a fatty layer of tissue above the subcutaneous layer.

Critical Decision Point: Piercing a blood vessel during a subcutaneous injection is very rare, so aspiration is not necessary when administering subcutaneous injections.

STEPS	RATIONALE
(4) Inject the medication slowly (see Step 21A(4) illustration).	• Injecting slowly minimizes the client's discomfort.
B. Intramuscular injection	
(1) Position your nondominant hand at the proper anatomical landmarks and pull the skin down approximately 2.5–3.5 cm or laterally with the ulnar side of your hand to administer the injection in a Z-track. Hold this position until the medication is injected. Use your dominant hand to insert the needle quickly at a 90-degree angle into the muscle.	• The Z-track creates a zigzag path through the tissues to seal the needle track and avoid tracking of the medication. The Z-track should be used for all intramuscular injections (Nicoll & Hesby, 2002).
(2) If the client's muscle mass is small, grasp a body of muscle between your thumb and fingers.	• Grasping the muscle ensures the medication reaches the muscle mass (Hockenberry & Wilson, 2007).
(3) After the needle pierces the skin, grasp the lower end of the syringe barrel with your nondominant hand to stabilize the syringe. Continue to hold the skin tightly with your nondominant hand. Move your dominant hand to the end of the plunger. Do not move the syringe.	• Smooth manipulation of the syringe reduces the client's discomfort from needle movement. The skin must remain pulled until after the drug is injected to ensure Z-track administration.

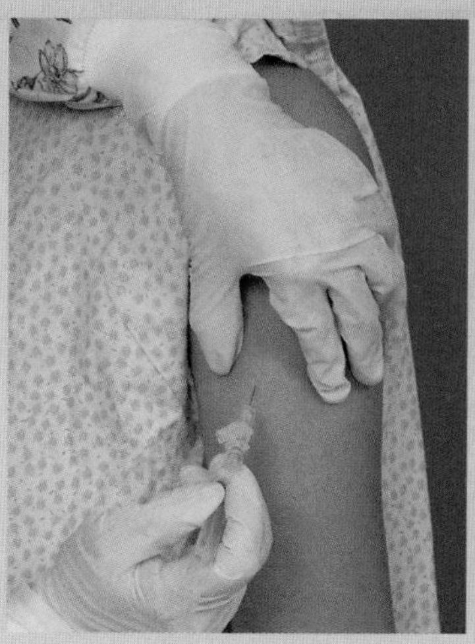

Step 20A Hold the syringe as if grasping a dart.

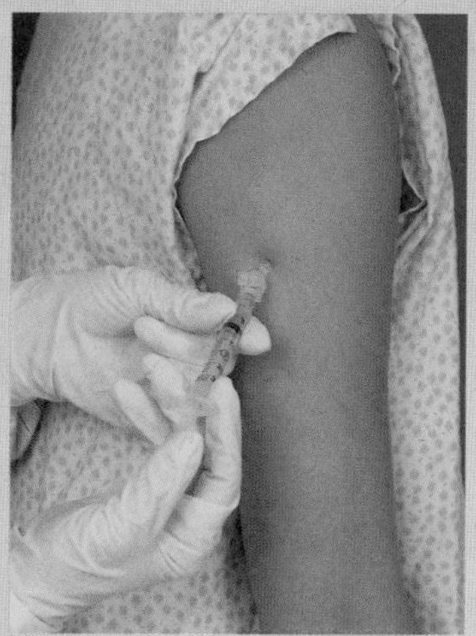

Step 21A(4) Inject the medication slowly.

Continued

➤ SKILL 34-5 Administering Injections *continued*

STEPS	RATIONALE
(4) Pull back on the plunger. If no blood appears, inject the medicine slowly, at a rate of 1 mL per 10 seconds.	• Aspiration of blood into the syringe indicates intravenous placement of the needle. A slow injection rate reduces the chance of pain and tissue trauma (Nicoll & Hesby, 2002).

Critical Decision Point: If blood appears in the syringe, remove the needle and dispose of the medication and syringe properly. Prepare another dose of medication for injection.

STEPS	RATIONALE
(5) Wait 10 seconds, and then smoothly and steadily withdraw the needle and release the skin. Apply gentle pressure with dry gauze if desired.	• A wait of 10 seconds allows time for the medication to absorb into the muscle before you remove the syringe and prevents the medication from leaking back out through the track created by the needle (Nicoll & Hesby, 2002).
C. Intradermal injection	
(1) With your nondominant hand, stretch the skin over the injection site with your forefinger or thumb.	• The needle pierces tight skin more easily than loose skin.
(2) With the needle almost against the client's skin, insert it slowly with the bevel pointed up at a 5- to 15-degree angle until resistance is felt. Advance the needle through the epidermis to approximately 3 mm below the skin surface. The needle tip can be seen through skin.	• This technique ensures the needle tip is in the dermis.
(3) Inject the medication slowly. Normally, resistance is felt. If resistance is not felt, the needle is in too deep; remove and begin again. Your nondominant hand can stabilize the needle during the injection.	• Slow injection minimizes the discomfort at the injection site. The dermal layer is tight and does not expand easily when the solution is injected. Stabilizing the needle prevents unnecessary movements and decreases the client's discomfort.
(4) While injecting medication, notice that a small bleb of approximately 6 mm in diameter (resembling a mosquito bite) appears on the skin's surface (see Step 21C(4) illustration). Instruct the client that this bleb is a normal finding.	• The bleb indicates the medication is deposited in the dermis.
22. Withdraw the needle while wiping an alcohol swab or gauze gently over the injection site.	• Support of tissue around the injection site minimizes the client's discomfort during withdrawal of the needle. Dry gauze may minimize the client's discomfort associated with the use of alcohol on nonintact skin.
23. Apply gentle pressure. Do not massage the injection site. Put on a bandage if needed.	• Massage may cause underlying tissue damage. Massage of the intradermal site may disperse the medication into underlying tissue layers and thereby alter the test results.
24. Assist the client to a comfortable position.	• Helping to client to a comfortable position gives the client a sense of well-being.
25. Discard into a puncture- and leak-proof receptacle the uncapped needle or the needle enclosed in safety shield and attached to the syringe. Do *not* recap the needle.	• Proper needle disposal prevents injury to clients and health care personnel. Recapping the needle increases the risk of needle-stick injury (Health Canada, 1997).
26. Remove disposable gloves and perform hand hygiene.	• Proper hygiene reduces the transmission of microorganisms.
27. Stay with the client for 3–5 minutes to observe for any allergic reactions.	• Severe anaphylactic reaction is characterized by dyspnea, wheezing, and circulatory collapse and is a life-threatening emergency.
28. Periodically return to the client's room to ask whether the client feels any acute pain, burning, numbness, or tingling at the injection site.	• Continued discomfort may indicate injury to underlying bones or nerves.

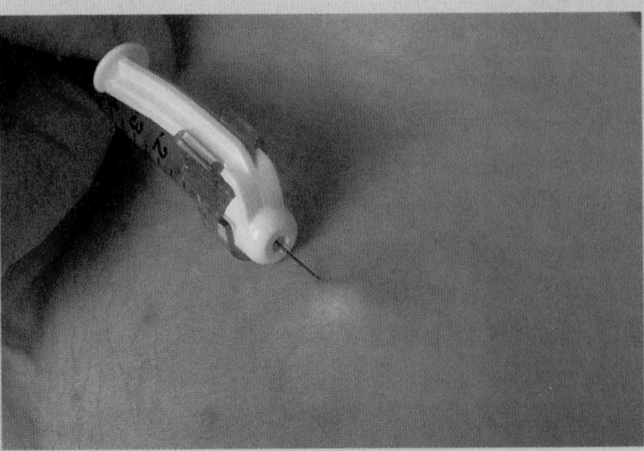

Step 21C(4) The injection creates a small bleb.

➤ SKILL 34-5 Administering Injections *continued*

STEPS	RATIONALE
29. Inspect the injection site, noting any bruising or induration.	• Bruising or induration indicates a complication associated with the injection. Document your findings and notify the client's health care professional. Provide a warm compress to the site.
30. Observe the client's response to medication at times that correlate with the medication's onset, peak, and duration.	• Intramuscular medications are rapidly absorbed. Adverse effects of parenteral medications may develop rapidly. Your observations evaluate the efficacy of the medication action.
31. Ask the client to explain the purpose and effects of the medication.	• Questioning the client will help to evaluate the client's understanding of the information you have taught.
32. For intradermal injections, use a skin pencil and draw a circle around the perimeter of the injection site. Read the site within an appropriate amount of time, which is determined by the type of medication or skin test administered.	• The pencil mark makes the injection site easy to find. Results of skin testing are read at various times, on the basis of the type of medication used or the type of skin test completed. Refer to the manufacturer's directions to determine when to read the test's results.

Unexpected Outcomes and Related Interventions

Raised, Reddened, or Hard Zone (Induration) Around Intradermal Test Site

- Notify the client's health care professional.
- Document the client's sensitivity to the injected allergen or the positive test if tuberculin skin testing was completed.

Hypertrophy of Skin, Resulting From Repeated Subcutaneous Injections

- Do not use this site for future injections.
- Instruct client not to use the injection site for 6 months.

Signs and Symptoms of Allergy or Side Effects

- Follow the institutional policy or guidelines for the appropriate response to adverse drug reactions.
- Notify the client's health care professional immediately.
- Add allergy information to the client's medical record.

Complaints of Localized Pain, Numbness, Tingling, or Burning Sensation at Injection Site, Indicating Possible Injury to Nerve or Tissues

- Assess the injection site.
- Document your findings.
- Notify the client's health care professional.

Recording and Reporting

- Chart the medication dose, route, site, time, and date of injection on the MAR immediately after giving medication, as per agency policy.
- Document if the scheduled medication is withheld and record the reason as per agency policy.
- Report any undesirable effects from the medication to the prescriber.
- Record the client's response to medications in the nurses' notes and report to prescriber if required.

Home Care Considerations

- Assess the client's readiness to learn before instructing him or her on how to administer self-injections. Some clients are hesitant to administer injections to themselves; relieve any anxiety before teaching this skill to a client.
- Clients can often purchase or obtain sharps boxes for home use. If this purchase is not feasible, a hard plastic bottle that is nontransparent (e.g., a fabric softener bottle or a detergent bottle) may be used to safely store syringes after use. Disposal of needles used in the home varies among communities. Check with local authorities to verify how to appropriately dispose of needles.

at least 1 month. The rate of insulin absorption varies depending on the site: the abdomen has the quickest absorption, followed by the arms, thighs, and buttocks (American Diabetes Association, 2004; Canadian Diabetes Association, 2008). For subcutaneous injections of insulin, pinch the skin and insert the needle at a 90-degree angle; inject the insulin, then release the pinched skin, count 5 to 6 seconds and remove the needle.

Only small doses (0.5 to 1 mL) of water-soluble medications should be given subcutaneously because the tissue is sensitive to irritating solutions and large volumes of medications. Medications can collect within the tissues to cause sterile abscesses, which appear as hardened, painful lumps under the skin.

A client's body weight indicates the depth of the subcutaneous layer. Therefore, choose the needle length and angle of insertion based on the client's weight and an estimation of the amount of subcutaneous tissue (Annersten & Willman, 2005). In general, medications can be injected in the subcutaneous tissue of a normal-size client using a 25-gauge 1.6-cm needle inserted at a 45-degree angle (Figure 34–23) or a 1.3-cm needle inserted at a 90-degree angle. A child may require only a 1.3-cm needle. If the client is obese, pinch the tissue and use a needle long enough to insert through the fatty tissue at the base of the skinfold. The preferred needle length is one-half the width of the skinfold; the angle of insertion may be between 45 and 90 degrees. Thin clients may have insufficient tissue for subcutaneous injections; the upper abdomen is the best injection site for these clients. To ensure a subcutaneous medication reaches the subcutaeous tissue, follow this rule: If you can grasp 5 cm of tissue, insert the needle at a 90-degree angle; if you can grasp 2.5 cm of tissue, insert the needle at a 45-degree angle (Rushing, 2004).

Intramuscular Injections. The intramuscular (IM) route provides faster medication absorption than the subcutaneous route because of a muscle's greater vascularity; however, intramuscular injections are associated with many risks. Therefore, when administering a medication by the intramuscular route, you must first verify that the injection is justified (Nicoll & Hesby, 2002; WHO, 2005). In many cases, such as influenza and pneumonia vaccinations, no alternative routes exist to administer the medication.

Use a longer and heavier-gauge needle to pass through the subcutaneous tissue and penetrate the deep muscle tissue (see Skill 34–5). The client's body weight and the amount of adipose tissue can influence the selection of a needle size. For example, an obese client

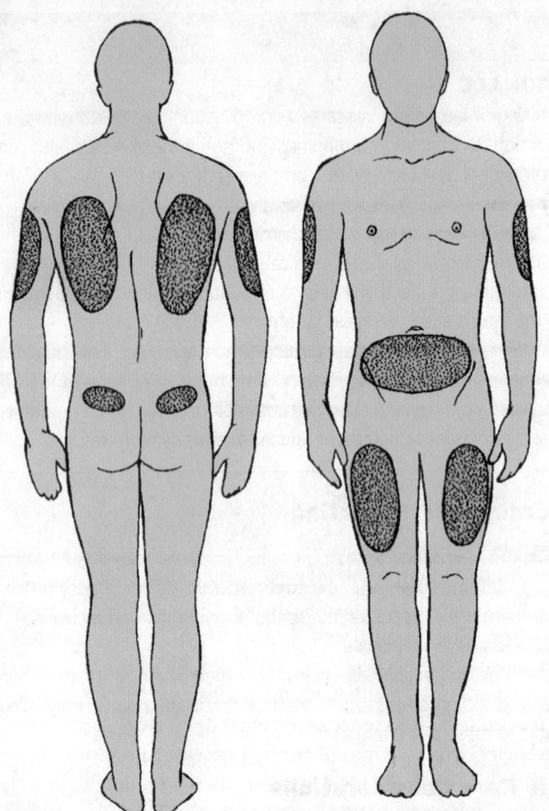

Figure 34-21 Sites recommended for subcutaneous injections

may require a needle 7.5 cm long, whereas a thin client may require a 1.3- to 2.5-cm needle.

The angle of insertion for an intramuscular injection is 90 degrees (see Figure 34–23). Muscle is less sensitive to irritating and viscous medications. A normal, well-developed client can tolerate 3 mL of medication into a larger muscle without severe muscle discomfort. A larger volume of medication is unlikely to be absorbed properly. Children, older adults, and thin clients can tolerate only 2 mL of an intramuscular injection. Do not give more than 1 mL to small children and older infants, and do not give more than 0.5 mL to smaller infants (Hockenberry & Wilson, 2007).

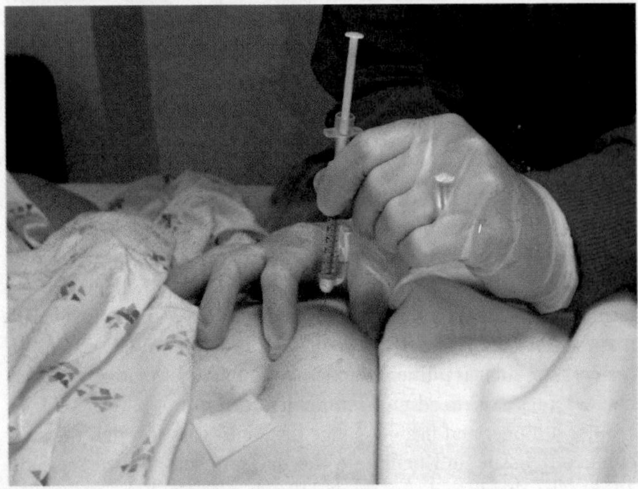

Figure 34-22 Giving subcutaneous heparin in the abdomen.

Assess the muscle integrity of the selected site before giving an injection. The muscle should be free of tenderness. Repeated injections in the same muscle can cause severe discomfort. Ensure that the client is relaxed, then palpate the muscle to rule out any hardened lesions. You can minimize discomfort during an injection by helping the client to assume a position that will help reduce muscle strain. Other interventions, such as distraction and applying pressure to the intramuscular site, may be used to decrease pain during an intramuscular injection.

Sites. When selecting an intramuscular site, consider the following: Is the area free of infection or necrosis? Do local areas show signs of bruising or abrasions? Where is the location of underlying bones, nerves, and major blood vessels? What volume of medication is to be administered? Each site has certain advantages and disadvantages. The characteristics of each intramuscular site and the indications for use of each site are listed in Box 34–24.

safety alert Researchers who have investigated complications associated with intramuscular injection sites indicate that the ventrogluteal site is the preferred site for most injections administered to adults and children, including infants of any age (Cook & Murtagh, 2006; Hockenberry & Wilson, 2007; Nicoll & Hesby, 2002).

Locate the ventrogluteal muscle by placing the heel of your hand over the greater trochanter of the client's hip with the wrist perpendicular to the femur. Use your right hand for the left hip, and your left hand for the right hip. Point your thumb toward the client's groin and point your fingers toward the client's head; point your index finger to the anterior superior iliac spine, and extend your middle finger back along the iliac crest toward the buttocks. The index finger, the middle finger, and the iliac crest form a V-shaped triangle; the injection site is the centre of the triangle (Figure 34–24). The client may lie on his or her side or back. Flexing of the knee and hip helps the client to relax this muscle.

➤ BOX 34-24 Characteristics of Intramuscular Sites and Indications for Usage

Vastus Lateralis Muscle

- Lacks major nerves and blood vessels
- Facilitates rapid drug absorption
- Used frequently with infants (younger than 12 months old) receiving immunizations
- May also be used in older children and toddlers receiving immunizations

Ventrogluteal Muscle

- Offers a deep site, situated away from major nerves and blood vessels
- Offers less chance of contamination in incontinent clients and infants
- Identified easily by prominent bony landmarks
- Is preferred site for medications (e.g., antibiotics) that are larger in volume, more viscous, and irritating for adults, children, and infants

Deltoid Muscle

- Is easily accessible but the muscle is not well-developed in most clients
- May be used for small amounts of medications
- Not used in infants or children with underdeveloped muscles
- Use of the muscle involves potential for injury to the brachial artery, and to the radial and ulnar nerves
- May be used for immunizations of toddlers, older children, and adults
- Recommended site for hepatitis B vaccine and rabies injections

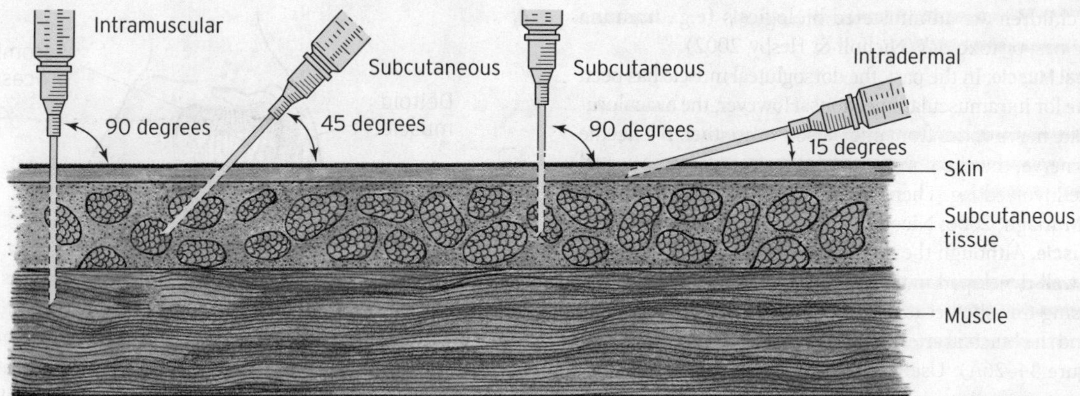

Figure 34-23 Comparison of angles of insertion for intramuscular (90 degrees), subcutaneous (45 and 90 degrees), and intradermal (15 degrees) injections.

Ventrogluteal Muscle. The ventrogluteal muscle, which involves the gluteus medius, is situated deep and away from major nerves and blood vessels. It is a safe site for all clients because it is a large muscle that is well-developed in adults and young children, including those who do not walk (Nicoll & Hesby, 2002). Research shows that injuries such as fibrosis, nerve damage, abscess, tissue necrosis, muscle contraction, gangrene, and pain have been associated with all of the common intramuscular sites except the ventrogluteal site. The only published case study of a complication at the ventrogluteal site reported a local reaction to the medication, which is not a complication associated with the site itself (Nicoll & Hesby, 2002).

Vastus Lateralis Muscle. This thick and well-developed muscle is located on the anterior lateral aspect of the thigh and extends in an adult from a handbreadth above the knee to a handbreadth below the greater trochanter of the femur (Figure 34–25). Use the middle third of the muscle for injection. The width of the muscle usually extends from the midline of the thigh to the midline of the thigh's outer side. When administering injections to young children or cachectic clients, grasp the body of the muscle during injection to ensure the medication is deposited in the muscle tissue. To help relax the muscle, ask the client to assume a sitting position or to lie flat with the knee slightly flexed. The vastus lateralis site is often used when infants,

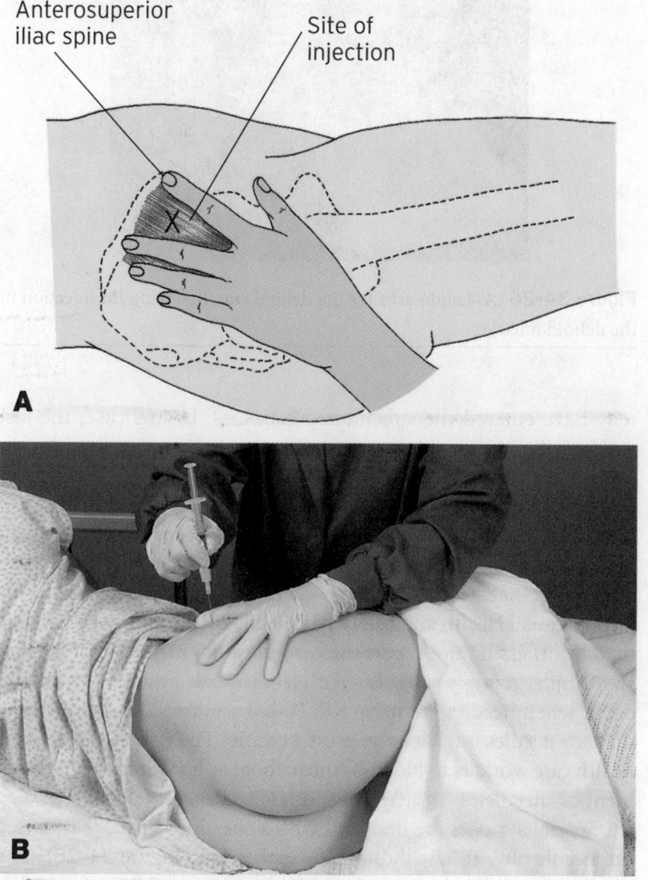

Figure 34-24 A, Landmarks for the ventrogluteal site. B, Giving IM injection in the ventrogluteal muscle.

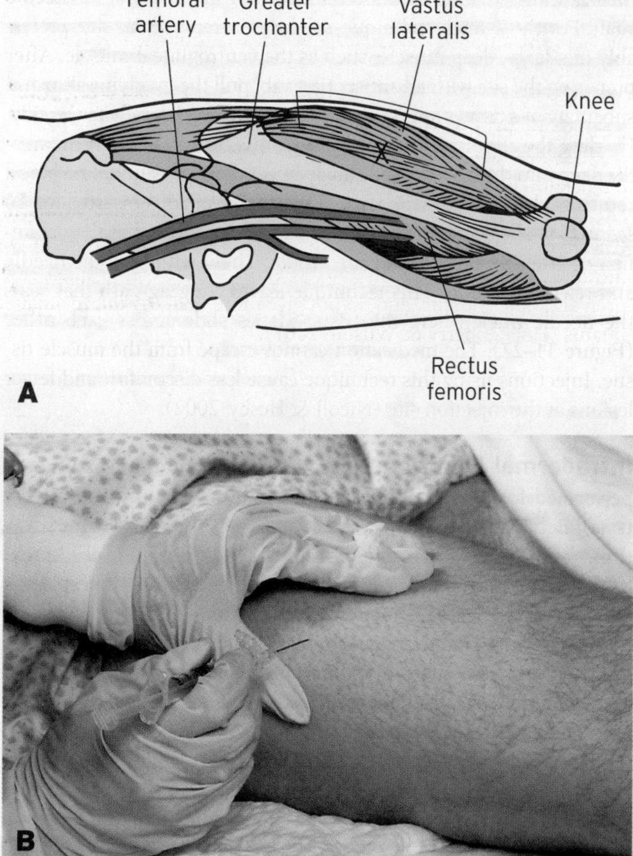

Figure 34-25 A, Landmarks for the vastus lateralis site. B, Giving IM injection in the vastus lateralis muscle.

toddlers, and children are administered biologicals (e.g., immune globulins, vaccines, or toxoids) (Nicholl & Hesby, 2002).

Dorsogluteal Muscle. In the past, the dorsogluteal muscle has been a traditional site for intramuscular injections. However, the exact location of the sciatic nerve varies from one person to another. If a needle hits the sciatic nerve, the client may experience permanent or partial paralysis of the involved leg. Therefore, do *not* use the ventrogluteal site (Cook & Murtagh, 2006; Nicoll & Hesby, 2002; Small, 2004).

Deltoid Muscle. Although the deltoid site is easily accessible, the muscle is not well-developed in many clients. A potential for injury exists when using this site because the axillary, radial, brachial, and ulnar nerves and the brachial artery lie within the upper arm along the humerus (Figure 34–26A). Use this site only for small medication volumes, when giving immunizations, or when other sites are inaccessible because of dressings or casts (Nicoll & Hesby, 2002).

To locate the deltoid muscle, fully expose the client's upper arm and shoulder. Do not roll up a tight-fitting sleeve. Have the client relax the arm at the side and flex the elbow. The client may sit, stand, or lie down (Figure 34–26B). Palpate the lower edge of the acromion process, which forms the base of a triangle in line with the midpoint of the lateral aspect of the upper arm. The injection site is in the centre of the triangle, approximately 3 to 5 cm below the acromion process (Nicoll & Hesby, 2002). You may also locate the site by placing four fingers across the deltoid muscle, with your top finger along the acromion process. The injection site is then three fingerwidths below the acromion process.

Technique for Intramuscular Injections. When administering IM injections, the **Z-track method** is recommended because it minimizes local skin irritation by sealing the medication in the muscle tissue. Insert a new needle into the syringe after preparing the medication so that no solution remains on the outside of the needle shaft. For the Z-track technique, select an intramuscular site, preferably in a large, deep muscle, such as the ventrogluteal muscle. After preparing the site with an antiseptic swab, pull the overlying skin and subcutaneous tissues approximately 2.5 to 3.5 cm laterally to the side. Holding the skin taut with your nondominant hand, insert the needle deep into the muscle, and slowly inject the medication if no blood return is observed on aspiration. The needle remains inserted for 10 seconds to allow the medication to disperse evenly rather than channelling back up the track of the needle. Then, withdraw the needle and release the skin. This technique leaves a zigzag path that seals the needle track where the tissue planes slide across each other (Figure 34–27). The medication cannot escape from the muscle tissue. Injections using this technique cause less discomfort and fewer lesions at the injection site (Nicoll & Hesby, 2002).

Intradermal Injections. Intradermal injections are commonly performed for skin testing (e.g., tuberculin screening and allergy tests). Because these medications are potent, they are injected into the dermis, where blood supply is reduced and medication absorption occurs slowly. If the medications enter the circulation too rapidly, a client may have a severe anaphylactic reaction.

For accurate skin testing, you must be able to see the injection site clearly to detect changes in colour and tissue integrity. Intradermal sites should be lightly pigmented, free of lesions, and relatively hairless. The inner forearm and upper back are ideal locations.

Use a tuberculin or small hypodermic syringe for skin testing. The angle of insertion for an intradermal injection is 5 to 15 degrees (see Figure 34–23), with the bevel of the needle pointed up. As you inject the medication, a small bleb resembling a mosquito bite should appear on the skin's surface (see Skill 34–5). If a bleb does not appear or if the site bleeds after you withdraw the needle, the medication may have entered the subcutaneous tissues. In this case, the test results will not be valid.

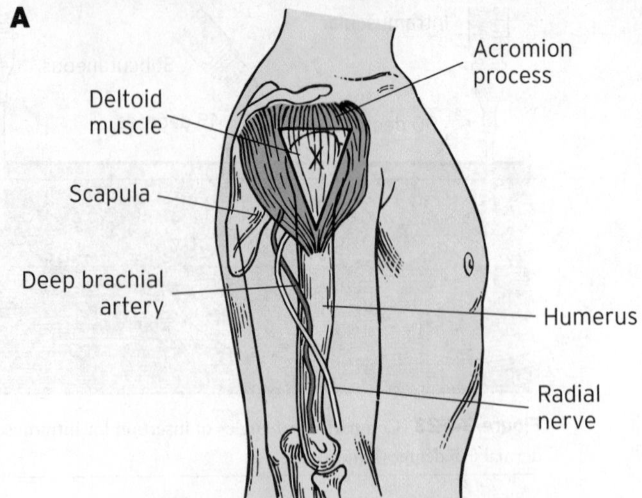

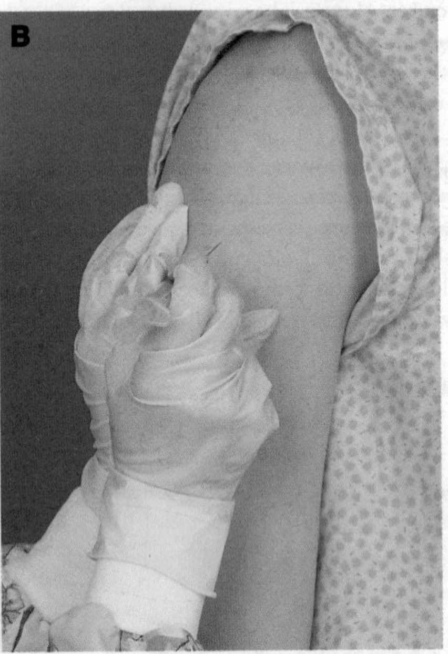

Figure 34-26 A, Landmarks for the deltoid site. B, Giving IM injection in the deltoid muscle.

Safety in Administering Medications by Injection

Needleless Devices. Needle-stick injuries occur frequently in all health care settings. Some hospitals report that one-third of nursing staff suffer needle-stick injuries each year (Canadian Centre for Occupational Health and Safety [CCOHS], 2005). However, because many workers do not report their injuries, the incidence of needle-stick injuries is probably higher. Needle-stick injuries commonly occur when needles are recapped, IV lines and needles are mishandled, or needles are left at a client's bedside. The risk of exposure of health care workers to blood-borne pathogens has led to the development of "needleless devices" or special needle safety devices.

Special syringes are designed with a sheath or guard that covers the needle after it is withdrawn from the skin (Figure 34–28). The needle is immediately covered to eliminate the possibility of a needle-stick injury. The syringe and sheath are disposed of together in a

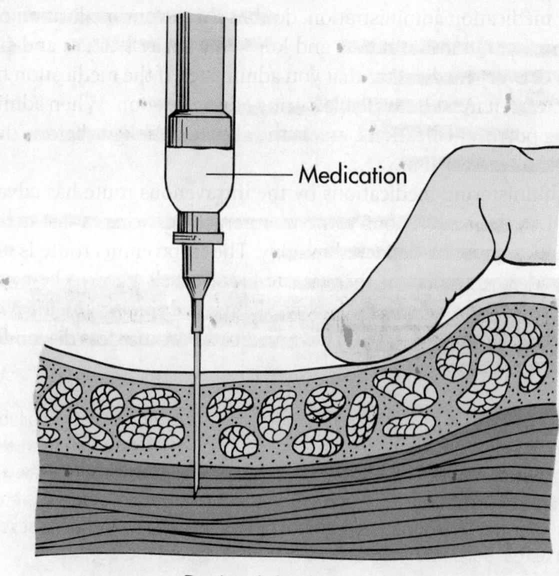

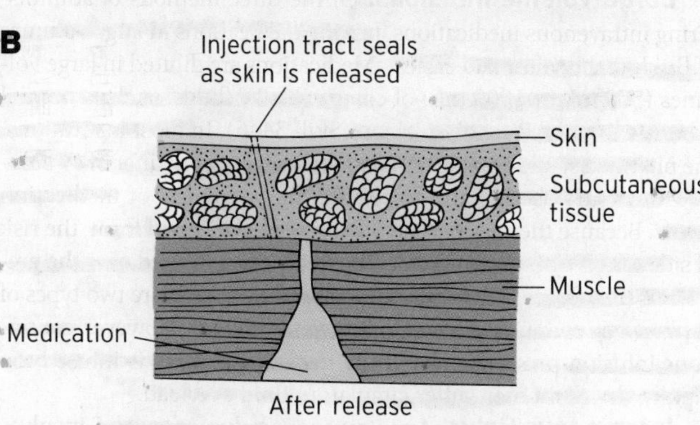

Figure 34-27 A, Pulling on the overlying skin during IM injection moves tissue to prevent later tracking. B, The Z-track left after injection prevents the deposit of medication through sensitive tissue.

receptacle. Needleless devices should be used whenever possible to reduce the risk of injury from needle sticks and sharps (CCOHS, 2005; Health Canada, 1997, 1999; Wilburn & Eijkemans, 2004).

Needles and other instruments that are considered "sharps" are always disposed of into clearly marked containers that are puncture-proof and leadk-proof (Figure 34–29). A needle should never be forced into a needle disposable receptacle that is full. Never place used needles and syringes in a wastebasket, in your pocket, on a client's meal tray, or at the client's bedside. Box 34–25 summarizes recommendations for the prevention of needle-stick injuries.

Intravenous Administration. Medications are administered intravenously by the following methods:

1. As mixtures within large volumes of intravenous fluids
2. By injection of a bolus, or small volume, of medication through an existing intravenous infusion line or intermittent venous access (heparin or saline lock)
3. By "piggyback" infusion of a solution containing the prescribed medication and a small volume of intravenous fluid through an existing intravenous line

In all three methods, the client has either an existing intravenous infusion line or an intravenous access site (sometime called a heparin

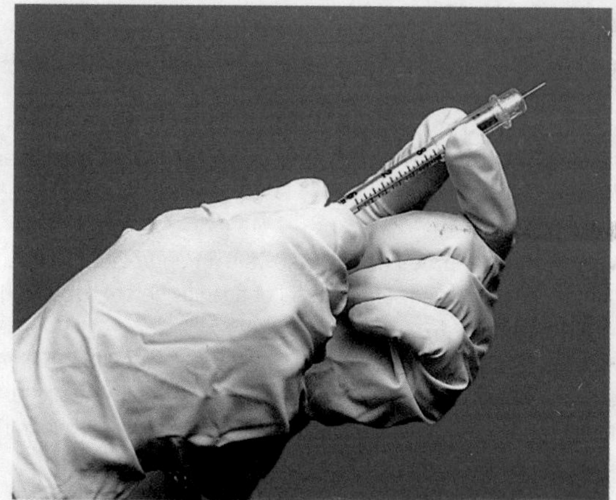

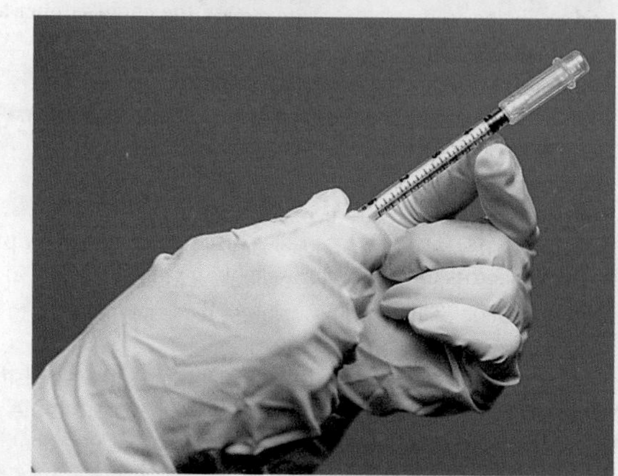

Figure 34-28 Needle with plastic guard to prevent needle sticks. A, Position of guard before injection. B, After injection, the guard locks in place, covering the needle.

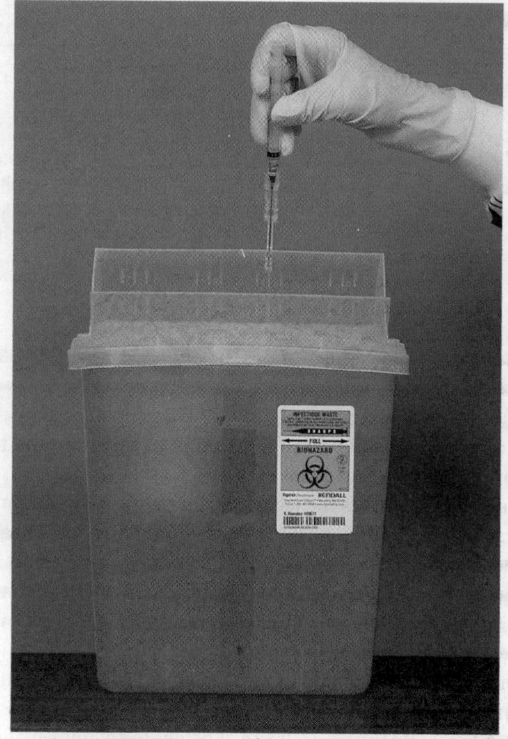

Figure 34-29 Sharps disposal using only one hand.

➤ BOX 34-25 Recommendations for the Prevention of Needle-Stick Injuries

- Avoid using needles when effective needleless systems or sharps with engineered sharps injury protections (SESIP) safety devices are available.
- Never recap needles.
- Never move an exposed needletip toward an unprotected hand.
- Plan safe handling and safe disposal of needles before beginning the procedure.
- Immediately dispose of needles, needleless systems, and SESIP into puncture-proof disposal containers located near the area of use.
- Maintain occupational health and safety standards that include the following:
  - Assessment and implementation of innovations in procedures and technological developments to reduce risks of exposure to contaminated sharps
  - Employee training to address the risks, hazards, and recommended precautions, and the importance of hepatitis B vaccination where appropriate
  - Documentation of consideration and use of appropriate, commercially available, and effective safer devices
  - Selection of devices that do not jeopardize client or employee safety and are determined to be medically advisable
  - Documentation of input from employees regarding methods to reduce exposure
  - Annual re-examination of occupational health and safety standards
- Maintain a needle-stick injury reporting protocol that protects the privacy of persons who have had sharps injuries and includes the following information:
  - Type and brand of device involved in the incident
  - Location of the incident (e.g., name of the department or work area)
  - Description of the incident
  - Protection of privacy for both the employee and client involved in the needle-stick injury

Data from Canadian Centre for Occupational Health and Safety. (2005). *Needlestick injuries,* Retrieved May 1, 2008, from http://www.ccohs.ca/oshanswers/diseases/needlestick_injuries.html; Occupational Safety and Health Administration. (2001). Occupational exposure to bloodborne pathogens: Needlestick and other sharp injuries—Final Rule (CFR 29, part 1910). Federal Register, 66, 5317; and National Institute for Occupational Safety and Health. (1999). *NIOSH alert: Preventing needle-stick injuries in health care settings* (U.S. Department of Health and Human Services [NIOSH] Publication No. 2000-108). Cincinnati, OH: Author.

or saline lock). In most institutions, policies and procedures list the persons who may give intravenous medications and the situations in which these medications may be given. These policies are based on the medication, capability, and availability of staff, and the type of monitoring equipment available.

Chapter 40 describes the technique for performing venipuncture and establishing continuous intravenous fluid infusions. Medication administration is only one reason for supplying intravenous fluids. Intravenous fluid therapy is used primarily for fluid replacement in clients unable to take oral fluids and as a means of supplying the client with electrolytes and nutrients.

When using any method of intravenous medication administration, observe clients closely for symptoms of adverse reactions. After a medication enters the bloodstream, it begins to act immediately, and its action cannot be stopped. Thus, take special care to avoid errors in dose calculation and preparation. Carefully follow the seven rights of safe medication administration, double-check your medication calculations with another nurse, and know the desired action and side effects of every medication that you administer. If the medication has an antidote, it must be available during administration. When administering potent medications, assess the client's vital signs before, during, and after infusion.

Administering medications by the intravenous route has advantages. Use the intravenous route in emergencies when a fast-acting medication must be delivered quickly. The intravenous route is also preferred when constant therapeutic blood levels need to be established. Some medications are highly alkaline and irritating to the muscle and subcutaneous tissue. These medications cause less discomfort when given intravenously.

safety alert Because IV medications are immediately available to the bloodstream after they are administered, verify the prescribed rate of administration with a drug reference manual or a pharmacist before giving any IV medication. This step ensures the medication is administered safely over the appropriate amount of time. Clients can experience severe adverse reactions if IV medications are administered too quickly.

Large-Volume Infusions. Of the three methods of administering intravenous medications, mixing medications in large volumes of fluids is the safest and easiest. Medications are diluted in large volumes (500 mL or 1000 mL) of compatible IV fluids, such as normal saline or lactated Ringer's solution (Skill 34–6). In most institutions, the pharmacist adds medications to the primary container of IV solution to ensure asepsis and to reduce the possibility of medication errors. Because the medication is not in a concentrated form, the risk of side effects or fatal reactions is minimal when infused over the prescribed time frame. Vitamins and potassium chloride are two types of medications commonly added to intravenous fluids. However, continuous infusion presents risks: if the intravenous fluid is infused too rapidly, the client may suffer circulatory fluid overload.

Intravenous Bolus. An intravenous bolus, or "push," involves the introduction of a concentrated dose of a medication directly into the client's systemic circulation (Skill 34–7). A bolus has the advantage of requiring only a small amount of fluid to deliver the medication; therefore, the bolus is useful when the client is on restricted fluids. However, an intravenous bolus, or "push," is the most dangerous method for administering medications because you have no time to correct an error. Also, a bolus may cause direct irritation to the lining of the blood vessels. Before administering a bolus, confirm the placement of the IV line by obtaining a blood return through the intravenous catheter or needle. The inability to obtain a blood return suggests that the needle or catheter is in the client's tissues or is resting against the vein wall. Never give a medication intravenously if the insertion site appears puffy or edematous or if the intravenous fluid cannot flow at the proper rate. Accidental injection of a medication into the tissues around a vein can cause pain, sloughing of tissues, and abscesses, depending on the medication's composition.

Determine the rate of administration of an intravenous bolus medication by the amount of medication that can be given per minute. For example, if a client is to receive 4 mL of a medication over 2 minutes, give 2 mL of the intravenous bolus medication every minute. Research each medication to determine the recommended concentration and rate of administration. When delivering a medication intravenous push, consider the purpose for which a medication is prescribed and any potential adverse effects related to the rate or route of administration.

Volume-Controlled Infusions. IV medications can also be administered through small amounts (50 to 100 mL) of compatible IV fluids. The fluid is within a secondary fluid container separate from the primary fluid bag. The container connects directly to the primary

➤ SKILL 34-6 Adding Medications to Intravenous Fluid Containers

Delegation Considerations

Adding medications to IV fluid containers cannot be delegated to unregulated care providers (UCPs). (In some institutions, the pharmacist may add medications to the primary containers of IV solutions to promote safe medication administration and ensure asepsis.)

Equipment

- Vial or ampule of prescribed medication
- Syringe of appropriate size (5–20 mL)
- Sterile needle (2.5–3.8 cm, 19–21 gauge) with special filters (if required)
- Diluent as indicated (e.g., sterile water, normal saline)
- Sterile IV fluid container (bag or bottle, 25–1000 mL in volume)
- Alcohol or antiseptic swab
- Label to attach to IV bag or bottle
- Medication administration record (MAR) or computer printout

STEPS	RATIONALE
1. Check the accuracy and completeness of each MAR or computer printout against the prescriber's original medication order. Check the client's name and the medication name, route, dosage, and time of administration. Copy or rewrite any portion of the MAR that is difficult to read.	
2. Assess the client's medical history.	
3. Collect information necessary to administer the drug safely, including the medication's action, purpose, side effects, normal dose, time of peak onset, and nursing implications.	
4. When more than one medication is to be added to the IV solution, assess for compatibility of the medications.	• Medications often are incompatible when mixed together. Chemical reactions that occur result in clouding or crystallization of IV fluids. Check the hospital policy for a list of approved medication compatibilities.
5. Assess the client's systemic fluid balance, as evidenced by skin hydration and turgor, body weight, pulse, blood pressure, and ratio of fluid intake to urinary output.	• Continuous IV infusions can lead to fluids that infuse too rapidly, thereby causing circulatory overload, especially in children and older adults (Ebersole et al., 2004; Hockenberry & Wilson, 2007).
6. Assess the client's history of medication allergies.	• The IV administration of medications causes rapid effects. Allergic response can be immediate.
7. Perform hand hygiene.	
8. Assess the IV insertion site for signs of infiltration or phlebitis (see Chapter 40).	• An intact, properly functioning site ensures medication is given safely.
9. Assess the client's understanding of the purpose of the medication therapy.	
10. Prepare the prescribed medication (see Skill 34–4); use aseptic techniques. Ensure that you compare the label of the medication with the MAR two times while preparing the medication.	• Proper technique ensures the medication is sterile; preparation techniques differ for ampules and vials.
11. Perform hand hygiene.	
12. Compare the labels of the medication and the IV fluid bag with the MAR or computer printout.	• Checking the labels ensures the correct medication is injected into the correct IV fluid.
13. Add the medication to a new container (usually in the medication room or at medication cart):	
A. *Solution in a bag:* Locate the medication injection port on the plastic IV solution bag. The port has small rubber stopper at the end. Do not select the port for the IV tubing insertion or the air vent.	• The medication injection port is self-sealing to prevent introduction of microorganisms after repeated use.
B. *Solution in a bottle:* Locate the injection site on the IV solution bottle, which is often covered by a metal or plastic cap.	• Accidental injection of medication through the main tubing port or the air vent can alter the pressure within the bottle and cause fluid leaks through the air vent. The cap seals the bottle to maintain its sterility.
C. Wipe the port or injection site with alcohol or an antiseptic swab (see Step 13C illustration).	• Cleaning the port of injection site reduces the risk of introducing microorganisms into the bag during needle insertion.
D. Remove the needle cap or sheath from the syringe and insert the needle of the syringe or the needleless device through the centre of injection port or site; inject the medication (see Step 13D illustration).	• Injection of the needle into the sides of the port may cause a leak and lead to fluid contamination.
E. Withdraw the syringe from the bag or bottle.	• When the syringe is withdrawn, the injection port self-seals to prevent the introduction of microorganisms.

Continued

➤ SKILL 34-6 Adding Medications to Intravenous Fluid Containers ***continued***

STEPS	RATIONALE
F. Mix the medication and the IV solution by holding the bag or bottle and turning it gently end to end.	• Gently turning the bag or bottle allows even distribution of the medication.
G. Complete the medication label by printing the name and dose of the medication, the date and time of administration, and your initials. Apply the label to the bottle or bag, being careful not to cover any essential information preprinted on the bottle or bag. Spike the bag or bottle with the IV tubing.	• The label informs other health care professionals of the contents of the bag or bottle. • Concealing important information on the IV bag can lead to medication errors.
14. Take the assembled items to the client's bedside at the right time; perform hand hygiene.	
15. Identify the client using at least two client identifiers. Compare the client's name and one other identifier (e.g., the hospital identification number) on the MAR, computer printout, or computer screen against information on the client's identification bracelet. Ask the client to state his or her name if possible, for a third identifier.	
16. Prepare the client by explaining that the medication is to be given through the existing IV line or a new line that will be started. Explain that no discomfort should be felt during the medication infusion. Encourage the client to report symptoms of discomfort.	• Most IV medications do not cause discomfort when diluted; however, potassium chloride is irritating. Pain at the insertion site may be an early indication of infiltration.
17. Connect the infusion tubing or spike container to the existing tubing. Regulate the infusion at the ordered rate.	• Properly regulated infusion prevents rapid infusion of fluid.

Critical Decision Point: Some medications (e.g., potassium chloride) can cause serious adverse reactions, including fatal cardiac dysrhythmias. These medications should be infused on an IV pump. Check the institutional guidelines or policies indicating which IV medications require administration on an IV pump.

18. Add the medication to the existing container.

Critical Decision Point: Because you cannot know exactly how much IV fluid remains in an existing hanging IV container, you are unable to determine the exact concentration of the medication in the IV solution. Therefore, it is recommended that medications be added to new IV fluid containers whenever possible.

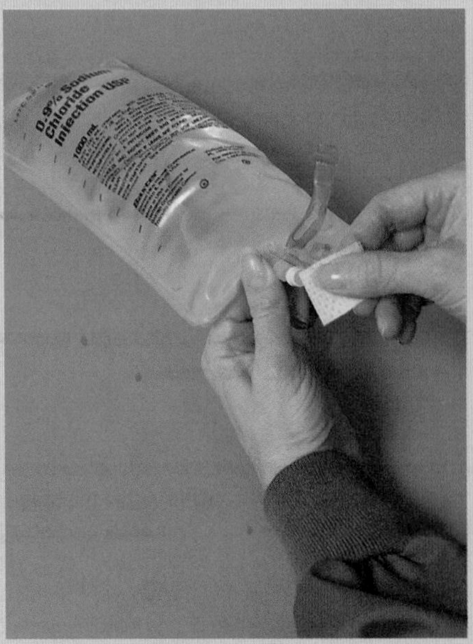

Step 13C Clean the injection port with an antiseptic swab.

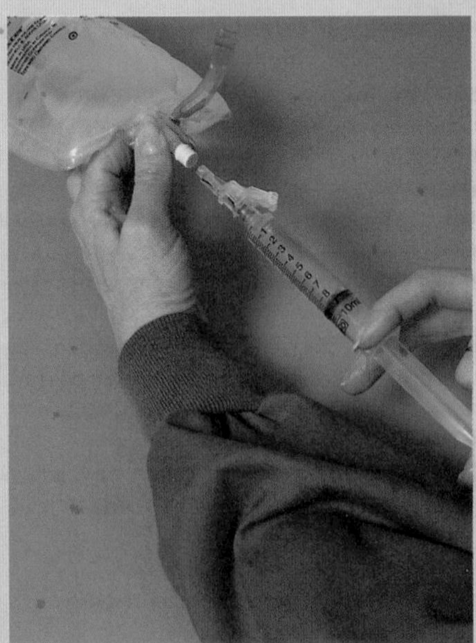

Step 13D Inject the medication through the port.

➤ SKILL 34-6 Adding Medications to Intravenous Fluid Containers *continued*

STEPS	RATIONALE
A. Prepare a vented IV bottle or plastic bag:	
(1) Check the volume of the solution remaining in the bottle or bag.	• Proper minimal volume (see drug insert) is needed to dilute the medication adequately.
(2) Close off the IV infusion clamp.	• Closing the clamp prevents medication from directly entering the client's circulation system when it is injected into the bag or bottle.
(3) Wipe the medication port with an alcohol or antiseptic swab.	• Cleaning the port mechanically removes microorganisms that could enter container during needle insertion.
(4) Remove the needle cap or sheath from the syringe; insert the syringe needle or needleless device through the injection port and inject the medication.	• The injection port is self-sealing and prevents fluid leaks.
(5) Withdraw the syringe from the bag or bottle.	
(6) Lower the bag or bottle from the IV pole and gently mix the medication and the IV solution by holding the bag or bottle and turning it gently end to end. Rehang the bag or bottle.	• Gently turning the bag or bottle ensures the medication is evenly distributed.
B. Complete the medication label and apply it to the unprinted side of the IV solution bag or bottle. Do not cover the imprinted label of the solution.	• The label informs other health care professionals of the contents of the bag or bottle. Concealing important information on the IV bag can lead to medication errors.
C. Regulate the infusion to the desired rate. Use an IV pump if indicated.	• Proper regulated infusion prevents rapid infusion of fluid.
19. Properly dispose of equipment and supplies. Do not recap the needle or syringe. Discard the specially sheathed needles as a unit with the needle covered.	• Proper disposal of the needle prevents injury to both you and the client. Capping of needles increases risk of needle-stick injuries.
20. Perform hand hygiene.	
21. Observe the client for signs or symptoms of medication reaction.	• IV medications can cause rapid effects.
22. Observe the client for signs and symptoms of fluid volume excess.	• Rapid uncontrolled infusion can cause circulatory overload.
23. Periodically return to the client's room to assess the IV insertion site and the rate of infusion.	• Over time, the IV site may become infiltrated or the needle may become malpositioned. The flow rate may change according to the client's body position or the volume of solution left in the container.
24. Observe the client for signs or symptoms of IV infiltration.	• Infiltrated medications can injure tissue.
25. Ensure that a label is applied to the IV tubing; the label must state the date and time that the IV tubing was opened and must be attached to the IV infusion system. Consult with agency policy regarding frequency of changing the IV tubing.	• Most agencies have policies indicating that IV tubing should be changed every 72 hours. The frequency of changing IV tubing may increase on the basis of the solution being administered (e.g., antibiotics, or total parental nutrition [TPN]) or the type of in-dwelling IV catheter (e.g., central line). Changing the IV tubing helps to prevent nosocomial infections.
26. Assess the IV tubing frequently for integrity and occlusions.	• Disruptions in the integrity of the IV tubing can lead to the client not receiving the required IV therapy or medication and may lead to infection.
27. Ask the client to explain the purpose and effects of the medication therapy.	

Unexpected Outcomes and Related Interventions

Adverse or Allergic Reaction to Medication

- Follow institutional policy or guidelines for your appropriate response to and reporting of adverse drug reactions.
- Notify the client's health care professional immediately.
- Add the allergy information to the client's medical record.

Signs of Fluid Volume Overload (e.g., Abnormal Breath Sounds, Shortness of Breath, Intake Greater Than Output)

- Assess the client for compromised circulatory regulation (vital signs, input:output, focused respiratory and cardiac assessments).
- Stop the IV infusion.
- Notify the client's health care professional immediately.

Swelling, Warmth, Redness, and Tenderness at Intravenous Site, Indicating Phlebitis (see Chapter 40)

- Stop IV infusion and discontinue IV.
- Treat the IV site as indicated by institutional policy.
- If continuation of IV therapy is indicated, insert a new IV site.

Coolness, Pallor, and Swelling at Intravenous Site, Indicating Infiltration (see Chapter 40)

- Some IV medications are extremely harmful to the subcutaneous tissue.
- Provide IV extravasation care as indicated by institutional policy, or use a medication reference manual or consult a pharmacist to determine the appropriate follow-up care.

Recording and Reporting

- Record the solution and medication added to parenteral fluid on the appropriate form.
- Report any adverse effects to the client's health care professional, and document adverse effects according to institutional policy.

SKILL 34-7 Administering Medications by Intravenous Bolus

Delegation Considerations

The administration of medications by IV bolus cannot be delegated to unregulated care providers (UCPs). Instruct UCPs to report immediately any unexpected drug reactions, discomfort at the infusion site, and changes in any required vital signs.

Equipment

- A watch with a second hand
- Medication administration record (MAR) or computer printout
- Clean gloves
- Antiseptic swab
- IV push (existing line):
  - Medication in a vial or ampule
  - Syringe for medication preparation
  - Needleless device or sterile needle (21–25 gauge)
- IV lock:
  - Syringe and needleless device (21–25 gauge) for medication preparation
  - Vial of the appropriate flush solution (saline is most common, but heparin may also be used; if heparin is used, the most common concentration is 10 to 100 units; check agency policy)

STEPS	RATIONALE
1. Check the accuracy and completeness of each MAR or computer printout against the prescriber's original medication order. Check the client's name and the medication name, route, dosage, and time of administration. Copy or rewrite any portion of the MAR that is difficult to read.	

Critical Decision Point: Some IV medications can only be pushed safely when the client is being continuously monitored for dysrhythmias, blood pressure changes, or other adverse effects. Therefore, some medications can only be pushed in specific areas within a health care agency. Confirm the institutional guidelines regarding requirements for special monitoring and verify that these requirements are available before giving medication.

STEPS	RATIONALE
2. Collect the information necessary to administer the medication safely, including action, purpose, side effects, normal dose, time of peak onset, the pace at which to give the medication, and nursing implications, such as the need to dilute the medication or to administer it through a filter.	
3. If pushing the medication into an IV line, determine the compatibility of the medication both with the IV fluids and any additives in the IV solution.	• Intravenous medications are not always compatible with IV solutions and additives.
4. Perform hand hygiene. Assess the IV or saline (heparin) lock insertion site for signs of infiltration or phlebitis (see Chapter 40).	• Confirming the placement of the IV catheter and the integrity of the surrounding tissue ensures the medication is administered safely.
5. Check the client's medical history and allergies.	• The intravenous bolus delivers medication rapidly. Allergic reactions can be fatal.
6. Check the date of expiration for the medication vial or ampule.	• Drug potency sometimes increases or decreases when medications are expired.
7. Assess the client's understanding of the purpose of medication therapy.	
8. Prepare the ordered medication from the vial or ampule using aseptic technique (see Skill 34–3). Check the label of the medication carefully with the MAR two times. Apply a removable label indicating the client's name and the medication name and dosage to the removable needle cap.	

Critical Decision Point: Some IV medications require dilution before administration. Verify the dilution requirements with the agency policy. If a small amount of medication is given (e.g., less than 1 mL), dilute the medication in 5 to 10 mL of normal saline or sterile water so that the medication does not collect in the "dead spaces" (e.g., the Y-site injection port or IV cap) of the IV delivery system.

STEPS	RATIONALE
9. Take the medication to the client at the correct time.	
10. Identify the client using at least two client identifiers. Compare the client's name and one other identifier (e.g., the hospital identification number) on the MAR, computer printout, or computer screen against information on the client's identification bracelet. Ask the client to state his or her name if possible, for a third identifier.	
11. Compare the label of the medication with the MAR at the client's bedside.	• The *third check* of the medication label against the MAR at bedside reduces medication administration errors.
12. Explain the procedure to the client. Encourage the client ro report symptoms of discomfort at the IV site.	• Asking the client to report symptoms of discomfort helps in early identification of infiltration.

➤ SKILL 34-7 Administering Medications by Intravenous Bolus *continued*

STEPS	RATIONALE
13. Perform hand hygiene. Apply gloves.	• Hand hygiene reduces the transmission of infection. During IV bolus administration, the risk of blood exposure is low. However, you may need to manipulate the IV dressing or expose the site while you complete other activities. Gloves reduce your exposure.
14. Administer the medication by IV push (through the existing IV line):	
A. Select the injection port of the IV tubing closest to client. Whenever possible, the injection port should accept a needleless syringe. Use the IV filter if required by a medication reference manual or agency policy.	• The WHO (2005; Wilburn & Eiijkemans, 2004), Health Canada (1999), the CCOHS (2005), and the National Institute for Occupational Safety and Health (NIOSH) (1999), which is part of the Centers for Disease Control and Prevention (CDC), strongly recommend that all IV injection sites be needleless to prevent needle-stick injuries.
B. Wipe the injection port with an antiseptic swab. Allow to dry.	• Wiping with an antiseptic swab prevents the introduction of micro-organisms during needle insertion.
C. Connect the syringe to the IV line. Insert the needleless tip or a small-gauge needle of a syringe containing the prepared drug through the centre of the injection port (see Step 14C illustration).	• This procedure prevents damage to the port's diaphragm and subsequent leakage.
D. Occlude the IV line by pinching the tubing just above the injection port (see Step 14D illustration). Pull back gently on the syringe's plunger to aspirate the blood return.	• This step is the *final check* that the medication is being delivered into the bloodstream.

Critical Decision Point: In some cases, especially with a smaller gauge IV needle or a needleless device, the blood return may not be aspirated, even if the IV is patent (open and unblocked). If the IV site does not show signs of infiltration, and the IV fluid is infusing without difficulty, proceed with the IV push.

STEPS	RATIONALE
E. Release the tubing and inject the medication within the amount of time recommended by institutional policy, the pharmacist, or a medication reference manual. Use your watch to time the administration (see Step 14E illustration). The IV line may be pinched while pushing medication and released when not pushing medication (see Step 14E illustration). Allow the IV fluids to infuse when the medication is not being pushed.	• Following the proper procedure ensures safe medication infusion. Rapid injection of IV medication can prove fatal. Allowing the IV fluids to infuse while not pushing the IV drug enables medications to be delivered to the client at a prescribed rate.

Critical Decision Point: If the IV medication is incompatible with IV fluids, stop the IV fluids, clamp the IV line, flush with 10 mL of normal saline or sterile water, give the IV bolus over the appropriate amount of time, flush with another 10 mL of normal saline or sterile water at the same rate as the medication was administered, and then restart the IV fluids at the prescribed rate. If the IV that is currently hanging is a medication, disconnect the IV, and administer the IV push as outlined in Step 14. This step avoids giving the client a sudden bolus of the medication in the existing IV line and avoids creating potential risks associated with IV incompatibilities. Some IV medications and fluids cannot be stopped. Verify the institutional policy regarding the temporary stopping of IV fluids or continuous IV medications. If unable to stop the IV infusion, start a new IV site (see Chapter 40) and administer the medication using the IV lock method.

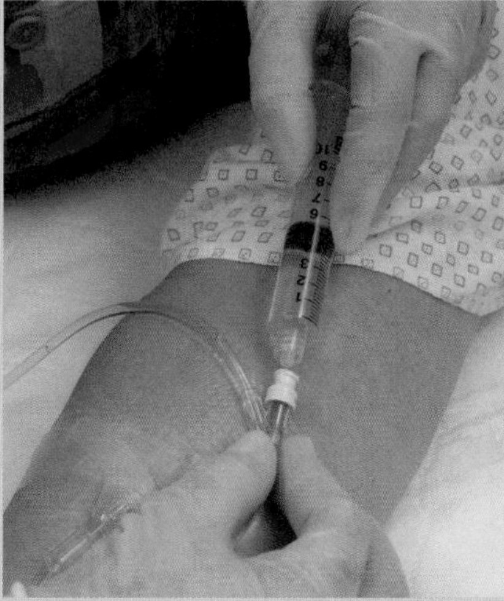

Step 14C Connecting the syringe to the IV line with a blunt needleless cannula tip.

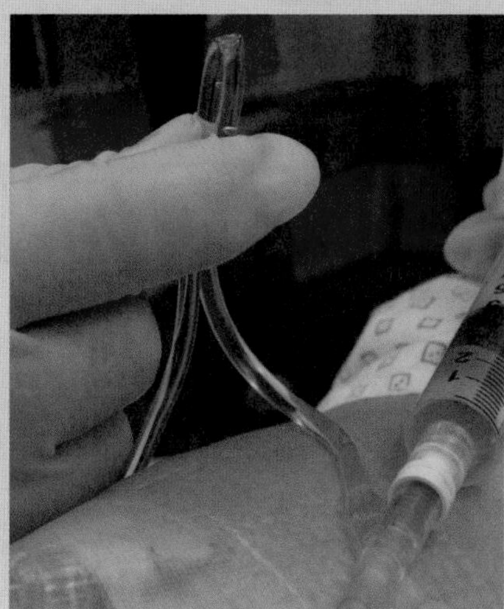

Step 14D Intravenous line pinched above the injection port for medication infusion.

Continued

➤ SKILL 34-7 Administering Medications by Intravenous Bolus *continued*

STEPS	RATIONALE
F. After injecting the medication, release the tubing, withdraw the syringe, and recheck the fluid infusion rate.	• Injection of the bolus may alter the rate of fluid infusion. Rapid fluid infusion can cause circulatory overload.
15. Administer medications by IV push (IV lock or a needleless system):	
A. Prepare the flush solutions according to agency policy. Ensure that a syringe with the correct barrel width is used. Consult with agency policy regarding syringes for delivering IV bolus medications.	• Small syringes with narrow bores (e.g., 1 mL or 3 mL) create greater pressure per square inch (PSI) when used to inject solutions into an IV line. A high PSI can damage the lumen of certain types on in-dwelling IV catheters (central lines and peripherally inserted central catheter [PICC] lines). Ensure that you consult with agency policy to ensure safe maintenance of these lines.
(1) *Saline flush method (preferred method):*	• Normal saline has been found to be effective in keeping IV locks patent and is compatible with a wide range of medications.
(a) Prepare two syringes with 2–3 mL of normal saline (0.9%) in a syringe.	
(2) *Heparin flush method (traditional method):*	
(a) Prepare one syringe with the ordered amount of heparin flush solution.	
(b) Prepare two syringes with 2–3 mL of normal saline.	
B. Administer medication:	
(1) Wipe the lock's injection port with an antiseptic swab.	• Wiping the injection port prevents introduction of microorganisms during the needle insertion.
(2) Insert a syringe containing normal saline into the injection port of the IV lock (see Step 15B2 illustration).	

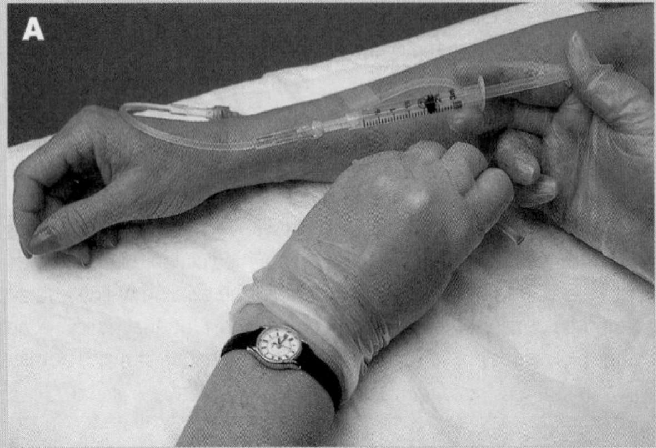

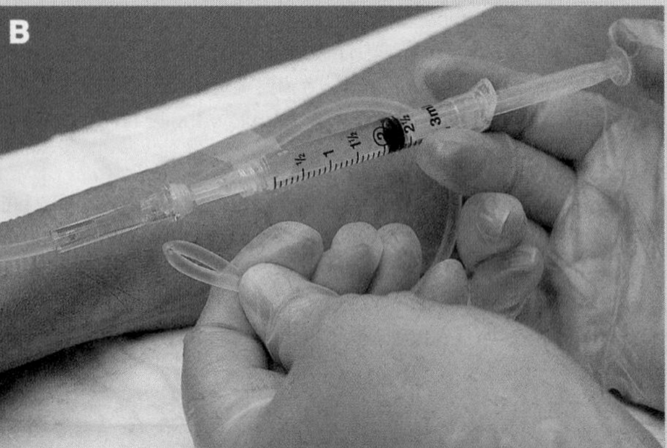

Step 14E A, Timing the IV push medication. **B,** The IV line is pinched off for medication infusion (optional).

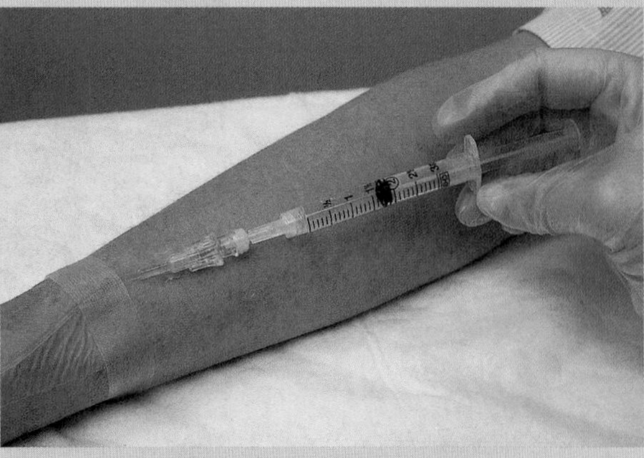

Step 15B(2) Syringe inserted into the injection port.

➤ SKILL 34-7 Administering Medications by Intravenous Bolus *continued*

STEPS	RATIONALE
(3) Pull back gently on the syringe plunger and look for blood return.	• This step determines whether the IV needle or catheter is positioned in the vein.

Critical Decision Point: Sometimes a saline (or heparin) lock will not yield a blood return even though the lock is patent. If the IV site does not show signs of infiltration, proceed with the IV push.

STEPS	RATIONALE
(4) Flush the IV lock with normal saline by pushing slowly on the plunger.	• Flushing the IV lock clears it of blood.

Critical Decision Point: Observe closely the area of skin above the IV catheter. As the IV lock is flushed, note any puffiness or swelling, which could indicate infiltration into the vein, and thereby require removal of the catheter.

STEPS	RATIONALE
(5) Remove the saline-filled syringe.	
(6) Clean the lock's injection port with an antiseptic swab.	• Cleaning the injection port prevents transmission of infection.
(7) Insert the syringe containing the prepared medication into the injection port of the IV lock.	
(8) Inject the medication within the amount of time recommended by institutional policy, the pharmacist, or a medication reference manual. Use a watch to time the administration.	• Rapid injection of the IV medication can result in death. Following the guidelines for IV push rates promotes patient safety (Karch & Karch, 2003).
(9) After administering the bolus, withdraw the syringe.	
(10) Clean the lock's injection port with an antiseptic swab.	• Cleaning the injection port prevents transmission of microorganisms.
(11) Attach the syringe with normal saline and inject the normal saline flush at the same rate that the medication was delivered.	• Irrigation with saline prevents occlusion of the IV access device and ensures all medication is delivered. Flushing the IV site at the same rate as the medication ensures that any medication remaining within the IV needle is delivered at the correct rate.
(12) *Heparin flush option:* Insert the needle of the syringe containing the heparin through the diaphragm.	• Inserting the needle through the diaphragm maintains the patency of the IV catheter and tubing by inhibiting clot formation. Use the SASH method: **S**aline, **A**dministration of medication, **S**aline, **H**eparin.
16. Dispose of uncapped needles and syringes in puncture-proof and leak-proof container.	• Proper disposal reduces the risk of accidental needle sticks.
17. Remove and dispose of gloves. Perform hand hygiene.	• Proper hygiene reduces the transmission of microorganisms.
18. Observe the client closely for adverse reactions while the medication is administered and for several minutes thereafter.	• IV medications act rapidly.
19. Observe the IV site during injection for sudden swelling.	• Swelling indicates infiltration into tissues surrounding the vein.
20. Observe the client's status after adminstering the medication to evaluate the effectiveness of medication.	• IV bolus medications often cause rapid changes in the client's physiological status. Some medications require careful monitoring and assessment and possible laboratory testing (e.g., vasopressors require the monitoring of blood pressure and heart rate; dilantin requires laboratory studies to determine whether it is at a therapeutic level).
21. Consult with agency policy with regard to the frequency of saline flushes.	• To maintain patency of intravenous catheters (peripheral or central), IV devices require routine flushing. Short-term peripheral angiocatheters are flushed every 12 hours with a normal saline solution. Consult with agency policy with regard to protocols for flushing central lines.
22. Ask the client to explain the medication's purposes and side effects.	

Unexpected Outcomes and Related Interventions

Adverse Reaction to Medication

- Stop delivering medication immediately and follow institutional policy or guidelines for the appropriate response and reporting of adverse drug reactions.
- Notify the client's health care professional of adverse effects immediately.
- Add allergy information to the client's medical record.

Symptoms of Infiltration or Phlebitis at Intravenous Site

- Immediately discontinue administration of the injection and discontinue use of the site.
- Follow institutional guidelines on appropriate extravasation care.

Recording and Reporting

- Record the medication, dose, time, and route on the appropriate form (MAR) or in computer record.
- Report any adverse reactions immediately to the health care professional because the reactions could be life-threatening. The client's response may indicate the need for additional medical therapy.
- Record the client's response to medication in the nurses' notes.

IV line or to separate tubing that inserts into the primary line. Three types of containers are volume-control administration sets (e.g., Volutrol or Pediatrol): piggyback sets, tandem sets, and mini-infusors. The use of volume-controlled infusions has several advantages:

- The risk of rapid-dose infusion by IV push is reduced. Medications are diluted and infused over longer time intervals (e.g., 30 to 60 minutes).
- Medications that are stable for only a limited time in solution (e.g., antibiotics) can be administered.
- IV fluid intake can be controlled.

Volume-Control Administration. Volume-control administration (e.g., Volutrol, Buretrol, Pediatrol) sets are small (50 to 150 mL) containers that attach just below the primary infusion bag or bottle. The set is attached and filled in a manner similar to the procedure used with a regular intravenous infusion; however, the priming or filling of the set is different and depends on the type of filter (floating valve or membrane). A Buretrol or Volutrol is used to deliver IV fluids in a safe manner to children in many agencies even when infusion pumps are used. Follow package directions for priming sets (see Chapter 40).

Piggyback. A piggyback is a small (25 to 250 mL) IV bag or bottle that connects to short tubing lines that, in turn, connect to the upper Y-port of a primary infusion line or to an intermittent venous access (Figure 34–30). The piggyback tubing is a microdrip or macrodrip system (see Chapter 40). The set is called a piggyback because the small bag or bottle is set higher than the primary infusion bag or bottle. In the piggyback setup, the main line does not infuse when the piggybacked medication is infusing. The port of the primary IV line contains a back-check valve that automatically stops flow of the primary infusion when the piggyback infusion flows. After the piggyback solution infuses and the solution within the tubing falls below the level of the primary infusion drip chamber, the back-check valve opens and the primary infusion again flows.

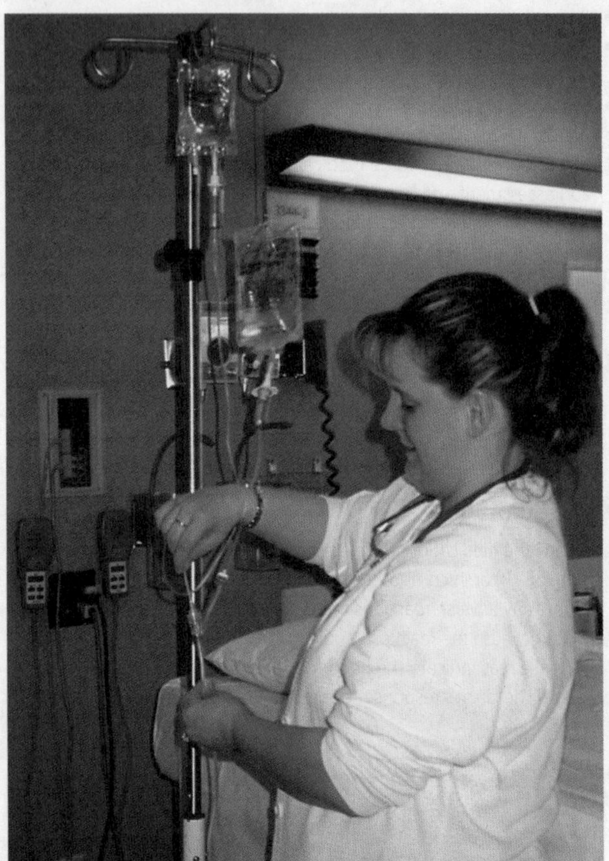

Figure 34-30 Piggyback setup.

Tandem. A tandem setup is a small (25 to 100 mL) IV bag or bottle connected to a short tubing line that connects to the lower Y-port of a primary infusion line or to an intermittent venous access. The tandem set is placed at the same height as the primary infusion bag or bottle. In the tandem setup, the tandem and the main line infuse simultaneously. Monitor the tandem setup closely. If it is not immediately clamped when the medication is infused, the IV solution from the primary line will back up into the tandem line.

Mini-Infusion Pump. The mini-infusion pump is battery operated and allows medications to be given in very small amounts (5 to 60 mL) within controlled infusion times using standard syringes (Skill 34–8).

Intermittent Venous Access. An intermittent venous access (commonly called a heparin lock or saline lock) is an IV catheter with a small chamber covered by a rubber diaphragm or a specially designed cap (Figure 34–31). Special rubber-seal injection caps accept the needle safety devices and can be inserted into most IV catheters (see Chapter 40). Advantages to intermittent venous access include the following:

- Reduced risk of the client developing fluid volume excess
- Increased mobility, safety, and comfort for the client

Before administering an IV bolus or piggyback medication, assess the patency and placement of the IV site. After the medication has been administered through an intermittent venous access, the access must be flushed with a solution to keep it patent. In general, normal saline is an effective flush solution for peripheral catheters. Some institutions require the use of heparin. Verify and follow the institution's policies regarding the care and maintenance of the IV site.

Administration of IV Therapy in the Home. Sometimes clients may be discharged from an acute care setting and continue to receive IV therapy in the home setting. Medications such as antibiotics, chemotherapy, total parenteral nutrition, pain medications, and blood transfusions may be given in the home. Most clients who have home IV therapy will have a central venous catheter inserted before their discharge (see Chapter 40). In addition, clients who need to receive IV therapy in the home have home care nurses who assist in the management of the IV therapy.

However, clients and their families need to be carefully assessed for their ability to manage this therapy at home. Instruction on IV care management must be provided while the client is still in the hospital. Clients and their families need to be taught how to recognize problems and what to do when these problems occur. It is important for the client's family to recognize signs of infection and complications and to know that when these signs occur, the home care nurse or physician must be notified. In addition, clients and their families need information regarding the maintenance of IV administration equipment, including the infusion pump.

Subcutaneous Butterfly Catheters. Subcutaneous butterfly catheters provide a route for both subcutaneous medication administration and hypodermoclysis (Box 34–26). As a route for medication administration, subcutaneous butterfly catheters reduce the frequency of breaking the skin barrier to inject a medication. This route is used for clients requiring longer-term therapy with medication that is administered via subcutaneous injection. **Hypodermoclysis** is the administration of fluids through a butterfly catheter and is commonly used for clients with limited intravenous access, palliative care clients, and clients at risk for or with mild dehydration.

➤ SKILL 34-8 Administering Intravenous Medications by Piggyback, Intermittent Intravenous Infusion Sets, and Mini-Infusion Pumps

Delegation Considerations

The administration of medications by IV fluid by piggyback, intermittent IV infusion sets, and mini-infusion pumps cannot be delegated to unregulated care providers (UCPs). Instruct UCPs to report any unexpected drug reactions or discomfort at the infusion site as soon as possible.

Equipment

- Antiseptic swab
- IV pole
- Medication administration record (MAR) or computer printout
- Medication labels
- Piggyback, tandem, or mini-infusion pump:
  - Medication prepared in 5- to 150-mL labelled infusion bag or syringe
  - Short microdrip or macrodrip tubing set for piggyback (may have needleless system attachment)
  - Needleless device or stopcocks if available
  - Needles (21 or 23 gauge, only if stopcocks or other needleless methods are not available)
  - Mini-infusion pump
  - Adhesive tape (optional)
- Volume-control administration set
  - Volutrol, Buretrol, or Pediatrol
  - Infusion tubing (may have needleless system attachment)
  - Syringe (1–20 mL)
  - Vial or ampule of ordered medication

STEPS	RATIONALE
1. Check the accuracy and completeness of each MAR or computer printout against the prescriber's original medication order. Check the client's name and the medication name, route, dosage, and time of administration. Copy or rewrite any portion of the MAR that is difficult to read.	• The order sheet is the most reliable source and only legal record of medications clients are to receive. Checking the accuracy of the medication order ensures that the client receives the correct medications. Illegible MARs are a source of medication errors.
2. Determine the client's medical history.	
3. Collect the information necessary to administer the medication safely, including the action, purpose, side effects, normal dose, time of peak onset, and nursing implications.	• Information about the medication indicates the type of appropriate IV solution to use and helps to ensure safe and accurate medication administration.
4. Assess the compatibility of the drug with the existing IV solution.	• Drugs that are incompatible with IV solutions may result in clouding or crystallization of the solution in IV tubing, which may harm the client.

Critical Decision Point: Never administer IV medications through tubing that is infusing blood, blood products, or parenteral nutrition solutions.

STEPS	RATIONALE
5. Assess the patency of the client's existing IV infusion line by noting the infusion rate of the main IV line.	• The IV line must be patent and fluids must infuse easily for medication to reach the venous circulation effectively.

Critical Decision Point: If the client's IV site is saline locked, clean the port with alcohol and assess the patency of the IV line by flushing it with 2–3 mL of sterile normal saline. Attach the appropriate IV tubing to the saline lock and administer the medication via piggyback, tandem, mini-infusion, or volume-control administration set. When the infusion is completed, disconnect the tubing, clean the port with alcohol, and flush the IV line with 2–3 mL sterile normal saline. Maintain sterility of the IV tubing between intermittent infusions.

STEPS	RATIONALE
6. Perform hand hygiene. Assess the IV insertion site for signs of infiltration or phlebitis: redness, pallor, swelling, tenderness on palpation.	• Confirmation of placement of IV needle or catheter and integrity of surrounding tissues ensures medication is administered safely.
7. Assess the client's history of medication allergies.	• The effects of medications can develop rapidly after IV infusion. You should be aware of clients who are at risk for an allergic reaction.
8. Assess the client's understanding of purpose of medication therapy.	
9. Prepare the medication. Ensure that you compare the label of the medication with the MAR two times while preparing the medication.	• Ensure that correct medication is given to client. *First and second checks for accuracy ensure that the correct medication is administered.*
10. Assemble the supplies at the bedside. Prepare the client by explaining that the medication will be given through the IV equipment.	
11. Perform hand hygiene.	
12. Identify the client using at least two client identifiers. Compare the client's name and one other identifier (e.g., the hospital identification number) on the MAR, computer printout, or computer screen against information on the client's identification bracelet. Ask the client to state his or her name, if possible, for a third identifier.	• This process complies with The Joint Commission's (2007) requirements and improves medication safety. In acute care settings, the client's name and identification number on an armband and the MAR are usually used to identify clients. Identification bracelets are made at the time of the client's admission and are the most reliable source of information. The client's room number is *not* an acceptable identifier.
13. Compare medication label with MAR at client's bedside.	• *This is the third accuracy check.*
14. Explain to the client the purpose of the medication and its side effects. Encourage the client to report symptoms of discomfort at the injection site.	• Communication with the client keeps the client informed of planned therapies. Clients who can verbalize pain at the IV site can help detect IV infiltrations early, reducing the possibility of damage to the surrounding tissues.

Continued

➤ SKILL 34-8 Administering Intravenous Medications by Piggyback, Intermittent Intravenous Infusion Sets, and Mini-Infusion Pumps *continued*

STEPS	RATIONALE
15. Administer the infusion:	
A. Piggyback or tandem infusion	
(1) Connect the infusion tubing to the medication bag (see Chapter 40). Allow the solution to fill the tubing by opening the regulator flow clamp. Once the tubing is full, close the clamp and cap the end of the tubing.	• The infusion tubing should be filled with solution and free of air bubbles to prevent an air embolus.
(2) Hang the piggyback medication bag above the level of the primary fluid bag. (A hook may be used to lower the main bag.) Hang the tandem infusion at same level as the primary fluid bag.	• The height of the fluid bag affects the rate of medication flow to the client.
(3) Connect the tubing of the piggyback or tandem infusion to the appropriate connector on the primary infusion line:	
(a) *Stopcock:* Wipe the stopcock port with an alcohol swab and connect the tubing. Turn the stopcock to the open position.	
(b) *Needleless system:* Wipe the needleless port, and insert the tip of the piggyback or tandem infusion tubing (see Step 15A(3)(b) illustrations).	• The WHO (2005; Wilburn & Eijkemans, 2004); Health Canada (1999), the CCOHS (2005), and the CDC (NIOSH, 1999) strongly recommend that all IV injection sites be needleless to prevent needle-stick injuries The needleless system establishes the route for IV medication to enter the main IV line.
(c) *Tubing port:* Connect the sterile needle to the end of the piggyback or tandem infusion tubing, remove the cap, clean the injection port on the main IV line, and insert the needle or needleless access device through the centre of the port. Secure by taping the connection.	• Use this step *only* if the needleless system is not available. The tubing port prevents the introduction of microorganisms during needle insertion.
(4) Regulate the flow rate of the medication solution by adjusting the regulator clamp. (Infusion times vary. Refer to a medication reference manual or institutional policy for the safe flow rate.)	• The proper flow rate provides a slow, intermittent infusion of medication and maintains therapeutic blood levels.
(5) After medication has infused, check the flow regulator on the primary infusion. The primary infusion should automatically begin to flow after the piggyback or tandem solution is empty.	• The back-check valve on the piggyback stops the flow of the primary infusion until the second medication infuses. The tandem and primary infusions flow together until the tandem set empties. Monitoring the flow rate ensures the proper administration of IV fluids.
(6) Regulate the main infusion line to the desired rate, if necessary.	• The infusion of the piggyback may interfere with the main line infusion rate.
(7) Leave the IV piggyback bag and tubing in place for future medication administration or discard in appropriate containers.	• The establishment of a secondary line produces a route for microorganisms to enter the main line. Repeated changes in the tubing increase the risk of infection transmission (check agency policy).
B. Volume-control administration set (e.g., Volutrol)	
(1) Assemble the supplies in the medication room.	• Use of the medication room controls the risk of contaminating the IV solution.
(2) Prepare medication from a vial or ampule (see Skill 34–3).	• Following proper procedure ensures the medication is sterile.
(3) Fill the Volutrol with the desired amount of fluid (50–100 mL) by opening the clamp between the Volutrol and the main IV bag (see Step 15B(3) illustration).	• Use of a small volume of fluid dilutes the IV medication and reduces the risk of too-rapid infusion.

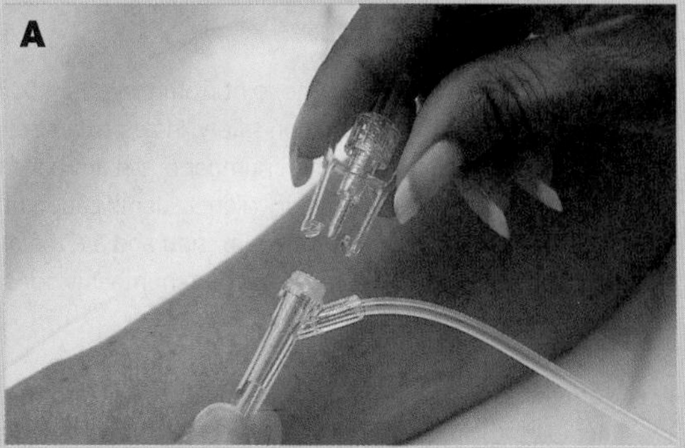

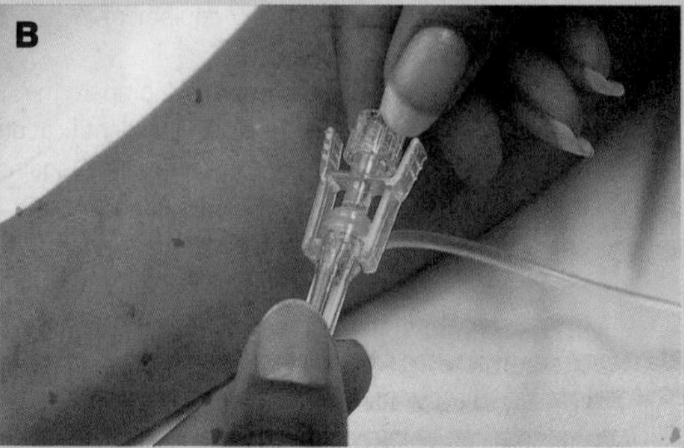

Step 15A(3)(b) **A,** Needleless lever lock cannula system. **B,** The blunt-ended cannula inserts into the port and locks.

➤ SKILL 34-8 Administering Intravenous Medications by Piggyback, Intermittent Intravenous Infusion Sets, and Mini-Infusion Pumps ***continued***

STEPS	RATIONALE
(4) Close the clamp and ensure the clamp on the air vent of the Volutrol chamber is open.	• Prevents additional leakage of fluid into the Volutrol. The air vent allows fluid in the Volutrol to exit at regulated rate.
(5) Clean the injection port on the top of the Volutrol with an antiseptic swab.	• Cleaning the injection port prevents the introduction of microorganisms during needle insertion.
(6) Remove the needle cap or sheath and insert the syringe needle through the port, then inject the medication (see Step 15B(6) illustrations). Gently rotate the Volutrol between your hands.	• Rotating mixes the medication with the solution in the Volutrol to ensure equal distribution.
(7) Regulate the IV infusion rate to allow the medication to infuse in the time recommended by institutional policy, a pharmacist, or a medication reference manual.	• For optimal therapeutic effect, the medication should infuse in the prescribed time interval.
(8) Label the Volutrol with the name of the medication, the dosage, the total volume (including the diluent), and the time of administration.	• Proper labelling alerts nurses to medication being infused and prevents other medications from being added to the Volutrol.
(9) Dispose of the uncapped needle or the needle enclosed in safety shield and syringe in a proper container. Perform hand hygiene.	• Proper disposal prevents accidental needle-stick injuries. Hand hygiene reduces the transmission of microorganisms.
C. Mini-infusion administration	
(1) Connect the prefilled syringe to the mini-infusion tubing.	• The special tubing is designed to fit the syringe to deliver the medication to the main IV line.
(2) Carefully apply pressure to the syringe plunger, allowing the tubing to fill with medication.	• Applying pressure ensures the tubing is free of air bubbles to prevent an air embolus.
(3) Place the syringe into a mini-infusor pump (follow product directions). Ensure the syringe is secure (see Step 15C(3) illustration).	
(4) Connect the mini-infusion tubing to the main IV line.	
(a) *Stopcock:* Wipe the stopcock port with an alcohol swab and connect the tubing. Turn the stopcock to the open position.	• Use of the stopcock reduces the risk of needle-stick injuries.
(b) *Needleless system:* Wipe the needleless port and insert the tip of the mini-infusor tubing.	
(c) *Tubing port:* Connect the sterile needle to the mini-infusion tubing, remove the cap, clean the injection port on the main IV line, and insert the needle through the centre of the port. Consider placing tape where the IV tubing enters the port to secure the connection.	• Cleaning reduces the transmission of microorganisms.

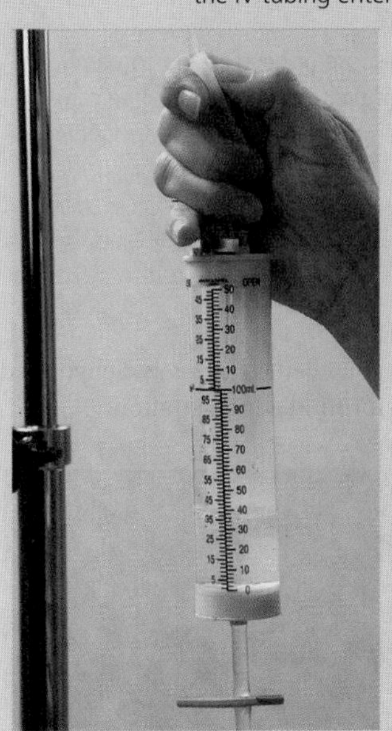

Step 15B(3) Filling the volume-control administration device.

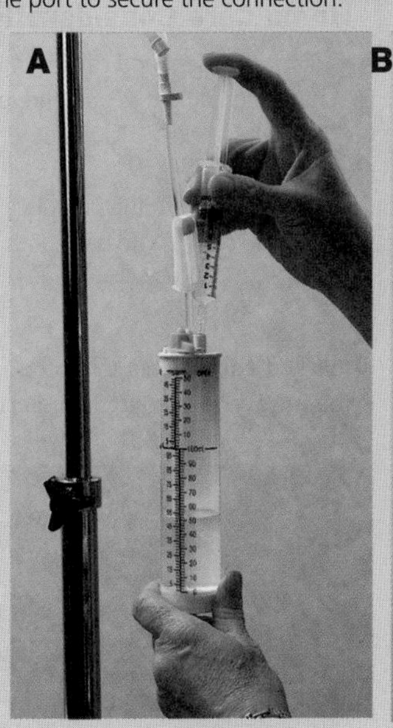

Step 15B(6) A, Medication injected into the device. **B,** The prepared device.

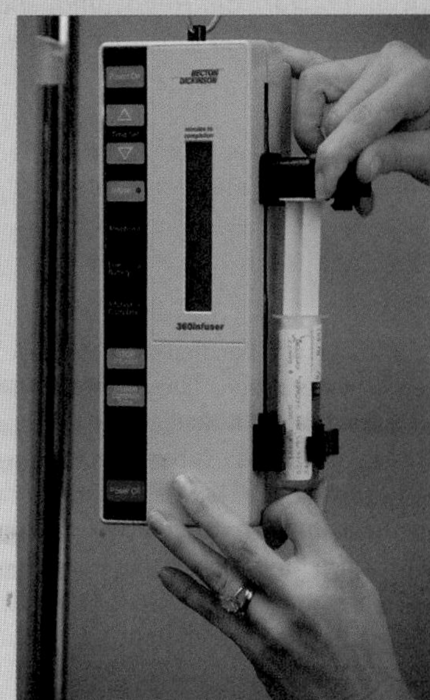

Step 15C(3) Securing the syringe into a mini-infusor.

Continued

➤ SKILL 34-8 Administering Intravenous Medications by Piggyback, Intermittent Intravenous Infusion Sets, and Mini-Infusion Pumps *continued*

STEPS	RATIONALE
(5) Explain the purpose of the medication and the side effects to the client and explain that the medication is to be given through the existing IV line. Ask the client to report any symptoms of discomfort at the injection site.	• Proper communication informs the client of planned therapies.
(6) Hang the infusion pump with the syringe on the IV pole alongside the main IV bag. Set the pump to deliver medication within the time recommended by institutional policy, the pharmacist, or a medication reference manual. Press the button on the pump to begin infusion. Optional: Set the alarm.	• The pump automatically delivers medication at a safe, constant rate, on the basis of the volume in the syringe. (An alarm is used if the medication is delivered into a heparin or saline lock.)
(7) After medication has infused, check the flow regulator on the primary infusion. The infusion should automatically begin to flow once the pump stops. Regulate the main infusion line to the desired rate as needed. (Note: If the stopcock is used, turn off the mini-infusion line.)	• Proper flow maintains the patency of primary IV line.
16. Observe the client for signs of adverse reactions.	• IV medications act rapidly.
17. During infusion, periodically check the infusion rate and the condition of the IV site.	• The IV must remain patent for proper medication administration. If infiltration develops, discontinue the infusion.
18. Ask the client to explain the purpose and side effects of the medication.	• Asking the client about the medication evaluates the client's understanding of the instructions.

Unexpected Outcomes and Related Interventions

Adverse Drug Reaction

- Stop medication infusion immediately.
- Follow institutional policy or guidelines for the appropriate response, assessments, and reporting of adverse drug reactions.
- Notify the client's health care professional of adverse effects immediately.
- Document the allergy in the client's medical record.

Medication Does Not Infuse Over Desired Period

- Determine the reason for the lack of infusion (e.g., improper calculation of flow rate, wrong positioning of the IV needle at the insertion site, or infiltration).
- Take corrective action as indicated.

Swelling, Warmth, Reddening, and Tenderness at Intravenous Site, Indicating Phlebitis (see Chapter 40)

- Stop IV infusion.
- Discontinue IV.
- Treat the IV site as indicated by the institutional policy.
- Insert a new IV site if continuation of therapy is indicated.

Coolness, Pallor, and Swelling at Intravenous Site (see Chapter 40)

- Signs of infiltration are indicated.
- Some IV medications are extremely harmful to subcutaneous tissue.
- Provide IV extravasation care as indicated by institutional policy; or use a medication reference manual or consult a pharmacist to determine the appropriate follow-up care.

Recording and Reporting

- Record the medication, dose, route, and time administered on the MAR or computer printout.
- Record on the intake and output form the volume of fluid in the medication bag or Volutrol.
- Report any adverse reactions to the nurse in charge or the physician.

Home Care Considerations

- Teach the client and caregiver to dispose of needles and contaminated equipment in puncture-proof containers (e.g., a coffee can).
- Instruct the client's family about community resources for obtaining supplies.
- Collaborate with the interdisciplinary team to facilitate access to supplies for clients who have both physical and geographical barriers.

A fine-gauge needle (e.g., 24 gauge) is inserted into the client's subcutaneous tissue. The preferred site for subcutaneous butterfly catheters is the subcutaneous tissue of the abdomen. Other appropriate sites include the subcutaneous tissue of the upper arms, upper back (scapular area), anterior thighs, and the anterior upper chest (avoiding the breast and axilla). Do not insert a subcutaneous butterfly catheter into tissues that have recently been irradiated or where a rash, bruising, or scar tissue is present. After inserting a subcutaneous butterfly catheter, only one type of medication can be injected (e.g., morphine).

Contraindications to using the hypodermoclysis route for IV fluid administration include cardiac failure, prerenal or renal failure, low platelet or coagulation disorders, and existing fluid overload or marked edema (see Chapter 40). If a client is severely dehydrated, the intravenous route is preferred for fluid administration.

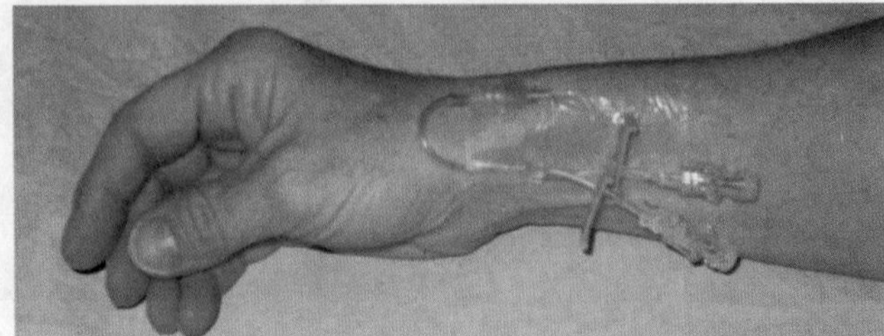

Figure 34-31 Intermittent lock covered with a rubber diaphragm.

➤ BOX 34-26 Procedural Guidelines

Subcutaneous Butterfly Catheters and Hypodermoclysis

Delegation Considerations: The insertion of subcutaneous butterfly catheters cannot be delegated. Instruct unregulated care providers to report the occurrence of side effects of medications immediately.

Equipment:

- Butterfly catheter with 24-gauge, 19-mm needle (the smallest and shortest gauge should be used)
- Interline injection site
- Antiseptic swab
- Occlusive dressing (Tegaderm™ or Opsite™)
- Tape
- Clean gloves

Subcutaneous Medication Administration

- Ordered medication
- Syringe and needleless access device

Hypodermoclysis

- Ordered IV fluid
- IV administration set

Procedure

1. Check the accuracy and completeness of each medication administration record (MAR) or computer printout against the prescriber's original medication order. Check the client's name and the medication name, route, dosage, and time of administration. Copy or rewrite any portion of the MAR that is difficult to read.
2. Assess the client's medical history, medication history, and history of allergies; know the substances the client is allergic to and the allergic reaction.
3. Check the date of expiration for the medication.
4. Assess the adequacy of adipose tissue and any contraindications, such as rash, bruising, or scar tissue.
5. Remove the butterfly catheter from the package (see Step 5 illustration). Replace the existing cap with an interlink injection site.

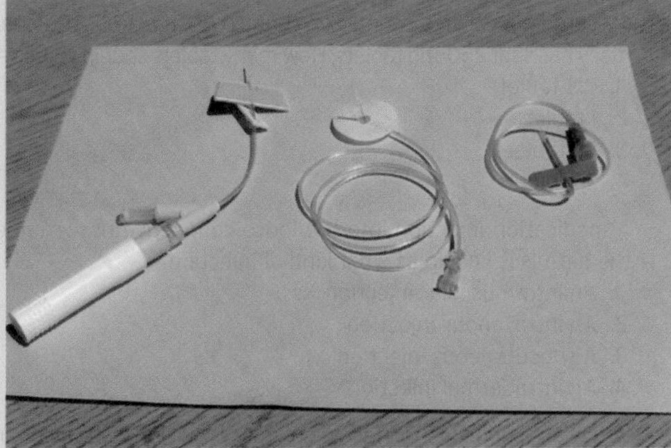

Step 5 Subcutaneous butterfly catheters. **Source:** Courtesy Lynne Thibeault, Confederation College. Thunder Bay, ON.

6. *Subcutaneous medication administration:* Aseptically prepare the correct medication dose from an ampule or vial (see Skill 34–3). Ensure all air is expelled. Check the label of the medication with the MAR two times while preparing the medication. Replace the needle with a needleless injection device, clean the interlink injection port with an aseptic swab, and prime the subcutaneous catheter tubing. *Hypodermoclysis:* Attach the IV line to the interlink injection site on the subcutaneous butterfly catheter device and prime the unit.
7. Take the medication to the client at the right time and perform hand hygiene.
8. Close the room curtain or door to provide privacy.
9. Identify the client using at least two identifiers. Compare the client's name and one other identifier (e.g., the hospital identification number) on the MAR, computer printout, or computer screen against information on the client's identification bracelet. Ask the client to state his or her name, if possible, as a third identifier.
10. Compare the label of the medication with the MAR one more time at the client's bedside.
11. Explain to the client the steps of the procedure and the sensations to expect, including a slight burning or stinging when the catheter is inserted. Inform the client that the catheter will remain and will be used for medication administration of a particular medication.
12. Keep a sheet or gown draped over the body parts not requiring exposure.
13. Apply clean gloves.
14. Select an appropriate injection site. Inspect the skin surface over the sites for bruises, inflammation, or edema.
15. Palpate the sites for masses or tenderness. Avoid these areas.
16. Assist the client into a comfortable position; have the client relax the abdomen, thigh, or upper arm, depending on selected site.
17. Locate the site using appropriate anatomical landmarks.
18. Clean the site with an antiseptic swab. Apply the swab at the centre of the site and rotate outward in a circular direction for about 5 cm.
19. Remove the sheath from the catheter needle by pulling it straight off.
20. Hold the subcutaneous butterfly wings between the thumb and forefinger of your dominant hand with the palm down.
21. Ensure the bevel of the needle is pointed upward.
22. Using the thumb and index finder of your nondominant hand, gently pinch the client's skin around the selected injection site to create a roll of skin 1.25 to 2.5 cm in diameter.
23. Insert the full length of the needle through the skin at a 30-degree angle.
24. Assess for blood return into the catheter tubing. If blood return occurs, withdraw the needle and repeat the procedure at a new site.
25. Release the catheter wings and stabilize them on the skin surface with your thumb and index finger.
26. Apply an occlusive dressing (e.g., Tegaderm™ or Opsite™) over the insertion site and some of the tubing. Reinforce the dressing with tape.
27. Apply a label to the occlusive dressing that shows the date and time of administration and your initials.
28. *Subcutaneous medication administration:* Wipe the interlink injection port with an antiseptic swab and administer the medication. *Hypodermoclysis:* Adjust the flow rate of IV fluids according to the physician's order.
29. Dispose of the syringe with the needleless injection device into a sharps container.
30. Remove gloves and discard. Perform hand hygiene.
31. Document the procedure, including the site, type and gauge of subcutaneous butterfly catheter; the date and time of insertion; the client's response to the insertion; and your initials.

* KEY CONCEPTS

- Learning the medication classifications improves your understanding of nursing implications for administering medications with similar characteristics.
- Federal medication legislation regulates the production, distribution, prescription, and administration of medications.
- All controlled substances are handled according to strict procedures that account for each medication.
- Apply your understanding of the physiology of medication action when physically assessing a client before medication, timing the administration, selecting routes, initiating actions to promote medication efficacy, and observing responses to medications.
- The older adult's body undergoes structural and functional changes that alter medication actions and influence the way in which medication therapy is provided.
- Children's medication doses are computed on the basis of body surface area and weight.
- Medications given parenterally are absorbed more quickly than medications administered by other routes.
- Each medication order should include the client's name; the order date; the medication name, dosage, route, time of administration, and indication; and the prescriber's signature.
- A medication history reveals allergies, medications that the client is taking, and the client's compliance with therapy.
- The nursing process should be used when administering medication.
- The seven rights of medication administration ensure accurate preparation and administration of medication doses.
- The seven rights of medication administration are the right medication, right dose, right client, right route, right time, right documentation, and right reason.
- Administer only the medications that you prepare; never leave prepared medications unattended.
- Avoid distractions and follow the same routines when preparing medications to reduce the chance of medication errors.
- Never recap needles.
- To prevent medication errors, document immediately all medications you administer.
- Use your clinical judgement to determine the best time to administer "prn" (when needed) medications.
- Report medication errors immediately.
- When preparing medications, check the medication container label against the medication administration record three times.
- The Z-track method for intramuscular injections protects the subcutaneous tissues from irritating parenteral fluids.
- Failure to select injection sites by anatomical landmarks may lead to tissue, bone, or nerve damage.

* CRITICAL THINKING EXERCISES

1. Mrs. Nguyen, a 69-year-old woman, has recently experienced a stroke and has right-sided weakness. The neurological clinical nurse specialist wrote orders to start oral medications today. What steps do you take to ensure that this client can safely receive her oral medications? What do you do if the client is unable to swallow?
2. Marissa is a 25-year-old woman who recently delivered a healthy infant. She is to receive RhoGAM 300 mcg IM today. What size needle and which injection site and technique do you use to administer this medication?
3. Jack, a 70-year-old retired farmer, has been experiencing new respiratory difficulties. His physician has ordered him to start using an albuterol inhaler with a spacer. What steps do you take to ensure that he can self-administer his metered-dose inhaler?
4. You receive an order to give furosemide (Lasix) 40 mg IV push. You have never given this medication on this unit. What steps do you take before administering the Lasix?

* REVIEW QUESTIONS

1. Which of the following rights has been added to the seven rights of medication administration?
   1. Right documentation
   2. Right route
   3. Right medication
   4. Right reason
2. You are having difficulty reading a physician's order for a medication. You know the physician is very busy and does not like to be called. What do you do?
   1. Call a pharmacist to interpret the order.
   2. Call the physician to have the order clarified.
   3. Consult the unit manager to help interpret the order.
   4. Ask the unit secretary to interpret the physician's handwriting.
3. A client has a gastrointestinal alteration. Which method of medication administration should NOT be used?
   1. Oral
   2. Topical
   3. Inhalation
   4. Injection
4. Most medication errors occur when the nurse
   1. Fails to follow routine procedures
   2. Is responsible for administering numerous medications
   3. Is caring for too many clients
   4. Is administering unfamiliar medications
5. A client is to receive cephalexin (Keflex) 500 mg PO. The pharmacy has sent 250-mg tablets. How many tablets should you give?
   1. 0.5 tablet
   2. 1 tablet
   3. 1.5 tablets
   4. 2 tablets
6. A medication injection into the loose connective tissue under the dermis is known as what kind of injection?
   1. An intramuscular injection
   2. An intravenous injection
   3. A subcutaneous injection
   4. An intradermal injection
7. You are responsible for following legal provisions when administering controlled substances or narcotics. What may be the result of your failure to comply?
   1. Fines, imprisonment, and loss of nurse licensure
   2. Loss of employment
   3. Medication errors
   4. Poor health outcomes resulting from narcotic use

8. Pharmacokinetics is the study of how medications
   1. Are derived from plants
   2. Enter the body, reach their site of action, are metabolized, and exit the body
   3. Are used for certain disease processes
   4. Are manufactured and distributed to pharmaceutical companies
9. Which of the following is an official publication that sets standards for medication strength, quality, purity, packaging, safety, labelling, and dose form?
   1. *Physicians Reference Guide*
   2. *Nurse's Drug Guide*
   3. *Narcotic Control Act*
   4. *The Canadian Formulary* (*CF*)
10. Who is responsible for the administration of the *Food and Drugs Act* and the *Controlled Drugs and Substances Act*?
    1. Health Protection Branch (HPB)
    2. Nurse or physician dispensing and prescribing medications
    3. Canadian Formulary
    4. Health care institutions

* RECOMMENDED WEB SITES

Canadian Pharmacists Association: http://www.pharmacists.ca
The Canadian Pharmacists Association (CPhA) is a national organization of pharmacists. CPhA's Web site provides links to drug information, client information, and resources.

Health Canada: Drug Products: http://www.hc-sc.gc.ca/dhp-mps/prodpharma/databasdon/index-eng.php/
This Web site provides access to government reports, resources, and programs about the safety and effectiveness of pharmaceutical drugs and other therapeutic products.

Health Canada Therapeutic Products Directorate: http://www.hc-sc.gc.ca/ahc-asc/branch-dirgen/hpfb-dgpsa/tpd-dpt/index-eng.php
Health Canada's Therapeutic Products Directorate is the Canadian federal authority that regulates pharmaceutical drugs and medical devices for human use. This Web site provides access to information on reporting adverse reaction information.

Saskatchewan Drug Information Service: http://druginfo.usask.ca/
The Saskatchewan Drug Information Service (SDIS), operating from the University of Saskatchewan, aims to provide health care professionals and laypersons with access to objective and concise information on drugs and drug therapy.

35

Complementary and Alternative Therapies

Original chapter by Steven Kilkus, RN, MSN

Canadian content written by Jean McClennon-Leong, RN, MN, APNP

objectives

Mastery of content in this chapter will enable you to:

- Define the key terms listed.
- Differentiate between complementary and alternative therapies.
- Discuss the relaxation response and its effect on somatic ailments.
- Identify the principles and effectiveness of imagery, meditation, and breathwork.
- Describe the purpose and principles of biofeedback.
- Describe the methods of and psychophysiological responses to therapeutic touch.
- Explain the scope of chiropractic therapy.
- Discuss the principles and applications of acupuncture.
- Describe the effect of nutrition on disease prevention and health promotion.
- Describe safe and unsafe herbal therapies.

key terms

media resources

evolve Web Site

- Animations
- Audio Chapter Summaries
- Glossary
- Multiple-Choice Review Questions
- Skills Performance Checklists
- Student Learning Activities
- Video Clips
- Weblinks

Companion CD

- Glossary
- Interactive Learning Activities
- Fluids and Electrolytes Tutorial
- Test-Taking Skills

Since 1900, the health of North Americans has steadily improved. Scientific and medical changes have provided the knowledge and technology to successfully alter the course of many illnesses. However, despite the success of traditional Western medicine, known as **allopathic medicine**, many conditions are difficult to treat—for example, arthritis, chronic back pain, gastrointestinal problems, allergies, headaches, and insomnia. Thus, more clients are exploring alternative methods to relieve their symptoms. Up to three-quarters of clients visit primary care practitioners for stress, pain, and health conditions that have no known causes or cures (Andrews & Boon, 2005; Mulkins et al., 2003; Rakel & Faass, 2006). Allopathic medicine effectively treats numerous physical ailments, such as bacterial infections, structural abnormalities, and acute emergencies; however, it is less effective in preventing disease, decreasing stress-induced illnesses, managing chronic disease, and caring for individuals' emotional and spiritual needs.

Clients increasingly seek unconventional treatments, in part because treatments offered by allopathic professionals are not always perceived as being effective, and the primary focus of these health care professionals is acute disease, trauma, and end-stage malfunction. Also, many clients are attracted to holistic approaches that focus on the mind, body, and spiritual components of health (Rakel & Faass, 2006). Holistic health care philosophy regards the client as an active partner who takes personal responsibility for wellness and disease prevention. Today, the public has greater access to information about their personal health through the Internet and through journals such as the *Annals of Behavioral Medicine, Alternative Therapies in Health and Medicine,* and *Journal of Alternative and Complementary Medicine,* and through organizations such as the Canadian Holistic Nurses Association.

Complementary and Alternative Medicine Therapies in Health Care

Unconventional therapies are frequently referred to as complementary and alternative medicine (CAM) therapies. **Complementary therapies** are therapies that are used in addition to conventional treatment recommended by the client's health care professional. As its name implies, complementary therapies complement, or contribute to and enhance, conventional health care treatment. Many complementary therapies, such as acupuncture, require diagnostic and therapeutic methods specific to their field, whereas other complementary therapies, such as imagery and breathwork, are, in general, easily learned and applied. Complementary therapies also include relaxation; exercise; massage (Figure 35–1); reflexology; prayer; biofeedback; hypnotherapy; shamanism; creative therapies, including art, music, and dance (Figure 35–2); acupuncture and Chinese medicine; Ayurveda and naturopathic medicine; meditation; chiropractic therapy; osteopathy; herbalism; and homeopathy (Fontaine, 2005). You need to become knowledgeable about the safety and efficacy of these various therapies in order to advise clients effectively and wisely.

Alternative therapies may include the same interventions as complementary therapies but frequently become the primary treatment that replaces allopathic medical care. Both complementary and alternative therapies vary in their compatibility with allopathic medicine. For example, chiropractic and Feldenkrais (gentle body-movement therapy) practitioners frequently use diagnostic terminology and methods similar to those used by allopathic practitioners. These practitioners base their interventions on conventional pathophysiology, anatomy, and kinesiology but explore mind–body connections that may cause or contribute to the physiological condition. Some alternative therapies are not supported by scientific data, such as the use of shark cartilage and coffee enemas, and must be regarded with caution. Even established therapies have been tested on only small or limited populations. You need to make well-informed decisions when considering alternative therapies.

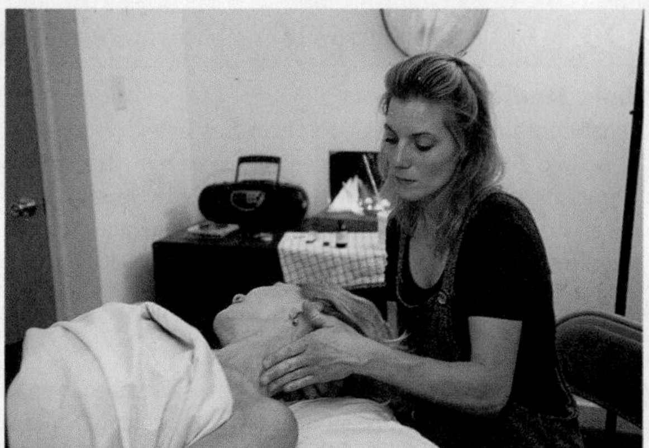

Figure 35-1 Massage therapy can effectively relieve tension.

Complementary and alternative therapies are often organized into five categories that researchers find useful (Box 35–1). Some types of complementary and alternative therapies are presented in Table 35–1. This list is not exhaustive and does not address issues of safety and efficacy.

Public Interest in Complementary and Alternative Medicine Therapies

Increasingly, the boundaries between CAM and allopathic medicine are being eroded. The interest in CAM is evident in the increased number of articles about it in respected medical journals and the development of several journals specific to CAM. Some universities are adding courses about CAM therapies to their medical and nursing curricula, and colleges offer certificate courses in a variety of alternative therapies (University of York Department of Health Sciences, 2008). **Integrative medical programs** are being developed to provide

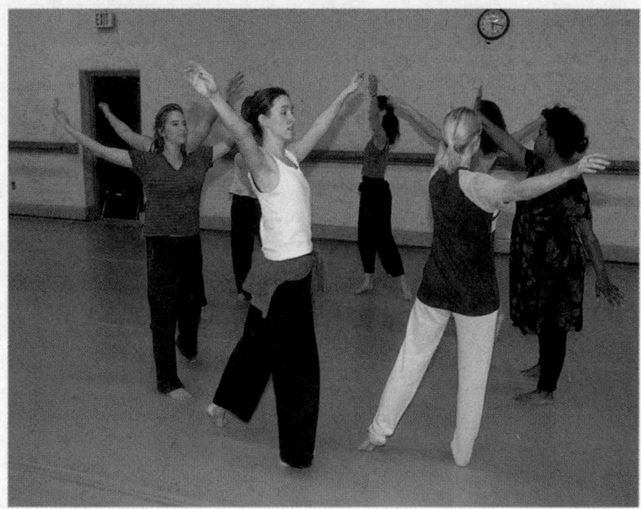

Figure 35-2 Young adults participating in dance therapy.

BOX 35-1 Categories of Complementary and Alternative Medicine (CAM) Therapies

Whole Medical Systems

Alternative medical systems encompass both theories and practices. Often, they evolved earlier than the conventional Western medical approach. Examples of alternative medical systems that have developed in Western cultures include homeopathic medicine and naturopathic medicine. Systems that have developed in non-Western cultures include traditional Chinese medicine and Ayurveda (which originated in India).

Mind–Body Interventions

Mind–body interventions use a variety of techniques designed to enhance the mind's capacity to affect bodily function and symptoms. Some techniques that were considered CAM in the past have become mainstream (e.g., client support groups and cognitive-behavioural therapy). Other mind–body techniques that are still considered CAM include meditation, prayer, mental healing, art therapy, music therapy, and dance therapy.

Biologically Based Therapies

Biologically based therapies use substances found in nature, such as herbs, foods, and vitamins. Examples include dietary supplements, herbal products, and other so-called natural but as yet scientifically unproven therapies (e.g., shark cartilage to treat cancer). Some uses of dietary supplements have been incorporated into conventional medicine. For example, folic acid is used to prevent certain birth defects, and a regimen of vitamins and zinc can slow the progression of age-related macular degeneration, an eye disease that can lead to vision loss.

Manipulative and Body-Based Therapies

Manipulative and body-based therapies are based on manipulation or movement of one or more parts of the body. Examples include massage therapy and chiropractic or osteopathic manipulation.

Energy Medicine

Energy therapies involve the use of energy fields. Energy therapies can be divided into two types:

- Biofield therapies are intended to affect the energy fields that purportedly surround and penetrate the human body. The existence of such fields has not been scientifically proven. Biofield therapies involve applying pressure or manipulating the body by placing the hands in or through these fields. Examples of biofield therapies are qigong, reiki, and therapeutic touch.
- Bioelectromagnetism-based therapies involve the unconventional use of electromagnetic fields, such as pulsed, magnetic, or alternating or direct current fields.

From National Institutes of Health, National Center for Complementary and Alternative Medicine. (Updated February, 2007). *What Is Complementary and Alternative Medicine?* (NCCAM publication no. D347). Retrieved January 12, 2009, from http://nccam.nih.gov/health/whatiscam/

TABLE 35-1 Complementary and Alternative Therapies

Types	Mechanism or Philosophy of Action
Whole Medical Systems	
Ayurveda	This traditional Hindu system of medicine dates to ancient India. Ayurveda practitioners use a combination of remedies, such as herbs, purgatives, and oils, to treat disease.
Latin American practices	The curanderismo medical system includes a humoral model (the model used by Hippocrates to explain disease) for classifying food, activity, drugs, illnesses, and a series of folk illnesses.
Traditional Aboriginal medicine	This healing practice promotes harmony within a community and in the physical and spiritual worlds through sweating and purging, herbal remedies, and shamanic healing.
Naturopathic medicine	This system of therapeutics is based on natural foods, light, warmth, massage, fresh air, regular exercise, and avoidance of medications. Naturopathic medicine recognizes the body's inherent healing abilities. The treatments integrate traditional natural therapies with modern diagnostic sciences and may include botanical (plant) medicine.
Traditional Chinese medicine	These traditional and systematic techniques and methods promote health and treat disease through acupuncture, herbal remedies, massage, acupressure, qigong (balancing energy flow through movement), and moxibustion (the use of heat from burning herbs). The fundamental concepts of traditional Chinese medicine are embedded in Taoism, Confucianism, and Buddhism.
Biologically Based Therapies (Natural Health Products)	
Herbal remedies	These supplements contain a plant, plant part, or herb that is used singly or in mixtures to convey a health or therapeutic benefit.
Homeopathic medicines	This system of medicinal treatments is based on the theory that certain diseases can be cured with small doses of substances that, in a healthy person, would produce symptoms similar to the symptoms of disease. The prescribed remedies are made from naturally occurring plant, animal, or mineral substances.
Vitamins and minerals (megavitamin therapy)	This therapy promotes the increased intake of nutrients, such as vitamin C and beta carotene. The treatment focus is on cancer, schizophrenia, and certain chronic diseases, such as hypercholesterolemia and coronary artery disease.
Traditional medicines (Ayurvedic remedies) (traditional Chinese herbal remedies)	Ayurvedic remedies: Combinations of herbs, purgatives, and rubbing oils are used to treat disease. Herbs are considered the backbone of medicine. More than 50,000 medicinal plant species exist, many of which have been studied extensively.
Probiotics	These live microorganisms are orally administered to confer a protective benefit upon the immune system of the small intestine.

Continued

TABLE 35-1 Complementary and Alternative Therapies *continued*

Biologically Based Therapies (Natural Health Products) continued	
Amino acids, essential fatty acids (EFAs), and antioxidant supplements	These products are packaged as tablets or capsules that may have a beneficial effect on reducing the body's inflammatory response and limiting oxidative stress within the body.
Nutrition as Medicine	
Gerson therapy	This therapy advocates a low-salt, high-potassium organic diet of fruit juices, raw vegetables, and nutritional supplements, plus coffee enemas for detoxification. According to this therapy, disease is believed to be caused by the accumulation of toxic substances that disrupt the body's immune system. Gerson therapy is used primarily in the treatment of cancer.
Macrobiotic diet	This predominantly vegan diet (white meat fish, occasional fruits, seeds, and nuts) is believed to have anticancer properties. The diet consists of 40%–60% whole cereal grain, 20%–30% vegetables, 5%–10% beans.
Mediterranean diet	This diet, characteristic of persons living in the Mediterranean region, is high in whole grains, nuts, fruits, vegetables, and omega-3 essential fatty acids. Following this diet is believed to produce a protective benefit for cardiac health and various inflammatory diseases.
Manipulative and Body-Based Therapies	
Acupressure	In this therapeutic technique, digital pressure is applied in a specified way on designated body points to relieve pain, produce analgesia, or regulate bodily function.
Chiropractic medicine	This therapy involves the manipulation of the spinal column and may include physiotherapy and diet therapy.
Feldenkrais method	This therapy is based on establishing good self-image through awareness and correction of body movements. The technique integrates the impact of physics on body movement patterns with how people move, behave, and interact.
Tai chi	This technique incorporates breath, movement, and meditation to cleanse, strengthen, and circulate vital energy and blood. Tai chi helps to stimulate the immune system and maintain balance.
Massage therapy	The manipulation of soft tissue through stroking, rubbing, or kneading increases the body's circulation and improves muscle tone and relaxation.
Simple touch	Touching the client in appropriate, gentle ways stimulates connection, displays acceptance, and gives appreciation.
Mind-Body Interventions	
Aromatherapy	Essential plant oils are used to promote relaxation or stimulation, thereby enhancing overall well-being.
Art therapy	Art is used to reconcile emotional conflicts, foster self-awareness, and express frequently subconscious concerns.
Biofeedback	Instruments are used to provide a person with visual or auditory information about autonomic physiological body functions, such as muscle tension, skin temperature, and brain wave activity.
Breathwork	A variety of breathing patterns are used to relax, invigorate, or open the emotional channels.
Dance therapy	Dance is used to treat social, emotional, cognitive, or physical problems.
Hypnotherapy	The induction of trance states and the use of therapeutic suggestion are used to treat paralysis, headaches, addictions, pain, and phobias.
Imagery	This therapeutic technique is used to treat pathological conditions by concentrating on an image or series of images.
Labyrinth meditation	Labyrinths are ancient spiritual symbols found in almost every religious tradition. Walking the labyrinth is regarded as an ancient spiritual act of meditation, a time for reflection and prayer, and a pilgrimage.
Meditation	This self-directed practice relaxes the body and calms the mind by focusing on rhythmic breathing.
Music therapy	Music meets the physical, psychological, cognitive, and social needs of persons with disabilities and illness. Music therapy is used to manage pain and to improve physical movement, communication, emotional expression, and memory.
Prayer therapies	A variety of techniques are used in multiple cultures to incorporate caring, compassion, love, and empathy. Prayer can be verbal or silent, a solitary or group activity, and can include chanting, visualizations, and rituals.
Psychotherapy	Mental and emotional disorders are treated by the use of psychological techniques.
Yoga	Exercise, postures, regulated breathing, and meditation are used to attain physical and mental well-being. The practice focuses on the body's musculature, posture, breathing, and consciousness.
Energy Medicine	
Qigong	Qigong is derived from the ancient Chinese practice of breathing, movement, and meditation and involves the assuming of basic postures. This practice is believed to promote strength, balance, and optimal body functioning. Qigong is used to treat stress-related conditions, fatigue, and musculoskeletal stiffness.
Reiki therapy	Derived from ancient Buddhist practices in which a practitioner places a hand on or above the body and transfers "universal life energy" to the client, this energy provides strength, harmony, and balance to treat health issues.
Therapeutic touch	In this therapy, a practitioner directs his or her balanced energies toward the energies of a client by laying the hands on or close to a client's body.

health care consumers with access to both allopathic and complementary practitioners. In some institutions, for example, nurses practise massage, reiki, and therapeutic touch.

In Canada and worldwide, demand is growing for alternative medicines and the services of alternative health care providers (Andrews & Boon, 2005; University of York Department of Health Sciences, 2008). A study released by the Fraser Institute (2007) indicated that 54% of respondents had used at least one form of complementary or alternative therapy and that 74% of Canadians had used CAM at some point during their lifetimes. Commonly used therapies included massage, prayer, chiropractic care, relaxation techniques, and herbal therapies. In another study, 40% to 80% of Canadians with the human immunodeficiency virus (HIV) or acquired immune deficiency syndrome (AIDS) reported using complementary therapies. The main reasons for use were to enhance the immune response, improve nutrition, and prevent infection (Pawluch et al., 1998, as cited in University of York Department of Health Sciences, 2008). Recent Canadian research has focused on aging and the use of CAM by persons who have received a diagnosis of cancer (Mulkins et al., 2003; Willison & Andrews, 2004).

Although CAM therapies are less expensive and less invasive than allopathic medicine, and their use could save the health care system money, clients (or their private insurance plans) must pay for these therapies. Therefore, many clients cannot afford CAM therapies. The persons who use CAM therapies typically are women with a post–high school or college-equivalent education (Bardia et al., 2007).

Complementary and Alternative Medicine Therapies and Holistic Nursing

The practice of holistic nursing regards and treats the client's mind, body, and spirit. Nurses can use holistic interventions such as relaxation therapy, imagery, music therapy, simple touch (especially helpful with older clients; Box 35–2), massage, and prayer (Box 35–3). Such interventions affect the whole person and are economical, noninvasive, nonpharmacological complements to traditional medical care. Holistic interventions can augment standard treatments, replace ineffective or debilitating interventions, and promote and maintain health (Patterson et al., 2003). The Canadian Holistic Nurses Association develops standards of practice for holistic nursing and promotes holistic nursing practice, education, research, and administration (Canadian Holistic Nurses Association, 2006).

Growing appreciation for the importance of healing both the spirit and the body has influenced the development of such hospital programs as music therapy, art therapy, and recreation therapy. At the University of Alberta Hospital, in Edmonton, the Artists on the Wards program connects local artists with individual clients at the bedside. This program helps clients develop their creativity, which may aid physical, spiritual, emotional, and mental healing. The hospital also houses the McMullen Art Gallery (Figure 35–3). Many hospitals now provide space for spiritual practice, and chaplains are widely regarded as part of the health care team. For instance, the University of Alberta Hospital offers clients and their families both a chapel and a teepee. The teepee, built specifically for Aboriginal clients and their families, is used for prayer, reflection, and healing ceremonies (Figure 35–4). A few hospitals have or are considering the construction of labyrinths on their grounds. Clients and visitors can use these labyrinths for walking, meditation, and prayer (see Table 35–1).

The following sections discuss several types of complementary and alternative medicine therapies. The therapies are organized into two types. The first are nursing-accessible therapies. These are therapies that you can begin to learn and apply in client care. The second

BOX 35-3 RESEARCH HIGHLIGHT

Use of Prayer

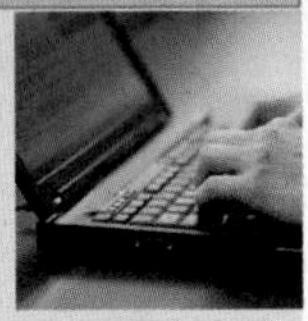

Research Focus

Individuals use prayer to cope with distressing symptoms, anxiety-provoking medical procedures, and the illness experience in general. No research, however, has explored the lived experience of using prayer to cope with illness. Some studies suggest that prayer is highly valued by those who use it, but minimal empirical knowledge is available about clients' prayer experiences and the perspectives that nurses can use to support their clients.

Research Abstract

Because prayer appears to be a significant coping strategy for persons with cancer, Taylor and Outlaw (2007) sought to describe the experience of prayer among persons with cancer. Thirty persons with cancer were interviewed about why, when, and how they prayed; what they prayed for; and what they expected their prayers to achieve. The research findings detailed how persons with cancer used prayer to ease the physical, emotional, and spiritual distress of illness. Researchers observed a range of approaches to prayer and of topics for prayer, which were often determined by the circumstances of the illness.

Evidence-Informed Practice

- Nurses can promote coping by recognizing and facilitating the client's use of prayer.
- Clients are likely to pray at times of symptom distress, emotional distress, and during diagnostic and therapeutic processes. At such times, nurses can help clients by fostering conditions and an environment conducive to prayer.
- Although all experiences of prayer share some aspects, the nature of prayer is typically unique to individuals. Therefore, nursing strategies for facilitating prayer must be designed with sensitivity to the uniqueness of each client.
- Nurses can provide an atmosphere that is supportive of prayer by helping the client to relax, offering spiritual reading material, placing the client near a view of nature, or offering a notebook for journal writing.

References: Taylor, E. J., & Outlaw, F. H. (2002). Use of prayer among persons with cancer. *Holistic Nursing Practice, 16*(3), 46–60.

BOX 35-2 FOCUS ON OLDER ADULTS

- Touch is a primary need and is as necessary to humans as food, growth, and shelter. Touch refers to a broad range of techniques for the purpose of assisting the recipient toward optimal health (Keegan & Shames, 2005).
- Older adults need touch as much as, or more than, any other age group. However, skin hunger or poverty of touch can be acute among older adults, who often have fewer family members or friends to touch them.
- Simple touch can be an enhanced form of communication when the other senses are reduced (Dossey et al., 2005).
- Simple touch helps older adult clients feel more connected to their environment and accepted by those around them. The act of touching can enhance the older client's self-esteem and sense of worth.

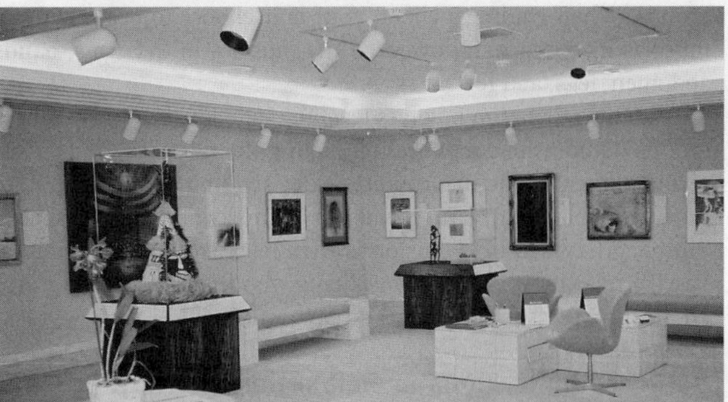

Figure 35-3 McMullen Art Gallery, University of Alberta Hospital, is open to visitors, staff, and clients. **Source:** Courtesy of the University of Alberta Hospital, Edmonton, Alberta.

type includes training-specific therapies, such as chiropractic therapy or acupressure, which a nurse cannot perform without additional training. Some of these therapies also require certification.

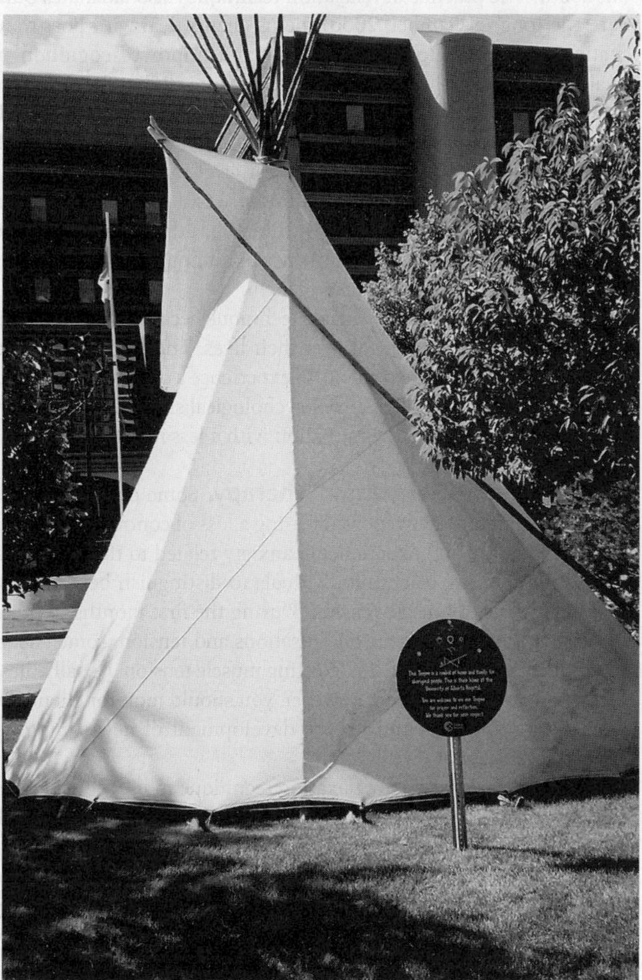

Figure 35-4 This teepee outside the University of Alberta Hospital in Edmonton is available for prayer, meditation, and sacred ceremony. **Source:** Courtesy of the University of Alberta Hospital, Edmonton, Alberta.

Nursing-Accessible Therapies

Some CAM therapies and techniques use natural processes, such as breathing, concentration, and simple touch, to help clients feel better and cope with their chronic conditions. You can learn these techniques with minimum preparation, and many of these procedures can be used with clients as an independent nursing practice (Dossey et al., 2005). Adequate assessment and the client's permission are prerequisites for implementing these therapies. Some CAM therapies may alter physiological responses such that physician-prescribed therapies (e.g., drug doses) may need to be changed. CAM therapies should be chosen according to the client's functional status, beliefs or religious perspectives, access to health care, and insurance coverage (Box 35–4).

These therapies are designed to teach clients how they can change their behaviour to alter their physical responses to stress and relieve such symptoms as muscle tension, gastrointestinal discomfort, pain, and sleep disturbances. One of the principles of these therapies is that the individual must be actively involved in the treatment. Clients achieve better responses if they practise the techniques or exercises daily. The client must commit to implementing and maintaining the therapy until a desired outcome is achieved.

Relaxation Therapy

People are exposed to stressful situations in everyday life that evoke the **stress response** (see Chapter 26). The biochemical functions of major organ systems are modulated by the mind. Thoughts and feelings influence the production of chemicals (i.e., neurotransmitters, neurohormones, and peptides) that circulate in the body and convey messages to various body systems. Physiologically, the stress response can cause increased heart, respiratory, and metabolism rates; tightened muscles; and a general sense of foreboding, fear, nervousness, irritability, and negative mood. Other physiological responses include elevated blood pressure, dilated pupils, stronger cardiac contractions, and increased levels of blood glucose, serum cholesterol, circulating free fatty acids, and triglycerides. Although these responses effectively prepare a person for short-term stress, long-term stress can cause structural damage and chronic illness, such as angina, tension headaches, cardiac arrhythmias, pain, ulcers, and atrophy of immune system organs (Dossey et al., 2005).

Relaxation is a state of overall decreased cognitive, physiological, and behavioural arousal. The process of relaxation elongates the muscle fibres and reduces the neural impulses sent to the brain, thus decreasing the brain's activity. Relaxation is characterized by decreases in heart and respiratory rates, blood pressure, and oxygen consumption and increases in alpha-wave brain activity and peripheral skin temperature. Relaxation can be achieved by using a variety of techniques that incorporate a repetitive mental focus and the adoption of a calm, peaceful attitude (Benson, 1975). Teaching strategies for relaxation are listed in Box 35–5.

Relaxation helps individuals develop cognitive skills to reduce negative responses to situations. Cognitive skills include focus (the ability to identify, differentiate, and return attention to simple stimuli for an extended period), passivity (the ability to stop unnecessary goal-directed and analytical activity), and receptivity (the ability to tolerate and accept experiences that may be uncertain, unfamiliar, or paradoxical). By practising relaxation therapy, the client learns to monitor and consciously release tension.

Progressive relaxation involves teaching individuals to effectively rest and to reduce their physical tension. The client learns to detect subtle localized sensations of muscle tension in one muscle group (e.g., the forearm muscle). In addition, the client learns to differentiate between high-intensity tension (strong fist clenching) and subtle tension (Dossey et al., 2005). Progressive relaxation is then practised using different muscle groups. One active progressive relaxation technique involves the use of slow, deep abdominal breathing while tightening and relaxing an ordered succession of muscle groups. When guiding a client, your may choose to begin with the muscles in the face, followed by the muscles in the arms, hands, abdomen, legs, and feet.

Passive relaxation involves teaching individuals to relax muscle groups without first actively contracting the muscles. One passive relaxation technique incorporates slow, abdominal breathing exercises with imagining warmth and relaxation flowing through specific muscle groups; muscle tension is then released during expiration. Passive relaxation is useful for clients who find that active muscle contracting leads to discomfort or exhaustion.

BOX 35-4 NURSING STORY

A Holistic Approach to Health

At the Integrative Medicine clinic, you are the nurse responsible for completing initial assessments and for counselling and advising new clients about complementary and alternative therapies during their first visit. Today, you meet Mrs. L., a 48-year-old woman, who is employed as a teacher. She has come to the clinic after multiple unsuccessful attempts to lose weight. Her current body mass index (BMI) is 32, which indicates obesity. She decided to visit the clinic after discovering that her latest serum glucose and cholesterol levels are elevated. She is considering gastric bypass surgery for permanent weight loss. Her primary reason for visiting the clinic is to learn what she can do to lose weight and to gain control of her health without undergoing a surgical intervention.

Key Points

Past history: Mother has hypertension and diabetes.

Social history: Relationships with her children and husband are strong. She attends church regularly and feels strongly connected to her faith.

Medications: She takes multiple herbal remedies and supplements for weight loss.

Attitude toward health: She cries during the interview and expresses anger about her perceived inability to take control of her health. She finds her occupation and family activities stressful; she has little time or energy left at the end of the day.

Approaches

First, ask some important questions. What is the client's medical diagnosis? Is it correct? Could other medical problems be contributing to her obesity? Have all the conventional medical therapies been thoroughly explored or considered? Has she discussed with her primary health care professional any other treatment plans? It is important to explore the client's attitude, frame of mind, coping strategies, support systems, and goals. You also need to assess safer alternatives for achieving weight loss and her willingness to participate in them. One key element in her social history is her strong relationships with her family members and her faith. She will need to connect with those support systems to meet her weight loss goals within the larger context of improving the family's nutrition and health. Together with Mrs. L., you can explore practical steps that her family can take to help her meet her weight loss goals, such as purchasing groceries, planning and contributing to the preparation of healthy meals, and making time to exercise regularly. These elements must be combined with realistic weight loss guidelines, including a structured follow-up. Review the herbal and dietary supplements she uses and emphasize the importance of sharing this information with her primary health care professional to determine whether the supplements are beneficial or harmful to her health. You have a good opportunity to inform Mrs. L. about how to choose her supplements wisely. In developing her plan of care, develop a realistic weight loss program that combines the benefits of exercise and other mind–body therapies, including journal writing, guided imagery with visualization, meditation (e.g., through a prayer group at her church), and other group supports for stress reduction and weight loss support. Other helpful resources might include appropriate self-help books, weight loss and recipe books, and Web site resources that can provide her with more insight and information into the psychological, physical, and lifestyle challenges associated with losing weight effectively and permanently.

Clinical Applications of Relaxation Therapy. Relaxation techniques can lower heart rate and blood pressure, decrease muscle tension, improve perceived well-being, and reduce symptom distress in persons experiencing a variety of situations (e.g., complications from medical treatment or grieving the loss of a significant other) (Hui et al., 2006; Kaushik et al., 2006). The type of relaxation intervention should be matched to the individual's functional status, the energy expenditure of the relaxation technique, and the motivation of the individual for frequent practice.

Relaxation therapy, either alone or in combination with deep breathing, imagery, yoga (Figure 35–5), and music, has been shown to reduce pain (Gustavsson & von Koch, 2006; Medlicott & Harris, 2006; Norrbrink et al., 2006), alleviate tension headaches (Kanji et al., 2006), and help to diminish anxiety related to HIV (Kemppainnen et al., 2006). The practice of relaxation techniques also facilitates burn care (de Jong & Gambel, 2006), helps clients deal with post-traumatic stress (Stapleton et al., 2006), and improves cognition in healthy aging adults (Galvin et al., 2006). More studies, however, are needed to validate the effects of relaxation therapy. For example, studies could test other variables or activities that may also lead to both reduced physiological activity and lower levels of pain to determine whether an individual's improved response is due to the relaxation therapy alone. Such variables may include a healthy support network, a positive attitude that includes the use of humour, and other behavioural therapies, such as yoga and tai chi.

Relaxation therapy is a valuable technique because it enables individuals to exert some control over their lives. The practice of relaxation techniques may help clients to experience a decreased feeling of helplessness and a more positive psychological state overall, thereby helping them to regard their situation with a less negative view.

Limitations of Relaxation Therapy. Some clients who use relaxation therapy have reported fearing a loss of control, feeling like they are floating, and experiencing anxiety related to these feelings. Relaxation training teaches individuals to distinguish between low and high levels of muscle tension. During the first months of training, when learning to focus on sensations and tension, some clients report increased sensitivity in detecting muscle tension. Usually these feelings abate with training; however, you should monitor clients for worsening symptoms and for the development of new symptoms (Dossey et al., 2005).

When choosing which relaxation technique to use, consider the physiological and psychological status of the client. Clients with advanced diseases, such as cancer, may seek relaxation training to reduce their stress response; however, techniques such as active progressive relaxation training require a moderate expenditure of energy, which can amplify a person's existing fatigue and limit the ability to complete individual relaxation sessions and practice. Therefore, active progressive relaxation is not appropriate for clients with advanced disease or with decreased energy reserves. For these individuals, passive relaxation or imagery is more appropriate.

BOX 35-5 CLIENT TEACHING

Relaxation

Objective

- The client will demonstrate decreased anxiety, tension, and other manifestations of the stress response as a result of the relaxation intervention.

Teaching Strategies

Meditation and Rhythmic Breathing (Eliciting the Relaxation Response)

1. Provide a quiet environment.
2. Help the client to a comfortable position, either seated or lying on the back. Have the client remain as still as possible and encourage movement only if necessary to remain comfortable.
3. Instruct the client to close the eyes and to maintain a receptive attitude: for example, by repeating silently, "Nothing is more important for me to do for the next 15 minutes" or "What will be, will be."
4. Instruct the client to breathe in and out, slowly and deeply, by using the abdominal muscles and keeping the chest still.
5. At the beginning of every exhalation, have client repeat the number "1" silently in his or her mind. Continue for a period of meditation.
6. Explain that when the mind wanders, the client should, without judgement, refocus his or her attention by again slowly counting on the exhalation.
7. Have the client practise for 5, 10, 15, or 20 minutes per session. Practise daily for at least one session.

Progressive Relaxation

1. Follow steps 1, 2, 3, and 4 of meditation and rhythmic breathing.
2. When the client is breathing slowly and comfortably, instruct the client to tighten and relax an ordered succession of muscle groups, tensing them and then relaxing them, while being aware of each part relaxing.
3. Instruct the client to tense and then relax the calves, then the knees, and so on.

Relaxation by Sensory Pacing

1. Follow steps 1, 2, 3, and 4 of meditation and rhythmic breathing.
2. Instruct the client to slowly repeat and finish each of the following sentences, either in a low voice or silently:
   Now I am aware of seeing . . . .
   Now I am aware of feeling . . . .
   Now I am aware of hearing . . . .
3. Instruct the client to repeat and complete each sentence four times, then three times, then twice, and finally once.

Relaxation by Colour Exchange

1. Follow steps 1, 2, 3, and 4 of meditation and rhythmic breathing.
2. Instruct the client to notice any tension, tightness, aches, or pains in the body and to give that sensation the first colour that comes to mind.
3. Instruct the client to breathe in pure white light from the universe and to send the light to a tense or painful place in the body, letting the white light surround the colour of the discomfort.
4. Instruct the client to exhale the colour of the discomfort and let the white light take its place.
5. Instruct the client to continue breathing in the white light and exhaling the colour of the discomfort, allowing the white light to fill the entire body and bring about a sense of peace, well-being, and energy.

Modified Autogenic Relaxation

1. Follow steps 1, 2, 3, and 4 of meditation and rhythmic breathing.
2. Instruct the client to repeat each of the following phrases silently four times, saying the first part of the phrases while inhaling for 2–3 seconds, holding the breath for 2–3 seconds, then saying the last part of the phrases while exhaling for 2–3 seconds.

Breathing in	Breathing out
I am	relaxed.
My arms and legs	are heavy and warm.
My heartbeat	is calm and regular.
My breathing	is free and easy.
My abdomen	is loose and warm.
My forehead	is cool.
My mind	is quiet and still.

Relaxing With Music

- Provide the client with a CD player and headset.
- Ask the client to select a favourite CD of slow, quiet music.
- Instruct the client to find a comfortable position (either sitting or lying down but with arms and legs uncrossed) and to close the eyes and listen to the music through the headset.
- Instruct the client to imagine floating or drifting with the music.

Evaluation

- Assess the client's vital signs, particularly the respiratory pattern.
- Ask the client to describe the level of tension or uneasiness felt.
- Observe the client for the presence of behaviours that display anxiety.

Meditation and Breathing

Meditation is any activity that limits stimulus input by directing the attention to a single unchanging or repetitive stimulus (Rakel & Faass, 2006). Meditation is a general term that refers to a range of practices that relax the body and still the mind. The root word, *meditari*, means "to consider." In 1975, Dr. Herbert Benson's book, *The Relaxation Response,* drew the attention of Western health care practitioners to the physical and psychological benefits of relaxation. As Benson noted, the components of meditation are simple: a quiet space, a comfortable position, a receptive attitude, and a focus of attention. He described meditation as a process that anyone can use to calm down, to cope with stress, and, for those with spiritual inclinations, to feel at one with God or the universe. Meditation is compatible with most religious traditions and can be practised alone or in groups. Most meditation techniques involve slow, relaxed, deep, usually abdominal, breathing (see Box 35–5). Meditation evokes a restful state, lowers oxygen consumption, reduces respiratory and heart rates, and decreases anxiety.

Clinical Applications of Meditation. Many conditions are indications for meditation (Box 35–6). Evidence has shown that meditation improves breathing patterns in clients with asthma, manages stress-related illnesses, and lowers blood pressure (Paul-Labrador et al., 2006; Walton et al., 2002). AIDS clients use meditation to reduce stress and anxiety (Brazier et al., 2006). Also benefiting from meditation are cancer clients (Zaza et al., 2005) and persons with depression (Brown & Gerbarg, 2005). Battered women benefit from a meditation practice (Kane, 2006), as do persons who have chronic low back

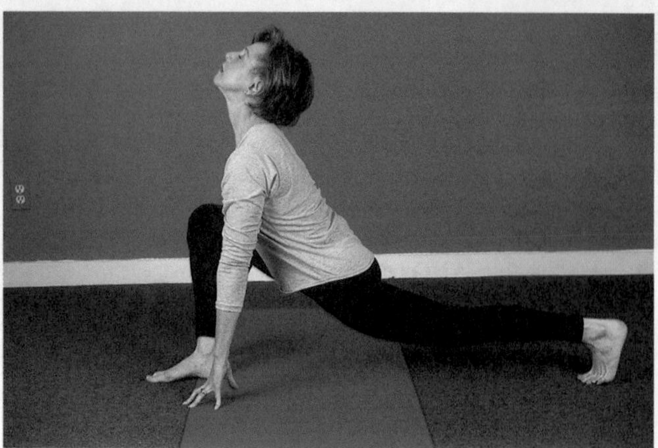

Figure 35-5 Yoga focuses on muscles, posture, breathing, and consciousness.

pain (Mehling et al., 2005). Meditation also increases a person's productivity and sense of self, improves mood, and reduces irritability (Dossey et al., 2005).

When considering the use of meditation for a client, consider the client's degree of self-discipline, although meditation actually requires less self-discipline than most other behavioural therapies.

Limitations of Meditation. Although meditation can lead to numerous physiological and psychological benefits, it may be contraindicated in some clients. For example, a client with a strong fear of losing control may perceive meditation as a form of mind control and thus may be resistant to learning the technique. Some clients respond well to meditation and require shorter sessions than the typical 15 to 20 minutes.

Meditation can also augment the effects of certain drugs. For example, individuals taking medications to treat hypertension, overactive or underactive thyroid glands, depression, or anxiety should be monitored. Prolonged practice of meditation techniques may, in some cases, lead to the reduced need for certain medications, and some doses of medications may need to be adjusted. Individuals learning meditation, therefore, should be monitored closely for physiological changes with respect to their medications.

Imagery

Imagery or visualization techniques, which are frequently used with relaxation training, help create mental images to stimulate physical changes, improve perceived well-being, and enhance self-awareness. Imagery can be either self-directed or guided by a practitioner (Dossey et al., 2005). For example, the client may be directed to begin slow, abdominal breathing while focusing on the rhythm of the breath. The client is then guided to visualize ocean waves washing onto a shore with each inhalation, then receding with each exhalation. Next, the client is encouraged to notice the smells, sounds, and temperatures that he or she is experiencing. As the session progresses, the client may be instructed to visualize warmth entering the body during inspiration and tension leaving the body during expiration. Imagery scenarios can be individualized for each client or left to the client to develop.

Imagery can evoke powerful psychophysiological responses, such as alterations in the immune function (Fontaine, 2005). Many imagery techniques involve visual imagery, but they can also include the auditory, proprioceptive, gustatory, and olfactory senses. For example, visualizing a lemon being sliced in half and squeezing the lemon juice under the tongue has been observed to produce increased salivation as effectively as the actual event. People typically respond to their environment according to the way they perceive it and according to their own visualizations and expectatations. Therefore, individuals can learn to self-regulate their visualization experiences by selecting appropriate visualizations and expectations (Dossey et al., 2005).

Creative visualization is a form of self-directed imagery that is based on the principle of mind–body connectivity (i.e., every mental image leads to physical or emotional responses; Gawain, 2002). Client teaching strategies for creative visualization are listed in Box 35–7.

Clinical Applications of Imagery. Imagery is used to control or relieve pain, to achieve calmness and serenity, and to visualize cancer cells being destroyed by immune system cells. Imagery is also used in the treatment of chronic conditions, such as asthma, hypertension, functional urinary disorders, menstrual and premenstrual syndromes, rheumatoid arthritis, and gastrointestinal disorders, such as irritable bowel syndrome (Dossey et al., 2005; Fontaine, 2005).

Limitations of Imagery. Imagery has few side effects; however, it is probably one of the least clearly defined interventions and can range from being highly structured to consisting of spontaneous daydreams (Rakel & Faass, 2006).

BOX 35-6 Indications for Meditation

Anxiety or tension
Chronic bereavement
Chronic fatigue syndrome
Chronic pain
Drug abuse, alcohol abuse, tobacco use
Hypertension
Irritability
Low self-esteem; self-blame
Mild depression
Psychophysiological disorders
Sleep disorders

BOX 35-7 CLIENT TEACHING

Creative Visualization

Objective

The client will demonstrate skills in creative visualization.

Teaching Strategies

- Set goals that can be accomplished because confidence and increased self-esteem are achieved through success.
- Create clear images described in the present tense (e.g., imagine you are floating on a soft, white cloud).
- Frequently visualize the image. Visualization should be practised throughout the day but especially upon awakening or before sleep, when the mind is usually more relaxed.
- While focusing on the image, repeat encouraging statements, such as positive affirmations to alleviate doubts about the ability to achieve goals.

Evaluation

- Observe the client for anxiety.
- Ask the client whether the experience was helpful.
- Ask the client whether he or she uses positive self-dialogue with visualization (e.g., "I am feeling stronger").
- Note whether the client reports images of desired health habits, desired feelings, and desires for healing.
- Note whether the client reports improved coping with daily stressors.

Training-Specific Therapies

Training-specific therapies are CAM treatments that may be administered by nurses but only after the completion of a specific course of study and training. A nurse must have a certification, degree, or licence beyond a registered nursing degree to administer most of these therapies. Several training-specific therapies are recognized as being effective and are recommended by Western health care practitioners (e.g., biofeedback and therapeutic touch). Many other therapies have not yet been studied in a systematic way to establish their effectiveness. Many of these unproven techniques are very popular in our society and are used by many persons from other cultures who now live in Canada. Many therapies have positive effects, but some have negative effects, too. Some may have harmful results when used with standard Western medical therapies. Therefore, you need to acquire knowledge of such treatments and to be aware of their possible harmful interactions.

Biofeedback

Biofeedback techniques are frequently used in addition to relaxation interventions to assist individuals in learning how to control specific autonomic nervous system responses. **Biofeedback** is a group of therapeutic procedures that use electronic or electromechanical instruments to measure, process, and provide information about neuromuscular and autonomic nervous system activity (Figure 35–6). This information, or feedback, is provided in physical, physiological, auditory, and visual measurements through a pneumograph. For example, clients may hear a sound if their pulse rate or blood pressure increases out of their therapeutic zone. Biofeedback practitioners help clients to develop awareness of and voluntary control over physiological responses (Rakel & Faass, 2006).

Biofeedback is considered to complement traditional relaxation programs because it can immediately demonstrate to clients their ability to control some physiological responses. Biofeedback also helps individuals to focus on and monitor responses in specific body parts. By providing immediate feedback for the stress relaxation behaviours that work most effectively, clients learn to control the physiological functions that are most difficult to control. Eventually, the client will be aware of positive physiological changes without the need for instrument feedback. Biofeedback demonstrates to the client the relationships between thoughts, feelings, and physiological responses.

Clinical Applications of Biofeedback. Biofeedback has numerous applications. It has successfully treated migraine headaches (Damen et al., 2006), other pain (Breuhl & Chung, 2006), stroke (Cristea et al., 2006), and a variety of gastrointestinal and urinary tract disorders (Chiarioni et al., 2005).

One of the most critical components of any behavioural program is adherence to the treatment regimen. Clients who are compliant with appointments, practice times, and goal setting tend to be the most successful.

Limitations of Biofeedback. Although biofeedback has demonstrated effectiveness in a number of client populations, several precautions should be noted. During relaxation therapy and biofeedback sessions, repressed emotions or feelings may emerge, and clients may find they cannot cope with these emotions alone. For this reason, practitioners should be trained in traditional psychological methods or be able to refer clients to qualified professionals.

Therapeutic Touch

Therapeutic touch (TT) is a training-specific therapy that was developed in the 1970s by a nurse, Dr. Dolores Krieger. Although the philosophical and religious assumptions of TT differ from those of other Eastern healing modalities, both practices involve trained practitioners who attempt to direct their own balanced energies in an intentional and motivated manner toward the client (Krieger et al., 1979).

TT consists of the practitioner's hands being placed either on or close to a person's body (Figure 35–7). The practitioner scans the client's body and diagnoses areas of accumulated tensions. The practitioner then attempts to redirect these energies to bring the person's energy back into balance (Krieger, 1975; Krieger et al., 1979).

TT consists of five phases: centring, assessment, unruffling, treatment, and evaluation. Centring is the process whereby the practitioner becomes aware and fully present during the entire treatment. The next phase, assessment of the client, involves the practitioner moving his or her hands (roughly 5 to 15 cm from the body) in a rhythmic and symmetrical movement from the head to the toes. During this phase, the practitioner notices the quality of **energy flow** and detects accumulations of energy. Physiological indicators of energy imbalance are perceived as congestion, pressure, warmth, coolness, blockage, pulling or drawing, or static or tingling (Krieger, 1975). During the third phase, the practitioner "unruffles" the energy flow or facilitates the symmetrical and rhythmical flow of energy

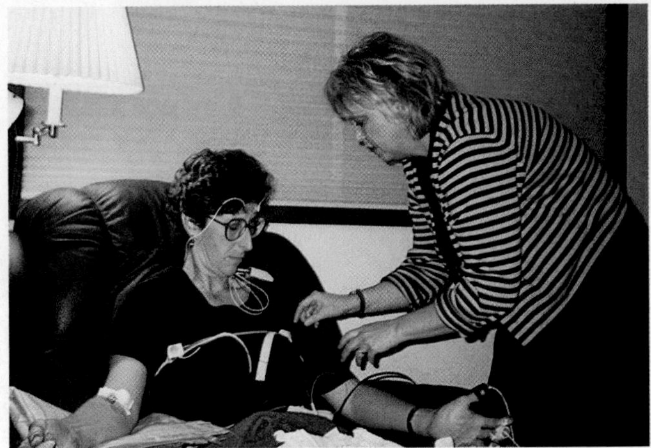

Figure 35-6 Biofeedback monitoring. Electrodes are placed on the frontalis and trapezius muscles and on the fingers of the left hand. Pneumograph measurements are also made.

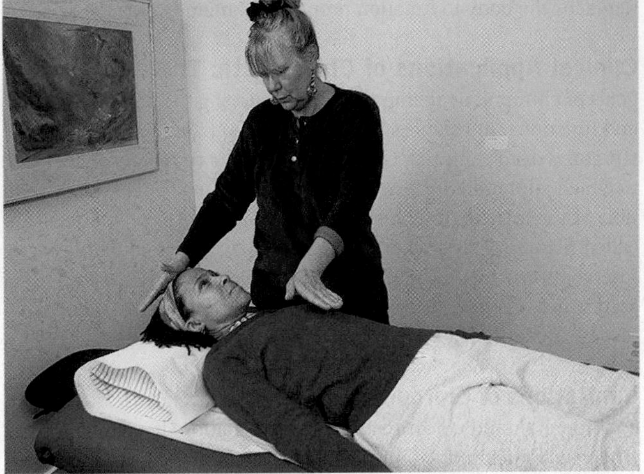

Figure 35-7 In therapeutic touch, the practitioner's own energy is directed to help or heal another person.

through the body with long downward strokes over the energy field located over the entire body. This rebalancing of energy is achieved either by the practitioner touching the body or by maintaining the hands in a position a few centimetres away from the body. The final phase consists of an evaluation of the client and a reassessment of the energy field. If rebalance is achieved, the practitioner detects a more symmetrical, freely flowing energy field (Krieger et al., 1979).

Clinical Applications of Therapeutic Touch. Early studies found that TT was able to increase hemoglobin levels in several clients (Krieger, 1975; Krieger et al., 1979). This same positive result was found in a recent study (Movaffaghi et al., 2006). Other studies have found that TT reduced headache pain, improved the mood of bereaved adults, and reduced anxiety levels in hospitalized clients with cardiovascular disease (Krieger, 1975; Krieger et al., 1979). Research has also shown that TT reduces chemical dependency in pregnant women (Larden et al., 2004).

Limitations of Therapeutic Touch. Although some studies have demonstrated that TT produces positive outcomes, others have not. TT may be contraindicated in certain client populations. For example, clients who are sensitive to human interaction and touch (e.g., persons who have been physically abused or have psychiatric disorders) may misinterpret the intent of the treatment and may feel threatened and anxious. Other clients who are sensitive to energy repatterning may also need to avoid TT. These clients include premature infants, newborns, children, pregnant women, older or debilitated people, and clients who are in critical, unstable conditions (Fontaine, 2005).

Chiropractic Therapy

Chiropractic therapy was developed in 1895 and has become the third-largest independently practised health profession in the Western world (Rakel & Faass, 2006). Chiropractors graduate from well-established preparatory programs similar to medical schools. The central tenet of the chiropractic profession is spinal manipulation directed at specific joints. Manipulation is defined as the forceful passive movement of a joint beyond its active limit of motion. Practitioners use either their hands or an instrument to manipulate the spine. Chiropractic therapy is considered a holistic therapy that does not typically use drugs or surgery.

The basic principles of chiropractic therapy incorporate the idea that human beings have an innate healing potential; harnessing this potential is the goal of this healing profession. Chiropractic therapy promotes both a natural diet and regular exercise as essential components for the body to function properly (Fontaine, 2005).

Clinical Applications of Chiropractic Therapy. The basic goals of chiropractic therapy focus on restoring the body's structural and functional imbalances that may result in pain. One of the major structural distortions that chiropractors treat is vertebral subluxation, in which joint mobility is decreased due to slight changes in the position of the articulating bones. A more severe form of subluxation, called fixation, exists when joint motion is restricted. Chiropractic interventions treat musculoskeletal abnormalities, headaches, dysmenorrhea, disorders of blood pressure, vertigo, tinnitus, and visual disorders (Rakel & Faass, 2006).

Limitations of Chiropractic Therapy. Several diseases or joint conditions should not be treated by manipulation. If a malignancy is suspected or determined through diagnostic testing, the client should be referred to a medical physician for further evaluation and treatment. Bone and joint infections also require pharmaceutical or surgical intervention, and the structural integrity of the bone may be compromised if excessive force is used. Contraindications for chiropractic therapy include acute myelopathy, fractures, dislocations, rheumatoid arthritis, and osteoporosis. Severe complications secondary to neck and spine manipulation are rare; however, some research suggests avoiding this type of manipulation on infants and children (Stewart et al., 2002).

Traditional Chinese Medicine

Traditional Chinese medicine (TCM) comprises several healing modalities, including herbal remedies, acupuncture, moxibustion, diet, exercise, and meditation. TCM is several thousand years old. A major concept in Chinese medicine is the **yin and yang**, which represent opposing, yet complementary, phenomena that exist in a state of dynamic equilibrium. Examples of yin and yang are night and day, hot and cold, and shady and sunny. Yin represents shade, cold, and inhibition, whereas yang represents fire, light, and excitement. Yin also represents the inner part of the body, specifically the viscera, liver, heart, spleen, lungs, and kidneys; whereas yang represents the outer part, specifically the bowels, stomach, and bladder. According to TCM, when an imbalance occurs in these paired opposites, disease can emerge (Fontaine, 2005).

Qi (pronounced *chee*) is defined as the body's vital energy. Disease is classified into three major categories: external causes, internal causes, and neither internal nor external causes (Table 35–2). Regardless of the cause, when yin and yang are out of balance, the movement of qi is altered. The body has several forms of qi that directly influence its physiological functions and help maintain homeostasis.

Channels of energy run in regular patterns throughout the body and over its surface. These channels, called **meridians**, are like rivers flowing through the body. An obstruction of these meridians functions like a dam, by backing up the flow in one part of the body and restricting the flow in other parts, eventually leading to disease. Located along the channels are **acupoints**, or holes through which qi can be influenced by the insertion of needles, a process known as **acupuncture.**

Another important component of Chinese medicine involves five elements: earth, metal, water, wood, and fire. Various health phenomena are organized according to these elements and interact with each other. In Chinese medicine, outward manifestations reflect the internal environment. Two primary areas are assessed in Chinese medicine: the tongue and several pulses. The colour, shape, and coating of the tongue reflect the general condition of the internal organs.

TABLE 35-2 Three Causes of Disease According to Traditional Chinese Medicine

Cause of Disease	Influences
External causes, or "the six evils"	Wind, cold, fire, damp, summer heat, dryness
Internal causes, or internal damage by seven effects	Joy, anger, anxiety, thought, sorrow, fear, fright
Nonexternal, noninternal causes	Dietary irregularities, excessive sexual activity, fatigue, trauma, parasites

The pulses provide information about the condition and balance of qi, blood, yin and yang, and the internal organs (Fontaine, 2005).

Acupuncture

Acupuncture is a method of stimulating certain points (acupoints) on the body by the insertion of special needles to modify the perception of pain, normalize physiological functions, or treat or prevent disease (Figure 35–8). Acupuncture is used to regulate the flow of qi. According to Chinese traditional medicine, acupuncture needles unblock obstructed energy and re-establish the flow of qi through the meridians, thereby stimulating and activating the body's self-healing abilities. The effects of the acupuncture needles may be enhanced by applying heat or weak electrical currents to the needles (Fontaine, 2005).

Clinical Applications of Acupuncture. Acupuncture is the primary treatment used by practitioners of Chinese medicine. Many allopathic physicians and health care professionals are also trained and certified in acupuncture.

Acupuncture is used to treat low back pain, myofascial pain, headaches, tennis elbow, osteoarthritis, whiplash, and musculoskeletal sprains. Other problems that have been successfully treated include sinusitis, gastrointestinal disorders, menstrual symptoms, neurological disorders, chronic pulmonary diseases (including asthma), hypertension, smoking and other addictions, and clinical depression (Rakel & Faass, 2006).

Limitations of Acupuncture. Acupuncture is considered a safe therapy when the practitioner has successfully completed the appropriate training and uses sterilized needles. Although complications have been noted, they are rare if appropriate steps are taken to ensure the safety of the equipment and the client. These complications include the puncture of an internal organ, bleeding, fainting, seizures, miscarriage, post-treatment drowsiness, and infections from contaminated or broken needles or from needles that have been left in place for an extended length of time.

Acupuncture should be used with caution in pregnant clients and clients who have a history of seizures, are hepatitis carriers, or are infected with HIV. Acupuncture treatment is contraindicated in people with bleeding disorders, thrombocytopenia, or skin infections.

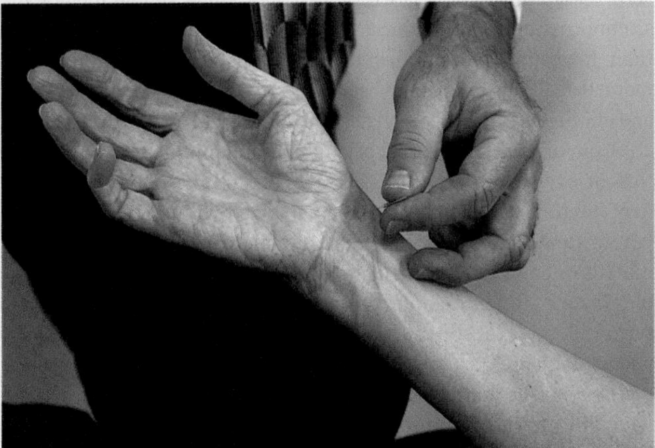

Figure 35-8 Acupuncture involves the insertion of special needles to regulate the flow of energy.

Electroacupuncture should be avoided in people who have pacemakers, are pregnant, or have cardiac arrhythmias or epilepsy (Fontaine, 2005).

Role of Nutrition in Disease Prevention and Health Promotion

A growing body of scientific evidence over the past few decades has been exploring the relationship between **nutrition** and its preventive effect on disease. Substantial evidence from epidemiological studies indicates that the relationship between nutrition and cancer, diabetes, and cardiovascular disease is often directly linked to lifestyle and nutritional choices.

Current scientific research relates diet and nutrition to cancer risk (Berkow et al., 2007; Chan et al., 2006; Peeters et al., 2003; Webb & McCullough, 2005). The research findings are conclusive enough for some investigators to suggest that further research should focus on developing protective nutritional strategies against cancer, especially because of people's increasing exposure to environmental carcinogenic agents and because of the aging of populations worldwide (Dinkova-Kostova, 2007; Thorogood et al., 2007). Canadians typically consume a diet lacking in foods of plant origin (fruits and vegetables) and high in fat, including refined and processed foods with little or no nutrient value. Consequently, rates of obesity are rising in our country, particularly for young children. The prevalence of diseases such as type 2 diabetes, which previously was rarely seen in young children, is now increasing in this population (Katzmarzyk & Ardern, 2004).

Studies show that increased intake of whole grains and dietary fibre is inversely associated with insulin resistance and type 2 diabetes (McKeown, et al., 2004). Coronary heart disease is a leading cause of death and is related to lifestyle choices, including overeating, inactivity, and poor diet choices. The value of nutrition has become clear, evidenced by studies that have found strong correlations between what researchers identify as Western diseases: for example, coronary artery disease, obesity, and unhealthy dietary habits (Berkow, et al., 2007; Parkin et al., 1999). Research has shown that the Mediterranean diet is rich in omega-3 fatty acids, which reduce inflammatory markers associated with coronary artery disease (Esposito et al., 2004). Dean Ornish (1998) determined that intensive lifestyle and dietary changes could, in fact, reverse coronary artery disease. Research is ongoing, but numerous studies indicate that attention to diet and to factors such as weight and exercise has been proven to reduce cancer risk. In addition, current research is examining the complex relationships between specific food components and their health effects. Whole foods (foods that are raw, unrefined, and minimally processed) provide more nutrients than can be obtained from supplements. A single fruit or vegetable contains many protective chemicals and nutrients that cannot be sourced from a supplement alone. These plant chemicals, commonly called *phytochemicals*, work together to provide better defence against disease. Phytochemicals provide pigment and flavour; they give garlic its pungent taste and give fruits and vegetables their bright and varied colors (Bragdon & Scroggs, 2006).

Phytochemicals are antioxidants, which are compounds that protect cells from damage. Antioxidants destroy free radicals, which are chemicals that are produced when the body uses oxygen. Free radicals can damage cells, thereby leading to the mutations that cause cancer. Several phytochemicals are being studied to determine how they influence the cancer process (Bragdon & Scroggs, 2006; Milner, 2006).

The Canadian Cancer Society (2007) addresses some key dietary sources of phytochemicals that are optimal for health and disease prevention and advise choosing a food from each colour group every day. Colour groups and some examples of their foods include dark green and orange (carrots, spinach, oranges); red and blue or purple (beets, red peppers, blueberries); and white, brown, and tan (cauliflower, garlic, bananas). In association with the Canadian Cancer Society, Beliveau and Gingras (2006) have written a book that addresses how a healthy diet can prevent disease and offers recipes geared toward preventing cancer.

Despite the lack of conclusive data that dietary changes can prevent cancer, sufficient evidence exists to suggest that cancer risk can be reduced by eating more fruit, vegetables, and whole foods. Cancer is a complex group of diseases with many causes not related to diet alone but to a combination of individual and general risk factors. Because of the relationship of diet to many other lifestyle diseases, the best approach to nutrition may be to focus on a well-balanced, whole-food approach rich in disease-fighting phytochemicals.

Herbal Therapies

An estimated 25,000 plant species are used medicinally throughout the world. **Herbal therapy** is the oldest form of medicine; archeological evidence suggests that Neanderthals used herbal remedies 60,000 years ago. Herbal therapy was widespread for thousands of years, but its popularity declined with the development of modern scientific medicine in the early eighteenth century. However, because approximately 80% of the world's population live in developing countries, herbal medicine constitutes a prominent approach to health care worldwide. In countries that use predominantly allopathic medicine, an increased interest in herbal medicine has developed from consumer interest in natural foods and growing concern about the complications and limitations of scientific medicine (Fontaine, 2005).

Herbal substances are extracted from plants, animals, and minerals. The active ingredients are prepared in tinctures or extracts, elixirs, syrups, capsules, pills, tablets, lozenges, powders, ointments or creams, drops, and suppositories. Many people think, incorrectly, that because herbs are natural plants, they cannot cause harm or side effects. As with other medications, some herbal substances contain powerful chemicals and should be examined for interaction and compatibility with other prescribed or unprescribed substances. As well, many herbs are sold with claims that they can "cure" certain ailments when their efficacy has not been determined through clinical trials. In a recent study on herbal remedies for psoriasis (Steele et al., 2007), the magnitude of information on the Internet (more than 1 million sites offered by Yahoo versus 31 articles found in the medical literature) illustrates the lack of scientific evidence to support the many uses of herbal remedies. Herbs are, in general, classified as beneficial, harmful, or neutral, in which case they have no effects on the specific ailment.

The philosophy of herbal therapy differs from the philosophy of conventional drug therapy. The goal of herbal therapy is to restore balance within the individual by facilitating the self-healing ability. Drug therapy, on the other hand, is aimed at the treatment of a specific disease or symptoms. Herbal therapy is also prescribed on an individual basis with unique herbal concoctions tailored for each person (Kuhn & Winston, 2001). Many herbal medicines are sold as food, food supplements, or natural health products in health food stores and through private companies.

According to the Canadian *Food and Drugs Act*, all drugs must be proven safe and effective before being sold to the public. A 2002 Canadian study revealed that of 1,543 persons surveyed, nearly 50% of the women and 33% of the men had used a natural health product in a 24-hour period (Troppmann et al., 2002). In 2004, Health Canada launched a 6-year program to regulate all over-the-counter natural health products (NHPs). NHPs are considered to be any product derived from a plant, animal, or microorganism (e.g., herbs, essential fatty acids) and vitamins, minerals, and homeopathics that are, in the words of the *Act,* used to "diagnose, treat, prevent disease; restore or correct function, maintain or promote health." These new regulations include good manufacturing practices and guidelines for obtaining a product licence. NHPs that have been approved for sale under the new regulations have been assigned a drug identification number (DIN; DIN-HM for homeopathic medicines) or natural product number (NPN). These numbers certify that the product has passed a review of its formulation, labelling, and instructions for use. Health Canada advises Canadians to use only health products that carry a DIN, DIN-HM, or NPN on the label.

Clinical Applications of Herbal Therapy. Numerous natural health products have been determined to be safe and effective for a variety of conditions (Table 35–3). Milk thistle, for example, can effectively treat certain liver and gallbladder conditions; its antioxidant properties are believed to protect the liver and facilitate regeneration of liver cells. St. John's wort has been found to be effective as a tricyclic antidepressant agent and more effective than placebo (Linde et al., 2008).

Limitations of Herbal Therapy. Although herbal medicine has been shown to provide beneficial effects for a variety of conditions, a number of problems may exist. Concentrations of active ingredients can vary considerably, and contamination may occur with other herbs or chemicals, including pesticides and heavy metals. Some herbs have also been found to contain toxic products that can cause cancer. Comfrey, for example, has been used for its wound-healing properties; however, various species of comfrey contain highly carcinogenic pyrrolizidine alkaloids and have produced liver cancer in small animals. Other unsafe herbs are listed in Table 35–4.

Not all companies follow strict quality control and manufacturing guidelines, which set standards for acceptable levels of pesticides, residual solvents, bacterial levels, and heavy metals. For this reason, herbal medicine should be purchased only from reputable manufacturers (Box 35–8). In addition, labels on herbal products should include the scientific name of the botanical, the name and address of the manufacturer, the batch or lot number, the date of manufacture, and the expiration date. If the product has been assessed by Health Canada for safety and effectiveness, it will also have a DIN, DIN-HM, or NPN on its label.

Concurrent use of herbal or other natural products with prescription or over-the-counter medications should be monitored. Herbs may interfere with medications metabolized within a narrow therapeutic range. Pharmacokinetic interactions occur when an herb inhibits or enhances a particular medication's site of action. For example, theophylline in combination with St. John's wort may elevate serum blood levels of theophylline, leading to negative side effects (Bonakdar, 2003).

Despite the increased use of herbal products, reports of toxicity have not increased commensurately. Nonetheless, herbal products should be either avoided or used with extreme caution in pregnant women, nursing mothers, infants or young children, and older adults with liver or cardiovascular disease (Fontaine, 2005).

TABLE 35-3 Natural Health Products in Common Use and Considered Safe

Common Name	Effects	Indications	Warnings*	Other
Black cohosh	Acts centrally via the dopaminergic system	Menopausal hot flashes Premenstrual syndrome	Significant estrogenic activity has not been found	Safely used in studies lasting up to 6 months Many active constituents, including glycosides, tannins, and sugars Is promising for the relief of hot flashes related to menopause
Chamomile (German or Hungarian)	Topically: Anti-inflammatory, aids wound healing Orally: Antidiarrheal, antispasmodic, anti-inflammatory	Eczema Eye irritation Throat discomfort Hemorrhoids Gastrointestinal spasms Inflammatory conditions Insomnia Menstrual disorders Migraines	Contraindicated if allergies to the daisy family May potentiate the effect of anticoagulants	
Echinacea	Topically: Anaesthetic and anti-inflammatory, wound healing Orally: Stimulates the immune system	Upper respiratory infections Colds Urinary tract infections Septicemia Boils	Contraindicated in clients receiving cancer treatments and for people with autoimmune diseases, multiple sclerosis, tuberculosis, diabetes, asthma, leukemia, HIV/AIDS, lupus, or allergies to the daisy family Not to be used longer than 8 weeks	Chemical constituents differ among roots, leaves, and flowers and between species
Evening primrose oil	Anti-inflammatory May lower blood pressure	Atopic dermatitis Premenstrual syndrome Menopausal hot flashes Rheumatoid arthritis Raynaud's disease	Contraindicated in clients with seizure disorders Large doses may cause loose stools and abdominal pain	Active ingredient is omega-6 essential fatty acid, gamma-linoleic acid Studies have shown positive effects on atopic dermatitis
Fish oil	Omega-3 essential fatty acids are believed to have anti-inflammatory properties	Inflammation in rheumatoid arthritis Prevents cardiovascular disease and cancer	Possible increase of INR with warfarin Quality of product should be monitored for cancer-causing pollutants, such as dioxin and PCBs	Studies indicate its effectiveness in reducing cardiovascular disease The Mediterranean diet, which is rich in fish, has been associated with lower rates of cancers
Garlic	Lowers blood pressure and blood lipids Stimulates the immune system Inhibits platelet aggregation Antibacterial	Hypertension Cold and flu prevention Athlete's foot (topically)	May prolong bleeding time Possible interactions with anticoagulants	Not recommended for use during pregnancy due to its effect on bleeding time

Continued

TABLE 35-3 Natural Health Products in Common Use and Considered Safe *continued*

Common Name	Effects	Indications	Warnings*	Other
Ginger	Antiemetic	Motion sickness Nausea and vomiting	May enhance the effects of warfarin, aspirin, and NSAIDs	
Ginkgo biloba	Inhibits the platelet-activating factor Antimicrobial Antitumour Bronchodilator Arterial and vasodilator Decreases capillary fragility Antioxidant	Dementia Poor circulation Poor memory Tinnitus	Ingestion may increase the risk of serious bleeding, especially in clients taking anticoagulants or NSAIDs Can cause contact dermatitis	Recent studies show promise in enhancing cognitive functions in people with dementia
Glucosamine	Naturally occurring substance that stimulates the synthesis of chitin and mucoproteins	Joint pain Osteoarthritis	No known drug reactions Considered to have no significant adverse side effects	Mounting evidence for pain reduction and disease-modifying effects in osteoarthritis
Milk thistle	Antioxidant Protects liver cells Anti-inflammatory Anticarcinogenic Inhibits hepatic cholesterol synthesis	Chronic hepatitis Cirrhosis Alcohol liver disease	No known contraindications	
Saw palmetto	Androgen receptor blocker Anti-inflammatory	Benign prostatic hyperplasia Urinary problems	May interact with oral contraceptives	Evidence suggests that it provides mild to moderate improvement for urinary problems
St. John's wort	Antidepressant Antiviral Wound healing (topical)	Mild to moderate depression Sedative	Not appropriate for severe depression May enhance the effects of SSRIs and other antidepressants May decrease digoxin levels	Studies support its use in treating mild to moderate depression
Valerian	Smooth muscle relaxant Vasodilator in angina Possible antidepressant	Muscle spasms Sleep disorders Restlessness	May cause headaches or gastrointestinal disturbances	Studies support its use in treating insomnia Client must avoid using concurrently with other sedatives

*Data do not support the use of these herbs in infants or children, or during pregnancy or lactation.
INR, international normalized ratio; NSAIDs, nonsteroidal anti-inflammatory drugs; PCBs, polychlorinated biphenyls; SSRIs, selective serotonin reuptake inhibitors.

Adapted from Skidmore-Roth, L. (2006). *Skidmore-Roth Mosby's herbs and natural supplements* (3rd ed.). St. Louis: Mosby; Chandler, F. (Ed.). (2000). *Herbs: Everyday reference for health professionals.* Ottawa: Canadian Pharmacists Association and the Canadian Medical Association; and The Pharmacists Letter. (2003). *Natural medicines comprehensive database* (5th ed.). Stockton, CA: Therapeutic Research Faculty Staff.

TABLE 35-4 Unsafe Herbs

Common Name	Effects	Comments
Aristolochia (also known as birthwort, snakeroot, snakeweed, sangree root)	Appetite stimulant Promotion of menstruation Aphrodisiac	Contains aristocholic acid, which causes kidney damage and cancer
Borage	Diuretic Antidiarrheal	Contains toxic pyrrolizidine alkaloids
Chaparral	Anticancer	No proven efficacy May induce severe liver toxicity
Comfrey	Wound healing	Contains large number of toxic pyrrolizidine alkaloids May induce venoocclusive disease
Ephedra (*ma huang*)	Central nervous system stimulant Anorectic Bronchodilator Cardiac stimulation	Unsafe for people with hypertension, diabetes, or thyroid disease Avoid consumption with caffeine
Kava	Used to treat nervous anxiety and stress Sleep aid	Hepatotoxicity and liver failure in at least 68 documented cases of liver toxicity after use Issues related to contaminants in product
Life root (ragwort)	Menstrual flow stimulant	Hepatotoxic Contains toxic pyrrolizidine alkaloids
Sassafras	Stimulant and tonic Antispasmodic Antirheumatic	Volatile oil Contains safrole, a liver carcinogen
Yohimbe	Used to treat impotence, as an aphrodisiac	May cause kidney damage, cancer, hypertension, and cardiac conduction disorders

Adapted from Kirn, T. (2004). Group rates efficacy of herbs. *Family Practice News, 34*(8), 26; The Pharmacists Letter. (2003). *Natural medicines comprehensive database* (5th ed.). Stockton, CA: Therapeutic Research Faculty Staff; and Bonakdar, R. A. (2003). Herb–drug interactions: What physicians need to know. *Patient Care, 37*(1), 58–69.

BOX 35-8 FOCUS ON PRIMARY HEALTH CARE

Educating Clients About Purchasing Herbal Remedies

Many people who buy herbal products are unaware of the lack of regulation regarding the manufacturing and sale of such products. It is difficult to make informed decisions when faced with hundreds of products. When clients choose to use herbal therapies, they should purchase these products only from reputable manufacturers to ensure safety, appropriate use, and response.

You can help clients make informed choices about herbal products by offering these guidelines:

- Avoid hype: Be wary of supplements that offer a "cure" or a "secret formula."
- All product labels should indicate the following:
    - The scientific name of the botanical
    - The quantity, concentration, expiration date, and manufacturer's name
    - The purpose, dosage form, route of administration, and warnings or possible adverse reactions
    - The names of other key ingredients
    - The natural product number (NPN) or drug identification number (DIN), which indicates that Health Canada has reviewed its formulation

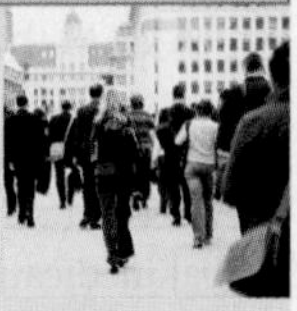

- Ensure the product is supported by published research. Avoid "multi-ingredient" formulations when possible; otherwise, determining potential reactions with other medicines will be difficult. Consumers often pay more for secondary products that may not be present in established therapeutic levels.
- Look for well-educated service staff who can answer consumers' questions.
- Be cautious about "mega" doses of anything: Even excess ingestion of certain vitamins can be toxic.
- Be sceptical about cheap herbal remedies. Consumers must pay for the manufacturer's investments in ensuring quality and purity. Very inexpensive herbal products are often of inferior quality.

Nursing Role in Complementary and Alternative Therapies

The integrative medicine approach is consistent with the holistic approach nurses learn to practise. Indeed, many nurses already practise the use of simple touch. This therapy is an example of a holistic approach to care that includes a variety of practice modalities designed to promote the health and well-being of the client. The use of these practice modalities is based on the assumption that nurses practise within the Scope of Practice, as defined by the Canadian Nurses Association (Canadian Holistic Nursing Practice Standards, 2006). As essential participants, nurses who provide CAM therapies must have the knowledge and skill necessary to provide care safely and ethically through self-study, certificate courses offered by community colleges, or study with expert practitioners. Nurses should understand provincial and territorial legislation regarding complementary therapies, practise within the scope of these laws, and be able to make appropriate recommendations about CAM therapies to allopathic primary care providers. Various nursing resources on CAM are available through the Canadian Holistic Nurses Association. The College of Registered Nurses of Nova Scotia (2005) has developed a guide for registered nurses. These resources help you to understand your professional responsibilities, the ethics related to implementation and advisement of CAM, and the general implications for nurses.

You also need to keep abreast of the current research in the field of CAM therapy to provide accurate information to clients and other health care professionals. For example, the Canadian Interdisciplinary Network for Complementary and Alternative Medicine Research has been created to foster excellence in CAM research (Andrews & Boon, 2005).

You should advise clients about the appropriate times to use conventional or CAM therapy. Consumers often look to you for advice on the use of different therapies; therefore, you need to have knowledge of both the potential benefits and the risks associated with these therapies. For example, if a client complains of right lower abdominal pain, nausea, and vomiting—signs of appendicitis—you should recommend an allopathic assessment. However, if the client has a chronic gastrointestinal disorder and is diagnosed with irritable bowel syndrome, you may suggest the client could benefit from relaxation therapy and herbal therapy. Because you work very closely with your clients, you are in a unique position to become familiar with clients' religious and cultural viewpoints. You may be able to determine which CAM therapies would be best suited to individual beliefs.

You should encourage clients to inform all caregivers, including other health care professionals, about the medications and therapies they receive. In particular, complete information about the use of herbal medication should be added to the medical record to prevent potential drug and herb interactions.

* KEY CONCEPTS

- Complementary therapy is used in conjunction with allopathic medicine, whereas alternative therapy is generally used without the addition of conventional health care methods.
- Integrative medical programs use a multidisciplinary (both allopathic and complementary) treatment approach.
- Stress is an adaptive response that allows individuals to react to demanding situations.
- Chronic stress may be maladaptive, thereby leading to chronic muscle tension and changes in mood and immunity.
- Relaxation is a beneficial state characterized by improved mood, relaxed muscle tension, lowered blood pressure, and slower pulse and respiratory rates.
- To be most effective and to have prolonged beneficial outcomes, complementary and alternative medicine therapies require the client's commitment and regular involvement.
- Complementary and alternative medicine therapies should be chosen according to the client's functional status, belief or religious perspectives, access to health care, and insurance coverage.
- Some complementary and alternative medicine therapies may alter physiological responses, thereby requiring changes in routine medication doses.
- Imagery is usually visual but can also involve the auditory, proprioceptive, gustatory, and olfactory senses.
- Many complementary and alternative medicine therapies lack a scientific basis but are thought to be effective on the basis of observed positive outcomes in a number of clients. Some complementary and alternative medicine therapies are supported by research published in professional nursing and medical journals.
- Current research supports various nutritional practices that limit the development of lifestyle-specific diseases.
- Not all herbal therapies are safe.

* CRITICAL THINKING EXERCISES

Client profile: Margaret is a 76-year-old Catholic woman who has received a diagnosis of a slow-growing renal tumour. Surgery is scheduled in 2 weeks, and Margaret is afraid of both the procedure and the outcome. Is it cancer? Will the surgery result in a disability?

1. What specific nursing-accessible complementary and alternative medicine interventions can you offer Margaret to prepare her for the surgery and reduce her anxiety?
2. After surgery, Margaret becomes depressed. What complementary and alternative medicine therapies may be appropriate to help her deal with her depression?

* REVIEW QUESTIONS

1. Despite the success of allopathic medicine (traditional Western medicine), many clients find complementary therapies provide relief for which of the following conditions?
   1. Heart disease and pancreatitis
   2. Ulcers and hepatitis
   3. Chronic back pain and arthritis
   4. Lupus and diabetes
2. Many complementary therapies, such as acupuncture, have diagnostic and therapeutic methods specific to their field. Which therapies can be easily learned and used as part of independent nursing practice?
   1. Massage therapy
   2. Chinese medicine
   3. Shamanism
   4. Breathwork and imagery
3. Which of the following statements best describes the experience of the estimated 50% of Canadians who have used a complementary and alternative medicine therapy within the last year?
   1. Most used complementary and alternative medicine therapy to prevent illness or maintain wellness.
   2. Few found these therapies helpful.
   3. Most had their complementary and alternative medicine therapy financed by Medicare.
   4. Most are from lower socioeconomic backgrounds.

4. Which of the following does holistic nursing regard and treat?
   1. Mind, body, and spirit
   2. Disease, spirit, and family
   3. Desires and emotions
   4. Muscles, nerves, and spine disorders
5. After you complete your assessment of the client, whose permission is required before you can implement a complementary and alternative medicine therapy?
   1. The client's
   2. The physician's
   3. The family's
   4. No permission is required.
6. According to one of the principles of complementary and alternative medicine therapies, which of the following statements best describes the individual who receives treatment?
   1. Actively involved in the treatment
   2. A total believer in what is being taught
   3. Submissive to the practitioner
   4. Less competent in his or her own care
7. Which of the following describes the most effective use of St. John's wort?
   1. Antioxidant
   2. Anti-inflammatory
   3. Mild antidepressant
   4. Vasodilator
8. Meditation may augment the effects of which of the following medications?
   1. Antihypertensive and thyroid-regulating medications
   2. Insulin and vitamins
   3. Prednisone
   4. Cough syrups and aspirin
9. Biofeedback techniques are frequently used in addition to relaxation interventions to assist individuals to do which of the following?
   1. Eat less food
   2. Learn to control specific autonomic nervous system responses
   3. Control diabetes
   4. Live longer with human immunodeficiency virus (HIV)
10. Therapeutic touch is a training-specific therapy that was developed by which of the following?
    1. Physician
    2. Nurse
    3. Physiotherapist
    4. Ancient Scandinavian culture

* RECOMMENDED WEB SITES

Canadian College of Naturopathic Medicine: http://www.ccnm.edu

The Web site of the Canadian College of Naturopathic Medicine (CCNM) provides detailed information about Canada's only four-year, full-time professional college of naturopathic medicine. The Web site also includes job postings and a resource centre with links to CCNM and other free journals.

Canadian Interdisciplinary Network for Complementary and Alternative Research: http://www.incamresearch.ca/

This initiative was created to facilitate research and promote knowledge and education in complementary and alternative medicine. The Web site provides links to other associated networks and institutions.

Chinese Medicine and Acupuncture Association of Canada: http://www.cmaac.ca

This organization aims to raise the profile and reputation of Chinese medicine and acupuncture. Its Web site includes the organization's history and a Canada-wide members' index.

College of Nurses of Ontario: Practice Guideline: Complementary Therapies: http://www.cno.org/docs/prac/41021_CompTherapies.pdf

This document is a helpful resource on complementary therapies and their application to nursing practice in Ontario, including guidelines for practice.

ConsumerLab: http://www.consumerlab.com/

This Web site provides information about independent testing of the quality and quantity of ingredients in various brands of natural health products. General use is free, but a small yearly fee is required to access the entire database.

Memorial Sloan-Kettering Cancer Center: Integrative Medicine: http://www.mskcc.org/mskcc/html/1979.cfm

This Web page provides updated information on therapies and supplements used by cancer clients. Information is also available on cancer treatment frauds.

M. D. Anderson Cancer Center: http://www.mdanderson.org/departments/cimer

The M. D. Anderson Cancer Center Complementary/Integrative Medicine Education Resources (CIMER) Web site offers information to both health care professionals and the public about complementary medicine and how it can be integrated with allopathic medicine.

National Center for Complementary and Alternative Medicine: http://nccam.nih.gov/

This extensive index provides information on various natural health products, research, and ongoing clinical trials related to complementary and alternative medicines. The Web site also has links to a variety of other resources and institutions related to complementary and alternative medicines.

Natural Health Products Directorate: http://www.hc-sc.gc.ca/ahc-asc/branch-dirgen/hpfb-dgpsa/nhpd-dpsn/index_e.html

The Natural Health Products Directorate is Health Canada's regulating authority for natural health products for sale in Canada. Its Web site includes information on the regulatory practices, definitions related to natural health products, and an index of various health-related issues.

Public Health Agency of Canada: http://www.phac-aspc.gc.ca/chn-rcs/index-eng.php

The Public Health Agency of Canada is focused on more effective efforts to prevent chronic diseases, such as cancer and heart disease; prevent injuries; and respond to public health emergencies and infectious disease outbreaks. The agency works closely with provinces and territories to keep Canadians healthy and help reduce pressures on the health care system.

36

Activity and Exercise

Written by Ann Brokenshire, RN, BScN, MEd

Based on the original chapter by Rita Wunderlich, BSN, MSN(R), PhD

objectives

Mastery of content in this chapter will enable you to:

- Define the key terms listed.
- Describe the role of the musculoskeletal and nervous systems in the regulation of movement.
- Discuss physiological and pathological influences on body alignment and joint mobility.
- Describe how to use proper body mechanics and ergonomics to prevent musculoskeletal injuries.
- Describe how exercise and activity benefit physiological and psychological functioning.
- Describe the benefits of implementing an exercise program for the purpose of health promotion.
- Describe the benefits of implementing exercise and activity during the acute, restorative, and continuing care of clients.
- Describe important factors to consider when planning an exercise program for clients across the lifespan and for those with specific chronic illnesses.
- Assess clients for impaired mobility and activity intolerance.
- Formulate nursing diagnoses for clients who experience mobility and activity tolerance.
- Write a nursing care plan for a client with impaired mobility and activity intolerance.
- Describe the interventions for maintaining activity tolerance and mobility during the acute, restorative, and continuing care of clients.
- Evaluate the nursing care plan for maintaining activity and exercise for clients across the lifespan and with specific chronic illnesses.

key terms

Activities of daily living (ADLs), p. 775
Activity tolerance, p. 776
Antagonistic muscles, p. 779
Antigravity muscles, p. 779
Body mechanics, p. 775
Cartilage, p. 776
Cartilaginous joints, p. 776
Centre of gravity, p. 775
Concentric tension, p. 779
Eccentric tension, p. 779
Egonomics, p. 775
Exercise, p. 775
Fibrous joints, p. 775
Flat bones, p. 777
Friction, p. 776
Gait, p. 784
Gait belt, p. 792
Hemiparesis, p. 784
Hemiplegia, p. 780
Immobility, p. 790
Irregular bones, p. 777
Isometric contraction, p. 777
Isotonic contraction, p. 776
Joint, p. 775
Ligaments, p. 776
Long bones, p. 777
Mobility, p. 784
Muscle tone, p. 775
Pathological fractures, p. 777
Posture, p. 775
Proprioception, p. 779
Range of motion (ROM), p. 777
Short bones, p. 777
Synarthrotic joint, p. 777
Synergistic muscles, p. 779
Synovial joints, p. 776
Tendons, p. 776
Transfer belt, p. 792

media resources

evolve Web Site

- Audio Chapter Summaries
- Glossary
- Multiple-Choice Review Questions
- Student Performance Checklists
- Student Learning Activities
- Video Clips
- Weblinks

Companion CD

- Glossary
- Interactive Learning Activities
- Fluids and Electrolytes Tutorial
- Test-Taking Skills

When providing nursing care, you will walk, turn, lift, and transfer. You use muscles and leverage when carrying out these activities. To reduce the risk of injury to the client or yourself, you must understand and practise proper **body mechanics**, as well as use safe lifting and moving techniques. To prevent injury to yourself when performing other nursing tasks, such as pushing medication carts or stretchers, using the telephone, and documenting client care, attention to **ergonomics** is equally important. Understanding both body mechanics and ergonomics includes knowledge of the actions of various muscle groups, knowledge of the factors involved in the coordination of body movement, and familiarity with the integrated functioning of the skeletal, muscular, and nervous systems. This chapter focuses on body mechanics and you, the nurse, whereas Chapter 46 discusses body mechanics in relation to the client.

Nurses must promote activity and **exercise** because of the beneficial impact they have on wellness, prevention of illness, and restoration of optimal functioning. A program of regular physical activity and exercise has the potential to enhance all dimensions of wellness (Box 36–1). This chapter provides you with information about exercise and activity as it relates to health promotion, to the acute phase of illness, and to the restorative and continuing care of clients. Nursing strategies are included to help plan an individualized exercise and activity program for a variety of clients with specific disease entities and needs. The discussion of activity and exercise is equally important to you as the nurse.

BOX 36-1 The Gift of Exercise

The other day I was looking for a gift to give to a friend. This friend is very important to me and I want her to be around for a long time. I want her to live a long and healthy life. I thought how great it would be if I could give her a gift that would improve the quality of her life.

So I sat down and made a list of what I would look for in this special gift:

It would help her to be stronger, firmer, leaner, more flexible, and energetic.

It would help lower her risk of dying from heart disease, help lower blood pressure and improve lipid profile, control blood glucose level, fight obesity, and help her to age more gracefully.

It would help improve immune function, concentration and task performance, and the quality of sleep.

It would help reduce stress, improve mood, enhance self-esteem, and increase optimism and confidence.

It would help to increase self-awareness and control over the choices in her life.

It would be fun but also challenging.

It would allow for socialization but also time alone, depending on her needs.

It would come in all different modes and styles and adapt to various environments and weather conditions.

Finally, it would have a solid *Consumer Reports* rating, supported by scientific data from reputable sources.

After completing my list, I realized that the only gift that meets all the above criteria is the gift of exercise. Have a happy and healthy life, my friend.

From Huddleston, J. S. (2006). Exercise. In C. L. Edelman & C. L. Mandle (Eds.), *Health promotion throughout the lifespan* (6th ed.).St. Louis, MO: Mosby.

Scientific Knowledge Base

Activity and exercise are important to the well-being of all persons. However, you will be able to provide a more individualized approach to care by knowing the physiology and regulation of body mechanics, exercise, and activity.

Overview of Body Mechanics, Exercise, and Activity

The coordinated efforts of the musculoskeletal and nervous systems to maintain body alignment, balance, and **posture** during lifting, bending, moving, and performing **activities of daily living (ADLs)** provide the foundation for body mechanics. It is essential to implement these activities properly to reduce the risk of injury to the musculoskeletal system and to facilitate body movements, allowing physical mobility without muscle strain or excessive use of muscle energy.

Body Alignment. Body alignment refers to the relationship of one body part to another body part along a horizontal or vertical line. Correct alignment reduces the strain on musculoskeletal structures, maintains adequate **muscle tone**, and contributes to balance. The nervous system is responsible for muscle tone and regulates and coordinates the amount of pull exerted by individual muscles (Thibodeau & Patton, 2007). This is discussed in more depth in Chapter 46.

Body Balance. Body balance is achieved when a relatively low centre of gravity is balanced over a wide, stable base of support and a line falls from the **centre of gravity** vertically through the base of support. The base of support is the foundation. When the line from the centre of gravity does not fall vertically through the base of support (that is, when the line is on an angle other than 90 degrees), the body loses balance. Body balance is also enhanced by proper posture, or the body position that most favours function, requires the least muscular work to maintain, and places the least strain on muscles, ligaments, and bones (Thibodeau & Patton, 2007).

Use balance to maintain proper body alignment and posture by taking two simple actions. First, widen the base of support by separating your feet to a comfortable distance. Second, to increase your balance, bring the centre of gravity closer to the base of support; do this by bending your knees and flexing your hips until you are squatting yet maintaining proper back alignment by keeping your trunk erect.

Skeletal System

Bones. Bones perform five functions in the body: support, protection, movement, mineral storage, and hematopoiesis (blood cell formation). In a discussion of body mechanics (see Box 36–3), two of these functions—support and movement—are most important. In support, bones serve as the body's framework and contribute to the shape, alignment, and positioning of body parts. In movement, bones, together with their joints, act as levers and are sites for muscle attachment. As muscles contract and shorten, they pull on bones, producing joint movement (Thibodeau & Patton, 2007).

Joints. An articulation, or **joint**, is the connection between bones. Each joint is classified according to its structure and degree of mobility. Depending on the connective structures, joints are classified as fibrous, cartilaginous, synovial, or synarthrotic (Huether & McCance, 2008). **Fibrous joints** fit closely together and are fixed, permitting little if any movement—for example, the syndesmosis (united by ligaments) between the tibia and fibula. **Cartilaginous joints** have little movement but are elastic—for example, the synchondrosis (united by cartilage) that attaches the ribs to the costal cartilage. **Synovial joints**, or true joints, are freely movable and are the body's most mobile, numerous, and anatomically complex joints—for example, the hinged joint at the elbow.

Ligaments, Tendons, and Cartilage. Ligaments, tendons, and cartilage are structures that support the skeletal system (see Chapter 46). **Ligaments** are white, shiny, flexible bands of fibrous tissue that bind joints and connect bones and cartilage; they are elastic and aid joint flexibility and support. **Tendons** are white, glistening, fibrous bands of tissue that connect muscle to bone. **Cartilage** is nonvascular, a supporting connective tissue with a flexibility similar to that of firm plastic. The gristlelike nature of cartilage permits it to sustain weight and to serve as a shock absorber between articulating bones.

Skeletal Muscle. Walking, talking, running, breathing, and participating in physical activity require the contraction of skeletal muscles. The body has more than 600 skeletal muscles. In addition to facilitating movement, these muscles determine the form and contour of the body. Most muscles span at least one joint and attach to both articulating bones. When contraction occurs, one bone is fixed and the other moves. The origin is the point of attachment that remains still; the insertion is the point that moves when the muscle contracts (Thibodeau & Patton, 2007).

Friction. Friction is a physical force, the resistance encountered during the act of rubbing one object against another (Myers, 2006). Because it opposes movement, you are more likely to experience a musculoskeletal injury as a result of friction (and the client may suffer a friction abrasion) if you are not careful. To minimize the chance of such injuries, reduce friction by following some basic principles:

- Avoid lifting or moving clients manually. Using a mechanical lift completely prevents friction.
- In situations when you must assist manually:
  - Friction can be reduced by lifting rather than pushing a client. Lifting has an upward component and decreases the pressure between the client and the bed or the chair. To move the client more easily along the bed's surface, use a special slide sheet, slide board, or transfer board to reduce friction.
  - Because a passive or immobilized client produces greater friction to movement (see Chapter 46), when possible, use some of the client's strength and mobility when lifting, transferring, or moving the client up in bed. For instance, if clients can bend their knees as you assist them in moving up in bed, friction is decreased. Explain the procedure and tell the client when to move.
  - The greater the surface area of the object to be moved, the greater the friction. If a client is unable to assist in moving up in bed, placing the client's arms across the chest decreases surface area and therefore reduces friction.

Exercise and Activity. Exercise is physical activity for the purpose of conditioning the body, improving health, and maintaining fitness, or it may be used as a therapeutic measure. When a person exercises, physiological changes occur in body systems (Box 36–2). The exercise program chosen and developed for a client depends on that individual's **activity tolerance**, or the kind and amount of exercise or activity that the individual is able to perform. Physiological, emotional, and developmental factors influence the client's activity tolerance.

A program of regular physical activity and exercise promotes physical and psychological health. An active lifestyle is important for promoting and maintaining health, and is also an essential treatment modality for chronic illnesses (Warburton et al., 2006, 2007). Regular physical activity and exercise enhance functioning of all body systems, including cardiopulmonary functioning (endurance), musculoskeletal fitness (strength, flexibility, and bone integrity), weight control and maintenance, and psychological well-being (body image) (Bloomfield, 2005; Huddleston, 2006).

The best program of physical activity includes a combination of exercises that produce different physiological and psychological benefits. Isotonic, isometric, and resistive isometric are three categories of exercise classified according to the type of muscle contraction involved. Isotonic exercises cause muscle contraction and changes in muscle length (**isotonic contraction**). Walking, swimming, dance aerobics, jogging, bicycling, and moving arms and legs with light resistance are examples of isotonic exercises. The benefits of isotonic exercises include increased circulatory and respiratory functioning, increased osteoblastic activity (activity by bone-forming cells) to combat osteoporosis, and increased muscle tone, mass, and strength.

➤ BOX 36-2 Effects of Exercise

Cardiovascular System
- Increased cardiac output
- Improved myocardial contraction, thereby strengthening cardiac muscle
- Decreased resting heart rate
- Improved venous return

Pulmonary System
- Increased respiratory rate and depth followed by a quicker return to resting state
- Improved alveolar ventilation
- Decreased work of breathing
- Improved diaphragmatic excursion

Metabolic System
- Increased basal metabolic rate
- Increased use of glucose and fatty acids
- Increased triglyceride breakdown
- Increased gastric motility
- Increased production of body heat

Musculoskeletal System
- Improved muscle tone
- Increased joint mobility
- Improved muscle tolerance to physical exercise
- Possible increase in muscle mass
- Reduced bone loss

Activity Tolerance
- Improved tolerance
- Decreased fatigue

Psychosocial Factors
- Improved tolerance to stress
- Reports of "feeling better"
- Reports of decrease in illness (e.g., colds, influenza)

Data from Huether, S. E., & McCance, K. L. (2008). *Understanding pathophysiology* (2nd ed.). St. Louis, MO: Mosby; and Hoeman, S. P. (2008). *Rehabilitation nursing: Process, application, and outcomes* (4th ed.). St. Louis, MO: Mosby.

Isometric exercises involve tightening a muscle and holding it for a number of seconds in a stationary position while maintaining the tension (**isometric contraction**). This form of exercise is ideal for clients who are unable to tolerate the increase in activity expected during isotonic exercises. Isometric exercises are especially helpful to people who are recovering from injuries that limit range of motion. For example, *quad setting*—pressing the knee toward the bed and holding—is used after knee surgery. The benefits of isometric exercises include minimized potential for muscle wasting by increasing muscle mass, tone, and strength; increased circulation to the involved body part; and increased osteoblastic activity.

Isometric exercises also may be resistive. Resistive isometric exercises are those in which the individual contracts the muscle while pushing against a stationary object or resisting the movement of an object (Hoeman, 2008). A gradual increase in the amount of resistance and in the length of time that the muscle contraction is held will increase muscle strength and endurance. The *plank* (for abdominal strengthening) and the *wall push-up* (for chest, tricep, and shoulder strengthening) are resistive isometric exercises with which you may be familiar. The client who is in a sitting position may do *hip lifting*, in which the hands push against a surface such as the seat of a chair to raise the hips. After hip surgery, *gluteal setting* is prescribed: in a supine position, keeping the legs straight, together, and in contact with the bed, with a loop or belt positioned around the thighs just above the knees, press legs outward against the belt and hold. Resistive isometric exercises help to promote muscle strength and provide sufficient stress against bone to promote osteoblastic activity.

Regulation of Movement

Coordinated body movement involves the integrated functioning of the skeletal, muscular, and nervous systems. Because these three systems cooperate so closely in the mechanical support of the body, they are often considered as a single functional unit.

Skeletal System. The skeleton provides attachment sites for muscles and ligaments and the leverage necessary for movement. It is the body's supporting framework and consists of four types of bones: long, short, flat, and irregular. **Long bones** contribute to height (e.g., the femur, fibula, and tibia in the leg) and length (e.g., the phalanges of the fingers and toes). **Short bones** occur in clusters and, when combined with ligaments and cartilage, permit movement of the extremities. Two examples of short bones are the tarsal bones in the foot and the patella in the knee. **Flat bones** provide structural contour, such as bones in the skull and the ribs in the thorax. **Irregular bones** make up the vertebral column and some bones of the skull, such as the mandible.

Bones are further characterized by firmness, rigidity, and elasticity. Firmness results from inorganic salts, such as calcium and phosphate, that are laid down in the bone matrix. Firmness is related to the bone's rigidity, which is necessary to keep long bones straight and enables bones to bear weight. In addition, bones have a degree of elasticity and flexibility that changes with age. For example, newborns have a large amount of cartilage and are highly flexible but their bones are unable to support weight. Toddler's bones are more pliable than those of older people and thus are better able to withstand falls. Older adults, especially women, are more susceptible to bone loss (resorption) and osteoporosis.

The skeletal system has several functions. Bones protect vital organs (e.g., the skull around the brain; the ribs around the heart and lungs). They also aid in calcium regulation, store calcium, and release calcium into the body's circulation as needed. Clients with decreased calcium regulation and metabolism are at risk for developing osteoporosis and **pathological fractures** (fractures caused by weakened bone tissue). In addition, the internal structure of bones contains bone marrow, participates in red blood cell (RBC) production, and acts as a reservoir for blood. Clients with altered bone marrow function or diminished RBC production are usually weakened and fatigue easily, which decreases their mobility and places them at risk of falling.

Joints, ligaments, tendons, and cartilage permit strength and flexibility of the skeleton. Strength enables the skeletal system to support the body.

Joints. Joints are the connections between bones. Each joint is classified according to its structure and degree of mobility. Joints are classified as four types: synarthrotic, cartilaginous, fibrous, and synovial. A person's flexibility is demonstrated through **range of motion (ROM)**, which is the range of normal movement for a joint.

In a **synarthrotic joint**, bones are jointed by bones. No movement is associated with this type of joint, and the bony tissue that forms between the bones provides strength and stability. The classic example of this type of joint is the sacrum, in which vertebrae are joined (Figure 36–1A).

The cartilaginous joint, or synchondrodial joint, has little movement but is elastic and uses cartilage to unite body surfaces. Cartilaginous joints are found when bones are exposed to constant pressure, such as the costosternal joints between the sternum and ribs (see Figure 36–1B).

The fibrous joint, or syndesmodial joint, is a joint in which two bony surfaces are united by a ligament or membrane. The fibres of ligaments are flexible and stretch, permitting a limited amount of movement. For example, the paired bones of the lower leg (tibia and fibula) are fibrous joints (Heuther & McCance, 2008) (see Figure 36–1C).

The synovial joint, or true joint, is a freely movable joint in which contiguous bony surfaces are covered by articular cartilage and connected by ligaments lined with a synovial membrane. Joining of the humeral radius and ulna by cartilage and ligaments forms a pivotal joint (see Figure 36–1D). Other types of synovial joints are the ball-and-socket joints (e.g., the hip joint) and the hinge joints (e.g., the interphalangeal joints of the fingers).

Ligaments. Ligaments are white, shiny, flexible bands of fibrous tissue that bind joints together and connect bones and cartilages. Ligaments are elastic and aid joint flexibility and support (Figure 36–2). In addition, some ligaments have a protective function. For example, ligaments between the vertebral bodies and the ligamentum flavum prevent damage to the spinal cord during movement of the back.

Tendons. Tendons are white, fibrous bands of tissue that connect muscle to bone. Tendons are strong, flexible, and inelastic, and they occur in various lengths and thicknesses. The Achilles tendon (tendo calcaneus) is the thickest and strongest tendon in the body. It begins near the middle of the posterior of the leg and attaches the gastrocnemius and soleus muscles in the calf to the calcaneal bone in the back of the foot (Figure 36–3).

Cartilage. Cartilage is nonvascular, supporting connective tissue located chiefly in the joints and thorax, trachea, larynx, nose, and ear. The fetus has a large amount of temporary cartilage, which is replaced by bone developed during infancy. Permanent cartilage is unossified (not hardened) except in advanced age and in diseases such as osteoarthritis.

Skeletal Muscle. Movement of bones and joints involves active processes that must be carefully integrated to achieve coordination. Skeletal muscles, because of their ability to contract and relax, are the working elements of movement. Contractile elements of the skeletal muscle are enhanced by anatomical structure and attachment to the skeleton. Adequate skeletal muscle is necessary for strength and flexibility.

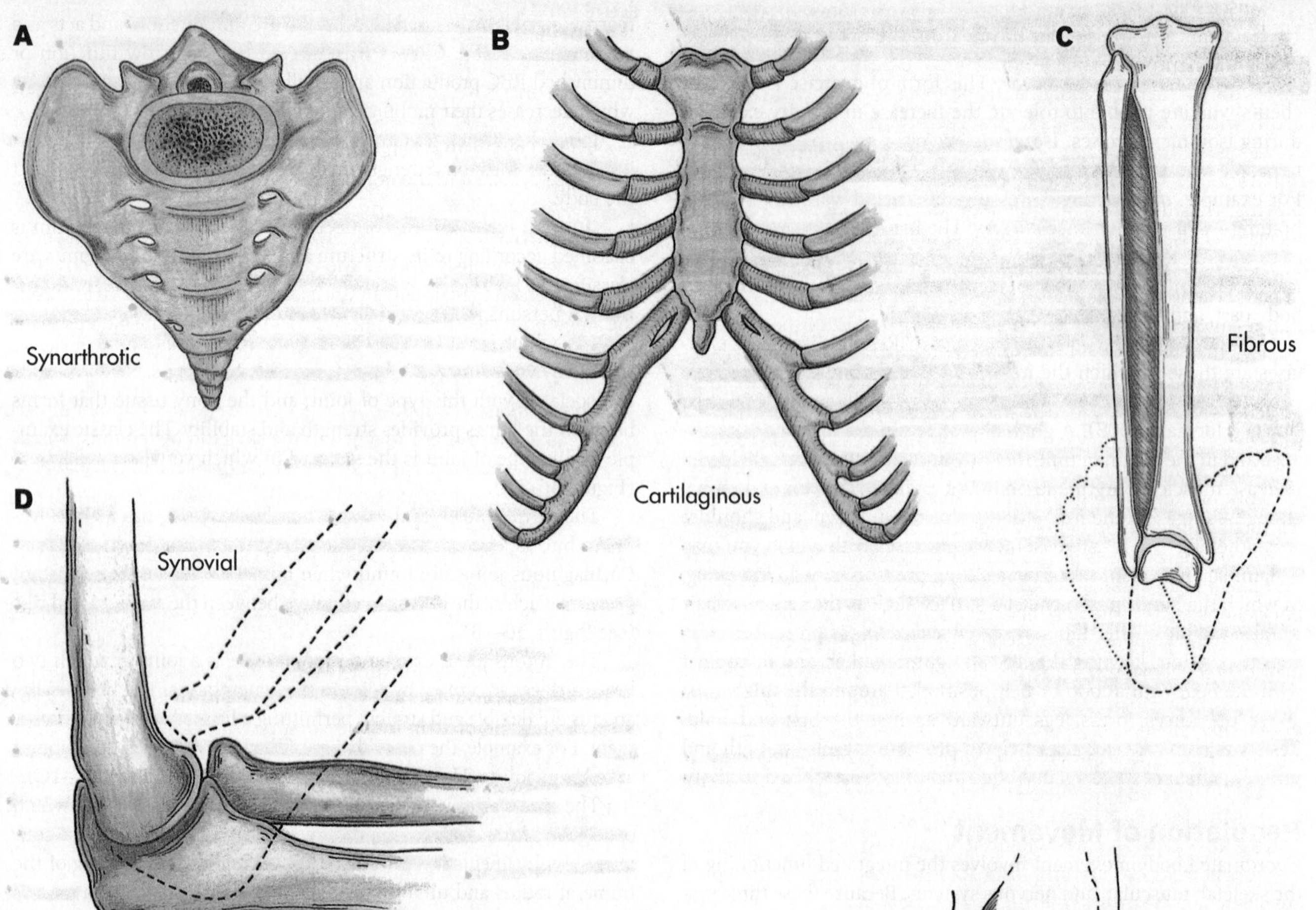

A
Synarthrotic
B
Cartilaginous
C
Fibrous
D
Synovial

Figure 36-1 Joint types. A, Synarthrotic. B, Cartilaginous. C, Fibrous. D, Synovial.

Figure 36-2 Ligaments of the hip joint.

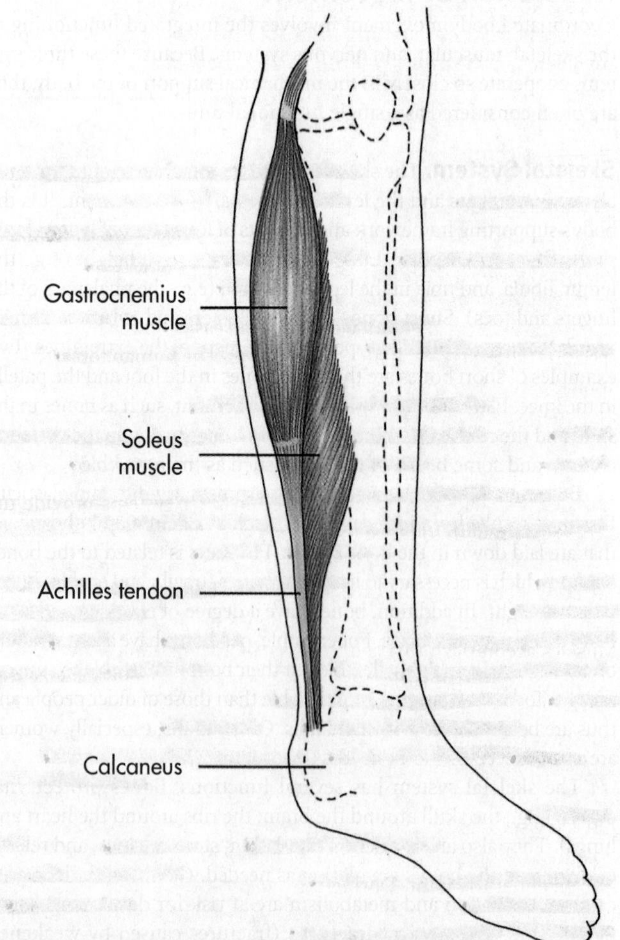

Figure 36-3 Tendons and muscles of the lower leg.

Muscles are made of fibres that contract when stimulated by an electrochemical impulse that travels from the nerve to the muscle across the neuromuscular junction. The electrochemical impulse causes the filaments (predominantly protein molecules of myosin and actin) within the fibre to slide past each other, with the filaments changing length.

Muscle contractions can be categorized by functional purpose: moving, resisting, or stabilizing body parts. In **concentric tension**, increased muscle contraction causes muscle shortening resulting in movement, such as when a client uses an overhead trapeze to pull up in bed. **Eccentric tension** helps to control the speed and direction of movement as the muscle lengthens. In the example of the overhead trapeze, the client should slowly lower to the bed. This lowering is controlled when the muscles lengthen. Concentric and eccentric muscle actions are necessary for active movement and are therefore referred to as dynamic or isotonic contraction. In contrast, isometric contraction (static contraction) causes an increase in muscle tension or muscle work but no shortening or active movement of the muscle (e.g., instructing the client in tightening and relaxing a muscle group, as in quadriceps set exercises or pelvic floor muscle exercises). Voluntary movement is a combination of isotonic and isometric contractions. For example, when you lift a client up in bed, the client's weight causes increased tension in the muscles of your arms until the tension (isometric) is equal to the weight to be lifted and the weight of your lower arms. When this equilibrium is reached, continued stimulation of the muscles results in muscle shortening (isotonic) and bending of the elbows (active movement), and the client is lifted off the bed.

Although isometric contractions do not result in muscle shortening, energy expenditure is increased. This type of muscle work is comparable to having a car in neutral while the driver continually depresses the accelerator and races the engine. The car is not going anywhere but the driver still expends a large amount of energy. You, as the nurse, must recognize the energy expenditure (increased respiratory rate and increased work on the heart) associated with isometric exercises because these types of exercises may be contraindicated in certain illnesses or conditions (e.g., myocardial infarction or chronic obstructive pulmonary disease).

Muscles Concerned With Movement. The muscles of movement are located near the skeletal region, where movement is caused by a lever system (Thibodeau & Patton, 2007). The lever system makes the work of moving a weight or load easier. In the human body, it occurs when specific bones act as a lever. The human forearm is an application of the lever: the elbow acting as the fulcrum, the weight held in the hand and being lifted acting as the resistance, and the pull of the muscles between the elbow and the hand acting as the effort. The mandible is another example of a lever system in the body. Muscles that attach to bones involved in lever systems provide the necessary strength to move the object.

Muscles Concerned With Posture. Gravity pulls on parts of the body all the time; the only way that the body can be held in position is for muscles to exert pull on bones in the opposite direction. Muscles accomplish this counterforce by maintaining a low level of sustained contraction. Because poor posture represents a stance that is less than optimal for counteracting the force of gravity, it places more work on muscles. This leads to fatigue and can eventually interfere with bodily functions and cause deformities.

Muscle Groups. The antagonistic, synergistic, and antigravity muscle groups are coordinated by the nervous system and maintain posture and initiate movement. **Antagonistic muscles** bring about movement at the joint. During movement, the active mover muscle contracts, and its antagonist relaxes. For example, during flexion of the arm, the active mover (the biceps brachii) contracts and its antagonist (the triceps brachii) relaxes. During extension of the arm, the active mover, now the triceps brachii, contracts and the new antagonist, the biceps brachii, relaxes.

Synergistic muscles contract to accomplish the same movement. When the arm is flexed, the strength of the contraction of the biceps brachii is increased by contraction of the synergistic muscle, the brachialis. Thus, with synergistic muscle activity, two active movers—the biceps brachii and the brachialis—contract, and the antagonistic muscle, the triceps brachii, relaxes.

Antigravity muscles are involved with joint stabilization. These muscles continuously oppose the effect of gravity on the body and permit a person to maintain an upright or sitting posture. In an adult, the antigravity muscles are the extensors of the leg—the gluteus maximus, the quadriceps femoris, and the soleus muscles—and the muscles of the back.

Skeletal muscles support posture and carry out voluntary movement. These muscles are attached to the skeleton by tendons, which provide strength and permit motion. The movement of the extremities is voluntary and requires coordination from the nervous system.

Nervous System. Movement and posture are regulated by the nervous system. The major voluntary motor area, located in the cerebral cortex, is the precentral gyrus, or motor strip. A majority of motor fibres descend from the motor strip and cross at the level of the medulla. Thus, the motor fibres from the right motor strip initiate voluntary movement for the left side of the body, and the motor fibres from the left motor strip initiate voluntary movement for the right side of the body.

Transmission of the impulse from the nervous system to the musculoskeletal system is an electrochemical event and requires a neurotransmitter. Neurotransmitters are chemicals (e.g., acetylcholine) that transfer the electrical impulse from the nerve across the myoneural junction to stimulate the muscle, causing movement.

Movement can be impaired by disorders that alter neurotransmitter production, as in Parkinson's disease; alter transfer from the neurotransmitter to the muscle, as in myasthenia gravis; or alter activation of muscle activity, as in multiple sclerosis (Huether & McCance, 2008).

Proprioception. Proprioception is the awareness of the position of the body and its parts (Huether & McCance, 2008). Position is monitored by proprioceptors located on nerve endings in muscles, tendons, and joints. Posture is regulated by the nervous system and requires coordination of proprioception and balance. As a person carries out ADLs, proprioceptors monitor muscle activity and body position. For example, the proprioceptors on the soles of the feet contribute to correct posture during standing or walking. During standing, pressure is continuous on the bottom of the feet. The proprioceptors monitor the pressure, communicating this information through the nervous system to the antigravity muscles. The standing person remains upright until deciding to change position. As a person walks, the proprioceptors on the bottom of the feet monitor pressure changes. Thus, when the bottom of the moving foot comes in contact with the walking surface, the individual automatically moves the stationary foot forward. The proprioceptors allow people to walk without having to watch their feet.

Balance. A person must have adequate balance when standing, running, lifting, or performing ADLs. Balance is controlled by the nervous system, specifically by the cerebellum and the inner ear. A major function of the cerebellum is to coordinate all voluntary movement, particularly highly skilled movements, such as those required in skiing.

Within the inner ear are the semicircular canals, three fluid-filled structures that assist in maintaining balance. Fluid within the canals has a certain inertia, and when the head is suddenly rotated in one direction, the fluid remains stationary for a moment, whereas the canal turns with the head. This allows a person to change position suddenly without losing balance.

Principles of Body Mechanics

Good body mechanics is the use of correct muscles to complete activities safely and efficiently, without unnecessary strain on any muscle or joint. Using principles of proper body mechanics during routine activities prevents injury (Box 36–3). In Ontario, 52% of nurses who lost work time experienced neck, shoulder, and back injuries; in the United States, 83% of nurse respondents to a survey reported experiencing back pain at work, mostly related to client-lifting tasks (Workers Health and Safety Centre, 2003). Whether you are assisting a client from the bed to the chair, lifting a client's limb, or teaching a client to carry out ADLs efficiently, knowledge of safe working posture (i.e., body mechanics) is crucial to prevent injury. When providing client care, incorporate your knowledge of physiological influences on body alignment and mobility.

Using principles of safe client transfer and positioning during routine care activities also decreases work effort (see Chapter 46). To increase and reinforce their knowledge, teach colleagues and clients' families how to transfer or position clients properly.

Keep in mind that nurses spend a good deal of time performing other tasks, ones not directly associated with their clients. Other activities often include standing or sitting at desks and computers to document care, collaborating with other members of the health team, and preparing equipment and supplies. All of these activities require as much attention to proper body mechanics as does hands-on client care.

Pathological Influences on Body Mechanics. Many pathological conditions affect body alignment and mobility. These conditions include congenital abnormalities; disorders of bones, joints, and muscles; central nervous system damage; and musculoskeletal trauma.

Congenital Abnormalities. Congenital abnormalities affect musculoskeletal alignment, balance, and appearance. For example, osteogenesis imperfecta is an inherited disorder characterized by bones that are porous, short, bowed, and deformed; as a result, children with this disorder experience curvature of the spine and shortness of stature (Hockenberry-Eaton & Wilson, 2008). Scoliosis is a structural curvature of the spine associated with vertebral rotation. Muscles, ligaments, and other soft tissues become shortened as a result. Balance and mobility are affected in proportion to the severity of abnormal spinal curvatures (Hockenberry-Eaton & Wilson, 2008).

➤ BOX 36-3 Principles of Body Mechanics

- The wider the base of support, the greater the stability.
- The lower the centre of gravity, the greater the stability.
- The equilibrium of an object is maintained as long as the line of gravity passes through its base of support.
- Facing the direction of movement prevents abnormal twisting of the spine.
- Dividing balanced activity between arms and legs reduces the risk of back injury.
- Leverage, rolling, turning, or pivoting requires less work than lifting.
- When friction is reduced between the object to be moved and the surface over which it is moved, less force is required to move it.
- Reducing the force of work reduces the risk of injury.
- Maintaining good body mechanics reduces fatigue of the muscle groups.
- Alternating periods of rest and activity helps to reduce fatigue.

Disorders of Bones, Joints, and Muscles. Osteoporosis is a well-known and well-publicized disorder of aging in which the density or mass of bone is reduced. The bone remains biochemically normal but has difficulty maintaining integrity and support. The cause is uncertain, and theories vary from hormonal imbalances to insufficient intake of nutrients, including calcium (Huether & McCance, 2008; Lewis et al., 2008).

Osteomalacia is an uncommon metabolic disease most often caused by lack of vitamin D. Because mineral calcification and deposition do not occur, bones are compact and spongy (Lewis et al., 2008).

Joint mobility can be altered by inflammatory and noninflammatory joint diseases and by articular disruption. Inflammatory joint disease (e.g., arthritis) is characterized by inflammation or destruction of the synovial membrane and articular cartilage and by systemic signs of inflammation. Noninflammatory diseases have none of these characteristics, and the synovial fluid is normal (Huether & McCance, 2008). Joint degeneration, which can occur with inflammatory and noninflammatory diseases, is marked by changes in articular cartilage combined with overgrowth of bone at the articular ends. Degenerative changes commonly affect weight-bearing joints.

Articular disruption may be as mild as a sprain or as severe as dislocation. It involves trauma to the articular capsules, such as a tear in a sprain or a separation in a dislocation. Articular disruption usually results from trauma but can also be congenital, as with developmental dysplasia of the hip (Hockenberry-Eaton & Wilson, 2008).

Central Nervous System Damage. Damage to any component of the central nervous system that regulates voluntary movement results in impaired body alignment and mobility. For example, the motor strip in the cerebrum can be damaged by trauma from a head injury. The amount of voluntary motor impairment is directly related to the amount of destruction of the motor strip. A client with a right-sided cerebral hemorrhage and damage to the right motor strip may have left-sided **hemiplegia.** However, another client with a right-sided head injury may have only cerebral edema (but not destruction) of the motor strip. With extensive physiotherapy, voluntary movement will gradually return to the left side.

Musculoskeletal Trauma. Musculoskeletal trauma can result in bruises, contusions, sprains, and fractures. A fracture is a disruption of bone tissue continuity. Fractures most commonly result from direct external trauma. They can also occur because of deformity of the bone, as with pathological fractures of osteoporosis (see Chapter 46).

safety alert The most crucial period of time for treating soft tissue injuries is during the first 6 to 12 hours (Lewis et al., 2008). Basic treatment of soft tissue injuries is summarized by the acronym RICES (Smeltzer & Bare, 2003):

- **R:** **R**est minimizes the potential for further damage to a joint already unstable because of injury.
- **I:** **I**ce reduces pain threshold; it should not be applied for longer than 30 minutes at a time.
- **C:** A wet elastic wrap is applied, with enough **c**ompression to hold ice in place.
- **E:** **E**levation of the injured part several centimetres above the heart facilitates venous return and reduces swelling.
- **S:** **S**upport: Usual initial treatment is immobilization by application of either a brace or a cast.

Nursing Knowledge Base

This section is concerned with knowledge from areas of nursing practice that enable you to meet the holistic needs of the client. Developmental changes, behavioural aspects, environmental issues, cultural and ethnic influences, and family and social support are important aspects of a person and must be incorporated into the plan of care, whether the client is seeking health promotion, acute care, or restorative and continuing care.

Developmental Changes

Throughout the lifespan, the body's appearance and functioning undergo change. The greatest change and impact on the maturational process are observed at both ends of the developmental spectrum.

Infants Through School-Age Children. The newborn infant's spine is flexed and lacks the anteroposterior curves of the adult. The first spinal curve occurs when the infant extends the neck from the prone position. As growth and stability increase, the thoracic spine straightens and the lumbar spinal curve appears, which allows sitting and standing.

The toddler's posture is awkward because of the slight swayback and protruding abdomen. As the child walks, the legs and feet are usually far apart and the feet are slightly everted. Toward the end of toddlerhood, posture appears less awkward, curves in the cervical and lumbar vertebrae are accentuated, and foot eversion disappears.

By the third year, the body is slimmer, taller, and better balanced. Abdominal protrusion is decreased, the feet are not as far apart, and the arms and legs have increased in length. The child appears more coordinated. The musculoskeletal system continues to grow and develop until adolescence (see Chapter 23).

Adolescence. The period of adolescence is usually initiated by a tremendous growth spurt. Growth is frequently uneven. As a result, the adolescent may appear awkward and uncoordinated. Adolescent girls usually grow and develop earlier than boys do. In girls, hips widen and fat is deposited in the upper arms, thighs, and buttocks. The adolescent boy's changes in shape are usually a result of long-bone growth and increased muscle mass (see Chapter 23).

Young to Middle-Age Adults. An adult who has correct posture and body alignment feels good, looks good, and generally appears self-confident. The healthy adult also has the necessary musculoskeletal development and coordination to carry out ADLs. Normal changes in posture and body alignment in adulthood occur mainly in pregnant women. These changes result from the body's adaptive response to weight gain and the growing fetus (see Chapter 24). When pregnant, the woman's centre of gravity shifts toward the anterior. As a result, the pregnant woman leans back and is slightly swaybacked. She may complain of back pain.

Older Adults. A progressive loss of bone mass occurs in the older adult. Some of the possible causes of this loss include physical inactivity, hormonal changes, and increased osteoclastic activity (activity by cells responsible for bone tissue absorption). The effect of bone loss is weaker bones, causing vertebrae to be softer and long shaft bones to be less resistant to bending.

In addition, older adults may walk more slowly and appear less coordinated. They also may take smaller steps, keeping their feet closer together, which decreases their base of support. Thus, body balance may become unstable, and they are at greater risk for falls and injuries (see Chapter 25).

Changes in muscle tissue also occur as adults age, beginning as early as during the twenties for men and during the forties for women. Muscle fibres shrink and have reduced tone and contractility. Strength and endurance change; fatigue occurs more readily, and overall energy may be reduced (Veterans Affairs Canada, 2003).

safety alert Falls and the resulting injuries are among the most debilitating medical problems that prevent the older adult from remaining independent. Regular exercise that promotes strengthening, flexibility, and balance can help prevent falls in the older adult (Fahlman et al., 2007; Huddleston, 2006; Robitaille et al., 2004; Rockwood et al., 2004).

Behavioural Aspects

Clients are more likely to incorporate an exercise program into their daily lives if it is supported and assisted by family and friends, nurses, physicians, and other members of the health care team. As the nurse, you should take into consideration the client's knowledge of exercise and activity, barriers to a program of exercise and physical activity, and current exercise habits. Clients are more open to developing an exercise program if they are at the stage of being ready to change their behaviour (Dacey, 2005). Information on the benefits of regular exercise may be helpful to the client who has not yet reached the stage of being ready to act. Clients' decisions to change behaviour and include a daily exercise routine in their lives may occur gradually with the provision of repeated information that is individualized to their needs and lifestyle (Box 36–4). Once the client has reached the stage of readiness, you must develop, in collaboration with the client, an exercise program that is customized to fit his or her needs. You then must provide continued follow-up support and assistance until the exercise program becomes a daily routine.

Environmental Issues

Work Sites. A common barrier for many clients is the lack of time that is needed to engage in a daily exercise program. Work sites have the potential to help their employees overcome the obstacle of time constraints by offering opportunities, reminders, and rewards for those committed to physical fitness (Health Canada, 2004; Box 36–5). Signs could be used to encourage employees to use the stairs instead of elevators. Rewards such as free parking or discounted parking fees could be given to employees who walk from distant lots (Canadian Fitness and Lifestyle Research Institute, 2006; Health Canada, 2004).

➤ BOX 36-4 General Strategies for Initiating and Maintaining an Exercise Program

An exercise program is most likely to be initiated and maintained when the individual:

- Perceives a net benefit
- Chooses an enjoyable activity
- Feels competent doing the activity
- Feels safe doing the activity
- Can easily access the activity on a regular basis
- Can fit the activity into the daily schedule
- Feels that the activity does not generate financial or social costs that he or she is unwilling to bear
- Experiences a minimum of negative consequences such as injury, loss of time, negative peer pressure, and problems with self-identity
- Is able to successfully address issues of competing time demands
- Recognizes the need to balance the use of labour-saving devices and sedentary activities with activities that involve a higher level of physical exertion

Data from Mayo Clinic Tools for Healthier Lives. (2005). *Fitness programs: Ready to get started?* Retrieved April 17, 2008, from http://www.mayoclinic.com/health/fitness/GQ00171

BOX 36-5 FOCUS ON PRIMARY HEALTH CARE

A Work Site Diabetes Prevention Program

Diabetes has so many potential complications, with associated economic and social costs, that all individuals, whether they are recognized as being at higher risk or not, should exercise as an essential primary prevention strategy.

In a recent study, prediabetic and previously undiagnosed diabetic employees participated in a 12-month diabetes prevention program at their work site. Registered nurses and a diabetic educator presented the three components of the program in both group and individual settings. Employees were encouraged to raise their level of physical activity, with membership in the employee fitness centre offered as an incentive. Dietary education focused especially on lowering fat intake. Behaviour change activities incorporated social support networks and consisted of identifying barriers to change in activity level and diet.

Aerobic fitness and a number of physiological measures improved significantly after 6 months and were maintained over the 12 months of the program. Significant improvement in glucose tolerance tests (GTT) and aerobic fitness continued for a full 24 months. More than half of the employees who participated in the study had normal GTT at 2 years.

The research by Aldana, et al. (2006) demonstrates that implementation of education and exercise programs by occupational health nurses can have a strong influence on the well-being of employees. By reducing blood glucose below prediabetic and diabetic levels, workplace diabetes prevention programs can help prevent the onset of diabetes.

Adapted from Aldana, S., Barlow, M., Smith, R., Yanowitz, F., Adams, T., Loveday, L., et al. (2006). A worksite diabetes prevention program: Two-year impact on employee health. *American Association of Occupational Health Nurses Journal, 54*(9), 389–396.

Schools. After many years of decreasing emphasis on physical education, it is increasingly clear that children are becoming less active, resulting in an increase in childhood obesity (Flynn et al., 2006). Recently, daily physical activity or physical education has been mandated in elementary schools across Canada, but secondary schools are not keeping up (Active Healthy Kids Canada, 2007). Only 18% of Canadian teenagers are accumulating enough daily activity to meet the international guidelines for optimal growth and development (Canadian Fitness and Lifestyle Research Institute, 2005). Schools can provide a foundation for lifetime commitment to exercise and physical fitness by incorporating physical activity into a child's daily routine. The Canadian Association for Health, Physical Education, Recreation and Dance (2008) recommends that all schools provide daily physical activity programs, not limited to competitive sports or physical education classes, that are appropriate for boys and girls of all skill levels and from diverse backgrounds.

Community. The community's support of physical fitness can be instrumental in promoting the health of its members. Examples of community involvement to promote physical fitness are the provision of walking trails and track facilities in community parks and physical fitness classes offered by trained professionals. Cost constraints may make availability of such amenities challenging. However, success in implementing physical fitness programs depends on a collaborative effort between public health agencies, parks and recreational associations, provincial and local government agencies, health care agencies, and community members.

Cultural and Ethnic Influences

Exercise and physical fitness is beneficial to all human beings. When developing a physical fitness program for culturally diverse populations, you must consider what is motivating and what is deemed appropriate and enjoyable. For example, South Asians living in Canada have reported that their physical exercise has been limited because of weather, lack of motivation, embarrassment over clothing or appearance, and not feeling comfortable participating in activities outside the home (South Asian Dietary Resource Working Group, 2007). Aerobic exercise in the form of dancing to songs from Bollywood movies is one culturally appropriate and community-based activity recommended for this population by the Working Group. Canadians from a traditional Chinese background value fitness activities based on Chinese culture—that is, activities that are gentle, soft, slow, relaxed, safe, and outdoor oriented (Lu, 2006).

You also must have knowledge of the specific disease entities that are associated with different cultural and ethnic populations (Box 36–6). Hyman (2004) found that, in Montreal, heart disease mortality rates vary by ethnicity, with Scandinavians and Africans having the highest rates and Asians and Latin Americans having the lowest

BOX 36-6 CULTURAL ASPECTS OF CARE

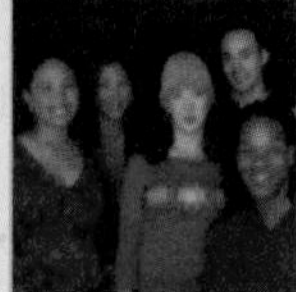

Epidemiological studies of ethnic groups indicate that physical inactivity is one of the risk factors associated with noninsulin-dependent diabetes mellitus (NIDDM). In Canada, NIDDM is between 3.6 and 5.3 times more prevalent within the Aboriginal population. Physical activity has been identified as playing an important role in the prevention and treatment of NIDDM, yet the Aboriginal population has a disproportionate number of poor, unemployed, and disadvantaged individuals who lack access to recreation and leisure activities.

Implications for Practice

- Because physical inactivity is a modifiable risk factor for the development of NIDDM, prevention and treatment programs need to focus heavily on exercise and to be tailored to the activity tolerance of the individual client.
- Motivational factors incorporated into the exercise program, such as providing a healthy snack or meal for participants and furnishing each client with a log to monitor weight loss and blood glucose levels, will enhance compliance.
- Promotion of physical activity should be supported by recognizing that a symbiotic relationship exists between cultural values and traditional leisure pursuits. Clients with a strong spiritual connection to the land may enjoy outdoor or wilderness recreation in the form of traditional games and activities, such as lacrosse and hunting.
- Ensure that members of Aboriginal groups collaborate in the planning and educational program initiatives.
- Development of an exercise or prevention program, or both, should attempt to remove potential barriers, such as transportation and cost, to facilitate commitment to the program.

Data from Huddleston, J. S. (2006). Exercise. In C. L. Edelman & C. L. Mandle (Eds.), *Health promotion throughout the lifespan* (6th ed.). St. Louis, MO: Mosby; Young, T. K., & Katzmarzyk, P. T. (2007). Physical activity of Aboriginal people in Canada. *Applied Physiology, Nutrition and Metabolism, 32*(Suppl. 2E), S148–S160; and Government of Alberta. (2007). *Cultural diversity: Including everyone in physical activity.* Retrieved April 17, 2008, from http://www.healthyalberta.com/HealthyPlaces/642.htm

rates. Women from Black African/Caribbean, Latin American, and South Asian ethnic backgrounds have been identified as having an increased risk of and vulnerability to type 2 diabetes (Health Council of Canada, 2007).

Family and Social Support

Social support can be used as a motivational tool to encourage and promote exercise and physical fitness. The client can engage a friend or a significant other to participate in a "buddy system" whereby they walk together each day at a specified time. This companionship provides for socialization and increases the enjoyment for some clients. It may lead to the development of a lifelong commitment to physical fitness. Parents can support their children in sports and physical activity by providing encouragement, praise, and transportation and by participating themselves (Health Canada, 2005).

Critical Thinking

Successful critical thinking requires a synthesis of knowledge, experience, information gathered from clients, critical thinking attitudes, and intellectual and professional standards. Clients' conditions are always changing. Clinical judgements require you to anticipate the information necessary, analyze the data, and make decisions regarding client care.

To understand activity tolerance and physical fitness and their impact on the client, you must integrate knowledge from nursing and other disciplines, previous experiences, and information gathered from clients. As you begin the process of problem solving for client care, a variety of concepts must be considered together to provide the best outcome for the client. The foundation for planning and decision making is knowledge of the musculoskeletal system and of health alterations that create problems for the client in the area of activity, exercise, and body mechanics. In addition, you must stay current on and incorporate various guidelines, such as those found at the Canadian Diabetes Association (2003) and in *Canada's Physical Activity Guide to Healthy Active Living*, developed by Health Canada (2003a) in conjunction with the Canadian Society for Exercise Physiology (Health Canada, 2002). Guidelines have also been created for children, youth, and older adults (Health Canada, 2003b, 2003c, 2005a, 2005b). Your experiences and your ability to think creatively and critically enhance your approach to each new client situation.

Any acquired or congenital condition that affects the structure of the musculoskeletal system or nervous system impairs to some degree activity, body alignment, or joint mobility. The impairment can be temporary, such as casting of an extremity, or permanent, as in contractures. For clients with limited ROM or mobility, develop the nursing care plan to include interventions that maintain the present level of alignment and joint mobility and increase the level of motor function.

Your experiences and your critical thinking attitude affect the problem-solving approach that is used with each new client. Remember that clients have the capacity for recovery in spite of the loss of some physical function. Restoration of functioning begins early in the care of clients who are experiencing disruption in their ability to perform self-care. Encouragement, support, commitment, and perseverance are important attitudes in critical thinking for these clients.

Perseverance is necessary when caring for clients who depend on you for assistance with positioning, turning, or ambulation. The repetition involved in the hourly responsibility for turning often leads to nurses losing sight of its importance. Perseverance is especialy important in delegating these tasks to other personnel. Making certain that the task is performed correctly is an essential nursing function. Problems with activity and mobility are often prolonged, so creativity is necessary when designing interventions aimed at improving activity tolerance and mobility skills.

Nursing Process

❖Assessment

Assessment of body alignment and posture is completed with the client standing, sitting, or lying down. Use assessment to determine normal physiological changes in growth and development; deviations related to poor posture, trauma, muscle damage, or nerve dysfunction; and any learning needs of clients. In addition, during assessment you can observe their posture and obtain important information about other factors that contribute to poor alignment, such as inactivity, fatigue, malnutrition, and psychological problems (see Box 36–7). To gather relevant information, ask questions related to the client's exercise and activity tolerance. During assessment (Figure 36–4), consider all of the elements that contribute to making appropriate nursing diagnoses.

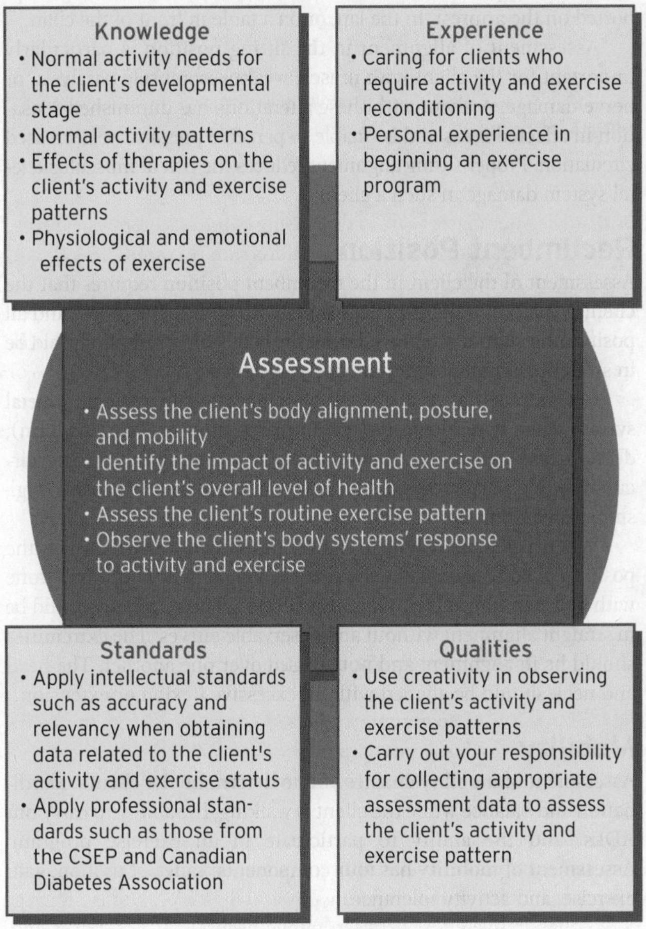

Knowledge
- Normal activity needs for the client's developmental stage
- Normal activity patterns
- Effects of therapies on the client's activity and exercise patterns
- Physiological and emotional effects of exercise

Experience
- Caring for clients who require activity and exercise reconditioning
- Personal experience in beginning an exercise program

Assessment
- Assess the client's body alignment, posture, and mobility
- Identify the impact of activity and exercise on the client's overall level of health
- Assess the client's routine exercise pattern
- Observe the client's body systems' response to activity and exercise

Standards
- Apply intellectual standards such as accuracy and relevancy when obtaining data related to the client's activity and exercise status
- Apply professional standards such as those from the CSEP and Canadian Diabetes Association

Qualities
- Use creativity in observing the client's activity and exercise patterns
- Carry out your responsibility for collecting appropriate assessment data to assess the client's activity and exercise pattern

Figure 36-4 Critical thinking model for activity and exercise assessment. CSEP, Canadian Society for Exercise Physiology.

Put the client at ease so that unnatural or rigid positions are not assumed. When assessing body alignment of an immobilized or unconscious client, remove pillows and positioning supports from the bed if not contraindicated, and place the client in the supine position.

Standing

Assessment of the standing client includes the following: the head should be erect and in the body's midline; body parts should be symmetrical; the spine should be straight with normal curvatures (cervical concave, thoracic convex, lumbar concave); the abdomen should be comfortably tucked; the knees should be in a straight line between the hips and ankles and should be slightly flexed; the feet should be flat on the floor and pointed directly forward and slightly apart to maintain a wide base of support; and the arms should hang comfortably at the sides (Figure 36–5). The client's centre of gravity is in the midline, and the line of gravity is from the middle of the forehead to a midpoint between the feet. Laterally, the line of gravity runs vertically from the middle of the skull to the posterior third of the foot (Wilson & Giddens, 2005).

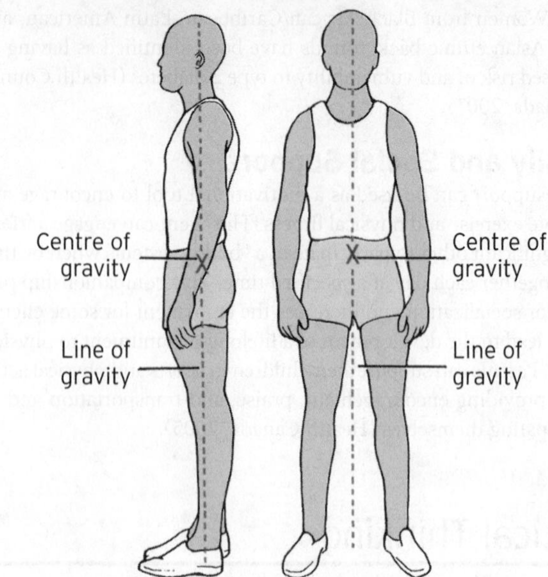

Figure 36-5 Correct body alignment when standing.

Sitting

Assessment of the client in the sitting position includes the following: the head should be erect and the neck and vertebral column in straight alignment; the body weight should be distributed on the buttocks and thighs; the thighs should be parallel and in a horizontal plane (be careful to avoid pressure on the popliteal nerve and blood supply); the feet should be supported on the floor; and the forearms should be supported on the armrest, in the lap, or on a table in front of the chair.

Assessment of alignment in the sitting position is particularly important for the client with muscle weakness, muscle paralysis, or nerve damage. A client with these alterations has diminished sensation in affected areas and is unable to perceive pressure or decreased circulation. Proper sitting alignment reduces the risk of musculoskeletal system damage in such a client.

Recumbent Position

Assessment of the client in the recumbent position requires that the client be placed in the supine position with all but one pillow and all positioning supports removed from the bed. The vertebrae should be in straight alignment without observable curves.

Conditions that create a risk of damage to the musculoskeletal system when lying down include impaired mobility (e.g., traction), decreased sensation (e.g., **hemiparesis** from a stroke), impaired circulation (e.g., diabetes), and lack of voluntary muscle control (e.g., spinal cord injuries).

When a client is unable to change position voluntarily, assess the position of body parts while the client is lying down. This is best done with you standing at the foot or head of bed. The vertebrae should be in straight alignment without any observable curves. The extremities should be in alignment and not crossed over one another. The head and neck should be aligned without excessive flexion or extension.

Mobility

Assessment of mobility enables you to determine the client's coordination and balance while the client is walking, the ability to carry out ADLs, and the ability to participate in an exercise program. Assessment of **mobility** has four components: range of motion, gait, exercise, and activity tolerance.

Range of Motion. Assessing range of motion (ROM) is one assessment technique used to determine the degree of damage or injury to a joint (see Chapter 32). These measurements enable you to answer questions about joint stiffness, swelling, pain, limitation of movement, and unequal movement. Limited ROM may indicate inflammation such as arthritis, fluid in the joint, altered nerve supply, or contractures. Increased mobility (beyond normal) of a joint may indicate connective tissue disorders, ligament tears, or possible joint fractures.

Gait. Gait, including rhythm, cadence, and speed, is the manner or style of walking. Walking with a limp is a gait. Propulsive, scissors, spastic, steppage, and waddling are descriptive names for other common gaits. Assessing gait allows you to draw conclusions about balance, posture, and the ability to walk without assistance. Note conformity; a regular, smooth rhythm; symmetry in the length of leg swing; smooth swaying related to the gait phase; and a smooth, symmetrical arm swing (Wilson & Giddens, 2005).

Exercise. Exercise is physical activity aimed at conditioning the body, improving health, maintaining fitness, or providing therapy to correct a deformity or restore the overall body to a maximal state of health. When a person exercises, physiological changes occur in body systems (see Box 36–2). Determine how much exercise and the types of exercise that the client receives regularly.

Activity Tolerance. Activity tolerance is the kind and amount of exercise or activity a person is able to perform. You need to assess activity tolerance when planning physical activity for health promotion and for clients with acute or chronic illness. This assessment provides the nurse with baseline data about the client's activity patterns and assists in determining which factors (physical, psychological, or motivational) are affecting activity tolerance. Box 36–7 lists factors that affect activity tolerance.

Client Expectations

In assessing the client's expectations concerning activity and exercise, you will first need insight into the client's perception of what is normal or acceptable with regard to physical fitness (Box 36–8). For example, one of the factors that affects physical activity is freedom from pain. If exercising is painful or fatiguing to the client, compli-

> **BOX 36-7 Factors That Affect Physical Activity Tolerance**
>
> **Physiological Factors**
>
> Skeletal abnormalities
> Muscular impairments
> Endocrine or metabolic illnesses (e.g., diabetes mellitus or thyroid disease)
> Hypoxemia
> Decreased cardiac function
> Decreased endurance
> Impaired physical stability
> Pain
> Sleep pattern disturbance
> Prior exercise patterns
> Infectious processes and fever
>
> **Emotional Factors**
>
> Anxiety
> Depression
> Chemical addictions
> Motivation
>
> **Developmental Factors**
>
> Age
> Gender
>
> **Pregnancy**
>
> Physical growth and development of muscle and skeletal support
>
> Adapted from Monohan, F. D., Sands, J. K., Neighbors, M., Marek, J. F., & Green-Nigro, C. J. (2007). *Phipps' medical-surgical nursing: Health and illness perspectives* (8th ed.). St. Louis, MO: Mosby.

ance with and commitment to the desired interventions may be lacking. Clients may be content with their present physical activity and fitness and may not perceive a need for improvement. Unless a real threat to health maintenance exists, forcing the client to accept your perspective is a breach of standards of care.

❖Nursing Diagnosis

Assessment of the client's activity tolerance, physical fitness, body alignment, and joint mobility provides related clusters of data or defining characteristics that help you identify a nursing diagnosis. You must be accurate when identifying diagnoses. For example, a client who reports being tired or weakened potentially could be diagnosed as having activity intolerance or fatigue. Use defining characteristics to lead to the definitive diagnosis. For example, a finding of abnormal heart rate or dyspnea would lead you to the diagnosis of activity intolerance, not to fatigue.

When activity and exercise are problems for a client, nursing diagnoses often focus on the individual's ability to move. The diagnostic label should direct nursing interventions. This requires the correct selection of the related factors. For example, activity intolerance related to excess weight gain requires very different interventions than if the related factor is prolonged bed rest. Box 36–9 provides an example of how the diagnostic process leads to accurate diagnosis selection. The following are examples of nursing diagnoses related to activity and exercise:

- *Health-seeking behaviours*
- *Readiness for enhanced self-care*
- *Activity intolerance*
- *Ineffective coping*
- *Impaired gas exchange*
- *Risk for injury*
- *Impaired physical mobility*
- *Imbalanced nutrition: more than body requirements*
- *Acute or chronic pain*

> **BOX 36-8 Nursing Assessment Questions**
>
> **Nature of the Problem**
>
> - What types of problems are you having with physical activities and exercise?
> - Why do you think your exercise and physical activity levels are inadequate?
> - Describe your typical daily exercise routine and level of physical activity.
> - What types of exercise do you prefer?
> - How long do you exercise at any given time?
>
> **Signs and Symptoms**
>
> - Do you experience muscular or joint pain during or after exercise?
> - Do you experience shortness of breath during physical activity?
> - Do you experience chest discomfort or pain during exercise or physical activity?
>
> **Onset and Duration**
>
> - Which physical activities cause you to become short of breath?
> - How long does it take to resume normal breathing after exercise or physical activity?
>
> **Severity**
>
> - How far do you walk before the pain in your legs begins?
> - On a scale of 0 to 10 (with 10 being the worst discomfort), rate your leg pain.
> - Describe your shortness of breath as minimal, moderate, or severe after physical activities or exercise, or both.
>
> **Barriers to Exercise and Activity**
>
> - Do you have any chronic illnesses that affect your ability to carry out activities of daily living (ADLs) or exercise?
> - Do you have any physical limitations that prevent you from exercising on a daily basis?
> - Do you have access to a community walking path or exercise equipment, or both?
> - What prevents you from exercising 30 minutes each day?
>
> **Effect on Client**
>
> - Has the lack of an exercise routine affected your weight?
> - Have you felt more fatigued since you have not been able to exercise on a routine basis?
> - Have you noticed any increase in shortness of breath when performing activities that require little exertion?

BOX 36-9 NURSING DIAGNOSTIC PROCESS

Impaired Physical Mobility

Assessment Activities	***Defining Characteristics***
Observe client's gait.	Shuffled gait Uncoordinated gait Client reports slower walking speed
Observe client performing tasks such as feeding, dressing, or recreational activities.	Uncoordinated movements Limited fine motor coordination
Measure range of joint motion.	Reduced joint motion in lower and/or upper extremeties Stiffness in joints

❖Planning

During planning, synthesize information from multiple resources (Figure 36–6). Your critical thinking ensures that the client's care plan integrates all client information. Best-practice guidelines are especially important to consider when you develop a care plan as these documents establish scientifically based guidelines for selecting effective nursing interventions.

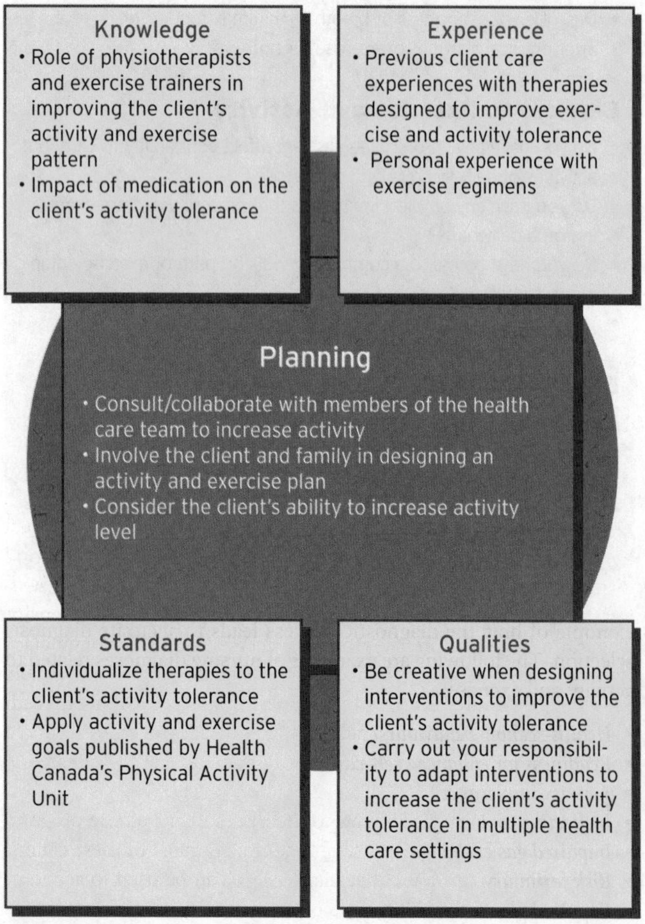

Figure 36-6 Critical thinking model for activity and exercise planning.

Concept maps assist in the planning of care. Figure 36–7 shows the relationship between a client's medical diagnosis of congestive heart failure and the identified nursing diagnosis.

Goals and Outcomes. Once you identify the nursing diagnoses, you and the client can set goals and expected outcomes to direct interventions. The plan should include consideration of pre-existing health concerns and of any risks of injury to the client. It is especially important to have knowledge of the client's home environment when planning therapies to maintain or improve activity, body alignment, and mobility. For some clients with alterations in joint mobility, family members may be the providers of care. Include the client's family in the care plan. The general goal related to exercise and activity is to improve or maintain the client's motor function and independence. The following are examples of outcomes for clients with deficits in activity and exercise (Ackley & Ladwig, 2008):

- Participates in prescribed physical activity while maintaining appropriate heart rate, blood pressure, and breathing rate.
- Shows an understanding of the need to increase activity gradually according to tolerance and symptoms.
- Expresses understanding of the need to balance rest and activity.

Setting Priorities. Care planning is individualized to the client, taking into consideration the client's most immediate needs. The immediacy of any problem is determined by the effect that the problem has on the client's mental and physical health. Because of the many skills, such as turning, transferring, and positioning, that are associated with the care of clients with activity intolerance, improper body mechanics, and impaired mobility, it is easy to overlook the complications associated with these health alterations. Therefore, to prevent complications and potential injury, be vigilant in monitoring the client and supervising unregulated care providers in carrying out activities.

Collaborative Care. Planning also involves understanding the client's need to maintain function and independence. Collaboration with other members of the health care team—for example, physiotherapists and occupational therapists—will be especially important for these clients. Long-term rehabilitation may be necessary, and you need to begin planning for discharge when a client enters the health care system. In addition, always individualize a care plan to meet the actual or potential needs of the client (see Box 36–10).

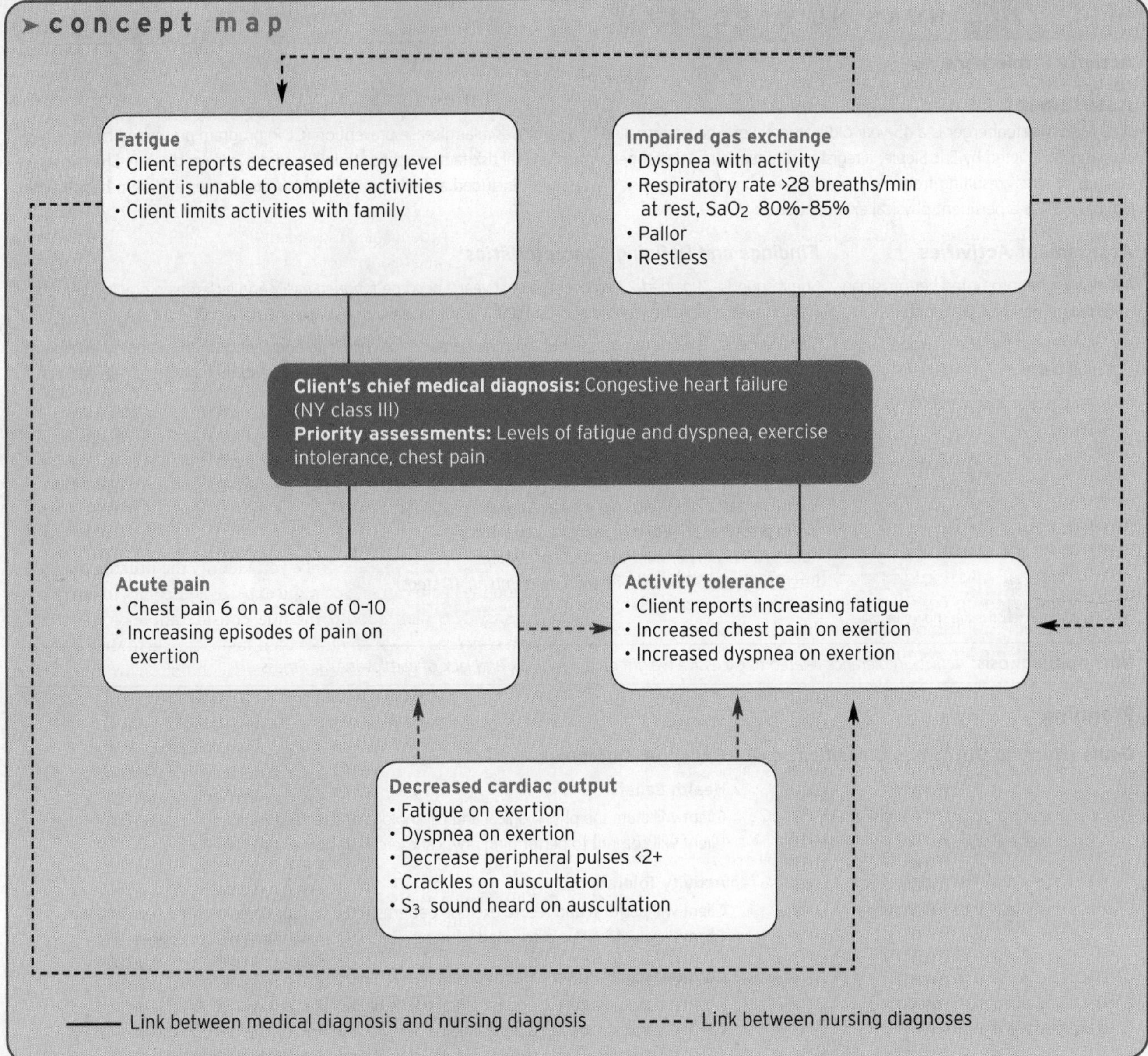

Figure 36-7 Concept map for a client with congestive heart failure and decreased activity.

❖Implementation

Health Promotion

A sedentary lifestyle contributes to the development of health-related problems. Promote health by encouraging clients to engage in a regular exercise program (Box 36–11). Take a holistic approach when developing and implementing a plan to enhance the client's overall physical fitness. Discuss the recommendations for physical activity and fitness with the client, and design a program of exercise in collaboration with the client (Box 36–12).

Before starting an exercise program, clients should calculate their maximum heart rate by subtracting their current age in years from 220 and then determine their target heart rate by calculating 60% to 90% of this maximum rate. Regardless of the exercise prescription implemented for the client, warm-up and cool-down periods must be included in the program (Gillespie, 2006). The warm-up period usually lasts 5 to 10 minutes and may include stretching, calisthenics, and subsequent aerobic activity performed at a lower intensity. The warm-up period prepares the body and decreases the potential for injury. The cool-down period follows the exercise routine and usually lasts 5 to 10 minutes. The cool-down period allows the body to readjust to baseline functioning gradually and provides an opportunity to combine movement such as stretching with relaxation-enhancing mind–body awareness (Gillespie, 2006).

Many clients find it difficult to incorporate an exercise program into their daily routines because of time constraints. For these clients, it is beneficial to reinforce that many ADLs can be used to accumulate the recommended 30 minutes or more per day of moderate-intensity physical activity (Box 36–13).

BOX 36-10 NURSING CARE PLAN

Activity Intolerance

Assessment

Mrs. Mary Wertenberger is a 45-year-old homemaker. She has enrolled in a cardiovascular disease prevention (CDP) program prescribed by her physician and conducted by Eric Sieple, a registered nurse. Mrs. Wertenberger has several risk factors associated with cardiovascular disease. She expresses feelings of stress resulting from excessive demands on her time. Eric's assessment included a discussion of Mrs. Wertenberger 's current health problems as well as a pertinent physical examination.

Assessment Activities	***Findings and Defining Characteristics****
Ask Mary what prompted her physician to recommend a CDP program.	She responds, "I *gained 23 kg* over the past year. I become *fatigued* easily and lack the energy to keep up with even simple household chores. I don't want to leave the house anymore."
Ask Mary about her exercise and eating habits.	She responds, "I want to exercise but with the demands of child care and caring for my aging parents, I just don't feel like it. I feel pulled in every direction, that increases my **stress**, and then I want to eat, eat, eat!"
Perform baseline assessment.	Height: 160 cm Weight: *102 kg* Blood pressure: *152/90 mm Hg (at rest)* Pulse: 96 beats per minute (at rest) Breathing rate: 20 breaths per minute (at rest) Blood pressure: *164/96 mm Hg (climbing 10 steps)* Pulse: *120 beats per minute (climbing 10 steps)* Breathing rate: *36 breaths per minute (climbing 10 steps)*

*Defining characteristics are shown in italics.

Nursing Diagnosis: *Activity intolerance related to excessive weight gain, inactivity, and lack of cardiovascular fitness*

Planning

Goals (Nursing Outcomes Classification)†	***Expected Outcomes***
	Health Beliefs
Client will develop a plan of exercise that incorporates isotonic and isometric exercises.	Client will state the physiological and psychological effects of exercise. Client will commit to performing physical exercise at home.
	Activity Tolerance
Client's activity tolerance will improve.	Client will perform and record exercise patterns three to four times over the next two weeks. Client's level of fatigue associated with exercise will remain the same or decrease.
	Cardiovascular Pump Effectiveness
Client's cardiopulmonary response to exercise will improve.	Client's resting diastolic blood pressure will be below 80 mm Hg. Client's systolic blood pressure will be below 140 mm Hg. Client's resting heart rate will range between 75 and 85 beats per minute.

†Outcome classification labels from Moorhead, S., Johnson, M., Maas, M. L., & Swanson, E. (Eds.). (2004). *Nursing Outcomes Classification (NOC)* (3rd ed.). St. Louis, MO: Mosby.

Interventions (Nursing Interventions Classification)‡

Exercise Promotion	***Rationales***
Instruct the client about the physiological benefits of a regular exercise program.	Physical activity and exercise protect against the development of cardiovascular disease (CVD) and decrease other risk factors associated with CVD, such as obesity, hypertension, and hyperlipidemia (Hamilton et al., 2007; Lloyd & Barnett, 2008; Sigal et al., 2006).
Instruct the client about the psychological benefits of a regular exercise program.	Physical activity and exercise increase self-esteem, feelings of enjoyment, self-confidence, and mood and decrease physical and psychological stress, anxiety, and depression (School of Physical and Health Education, 2004).
Develop a progressive plan of exercise with the client, such as 3 to 5 km of brisk walking and quadriceps, biceps, and gluteal muscle isometric exercises three to four times per week.	Cross-training (a combination of exercise activities) provides variety to combat boredom and increases potential for total body conditioning (Huddleston, 2006).
Instruct client to use an exercise log and to record the day, time, duration, and responses (pulse, feelings, shortness of breath, daily weight).	Keeping a log may increase adherence to exercise prescription.

➤ BOX 36-10 NURSING CARE PLAN *continued*

Interventions *continued*

Exercise Promotion	***Rationales***
Schedule weekly meetings with the client for follow-up and review of exercise log, progress, and barriers.	Clients are more likely to increase physical activity and remain compliant with an exercise program if they are counselled by a health care professional (Gillespie, 2006).

†Intervention classification labels from Dochterman, J. M., Butcher, H. K., & Bulechek, G. M. (Eds.). (2008). *Nursing Interventions Classification (NIC)* (5th ed.). St. Louis, MO: Mosby.

Evaluation

Nursing Actions	***Client Responses and Findings***	***Achievement of Outcomes***
Review client's exercise log at each visit.	She responds, "I make time to exercise because of this log. I hate missing a day and leaving a blank page; this represents failure. I want to succeed."	Client reports enjoying exercise, as well as observing some personal benefits of exercise.
	Exercise log documents activity four times per week.	The exercise log is facilitating adherence to the exercise prescription.
Record weight, blood pressure, and pulse.	Weight, 95 kg. Resting heart rate between 80 and 85 beats per minute. Blood pressure, 146/86 mm Hg.	Improved cardiovascular effects of exercise: • Heart rate is within normal range. • Blood pressure is lower but not at expected range. Monitor blood pressure as client continues to lose weight.
Ask client if exercise is helping to lower fatigue level.	She responds, "At first, finding time to exercise was hard, but once I started feeling less tired and even less stressed, it was easy to integrate exercise into my daily activities."	Achieved improved activity tolerance with exercise.

➤ BOX 36-11 Procedural Guidelines

Helping Clients Exercise

Encouraging and assisting clients to exercise is an important nursing activity. When a client has specialized rehabilitation needs, as in the case of those who have experienced a stroke or trauma, consult and collaborate with physiotherapists or occupational therapists to develop an exercise plan. Teach family members or unregulated care providers to help prepare the client for exercise (e.g., shoes, clothing, hygiene).

Procedure

1. Assess for any medical limitations (e.g., weight-bearing status, untreated fracture, cardiovascular disease).
2. Teach clients breathing skills to help reduce anxiety and to oxygenate tissues and expand lungs fully.
3. Assess for client's physiological and psychological limitations in terms of learning and implementing an exercise program.
4. Assess for joint limitations and do not force a muscle or a joint during exercise.
5. Encourage each client to move at his or her own pace.
6. Assess for proper posture, body alignment, and good body mechanics during exercise.
7. Monitor vital signs before, during, and after exercise.
8. Assess for pain, shortness of breath, or a change in vital signs. If present, stop exercise.
9. Ensure that the client wears rubber-soled shoes and comfortable clothing.
10. Assess prehospitalization mobility status.
11. Document client's progress and provide feedback as the client exercises.

Other clients may benefit from a prescribed exercise and physical fitness program carefully designed to meet their needs and expectations. A comprehensive exercise prescription incorporates a combination of aerobic exercise, stretching and flexibility exercises, and resistance training. Aerobic exercise includes such activities as walking, running, bicycling, aerobic dance, jumping rope, and cross-country skiing. Recommended frequency of aerobic exercise is three

➤ BOX 36-12 Recommendations for Exercise

Adults should accumulate 30 minutes or more a day of moderate-intensity (brisk) physical activity on most (or all) days of the week for a weekly total of 3 to 4 hours.

The activity does not need to be continuous; benefits can be realized with short bouts of activity (minimum of 10 minutes each) over the course of the day.

This amount of activity will expend about 150 to 200 calories per day (the equivalent of walking 3 km briskly), or 1000 to 1400 calories per week.

All types of physical activity can be applied to the daily total (e.g., raking leaves, dancing, gardening).

Lower-intensity activities should be carried out more often, for longer periods of time, or both. More vigorous activities should be performed for shorter periods of time or less frequently.

Data from Konradi, D. B., & Anglin, L. T. (2001). Moderate-intensity exercise: For our patients, for ourselves. *Orthopedic Nursing, 20*(1), 47–54; Health Canada. (2003). *Physical activity guide for older adults* [Electronic version]. Ottawa, ON: Author; and Huddleston, J. S. (2006). Exercise. In C. L. Edelman & C. L. Mandle (Eds.). *Health promotion throughout the lifespan* (6th ed.) St. Louis, MO: Mosby.

BOX 36-13 EVIDENCE-INFORMED PRACTICE GUIDELINE

Promoting Safe Handling of Clients and Prevention of Injury to Nurses and Their Clients

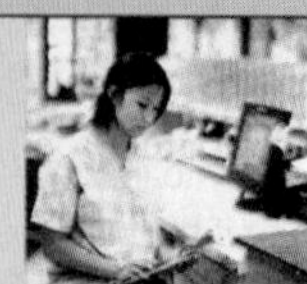

- Know your health care facility's safety information and training concerning the transfer, positioning, and lifting of clients.
- Use recommended back safety guidelines to prevent musculoskeletal injuries.
- Use current research, standards, and guidelines regarding safe positioning and transfer of clients.
- Use "lift teams" and client-handling equipment, such as mechanical lifts and transfer, to prevent injury to yourself and the client.

Data from WorkPlaceBC. (2006). *High risk manual handling of patients in healthcare.* Retrieved April 30, 2008, from http://www.worksafebc.com/publications/health_and_safety/by_topic/assets/pdf/handling_patients_bk97.pdf; and Nelson, A., Owen, B., Lloyd, J. D., Fragala, G., Matz, M. W., Amato, M., et al. (2003). Safe patient handling and movement. *American Journal of Nursing, 103*(3), 32–44.

to five times per week, or every other day. For a client who prefers to exercise every day, recommend cross-training. For example, the client may run one day and do yoga on the next day.

Stretching and flexibility exercises include active ROM exercises that allow for stretching of all muscle groups and joints. This form of exercise is ideal for warm-up and cool-down periods. Benefits include increased flexibility, improved circulation and posture, and an opportunity for relaxation.

Resistance training increases muscle strength and endurance and is associated with improved performance of daily activities and avoidance of injuries and disability. Formal resistance training includes weight training, but the same benefits can be obtained by performing ADLs such as pushing a vacuum cleaner, raking leaves, shovelling snow, and kneading bread. Some clients may use weight training to bulk up their muscles. However, the purpose of weight training from a health perspective is to develop tone and strength and to stimulate and maintain healthy bones (Katula et al., 2006).

Body Mechanics

The Canadian Centre for Occupational Health and Safety (2004) has published numerous guidelines related to ergonomic standards for preventing musculoskeletal injuries in the workplace. More than half of all back pain in health care settings is associated with manual lifting tasks (Workers Health and Safety Centre, 2003). The most common back injury is strain on the muscle group around the lumbar vertebrae. Injury to this area affects the ability to bend forward, backward, and from side to side. The ability to rotate the hips and lower back is also decreased. Relying on body mechanics alone does not provide sufficient protection from musculoskeletal injuries that can occur when lifting or transferring clients (Waters et al., 2006). Although safe lifting guidelines are in widespread use, all of them acknowledge that no particular weight is absolutely safe to lift (Workers Health and Safety Centre, 2003). Moreover, as has been stated, "The adult human form is an awkward burden to lift or carry. Weighing up to 200 pounds or more, it has no handles, it is not rigid, and is susceptible to severe damage if mishandled or dropped. When lying in a bed, a patient is placed inconveniently for lifting, and the weight and placement of such a load would be tolerated by few industrial workers" (Anonymous, 1965, p. 422).

Manual lifting should be the last resort, and is only used when it does not involve lifting most or all of the client's weight (Nelson & Baptiste, 2004). Before lifting, assess the weight to be lifted and determine the assistance needed and the resources available. Use safe client-handling equipment in conjunction with agency "lift teams" to reduce the risk of injury to the client and to members of the health care team (Table 36–1).

Lifting Techniques. Before lifting, assess the weight of the person being lifted and what assistance, if any, you need. If you need help, assess whether a second person will be adequate or whether mechanical assistance is needed. Once you have determined the amount of assistance required, follow these steps:

1. Tighten your gluteal, abdominal, pelvic, and leg muscles. Providing this balance and stability protects your back.
2. Bend at your knees. This helps to maintain your centre of gravity and allows the strong muscles of your legs to do the lifting (Figure 36–8).
3. Keep the person's weight as close to your body as possible. This places the weight in the same plane as yours, close to your centre of gravity, and helps with balance.
4. Keep your trunk erect and knees bent, so that multiple muscle groups work together in a synchronized manner (Occupational Health & Safety Agency for Healthcare in British Columbia, 2003).
5. Avoid twisting. Twisting can overload your spine and lead to serious injury.

Acute Care

Encourage hospitalized clients to do stretching and isometric exercises, active ROM exercises, and low-intensity walking, depending on their conditions. The longer the period of inactivity, or **immobility**, the greater the physiological changes are (see Chapter 46). For those clients who are unable to perform physical activity themselves, you are responsible for maintaining musculoskeletal function by implementing passive ROM exercises.

Musculoskeletal System. Encouraging the use of stretching and isometric-type exercises will help the client maintain the musculoskeletal system during acute care. Review the client's chart and collaborate with the physician to alert you to any possible contraindications before initiating isometric exercises. An isometric exercise program is designed for the specific needs of a client. For example, to prepare the client for walking with crutches, you may implement an exercise program that includes isometric exercises targetting the biceps and triceps. Tell the client to stop the activity if pain, fatigue, or discomfort is experienced, and reinforce this as necessary.

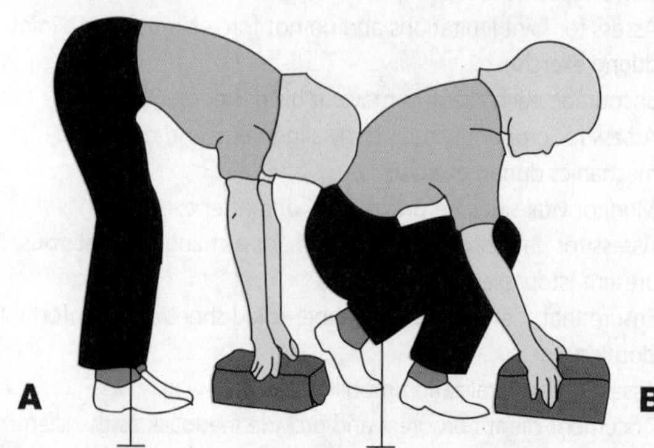

Figure 36-8 Incorrect (A) and correct (B) body positions for lifting.

TABLE 36-1 Preventing Lift Injuries in Health Care Workers

Action	Rationale
When planning to move a client, arrange for adequate help. If your institution has a lift team, use it as a resource.	A lift team is properly trained in techniques to prevent musculoskeletal injuries.
Use client-handling equipment and devices, such as height-adjustable beds, ceiling-mounted lifts, friction-reducing slide sheets, and air-assisted devices (Nelson & Baptiste, 2004).	These devices help to reduce the caregiver's muscular strain during client handling.
Encourage client to assist as much as possible.	This promotes client's independence and strength but minimizes workload.
Keep back, neck, pelvis, and feet aligned. Avoid twisting.	Reduces risk of injury to lumbar vertebrae and muscle groups. Twisting increases risk of injury.
Flex knees; keep feet wide apart.	A broad base of support increases stability.
Position yourself close to client (or object being lifted).	Reduces horizontal reach and stress on caregiver's back.
Use arms and legs (not back).	The leg muscles are stronger, larger muscles capable of greater work without injury.
Slide client toward yourself, using a pull sheet or slide board. When transferring a client onto a stretcher or bed, a slide board is more appropriate.	Sliding requires less effort than lifting. A pull sheet minimizes shearing forces, which can damage client's skin.
The person with the heaviest load coordinates efforts of the team involved by counting to 3.	Simultaneous lifting minimizes the load for any one lifter.
Perform manual lifting as a last resort and only if it does not involve lifting most or all of a client's weight (Nelson & Baptiste, 2004).	Lifting is a high-risk activity that causes significant biochemical and postural stressors.

From Markusic, J. (2003). Maintain a healthy spine using good body mechanics. *Spine Universe*. Retrieved August, 2008, from http://spineuniverse.com.

Generally, in an isometric exercise the muscle group is tightened (contracted) for 10 seconds and then completely relaxed for several seconds. Repetitions are gradually increased for each muscle group until the isometric exercise can be repeated 8 to 10 times. Instruct clients to perform the exercises slowly and to increase repetitions as their physical condition improves. Muscle groups used for walking (quadriceps and gluteal) should be exercised isometrically four times per day until the client is ambulatory (Hoeman, 2008).

Joint Mobility. The easiest intervention to maintain or improve joint mobility for clients, and one that can be coordinated with other activities, is the use of ROM exercises (see Chapter 46). In *active* ROM exercises, the client is able to move his or her joints independently. For clients who are unable to perform these exercises themselves, move each joint for *passive* ROM exercises. The use of ROM exercises enables you to systematically assess and improve the client's joint mobility.

Joints that are not moved periodically can develop contractures, a permanent shortening of a muscle followed by the eventual shortening of associated ligaments and tendons. Over time, the joint may become fixed in one position and the client will lose normal use of that joint. For the client who does not have voluntary motor control, passive ROM exercises are the exercises of choice.

Older adults often experience a decline in physical activity in association with musculoskeletal changes that may predispose them to problems with mobility. Recommend approaches to help older adults use proper body mechanics and prevent injury (Box 36–14).

Mechanical devices such as the continuous passive movement (CPM) machine are available to place specific joints in continuous passive ROM. The machine can be set to various degrees of joint mobility, with increased joint mobility or flexion as the goal. Clients who most commonly use the CPM machine are those who have undergone some form of joint replacement surgery (e.g., knee replacement).

Unless contraindicated, the nursing care plan should include exercising each joint through as nearly a full ROM as possible. Initiate passive ROM exercises as soon as the client loses the ability to move an extremity or joint. Chapter 46 details ROM exercises for each area and illustrates the motion of each joint.

Walking. Joint mobility is also increased by walking. Distances walked should be measured in metres instead of charting simply "ambulated to nurses' station and back." In good walking posture, the head is erect; the cervical, thoracic, and lumbar vertebrae are aligned; the hips and knees have appropriate flexion; and the arms swing freely in alternation with the legs. Illness or trauma can reduce activity tolerance, resulting in the need for assistance with walking or for the use of mechanical devices such as crutches, canes, or walkers. These aids are discussed in more detail in Chapter 46.

Helping a Client to Walk. Helping a client to walk requires preparation. Assess the client's activity tolerance, strength, coordination, and balance to determine the type of assistance needed. Also assess the client's orientation, motivation, and level of cooperation, and determine the presence of any signs of distress that might preclude attempts at ambulation.

BOX 36-14 FOCUS ON OLDER ADULTS

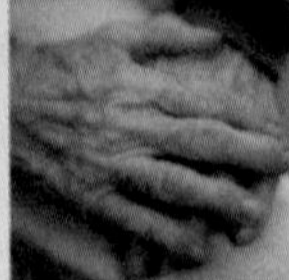

- Encourage the older client to avoid prolonged sitting and to get up and stretch. Frequent stretching diminishes the potential for joint contractures.
- Be sure that the older client maintains proper body alignment when sitting to minimize joint and muscle stress.
- Teach clients how to use stronger joints or larger muscle groups. Efficient distribution of the workload decreases joint stress and pain.
- Provide resources for planned exercise programs, such as Health Canada's (2003b) *Physical Activity Guide for Older Adults*. Weight-bearing and resistance exercise slow further bone loss and prevent fractures in older adults with osteoporosis (Monohan et al., 2007; Walker, 2008).
- Assure clients that gardening is an effective, as well as enjoyable, form of exercise. Promote plant therapy with clients who reside in assisted living settings.
- Recommend Tai Chi, a traditional Chinese conditioning exercise that increases balance and strength. This form of exercise has resulted in reduced fear of falling and an increased sense of well-being in older adults (Adler & Roberts, 2006).
- Advise clients that is never too late to begin an exercise program (Health Canada, 2003b; Huddleston, 2006). However, remind clients to consult a health care professional before beginning an exercise program, particularly if a client has heart or lung disease or other chronic illnesses.
- Exercise is extremely beneficial to older adults, but adjustments in an exercise program may need to be made for those in advanced age to prevent injuries.
- When developing an exercise program for older adults, consider not only their current activity level, range of motion, muscle strength and tone, and response to physical activity, but also their interests, capacities, and limitations.
- Older adults who are unable to participate in a formal exercise program can achieve the benefits of improved joint mobility and enhanced circulation simply by stretching and exaggerating movements during the performance of ADLs.

Evaluate the environment for safety before ambulation; this includes removing obstacles, ensuring that the floor is clean and dry, and identifying rest points in case the client's activity tolerance is less than expected or the client becomes dizzy. The client should also wear supportive, nonskid shoes.

Assist the client to a position of sitting at the side of the bed; let the client "dangle" for one to two minutes before standing. Some clients experience orthostatic hypotension, a drop in blood pressure that occurs when one's position changes from horizontal to vertical (Monohan et al., 2007) (see Chapter 31). Those at higher risk for orthostatic hypotension include immobilized clients, those undergoing prolonged rest, the older adult client, and clients with chronic illnesses such as diabetes mellitis and cardiovascular disease (Dingle, 2003). To dangle a client, advise the client to keep his or her head up, to take a deep breath or two, and to rotate the ankles a few times while sitting.

Several methods are used to assist a client with ambulation. Provide support at the waist using a gait belt, so that the client's centre of gravity remains at the midline. Do not hold the client's waist or rib cage, or the top of the client's trousers. A **gait belt** is a belt that is placed around the lower rib cage to provide stability; it has handles that you can hold while the client ambulates. The same belt may be called a **transfer belt** when it is used for lifts and transfers. The proper way to apply the belt is to keep two fingers between it and the patient's body. Tighten the belt until it has just enough room for your fingers. If the belt is too loose, it might slip upward and injure the client's chest (particularly in women) or increase your risk of dropping the client once weight is put on the belt.

If the client has a syncopal (fainting) episode or begins to fall, assume a wide base of support with one foot in front of the other, providing enough support of the client's body weight to prevent injury (Figure 36–9A). Protecting the client's head is the primary goal, but take care to avoid being injured yourself. To extend your front leg, move your back foot further away, and slide the client against your forward leg to ease him or her to the floor (see Figure 36–9B and 36–9C). Practise this technique with a friend or classmate before attempting it in a clinical setting. When the client attempts to ambulate again, proceed more slowly, monitoring for complaints of dizziness; also monitor the client's blood pressure before, during, and after ambulation. Do not attempt to lift a client manually from the floor, alone or with assistance. The best option is to allow the client to get up without help, if possible, or to use mechanical lifting equipment.

Restorative and Continuing Care

Restorative and continuing care involves implementing activity and exercise strategies to assist the client in ADLs after acute care is no longer needed. Restorative and continuing care also includes activities and exercises that restore and promote optimal functioning in clients with specific chronic illnesses, such as coronary heart disease (CHD), hypertension, chronic obstructive pulmonary disease (COPD), and diabetes mellitis.

Assistive Devices for Walking. In collaboration with other health care professionals such as physiotherapists, you can promote activity and exercise by teaching the proper use of canes, walkers, or crutches, depending on the assistive device most appropriate for the client's condition (see Chapter 46).

Restoration of Activity in Clients with Chronic Illness. Health Canada's (2003c) Physical Activity Unit addresses the role of physical activity in disease prevention and in the treatment of chronic disabling conditions. With this role in mind, care plans are designed to increase activity and exercise in clients with specific disease conditions and chronic illnesses (Box 36–15) such as CHD, hypertension, COPD, and diabetes mellitus.

Coronary Heart Disease (CHD). Activity and exercise have been shown to play a role in secondary prevention or recurrence of CHD. Cardiac rehabilitation is an integral part of comprehensive care of clients who have been diagnosed with CHD. Nurses are involved in many aspects of cardiac rehabilitation and assist clients in developing exercise programs that fit their needs and levels of functioning. Increased physical activity appears to benefit individuals with myocardial infarction, angina pectoris, or congestive heart failure, as well as those who have had a coronary artery bypass graft or percutaneous transluminal coronary angioplasty. Clients with CHD benefit from exercise and activity in terms of reduced mortality and morbidity, improved quality of life, increased psychological well-being, improved left ventricular function, increased functional capacity, and decreased blood lipids (Conroy et al., 2005; Villareal et al., 2006).

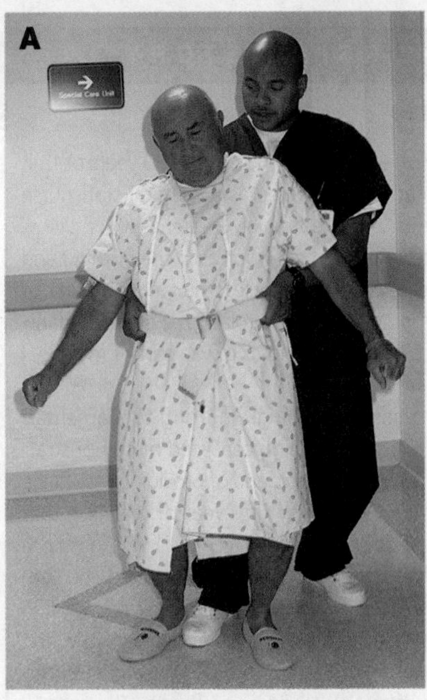

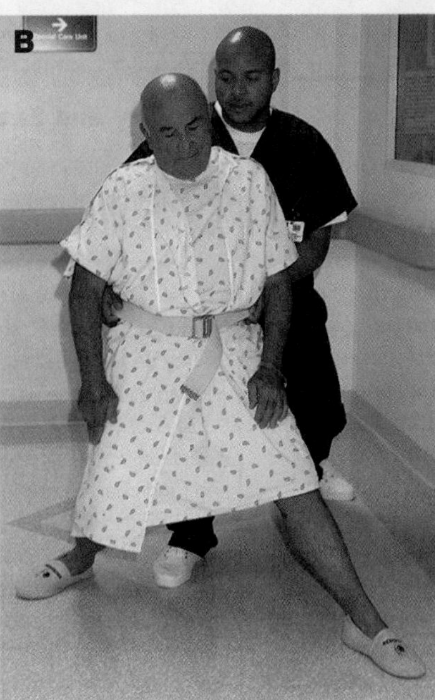

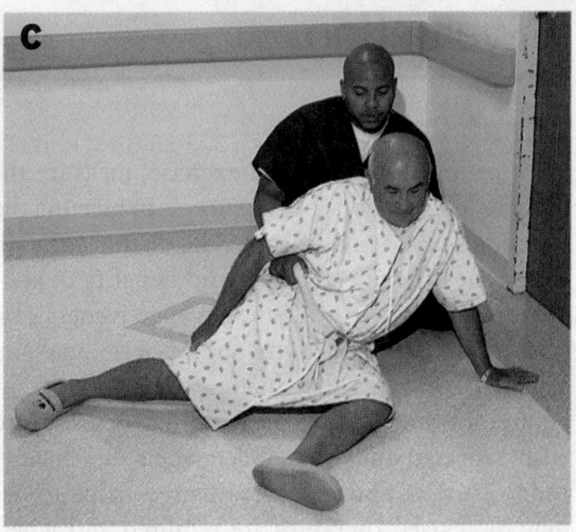

Figure 36-9 A, Stand with feet apart to provide a broad base of support. B, Extend one leg and let client slide against it to the floor. C, Bend knees to lower body as client slides to the floor.

Hypertension. Exercise is instrumental in the reduction of systolic and diastolic blood pressure readings. Low- to moderate-intensity aerobic exercise (e.g., brisk walking, bicycling) appears to be the most effective exercise in terms of lowering blood pressure, whereas weight training and high-intensity aerobics seem to have minimal benefits (Gillespie, 2006; Huddleston, 2006).

Chronic Obstructive Pulmonary Disease (COPD). Pulmonary rehabilitation is a beneficial therapeutic tool to help clients with COPD reach an optimal level of functioning. Some clients are fearful of participating in exercise because of the potential of worsening dyspnea (difficulty breathing). This aversion to physical activity sets up a progressive deconditioning in which minimal physical exertion results in dyspnea. A program of graded exercise for peripheral muscle conditioning improves exercise tolerance (Beers, 2000). Many people with COPD enjoy walking, water aerobics, and riding a stationary bike. Specific breathing techniques can reduce the work of breathing and can be applied in times of anxiety or stress when inefficient breathing patterns appear.

Diabetes Mellitus. Along with diet, glucose monitoring, and medication, exercise is an important component in the care of clients with diabetes mellitus. Individuals with type 1 diabetes are encouraged to exercise because exercise leads to improved cardiovascular fitness and psychological well-being. You can instruct the client with type 1 diabetes about certain risks and precautions regarding exercise. Instruction should include the need for a pre-exercise physical examination and precautions to monitor blood glucose immediately before and after exercise. You also can instruct clients to perform low- to moderate-intensity exercises, to carry a concentrated form of carbohydrates (e.g., sugar packets, hard candy), and to wear a medical alert bracelet. The client with type 2 diabetes who decides to participate in a regular program of exercise should incorporate low-intensity warm-up and cool-down periods; should include aerobic exercise at 50% to 75% of maximal oxygen uptake; and should exercise for 20 to 45 minutes, 3 days per week (Canadian Diabetes Association, 2003).

BOX 36-15 RESEARCH HIGHLIGHT

Energy Requirements of Tai Chi

Research Focus

Developing alternative exercise strategies for clients with very low functional capacities is a challenge because of the increased risk for complications and injuries. Tai Chi C'hih, a modified version of Tai Chi, may be an approach to health promotion in older adults and in clients with chronic illnesses.

Research Abstract

The purpose of the study conducted by Li, et al. (2004) was to determine the energy cost of Tai Chi C'hih, which is a form of exercise consisting of a series of slow, balanced movements and breathing. The objective of this study was to measure the energy costs and cardiovascular effects of Tai Chi C'hi to assist in the planning of a safe exercise regime for clients with very low energy reserves. Twenty-six adults participated in the completion of surveys to estimate functional capacity and exercise participation, in a select series of nine Tai Chi C'hih movements, and in oxygen consumption testing during the exercise program. The results of the study indicated that the energy requirements for this alternative form of exercise were comparable with low-level exercises suitable for people with low exercise tolerance.

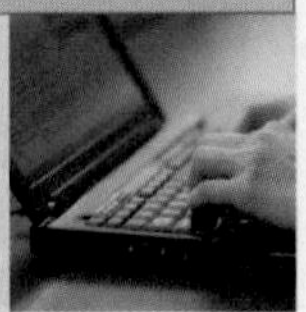

Evidence-Informed Practice

- Before initiating exercise, clients should consult a health care professional.
- Encouraging clients with chronic illnesses to exercise has the potential to maintain and improve activity tolerance.
- Tai Chi C'hih promotes feelings of relaxation and increased energy, thus making it an ideal alternative form of exercise for clients with chronic illnesses.

References: Li, F., Harmer, P., Fisher, K. J., & McAuley, E. (2004). Tai Chi: Improving functional balance and predicting subsequent falls in older persons. *Medicine and Science in Sports and Exercise, 36*(12), 2046–2052.

❖Evaluation

Client Care

With regard to activity and exercise, measure the effectiveness of nursing interventions by the success in meeting the client's expected outcomes and goals of care. The client is the only one who will experience the effectiveness and benefits of activity and exercise (Figure 36–10). To evaluate the effectiveness of nursing interventions in enhancing activity and exercise, make comparisons with baseline measures that include pulse, blood pressure, strength, endurance, and psychological well-being. Compare actual outcomes with expected outcomes to determine the client's health status and progression. Continuous evaluation helps to determine whether new or revised therapies are required and whether new nursing diagnoses have developed.

Client Expectations

To evaluate the client's perception of nursing care related to activity and exercise, you must first have assessed the client's perspective on what is most important and the client's expectations of the health care team. Working closely with the client will enable you to identify goals and strategies that can be met realistically within the limits of the client's priorities, capabilities, and health treatment (Box 36–16). Because the outcome you consider to be acceptable or anticipated may be different from that of the client and family members, it is important to ask clients if their expectations of care have been met.

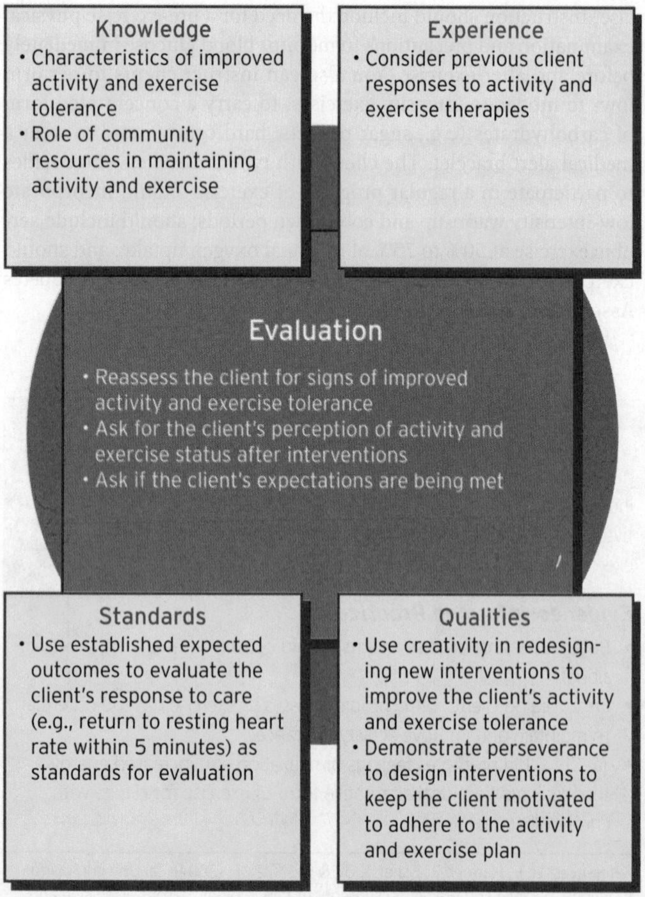

Knowledge
- Characteristics of improved activity and exercise tolerance
- Role of community resources in maintaining activity and exercise

Experience
- Consider previous client responses to activity and exercise therapies

Evaluation
- Reassess the client for signs of improved activity and exercise tolerance
- Ask for the client's perception of activity and exercise status after interventions
- Ask if the client's expectations are being met

Standards
- Use established expected outcomes to evaluate the client's response to care (e.g., return to resting heart rate within 5 minutes) as standards for evaluation

Qualities
- Use creativity in redesigning new interventions to improve the client's activity and exercise tolerance
- Demonstrate perseverance to design interventions to keep the client motivated to adhere to the activity and exercise plan

Figure 36-10 Critical thinking model for activity and exercise evaluation.

BOX 36-16 NURSING STORY

Activity and Exercise

I have been in nursing for over 40 years. For more than 30 years of that time, before moving into teaching, I worked as a hospital staff nurse providing direct care to clients. I worked mainly in areas where clients were unable to assist themselves very much, such as in the birthing and critical care units. As is the case with most nurses, the wear and tear of lifting, turning, and transferring clients took a toll on my body, primarily on my back, knees, and feet. But for as long as it was part of my role, I was able to do the work.

Several years later, after I began teaching a nursing fundamentals course, my physical activity related to nursing consisted of demonstrating fundamental skills in the labratory setting and of providing assistance to students with their practice. During my fifth year of teaching that course, I was taken by surprise at how difficult I found it to lift, position, or transfer my volunteer "clients," and at how extremely tired and sore I was at the end of each day. What was happening to me?

Upon reflection, I realized that two factors were involved. The first was a normal change resulting from aging: the decrease in strength and endurance that occurs after age 40 among women. The second factor was the relatively sedentary lifestyle I had led since I had left bedside nursing. Mine was a classic case of functional decline from disuse, a major concern as aging occurs. As I thought further about it, I remembered that I had noticed groceries becoming heavier and stair climbing feeling more difficult. At the rate I was changing, I had little hope of maintaining my independence well into old age. In the shorter term, if I expected to keep teaching for a few more years, I would need to do something about my fitness level quickly!

My strategies? To use my gym membership (neglected for months and never attended routinely) four times per week from June through August and at least three times per week throughout the academic year, and to walk for no less than 30 minutes every day. No more avoiding stairs, either! I decided to walk up one floor and down two or three until that became easier and then increase stair climbing from there.

How will I know whether my plan has been effective? Although I don't expect to be as strong as I once was as a clinical nurse, I will be able to accomplish my teaching activities and my normal daily routines effortlessly, with minimal backaches and energy to spare.

Although it was a shock to recognize that aging had affected my personal and professional life, the ingrained nursing habits of reflection and of establishing goals helped me feel confident that I could manage them.

* KEY CONCEPTS

- Exercise is physical activity for the purpose of conditioning the body, improving health, and maintaining fitness, or it may be used as a therapeutic measure.
- Careful attention to body mechanics and use of appropriate equipment is critical in the prevention of musculoskeletal injuries.
- Activity tolerance is the kind and amount of exercise or work that a person is able to perform.
- Physiological, emotional, and developmental factors influence the client's activity tolerance.
- The best program of physical activity includes a combination of exercises that produce different physiological and psychological benefits.

- Coordinated body movement to move, lift, bend, stand, sit, lie down, and complete daily activities requires integrated functioning of the skeletal system, skeletal muscles, and nervous system.
- Muscles primarily associated with movement are located near the skeletal region, where movement results from leverage, which is characteristic of the upper extremities.
- Coordination and regulation of muscle groups depend on muscle tone and activity of antagonistic, synergistic, and antigravity muscles.
- Balance is assisted by nervous system control in the cerebellum and by inner ear function.
- Body balance is achieved when a wide base of support exists, the centre of gravity is within the base of support, and the centre of gravity is vertically aligned with the base of support.
- Developmental changes, behavioural aspects, environmental issues, cultural and ethnic influences, and family and social support affect the client's perception of and motivation to engage in physical activity and exercise.
- Ability to engage in normal physical activity and exercise depends on intact and functioning nervous and musculoskeletal systems.
- Use the nursing process to provide care for clients who are experiencing or are at risk for activity intolerance and impaired physical mobility.
- After identifying nursing diagnoses, plan and implement interventions to increase activity and exercise, in collaboration with the client when possible.
- Range-of-motion (ROM) exercises incorporated into daily activities can include one or all of the body's joints.

* CRITICAL THINKING EXERCISES

1. Mr. Neel was bedridden for a lengthy period and is now ready to ambulate. What assessment parameters should be considered before this client ambulates? What precautions should you take before ambulating him for the first time?
2. Mrs. Wong has quadriplegia, weighs 72 kg, and requires total care. Her family has decided to care for her at home. As her nurse, you are responsible for instructing the family on several aspects of Mrs. Wong's care. Develop a list of basic principles that describes safe lifting and positioning to protect Mrs. Wong's family members from injury.

* REVIEW QUESTIONS

1. Nurses must know and practise safe lifting, positioning, and transfer techniques in order to
   1. Increase their muscle strength.
   2. Restore optimal client functioning.
   3. Reduce the risk of injury.
   4. Assess the body alignment of clients.
2. Proprioception is
   1. Awareness of the position of the body.
   2. Needed for antigravity.
   3. Located within the semicircular canals.
   4. The individual's perception of movement at a joint.
3. A client with a right-sided cerebral hemorrhage and damage to the right motor strip may have
   1. Left-sided hemiplegia.
   2. Right-sided hemiplegia.
   3. Bilateral hemiplegia.
   4. Degenerative hemiplegia.
4. Older adults are at greater risk for falls and injuries partly because
   1. They may take smaller steps, decreasing their base of support.
   2. Their centre of gravity shifts toward the anterior.
   3. They tend to walk more quickly, with wide strides.
   4. Total bone mass decreases.
5. Clients are more open to developing an exercise program if they
   1. Have been diagnosed with a chronic disease such as diabetes.
   2. Are ordered by a physician to begin an exercise program.
   3. Have had a family member request that they exercise.
   4. Are at the stage of being ready to change their behaviour.
6. Children becoming increasingly less physically active outside of school has resulted in
   1. An increase in juvenile arthritis.
   2. An increase in obesity.
   3. Improved school attendance and grades.
   4. An increase in school-based fitness activities.
7. A client begins to fall during ambulation. To prevent injury to the client, you should
   1. Call for assistance.
   2. Slide the client down your body and forward leg to the floor.
   3. Instruct the client to sit in the nearest chair.
   4. Allow the client to fall to prevent injury to yourself.

* RECOMMENDED WEB SITES

Active Living Alliance for Canadians with a Disability: http://www.ala.ca/content/home.asp
This organization is an alliance of individuals, agencies, and national associations that together promote, support, and enable Canadians with disabilities, across all settings and environments, to lead active and healthy lives.

Canadian Centre for Activity and Aging: http://www.uwo.ca/actage/
The Centre is a research and community resource institution whose mandate is to investigate the interrelationship of physical activity and aging and to develop strategies, based on research, to promote the independence of older adults.

Canadian Fitness and Lifestyle Research Institute: http://www.cflri.ca/
The Institute addresses the well-being of Canadians through research on and communication of information about physically active lifestyles to the public and private sectors.

Fitness Vancouver: http://www.fitnessvancouver.ca/
This Web site's Exercise Library contains an abundance of clearly described and well-illustrated exercises that any nurse could use to establish a fitness program.

Health Promotion Online: http://www.hc-sc.gc.ca/ahc-asc/activit/marketsoc/index-eng.php
This Web site, maintained by Health Canada, contains many useful health promotion resources and guides that will aid health care professionals and community leaders in encouraging Canadians to take a more active role in their health.

Public Health Agency of Canada: http://www.phac-aspc.gc.ca/chn-rcs/index.html
The role of this new federal agency is to protect the health and safety of Canadians, focusing on preventing chronic diseases, preventing injuries, and responding to public health emergencies such as outbreaks of infectious diseases.

37

Client Safety

Original chapter by Eileen Costantinou, RN, BC, MSN

Canadian content written by Daria Romaniuk, RN, MN, PhD(c)

objectives

Mastery of content in this chapter will enable you to:

- Define the key terms listed.
- Describe how the unmet basic physiological needs of oxygen, nutrition, temperature, and humidity can threaten clients' safety.
- Discuss the specific risks to safety related to each developmental stage.
- Discuss the least-restraint approach.
- Describe the four categories of risks in a health care agency.
- Describe assessment activities designed to identify clients' physical, psychosocial, and cognitive statuses as they pertain to clients' safety status.
- Identify nursing diagnoses associated with risks to safety.
- Develop care plans for clients whose safety is threatened.
- Describe nursing interventions specific to clients' age for reducing the risk of falls, fires, poisonings, and electrical hazards.
- Describe methods to evaluate interventions designed to maintain or promote safety.

key terms

Air pollution, p. 798
Ambularm, p. 817
Bed-Check, p. 817
Carbon monoxide, p. 797
Chemical restraint, p. 823
Environment, p. 797
Environmental restraints, p. 823
Food poisoning, p. 797
Hypothermia, p. 797
Immunization, p. 798
Land pollution, p. 798
Material Safety Data Sheets (MSDSs), p. 800
Noise pollution, p. 798
Pathogen, p. 798
Physical restraint, p. 817
Poison, p. 798
Pollutant, p. 798
Relative humidity, p. 797
Restraint, p. 816
Seizure, p. 800
Seizure precautions, p. 824
Water pollution, p. 798
Workplace Hazardous Materials Information System (WHMIS), p. 800

media resources

evolve Web Site

- Audio Chapter Summaries
- Glossary
- Multiple-Choice Review Questions
- Student Learning Activities
- Video Clips
- Weblinks

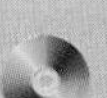

Companion CD

- Glossary
- Interactive Learning Activities
- Fluids and Electrolytes Tutorial
- Test-Taking Skills

Safety, often defined as freedom from psychological and physical injuries, is a basic human need that must be met. Health care provided in a safe manner and in a safe community environment are essential for a client's survival and well-being. While incorporating critical thinking skills when following the nursing process, you are also responsible for assessing the client and the environment for safety hazards as well as for planning and intervening appropriately to maintain a safe environment. By paying attention to client safety, you are not only functioning as a provider of safe care but also as an active participant in health promotion.

Scientific Knowledge Base

Environmental Safety

A client's **environment** includes the physical and psychosocial factors that influence or affect the life and survival of that client. This broad definition of environment crosses the continuum of care for settings in which you and clients interact (e.g., the home, community centre, school, clinic, hospital, and long-term care facility). Safety in health care settings reduces the incidence of illness and injury, shortens the length of treatment or hospitalization, improves or maintains a client's functional status, and increases the client's sense of well-being. A safe environment affords protection to the staff as well, allowing them to function at an optimal level. A safe environment is one in which basic needs are met, physical hazards are reduced, the transmission of pathogens is reduced, sanitation is maintained, and pollution is controlled. In addition, in a safe environment, a plan is in place to respond to a possible terrorist attack.

Basic Needs. Physiological needs, which include sufficient oxygen and nutrition and the optimal temperature and humidity, influence a person's safety.

Oxygen. Be aware of factors in a client's environment that decrease the amount of available oxygen. A common environmental hazard in the home is an improperly functioning heating system. A furnace that is not properly vented or a car left running inside a closed garage may introduce carbon monoxide into the environment. **Carbon monoxide** is a colourless, odourless, poisonous gas produced by the combustion of carbon or organic fuels. It binds strongly with hemoglobin, preventing the formation of oxyhemoglobin and thus reducing the supply of oxygen delivered to tissues (see Chapter 39). Exposure can cause nausea, headache, drowsiness, confusion, loss of consciousness, and death (Technical Standards and Safety Authority, 2004). Carbon monoxide detectors can be purchased for home use.

Nutrition. Meeting nutritional needs adequately and safely requires environmental controls and knowledge. In the home, the client needs a refrigerator with a freezer compartment to keep perishable foods fresh. An adequate clean water supply is needed for drinking and to wash dishes and fresh produce. Provisions for garbage collection are necessary to maintain sanitary conditions.

Foods that are inadequately prepared or stored, or are subject to unsanitary conditions, increase a client's risk for infections and food poisoning. Bacterial food infections result from eating food contaminated by bacteria such as *Escherichia coli* and *Salmonella, Shigella,* or *Listeria* organisms. **Food poisoning** is caused by the ingestion of bacterial toxins produced in food; staphylococcal and clostridial bacteria are the most common causes. Although most foodborne diseases are bacterial, the hepatitis A virus is spread by fecal contamination of food, water, or milk (Nix, 2005).

In illnesses caused by bacterial contamination, the onset of symptoms may be very rapid or take a week or even longer. For hepatitis A, the average incubation period is 28 to 30 days (Health Canada, 2004). Preventive measures include thorough handwashing before handling food, adequate cooking, and the proper storage and refrigeration of perishable foods.

For consumer protection, commercially processed and packaged foods are subject to the provisions of the *Food and Drug Act,* which regulates the manufacture, processing, and distribution of foods, drugs, and cosmetics. The act protects consumers from the sale of impure or dangerous substances. Ensuring safe food supplies for Canadians is a joint effort between Health Canada, the Canadian Food Inspection Agency, and provincial, territorial, and municipal organizations.

Temperature and Humidity. The comfort zone for environmental temperature varies among individuals, but the usual comfort range is between 18.3°C and 23.9°C. Temperature extremes that frequently occur during the winter and summer affect not only comfort and productivity but also safety.

Exposure to severe cold for prolonged periods may cause frostbite and hypothermia. Frostbite occurs when a surface area of the skin freezes as a result of exposure to extremely cold temperatures. **Hypothermia** occurs when the core body temperature is 35°C or below (see Chapter 31). Older adults; the young; clients with cardiovascular conditions; clients who have ingested drugs, alcohol, or other substances in excess; and the homeless are at high risk for hypothermia.

Exposure to extreme heat can raise the core body temperature, resulting in heatstroke or heat exhaustion. Chronically ill clients, older adults, and infants are at greatest risk for injury from extreme heat. These clients should avoid extremely hot, humid environments.

The relative humidity of the air in the environment may affect a client's health and safety. **Relative humidity** is the amount of water vapour in the air compared with the maximum amount of water vapour that the air could contain at that temperature. The comfort zone varies from person to person, but most persons are comfortable when the humidity is between 60% and 70%. Increasing the environmental humidity can have therapeutic benefits for clients with upper respiratory tract infections because humidity helps to liquefy pulmonary secretions and improve breathing. It is important to follow the manufacturer's directions regarding the cleaning and maintenance of home humidifiers to prevent water contamination.

Physical Hazards. Physical hazards in the environment place clients at risk for accidental injury and death. In Canada, accidental injuries are the leading cause of death for persons between the ages of 1 and 34 years (Public Health Agency of Canada, 2004). Accidental injuries are also a major cause of disability. Other causes of injury and death include poisoning, suffocation, drowning, fires, burns, and machinery accidents. Among adults aged 65 and over, falls are the most common cause of hospital admissions for trauma (Canadian Institute for Health Information [CIHI], 2006). Many physical hazards, especially those contributing to falls, can be minimized through adequate lighting, the reduction of obstacles, and the implementation of security measures.

Lighting. Adequate lighting reduces physical hazards by illuminating the areas in which a person moves and works. Outside the home, all walkways should have adequate lighting. Outdoor lighting also helps protect the home and its inhabitants from crime. Well-lit garages, walkways, and doorways discourage intruders from entering or lurking on the premises.

Inside the house, halls, staircases, and individual rooms should be adequately lit so that residents can safely carry out activities of daily living. Night lights in dark halls, bathrooms, and the rooms of children and older adults help maintain safety by reducing the risk of falls. A night light in a guest room can help orient an overnight guest who needs to get up in the middle of the night. Artificial lighting should be soft and nonglaring because glare is a major problem for older adults (Ebersole et al., 2004).

Obstacles. Injuries in the home frequently result from tripping over or coming into contact with common household objects, including doormats, small rugs on the stairs and floor, wet spots on the floor, and clutter on bedside tables, closet shelves, and bookshelves. The risk of falls from obstacles is present for all age groups; however, it is greatest for older adults. Falls are usually the result of a combination of intrinsic risk factors (e.g., illness, drug therapy, or alcohol use) and extrinsic or environmental factors. In some cases, an obstacle or extrinsic factor may be the only cause of a fall. Intrinsic factors may be difficult to modify or eliminate, but extrinsic factors are usually easily removed.

Fire. More than 50,000 residential fires occur each year in Canada (Canada Safety Council, 2006). Most fire deaths occur in the home and are due to smoke inhalation. The most common causes of fire are careless smoking and cooking accidents.

Poisoning. A **poison** is any substance that impairs health or destroys life when ingested, inhaled, or otherwise absorbed by the body. Individuals can be at risk for poisoning from substances including cleaning agents, medications, and plants. Specific antidotes or treatments are available for only some types of poisons. The capacity of body tissue to recover from the poison determines the reversibility of the effect. Poisons can impair the respiratory, circulatory, central nervous, hepatic, gastrointestinal (GI), and renal systems of the body.

Lead poisoning is an important safety concern. Individuals may be exposed to lead from various sources. Although Canadian regulations have restricted the lead content of paint since 1976, older homes may still have high lead levels because of old paint. Lead may also be found in contaminated water systems and in household articles such as vinyl blinds and candles. Exposure to lead may occur through oral ingestion, inhalation, or the skin. Fetuses, infants, and children are more vulnerable to lead poisoning than adults because lead is more easily absorbed into their growing bodies. As well, small children are more sensitive to the damaging effects of lead. Exposure to excessive levels of lead can lead to vomiting, headaches, anemia, weight loss, poor attention span, slowed speech development, and learning difficulties (Health Canada, 2008a).

Security. An insecure home places a client at risk for injury or burglary. Inadequate locks on doors and windows make the home susceptible to intruders. A lack of attention to personal safety can place the client at risk for injury away from home as well, for example, when walking or driving after dark.

Transmission of Pathogens. A **pathogen** is a microorganism capable of producing an illness. Medical asepsis reduces the transfer of organisms (see Chapter 33).One of the most effective methods of limiting pathogen transmission is the aseptic practice of hand hygiene. Clients must be instructed in proper hand-hygiene techniques and encouraged to use them frequently in the home and hospital.

The transmission of disease from person to person can also be reduced, and in some cases prevented, by immunization. **Immunization** is the process by which resistance to an infectious disease is produced or augmented. Active immunity is acquired by injecting a small amount of attenuated (weakened) or dead organisms or modified toxins from the organism (toxoids) into the body. Passive immunity occurs when antibodies produced by other persons or animals are introduced into a person's bloodstream for protection against a pathogen.

Human immunodeficiency virus (HIV)—the pathogen that causes acquired immunodeficiency syndrome (AIDS)—and hepatitis B virus are transmitted through blood and other body fluids. Substance abusers frequently share syringes and needles; this practice increases the risk of acquiring these viruses. Safer sex practices (see Chapter 27), including the correct use of condoms and engaging in monogamous relationships, reduce the risk for both of these diseases and for other sexually transmitted infections. You use standard precautions/routine practices when caring for all clients to prevent the spread of infection and contact with blood and body fluids (see Chapter 33).

At the community level, the transmission of disease is also controlled through the adequate disposal of human waste through the proper construction and repair of sewers and drains. Rodent and insect control (e.g., spraying for mosquitoes) is also necessary to reduce the transmission of disease.

Pollution. A healthy environment is free of pollution. A **pollutant** is a harmful chemical or waste material discharged into the water, soil, or air. Persons commonly think of pollution only in terms of air, land, or water pollution, but excessive noise can also be a form of pollution that presents health risks. **Air pollution** is the contamination of the atmosphere with a harmful chemical. Prolonged exposure to air pollution increases the risk of pulmonary disease. In urban areas, industrial waste and vehicle exhaust are common contributors to air pollution. Cigarette smoke is a common cause of air pollution. **Land pollution** can be caused by the improper disposal of radioactive and bioactive waste products (e.g., dioxin).

Water pollution is the contamination of lakes, rivers, and streams, usually by industrial pollutants. Water-treatment facilities filter harmful contaminants from the water, but these systems can contain flaws. If water becomes contaminated, the public must use bottled or boiled water for drinking and cooking. Flooding frequently causes damage to water-treatment stations, which also necessitates the use of bottled or boiled water. Another hazard is the contamination of water with nitrates, chemicals made up of nitrogen and oxygen. These chemicals occur naturally in soil and may also be added through the use of fertilizers; contamination of well water may occur when nitrates leach out of the soil into the water (Government of Saskatchewan, 2008). Nitrates pose a hazard to our health, particularly for pregnant women and infants, who are more susceptible to methemoglobinemia, an illness that occurs when ingested nitrates are converted to nitrites in the body (Government of Saskatchewan, 2008). The nitrites disrupt the oxygen-carrying capacity of the blood, causing cyanosis, shortness of breath, and fatigue. Routine testing of municipal water supplies for nitrates ensures that levels are maintained within the accepted limit of less than 10 mg/L nitrate–nitrogen. However, you may need to educate individuals with private wells about arranging for annual testing of their water (Government of Saskatchewan, 2008).

Noise pollution occurs when the noise level in an environment becomes uncomfortable to the inhabitants of the environment. Noise levels are measured in units of sound intensity called decibels. Tolerance for noise varies from individual to individual and is influenced by health status. Irreversible hearing loss may result from constant exposure to high sound intensity. Clients working in environments with high noise levels should wear protective devices to reduce hearing loss (Figure 37–1). Adolescents should limit their exposure to intense noise such as that encountered at rock concerts.

A health care facility can also be polluted by noise. The sounds of machines, persons talking, intercoms, and paging systems can create increased noise levels. Even when the noise level is not high enough to affect hearing acuity, it can produce a syndrome called sensory overload, which is a marked increase in the intensity of auditory and visual stimuli. It disrupts processing of information, and the client no longer perceives the environment in a meaningful way (see Chapter 48).

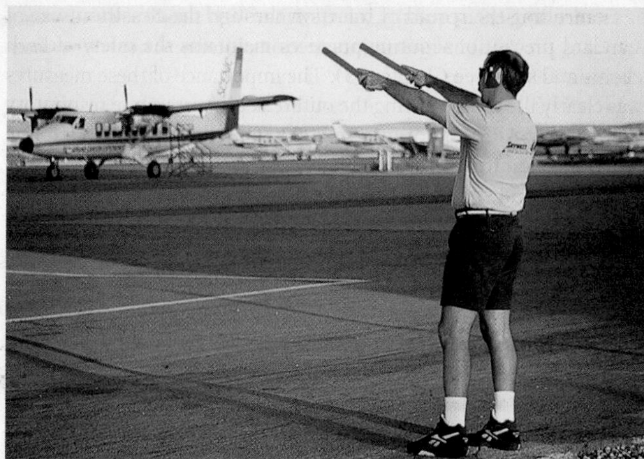

Figure 37-1 Protective device to reduce hearing loss.

Terrorism. A more recent potential environmental health threat is the possibility of a terrorist attack. The terrorist attacks in the United States on September 11, 2001, raised awareness of this threat for Canadians. If a terrorist health threat were to occur in Canada, Health Canada would work with provincial, territorial, and local health officials to address the situation. Health care facilities must have well-rehearsed plans to deal with such an attack (Kollek, 2003). Hospitals comprise one of several components of a community's emergency response plan (Christian et al., 2005). You must be prepared through education and training to respond to an attack by taking the necessary steps to participate in your agency's role in the community's emergency management plan.

Nursing Knowledge Base

In addition to being knowledgeable about the environment, you must be familiar with a client's developmental level; mobility, sensory, and cognitive statuses; and lifestyle choices. You must also be aware of common safety precautions and of the special risks to safety that are found in agency settings.

Risks at Developmental Stages

A client's developmental stage presents specific threats to safety. Clients throughout all developmental stages may be subject to abuse. Child abuse, domestic violence, and abuse of older adults are serious threats to safety. These topics are discussed in Chapters 23 and 32.

Infants and Children. Unintentional injuries are the leading cause of death in Canadian children between the ages of 1 and 14 years; each year 1 of every 230 children is hospitalized for treatment of unintentional injuries (Safe Kids Canada, 2007). The nature of the injuries sustained is related to normal growth and development. Small children are curious and trusting of their environment and do not perceive themselves to be in danger. The incidence of poisoning is highest in late infancy and toddlerhood because of children's increased level of oral activity and growing ability to explore the environment. Toddlers and preschoolers, who are attracted to water but do not perceive its dangers, are at a greater risk for drowning. Childhood injuries are also reflective of adults' perceptions of the causes of accidents and their ability to prevent them. For example, the incorrect use or lack of use of vehicle restraints for children aged 5 to 14 places these children at greater risk of death from injuries sustained in motor vehicle accidents (the leading cause of death from injury in this age group) (Safe Kids Canada, 2007).

Adolescents. As children enter adolescence, they develop greater independence and begin to develop a sense of identity and their own values. Adolescents start to separate emotionally from their families, and peers generally have a stronger influence on them. The struggle toward identity may cause a teenager to experience shyness, fear, and anxiety, with resulting dysfunction at home or school. In an attempt to relieve the tensions associated with physical and psychosocial changes, as well as peer pressures, adolescents may begin to act impulsively and engage in risk-taking behaviours such as smoking and substance use. In addition to the health risks posed by nicotine and other substances (e.g., alcohol, drugs, glue), the ingestion of such substances increases the incidence of accidents such as drowning and motor vehicle accidents.

Adults. Threats to an adult's safety are frequently related to lifestyle habits. For example, a client who consumes excessive alcohol is at greater risk for motor vehicle accidents. A long-term smoker has a greater risk of cardiovascular and pulmonary diseases. Likewise, an adult experiencing a high level of stress is more likely to have an accident or illnesses such as headaches, GI disorders, and infections.

Older Adults. The physiological changes that occur during the aging process increase a client's risk for injury (Box 37–1). Changes in vision, hearing, mobility, reflexes, circulation, and the ability to make quick judgements predispose older adults to falls (see Chapter 25). When a client is hospitalized, confusion, multiple medical problems, medications, immobility, urinary urgency, age-related sensory changes, postural instability, and an unfamiliar environment further contribute to the risk of falls (Meiner & Leuckenotte, 2006). Certain disease states common to older adults, such as arthritis and cerebrovascular accidents, also increase the chances of injury. In 2001 to 2002, 85% of injury hospitalizations for adults 65 years and older were due to falls (CIHI, 2004). Clients most often fall while transferring from beds,

➤ BOX 37-1 Changes Associated With Aging That Increase the Risk of Accidents

Musculoskeletal Changes

Muscle strength and function decrease, joints become less mobile, bones are more brittle due to osteoporosis, postural changes (e.g., kyphosis) are common, and range of motion is limited.

Nervous System Changes

All voluntary or automatic reflexes slow to some extent, the ability to respond to multiple stimuli decreases, and sensitivity to touch is decreased.

Sensory Changes

Peripheral vision and lens accommodation decrease, lenses may develop opacity (cataracts), the stimuli threshold for light touch and pain increases, the transmission of hot and cold impulses is delayed, and hearing is impaired as high-frequency tones become less perceptible.

Genitourinary Changes

Nocturia and occurrences of incontinence increase.

Adapted from Ebersole, P., & Hess, P. (2003). *Toward healthy aging* (6th ed.). St. Louis, MO: Mosby.

chairs, and toilets; while getting into or out of a bathtub; by tripping over carpet edges or doorway thresholds; by slipping on wet surfaces; and while descending stairs. Icy walkways and obstacles in the yard are also common causes of outdoor falls in older adults.

Individual Risk Factors

Other risk factors posing threats to safety include lifestyle, impaired mobility, sensory or communication impairment, and a lack of safety awareness.

Lifestyle. Lifestyle can increase safety risks. Persons who drive or operate machinery while under the influence of chemical substances, who work at inherently dangerous jobs, or who are risk takers are at greater risk of injury. In addition, persons experiencing stress, anxiety, fatigue, or alcohol or drug withdrawal and those taking prescribed medications may be more accident prone. These clients may also be too preoccupied to notice a source of potential accidents, such as cluttered stairs or a road intersection.

Impaired Mobility. Impaired mobility due to muscle weakness, paralysis, or poor coordination or balance is a major factor in client falls. Immobilization predisposes a client to additional physiological and emotional hazards, which can in turn further restrict mobility and independence.

Sensory or Communication Impairment. Clients with visual, hearing, tactile, or communication impairment, such as aphasia or a language barrier, are at greater risk for injury. Such clients may not be able to perceive a potential danger or express their need for assistance (see Chapter 48).

Lack of Safety Awareness. Some clients are unaware of safety precautions, such as keeping medicine or poisons away from children or observing the expiration date on food products. A complete nursing assessment, including a home inspection, helps you identify the client's level of knowledge regarding home safety so that deficiencies can be corrected with an individualized nursing care plan.

Risks in the Health Care Agency

Specific risks, including risks in the workplace and to client safety, exist in health care agencies and must also be addressed.

Workplace Risks. Various forms of chemicals used in health care settings are a source of environmental risk for both the client and the health care worker. Chemicals such as mercury and those found in some medications, anaesthetic gases, cleaning solutions, and disinfectants are potentially toxic if ingested or inhaled. The **Workplace Hazardous Materials Information System (WHMIS)** sets the standards for the control of hazardous substances in workplaces across Canada (Health Canada, 2008b). A hazardous substance is any product or material that could cause physical or medical problems. WHMIS consists of three main elements: worker education programs, cautionary labelling of products, and the provision of **Material Safety Data Sheets (MSDSs)**. Cautionary labels include information needed to safely handle the hazardous substance, including a description of physical and health hazards, safety and first aid measures, and hazard symbols, which depict the types of hazard that the product presents (Figure 37–2). MSDSs are available to provide detailed information about the substance, any health hazards imposed, precautions for safe handling and use, and steps to take if the substance is released or spilled. You must understand WHMIS labelling requirements and be aware of the location of MSDSs where you work.

Controlling the spread of infection through the consistent use of standard precautions/routine practices maintains the safety of both clients and staff (see Chapter 33). The importance of these measures was clearly illustrated during the outbreak of severe acute respiratory syndrome (SARS) in Toronto in 2003. The illness began with one individual admitted to an emergency department and spread to several clients and staff before its infectious nature was recognized and precautions were instituted. Maintaining the safety of staff caring for SARS-infected clients was a significant challenge during the outbreak (Hynes-Gay et al., 2003).

Risks to Client Safety. Specific risks to a client's safety within the health care environment include falls, client-inherent accidents, procedure-related accidents, and equipment-related accidents. You must assess for these four potential problem areas and, considering the developmental level of the client, take steps to prevent or minimize accidents. When an accident occurs, you must file an incident report (also called *adverse occurrence report*). This report is a confidential document that completely describes any client accident occurring on the premises of a health care agency (see Chapter 9). The report documents the accident, the client assessment, and interventions carried out for the client. In addition to completing the incident report, you must objectively document the incident in the client's medical record. Because this is a confidential document, the completion of the incident report should not be mentioned in the medical record because this eliminates the health care agency's protective clause.

Falls. Falls account for up to 90% of all reported incidents in hospitals. In addition to age, a history of previous falls, gait disturbance, balance and mobility problems, postural hypotension, sensory impairment, urinary and bladder dysfunction, and certain medical diagnostic categories (e.g., cancer and cardiovascular, neurological, and cerebrovascular diseases) increase the risk of falling. One of the more common factors precipitating a fall is a client's attempt to get out of bed to use the toilet. Drug use and drug interactions are also implicated in falls. Hip fractures are among the most serious fall-related injuries. Between April 2003 and March 2006, the rate of hip fracture in Canadian seniors during admission to hospital was close to one in 1000 (CIHI, 2007). Older adults with a hip fracture may have a long period of recovery and may not be able to return to their previous level of functioning, even losing their ability to live independently (SMARTRISK, 1998). Falls that result in injuries can extend a client's length of stay in the health care environment, placing the client at a greater risk for other complications.

Client-Inherent Accidents. Client-inherent accidents are accidents (other than falls) in which the client is the primary reason for the accident. Examples of client-inherent accidents are self-inflicted cuts, injuries, and burns; the ingestion or injection of foreign substances; self-mutilation or fire setting; and pinching fingers in drawers or doors. A client-inherent accident may occur as a result of a seizure. A **seizure** is a sudden and abnormal discharge of neurons in the brain leading to alterations in sensation, behaviour, movement, perception, or consciousness (Black & Hawks, 2005). Accidental injuries may occur during a seizure if clients hit themselves against an object such as a bed rail or the floor.

Procedure-Related Accidents. Procedure-related accidents are those that occur during therapy. They include medication and fluid administration errors, the improper application of external devices, and accidents related to the improper performance of procedures (e.g., incorrect Foley catheter insertion).

In a study of Canadian hospitals, Baker et al. (2004) found that 7.5% of clients were affected by medical errors during their hospital stay. The most common errors were related to surgical procedures

Symbol	Name	Description
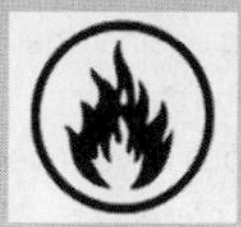	Flammable and combustible material	Product may catch fire when exposed to heat, sparks, or flame.
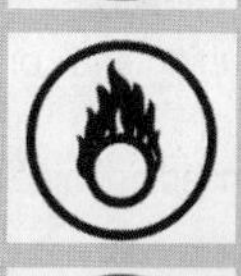	Oxidizing material	Product may cause a fire or explosion if exposed to combustible material.
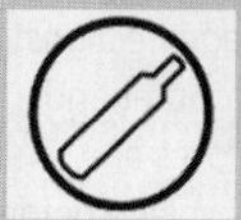	Compressed gas	Product is under high pressure. May explode or burst when heated, dropped, or damaged.
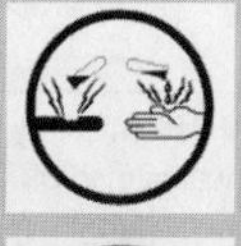	Corrosive material	Product can cause burns to eyes, skin, or respiratory system.
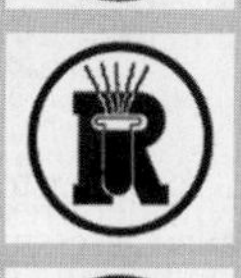	Dangerously reactive material	Product may react with light, heat, extreme temperatures, or vibration causing explosion, fire, or release of poisonous gases.
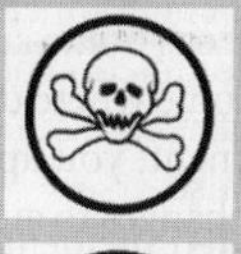	Poisonous and infectious material: immediate and serious toxic effects	Product may be fatal or cause serious or permanent damage if exposed to even once.
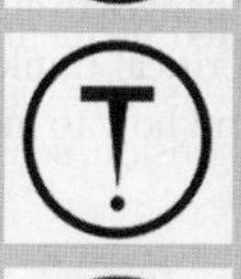	Poisonous and infectious material: other toxic effects	Product may cause cancer, birth defects, or other permanent damage if exposed to repeatedly.
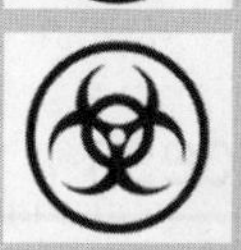	Poisonous and infectious material: biohazardous and infectious material	Product may cause disease, serious illness, or death.

Figure 37-2 Workplace Hazardous Materials Information System hazard symbols. **Source:** Adapted from the Canadian Centre for Occupational Health and Safety. (2001). *WHMIS labelling requirements*. Retrieved April 16, 2008, from http://www.ccohs.ca/oshanswers/legisl/msds_lab.html#

and drug or fluid administration. In 15.9% of these cases, the errors resulted in the death of a client. Etchells et al. (2008) stress that although medication errors cannot be avoided completely, systems can be designed to minimize the possibility and severity of errors. Providing safe care is an important concern for Canadian nurses, with individual and system factors influencing that care (Canadian Nurses Association & University of Toronto Faculty of Nursing, 2004). Nurses and health care facilities must build safety into processes of care and take a systems approach when taking on efforts to reduce medical errors.

You can prevent many procedure-related accidents (Box 37–2). For example, strictly following the procedure for administering medications prevents medication errors (see Chapter 34). The potential for infection is reduced when surgical asepsis is used for sterile dressing changes or any invasive procedure, such as insertion of a Foley catheter. Finally, the correct use of lifting devices reduces the risk of injuries when moving and lifting clients (see Chapter 46).

Equipment-Related Accidents. Equipment-related accidents result from the malfunction, disrepair, or misuse of equipment or from an electrical hazard. For example, a too-rapid infusion of intravenous (IV) fluids may result from a dysfunctional IV pump. To avoid accidents, do not operate monitoring or therapy equipment without instruction. A checklist should be used to assess potential electrical hazards to reduce the risk of electrical fires, electrocution, or injury from faulty equipment. In health care settings, clinical engineering staff make regular safety checks of equipment.

Critical Thinking

Successful critical thinking requires a synthesis of knowledge, experience, information gathered from clients, critical thinking qualities, and intellectual and professional standards. Clinical judgements require you to anticipate necessary information, analyze the data, and make decisions regarding client care. Critical thinking is an ongoing process. During assessment (Figure 37–3), you need to consider all critical thinking elements as well as information about the specific client to make appropriate nursing diagnoses.

In the case of safety, you integrate knowledge from nursing and other scientific disciplines, previous experiences in caring for clients who had an injury or were at risk, critical thinking qualities such as perseverance, and any standards of practice that are applicable. Agency guidelines and professional nursing associations provide

BOX 37-2 Nine Life-Saving Client Safety Solutions

- *Be aware of look-alike and sound-alike medication names.* Carefully review the medication orders of these drugs and use the six rights of medication safety.
- *Use client identification.* Use two forms of client identification, such as a hospital arm band and medical record number.
- *Communicate during client handover.* Communicate critical information, provide time for health care personnel to ask and resolve questions, and involve the client and family during a handover process.
- *Perform correct procedure at correct body site.* Mark the operative site and take a "time out" to verify that you have identified the correct client, operative site, and procedure before initiating the procedure.
- *Control concentrated electrolyte solutions.* Use the six rights of medication administration, and follow your agency's protocols for these solutions.
- *Ensure medication accuracy at transitions in care.* Perform medication reconciliation at each health care transition. During admission, transfer, and discharge, compare all medications a client is taking against the medical order and against the client's "home medication list."
- *Avoid catheter and tubing misconnections.* Be meticulous in your verification of the catheter and tubing connections, of the correct catheter, and of the correct connection tubing. Label tubing and connections when a client has multiple catheters.
- *Do not reuse single-use injection devices.* Never reuse needles, injection devices, or intravenous catheters.
- *Improve hand hygiene to prevent health care–associated infections.* Perform hand hygiene before and after each client encounter and after contact with contaminated objects (even when gloves are worn). Encourage family and visitors to perform hand hygiene before and after visits.

Courtesy of the World Health Organization Collaborating Centre for Patient Safety Releases. (2007, May 2). *Nine patient safety solutions.* Retrieved January 26, 2009, from http://www.who.int/mediacentre/news/releases/2007/pr22/en/index.html

standards for nursing activities such as medication administration, fall-prevention steps, and infection control to guide nurses in the provision of safe care. For example, the Registered Nurses Association of Ontario (2005) has published *Nursing Best Practice Guideline: Prevention of Falls and Fall Injuries in the Older Adult.* You refer to all this information and experience as you conduct a detailed assessment of a specific client. For example, while assessing a client's home environment, you consider typical locations within the home where dangers commonly exist. If a client has a visual impairment, you apply previous experience in caring for clients with visual changes to anticipate how to thoroughly assess the client's needs. Critical thinking directs you to anticipate what needs to be assessed and how to make conclusions about available data.

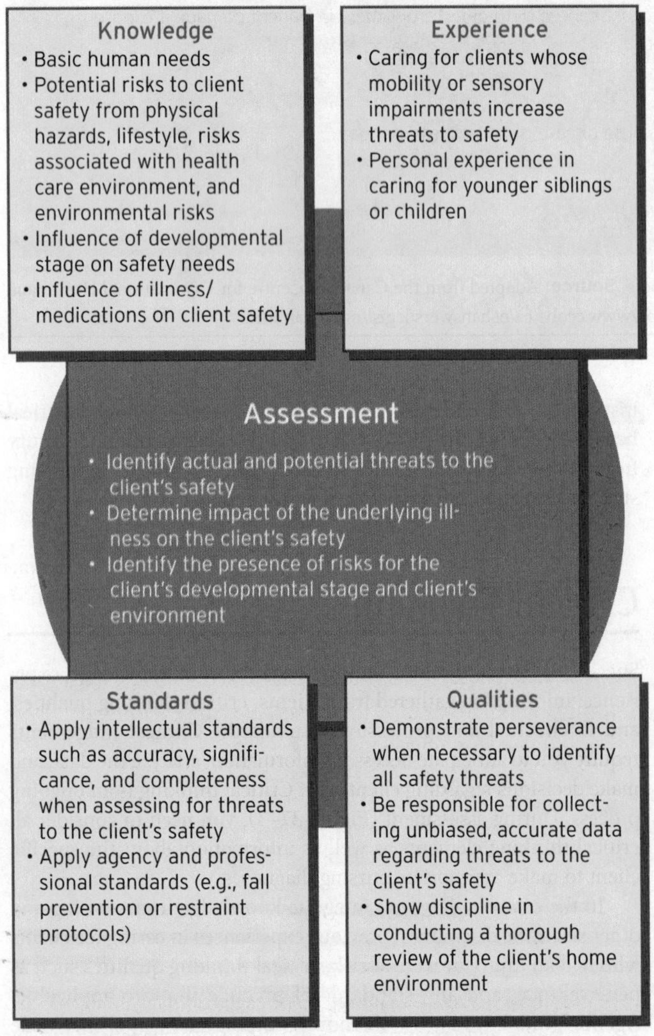

Knowledge
- Basic human needs
- Potential risks to client safety from physical hazards, lifestyle, risks associated with health care environment, and environmental risks
- Influence of developmental stage on safety needs
- Influence of illness/medications on client safety

Experience
- Caring for clients whose mobility or sensory impairments increase threats to safety
- Personal experience in caring for younger siblings or children

Assessment
- Identify actual and potential threats to the client's safety
- Determine impact of the underlying illness on the client's safety
- Identify the presence of risks for the client's developmental stage and client's environment

Standards
- Apply intellectual standards such as accuracy, significance, and completeness when assessing for threats to the client's safety
- Apply agency and professional standards (e.g., fall prevention or restraint protocols)

Qualities
- Demonstrate perseverance when necessary to identify all safety threats
- Be responsible for collecting unbiased, accurate data regarding threats to the client's safety
- Show discipline in conducting a thorough review of the client's home environment

Figure 37-3 Critical thinking model for safety assessment.

Safety and the Nursing Process

❖Assessment

To conduct a thorough client assessment, consider possible threats to a client's safety, including the client's immediate environment, as well as any individual risk factors.

Health History

By conducting a health history, you gather data about the client's level of wellness to determine if any underlying conditions exist that pose threats to safety. For example, you give special attention to assessing the client's gait, muscle strength and coordination, balance, and vision. A review of the client's developmental status must be considered as assessment information is analyzed. Also review whether the client has been exposed to any environmental hazards or is taking medications or undergoing procedures that pose risks. For example, the use of diuretics increases the frequency of voiding and may result in the client having to use toilet facilities more often. Falls often occur when clients get out of bed quickly because of urinary urgency.

Client's Home Environment

When caring for a client in the home, a home hazard assessment is necessary (Box 37–3). Walk through the home with the client and discuss how the client normally conducts daily activities. Key areas to inspect are the bathroom, kitchen, and areas with stairs. For example, when assessing the adequacy of the lighting, you inspect areas where the client moves and works, such as outside walkways, steps, interior halls, and doorways. Getting a sense of the client's routine helps you recognize less-obvious hazards.

BOX 37-3 Home Hazard Assessment

Home Exterior

Are sidewalks uneven?
Are steps in good repair?
Is ice and snow removal adequate?
Do steps and balconies have securely fastened railings?
Is lighting present and adequate?
Is outdoor furniture sturdy?
Are window screens in high-rise apartments properly secured?

Home Interior

Do all rooms, stairways, and halls have adequate, nonglare lighting?
Are night lights available?
Are area rugs secured?
Are wooden floors nonslippery?
Are floors where water accumulates covered by nonslip floor mats?
Is furniture placed appropriately to permit mobility? Is furniture sturdy enough to provide support for getting up and down?
Are temperature and humidity within normal ranges? Are any steps or thresholds present that may pose a hazard? Are step edges clearly marked with coloured tape? Are handrails available and secure?
In homes with young children, are window guards and electrical outlet covers installed?
Can all doors and windows with security gates and locks be opened from the inside without a key?

Kitchen

Are handwashing facilities available?
Is the pilot light on for the gas stove?
Are the stovetop and oven clean?
Are the dials on the stove readable?
Are storage areas within easy reach?
Are fluids such as cleaners and bleach in original containers and stored properly?
In homes with young children, are safety locks on cabinets and corner counter protectors installed?
Is the water temperature within a normal range?
Do clean areas for food storage and preparation exist? Is refrigeration adequate? Are the refrigerator and freezer temperatures correct?

Bathroom

Are handwashing facilities available?
Does the tub or shower have skid-proof strips or surfaces? Are bath mats secured?
Does the client need grab bars near the bathtub and toilet? Does the client need an elevated toilet seat?
Is the medicine cabinet well lit?
Are medications in their original containers?
If children live in the home or visit, are medication containers child resistant?
Have outdated medications been discarded?

Bedroom

Are beds of adequate height for getting on and off easily?
Is lighting adequate for both day and night?
Are floor coverings nonskid?
Does the client have a telephone nearby?
Are emergency numbers visible near the telephone?

Electrical and Fire Hazards

Are smoke and carbon monoxide detectors installed? Are the batteries for all detectors tested every month and changed twice a year?
Have the furnace, chimney, and stove been checked for proper ventilation?
Are extension cords in good condition and used appropriately?
Are appliances in good working order?
Are electrical appliances located away from water sources? Is a multipurpose fire extinguisher near the cooking area, and does client understand how to use it?
Are combustible items such as oil-based paints, gasoline, and oily rags stored in a garage or basement?
Are electrical outlets overloaded?
Are flashlights available?
Is a first aid kit available to the adult members of the household?
Does everyone in the family know the fire escape plan and have easy access to emergency phone numbers?

Adapted from Ebersole, P., Hess, P., & Luggen, A. (2004). *Toward healthy aging: Human needs and nursing response* (6th ed.). St. Louis, MO: Mosby; and McCullagh, M. C. (2006). Home modification: How to help patients make their homes safer and more accessible as their abilities change. *American Journal of Nursing, 106*(10), 54.

Assessment for the risk of food infection or poisoning involves obtaining a detailed dietary assessment for the previous week; conducting an examination of GI and central nervous system functions; observing for a fever; and analyzing the results of cultures of feces and vomitus. Suspected food and water sources are also studied. In addition, you should assess the client's handwashing practices. It is useful to ask clients when they routinely wash their hands. This question can then prompt a helpful discussion about the purpose and importance of handwashing.

An assessment of the environmental comfort of the client's home should include a review of when the client normally has heating and cooling systems serviced. Does the client have a functional furnace or space heater? Does the home have air conditioning or fans? Clients who use space heaters must be informed of the risk for fires.

When clients live in older homes, encourage an inspection for the presence of lead in paint, dust, or soil. Because lead can also come from the solder of plumbing fixtures in a home, water from each faucet should also be tested. Local health offices can assist a homeowner in locating a trained lead inspector who will take samples from various locations and have them analyzed at a laboratory for lead content.

Health Care Environment

When a client is cared for within a health care facility, you must determine if any hazards exist in the immediate care environment. Does the placement of equipment or furniture pose barriers to ambulation? Does the positioning of the client's bed allow the client to reach items on a bedside table? Does the client need assistance with ambulation? Is the client aware of activity restrictions? Has the client been taught to use the call bell, and is it within reach? Collaborate with clinical engineering staff to make sure that equipment has been assessed to ensure its proper function and condition.

Risk for Falls

Assessment of the client's fall risk factors is essential in determining specific needs and targeting interventions to prevent falls. Begin by asking the client if he or she has had a history of falls. A fall assessment tool (Table 37–1) can help you determine potential risks before accidents and injuries result. Familiarize yourself with the fall assessment tool used in your clinical area as such tools vary among agencies. The tool shown in Table 37–1 has weighted risk factors. A client's risk of falling increases as the number of risk factors increases. In this tool, a client with a history of falls receives a minimum score of 15 as the individual who has fallen once has a significantly higher risk of falling again. Initial and daily assessments of fall risk are important in identifying clients at risk of falling. In many cases, family members can be significant resources in assessing a client's fall risk. Families often are able to report on the client's level of confusion and ability to ambulate.

Risk for Medical Errors

Be alert to factors within your environment that create conditions in which medical errors are more likely to occur. Studies indicate that overwork and fatigue cause a significant decrease in alertness and concentration, leading to errors (Trinkoff et al., 2006). You need to be aware of these factors and include checks and balances when working under stressful conditions. For example, to reduce the potential for a medical error, it is essential for you to check the client's identification bracelet before beginning any procedure or administering any medication.

The National Steering Committee on Patient Safety (2002) made recommendations to improve the safety of Canada's health care system. At the core of these recommendations was the need to nurture a culture of safety within the system. The Canadian Patient Safety Institute (CPSI) was established in 2003 to provide leadership in the development of such a culture.

Client Expectations

Clients generally expect to be safe in their home and in the health care setting. However, a client's viewpoint of what is safe may differ from your viewpoint. For this reason, any assessment must include the client's understanding of his or her perception of risk factors. This information will be important later if you need to make changes in the client's environment. Clients usually do not purposefully put themselves in jeopardy. When clients are uninformed or inexperienced, threats to their safety can occur. Clients must always be consulted on ways to reduce hazards in their environment.

❖Nursing Diagnosis

After completing an assessment of a client's safety status, review any clusters of data to identify patterns suggesting that safety is threatened. Defining characteristics and related factors from the data guide you in identifying appropriate nursing diagnoses (Box 37–4).

The related factors become the basis for selecting nursing therapies. For example, *risk for injury related to impaired mobility* and *risk for injury related to barriers in the home environment* require different nursing interventions. The client with altered mobility may require ambulatory aids and physiotherapy. When the related factor is barriers in the home, you recommend changes that will create a safer environment. At times, as in the example in Box 37–4, multiple related factors may apply. Examples of nursing diagnoses that may apply for clients whose safety is threatened include the following:

- Impaired home maintenance—*risk for imbalanced body temperature*
- Impaired home maintenance—*risk for injury*
- Deficient knowledge—*risk for poisoning*
- Disturbed sensory perception—*risk for suffocation*
- Disturbed thought processes—*risk for trauma*

➤ TABLE 37-1 Fall Assessment Tool

Instructions: Circle the score for the risk factor(s) that corresponds to the client. The tool should be administered upon admission to the facility or agency and again at specified intervals and when warranted by changes in the client's health status. Scores of 15 and higher indicate high risk; preventive measures should be implemented for these clients.

Client Factors	**Date Admit**	**Initial Score**	**Date**	**Reassessed Score**
History of falls		15		15
Confusion		5		5
Age (over 65)		5		5
Impaired judgement		5		5
Sensory deficit		5		5
Unable to ambulate independently		5		5
Decreased level of cooperation		5		5
Increased anxiety/emotional lability		5		5
Incontinence/urgency		5		5
Cardiovascular/respiratory disease affecting perfusion and oxygenation		5		5
Medications affecting blood pressure or level of consciousness		5		5
Postural hypotension with dizziness		5		5
Environmental Factors				
First week on unit/facility/service, etc.		5		5
Attached equipment (e.g., intravenous pole, chest tubes, appliances, oxygen, tubing)		5		5

Adapted from Farmer, B. (2000). *Try this: Best practices in nursing care to older adults*. New York: The Hartford Institute for Geriatric Nursing, New York University.

BOX 37-4 NURSING DIAGNOSTIC PROCESS

Assessment Activities	*Defining Characteristics*	*Nursing Diagnosis*
Observe client's mobility and body alignment.	Uncoordinated gait Poor posture	*Risk for injury related to impaired mobility, decreased vision, poorly lit home, and cluttered environment*
Ask client about visual acuity.	Reports difficulty seeing at night Reports tripping over rugs and furniture	
Complete a home hazard appraisal.	Poorly lit home Rooms filled with small items Excessive amount of furniture for size of room Rugs not secure	

❖Planning

During planning, you critically synthesize information from multiple sources (Figure 37–4). Critical thinking ensures that the client's plan of care integrates all that you have learned about the client, as well as the key critical thinking elements. For example, reflect on knowledge regarding the services that other disciplines (e.g., occupational therapy) can provide in helping the client return home safely, as well as on any previous experience wherein a client benefited from safety interventions. Such experience helps you adapt approaches with a new client. Applying critical thinking qualities such as creativity helps you and the client collaborate in planning interventions that are relevant and most useful, particularly when changes are made in the home environment.

Goals and Outcomes

Planning and goal setting need to be done in collaboration with the client, family, and other members of the health care team (Box 37–5). The client who is an active participant in reducing threats to safety will be more alert to potential hazards. Goals and outcomes must be measurable and realistic, with consideration of the resources available to the client. The overall goal for a client with a threat to safety is to remain free from injury. The following are examples of expected outcomes that focus on a client's need for safety:

- Modifiable hazards will be reduced in the home environment by 100% within 1 month.
- The client will not suffer a fall or injury.
- The client will identify risks associated with visual impairment.

Setting Priorities

Nursing interventions are prioritized to provide safe and efficient care. For example, the client described in the concept map (Figure 37–5) has several nursing diagnoses. The client's mobility problem is an obvious priority because of its influence on skin integrity and the risk for falls. Plan individualized interventions based on the severity of risk factors and the client's developmental stage, level of health, lifestyle, and culture (Box 37–6). Planning also involves understanding the client's need to maintain independence within physical and cognitive capabilities. You and the client collaborate to establish ways of maintaining the client's active involvement within the home and health care environment. Educating the client and family is also an important intervention to reduce safety risks over the long term.

Continuity of Care

Clients need to learn how to identify and select resources within their community that enhance safety (e.g., block parent homes, local police departments, and neighbours willing to check on a client's well-being). Collaboration with the client and family and other disciplines such as social work and occupational and physiotherapy may become an important part of your plan of care. For example, a hospitalized

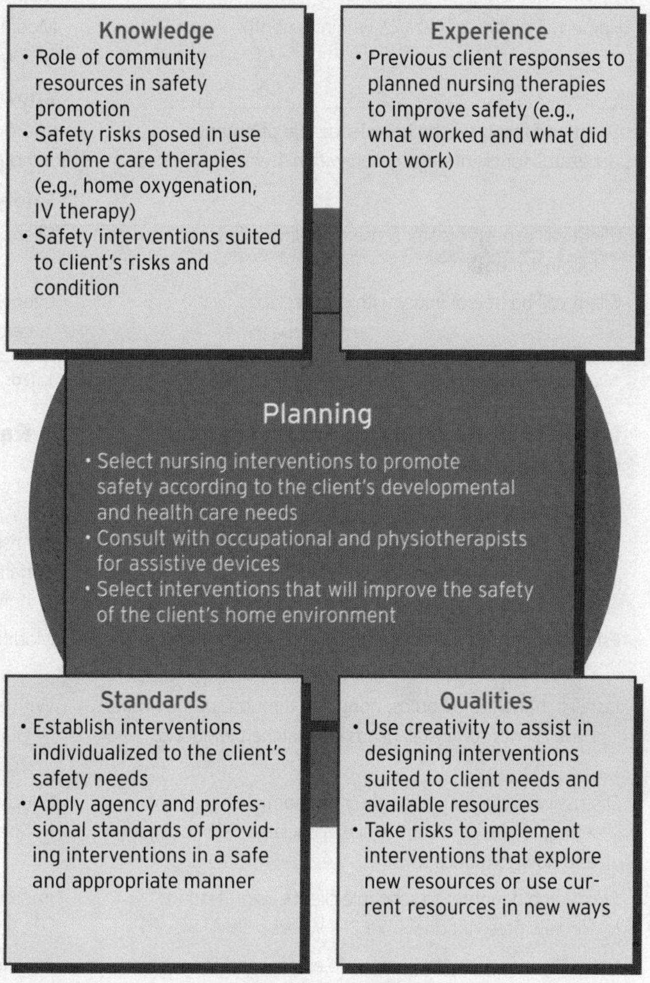

Knowledge
- Role of community resources in safety promotion
- Safety risks posed in use of home care therapies (e.g., home oxygenation, IV therapy)
- Safety interventions suited to client's risks and condition

Experience
- Previous client responses to planned nursing therapies to improve safety (e.g., what worked and what did not work)

Planning
- Select nursing interventions to promote safety according to the client's developmental and health care needs
- Consult with occupational and physiotherapists for assistive devices
- Select interventions that will improve the safety of the client's home environment

Standards
- Establish interventions individualized to the client's safety needs
- Apply agency and professional standards of providing interventions in a safe and appropriate manner

Qualities
- Use creativity to assist in designing interventions suited to client needs and available resources
- Take risks to implement interventions that explore new resources or use current resources in new ways

Figure 37-4 Critical thinking model for safety planning. IV, intravenous.

BOX 37-5 NURSING CARE PLAN

Risk for Injury

Assessment

Mr. Key, a visiting nurse, is seeing Ms. Cohen, an 85-year-old woman, at her home. The client has been recovering from a mild stroke affecting her left side. Ms. Cohen lives alone but receives regular assistance from her daughter and son, who both live within 16 km. Mr. Key's assessment includes a discussion of Ms. Cohen's health problem and how the stroke has affected her, as well as a pertinent physical examination.

Assessment Activities	***Findings and Defining Characteristics***
Ask Ms. Cohen how the stroke has affected her mobility.	She responds, "I bump into things, and I'm afraid I'm going to fall."
Conduct a home hazard assessment.	Cabinets in the kitchen are in disarray and full of breakable items that could fall out. Throw rugs are on floors; bathroom lighting is poor (40-W bulb); bathtub lacks safety strips or grab bars; and home is cluttered with furniture and small objects.
Observe Ms. Cohen's gait and posture.	Ms. Cohen has kyphosis and has a hesitant, uncoordinated gait. She frequently holds walls for support.
Assess Ms. Cohen's muscle strength.	The left arm and leg are weaker than the right.
Assess visual acuity with corrective lenses.	Ms. Cohen has trouble reading and seeing familiar objects at a distance while wearing current glasses.

Nursing Diagnosis: Risk for injury related to impaired mobility, decreased visual acuity, and physical environmental hazards

Planning

Goals (Nursing Outcomes Classification)*	***Expected Outcomes***
	Risk Control
Home will be free of hazards within 1 month.	Modifiable hazards in kitchen and hallway will be reduced in the home within 1 week. Revisions to bathroom will be completed in 1 month.
	Knowledge: Personal Safety
Client and family will be knowledgeable of potential hazards for client's age group within 1 week.	Client and her daughter will identify risks and the steps to avoid them in the home at the conclusion of a teaching session next week.
	Safety Behaviour: Fall Prevention
Client will express greater sense of feeling safe from falls in 1 month.	Client will report improved vision with the aid of new eyeglasses.
Client will be free of injury within 2 weeks.	Client will be able to safely ambulate throughout the home and perform personal care activities within 2 weeks.

*Outcome classification labels from Moorhead, S., Johnson, M., & Maas, M. L. (Eds.). (2004). *Nursing Outcomes Classification (NIC)* (3rd ed.). St. Louis, MO: Mosby.

Interventions (Nursing Interventions Classification)†	**Rationale**
Fall Prevention	
Review findings from home hazard assessment with client and her daughter.	Fall risks for homebound older adults include visual disturbances, unsteady gait, and postural changes (Meiner & Lueckenotte, 2006). Evaluation of home hazards will highlight extrinsic factors that may lead to falls.
Establish a list of priorities to modify. Have client's son assist in installing bathroom safety devices.	Modification of environment reduces fall risk (McCullagh, 2006).
Install lighting (75-W bulbs, nonglare) throughout the home. Have client's son install blinds over kitchen windows.	With aging, the pupil loses the ability to adjust to light, causing sensitivity to glare. Glare can make it difficult to clearly see a walking path (Meiner & Lueckenotte, 2006).
Discuss with client and daughter the normal changes of aging, effects of recent stroke, associated risks for injury, and how to reduce risks.	Education regarding hazards can reduce fear of falling (American Geriatrics Society, 2001).
Encourage daughter to schedule client's vision testing for new prescription within 2–4 weeks.	Improved visual acuity reduces incidence of falls (Edelman & Mandle, 2006).
Refer client to a physiotherapist to assess need for assistive devices for kyphosis, left-sided weakness, and gait.	Exercise often improves gait, balance, and flexibility. Modifying gait problems by increasing lower extremity strength reduces fall risk.

†Intervention classification labels from Dochterman, J. M. & Bulechek, G. M. (Eds.). (2004). *Nursing Interventions Classification (NIC)* (4th ed.). St. Louis, MO: Mosby.

BOX 37-5 NURSING CARE PLAN *continued*

Evaluation

Nursing Actions	*Client Response and Finding*	*Achievement of Outcome*
Ask client and family to identify risks.	Ms. Cohen and her daughter are able to identify risks during a walk through the home and expressed a greater sense of safety as a result of changes made.	Ms. Cohen and her daughter are more knowledgeable of potential hazards.
Observe environment for elimination of hazards.	Throw rugs have been removed. Lighting has been increased to 75 W, except in the bathroom and bedroom.	Environmental hazards have been partially reduced.
Reassess Ms. Cohen's visual acuity.	Ms. Cohen has new glasses and says she can read better and see distant objects more clearly.	Ms. Cohen's vision has improved, enabling her to ambulate more safely.
Observe Ms. Cohen's gait and posture.	Ms. Cohen's gait remains hesitant and uncoordinated; she reports that her daughter has not had time to take her to the physiotherapist.	The outcome of safe ambulation has not been totally achieved; continue to encourage Ms. Cohen and daughter to go to physiotherapy appointment.

concept map

Nursing diagnosis: Risk for falls related to left-sided paralysis
- Imbalanced gait
- Receiving diuretic
- Urinary incontinence
- Fell at home 1 month ago

Interventions
- Implement fall precautions
- Visit client hourly to determine needs
- Avoid late evening fluids
- Schedule toileting and hygiene activities

Nursing diagnosis: Risk for impaired skin integrity related to decreased sensation
- Sensory impairment left side
- Urinary incontinence
- Difficulty changing positions

Interventions
- Initiate skin care protocol
- Turn client every 1.5 hours
- Offer urinal/toilet every 2 hours

Client's chief medical diagnosis: 20 pack-year smoking history, left-sided paralysis from previous stroke, postoperative leg surgery
Priority assessments: Functional status, respiratory status, skin integrity

Nursing diagnosis: Impaired physical mobility related to left-sided paralysis
- Difficulty turning
- Reduced strength on left side
- Left-sided neglect

Interventions

- Range of joint motion
- Schedule short walks
- Occupational therapy for bathing, dressing, and other ADLs

Nursing diagnosis: Ineffective airway clearance related to retained thick pulmonary secretions
- Abnormal lung sounds in both lobes
- Dyspnea
- Coughs with difficulty

Interventions
- Teach ascade cough
- Increase fluids
- Assist client with coughing and deep breathing every hour

—— Link between medical diagnosis and nursing diagnosis

Figure 37-5 Concept map for a client with a cerebrovascular accident 3 months previously with left-sided paralysis; 2 days after right femoral–popliteal bypass. ADLs, activities of daily living.

BOX 37-6 CULTURAL ASPECTS OF CARE

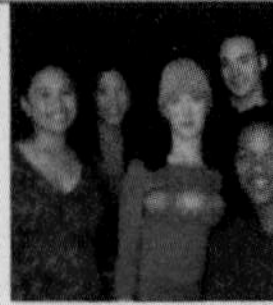

Cultural phenomena affecting health and safety include attitudes toward personal space, social organizations, communication, and environmental control. While conducting a home assessment for risks to safety, you must realize that you have entered the client's territory and that the client's attitude toward his or her residence and belongings must be appreciated. For example, clients from Western Europe and the British Isles may be considered aloof and distant in terms of personal space. It may be very difficult for them to have an outsider in their home who suggests changes regarding their personal belongings to reduce physical hazards. It is particularly difficult to determine a client's attitude toward his or her home environment when the client's primary language and that of the health care professional differ.

Another culturally sensitive issue involves the client's sense of environmental control. You must be aware of health beliefs and practices that will affect the outcome of interventions. For example, a reliance on family and religious organizations, as opposed to community resources, may affect the client's compliance with nursing interventions and referrals.

Learn to ask questions sensitively and to show respect for different cultural beliefs. Adapting to different cultural beliefs and practices requires flexibility. Respect for the belief systems of others and the effects of those beliefs on the client's well-being are critically important to competent health care. You must have the ability and knowledge to communicate about and to understand health behaviours influenced by culture.

Implications for Practice

- Resistance to change longstanding habits can interfere with a cultural group's acceptance of injury-prevention practices. Include family members who have a strong influence, such as a dominant man or older woman, when providing safety education.
- Evaluate the use of traditional ethnic remedies or foods that contain lead; these can increase a client's risk for lead poisoning.
- Remember that living in rural areas and in manufactured housing places the client at greater risk for fire-related injuries and death.
- Stress the importance of having fully functioning smoke detectors and a multipurpose fire extinguisher.
- Assess the client's smoking and drinking habits. Residential fire deaths are often attributed to the use of cigarettes and alcohol.
- Clients who live in poverty and have low educational levels are at greater risk for injury and disease. Assist the client and family in identifying community resources, such as the local health office or clinic.
- Be aware of family patterns and how the client and family interact with each other. Family disruption and weak intergenerational ties can increase a client's risk for injury from violent behaviour.

Adapted from Giger, J. N., & Davidhizar, R. (2002). The Giger and Davidhizar transcultural assessment model. *Journal of Transcultural Nursing 13*, 185.

client may need to go to a rehabilitation facility to gain strength and endurance before being discharged home. Be sure that the client and family understand the need for resources and are willing to make changes that will promote the client's safety.

❖Implementation

Nursing interventions are directed toward ensuring a client's safety in all settings and include health promotion, developmental interventions, environmental interventions, and limiting specific risks to client safety.

Health Promotion

To promote a client's health, it is necessary for the individual to be in a safe environment and to practise a lifestyle that minimizes the risk of injury. Edelman and Mandle (2006) described passive and active strategies aimed at health promotion. Passive strategies are implemented through public health and government legislative interventions (e.g., sanitation and clean water laws; see Chapter 4). Active strategies are those in which the individual is actively involved through changes in lifestyle (e.g., wearing a seat belt or installing outdoor lighting) and participation in wellness programs.

You can participate by supporting legislation and working in community-based settings. Because environmental and community values have the greatest influence on health promotion, community and home health nurses assess and recommend safety measures in the home (see Box 37–3), school, neighbourhood, and workplace.

Developmental Interventions

Accidents involving children are mostly preventable, and parents need to be aware of specific dangers at each stage of growth and development. Accident prevention thus requires health education for parents and the removal of dangers whenever possible. You are frequently in a position to educate parents or guardians about reducing the risks of injuries for young children (see Chapter 23). Nurses working in prenatal and postpartum settings can easily incorporate safety into the care plan of the child-bearing family. Community health nurses can assess the home and show parents how to promote safety in their homes (see Table 37–2 and Figures 37–7 and 37–8). The following discussion highlights some specific risks at different developmental stages.

Infants, Toddlers, and Preschoolers. Small children must be protected from accidental poisoning. Educate parents and guardians to use child-resistant caps, place medications and cleaning agents out of the reach of children, leave potentially poisonous materials in their original containers, and remove poisonous plants from the home—these steps can prevent the accidental ingestion of poisonous materials. Also ensure that parents and guardians are aware that poisoning can result from swallowing miniature button or disk batteries, which are commonly found in games, cameras, calculators, and watches. In any instance of accidental poisoning, guidelines for intervening (Box 37–7) should be adhered to. The poison control centre phone number should be visible on the telephone in homes with young children, and the centre should be called immediately if poisoning is suspected.

Educate parents that children under 5 years of age are also more susceptible to diseases such as measles, mumps, and chickenpox. Immunizations given before the age of 2 years and at recommended intervals can protect a child from life-threatening diseases.

School-Age Children. School-age children increasingly explore their environment (see Chapter 23). They may travel to and from school on foot or by school bus, and they may have friends outside their immediate neighbourhood. They may also become more active in extracurricular activities. Parents, teachers, and nurses must instruct children in safe practices to follow at school and play. Table 37–2 lists nursing interventions to help guide parents in providing for the safety of school-age children. Using examples when discussing safe practices is an effective way to teach school-age children.

Because school-age children participate in more activities outside their home and neighbourhood environments, they are at greater risk of injury from strangers. Children should be warned repeatedly not

BOX 37-7 Procedural Guidelines

Interventions for Accidental Poisoning

Procedure

1. Assess for airway patency, breathing, and circulation (ABCs) in all clients in whom accidental poisoning is suspected.
2. Remove any visible materials from areas such as the mouth and eyes to terminate exposure to the poison(s).
3. Identify the type and amount of substance ingested, if possible. This may help to determine the required antidote.
4. Call your local poison control centre before attempting any interventions.
5. If directed by a physician, give oral fluids to assist vomiting.
6. If directed, save the vomitus for laboratory analysis; this may assist with further treatment of the client.
7. Position the victim with the head to the side to prevent the aspiration of vomitus, and assist in keeping the airway open.
8. Never induce vomiting in an unconscious person or in a person experiencing convulsions because aspiration may occur.
9. Never induce vomiting if any of the following substances have been ingested: lye, household cleaners, hair care products, grease or petroleum products, or furniture polish. In the case of these substances, vomiting may increase internal burns.
10. If instructed, arrange for the victim to be taken to the emergency department. Call an ambulance—emergency equipment may be needed en route.
11. In the case of convulsions, cessation of breathing, or unconsciousness, call 911.
12. Do not administer syrup of ipecac to induce vomiting. It has not been proven effective in preventing poisoning.

From American Academy of Pediatrics. (2004). *Don't treat swallowed poison with syrup of ipecac says AAP* [News release]. Retrieved August, 2008, from www.aap.org/advocacy/releases/novpoison.htm

to accept candy, food, gifts, or rides from strangers. In addition, children need to know what to do if a stranger approaches. Frequently, neighbourhoods have a "block parent" program. The owner of a block parent home ensures that an adult is home during the times when children are walking to and from school. If a stranger approaches a child, the child can run to that home (identified by a sign), and the adult will protect the child and call the proper authorities. You may work with school systems or neighbourhoods to initiate such a system to protect children.

Sports safety is stressed in school sports, but parents and health care professionals can reinforce these safety tips by insisting that children wear protective gear while participating in sports such as skateboarding and snowboarding. For example, schools provide hard batting helmets for baseball games, and parents should also provide this equipment when children are playing baseball in their own backyards.

Bicycle- and scooter-related injuries are a major cause of death and disability among children. Children 5 to 14 years of age account for one-third of bicyclists hospitalized as a result of bicycle injuries (CIHI, 2004). Bikes should be in good working order and the proper size for the child. Children should be taught the rules of the road and cautioned not to engage in dangerous stunts or activities while bike riding. A properly fitted helmet should be worn. Because most fatalities from bicycle accidents are related to head injuries, most provinces have implemented laws requiring that children wear bicycle helmets while cycling (Figure 37–6).

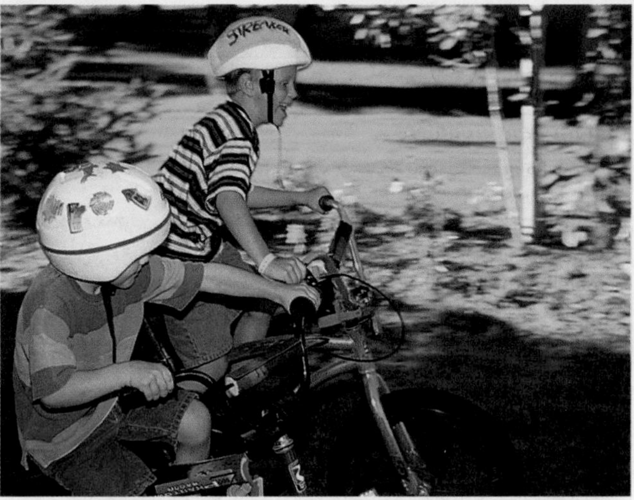

Figure 37-6 Proper bicycle safety equipment for school-age children.

Adolescents. Risks to the safety of adolescents involve many factors outside the home environment, particularly their almost constant involvement with their peers (see Chapter 23). Adults serve as role models for adolescents and, through providing examples, setting expectations, and providing education, can help adolescents minimize risks to their safety. This age group has a high incidence of suicide because of feelings of decreased self-worth and hopelessness. You should be aware of the risks posed at this time and be prepared to teach adolescents and their parents measures to prevent accidents and injury (Table 37–2).

When adolescents learn to drive, their environment expands and so does their risk for injury. The potential for motor vehicle accidents is higher among teen drivers than in any other age group. Teens are more likely to speed, run red lights, and drive while intoxicated. The young driver must be taught to comply with rules and regulations when using a car.

safety alert Reinforce to new drivers and their parents the need to consistently wear safety belts and to never ride in a car with a driver who may be intoxicated. Assist parents and their teen in developing a plan of action to be used if the teen finds himself or herself with a driver who has been drinking or has used other substances.

Because adolescence is a time when mature sexual physical characteristics develop, adolescents may begin to have physical relationships with others. They need prompt, accurate instruction about abstinence, safer sexual practices, and birth control (see Chapter 27).

Adults. Risks to young and middle-aged adults frequently result from lifestyle factors such as postpartum depression, high stress levels, inadequate nutrition, the use of firearms, excessive alcohol intake, and substance abuse (see Chapter 24). In our fast-paced society, there appears to be more expression of anger, which can quickly precipitate accidents (e.g., "road rage"). Adults need to have the opportunity to discuss the choices they have made in their life and the types of threats to safety that exist. Given information about threats to their well-being, adults may make the necessary modifications to their lifestyle practices. Useful resources are stress-management centres, employee-assistance programs, and health-promotion activities, which can be found in many communities and hospitals. In addition, neighbourhood centres, community clinics, and outpatient clinics are equipped to assist adults in modifying lifestyle habits that present risks to their health (e.g., smoking, overeating, lack of exercise, and alcoholism).

➤ TABLE 37-2 Interventions to Promote Safety for Children and Adolescents

Intervention	Rationale
Infants and Toddlers	
Ensure that infants sleep on their backs. Teach parents the mnemonic "back to sleep."	Sleeping on the back is associated with the lowest risk if sudden infant death syndrome (SIDS) (Canadian Pediatric Society, 2004).
Ensure that parents do not fill cribs with pillows, large stuffed toys, or comforters. Sheets should fit snugly.	Infants may become entwined in sheets and other bedding and suffocate.
Ensure that pacifiers are not attached to a string or ribbon and placed around a child's neck.	Choking may occur.
Ensure that all instructions for preparing and storing formula are being followed.	Proper formula preparation and storage prevents contamination. A formula may come in a concentrated form, or it may already be diluted and ready to use. Following directions ensures the proper concentration of the formula. Undiluted formula can cause fluid and electrolyte disturbances; very diluted formula does not provide sufficient nutrients.
Ensure that only large, soft toys without small parts such as buttons are being used.	Small parts can become dislodged, and choking and aspiration are possible.
Teach parents that playpens with mesh sides should not be left with a side down; spaces between crib slats should be <6 cm apart.	A child's head may become wedged in the lowered mesh side or between crib slats, and asphyxiation may occur.
Teach parents to never leave crib sides down or leave babies unattended on change tables or in infant seats, swings, strollers, or high chairs.	Infants and toddlers can roll or move and fall from change tables or out of accessories such as infant seats or swings.
Teach parents to discontinue using accessories such as infant seats and swings when the child becomes too active or physically too big.	When physically active or too big, the child can fall out of or tip over these accessories and suffer an injury.
Teach parents to never leave a child alone in the bathroom, in the tub, or near any water source (e.g., a pool).	Accidental drowning may occur.
Ensure that the home has been baby-proofed; small or sharp objects and toxic or poisonous substances, including plants, should be removed; safety locks should be installed on floor-level cabinets.	Babies explore their world with their hands and mouth. Choking and poisoning may occur.
Teach parents to remove plastic bags from the cleaners or grocery store from the home.	Suffocation may occur if plastic covers the nose and mouth.
Ensure that electrical outlets are protected by covers (Figure 37–7).	Crawling babies may insert objects into outlets and experience an electrical shock.
Ensure that window guards are on all windows.	Guards prevent children from falling out of windows.
Ensure that keyless locks (e.g., deadbolts) have been installed on doors above a child's reach (even when they are standing on a chair).	Keyless locks prevent a toddler from leaving the house and wandering off. Death from exposure, car accidents, and drowning may occur if a toddler wanders away. Keyless locks allow for rapid exit in the case of fire.
Teach parents that children weighing <36 kg or who are <8 years of age must always be in an age- and weight-appropriate car seat that has been installed according to the manufacturer's instructions (Figure 37–8). This includes car seats and booster seats. In cars with a passenger air bag, children under 12 years should be in the back seat. All passengers should wear their seat belts.	In case of a sudden stop or crash, an unrestrained child may suffer severe head injuries and death.

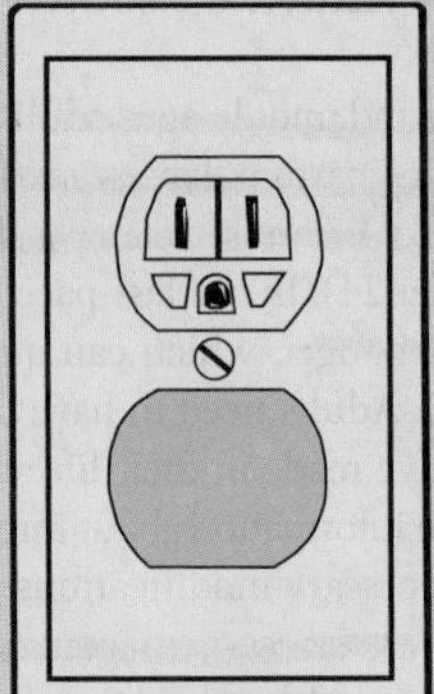

Figure 37-7 Safety covers for electrical outlets.

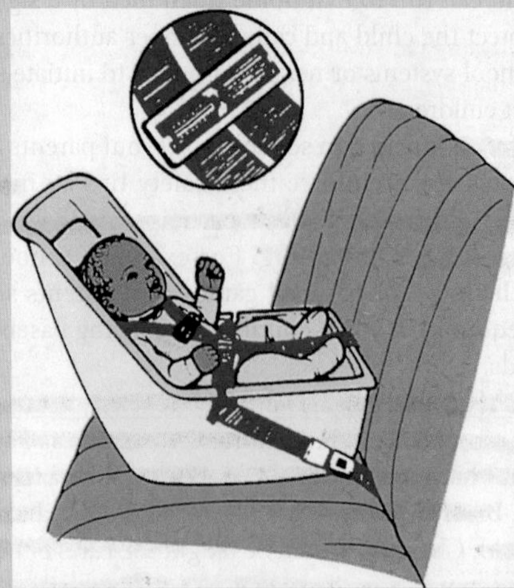

Figure 37-8 Infant car seat.

➤ TABLE 37-2 Interventions to Promote Safety for Children and Adolescents *continued*

Intervention	Rationale
Encourage caregivers to learn cardiopulmonary resuscitation and the Heimlich manoeuvre.	Caregivers should be prepared to intervene in acute emergencies, such as choking.
Preschoolers	
Encourage parents to teach children to swim at an early age, but always provide supervision near water.	Swimming is a useful skill that may someday save a child's life. However, all children need constant supervision near water.
Encourage parents to teach children how to cross streets and walk in parking lots. Instruct them to never run out into the street after a ball or toy.	Pedestrian accidents involving young children are common.
Encourage parents to teach children not to talk to, go with, or accept any item from a stranger.	This precaution reduces the risk of injury and abduction by a stranger.
Encourage parents to teach children basic physical safety rules, such as the proper use of safety scissors, never running with an object in their mouth or hand, and never attempting to use the stove or oven unassisted.	The risk of injury is lower if children are taught basic safety procedures.
Encourage parents to teach children not to eat items found in the street or grass.	Poisoning may occur.
Teach parents to remove doors from unused refrigerators and freezers and to instruct children not to play or hide in a car trunk or unused appliances.	If a child cannot freely exit from an appliance or car trunks, asphyxiation may occur.
School-Age Children	
Encourage parents to teach children the safe use of equipment for play and work.	Children need to learn the safe, appropriate use of implements to avoid injury.
Encourage parents to teach children proper bicycle safety, including the use of a helmet and rules of the road.	These safety precautions may reduce injuries from falling off a bike or being hit by a car.
Encourage parents to teach children proper techniques for specific sports, as well as the need to wear proper safety gear (e.g., eyewear or mouth guards).	The use of proper sports techniques, the correct equipment, and protective gear prevents injuries.
Encourage parents to teach children not to operate electrical equipment while unsupervised.	If an electrical mishap were to occur, no one would be available to help.
Teach parents that children should never have access to firearms or other weapons. All firearms should be kept in locked cabinets.	Children are often fascinated by firearms and weapons and may attempt to play with them.
Encourage parents to teach children safe use of the Internet.	Children are vulnerable to being exploited by predators over the Internet.
Adolescents	
Encourage enrolment in driver's education classes.	Many injuries in this age group are related to motor vehicle accidents.
Provide information about the effects of using alcohol, drugs, or other substances (e.g., glue, aerosols, or gasoline).	Adolescents are prone to risk-taking behaviours and are subject to peer pressure.
Provide sex education, emphasizing safer sex practices and abstinence.	Many adolescents begin sexual relationships. Pregnancy and sexually transmitted infections may result.
Refer adolescents to community and school-sponsored activities.	Adolescents need to socialize with peers yet need some supervision.
Encourage mentoring relationships between adults and adolescents.	Adolescents are in need of role models after whom they can pattern their behaviour.
Teach adolescents the safe use of the Internet.	Safe use of the Internet avoids overuse and possible exposure to inappropriate Web sites.

Adapted from Hockenberry, M. & Wilson, D. (2007). *Wong's nursing care of infants and children* (8th ed.). St. Louis, MO: Mosby.

Older Adults. Nursing interventions for older adults are designed to reduce the risk of falls and other accidents and to compensate for the physiological changes of aging (Box 37–8).

In older adults, diminished eyesight and impaired memory may result in the accidental ingestion of poisonous substances or in an accidental overdose of prescribed medications. To prevent medication errors on the part of clients in the home, recommend the use of medication organizers that are filled once a week by the client or family. These organizers have the day and time on each box so that the client knows when and what to take at any given time (Figure 37–9). This information is particularly useful for clients who may forget whether they have taken their medications. Medication not in use or out of date should be taken to a pharmacy or municipal waste disposal depot for proper disposal (Health Canada, 2005).

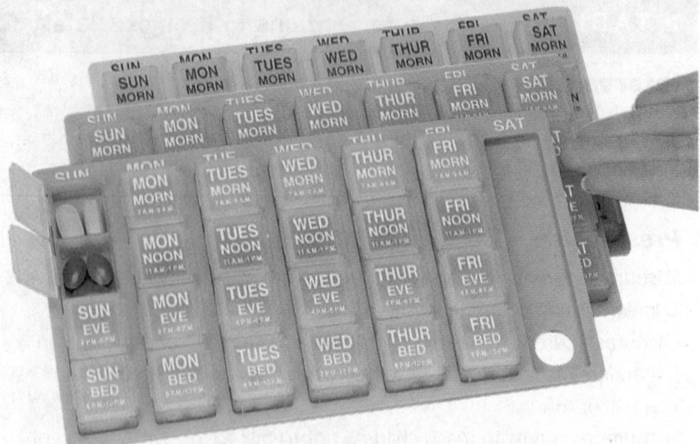

Figure 37-9 The One-Day-At-A-Time medicine organizer. **Source:** Courtesy Apothecary Products, Inc. Burnsville, MN.

BOX 37-8 FOCUS ON OLDER ADULTS

- Older adults experience alterations in vision and hearing. Encourage yearly vision and hearing examinations and frequent cleaning of glasses and hearing aids as a means of preventing falls and burns.
- Older adults may have slower reaction times. Teach clients safety tips for avoiding motor vehicle accidents. Driving may need to be restricted to daylight hours or suspended altogether.
- Range of motion, flexibility, and strength are decreased. Encourage supervised exercise classes for older adults and teach them to seek assistance with household tasks as needed. Assess whether safety features, such as grab bars in the bathroom, are needed.
- Reflexes are slowed, and the ability to respond to multiple stimuli is reduced. Provide adequate, meaningful stimuli but prevent sensory overload.
- Nocturia and incontinence are more frequent in older adults. Institute a regular toileting schedule for the client. A recommended frequency is every 3 hours. Diuretics are generally given in the morning; however, you should speak with your client about his or her response to the drug to determine the best timing. Assistance should be provided, along with adequate lighting, to clients who need to use the bathroom at night.
- Memory may be impaired. Clients should use medication organizers, which can be purchased at any drugstore at a very reasonable cost. These dispensers can be filled once a week with the proper medications to be taken at a specific time during the day.
- The family plays a significant role in the care of older adults. Often, family members serve as informal caregivers for older adults. Twenty-three percent of Canadians between the ages of 45 and 65 provide informal care to an older relative or friend with long-term health problems (Vanier Institute of the Family, 2004). Encourage the family to allow the older adult to remain as independent as possible and to provide help for only those things that are necessary.
- The high prevalence of chronic conditions in older adults results in the use of a high number of prescription and over-the-counter medications. Coupled with age-related changes in pharmacokinetics, this presents a greater risk of serious adverse effects. Medications typically prescribed for older adults include anticholinergics, diuretics, anxiolytic and hypnotic agents, antidepressants, antihypertensives, vasodilators, analgesics, and laxatives, all of which may themselves pose risks or interact with other medications to increase the risk for falls. Review the client's drug profile to ensure that any of the above-noted drugs are used cautiously, and assess the client regularly for any adverse effects that may increase the risk for falls.

Burns and scalds are also more apt to occur with older persons because they may forget to turn off the hot water faucet or become confused when turning the dials on a stove or other heating appliance. Nursing measures for preventing burns are designed to minimize the risk presented by impaired vision. Hot water faucets and dials can be colour coded to make it easier for the adult to know what has been turned on. Lowering the thermostat setting on the water heater reduces the risk of scalding.

Older adults are more likely to have motor vehicle accidents because of three specific physiological changes. First, changes in visual acuity, depth perception, and poor peripheral vision prevent these clients from quickly observing situations in which an accident is likely to occur. Second, decreased hearing acuity alters older adults' ability to hear emergency vehicle sirens or car and truck horns. Third, because of a decreased nervous system response, older adults may be unable to react as quickly as they once could to avoid an accident. A decline in these skills may account for the most common types of accidents, including right-of-way and turning accidents. Educate clients regarding safe driving (e.g., driving shorter distances or only in daylight, using side- and rear-view mirrors carefully, and looking back toward their "blind spot" before changing lanes). If hearing is a problem, clients might try keeping a window rolled down while driving or reducing the volume of the radio or compact disc or cassette player.

Eventually, counselling may be necessary to help a client make the decision of when to stop driving. This is often not an easy decision as it can have implications for the client's self-concept and self-esteem. It also has practical implications—the individual who has been accustomed to driving to daily activities will have to find alternative transportation. As a result, the client may resist giving up his or her driver's license and vehicle. You can support the decision to stop driving by offering anticipatory guidance when an illness with progressive impairment is diagnosed, working with family members to determine how to approach the issue with the client, and providing information about objective assessment of driver ability (DriveABLE, 2007). When your client makes this decision, you should help locate resources in the community that provide transportation.

Pedestrian accidents can be reduced for older adults and persons in all other age groups by persuading them to wear reflectors on garments when walking at night; to stand on the sidewalk and not in the street when waiting to cross; to always cross at corners and not in the middle of the block (particularly on a major street); to cross with the traffic light and not against it; and to look left, right, and left again before entering the street or crosswalk.

Environmental Interventions

You can implement specific interventions aimed at maintaining a safe environment. Particularly important are measures for preventing fires and dealing with them if they do occur. Other environmental interventions include those that address basic needs, physical hazards, and the transmission of pathogens.

Fires. A fire is always possible in the home or health care facility. Accidental home fires typically result from smoking in bed, placing cigarettes in trash cans, cooking accidents, or faulty wiring or appliances. Institutional fires typically result from electrical or anaesthetic-related causes. Although smoking is usually not allowed in the health care setting, smoking-related fires continue to pose a significant risk as a result of unauthorized smoking in bed.

The interventions described here are directed toward fires occurring in health care agencies, but the same principles apply for fires in the home (Box 37–9). Smoke detectors (Figure 37–10) should be placed strategically throughout the home and checked regularly. Multipurpose fire extinguishers should be installed near the kitchen and any workshop areas.

In the home, it is important to have a plan of action in the event of fire, including a route of exit, a location where family members will meet, and the identification of who will help individuals in need of assistance. A fire drill should be held to practise this plan once or twice each year. Although having an escape plan is necessary for all families, it is particularly important for families with disabled individuals. All clients, even young children, should be familiar with the phrase "stop, drop, and roll," which describes the actions to be followed when a client's clothing or skin are burning.

If a fire occurs in a health care agency, you protect clients from immediate injury, report the exact location of the fire, and contain the fire and extinguish it if possible. All personnel are mobilized to evacuate clients. Clients who are close to the fire, regardless of its size, are at risk of injury and should be moved to another area. If a client is receiving oxygen but not life support, discontinue the oxygen because it is combustible and can fuel an existing fire. If the client is on life support, you may need to maintain the client's respiratory status manually with an Ambu-bag (see Chapter 39) until the client is moved away from the fire and the ventilator can be restarted. Ambulatory clients can be directed to walk by themselves to a safe area and, in some cases, may be able to assist in moving clients in wheelchairs. Bedridden clients are generally moved from the scene of a fire on a stretcher, in their bed, or in a wheelchair. If none of these methods is appropriate, clients must be carried from the area. If a client must be carried, be careful not to overextend your physical limits for lifting because an injury to you can result in further injury to the client. If fire department personnel are on the scene, they can help evacuate clients.

After a fire has been reported and clients are out of danger, nurses and other personnel must take measures to contain or put out the fire, such as closing doors and windows, placing wet towels along the base of doors, turning off oxygen and electrical equipment, and using a fire extinguisher. Fire extinguishers are categorized as type A, used for ordinary combustibles (e.g., wood, cloth, paper, and many plastic items); type B, used for flammable liquids (e.g., gasoline, grease, paint, and anaesthetic gas); and type C, used for electrical equipment. The correct use of an extinguisher is discussed in Box 37–10 and demonstrated in Figure 37–11.

The best intervention is to prevent fires. Nursing measures include complying with your agency's smoking policies and keeping combustible materials away from heat sources. Some agencies have fire doors that are held open by magnets and close automatically when a fire alarm sounds. It is important to keep equipment away from these doors.

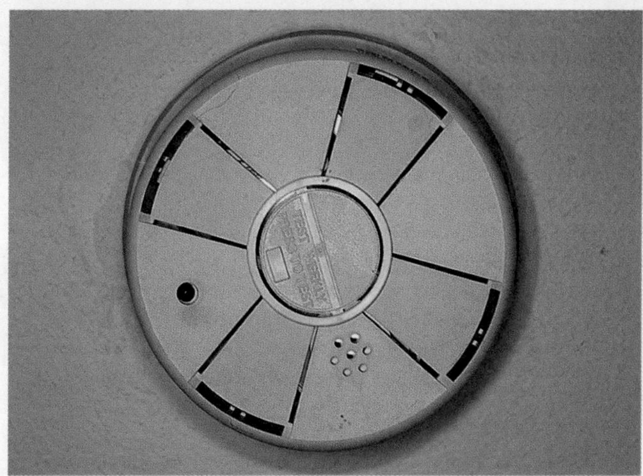

Figure 37-10 Smoke and fire detector.

> **BOX 37-9 Fire Intervention Guidelines for Nurses Working in Health Care Agencies**
>
> - Ensure that the phone number for reporting fires appears on the telephone and is visible at all times.
> - Know your agency's mnemonic (if any), fire drill, and evacuation plan.
> - Know the location of all fire alarms, exits, extinguishers, and the oxygen shut-off.
> - Use the mnemonic RACE to set priorities in case of fire:
>
>   **R**escue and remove all clients in immediate danger.
>
>   **A**ctivate the alarm. Always do this before attempting to extinguish even a minor fire.
>
>   **C**onfine the fire by closing doors and windows and turning off oxygen and electrical equipment.
>
>   **E**xtinguish the fire using an extinguisher (see Box 37–10).

Other Environmental Interventions. You can contribute to a safer environment by helping your clients meet basic needs related to oxygen, humidity, nutrition, and temperature. To ensure that oxygen availability is not threatened, recommend that clients living at home have annual inspections of the heating system, chimney, and appliances. Carbon monoxide detectors are available for home use at a reasonable cost but should not be considered a replacement for the proper use and maintenance of fuel-burning appliances. To achieve a comfortable level of humidity in the home, clients can attach a humidifier to the furnace or, in the case of clients who have upper respiratory tract infections, use a room humidifier where they sleep. Teach basic techniques for food handling (e.g., handwashing and checking for spoilage) and preparation (e.g., keeping food refrigerated before serving) so that nutritional needs are met safely. It is also helpful for family members to date leftovers. Older adults who have difficulty preparing their own food may benefit from Meals on Wheels, an organization that provides fresh, nutritious meals in the home. Client education for older adults and clients who enjoy outdoor activities should include ways to prevent and treat frostbite, hypothermia, heatstroke, and heat exhaustion (see Chapter 31).

Adequate lighting and security measures in and around the home, including the use of night lights, exterior lighting, and

BOX 37-10 CLIENT TEACHING

Correct Use of a Fire Extinguisher in the Home

Objectives

- Client will correctly place the extinguisher in the home.
- Client will describe when it is appropriate to use a home fire extinguisher.
- Client will demonstrate the correct technique when using a fire extinguisher.
- Client will state when fire extinguishers need to be replaced.

Teaching Strategies

- Discuss correct location of the fire extinguisher. It is recommended that one be placed on each level of the home, near an exit, in clear view, away from stoves and heating appliances, and above the reach of small children. Keep a fire extinguisher in the kitchen, near the furnace, and in the garage. The instructions should be read when the extinguisher is purchased and kept available for periodic review.
- Describe the steps to take before using the extinguisher. The client should attempt to fight the fire only after all occupants have left the home, the fire department has been called, the fire is confined to a small area, an exit route is readily available, the extinguisher is the right type for the fire (see the text for a description of extinguisher types), and the client knows how to use the extinguisher.
- Instruct the client to memorize the mnemonic PASS: **P**ull the pin to unlock handle; **A**im low at the base of the fire; **S**queeze the handle; and **S**weep the unit from side to side (see Figure 37–11).

Evaluation

- Observe the client correctly installing an extinguisher in the home.
- Ask the client to correctly list the steps to take before attempting to use an extinguisher.
- Ask the client to demonstrate the correct use of the extinguisher while reciting the instructions with the mnemonic PASS.

Adapted from National Safety Council. (2002). *Home fire prevention and preparedness fact sheet.* Itasca, IL: Author.

good-quality locks on windows and doors, enable clients to reduce the risk of injury from crime. Local police departments and community organizations often have safety classes available to teach residents how to take precautions to minimize the chance of becoming involved in a crime. Some useful tips include always parking the car near a bright light or in a busy public area, carrying a whistle attached to the car keys, keeping car doors locked while driving, and always paying attention while driving to notice if anyone starts to follow the car. Clients should be encouraged to join block associations and work closely with law enforcement personnel to reduce crime in their neighbourhoods.

To prevent the transmission of pathogens, you teach aseptic practices. Clients and family members need to learn thorough hand hygiene (handwashing or the use of hand rub) and when to use it (e.g., before and after caring for a family member, before food preparation, before preparing a medication for a family member, and after contacting any body fluids). When clients require dressing changes or the use of syringes and needles, families should be shown how to properly dispose of contaminated items in the home. Most communities have regulations for the disposal of biohazardous waste.

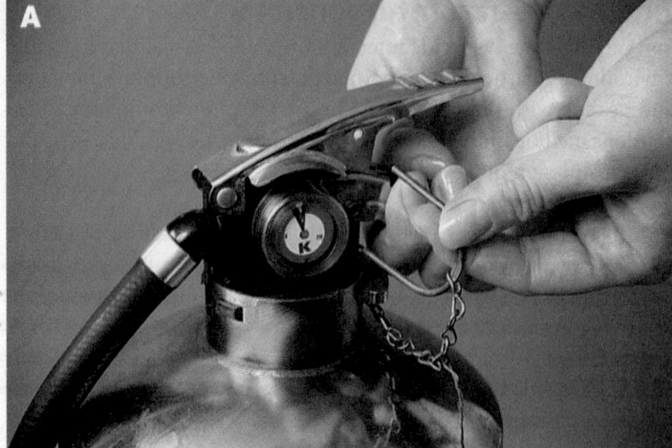

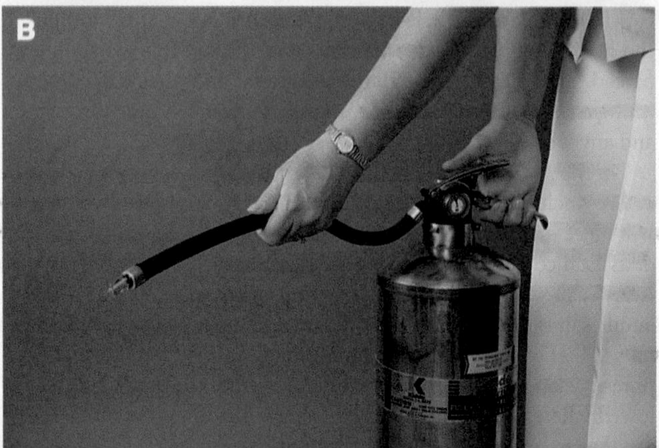

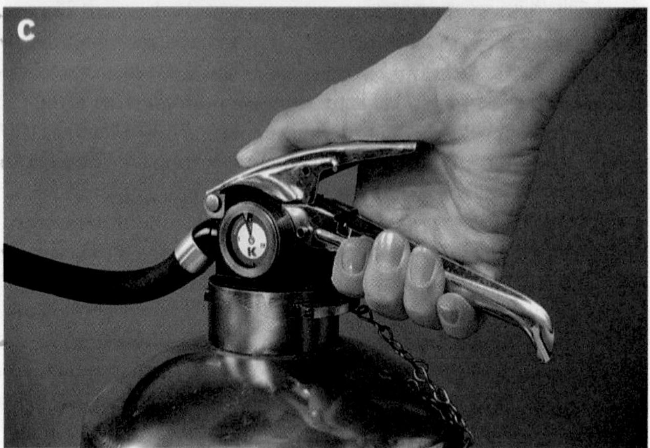

Figure 37-11 The correct use of a fire extinguisher. A, Pull the pin. B, Aim at the base of the fire. C, Squeeze the handle. Sweep from side to side to coat the area evenly. **Source:** Adapted from Sorrentino, S. A. (1999). *Mosby's assisting with patient care.* St. Louis, MO: Mosby.

Limiting Specific Risks to Client Safety

A number of specific safety measures are applicable to clients in the home or health care agency. Take actions to help clients avoid injuries related to falls, the use of restraints and side rails, electrical hazards, and radiation. Special precautions are necessary to prevent injury in clients susceptible to having seizures.

Falls. Easy modifications in the home and health care environment can reduce the risk of falls (Table 37–3). A heavy or debilitated client in a bed or wheelchair or on a toilet should be properly supported

➤ TABLE 37-3 Measures to Prevent Falls by Older Adults

Measure	Rationale
Stairs	
Install treads with a uniform depth of 22.5 cm and 22.5-cm risers (vertical face of steps).	If stairs are of uniform size, older adults do not need to continually adjust their vision.
Install uniform-textured or plain-coloured surfaces on each tread, and mark the edges of treads with a contrasting colour.	Uniform textures or colour help to decrease vertigo. Marking the edges of treads provides obvious visual cues to end of stairs.
Ensure proper lighting of each tread. Block glare from the sun or a light bulb with translucent shades or a screen, or use lower-wattage or nonglare bulbs.	Older adults' vision is unable to adjust quickly to changes in lighting.
Ensure adequate headroom so that clients do not have to duck to negotiate stairs.	Sudden changes in head position may result in dizziness.
Remove protruding objects from staircase walls.	Decreased peripheral vision may prevent the client from seeing an object.
Maintain outdoor walkways and stairs in good condition and free of holes, cracks, and splinters.	Decreased visual acuity can prevent the client from seeing any structural defect.
Handrails	
Install a smooth but slip-resistant handrail at least 5 cm from wall.	A 5-cm distance allows the client to grasp the handrail firmly for support.
Secure the handrail firmly so that the client's weight is supported, especially at bottom and top of stairway.	Older adults have the greatest risk of falling at top and bottom of stairs because their centre of gravity is being shifted and balance is unstable.
Install grab rails in bathroom near the toilet and tub. Install an elevated toilet seat with armrests and nonslip strips.	These measures enable the client to have support while rising from a sitting to standing position.
Floors	
Ensure that clients wear properly fitting shoes or slippers with a nonskid surface.	Such footwear reduces the chances of slipping.
Secure all carpeting, mats, and tiles; place nonskid backing under small rugs.	A sudden slip may cause dizziness and an inability to regain balance.
Place bath mats or nonskid, coloured strips on bathtub or shower stall floors and on the floor in front of the toilet.	Wet surfaces increase the risk of falling.
Secure electrical cords against the baseboards.	This measure prevents tripping.
Maintain proper illumination inside and outside where the client moves and walks.	This measure reduces the risk of falling due to eye strain.
Health Care Facility	
Orientation	
Place disoriented clients in a room near the nurses' station.	Proximity provides for more frequent observation by nursing staff.
Supervise confused clients closely.	Confused clients often attempt to wander out of bed or the room.
Show the client how to use the call light at the bedside and in the bathroom, and place it within easy reach.	The location and use of the call light are essential to client safety.
Place bedside tables and overbed tables close to the client.	This measure prevents the client from searching or overreaching for items such as eyeglasses, dentures, a hearing aid, or the telephone.
Remove clutter from bedside tables, hallways, bathrooms, and grooming areas.	This measure eliminates potential hazards and promotes client independence.
Leave one side rail up and one down on the side where the oriented and ambulatory client gets out of bed.	The client can use the side rail for support when getting in and out of bed and to position self once in bed.
Transport	
Lock beds and wheelchairs when transferring a client from a bed to a wheelchair or back to bed.	The locks provide stability and support during transfer.
Place side rails in the up position and secure safety straps around the client when transporting him or her by stretcher.	This measure prevents the client from rolling off the stretcher.

Modified from Chang, J. T., Morton, S. C., Rubenstein, L. Z., Mojica, W. A., Maglione, M., Suttorp, M. J., et al. (2004). Interventions for the prevention of falls in older adults: Systematic review with meta-analysis of randomized clinical trials. *British Medical Journal, 328*, 680.

and secured. Side rails may be necessary. Safety bars near toilets, locks on beds and wheelchairs, and call lights are additional safety features found in health care settings (Figures 37–12 and 37–13). Excess furniture and equipment should be removed. Weakened clients should wear rubber-soled shoes or slippers when walking or transferring. For clients who use assistive aids such as canes, crutches, or walkers, it is important to routinely check the condition of rubber tips and the integrity of the aid.

In the health care setting, injuries may occur when clients attempt to address self-care needs independently despite encouragement to call you for assistance. One way to minimize the occurrence of such incidents is to check in on clients frequently during the day. A formal routine of nursing rounds, during which nurses visit clients every hour and provide necessary assistance, has been found to decrease the incidence of falls and increase client satisfaction (Box 37–11).

The risk of injury in the home may be reduced by removing all obstacles from halls and other heavily travelled areas. Necessary objects such as clocks, glasses, tissues, and medications should remain on bedside tables within reach of the client but out of the reach of children. Care should also be taken to ensure that end tables are secure and have stable, straight legs. Nonessential items should be placed in drawers to eliminate clutter. If small area rugs are used, they should be secured with a nonslip pad or skid-resistant adhesive strips. Carpeting on the stairs should be secured with carpet tacks.

Restraints. A **restraint** is a physical, chemical, or environmental means of controlling an individual's behaviour or actions (College of Nurses of Ontario, 2005). The use of restraints is controversial as they have been associated with negative consequences including injury and death. You must be familiar with the legal aspects of restraint use. You also need to follow guidelines and standards provided by your provincial nursing governing body as well as policies and procedures set by your clinical practice setting. A least-restraint approach is recommended to ensure highest-quality care. This approach ensures that all alternative interventions are attempted before moving to the use of restraints, and that the form of restraint selected is the one that addresses a client's needs in the least restrictive way (College of Nurses of Ontario, 2005).

It is imperative that you try alternative measures (Box 37–12) as the application of a restraint should always be a measure of last resort. The use of restraints must be guided by a client's needs and requires a thorough assessment by you and other members of the multidisciplinary team involved in the client's care. A restraint-use algorithm provides evidence-informed guidelines for determining whether a restraint is appropriate and what interventions might be used (Figure 37–14).

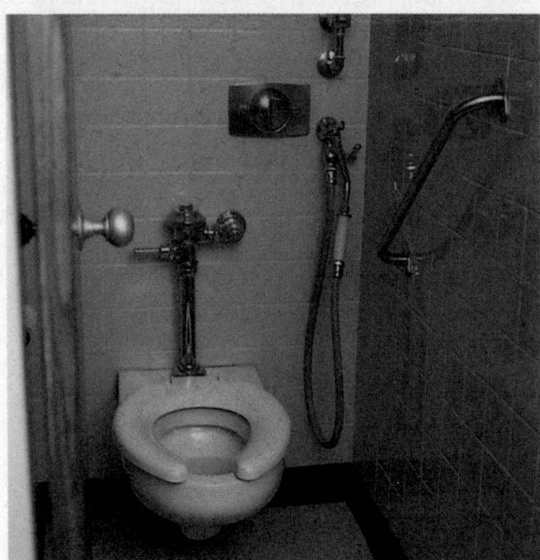

Figure 37-12 Safety bars beside a toilet and shower.

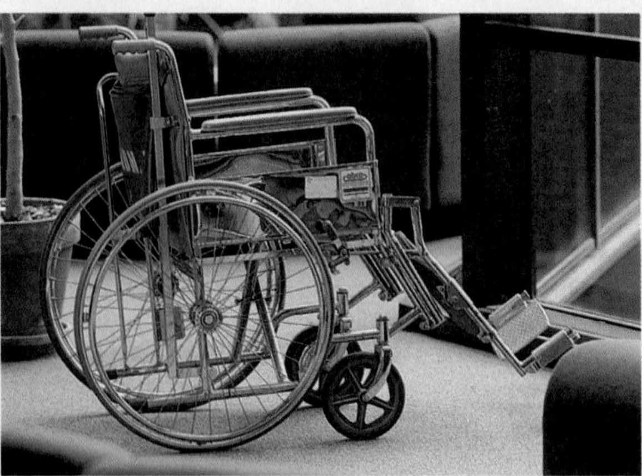

Figure 37-13 Safety locks on a wheelchair.

BOX 37-11 RESEARCH HIGHLIGHT

Effects of Nursing Rounds

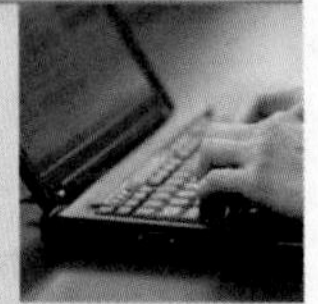

Research Focus

Hospitalized clients often require assistance with basic activities of daily living such as eating, toileting, and ambulating. Clients usually communicate their needs by use of a call light. Not meeting a client's needs in a timely fashion decreases client satisfaction and places him or her at greater risk for injury. You play a key role in the prevention of falls and injuries related to falls.

Research Abstract

Meade, Bursell and Ketelsen (2006) wanted to know if making nursing rounds every 1 or 2 hours would reduce call light usage, increase client satisfaction, and reduce the frequency of client falls. During rounds, the following actions were performed for each client: pain management, toileting, positioning, and placing items such as the call light, telephone, television remote, bed light switch, tissues, and water within reach and the garbage can next to bed. In addition, before leaving the room, the nurse asked, "Is there anything else I can do for you before I leave? I have time while I'm here in the room." The client was also told that a staff member would be back in 1 (or 2) hours.

A 6-week quasi-experimental study was conducted on 27 nursing units in 14 hospitals. Researchers took baseline data on call light usage during the initial 2 weeks. Performing rounds at set intervals, including specific nursing actions, was associated with statistically significant reduced client call light usage, increased client satisfaction, and, in the group receiving rounds hourly, decreased client falls.

Evidence-Informed Practice

- Nursing rounds performed at set intervals positively affect client satisfaction and safety and lead to fewer distractions for the staff.
- Nurses' ability to meet clients' needs affects clients' perception of the quality of nursing care.
- Nurses can anticipate client needs by performing rounds, including specific nursing actions, at 1-hour intervals.

References: Meade, C. M., Bursell, A. L., & Ketelsen, L. (2006). Effects of nursing rounds on patients' call light use, satisfaction, and safety. *American Journal of Nursing*, *106*(9), 58–70.

> **BOX 37-12 Alternatives to Restraints**
>
> - Orient clients and families to their environment; explain all procedures and treatments.
> - Provide companionship and supervision; use trained sitters or adjust staffing.
> - Offer diversionary activities, such as listening to music or having something to hold; enlist support and input from the family.
> - Assign confused or disoriented clients to rooms near the nurses' station; observe these clients frequently.
> - Use calm, simple statements and physical cues as needed.
> - Use de-escalation, time outs, and other verbal intervention techniques when managing aggressive behaviours.
> - Provide appropriate visual and auditory stimuli (e.g., family pictures, a clock, or a radio).
> - Remove cues that promote leaving (e.g., sight of elevators, stairs, or street clothes).
> - Promote relaxation techniques and normal sleep patterns.
> - Institute exercise and ambulation schedules as allowed by clients' conditions; consult a physiotherapist for mobility and exercise programs.
> - Attend to the client's toileting, food, and fluid needs.
> - Camouflage IV lines with clothing, a stockinette, or a Kling dressing.
> - Evaluate all medications the clients are receiving, and ensure effective pain management.
> - Reassess the physical status of clients, and review laboratory findings connected with their health.
>
> Adapted from Joint Commission Resources. (2006). *Strategies for avoiding restraint related errors*. Retrieved from http://www.jcrinc.com; and American Nurses Association. (2006). Geriatric nursing resources for care of older adults. *Physical restraints*. Retrieved from http://www.geronurseonline.org/index

The use of any type of restraint involves a psychological adjustment for the client and family. If restraints must be used, assist family members and the client by explaining the purpose of the restraints, the client's expected care while restrained, the precautions to be taken to avoid injury, and the temporary and protective aspects of restraints. Informed consent from family members may also be required before using restraints, as is the case in long-term care settings. The nursing story in Box 37–13 demonstrates family involvement in a decision about restraint.

A **physical restraint** is a mechanical or physical device that is used to immobilize a client or extremity, restricts the freedom of movement or normal access to a person's body, and is not a usual part of treatment plans indicated by the person's condition or symptoms (Zusman, 2001). The optimal goal with all clients is to avoid the use of physical restraints, and alternatives must always be considered. However, clients who are at risk for injury to self or others may need physical restraints temporarily. Alternative forms of restraint should always be considered as well. Physical restraints do not prevent falls or injury and may actually increase the severity of an injury (Registered Nurses Association of Ontario, 2005).

Whenever clients are physically restrained, there is a natural tendency for them to try to remove the restraint, and this can lead to injury. Restrained clients can easily become entangled in a restraint device when attempting to get out of it. In some cases, death has resulted from strangulation or asphyxiation. As a result, long-term care facilities and many health care facilities have banned the use of the jacket (vest) restraint. The use of any physical restraint is also associated with serious complications, including pressure ulcers; constipation; pneumonia; urinary and fecal incontinence; and urinary retention (see Chapter 46). Contractures, nerve damage, and circulatory impairment are also potential hazards. In addition, restrained clients can experience humiliation, fear, anger, and a loss of self-esteem.

> **safety alert** Routine assessment of a client in a physical restraint is critical to prevent injury. The restraint must be moved and the client repositioned at regular intervals, according to your agency's policy. Restraints should be used only after other alternatives have been tried, and the least restrictive method of restraint should be used. The use of restraints must be part of the client's medical treatment. Restraints are considered a short-term intervention, and once they have been applied, regular assessments are needed to determine whether they should be continued. All assessments and interventions must be clearly documented according to your agency's policy.

For legal purposes, you must know your agency's policy and procedures for the appropriate use and monitoring of physical restraints. The use of a restraint must be clinically justified and be a part of the client's prescribed medical treatment and care plan. A physician's order may be required, depending on provincial or territorial legislation and agency policy—in some settings, you may order restraints. Requirements for ordering restraints may vary depending on the circumstances of a client's situation and the type of restraint needed; you must comply with your agency's policies. Assessment of clients who are restrained must be ongoing. Proper documentation, including the behaviours that necessitated the application of restraints, the procedure used in restraining, the condition of the body part restrained (e.g., circulation to the client's hand), and the evaluation of the client response, is essential. Remove the restraints periodically and assess the client to determine if the restraints continue to be needed.

Skill 37–1 includes guidelines for the proper use and application of restraints. Use of restraints must meet the following objectives:

- Reduce the risk of client injury
- Prevent the interruption of therapy, such as traction, IV infusion, nasogastric tube feeding, or Foley catheterization
- Prevent the confused or combative client from removing life-support equipment
- Reduce the risk of injury to others by the client

In keeping with current trends toward health promotion, improved assessment techniques and modifications of the environment are offered as alternatives to physical restraints. An **Ambularm** is a device worn on the leg that signals when the leg is in a dependent position, such as over the side rail or on the floor (Figure 37–15). The device is used for clients who tend to climb out of bed unassisted but are in danger of falling. The **Bed-Check** bed exit alarm system (Figure 37–16) uses a weight-sensitive sensor mat that can be placed on the client's mattress or chair. This device sounds an audible alarm at the bedside when pressure is released off the sensor mat; it can be designed to signal at the central nurses' station so that staff are alerted quickly when the client is out of bed. There are also alarms that can be placed on doors to alert staff or family members when a confused or disoriented client, prone to wandering, opens a door.

Another alternative form of restraint is the Posey Bed Enclosure (Figure 37–17), a soft-sided, self-contained enclosed bed. It allows for freedom of movement and thus reduces the side effects caused by physical restraints such as pressure ulcers and loss of dignity. A vinyl top covers the padded upper frame of the bed, and a nylon-net canopy surrounds the mattress and completely encloses the client in the bed. Zippers on the four sides of the enclosure provide access to the client. The Posey Bed Enclosure works well for clients who are restless and unpredictable, cognitively impaired, and at risk for injury if they were to fall or get out of bed, such as clients on anticoagulant therapy at risk for intracranial bleed. The bed may also be a safer alternative to side rails.

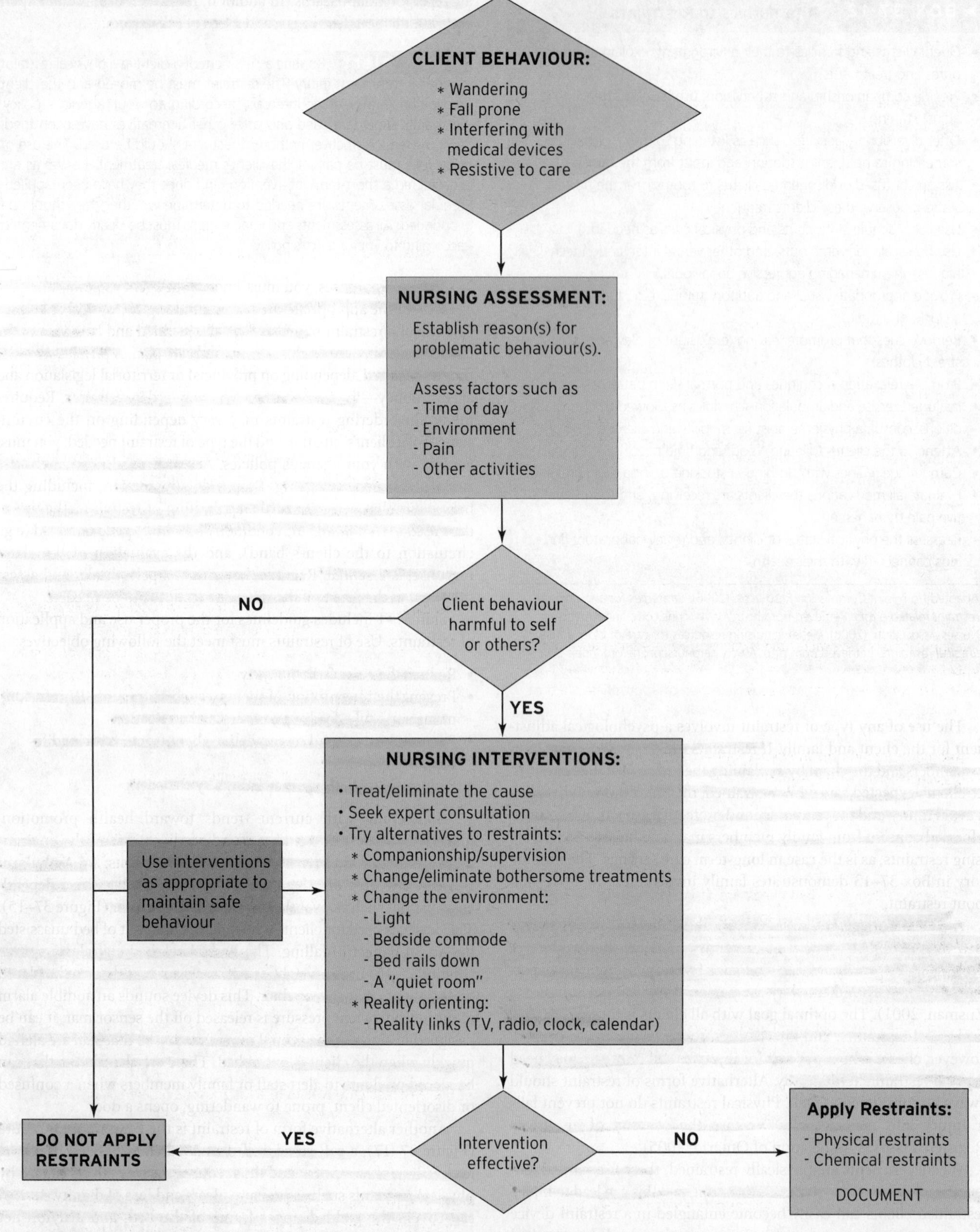

Figure 37-14 Algorithm for the use of restraints. **Source:** Developed from Ledford, L., & Mentals, J. (Written 1996; revised November 2005). *"Restraints"—A research-based protocol.* Iowa City, IA: University of Iowa Gerontological Nursing Interventions Research Center. © The University of Iowa Gerontological Nursing Interventions Research Center, Research Translation and Dissemination Core.

BOX 37-13 NURSING STORY

David's Mittens

Katherine has been caring for David, a 6-month-old boy who has been hospitalized for several weeks. David has a complex health problem and is currently experiencing severely dry, itchy skin associated with his illness. Katherine has noticed that anti-itch medications seem to decrease David's discomfort but do not eliminate the itch entirely. As a result, he continues to scratch, and even with regularly trimmed nails, he has scratched himself hard enough to cause bleeding. David's mother plays with him to distract him from the itch, and when he tries to scratch, she gently holds his hands. However, she cannot be with David at all times in the hospital. Another concern is that David scratches his skin while sleeping.

Katherine discusses the situation with David's mom, and they decide to use mitten restraints to protect David's skin. They agree to use the restraints when David sleeps and when he is awake and alone. Katherine notes this decision in David's care plan, implements the required documentation according to her hospital's policy, and applies the restraints according to the proper procedure.

Katherine returns to work after 2 days off and finds that David's restraints have been applied improperly, leaving him at risk for injury. Recognizing that this may reflect a knowledge gap on the part of staff involved in David's care, she places a copy of the instructions for the proper application of restraints at David's bedside, where they will be more easily seen. Katherine also notes in David's care plan the need for proper use of restraints.

Reassessment of the need for the mitten restraints is performed daily and includes feedback from David's mother. Volunteers arrange to visit him at the times he is most likely to be awake and alone, thus minimizing the need for restraints. Regular assessment and documentation are maintained according to the hospital's protocol. With continued treatment of David's illness, his skin condition improves, and within 5 days, the mitten restraints are discontinued.

Katherine and David's mom are pleased to see that David sustained no further scratch injuries once the restraints were implemented. David's mom states that although she does not like to see her baby restrained, she knows it is in his best interest. She appreciates the volunteers' efforts to spend time with David as well as everyone's diligence in applying the restraints properly. Katherine reflects upon this situation and decides that the next time she implements the use of restraints, she will post instructions for their use at the bedside immediately upon implementation.

➤ SKILL 37-1 Applying Physical Restraints

Delegation Considerations

The application of physical restraints can be delegated to trained unregulated care providers (UCPs). However, you are always responsible for the assessment of a client's safety needs, selection of appropriate alternative interventions, evaluation of the effectiveness of restraint, and ongoing assessment to prevent complications of restraint use.

- Ask the UCP to inform you of any redness, excoriation, or constriction of circulation under the restraint.
- Ask the UCP to request assistance if the client has any mobility restrictions that might affect how to remove or reapply a restraint.
- Instruct the UCP when and how to change the client's position and to provide range of motion exercises, skin care, toileting, and opportunities for socialization.

Equipment

- Proper restraint: mitten, belt, extremity
- Padding (if needed)

Procedure

STEPS	RATIONALE
1. Assess whether the client needs a restraint. Does the client continually try to interrupt needed therapy? Is the client at risk for injuring self or others?	• Restraints are used only when other measures have failed to prevent the interruption of therapy such as traction, IV infusions, or nasogastric tube feedings; to prevent a confused or combative client from self-injury by falling out of bed or a wheelchair; to prevent a client from removing a urinary catheter, surgical drain, or life-support equipment; and to reduce the risk of injury to others by the client.
2. Assess the client's behaviour, such as confusion, disorientation, agitation, restlessness, combativeness, or inability to follow directions. Consult with a gerontological nurse specialist if available.	• If client's behaviour continues despite attempts to eliminate the cause of behaviour, use of physical restraint may be necessary.
3. Review your agency's policies regarding restraints. Consider the purpose, type, location, and duration of restraint. Determine whether signed consent for the use of restraint is needed.	• The least restrictive type of restraint must be ordered. A physician's order may be necessary—check provincial or territorial legislation and agency policy. Because restraints limit the client's ability to move freely, you must make clinical judgements appropriate to the client's condition and the agency policy.
4. Review manufacturer's instructions before entering the client's room. Determine the most appropriate size restraint.	• You should be familiar with all devices used for client care and protection. Incorrect application of a restraining device may result in client injury or death.
5. Perform hand hygiene and gather equipment.	• Reduces transmission of microorganisms; promotes organization.
6. Introduce yourself to the client and family. Assess their feelings about restraint use. Explain that restraint is temporary and designed to protect the client from injury.	• Helps minimize client anxiety during the application of the device, and helps minimize family concern during the maintenance of restraint.

Continued

➤ SKILL 37-1 Applying Physical Restraints *continued*

STEPS	RATIONALE
7. Inspect the area where the restraint is to be placed. Assess the condition of skin underlying where the restraint is to be applied.	• Restraints may compress and interfere with the functioning of devices or tubes. Inspection provides baseline assessment data regarding skin integrity.
8. Approach the client in a calm, confident manner. Check the client's identification using two identifiers. Explain what you plan to do.	• Reduces client anxiety and promotes cooperation.
9. Adjust the bed to proper height, and lower the side rail on the side of client contact.	• Allows you to use proper body mechanics and prevent injury.
10. Provide privacy. Make sure the client is comfortable and in proper body alignment. Drape client as needed.	• Privacy protects self-esteem. Proper body alignment promotes comfort and prevents contractures and neurovascular injury.
11. Pad the skin and bony prominences (if necessary) before applying restraints.	• Padding reduces friction and pressure on skin and underlying tissues.
12. Apply the appropriate-size restraint, making sure it is not over an IV line or other device (e.g., dialysis shunt) and that it does not cover the client's identification or allergy bracelet.	• IV lines and other therapeutic devices may become occluded. The client's ID and allergy information must always be visible and accessible.
A. **Belt restraint:** This device secures the client to a bed or stretcher. Apply it over the client's clothes or gown. Remove wrinkles from the front and back of the restraint while placing it around the client's waist. Bring ties through slots in the belt. Avoid placing the belt across the chest or too tightly across the abdomen (see Step 12A illustration).	• Restrains centre of gravity and prevents the client from rolling off the stretcher or sitting up while on stretcher or from falling out of bed. Tight application may interfere with ventilation.
B. **Extremity (ankle or wrist) restraint:** This restraint is designed to immobilize one or all extremities. Commercially available limb restraints are composed of sheepskin or foam padding (see Step 12B illustration). The limb restraint is wrapped around the wrist or ankle with the soft part toward the skin and is secured snugly in place with Velcro straps.	• Maintains immobilization of the extremity to protect the client from injury from a fall or accidental removal of a therapeutic device (e.g., IV tube or Foley catheter). Tight application may interfere with circulation.

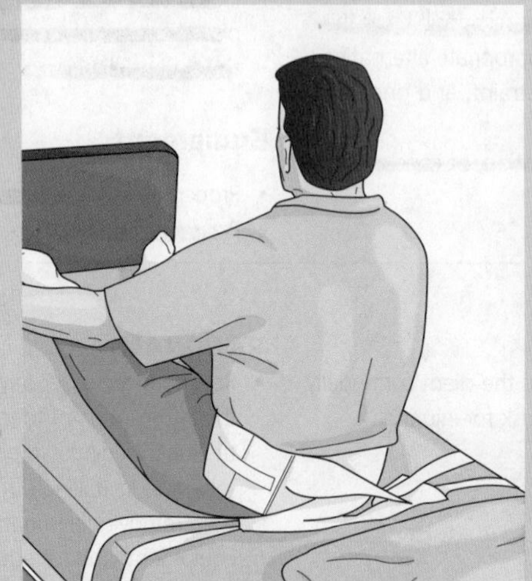

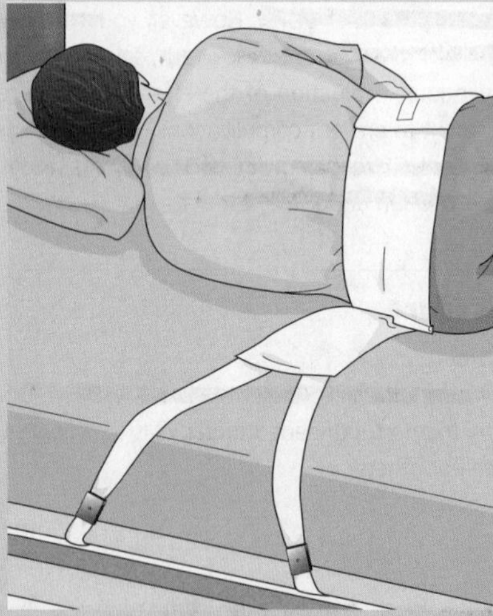

Step 12A Belt restraint is tied to the bed frame and to an area that does not cause the restraint to tighten when the side rail is raised or lowered. **Source:** From Sorrentino, S. A. (2004). *Mosby's textbook for nursing assistants* (6th ed., p. 4). St. Louis, MO: Mosby.

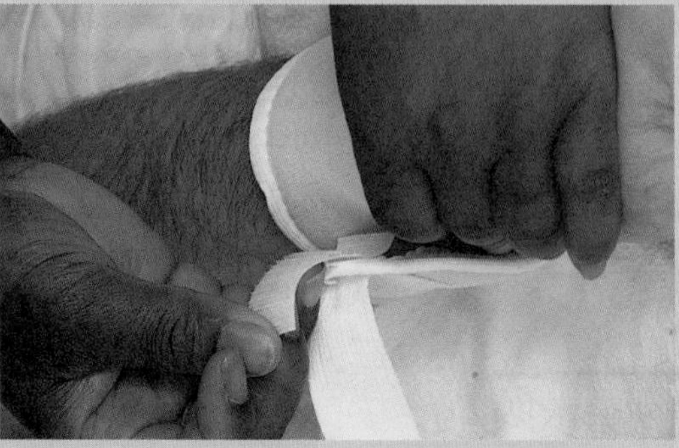

Step 12B Extremity restraint being applied to the wrist.

➤ SKILL 37-1 Applying Physical Restraints *continued*

STEPS	RATIONALE
C. **Mitten restraint:** This thumbless mitten device is used to restrain the client's hands (see Step 12C illustration). Place a hand in the mitten, being sure the mitten end is brought all the way over the wrist.	• Prevents clients from dislodging invasive equipment, removing dressings, or scratching, yet allows greater movement than a wrist restraint.
D. **Elbow restraint:** This piece of fabric with slots has tongue blades placed so that the elbow joint remains rigid (see Step 12D illustration).	• Commonly used with infants and children to prevent elbow flexion (e.g., when an IV line is in place).
E. **Mummy restraint:** The mummy restraint consists of a blanket or sheet. It is opened on the bed or crib with one corner folded toward the centre. The child is placed on the blanket with shoulders at the fold and feet toward the opposite corner (see Step 12E-1 illustration). With the child's right arm straight down against body, the right side of blanket is pulled firmly across the right shoulder and chest and secured beneath the left side of body (see Step 12E-2 illustration). The left arm is placed straight against the body, and the left side of the blanket is brought across the shoulder and chest and locked beneath child's body on the right side (see Step 12E-3 illustration). The lower corner is folded and brought over the body and tucked or fastened securely with safety pins (see Step 12E-4 illustration).	• Maintains short-term restraint of small child or infant for an examination or treatment involving the head and neck. Effectively controls movement of torso and extremities.

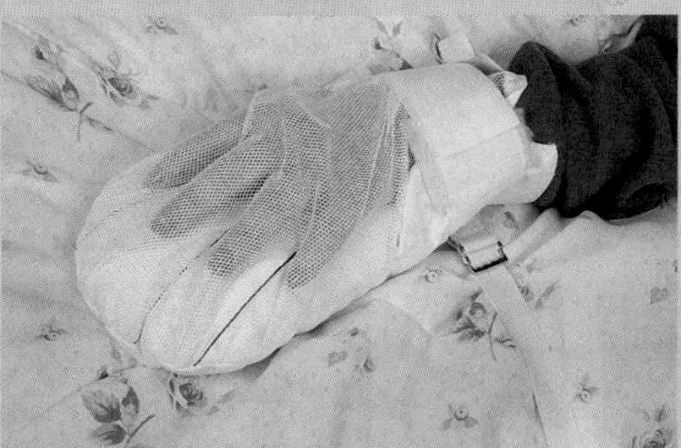

Step 12C Mitten restraint.

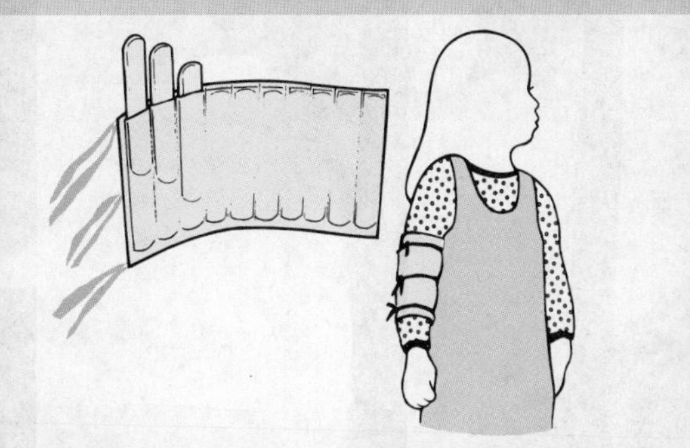

Step 12D Elbow restraint.

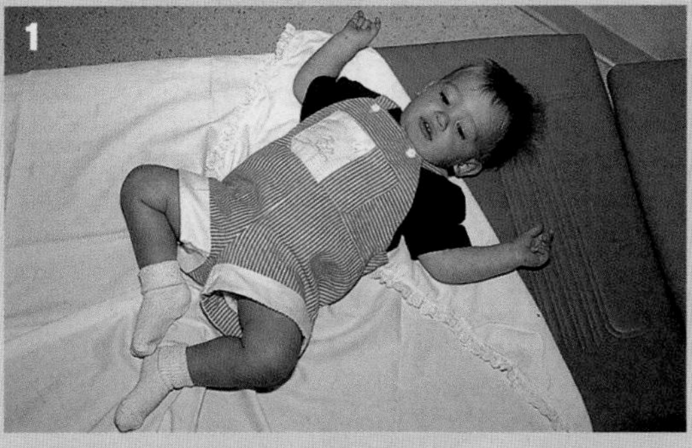

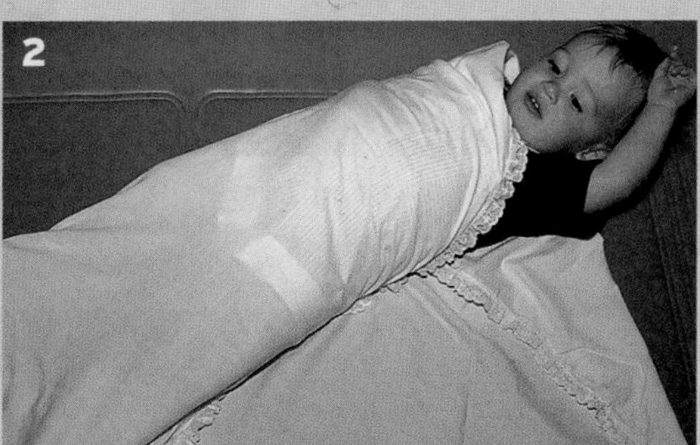

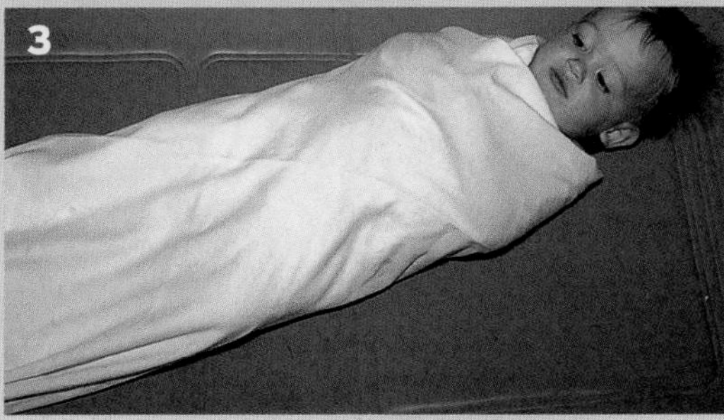

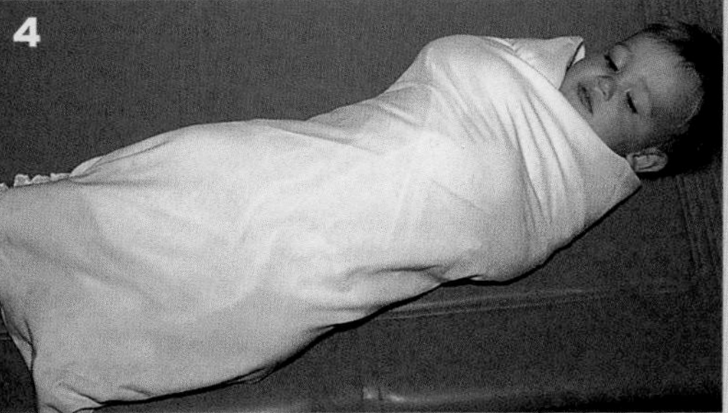

Step 12E Mummy restraint.

Continued

➤ SKILL 37-1 Applying Physical Restraints *continued*

STEPS	RATIONALE
13. Attach restraints to the bed frame, which moves when the head of the bed is raised or lowered (see Step 13 illustration).	• Client may be injured if restraint is secured to side rail and it is lowered.
Critical Decision Point: Do not attach end of restraint to side rails.	
14. Secure restraints with a quick-release tie (see Step 14 illustration). Do not tie in a knot.	• Allows for quick release in an emergency.
15. Insert two fingers under the secured restraint (see Step 15 illustration).	• A tight restraint may cause constriction and impede circulation. Checking for constriction prevents neurovascular injury.
16. The proper placement of the restraint, skin integrity, pulses, temperature, colour, and sensation of the restrained body part should be assessed at least every hour or according to your agency's policy.	• Frequent assessments prevent complications, such as suffocation, skin breakdown, and impaired circulation.
17. Restraints should be removed at regular intervals (see agency policy). If the client is violent and noncompliant, remove one restraint at a time or have staff assist while removing the restraints. The client should not be left unattended at this time.	• Provides opportunity to change client's position and perform full range of motion, toileting, and exercise and to provide food or fluids.

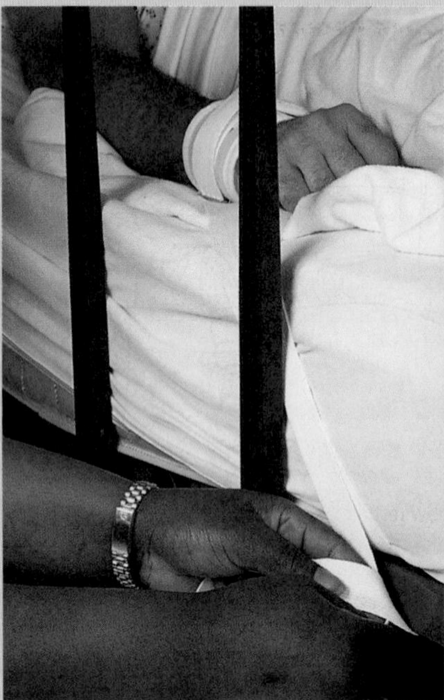

Step 13 Tie restraint strap to the bed frame.

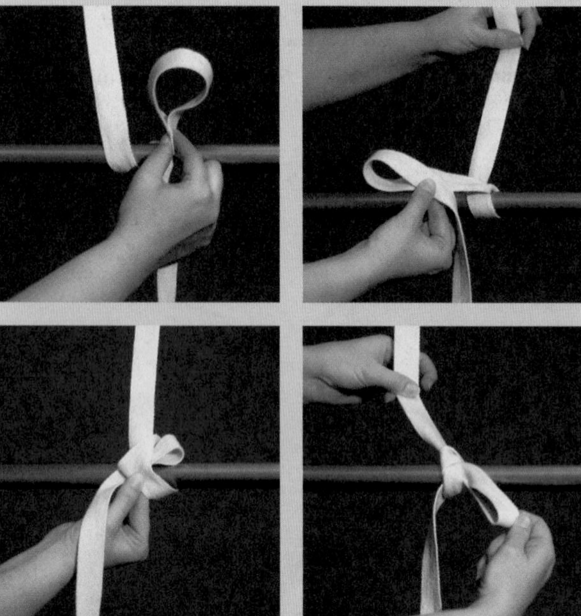

Step 14 The Posey quick-release tie. **Source:** Courtesy JT Posey Co., Arcadia, CA.

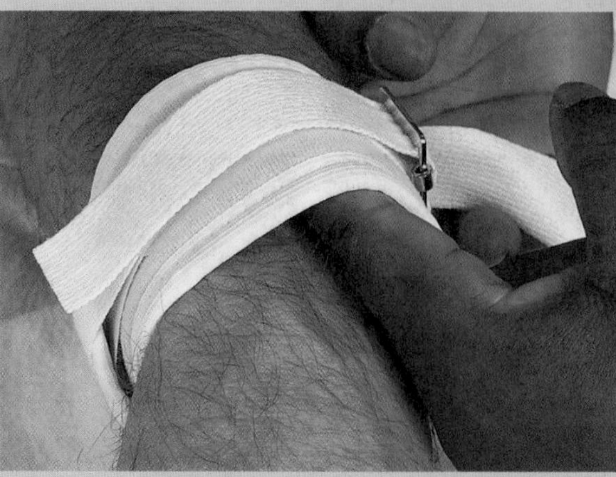

Step 15 Place two fingers under the restraint to check tightness.

SKILL 37-1 Applying Physical Restraints continued

Steps	Rationale
18. Secure a call light or intercom system within the client's reach.	• Allows client, family, or caregiver to obtain assistance quickly.
19. Leave the bed or chair with wheels locked. The bed should be in its lowest position.	• Locked wheels prevent the bed or chair from moving if the client attempts to get out. If the client falls when the bed is in lowest position, the chances of injury are reduced.
20. Perform hand hygiene.	• Reduces transmission of microorganisms.
21. Reassess the client's status and needs.	
A. Inspect the client for any injuries, including all hazards of immobility, while restraints are in use.	• Client should be free of injury and not exhibit any signs of immobility complications.
B. Observe IV catheters, urinary catheters, and drainage tubes to ensure that they are positioned correctly and that therapy remains uninterrupted.	• Reinsertion can be uncomfortable and can increase the risk of infection or interrupt therapy.
C. Regularly reassess the client's need for continued use of the restraint (for medical or surgical reason) with the intent of discontinuing the restraint at the earliest possible time (see agency-specific policy).	• Use of restraints should be seen as a temporary measure and discontinued as soon as possible (College of Nurses of Ontario, 2005).
D. Provide appropriate sensory stimulation and reorient client as needed.	• Use of restraints can further increase disorientation.

Unexpected Outcomes and Related Interventions

Client Has Signs of Impaired Skin Integrity

- Assess skin and provide appropriate therapy.
- Notify the physician and reassess the need for continued use of the restraint.
- Ensure the correct application of restraint. Pad the skin under the restraint, and remove restraint more often.

Client Has Altered Neurovascular Status in an Extremity (Cyanosis, Pallor, Coldness of Skin, or Complaints of Tingling, Pain, or Numbness)

- Remove the restraint immediately, stay with the client, and notify the physician.
- Protect the extremity from further injury (e.g., pressure from tubing or encumbrance, positioning).

Client Is Increasingly Confused, Disoriented, or Agitated

- Identify the reason for this change in behaviour, and attempt to eliminate the cause.
- Attempt a restraint alternative.

Client Escapes From Restraint Device and Suffers Fall or Injury

- Attend to the client's immediate physical needs, and inform the physician.
- Reassess the type of restraint used, the correct application, and if alternatives can be used.

Recording and Reporting

- Record behaviours that place client at risk for injury.
- Describe restraint alternatives attempted and client's response.
- Record client's and family's understanding of and consent to restraint application.
- Record type and location of the restraint and time applied.
- Record time of assessments and releases.
- Document the client's behaviour after the application of the restraint.
- Document specific assessments related to orientation, oxygenation, skin integrity, circulation, and positioning.
- Describe the client's response when restraints were removed.

Home Care Considerations

- Plan care with family. If possible, use of an Ambularm may free client from physical restraints.
- Instruct family members (or other caregivers) in the use of alternatives to restraints (see Box 37–12).
- A physical restraint may require a physician order. The restraint should not be sent home with family unless the device is needed to protect the client from injury. If physical restraints are necessary, the family members (or other caregivers) must be instructed in its proper application, the care needed while in restraints, and the complications for which to look. Also inform caregivers whom to contact if any abnormal findings occur.
- A client who needs to be restrained in bed should have a hospital bed and will require constant supervision in the home.

A long-term care setting may be designed to include **environmental restraints**, such as locked nursing units. Residents with dementia may be at risk for injury if they wander away from their unit or building. A locked nursing unit can be designed to permit individuals the freedom to wander safely around their unit and can include exits to secure, enclosed outdoor spaces when weather permits. A locked unit is still a form of restraint and should only be implemented after alternatives to restraint have proven unsuccessful.

In some situations, chemical restraints may be indicated. **Chemical restraint** is defined as "any form of psychoactive medication used, not to treat illness, but to intentionally inhibit a particular behaviour or movement" (College of Nurses of Ontario, 2005, p. 4). For example, it may be necessary to sedate a client who is consistently pulling out a nasogastric tube. As with any other restraint, chemical restraints should be implemented only after nonrestraining measures (e.g., distraction, use of a sitter) have proven ineffective and with the informed consent of the clients or their substitute decision maker. Proper adherence to medication administration guidelines is vital to the safe use of chemical restraints, and the clients' response to and need for these medications must be assessed on a regular basis.

Side Rails. Side rails may help to increase a client's mobility and stability when in bed or when moving from the bed to a chair. Side rails also help prevent the unconscious client from falling out of bed or off a stretcher (Figure 37–18). However, raised side rails that cannot be opened by the client are considered a restraint (College of Nurses

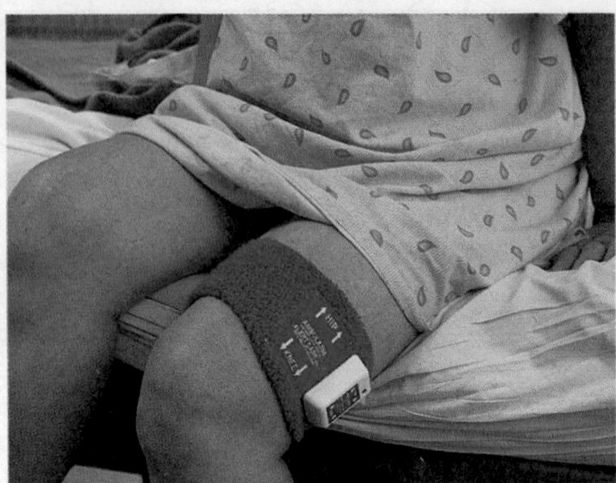

Figure 37-15 Client wearing an Ambularm device.

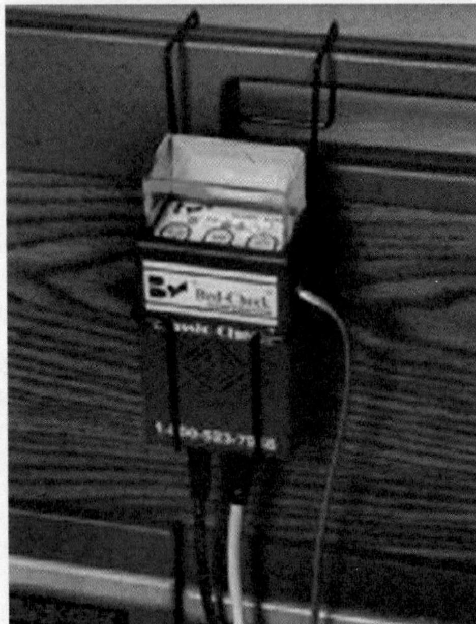

Figure 37-16 The Bed-Check bed exit alarm. **Source:** Courtesy Bed-Check Corp.

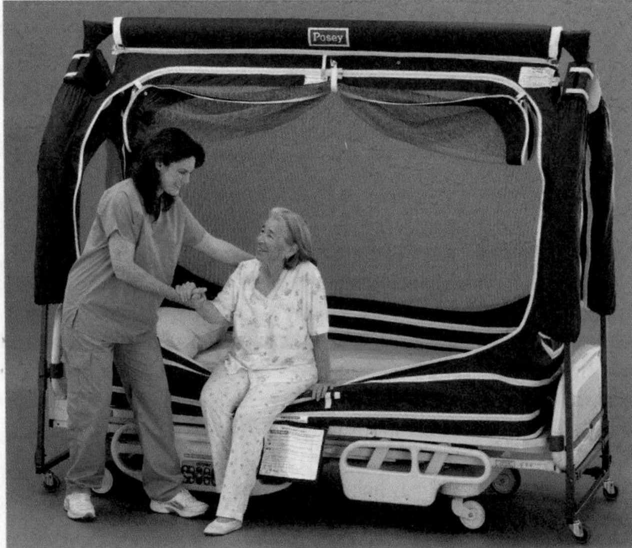

Figure 37-17 The Posey Bed Enclosure. **Source:** Courtesy J. T. Posey Co., Arcadia, CA.

of Ontario, 2005). The use of side rails alone for a disoriented client may cause more confusion and further injury. A confused client who is determined to get out of bed attempts to climb over the side rail or climbs out at the foot of the bed. Either attempt usually results in a fall or injury. Nursing interventions to reduce a client's confusion should first focus on the cause of the confusion. Frequently a client's attempt to explore his or her environment or to self-toilet is mistaken as confusion. A thorough assessment is essential. Whenever side rails are used, the bed should be maintained in the lowest position possible.

safety alert Side rails have the potential to trap the head and body, especially in older adult clients who are confused and restless. Entrapment in side rails can result in serious injury and death (College of Nurses of Ontario, 2005). Hazards can be prevented by assessing for excessive gaps and openings between the bed frame and mattress and using side rail netting, protective padding, or antiskid mats to prevent the mattress from being pushed to one side.

Electrical Hazards. Electrical equipment must be maintained in good working order and should be grounded. The third (longer) prong in an electrical plug is the ground. Theoretically, the ground prong carries any stray electrical current back to the ground—hence, its name. The other two prongs carry the power to the piece of electrical equipment. Improperly grounded or malfunctioning electrical equipment increases the risks of electrical injury and fire. Educating both the client and the family can reduce the risk for electrical hazards in the home environment (Box 37–14).

If a client receives an electrical shock in a health care setting, immediately determine whether the client has a pulse. If the client has no pulse, cardiopulmonary resuscitation should be initiated and emergency personnel should be notified. If the client has a pulse and remains alert and oriented, quickly obtain vital signs and assess the skin for signs of thermal injury. The client's physician must be notified. If an electrical shock occurs in the home, follow the same procedure but have the client go to the emergency department and then notify the client's physician.

Seizures. Clients with a history of seizures and those who have experienced some form of neurological injury or metabolic disturbance may be at risk for a seizure. **Seizure precautions** are nursing interventions during and after a seizure and include protecting the client from traumatic injury, positioning the client for adequate ventilation and drainage of oral secretions, and providing privacy and support following the seizure (Skill 37–2). It is important that you observe the client carefully before, during, and after the seizure and document assessments accurately.

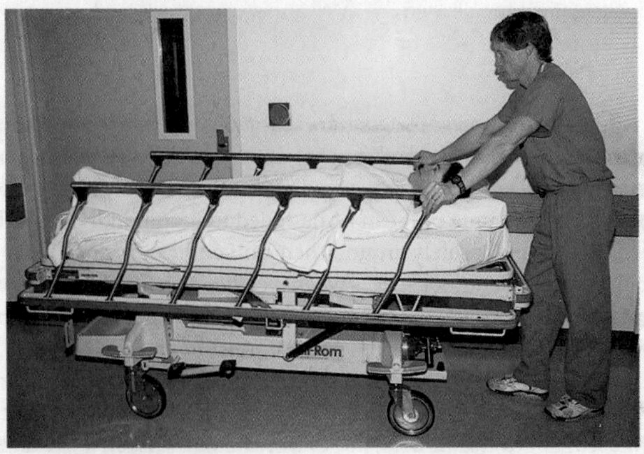

Figure 37-18 Side rails in the up position on a stretcher.

BOX 37-14 CLIENT TEACHING

Prevention of Electrical Hazards in the Home

Objective

- Client will recognize electrical hazards in the home and eliminate them.

Teaching Strategies

- Discuss grounding appliances and other equipment.
- Provide examples of common hazards: frayed cords, damaged equipment, and overloaded outlets.
- Discuss guidelines to prevent electrical shocks:
  - Use extension cords only when necessary, and use electrical tape to secure the cord to the floor where it will not be stepped on.
  - Do not run wires under carpeting.
- Teach the client to grasp the plug, not the cord, when unplugging items.
- Teach the client to keep electrical items away from water.
- Teach the client not to operate equipment with which he or she is unfamiliar.
- Teach the client to disconnect items before cleaning them.

Evaluation

- Have client list electrical hazards existing in the home.
- Review with the client the steps he or she will take to eliminate these hazards.
- Reassess the home after the client has had an opportunity to eliminate the hazards.

SKILL 37-2 Seizure Precautions

Delegation Considerations

Assessment of a client's need for seizure precautions cannot be delegated to an unregulated care provider (UCP). If a seizure occurs, you must constantly assess the client's airway patency, adequacy of breathing, and circulatory status. Clinical judgements must be made quickly. The tasks of setting up seizure precautions and protecting clients at risk for seizures may be delegated to UCP:

- Have the UCP protect at-risk clients from falls by assisting with ambulation and transfer.
- Caution the UCP against any attempt to restrain the client's extremities during a seizure.

Equipment

- Oral airway
- Padding for side rails and headboard
- Suction machine, oral suction equipment
- Disposable gloves

Procedure

STEPS	RATIONALE
1. Assess seizure history, noting the frequency of seizures, presence of aura, and sequence of events, if known. Assess for medical and surgical conditions that may lead to seizures or exacerbate existing seizure condition. Assess medication history.	• Enables you to anticipate the onset of seizure activity. Seizure medications must be taken as prescribed and not stopped suddenly because this may precipitate seizure activity.
2. Inspect the client's environment for potential safety hazards if risk for seizure exists, such as a bedside stand or table, an IV pole, or other medical equipment.	• Prevents client from sustaining injury by striking head or body on furniture or equipment.
3. Perform hand hygiene and prepare bed with padded side rails and headboard. Set the bed in the low position, and place the client in side-lying position when possible (see Step 3 illustration).	• Minimizes risks associated with seizure activity.
4. For clients with a history of seizures ensure that items such as an airway (see Step 4 illustration), suction apparatus, disposable gloves, and pillows are visible in the hospital setting for immediate use.	• Ensures a prompt, organized intervention.

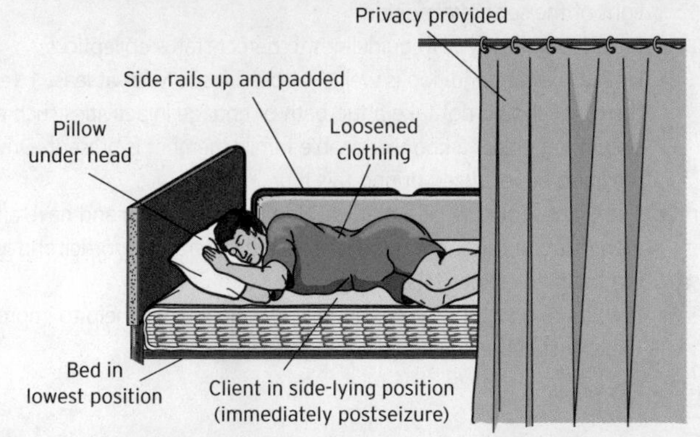

Step 3 Provide client privacy. Put bed in lowest position with side rails up and padded. Position client in side-lying position, with pillow under head, and loosen clothing.

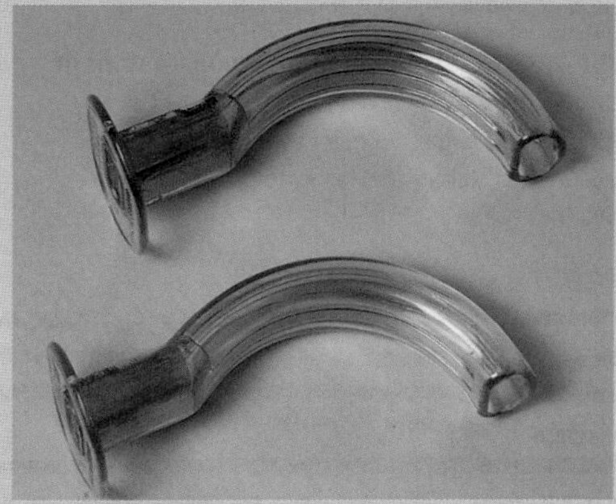

Step 4 Oral airways.

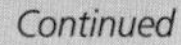
Continued

➤ SKILL 37-2 Seizure Precautions *continued*

STEPS	RATIONALE
5. When a seizure begins, position client safely. If client is standing or sitting, guide the client to floor and protect his or her head by cradling it in your lap or placing a pillow under the head. Clear the surrounding area of furniture. If the client is in bed, raise the side rails, add padding, and put the bed in low position.	• Protects client from traumatic injury, especially a head injury.
6. Provide privacy.	• Embarrassment is common after a seizure, especially if others witness the seizure.
7. If possible, turn client on side, with head flexed slightly forward.	• Prevents tongue and dentures from blocking the airway and promotes drainage of secretions, thus reducing the risk of aspiration.
8. Do not restrain client. Loosen client's clothing.	• Prevents musculoskeletal injury.
9. Do not put anything into the client's mouth such as fingers, tongue depressor, or medicine.	• Putting something in the client's mouth could result in injury to the client.

Critical Decision Point: Objects in the client's mouth could cause injury to the jaw, tongue, or teeth and cause stimulation of the gag reflex, causing vomiting, aspiration, and respiratory distress (Epilepsy Canada, 2005).

STEPS	RATIONALE
10. Stay with the client, observing the sequence and timing of seizure activity.	• Continued observation is necessary to ensure adequate ventilation during and following seizure activity. Accurate, specific observations will assist in the documentation, diagnosis, and treatment of the seizure disorder.
11. After the seizure is over, explain what happened and answer the client's questions. Foster an atmosphere of acceptance and respect.	• Informing clients of the type of seizure activity experienced assists them in participating knowledgeably in their care.
12. Following the seizure, assist the client to a position of comfort in bed with padded side rails up and the bed in low position. Place a call light within reach, and provide a quiet, nonstimulating environment. Perform hand hygiene before leaving the room.	• Provides for continued safety. Clients are often confused and sleepy following a seizure.

Status Epilepticus

For a client experiencing status epilepticus, the following actions are required:

STEPS	RATIONALE
13. Put on disposable gloves and insert an oral airway (see Step 4 illustration) when the jaw is relaxed between seizure activities. Hold the airway with curved side up, insert downward until airway reaches back of throat, then rotate and follow natural curve of the tongue. Do not place fingers near or in the client's mouth.	• Prevents transmission of infection. Client is in continual seizure state and requires oral airway to ensure airway patency. Client may inadvertently bite fingers during a seizure if caution is not used.
14. Access oxygen and suction equipment. Prepare for IV insertion.	• Intensive monitoring and treatment are required for this medical emergency.
15. Use pillows or pads to protect the client from injuring self.	• Traumatic injury is avoided.

Unexpected Outcomes and Related Interventions

Client Suffers Traumatic Injury

- Continue to protect the client from further injury.
- Notify the physician immediately.
- Ensure the environment is free of safety hazards.

Client Verbalizes Feelings of Embarrassment and Humiliation

- Offer support and allow client to verbalize feelings.
- Encourage the client and family to participate in decision making and planning care.

Recording and Reporting

- Record the timing of seizure activity and the sequence of events. Record the presence of aura (if any), level of consciousness, posture, colour, movements of extremities, incontinence, and patterns of sleep following the seizure.
- Document client's response and expected or unexpected outcomes.
- Report to the physician immediately as seizure begins. Status epilepticus is an emergency situation requiring immediate medical management.

Home Care Considerations

- Communicate with the client and family to identify precipitating factors.
- Teach the family to care for the client during a seizure.
- The client's home should be assessed for environmental hazards in light of the seizure condition.
- Provide the family with guidelines to detect status epilepticus.
- Until a seizure condition is well controlled (usually for at least 1 year), the client should not take a tub bath or engage in activities such as swimming unless a knowledgeable family member is present. Driving may also be restricted during this time.
- The client should wear a medical alert bracelet or tag and have an identification card noting the presence of a seizure disorder and listing the medications taken.
- Referral to a support group or Epilepsy Canada may help to improve the client's self-esteem and coping ability.

Radiation. Radiation is a health hazard in the health care setting and the community. Radiation and radioactive materials are used in the diagnosis and treatment of clients. Hospitals have strict guidelines on the care of clients who are receiving radiation and radioactive materials. Familiarize yourself with your agency's established protocols. Exposure to radiation can be reduced by limiting the time spent near the source, making the distance from the source as great as possible, and using shielding devices such as lead aprons. Staff working near radiation wear devices that track accumulative exposure to radiation.

The community can be at risk for radiation exposure if there has been incorrect disposal and transportation of radioactive waste products. The Canadian Nuclear Safety Commission ensures that the disposal of radioactive waste does not pose a danger for the public or the environment. If a radioactive leak occurs, this commission institutes measures to prevent the exposure of surrounding neighbourhoods, to clean up radioactive leaks as quickly as possible, and to ensure that injured parties receive prompt medical care.

❖Evaluation

Client Care

The components of critical thinking are applied to the evaluation step of the nursing process (Figure 37–19). The actual care delivered by the health care team is evaluated on the basis of expected outcomes. If the client's goals have been met, the nursing interventions can be considered effective and appropriate. If not, determine whether new risks to the client have developed or whether previous risks remain. The client and family need to participate to find permanent ways to reduce risks to safety. Continually assess the client's and family's need for additional support services, such as home care, physiotherapy, counselling, and further teaching.

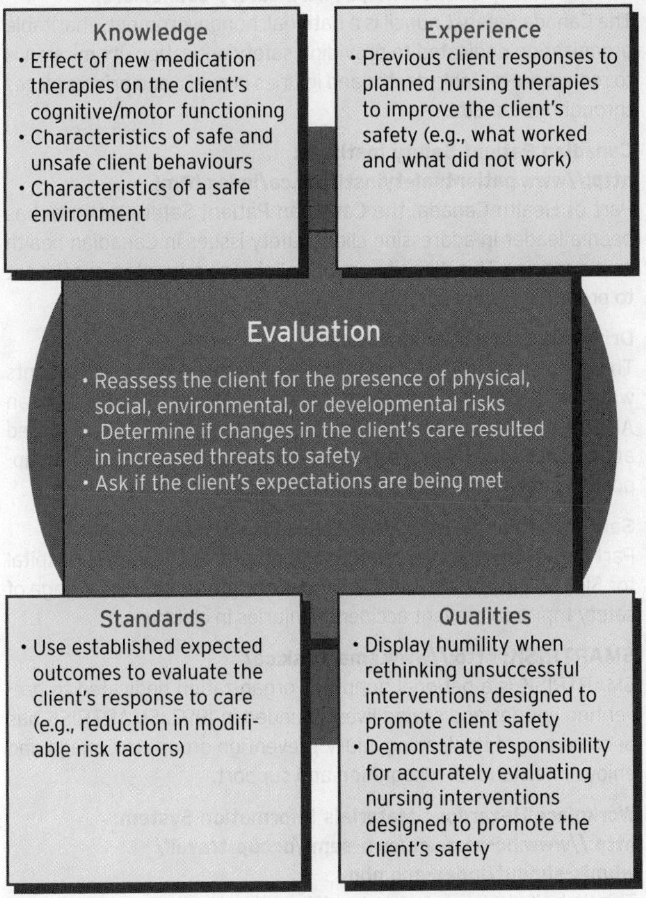

Figure 37-19 Critical thinking model for safety evaluation.

Client Expectations

When you have developed a good relationship with a client and the client feels safe and secure in the environment, he or she will most likely demonstrate satisfaction. You must determine, however, if client expectations have been met. Is the client satisfied with any changes made to the environment? Does the client believe that his or her safety is ensured? If client expectations have not been met, you must reassess not only the client and the environment, but also the client's expressed desires.

✻ KEY CONCEPTS

- A safe environment is essential to promoting, maintaining, and restoring health.
- In the community, a safe environment is one in which basic needs are achievable, physical hazards are reduced, the transmission of pathogens is reduced, pollution is controlled, and sanitation is maintained.
- In a health care agency, a safe environment is one that minimizes falls, client-inherent accidents, procedure-related accidents, and equipment-related accidents.
- A factor that reduces atmospheric oxygen is the presence of high carbon monoxide levels, which may result from an improperly functioning furnace.
- Prolonged exposure to extreme environmental temperatures can cause client injury or even death.
- The reduction of physical hazards in the environment includes providing adequate lighting, decreasing clutter, and securing the home.
- The transmission of pathogens is reduced through medical and surgical asepsis, immunization, adequate food sanitation, insect and rodent control, and the appropriate disposal of human waste.
- Children less than 5 years of age are at the greatest risk for home accidents that may result in severe injury and death.
- The school-age child is at risk for injury at home, at school, and while travelling to and from school.
- Adolescents are at risk for injury from automobile accidents, suicide, and substance abuse.
- Threats to an adult's safety are frequently associated with lifestyle habits.
- Risks of injury for older clients are directly related to the physiological changes of the aging process; falls are the greatest cause of accidental injury in older adults.
- By incorporating critical thinking skills in the application of the nursing process, you assess the client and the environment to determine risk factors for injury; cluster risk factors; formulate a nursing diagnosis; and plan specific interventions, including client education.
- Nursing interventions for promoting safety are individualized for developmental stage, lifestyle, and environment.
- Nursing interventions are developed to modify the environment for protection from falls, fires, poisoning, and electrical hazards.
- The expected outcomes include a safe physical environment, a client whose expectations have been met and who is knowledgeable about safety factors and precautions, and a client free of injury.

* CRITICAL THINKING EXERCISES

1. Mrs. Santiago, who is 88 years old and has been functioning independently at home, was recently admitted to the hospital. Through your admission assessment, you learn that she experiences urinary frequency and urgency, walks with an unsteady gait, and is very anxious about being in the hospital. Use the Fall Assessment Tool (see Table 37-1) to determine Mrs. Santiago's risk for a fall, and design specific interventions to ensure her safety in the hospital.
2. Mrs. Patel, a 76-year-old long-term care resident with Alzheimer's disease, has been refusing food and fluids for the past month. The family has agreed to the placement of a nasogastric tube to improve her fluid and nutritional statuses. Shortly after the first tube feeding was started, Mrs. Patel became more restless, and she has been picking at the tube.
   a. What might be precipitating Mrs. Patel's behaviour of picking at the tube?
   b. What approaches can be used to eliminate interference with the treatment?
   c. If a restraint is necessary to avoid the disruption of therapy, what interventions are required to ensure the client's safety while in restraints?
3. A family member of a client reports that, just a few minutes ago, a lit cigarette dropped on the client's mattress but that the small fire was put out. What actions are needed to ensure the safety of this client?

* REVIEW QUESTIONS

1. The following pollutant could occur in a health care facility:
   1. Air pollution
   2. Water pollution
   3. Noise pollution
   4. Bioactive waste pollution
2. Accidental injuries are the leading cause of death for which age group?
   1. 1 to 12 months
   2. 1 to 34 years
   3. 45 to 64 years
   4. 65 years and over
3. Adolescents are at a greater risk for injury from
   1. Poisoning, drowning, motor vehicle accidents
   2. Motor vehicle accidents, suicide, and substance abuse
   3. Home accidents, motor vehicle accidents, fire
   4. Falls, suicide, drowning
4. The physiological changes caused by aging increase the older client's risk for
   1. Falls
   2. Suicide
   3. Alcoholism
   4. Seizures
5. WHMIS is a system to control hazardous substances in the workplace and includes
   1. Environmental interventions and cautionary labelling of products
   2. Worker education programs and the provision of MSDSs
   3. Client education programs and worker education programs
   4. Risk assessment and the provision of MSDSs
6. Medication and fluid administration errors and the improper application of external devices are examples of
   1. Client-inherent accidents
   2. Procedure-related accidents
   3. Equipment-related accidents
   4. Environmental-related accidents
7. Which of the following statements about restraints is *not* true?
   1. Restraints are used only after other alternatives have been tried.
   2. The least-restrictive method of restraint should be used.
   3. Restraints are considered a long-term intervention.
   4. If a restraint is used, it must be part of the client's medical treatment.
8. When teaching parents about responding to poisoning in children, you should instruct them to
   1. Give oral fluids
   2. Induce vomiting
   3. Call the local poison control centre
   4. Drive the child to the emergency department
9. All of the following are acceptable alternatives to the use of restraints, *except*
   1. Attending to needs for toileting, food, and liquid
   2. Offering diversionary activities, such as music or something to hold
   3. Camouflaging IV lines with clothing or a Stockinette
   4. Ensuring that a family member is with the client at all times

* RECOMMENDED WEB SITES

Canada Safety Council: http://www.safety-council.org/
The Canada Safety Council is a national, nongovernment, charitable organization dedicated to providing safety education. Its mission is to reduce preventable deaths and injuries in public and private places throughout Canada.

Canadian Patient Safety Institute: http://www.patientsafetyinstitute.ca/index.html
Part of Health Canada, the Canadian Patient Safety Institute has been a leader in addressing client safety issues in Canadian health care agencies. This Web site provides links to various topics relevant to promoting client safety.

DriveABLE: http://driveable.com/
This Web site is a useful resource for nurses working with clients who need to make a decision to stop driving. DriveABLE is an Alberta-based company that provides objective and evidence-based approaches to assessing driver ability, as well as resources for supporting individuals and families through this process.

Safe Kids Canada: http://www.sickkids.ca/safekidscanada/
Part of the national injury prevention program at Toronto's Hospital for Sick Children, Safe Kids Canada offers information on a range of safety topics to prevent accidental injuries in children.

SMARTRISK: http://www.smartrisk.ca/
SMARTRISK is a national nonprofit organization dedicated to preventing injuries and saving lives. Founded in 1992, SMARTRISK has become one of the leading injury-prevention groups in Canada and enjoys international recognition and support.

Workplace Hazardous Materials Information System: http://www.hc-sc.gc.ca/ewh-semt/occup-travail/whmis-simdut/index-eng.php
This Web site is developed and maintained by Health Canada's WHMIS Division and includes policies and information related to WHMIS.

38

Hygiene

Original chapter by Sylvia K. Baird, RN, BSN, MM
Canadian content written by Yvonne G. Briggs, RN, BScN, MN

objectives

Mastery of content in this chapter will enable you to:

- Define the key terms listed.
- Describe factors that influence personal hygiene practices.
- Discuss the role that critical thinking plays in the provision of hygiene care.
- Conduct a comprehensive assessment of a client's total hygiene needs.
- Discuss conditions that place clients at risk for impaired skin integrity.
- Discuss factors that influence the condition of the nails and feet.
- Explain the importance of foot care for the diabetic client.
- Discuss conditions that place clients at risk for impaired oral mucous membranes.
- List common hair and scalp problems and their related interventions.
- Describe how hygiene care for the older client may differ from that for the younger client.
- Discuss the different approaches used in maintaining a client's comfort during hygiene care.
- Successfully perform hygiene procedures for care of the skin; perineum; feet, hands, and nails; mouth; and eyes, ears, and nose.

key terms

Acne, p. 836
Alopecia, p. 835
Buccal glands, p. 831
Cerumen, p. 836
Complete bed bath, p. 846
Cuticle, p. 831
Dermis, p. 830
Enucleation, p. 866
Epidermis, p. 830
Gingivitis, p. 832
Halitosis, p. 834
Lunula, p. 831
Mastication, p. 832
Neuropathy, p. 831
Ophthalmologist, p. 867
Optometrist, p. 867
Partial bed bath, p. 846
Perineal care, p. 854
Stomatitis, p. 859

media resources

evolve Web Site

- Audio Chapter Summaries
- Glossary
- Multiple-Choice Review Questions
- Student Learning Activities
- Video Clips
- Weblinks

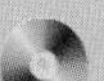
Companion CD

- Glossary
- Interactive Learning Activities
- Fluids and Electrolytes Tutorial
- Test-Taking Skills

Personal hygiene affects an individual's comfort, safety, and physical and psychological well-being. Individuals who are well are capable of meeting their own hygiene needs, but those who are ill or have disabilities may require various levels of assistance. Many personal, social, and cultural factors can influence hygiene practices. In agency or home care settings, determine a client's ability to perform self-care and provide hygiene care according to the client's needs and preferences. In the home setting, assist in helping the client and family to adapt hygiene techniques and approaches.

Because hygiene care requires close contact with the client, therapeutic communication skills should be used (see Chapter 18) to build and promote a caring therapeutic relationship and to assist you in providing the client with teaching regarding hygiene care. Other nursing activities can be integrated during hygiene care, including client assessment and interventions, such as range-of-motion exercises, the application of dressings, and the inspection and care of intravenous (IV) sites. During hygiene care, the client's independence is encouraged and promoted as much as possible, privacy is ensured, respect is conveyed, and physical comfort is maintained and supported.

Scientific Knowledge Base

Proper hygiene care requires an understanding of the anatomy and physiology of the integument, oral cavity, eyes, ears, nose, hands, feet, and nails. The skin and mucosal cells exchange oxygen, nutrients, and fluids with underlying blood vessels. The cells require adequate nutrition, hydration, and circulation to resist injury and disease. Good hygiene techniques assist in promoting the normal structure and function of body tissues.

In addition, knowledge of pathophysiology is applied to provide good preventive hygiene care. Learn to recognize disease states that create changes in the integument, oral cavity, and sensory organs. For example, diabetes mellitus results in chronic vascular changes that impair healing of the skin and mucosa. In the early stages of acquired immune deficiency syndrome (AIDS), fungal infections of the oral cavity are common. Stroke can result in paralysis of the trigeminal nerve, which eliminates the blink reflex, increasing the risk for corneal drying. In the presence of conditions such as these, hygiene practices are adapted to anticipate client needs and minimize harmful effects. By integrating knowledge of anatomy, physiology, and pathophysiology during hygiene care, you can recognize abnormalities and initiate appropriate actions to prevent further injury.

The Skin

The skin is an active organ with the functions of protection, secretion, excretion, temperature regulation, and sensation (Table 38–1). The skin has three primary layers: epidermis, dermis, and subcutaneous. The **epidermis** (outer layer) is composed of several thin layers of cells undergoing different stages of maturation. It shields underlying tissue against water loss and injury and prevents the entry of disease-producing microorganisms. The innermost layer of the epidermis generates new cells to replace the dead cells that are continuously shed from the skin's outer surface. Bacteria commonly reside on the outer epidermis. These resident bacteria are normal flora (see Chapter 33)—they do not cause disease but instead inhibit the multiplication of disease-causing microorganisms.

The **dermis** is a thicker skin layer containing bundles of collagen and elastic fibres to support the epidermis. Nerve fibres, blood vessels, sweat glands, sebaceous glands, and hair follicles course through the

TABLE 38-1 Function of the Skin and Implications for Care

Function and Description	Implications for Care
Protection	
The epidermis is a relatively impermeable layer that prevents the entrance of microorganisms. Although microorganisms reside on the skin surface and in hair follicles, the relative dryness of skin's surface inhibits bacterial growth. Sebum removes bacteria from hair follicles. The acidic pH of skin further retards bacterial growth.	Weakening of the epidermis occurs by scraping or stripping its surface (e.g., through the use of dry razors, tape removal, or improper turning or positioning techniques). Excessive dryness causes cracks and breaks in the skin and mucosa that allow bacteria to enter. Emollients soften the skin and prevent moisture loss, and hydration of the mucosa prevents dryness. Constant exposure of skin to moisture can cause maceration (softening), which interrupts dermal integrity and promotes ulcer formation and bacterial growth. Bed linen and clothing should be kept dry. Misuse of soap, detergents, cosmetics, deodorant, and depilatories can cause chemical irritation. Alkaline soaps neutralize the protective acid condition of skin. Cleansing of skin removes excess oil, sweat, dead skin cells, and dirt that can promote bacterial growth. Bath water should not be excessively hot or cold.
Sensation	
The skin contains sensory organs for touch, pain, heat, cold, and pressure.	Friction should be minimized to avoid the loss of the stratum corneum, which can result in the development of pressure ulcers. Smoothing linen removes sources of mechanical irritation. To prevent accidental injury of the client's skin, nurses should remove their own jewellery before giving care.
Temperature Regulation	
Body temperature is controlled by radiation, evaporation, conduction, and convection.	Factors that interfere with heat loss can alter temperature control. Wet bed linens or gowns interfere with convection and conduction. Excess blankets or bed coverings can interfere with heat loss through radiation and conduction. Coverings can promote heat conservation.
Excretion and Secretion	
Sweat promotes heat loss by evaporation. Sebum lubricates the skin and hair.	Perspiration and oil can harbour microorganisms. Bathing removes excess body secretions; however, excessive bathing can cause drying of the skin.

dermal layers. Sebaceous glands secrete sebum, an oily, odorous fluid, into the hair follicles.

The subcutaneous tissue layer contains blood vessels, nerves, lymph, and loose connective tissue filled with fat cells. The fatty tissue is a heat insulator for the body. Subcutaneous tissue also supports upper skin layers to withstand stresses and pressure without injury. Very little subcutaneous tissue underlies the oral mucosa.

The skin often reflects a change in physical condition by alterations in colour (Box 38–1), thickness, texture, turgor, temperature, and hydration (see Chapter 32). As long as the skin remains intact and healthy, its physiological function remains optimal.

The Feet, Hands, and Nails

The feet, hands, and nails often require special attention to prevent infection. Any injury or deformity to the foot, including growths or injuries to the overlying skin, can be painful and thus interfere with a client's normal ability to walk and bear weight.

The hand, in contrast to the foot, is constructed largely for manipulation rather than support. Dexterity exists in the hand because of the wide range of movement between the thumb and fingers. Any condition that interferes with the movement of the hand (e.g., superficial or deep pain or joint inflammation) can impair a client's self-help abilities.

The nails are epithelial tissues that grow from the root of the nail bed, which is located in the skin at the nail groove and hidden by the fold of skin called the **cuticle**. The visible part of the nail is the nail body. It has a crescent-shaped white area known as the **lunula**. Under the nail lies a layer of epithelium called the nail bed (Figure 38–1). In light-skinned individuals, a healthy nail is transparent, smooth, and convex, with a pink nail bed and translucent white tip. Disease processes can cause changes in the shape, thickness, and curvature of the nail (see Chapter 32).

The Oral Cavity

The oral cavity is lined with mucous membranes continuous with the skin. The oral or buccal cavity consists of the lips surrounding the opening of the mouth, the cheeks running along the side walls of the cavity, the tongue and its muscles, and the hard and soft palates. The oral mucosa is normally light pink and moist. The floor of the mouth and the undersurface of the tongue are richly supplied with blood vessels. Any type of ulceration or trauma can result in significant bleeding. Three pairs of salivary glands secrete about 1 L/day of saliva. The **buccal glands**, found in the mucosa lining the cheeks and mouth, maintain the hygiene and comfort of oral tissues. Salivary secretion in the mouth can be impaired by the effects of medications, exposure to radiation, and mouth breathing.

BOX 38-1 CULTURAL ASPECTS OF CARE

Identifying changes in skin colour and determining whether these changes are normal reactive hyperemia or abnormal reactive hyperemia are important in evaluating clients' risks for pressure ulcers (see Chapter 47). When a client's natural skin contains more melanin, it is more difficult to determine abnormal reactive hyperemia and cyanosis. Some hyperpigmentation areas are normal, such as mongolian spots, which may be on the sacrum of African, Aboriginal, and Asian clients. These areas should not be confused with skin colour changes such as abnormal reactive hyperemia or cyanosis.

Implications for Practice

- For dark-skinned clients, assess baseline skin tone by asking the client or family to point out an area of baseline skin colour for that person.
- Frequently assess skin for changes in baseline skin tone and skin temperature over pressure areas.
- Use natural light sources when possible because fluorescent light sources cast a bluish hue on darkly pigmented skin tones.
- Examine the body sites with the least amount of melanin for underlying skin colour identification.

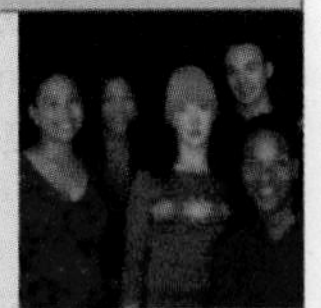

Data from Gaskin, F. C. (1986). Detection of cyanosis in the person with dark skin. *Journal of National Black Nurses' Association, 1*, 52–60; Bennet, M. A. (1995). Report of the Task Force on the Implications for Darkly Pigmented Intact Skin in the Prediction and Prevention of Pressure Ulcers. *Advances in Wound Care, 8*(6), 34–35; and Henderson, C. T., Ayello, E. A., Sussman, C., Leiby, D. M., Bennett, M. A., Dungog, E. F., et al. (1997). Draft definition of stage I pressure ulcers: Inclusion of persons with darkly pigmented skin. *Advances in Wound Care, 10*(5), 16–19.

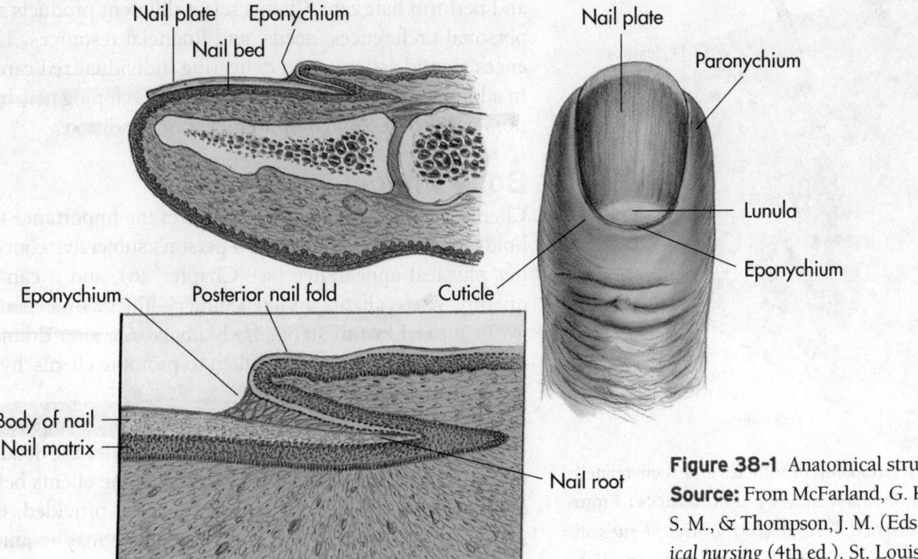

Figure 38-1 Anatomical structure of a normal nail. **Source:** From McFarland, G. K., Hirsch, J. E., Tucker, S. M., & Thompson, J. M. (Eds.). (1997). *Mosby's clinical nursing* (4th ed.). St. Louis, MO: Mosby.

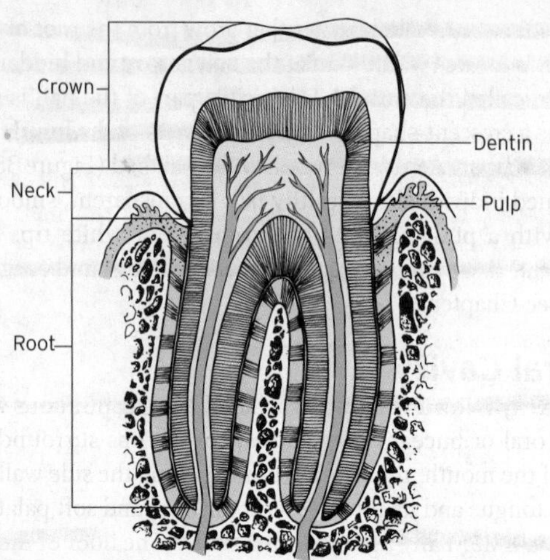

Figure 38-2 A normal tooth.

The teeth are the organs of chewing, or **mastication**. They are designed to cut, tear, and grind ingested food so that it can be mixed with saliva and swallowed. A normal tooth consists of a crown, neck, and root (Figure 38–2). The periodontal membrane lies just below the gum margins, surrounds a tooth, and holds it firmly in place. Healthy teeth appear white, smooth, shiny, and properly aligned.

Difficulty in chewing can develop when gum tissues become inflamed or infected or when teeth are lost or become loose. Regular oral hygiene is necessary to maintain the integrity of tooth surfaces and to prevent **gingivitis**, or gum inflammation.

The Hair

Hair growth, distribution, and pattern can indicate a person's general health status. Hormonal changes, emotional and physical stresses, aging, infection, and certain illnesses can affect hair characteristics. The hair shaft itself is inert and cannot be directly affected by physiological factors. However, changes in its colour or condition are caused by hormonal or nutrient deficiencies of the hair follicle (Figure 38–3).

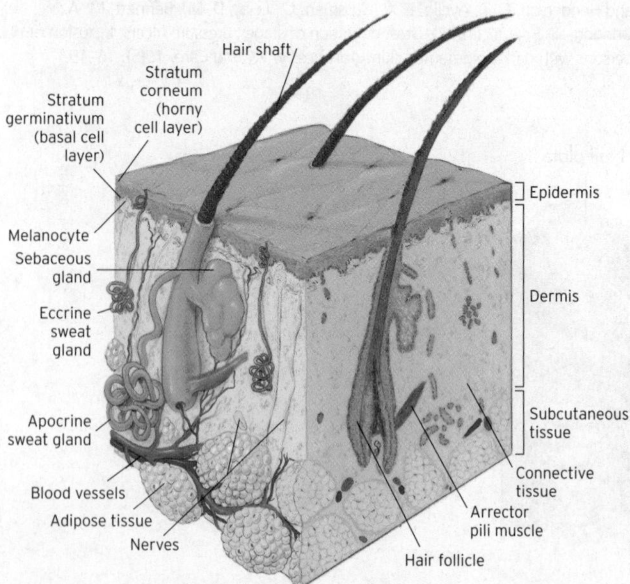

Figure 38-3 Hair follicles and relationship of follicles and their related structures to the epidermal and dermal layers of the skin. **Source:** From Lewis, S. M., Heitkemper, M. M., Dirksen, R. R., et al. (2007). *Medical–surgical nursing: Assessment and management of clinical problems* (7th ed., p. 450, Fig. 23-1). St. Louis, MO: Mosby.

The Eyes, Ears, and Nose

The eyes, ears, and nose require careful attention during the provision of hygiene. Chapter 32 describes the structure and function of these organs. Cleansing of the sensitive sensory tissues should be done in a way that prevents injury and discomfort for the client, such as being careful not to get soap in the client's eyes. In addition, the time that is spent with a client during hygiene provides an excellent opportunity to ask whether he or she has experienced any changes in vision, hearing, or sense of smell.

Nursing Knowledge Base

A client's personal preferences for hygiene are influenced by a number of factors. No two individuals perform hygiene in the same manner, and it is important to individualize care from knowledge about the client's unique hygiene practices and preferences.

Hygiene care is never routine; the care requires intimate contact with clients and good communication skills are necessary in order to build and promote a therapeutic relationship. While providing hygiene care, you can learn about clients' health-promotion practices and needs, emotional needs, and needs pertaining to health care education.

Social Practices

Social groups influence hygiene preferences and practices, including the type of hygiene products used and the nature and frequency of personal care. During childhood, hygiene is influenced by family customs, including, for example, the frequency of bathing, the time of day bathing is performed, and the type of oral hygiene practised. As children enter their adolescent years, personal hygiene may be influenced by peer group behaviour and they may become more interested in their personal appearance. For example, girls may begin to wear makeup, and boys may begin shaving. During the adult years, involvement with friends and work groups shapes the expectations individuals have about their personal appearance. Older adults' hygiene practices may change because of living conditions, health status, and available resources.

Personal Preferences

Each client has individual preferences about when to bathe, shave, and perform hair care. Clients select different products according to personal preferences, needs, and financial resources. These preferences should assist you in delivering individualized care for clients. In addition, you should assist clients in developing new hygiene practices when necessitated by an illness or condition.

Body Image

Clients' general appearance may reflect the importance that hygiene holds for them. Body image is a person's subjective concept of his or her physical appearance (see Chapter 26), and it can change frequently. When clients undergo surgery, illness, or a change in physical or mental health status, body image can alter dramatically. For this reason, effort should be taken to promote clients' hygienic comfort and appearance.

Body image affects the way in which hygiene is maintained. If clients are neatly groomed, you should consider the details of grooming when planning care and consult with the clients before making decisions about how hygiene care is to be provided. Clients who appear unkempt or uninterested in hygiene may require an assessment of their hygiene practices or additional education about the importance of hygiene.

Socioeconomic Status

A person's economic resources can influence the type and extent of hygiene practices used. You should be sensitive in considering whether a client's economic status influences his or her ability to regularly maintain hygiene. When clients have the added problem of a lack of socioeconomic resources, it becomes difficult to participate and take a responsible role in health-promotion activities such as basic hygiene.

When basic care items are not affordable, alternatives need to be considered. It is also important to assess whether the use of these products is an acceptable practice among clients' social or cultural group. For example, not all clients may choose to use deodorant or cosmetics.

Health Beliefs and Motivation

Knowledge about the importance of hygiene and its implications for well-being influences hygiene practices. However, knowledge alone is not enough. According to Pender et al. (2006), individual characteristics such as personal factors (psychological, sociocultural, and biological) directly influence an individual's health-promotion activities.

It is important to know, for example, whether clients perceive that they are at risk for dental disease, that dental disease is serious, and that brushing and flossing are effective in reducing this risk. When clients recognize that a risk is present and that reasonable action can be taken to reduce the risk, they are more receptive to counselling and teaching efforts.

Cultural Variables

Clients' cultural beliefs and personal values can influence hygiene care (Box 38–2). Individuals from diverse cultural backgrounds follow different self-care practices (see Chapter 10). Feelings of disapproval must not be conveyed when caring for clients whose hygienic practices are different from your own. In some cultures, it is customary to bathe once a week; in North America, it is common to bathe or shower daily.

Physical Condition

Clients with certain types of physical limitations, disabilities, or pain often lack the physical energy, dexterity, and range of motion to perform hygiene care. A client in traction or a cast or who has an IV line or other device connected to the body needs assistance with hygiene. Clients under the effects of sedation do not have the mental clarity or coordination to perform self-care. Chronic illnesses, such as cardiac disease, cancer, neurological disorders, and certain psychiatric conditions, may exhaust or incapacitate a client. A weakened grasp resulting from arthritis, stroke, or muscular disorders can prevent a client from using a toothbrush, washcloth, or comb.

Critical Thinking

Successful critical thinking requires the synthesis of knowledge, experience, information gathered from clients, critical thinking qualities, and intellectual and professional standards. Clinical judgments require you to anticipate the information necessary to analyze data and make decisions regarding client care. Clients' conditions are always changing, requiring ongoing critical thinking. During assessment, you must consider all contributing factors needed to make a nursing diagnosis (Figure 38–4).

Because hygiene care is so important for clients to feel comfortable, refreshed, and renewed, you should avoid making hygiene care a simple routine. Instead, integrate knowledge from nursing and other disciplines, previous experiences, and information gathered from clients. In addition, use attributes such as curiosity and humility when designing a plan of care that will meet the clients' hygiene needs. Agency and professional nursing standards and guidelines, such as those from the Canadian Diabetes Association (2003), are used when planning care to meet the client's hygiene needs.

➤ BOX 38-2 Cultural Influences on Hygiene

Clients need a culturally competent plan for hygiene care. For some, hygiene practices are influenced by culture and are a potential source of conflict and stress in a hospital environment. Hygiene is a very personal matter and bathing, perineal hygiene, and hair care practices can be sensitive issues.

Implications for Practice

- Maintain privacy, especially for women from cultures that value female modesty.
- Be aware that in some cultures, touching between unrelated males and females is taboo.
- Provide gender-congruent caregivers as needed or requested. If a gender-congruent caregiver is not available, ask the family for assistance.
- Do not cut or shave a client's hair without prior discussion with the client or family (Galanti, 2004).
- Be aware that some cultures (e.g., Chinese and Filipino) discourage bathing for 7–10 days after childbirth (Galanti, 2004).
- Bear in mind that some cultures (e.g., Chinese, Japanese, Koreans, and Hindus) consider the top parts of the body cleaner than the lower parts.
- Be aware that among Hindus and Muslims, the left hand is used for cleaning and the right hand is used for eating and praying.

Knowledge
- Anatomy and physiology of integument, oral cavity, and sense organs
- Principles of comfort and safety
- Communication principles that convey caring
- Risk factors posing hygiene problems
- Knowledge of cultural variations in hygiene

Experience
- Prior experience caring for clients requiring assistance with hygiene
- Personal hygiene practices

Assessment
- Observe the client's physical condition and integrity of integument, oral cavity, and sense organs
- Explore any developmental factors influencing the client's hygiene needs
- Note the client's self-care ability and hygiene practices
- Determine the client's cultural preferences

Standards
- Apply Canadian Diabetes Association's practice standards for foot care
- Apply AHCPR and RNAO guidelines on prevention and management of pressure ulcers
- Assess any skin alterations using accurate and consistent measurements

Qualities
- Display curiosity; be thorough in assessing the condition of the client's tissues; changes may indicate signs of disease
- Display humility; hygiene care is not the same for all clients; know when to learn more about the client's preferences

Figure 38-4 Critical thinking model for hygiene assessment. AHCPR, Agency for Health Care Policy and Research; RNAO, Registered Nurses Association of Ontario. These guidelines are still relevant.

Nursing Process

❖Assessment

Nursing assessment is an ongoing process. Not all body regions need to be assessed before administering hygiene; however, routine assessment of a client's condition is undertaken whenever client care is given. For example, during oral care, the condition of the teeth and mucosa can be inspected. If the client has had a repeated problem (e.g., dry skin or inflamed oral mucosa), then it is important to conduct an assessment before care is administered because variations in technique may be necessary. Hygiene care is an opportunity for you to make assessment findings for a variety of health care problems and thus help set health care priorities.

Physical Examination

While assisting a client with personal hygiene, carefully assess the integument, oral cavity structures, and the eyes, ears, and nose (see Chapter 32). Using the skills of inspection and palpation, look for alterations in the integrity and function of tissues. Your assessment also reveals the type and extent of hygiene care required. Special attention should be given to the structures most influenced by hygiene measures. Is the skin intact, especially over bony prominences? Is the skin dry from too much bathing? Are calluses present on the feet, which may benefit from soaking? Is a coating of the tongue present, which necessitates frequent brushing and hydration? Over time, your assessment provides the baseline for determining whether hygienic measures maintain or improve the client's condition.

The Skin. While inspecting the skin, thoroughly examine its colour, texture, thickness, turgor, temperature, and hydration. The skin should be smooth, warm, supple, and have good turgor. Pay special attention to the presence and condition of any lesions (see Chapter 32), and assess for dryness indicated by flaking, redness, scaling, and cracking. Certain common skin problems affect how hygiene is administered (Table 38–2). Careful attention should be paid in assessing less obvious or difficult-to-reach skin surfaces, such as under the female client's breasts, under the male client's scrotum, or around the female's perineal tissues. Observed skin problems should be explained to the client, and instruction on proper skin care and specific hygiene techniques should also be discussed with the client.

Certain conditions place clients at risk for impaired skin integrity (Box 38–3). You must be particularly alert when assessing clients with reduced sensation, vascular insufficiency, or immobility. Make sure to assess both extremities and assist clients in turning so that skin surfaces can be fully viewed. The development of pressure ulcers is a common complication that can extend hospital stays and threaten the well-being of long-term care clients. Tools such as the Braden Scale (Gulanick & Myers, 2007) are available to determine those clients who may be at risk for impaired skin integrity. When caring for clients with darkly pigmented skin, you should be aware of assessment techniques and skin characteristics unique to highly pigmented skin (Box 38–4).

The Feet and Nails. When assessing the feet, perform a thorough examination of all skin surfaces, including the areas between the toes and over the soles of the feet. The heels, soles, and sides of the feet are prone to irritation from poorly fitting shoes. In addition, inspect the shape and size of the toes, as well as the shape of the foot. The toes are normally straight and flat. The feet should be in straight alignment with the ankle and tibia. Inspect the feet for lesions and note areas of dryness, inflammation, or cracking.

Assess the client's gait. Painful foot disorders or decreased sensation can cause limping or an unnatural gait. Inquire whether the client has foot discomfort and determine factors that aggravate the pain. Foot problems may result from bone or muscular alterations or wearing poor-fitting footwear, rather than skin disorders.

Clients with peripheral vascular disease, diabetes mellitus, and other diseases that affect peripheral circulation and sensation should be assessed for the adequacy of circulation to the feet (see Chapter 32). Inspection and daily foot care can help prevent the development of a foot ulcer, which has been found to be the most common single precursor to lower extremity amputations in individuals with diabetes mellitus (Canadian Diabetes Association, 2003; Moulik et al., 2003). Palpation of the dorsalis pedis and posterior tibial pulses indicates whether adequate blood flow is reaching peripheral tissues. Edema and changes in skin colour, texture, and temperature can indicate whether clients require special hygiene care. Individuals with diabetes mellitus should also be checked for **neuropathy**—degeneration of the peripheral nerves characterized by a loss of sensation. Assess clients' sensation to light touch, pinprick, and temperature.

Inspect the condition of the fingernails and toenails, looking for lesions, dryness, inflammation, and cracking (Table 38–3). The nail is surrounded by a cuticle, which slowly grows over the nail and must be regularly pushed back. The skin around the nail beds and cuticles should be smooth and without inflammation. You should ask women whether they frequently polish their nails and use polish remover because chemicals in these products can cause excessive nail dryness. Disease can change the shape and curvature of the nails. Inflammatory lesions and fungus of the nail bed can cause thickened, horny nails, which can separate from the nail bed.

The Oral Cavity. Inspect all areas of the oral cavity carefully for colour, hydration, texture, and lesions (see Chapter 32). Clients who do not follow regular oral hygiene practices may have receding gum tissue, inflamed gums, a coated tongue, discoloured teeth (particularly along the gum margins), dental caries, missing teeth, and **halitosis** (bad breath). Localized pain and infection are common symptoms of gum disease and certain tooth disorders.

Some clients in acute care settings require a complete oral assessment. The identification of risks for infection and other conditions identify the type and frequency of oral care. Proper oral care has been shown to decrease the risk of aspiration and nosocomial infections in ventilated clients (Smeltzer & Bare, 2004). Ebersole et al. (2008) posit that Gram-negative bacteria (e.g., *Pseudomonas aeruginosa*) found in dental plaque can result in pneumonia in hospitalized older adults. It is especially important to examine the oral cavity of clients receiving radiation or chemotherapy. Both treatments can reduce the amount of saliva, resulting in drying and inflammation of the oral mucosal tissues. The assessment serves as a basis for preventive care for clients as they undergo treatment.

The Hair. Before performing hair care, assess the condition of the hair and scalp. Healthy hair is clean, shiny, and untangled; the scalp is clear of lesions. The hair of dark-skinned clients is usually thicker, drier, and curlier than that of lighter-skinned clients. Table 38–4 summarizes hair and scalp problems that may be identified during the assessment. In community and home care settings, it is particularly important to inspect the hair for pediculosis capitis (head lice) so that the appropriate treatment can be provided. If head lice is suspected, you guard against self-infestations by handwashing and using gloves or tongue blades to inspect the client's hair. A loss of hair (**alopecia**) can result from the effects of chemotherapy medications, hormonal changes, or improper hair care practices. Clients at risk for scalp problems are those who have experienced head trauma and those who practise poor hygiene.

The Eyes, Ears, and Nose. Examine the condition and function of the eyes, ears, and nose (see Chapter 32). Normally the eyes are free of infection and irritation. The sclerae are visible anteriorly as the white portion of the eye. The conjunctivae (the lining of the eyelids) are clear, pink, and without inflammation. The eyelid margins are in close approximation with the eyeball, and the lashes are turned outward. The lid margins are without inflammation, drainage, or lesions. The eyebrows are symmetrical.

TABLE 38-2 Common Skin Problems

Characteristics	Implications	Interventions
Dry Skin		
Flaky, rough texture on exposed areas such as hands, arms, legs, or face	Skin may become infected if epidermal layer is allowed to crack.	Ask client to bathe less frequently and to rinse body of all soap because residue left on the skin can cause irritation and breakdown. Add moisture to air through the use of a humidifier. Increase fluid intake when the skin is dry. Use a nonallergenic moisturizing cream to aid healing—cream can form a protective barrier and assist with keeping fluid within the skin. Use creams to clean skin that is dry or if client is allergic to soaps and detergents.
Acne		
Inflammatory, papulopustular skin eruption, usually involving bacterial breakdown of sebum; appears on face, neck, shoulders, and back	Infected material within pustule can spread if area is squeezed or picked. Permanent scarring can result.	Wash hair and skin thoroughly each day with soap to remove oil. Use cosmetics sparingly because oily cosmetics and creams accumulate in pores and tend to make the condition worse. Use prescribed topical or oral antibiotics for severe forms of acne.
Skin Rashes		
Skin eruption that may result from overexposure to sun or moisture or from an allergic reaction (may be flat or raised, localized or systemic, pruritic or nonpruritic)	If skin is continually scratched, inflammation and infection may occur. Rashes can also cause discomfort.	Wash the area thoroughly and apply an antiseptic spray or lotion to prevent further itching and aid in the healing process. Apply warm or cold soaks to relieve inflammation, if indicated.
Contact Dermatitis		
Inflammation of skin characterized by abrupt onset with erythema, pruritus, pain, and appearance of scaly oozing lesions (seen on face, neck, hands, forearms, and genitalia)	Dermatitis is often difficult to eliminate because the person is usually in continual contact with the substance causing the skin reaction, and it may be hard to identify this substance.	Avoid causative agents (e.g., cleansers and soaps).
Psoriasis		
Noncontagious, chronic skin condition characterized by an abnormal growth of keratinocytes (a type of skin cell) and an inflammatory reaction that results in the formation of thick, silvery, scaly, inflamed patches of skin; commonly seen on the scalp, knees, elbows, and chest	The cause of psoriasis is unknown, and no cure exists. It is often difficult to diagnosis as it has similar symptoms to eczema and atopic dermatitis.	Treatment options are aimed at reducing the extent and severity of the condition and improving quality of life. The client should avoid trigger agents such as smoking, stress, excessive alcohol, and skin injury (e.g., sunburn).
Abrasion		
Scraping or rubbing away of epidermis that may result in localized bleeding and later weeping of serous fluid	Infection occurs easily because of the loss of this protective skin layer.	Take care not to scratch client with jewellery or fingernails. Wash abrasions with mild soap and water; dry thoroughly and gently. Observe for retained moisture in dressings or bandages—excess moisture can increase the risk of infection.

BOX 38-3 Risk Factors for Skin Impairment

Immobilization

When restricted from moving freely, clients' dependent body parts are exposed to pressure, reducing circulation to the affected body parts. You should know which clients require assistance to turn and change positions.

Reduced Sensation

Clients with paralysis, circulatory insufficiency, or local nerve damage are unable to sense an injury to the skin. While bathing a client, assess the status of sensory nerve function by checking for pain, tactile sensation, and temperature sensation.

Nutrition and Hydration Alterations

Clients with limited caloric and protein intake can develop thinner, less elastic skin, with a loss of subcutaneous tissue. This can result in impaired or delayed wound healing.

Secretions and Excretions on the Skin

Moisture on the skin's surface serves as a medium for bacterial growth and can cause irritation, soften epidermal cells, and lead to skin breakdown. The presence of perspiration, urine, watery fecal material, or wound drainage on the skin can also result in breakdown or infection, or both.

Vascular Insufficiency

Inadequate arterial supply to tissues and impaired venous return decrease the circulation to the extremities. Inadequate blood flow can cause ischemia and tissue breakdown. The risk of infection also exists because the delivery of nutrients, oxygen, and white blood cells to injured tissues is inadequate.

External Devices

An external device applied to or around the skin exerts pressure and friction on the skin. Assess all surfaces exposed to casts, cloth restraints, bandages and dressings, tubing, or orthopedic braces.

Determine whether the client wears contact lenses. This is especially significant for clients who enter hospitals or other agencies unresponsive or in a confused state. To determine whether a contact lens is present, stand to the side of the client's eye and observe the cornea for the presence of a soft or rigid lens; if you do not see one, observe the sclera to detect whether a contact lens has shifted off the client's cornea. An undetected lens can cause severe corneal injury if left in place too long.

Inspect the external ear structures (auricle, helix, and earlobe), and use an otoscope to inspect the external auditory canal, and tympanic membrane. While performing hygiene measures, you are most concerned with noting the presence of accumulated **cerumen** or drainage in the ear canal, local inflammation, tenderness on palpation, or the client's report of pain (see Chapter 32).

Inspect the nares for signs of inflammation, discharge, lesions, edema, and deformity (see Chapter 32). The nasal mucosa is normally pink and clear and has little or no discharge. A clear, watery discharge may be the result of allergies. If clients have any form of tubing exiting the nose (e.g., nasogastric tube), inspect the naris surfaces that come in contact with the tubing for tissue sloughing, localized tenderness, inflammation, and bleeding.

Developmental Changes

The normal process of aging influences the condition of body tissues and structures and, thus, the manner in which hygiene measures are performed. Chapter 48 addresses the changes in hearing, vision, and olfaction across the lifespan as a result of growth and development.

The Skin. Neonates' skin is relatively immature at birth. The epidermis and dermis are loosely bound together, and the skin is very thin. Friction against the skin layers can cause bruising, so neonates must be handled carefully during bathing. Any break in the skin can easily lead to infection.

Toddlers' skin layers are more tightly bound together. Thus, children have a greater resistance to infection and skin irritation. However, because of children's active play and the absence of established hygiene habits, greater attention is needed from parents and caregivers to provide thorough hygiene and to begin teaching good hygiene habits.

During adolescence, the growth and maturation of the integument increases. In girls, estrogen secretion causes the skin to become soft, smooth, and thicker, with increased vascularity. In boys, male hormones produce an increased thickness of the skin with some darkening in colour. Sebaceous glands become more active, predisposing adolescents to **acne**. Eccrine and apocrine sweat glands become fully functional during puberty. Adolescents usually begin to use deodorants, and more-frequent bathing and shampooing become necessary to reduce body odours and eliminate oily hair. Sweating is usually more pronounced in boys.

The condition of adults' skin depends on hygiene practices and exposure to environmental irritants. Normally, the skin is elastic, well hydrated, firm, and smooth. When adults practise frequent bathing or

BOX 38-4 Skin Assessment for the Client With Darkly Pigmented, Intact Skin

Assess localized skin changes:

- Colour darker than surrounding skin colour; purplish, bluish, eggplant
- Taut skin
- Shiny skin
- Induration (hardening of the tissues)

Assess for edema (nonpitting, pitting):

- Importance of lighting for skin assessment:
  - Use natural or halogen light.
  - Avoid fluorescent lamps, which can give the skin a bluish tone.

Assess skin temperature, using the back of your hand and fingers; if the client's condition allows, do not use gloves when doing this assessment:

- Initially may feel warmer than surrounding skin
- Subsequently may feel cooler than surrounding skin

Data from Estes, M. E., & Buck, M. (2008). *Health assessment and physical examination* (1st Canadian ed., pp. 295, 315). Toronto, ON: Thomson Nelson; and Smeltzer, S. C., & Bare, B. (2004). *Brunner and Suddarth's textbook of medical–surgical nursing* (10th ed., pp. 1645–1647). Philadelphia, PA: Lippincott Williams & Wilkins.

➤ TABLE 38-3 Common Foot and Nail Problems

Characteristics	Implications	Interventions
Callus A callus is a thickened portion of the epidermis consisting of a mass of horny, keratotic cells. A callus is usually flat, painless, and found on the undersurface of the foot or on the palm of the hand. Problems are caused by local friction or pressure.	The condition may cause discomfort when wearing tight shoes.	Advise the client to wear gloves when using tools or objects that may create friction on palmar surfaces, and to wear soft-soled shoes with insoles. Soak callus in warm water and magnesium sulphate (Epsom salts) to soften the cell layers. Apply cream or lotion to reduce reformation. Encourage the client to see a podiatrist.
Corn Keratosis (a corn) is caused by friction and pressure from ill-fitting or loose shoes. It is seen mainly on or between toes or over a bony prominence. A corn is usually cone shaped, round, and raised. Soft corns are macerated.	The conical shape compresses the underlying dermis, making it thin and tender. The pain worsens when tight shoes are worn. The tissue can become attached to bone if allowed to grow. The client may suffer an alteration in gait resulting from pain.	Surgical removal may be necessary, depending on the severity of pain and size of the corn. Avoid the use of oval corn pads, which can increase the pressure on toes and reduce circulation. Use warm water soaks to soften the corns before gentle rubbing with a callus file or pumice stone (consult with physician). Wider and softer shoes are suggested.
Plantar Wart A plantar wart is a fungating lesion caused by the papillomavirus that appears on the sole of foot.	Warts may be contagious. They are painful and make walking difficult.	Treatment ordered by a physician may include applications of salicylic acid, electrodessication (burning with electrical spark), or freezing with solid carbon dioxide.
Athlete's Foot (Tinea Pedis) Athlete's foot is a fungal infection of the foot; scaliness and cracking of skin occurs between the toes and on the soles of feet. Small blisters containing fluid may appear. The problem can be induced by wearing constricting footwear.	Athlete's foot can spread to other body parts, especially the hands. It is contagious and frequently recurs.	Feet should be well ventilated. Drying feet well after bathing and applying powder helps to prevent infection. Wearing clean socks or stockings reduces the incidence. The physician may treat the condition with antifungal topical applications.
Ingrown Nail An ingrown toenail or fingernail is one that grows inward into the soft tissue around nail. An ingrown nail often results from improper nail trimming.	Ingrown nails can cause localized pain when pressure is applied.	Treatment is frequent hot soaks in an antiseptic solution and removal of the portion of nail that has grown into skin. Instruct the client regarding proper nail-trimming techniques, and provide a referral to a podiatrist. (Ensure that the client is aware of the associated cost.)
Ram's Horn Nail A ram's horn nail is an unusually long, curved nail.	Attempts to cut ram's horn nails may result in damage to the nail bed with a risk of infection.	Refer the client to a podiatrist. (Ensure that the client is aware of the associated cost.)
Paronychia Paronychia is the inflammation of tissue surrounding the nail, after a hangnail or other injury. It occurs in individuals who frequently have their hands in water and is common in clients with diabetes.	The area can become infected.	Treatment is hot compresses or soaks and local application of antibiotic ointments. Paronychia can be prevented by careful manicuring.
Foot Odour Foot odour is the result of excess perspiration, promoting microorganism growth.	The condition may cause discomfort because of excess perspiration.	Frequent washing, using foot deodorants and powders, and wearing clean footwear prevents or reduces the problem.

are exposed to an environment with low humidity, the skin can become very dry and flaky.

With aging, the skin loses its resiliency and moisture, and sebaceous and sweat glands become less active. The epithelium thins, and elastic collagen fibres shrink, making the skin fragile and subject to bruising and breaking. These changes warrant caution when turning and repositioning older adults (Meiner & Lueckenotte, 2006). Typically, older adults' skin becomes drier and wrinkled. Because the skin may be excessively dry, older adults should avoid bathing daily and using very hot water or harsh soaps.

The Feet and Nails. When we stand, the feet provide body support and absorb shock. With aging, they begin to show signs of wear and tear. This may occur earlier if individuals have failed to wear comfortable, supportive footwear. The cushioning layer of fat on the soles of the feet becomes thin.

TABLE 38-4 Problems of Head and Body Hair and Scalp

Characteristics	Implications	Interventions
Dandruff		
Scaling of the scalp is accompanied by itching. In severe cases, dandruff can be found on eyebrows.	Dandruff causes individuals embarrassment. If dandruff enters the eyes, conjunctivitis may develop.	Shampoo regularly with a medicated shampoo. In severe cases, obtain a physician's advice.
Ticks		
Small, grey–brown parasites burrow into the skin and suck the blood.	Ticks transmit several diseases to individuals. The most common are Rocky Mountain spotted fever, tularemia, and Lyme disease.	Do not pull ticks from the skin because their sucking apparatus remains and may cause infection. Suffocate the tick by placing a drop of oil on it or by covering it with petrolatum for ease of removal.
Pediculosis Capitis (Head Lice)		
Head lice require a source of human blood to survive. Transmission is by direct contact (e.g., head to head). The parasite is found near the scalp attached to hair strands. Eggs look like oval particles, similar to dandruff. Bites or pustules may be observed behind the ears and at the hairline. Itching at the hairline is the most common symptom.	Contacts of the clients (e.g., family members and classmates) should be examined and treated. Although no current evidence exists of transmission by shared articles, families may wish to wash bedding and combs in hot water. Dry cleaning or storing items in plastic bags for 10 days is also effective (Infectious Diseases and Immunization Committee, Canadian Pediatric Society, 2003).	Check the entire scalp. Use a medicated shampoo to eliminate lice. Follow the product directions carefully; a repeat application is required 7–10 days later to ensure that surviving eggs are killed. Seek physician advice if treatment is ineffective; a new medication may be required for effective chemical eradication. Some products can cause neurotoxicity and should not be used with children under 6 years of age. Caution is advised against use of products containing lindane. This product has been withdrawn for use in some countries. Use a fine-toothed comb to assist with the manual removal of nits (the empty eggshell) and lice.
Pediculosis Corporis (Body Lice)		
Body lice differ from head lice in that body lice tend to cling to clothing and may not be easily seen. They suck blood and lay eggs on clothing and furniture.	The client itches constantly. Scratches seen on the skin may become infected. Hemorrhagic spots may appear on skin where lice are sucking blood.	Ask the client to bathe or shower thoroughly. After the skin is dried, apply a recommended pediculicide lotion. After 8–12 hours, have the client take another bath or shower. Bag infested clothing or linen until laundered in hot water. Vacuum rooms thoroughly and throw away the bag after completion.
Pediculosis Pubis (Crab Lice)		
Crab lice parasites are found in pubic hair. Crab lice are greyish white with red legs.	Lice may be spread via bed linen, clothing, or furniture, or between persons via sexual contact.	Cleanse as for body lice. The treatment of sexual partners is recommended.
Hair Loss (Alopecia)		
Alopecia occurs in individuals of all races. Balding patches are seen at the periphery of the hairline. Hair becomes brittle and broken. The condition is caused by genetics and the use of hair curlers, hot combs, and hair picks and by tight braiding.	Patches of uneven hair growth and loss alter the client's appearance.	Advise the client to stop any hair-care practices that might be further damaging the hair.

Chronic foot problems are a common result of poor foot care, improperly fitting footwear, aging, and systemic disease. Older adults often have dry feet because of a decrease in sebaceous gland secretion, dehydration of epidermal cells, and poor condition of footwear. Fissures that develop as a result of dry skin can lead to foot ulcers (Smeltzer & Bare, 2004). Painful feet can be the result of congenital deformities, weak structure, injuries, and diseases such as diabetes, rheumatoid arthritis, or osteoarthritis. After 55 years of age, arthritis is a common cause of changes in the feet. Additional common foot problems include hammer toes, a loss of sensation, and pathological nail conditions (Smeltzer & Bare, 2004).

Fungal infections can occur under toenails, causing dark yellow streaks or total discoloration. The nails can also become opaque, scaly, and hypertrophied. If foot or nail problems stay unresolved, clients can easily become disabled. You must apply knowledge of typical changes in the feet and nails when anticipating the type of hygiene that clients will require.

The Oral Cavity. Infants begin teething at approximately 6 to 8 months of age (Hockenberry & Wilson, 2007). The first permanent (secondary) teeth erupt at about 6 years of age. From adolescence, when all of the permanent teeth are in place, through middle adulthood, the teeth and gums remain healthy if individuals avoid fermentable carbohydrates and sticky sweets. Regular dental care and hygiene practices such as brushing and flossing help to prevent caries and periodontal disease.

As individuals grow older, numerous factors can result in poor oral care. These include age-related changes of the mouth, chronic disease such as diabetes, physical disabilities involving hand grasp or strength affecting the ability to perform oral care, lack of attention to oral care, and prescribed medications that have oral side effects. Aging teeth become brittle, drier, and darker. Teeth can become uneven, jagged, and fractured. Gums lose vascularity and tissue elasticity, which can cause dentures to fit poorly. Many older adults are edentulous and wear complete or partial dentures. It is important to determine whether older clients wear dentures and the condition of underlying supportive gum tissue.

The Eyes, Ears, and Nose. Although the structure of the eyes do not have marked developmental changes, altered visual acuity can occur at several points during the aging process; for example, when children start school or when clients reach middle age, visual acuity may change. As clients age, they are also at risk for changes in visual clarity (e.g., caused by glaucoma or cataracts) and visual field losses (e.g., caused by macular degeneration or glaucoma).

Structures of the ears do not change as clients age; however, changes in hearing acuity or balance may occur with aging. In young children, changes in hearing acuity may result from a foreign object being placed in the ear—this may be a temporary change, resolved once the object is removed. Changes may also result from repeated ear infections or exposure to loud noise, such as when children listen to loud music on headphones.

Older adults may have changes in the structure and function of the small bones in the inner ear that affect hearing acuity. Aging may result in increased cerumen production, which can also impede hearing acuity. In addition, the movement of fluid through the semicircular canals may change with age, and clients may experience positional dizziness or balance problems.

Although changes in the sense of smell can occur at any time, they seem to be more common in older adults. These changes may also affect taste and clients' appetite.

New and acute changes in the structure and function of the eyes, ears, and nose must be fully assessed and evaluated. Timely evaluation of these changes may confirm that they are age related or identify other illnesses.

Use of Sensory Aids

When clients wear eyeglasses, contact lenses, artificial eyes, or hearing aids, assess their knowledge and ask them to describe the methods that are used for routine care (Box 38–5). Compare information gathered from clients with the proper care technique for these devices. Any differences in client practice with standard practice may indicate a need for client education.

Self-Care Ability

Clients with physical or cognitive impairments need assistance with all or some aspects of personal hygiene. Assessment of clients' physical and cognitive statuses determines specifically which aspects of hygiene care can be performed independently, which require some assistance, and which require total assistance.

The assessment must include the measurement of clients' muscle strength, flexibility and dexterity, balance, coordination, and activity tolerance—these qualities are needed to perform activities such as bathing, brushing teeth, and bending over to inspect the feet. The degree of assistance needed by clients during hygiene care may also depend on vision, their ability to sit without support, their hand grasp strength, the range of motion in their extremities, or the presence of equipment such as an IV line, dressings, or traction. Painful conditions of the upper extremities pose special problems. Assess

➤ BOX 38-5 Assessing a Client's Use of Sensory Aids

Eyeglasses

- Ask about purpose for wearing glasses (e.g., reading, distance, or both)
- Ask about methods used to clean glasses
- Ask about presence of symptoms (e.g., blurred vision, photophobia, headaches, or irritation)

Contact Lenses

- Determine type of lens worn
- Ask about frequency and duration of time lenses are worn (including sleep time)
- Ask about presence of symptoms (e.g., burning, excess tearing, redness, irritation, swelling, or sensitivity to light)
- Ask about techniques used by the client to cleanse, store, insert, and remove lenses
- Ask about use of eye drops or ointments
- Determine whether client has an emergency identification bracelet or card that alerts others to remove client's lenses in case of emergency

Artificial Eye

- Ask about method used to insert and remove eye
- Ask about method for cleansing eye
- Ask about presence of symptoms (e.g., drainage, inflammation, or pain involving the orbit)

Hearing Aid

- Ask about type of aid worn
- Ask about methods used to cleanse aid
- Ask about client's ability to change battery and adjust hearing aid volume

self-care ability by asking clients to perform activities such as brushing their teeth or combing their hair. Observe them carefully and note whether the clients can perform the task thoroughly and correctly (Figure 38–5).

When a client has self-care limitations, part of the assessment is to determine whether family or friends are available to assist. Assisting with hygiene measures can at times be unpleasant, so the assessment should include how the family members assist, how often this assistance is provided, and what their feelings are about being a caregiver. In addition, assess the home environment and its influence on the client's hygiene practices. Does the home environment contain barriers that may affect the client's self-care abilities? Water faucets that are too tight to easily adjust, bathtubs with high sides, and a bathroom too small to fit a wheelchair or walker in front of a sink are a few examples.

Hygiene Practices

An assessment of hygiene practices reveals a client's grooming preferences. For example, a client may choose to groom the hair in a certain style or to trim nails a certain way. When a client has a physical disability, special precautions may be needed to perform grooming without injury. Asking the client to assist or teach how to perform preferred grooming practices gives the client a greater sense of independence and helps you to avoid causing the client discomfort or injury.

Cultural Factors

A client's cultural background is an influential factor when determining hygiene needs. Culture plays a role not only in hygiene practices and preferences but also in sensitivity regarding personal space (see Chapter 10). For example, some clients may view tasks associated with closeness and touch as being offensive or impolite. Ask clients what would make them feel most comfortable during a bath. Instead of a full bath, perhaps a client would prefer only a partial bath, with a family member performing the bathing of private body areas. The client may also defer part of the hygiene care. If, in your judgement, hygiene is critical to prevent developing or worsening problems, such as skin breakdown, you must take the time to understand the client's concerns and negotiate a mutually satisfactory solution to the problem.

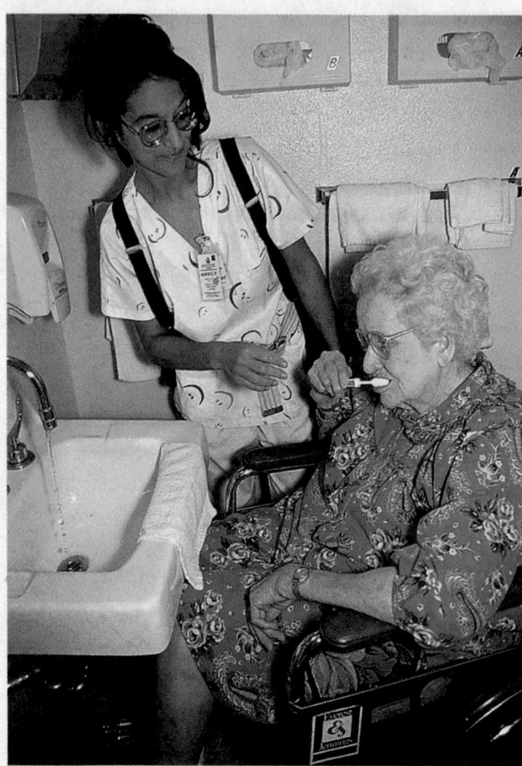

Figure 38-5 Observe client brushing the teeth. Observation allows you to determine how much assistance the client may need.

Clients at Risk for Hygiene Problems

Some clients present risks that require more attentive and rigorous hygiene care (Table 38–5). These risks may result from side effects of medications, a lack of knowledge, an inability to perform hygiene, or a physical condition that potentially injures the skin or other structures. An immobilized client who has a fever, for example, requires more frequent bathing to minimize perspiration on the skin, and more frequent turning and positioning to reduce the risk of skin breakdown.

Anticipate whether a client is predisposed to such risks and follow through with a complete assessment. For example, if a client is receiving chemotherapy, the treatment has a risk of destroying the normal flora in the mouth, allowing for the overgrowth of opportunistic bacteria. Therefore, the oral examination should be more thorough and detailed, involving all surfaces of the tongue and mucosa. If a client is diaphoretic, special attention should be given to body areas such as underneath the breasts and the perineal area, where moisture may collect and irritate skin surfaces. You should anticipate problems created by these risks and provide appropriate preventive care. Your assessment should include a review of the client's medical and surgical histories, medications, and specific risk factors.

Special Considerations in Hygiene Assessment

Depending on the type of hygiene you are planning to provide, you should conduct certain focused assessments. Before giving foot care, you should assess the type of footwear worn by a client. Children or young adults who frequently fail to wear socks may have excess perspiration that promotes fungal growth. Tight or poorly fitting shoes, socks, garters, or knee-high nylon stockings may cause skin irritation and interfere with circulation to the feet. You should also assess whether clients wear clean footwear daily because repeated use of soiled footwear can lead to infection. If clients have diabetes mellitus or another peripheral vascular disease, it is extremely important that they wear appropriate footwear. Extra-wide and extra-deep shoes accommodate bunions or hammer toes. Cushioned inner soles help redistribute pressure on the metatarsal head. Clients may need to be referred to a podiatrist and orthotic footwear specialist.

It is also important to assess clients' eating patterns before providing oral care. Ask clients whether problems are noted with chewing, swallowing, or the fit of their dentures, if any. Clients may have changed the type of food in their diet as a result of chewing difficulties. The presence of an ulcer or irritation may impair chewing and cause clients to avoid eating. This is common in older adults with poorly fitting dentures.

Client Expectations

As is the case in any nursing assessment, it is important to know what clients expect from nursing care. For hygiene care, clients may simply expect to have hygiene preferences and practices applied in the health care setting. You can assess clients' expectations by asking questions such as, "To make you most comfortable and feeling at home, how can I best perform your bath and personal care?" or "How can we help you care for your teeth, nails, and hair, now that you are at home?"

Understanding your clients' expectations and applying them in practice is important in establishing a caring relationship. Truly

TABLE 38-5 Health Risks and Implications for Hygiene

Risks	Hygiene Implications
Oral Problems	
Inability to use upper extremities due to paralysis, weakness, or restriction (e.g., cast or dressing)	Client lacks upper extremity strength or dexterity needed to brush teeth (Miller, 2009).
Dehydration, inability to take fluids or food by mouth	Dehydration causes excess drying and fragility of the mucosa, and increases the accumulation of secretions on the tongue and gums.
Presence of nasogastric or oxygen tubes; mouth breathers	These cause drying of the mucosa.
Chemotherapeutic drugs	Drugs kill rapidly multiplying cells, including normal cells lining the oral cavity. Ulcers and inflammation can develop.
Over-the-counter lozenges, cough drops, antacids, and chewable vitamins	Medications may contain large amounts of sugar. Repeated use increases sugar or acid content in mouth.
Radiation therapy to head and neck	Radiation therapy reduces salivary flow and lowers the pH of saliva; this can lead to stomatitis and tooth decay (Smeltzer & Bare, 2004).
Oral surgery, trauma to mouth, placement of an oral airway	These cause trauma to the oral cavity with swelling, ulcerations, inflammation, and bleeding.
Immunosuppression; altered blood clotting	These conditions predispose to inflammation and bleeding gums.
Diabetes mellitus	Clients with diabetes are prone to dryness of the mouth, gingivitis, periodontal disease, and tooth loss.
Skin Problems	
Immobilization	Dependent body parts are exposed to pressure from underlying surfaces. The inability to turn or change position increases the risk for pressure ulcers.
Reduced sensation due to stroke, spinal cord injury, diabetes, local nerve damage	Client does not receive the normal transmission of nerve impulses when excessive heat or cold, pressure, friction, or chemical irritants are applied to skin.
Limited protein or caloric intake and reduced hydration (e.g., caused by fever, burns, gastrointestinal alterations, poorly fitting dentures)	Limited caloric and protein intakes predispose to impaired tissue synthesis. The skin becomes thinner, less elastic, and smoother, with a loss of subcutaneous tissue. Poor wound healing may result. Reduced hydration impairs skin turgor.
Excessive secretions or excretions on the skin from perspiration, urine, watery fecal material, and wound drainage	Moisture is a medium for bacterial growth and can cause local skin irritation, softening of epidermal cells, and skin maceration.
Presence of external devices (e.g., casts, restraint, bandage, dressing)	A device can exert pressure or friction against the skin's surface.
Vascular insufficiency	Arterial blood supply to tissues is inadequate, or venous return is impaired, causing decreased circulation to the extremities. Tissue ischemia and breakdown may occur. The risk for infection is high.
Foot Problems	
Inability to bend over or see clearly	Client is unable to fully visualize the entire surface of each foot, impairing his or her ability to adequately assess the condition of skin and nails.
Eye Care Problems	
Reduced dexterity and hand coordination	Physical limitations create an inability to safely insert or remove contact lenses.

individualizing hygiene care shows respect for your clients' needs. As you learn what each client expects, this information can be incorporated into the individual's plan of care (see "Planning" section later).

❖Nursing Diagnosis

Your assessment reveals the condition of the skin, oral cavity, and other tissues, as well as a client's need for and ability to meet personal hygiene needs. As you review all data gathered, consider previous clients cared for, review your knowledge pertaining to pre-existing conditions, and then look for clusters of data suggesting a problem trend. For example, an older adult with degenerative arthritis can present with pain in the joints, weakness, mobility limitations in the dominant hand, and a generally unkempt appearance. A closer review of assessment data reveals defining characteristics of an inability to wash body parts and difficulty turning and regulating a water faucet. The nursing diagnosis of *bathing/hygiene self-care deficit* is supported and becomes part of the plan of care. The accurate selection of nursing diagnoses requires critical thinking to identify actual or potential health problems. Assessment activities must be thorough in identifying all appropriate defining characteristics so that an accurate diagnosis can be made (Box 38–6).

The focus of nursing interventions depends on whether a client has an actual alteration (e.g., impaired tissue integrity) or is at risk for a problem (e.g., risk for impaired oral mucous membrane). The client with an actual alteration requires extensive hygiene care, which is often more thorough than routine care. For example, if the client has skin breakdown, you must initiate care more frequently to keep intact skin surfaces clean and dry and to eliminate factors such as moisture or drainage that can worsen the condition of the skin. You also provide

BOX 38-6 NURSING DIAGNOSTIC PROCESS

Assessment Activities	Defining Characteristics	Nursing Diagnosis
Observe client's attempt to bathe self either in bed or at bathroom sink. (*Note:* Be sure positioning does not restrict potential movement.)	Unable to wash body or body parts	*Self-care deficit in bathing or hygiene related to upper extremity weakness and generalized fatigue*
Assess client's upper extremity strength, range of motion, and coordination.	Restricted upper extremity range of motion and strength Coordination adequate	
Ask client about level of fatigue after bathing.	Complains of fatigue and needs to rest after bathing	
Obtain vital signs before and after bathing.	Pulse elevated from 90–110 beats per minute, blood pressure stable, respirations elevated from 16–22 breaths per minute	

care to promote healing of injured skin surfaces (see Chapter 47). If the client is at risk for a problem, you institute preventive measures. In the case of risk for impaired oral mucous membranes, you keep the mucosa well hydrated, minimize foods irritating to tissues, and provide cleansing that soothes and reduces tissue inflammation.

The identification of related factors guides in the selection of nursing interventions. Diagnoses of *impaired oral mucous membrane related to malnutrition* and *impaired oral mucous membrane related to chemical trauma* require very different interventions. When malnutrition is a causal factor, you confer with a dietitian for appropriate dietary supplements and incorporate client education into the plan. When mucosa are injured as a result of chemical trauma from chemotherapy, techniques for cleansing and hydrating inflamed tissues and eliminating sources of irritation are the focus of nursing care. Although many nursing diagnoses associated with hygiene problems are possible, the following are a few of the more common diagnoses:

- *Impaired dentition*
- *Fatigue*
- *Ineffective health maintenance*
- *Risk for infection*
- *Deficient knowledge about hygiene practices*
- *Impaired physical mobility*
- *Impaired oral mucous membrane*
- *Self-care deficit, bathing/hygiene, dressing/grooming, toileting*
- *Chronic low self-esteem*
- *Risk for impaired skin integrity*
- *Ineffective tissue perfusion*

❖Planning

During planning, you synthesize information from multiple resources (Figure 38–6). Critical thinking ensures that the client's plan of care integrates all that you know about the individual client and key critical thinking elements.

Certain clients have multiple nursing diagnoses. The concept map (Figure 38–7) shows graphically how numerous nursing diagnoses can be interrelated.

Previous experience with other clients can be very useful in knowing how to adapt hygiene techniques for special needs. Professional nursing standards and evidence-informed clinical guidelines are especially important to consider when developing a care plan. For example, the clinical practice recommendations of the Canadian Diabetes Association (2006a, 2006b) offer valuable foot care guidelines for diabetic clients.

Goals and Outcomes

You and the client work together to identify goals and expected outcomes and to develop an individualized care plan based on the client's nursing diagnoses (Box 38–7). Goals are established with the client's self-care abilities and resources in mind and focus on maintaining or improving the condition of the skin and mucosa, oral mucosa, or dental hygiene, for example. Outcomes should be measurable and achievable within client limitations. Further collaborate with the client to then select hygiene measures that are appropriate and realistic.

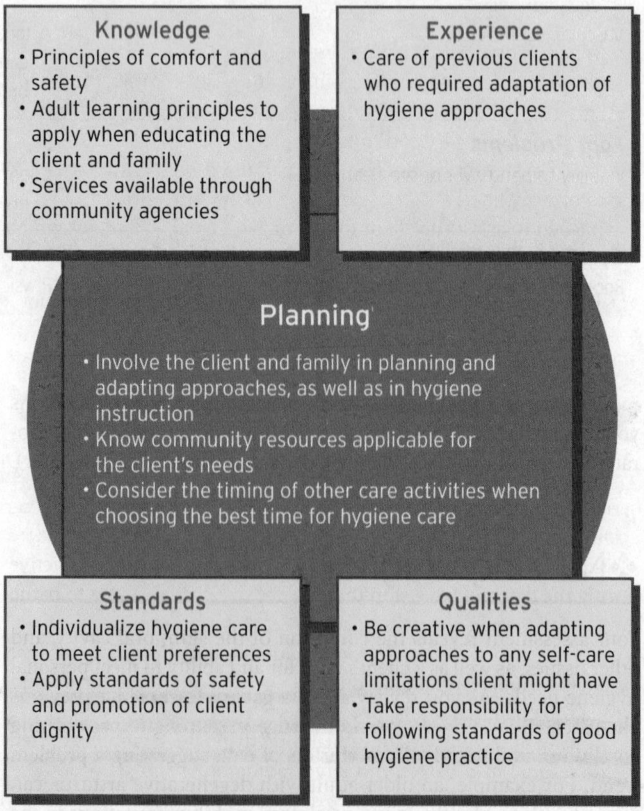

Figure 38-6 Critical thinking model for hygiene planning.

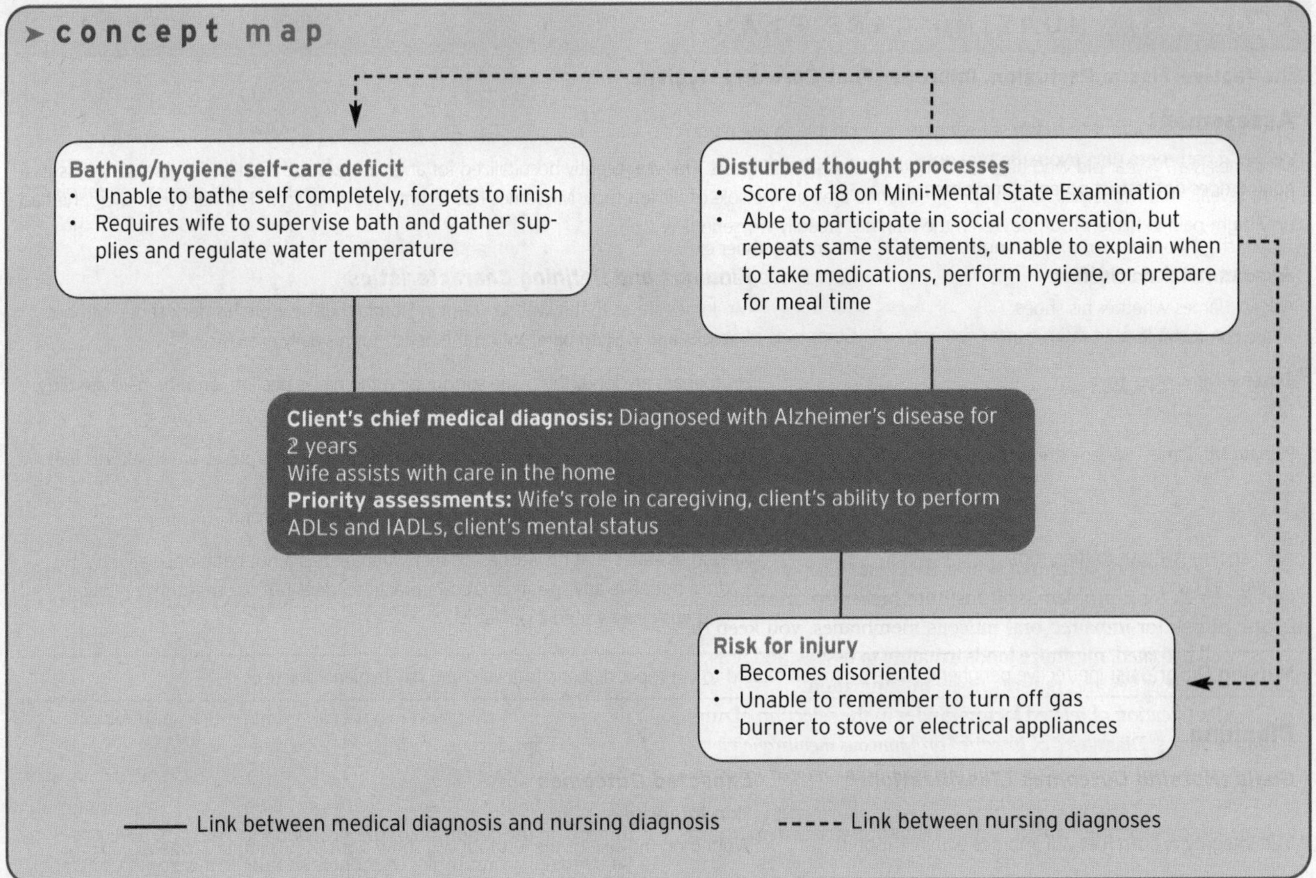

Figure 38-7 Concept map for a client with Alzheimer's disease and hygiene needs. ADLs, activities of daily living; IADLs, instrumental activities of daily living.

When providing for client hygiene, you care for a variety of clients with different self-care abilities and needs. For example, for a client who has hemiparesis after a cerebral vascular accident, you and the client might develop the following goal: "Client's musculoskeletal system remains free of breakdown or contractures." A series of realistic individualized expected outcomes would then be established to assist the client in meeting this goal. These outcomes may include the following:

- Client's skin is clean, dry, and intact without signs of inflammation.
- Client's skin remains elastic and well hydrated.
- Client's range of joint motion remains within normal limits on both affected and unaffected sides.

Setting Priorities

The client's condition influences the plan for delivering hygiene. A seriously ill client usually needs a daily bath because body secretions accumulate. An older client at home may require a visit from a home care aide to assist with a tub bath. Clients who are normally inactive during the day and have skin that tends to be dry may need to bathe only twice a week. You must plan for necessary assistance for clients who are weakened or possess poor coordination. For example, a client who has hemiparesis and has difficulty getting out of the tub should have a tub chair, handrails, or extra personnel available for help.

Timing is also important in planning hygiene. Being interrupted in the middle of a bath to undergo radiography can frustrate and embarrass a client. After extensive diagnostic tests (e.g., a stress test), it may be best to delay hygiene and allow a client to rest.

Continuity of Care

It is important to plan for care throughout the hospital stay, in discharge to a rehabilitation facility, and at home. When a client needs assistance as a result of a self-care limitation, the family becomes a valuable resource. Family members can usually assist with hygiene measures but may need support and guidance in adapting techniques to fit client limitations. You must be aware of equipment and procedures that were used while the client was in the hospital or facility so that the client and family are knowledgeable about the care, have the skill needed to provide the care, and have access to necessary equipment. In addition, various community resources may be needed. For example, if you are involved in the care of a homeless client, you may need to be aware of the location of clothing distribution centres for basic hygiene supplies or a shelter where bathing facilities are available. Forming partnerships with social workers or staff in local area churches and schools can assist in ensuring that clients have the resources they need to maintain hygiene.

❖Implementation

Providing hygiene is a very basic part of a client's care. The use of caring practices helps to alleviate the client's anxiety and promote comfort and relaxation while you perform each hygiene measure. For example, while giving a client a bath and changing a gown, use a gentle approach in turning and repositioning the client. Using a soft,

BOX 38-7 NURSING CARE PLAN

Ineffective Tissue Perfusion, Improper Foot Care and Hygiene

Assessment

Mr. James is a 77-year-old who has had diabetes mellitus for 20 years. He was recently hospitalized for an acute exacerbation of the disease. An assessment reveals that Mr. James has an open, reddened area on the sole of his left foot. Mr. James has recently returned from Florida. While there, he had only slight pain in his left foot; however, the pain has steadily worsened.

Assessment Activities	*Findings and Defining Characteristics*
Ask Mr. James whether his shoes are comfortable.	Mr. James states that it was so warm in Florida that he wore his deck shoes without socks and walked barefoot on the beach for his daily exercise.
Observe Mr. James' feet.	His toenails are long, the tissue surrounding the nail is peeling, and the nails are dirty. A small laceration is present on the bottom of his left foot.
Palpate Mr. James' lower extremities.	His popliteal pulses are within normal limits. Dorsalis pedis pulses are weak. His feet are pale and cool to the touch. His capillary refill time is increased in his left foot at >2 seconds.
Ask Mr. James about routine foot and nail care.	Mr. James states that he washes his feet when he has a hot bath, once a week. He does not have any specific foot care practices, does not use moisturizing lotion, and has never visited a podiatrist.

Nursing Diagnosis: Ineffective peripheral tissue perfusion related to improper diabetic foot care and nail hygiene practices

Planning

*Goals (Nursing Outcomes Classification)**	*Expected Outcomes*
	Skin Integrity
Skin integrity in both feet will improve within 1 month.	Wound on the sole of the left foot will show signs of healing in 2 weeks.
	Tissue Perfusion: Peripheral
Client will have improved peripheral circulation to both feet.	Within 3 months, capillary refill time will show improvement.
	Deficient Knowledge: Treatment Regimen
Proper hygiene is encouraged and client will be able to complete diabetic foot care independently.	Client is able to accurately inspect tissue integrity of feet and toenails within 1 month. Client describes correct preventive diabetic foot care practices. Client has improved diabetic foot care and nail hygiene within 2 weeks.

*Outcome classification labels from Moorhead, S., Johnson, M., & Maas, M. (Eds.). (2004). *Nursing Outcomes Classification (NOC)* (3rd ed.). St. Louis, MO: Mosby.

Interventions (Nursing Intervention Classification)†	**Rationale**
Skin Surveillance	
Review with client how to assess feet for breaks in the skin (blisters, abrasions, ulcers), friction from shoes (reddened or swollen areas), and how to avoid foot injury.	Injury to a diabetic foot from improper nail care or friction from poorly fitting shoes can cause redness and swelling; minor injuries to the foot can increase the client's risk for infection, impaired mobility, and amputation (Smeltzer & Bare, 2004).
Skin Care	
Show client how to clean and apply moisturizers and other skin care products to feet daily.	Proper foot care practices include daily cleaning and moisturizing of the feet (Smeltzer & Bare, 2004).
Demonstrate to client how to apply moleskin over blistered areas.	Moleskin preparations are useful in relieving pressure and friction and allow the area to heal.
Explain that the client should visit a podiatrist every 4–6 weeks for toenail care.	In addition to regular nail care, callus removal, and inspection of feet, the client should have his feet examined by a professional at least once a year or more often, depending on risk factors (Smeltzer & Bare, 2004).
Refer client to orthotic footwear specialist.	Orthotic footwear specialists can evaluate a client's walk patterns and create footwear individualized to the client's walk, weight, and other individual needs. Specialized footwear can reduce the risk of impaired skin integrity of the feet.

†Intervention classification labels from Dochterman, J. M., & Bulechek, G. M. (Eds.). (2004). *Nursing Interventions Classification (NIC)* (4th ed.). St. Louis, MO: Mosby.

➤ BOX 38-7 NURSING CARE PLAN *continued*

Evaluation

Nursing Actions	*Client Response and Finding*	*Achievement of Outcome*
Observe client's feet.	The laceration is healed.	The resolution of the left foot laceration has been achieved.
	Toenails are clean and properly trimmed, and no cracks around the nail tissue are observed.	Mr. James has improved diabetic foot and nail hygiene.
Palpate lower extremities.	Pulses are equal bilaterally; capillary refill is still sluggish.	Tissue perfusion to the feet has not improved greatly.
Ask client about frequency of foot inspection.	Mr. James states he observes his feet daily after removing his shoes and immediately before bed.	Mr. James inspects his feet daily; because no new foot injuries are observed, Mr. James appears to have achieved this outcome.
Observe client's foot care practice.	Mr. James correctly washed and moisturized his feet but was not wearing socks with his shoes. He states that he does not consistently wear socks.	Mr. James is able to perform diabetic foot hygiene practice but is not consistent in preventive practice.
Ask client about podiatrist appointment.	Mr. James has been to the podiatrist twice and will be returning every 6 weeks for toenail trimming and care.	Mr. James has improved diabetic foot and nail hygiene practice.

gentle voice while conversing with the client helps to relieve any fears or concerns. For clients with symptoms such as pain or nausea, administering symptom relief therapies before starting hygiene care helps to prepare the client for the procedure.

Another important part of implementation is assisting clients to administer their own hygiene. This includes educating clients on proper hygiene techniques and connecting clients with the community resources necessary to enable them to perform hygiene care. The same clients at risk for hygiene problems are those in greatest need of understanding their risks, knowing the implications, and having the information they need to make choices about when and how hygiene is performed.

Health Promotion

In primary health care settings, educate and counsel clients and families on proper hygiene techniques. A new mother needs assistance in learning how to bathe her newborn infant. An older adult needs to become informed about the importance of regular ear care to avoid hearing deficits resulting from accumulated cerumen. When assisting clients, maintain the standards for hygiene illustrated in this chapter and incorporate adaptations as needed to their lifestyle, living arrangements, and preferences. Guidelines to assist you in educating clients about hygiene are presented in Box 38–8.

Acute and Restorative Care

Nursing knowledge and skills needed for performing hygiene care are consistent across all health care settings where acute and restorative care are provided. In addition, some of the skills in this section are applicable in areas of health promotion.

In health care settings where clients receive direct nursing care, a variety of scheduled hygiene measures are provided (Box 38–9). Times may change because of factors affecting your organization or scheduling of care such as planned diagnostic and treatment procedures, the client's need for more hygiene, or your work assignment. In long-term care facilities, the schedule for hygiene may be less frequent.

Bathing and Skin Care

Bathing and skin care are a part of total hygiene. The extent of clients' bath and the methods used for bathing depend on their physical abilities, health problems, and the degree of hygiene required. If clients are physically dependent or cognitively impaired, increase skin

➤ BOX 38-8 Educating Clients About Hygiene Care

- Make instructions relevant. After assessing a client's knowledge, motivation, and health beliefs, provide information that relates to the client's situation and will be most useful in resolving the client's problem. For example, when offering foot care instruction to a client with diabetes mellitus, explain how the circulation to the feet can be impaired and how that poses a risk for poor healing and infection should the skin become cut or broken.
- Adapt teaching of techniques to the client's personal bathing facilities. Not all clients will have the ideal situation that exists in a health care setting (e.g., easily accessible shower or a bedside table to place over a bed). Use the facilities or equipment that the client has so that personal care items are easy to reach, the client's safety is ensured, and the client feels comfortable when performing hygiene. For example, a young mother may feel more comfortable bathing an infant in a baby bath chair.
- Teach the client steps to take to avoid injury. Almost any hygiene procedure can pose risks (e.g., cutting a nail too close to the skin, failing to adjust the water temperature of a bath, or using tap water for contact lens care). Any instruction you provide must clearly outline safety risks.
- Reinforce infection-control practices. Damage to the skin, mucosa, eyes, or other tissues creates an immediate risk for infection. Be sure the client understands the relationship between healthy and intact skin and tissues, hand hygiene practices, and the prevention of infection.

➤ BOX 38-9 Hygiene Care Schedule in Acute and Long-Term Care Settings

Early Morning Care

If you work the night shift, you may be required to provide basic hygiene to clients getting ready for breakfast, scheduled tests, or early morning surgery. Early morning care (often referred to as "A.M. care") includes offering a bedpan or urinal if the client is not ambulatory, washing the client's hands and face, and assisting with oral care.

Routine Morning Care

Before or after breakfast, assist by offering a bedpan or urinal to clients confined to bed; providing a bath or shower; providing perineal care; providing oral, foot, nail, and hair care; giving a back rub; changing the client's gown or pyjamas; changing the bed linens; and straightening the client's bedside unit and room. This is often referred to as "complete A.M. care."

Afternoon Care

Hospitalized clients often undergo many exhausting diagnostic tests or procedures in the morning. In rehabilitation centres, clients may participate in physiotherapy during the morning. Afternoon hygiene care includes washing the hands and face, assisting with oral care, offering a bedpan or urinal to those clients who are not ambulatory, and straightening bed linen.

Evening, or Hour-Before-Sleep, Care

Before bedtime, offer personal hygiene care that helps a client relax to promote sleep. Evening care, or P.M. care, may include changing soiled bed linens, gowns, or pyjamas; assisting the client in washing the face and hands; providing oral hygiene; giving a back massage; and offering a bedpan or urinal to nonambulatory clients. Ask clients if they would like a beverage, such as juice.

assessment and provide skin care directed toward reducing the risk for skin breakdown. When bathing cognitively impaired clients, consider their special needs and challenges (Box 38–10). These clients can easily become afraid, may use physical and verbal aggressive behaviours to avoid bathing, and may also display self-injurious behaviours (Miller, 2009).

A **complete bed bath** is used with clients who are totally dependent and require total hygiene care (Skill 38–1). It is an activity that can be exhausting for clients, even if you provide all the care. You must anticipate and assess whether clients are physically able to tolerate a complete bath. Measuring clients' vital signs before, during, and after the bath provides a measure of their physical tolerance. A **partial bed bath** involves bathing only those body parts that would cause discomfort or odour if not bathed, and those areas not easily reached by the client. This includes perineal care. Aging or dependent clients in need of only partial hygiene and self-sufficient bedridden clients unable to reach all body parts receive partial bed baths. Carefully assess these clients to determine that they can sufficiently bathe other body parts on their own.

It is important when administering a complete or partial bath to assess the condition of the skin to determine which type of cleansing product is necessary or whether the client requires daily bathing. Clients with excessively dry skin are predisposed to skin impairment. You may decide to skip a bath for a day or bathe only badly soiled areas. The use of a soap that contains emollients is another option. Lubricating the skin with lotion can also help reduce dryness.

The tub bath or shower can be used to give a more thorough bath than a bed bath. Safety is of primary concern because the surface of a tub or shower stall is slippery. In some settings, it is necessary to obtain a physician's order for a shower or tub bath. In some agencies, showers are equipped with a chair for clients with weakness or poor balance. Both tubs and showers should be equipped with grab bars for clients to hold on to during their entry and exit and when manoeuvring. Clients vary in how much assistance they need. Regardless of the type of bath the client receives, the following guidelines should be used:

- *Provide privacy.* Close the door or pull the room curtains around the bathing area. While bathing the client, expose only the areas being bathed.
- *Maintain safety.* Keep the side rails up while away from the client's bedside. This is critical for dependent, debilitated, and unconscious clients. (*Note:* When side rails are used as a restraint, a physician's order may be needed. Check your agency's policy.) Place the call light within the client's reach if you are leaving the room temporarily.
- *Maintain warmth.* The room should be kept warm because the client is partially uncovered and may easily be chilled. Wet skin causes an excess loss of heat through convection. Control drafts. Keep the client covered, exposing only the body part being washed during the bath.
- *Promote independence.* Encourage the client to participate in as much of the bathing activities as possible. Offer assistance when needed.
- *Anticipate needs.* Bring a new set of clothing and hygiene products to the bedside or bathroom.

✱ BOX 38-10 EVIDENCE-INFORMED PRACTICE GUIDELINE

Bathing Clients With Dementia

Provide individualized and flexible client-centred care:

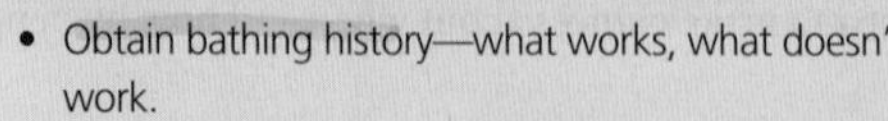

- Obtain bathing history—what works, what doesn't work.

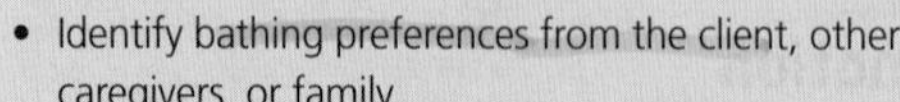

- Identify bathing preferences from the client, other caregivers, or family.
- Determine the method that is least distressing to the client (e.g., soaking feet in the bathtub).
- Prepare the bath environment in advance.
- Minimize the time the client is unclothed.
- Use distraction and negotiation instead of demands (e.g., give the client a washcloth to keep hands occupied).
- Minimize noise in the bathing area.
- Be sure the bathing environment is warm.
- Assess whether the client requires glasses or a hearing aid, which can assist with communication (remove aids as required during bathing after communicating your intent to the client).
- Set priorities regarding which body parts need bathing and which can be "skipped" (e.g., separate hair washing from bathing).
- Use as few staff as possible.
- If client fears water, try using coloured water or drawing a bubble bath.
- Reward client after bathing; praise and rewards should be realistic.

Adapted from Alzheimer Society of Canada. (2003). Understanding Alzheimer disease: The link between brain and behaviour. In *The Alzheimer Journey* [Module 4 in video and workbook series]. Retrieved May 30, 2004, from http://www.alzheimer.ca/english/disease/whatisit-video.htm; and Hall, G. R., & Buckwalter, K. C. (2001). Research-based protocol: Bathing persons with dementia. In M. G. Titler (Series Ed.), *Series on evidence-based practice for older adults.* Iowa City, IA: The University of Iowa College of Nursing Gerontological Nursing Interventions Research Center, Research Dissemination Core.

➤ SKILL 38-1 Bathing a Client

video

Delegation Considerations

Skills of bathing may be delegated to an unregulated care provider. Instructions about the following should be provided:

- The importance of not massaging reddened skin areas
- The clarification of early signs of impaired skin integrity
- The importance of reporting changes in the client's skin
- Proper positioning of an in-dwelling catheter during perineal care
- The importance of reporting any perineal drainage, excoriation, or rash observed

Equipment

- Washcloths and bath towels
- Wash basin
- Bath blanket (warm, if possible)
- Cleansing solution (agency or client specific)
- Personal hygiene items (deodorant, powder, lotion, unscented)
- Clean hospital gown or client's own pyjamas or gown
- Bed linen
- Linen bag
- Disposable gloves
- Disposable wipes
- Bedpan or urinal

Procedure

STEPS	RATIONALE
General Instructions	
1. Review orders for specific safety measures concerning the client's movement, positioning, or isolation precautions.	• Prevents accidental injury to the client during bathing activities. • Determines level of assistance required by the client.
2. Explain procedure, and ask client for suggestions on how to prepare supplies. Encourage and promote independence by asking the client how much of the bath he or she wishes to complete.	• Promotes client's cooperation and participation.
3. *Assess client's ability to perform self-care and allow client to perform as much of the bath as possible.*	• Client participates in plan of care. Promotes client's comfort and provides an opportunity to include cultural or personal hygiene preferences in hygiene care.
4. *Assess client's tolerance for activity, comfort level, cognitive ability, and musculoskeletal function.*	• Determines client's ability to perform self-care and level of assistance required. Also determines type of bath to administer (e.g., tub bath or partial bed bath).

Critical Decision Point: Clients whose level of independence and mobility change frequently may require more or less assistance during bathing.

STEPS	RATIONALE
5. Assess client's bathing preferences: frequency, type of hygiene products, and other factors related to client preferences.	• Encourages and promotes client participation.
6. Ask whether client has noticed any problems or unusual marks on skin. Observe the skin throughout the procedure, paying particular attention to areas that were previously soiled, reddened, or showed early signs of breakdown.	• Provides information to direct physical assessment of skin during bathing.
7. Begin complete or partial bed bath, or tub/whirlpool bath or shower.	
A. **Complete or partial bed bath**	
(1) Close room doors and draw the room divider curtain.	• Privacy ensures client's mental and physical comfort.
(2) Prepare equipment and supplies.	• Reduces transmission of microorganisms and avoids interrupting the procedure or leaving the client unattended to retrieve missing equipment.
(3) For nonambulatory clients, offer a bedpan or urinal. Provide a towel and washcloth for perineal care afterward.	• Client will feel more comfortable after voiding. Prevents the interruption of bath.
(4) Perform hand hygiene. If client's skin is soiled with drainage or body secretions, put on disposable gloves. Ensure the client is not allergic to latex.	• Reduces transmission of microorganisms.
(5) Place hospital bed at appropriate level, lower side rail closest to you. Assist client in assuming a comfortable position, preferably supine. Bring or have the client move toward side closest to you.	• Raising the height of the bed to the appropriate position facilitates proper body mechanics. Maintains client's comfort throughout procedure. Minimizes strain on back muscles because you do not have to reach across bed.
(6) Loosen the top covers. Place bath blanket over the top sheet. Remove top sheet from under the blanket. If possible, have client hold bath blanket while you withdraw sheet. Optional: Use the top sheet when a bath blanket is not available.	• Removal of top linens prevents them from becoming soiled or moist during the bath. Blanket provides warmth and privacy. The client is not exposed unnecessarily.
(7) If top sheet is to be reused, fold it for replacement later. If not, dispose in linen bag, taking care not to allow linen to contact uniform.	• Proper disposal prevents transmission of microorganisms.
(8) Assist client with oral hygiene. See Skill 38–3.	

Continued

➤ SKILL 38-1 Bathing a Client *continued*

STEPS	RATIONALE
(9) Remove client's gown or pyjamas. If the client has an IV infusing and the gown has snaps, simply unsnap and remove the gown without disconnecting the IV tubing. If the gown does not have snaps, remove gown from the arm without IV first; then lower the IV container or remove from the pump and slide the gown covering the affected arm over the tubing and container. Rehang IV container and check flow rate (see Step 7A(9) illustrations) or reset pump rate. Do not disconnect the tubing. If an extremity is injured or has reduced mobility, begin removal from the unaffected side.	• Provides full exposure of body parts during bathing. Undressing unaffected side first allows easier manipulation of gown over body part with reduced range of motion (ROM). • Manipulation of IV tubing and container will possibly disrupt flow rate.

Critical Decision Point: If available, be sure that clients with an IV or upper extremity injury have a gown with snap or tie sleeves; this ensures easy access to the upper extremities during hygiene.

Critical Decision Point: When an IV pump is used, it may be appropriate to manually adjust the IV flow rate to a keep-vein-open (KVO) and remove the IV tubing from the pump (check agency policy). Once the gown has been removed, reset the pump to the prescribed IV flow rate (see Chapter 40).

STEPS	RATIONALE
(10) Raise the side rail. Fill a wash basin two-thirds full with warm water. Have client place fingers in water to test temperature tolerance. Change the water as necessary throughout the bath.	• Raising side rail maintains the client's safety as you leave the bedside. Warm water promotes comfort, relaxes muscles, and prevents unnecessary chilling. Testing the temperature prevents accidental burns.
(11) Remove pillow, if allowed, and raise head of the bed 30–45 degrees. Place bath towel under the client's head. Place a second bath towel over client's chest.	• Removal of the pillow makes it easier to wash the client's ears and neck. The placement of towels prevents soiling of the bed linen and bath blanket.

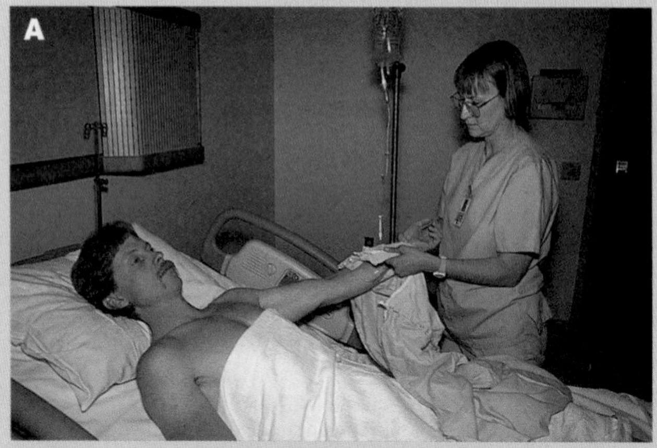

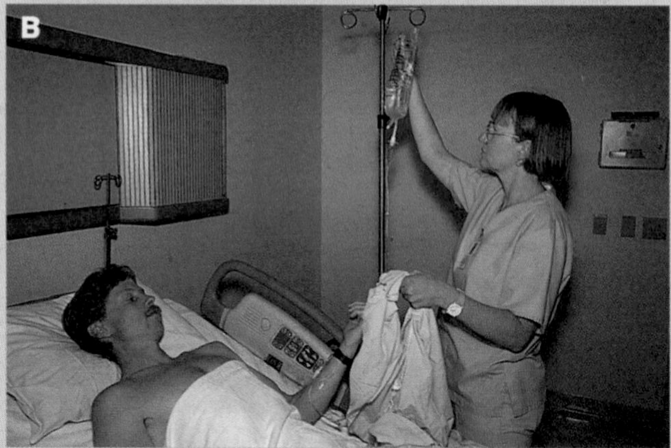

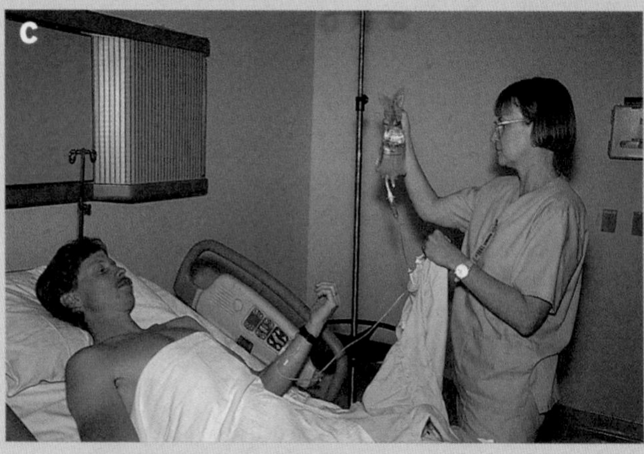

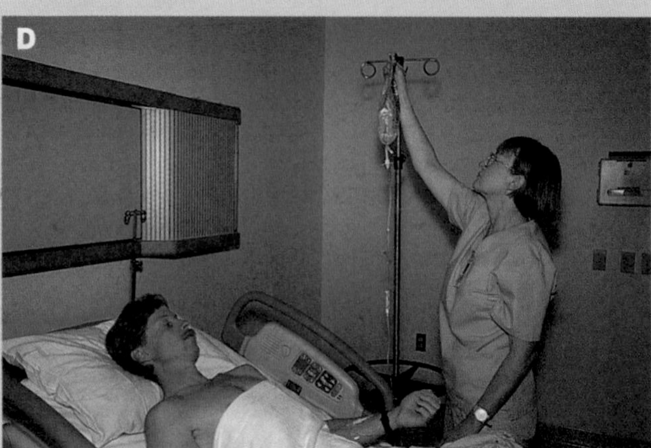

Step 7A(9) **A,** Remove client's gown. **B,** Remove IV from pole. **C,** Slide IV tubing through arm of client's gown. **D,** Rehang IV bag and check flow rate.

➤ SKILL 38-1 Bathing a Client *continued*

STEPS	RATIONALE
(12) Immerse washcloth in water and wring thoroughly. If desired, fold the washcloth around the fingers of your hand to form a mitt (see Step 7A(12) illustration).	• A mitt retains water and heat better than a loosely held washcloth; prevents splashing and cold edges from brushing against the client.
(13) Inquire whether the client is wearing contact lenses. Wash client's eyes with plain warm water. Use a different section of mitt for each eye. Move mitt from inner to outer canthus (see Step 7A(13) illustration). Soak any crusts on eyelid for 2–3 minutes with damp cloth before attempting removal. Dry eyes thoroughly but gently.	• Soap irritates eyes. The use of separate sections of mitt reduces infection transmission. Bathing the eye from inner to outer canthus prevents secretions from entering nasolacrimal duct. Pressure can cause internal injury.
(14) Ask whether client prefers to use soap on his or her face. Wash, rinse, and thoroughly dry all areas of the face, neck, and ears. (Men may wish to shave at this point or after the bath.)	• Soap tends to dry the face, which is exposed to air more than other body parts.
(15) Expose client's arm that is farthest from you and place bath towel lengthwise under the arm.	• Prevents soiling of bed. Washing far side first eliminates contaminating clean areas once they are washed.
(16) Bathe arm using long, firm strokes from distal to proximal areas (fingers to axilla). Raise and support arm as needed while thoroughly washing the axilla (see Step 7A(16) illustration).	• Soap lowers the surface tension of the skin and facilitates the removal of debris and bacteria when friction is applied during washing. Long, firm strokes stimulate circulation. Movement of the arm exposes the axilla and exercises the joint's normal ROM.
(17) Rinse and dry arm and axilla thoroughly. If client uses deodorant or talcum powder, apply it.	• Excess moisture causes skin maceration or softening. Deodorant controls body odour.
(18) Fold bath towel in half and lay it on the bed beside the client. Place a basin on the towel. Immerse client's hand in water. Allow hand to soak for 3–5 minutes before washing hand and fingernails (see Skill 38–2). Remove basin and dry hand well.	• Soaking softens cuticles and calluses of the hand, loosens debris beneath nails, and enhances the feeling of cleanliness. Thorough drying removes moisture from between fingers. *Note:* Do not soak if the client is diabetic or is cognitively impaired and unable to understand the procedure.
(19) Cover the arm with bath blanket or towel. Repeat steps 15–18 for the other arm.	

Critical Decision Point: If a client is at risk for falls, be sure the two side rails are up before obtaining fresh water or other supplies. Remember, side rails cannot be used as a restraint unless ordered.

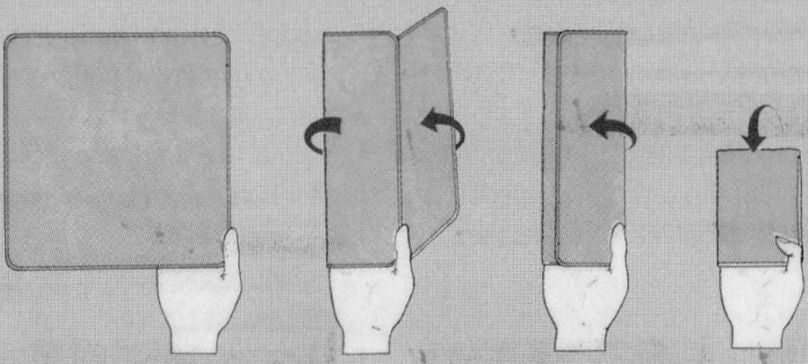

Step 7A(12) Steps for folding washcloth to form a mitt.

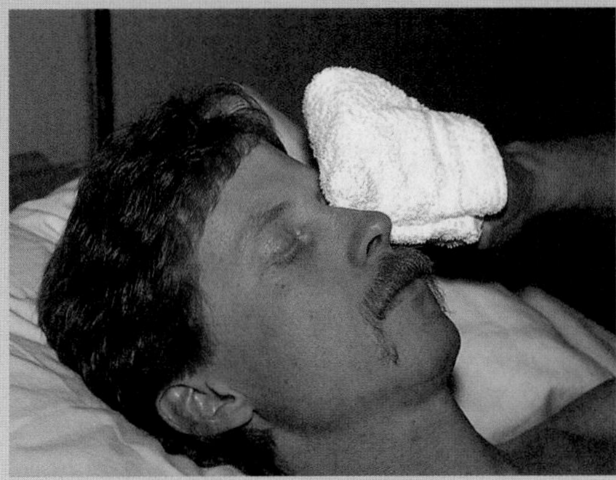

Step 7A(13) Wash eye from inner to outer canthus.

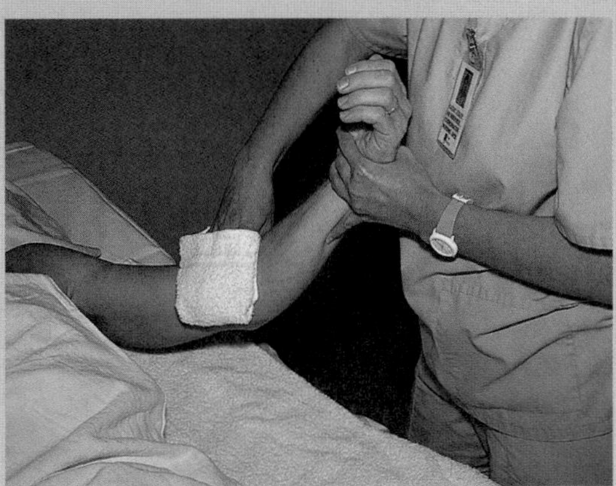

Step 7A(16) Washing from fingers to axilla.

Continued

➤ SKILL 38-1 Bathing a Client *continued*

STEPS	RATIONALE
(20) Cover client's chest with a bath towel, and fold bath blanket down to the umbilicus. With one hand, lift edge of towel away from client's chest. With washcloth or mitted hand, bathe chest using long, firm strokes. Take special care to wash skinfolds under the client's breasts. Keep client's chest covered between wash and rinse periods. Dry well.	• Draping prevents unnecessary exposure of body parts. The towel maintains warmth and privacy. Secretions and dirt collect easily in areas of tight skinfolds. Skinfolds are susceptible to excoriation if not cleaned and dried properly.
(21) Place bath towel lengthwise over client's chest and abdomen. (Two towels may be needed.) Fold blanket down to just above the pubic region.	• Prevents chilling and unnecessary exposure of body parts.
(22) With one hand, lift the bath towel. With mitted hand, bathe the abdomen, giving special attention to bathing the umbilicus and abdominal folds. Keep the abdomen covered between washing and rinsing. Dry well.	• Moisture and sediment that collect in skinfolds predisposes skin to maceration and irritation.
(23) Cover client's chest and abdomen with top of the bath blanket or bath towels. Expose far leg by folding blanket toward midline. Be sure other leg and perineum are covered.	• Maintains client's warmth and comfort. Prevents chilling and unnecessary exposure.
(24) Place bath towel lengthwise under the far leg and, using firm strokes (unless contraindicated), wash, rinse, and dry thoroughly. Support the leg with one hand if client is unable to support it.	• Promotes venous return.

Critical Decision Point: Clients with a history of deep vein thrombosis (DVT) or hypercoagulation disorders *should not* have their lower extremities washed with long firm strokes.

STEPS	RATIONALE
(25) Cleanse the foot, making sure to bathe between toes. Clean and clip nails as per physician orders (see Skill 38–2). Dry well. If skin is dry, apply lotion.	• Secretions and moisture may be present between toes. Lotion helps retain moisture and soften the skin. • Client's own nail clippers should be used to avoid the transmission of microorganisms.

Critical Decision Point: Do not massage any reddened area on the client's skin because massaging causes breaks in the skin's surface capillaries and increases the risk of skin breakdown (Smeltzer & Bare, 2004).

STEPS	RATIONALE
(26) Repeat Steps 23–25 for the other leg and foot.	
(27) Assist client in assuming a prone or side-lying position (as applicable). Place the towel lengthwise along the client's side. Put on disposable gloves if not done so already.	• Exposes back and buttocks for bathing. Prevents contact with microorganisms in body secretions.
(28) Wash, rinse, and dry client's back from neck to buttocks using long, firm strokes (see Step 7A(28) illustration). Pay special attention to folds of the buttocks and the anus for redness or skin breakdown. Give a back rub (see Chapter 42). Change bath water if necessary and put on disposable gloves.	• Maintains warmth and prevents unnecessary exposure. Skinfolds near buttocks and anus may contain fecal secretions that harbour microorganisms. • Prolonged pressure on the sacral area or other bony prominences may lead to the development of pressure ulcers. • Changing the water prevents the transfer of microorganisms from the anal area to genitalia.

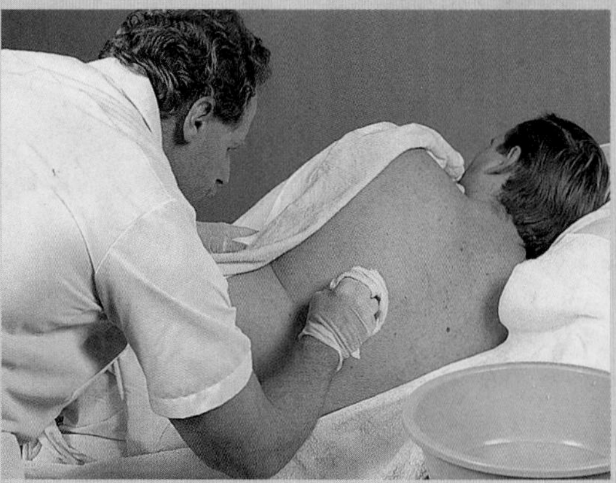

Step 7A(28) Washing client's back.

➤ SKILL 38-1 Bathing a Client *continued*

STEPS	RATIONALE
(a) **Female perineal care**	
(a1) Assist client in assuming a dorsal recumbent position, if not contraindicated. Cover chest and upper extremities with a towel and lower extremities with a bath blanket. Expose only the genitalia. (If client can wash, covering entire body with a bath blanket may be preferable.) Clean the perineal area. Pay special attention to skinfolds. Clients at risk for infection of the genitalia, urinary tract, or reproductive tract include those with in-dwelling catheters or fecal or urinary incontinence. If fecal material is present, enclose in a fold of underpad and remove with disposable wipes.	• Provides easy access to genitalia. • Clients capable of performing partial bath usually prefer to wash their own genitalia. • Secretions that accumulate on surface of skin surrounding genitalia act as reservoir for infection. • Cleansing reduces transmission of microorganisms from the anus to the urethra or genitalia.
(a2) Wash labia majora. Wipe from the perineum to the rectum. Repeat on the opposite side using a different section of the washcloth.	• Wiping from the perineum to the rectum reduces the chance of transmitting fecal organisms to the urinary meatus.
(a3) Separate the labia with your nondominant hand, exposing the urethral meatus and vaginal orifice. Wash downward from the pubic area toward the rectum in one smooth stroke (see Step 7A(28)(a3) illustration). Use a separate section of cloth for each stroke. Cleanse thoroughly around the labia minora, clitoris, and vaginal orifice.	• Cleansing method reduces the risk of transferring of microorganisms to the urinary meatus. (For menstruating women or clients with in-dwelling urinary catheters, cleanse with disposable wipes.)
(a4) Assist client to a comfortable position.	
(a5) Remove disposable gloves and perform hand hygiene.	• Prevents the transmission of infection.
(b) **Male perineal care**	
(b1) Lower the side rails, and assist client to a supine position. Note restriction in mobility. Clients at risk for infection of the genitalia, urinary tract, or reproductive tract include uncircumcised males and clients with in-dwelling catheters or fecal or urinary incontinence.	• Provides full exposure of male genitalia. • Clients capable of performing partial bath usually prefer to wash their own genitalia.
(b2) Gently raise the penis, and place a bath towel underneath. Gently grasp the shaft of penis. If the client is uncircumcised, retract the foreskin (see Step 7A(28)(b2) illustration). If the client has an erection, defer perineal care until later.	• Gentle but firm handling reduces the chance of the client having an erection. Secretions capable of harbouring microorganisms collect underneath foreskin. Cleansing the penis can lead to an erection, which can embarrass both the client and you.
(b3) Wash tip of the penis at the urethral meatus first using a circular motion. Cleanse from the meatus outward. Rinse and dry gently.	• The direction of the cleansing moves from areas of least contamination to most contamination, preventing microorganisms from entering urethra.
(b4) *Return foreskin to its natural position.*	• Tightening of the foreskin around the shaft of the penis can cause local edema and discomfort.
(b5) Wash the shaft of the penis with gentle but firm downward strokes. Pay special attention to the underlying surface of the penis. Rinse and dry thoroughly.	• The underlying surface of penis may have a greater accumulation of secretions.
(b6) Gently cleanse scrotum, making sure to wash underlying skinfolds. Rinse and dry thoroughly.	• Pressure on scrotal tissue can be painful to the client. Secretions collect between skinfolds.

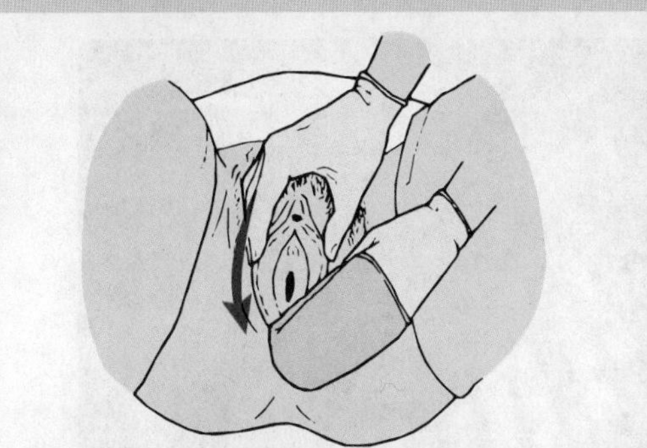

Step 7A(28)(a3) Cleanse from perineum to rectum (front to back).

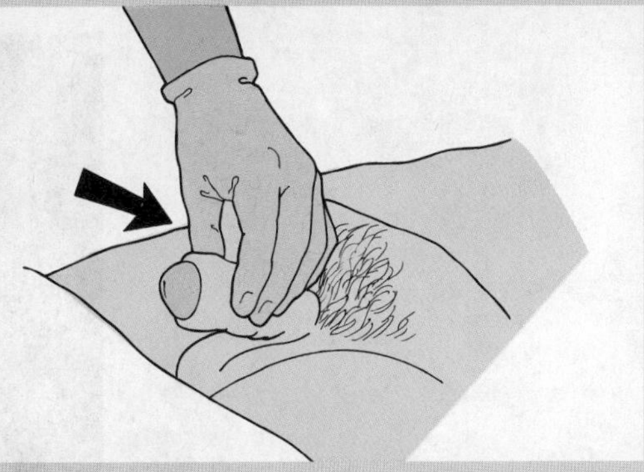

Step 7A(28)(b2) Retract foreskin.

Continued

➤ SKILL 38-1 Bathing a Client *continued*

STEPS	RATIONALE
(b7) Inspect the surface of external genitalia after cleansing.	• Thick secretions may cover underlying skin lesions or areas of breakdown. Evaluation determines the need for additional hygiene.
(b8) If the client has bowel or urinary incontinence, apply a thin layer of skin barrier cream to the buttock, anus, and perineal area.	• Protects skin from excess moisture and toxins from urine and stool.
(b9) Assist client to a comfortable position and cover with bath blanket.	
(29) Assist client in dressing. Comb client's hair. Women may want to apply makeup, and men may wish to shave at this point. Assist client to a chair or wheelchair.	• Promotes client's body image.
(30) Make the client's bed (see Skill 38–5).	• Provides a clean environment.
(31) Remove soiled linen and place it in linen bag. Clean and replace the bathing equipment. Replace the call light and personal possessions. Leave the room as clean and comfortable as possible.	• Prevents the transmission of microorganisms. A clean environment promotes the client's comfort. Keeping the call light and articles of care within reach promotes the client's safety.
(32) Remove disposable gloves (if applied) and perform hand hygiene.	• Reduces the transmission of microorganisms.
B. Tub or whirlpool bath or shower (verify with agency policy whether a physician's order is needed)	
(1) Check tub or shower for cleanliness. Use cleaning techniques outlined in agency policy. Place rubber mat on tub or shower bottom. Place disposable bath mat or towel on the floor in front of the tub or shower.	• Cleaning prevents the transmission of microorganisms. Mats prevent slipping and falling.
(2) Collect all hygienic aids, toiletry items, and linens requested by the client. Place within easy reach of the tub or shower.	• Placing items close at hand prevents possible falls when client reaches for equipment.
(3) Assist client to the bathroom if necessary. Have client wear a robe and slippers to bathroom.	• Assistance prevents accidental falls. Wearing a robe and slippers prevents chilling and provides for privacy and comfort.
(4) Demonstrate how to use the call signal for assistance.	• Bathrooms are equipped with signalling devices in case a client feels faint or weak or needs immediate assistance. Clients prefer privacy during bathing if safety is not jeopardized.
(5) Place an "occupied" sign on bathroom door.	• Maintains the client's privacy.
(6) Provide a shower seat or tub chair if needed (see Step 7B(6) illustration). Fill the bathtub halfway with warm water. If client's sensation is normal, ask client to test the water, and adjust the temperature if the water is too warm. Explain which faucet controls hot water. If client is taking shower, turn it on and adjust the water temperature before client enters the shower stall.	• The use of assistive devices facilitates bathing and minimizes physical exertion. Adjusting water temperature prevents accidental burns. Older adults and clients with neurological alterations (e.g., spinal cord injury) are at high risk for burns as a result of reduced sensation.
(7) Instruct the client to use safety bars when getting in and out of the tub or shower. Caution the client against use of bath oil in tub water.	• Prevents slipping and falling. Oil causes tub surfaces to become slippery.
(8) Instruct the client not to remain in tub >20 minutes. Check on client every 5 minutes. Observe ROM during bath.	• Prolonged exposure to warm water may cause vasodilation and pooling of blood, leading to light-headedness or dizziness. Measures joint mobility.

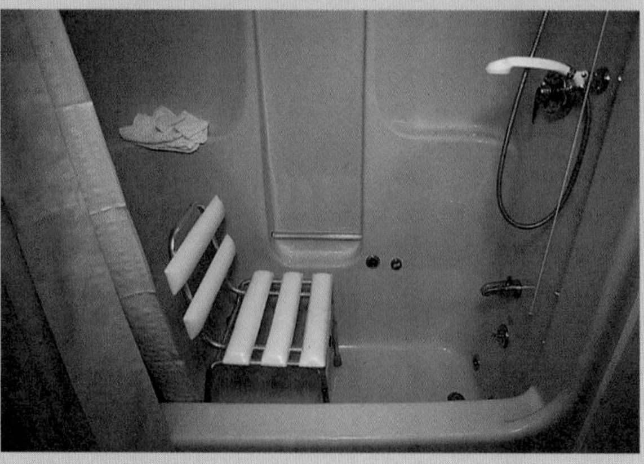

Step 7B(6) Shower seat for client safety.

➤ SKILL 38-1 Bathing a Client *continued*

STEPS	RATIONALE
(9) Return to the bathroom when the client signals, and knock before entering.	• Provides privacy.
(10) For the client who is unsteady, drain the tub of water before client attempts to get out of it. Place a bath towel over client's shoulders. Assist client in getting out of tub as needed, and assist with drying. If the client is weak or unstable, have another person assist.	• Prevents accidental falls. Client may become chilled as water drains.

Critical Decision Point: Weak or unstable clients need extra assistance in getting out of a tub. Planning for additional personnel is essential before attempting to assist a client from tub.

STEPS	RATIONALE
(11) Observe client's skin, paying particular attention to areas that were previously soiled, reddened, or showed early signs of breakdown.	• Techniques used during bathing should leave skin clean and clear.
(12) Assist client as needed in donning a clean gown or pyjamas, slippers, and robe. (In a home setting, the client may don regular clothing.)	• Maintains warmth to prevent chilling.
(13) Assist client to his or her room and a comfortable position in a bed or chair.	• Maintains relaxation gained from bathing.
(14) Clean the tub or shower according to agency policy. Whirlpool baths may require special cleaning. Remove soiled linen and place it in a linen bag. Discard disposable equipment in the proper receptacle. Place an "unoccupied" sign on the bathroom door. Return supplies to the storage area.	• Prevents the transmission of infection through soiled linen and moisture.
(15) Perform hand hygiene.	• Reduces the transfer of microorganisms.

Unexpected Outcomes and Related Interventions

Areas of Excessive Dryness, Rashes, or Irritation, or Signs of Pressure Ulcer on Client's Skin

- Review your agency's skin care policy regarding special cleansing and moisturizing products.
- Limit the frequency of complete baths.
- Complete a pressure ulcer assessment (see Chapter 47).
- Obtain a special bed surface if client is at risk for skin breakdown.

Inflammation of Skin and Genitalia, With Localized Tenderness, Swelling, and Presence of Foul-Smelling Discharge

- Bathe the area frequently to keep it clean and dry.
- Obtain an order for a sitz bath.
- Apply a protective barrier.
- Notify the physician and apply prescribed antibacterial or antifungal ointment or cream.

Client Expresses Perineal Discomfort

- Increase the frequency of perineal care.
- Assess the perineum for signs of irritation or discharge.

Client Unable to Perform Perineal Care Correctly

- Review perineal care with the client.
- Position the client and have client observe the cleansing procedure.

Client Becomes Excessively Fatigued and Unable to Cooperate or Participate in Bathing

- Reschedule bathing to a time when the client is more rested.
- Clients with cardiopulmonary conditions and breathing difficulties require a pillow or elevated head of the bed during bathing.
- Notify the physician about changes in the client's fatigue level.
- Schedule rest periods.

Client Seems Unusually Restless or Complains of Discomfort

- Consider analgesia before bathing.
- Schedule rest periods before bathing.

Recording and Reporting

- Record the condition of skin and any significant findings (e.g., reddened areas, bruises, nevi, or joint or muscle pain).
- Report any evidence of alterations in skin integrity or increased wound secretions to the person in charge or the physician.
- Record the presence of any abnormal findings (e.g., the character and amount of discharge or condition of the genitalia), and record any related procedure you perform.
- Record the appearance of a suture line, if present.
- Report any break in a suture line or the presence of abnormalities to the person in charge or the physician.
- Record all procedures performed, the amount of assistance provided, and the extent of the client's participation.

Home Care Considerations

- Assess the client's tub and shower area for the need for safety devices (e.g., grab bars, bath mats).
- Assess the client for the need for assistive bathing devices (e.g., shower chair, hand-held shower).
- Instruct caregivers to assess the client's perineal area daily for signs of infection and skin breakdown.

Older Adult Considerations

- Check the temperature of water carefully as the client's sensitivity to temperature may be impaired.
- Continent clients may not require bathing every day, especially if dry skin is a problem.

Bag Baths. An innovative approach to the traditional bed bath was developed because of concern for clients who are predisposed to dry skin and the risk for infection. When wash basins are not cleaned and dried completely after use, contamination with Gram-negative organisms may occur. Successive uses of the basin may cause a client's skin to harbour more Gram-negative organisms. The "bag bath" (Figure 38–8) is a specially prepared package containing 10 washcloths that are premoistened with a mixture of water and a nonrinsable cleanser. The bag bath package is warmed in a microwave before use, and a different cloth is used for each part of the client's body. With this technique, the skin air-dries because towel drying removes the emollient that is left behind after the water–cleanser solution evaporates. Staff members who have used the bag bath report shorter bathing times and increased client and nurse satisfaction (Larson et al., 2004).

Perineal Care. Perineal care is usually part of a complete bed bath (see Skill 38–1). Clients most in need of perineal care are those at greatest risk for acquiring an infection (e.g., clients who have indwelling urinary catheters, clients who are recovering from rectal or genital surgery or childbirth, uncircumcised males, clients who are incontinent, or clients who are morbidly obese). In addition, women who are having a menstrual period require good perineal care. Clients who are able to perform self-care should be encouraged to do so. Sometimes you can feel embarrassed when providing perineal care, particularly for clients of the opposite sex. Similarly, clients may feel embarrassed, but this should not cause you to overlook clients' hygiene needs. A professional, dignified, and sensitive approach can reduce embarrassment and put the clients at ease.

If clients perform self-care, various problems such as vaginal and urethral discharge, skin irritation, and unpleasant odours may go unnoticed. You must be alert for complaints of burning during urination or localized soreness, excoriation, or pain in the perineum. You should also inspect your clients' bed linen for signs of discharge.

Back Rub. A back rub or massage is usually performed after a client's bath. It promotes relaxation, relieves muscular tension, stimulates circulation, and improves sleep (Ebersole et al., 2008). Zullino et al. (2005) posit that massage is associated with a reduction in blood pressure, a reduction in pain, and decreases anxiety and depression. Clients generally report that they are more comfortable after a back rub or massage and find the experience pleasant, regardless of the length of the massage.

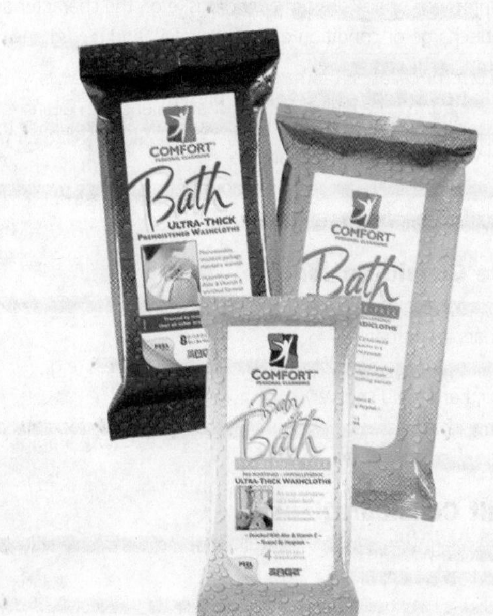

Figure 38-8 Commercial bath cleansing pack. **Source:** From Sage Products, Cary, IL. (2009). Retrieved January 7, 2008, from http://www.comfortbath.com

When providing a back rub, relaxation can be enhanced by reducing any noise and ensuring that the client is comfortable. Because some individuals may dislike physical contact, it is important to ask the client whether he or she would like a back rub and whether gentle or deep massage is preferred. The client's medical record should be reviewed for any contraindications to massage (e.g., fractured ribs, burns of the skin, or heart surgery).

Foot and Nail Care. Foot and nail care should be incorporated into a person's regular hygiene routine. Routine care involves soaking to soften the cuticles, thorough cleansing, drying, and proper nail trimming. The exception involves clients with diabetes mellitus, who do not soak their feet because of the risk of infection. When providing foot and nail care, clients may remain in bed or sit in a chair (Skill 38–2). In some settings or with specific clients, such as a person with diabetes mellitus, a physician's order is needed to trim the toenails. Before implementing this procedure, check your agency's policy.

During the procedure, time is taken to teach the clients and family members the proper techniques for cleaning and nail trimming. Measures to prevent infection and promote good circulation should be stressed. Clients learn to protect their feet from injury, keep their feet clean and dry, and wear footwear that fits properly. Clients are instructed on the proper way to inspect all surfaces of the feet and hands for lesions, dryness, and signs of infection. It is important for clients to know the appearance of any abnormalities and the importance of reporting these conditions to their caregiver.

Clients with diabetes mellitus or peripheral vascular disease are at risk for foot and nail problems as a result of poor peripheral blood supply to the feet. In addition, sensation in the feet can be reduced. These clients are especially at risk for the development of chronic foot ulcers. These lesions typically heal very slowly and, once present, are difficult to treat. Over time, circulation can become compromised enough to cause ischemia and sloughing of tissue. Although ongoing foot care can help prevent toe amputation, studies show that many clients have not learned or do not practise proper care (Box 38–11) (Canadian Diabetes Association, 2003; Neil, 2002; Smeltzer & Bare, 2004).

Clients with diabetes mellitus or peripheral vascular disease must be given information to understand how circulation directly affects the health and integrity of tissues. These clients should be advised to use the following guidelines in a routine foot and nail care program (Canadian Diabetes Association, 2003; Smeltzer & Bare, 2004):

- Inspect the feet daily, including the tops and soles of the feet, the heels, and the areas between the toes. Use a mirror to help inspect the feet thoroughly or ask a family member to check daily.
- If you have diabetes mellitus, you should receive a thorough foot examination at least once a year. If you have one or more high-risk foot conditions, you should be evaluated more frequently and referred to a specialist as necessary (Canadian Diabetes Association, 2003).
- Wash the feet daily using lukewarm water; *do not soak*. If you have reduced sensation, you may want to use a bath thermometer at home to test the water temperature. Thoroughly pat the feet dry, and dry well between toes.
- Do not cut corns or calluses or use commercial removers. Consult a physician or podiatrist.
- If your feet perspire excessively, apply a nonallergenic foot powder.

➤ SKILL 38-2 Performing Nail and Foot Care

Delegation Considerations

The skill of nail and foot care for the nondiabetic client can be delegated to an unregulated care provider; however, this skill should not be delegated if the client is diabetic. It is important to discuss the following:

- That nail clipping must be performed by you
- Any special considerations for client positioning

Equipment

- Wash basin
- Emesis basin
- Washcloth and bath towel
- Nail clippers (the client's)
- Orange stick
- Emery board or nail file
- Body lotion, unscented
- Disposable bath mat
- Paper towels
- Disposable gloves

Procedure

STEPS	RATIONALE
1. Identify client's at risk for foot or nail problems:	• Certain conditions increase the likelihood of foot or nail problems.
A. Older adult	• Poor vision, lack of coordination, or inability to bend over contributes to difficulty in performing foot and nail care. Normal physiological changes of aging also result in nail and foot problems (Smeltzer & Bare, 2004).
B. Diabetes mellitus	• Vascular changes associated with diabetes mellitus reduce blood flow to peripheral tissues. Breaks in the skin integrity place a diabetic client at high risk for a skin infection. Meticulous foot assessment reduces the diabetic client's risk of debilitating foot problems (Canadian Diabetes Association, 2003).
C. Heart failure or renal disease	• Both conditions can increase tissue edema, particularly in dependent areas (e.g., feet). Edema reduces blood flow to neighbouring tissues.
D. Cerebrovascular accident (stroke)	• The presence of residual foot or leg weakness or paralysis results in altered walking patterns. An altered gait pattern increases friction and pressure on feet.
2. Assess client's knowledge of foot and nail care practices.	• Determines client's need for health teaching.
3. Ask female clients about whether they use nail polish and polish remover frequently.	• Chemicals in these products can cause excessive dryness.
4. Assess client's ability to care for nails or feet: consider visual alterations, fatigue, and musculoskeletal weakness.	• Demonstrates client's knowledge of proper foot care. Determines the amount of assistance and teaching required.
5. Assess the types of home remedies (e.g., aloe vera, herbal preparations; Miller, 2009) that the client uses for existing foot problems:	• Some liquid preparations can cause burns and ulcerations. • Certain preparations or applications may cause injury to soft tissue (Neil, 2002).
A. Over-the-counter liquid preparations to remove corns	• Liquid preparations can cause burns and ulcerations.
B. Cutting of corns or calluses with razor blade or scissors	• Cutting of corns or calluses may result in an infection caused by a break in skin integrity. The diabetic client or any client with decreased peripheral circulation has an increased risk for infection secondary to a break in skin integrity (Canadian Diabetes Association, 2003).
C. Use of oval corn pads	• Oval pads may exert pressure on the toes, thereby decreasing circulation to surrounding tissues.
D. Application of adhesive tape	• The skin of older adults is thin and delicate and prone to tearing when adhesive tape is removed.
6. Assess the type of footwear worn by clients: Are socks worn? Are shoes tight or ill fitting? Are garters or knee-high nylons worn? Is footwear clean?	• Types of shoes and footwear may predispose client to foot and nail problems (e.g., infection, areas of friction, ulcerations). These conditions decrease mobility and increase the risk for amputation in the diabetic client (Smeltzer & Bare, 2004).
7. Observe client's walking gait. Have the client walk down a hall or in a straight line (if able).	• Structural as well as painful disorders of the feet can cause limping or an unnatural gait.
8. Assist an ambulatory client to sit in a bedside chair. Help a bed-bound client to a supine position with head of the bed elevated. Place disposable bath mat on the floor under client's feet or place a towel on the mattress.	• Sitting in a chair facilitates immersing feet in basin. The bath mat protects feet from exposure to soil or debris.
9. Obtain a physician's order for cutting nails if agency policy requires it.	• The client's skin may be accidentally cut. Certain clients are more at risk for infection, depending on their medical condition.

Continued

➤ SKILL 38-2 Performing Nail and Foot Care *continued*

STEPS	RATIONALE
10. Explain the procedure to the client, including fact that proper soaking requires several minutes.	• Client must be willing to place fingers and feet in basins for 10–20 minutes. Client may become anxious or fatigued.
Critical Decision Point: Clients with diabetes do not soak hands and feet. Soaking increases their risk of infection due to maceration of the skin.	
11. Perform hand hygiene. Arrange equipment on an overbed table.	• Reduces transmission of microorganisms. Easy access to equipment prevents delays.
12. Fill wash basin with warm water. Test water temperature.	• Warm water softens nails and thickened epidermal cells, reduces inflammation of the skin, and promotes local circulation. Proper water temperature prevents burns.
13. Place basin on bath mat or towel.	• Avoids spills; this maintains the safety of the care provider and the client.
14. Fill emesis basin with warm water, and place basin on paper towels on overbed table.	• Warm water softens nails and thickened epidermal cells.
15. Pull curtain around the bed or close the room door (if desired).	• Maintaining the client's privacy reduces anxiety.
16. Inspect all surfaces of the fingers, toes, feet, and nails. Pay particular attention to areas of dryness, inflammation, or cracking. Also inspect the areas between toes, heels, and soles of feet.	• The integrity of feet and nails determines the frequency and level of hygiene required. Heels, soles, and sides of the feet are prone to irritation from ill-fitting shoes.
Critical Decision Point: Clients with peripheral vascular diseases or diabetes mellitus, older adults, and clients whose immune system is suppressed may require nail care from a specialist to reduce the risk of infection.	
17. Assess the colour and temperature of toes, feet, and fingers. Assess capillary refill. Palpate radial and ulnar pulses of each hand and dorsalis pedis pulses of feet; (see Chapter 32).	• Assesses the adequacy of blood flow to extremities. Peripheral vascular disease can contribute to poor wound healing. Immunocompromised and diabetic clients are at greater risk of developing infections (Smeltzer & Bare, 2004).
18. Instruct client to place his or her fingers in the emesis basin and place arms in a comfortable position.	• Prolonged positioning can cause discomfort unless normal anatomical alignment is maintained.
Assist the client to place feet in the basin.	• Clients with muscular weakness may have difficulty positioning their feet.
19. Allow client's feet and fingernails to soak for 10–20 minutes (unless the client has diabetes). Rewarm the water after 10 minutes.	• Softening of corns, calluses, and cuticles ensures easy removal of dead cells and easy manipulation of cuticles.
20. Clean gently under the fingernails with an orange stick or the wooden end of a cotton-tipped swab while fingers are immersed (see Step 20 illustration). Remove fingers from the emesis basin, and dry thoroughly.	• The orange stick removes debris under nails that harbours microorganisms. Thorough drying impedes fungal growth and prevents maceration of the tissues.
21. Using nail clippers, clip fingernails straight across and even with the tops of fingers (see Step 21 illustration). Using a file, shape the nails straight across. If client has circulatory problems, do not cut the nail; only file the nail.	• For infection-control purposes, use the client's own nail clippers. Cutting straight across prevents splitting of the nail margins and the formation of sharp nail spikes that can irritate lateral nail margins. Filing prevents cutting the nail too close to the nail bed.
22. Push cuticle back gently with the orange stick. Thoroughly dry the hands.	• Reduces incidence of inflamed cuticles. Thorough drying impedes fungal growth and prevents maceration of the tissues.
23. Move the overbed table away from the client.	• Provides easier access to the feet.

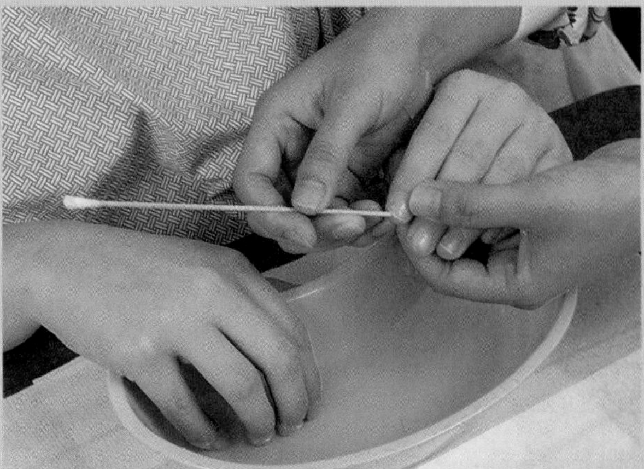

Step 20 Clean fingernails with the end of a cotton-tipped swab or an orange stick.

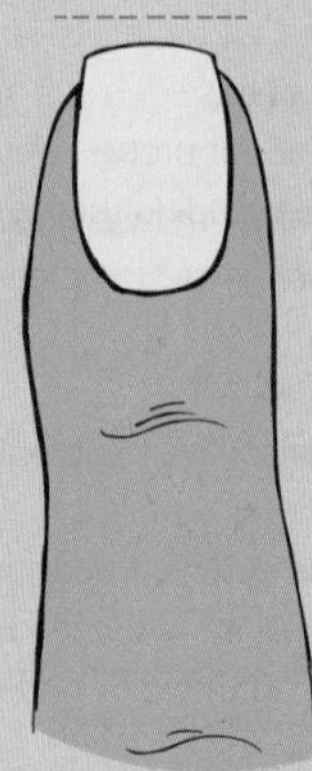

Step 21 Using nail clippers, trim nails straight across.

➤ SKILL 38-2 Performing Nail and Foot Care *continued*

STEPS	RATIONALE
24. Put on disposable gloves, and scrub callused areas of the feet with a washcloth.	• Gloves prevent the transmission of fungal infection. Friction removes dead skin layers.
25. Clean gently under nails with an orange stick. Remove feet from basin, and dry them thoroughly.	• Removal of debris and excess moisture reduces chances of infection.
26. Clean and trim the toenails using the procedures in Steps 21 and 22. Do not file the corners of toenails.	• For infection control purposes, use the client's own nail clippers. Shaping corners of toenails may damage tissues.
27. Apply lotion to feet and hands, and assist client back to bed and into a comfortable position.	• Lotion lubricates dry skin by helping to retain moisture.
28. Remove disposable gloves and place in a receptacle. Clean and return the equipment and supplies to the proper place. Dispose of soiled linen in a hamper. Perform hand hygiene.	• Reduces the transmission of infection.
29. Inspect the nails and surrounding skin surfaces after soaking and nail trimming.	• Determines the condition of skin and nails. Allows you to note any remaining rough nail edges.
30. Ask client to explain or demonstrate nail care.	• Evaluates client's level of learning techniques.
31. Observe client's walk after toenail care.	• Evaluates the level of comfort and mobility achieved.

Unexpected Outcomes and Related Interventions

Inflammation and Tenderness of Cuticles and Surrounding Tissues

- Repeated soakings may be needed to relieve inflammation and loosen layers of cells from calluses or corns.
- Client with diabetes or peripheral vascular disease may require referral to a podiatrist.
- Antifungal cream may be needed.

Localized Areas of Tenderness on Feet, with Calluses or Corns at Points of Friction

- Change in footwear may be needed.
- Refer to a podiatrist.

Appearance of Ulcer Between Toes or Other Pressure Areas in Foot

- Notify physician.
- Refer to a podiatrist.
- Increase frequency of foot assessment and hygiene.

Recording and Reporting

- Document the procedure and any observations (e.g., breaks in the skin, inflammation, ulcerations) on the client's record sheets using the forms provided by your agency or facility.
- Report any breaks in the skin or ulcerations to the person in charge or the physician. These breaks are serious in clients with diabetes, peripheral vascular disease, and illnesses that impair circulation. Special foot care treatments may be needed.

Home Care Considerations

- If the client has diabetes or decreased peripheral circulation, alternative therapies or foot soaking should only be done after consulting with a physician.
- An alternative therapy is moleskin applied to areas of the feet that are under friction—this is less likely to cause pressure than corn pads. Spot adhesive bandages can guard against friction, but they do not have padding to protect against pressure.
- If the client is ambulatory, instruct him or her to soak feet in a bathtub.
- If the client's mobility is limited, a large basin or pan can be used for soaking.

✱ BOX 38-11 RESEARCH HIGHLIGHT

Foot Care Practices of Adults in Rural Settings

Research Focus

Foot injuries are debilitating and painful; however, to the diabetic population, foot injuries, even minor ones, can result in long-term disability or even death. When clients are taught proper foot care practices and they implement them, the risks for developing foot ulcers and the subsequent complications are greatly reduced.

Research Abstract

The purpose of Neil's (2002) study was to determine the knowledge about foot care practices in a sample of adults who had either type 1 or type 2 diabetes mellitus. These adults all lived in an impoverished rural area that offered little access to health care, and where going barefoot and wading in local streams were normal activities. Thirty-seven of the adults were ulcer free, whereas the remaining adults had a foot ulcer present. Factors surveyed included foot inspection, foot cleaning, nail care, and the use of proper footwear. The scores of both groups were low, and it appeared to the investigators that the foot care practices for both groups were the same. These two groups of clients were inconsistent in preventive foot care practices, but the lowest scores were found for foot inspection and wearing proper footwear. The investigators concluded that ongoing assessment and the use of preventive practices were necessary to reduce the risk of foot ulcers in this high-risk population. In addition, the assessment of these practices at the point of client contact, either in the home or clinic environment, was essential in increasing clients' adherence to foot care practice protocols.

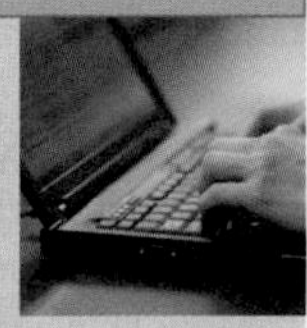

Evidence-Informed Practice

- Use of an assessment designed to evaluate foot care practices helps to increase clients' awareness of potential disease-related complications.
- Reinforce foot care practices at each point of client contact.
- When possible, conduct an assessment of foot care practices in the clients' home environment to assist in determining true foot care practices and in correcting any client misconceptions.

References: Neil, J. A. (2002). Assessing foot care knowledge in a rural population with diabetes. *Ostomy/Wound Management, 48*(1), 50–56.

- If you note dryness along the sides of the feet, rub a nonallergenic lotion gently into the skin, wiping off any excess. *Do not apply lotion between the toes, as excessive moisture can result in infection* (Canadian Diabetes Association, 2006a, 2006b).
- File the toenails straight across and square; do not use scissors or clippers. Consult a podiatrist as needed.
- Do not use over-the-counter preparations to treat athlete's foot or ingrown toenails. Consult a physician or podiatrist.
- Avoid elastic stockings, knee-high hose, constricting garters, and crossing the legs while sitting; these can cause impaired circulation to the lower extremities.
- Wear clean socks or stockings daily. Change socks twice a day if feet perspire heavily. Socks should be dry and free of holes or repairs that might cause pressure on the tissue.
- Do not walk barefoot.
- Wear properly fitted shoes with porous uppers if possible. The soles of shoes should be flexible and nonslipping. Shoes should be sturdy, closed in, and not restrictive to the feet. Clients with increased plantar pressure (e.g., due to erythema or callus) should use footwear that cushions and redistributes pressure. Clients with bony deformity (e.g., a bunion or Charcot's joint) may need extra-wide or extra-deep shoes with cushioned insoles.
- Do not wear high-heeled, open-toed, or pointed-toe shoes (Canadian Diabetes Association, 2006a, 2006b).
- Do not wear new shoes for an extended time. Wear them for short periods over several days to break them in.
- Exercise regularly to improve circulation to the lower extremities. Walk slowly and elevate, rotate, flex, and extend the feet at the ankles. Dangle the feet over the side of the bed for 1 minute, then extend both legs and hold them parallel to the bed while lying supine for 1 minute, and, finally, rest for 1 minute.
- Do not apply hot water bottles or heating pads to the feet; use extra coverings instead.
- Wash minor cuts immediately and dry them thoroughly. Use only mild antiseptics (e.g., Neosporin ointment). Avoid iodine or merbromin (Mercurochrome). Contact a physician to treat cuts or lacerations.

Any clients who require regular, thorough foot care should have a caregiver or family member able to provide care during times when the client is incapacitated. Clients with visual difficulties, physical constraints preventing movement, or cognitive problems that impair their ability to assess the condition of the feet need caregiver or family assistance (Canadian Diabetes Association, 2003; Smeltzer & Bare, 2004).

Oral Hygiene

Oral hygiene helps to maintain the healthy state of the mouth, teeth, gums, lips, and tongue (Canadian Dental Association, 2005). Brushing cleans the teeth of food particles, plaque, and bacteria. It also massages the gums and relieves any discomfort resulting from unpleasant odours and tastes. Flossing helps to further remove plaque and bacteria from between the teeth to reduce gum inflammation and infection. Complete oral hygiene enhances well-being and comfort and stimulates the appetite.

Clients also benefit from a proper diet, which excludes foods that promote plaque formation and tooth decay and which promotes healthy periodontal structures (Canadian Dental Association, 2005). Plaque-forming foods include carbonated beverages, breads, and starches. Oral hygiene immediately after a meal further reduces plaque. You can assist clients in maintaining good oral hygiene by teaching them the importance of correct techniques and a routine daily schedule.

Clients of all ages should be advised to have a dental checkup at least every 6 months. Education about common gum and tooth disorders and methods of prevention can motivate clients to follow good oral hygiene practices. Provide assistance with oral hygiene for weakened or disabled clients. When clients have variations in oral mucosal integrity, adapt hygiene techniques to ensure thorough and effective care (Box 38–12).

Brushing and Flossing. Thorough tooth brushing at least four times a day (after meals and at bedtime) is basic to an effective oral hygiene program. If clients are unable to perform oral care four times per day then they should do it at least once during the day and always at night. All tooth surfaces should be brushed thoroughly with a fluoride toothpaste. A toothbrush should have a straight handle and a brush small enough to reach all areas of the mouth. A toothbrush with soft, rounded bristles should be used to stimulate gums without causing bleeding. Toothbrushes should be replaced every 3 months (Canadian Dental Association, 2005). Older adult clients with reduced dexterity and grip may require an enlarged handle with an easier grip or an electric toothbrush (Miller, 2009). One simple way to make an enlarged brush handle is to pierce a soft rubber ball and push the brush handle through it or glue a short piece of plastic tubing around the handle. Commercially made foam rubber toothbrushes are useful for clients with sensitive gums. However, swabbing fails to cleanse teeth adequately because plaque accumulates around the base of the teeth. Foam rubber swabs should be used in moderation. Electric toothbrushes can be used, but consult your agency's policy to ascertain whether their use is permitted. Lemon–glycerine sponges should not be used because they dry mucous membranes and

BOX 38-12 FOCUS ON OLDER ADULTS

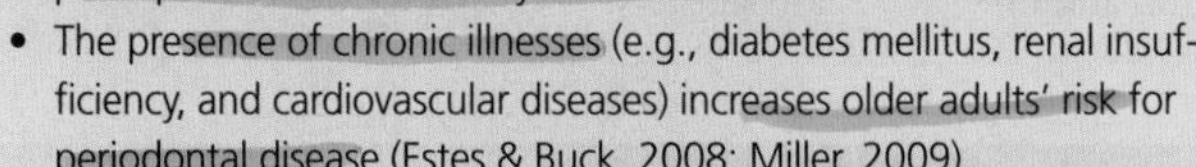

- Many older adults are edentulous (without teeth), and the teeth that are present are often diseased or decayed (Meiner & Lueckenotte, 2006).
- The periodontal membrane weakens, making it more prone to infection; periodontal disease can predispose older adults to systemic infection.
- The presence of chronic illnesses (e.g., diabetes mellitus, renal insufficiency, and cardiovascular diseases) increases older adults' risk for periodontal disease (Estes & Buck, 2008; Miller, 2009).
- Dentures or partial plates may not fit properly, causing pain and discomfort; this can, in turn, affect digestive processes, the enjoyment of food, and nutritional status (Ebersole et al., 2008).
- Weaker jaw muscles and shrinkage of the bony structure of the mouth may increase the work of chewing and lead to increased fatigue when eating (Meiner & Lueckenotte, 2006).
- Dry mouth can be caused by an age-related decline in saliva secretion, as well as by medications that are frequently used by older adults (e.g., antihypertensives, diuretics, anti-inflammatories, and antidepressants) (Smeltzer & Bare, 2004).
- Poor nutritional status in some older adults can increase the risk for and severity of dental problems (e.g., caries, periodontal disease, receding gums, and tooth degeneration) (Miller, 2009).
- An inability or unwillingness to access dental care and the belief that tooth loss is a natural outcome of aging are reasons why some older adults do not seek dental care (Ebersole et al., 2008).
- Financial limitations and the belief that dentures eliminate the need for routine dental care are also reasons why some older adults do not seek dental care (Eliopoulos, 2005).

erode teeth enamel. Moi-Stir is a salivary supplement that improves moisture and the texture of the tongue and mucosa (Miller, 2009).

When teaching clients about mouth care, you should recommend that they do not share toothbrushes with family members or drink directly from a bottle of mouthwash. Cross-contamination occurs easily. The use of disclosure tablets or drops to stain the plaque that collects at the gum line can be useful for showing clients how effectively they brush.

Clients experience conditions that threaten the integrity of the oral mucosa. For example, mucosal changes associated with aging, use of chemotherapeutic drugs, or dehydration require adaption to oral hygiene approaches. More frequent mouth care and use of anti-infective agents are examples of ways you can revise approaches to meet client needs. Unconscious clients and those with artificial airways (e.g., endotracheal or tracheal tubes) need more frequent and specialized oral hygiene. These clients have an increased risk of aspiration and, subsequently, aspiration pneumonia, and they also have more problems with dry and inflamed oral mucosa.

The amount of assistance needed by the client when brushing the teeth may vary. Many clients can perform their own oral care and should be encouraged to do so. You should observe clients to be sure proper techniques are used. When assisting with or providing oral hygiene, you must determine the amount of assistance needed and the individuals' oral hygiene preferences (Skill 38–3).

Flossing. Dental flossing removes plaque and bacteria from between teeth. Flossing involves inserting waxed or unwaxed dental floss between all tooth surfaces, one space at a time. Flossing at least once a day is sufficient (Canadian Dental Association, 2005). To prevent bleeding, clients who are receiving chemotherapy or radiation or who are on anticoagulant therapy should use unwaxed floss and avoid vigorous flossing near the gum line. If toothpaste is applied to the teeth before flossing, this allows fluoride to come in direct contact with tooth surfaces, aiding in cavity prevention. Because it is important to clean all tooth surfaces thoroughly, you should not rush flossing. Placing a mirror in front of the client helps you to demonstrate the proper method for holding the floss and cleaning between the teeth. Flossing a client's teeth is not realistic or appropriate in all care settings. However, flossing may be done more frequently in rehabilitation and long-term care settings.

Clients With Special Needs. Some clients require special oral hygiene methods because of their level of dependence on the care provider or the presence of oral mucosa problems. Unconscious clients are susceptible to drying of mucous-thickened salivary secretions because they are unable to eat or drink, frequently breathe through the mouth, and often receive oxygen therapy. Unconscious clients also cannot swallow salivary secretions that accumulate in the mouth. These secretions often contain Gram-negative bacteria that can cause pneumonia if aspirated into the lungs. While providing hygiene to unconscious clients, you must protect them from choking and aspiration. While cleansing the oral cavity, you should never use your fingers to hold the client's mouth open as a human bite is highly contaminated. It may be necessary to perform mouth care at least every 2 hours for the unconscious client. Research shows that the use of chlorhexidine with oral hygiene reduces the risk of ventilator-associated pneumonia (Berry et al., 2007; Munro et al., 2006). Explain the steps of mouth care, the sensations the client will feel, and when the procedure is completed (Skill 38–4).

Clients who receive chemotherapy, radiation, or nasogastric tube intubation or who have an infection of the mouth can suffer from **stomatitis,** an inflammation of the oral mucosa that can cause burning, pain, and a change in food tolerance. Gentle brushing and flossing are important in preventing bleeding of the gums. Clients should be advised to avoid alcohol and commercial mouthwash and to stop smoking. Normal saline rinses (approximately 30 mL) used upon awaking in the morning, after each meal, and at bedtime can effectively clean the oral cavity. The rinses can be increased to every 2 hours if necessary. The physician may order a mild oral analgesic for pain control.

Clients with diabetes mellitus frequently have periodontal disease. Visits to the dentist are needed every 3 to 4 months. All tissues should be handled gently with a minimum of trauma. Clients should learn to follow rigid cleansing schedules, at least four times a day.

Denture Care. Clients should be encouraged to clean their dentures on a regular basis to avoid gingival infection and irritation. When clients become disabled, the care provider or family caregiver can assume responsibility for denture care (Box 38–13). Dentures are clients' personal property and need to be handled with care because they can be easily broken. They must be removed at night to give the gums a rest and prevent bacterial buildup. Dentures should be kept covered in water when they are not worn to prevent warping, and they should always be stored in an enclosed, labelled cup and placed in the clients' bedside stand. Discourage clients from removing their dentures and placing them on a napkin or tissue because they could be easily thrown away.

Hair and Scalp Care

A person's appearance and feeling of well-being can often depend on the way his or her hair looks and feels. Illness or disability may prevent clients from maintaining daily hair care. Immobilized clients' hair soon becomes tangled. Dressings may leave sticky blood or antiseptic solutions on the hair. In the clinic and home care setting, you may encounter clients who have head lice. Proper hair care is important to clients' body image. Brushing, combing, and shampooing are basic hygiene measures for all clients.

Brushing and Combing. Frequent brushing helps to keep hair clean and distributes oil evenly along hair shafts. Combing prevents hair from tangling. Clients should be encouraged to maintain routine hair care. However, clients with limited mobility or weakness and those who are confused require assistance. Clients in a hospital or long-term care facility appreciate the opportunity to have their hair brushed and combed before being seen by others.

When caring for clients from different cultures, it is important to learn as much as possible from them or their family about their preferred hair care practices. Cultural preferences affect how hair is combed and styled.

Long hair can easily become matted when clients are confined to bed, even for a short period. When lacerations or incisions involve the scalp, blood and topical medications can also cause tangling. Frequent brushing and combing keeps long hair neatly groomed. Braiding can help to avoid repeated tangles; however, braids should be unbraided periodically and the hair combed to ensure good hygiene. Braids made too tightly can result in bald patches. Always obtain permission from the clients, if conscious, before braiding their hair.

To brush the hair, part it into two sections and separate each into two more sections. It is easier to brush smaller sections of hair. Brushing from the scalp toward the hair ends minimizes pulling. Moistening the hair with water or alcohol frees tangles for easier combing. Never cut a client's hair without written consent.

Clients who develop head lice require special considerations in the way combing is performed. The lice are small, about the size of a sesame seed. Bright light or natural sunlight is necessary for the lice

➤ SKILL 38-3 Providing Oral Hygiene

video

Delegation Considerations

The skill of brushing teeth can be delegated to an unregulated care provider. It is important to discuss the following with him or her:

- How to adapt the procedure for a client who is at risk of aspiration. These clients include those with an impaired level of consciousness or impaired swallowing, and those who are confused.
- To immediately report excessive client coughing or choking during or after oral hygiene
- To report any bleeding of the oral mucosa or gums, lesions, or client report of pain

Equipment

- Soft-bristled toothbrush
- Nonabrasive fluoride toothpaste or dentifrice
- Dental floss
- Water glass with cool water
- Normal saline or an essential oil antiseptic mouthwash (optional; follow client's preference)
- Emesis basin
- Tongue blade
- Face towel
- Paper towels
- Disposable gloves

Procedure

STEPS	RATIONALE
1. Determine client's oral hygiene practices:	• Allows you to identify errors in technique, deficiencies in preventive oral hygiene, and client's level of knowledge regarding dental care.
A. Frequency of toothbrushing and flossing B. Type of toothpaste or dentifrice used C. Last dental visit D. Frequency of dental visits	
E. Type of mouthwash or moistening preparation such as over-the-counter saliva substitutes or sugar-free gum with xylitol (Miller, 2009).	• Mouthwash provides a pleasant aftertaste but can dry mucosa after extended use if it has an alcohol base.
2. Assess risk for oral hygiene problems (see Table 38–5).	• Certain conditions increase the likelihood of impaired oral cavity integrity and the need for preventive care.
3. Assess client's risk for aspiration: impaired swallowing, reduced gag reflex.	• An accumulation of secretions and dentifrice can increase the client's risk for aspiration if the client's ability to control oral secretions is impaired.
4. Assess client's ability to grasp and manipulate a toothbrush. (For older adults, try a 30-second toothbrushing assessment.)	• A toothbrush test is useful in assessing dexterity and strength. Determines level of assistance required.
5. Prepare equipment at bedside.	• Avoids interrupting the procedure or leaving the client unattended to retrieve missing equipment.
6. Perform hand hygiene and put on disposable gloves.	• Reduces the transmission of microorganisms.
7. Inspect the integrity of the lips, teeth, buccal mucosa, gums, palate, and tongue (see Chapter 32).	• Determines status of client's oral cavity and the extent of need for oral hygiene.
8. Identify the presence of common oral problems:	• Helps determine type of hygiene client requires and information client requires for self-care.
A. Dental caries—chalky white discoloration of a tooth or the presence of brown or black discoloration B. Gingivitis—inflammation of gums	
C. Periodontitis—receding gum lines, inflammation, gaps between teeth	• Receding gums occur with aging, and as a result older clients require meticulous oral hygiene.
D. Halitosis—bad breath E. Cheilosis—cracking of the lips	
F. Stomatitis—inflammation of the mouth G. Dry, cracked, coated tongue	• Clients receiving immunosuppressive chemotherapy (e.g., cancer chemotherapy, antirejection medication after receiving an organ transplant) and clients with suppressed immune function are at risk for stomatitis (Smeltzer & Bare, 2004).
9. Explain the procedure to the client and discuss preferences regarding the use of hygiene aids.	• Some clients feel uncomfortable about having you care for their basic needs. Client involvement with procedure minimizes anxiety.
10. Raise the bed to a comfortable working position. Raise head of the bed (if allowed) and lower the side rail. Move the client, or help client move closer. A side-lying position can be used.	• Raising the bed and re-positioning the client prevents straining of muscles. A semi-Fowler position helps prevent client from choking or aspirating.
11. Place paper towels on an overbed table, and arrange other equipment in easy reach.	• Prevents soiling of the tabletop. Equipment prepared in advance ensures a smooth, safe procedure.
12. Place a towel over client's chest.	• Prevents soiling of bed linen.
13. Apply toothpaste to brush, holding brush over the emesis basin. Pour a small amount of water over toothpaste.	• Moisture aids in the distribution of toothpaste over tooth surfaces.

➤ SKILL 38-3 **Providing Oral Hygiene** ***continued***

STEPS	RATIONALE
14. Client may assist by brushing. Hold toothbrush bristles at 45-degree angle to gum line (see Step 14 illustration, part A). Be sure tips of bristles rest against and penetrate under gum line. Brush inner and outer surfaces of upper and lower teeth by brushing from gum to crown of each tooth. Clean biting surfaces of teeth by holding top of bristles parallel with teeth and brushing gently back and forth (see Step 14 illustration, part B). Brush sides of teeth by moving bristles back and forth (see Step 14 illustration, part C).	• Angle allows brush to reach all tooth surfaces and to clean under gum line where plaque and bacteria accumulate. Back-and-forth motion dislodges food particles caught between teeth and along chewing surfaces.
15. Have client hold brush at 45-degree angle and lightly brush over surface and sides of tongue (see Step 15 illustration). Avoid initiating gag reflex.	• Microorganisms collect and grow on tongue's surface and contribute to bad breath. Gagging may cause aspiration of toothpaste. Evaluates client's ability to use correct technique.
16. Allow client to rinse mouth thoroughly by taking several sips of water, swishing water across all tooth surfaces, and spitting into the emesis basin.	• Irrigation removes food particles.
17. Allow client to gargle and rinse mouth with mouthwash as desired.	• An essential oil antiseptic mouthwash can be effective in reducing plaque and gingivitis (Bauroth et al., 2003).
18. Assist in wiping client's mouth.	• Promotes sense of comfort.
19. Allow client to floss.	• Reduces tartar on tooth surfaces.
20. Allow client to rinse mouth thoroughly with cool water and spit into emesis basin. Assist in wiping client's mouth.	• Irrigation removes plaque and tartar from the oral cavity.
21. Ask client whether any area of oral cavity feels uncomfortable or irritated. Inspect the oral cavity.	• Pain *can* indicate a chronic problem.
22. Assist client to comfortable position, remove emesis basin and bedside table, raise side rail, and lower the bed to the original position.	• Provides for client comfort and safety.
23. Wipe off overbed table, discard soiled linen and paper towels in appropriate containers, remove soiled gloves, and return equipment to the proper place.	• Proper disposal of soiled equipment prevents the spread of infection.
24. Remove gloves and perform hand hygiene.	• Reduces the transmission of microorganisms.
25. Ask client to describe proper hygiene techniques.	• Evaluates client's learning.

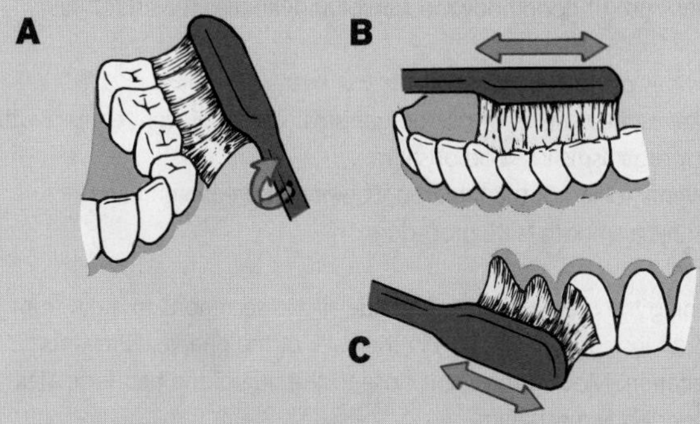

Step 14 Direction for toothbrush placement. **A,** A 45-degree angle brushes gum line. **B,** Parallel position brushes biting surfaces. **C,** Lateral position brushes sides of teeth.

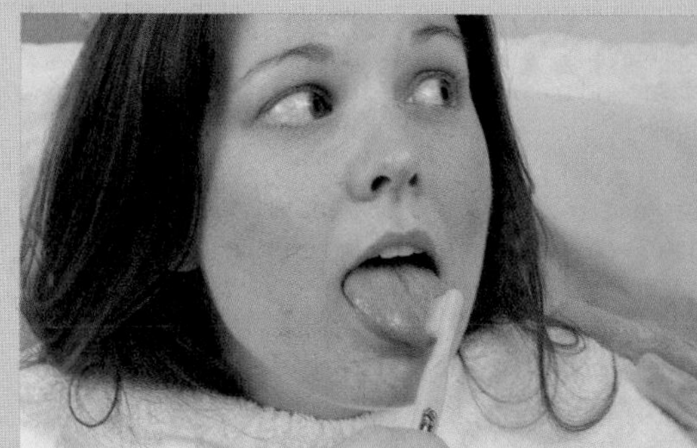

Step 15 Assisting client with brushing tongue.

Unexpected Outcomes and Related Interventions

Dryness and Inflammation of Oral Mucosa

- Increase frequency of oral hygiene.
- Increase client's hydration.
- Apply protectant to the client's lips.

Retraction of Gum Margins From Teeth, Localized Areas of Inflammation, and Bleeding Around Gum Margins

- Determine whether client has an underlying bleeding tendency (e.g., anticoagulant therapy).
- Report findings to the physician.
- Use a soft-bristled toothbrush.
- Increase frequency of oral hygiene.

Signs of Dental Caries

- Refer client to a dentist.
- Teach client oral hygiene techniques.

Recording and Reporting

- Record all procedures on a flow sheet provided by your agency or facility. Note the condition of the oral cavity in the client care notes.
- Report any bleeding or the presence of lesions to the person in charge or the physician.

Home Care Considerations

- Teach the client and caregiver to assess the oral cavity daily to determine any effects of medications on the oral cavity (e.g., reddened, inflamed gums).

➤ SKILL 38-4 Performing Mouth Care for an Unconscious or Debilitated Client

video

Delegation Considerations

The skill of brushing teeth of an unconscious or debilitated client can be delegated to an unregulated care provider. You must first assess the client for the gag reflex and determine whether the person providing assistance can safely use oral suctioning for clearing the client's oral secretions (see Chapter 39). When delegating tasks to an unregulated care provider it is important to instruct him or her about the following:

- The proper way to position the client for mouth care
- How to safely use oral suctioning for clearing oral secretions (see Chapter 39)
- To report to any bleeding of the mucosa or gums, any painful reaction by the client, or excessive coughing or choking

Equipment

- Anti-infective solution (e.g., commercial diluted hydrogen peroxide solution) that loosens crusts
- Small soft-bristled toothbrush
- Sponge swab (e.g., Toothette swab) or tongue blade wrapped in a single layer of gauze
- Oral airway
- Padded tongue blade
- Face towel
- Paper towels
- Emesis basin
- Water glass with cool water
- Water-soluble lip lubricant
- Small-bulb syringe (optional)
- Suction equipment
- Disposable gloves

Procedure

STEPS	RATIONALE
1. Assess client's risk for oral hygiene problems (see Table 38–5).	• Oral care is provided frequently to intubated clients who also have a nasogastric tube and who are at risk of aspiration, which can lead to pneumonia (Smeltzer & Bare, 2004).
2. Explain procedure to client.	• Allows debilitated client to anticipate procedure without anxiety. Unconscious clients retain ability to hear.
3. Test for the presence of a gag reflex by placing a tongue blade on back half of the client's tongue.	• Reveals whether client is at risk for aspiration.

Critical Decision Point: Clients with an impaired gag reflex require oral care as well. You must determine the type of suction apparatus needed at the bedside to protect the client's airway against aspiration.

STEPS	RATIONALE
4. Raise bed to the appropriate height; lower head of the bed and then lower the side rail.	• Allows use of good body mechanics and reduces the risk of injury.
5. Pull curtain around the bed, or close the room door.	• Provides privacy.
6. Perform hand hygiene and put on disposable gloves.	• Reduces the transfer of microorganisms. Gloves prevent contact with microorganisms in blood or saliva.
7. Place paper towels on an overbed table and arrange equipment. If needed, turn on a suction machine and connect tubing to the suction catheter.	• Prevents soiling of the tabletop. Equipment prepared in advance ensures a smooth, safe procedure.
8. Position client on side (Sims' position) with head turned well toward dependent side. Move client close to side of the bed. Raise the side rail.	• Turning the client's head to the side allows secretions to drain from mouth instead of collecting in the back of the pharynx. Prevents aspiration. Moving the client close to the side of the bed facilitates proper body mechanics.
9. Place a towel under client's head and an emesis basin under the chin.	• Prevents soiling of bed linen.
10. Carefully separate upper and lower teeth with padded tongue blade by inserting blade, quickly but gently, between back molars. Insert blade when client is relaxed, if possible. Do not use force (see Step 10 illustration).	• Prevents client from biting down on your fingers and provides access to oral cavity.

Critical Decision Point: Never use fingers to separate the client's teeth.

STEPS	RATIONALE
11. Inspect condition of the oral cavity (see Chapter 32).	• Determines condition of the oral cavity and the need for hygiene.
12. Clean mouth using brush or sponge Toothette swabs moistened with chlorhexidine solution if client condition can tolerate it; otherwise, moisten with water. Clean chewing and inner and outer tooth surfaces. Swab roof of mouth, gums, and inside cheeks. Gently swab or brush tongue, but avoid stimulating gag reflex (if present). Moisten clean swab or Toothette swab with water to rinse. (Bulb syringe may also be used to rinse.) Repeat rinse several times.	• Brushing action removes food particles between teeth and along chewing surfaces. Swabbing helps remove secretions and crusts from mucosa and moistens mucosa. Rinsing removes any debris and cleansing agent, and provides for client comfort.
13. Suction secretions as they accumulate, if necessary.	• Suction removes secretions and fluid that can collect in the posterior pharynx.

➤ SKILL 38-4 Performing Mouth Care for an Unconscious or Debilitated Client ***continued***

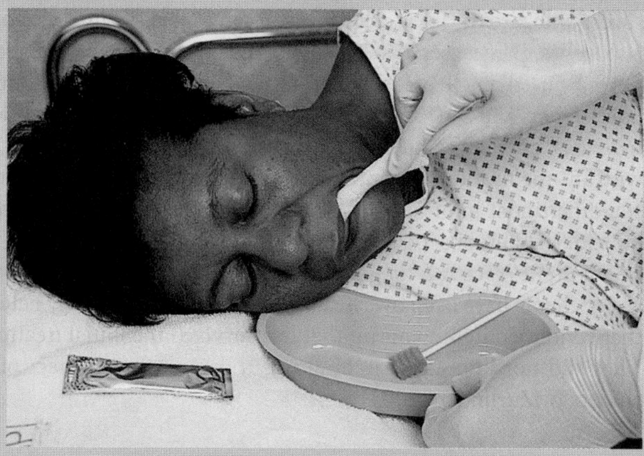

Step 10 Separate upper and lower teeth with padded tongue blade.

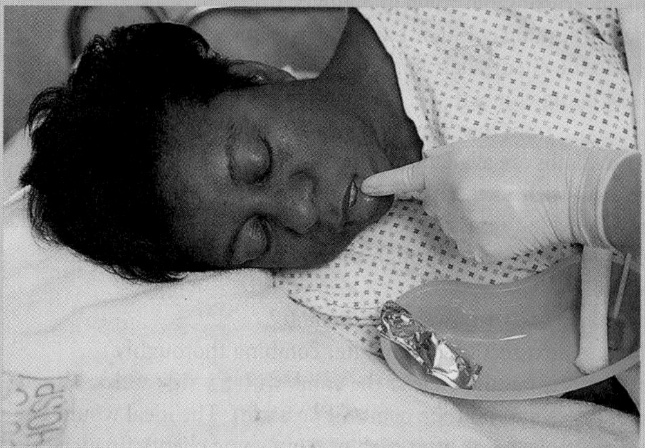

Step 14 Application of water-soluble moisturizer to lips.

STEPS	RATIONALE
14. Apply a thin layer of water-soluble jelly to lips (see Step 14 illustration).	• Lubricates lips to prevent drying and cracking.
15. Inform client that procedure is completed.	• Provides meaningful stimulation to unconscious or less-responsive client.
16. Put on clean gloves, and inspect oral cavity.	• Determines efficacy of cleansing. Once thick secretions are removed, underlying inflammation or lesions may be revealed.
17. Ask debilitated client whether mouth feels clean.	• Evaluates level of comfort.
18. Reposition client comfortably, raise side rail as appropriate or as ordered, and return the bed to original position.	• Maintains client's comfort and safety. Raising all four side rails may be considered a restraint, and a physician's order is needed.
19. Clean equipment and return to its proper place. Place soiled linen in the proper receptacle.	• Proper disposal of soiled equipment prevents the spread of infection.
20. Remove and discard gloves. Perform hand hygiene.	• Reduces the transmission of microorganisms.
21. Assess client's respirations on an ongoing basis.	• Ensures early recognition of aspiration.

Unexpected Outcomes and Related Interventions

Secretions or Crusts Remaining on Oral Mucosa, Tongue, or Gums

- Increase frequency of oral hygiene.
- Try using a pediatric-size toothbrush—it may provide better hygiene.

Localized Inflammation of Gums or Mucosa

- Increase frequency of oral hygiene with a soft-bristled toothbrush.
- Apply moisturizing gel on the oral mucosa.
- Chemotherapy and radiation can cause stomatitis. To provide relief and promote oral hygiene, topical anti-inflammatories and anaesthetics may be prescribed (Smeltzer & Bare, 2004).

Aspiration of Secretions

- Suction oral airway.
- Perform tracheal bronchial suctioning.
- Notify the physician.

Recording and Reporting

- Record the procedure, including pertinent observations (e.g., the presence of bleeding gums, dry mucosa, ulcerations, or crusts on the tongue).
- Report any unusual findings to the person in charge or the physician.

Home Care Considerations

- Cavity should be irrigated with bulb syringe.
- Mouth care should be given at least twice a day. Caregivers can buy nonprescription oral care solutions (e.g., chlorhexidine solutions) at most pharmacies.
- Have caregivers demonstrate positioning of the client to prevent aspiration.

to be seen. Thorough combing is recommended and may remove nits (empty eggshells) if infestation is extensive. Follow these steps:

- Put on a disposable gown and gloves.
- Use a grooming comb or hairbrush to remove any tangles.
- Divide the client's hair in sections and fasten off the hair that is not being combed.
- Comb out from the scalp to the end of the hair (special fine-tooth combs are available in drugstores).
- Between each pass, dip the comb in a cup of water or use a paper towel to remove nits.
- After combing, look through the hair carefully for attached live lice.
- Catch live lice with tweezers or comb.
- Move to next section of hair after combing thoroughly.
- Instruct the family to clean the comb with an old toothbrush and dental floss and boil the comb (if possible). The ideal would be to discard the comb after each use, but some client's financial situations may prevent the purchase of multiple combs.
- Instruct the family to comb and screen for lice daily.
- Instruct the family to contain the client's clothes and then wash them in hot water.
- Instruct caregivers on how to prevent the transmission of lice:
  - Do not share bed linens.
  - Avoid placing your bare hand on client's head.
  - Immediately wash your hands after providing hair care.
  - Contain all hair care products.

If a pediculicidal shampoo is ordered, instruct the client and caregiver on the proper use of shampoo. These shampoos may have neurological side effects. The very young and very old have increased susceptibility to the toxic effects, which can lead to seizures, dizziness, headaches, paraesthesia, and death. This type of medication should never be used on clients who have tested positive for human immunodeficiency virus (HIV), clients with neurological conditions, neonates, or clients who weigh less than 50 kg (Zurlinden, 2003). As with any medication preparation, it is important to review and understand pertinent information. Most side effects associated with pediculicidal shampoos occur from applying too much, leaving the shampoo in place too long, or repeating the shampooing too soon. Many clients have been overtreated because they incorrectly believed that continued itching meant that lice survived the initial treatment. They did not know that itching was a common side effect of the shampoo (Zurlinden, 2003).

Shampooing. Frequency of shampooing depends on clients' daily routines and the condition of their hair. You should remind clients in hospitals or long-term care facilities that staying in bed, perspiring excessively, or undergoing treatments that leave blood or solutions in the hair may result in a need more frequent shampooing.

For clients at home who have limited mobility, it is challenging to find ways that they can shampoo their hair without causing injury. If clients are able to take a shower or bath, their hair can usually be shampooed without difficulty. A shower or tub chair may be used for

➤ BOX 38-13 Procedural Guidelines

Care of Dentures

Delegation Considerations: The skill of denture care can be delegated to an unregulated care provider. It is important to discuss the following with him or her:

- To report any cracks found in the dentures
- To report any client complaints of oral discomfort

Equipment:

- Soft-bristled toothbrush or denture toothbrush
- Denture cleaning agent or toothpaste
- Denture adhesive (optional)
- Glass of water
- Emesis basin or sink
- Washcloth
- Disposable gloves
- Denture cup (if dentures are to be stored after cleaning)

Procedure

1. Ask client whether dentures fit and whether the gums or mucous membranes are tender or irritated.
2. Ask client about preferences for denture care and products used. If client is unable to care for own dentures, you must provide this care. Clean dentures for the client during routine mouth care.
3. Fill emesis basin with tepid water or, if using sink, place washcloth in bottom of sink and fill sink with 2.5 cm of water.
4. Remove dentures. If client is unable to do this independently, perform hand hygiene and put on gloves, grasp upper plate at front with thumb and index finger wrapped in gauze, and pull downward. Gently lift lower denture from jaw, and rotate one side downward to remove from client's mouth. Place dentures in emesis basin or sink.
5. Apply cleaning agent to brush and brush surfaces of dentures (see Step 5 illustration). Hold dentures close to water. Hold the brush horizontally, and use a back-and-forth motion to cleanse biting surfaces. Use short strokes from the top of the denture to biting surfaces to clean outer and inner teeth surfaces. Hold the brush vertically, and use short strokes to clean inner tooth surfaces. Hold the brush horizontally, and use a back-and-forth motion to clean the undersurface of dentures.
6. Rinse thoroughly in tepid water.
7. Some clients use an adhesive to seal dentures in place. If so, apply a thin layer to the undersurface before inserting.
8. If client needs assistance with the insertion of dentures, moisten the upper denture and press firmly to seal it in place. Then insert moistened lower denture. Ask whether dentures feel comfortable.
9. Dentures should be removed at night and the gums cleaned gently. Dentures should be stored in a denture container that is labelled with the client's name and placed in the bedside table to prevent loss.
10. Remove and discard gloves and perform hand hygiene.

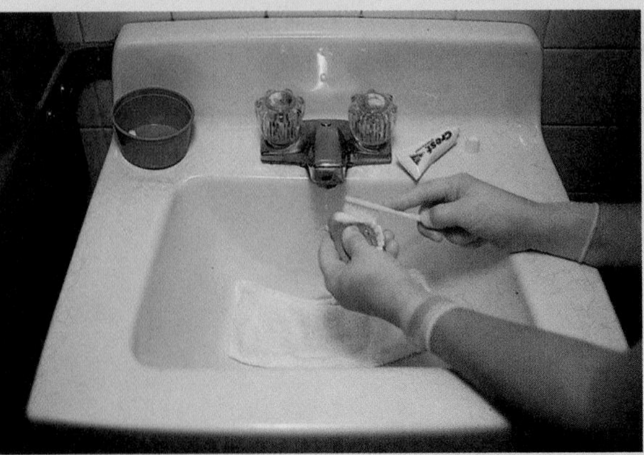

Step 5 Brushing dentures.

ambulatory, weight-bearing clients who become tired or faint. Hand-held shower nozzles allow clients to easily wash their hair in the tub or shower. Clients allowed to sit in a chair may choose to be shampooed in front of a sink or over a wash basin. However, bending is limited or contraindicated in certain conditions (e.g., eye surgery or neck injury). In these situations, you need to teach the clients and their family members the degree of bending allowed.

If clients are unable to sit but can be moved, you may transfer them to a stretcher for transportation to a sink or shower equipped with a hand-held nozzle. This equipment is commonly found in long-term care facilities. Caution is again needed when the clients' head and neck are positioned, particularly in clients with any form of head or neck injury.

If clients are unable to sit in a chair or be transferred to a stretcher, shampooing must be done while the clients are in bed (Box 38–14). A special shampoo trough can be positioned under the client's head to catch water and suds. After shampooing, clients like having their hair styled and dried. Dry shampoos that reduce the need to wet the clients' hair are also available but are not highly effective. These dry shampoo preparations vary, and the application procedures, listed on the container, should be followed exactly. In some agencies, a physician's order is necessary to shampoo the dependent client.

Shaving. Shaving facial hair can be done after a bath or shampoo. Women may prefer to shave their legs or axillae while bathing. When assisting a client, you should take care to avoid cutting the client with a razor blade. Clients prone to bleeding (e.g., those receiving anticoagulants or high doses of aspirin or those with low platelet counts) must use an electric razor. Before the use of an electric razor, you should check for frayed cords and other electrical hazards, as well as

➤ BOX 38-14 Procedural Guidelines

Shampooing the Hair of a Bed-Bound Client

Delegation Considerations: The skill of shampooing hair can be delegated to an unregulated care provider. It is important to discuss the following with him or her:

- To follow any precautions necessary in positioning the client
- To report any client complaints of neck pain
- To report any new skin lesions

Equipment:

- Bath towels
- Washcloths
- Shampoo
- Hair conditioner (optional)
- Water pitcher with warm water
- Plastic shampoo trough
- Wash basin
- Bath blanket
- Waterproof pad
- Clean comb and brush
- Hair dryer (optional)
- Disposable gloves (optional)

Procedure

1. Before washing the client's hair, ensure that this procedure is not contraindicated for the client. Certain medical conditions, such as head and neck injuries, spinal cord injuries, and arthritis, could place client at risk for injury during shampooing because of positioning and manipulation of the client's head and neck.
2. Put on gloves if needed. Inspect the hair and scalp before initiating the procedure to determine the presence of any conditions that may require the use of special shampoos or treatments (e.g., for dandruff or the removal of dried blood).
3. Place waterproof pad under client's shoulders, neck, and head (see Step 3 illustration). Position client supine, with head and shoulders at top edge of the bed. Place a plastic trough under client's head and a wash basin at end of trough. Be sure the trough spout extends beyond edge of the mattress.
4. Place rolled towel under client's neck and bath towel over client's shoulders.
5. Brush and comb client's hair.
6. Obtain warm water.
7. Offer client the option of holding a face towel or washcloth over the eyes.
8. Slowly pour water from a water pitcher over hair until it is completely wet (see Step 8 illustration). If hair contains matted blood, don gloves, apply peroxide to dissolve the clots, and then rinse the hair with saline. Apply small amount of shampoo.
9. Work up lather with both hands. Start at the hairline and work toward back of the neck. Lift head slightly with one hand to wash back of the head. Shampoo sides of the head. Massage scalp by applying pressure with fingertips.
10. Rinse hair with water. Make sure water drains into basin. Repeat rinsing until hair is free of soap.
11. Apply conditioner or cream rinse, if requested, and rinse hair thoroughly.
12. Wrap client's head in bath towel. Dry client's face with cloth used to protect eyes. Dry off any moisture along the neck or shoulders.
13. Dry client's hair and scalp. Use a second towel if first becomes saturated.
14. Comb hair to remove tangles, and dry with dryer if desired (not available in all agencies or facilities).
15. Apply oil preparation or conditioning product to hair, if desired by client.
16. Assist client to a comfortable position, and complete styling of hair.

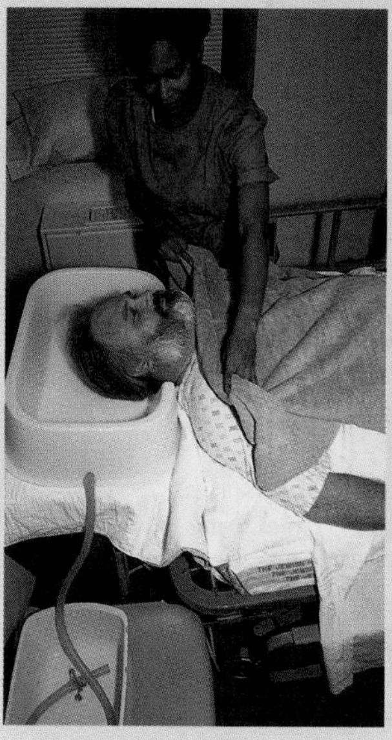

Step 3 Pad has been placed under shoulders, neck, and head.

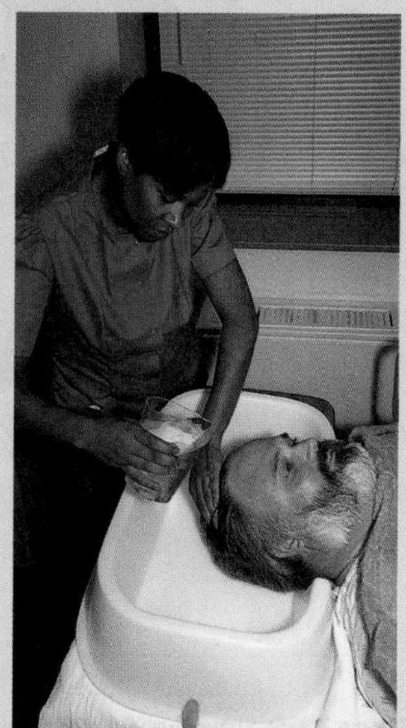

Step 8 Pour water over hair.

your agency's policy with respect to the use of these razors. Each razor blade or electric razor should be used on only one client because of infection-control considerations.

Before a razor blade is used for shaving, the skin must be softened to prevent pulling, scraping, or cuts. Place a warm washcloth over the male client's face for a few seconds, then apply shaving cream or lather a mild soap to soften the skin. If the client is unable to shave, you may perform the task. To avoid causing discomfort or razor cuts, gently pull the skin taut and use short, firm razor strokes in the direction in which the hair grows (Figure 38–9). Short downward strokes work best to remove hair over the upper lip. A client usually can explain the best way to move the razor across the skin. In dark-skinned clients, facial hair tends to be curly and can become ingrown unless shaved close to the skin.

Moustache and Beard Care

Clients with moustaches or beards require daily grooming. Keeping these areas clean is important because food particles and mucus can easily collect in the hair. If the client is unable to carry out self-care, you must perform this care for the client. Beards can be gently combed out. A shaggy or unkempt moustache or beard can be trimmed, with consent from the client or family. For cultural or religious reasons, trimming or shaving off a moustache or beard cannot be performed without the client's or family's consent.

Hair and Scalp Health

To best promote and restore hair and scalp health, clients should be instructed to keep hair clean, combed, and brushed regularly. Clients may also need to know how to check for and remove parasites, such as lice (see Table 38–4). You should inform clients that they need to notify their primary caregiver of changes in the texture and distribution of hair, which may indicate a serious systemic problem.

Care of the Eyes, Ears, and Nose

Special attention is given to cleansing the eyes, ears, and nose during a routine bath and when drainage or discharge accumulates. This aspect of hygiene not only makes clients more comfortable, it also improves sensory reception (see Chapter 48). Care focuses on preventing infection and maintaining normal sensory function and requires approaches that consider clients' special needs.

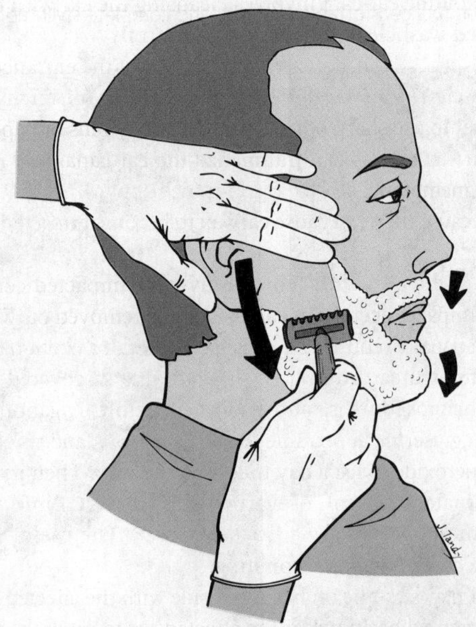

Figure 38-9 Shave in the direction of hair growth. Use longer strokes on the larger areas of the face. Use short strokes around the chin and lips. **Source:** From Sorrentino, S. A. (1999). *Assisting with patient care.* St. Louis, MO: Mosby.

Basic Eye Care. Cleansing the eyes simply involves washing them with a clean washcloth moistened in water. Soap may cause burning and irritation (see Skill 38–1). Direct pressure should never be applied over the eyeball because it may cause serious injury. When cleansing a client's eyes, you use a clean washcloth and cleanse from the inner to outer canthus. Use a different section of the washcloth for each eye. Unconscious clients often require more frequent eye care.

Secretions may collect along the lid margins and inner canthus when the blink reflex is absent or an eye does not close completely. It may be necessary to place an eye patch over the involved eye to prevent corneal drying and irritation. Lubricating eye drops may be given according to the physician's orders.

Eyeglasses. Glasses are made of hardened glass or plastic that is impact resistant to prevent shattering. Nevertheless, because of their cost, extra care should be taken when cleaning glasses and they should be protected from breakage or other damage when they are not worn. Glasses should be put in a case in a drawer of the bedside table when not in use and labelled with the client's name.

Cool water is sufficient for cleaning glass lenses. A soft cloth is best for drying to prevent scratching the lens; paper towels can scratch a lens. Plastic lenses in particular are scratched easily, and special cleansing solutions and drying tissues are available for them. Use whatever the client's eye care specialist recommends.

Contact Lenses. A contact lens is a small, round, transparent, and sometimes coloured disc that fits directly over the cornea of the eye. Contact lenses are designed specifically to correct refractive errors of the eye or abnormalities in the cornea's shape. They are relatively easy to apply and remove.

Contact lenses are available in daily-wear, extended-wear, and disposable varieties. All lenses must be removed periodically to prevent ocular infection and corneal ulcers or abrasions. Common infectious agents are *Pseudomonas aeruginosa* and *Staphylococcus*. Client education must include a discussion of proper lens care techniques (Box 38–15).

Daily-wear lenses should be removed overnight for cleaning and disinfecting; extended-wear lenses can be worn for up to 30 days without being removed (Health Canada, 2006). Disposable lenses are available in daily-wear and extended-wear varieties. Extended-wear disposable lenses are usually replaced every 1 to 2 weeks. Pain, tearing, discomfort, and redness of the conjunctivae may be symptoms of lens overwear. The persistence of symptoms after lens removal may indicate serious ocular injury.

Contact lenses accumulate secretions and foreign matter while they are being worn. These materials deteriorate and then irritate the eye, causing distorted vision and the risk for infection. Contact lenses should be cleaned and thoroughly disinfected once removed. Clients should be cautioned to never use saliva, homemade saline, or tap water when cleaning lenses as these solutions may contain microorganisms that can cause serious infections.

Artificial Eyes. Clients with artificial eyes have had an **enucleation**, or removal, of an entire eyeball as a result of a tumour growth, severe infection, or eye trauma. Some artificial eyes are permanently implanted, whereas others can be removed for routine cleaning. Clients with an artificial eye usually prefer to care for their own eye. You should respect the client's wishes and assist by assembling needed equipment.

BOX 38-15 CLIENT TEACHING

Contact Lens Care

Objectives

- Client will be able to identify warning signs of corneal irritation and eye infection.
- Client will be able to clean and care for contact lenses correctly.

Teaching Strategies

Encourage the client to see a vision care specialist (**ophthalmologist** or **optometrist**) regularly: every 3–5 years before the age of 40 years, every 2 years after age 40, and yearly after age 65. Teach the client the following facts about contact lens care:

- Special cleaning solutions should be used when cleaning and disinfecting contact lenses.
- Never use fingernail on a lens to remove dirt or debris that does not loosen during washing with cleaning solutions.
- Follow the recommendations of lens manufacturer or your eye care practitioner when cleaning and disinfecting lenses.
- Remember the mnemonic RSVP: *redness, sensitivity, vision problems,* and *pain* (Health Canada, 2006). If one of these problems occurs, remove the contact lenses immediately. If problems continue, contact a vision care specialist.
- Lenses become very slippery once cleaning solution is applied.
- If a lens is dropped on a hard surface, moisten your finger with the cleaning or wetting solution and gently touch the lens to pick it up. Then clean, rinse, and disinfect the lens.
- Lenses should be kept moist or wet when not worn.
- Use fresh solution daily when storing and disinfecting lenses.
- Do not wipe the lens with a tissue or towel.
- Thoroughly wash and rinse the lens storage case on a daily basis. Clean it periodically with soap or liquid detergent; rinse it thoroughly with warm water and air-dry it.
- To avoid a mix-up, always start with the same lens when removing or inserting lenses.
- Throw away disposable or planned replacement lenses after the prescribed wearing period.

Evaluation

- Ask the client to identify the warning signs of corneal irritation and eye infection.
- Ask the client to describe methods of poor contact lens handling that can lead to infection.
- Ask the client to describe the techniques required to clean and store contact lenses.

A

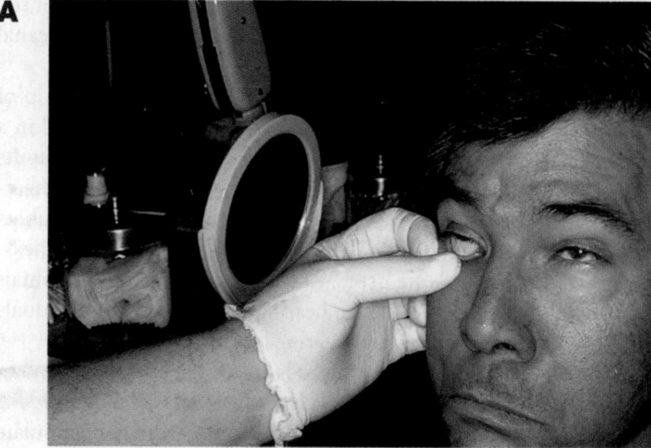

B

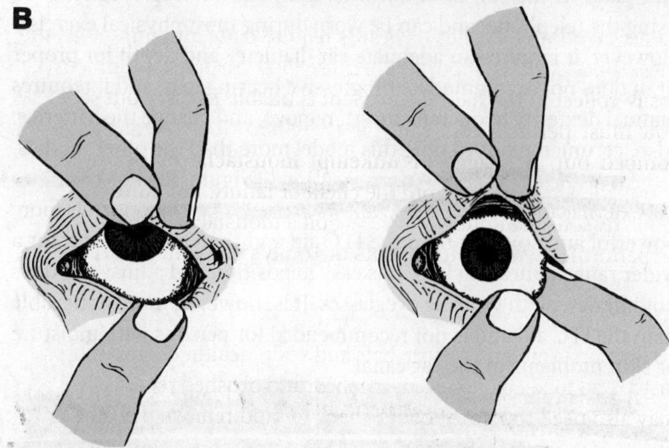

Figure 38-10 Removal of a prosthetic eye.

Clients may at times require assistance in prosthesis removal and cleansing. To remove an artificial eye, you retract the lower eyelid and exert slight pressure just below the eye (Figure 38–10). This action causes the artificial eye to rise from the socket because the suction holding the eye in place has been broken. You may also use a small, rubber bulb syringe or medicine dropper bulb to create a suction effect. The suction created by placing the bulb tip directly over the eye and squeezing lifts the artificial eye from the socket.

The artificial eye is usually made of glass or plastic. You use warm normal saline to cleanse the prosthesis. You should also cleanse the edges of the eye socket and surrounding tissues with soft gauze moistened in saline or clean tap water. Signs of infection should be reported immediately because bacteria can spread to the neighbouring eye, underlying sinuses, or even underlying brain tissue. To reinsert the eye, retract the upper and lower lids and gently slip the eye into the socket, fitting it neatly under the upper eyelid. An artificial eye may be stored in a labelled container filled with tap water or saline.

Ear Care. Routine ear care involves cleansing the ear with the end of a moistened washcloth, rotated gently into the ear canal. When cerumen is visible, gentle, downward retraction at the entrance of the ear canal may cause the wax to loosen and slip out. You should warn clients to never to use sharp objects such as bobby pins or paper clips to remove earwax as this can traumatize the ear canal and rupture the tympanic membrane. Use of cotton-tipped applicators should also be avoided because they can cause earwax to become impacted within the canal.

Children and older adults commonly have impacted cerumen. Excessive or impacted cerumen can usually be removed only by irrigation, which usually requires a physician's order. If a client has a history of a perforated eardrum or if perforation is discovered during assessment, the procedure is contraindicated. Before irrigation, instill three drops of glycerine at bedtime to soften the wax and three drops of hydrogen peroxide twice a day to loosen the wax. Then irrigation with approximately 250 mL of warm water (at 37°C) into the ear canal mechanically washes away loosened wax. The use of cold or hot water can cause nausea or vomiting.

The client may sit or lie on his or her side with the affected ear up. Place a small curved basin under the affected ear to catch the irrigating solution. You can use a bulb-irrigating syringe . The tip of the syringe should not occlude the ear canal to avoid exerting pressure against the tympanic membrane. Direct gentle irrigation at the top of the canal to loosen the cerumen from the sides of the canal. After the canal is clear, wipe off any moisture from the ear and inspect the canal for remaining cerumen.

Hearing Aid Care. Hearing aids are instruments made up of miniature parts working together as a system to amplify sound in a controlled manner. Aids receive normal low-intensity sound inputs and deliver them to the ear as louder outputs. The new class of hearing aids can reduce background noise interference. Computer chips placed in the aids allow for fine adjustments to a specific client's hearing needs. Hearing aids are used by both hard-of-hearing individuals (those with a slight or moderate hearing loss) and deaf individuals (those with severe or profound hearing loss).

Three popular types of hearing aids are available. An *in-the-canal (ITC) aid* is the newest, smallest, and least visible hearing aid and fits entirely in the ear canal. It has cosmetic appeal, is easy to manipulate and place in the ear, does not interfere with wearing eyeglasses or using the telephone, and can be worn during most physical exercise. However, it requires an adequate ear diameter and depth for proper fit. It does not accommodate progressive hearing loss, and it requires manual dexterity to operate, insert, remove, and change the batteries. Also, cerumen tends to plug this model more than the other models.

An *in-the-ear (ITE, or intra-aural) aid* (Figure 38–11A) fits into the external auditory canal and allows for better fine-tuning. It is more powerful and stronger than the ITC aid and therefore is useful for a wider range of hearing loss. It is easy to position and adjust and does not interfere with wearing eyeglasses. It is, however, more noticeable than the ITC aid and is not recommended for persons with moisture or skin problems in the ear canal.

A *behind-the-ear (BTE, or postaural) aid* (Figure 38–11B) hooks around and behind the ear and is connected by a short, clear, hollow plastic tube to an ear mould inserted into the external auditory canal. It allows for fine-tuning. It is the largest of the three aids and is useful for clients with rapidly progressive hearing loss or manual dexterity difficulties and those who find partial ear occlusion intolerable. Disadvantages are that it is more visible, may interfere with wearing eyeglasses and using a phone, and is more difficult to keep in place during physical exercise. Box 38–16 reviews client education guidelines for the care and use of a hearing aid.

Nasal Care. The client can usually remove secretions from the nose by gently blowing into a soft tissue. Caution the client against harsh blowing; this can create pressure capable of injuring the eardrum, nasal mucosa, and even sensitive eye structures. Bleeding from the nares is a sign of harsh blowing.

If the client is unable to remove nasal secretions, assist by using a wet washcloth or a cotton-tipped applicator moistened in water or saline. The applicator should never be inserted beyond the length of the cotton tip. Excessive nasal secretions can also be removed by gentle suctioning.

When clients have a nasogastric, feeding, or endotracheal tube inserted through the nose, you should change the tape anchoring the tube at least once a day. When tape becomes moist from nasal secretions, the skin and mucosa can easily become macerated. Friction from the tube can cause tissue sloughing. After carefully removing the tape, maintain your hold of the tubing and thoroughly cleanse and dry the nasal surface (see Chapter 43).

Client's Room Environment

Attempting to make a client's room as comfortable as possible is an important priority. The client's room should be comfortable, safe, and large enough to allow the client and visitors to move about freely. Room temperature and ventilation are difficult to control; however, noise and odours can be controlled to create a more comfortable environment. Keeping the room neat and orderly also contributes to the client's sense of well-being.

Maintaining Comfort. The nature of what constitutes a comfortable environment depends on the client's age, severity of illness, and level of daily activity. Depending on the client's age and physical condition, the room temperature should be maintained between 20°C and 23°C. if possible. Infants, older adults, and the acutely ill may need a warmer room. However, certain acutely ill clients (e.g., clients with head injuries) benefit from cooler room temperatures to lower the body's metabolic demands.

A good ventilation system keeps stale air and odours from lingering in the room. The acutely ill, infants, and older adults must be protected from drafts by ensuring that they are adequately dressed and covered with a lightweight blanket.

Good ventilation also reduces lingering odours caused by draining wounds, vomitus, bowel movements, and unemptied urinals. Room deodorizers can help remove many unpleasant odours but should be used with discretion in consideration of the client's possible embarrassment. Before using room deodorizers, it is important to determine that the client is not allergic or sensitive to the deodorizer itself. Bedpans and urinals should be emptied and rinsed promptly. Thorough hygiene measures are the best way to control body or breath odours.

Ill clients seem to be more sensitive to common hospital noises (e.g., IV pump alarms, suction apparatus, or stretchers exiting an

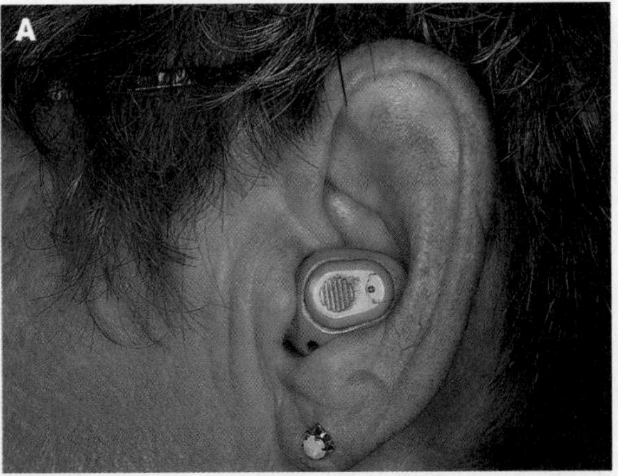

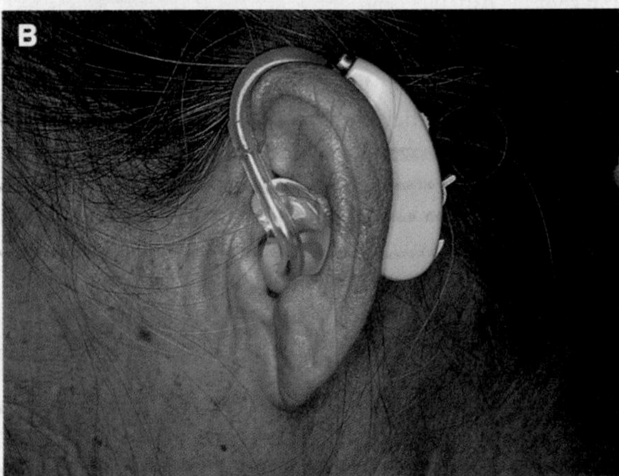

Figure 38-11 Two common types of hearing aids. A, In the ear. B, Behind the ear.

> **BOX 38-16 Care and Use of Hearing Aids**
>
> - Initially wear a hearing aid for short periods; then gradually increase the wearing time to 10–12 hours.
> - Once inserted, turn the aid slowly to one-third to one-half volume.
> - Remember that a whistling sound indicates too high a volume, incorrect ear mould insertion, an improper fit of the aid, or a buildup of earwax or fluid.
> - Adjust the volume to a comfortable level for talking at a distance of 1 m.
> - Do not wear the aid under heat lamps, while using a hair dryer, or in very wet, cold weather.
> - Keep in mind that batteries can last 70–85 hours—1 week with daily wearing of 10–12 hours.
> - Remove or disconnect the battery when not in use.
> - Replace ear moulds every 2–3 years.
> - Routinely check the battery compartment: Is it clean? Are batteries inserted properly? Is the compartment shut all the way?
> - Remember that dials on the hearing aid should be clean and easy to rotate, creating no static during adjusting.
> - Keep the aid clean.
> - Aids are usually cleaned with a soft cloth and warm soapy water; see the manufacturer's instructions.
> - Avoid the use of hairspray and perfume while wearing the hearing aid; the residue from the spray can cause the aid to become oily and greasy.
> - Do not submerse the aid in water.
> - Routinely check the cord or tubing (depending on type of aid) for cracking, fraying, and poor connections.
> - Follow-up with an audiologist routinely to evaluate the effectiveness of the current aid.
> - Remember that the frequencies of newer computerized hearing aids can be easily adjusted.
>
> Data from Ebersole, P., Hess, P., Touhy, T. A., Jett, K., & Luggen, A. (2008). *Toward healthy aging: Human needs and nursing response* (7th ed.). St. Louis, MO: Mosby; Eliopoulous, C. (2005). *Gerontological nursing* (6th ed.). Philadelphia, PA: Lippincott Williams & Wilkins; and Miller, C. A. (2009). *Nursing for wellness in older adults* (5th ed.). Philadelphia, PA: Lippincott Williams & Wilkins.

elevator). You should explain the source of any unfamiliar noise to the client and family members. Until the client is familiar with hospital noises, the noise level should be controlled as much as possible. This can also help the client sleep (see Chapter 41).

Proper lighting is necessary for everyone's safety and comfort. A brightly lit room is usually stimulating, and a darkened room is best for rest and sleep. Room lighting can be adjusted by closing or opening drapes, regulating overbed lights, and closing or opening room doors. When entering a client's room at night, refrain from abruptly turning on an overhead light unless necessary.

Room Equipment. Although variations in hospital rooms exist across health care settings, a typical hospital room contains the following basic pieces of furniture: an overbed table, a bedside stand, chairs, and a bed (Figure 38–12). Long-term care and rehabilitation facilities may have similar equipment. The overbed table rolls on wheels and can be adjusted to various heights over the bed or a chair. The table provides an ideal working space for performing procedures. It also provides a surface on which to place meal trays, toiletry items, and objects frequently used by the client. The bedpan and urinal should not be placed on the overbed table. The bedside stand is used to store the client's personal possessions and hygiene equipment. A telephone (if supplied), water pitcher, and drinking cup are commonly found on top of the bedside stand.

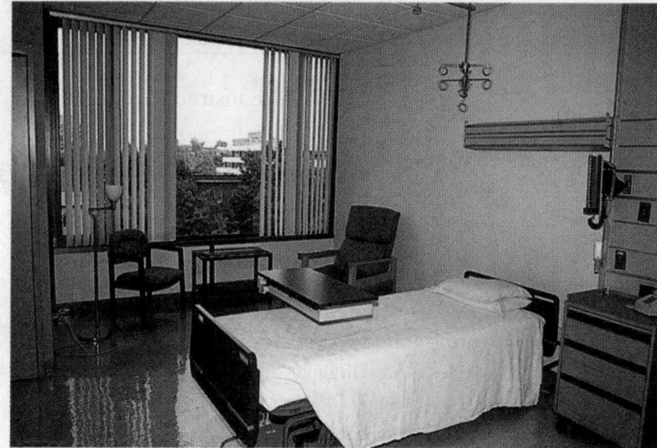

Figure 38-12 A typical hospital room.

Most hospital rooms contain an armless straight-backed chair or an upholstered lounge chair with arms. Straight-backed chairs are convenient to use when temporarily transferring the client from the bed, such as during bed making. Lounge chairs tend to be more comfortable when a client is willing and able to sit for an extended period.

Each room usually has an overbed light. Additional portable lighting can be used to provide extra light during bedside procedures. Other equipment usually found in a client's room includes a call bell, a television set (not available in all agencies and facilities), a wall-mounted blood pressure gauge, oxygen and vacuum wall outlets, and personal care items. Special equipment designed for comfort or positioning clients includes foot boots, special mattresses, and bed boards (see Chapters 46 and 47). Check your agency's policy and the manufacturers' directions before using comfort and positioning equipment.

Beds. Seriously ill clients may remain in bed for a long time. Because a bed is the piece of equipment used most by a hospitalized client, it should be designed for comfort, safety, and adaptability for changing positions. The typical hospital bed has a firm mattress on a metal frame that can be raised and lowered horizontally. Many hospitals are converting the standard hospital bed to one in which the mattress surface can be electronically adjusted for client comfort. Different bed positions are used to promote client comfort, minimize symptoms, promote lung expansion, and improve access during certain procedures (Table 38–6).

The position of a bed is usually changed by electrical controls incorporated into the client's call light and in a panel on the side or foot of the bed (Figure 38–13). However, some facilities do have hospital beds that are manually controlled. It is important to become familiar with the use of the bed controls. Ease in raising and lowering a bed and in changing the position of the bed head and foot eliminates undue musculoskeletal strain on the care provider. Instructions should be provided to the clients on the proper use of controls; caution them against raising the bed to a position that might cause harm.

Beds contain safety features such as locks on the wheels or casters, and alarms. Wheels should be locked when the bed is stationary to prevent accidental movement. Alarms should be turned on to protect clients at risk for falls when getting out of bed without assistance. Side rails protect clients from accidental falls. The headboard can be removed from most beds. This is important when the medical team must have easy access to the client's head, such as during cardiopulmonary resuscitation.

TABLE 38-6 Common Bed Positions

Position	Description	Uses
Fowler's	Head of bed raised to angle of 45 degrees or more; semisitting position; foot of bed may also be raised at knee	Is preferred while client eats Is used during nasogastric tube insertion and nasotracheal suction Promotes lung expansion
Semi-Fowler	Head of bed raised approximately 30 degrees; inclination less than Fowler's position; foot of bed may also be raised at knee	Promotes lung expansion Is used when clients receive gastric feedings to reduce regurgitation and risk of aspiration
Trendelenburg's	Entire bed frame tilted with head of bed down	Is used for postural drainage Facilitates venous return in clients with poor peripheral perfusion
Reverse Trendelenburg's	Entire bed frame tilted with foot of bed down	Is used infrequently Promotes gastric emptying Prevents esophageal reflux
Flat	Entire bed frame horizontally parallel with floor	Is used for clients with vertebral injuries and in cervical traction Is used for clients who are hypotensive Is generally preferred by clients for sleeping

Bed Making. A client's bed should be kept clean and comfortable. This requires frequent inspections to be sure linen is clean, dry, and free of wrinkles. When clients are diaphoretic, have draining wounds, or are incontinent, you should check frequently for soiled linen.

The bed is usually made in the morning after the client's bath or while the client is in the shower, sitting in a chair eating, or out of the room for procedures or tests. Throughout the day, bed linens should be straightened when they become loose or wrinkled. The bed linen should also be checked for food particles after meals and for wetness or soiling. Linen that are soiled or wet should be changed.

When changing bed linen, follow the principles of medical asepsis by keeping soiled linen away from your uniform (Figure 38–14). Soiled linen is placed in special linen bags before discarding it in a hamper. To avoid air currents, which can spread microorganisms, bed

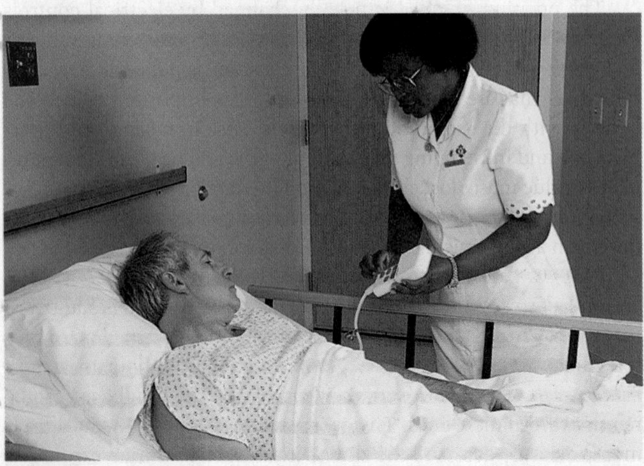

Figure 38-13 Instruct client in use of call light and bed controls.

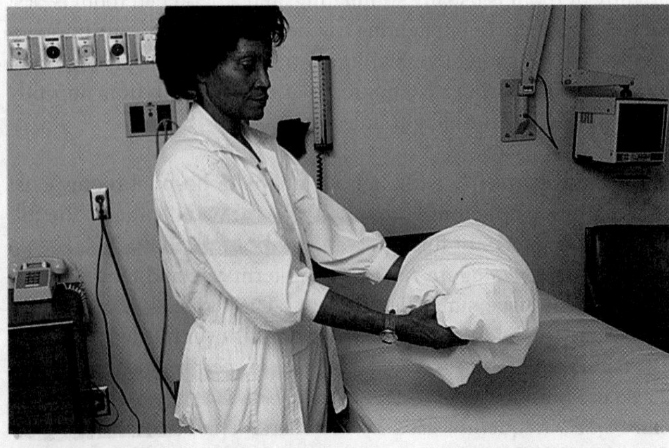

Figure 38-14 Holding linen away from the uniform prevents contact with microorganisms.

➤ SKILL 38-5 **Making an Occupied Bed** video

Delegation Considerations

The skill of making an occupied bed can be delegated to an unregulated care provider. It is important to discuss the following with him or her:

- Any precautions or activity restrictions for the client
- What to do if wound drainage, dressing material, drainage tubes, or IV tubing becomes dislodged or is found in the linens
- What to do if the client becomes fatigued

Equipment

See Figure 38-15.

- Linen bag(s)
- Bottom sheet (flat or fitted)
- Drawsheet (optional)
- Top sheet
- Blanket
- Bedspread
- Waterproof pads or soaker pad (optional)
- Pillowcases
- Bedside chair or table
- Disposable gloves (optional)
- Towel
- Disinfectant

Procedure

STEPS	RATIONALE
1. Assess potential for client incontinence or excess drainage on bed linen.	• Determines the need for protective waterproof pads or extra bath blankets on the bed.
2. Check chart for orders or specific precautions concerning movement and positioning.	• Ensures client safety and the use of proper body mechanics.
3. Explain procedure to the client, noting that he or she will be asked to turn on side and roll over linen.	• Minimizes anxiety and promotes cooperation.
4. Perform hand hygiene and put on gloves. (Gloves are worn only if linen is soiled or if contact with body secretions is possible.)	• Reduces the transmission of microorganisms.
5. Assemble equipment and arrange it on a bedside chair or table. Remove unnecessary equipment such as a dietary tray or items used for hygiene.	• Assembling all equipment provides for a smooth procedure and assists in increasing client's comfort. Placing linen on clean surface minimizes spread of infection.
6. Draw room curtain around bed or close room door.	• Maintains client's privacy.
7. Adjust bed height to a comfortable working position. Lower any raised side rail on one side of bed. Remove the call light.	• Minimizes strain on the back. It is easier to remove and put on linen evenly to bed in a flat position. Provides easy access to bed and linen.
8. Loosen top linen at foot of the bed.	• Makes linen easier to remove.
9. Remove bedspread and blanket separately. If bedspread and blanket are soiled, place them in a linen bag. Keep soiled linen away from your uniform.	• Reduces the transmission of microorganisms.
10. If blanket and bedspread are to be reused, fold them by bringing the top and bottom edges together. Fold the farthest side over onto nearer bottom edge. Bring top and bottom edges together again. Place folded linen over back of chair.	• Folding method facilitates replacement and minimizes wrinkles.

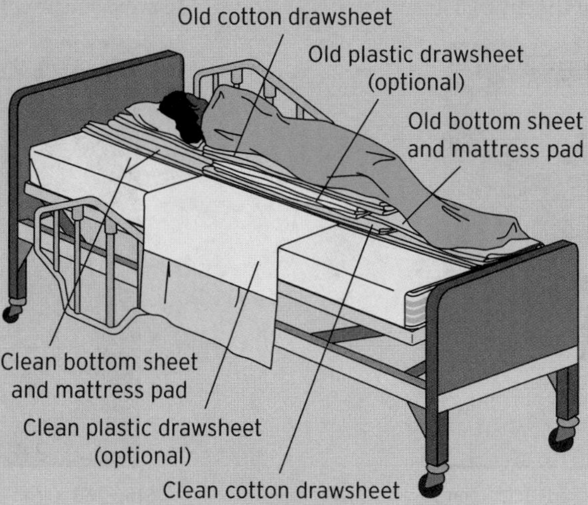

Figure 38-15 Equipment for making an occupied bed.

Continued

➤SKILL 38-5 Making an Occupied Bed *continued*

STEPS	RATIONALE
11. Cover client with a bath blanket in the following manner: Unfold bath blanket over top sheet. Ask client to hold top edge of the bath blanket. If client is unable to help, tuck top of bath blanket under client's shoulder. Grasp top sheet under bath blanket at client's shoulders and bring sheet down to foot of bed. Remove the sheet and discard in a linen bag.	• Bath blanket provides warmth and keeps body parts covered during linen removal.
12. With assistance from another, slide mattress toward head of the bed.	• If mattress slides toward foot of the bed when head of the bed is raised, it is difficult to tuck in linen. In addition, it is uncomfortable for the client because the client's feet may be pressed against or hang over the foot of the bed.
13. Position the client on the far side of the bed, turned onto his or her side and facing away from you. Be sure side rail in front of client is up. Adjust pillow under client's head.	• Turning client onto side provides space for placement of clean linen. Side rail ensures client's safety from forward falls from the bed surface and helps client in moving.
14. Loosen bottom linens, moving from head to foot. With seam side down (facing the mattress), fanfold bottom sheet and drawsheet toward client—first drawsheet, then bottom sheet. Tuck edges of linen just under buttocks, back, and shoulders. Do not fanfold mattress pad if it is to be reused (see Step 14 illustration).	• Prepares for removal of all bottom linen simultaneously. Provides maximum workspace for placing clean linen. Later, when client turns to other side, soiled linen can be removed easily.
15. Wipe off any moisture on exposed mattress with towel and appropriate disinfectant.	• Reduces the transmission of microorganisms.
16. Put on clean linen to exposed half of the bed:	
A. Place clean mattress pad on bed by folding it lengthwise with centre crease in middle of bed. Fanfold top layer over mattress. (If pad is reused, simply smooth out any wrinkles.)	• Putting on linen over bed in successive layers minimizes energy and time used in bed making.
B. Unfold bottom sheet lengthwise so that centre crease is situated lengthwise along centre of bed. Fanfold sheet's top layer toward centre of bed alongside the client. Smooth bottom layer of sheet over mattress, and bring the edge over closest side of the mattress. Pull fitted sheet smoothly over mattress ends. Allow edge of flat unfitted sheet to hang about 25 cm over mattress edge. Lower hem of bottom flat sheet should lie seam down and even with bottom edge of mattress (see Step 16B illustration).	• Proper positioning of linen on one side ensures that adequate linen will be available to cover opposite side of bed. Keeping seam edges down eliminates irritation to client's skin.
17. Mitre bottom flat sheet at head of bed:	• Mitred corner cannot be loosened easily even if client moves frequently in bed.
A. Face head of bed diagonally. Place hand away from head of bed under top corner of mattress, near mattress edge, and lift.	
B. With other hand, tuck top edge of bottom sheet smoothly under mattress so that side edges of sheet above and below the mattress would meet if brought together.	

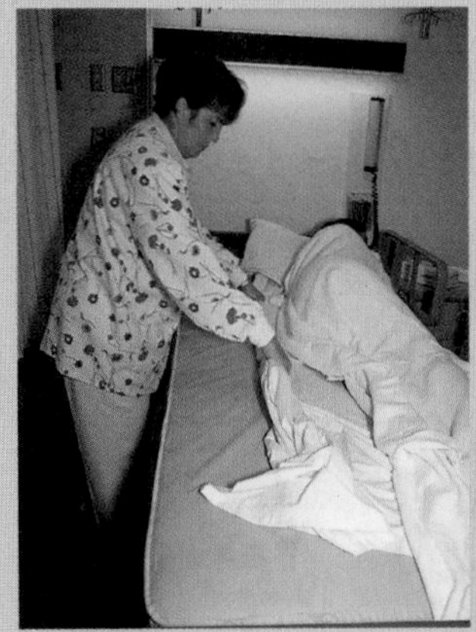

Step 14 Old linen tucked under client.

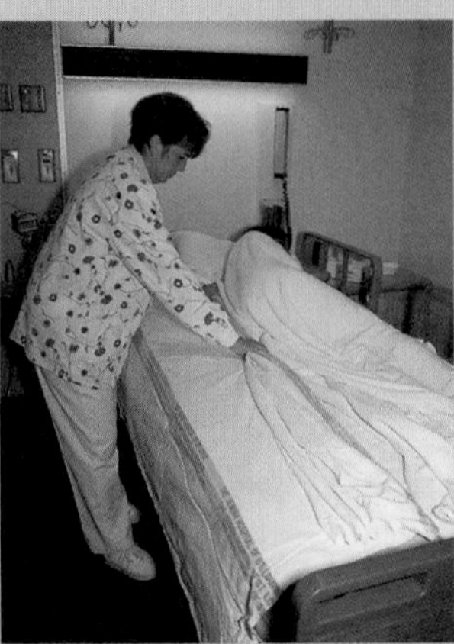

Step 16B Clean linen applied to bed.

➤ SKILL 38-5 Making an Occupied Bed *continued*

STEPS	RATIONALE
C. Face side of the bed and pick up top edge of sheet at approximately 45 cm from top of mattress (see Step 17C illustration).	
D. Lift sheet, and lay it on top of mattress to form a neat triangular fold, with lower base of the triangle even with the mattress side edge (see Step 17D illustration).	
E. Tuck lower edge of sheet, which is hanging free below the mattress, under the mattress. Tuck with palms down, without pulling triangular fold (see Step 17E illustration).	
F. Hold portion of sheet covering side of mattress in place with one hand. With the other hand, pick up top of triangular linen fold and bring it down over side of the mattress (see Step 17F illustrations). Tuck this portion under mattress (see Step 17F illustrations).	
18. Tuck remaining portion of sheet under the mattress, moving toward foot of the bed. Keep linen smooth.	• Folds of linen are source of irritation.
19. *(Optional)* Open drawsheet so that it unfolds in half. Lay centrefold along middle of bed lengthwise, and position sheet so that it will be under the client's buttocks and torso (see Step 19 illustration). Fanfold top layer toward client, with edge along the client's back. Smooth bottom layer out over the mattress, and tuck excess edge under mattress (keep palms down).	• Drawsheet is used to lift and reposition the client. Placement under client's torso distributes most of the client's body weight over the sheet.
20. Place waterproof pad over drawsheet, with centrefold against client's side. Fanfold top layer toward client.	• Protects bed linen from being soiled.
21. Have client roll slowly toward you, over the layers of linen. Raise side rail on working side, and go to other side of the bed.	• Positions client for removal and placement of linens. Maintains client's safety and body alignment during turning.
22. Lower side rail. Assist client in positioning on other side, over folds of linen (see Step 22 illustration). Loosen edges of soiled linen from under mattress.	• Exposes opposite side of bed for removal of soiled linen and placement of clean linen. Makes linen easier to remove.
23. Remove soiled linen by folding it into a bundle or square, with soiled side turned in. Discard in linen bag. If necessary, wipe mattress with antiseptic solution, and dry mattress surface before putting on new linen.	• Reduces the transmission of microorganisms.

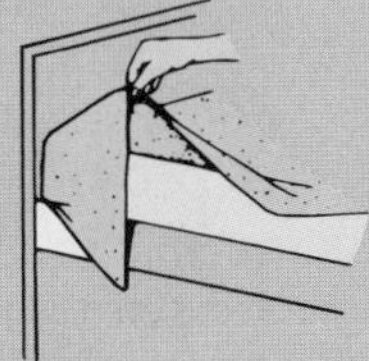

Step 17C Pick up top edge of sheet.

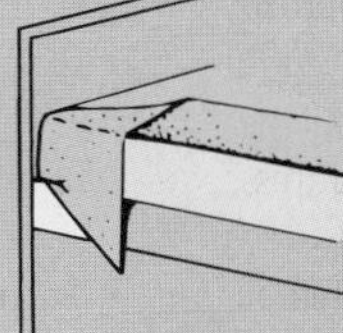

Step 17D Sheet on top of mattress in a triangular fold.

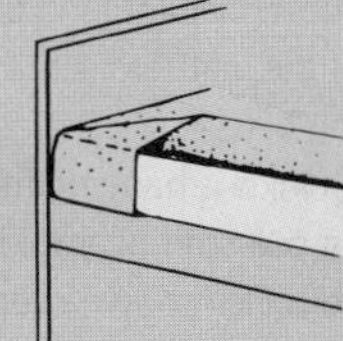

Step 17E Lower edge of sheet tucked under mattress.

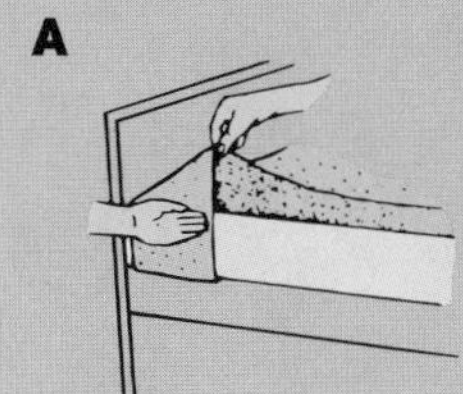

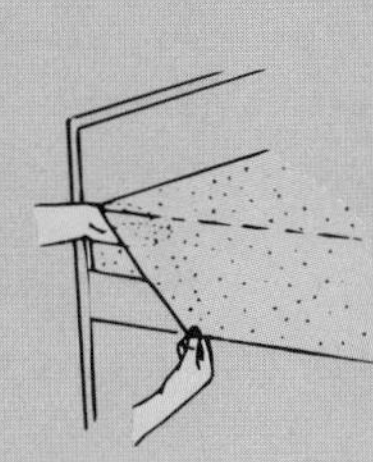

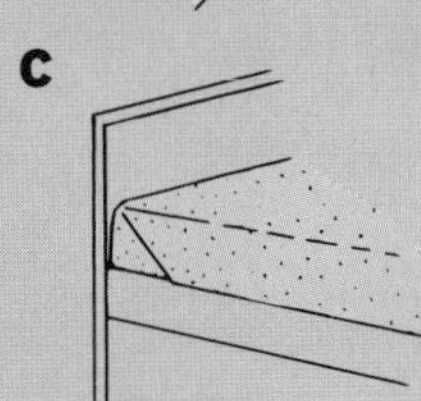

Step 17F **A** and **B,** Triangular fold placed over side of mattress. **C,** Linen tucked under mattress.

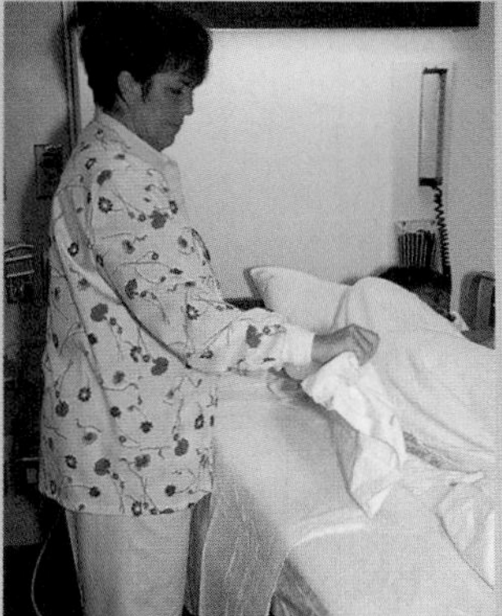

Step 19 Optional drawsheet.

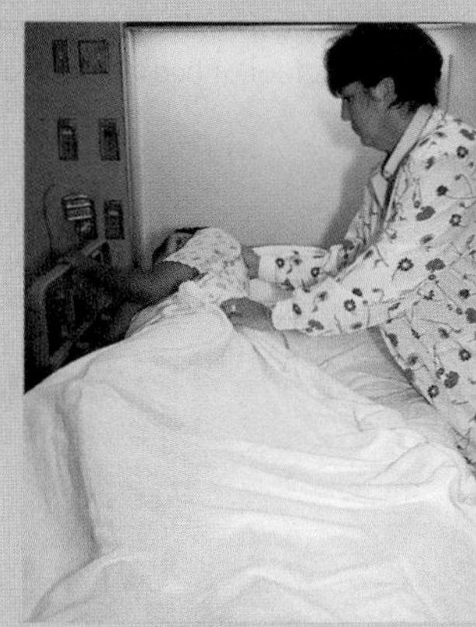

Step 22 Assist client to roll over folds of linen.

Continued

➤ SKILL 38-5 Making an Occupied Bed *continued*

STEPS	RATIONALE
24. Pull clean, fanfolded linen smoothly over edge of mattress from head to foot of bed.	• Smooth linen will not irritate client's skin.
25. Assist client in rolling back into supine position. Reposition pillow.	• Maintains client's comfort.
26. Pull fitted sheet smoothly over mattress ends. Mitre top corner of bottom sheet (see Step 17). When tucking corner, be sure that sheet is smooth and free of wrinkles.	• Wrinkles and folds can cause irritation to the skin.
27. Facing side of the bed, grasp remaining edge of bottom flat sheet. Lean back; keeping back straight, pull while tucking excess linen under mattress. Proceed from head to foot of the bed. (Avoid lifting mattress during tucking to ensure fit.)	• Proper use of body mechanics while tucking linen prevents injury.
28. Smooth fanfolded drawsheet out over bottom sheet. Grasp edge of the sheet with palms down, lean back, and tuck sheet under mattress. Tuck from middle to top and then to bottom.	• Tucking first at top or bottom may pull sheet sideways, causing poor fit.
29. Place top sheet over client with centrefold lengthwise down middle of bed. Open sheet from head to foot, and unfold over client.	• Sheet should be equally distributed over bed by correctly positioning centrefold.
30. Ask client to hold clean top sheet, or tuck sheet around client's shoulders. Remove the bath blanket and discard in linen bag.	• Sheet prevents exposure of body parts. Having client hold sheet encourages client participation in care.
31. Place blanket on bed, unfolding it so that crease runs lengthwise along middle of bed. Unfold blanket to cover client. Top edge should be parallel with edge of top sheet and 15–20 cm from top sheet's edge.	• Blanket should be placed to cover client completely and provide adequate warmth.
32. Place bedspread over bed according to Step 31. Be sure that top edge of bedspread extends about 2.5 cm above blanket's edge. Tuck top edge of bedspread over and under top edge of blanket.	• Gives bed neat appearance and provides extra warmth.
33. Make cuff by turning edge of top sheet down over top edge of the blanket and bedspread.	• Protect client's face from rubbing against blanket or bedspread.
34. Standing on one side at foot of the bed, lift mattress corner slightly with one hand and tuck linens under mattress. Tuck top sheet and blanket under together. Be sure that linens are loose enough to allow movement of client's feet. Making a horizontal toe pleat is an option (see Step 34 illustration).	• Makes neat-appearing bed. Pressure ulcers can develop on client's toes and heels from feet rubbing against tight-fitting bed sheets.
35. Make modified mitred corner with top sheet, blanket, and bedspread (see Box 38–17, Step 20 illustration):	• Ensures top covers will not loosen easily.
A. Pick up side edge of top sheet, blanket, and bedspread approximately 45 cm from foot of the mattress. Lift linen to form triangular fold, and lay it on bed.	
B. Tuck lower edge of sheet, which is hanging free below mattress, under the mattress. Do not pull triangular fold.	
C. Pick up triangular fold, and bring it down over mattress while holding linen in place along side of the mattress. Do not tuck tip of triangle.	• Secures top linen but keeps even edge of blanket and top sheet draped over mattress.
36. Raise side rail. Make other side of bed; spread sheet, blanket, and bedspread out evenly. Fold top edge of bedspread over the blanket and make cuff with top sheet (see Step 33); make modified mitred corner at foot of bed (see Step 35).	• Side rail protects client from accidental falls.

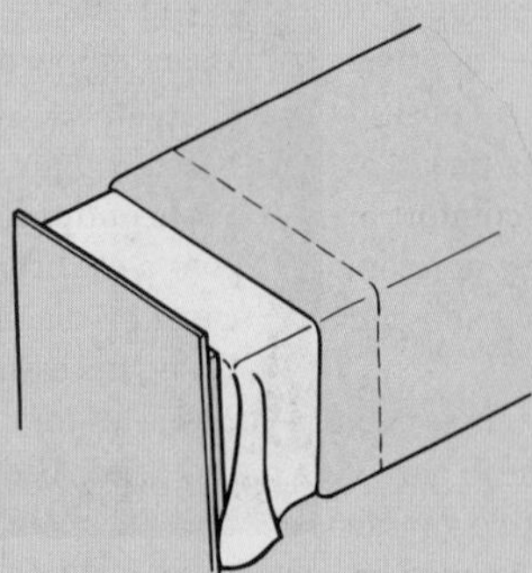

Step 34 Optional toe pleat.

➤ SKILL 38-5 Making an Occupied Bed ***continued***

STEPS	RATIONALE
37. Change pillowcase:	
A. Have client raise his or her head. While supporting client's neck with one hand, remove pillow. Allow client to lower head.	• Support of neck muscles prevents injury during flexion and extension of neck.
B. Remove soiled case by grasping pillow at open end with one hand and pulling case back over pillow with the other hand. Discard case in linen bag.	• Pillows slide out easily, thus minimizing contact with soiled linen.
C. Grasp clean pillowcase at centre of closed end. Gather case, turning it inside out over the hand holding it. With the same hand, pick up the middle of one end of the pillow. Pull pillowcase down over pillow with the other hand.	• Eases sliding of pillowcase over pillow.
D. Be sure pillow corners fit evenly into corners of the pillowcase. Place pillow under the client's head.	• Poorly fitting case constricts fluffing and expansion of the pillow and interferes with client comfort.
38. Place call bell within the client's reach, and return the bed to comfortable position.	• Ensures client safety and comfort.
39. Open room curtains, and rearrange furniture. Place personal items within easy reach on overbed table or bedside stand. Return bed to a comfortable height.	• Promotes sense of well-being.
40. Discard dirty linen in a hamper or chute, remove your gloves, and perform hand hygiene.	• Prevents the transmission of microorganisms.
41. Ask whether client feels comfortable.	• Ensures bed linens are clean and smooth.
42. While you are performing this skill, inspect the skin for areas of irritation.	• Folds in linen can cause pressure on the skin.
43. Observe the client for signs of fatigue, dyspnea, pain, or discomfort throughout the skill.	• Provides data about client's level of activity tolerance and ability to participate in other procedures.

Unexpected Outcomes and Related Interventions

Discomfort Caused by Linen Fold

- Tighten sheets.
- Change client's position frequently.

Signs of Breakdown of Client's Skin

- Institute skin care measures to reduce risk of pressure ulcer (see Chapter 47).
- Change client's position frequently.

Recording and Reporting

- Making an occupied bed need not be recorded.

linens should never be shaken. To avoid transmitting infection, do not place soiled linen on the floor. If clean linen touches the floor, it should be immediately discarded.

During bed making, use proper body mechanics (see Chapter 36). You should always raise the bed to the appropriate height before changing linen so that you do not have to bend or stretch over the mattress. You should also move back and forth to opposite sides of the bed while putting on new linen. Body mechanics is also important when turning or repositioning the client in bed.

When clients are confined to a bed, organize bed-making activities to conserve time and energy (Skill 38–5). The client's privacy, comfort, and safety are all important. Using side rails to aid positioning and turning, keeping a call light within the client's reach, and maintaining the proper bed position help to promote comfort and safety. After making a bed, always return it to the lowest horizontal position to prevent accidental falls should the client get in and out of the bed alone.

When possible, a bed should be made while it is unoccupied (Box 38–17). Clinical judgement is used regarding the best time to have the client sit up in a chair while the bed is made. When making an unoccupied bed, follow the basic principles for making an occupied bed.

An unoccupied bed can be open or closed. In an open bed, the top covers are folded back so that a client can easily get into bed. In a closed bed, the top sheet, blanket, and bedspread are drawn up to the head of the mattress and under the pillows. A closed bed is prepared in a hospital room before a new client is admitted to that room.

A surgical, recovery, or postoperative bed is a modified version of the open bed. The top bed linen is arranged for easy transfer of the client from a stretcher to the bed. The top sheets and bedspread are not tucked or mitred at the corners. Instead, the top sheets are folded to one side or to the bottom third of the bed (Figure 38–16). This makes it easier to transfer the client into the bed.

Linens. In any health care agency, it is important to have an adequate supply of linen to care appropriately for clients. Many agencies have "nurse servers," either within or just outside a client's room, where a daily supply of linen is stored. Because of the emphasis on cost control in health care, it is important to not bring excess linen into a client's room. Linen brought into a client's room, if unused, must be discarded for laundering, which can increase an agency's costs. Excess linen lying around a client's room creates clutter and obstacles for client care activities.

Before bed making, it is important to collect necessary bed linens and the client's personal items. In this way, you have all equipment accessible to prepare the bed and room. Linens are pressed and folded to prevent the spread of microorganisms and to make bed making easier. When fitted sheets are not available, flat sheets usually are

➤ BOX 38-17 **Procedural Guidelines**

Making an Unoccupied Bed

Delegation Considerations: The skill of making an unoccupied bed can be delegated to an unregulated care provider.

Equipment:
- Linen bag
- Bottom sheet (flat or fitted)
- Drawsheet (optional)
- Top sheet
- Blanket
- Bedspread
- Waterproof pads or soaker pad (optional)
- Pillowcases
- Bedside chair or table
- Disposable gloves (if linen is soiled)
- Washcloth
- Antiseptic cleanser

Procedure
1. Determine whether client has been incontinent or whether excess drainage is on linen. Gloves will be necessary.
2. Assess activity orders or restrictions in mobility to plan whether client can get out of bed for the procedure. If so, assist client to bedside chair or recliner.
3. Raise bed to a comfortable working position. Lower the side rails on both sides of the bed.
4. Remove soiled linen and place in linen bag. Avoid shaking or fanning linen.
5. Reposition mattress and wipe off any moisture using a washcloth moistened in antiseptic solution. Dry thoroughly.
6. Put on all bottom linen on one side of bed before moving to opposite side.
7. Be sure fitted sheet is placed smoothly over mattress. To put on a flat unfitted sheet, allow about 25 cm to hang over mattress edge. Lower hem of the sheet should lie seam down, even with bottom edge of the mattress. Pull remaining top portion of sheet over top edge of the mattress.
8. While standing at head of the bed, mitre top corner of bottom sheet (see Skill 38–5, Step 17).
9. Tuck remaining portion of unfitted sheet under the mattress.
10. *Optional and agency or facility specific:* Put on a drawsheet, laying centre fold along middle of the bed lengthwise. Smooth drawsheet over the mattress and tuck excess edge under mattress, keeping palms down.
11. Move to opposite side of the bed, and spread bottom sheet smoothly over edge of mattress from head to foot of the bed.
12. Put on fitted sheet smoothly over each mattress corner. For an unfitted sheet, mitre the top corner of bottom sheet (see Skill 38–5, Step 17), making sure corner is taut.
13. Grasp remaining edge of unfitted bottom sheet and tuck tightly under the mattress while moving from head to foot of the bed. Smooth folded drawsheet over the bottom sheet and tuck under mattress, first at middle, then at top, and then at bottom.
14. If needed, put on a waterproof pad or soaker pad over bottom sheet.
15. Place top sheet over bed with vertical centre fold lengthwise down middle of the bed. Open sheet out from head to foot, being sure top edge of the sheet is even with top edge of the mattress.
16. Make horizontal toe pleat: Stand at foot of bed and fanfold in sheet 5–10 cm across bed. Pull sheet up from bottom to make fold approximately 15 cm from bottom edge of the mattress (see Skill 38–5, Step 34).
17. Tuck in remaining portion of the sheet under foot of mattress. Place blanket over the bed with top edge parallel to top edge of sheet and 15–20 cm down from edge of sheet. (*Optional:* Put on additional bedspread over bed.)
18. Make cuff by turning edge of top sheet down over top edge of the blanket and bedspread.
19. Standing on one side at foot of the bed, lift mattress corner slightly with one hand, and with the other hand tuck top sheet, blanket, and bedspread under the mattress. Be sure toe pleats are not pulled out.
20. Make modified mitred corner with top sheet, blanket, and bedspread. After triangular fold is made, do not tuck tip of triangle (see Step 20 illustration).
21. Go to other side of the bed. Spread sheet, blanket, and bedspread out evenly. Make cuff with top sheet and blanket. Make modified corner at foot of the bed.
22. Put on clean pillowcase.
23. Place call light within client's reach on a bed rail or pillow and return bed to height allowing for client transfer. Assist the client to get into bed.
24. Arrange client's room. Remove and discard supplies. Perform hand hygiene.

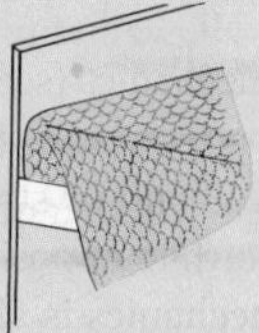

Step 20 Modified mitred corner.

pressed with a centre crease to be placed down the centre of the bed. The linens unfold easily to the sides, with creases often fitting over the mattress edge. A complete linen change is not always necessary. The sheet, blanket, and bedspread may be reused for the same client if they are not wet or soiled.

Disposal of linen must be done to minimize the spread of infection (see Chapter 33). Agency policies provide guidelines for the proper way to bag and dispose of soiled linen. After a client is discharged, all bed linen is sent to the laundry, the mattress and bed are cleaned by housekeeping staff, and new bed linen is applied.

❖Evaluation

Client Care

Evaluation of hygiene measures occurs both during and after each particular skill. For example, while bathing a client, closely inspect the skin to determine whether drainage or other soiling has been effectively removed from the skin's surface. Once the bath is completed, ask the client whether his or her comfort and relaxation have improved. When evaluating for the effectiveness of hygiene measures,

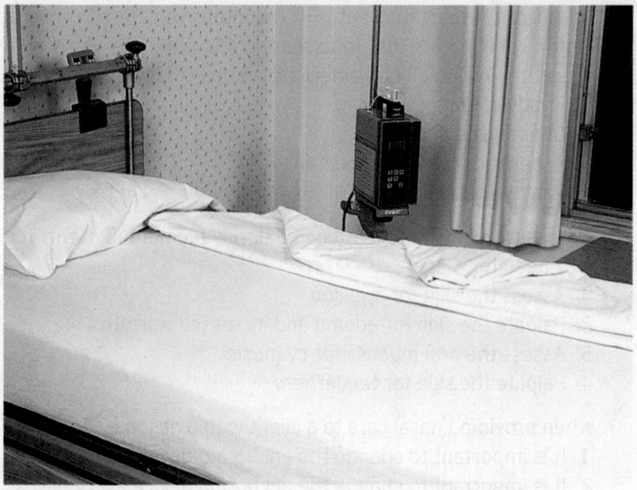

Figure 38-16 Surgical or recovery bed.

observe for changes in the client's behaviour. Does the client assume a more relaxed position? Is the client free of body odour? Is the client able to fall asleep? Does the client's facial expression convey a sense of comfort?

Frequently, it takes time for hygiene care to result in an improvement in a client's condition. The presence of oral lesions, a scalp infestation, or skin excoriation often requires repeated measures and a combination of nursing interventions. Evaluate for improvement in the client's condition over time and determine whether existing therapies are effective.

Throughout evaluation, consider the goals of care and evaluate whether expected outcomes are achieved. A critical thinking approach ensures that consideration is given to all factors when evaluating a client's care (Figure 38–17). Knowledge base and experience provide important perspectives when analyzing observations made about a client. For example, once you have seen how dehydration of the oral mucosa clears with repeated hygiene, it helps you to recognize when progress in another client is slow. The standards for evaluation are the expected outcomes established in the planning stage of the client's care. If outcomes are not met, the care plan may need to be revised. Continual application of critical thinking and clinical judgement is necessary when considering all evaluation findings.

Client Expectations

The final portion of the evaluation considers whether or not a client's expectations have been met through hygiene care. You might ask the client, "Do you feel your bath and back rub helped to make you comfortable?" "Can you suggest ways in which we can improve your foot care?" "What further measures do you think are necessary to keep your mouth clean and refreshed?"

Clients' expectations are important guidelines in determining client satisfaction. As the care provider, you must feel comfortable in addressing your clients' concerns and expectations. A caring approach can facilitate a discussion of these issues.

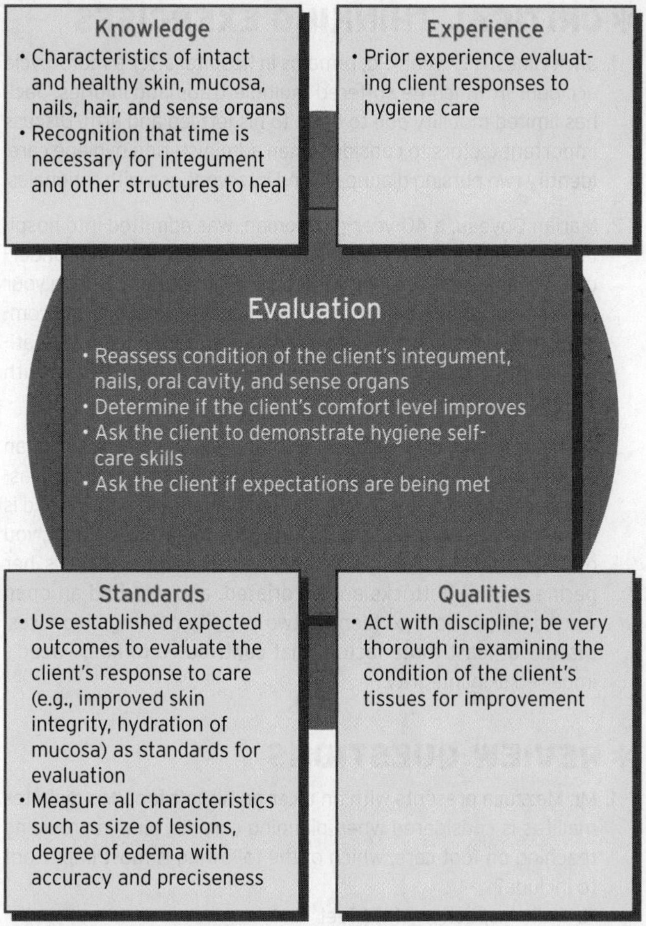

Knowledge
- Characteristics of intact and healthy skin, mucosa, nails, hair, and sense organs
- Recognition that time is necessary for integument and other structures to heal

Experience
- Prior experience evaluating client responses to hygiene care

Evaluation
- Reassess condition of the client's integument, nails, oral cavity, and sense organs
- Determine if the client's comfort level improves
- Ask the client to demonstrate hygiene self-care skills
- Ask the client if expectations are being met

Standards
- Use established expected outcomes to evaluate the client's response to care (e.g., improved skin integrity, hydration of mucosa) as standards for evaluation
- Measure all characteristics such as size of lesions, degree of edema with accuracy and preciseness

Qualities
- Act with discipline; be very thorough in examining the condition of the client's tissues for improvement

Figure 38-17 Critical thinking model for hygiene evaluation.

* KEY CONCEPTS

- Determine a client's ability to perform self-care and provide hygiene care according to the client's needs and preferences.
- During hygiene, integrate other activities such as physical assessment, wound care, and ROM exercises.
- While providing daily hygiene needs, use teaching and communication skills in developing a caring relationship with the client.
- Various personal, sociocultural, socioeconomic, and developmental factors influence clients' hygiene practices.
- Clients' health beliefs predict the likelihood of their assuming health-promoting behaviour, such as the maintenance of good hygiene.
- You might not assess all body regions before administering hygiene; however, routine assessment of the client's condition is undertaken whenever care is given.
- Clients with reduced sensation, vascular insufficiency, and immobility are at greater risk for impaired skin integrity.
- You must perform an assessment of each client's physical and cognitive abilities to perform basic hygiene measures, including muscle strength, flexibility and dexterity, balance, coordination, activity tolerance, and ability to comprehend. For clients suffering symptoms such as pain or nausea, administering symptom relief therapies before performing hygiene procedures better prepares the client.
- Clients with diabetes mellitus require special nail and foot care.
- When administering oral care to unconscious clients, measures must be taken to prevent aspiration.
- A client's room should be comfortable, safe, and uncluttered to provide for client comfort and safety.
- An evaluation of hygiene care is based on the client's sense of comfort, relaxation, well-being, and understanding of hygiene techniques.

✻ CRITICAL THINKING EXERCISES

1. Jack Hines, a 19-year-old, remains in hospital after a motorcycle accident in which he suffered multiple traumatic injuries. Jack has limited mobility due to casts to his left leg and arm. Discuss important factors to consider when administering hygiene care. Identify two nursing diagnoses and interventions with rationales.
2. Marian Goyeau, a 40-year-old woman, was admitted into hospital for treatment of a malignant breast lesion. Marian is undergoing chemotherapy along with radiation treatment. During your assessment, she complains of a loss of appetite, nausea and vomiting, and sores in her mouth. Marian is suffering from stomatitis. Identify two nursing diagnoses and interventions with rationales.
3. Michelle Tweed, a 78-year-old woman, was transferred from an acute care hospital to a rehabilitation facility after a cerebrovascular accident. She exhibits right hemiparesis and aphasia and is incontinent of urine and stool. During the initial assessment, you discover that Mrs. Tweed has reddened areas on both heels, her perineum and buttocks are excoriated, and you find an open wound on her coccyx. Identify two priority nursing diagnoses. Discuss at least three factors that contributed to Mrs. Tweed's impaired skin integrity.

✻ REVIEW QUESTIONS

1. Mr. Mazzuca presents with an ulcer on his left foot. His diabetes mellitus is considered when planning care for him. In providing teaching on foot care, which of the following is most important to include?
   1. Daily inspection of his feet
   2. Application of lotion to his feet and between his toes daily
   3. Daily soaking of his feet in hot water
   4. Cutting his toenails in the shape of a curve
2. A 35-year-old man is interested in obtaining information about the cause of his psoriasis. You would share with him that psoriasis
   1. Is contagious
   2. Can be related to poor hygiene
   3. Is not contagious
   4. Can be cured
3. A 75-year-old woman who has a history of diabetes and peripheral vascular disease has been trying to remove a corn from the bottom of her foot with a pair of scissors. Client teaching will include the following:
   1. With her diabetes, she has increased circulation in her foot, and this action could cause severe bleeding
   2. Her peripheral vascular disease increases her risk of developing more corns
   3. With her chronic disease, she could be at an increased risk for infection
   4. Her chronic disease limits her range of motion, and she may not be able to safely see or reach the corn
4. A thorough skin assessment is very important because the skin can provide information about
   1. Support systems
   2. Circulatory status
   3. Psychological wellness
   4. Fundamental skills
5. An African American client is in the intensive care unit after a motor vehicle collision. In assessing for cyanosis, you would expect to find which characteristics in this client's skin?
   1. Ruddy colour
   2. Generalized pallor
   3. Ashen, grey, or dull appearance
   4. Patchy areas of pallor
6. When assessing inflammation in a darkly pigmented client, you may need to
   1. Assess the skin for swelling
   2. Palpate the skin for edema and increased warmth
   3. Assess the oral mucosa for cyanosis
   4. Palpate the skin for tenderness
7. When providing nasal care to a client with a nasogastric tube,
   1. It is important to change the anchoring device as necessary
   2. It is important to change the anchoring device every day
   3. It is not necessary to change the anchoring device
   4. It is important to change the anchoring device every other day
8. When providing hair care for a client, it is important to consider all of the following, except
   1. Caregiver preferences
   2. Family preferences
   3. Cultural preferences
   4. Client preferences
9. When providing eye care,
   1. Eyes should be cleansed from the outer to the inner canthus
   2. Eyes should be cleansed from the inner to the outer canthus
   3. Eye hygiene is not necessary
   4. It is acceptable to cleanse eyes from either direction
10. In providing hygiene care for clients, it is important to
    1. Use communication skills that promote a caring therapeutic relationship
    2. Provide privacy, convey respect, and promote independence
    3. Provide an environment that promotes the client's physical and mental comfort
    4. All of the above

✻ RECOMMENDED WEB SITES

Alzheimer's Society of Canada: http://www.alzheimer.ca
The Alzheimer's Society of Canada Web site offers important information on Alzheimer's disease and other dementias, treatment, research, support, and services.

Canadian Dental Association: http://www.cda-adc.ca
The Canadian Dental Association Web site offers information on maintaining optimal oral health, including oral hygiene for older adults.

Canadian Diabetes Association: http://www.diabetes.ca
The Canadian Diabetes Association Web site offers information on the different types of diabetes, treatment, research, and services.

Public Health Agency of Canada: http://www.publichealth.gc.ca
This Web site is a valuable and unique resource offering information on healthy living, disease, and injury prevention.

39

Cardiopulmonary Functioning and Oxygenation

Original chapter by Anne G. Perry, RN, EdD, FAAN
Canadian content written by Giuliana Harvey RN, MN

objectives

Mastery of content in this chapter will enable you to:

- Define the key terms listed.
- Describe the structure and function of the cardiopulmonary system.
- Identify the physiological processes of cardiac output, myocardial blood flow, and coronary artery circulation.
- Diagram the electrical conduction system of the heart.
- Describe the relationship among cardiac output, preload, afterload, contractility, and heart rate.
- Identify the physiological processes involved in ventilation, perfusion, and exchange of respiratory gases.
- Describe the neural and chemical regulation of respiration.
- Describe the impact of a client's level of health, and age, lifestyle, and environment on tissue oxygenation.
- Identify and describe clinical outcomes as a result of disturbances in conduction, altered cardiac output, impaired valvular function, myocardial ischemia, and impaired tissue perfusion.
- Identify and describe clinical outcomes of hyperventilation, hypoventilation, and hypoxemia.
- Identify nursing care interventions in the primary care, acute care, and restorative and continuing care settings that promote oxygenation.

key terms

Afterload, p. 881
Anemia, p. 884
Angina pectoris, p. 888
Asystole, p. 888
Atelectasis, p. 889
Atrial fibrillation, p. 885
Bronchoscopy, p. 893
Cardiac index (CI), p. 881
Cardiac output, p. 881
Cardiopulmonary rehabilitation, p. 927
Cardiopulmonary resuscitation (CPR), p. 927
Chest physiotherapy (CPT), p. 904
Chest tube, p. 920
Cor pulmonale, p. 883
Cyanosis, p. 889
Diaphragmatic breathing, p. 928
Diffusion, p. 883
Dyspnea, p. 892
Dysrhythmias, p. 885
Electrocardiogram (ECG), p. 881
Expiration, p. 883
Hematemesis, p. 893
Hemoptysis, p. 893
Hemothorax, p. 920
High-flow device, p. 924
Humidification, p. 904
Hyperventilation, p. 889
Hypoventilation, p. 889
Hypovolemia, p. 884
Hypoxia, p. 889
Incentive spirometry, p. 913
Inspiration, p. 883
Low-flow device, p. 924
Myocardial contractility, p. 881
Myocardial infarction (MI), p. 888
Myocardial ischemia, p. 888
Nasal cannula, p. 924
Nebulization, p. 904
Normal sinus rhythm (NSR), p. 881
Orthopnea, p. 893
Pneumothorax, p. 920
Postural drainage, p. 905
Preload, p. 881
Pulse oximeter, p. 898
Pursed-lip breathing, p. 928
Stroke volume, p. 881
Ventilation, p. 882
Ventricular fibrillation, p. 888
Ventricular tachycardia, p. 885
Wheezing, p. 893

media resources

evolve Web Site

- Animations
- Audio Chapter Summaries
- Glossary
- Multiple-Choice Review Questions
- Skills Performance Checklists
- Student Learning Activities
- Video Clips
- Weblinks

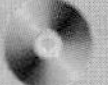
Companion CD

- Glossary
- Interactive Learning Activities
- Fluids and Electrolytes Tutorial
- Test-Taking Skills

Oxygen is required to sustain life. The cardiac and respiratory systems function to supply the body's oxygen demands. Blood is oxygenated through the mechanisms of ventilation, perfusion, and transport of respiratory gases. Neural and chemical regulators control the rate and depth of respiration in response to tissue's changing oxygen demands.

Scientific Knowledge Base

Cardiovascular Physiology

Cardiopulmonary physiology involves delivery of (a) deoxygenated blood (blood high in carbon dioxide and low in oxygen) to the right side of the heart and to the pulmonary circulation and (b) oxygenated blood from the lungs to the left side of the heart and the tissues. The cardiac system delivers oxygen, nutrients, and other substances to the tissues and removes the waste products of cellular metabolism through the cardiac pump, the circulatory vascular system, and the integration of other systems (e.g., respiratory, digestive, and renal) (McCance & Huether, 2005).

Structure and Function. The right ventricle pumps blood through the pulmonary circulation. The left ventricle pumps blood to the systemic circulation (Figure 39–1). The circulatory system exchanges respiratory gases, nutrients, and waste products between the blood and the tissues.

Myocardial Pump. The pumping action of the heart is essential to maintaining oxygen delivery. Coronary artery disease and cardiomyopathic (enlarged heart) conditions result in a diminished stroke volume (i.e., the volume of blood ejected from the ventricles) and decreased pump effectiveness. Hemorrhage and dehydration decrease pump effectiveness by decreasing the amount of blood ejected from the ventricles, thereby reducing circulating blood volume. The four chambers of the heart fill with blood during diastole and empty during systole.

The myocardial (cardiac muscle) fibres have contractile properties that enable them to stretch during filling. In a healthy heart, this stretch is proportionally related to the strength of contraction. As the myocardium stretches, the strength of the subsequent contraction increases; this is known as the Frank–Starling (Starling's) law of the heart. In the diseased heart, Starling's law does not apply because the stretch of the myocardium is beyond the heart's physiological limits. The subsequent contractile response results in insufficient ventricular ejection (volume), and blood begins to "back up" in the pulmonary (left heart failure) or systemic circulation (right heart failure).

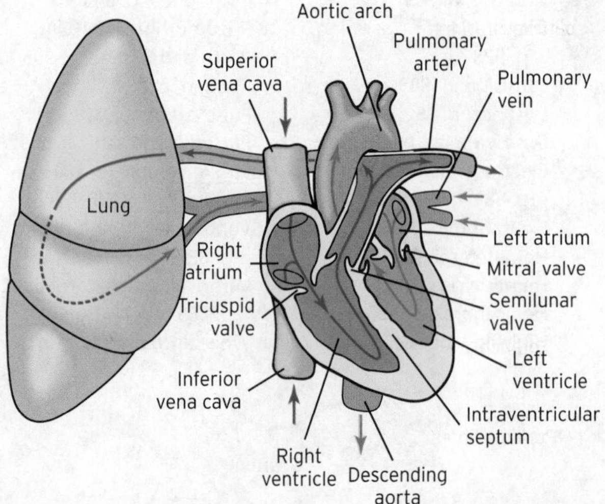

Figure 39-1 Schematic representation of blood flow through the heart. Arrows indicate direction of flow. **Source:** From Lewis, S. M., Heitkemper, M. M., & Kirksen, S. R. (2000). *Medical-surgical nursing: Assessment and management of clinical problems* (5th ed.). St. Louis: Elsevier Mosby.

Myocardial Blood Flow. To maintain adequate blood flow to the pulmonary and systemic circulation, myocardial blood flow must supply sufficient oxygen and nutrients to the myocardium itself. Blood flow through the heart is unidirectional. There are four heart valves that ensure this forward blood flow (see Figure 39–1). During ventricular diastole, the atrioventricular (mitral and tricuspid) valves open and blood flows from the higher-pressure atria into the relaxed ventricles. This represents S_1, or the first heart sound. After ventricular filling, the systolic phase begins.

During the systolic phase, semilunar (aortic and pulmonic) valves open and blood flows from the ventricles into the aorta and pulmonary artery. Closure of aortic and pulmonic valves represents S_2, or the second heart sound. Clients with valvular disease may have backflow or regurgitation of blood through the incompetent valve, causing a murmur that is heard on auscultation (see Chapter 32).

Coronary Artery Circulation. Blood in the atria and ventricles does not supply oxygen and nutrients to the myocardium itself. The coronary circulation is the branch of the systemic circulation that supplies the myocardium with oxygen and nutrients and removes waste. The coronary arteries fill during ventricular diastole (McCance & Huether, 2005). The right and left coronary arteries arise from the aorta just above and behind the aortic valve through openings called the coronary ostia (coronary openings). The left coronary artery, the most abundant blood supply, feeds the left ventricular myocardium, which is more muscular and does most of the heart's work (Box 39–1).

Systemic Circulation. The arteries and veins of the systemic circulation deliver nutrients and oxygen to and remove waste from the tissues. Oxygenated blood flows from the left ventricle by way of the aorta and into large systemic arteries. These arteries branch into

> **BOX 39-1 Coronary Arteries**
>
> **Right Coronary Artery**
>
> ***Right Atrium, Anterior Right Ventricle***
>
> **Supplies**
> - Posterior aspect of septum (90% of population)
> - Posterior papillary muscle
> - Sinus and atrioventricular nodes (80%–90% of population)
> - Inferior aspect of left ventricle
>
> **Left Coronary Arteries**
>
> ***Left Anterior Descending Artery***
>
> **Supplies**
> - Anterior left ventricular wall
> - Anterior interventricular septum (septal branches supply conduction system, bundle of His, and bundle branches)
> - Anterior papillary muscle
> - Left ventricular apex
> - Right ventricle
>
> **Circumflex Artery**
>
> **Supplies**
> - Left atrium
> - Posterior surfaces of left ventricle
> - Posterior aspects of septum

smaller arteries, into arterioles, and finally into the smallest vessels, the capillaries. At the capillary level, the exchange of respiratory gases, nutrients, and wastes occurs, and the tissues are oxygenated. The waste products exit the capillary network by way of the venules that join to form veins. These veins form larger veins, which carry deoxygenated blood to the right side of the heart, where it is returned to pulmonary circulation.

Blood Flow Regulation. The amount of blood ejected from the left ventricle each minute is the **cardiac output**. The normal cardiac output is 4 to 6 L/minute in the healthy 68-kg adult at rest. The circulating volume of blood changes according to the oxygen and metabolic needs of the body. For example, during exercise, pregnancy, and fever, the cardiac output increases, but during sleep it decreases. Cardiac output is represented by the following formula:

Cardiac output (CO) = Stroke volume (SV) × Heart rate (HR)

Cardiac output in the older adult may be affected by increased arterial wall tension and moderate myocardial hypertrophy due to an increased systolic blood pressure.

Cardiac index (CI) is the adequacy of the cardiac output for an individual. It takes into account the body surface area (BSA) of the client. The CI is determined by dividing the cardiac output by the BSA. The normal range is 2.5 to 4 L/minute/m^3. Both cardiac output and the CI are measured with invasive pulmonary artery catheters.

Stroke volume is the amount of blood ejected from the left ventricle with each contraction. It can be affected by the amount of blood in the left ventricle at the end of diastole (preload), the resistance to left ventricular ejection (afterload), and myocardial contractility.

Preload is essentially the end-diastolic volume. The ventricles stretch when filling with blood. The more stretch on the ventricular muscle, the greater the contraction and the greater the stroke volume (Starling's law). In clinical situations, the preload and subsequent stroke volume can be manipulated by changing the amount of circulating blood volume. For example, in the client with hemorrhagic shock, fluid therapy and replacement of blood increases volume, thus increasing the preload and cardiac output. If volume is not replaced, preload decreases, the cardiac output decreases, and, ultimately, the venous return to the right atrium decreases, further decreasing preload and cardiac output.

Afterload is the resistance to left ventricular ejection—the work that the heart must overcome to fully eject blood from the left ventricle. The diastolic aortic pressure is a good clinical measure of afterload. In a client with an acute hypertensive crisis, the afterload is greater than normal, increasing the cardiac workload. Afterload in this situation can be manipulated by decreasing systemic blood pressure.

The measurement and monitoring of these cardiopulmonary hemodynamics is usually performed in critical care units. Some step-down or special care units may also have the capability to measure and monitor hemodynamics.

Myocardial contractility also affects stroke volume and cardiac output. Poor contraction decreases the amount of blood ejected by the ventricles during each contraction. Drugs that can increase the force of myocardial contraction include digitalis preparations, epinephrine, and sympathomimetic drugs (drugs that mimic the effects of the sympathetic nervous system). Injury to the myocardial muscle, such as an acute myocardial infarction (AMI), can cause a decrease in myocardial contractility. The myocardium of the older adult is more rigid and slower in recovering its contractility (Meiner & Leuckenotte, 2006).

Heart rate affects blood flow because of the interaction between rate and diastolic filling time. With a sustained heart rate greater than 160 beats per minute, diastolic filling time decreases, decreasing stroke volume and cardiac output. The heart rate of the older adult is slow to increase under stress (Meiner & Leuckenotte, 2006).

Conduction System. The rhythmic relaxation and contraction of the atria and ventricles depend on continuous, organized transmission of electrical impulses. These impulses are generated and transmitted by way of the cardiac conduction system (Figure 39–2).

The heart's conduction system generates the necessary action potentials that conduct the impulses required to initiate the electrical chain of events resulting in the heartbeat. The autonomic nervous system influences the rate of impulse generation, the speed of transmission through the conductive pathway, and the strength of atrial and ventricular contractions. Sympathetic nerve fibres, which increase the rate of impulse generation and the speed of impulse transmission, innervate all parts of the atria and ventricles. The parasympathetic fibres originating from the vagus nerve decrease the rate and innervate all parts of the atria and ventricles, as well as the sinoatrial (SA) and atrioventricular (AV) nodes (McCance & Huether, 2005).

The conduction system originates with the SA node, the "pacemaker" of the heart. The SA node is in the right atrium next to the entrance of the superior vena cava. Impulses are initiated at the SA node at an intrinsic rate of 60 to 100 beats per minute. The resting adult rate is approximately 75 beats per minute.

The electrical impulses are then transmitted through the atria along intra-atrial pathways to the AV node. The AV node mediates impulses between the atria and the ventricles. The intrinsic rate of the normal AV node is 40 to 60 beats per minute. The AV node assists atrial emptying by delaying the impulse before transmitting it through the bundle of His and the ventricular Purkinje network. The intrinsic rate of the bundle of His and the ventricular Purkinje network is 20 to 40 beats per minute.

An **electrocardiogram (ECG)** reflects the electrical activity of the conduction system. An ECG monitors the regularity and path of the electrical impulse through the conduction system; however, it does not reflect muscular work of the heart. The normal sequence on the ECG is called **normal sinus rhythm** (NSR; Figure 39–3).

NSR implies that the impulse originates at the SA node and follows the normal sequence through the conduction system. The P wave represents the electrical conduction through both atria. Atrial contraction follows the P wave. The PR interval represents the impulse travel

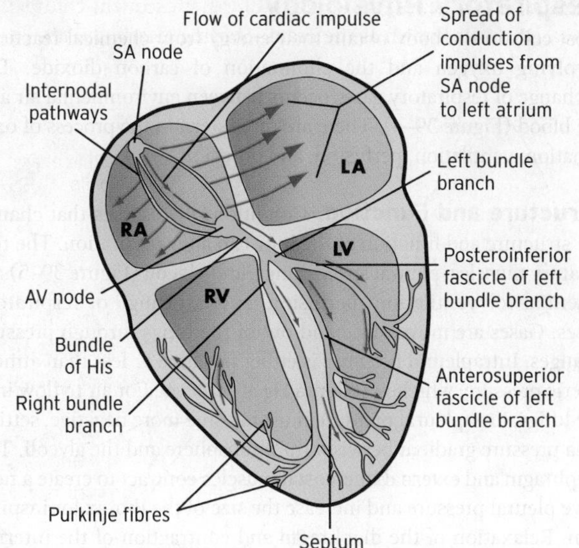

Figure 39–2 Conduction system of the heart. AV, atrioventricular; LA, left atrium; LV, left ventricle; RA, right atrium; RV, right ventricle; SA, sinoatrial. **Source:** From Lewis, S. M., Heitkamper, M. M., & Dirksen, S. R. (2000). *Medical-surgical nursing: assessment and management of clinical problems* (5th ed.). St. Louis: Mosby.

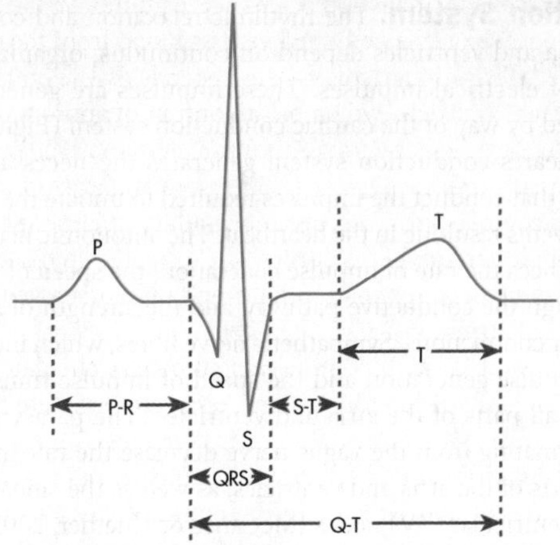

Figure 39-3 Normal ECG waveform.

time through the AV node, through the bundle of His, and to the Purkinje fibres. The normal length for the PR interval is 0.12 to 0.20 seconds. An increase in the time (i.e., >0.20 seconds) indicates that there is a block in the impulse transmission through the AV node; a decrease (i.e., <0.12 seconds) indicates the initiation of the electrical impulse from a source other than the SA node.

The QRS complex indicates that the electrical impulse has travelled through the ventricles. Normal QRS duration is 0.06 to 0.12 seconds. An increase in QRS duration indicates a delay in conduction time through the ventricles. Ventricular contraction usually follows the QRS complex.

The QT interval represents the time needed for ventricular depolarization and repolarization. The normal QT interval is 0.12 to 0.42 seconds. Changes in electrolyte values, such as in hypocalcemia or during therapy with drugs such as disopyramide, amiodarone, and theophylline (Theo-Dur), can increase the QT interval. Shortening of the QT interval occurs with digitalis therapy, hyperkalemia, and hypercalcemia.

Respiratory Physiology

Most cells in the body obtain their energy from chemical reactions involving oxygen and the elimination of carbon dioxide. The exchange of respiratory gases occurs between environmental air and the blood (Figure 39–4). There are three steps in the process of oxygenation: ventilation, perfusion, and diffusion.

Structure and Function. Conditions or diseases that change the structure and function of the lung can alter respiration. The respiratory muscles, pleural space, lungs, and alveoli (Figure 39–5) are essential for ventilation, perfusion, and exchange of respiratory gases. Gases are moved into and out of the lungs through pressure changes. Intrapleural pressure is either negative or less than atmospheric pressure, which is 760 mm Hg at sea level. For air to flow into the lungs, intrapleural pressure must become more negative, setting up a pressure gradient between the atmosphere and the alveoli. The diaphragm and external intercostal muscles contract to create a negative pleural pressure and increase the size of the thorax for inspiration. Relaxation of the diaphragm and contraction of the internal intercostal muscles allows air from the lung to escape. The coordination of the respiratory muscles is essential for effective respiration and gas exchange. The lung transfers oxygen from the atmosphere into the alveoli, where the oxygen is exchanged for carbon dioxide. The alveoli transfer oxygen and carbon dioxide to and from the blood through the alveolar membrane.

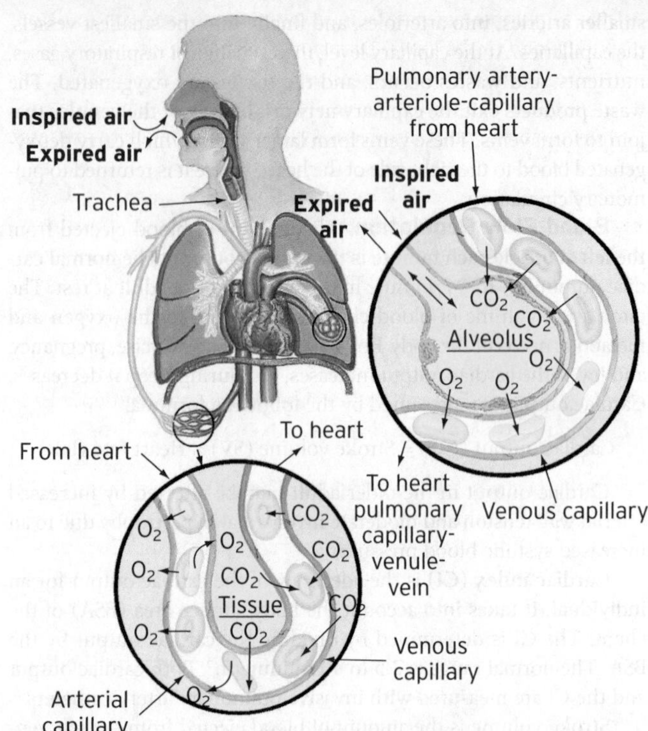

Figure 39-4 Structures of the pulmonary system. The circle denotes the alveoli. **Source:** From Thompson, J. M., McFarland, G. K., Hirsch, J. E., Tucker, S. M., & Bowers, A. C. (Eds.). (1993). *Mosby's clinical nursing* (3rd ed.). St. Louis, MO: Mosby-Year Book.

Ventilation is the process of moving gases into and out of the lungs. Ventilation requires coordination of the muscular and elastic properties of the lung and thorax, as well as intact innervation. The major inspiratory muscle of respiration is the diaphragm. It is innervated by the phrenic nerve, which exits the spinal cord at the fourth cervical vertebra. Perfusion relates to the ability of the cardiovascular

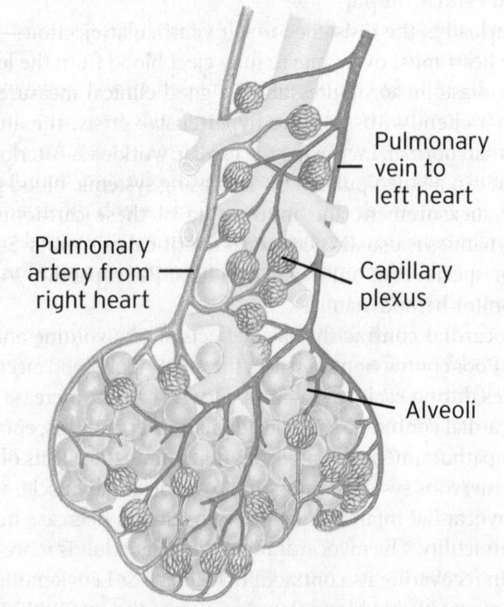

Figure 39-5 Alveoli at the terminal end of the lower airway. **Source:** From Thompson, J., M., McFarland, G. K., Hirsch, J. E., Tucker, S. M., & Bowers, A. C. (Eds.). (1993). *Mosby's clinical nursing* (3rd ed.).St. Louis, MO: Mosby-Year Book.

system to pump oxygenated blood to the tissues and return deoxygenated blood to the lungs. Diffusion is responsible for moving the molecules from one area to another. For the exchange of respiratory gases to occur, the organs, nerves, and muscles of respiration must be intact and the central nervous system able to regulate the respiratory cycle.

Work of Breathing. Breathing is the effort required for expanding and contracting the lungs. In the healthy individual, breathing is quiet and accomplished with minimal effort. The amount of energy expended on breathing depends on the rate and depth of breathing, the ease with which the lungs can be expanded (compliance), and airway resistance (Jevon & Ewens, 2001).

Inspiration is an active process, stimulated by chemical receptors in the aorta. **Expiration** is a passive process that depends on the elastic-recoil properties of the lungs, requiring little or no muscle work. Elastic recoil is produced by elastic fibres in lung tissue and by surface tension in the fluid film lining the alveoli. Surfactant is a chemical produced in the lungs that maintains the surface tension of the alveoli and keeps them from collapsing. Clients with advanced chronic obstructive pulmonary disease (COPD) lose the elastic recoil of the lungs and thorax. As a result, the client's work of breathing is increased. In addition, clients with certain pulmonary diseases can have decreased surfactant production and may, in turn, develop atelectasis.

Accessory muscles of respiration can increase lung volume during inspiration. Clients with COPD, especially emphysema, frequently use these muscles to increase lung volume. Prolonged use of the accessory muscles of respiration does not promote effective ventilation and causes fatigue. During assessment, observe elevation of the client's clavicles during inspiration.

Compliance is the ability of the lungs to distend or expand in response to increased intra-alveolar pressure. Compliance is decreased in diseases such as pulmonary edema, interstitial and pleural fibrosis, and congenital or traumatic structural abnormalities such as kyphosis or fractured ribs.

Airway resistance is the pressure difference between the mouth and the alveoli in relation to the rate of flow of inspired gas. Airway resistance can be increased by an airway obstruction, small airway disease (such as asthma), and tracheal edema. When resistance is increased, the amount of air travelling through the anatomical airways is decreased.

Decreased lung compliance, increased airway resistance, active expiration, or the use of accessory muscles increases the work of breathing, resulting in increased energy expenditure. To meet this expenditure, the body increases its metabolic rate, and the need for oxygen, as well as for the elimination of carbon dioxide, increases. This sequence is a vicious cycle for a client with impaired ventilation, causing further deterioration of respiratory status and the ability to oxygenate adequately.

Lung Volumes and Capacities. Spirometry is used to measure the volume of air entering or leaving the lungs. Variations in lung volumes may be associated with health states such as pregnancy, exercise, obesity, or obstructive and restrictive conditions of the lungs. The amount of surfactant, degree of compliance, and strength of respiratory muscles can affect pressures and volumes within the lungs.

Pulmonary Circulation. The primary function of the pulmonary circulation is to move blood to and from the alveolocapillary membrane in order for gas exchange to occur. The pulmonary circulation serves as a reservoir for blood so that the lung can increase its blood volume without large increases in pulmonary artery or venous pressures. The pulmonary circulation also acts as a filter, removing small thrombi before they can reach vital organs.

The pulmonary circulation begins at the pulmonary artery, which receives poorly oxygenated mixed venous blood from the right ventricle. Blood flow through this system depends on the pumping ability of the right ventricle, which has an output of approximately 4 to 6 L/minute. The flow continues from the pulmonary artery through the pulmonary arterioles to the pulmonary capillaries, where blood comes in contact with the alveolocapillary membrane and the exchange of respiratory gases occurs. The oxygen-rich blood then circulates through the pulmonary venules and pulmonary veins, returning to the left atrium.

Pressure and resistance within the pulmonary circulatory system is lower than that within the systemic circulatory system. The walls of the pulmonary vessels are thinner and contain less smooth muscle. The lung accepts the total cardiac output from the right ventricle and, except in cases of alveolar hypoxia or cor pulmonale, does not direct blood flow from one region to another. **Cor pulmonale** is a condition in which the right ventricle is enlarged, secondary to diseases of the lung, thorax, or pulmonary circulation.

Respiratory Gas Exchange. Respiratory gases are exchanged in the alveoli and the capillaries of the body tissues. Oxygen is transferred from the lungs to the blood, and carbon dioxide is transferred from the blood to the alveoli to be exhaled as a waste product. At the tissue level, oxygen is transferred from the blood to tissues, and carbon dioxide is transferred from tissues to the blood to return to the alveoli and be exhaled. This transfer is dependent on the process of diffusion.

Diffusion is the movement of molecules from an area of higher concentration to an area of lower concentration. Diffusion of respiratory gases occurs at the alveolocapillary membrane, and the rate of diffusion can be affected by the thickness of the membrane. Increased thickness of the membrane impedes diffusion because gases take longer to transfer across. Clients with pulmonary edema, pulmonary infiltrates, or a pulmonary effusion have an increased thickness of the alveolocapillary membrane, resulting in slowed diffusion, slowed exchange of respiratory gases, and impaired delivery of oxygen to tissues. The surface area of the membrane can be altered as a result of chronic disease (e.g., emphysema), acute disease (e.g., pneumothorax), or surgical process (e.g., lobectomy). The alveolocapillary membrane can be destroyed or may thicken, changing the rate of diffusion. When fewer alveoli are functioning, the surface area is decreased.

Oxygen Transport. The oxygen transport system consists of the lungs and cardiovascular system. Delivery depends on the amount of oxygen entering the lungs (ventilation), blood flow to the lungs and tissues (perfusion), rate of diffusion, and oxygen-carrying capacity. The capacity of the blood to carry oxygen is influenced by the amount of dissolved oxygen in the plasma, amount of hemoglobin, and tendency of hemoglobin to bind with oxygen. Only a relatively small amount of required oxygen, less than 1%, is dissolved in the plasma. Most oxygen is transported by hemoglobin, which serves as a carrier for oxygen and carbon dioxide. The hemoglobin molecule combines with oxygen to form oxyhemoglobin. The formation of oxyhemoglobin is easily reversible, allowing hemoglobin and oxygen to dissociate, which frees oxygen to enter tissues.

Carbon Dioxide Transport. Carbon dioxide diffuses into red blood cells and is rapidly hydrated into carbonic acid (H_2CO_3) because of the presence of carbonic anhydrase. The carbonic acid then dissociates into hydrogen (H^+) and bicarbonate (HCO_3^-) ions. The hydrogen ion is buffered by hemoglobin, and the HCO_3^- diffuses into the plasma (see Chapter 40). In addition, some of the carbon dioxide in red blood cells reacts with amino acid groups, forming carbamino compounds. This reaction can occur rapidly without the presence of an enzyme. Reduced hemoglobin (deoxyhemoglobin) can combine with carbon dioxide more easily than oxyhemoglobin, thus venous blood transports most of the carbon dioxide.

Regulation of Respiration. Regulation of respiration is necessary to ensure sufficient oxygen intake and carbon dioxide elimination to meet the body's demands (e.g., during exercise, infection, or pregnancy). Neural and chemical regulators control the process of respiration. Neural regulation includes the central nervous system control of respiratory rate, depth, and rhythm. Chemical regulation involves the influence of chemicals such as carbon dioxide and hydrogen ions on the rate and depth of respiration (Box 39–2).

Factors Affecting Oxygenation

Adequacy of circulation, ventilation, perfusion, and transport of respiratory gases to the tissues is influenced by four types of factors: (1) physiological, (2) developmental, (3) lifestyle, and (4) environmental. Developmental, lifestyle, and environmental factors will be presented in a later section.

Physiological Factors. Any condition that affects cardiopulmonary functioning directly affects the body's ability to meet oxygen demands. The general classifications of cardiac disorders include disturbances in conduction, impaired valvular function, myocardial hypoxia, cardiomyopathic conditions, and peripheral tissue hypoxia. Respiratory disorders include hyperventilation, hypoventilation, and hypoxia.

Other physiological processes affecting a client's oxygenation include alterations that affect the oxygen-carrying capacity of blood, such as anemia, increases in the body's metabolic demands (e.g., pregnancy, fever, infection), and alterations that affect chest wall movement or the central nervous system (Table 39–1).

Decreased Oxygen-Carrying Capacity. Hemoglobin carries most of the oxygen to tissues. Anemia and inhalation of toxic substances decrease the oxygen-carrying capacity of blood by reducing the amount of available hemoglobin to transport oxygen. **Anemia**, a hemoglobin level lower than normal, is a result of decreased hemoglobin production, increased red blood cell destruction, blood loss, or a combination of these factors. Clients will have complaints of fatigue, decreased activity tolerance, and increased breathlessness, as well as pallor (especially seen in the conjunctiva of the eye) and an increased heart rate.

➤ BOX 39-2 Physiological Processes of Oxygenation

Neural Regulation

Maintains rhythm and depth of respiration and balance between inspiration and expiration.

Cerebral Cortex

Voluntary control of respiration delivers impulses to the respiratory motor neurons by way of the spinal cord; accommodates speaking, eating, and swimming.

Medulla Oblongata

Automatic control of respiration occurs continuously.

Chemical Regulation

Maintains appropriate rate and depth of respirations according to changes in the blood's carbon dioxide (CO_2), oxygen (O_2), and hydrogen ion (H+) concentration.

Chemoreceptors

Located in the medulla, aortic body, and carotid body. Changes in chemical content of O_2, CO_2, and H+ stimulate chemoreceptors, which in turn stimulate neural regulators to adjust the rate and depth of ventilation to maintain normal arterial blood gas levels. Chemical regulation can occur during physical exercise and with some illnesses. It is a short-term adaptive mechanism.

➤ TABLE 39-1 Physiological Processes Affecting Oxygenation

Process	Effect on Oxygenation
Anemia	Decreases oxygen-carrying capacity of blood
Toxic inhalant	Decreases oxygen-carrying capacity of blood
Airway obstruction	Limits delivery of inspired oxygen to alveoli
High altitude	Atmospheric oxygen concentration is lower and inspiratory oxygen concentration decreases
Fever	Increases metabolic rate and tissue oxygen demand
Decreased chest wall motion (e.g., from musculoskeletal impairments)	Prevents lowering of diaphragm and reduces anteroposterior diameter of thorax on inspiration, reducing volume of air inspired

Carbon monoxide is the most common toxic inhalant that decreases the oxygen-carrying capacity of blood. The affinity for hemoglobin to bind with carbon monoxide is greater than 200 times its affinity to bind with oxygen, creating a functional anemia. Because of the bond's strength, carbon monoxide is not easily dissociated from hemoglobin, making the hemoglobin unavailable for oxygen transport.

Decreased Inspired Oxygen Concentration. When the concentration of inspired oxygen declines, the blood has less oxygen-carrying capacity. Decreases in the fraction of inspired oxygen concentration (FiO_2) can be caused by an upper or lower airway obstruction limiting delivery of inspired oxygen to alveoli; decreased environmental oxygen, such as at high altitudes; or decreased inspiration as a result of an incorrect oxygen concentration setting on respiratory therapy equipment.

Hypovolemia. Hypovolemia is caused by conditions such as shock and severe dehydration resulting from extracellular fluid loss and reduced circulating blood volume. With a significant fluid loss, the body tries to adapt by increasing the heart rate and peripheral vasoconstriction to increase the volume of blood returned to the heart and, in turn, increase the cardiac output.

Increased Metabolic Rate. Increased metabolic activity causes increased oxygen demand. When body systems are unable to meet this increased demand the level of oxygenation declines. An increased metabolic rate is a normal physiological response to pregnancy, wound healing, and exercise because the body is building tissue. Most people can meet the increased oxygen demand and do not display signs of oxygen deprivation. Fever increases the tissues' need for oxygen, and as a result, carbon dioxide production also increases.

If the febrile state persists, the metabolic rate remains high and the body begins to break down protein stores, resulting in muscle wasting and decreased muscle mass. Respiratory muscles such as the diaphragm and intercostal muscles are also wasted. The body attempts to adapt to the increased carbon dioxide levels by increasing the rate and depth of respiration. The client's work of breathing increases, and the client will eventually display signs and symptoms of hypoxemia. Clients with pulmonary diseases are at greater risk for hypoxemia and hypercapnia. Assessment findings include an increased rate and depth of respiration, use of the accessory muscles of respiration, pursed-lip breathing, and decreased activity tolerance.

Conditions Affecting Chest Wall Movement. Any condition that reduces chest wall movement can result in decreased ventilation. If the diaphragm cannot fully descend with breathing, the volume of inspired air decreases and less oxygen is delivered to the alveoli and subsequently to tissues.

Pregnancy. As the fetus grows during pregnancy, the greater size of the uterus pushes abdominal contents upward against the diaphragm. In the last trimester of pregnancy, the inspiratory capacity declines, resulting in dyspnea on exertion and increased fatigue.

Obesity. Morbidly obese clients have reduced lung volumes as a result of the heaviness of the lower thorax and abdomen, particularly when in the recumbent and supine positions. These clients have a reduction in compliance as a result of encroachment of the abdomen into the chest, increased work of breathing, and decreased lung volumes, and they may experience fatigue and have carbon dioxide retention. In some clients, an obesity–hypoventilation syndrome develops in which oxygenation is decreased and carbon dioxide is retained, resulting in daytime sleepiness. Morbidly obese clients may also develop obstructive sleep apnea, characterized by excessive daytime somnolence and loud snoring and apneic periods during sleep. The obese client is also susceptible to pneumonia after an upper respiratory tract infection because the lungs cannot fully expand and pulmonary secretions are not mobilized in the lower lobes.

Musculoskeletal Abnormalities. Musculoskeletal impairments in the thoracic region reduce oxygenation. Such impairments may result from abnormal structural configurations, trauma, muscular diseases, and diseases of the central nervous system. Abnormal structural configurations impairing oxygenation include those that affect the rib cage, such as pectus excavatum (an indentation of the lower sternum), and those that affect the vertebral column, such as kyphosis, lordorsis, or scoliosis.

Trauma. The person with multiple rib fractures can develop a flail chest, a condition in which fractures cause instability in part of the chest wall. The unstable chest wall allows the lung underlying the injured area to contract on inspiration and bulge on expiration, resulting in hypoxia. Chest wall or upper abdominal incisions may also decrease chest wall movement as the client uses shallow respirations to minimize chest wall movement to avoid pain. Excessive or high doses of narcotic analgesics may depress the respiratory centre, further decreasing respiratory rate and chest wall expansion.

Neuromuscular Diseases. Diseases such as muscular dystrophy affect oxygenation of tissues by decreasing the client's ability to expand and contract the chest wall. Ventilation is impaired, and atelectasis, hypercapnia, and hypoxemia can occur. Myasthenia gravis, Guillain-Barré syndrome, and poliomyelitis affect respiratory functioning and result in hypoventilation. Myasthenia gravis interferes with normal transmission of impulses from nerves to muscles, involving the whole body, including muscles of respiration. Guillain-Barré syndrome and poliomyelitis cause inflammation and paralysis of muscle groups. Guillain-Barré syndrome usually results in an ascending pattern of paralysis. Respiratory muscles become paralyzed as paralysis ascends to the thoracic region. Poliomyelitis may lead to general or local paralysis. Both disorders may reverse, but poliomyelitis usually results in more residual paralysis.

Central Nervous System Alterations. Diseases or trauma involving the medulla oblongata and spinal cord may result in impaired respiration. When the medulla oblongata is affected, neural regulation of respiration is damaged and abnormal breathing patterns may develop. If the phrenic nerve is damaged, the diaphragm may not descend, thus reducing inspiratory lung volumes and causing hypoxemia. Cervical trauma at C3 to C5 can result in paralysis of the phrenic nerve. Spinal cord trauma below the fifth cervical vertebra usually leaves the phrenic nerve intact but damages nerves that innervate the intercostal muscles, preventing anteroposterior chest expansion.

Influences of Chronic Disease. Oxygenation can be decreased as a direct consequence of chronic disease. It can also be decreased as a secondary effect, as with anemia. The physiological response to chronic hypoxemia is the development of a secondary polycythemia. This adaptive response is the body's attempt to increase the amount of circulating hemoglobin to increase the available oxygen-binding sites.

Alterations in Cardiac Functioning

Illnesses and conditions that affect cardiac rhythm, strength of contraction, blood flow through the chambers, myocardial blood flow, and peripheral circulation cause alterations in cardiac functioning. Older adults experience alterations in cardiac function due to calcification of the conduction pathways, thicker and stiffer heart valves from lipid accumulation and fibrosis, and a decrease in the number of pacemaker cells in the SA node (Meiner & Leuckenotte, 2006).

Disturbances in Conduction. Some disturbances in conduction are a result of electrical impulses that do not originate from the SA node. These rhythm disturbances are called **dysrhythmias**, meaning a deviation from the normal sinus heart rhythm (Table 39–2). Dysrhythmias may occur as a primary conduction disturbance; as a response to ischemia, valvular abnormality, anxiety, or drug toxicity; as a result of caffeine, alcohol, or tobacco use; or as a complication of acid–base or electrolyte imbalance (see Chapter 40). Such disturbances may be alleviated by the use of automated external defibrillators (Box 39–3).

Dysrhythmias are classified by cardiac response and site of impulse origin. Cardiac response can be tachycardiac (>100 beats/minute), bradycardiac (<60 beats/minute), a premature (early) beat, or a blocked (delayed or absent) beat. Tachydysrhythmias and bradydysrhythmias can lower cardiac output and blood pressure. Tachydysrhythmias reduce cardiac output by decreasing diastolic filling time. Bradydysrhythmias lower cardiac output because of the decreased heart rate.

Atrial fibrillation is a common type of dysrhythmia in older adults. The electrical impulse in the atria is chaotic and originates from multiple sites. The rhythm is irregular because of the multiple pacemaker sites and the unpredictable conduction to the ventricles. The QRS complex is normal; however, it occurs at irregular intervals. Atrial fibrillation is often described as an irregularly irregular rhythm.

Abnormal impulses originating above the ventricles are referred to as supraventricular dysrhythmias. The abnormality on the waveform is the configuration and placement of the P wave. Ventricular conduction usually remains normal, and a normal QRS complex is observed.

Ventricular dysrhythmias represent an ectopic site of impulse formation within the ventricles. It is ectopic in that the impulse originates in the ventricle, not the SA node. The configuration of the QRS complex is usually widened and bizarre. P waves may or may not be present; often they are buried in the QRS complex. **Ventricular tachycardia**

TABLE 39-2 Common Basic Cardiac Dysrhythmias

Rhythm Characteristics and Etiology	Clinical Significance and Management
Sinus Tachycardia	
Regular rhythm, rate 100–180 beats/minute (higher in infants), normal P wave, normal QRS complex. Rate increase may be a normal response to exercise, emotion, or stressors such as pain, fever, pump failure, hyperthyroidism, and certain drugs (e.g., caffeine, nitrates, epinephrine, nicotine). 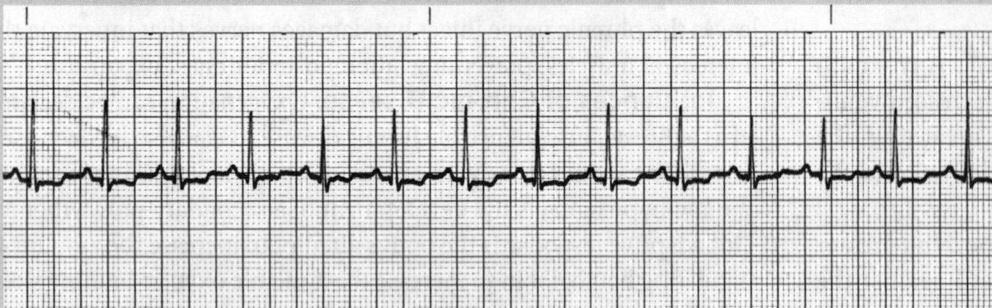	Client with damaged heart may not be able to sustain increased myocardial oxygen consumption by increased heart rate. Correct underlying factors; discontinue drugs producing the side effect.
Sinus Bradycardia	
Regular rhythm, rate <60 beats/minute, normal P wave, normal PR interval, normal QRS complex. Rate decrease may be a normal response to sleep or in well-conditioned athlete; abnormal drops in rate may be caused by diminished blood flow to SA node, vagal stimulation, hypothyroidism, increased intracranial pressure, or pharmacological agents (e.g., digoxin, propranolol, quinidine, procainamide). 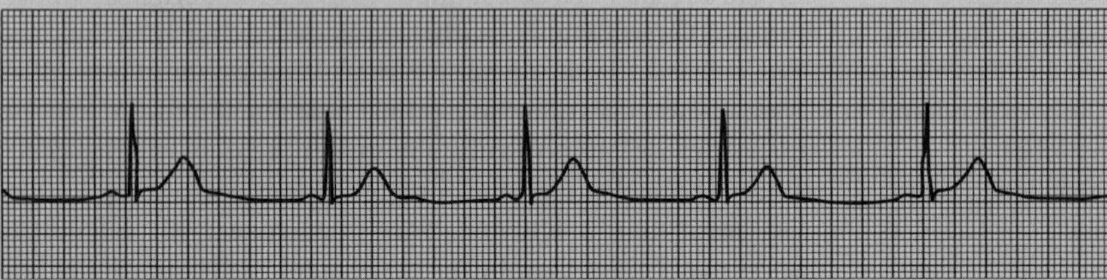	No clinical significance unless associated with signs and symptoms of reduced cardiac output such as dizziness or syncope or presence of chest pain. Bradycardia with hypotension and decreased cardiac output is treated with atropine; a pacemaker may be required.
Atrial Fibrillation (A-fib)	
Chaotic, irregular atrial activity resulting in an irregular ventricular response. No identifiable P waves. Irregular ventricular response resulting in an irregular cardiac rate and rhythm. The rate is determined by the conduction of the multiple atrial impulses across the AV node. A-fib is caused by aging, calcification of the SA node, or changes in myocardial blood supply. 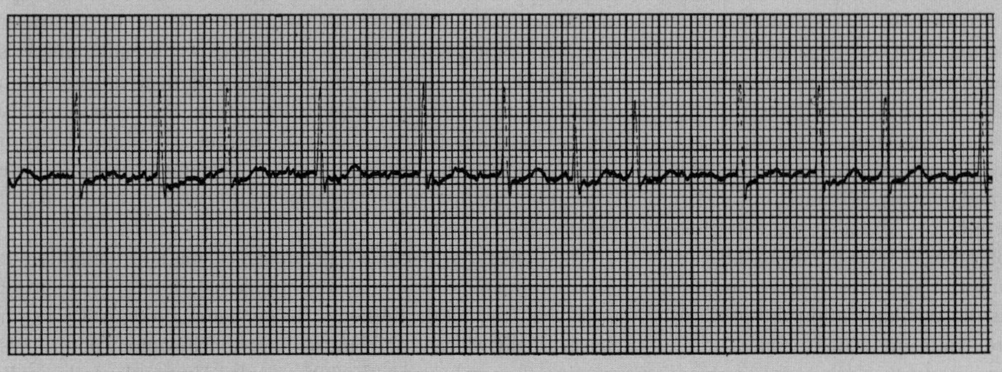	There is a loss of the atrial kick (portion of the cardiac output squeezed in the ventricles with a coordinated atrial contraction), pooling of blood in the atria, and development of microemboli. The client may complain of fatigue, a fluttering in the chest, or shortness of breath if the ventricular response is rapid. A-fib is a commonly occurring dysrhythmia in the aging and older adult. Anticoagulants such as warfarin (Coumadin) may be used to reduce the risk of stroke. Warfarin is prescribed on the basis of the International Normalized Ratio (INR) and thus dose adjustments are based on daily INR results.

➤ TABLE 39-2 Common Basic Cardiac Dysrhythmias *continued*

Rhythm Characteristics and Etiology	Clinical Significance and Management
Ventricular Tachycardia	
Rhythm slightly irregular, rate 100–200 beats/minute, P wave absent, PR interval absent, QRS complex wide and bizarre, >0.12 seconds. Caused by changes in the normal pacemaker of the heart, such as decrease in blood flow, ischemia, or embolus.	Results in a decreased cardiac output due to decreased ventricular filling time; may lead to severe hypotension and loss of pulse and consciousness. If refractory to defibrillation, amiodarone 300 mg IV followed by an additional 150 mg IV in 3–5 minutes (American Heart Association [AHA], 2005).
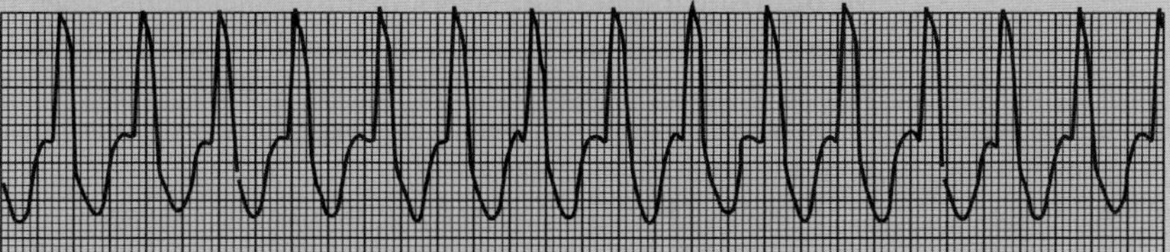	
Ventricular Fibrillation	
Uncoordinated electrical activity. No identifiable P, QRS, or T wave. Causes include sudden cardiac death, electrical shock, acute myocardial infarction, drowning, or trauma.	Acute loss of pulse and respiration. Immediate defibrillation after assessment of airway, breathing, and circulation (ABCs) of cardiopulmonary resuscitation (CPR). Availability of automated external defibrillator is recommended in public and private places where large numbers of people gather or where there are people who are at high risk for heart attack (AHA, 2005, 2006; see Box 39–3).
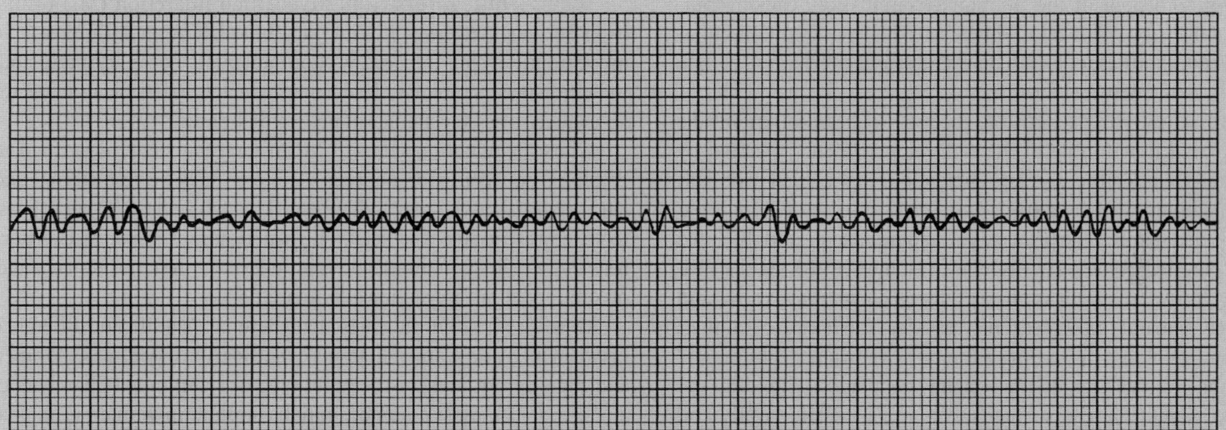	
Asystole	
Classically referred to as a "flat line." There are no electrical impulses and therefore no QRS complex, no contraction, and no cardiac output. Possible causes include hypoxia, hyperkalemia and hypokalemia, pre-existing acidosis, drug overdose, and hypothermia.	The unresponsive client will have no pulse, blood pressure, or respirations. The management of asystole consists of CPR, administering epinephrine and atropine, and correction of the underlying cause.
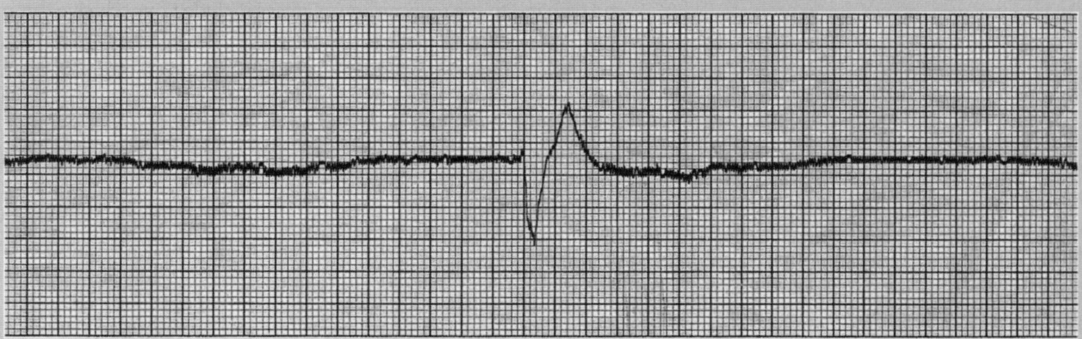	

Table adapted from Canobbio, M. M. (1990). *Cardiovascular disorders.* St. Louis, MO: Mosby. Diagrams "sinus tachycardia" and "asystole" from Ignatavicius, D. D., & Workman, M. L. (2006). *Medical-surgical nursing: Critical thinking for collaborative care* (5th ed.) (pp. 718 and 731). Philadelphia: W. B. Saunders.

and **ventricular fibrillation** are life-threatening rhythms that require immediate intervention. Ventricular tachycardia is considered a life-threatening dysrhythmia because of the decreased cardiac output and the potential to deteriorate into ventricular fibrillation (Black & Hawks, 2005).

Asystole is a lethal rhythm associated with no apparent electrical activity. The client has no cardiac output and thus no palpable pulse. If the client is on a cardiac monitor, the lack of electrical activity is noted by an absent rhythm. Asystole can occur as a primary event, it may follow ventricular fibrillation, or can occur in clients with complete heart block (Black & Hawks, 2005). Asystole must be treated immediately.

Altered Cardiac Output. Failure of the myocardium to eject sufficient volume to the systemic and pulmonary circulations can result in heart failure. Primary coronary artery disease, cardiomyopathic conditions, valvular disorders, and pulmonary disease lead to myocardial pump failure.

Left-Sided Heart Failure. Left-sided heart failure is an abnormal condition characterized by impaired functioning of the left ventricle as a result of elevated pressures and pulmonary congestion. If left ventricular failure is significant, the amount of blood ejected from the left ventricle drops greatly, resulting in decreased cardiac output. Assessment findings may include decreased activity tolerance, breathlessness, dizziness, and confusion as a result of tissue hypoxia from the diminished cardiac output. As the left ventricle continues to fail, blood begins to pool in the pulmonary circulation, causing pulmonary congestion. Clinical findings include crackles on auscultation, hypoxia, shortness of breath on exertion and often at rest, cough, and paroxysmal nocturnal dyspnea.

Right-Sided Heart Failure. Right-sided heart failure results from impaired functioning of the right ventricle characterized by venous congestion in the systemic circulation. Right-sided heart failure more commonly results from pulmonary disease or from long-term left-sided failure. The primary pathological factor in right-sided failure is elevated pulmonary vascular resistance (PVR). As the PVR continues to rise, the right ventricle must generate more work, and the oxygen demand of the heart increases. As the failure continues, the amount of blood ejected from the right ventricle declines, and blood begins to "back up" in the systemic circulation. Clinically, the client has weight gain, distended neck veins, hepatomegaly and splenomegaly, and dependent peripheral edema.

Impaired Valvular Function. Valvular heart disease is an acquired or congenital disorder of a cardiac valve characterized by stenosis and obstructed blood flow or valvular degeneration and regurgitation of blood. When stenosis occurs in the semilunar valves (aortic and pulmonic valves), the adjacent ventricles must work harder to move the ventricular volume beyond the stenotic valve. Over time, the stenosis can cause the ventricle to hypertrophy (enlarge), and if the condition is left untreated, left- or right-sided heart failure can occur. If stenosis occurs in the atrioventricular valves (mitral and tricuspid valves), the atrial pressure rises, causing the atria to hypertrophy. When regurgitation occurs, there is a backflow of blood into an adjacent chamber. For example, in mitral regurgitation, the mitral leaflets do not close completely. When the ventricles contract, blood escapes back into the atria, causing a murmur, or "whooshing" sound (see Chapter 32).

> **BOX 39-3 Automated External Defibrillator (AED)**
>
> - An automated external defibrillator is a device used to administer an electrical shock through the chest wall to the heart.
> - Built-in computers assess the victim's heart rhythm and determine if defibrillation is needed.
> - The AED delivers a shock to the victim.
> - It can be used by nonmedical personnel.
> - It is used to strengthen the chain of survival. Every minute of a sudden cardiac arrest without defibrillation decreases the survival rate by 7%–10% (AHA, 2003, 2005).

Myocardial Ischemia. **Myocardial ischemia** results when the supply of blood to the myocardium from the coronary arteries is insufficient to meet the oxygen demands of the organ. Common manifestations of this ischemia include angina pectoris, myocardial infarction, and acute coronary syndrome.

Angina Pectoris. **Angina pectoris** is usually a transient imbalance between myocardial oxygen supply and demand. The condition results in chest pain that is aching, sharp, tingling, or burning, or that feels like pressure. The chest pain may be left sided or substernal and may radiate to the left or both arms, and to the jaw, neck, and back. In some clients, anginal pain may not radiate. The pain can last from 1 to 15 minutes. Clients report that pain is often precipitated by activities that increase myocardial oxygen demand (e.g., exercise, anxiety, or stress). The pain is usually relieved with rest and coronary vasodilators, the most common being a nitroglycerine preparation.

Myocardial Infarction. **Myocardial infarction (MI)** results from sudden decreases in coronary blood flow or an increase in myocardial oxygen demand without adequate coronary perfusion. Infarction occurs because of ischemia (which is reversible) and necrosis (which is not reversible) of myocardial tissue.

Chest pain associated with MI in men is usually described as crushing, squeezing, or stabbing. The pain may be retrosternal and left precordial, and it may radiate down the left arm to the neck, jaws, teeth, epigastric area, and back. The pain occurs at rest or on exertion, lasts more than 30 minutes, and is unrelieved by rest, position change, or sublingual nitroglycerine administration.

Current research indicates that there is a significant difference between men and women in terms of coronary artery disease. Women and men do not present the same type of symptoms (Chambers et al., 2007). The most common initial symptom in women is angina. However, women may also present with atypical symptoms such as fatigue, "indigestion," vasospasm, shortness of breath, or back or jaw pain (Denke, 2001; Shaw et al., 2006). Compared to men, women tend to have fewer Q waves and ST-segment changes with chest pain.

Acute Coronary Syndrome. Acute coronary syndrome (ACS) includes unstable angina, non-ST-segment elevation MI, and ST-segment elevation MI. There is an imbalance in the oxygen supply and demand to the myocardium. Causes include nonocclusive thrombus on pre-existing plaque, coronary vasospasm, arterial narrowing from atherosclerosis, inflammation or infection, and secondary unstable angina from anemia, fever, or hypoxemia (Granger & Miller, 2001). Symptoms may not be constant and may present atypically. Clients with classic AMI symptoms are more easily identified. Intermediate risk factors for ACS include male gender, age greater than 70 years with diabetes mellitus, extracardiac vascular disease, fixed Q waves, and previous abnormal ST segment and T-wave changes (Granger & Miller, 2001).

Alterations in Respiratory Functioning

Illnesses and conditions that affect ventilation or oxygen transport cause alterations in respiratory functioning. The three primary alterations are hyperventilation, hypoventilation, and hypoxia.

The goal of ventilation is to produce a normal arterial carbon dioxide tension ($PaCO_2$) between 35 and 45 mm Hg and maintain a normal arterial oxygen tension (PaO_2) between 80 and 100 mm Hg. Hyperventilation and hypoventilation refer to alveolar ventilation and not to the client's respiratory rate. Arterial oxygen levels can be monitored using a noninvasive oxygen saturation monitor. The normal range is 95% to 100%. Hypoxia refers to a decrease in the amount of arterial oxygen.

Hyperventilation. **Hyperventilation** is a state of ventilation in excess of that required to eliminate the normal venous carbon dioxide produced by cellular metabolism. Anxiety, infections, drugs, or an acid–base imbalance can induce hyperventilation, as well as hypoxia associated with pulmonary embolus or shock. Acute anxiety can lead to hyperventilation and may cause loss of consciousness from excess carbon dioxide exhalation. Fever can cause hyperventilation. As a client's body temperature increases, there is an increase in the metabolic rate, thereby increasing carbon dioxide production. The clinical response is an increased rate and depth of respiration.

Hyperventilation may also be chemically induced. Salicylate (aspirin) poisoning causes excessive stimulation of the respiratory centre as the body attempts to compensate for excess carbon dioxide. Amphetamines also increase ventilation by raising carbon dioxide production. Hyperventilation can also occur as the body tries to compensate for metabolic acidosis by producing a respiratory alkalosis. For example, the diabetic client who has gone into diabetic ketoacidosis is producing large amounts of metabolic acids. The respiratory system tries to correct the acid–base balance by over-breathing. Ventilation increases to reduce the amount of carbon dioxide available to form carbonic acid (see Chapter 40). Hemoglobin does not release oxygen to tissues as readily, and tissue hypoxia results. As symptoms worsen, the client may become more agitated, which further increases the respiratory rate and can result in respiratory alkalosis.

Hypoventilation. **Hypoventilation** occurs when alveolar ventilation is inadequate to meet the body's oxygen demand or to eliminate sufficient carbon dioxide. As alveolar ventilation decreases, $PaCO_2$ is elevated. Severe atelectasis can produce hypoventilation. **Atelectasis** is a collapse of the alveoli that prevents normal respiratory exchange of oxygen and carbon dioxide. As alveoli collapse, less of the lung can be ventilated and hypoventilation occurs.

In clients with COPD, the inappropriate administration of excessive oxygen can result in hypoventilation. These clients have adapted to a high carbon dioxide level, and their carbon dioxide–sensitive chemoreceptors are essentially not functioning. Their stimulus to breathe is a decreased PaO_2. If excessive oxygen is administered, the oxygen requirement is satisfied and the stimulus to breathe is negated. High concentrations of oxygen (e.g., >24%–28% [1–3 L/minute]) prevent the PaO_2 from falling and obliterate the stimulus to breathe, resulting in hypoventilation. The excessive retention of carbon dioxide may lead to respiratory arrest.

Signs and symptoms of hypoventilation include mental status changes, dysrhythmias, and potential cardiac arrest. Treatment requires improving tissue oxygenation, restoring ventilatory function, treating the underlying cause of the hypoventilation, and achieving acid–base balance. If untreated, the client's status can rapidly decline, leading to convulsions, unconsciousness, and death.

Hypoxia. **Hypoxia** is inadequate tissue oxygenation at the cellular level. This can result from a deficiency in oxygen delivery or oxygen utilization at the cellular level. Hypoxia can be caused by (a) a decreased hemoglobin level and lowered oxygen-carrying capacity of the blood; (b) a diminished concentration of inspired oxygen, which may occur at high altitudes; (c) the inability of the tissues to extract oxygen from the blood, as with cyanide poisoning; (d) decreased diffusion of oxygen from the alveoli to the blood, as in pneumonia; (e) poor tissue perfusion with oxygenated blood, as with shock; and (f) impaired ventilation, as with multiple rib fractures or chest trauma.

The clinical signs and symptoms of hypoxia include apprehension, restlessness, inability to concentrate, declining level of consciousness, dizziness, and behavioural changes. The client with hypoxia is unable to lie down and appears fatigued and agitated. Vital-sign changes include an increased pulse rate and increased rate and depth of respiration. The client with a narcotic overdose, such as a heroin overdose, may display signs of hypoventilation. During early stages of hypoxia, the blood pressure is elevated unless the condition is caused by shock. As the hypoxia worsens, the respiratory rate may decline as a result of respiratory muscle fatigue.

Cyanosis, or blue discoloration of the skin and mucous membranes caused by the presence of desaturated hemoglobin in capillaries, is a late sign of hypoxia. The presence or absence of cyanosis is not a reliable measure of oxygenation status. Central cyanosis, observed in the tongue, soft palate, and conjunctiva of the eye, where blood flow is high, indicates hypoxemia. Peripheral cyanosis, seen in the extremities, nail beds, and earlobes, is often a result of vasoconstriction and stagnant blood flow. Hypoxia is a life-threatening condition. Untreated, it can produce cardiac dysrhythmias that result in death. Hypoxia is managed by administration of oxygen and treatment of the underlying cause, such as airway obstruction.

Nursing Knowledge Base

Developmental Factors

The developmental stage of the client and the normal aging process can affect tissue oxygenation.

Infants and Toddlers. Infants and toddlers are at risk for upper respiratory tract infections as a result of frequent exposure to other children and exposure to second-hand smoke. In addition, during the teething process, some infants develop nasal congestion, which encourages bacterial growth and increases the potential for respiratory tract infection. Upper respiratory tract infections are usually not dangerous, and infants or toddlers recover with little difficulty.

School-Age Children and Adolescents. School-age children and adolescents are exposed to respiratory infections and respiratory risk factors such as second-hand smoke and cigarette smoking. A healthy child usually does not have adverse pulmonary effects from respiratory infections. A person who starts smoking in adolescence and continues to smoke into middle age, however, has an increased risk for cardiopulmonary disease and lung cancer.

Young and Middle-Aged Adults. Young and middle-aged adults are exposed to multiple cardiopulmonary risk factors: an unhealthy diet, lack of exercise, stress, over-the-counter and prescription drugs not used as intended, illegal drugs, and smoking. By reducing these modifiable factors clients may decrease their risk for cardiac or pulmonary diseases. During youth and middle age, lifelong habits and lifestyles are established. It is thus important to help these clients make good choices and informed decisions about the rest of their lives and their health care practices.

Older Adults. The cardiac and respiratory systems undergo changes throughout the aging process (Box 39–4). The changes are associated with calcification of the heart valves, SA node, and costal cartilages. The arterial system develops atherosclerotic plaques. Osteoporosis leads to changes in the size and shape of the thorax.

The trachea and large bronchi become enlarged from calcification of the airways. The alveoli enlarge, decreasing the surface area available for gas exchange. The number of functional cilia is reduced, causing a decrease in the effectiveness of the cough mechanism, putting the older adult at increased risk for respiratory infections (Meiner & Leuckenotte, 2006). Ventilation and transfer of respiratory gases decline with age because the lungs are unable to expand fully, leading to lower oxygenation levels.

Lifestyle Risk Factors

Lifestyle modifications that influence cardiopulmonary functioning are frequently difficult because a client is being asked to change a habit or behaviour that may be enjoyed, such as cigarette smoking or eating certain foods; however, these changes can be achieved with encouragement, support, and time (Box 39–5). Risk factor modification is important, including smoking cessation, weight reduction, a low-cholesterol and low-sodium diet, management of hypertension, and moderate exercise. Although it may be difficult to get older adults to change long-term behaviour, developing healthy behaviours can slow or halt the progression of their cardiopulmonary disease (Meiner & Leuckenotte, 2006).

Poor Nutrition. Nutrition affects cardiopulmonary function in several ways. Severe obesity decreases lung expansion, and the increased body weight increases oxygen demands to meet metabolic needs. The malnourished client may experience respiratory muscle wasting, resulting in decreased muscle strength and respiratory excursion. Cough efficiency is reduced secondary to respiratory muscle weakness, putting the client at risk for retention of pulmonary secretions. Diets high in fat increase cholesterol and atherogenesis in the coronary arteries.

Clients who are morbidly obese, malnourished, or both are at risk for anemia. Diets high in carbohydrates may play a role in increasing the carbon dioxide load for clients with carbon dioxide retention. As carbohydrates are metabolized, an increased load of carbon dioxide is created and excreted via the lungs.

Dietary restriction of sodium has been shown to be beneficial in reducing antihypertensive medication requirements and may cause left ventricular hypertrophy to regress (Joint National Committee [JNC], 2003). Diets high in potassium may prevent hypertension and help improve control in clients with hypertension. A 2000-calorie diet high in fibre, potassium, calcium, and magnesium, with an emphasis on fruits, vegetables, and low-fat dairy foods and low in saturated and total fat, is recommended to help prevent and reduce the effects of hypertension (JNC, 2003).

Inadequate Exercise. Exercise increases the body's metabolic activity and oxygen demand. The rate and depth of respiration increase, enabling the person to inhale more oxygen and exhale excess carbon dioxide. A physical exercise program has many benefits (see Chapter 36). People who exercise for 1 hour daily have a lower pulse rate and blood pressure, decreased cholesterol level, increased blood flow, and greater oxygen extraction by working muscles. Fully conditioned people can increase oxygen consumption by 10% to 20% because of increased cardiac output and increased efficiency of the myocardial muscle (JNC, 2003).

Smoking. Cigarette smoking is associated with a number of diseases, including heart disease, chronic obstructive lung disease, and lung cancer. Cigarette smoking can worsen peripheral vascular and coronary artery diseases (JNC, 2003). Inhaled nicotine causes vasoconstriction of peripheral and coronary blood vessels, increasing blood pressure and decreasing blood flow to peripheral vessels. Women who take birth control pills and smoke cigarettes are at increased risk for cardiovascular problems such as thrombophlebitis and pulmonary emboli.

BOX 39-4 FOCUS ON OLDER ADULTS

- The tuberculin skin test is an unreliable indicator of tuberculosis in older clients. They frequently display false-positive or false-negative skin test reactions.
  - Older clients are at an increased risk for reactivation of dormant organisms that have been present for decades, as a result of age-related changes in the immune system.
  - The standard 5-TU Mantoux test is given and repeated or repeated with the 250-TU strength to create a booster effect.
  - If the older client has a positive reaction, a complete history is necessary to determine any risk factors.
- Older adults have more atypical signs and symptoms of coronary artery disease (Meiner & Leuckenotte, 2006).
- The incidence of atrial fibrillation increases with age and is the leading contributing factor for stroke in the older adult (Meiner & Leuckenotte, 2006).
- Mental status changes are often the first signs of respiratory problems and may include forgetfulness and irritability.
- Older adults may not complain of dyspnea until it affects the activities of daily living that are important to them.
- Changes in the older adult's cough mechanism may lead to retention of pulmonary secretions, airway plugging, and atelectasis, if cough suppressants are not used with caution.

BOX 39-5 FOCUS ON PRIMARY HEALTH CARE

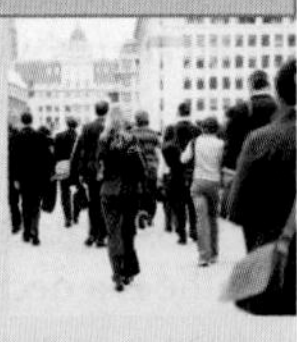

Positive Lifestyle Practices for Cardiopulmonary Health Promotion

As part of a primary health care focus, it is important to educate young to older adults about the following lifestyle practices that promote cardiopulmonary health:

- Maintain ideal body weight.
- Eat a low-fat, low-salt, calorie-appropriate diet.
- Engage in regular aerobic exercise 1 hour daily.

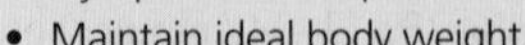

- Use a filter mask when exposed to occupational hazards.
- Use stress-reduction techniques.
- Reduce exposure to secondary infections.
- Do not smoke.
- Avoid second-hand smoke and other pollutants.
- Have annual visits with a health care professional.
- Monitor blood pressure.
- Monitor cholesterol and triglyceride levels.
- Request an annual influenza vaccine, especially if at risk for the development of influenza.
- Request a pneumococcal vaccine, if appropriate.

Cigarette smoking is the major cause of lung cancer, accounting for 85% of all new cases of lung cancer in Canada (Health Canada, 2008). Regular exposure to second-hand smoke increases the chances of contracting lung disease by 25% and heart disease by 10% (Health Canada, 2007). Lung cancer is the leading cause of death for both men and women (National Cancer Institute of Canada, 2008). It is estimated that 1 in 12 men and 1 in 16 women will develop lung cancer in their lifetime (Canadian Cancer Society, 2007). The 5-year survival rate (2001–2003) for all clients with lung cancer is only 15%, regardless of the diagnosis (National Cancer Institute of Canada, 2008). If lung cancer is detected when the disease is still localized, the survival rate is 49%. However, lung cancer is often diagnosed only when it has reached an advanced stage.

Substance Abuse. Excessive use of alcohol and other drugs can impair tissue oxygenation in two ways. First, the person who chronically abuses substances often has a poor nutritional intake. With the resultant decrease in intake of iron-rich foods, hemoglobin production declines. Second, excessive use of alcohol and certain other drugs can depress the respiratory centre, reducing the rate and depth of respiration and the amount of inhaled oxygen. Substance abuse by either smoking or inhaling, such as crack cocaine or inhaling fumes from paint or glue cans, causes direct injury to lung tissue that can lead to permanent lung damage and impaired oxygenation.

Stress. A continuous state of stress or severe anxiety increases the body's metabolic rate and the oxygen demand. The body responds to anxiety and other stresses with an increased rate and depth of respiration. Most people can adapt, but some, particularly those with chronic illnesses or acute life-threatening illnesses such as a myocardial infarction, cannot tolerate the oxygen demands associated with anxiety (see Chapter 30).

Environmental Factors

The environment can also influence oxygenation. The incidence of pulmonary disease is higher in smoggy, urban areas than in rural areas. In addition, the client's workplace may increase the risk for pulmonary disease. Occupational pollutants include asbestos, talcum powder, dust, and airborne fibres. Asbestosis is an occupational lung disease that develops after exposure to asbestos. The lung in asbestosis is characterized by diffuse interstitial fibrosis, creating a restrictive lung disease. It can also cause pleural mesotheliomas and pleural plaques. Clients at risk for developing asbestosis include those working with textiles, fireproofing, or milling, or in the production of paints, plastics, or some prefabricated construction. Clients exposed to asbestos who also smoke are at increased risk of developing lung cancer.

Critical Thinking

Successful critical thinking requires a synthesis of knowledge, experience, information gathered from clients, critical thinking qualities, and intellectual and professional standards. Clinical judgments require you to anticipate the information necessary, analyze the data, and make decisions regarding the client's care. During the assessment, consider all elements that build toward making an appropriate nursing diagnosis (Figure 39–6).

To understand the oxygen demands of a client and the ability of the client's body to meet those demands, you need to integrate knowledge from nursing and other disciplines, previous experiences, and information gathered from clients. The use of professional standards, such as those developed by the Heart and Stroke Foundation of Canada, the Canadian Lung Association, the Canadian Thoracic Society, and the Canadian Infectious Diseases Society, provide valuable guidelines for care and management of clients with altered oxygenation.

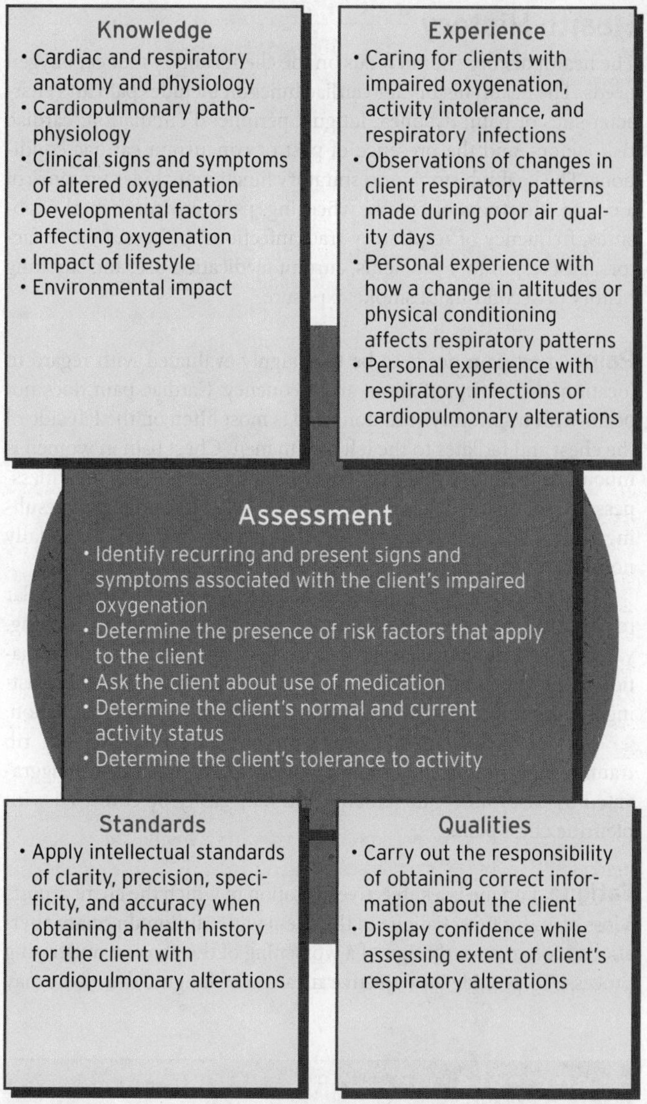

Knowledge
- Cardiac and respiratory anatomy and physiology
- Cardiopulmonary pathophysiology
- Clinical signs and symptoms of altered oxygenation
- Developmental factors affecting oxygenation
- Impact of lifestyle
- Environmental impact

Experience
- Caring for clients with impaired oxygenation, activity intolerance, and respiratory infections
- Observations of changes in client respiratory patterns made during poor air quality days
- Personal experience with how a change in altitudes or physical conditioning affects respiratory patterns
- Personal experience with respiratory infections or cardiopulmonary alterations

Assessment
- Identify recurring and present signs and symptoms associated with the client's impaired oxygenation
- Determine the presence of risk factors that apply to the client
- Ask the client about use of medication
- Determine the client's normal and current activity status
- Determine the client's tolerance to activity

Standards
- Apply intellectual standards of clarity, precision, specificity, and accuracy when obtaining a health history for the client with cardiopulmonary alterations

Qualities
- Carry out the responsibility of obtaining correct information about the client
- Display confidence while assessing extent of client's respiratory alterations

Figure 39-6 Critical thinking model for oxygenation assessment.

Nursing Process

❖Assessment

The nursing assessment of a client's cardiopulmonary functioning includes an in-depth history of the client's normal and present cardiopulmonary function, past impairments in circulatory or respiratory functioning, and measures that the client uses to optimize oxygenation. The history should include a review of drug, food, and other allergies, such as pet dander, mould, and environmental triggers.

Physical examination of the client's cardiopulmonary status reveals the extent of existing signs and symptoms. A review of laboratory and diagnostic test results provides valuable data on respiratory and ventilatory parameters.

Health History

The health history should focus on the client's ability to meet oxygen needs. The health history for cardiac function includes pain and characteristics of pain, dyspnea, fatigue, peripheral circulation, cardiac risk factors, and the presence of past or concurrent cardiac conditions. The health history for respiratory function includes presence of a cough, shortness of breath, wheezing, pain, environmental exposures, frequency of respiratory tract infections, pulmonary risk factors, past respiratory problems, current medication use, and smoking history or second-hand smoke exposure.

Pain. Chest pain needs to be thoroughly evaluated with regard to location, duration, radiation, and frequency. Cardiac pain does not occur with respiratory variations and is most often on the left side of the chest and radiates to the left arm in men. Chest pain in women is much less definitive and may be a sensation of choking, breathlessness, or pain that radiates through to the back. Pericardial pain resulting from an inflammation of the pericardial sac is usually nonradiating and may occur with inspiration.

Pleuritic chest pain is peripheral and may radiate to the scapular regions. It is worsened by inspiratory manoeuvres, such as coughing, yawning, and sighing. Pleuritic pain is often caused from an inflammation or infection in the pleural space and is described as knifelike, lasting from a minute to hours and always in association with inspiration.

Musculoskeletal pain may be present following exercise, rib trauma, and prolonged coughing episodes. This pain is also aggravated by inspiratory movements and may easily be confused with pleuritic chest pain.

Fatigue. Fatigue is a subjective sensation in which the client reports a loss of endurance. Fatigue in the client with cardiopulmonary alterations is often an early sign of a worsening of the chronic underlying process. To provide an objective measure of fatigue, the client may be asked to rate the fatigue on a scale of 0 to 10, with 10 being the worst level of fatigue and 0 representing no fatigue.

Smoking. It is important to determine clients' direct and secondary exposure to cigarette smoke. Ask the client about any history of smoking; include the number of years smoked and the number of packages smoked per day. This is recorded as pack-year history. For example, if a client smoked two packs a day for 20 years, the client would have a 40 pack-year history (packages per day • years smoked).

It is also important to determine if the client is exposed to second-hand smoke from family or coworkers. Exposure to second-hand smoke increases the client's risk for chronic lung or cardiac diseases.

Dyspnea. **Dyspnea** is a clinical sign of hypoxia and manifests as breathlessness. It is the subjective sensation of difficult or uncomfortable breathing (Box 39–6). Dyspnea is shortness of breath associated with exercise or excitement, but in some clients dyspnea may be present without any relation to activity or exercise. Dyspnea is associated with many conditions, such as pulmonary diseases, cardiovascular diseases, neuromuscular conditions, and anemia. In addition, dyspnea may occur in the pregnant woman in the final months of pregnancy. Environmental factors, such as pollution, cold air, and smoking, may also cause or worsen dyspnea.

Dyspnea can be associated with clinical signs such as exaggerated respiratory effort, use of the accessory muscles of respiration, nasal flaring, and marked increases in the rate and depth of respirations (Jevon & Ewens, 2001). The use of a visual analog scale (VAS) can help clients make an objective assessment of their dyspnea. The VAS is a 100-mm vertical line with end points of 0 and 10. Zero is equated with no dyspnea and 10 is equated with the worst breathlessness the client has experienced. Studies have validated the use of the VAS to evaluate a client's dyspnea in the clinical setting. Evaluate the effectiveness of nursing interventions by monitoring the client's assessment of their dyspnea.

BOX 39-6 RESEARCH HIGHLIGHT

The Efficacy of Exercise Training in Clients With Dyspnea

Research Focus

Clients with dyspnea often have a difficult time controlling their breathing. Assisting clients with dyspnea self-management may improve their quality of life. Knowing what interventions are helpful will be beneficial in developing a plan of care.

Research Abstract

The purpose of the study by Stulbarg et al. (2002) was to determine (a) whether exercise training adds benefit to dyspnea self-management and (b) whether there is a response to supervised exercise training sessions in dyspnea, to exercise performance, and to health-related quality of life. Subjects with COPD, aged 58 to 74 years, with a forced expiratory volume at 1 second (FEV_1) ranging from 30.8% to 58.8% of predicted, were randomized into three groups. All three groups participated in a dyspnea self-management program, which included individualized education about dyspnea management strategies, a home-walking prescription, and daily logs. One group received no additional exercise supervision, another group had exposure to exercise (30 minutes every other week for 8 weeks), and the third group had supervised exercise training (30 minutes, 3 times per week for 8 weeks). Outcomes were measured at baseline and at every 2-month interval as part of a 1-year longitudinal randomized clinical trial using the Chronic Respiratory Questionnaire (CRQ), Shortness of Breath Questionnaire, and Baseline/Transitional Dyspnea Index. Outcomes measured included dyspnea during laboratory exercise and with activities of daily living, exercise performance and endurance testing, a 6-minute walk, and a quality-of-life survey (Short Form-36 [SF-36]). The group that received supervised exercise training had a significantly greater improvement in dyspnea management than did the group that received no exercise training.

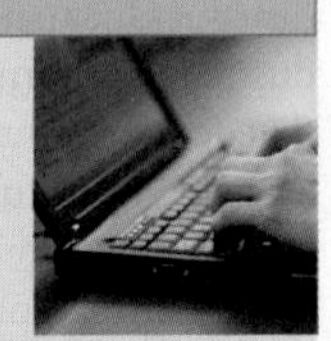

Evidence-Informed Practice

- Supervised exercise (rehabilitation) programs improve dyspnea management for clients with COPD.
- Simply providing information on dyspnea self-management techniques does not have a significant impact on clients' ability to manage their condition.
- A prescription for exercise is not an effective tool in helping clients with COPD learn to manage their dyspnea.
- Individualized programs for dyspnea self-management lead to better management of the client's dyspnea and improvement in quality of life.

References: Stulbarg, M. S., Carrieri-Kohlman V., Demir-Deviren S., Nguyen H. Q., Admas, L., Tsang, A. H., et al. (2002). Exercise training improves outcomes of a dyspnea self-management program. *Journal of Cardiopulmonary Rehabilitation, 22*(2), 109–121.

If the client has a history of dyspnea, determine the circumstances under which it occurred, such as with exertion, stress, or respiratory tract infection. Determine whether the client's perception of dyspnea affects the ability to lie flat. **Orthopnea** is an abnormal condition in which the person must use multiple pillows when lying down or must sit with the arms elevated and leaning forward to breathe. The number of pillows required for sleeping, such as two- or three-pillow orthopnea, usually quantifies the presence of orthopnea.

Cough. Cough is a sudden, audible expulsion of air from the lungs. The person breathes in, the glottis is partially closed, and the accessory muscles of expiration contract to expel the air forcibly. Coughing is a protective reflex to clear the trachea, bronchi, and lungs of irritants and secretions. The carina, the point of bifurcation of the right and left mainstem bronchus, is the most sensitive area for cough production. A cough is difficult to evaluate, and almost everyone has periods of coughing. Clients with a chronic cough tend to deny, underestimate, or minimize their coughing, often because they are so accustomed to it that they are unaware of how frequently it occurs.

Coughing is classified according to the time when the client most frequently coughs. Clients with chronic sinusitis may cough only in the early morning or immediately after rising from sleep. This clears the airway of mucus resulting from sinus drainage. Clients with chronic bronchitis generally produce sputum all day, although greater amounts are produced after rising from a semi-recumbent or flat position. This is a result of the dependent accumulation of sputum in the airways and is associated with reduced mobility (see Chapter 46). When a client has a cough, determine its frequency and if it is productive or nonproductive. A productive cough results in sputum production, material coughed up from the lungs that may be swallowed or expectorated. Sputum contains mucus, cellular debris, and microorganisms, and it may contain pus or blood. Collect data about the type and quantity of sputum. Instruct the client to try to produce some sputum, being careful not to simply clear the throat to produce a sample of saliva. Then inspect it for colour, consistency, odour, and amount (Box 39–7).

If **hemoptysis** (bloody sputum) is reported, determine if it is associated with coughing and bleeding from the upper respiratory tract, from sinus drainage, or from the gastrointestinal tract (**hematemesis**). In addition, the hemoptysis should be described according to amount, colour, and duration and whether it is mixed with sputum. When the client reports bloody or blood-tinged sputum, diagnostic tests, such as examination of sputum specimens, chest X-ray examinations, **bronchoscopy**, and other X-ray studies, should be performed.

BOX 39-7 Sputum Characteristics

Colour
Clear
White
Yellow
Green
Brown
Red
Streaked with blood

Changes in Colour
Same colour throughout the day
Clearing with coughing
Progressively darker

Odour
None
Foul

Quantity
Same as usual
Increased
Decreased

Consistency
Frothy
Watery
Tenacious, thick

Presence of Blood
Occasional
Early morning
Bright or dark red
Blood tinged

Wheezing. Wheezing is characterized by a high-pitched musical sound caused by high-velocity movement of air through a narrowed airway. Wheezing may be associated with asthma, acute bronchitis, or pneumonia. Wheezing can occur on inspiration, expiration, or both. Determine if there are any precipitating factors, such as respiratory infection, allergens, exercise, or stress.

Environmental or Geographical Exposures. Environmental exposure to many inhaled substances is closely linked with respiratory disease. Investigate exposures in the client's home and workplace. The most common environmental exposures in the home are cigarette smoke, carbon monoxide, and radon. In addition, determine whether a client who is a nonsmoker is passively exposed to smoke.

Carbon monoxide poisoning can result from a blocked furnace flue or fireplace. The client may have vague complaints of general malaise, flu-like symptoms, and excessive sleepiness. Clients are particularly at risk in the late fall when they turn the heat on or begin to use the fireplace again. Radon gas, a radioactive substance that can damage lung tissue and cause lung cancer, enters homes through the ground. When homes are underventilated, this gas is not able to escape into the atmosphere and becomes trapped in the home.

Obtain an employment history to assess exposure to substances such as asbestos, coal, cotton fibres, fumes, or chemical inhalants. This is particularly important with middle-aged and older adults, who may have worked in places without regulations to protect workers from carcinogens such as asbestos.

Exposure to pathogens may occur during travel. Schistosomiasis can be acquired in Asia, Africa, the Caribbean, and South America. This is infection of a human with a species of fluke found in fresh water that has been contaminated by human feces. Coccidioidomycosis is a fungal disease caused by inhalation of *Coccidioides immitis*, a wind-borne spore carried on dust particles.

Respiratory Infections. A health history should contain information about the client's frequency and duration of respiratory tract infections. Although everyone occasionally experiences a cold, for some people it can result in bronchitis or pneumonia. On average, clients will have four colds per year. Determine if the client has had a pneumococcal or flu vaccine in the past and ask about any known exposure to tuberculosis (TB) and the results of the tuberculin skin test.

Determine the client's risk for human immunodeficiency virus (HIV) infection. Clients with a history of intravenous (IV) drug use and multiple unprotected sexual partners are at risk of developing HIV infection. Clients may not display any symptoms of HIV infection until they present with *Pneumocystis carinii* (PCP) or *Mycoplasma* pneumonia. Presentation with PCP or *Mycoplasma* pneumonia indicates a significant depression of the client's immune system and progression to acquired immune deficiency syndrome (AIDS).

Allergies. When obtaining a respiratory system history, inquire about airborne allergens. The client's allergic response may be watery eyes, sneezing, runny nose, or respiratory symptoms, such as cough or wheezing. Ask the client specific questions about the type of allergens, response to these allergens, and successful and unsuccessful relief measures. In addition, determine the impact that environmental air quality and second-hand smoke exposure has on the client's allergy and symptoms.

Safe nursing practice also includes obtaining information about food, drug, or insect-sting allergies. These data are usually obtained on initial history and physical. However, always double-check this information with the client, especially when obtaining information about respiratory allergens.

Health Risks. Investigate familial risk factors, such as a family history of lung cancer or cardiovascular disease. Documentation should include which blood relatives have had the disease and their present level of health or age at time of death. Other family risk factors include the presence of infectious diseases, particularly TB. It is important to determine who in the client's household has been infected and the status of treatment.

Medications. The health history should also list medications the client is using. These include prescribed, over-the-counter, folk medicine, herbal medicines, alternative therapies, and illicit drugs and substances. Such medications may have adverse effects by themselves or through interactions with other drugs. A person using a prescribed bronchodilator drug, for example, may decide that using an over-the-counter inhalant as well will be beneficial. Many of these contain ephedrine or ma huang, a natural chemical that acts like epinephrine. This product may react with the prescribed medication by potentiating or decreasing the effect of the prescribed medication. Clients taking warfarin (Coumadin) for blood thinning will prolong the prothrombin time (international normalized ratio [INR]) results if they are taking gingko biloba, garlic, or ginseng with the anticoagulant. The drug interaction could precipitate a life-threatening bleed.

safety alert During history taking, ask clients to list all of the over-the-counter and herbal supplements they are taking to ensure that medication interactions do not develop.

When clients are prescribed drugs for which toxic levels can be monitored by blood analyses, you need to review these laboratory values. Common drugs that can be monitored include theophylline (theophylline levels), digitalis preparations (digitalis levels), anticoagulants such as warfarin (Coumadin; INR level), and phenobarbital (phenobarbital levels). Toxic effects of these medications can impair cardiopulmonary functioning.

It is important to determine whether a client uses illicit drugs. These drugs, particularly parenterally administered narcotics, which are often diluted with talcum powder, can cause pulmonary disorders resulting from the irritant effect of the powder on lung tissues.

As with all medication, assess the client's knowledge and ability to self-administer medications correctly (see Chapter 34). Of particular importance is the assessment of the client's understanding of potential side effects of the medications. Clients should be able to recognize adverse reactions and be aware of the dangers in combining prescribed medications with over-the-counter drugs.

Physical Examination

The physical examination performed to assess the client's level of tissue oxygenation includes evaluation of the cardiopulmonary system (see Chapter 32). Special consideration should be given when assessing the older client because changes in the cardiopulmonary system occur with the aging process (Table 39–3). These changes may result

TABLE 39-3 Assessment Findings in the Aging Cardiopulmonary System

Function	Pathophysiological Change	Key Clinical Findings
Heart		
Muscle contraction	Thickening of the ventricular wall, increased collagen and decreased elastin in the heart muscle	Decreased cardiac output Diminished cardiac reserve
Blood flow	Heart valves become thicker and stiffer, more often in the mitral and aortic valves.	Systolic ejection murmur
Conduction system	The SA node becomes fibrotic from calcification; the number of pacemaker cells in the SA node decreases.	Increased PR, QRS, and Q-T intervals, decreased amplitude of the QRS complex
Arterial vessel compliance	Vessels become calcified, loss of arterial distensibility, decreased elastin in the vessel walls, more bends and twists (tortuous) in the vessels	Hypertension, with an increase in systolic blood pressure Fluctuation in blood pressure
Lungs		
Breathing mechanics	Decreased chest wall compliance, loss of elastic recoil Decreased respiratory muscle mass/strength	Prolonged exhalation phase Decreased vital capacity
Oxygenation	Increased ventilation–perfusion mismatch Decreased alveolar surface area Decreased carbon dioxide diffusion capacity	Decreased PaO_2 (arterial oxygen tension) Decreased cardiac output Slightly increased $PaCO_2$ (arterial carbon dioxide tension)
Breathing control/breathing pattern	Decreased responsiveness of central and peripheral chemoreceptors to hypoxemia and hypercapnia	Increased respiratory rate Decreased tidal volume
Lung defence mechanisms	Decreased number of cilia Decreased IgA production and humoral and cellular immunity	Decreased airway clearance Diminished cough reflex
Sleep and breathing	Decreased respiratory drive Decreased tone of upper airway muscles	Increased risk of aspiration and infection Decreased PaO_2 Snoring, obstructive sleep apnea

in changes in the client's activity tolerance, level of fatigue, or transient changes in vital signs and may not be associated with a specific cardiopulmonary disease.

Inspection. Using inspection techniques, perform a head-to-toe observation of the client for skin and mucous membrane colour, general appearance, level of consciousness, adequacy of systemic circulation, breathing patterns, and chest wall movement (Table 39–4). Any abnormalities should be investigated during palpation, percussion, and auscultation.

➤ TABLE 39-4 Inspection of Cardiopulmonary Status

Abnormality	Cause
Eyes	
Xanthelasma (yellow lipid lesions on eyelids)	Hyperlipidemia
Corneal arcus (whitish opaque ring around junction of cornea and sclera)	Hyperlipidemia in young to middle-aged adults, normal finding in older adults with arcus senilis
Pale conjunctivae	Anemia
Cyanotic conjunctivae	Hypoxemia
Petechiae on conjunctivae	Fat embolus or bacterial endocarditis
Mouth and Lips	
Cyanotic mucous membranes	Decreased oxygenation (hypoxia)
Pursed-lip breathing	Associated with chronic lung disease
Neck Veins	
Distension	Associated with right-sided heart failure
Nose	
Flaring nares	Air hunger, dyspnea
Chest	
Retractions	Increased work of breathing, dyspnea
Asymmetry	Chest wall injury
Skin	
Peripheral cyanosis	Vasoconstriction and diminished blood flow
Central cyanosis	Hypoxemia
Decreased skin turgor	Dehydration (normal finding in older adults as a result of decreased skin elasticity)
Dependent edema	Associated with right- and left-sided heart failure
Periorbital edema	Associated with kidney disease
Fingertips and Nail Beds	
Cyanosis	Decreased cardiac output or hypoxia
Splinter hemorrhages	Bacterial endocarditis
Clubbing	Chronic hypoxemia

From Potter, P. A., & Weilitz, P. B. (2003). *Health assessment: Pocket guide series* (6th ed.). St. Louis, MO: Mosby.

Inspection includes observations of the nails for clubbing. Clubbed nails, obliteration of the normal angle between the base of the nail and the skin, are seen in clients with prolonged oxygen deficiency, endocarditis, and congenital heart defects.

Observe the chest wall movement for retraction, sinking in of soft tissues of the chest between the intercostal spaces. Also observe for paradoxical breathing, asynchronous breathing, and the client's breathing pattern (Table 39–5). In paradoxical breathing, the chest wall contracts during inspiration and expands during exhalation. Infants can experience sternal and substernal chest wall retractions with only a slight inspiratory effort because of the pliability of the chest wall. Note the anteroposterior diameter of the chest wall. Conditions such as emphysema, advancing age, and COPD can cause the chest to assume a rounded shape.

Palpation. Palpation of the chest provides assessment data in several areas. It documents the type and amount of thoracic excursion, elicits any areas of tenderness, and can identify tactile fremitus, thrills, heaves, and the cardiac point of maximal impulse (PMI). Palpation also aids in detecting abnormal masses or lumps in the axilla and breast tissue. Palpation of the extremities provides data about the peripheral circulation, the presence and quality of peripheral pulses, skin temperature, colour, and capillary refill (see Chapter 32).

Palpation should also include the feet and legs to assess the presence or absence of peripheral edema. Clients with alterations in their cardiac function, such as those with congestive heart failure or hypertension, often have pedal or lower extremity edema. Edema is graded from 1+ to 4+, depending on the depth of visible indentation after firm application of a finger (see Chapter 32).

Palpation of the pulses in the neck and extremities is performed to assess arterial blood flow (see Chapter 32 and Box 39–8). A scale of 0 (absent pulse) to 3+ (full, bounding pulse) is used to describe what is palpated. The normal pulse is graded at 2+, and a weak, thready pulse is graded as 1+.

Percussion. Percussion is used to detect the presence of abnormal fluid or air in the lungs. It also aids in determining diaphragmatic excursion (see Chapter 32).

Auscultation. Auscultation helps in identifying normal and abnormal heart and lung sounds (see Chapter 32). Auscultation of the cardiovascular system should include assessment for normal S_1 and S_2 sounds, the presence of abnormal S_3 and S_4 sounds (gallops), and murmurs or rubs. Auscultation is also used to identify a bruit over the carotid arteries, abdominal aorta, and femoral arteries.

Auscultation of lung sounds involves listening for movement of air throughout all lung fields: anterior, posterior, and lateral. Adventitious breath sounds occur with collapse of a lung segment, fluid in a lung segment, or narrowing or obstruction of an airway. Auscultation also evaluates the client's response to interventions for improving the respiratory status.

Diagnostic Tests

There are a variety of diagnostic tests to monitor cardiopulmonary functioning. Some of these tests can be obtained through screening, simple blood specimens, X-ray films, or other noninvasive means. One such screening mechanism is TB skin testing (Box 39–9). This is a simple test that is usually required annually for health care workers to monitor possible TB exposure. In contrast, invasive diagnostic tests, such as a thoracentesis, can be quite painful, depending on the client's tolerance for pain.

Tables 39–6 and 39–7 and Box 39–10 summarize diagnostic testing used in the assessment and evaluation of clients with cardiopulmonary

➤ TABLE 39-5 Assessment of Breathing Pattern

Pattern and Rate (Breaths/Minute)	Clinical Significance
Eupnea (12–20)	Normal rate in the adult
Tachypnea (>35)	Can result from anxiety or response to pain or fever, respiratory failure, shortness of breath, or a respiratory infection. May lead to respiratory alkalosis, paresthesia, tetany, and confusion
Bradypnea (<10)	Results from sleep, respiratory depression, drug overdose, or central nervous system lesion
Apnea (absence of respiration >15 seconds)	May be intermittent, such as in sleep apnea, or prolonged, as in a respiratory arrest
Kussmaul's respirations (usually >35, may be slow or normal)	Tachypnea pattern associated with metabolic imbalance such as diabetic ketoacidosis, metabolic acidosis, or renal failure

alterations. Explain the procedure and tell the client what to expect, to reduce the client's anxiety. The client must understand the importance of following instructions, such as holding the breath as requested and not coughing during the procedure. After any procedure, monitor the client for signs of changes in cardiopulmonary functioning, sudden shortness of breath, pain, oxygen desaturation, and anxiety. Promote the client's comfort and encourage the client to rest after the test, because many clients find these tests to be tiring.

BOX 39-8 NURSING STORY

My First Maternal–Child Clinical Experience

It was one of my first clinical experiences as a student nurse. I was placed on a maternity unit with seven other students. Because I was so nervous, I asked another student colleague to accompany me while I recorded vital signs on a newborn baby. I entered the room, introduced myself to the baby's mother, and grasped for the baby's wrist to check the heart rate. I had a hard time finding the pulse; it felt like hours before I finally felt what I hoped was the pulse. As I began counting each heart beat, the responsible registered nurse entered the room and said, "Oh, are you trying to get the heart rate?" I was relieved that help had arrived. She indicated, "You need to use your stethoscope to listen to the apical pulse." I was so embarrassed, and even more nervous. I immediately put the stethoscope on the baby's chest. Confused, I told the student standing next to me, "I still can't hear anything." She smiled and pointed to the earpieces, which were sitting around my neck instead of in my ears.

➤ BOX 39-9 Tuberculosis Skin Testing

- Skin testing is used to determine past exposure to *Mycobacterium tuberculosis*.
- Tuberculosis skin testing (TST) is performed by administering an intradermal injection of 0.1 mL of tuberculin-purified protein derivative on the inner surface of the forearm. The injection produces a pale elevation of the skin 6–10 mm in diameter. Afterward, the injection site may be circled, and the client is instructed not to wash off the circle.
- Tuberculin skin tests are read 48–72 hours after injection. If the site is not read within 72 hours, the client must undergo another skin test.
- Positive results are indicated by a palpable, elevated, hardened, reddened area around the injection site, caused by edema and inflammation from the antigen–antibody reaction. The site is measured in millimetres. A positive test result occurs when the site is ‡ 10 mm.
- Reddened flat areas are ***not*** positive reactions and are not measured.
- TST in older adults is less reliable (see Box 39–3).

Client Expectations

Ask clients what they expect from the encounter and what their priority is for management of their health. In identifying expectations, you involve clients in the decision-making process and allow them to participate in their care and know what will happen to them. For example, if you plan a smoking cessation or weight-reduction program for a client who is not ready for the change, both you and the client will become frustrated. Establish short-term, realistic goals that build to a larger goal. For example, reducing the fat in the client's diet might start out with replacing food such as whole milk with 2% milk and gradually introducing skim milk. A sudden change from whole to skim milk will most likely fail, because the change is too much. A plan for adding exercise to the client's lifestyle could start with a commitment to exercise once a week for 20 minutes, or the client could commit to a weight-reduction plan of 2 kg per month.

Remember that your goals and expectations may not always coincide with those of your client. By addressing the client's concerns and expectations, you will establish a relationship that can address other health care goals and expected outcomes. Knowing the mindset of clients and respecting their wishes will go a long way toward helping clients make significant lifestyle changes to benefit their health.

➤TABLE 39-6 Cardiopulmonary Diagnostic Blood Studies

Test and Normal Values	Interpretation
Complete Blood Count (CBC)	
Normal values for a CBC vary with age and gender.	A CBC determines the number and type of red and white blood cells per cubic millimetre of blood.
Cardiac Enzymes	
Creatine kinase (CK) levels begin to rise approximately 3–12 hours after an acute myocardial infarction, peak in 24 hours, and then return to normal within 2–3 days. Male normal: <195 IU/L Female normal: <170 IU/L	Cardiac enzymes are used to diagnose acute myocardial infarcts.
The CK enzyme may be fractionated into bands, including the MB band. Depending on the individual laboratory, MB bands >3% indicate a myocardial infarction (Lewis et al., 2006).	The MB band is specific to the myocardial cell and may quantify myocardial damage.
Plasma cardiac troponin I <0.1–3.1 μg/L	Often remains elevated for 7–10 days.
Plasma cardiac troponin T <0.1 μg/L	Often remains elevated for 10–14 days.
Serum Electrolytes	
Potassium (K^+) 3.5–5 mmol/L	Clients on diuretic therapy are at risk for hypokalemia (low potassium). Clients receiving angiotensin-converting enzyme inhibitors are at risk for hyperkalemia (elevated potassium).
Cholesterol	
Fasting cholesterol 3.6–5.2 mmol/L	Contributing factors include sedentary lifestyle, intake of saturated fatty acids, and familial hypercholesterolemia.
Low-density lipoprotein (LDL) cholesterol (bad cholesterol) <3.4 mmol/L	High LDL cholesterol (hypercholesterolemia) is caused by excessive intake of saturated fatty acids, dietary cholesterol intake, and obesity. Familial hypercholesterolemia and hyperlipidemia are also contributing factors, as are hypothyroidism, nephrotic syndrome, and diabetes mellitus.
High-density lipoprotein (HDL) cholesterol (good cholesterol) Male: >1.2 mmol/L Female: >1.4 mmol/L	Low HDL cholesterol is caused by cigarette smoking, obesity, lack of regular exercise, β-adrenergic blocking agents, genetic disorders of HDL metabolism, hypertriglyceridemia, and type 2 diabetes.
Triglycerides 0.45–1.69 mmol/L	Obesity, excessive alcohol intake, diabetes mellitus, β-adrenergic blocking agents, and genetic predisposition cause hypertriglyceridemia.

From Pagana, K. D., & Pagana, T. J. (2005). *Mosby's diagnostic and laboratory test reference* (7th ed.). St. Louis, MO: Mosby.

TABLE 39-7 Cardiac Function Diagnostic Tests

Test	Significance
12-Lead electrocardiogram (ECG)	Graphic recording of the electrical activity of the heart, used to detect abnormal electrical activity and the electrical position of the heart. The ECG includes 12 leads: I, II, III, AVR, AVL, AVF, and V1–6. It provides a 360-degree view of the heart.
Holter monitor	Portable ECG worn by the client. The test produces a continuous ECG tracing over a period of time. Clients keep a diary of activity, noting when they experience rapid heartbeats or dizziness. Evaluation of the ECG recording along with the diary provides information about the heart's electrical activity during activities of daily living.
ECG exercise stress test	ECG is monitored while the client walks on a treadmill at a specified speed and duration of time. Used to evaluate the cardiac response to physical stress. The test is not a valuable tool for evaluation of cardiac response in women because of increased false-positive findings among women.
Thallium stress test	An ECG stress test with the addition of talliuym-201-injected IV. The test determines coronary blood flow changes with increased activity.
Electrophysiological study (EPS)	Invasive measure of intracardiac electrical pathways. Provides more specific information about difficult-to-treat dysrhythmias. EPS assesses the adequacy of antidysrhythmic medication.
Echocardiography	Noninvasive measure of heart structure and heart wall motion. Graphically demonstrates overall cardiac performance.
Scintigraphy	Radionuclide angiography. Used to evaluate cardiac structure, myocardial perfusion, and contractility.
Cardiac catheterization and angiography	Used to visualize cardiac chambers, valves, the great vessels, and coronary arteries. Pressures and volumes within the four chambers of the heart can also be measured.

BOX 39-10 Common Respiratory Tests and Methods

Oxygenation Tests

- *Pulse oximetry:* A **pulse oximeter** is a device used to measure pulse rate and oxygen concentration in arterial blood (SaO_2). A sensor is attached to the client's finger, toe, nose, earlobe, or forehead. Accuracy is directly related to the perfusion of the probe area, a systolic blood pressure >90 mm Hg, and the hemoglobin level. Decreased levels correlate well with arterial oxygen levels and are used to trend oxygenation over time. Normal SaO_2 values are 98%–100%. An SaO_2 below 70% is life threatening.
- *Arterial blood gas:* A radial or femoral artery is punctured to obtain arterial blood. Tests measure the oxygen concentration in the blood, the hydrogen ion concentration (pH), partial pressure of carbon dioxide ($PaCO_2$), and the partial pressure of oxygen (PaO_2). Normal values are as follows:
  - pH 7.35–7.45
  - $PaCO_2$ 35–45 mm Hg
  - PaO_2 80–100 mm Hg
  - SaO_2 95%–100%

Pulmonary Function Tests

Pulmonary function tests measure lung volume (the amount of air moving into and out of the lungs) and capacity (how much air the lungs can hold). Respiratory therapists usually conduct these tests. The client takes as deep a breath as possible and forcefully exhales into a mouthpiece attached to a machine. Pulmonary readings are recorded and compared with previous readings and with average normal values, which vary depending on the client's age, gender, weight, height, and race. These tests are used to diagnose and monitor pulmonary disease and conditions (e.g., asthma, emphysema). They are also used to evaluate postoperative lung conditions.

Imaging

- *Chest X-ray examination:* Usually posteroanterior and lateral films are taken to adequately visualize all of the lung fields. A radiograph of the thorax is used to observe the lung fields for fluid, infiltrates (e.g., pneumonia), masses (e.g., lung cancer), fractures, pneumothorax, and other abnormal processes.
- *Computed tomography (CT) scan:* A CT scan provides visualization of fine detail of the lungs and other structures in the thorax. It is often used as part of the assessment of clients with pneumonia, lung masses, and suspected pulmonary emboli.
- *Ventilation/perfusion (nuclear medicine) lung scan:* This scan is used to detect pulmonary emboli. The results from two separate scans are compared: the perfusion scan uses an injected radioactive tracer to measure pulmonary blood flow, and the ventilation scan shows the pulmonary distribution of a different inhaled tracer. Mismatches (areas of ventilation without corresponding perfusion or blood flow) indicate pulmonary emboli.

Methods of Obtaining Respiratory Specimens for Analysis

Specimens are cultured so they can be used to detect the presence of blood, microbes, and abnormal cells. A variety of methods are used to obtain respiratory specimens.

- *Sputum tests:* Sputum is mucus from the respiratory system that is expectorated through the mouth. Sputum specimens are obtained when the client coughs up sputum from the bronchi and trachea; specimens are easier to obtain in the morning when the secretions are coughed up upon awakening. Sputum tests include (a) *sputum culture and sensitivity (C and S)* test, used to identify a specific

BOX 39-10 Common Respiratory Tests and Methods *continued*

microorganism growing in the sputum and to identify drug resistance and sensitivities; (b) *sputum for acid-fast bacillus (AFB)*, a test used to screen for the presence of AFB for detection of TB by early-morning specimens on 3 consecutive days; and (c) *sputum for cytology*, used to identify abnormal lung cancer and differentiates the type of cancer cells (small cell, oat cell, large cell).

- *Tracheal aspiration via endotracheal tube in intubated clients:* Secretions are collected by passing a flexible suction catheter through the endotracheal tube.
- *Bronchoscopy:* A narrow, flexible, fibre-optic scope is passed into the trachea and bronchi to enable visual examination of the tracheobronchial tree. The procedure is performed to obtain fluid, sputum, or biopsy samples, and to remove mucous plugs or foreign bodies.
- *Thoracentesis:* This involves surgical perforation of the chest wall and pleural space with a needle to aspirate fluid for diagnostic or therapeutic purposes or to remove a specimen for biopsy. The procedure is performed using aseptic technique and local anaesthetic. The client usually sits upright with the anterior thorax supported by pillows or an overbed table.
- *Nasopharyngeal aspirate or swab:* This swab is used to detect respiratory viruses. Aspirates are the best specimens from young children, whereas swabs can be used for obtaining samples from older children and adults.

❖Nursing Diagnosis

Clients with an altered level of oxygenation can have nursing diagnoses that are primarily from a cardiovascular or pulmonary origin. Each nursing diagnosis is based on specific defining characteristics and the related etiology (Box 39–11). Use the information gathered in the nursing assessment to identify and cluster the defining characteristics. The clustered defining characteristics support the nursing diagnosis.

Nursing diagnoses appropriate for the client with alterations in oxygenation include, but are not limited to, the following:

- *Activity intolerance*
- *Risk for activity intolerance*
- *Ineffective airway clearance*
- *Anxiety*
- *Ineffective breathing pattern*
- *Decreased cardiac output*
- *Impaired comfort*
- *Impaired verbal communication*
- *Ineffective individual coping*
- *Fatigue*
- *Fear*
- *Risk for imbalanced fluid volume*
- *Impaired gas exchange*
- *Ineffective health maintenance*
- *Risk for infection*
- *Deficient (specify) knowledge*
- *Risk for impaired skin integrity*
- *Disturbed sleep pattern*
- *Ineffective tissue perfusion*
- *Impaired spontaneous ventilation*

BOX 39-11 NURSING DIAGNOSTIC PROCESS

Assessment Activities	***Defining Characteristics***	***Nursing Diagnosis***
Ask client or family about client's mood, attentiveness, memory, and activity level.	Confusion Decreased activity Fatigue Irritability Restlessness Sleepiness	*Impaired gas exchange related to decreased lung expansion*
Observe client's respirations.	Dyspnea Impaired gas exchange related to collapsed alveoli Nasal flaring Tachypnea Use of accessory muscles	
Inspect skin and mucous membranes.	Diaphoresis Pallor Moist skin	
Auscultate chest.	Decreased respiratory excursion Abnormal, distant lung sounds	

❖Planning

During planning, use critical thinking skills to synthesize information from multiple sources (Figure 39–7). Critical thinking ensures that your plan of care integrates individualized client needs. Professional standards are especially important to consider when developing a care plan. These standards often establish scientifically proven guidelines for selecting effective nursing interventions.

Goals and Outcomes

Develop an individualized care plan for each nursing diagnosis (Box 39–12). In collaboration with your client, set realistic expectations for care. Goals should be individualized and realistic with measurable outcomes.

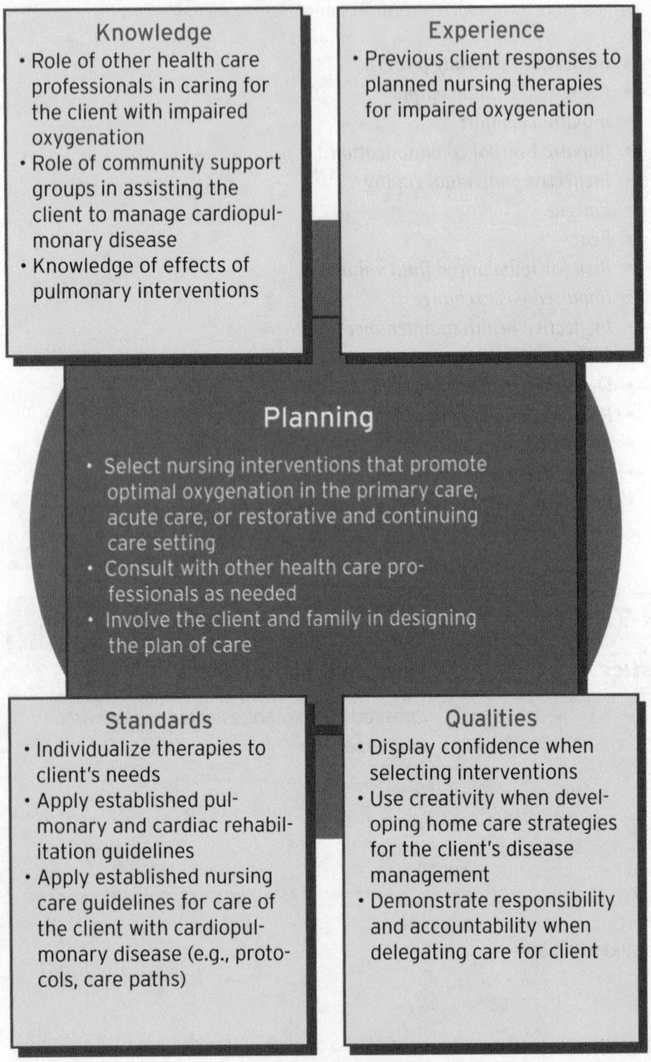

Figure 39-7 Critical thinking model for oxygenation planning.

Clients with impaired oxygenation require a nursing care plan directed toward meeting the actual or potential oxygenation needs of the client. Individual outcomes are derived from client-centred needs. For example, the goal of maintaining a patent airway can be evaluated by specific outcomes for the client. These might include the following expected outcomes:

- Client's lungs are clear to auscultation.
- Client achieves maintenance and promotion of bilateral lung expansion.
- Client coughs productively.
- Tissue oxygenation (SaO_2) is maintained or improved.

Often a client with cardiopulmonary disease has multiple nursing diagnoses (Figure 39–8). In this case, identify when goals or outcomes apply to more than one diagnosis. The presence of multiple diagnoses also makes priority setting a critical activity.

Setting Priorities

The client's level of health, age, lifestyle, and environmental risks affect the level of tissue oxygenation. Clients with severe impairments in oxygenation frequently require nursing interventions in multiple areas. Consider what the most important goal is during the limited amount of time the client is seen in the hospital or primary care setting. For example, in an acute care setting, maintaining a patent airway has a higher priority than improving the client's exercise tolerance. The need for a patent airway is an immediate need. In a second example, when caring for a client who has an abdominal incision, pain control may have a greater priority than coughing and deep breathing. Again, in this situation, controlling the client's pain ultimately will facilitate coughing and deep breathing.

However, in a community-based or primary setting, the priority may focus on smoking cessation, exercise, diet modifications, or a combination of these activities. Both you and the client need to be focused on the same goal and expected outcomes to be successful. In addition to being individualized, each goal should be realistic and attainable for the client.

Collaborative Care

The time spent with the client in any setting is limited. Therefore, collaborate with family members, colleagues, and other specialists to accomplish the goals and outcomes that have been determined. Some clients may need to improve their exercise and activity tolerance; for some clients their continuity of care may involve enrolling in a community-based cardiopulmonary rehabilitation program. Another client may have the same health care need but is unable to leave the home, and home physiotherapy is needed.

Collaboration with physiotherapists, nutritionists, and community-based nurses may be valuable for a client with congestive heart failure or chronic lung conditions and is an essential component of primary health care. These professionals work with the client and the community to optimize resources to assist the client in attaining the highest level of wellness. In addition, professionals can help to identify community resources and support systems for both the client and family in preventing and managing symptoms related to cardiopulmonary diseases.

BOX 39-12 NURSING CARE PLAN

Ineffective Airway Clearance/Retained Secretions

Assessment

Mr. Edwards, an older adult with a history of COPD, comes to the primary care office with complaints of continued coughing. He continues to smoke 2 to 3 cigarettes a day, an improvement from his previous 10 to 15 per day.

Assessment Activities	*Findings and Defining Characteristics*
Ask Mr. Edwards how long he has had this cough.	He replies, "I have a morning cough every day, but this cough is different. It started about a week ago."
Ask Mr. Edwards what is different about this cough.	He replies, "My ribs are getting sore. I can't cough up anything, my mouth is dry, and I have become more fatigued over the past week."
Observe Mr. Edwards's skin and mucous membranes.	His skin and mucous membranes are dry.
Auscultate lung fields.	Abnormal lung sounds in the upper lobes. The lower lobes are clear.
Ask Mr. Edwards how many glasses of water he drinks daily.	Over the last week he has drunk two to three glasses a day.
Ask Mr. Edwards to produce a sputum sample.	He is unable to produce a sputum sample for evaluation.

Nursing Diagnosis: Ineffective airway clearance related to retained secretions and reduced fluid intake

Planning

*Goals (Nursing Outcomes Classification)**	*Expected Outcomes*
	Respiratory Status: Airway Patency
Client will be able to effectively clear secretions.	Lung sounds will be normal in 48 hours. Sputum will be thin, white, and watery. Respiratory rate will be within 20–24 breaths/minute in 48 hours. Client will be able to clear airway by coughing.
Client will increase oral hydration to 1000 mL of water every 24 hours.	Oral mucous membranes will be pink and moist. Client will verbalize that his mouth is not dry. Client will notice an increase in ease of sputum production. Client will report that his sputum is thin, white, and watery.

*Outcome classification labels from Moorhead, S., Johnson, M., & Maas, M. (Eds.). (2004). *Nursing Outcomes Classification (NOC),* (3rd ed.). St. Louis, MO: Mosby.

Interventions (Nursing Interventions Classification)†

Airway Management	**Rationale**
Increase fluids to 1000 mL in 24 hours if not contraindicated by cardiovascular disease (Lewis et al., 2000).	Fluids help to liquefy secretions and promote ease of removal (Snow et al., 2001). Fluids will relieve oral mucosa and skin dryness.
Have client deep breathe and cough every 2 hours four to five times (Lewis et al., 2000).	Retained secretions predispose client to atelectasis and pneumonia (Day et al., 2002).
Teach client effective cough techniques.	Coughing techniques will help to clear the airway effectively and decrease fatigue from ineffective coughing (Snow et al., 2001).
Consider chest physiotherapy (CPT) if there is evidence of infiltrates on chest X-ray film.	Standards for CPT include sputum production >30 mL/day or infiltrates on chest X-ray film.

†Intervention classification labels from Dochterman, J. M., & Bulechek, G. M. (Eds.). (2004). *Nursing Interventions Classification (NIC),* (4th ed.). St. Louis, MO: Mosby.

Evaluation

Nursing Actions	*Client Response and Findings*	*Achievement of Outcome*
Ask Mr. Edwards if he can deep breathe and cough.	Mr. Edwards reports, "It is easier to cough up my secretions now."	Client is able to clear airway by coughing.
Assess the chest for adventitious lung sounds.	Mr. Edwards reports that he has not heard any wheezing or rattling in his chest.	Lungs clear to auscultation in all fields.
Assess respiratory rate.	No use of accessory muscles of respiration. Normal breathing pattern and respiratory rate	Respiratory rate is between 20 and 24 breaths/minute.
Assess client's level of hydration.	Mucous membranes are moist. Mr. Edwards reports, "My mouth isn't so dry anymore."	Oral mucous membranes are pink and moist.
Observe appearance of sputum.	Sputum is thin, white, and watery.	Sputum is thin, white, and watery.

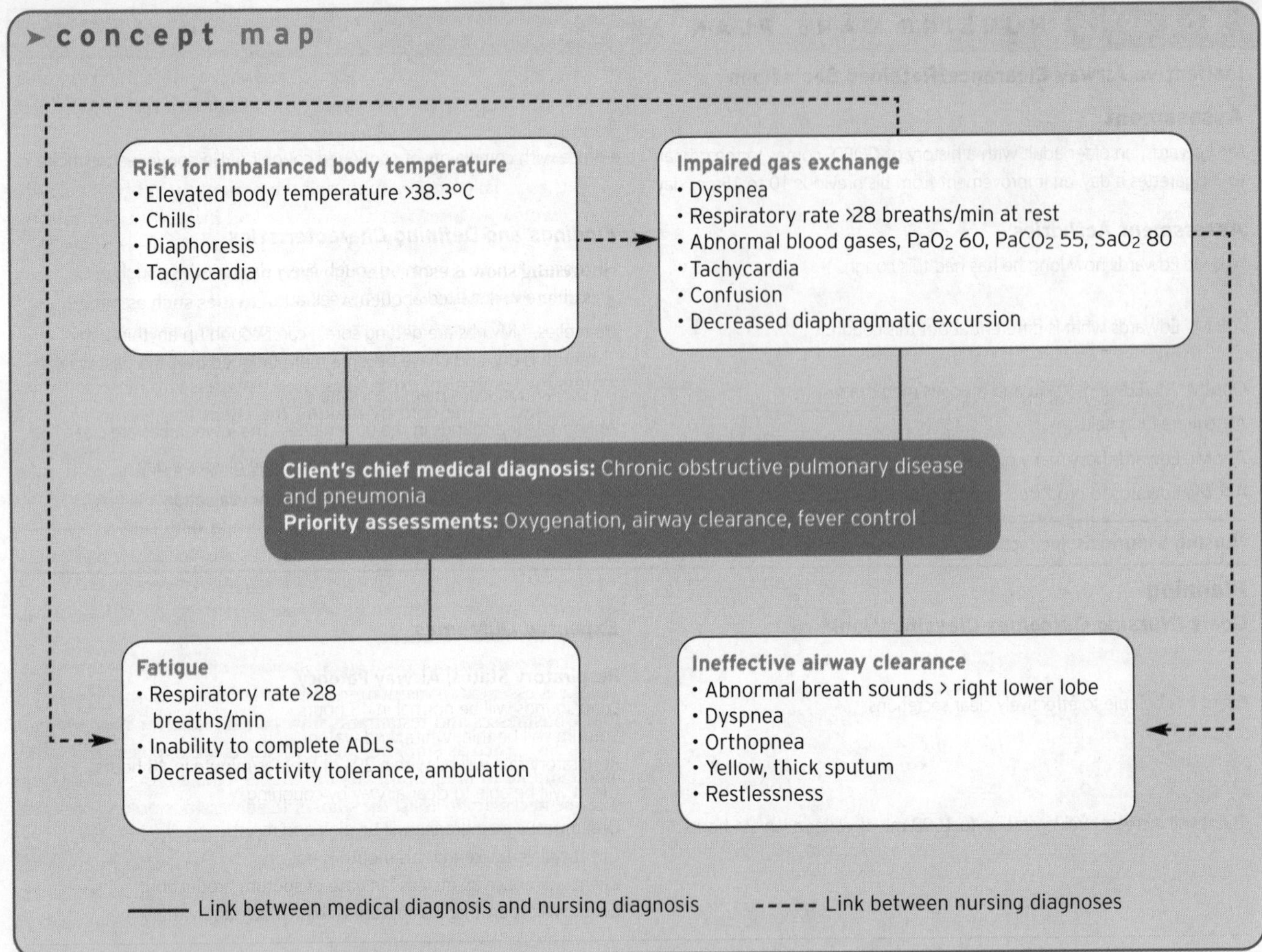

Figure 39-8 Concept map for a client with chronic obstructive pulmonary disease and pneumonia. ADLs, activities of daily living.

❖Implementation

Nursing interventions for promoting and maintaining adequate oxygenation include independent nursing actions such as health-promotion and disease-prevention behaviours, positioning, and coughing techniques. Interdependent or dependent interventions include oxygen therapy, lung inflation techniques, hydration, medication administration, and chest physiotherapy (CPT).

Health Promotion

Maintaining the client's optimal level of health is important in reducing the number and severity of respiratory symptoms. Prevention of respiratory infections is foremost in maintaining optimal health. Providing cardiopulmonary-related health information (Box 39–13) is an important nursing responsibility and part of a primary health care model.

Vaccinations. Annual influenza vaccines are recommended for children 6 to 23 months of age, older clients, and clients with chronic illnesses (Health Canada, 2005). This includes clients older than 65 years of age; clients of any age with chronic disease of the heart, lung, or kidneys; clients with diabetes; and clients with immunosuppression or severe forms of anemia. The vaccine is also recommended for people in close or frequent contact with anyone in the high-risk groups. In Canada, flu season occurs from November to April, and it is estimated that 10% to 25% of Canadians may get the flu each year (Health Canada, 2005). Although most individuals recover completely, an estimated 4000 to 8000 Canadians, mostly older adults, die every year from pneumonia related to the flu (Health Canada, 2005). Many others may die from other serious complications of the flu (Health Canada, 2005). After the vaccination, antibodies develop against the strains of the virus (Health Canada, 2005). The antibodies are effective for 4 to 6 months (Health Canada, 2005). The vaccine is most effective in reducing the severity of illness and the risk of serious complications and of death (Centers for Disease Control [CDC], 2006).

The value of vaccination of immunocompromised clients is not completely understood. HIV-positive clients may receive the flu vaccine; however, they may require a second vaccine to gain protection. People who should not be vaccinated include those with a known hypersensitivity to eggs or other components of the vaccine and adults with an acute febrile illness. The vaccines are formulated annually on the basis of worldwide surveillance data.

Pneumococcal vaccine is recommended for clients at increased risk of developing pneumonia, those with chronic illnesses or immunosuppression (such as HIV/AIDS), those living in special environments such as long-term care facilities, and clients over the age of 65 years (CDC, 2006).

BOX 39-13 CLIENT TEACHING

Cardiovascular Disease

Objectives

- Client will be able to describe the risk factors associated with cardiovascular disease.
- Client will be able to demonstrate health promotion behaviours.

Teaching Strategies

- Explain to the client about modifying risk factors, such as quitting smoking, reducing alcohol intake, and modifying high-fat and high-carbohydrate diets.
- Inform the client about other risk factors for cardiovascular disease, such as diabetes, obesity, physical inactivity, stress, and oral contraceptives.
- Discuss with the client the importance of regular blood pressure and blood cholesterol monitoring (total cholesterol, high-density lipoprotein, low-density lipoprotein, and triglyceride levels).
- Educate the client about low-fat, low-salt, and calorie-appropriate diets. Provide sample menus.
- Educate the client about the benefits of exercising for 30–60 minutes a day to help reduce weight and lower blood pressure. Help the client develop an exercise program.

Evaluation

- Ask the client to describe the modifiable and nonmodifiable risk factors for cardiovascular disease.
- Ask the client to verbalize strategies for balanced nutrition.
- Obtain client's weight and blood pressure.
- Monitor the client's serum cholesterol (total, high- and low-density lipids) and triglyceride levels.

Both the influenza vaccine and pneumococcal vaccine can be administered to pregnant women after the first trimester. However, in all cases, it is important to consult the client's obstetrician before administering either vaccine.

Healthy Lifestyle Behaviour. Identification and elimination of risk factors for cardiopulmonary disease is an important part of primary health care. Encourage clients to eat a healthy, low-fat, high-fibre diet; monitor their cholesterol, triglyceride, high-density lipoprotein (HDL), and low-density lipoprotein (LDL) levels; reduce stress; exercise; and maintain a body weight in proportion to their height.

Elimination of cigarettes and other tobacco products, reduction of pollutants, monitoring of air quality, and adequate hydration are additional healthy behaviours. Clients should be encouraged to examine their habits and make changes to achieve their goals.

Exercise is a key factor in promoting and maintaining a healthy heart and lungs. Clients should be encouraged to exercise three to four times a week for 20 to 30 minutes. Aerobic exercise is necessary to improve lung function, strengthen muscles, and achieve the desired outcome. Walking is one of the most efficient ways to achieve a good aerobic workout. Many shopping malls have programs that allow people to enter the mall before the shops open and use the enclosed area for walking. Some even have measured the distances to help people plan their activity and measure their progress. Clients should be taught how to take their pulse and pace themselves. It is better to walk 15 minutes every day than to walk to exhaustion to achieve a goal. Clients should plan a time interval and walk for the designated time. Gradually, they will notice that the distance increases as their endurance and fitness improve.

Clients with cardiopulmonary alterations need to minimize their risk for infection, especially during the winter months. Teach clients to avoid large, crowded places; to keep their mouth and nose covered; and to be sure to dress warmly, including a scarf, hat, and gloves. This is especially important during the peak of the influenza season.

Clients with known cardiac disease and those with multiple risk factors should be cautioned to avoid exertion in cold weather. Shovelling snow is especially risky and has been known to precipitate a cardiac event in many clients. Other activities such as hanging holiday lights and decorations in the extreme cold can precipitate chest pain and bronchospasm. Advise clients to avoid alcohol, because it blunts the respiratory drive when used in excess and may contribute to exposure to the cold by making the client feel warm when the client is really not protected.

Clients should also be taught to plan for the hot summer months. Activities should be limited to early in the day or late in the evening, when temperatures are lower. Clients should take care to maintain adequate hydration and sodium intake; this is especially true for those clients taking diuretics. Caffeinated and alcoholic beverages should be limited or avoided completely, because they act as diuretics and can contribute to dehydration.

Environmental Pollutants. Avoiding exposure to second-hand smoke is essential to maintaining optimal cardiopulmonary function. Most businesses and restaurants now ban smoking or have separate areas designated as smoking areas. If clients are exposed to second-hand smoke in their home environments, counselling and support may be necessary to assist the smoker in successful smoking cessation or alterations in behaviour patterns, such as smoking outside.

Exposure to chemicals and pollutants in the work environment must also be considered. Clients such as farmers, painters, carpenters, and others benefit from the use of particulate filter masks to reduce inhalation of particles.

Acute Care

Clients with acute pulmonary illnesses require nursing interventions directed toward halting the pathological process (e.g., respiratory tract infection), shortening the duration and severity of the illness (e.g., hospitalization with pneumonia), and preventing complications from the illness or treatments (e.g., nosocomial infection resulting from invasive procedures).

Dyspnea Management. Dyspnea is difficult to quantify and to treat. Treatment modalities need to be individualized for each client, and more than one therapy is usually implemented. The underlying process that causes or worsens dyspnea must be treated and stabilized initially, then four additional therapies—pharmacological measures, oxygen therapy, physical techniques, and psychosocial techniques—are implemented. Pharmacological agents may include bronchodilators, steroids, mucolytics, and low-dose antianxiety medications. Oxygen therapy can reduce dyspnea associated with exercise. Physical techniques, such as cardiopulmonary reconditioning through exercise, breathing techniques, and cough control, can help to reduce dyspnea. Relaxation techniques, biofeedback, and meditation are physiological measures that the client can use to help lessen the sensation of dyspnea.

Airway Maintenance. The airway is patent when the trachea, bronchi, and large airways are free from obstruction. Airway maintenance requires adequate hydration to prevent thick, tenacious secretions. Proper coughing techniques remove secretions and keep the airway open. A variety of interventions, such as suctioning, chest physiotherapy, and nebulizer therapy, assist the client in managing alterations in airway clearance.

Mobilization of Pulmonary Secretions. The ability of a client to mobilize pulmonary secretions may make the difference between a short-term illness and a long recovery involving complications. Nursing interventions that promote mobilization of pulmonary secretions help the client to achieve and maintain a clear airway, and encourage lung expansion and gas exchange.

Humidification. **Humidification** is the process of adding water to gas. Temperature is the most important factor affecting the amount of water vapour a gas can hold. The percentage of water in the gas in relation to its capacity for water is the relative humidity. Air or oxygen with a high relative humidity keeps the airways moist and helps loosen and mobilize pulmonary secretions. Humidification is necessary for clients receiving oxygen therapy at >4 L/minute. Bubbling oxygen through water can add humidity to the oxygen delivered to the upper airways, as with a nasal cannula or face mask.

An oxygen hood is used for infants and a humidity tent is used for children with illnesses such as croup and tracheitis to liquefy secretions and assist in the reduction of fever (Hockenberry & Wilson, 2007). To prevent nonhumidified air or oxygen from entering the tent, the nebulizer at the top of the humidity tent remains filled with water. Air in the humidity tent can become cool and may fall below 20°C, thus causing the child to become chilled. Children in humidity tents require frequent changes of clothing and bed linen to remain dry and warm.

Nebulization. **Nebulization** is a process of adding moisture or medications to inspired air by mixing particles of varying sizes with the air. A nebulizer uses the aerosol principle to suspend a maximum number of water drops or particles of the desired size in inspired air. The moisture added to the respiratory system through nebulization improves clearance of pulmonary secretions. Nebulization is often used for administration of bronchodilators and mucolytic agents.

When the thin layer of fluid that supports the mucous layer over the cilia is allowed to dry, the cilia are damaged and cannot adequately clear the airway. Humidification through nebulization enhances mucociliary clearance, the body's natural mechanism for removing mucus and cellular debris from the respiratory tract.

Chest Physiotherapy. **Chest physiotherapy (CPT)** is a group of therapies used in combination to mobilize pulmonary secretions. These therapies include postural drainage, chest percussion, and vibration. CPT should be followed by productive coughing and suctioning of the client who has a decreased ability to cough. CPT is recommended for clients who produce greater than 30 mL of sputum per day or have evidence of atelectasis by chest X-ray examination. This procedure can be safely used with infants and young children; however, conditions and diseases unique to children may at times contraindicate this procedure. CPT is used for a select group of clients. Box 39–14 describes the guidelines for determining if CPT is indicated for the client.

Chest percussion involves striking the chest wall over the area being drained. The hand is positioned so that the fingers and thumb touch and the hands are cupped (Figure 39–9). Percussion on the surface of the chest wall sends waves of varying amplitude and frequency through the chest, changing the consistency and location of the sputum. Chest percussion is performed by striking the chest wall alternately with cupped hands (Figure 39–10). Percussion is performed over a single layer of clothing, not over buttons, snaps, or zippers. The single layer of clothing prevents slapping the client's skin. Thicker or multiple layers of material dampen the vibrations.

Percussion is contraindicated in clients with bleeding disorders, osteoporosis, or fractured ribs. It is important to percuss the lung

➤ BOX 39-14 Guidelines for Chest Physiotherapy

Nursing care and selection of chest physiotherapy (CPT) skills are based on specific assessment findings. The following guidelines are designed to help in physical assessment and subsequent decision making:

- Know the client's normal range of vital signs. Conditions such as atelectasis and pneumonia requiring CPT can affect vital signs. The degree of change is related to the level of hypoxia, overall cardiopulmonary status, and tolerance to activity.
- Know the client's medications. Certain medications, particularly diuretics and antihypertensives, cause fluid and hemodynamic changes. These changes may decrease the client's tolerance to the positional changes of postural drainage. Steroid medications increase the client's risk of pathological rib fractures and often contraindicate rib shaking.
- Know the client's medical history. Certain conditions such as increased intracranial pressure, spinal cord injuries, and abdominal aneurysm resection contraindicate the positional changes of postural drainage. Thoracic trauma or surgery may also contraindicate percussion, vibration, and rib shaking.
- Know the client's level of cognitive function. Participation in controlled coughing techniques requires the client to follow instructions. Congenital or acquired cognitive limitations may alter the client's ability to learn and participate in these techniques.
- Be aware of the client's exercise tolerance. CPT manoeuvres are fatiguing. When the client is not used to physical activity, initial tolerance for the manoeuvres may be decreased. However, with gradual increases in activity and planned CPT, client tolerance for the procedure will improve.

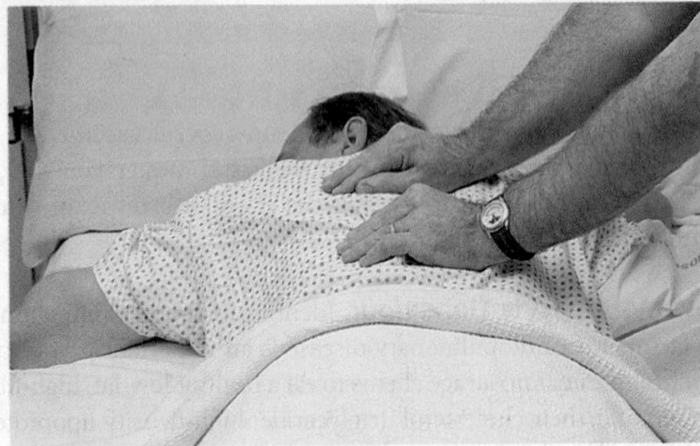

Figure 39-9 Hand position for chest wall percussion during chest physiotherapy.

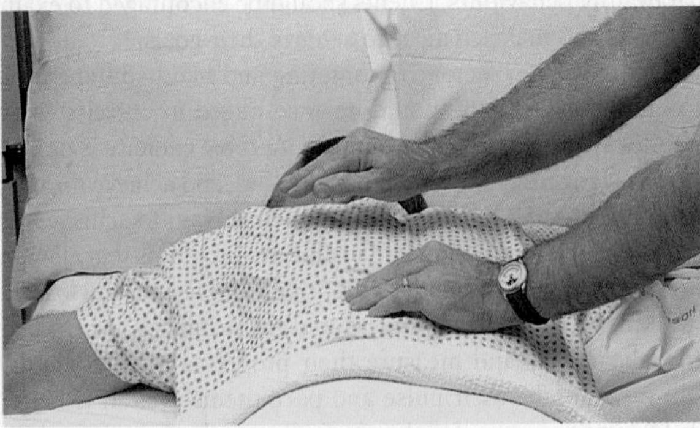

Figure 39-10 Chest wall percussion, alternating hand clapping against the client's chest wall.

fields and not the scapular regions, or trauma may occur to the skin and underlying musculoskeletal structures.

Vibration is a fine, shaking pressure applied to the chest wall only during exhalation. This technique is thought to increase the velocity and turbulence of exhaled air, facilitating secretion removal. Vibration increases the exhalation of trapped air and may shake mucus loose and induce a cough.

Postural drainage is the use of positioning techniques that draw secretions from specific segments of the lungs and bronchi into the trachea. Coughing or suctioning normally removes secretions from the trachea. The procedure for postural drainage can include most lung segments (Table 39–8). Because clients may not require postural drainage of all lung segments, the procedure is based on clinical assessment findings. For example, clients with left lower lobe atelectasis may require postural drainage of only the affected region, whereas a child with cystic fibrosis may require postural drainage of all lung segments.

Suctioning Techniques. Suctioning is necessary when a client is unable to clear respiratory tract secretions with coughing. The suctioning techniques include oropharyngeal and nasopharyngeal suctioning, orotracheal and nasotracheal suctioning, and suctioning of an artificial airway.

These techniques are based on common principles. In most cases, use sterile technique for suctioning because the oropharynx and trachea are considered sterile. The mouth is considered clean, thus the suctioning of oral secretions should be performed after suctioning of the oropharynx and trachea. Each type of suctioning requires the use of a rounded-tipped catheter with a number of side holes at the distal end of the catheter. Frequency of suctioning is determined by client assessment and need. If secretions are identified by inspection or auscultation techniques, suctioning is required. Because sputum is not produced continuously or every 1 or 2 hours but occurs as a response to a pathological condition, there is no rationale for routine suctioning of all clients every 1 to 2 hours. In addition, suctioning reduces the amount of the available dead space in the oropharynx and trachea, often resulting in significant desaturation. Be careful to monitor the client to ensure adequate oxygenation. Too-frequent suctioning can put the client at risk for development of hypoxemia, hypotension, arrhythmias, and possible trauma to the mucosa of the lungs (Day et al., 2002).

Oropharyngeal and Nasopharyngeal Suctioning. The oropharynx extends behind the mouth from the soft palate above the level of the hyoid bone and contains the tonsils. The nasopharynx is located behind the nose and extends to the level of the soft palate. Oropharyngeal or nasopharyngeal suctioning is used when the client is able to cough effectively but is unable to clear secretions by expectorating or swallowing. The suction procedure is used after the client has coughed (Skill 39–1). As the amount of pulmonary secretions is reduced and the client is less fatigued, the client may be able to expectorate or swallow the mucus, and suctioning is no longer required.

Orotracheal and Nasotracheal Suctioning. Orotracheal or nasotracheal suctioning is necessary when the client with pulmonary secretions is unable to manage secretions by coughing and does not have an artificial airway (see Skill 39–1). A catheter is passed through the mouth or nose into the trachea. The nose is the preferred route because stimulation of the gag reflex is minimal. The procedure is similar to nasopharyngeal suctioning, but the catheter tip is moved farther into the client's trachea. The entire procedure from catheter passage to its removal should be done quickly, lasting no longer than 15 seconds (American Association of Respiratory Care [AARC], 2004). Unless in respiratory distress, the client should be allowed to rest between passes of the catheter. If the client is using supplemental oxygen, the oxygen cannula or mask should be replaced during rest periods.

Tracheal Suctioning. Tracheal suctioning is accomplished through an artificial airway such as an endotracheal tube or tracheostomy tube (see Skill 39–1). The suction catheter should be no greater than one-half the size of the internal diameter of the artificial airway (Moore, 2003). Secretion removal should be as atraumatic as possible. To avoid trauma to the mucosa of the lung, never apply suction pressure while inserting the catheter, and maintain suction pressure between 120 and 150 mm Hg (AARC, 2004). Apply suction intermittently as the catheter is withdrawn. Rotating the catheter will enhance removal of secretions that have adhered to the sides of the endotracheal tube. Apply a mask and goggles, and wear a barrier gown to prevent splashes with body fluids.

The practice of normal saline instillation (NSI) into artificial airways to improve secretion removal is inconclusive. Clinical studies comparing suctioning after NSI with standard suctioning have not demonstrated any clinical or significant results (Akgul & Akyolcu, 2002; Moore, 2003). More recently, some clinicians have recommended that instillation of isotonic sodium chloride before suctioning of an endotracheal tube not be used as routine or standard clinical practice (Akgul & Kanan, 2006). There are anecdotal results supporting the theory that NSI stimulates the client to cough, thus loosening and dislodging the airway secretions. However, the practice of NSI via an endotracheal tube may decrease oxygen saturation, increase intracranial pressure and arterial blood pressure, and cause cardiac dysrhythmias, cardiac arrest, respiratory arrest, and nosocomial infection (Akgul & Kanan, 2006).

The two current methods of suctioning are the open and closed methods. Open suctioning involves a sterile catheter that is opened at the time of suctioning. Wear sterile gloves to perform the suction procedure. Closed suctioning involves a multiple-use suction catheter encased in a plastic sheath (Figure 39–11). Closed suctioning is most often used on clients who require mechanical ventilation to support their respiratory efforts, because it permits continuous delivery of oxygen while suction is performed, thus reducing the risk of oxygen desaturation. Although sterile gloves are not required in this procedure, at least nonsterile (i.e., disposable) gloves are recommended to prevent contact with splashes from body fluids.

Artificial Airways. An artificial airway is indicated for clients with a decreased level of consciousness or an airway obstruction and to aid in the removal of tracheobronchial secretions.

Oral Airway. The oral airway, the simplest type of artificial airway, prevents obstruction of the trachea by displacement of the tongue into the oropharynx (Figure 39–12). The oral airway extends from the teeth to the oropharynx, maintaining the tongue in the normal position. The correct-size airway must be used. Proper oral airway size is determined by measuring the distance from the corner of the mouth to the angle of the jaw just below the ear. The length is equal to the distance from the flange of the airway to the tip. If the airway is too small, the tongue is not held in the anterior portion of the mouth; if the airway is too large, it may force the tongue toward the epiglottis and obstruct the airway.

Insert the airway by turning the curve of the airway toward the cheek and placing it over the tongue. When the airway is in the oropharynx, turn it so that the opening points downward. When correctly placed, the airway moves the tongue forward away from the oropharynx, and the flange, the flat portion of the airway, rests against the client's teeth. Incorrect insertion merely forces the tongue back into the oropharynx.

➤ TABLE 39-8 Positions for Postural Drainage

Lung Segment	Position of Client
Adult	
Bilateral	High-Fowler's position
Apical segments Right upper lobe—anterior segment	Supine with head of bed elevated 15–30 degrees
Left upper lobe—anterior segment	Supine with head elevated
Right upper lobe—posterior segment	Side lying with right side of chest elevated on pillows
Left upper lobe—posterior segment	Side lying with left side of chest elevated on pillows
Right middle lobe—anterior segment	Three-fourths supine position with dependent lung in Trendelenburg's position
Right middle lobe—posterior segment	Prone with thorax and abdomen elevated
Both lower lobes—anterior segments	Supine in Trendelenburg's position
Left lower lobe—lateral segment	Right side lying in Trendelenburg's position
Right lower lobe—lateral segment	Left lateral in Trendelenburg's position
Right lower lobe—posterior segment	Prone in Trendelenburg's position with abdomen and thorax elevated
Both lower lobes—posterior segments	Prone in Trendelenburg's position with abdomen and thorax elevated
Child	
Bilateral—apical segments	Sitting on nurse's lap, leaning slightly forward, flexed over pillow
Bilateral—middle anterior segments	Sitting on nurse's lap, leaning against nurse
Bilateral lobes—anterior segments	Lying supine on nurse's lap, back supported with pillow

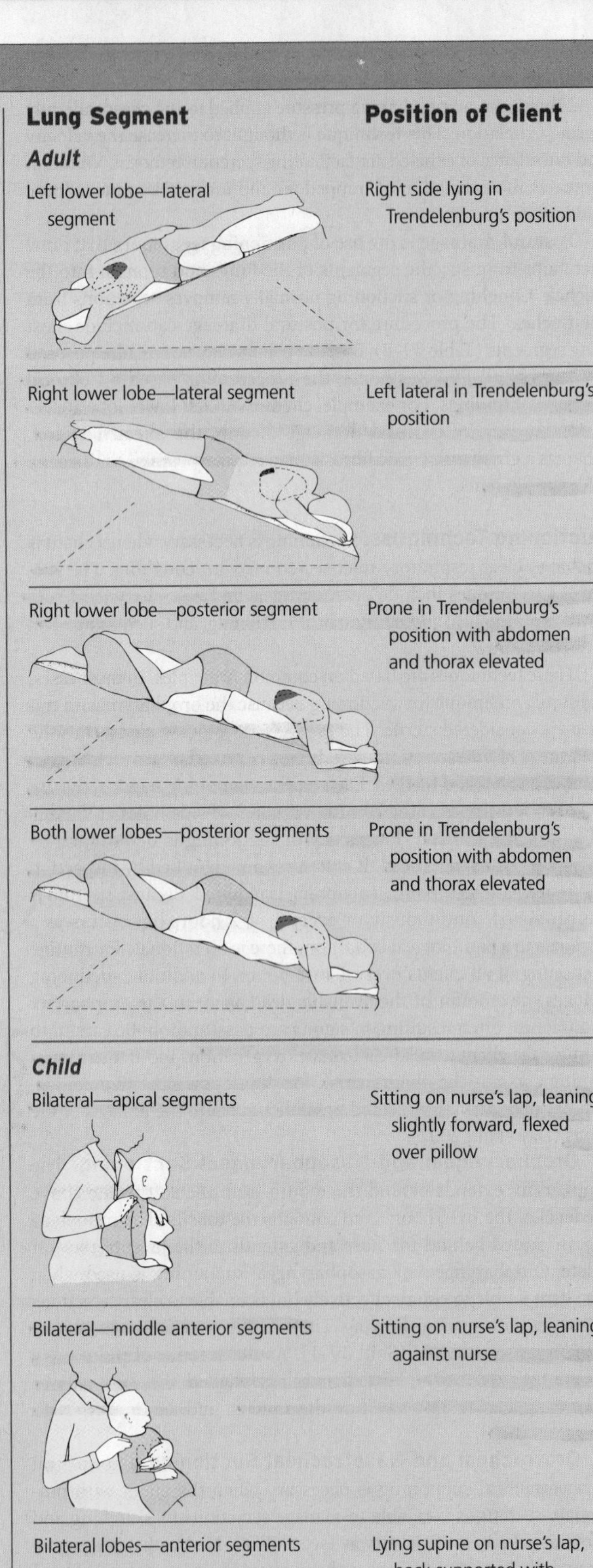

➤ SKILL 39-1 Suctioning

video

Delegation Considerations

This skill may be delegated to unregulated care providers (UCPs) in special situations. When you determine that the client is stable, the skill of performing suctioning of an established tracheostomy can be delegated to a UCP when the client has a permanent tracheostomy tube or is receiving home mechanical ventilation. Before delegating this skill, you must do the following:

- Discuss with the care provider any unique modifications of the skill, such as the need to reapply any supplemental oxygen equipment following the procedure.
- Instruct the UCP to report any change in the client's respiratory status, secretion colour or volume, or unresolved coughing or gagging.
- Instruct the UCP to report any change in client's colour, vital signs, or complaints of pain.

Equipment

- Appropriate-size suction catheter (smallest diameter that will remove secretions effectively) or Yankauer catheter (oral suction)
- Nasal or oral airway (if indicated)
- Two sterile gloves or one sterile and one clean disposable glove (refer to technique)
- Clean towel or paper drape
- Portable or wall suction
- Mask or face shield
- Connecting tube (1.8 metres)
- Pulse oximeter and stethoscope

Equipment for Procedure Without Closed-Suction Catheter

- Small Y adapter (if catheter does not have a suction-control port)
- Water-soluble lubricant
- Sterile basin
- Sterile normal saline solution or water (approximately 100 mL)

Procedure

STEPS	RATIONALE
1. Assess for signs and symptoms of upper and lower airway obstruction requiring nasotracheal or orotracheal suctioning, abnormal respiratory rate, adventitious sounds, nasal secretions, gurgling, drooling, restlessness, gastric secretions, or vomitus in mouth, and coughing without clearing secretions from airway.	• Physical signs and symptoms result from decreased oxygen to tissues, as well as pooling of secretions in upper and lower airways. Complete assessment before and after suction procedure (Moore, 2003).
2. Assess signs and symptoms associated with hypoxia and hypercapnia: decreased SpO_2, increased pulse and blood pressure, increased respiratory rate, apprehension, anxiety, decreased ability to concentrate, lethargy, decreased level of consciousness (especially acute), increased fatigue, dizziness, behavioural changes (especially irritability), dysrhythmias, pallor, and cyanosis.	• Physical signs and symptoms resulting from decreased oxygen to tissues indicate need for suctioning.
3. Determine factors that normally influence upper or lower airway functioning:	
• Fluid status	• Fluid overload may increase amount of secretions. Dehydration promotes thicker secretions.
• Lack of humidity	• The environment influences secretion formation and gas exchange, necessitating airway suctioning when the client cannot clear secretions effectively.
• Pulmonary disease, chronic obstructive pulmonary disorder, pulmonary infection	• Increases client's risk for retaining pulmonary secretions. Clients with respiratory infections are prone to increased secretions that are thicker and sometimes more difficult to expectorate.
• Anatomy	• Abnormal anatomy can impair normal drainage of secretions. For example, nasal swelling, a deviated septum, or facial fractures may impair nasal drainage. Tumours in or around the lower airway may impair secretion removal by occluding or externally compressing the lumen of the airway.
• Changes in level of consciousness	• Impairs client's ability to cough independently or follow instructions to cough and clear airway.
• Decreased cough or gag reflex	• Increases client's risk for aspiration and subsequent pulmonary infection.
4. Identify contraindications to nasotracheal suctioning: occluded nasal passages; nasal bleeding, epiglottitis, or croup; acute head, facial, or neck injury or surgery, coagulopathy, or bleeding disorder; irritable airway or laryngospasm or bronchospasm; gastric surgery with high anastomosis; myocardial infarction (American Association of Respiratory Care [AARC], 2004).	• These conditions are contraindicated because the passage of the catheter through the nasal route causes trauma to existing facial trauma or surgery, increases nasal bleeding, or causes severe bleeding in the presence of bleeding disorders. With epiglottitis, croup, laryngospasm, or irritable airway, the entrance of a suction catheter via the nasal route causes intractable coughing, hypoxemia, and severe bronchospasm, necessitating emergency intubation or tracheostomy (Moore, 2003).

Continued

➤ SKILL 39-1 Suctioning *continued*

STEPS	RATIONALE
5. Examine sputum microbiology data.	• Certain bacteria are easier to transmit or require isolation because of virulence or antibiotic resistance.
6. Assess client's understanding of the procedure.	• Reveals need for client instruction and encourages cooperation.
7. Obtain physician's order if indicated by agency policy.	• Some institutions require a physician's order for tracheal suctioning.
8. Explain to client how the procedure will help clear the airway and relieve breathing problems and that temporary coughing, sneezing, gagging, or shortness of breath is normal. Encourage client to cough out secretions. Have client practice coughing, if able. Splint surgical incisions, if necessary.	• Encourages cooperation and minimizes risks, anxiety, and pain.
9. Explain the importance of coughing and encourage coughing during procedure.	• Facilitates secretion removal and may reduce frequency and duration of future suctioning.
10. Help client to assume a position comfortable for you and the client (usually semi-Fowler's or sitting upright with head hyperextended, unless contraindicated).	• Reduces stimulation of gag reflex, promotes client comfort and secretion drainage, and prevents aspiration. Position lessens strain on the nurse's back. Hyperextension facilitates insertion of the catheter into the trachea.
11. Place pulse oximeter on client's finger. Take reading and leave pulse oximeter in place.	• Provides baseline oxygen level to determine client's response to suctioning.
12. Place towel across client's chest.	• Reduces transmission of microorganisms by protecting gown from secretions.
13. Perform hand hygiene. Apply a face shield if splashing is likely.	• Reduces transmission of microorganisms.
14. Connect one end of connecting tubing to suction machine and place the other end in a convenient location near client. Turn suction device on and set vacuum regulator to appropriate negative pressure (120–150 mm Hg) (AARC, 2004). Appropriate pressure may vary; check institutional policy.	• Excessive negative pressure damages nasal pharyngeal and tracheal mucosa and induces greater hypoxia. • Negative pressures should not exceed 150 mm Hg, as higher pressures increases risk for airway trauma and atelectasis, and can induce greater hypoxia (AARC, 2004).
15. If indicated, increase supplemental oxygen therapy to 100% or as ordered by physician. Encourage client to deep breathe.	• Hyperoxygenation provides some protection from suction-induced decline in oxygenation. Hyperoxygenation is most effective in the presence of hyperinflation, such as when encouraging the client to deep breathe or to increase ventilator tidal volume settings (Bourgault et al., 2006; Moore, 2003).
16. Preparation for all types of suctioning:	
A. Open suction kit or catheter with use of aseptic technique. If a sterile drape is available, place it across the client's chest or on the overbed table. Do not allow the suction catheter to touch any nonsterile surfaces.	• Prepares catheter and prevents transmission of microorganisms. A sterile drape provides sterile surface on which to lay the suction catheter between passes, if needed.
B. Unwrap or open sterile basin and place on bedside table. Fill basin or cup with approximately 100 mL of sterile normal saline solution or water (see Step 16B illustration).	• Normal saline or water to flush catheter and tubing after each suction pass.
C. Turn on suction device. Set regulator to appropriate negative pressure: 100–150 mm Hg for adults (AARC, 2004).	

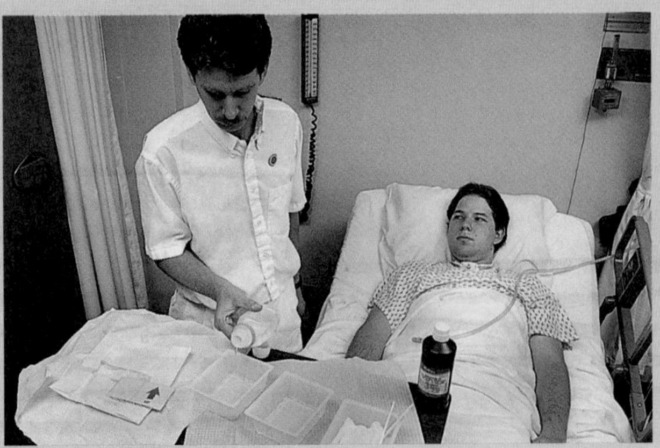

Step 16B Pouring sterile saline into basin.

➤ SKILL 39-1 **Suctioning** ***continued***

STEPS	RATIONALE
17. Suction airway.	
A. **Oropharyngeal suctioning**	
(1) Apply clean disposable glove to dominant hand. Apply mask or face shield.	• Suction of oral cavity does not require use of sterile gloves. Suction may cause splashing of body fluids.
(2) Attach suction catheter to connecting tubing. Check that equipment is functioning properly by suctioning a small amount of water or normal saline from the cup or basin.	
(3) Remove oxygen mask if present. Keep oxygen mask near client's face. Nasal cannula may remain in place (if present).	• Allows access to client's mouth. Reduces chances of hypoxia.

Critical Decision Point: Be prepared to quickly reapply oxygen mask if SpO_2 falls or respiratory distress develops during or at the end of suctioning.

STEPS	RATIONALE
(4) Insert catheter into the client's mouth. With suction applied, move catheter around mouth, including pharynx and gum line, until secretions are cleared.	• If catheter does not have a suction control to apply intermittent suction, take care not to allow suction tip to invaginate oral mucosal surfaces with continuous suction (Moore, 2003).
(5) Encourage client to cough, and repeat suctioning if needed. Replace oxygen mask if used.	• Coughing moves secretions from lower to upper airways into mouth.
(6) Suction water from basin through catheter until catheter is cleared of secretions.	• Clearing secretions before they dry reduces the probability of transmission of microorganisms and enhances delivery of preset suction pressures.
(7) Place catheter in a clean, dry area for reuse, with suction turned off, or within client's reach, with suction on, if client is capable of suctioning self.	• Facilitates prompt removal of airway secretions when suctioning is needed in the future.
B. **Nasopharyngeal and nasotracheal suctioning**	
(1) Open lubricant. Squeeze small amount onto open sterile catheter package without touching package.	• Prepares lubricant while maintaining sterility. Water-soluble lubricant is used to avoid lipoid aspiration pneumonia. Excessive lubricant can occlude the catheter.
(2) Apply sterile glove to each hand, or apply nonsterile glove to nondominant hand and sterile glove to dominant hand.	• Reduces transmission of microorganisms and allows nurse to maintain sterility of suction catheter.

Critical Decision Point: A clean technique is used in selected settings, such as the home or long-term care facility, and with clients with an established tracheostomy who do not have an airway infection.

STEPS	RATIONALE
(3) Pick up suction catheter with dominant hand without touching nonsterile surfaces. Pick up connecting tubing with nondominant hand. Secure catheter to tubing (see Step 17B(3) illustration).	• Maintains catheter sterility. Connects catheter to suction.
(4) Check that the equipment is functioning properly by suctioning a small amount of normal saline solution from the basin.	• Ensures equipment function; lubricates catheter and tubing.
(5) Lightly coat distal 6–8 cm of catheter with water-soluble lubricant.	• Lubricates catheter for easier insertion.
(6) Remove oxygen delivery device, if applicable, with non-dominant hand. *Without applying suction* and using dominant thumb and forefinger, gently insert catheter into naris during inhalation.	• Application of suction pressure while introducing catheter into nasopharyngeal tissues increases risk of damage to mucosa. When advanced into trachea, suction could damage mucosa and increase risk of hypoxia.

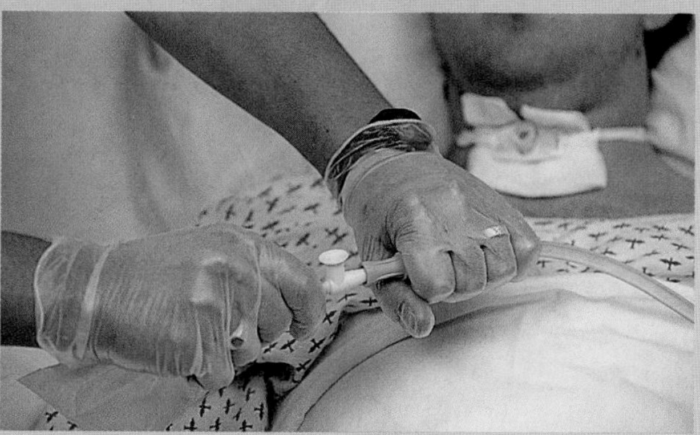

Step 17B(3) Attaching catheter to suction.

Continued

➤ SKILL 39-1 Suctioning *continued*

STEPS	RATIONALE
(7) *Nasopharyngeal:* Follow natural course of naris; slightly slant catheter downward and advance to back of pharynx. In adults, insert catheter about 16 cm; in older children, 8–12 cm; in infants and young children, 4–8 cm. The rule of thumb is to insert catheter a distance from tip of nose (or mouth) to base of earlobe.	• Proper placement ensures removal of pharyngeal secretions.
(a) Apply intermittent suction for up to 10–15 seconds by placing and releasing nondominant thumb over catheter vent. Slowly withdraw catheter while rotating it back and forth between thumb and forefinger.	• Intermittent suction safely removes pharyngeal secretions. Suction time of >15 seconds increases risk for suction-induced hypoxemia (Oh & Seo, 2003).
(8) *Nasotracheal:* Follow natural course of naris and advance catheter slightly slanted and downward to just above entrance into trachea. Allow client to take a breath. Quickly insert catheter approximately 16–20 cm (in adult) into trachea (see Step 17B(8) illustration). Client will begin to cough. *Note:* In older children, advance 14–20 cm; in young children and infants, 8–14 cm.	• Ensures catheter will be inserted into trachea with minimum stress to client.

Critical Decision Point: Insert catheter during client inhalation, especially if inserting catheter into trachea because epiglottis is open. *Do not insert during swallowing* or catheter will most likely enter the esophagus. *Never* apply suction during insertion. Client should cough. If client gags or becomes nauseated, catheter is most likely in the esophagus and must be removed.

(a) *Positioning option for nasotracheal suctioning:* In some instances, turning the client's head to the right will help you suction the left mainstem bronchus; turning head to the left will help you suction the right mainstem bronchus. If resistance is felt after insertion of catheter for maximum recommended distance, the catheter has probably hit carina. Pull the catheter back 1–2 cm before applying suction.	• Turning the client's head to the side elevates the bronchial passage on the opposite side and facilitates passage of the catheter.

Critical Decision Point: Use nasal approach and perform tracheal suctioning before pharyngeal suctioning whenever possible. The mouth and pharynx contain more bacteria than the trachea does. If copious oral secretions are present before beginning the procedure, suction the mouth with an oral suction device.

(b) Apply intermittent suction for up to 10–15 seconds by placing and releasing nondominant thumb over vent of catheter and slowly withdrawing catheter while rotating it back and forth between dominant thumb and forefinger. Encourage client to cough. Replace oxygen device, if applicable.	• Intermittent suction and rotation of catheter prevent injury to mucosa. If the catheter "grabs" mucosa, remove thumb to release suction. Suctioning longer than 10 seconds can cause cardiopulmonary compromise, usually from hypoxemia or vagal overload.

Critical Decision Point: If ordered to monitor client's vital signs and oxygen saturation during the procedure, note if there is a change of 20 beats/minute (either increase or decrease) or if pulse oximetry falls below 90% or 5% from baseline (Akgul & Akyolcu, 2002).

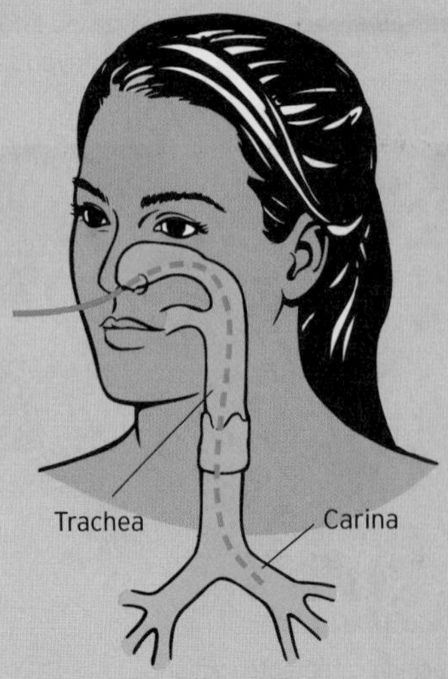

Step 17B(8) Distance of insertion of nasotracheal catheter.

➤ SKILL 39-1 Suctioning *continued*

STEPS	RATIONALE
(9) Rinse catheter and connecting tubing with normal saline or water until cleared.	• Removes secretions from catheter. Secretions that remain in suction catheter or connecting tubing decrease suctioning efficiency.
(10) Assess for need to repeat suctioning procedure. Allow adequate time (1–2 minutes) between suction passes for ventilation and oxygenation. Ask client to deep breathe and to cough.	• Observe for alterations in cardiopulmonary status. Suctioning can induce hypoxemia, dysrhythmias, laryngospasm, and bronchospasm. Deep breathing reventilates and reoxygenates alveoli and reduces the risk for suction-induced hypoxemia (Bourgault et al., 2006). Repeated passes clear the airway of excessive secretions but can also remove oxygen and may induce laryngospasm.
C. **Artificial airway suctioning**	
(1) Apply face shield.	• Reduces transmission of microorganisms.
(2) Apply one sterile glove to each hand, or apply nonsterile glove to nondominant hand and sterile glove to dominant hand.	• Reduces transmission of microorganisms and allows nurse to maintain sterility of suction catheter.
(3) Pick up suction catheter with dominant hand without touching nonsterile surfaces. Pick up connecting tubing with nondominant hand. Secure catheter to tubing.	• Maintains catheter sterility. Establishes suction.
(4) Check that equipment is functioning properly by suctioning a small amount of saline from the basin.	• Ensures equipment function; lubricates catheter and tubing.
(5) Hyperinflate or hyperoxygenate client, or do both, before suctioning, using manual resuscitation Ambu-bag connected to oxygen source on mechanical ventilator. Some mechanical ventilators have a button that, when pushed, delivers oxygen for a few minutes and then resets to the previous value.	• Hyperinflation decreases risk for atelectasis caused by negative pressure of suctioning (Moore, 2003). Preoxygenation converts a large proportion of resident lung gas to 100% oxygen to offset the amount used in metabolic consumption while ventilator or oxygenation is interrupted, and to offset volume lost during suction procedure (Bourgault et al., 2006; Day et al., 2002; Oh & Seo, 2003).
(6) If client is receiving mechanical ventilation, open swivel adapter or, if necessary, remove oxygen or humidity delivery device with nondominant hand.	• Exposes artificial airway.
(7) Without applying suction, gently but quickly insert catheter using dominant thumb and forefinger into artificial airway (it is best to time catheter insertion with inspiration) until resistance is met or client coughs, then pull back 1 cm.	• Application of suction pressure while introducing catheter into the trachea increases risk of damage to tracheal mucosa and greater hypoxia through removal of entrained oxygen present in airways. The action of pulling back stimulates cough and removes catheter from mucosal wall so that catheter is not resting against tracheal mucosa during suctioning.

Critical Decision Point: If unable to insert catheter past the end of the endotracheal tube, the catheter is probably caught in the Murphy eye (i.e., side hole at the distal end of the endotracheal tube that allows for collateral airflow in the event of main stem intubation). If this happens, rotate catheter to reposition it away from the Murphy eye, or withdraw it slightly and reinsert with the next inhalation. Usually the catheter meets resistance at the carina. One indication that the catheter is at the carina is acute onset of coughing, because the carina contains many cough receptors. The catheter should be pulled back 1 cm.

STEPS	RATIONALE
(8) Apply intermittent suction by placing and releasing nondominant thumb over vent of catheter; slowly withdraw catheter while rotating it back and forth between dominant thumb and forefinger (see Step 17C(8) illustration). Encourage client to cough. Watch for respiratory distress.	• Intermittent suction and rotation of catheter prevent injury to tracheal mucosal lining. If catheter "grabs" mucosa, remove thumb to release suction.

Critical Decision Point: If client develops respiratory distress during suction procedure, immediately withdraw catheter and supply additional oxygen and breaths as needed. Oxygen can be administered directly through the catheter in an emergency. Disconnect suction and attach oxygen at prescribed flow rate through the catheter.

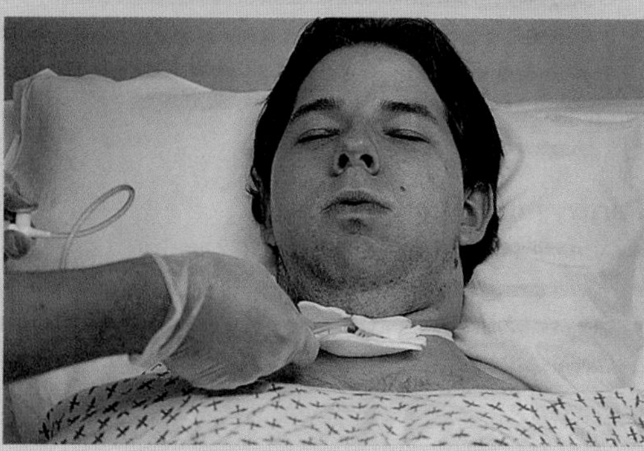

Step 17C(8) Suctioning tracheostomy.

Continued

➤ SKILL 39-1 Suctioning *continued*

STEPS	RATIONALE
(9) If client is receiving mechanical ventilation, close swivel adapter or replace oxygen delivery device.	• Re-establishes the artificial airway.
(10) Encourage client to deep breathe, if able. Some clients respond well to several manual breaths from the mechanical ventilator or Ambu-bag.	• Reoxygenates and re-expands alveoli. Suctioning can cause hypoxemia and atelectasis.
(11) Rinse catheter and connecting tubing with normal saline until clear. Use continuous suction.	• Removes catheter secretions. Secretions left in tubing decrease suction and provide environment for microorganism growth. Secretions left in connecting tube decrease suctioning efficiency.
(12) Assess client's cardiopulmonary status for secretion clearance and complications. Repeat Steps 17C(5) through 17C(11) once or twice more to clear secretions. Allow adequate time (at least 1 full minute) between suction passes for ventilation and reoxygenation. Perform oropharyngeal and nasopharyngeal suctioning (Steps 17A, 17B). After oropharyngeal and nasopharyngeal suctioning is performed, catheter is contaminated; do not reinsert into endotracheal or tracheostomy tube.	• Suctioning can induce dysrhythmias, hypoxia, and bronchospasm and impair cerebral circulation or adversely affect hemodynamics (Akgul & Akyolcu, 2002; Kerr et al., 1999). Repeated passes with suction catheter clear airway of excessive secretions and promote improved oxygenation. • The upper airway is considered clean and lower airway is considered sterile. Therefore, the same catheter can be used to suction from sterile to clean areas, but not from clean to sterile areas.
18. Complete procedure:	
A. Disconnect catheter from connecting tubing. Roll catheter around fingers of dominant hand. Pull glove off inside out so that catheter remains in glove. Pull off other glove over first glove in same way to contain contaminants. Discard into appropriate receptacle. Turn off suction device.	• Reduces transmission of microorganisms. Clean equipment should not be touched with contaminated gloves.
B. Remove towel and place in laundry or remove drape and discard in appropriate receptacle.	
C. Reposition client as indicated by condition. You may need to reapply clean gloves for client's personal care (e.g., oral hygiene).	• Proper positioning based on client's condition promotes comfort, encourages secretion drainage, and reduces risk of aspiration.
D. If indicated, readjust oxygen to original level.	• Helps client's blood oxygen level return to baseline.
E. Discard remainder of normal saline into appropriate receptacle. If basin is disposable, discard into appropriate receptacle. If basin is reusable, rinse and place in soiled utility room.	• Solution is contaminated.
F. Remove and discard face shield, and perform hand hygiene.	• Reduces transmission of microorganisms.
G. Place unopened suction kit on suction machine table or at head of bed according to institution preference.	• Provides for immediate access of suction catheter and equipment in the event of an emergency or for the next suctioning procedure.
19. Compare client's vital signs and SpO_2 saturation before and after suctioning.	• Identifies physiological effects of suction procedure to restore airway patency.
20. Ask client if breathing is easier and if congestion is decreased.	• Provides subjective confirmation that airway obstruction is relieved with suctioning procedure.
21. Observe airway secretions.	• Provides data to document presence or absence of respiratory tract infection.

Unexpected Outcomes and Related Interventions

Worsening Respiratory Status

- Limit length of suctioning.
- Determine need for more frequent suctioning, possibly of shorter duration.
- Notify physician.

Return of Bloody Secretions

- Determine amount of suction pressure used. It may need to be decreased.
- Evaluate suctioning frequency.
- Provide more frequent oral hygiene.

Unable to Pass Suction Catheter Through First Naris Attempted

- Try other naris or oral route.
- Insert nasal airway, especially if suctioning through client naris frequently.
- Guide catheter along naris floor to avoid turbinates.
- If obstruction is mucus, apply suction to relieve obstruction, but do not apply suction to mucosa. If obstruction is thought to be a blood clot, consult physician.
- Increase lubrication of catheter.

Paroxysms of Coughing

- Administer supplemental oxygen.
- Allow client to rest between passes of suction catheter.
- Consult physician regarding need for inhaled bronchodilators or topical anaesthetics.

➤ SKILL 39-1 **Suctioning** *continued*

No Secretions Obtained

- Evaluate client's fluid status.
- Assess for signs of infection.
- Determine need for chest physiotherapy.
- Assess adequacy of humidification on oxygen delivery device.

Recording and Reporting

- Record the amount, consistency, colour, and odour of secretions and client's response to procedure; document client's pre-suctioning and post-suctioning cardiopulmonary status.

Home Care Considerations

- You need to adhere to best practices for infection control while weighing cost-effectiveness in the setting of a chronic situation. If the client has an established tracheostomy or requires long-term nasotracheal suctioning and infection is not present, clean suction technique is appropriate.
- Instruct the client and family in infection-control measures for emptying the secretion jar. These secretions should be emptied in the toilet but they have a splash risk. Instruct the caregiver to apply a mask (shield if available) and gloves and bring the secretion jar as close to the toilet bowel as possible to decrease the risk of splash.

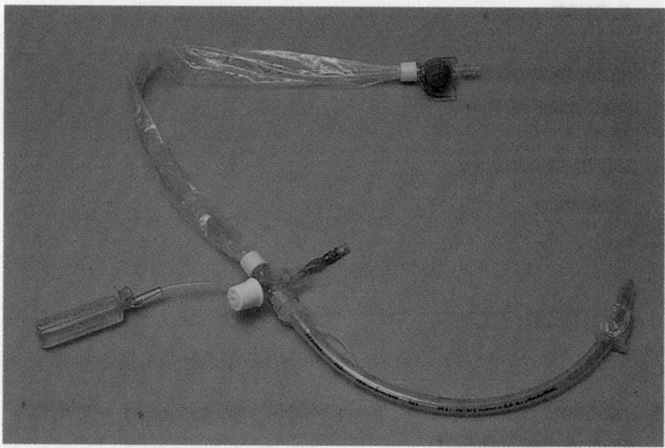

Figure 39-11 Ballard tracheal care, closed suction.

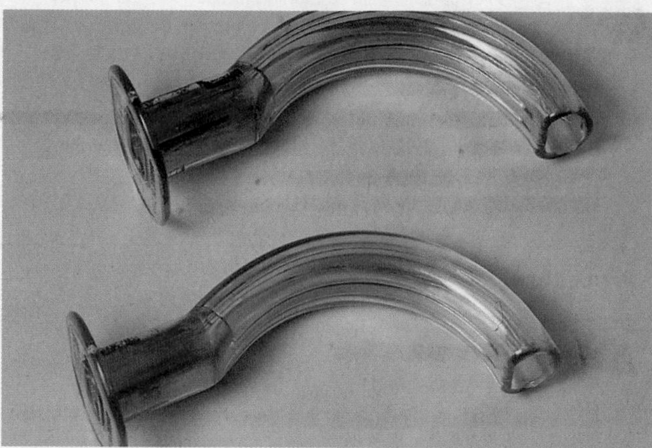

Figure 39-12 Artificial oral airways.

Endotracheal and Tracheal Airway. The presence of an artificial airway places the client at high risk for infection and airway injury. Use sterile technique in caring for and maintaining an artificial airway to prevent nosocomial infections. Artificial airways need to be cared for and maintained in the correct position to prevent airway damage (Skill 39–2).

Endotracheal (ET) tubes are used as short-term artificial airways to administer mechanical ventilation, relieve upper airway obstruction, protect against aspiration, or clear secretions. ET tubes are generally removed within 14 days; however, they may be used for a longer period of time if the client is showing progress toward weaning from mechanical ventilation and extubation.

If the client requires long-term assistance from an artificial airway, a tracheostomy is considered. A surgical incision is made into the trachea, and a short artificial airway (a tracheostomy tube) is inserted.

Maintenance and Promotion of Lung Expansion. Nursing interventions to maintain or promote lung expansion include noninvasive and invasive techniques. Noninvasive techniques include positioning and incentive spirometry. Invasive procedures include management of a chest tube.

Positioning. In the healthy, completely mobile person, adequate ventilation and oxygenation are maintained by frequent position changes during daily activities. However, when a person's illness or injury restricts mobility, there is an increased risk for respiratory impairment. Frequent changes of position are simple and cost-effective methods for reducing the risks of stasis of pulmonary secretions and decreased chest wall expansion.

The most effective position for clients with cardiopulmonary diseases is the 45-degree semi-Fowler's position, using gravity to assist in lung expansion and reduce pressure from the abdomen on the diaphragm. When the client uses this position, ensure that the client does not slide down in bed, which could reduce lung expansion. A client with unilateral lung disease (e.g., pneumothorax, atelectasis, pneumonia, thoracotomy, multiple trauma affecting one lung) should be positioned with the unaffected lung down ("good lung down"). This promotes better perfusion of the healthy lung, improving oxygenation. In the presence of pulmonary abscess or hemorrhage, the client should be placed with the affected lung down to prevent drainage toward the unaffected (healthy) lung.

Incentive Spirometry. **Incentive spirometry** is a method of encouraging voluntary deep breathing by providing visual feedback to clients about inspiratory volume. Incentive spirometry is used to promote deep breathing and to prevent or treat atelectasis in the post-operative client. The use of an incentive spirometer to promote lung expansion and thus prevent postoperative pulmonary complications following abdominal surgery is supported by research (Lawrence et al., 2006).

➤ SKILL 39-2 Care of an Artificial Airway

Delegation Considerations

This skill should not be routinely delegated to unregulated care providers (UCPs). It is your responsibility to perform endotracheal care. In some settings, clients who have well-established tracheostomy tubes may have the care delegated to UCPs. It is your responsibility to assess and ensure that proper artificial airway care is provided. In addition, UCPs may perform other aspects of the client's care. You must instruct the UCP about the following:

- To report any changes in the client's respiratory status, level of consciousness, confusion, or pain
- Emergency procedures in case the tracheostomy tube inadvertently becomes dislodged when ties are changed
- Expected drainage from tracheostomy

Equipment

Endotracheal (ET) Tube Care

- Towel
- ET and oropharyngeal suction equipment
- 2.5- to 3-cm adhesive or waterproof tape (not paper tape) or commercial ET tube holder (follow manufacturer's instructions for securing)
- Two pairs of disposable (nonsterile) gloves
- Adhesive remover swab or acetone on a cotton ball
- Mouth care supplies (e.g., toothbrush, toothpaste, mouth swabs)
- Face cleanser (e.g., wet washcloth, towel, soap, shaving supplies)
- Clean 2 × 2 gauze
- Tincture of benzoin or liquid adhesive
- Face shield (if indicated)

Tracheostomy Care

- Towel
- Tracheostomy suction supplies
- Sterile tracheostomy care kit, if available, or three sterile 4 × 4 gauze pads
- Sterile cotton-tipped applicators
- Sterile tracheostomy dressing
- Sterile basin
- Small sterile brush (or disposable cannula)
- Tracheostomy ties (e.g., twill tape, manufactured tracheostomy ties, Velcro tracheostomy ties)
- Hydrogen peroxide
- Normal saline (NS)
- Scissors
- Two sterile gloves
- Face shield, if indicated

Procedure

STEPS	RATIONALE
1. Perform pulmonary assessment:	
A. Auscultate lung sounds.	• Provides baseline information.
B. Assess condition and patency of airway and surrounding tissues.	• Indicates if additional skin care to irritated areas is needed. Identifies potential pressure areas.
C. Note type and size of tube, movement of tube, and cuff size.	• Movement of tube predisposes the client to tracheal trauma or tube dislodgement and may indicate the need for another size airway. Cuff size indicates the amount of air needed to properly inflate cuff. An underinflated cuff increases the client's risk for aspiration.
2. Explain procedure to the client and family.	• Reinforces information given to client and family and provides an opportunity for them to ask additional questions.
3. Position client. Clients usually prefer to be lying down. A client with a long-term well-established tracheostomy may be seated.	• Provides access to the site and facilitates completion of the procedure.
4. Place towel across client's chest.	• Reduces transmission of microorganisms and protects linens and bedclothes.
5. Perform hand hygiene.	• Reduces transmission of microorganisms.
6. Perform airway care.	
A. **Endotracheal tube care**	
(1) Observe for signs and symptoms of need to perform care of the artificial airway: (a) Soiled or loose tape (b) Pressure sores on nares, lip, or corner of mouth (c) Unstable tube (d) Excessive secretions	• A client with an artificial airway is at increased risk because of the inability to control secretions or difficulty in controlling them, and because of pressure points of the artificial airway.
(2) Identify factors that increase the risk of complications from ET tubes: (a) Type and size of tube (b) Movement of tube up and down trachea (c) Cuff size (d) Duration of placement	• A tube moving up and down the trachea predisposes the client to tracheal trauma or dislodgement. Cuff underinflation may allow aspiration, whereas overinflation causes tracheal mucosa injury (Hess, 2005).
(3) Suction ET tube (see Skill 39–1):	• Removes secretions. Diminishes client's need to cough during procedure.

Critical Decision Point: An oral airway should be immediately accessible in the event that the client bites down and obstructs the ET tube.

➤ SKILL 39-2 Care of an Artificial Airway *continued*

STEPS	RATIONALE
(a) Instruct client not to bite or move ET tube with tongue or pull on tubing; removal of tape can be uncomfortable.	• Prepares client for procedure and what to expect.
(b) Leave Yankauer suction catheter connected to suction source.	• Prepares for oropharyngeal suctioning.
(4) Prepare method to secure endotracheal tube (check agency policy).	• Adhesive tape must be placed around the head from cheek to cheek below the ears. Avoid placing it over the ears, as this may result in a pressure sore.
(a) *Tape method:* Cut piece of tape long enough to go completely around client's head from naris to naris plus 15 cm: for an adult, approximately 30–60 cm. Lay adhesive side up on bedside table. Cut and lay 8–15 cm of tape, adhesive side down, in centre of long strip to prevent tape from sticking to hair.	
(b) *Commercially available endotracheal tube holder:* Open package per manufacturer's instructions. Set device aside with the head guard in place and the Velcro strips open.	
(5) Apply gloves, and instruct assistant to apply gloves and hold ET tube firmly at client's lips. Note the number marking on the ET tube at the gum line.	• Reduces transmission of microorganisms. Maintains proper tube position and prevents accidental extubation.
(6) Remove old tape or device.	• Provides access to skin under tape for assessment and hygiene. Reduces transmission of microorganisms.
(a) *Tape:* Carefully remove tape from ET tube and client's face. If tape is difficult to remove, moisten it with water or adhesive tape remover. Discard tape in appropriate receptacle if nearby. If not, place soiled tape on bedside table or on distant end of towel.	
(b) *Commercially available device:* Remove Velcro strips from ET tube, and remove ET tube holder from client.	• Devices are latex free, fast, and convenient. They do not require tape, are easy to apply in the presence of facial hair, and reduce the risk of skin irritation. The Velcro strips secure the ET tube in place.
(7) Remove excess secretions or adhesive left on client's face.	• Promotes hygiene. Retained adhesive can cause damage to skin and prevent adhesion of new tape.
(8) Remove oral airway or bite block if present.	• Provides access and complete observation of client's oral cavity.

Critical Decision Point: Do not remove oral airway if client is actively biting. Wait until tape or device is partially or completely secured to ET tube.

STEPS	RATIONALE
(9) Clean mouth, gums, and teeth opposite ET tube with mouthwash solution and 4 × 4 gauze, sponge-tipped applicators, or saline swabs. Brush teeth as indicated. If necessary, administer oropharyngeal suctioning with Yankauer catheter.	• Provides oral hygiene and allows for observation of any pressure ulcers.
(10) Note "cm" ET tube marking at lips or gums. With help of assistant, move ET tube to opposite side or centre of mouth. Do not change tube depth.	• Prevents formation of pressure sores at sides of client's mouth. Ensures correct position of tube and allows for quick visual scan of displaced tube.
(11) Repeat oral cleaning as in Step (9) on opposite side of mouth.	• Removes secretions from mouth and oropharynx.
(12) Clean face and neck with soapy washcloth; rinse and dry. Shave male client as necessary.	• Moisture and beard growth prevent adhesive tape adherence.
(13) Use small amount of skin protectant or liquid adhesive on clean 2 × 2 gauze and dot on upper lip (oral ET tube) or across nose (nasal ET tube) and cheeks to ear. Allow tincture to dry completely.	• Protects and makes skin more receptive to tape.
(14) Secure ET tube.	
(a) *Tube method:*	
(a1) Slip tape under client's head and neck, adhesive side up. Do not twist tape or catch hair, or allow tape to stick to itself. It helps to stick tape gently to the tongue blade, which serves as a guide as tape is passed behind the client's head. Centre tape so that double-faced tape extends around the back of the neck from ear to ear.	• Positions tape to secure ET tube in proper position.

Continued

➤ SKILL 39-2 Care of an Artificial Airway *continued*

STEPS	RATIONALE
(a2) On one side of face, secure tape from ear to naris (nasal ET tube) or edge of mouth (oral ET tube). Tear remaining tape in half lengthwise, forming two pieces that are 1–2 cm wide. Secure bottom half of tape across upper lip (oral ET tube) or across top of nose (nasal ET tube; see Step 6A(14)(a2) illustration, part A). Wrap top half of tape around tube (see Step 6A(14)(a2) illustration, part B).	• Secures tape to face. Using top tape to wrap tube prevents downward drag on ET tube.
(a3) Gently pull other side of tape firmly to pick up slack, and secure it to remaining side of face (see Step 6A(14)(a3) illustration). Have assistant release hold when tube is secure. You may want the assistant to help reinsert the oral airway.	• Secures tape to face and ET tube. Tube should be at same depth at the lips. Check earlier assessment for verification of tube depth in centimetres.
(b) *Commercially available device:*	
(b1) Place ET tube through opening designed to secure ET tube. Ensure that pilot balloon to the ET tube is accessible.	• Commercially available holders have a slit in the front of the holder designed to secure the ET tube.
(b2) Place Velcro strips of ET holder under client at occipital region of the head.	• Ensures that the ET tube remains at the correct depth as determined during assessment.
(b3) Verify that ET tube is at the established position using the lip or gum line as a guide.	• The ET tube needs to be secure so that the position of the tube remains at the correct depth.
(b4) Secure Velcro strips at base of the client's head. Leave 1 cm slack in the strips.	
(b5) Verify that tube is secure, that it does not move forward from client's mouth or backward down into client's throat. Ensure that there are no pressure areas on oral mucosa or occipital region of the head.	
(15) Clean oral airway in warm, soapy water and rinse well. Hydrogen peroxide can aid in removal of crusted secretions. Shake excess water from oral airway.	• Promotes hygiene. Reduces transmission of microorganisms.
(16) For unconscious client, reinsert oral airway without pushing tongue into oropharynx.	• Prevents client from biting ET tube and allows access for oropharyngeal suctioning. An oral airway in a conscious, cooperative client may cause excessive gagging and pressure ulcers to the mouth and tongue.
B. Tracheostomy care	
(1) Observe for signs and symptoms of need to perform tracheostomy care: (a) Soiled or loose ties or dressing (b) Nonstable tube (c) Excessive secretions	• A client with a tracheostomy tube is at increased risk because of loss of natural airway protection of the upper airway.
(2) Suction tracheostomy (see Skill 39–1). Before removing gloves, remove soiled tracheostomy dressing and discard in glove with coiled catheter.	• Removes secretions so as not to occlude outer cannula while inner cannula is removed. Reduces need for client to cough. Prevents aspiration of retained secretions. • Disposal method helps to contain microorganisms.

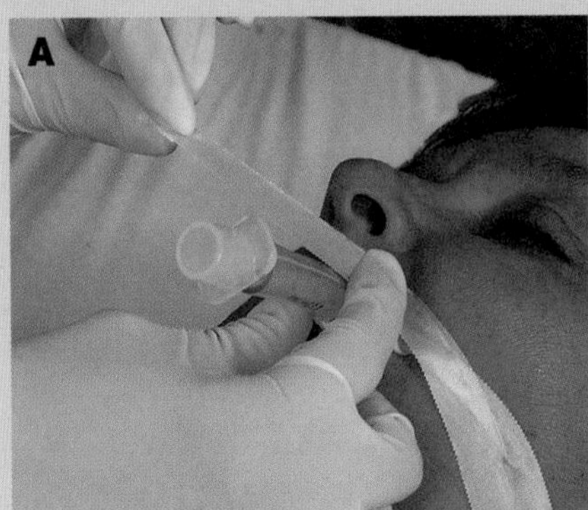

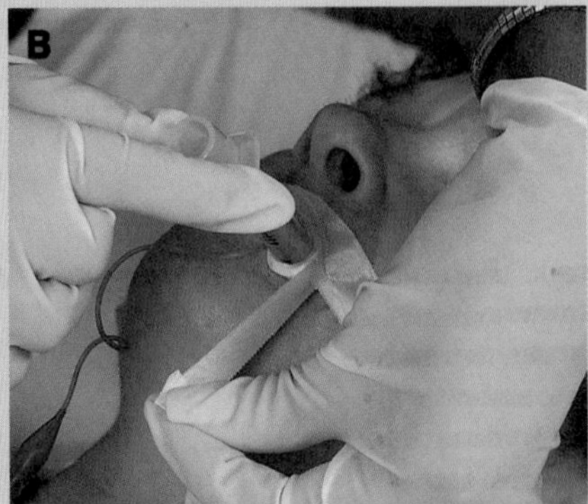

Step 6A(14)(a2) **A,** Securing bottom half of tape across client's upper lip. **B,** Securing top half of tape around tube.

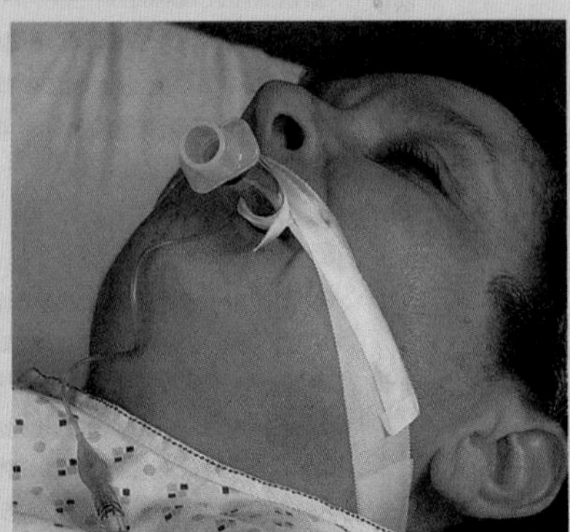

Step 6A(14)(a3) Tape securing ET tube.

➤ SKILL 39-2 Care of an Artificial Airway *continued*

STEPS	RATIONALE
(3) Prepare equipment:	
(a) Open sterile tracheostomy kit. Open three 4 × 4 inch gauze packages using aseptic technique, and pour normal saline (NS) on one package and hydrogen peroxide on another. Leave third package dry. Open two packages of cotton-tipped swabs and pour NS on one package and hydrogen peroxide on the other. Do not recap hydrogen peroxide and NS.	• Preparation and organization of equipment allows for efficient tracheostomy care and reconnecting of the client to an oxygen source in a timely manner.
(b) Open sterile tracheostomy dressing package.	
(c) Unwrap sterile basin and pour approximately 0.5–2 cm of hydrogen peroxide into it.	
(d) Open small sterile brush package and place aseptically into sterile basin.	
(e) Prepare length of twill tape long enough to go around client's neck two times, approximately 60–75 cm for an adult. Cut ends on diagonal. Lay aside in dry area.	• Cutting ends of tie on diagonal aids in inserting tie through eyelet.
(f) If using commercially available tracheostomy tube holder, open package according to manufacturer's directions.	
(4) Apply gloves. Keep dominant hand sterile throughout procedure.	• Reduces transmission of microorganisms.
(5) Remove oxygen source. Apply oxygen source loosely over tracheostomy if client desaturates during procedure.	• Helps reduce amount of desaturation.

Critical Decision Point: It is important to stabilize the tracheostomy tube at all times during tracheostomy care to prevent injury and unnecessary discomfort.

STEPS	RATIONALE
(6) If a *nondisposable inner cannula* is used:	
(a) While touching only the outer aspect of the tube, remove inner cannula with nondominant hand. Drop inner cannula into hydrogen peroxide basin.	• Removes inner cannula for cleaning. Hydrogen peroxide loosens secretions from inner cannula.
(b) Place tracheostomy collar or T tube and ventilator oxygen source over or near outer cannula. (*Note:* T tube and ventilator oxygen devices cannot be attached to all outer cannulas when inner cannula is removed.)	• Maintains supply of oxygen to client.
(c) To prevent oxygen desaturation in affected clients, quickly pick up inner cannula and use small brush to remove secretions inside and outside cannula (see Step 6B(6)(c) illustration).	• Tracheostomy brush provides mechanical force to remove thick or dried secretions.
(d) Hold inner cannula over basin and rinse with NS, using nondominant hand to pour.	• Removes secretions and hydrogen peroxide from inner cannula.
(e) Replace inner cannula and secure "locking" mechanism (see Step 6B(6)(e) illustration). Reapply ventilator or oxygen sources.	

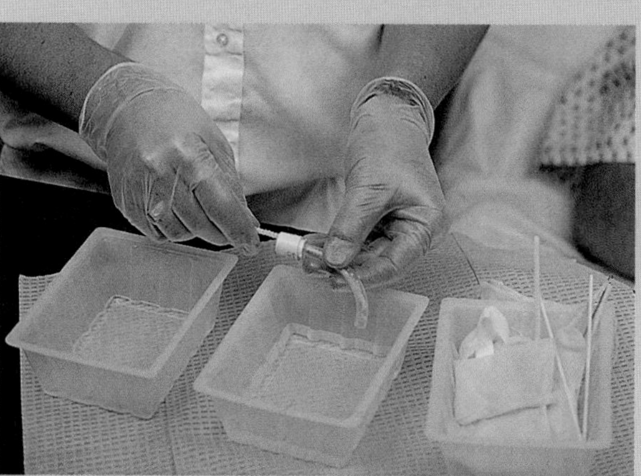

Step 6B(6)(c) Cleaning the tracheostomy inner cannula.

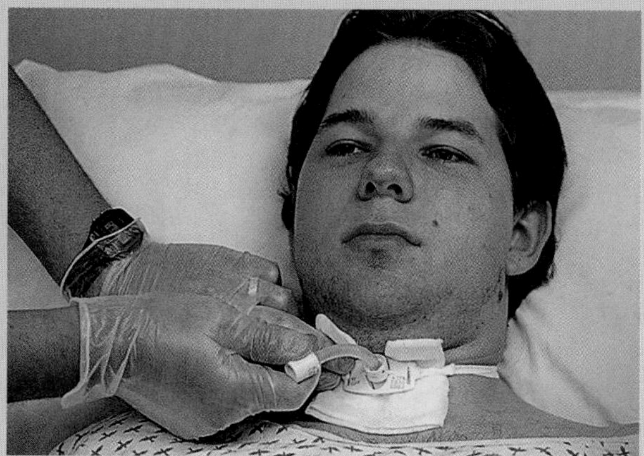

Step 6B(6)(e) Reinserting the inner cannula.

Continued

➤ SKILL 39-2 Care of an Artificial Airway *continued*

STEPS	RATIONALE
(7) If a *disposable inner cannula* is used:	
(a) Remove cannula from manufacturer's packaging.	
(b) While touching only the outer aspect of the tube, withdraw inner cannula and replace with new cannula. Lock into position.	
(c) Dispose of contaminated cannula in appropriate receptacle and apply oxygen source.	• Prevents unnecessary oxygen desaturation.
(8) Using hydrogen peroxide–prepared cotton-tipped swabs and 4 × 4 gauze, clean exposed outer cannula surfaces and stoma under faceplate, extending 5–10 cm in all directions from stoma (see Step 6B(8) illustration). Clean in circular motion from stoma site outward, using dominant hand to handle sterile supplies.	• Aseptically removes secretions from stoma site. Unless there are excessive tracheal secretions or drainage from the stoma, cleaning 1 or 2 times a day is sufficient (Lewarski, 2005).
(9) Using NS-prepared cotton-tipped swabs and 4 × 4 gauze, rinse hydrogen peroxide from tracheostomy tube and skin surfaces.	• Rinses hydrogen peroxide from surfaces, preventing possible irritation.
(10) Using dry 4 × 4 gauze, pat lightly at skin and exposed outer cannula surfaces.	• Dry surfaces prevent formation of moist environment conducive to growth of microorganisms and prevent skin excoriation.
(11) Secure tracheostomy.	
(a) *Tracheostomy tie method:*	
(a1) Instruct assistant, if available, to hold tracheostomy tube securely in place while ties are cut.	• Promotes hygiene, reduces transmission of microorganisms, and secures tracheostomy tube.

Critical Decision Point: Assistant must not release hold on tracheostomy tube until new ties are firmly tied to reduce risk of accidental extubation. If no assistant is present, do not cut old ties until new ties are in place and securely tied.

(a2) Take prepared tie and insert one end of tie through faceplate eyelet, and pull ends even (see Step 6B(11)(a2) illustration).

Critical Decision Point: Tracheostomy obturator should be kept at bedside with a fresh tracheostomy to facilitate reinsertion of the outer cannula, if dislodged. An additional tracheostomy tube of the same size and shape should be kept on hand for emergency replacement.

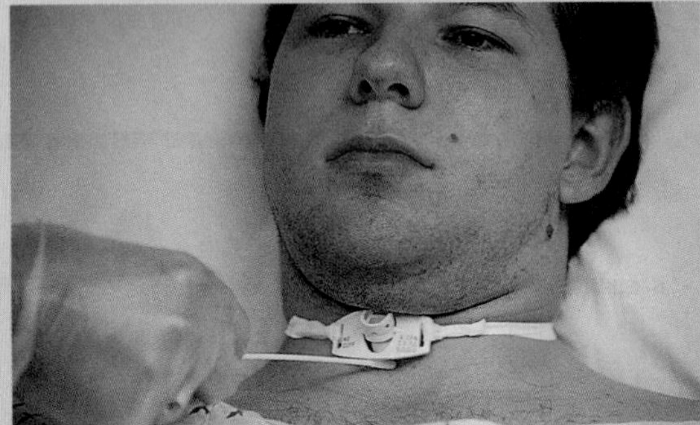

Step 6B(8) Cleansing around stoma.

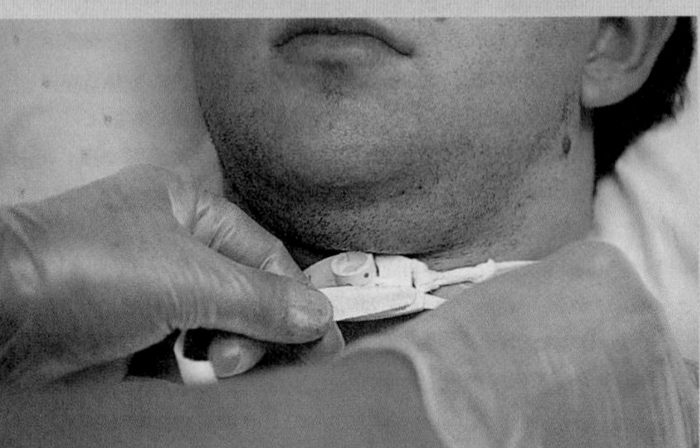

Step 6B(11)(a2) Replacing tracheostomy ties when an assistant is not available. Do not remove old tracheostomy ties until new ones are secure.

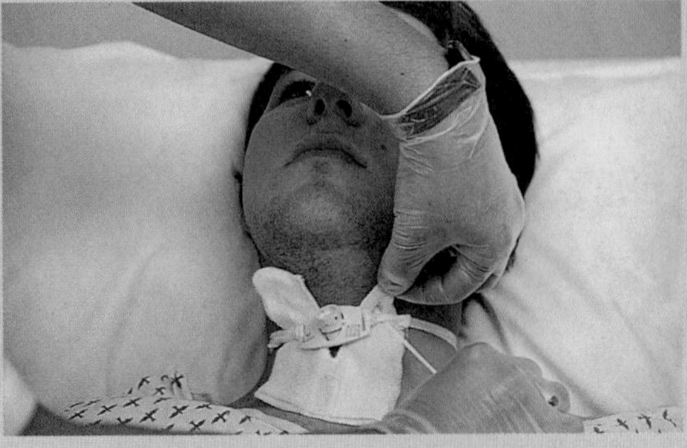

Step 6B(11)(a6) Applying tracheostomy dressing.

➤ SKILL 39-2 Care of an Artificial Airway ***continued***

STEPS	RATIONALE
(a3) Slide both ends of tie behind head and around neck to other eyelet, and insert one tie through second eyelet.	
(a4) Pull snugly.	• Secures tracheostomy tube in place.
(a5) Tie ends securely in double square knot, allowing space for only one finger in tie.	• One-finger slack prevents ties from being too tight when tracheostomy dressing is in place.
(a6) Insert fresh tracheostomy dressing under clean ties and faceplate (see Step 6B(11)(a6) illustration).	• Absorbs drainage. Dressing prevents pressure on clavicle heads.
(b) *Tracheostomy tube holder method:*	
(b1) While wearing gloves, maintain secure hold on tracheostomy tube. This can be done with an assistant, or, when an assistant is not available, by leaving the old tracheostomy tube holder in place until new device is secure.	• Prevents accidental displacement of tube.
(b2) Align strap under client's neck. Ensure that Velcro attachments are positioned on either side of tracheostomy tube.	
(b3) Place narrow end of ties under and through faceplate eyelets. Pull ends even, and secure with Velcro closures.	
(b4) Verify that there is space for only one loose or two snug finger width(s) under neck strap.	• Prevents skin necrosis.
7. Position client comfortably and assess respiratory status.	• Promotes comfort. Some clients may require post-tracheostomy care suctioning.
8. Replace any oxygen delivery devices.	• Maintains oxygen therapy.
9. Remove and discard gloves. Replace cap on hydrogen peroxide and normal saline. Perform hand hygiene.	• Reduces transmission of infection. Once opened, NS can be considered if free of bacteria for 24 hours, after which it should be discarded.
10. Compare respiratory assessments before and after procedure.	• Identifies any changes in presence and quality of breath sounds after procedure.
11. Observe depth and position of tubes.	• Verifies that position of tube is correct.
12. Assess security of tape or commercial ET or tracheostomy tube holder by tugging at tube.	• Artificial airway should not move. Client may cough.
13. Assess skin around mouth and oral mucosa (ET tube) and tracheostomy stoma for drainage, pressure, and signs of irritation.	• Skin breakdown or irritation should not be present.

Unexpected Outcomes and Related Interventions

Accidental Extubation

- Call for assistance.
- Maintain patent airway. Replace old tracheostomy tube with new tube.
- Observe vital signs and signs of respiratory distress.

Breath Sounds Not Equal Bilaterally With ET Tube in Place

- Evaluate ET tube for proper depth. If incorrect, arrange for ET tube to be repositioned as allowed by institution.
- Obtain order for chest X-ray study to verify placement, if applicable.

Hard, Reddened Areas With or Without Excessive or Foul-Smelling Secretions

- This indicates infection. Notify physician.
- Increase frequency of tube care.
- Remove inner cannula, if applicable, for cleaning and suctioning.

Insecure Tube, Artificial Airway Moves In or Out, Coughed Out by Client

- Assess client's respiratory status and observe for the presence of mucus plugs.
- Adjust or apply new ties.

Breakdown, Pressure Areas, or Stomatitis (Tracheostomy Tube)

- Increase frequency of tube care.
- Make sure skin areas are clean and dry.

Recording and Reporting

- Record respiratory assessments before and after care.
- Record ET tube care: depth of ET tube, frequency and extent of care, client tolerance, and any complications related to presence of the tube.
- Record tracheostomy care: type and size of tracheostomy tube, frequency and extent of care, client tolerance, and any complications related to presence of the tube.

Home Care Considerations (Tracheostomy Only)

- Instruct caregivers on how to obtain supplies.
- Instruct caregivers on signs and symptoms of respiratory distress, tube dysfunction, and respiratory and stoma infections.

Flow-oriented incentive spirometers consist of one or more plastic chambers containing freely moving coloured balls. The client inhales slowly and with an even flow to elevate the balls and keep them floating as long as possible to ensure a maximally sustained inhalation.

Volume-oriented incentive spirometry devices have a bellows that is raised to a predetermined volume by an inhaled breath (Figure 39–13). An achievement light or counter is used to provide feedback. Some devices are constructed so that the light will not turn on unless the bellows is held at a minimum desired volume for a specified period to enhance lung expansion.

The aim of incentive spirometry is to encourage clients to breathe to their normal inspiratory capacities. A postoperative inspiratory capacity one half to three fourths of the preoperative volume is acceptable because of postoperative pain. Administration of pain medications before incentive spirometry will help the client achieve deep breathing by reducing pain and splinting (see Chapter 49).

Chest Tubes. Chest tubes are inserted to remove air and fluids from the pleural space, prevent air or fluid from re-entering the pleural space, and re-establish normal intrapleural and intrapulmonic pressures. A **chest tube** is a catheter inserted through the thorax to remove fluid or air. There are a variety of chest tubes on the market. In addition to the usual disposable waterless system, the traditional reusable-glass, three-bottle systems may still be used. The newest systems available are the mobile chest drain and the dry chest drainage system.

Mobile systems rely on gravity, not suction, for drainage. In specific clients these mobile drains reduce the length of time needed for the chest tube, improve ambulation, and decrease the length of time in the hospital (Carroll, 2005). Mobile chest drains are lighter and smaller, thus the client is able to move more easily (Carroll, 2005).

The dry chest drainage system does not use water in the suction chamber. An automated control valve (ACV) is located inside the regulator and continuously balances the force of the suction with the atmosphere. As a result, the ACV responds to and adjusts to changes in client air leaks and fluctuations in suction source vacuum to deliver accurate suction. Pressure is set between -10 cm H_2O and -40 cm H_2O (Roman & Mercado, 2006).

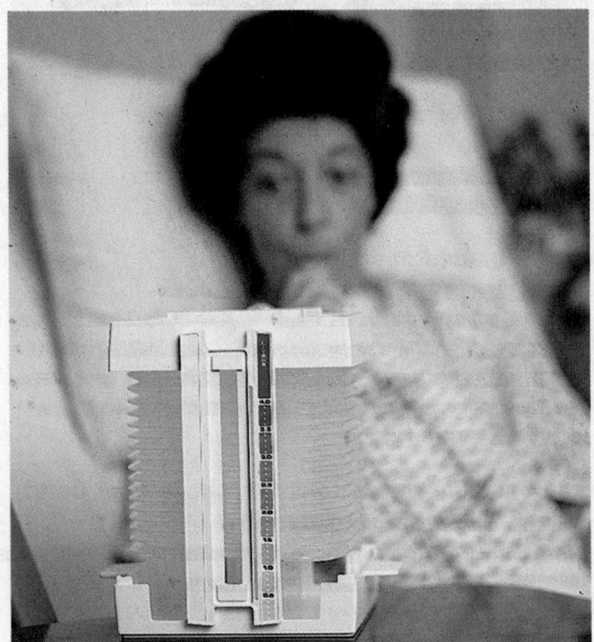

Figure 39-13 Volume-oriented spirometer.

Regardless of the system used, the principles of client management are the same (Carroll, 2002). Chest tubes are commonly used after chest surgery and chest trauma and for pneumothorax or hemothorax to promote lung re-expansion (Skill 39–3).

A **pneumothorax** is a collection of air in the pleural space. The loss of negative intrapleural pressure causes the lung to collapse. There are a variety of mechanisms for a pneumothorax. It may occur spontaneously or as a result of chest trauma, such as a stabbing or the chest striking the steering wheel in a motor vehicle accident. A pneumothorax may also result from the rupture of an emphysematous bleb on the surface of the lung (a large bulla resulting from the destruction caused by emphysema) or from an invasive procedure, such as insertion of a subclavian IV line.

A client with a pneumothorax usually feels pain as atmospheric air irritates the parietal pleura. The pain may be sharp and pleuritic. Dyspnea is common and worsens as the size of the pneumothorax increases.

A **hemothorax** is an accumulation of blood and fluid in the pleural cavity between the parietal and visceral pleurae, usually as a result of trauma. It produces a counterpressure and prevents the lung from full expansion. A hemothorax can also be caused by rupture of small blood vessels from inflammatory processes, such as pneumonia or TB. In addition to pain and dyspnea, signs and symptoms of shock can develop if blood loss is severe.

A disposable system, such as a Thora-Sene III or Pleur-Evac chest drainage system (DeKnatel), is a one-piece moulded plastic unit that provides for a single- or multiple-chamber closed drainage system (Figure 39–14). The disposable units appear to be the system of choice because they are cost-effective and some facilitate autotransfusion, a common practice in open-heart surgeries. Knowledge of the basics of chest tube management and troubleshooting manoeuvres reduces the client's risk of complications.

The simplest closed drainage system is the use of a single chamber. The chamber serves as a collector and a water seal. During normal respiration, the fluid will ascend with inspiration and descend with expiration. A single chamber is used for smaller amounts of drainage, such as an empyema—a collection of infected fluid or pus in the pleural space.

The use of two chambers permits the liquid to flow into the collection chamber as air flows into the water-sealed chamber. Fluctuations in the water-seal tube are still anticipated. Use of two chambers enables more accurate measurement of chest drainage and is used when larger amounts of drainage are expected.

When a volume of air or fluid needs to be evacuated with controlled suction, all three chambers are used. The suction control is marked with centimetre readings to adjust the amount of suction. Usually 15 to 20 cm of water is used for adults. This means that the chamber is filled with sterile water to the 15- or 20-cm water level (Roman & Mercado, 2006).

Special Considerations. Clamping a chest tube at any time is inadvisable. Handle the chest drainage unit carefully and maintain the drainage device below the client's chest. If the tubing disconnects from the drainage unit, instruct the client to exhale as much as possible and to cough. This manoeuvre rids the pleural space of as much air as possible. Cleanse the tips of the tubing and reconnect them quickly. If the drainage unit is broken, the end of the chest tube can be quickly submerged in a container of sterile water to re-establish the seal. Clamping the chest tube may result in a tension pneumothorax. Air pressure builds in the pleural space, collapsing the lung and creating a life-threatening event.

➤ SKILL 39-3 Care of Clients With Chest Tubes

Delegation Considerations

This skill should not be delegated to unregulated care providers (UCPs). However, a UCP may assist with other aspects of the client's care. It is important to inform the UCP of the following:

- Proper positioning of the client with chest tubes to facilitate chest tube drainage and optimal function of the system
- How to ambulate and transfer a client with chest drainage
- Appropriate setup of drainage equipment for the type of system to be used
- To report to the nurse any changes in vital signs, chest pain, sudden shortness of breath, or excessive bubbling in the water-seal chamber
- To immediately report to the nurse a disconnection of the system, any change in type and amount of drainage, sudden bleeding, or sudden cessation of bubbling.

Equipment

- Disposable chest drainage system (see Figure 39–14)
- Suction source and setup (wall canister or portable)
- Disposable (nonsterile) gloves
- 5-cm tape
- Sterile gauze sponges
- Two shodded hemostats

Procedure

STEPS	RATIONALE
1. Perform hand hygiene and assess client.	• Signs and symptoms should reflect improvement in respiratory distress and chest pain after insertion of chest tube.
A. Pulmonary status: Assess for respiratory distress, chest pain, breath sounds over affected lung area, and stable vital signs (see Chapter 31). Signs and symptoms of increased respiratory distress or chest pain include decreased breath sounds over the affected and nonaffected lungs, marked cyanosis, asymmetrical chest movements, presence of subcutaneous emphysema around tube insertion site or neck, hypotension, and tachycardia (Carroll, 2002).	• Notify physician immediately.
B. Vital signs and SpO_2.	• Changes in pulse and blood pressure may indicate infection, respiratory distress, or pain.
C. Pain: If possible, ask client to rate level of pain on a scale of 0 to 10.	• Chest tubes can be painful and interfere with a client's mobility, coughing and deep breathing, and rehabilitation.
2. Observe:	
A. Chest tube dressing and site surrounding tube insertion.	• Ensures that dressing is intact and occlusive seal remains without air or fluid leaks and that area surrounding insertion site is free of drainage or skin irritation (Carroll, 2002).
B. Tubing for kinks, dependent loops, or clots.	• Maintains a patent, freely draining system, preventing fluid accumulation in the chest cavity. The presence of kinks, dependent loops, or clotted drainage increases the client's risk for infection, atelectasis, and tension pneumothorax (Allibone, 2003).
C. Chest drainage system, which should be upright and below level of tube insertion.	• Facilitates drainage; the system must be in this position to function properly.
3. Provide two shodded hemostats or approved clamps for each chest tube, attached to the top of client's bed with adhesive tape. Chest tubes are only clamped under specific circumstances per physician order or nursing policy and procedure: A. To assess air leak. B. To quickly empty or change disposable systems; performed by a nurse who has received education in the procedure. C. If there is an accidental disconnection of drainage tubing from the drainage collection device or damage to the device. D. To assess if client is ready to have the chest tube removed (which is done by physician's order); monitor the client for recurrent pneumothorax.	• Shodded hemostats have a covering to prevent hemostat from penetrating the chest tube once changed. The use of these shodded hemostats or other clamp prevents air from re-entering the pleural space (Allibone, 2003).
4. Position client.	• Permits optimal drainage of fluid and air.
A. Semi-Fowler's position to evacuate air (pneumothorax).	• Air rises to the highest point in the chest. Pneumothorax tubes are usually placed on the anterior aspect at the midclavicular line, second or third intercostal space.
B. High-Fowler's position to drain fluid (hemothorax, effusion).	• Permits optimal drainage of fluid. Posterior tubes are placed on the midaxillary line, eighth or ninth intercostal space.

Continued

➤ SKILL 39-3 Care of Clients With Chest Tubes ***continued***

STEPS	RATIONALE
5. Maintain tube connection between chest and drainage tubes; ensure that it is intact and taped.	• Secures chest tube to drainage system and reduces risk of air leak causing breaks in airtight system.
A. Water-sealed vent must be without occlusion.	• Permits displaced air to pass into atmosphere.
B. Suction-control chamber vent must be without occlusion when suction is used.	• Provides safety factor of releasing excess negative pressure into the atmosphere. Too little suction prevents lung re-expansion and increases client risk for infection, atelectasis, and tension pneumothorax. Too much suction damages the lung tissue and perpetuates existing air leaks (Allibone, 2003).
6. Avoid excess tubing; the tubing should be laid horizontally across the client bed or chair before dropping vertically into the drainage bottle. If the client is in a chair and the tubing is coiled, the tubing should be lifted every 15 minutes to promote drainage.	• The length of tubing should be tailored to each client to avoid excessive coiling or loop formation. Coiled, looped, or clotted tubing impedes chest tube drainage (Allibone, 2003).
7. Adjust tubing to hang in a straight line from top of mattress to drainage chamber. If chest tube is draining fluid, indicate time (e.g., 0900) that drainage was begun on drainage bottle's adhesive tape or on write-on surface of disposable commercial system.	• Provides a baseline for continuous assessment of type and quality of drainage.

Critical Decision Point: Currently, no evidence exists in support of manipulation of chest tubes to promote chest tube patency or mediastinal drainage (Halm, 2007). Chest tube stripping increases negative intrathoracic pressure that could prolong the client's recovery (Halm, 2007).

STEPS	RATIONALE
8. Perform hand hygiene.	• Reduces transmission of infection.
9. Evaluate:	
A. Monitor vital signs and pulse oximetry as ordered or if client's condition changes.	• Provides ongoing data about the client's level of oxygenation.
B. Chest tube dressing.	• Appearance of drainage may be due to tube occlusion, causing drainage to exit around tube.

Critical Decision Point: Check the dressing carefully because it must remain occlusive. It can come loose from the skin, although this may not be readily apparent.

STEPS	RATIONALE
C. Tubing: it should be free of kinks and dependent loops.	• Straight and coiled drainage tube positions are optimal for pleural drainage. However, when a dependent loop is unavoidable, periodic lifting and drainage of the tube will promote pleural drainage.
D. Chest drainage system: it should be upright and below level of tube insertion. Note presence of clots or debris in tubing.	• The system must be in the upright position to function and facilitate proper drainage.
E. Water seal for fluctuations with client's inspiration and expiration.	
(1) Waterless system: diagnostic indicator for fluctuations for client's inspirations and expirations.	• In the non-mechanically ventilated client, fluid should rise in the water seal or diagnostic indicator with inspiration and fall with expiration. The opposite occurs in the client who is mechanically ventilated. This indicates that the system is properly functioning.
(2) Water-seal system: bubbling in the water-seal chamber.	• When system is initially connected to client, bubbles are expected from the chamber. These are from air that was present in the system and in the client's intrapleural space. After a short time, the bubbling stops. Fluid will continue to fluctuate in the water seal on inspiration and expiration until the lung is re-expanded or the system becomes occluded.
(3) Water-seal system: bubbling in the suction-control chamber (when using suction).	• The suction-control chamber has constant gentle bubbling. Tubing remains free of obstruction and the suction source is turned to the appropriate setting.
F. Waterless system: bubbling in diagnostic indicator.	• Mechanism to observe for the presence of tidaling.
G. Type and amount of fluid drainage: Note colour and amount of drainage, client's vital signs, and skin colour. The normal amount of drainage is as follows:	
(1) In the adult: <50–200 mL/hour immediately after surgery in a mediastinal chest tube; approximately 500 mL in first 24 hours.	• Dark-red drainage is expected only in the postoperative period, turning serous with time.

➤SKILL 39-3 Care of Clients With Chest Tubes *continued*

STEPS	RATIONALE
(2) Between 100 and 300 mL of fluid may drain in a pleural chest tube in an adult during the first 3 hours after insertion. This rate will decrease after 2 hours; 500–1000 mL can be expected in the first 24 hours. Drainage is grossly bloody during the first several hours after surgery and then changes to serous. Remember that a sudden gush of drainage may be retained blood and not active bleeding. This increase in drainage can result from client position changes.	• Re-expansion of lungs forces drainage into the tube. Coughing can also cause large gushes of drainage or air. • Excessive amounts or continued presence of frank, bloody drainage during the first several hours after surgery should be reported to the physician, along with client's vital signs and respiratory status.

Critical Decision Point: Inform the physician if drainage suddenly increases or if there is >100 mL/hour of blood drainage (except for the first 3 hours postoperative) (Allibone, 2003).

STEPS	RATIONALE
H. Waterless system: The suction control (float ball) indicates the amount of suction that the client's intrapleural space is receiving.	• The suction float ball dictates the amount of suction in the system. The float ball allows no more suction than allowed by its setting. If the suction source is set too low, the suction float ball cannot reach the prescribed setting. In this case, the suction must be increased for the float ball to reach the prescribed setting.
I. Observe client for decreased respiratory distress and chest pain, auscultate lung sounds over affected area, and monitor SpO_2.	• Breath sounds should be equal. Decreased breath sounds on the affected side may indicate that air or fluid has reaccumulated in the pleural space. Increasing respiratory distress, decreased breath sounds, cyanosis, asymmetrical chest wall motion, and declining vital signs may indicate a tension pneumothorax (Carroll, 2002). This must be reported immediately to the client's health care professional.
J. Pain: Ask client to evaluate pain on a level of 0 to 10.	• May indicate the need for medication for pain.

Unexpected Outcomes and Related Interventions

Continuous Bubbling in Water-Sealed Chamber

- This indicates a leak between the client and water seal.
- Assess all connections between the client and drainage system, and tighten any loose connections (Cerfolio, 2005).
- Cross-clamp chest tube close to client's chest. If bubbling stops, air leak is inside client's thorax or at chest tube insertion site. Unclamp tube, and notify physician immediately. Reinforce chest dressing. Leaving a chest tube clamped causes a tension pneumothorax and mediastinal shift.
- Gradually move clamps down drainage tubing away from the client and toward the drainage chamber, moving one clamp at a time. When bubbling stops, the leak is in a section of tubing or connection distal to the clamp. Replace tubing or secure connection and release clamp.

Leak in Drainage System

- Change drainage system.

Tension Pneumothorax

- Determine that chest tubes are not clamped, kinked, or occluded. Obstructed chest tubes trap air in the intrapleural space when an air leak originates within the client.
- Notify physician immediately.
- Prepare immediately for another chest tube insertion; obtain a flutter (Heimlich) valve or large-gauge needle for short-term emergency release of air in the intrapleural space. Have emergency equipment (e.g., oxygen, code cart) near client.

Trapped Fluid in Dependent Loops of Drainage Tubing

- Drain tubing contents into drainage bottle. Coil excess tubing onto mattress, and secure in place or place in a straight line down the length of the bed.

Recording and Reporting

- Record in nurse's notes patency of chest; presence, type, and amount of drainage; presence of fluctuations; client's vital signs; chest dressing status, amount of suction and water seal; and level of comfort.

Home Care Considerations

- Clients with chronic conditions (e.g., uncomplicated pneumothorax, effusions, empyema) that require a chest tube may be discharged home with smaller mobile chest drains. These systems do not have a suction-control chamber and use a mechanical one-way valve instead of a water-seal chamber (Carroll, 2002, 2005).
- Instruct client in how to ambulate and remain active with a home chest tube drainage system.
- Provide client with information on when to contact health care professionals regarding changes in drainage system (e.g., chest pain, breathlessness, change in drainage).

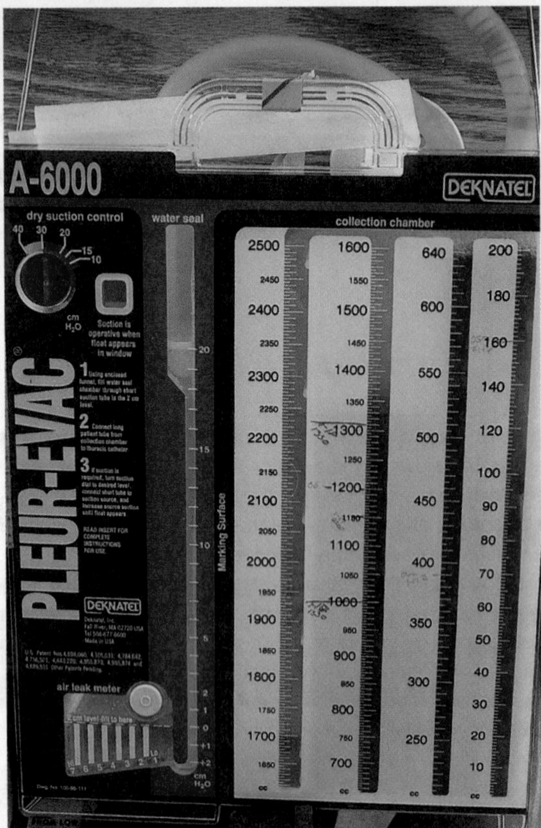

Figure 39–14 Disposable, commercial chest drainage system.

Removal of chest tubes requires client preparation. Clients report various sensations during chest tube removal. The most frequent sensations include burning, pain, and a pulling sensation.

Maintenance and Promotion of Oxygenation. Promotion of lung expansion and of mobilizing secretions and maintaining a patent airway assists the client in meeting oxygenation needs. Some clients, however, also require oxygen therapy to keep a healthy level of tissue oxygenation.

Oxygen Therapy. Oxygen therapy is cheap, widely available, and used in a variety of settings to relieve or prevent tissue hypoxia (Thomson et al., 2002). The goal of oxygen therapy is to prevent or relieve hypoxia. Any client with impaired tissue oxygenation can benefit from controlled oxygen administration. Oxygen is not a substitute for other treatment, however, and should be used only when indicated. Oxygen should be treated as a drug. It has dangerous side effects, such as atelectasis or oxygen toxicity (Thomson et al., 2002). As with any drug, the dosage or concentration of oxygen should be continuously monitored. Routinely check the physician's orders to verify that the client is receiving the prescribed oxygen concentration. The seven rights of medication administration also pertain to oxygen administration (see Chapter 34).

Safety Precautions. Oxygen is a highly combustible gas. Although it will not spontaneously burn or cause an explosion, it can easily cause a fire to ignite in a client's room if it contacts a spark from an open flame or electrical equipment. With increasing use of home oxygen therapy, clients and health care professionals must be aware of the dangers of combustion.

safety alert Oxygen in high concentrations has a great combustion potential and readily fuels fire.

Promote oxygen safety by using the following measures:

- Inform the client, visitors, roommates, and all personnel that smoking is not permitted in areas where oxygen is in use.
- Ensure that all electrical equipment in the room is functioning correctly and is properly grounded (see Chapter 37). An electrical spark in the presence of oxygen can result in a serious fire.
- Locate the closest fire extinguisher.
- Know the fire procedures and the evacuation route for the area.
- Check the oxygen level of portable tanks before transporting a client to ensure that enough oxygen in the tank exists to complete the transport.

Supply of Oxygen. Oxygen is supplied to the client's bedside either by oxygen tanks or through a permanent wall-piped system. Oxygen tanks are transported on wide-based carriers that allow the tank to be placed upright at the bedside. Regulators are used to control the amount of oxygen delivered. One common type is an upright flowmeter with a flow adjustment valve at the top. A second type is a cylinder indicator with a flow adjustment handle. In the home setting, oxygen therapy is also supplied in a variety of methods, including refillable cylinders (Cuvelier et al., 2002).

In the hospital or home, oxygen tanks are delivered with the regulator in place. In the hospital, the respiratory care department usually connects the regulator to the oxygen source. Home care vendors are usually responsible for connecting the oxygen tank to the regulator for home use.

Methods of Oxygen Delivery. Oxygen delivery devices can be considered low-flow or high-flow systems. **Low-flow devices** such as nasal cannulas, simple face masks, and reservoir masks provide oxygen in concentrations that vary with the person's respiratory pattern (Pruitt & Jacobs, 2003). **High-flow devices** deliver oxygen rates above the normal inspiratory flow rate and maintain a fixed FiO_2 (fraction of inspired oxygen) regardless of the client's inspiratory flow and breathing pattern (Pruitt & Jacobs, 2003). The venturi mask is an example of a high-flow device (Pruitt & Jacobs, 2003).

Nasal Cannula. A **nasal cannula** is a low-flow device used for oxygen delivery (Skill 39–4). The two cannulas, approximately 1.5 cm long, protrude from the centre of a disposable tube and are inserted into the nares (Figure 39–15). Oxygen is delivered via the cannulas with a flow rate of up to 6 L/minute. Flow rates greater than 4 L/minute are not often used because of the drying effect on the mucosa and the relatively little increase in delivered oxygen concentration. Know what flow rate produces a given percentage of inspired oxygen concentration (FiO_2; Table 39–9). Also be alert for skin breakdown over the ears and in the nares from too tight an application of the nasal cannula.

Oxygen Masks. An oxygen mask is a device used to administer oxygen, humidity, or heated humidity. It is shaped to fit snugly over the mouth and nose and is secured in place with a strap.

The simple face mask (Figure 39–16) is used for short-term oxygen therapy. It fits loosely and delivers oxygen concentrations from 30% to 60%. The mask is contraindicated for clients with carbon dioxide retention because retention can be worsened.

The partial rebreathing mask and the non-rebreathing mask are low-flow devices with a reservoir bag (Figure 39–17). The partial rebreather mask provides an oxygen concentration of 35% to 60% with a flow rate of 6 to 10 L/minute (Rhoads & Meeker, 2008). The non-rebreather provides the highest concentration of oxygen at 60% to 100% with a flow rate of 6 to 10 L/minute (Rhoads & Meeker, 2008). Oxygen flows into the reservoir bag and mask during inhalation; a valve on the non-rebreather mask prevents expired air from flowing back into the bag. Frequently inspect the bag to make sure it is inflated. If it is deflated, the client may be breathing large amounts of exhaled carbon dioxide.

➤ SKILL 39-4 Applying a Nasal Cannula or Oxygen Mask

Delegation Considerations

This skill cannot be delegated to unregulated care providers (UCPs). You are responsible for assessing the client and providing safe and accurate oxygen therapy, including adjustment of oxygen flow rate and evaluation of client response. It is important to instruct the UCP about the following:

- Correct placement and adjustment of delivery device
- The type of equipment and the oxygen flow rate
- Unexpected outcomes associated with the oxygen delivery device (e.g., increased rate of breathing, decreased level of consciousness, increased confusion, pain) and the need to inform you if any of these outcomes occur

Equipment

- Nasal cannula or oxygen mask
- Oxygen tubing
- Humidifier, if indicated
- Sterile water for humidification, if indicated
- Oxygen source
- Oxygen flowmeter
- Appropriate room signs

Procedure

STEPS	RATIONALE
1. Inspect client for signs and symptoms associated with hypoxia and presence of airway secretions.	• Left untreated, hypoxia can produce cardiac dysrhythmias and death. Presence of airway secretions decreases the effectiveness of oxygen delivery.

Critical Decision Point: Clients with sudden changes in their vital signs, level of consciousness, or behaviour may be experiencing profound hypoxia. Clients who demonstrate subtle changes over time may have worsening of a chronic or existing condition or have a new medical condition (Jevon & Ewens, 2001).

STEPS	RATIONALE
2. Obtain client's most recent SpO_2 or arterial blood gas (ABG) values.	• Provides objective baseline data to use to compare outcome of oxygen therapy.
3. Explain to the client and family what the procedure entails and the purpose of oxygen therapy.	• Decreases client's anxiety, which reduces oxygen consumption and increases client cooperation.
4. Perform hand hygiene.	• Reduces transmission of infection.
5. Attach nasal cannula to oxygen tubing and attach to humidified oxygen source adjusted to prescribed flow rate (see Step 5 illustration).	• Prevents drying of nasal and oral mucous membranes and airway secretions.
6. Place tips of cannula into client's nares, and adjust elastic headband or plastic slide until cannula fits snugly and comfortably (see Step 6 illustration).	• Directs flow of oxygen into client's upper respiratory tract. Client is more likely to keep cannula in place if it fits comfortably.
7. Maintain sufficient slack on oxygen tubing and secure to client's clothes.	• Allows client to turn head without dislodging cannula and reduces pressure on tips of nares.

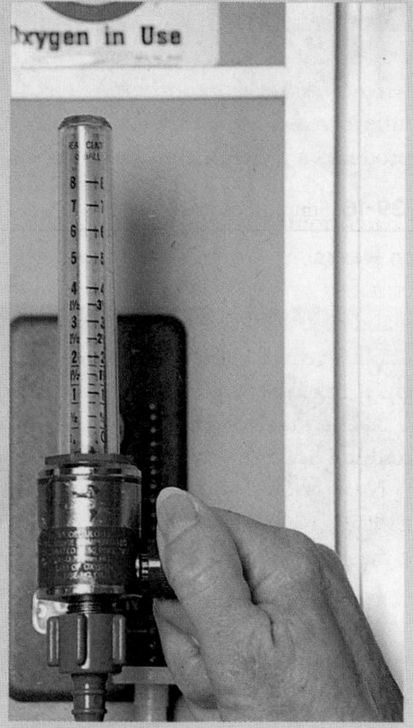

Step 5 Adjusting flowmeter to prescribed oxygen flow rate.

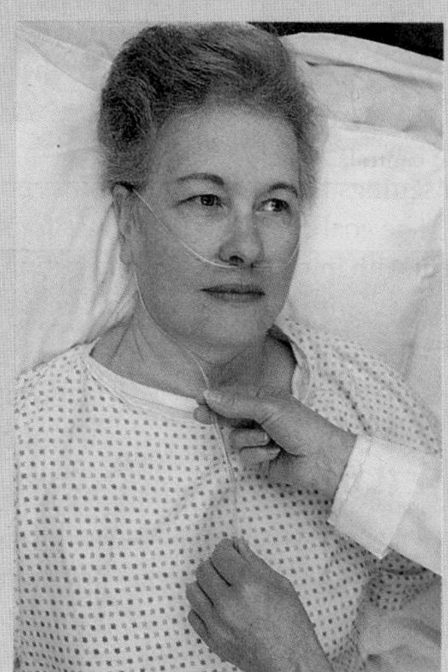
Step 6 Adjusting nasal cannula to fit client and ensure comfort.

Continued

➤ SKILL 39-4 Applying a Nasal Cannula or Oxygen Mask *continued*

STEPS	RATIONALE
8. Check cannula every 8 hours. Keep humidification jar filled at all times.	• Ensures patency of cannula and oxygen flow. Prevents inhalation of dehumidified oxygen.
9. Observe client's nares and superior surface of both ears for skin breakdown.	• Oxygen therapy can cause drying of nasal mucosa. Pressure on ears from cannula tubing or elastic can cause skin irritation.
10. Perform hand hygiene.	• Reduces transmission of microorganisms.
11. Check oxygen flow rate and physician's orders every 8 hours.	• Ensures delivery of prescribed oxygen flow rate and patency of cannula.
12. Inspect client for relief of symptoms associated with hypoxia.	• Indicates that hypoxia is corrected or reduced.

Unexpected Outcomes and Related Interventions

Worsening Respiratory Status

- Check that oxygen delivery device is patent, not kinked, and attached to the oxygen flowmeter.
- Check oxygen level set on flowmeter; determine if delivered amount is consistent with physician order.
- If not using wall oxygen, determine if the oxygen source contains enough oxygen to deliver the prescribed oxygen amount.
- Notify physician.

Dry Nasal and Upper Airway Mucosa

- If oxygen flow rate is >4 L/minute, determine the need for humidification.
- Assess the client's fluid status and increase fluids if appropriate.
- Provide frequent oral care.
- Obtain physician order for use of sterile nasal saline intermittently.

Skin Breakdown Over Ears

- Adjust tightness of elastic strap to looser level.
- Use good hygiene and skin care around the ears.
- Place soft, woven 4 × 4 gauze pads between elastic and ears.
- Reposition elastic strap frequently.

Recording and Reporting

- Record oxygen delivery device and litre flow in medical record. Document client and family education. Report oxygen delivery device, litre flow, and response to changes in therapy to oncoming shift.

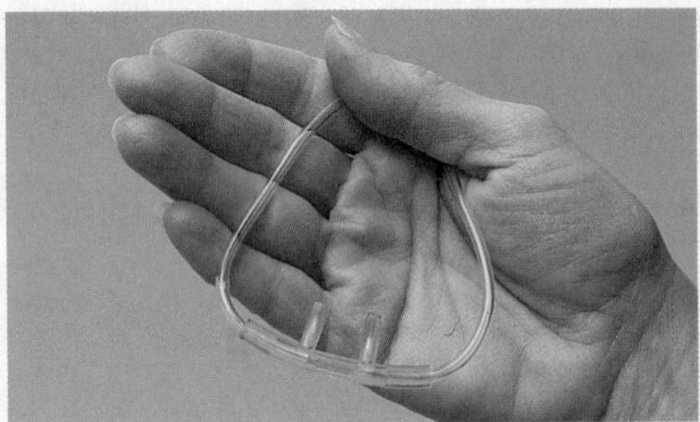

Figure 39-15 Nasal cannula.

Figure 39-16 Simple face mask.

➤ TABLE 39-9 Approximate FiO_2 With Different Oxygen Delivery Devices

Oxygen Delivery Device	Required Litre Flow (L/minute)	Approximate Percent Oxygen
Nasal cannula	1–2	24–28
	3–4	32–36
	5–6	40–44
Simple face mask	5–6	40
	6–7	50
	7–8	60
Venturi mask	4	24–28
	8	35–40
	12	50–60

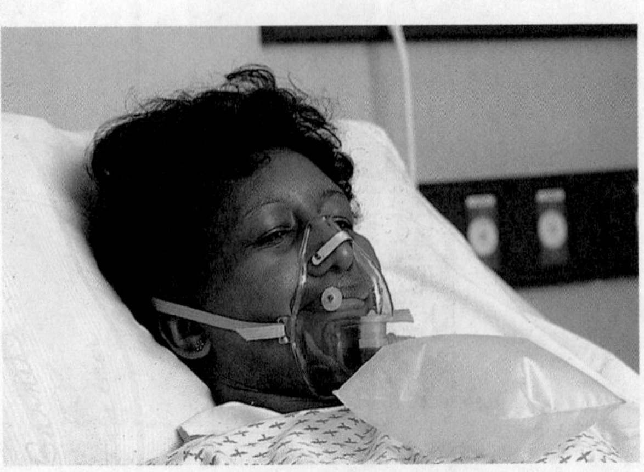

Figure 39-17 Plastic face mask with reservoir bag.

The Venturi mask (Figure 39–18), a high-flow device, can be used to deliver oxygen concentrations of 24% to 60% with oxygen flow rates of 4 to 12 L/minute, depending on which flow-control meter is selected (see Table 39–9). This mask entrains room air to achieve a consistent and precise oxygen concentration. The venturi mask is helpful for clients with COPD who require low, constant oxygen concentrations.

Home Oxygen Therapy. Indications for home oxygen therapy include a PaO_2 of 55 mm Hg or less or an SaO_2 of 88% or less on room air at rest, on exertion, or with exercise. Clients with a PaO_2 from 56 to 59 mm Hg may also receive oxygen if there is also evidence of cor pulmonale, pulmonary hypertension, erythrocytosis, central nervous system dysfunction, impaired mental status, or increasing hypoxemia with exertion.

Home oxygen therapy has beneficial effect with clients with chronic cardiopulmonary diseases (Snow et al., 2001). This therapy improves clients' exercise tolerance and fatigue levels and in some situations assists in the management of dyspnea (Fujimoto et al., 2002). When home oxygen is required, it is usually delivered by nasal cannula. When a client has a permanent tracheostomy, however, a T tube or tracheostomy collar is necessary. Three types of oxygen are used: compressed oxygen, liquid oxygen (Figure 39–19), and oxygen concentrators. The advantages and disadvantages (Table 39–10) of each type are assessed, along with the client's needs and community resources, before placing a certain delivery system in the home. In the home, the major consideration is the oxygen delivery source.

Clients requiring home oxygen need extensive teaching to be able to continue oxygen therapy at home efficiently and safely (Skill 39–5). This includes oxygen safety, regulation of the amount of oxygen, and how to use the prescribed home oxygen delivery system. It is important to coordinate the efforts of the client and family, home care nurse, home respiratory therapist, and home oxygen equipment vendor. The social worker usually assists with arranging for the home care nurse and oxygen vendor. Assist the client and family in learning about home oxygen and ensure their ability to maintain the oxygen delivery system.

Restoration of Cardiopulmonary Functioning. If a client's hypoxia is severe and prolonged, cardiac arrest may result. A cardiac arrest is a sudden cessation of cardiac output and circulation. When this occurs, oxygen is not delivered to tissues, carbon dioxide is not transported from tissues, tissue metabolism becomes anaerobic, and metabolic and respiratory acidosis occurs. Permanent heart, brain, and other tissue damage occurs within 4 to 6 minutes.

Cardiopulmonary Resuscitation. Cardiac arrest is characterized by an absence of pulse and respiration. If you determine that the client has had a cardiac arrest, **cardiopulmonary resuscitation (CPR)** must be initiated. CPR is a basic emergency procedure of artificial respiration and manual external cardiac massage. Most nursing students are required to have successfully completed a CPR course before their clinical experiences.

The "ABCs" of CPR are to establish an Airway, initiate Breathing, and maintain Circulation. When an airway cannot be established, reassess proper head position and assess for airway obstruction. There is no clinical benefit to cardiac compressions if an airway cannot be established. The purpose of CPR is to circulate oxygenated blood to the brain to prevent permanent tissue damage (AHA, 2005).

Restorative and Continuing Care

Restorative and continuing care may emphasize cardiopulmonary reconditioning as a structured rehabilitation program. **Cardiopulmonary rehabilitation** is actively helping the client to achieve and maintain an optimal level of health through controlled physical exercise, nutrition counselling, relaxation and stress management techniques, prescribed medications and oxygen, and compliance. As physical reconditioning occurs, the client's complaints of dyspnea, chest pain, fatigue, and activity intolerance should decrease. The client's anxiety, depression, or somatic concerns also often decrease. The client and the rehabilitation team define the goals of rehabilitation.

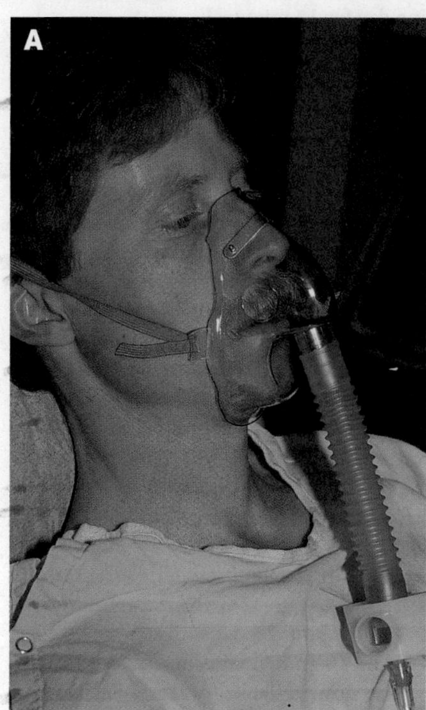

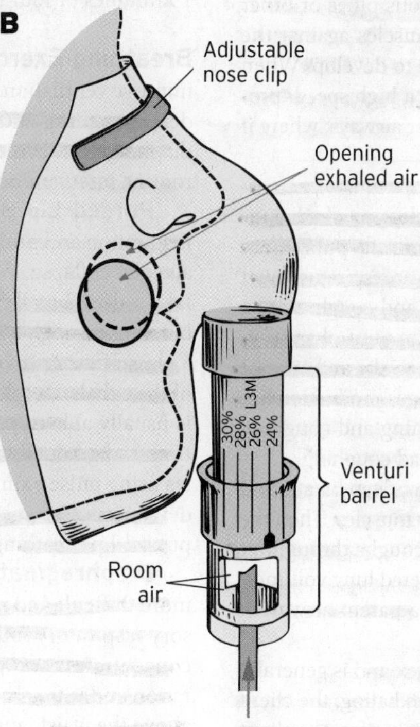

Figure 39-18 Venturi mask.

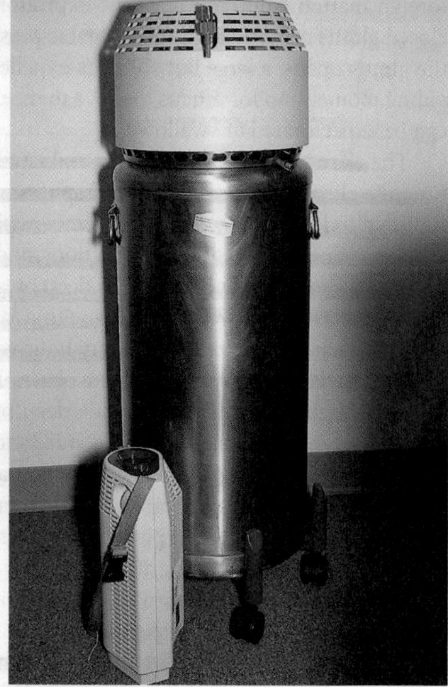

Figure 39-19 Primary and portable liquid oxygen source for ambulation.

➤ TABLE 39-10 Home Oxygen Systems

Primary Use	Advantages	Disadvantages
Compressed Gas Cylinders		
Intermittent therapy Used for exercise or sleep only	100% oxygen, relatively inexpensive, no loss of gas during storage, relatively portable, delivery of up to 15 L/minute	Bulky, possibly unsightly, frequent refilling necessary with continuous use
Liquid Oxygen Systems *(see Figure 39-19)*		
Used with active clients	100% oxygen, conveniently portable, portable units refilled at home, delivery of up to 6 L/minute	Usually weekly delivery necessary for refill, evaporates if not used, potential for frostbite at connections and if liquid is spilled
Oxygen Concentrators		
Homebound clients with limited mobility inside or outside home	Fixed monthly cost, minimal interruption of household by supplier, no refills of "main tank," most units with delivery of up to 4 or 5 L/minute	Oxygen concentration decreases as litre flow increases (usually 85%–90%), power supply needed, electric bill increase, second system needed for portability, usually E tank gas cylinders

Hydration. Maintenance of adequate systemic hydration keeps mucociliary clearance normal. In clients with adequate hydration, pulmonary secretions are thin, white, watery, and easily removable with minimal coughing. Excessive coughing to clear thick, tenacious secretions is fatiguing and energy depleting. The best way to maintain thin secretions is to provide a fluid intake of 1500 to 2000 mL/day unless contraindicated by cardiac status. The colour, consistency, and ease of secretion expectoration can determine adequacy of hydration.

Coughing Techniques. Coughing is effective for maintaining a patent airway. Coughing enables the client to remove secretions from both the upper and lower airways. The normal series of events in the cough mechanism are deep inhalation, closure of the glottis, active contraction of the expiratory muscles, and glottis opening. Deep inhalation increases the lung volume and airway diameter, allowing the air to pass through partially obstructing mucous plugs or other foreign matter. Contraction of the expiratory muscles against the closed glottis causes a high intrathoracic pressure to develop. When the glottis opens, a large flow of air is expelled at a high speed, providing momentum for mucus to move to the upper airways, where it can be expectorated or swallowed.

The effectiveness of coughing is evaluated by sputum expectoration, the client's report of swallowed sputum, or clearing of adventitious sounds by auscultation. Clients with chronic pulmonary diseases, upper respiratory tract infections, and lower respiratory tract infections should be encouraged to deep breathe and cough at least every 2 hours while awake. Clients with a large amount of sputum should be encouraged to cough every hour while awake and every 2 to 3 hours while asleep until the acute phase of mucus production has ended. Coughing techniques include deep breathing and coughing for the postoperative client, cascade, huff, and quad coughing.

With the *cascade cough,* the client takes a slow, deep breath and holds it for 2 seconds while contracting expiratory muscles. Then the client opens the mouth and performs a series of coughs throughout exhalation, thereby coughing at progressively lowered lung volumes. This technique promotes airway clearance and a patent airway in clients with large volumes of sputum.

The *huff cough* stimulates a natural cough reflex and is generally effective only for clearing central airways. While exhaling, the client opens the glottis by saying the word "huff." With practice, the client inhales more air and may be able to progress to the cascade cough.

The *quad cough* technique is used for clients without abdominal muscle control, such as those with spinal cord injuries. While the client breathes out with a maximal expiratory effort, the client or nurse pushes inward and upward on the abdominal muscles toward the diaphragm, causing the cough.

Respiratory Muscle Training. Respiratory muscle training improves muscle strength and endurance, resulting in improved activity tolerance. Respiratory muscle training may prevent respiratory failure in clients with COPD.

One method for respiratory muscle training is the incentive spirometer resistive breathing device (ISRBD). Resistive breathing is achieved by placing a resistive breathing device into a volume-dependent incentive spirometer. Muscle training is achieved when the client uses the ISRBD on a scheduled routine (e.g., twice a day for 15 minutes or four times a day for 15 minutes).

Breathing Exercises. Breathing exercises include techniques to improve ventilation and oxygenation. The three basic techniques are deep breathing and coughing exercises, pursed-lip breathing, and diaphragmatic breathing. Deep breathing and coughing exercises are routine interventions for postoperative clients (see Chapter 49).

Pursed-Lip Breathing. **Pursed-lip breathing** involves deep inspiration and prolonged expiration through pursed lips to prevent alveolar collapse. While the client is sitting up, instruct the client to take a deep breath and to exhale slowly through pursed lips, as if blowing through a straw. Have the client blow through a straw into a glass of water to learn the technique. Clients need to gain control of the exhalation phase so that it is longer than inhalation. The client is usually able to perfect this technique by counting the inhalation time and gradually increasing the count during exhalation. In studies using pulse oximetry as a feedback tool, clients have been able to demonstrate an increase in their arterial oxygen saturation during pursed-lip breathing.

Diaphragmatic Breathing. **Diaphragmatic breathing** is more difficult and requires the client to relax intercostal and accessory respiratory muscles while taking deep inspirations. The client concentrates on expanding the diaphragm during controlled inspiration and is taught to place one hand flat below the breastbone and above the waist, and the other hand 2 to 3 cm below the first hand. The client is asked to inhale while the lower hand moves outward

➤ SKILL 39-5 Using Home Oxygen Equipment

Delegation Considerations

This skill should not be delegated to unregulated care providers (UCPs). However, once the client is stable on home oxygen therapy, UCPs may perform certain aspects of care. You are responsible for assessing the client, checking the device setup, and providing safe and accurate oxygen therapy. You must instruct the UCP about the following:

- Unique needs of the client (e.g., amount of assistance in applying home nasal cannula or mask) and any assistance needed in filling liquid canisters
- The type of equipment that the client should have in the home and the oxygen flow rate
- Unexpected outcomes associated with the oxygen delivery device (e.g., increased rate of breathing, decreased level of consciousness, increased confusion, pain), and the need to inform you if any occur

Equipment

- Nasal cannula equipment (see Skill 39–4)
- Oxygen tubing
- Home oxygen delivery system with appropriate equipment

Procedure

STEPS	RATIONALE
1. While client is in the hospital, determine client's or family's ability to use oxygen equipment correctly. In the home setting reassess for appropriate use of equipment.	• Physical or cognitive impairments of client necessitate instructing a family member or significant other how to operate home oxygen equipment. Ongoing assessment enables nurse to determine specific components of skill that the client or family easily complete.
2. Assess home environment for adequate electrical service if oxygen concentrator is used.	• Oxygen concentrators require electricity to work. Continuous oxygen therapy must not be interrupted.
3. Assess client's and family's ability to observe for signs and symptoms of hypoxia.	• Hypoxia occurs at home despite use of oxygen therapy. Worsening of a client's physical condition or another underlying condition such as a change in respiratory status can cause hypoxia.
4. Determine appropriate resources in the community for equipment and assistance, including maintenance and repair services, and medical equipment supplier.	• Ensure readily available assistance for clients with home oxygen systems.
5. In case of power failure, determine appropriate backup system when using a compressor. Have a spare oxygen tank available.	• Many municipalities require that clients with home oxygen equipment notify emergency medical services (EMS) before bringing the equipment home. When there is a power outage, EMS calls the home, and in some cases the home is on a priority list for having power restored.
6. Perform hand hygiene.	• Reduces transmission of infection.
7. Place oxygen delivery system in a clutter-free environment that is well ventilated; away from walls, drapes, bedding, combustible materials; and at least 8 feet from heat source.	• Prevents injury from improper placement of oxygen equipment.
8. Demonstrate steps for preparation and completion of oxygen therapy.	
A. Compressed oxygen system	• Teaches psychomotor skills and enables a client to ask questions.
(1) Turn cylinder valve counterclockwise two to three turns with wrench. Store wrench with oxygen tank.	• Turns on oxygen. Keep wrench available.
(2) Check cylinders by reading amount on pressure gauge.	• Verifies adequate oxygen supply for client use.
B. Oxygen concentrator system	
(1) Plug concentrator into appropriate outlet.	• Provides power source.
(2) Turn on power switch.	• Starts concentrator motor.
(3) Alarm will sound for a few seconds.	• Alarm turns off when desired pressure inside concentrator is reached.
C. Liquid oxygen system	
(1) Check liquid system by depressing button at lower right corner and reading the dial on the stationary oxygen reservoir or ambulatory tank.	• Verifies adequate oxygen supply.
(2) Collaborate with medical equipment provider to provide instruction on refilling ambulatory tank.	• Ambulatory tanks of liquid oxygen must be filled when empty.

Critical Decision Point: Only fill ambulatory tanks when they are empty. Liquid oxygen is stored at or below –297°F inside the reservoir, and the temperature inside the ambulatory tank is warmer. If cold oxygen from the reservoir mixes with warmer oxygen left in the ambulatory tank, the ambulatory tank may malfunction.

STEPS	RATIONALE
(3) Refilling oxygen tank:	
(a) Wipe both filling connectors with a clean, dry, lint-free cloth.	• Removes dust and moisture from system.
(b) Turn off flow selector of ambulatory unit.	

Continued

➤ SKILL 39-5 Using Home Oxygen Equipment *continued*

STEPS	RATIONALE
(c) Attach ambulatory unit to stationary reservoir by inserting adapter from ambulatory tank into adapter of stationary reservoir.	• Secures connections.
(d) Open fill valve on ambulatory tank, and apply firm pressure to top of stationary reservoir (see Step 8C(3)(d) illustration). Stay with unit while it is filling. You will hear a loud hissing noise. The tank fills in about 2 minutes.	• Prevents leaking of oxygen during filling process. If oxygen leaks during filling process, the connection between ambulatory tank and reservoir will ice up and stick together.
(e) Disengage ambulatory unit from stationary reservoir when hissing noise changes and vapor cloud begins to form from stationary unit.	• Overfilling causes the ambulatory unit to malfunction from high pressure in the tank.
(f) Wipe both filling connectors with a clean, dry, lint-free cloth.	• Ice sometimes forms during filling. Wiping removes moisture from oxygen system.

Critical Decision Point: If ambulatory unit does not separate easily, valves from the reservoir and ambulatory unit may be frozen together. Wait until the valves warm to disengage (about 5–10 minutes). Do not touch any frosted areas because contact with skin may cause skin damage from frostbite.

STEPS	RATIONALE
9. Connect oxygen delivery device to oxygen system.	• Connects oxygen source to delivery system.
10. Adjust to prescribed flow rate (L/min).	• Ensures appropriate oxygen prescription.
11. Place oxygen delivery device on client.	• Delivers oxygen to client.
12. Perform hand hygiene.	• Reduces transmission of microorganisms.
13. Instruct client and family not to change oxygen flow rate.	
14. Guide the client and family as they perform each step. Provide written material for reinforcement and review.	• Allows nurse to correct errors in technique and discuss their implications.
15. Instruct the client or family to notify physician if signs or symptoms of hypoxia or respiratory tract infection occur.	• Respiratory tract infections increase oxygen demand and may affect oxygen transfer from lungs to blood. They may cause severe exacerbation of client's pulmonary disease.
16. Discuss emergency plan for power loss, natural disaster, and acute respiratory distress. Have client or family call 911 and notify physician and home care agency.	• Ensures appropriate response and can prevent worsening of client's condition.
17. Instruct client in safe home oxygen practices including not allowing smoking in the home, keeping oxygen tanks away from open flames, and storing tanks upright.	• Ensures safe use of oxygen in the home and prevents injury to client and family.
18. Monitor rate of oxygen delivery.	• Determines if client is regulating oxygen at prescribed rate.

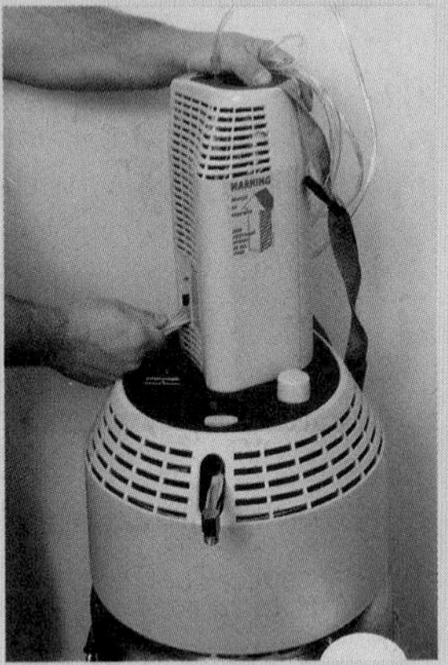

Step 8C(3)(d) Fill valve on ambulatory tank is open while applying firm pressure to top of ambulatory unit.

Unexpected Outcomes and Related Interventions

Client Reports No Oxygen Flow

- Check tank pressure gauge. If level of oxygen is low, refill tank if portable, or provide alternate source of oxygen, such as concentrator or H cylinder.
- Notify home oxygen supplier of need for refill.
- Reassure client and family.

Unable to Fill Portable Liquid Oxygen From Main Source

- Check to see that portable tank is connected correctly.
- Determine if valve is frozen.
- Contact home oxygen supplier for service visit.
- Provide alternate oxygen source if necessary.

Recording and Reporting

- Record the client's and family's ability to safely use the home oxygen equipment. Report the type of home oxygen equipment to be used, the client's and family's understanding of how to use the equipment, knowledge of safety guidelines and unexpected outcomes, and ability to demonstrate proper use of the oxygen delivery device.

during inspiration. The client observes for inward movement as the diaphragm ascends. These exercises are initially taught with the client in the supine position and then practised while the client sits and stands. The exercise is often used with the pursed-lip breathing technique.

Diaphragmatic breathing is also useful for clients with pulmonary disease, for postoperative clients, and for women in labour to promote relaxation and provide pain control. The exercise improves efficiency of breathing by decreasing air trapping and reducing the work of breathing.

❖Evaluation

Nursing interventions and therapies are evaluated by comparing the client's progress with the goals and expected outcomes of the nursing care plan. Evaluate the actual care given to the client by the health care team on the basis of the expected outcomes (Figure 39–20).

Client Care

The client is the only one who can evaluate his or her degree of breathlessness. The client should be asked to rate breathlessness on a scale of 1 to 10, with 1 being no shortness of breath and 10 being severe shortness of breath. Arterial blood gas levels, pulmonary function tests, vital signs, ECG tracings, and physical assessment data provide objective measurement of the success of therapies and treatments. Outcomes are compared with expected outcomes to determine the client's health status. Continuous evaluation helps to determine whether new or revised therapies are required and if new nursing diagnoses have developed and require a new plan of care.

When nursing measures directed to improve oxygenation are unsuccessful, immediately modify the nursing care plan. Do not hesitate to notify the physician about a client's deteriorating oxygenation status. Prompt notification can avoid an emergency situation or even the need for CPR.

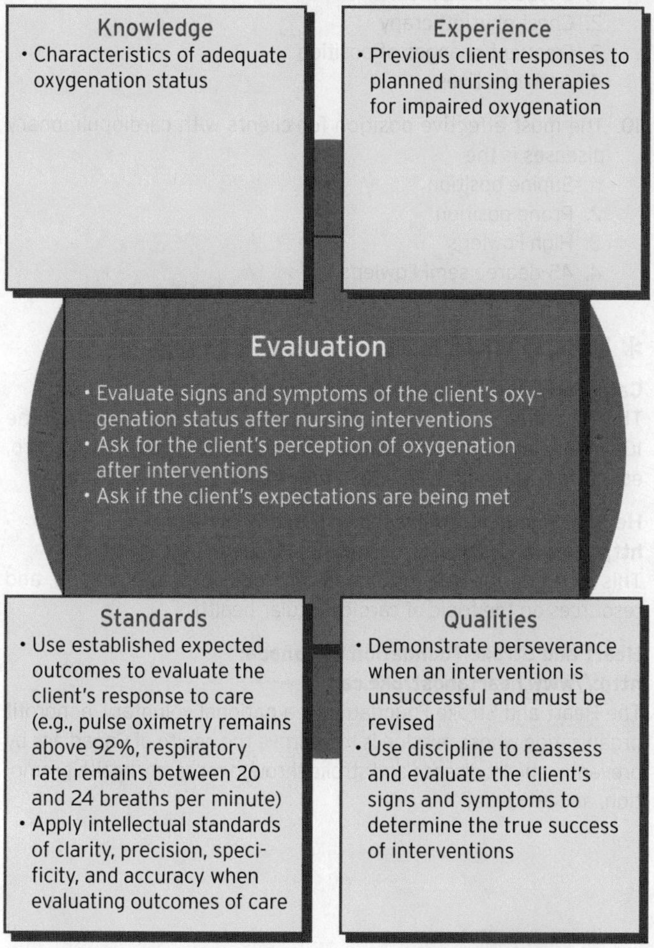

Client Expectations

It is important to ask clients if their expectations of care have been met. For example, you can ask the client, "Do you feel like you will be able to use the breathing techniques we have practised at home?" If the client does not think this will work at home, then the client's expectations for care management have not been met.

You should ask the client whether all questions and needs have been met. If not, spend more time understanding what the client wants and needs to meet his or her expectations. Working closely with the client will enable you to redefine those client expectations that can be realistically met within the limitations of the client's condition and treatment.

Knowledge
- Characteristics of adequate oxygenation status

Experience
- Previous client responses to planned nursing therapies for impaired oxygenation

Evaluation
- Evaluate signs and symptoms of the client's oxygenation status after nursing interventions
- Ask for the client's perception of oxygenation after interventions
- Ask if the client's expectations are being met

Standards
- Use established expected outcomes to evaluate the client's response to care (e.g., pulse oximetry remains above 92%, respiratory rate remains between 20 and 24 breaths per minute)
- Apply intellectual standards of clarity, precision, specificity, and accuracy when evaluating outcomes of care

Qualities
- Demonstrate perseverance when an intervention is unsuccessful and must be revised
- Use discipline to reassess and evaluate the client's signs and symptoms to determine the true success of interventions

Figure 39-20 Critical thinking model for oxygenation evaluation.

✻ KEY CONCEPTS

- The primary function of the heart is to deliver deoxygenated blood to the lungs for oxygenation and to deliver oxygen and nutrients to the tissues.
- Preload, afterload, contractility, and heart rate alter cardiac output.
- Cardiac dysrhythmias are classified by cardiac activity and site of impulse origin.
- The primary function of the lungs is to transfer oxygen from the atmosphere into the alveoli and to transfer carbon dioxide out of the body as a waste product.
- Ventilation is the process of providing adequate oxygenation from the alveoli to the blood.
- Compliance, or the ability of the lungs to expand and contract, depends on the function of musculoskeletal and neurological systems and on other physiological factors.
- The process of inspiration (active process) and expiration (passive process) is caused by changes in intrapleural and intra-alveolar pressures and lung volumes.
- Respiration is controlled by the central nervous system and by chemicals within the blood.
- Decreased hemoglobin levels alter the client's ability to transport oxygen.
- Impaired chest wall movement reduces the level of tissue oxygenation.
- Hyperventilation is a respiratory rate greater than that required to maintain normal levels of carbon dioxide.
- Hypoventilation causes carbon dioxide retention.
- Hypoxia occurs if the amount of oxygen delivered to tissues is too low.
- The health history and assessment includes information about the client's cough, dyspnea, fatigue, wheezing, chest pain, environmental exposures, respiratory infection, cardiopulmonary risk factors, and use of medications.
- Diagnostic and laboratory tests may be needed to complete the database for a client with decreased oxygenation.
- Breathing exercises improve ventilation, oxygenation, and sensations of dyspnea.

- Nebulization delivers small drops of water or particles of medication to the airways.
- Chest physiotherapy includes postural drainage, percussion, and vibration to mobilize pulmonary secretions.
- Coughing and suctioning techniques are used to maintain a patent airway.
- Oxygen therapy is used to improve levels of tissue oxygenation and is delivered by a nasal cannula, various oxygen masks, or the use of an artificial airway.

* CRITICAL THINKING EXERCISES

1. Ms. Delgado is a 56-year-old postmenopausal woman with a history of hypertension. She presents to her primary care office with complaints of nausea, indigestion, increased fatigue, and shortness of breath with increased activity for the past 16 hours. What questions would you ask Ms. Delgado in the nursing health history?
2. Mr. Kwan has recently immigrated to Canada. He comes to the clinic because he has been increasingly fatigued, has a persistent cough, has been losing weight, and awakens at night with sweats. What questions would be important to ask when completing the nursing health history?
3. Mrs. Leblanc, age 45 years, has been admitted to the hospital with community-acquired pneumonia. She has a productive cough, fever, chills, crackles and wheezes on auscultation of her chest, and a heart rate of 104 beats per minute. What nursing diagnosis would you consider for this client? What nursing interventions would be appropriate for her? What health promotion interventions need to be initiated before discharge from the hospital?
4. Mr. Chen Lee, age 72 years, is on a medical unit for a recent diagnosis of COPD. He uses his call bell to indicate that he feels short of breath. His respiratory rate is 32 breathes per minute and oxygen saturation is 86% on room air. What immediate nursing interventions would you initiate?

* REVIEW QUESTIONS

1. Clients with anemia may complain of
   1. Fatigue
   2. Increased activity tolerance
   3. Decreased breathlessness
   4. Increased appetite
2. The most common toxic inhalant that decreases the oxygen-carrying capacity of blood is
   1. Carbon dioxide
   2. Carbon monoxide
   3. Nitrogen
   4. Mustard gas
3. Conditions such as shock and severe dehydration resulting from extracellular fluid loss and reduced circulating blood volume cause
   1. Hypovolemia
   2. Hypervolemia
   3. Uncontrolled bleeding
   4. Hypoxia
4. Fever increases the tissues' need for oxygen, and as a result
   1. Carbon dioxide decreases
   2. Cyanosis occurs
   3. Carbon dioxide increases
   4. Muscle mass increases
5. Left-sided heart failure is an abnormal condition characterized by
   1. Impaired functioning of the left ventricle
   2. Impaired functioning of the left atrium
   3. Lowered cardiac pressures
   4. Increased cardiac output
6. Right-sided heart failure results from
   1. Impaired functioning of the right ventricle
   2. Impaired functioning of the right atrium
   3. Severe weight loss
   4. Lowered pulmonary vascular resistance
7. Cyanosis, the blue discoloration of the skin and mucous membranes caused by the presence of desaturated hemoglobin in capillaries, is a(an)
   1. Early sign of hypoxia
   2. Late sign of hypoxia
   3. Reliable measure of oxygenation status
   4. Non-life-threatening event
8. A person who starts smoking in adolescence and continues to smoke into middle age
   1. Has an increased risk for cardiopulmonary disease and lung cancer
   2. Has an increased risk for obesity and diabetes
   3. Has an increased risk for stress-related illnesses
   4. Has an increased risk for alcoholism
9. A simple and cost-effective method for reducing the risks of stasis of pulmonary secretions and decreased chest wall expansion is
   1. Oxygen humidification
   2. Chest physiotherapy
   3. Frequent changes of position
   4. Anti-infectives
10. The most effective position for clients with cardiopulmonary diseases is the
    1. Supine position
    2. Prone position
    3. High Fowler's
    4. 45-degree semi-Fowler's

* RECOMMENDED WEB SITES

Canadian Lung Association: http://www.lung.ca/
The Canadian Lung Association is the umbrella group for the 10 provincial lung associations. Its goal is to promote research, education, and healthy living in order to combat lung disease.

Health Canada—Cardiovascular Disease Division: http://www.hc-sc.gc.ca/dc-ma/heart-coeur/index_e.html
This Web site for Health Canada provides links, information, and resources on the topic of cardiovascular health.

Heart and Stroke Foundation of Canada: http://www.heartandstroke.ca
The Heart and Stroke Foundation is a national voluntary, nonprofit organization whose mission is to improve the health of Canadians by preventing heart disease and stroke through research, health promotion, and advocacy.

40

Fluid, Electrolyte, and Acid–Base Balances

Written by Darlaine Jantzen, RN, MA
and Anita Molzahn, RN, MN, PhD
Based on the original chapter by
Wendy Ostendorf, BSN, MS, EdD

objectives

Mastery of content in this chapter will enable you to:

- Define the key terms listed.
- Describe the distribution, composition, movement, and regulation of body fluids.
- Describe the regulation and movement of major electrolytes.
- Describe the processes involved in acid–base balance.
- Identify factors that affect normal fluid, electrolyte, and acid–base balances.
- Discuss the clinical assessments for fluid, electrolyte, and acid–base balances.
- Describe laboratory studies associated with fluid, electrolyte, and acid–base balances.
- Identify and discuss nursing interventions for clients with fluid, electrolyte, and acid–base imbalances.
- Discuss the purpose of and procedure for initiating, maintaining, and discontinuing intravenous therapy.
- Calculate the intravenous flow rate.
- Discuss complications associated with intravenous therapy.
- Discuss the purpose of and procedure for initiating a blood transfusion and interventions to manage a transfusion reaction.

key terms

Active transport, p. 936
Aldosterone, p. 937
Anion gap, p. 942
Anions, p. 934
Antidiuretic hormone (ADH), p. 937
Arterial blood gas (ABG), p. 942
Autologous transfusion, p. 978
Base excess, p. 942
Buffer, p. 938
Cations, p. 934
Colloid, p. 955
Colloid osmotic pressure, p. 935
Concentration gradient, p. 935
Crystalloid, p. 955
Dehydration, p. 936
Diffusion, p. 935
Edema, p. 935
Electrolytes, p. 934
Extracellular fluid (ECF), p. 934
Filtration, p. 935
Fluid volume deficit (FVD), p. 945
Fluid volume excess (FVE), p. 954
Hemolysis, p. 979
Homeostasis, p. 936
Hydrostatic pressure, p. 935
Hypercalcemia, p. 939
Hyperchloremia, p. 939
Hyperkalemia, p. 939
Hypermagnesemia, p. 939
Hypernatremia, p. 939
Hypertonic, p. 935
Hypocalcemia, p. 939
Hypochloremia, p. 939
Hypokalemia, p. 939
Hypomagnesemia, p. 939
Hyponatremia, p. 939
Hypotonic, p. 935
Hypovolemia, p. 936
Infiltration, p. 973
Infusion pump, p. 957
Insensible water loss, p. 937
Interstitial fluid, p. 934
Intracellular fluid (ICF), p. 934
Intravascular fluid, p. 934
Ions, p. 934
Isotonic, p. 935
Metabolic acidosis, p. 942
Metabolic alkalosis, p. 942
Osmolality, p. 935
Osmolarity, p. 935
Osmoreceptors, p. 936
Osmosis, p. 935
Osmotic pressure, p. 935
Oxygen saturation, p. 942
Phlebitis, p. 973
Respiratory acidosis, p. 942
Respiratory alkalosis, p. 942
Sensible water loss, p. 937
Solutes, p. 934
Solution, p. 934
Solvent, p. 934
Transcellular fluid, p. 934
Transfusion reaction, p. 978
Vascular access devices, p. 955

media resources

evolve Web Site

- Audio Chapter Summaries
- Glossary
- Multiple-Choice Review Questions
- Skills Performance Checklists
- Student Learning Activities
- Video Clips
- Weblinks

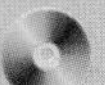
Companion CD

- Glossary
- Interactive Learning Activities
- Fluids and Electrolytes Tutorial
- Test-Taking Skills

Fluid, electrolyte, and acid–base balances within the body are essential for normal body function. These balances are maintained by respiration and the ingestion, distribution, and excretion of water and electrolytes. Within the body, these balances are regulated by the renal, pulmonary, and buffer systems. Imbalances may result from many factors, including altered intake, illness, or excessive losses, such as exercise-induced diaphoresis. These imbalances impact physiological processes at the cellular, tissue, and system levels of the body (Box 40–1). Therefore, knowledge and understanding of the mechanisms that contribute to fluid, electrolyte, and acid–base balances are essential.

Scientific Knowledge Base

Water is the largest single component of the body. Although 60% of the average adult's weight is fluid, this amount varies with age, gender, and weight. A healthy, mobile, well-oriented adult can usually maintain normal fluid, electrolyte, and acid–base balances because of the body's adaptive physiological mechanisms.

> **BOX 40-1 NURSING STORY**
>
> **Harold's Water Works**
>
> Susanne Walter works on a medical unit in a small city in the Maritimes. One evening, Harold Short was admitted to Susanne's unit after his friends found him at home weak and confused after not showing up at his weekly bridge club meeting. Harold had been managing well on his own, still caring for his home and garden with only occasional assistance with heavy jobs from his son. Harold's wife had passed away 4 years previously, after complications from minor surgery. Harold was known to his physician but rarely made appointments, which were usually focused on maintaining his driver's licence. Over the fall, Harold's friends had noted that he complained about problems with his "water works" but was otherwise well.
>
> On Susanne's initial assessment, she determined that Harold had been minimizing his fluid intake to avoid having to get up "every 10 minutes" at night. Over the 24 hours before admission, he had not been able to get out of his bedroom because of weakness and "the other people rambling around." Susanne observed that Harold had moments of uncharacteristic confusion during his interview. On physical assessment, Susanne assessed Harold's venous filling because assessing skin turgor is less reliable in older adults. His blood pressure was low, and his heart rate was elevated. His laboratory tests revealed hypernatremia (sodium 148 mmol/L) with elevated blood urea nitrogen (BUN) (18.0 mmol/L) and creatinine (130 mmol/L). Harold's provisional diagnosis was dehydration. On further assessment, Susanne palpated a distended bladder, conducted a bladder scan, and was able to determine that Harold had urinary retention, which was the root cause of his behavioural changes, including avoiding fluids.
>
> Harold was catheterized and treated with intravenous and oral fluids; his blood work and mental status returned to normal. Susanne cared for Harold over her four shifts and developed a therapeutic nurse–client relationship. Before Harold's discharge, Susanne was able to educate Harold about the importance of fluid for his well-being. She also educated Harold's family and friends regarding how to increase Harold's access to fluids during the day, the importance of drinking earlier in the day to avoid having to get up as often at night, and the signs and symptoms of fluid and electrolyte imbalances. In addition, Susanne advocated for a urology consultation regarding his urinary retention. Although Harold refused to "carry around a drinking bottle like those young folks," he expressed clear understanding regarding his fluid and electrolyte health.

Distribution of Body Fluids

Body fluids are distributed in two distinct compartments, one containing intracellular fluids and the other containing extracellular fluids. **Intracellular fluid (ICF)** comprises all fluid within body cells, accounting for approximately 66% of total body water and 40% of body weight (Porth, 2005).

Extracellular fluid (ECF), all the fluid outside cells, is divided into three smaller compartments: interstitial fluid, intravascular fluid, and transcellular fluids. **Interstitial fluid**, including lymph, is the fluid between the cells and outside the blood vessels, whereas **intravascular fluid** is blood plasma. **Transcellular fluids**, separated from other fluid by epithelium, include cerebrospinal, pleural, peritoneal, and synovial fluids and the fluids in the gastrointestinal tract (Porth, 2005).

Composition of Body Fluids

Electrolytes are important **solutes** in all body fluids. An electrolyte, when dissolved in an aqueous solution, separates into **ions** and is able to carry an electrical current (Martini & Nath, 2009). Positively charged electrolytes are **cations** (e.g., sodium [Na^+], potassium [K^+], calcium [Ca^{2+}]). Negatively charged electrolytes are **anions** (e.g., chloride [Cl^-], bicarbonate [HCO_3^-], sulphate [SO_4^-]). Electrolytes are vital to many body functions.

The body carefully regulates electrolyte concentration (Table 40–1). The value millimoles per litre (mmol/L) represents the amount of the specific electrolyte (solute) dissolved in a litre of fluid (**solution**). The solution in which a solute is dissolved is called a **solvent**. Electrolyte concentration within fluid compartments is influenced by electrical charge. During normal physiological processes, ions are exchanged for other ions with the same electrical charge.

Electrolytes are ingested, often in the form of bulk and trace minerals or salts, and then utilized for basic physiological processes, stored for future use, or excreted. These electrolytes are important for maintaining osmotic concentrations in body fluids. They are also necessary for enzyme reactions, nerve impulses, muscle contraction, and metabolism. In addition, some minerals contribute to the regulation of hormone production and strengthening of skeletal structures.

TABLE 40-1 Electrolyte Concentration in Extracellular Fluid

Electrolyte	Extracellular Fluid Concentration (mmol/L)
Sodium (Na^+)	135–145
Potassium (K^+)	3.5–5.0
Calcium (Ca^{2+})	2.25–2.74
Bicarbonate (HCO_3^-)	22–26 (arterial), 24–30 (venous)
Chloride (Cl^-)	95–105
Magnesium (Mg^{2+})	0.6–1.0
Phosphate (PO_4^{3-})	1.0–1.5

Movement of Body Fluids

Fluids and electrolytes constantly shift between compartments to facilitate body processes such as tissue oxygenation, acid–base balance, and urine formation. Because cell membranes separating the body fluid compartments are selectively permeable, water can pass through them easily. However, most ions and molecules pass through them more slowly. Fluids and solutes move across these membranes by four processes: osmosis, diffusion, filtration, and active transport.

Osmosis. Osmosis is the movement of a pure solvent, such as water, through a semi-permeable membrane from an area of lesser solute concentration to an area of greater solute concentration in an attempt to equalize concentrations on both sides of the membrane (Figure 40–1). A semi-permeable membrane allows water to pass through while remaining impermeable to most solutes. The rate of osmosis depends on the concentration of the solutes in the solution, temperature of the solution, electrical charges of the solutes, and differences between the osmotic pressures exerted by the solutions. The concentration of a solution is measured in osmols, which reflect the amount of a substance in solution in the form of molecules, ions, or both. One example of osmosis is the action of osmotic laxatives. These laxative salts are poorly absorbed through the intestinal lining and therefore draw water into the intestinal lumen, causing an accumulation of water and therefore softened stool. The swelling also stretches the intestine, stimulating peristalsis (Lehne, 2007).

Osmotic pressure is the drawing power for water and depends on the number or concentration of molecules in solution. A solution with a high solute concentration has a high osmotic pressure and draws water into itself. If the concentration of the solute is greater on one side of the semipermeable membrane, the rate of osmosis is faster, and solvent rapidly transfers across the membrane. This continues until equilibrium is reached. The osmotic pressure of a solution is called its osmolality, which is expressed in osmols or milliosmols per kilogram (mOsm/kg) of water (Goertz, 2006). **Osmolality** is the measure used to evaluate serum and urine in clinical practice. The normal serum osmolality is 275 to 295 mOsm/kg (Porth, 2005). Changes in extracellular osmolality may result in changes in both ECF and ICF volume.

Solutions are classified as **hypertonic, isotonic,** or **hypotonic. Osmolarity**, reflecting the osmolar concentration in 1 L of solution (mOsm/L), is most often used to describe fluids outside the body (Porth, 2005). A solution with the same osmolarity as blood plasma is called isotonic. A hypertonic solution (a solution of higher osmotic pressure), such as 3% sodium chloride, pulls fluid from cells, causing them to shrink. An isotonic solution (a solution of same osmotic pressure), such as 0.9% sodium chloride, expands the body's fluid volume without causing a fluid shift from one compartment to another. A hypotonic solution (a solution of lower osmotic pressure), such as 0.45% sodium chloride, moves fluid into the cells, causing them to enlarge. Each of these actions occurs through osmosis.

Plasma proteins affect the blood's osmotic pressure. The three main classes of plasma proteins are albumins, globulins, and fibrinogen (Martini & Nath, 2009). Because albumin, produced in the liver, comprises the greatest proportion of plasma proteins, it exerts **colloid osmotic pressure** or oncotic pressure, which tends to keep fluid in the intravascular compartment by pulling water from the interstitial space back into the capillaries.

Diffusion. Diffusion is the movement of ions and molecules in a solution across a semi-permeable membrane from an area of higher concentration to an area of lower concentration (Figure 40–2). The result is an even distribution of the solute in a solution. The rate of diffusion is affected by the molecule size, concentration, and temperature of a solution. The larger the molecule is and the cooler the solution is, the slower the rate of diffusion is. The difference between the two concentrations is known as a **concentration gradient**. Perfume permeating a room and a drop of food colouring moving through a glass of water are common examples of diffusion. A physiological example is the movement of oxygen (O_2) and carbon dioxide (CO_2) between the alveoli and blood vessels in the lungs.

Filtration. Filtration is the process by which water and diffusible substances move together in response to fluid pressure, moving from an area of higher pressure to one of lower pressure. This process is active in capillary beds, where **hydrostatic pressure** differences determine the movement of water (Figure 40–3). Problems occur when hydrostatic pressure is increased on the venous side of the capillary bed, as occurs in congestive heart failure, such that the normal movement of water from the interstitial space into the intravascular space by filtration is reversed, resulting in an accumulation of excess fluid in the interstitial space, known as **edema**. Filtration is also very important for urine formation as water and solutes are carried across the wall of the glomerular capillaries by hydrostatic or blood pressure. Falling blood pressure impacts this process.

Semi-permeable membrane

Before osmosis

After osmosis

Figure 40-1 Osmosis through a semi-permeable membrane. **Source:** From Lewis, S. L., Heitkemper, M. M., Dirksen, S. R., O'Brien, P. G., & Bucher, L. (2007). *Medical-surgical nursing: Assessment and management of clinical problems* (7th ed., p. 317, Fig. 17-6). St. Louis, MO: Mosby.

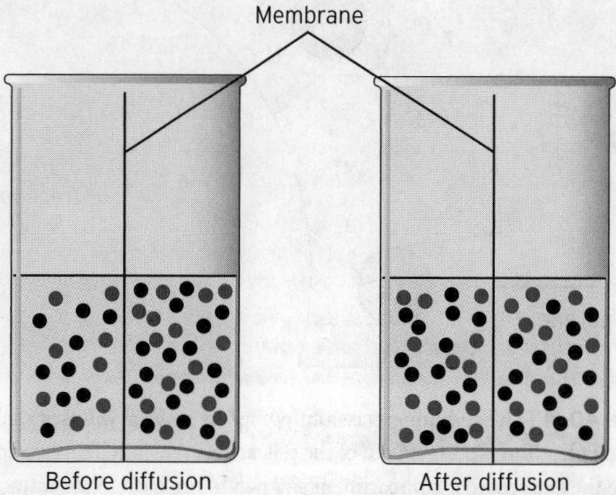

Figure 40-2 Diffusion across a semi-permeable membrane. **Source:** From Lewis, S. L., Heitkemper, M. M., Dirksen, S. R., O'Brien, P. G., & Bucher, L. (2007). *Medical-surgical nursing: Assessment and management of clinical problems* (7th ed., p. 317, Fig. 17-4). St. Louis, MO: Mosby.

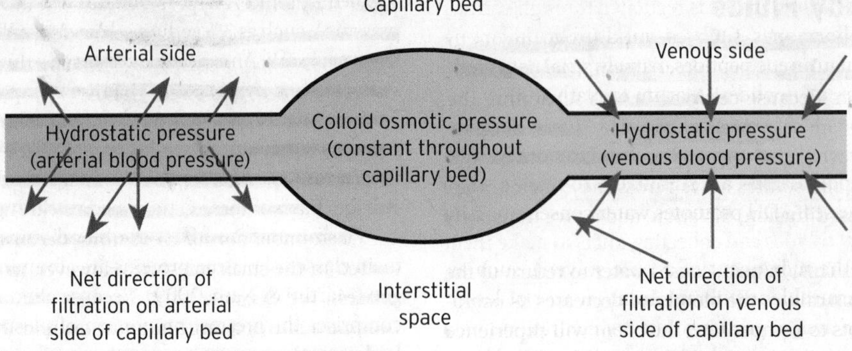

Figure 40-3 An example of filtration and hydrostatic pressure.

Active Transport. Active transport requires the metabolic activity and expenditure of energy to move materials across cell membranes, allowing cells to admit larger molecules than they would otherwise be able to admit or to move molecules from areas of lesser concentration to areas of greater concentration "uphill" (Figure 40–4). An example of active transport is the sodium–potassium pump. Sodium is pumped out of the cell and potassium is pumped in against the concentration gradient. This process enables a higher concentration of potassium in the ICF and a higher concentration of sodium in the ECF.

Active transport is enhanced by carrier molecules within a cell, which bind to incoming molecules. For example, glucose is able to enter cells after it binds with the transport vehicle insulin. Active transport is the mechanism by which cells absorb glucose and other substances to carry out metabolic activities.

Regulation of Body Fluids

Body fluids are regulated by fluid intake, hormonal controls, and fluid output, in order to maintain **homeostasis**. Homeostasis, or internal balance, is essential for survival despite changes in the external environment (Clancy & McVicar, 2007a). In health, the body is able to respond to disturbances in fluids and electrolytes to prevent and repair damage. This involves autoregulation, or intrinsic regulation, and extrinsic regulation through the nervous and endocrine systems.

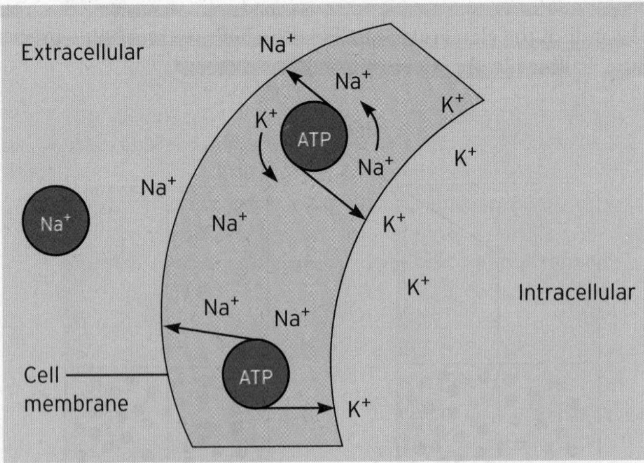

Figure 40-4 The sodium–potassium pump. As sodium diffuses into the cell and potassium is pumped out of the cell, active transport delivers sodium back to the extracellular compartment and potassium back to the intracellular compartment. ATP, adenosine triphosphate. **Source:** From Lewis, S. L., Heitkemper, M. M., Dirksen, S. R., O'Brien, P. G., & Bucher, L. (2007). *Medical-surgical nursing: Assessment and management of clinical problems* (7th ed., p. 317, Fig. 17-5). St. Louis, MO: Mosby.

Fluid Intake. Fluid intake is regulated primarily through the thirst mechanism. The thirst control centre is located within the brain's hypothalamus. Thirst is one of the major factors that determines fluid intake (Porth, 2005). **Osmoreceptors** continually monitor the serum osmotic pressure, and when osmolality increases, the thirst centre in the hypothalamus is stimulated (Martini & Nath, 2009). An increase in plasma sodium increases the osmotic pressure and stimulates the thirst mechanism. Increased plasma osmolality can occur with any condition that interferes with the oral ingestion of fluids, or it can occur with the intake of hypertonic fluids. The hypothalamus will also be stimulated when excess fluid is lost and **hypovolemia** occurs, as in excessive vomiting and hemorrhage. In addition, stimulation of the renin–angiotensin–aldosterone mechanism, potassium depletion, psychological factors, and oropharyngeal dryness initiate the sensation of thirst (Figure 40–5).

The average adult's fluid intake is about 2200 to 2700 mL per day; oral intake accounts for 1100 to 1400 mL, solid foods for about 800 to 1000 mL, and oxidative metabolism for 300 mL daily (Porth, 2005). Water oxidation (oxidative metabolism) is the by-product of cellular metabolism of ingested solid foods. For fluid intake, clients must be in an alert state. Infants, clients with neurological or psychological problems, and some older adults who are unable to perceive or respond to the thirst mechanism are at risk for **dehydration**.

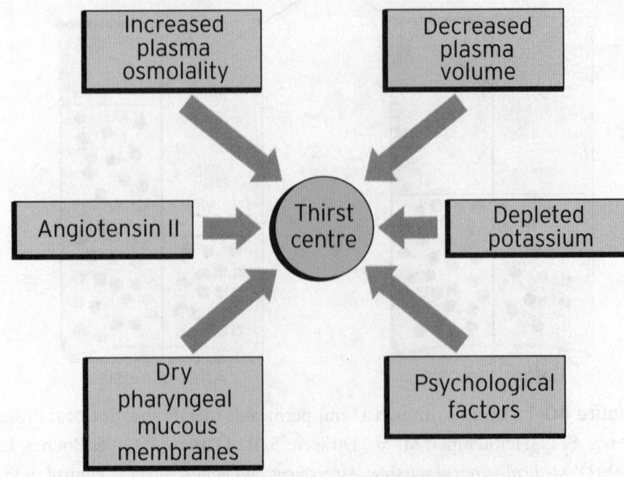

Figure 40-5 Stimuli affecting the thirst mechanism.

Hormonal Regulation. Fluid intake is regulated through various mechanisms involving hormones such as antidiuretic hormone (ADH), aldosterone, and natriuretic peptides, namely atrial natriuretic peptides and brain natriuretic peptides (Martini & Nath, 2009).

Antidiuretic hormone (ADH) is stored in the posterior pituitary gland and is released in response to changes in blood osmolality. The osmoreceptors in the hypothalamus are stimulated to release ADH when the osmolality increases. ADH promotes water conservation by acting directly on the renal tubules and collecting ducts to make them more permeable to water. This, in turn, causes water to return to the systemic circulation, which dilutes the blood and decreases its osmolality. As the body attempts to compensate, the client will experience a temporary decrease in urinary output. When the blood has been sufficiently diluted, the osmoreceptors stop the release of ADH and urinary output is restored. ADH also stimulates the thirst centre to promote fluid intake.

Aldosterone is released by the adrenal cortex in response to increased plasma potassium or falling sodium levels or as part of the renin–angiotensin–aldosterone system to counteract hypovolemia. To resolve hypovolemia, renin is released from the kidney in response to sympathetic nervous system stimulation and decreased renal blood flow, initiating a cascade of physiological and endocrine processes, one of which is the release of aldosterone. Aldosterone acts on the distal portion of the renal tubule to increase the reabsorption (saving) of sodium and the secretion and excretion of potassium and hydrogen.

Natriuretic peptides respond to increases in circulating blood volume. They are released from cardiac muscle cells and act on the peripheral vasculature, other hormones, and the kidney to facilitate diuresis. Natriuretic peptides increase sodium excretion and fluid loss while reducing thirst and blocking the release of ADH and aldosterone.

Fluid Output Regulation. Fluid output occurs through four organs of water loss: the kidneys, the skin, the lungs, and the gastrointestinal tract. The kidneys are the major regulatory organs of fluid balance. They receive approximately 180 L of plasma to filter each day and produce 1200 to 1500 mL of urine (Table 40–2).

Insensible water loss is continuous, gradual movement of water from the respiratory and skin epitheliums, amounting to about 20 to 25 mL/hour (Martini & Nath, 2009). The lungs expire about 400 mL of water daily, whereas insensible skin perspiration losses are approximately 600 mL/day. This insensible water loss may increase in response to changes in respiratory rate and depth. In addition, devices for giving oxygen can increase insensible water loss from the lungs.

➤ TABLE 40-2 Adult Average Daily Fluid Gains and Losses

Type of Fluid	Change (mL)
Fluid Gains	
Oral fluids	1100–1400
Solid foods	800–1000
Metabolism	300
Total gains	2200–2700
Fluid Losses	
Kidneys	1200–1500
Skin	500–600
Lungs	400
Gastrointestinal tract	100–200
Total losses	2200–2700

Fever may increase insensible water loss. Visible or **sensible water loss** from the skin varies greatly depending on the sweat glands. Water loss from the skin is regulated by the sympathetic nervous system, which activates sweat glands.

The gastrointestinal tract plays a vital role in fluid regulation. Approximately 8 L fluid is moved into the gastrointestinal tract and then returns to the ECF daily (Day et al., 2007). Of the 3 to 6 L that the average adult loses each day, only 100 to 200 mL is lost through the feces, under normal conditions, because most of the fluid is reabsorbed in the small intestine. However, in the presence of a disease process, for example with diarrhea, the gastrointestinal tract may become a site of a large amount of fluid loss. This loss may have a significant impact on maintaining normal fluid regulation.

Regulation of Electrolytes

For normal cell function and human well-being, the body maintains a normal balance of electrolytes in the ECF and ICF in spite of changes in intake and loss. This is accomplished primarily through regulation of absorption in the gastrointestinal tract and of excretion through the kidneys. Although fluid and electrolyte balances are inextricably linked, it is important to explore electrolyte balance separately.

Cations. Major cations within the body fluids include sodium, potassium, calcium, and magnesium (Mg^{2+}). Cations interchange when one cation leaves the cell and is replaced by another. This occurs because cells tend to maintain electrical neutrality.

Sodium Regulation. Sodium is the most abundant cation (90%) in ECF and therefore exerts the greatest influence on the ECF osmotic concentration and water balance. Normally, the intake and output of sodium is between 48 and 144 mmol/L daily. With an increase in sodium intake, and therefore an increase in ECF sodium content, water enters the ECF by osmosis, primarily from the digestive tract. Therefore, increased sodium intake results in increased blood volume rather than significant changes in ECF sodium concentration.

The body continually responds to small changes in sodium content. Fluid moves from the ICF into the ECF, and ADH alters water loss and the thirst mechanism. Excessive perspiration and oral intake of water, for example, result in high sodium loss. When this occurs, ADH is reduced in order to maintain homeostasis, and water excretion increases in order to maintain osmotic concentration. However, if, to regulate sodium concentration, a large change in ECF volume occurs, baroreceptors are stimulated to regulate fluid volumes (Martini & Nath, 2009). A reduction in ECF volume is sensed by baroreceptors; this reduction stimulates the renin–angiotensin–aldosterone system to increase aldosterone and ADH production, reducing water and sodium loss and increasing water intake. With an increase in ECF volume, natriuretic peptides decrease aldosterone and ADH, resulting in increased water and sodium loss and decreased water intake.

Sodium ions are also major contributors to nerve impulse transmission, regulation of acid–base balance, and cellular chemical reactions. The normal extracellular sodium concentration is 135 to 145 mmol/L. Sustained or severe problems with sodium concentration result in high sodium, above 145 mmol/L (hypernatremia), or low sodium, below 135 mmol/L (hyponatremia).

Potassium Regulation. Potassium is the major electrolyte and principal cation in the intracellular compartment (Martini & Nath, 2009). The majority (98%) of potassium content is in the ICF. Because the potassium concentration of ECF is relatively low, the cells expend energy to maintain the potassium content of ICF. Potassium is regulated by dietary intake and strongly affected by aldosterone. Extracellular potassium concentration is affected by many complex mechanisms, including those of dietary intake and renal excretion. Renal excretion is regulated by changes in potassium concentration;

changes in the acidity or alkalinity of a fluid (pH measurements), sodium reabsorption, and aldosterone levels (Martini & Nath, 2009). The body conserves potassium poorly, so any condition that increases urine output decreases the serum potassium concentration.

Potassium regulates many metabolic activities and is necessary for glycogen deposits in the liver and skeletal muscle, transmission and conduction of nerve impulses, normal cardiac conduction, and skeletal and smooth muscle contraction. The normal range for serum potassium concentrations is 3.5 to 5 mmol/L.

Calcium Regulation. Calcium is stored in bone, plasma, and body cells. Ninety-nine percent of calcium is located in bone, and only 1% is located in ECF. Approximately 50% of calcium in the plasma is bound to protein, primarily albumin, and 40% is free ionized calcium. The remaining small percentage is combined with non-protein anions such as phosphate (PO_4^{3-}), citrate, and carbonate (Porth, 2005). Normal serum ionized calcium is 1.0 to 1.2 mmol/L. Normal total calcium is 2.25 to 2.74 mmol/L. Calcium is necessary for bone and teeth formation, blood clotting, hormone secretion, cell membrane integrity, cardiac conduction, transmission of nerve impulses, and muscle contraction.

Magnesium Regulation. Magnesium, the second most abundant intracellular cation, is essential for many intracellular activities, such as enzyme reactions. Magnesium, with a plasma concentration of 1.4 to 2.1 mmol/L, is important for bone structure and neuromuscular function, including skeletal and cardiac muscle excitability. Serum magnesium is regulated by dietary intake, renal mechanisms, and actions of the parathyroid hormone.

Anions. The three major anions of body fluids are chloride, bicarbonate, and phosphate ions.

Chloride Regulation. Chloride is the major anion in ECF. The transport of chloride follows sodium. Normal concentrations of chloride range from 97 to 107 mmol/L. Serum chloride is regulated by dietary intake and the kidneys. A person with normal renal function who has a high chloride intake will excrete a higher amount of urine chloride.

Bicarbonate Regulation. Bicarbonate is the major chemical base buffer within the body. The bicarbonate ion is found in ECF and ICF. The bicarbonate ion is an essential component of the carbonic acid–bicarbonate buffering system, which is essential to acid–base balance. The kidneys regulate bicarbonate. Normal arterial bicarbonate levels range between 22 and 26 mmol/L; venous bicarbonate is measured as carbon dioxide content, and the normal value is 24 to 30 mmol/L.

Phosphate Regulation. Phosphorus is the major anion in the ICF; however, nearly all the phosphorus in the body exists in the form of phosphate. Phosphate's most important role is within the ICF, where it assists in the formation of high-energy compounds, such as adenosine triphosphate (ATP) and nucleic acids, and in enzyme activity. Similar to magnesium and calcium, phosphate is used and stored in the skeleton. It also functions with calcium to develop and maintain teeth. Calcium and phosphate are inversely proportional; if one rises, the other falls. Phosphate also assists in acid–base regulation, promotes normal neuromuscular action, and participates in carbohydrate metabolism. Phosphate is normally absorbed through the gastrointestinal tract and is regulated by dietary intake, renal and intestinal excretion, and parathyroid hormone. The normal serum phosphorus level is 0.9 to 1.45 mmol/L.

Regulation of Acid–Base Balance

Acid–base balance exists when the rate at which the body produces and gains acids or bases, through cellular metabolism and gastrointestinal absorption, equals the rate at which acids or bases are excreted. This balance results in a stable concentration of hydrogen ions (H^+) in body fluids that is expressed as the pH value. Hydrogen ions are primarily excreted by the kidneys. A normal hydrogen ion level is necessary to maintain cell membrane integrity and the speed of cellular enzymatic actions. The pH is a scale for measuring the acidity or alkalinity of a fluid. A pH value of 7 is neutral; below 7, acid; and above, 7 alkaline. Arterial blood pH ranges from 7.35 to 7.45.

Arterial blood pH is inversely proportional to the hydrogen ion concentration (i.e., the greater the concentration, the more acidic the solution is and the lower the pH is; the lower the concentration, the more alkaline the solution is and the higher the pH is). The pH is also a reflection of the balance between carbon dioxide, which is regulated by the lungs, and bicarbonate, a base regulated by the kidneys. Because hydrogen, carbon dioxide, and bicarbonate are excreted a significant distance from where they are produced, normal pH is maintained by **buffers** and buffer systems. A buffer is a substance or a group of substances that can absorb or release hydrogen ions to stabilize pH. In addition to buffering by weak acids and bases throughout the body, homeostasis is maintained by buffer systems and regulatory mechanisms in the lungs and the kidneys.

Buffers. Buffer systems are combinations of a weak acid and a weak base and are the short-term regulators of acid–base balance. The four main types of buffer systems are protein (amino acids, plasma proteins), hemoglobin (also a protein but unique in its buffering role), carbonic acid (H_2CO_3) and bicarbonate, and phosphate. Other types include the ammonia buffer system, a complex system that occurs in ICF, and the tubular system in the kidneys. All of these buffers bind hydrogen ion until it can be permanently removed through the regulatory mechanisms in the lungs and the kidneys.

The carbonic acid–bicarbonate buffer system (Figure 40–6) is used to evaluate acid–base balance, using the arterial blood gas (ABG) test. This system can be expressed as the following:

$$CO_2 + H_2O \leftrightarrow H_2CO_3 \leftrightarrow H^+ + HCO_3^-$$

Carbon dioxide + Water ↔ Carbonic acid ↔
Hydrogen ion + Bicarbonate

The carbonic acid–bicarbonate buffer system is the principal buffering system to react to change in the pH of ECF, and it reacts within seconds. The previous equation demonstrates how hydrogen ions and carbon dioxide concentrations are directly related to each other. Whenever carbon dioxide increases, an increase in hydrogen ions is produced, and whenever hydrogen ions are produced, more carbon dioxide is produced (Clancy & McVicar, 2007b). The lungs

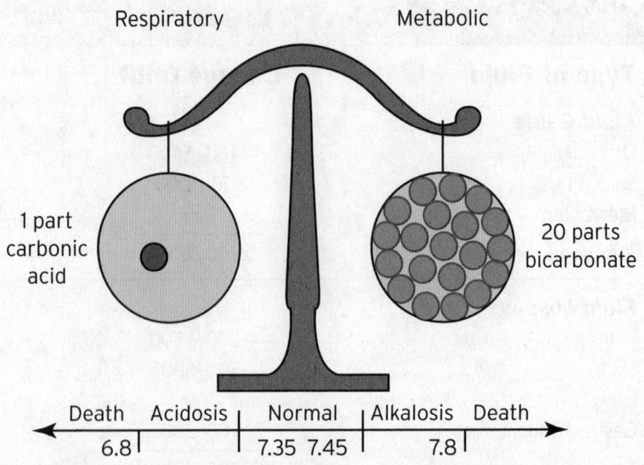

Figure 40-6 Carbonic acid-to-bicarbonate ratio and pH.

control the excretion of carbon dioxide, and the kidneys control the excretion of hydrogen and bicarbonate ions.

Another buffer system is the hemoglobin–oxyhemoglobin system within red blood cells (RBCs). This buffer system can have an immediate effect on pH because carbon dioxide diffuses readily into the RBC and forms carbonic acid. The carbonic acid dissociates into hydrogen and bicarbonate ions, the latter of which diffuse into the plasma in exchange for chloride. The hydrogen ions attach to hemoglobin, whereas the carbon dioxide is carried to the lungs, where the reaction is reversed.

Regulatory Mechanisms. When the ability of buffer systems is exceeded, acid–base homeostasis is regulated by the lungs and the kidneys. The lungs adapt rapidly to an acid–base imbalance. Ordinarily, increased levels of hydrogen ions and carbon dioxide provide the stimulus for respiration. When the concentration of hydrogen ions is altered, the lungs react to correct the imbalance by altering the rate and depth of respiration. For example, when metabolic acidosis is present, respirations are increased, resulting in a greater amount of carbon dioxide being exhaled, which results in a decrease in the acidic level; when metabolic alkalosis is present, the lungs retain carbon dioxide by decreasing the respirations, thereby increasing the acidic level (Martini & Nath, 2009).

The kidneys take from a few hours to several days to regulate acid–base imbalance. They regenerate or reabsorb bicarbonate in cases of acid excess and excrete it in cases of acid deficit. In addition, the kidneys use a phosphate ion to excrete hydrogen ions by forming phosphoric acid (H_3PO_4); sulphuric acid (H_2SO_4) may also be excreted. Finally, the kidneys use the ammonia mechanism to regulate acid–base balance. In this mechanism, certain amino acids are chemically changed within the renal tubules into ammonia, which, in the presence of hydrogen ions, forms ammonium and is excreted in the urine, hence releasing hydrogen ions from the body (Monahan et al., 2007).

Disturbances in Electrolyte, Fluid, and Acid-Base Balances

Disturbances in electrolyte, fluid, or acid–base balance seldom occur alone and can disrupt normal body processes. For example, when body fluids are lost because of burns, illness, or trauma, the client is also at risk for electrolyte imbalances. In addition, some untreated electrolyte imbalances (e.g., potassium loss) contribute to acid–base disturbances.

Electrolyte Imbalances. Table 40–3 provides a list of the causes, signs, and symptoms of electrolyte imbalances.

Sodium Imbalances. **Hyponatremia** is a lower-than-normal concentration of sodium in the blood (serum), which can occur with a net sodium loss or net water excess (see Table 40–3). It occurs frequently in seriously ill clients and is the most common electrolyte disturbance among older adults (Woodrow, 2003a, 2003b). Clinical indicators and treatment depend on the cause of hyponatremia and whether it is associated with a normal, decreased, or increased ECF volume (Heitz & Horne, 2005). The usual situation is a loss of sodium without a loss of fluid, which results in a decrease in the osmolality of ECF. Sodium and chloride are not stored in the body; therefore, they must be consumed daily or provided through IV solutions in the ill.

Hypernatremia is a greater-than-normal concentration of sodium in ECF that can be caused by excess water loss or overall sodium excess (see Table 40–3). When the cause of hypernatremia is an increased aldosterone secretion, sodium is retained and potassium is excreted. When hypernatremia occurs, the body attempts to conserve as much water as possible through renal reabsorption.

Potassium Imbalances. **Hypokalemia** is one of the most common electrolyte imbalances, in which an inadequate amount of potassium circulates in ECF (see Table 40–3). Hypokalemia, with potassium levels less than 3.5 mmol/L, results in cardiac arrhythmias, fatigue, and altered muscle activity throughout the body (Day et al., 2007). Because the normal amount of serum potassium is so small, little tolerance for fluctuations exists. The most common cause of hypokalemia is the use of potassium-wasting diuretics such as thiazide and loop diuretics.

Hyperkalemia is a greater-than-normal amount of potassium in the blood. Lethal cardiac arrhythmias result from potassium levels over 5.0 mmol/L, as well as skeletal muscle weakness and paralysis (see Table 40–3). The primary cause of hyperkalemia is renal failure because any decrease in renal function diminishes the amount of potassium the kidney can excrete. Elevations in potassium may also be seen in crush injuries, in which cells are broken and potassium is released from within the cells.

Calcium Imbalances. **Hypocalcemia** represents a drop in serum or ionized calcium. It can result from several illnesses, some of which directly affect the thyroid and parathyroid glands (see Table 40–3). Other causes include prolonged bed rest and renal insufficiency (in which the kidneys' inability to excrete phosphorus causes the phosphorus level to rise and the calcium level to decline). Signs and symptoms can be related to diminished functioning of the neuromuscular, cardiac, and renal systems.

Hypercalcemia is an increase in the total serum concentration of calcium or ionized calcium. Hypercalcemia is frequently a symptom of an underlying disease, such as malignancy or hyperparathyroidism, resulting in excess bone reabsorption with release of calcium (Porth, 2005).

Magnesium Imbalances. Disturbances in magnesium levels are summarized in Table 40–3. Symptoms are the result of changes in neuromuscular excitability. **Hypomagnesemia**, a drop in serum magnesium below 0.65 mmol/L, occurs with malnutrition, malabsorption disorders, diarrhea, and alcohol withdrawal and may cause neuromuscular symptoms, seizures, or cardiac arrhythmias. **Hypermagnesemia**, an increase in serum magnesium levels, more than 1.05 mmol/L, depresses skeletal muscles and nerve function. Magnesium may inhibit acetylcholine, thereby causing a sedative effect.

Chloride Imbalances. **Hypochloremia** occurs when the serum chloride level falls below normal. Vomiting or prolonged and excessive nasogastric or fistula drainage can result in hypochloremia because of the loss of hydrochloric acid. The use of loop and thiazide diuretics also results in increased chloride loss as sodium is excreted. When serum chloride levels fall, metabolic alkalosis results as the body adapts by increasing reabsorption of the bicarbonate ion to maintain electrical neutrality.

Hyperchloremia occurs when the serum chloride level rises above normal, which usually occurs when the serum bicarbonate value falls or the sodium level rises. Hypochloremia and hyperchloremia rarely occur as single disease processes but are commonly associated with acid–base imbalance. No single set of symptoms is associated with these two alterations.

Fluid Disturbances. The basic types of fluid imbalances are isotonic and osmolar. Isotonic deficit and excess exist when water and electrolytes are gained or lost in equal proportions. In contrast, osmolar imbalances are losses or excesses of only water, so the concentration (osmolality) of the serum is affected. It is important to recognize that maintaining fluid homeostasis is primarily related to circulatory volume. Hemodynamics respond quickly to changes in the intravascular compartment, followed more slowly by sodium and water balance mechanisms (Porth, 2005). Table 40–4 lists the causes and signs and symptoms of common fluid disturbances.

➤ TABLE 40-3 Electrolyte Imbalances

Imbalance and Related Causes	Signs and Symptoms
Hyponatremia GI losses: vomiting, diarrhea, nasogastric suction Renal loss: kidney disease resulting in salt wasting; diuretics; adrenal insufficiency Skin loss: excessive perspiration; burns Psychogenic polydipsia Syndrome of inappropriate antidiuretic hormone (SIADH)	*Physical examination:* apprehension, personality change, postural hypotension, postural dizziness, abdominal cramping, nausea and vomiting, diarrhea, tachycardia, dry mucous membranes, convulsions, and coma *Laboratory findings:* serum sodium level <135 mmol/L, serum osmolality <285 mmol/kg, and urine specific gravity <1.010 (if not caused by SIADH)
Hypernatremia Excess salt intake: ingestion of large amounts of concentrated salt solutions; iatrogenic administration of hypertonic saline solution parenterally Excess aldosterone secretion Diabetes insipidus Increased sensible and insensible water losses Water deprivation	*Physical examination:* extreme thirst, dry and flushed skin, dry and sticky tongue and mucous membranes, postural hypotension, fever, agitation, convulsions, restlessness, and irritability *Laboratory findings:* serum sodium levels >145 mmol/L, serum osmolality >300 mmol/kg, and urine specific gravity >1.030 (if not caused by diabetes insipidus)
Hypokalemia Use of potassium-wasting diuretics Diarrhea, vomiting, or other GI losses Alkalosis Excess aldosterone secretion Polyuria Extreme sweating Excessive use of potassium-free intravenous solutions Treatment of diabetic ketoacidosis with insulin	*Physical examination:* weakness and fatigue, muscle weakness, nausea and vomiting, intestinal distension, decreased bowel sounds, decreased deep tendon reflexes, ventricular dysrhythmias, paraesthesias, and weak, irregular pulse *Laboratory findings:* serum potassium level <3.5 mmol/L; ECG abnormalities (flattened T wave, ST segment depression, U wave); potentiated digoxin effects (e.g., ventricular dysrhythmias)*
Hyperkalemia Renal failure Fluid volume deficit Massive cellular damage such as from burns and trauma Iatrogenic administration of large amounts of potassium intravenously Adrenal insufficiency Acidosis, especially diabetic ketoacidosis Rapid infusion of stored blood Use of potassium-sparing diuretics Ingestion of K^+ salt substitutes	*Physical examination:* anxiety, dysrhythmias, paraesthesia, weakness, abdominal cramps, and diarrhea *Laboratory findings:* serum potassium level >5.0 mmol/L; ECG abnormalities (peaked T wave and widened QRS complex [bradycardia, heart block, dysrhythmias]; eventually, QRS pattern widens and cardiac arrest occurs*)
Hypocalcemia Rapid administration of blood transfusions containing citrate Hypoalbuminemia Hypoparathyroidism Vitamin D deficiency Pancreatitis Alkalosis Chronic renal failure Chronic alcoholism	*Physical examination:* numbness and tingling of fingers and circumoral (around mouth) region, hyperactive reflexes, positive Trousseau's sign (carpopedal spasm with hypoxia), positive Chvostek's sign (contraction of facial muscles when facial nerve is tapped), tetany, muscle cramps, and pathological fractures (chronic hypocalcemia) *Laboratory findings:* serum ionized calcium level <1.05 mmol/L or total serum calcium level <2.25 mmol/L; ECG abnormalities (ventricular tachycardia)
Hypercalcemia Hyperparathyroidism Osteometastasis Paget's disease Osteoporosis Prolonged immobilization Acidosis Thiazide diuretics	*Physical examination:* anorexia, nausea and vomiting, weakness, hypoactive reflexes, lethargy, flank pain (from kidney stones), decreased level of consciousness, personality changes, and cardiac arrest *Laboratory findings:* serum ionized calcium level >1.30 mmol/L or total serum calcium level >2.75 mmol/L; abnormalities visible on X-ray examination (generalized osteoporosis, widespread bone cavitation, radiopaque urinary stones); elevated blood urea nitrogen level >7.1 mmol/L and elevated creatinine level >106 mmol/L, caused by fluid volume deficit or renal damage caused by urolithiasis; ECG abnormalities (heart block)

TABLE 40-3 Electrolyte Imbalances *continued*

Imbalance and Related Causes	Signs and Symptoms
Hypomagnesemia	
Inadequate intake: malnutrition and alcoholism Inadequate absorption or loss: diarrhea, vomiting, nasogastric drainage, fistulas, diseases of small intestine Excessive loss resulting from thiazide diuretics Aldosterone excess Polyuria	*Physical examination:* muscular tremors, hyperactive deep tendon reflexes, confusion and disorientation, tachycardia, hypertension, dysrhythmias, and positive Chvostek's and Trousseau's signs *Laboratory findings:* serum magnesium level <0.65 mmol/L
Hypermagnesemia	
Renal failure Excess oral or parenteral intake of magnesium	*Physical examination:* acute elevations in magnesium levels: hypoactive deep tendon reflexes, decreased depth and rate of respirations, hypotension, and flushing *Laboratory findings:* serum magnesium level >1.05 mmol/L; ECG abnormalities (prolonged QT interval, atrioventricular block)

ECG, electrocardiogram; GI, gastrointestinal.

*Data from Heitz, U. E., & Horne, M. M. (2005). *Mosby's pocket guide series: Fluid, electrolyte, and acid-base balance* (5th ed.). St. Louis, MO: Mosby.

TABLE 40-4 Fluid Disturbances

Imbalance and Related Causes	Signs and Symptoms
Isotonic Imbalances	
Fluid Volume Deficit: Water and Electrolytes Lost in Equal or Isotonic Proportions	
GI losses such as diarrhea, vomiting, or drainage from fistulas or tubes Loss of plasma or whole blood, such as burns or hemorrhage Excessive perspiration Fever Decreased oral intake of fluids Confusion or depression Use of diuretics	*Physical examination:* postural hypotension, tachycardia, dry mucous membranes, poor skin turgor, thirst confusion, rapid weight loss, slow vein filling, flat neck veins, lethargy, oliguria (<30 mL/hr), weak pulse *Laboratory findings:* urine specific gravity >1.030, increased hematocrit level >50%, and increased BUN level >7.1 mmol/L (see Appendix B) (hemoconcentration)
Fluid Volume Excess: Water and Sodium Retained in Isotonic Proportions	
Congestive heart failure Renal failure Cirrhosis of the liver Increased serum aldosterone and steroid levels Excessive sodium intake or administration	*Physical examination:* rapid weight gain, edema (especially in dependent areas), hypertension, polyuria (if renal mechanisms are normal), neck vein distension, increased blood venous pressure, crackles in lungs, confusion *Laboratory findings:* decreased hematocrit level <30% and decreased BUN level <3.6 mmol/L (hemodilution)
Osmolar Imbalances	
Hyperosmolar Imbalance: Dehydration	
Diabetes insipidus Interruption of neurologically driven thirst drive Diabetic ketoacidosis Osmotic diuresis Administration of hypertonic parenteral fluids or tube-feeding formulas	*Physical examination:* dry and sticky mucous membranes, flushed and dry skin, thirst, elevated body temperature, irritability, convulsions, coma *Laboratory findings:* increased serum sodium level >145 mmol/L and increased serum osmolality >300 mmol/kg
Hypo-osmolar Imbalance: Water Excess	
Syndrome of inappropriate antidiuretic hormone (SIADH) Excess water intake	*Physical examination:* decreased level of consciousness, convulsions, coma *Laboratory findings:* decreased serum sodium level <135 mmol/L and decreased serum osmolality <275 mmol/kg

BUN, blood urea nitrogen; GI, gastrointestinal.

Acid-Base Balance. Arterial blood gas (ABG) analysis is the best way to evaluate acid–base balance and is based on the carbonic acid–bicarbonate buffer system. Measurement of ABGs involves analysis of six components: pH, $PaCO_2$, PaO_2, oxygen saturation, base excess, and bicarbonate. Deviation from a normal value will indicate that the client is experiencing an acid–base imbalance.

Measurements of Acidity or Alkalinity of Fluids. The pH reflects hydrogen ion concentration in the body fluids. Even a slight change can be potentially life-threatening. An increase in concentration of hydrogen ion makes a solution more acidic; a decrease makes the solution more alkaline. Normal pH value is 7.35 to 7.45; therefore, a pH value below 7.35 is acidic, and one above 7.45 is alkalotic.

$PaCO_2$. $PaCO_2$ is the partial pressure of carbon dioxide in arterial blood and is a reflection of the depth of pulmonary ventilation. The normal range is 35 to 45 mm Hg. A $PaCO_2$ less than 35 mm Hg is an indication that hyperventilation has occurred. As the rate and depth of respiration increase, more carbon dioxide is exhaled, and the carbon dioxide concentration decreases. When the $PaCO_2$ is more than 45 mm Hg, hypoventilation has occurred. As the rate and the depth of respiration decrease, less carbon dioxide is exhaled and more is retained, increasing the concentration of carbon dioxide.

PaO_2. PaO_2 is the partial pressure of oxygen in arterial blood. It has no primary role in acid–base regulation if it is within normal limits. A PaO_2 less than 60 mm Hg can lead to anaerobic metabolism, resulting in lactic acid production and metabolic acidosis. A reduction in vital capacity (Martini & Nath, 2009) may contribute to a reduction in PaO_2 in older adults. The normal range is 80 to 100 mm Hg.

Oxygen Saturation. **Oxygen saturation** is the point at which hemoglobin is saturated by oxygen. When a client is hypoxic and uses up readily available oxygen, the reserve oxygen (oxygen attached to hemoglobin) is drawn upon to provide oxygen to the tissues (Ignatavicius & Workman, 2005). Oxygen can be affected by changes in temperature, pH, and $PaCO_2$. When the PaO_2 falls below 60 mm Hg, a large drop in saturation results (Heitz & Horne, 2005). The normal range is 95% to 99%.

Base Excess. Base excess refers to the buffering systems discussed previously, with a normal range of +2 to −2. Base excess reflects deviations from a serum pH of 7.4 (neutral). Higher values of **base excess**, indicate alkalosis. Negative values of base excess indicate acidosis, usually the result of the elimination of too many bicarbonate ions.

Bicarbonate. Serum bicarbonate is excreted or retained by the kidneys to maintain a normal acid–base environment. It is also the principal buffer of the ECFs of the body. A normal pH is maintained with a bicarbonate ratio 20 times that of the fluid concentration of carbonic acid (Porth, 2005). The normal range is 22 to 26 mmol/L. Less than 22 mmol/L of bicarbonate usually indicates metabolic acidosis, whereas more than 26 mmol/L indicates metabolic alkalosis.

Types of Acid-Base Imbalances. The four primary types of acid–base imbalance are respiratory acidosis, respiratory alkalosis, metabolic acidosis, and metabolic alkalosis (Table 40–5).

Respiratory Acidosis. **Respiratory acidosis** is marked by an increased $PaCO_2$, excess carbonic acid, and an increased hydrogen ion concentration (decreased pH). This occurs when respirations are not effective in excreting carbon dioxide, thereby resulting in an increase in hydrogen concentration. With respiratory acidosis, carbon dioxide crosses the blood–brain barrier, causing neurological changes, such as headaches, irritability, and, ultimately, impaired consciousness. Hypoxemia occurs simultaneously because of respiratory depression, resulting in further neurological impairment. Electrolyte changes such as hyperkalemia and hypercalcemia may accompany the acidosis. The renal system compensates by increasing bicarbonate and eliminating hydrogen ion.

Example: Mr. Butler comes to the emergency department short of breath. The first set of ABGs includes the following: pH = 7.26, $PaCO_2$ = 55 mm Hg, and bicarbonate = 23 mmol/L. His body has not yet compensated for his respiratory insufficiency. A person with chronic lung disease may present with greater compensation and a pH that is closer to normal.

Respiratory Alkalosis. **Respiratory alkalosis** is marked by decreased $PaCO_2$ and increased pH. Respiratory alkalosis can begin outside the respiratory system (e.g., anxiety with hyperventilation) or within the respiratory system (e.g., the initial phase of an asthma attack). Usually, the respiratory system corrects imbalances before compensatory changes are required.

Example: Janet is hyperventilating when she comes into the emergency department. Her ABGs are as follows: pH = 7.52, $PaCO_2$ = 30 mm Hg, bicarbonate = 24 mmol/L, and base excess = 2.5 mmol/L. Her kidneys have not had time to compensate and lower the bicarbonate level.

Metabolic Acidosis. **Metabolic acidosis** results from a decrease in serum bicarbonate or the production of organic or fixed acids. An analysis of serum electrolytes to detect an anion gap may be helpful in attempting to identify the cause of the metabolic acidosis. An **anion gap** reflects unmeasurable anions present in plasma and is calculated by subtracting the sum of chloride and bicarbonate from the amount of plasma sodium concentration (Table 40–6). Compensation for metabolic acidosis involves an increase in respiratory rate and depth to eliminate carbon dioxide initially, followed by renal mechanisms such as increased hydrogen ion excretion and generation and release of bicarbonate into the ECF.

Example: Ms. Jane Smith is admitted to hospital after having run her first marathon. Her electrolytes are as follows: sodium = 131 mmol/L, bicarbonate = 9 mmol/L, and chloride = 86 mmol/L. You would calculate the anion gap as follows: $Na - (HCO_3^- + Cl^-) = 131 - (9 + 86) = 36$ mmol/L. The normal anion gap is less than 16 mmol/L (so her anion gap is high). Ms. Smith receives a diagnosis of lactic acidosis because of tissue hypoxia.

Metabolic Alkalosis. **Metabolic alkalosis** is marked by the heavy loss of acid from the body or by increased levels of bicarbonate. The most common causes are vomiting and gastric suction, as well as potassium deficiency, hyperaldosteronism, and diuretic therapy (Porth, 2005). The body attempts to compensate by increasing the excretion of bicarbonate and decreasing the rate and the depth of respirations. Symptoms associated with metabolic alkalosis are depressed respirations and tingling of the fingers and dizziness related to secondary low calcium (Day et al., 2007). In serious metabolic alkalosis, cardiac arrhythmias can occur.

Example: Mr. Jones comes into the clinic with persistent vomiting. His ABGs are as follows: pH = 7.63, bicarbonate = 45 mmol/L, $PaCO_2$ = 48 mm Hg, and base excess = 16 mmol/L. He is in metabolic alkalosis.

➤ TABLE 40-5 Acid-Base Imbalances

Imbalance and Related Causes	Signs and Symptoms
Respiratory Acidosis	
Hypoventilation Resulting From Primary Respiratory Problems	
Atelectasis (obstruction of small airways, often caused by retained mucus) Pneumonia Cystic fibrosis Respiratory failure Airway obstruction Chest wall injury	*Physical examination:* confusion, dizziness, lethargy, headache, ventricular dysrhythmias, warm and flushed skin, muscular twitching, convulsions, and coma *Laboratory findings:* arterial blood gas alterations: pH <7.35, $PaCO_2$ >45 mm Hg, PaO_2 <80 mm Hg, and bicarbonate level normal (if uncompensated) or >26 mmol/L (if compensated)
Hypoventilation Resulting From Factors Outside the Respiratory System	
Drug overdose with a respiratory depressant Paralysis of respiratory muscles caused by various neurological alterations Head injury Obesity	*Physical examination:* confusion, dizziness, lethargy, headache, ventricular dysrhythmias, warm and flushed skin, muscular twitching, convulsions, and coma *Laboratory findings:* arterial blood gas alterations: pH <7.35, $PaCO_2$ >45 mm Hg, PaO_2 <80 mm Hg, and bicarbonate level normal (if uncompensated) or >26 mmol/L (if compensated)
Respiratory Alkalosis	
Hyperventilation Resulting From Primary Respiratory Problems	
Asthma Pneumonia Inappropriate mechanical ventilator settings	*Physical examination:* dizziness, confusion, dysrhythmias, tachypnea, numbness and tingling of extremities, convulsions, and coma *Laboratory findings:* arterial blood gas alterations: pH >7.45, $PaCO_2$ <35 mm Hg, PaO_2 normal, and bicarbonate level normal (if short-lived or uncompensated) or <22 mmol/L (if compensated)
Hyperventilation Resulting From Factors Outside the Respiratory System	
Anxiety Hypermetabolic states (fever, exercise) Disorders of the central nervous system (head injuries, infections) Salicylate overdose	*Physical examination:* dizziness, confusion, dysrhythmias, tachypnea, numbness and tingling of extremities *Laboratory findings:* arterial blood gas alterations: pH >7.45, $PaCO_2$ <35 mm Hg, PaO_2 normal, and bicarbonate level normal (if short-lived or uncompensated)
Metabolic Acidosis	
High Anion Gap	
Starvation Diabetic ketoacidosis Renal failure Lactic acidosis from heavy exercise Use of drugs (e.g., methanol, ethanol, formic acid, paraldehyde, aspirin)	*Physical examination:* headache, lethargy, confusion, dysrhythmias, tachypnea with deep respirations, abdominal cramps, and flushed skin *Laboratory findings:* arterial blood gas alterations: pH <7.35, $PaCO_2$ normal (if uncompensated) or <35 mm Hg (if compensated), PaO_2 normal or increased with rapid, deep respirations, bicarbonate level <22 mmol/L, and oxygen saturation normal
Normal Anion Gap	
Renal tubular acidosis Diarrhea	*Physical examination:* headache, lethargy, confusion, dysrhythmias, tachypnea with deep respirations, abdominal cramps, and flushed skin *Laboratory findings:* arterial blood gas alterations: pH <7.35, $PaCO_2$ normal (if uncompensated) or <35 mm Hg (if compensated), PaO_2 normal or increased with rapid, deep respirations, anion gap (difference between positive ions and negative ions) of greater than 12 mmol/L
Metabolic Alkalosis	
Excessive vomiting Prolonged gastric suctioning Hypokalemia or hypercalcemia Excess aldosterone Use of drugs (steroids, sodium bicarbonate, diuretics)	*Physical examination:* dizziness; dysrhythmias; numbness and tingling of fingers, toes, and circumoral region; muscle cramps; tetany *Laboratory findings:* arterial blood gas alterations: pH >7.45, $PaCO_2$ normal (if uncompensated) or >45 mm Hg (if compensated), PaO_2 normal, and bicarbonate level >26 mmol/L

$PaCO_2$, partial pressure of carbon dioxide in arterial blood; PaO_2, partial pressure of oxygen in arterial blood; pH, measurement of the acidity or alkalinity of a fluid.

TABLE 40-6 Anion Gap

Anion Gap Type	Value (mmol/L)	Causes
Normal	12 (±2)	Diarrhea, renal tubular acidosis, or pancreatic fistula causing a direct loss of HCO_3^-: addition of chloride-containing acids
Increased	>14	Lactic acidosis, uremia, diabetic ketoacidosis, or salicylate and methanol toxicity, resulting in accumulation of nonvolatile acids with a decrease in (HCO_3^-)

From Adams, B. D., Bonzani, T. A., & Hunter, C. J. (2006). The anion gap does not accurately screen for lactic acidosis in emergency department clients. *Emergency Medicine Journal, 23*, 179–182; and Heitz, U. E., & Horne, M. M. (2005). *Mosby's pocket guide series: Fluid, electrolyte, and acid–base balance* (5th ed.). St. Louis, MO: Mosby.

Knowledge Base of Nursing Practice

The essential functions of fluid, electrolyte, and acid–base balances are important aspects of the scientific knowledge base of nursing practice. In all areas of nursing practice, nurses attend to the relationship between healthy water and human health (Davidhizar et al., 2004). Regardless of the area of practice, all nurses will be involved in assessment, planning, and interventions in relation to water, electrolytes, and factors that influence acid–base balance. Certain clients are particularly vulnerable to imbalances, including infants, severely ill clients, disoriented or immobile clients, and older adults because they cannot respond independently to early symptoms. If untreated, over time, the body can no longer maintain fluid and electrolyte or acid–base balances adequately, and the client's health becomes compromised. Prolonged or severe compromises may lead to irreversible chronic health problems (Box 40–2). Good nursing care involves informed assessment in relation to fluid, electrolyte, and acid–base balances.

BOX 40-2 Risk Factors for Fluid, Electrolytes, and Acid-Base Imbalances

Age
Very young
Very old

Gender
Women

Environment
Diet
Exercise
Hot weather and sweating

Chronic Diseases
Cancer
Cardiovascular disease, such as congestive heart failure
Endocrine disease such as Cushing's disease and diabetes mellitus
Malnutrition
Chronic obstructive pulmonary disease
Renal disease

Trauma
Crush injuries
Head injuries
Burns

Therapies
Diuretics
Steroids
Intravenous therapy
Total parenteral nutrition (TPN)

Gastrointestinal Losses
Gastroenteritis
Nasogastric suctioning
Fistulas

Critical Thinking

Successful critical thinking requires a synthesis of knowledge, experience, information gathered from clients, critical thinking qualities and intellectual and professional standards. You must use clinical judgements to anticipate the information necessary, analyze the data, and make decisions regarding client care. You must also adapt critical thinking to the changing needs of the client. During assessment (Figure 40–7), you must consider all elements that contribute to making appropriate nursing diagnoses.

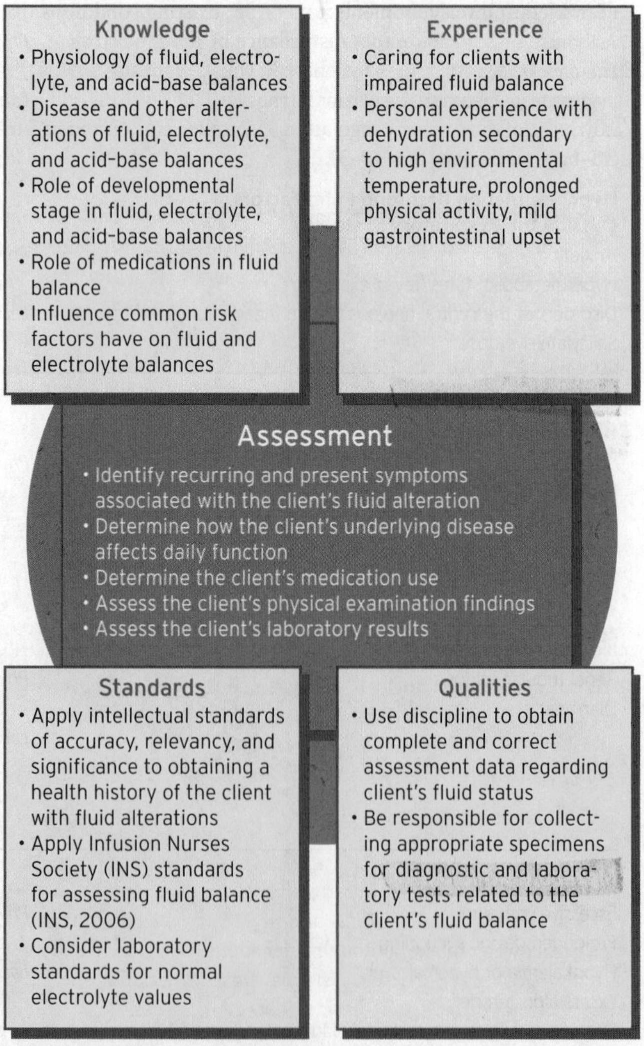

Knowledge
- Physiology of fluid, electrolyte, and acid-base balances
- Disease and other alterations of fluid, electrolyte, and acid-base balances
- Role of developmental stage in fluid, electrolyte, and acid-base balances
- Role of medications in fluid balance
- Influence common risk factors have on fluid and electrolyte balances

Experience
- Caring for clients with impaired fluid balance
- Personal experience with dehydration secondary to high environmental temperature, prolonged physical activity, mild gastrointestinal upset

Assessment
- Identify recurring and present symptoms associated with the client's fluid alteration
- Determine how the client's underlying disease affects daily function
- Determine the client's medication use
- Assess the client's physical examination findings
- Assess the client's laboratory results

Standards
- Apply intellectual standards of accuracy, relevancy, and significance to obtaining a health history of the client with fluid alterations
- Apply Infusion Nurses Society (INS) standards for assessing fluid balance (INS, 2006)
- Consider laboratory standards for normal electrolyte values

Qualities
- Use discipline to obtain complete and correct assessment data regarding client's fluid status
- Be responsible for collecting appropriate specimens for diagnostic and laboratory tests related to the client's fluid balance

Figure 40-7 Critical thinking model for assessment of fluid, electrolyte, and acid–base balances.

To understand how fluid, electrolyte, and acid–base imbalances affect the client, you must integrate knowledge of physiology, pathophysiology, and pharmacology with previous experiences and information gathered from the client. Critical thinking qualities such as discipline and integrity are also necessary to identify diagnoses and plan interventions. Professional standards provide valuable guidelines for comprehensive assessment and intelligent planning and intervention.

Nursing Process

❖Assessment

Client care begins with informed assessment, including data regarding the status of the client's fluid, electrolyte, and acid–base balances. Assessment is informed by knowledge of risk factors, physiology, and developmental considerations and by critical thinking. By gathering data through a health history and physical examination, you will identify clients at risk and then identify all appropriate nursing diagnoses.

Health History

The nursing assessment begins with a nursing health history, which is designed to reveal any risk factors or pre-existing conditions that may cause or contribute to a disturbance of fluid, electrolyte, and acid–base balances. With the client, you will explore any factors that may cause a disturbance and will integrate the information with knowledge of fluid volume regulation, electrolyte concentration, and acid–base regulation (Box 40–3).

Age. First consider the client's age. An infant's proportion of total body water, approximately 75%, is greater than that of children or adults. Infants also are more vulnerable to alterations in dietary intake of electrolytes because they have smaller reserves (Martini & Nath, 2009). Infants are not protected from fluid loss because they ingest and excrete a relatively greater daily water volume than do adults (Hockenberry & Wilson, 2007). Therefore, infants are at a greater risk for **fluid volume deficit (FVD)** and hyperosmolar imbalance because body water loss is proportionately greater per kilogram of weight.

Children ages 2 through 12 years have less stable regulatory responses to imbalance and in childhood illnesses tend to have less tolerance for large changes. Children frequently respond to illnesses with fevers of higher temperatures and longer duration than those of adults. At any age, fever can increase the rate of insensible water loss. Adolescents have increased metabolic processes and increased water production because of the major rapid changes that occur in the anatomical and physiological processes. Changes in fluid balance are greater in adolescent girls because of hormonal changes associated with the menstrual cycle.

Aging has a significant impact on fluid, electrolyte, and acid–base balances and on compensatory mechanisms. Total body water proportion gradually declines with age, in general after age 40 (Martini & Nath, 2009). With normal aging, the glomerular filtration rate is reduced, along with the number and functional capacity of nephrons. Changes in the skin and skeletal and muscle mass result in the need for a higher water intake, although older adults have a decreased thirst sensation. Also, a reduction in taste may limit the amount of oral fluids consumed, resulting in older adults not meeting their daily requirements (Box 40–4). Older adults have a reduction in aldosterone, which increases sodium excretion and may result in hyponatremia. Because older adults are more susceptible to dehydration, and have a higher rate of mortality from dehydration, early detection of infection and disorders in fluid balance is very important (Davidhizar et al., 2004).

Reduced respiratory lung capacity, compounded by arthritic changes, impairs the ability of older adults to compensate for acid–base imbalances and maintain oxygen requirements. With increased age, clients are at risk for disorders of other body systems, including the cardiovascular, renal, and endocrine systems, which have an impact on fluid, electrolyte, and acid–base balances. In addition, older adults have a decreased ability to excrete medications.

Older adults are frequently on diuretics. Nicholls and Sani (2004) recommend lower initial doses because of reduced renal function with normal aging, which causes slower excretion of medication and the potential for increased side effects. Long-term diuretic therapy should include potassium-sparing diuretics, such as spironolactone, to avoid hypokalemia.

➤BOX 40-3 Nursing Assessment Questions

Nature of the Problem

- Are you currently under the care of a health care professional for management of any ongoing health problems, such as kidney, heart, or endocrine disease or blood pressure problems?
- Describe any new-onset problems, such as vomiting, diarrhea, or a surgical procedure.
- Do you regularly take any medications, such as salt substitutes, antacids, diuretics, antihypertensives, or calcium or potassium supplements?

Signs and Symptoms

- In the past several weeks, have you lost or gained any weight without trying?
- Do you feel thirsty, have a dry mouth or skin, or notice a lack of tears?
- Have you noticed a change in your urine output: decreased volume, dark colour, or concentrated appearance?
- Have you had any recent problems with vomiting or diarrhea? If so, for how long?
- Are you experiencing any problems with swelling of your hands, feet, ankles, or lower legs?
- Do you have problems breathing when you lie down at night?
- Have you noticed any dizziness, weakness, cramps, or unusual sensations, such as tingling?

Severity

- How many times a day do you urinate?
- Do you continue to feel thirsty no matter how much fluid you drink?
- Are you experiencing these symptoms more at night than in the morning?
- Are you having difficulty concentrating, or do you feel confused?
- How does this compare with what is normal or usual for you?

Predisposing Factors

- How much do you usually drink every day? What type of fluids do you drink?
- Describe your normal diet. Do you frequently eat processed, canned, or frozen foods? Do you use a salt substitute?
- Are you following any weight loss program?
- Have you had any recent changes in taste or appetite?

Effect on the Client

- How have these symptoms affected you?
- Are you losing sleep, feeling irritable, or having difficulty performing your usual daily tasks?

Environmental Factors. You should also include certain environmental factors in the health history. Clients who have participated in vigorous exercise or who have become exposed to temperature extremes may have clinical signs of fluid and electrolyte alterations. Exposure to environmental temperatures exceeding 28°C to 30°C results in excessive sweating with weight loss. A body weight loss over 7% decreases the ability of the cooling mechanism to conserve water. Loss of fluid from sweating varies and can reach up to 1 to 3 L/hour (Porth, 2005). Inadequate fluid replacement can lead to fluid and electrolyte disturbances.

Diet. A client's current dietary history is an important component of nursing assessment. Dietary intake of fluids, salt, potassium, calcium, magnesium, and necessary carbohydrates, fats, and protein helps maintain normal fluid, electrolyte, and acid–base homeostasis. Recent changes in appetite or the ability to chew and swallow can affect nutritional status and fluid hydration. When nutritional intake is inadequate, the body tries to preserve its protein stores by breaking down glycogen and fat stores. When excess free fatty acids are released, metabolic acidosis can occur because the liver converts free fatty acids to ketone, a strong acid. With high-protein diets, ketosis can also occur. After fat and carbohydrate resources are depleted, the body begins to destroy protein stores. Hypoalbuminemia occurs when serum protein levels drop below normal. In hypoalbuminemia, the serum colloid osmotic pressure is decreased, and fluid shifts from the circulating blood volume and enters the interstitial fluid space in the peritoneal cavity.

Lifestyle. Lifestyle factors should also be included in the client's health history. Pre-existing medical risks, such as a history of smoking or alcohol consumption, can further impair the client's ability to adapt to fluid, electrolyte, and acid–base alterations. For example, the consistent use of alcohol and tobacco can ultimately cause respiratory depression, which can result in respiratory acidosis and alteration in maintaining adequate fluid and electrolyte balances.

Medication. A final category to include in the nursing assessment is a history of medication use (Box 40–5). If the assessment reveals a medication that is likely to cause an electrolyte or acid–base disorder, you will need to examine laboratory values closely. In addition, you will assess the client's knowledge of side effects and adherence to medication schedules and the client's knowledge of the potential side effects of over-the-counter medications on fluid, electrolyte, and acid–base balances.

Prior Medical History

Acute Illness. Recent surgery, head and chest trauma, shock, and second- or third-degree burns are conditions that place clients at high risk for fluid, electrolyte, and acid–base alterations. In addition, the client continues to be at risk during the acute phase until the underlying process is resolved. For example, the stress response of surgery may cause fluid–balance changes on the second to fifth postoperative day, when aldosterone, glucocorticoids, and ADH are increasingly secreted, causing sodium and chloride retention, potassium excretion, and decreased urinary output.

Surgery. The more extensive the surgery and fluid loss are during the surgical procedure, the greater the body's response is to the surgical trauma. After surgery, clients can exhibit many acid–base changes. The client who is reluctant to breathe deeply and cough may develop respiratory acidosis as a result of retained $PaCO_2$. The client with nasogastric suction may develop metabolic alkalosis as a result of the loss of gastric acid, fluids, and electrolytes.

Burns. The greater the body surface burned, the greater the fluid loss is. The burned client loses body fluids by one of five routes. First, plasma leaves the intravascular space and becomes trapped edema. This is also called the plasma-to-interstitial fluid shift. It is accompanied by a loss of serum proteins. Second, plasma and interstitial fluids are lost as burn exudate. Third, water vapour and heat are lost in proportion to the amount of skin that is burned away. Fourth, blood leaks from damaged capillaries, adding to the loss of intravascular fluid volume. Last, sodium and water shift into the cells, further compromising ECF volume (Monahan et al., 2007).

Respiratory Disorders. Many alterations in respiratory function predispose the client to respiratory acidosis. For example, the changes involved in pneumonia, sedative overdose, and exacerbated

✱ BOX 40-4 EVIDENCE-INFORMED PRACTICE GUIDELINE

Determining Adequate Oral Intake for Older Adults

- Initial assessment of hydration status should include physiological measures, including urine specific gravity, urine colour, 24-hour intake and output, patterns of fluid intake, and treatments.
- Evaluate acute losses such as vomiting, medical issues such as diabetes or malnutrition, use of medications such as diuretics, cognitive level, and functional status. These factors, especially in clients older than 85 years, may contribute to dehydration.
- Acute management requires close monitoring of high-risk clients, implementing intake and output measurement, and providing additional fluids.
- Ongoing management consists of daily fluid goals, comparing current intake with physiological needs, and provision of fluids.
- Documentation is more accurate when alert and oriented clients participate in fluid management.

Modified from Mentes, J. C. (2004). Hydration management. In Titler, M. (Ed.). *Series on evidence-based practice for older adults.* Iowa City: University of Iowa Gerontological Nursing Interventions Research Center.

➤ BOX 40-5 Medications That Cause Fluid, Electrolyte, and Acid-Base Disturbances

- Diuretics: Metabolic alkalosis, hyperkalemia, and hypokalemia
- Steroids: Metabolic alkalosis
- Potassium supplements: Gastrointestinal disturbances, including intestinal and gastric ulcers and diarrhea
- Respiratory centre depressants (e.g., opioid analgesics): Decreased rate and depth of respirations, resulting in respiratory acidosis
- Antibiotics: Nephrotoxicity (e.g., vancomycin, methicillin, aminoglycosides); hyperkalemia or hypernatremia (e.g., azlocillin, carbenicillin, piperacillin, ticarcillin, ampicillin sodium–sulbactam sodium [Unasyn])
- Calcium carbonate (Tums): Mild metabolic alkalosis with nausea and vomiting
- Magnesium hydroxide (Milk of Magnesia): Hypokalemia
- Nonsteroidal anti-inflammatory drugs: Nephrotoxicity

Data from McKenry, L., Tessier, E., & Hogan, M. A. (2006). *Mosby's pharmacology in nursing* (22nd ed.). St. Louis, MO: Mosby.

chronic airflow limitation interfere with the elimination of carbon dioxide as the client retains carbon dioxide during hypoventilation. As the carbon dioxide continues to build up in the bloodstream, the body's compensatory mechanisms can no longer adapt, and the pH decreases. Likewise, hyperventilation that occurs with conditions such as fever or anxiety causes the client to experience respiratory alkalosis by expelling too much carbon dioxide with the increased respiratory rate.

Gastrointestinal Disturbances. Gastroenteritis and nasogastric suctioning result in a loss of fluid, potassium, and chloride ions. Hydrogen ions are also lost, resulting in metabolic alkalosis. Timely education of infant and child caregivers is necessary to prevent dehydration when the infant or child is experiencing diarrhea. Gastrointestinal fistulas can also result in a loss of potassium, resulting in an increased risk for hypokalemia. The loss of potassium increases the risk for acid–base disturbances as well.

Head Injury. Head injury can result in cerebral edema. Occasionally, this edema creates pressure on the pituitary gland, and, as a result, ADH secretion is changed. Two alterations can occur. Diabetes insipidus occurs when too little ADH is secreted and the client excretes large volumes of diluted urine with a low specific gravity. The second alteration is the syndrome of inappropriate antidiuretic hormone (SIADH), the continued inappropriate secretion of ADH. This results in water intoxication characterized by fluid volume expansion and hyponatremia, as well as hypotonicity of fluids as a result of high urine osmolality and low serum osmolality (Monahan et al., 2007).

Chronic Illness. Chronic disease (e.g., cancer, congestive heart failure, or renal disease) comprises a variety of conditions that can create fluid, electrolyte, and acid–base imbalances. You must review the normal course of the client's chronic disease in order to understand how fluid, electrolyte, and acid–base status may be affected.

Cancer. The types of fluid and electrolyte imbalances that are observed in a client with cancer depend on the type and progression of the cancer. The range of potential electrolyte imbalances results from anatomical distortion and functional impairment from tumour growth and tumour-caused metabolic and endocrine abnormalities. In addition, clients with cancer are at risk for fluid and electrolyte imbalances related to the side effects (e.g., diarrhea and anorexia) of their chemotherapeutic and radiological treatments.

Cardiovascular Disease. In the client with cardiovascular disease, diminished cardiac output reduces kidney perfusion, causing the client to experience a decrease in urinary output. The client will retain sodium and water, resulting in circulatory overload, and run the risk of developing pulmonary edema. Fluid and electrolyte imbalances associated with heart disease can be controlled for a time with medications and with fluid and sodium restrictions. The goal of fluid reduction is to decrease the workload of the left ventricle by reducing the excess circulating fluid volume.

Renal Disorders. Kidney disease alters fluid and electrolyte balances by the abnormal retention of sodium, chloride, potassium, and water in the extracellular compartment. The plasma levels of metabolic waste products such as BUN and creatinine are elevated because the kidneys are unable to filter and excrete the waste products of cellular metabolism. This elevation is toxic to cellular processes. Metabolic acidosis results when hydrogen ions are retained because of decreased renal function. Because of the renal disorder, the usual renal compensatory mechanisms, such as bicarbonate reabsorption, are not available; therefore, the body's ability to restore normal acid–base balance is limited.

The severity of fluid and electrolyte imbalance is proportional to the degree of renal failure. Acute renal failure or a decrease in ECF may be reversible. Although chronic renal failure is progressive, the client may be treated successfully with dietary control of protein and salt intake, diuretic medications, and fluid restrictions. In later stages, treatment with dialysis, transplantation, or both may be required.

Gastrointestinal Disorders. Chronic gastrointestinal disorders can have a serious impact on fluid, electrolyte, and acid–base balances. Inflammatory bowel diseases, such as ulcerative colitis, regional enteritis, and celiac disease, are relatively common (Day et al., 2007). Clients with liver failure may have a number of imbalances, including metabolic acidosis, ECF shifts in the case of ascites, and electrolyte disturbances. Key assessments include the length of the illness, the presence of exacerbations in the case of inflammatory bowel disease, and the type of treatment currently being administered. In addition to chronic health problems, determine whether the client has a history of new-onset acute illnesses such as diarrhea or vomiting because any condition that results in the loss of gastrointestinal fluids predisposes the client to the development of dehydration and a variety of electrolyte disturbances.

Human Immunodeficiency Virus (HIV) and Acquired Immune Deficiency Syndrome (AIDS). The types of fluid and electrolyte imbalances that are observed in clients with HIV and AIDS depend on the stage of the disease and manifestations of the illness, complications (e.g., nephropathy, malignancy, and opportunistic infections), and the side effects of antiretroviral therapy. Electrolyte and acid–base imbalances can occur as a result of anorexia, nausea, vomiting, diarrhea, and malignancies. Treatment should focus on improving food and fluid intake, providing comfort measures, and addressing the cause of the imbalance.

Physical Assessment

A thorough physical examination (see Chapter 32) is necessary because fluid and electrolyte imbalances or acid–base disturbances can affect all body systems. When conducting a physical examination, incorporate knowledge regarding the signs and symptoms of fluid, electrolyte, and acid–base imbalances; disease processes that may impact these balances; developmental considerations; and common risk factors. For example, an examination of the oral cavity may reveal signs of dehydration. Table 40–7 summarizes possible physical findings for clients with fluid, electrolyte, and acid–base imbalances.

Measuring Fluid Intake and Output. Assessing fluid balance involves knowledge of normal fluid requirements and accurate measurement techniques (Chapelhow & Crouch, 2007). Measuring and recording all liquid intake and output during a 24-hour period is one key component of client assessment. Recognition of trends in intake and output is also important (e.g., a gradually decreasing urine output may signal FVD or hyperosmolar fluid imbalance). Daily weight is considered the most accurate means to evaluate fluid balance (Day et al., 2007). Weigh the client at the same time each day with the same scale after the client voids. Calibrate the scale routinely. The client should wear the same clothes (or clothes that weigh the same); if you are using a bed scale, use the same number of sheets on the scale with each weighing. Accurate fluid balance measurements can be used to identify both clients at risk for and clients who are experiencing fluid, electrolyte, and acid–base disturbances.

For clients in health care settings, intake and output measurement is a routine nursing assessment of clients after a procedure, clients who are febrile, clients with restricted fluids, or clients who receive diuretic or intravenous therapy. Measure intake and output for clients with chronic cardiopulmonary or renal illnesses and clients whose health status has deteriorated or has become unstable.

Intake includes all liquids taken by mouth (e.g., gelatin, ice cream, soup, juice, and water) or through nasogastric or jejunostomy

TABLE 40-7 Physical and Behavioural Nursing Assessment for Fluid, Electrolyte, and Acid-Base Imbalances

Assessment	Imbalance
Weight Changes	
2%–5% loss	Mild FVD
5%–8% loss	Moderate FVD
8%–15% loss	Severe FVD
>15% loss	Death
2% gain	Mild FVE
5%–8% gain	Moderate to severe FVE
Head	
History	
Headache	FVD,* metabolic or respiratory acidosis, metabolic alkalosis
Dizziness	FVD, respiratory acidosis or alkalosis, hyponatremia
Observation	
Irritability	Metabolic or respiratory alkalosis, hyperosmolar imbalance, hypernatremia, hypokalemia
Lethargy	FVD, metabolic acidosis or alkalosis, respiratory acidosis, hypercalcemia
Confusion, disorientation	FVD, hypomagnesemia, metabolic acidosis, hypokalemia
Eyes	
History	
• Blurred vision	FVE
Inspection	
• Sunken, dry conjunctivae, decreased or absent tearing	FVD
• Periorbital edema, papilledema	FVE
Throat and Mouth	
Inspection	
• Sticky, dry mucosa, dry cracked lips, decreased salivation, longitudinal tongue furrows	FVD, hypernatremia
Cardiovascular System	
Inspection	
Flat neck veins	FVD
Distended neck veins	FVE
Dependent body parts: legs, sacrum back	FVD
Slow venous filling	FVD
Palpation	
Edema: dependent body parts (legs, sacrum, back)	FVE
Dysrhythmias (also noted as ECG changes)	Metabolic acidosis, respiratory alkalosis and acidosis, potassium imbalance, hypomagnesemia
Increased pulse rate	Metabolic alkalosis, respiratory acidosis, hyponatremia, FVD, FVE, hypomagnesemia
Decreased pulse rate	Metabolic alkalosis, hypokalemia
Weak pulse	FVD, hypokalemia
Decreased capillary filling	FVD
Bounding pulse	FVE
Auscultation	
Blood pressure low or with orthostatic changes	FVD, hyponatremia, hyperkalemia, hypermagnesemia
Third heart sound (except in young children)	FVE
Hypertension	FVE
Respiratory System	
Inspection	
Increased rate	FVE, respiratory alkalosis, metabolic acidosis
Dyspnea	FVE
Auscultation	
Crackles	FVE
Gastrointestinal System	
History	
Anorexia	Metabolic acidosis
Abdominal cramps	Metabolic acidosis
Inspection	
Sunken abdomen	FVD
Distended abdomen	Third-space syndrome
Vomiting	FVD, hypercalcemia, hyponatremia, hypochloremia, metabolic alkalosis
Diarrhea	Hyponatremia, metabolic acidosis
Auscultation	
Loud "growling" sounds from hyperperistalsis with diarrhea or no sounds from hypoperistalsis	FVD, hypokalemia
Renal System	
Inspection	
Oliguria or anuria	FVD, FVE
Diuresis (if kidneys are normal)	FVE
Increased urine specific gravity	FVD
Neuromuscular System	
Inspection	
Numbness, tingling	Metabolic alkalosis, hypocalcemia, potassium imbalance
Muscle cramps, tetany	Hypocalcemia, metabolic or respiratory alkalosis
Coma	Hyperosmolar or hypo-osmolar imbalances, hyponatremia
Tremors	Respiratory acidosis, hypomagnesemia
Palpation	
Hypotonicity	Hypokalemia, hypercalcemia
Hypertonicity	Hypocalcemia, hypomagnesemia, metabolic alkalosis
Skin	
Body temperature	
Increased	Hypernatremia, hyperosmolar imbalance, metabolic acidosis
Decreased	FVD
Inspection	
Dry, flushed	FVD, hypernatremia, metabolic acidosis
Palpation	
Inelastic skin turgor, cold, clammy skin	FVD

ECG, electrocardiogram; FVD, fluid volume deficit; FVE, fluid volume excess.

*Data from Heitz, U. E., & Horne, M. M. (2005). *Mosby's pocket guide series: Fluid, electrolyte, and acid–base balance* (5th ed.). St. Louis, MO: Mosby.

feeding tubes (see Chapter 43), intravenous fluids (including both continuous and intermittent intravenous fluids), and blood or its components. Occasionally, clients receive a specific amount of a liquid medication every 1 to 2 hours. A client receiving tube feedings may receive numerous liquid medications, and water may be used to flush the tube for the medications. Over a 24-hour period, these liquids can amount to significant intake and should always be recorded on the intake and output record. Output includes urine, diarrhea, vomitus, gastric suction, and drainage from postsurgical wounds or other tubes (see Chapter 49). Daily intake should equal output plus 500 mL (to cover for insensible fluid losses).

Ambulatory clients are instructed to save their urine in a calibrated receptacle that attaches to the rim of the toilet bowl (Figure 40–8). When a client has an in-dwelling Foley catheter, drainage tube, or suction, output is recorded either for the nursing shift or hourly, depending on the client's condition. Client and family cooperation is essential for accurate intake and output measurements. Teach the client and the family the purpose of the measurements and instruct them either to notify you when urine is in the receptacle or how to measure the urine and empty the container themselves.

Recording intake and output is essential for obtaining an accurate database. This information helps maintain an ongoing evaluation of the client's hydration status to prevent severe imbalances. In the hospital, forms for recording intake and output are attached to the bedside chart or room door (Figure 40–9). The 24-hour total is calculated as directed by agency policy. You may delegate intake and output recording to unregulated care providers with competent skills in measurement and calculation. Estimation is not acceptable.

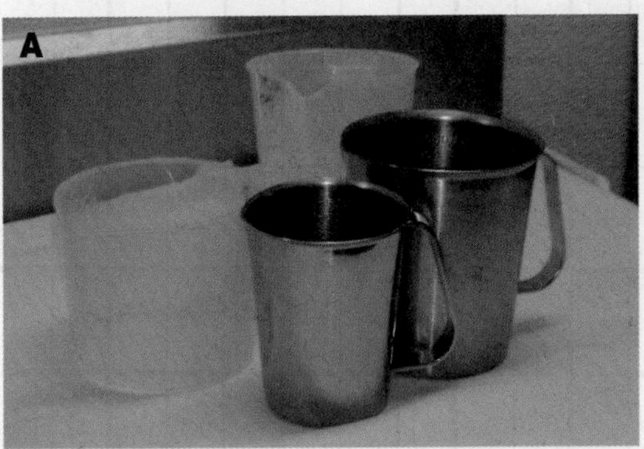

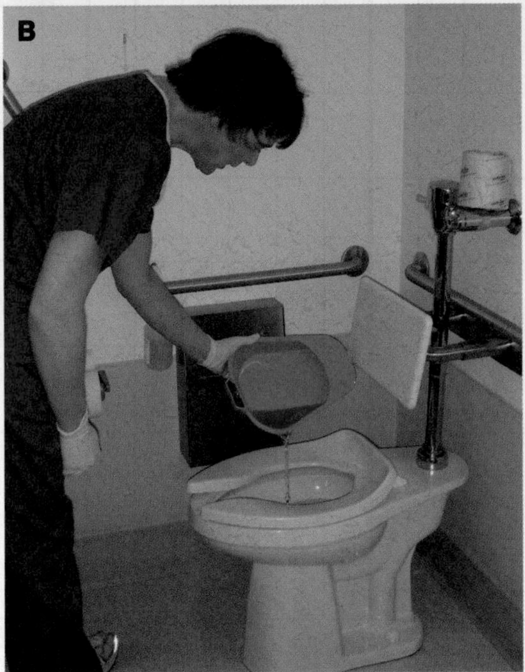

Figure 40-8 A, Graduated measuring containers. B, Emptying collected urine. **Source:** Courtesy Darlaine Jantzen.

Laboratory Studies. Review laboratory tests to obtain further objective data about fluid, electrolyte, and acid–base balances. These tests include serum and urinary electrolyte levels, hematocrit, blood creatinine level, BUN levels, urine specific gravity, and ABG readings (Box 40–6). Serum electrolyte levels are measured to determine the hydration status, the electrolyte concentration of the blood plasma,

➤ BOX 40-6 Laboratory Data for Fluid, Electrolyte, and Acid-Base Imbalances

Fluid and Electrolytes

Alterations in sodium, potassium, magnesium, calcium, phosphates, chloride, and bicarbonate (venous carbon dioxide concentrations)
Increase in hematocrit, BUN, sodium, and osmolality in serum (related to loss of ECF or gain of solutes)
Decrease in hematocrit, BUN, sodium, and osmolality in serum (related to gain of ECF or loss of solutes)
Concentrated urine demonstrated by urine specific gravity of 1.030
Dilute urine demonstrated by a specific gravity of 1.010

Metabolic Alkalosis

pH: 7.45
$PaCO_2$: normal or <45 mm Hg if lungs are compensating
PaO_2: normal
Oxygen saturation: normal
Bicarbonate: 23–26 mmol/L
Potassium: 3.5 mmol/L

Metabolic Acidosis

pH: 7.35
$PaCO_2$: normal or <35 mm Hg if lungs are compensating
PaO_2: normal
Oxygen saturation: normal
Bicarbonate: 22 mmol/L
Potassium: 5.0 mmol/L

Respiratory Alkalosis

pH: 7.45
$PaCO_2$: 35 mm Hg
PaO_2: normal
Oxygen saturation: normal
Bicarbonate: 22 mmol/L
Potassium: 3.5 mmol/L

Respiratory Acidosis

pH: 7.35
$PaCO_2$: 45 mm Hg
PaO_2: normal or <80 mm Hg, depending on cause of acidosis
Oxygen saturation: normal or 95%, depending on cause of acidosis
Bicarbonate: normal if early respiratory acidosis or >26 mmol/L if kidneys are compensating
Potassium: 5.0 mmol/L

BUN, Blood urea nitrogen; ECF, extracellular fluid; $PaCO_2$, partial pressure of carbon dioxide in arterial blood; PaO_2, partial pressure of oxygen in arterial blood; pH, measurement of acidity or alkalinity of a fluid.

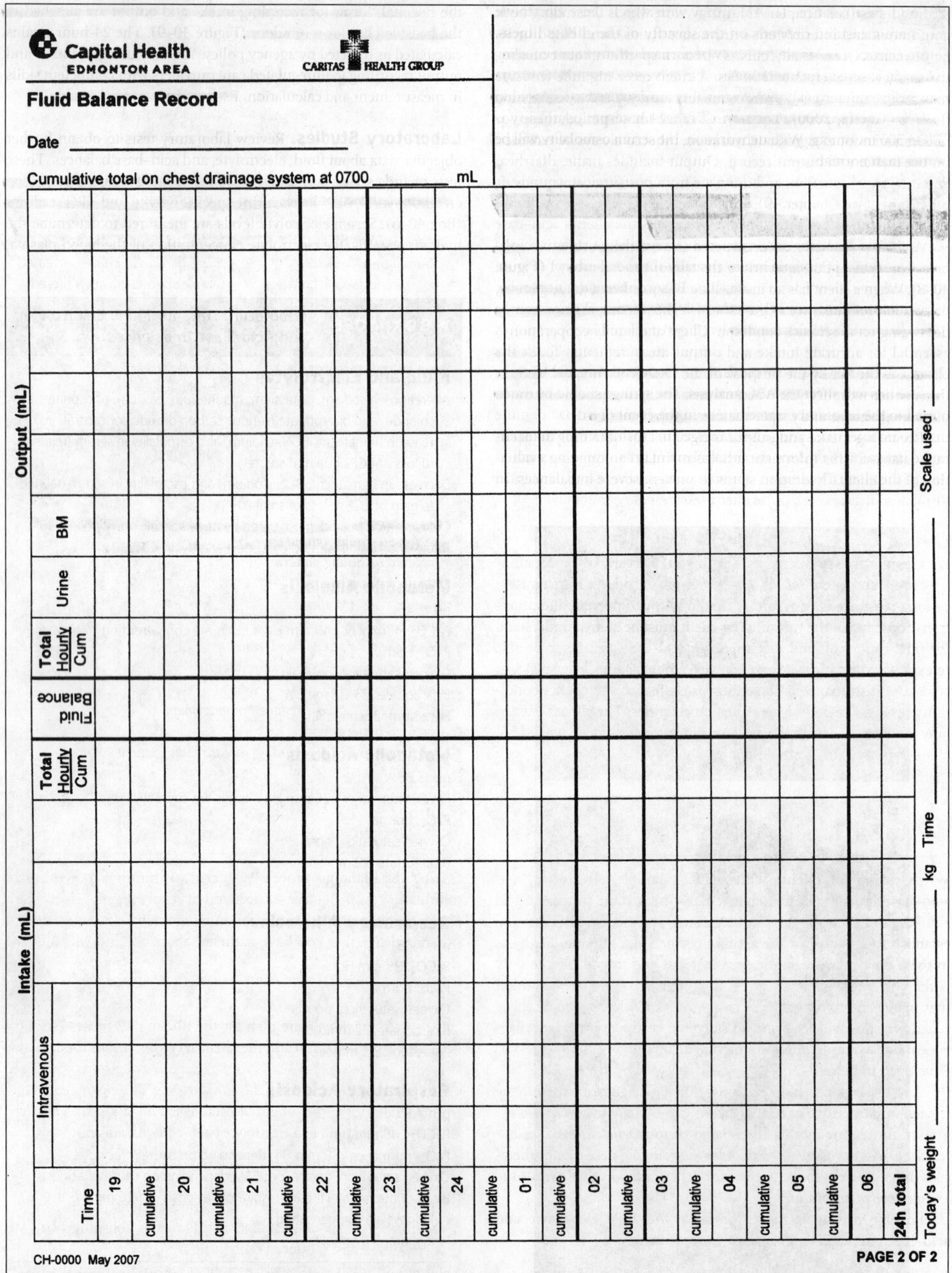

Capital Health
EDMONTON AREA

CARITAS HEALTH GROUP

Fluid Balance Record

Date

Cumulative total on chest drainage system at 0700 ________ mL

Time	Intravenous	Intake (mL)			Total Hourly Cum	Fluid Balance	Total Hourly Cum	Urine	BM	Output (mL)	
19											
cumulative											
20											
cumulative											
21											
cumulative											
22											
cumulative											
23											
cumulative											
24											
cumulative											
01											
cumulative											
02											
cumulative											
03											
cumulative											
04											
cumulative											
05											
cumulative											
06											
cumulative											
24h total											

Today's weight ________ kg Time ________ Scale used ________

CH-0000 May 2007

PAGE 2 OF 2

Figure 40-9 Twenty-four-hour intake and output record. **Source:** Courtesy Capital Health, Edmonton, Alberta.

and acid–base balance. The frequency with which these electrolyte levels are measured depends on the severity of the client's illness. Serum electrolyte tests are routinely performed on any client entering a hospital to screen for alterations and to serve as a baseline for future comparisons. Serum and urine osmolality are also used to assess fluid balance (Goertz, 2006). The normal range for serum osmolality is 280 to 300 mOsm/kg. With dehydration, the serum osmolality will be higher than normal.

Arterial Blood Gases. To determine ABG levels. a sample of blood from an artery must be taken to assess the client's acid–base status and the adequacy of ventilation and oxygenation. Arterial blood is drawn from a peripheral artery (usually the radial artery) or from an arterial line inserted by a physician. In some agencies, nurses are responsible for radial artery punctures. Beginning nursing students do not draw arterial samples but frequently assist in the sampling process and care for the client after the procedure. After the specimen is obtained, care is taken to prevent air from entering the syringe because this will affect the ABG analysis. The syringe should be transported to the laboratory immediately. In the event of a delay of more than 20 minutes, the syringe is submerged in crushed ice for transport to the laboratory to reduce the metabolism of cells. Apply pressure to the puncture site for at least 5 minutes to reduce the risk of hematoma formation. Reassess the pulse after pressure has been removed.

Client Expectations

If a client is able to discuss care with you, a review of expectations may reveal short-term needs (e.g., provision of comfort from nausea) or long-term needs (e.g., understanding how to prevent alterations from occurring in the future). The client must be able to understand the implications of fluid, electrolyte, or acid–base changes to be able to express expectations of care. However, often a fluid, electrolyte, or acid–base disturbance is so serious or acute that the client's condition prevents a review of his or her expectations. The client's trust in you is strengthened through your competent response to sudden changes in the client's condition.

❖Nursing Diagnosis

When caring for clients with suspected fluid, electrolyte, and acid–base imbalances, it is particularly important to use critical thinking to formulate nursing diagnoses. The assessment data that establish the risk for or the actual presence of a nursing diagnosis in these areas may be subtle, and patterns and trends emerge only when you conscientiously assess for them. You must keep in mind that many body systems may be involved. Clustering of defining characteristics will lead you to selection of the appropriate diagnoses. For example, the nursing diagnosis *deficient fluid volume* is developed in Box 40–7.

An important part of formulating nursing diagnoses is identifying the relevant causative or related factor. The nursing interventions are chosen to treat or modify the related factor. *Deficient fluid volume related to loss of gastrointestinal fluids via vomiting* necessitates therapies different from those needed for *deficient fluid volume related to elevated body temperature.*

Possible nursing diagnoses for clients with fluid, electrolyte, and acid–base alterations may include the following:

- *Actual or risk of deficient fluid volume*
- *Actual or risk of excess fluid volume*

BOX 40-7 NURSING DIAGNOSTIC PROCESS

Assessment Activities	Defining Characteristics
Assess blood pressure and pulse	Client is hypotensive, with increased heart rate
Obtain daily weight measurements	Client experiences sudden weight loss
Observe volume of urine output and measure intake and specific gravity	Decreased volume of output in comparison to intake; increased urine specific gravity is present
Assess skin turgor	Inelastic skin turgor noted
Ask if client is thirsty or weak	Client verbalizes thirst and weakness
Inspect mucous membranes for degree of moisture	Dry mucous membranes are noted

- *Decreased cardiac output*
- *Impaired breathing pattern*
- *Impaired gas exchange*
- *Impaired tissue perfusion*
- *Acute confusion*
- *Impaired oral mucous membrane*
- *Actual or risk of impaired skin integrity*
- *Impaired mobility*
- *Ineffective therapeutic regimen management*
- *Impaired tissue integrity*
- *Deficient knowledge regarding disease management*

❖Planning

During the planning process, use critical thinking to synthesize information from multiple sources and to ensure that the client's care plan integrates both scientific and nursing knowledge, as well as all the knowledge that you have gathered about the individual client (Figure 40–10).

Goals and Outcomes

Develop an individual care plan for the nursing diagnoses (see Box 40–7 and Box 40–8). You and the client set expectations for care that are individualized and realistic, with measurable outcomes. Goals are designed to achieve and maintain homeostasis. For example, the following related outcomes might be established for this goal: *The client will have normal fluid and electrolyte balance at discharge*:

- The client will be free of complications associated with the intravenous therapy.
- The client will demonstrate fluid balance by moist, mucous membranes and good skin turgor and by re-establishing a balanced intake and output or daily weight.
- The client will have serum electrolytes within the normal range within 48 hours.

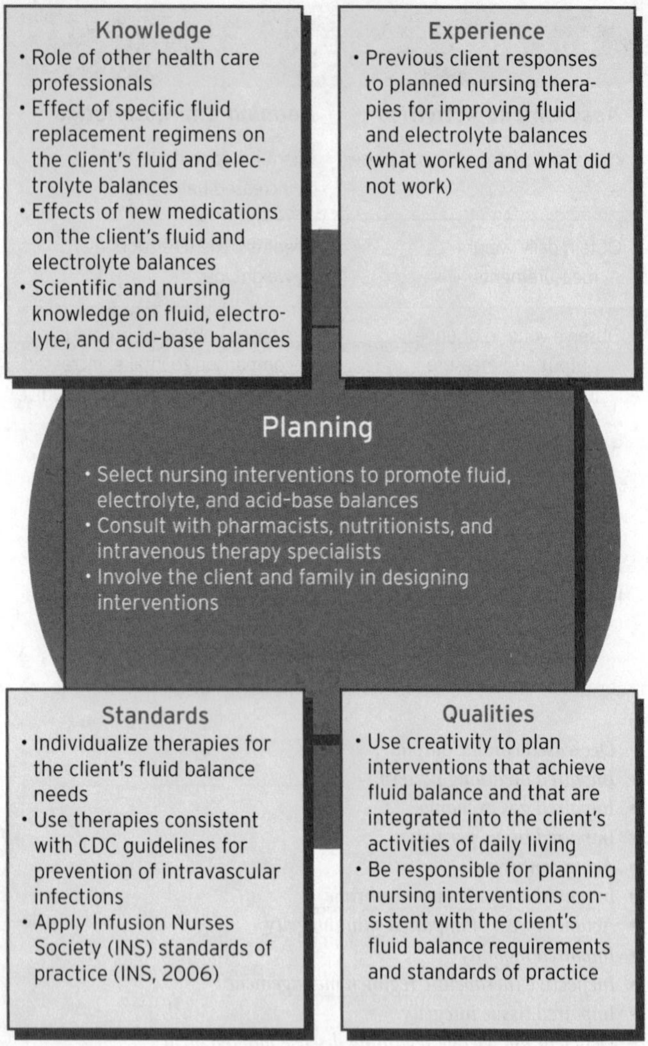

Knowledge
- Role of other health care professionals
- Effect of specific fluid replacement regimens on the client's fluid and electrolyte balances
- Effects of new medications on the client's fluid and electrolyte balances
- Scientific and nursing knowledge on fluid, electrolyte, and acid-base balances

Experience
- Previous client responses to planned nursing therapies for improving fluid and electrolyte balances (what worked and what did not work)

Planning
- Select nursing interventions to promote fluid, electrolyte, and acid-base balances
- Consult with pharmacists, nutritionists, and intravenous therapy specialists
- Involve the client and family in designing interventions

Standards
- Individualize therapies for the client's fluid balance needs
- Use therapies consistent with CDC guidelines for prevention of intravascular infections
- Apply Infusion Nurses Society (INS) standards of practice (INS, 2006)

Qualities
- Use creativity to plan interventions that achieve fluid balance and that are integrated into the client's activities of daily living
- Be responsible for planning nursing interventions consistent with the client's fluid balance requirements and standards of practice

Figure 40-10 Critical thinking model for planning fluid, electrolyte, and acid–base balances.

Setting Priorities

The client's clinical condition will determine which diagnosis takes the greatest priority. Many nursing diagnoses in the area of fluid, electrolyte, and acid–base balances are of highest priority because the consequences for the client can be serious or even life-threatening. For example, in the concept map for the client with gastroenteritis and dehydration (Figure 40–11), nausea and diarrhea have caused a deficient fluid volume and electrolyte imbalances. Without treating the cause to resolve the client's nausea and diarrhea, the fluid, electrolyte, and acid–base imbalances will progress.

Consultation with the client's physician may assist in setting realistic time frames for the goals of care, particularly when the client's physiological status is unstable. During planning, collaborate as much as possible with the client, family, and other members of the health care team. The family can be particularly helpful in identifying subtle changes in a client's behaviour associated with imbalances (e.g., anxiety, confusion, or irritability).

Continuity of Care

For clients with acute disturbances, discharge planning must begin early. You must ensure that care can continue in the home or long-term care setting with few disruptions. For example, when a client is discharged on intravenous therapy, you must determine the knowledge and skills of the person who is to assume caregiving responsibilities and make a referral for home intravenous therapy as soon as possible. You must also collaborate closely with other members of the health care team, such as the physician, dietitian, and pharmacist. In consultation with a dietitian, you can recommend foods to increase intake of certain electrolytes or reduce intake as necessary (see Chapter 43). The pharmacist can help identify medications likely to cause electrolyte or acid–base disturbances and describe possible side effects of the client's prescribed drugs. The physician directs the treatment of any fluid, electrolyte, or acid–base alteration.

❖Implementation

Health Promotion

Health promotion activities in the area of fluid, electrolyte, and acid–base imbalances include client education regarding fluid and electrolyte requirements, promotion of healthy environments affecting hydration, particularly for vulnerable clients, and advocating for secure access to safe water as a universal need and human right (International Council of Nurses [ICN], 2002).

Clients and caregivers need to recognize risk factors for these imbalances and implement appropriate preventive measures. For example, parents of infants need to understand that gastrointestinal losses can quickly lead to serious imbalances; therefore, when an infant is vomiting or has diarrhea, the parent must recognize the risk and promptly seek health care to restore normal balance. Even the healthy adult is at risk for developing imbalances when subjected to high temperatures. Advise clients to increase water intake, maintain adequate ventilation, and refrain from excessive activity during heat waves. Davidhizar et al. (2004) highlighted the importance of adequate staffing and supervision for older adults in relation to hydration.

All clients with a chronic health alteration are at risk for developing changes in their fluid, electrolyte, and acid–base balances. They need to understand their own risk factors and the measures to be taken to avoid imbalances. For example, clients with renal failure must avoid excess intake of fluid, sodium, potassium, and phosphorus. Through diet education, these clients learn the types of foods to avoid and the suitable volume of fluid they are permitted daily (Box 40–9; see Chapter 43). Clients with chronic health conditions need to be made aware of early signs and symptoms of fluid, electrolyte, and acid–base imbalances. A client with heart disease should be instructed to obtain an accurate body weight each day at approximately the same time and to inform the health care professional of significant changes in weight from one day to another. Increase in weight, shortness of breath, orthopnea, and dependent edema are all associated with fluid retention.

Acute Care

Fluid, electrolyte, and acid–base imbalances can occur in all settings, although many clients are cared for in acute care settings. Although you must manage the client's complex medical care in a short span of time, while performing difficult technological skills, advances in technology, such as infusion pumps and peripherally inserted central catheters (PICC lines), in surgical techniques (laparoscopic procedures), and in pharmacology have all contributed to positive health outcomes for many people.

Enteral Replacement of Fluids. Oral replacement of fluids and electrolytes is appropriate as long as the client is not so physiologically compromised that oral fluids cannot be replaced rapidly. Clients

➤ BOX 40-8 NURSING CARE PLAN

Fluid Volume Deficit

Assessment

Mrs. Hilda Topping is a 72-year-old who presented to her health care professional this morning concerned about two days of vomiting and diarrhea. She initially thought that she had food poisoning, but the symptoms have not abated, and she now feels very weak and dizzy and has a headache. After an initial assessment, Mrs. Topping's physician admits her to a medical unit with a diagnosis of dehydration secondary to gastroenteritis. She had an abdominal X-ray to rule out bowel obstruction and blood work. The significant findings are an elevated hematocrit at 56%, elevated hemoglobin (160 g/L), hypernatremia (sodium 146 mmol/L), and elevated BUN and creatinine.

Assessment Activities	***Findings and Defining Characteristics***
Ask Mrs. Topping to describe her activities before onset of her symptoms, including any recent travel.	Mrs. Topping states that she has been caring for her great-grandchildren for the past week during their school break. She is aware that one of the children had had a "tummy upset." In addition, she reports that she had taken them to a fast-food restaurant for a treat. She has not been travelling.
Have Mrs. Topping describe her symptoms, including the frequency and quality of her bowel movements and emesis.	Mrs. Topping describes up to 10 liquid stools per day, accompanied by waves of nausea. With nausea, she often vomits bile-coloured liquid in very small amounts. She had taken a cup of tea twice over the previous day but was "unable to keep [it] down." She describes acute cramping pain with her stools.
Assess her vital signs, bowel sounds, skin turgor, and the characteristics of her urine and output.	Mrs. Topping's vital signs are as follows: temperature = 39°C, pulse = 118, blood pressure = 100/50 mm Hg, and respiration rate = 24/minute. She has increased bowel sounds throughout her abdomen. Her mucous membranes are dry, her tongue is coated, and her lips are cracked. Her urine is dark amber, and she voided only 100 mL on request for a sample.
Evaluate her ABGs.	ABG results show metabolic alkalosis. Her pH = 7.5, bicarbonate = 45 mmol/L, $PaCO_2$ = 48 mm Hg, and base excess = 11 mmol/L.

Nursing Diagnosis: FVD from excessive loss of fluid and electrolytes through increased gastrointestinal loss

Planning

Goals (Nursing Outcomes Classification)*	***Expected Outcomes***
	Electrolyte and Acid–Base Balances
The client will maintain fluid balance as evidenced by balanced intake and output, maintenance of adequate hydration, and absence of manifestations of dehydration.	Client's vital signs will return to normal and remain stable. ABG levels will be within normal limits in 24 hours. Electrolyte values and any other abnormal blood work values will return to normal within 24 hours.
	Fluid Balance Urinary output will increase to 60 mL/hour within 24 hours. Client's fluid volume will return to normal and remain within normal limits throughout hospital stay. Mucous membranes will remain moist.
The client will report relief of abdominal pain.	**Abdominal Pain** Client will have a reduction in abdominal cramping within two hours.

*Outcome classification labels from Moorhead, S., Johnson, M., & Maas, M. L. (Eds.). (2004). *Nursing Outcomes Classification (NOC)* (3rd ed.). St. Louis, MO: Mosby.

Interventions (Nursing Interventions Classification)[†]	**Rationale**
Fluid, Electrolyte, and Acid-Base Management	
Initiate and administer intravenous solution per physician's order.	Administering parenteral fluids is an effective way to restore fluid balance when oral ingestion of fluid is contraindicated.
Maintain client on nothing by mouth (NPO). Provide ice chips and lip cream to relieve symptoms of mouth dryness.	Maintaining client on NPO allows the gut to rest.
Increase fluid intake when gastrointestinal symptoms have resolved, beginning with clear fluids and advancing to full fluids and light meals. Prepare the client for the diagnostic tests and possible antibiotic therapy.	When symptoms have resolved, beginning with clear fluids prevents recurrence of distress and minimizes gastrointestinal pain.
Pain Management	
Administer anti-emetics and analgesics for the first 24 hours and re-evaluate.	Pharmacotherapy is important for treating nausea, emesis, and pain.
Place a warm blanket on the client's abdomen.	Other comfort measures, such as using warm blankets, are important complementary pain management strategies.

[†]Intervention classification labels from Dochterman, J. M., & Bulechek, G. M. (Eds.). (2004). *Nursing Interventions Classification (NIC)* (4th ed.). St. Louis, MO: Mosby.

Continued

BOX 40-8 NURSING CARE PLAN *continued*

Evaluation

Nursing Actions	*Client Response and Finding*	*Achievement of Outcome*
Monitor ABG levels, vital signs, intake and output, daily weight and bowel sounds.	ABG analysis: pH = 7.36, PaO_2 = 95, bicarbonate = 35, $PaCO_2$ = 38.	Mrs. Topping's acid–base balance returns to normal. Her intake and output measurements are balanced. Her daily weight remains stable.
Assess mucous membranes.	Mucous membranes are moist.	She is able to take clear fluids, and her intravenous rate is reduced.

ABG, arterial blood gas; $PaCO_2$, partial pressure of carbon dioxide in arterial blood; PaO_2, partial pressure of oxygen in arterial blood; pH, measurement of the acidity or alkalinity of a fluid.

concept map

Nursing diagnosis: Nausea
- Client reports feeling "sick to stomach"
- Abdominal pain
- Unable to tolerate oral intake

Interventions
- Administer ordered antiemetics
- Provide comfortable environment: keep room cool, keep linen clean; reduce noise
- Provide oral care

Nursing diagnosis: Deficient fluid volume
- Elevated body temperature >38.9°C
- Decreased urine output <50 mL/hr
- Abnormal serum sodium and potassium
- Tachycardia
- Decreased skin turgor

Interventions
- Initiate ordered peripheral IV line, administer 1000 mL D5NS over 8 hours
- Weigh client
- Measure I&O
- Obtain serum blood sample for electrolytes
- Administer skin care, apply hydrating lotion

Client's chief medical diagnosis: Gastroenteritis and dehydration
Priority assessments: Fluid balance, elimination function, comfort

Nursing diagnosis: Risk for impaired skin integrity
- Skin intact, area of redness, 3-cm diameter over perianal area
- Skin exposed to diarrheal stool
- Decreased skin turgor

Interventions
- Administer skin care, apply moisture barrier to skin
- Position off inflamed area

Nursing diagnosis: Diarrhea
- Hyperactive bowel sounds on auscultation in all four quadrants
- Loose watery stools >6/day
- Abdominal cramping

Interventions
- Administer ordered antidiarrheal agents
- Measure stool output
- Diet: NPO

——— Link between medical diagnosis and nursing diagnosis - - - - Link between nursing diagnoses

Figure 40-11 Concept map for a client with gastroenteritis and dehydration. D5NS, dextrose 5% in 0.9% sodium chloride; I&O, intake and output; NPO, nothing by mouth.

unable to tolerate solid foods may still be able to ingest fluids. Use strategies to encourage fluid intake such as frequently offering small sips of fluid, ice pops, and ice chips. Ice chips should be included in the intake and output measurements, at one-half the volume of the chips (i.e., 250 mL of ice chips = 125 mL). Hartling et al. (2006) conducted a systematic review and concluded that oral hydration is effective and safe in treating dehydration in children with gastroenteritis, particularly with low-osmolarity solutions, in keeping with World Health Organization (WHO) recommendations. A key nursing role is to encourage children and their caregivers regarding oral rehydration and to assess for bowel sounds.

When replacing fluids by mouth in a client who has a fluid deficit, it is wise to choose fluids with adequate calories and electrolyte content (e.g., fruit juices, gelatin, and replacements such as Pedialyte and Gastrolyte). However, liquids containing lactose, caffeine, or low-sodium content may not be appropriate when the client has diarrhea. Oral replacement of fluids is contraindicated if the client has a mechanical obstruction of the gastrointestinal tract, is at risk for aspiration, or has impaired swallowing. In some cases, a feeding tube may be appropriate, such as when the client's gastrointestinal tract is healthy, but the client cannot ingest fluids (e.g., after oral surgery or with impaired swallowing). Fluids can also be replaced through a gas-

BOX 40-9 CLIENT TEACHING

Primary Health Care and Client Teaching: Preventing and Managing Chronic Kidney Disease

Chronic kidney disease is a major burden for both individuals and the health care system to carry. The accumulation of waste products and the fluid, electrolyte, and acid–base imbalances associated with this disease have many negative results. Primary health care for clients with chronic kidney disease can alleviate some of the morbidity, early mortality, and psychosocial and financial challenges for clients and their families.

Cardiovascular disease is a major cause of death of people with chronic kidney disease. Clients should be taught that the progression of kidney disease can be slowed and cardiovascular risk reduced through the following measures:

- Smoking cessation
- Control of blood pressure
- Control of blood sugar for clients with diabetes
- Control of lipids, antiplatelet therapy
- Renin–angiotensin system antagonism
- Management of anemia
- Control of calcium and phosphate levels

Data from Barrett, B. J. (2003). Applying multiple interventions in chronic kidney disease. *Seminars in Dialysis, 16,* 157–164; and Curtis, B. M., Levin A., & Parfrey, P. S. (2005). Multiple risk factor intervention in chronic kidney disease: Management of cardiac disease in chronic kidney disease patients. *Medical Clinics of North America, 89,* 511–523.

trostomy or jejunostomy feeding tube or administered via a small-bore nasoenteral feeding tube.

Restriction of Fluids. Clients who retain fluids and have **fluid volume excess** (FVE) require restricted fluid intake. Fluid restriction is often difficult for clients, particularly if they take drugs that dry the oral mucous membranes or if they breathe through the mouth and experience thirst. You should explain the reason that fluids are restricted. In addition, the client needs to know the amount of fluid permitted orally and should understand that ice chips, gelatin, and ice cream are considered fluid. The client should help decide the amount of fluid with each meal, between meals, before bed, and with medications. Frequently, clients on fluid restriction can swallow a number of pills with as little as 30 mL of liquid.

In general, when restricting fluids, allow half of the allotted total oral fluids between 7 A.M. and 3 P.M., the period when clients usually are more active, receive two meals, and take most of their oral medications. Clients on fluid restriction require mouth care frequently to moisten mucous membranes, decrease the chance of mucosal drying and cracking, and maintain comfort.

Interventions for Acid-Base Imbalances. Nursing interventions to promote acid–base balance support prescribed medical therapies and are aimed at reversing the acid–base imbalance. Such imbalances can be life-threatening and require rapid correction. You must maintain a functional intravenous line and frequently check the physician's orders for new medications or fluids. Prescribed drugs, such as insulin or sodium bicarbonate, and fluid and electrolyte replacement should be given promptly. In Chapter 39, appropriate therapies for clients with respiratory acidosis are reviewed. You also monitor clients closely for changes in acid–base balance. Clients with acid–base disturbances usually require repeated ABG analysis.

Parenteral Replacement of Fluids and Electrolytes. Fluid and electrolytes may be replaced through infusion directly into the blood rather than via the digestive system. Parenteral replacement includes administration of **crystalloids**, **colloids**, and TPN. TPN is a nutritionally adequate hypertonic solution consisting of glucose, other nutrients, and electrolytes administered through an in-dwelling or central intravenous catheter, which can be inserted peripherally or percutaneously, implanted, or tunnelled. See Chapter 43 for important information regarding initiation and administration of TPN.

The goal of intravenous fluid administration is to maintain fluid, electrolyte, and energy demands when clients are limited in their intake and to correct or prevent fluid and electrolyte disturbances from excess losses. Intravenous fluid administration allows for direct access to the vascular system, permitting the continuous infusion of fluids over a period of time. Intravenous fluid therapy must be continuously regulated because of ongoing changes in the client's fluid and electrolyte balances. When clients require intravenous fluid administration, knowledge of the correct ordered solution, the equipment needed, the procedures required to initiate an infusion, how to regulate the infusion rate and maintain the system, how to identify and correct problems, and how to discontinue the infusion is necessary for safe and appropriate therapy. Because of the risk of transmission of infectious diseases (e.g., HIV, hepatitis B virus), standard precautions/routine practices must be followed when administering parenteral fluids (see Chapter 33).

The two main categories of intravenous fluids are crystalloids and colloids. Crystalloids are used most commonly and include glucose, sodium chloride, and lactated Ringer's solutions. These solutions contain solutes that mix, dissolve, and cross semi-permeable membranes. They vary in their tonicity. Colloids contain protein or starch (Phillips, 2005). The protein or starch does not cross semi-permeable membranes and therefore remains suspended and distributed in the extracellular space, primarily the intravascular space, for up to several days. Therefore, colloids are used to increase the osmotic pressure in the intravascular space and then draw fluid to increase vascular volume, such as following acute blood loss. Colloids are either semi-synthetic, such as dextran, pentastarch, or hetastarch, or human plasma derivatives, such as albumin, plasma proteins, or blood (Chavin & Chow, 2008).

Vascular Access Devices. **Vascular access devices** are catheters, cannulas, or infusion ports designed for repeated access to the vascular system. Peripherally placed catheters (PICCs) are designed for short-term use (e.g., postoperative fluid restoration and short-term antibiotic administration). Devices such as central line catheters or central venous catheters (CVCs), PICCs, and implanted ports (Figure 40–12) are for long-term use or for administration of medications or solutions that are irritating to veins. Other reasons for use of central lines include limited or poor peripheral veins, the need

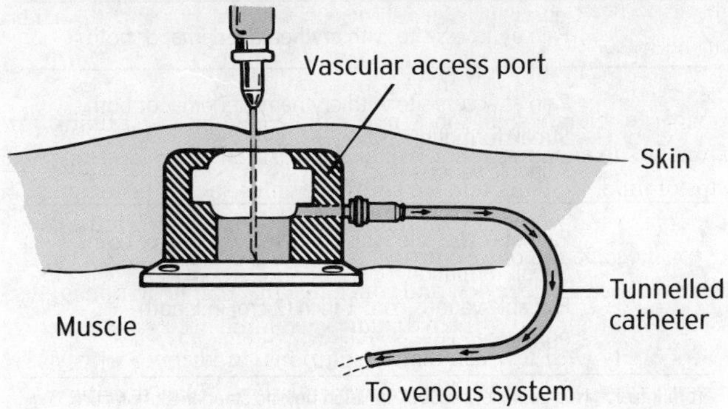

Figure 40-12 Example of an implantable vascular access device.

for good access to administer large volumes of fluid, and the need for reliable measurement (Hamilton, 2004).

You play an important role in education of clients and advocating for and facilitating discussions with the client and family regarding venous access device selection (Registered Nurses Association of Ontario [RNAO], 2005). Many factors are involved in device selection, including safety concerns, treatment goals and duration, access to services such as home intravenous programs, and physical assessments. Comprehensive assessment is the first step in initiating any intravenous therapy (Hamilton, 2006a) (see Skill 40–1, Steps 2 to 7). Most treatments requiring intravenous access for more than 1 week are best suited to midline, PICC, or implanted ports (RNAO, 2005). These lines are inserted by specially trained health care professionals. Increasingly, you will be required to care for clients with CVCs or PICCs in many settings.

A CVC is a venous access device with a tip that terminates in a great vessel (Brungs & Render, 2006), mostly commonly in the lower third of the superior vena cava (Hamilton, 2006a). The catheters are available in a variety of lengths, sizes, and numbers of lumens and are often made of silicone or polyurethrane. The type of catheter selected is often determined by the length of time it will be used. For example, for clients undergoing chemotherapy, the CVC may remain in place for many months. The most common insertion sites are the internal jugular and subclavian veins; the right internal jugular vein is considered the best option (Hamilton, 2004). Although inserted through a peripheral vein, such as the basilic, median cubital, or cephalic vein, PICCs are considered CVCs (Hamilton, 2006a).

You need to be aware of potential complications and strategies to prevent these complications when caring for clients with a CVC. You need to be able to recognize the following complications: pneumothorax, arterial puncture, hemorrhage, cardiac tamponade, air embolus, hemothorax, hydrothorax, infection, catheter occlusion, and phlebitis (Table 40–8). Aseptic technique is critical, including hand hygiene, preparation of the insertion site with chlorhexidine, and maximal barrier precautions during insertion. It is also important to ensure airtight connections, secure the dressing, minimize movement of the catheter, and adhere to the manufacturer's guidelines for maintenance of the line. Current recommendations for flushing CVCs and PICCs are available in the RNAO *Best Practice Guidelines Supplement* on the RNAO Web site (RNAO, 2008). A 10 mL or larger syringe should be used for flushing CVCs. Specialized teams are recommended for the care of PICCs and CVCs (Brungs & Render, 2006; Hamilton, 2006b).

➤ TABLE 40-8 Phlebitis Scale

Grade	Clinical Criteria
0	No symptoms
1	Erythema at access site with or without pain
2	Pain at access site with erythema, edema, or both
3	Pain at access site with erythema, edema, or both Streak formation Palpable venous cord
4	Pain at access site with erythema, edema, or both Streak formation Palpable venous cord 1 inch (2 cm) in length Purulent drainage

From Infusion Nurses Society. (2006). Infusion nursing standards of practice. *Journal of Infusion Nursing, 29*(1 Suppl.), S59.

Administration of Intravenous Therapy

Types of Solutions. Many prepared intravenous solutions are available for use (Table 40–9). Intravenous solutions fall into the following categories: isotonic, hypotonic, and hypertonic. Isotonic solutions are those that have the same effective osmolality as body fluids. Hypotonic solutions are those that have an effective osmolality that is less than that of body fluids. Hypertonic solutions are those that have an effective osmolality that is greater than that of body fluids (Heitz & Horne, 2005).

In general, isotonic fluids are used most commonly for extracellular volume replacement (e.g., FVD after prolonged vomiting). The decision to use a hypotonic or a hypertonic solution is based on the specific fluid and electrolyte imbalances. For example, the client with a hypertonic fluid imbalance will in general receive a hypotonic intravenous solution to dilute the ECF and rehydrate the cells. All intravenous fluids should be given carefully, especially hypertonic solutions, because these pull fluid into the vascular space by osmosis, resulting in an increased vascular volume that can lead to pulmonary edema, particularly in clients with heart or renal failure. Certain additives, most commonly vitamins and potassium chloride, are frequently added to intravenous solutions.

safety alert Under no circumstances should potassium chloride (KCl) be given by intravenous push. Direct intravenous infusion of KCl may cause death. If an intravenous fluid requires additives, a physician's order must specify the required additives: for example, "1000 mL D51/2 NS with 20 mmol/L KCl at 125 mL/hour."

Clients with normal renal function who are receiving nothing by mouth should have potassium added to intravenous solutions. The body cannot conserve potassium, and even when the serum level falls, the kidneys continue to excrete potassium. Without oral or parenteral potassium intake, hypokalemia can develop quickly. Conversely, you should verify that the client has adequate renal function before administering an intravenous solution containing potassium because hyperkalemia can develop quickly.

Equipment. Correct selection and preparation of intravenous equipment are necessary for safe and quick placement of an intravenous line (Figure 40–13). Because fluids are instilled into the bloodstream, sterile technique is necessary; have all equipment organized for efficient insertion (Skill 40–1). Intravenous cannulas are available in a variety of gauges; the 22-gauge cannula is preferred in most situations, with the exception of blood administration. (The larger the gauge, the smaller the diameter of the cannula is.) These cannulas are plastic tubing threaded over a needle. Once the cannula is inserted into the vein, the needle is withdrawn, leaving the cannula in place. Intravenous tubing or an intermittent infusion device, such as a needleless port, is then connected.

safety alert Intravenous pumps or volume control devices ensure a prescribed rate of infusion. A prescribed rate of infusion is vital for children, clients with renal or cardiac failure, and critically ill clients. Intravenous pumps are also used for medications that require precise rates of administration. Some agencies use these devices routinely in most clients.

Initiating an Intravenous Line. A venipuncture is a technique in which a vein is punctured through the skin by a sharp rigid stylet (e.g., butterfly needle or metal needle), a partially covered plastic catheter (over-the-needle catheter), or a needle attached to a syringe. Catheters placed into a central vein such as the subclavian or superior vena cava vein are used to deliver large volumes of fluids and TPN or

TABLE 40-9 Intravenous Solutions

Solution	Concentration	Other Names
Dextrose in Water Solutions		
Dextrose 5% in water*	Isotonic	D5W
Dextrose 10% in water	Hypertonic	D10W
Saline Solutions		
0.45% sodium chloride (half normal saline)	Hypotonic	1/2 NS 0.45% NS
0.33% sodium chloride (one-third normal saline)	Hypotonic	1/3 NS
0.9% sodium chloride† (normal saline)	Isotonic	NS 0.9% NS 0.9% NaCl
3%–5% sodium chloride	Hypertonic	3%–5% NS 3%–5% NaCl
Dextrose in Saline Solutions		
Dextrose 5% in 0.9% sodium chloride	Hypertonic	D50.9% NaCl D50.9% NS D5NS
Dextrose 5% in 0.45% NaCl sodium chloride	Hypertonic	D50.45% NaCl D50.45% NS D51/2 NS
Multiple Electrolyte Solutions		
Lactated Ringer's solution‡	Isotonic	LR
Dextrose 5% in lactated Ringer's solution	Hypertonic	D5LR

*Dextrose is quickly metabolized, leaving free water to be distributed evenly in all fluid compartments (Heitz & Horne, 2005).
†Although it is isotonic because the total concentration of electrolytes equals plasma concentration, sodium chloride contains 154 mmol of both sodium and chloride, which is a higher concentration of these electrolytes than is found in the plasma, which can cause fluid volume excess (Heitz & Horne, 2005).
‡Contains sodium, potassium, calcium, chloride, and lactate.

to administer irritating medications. PICCs may be placed by nurses; however, central line catheters require insertion by physicians. Both types of cannulas require careful monitoring and maintenance. When veins are fragile or collapse, venipuncture may become extremely difficult, but it may be a life-saving measure as well. For these difficult cases, venipuncture should be performed by an experienced practitioner. The general purposes of venipuncture are to collect a blood specimen, instill a medication, start an intravenous infusion, or inject a radiopaque or radioactive tracer for special examinations. Skill 40–1 describes venipuncture for intravenous fluid infusion.

Venipuncture Site. After the equipment is collected at the bedside, prepare to place the intravenous line by assessing the client for a venipuncture site (see Skill 40–1, Step 25A). Common intravenous puncture sites include the hand and the arm (Figure 40–14). The use of the foot for an intravenous site is common with children but is avoided in the adult because of the danger of thrombophlebitis (INS, 2006).

When assessing the client for potential venipuncture sites for intravenous infusion, you should consider conditions and contraindications that exclude certain sites. Because children and older adults have fragile veins, you should avoid sites that are easily moved or bumped, such as those on the dorsal surface of the hand. Venipuncture is contraindicated in a site that has signs of infection, infiltration, or thrombosis. An infected site is red, tender, swollen, and possibly warm to the touch, and exudate may be present. An infected site is not used because of the danger of introducing bacteria from the skin surface into the bloodstream. Arms on the side of a mastectomy and extremities with an arteriovenous graft or fistula for dialysis should be avoided. It is important to place intravenous devices at the most distal point when possible as this allows for the use of proximal sites later if the client needs a venipuncture site change. See Box 40–10 for guidelines related to the older adult.

Regulating the Infusion Flow Rate. After the intravenous infusion is secured and the line is patent, you must regulate the rate of infusion according to the prescriber's orders (Skill 40–2). An infusion rate that is too slow can lead to further cardiovascular and circulatory collapse in a critically ill client. An intravenous fluid that is running too slowly can also clot more easily. An infusion rate that is too rapid can result in FVE. Calculate the infusion rate to prevent too slow or too rapid administration of the intravenous fluids. Numerous methods are used to ensure an accurate hourly infusion rate for intravenous therapy. Fluids that run by gravity are adjusted through use of a flow control or regulator clamp. Fluids infused by an electronic infusion device or rate controller are regulated by a mechanical mechanism set at the prescribed rate. Regardless of the device in use, the client requires close monitoring to verify the correct infusion of the intravenous solution and to detect the occurrence of any complication.

Electronic **infusion pumps** are necessary when administering low hourly volumes (e.g., less than 20 mL/hour) and for clients who are at risk for volume overload, such as neonatal, pediatric, and geriatric clients. In addition, when infusing high volumes of intravenous fluids (more than 150 mL/hour) to clients with impaired renal clearance, older adults, or children, or when infusing drugs or intravenous fluids that require specific hourly volumes, electronic infusion devices permit accurate infusion. Electronic infusion pumps deliver the infusion via positive pressure. A rate controller used on gravity infusions regulates the infusion but, unlike the electronic pump, is affected by

➤ SKILL 40-1 Initiating a Peripheral Intravenous Infusion

Delegation Considerations

In many provinces, monitoring intravenous therapy is included within the scope of practice for licensed and registered practical nurses. However, the delegating nurse is ultimately responsible for assessment and monitoring of the intravenous device. *The skill of initiating intravenous therapy should not be delegated to unregulated care providers (UCPs).* Other aspects of the client's care may be delegated to UCPs. Instruct the UCP about the following:

- To inform the nurse if the client complains of burning sensation, bleeding, swelling, or coolness at the catheter insertion site
- The prescribed flow rate and to report if the rate has slowed or increased
- To inform the nurse if the intravenous dressing becomes wet or if an electronic infusion device (EID) sounds
- To inform the nurse if the volume of fluid in the intravenous bag is low

Equipment

- Correct intravenous solution (with time tape attached)
- Proper catheter for venipuncture (the gauge will vary with the client's body size and the reason for intravenous fluid administration). In an adult, a 22-gauge catheter is appropriate for fluid maintenance (Schelper, 2003).
- Intravenous start kit (if available): may contain a sterile drape to place under the client's arm, a tourniquet, cleansing and antiseptic preparations, dressings, and a small roll of sterile tape
- Local anaesthetic (optional)

For Intravenous Fluid Infusion

- Administration set (the choice depends on the type of solution and the rate of administration; infants and children, clients with cardiac or renal disease, and certain medications require microdrip tubing, which provides 60 gtt/mL)
- 0.22-μm filter (if required by agency policy or if particulate matter is likely; the size appropriate to the type of solution)
- Extension tubing (used when a longer intravenous line is necessary or to avoid manipulation of the catheter insertion site with frequent tubing changes)
- Antiseptic swabs or sticks (chlorhexidine, povidone–iodine, alcohol)
- Disposable gloves
- Tourniquet (Determine the type of tourniquet on the basis of the client assessment, e.g., a blood pressure [BP] cuff [older adult] or a rubber band [infants]. Tourniquets can be a source of contamination; use a single-use product.)
- Arm board and protective cover, if needed (used to maintain wrist or elbow joint position when an over-the-needle catheter [ONC] is placed close to or over a joint; will help prevent infiltration of the intravenous line and mechanical phlebitis).
- Nonallergenic tape and sterile tape (for use under the dressing)
- Waterproof pad (to place under client's hand or arm)
- Intravenous pole, rolling or ceiling mounted
- Special client gown with snaps at shoulder seams if available (makes removal with intravenous tubing easier)
- Needle disposal container (also called sharps container)
- Intravenous site protection device (optional)

For Normal Saline Lock

- Injection cap (also called intravenous plug, adapter)
- Intravenous loop or short piece of extension tubing, if necessary
- 1 to 3 mL of sterile normal saline
- Syringes and 25-gauge needles

Gauze Dressing Only

- 2 × 2 (5-cm × 5-cm) or 4 × 4 (10-cm × 10-cm) sterile gauze sponge

Transparent Dressing Only

- Transparent dressing

Procedure

STEPS	RATIONALE
1. Review physician's order for type and amount of intravenous fluid, rate of fluid administration, and purpose of infusion. Follow seven rights for administration of medications (see Chapter 34).	• An order requesting the initiation of a peripheral intravenous access and administration of an intravenous solution must be made by a physician before implementation of this procedure. Assists in decision making for selection of appropriate access device.

Critical Decision Point: Health care professionals do not write orders to "initiate peripheral access" or "perform venipuncture." "Start IV" may be written, followed by the exact intravenous therapy order. The order to perform venipuncture is implied. If the order is confusing or in question, clarify it with the health care professional before proceeding.

STEPS	RATIONALE
2. Observe for signs and symptoms indicating fluid or electrolyte imbalances that may be affected by intravenous fluid administration:	• Provides baseline data for later evaluation of change in fluid and electrolyte status.
A. Peripheral edema	• Indicates expanded interstitial fluid volume, evident in dependent body parts (e.g., feet and ankles). Excess intravenous fluids will worsen this condition.
B. Greater than 20% change in body weight	• Daily weights assist in documenting fluid retention or loss. Change in body weight of 1 kg corresponds to 1 L of fluid retention or loss.
C. Dry skin and mucous membranes	• Frequently associated with FVD.
D. Distended neck veins	• Frequently associated with FVE or cardiovascular alterations.
E. BP changes	• Elevations in BP may indicate volume excess, and decreased pressure may indicate FVD. These changes can be more sudden and pronounced in those clients with underlying cardiopulmonary disease.

➤ SKILL 40-1 Initiating a Peripheral Intravenous Infusion *continued*

STEPS	RATIONALE
F. Irregular pulse rhythm; tachycardia	• Rate and rhythm change can occur with changes in intravascular volume, as well as changes in potassium, calcium, or magnesium. Tachycardia may indicate cardiac compensation for reduced circulating volume, whereas irregular pulse may indicate arrhythmias secondary to electrolyte imbalance.
G. Auscultation of abnormal lung sounds	• With FVE, the cardiovascular system is unable to compensate for this excess and fluid builds up in the lungs, creating abnormal lung sounds.
H. Decreased skin turgor	• With decreased fluid volume, the skin when pinched remains in that state for several seconds. This is called "tenting."

Critical Decision Point: Changes in skin turgor are a less reliable indicator for older adult clients because of the natural loss in skin elasticity caused by the normal aging process.

STEPS	RATIONALE
I. Thirst	• Symptomatic of FVD. Very young, confused, and severely debilitated clients may not be able to indicate their thirst.
J. Anorexia, nausea, and vomiting	• May be present with FVE or FVD. These symptoms may also be present with the client's underlying disease.
K. Decreased urine output	• During dehydration, the kidneys attempt to restore fluid balance by reducing urine production.
L. Behavioural changes	• May occur with FVD and acid–base imbalance. In addition, behavioural changes may be due to fever, the underlying condition, or pre-existing disease.
3. Assess client's previous or perceived experience with intravenous therapy and arm placement preference.	• Determines level of emotional support and instruction necessary. If hypersensitive to venipunctures, a local anaesthetic may be indicated. Anaesthetic cream needs to be applied for 60 minutes. Transdermal anaesthetic may be administered before venipuncture.
4. Determine whether client is to undergo any planned surgeries or is to receive blood infusion later.	• Allows nurse to place an adequate-size catheter (i.e., 18 or 16 gauge for surgery) and avoids placement in an area that will interfere with medical procedures.
5. Assess laboratory data and client's history of allergies.	• May reveal information that affects insertion of devices, such as FVD, anemia, or allergy to iodine, adhesive, or latex.
6. Assess for the following risk factors: child or older adult, presence of heart failure or renal failure, or low platelet count.	• Fluid imbalances develop more rapidly in extremely young clients (infants) and older clients because such clients have proportionately larger ECF volume, clients with heart failure may require fluid restriction and cannot adapt to sudden increases in vascular volume, and clients with renal failure cannot eliminate excess ECF. A low platelet count predisposes clients to bleeding at intravenous site.
7. Prepare client and family by explaining the procedure, its purpose, and what is expected of the client.	• Decreases anxiety and promotes cooperation.
8. Perform hand hygiene.	• Reduces transmission of microorganisms.
9. Assist client to comfortable sitting or supine position.	• Enables client to extend arm.
10. Organize equipment on clean, clutter-free bedside stand or overbed table.	• Reduces risk of contamination and accidents.
11. Change client's gown to the more easily removed gown with snaps at the shoulder, if available.	• Use of a special intravenous gown facilitates safe removal of the gown.
12. Open sterile packages using sterile aseptic technique.	• Maintains sterility of equipment and reduces spread of microorganisms.
13. Check intravenous solution, using the rights of drug administration (see Chapter 34). Make sure prescribed additives, such as potassium and vitamins, have been added. Check solution for colour, clarity, and expiration date. Check bag for leaks, which is best if done before reaching the bedside.	• Intravenous solutions are medications and should be carefully checked to reduce the risk of error. Solutions that are discoloured, contain particles, or are expired are not to be used. (Some solutions may have slight discoloration [e.g., be pink-tinged] and still be suitable for use.) Leaky bags present an opportunity for infection and must not be used.
14. Open the infusion set, maintaining sterility of both ends of tubing. Many sets allow for priming of tubing without removal of end cap.	• Prevents bacteria from entering infusion equipment and bloodstream.

Continued

➤ SKILL 40-1 Initiating a Peripheral Intravenous Infusion *continued*

STEPS	RATIONALE
15. Place roller clamp about 2 to 5 cm below drip chamber and move roller clamp to closed position (see Step 15 illustrations).	• Close proximity of roller clamp to drip chamber allows more accurate regulation of flow rate. Moving clamp to closed position prevents accidental spillage of fluid.
16. Remove protective sheath over intravenous tubing port on plastic intravenous solution bag (see Step 16 illustration). For bottled intravenous solution, remove metal cap and metal and rubber discs beneath cap. Use caution to avoid touching exposed opening.	• Provides access for insertion of infusion tubing into solution.
17. Insert infusion set into fluid bag or bottle by removing protector cap from tubing insertion spike (keeping spike sterile) and inserting spike into opening of intravenous bag (see Step 17 illustration). Cleanse rubber stopper on glass-bottled solution with antiseptic and insert spike into black rubber stopper of intravenous bottle. Hang solution container on intravenous pole at a minimum height of 90 cm above planned insertion site.	• Prevents contamination of solution from contaminated insertion spike. • Container heights of approximately 1 m are usually sufficient to overcome venous pressure and other resistance from tubing and catheter.
18. Compress drip chamber and release, allowing it to fill one-third to one-half full (see Step 18 illustration). Open clamp and prime infusion tubing by filling with intravenous solution, carefully inverting valves and ports in sequence as the solution moves through the tubing.	• Creates vacuum effects; fluid enters drip chamber to prevent air from entering tubing. By inverting valves and ports, you allow them to fill with fluid, minimizing air bubbles.

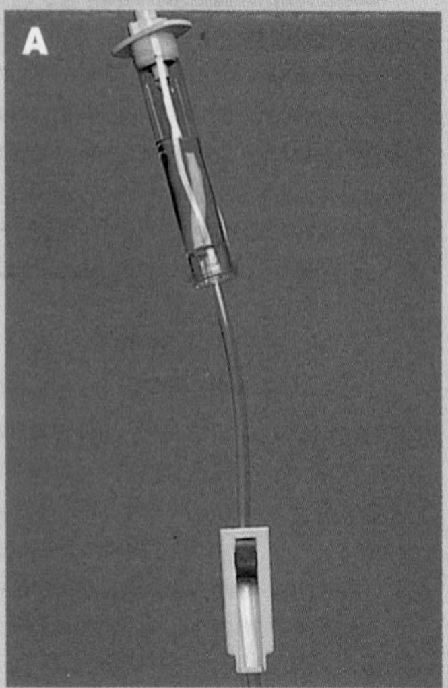

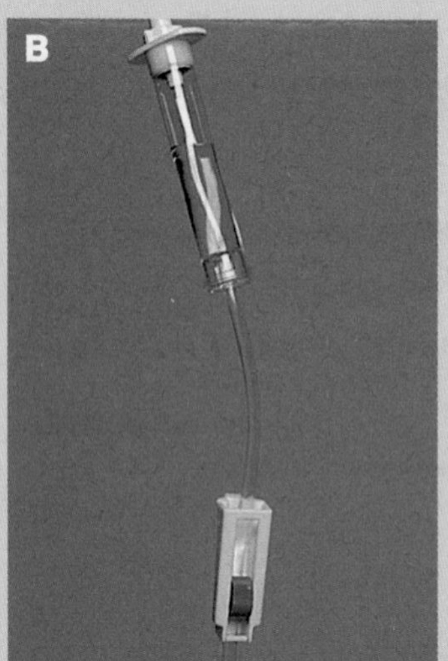

Step 15 **A,** Roller clamp in open position. **B,** Roller clamp in closed position.

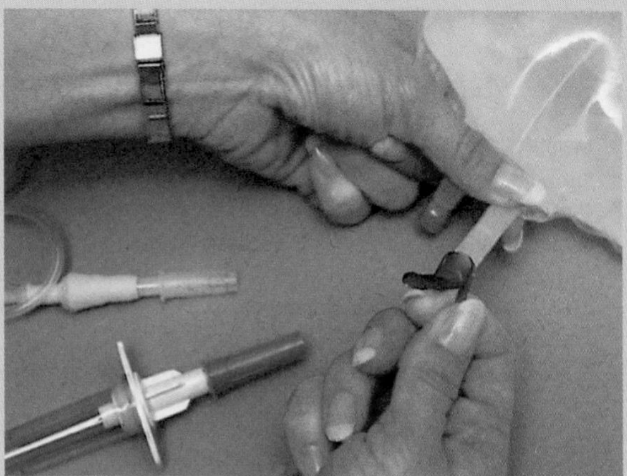

Step 16 Removing protective sheath from intravenous bag port.

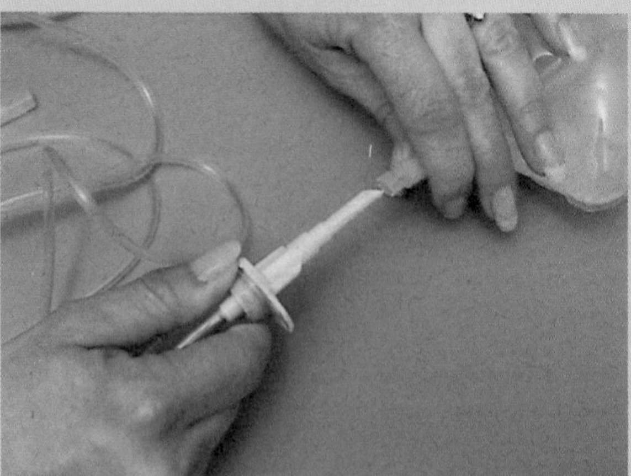

Step 17 Inserting spike into intravenous bag.

➤ SKILL 40-1 Initiating a Peripheral Intravenous Infusion *continued*

STEPS	RATIONALE
19. Remove tubing protector cap (some tubing can be primed without removal) and slowly release roller clamp to allow fluid to travel from drip chamber through tubing to needle adapter. Return roller clamp to closed position after tubing is primed (filled with intravenous fluid).	• Slow filling of tubing decreases turbulence and chance of bubble formation. Removes air from tubing and permits tubing to fill with solution. Closing the clamp prevents accidental loss of fluid.
20. Be certain tubing is clear of air and air bubbles. To remove small air bubbles, firmly tap intravenous tubing where air bubbles are located. Check entire length of tubing to ensure that all air bubbles are removed (see Step 20 illustration).	• Large air bubbles can act as emboli. Air bubbles may contribute to anxiety related to intravenous therapy.

Critical Decision Point: Do not touch spike. It is sterile. If contamination occurs (e.g., spike is accidentally dropped on the floor), then discard intravenous tubing and obtain a new one.

Critical Decision Point: Extra extension tubing may be added to intravenous tubing to allow for more length, which will enable the client to move more freely while still keeping the intravenous line stable. But remember, adding extensions increases risk for infection.

STEPS	RATIONALE
21. Replace tubing cap protector on end of tubing.	• Maintains system sterility.
22. *Optional:* Prepare normal saline lock for infusion. If a loop or short extension tubing is needed, use sterile technique to connect the intravenous plug to the loop or short extension tubing. Inject 1 to 3 mL normal saline through the plug and through the loop or short extension tubing.	• Removes air to prevent introduction into the vein. Do the same with the saline plug.
23. Apply disposable gloves. Eye protection and mask may be worn (see agency policy) if splash or spray of blood is possible. *Note:* Gloves can be left off to locate vein but must be applied before preparing site.	• Reduces transmission of microorganisms. Decreases exposure to HIV, hepatitis, and other bloodborne organisms (Infusion Nurses Society [INS], 2006).

Critical Decision Point: Do not shave area with a razor. Shaving may cause microabrasions and predispose client to infection (INS, 2006). Clipping excess hair is appropriate.

STEPS	RATIONALE
24. Identify accessible vein for intravenous placement. Apply tourniquet 10 to 15 cm above the proposed insertion site (see Step 24 illustration). Position tourniquet so that ends are away from proposed venipuncture site. Check for presence of radial pulse. OPTION: Apply BP cuff instead of tourniquet. Inflate to a level just below client's normal diastolic pressure. Maintain inflation at that pressure until venipuncture is completed.	• Tourniquet should be tight enough to impede venous return but not occlude arterial flow.

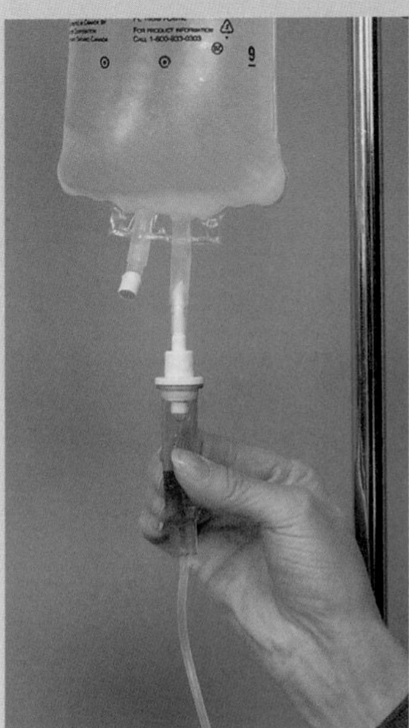

Step 18 Squeezing drip chamber to fill with fluid.

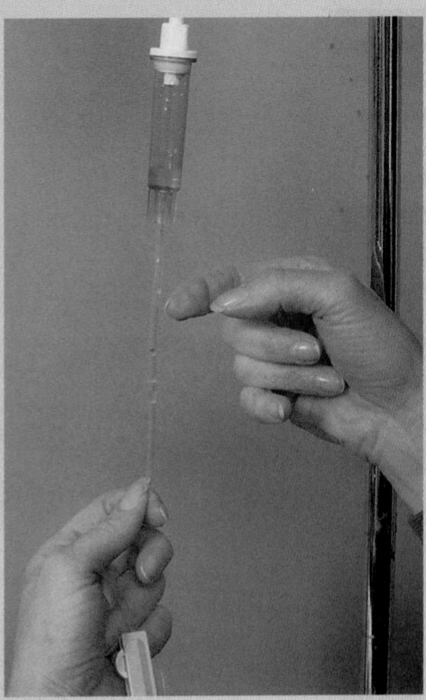

Step 20 Removing air bubbles from tubing.

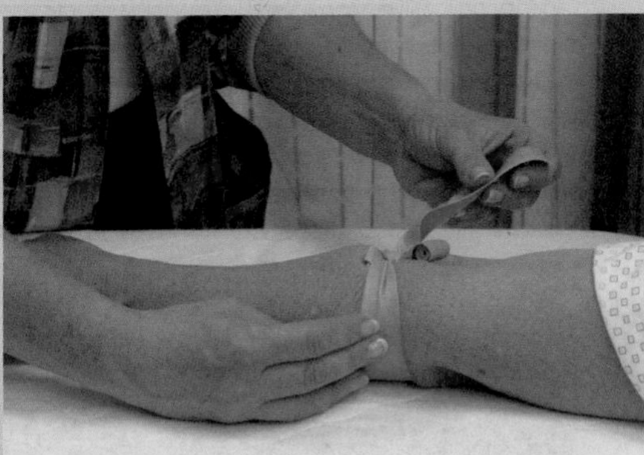

Step 24 Apply tourniquet.

Continued

➤SKILL 40-1 Initiating a Peripheral Intravenous Infusion *continued*

STEPS	RATIONALE
25. Select the vein. Common intravenous sites for the adult include cephalic, basilic, and median cubital veins (see Figure 40–14).	
A. Use the most distal site in the nondominant arm, if possible.	• Venipuncture should be performed distal to proximal, which increases the availability of other sites for future intravenous therapy.
B. Avoid areas that are painful to palpation.	• May indicate inflamed vein.
C. Select a vein large enough for catheter placement.	• Prevents interruption of venous flow while allowing adequate blood flow around the catheter.
D. Choose a site that will not interfere with client's activities of daily living or planned procedures.	• Selection of an appropriate site will minimize risk of injury and loss of the IV.
E. Use the fingertips to palpate the vein by pressing downward and noting the resilient, soft, bouncy feeling as the pressure is released (see Step 25E illustration).	• Fingertips are more sensitive and are better to assess vein condition.
F. Promote venous distension by instructing the client to open and close the fist several times, lowering the client's arm in a dependent position, applying warmth to the arm for several minutes, and rubbing or stroking the client's arm from distal to proximal below proposed site.	• These activities increase blood flow to the area of insertion. When these techniques are properly used, they foster venous dilation and access to the vein.

Critical Decision Point: Avoid vigorous rubbing and multiple tapping of client's veins. These techniques may cause injury to the vein, such as a hematoma, or cause venous constriction.

STEPS	RATIONALE
G. Avoid sites distal to previous venipuncture site, sclerosed or hardened cordlike veins, infiltrated site or phlebotic vessels, bruised areas, and areas of venous valves or bifurcation. Avoid veins in antecubital fossa and ventral surface of the wrist.	• Such sites increase the risk of infiltration of newly placed intravenous line and excessive vessel damage. • Veins in the antecubital fossa are used for blood draws, and placement in this area limits mobility. Inner wrist contains numerous tendons that could be damaged.
H. Avoid fragile dorsal veins in older adults and vessels in an extremity with compromised circulation (e.g., in cases of mastectomy, dialysis graft, or paralysis).	• Venous alterations can increase risk of complications (e.g., infiltration and decreased catheter dwelling time).
26. Release tourniquet temporarily and carefully. Clip arm hair with scissors (if necessary). Do not shave area.	• Hair impedes venipuncture and adherence of dressing. Shaving can cause microabrasions and predispose client to infection.
27. (If area of insertion appears to need cleansing, use soap and water first.) Cleanse insertion site using firm, circular motion (centre to outward) in concentric circles 5 to 7.5 cm from insertion site. Use antiseptic preparation as a single agent or in combination, according to agency policy. Two percent chlorhexidine gluconate is the antiseptic cleansing agent of choice (RNAO, 2005). Povidone–iodine is a topical anti-infective agent that reduces skin surface bacteria; 70% alcohol is another antiseptic cleansing agent. Povidone–iodine must dry to be effective in reducing microbial counts (Millam & Hadaway, 2003). Avoid touching the cleansed site. Allow the site to dry for at least 2 minutes (see Step 27 illustration). If skin is touched after cleansing, repeat cleansing procedure.	• Air-drying prevents chemical reactions between agents and allows time for maximum microbicidal activity of agents (INS, 2006). • Touching the cleansed area would introduce organisms from nurse's hand to the site.

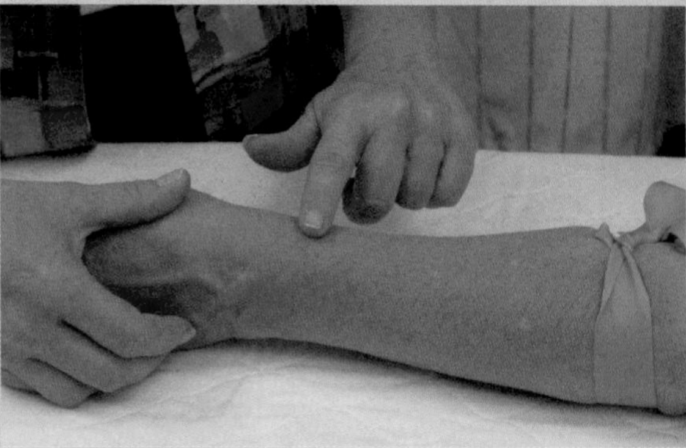

Step 25E Palpate vein for resilience.

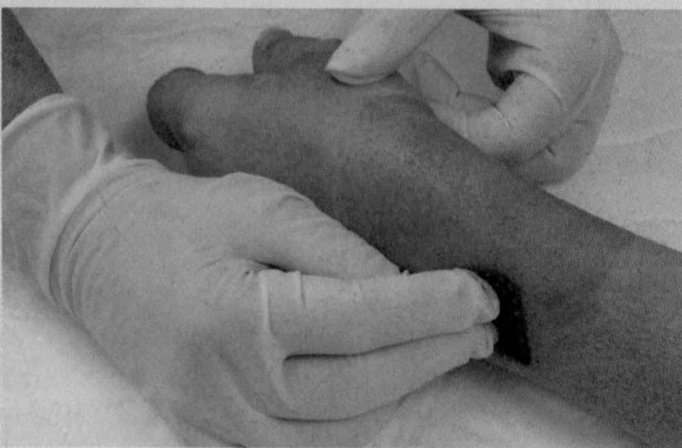

Step 27 Cleanse site chosen for insertion.

➤ SKILL 40-1 Initiating a Peripheral Intravenous Infusion *continued*

STEPS	RATIONALE
28. Reapply tourniquet or BP cuff.	
Critical Decision Point: Do not use povidone–iodine if the client is allergic to iodine; use an alternative cleansing agent.	
29. Perform venipuncture. Anchor vein by placing thumb over vein beneath insertion site and by stretching the skin against the direction of insertion 5 to 7.5 cm distal to the site (see Step 29 illustration). Warn client of a sharp stick. Puncture skin and vein, holding catheter at 10- to 30-degree angle with the bevel pointed upward. A. **Butterfly needle:** Hold needle at 10- to 30-degree angle with bevel up slightly distal to actual site of venipuncture. B. **Needleless ONC safety device:** Insert ONC (see Step 29B illustration) with bevel up at 10- to 30-degree angle slightly distal to actual site of venipuncture in the direction of the vein.	• The vascular access device selected should be the smallest gauge and shortest length that will accommodate the therapy (INS, 2006). • Places needle parallel to vein. When vein is punctured, risk of puncturing posterior vein wall is reduced. • Superficial veins require a smaller angle; deeper veins require a greater angle.
Critical Decision Point: No more than two attempts at inserting an intravenous line should be made by a single nurse (INS, 2006).	
30. Look for blood return through tubing of butterfly needle or flashback chamber of ONC, indicating that needle has entered vein (see Step 30 illustration, part A). Lower catheter or needle until almost flush with skin. Advance butterfly needle until hub rests at venipuncture site. Advance ONC 0.5 cm into vein and then loosen stylet. Advance catheter off the stylet into vein until hub rests at venipuncture site (see Step 30 illustration, part B). Do not reinsert the stylet once it is loosened. (Advance the safety device by using push-tab to thread the catheter.)	• Increased venous pressure from tourniquet increases backflow of blood into catheter or tubing. • Lowering the angle and advancing the cannula slightly allow for full penetration of vein wall, placement of catheter within vein's inner lumen, and easy advancement of catheter off stylet. • Threading catheter up to hub reduces the risk of introduction of infectious organisms along the catheter length. Reinsertion of the stylet can cause catheter damage and potential catheter embolization.

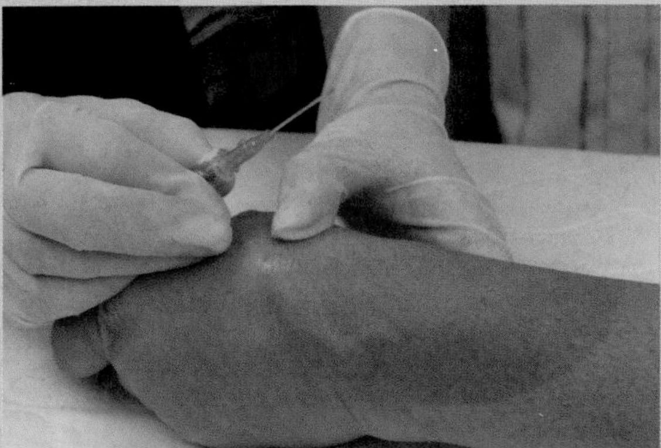

Step 29 Stabilize vein below insertion site with skin taut.

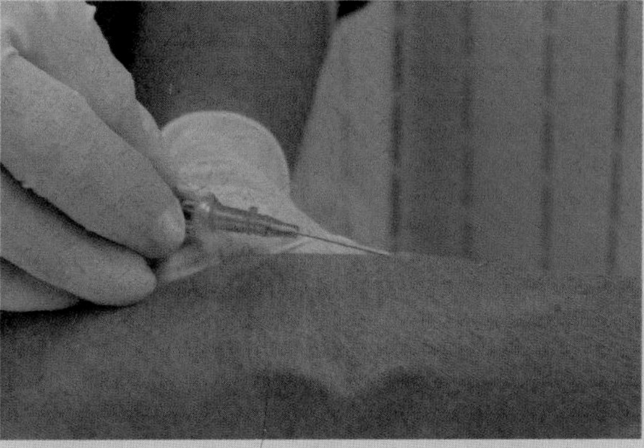

Step 29B Puncture skin with catheter at 10- to 30-degree angle. Catheter enters vein.

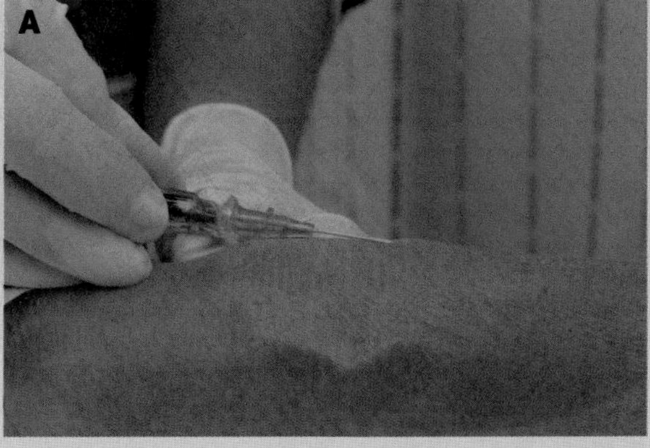

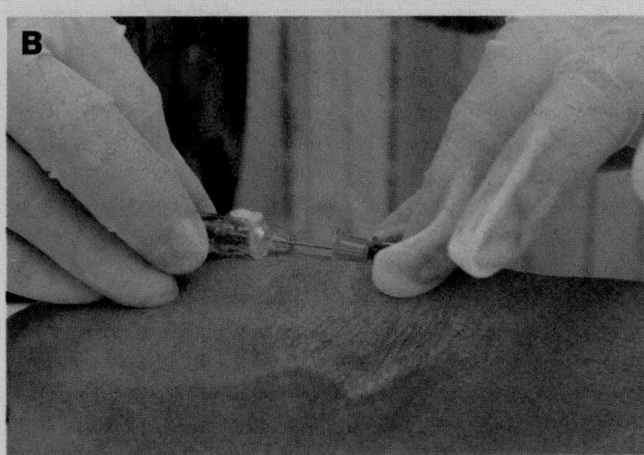

Step 30 **A,** Blood return in flashback chamber, catheter lowered flush with skin. **B,** Advance catheter into vein; use safety device push-tab.

Continued

➤ SKILL 40-1 Initiating a Peripheral Intravenous Infusion *continued*

STEPS	RATIONALE
31. Stabilize the catheter. Apply gentle but firm pressure with the index finger of nondominant hand 3 cm above insertion site (see Step 31 illustration, part A). Release tourniquet or BP cuff with dominant hand and retract stylet from ONC (see Step 31 illustration, part B). Do not recap the stylet. For a safety device, slide the catheter off the stylet while gliding the protective guard over the stylet. A click indicates the device is locked over the stylet.	• Permits venous flow, reduces backflow of blood, and prevents accidental withdrawal or dislodgement.
32. Quickly connect adapter of primed fluid administration set (see Step 32 illustration) or saline lock to hub of ONC or butterfly tubing. Be sure connection is secure. Do not touch point of entry of adapter.	• Prompt connection of infusion set maintains patency of vein. • Maintains sterility.
33. Release roller clamp slowly to begin infusion at a rate to maintain patency of intravenous line.	• Permits venous flow and prevents clotting of vein and obstruction of flow of intravenous solution.
A. *Intermittent infusion:* Continue to stabilize catheter with nondominant hand and attach injection cap of adapter. Insert prefilled flush solution into injection cap. Flush slowly (see Step 33A illustration). Maintain thumb pressure on syringe during withdrawal or close clamp on extension tubing of injection cap while still flushing last 0.2 to 0.4 mL of flush solution.	• Positive pressure in the catheter prevents reflux of blood into the catheter lumen (Phillips, 2005).

Critical Decision Point: Be sure to calculate rate so as not to infuse intravenous solution too rapidly or too slowly.

STEPS	RATIONALE
34. Tape or secure catheter.	
A. **If applying transparent dressing,** secure catheter with nondominant hand while preparing to apply dressing.	• Securing the catheter and tubing prevents movement and tension on the device, reducing mechanical irritation and possible phlebitis or infection.

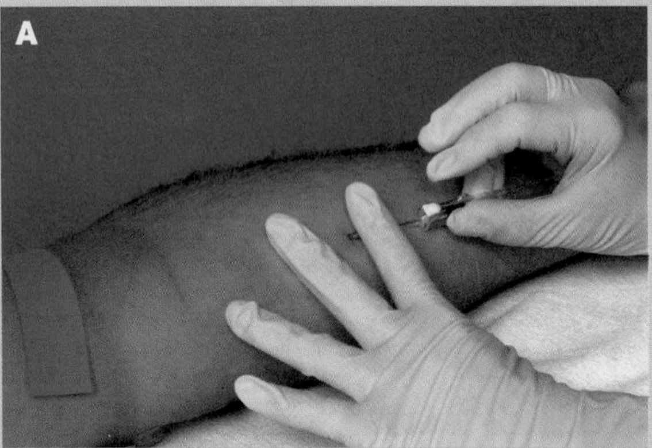

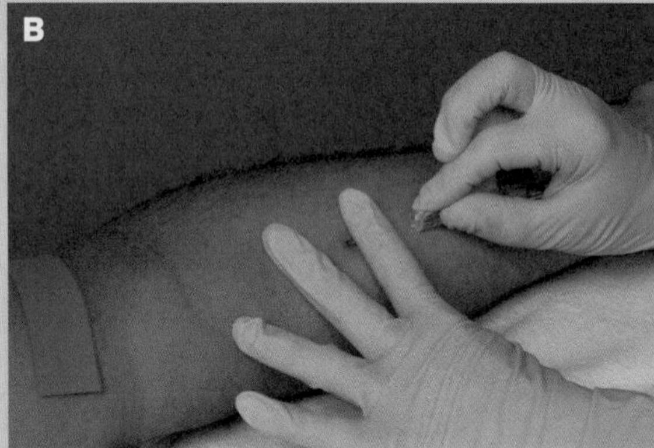

Step 31 **A,** Apply pressure above insertion site with index finger of nondominant hand. **B,** Retract the stylet by pushing safety tab.

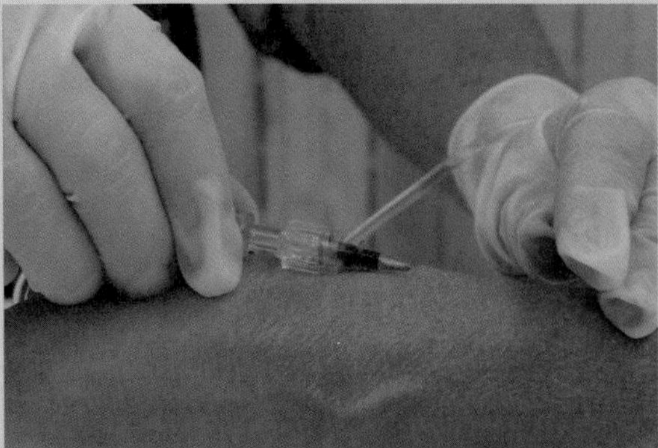

Step 32 Connect end of intravenous tubing to catheter tubing. Secure connector.

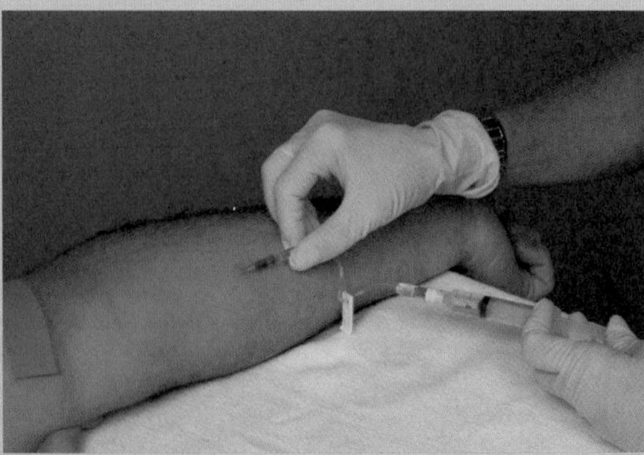

Step 33a Flush injection cap slowly.

➤ SKILL 40-1 Initiating a Peripheral Intravenous Infusion *continued*

STEPS	RATIONALE
B. **If applying a gauze dressing:**	
(1) Tape the intravenous catheter. Place narrow piece (1-cm wide) of sterile tape under hub of catheter with adhesive side up (see Step 34B(1) illustration, part A) and criss-cross tape over hub to form a chevron (see Step 34B(1) illustration, part B).	• Securing the catheter and tubing prevents movement and tension on the device, reducing mechanical irritation and possible phlebitis or infection. Tape placed underneath the dressing should be sterile; nonsterile tape is a potential source of pathogenic bacteria.
(2) Place tape only on the catheter, never over the insertion site. Secure the site to allow easy visual inspection and early recognition of infiltration and phlebitis. Avoid applying tape around the extremity.	• Taping around extremity could result in a "tourniquet effect" and impede venous return.
C. **Observe site for swelling.**	
35. Apply sterile dressing over site.	
A. **Transparent dressing**	
(1) Carefully remove adherent backing. Apply one edge of dressing and then gently smooth remaining dressing over site, leaving end of catheter hub uncovered (see Step 35A(1) illustration). Refer to manufacturer's directions.	• Transparent dressings are occlusive to moisture and microorganisms. • Transparent dressings allow continuous inspection of the intravenous site, are more comfortable, and permit clients to bathe and shower without saturating the dressing (Phillips, 2005).
(2) Take a 2.5-cm piece of tape and place it from end of hub of the catheter to insertion site, over transparent dressing (see Step 35A(2) illustration).	
(3) Then apply chevron and place only over tape, not the transparent dressing (see Step 35A(3) illustration).	

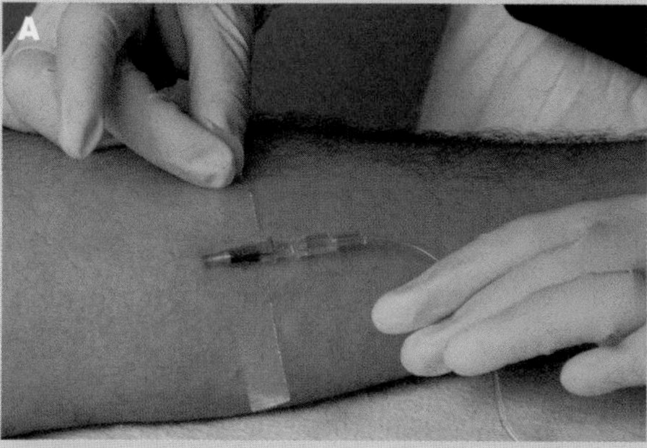

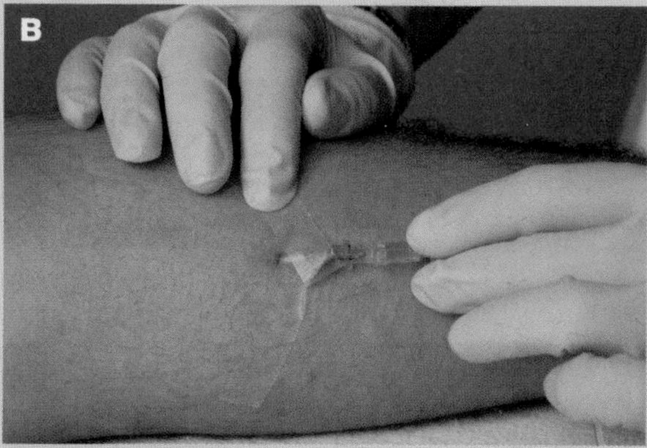

Step 34B(1) **A,** Place tape under catheter hub. **B,** Criss-cross ends of tape over hub.

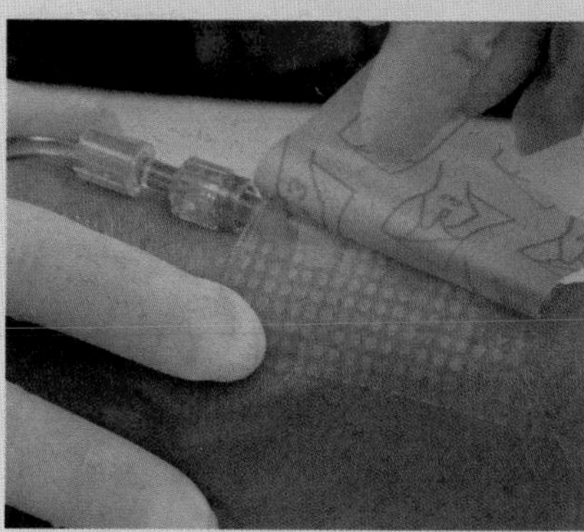

Step 35A(1) Apply transparent dressing.

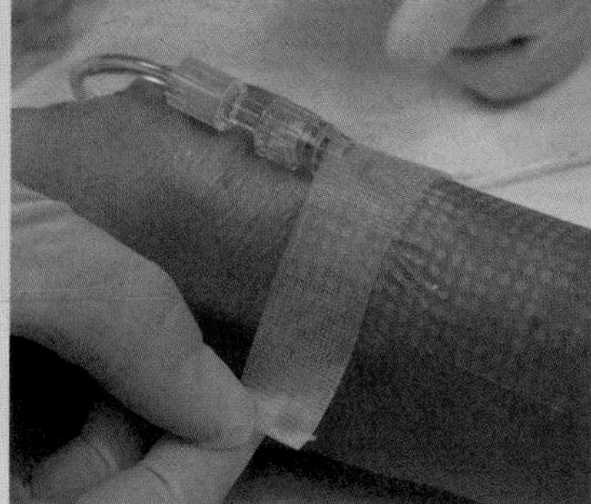

Step 35A(2) Place tape over transparent dressing.

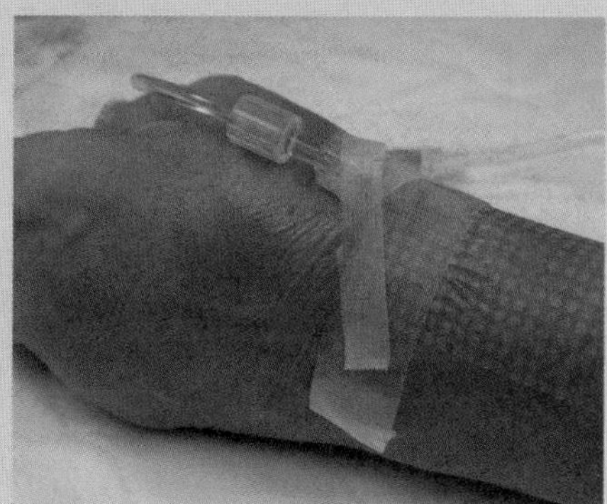

Step 35A(3) Apply chevron over tape.

Continued

➤ SKILL 40-1 Initiating a Peripheral Intravenous Infusion *continued*

STEPS	RATIONALE
B. Sterile gauze dressing	
(1) Fold a 2 × 3 × 2 gauze in half and cover with a 2.5-cm-wide piece of sterile tape extending about 2.5 cm from each side. Place it under the tubing–catheter hub junction (see Step 35B(1) illustration).	• Tape on top of tape makes it easier to access hub–tubing junction. Securing loop of tubing reduces risk of dislodging catheter from accidental pull. • Gauze is less expensive than transparent dressing and may also be useful for bleeding or excessive moisture at the site.
(2) Curl a loop of tubing alongside the arm and place a second piece of tape directly over the padded 2 × 2 gauze, securing tubing in two places (see Step 35B(2) illustrations).	
36. Prepare the equipment according to expected frequency of use.	
A. *For intravenous fluid administration:* Adjust flow rate to correct drops per minute or connect to EID (see Skill 40–2, Steps 9 to 15).	• Maintains correct rate of flow for intravenous solution. Flow can fluctuate; therefore, it must be checked at intervals.
B. *For intermittent use:* Saline lock. Flush with 3 mL of sterile normal saline at prescribed frequency or agency policy.	• Maintains patency of intravenous catheter. While some authors recommend heparin lock, the RNAO (2008) recommends use of saline for flushing and locking peripheral short catheters, after each use and daily if not in use.
37. Label dressing with date, time, gauge size and length of catheter, and your initials (see Step 37 illustration).	• Allows for easy recognition of type of device and time interval for site rotation. INS standard for site rotation of peripheral intravenous access device is every 72 hours (INS, 2006).

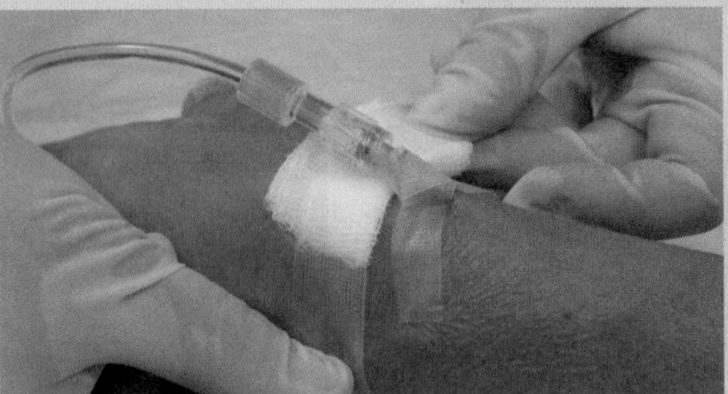

Step 35B(1) Place and tape gauze under catheter hub.

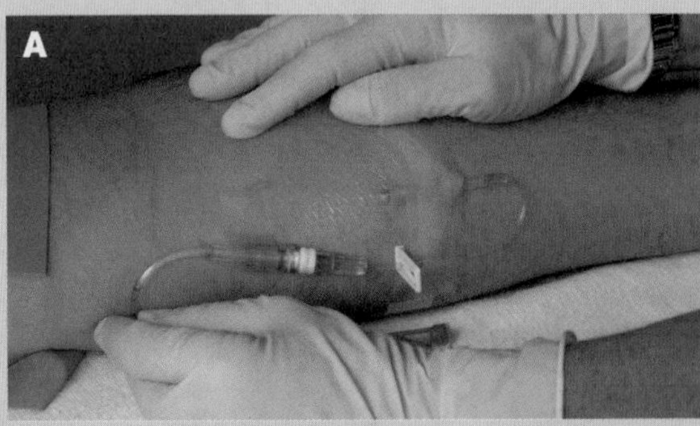

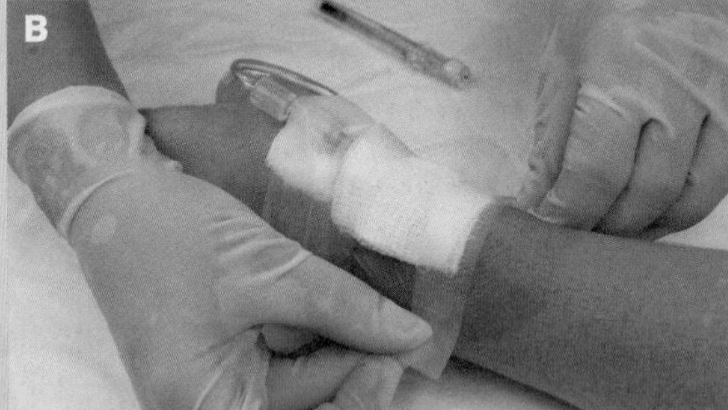

Step 35B(2) **A,** Loop and secure tubing. **B,** Apply 2 × 2 gauze.

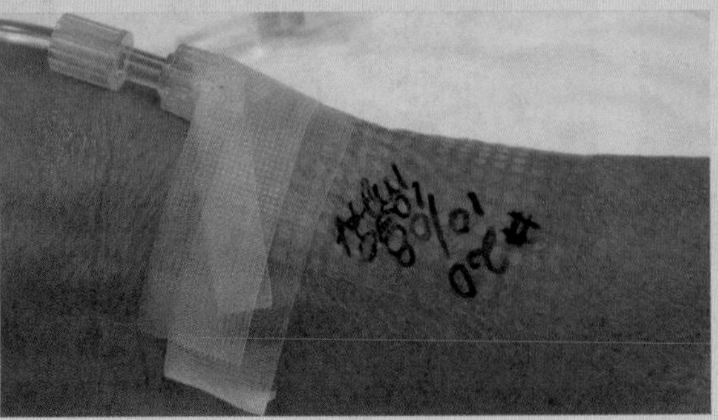

Step 37 Dressing labelled with date and time.

➤ SKILL 40-1 Initiating a Peripheral Intravenous Infusion *continued*

STEPS	RATIONALE
38. Dispose of used needles in appropriate sharps container. Discard supplies. Remove gloves and perform hand hygiene.	• Reduces transmission of microorganisms and protects staff from injury.
39. Observe client every hour to determine whether fluid is infusing correctly: A. Check whether correct amount of solution is infused as prescribed by looking at time tape. B. Count flow rate or check rate on infusion pump. C. Check patency of intravenous catheter or needle. D. Observe client for signs of discomfort. E. Inspect insertion site for absence of phlebitis (see Table 40–8), infiltration (see Table 40–10), or inflammation.	• Correct administration of fluid volume prevents fluid imbalance. • Accurate monitoring of rate furthers ensures correct volume administration.
40. Observe client every hour to determine response to therapy (i.e., measure vital signs, conduct postprocedure assessments).	• Provides continuous evaluation of type and amount of fluid delivered to client. Hourly inspection prevents accidental fluid overload or inadequate infusion rate and identifies early incidence of vein inflammation or tissue damage. Intravenous fluids and additives are given to maintain or restore fluid and electrolyte balance. They can also cause unexpected effects, which can be serious.

Unexpected Outcomes and Related Interventions

FVD, as Manifested by Decreased Urine Output, Dry Mucous Membranes, Hypotension, and Tachycardia

- Notify physician; may require readjustment of infusion rate.

FVE, as Manifested by Crackles in Lungs, Shortness of Breath, and Edema

- Reduce intravenous flow rate if symptoms appear and notify physician.

Electrolyte Imbalances, as Manifested by Abnormal Serum Electrolyte Levels; Changes in Mental Status, Neuromuscular Function, and Vital Signs; and Other Signs and Symptoms

- Notify physician. Additives in intravenous or type of intravenous fluid may be adjusted.

Infiltration, as Indicated by Swelling and Possible Pitting Edema, Pallor, Coolness, Pain at Insertion Site, and Possible Decrease in Flow Rate

- Stop infusion and discontinue intravenous therapy. Elevate affected extremity. Restart new intravenous line if continued therapy is necessary.

Phlebitis, as Indicated by Pain, Increased Skin Temperature, and Erythema Along Path of Vein

- Stop infusion and discontinue intravenous therapy. Restart new intravenous line if continued therapy is necessary.
- Place moist, warm compress over area of phlebitis.

Bleeding at Venipuncture Site

- Bleeding from vein is usually slow, continuous seepage. Common in clients who have received heparin or have a bleeding disorder or if the intravenous site is over bend in arm or hand.
- If bleeding occurs around venipuncture site and catheter is within vein, gauze dressing may be applied over site. Eventually, intravenous therapy may need to be discontinued.
- Blood on the dressing can result when the administration set becomes disconnected from the catheter's hub. When blood appears on the dressing, verify that the system is intact and change the dressing.

Recording and Reporting

- Record in nurses' notes number of attempts for insertion, type of fluid, insertion site by vessel, flow rate, size and type of catheter or needle, and when infusion was begun. A special parenteral therapy flow sheet may be used.
- Record client's response to intravenous fluid, amount infused, and integrity and patency of system every 4 hours or according to agency policy.
- Report the following to oncoming nursing staff: type of fluid, flow rate, status of venipuncture site, amount of fluid remaining in present solution, expected time to hang next intravenous bag or bottle, and any side effects.

Home Care Considerations

- Teach caregiver to apply pressure with sterile gauze if catheter falls out and, if client is on anticoagulant therapy, to tape several pieces of sterile gauze in place for at least 20 minutes with pressure or until bleeding stops.
- Teach client and caregiver to perform tub bath without getting intravenous tubing wet and to unplug pump first if one is used. For showering, the client must protect the intravenous site and dressing from getting wet by covering them completely with plastic.
- Teach client and family to monitor intake and output using measuring devices.
- Teach client and family to dispose of open and sheathed needles into sharps container. All sharps containers must be stored in safe area away from children.

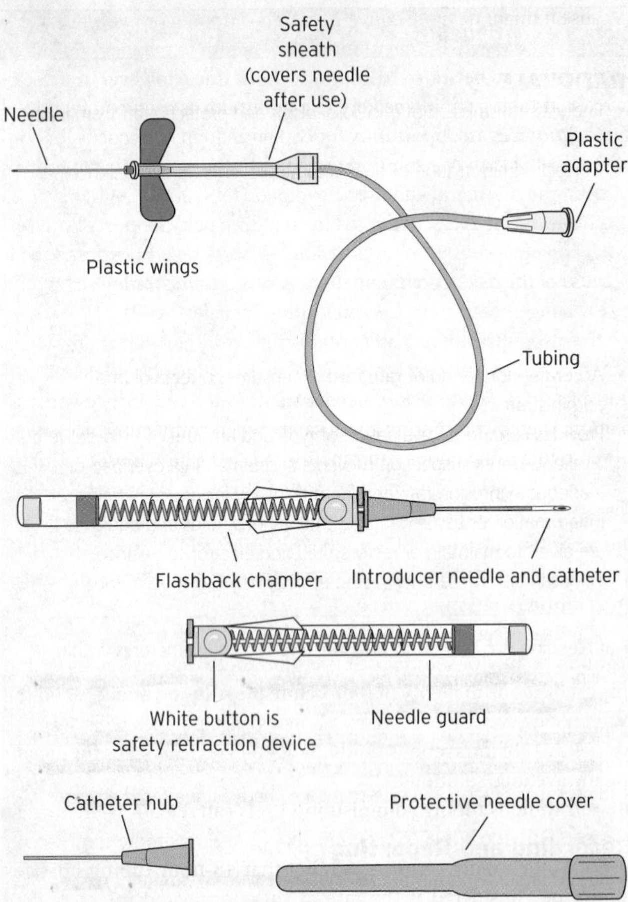

Figure 40-13 Options for intravenous access device.

many mechanical and client factors. Recent advances in infusion technology have resulted in a variety of devices available for use to ensure accurate delivery.

Many devices have operating and programming capabilities that allow for single- and multiple-solution infusions at different rates. A variety of detectors and alarms respond to air in intravenous lines, completion of infusion, high and low pressure, low battery power, occlusion, and the inability to deliver at a preset rate.

safety alert An anti–free-flow safeguard (preventing bolus infusion in the event of machine malfunction) is an important element of an electronic infusion device and is required. The manufacturer's recommendations for specific device features should always be checked.

Patency of the intravenous needle or catheter means that the tip of the needle or catheter has no clots and that the catheter or needle tip is not against the vein wall. A blocked catheter or needle can affect the rate of infusion of the intravenous fluids. Intravenous flow rates can also be affected by infiltration, a knot or kink in the tubing, the height of the solution, a restrictive intravenous dressing, and the position of the client's extremity. One way to assess patency is by lowering the intravenous bag below the level of the intravenous insertion site and observing for a blood return; however, this method does not confirm patency. If no blood return occurs and fluid does not flow easily from the drip chamber when the roller clamp is opened, you should assess potential causes: a clot may be occluding the cannula of the intravenous catheter, the catheter tip may be occluded against the wall of the vein, or the intravenous dressing may be too tight, thereby impeding the flow. The tubing and area around the insertion site should be inspected for anything that could obstruct the flow of intravenous fluids. A knot or kink in the tubing can decrease the flow rate. Occasionally, the tubing is kinked under a dressing; remove the dressing to locate the problem. The client may also occlude the tubing by lying or sitting on it. The flow rate frequently resumes after the tubing is straightened. The height of the intravenous bag can also affect flow rates. Raising the bag usually increases the rate because of increased hydrostatic pressure.

The position of the extremity, particularly at the wrist or elbow, can decrease flow rates. Occasionally, the use of an arm board helps keep the joint extended (Figure 40–15). The arm board also provides some protection to the intravenous site and tubing. Sometimes it is more comfortable for the client to have an infusion started in a new location rather than relying on a site that causes problems. However, before discontinuing the infusion hampered by an extremity position, you should start the infusion in another site to verify that the client has other accessible veins.

Children, older adults, clients with severe head trauma, and clients susceptible to volume overload must be protected from sudden increases in infusion volumes. When certain intravenous controller devices are opened, the intravenous fluid will infuse rapidly. If this is not controlled, an excessive amount of solution can infuse.

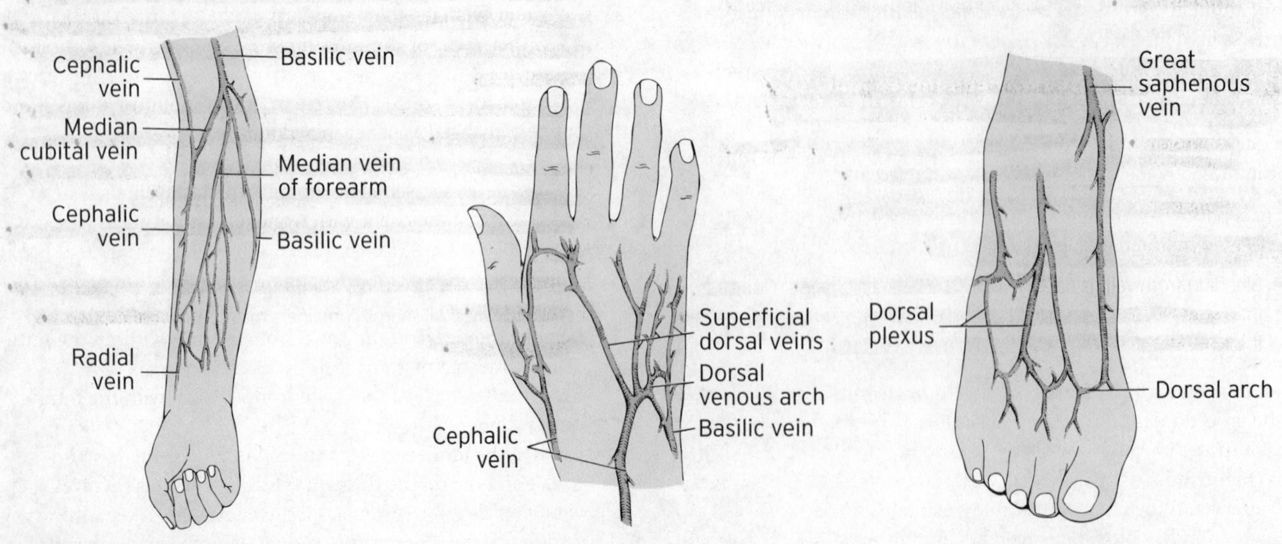

Figure 40-14 Common intravenous sites.

BOX 40-10 FOCUS ON OLDER ADULTS

Protection of Skin and Veins

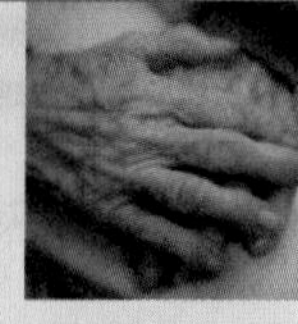

- Use the smallest gauge cannula or needle possible (e.g., 22 to 24 gauge). Veins are very fragile, and a smaller gauge allows better blood flow to provide increased hemodilution of the intravenous fluids or medications (Schelper, 2003).
- Avoid the back of the hand, which may compromise the client's need for independence and mobility.
- Impaired skin integrity may lead to susceptibility for tearing, venous sclerosis, and difficulty detecting complications.
- Avoid placement of an intravenous line in veins that are easily bumped because less subcutaneous support tissue is present.
- If the client has fragile skin and veins, use minimal or no tourniquet pressure.
- After applying a tourniquet, venous pressure rises rapidly, the vein is overstretched, and puncture with even a thin needle can rupture the wall of the vein (Millam & Hadaway, 2003).
- If using a tourniquet, place it over the client's sleeve to decrease shearing of fragile skin.
- With loss of supportive tissue, veins tend to lie more superficially; lower the insertion angle for venipuncture to 5 to 15 degrees (Coulter, 2004; INS, 2006; Rosenthal, 2005).
- If the client has lost subcutaneous tissue, the veins lose stability and will roll away from the needle. To stabilize the vein, apply traction to the skin below the projected insertion site.
- Secure the device with mesh dressing or a securement device for protection (Coulter, 2004).
- Nutritional deficiencies promote fluid to migrate into tissues surrounding vessels, making intravenous access more difficult.
- Multiple medication usage (e.g., anticoagulants, antibiotics, and steroids) increases the likelihood of fragile, transparent skin that bruises and bleeds easily.
- Dehydration related to a lower percentage of body weight as water and diminished thirst mechanism contribute to difficult intravenous access (Grandjean et al., 2003; Rosenthal, 2005).

Sudden increases can occur accidentally. For example, a restless client may loosen the roller clamp with a sudden movement and increase the flow rate, or the flow rate may be accidentally increased if the client ambulates. A sudden increase in the intravenous infusion rate causes a rapid increase in vascular volume, which can make the client critically ill or even cause death. Volume control devices, such as a Volutrol burette, can prevent sudden excessive increases in the volume of intravenous solution infused.

Maintaining the System. After the intravenous line is in place and the flow rate is regulated, you must maintain the system. Keep agency policy regarding the maintenance of intravenous lines in mind. Line maintenance is achieved by (1) keeping the system sterile; (2) changing solutions, tubing, and site dressings; and (3) assisting the client with self-care activities so as not to disrupt the system.

You play an important role in maintaining the integrity of an intravenous line to prevent infection from developing. The client's microflora and contamination by insertion are initially controlled for in the procedure for intravenous insertion. However, the other factors are controlled through conscientious use of infection control principles (Figure 40–16). This begins with thorough hand hygiene before and after handling any component of the intravenous system.

The integrity of the intravenous system must always be maintained. Never disconnect tubing because it becomes tangled or because it might be more convenient in positioning or moving a client or applying a gown. If a client needs more room to manoeuvre, extension tubing can be added to an intravenous line. However, the use of extension tubing should be kept to a minimum as each connection of tubing provides an opportunity for contamination. Stopcocks for connecting more than one solution to a single intravenous site are sources of contamination and should be avoided (INS, 2006). Whenever an intravenous line is disconnected from a stopcock, the port should be plugged with a sterile cap. A port should never remain exposed to air because of the risk of contamination. A new administration set should be exchanged with the subsequent fluid change.

Intravenous tubing also contains injection ports through which adapters can be inserted for medication injections. Needleless injection ports reduce the risk of needle-stick injury and reduce contamination, thereby promoting client safety when connecting, accessing, or removing intravenous equipment (Casey & Elliot, 2007a, 2007b). This risk is further minimized by using alcohol–chlorhexidine gluconate solution or povidone–iodine for cleansing the port both before and after use (Casey & Elliott, 2007b). Kaler and Chinn (2007) recommend using pressure and friction with a cleansing swab for 15 seconds for preparation of a needleless port.

Clients receiving intravenous therapy over several days will require a change of solutions. It is important to organize tasks so that this can be done in plenty of time before the solution empties and the cannula becomes clotted. Many agencies have policies regarding the "hang time" of intravenous fluids. Skill 40–3 reviews steps for changing intravenous solutions.

Intravenous tubing administration sets can remain sterile for 72 hours (CDC, 2002; INS, 2006). The INS (2006) recommends 72-hour intervals for tubing changes, adding that 48-hour tubing changes should be considered if the rate of catheter-related infection and phlebitis in an agency exceeds 5%. The exception is tubing containing blood, TPN, blood products, and lipid emulsions, which are more likely to promote bacterial growth. Agency policy may require more frequent tubing changes (e.g., every 24 hours). Whenever possible, schedule tubing changes when it is time to hang a new container to promote aseptic technique. To prevent entry of bacteria into the bloodstream, maintain sterility during tubing and solution changes.

The dressings over intravenous sites are applied to reduce the entrance of bacteria into the insertion site. The two forms of dressings are transparent and gauze. Transparent dressings reliably secure the intravenous device, allow continuous visual inspection of the intravenous site, become less easily soiled or moistened, and require less frequent changes than standard gauze (CDC, 2002; Hindley, 2004). Either form of dressing must be changed when the intravenous device is removed or replaced or when the dressing becomes damp, loosened, or soiled (INS, 2006). Intravenous dressings should be routinely changed as per agency policy (e.g., every 48 to 72 hours; Skill 40–4).

To prevent the accidental disruption of an intravenous system, you may need to assist the client with hygiene, comfort measures, meals, and ambulation. Using a gown specifically made with snaps along the top sleeve seam helps facilitate changing the gown without disturbing the venipuncture site. Regular gowns are changed as follows:

1. Remove the sleeve of the gown from the arm without the intravenous line, maintaining the client's privacy.
2. Remove the sleeve of the gown from the arm with the intravenous line.
3. Remove the intravenous solution container from its stand and pass it and the tubing through the sleeve. (If this involves removing the tubing from an intravenous electronic infusion device, use the roller clamp to slow the infusion to prevent the accidental infusion of a large volume of solution or medication.)

4. Place the intravenous solution container and tubing through the sleeve of the clean gown and hang it on its stand. (If the intravenous line is connected to an electronic infusion device, open the roller clamp. Turn on the pump.)
5. Place the arm with the intravenous line through the gown sleeve.
6. Place the arm without the intravenous line through the gown sleeve. (Breaking the integrity of an intravenous line to change a gown leads to contamination.)

➤ SKILL 40-2 Regulating Intravenous Flow Rates

video

Delegation Considerations

In many provinces, regulating and monitoring intravenous therapy is included within the scope of practice for licensed and registered practical nurses. The skill of regulating intravenous therapy should not be delegated to unregulated care providers (UCPs). Refer to Skill 40–1 for important information to instruct the UCP.

Equipment

- Watch with second hand
- Paper and pencil or calculator
- Intravenous electronic infusion controller or pump (optional)
- Volume control device (optional)
- Time indicator tape

Procedure

STEPS	RATIONALE
1. Check client's medical record for correct solution, additives, and time of infusion. Usual order includes solution for 24 hours, usually divided into 2 or 3 L. Occasionally, intravenous order contains only 1 L to keep vein open (KVO). Order also indicates time over which each litre is to infuse.	• Use principles of drug administration to ensure correct fluids are given to correct client.

Critical Decision Point: It is common for health care professionals to write an abbreviated intravenous order such as "D_5W with 20 mmol KCl 125 mL/hr continuous." This order implies that the intravenous fluid should be maintained at this rate until order has been written for intravenous line to be discontinued.

STEPS	RATIONALE
2. Perform hand hygiene. Observe for patency of intravenous line and needle or catheter.	• For fluid to infuse at proper rate, intravenous line and needle must be free of kinks, knots, and clots.
A. Open drip regulator and observe for rapid flow of fluid from solution into drip chamber and then close drip regulator to prescribed rate.	• Rapid flow of fluid into drip chamber indicates patency of intravenous line. Closing drip chamber to prescribed rate prevents fluid overload.
3. Check client's knowledge of how positioning of the intravenous site affects flow rate.	• Fosters client participation in maintaining most effective position of arm with intravenous equipment.
4. Verify with client how venipuncture site feels (e.g., determine whether the client is experiencing pain or burning sensation).	• Includes client in decision making. Pain or burning sensation may be early indication of phlebitis.
5. Have paper and pencil or calculator to calculate flow rate or use calculator.	• The beginning student is unfamiliar with intravenous fluid rates and should use mathematical calculations to obtain correct rate.
6. Know calibration (drop factor) in drops per millilitre (gtt/mL) of infusion set: A. **Microdrip:** 60 gtt/mL B. **Macrodrip:** 15 gtt/mL or 10 gtt/mL depending on manufacturer (will state on package)	• Microdrip tubing, also called pediatric tubing, universally delivers 60 gtt/mL and is used when small or very precise volumes are to be infused. However, different commercial parenteral administration sets for macrodrip tubing are available. Macrodrip tubing should be used when large quantities or fast rates are necessary.

Critical Decision Point: Know which company's infusion set your agency uses.

STEPS	RATIONALE
7. Calculate flow rate (hourly volume) of prescribed infusion. Flow rate mL/hr = total infusion (volume in mL)/hours of infusion (time to be infused). Example: 1000 mL/8 hr = 125 mL/1 hr	• Once hourly rate has been determined, these formulas give correct flow rate.
8. Read physician's orders and follow seven rights for correct solution and proper additives.	• Intravenous fluids are medications; following seven rights decreases chance of medication error.
9. Intravenous fluids are usually ordered by rate, such as 100 mL/hr. However, occasionally, intravenous fluids are ordered over a period of time, such as 1000 mL D_5W with 20 mmol KCl over 8 hr.	• Determines volume of fluid that should infuse hourly.
10. Place adhesive or fluid indicator tape on intravenous bottle or bag next to volume markings (see Step 10 illustration).	• Time taping intravenous bag gives visual cue as to whether fluids are being administered over correct period of time. Time tapes may be required for all intravenous infusions, including those on therapies infused via electronic infusion devices (EIDs). Check agency policy.

Critical Decision Point: Do not use felt-tipped pens or permanent markers on intravenous bags made of polyvinyl chloride because ink could contaminate the solution (Millam & Hadaway, 2003).

➤ SKILL 40-2 Regulating Intravenous Flow Rates *continued*

STEPS	RATIONALE
11. Select one of the following formulas to calculate minute flow rate (drops/min) on the basis of the drop factor of infusion set:	• Formulas compute correct flow rate over a minute.
A. mL/hr/60 min = mL/min and Drop factor × mL/min = drops/min	• Total volume × Drop factor/infusion time in minutes • Volume is multiplied by drop factor, and the product is divided by time (in minutes).
B. Alternative: mL/hr × drop factor/60 min = drops/min Using formula B above, calculate minute flow rate for bottle 1:1000 mL with 20 mmol KCl *Microdrip:* 125 mL/hr × 60 gtt/mL = 7500 gtt/hr 7500 gtt ÷ 60 minutes = 125 gtt/min *Macrodrip:* 125 mL/hr × 15 gtt/mL = 1875 gtt/hr 1875 gtt ÷ 60 minutes = 31 gtt/min	• When using microdrip, mL/hr always equals gtt/minute.
12. Establish flow rate by counting drops in drip chamber for 1 minute by watch; then adjust roller clamp to increase or decrease rate of infusion (see Step 12 illustration).	• Determines whether fluids are administered too slowly or too quickly.
13. Follow this procedure for infusion controller or pump:	
A. Place electronic eye on half-filled drip chamber below origin of drop and above fluid level in chamber or consult manufacturer's directions for setup of the infusion (see Step 13A illustration). If a controller is used, ensure that intravenous bag is 1 m above the intravenous site.	• The electronic eye counts the number of drops flowing from administration set to ensure that proper rate infuses. Intravenous controller works by gravity.

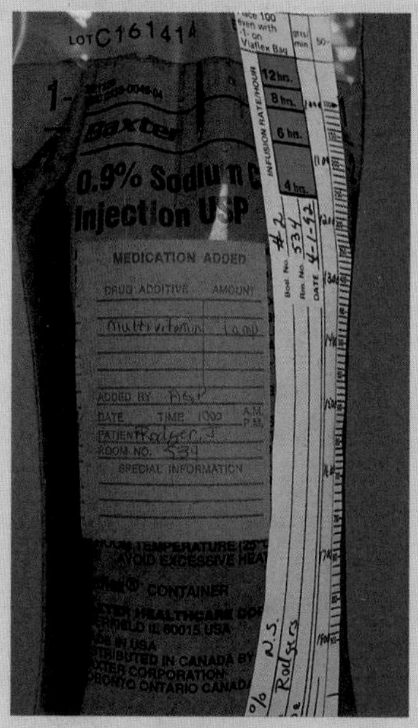

Step 10 Intravenous fluid bag with time tape.

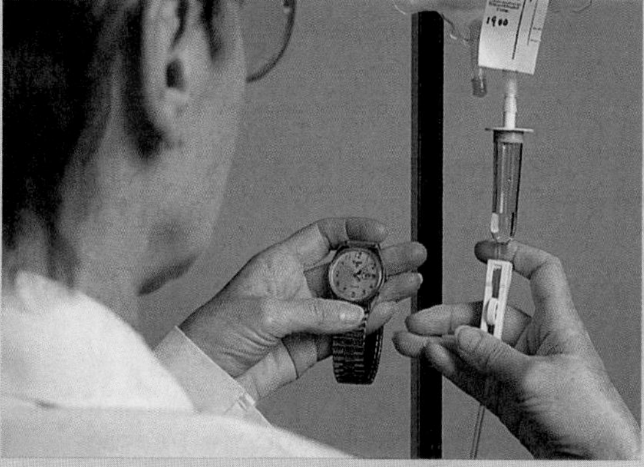

Step 12 Counting intravenous drip rate.

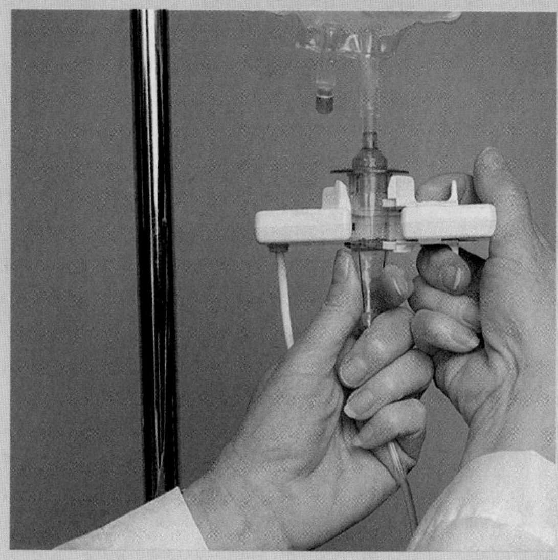

Step 13A Place electronic eye above fluid level in drip chamber.

Continued

➤ SKILL 40-2 Regulating Intravenous Flow Rates *continued*

STEPS	RATIONALE
B. Place intravenous infusion tubing within ridges of control box in direction of flow (i.e., portion of tubing nearest intravenous bag at top and portion of tubing nearest client at bottom) or consult manufacturer's directions for use of pump (see Step 13B illustrations). Some devices require securing tubing through "air in line" alarm system. Close control chamber door. Turn on pump. Required drops per minute or volume per hour and volume to be infused are selected. Open rate control clamp and press start button.	• Infusion pumps move fluid by compressing and milking intravenous tubing, thus propelling fluid through tubing. • Rate control clamp should be open completely while infusion controller or pump is in use.

Critical Decision Point: Special infusion tubing is required for some pumps (check manufacturer's directions).

STEPS	RATIONALE
C. Monitor infusion rates and intravenous site for complications according to agency policy.	• Infusion controllers or pumps are not infallible and do not replace frequent, accurate nursing assessments. Infusion pumps may continue to infuse intravenous fluids after an infiltration has begun. All EIDs must have free-flow protector device.
D. Assess patency and integrity of system when alarm sounds.	• Alarm indicates that electronic eye has not noted precise number of drops from drip chamber, the solution bag or bottle is empty, or flow is obstructed (e.g., kink in tubing, closed drip regulator, infiltrated or clotted needle, or air in the tubing).
14. Follow this procedure for volume control device:	
A. Place volume control device (see Step 14A illustration) between intravenous bag and insertion spike of infusion set using sterile technique.	• Reduces risk of sudden increase in fluid volume.
B. Place 2 hours of fluid allotment into chamber device.	• Prevents intravenous line from running dry if nurse does not return in exactly 60 minutes. In addition, if an accidental increase in flow rate occurs, client receives at most only a 2-hour allotment of fluid.
C. Assess system at least hourly; add fluid to volume control device. Regulate flow rate.	• Maintains patency of system.
15. Observe client for response to therapy. Refer to Skill 40–1, Steps 39 and 40.	• Signs and symptoms of dehydration or overhydration warrant changing rate of fluid infused.
16. Evaluate infusion site for signs of infiltration, inflammation, clot in catheter, or kink or knot in infusion tubing.	• Prevents decrease in or cessation of flow rate.

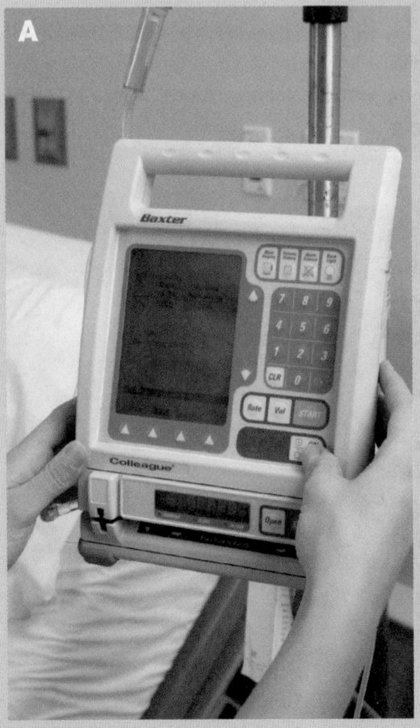

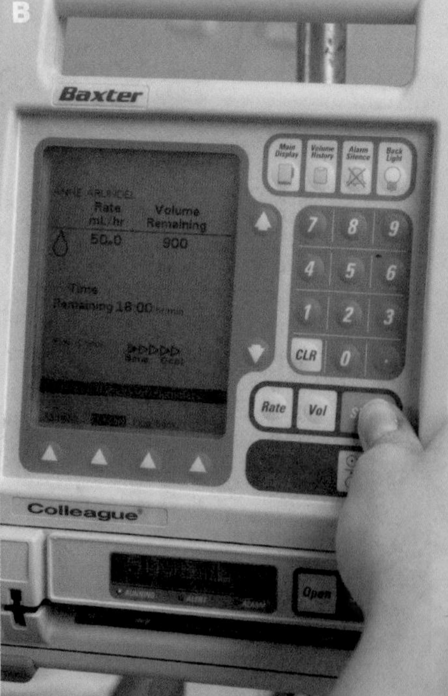

Step 13B **A,** Place infusion tubing within ridges of pump. **B,** Press start button to begin infusion.

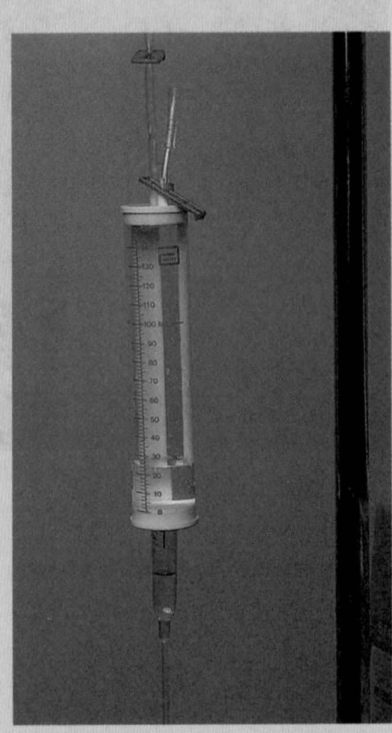

Step 14A Volume control device.

SKILL 40-2 Regulating Intravenous Flow Rates *continued*

Unexpected Outcomes and Related Interventions

Sudden Infusion of Large Volume of Solution, With Symptoms of Dyspnea, Crackles in Lungs, and Increased Urine Output, Indicating Fluid Overload

- Slow infusion to KVO rate and notify physician immediately. New intravenous orders will be required. Client may require diuretics.

Intravenous Fluid Bag Runs Empty, With Subsequent Loss of Intravenous Line Patency

- Intravenous therapy will be restarted.
- The intravenous infusion is slower than ordered.
- Check client for positional change that might affect infusion rate, height of intravenous bag, kinking of tubing.
- An infiltration may be developing at intravenous site. Check condition of site.
- If volume infused is deficient, consult physician for new order to provide necessary fluid volume.

Recording and Reporting

- Record name of solution, rate of infusion, drops/minute, and mL/hour in nurses' notes or flow sheet every 4 hours or according to agency policy.
- Immediately record in nurses' notes or flow sheet any new intravenous fluid rates.
- Document use of any EID or controlling device and number on that device.
- At change of shift or when leaving on break, report rate of infusion to nurse in charge or next nurse assigned to care for client.

Home Care Considerations

- Ensure that client is able and willing to operate the EID (if applicable) and administer intravenous therapy or that a reliable caregiver or nursing support personnel is at home to provide this intravenous therapy care.
- Teach client and primary caregiver to time drops per minute using watch with second hand.
- Ensure that electrical outlets are functioning properly and grounded and infusion device has backup power, if required by type of infusate.

Protective devices designed to prevent accidental dislodgement of an intravenous catheter (Figure 40–17) are now available. The device fits comfortably around a client's hand or arm and provides a plastic shield to cover the intravenous device. Protective devices extend the time a catheter remains in the vein and minimize repeated venipuncture (Rosenthal, 2005).

The client with an arm or a hand infusion is able to walk, unless contraindicated. A portable intravenous pole (a standard intravenous pole with wheels) is needed. Help the client get out of bed and place the pole next to the involved arm. The client is instructed to hold on to the pole and push it while walking. Assess the equipment to make sure that the intravenous bag is at the proper height, that the tubing is not tense, that the flow rate is correct, and that the tubing does not get contaminated. Instruct the client to report any blood in the tubing, a stoppage in the flow, or increased discomfort. Intravenous medications, especially antibiotics and potassium, can cause discomfort and burning sensations at the intravenous site. Although discomfort may be relieved by repositioning the extremity, the source of discomfort must always be carefully evaluated and may necessitate starting a new intravenous line in a larger vein.

Figure 40-15 Intravenous arm board.

Complications of Intravenous Therapy. An **infiltration** occurs when intravenous fluids enter the surrounding space around the venipuncture site (Table 40–10). This is manifested as swelling (from increased tissue fluid) and pallor and coolness (caused by decreased circulation) around the venipuncture site. Fluid may be flowing through the intravenous line at a decreased rate or may have stopped flowing. Pain may also be present and usually results from edema. This pain increases proportionately as the infiltration continues.

When infiltration occurs, the infusion must be discontinued, and if intravenous therapy is still necessary, a new cannula is inserted into a vein in another extremity. To reduce discomfort and edema, raise the extremity, which promotes venous drainage. Wrapping the extremity in a warm, moist towel for 20 minutes while keeping it elevated on a pillow also promotes venous return, increases circulation, and reduces pain and edema. This can be repeated three to four times per day until resolved.

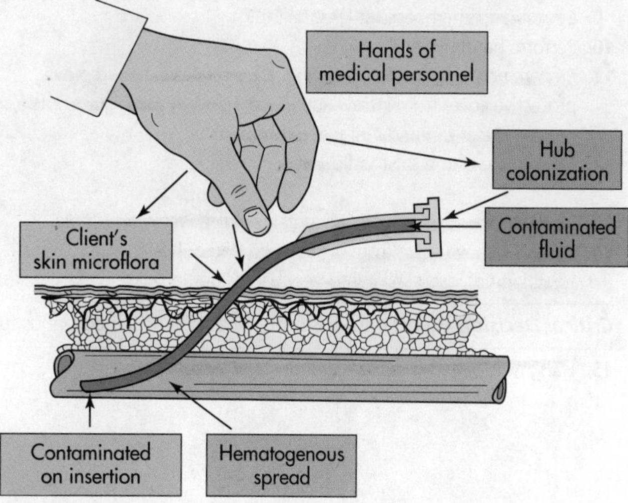

Figure 40-16 Potential sites for contamination of an intravenous device.

➤ SKILL 40-3 Maintenance of Intravenous System

video

Delegation Considerations

In many provinces, this skill is included within the scope of practice for licensed and registered practical nurses. The skill of changing intravenous solutions and tubing should not be delegated to unregulated care providers (UCPs). UCPs may be delegated the tasks of collecting supplies, assisting with comfort measures, and distracting the client during the procedure.

Equipment

Intravenous Infusion

- Bottle or bag of intravenous solution as ordered by physician
- Time tape
- Infusion tubing and tubing label
- Filter (size appropriate to solution) and extension tubing (if necessary)

Intermittent Saline Lock

- Injection cap, loop, or short extension tubing (if necessary)

Normal Saline Flush

- Syringe filled with normal saline
- 2 sterile 2 × 2 (5-cm × 5-cm) gauze pads
- Tape
- Disposable gloves

Discontinuation of Intravenous Line

- Disposable gloves
- Alcohol swabs
- Sterile 2 × 2 (5-cm × 5-cm) gauze
- Tape

Procedure

STEPS	RATIONALE
Changing Intravenous Solution	
1. Check physician's orders.	• Ensures that correct solution will be used. Intravenous therapy requires the seven rights of medication administration.
2. If order is written for keep vein open (KVO) or to keep open (TKO), contact physician for clarification of the rate of the infusion. Note date and time when solution was last changed.	• Orders for KVO do not provide complete information and can result in fluid overload or deficit and electrolyte imbalance. A KVO order should contain a specific infusion rate (INS, 2006). Refer to agency policy. Intravenous tubing and solution should be changed at the same time.
3. Determine the compatibility of all intravenous fluids and additives by consulting appropriate literature or the pharmacy.	• Incompatibilities may lead to precipitate formation and can cause physical, chemical, and therapeutic client changes. Precipitation may occlude patency of catheter.
4. Determine client's understanding of need for continued intravenous therapy.	• Reveals need for client instruction.
5. Assess patency of current intravenous access site.	• If patency is occluded, a new intravenous access site may be needed. Notify physician.
6. Have next solution prepared and accessible at least 1 hour before needed. Check that solution is correct and properly labelled. Check solution expiration date and for presence of precipitate and discoloration.	• Adequate planning reduces risk of clot formation in vein caused by empty intravenous bag. Checking prevents medication error.
7. Prepare to change solution when less than 50 mL of fluid remains in bottle or bag or when a new type of solution is ordered.	• Prevents air from entering tubing and vein from clotting from lack of flow.
8. Prepare client and family by explaining the procedure, its purpose, and what is expected of client.	• Decreases anxiety and promotes cooperation.
9. Be sure drip chamber is at least half full.	• Provides fluid to vein while bag is changed.
10. Perform hand hygiene.	• Reduces transmission of microorganisms.
11. Prepare new solution for changing. If using plastic bag, remove protective cover from intravenous tubing port. If using glass bottle, remove metal cap and metal and rubber discs.	• Permits quick, smooth, and organized change from old to new solution.
12. Move roller clamp to stop flow rate.	• Prevents solution remaining in drip chamber from emptying while changing solutions.
13. Remove old intravenous fluid container from intravenous pole.	• Brings work to nurse's eye level.
14. Quickly remove spike from old solution bag or bottle and, without touching tip, insert spike into new bag or bottle.	• Reduces risk of solution in drip chamber running dry and maintains sterility.

Critical Decision Point: If spike is contaminated, a new intravenous tubing set is required.

15. Hang new bag or bottle of solution on intravenous pole.	• Gravity assists with delivery of fluid into drip chamber.

➤ SKILL 40-3 Maintenance of Intravenous System *continued*

STEPS	RATIONALE
16. Check for air in tubing. If bubbles form, they can be removed by closing the roller clamp, stretching the tubing downward, and tapping the tubing with the finger (the bubbles rise in the fluid to the drip chamber; see Step 16 illustration). For larger amounts of air, swab injection port below the air with alcohol and allow to dry. Connect a syringe to this port and aspirate the air into the syringe. Reduce air in tubing by priming slowly instead of allowing a wide-open flow.	• Reduces risk of air embolus. Use of an air-eliminating filter also reduces this risk.
17. Make sure drip chamber is one-third to one-half full. If the drip chamber is too full, pinch off tubing below the drip chamber, invert the container, squeeze the drip chamber (see Step 17 illustration), hang up the bag, and release the tubing.	• Reduces risk of air entering tubing.
18. Regulate flow to prescribed rate.	• Maintains measures to restore fluid balance and deliver intravenous fluid as ordered.
19. Mark time on label tape and place on bag. Do not use felt-tipped pens or permanent markers on intravenous bags.	• Ink from markers may leach through polyvinyl chloride containers.
20. Observe client for signs of overhydration or dehydration to determine response to intravenous fluid therapy.	• Provides ongoing evaluation of client's fluid and electrolyte status.
21. Observe intravenous system for patency and development of complications (e.g., infiltration or phlebitis).	• Provides ongoing evaluation of intravenous system.
Changing Intravenous Tubing	
22. Determine when new infusion set is needed:	• Note that usually the tubing and the bag, and even the site, are changed at the same time. (Refer to Steps 13–22, 33, and 34, to change bag *and* tubing.)
A. Agency policy will indicate frequency of routine change for intravenous administration sets and saline flush tubing.	• The Centers for Disease Control and Prevention (CDC) (O'Grady et al., 2002) and INS (2006) recommend changing tubing for primary infusions no more frequently than 72-hour intervals or whenever tubing has been compromised.
B. Puncture of infusion tubing requires immediate change.	• Punctured tubing results in fluid leakage and bacterial contamination.
C. Contamination of tubing requires immediate change.	• Contamination of tubing allows entry of bacteria into client's bloodstream.
D. Occlusions in existing tubing can occur after infusion of packed red blood cells, whole blood, albumin, or other blood components.	• Whole blood or blood component product can occlude or partially occlude tubing because viscous solutions adhere to walls of tubing and decrease the size of the lumen.

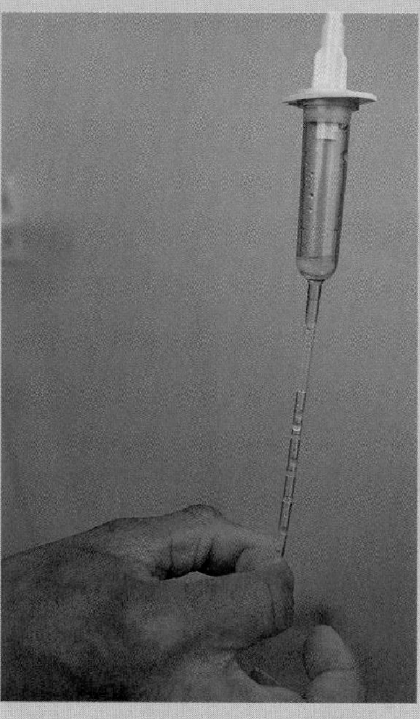

Step 16 Tap tubing to cause air bubbles to rise up to drip chamber.

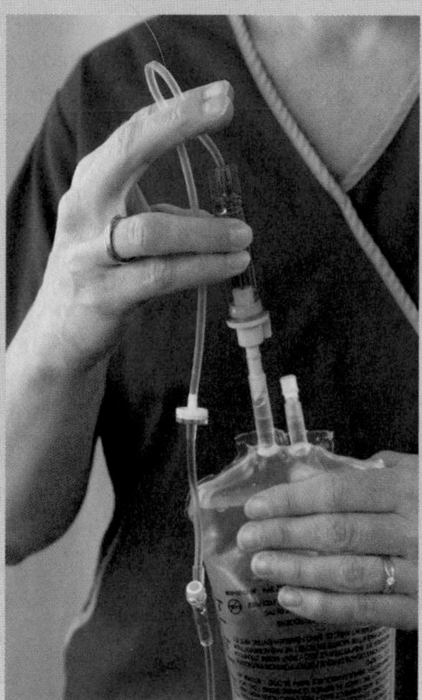

Step 17 Pinch tubing, invert chamber, and squeeze drip chamber to remove a portion of fluid. **Source:** Courtesy Darlaine Jantzen.

Continued

➤ SKILL 40-3 Maintenance of Intravenous System *continued*

STEPS	RATIONALE
23. Prepare client and family by explaining the procedure, its purpose, and what is expected of client.	• Decreases anxiety, promotes cooperation, and prevents sudden movement of extremity, which could dislodge intravenous needle or catheter.
24. Perform hand hygiene.	• Reduces transmission of microorganisms.
25. Open new infusion set, keeping protective coverings over infusion spike and distal adapter. Secure all junctions with Luer-Loks, clasping devices, or threaded devices.	• Provides nurse with ready access to new infusion set and maintains sterility of infusion set.
26. Apply nonsterile, disposable gloves.	• Reduces risk of exposure to HIV, hepatitis, and other bloodborne pathogens.
27. If needle or catheter hub is not visible, remove intravenous dressing while maintaining stability of catheter. If transparent dressing has to e removed, place small piece of sterile tape across hub temporarily to anchor catheter during disconnection. Do not remove tape securing needle or catheter to skin with gauze dressing.	• Needle hub must be accessible to provide smooth transition when removing old and inserting new tubing.
28. For intravenous continuous infusion:	
A. Move roller clamp on new intravenous tubing to closed position.	• Prevents spillage of solution after bag or bottle is spiked.
B. Slow rate of infusion by regulating drip rate on old tubing. Be sure rate is at KVO rate.	• Prevents complete infusion of solution that remains in tubing, which can increase risk of occlusion of intravenous catheter or needle.
C. Compress and fill drip chamber of old tubing.	• Provides surplus of fluid in drip chamber so enough fluid is available to maintain intravenous patency while changing tubing.
D. Remove intravenous container from pole, invert container, and remove old tubing from container. Carefully hold container while hanging or taping drip chamber on intravenous pole 1 m above intravenous site.	• Fluid in drip chamber will run slowly to keep catheter patent.
E. Place insertion spike of new tubing into old solution bag opening and hang solution bag on intravenous pole.	• Permits flow of fluid from solution into new infusion tubing.
F. Compress and release drip chamber on new tubing; fill drip chamber one-third to one-half full.	• Allows drip chamber to fill and promotes rapid, smooth flow of solution through new tubing.
G. Slowly open roller clamp, remove protective cap from needle adapter (if necessary), and flush new tubing with solution. Replace cap.	• Removes air from tubing and replaces it with fluid.
H. Turn roller clamp on old tubing to closed position.	• Prevents spillage of fluid as tubing is removed from needle hub.
29. For saline lock:	
A. If a loop or short extension tubing is needed because of an awkward intravenous site placement, use sterile technique to connect the new injection cap to the loop or tubing.	
B. Swab injection cap with alcohol, povidone–iodine, or chlorhexidine. Insert syringe with 1 to 3 mL saline and inject through the injection cap into the loop or short extension tubing (see Step 30B illustrations).	• Removes air to prevent introduction into the vein.

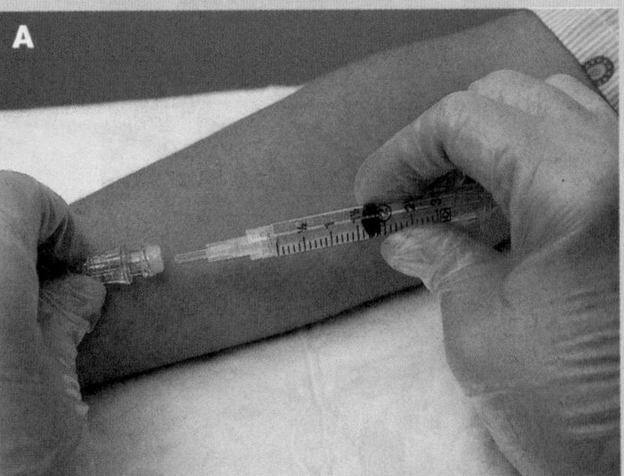

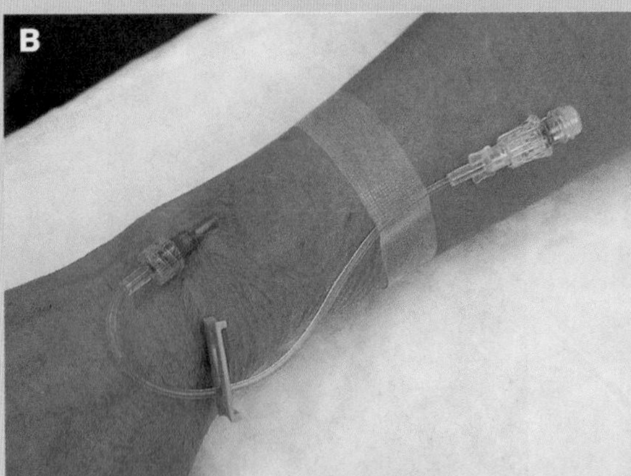

Step 30B **A,** Inject saline into injection cap. **B,** Connect to saline lock extension tube. **Source:** Courtesy Darlaine Jantzen.

➤SKILL 40-3 Maintenance of Intravenous System *continued*

STEPS	RATIONALE
30. Stabilize hub of catheter and apply pressure over vein just above catheter tip at least 3 cm above insertion site. Gently disconnect old tubing from catheter hub (see Step 31 illustration, part A). Maintain stability of hub and quickly insert adapter of new tubing or saline lock into hub (see Step 31 illustrations, parts B and C).	• Prevents accidental displacement of catheter or needle. • Prevents clot formation in catheter or needle and backflow of blood.
31. Open roller clamp on new tubing. Allow solution to run rapidly for 30 to 60 seconds.	• Permits intravenous solution to enter catheter to prevent catheter occlusion.
32. Regulate intravenous drip according to physician's orders and monitor rate hourly.	• Maintains infusion flow at prescribed rate.
33. Apply new dressing, if needed.	• Reduces risk of bacterial infection from skin.
34. Discard old tubing in proper container.	• Reduces accidental transmission of microorganisms.
35. Remove and dispose of gloves. Perform hand hygiene.	• Reduces transmission of microorganisms.
36. Evaluate flow rate and observe connection site for leakage.	• Maintains prescribed rate of flow of intravenous fluid and determines if fit is secure.
Discontinuing Peripheral Intravenous Access	
37. Check physician's order for discontinuation of intravenous therapy.	• Order is required for discontinuation of fluids or medication.
38. Explain procedure to client. Explain that affected extremity must be held still and how long procedure will take.	• Minimizes client's anxiety and discomfort.
39. Perform hand hygiene and apply disposable gloves.	• Reduces transmission of microorganisms.
40. Turn intravenous tubing roller clamp to closed position. Remove tape securing tubing.	
41. Remove intravenous site dressing and tape while stabilizing catheter.	• Movement of catheter will cause discomfort.
42. With dry gauze or alcohol swab held over site, apply light pressure and withdraw the catheter, using a slow steady movement, keeping the hub parallel to the skin (see Step 43 illustration).	• Changing the angle of the catheter inside the vein could cause additional vein irritation, increasing the risk of postinfusion phlebitis.

Critical Decision Point: If client has received anticoagulants (e.g., low-dose aspirin, warfarin sodium [Coumadin], heparin) or has a low platelet count, apply steady pressure for 5 to 10 minutes and assess bleeding.

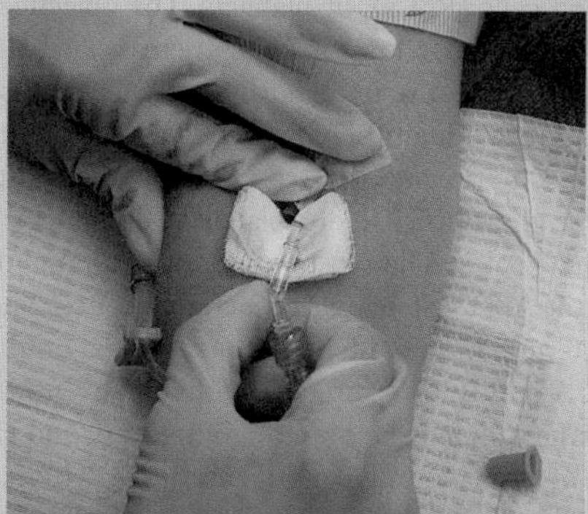

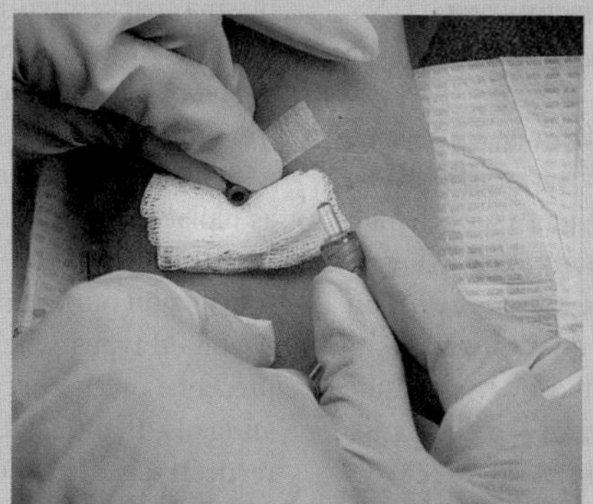

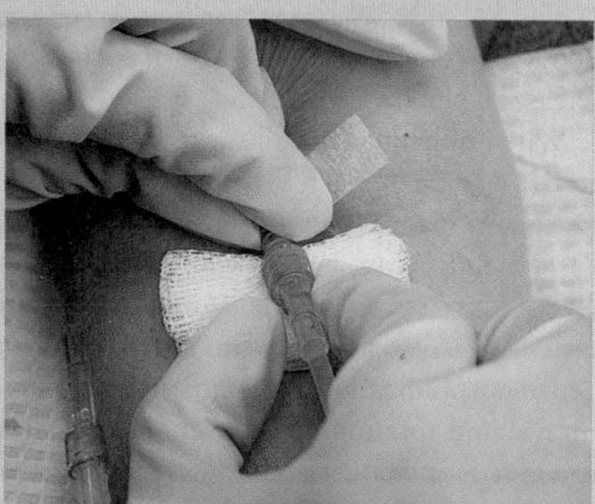

Step 31 **A,** Maintain stability of catheter hub while removing old tubing. **B,** Connect new infusion tubing. **C,** Be sure connection at hub is secure.

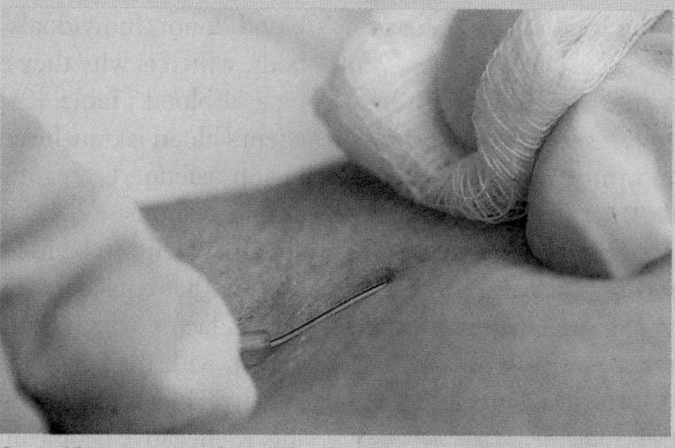

Step 43 Remove catheter slowly, keeping it parallel to the vein.

Continued

➤ SKILL 40-3 Maintenance of Intravenous System *continued*

STEPS	RATIONALE
43. Apply pressure to the site for 2 to 3 minutes, using the dry, sterile gauze pad. Secure with tape.	• Dry pad causes less irritation to the puncture site. Subcutaneous hematoma is a common complication. When needle is removed, vein wall contracts to stop bleeding. Contraction is enhanced by pressure to site for at least 2 to 3 minutes (Chukhraev & Grekov, 2000).
44. Inspect the catheter for intactness, noting tip integrity and length.	• Tips of catheter can break off, causing an embolus, an emergency situation. Notify physician if tip is broken.
45. Discard used supplies.	
46. Remove and discard gloves and perform hand hygiene.	
47. Instruct client to report any redness, pain, drainage, or swelling that may occur after catheter removal.	• Postinfusion phlebitis may occur within 48 to 96 hours after catheter removal.

Unexpected Outcomes and Related Interventions

Incorrect Flow Rate; Client Receives Too Little or Too Much Fluid

- Readjust infusion rate to ordered rate; evaluate client for adverse effects; notify physician.

Decreased or Absent Flow of Intravenous Fluid

- Assess intravenous infusion system for patency.
- Recalibrate drip rate on new tubing.
- Assess intravenous site for infiltration.

Recording and Reporting

- Record changing of tubing and solution on client's record. A special parenteral therapy flow sheet may be used.
- Place a piece of tape or preprinted label with the date and time of tubing change and attach to tubing below the level of drip chamber.

Home Care Considerations

- Emphasize to client and family the importance of changing solutions when intravenous tubing still contains fluid.

Phlebitis is inflammation of the vein. Selected risk factors for phlebitis include the type of catheter material, chemical irritation of additives and drugs given intravenously (e.g., antibiotics), and the anatomical position of the catheter. Signs and symptoms may include pain, edema, erythema, increased skin temperature over the vein, and, in some instances, redness travelling along the path of the vein (INS, 2006). Dehydration may also be a contributing factor because of the increase in blood viscosity.

When phlebitis develops, the intravenous line must be discontinued and a new line inserted in another vein. Warm, moist heat on the site of phlebitis can offer some relief to the client (see Chapter 47). Phlebitis can be dangerous because blood clots (thrombophlebitis) can occur and in some cases may result in emboli. This may result in permanent damage to veins and in prolonging the client's hospitalization. Phlebitis may be prevented by the routine removal and rotation of intravenous sites. The CDC recommends replacing peripheral venous catheters and rotating sites at least every 72 hours (CDC, 2002; Rosenthal, 2005).

FVE may occur if a client receives a larger volume of fluids over a shorter period than is therapeutic. The assessment findings include shortness of breath, crackles in the lungs, and tachycardia. Slow the rate of infusion, notify the physician, raise the head of the bed, and monitor vital signs.

Bleeding can occur around the venipuncture site during the infusion or through the catheter needle or tubing if these become inadvertently disconnected. Bleeding is common in clients who have received heparin or who have a bleeding disorder (e.g., leukemia or thrombocytopenia). If bleeding occurs around the venipuncture site and the catheter is within the vein, a pressure dressing may be applied over the site to control the bleeding. Bleeding from a vein is usually a slow, continuous seepage and is not serious.

Discontinuing Intravenous Infusions. Discontinuing an infusion is necessary after the prescribed amount of fluid has been infused, when an infiltration occurs, if phlebitis is present, or if the infusion catheter or needle develops a clot at its tip. Refer to Skill 40–3, Steps 38 to 48.

Blood Replacement. Blood replacement or transfusion is the intravenous administration of whole blood or a component such as plasma, packed red blood cells (RBCs), or platelets. The objectives for blood transfusions include the following: (1) to increase circulating blood volume after surgery, trauma, or hemorrhage; (2) to increase the number of RBCs and to maintain hemoglobin levels in clients with severe anemia; and (3) to provide selected cellular components as replacement therapy (e.g., clotting factors, platelets, albumin).

Blood Groups and Types. The most important grouping for transfusion purposes is the ABO system, which includes A, B, O, and AB blood types. The determination of blood groups is based on the presence or absence of A and B RBC antigens. Individuals with A antigens, B antigens, or no antigens belong to groups A, B, and O, respectively. The person with A and B antigens has AB blood. Individuals with type A blood naturally produce anti-B antibodies in their plasma. Similarly, individuals with type B blood naturally produce anti-A antibodies. An individual with type O blood has neither type A nor type B antigen and thus is considered a universal blood donor. Individuals with type AB blood produce neither antibody, which is why they can be universal recipients and receive any type of blood (Table 40–11). If blood that is mismatched with the client's blood is transfused, a **transfusion reaction** occurs. The transfusion reaction is an antigen–antibody reaction and can range from a mild response (e.g., faintness, dizziness) to severe anaphylactic shock, which can be life-threatening (Davis et al., 2005–2006).

Another consideration when matching for blood transfusions is the Rh factor, which is an antigenic substance in the erythrocytes. A person with the factor is Rh positive, and a person without it is Rh negative. Blood must be matched for Rh factor as well as ABO grouping. Rh negative people must only receive Rh negative blood, whereas Rh positive people can receive either Rh negative or Rh positive blood.

Autologous Transfusion. **Autologous transfusion** or autotransfusion is the collection of a client's own blood. The blood for an autologous transfusion can be obtained by preoperative donation up to 5 weeks before the planned surgery (e.g., heart, orthopedic, plastic, or gynecological). Clients can donate 1 to 5 units of their own blood depending on the type of surgery and the ability of the client to maintain an acceptable hematocrit. The blood will be tested for HIV and hepatitis B virus. Another way to collect blood for an autologous transfusion is during perioperative blood salvage (e.g., during vascular and orthopedic surgery, organ transplant surgery, and traumatic injuries). The blood that has been salvaged is then reinfused during the surgery. Blood can also be salvaged postoperatively from mediastinal and chest tube drainage and after joint and spinal surgery. Autologous transfusions decrease the risk of complications such as mismatched blood and exposure to bloodborne infectious agents.

Blood Transfusions. When transfusing blood or blood components, assessment is required before, during, and after the transfusion and for regulation of the transfusion because of the risk of allergic reactions. If the client has an intravenous line in place, assess the venipuncture site for signs of infection or infiltration and patency. Determine the appropriate gauge of the intravenous catheter. A large catheter, such as 18 to 20 gauge, is recommended because blood is thicker and stickier than intravenous fluids (Millam & Hadaway, 2003). Blood administration tubing has an in-line filter (Figure 40–18). When priming blood administration tubing, 0.9% normal saline should be used to prevent **hemolysis**, or breakdown of RBCs.

Pretransfusion assessment also includes obtaining information from the client. Ask whether the client knows the reason for the blood transfusion and whether the client has ever had a previous transfusion or transfusion reaction. A client who has had a transfusion reaction is usually at no greater risk for a reaction with a subsequent

SKILL 40-4 Changing a Peripheral Intravenous Dressing

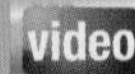

Delegation Considerations

In many provinces, the skill of changing a peripheral intravenous dressing is included within the scope of practice for licensed and registered practical nurses. This skill should not be delegated to unregulated care providers (UCPs). UCPs may be delegated the tasks of collecting supplies, assisting with comfort measures, and distracting the client during the procedure.

Equipment

- Antiseptic swab stick (chlorhexidine, povidone–iodine, or 70% alcohol, as recommended by the agency)
- Alcohol swab stick
- Adhesive remover (if needed)
- Strips of nonallergenic sterile tape for use underneath the dressing
- Disposable gloves
- Arm board or housing device (if needed)
- For gauze dressing:
  - Sterile 2 × 2 (5-cm × 5-cm) gauze pad OR
  - Sterile 4 × 4 (10-cm × 10-cm) gauze pad
- For transparent dressing:
  - Sterile transparent dressing

Procedure

STEPS	RATIONALE
1. Determine when dressing was last changed. Many institutions require that the nurse records the date and time on the dressing when the device is first placed.	• Provides information regarding length of time present dressing has been in place. The CDC recommends that, whenever possible, peripheral intravenous dressings should be scheduled when intravenous system is changed.
2. Perform hand hygiene. Observe present dressing for moisture and intactness.	• Moisture is a medium for bacterial growth and renders dressing contaminated.
3. Observe intravenous system for proper functioning or complications: kinks in infusion tubing or intravenous catheter. Palpate the catheter site through the intact dressing for inflammation or subjective complaints of pain or burning sensation.	• Unexplained decrease in flow rate requires investigation of placement and patency of the intravenous catheter. Pain can be associated with both phlebitis and infiltration.
4. Inspect exposed catheter site for swelling or blanching.	• Indicates fluid infusing into surrounding tissues. Will require removal of intravenous catheter.
5. Assess client's understanding of need for continued intravenous infusion.	• Determines need for client instruction.
6. Explain procedure and purpose to client and family. Explain that affected extremity must be held still and how long procedure will take.	• Decreases anxiety, promotes cooperation, and gives client time frame around which personal activities can be planned.
7. Apply disposable gloves	• Reduces transmission of microorganisms.
8. Remove tape, gauze, or transparent dressing from old dressing one layer at a time, leaving tape (if present) that secures intravenous catheter in place. Be cautious if catheter tubing becomes tangled between two layers of dressing. When removing transparent dressing, hold catheter hub and tubing with nondominant hand.	• Prevents accidental displacement of catheter or needle.
9. Observe insertion site for signs and symptoms of infection (redness, swelling, and exudate). If present, remove catheter and insert a new intravenous line in another site.	• Presence of infection or complication indicates need to remove VAD at current site.

Continued

➤ SKILL 40-4 Changing Peripheral Intravenous Dressing *continued*

STEPS	RATIONALE
10. If infiltration, phlebitis, or clot occurs or if ordered by physician, stop infusion and discontinue intravenous therapy. Restart new intravenous line if continued therapy is necessary. Place moist, warm compress over area of phlebitis (see Tables 40–8 and 40–10).	
11. If intravenous fluid is infusing properly, gently remove any tape securing catheter. Stabilize needle or catheter with one hand. Use adhesive remover to cleanse skin and remove adhesive residue, if needed.	• Exposes venipuncture site. Stabilization prevents accidental displacement of catheter or needle. Adhesive residue decreases ability of new dressing to adhere tightly to skin.
12. Stabilize catheter at all times with one finger over catheter until tape or dressing is replaced.	• Prevents decannulation from vein.
13. Using circular motion, cleanse peripheral intravenous insertion site with antiseptic swab starting at insertion site and working outward, creating concentric circles (see Step 13 illustration). Allow swab solution to air-dry completely.	• Circular motion prevents cross-contamination from skin bacteria near venipuncture site. Antiseptics may include chlorhexidine, povidone–iodine, and alcohol. RNAO (2005) recommends 2% chlorhexidine-based solution. Povidone–iodine is a topical anti-infective agent that reduces skin surface bacteria; the solution must be dry to be effective in reducing microbial counts (CDC, 2002). If antiseptic agents are used in combination, allow each to dry separately.

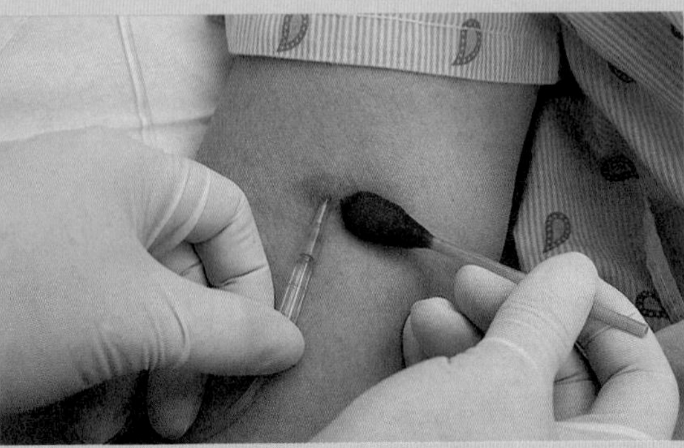

Step 13 Cleanse peripheral insertion site.

Critical Decision Point: Do not tape over connection of access tubing or port to intravenous catheter.

STEPS	RATIONALE
14. Apply new transparent or gauze dressing (see Skill 40–1, Step 35B).	• Ensures protection of intravenous site and reduces chance of infection.
15. Remove and discard gloves.	
16. Anchor intravenous tubing with additional pieces of tape. When using transparent polyurethane dressing, minimize the tape placed over dressing.	• Prevents accidental displacement of intravenous needle or catheter or separation of intravenous tubing from needle adapter.
17. Place insertion date, date and time of dressing change, size and gauge of catheter, and your initials directly on dressing. Apply arm board, commercial housing device, or both if site is affected by joint motion.	• Documents dressing change.
18. Discard used equipment and perform hand hygiene.	• Reduces transmission of microorganisms.
19. Observe functioning and patency of intravenous system in response to changing dressing.	• Validates that intravenous line is patent and functioning correctly.
20. Monitor client's body temperature.	• Elevated temperature indicates an infection that may be associated with bacterial contamination of the venipuncture site.

Unexpected Outcomes and Related Interventions

Infiltration of Intravenous Catheter, as Evidenced by Decreased Flow Rate or Edema, Pallor, or Decreased Temperature Around Insertion Site

- Stop infusion and discontinue intravenous therapy. Restart new intravenous line in other extremity if continued therapy is necessary.
- Elevate affected extremity.

Phlebitis, as Evidenced by Erythema and Tenderness Along Vein Pathway

- Stop infusion and discontinue intravenous therapy. Restart new intravenous line in other extremity if continued therapy is necessary.
- Apply warm, moist compress to area of phlebitis.

Accidental Removal of Intravenous Catheter or Needle

- Restart intravenous infusion if continued therapy is needed.

Elevated Body Temperature

- Notify physician. Intravenous line may be removed and restarted. Client will be evaluated for source of infection.

Red, Edematous, or Painful Insertion Site or Presence of Exudates, Indicating Infection at Venipuncture Site

- Discontinue intravenous infusion. Antibiotic therapy may begin.
- Apply warm, moist compress to area of inflammation.

Recording and Reporting

- Record appearance of intravenous site, type of dressing, and status of intravenous fluid infusion.
- A special parenteral fluid flow sheet may be used for recording.

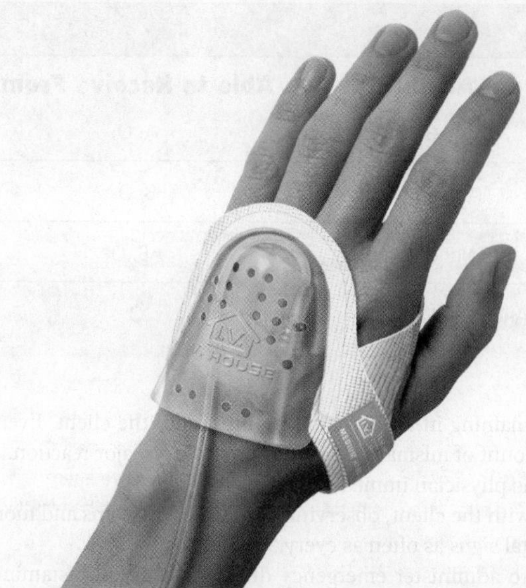

Figure 40-17 IV House protective device. **Source:** Courtesy IV House, St. Louis, MO.

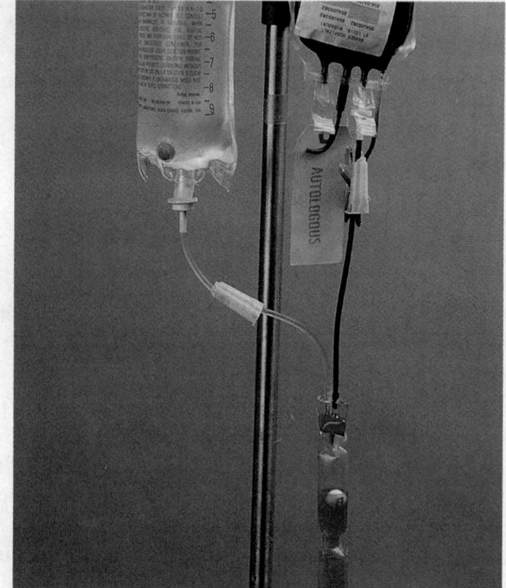

Figure 40-18 Blood administration tubing.

transfusion. However, the client may be anxious about the transfusion. Before giving a transfusion, explain the procedure and instruct the client to report any side effects (e.g., chills, dizziness, or fever) once the transfusion begins. Check to be sure the client has signed an informed consent form. Clients with certain cultural backgrounds may abstain from blood transfusions (Box 40–11).

Because of the danger of transfusion reactions, it is very important to use specific precautions in administering blood or blood products. Obtain the client's baseline vital signs before the transfusion begins. This allows you to determine when changes in vital signs occur, which can indicate that a transfusion reaction is developing. A thorough check of the blood product, the client, and the compatibility of the blood and the client ensures that the right client receives the correct type of blood or blood product. Although you are not involved in the blood labelling process, you are responsible for determining that the blood delivered to the client corresponds to the blood type listed in the client's medical record. Two registered nurses or one

TABLE 40-10 Infiltration Scale

Grade	Clinical Criteria
0	No symptoms
1	Skin blanched Edema, 2.5 cm in any direction Cool to touch With or without pain
2	Skin blanched Edema 2.5–15.2 cm in any direction Cool to touch With or without pain
3	Skin blanched, translucent Gross edema 15.2 cm in any direction Cool to touch Mild to moderate pain Possible numbness
4	Skin blanched, translucent Skin tight, leaking Skin discoloured, bruised, swollen Gross edema 15.2 cm in any direction Deep pitting tissue edema Circulatory impairment Moderate to severe pain Infiltration of any amount of blood product, irritant, or vesicant

From Infusion Nurses Society. (2006). Infusion nursing standards of practice. *Journal of Infusion Nursing, 29*(1 Suppl.), S60.

BOX 40-11 CULTURAL ASPECTS OF CARE

Preinfusion Assessments

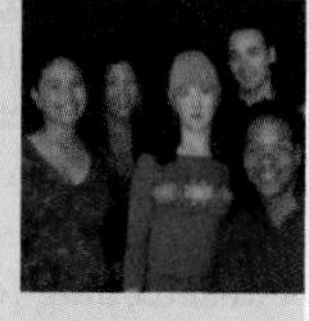

When a client's natural skin contains more melanin, it becomes more difficult to identify colour changes. Intravenous complications such as phlebitis and infiltration may not be easily detected. Clients with some cultural backgrounds have fear related to the donor process for blood. Clients with certain religious or personal beliefs may abstain from receiving blood transfusions or medications.

Implications for Practice

- Establish communication. Understand the values of family elders and know whom to speak with about intravenous procedures.
- Assess clients individually to determine their acceptance of or abstinence from therapeutic regimens.
- Appreciate clients' choice related to their therapy.
- Although some clients will abstain from receiving whole blood or packed RBCs, they will accept other blood products or alternatives.

Adapted from Rudnicke, C. (2003). Transfusion alternatives. *Journal of Infusion Nursing, 26*(3), 29.

TABLE 40-11 Blood Groups and Compatibility

Blood Type	Antigens on Cell	Able to Donate	Serum Antibodies	Able to Receive From
A	A	A, AB	Anti-B	A, O
B	B	B, AB	Anti-A	B, O
AB	A and B	AB	None	AB, O
O	None	A, B, AB, O	Anti-A and anti-B	O

registered nurse and a licensed practical nurse (see agency policy) must together check the label on the blood product against the client's identification number, blood group, and complete name. If even a minor discrepancy exists, the blood should not be given and the blood bank should be notified immediately.

Initiation of a transfusion begins slowly to allow for the early detection of a transfusion reaction. Maintain the infusion rate, monitor for side effects, assess vital signs, and promptly record all findings. Stay with the client during the first 15 minutes, the time when a reaction is most likely to occur. Continue to monitor the client and obtain vital signs periodically during the transfusion as directed by agency policy.

The rate of transfusion is usually specified in the health care professional's orders. Ideally, a unit of whole blood or packed RBCs is transfused in 2 hours. This time can be lengthened to 4 hours if the client is at risk for FVE. Beyond 4 hours, bacterial contamination of the blood is a risk (Davis et al., 2005–2006). When clients have a severe blood loss, such as with hemorrhage, they may receive rapid transfusions through a CVC. A blood-warming device is often necessary because the tip of the central venous cannula lies in the superior vena cava, above the right atrium. Rapid administration of cold blood can result in cardiac dysrhythmia (Burgess, 2006).

Transfusion Reactions. A transfusion reaction is a systemic response by the body to incompatible blood. Causes include RBC incompatibility or allergic sensitivity to the components of the transfused blood or to the potassium or citrate preservative in the blood. Several types of acute reactions can result from blood transfusions (Table 40–12). If a transfusion reaction is anticipated or suspected, monitor vital signs more frequently (see Table 40–12).

A second category of transfusion reactions includes diseases transmitted by infected blood donors who are asymptomatic. Diseases transmitted through transfusions are malaria, hepatitis, and AIDS. Because all units of blood collected must undergo serological testing and screening for HIV and hepatitis B virus, the risk of acquiring bloodborne infections from blood transfusions is reduced.

Circulatory overload is a risk when a client receives large volumes of whole blood or packed RBC transfusions for massive hemorrhagic shock or when a client with normal blood volume receives blood. Clients particularly at risk for circulatory overload are older adults and those with cardiopulmonary diseases.

Blood transfusion reactions are life-threatening, but prompt nursing intervention can maintain the client's physiological stability.

safety alert If a blood reaction is suspected, stop the transfusion immediately.

- Keep the intravenous line open by "piggybacking" 0.9% normal saline directly into the intravenous line and running the saline.
- Do not turn off the blood and simply turn on the 0.9% normal saline that is connected to the Y-tubing infusion set. This would cause blood remaining in the Y-tubing to infuse into the client. Even a small amount of mismatched blood can cause a major reaction.
- Notify the physician immediately.
- Remain with the client, observing signs and symptoms and monitoring vital signs as often as every 5 minutes.
- Prepare to administer emergency drugs such as antihistamines, vasopressors, fluids, and steroids as per physician order or protocol.
- Prepare to perform cardiopulmonary resuscitation.
- Obtain a urine specimen and send it to the laboratory to determine the presence of hemoglobin as a result of RBC hemolysis.
- Save the blood container, tubing, attached labels, and transfusion record, and return them to the laboratory.

Restorative Care

After experiencing acute alterations in fluid, electrolyte, or acid–base balance, clients often require ongoing maintenance to prevent a recurrence of health alterations. Older adults and the chronically ill require special considerations to prevent complications from developing.

Home Intravenous Therapy. Intravenous therapy is often continued in the home setting for clients who are discharged from the hospital and have not completed their prescribed treatment or who require long-term therapy. Ideally, a family member will be available at home if the client suddenly cannot manage the intravenous system or if a problem develops. A home care nurse will work closely with the client and family to ensure that a sterile intravenous system is maintained and that complications are avoided or recognized promptly. Box 40–12 summarizes client education guidelines for home intravenous therapy.

Nutritional Support. Most clients who have had electrolyte disorders or metabolic acid–base disturbances require ongoing nutritional support. Depending on the type of disorder, fluid or food intake may be encouraged or restricted. Depending on the type of disorder, fluid or food intake may be encouraged or restricted (see Chapter 43). If clients are still responsible for meal preparation, they should learn to understand nutritional content of foods and to read the labels of commercially prepared foods.

Medication Safety. Numerous medications and over-the counter drugs contain components or create potential side effects that can alter fluid and electrolyte balances. Clients with chronic disease who are receiving multiple medications and those with renal or liver disorders are at significant risk for alterations in fluid and electrolyte status (Box 40–13). Once clients return to a restorative care setting, whether in their home or in a residential care home, drug safety becomes very important. Client and family education is essential to providing information regarding potential drug interactions and what side effects they cause. Review all medications with clients and encourage them to consult with their local pharmacist, especially if they try a new over-the-counter medication.

TABLE 40-12 Acute Transfusion Reactions

Reaction	Cause	Clinical Manifestations	Management	Prevention
Acute hemolytic	Infusion of ABO-incompatible whole blood, RBCs, or components containing 10 mL or more of RBCs Antibodies in the recipient's plasma attach to antigens on transfused RBCs, causing RBC destruction	Chills, fever, low back pain, flushing, tachycardia, tachypnea, hypotension, vascular collapse, hemoglobinuria, hemoglobinemia, bleeding, acute renal failure, shock, cardiac arrest, death	Stop transfusion. Treat shock, if present. Draw blood samples for serological testing slowly to avoid hemolysis from the procedure. Send urine specimen to the laboratory. Maintain BP with intravenous colloid solutions. Give diuretics as prescribed to maintain urine flow. Insert in-dwelling catheter or measure voided amounts to monitor hourly urine output. Dialysis may be required if renal failure occurs. Do not transfuse additional RBC-containing components until transfusion service has provided newly cross-matched units.	Meticulously verify and document client identification from sample collection to component infusion.
Febrile, nonhemolytic (most common)	Sensitization to donor white blood cells, platelets, or plasma proteins	Sudden chills and fever (rise in temperature of greater than 1°C), headache, flushing, anxiety, muscle pain	Give antipyretics as prescribed—avoid aspirin in clients with thrombocytopenia. *Urgent:* Do not restart transfusion.	Consider leukocyte-poor blood products (filtered, washed, or frozen).
Mild allergic	Sensitivity to foreign plasma proteins	Flushing, itching, urticaria (hives)	Give antihistamine as directed. If symptoms are mild and transient, transfusion may be restarted slowly. *Urgent:* Do not restart transfusion if fever or pulmonary symptoms develop.	Treat prophylactically with antihistamines.
Anaphylactic	Infusion of IgA proteins to IgA-deficient recipient who has developed IgA antibody	Anxiety, urticaria, wheezing, progressing to cyanosis, shock, possible cardiac arrest	Initiate CPR, if indicated. Have epinephrine ready for injection (0.4 mL of a 1:1000 solution subcutaneously or 0.1 mL of 1:1000 solution diluted to 10 mL with saline for intravenous use). *Urgent:* Do not restart transfusion.	Transfuse extensively washed RBC products, from which all plasma has been removed. Alternately, use blood from IgA-deficient donor.
Circulatory overload	Fluid administered faster than the circulation can accommodate	Cough, dyspnea, pulmonary congestion (rales), headache, hypertension, tachycardia, distended neck veins	Place client upright with feet in dependent position. Administer prescribed diuretics, oxygen, morphine. Phlebotomy may be indicated.	Adjust transfusion volume and flow rate on the basis of client size and clinical status. Have transfusion service divide unit into smaller aliquots for better spacing of fluid input.
Sepsis	Transfusion of contaminated blood components	Rapid onset of chills, high fever, vomiting, diarrhea, and marked hypotension and shock	Obtain culture of client's blood and send bag with remaining blood to transfusion service for further study. Treat septicemia as directed—antibiotics, intravenous fluids, vasopressors, steroids.	Collect, process, store, and transfuse blood products according to blood banking standards and infuse within 4 hours of starting time.

ABO, blood group consisting of groups A, AB, B, and O; BP, blood pressure; CPR, cardiopulmonary resuscitation; IgA, immunoglobulin A; RBCs, red blood cells.

Data from Brecher, M. (Ed.). (2005). *AABB technical manual* (15th ed.). Bethesda, MD: American Association of Blood Banks; and Goodnough, L. T. (2005). Risks of blood transfusions. *Anesthesiology Clinics of North America, 23,* 241.

BOX 40-9 CLIENT TEACHING

Home Intravenous Therapy

Objectives

- The client, the primary caregiver, or both will demonstrate understanding and competence with intravenous therapy for safe delivery of medication in the home setting.

Teaching Strategies

- Explain to the client and the primary caregiver the importance of intravenous therapy in maintaining hydration and access for the delivery of medications.
- Ensure that the client and primary caregiver understand the risks involved when the intravenous system is not kept sterile.
- Be sure that the client, the primary caregiver, or both can manipulate the required equipment.
- Instruct the client and the primary caregiver in aseptic technique and hand hygiene when the handling of all intravenous equipment.
- Instruct the client and the primary caregiver in how to change intravenous solutions, tubing, and dressings when they become soiled or dislodged. (Note: The home care nurse may be able to visit frequently enough to perform scheduled tubing and dressing changes.)
- Instruct the client and the primary caregiver in procedures for safe disposal, in appropriate containers, of all sharps and intravenous materials exposed to blood.
- Instruct the client and the primary caregiver about signs and symptoms of infiltration, phlebitis, and infection and about reporting symptoms immediately.
- Instruct the client, the primary caregiver, or both to report slowing or cessation of the infusion or to report the presence of blood in the tubing.
- Teach the client, with the primary caregiver's assistance, how to ambulate, perform hygiene, and participate in other activities of daily living without dislodging or disconnecting cannula and tubing.

Evaluation

- Ask the client and the primary caregiver why it is necessary to maintain hydration and intravenous access for the delivery of medications.
- Ask the client and the primary caregiver what to do if intravenous fluid stops.
- Ask the client and the primary caregiver to describe signs and symptoms of complications and the actions they should take.
- Observe the client, the primary caregiver, or both changing the intravenous container, tubing, and dressing.
- Observe the client ambulating and participating in activities of daily living to see how he or she protects and manipulates the intravenous cannula and apparatus.

BOX 40-13 RESEARCH HIGHLIGHT

Managing Chronic Kidney Disease

Research Focus

Prevention of complications associated with chronic kidney disease requires attention to many biochemical parameters. In nurse-run clinics, nurses, with the guidance of physicians, are able to successfully manage these parameters through client-centred care, health promotion, teaching, dealing with problems, time, protocols, consultations or referrals, logistics, paperwork or documentation, and nurse–physician collaboration.

Research Abstract

The purpose of the study conducted by Molzahn, et al. (2008) was to describe the nature of the care provided to people with chronic kidney disease in a larger study of nurse-run, physician-monitored clinics and to describe how clients, nurses, and nephrologists described their experience with the clinics. Seven nurses, five physicians, and 22 clients participated in interviews, which were tape-recorded and transcribed. In addition to interviews, data collection involved review of 40 randomly selected charts. Themes identified related to the characteristics of the nurse, client-centred care, health promotion, teaching, dealing with problems, time, protocols, consultations or referrals, logistics, paperwork or documentation, and nurse–physician collaboration. Challenges and outcomes were also described as part of the experience with the clinic. Clients were actively engaged in self-management and reported high levels of satisfaction with care, as well as improvements in selected outcomes. Overall, the perceptions about this model of care were positive, and the approach warrants further exploration.

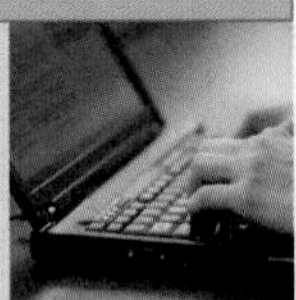

Evidence-Informed Practice and Primary Health Care

- Regular assessment and management by nurses can be used to prevent cardiovascular disease and other complications of chronic kidney disease.
- Client-centred care, teaching, and health promotion are important processes in caring for the client with chronic kidney disease.
- Many people with chronic kidney disease are able and willing to self-manage their illness.

References: Molzahn, A. E., Pelletier Hibbert, M., Gaudet, D., Starzomski, R., Barrett, B., & Morgan, J. (2008). Managing chronic kidney disease in a nurse-run, physician monitored clinic: The CanPREVENT experience. *Canadian Journal of Nursing Research, 40,* 96–112.

❖Evaluation

Client Care

The evaluation of a client's clinical status is especially important if an acute fluid and electrolyte or acid–base disturbance exists. The client's condition can change very quickly, and you must be able to recognize the signs and symptoms of impending problems by being aware of health alterations, the effects of medications and fluids, and the client's presenting clinical status (Figure 40–19).

You determine whether changes have occurred from the last client assessment, and you assess such changes. For example, the physical signs and symptoms of the assessed condition begin to disappear or lessen in intensity.

For clients with less acute alterations, evaluation likely occurs over a longer period of time. In this situation, your evaluation may be focused more on behavioural changes (e.g., the client's ability to follow dietary restrictions and medication schedules). The family's ability to anticipate alterations and prevent problems from recurring is also an important element of evaluation.

The client's level of progress determines whether you need to continue or revise the care plan. If goals are not met, you may need to consult with a physician and discuss additional methods, such as increasing the frequency of an intervention (e.g., provide more fluids to a dehydrated client), introducing a new therapy (e.g., initiate insertion of an intravenous line), or discontinuing a particular therapy. Once outcomes have been met, you can resolve the nursing diagnosis and focus on other priorities.

Client Expectations

You routinely review with the client his or her success in meeting expectations of care. "Tell me if I have helped you feel more comfortable" is a question you might raise if the client's expectations revolve around comfort and symptom management. If the client's concerns involve having a better understanding of a chronic problem, your evaluation might focus on the client's satisfaction with educational offerings. Often the client's level of satisfaction with care also depends on your success in involving family and friends. If the client has concerns about returning home or to a different care setting, it will be important to evaluate if the client feels prepared for the transition from acute care.

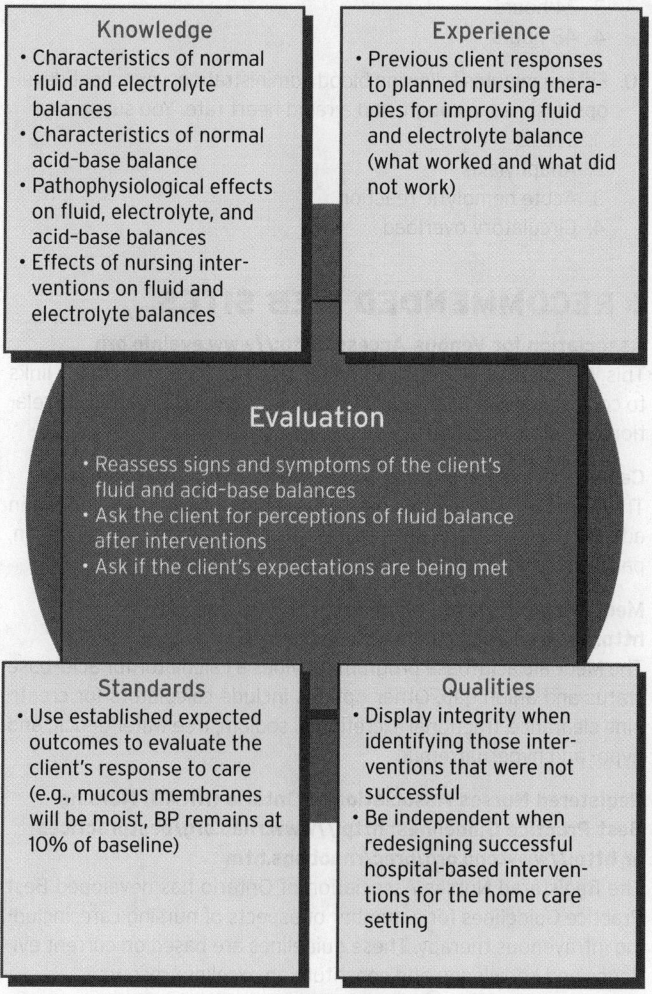

Knowledge
- Characteristics of normal fluid and electrolyte balances
- Characteristics of normal acid-base balance
- Pathophysiological effects on fluid, electrolyte, and acid-base balances
- Effects of nursing interventions on fluid and electrolyte balances

Experience
- Previous client responses to planned nursing therapies for improving fluid and electrolyte balance (what worked and what did not work)

Evaluation
- Reassess signs and symptoms of the client's fluid and acid-base balances
- Ask the client for perceptions of fluid balance after interventions
- Ask if the client's expectations are being met

Standards
- Use established expected outcomes to evaluate the client's response to care (e.g., mucous membranes will be moist, BP remains at 10% of baseline)

Qualities
- Display integrity when identifying those interventions that were not successful
- Be independent when redesigning successful hospital-based interventions for the home care setting

Figure 40-19 Critical thinking model for evaluation of fluid, electrolyte, and acid–base balances. BP, blood pressure.

* KEY CONCEPTS

- Body fluids are distributed in ECF and ICF compartments.
- Body fluids are composed of electrolytes, minerals, cells, and water.
- Body fluids are regulated through fluid intake, fluid output, and hormonal regulation.
- Volume disturbances include isotonic and osmolar deficits and excesses.
- Electrolytes are regulated by dietary intake and hormonal controls.
- Acid-base imbalances are buffered by chemical, biological, and physiological buffering, especially the lungs and kidneys.
- Chronic and serious illnesses increase the risk of fluid, electrolyte, and acid-base imbalances.
- Clients who are very young or very old are at greater risk for fluid, electrolyte, and acid-base imbalances.
- Assessment for fluid, electrolyte, and acid-base alterations includes the nursing health history, physical and behavioural assessments, measurements of intake and output, daily weights, and specific laboratory data.
- Osmolar imbalances and FVD can be corrected by enteral or parenteral administration of fluid.
- Common complications of intravenous therapy include infiltration, phlebitis, infection, FVE, and bleeding at the infusion site.
- Blood transfusions are given to replace fluid volume loss from hemorrhage, treat anemia, or replace coagulation factors.
- Blood transfusions can be obtained from a donor, autologous, or obtained through perioperative salvage.
- Administration of blood or blood products requires the nurse to follow a specific procedure to identify transfusion reactions quickly.
- In addition to transfusion reactions, the risks of transfusion also include hyperkalemia, hypocalcemia, FVE, and infection.
- Treatment for electrolyte disturbances includes dietary and pharmacological interventions.
- The body's chemical buffering system responds first to acid-base abnormalities.
- The goals of therapy for acid-base imbalances are to treat the underlying illness and to restore the arterial blood pH to normal.

* CRITICAL THINKING EXERCISES

1. Mrs. Emanuele is an 81-year-old woman admitted to the hospital with a 3-day history of vomiting and diarrhea. She has had only ice chips since the first episode of vomiting and is now complaining of malaise, cramping muscles, and a temperature of 39°C. Which laboratory findings would you expect to be abnormal on the basis of her complaints? What interventions would you expect the physician to order?

2. Caroline, a nurse, has just received a new client on her unit who is to receive 1 unit of RBCs within the next hour. What nursing actions are necessary before administering blood? Can Caroline delegate the administration of blood to a licensed practical nurse or an unregulated care provider?

3. Carlos is caring for Mr. Rossi, a 52-year-old man who has been seen in the emergency department following a motor vehicle accident. Mr. Rossi is complaining of difficulty breathing and has a respiratory rate of 40 breaths per minute. He is transferred to the intensive care unit, intubated, and placed on a ventilator. A nursing student asks Carlos to interpret Mr. Rossi's last ABG results: pH = 7.30; PaO_2 = 70; $PaCO_2$ = 50; bicarbonate = 24 mmol/L. What

interpretation will Carlos give to the student nurse? What is the relationship between the ABG results and Mr. Rossi being intubated and ventilated?

4. Janelle is the nurse caring for Mrs. Kwan, a 59-year-old woman who has just had a total knee replacement. The physician has ordered cefazolin (Ancef) 1 g in 50 mL to run over 30 minutes intravenous piggyback three times daily. Mrs. Kwan has a continuous infusion of Ringer's lactate at 75 mL/hour in the left forearm. What type of tubing will Janelle use to administer the intravenous piggyback medication? Calculate the drops per minute of the piggyback using both microtubing (60 drops/mL) and macrotubing (15 drops/mL).

5. Mrs Yoe is on a surgical unit following a total abdominal hysterectomy. She experienced postoperative bleeding and requires blood products; however, because of religious and cultural reasons, she has refused blood products. What are the key principles in providing care for Mrs Yoe? How does a health promotion perspective inform your care? What other options are available, and how realistic or viable are these options?

6. A 24-year-old tennis professional was admitted to the clinic with a temperature of 41ºC. He has a history of playing in a 5-hour tennis match in 38ºC heat. His coach brought him to the clinic because he was weak and lethargic. What assessment findings would you expect to find? What interventions would be necessary? Describe a teaching plan for this client upon discharge.

* REVIEW QUESTIONS

1. One of the most common electrolyte imbalances is
   1. Hypokalemia
   2. Hyperkalemia
   3. Hyponatremia
   4. Hypocalcemia

2. The client most at risk for FVDs is a(n)
   1. Older adult
   2. Young to middle adult
   3. Child
   4. Infant

3. One reason that older adults experience fluid and electrolyte imbalance and acid-base imbalances is that they
   1. Eat poor-quality food
   2. Have a decreased thirst sensation
   3. Have a more severe stress response
   4. Have an overly active thirst response

4. Output recorded on an intake and output record includes
   1. Urine, vomitus, diarrhea, and drainage from wounds
   2. Diarrhea, gastric suction, and drainage from wounds
   3. Medications, juices, and water
   4. Urine, diarrhea, vomitus, gastric suction, and drainage from wounds or tubes

5. Health promotion activities in the area of fluid and electrolyte imbalances focus primarily on
   1. Client teaching
   2. Dietary intake
   3. Medication regimen
   4. Physician involvement in care

6. The nurse is aware that the following medication is never given directly intravenously:
   1. Potassium chloride (KCl)
   2. Furosemide (Lasix)
   3. Dextrose
   4. Calcium gluconate

7. Many factors are initially controlled for in the intravenous insertion procedure. The nurse understands that this begins with
   1. Hand hygiene
   2. Checking the sterility of supplies
   3. Ensuring the seven rights of medication administration
   4. Carefully checking the order for the intravenous therapy

8. Indications of intravenous fluid infiltration include
   1. Phlebitis and coolness
   2. Edema and erythema
   3. Pallor and coolness
   4. Pain and erythema

9. The CDC recommends that replacing peripheral venous catheters and rotating sites should occur at least every
   1. 96 hours
   2. 72 hours
   3. 24 hours
   4. 48 hours

10. Fifteen minutes following blood administration, your client develops dyspnea, a cough, and a rapid heart rate. You suspect
    1. Sepsis
    2. Anaphylaxis
    3. Acute hemolytic reaction
    4. Circulatory overload

* RECOMMENDED WEB SITES

Association for Venous Access: http://www.avainfo.org
This Web site for the Association for Venous Access has many links to conferences and national and international organizations in relation to venous access.

Canadian Vascular Access Association: http://www.cvaa.info/
The Canadian Vascular Access Association provides leadership in advocating for safe, quality vascular access by promoting education, partnerships, knowledge, and research.

MedCalc: Acid-Base Calculator: http://www.medcalc.com/acidbase.html
The MedCalc acid-base program provides a calculator for acid-base status and anion gap. Other options include calculators for creatinine clearance, fractional excretion of sodium, free water deficit, and hypo- and hypernatremia.

Registered Nurses Association of Ontario (RNAO) Nursing Best Practice Guidelines: http://www.rnao.org/bestpractices or http://www.cno.org/prac/rnaobpgs.htm
The Registered Nurses Association of Ontario has developed Best Practice Guidelines for a number of aspects of nursing care, including intravenous therapy. These guidelines are based on current evidence and knowledge and constitute an excellent resource.

41

Sleep

Original chapter by Patricia A. Stockert, RN, BSN, MS, PhD

Canadian content written by

Kathryn A. Smith Higuchi, RN, BScN, MEd, PhD

objectives

Mastery of content in this chapter will enable you to:

- Define the key terms listed.
- Compare the characteristics of rest and sleep.
- Explain the effect of the 24-hour sleep–wake cycle on biological functions.
- Discuss the mechanisms that regulate sleep.
- Describe the stages of a normal sleep cycle.
- Explain the functions of sleep and rest.
- Compare the sleep requirements of different age groups.
- Identify factors that normally promote sleep and factors that normally disrupt sleep.
- Discuss the characteristics of common sleep disorders.
- Conduct a sleep history for a client.
- Identify nursing diagnoses appropriate for clients with sleep alterations.
- Identify nursing interventions designed to promote normal sleep cycles for clients of all ages.
- Describe ways to evaluate sleep therapies.

key terms

Biological clocks, p. 988
Cataplexy, p. 992
Circadian rhythm, p. 988
Emotional stress, p. 995
Excessive daytime sleepiness (EDS), p. 992
Hypersomnolence, p. 991
Hypnotics, p. 1006
Insomnia, p. 992
Narcolepsy, p. 992
Nocturia, p. 990
Nonrapid eye movement (NREM) sleep, p. 989
Parasomnias, p. 991
Polysomnogram, p. 992
Rapid eye movement (REM) sleep, p. 989
Rest, p. 993
Sedatives, p. 1006
Sleep, p. 988
Sleep apnea, p. 992
Sleep deprivation, p. 993
Sleep hygiene, p. 992

media resources

evolve Web Site

- Audio Chapter Summaries
- Glossary
- Multiple-Choice Review Questions
- Student Learning Activities
- Video Clips
- Weblinks

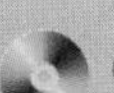

Companion CD

- Glossary
- Interactive Learning Activities
- Fluids and Electrolytes Tutorial
- Test-Taking Skills

Proper rest and sleep are as important to good health as are good nutrition and adequate exercise. Everyone needs different amounts of sleep and rest. Physical and emotional health depends on the ability to fulfill these basic human needs. A lack of the proper amounts of rest and sleep increases irritability and decreases the ability to concentrate, make judgements, and participate in daily activities.

To help clients by identifying and treating their sleep pattern disturbances, you need to first understand the nature of sleep, the factors influencing sleep, and clients' sleep habits. Clients require an individualized approach that is formed on the basis of their personal habits and patterns of sleep and addresses the particular problem that is disrupting their sleep. Nursing interventions are often effective in resolving short- and long-term sleep disturbances.

Sleep provides healing and restoration (McCance & Huether, 2006). Achieving the best possible sleep quality contributes to the promotion of good health and to recovery from illness. Ill clients often require more sleep and rest than healthy clients. The nature of illness, however, often prevents some clients from getting adequate rest and sleep. Sleep can also be made difficult by the environment of a hospital or long-term care facility and the activities of health care professionals. Some clients have pre-existing sleep disturbances, whereas other clients develop sleep problems as a result of illness or hospitalization.

Scientific Knowledge Base

Physiology of Sleep

Sleep is a cyclical physiological process that alternates with longer periods of wakefulness. The sleep–wake cycle influences and regulates physiological function and behavioural responses.

Circadian Rhythms

People experience cyclical rhythms as part of their everyday life. The most familiar rhythm is the 24-hour, day–night cycle known as the diurnal or **circadian rhythm** (derived from the Latin *circa*, meaning "about," and from *dies*, meaning "day"). Circadian rhythms influence the pattern of major biological and behavioural functions. The predictable change of body temperature, heart rate, blood pressure, hormone secretion, sensory acuity, and mood depend on the maintenance of the 24-hour circadian cycle (Izac, 2006).

Factors that affect circadian rhythms and daily sleep–wake cycles include light and temperature, social activities, and work routines. All persons have **biological clocks** that synchronize their sleep cycles, which explains why some individuals fall asleep at 9 P.M., whereas others go to bed at midnight. Different individuals also function at their best at different times of the day.

Hospitals or extended care facilities usually do not adapt care to an individual's sleep–wake cycle preferences. Typical hospital routines often interrupt sleep or prevent clients from falling asleep at their usual time. A person has poor quality of sleep if his or her sleep–wake cycle changes significantly. A serious illness is often indicated by reversals in the sleep–wake cycle, such as falling asleep during the day (or vice versa for people who work nights).

The biological rhythm of sleep frequently synchronizes with other body functions. Changes in body temperature, for example, correlate with sleep patterns. Normally, a person's body temperature peaks in the afternoon, decreases gradually, and then drops sharply after a person falls asleep. When the sleep–wake cycle is disrupted (e.g., by working rotating shifts), other physiological functions can also change. For example, the person may experience a decreased appetite and lose weight or may experience other common symptoms of sleep cycle disturbances, such as anxiety, restlessness, irritability, and impaired judgement. Failure to maintain the usual sleep–wake cycle can negatively influence the client's overall health.

Sleep Regulation. Sleep involves a sequence of physiological states maintained by highly integrated central nervous system (CNS) activity, which is associated with changes in the peripheral nervous, endocrine, cardiovascular, respiratory, and muscular systems (McCance & Huether, 2006). Each sequence of physiological states is identified by specific physiological responses and patterns of brain activity. Special instruments provide information about the structural and physiological aspects of sleep: for example, the electroencephalogram (EEG) measures electrical activity in the cerebral cortex, the electromyogram (EMG) measures muscle tone, and the electro-oculogram (EOG) measures eye movements.

Current theory suggests that sleep is an active multiphase process. The body's major sleep centre is the hypothalamus. The hypothalamus secretes hypocreatins (orexins) that promote wakefulness and rapid eye movement sleep. Prostaglandin D_2, L-tryptophan, and growth factors control sleep (McCance & Heuther, 2006).

Researchers believe the ascending reticular activating system (RAS), located in the upper brain stem, contains special cells that maintain alertness and wakefulness. The RAS receives visual, auditory, pain, and tactile sensory stimuli. Activity from the cerebral cortex (e.g., emotions and thought processes) also stimulates the RAS. Arousal, wakefulness, and maintenance of consciousness result from neurons in the RAS that release catecholamines, such as norepinephrine (Izac, 2006).

Researchers hypothesize that the release of serotonin from specialized cells in the raphe nuclei sleep system of the pons and medulla produces sleep. This area of the brain is also called the bulbar synchronizing region (BSR). Whether a person remains awake or falls asleep depends on a balance of impulses received from higher centres (e.g., thoughts), peripheral sensory receptors (e.g., sound or light stimuli), and the limbic system (e.g., emotions) (Figure 41–1). As a person tries to fall asleep, the eyes close and the body assumes a relaxed position. Stimuli to the RAS decline. If the room is dark and

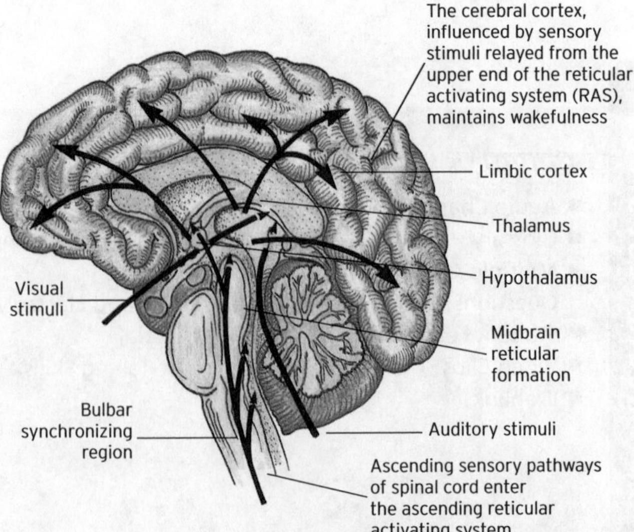

Figure 41-1 The reticular activating system and the bulbar synchronizing region control sensory input by intermittently activating and suppressing the brain's higher centres to control sleep and wakefulness.

quiet, activation of the RAS further declines. At some point, the BSR takes over, causing sleep.

Stages of Sleep. Changes in brainwave activity, muscle tone, and eye movements are associated with different stages of sleep (Izac, 2006). Normal sleep involves two phases: **nonrapid eye movement (NREM) sleep** and **rapid eye movement (REM) sleep** (Box 41–1). During NREM, a sleeper progresses through four stages during a typical 90-minute sleep cycle. The quality of sleep from stage 1 through stage 4 becomes increasingly deeper. Lighter sleep is characteristic of stages 1 and 2, when a person can be more easily aroused. Stages 3 and 4 involve a deeper sleep, called slow-wave sleep. REM sleep is the phase at the end of each sleep cycle. Different factors promote or interfere with various stages of the sleep cycle. It is important to choose therapies that foster sleep and eliminate factors that disrupt it.

> **BOX 41-1 Stages of the Sleep Cycle**
>
> **Stage 1: Non-Rapid Eye Movement**
>
> This stage represents the lightest level of sleep.
> Physiological activity begins to decrease, accompanied by a gradual fall in vital signs and metabolism.
> Persons are easily aroused by sensory stimuli, such as noise.
> When awakened from this stage, a person feels as though he or she had been daydreaming.
> This stage lasts a few minutes.
>
> **Stage 2: Non-Rapid Eye Movement**
>
> This stage is a period of sound sleep.
> Relaxation progresses.
> Persons are relatively easy to arouse.
> Body functions continue to slow.
> This stage lasts 10–20 minutes.
>
> **Stage 3: Non-Rapid Eye Movement**
>
> This stage begins the initial period of deep sleep.
> The sleeper is difficult to arouse and rarely moves.
> The muscles are completely relaxed.
> The vital signs decline but remain regular.
> This stage lasts 15–30 minutes.
>
> **Stage 4: Non-Rapid Eye Movement**
>
> This stage is the deepest period of sleep.
> The sleeper is very difficult to arouse.
> If sleep loss has occurred, the sleeper will spend a considerable portion of the sleep period in this stage.
> The vital signs are significantly lower than during waking hours.
> Sleepwalking and enuresis (bedwetting) sometimes occur.
> This stage lasts approximately 15–30 minutes.
>
> **Rapid Eye Movement Sleep**
>
> Vivid, full-colour dreaming occurs.
> Less vivid dreaming occurs in other stages.
> This stage usually begins about 90 minutes after sleep has begun.
> This stage is typified by the autonomic responses of rapidly moving eyes, fluctuating heart and respiratory rates, and increased or fluctuating blood pressure.
> Loss of skeletal muscle tone occurs.
> Gastric secretions increase.
> The sleeper is very difficult to arouse.
> The duration of REM sleep increases with each cycle and averages 20 minutes.

Sleep Cycle. The normal sleep pattern for an adult begins with a presleep period during which the person is aware of only gradually developing sleepiness. This period normally lasts 10 to 30 minutes, but if a person has difficulty falling asleep, it can last an hour or longer. Once asleep, the person usually passes through four to five complete sleep cycles per night, each consisting of four stages of NREM sleep and a period of REM sleep (McCance & Huether, 2006). Each cycle lasts approximately 90 to 100 minutes. The cyclical pattern usually progresses from stage 1 through stage 4 of NREM, followed by a reversal from stage 4 to stage 3 to stage 2, ending with a period of REM sleep (Figure 41–2). A person usually reaches REM sleep about 90 minutes into the sleep cycle. Of the total sleep time, 75 to 80% is spent in NREM sleep. With each successive cycle, stages 3 and 4 shorten, and the period of REM sleep lengthens. During the last sleep cycle, REM sleep can last up to 60 minutes. Not all people progress consistently through the stages of sleep. For example, a sleeper may move back and forth for short intervals between the NREM stages 2, 3, and 4 before entering the REM stage. The amount of time spent in each stage varies over a person's lifespan. Newborns and children spend more time in deep sleep. As individuals age, sleep becomes more fragmented and more time is spent in the lighter stages of sleep (Ferebee, 2006). Shifts from one stage of sleep to another tend to accompany body movements. Shifts to a light sleep or to wakefulness tend to occur suddenly, whereas shifts to deep sleep tend to be gradual (Izac, 2006). The number of sleep cycles depends on the total amount of time that the person spends sleeping.

Functions of Sleep

The purpose of sleep remains unclear. Sleep contributes to physiological and psychological restoration. NREM sleep contributes to body tissue restoration (McCance & Huether, 2006). During NREM sleep, biological functions slow. A healthy adult's normal heart rate throughout the day averages 70 to 80 beats per minute, or less if the individual is in excellent physical condition; however, during sleep, the heart rate falls to 60 beats per minute or less. Thus, the heart beats 10 to 20 fewer times each minute during sleep, or 60 to 120 fewer beats each hour. Clearly, restful sleep is beneficial in preserving cardiac function. Other biological functions also decrease during sleep: for example, respirations, blood pressure, and muscle tone (McCance & Huether, 2006).

The body needs sleep to routinely restore biological processes. During deep slow-wave (NREM stage 4) sleep, the body releases human growth hormone for the repair and renewal of epithelial and specialized cells, such as brain cells (Jones, 2005). During rest and sleep, protein synthesis and cell division occur for renewal of tissues

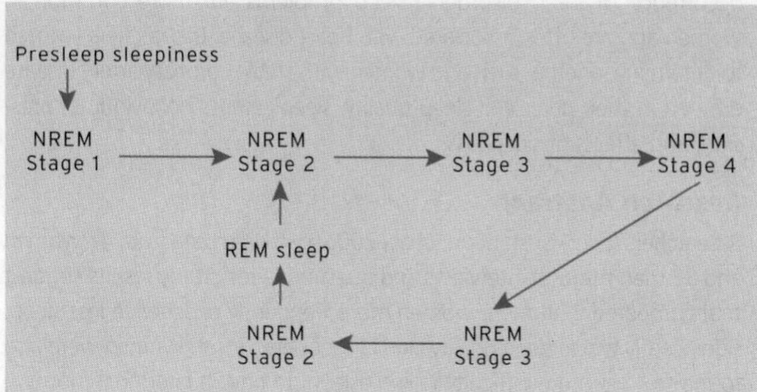

Figure 41-2 The stages of the adult sleep cycle.

such as the skin, bone marrow, gastric mucosa, and the brain. NREM sleep is especially important in children, who experience more stage 4 sleep. It is also believed that the body conserves energy during sleep. The skeletal muscles relax progressively, and the absence of muscular contraction preserves chemical energy for cellular processes. Lowering of the basal metabolic rate further conserves the body's energy supply (Izac, 2006).

REM sleep is necessary for brain tissue restoration and appears to be important for cognitive restoration (Buysse, 2005). REM sleep is associated with changes in cerebral blood flow, increased cortical activity, increased oxygen consumption, and epinephrine release. This association assists with memory storage and learning (McCance & Huether, 2006). During sleep, the brain filters stored information about the day's activities. The benefits of sleep on behaviour often go unnoticed until a problem develops as a result of sleep deprivation. A loss of REM sleep leads to feelings of confusion and suspicion.

Various body functions (e.g., mood, motor performance, memory, and equilibrium) are altered when sleep loss is prolonged (National Sleep Foundation, 2002a). Changes in the natural and cellular immune function also occur with moderate to severe sleep deprivation (Buysse, 2005). Researchers suggest that people who report sleeping for less than 5 hours are more likely to have diabetes (Gangwisch et al., 2007). Sleep deprivation can lead to traffic collisions, injuries in the home, and work-related accidents, all of which cost billions of dollars a year in lost productivity and incurred health care costs (Irwin et al., 2006).

Dreams Although dreams occur during both NREM and REM sleep, the dreams of REM sleep are more vivid and elaborate, and some believe these dreams are functionally important to learning, memory processing, and adaptation to stress (Stickgold, 2005). REM dreams progress in content throughout the night, from dreams about current events, to emotional dreams of childhood or past events. Personality influences the quality of dreams; for example, a creative person has elaborate and complex dreams, whereas a depressed person dreams of helplessness.

Most people dream about their immediate concerns, such as an argument with a spouse or worries over work. Sometimes a person is unaware of the fears represented in bizarre dreams. Clinical psychologists can try to analyze the symbolic nature of dreams as part of a client's psychotherapy. The ability to describe a dream and interpret its significance sometimes helps resolve personal concerns or fears.

According to another theory, dreams erase certain fantasies or nonsensical memories. Because most persons forget their dreams, few have dream recall and many do not believe they dream at all. To remember a dream requires a person to consciously think about the dream on awakening. Persons who recall dreams vividly usually awake just after a period of REM sleep.

Physical Illness

Any illness that causes pain, physical discomfort, or mood problems, such as anxiety or depression, often results in sleep problems. Persons with such alterations frequently have trouble falling asleep or staying asleep. Illnesses can also force clients to sleep in unfamiliar positions. For example, when an arm or leg is in traction, clients have a difficult time finding a comfortable position for sleep.

Respiratory disease often interferes with sleep. Clients with chronic lung disease, such as emphysema, are short of breath and frequently cannot sleep without two or three pillows to raise their head. Asthma and bronchitis alter the rhythm of breathing and disturb sleep. People with allergic rhinitis are also at greater risk for sleep disorders because of increased nasal airway resistance as a result of congestion from increased nasal discharge and edema of the nasal mucosa (Craig et al., 2004; Santos et al, 2006).

Heart disease is related to the quality of sleep and to sleep disorders (Box 41–2). Sleep-related breathing disorders are linked to increased incidence of nocturnal angina (chest pain), increased heart rate, electrocardiogram changes, high blood pressure, and risk of heart diseases and stroke (McCance & Huether, 2006). Hypertension often causes early morning awakening and fatigue. Research also suggests an increased risk of sudden cardiac death in the first hours after wakening. Hypothyroidism decreases stage 4 sleep, whereas hyperthyroidism causes persons to take more time to fall asleep.

Nocturia, or urination during the night, disrupts sleep and the sleep cycle. This condition is most common in older people with reduced bladder tone or persons who have cardiac disease, diabetes, urethritis, or prostatic disease. After a person awakens repeatedly to urinate, returning to sleep is difficult.

Older adults often experience restless leg syndrome (RLS), which occurs before sleep onset. Persons with RLS experience recurrent,

BOX 41-2 RESEARCH HIGHLIGHT

Sleep Disorders in Clients With Coronary Artery Disease

Research Focus

Prior research shows a relationship between heart disease, sleep, and the occurrence of sleep disorders. Sleep problems are more common in women and are often associated with heart disease. Researchers wanted to determine whether men and women with stable coronary artery disease differed in their perceived sleep quality, sleeplessness behaviour, depression, and effects of sleep loss.

Research Abstract

Researchers (Edell-Gustafsson, et al., 2006) gathered data from 47 women and 88 men through interviews and questionnaires. Study results suggest that compared with men, women more frequently experience less sleep, significantly worse sleep quality, and longer sleep onset. Women were also found to have more difficulty falling asleep, to have a later final morning awakening time, and to more frequently use hypnotics to aid their sleep.

Evidence-Informed Practice

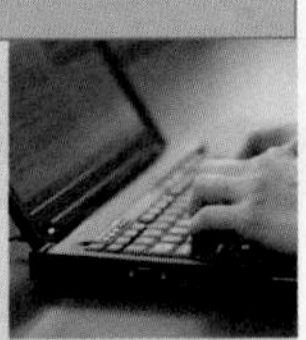

- Be aware that women with coronary artery disease experience different sleep problems from men with coronary artery disease.
- During your assessment of a client's health problems, ensure you ask questions related to sleep quality and sleep patterns.
- If the client indicates a problem with sleep, conduct a thorough sleep history.
- Reinforce good sleep hygiene habits.
- Encourage clients to notify their health care professional if they begin to experience sleep problems.

References: Edell-Gustafsson, U., Svanborg, E., & Swahn, E. (2006). A gender perspective on sleeplessness behavior, effects of sleep loss, and coping resources in patients with stable coronary artery disease. *Heart and Lung, 35*, 75–89.

rhythmical movements of the feet and legs and feel an itching sensation deep in their muscles. Relief comes only from moving the legs, which prevents relaxation and, consequently, sleep. RLS is sometimes a relatively benign condition depending on how severely sleep is disrupted. Primary restless leg syndrome is a central nervous system disorder, whereas secondary RLS is associated with pregnancy, uremia, and lower levels of iron (National Heart, Lung, and Blood Institute Working Group on Restless Legs Syndrome, 2000).

Persons with peptic ulcer disease often awaken in the middle of the night. Research studies showing a relationship between gastric acid secretion and stages of sleep are conflicting. One consistent finding is that persons with duodenal ulcers fail to suppress acid secretions in their first 2 hours of sleep (Orr, 2005).

Sleep Disorders

Sleep disorders are conditions that, if untreated, can cause disturbed nighttime sleep that results in one of three problems: insomnia, abnormal movements or sensations (during sleep or when awakened at night), or excessive daytime sleepiness (Malow, 2005). Many adults have significant sleep problems as a result of inadequacies in either the quantity or quality of their nighttime sleep, and thereby experience **hypersomnolence** on a daily basis (National Sleep Foundation, 2002a). The American Academy of Sleep Medicine developed the International Classification of Sleep Disorders version 2 (ICSD-2), which classifies sleep disorders into eight major categories (Box 41–3).

The insomnias are primary disorders related to difficulty falling asleep. Individuals with sleep-related breathing disorders have disordered respirations during sleep. Hypersomnia not due to sleep-related breathing disorders is a group of disorders that are not caused by disturbances in circadian rhythms or in nocturnal sleep. The **parasomnias** are undesirable behaviours that usually occur during sleep. Sleep disturbances and wake disturbances are associated with many medical and psychiatric sleep disorders, including psychiatric, neurological, and other medical disorders. The circadian rhythm sleep disorders are caused by a misalignment between the timing of sleep and the societal norm or the desires of the individual. In sleep-related movement disorders, the person experiences movements such as leg cramps or teeth grinding that disturb sleep. The category of isolated symptoms,

➤ BOX 41-3 Classification of Sleep Disorders

Insomnias
Adjustment sleep disorder (acute insomnia)
Inadequate sleep hygiene
Paradoxical insomnia
Insomnia due to a mental disorder
Behavioural insomnia of childhood
Idiopathic insomnia
Insomnia due to a medical condition

Sleep-Related Breathing Disorders
Central Sleep Apnea Syndromes
Primary central sleep apnea
Central sleep apnea due to a drug or substance
Central sleep apnea due to a medical condition
Obstructive sleep apnea syndromes

Hypersomnias Not Due to a Sleep-Related Breathing Disorder
Narcolepsy (four specified types)
Menstrual-related hypersomnia
Idiopathic hypersomnia with long sleep time
Behaviourally induced insufficient sleep syndrome
Hypersomnia due to a medical condition

Parasomnias
Disorders of Arousal
Sleepwalking
Sleep terrors

Parasomnias Usually Associated With REM Sleep
Nightmare disorder
REM sleep behaviour disorder
Sleep paralysis

Other Parasomnias
Sleep-related groaning
Sleep-related hallucinations
Sleep-related eating disorder
Sleep-related enuresis (bedwetting)

Circadian Rhythm Sleep Disorders
Primary Circadian Rhythm Sleep Disorders
Delayed sleep phase type
Advanced sleep phase type

Behaviourally Induced Circadian Rhythm Sleep Disorders
Jet lag type
Shift work type
Delayed sleep phase type
Drug or substance use

Sleep-Related Movement Disorders
Restless leg syndrome
Periodic limb movements
Sleep-related leg cramps
Sleep-related bruxism (teeth grinding)

Isolated Symptoms, Apparently Normal Variants, and Unresolved Issues
Long sleeper
Short sleeper
Snoring
Sleep talking
Benign sleep myoclonus of infancy

Other Sleep Disorders
Physiological (organic) sleep disorders
Environmental sleep disorder
Sleep disorder not due to a substance or physiological condition

Adapted from American Academy of Sleep Medicine: International classes of diseases and international classification of sleep disorders, as cited in Thorpy, M. (2005). Classification of sleep disorders. In M. Kryger, T. Roth, & W. C. Dement (Eds.), *Principles and practice of sleep medicine* (4th ed., pp. 615–625). Philadelphia, PA: Elsevier.

apparently normal variants, and unresolved issues includes sleep-related symptoms that fall between normal and abnormal sleep. The other sleep disorders category contains sleep problems that do not fit into other categories.

Sleep laboratory studies are often used to diagnose a sleep disorder (Buysse, 2005; Cohen, 2004). A **polysomnogram** involves the use of EEG, EMG, and EOG to monitor stages of sleep and wakefulness during nighttime sleep. The Multiple Sleep Latency Test (MSLT) provides objective information about sleepiness and selected aspects of sleep structure by measuring eye movements, muscle tone changes, and brain electrical activity during at least four napping opportunities spread throughout the day. The MSLT takes 8 to 10 hours to complete. Clients wear an Actigraph device on the wrist to measure sleep–wake patterns over an extended period of time. Actigraphy data provides information such as sleep time, number and duration of awakenings, and levels of activity and rest (Buysse, 2005; Cohen, 2004).

Insomnia. Clients experience the symptom of **insomnia** when they have chronic difficulty falling asleep, frequent awakenings from sleep, a short sleep, or nonrestorative sleep (Edinger & Means, 2005). Insomnia is the most common sleep-related complaint. Persons with insomnia report excessive daytime sleepiness and insufficient quantity and quality of sleep. Frequently, however, the client sleeps for longer than he or she realizes. Insomnia often signals an underlying physical or psychological disorder. Insomnia occurs more frequently in women and is the most common sleep problem for women.

Persons experience transient insomnia as a result of situational stresses, such as worries about family, work, or school; jet lag; illness; or loss of a loved one. Insomnia sometimes recurs, but the client is able to sleep well between episodes. However, a temporary case of insomnia due to a stressful situation can lead to chronic difficulty in obtaining sufficient sleep, sometimes the result of the worry and anxiety that develops about obtaining adequate sleep.

Insomnia is often associated with poor **sleep hygiene**, which refers to the practices or habits the client associates with sleep. If insomnia continues, the fear of not being able to sleep is enough to cause wakefulness. During the day, persons with chronic insomnia feel sleepy, fatigued, depressed, and anxious. Treatment is symptomatic, including improved sleep hygiene measures, biofeedback, cognitive techniques, and relaxation techniques. Behavioural and cognitive therapies have few adverse effects and show evidence of sustained improvement in sleep over a 6-month period (Morin et al., 2007).

Sleep Apnea. **Sleep apnea** is a disorder characterized by the lack of airflow through the nose and mouth for periods of 10 seconds or longer during sleep. The most common form of sleep apnea is obstructive sleep apnea (OSA). An estimated 24% of middle-aged men and 9% of middle-aged women have OSA (Tsai, 2003). Risk factors for developing OSA include obesity, smoking, alcohol, and a positive family history of OSA (Redline, 2005). OSA may affect middle-aged men more frequently, particularly when they are obese (Groth, 2005). Obstructive sleep apnea is also common in postmenopausal women and in younger women and children (Mendez & Olson, 2006a).

OSA occurs when the muscles or structures of the oral cavity or throat relax during sleep. The upper airway becomes partially or completely blocked, thereby diminishing the nasal airflow (hypopnea) or stopping it (apnea) for as long as 30 seconds (Guilleminault & Bassiri, 2005). The person still attempts to breathe; chest and abdominal movements continue and often result in loud snoring and snorting sounds. When breathing is partially or completely diminished, each successive diaphragmatic movement becomes stronger until the obstruction is relieved. Structural abnormalities such as a deviated septum, nasal polyps, certain jaw configurations, or enlarged tonsils predispose a client to obstructive sleep apnea. The effort to breathe during sleep results in arousals from deep sleep often to the stage 2 cycle. In severe cases, hundreds of hypopnea or apnea episodes occur every hour, resulting in severe interference with deep sleep.

Excessive daytime sleepiness (EDS) and fatigue are the most common complaints of persons who have OSA (Holman, 2005). Persons who have severe OSA often report taking daytime naps and experience a disruption in their daily activities because of sleepiness (National Sleep Foundation, 2002b). Feelings of sleepiness are usually most intense when waking up, right before going to sleep, and approximately 12 hours after the mid-sleep period. EDS often results in impaired waking function, poor work or school performance, accidents while driving or using equipment, and behavioural or emotional problems.

Obstructive sleep apnea causes a serious decline in the saturation level of arterial oxygen. Clients with OSA are at risk for cardiac dysrhythmias, right heart failure, pulmonary hypertension, angina attacks, stroke, and hypertension. Sleep apnea contributes to high blood pressure and increased risk for heart attack and stroke (National Sleep Foundation, 2002b).

Clients who have OSA rarely achieve deep sleep. In addition to reports of excessive daytime sleepiness, common symptoms include fatigue, morning headaches, irritability, depression, difficulty concentrating, and decreased sex drive (White, 2005). OSA affects marital relationships and interactions within and outside the family, and is an embarrassment to the client (Reishtein et al., 2006). Treatment for OSA includes therapy to address the underlying cardiac or respiratory complications and emotional problems that occur as a result of the symptoms of this disorder.

Narcolepsy. **Narcolepsy** is a dysfunction of the mechanisms that regulate the sleep and wake states. Excessive daytime sleepiness is the most common complaint associated with narcolepsy. During the day, a person who has narcolepsy may suddenly feel an overwhelming wave of sleepiness and fall asleep; REM sleep occurs within 15 minutes of falling asleep. Symptoms of narcolepsy include cataplexy, vivid dreams and sleep paralysis. **Cataplexy**, or sudden muscle weakness during intense emotions, such as anger, sadness, or laughter, can occur at any time during the day. If the cataplectic attack is severe, the client loses voluntary muscle control and falls to the floor. A person with narcolepsy often has vivid dreams that occur as the person is falling asleep. These dreams are difficult to distinguish from reality. Sleep paralysis, or the feeling of being unable to move or talk just before waking or falling asleep, is another symptom (Guilleminault & Fromberz, 2005). Some studies show a genetic link for narcolepsy (Mignot, 2005).

A person who has narcolepsy has the problem of falling asleep uncontrollably at inappropriate times. When others do not understand this disorder, they may mistake a sleep attack for laziness, lack of interest in activities, or drunkenness. Typically, the symptoms first begin to appear in adolescence and are often confused with the excessive daytime sleepiness that commonly occurs in teenagers. Clients with narcolepsy are treated with stimulants that often only partially increase their wakefulness and reduce the frequency of sleep attacks. These clients are also treated with antidepressant medications that suppress cataplexy and other REM-related symptoms. Brief daytime naps no longer than 20 minutes help to reduce subjective feelings of sleepiness. Drugs classified as wakefulness-promoting agents, such as modafinil, are available to treat narcolepsy. Other management methods include following a regular exercise program, avoiding shifts in sleep, strategically timed daytime naps (if possible), eating light meals that are high in protein, practising deep breathing, chewing gum, and taking vitamins (Guilleminault & Fromberz, 2005). Clients who have narcolepsy need to avoid factors that increase drowsiness (e.g., alcohol, heavy meals, exhausting activities, long-distance driving, and extended periods of sitting in hot, stuffy rooms).

Parasomnias. Parasomnias are sleep problems that occur while falling asleep, between sleep phases, or during transitions from sleep to wakefulness. Parasomnias are more common in children than in adults. Some researchers have hypothesized that one parasomnia, sudden infant death syndrome (SIDS), is related to sleep apnea, hypoxia, and cardiac arrhythmias caused by abnormalities in the autonomic nervous system that are manifested during sleep (Verrier & Josephson, 2005). The Canadian Sleep Society recommended that parents place healthy infants on their backs for sleep because this position is associated with the lowest risk of SIDS (Driver, 2003).

Parasomnias that occur among older children include somnambulism (sleepwalking), night terrors, nightmares, nocturnal enuresis (bedwetting), body rocking, and bruxism (teeth grinding). When adults experience these symptoms, more serious disorders are often indicated. Specific treatment for these disorders varies; however, in all cases clients need to be supported and their safety maintained.

Sleep Deprivation. Sleep deprivation is experienced by many clients as a result of other conditions. Causes include illness (e.g., fever, difficulty breathing, or pain), emotional stress, certain medications, environmental disturbances (e.g., frequent nursing care), and variability in the timing of sleep due to shift work. Physicians and nurses are particularly prone to sleep deprivation due to their long work schedules and rotating shifts (Basner, 2005; Blachowicz & Letizia, 2006; Scott et al, 2007; Shen et al., 2006). Hospitalization, especially in intensive care units (ICUs), makes clients particularly vulnerable to the extrinsic and circadian sleep disorders that cause the "ICU syndrome of sleep deprivation" (Dines-Kalinowski, 2002; Honkus, 2003). Constant environmental stimuli within the ICU, such as strange noises from equipment, the frequent monitoring and care given by nurses, and ever-present lights, confuse clients. Repeated environmental stimuli and the client's poor physical status lead to sleep deprivation (Olson et al., 2001).

A person's response to sleep deprivation is highly variable. Clients exhibit a variety of physiological and psychological symptoms (Box 41–4). The severity of symptoms is often related to the duration of sleep deprivation. The most effective treatment for sleep deprivation is elimination or correction of factors that disrupt the sleep pattern. You play an important role in identifying clients' treatable sleep deprivation problems.

> **BOX 41-4 Sleep Deprivation Symptoms**
>
> **Physiological Symptoms**
> Ptosis, blurred vision
> Clumsiness in fine motor skills
> Decreased reflexes
> Slowed response time
> Decreased reasoning and judgement
> Decreased auditory and visual alertness
> Cardiac arrhythmias
>
> **Psychological Symptoms**
> Confusion and disorientation
> Increased sensitivity to pain
> Irritability, withdrawal, apathy
> Excessive sleepiness
> Agitation
> Hyperactivity
> Decreased motivation

Nursing Knowledge Base

Sleep and Rest

When persons are at **rest**, they usually feel mentally relaxed, free from anxiety, and physically calm. Rest does not imply inactivity, although rest is often thought of as the act of settling down in a comfortable chair or lying in bed. When persons are at rest, they are in a state of mental, physical, and spiritual activity that leaves them feeling refreshed, rejuvenated, and ready to resume the activities of the day. Individuals have their own habits for obtaining rest and can adjust to new environments or conditions that affect their ability to rest. Rest is gained from reading a book, practising a relaxation exercise, listening to music, taking a long walk, or sitting quietly.

Illness and unfamiliar health care routines can easily affect the usual rest and sleep patterns of persons entering a hospital or other health care facility. You may frequently care for clients on bedrest, which confines clients to the bed to reduce the physical and psychological demands on their body. Clients may not necessarily feel rested because they may still have emotional worries that prevent complete relaxation. For example, concern over physical limitations or a fear of being unable to return to their usual lifestyle can cause clients to feel stressed and unable to relax. You must always be aware of the client's need for rest. Long periods without rest can lead to illness or to the worsening of an existing illness.

Normal Sleep Requirements and Patterns

Individual requirements for sleep duration and quality vary among persons of all age groups. For example, one person may feel adequately rested after 6 hours of sleep, whereas another person may require 10 hours of sleep.

Neonates. The neonate up to the age of 3 months averages about 16 hours of sleep a day, sleeping almost constantly during the first week. The sleep cycle is generally 40 to 50 minutes with waking occurring after one to two sleep cycles. Approximately 50% of this sleep is REM sleep, which stimulates the higher brain centres. REM sleep is essential for development because the neonate is not awake long enough for significant external stimulation.

Infants. Infants usually develop a nighttime pattern of sleep by 3 months of age. The infant normally takes several naps during the day but usually sleeps an average of 8 to 10 hours during the night for a total daily sleep time of 15 hours. About 30% of sleep time is in the REM cycle. Awakening commonly occurs early in the morning, although awakening during the night is not unusual.

Toddlers. By 2 years of age, children usually sleep through the night and take daily naps. Total sleep time averages 12 hours a day. After 3 years of age, children often give up daytime naps (Hockenberry & Wilson, 2007). Awakening during the night is common for toddlers. The percentage of REM sleep continues to fall. Toddlers may be unwilling to go to bed at night either because of their need for autonomy or a fear of separation from their parents.

Preschoolers. A preschooler sleeps about 12 hours a night (about 20% of which is REM sleep). By 5 years of age, the preschooler rarely takes daytime naps, except in cultures where siestas are the custom

(Hockenberry & Wilson, 2007). The preschooler usually has difficulty relaxing or quieting down after long, active days and may experience bedtime fears, waking during the night, or nightmares. Partial wakening, followed by a normal return to sleep is frequent (Hockenberry & Wilson, 2007). In the waking period, the child may exhibit brief episodes of crying, walking aimlessly, unintelligible speech, sleepwalking, or bedwetting.

School-Age Children. The amount of sleep needed varies during the school-age years. A 6-year-old averages 11 to 12 hours of sleep nightly, whereas an 11-year-old sleeps 9 to 10 hours (Hockenberry & Wilson, 2007). The 6- or 7-year-old will usually go to bed with some encouragement or after participating in quiet activities. The older child often resists sleeping because of an unawareness of fatigue or a need to be independent.

Adolescents. Teenagers require about 9 hours of sleep per night, but half receive less than 8 hours per night (Gibson & Trajanovic, 2005). The typical adolescent is subject to a number of outside influences, such as school demands, after-school social activities, and part-time jobs, which reduce the time spent sleeping (National Sleep Foundation, 2006a). This shortened sleep time often results in excessive daytime sleepiness (EDS). As a result of EDS due to insufficient sleep, adolescents may experience reduced performance in school, vulnerability to accidents, behaviour and mood problems, and increased use of alcohol (Spilsbury et al., 2004; Walsh et al., 2005).

Young Adults. Most young adults average 6 to 8.5 hours of sleep per night. Approximately 20% of sleep time is REM sleep, which remains consistent throughout life. The stresses of the job, family relationships, and social activities frequently lead to both insomnia and the use of medications to aid sleep. Daytime sleepiness contributes to an increased number of accidents, decreased productivity, and interpersonal problems in this age group. Pregnancy increases the need for sleep and rest. During the third trimester of pregnancy, women may experience insomnia, periodic limb movements, restless leg syndrome, and sleep disordered breathing (Driver, 2005; Wolfson & Lee, 2005).

Middle Adults. During middle adulthood, the total time spent sleeping at night begins to decline. The amount of stage 4 sleep begins to fall and continues to fall with advancing age. Insomnia is particularly common, probably because of the changes and stresses experienced in middle age. Anxiety, depression, and certain physical illnesses cause sleep disturbances. Women who have menopausal symptoms often experience insomnia (Driver, 2005).

Older Adults. Complaints of sleeping difficulties increase with age. More than 50% of adults aged 65 years or older report problems with sleep (Hoffman, 2003). Episodes of REM sleep tend to shorten. Stages 3 and 4 NREM sleep decrease progressively; some older adults have almost no stage 4, or deep sleep. An older adult awakens more often during the night and takes more time to fall asleep again (Ferebee, 2006). The tendency to nap seems to increase progressively with age because of the frequent awakenings experienced at night. The presence of chronic illness often results in sleep disturbances for the older adult. For example, an older adult with arthritis frequently has difficulty sleeping because of joint pain. Changes in sleep pattern are often due to changes in the central nervous system (CNS) that affect the regulation of sleep. Sensory impairment reduces an older person's sensitivity to time cues that maintain circadian rhythms.

Factors Affecting Sleep

Often, multiple factors alter the quality and quantity of sleep, such as physiological, psychological, and environmental influences.

Drugs and Substances. Sleepiness, insomnia, and fatigue often result as a direct effect of commonly prescribed medications (Box 41–5). These medications alter sleep and weaken daytime alertness, which can be problematic for individuals (Schweitzer, 2005). Medication prescribed for sleep often causes more problems than benefits. Many older adults take a variety of drugs to control or treat chronic illness, and the combined effects of several drugs can seriously disrupt sleep. One substance that promotes sleep in many people is L-tryptophan, a natural protein found in milk, cheese, and meats.

Lifestyle. A person's daily routine influences sleep patterns. An individual working a rotating shift (e.g., 2 weeks of day shifts followed by a week of night shifts) often has difficulty adjusting to the

➤ BOX 41-5 Drugs and Their Effect on Sleep

Hypnotics
- Interfere with reaching deeper sleep stages
- Provide only temporary (1 week) increase in the quantity of sleep
- Eventually cause "hangover" during the day, excess drowsiness, confusion, decreased energy
- May worsen sleep apnea in older adults

Diuretics
- Nighttime awakenings caused by nocturia

Antidepressants and Stimulants
- Suppress REM sleep
- Decrease total sleep time

Alcohol
- Speeds onset of sleep
- Reduces REM sleep
- Interrupts sleep during the night and makes returning to sleep difficult

Caffeine
- Prevents the onset of sleep
- Interrupts sleep during the night
- Interferes with REM sleep

Beta-Adrenergic Blockers
- Cause nightmares
- Cause insomnia
- Interrupt sleep

Benzodiazepines
- Alter REM sleep
- Increase sleep time
- Increase daytime sleepiness

Narcotics
- Suppress REM sleep
- Cause increased daytime drowsiness

Anticonvulsants
- Decrease REM sleep time
- May cause daytime drowsiness

altered sleep schedule (Van Dongen, 2006). For example, the body's internal clock for bedtime is set at 11 P.M., but the work schedule instead forces sleep at 9 A.M. The individual is able to sleep only 3 or 4 hours because the body's clock perceives that the morning is the time to be awake and active. Difficulties with maintaining alertness during work time result in decreased and even hazardous performance (Scott et al., 2007). After several weeks of working a night shift, a person's biological clock usually does adjust. Other alterations in routines that disrupt sleep patterns include performing unaccustomed heavy work, engaging in late-night social activities, and changing the evening mealtime.

Usual Sleep Patterns. In the past century, the amount of sleep obtained nightly has decreased by more than 20% (National Sleep Foundation, 2003), which indicates that many adults are sleep deprived and experience excessive sleepiness during the day. Sleepiness becomes pathological when it occurs at times when individuals need to or want to be awake. Persons who experience temporary sleep deprivation as a result of an active social evening or a lengthened work schedule usually feel sleepy the next day. However, they are usually able to overcome these feelings despite the difficulty they experience in performing tasks and remaining attentive. Much more serious than temporary sleep deprivation is chronic lack of sleep, which causes serious alterations in the ability to perform daily functions. Sleepiness tends to be most difficult to overcome during the performance of sedentary (inactive) tasks. For example, single-vehicle accidents related to a driver falling asleep at the wheel occur most often between 2 A.M. and 5 A.M., as a result of the sleepiness that occurs when persons are awake during what is their normal period of sleep (Sitzman, 2005).

Emotional Stress. Sleep is frequently disrupted by worry over personal problems or a personal situation. **Emotional stress** causes a person to be tense and often leads to frustration when sleep does not occur. Stress also causes a person to try too hard to fall asleep, to awaken frequently during the sleep cycle, or to oversleep. Continued stress can lead to poor sleep habits.

Older clients frequently experience personal losses, such as retirement, physical impairment, or the death of a loved one, all of which can lead to emotional stress. Older adults and other individuals who live with depressive mood problems may experience delays in falling asleep, the earlier appearance of REM sleep, frequent awakening, increased total bed time, feelings of having slept poorly, and early awakening (National Sleep Foundation, 2006b).

Environment. The physical environment in which a person sleeps can significantly influence the ability to fall asleep and remain sleep. Good ventilation is essential for restful sleep. The size, firmness, and position of the bed also affect the quality of sleep. If a person usually sleeps with another individual, sleeping alone often causes wakefulness. On the other hand, sleeping with a restless or snoring bed partner disrupts sleep.

In hospitals and other inpatient facilities, noise creates a problem for clients. Noise in hospitals is usually new or strange and often loud, and clients wake easily. This problem is greatest the first night of hospitalization, when clients often experience increased total wake time, increased awakenings, and decreased REM sleep and total sleep time. People-induced noises (e.g., nursing activities) are sources of increased sound levels. Intensive care units are sources for high noise levels as the result of staff consultations, monitor alarms, and equipment sounds. The environment is unpleasant for sleeping because of the close proximity of clients, noise from confused and ill clients, the ringing of alarm systems and telephones, and disturbances caused by emergencies. Noise contributes to hearing loss, delays healing, impairs the immune function, and increases blood pressure, heart rate, and stress (Cmiel et al., 2004).

The level of light in a room affects the ability to fall asleep. Some clients prefer a dark room for sleep, whereas others, such as children or older adults, often prefer soft lighting during sleep. Clients may also have trouble sleeping because of the temperature of a room. A room that is too warm or too cold often causes a client to become restless.

Exercise and Fatigue. A person who is moderately fatigued usually achieves restful sleep, especially when the fatigue is the result of enjoyable work or exercise. Exercising that is completed 2 hours or more prior to bedtime allows the body enough time to cool down and maintains a state of fatigue that promotes relaxation. However, excess fatigue resulting from exhausting or stressful work makes falling asleep difficult. Excess fatigue is a common problem for grade-school children and adolescents.

Food and Caloric Intake. Following good eating habits is important for proper sleep. Eating a large, heavy meal or a spicy meal at night often leads to indigestion that interferes with sleep. Insomnia can result from caffeine, alcohol, or nicotine consumed in the evening. Coffee, tea, cola, and chocolate contain caffeine and xanthines that cause sleeplessness. Persons who have insomnia can improve their sleep by drastically reducing or by completely avoiding these substances. Some food allergies cause insomnia. In infants, a milk allergy sometimes causes nighttime waking and crying, or colic.

Both weight loss and weight gain influence sleep patterns. Weight gain contributes to obstructive sleep apnea because of the increased size of the soft tissue structures in the upper airway (Schwab, 2005). Weight loss causes insomnia and decreased amounts of sleep (Benca & Schenck, 2005). Certain sleep disorders are the result of the semi-starvation diets popular in a weight-conscious society.

Critical Thinking

Successful critical thinking requires a synthesis of knowledge, including information gathered from clients, past experience, critical thinking qualities, and intellectual and professional standards. Clinical judgements require you to anticipate the required information, analyze the data, and make decisions regarding client care. You adapt your critical thinking to the changing needs of the client. During assessment (Figure 41–3), consider all elements to make appropriate nursing diagnoses.

In the case of sleep, you will integrate knowledge from nursing and from disciplines such as pharmacology and psychology. Your personal experience with a sleep problem and your experience with clients who have sleep problems will prepare you to know effective forms of sleep therapies. You will need to use critical thinking qualities, such as perseverance, confidence, and discipline to complete a comprehensive assessment and to develop a plan of care that can successfully manage the sleep problem. The framework for practice developed by the Canadian Nurses Association (2007) and standards of practice developed by each provincial and territorial nursing organization identify your role as a nurse in client care. In addition, clinical guidelines such as those in *Excessive Sleepiness* (Chasens et al., 2008) provide specific instructions for assessing and addressing the needs of older clients with sleep disorders.

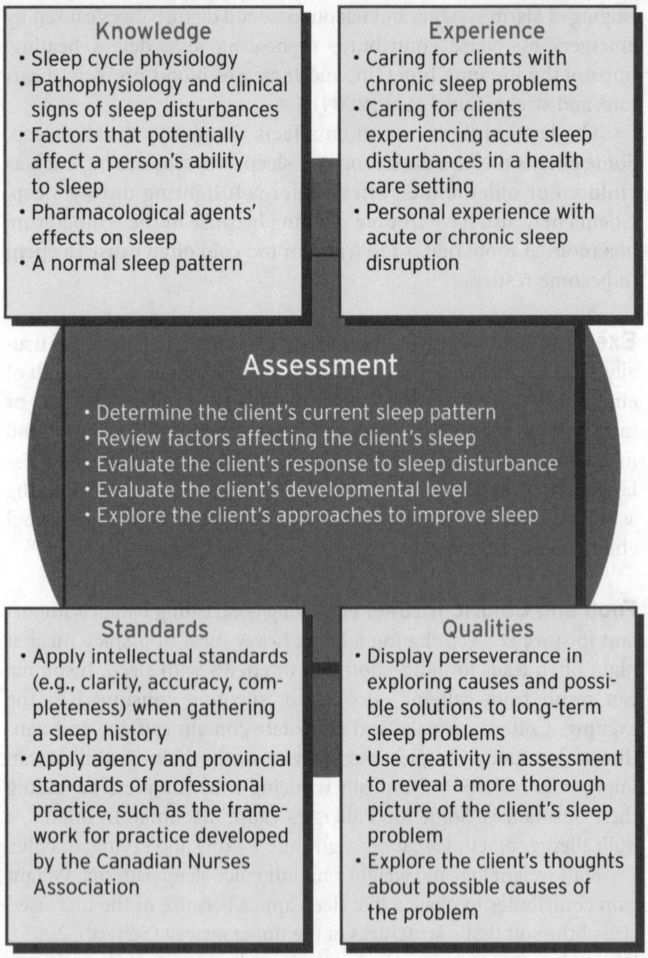

Figure 41-3 Critical thinking model for sleep assessment.

Nursing Process

❖Assessment

Assess clients' sleep patterns by using the nursing history to gather information about factors that usually influence sleep. Because sleep is a subjective experience, only the client is able to report whether it is sufficient and restful. If the client is satisfied with the quantity and quality of sleep received, you will consider it normal, and the nursing history is brief. If, however, a client reports or suspects a sleep problem, you need to conduct a detailed history.

Sleep Assessment

Most persons are able to provide a reasonably accurate estimate of their sleep patterns, particularly if any changes have occurred. In your assessment, focus on understanding the characteristics of the client's sleep problem and usual sleep habits so that your nursing care strategies to promote sleep are individualized. For example, if the nursing history reveals that a client always reads before falling asleep, then offer reading material at bedtime.

Sources for Sleep Assessment. Usually, clients are the best resource for describing their sleep problems and how these problems differ from their usual sleep and waking patterns. The client often knows the cause of sleep problems, such as a noisy environment or worry over a relationship. In addition, bed partners are able to provide information on the client's sleep patterns that help to reveal the nature of certain sleep disorders. For example, partners of clients with sleep apnea often complain that the client's snoring disturbs their sleep. Often the partners must sleep in a different bed or move to another room to obtain adequate sleep. Ask bed partners whether clients have pauses of breathing during sleep and how frequently these pauses occur. Some partners mention becoming fearful when clients stop breathing during sleep.

When caring for children, seek information about sleep patterns from the parents, who are usually a reliable source of information about their child's trouble with sleeping.

An infant's difficulty in falling asleep or frequent awakenings during the night are often the result of hunger, excessive warmth, or separation anxiety. Parents of infants need to keep a 24-hour log of their infant's waking and sleeping behaviour for several days to determine the cause of the problem. Ask the parents to describe the infant's eating pattern and sleeping environment, both of which can influence sleeping behaviour. Older children often are able to verbalize the fears or worries that inhibit their ability to fall asleep. If children frequently awaken in the middle of bad dreams, parents are able to identify the problem, although they may not be able to understand the meanings of the dreams. Ask parents to describe the typical behaviour patterns that foster or impair sleep. For example, excessive stimulation from active play or from visiting friends will predictably impair sleep. In the case of a child who experiences chronic sleep problems, ask the parents to describe the duration of the problem, its progression, and the child's responses.

Tools for Sleep Assessment. Subjective reports of sleep are reliable and valid measures of sleep (Cohen, 2004). One effective, brief method for assessing sleep quality is the use of a visual analog scale (Cohen, 2004). Draw a straight horizontal line 100 mm long. At the opposite ends of the line, print two opposing statements, such as "best night's sleep" and "worst night's sleep." Ask clients to mark a point on the horizontal line that corresponds to their perception of the previous night's sleep. Measure the distance of the mark along the line in millimetres; this number is a numerical value for satisfaction with sleep. Use the scale repeatedly to show change over time. Such a scale is useful to assess an individual client, not to compare clients.

Another brief subjective method to assess sleep is a numeric scale with a 0 to 10 sleep rating (Cohen, 2004). Instruct clients to first rate their sleep quantity, then their quality of sleep on a scale of 1 to 10, with 0 being the worst sleep and 10 being the best sleep.

Sleep History

When a client reports having received adequate sleep, a sleep history is usually brief. The information needed for you to plan care conducive to sleep includes the following: the usual bedtime, normal bedtime rituals, the preferred environment for sleeping, and the time the client usually rises. When you suspect a sleep problem, explore the quality and characteristics of sleep in greater depth by asking clients to describe the nature of their sleep, including recent changes in their sleep pattern, sleep symptoms experienced during waking hours, use of sleep medications and other prescribed or over-the-counter medications, diet and intake of substances such as caffeine or alcohol that influence sleep, and recent life events that may have affected the client's mental and emotional status.

Description of Sleeping Problems. When a client reports a sleep problem, you need to conduct a more detailed history. A detailed assessment ensures that the appropriate therapeutic care is provided. Open-ended questions help a client to describe the problem more fully. After the client provides a general description of the problem, you can ask some focused questions, which will usually reveal specific characteristics that are useful in planning therapies. To begin, you need to understand the nature of the sleep problem, its signs and symptoms, its onset and duration, its severity, any predisposing factors or causes, and the overall effect on the client. Ask specific questions related to the sleep problem (Box 41–6).

Proper questioning helps to determine the type of sleep disturbance and the nature of the problem. Box 41–7 gives examples of additional questions for you to ask the client when you suspect specific sleep disorders. The questions assist in selecting specific sleep therapies and the best time for implementation.

As an adjunct to the sleep history, have the client and the client's bed partner keep a sleep–wake log for 1 to 4 weeks (Cohen, 2004). The client completes the sleep–wake log daily to provide information on day-to-day variations in sleep–wake patterns over extended periods. Entries in the log can include 24-hour information about various waking and sleeping health behaviours, such as physical activities, mealtimes, type and amount of alcohol and caffeine consumed, time and length of daytime naps, evening and bedtime routines, the time the client tries to fall asleep, the time of nighttime awakenings, and the time of morning awakening. A partner helps to record the estimated times the client falls asleep or awakens. Although the log is helpful, the client needs to be motivated to participate in recording the entries.

Usual Sleep Pattern. Normal sleep is difficult to define because individuals vary in their perception of the adequate quantity and quality of sleep. Clients need to describe their usual sleep pattern to determine the significance of the changes caused by a sleep disorder. Knowing a client's usual, preferred sleep pattern allows you to try to match the sleeping conditions in a health care setting to the sleeping conditions in the home. Ask the following questions to determine a client's sleep pattern:

1. What time do you usually go to bed each night?
2. What time do you usually fall asleep? Do you do anything special to help you fall asleep?
3. How many times do you awaken during the night? Why?
4. What time do you typically wake in the morning?
5. What is the average number of hours you sleep each night?

Compare the client data with the predominant sleep pattern for other clients of the same age. On the basis of this comparison, you can begin to assess for identifiable patterns, which may indicate a specific sleep disturbance, such as insomnia.

➤ BOX 41-6 Nursing Assessment Questions

Nature of the Problem

What type of problem are you having with your sleep?
Why do you think your sleep is inadequate?
Describe for me a recent typical night's sleep. How is this sleep different from what you are accustomed to?

Signs and Symptoms

Do you have difficulty falling asleep, staying asleep, or waking up?
Have you been told that you snore loudly?
Do you have headaches when awakening? Does your child awaken from nightmares?

Onset and Duration

When did you notice the problem?
How long has this problem lasted?

Severity

How long does it take you to fall asleep?
How often during the week do you have trouble falling asleep?
How many hours of sleep a night did you get this week?
How does this amount of sleep compare to what is usual for you?
What do you do when you awaken during the night or when you awaken too early in the morning?

Predisposing Factors

What do you do just before you go to bed?
Have you recently had any changes at work or at home?
How is your mood? Have you noticed any changes in your mood recently?
What medications or recreational drugs do you take on a regular basis?
Are you taking any new prescription or over-the-counter medications?
Do you eat food (spicy or greasy foods) or drink substances (alcohol or caffeinated beverages) that interfere with your sleep?
Do you have a physical illness that interferes with your sleep?
Does anyone in your family have a history of sleep problems?

Effect on the Client

How has the loss of sleep affected you?
Do you feel excessively sleepy or irritable? Do you have trouble concentrating during waking hours?
Do you have trouble staying awake? Have you fallen asleep at inappropriate times, for example, while driving, sitting quietly in a meeting, or watching TV?

➤ BOX 41-7 Questions to Ask to Assess for Specific Sleep Disorders

Insomnia

How easily do you fall asleep?
After you fall asleep, do you have difficulty staying asleep? How many times do you awaken?
What time do you awaken in the morning? What causes you to awaken early?
What do you do to prepare for sleep? What do you do to improve your sleep?
What do you think about as you try to fall asleep?
How often do you have trouble sleeping?

Sleep Apnea

Do you snore loudly? Does anyone else in your family snore loudly?
Has anyone (e.g., spouse, bed partner, roommate) ever told you that you stop breathing for short periods during your sleep?
Do you experience headaches after awakening?
Do you have difficulty staying awake during the day?

Narcolepsy

Do you fall asleep at inopportune times? (Friends or relatives may report any occurrences.)
Have you ever had an episode of losing muscle control or falling to the floor?
Have you ever had the feeling of being unable to move or talk just before falling asleep?
Do you have vivid lifelike dreams when going to sleep or waking up?

Clients with sleep problems frequently show patterns that differ drastically from their usual sleep pattern, or sometimes the change is relatively minor. Hospitalized clients usually need or want more sleep as a result of their illness; however, some clients require less sleep because they are less active. Some clients who are ill think that they need to try to sleep more than their usual amount of sleep, a perception that eventually makes sleeping difficult.

Physical and Psychological Illness. Determine whether the client has any pre-existing health problems that interfere with sleep. A history of psychiatric problems can also contribute to sleep disturbances. For example, a bipolar, or manic-depressive, client sleeps more when depressed than when manic. A depressed client often experiences an inadequate amount of fragmented sleep. Chronic diseases, such as chronic obstructive pulmonary disease, and painful disorders, such as arthritis, interfere with sleep. Assess the client's medication history, including a description of over-the-counter and prescribed drugs. If a client takes medications to aid sleep, gather information about the type and amount of medication that the client uses. Also assess the client's daily caffeine intake.

If the client has recently undergone surgery, expect the client to experience some disturbance in sleep. During the first night after surgery, clients usually awaken frequently and receive little deep sleep, or REM sleep. Depending on the type of surgery, several days to months may pass before a normal sleep cycle returns.

Current Life Events. During your assessment, ask whether the client is experiencing any changes in lifestyle that could disrupt sleep. A person's occupation often offers a clue to the nature of the sleep problem. Changes in job responsibilities, rotating shifts, or long hours contribute to a sleep disturbance. You can question the client about social activities, recent travel, or mealtime schedules to help clarify the sleep assessment.

Emotional and Mental Status. The client's emotions and mental status affect the ability to sleep. For example, insomnia often results when the client is experiencing anxiety, emotional stress related to illness, or a situational crisis, such as the loss of a job or the death of a loved one. Clients with psychiatric disorders may need mild sedation to obtain adequate rest. Assess the effectiveness of any medication and its effect on daytime function.

Bedtime Routines. Ask clients what they do to prepare for sleep. For example, the client may drink a glass of milk, take a sleeping pill, eat a snack, or watch television. Note the habits that are beneficial compared with those that disturb sleep. For example, watching television may promote sleep for one person, whereas watching TV may stimulate another person to stay awake. Sometimes pointing out that a particular habit is interfering with sleep helps clients to find ways to change or eliminate that habit.

Pay special attention to a child's bedtime rituals. Parents need to report whether it is necessary, for example, to read the child a bedtime story, rock the child to sleep, or engage in quiet play. Some young children need a special blanket or stuffed animal when going to sleep.

Bedroom Environment. During your assessment, ask the client to describe the preferred bedroom conditions. These preferences may include the lighting in the room, music or television in the background, or the need to have the bedroom door open or closed. Some children require the company of a parent to fall asleep. In a health care environment, environmental distractions often interfere with sleep, such as a roommate's television, an electronic monitor in the hallway, a noisy nurses' station, or another client who cries out at night. Identify strategies that you or the client can use to reduce the effects of the distractions or to control the environment.

Behaviours of Sleep Deprivation. Some clients are unaware of how their sleep problems affect their behaviour. Observe the client for behaviours such as irritability, disorientation (similar to a drunken state), frequent yawning, and slurred speech. If sleep deprivation has lasted a long time, psychotic behaviour, such as delusions and paranoia, sometimes develop. For example, a client may report seeing strange objects or colours in the room, or the client may act afraid when a nurse enters the room.

Client Expectations

When a client experiences a poor night's sleep, a vicious cycle of anticipatory anxiety may begin. The client may fear that sleep will again be disturbed and will try harder and harder to sleep (Attarian, 2000). When assessing the client's sleep needs, use a skilled, individualized, and caring approach. Always ask clients what they expect regarding their sleep, the interventions they currently use, and the success of the interventions. Also ask clients which other interventions they prefer, and how they could be implemented. It is important to understand the clients' expectations regarding their sleep pattern. When clients ask for assistance because of sleep disturbances, they typically expect a nurse to respond promptly to assist them in improving their quantity and quality of sleep.

❖Nursing Diagnosis

Review your assessment to identify clusters of data that characterize a sleep pattern disturbance. If you identify a sleep pattern disturbance, specify the condition. By specifying the nature of a sleep disturbance, you are able to design more effective interventions. For example, you choose different therapies for clients with insomnia than for clients with sleep apnea. Box 41–8 demonstrates how to use nursing assessment activities to identify and cluster defining characteristics to make an accurate nursing diagnosis.

Your assessment identifies the probable cause of or factors related to the sleep disturbance, such as a noisy environment or a high intake of caffeinated beverages in the evening. These causes become the focus of interventions for minimizing or eliminating the problem. For example, if a client is experiencing insomnia as a result of a noisy health care environment, use strategies to promote sleep, such as controlling the noise of hospital equipment, reducing interruptions, or keeping doors closed. If the insomnia is related to worry over a threatened marital separation, introduce coping strategies, and create an environment for sleep. If you incorrectly identify the probable cause or related factors, the client will not benefit from the strategies to minimize or eliminate the presumed sources of disruption.

Sleep problems affect clients in other ways. For example, you may find that a client with sleep apnea is in conflict with a spouse who is tired of and frustrated over the client's snoring. In addition, the spouse may be concerned that the client is breathing improperly and thus is in danger. The nursing diagnosis of *compromised family coping* indicates that you need to provide support to both the client and the client's spouse so that they both understand sleep apnea and obtain the medical treatment needed. Examples of nursing diagnoses for clients with sleep problems include the following:

- *Anxiety*
- *Ineffective breathing pattern*
- *Acute confusion*
- *Compromised family coping*

> BOX 41-8 NURSING DIAGNOSTIC PROCESS

Insomnia

Assessment Activities	*Defining Characteristics*
Ask the client to explain the nature of the sleep problem.	The client reports difficulty in falling asleep, which sometimes takes up to 1 hour. The client reports awakening two to three times nightly, followed by difficulty returning to sleep.
Observe the client's behaviour, and ask the client's spouse whether the client is experiencing behavioural changes.	The client reports not feeling well rested. The spouse describes times when the client was lethargic and irritable.
Determine whether the client has experienced recent lifestyle changes.	The spouse reports the client recently lost his or her job and is concerned about finding a new position.

- *Ineffective coping*
- *Fatigue*
- *Ineffective protection*
- *Insomnia*
- *Disturbed sensory perception*
- *Sleep deprivation*

❖Planning

Goals and Outcomes

During your planning of a strategy of care, you again synthesize information from multiple resources to develop an individualized plan of care (Figure 41–4, Box 41–9). Ensure you consider standards of nursing practice and clinical guidelines when developing a care plan. Clinical guidelines are based on a systematic review of research, other guidelines and expert practice recommendations. For example general nursing care strategies need to be individualized and based on a thorough sleep assessment of the client and family (Chasens et al 2008).

As you plan care for the client with sleep disturbances, you can create a concept map to help develop a holistic approach to client-centred care (Figure 41–5). Create the concept map after identifying the relevant nursing diagnoses from the assessment database. In this example, the nursing diagnoses are linked to the client's medical diagnosis of depression following the death of her spouse. The concept map shows the relationships between the nursing diagnoses *dysfunctional grieving, disturbed sleep pattern,* and *impaired social interaction.* This approach to planning care can assist you in recognizing relationships between planned interventions. For this client, interventions and successful outcomes for one nursing diagnosis affect the resolution of another nursing diagnosis.

When developing goals and outcomes, you and the client need to collaborate. As a result, you will be more likely to set realistic goals and measurable outcomes. An effective plan includes outcomes that focus on the goal of improving the quantity and quality of sleep in the home over a realistic period of time. Family members are often very helpful in contributing to the plan. A sleep promotion plan frequently requires many weeks to accomplish. The following is an example of a goal with client outcomes:

Goal: The client will control the environmental sources that disrupt sleep within 1 month.

Outcomes:

- The client will identify factors in the immediate home environment that disrupt sleep within 2 weeks.
- The client will report having a discussion with family members about environmental barriers to sleep within 2 weeks.
- The client will report changes made in the bedroom to promote sleep within 4 weeks.
- The client will report having fewer than two awakenings per night within 4 weeks.

Setting Priorities

Work with the client to establish the priority outcomes and interventions. Sleep disturbances are frequently the result of other health problems. For example, when physical symptoms are interfering with sleep, management of the symptoms is your first priority. Once the

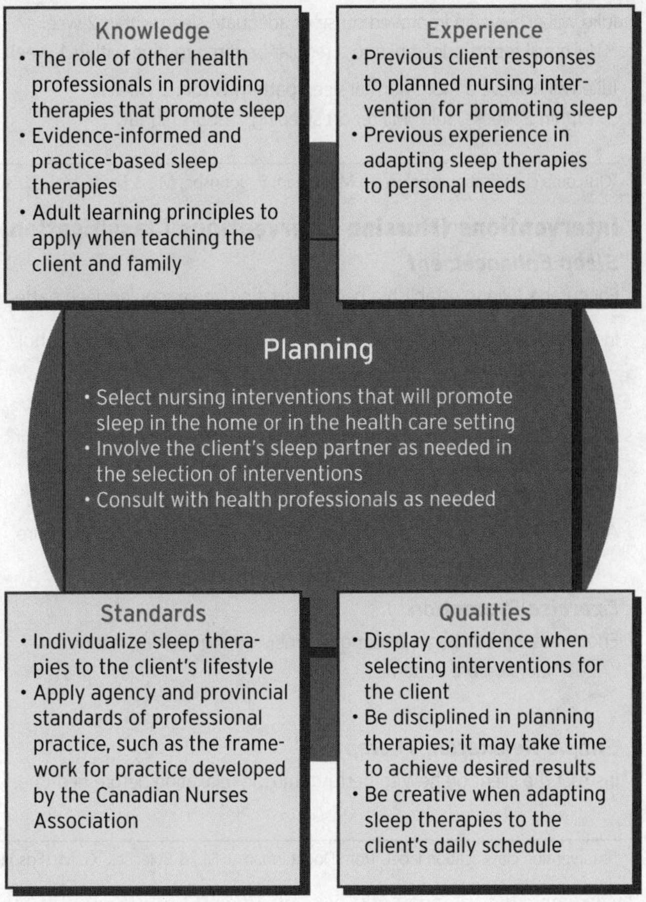

Knowledge
- The role of other health professionals in providing therapies that promote sleep
- Evidence-informed and practice-based sleep therapies
- Adult learning principles to apply when teaching the client and family

Experience
- Previous client responses to planned nursing intervention for promoting sleep
- Previous experience in adapting sleep therapies to personal needs

Planning
- Select nursing interventions that will promote sleep in the home or in the health care setting
- Involve the client's sleep partner as needed in the selection of interventions
- Consult with health professionals as needed

Standards
- Individualize sleep therapies to the client's lifestyle
- Apply agency and provincial standards of professional practice, such as the framework for practice developed by the Canadian Nurses Association

Qualities
- Display confidence when selecting interventions for the client
- Be disciplined in planning therapies; it may take time to achieve desired results
- Be creative when adapting sleep therapies to the client's daily schedule

Figure 41-4 Critical thinking model for sleep planning.

BOX 41-9 NURSING CARE PLAN

Disturbed Sleep Pattern

Assessment

Julie Arnold, a 42-year-old lawyer, is the first client of the day at the neighbourhood health clinic where you work. When you ask her how she is doing, she tells you she is having difficulty sleeping. Julie is married and has two school-age children. Julie's assessment includes a thorough sleep history and a discussion of how the sleep problem is affecting her life. A physical examination is also completed.

Assessment Activities	***Findings and Defining Characteristics***
Ask Julie to explain the nature of her sleep problem.	Julie says she wakes up once or twice a night. She states, *"I feel tired when I wake up, and I have trouble concentrating at work in the afternoon."* She also *reports* that she has less patience with her children.
Ask Julie whether she has had any recent changes in her life.	Julie says she is feeling pressured at work to complete an important case that she started 2 weeks ago. She also reports that she has *stopped* her routine of walking 2–4 km daily because of her heavy workload.
Ask Julie to describe her bedtime routine.	Julie reports she is going to bed between midnight and 1 A.M., which is 2 hours later than her usual bedtime. *It takes her an hour to fall asleep.* In the past, she received 7–8 hours of sleep each night, but now *it is closer to 5–6 hours.* She drinks two to three cups of coffee after dinner while she is working on her case. Julie reports drinking a glass of wine before bedtime to help her relax because she has been having trouble falling asleep.
Assess Julie for signs of sleep problems.	During your examination, you note that Julie has dark circles under her eyes; she shifts her position in her chair multiple times and yawns frequently.

*Defining characteristics are in italic type.

Nursing Diagnosis: Insomnia related to psychological stress from job pressures.

Planning

Goals (Nursing Outcomes Classification)[†]	***Expected Outcomes***
Sleep	
Julie will achieve an improved sense of adequate sleep within 2 weeks.	Julie will report waking less frequently during the night and feeling rested within 2 weeks.
Julie will report adherence to a regular bedtime routine within 1 week.	
Julie will achieve a more normal sleep pattern within 2 weeks.	Within 2 weeks, Julie will fall asleep within 30 minutes of going to bed.
Within 2 weeks, Julie will report sleeping 7 hours nightly.	

[†]Outcome classification labels from Moorhead, S., Johnson, M., & Maas, M. L. (Eds.). (2004). *Nursing Outcomes Classification (NOC)* (3rd ed.). St. Louis, MO: Mosby.

Interventions (Nursing Interventions Classification)[‡]	**Rationale**
Sleep Enhancement	
Encourage Julie to establish a bedtime routine and a regular sleep pattern.	Maintaining a consistent schedule helps induce sleep (Morin, 2003).
Instruct Julie to limit her consumption of caffeine, nicotine, and alcohol before bedtime.	Caffeine and nicotine are stimulants and cause difficulty in falling asleep. Alcohol has the effect of lightening and fragmenting sleep (Morin, 2003).
Assist Julie in identifying ways to eliminate stressful concerns about work before bedtime (e.g., taking time before actual sleep time to read a light novel).	Excess worry and intense activities before bedtime may stimulate the client and prevent sleep (Robinson et al., 2005).
Adjust the sleep environment: have Julie control the noise, temperature, and light in the bedroom.	Develop an environment conducive to sleep (Morin et al., 2007).
Exercise Promotion	
Encourage Julie to begin walking routinely during the day, but not 2–3 hours before bedtime.	Regular exercise increases activity levels and improves sleep quality. When exercise occurs just before bedtime, it can act as a stimulant that prevents sleep (Hoffman, 2003).
Simple Relaxation Therapy	
Instruct the client on how to perform muscle relaxation before bedtime.	Relaxation therapy can help to reduce anxiety, which interferes with sleep (Richardson, 2003).

[‡]Intervention classification labels from Dochterman, J. M., & Bulechek, G. M. (Eds.) (2004). *Nursing Interventions Classification (NIC)* (4th ed.). St. Louis, MO: Mosby.

➤ BOX 41-9 NURSING CARE PLAN *continued*

Evaluation

Nursing Actions	*Client Response and Finding*	*Achievement of Outcome*
Ask Julie whether she is able to fall asleep and stay asleep.	Julie responds, "It usually takes me 15–20 minutes to fall asleep, and I woke up once at night twice last week."	Julie reports she falls asleep within 30 minutes, and wakes up less frequently during the night.
Ask Julie to describe her waking behaviours at work and home during the day.	Julie responds that she has completed her case at work and feels less pressure. She has restarted her walking routine. She reports that she is better able to cope with her children. She is able to concentrate at work more.	Julie reports feeling more rested.
Observe Julie's waking nonverbal expressions and behaviour.	Julie sits in the chair without shifting position. She does not yawn during the interview. The circles under her eyes are almost gone.	Julie says she sleeps for an average of 7 hours a night.

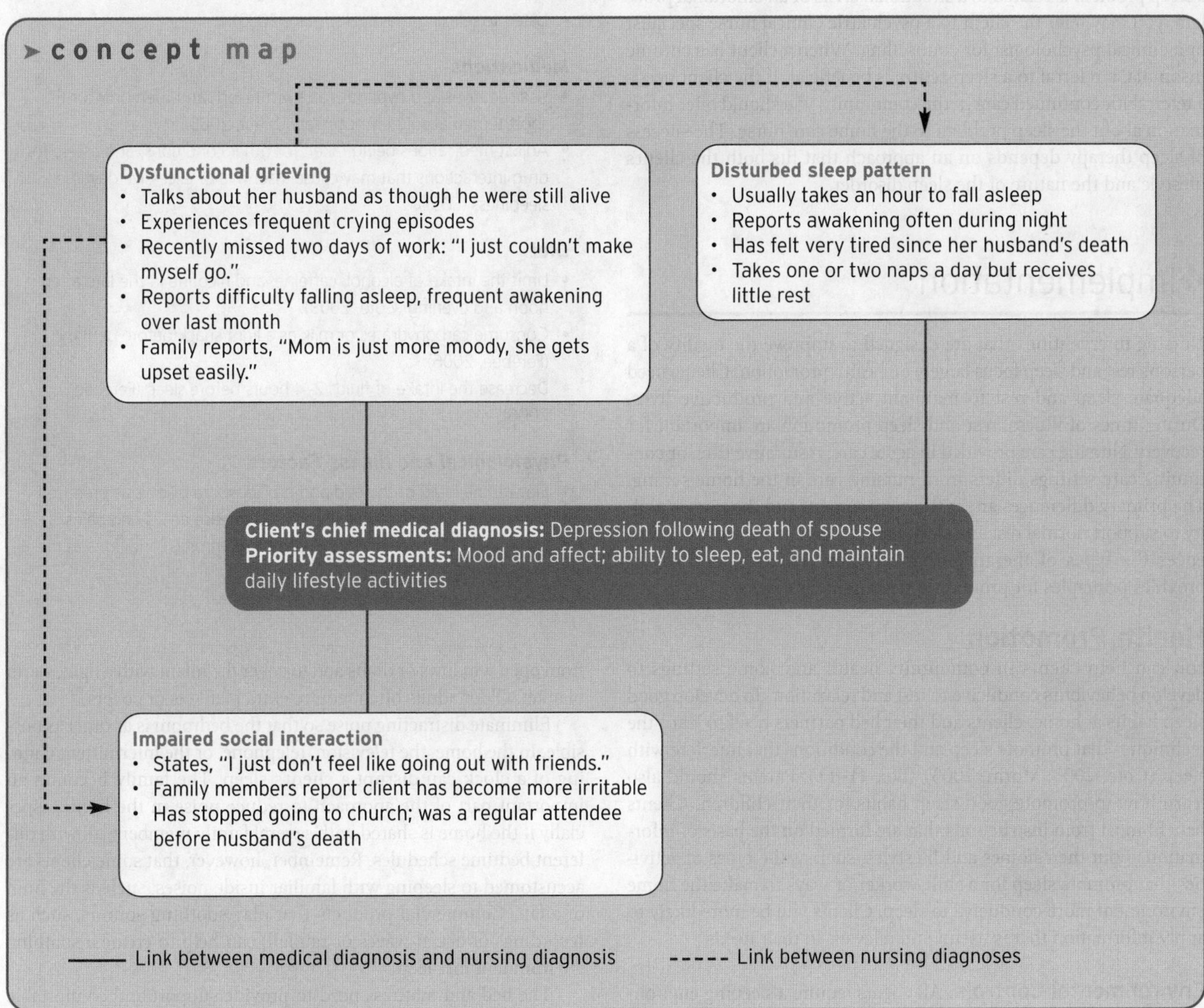

Figure 41-5 Concept map for a client who has depression following the death of her spouse.

symptoms are relieved, you can then focus on sleep therapies. Clients are helpful resources in determining which interventions hold priority. For example, after clients understand the factors that disrupt sleep, they can make choices regarding the changes they would like to make in their lifestyle or sleeping environment.

Collaborative Care

Partner closely with the client and the client's significant others to ensure that any therapies, such as a change in the sleep schedule or changes to the bedroom environment, are realistic and achievable. In a health care setting, plan the treatments or routines so that the client is able to rest. For example, in the intensive care unit, use available electronic monitors to track trends in vital signs without awakening the client each hour. Other staff members need to be aware of the care plan so they can cluster activities at certain times to reduce the number of awakenings. In a nursing home, the focus of the plan involves better planning of rest periods around the activities of the other residents. Often, clients' roommates have very different schedules that need to be taken into account.

The nature of the sleep disturbance determines whether referrals are necessary to additional health care professionals. For example, if a sleep problem is related to a situational crisis or an emotional problem, you may refer the client to a psychiatric clinical nurse specialist or a clinical psychologist for counselling. When a client has chronic insomnia, a referral to a sleep centre is beneficial. If the client needs a referral for continued care in the community, you should offer information about the sleep problem to the home care nurse. The success of sleep therapy depends on an approach that fits both the client's lifestyle and the nature of the sleep disorder.

BOX 41-10 FOCUS ON OLDER ADULTS

Promoting Sleep

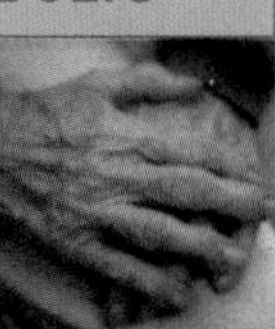

Sleep-Wake Pattern

- Maintain a regular bedtime and wake-up schedule (Cote, 2003).
- Eliminate naps unless they are a routine part of the schedule.
- If naps are used, limit them to 20 minutes or less, twice a day.
- Go to bed when sleepy.
- Use a warm bath and relaxation techniques to promote sleep (Cote, 2003; Ferebee, 2006).
- If unable to sleep within 15–30 minutes, get out of bed.

Environment

- Sleep where you sleep best.
- Keep noise to a minimum; use soft music to mask noise if necessary.
- Use a night light and keep the path to the bathroom free of obstacles.
- Set the room temperature to your preference; use socks to promote warmth.
- Listen to relaxing music (Hoffman, 2003).

Medications

- Use sedatives and hypnotics as a last resort, and then only for the short term if absolutely necessary (Maur, 2005).
- Adjust medications being taken for other conditions, and assess for drug interactions that may cause insomnia or excessive daytime sleepiness (EDS).

Diet

- Limit the intake of alcohol, caffeine, and nicotine in the late afternoon and evening (Cote, 2003).
- Consume carbohydrates or milk as a light snack before bedtime (Ferebee, 2006).
- Decrease the intake of fluids 2–4 hours before sleep (Ferebee, 2006).

Physiological and Illness Factors

- Elevate the head of the bed and provide extra pillows as preferred.
- Use analgesics 30 minutes before bed to ease aches and pains.
- Use therapeutics to control symptoms of chronic conditions as prescribed (Maur, 2005).

❖Implementation

Nursing interventions that are designed to improve the quality of a person's rest and sleep focus largely on health promotion. Clients need adequate sleep and rest to maintain active and productive lives. During times of illness, rest and sleep promotion are important for recovery. Nursing care provided in acute care, restorative care, or continuing care settings differs from nursing care in the home setting. The primary differences are in the environment and the nurse's ability to support normal rest and sleep habits. The client's age also influences the types of therapies that are most effective. Box 41–10 provides principles for promoting sleep in older clients.

Health Promotion

You can help clients in community health and home settings to develop behaviours conducive to rest and relaxation. To develop good sleep habits at home, clients and their bed partners need to learn the techniques that promote sleep and the conditions that interfere with sleep (Cote, 2003; Morin, 2003) (Box 41–11). Parents should also learn how to promote good sleep habits for their children. Clients benefit most from instructions that are formed on the basis of information about their homes and lifestyles, such as the types of activities that promote sleep for a shift-worker or ways to make the home environment more conducive to sleep. Clients will be more likely to apply information that is useful and relevant to their needs.

Environmental Controls. All clients require a sleeping environment with a comfortable room temperature, proper ventilation, minimal noise, a comfortable bed, and proper lighting (Dochterman & Bulechek, 2004). Children and adults vary in their preferences for a comfortable room temperature. Instruct parents to position cribs away from open windows or drafts and to cover the infant with a light, warm blanket. Older adults often require extra blankets or covers.

Eliminate distracting noise so that the bedroom is as quiet as possible. In the home, the television, telephone, or the intermittent chiming of a clock can disrupt a client's sleep. The family becomes an important part of the approach to reduce noise in the home, especially if the home is shared with several family members, all with different bedtime schedules. Remember, however, that some clients are accustomed to sleeping with familiar inside noises, such as the hum of a fan. Commercial products that play soothing sounds, such as recordings of ocean waves or rainfall, can help to create a soothing environment for sleep.

The bed and mattress need to provide support and comfortable firmness. Bed boards can be placed under mattresses to provide additional support. Sometimes extra pillows can help to position a person comfortably in bed. For some clients, the position of the bed in the room also makes a difference.

BOX 41-11 CLIENT TEACHING

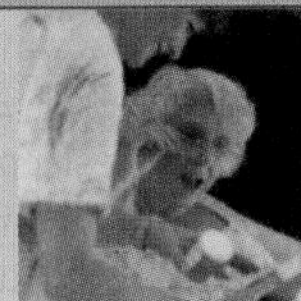

Sleep Hygiene Habits

Objective

- Client will follow proper sleep hygiene habits at home.

Teaching Strategies

- Instruct the client to try to exercise daily, preferably in the morning or afternoon, and to avoid vigorous exercise within 2 hours of bedtime.
- Caution the client against sleeping long hours during weekends or holidays to prevent disturbance of the normal sleep–wake cycle.
- Explain that the client should not use the bedroom for intensive studying, snacking, TV watching, or other nonsleep activity, besides sex.
- Encourage the client to try to avoid worrisome thinking when going to bed and to practise relaxation exercises.
- If the client does not fall asleep within 30 minutes of going to bed, advise the client to get out of bed and do some quiet activity until the client feels sleepy enough to go back to bed.
- Recommend the client limit caffeine intake to a morning coffee and limit alcohol intake (more than 1–2 drinks a day interrupts the sleep cycle).
- Ask the client to examine the sleeping environment. If noise or light is an issue, suggest the use of earplugs or eyeshades.
- Instruct the client to avoid heavy meals for 3 hours before bedtime; the client may have a light snack before bedtime.

Evaluation

- Ask the client to complete a sleep–wake and activity diary for 1 week, and compare it with the previous week's diary.
- Ask the client to periodically complete a visual analog or sleep rating scale to record perceptions of quality of sleep.

Clients vary in their preference for the amount of light they can tolerate in the bedroom. Infants and older adults sleep best in softly lit rooms. Light should not shine directly on their eyes. Small table lamps can be used to prevent total darkness. For older adults, proper lighting reduces the chance of confusion and prevents falls while walking to the bathroom. Heavy shades, drapes, or slatted blinds are helpful if streetlights shine through windows, or if clients nap during the day.

Promoting Bedtime Routines. Bedtime routines help to relax clients in preparation for sleep (Dochterman & Bulechek, 2004). Persons should to go to bed when they feel fatigued or sleepy. Going to bed while fully awake and thinking about other things often leads to insomnia and interferes with the perception of the bed as a stimulus for sleep. Newborns and infants sleep through so much of the day that a specific routine is hardly necessary. However, quiet activities, such as holding them snugly in blankets, singing or talking softly, and gentle rocking, help infants to fall asleep.

Parents need to reinforce short, predictable routines associated with preparing for bedtime (Weiss, 2005). A bedtime routine that is used consistently (e.g., the same hour for bedtime, eating a snack, or pursuing a quiet activity) helps young children to avoid delaying sleep. Bedtime routines can include quiet activities such as reading stories, colouring, allowing children to sit in a parent's lap while listening to music, or listening to a prayer.

Adults need to avoid excessive mental stimulation just before bedtime. Reading a light novel, watching an enjoyable television program, or listening to music can help a person to relax. Relaxation exercises, such as slow, deep breathing for 1 or 2 minutes, can help to relieve tension and prepare the body for rest (see Chapter 36). Guided imagery and praying also promote sleep for some clients.

At home, discourage clients from trying to finish office work or to resolve family problems before bedtime. The bedroom is not a place to work, and clients need to always associate the bedroom with sleep. Working toward a consistent time for sleeping and wakening helps most clients to gain a healthy sleep pattern and to strengthen the rhythm of their sleep–wake cycle.

Promoting Safety. For any client prone to confusion or falls, safety is critical. A small night light can assist the client in orienting to the room environment before going to the bathroom. Beds set lower to the floor reduce the chance of a person falling when first standing. Instruct clients to remove clutter and small rugs from the path used to walk from the bed to the bathroom. If a client needs assistance in ambulating from a bed to the bathroom, place a small bell at the bedside to call family members. Sleepwalkers are unaware of their surroundings and are slow to react, which increases their risk of falls. Do not startle sleepwalkers but instead gently awaken them and lead them back to bed.

Infants' beds need to be safe. To reduce the chance of suffocation, do not place pillows, stuffed toys, or the ends of loose blankets in cribs. Loose-fitting plastic mattress covers are dangerous because infants can pull them over their face and suffocate. Parents should place infants on their back to prevent sudden infant death syndrome (SIDS) (Driver, 2003).

Promoting Comfort. People fall asleep only after feeling comfortable and relaxed (Dochterman & Bulechek, 2004). Minor irritants often keep clients awake. Soft cotton nightclothes keep infants or small children warm and comfortable. Instruct clients to wear loose-fitting nightwear. An extra blanket is sometimes all that is necessary to prevent a person from feeling chilled and thus being unable to fall asleep. Clients need to void before retiring so they are not kept awake by a full bladder.

Establishing Periods of Rest and Sleep. Encourage clients living at home to stay physically active during the day so that they will be more likely to sleep at night. Increasing daytime activity reduces the likelihood of having problems with falling asleep. In the home setting, nurses frequently care for clients with chronic debilitating disease. The nursing care plan includes having clients set aside afternoons for rest to promote optimal health. To provide uninterrupted rest periods, adjust clients' medication schedules, instruct clients to void before rest periods, and suggest unplugging the telephone.

Stress Reduction. The inability to sleep because of emotional stress can make a person feel irritable and tense. When clients feel emotionally upset, encourage them not to force sleep. Otherwise, insomnia can develop, and bedtime is soon associated with the inability to relax. Encourage a client who has difficulty falling asleep to get up and pursue a relaxing activity, such as reading, rather than staying in bed and thinking about sleep.

Preschoolers have bedtime fears (e.g., fear of the dark or fear of strange noises) and frequently awaken during the night or have nightmares. When a child experiences a nightmare, the parent should enter the child's room immediately and talk to the child briefly about fears to provide a cooling-down period. One approach is to comfort children and leave them in their own beds so that their fears are not used as an excuse to delay bedtime. Keeping a light turned on in the room will also help some children. Cultural tradition causes families to approach sleep practices differently (Box 41–12).

BOX 41-12 CULTURAL ASPECTS OF CARE

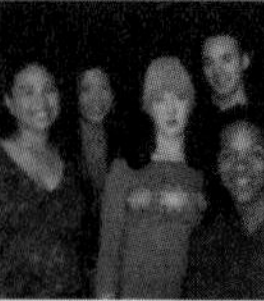

Practices and patterns of sleep and rest vary among cultures. Culture and biology influence the development of sleep problems in children. Sleep patterns, bedtime routines, sleep aids, and sleep arrangements are a component of the cultural practices related to the use of space and the perception of comfortable distances for interactions with others. Sleep experts traditionally recommend having infants and children sleep in their own beds. Co-sleeping (i.e., the practice of infants and children sleeping with their parents) is a culturally preferred habit and is common in nonindustrialized countries. Health care professionals in Canada frequently discourage this practice because of safety issues. The Canadian culture promotes independence in childhood. Because co-sleeping does not promote this independence, health care workers discourage it. As a nurse, you need to be culturally sensitive when discussing co-sleeping practices with parents and developing sleeping plans for children.

Implications for Practice

- Complete a thorough sleep assessment of the child and the family.
- Discuss the risks of the child sleeping with the parents. During the discussion, remain culturally sensitive and respectful of the parents' views.
- Co-sleeping affects the infant's normal sleep pattern by decreasing slow-wave sleep and increasing the number of nighttime arousals.
- Co-sleeping has been linked to an increased risk of sudden infant death syndrome (SIDS) under certain conditions, such as parental smoking and alcohol or drug use.
- Instruct parents who practise co-sleeping to avoid using alcohol or drugs that impair arousal. Decreased arousal prevents the parents from awakening if the child experiences problems.
- Co-sleeping should occur only with parents and not with another adult or child.
- Encourage the parents who co-sleep to use light sleeping clothes, to keep the room temperature comfortable, and to not bundle the child tightly or in too many clothes.

Data from Andrews, M. M., & Boyle, J. S. (2003). *Transcultural concepts in nursing care* (4th ed.). Philadelphia: Lippincott; Davis, K. F., Parker, K. P., & Montgomery, G. L. (2004). Sleep in infants and young children. Part I: Normal sleep, *Journal of Pediatric Health Care, 18* (2), 65–71; Giger, J. N., & Davidhizar, R. E. (2004). *Transcultural nursing: Assessment and intervention* (4th ed.). St. Louis: Mosby; Jenni, O. G., & O'Connor, B. B. (2005). Children's sleep: An interplay between culture and biology. *Pediatrics, 115*, 204–216.

Bedtime Snacks. Some persons enjoy bedtime snacks, whereas others cannot sleep after eating. A dairy product snack, such as warm milk or cocoa, contains L-tryptophan and is often helpful in promoting sleep. A full meal before bedtime often causes gastrointestinal upset and can interfere with the ability to fall asleep.

Encourage clients to avoid drinking or ingesting caffeine before bedtime. Because coffee, tea, cola, and chocolate act as stimulants, they can cause a person to stay awake or to awaken throughout the night (Morin, 2003). Infants require special measures to minimize their nighttime awakenings for feeding. Children commonly need a middle-of-the-night bottle or to breastfeed at night. Hockenberry and Wilson (2007) recommend offering the last feeding as late as possible. Instruct parents not to give infants bottles in bed.

Pharmacological Approaches. Melatonin is a neurohormone produced in the brain that helps control circadian rhythms and promote sleep (Scheer et al., 2005). Melatonin is a popular nutritional supplement to aid sleep. The recommended dosage is 0.3 to 1 mg taken 2 hours before bedtime. Older adults who have decreased levels of melatonin find taking melatonin to be beneficial as a sleep aid (Scheer et al., 2005). Several other herbal products also assist in promoting sleep. Valerian is effective in mild insomnia. It effects the release of neurotransmitters and produces a very mild sedation (Buysse et al., 2005). Kava helps promote sleep in clients who have sleep problems related to anxiety but needs to be used cautiously because of its potential toxic effects on the liver (Morin et al., 2007). Chamomile, passion flower, lemon balm, and lavender are other herbal products that have mild sedative effects (Elliott, 2001). Caution clients about the dosage and use of herbal compounds. Because some herbal compounds interact with prescribed medication, clients should avoid using these treatments together (Ferebee, 2006) (see Chapter 35).

The use of nonprescription sleeping medications is not advisable. Clients need to learn the risks of such drugs. Although these drugs initially seem to be effective, over the long term, they can lead to further sleep disruption. Help clients to use behavioural and proper sleep hygiene habits to establish sleep patterns that do not require the use of drugs.

Acute Care

Clients in an acute care setting frequently have their normal rest and sleep routines disrupted, which, in general, leads to sleep problems. In this setting, nursing interventions focus on controlling factors in the environment that disrupt sleep, relieving physiological or psychological disruptions to sleep, and providing uninterrupted rest and sleep periods for the client.

Environmental Controls. In a hospital setting, nurses can control the environment in several ways. In semiprivate rooms, the curtains should be closed between clients. The lights on a hospital nursing unit should be dimmed at night. Noise levels can be reduced by conducting conversations and reports in a private area away from client rooms and by keeping necessary conversations to a minimum, especially at night (Cmiel et al., 2004). Additional ways to control noise in the hospital are listed in Box 41–13.

Promoting Comfort. Compared with beds at home, hospital beds are often harder and of a different height, length, or width. Keeping beds clean and dry and in a comfortable position helps clients to relax. Some clients who have painful illnesses require special comfort measures, such as the application of dry or moist heat, use of supportive dressings or splints, or proper positioning before retiring (Figure 41–6).

BOX 41-13 Control of Noise in the Hospital

- Close the doors to clients' rooms when possible.
- Keep the doors to work areas on the unit closed when in use.
- Reduce the volume of nearby telephone and paging equipment.
- Wear soft-soled shoes.
- Turn off bedside oxygen and other equipment that is not in use.
- Turn down alarms and beeps on bedside monitoring equipment.
- Turn off the room's TV and radio unless the client prefers soft music.
- Avoid abrupt loud noises, such as flushing a toilet unnecessarily or moving a bed if it can wait until morning.
- Keep necessary conversations at a quiet level, particularly at night.
- Conduct conversations and oral reports in a private area away from client rooms.

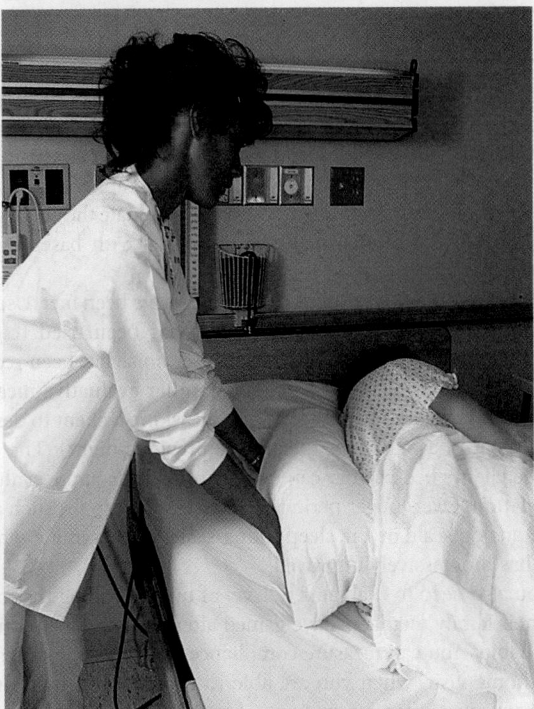

Figure 41-6 Positioning a client for sleep.

Establishing Periods of Rest and Sleep. In a hospital or long-term care setting, it is sometimes difficult to provide clients with the time needed to rest and sleep. However, you should plan your nursing care to avoid awakening clients for nonessential tasks. When possible, schedule assessments, treatments, procedures, and routines for times when clients are awake. For example, if a client's physical condition has been stable, avoid awakening the client to check vital signs. Allowing clients to determine the timing and methods of delivery of personal care measures will promote rest. Do not choose to give baths and routine hygiene measures during the night because that timing may be most convenient for the nursing staff. Draw blood samples at a time when the client is awake. Unless maintaining a drug's therapeutic blood level is essential, give medications during waking hours. Work with the radiology department and other support services to schedule diagnostic studies and therapies at intervals that allow clients time for rest. Always try to provide the client with 2 to 3 hours of uninterrupted sleep during the night (Cmiel et al., 2004).

When the client's condition demands more frequent monitoring, schedule activities to allow the client to have extended rest periods. Plan activities to ensure both that health care personnel will avoid returning to the room every few minutes and that the client will have up to an hour or more to rest quietly. For example, if a client needs frequent dressing changes, is receiving intravenous therapy, and has drainage tubes from several sites, do not make a separate trip into the room to attend to each task. Instead use a single visit to change the dressing, regulate the intravenous system, and empty the drainage tubes. Become the client's advocate for promoting optimal sleep by postponing or rescheduling visits by family, asking consultants to reschedule visits, or questioning the frequency of certain procedures.

Promoting Safety. Clients with obstructive sleep apnea are at risk for complications while in the hospital. Surgery and anaesthesia disrupt the clients' normal sleep patterns. Postoperatively, these clients reach deep levels of REM sleep. This deep sleep causes muscle relaxation that can lead to obstructive sleep apnea (Cullen, 2001). Clients with OSA who are given opioid analgesics after surgery have an increased risk of developing airway obstruction because these medications suppress the normal arousal mechanisms (Cullen, 2001). Monitor the client's airway, respiratory rate, depth, and breath sounds frequently after surgery.

Recommend lifestyle changes to clients with OSA, including sleep hygiene improvements, alcohol moderation, smoking cessation, and a weight-loss program (Mendez & Olson, 2006b). Teach the client to prevent sleeping in the supine position by wearing a fanny pack or tight shirt with a tennis ball on the back or by elevating the head of the bed 30 to 45 degrees (Holman, 2005). One of the most effective therapies is use of a nasal continuous positive airway pressure (CPAP) device at night, which requires a client to wear a mask over the nose. The mask delivers room air at a high pressure and the air pressure prevents airway collapse. The CPAP device is portable and is effective particularly for obstructive sleep apnea.

Another treatment option is the use of an oral appliance. These appliances advance the mandible or tongue to relieve pharyngeal obstruction (Mendez & Olson, 2006b). In cases of severe sleep apnea, the tonsils, uvula, or portions of the soft palate are surgically removed. Success with surgical procedures is variable.

Stress Reduction. Clients who are hospitalized for extensive diagnostic testing often have difficulty resting or sleeping because of uncertainty about their state of health. Giving clients control over their health care minimizes uncertainty and anxiety. Providing information about the purpose of procedures and routines, and answering questions will give clients the peace of mind they need to rest or to fall asleep. During the night shift, take time to sit and talk with clients who are unable to sleep. You may be able to determine the factors preventing clients from sleeping. Back rubs also help clients relax more thoroughly. If a sedative is indicated, confer with the physician to ensure the lowest dosage is used initially. Discontinue a sedative as soon as possible to prevent a dependence that can seriously disrupt the normal sleep cycle. Be aware that the metabolism of drugs in older adults is slower, making them more vulnerable to the side effects of sedatives, hypnotics, antianxiety drugs, and analgesics.

Restorative or Continuing Care

Nursing interventions implemented in the acute care setting are also used in the restorative or continuing care environment. Important considerations include controlling the environment, especially the noise level; establishing periods of rest and sleep; and promoting comfort. Nursing interventions related to stress reduction and the control of physiological disturbances are also implemented in these settings. Helping a client achieve restful sleep in this environment sometimes takes a period of time.

Promoting Comfort. Providing for personal hygiene improves a client's sense of comfort. A warm bath or shower before bedtime is relaxing. Offer clients who are restricted to bed the opportunity to void and wash their face and hands. Brushing teeth and care of dentures also help to prepare the client for sleep. Position the client so that the dependent body parts are supported and protect the pressure points. Offer a massage to aid in muscle relaxation just before the client prepares to sleep (Robinson et al., 2005) (see Chapter 42).

Controlling Physiological Disturbances. For clients with physical illness, you can help to control the symptoms that disrupt sleep. For example, a client with respiratory abnormalities sleeps with two pillows or in a semi-sitting position to ease the effort to breathe.

The client benefits from taking prescribed bronchodilators before sleep to prevent airway obstruction. A client with a hiatal hernia also needs special care. After meals, the client often experiences a burning sensation as a result of gastric reflux. To prevent sleep disturbances, have the client eat a small meal several hours before bedtime and sleep in a semi-sitting position. Clients with pain, nausea, or other recurrent symptoms should be given any symptom-relieving medication at an appropriate time so that the drug takes effect at bedtime. Remove or change any irritants against the client's skin, such as moist dressings or drainage tubes.

Pharmacological Approaches. The liberal use of drugs to manage insomnia is common. Central nervous system (CNS) stimulants, such as amphetamines, caffeine, nicotine, terbutaline, theophylline, and pemoline, need to be used sparingly and only under medical management (McKenry & Salerno, 2003). In addition, withdrawal from CNS depressants, such as alcohol, barbiturates, tricyclic antidepressants (amitriptyline, imipramine, and doxepin), and triazolam can cause insomnia. You will need to manage these medications carefully.

Medications that induce sleep are called **hypnotics. Sedatives** are medications that produce a calming or soothing effect (McKenry & Salerno, 2003). Hypnotics and sedatives can be used as sleep medications and will help, if used correctly. A client who takes sleep medications needs to understand their proper use, their risks, and their possible side effects. Long-term use of antianxiety, sedative, or hypnotic agents, however, can disrupt sleep and lead to more serious problems.

One group of drugs considered to be relatively safe is the benzodiazepines. The benzodiazepines cause relaxation, antianxiety, and hypnotic effects by facilitating the action of neurons in the CNS that suppress responsiveness to stimulation, thereby decreasing the levels of arousal (Mendelson, 2005). Unlike sedatives and hypnotics, benzodiazepines do not cause general CNS depression, and they also have a lower potential for abuse. These drugs are frequently prescribed because antianxiety effects occur at safe, nontoxic doses. In the older adult, short-acting benzodiazepines, such as temazepam and triazolam are used before long-acting drugs, and the drug should not be used for more than 10 consecutive days in any 30-day period (McKenry & Salerno, 2003).

Administer benzodiazepines cautiously with children younger than 12 years of age. These medications are contraindicated in infants younger than 6 months. Pregnant women need to avoid benzodiazepines because their use is associated with the risk of congenital anomalies. Nursing mothers do not receive these drugs because they are excreted in breast milk. Initial doses are small, and increments are added gradually, on the basis of client response, for a limited period of time. Warn clients not to take more than the prescribed dose, especially if the medication seems to become less effective after the initial use. If older clients who were continent, ambulatory, and alert suddenly become incontinent, confused, or demonstrate impaired mobility, the use of benzodiazepines needs to be considered as a possible cause. Regular use of any sleep medication often leads to drug tolerance. Rebound insomnia is a problem that can be experienced after stopping the medication. Immediately administering a sleeping medication when a hospitalized client complains of being unable to sleep will do the client more harm than good. Consider alternative approaches to promote sleep. Routine monitoring of the client's response to sleeping medications is also important.

❖Evaluation

The client is an important source of information for evaluating outcomes related to sleep and rest. Each client has a unique need for sleep and rest, and only the client will know whether sleep problems have improved, and which interventions or therapies are most successful in promoting sleep (Figure 41–7). To evaluate the effectiveness of nursing interventions, make comparisons with baseline sleep assessment data.

Determine whether expected outcomes have been met. Use evaluative measures shortly after a therapy has been tried (e.g., by observing whether a client falls asleep after noise has been reduced and the room has been darkened). Use other evaluative measures after a client awakens from sleep (e.g., by asking a client to describe the number of awakenings during the previous night). The client and the client's bed partner can usually provide accurate evaluative information. Over longer periods, use assessment tools, such as the visual analog scale or the sleep rating scale, to determine whether sleep has progressively improved.

You also need to evaluate the level of understanding that clients and their family members have gained after receiving instruction in sleep habits. You can measure compliance with these practices during a home visit, when you are able to observe the environment. When expected outcomes are not met, revise the nursing measures or expected outcomes, on the basis of the client's needs or preferences. When outcomes are not met, ask questions such as "Do you feel as

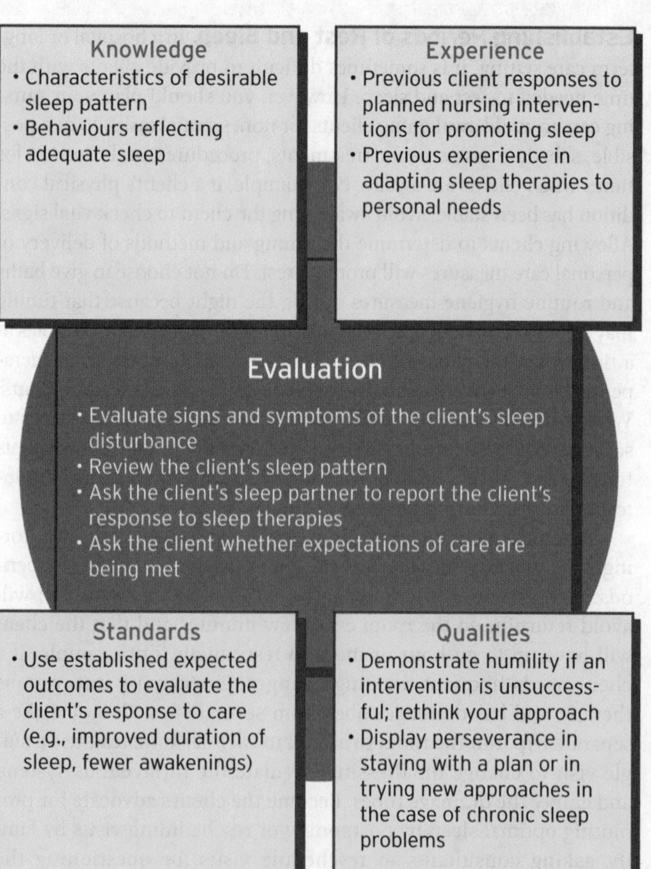

Figure 41-7 Critical thinking model for sleep evaluation.

though you slept better when you exercised?" or "Do you feel rested when you wake up?"

When nurses successfully develop good relationships with clients and when they have developed therapeutic plans of care, subtle behaviours often indicate the clients' levels of satisfaction. Note the absence of signs of sleep problems, such as lethargy, frequent yawning, or position changes. Ask the client whether his or her sleep needs have been met. For example, ask the client, "Are you feeling more rested?" or "Can you tell me if you feel we have done all we can to help improve your sleep?" If the client's expectations have not been met, you will need to spend more time trying to understand the client's needs and preferences. Working closely with the client and the client's bed partner will enable you to redefine the expectations that can be realistically met within the limits of the client's condition and treatment.

* KEY CONCEPTS

- Sleep provides physiological and psychological restoration.
- The 24-hour sleep-wake cycle is a circadian rhythm that influences physiological function and behaviour.
- The control and regulation of sleep depends on a balance between regulators within the central nervous system.
- During a typical night's sleep, a person passes through four to five complete sleep cycles. Each sleep cycle contains four nonrapid eye movement (NREM) stages of sleep and a period of rapid eye movement (REM) sleep.
- The most common type of sleep disorder is insomnia.
- The sleep pattern is frequently disrupted by the hectic pace of a person's lifestyle, emotional and psychological stress, and alcohol ingestion.
- If a client's sleep is adequate, assess the client's usual bedtime, normal bedtime ritual, preferred environment for sleeping, and usual rising time.
- When a client reports a sleep problem, conduct a complete sleep history. Diagnosing sleep problems depends on identifying the factors that impair sleep.
- When planning interventions to promote sleep, consider the characteristics of the client's home environment and normal lifestyle.
- A regular bedtime routine of relaxing activities prepares a person physically and mentally for sleep.
- An environment with a darkened room, reduced noise, comfortable bed, and good ventilation promotes sleep.
- Important nursing interventions for promoting sleep in the hospitalized client are controlling noise levels and establishing periods for uninterrupted sleep and rest.
- Pain or other disease symptom control is essential in promoting the ability to sleep.
- Long-term use of sleeping pills often leads to difficulty in initiating and maintaining sleep.

* CRITICAL THINKING EXERCISES

1. Julie returns to the neighbourhood health clinic with her husband, David, for a follow-up visit. Julie tells you that since she started her sleep hygiene plan she feels more rested but is still having some problems sleeping because of her husband's loud snoring. In addition to Julie's report of David's snoring, you note that he is overweight. On the basis of Julie's report of David's snoring, what additional assessment data should you gather from David?
2. On the basis of David's reported symptoms, what problem do you suspect he might have?
3. What action do you take at this time?
4. Julie and David also tell you that they are concerned about their 15-year-old daughter. Her grades in school are getting worse, and she says she is always tired. What do you need to know about their daughter's sleep patterns?
5. What would you recommend to Julie and David about their daughter?

* REVIEW QUESTIONS

1. You are gathering a sleep history from a client who is being evaluated for obstructive sleep apnea. What symptom is the client most likely to report?
   1. Headache
   2. Early wakening
   3. Impaired reasoning
   4. Excessive daytime sleepiness
2. When preparing a plan of care to promote sleep for a hospitalized client, which of the following priority nursing interventions would you incorporate?
   1. Ensure that the client follows hospital routines.
   2. Avoid awakening the client for nonessential tasks.
   3. Give prescribed sleeping medications at dinner.
   4. Turn the TV volume down, to late-night programming.
3. Older adults are cautioned about the use of nonprescription sleeping medications because these medications are characterized by which of the following statements?
   1. They cause headaches and nausea.
   2. They are expensive and difficult to obtain
   3. They cause severe depression and anxiety
   4. They can lead to further sleep disruption even when they initially seemed to be effective
4. You are providing health teaching for a client using herbal compounds, such as valerian, to aid sleep. Key information about the use of herbal compounds would include the following:
   1. It can cause urinary retention.
   2. It may cause diarrhea and anxiety.
   3. It may interfere with prescribed medications.
   4. It can lead to further sleep problems over time.
5. A client reports having vivid dreams. Through your understanding of the sleep cycle, you recognize that vivid dreaming occurs during which sleep phase?
   1. REM sleep
   2. Stage 1 NREM sleep
   3. Stage 4 NREM sleep
   4. Transition period from NREM to REM sleep
6. You are providing instruction for a client who is having difficulty falling asleep. You identify the need for further instruction when the client says which of the following statements?
   1. I should avoid having drinks with caffeine before going to bed.
   2. If I can't get to sleep right away, I should get up and read a book.
   3. I should have an alcoholic drink before bedtime to help me relax.
   4. I should avoid exercising just before going to bed.

7. Which of the following interventions is appropriate to include in a care plan for improving sleep in the older adult?
   1. Decrease fluids 2–4 hours before sleep.
   2. Exercise in the evening to increase fatigue.
   3. Allow the client to sleep as late as possible.
   4. Take a nap during the day to make up for lost sleep.

8. Which statement made by a mother being discharged to home with her newborn infant indicates a need for further teaching?
   1. I won't put the baby to bed with a bottle.
   2. For the first few weeks, we are putting the cradle in our room.
   3. My grandmother told me that babies sleep better on their stomachs.
   4. I know I will have to get up during the night to feed the baby when he wakes up.

9. You are developing a plan of care for a client experiencing narcolepsy. Which of the following interventions is appropriate to include in the plan?
   1. Increase the amount of carbohydrates in the diet.
   2. Limit fluid intake 2 hours before bedtime.
   3. Preserve energy by limiting exercise to morning hours.
   4. Take one or two 20-minute naps during the day.

10. Which of the following nursing measures promotes sleep in school-age children?
    1. Encourage evening exercise.
    2. Encourage television viewing.
    3. Ensure the room is dark and quiet.
    4. Encourage quiet activities before bedtime.

* RECOMMENDED WEB SITES

Canadian Lung Association: http://www.lung.ca
This Web site includes educational information on sleep apnea.

Canadian Paediatric Society: http://www.cps.ca
This Web site includes educational information about reducing the risk of sudden infant death syndrome (SIDS).

Canadian Sleep Society: http://www.css.to
This organization is a professional association for health care professionals and researchers who are interested in sleep-related conditions. The Web site also includes information for the public on sleep-related topics and links to other sleep-related organizations and services.

Public Health Agency of Canada: Division of Aging and Seniors: http://www.phac-aspc.gc.ca/seniors-aines/index_pages/whatsnew_e.htm
This government Web site includes publications that are of interest to older adults and health care professionals who work with them. Some sleep-related publications are listed in the publications section under the category Medication Use.

National Sleep Foundation (US): http://www.sleepfoundation.org
This organization is for health care professionals and laypersons interested in sleep-related topics. The Web site includes sleep-related educational material and research reports.

42

Pain and Comfort

Original chapter by Joan Wentz, RN, MSN

Canadian content written by Fay F. Warnock, RN, PhD

objectives

Mastery of content in this chapter will enable you to:

- Define the key terms listed.
- Discuss common misconceptions about pain.
- Describe the physiology of pain.
- Identify components of the pain experience.
- Explain how the physiology of pain relates to selecting interventions for pain relief.
- Describe the components of pain assessment.
- Perform an assessment of a client experiencing pain.
- Explain how cultural factors influence the pain experience.
- Describe the appropriate nursing diagnoses, outcomes, and interventions for a client with pain.
- Describe guidelines for selecting and individualizing pain interventions.
- Explain the various pharmacological approaches to treating pain.
- Describe applications for the use of nonpharmacological pain interventions.
- Discuss nursing implications for administering analgesics.
- Identify barriers to effective pain management.
- Evaluate a client's response to pain interventions.

key terms

Acupressure, p. 1030
Acupuncture, p. 1030
Acute pain, p. 1013
Addiction, p. 1038
Adjuvants, p. 1033
Anaesthetics, p. 1016
Analgesics, p. 1016
Biofeedback, p. 1030
Breakthrough pain, p. 1036
Chordotomy, p. 1035
Chronic pain, p. 1013
Cutaneous stimulation, p. 1030
Dorsal rhizotomy, p. 1035
Drug tolerance, p. 1038
Epidural analgesia, p. 1034
Epidural space, p. 1034
Guided imagery, p. 1029
Idiopathic pain, p. 1014
Local anaesthesia, p. 1034
Modulation, p. 1011
Nociceptor, p. 1010
Opioids, p. 1032
Pain, p. 1010
Pain threshold, p. 1012
Pain tolerance, p. 1012
Patient-controlled analgesia (PCA), p. 1033
Perception, p. 1011
Physical dependence, p. 1038
Placebos, p. 1039
Pruritus, p. 1035
Pseudoaddiction, p. 1013
Regional anaesthesia, p. 1034
Relaxation, p. 1029
Transcutaneous electrical nerve stimulation (TENS), p. 1030
Transduction, p. 1010

media resources

evolve Web Site

- Audio Chapter Summaries
- Glossary
- Multiple-Choice Review Questions
- Student Learning Activities
- Video Clips
- Weblinks

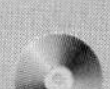
Companion CD

- Glossary
- Interactive Learning Activities
- Fluids and Electrolytes Tutorial
- Test-Taking Skills

Pain is the most common reason people seek health care. Despite being a commonly occurring symptom experienced by even the tiniest of babies, pain is not well understood. A person in pain feels distress or suffering and seeks relief. However, you cannot see or feel the client's pain. Pain is subjective; no two people will experience, feel, or respond to pain in the same way. The International Association for the Study of Pain Subcommittee on Taxonomy (1979) defines pain as "an unpleasant, subjective sensory *and* emotional experience associated with actual or potential tissue damage, or described in terms of such damage" (pp. 209–214). Thus, physical pain can cause psychological pain, and vice versa.

Comfort is central to nursing. As Donahue (1989) summarized, "Through comfort and comfort measures . . . nurses provide strength, hope, solace, support, encouragement, and assistance" (p. 27). Comfort, like pain, is highly subjective. Each person has physiological, social, spiritual, psychological, and cultural characteristics that influence how comfort is interpreted and experienced. The concept of comfort thus provides an important context for how nurses can come to understand the complexity of pain and how to effectively assess and manage pain.

You should not assume that suffering is a natural part of a hospital stay or of being ill. The relief from pain is considered a basic human right, and is incorporated into the Canadian Pain Society's Patient Pain Manifesto (2001). Yet, in Canada, pain continues to be a major health issue. Acute pain in hospitalized infants (Johnston et al., 1997) and children (Taylor et al., 2008), cancer pain in adults (MacDonald et al., 2002), and chronic pain in oder adults (Lansbury, 2000) continue to be poorly assessed and treated. As a nurse, you are ethically responsible for managing pain and relieving suffering. You are also legally and ethically obligated to advocate for change in the care plan when pain relief is inadequate (Registered Nurses' Association of Ontario [RNAO], 2002).

An important way for a nurse to respectfully respond to a client in pain is to understand McCaffery's definition of pain (1979): "Pain is whatever the experiencing person says it is, existing whenever he says it does" (cited in Herr et al., 2006, p. 44). Listen to what the client is telling you, and consider using a variety of *evidence-informed* interventions that include scientifically based sources of knowledge as well as effective nursing knowledge. Responsive, evidence-informed pain management not only reduces physical discomfort, but also improves quality of life and promotes earlier mobilization and return to work, resulting in fewer hospital and clinic visits, shortened hospital stays, and reduced health care costs.

Scientific Knowledge Base

Pain is part of the human experience. In the past, pain was viewed simply as a symptom of an illness or condition. Pain itself is now considered to be a separate disease.

Nature of Pain

Pain is much more than a physical sensation caused by a specific stimulus. An individual's perception of pain has important *affective* (emotional), cognitive, behavioural, and sensory components that are shaped by cultural and situational factors. The stimulus for pain can be physical, mental, or a combination of both, in nature.

Physiology of Pain

Nociceptive (normal) pain is experienced in four processes: transduction, transmission, perception, and modulation (McCaffery & Pasero, 1999). A client in pain cannot discriminate among the processes. However, understanding each process will help you to recognize factors that can cause pain, symptoms that accompany pain, and the rationale and actions of select therapies.

Pain is usually caused by thermal, chemical, or mechanical stimuli. The energy of these stimuli is converted to electrical energy. This energy conversion is known as **transduction.** Transduction begins in the periphery when a pain-producing stimulus sends an impulse across a peripheral pain nerve fibre (**nociceptor**), initiating an action potential. Once transduction is complete, transmission of the pain impulse begins.

All cellular damage caused by thermal, mechanical, or chemical stimuli results in the release of excitatory neurotransmitters such as prostaglandins, bradykinin, potassium, histamine, and substance P (Box 42–1). These pain-sensitizing substances surround the pain fibres in the extracellular fluid, creating the spread of the pain message and causing an inflammatory response (Paice, 1994). The pain fibre enters the spinal cord and travels one of several routes until ending within the grey matter of the spinal cord. Within the dorsal horn, substance P is released, causing a synaptic transmission from the *afferent* (sensory) peripheral nerve to spinothalamic tract nerves (Wall & Melzack, 1999; Figure 42–1).

Nerve impulses resulting from the painful stimulus travel along afferent peripheral nerve fibres. Two types of peripheral nerve fibres conduct painful stimuli: the fast, myelinated A-delta fibres, and the very small, slow, unmyelinated C fibres. The A fibres send sharp, localized, and distinct sensations that focus the source of the pain and detect its intensity. The C fibres relay impulses that are poorly

➤ BOX 42-1 Neurophysiology of Pain: Neuroregulators

Neurotransmitters (Excitatory)

Substance P

Found in the pain neurons of the dorsal horn (excitatory peptide)
Needed to transmit pain impulses from the periphery to the higher brain centre
Causes vasodilation and edema

Serotonin

Released from the brain stem and dorsal horn to inhibit pain transmission

Prostaglandins

Generated from the breakdown of phospholipids in cell membranes
Believed to increase sensitivity to pain

Neuromodulators (Inhibitory)

Endorphins and Dynorphins

Function as the body's natural supply of morphine-like substances
Activated by stress and pain
Located within the brain, spinal cord, and gastrointestinal tract
Cause analgesia when they attach to opiate receptors in the brain
Present in higher levels in people who have less pain than others with a similar injury

Bradykinin

Released from plasma that leaks from surrounding blood vessels at the site of tissue injury
Binds to receptors on peripheral nerves, increasing pain stimuli
Binds to cells that cause the chain reaction-producing prostaglandins

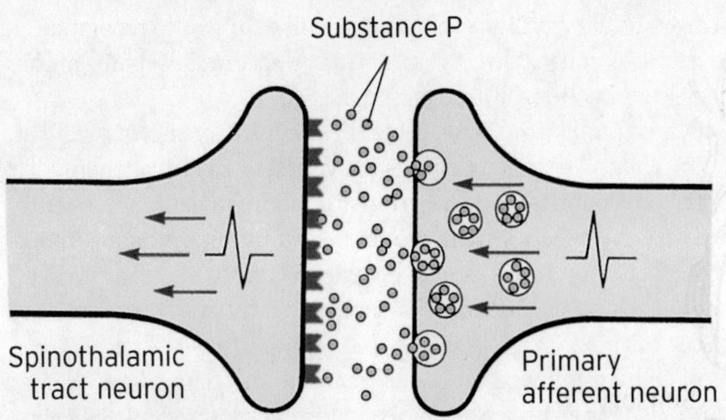

Figure 42-1 Substance P and other neurotransmitters are released from primary afferent fibres that terminate in the dorsal horn of the spinal cord. **Source:** From Paice, J. A. (1991). Unraveling the mystery of pain. *Oncology Nursing Forum, 18*(5), 843.

localized, burning, and persistent (Wall & Melzack, 1999). For example, after stepping on a nail, a person initially feels a sharp, localized pain, which is a result of A-fibre transmission. Within a few seconds, the pain becomes more diffuse and widespread, until the whole foot aches, because of C-fibre innervation.

Transmission of the pain stimulus continues along the afferent nerve fibres until they end in the dorsal horn of the spinal cord. Pain stimuli continue to travel through nerve fibres in the spinothalamic tracts that cross to the opposite side of the spinal cord. Pain impulses then travel up the spinal cord. Figure 42–2 shows the normal pain reception pathway. After the pain impulse ascends the spinal cord, information is quickly transmitted by the thalamus to higher centres in the brain. These centres include the reticular formation, limbic system, somatosensory cortex, and association cortex.

Once a pain stimulus reaches the cerebral cortex, the brain interprets the quality of the pain and uses information from past experiences, knowledge, and cultural associations to process the perception of the pain (McCaffery & Pasero, 1999). **Perception** is the point at which a person is aware of pain. The somatosensory cortex identifies the location and intensity of the pain, and the association cortex determines how we feel about the pain. Certain cells within the limbic system are believed to control emotion, particularly anxiety. Thus the limbic system may play an active role in processing the emotional reaction to pain and the memory of the pain experience. However, the human ability to experience and remember pain does not depend on *cognitive ability* (explicit memory).The experience of pain is remembered by even the youngest of infants, including those born prematurely (Anand & Scalzo, 2000). Pain studies using animal models (Fitzgerald, 1995) show that significant exposure to pain can permanently alter a developing organism's pain mechanism. This suggests that physiological and implicit forms of pain memory take place in the first days of life.

As a person becomes aware of pain, a complex reaction unfolds. Psychological and cognitive factors interact with neurophysiological factors in the perception of pain. Perception gives awareness and meaning to pain so that a person can then react. The reaction to pain is the physiological and behavioural responses that occur after pain is perceived.

Once the brain perceives the pain, inhibitory neurotransmitters are released (see Box 42–1); these include endogenous opioids (endorphins and enkephalins), serotonin, norepinephrine, and gamma aminobutyric acid, which work to hinder the transmission of pain and help produce an analgesic effect (McCaffery & Pasero, 1999). This inhibition of the pain impulse is the fourth phase of the nociceptive process, known as **modulation**.

A protective reflex response may also occur with pain reception (Figure 42–3). A-delta fibres send sensory impulses to the spinal cord, where they synapse with spinal motor neurons. The motor impulses travel via a reflex arc along *efferent* (motor) nerve fibres back to a peripheral muscle near the site of stimulation, thus bypassing the brain. Contraction of the muscle leads to a protective withdrawal from the source of pain. For example, when a person touches a hot iron, a burning sensation is felt, but the hand also reflexively withdraws from the iron's surface. When superficial fibres in the skin are stimulated, a person moves away from the pain source. If internal tissues such as muscle or mucous membranes become stimulated, tightening and guarding of muscles occur. This reflex is usually absent below the injury in clients with spinal cord injuries. However, clients with spinal cord injuries can still experience pain above the level of injury (Finnerup & Jensen, 2004).

Gate-Control Theory of Pain. No specific pain centre exists in the nervous system. Melzack and Wall's gate-control theory (1965) was the first to suggest that in addition to the physical sensation, pain has emotional and cognitive dimensions and that pain impulses can

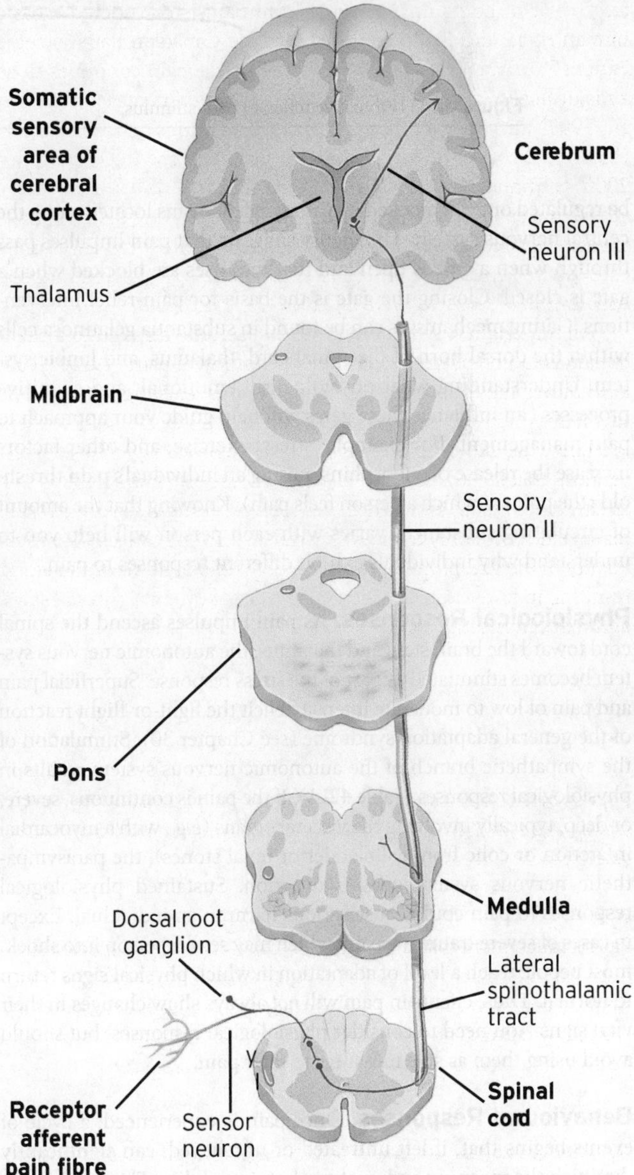

Figure 42-2 Spinothalamic pathway that conducts pain stimuli to the brain.

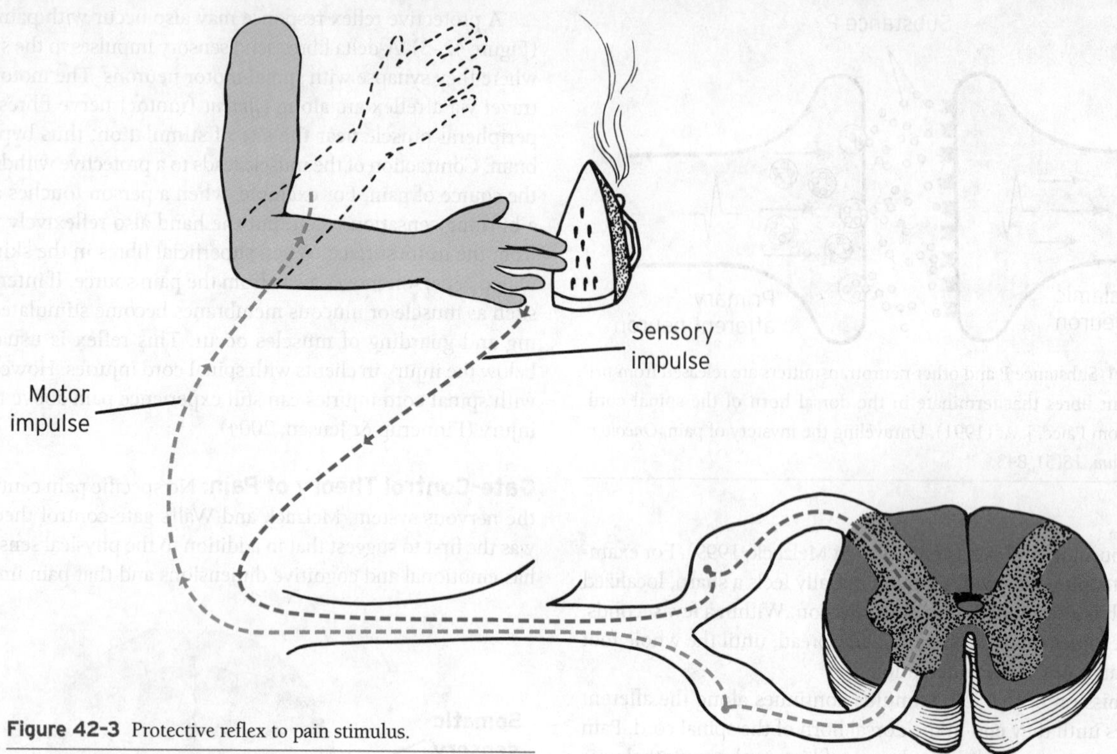

Figure 42-3 Protective reflex to pain stimulus.

be regulated or even blocked by gating mechanisms located along the central nervous system. The theory suggests that pain impulses pass through when a gate is open and that impulses are blocked when a gate is closed. Closing the gate is the basis for pain-relief interventions. Gating mechanisms can be found in substantia gelatinosa cells within the dorsal horn of the spinal cord, thalamus, and limbic system. Understanding what physiological, emotional, and cognitive processes can influence these gates will help guide your approach to pain management. For example, stress, exercise, and other factors increase the release of endorphins, raising an individual's **pain threshold** (the point at which a person feels pain). Knowing that the amount of circulating substances varies with each person will help you to understand why individuals exhibit different responses to pain.

Physiological Responses. As pain impulses ascend the spinal cord toward the brain stem and thalamus, the autonomic nervous system becomes stimulated as part of the stress response. Superficial pain and pain of low to moderate intensity elicit the fight-or-flight reaction of the general adaptation syndrome (see Chapter 30). Stimulation of the sympathetic branch of the autonomic nervous system results in physiological responses (Table 42–1). If the pain is continuous, severe, or deep, typically involving the visceral organs (e.g., with a myocardial infarction or colic from gallbladder or renal stones), the parasympathetic nervous system goes into action. Sustained physiological responses to pain could cause serious harm to an individual. Except in cases of severe traumatic pain, which may send a person into shock, most people reach a level of adaptation in which physical signs return to normal. Thus, clients in pain will *not* always show changes in their vital signs. You need to consider physiological responses, but should avoid using them as sole measures to infer pain.

Behavioural Responses. Once pain is experienced, a cycle of events begins that, if left untreated or unrelieved, can significantly diminish the meaning and quality of a person's life. The dominating nature of pain can also interfere with the ability to care for oneself, as well as how one interacts with his or her environment and other people. This component of pain reaction helps to explain why the management of pain can be such a challenge.

Pain threatens physical and psychological well-being. Some clients will endure severe pain without asking for assistance. Clients may choose not to report pain if they believe their pain would inconvenience others or signal a loss of self-control. To ensure optimal health outcomes, encourage such a client to accept pain-relieving measures so that activity or nutritional intake is not seriously compromised. You also need to educate the client about the benefits of maintaining his or her blood level with analgesics in order to prevent pain *before* it occurs. Remember that a client's ability to tolerate pain may significantly influence what you perceive his or her degree of discomfort to be. Clients deemed to have a low **pain tolerance** (the level of pain a person is willing to put up with) may be perceived as whiners. Acknowledge your own views, and avoid making judgements about another's pain. Teach clients the importance of self-reporting. Consider the immediate context in which a client is experiencing pain, as well as their past experiences of pain. Base your pain assessment and pain care decision making on a variety of sources and observations (such as client self-reporting, family feedback, the client's behaviour and physiology, and internal and external environmental factors).

Typical body movements and facial expressions that indicate pain include clenching the teeth, holding the painful part, bent posture, and grimaces. A client may cry or moan, be restless, or make frequent requests. You will learn to recognize common behaviour patterns that reflect pain, but remain flexible in your conclusions. Lack of pain expression does not necessarily mean that a person has no pain. Premature and full-term infants sometimes do not cry, and they exhibit few motor movements after excessive and repeated exposure to pain (Johnston et al., 1999; Warnock & Sandrin, 2004).

Types of Pain

Pain may be categorized by duration or pathology. Acute and chronic pain are categorized by duration.

TABLE 42-1 Physiological Reactions to Pain

Response	Cause or Effect
Sympathetic Stimulation*	
Dilation of bronchial tubes and increased respiratory rate	Provides increased oxygen intake
Increased heart rate	Provides increased oxygen transport
Peripheral vasoconstriction (pallor, elevation in blood pressure)	Elevates blood pressure with shift of blood supply from periphery and viscera to skeletal muscles and brain
Increased blood glucose level	Provides additional energy
Diaphoresis	Controls body temperature during stress
Increased muscle tension	Prepares muscles for action
Dilation of pupils	Affords better vision
Decreased gastrointestinal motility	Frees energy for more immediate activity
Parasympathetic Stimulation†	
Pallor	Causes blood supply to shift away from periphery
Muscle tension	Results from fatigue
Decreased heart rate and blood pressure	Results from vagal stimulation
Rapid, irregular breathing	Causes body defences to fail under prolonged stress of pain
Weakness or exhaustion	Results from expenditure of physical energy

*Superficial pain and pain of low to moderate intensity.
†Severe or deep pain.

Acute Pain. Acute **pain** is protective, has an identifiable cause, is of short duration (usually less than 6 months), and causes limited tissue damage and emotional response. Acute pain eventually resolves with or without treatment after a damaged area heals. Because acute pain has a predictable ending (healing) and an identifiable cause, health care professionals are usually willing to treat acute pain aggressively. Evidence, however, suggests that unrelieved acute pain may have development- and age-related consequences.

Significant and repeated exposure to acute pain during epochs of rapid early infant brain development may alter an infant's pain mechanism (Anand & Scalzo, 2000). Untreated or poorly treated intraoperative and postoperative pain and stress can also increase infant mortality and morbidity (Anand et al., 1987).

In the older adult, unrelieved acute pain can seriously threaten recovery, resulting in prolonged hospitalization, increased risks of complications from immobility (see Chapter 46), and delayed rehabilitation. Physical or psychological progress cannot be made as long as acute pain persists, because all energy is focused on pain relief. Your efforts to teach self-care will also be ineffective until the pain is successfully managed. Complete pain elimination may not be achievable, but reducing pain to an acceptable level is realistic. Your primary goals should be to *prevent* pain and to provide pain relief that allows clients to participate in their recovery.

Chronic Pain. Unlike acute pain, **chronic pain** is not considered protective, and thus serves no purpose. Chronic pain is generally defined as pain that has been present for at least 6 months, persists beyond the normal time of healing, may not have an identifiable cause, serves no biological benefit, and leads to great personal suffering (Jovey et al., 2003). Chronic pain can be experienced at any point in life, including early infancy and childhood (McGrath & Finley, 1999). Chronic pain may be noncancerous or cancerous. Chronic noncancer pains are usually not life-threatening, and include arthritis, low back pain, myofascial pain, headache, and peripheral neuropathy (McCaffery & Pasero, 1999). However, clients with chronic noncancer pains are often frustrated because they never know how they will feel from day to day. The pain may be unrelenting, and its cause may be difficult to identify. It may stem from an injured area that healed long ago but continues to provide pain that is nonresponsive to treatment. Chronic noncancer pain is often experienced along with other symptoms such as sleep disturbances, depression, anxiety, and anger (Fernandez, 2002). This type of pain is a major cause of psychological and physical disability, leading to problems such as job loss, the inability to perform simple daily activities, sexual dysfunction, and social isolation from family and friends.

In 1998, the Canadian Pain Society approved a consensus statement and developed guidelines to support the use of opioid analgesics for the management of chronic noncancer pain (Jovey et. al, 2003). However, health care professionals are usually reluctant to treat this type of pain with opioids. Often, clients with chronic noncancer pain who "doctor shop" are labelled as drug seekers, although they are actually seeking pain relief. This behaviour is known as **pseudoaddiction.** To break the cycle of poor pain management, inform the client about the issues raised by having multiple health care professionals, and refer him or her to pain experts.

The beliefs and coping strategies used by individuals with chronic pain may determine how they will function with and adjust to their pain. Jensen et al. (1991) found that individuals who believed they could control their pain, who avoided viewing their condition as a tragedy, and who believed that they were not severely disabled appeared to function better than those who did not. You should emphasize to the client that pain can be successfully managed, although not necessarily cured. Make use of a comprehensive approach that includes both nonpharmacological and pharmacological strategies. Help strengthen the individual's confidence in his or her ability to control the pain, and suggest referral for treatment of possible depression, if necessary. Keep yourself updated about the best examples of adaptive coping strategies, such as cognitive behaviour therapy, by conducting a search of health databases.

Cancer Pain. Not all clients with cancer experience pain. But for those who do, the Agency for Healthcare Research and Quality (AHRQ), formerly the Agency for Health Care Policy and Research (AHCPR), reports that up to 90% can have their pain managed (Jacox et al., 1994). Pain in a client with cancer may be acute, chronic, or both. The pain may also be nociceptive, neuropathic, or both. Cancer pain may be caused by tumour progression and its related pathological process, invasive procedures, toxicities of treatment, infection, and physical limitations. It can be sensed at the actual site of the tumour or distant to the site, which is called *referred pain.* A new report of pain by a client with existing pain needs to be investigated. Although the need for treatment of cancer pain has become more visible, the issue of undertreatment continues. In a study conducted in a hospice setting, of those clients with pain, only 42% stated they had pain-relief scores of 5 or more on a scale of 1 to 10 (where 1 means no relief and 10 means complete relief) (McMillan, 1996). Many individuals with cancer pain live in community settings, and pain relief is often provided by their families. Findings suggest that accessing community resources may be difficult for these families (Whelan et al., 2000) and that the stress of caring for a loved one with cancer pain can impact the health of family caregivers (Grunfeld et al., 2004). The importance of establishing an organized, systematic, and comprehensive approach to pain assessment and treatment, as well as communicating with and supporting clients' families, cannot be overemphasized; nurses have the potential to play pivotal roles in these endeavours.

Pain by Inferred Pathology Process. Identifying the cause of pain is the first step in successfully treating pain. Nociceptive, or normal, pain is subdivided into *somatic* (musculoskeletal) and *visceral* (internal organ) pain. Neuropathic pain arises from abnormal or damaged pain nerves (Table 42–2). Each of these pathological processes has distinct pain characteristics that are discussed under pain assessment.

Idiopathic Pain. Because not all pain has an identifiable cause, a third category is necessary: **idiopathic pain**. Idiopathic pain is chronic pain present in the absence of an identifiable physical or psychological cause, or pain perceived as excessive for the extent of the organic pathological condition. An example of idiopathic pain is complex regional pain syndrome (CRPS), previously known as reflex sympathetic dystrophy (RSD) or causalgia.

Nursing Knowledge Base

In *Notes on Nursing: What It Is and What It Is Not,* Florence Nightingale (1859;1969) stated that "pain . . . perpetuates and intensifies itself." Thus, nurses have a long history of dealing with the effects of pain on clients. In this section, factors that influence pain are explored.

Knowledge, Attitudes, and Beliefs

When no obvious source of pain can be found (e.g., the client with chronic low back pain or neuropathies), nurses and physicians may not believe that clients are in discomfort, and may stereotype pain sufferers as complainers or "difficult" clients. These attitudes about pain are remnants of the traditional medical model of illness, which suggests that physical problems result from physical causes. Viewed from this perspective, pain is seen only as a physical response to organic dysfunction; the baseline knowledege, attitudes, and preferences of health care professionals will influence pain care decision making and actions.

McCaffery et al. (2000) studied nurses' attitudes to pain management, and found that the nurse's personal opinion about the client's report of pain affected the pain assessment and titration of opioid doses. Puntillo et al. (2001), when comparing nurse and client pain intensity scores, found 50% or less agreement across the disease conditions examined. Tesler et al. (1994) also found that nurses underrated postoperative pain in children compared to the pain ratings received from children themselves. Although inaccurate pain

➤TABLE 42-2 Classification of Pain by Inferred Pathology

Nociceptive Pain	Neuropathic Pain
Normal processing of stimuli that damages normal tissues or has the potential to do so if prolonged; usually responsive to non-opioids, opioids, or both. A. Somatic pain: Arises from bone, joint, muscle, skin, or connective tissue. It is usually aching or throbbing in quality, and is well localized. B. Visceral pain: Arises from visceral organs, such as the gastrointestinal tract and pancreas. This may be subdivided into: 1. Tumour involvement of the organ capsule, which causes aching and fairly well-localized pain. 2. Obstruction of hollow viscus, which causes intermittent cramping and poorly localized pain.	Abnormal processing of sensory input by the peripheral or central nervous system; treatment usually includes adjuvant analgesics. A. Centrally generated pain. 1. Deafferentation pain: Injury to either the peripheral or central nervous system. *Examples:* Phantom pain may reflect injury to the peripheral nervous system; burning pain below the level of a spinal cord lesion reflects injury to the central nervous system. 2. Sympathetically maintained pain: Associated with dysregulation of the autonomic nervous system. *Examples:* Pain associated with reflex sympathetic dystrophy, or causalgia (complex regional pain syndrome, type I, type II). B. Peripherally generated pain. 1. Painful polyneuropathies: Pain is felt along the distribution of many peripheral nerves. *Examples:* Diabetic neuropathy, alcohol-nutritional neuropathy, and those associated with Guillain-Barré syndrome. 2. Painful mononeuropathies: Usually associated with a known peripheral nerve injury; pain is felt at least partly along the distribution of the damaged nerve. *Examples:* Nerve root compression, nerve entrapment, trigeminal neuralgia.

Adapted from McCaffery, M., & Pasero, C. (1999). *Pain: Clinical manual* (2nd ed.). St. Louis, MO: Mosby. Data from Max, M. B., & Portenoy, R. K. (1993). Methodological challenges for clinical trials of cancer pain treatments. In C. R. Chapman & K. M. Foley (Eds.), *Current and emerging issues in cancer pain: Research and practice*. New York: Raven Press; and Portenoy, R. K. (1996). Neuropathic pain. In R. K. Portenoy & R. M. Kanner (Eds.), *Pain management: Theory and practice*. Philadelphia: F. A. Davis. Also see Loeser, J. D., & Melzack, P. (1999). Pain: An overview. *The Lancet, 353*, 1607–1609.

assessment in infants and children may be rooted in the nurse's personal biases or lack of knowledge (Porter et al., 1997), differences in pain ratings may also result from nurse preference in the type of tool they select for pain asssessment (Chambers et al., 2003). For example, nurses who use pain scales that incorporate a "happy face" rate pain lower than do nurses who use a visual analog scale (VAS). It is important to acknowledge your biases, and to avoid selecting pain assessment tools for personal reasons.

Making assumptions about clients in pain may seriously limit your ability to offer pain relief. Too often, nurses allow misconceptions about pain (Box 42–2) to affect their willingness to intervene. Some even avoid acknowledging a client's pain because of their own fear and denial. Nurses are entitled to their personal beliefs; however, they must accept the client's report of pain and act according to professional guidelines, standards, position statements, policies and procedures, and evidence-informed research findings. View the experience of pain from the client's perspective. Become an active, knowledgeable observer of a client in pain. This will not only help you to be more objective, it will allow you to provide a more holistic and effective approach to your pain care decision making and actions. These expressions of professionalism will be meaningful to the individual, and improve his or her pain outcomes. The client makes the diagnosis that pain is present, and you apply techniques and skills that ultimately give relief.

Factors Influencing Pain

Pain is complex, and involves physiological, social, spiritual, psychological, and cultural influences. Each individual's pain experience is different. Consider all factors that affect the client in pain.

Physiological Factors

Age. Age is an important variable that influences pain, particularly in infants and older adults. Developmental differences among these age groups influence how children and older adults react to pain. Young children have difficulty understanding the procedures that you administer that may cause pain. Cognitively, toddlers and preschoolers are often unable to recall explanations about pain, or associate pain with experiences that can occur in various situations. They may also have difficulty expressing their pain, or may use verbal descriptors that differ from those used by older individuals. Consider adapting your approaches when assessing pain in a child (including what to ask and the behaviours to observe). Help prepare the child for a painful procedure. Ask the child about the terms he or she most often uses to define pain and pain treatment, and then use those terms when communicating about pain with the child.

Pain is not an inevitable part of aging. Older adults with pain are at increased risk for developing serious impairments in their functional status. Mobility, activities of daily living (ADLs), social activities outside the home, and activity tolerance can all be reduced. Pain in an older adult requires aggressive assessment, diagnosis, and management (Box 42–3).

The ability of older clients to interpret pain can be complicated by the presence of multiple diseases with vague symptoms that affect similar parts of the body. You will need to undertake a detailed assessment when a client has more than one source of pain (Herr, 2002a, 2002b). The manifestations of different diseases can cause atypical presentations of painful conditions. Different diseases can also cause similar symptoms. For example, chest pain does not always indicate a heart attack; it may be a symptom of arthritis of the spine or of an abdominal disorder. Not all older adults experience cognitive impairment. However, when older adults are confused, they may not be able to recall and explain details of pain experiences. Misconceptions about pain management in the very young and in older adults may seriously hamper pain intervention for these populations, as illustrated in Tables 42–3 and 42–4.

Fatigue. Fatigue heightens pain perception, intensifies pain, and decreases coping abilities. This is a common problem for clients with long-term illnesses or with fatigue as a result of treatment. If fatigue occurs along with sleeplessness, the perception of pain may be even greater. Less pain is often experienced after a restful sleep than at the end of a long day.

Genes. Recent research on animal models suggests that genetic information passed on by parents might increase or decrease sensitivity to pain. What was historically described as pain threshold or pain

BOX 42-2 Common Biases and Misconceptions About Pain

The following statements are false:

- Drug abusers and alcoholics overreact to discomfort.
- Clients with minor illnesses have less pain than do those with severe physical alterations.
- Regular administration of analgesics will lead to drug addiction.
- The amount of tissue damage in an injury can accurately indicate pain intensity.
- Health care professionals are the best authorities on the nature of a client's pain.
- Psychogenic pain is not real.
- Chronic pain is psychological.
- Clients should expect to have pain during a hospital stay.
- Clients who cannot speak do not feel pain.

BOX 42-3 FOCUS ON OLDER ADULTS

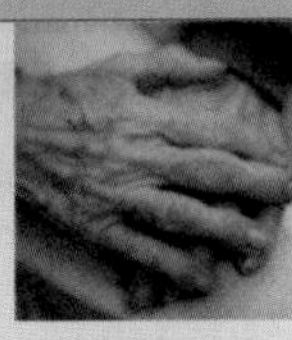

- With aging, muscle mass decreases, body fat increases, and the percentage of body water decreases. This results in an increased concentration of water-soluble drugs, such as morphine. Also, the volume of distribution for fat-soluble drugs, such as fentanyl, increases (Popp & Portenoy, 1996).
- Older adults frequently eat poorly, resulting in low serum albumin levels. Many drugs are highly protein bound. In the presence of low serum albumin, more of a drug (active form) remains unbound, which increases the risk for side effects, toxic effects, or both (Lehne, 2001).
- Decline of liver and renal function is a natural occurrence with aging. This results in reduced metabolism and excretion of drugs. Hence, older adults often experience a greater peak effect and longer duration of analgesics (Kelly, 2003).
- Age-related changes in the skin, such as thinning and loss of elasticity, could affect the absorption rate of topical analgesics.
- Patient-controlled analgesia (PCA) and regional analgesia are not contraindicated in older adults, but frequent assessments of pain, the side effects of analgesics, and cognition are necessary to ensure the efficacy and safety of PCA.
- The loss of the efficiency of homeostatic mechanisms puts older adults at risk for falls or delirium after the administration of sedative drugs or regional anaesthesia (Aubrun, 2005).

➤TABLE 42-3 Pain in Infants

Misconception	Correction
Infants are incapable of feeling pain.	By mid to late gestation, infants possess the anatomical and functional requirements for pain processing.
Infants are less sensitive to pain than older children and adults.	Preterm and full-term neonates may have a *greater* sensitivity to pain than older infants and children. This is because of their small skin surface area, the high density of cutaneous nerve fibres, and their developing, but still immature, ability to inhibit transmission of sensory nerve impulses. Older infants are as sensitive as children and adults.
Infants are incapable of expressing pain.	Although infants cannot verbalize pain, they respond with behavioural cues and physiological indicators that can be observed by others.
Infants must learn about pain from previous painful experiences.	Pain is present with the first insult; it need not be learned from an earlier painful experience (Anand & Craig, 1996).
Pain cannot be accurately assessed in infants.	Behavioural cues (i.e., facial expressions, cries, body movements) and physiological indicators of pain can be reliably and validly assessed, either alone or in combination. Pain assessment should be based on the use of tools that incorporate composite pain measures (Stevens & Koren, 1998). Inclusive approaches to infant pain assessment include not only taking into consideration the behavioural and physiological responses of the infant, but also assessing the pain context and how the infant is interacting, or failing to interact, with the immediate environments (Warnock, 2003).
Because infants cannot demonstrate cognitive awareness, they are insensible and lack memory for pain.	Early and repeated exposure to noxious stimuli is likely to affect the infant's future responses to painful events (Grunau et al., 1994).
Analgesics and anaesthetics cannot be safely given to infants and neonates because of their immature capacity to metabolize and eliminate drugs, as well as their sensitivity to opioid-induced respiratory depression.	Infants older than 1 month of age metabolize drugs in the same manner as older infants and children. Careful selection of the agent, dosage, administration route, and time; frequent monitoring for desired and undesired effects; and drug titration and weaning can minimize the adverse effects of opioids and non-opioids for pain management in neonates (Stevens, 1998).

Adapted from McCaffery, M., & Pasero, C. (1999). *Pain: Clinical manual* (2nd ed.). St. Louis, MO: Mosby.

tolerance may, in fact, be determined by genetic makeup. In addition, exposure to pain at a young age may increase sensitivity to pain (Ruda et al., 2000).

Neurological Function. A client's neurological function can influence the pain experience. Any factor that interrupts or influences normal pain reception or perception affects the client's awareness of and response to pain. For example, clients who have a spinal cord injury, peripheral neuropathy (as in the case of diabetes mellitus), or a neurological disease (e.g., multiple sclerosis) experience altered pain sensation. Certain pharmacological agents influence pain perception and response. **Analgesics** (medications that relieve pain), sedatives, and **anaesthetics** (medications that cause temporary loss of sensation) depress functions of the central nervous system. Because clients at risk for pain insensitivity could suffer injury, they require preventive nursing care that includes neurological assessment (see Chapter 32).

Social Factors

Attention. The degree to which a client focuses on pain can influence pain perception. Increased attention has been associated with increased pain, whereas distraction has been associated with a diminished pain response (Carroll & Seers, 1998). This is a concept that nurses use when applying pain-relief interventions such as relaxation and massage. By focusing a client's attention and concentration on other stimuli, his or her awareness of pain declines.

Previous Experience. Prior painful experiences may shape how a client reponds to subsequent painful events. If a person has had frequent episodes of pain without relief or has had bouts of severe pain, anxiety or fear may recur. In contrast, if a person has had repeated experiences with the same type of pain but the pain has been successfully relieved, it becomes easier to interpret the pain sensation. As a result, the client is better prepared to take actions to relieve the pain.

When clients have had no prior exposure to a particular pain-inducing event, they may be unprepared, and this may impair their coping abilities. For example, severe incisional pain is common after abdominal surgery. Unless clients know to expect pain, they may view their incisional pain as a serious complication. As a result, they may tense up and breathe shallowly. Inform clients of the type of pain that might be experienced, and methods to reduce it.

Family and Social Support. People in pain often depend on family or friends for support, assistance, or protection. A loved one can help minimize loneliness and fear. An absence of support can make the pain experience more stressful. The presence of parents is especially important for children with pain. Explain to the parent that children typically want their parents with them during a pain event,

➤ TABLE 42-4 Pain in Older Adults

Misconception	Correction
Pain is a natural outcome of growing old.	Older adults are at greater risk (as much as twofold) than younger adults for many painful conditions; however, pain is not an inevitable result of aging.
Pain perception, or sensitivity, decreases with age.	This assumption is unsafe. No scientific evidence exists that pain perception decreases with age, or that age dulls sensitivity to pain.
If the older client does not report pain, he or she does not have pain.	Older clients commonly under-report pain. Reasons include expecting to have pain with increasing age; not wanting to alarm loved ones; being fearful of losing independence; not wanting to distract, anger, or bother caregivers; and believing that caregivers know that the older client has pain and are doing all that can be done to relieve it. The absence of a report of pain does not mean the absence of pain.
If an older client appears to be occupied, asleep, or otherwise distracted from pain, he or she does not have pain.	Older clients often believe it is unacceptable to show pain and have learned to use a variety of ways to cope with it instead (e.g., many clients use distraction successfully for short periods of time). Sleeping may be a coping strategy or may indicate exhaustion, not pain relief. Assumptions about the presence or absence of pain cannot be made solely on the basis of a client's behaviour.
The potential side effects of opioids make them too dangerous to use to relieve pain in older adults.	Opioids may be used safely in older adults. Although the opioid-naive older adult may be more sensitive to opioids, this does not justify withholding their use in pain management for this population. The key to the use of opioids in the older adult is to "start low and go slow." Potentially dangerous opioid-induced side effects can be prevented with slow titration; regular, frequent monitoring and assessment of the client's response; and adjustment of dose and interval between doses when side effects are detected. If necessary, clinically significant respiratory depression can be reversed by an opioid antagonist drug.
Clients with Alzheimer's disease and other cognitive impairments do not feel pain, and their reports of pain are most likely invalid.	No evidence exists that cognitively impaired older adults experience less pain or that their reports of pain are less valid than those of individuals with intact cognitive function. It is probable that clients with dementia or other deficits of cognition suffer significant unrelieved pain and discomfort. Assessment of pain in these clients is challenging, but possible. The best approach is to accept the client's report of pain and treat the pain as it would be treated in an individual with intact cognitive function.
Older clients report more pain as they age.	Even though older clients experience a higher incidence of painful conditions than younger clients (e.g., arthritis, osteoporosis, peripheral vascular disease, and cancer), studies have shown that older adults under-report pain. Many older clients grew up valuing the ability to "grin and bear it," and, unfortunately, have been heavily influenced by the "Just Say No To Drugs" campaign.

Adapted from McCaffery, M., & Pasero, C. (1999). *Pain: Clinical manual* (2nd ed.). St. Louis, MO: Mosby. Data from Butler, R. N., & Gastel, B. (1992). Care of the aged: Perspectives on pain and discomfort. In D. C. Turk & R. Melzack (Eds.), *The handbook of pain assessment*. New York: Guilford Press; Harkins, S. W., & Price, D. D. (1993). Are there special needs for pain assessment in the elderly? *American Pain Society Bulletin, 3*, 4–6; Harkins, S. W., Price, D. D., Bush, F. M., & Small, R. E. (1999). Geriatric pain. In P. D. Wall & R. Melzack (Eds.), *Textbook of pain*. London: Churchill Livingstone; and American Geriatrics Society. (2002). The management of persistent pain in older persons. *Journal of the American Geriatrics Society, 50*(Suppl. 6), 205–224.

but warn them that a parent's own anxiety and responses may influence how the child experiences and responds to pain (LaMontagne et al., 2001). Provide parents with information about the procedure, and involve them by explaining how they can use pain-related distraction strategies with their child during the child's procedure.

Spiritual Factors. Spiritual questions may include, "Why has this happened to me?" "Why am I suffering?" "Why has God done this to me?" "Is this suffering teaching me something?" People may worry about losing their independence and becoming a burden to family (Otis-Green et al., 2002). Spiritual assessment tools such as FICA (Faith, Belief, Meaning; Importance and Influence; Community; and Address/Action in Care) are available (Maxwell et al., 2005). Emphasize to the client that their pain and suffering matters. Consider requesting a member of the clergy visit a client with chronic pain. Recall that pain is an experience that has both physical and emotional components. Providing interventions designed to treat both aspects is essential for the best possible pain management.

Psychological Factors

Anxiety. The relationship between pain and anxiety is complex. Anxiety often heightens the perception of pain, and pain may cause anxiety. Painful stimuli activate the portion of the limbic system believed to control emotion, particularly anxiety (Wall & Melzack,

1999). The limbic system may process the emotional reaction to pain, aggravating or relieving it.

Critically ill clients, who feel that they have lost control of their situation and care, are often anxious. When anxiety goes unnoticed, it may be difficult to manage pain effectively. The management of anxiety through the use of pharmacological and nonpharmacological approaches is appropriate. However, anxiolytic medications should not be used as a substitute for analgesia.

Coping Style. Coping style influences the ability to deal with pain. People with internal loci of control perceive themselves as being able to control their environment and the outcome of events (Gil, 1990). People with external loci of control perceive other factors in their environments, such as nurses, as being responsible for the outcome of events. The perception of self-control is key to pain management. For example, clients in acute pain who self-administer small doses of intravenous (IV) pain medication achieve pain control more quickly than those who receive intermittent doses of pain medication from nurses.

Meaning of Pain. The meaning of pain affects the experience of pain and how one adapts to it. A person will perceive pain differently if it suggests a threat, loss, punishment, or challenge. For example, a woman in labour may perceive pain differently than a woman with a history of cancer who is experiencing a new pain and is fearing recurrence.

Cultural Factors. Culture shapes an individual's responses, behaviours, and attitudes about pain, and how they react to and deal with pain. People learn what is expected and accepted by their culture. Based on your own cultural beliefs, as a nurse you may also expect that others will or should respond to pain in a particular manner. However, by understanding that pain has different meanings for different cultures, you can design culturally sensitive care.

Some cultures are demonstrative about pain; others are introverted. Your knowledge of the level of a client's assimilation into Canadian society may be helpful. For example, if several generations of an Asian client's family have lived in Canada, the influence of the Asian culture may be limited. In contrast, a recent immigrant from another culture may have different beliefs from those of the larger Canadian population. Explore the impact of cultural differences on the client's pain experience, and adjust the plan of care (Box 42–4). Work with the client and family to facilitate communication about the assessment and management of pain. Find a culturally appropriate assessment tool, and communicate the use of that tool to other health care professionals.

BOX 42-4 CULTURAL ASPECTS OF CARE

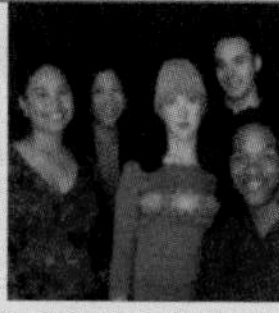

Culturally acquired patterns of pain responses may also influence the neurophysiological processing of pain information as well as psychological and verbal responses to pain. A client's expectations concerning pain may influence how much pain can be tolerated. Response to pain may be limited by language used to describe or report pain. The degree of pain expression does not necessarily correlate with pain intensity. Preferences for pain-coping strategies are usually determined by culture; thus, nontraditional interventions to manage pain need to be explored with the client. How people view and respond to pain may influence your choice of interventions.

Implications for Practice

- Be aware of perceived causal factors of pain (fate, lifestyle, punishment, witchcraft).
- Emotional responses to pain (overt, stoic) vary between and within cultures.
- Words used to express pain vary among cultures (hurt, ache, discomfort).
- Personal and social meanings of pain and past pain experiences affect pain perception.
- Definitions of pain change the perception of pain intensity.
- Feelings about pain direct treatment.
- Health care professional beliefs and expectations regarding pain expression sway pain management strategies.
- Therapeutic goals of pain management are influenced by cultural beliefs.

Data from Lasch, K. (2000). Culture, pain, and culturally sensitive pain care. *Pain Management Nursing, 1*(3 Suppl. 1), S16–22; Steefel, L. (2002). Treat pain in any culture. *Nursing Spectrum, 6*(5), 8; Rosmus, C., Johnston, C. C., Chan-Yip, A., & Yang, F. (2000). Pain response in Chinese and non-Chinese Canadian infants: Is there a difference? *Social Science & Medicine, 51,* 175–184; Patterson, C., Molloy, W., Jubelius, R., Guyatt, G. H., & Bédard, M. (1997). Provisional educational needs of health care providers in palliative care in three nursing homes in Ontario. *Journal of Palliative Care, 13*(3), 13–17; and Ramer, L., Richardson, J. L., Cohen, M. Z., Bedney, C., Danley, K. L., & Judge, E. A. (1999). Multimeasure pain assessment in an ethnically diverse group of patients with cancer. *Journal of Transcultural Nursing, 10*(2), 94–101.

Critical Thinking

Critical thinking requires synthesizing knowledge, experience, information from clients, critical thinking attitudes, and professional standards. Clinical judgements require that you anticipate the information you need, analyze the data, and make decisions about client care. A client's condition or situation is always changing. During assessment, consider all critical elements that will enable you to make a nursing diagnosis.

Knowledge about pain physiology and factors that influence pain will help you to manage clients' pain effectively. With experience, you will become more skilled at assessing pain and choosing effective therapies. Successful pain management does not necessarily mean pain elimination, but rather the attainment of mutually agreed upon pain-relief goals that allow clients to control their pain instead of the pain controlling them.

Nursing Process and Pain

The nursing process provides you with a systematic approach to understanding and treating a client's pain. An important aspect of effective pain management is establishing a trusting relationship with the client and family. Pain management extends beyond pain relief; it encompasses the client's quality of life and ability to work productively, to enjoy recreation, and to function normally within the family and society (Jacox et al., 1994).

Your application of the nursing process can be optimized by framing it around readily available clincial pain guidelines, which are based on best evidence and are continuously updated (see the "Recommended Web Sites" suggestions at the end of this chapter).

❖Assessment

Pain assessment is the basis of all pain management. In some institutions, pain is regarded as the fifth vital sign. Monitor the client's pain consistently along with temperature, pulse, respirations, and blood pressure. Place the person suffering from pain at the centre and consider the context in which he or she experiences pain, the course of his or her pain, and his or her ability to recover from pain.

Establishing a nursing diagnosis, deciding on appropriate interventions, and evaluating the client's response (outcomes) to the interventions are contingent on a timely and accurate pain assessment (Figure 42–4). Effective and unbiased pain assessment is best achieved if you make use of validated pain assessment instruments appropriate to the client (RNAO, 2002). The goal in using these tools is not to identify how much pain the client can tolerate; rather, it is to gauge the effects of pain treatment in order to optimize client function. It is important to understand that pain assessment is *not* simply a number. Relying solely on a number is unsafe (Vila et al., 2005).

The AHRQ has established guidelines for assessing clients with acute and cancer pain. The focus is on planning pain management interventions before pain is experienced. Because it involves collaboration, the AHRQ pain treatment flow chart (Figure 42–5) is a useful conceptual approach to acute pain control. However, clients must understand that reporting of pain is necessary if the health care team is to manage the pain effectively.

You should be sensitive to the client's level of discomfort when assessing pain. You will come across many pain assessment instruments; select those that are developmentally appropriate, reliable, valid, and applicable for clinical use. Behavioural pain assessment tools identify the presence of pain, whereas the visual analogue scale (VAS) assesses the intensity of pain. The VAS has been translated into several languages in order to aid the nurse when an interpreter or family member is not present (McCaffery & Pasero, 1999). Ask the client what level of pain will allow him or her to function. For example, you might ask, "What is an acceptable level of pain for you?"

Knowledge
- Physiology of pain
- Factors that potentially increase or decrease responses to pain
- Pathophysiology of conditions causing pain
- Awareness of biases affecting pain assessment and treatment
- Cultural variations in how pain is expressed
- Knowledge of nonverbal communication

Experience
- Caring for clients with acute, chronic, and cancer pain
- Caring for clients who experienced pain as a result of a health care therapy
- Personal experience with pain

Assessment
- Determine the client's perspective of pain including history of pain; its meaning; and physical, emotional, and social effects
- Measure objectively the characteristics of the client's pain
- Review potential factors affecting the client's pain

Standards
- Refer to AHCPR guidelines for acute pain management
- Apply intellectual standards (e.g., clarity, specificity, accuracy, and completeness when gathering assessment)
- Refer to RNAO Nursing Best Practice Guidelines: *Assessment and Management of Pain*

Qualities
- Persevere in exploring causes and possible solutions for chronic pain
- Display confidence when assessing pain to relieve the client's anxiety
- Display integrity and fairness to prevent prejudice from affecting assessment

Figure 42-4 Critical thinking model for pain and comfort assessment.

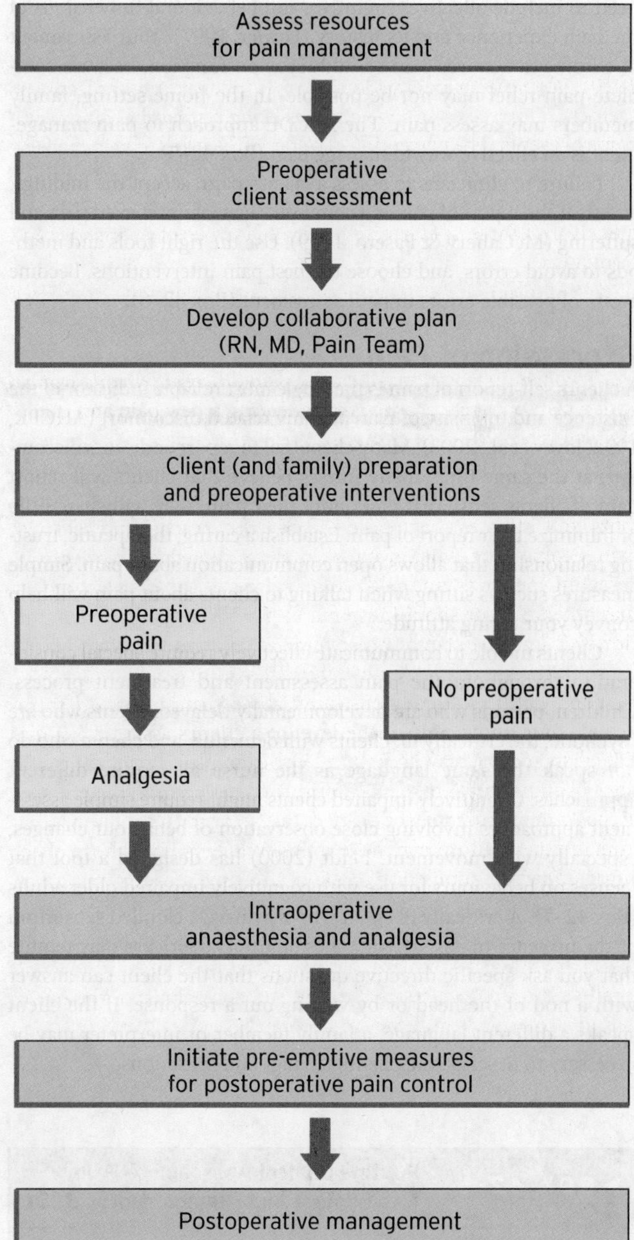

Figure 42-5 Pain treatment flow chart: preoperative and intraoperative phases. **Source:** From Agency for Health Care Policy and Research (AHCPR), Acute Pain Management Guideline Panel. (1992). *Acute pain management: Operative or medical procedures and trauma. Clinical practice guideline.* AHCPR Publication No. 92-0032. Rockville, MD: Agency for Health Care Policy and Research, Public Health Service, United States Department of Health and Human Services; and Jacox, A., Carr, D., Payne, R., Berde, C., Breitbart, W., Cain, J., et al. (1994). Management of cancer pain. *Clinical practice guideline No. 9.* AHCPR Publication No. 94-0592. Rockville, MD: Agency for Health Care Policy and Research, Public Health Service, United States Department of Health and Human Services.

The client might answer that a level 2 pain (on a scale of 0 to 10, with 0 being no pain and 10 being the worst pain imaginable) is acceptable. You then focus on decreasing the pain to at least that level. If pain is acute or severe, the client probably cannot describe the experience in detail. During an episode of acute pain, primarily assess the location, severity, and quality of the pain. Collect more information when the client is more comfortable.

For clients with chronic pain, thorough assessment of pain will need to include affective, cognitive, and behavioural dimensions of the pain experience and its history (Lawler, 1997). Your assessment of chronic noncancer pain should focus on function, because complete pain relief may not be possible. In the home setting, family members may assess pain. The ABCDE approach to pain management is an effective way to manage pain (Box 42–5).

Failure of clinicians to assess a client's pain, accept the findings, and treat the report of pain is a common cause of unrelieved pain and suffering (McCaffery & Pasero, 1999). Use the right tools and methods to avoid errors, and choose the best pain interventions. Become aware of possible errors in pain assessment (Box 42–6).

Expression of Pain

A client's self-report of pain is the single most reliable indicator of the existence and intensity of pain and any related discomfort (AHCPR, 1992; Jovey et al., 2003). Many clients fail to report or discuss discomfort; at the same time, many nurses believe that clients will report pain. If clients sense that you doubt their pain, they will share little or minimize their report of pain. Establish a caring, therapeutic, trusting relationship that allows open communication about pain. Simple measures such as sitting when talking to clients about pain will help convey your caring attitude.

Clients unable to communicate effectively require special consideration throughout the pain assessment and treatment process. Children, persons who are developmentally delayed, clients who are psychotic, the critically ill, clients with dementia, and clients who do not speak the same language as the nurse all require different approaches. Cognitively impaired clients might require simple assessment approaches involving close observation of behaviour changes, especially with movement. Feldt (2000) has designed a tool that focuses on behaviours for use with cognitively impaired older adults (Box 42–7). A critically ill client who may have a clouded sensorium or the presence of nasogastric tubes or artificial airways may require that you ask specific directive questions that the client can answer with a nod of the head or by writing out a response. If the client speaks a different language, a family member or interpreter may be necessary to describe the client's feelings and sensations.

➤ BOX 42-5 Routine Clinical Approach to Pain Assessment and Management: ABCDE

A: *Ask* about pain regularly. Assess pain systematically.
B: *Believe* the client and family in their report of pain and what relieves it.
C: *Choose* pain control options appropriate for the client, family, and setting.
D: *Deliver* interventions in a timely, logical, and coordinated fashion.
E: *Empower* clients and their families. Enable them to control their course to the greatest extent possible.

From Jacox, A., Carr, D., Payne, R., Berde, C., Breitbart, W., Cain, J., et al. (1994). Management of cancer pain. *Clinical practice guideline No. 9.* AHCPR Publication No. 94-0592. Rockville, MD: Agency for Health Care Policy and Research, Public Health Service, United States Department of Health and Human Services.

➤ BOX 42-6 Possible Sources of Error When Assessing Pain

- Bias, which causes nurses to consistently overestimate or underestimate their clients' pain
- Unclear assessment questions, which lead to unreliable assessment data
- Use of pain assessment tools that have no established reliability or validity
- Expecting self-reports of pain from individuals who cannot rate their pain using a pain scale or who cannot provide a complete verbal account of their pain
- Not considering the pain context and the trajectory or change in an individual's expression of pain over time

Characteristics of Pain

Assessment of common pain characteristics will help you to understand the type and pattern of pain, and aid in choosing interventions. When you assess pain, and when you ask the client for his or her self-report of pain, it is important to remember that using instruments to quantify the extent and degree of pain depends on a client being sufficiently cognitively alert to be able to understand your instructions.

Onset and Duration. Ask questions to determine the onset, duration, and sequence of pain. When did the pain begin? How long has it lasted? Does it occur at the same time each day? How often does it recur? Does the client have frequent breakthrough pain or prolonged pain recovery?

Certain types of headaches are characterized by the time of day when they occur. Sudden and severe pain is easier to assess than gradual, mild discomfort. Understanding the time cycle of pain will enable you to intervene before the pain occurs or worsens. Preventing recurrent pain is key.

Location. To assess location, ask the client to describe or point to all areas of discomfort. Do not assume that pain will always occur in the same location. When describing pain location, use anatomical landmarks and descriptive terminology. The statement "The pain is localized in the upper right abdominal quadrant" is more specific than "The client states that the pain is in the abdomen." Pain, classified by location, may be superficial or cutaneous, deep or visceral, referred, radiating, or neuropathic (Table 42–5). Examples of common pain medications are provided in Table 42–5 and explained elsewhere in this chapter. It is critical that you check the type of pain diagnosed, as pharmacological treatments will vary.

Intensity. One of the most subjective, and therefore most useful, characteristics for the reporting of pain is its severity, or intensity. Examples of pain intensity scales include the verbal descriptor scale (VDS), the numerical rating scale (NRS), and the visual analogue scale (VAS) (Figure 42–6). When scales are used to rate pain, a 10-cm baseline is recommended (AHCPR, 1992).

A verbal descriptor scale (VDS) consists of a line with three- to five-word descriptors equally spaced along the line. The descriptors are ranked from "no pain" to "unbearable pain." Ask the client to choose the descriptor, category, number, or place on the line that best reflects his or her current pain. A numerical rating scale (NRS) may be used instead of word descriptors. In this case, the client would rate his or her current pain on a scale of 0 to 10. It is generally assumed that a pain score of 0 to 3 indicates mild pain, 4 to 6 indicates moderate

BOX 42-7 RESEARCH HIGHLIGHT

Non-Verbal Pain Indicators in Cognitively Impaired Older Adults

Research Focus

Assessing pain in a nonverbal client is difficult. Nurses encounter many clients who are unable to express their pain, although this does not mean they do not feel pain. Increasingly, Canadian researchers are contibuting to the development of pain assessment instruments for use with cognitively impaired teenagers (Oberlander et al., 1999), children (Stallard et al., 2001), and older adults with limited ability to communicate (Fuchs-Lacelle & Hadjistavropoulos, 2004). Continuously keeping abreast of new research will help inform your thinking and help ground your practice in evidence. The following abstract illustrates how a pain assessment tool developed for use with cognitively impaired adults was initially tested for its clinical applicability.

Research Abstract

The purpose of the study by Feldt (2002) was to pilot test the Checklist of Nonverbal Pain Indicators (CNPI) as a measure of pain behaviours in cognitively impaired older adults. Nonverbal behaviours studied were vocalizations, grimaces, bracing, rubbing, and restlessness. The instrument was tested on cognitively intact and impaired older adults with hip fractures. Cognitively intact older adults showed fewer nonverbal indications of pain, both at rest and with movement, than did the impaired clients. Facial grimaces were the most common observed pain behaviour in both impaired and unimpaired clients at rest. CNPI indicators were observed more frequently with movement. Over half of the sample (56%) showed no nonverbal indications of pain at rest. The CNPI proved to be a reliable and simple tool for assessing pain in post-operative cognitively impaired older adults. The tool was more accurate in assessing pain during client movement.

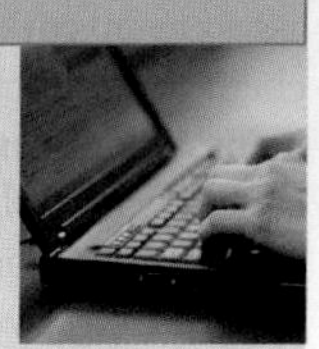

Evidence-Informed Practice

- Nonverbal clients require focused, around-the-clock pain assessment.
- Impaired clients may forget about painful areas when resting, thus requesting pain medication less frequently.
- Observe for pain behaviours and activity in cognitively impaired older adults.
- Do not assess pain in cognitively impaired older adults when they are resting, as this may give misleading cues about their pain.
- Make use of research-based pain assessment tool for nonverbal clients, as this will result in accurate pain assessment and better pain relief.

References: Feldt, K. S. (2000). The checklist of nonverbal pain indicators (CNPI). *Pain Management Nursing, 1*(1), 13–21.

pain, and 7 to 10 indicates severe pain (Miaskowski, 2005). The scales work best when assessing pain intensity before and after therapeutic interventions. Before applying these pain intensity scales, ensure that you are proficient in their use, and that you instruct the client on how to use these tools if you expect him or her to use them to provide a self-report of pain. Consider the ratings over a 24-hour period in order to get a sense of both the average and worst pain.

The visual analogue scale (VAS) does not have labelled subdivisions. It consists of a straight line, representing a continuum of intensity, and has verbal descriptors at each end. This scale gives the client total freedom in identifying the severity of pain. Although the VAS is less biased, it may not be as practical for daily use as an NRS (McCaffery & Pasero, 1999).

Assessing pain intensity in children requires special techniques. Children's verbal statements are most important (Hockenberry & Wilson, 2007). Because young children may not know what the word "pain" means, you will need to to use words such as *owie*, *boo-boo*, or *hurt*. Some tools measure pain intensity, while others measure pain affect in children. Beyer et al. (1992) have developed the "Oucher," which consists of two separate scales: a 0 to 100 scale on the left for older children, and a six-picture photographic scale on the right for younger children (Figure 42–7). Photographs of the face of a child (in increasing levels of discomfort) cue children into understanding what pain is and its severity; a child simply points to the selection. Ethnic versions of the tool are available. Wong and Baker (1988) developed the FACES scale to assess pain affect in children (Figure 42–8). The scale consists of six cartoon faces ranging from a smiling face ("no hurt") to increasingly less happy faces, to a final sad, tearful face ("hurts worst"). Children as young as 3 years of age can use the scale. Whatever tool is chosen, instruct the child on how to use the tool and ensure this understanding by having the child demonstrate his or her ability to use it (Fowler-Kerry & Lander, 1987). For full-term and premature infants and nonverbal toddlers, objective pain assessment tools such as the Premature Infant Pain Profile (PIPP) and the Neonatal Infant Pain (NIP) Scale (Stevens & Koren, 1998) are available. These tools are termed *composite pain scales*, meaning that they allow assessment of behavioural and physiological responses together rather than separately.

A pain scale should be easy to use and should not be time-consuming for the client to complete. Descriptive scales are used both to assess pain severity and to evaluate changes in a client's condition. You can use the scales after an intervention or when symptoms become aggravated in order to evaluate whether the pain has decreased or increased. Recall that you must select and consistently use the same scale for the same client. A pain scale cannot be used to compare the pain of one client to that of another client. A rating of 7 or more on a 0 to 10 scale requires immediate attention. However, a numerical value has limited meaning; effective pain assessment requires various approaches, not just a pain assessment tool. Box 42–8 (on p. 1024) describes one nurse's effective solutions in caring for a young client with burn injuries.

Quality. Another subjective characteristic of pain is its quality. Because no common or specific pain vocabulary exists, words used to describe pain vary. Clients may use "hurt" and "ache," but reserve the word "pain" for severe discomfort. The nurse should use words other than "pain" to obtain an accurate report. For example, you might say, "Tell me what your discomfort feels like." The client may describe the pain as crushing, throbbing, sharp, or dull. Although a list of descriptive terms is available, the client's own words are most accurate.

People describe certain types of pain fairly consistently. They often describe pain associated with a myocardial infarction as crushing or vise-like, and the pain of a surgical incision as dull, aching, and throbbing, indicating nociceptive pain. Neuropathic pain is usually described as burning, shooting, or electric-like (Williams, 2006). When the client's descriptions fit the pattern forming in the nurse's mind, a clearer analysis can be made. This will lead to better pain management, because nociceptive and neuropathic pain are treated differently.

Pain Pattern. Various factors affect the pain pattern. It helps to assess events or conditions that precipitate or aggravate pain. Ask the client to describe activities that cause pain, such as physical movement, and to demonstrate actions that cause pain, such as turning a certain way. In the example of a ruptured intravertebral disc, the low back pain and radiation down the leg are usually aggravated by bending or lifting. Swallowing and talking typically aggravate the pain of pharyngitis. Asking the client if the pain is worse at certain times of day, or if it is intermittent, constant, or a combination of both, will help you to plan effective interventions.

Relief Measures. Ask the client what pain relief measures they use, such as changing position, ritualistic behaviour (pacing, rocking, rubbing), or applying heat or cold to the painful site. The client's

TABLE 42-5 Classification of Pain by Location

Location	Characteristics	Examples of Causes	Examples of Common Medications
Superficial or Cutaneous			
Pain resulting from stimulation of skin	Pain is localized and of short duration. It is usually a sharp sensation.	Needle stick; small cut or laceration	Topical analgesics and anaesthetics (e.g., EMLA patch for children older than 1 year of age, Lidoderm patch for cutaneous neuropathic pain in adults)
Deep or Visceral			
Pain resulting from stimulation of internal organs	Pain is diffuse and may radiate in several directions. Duration varies, but it usually lasts longer than superficial pain. Pain may be sharp, dull, or unique to organ involved.	Crushing sensation (e.g., angina pectoris); burning sensation (e.g., gastric ulcer)	Demerol, morphine
Referred			
Common phenomenon in visceral pain because many organs themselves have no pain receptors; entrance of sensory neurons from affected organ into same spinal cord segment as neurons from areas where pain is felt; perception of pain is in unaffected areas	Pain is felt in a part of the body separate from the source of pain, and may assume any characteristic.	Myocardial infarction, which may cause referred pain to jaw, left arm, and left shoulder; kidney stones, which may refer pain to groin	Opioids (morphine) for acute MI by physician
Radiating			
Sensation of pain extending from initial site of injury to another body part	Pain feels as though it travels down or along the body part. It may be intermittent or constant.	Low-back pain from ruptured intravertebral disc, accompanied by pain radiating down leg from sciatic nerve irritation	Temporary treatment with one-time epidural injection of a steroid; injections of anaesthetics (e.g., xylocaine or bupivacaine)
Neuropathic			
Arises from abnormal or damaged pain nerves as a result of prior injury or disease; certain nerves may continue to send pain messages to brain even though no ongoing tissue damage is present (see Table 42–2)	Pain is usually described as burning, shooting, numbing, or electric-like.	Consequence of disease or prior injury to either the peripheral or central nervous system Complex regional pain syndrome, type I, type II, stroke, spinal cord injury, multiple sclerosis; diabetic neuropathy, alcohol-nutritional neuropathy, and those associated with Guillain-Barré syndrome; nerve root compression, nerve entrapment, trigeminal neuralgia; post- thoracotomy, herniorrhaphy, mastectomy; herpes zoster	Opioids, tricyclic antidepressants (e.g., nortriptyline), anticonvulsants (e.g., gabapentin), lidocaine patch

"Neuropathic section" based on Charlton, E. J. (Ed.). (2005). Neuropathic pain. *Core curriculum for professional education in pain* (pp. 1–8). Seattle, WA: IASP Press.

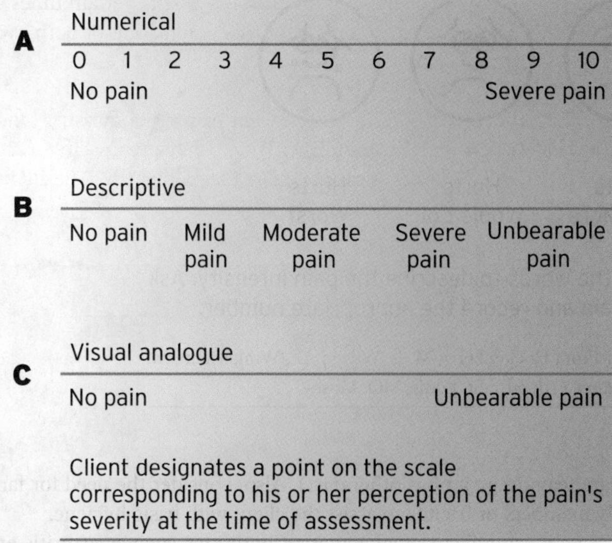

Figure 42-6 Sample pain scales. A, Numerical rating scale. B, Verbal descriptive scale. C, Visual analogue scale.

methods often work best. Clients gain comfort from knowing that you are willing to try their techniques. They also gain a sense of control over the pain instead of feeling that the pain is controlling them (Haythornthwaite et al., 1998). You should also identify practitioners whose services the client has used (e.g., orthopedist, acupuncturist, chiropractor).

Contributing Symptoms. Some symptoms (depression, anxiety, fatigue, sedation, anorexia, sleep disruption, spiritual distress, or guilt) may cause pain to worsen. You need to assess for these associated symptoms and evaluate their effects on the client's pain perception. Reporting and treating these symptoms contributes to effective pain management.

Effects of Pain. Pain is stressful, and chronic stress can worsen pain to the extent that it alters lifestyle and emotional health, and depletes energy levels. When a client is in pain, assess vital signs, conduct a focused physical examination, and observe for nonverbal responses to pain (e.g., posturing, grimacing, crying, or guarding). Examine the painful area to see if palpation or manipulation of the site increases pain (Jacox et al., 1994). If pain is unrelieved, look for signs of physical exhaustion.

Behavioural Effects. When a client has pain, assesses verbalization, vocal response, facial and body movements, and social interaction. A verbal report of pain is vital to assessment. You need to be willing to listen and understand. Many clients cannot verbalize discomfort (e.g., infants, clients who are unconscious, disoriented, confused, or aphasic, and clients who speak a foreign language). In these cases, you need to be alert to behaviours that indicate pain (Box 42–9).

Some nonverbal expressions characterize sources of pain. A person with chest pain often grabs or holds the chest. A person with severe abdominal pain often assumes a fetal position. The nonverbal expression of pain may support or contradict other information about pain. If a woman reports that her labour pains are occurring more frequently and begins to massage her abdomen more frequently, her report is confirmed. If a client complains of severe abdominal pain but grasps the chest, a more detailed assessment may be necessary. For some clients, vocalizations are culturally acceptable ways to communicate, and do not necessarily indicate a higher severity of pain or reduced pain tolerance.

Premature and full-term infants in pain often display characteristic facial actions. The Neonatal Facial Coding System (NFCS) (Grunau & Craig, 1987) is a coding tool for assessing pain-related changes in facial actions, such as brow lowering, eyes squeezing shut, chin quivering, mouth stretching vertically or horizontally, and lip pursing. Infants in pain may also show a complete lack of response, including no crying or movement (Johnston et al., 1999). This lack of pain response may also occur in older children and adults. Pain causes the person to attend to the discomfort and fight it, or to give in to the discomfort and withdraw socially.

Influence on Activities of Daily Living. Clients who have daily pain may not be able to carry out routine activities. Inactivity leads to physical deconditioning. The primary goal should be to improve client function. Ask clients if pain interferes with their sleep, awakens them, or keeps them awake (see Chapter 41). Sleeping pills or other medications may be needed to induce sleep.

Depending on the location of the pain, the client may have difficulty performing activities of daily living, including normal hygiene and dressing and grooming activities. For example, clients with severe arthritis may experience pain when grasping eating utensils or lowering themselves to a toilet seat. Assess the client's need for assistance with self-care activities, and collaborate with members of the health

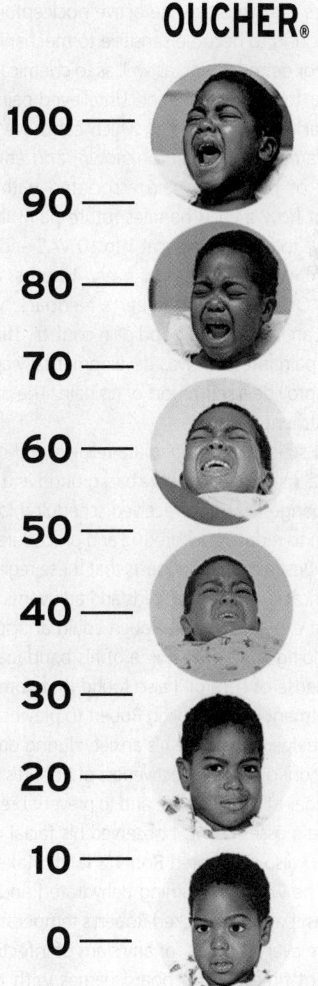

Figure 42-7 The Oucher pain scale. **Source:** Copyright Denyes, Villarrael, 1990.

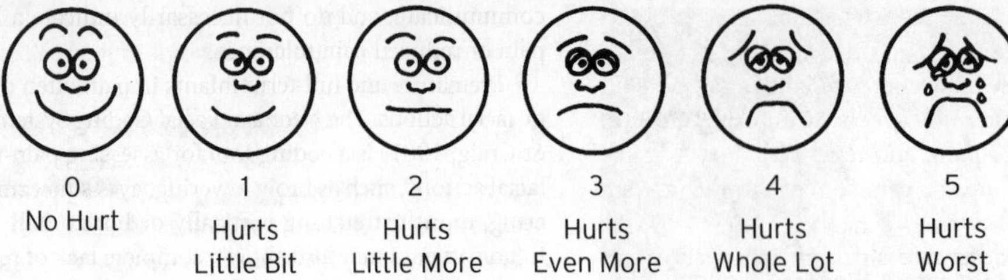

Brief word instructions: Point to each face using the words to describe the pain intensity. Ask the child to choose face that best describes own pain and record the appropriate number.

Figure 42-8 Wong-Baker FACES pain rating scale. **Source:** From Hockenberry, M. J., Wilson, D., Winkelstein, M. L., & Kline, N. E. (2003). *Wong's nursing care of infants and children* (7th ed.). St. Louis, MO: Mosby.

BOX 42-8 NURSING STORY

Relieving Robert's Burn Pain

I was responsible for caring for 12-year-old Robert, who had extensive burns to both of his legs. His treatment involved daily dressing changes. His family lived in a rural area and were not able to visit their child during his hospitalization.

In my plan of care, I focused on managing Robert's pain. Burn injuries are associated with an intense inflammatory response. The release of chemical mediators that sensitize the active nociceptors at the site of injury cause the wound to become sensitive to mechanical stimuli such as touch, rubbing, or debridement, as well as to chemical stimuli such as antiseptics or other topical applications. Unrelieved pain delays healing at both the cellular and tissue levels, which can have lasting effects. Separation from family, fear of the unknown, and anxiety increase a child's perception of pain, and pain associated with daily dressing changes can affect how a child handles future painful events. Robert was instructed how to use a numerical 1 to 10 VAS and how to keep a pain diary. The VAS was administered every 4 hours, as well as after dressing changes. On the basis of Robert's feedback, we aimed for a VAS target of 2 as an indicator of good pain control. This VAS was suitable for assessing pain intensity, was developmentally appropriate, and enabled Robert to provide a self-report of his pain. The pain diary helped to adjust pain treatment.

Robert received scheduled, immediate-release oral morphine and a titrated bolus of oral morphine to relieve background and procedural pain before dressing changes. He also received scheduled lorazepam and a bolus of lorazepam to reduce background and procedural anxiety before dressing changes. Best evidence suggests that these regimens contribute to the safe and efficacious use of opioids and adjuvants in children with burns. I found that explaining what Robert could anticipate, and giving him the job of helping to remove some of his bandages, increased his involvement and sense of control. I also found that combining pharmacological pain treatment with allowing Robert to play his favourite interactive videogame helped to reduce his anxiety during dressing changes.

I continuously monitored the effectiveness of Robert's pain medication in order to guard against oversedation and to prevent breakthrough pain. As part of each pain assessment, I observed his facial expressions and motor movement. I also monitored Robert's fluid intake and urine output to make sure he wasn't becoming dehydrated and to help reduce opioid-related constipation. I checked Robert's temperature, respiration, and blood pressure every 4 hours for any signs of infection. I listened to his concerns, spent time playing board games with him, and spoke biweekly with his family over the phone to discuss his care and progress.

care team (e.g., a physiotherapist). Also, consider the need for family members or friends to assist the client with basic hygiene.

Pain can affect sexual activity. Conditions such as arthritis and chronic back pain make it difficult to assume positions for intercourse. Prolonged use of opioids for cancer pain affects sexual function and libido (Jacox et al., 1994). Using discretion, ask the client if they are physically unable to participate in, or if pain has reduced their desire for, sexual intercourse.

Pain also affects the ability of the client to work. The more physical activity required in a job, the greater the risk of discomfort when the pain is associated with musculoskeletal and certain visceral

BOX 42-9 Behavioural Indicators of Pain

Vocalizations
- Moaning
- Crying
- Gasping
- Grunting

Facial Expressions
- Grimacing
- Clenched teeth
- Wrinkled forehead
- Tightly closed or widely opened eyes
- Lip biting

Body Movement
- Restlessness
- Immobilization
- Muscle tension
- Increased hand and finger movements
- Pacing activities
- Rhythmic or rubbing motions
- Protective movement of body parts

Social Interaction
- Avoidance of conversation
- Focused only on activities for pain relief
- Avoidance of social contacts
- Reduced attention span
- Despondent—failure to interact purposefully and meaningfully with immediate environment

alterations. Pain may increase if the job is stressful. Inquire about the client's work, and assess whether pain impacts his or her ability to function in the job. Assess the daily chores of homemakers in the same manner. Also assess whether it is necessary for clients to stop activity occasionally because of pain, and then help clients select ways of minimizing or controlling the pain so that they are able to remain productive.

It is also important to include an assessment of the effect of pain on social activities. The pain may be so debilitating that the client becomes too exhausted to socialize. Identify the client's normal social activities, the extent to which they have been disrupted, and the client's desire to participate.

Client Expectations

Clients who seek health care assistance with pain as a major symptom may have experienced the pain for many hours or days. Hospitalized clients may expect and even accept some pain. Asking clients to describe an acceptable comfort level is a first step in encouraging them to take control of their pain. Assessing previous pain experiences and effective home interventions provides a foundation on which you can build. Clients expect that nurses will believe their reports of pain and be prompt in meeting their pain needs.

❖Nursing Diagnosis

Do not diagnose pain simply because you assume that a client will have discomfort. You will make an accurate diagnosis only after you have performed a complete assessment. The development of an accurate nursing diagnosis of pain results from thorough data collection and analysis (Box 42–10). Careful assessment, which should include an examination of the client's history for recent procedures or pre-existing painful conditions, will reveal the presence of or potential for pain.

The nursing diagnosis focuses on the nature of the pain so that the nurse can identify the best interventions for relieving pain and minimizing its effect on function. Accurate identification of related factors ensures that appropriate nursing interventions will be chosen. For example, *acute pain related to physical trauma* versus *acute pain related to natural low-risk childbirth processes* require very different nursing interventions, such as "monitoring of vital signs for possible shock" versus "controlled breathing techniques." Examples of other diagnoses that may be applicable to clients at risk for pain include the following:

- *Anxiety*
- *Ineffective coping*
- *Fatigue*
- *Fear*
- *Hopelessness*
- *Impaired physical mobility*
- *Imbalanced nutrition: less than body requirements*
- *Acute pain*
- *Chronic pain*
- *Powerlessness*
- *Ineffective role performance*
- *Self-care deficit*
- *Chronic low self-esteem*
- *Situational low self-esteem*
- *Risk for situational low self-esteem*
- *Sexual dysfunction*
- *Disturbed sleep pattern*
- *Impaired social interaction*
- *Spiritual distress*

❖Planning

The care plan integrates key client information, critical thinking elements (Figure 42–9), and professional standards, which provide scientifically proven guidelines for selecting nursing interventions (Box 42–11). Professional standards of care regarding pain management are available as agency policies or through professional organizations such as the RNAO or the Canadian Pain Society and its affiliated special interest groups.

A concept map helps with care planning. Clients in pain frequently have interrelated problems. As one problem worsens, others also change. The concept map shows how nursing diagnoses link to one another and to medical diagnoses. For example, when planning care for the client with arthritis, the nurse notes the relationships between *acute pain, impaired physical mobility, self-care,* and *fatigue* (Figure 42–10). Understanding these relationships helps the nurse to develop a holistic and client-centred care plan.

BOX 42-10 NURSING DIAGNOSTIC PROCESS

Assessment Activities	Defining Characteristics	Nursing Diagnosis
Have client describe pain intensity.	Pain is constant; 5 out of 10	*Chronic pain related to chronic physical disability*
Assess onset and location of pain.	Present for 7 months in lower lumbar area	
Observe client behaviours.	Grimaces and grunts with movement, rubs flanks frequently; reduced movement	
Assess effect of pain on activities of daily living (ADLs).	Appetite poor; gets little sleep; difficulty dressing	
Review medical history.	Previous trauma; previous exposure to opioids	

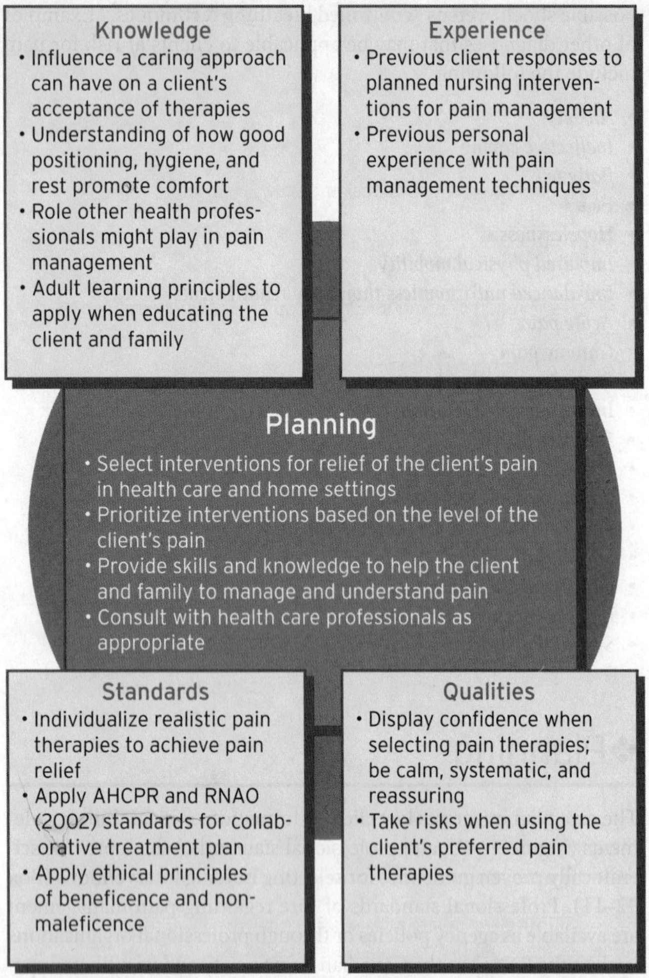

Figure 42-9 Critical thinking model for comfort planning.

Goals and Outcomes

Pain management goals permit the client to function to the best possible extent. Determine with the client what the pain has prevented the client from doing. Then, decide on a mutually acceptable level of pain that will allow a return of function. Success is determined through attainment of goals and outcomes. For example, if the goal is "the client will achieve a satisfactory level of pain relief within 24 hours," the following are possible outcomes:

- Reporting that pain is a 3 or less on a scale of 0 to 10, or does not interfere with ADLs
- Identifying factors that intensify pain, and modifying behaviour accordingly
- Using pain-relief measures safely

Setting Priorities

When setting priorities in pain management, consider the type of pain the client is experiencing and the effects pain has on various body functions. Discuss the selected interventions appropriate for the nature and effects of the pain with the client. For example, if a client has had acute pain but an analgesic has brought relief, centre your attention on how the pain is influencing activity, appetite, and sleep. In contrast, when a client's pain continues to be severe, preventing you from implementing other interventions, immediate pain relief is the obvious priority. Your priorities will change as the client's pain experience changes. Plans should take into account expected occurrences of pain.

Collaborative Pain Care

A comprehensive plan includes a variety of resources for pain control, including nurse specialists, pharmacologists, physiotherapists, occupational therapists, and clergy. An oncology nurse specialist knows the pharmacological and nonpharmacological interventions that work best for chronic cancer and noncancer pain. Pharmacologists are knowledgeable about pharmacological treatments for pain. Physiotherapists can plan exercises that strengthen muscle groups and lessen

➤ BOX 42-11 NURSING CARE PLAN

Acute Pain

Assessment

Mrs. Mays was diagnosed with a cancerous tumour in her left lung 8 months ago. After treatment, she was taking oral analgesics on a prn basis. She can no longer tolerate taking medications orally, and is now hospitalized with uncontrollable chest pain and possible pneumonia. Her husband is with her. A PCA of morphine 0.5 mg on-demand dose with a 10-minute lockout is begun.

Assessment Activities	*Findings and Defining Characteristics*
Ask Mrs. Mays what she did at home to control her pain.	Her pain escalated from a 3 to a 10, so she doubled her medication and went to bed. This did not help.
Ask Mrs. Mays what her pain intensity is now.	On a scale of 0 to 10, she reports a 9.
Ask Mrs. Mays what her pain has prevented her from doing.	She responds that she is unable to complete her own hygiene activities or sleep well.
Observe Mrs. Mays's nonverbal behaviour.	She is restless, unfocused, and is very still during the history-taking.
Ask Mrs. Mays her pain intensity goal (out of 10).	She says that a pain intensity of 5 out of 10 would help her function better now. A goal of 3 would be preferred.

Nursing Diagnosis: Acute pain related to a biological injuring agent (tumour).

BOX 42-11 NURSING CARE PLAN *continued*

Planning

*Goals (Nursing Outcomes Classification)**	*Expected Outcomes*
Pain Control	
Client will obtain an acceptable level of comfort before discharge.	Client will report pain at stated goal or below.
Husband will assist in restoring Mrs. Mays to a pain-free state.	Husband will provide slow-stroke massage to Mrs. Mays before bedtime.
Pain: Disruptive Effects	
Client will actively participate in ADLs.	Mrs. Mays will report sleeping for 5 to 6 hours without interruption from pain. She will complete her own hygiene with minimal assistance. She will walk the hallway with her husband every 4 hours for 15 minutes.
Medication Response	
Mrs. Mays will not experience unmanageable opioid side effects.	Mrs. Mays will report having a normal bowel movement every other day.

*Outcome classification labels from Moorhead, S., Johnson, M., & Maas, M. L. (Eds.). (2004). *Nursing Outcomes Classification (NOC)* (3rd ed.). St. Louis, MO: Mosby.

Interventions (Nursing Interventions Classification)†	**Rationale**
Pain Management	
Begin PCA at ordered dose. Explain to client and spouse how to use the PCA. Emphasize the importance of only the client pushing the button, not the husband.	Client is experiencing an acute episode of her cancer pain. Discouraging the husband from pushing the button will minimize potential toxic effects of the opioid because client must be awake to perceive the pain and push the button (Reiff & Nizolek, 2001).
Monitor IV PCA morphine use. Explain to client and spouse the action of the medication, potential side effects, and the importance of reporting if the pain is not relieved.	Pain is easier to prevent than to treat. Side effects are usually transient, except for constipation. Calculating a 24-hour dose of the opioid helps determine the appropriate oral dose (McCaffery & Pasero, 1999).
Have client select nonpharmacological interventions that have relieved pain in the past (e.g., distraction, music, simple relaxation therapy).	Personal control allows a client to shape immediate circumstances through his or her own actions (Salerno & Willens, 1996). Nonpharmacological interventions augment pharmacological strategies, but should not be used in place of analgesics (McCaffery & Pasero, 1999).
Teach her spouse how to perform slow-stroke back massage.	Slow-stroke back massage is easy to do, takes a brief amount of time, and has been shown to induce relaxation (Meek, 1993).

†Intervention classification labels from Dochterman, J. M., & Bulechek, G. M. (Eds.). (2004). *Nursing Interventions Classification (NIC)* (4th ed.). St. Louis, MO: Mosby.

Evaluation

Nursing Actions	*Client Response and Finding*	*Achievement of Outcome*
Ask Mrs. Mays if she attained her pain relief goal most of the time.	She responds, "My pain usually runs around a 3, which is my goal, except when I start walking."	Mrs. Mays reports an acceptable level of comfort, which is a change from the level that indicated unacceptable pain. Instruct her to push her button before ambulating.
Observe Mrs. Mays's ability to perform ADLs, walk, and sleep.	She is dressed for breakfast, and is walking the hallway every 4 hours with her husband. The night nurse's notes indicate Mrs. Mays slept through the night.	Ability to perform ADLs and sleep has improved. Continue to monitor.
Ask Mr. Mays if he was able to give his wife a back rub.	He reported that she did not want a back rub but preferred to have her feet rubbed, which he was happy to do. "She said it made her feel more relaxed."	Nonpharmacological intervention was successful, but the change from back rub to foot rub needs to be indicated in the nursing care plan.
Ask Mrs. Mays the time and consistency of her last bowel movement.	She has not had a bowel movement in 3 days (since starting the morphine PCA).	Assess her abdomen for bowel sounds and distension. Consult with her physician about starting a stimulant laxative once intestinal obstruction is ruled out (McCaffery & Pasero, 1999).

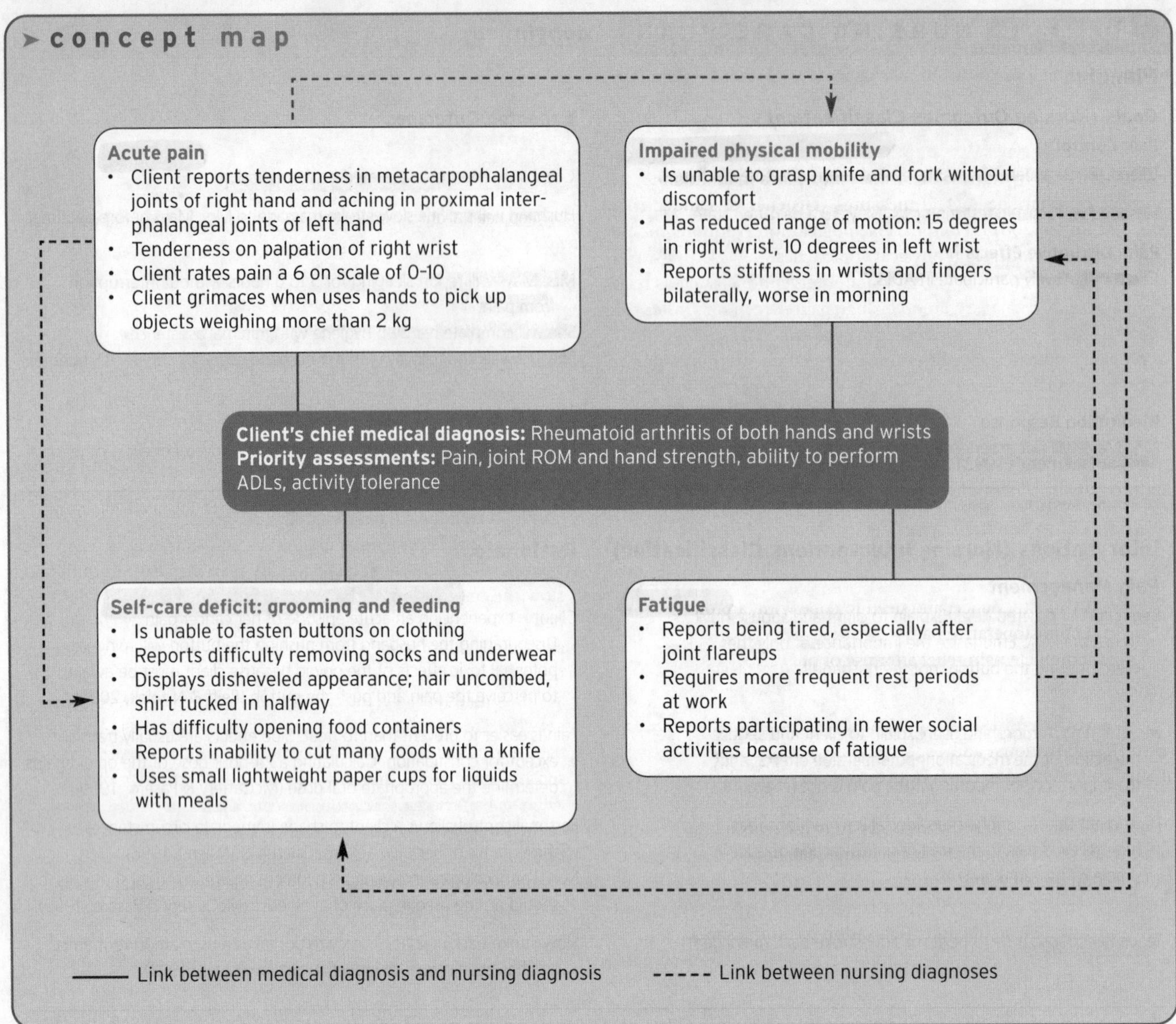

Figure 42-10 Concept map for client with pain related to rheumatoid arthritis.

pain in affected areas. Occupational therapists can devise splints to support painful body parts. Clergy members can help clients resolve spiritual pain. The family should also be involved in the care plan because they may need to administer care in the home after discharge. If the pain management plan is not successful, you should talk with the physician about changing the plan. Consultation with pain experts might be necessary.

❖Implementation

The nature of the pain and how much it affects well-being determines the choice of interventions. Pain therapy requires an *individualized* approach, perhaps more so than any other client problem. You, the client, and the family must be partners in using pain-control measures. Administer and monitor pain treatments ordered by a physician, but consider using other complementary comfort measures. Client remedies are often most successful, especially when the client has already had experience with pain. Generally, the least invasive or safest therapy should be tried first.

Health Promotion

The Ottawa Charter for Health Promotion (https://www.who.int/healthpromotion/conferences/previous/ottawa/en/) defines health promotion as the process of enabling individuals to gain control over and to improve their health and well-being (World Health Organization, 1990). Chronic pain and suffering diminishes quality of life; thus, relieving pain and promoting self-control becomes important. Once pain is controlled to an acceptable level, provide clients and their families with education and information about pain so that they can participate in the pain care decision-making process. This will help reduce anxiety and increases a client's sense of control. For example, clients who are in hospital for the first time may know that they require tests, but do not understand them. As a result, they may become anxious and fearful. Fear increases the perception of painful stimuli. Remember, however, that health promotion goes beyond teaching. Using pain management techniques from the Ottawa

Charter for Health will help you to develop your own skills in creating a supportive environment, using the strategies of enabling, mediating, and advocating for better pain-management services.

Nonpharmacological Pain-Relief Interventions. Several nonpharmacological interventions do not need a physician's order, but are initiated by nurses. Use these approaches in addition to, not in place of, pharmacological measures (Gruener & Lande, 2006, Titler & Rakel, 2001). Nonpharmacological interventions include cognitive–behavioural and physical approaches.

The goals of cognitive–behavioural interventions, such as relaxation and guided imagery, are to change pain perceptions, alter pain behaviour, and provide a greater sense of control. Physical agents aim to provide comfort, correct physical dysfunction, alter physiological responses, and reduce fears associated with pain-related immobility. Complementary and alternative medicine (CAM) therapies, such as herbal products, are also available. The AHCPR guidelines for acute pain management (1992) cite nonpharmacological interventions as appropriate for clients who meet the following criteria:

- Find such interventions appealing
- Express anxiety or fear
- May benefit from avoiding or reducing drug therapy
- Are likely to experience, and need to cope with, a prolonged interval of postoperative pain
- Have incomplete pain relief after use of pharmacological interventions

Relaxation and Guided Imagery. These techniques can alter affective-motivational and cognitive pain perception. **Relaxation** is mental and physical freedom from tension or stress. Relaxation techniques provide clients with self-control, and can be used at any phase of health or illness. Clients who successfully use relaxation techniques experience physiological and behavioural changes such as decreased pulse, blood pressure, and respirations; heightened global awareness; decreased oxygen consumption; a sense of peace; and decreased muscle tension and metabolic rate. Relaxation techniques include meditation, yoga, Zen, guided imagery, and progressive relaxation exercises (see Chapter 35).

For effective relaxation, clients must be in a state that will enable them to participate and cooperate. Relaxation is not taught to clients in severe pain because they may not be able to focus and concentrate. Explain the technique and describe common sensations that the client may experience (e.g., a decrease in temperature or numbness of a body part). The client should use these sensations as feedback. Coach and guide the client slowly through the steps of the exercise. The environment should be quiet and free of stimuli. The client may sit in a comfortable chair or lie in bed (Box 42–12). A light sheet or blanket may help the client feel more comfortable. Guided imagery and relaxation exercises may be done together or separately.

Progressive relaxation of the entire body takes about 15 minutes. The client pays attention to the body, noting areas of tension. Warmth and relaxation replace tension in these areas. Some clients relax better with their eyes closed. Soft background music can help.

Progressive relaxation exercises involve controlled breathing exercises and a series of contractions and relaxation of muscle groups. The client begins by breathing slowly and diaphragmatically, allowing the abdomen to rise slowly and the chest to expand fully. When the client establishes a regular breathing pattern, you can coach the client to locate any area of muscular tension, to think about how it feels, to tense muscles fully, and then to relax them completely. This creates the sensation of removing all discomfort and stress. Gradually the client can relax the muscles without first tensing them. When full relaxation is achieved, pain perception is lowered and anxiety about pain becomes minimal. Chapter 35 offers several relaxation exercise approaches.

BOX 42-12 Body Positions for Relaxation

Sitting

Sit with entire back resting against back of chair.
Place feet flat on floor.
Keep legs separated.
Hang arms at the side or rest on chair arms.
Keep head aligned with spine.

Lying

Keep legs separated with toes pointed slightly outward.
Rest arms at sides without touching sides of body.
Keep head aligned with spine.
Use thin, small pillow under head.

If a client becomes agitated or uncomfortable, it is best to stop the exercise. If the client has difficulty relaxing any part of the body, slow the progression of the exercise and concentrate on the tensed body part. The client must know that the exercise can be stopped at any time. With practice, the client can soon perform relaxation exercises independently.

In **guided imagery**, the client creates an image in his or her mind, concentrates on that image, and gradually becomes less aware of pain. Coach the client in forming the image and concentrating on the sensory experience. Initially, ask the client to think of a pleasant scene or experience that promotes the use of all of the senses. The client may describe the image, which you may record for use during later exercises. Use the information the client gives you, and do not change the client's image. The following is an example of part of a guided imagery exercise:

Imagine you are lying on a cool bed of grass with the sounds of rushing water from a nearby stream. It's a balmy day. You turn to see a patch of blue wildflowers in bloom and can smell their fragrance.

Sit close enough to be heard, and speak in a calm, soft voice. While relaxing, the client focuses on the image, and it will become unnecessary for you to speak continuously. If the client shows signs of agitation, restlessness, or discomfort, stop the exercise and try again when the client is more at ease.

Distraction. The reticular activating system inhibits painful stimuli if a person receives sufficient or excessive sensory input. People who are bored or in isolation tend to focus on their pain, and thus perceive it more acutely. Pleasurable stimuli cause the release of endorphins that help a person ignore or become unaware of pain. Distraction, particularly effective for young children, directs attention to something else, thus reducing pain awareness and increasing tolerance. It works best for short, intense pain lasting a few minutes, such as during an invasive procedure or while waiting for an analgesic to work. Examples include praying, describing photos or pictures aloud, listening to music, and playing games. Most distractions can be used in a hospital, home, or long-term care facility.

Music. Music can decrease physiological pain, stress, and anxiety by diverting attention away from pain and creating a relaxation response. It produces an altered state of consciousness through sound, silence, space, and time. All forms of music are used in music therapy. Music must be listened to for at least 15 minutes to be therapeutic.

Clients should select the music they prefer. Earphones can help concentration. Popular music does not usually produce deep relaxation because it is short, and has words and a steady beat. In an acute-care setting, listening to music can significantly reduce a client's postoperative pain. Help create a relaxing setting so that music can be listened to uninterrupted. If pain becomes acute, suggest increasing the music's volume until the pain subsides.

Clients with Alzheimer's disease often experience agitation, which worsens with pain. Music may be used to communicate with these clients even if they cannot understand speech and have problems interpreting environmental stimuli.

Biofeedback. **Biofeedback** is a behavioural therapy that involves giving individuals information about physiological responses (e.g., blood pressure or tension) and ways to exercise voluntary control over those responses (McGrady et al., 1994). It is used to produce deep relaxation, and is especially effective for muscle tension and migraine headaches. In the treatment of headaches, electrodes are attached externally over each temple. The electrodes measure skin tension in microvolts. A polygraph machine visibly records the tension level for the client to see. The client learns to achieve optimal relaxation by lowering the actual level of tension experienced, using feedback from the polygraph. The therapy takes several weeks to learn. Chapter 35 describes the benefits and limitations of biofeedback.

Acupuncture. **Acupuncture** may help reduce chronic and acute pain. The mechanism of action is similar to that of counterirritation-induced analgesia. Kotani et al. (2001) found that clients who had intradermal needles placed in their abdomens before abdominal surgery required less IV morphine and had less postoperative nausea than did the group that did not receive acupuncture.

Cutaneous Stimulation. **Cutaneous stimulation** is the stimulation of the skin to relieve pain. A massage, warm bath, ice bag, and transcutaneous electrical nerve stimulation (TENS) are simple ways to reduce pain perception. How cutaneous stimulation works is unclear. One suggestion is that it causes the release of endorphins, thus blocking the transmission of painful stimuli. The gate-control theory suggests that cutaneous stimulation activates larger, faster-transmitting A-beta sensory nerve fibres. This decreases pain transmission through small-diameter A-delta and C fibres. Synaptic gates close to the transmission of pain impulses. In a review by O'Mathuna (2000), touch and massage influenced autonomic nervous system activity. When a person perceives touch to be relaxing, the relaxation response is elicited.

An advantage to cutaneous stimulation is that the measures can be used in the home, giving clients and families some control over pain symptoms and treatment. The proper use of cutaneous stimulation can reduce pain perception and help to reduce muscle tension that might otherwise increase pain. When using cutaneous stimulation methods, conduct them in a noise-free room. Help the client to assume a comfortable position, and explain the purpose of the therapy. Cutaneous stimulation should not be used directly on sensitive skin areas (e.g., burns, bruises, skin rashes, inflammation, and underlying bone fractures).

Massage has been used by nurses for many years as a safe and effective way to produce physical and mental relaxation, reduce pain, and enhance the effectiveness of pain medications (Figure 42–11). Massaging the back and shoulders or the hands and feet for 3 to 5 minutes can help relax muscles and promote sleep and comfort (Grealish et al., 2000). Cassileth and Vickers (2004) reported a 50% reduction in pain, fatigue, stress, anxiety, nausea, and depression in clients with cancer who systematically used massage therapy. Massages communicate caring, and are easy for family members or other health care professionals to learn (Box 42–13).

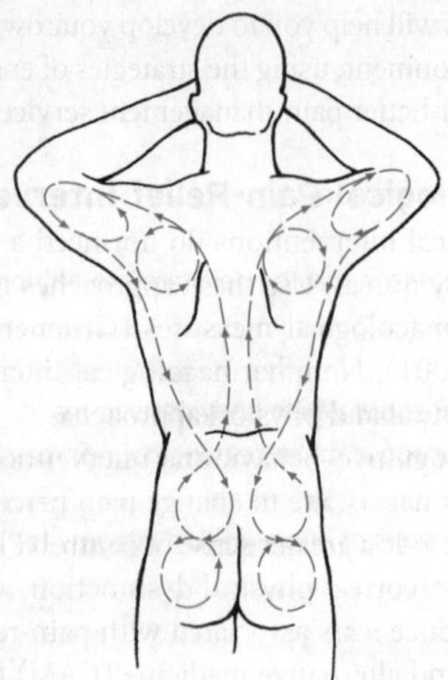

Figure 42-11 Back massage pattern.

Cold and heat applications (see Chapter 46) relieve pain and promote healing. The choice of heat or cold varies with clients' conditions. Moist heat can help relieve pain from a tension headache, and cold applications can reduce acute pain from inflamed joints. To avoid injury, check the temperature and avoid direct application of cold or heat to the skin. Clients at most risk for such injury include those with spinal cord or other neurological injury, older adults, and confused clients.

Ice massage and application of cold packs are particularly effective for pain relief. Ice massage involves the use of a large ice cube or a small paper cup filled with water and frozen (water rises out of the cup as it freezes to create a smooth surface of ice for massage). The massage is simple. You or the client can apply the ice with firm pressure to the skin, followed by a slow, steady, circular massage over the area. Cold may be applied near the pain site, on the opposite side of the body corresponding to the pain site, or on a site located between the brain and the pain site. It takes 5 to 10 minutes to apply cold. Each client responds differently to the site of application that is most effective. Application near the actual site of pain tends to work best. A client feels cold, burning, and aching sensations, as well as numbness. When numbness occurs, the ice should be removed. Cold is particularly effective for tooth or mouth pain when ice is placed on the web of the hand between the thumb and index finger. This point on the hand is an **acupressure** point that apparently influences nerve pathways to the face and head. Cold applications are also effective before invasive needle punctures.

Heat application might work better for some clients. Heating pads or hot water bottles may be used, but clients should be taught not to lie on the heating element to avoid burns. Commercial pillows that can be warmed in the microwave and that contour to the body can also be used.

Another form of cutaneous stimulation, sometimes called counterstimulation, is **transcutaneous electrical nerve stimulation (TENS)**. TENS involves stimulation of the skin with a mild electrical current passed through external electrodes (Melzack & Wall, 2003). This therapy requires a physician's order. The TENS unit consists of a battery-powered transmitter, lead wires, and electrodes. The electrodes are placed directly over or near the site of pain. Hair or skin preparations should be removed before attaching the electrodes. When a client feels pain, the transmitter is turned on and a buzzing or tingling sensation is created. The client may adjust the intensity and quality of skin stimulation. The tingling sensation can be applied

> ➤ BOX 42-13 **Procedural Guidelines**
>
> ## Massage
>
> **Delegation Considerations:** The nurse is responsible for assessing any possible contraindication or client response to massage. The skill of administering a massage may be delegated to an unregulated care provider (UCP), providing that the client is stable. Before delegation, you must:
>
> - Instruct the UCP about which body parts to massage.
> - Instruct the UCP about the importance of not massaging reddened skin areas.
> - Clarify the early signs of impaired skin integrity for select clients, and instruct the UCP to report changes in the client's skin.
>
> **Equipment**
>
> - Moisturizing lotion
> - Bath towel or blanket
>
> **Procedure**
>
> 1. Assist client to assume comfortable position.
> 2. Dim room lights, turn on soft music, or both, according to client preference.
> 3. Perform hand hygiene. Warm lotion in hands or place container in warm water.
> 4. Adjust or remove client's bed clothing.
> 5. Place small amount of lotion in your hands.
> 6. Massage each body part for at least 10 minutes.
>   A. *Back:* Begin a sacral area massage with a circular motion (see Figure 42–11), moving upward from buttocks to shoulders. Use a firm, smooth stroke over the scapula. Continue in one smooth stroke to upper arms and laterally along sides of back, down to iliac crests. Use long, gliding strokes along muscles of spine. Knead any muscles that feel tense or tight. Knead skin by gently grasping tissue between thumb and fingers. Knead upward along one side of the spine from buttocks to shoulders, around nape of neck. Knead or stroke downward toward sacrum. Repeat along other side of back.
>   B. *Neck:* Support neck at the hairline with one hand and massage upward with a gliding stroke. Knead muscles on one side. Switch hands to support neck, and knead other side. Stretch the neck slightly, with one hand at the top and the other at the bottom.
>   C. *Arms:* Use a gliding stroke to massage upwards from client's wrist or forearm. With thumb and forefinger of both hands, knead muscles from forearm to shoulder. Continue kneading bicep, deltoid, and tricep muscles. Finish with gliding strokes from wrists to shoulder.
>   D. *Hands:* Slowly open client's palm, and glide fingers over the palmar surface. Use thumbs to apply friction to palm and move thumbs in a circular motion. Stretch the palm outward. Massage each finger, using a corkscrew-like motion from the base of the finger to the tip. Gently knead each muscle in client's fingers. Glide hands smoothly from fingertips to wrists. Repeat for other hand.
>   E. *Feet:* Gently massage top and bottom of each foot. Using gliding motion, massage from heel to toe. Gently massage the dorsal surface of the foot and each toe. Repeat for other foot.
> 7. Wipe excess lotion off client's back, neck, or extremity. If necessary, gown or assist with pyjamas, and assist client to comfortable position.
> 8. Ask client about level of comfort. Note any areas of muscle pain or tension.

until pain relief occurs. TENS is effective for postsurgical pain control and reduction of pain caused by postoperative procedures.

Herbals. Although herbals have not been sufficiently studied to recommend for pain relief, many clients self-medicate using herbals such as echinacea, ginseng, ginkgo biloba, and garlic supplements (Wirth et al., 2005). Some herbal products may interact with prescribed analgesics, and ginkgo biloba may decrease the ability of blood to clot after surgery. Ask the client to report all substances taken to relieve pain (Yoon & Schaffer, 2006) (see Chapter 35).

Reducing Pain Perception. One simple way to promote comfort is to remove or prevent painful stimuli (Box 42–14). This is especially important for clients who are immobilized or have difficulty in expressing themselves. Take steps to reduce the individual's pain by paying attention to the way you perform procedures. Consider the client's condition and the aspects of the procedure that are uncomfortable. Use techniques to avoid pain-producing situations. For example, in a client with severe arthritic knee pain, know that extreme flexion of the knee can cause pain. Before walking the client to the bathroom, make sure that an elevated toilet seat is available. The client can then be seated and can rise with minimal discomfort.

Acute Care

Acute Pain Management. Some clients have acute pain from invasive procedures (e.g., surgery or endoscopy) or trauma. The AHCPR (1992) has a pain treatment flow chart (see Figure 42–15 on page 1037) for the aggressive treatment of postoperative pain and pain from medical procedures and trauma. A systematic approach ensures a quick response to client discomfort. The key to success in pain relief is the ongoing evaluation of interventions: Is relief obtained? Do the medications cause any unacceptable side effects? It is the responsibility of the health care team to collaborate in order to find the combination of therapy that works best for a client.

> ➤ BOX 42-14 **Controlling Painful Stimuli in the Client's Environment**
>
> Tighten and smooth wrinkled bed linen.
> Loosen constricting bandages (unless specifically applied as a pressure dressing).
> Change wet dressings and linens.
> Position client in anatomical alignment.
> Check temperature of hot or cold applications, including bath water.
> Lift client in bed—do not pull.
> Position client correctly on bedpan.
> Avoid exposing skin or mucous membranes to irritants (e.g., urine, stool, wound drainage).
> Prevent urinary retention by keeping Foley catheters patent and free flowing.
> Prevent constipation with stool softeners, fluids, diet, and exercise.
> Reduce lighting and ambient sound.

Pharmacological Pain-Relief Interventions. The ideal analgesic has yet to be developed, but several pain-relieving pharmacological agents are available. Most require a physician's order.

safety alert Your critical thinking and judgement in the selection and adminstration of analgesics help ensure safe and effective pain relief.

- Be cognizant of the pain diagnosis, the client's physical characteristics (e.g., age), and severity of the illness; know that some analgesics will be contraindicated
- Employ the seven rights (person, drug, dose, route, time, documentation, and reason) of medication adminstration
- When dispensing narcotics, be sure to check the dose and drug type, as the names of some common medications sound alike
- Administer all analgesics using standardized guidelines

Analgesics. Analgesics are the most common method of pain relief. Although analgesics can effectively relieve pain, recall that nurses and physicians still tend to undertreat clients because of incorrect drug information, concerns about addiction, anxiety over errors in using opioid analgesics, and administration of less medication than was ordered.

Three types of analgesics exist: (1) nonsteroidal anti-inflammatory drugs (NSAIDs) and nonopioids, (2) **opioids** (traditionally called narcotics), and (3) coanalgesics, a variety of medications that enhance analgesics or have analgesic properties that were originally unknown.

Acetaminophen (Tylenol) has no anti-inflammatory or antiplatelet effects. It works peripherally and centrally, but its action is unknown. Its major adverse effect is hepatotoxicity. It is in a variety of over-the-counter (OTC) cold, flu, and allergy remedies. The maximum 24-hour dose is 4 g (the same dose limitation as aspirin). It is often combined with opioids (e.g., Percocet, Vicodin, Lortab, and Ultracet) because it reduces the dose of opioid needed to achieve successful pain control. Overdoses of acetaminophen are treated with acetylcysteine (Mucomyst).

Nonselective NSAIDs, such as aspirin and ibuprofen, provide relief for mild to moderate acute intermittent pain, such as the pain associated with a headache or muscle strain. Treatment of mild to moderate postoperative pain begins with an NSAID unless contraindicated (AHCPR, 1992). NSAIDs are believed to act by inhibiting the synthesis of prostaglandins (Williams, 2005) and thus the cellular responses to inflammation. Most NSAIDs act on peripheral nerve receptors to reduce transmission of pain stimuli. Unlike opioids, NSAIDs do not depress the central nervous system, nor do they interfere with bowel or bladder function (AHCPR, 1992). Chronic NSAID use in the older client, however, is associated with more frequent adverse effects (e.g., gastrointestinal bleeding and renal insufficiency) and should be avoided. Mild to moderate musculoskeletal pain in older adults is effectively managed with the nonopioid acetaminophen (American Geriatrics Society [AGS], 2002).

Nonselective NSAIDs have been found to be safe when taken for short periods of time. Selective COX-2 inhibitors have caused heart attack and stroke, and have been withdrawn from the market. Celebrex is the only selective COX-2 inhibitor currently available; however, it should not be used in clients with a sulfa allergy. Some clients with asthma or an allergy to aspirin are also allergic to NSAIDs (Williams, 2005). Some NSAIDs are available OTC; advise clients to discuss using OTC NSAIDs for managing pain with their primary health care professional (D'Arcy, 2006).

Opioid or opioid-like analgesics are generally prescribed for moderate to severe pain. These analgesics act on higher centres of the brain and spinal cord by binding with opiate receptors to modify the perception of pain. A rare adverse effect of opioids in opioid-naive clients is respiratory depression (Wheeler et al., 2002). Respiratory depression is only clinically significant if the rate *and* depth of respirations decrease from the client's baseline measurements (McCaffery & Pasero, 1999). Clients who are breathing deeply rarely have clinical respiratory depression. It is important to note that another adverse effect of opioids, sedation, *always* occurs before respiratory depression. Therefore, closely monitor for sedation in opioid-naive clients (Pasero & McCaffery, 2002).

If a client experiences respiratory depression, naloxone (0.4 mg diluted with 9 mL of saline) intravenous push (IVP) at a rate of 0.5 mL is administered by a physician or ordered as policy every 2 minutes until the respiratory rate is greater than 8 breaths per minute with good depth. A too-fast administration will reverse the analgesic effect, and possibly cause pulmonary edema (American Pain Society, 2003). Reassess clients taking naloxone every 15 minutes for 2 hours after drug administration because of the risk of renarcotization and the return of respiratory depression.

Additional adverse effects of opioids include nausea, vomiting, constipation, itching, urinary retention, myoclonus, and altered mental processes (Ersek et al., 2004). Except for constipation, these side effects usually stop once the client receives an opioid around the clock (ATC) for 4 to 10 days. A client is considered **opioid-naive** before, and **opioid-tolerant** after, this period of ATC opioid dosing. One way to maximize pain relief while potentially decreasing drug use is to administer analgesics on an ATC basis rather than on a prn basis. Paice et al. (2005) found that clients receiving ATC opioids reported lower pain intensity scores than clients receiving prn opioids.

The American Pain Society (APS) (2003) states that if pain is anticipated for the majority of the day, ATC administration should be considered. The American Geriatrics Society (AGS) (2002) states that older adults are not treated with opioids frequently enough. The AGS suggests a "start low" (dose) and "go slow" (upward dose titration) philosophy. Furthermore, the AGS discourages the use of meperidine or propoxyphene in older adults (AGS, 2002; Fick et al., 2003; Willens, 2006). Meperidine is not recommended as an analgesic at any age because of its toxic metabolite, normeperidine, which can cause seizures (APS, 2003).

The proper use of analgesics requires careful assessment and critical thinking in the application of pharmacological principles and logic. A person's response to an analgesic is highly individualized. An NSAID can be as effective, or more effective, than an opioid for some clients if the pain is caused by inflammation. An orally administered analgesic usually has a longer onset and duration of action than an injectable form. In addition, controlled- or extended-release opioid formulations (MS Contin, OxyContin, Kadian, Avinza, and methadone) are available for administration every 8 to 12 hours ATC. Physicians should not order these long-acting formulations prn.

You need to know the comparative potencies of analgesics in both oral and injectable forms. In addition, know the route of administration most effective for a client so that you can achieve controlled, sustained pain relief. If nurses on succeeding shifts choose different routes for the same doses, the client will not receive the same level of analgesia, and pain control will be poor. Equianalgesic charts are charts that convert one opioid to another (e.g., morphine to hydromorphone), or parenteral forms of opioids to oral forms (or vice versa). They are available on most nursing units, or by contacting pharmacy team members. To see an example of an equianalgesic chart developed by the Mass Pain Initiative in partnership with the American Cancer Society, visit http://www.masspaininitiative.org/PDFs/PocketTool_June05.pdf.

Before administering opioids, it is important to consider the client's situation, including current treatments, diseases and conditions, and organ (kidney and liver) function. Opioid doses often need adjusting up or down according to client circumstances. Situations requiring special considerations include breast feeding mothers, clients on dialysis, those with neurological or respiratory conditions, and clients with recent abdominal surgery.

The Joint Commission (2009) requires health care agencies to have range order policies in place to help guide nurses in selecting the most appropriate dose of a medication: "Range orders are medication orders in which the dose varies over a prescribed range depending on the situation or the patient's status" (Manworren, 2006). "Administer 5 to 10 mg morphine sulfate IVP for acute pain" is an example of a range order. Such an order is dangerous when real clinical guidelines for selecting the exact dose do not exist. Pain severity assessment is not simply a number; therefore, it is important that analgesic doses not be solely dependent on a client's report of pain. For examples of clinical guidelines to use for range orders, see the position statements of Manworren (2006) and the American Society for Pain Management Nursing (n.d.).

Adjuvants, or co-analgesics, are drugs that were originally developed to treat conditions other than pain but have been shown to have analgesic properties. For example, tricyclic antidepressants (e.g., nortriptyline) and anticonvulsants (e.g., gabapentin [Neurontin]) successfully treat neuropathic pain (Gordon & Love, 2004), as does infusional lidocaine (Ferrini & Paice, 2004). Corticosteroids relieve pain associated with inflammation and bone metastasis. Other examples of adjuvants are bisphosphonates and calcitonin given for bone pain (Jacox et al., 1994). Sedatives, anti-anxiety agents, and muscle relaxants have *no* analgesic effects; however, they *can* cause drowsiness and impaired coordination, judgement, and mental alertness, and contribute to respiratory depression. It is important to avoid attributing these adverse effects solely to the opioid; you need to conduct a thorough reassessment.

Patient-Controlled Analgesia. Clients benefit from having control over pain therapy. When clients depend on nurses for prn analgesia, an erratic cycle of alternating pain and analgesia often occurs. The client feels pain and asks for medication, but the nurse must first assess the client and then prepare the medication. Within an hour, analgesia finally occurs, but pain relief may last only 30 minutes. The client's discomfort then gradually escalates, and the cycle is repeated. The client is constantly going in and out of analgesic therapeutic range.

A drug delivery system called **patient-controlled analgesia (PCA)** is a safe method for postoperative and cancer pain management that most clients prefer. It is a drug delivery system that allows clients to self-administer opioids (e.g., morphine, hydromorphone, fentanyl) with minimal risk of overdose. The goal is to maintain a constant plasma level of analgesic so that the problems of prn dosing are avoided. Systemic PCA usually involves IV drug administration, but it can also be given subcutaneously. PCAs are portable infusion pumps (usually computerized), containing a chamber for a syringe (Figure 42–12) or bag that delivers a small, preset dose of medication. To receive a demand dose, the client pushes a button attached to the PCA device. To avoid overdoses, the system is designed to deliver no more than a specified number of doses, either every hour or every 4 hours (depending on the pump). A typical PCA prescription relies on a series of "loading" doses (e.g., 3 to 5 mg of morphine) repeated every 5 minutes until initial postoperative pain diminishes. On-demand doses typically add 1 mg of morphine every 6 minutes, with a total hourly limit of 6 mg (AHCPR, 1992; APS, 2003). Most pumps have locked safety systems that prevent tampering by clients or their family members, and are generally safe to be managed in the home. For clients with cancer pain, a low-dose continuous infusion (basal rate) of 0.5 to 1 mg/hour may be programmed to deliver a steady dose of continuous medication.

safety alert PCA basal doses are not recommended for opioid-naive clients after surgery because of the possibility for respiratory depression.

PCA use is beneficial in many ways. The client gains control over his or her pain, and pain relief does not depend on nurse availability. Clients can also access medication when they need it. This can decrease anxiety and lead to decreased medication use. Small doses of medications are delivered at short intervals, stabilizing serum drug concentrations for sustained pain relief.

Clients who do not favour PCA are those who feel they do not understand how to use the technology, while nurses view PCA as a disadvantage when it is ordered for clients with short-term memory loss or states of confusion (King & Walsh, 2007). Client suitability,

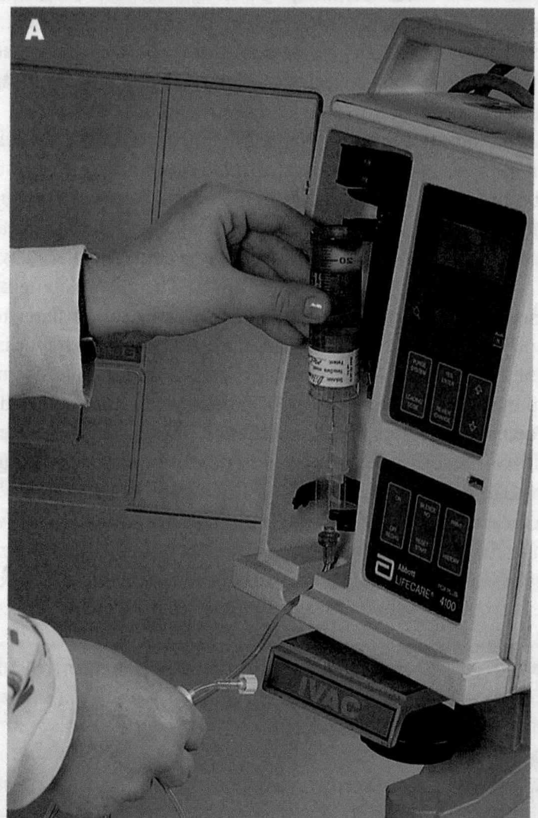

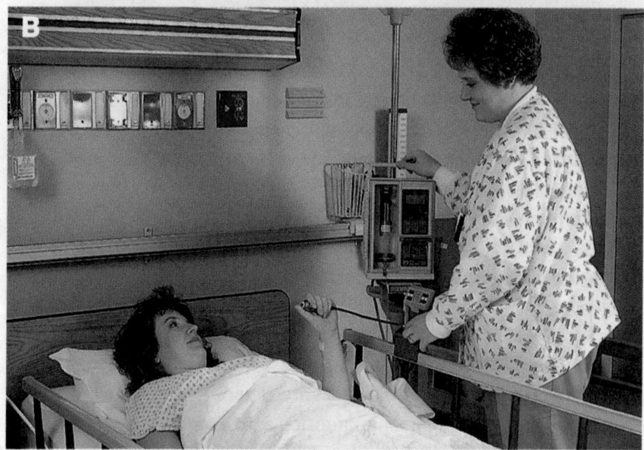

Figure 42-12 A, Patient-controlled analgesia (PCA) pump with syringe chamber. B, Client learns to use PCA pump.

preparation, and teaching is therefore critical to the safe and effective use of PCA devices (Box 42–15). Teach clients how to use the technology and determine if they are physically able to locate and press the button to deliver the dose. Remind family members they must not press the button for clients, as this could cause toxic effects (Reiff & Nizolek, 2001). Nurse-controlled analgesia may be implemented in lieu of client-controlled analgesia, with physician approval, after assessing the client.

Check the IV line and PCA device regularly to ensure proper functioning. Even though clients control administration of analgesics, programmable PCA errors do occur. In opioid-naive clients, do not simultaneously increase demand or basal dose *and* shorten the interval time because this will increase the risk for oversedation and respiratory depression. Document drug dosages, and track any waste of medications according to agency policy (Pasero, 2003).

The first controlled analgesia device for oral medications, Medication on Demand (MOD), recently became available. This device allows clients access to their own oral prn mediations, including opioids and other analgesics, anti-emetics, and anxiolytics, at the bedside (Avancen, 2006).

Local Analgesic Infusion Pump. After orthopedic surgery, to avoid systemic effects of oral analgesics, an application of a local anaesthetic may be appropriate. A catheter from the wound placed during surgery is connected to a pump containing a local anaesthetic (Marcaine). The pump may be set to either demand or continuous modes. The device is usually left in place for 48 hours. The client is taught how to discontinue the pump at home and to bring the catheter to the next physician visit. Oral analgesics may still be needed by the client, but the total dose is often reduced (Pasero, 2000). Safe use of the pump in non-orthopedic surgeries has not yet been established.

Topical Analgesics and Anaesthetics. Topical analgesics such as ELA-Max/LMX and EMLA (eutectic mixture of local anaesthetics) are available for children. Apply EMLA to the skin, via a disc or as thick cream, 30 to 60 minutes before minor procedures (e.g., IV start) or anaesthetic infiltration of soft tissue. Do not place EMLA around the eyes, on the tympanic membrane, or over large skin surfaces.

> **BOX 42-15 Preparation for Patient-Controlled Analgesia (PCA)**
>
> **Objectives**
> - Client will be able to explain the purpose of PCA in managing pain.
> - Client will use the PCA device correctly.
> - Client will achieve pain control.
>
> **Teaching Strategies**
> - Teach the use of PCA before any procedure so that clients can understand how to use it after awakening from anaesthesia or sedation. Reinforce as needed.
> - Instruct client on the purpose of PCA, emphasizing that the client controls medication delivery.
> - Explain that the pump prevents the risk of overdose.
> - Tell family members or friends that they should not operate the PCA device for the client.
> - Ask the client to demonstrate use of the PCA delivery button.
>
> **Evaluation**
> - Ask client to tell you the purpose of the PCA device.
> - Observe the client administering a dose.
> - Evaluate the severity of the client's pain 15 to 20 minutes after use of the PCA device.

The Lidoderm patch is a topical analgesic effective for cutaneous neuropathic pain in adults. Place three patches, cut to size, on and around the pain site using a 12-hour-on, 12-hour-off schedule to avoid lidocaine toxicity. Other topical analgesics include ketoprofen patches and capsaicin lotion.

Local and Regional Anaesthetics and Analgesics. **Local anaesthesia** is the infiltration of a local anaesthetic medication to induce loss of sensation to a localized body part. Physicians use local anaesthesia during brief surgical procedures, such as the removal of a skin lesion or suturing a wound. Apply the local anaesthetics topically on skin and mucous membranes, or inject subcutaneously or intradermally to anaesthetize a body part. The drugs produce temporary loss of sensation by inhibiting nerve conduction. Local anaesthetics can also block motor and autonomic functions, depending on the amount used and the location and depth of an injection. Smaller sensory nerve fibres are more sensitive to local anaesthetics than are large motor fibres. As a result, the client loses sensation before losing motor function, and, conversely, motor activity returns before sensation.

Local anaesthetics can cause side effects, depending on their absorption into the circulation. Itching or burning of the skin or a localized rash is common after topical applications. Application to vascular mucous membranes increases the chance of systemic effects, such as a change in heart rate.

Regional anaesthesia is the injection of a local anaesthetic to block a group of sensory nerve fibres. Tissues are anaesthetized layer by layer, as the surgeon or anaesthesiologist introduces the agent into deeper structures of the body. Kinds of regional anaesthesia include epidural anaesthesia, pudendal blocks, and spinal anaesthesia.

Whereas epidural anaesthesia induces temporary loss of sensation, **epidural analgesia** permits control or reduction of severe pain, without the more serious sedative effects of parenteral or oral narcotics. Epidural analgesia is commonly used for the treatment of acute postoperative pain, labour and delivery pain, and chronic pain, especially that associated with cancer (Roman & Cabaj, 2005). However, intraspinal morphine can produce the same side effects of nausea, mental clouding, and sedation, because it is absorbed via the cerebrospinal fluid into the circulation of the epidural vascular plexus. Epidural analgesia can be short- or long-term, depending on the client's condition and life expectancy. Short-term therapy is used for pain after intrathoracic, abdominal, and orthopedic surgery. Long-term therapy is used for intractable pain in the lower part of the body, particularly when it is bilateral (Du Pen & Williams, 1992).

Epidural analgesia is administered into the spinal **epidural space** (Figure 42–13). The physician inserts a blunt-tip needle into the level of the vertebral interspace nearest to the area requiring analgesia. When the needle reaches the space, solutions may be freely injected and small catheters may be passed into it. Once a catheter is advanced into the epidural space and the needle is removed, the remainder of the catheter is secured with a dressing and taped along the back of the client (Figure 42–14). If the catheter is only temporary, it is connected to tubing positioned along the spine and over the client's shoulder. The end of the catheter can then be placed on the client's chest for the nurse's access. Epidural analgesia may be anaesthesiology- or nurse-controlled, depending on agency policy. Clients may also be given control of the demand dose, which is known as patient-controlled epidural analgesia (PCEA).

Nursing Implications. You can provide emotional support to clients receiving local or regional anaesthesia by explaining insertion or application sites and warning clients that they will temporarily lose sensory function. In the case of regional anaesthesia, prepare the client for the type, as well as when motor and autonomic function (bowel and bladder control) are expected to be temporarily lost. Clients commonly fear paralysis because epidural and spinal

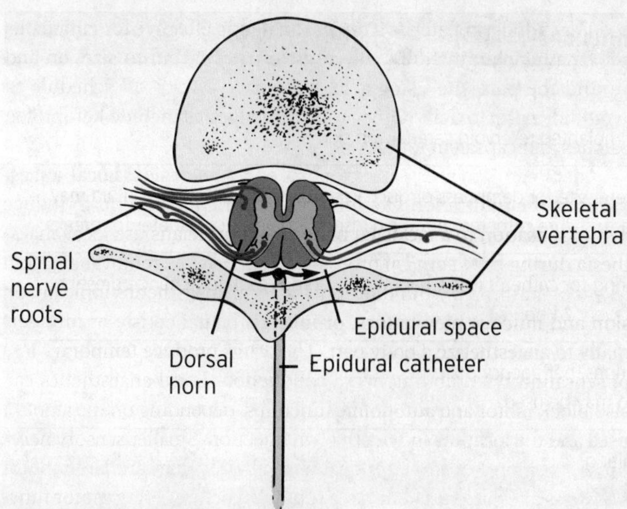

Figure 42-13 Anatomical drawing of epidural space.

injections come close to the spinal cord. To reassure the client, explain that numbness, tingling, and coldness are common. Catheter insertion is painful unless the primary health care professional first numbs the injection site. Prepare clients for such discomfort. Before a client receives an analgesic, check for allergies and assess vital signs to monitor systemic effects.

After administration of a local anaesthetic, protect the client from injury until full sensory and motor function return. Clients are at risk for injuring the anaesthetized body part without knowing it. For example, after an injection into a joint, warn the client to avoid using the joint until function returns. For clients with topical anaesthesia, avoid applying heat or cold to numb areas. After spinal anaesthesia, instruct the client to stay in bed until sensory and motor function return.

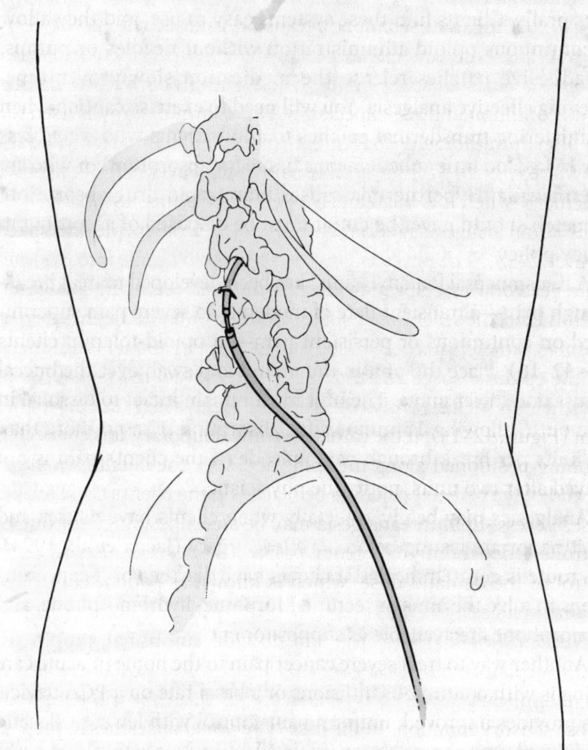

Figure 42-14 Epidural catheter taped in place.

Assist the client during the first attempt at getting out of the bed.

When managing epidural infusions, connect the catheter to an infusion pump, a port, or a reservoir, or cap it off for bolus injections. To reduce the risk of accidental epidural injection of drugs intended for IV use, clearly label the catheter as an "epidural catheter." Always administer continuous infusions through electronic infusion devices for proper control. Because of the catheter location, use surgical asepsis to prevent a serious and potentially fatal infection. Notify the physician immediately of any signs or symptoms of infection or pain at the insertion site. Thorough hygiene is necessary during nursing procedures to keep the catheter system clean and dry.

The nursing implications for managing epidural analgesia are numerous (Table 42–6). Supplemental doses of opioids or sedatives (hypnotics) are avoided because they have additive effects that can be detrimental to the central nervous system. Monitoring of medications' effects differs, depending on whether infusions are intermittent or continuous. Complications of epidural opioid use include nausea and vomiting, urinary retention, constipation, respiratory depression, and **pruritus** (itching) (Cox, 2001). When clients are receiving epidural analgesia, you will need to assess and monitor respiratory rate, respiratory effort, and skin colour every 15 minutes. Once stabilized, monitoring can move to every hour (refer to agency policy).

The client must receive thorough education about epidural analgesia in terms of the action of the medication and its advantages and disadvantages. Instruct clients about potential side effects, and that they should notify a health care professional if they develop. If the client requires long-term epidural use, inform the client that a permanent catheter may be tunnelled through the skin and exit at the client's side. Teach clients on long-term therapy how to safely administer infusions in the home with minimal ongoing intervention by the nurse.

Invasive Interventions for Pain Relief. When pain is severe, invasive interventions may give relief when more conservative treatment is neither tolerated nor effective (Jacox et al., 1994). These interventions include intrathecal implantable pumps or injections, spinal cord stimulators, deep brain stimulation, neuroablative procedures (e.g., **chordotomy, dorsal rhizotomy**, thalamotomy), trigger point injections, radiofrequency ablation, cryoablation, intradiscal electrothermal (IDET) annuloplasty, vertebroplasty, intraspinal medications (e.g., opioids, steroids, local anaesthetics, alpha agonists), and others. It is not acceptable to tell a client with severe unrelieved pain that "there is nothing more we can do for you." Clients with pain unresponsive to medications need consultation with a pain expert.

Procedure Pain Management.

The Thunder Project II (Puntillo et al., 2001) identified several procedures in critical-care clients that cause pain:

- Turning
- Wound drain removal
- Tracheal suctioning
- Femoral catheter removal
- Placement of central line
- Changing of nonburn wound dressings

Premedicating clients before painful procedures allows clients to cooperate more fully and reduces the experience of pain. This is also true for clients who present in the emergency department with abdominal pain. The APS (2003) recommends medicating the client in pain before conducting an extensive physical examination or diagnostic procedures.

Cancer Pain Management.

Cancer pain is either chronic or acute. The AHCPR released clinical practice guidelines for the management of cancer pain (Jacox et al., 1994). The guidelines are

➤ TABLE 42-6 Nursing Care for Clients With Epidural Infusions

Goal	Actions
Prevent catheter displacement.	Secure catheter (if not connected to implanted reservoir) carefully on skin.
Maintain catheter function.	Check external dressing around catheter site for dampness or discharge. (Leak of cerebrospinal fluid may develop.) Use transparent dressing to secure catheter and to aid inspection. Inspect catheter for breaks.
Prevent infection.	Use strict aseptic technique when caring for catheter (see Chapter 33). Do not routinely change dressing over site. Change infusion tubing every 24 hours.
Monitor for respiratory depression.	Monitor vital signs, especially respirations, per agency policy. Pulse oximetry and apnea monitoring may be used.
Prevent complications.	Assess for pruritus, nausea, and vomiting. Administer anti-emetics as ordered.
Maintain urinary and bowel function.	Monitor intake and output. Assess for bladder and bowel distension. Assess for discomfort, frequency, and urgency.

designed to treat cancer pain in a more comprehensive and aggressive manner. Similarly, they provide clients and families more options for pain relief. Figure 42–15 is a flow chart depicting cancer pain management from assessment to various treatment options. The best choice of treatment often changes as the client's condition and the characteristics of pain change, and is best achieved when pharmacological and nonpharmacological pain interventions are used together.

Various medications and routes of administration provide relief for clients with cancer pain. Long-acting or controlled-release medications have been very successful in managing all types of chronic pain. These controlled-released medications (e.g., MS Contin, Roxanol SR, and OxyContin) relieve pain for 8 to 12 hours. A 72-hour fentanyl patch is also available. You can manage most chronic pain by using oral or patch medications.

Estimates of addiction in clients with chronic pain range from 1% to 24% (Passik et al., 2003). Clients with persistent pain requiring prolonged opioid administration sometimes develop an opioid tolerance. As a result, higher doses of opioids are required to attain pain relief. The higher opioid dose is not lethal because clients also develop a tolerance to respiratory depression. For clients with chronic pain, it is necessary to give required analgesics on a regular basis. Prescribing analgesics on a prn basis for chronic pain is ineffective and causes more suffering. The client with chronic pain needs to take an analgesic ATC, even when the pain subsides. Regular administration maintains therapeutic drug blood levels for ongoing pain control. Your understanding of this issue and heightening the client's awareness will help prevent breakthrough pain and loss of pain control.

Administering analgesics to treat chronic noncancer and cancer pain requires principles different from those used to treat acute pain. The World Health Organization (1990) recommended a three-step approach to managing cancer pain (Figure 42–16). Therapy begins with using NSAIDs, adjuvants, or both, and progresses to strong opioids if pain persists. However, when a client with cancer first experiences pain, it is best to begin with a higher dosage than will be needed for continued pain relief. The physician can slowly decrease the dosage to the amount needed, thus providing the client with immediate pain relief. Side effects of analgesia, such as nausea and constipation, can be aggressively treated so that analgesia can be continued. Clients can become tolerant to the side effects of nausea, but not to the constipating effects of analgesics. Stimulant laxatives, not simple stool softeners, should be routinely administered both to prevent and to treat constipation.

Transdermal drug systems administer fentanyl at predetermined doses for up to 48 to 72 hours. Fentanyl is about 100 times more potent than morphine.

safety alert Fentanyl should only be used in clients who are opioid-tolerant.

The transdermal route is useful when clients are unable to take drugs orally. Clients find these systems easy to use, and they allow for continuous opioid administration without needles or pumps. Self-adhesive patches release the medication slowly over time, achieving effective analgesia. You will need to exercise caution when administering transdermal patches to adult clients who weigh less than 45 kg (too little subcutaneous tissue for absorption) or who are hyperthermic. Hyperthermia causes more rapid drug absorption. The patch should never be cut; it must be disposed of according to agency policy.

A transmucosal fentanyl "unit" has been developed to treat **breakthrough pain**—a transient flare of moderate to severe pain superimposed on continuous or persistent pain—in opioid-tolerant clients (Box 42–16). Place the unit in the mouth and swab over the buccal mucosa and lower gums. The unit must remain intact to dissolve in the mouth, allowing 15 minutes for absorption. Use no more than two units per breakthrough pain episode. If the client's pain is not relieved after two units, notify the physician.

Analgesics may be given rectally when clients have nausea and vomiting, or are fasting before or after surgery (Jacox et al., 1994). This route is contraindicated if clients have diarrhea or if cancerous lesions involve the anus or rectum. Morphine, hydromorphone, and oxymorphone are available as suppositories.

Another way to treat severe cancer pain in the home or acute care setting is with continuous infusions or a basal rate on a PCA device. This provides improved, uniform pain control with fewer peaks and valleys in plasma concentration, more effective drug action, and lower drug dosages overall. Candidates for continuous infusions include clients with severe pain for whom oral and injectable medications

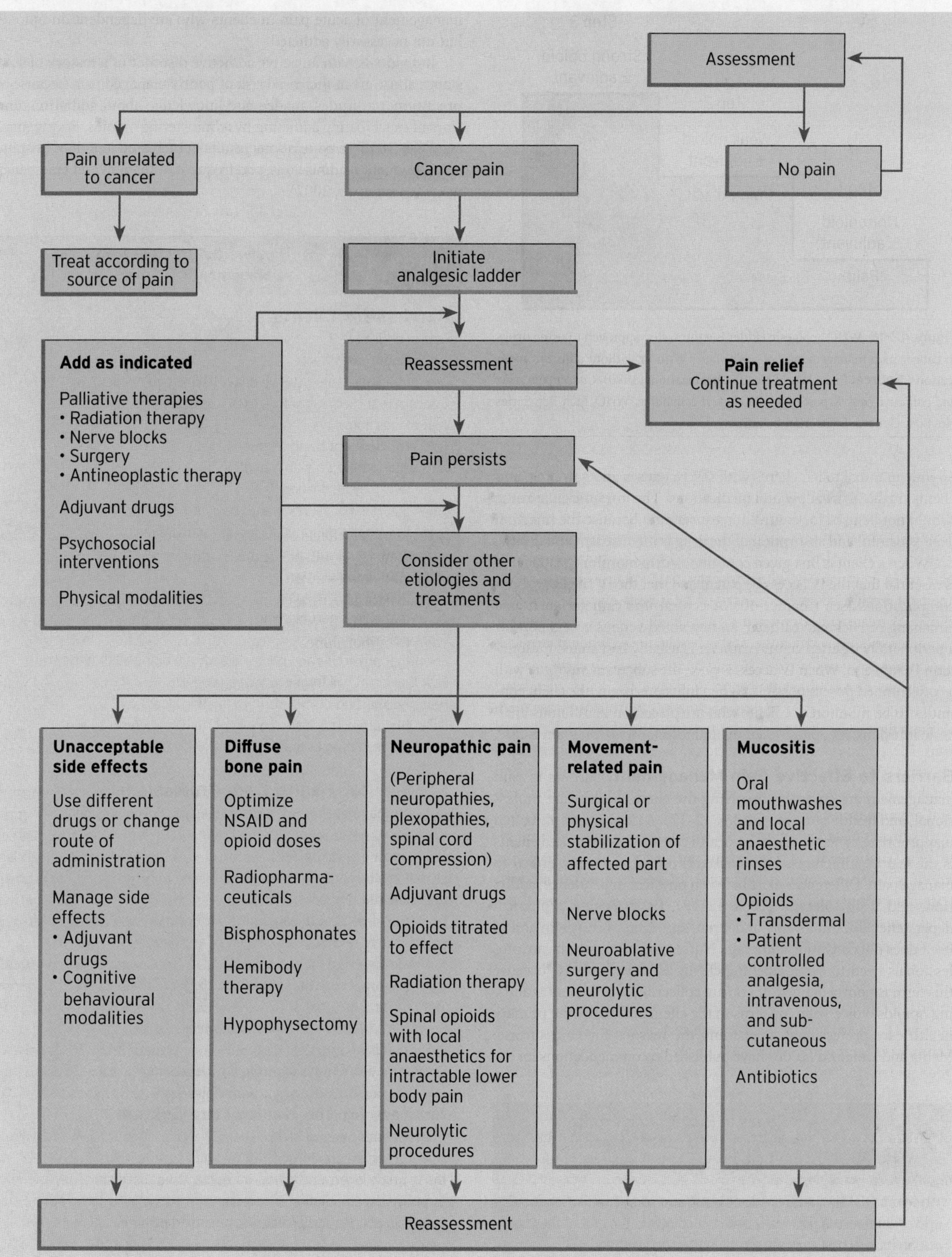

Figure 42-15 Flow chart: continuing pain management in clients with cancer. **Source:** From Jacox, A., Carr, D., Payne, R., Berde, C., Breitbart, W., Cain, J., et al. (1994). *Management of cancer pain. Clinical practice guideline No. 9*. AHCPR Publication No. 94-0592. Rockville, MD: Agency for Health Care Policy and Research, Public Health Service, United States Department of Health and Human Services.

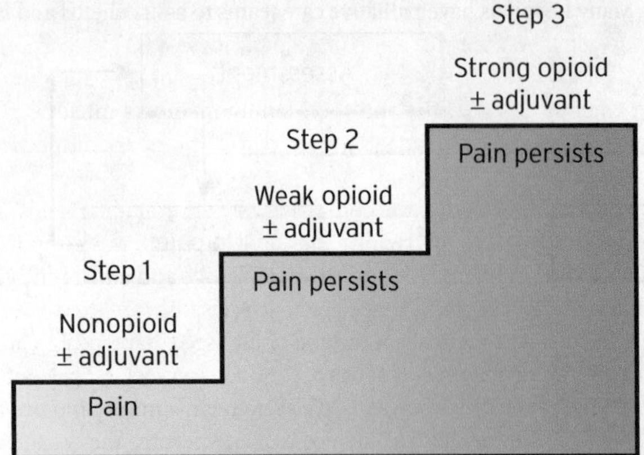

Figure 42-16 WHO analgesic ladder is a three-step approach to using drugs in cancer pain management. "*+/– adjuvant*," With or without adjuvant medications. **Source:** From World Health Organization. (1990). *Cancer pain relief and palliative care: Report of a WHO expert committee.* WHO Tech Rep Series No. 804. Geneva, Switzerland: Author.

provide minimal relief, clients with severe nausea and vomiting, and clients unable to swallow oral medications. The intramuscular route should not be used for controlling cancer pain because the injection itself is painful and absorption of the drug is inconsistent and erratic.

When a client is first given continuous-drip morphine sulphate, it is essential that the IV access be patent and that the IV site be without complications (see Chapter 40). A central line catheter such as a Groshong or Hickman catheter, an implanted venous access port, or a peripherally inserted central catheter is usually best suited for long-term IV infusion. When IV access is poor, the subcutaneous route with a concentrated dose is possible. When infusions begin, the client continues to be monitored. Clients who are placed on continuous analgesic infusions are opioid-tolerant, and respiratory depression is rare.

Barriers to Effective Pain Management. Barriers to pain management are complex, involving the client, health care professional, and health care system (Box 42–17). A deep-seated and often inappropriate concern shared by health care professionals and clients is the fear of addiction when long-term opioid use is prescribed to manage pain. Differences exist between **physical dependence, addiction,** and **drug tolerance** (Box 42–18). Experiencing a physical dependency does not imply addiction, and drug tolerance in and of itself does not constitute addiction. Nurses and other health care professionals need to avoid labelling clients as "drug seeking" because this term is poorly defined. If you are concerned that a client is abusing opioids, voice your concerns to the client and notify the primary health care professional, explaining the reasons for your unease. Mehta and Langford (2006) have published recommendations for the management of acute pain in clients who are dependent on opioids but not necessarily addicted.

Individuals with an active addictive disorder or a history of substance abuse are at increased risk of poorly managed pain because of practitioner attitudes, inadequate knowledge about addiction, and fears of exacerbating addiction by adminstering opioids. Poorly managed pain in these populations results in increased length of hospital stays, frequent readmissions, and frequent outpatient and emergency visits (Grant et al., 2007).

➤ BOX 42-16 Types of Breakthrough Pain: Pain That Extends Beyond Treated Steady Chronic Pain

Incident pain: Pain that is predictable and elicited by specific behaviours
End-of-dose failure pain: Pain that occurs toward the end of the usual dosing interval of a regularly scheduled analgesic
Spontaneous pain: Pain that is unpredictable and not associated with any activity or event

➤ BOX 42-17 Barriers to Effective Pain Management

Barriers for Clients

Fear of addiction
Worry about side effects
Fear of tolerance (drug will be unavailable when needed)
Concern that client takes too many pills already
Fear of injections
Concern about not being a "good" client
Not wanting to worry family and friends
More tests may be needed
Belief that one needs to suffer to be cured
Belief that pain is punishment for past indiscretions
Inadequate education
Reluctance to discuss pain
Belief that pain is inevitable
Belief that pain is part of aging
Fear of disease progression
Belief that physicians and nurses already are doing all that they can
Fear that client will forget to take analgesics
Fear of distracting physicians from treating illness
Belief that physicians have more important or ill clients to see
Belief that suffering in silence is noble and expected

Barriers for Health Care Professionals

Concern that client did not receive adequate pain assessment
Concern about addiction
Opiophobia (fear of opioids)
Fear of legal repercussions
No visible cause of pain exists
Belief that clients must learn to live with pain
Reluctance to deal with side effects of analgesics
Not believing client's report of pain
Fear of giving a dose that will kill the client
Time constraints
Belief that opioids may "mask" symptoms
Belief that pain is part of aging
Overestimation of rates of respiratory depression

Barriers for the Health Care System

Concern with creating "addicts"
Ability to fill prescriptions
Nurse practitioners and physician assistants not used efficiently
Extensive documentation requirements
Poor pain policies and procedures regarding pain management
Lack of money
Inadequate access to pain clinics
Poor understanding of economic impact of unrelieved pain

> **BOX 42-18 Definitions Related to the Use of Opioids for Pain Treatment**
>
> **Physical Dependence**
> A state of adaptation that is manifested by a drug class-specific withdrawal syndrome that can be produced by abrupt cessation, rapid dose reduction, decreasing blood level of the drug, or administration of an antagonist.
>
> **Drug Tolerance**
> A state of adaptation in which exposure to a drug induces changes that result in a diminution of one or more of the drug's effects over time.
>
> **Addiction**
> A primary, chronic, neurobiological disease, with genetic, psychosocial, and environmental factors influencing its development and manifestations. It is characterized by behaviours that include one or more of the following: impaired control over drug use, compulsive use, continued use despite harm, and craving.
>
> **Pseudoaddiction**
> Client behaviours (drug seeking) that may occur when pain is undertreated.
>
> **Pseudotolerance**
> Need to increase opioid dose for reasons other than opioid tolerance: progression of disease, onset of new disorder, increased physical activity, lack of adherence, change in opioid formulation, drug–drug interaction, or drug–food interaction (Wall & Melzack, 1999).
>
> Approved by the Boards of Directors of the American Academy of Pain Medicine, The American Pain Society, and the American Society of Addiction Medicine. February 2001.
>
> See also Health Canada (1992). *Therapeutic products directorate guidelines: The use of opioids in the management of opioid dependence.* Retrieved October 30, 2008, from http://dsp-psd.communication.gc.ca/Collection/H42-2-57-1992E.pdf; and Pereira, J., & Bruera, E, (Eds.) (2001). Appendix F: Opioid analgesics—Pharmacokinetics. In *Alberta hospice palliative care resource manual* (2nd ed., p. 80) [Electronic version]. Calgary, AB: Alberta Cancer Board. Retrieved October 30, 2008, from http://www.palliative.org/PC/ClinicalInfo/ACB%20PC%20resource%20manual.pdf

Placebos are "sugar pills" with no active ingredients, but they can produce positive or negative responses in 30% to 50% of people who take them (Thompson, 2000). The use of placebos to treat pain is discouraged by many professional organizations. Administering placebos is considered unethical and deceitful (Tucker, 2001), jeopardizing the trust between clients and health care professionals. If a placebo is ordered, you must question the order and ask, "Why?" Many health care agencies have policies that limit placebo use only to research.

Restorative and Continuing Care

Pain Clinics, Palliative Care, and Hospices. In recent years, health care professionals have recognized pain as a significant health problem (The SUPPORT Principal Investigators, 1995), and, as a result, programs have been designed for pain management. Pain clinics may offer several options. A comprehensive pain centre can treat clients on an inpatient or outpatient basis, conduct research into new treatments, and train professionals. Health care professionals from various disciplines, such as nursing, medicine, physiotherapy, pastoral care, and dietetics, work with clients to find effective pain-relief measures.

Many hospitals have palliative care teams to assist clients and families to manage their diseases (Ferrell & Coyle, 2001). Learning to live life fully with an incurable condition is the goal of palliative care (see Chapter 29). Clients and their family members must be given ongoing assistance in managing their pain at home (Schumacher et al., 2002).

In Canada, palliative and end-of-life care are emerging fields. The Canadian Institutes of Health Research (CIHR) are supporting research and program development in palliative and end-of-life care, including those programs associated with hospice care. Hospices are programs for care of clients at the end of life (see Chapter 29). Clients at the end of life may seek quality of life over quantity. Hospices help terminally ill clients continue to live at home in comfort and privacy. Pain control is a priority for hospices. Clients receive the dosage and form of analgesics that provide pain relief (Whitecar et al., 2004). Under the guidance of hospice nurses, families learn to monitor clients' symptoms and become their primary caregivers. A hospice client may become hospitalized in the event of a brief, acute care crisis or family problem.

Hospice programs help nurses overcome their fears of contributing to a client's death when administering large doses of opioids. Recent research suggests that moderate opioid dose increases in terminally ill clients at the end of life do not hasten death (Vitetta et al., 2005). The client's disease, not the opioid, is killing the client.

❖Evaluation

Client Care

Evaluating pain is one of many nursing responsibilities that require critical thinking (Figure 42–17). The client's behavioural responses to pain-relief interventions are not always obvious. Evaluating the effectiveness of a pain intervention requires that you be an intent observer and know what responses to anticipate on the basis of the type of pain, the type of intervention, the timing of the intervention, the physiological nature of the injury or disease, and the client's previous responses. Your evaluation involves psychological as well as physiological responses to pain.

If a client continues to have discomfort after an intervention, try a different approach. For example, if an analgesic provides only partial relief, consider adding relaxation or guided-imagery exercises. Consult with the physician about increasing the dosage, decreasing the interval between doses, or trying different analgesics. Also evaluate tolerance to therapy and the overall relief obtained. If an intervention aggravates discomfort, stop it immediately and seek an alternative. Time and patience are necessary to maximize the effectiveness of pain management. Evaluate the entire pain experience to determine the most effective interventions and times for administration.

Client Perceptions

The client, if able, is the best resource for evaluating the effectiveness of pain-relief measures. You must continually assess whether the character of the client's pain changes. The family can be a valuable resource, particularly if the client has cancer and may not be able to express discomfort during the latter stages of terminal illness. You are successful in treating pain when the client's expectations of pain relief are met. Recall, however, that some clients may experience pain needlessly because they accept suffering and because they lack knowledge of available pain-relief interventions.

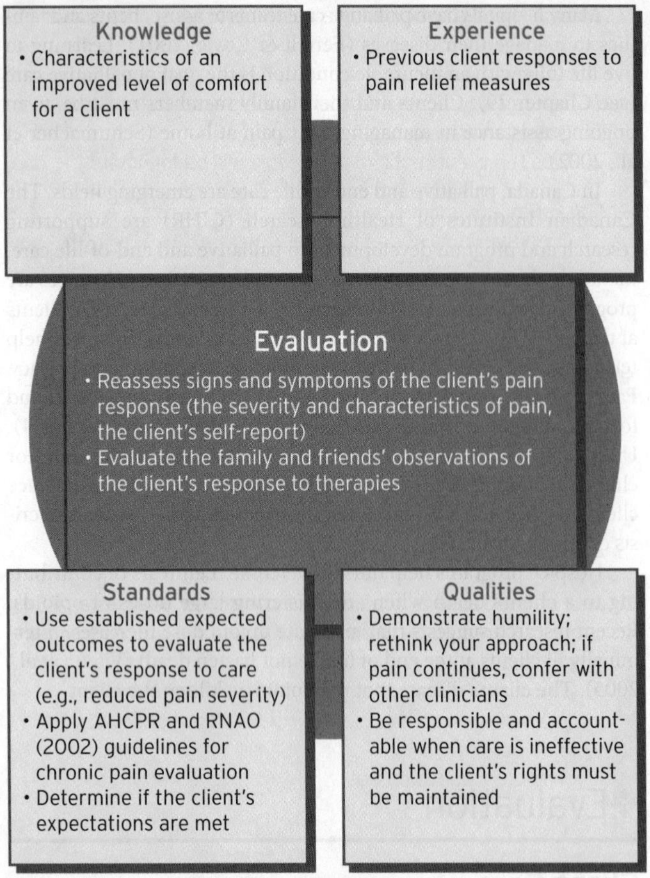

Knowledge
- Characteristics of an improved level of comfort for a client

Experience
- Previous client responses to pain relief measures

Evaluation
- Reassess signs and symptoms of the client's pain response (the severity and characteristics of pain, the client's self-report)
- Evaluate the family and friends' observations of the client's response to therapies

Standards
- Use established expected outcomes to evaluate the client's response to care (e.g., reduced pain severity)
- Apply AHCPR and RNAO (2002) guidelines for chronic pain evaluation
- Determine if the client's expectations are met

Qualities
- Demonstrate humility; rethink your approach; if pain continues, confer with other clinicians
- Be responsible and accountable when care is ineffective and the client's rights must be maintained

Figure 42-17 Critical thinking model for pain relief evaluation.

Pain assessment and responses to intervention should be accurately and thoroughly documented so that they can be communicated to others caring for the client. Communication occurs from nurse to nurse, shift to shift, and nurse to other health care professionals. The nurse caring for the client is responsible for reporting what has been effective for managing pain; the client is not responsible for communicating this information. Various bedside tools, such as a pain flow sheet, help centralize information about pain management. Clients expect nurses to be sensitive to their pain and to be diligent in managing that pain. Because pain relief is a team effort, communicate effectively with physicians (Box 42–19).

➤ BOX 42-19 Nurse-Physician Pain Communication

1. Identify the physician by name.
2. Give your name.
3. State the general nature of the call.
4. Identify the client by name and diagnosis.
5. State the pain management goal: rating and activities.
6. Summarize the current pain rating, and the effect of pain on activities.
7. List the current analgesic doses and relevant side effects.
8. Identify nonpharmacological strategies used.
9. Suggest a solution (on the basis of a clinical practice guideline, if possible).

Adapted from McCaffery, M., & Pasero, C. (1999). *Pain: Clinical manual* (2nd ed.). St. Louis, MO: Mosby.

✻ KEY CONCEPTS

- Pain is a purely subjective physical and psychosocial experience.
- A nurse's misconceptions about pain often result in doubt about the degree of the client's suffering and in unwillingness to provide relief.
- Knowledge of the nociceptive pain processes of the pain experience—transmission, transduction, perception, and modulation—will provide you with guidelines for determining pain-relief measures.
- An interaction of psychological and cognitive factors affects pain perception.
- A person's cultural background influences the meaning of pain and how it is expressed.
- It is common for older clients not to report pain.
- Clients who have chronic pain are unlikely to show behavioural changes.
- The difference between acute and chronic pain involves the concept of harm. Acute pain is protective, thus preventing harm; chronic pain is no longer protective.
- Do not collect an in-depth pain history when the client is experiencing severe discomfort.
- Pain can cause physical signs and symptoms similar to the signs and symptoms of other diseases.
- Clients waiting to undergo invasive tests may gain some pain relief from anticipatory guidance.
- Individualize your pain interventions by collaborating closely with the client, using assessment findings, and trying a variety of interventions.
- Eliminating sources of painful stimuli is a basic nursing measure for promoting comfort.
- Use a regular schedule for analgesic administration, as this is more effective than an as-needed schedule in controlling pain.
- A patient-controlled analgesic device gives clients pain control, with low risk of overdose.
- While caring for a client who receives local anaesthesia, protect the client from injury.
- When administering epidural analgesia, take steps to prevent infection and monitor closely for respiratory depression.
- Your goal in pain management is to anticipate and prevent pain, rather than to treat it.
- In evaluating the effectiveness of a pain intervention, consider the changing character of pain, the client's response to the intervention, and the client's perceptions of a therapy's effectiveness.

✻ CRITICAL THINKING EXERCISES

1. Mrs. Gorsky is a frail 83-year-old woman who sustained an injury to the lumbar region of her back during a fall 8 months ago. She is 180 cm tall and weighs 45 kg. She reports her pain intensity as a 5 (on a VAS scale of 0 to 10), increasing with activity; she has limited flexibility and is unable to get out of bed without assistance. What pain interventions and approaches might you use?

2. Alexis, aged 3 years, is admitted to the pediatric unit for a third-degree burn to her right lower extremity. How would you proceed in assessing this child's pain?

3. You are caring for an unconscious client who was involved in an automobile accident and sustained multiple injuries. The client has several lacerations, wounds, and surgical incisions, as well as multiple lines and tubes. What measures might you take to promote the client's comfort?

4. Madeleine Tremblay, a 55-year-old woman with metastatic breast cancer to the bone, has been receiving IV morphine sulphate (MSO_4) for a week for severe back and leg pain. Her frequently increased infusion of MSO_4 is not reducing her pain to an acceptable level, and she is becoming increasingly sedated. What other pharmacological interventions might be considered?

5. Ms. Wilkins, aged 65 years, returns from surgery after a small-bowel resection. The physician orders a 25-mcg fentanyl patch applied to help manage the postoperative pain. Ms. Wilkins received one dose of morphine 4 mg IV push in the recovery room 1 hour ago, which relieved her pain. What actions would be appropriate for you to take at this time?

✻ REVIEW QUESTIONS

1. Pain is viewed as:
   1. A separate disease
   2. A symptom of an illness
   3. A symptom of a condition
   4. An objective finding

2. This type of pain lasts longer than anticipated and a minimum of 6 months, may not have an identifiable cause, and leads to great personal suffering:
   1. Cancer pain
   2. Chronic pain
   3. Acute pain
   4. Idiopathic pain

3. One of the reasons that many nurses avoid acknowledging a client's pain is:
   1. Inadequate pain management skills
   2. Insufficient time to respond to the client
   3. Fear that the intervention may cause addiction
   4. Inability to manage their client load

4. Cognitively, this age group is unable to recall explanations about pain, or associate pain with experiences that can occur in various situations:
   1. Preschoolers
   2. Adolescents
   3. Young adults
   4. Older adults

5. An 82-year-old man with Alzheimer's disease is restless and moaning. The client's daughter states that the client did not sleep well most of the night. The nurse's first response would be to:
   1. Recommend giving the client sleeping medication
   2. Obtain a psychiatric evaluation
   3. Administer pain medication as ordered
   4. Assess and document physical and behavioural data

6. The client requests medication for her abdominal incision pain, which she rates as 5 (scale of 0 to 10, with 10 being the worst pain). One hour after administration of her pain medication, she is able to walk in the hall for 10 minutes, and rates her pain as a 7. This indicates that the dosage of pain medication was:
   1. Adequate
   2. Excessive
   3. Insufficient
   4. Unnecessary

7. When a client is anticipating a painful procedure, the nurse:
   1. Teaches about the procedure, avoiding focusing on the associated discomfort
   2. Teaches about the procedure and its associated discomfort
   3. Orders an analgesic
   4. Tells the client that the discomfort will be minimal

8. Relaxation and guided imagery are examples of:
   1. Cognitive-behavioural interventions
   2. Physical interventions
   3. Pharmacological interventions
   4. Adjuvants

9. The Canadian Pain Society recommends that if pain is anticipated for the majority of the day, health care professionals should consider administering opioids:
   1. On an as-needed (prn) basis
   2. With complementary therapies
   3. On an around-the-clock (ATC) basis
   4. When the pain tolerance level is exceeded

10. One of the reasons that patient-controlled analgesia (PCA) pumps are frequently used for postoperative and cancer pain management is to:
    1. Enable family members to control the drug doses
    2. Enable improved nursing control over drug doses
    3. Enable sustained pain relief, with the client in control
    4. Increase medication use

✻ RECOMMENDED WEB SITES

Health Canada: Record of Proceedings: Scientific Advisory Panel on Neuropathic Pain: http://www.hc-sc.gc.ca/dhp-mps/prodpharma/activit/sci-consult/neuropath/sapnp_rop_gcsdn_crd_2004-12-02-eng.php

Health Canada provides an extensive listing of clinical guidelines for nurses in primary care. It provides the public, clinicians, and researchers with information on pain and other public health concerns, such as this document outlining questions, issues, and research surrounding neuropathic pain.

Canadian Pain Society:
http://www.canadianpainsociety.ca/index.html

The Canadian Pain Society is an association whose members include physicians, nurses, and other clinicians involved with the management of pain. Its aim is to foster and encourage research on pain, and to improve the management of clients with acute and chronic pain.

The University of Toronto Centre for the Study of Pain:
http://www.utoronto.ca/pain/

The University of Toronto Centre for the Study of Pain is a partnership involving the faculties of dentistry, medicine, nursing, and pharmacy. The mission of the Centre is to lead, both nationally and internationally, in the areas of pain research, education, and clinical activity.

Pediatric Pain–Science Helping Children:
http://www.pediatric-pain.ca/

The Centre for Pediatric Pain Research, located in Halifax, Nova Scotia, offers online research and client education resources for health care professionals, as well as pain management guides for parents and children.

International Association for the Study of Pain (IASP): http://www.iasp-pain.org/
The IASP is the largest multidisciplinary international association in the field of pain. One of the purposes of this site is to call attention to the importance of pain as a field for multidisciplinary scientific enquiry, and to promote pain prevention and relief as a priority for health care delivery.

Canadian Hospice Palliative Care Association: http://www.chpca.net/home.htm
This site is intended as an educational resource for professional and informal caregivers and interest groups. It includes an extensive listing of online resources for those interested in palliative and end-of-life care, including cancer, clinical, and research sites.

Registered Nurses' Association of Ontario: Assessment and Management of Pain: http://www.rnao.org/Page.asp?PageID=924&ContentID=720
The Registered Nurses' Association of Ontario's site is specific to nursing, and is available in English and French. It features a number of best practice clinical guidelines, including those for the assessment and management of pain.

43

Nutrition

Written by Kathryn Weaver, RN, PhD

Based on the original chapter by

Patricia A. Stockert, RN, BSN, MS, PhD

objectives

Mastery of content in this chapter will enable you to:

- Define the key terms listed.
- Explain why each major nutrient is necessary for proper nutrition.
- Explain the importance of maintaining a balance between energy intake and energy requirements.
- List the end products of carbohydrate, protein, and fat metabolism.
- Explain the significance of saturated, unsaturated, polyunsaturated, and trans fats.
- Describe *Eating Well with Canada's Food Guide* and discuss its value in planning nutritious meals.
- Explain recommended dietary intake to ensure that clients include essential vitamins and minerals in their diets.
- Explain the variance in nutritional requirements throughout human growth and development.
- Discuss the major methods of nutritional assessment.
- Identify three major nutritional problems and describe clients at risk for them.
- Formulate a plan of care to help meet the specific nutritional needs of infants, toddlers, preschoolers, school-age children, adolescents, young adults, middle-aged persons, and older adults.
- Identify the potential nutritional deficits associated with vegetarian clients, with special consideration to clients who follow vegan or ovo-lactate diets.
- Discuss diet counselling and client teaching in relation to client expectations.

media resources

evolve Web Site

- Animations
- Audio Chapter Summaries
- Glossary
- Multiple-Choice Review Questions
- Skills Performance Checklists
- Student Learning Activities
- Video Clips
- Weblinks

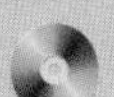

Companion CD

- Glossary
- Interactive Learning Activities
- Fluids and Electrolytes Tutorial
- Test-Taking Skills

key terms

Amino acids, p. 1045
Anabolism, p. 1048
Anorexia, p. 1067
Anorexia nervosa, p. 1054
Anthropometry, p. 1057
Aquaporins, p. 1046
Aspiration, p. 1046
Basal metabolic rate (BMR), p. 1044
Body mass index (BMI), p. 1058
Bulimia nervosa, p. 1054
Carbohydrates, p. 1045
Catabolism, p. 1048
Cholesterol, p. 1045
Chyme, p. 1047
Complementary proteins, p. 1045
Complex carbohydrates, p. 1045
Dietary reference intakes (DRIs), p. 1048
Dysphagia, p. 1046
Enzymes, p. 1046
Essential amino acids, p. 1045
Fat-soluble vitamins, p. 1046
Fatty acids, p. 1045
Food security, p. 1051
Gluconeogenesis, p. 1048
Glycemic index, p. 1045
Glycogenesis, p. 1048
Glycogenolysis, p. 1048
Hypervitaminosis, p. 1046
Ideal body weight (IBW), p. 1058
Ketones, p. 1048
Lipids, p. 1045
Macrominerals, p. 1046
Metabolism, p. 1048
Minerals, p. 1046
Monounsaturated fatty acids, p. 1045
Nitrogen balance, p. 1045
Nonessential amino acids, p. 1045
Nutrient density, p. 1044
Nutrients, p. 1044
Nutritional assessment, p. 1057
Nutritional screening, p. 1056
Peristalsis, p. 1046
Polyunsaturated fatty acids, p. 1045
Resting energy expenditure (REE), p. 1044
Saccharides, p. 1045
Saturated (fatty acids), p. 1045
Simple carbohydrates, p. 1045
Trace elements, p. 1046
Trans fatty acids, p. 1045
Triglycerides, p. 1045
Unsaturated (fatty acids), p. 1045
Vegetarianism, p. 1056
Vitamins, p. 1046
Waist circumference, p. 1059
Water-soluble vitamins, p. 1046

Although Canada has a wealth of abundant natural and physical resources, its greatest resource lies not in these riches but in the health of its people. In turn, the greatest resource for maintaining good health, in Canada and around the world, is the food that people eat. Food nourishes the body so that it can accomplish everyday activities, while providing amazing powers to prevent the contraction of certain diseases and to aid in the recovery from other diseases. Ensuring that the body receives the food substances needed to supply energy to conduct activities, to build and repair tissues, and to regulate organs and systems is the important work of all health care professionals and of all citizens.

Sustenance and health are but two of the important purposes related to the food we eat. Food also holds symbolic meaning for many cultures and communities. Ceremonies, social gatherings, holiday traditions, religious events, the celebration of births, and the mourning of deaths all happen within the background of giving or taking food significant to the event. With such a complexity of meanings embedded in food, it is no wonder that the withholding of food carries significant implications. This becomes acutely evident in palliative care settings when decisions to withhold food, even in the form of intravenous (IV) nutrients, during a terminal illness reflect the symbolic power that food has over life and death.

As nurses, our role in promoting proper nutrition, diet therapy, and health is vital to our clients. Over a century ago, the mother of modern nursing, Florence Nightingale (1858), instructed nurses to have a keen knowledge of a client's diet: "consider, remember how much he [or she] has had, and how much he [or she] ought to have today" (p. 39). We must pay as much attention to a client's diet as to his or her illness, treatments, and therapies. With the advent of technological tools, the study of nutrition as a science, and the explosion of media attention on weight and fitness, our role in addressing diet-related issues has expanded. For example, in illnesses such as type I diabetes mellitus, a common health concern across Western nations, diet can be a major treatment and nurses the key professionals responsible for educating clients and families about food choices that influence the course of the disease. Nurses are also instrumental in teaching effective ways to use the technology available to assist clients in self-care management (e.g., insulin pumps) (Canadian Diabetes Association [CDA], 2003). Along with type I diabetes, many other conditions, such as type II diabetes, hypertension, and inflammatory bowel disease, raise complex issues and greater responsibilities in nursing care. Such conditions may require highly specialized nutritional support protocols, including diets low in sugars, cholesterol, or salt (Touz et al., 2004).

Overall, the nutritional health of Canadians is rated good in comparison to that of other developed countries. This story may be changing, however, because of a series of challenges brought on by evolving demographic and economic issues that result in less time and fewer resources available for food-related activities. These issues include the rising poverty rate among young families, a decline in resources available to rural communities, the aging of the population, and the social isolation or marginalization of certain groups of citizens. Rates of stay-at-home spouses have dropped significantly to a mere 10% of Canadian households, leaving the majority of preschool children in day care or in school while parents work. Unemployment rates have risen, and reduced-income earners now reflect a Canadian population facing economic difficulties such as accumulated debt, household budget deficits, and restricted choices for purchasing power. Statistics Canada (2007) has indicated that a larger portion of the Canadian population is reaching retirement age, and these older adults are choosing to stay in their own homes longer, placing them at risk for poor nutrition associated with mobility impairments and with social isolation. In addition, between 1996 and 2001, national statistics showed that Aboriginal populations increased by 22% and that Aboriginal children account for 5.6% of all children in Canada. Shifts in cultural diversity are the norm in Canada, with the population composition no longer being predominantly White; since the late 1990s, an average of 218,346 people (most of whom are Chinese and South Asian) per year were accepted into Canada as permanent residents. All of these factors, along with the larger international issues arising from free trade and globalization, seriously affect the diets and health of Canadians.

One trend that has taken on alarming proportions is the increase in the conditions of being overweight or obese. In 2004 alone, approximately 58.8% of adult Canadians were overweight or obese (Statistics Canada, 2004). Likewise, the prevalence of being overweight or obese in children has soared to numbers and percentages of the population that were never before imagined. Type II diabetes is now being diagnosed in children in Canada as young as 5 and 8 years old (Public Health Agency of Canada, 1999; Young et al., 2000), an illness largely preventable through healthy eating and weight management and that in the past occurred mainly in older persons (Canadian Paediatric Society, 2005). Rates of type II diabetes among Aboriginal people are three to five times higher than those of the general population (Health Canada, 2007d; Saylor, 2005). Factors adversely affecting the nutritional health of Canadians are serious, and the resultant conditions are bordering on epidemic proportions in today's society. Thus it is critical that nurses acquire nutritional knowledge to apply to the complexities of diseases, diverse populations, and current demographics (age, gender, income level, and culture).

Scientific Knowledge Base

Nutrients: The Biochemical Units of Nutrition

The body requires fuel to provide energy for the chemical reactions that enable cellular growth and repair, organ function, and body movement. The energy requirement of a person at rest is called the **basal metabolic rate (BMR).** This is the energy needed to maintain life-sustaining activities (breathing, circulation, heart rate, and temperature) for a specific period of time. The **resting energy expenditure (REE)** is a measurement that accounts for BMR plus energy to digest meals and perform mild activity. REE is a baseline of energy requirement that accounts for approximately 60% to 75% of our daily needs. Factors such as age, body mass, gender, presence of fever, environmental temperature, starvation, stress, illness, injury, infection, activity level, or thyroid function may affect energy requirements. Factors that affect metabolism include illness, pregnancy, lactation, activity level, and the use of certain drugs.

In general, when energy requirements are completely met by kilocalorie (kcal) intake in food, weight does not change. When the kilocalories ingested exceed energy demands, a person gains weight. If the kilocalories ingested fail to meet energy requirements, a person loses weight.

Nutrients are the elements supplied by food that are necessary for body processes and function. Energy needs are met from three categories of nutrients: carbohydrates, proteins, and fats. Other nutrients include water, vitamins, and minerals. Water acts as a solvent for metabolic processes. Vitamins and minerals do not provide energy but contribute to metabolic processes, including acid–base balance. A nutrient is considered essential if the body cannot manufacture it in a sufficient quantity to meet metabolic demands.

Foods are also described according to their **nutrient density,** the proportion of essential nutrients to the number of kilocalories, the unit of energy required to raise 1 kilogram of water by 1° C (referred to as "calories" by the general public). High nutrient-density foods, such as fruits and vegetables, provide a large number of nutrients in relation to kilocalories. Low nutrient-density foods, such as alcohol or refined sugar, are high in kilocalories but nutrient poor.

Carbohydrates. **Carbohydrates** are the recommended main source of energy in the diet. Each gram of carbohydrate produces 4 kcal and serves as the main source of fuel (glucose) for the brain, for skeletal muscles during exercise, for red and while blood cell production, and for cell function of the renal medulla. Carbohydrates are obtained primarily from plant foods, except for lactose (milk sugar), and are classified according to their carbohydrate units, or **saccharides.**

Monosaccharides such as glucose (dextrose) or fructose (fruit sugar) are the building blocks of all other carbohydrates and cannot be broken down into a more basic carbohydrate unit. Disaccharides such as sucrose, lactose, and maltose are composed of two monosaccharides minus one unit of water. Both monosaccharides and disaccharides are classified as **simple carbohydrates** called *sugars.* Polysaccharides are composed of many carbohydrate units and are classified as **complex carbohydrates.** They include starch (stored form of glucose in plants) and glycogen (stored glucose in animals and humans). Some polysaccharides cannot be digested because humans do not have enzymes capable of breaking them down. Insoluble fibres are not digestible and include cellulose, hemicellulose, and lignin. Soluble fibres include pectin, guar gum, and mucilage. Dietary fibre is important to disease prevention, as it decreases the total and low-density lipoprotein (LDL) cholesterol associated with the development of heart disease (Schlenker & Long, 2007). Ingestion of fibre also helps prevent diarrhea in tube-fed clients (Cabré, 2004).

Carbohydrate-rich foods are ranked according to their **glycemic index**, the effect on blood glucose levels and insulin response (Canadian Diabetes Association, 2005). Carbohydrates that release glucose rapidly into the bloodstream (e.g., white bread, candy) have a high glycemic index. Carbohydrates that have a low glycemic index (e.g., barley, lentils), those that produce only small fluctuations in blood glucose, have the long-term health benefits of sustaining weight loss, prolonging physical endurance, and reducing risks associated with heart disease and diabetes.

Proteins. Proteins are essential for synthesis (building) of body tissue in growth, maintenance, and repair. Collagen, hormones, enzymes, immune cells, DNA, and RNA are all composed of protein. In addition, blood clotting, fluid regulation, and acid–base balance require proteins. Nutrients and many pharmacological substances are transported in the blood by proteins.

The simplest form of protein is the amino acid. As with other nutrients, **essential amino acids** are those that the body cannot synthesize but must have provided in the diet. Examples of essential amino acids are lysine and phenylalanine. **Nonessential amino acids** can be synthesized by the body. Examples of nonessential amino acids are alanine and glutamic acid. **Amino acids** can be linked together by peptide bonds to form larger protein molecules called polypeptides. Albumin and insulin are simple proteins because they contain only amino acids or their derivatives. The combination of a simple protein with a nonprotein substance produces a more complex protein, such as lipoprotein, formed by a combination of a lipid (fat) and a simple protein.

Protein quality is determined by the balance of essential amino acids. Incomplete proteins lack a sufficient quantity of one or more essential amino acids and include cereals, legumes (beans, peas), and vegetables. A complete protein contains all of the nine essential amino acids in sufficient quantity to support growth and maintain nitrogen balance—its most important function in the body. Examples of foods that contain complete proteins are chicken, soybeans, fish, and cheese. Complete proteins are referred to as high-quality proteins. **Complementary proteins** are pairs of incomplete proteins that, when combined, supply the total amount of protein provided by complete protein sources.

Protein is the only major nutrient that contains nitrogen (it is 16% nitrogen) and is the only source of nitrogen for the body. Thus nitrogen can be used to determine protein balance in the body. **Nitrogen balance** is achieved when the intake and output of nitrogen are equal. When the intake of nitrogen exceeds the output, the body is in positive nitrogen balance, which is required for growth, normal pregnancy, maintenance of lean muscle mass and vital organs, and wound healing. The nitrogen retained by the body is used for the building, repair, and replacement of body tissues. Negative nitrogen-balance occurs when the body loses more nitrogen than the body gains, for example, with severe infection, burns, fever, starvation, head injury, and trauma. The increased nitrogen loss is the result of body tissue destruction or loss of nitrogen-containing body fluids through urine, feces, sweat, and, at times, bleeding or vomiting. Nutrition during this period must provide nutrients to put clients into positive balance for healing.

Protein can be used to provide energy (4 kcal/g), but because of protein's essential role in growth, maintenance, and repair, adequate kilocalories should be provided in the diet from nonprotein sources. Protein is spared as an energy source when carbohydrate in the diet is sufficient to meet the energy needs of the body.

Fats. Fats (**lipids**) are the most calorically dense nutrient, providing 9 kcal/g. In addition to serving as fuel that supplies energy, fat cushions vital organs, lubricates body tissue, insulates, and protects cell membranes. Fats are composed of glycerol and fatty acids. **Triglycerides** circulate in the blood and are made up of three fatty acids attached to a glycerol. **Fatty acids** are composed of chains of carbon and hydrogen atoms with an acid group on one end of the chain and a methyl group at the other. Fatty acids can be **saturated**, in which each carbon in the chain has two attached hydrogen atoms, or **unsaturated**, in which an unequal number of hydrogen atoms are attached and the carbon atoms attach to each other with a double bond. **Monounsaturated fatty acids** have one double bond, whereas **polyunsaturated fatty acids** have two or more double carbon bonds. Most animal fats have high proportions of saturated fatty acids, whereas vegetable fats have higher amounts of monounsaturated and polyunsaturated fatty acids. The various types of fatty acids have significance for health and the incidence of disease and are referred to in the dietary guidelines from the Heart and Stroke Foundation, The Canadian Cancer Society, and the Canadian Diabetes Association.

More recently, trans fatty acids have received attention for their role in the development of coronary artery disease, diabetes, infertility in women, and prostate cancer in men (Merchant et al., 2008; Salmerón et al., 2001). **Trans fatty acids** are formed by the partial hydrogenation of vegetable oils and are mostly found in prepared foods, snack foods, and margarines. Increased research and consumer awareness led to mandatory nutrition labelling of trans fats in Canada since 2005 and in the United States since 2006 (Tonn, 2007). The acceptable macronutrient distribution range (AMDR), the range associated with reduced risk of chronic illness while providing essential intakes of total fat, is 25% to 35% for adults (Trumbo et al., 2002). However, it is recommended that Canadians decrease their intake of the proportion of saturated and trans fatty acids.

Cholesterol is often discussed in connection with fats, although it is a sterol, not a triglyceride (Schlenker & Long, 2007). It occurs naturally in animal foods but is also synthesized by the liver. Cholesterol deposits in blood vessel walls cause atherosclerosis, which is the underlying cause of coronary artery disease.

Water. Water is a critical component of the body because cell function depends on a fluid environment. Water composes 60% to 70% of total body weight. The percentage of total body water is greater for lean people than for obese people because muscle contains more water than any other tissue except blood. Infants have the greatest percentage of total body water, and older people have the least. When deprived of water, a person cannot survive for more than a few days. Water helps regulate body temperature and acts as a solvent for nutrients and waste products. Water passes freely through membranes that separate body fluids inside (intracellular) and outside (extracellular) cells. Various water-transport proteins called **aquaporins** function as water-selective channels in many cells, altering the speed at which water crosses cell membranes, and influence conditions such as cataract formation and hypertension (Verkman, 2005).

Fluid needs are met by ingesting liquids and solid foods high in water content, such as fresh fruits and vegetables. Water is also produced during digestion when food is oxidized. In a healthy individual, fluid intake from all sources equals fluid output through elimination, respiration, and sweating (see Chapters 36 and 40). An ill person can have an increased need for fluid (e.g., with fever or gastrointestinal losses). An ill person can also have a decreased ability to excrete fluid (e.g., with cardiopulmonary or renal disease), which may lead to the need to restrict fluid intake.

Vitamins. **Vitamins** are organic substances that are essential to normal metabolism. Small amounts of vitamins are present in foods. However, the body is unable to synthesize most vitamins in the required amounts and depends on dietary intake. The quantity of vitamins in food is affected by food processing, storage, and preparation. Vitamin content is usually highest in fresh foods used quickly after minimal exposure to heat, air, or water. Certain vitamins are currently of considerable interest regarding their role as antioxidants that neutralize substances called free radicals, which are thought to produce oxidative damage to body cells and tissues. It is believed that oxidative damage increases a person's risk for various cancers. Vitamins with antioxidant properties include water-soluble vitamin C, and fat-soluble beta-carotene and vitamins A and E (Schlenker & Long, 2007).

Fat-Soluble Vitamins. The **fat-soluble vitamins** (A, D, E, and K) can be stored in the body. With the exception of vitamin D, these vitamins are provided only through dietary intake. Vitamin D is provided by both dietary intake and synthesis in the body with exposure to sunlight. Canada's food guide recommends that adults consume 500 mL (2 cups) of milk each day in order to receive adequate vitamin D. Yet because vitamin D needs increase after the age of 50 and obtaining adequate vitamin D from the diet alone is very difficult, Health Canada (2007b) recommends that all adults over the age of 50 take a daily vitamin D supplement of 10 micrograms (μg; 400 IU) in addition to following Canada's Food Guide. The body can store fat-soluble vitamins; therefore, **hypervitaminosis** can result from megadoses (intentional or unintentional) of supplemental vitamins, ingesting excessive amounts of vitamins in fortified food, and consuming excessive fish oils.

Water-Soluble Vitamins. The **water-soluble vitamins** are vitamins C and B complex (which consists of eight vitamins: thiamine, riboflavin, niacin, vitamin B_6, folate, vitamin B_{12}, pantothenic acid, and biotin). Another element, choline, is sometimes classified as a B vitamin. Water-soluble vitamins are easily destroyed by cooking and must be provided in the daily food intake. Although water-soluble vitamins are not stored in the body, toxicity may still occur with vitamin megadoses.

Minerals. **Minerals** are inorganic elements essential to the body as catalysts in biochemical reactions. Minerals become part of the structure of the body and its enzymes. For example, iron becomes attached to protein globin to form hemoglobin, which enhances oxygen-carrying capacity. Minerals are classified as **macrominerals** when the daily requirement is 100 mg or more and as microminerals or **trace elements** when less than 100 mg is needed daily. The macrominerals are calcium, sodium, potassium, phosphorus, magnesium, sulphur, and chloride. Trace minerals include iron, iodine, fluoride, zinc, selenium, chromium, copper, manganese, cobalt, and molydenum. Additionally, other trace minerals such as aluminum, cadmium, arsenic, and boron have possible but not clearly delineated nutritional functions. Arsenic, aluminum, and cadmium have toxic effects.

Anatomy and Physiology of the Digestive System

Digestion. Digestion of food consists of mechanical breakdown that results from chewing, churning, and mixing with fluid, as well as chemical reactions by which food is reduced to its simplest form. Each part of the gastrointestinal system has an important digestive or absorptive function (Figure 43–1).

Enzymes are an essential component of the chemistry of digestion. Enzymes are proteinlike substances that act as catalysts to speed up chemical reactions. Most enzymes have one specific function and function best at a specific pH. The secretions of the gastrointestinal tract have vastly different pH levels. For example, saliva is relatively neutral, gastric juice is highly acidic, and the secretions of the small intestine are alkaline.

The mechanical, chemical, and hormonal activities of digestion are interdependent. Enzyme activity depends on the mechanical breakdown of food to increase the surface area for chemical action. Hormones regulate the flow of digestive secretions needed for enzyme supply. The secretion of digestive juices and the motility of the gastrointestinal tract are also regulated by physical, chemical, and hormonal factors. Action in the gastrointestinal tract is increased by nerve stimulation from the parasympathetic nervous system (e.g., the vagus nerve).

Digestion begins in the mouth, where chewing mechanically breaks down food. The food is mixed with saliva, which contains ptyalin (salivary amylase), an enzyme that acts on cooked starch to begin its conversion to maltose. The longer food is chewed, the more starch digestion occurs in the mouth. Proteins and fats are broken down physically but remain unchanged chemically because enzymes in the mouth do not react with these nutrients. Because simple sugars (monosaccharides) require no digestion, they may be absorbed from the mouth. Chewing reduces food particles to a size suitable for swallowing, and saliva provides lubrication to further ease swallowing of the food. The epiglottis is a flap of skin that closes over the trachea during swallowing to prevent **aspiration**. The tongue manoeuvres the mass of chewed food into the pharynx, which activates the swallowing reflex. Swallowed food enters the esophagus and is moved along by wavelike muscular contractions (**peristalsis**) to the base of the esophagus, above the cardiac sphincter. Pressure from a bolus of food at the cardiac sphincter causes it to relax, allowing the food to enter the fundus (uppermost portion) of the stomach. Difficulty swallowing is referred to as **dysphagia**.

In the stomach, pepsinogen is secreted by chief cells and then converted by hydrochloric acid (HCl) to pepsin, a protein-splitting enzyme. Gastric lipase and amylase are produced to begin fat and starch digestion, respectively. The stomach's pyloric glands secrete gastrin, a hormone that triggers parietal cells to secrete intrinsic factor (IF) and HCl. IF is necessary for absorption of vitamin B_{12} in the ileum. HCL also destroys bacteria, increases the absorbability of iron and calcium, and maintains the pH of the gastric juice. The lining of the stomach is protected from autodigestion by a thick layer of

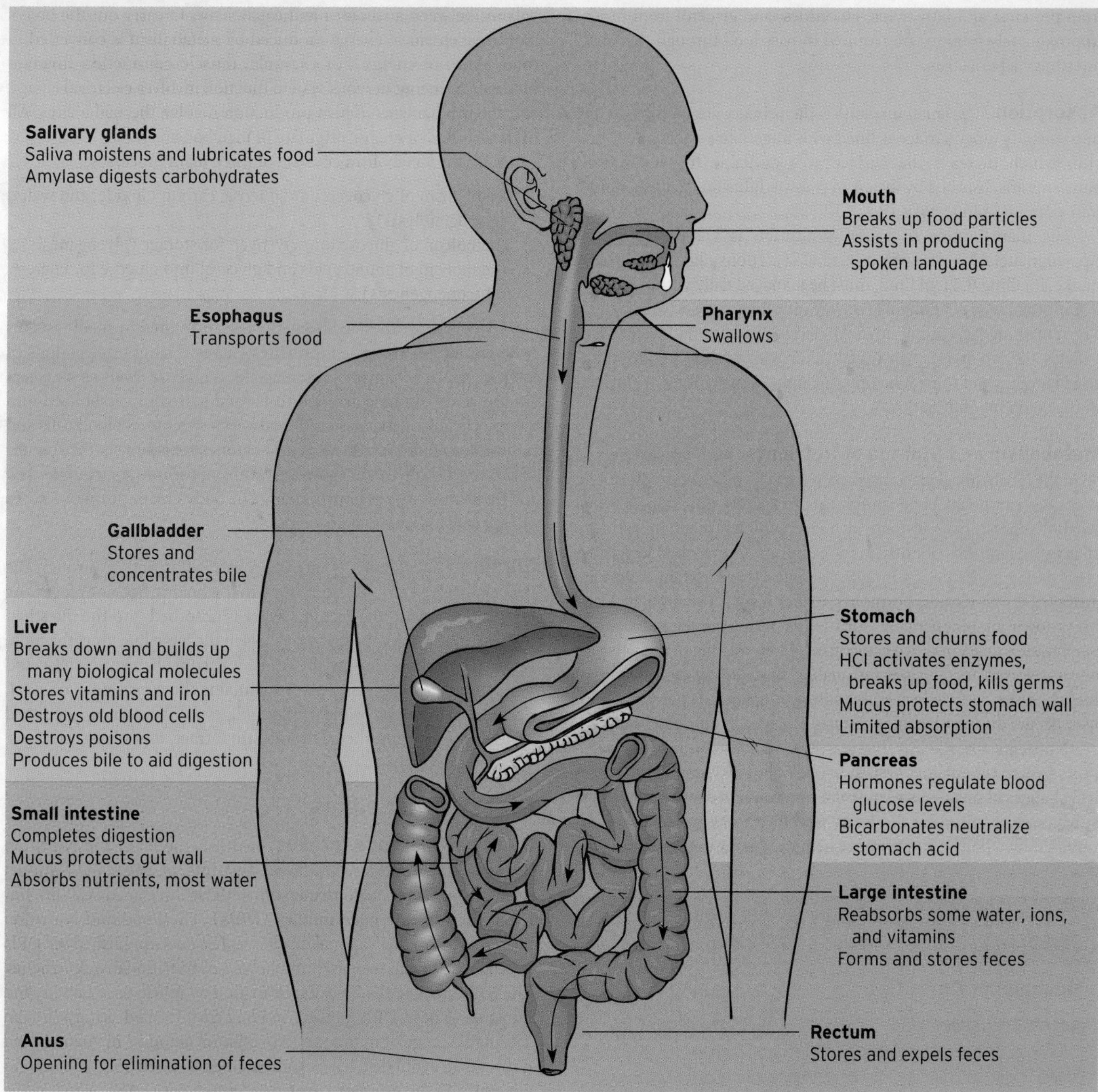

Figure 43-1 Summary of digestive system anatomy and organ function. **Source:** From Rolin Graphics.

mucus. Alcohol and aspirin are two substances directly absorbed through the lining of the stomach. The muscular walls of the stomach produce a churning action that continues mechanical digestion. The stomach acts as a reservoir where food remains for approximately 3 hours, within a range of 1 to 7 hours.

Food leaves the antrum, or distal stomach, via the pyloric sphincter and enters the duodenum. Food has now become an acidic, liquefied mass called **chyme.** Chyme flows into the duodenum and is quickly mixed with bile, intestinal juices, and pancreatic secretions. Secretin and cholecystokinin (CCK) are hormones secreted by the mucosa of the small intestine. Secretin activates release of bicarbonate from the pancreas, raising the pH of chyme. CCK inhibits further gastrin secretion and initiates the release of additional digestive enzymes from the pancreas and gallbladder.

Bile is manufactured in the liver and stored in the gallbladder. Bile acts as a detergent, as it emulsifies fat to permit enzyme action while suspending fatty acids in solution. Pancreatic secretions contain six enzymes: amylase to digest starch; lipase to break down emulsified fats; and trypsin, elastase, chymotrypsin, and carboxypeptidase to break down proteins.

Peristalsis continues in the small intestine, mixing the secretions with the chyme. The mixture becomes increasingly alkaline, inhibiting the action of the gastric enzymes and promoting the action of the duodenal secretions. Epithelial cells in the inner walls of the small intestine secrete enzymes to facilitate digestion. These enzymes include sucrase, lactase, maltase, lipase, and peptidase. The major portion of digestion occurs in the small intestine, producing glucose, fructose, and galactose from carbohydrates; amino acids and dipeptides from proteins; and fatty acids, glycerides, and glycerol from lipids. Approximately 5 hours are required to pass food through the small intestine via peristalsis.

Absorption. The small intestine is the primary absorption site for nutrients. Its inner surface is lined with fingerlike projections called villi, which increase the surface area available for absorption. Nutrients are absorbed by means of passive diffusion, osmosis, active transport, and pinocytosis (Box 43–1).

The main source of water absorption is via the intestine. Approximately 7 L of gastrointestinal secretions and 1.2 L of oral intake, totalling 8.2 L of fluid, must be managed daily within the gastrointestinal tract. The small and large intestines reabsorb 8.1 L a day. The remaining 0.1 L is eliminated in feces. In addition to water, electrolytes and minerals are absorbed, and bacteria in the colon synthesize vitamin K and some B-complex vitamins. Finally, feces are formed in the colon for elimination.

Metabolism and Storage of Nutrients. **Metabolism** refers to all of the biochemical reactions within the cells of the body. Metabolic processes can be anabolic (building) or catabolic (breaking down). **Anabolism** is the production of more complex biochemical substances by synthesis of nutrients. Anabolism occurs when lean muscle is added to the body through diet and exercise. Amino acids are anabolized into tissues, hormones, and enzymes. **Catabolism** is the breakdown of biochemical substances into simpler substances. Starvation is an example of catabolism, when wasting of body tissues occurs. Normal metabolism and anabolism are physiologically possible when the body is in positive nitrogen balance, whereas catabolism occurs during physiologic states of negative nitrogen balance.

Nutrients absorbed in the intestines, including water, are transported via the circulatory system to body tissues. Through the chemical changes of metabolism, nutrients are converted into a number of substances required by the body. Carbohydrates, protein, and fat undergo metabolism to produce chemical energy and to maintain a balance between anabolism and catabolism. To carry out the body's work, the chemical energy produced by metabolism is converted to other types of energy. For example, muscle contraction involves mechanical energy, nervous system function involves electrical energy, and the mechanisms of heat production involve thermal energy. All of these forms of energy originate in metabolism.

Nutrient metabolism consists of three main processes:

1. Catabolism of glycogen into glucose, carbon dioxide, and water (**glycogenolysis**).
2. Anabolism of glucose into glycogen for storage (**glycogenesis**).
3. Catabolism of amino acids and glycerol into glucose for energy (**gluconeogenesis**).

Glycogen, synthesized from glucose and stored in small reserves in liver and muscle tissue, provides energy during brief periods of fasting. This mechanism maintains blood glucose levels as we sleep. Amino acids can be converted to fat and stored or catabolized into energy via gluconeogenesis. All body cells except red blood cells and neurons can oxidize fatty acids into **ketones** for energy in the absence of dietary carbohydrates (glucose). Some of the nutrients required by the body are stored in body tissues. The body's major form of reserve energy is fat, stored as adipose tissue.

Elimination. Chyme is moved by peristaltic action through the ileocecal valve into the large intestine, where it becomes feces. As feces move toward the rectum, water is absorbed into the intestinal mucosa. The longer the material stays in the large intestine, the more water is absorbed, causing the feces to become firmer. Exercise and fibre stimulate peristalsis; water maintains the consistency of stool. Feces contain cellulose and similar indigestible substances, sloughed epithelial cells from the gastrointestinal tract, digestive secretions, water, and microbes.

➤ BOX 43-1 Mechanisms for Intestinal Absorption of Nutrients

Mechanism Definition

Active Transport

In this energy-dependent process, particles move from an area of greater concentration to an area of lesser concentration. A special "carrier" is needed to move the particle across the cell membrane.

Passive Diffusion

The force by which particles move outward from an area of greater concentration to lesser concentration constitutes passive diffusion. The particles do not need a special "carrier" to move outward in all directions.

Osmosis

In this process, water moves through a membrane that separates solutions of different concentrations. Water moves to equalize the concentration pressures on both sides of the membrane.

Pinocytosis

Large molecules of nutrients are engulfed by the absorbing cell when the molecule attaches to the absorbing cell membrane.

Data from Nix, S. (2005). *Williams' basic nutrition and diet therapy* (12th ed.). St. Louis, MO: Mosby; and Williams, S. D., & Schlenker, E. D. (2003). *Essentials of nutrition and diet therapy* (8th ed.). St. Louis, MO: Mosby.

Dietary Guidelines

Dietary Reference Intakes. In 1997, the Food and Nutrition Board of the American National Institute of Medicine/National Academy of Sciences, in partnership with Health Canada (2006), initiated **dietary reference intakes (DRIs)**. The Food and Nutrition Board (1997) of the National Academy of Sciences published the DRIs in response to the increased public use of nutritional supplements. The DRIs broaden the base of information on nutrients, vitamins, and minerals. These DRIs present evidenced-informed criteria for an acceptable range of minimum to maximum amounts of vitamins and nutrients to avoid deficiencies or toxicities. The DRIs have four components: (1) the estimated average requirement (EAR), which is the recommended amount of a nutrient sufficient to maintain a specific body function for 50% of the population based on age and gender; (2) the recommended dietary allowance (RDA), which is the average needs of 98% of the population, not the exact needs of an individual (Murphy et al., 2006); (3) the upper intake level (UL), which is the highest level believed to pose no risk of adverse health events but is not a recommended level of intake (Beaton, 2006); and (4) the adequate intake (AI), which is the suggested intake for individuals based on observed or scientifically determined estimates of nutrient intakes and is used when insufficient evidence exists to set the RDA. Because this evidence is continually evolving, clinicians should consult current resources, such as Health Canada Web pages and other evidence-informed literature, when determining a client's specific nutrition needs or supplementation.

Food Guidelines. In 1942, Health Canada developed Canada's first food guide, *Canada's Official Food Rules*. Since then, the food guide has undergone many changes in name, appearance, and content.

However, its ultimate purpose to inform daily food choices and promote optimal nutritional health has not changed (Katamay et al., 2007). The current guide, called *Eating Well with Canada's Food Guide* (Health Canada, 2007b; Figure 43–2), is based on a range of scientific evidence, including results from focus groups, on-line consultations, regional meetings, and reviews of literature, about the environmental context in which Canadians make food choices. Input from stakeholders (e.g., health professional groups, nongovernmental organizations [NGOs], industry) and the public at large helped to ensure that the recommendations are scientifically sound and address those characteristics of the diet most relevant to the promotion of health and reduction of chronic disease (Health Canada, 2007b).

In developing Canada's Food Guide, food-group composites were used, and once nutrient goals (e.g., RDA, AI) were met for a given food intake pattern, additional testing was done to evaluate the adequacy of varied food choices consistent with the pattern. For example, a bagel, 375 mL of rice, and 30 g of breakfast cereal rather than 6 servings of a grain composite were used (Murphy & Barr, 2007). Random simulated diets were generated for every age and gender group. The prevalence of inadequacy was assessed for each nutrient with an EAR. If the prevalence of inadequacy was low, the recommended intake pattern was considered adequate in diets that deviated from the proportions of foods included in the composites. If the prevalence of inadequacy was high, the food intake pattern was revised. Therefore, most people following the intake pattern listed in Canada's Food Guide have a high probability of meeting their nutritional requirements and a low probability of nutrient excess, even if their individual food choices vary (Katamay et al., 2007; Murphy & Barr, 2007).

Included in the general guidelines of *Eating Well with Canada's Food Guide* are specific suggestions for food choices. Consumers are told to make at least half their grain selections whole grain; choose grains lower in fat; eat at least one dark green and one orange vegetable per day; and use vegetables and fruits more than juice, which contains a lower amount of fibre. Lower-fat dairy products and lean meats are also promoted. Choices from the lower-fat meat group (e.g., legumes, tofu) are suggested as well. The minimum intake of unsaturated fats is 30 to 45 mL. Two food-guide servings of fish each week are suggested on the basis of evidence relating fish consumption and reduced risk of cardiovascular disease. The Food Guide lists water as a calorie-free way to quench thirst and recommends that community water supplies be fluoridated to the level of 1 mg/L. Recommended intakes and nutritional values according to Canada's Food Guide are shown in Table 43–1.

Canada's Food Guide notes the importance of physical activity in maintaining energy balance and recommends that adults spend 30–60 minutes per day carrying out some physical activity and that children and youth spend at least 90 minutes per day. The guide provides advice on the use of vitamin and mineral supplementation when the recommended food intake pattern does not ensure adequate amounts. Although not specified in the guide, Canadians are advised to limit salt to "healthy" levels, to limit alcohol to no more than 5% of total energy, and to limit caffeine to no more than 400 to 450 mg (or approximately 4 cups of regular coffee per day) for nonpregnant, non-breastfeeding women and to no more than 2.5 mg/kg/day for children (Health Canada, 2003a).

Eating Well with Canada's Food Guide has been adapted for First Nations, Inuit, and Métis persons (Health Canada, 2007c). Examples

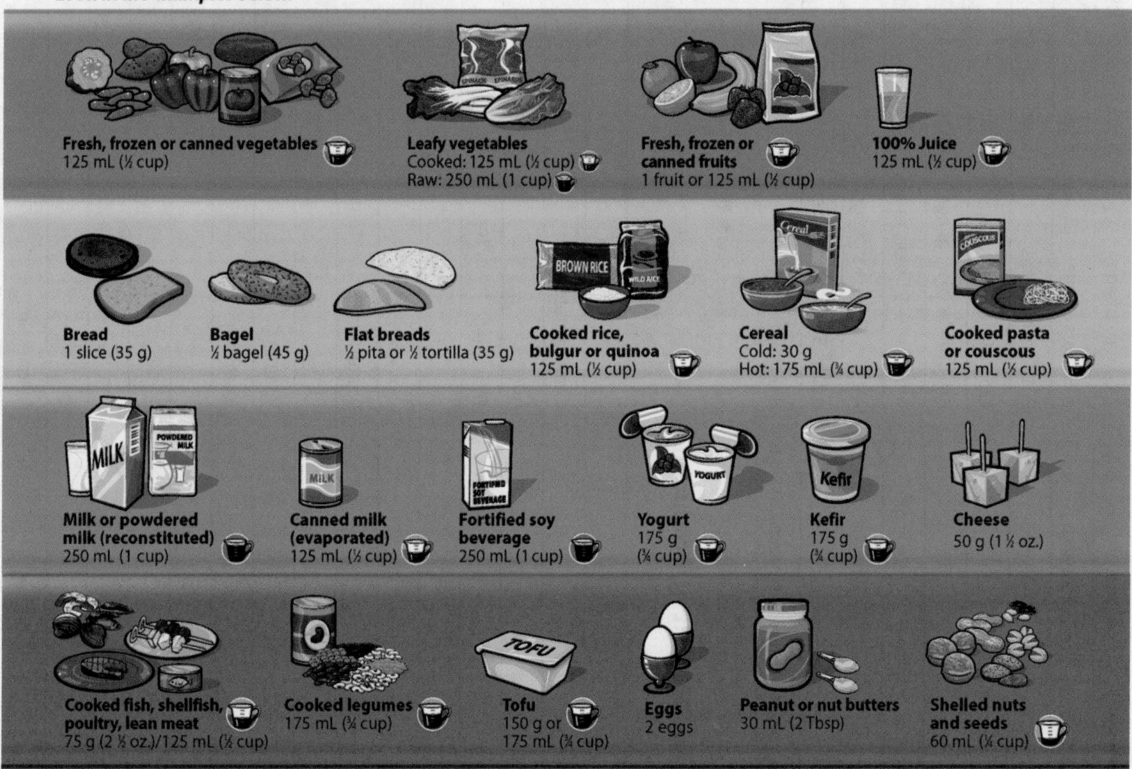

Figure 43-2 Extract from *Eating Well with Canada's Food Guide*. **Source:** From Health Canada. (2007). *Eating Well with Canada's Food Guide* (Catalogue No. H164-38/1-2007E). Ottawa, ON: Author. Retrieved August 22, 2008, http://www.hc-sc.gc.ca/fn-an/food-guide-aliment/index_e.html. Reproduced with permission of the Minister of Public Works and Government Services Canada.

➤ TABLE 43-1 Summary of Recommended Intakes and Nutritional Values According to *Eating Well with Canada's Food Guide*

Grain Products		Vegetables and Fruits		Milk Products		Meat and Alternatives	
2–3 years of age:	3 servings per day	2–3 years of age:	4 servings per day	2–3 years of age:	2 servings per day	2–8 years of age:	1 serving per day
4–8 years of age:	4 servings	4–8 years of age:	5 servings	4–8 years of age:	2 servings	9–13 years of age:	1–2 servings
9–13 years of age:	6 servings	9–13 years of age:	6 servings	9–13 years of age:	3–4 servings	Girls 14–18 years of age:	2 servings
Girls 14–18 years of age:	6 servings	Girls 14–18 years of age:	7 servings	14–18 years of age:	3–4 servings	Boys 14–18 years of age:	3 servings
Boys 14–18 years of age:	7 servings	Boys 14–18 years of age:	8 servings				
Women 19–51 years of age:	6–7 servings	Women 19–51 years of age:	7–8 servings				
Men 19–51 years of age:	7 servings	Men 19–51 years of age:	8–10 servings	19–51 years of age:	2 servings	Women 19–51 years of age:	2 servings
Women 51+ years of age:	6 servings	Adults 51+ years of age:	7 servings	Adults 51+ years of age:	3 servings	Men 19–51 years of age:	3 servings
Men 51+ years of age:	7 servings					Women 51+ years of age:	2 servings
						Men 51+ years of age:	3 servings

Nutritional Content of Products

Grain Products	Vegetables and Fruits	Milk Products	Meat and Alternatives
Protein		Protein	Protein
		Fat	Fat
Carbohydrate	Carbohydrate		
Fibre	Fibre		
Thiamine	Thiamine		Thiamine
Riboflavin		Riboflavin	Riboflavin
Niacin			Niacin
Folate	Folate		Folate
		Vitamin B_{12}	Vitamin B_{12}
	Vitamin C		
	Vitamin A	Vitamin A	
		Vitamin D	
		Calcium	
Iron	Iron		Iron
Zinc		Zinc	Zinc
Magnesium	Magnesium	Magnesium	Magnesium

Adapted from Health Canada. (2007). *Eating Well with Canada's Food Guide*. Ottawa, ON: Author. Retrieved August 22, 2008, http://www.hc-sc.gc.ca/fn-an/food-guide-aliment/index_e.html. Reproduced with permission of the Minister of Public Works and Government Services Canada.

of foods traditional to Canadian Aboriginal populations include wild plants and seaweed in the fruit and vegetable groups, bannock as a grain product, and wild game as a meat alternative. Included in the online Food Guide is a link to a government Web site for advice on limiting exposure to mercury from eating locally caught fish. Instructions are also given for including traditional fats in the diet such as seal and whale oil, ooligan grease, and bacon fat.

In the past, Canada's Aboriginal peoples subsisted on foods obtained from hunting, trapping, fishing, gathering, and agriculture. The resulting diet, high in animal protein and low in fat and carbohydrates, provided adequate energy and nutrients. In replacing traditional foods with contemporary market foods, the current diet of Aboriginal peoples is lower in iron, folacin, calcium, vitamins A and D, fibre, fruit, and vegetables and higher in fat and sugar intakes. Patterns of food consumption are further influenced by issues of **food security** (limited or uncertain ability to acquire acceptable foods), preferences in body size, individual taste preferences, unavailability of particular species for food, lack of knowledge of the nutritional deficits of store-bought food, and modification and contamination of the natural environment. Health problems including anemia, dental caries, obesity, heart disease, and diabetes are related to such beliefs and dietary practices (Willows, 2005).

To date, Canada's Food Guide has not been modified to recognize the nutritional concerns of Chinese Canadians or of other immigrant groups, although it has been translated into 10 languages other than English. This omission has implications for people living in Toronto, Vancouver, and Montreal since they are the primary destinations for new Canadians (Statistics Canada, 2003). In a study designed to explore the cultural relevance of a fruit-and-vegetable questionnaire for adults from Toronto's Chinese-, Portuguese-, and Vietnamese-speaking communities (Paisley et al., 2005), Chinese participants reported that they seldom included many of the vegetables and fruits listed on the questionnaire (e.g., raw vegetables, salads), that they would like to see common Chinese vegetables (e.g., lai kan, choy sum) on the list, and that the variety and composition of vegetable and fruit intake by Cantonese- and Mandarin-speaking people were not represented. Vietnamese-speaking participants asked why fresh herbs were not listed. Portuguese-speaking participants noted the absence of vegetables familiar to them such as collard greens. The need for further examples of culturally appropriate foods and portions will, no doubt be addressed through ongoing revisions to the Food Guide.

The Nutrition Label. Since December 12, 2007, mandatory nutrition labelling consisting of a nutrition facts table listing energy (calories) and 13 nutrients (fat, saturated fat, trans fat, cholesterol, sodium, carbohydrate, fibre, sugars, protein, vitamin A, vitamin C, calcium, and iron) has been required on most prepackaged foods in Canada. This easy-to-read table, which appears on food labels in a consistent appearance, provides consumers with the information necessary to make informed food choices and compare products (Figure 43–3). This information includes (a) the specific amount of the food item that comprises the serving size, an amount that may differ from the food guide serving size, and (b) the percent daily value (% DV), a general guideline of how the food's nutrient content contributes to daily diet. It is important to note that the % DV is based on a 2000–reference calorie adult diet and, as such, does not address recommended nutrient intake for those who are pregnant or breastfeeding. Diet-related health claims have also been established from recognized health and scientific information (Health Canada, 2007e). The permitted claims are about the following diet–health relationships:

- A healthy diet low in sodium and high in potassium may reduce high blood pressure risk.
- A healthy diet adequate in calcium and vitamin D may reduce the risk of osteoporosis.
- A healthy diet low in saturated fat and trans fat may reduce the risk of heart disease.
- A healthy diet rich in vegetables and fruit may reduce the risk of some types of cancer.

The Canadian government defines words used in nutritional claims that describe a product to allow consumers to associate claims with particular standards. New regulations regarding nutrient content claims include the following:

- *Free* indicates that the number of calories or the amount of a nutrient is nutritionally insignificant in a specified amount of food.
- Claims for *saturated fatty acids* include a restriction on levels of both saturated and trans fatty acids.
- The claim *(naming the percent) fat-free* is allowed only if accompanied by the statement *low fat* or *low in fat*.
- The nutrient content claim *light* is allowed only on foods that meet the criteria for either *reduced in fat* or *reduced in calories*.
- A statement that explains what makes the food light must accompany the use of *light*; this is also true if *light* refers to a sensory characteristic such as light in colour.
- The only nutrient content claims permitted for foods for children under 2 years of age are *source of protein, excellent source of protein, more protein, no added sodium,* and *no added sugar*.
- A claim of *reduced in calories* is allowed if the item has at least 25% fewer calories than the food to which it is compared.

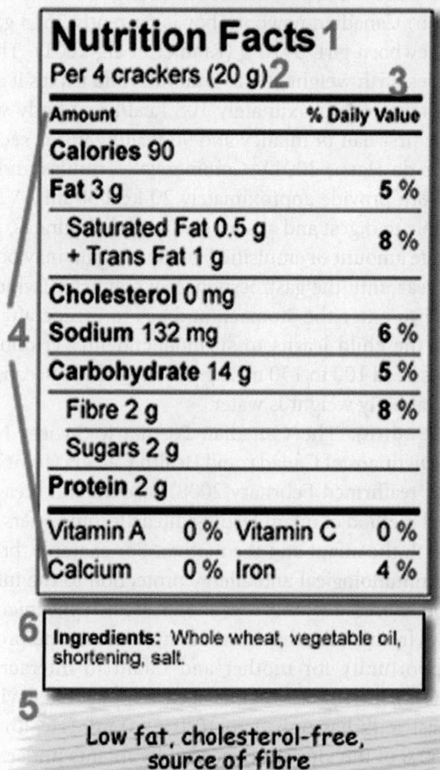

Figure 43-3 Example of food label. **Source:** Health Canada. (2007). *Interactive nutrition label: Get the facts*. Ottawa, ON: Author. Retrieved April 9, 2008, from http://www.hc-sc.gc.ca/fn-an/label-etiquet/nutrition/cons/inl_main_e.html. Reproduced with the permission of the Minister of Public Works and Government Services Canada.

Nutrition for Health: An Agenda for Action. In 1992, the World Health Organization (WHO) endorsed a World Declaration on Nutrition. This declaration set goals for each country to eliminate starvation, nutritional diseases, and disorders (e.g., iodine and vitamin deficiency disorders), and to promote nutritional well-being of all people. In 1996, Canada responded to this endorsement and devised *Nutrition for Health: An Agenda for Action* (Health Canada, 2002). This document is the combined work of multisectoral groups in Canada focused on stimulating and accelerating action by all sectors to achieving healthier people. The strategic directions recommended by the *Agenda for Action* have arisen from an analysis of Canada's current situation and from select high-priority, health-enhancing activities that build on the strength of previous activities. The challenge remains to motivate consumers to put the dietary recommendations into practice. The current Health Canada information on patterns of consumption indicates a move by most Canadians toward meeting the nutritional recommendations. Health professionals can play a key role in promoting healthy dietary practices.

Nursing Knowledge Base

Nutrition During Human Growth and Development

Infants Through School-Age Children. Infancy is marked by rapid growth with high protein, vitamin, mineral, and energy requirements. The average (50th percentile) birth weight of a full-term (40-week gestation) Canadian newborn boy is currently 3613 g; that for a Canadian newborn girl, 3470 g (Kramer et al., 2001). The infant usually doubles birth weight at 4 to 5 months and triples it at 1 year. An energy intake of approximately 108 kcal/kg of body weight is needed in the first half of infancy and 98 kcal/kg in the second half (Tontisirin & de Haen, 2001). Commercial formulas and human breast milk both provide approximately 20 kcal/30 mL. A full-term newborn is able to digest and absorb simple carbohydrates, proteins, and a moderate amount of emulsified fat. Spitting up may occur during the first year until the gastroesophageal sphincter (which opens to allow food to enter the stomach and gas to escape after meals) matures and the child learns to sit independently (Hobbie et al., 2000). Infants need 100 to 150 mL/kg per day of fluid because a large portion of total body weight is water.

Breastfeeding. The Canadian Paediatric Society Nutrition Committee, Dietitians of Canada, and Health Canada (Joint Working Group, 1998; reaffirmed February 2008) recommend breastfeeding as the optimal method of infant feeding. Breastfeeding offers multiple benefits to both the infant and the mother. For example, breastfeeding confers immunological and allergy protection to the infant during the period of breastfeeding, is economical and convenient (breast milk is always fresh and at the correct temperature), and provides an excellent opportunity for mother and infant to interact (Health Canada, 2004a). Breastfed infants need supplemental vitamin D because breast milk has only 1 to 10 IU/250 mL (Health Canada, 2004b), or 60% of the vitamin D needed by infants under 1 year of age. Other vitamin or mineral supplementation is not recommended for the first 6 months (Health Canada, 2004b).

Interdisciplinary promotion of breastfeeding has resulted in an increased initiation rate from 75% in 1982 to 87% in Ontario in 2003 (Millar & Maclean, 2005). However, duration of breastfeeding has decreased to only 60% and 30% of mothers still exclusively breastfeeding at 3 and 6 months, respectively. Many hospitals and communities have nurse lactation consultants who work individually with mothers for successful breastfeeding in the hospital and at home. The need for health practitioners to promote, protect, and support breastfeeding as the healthiest choice for both infant and mother is well recognized (Health Canada, 2004a; WHO, 2003).

Formula. Commercially prepared infant formulas, cow's milk based and iron fortified, are the most acceptable alternative to breast milk. Infant formulas are designed to contain the approximate nutrient composition of human milk. Protein in the formula is typically supplied as whey, soy, cow's milk base, casein hydrolysate, or elemental amino acids. The composition, processing, packaging, and labelling of all infant formulas are regulated under Canadian food and drug laws. Research shows that differences in the way certain constituents within formulas are absorbed may influence optimal growth and development. For example, infants fed formulas containing palm and palm olein (PO) oils as the main source of fat excreted more calcium in their stools and had significantly lower bone mineral content than did infants fed the PO-free formula. Infants fed formulas containing total potentially available nucleosides (TPAN), which mitigate against suppression of the immune system, increase resistance to some bacterial and fungal pathogens, and reduce the risk of diarrhea, experienced the same gastrointestinal tolerance as those receiving human milk (Health Odyssey International, 2008). Specialty formulas are indicated for infants with detected or suspected pathology. Health professionals caring for new mothers and their infants can address mothers' concerns about infant formulas and help them make informed choices when selecting the best substitute for human milk.

Health Canada (2004a) and WHO (2001) recommend the exclusive use of breast milk for the first 6 months of the infant's life. Regular cow's milk should not be used in infant formula before 9 to 12 months of age. It may cause gastrointestinal bleeding, is too concentrated for the infant's kidneys to manage, increases the risk of milk product allergies, and is a poor source of iron and vitamins C and E (Schlenker & Long, 2007). Honey is a potential source of botulism toxin and should not be used in the infant's diet, as the toxin can be fatal in children under 1 year of age (Schlenker & Long, 2007).

Introduction to Solid Food. Breast milk or formula provides sufficient nutrition for the first 6 months of the infant's life. After that, solids are introduced to meet the infant's nutrient needs, specifically, iron, zinc, and vitamin A. Cues indicating readiness for solid foods are the appearance of fine motor skills of the hand and fingers, hand-to-mouth movement, interest in adult food and self-feeding, increased milk consumption, ability to move food to the back of the mouth, and ability to sit alone in a high chair. Pureed smooth foods are typically the first semi-solid food to be introduced to an infant. The addition of foods to an infant's diet should be governed by the infant's nutrient needs and physical readiness to handle different forms of foods and by the need to detect and control allergic reactions. New foods should be introduced one at a time, early in the day, at 2-day intervals, or 4 to 7 days apart if the child is known to have allergies (Alberta Health and Wellness, 2008). It is best to introduce new foods before milk or other foods to avoid satiety (Health Canada, 2005b).

The growth rate slows during toddler years (ages 1–3 years). The toddler needs fewer kilocalories but an increased amount of protein in relation to body weight; consequently, appetite may decrease at about 18 months of age. Toddlers exhibit strong food preferences and become picky eaters. Small, frequent meals consisting of breakfast, lunch, and dinner, with three interspersed, high nutrient-density snacks, may improve nutritional intake (Hockenberry, 2004). Calcium and phosphorus are important for healthy bone growth. Whole milk should be used until the toddler reaches 2 years of age to help ensure adequate intake of fatty acids necessary for brain and neurological development. Toddlers and preschoolers need vitamin D supplementation until their diet includes at least 10 µg (400 IU) per day of vitamin D from other dietary sources (i.e., drinking 2 cups of milk daily and eating 1–2 servings of fish weekly). Toddlers who consume more than 720 mL of milk daily in lieu of other foods may develop milk anemia, as milk is a poor source of iron.

The oral health of infants and children needs to be focussed on preventing cavities. Children who sleep with a bottle are at particular risk of developing early childhood tooth decay (ECTD), a severe type of tooth decay that can affect baby teeth, especially the upper front teeth. The sugars from the milk, juice, and drinks left in the mouth combine with bacteria in plaque to create an acid that damages the enamel of a tooth. The longer and more often food is left in the mouth, the greater the chance of developing ECTD (Health Canada, 2005b). Dental visits should begin within 6 months of the eruption of the first tooth or at 1 year of age at the latest. From the age of 3 years, twice-yearly dental inspections are recommended. Children under 3 years of age should have their teeth brushed by an adult, and parents need to supervise children under 6 years of age during brushing (Canadian Dental Association, 2005).

Preschoolers' (3 to 5 years old) dietary requirements are similar to those of toddlers. They consume slightly more than toddlers, and nutrient density is more important than quantity. Encouragement of healthy eating among toddlers is an important goal of parenting, and to this end, parents should try to use fun, educational initiatives (Anonymous, 2005) and attractive food presentations rather than unhealthy food as a reward (Tucker et al., 2006). For both preschoolers and toddlers, certain foods such as hot dogs, candy, gum, cough drops, raisins, sunflower seeds, fish with bones, peanuts, peanut butter, marshmallows, nuts, grapes, raw vegetables, popcorn, and fruit gel snacks have been implicated in choking deaths and should be avoided or prepared in a safe manner (Qureshi & Mink, 2003).

School-age children, 6 to 12 years old, grow at a slower and steadier rate, with a gradual decline in energy requirements per unit of body weight. The school-age child gains 3 to 5 kg in weight and 6 cm in height per year until puberty. Despite better appetites and more varied food intake, school-age children's diets should be carefully assessed for adequate protein and vitamins A and C. School-age children frequently fail to eat a proper breakfast and have an unsupervised food intake at school. High amounts of fat, sugar, and salt can result from a liberal intake of commercially prepared snack foods.

Inappropriate nutrition may play an important role in childhood obesity. The prevalence of childhood obesity in Canada has increased by 200% to 300% between 1981 and 2001 (Starky, 2005). Data from the 2004 Canadian Community Health Survey (Statistics Canada, 2006) showed that 59% of Canadian children do not consume adequate fruits and vegetables and that these children are significantly more likely to be overweight and obese than those children who consume the recommended amounts of fruits and vegetables. In Prince Edward Island, Aboriginal children do not consume the minimum number of fruit and vegetable servings, and less than half of the 55 children in the study sample consumed the minimum number of milk products daily (Taylor et al., 2007).

Research by Tremblay and Willms (2003) indicates that children who watch more than 2 hours of television per day are at an increased risk for being overweight and obese. It is of concern therefore that 50% of Canadian children spend between 2 and 4 hours per day watching television (Active Healthy Kids Canada, 2008). Currently, 18.1% of all Canadian children are classified as overweight and an additional 8.2% as obese (Statistics Canada, 2006). Children who live in Atlantic Canada are twice as likely to be overweight as children in the Prairie Provinces (Willms et al., 2003). In First Nations' communities, the prevalence of pediatric and adolescent obesity is much higher (Kuperberg & Evers, 2006).

Considerable health risks are associated with being overweight or obese, including type 2 diabetes, sleep apnea, cardiovascular disease, gallbladder and liver disease, certain types of cancers, hypertension, osteoarthritis, and hypercholesterolemia (Starky, 2005). These diseases and disorders, traditionally limited to adults, are manifesting in Canadian youth (Tremblay, 2003). In addition, overweight and obese children encounter negative attitudes. A well-cited research study by Richardson and colleagues (1961) asked children in public schools and summer camps to rate six pictures of children with various conditions to determine which one they would most like to have as a friend. The majority of children ranked the obese child last, after children on crutches, in a wheelchair, with an amputated hand, or with facial disfigurement. This benchmark study was replicated in 2003 by Latner and Stunkard. Their results confirmed those found in 1961 and revealed that the stigmatization had become even stronger. The preference of liking the picture of the normal-weight child more than that of the obese child had increased by 40.8% since the original study.

Because juvenile obesity frequently continues into adulthood, it could lead to higher rates of morbidity and mortality. Thus the prevention and treatment of obesity in childhood and adolescence is a critical public health issue and, ultimately, an important determinant of long-term health. Obesity-prevention strategies recommended by family physicians include initiating obesity prevention during pregnancy, using a family approach, and encouraging increased physical activity and less television viewing (Plourde, 2006). Evidence exists also to suggest that school interventions may reduce childhood obesity and that the role of parents in this area is critical. Delegates to a Toronto think tank organized by the Canadian Council for Food and Nutrition agreed that ongoing input from experts and leaders of all sectors and fields is required to help effectively promote healthy lifestyles in schools and homes (Mendelson, 2007).

Nurses who work with children with type I diabetes need to be aware of the many implications such a diagnosis can have on a child. Beyond the illness and treatments, these children experience a range of emotions and are faced with issues of identity, autonomy, and belonging—all requiring a sensitive approach to support regarding nutrition and other interventions. The story that appears in Box 43–2 conveys a nurse's experiences with a young boy who had recently received a diagnosis of diabetes.

Adolescents. During adolescence, physiological age is a better guide to nutritional needs than chronological age. Energy needs to increase to meet the greater metabolic demands of growth. The daily requirement of protein also increases. Calcium and vitamin D are essential for the rapid bone growth that occurs during adolescence, and girls need a continuous source of iron to replace menstrual blood losses. Boys also need adequate iron for muscle development. In addition to meats and fish, greens, nuts, dried fruits, and whole grains are iron-rich foods (College of Family Physicians of Canada, 2007). Iodine supports increased thyroid activity, so it is important that adolescents use iodized table salt to ensure adequate intake. B-complex vitamins are needed to support heightened metabolic activity.

The adolescent's diet is influenced by many factors other than nutritional needs, including concern about body image and appearance, desire for independence, and fad diets. Nutritional and energy deficiencies may occur in adolescent girls as a result of dieting (Adolescent Health Committee, Canadian Pediatric Society, 2004; reaffirmed 2008) and use of oral contraceptives (Brown et al., 2005). In a recent analysis of Canadian women's magazines, the frequency of messages about body weight and dieting far outnumbered those about calcium. Because many Canadian girls and women use magazines as their primary source of nutrition information, this imbalance in coverage could result in promotion of a lifestyle that increases the risk for osteoporosis (Hassan et al., 2007). The adolescent boy's diet may be inadequate in total kilocalories, protein, iron, folic acid, B vitamins, and iodine.

At the same time, snacks provide approximately 25% of teenagers' total dietary intake. The consumption of fast foods has been associated with excess weight gain, which may be related to the higher energy and fat content of most of these foods. Fast-food restaurants also offer larger portions of food, so consumers are eating greater amounts (CTV National News with Lloyd Robinson, 2003). To counteract this trend among adolescents, health promotion initiatives are being implemented in schools to develop supportive environments for healthier eating (e.g., reducing the availability of junk foods in school cafeterias and in vending machines).

The onset of eating disorders such as **anorexia nervosa** or **bulimia nervosa** often occurs during early adolescence when individuals are establishing independence and autonomy. Dieting and weight control are viewed as a defense for feelings of inadequacy or ineffectiveness. In later adolescence, when facing the task of separation–individualization, similar conflicts may arise (Weaver, 2008). Recognition of eating disorders is essential for early intervention (Table 43–2).

Sports and regular moderate-to-intense exercise necessitate dietary modification to meet the increased energy needs of adolescents. Carbohydrates, both simple and complex, are the main source of energy. Protein needs increase to 1.0 to 1.5 g/kg per day; fat needs do not increase. Adequate hydration is very important for all athletes. They need to ingest water before and after exercise to prevent dehydration, especially in hot, humid environments. It is not necessary to supplement the diet with vitamins and minerals, but intake of iron-rich foods is required to prevent anemia (Croll et al., 2006).

Parents often have more influence over the adolescent diet than they believe they have. Effective strategies include limiting the amount of unhealthy foods kept at home and enhancing the appearance and taste of healthy foods. Making healthy foods more convenient and available and working to change social norms that determine what foods are "cool" are other ways to promote optimal nutritional health among adolescents (Contento et al., 2006).

Pregnancy occurring within 4 years of menarche may place the mother and fetus at risk because of the mother's anatomical and physiological immaturity. Malnutrition at the time of conception increases risk to the adolescent and her fetus. Most teenage girls do not want to gain weight, thus counselling adolescent girls on the nutritional needs associated with pregnancy may be difficult; suggestions are better tolerated than rigid directions. The diet of pregnant adolescents is often deficient in calcium, iron, and vitamins A and C. Prenatal vitamin and mineral supplements are recommended.

BOX 43-2 NURSING STORY

Counselling Children About Nutrition*

Thomas, a 10-year-old boy who had received a diagnosis of type I diabetes mellitus, was referred to the diabetes clinic for nutrition counselling when he started having difficulty making healthy food choices. As his nurse on the pediatric unit, I accompanied Thomas and his family to the clinic to provide ongoing support and guidance. Initially, Thomas appeared angry and upset, voicing his frustrations about being diabetic and its impositions on his lifestyle. Being viewed differently by his friends for having to "take needles every day to stay alive" worried him, "because nobody else I know has to do this. I can't do what *I* want when *I* want." Thomas needed help understanding type I diabetes so he could begin to dispel the myths he had heard and gain control over the diabetes. My first goal was for Thomas to understand what it meant to have type I diabetes and to understand its challenges to his health. With the use of illustrations and diagrams, Thomas was able to articulate what was happening in his body and what that meant to him. Irritated and constantly feeling "sick and tired," he wanted to feel better.

Our next goal was for Thomas to appreciate the value that proper nutrition plays in controlling blood sugars. Again, using visual images, Thomas was able to understand and describe in his own words the role of protein, fats, and carbohydrates in his body's metabolism. He was particularly quick to grasp the significance of the glycemic index (e.g., "Foods with high GIs will make me feel sicker!"). Thomas concluded that in order to feel better, he would need to expand his food choices within the recommended guidelines of *Eating Well with Canada's Food Guide* (Health Canada, 2007b). Yet, as a typical 10-year-old boy whose favourite foods were pepperoni pizza and bologna sandwiches on white bread, Thomas wanted to be able to continue to eat these foods and not appear different to his friends. He was relieved that whole grains could look like white bread and that the substitution of chicken for the bologna would likely not be noticed by others. I role-played with Thomas "cool" responses he could make if questioned about his food (e.g., "whole grain rocks—it helps keep sugar in line").

Thomas anticipated some difficulty in obtaining the required number of servings of fruits and vegetables. According to his mother, Thomas struggled with the textures of fruits and vegetables; he occasionally ate a banana or an apple if his mother peeled it for him. So we discussed the types of fruits and vegetables that his parents typically bought and the possibility of trying new foods with similar textures. The clinic dietician also referred Thomas and his parents to "diabetes-friendly" recipes, including those for muffins and fruit smoothies, which were an instant success. We talked further with Thomas about hiding vegetables in foods he enjoys—for example, pureeing cauliflower and mixing it with chicken to make chicken nuggets.

Thomas agreed to try these ideas and accepted as a challenge the need to alternate one new fruit and one new vegetable each day. He made a "score" chart for his bulletin board to record his efforts in taking control over the diabetes. At post-discharge visits, Thomas excitedly shared his accomplishments and was proud that he was "winning the battle with diabetes." Thomas and his parents thanked me and the clinic staff for helping him to feel better and to gain control over his health and wellness.

*By Bev Gaudet, BN, RN

Young and Middle-Aged Adults. The demands for most nutrients are reduced as the growth period ends. Adults need nutrients for energy, maintenance, and repair, although adults' energy needs usually decline over the years. Obesity may become a problem as a result of decreased physical exercise, frequent dining out, and the increased ability to afford more luxury foods. Women who use oral contraceptives may need extra vitamins. Iron and calcium intake continues to be important.

Maintaining good oral health is important throughout adulthood. Poor oral hygiene and periodontal disease are potential risk factors for systemic diseases such as bacteremia, endocarditis, cardiopulmonary disease, diabetes mellitus, and for adverse outcomes in pregnancy (WHO, 2008).

Pregnancy. Poor nutrition during pregnancy can cause low birth weight in infants and decrease their chances of survival. Generally, the fetus's needs are met at the expense of the mother. However, if nutrient sources are not available, both will suffer. The nutritional status of the mother at the time of conception is important because significant aspects of fetal growth and development often occur before pregnancy is even suspected.

The energy requirements associated with pregnancy are related to the mother's body weight and activity levels. Pregnant women need

➤ TABLE 43-2 Potential Assessment for Eating Disorders

Anorexia Nervosa

A. Body weight not maintained over a minimal normal weight for age and height, (e.g., weight loss leading to maintenance of body weight <85% of ideal body weight [IBW]); or failure to make expected weight gain during period of growth, leading to body weight <85% of that expected.
B. Intense fear of gaining weight or becoming fat, although underweight.
C. Disturbance in the way in which one's body weight, size, or shape is experienced (e.g., the person claims to "feel fat" even when obviously underweight).
D. In females, absence of at least 3 consecutive menstrual cycles when otherwise expected to occur (amenorrhea). (A woman is considered to have amenorrhea if her periods occur only following hormone administration.)

Bulimia Nervosa

A. Recurrent episodes of binge eating (rapid consumption of a large amount of food in a small period of time).
B. A feeling of lack of control over eating behaviour during the eating binges.
C. The person regularly engages in either self-induced vomiting, use of laxatives or diuretics, strict dieting or fasting, or vigorous exercise in order to prevent weight gain.
D. A minimum average of 2 binge eating episodes a week for at least 3 months.

From American Psychiatric Association. *Diagnostic and statistical manual of mental disorders* (4th revised ed.). Washington, DC: Author. Copyright 1994, American Psychiatric Association. Reprinted with permission.

100 kcal per day above the usual allowance during the first trimester and approximately 300 extra calories per day in the second and third trimesters. The extra nutrition should consist of a variety of foods from the four food groups to ensure adequate vitamin, mineral, and nutrient intake (Public Health Agency of Canada, 2008). Rigid recommendations about weight gain should be avoided because the quality of nutrition during pregnancy is more important than weight gain per se or than the number of kilocalories consumed per day. Food intake during the first trimester should include balanced portions of essential nutrients with emphasis on quality. *Canada's Food Guide* recommends that pregnant women get the additional nutrients needed for fetal growth by increasing their daily servings of milk and milk products, breads and cereals, and fruits and vegetables (Health Canada, 2007b). Supplementation may be recommended, along with dietary modification, to increase intake of folate, calcium, vitamin D, iron, and essential fatty acids (Health Canada, 1999).

Calcium intake is especially critical during the third trimester, when fetal bones are mineralized. Iron may be supplemented to provide for increased maternal blood volume, for fetal blood storage, and for maternal blood loss during delivery. Iodine needs increase 15% to 17% because of increased activity of the thyroid gland. Folic acid intake is particularly important for DNA synthesis and the growth of red blood cells. Inadequate intake may lead to fetal neural tube defects, anencephaly, or maternal megaloblastic anemia (Schlenker & Long, 2007). The role of folic acid supplementation is currently being reexamined in light of recent studies suggesting that folic acid may promote the progression of already existing, undiagnosed cancers (Kim, 2007). Prenatal care usually includes vitamin and mineral supplementation to ensure daily intakes; however, pregnant women should not take additional supplements beyond prescribed amounts. For example, vitamin A is essential to maternal and fetal health but is teratogenic (harmful to the growth and development of an embryo or fetus) when consumed in excess (Schlenker & Long, 2007). Pregnant women should drink at least eight glasses of water daily. Pregnant women should also avoid artificial sweeteners, alcohol, excessive caffeine, and all drugs not specifically ordered, as these substances pass through the placenta and affect the growing baby. Adequate fluid and fibre intake and moderate exercise help prevent constipation, which is commonly associated with pregnancy in response to the growing uterus, to pregnancy hormones, and to iron supplementation.

Lactation. Lactating women need 500 kcal per day above the usual allowance because the production of milk increases energy requirements. *Canada's Food Guide* suggests that lactating women ingest the same nutrient levels as recommended during pregnancy. The need for calcium remains the same as during pregnancy, but lactating women require additional vitamins A and C. Daily intake of water-soluble vitamins (B and C) is needed to ensure adequate levels in breast milk. Fluid intake should be adequate but need not be excessive. Caffeine, alcohol, and drugs are excreted in breast milk and thus should be avoided. It is recommended that nursing be postponed by at least 1 hour after consuming an alcoholic drink, as it takes an adult woman (55 kg) about 1.25 hours to metabolize the 10 g of alcohol contained in the average drink (Health Canada, 2007a). Tobacco use can decrease the mother's milk production (Myr, 2004).

Older Adults. Adults age 65 years and older have a decreased need for energy because the metabolic rate slows with age. However, vitamin and mineral requirements remain unchanged from middle adulthood.

Many factors influence the nutritional status of older adults (Box 43–3). Income is significant because for those living on a fixed income, the amount of money available to buy food may be reduced. A large number of older clients benefit from home-delivered or congregate meal services. Health status is another important factor. The older adult may be following a therapeutic diet; have difficulty eating because of physical symptoms, lack of teeth, or dentures; or be at risk for drug–nutrient interactions (Table 43–3). Thirst sensation may diminish, leading to inadequate fluid intake or dehydration (see Chapter 36). Meats may be avoided because of their cost or because they are difficult to chew. Cream soups and meat-based vegetable soups are nutrient-dense sources of protein; however, commercial soups and packaged meats contain a high salt content. Cheese, eggs, and peanut butter are also useful high-protein alternatives. Milk continues to be an important food for older adults, who need adequate calcium to protect against osteoporosis (a decrease of bone-mass density). Although research has shown that older men lag behind women by approximately a decade in developing osteoporosis, screening and treatment are necessary for older men as well as older women (Schlenker & Long, 2007). The diets of older adults should contain choices from all food groups and may require a vitamin and mineral supplement.

safety alert Homebound older adults with chronic illness have additional nutritional risks. Frequently, this group lives alone with little or no social resources to assist in obtaining or preparing nutritionally sound meals. Increased nutritional screening during regular medical visits may result in more timely recognition of potential nutritional deficiencies and subsequent treatment of these deficiencies (LaForest et al., 2007).

Alternative Food Patterns

Many people follow special patterns of food intake that are based on religion (Table 43–4), cultural background (Box 43–4) ethics, health beliefs, personal preference, or concern for the efficient use of land to produce food. Such special diets are not necessarily more or less nutritious than diets based on *Eating Well with Canada's Food Guide* or other nutritional guidelines because good nutrition depends on a balanced intake of all required nutrients.

Vegetarian Diet. **Vegetarianism** is the consumption of a diet consisting predominantly of plant foods. Vegetarians may be ovo-lacto vegetarians (avoid meat, fish, and poultry but eat eggs and milk), lacto-vegetarians (drink milk but avoid eggs), or vegans (consume only plant foods). Dietitians of Canada and the American Dietetic Association maintain that appropriately planned vegetarian diets can help prevent and treat certain diseases such as hypertension, type II diabetes, and prostate and colon cancer (Mangels et al., 2003). However, knowledge related to complementary use of complete and incomplete proteins, food sources of vitamin B_{12} (e.g., fortified breakfast cereal and soymilk), and nondairy sources of calcium is necessary (Messina et al., 2003). Vegan, Zen macrobiotic (consisting primarily of brown rice, other grains, and herb teas), and fruitarian (consisting of only fruit, nuts, honey, and olive oil) diets can be nutrient poor and can result in malnutrition. Children who follow a vegetarian diet are especially at risk for protein and vitamin deficiencies such as vitamin B_{12} (Mangels et al., 2003; Stabler & Allen, 2004). Canadian adolescent girls and women of reproductive age who are vegetarian are at greater risk for low iron stores because diets high in plant foods contain dietary iron inhibitors (Cooper et al., 2006).

The vegetarian food guide rainbow (Figure 43–4) is laid out in a format similar to that of *Eating Well with Canada's Food Guide*. The widest arc forms the foundation of the diet, vegetables and fruits are grouped separately to ensure choice from both, and dairy products are included in the legumes and nuts group as protein-rich sources to ensure that protein needs are met, regardless of whether dairy products are included. Dietary needs for iron can be met through choices from the grain and legumes and nuts groups, with the exception of dairy products, which are not sources of iron. To reduce cardiovascular risk, vegetarians who do not eat fish are advised to consume two servings per day of foods that contain omega-3 fats. Any one of the following is considered one serving: 5 mL flaxseed oil, 15 mL canola or soybean oil, 15 mL ground flaxseed, or 60 mL walnuts. The placement of calcium-rich food groups adjacent to each of the other groups emphasizes how calcium needs can be met by choosing a variety of foods across all the food groups (Messina et al., 2003).

BOX 43-3 FOCUS ON OLDER ADULTS

Factors Affecting Nutritional Status

- Age-related gastrointestinal changes that affect digestion of food and maintenance of nutrition include changes in the teeth and gums, reduced saliva production, atrophy of oral mucosal epithelial cells, increased taste threshold, decreased thirst sensation, reduced gag reflex, and decreased esophageal and colonic peristalsis (Brownie, 2006).
- Presence of other diseases, such as diabetes and cognitive impairments related to delirium, dementia, and depression, increase risk of poor nutrition (Watson et al., 2006).
- Malnutrition in older adults has multiple causes, such as low income, low educational level, lack of physical functional level to meet activities of daily living, loss, dependency, loneliness, and lack of transportation (Payette & Shatenstein, 2005).
- Nutrition awareness and motivation may be poor: Older adults may not read food labels or understand the nutrient value of foods (van Dillen et al., 2008).
- Medications may have adverse effects such as causing anorexia (loss of appetite), xerostomia (severe dryness of the mouth), early satiety, and impaired smell and taste perception. Older adults are more likely to be prescribed medications than younger persons (Watson et al., 2006).
- Intake of calcium, vitamin D, and phosphorus may be deficient, increasing the risk for osteoporosis. Vitamin B_{12} may not be synthesized because of lack of intrinsic factor (glycoprotein necessary for the absorption of vitamin B_{12}) in the terminal ileum, decreased lean muscle mass, and lower basic energy expenditure (Masse et al., 2004).

Critical Thinking

Critical thinking requires the gathering and synthesizing of knowledge, experience, information from clients that is gained through intellectual and professional standards and attitudes of open-mindedness, respect for client autonomy, and confidence. Clinical judgements involve the anticipation of the required information, analysis of the data, and openness to new ideas and multiple perspectives when making decisions regarding client care. Critical thinking is thus a dynamic process. During assessment (Figure 43–5), you must consider all elements that contribute to the rendering of appropriate nursing diagnoses.

When assessing nutrition, you must integrate knowledge from nursing and other disciplines, from previous experiences, from information gathered from clients and families about food preferences, from clinical observations, and from dietary history. Professional standards, such as the DRIs and *Eating Well with Canada's Food Guide* (Health Canada, 2007b), provide guidelines for assessing and maintaining clients' nutritional status. Other professional standards from the Heart and Stroke Foundation of Canada, the Canadian Cancer Society, Canadian Society for Clinical Nutrition, and the Canadian Dietetic Association are available. These standards are research based and are regularly updated to enhance optimal care.

Nursing Process and Nutrition

Nurses are in an excellent position to recognize signs of poor nutrition and to take steps to initiate change. Close contact with clients and their families enables nurses to make observations about physical status, food intake, weight changes, and responses to therapy.

❖Assessment

Early recognition of malnourished or at-risk clients has a strong, positive influence on both short- and long-term health outcomes. Studies have identified 20% to 50% of adult clients as being nutritionally at

TABLE 43-3 Sample Nutrient-Drug Interactions*

Drug	Effect
Analgesic	
Acetaminophen	Decreased drug absorption with food; overdose associated with liver failure
Aspirin	Absorbed directly through stomach; decreased drug absorption with food; decreased folic acid, vitamins C and K, and iron absorption
Antacid	
Aluminum hydroxide	Decreased phosphate absorption
Sodium bicarbonate	Decreased folic acid absorption
Antiarrhythmic	
Amiodarone	Taste alteration
Digitalis	Anorexia; decreased renal clearance in older persons
Antibiotic	
Penicillins	Decreased drug absorption with food; taste alteration
Cephalosporin	Decreased vitamin K
Rifampin	Decreased vitamin B_6, niacin, vitamin D
Tetracycline	Decreased drug absorption with milk and antacids; decreased nutrient absorption of calcium, riboflavin, vitamin C due to binding
Trimethoprim/ sulfamethoxazole	Decreased folic acid
Anticoagulant	
Coumarin	Acts as antagonist to vitamin K
Anticonvulsant	
Carbamazepine	Increased drug absorption with food
Phenytoin	Decreased calcium absorption; decreased vitamins D and K and folic acid; taste alteration; decreased drug absorption with food
Antidepressant	
Amitriptyline	Appetite stimulant
Clomipramine	Taste alteration; appetite stimulant
Fluoxetine (selective serotoin reuptake inhibitors [SSRIs])	Taste alteration; anorexia
Antihypertensive	
Capropril	Taste alteration; anorexia
Hydralazine	Enhanced drug absorption with food; decreased vitamin B_6
Labetalol	Taste alteration (weight gain for all β-blockers)
Methyldopa	Decreased vitamin B_{12}, folic acid, iron
Anti-inflammatory	
All steroids	Increased appetite and weight; increased folic acid; decreased calcium (osteoporosis with long-term use); promotes gluconeogenesis of protein
Antiparkinson	
Levodopa	Taste alteration; decreased vitamin B_6; and decreased drug absorption with food
Antipsychotic	
Chlorpromazine	Increased appetite
Thiothixene	Decreased riboflavin; increased need
Bronchiodilator	
Albuterol sulfate	Appetite stimulant
Theophylline	Anorexia
Cholesterol Lowering	
Cholestyramine	Decreased fat-soluble vitamins (A, D, E, K); vitamin B_{12}; iron
Diuretic	
Furosemide	Decreased drug absorption with food
Spironolactone	Increased drug absorption with food
Thiazides	Decreased magnesium, zinc, and potassium
Laxative	
Mineral oil	Decreased absorption of fat-soluble vitamins (A, D, E, K,), carotene
Platelet Aggregate Inhibitor	
Dipyridamole	Decreased drug absorption with food
Potassium Replacement	
Potassium chloride	Decreased vitamin B_{12}
Tranquilizer	
Benzodiazepines	Increased appetite

*Not intended to be an exhaustive or all-inclusive list. Always check pharmacology references before administering medications.

Data from McKenry, L. M., & Salerno, E. (2003). *Mosby's pharmacology in nursing* (21st revised ed.). St. Louis, MO: Mosby; and "Nutrient–drug interactions." (2006). *Nutrition and well-being A to Z.* Retrieved January 19, 2009, from http://www.faqs.org/nutrition/Met-Obe/Nutrient-Drug-Interactions.html

risk upon hospital admission and that such malnutrition increases hospital costs (Amarat et al., 2007; Kubrak & Jensen, 2007). Other studies have shown a relationship between malnutrition and adverse outcomes, including mortality (Stratton & Elias, 2006; Stratton et al., 2006). Moreover, the prevalence of malnutrition among special client populations (e.g., oncology clients) may range as high as 90% (Krubrack & Jensen, 2007). This high prevalence is associated with the interrelations between disease severity, disability, treatment, and self-care practices. Clearly, accurate assessment of nutritional status is necessary for nurses to help clients make significant differences in their health and quality of life.

Nutritional screening is part of an initial assessment of identifying malnutrition or risk of malnutrition. **Nutritional screening** involves identification of clients who are either malnourished or at risk of malnourishment (Green & Watson, 2005). The SCREEN (Figure 43–6) is a nutrition-risk screening index that consists of 15 questions about weight change, food and fluid intake, and risk factors associated with food and fluid intake. Five responses to questions are possible, with item scores ranging from 0 to 4; for example, the question "How would you describe your appetite?" can be rated as very good (4), good (3), fair (2), poor (1), or very poor (0). Low scores (<50) indicate increased nutritional risk.

TABLE 43-4 Religion-Based Dietary Restrictions and Guidelines

Islam	Christianity	Hinduism	Judaism	Church of Jesus Christ of Latter-Day Saints (Mormons)	Seventh-Day Adventists
Pork Alcohol Caffeine Ramadan fasting sunrise to sunset for 1 month Ritualized methods of animal slaughter required for meat ingestion	Minimal or no alcohol Holy-day observances may restrict meat	All meats Alcohol	Pork Predatory fowl Shellfish (eat only fish with scales) Rare meats Blood (blood sausage, etc.) Do not mix milk or dairy products with meat dishes Must adhere to kosher food preparation methods 24 hours of fasting on Yom Kippur, a day of atonement No leavened bread eaten during Passover (8 days) No cooking on the Sabbath (Saturday)	Alcohol Tobacco Caffeine Limit meat	Pork Shellfish Alcohol Vegetarian diet encouraged

Nutritional assessment goes beyond nutritional screening and involves five major areas: anthropometry, laboratory tests, dietary and health history, clinical observation and physical examination, and client expectations to determine nutritional status. Assess the client's nutritional status when a condition that interferes with the ability to ingest, digest, or absorb adequate nutrition exists. No single area or measurement accurately determines nutritional status, and a client's personal and social health context needs to be considered.

Anthropometry

Anthropometry is a measurement system of the size and makeup of the body. Height and weight are obtained for each client admission to any health care setting. If height cannot be measured with the client standing, position the client lying flat in bed as straight as possible, arms folded on the chest, and measure the client lengthwise. If possible, the client should be weighed at the same time each day, on the same scale, and with the same apparel. Serial measures over time provide more useful information than one-time measurement. An **ideal body weight (IBW)** provides an estimate of what a person should weigh. Rapid weight gain usually reflects fluid shifts. Five hundred millilitres of fluid equals 0.45 kg. For example, for a client with renal failure or congestive heart failure, a weight increase of 0.9 kg is significant, as it may indicate that the client has retained a litre of fluid. Recent weight changes should be documented.

Body mass index (BMI) measures weight corrected for height and serves as an alternative to traditional height–weight relationships.

BOX 43-4 CULTURAL ASPECTS OF CARE

Nutrition

Food patterns developed as a child, through habits and culture, interact to influence food intake. Culture also influences the meaning of food not related to nutrition. Eating is associated with sentiments and feelings such as "good" and "bad." For example, children are often rewarded for "being good" with a treat such as candy. They then associate candy with "being good."

The incidence of lactose intolerance around the world occurs in the following ethnic or racial groups: Asian-Pacific, African and African American, Native American, Mexican American, Middle Eastern, and Whites. This condition affects nutrient absorption, and calcium deficiency results. Calcium is necessary for maintaining bone mass density. The theory of "hot" and "cold" foods predominates in many cultures. The origin appears to be from Hippocratic beliefs concerning health and the four humors. Arabs were keepers of this knowledge during the Dark Ages and later influenced the Spanish to adopt this belief system in the late Middle Ages. The foundation of the theory is to keep harmony with nature, one must balance "cold," "hot," "wet," and "dry." Some cultures believe hot characterizes warmth, strength, and reassurance, whereas cold represents menace and weakness. Classification of a food has nothing to do with spiciness but is a symbolic representation of temperature.

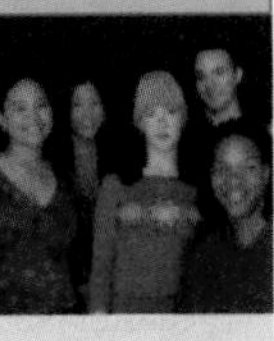

Implications for Practice

- Identify the meaning that certain types of food have for each client.
- Lactose and other food intolerances unique to specific cultures require diet adaptation to meet nutrient, mineral, and vitamin daily-intake requirements.
- When clients use hot and cold foods as part of their cultural health practices, dietary modifications are necessary.
- Hot foods include rice, grain cereals, alcohol, beef, lamb, chili peppers, chocolate, cheese, temperate-zone fruits, eggs, peas, goat's milk, cornhusks, oils, onions, pork, radishes, and tamales. By contrast, cold foods are considered to be beans, citrus fruits, tropical fruits, dairy products, most vegetables, honey, raisins, chicken, fish, and goat meat.
- In some cultures, specific conditions require hot foods. Menstruation, cancer, pneumonia, earache, colds, paralysis, headache, and rheumatism are "cold" illnesses requiring hot foods.
- Other conditions, such as pregnancy, fever, infections, diarrhea, rashes, ulcers, liver problems, constipation, kidney problems, and sore throats, are "hot" conditions requiring cold foods.

Adapted from Giger, J. N., & Davidhizar, R. E. (2004). *Transcultural nursing: assessment and intervention* (3rd ed.). St. Louis, MO: Mosby.

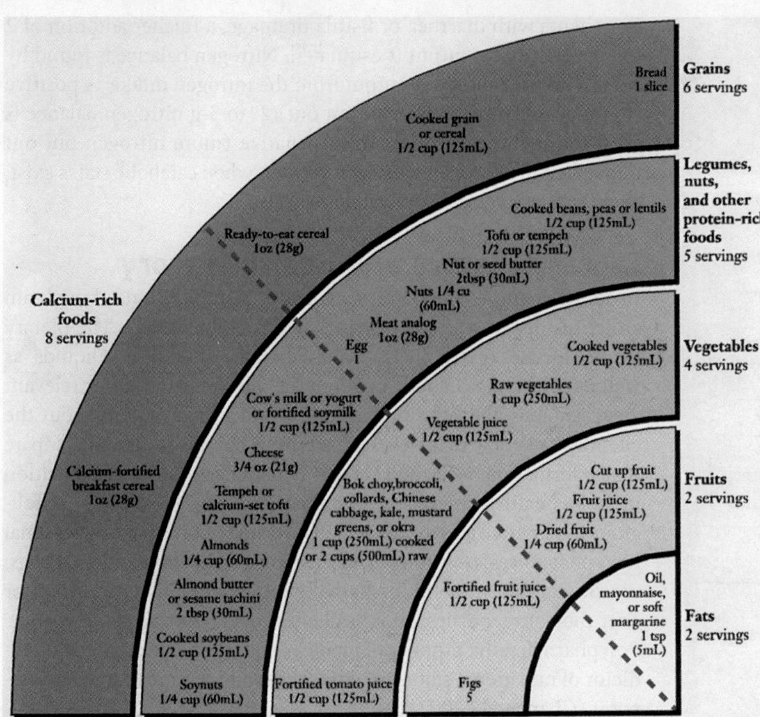

Figure 43-4 Vegetarian food guide rainbow. **Source:** From Messina, V., Melina, V., & Mangels, A. R. (2003). A new food guide for North American vegetarians. *Canadian Journal of Dietetic Research and Practice, 64*(2), p. 85. Copyright 2003. Dieticians of Canada. Used with permission.

Calculation of BMI is achieved by dividing the client's weight in kilograms by height in metres squared: Weight (kg)/Height^2 (m^2). The BMI nomogram is available on Health Canada's Web site at: http://www.hc-sc.gc.ca/fn-an/nutrition/weights-poids/guide-ld-adult/bmi_chart_java-graph_imc_java-eng.php. A BMI measuring between 25 and 30 indicates being overweight, and greater than 30 defines obesity (Health Canada, 2003b). The BMI is a valid measurement of weight in relation to health; however, it is not recommended for use as the sole measurement of body composition or level of fitness because it does not differentiate between excess fat and muscle or bone, and does not consider age, gender, or ethnicity (Scheier, 2004). Health Canada has established its own standards for adult obesity but not for child obesity (He & Beynon, 2006). Thus different cutoff points have been used to calculate BMIs for children (e.g., US Centres for Disease Control and Prevention [CDC], Cole's International references). Care must be taken when interpreting overweight and obesity results.

New Heart and Stroke Foundation research indicates that for most people, the **waist circumference** (WC) measurement may be used to determine health risk. Overweight people who carry excess pounds around the waist are at greater risk of heart disease and stroke than those who carry it on their hips, thighs, and buttocks. The WC is measured at the part of the trunk located midway between the lower costal margin (bottom of lower rib) and the iliac crest (top of pelvic bone) while the person is standing, with feet somewhat apart. The person doing the measuring should stand beside the individual and fit the tape snugly, without compressing any underlying soft tissues. The circumference should be measured to the nearest 0.5 cm, at the end of a normal expiration. In men a WC of 102 cm (40 inches) or greater places them at significant increased risk for heart disease and stroke. In women this measurement is 88 cm (35 inches) or more (Health Canada, 2003b; Heart and Stroke Foundation of Canada, 2008).

Laboratory and Biochemical Tests

No single laboratory or biochemical test can be used to diagnose malnutrition. Factors that may alter test results include fluid balance, liver function, kidney function, and the presence of disease. Common

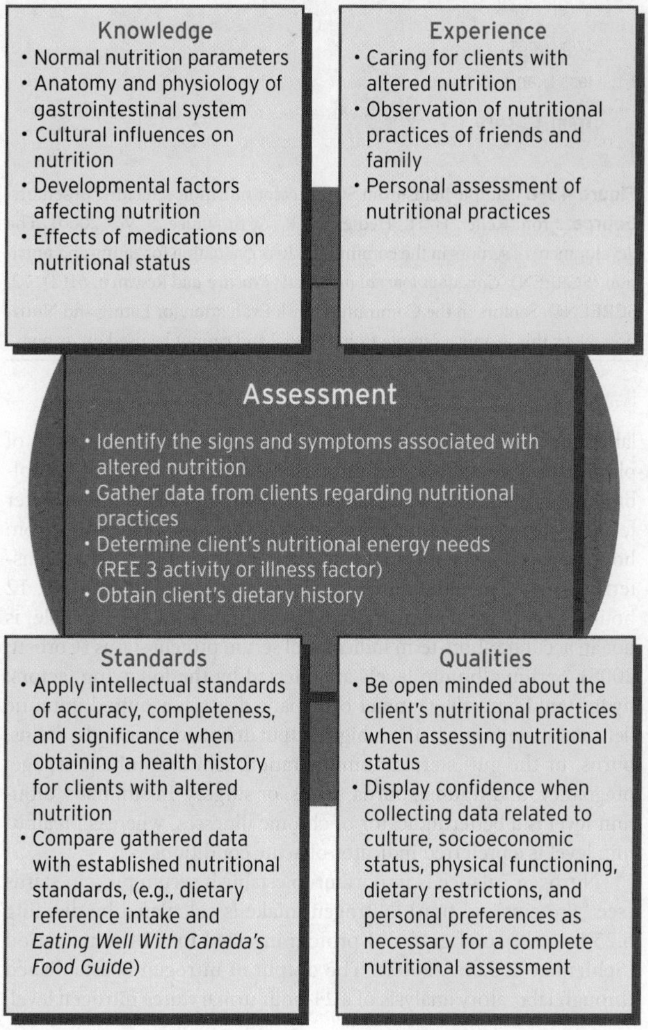

Knowledge
- Normal nutrition parameters
- Anatomy and physiology of gastrointestinal system
- Cultural influences on nutrition
- Developmental factors affecting nutrition
- Effects of medications on nutritional status

Experience
- Caring for clients with altered nutrition
- Observation of nutritional practices of friends and family
- Personal assessment of nutritional practices

Assessment
- Identify the signs and symptoms associated with altered nutrition
- Gather data from clients regarding nutritional practices
- Determine client's nutritional energy needs (REE 3 activity or illness factor)
- Obtain client's dietary history

Standards
- Apply intellectual standards of accuracy, completeness, and significance when obtaining a health history for clients with altered nutrition
- Compare gathered data with established nutritional standards, (e.g., dietary reference intake and *Eating Well With Canada's Food Guide*)

Qualities
- Be open minded about the client's nutritional practices when assessing nutritional status
- Display confidence when collecting data related to culture, socioeconomic status, physical functioning, dietary restrictions, and personal preferences as necessary for a complete nutritional assessment

Figure 43-5 Critical thinking model for nutrition assessment.

Sample Items from SCREEN
(Please choose only 1 response)

1. **Weight Change**
In the past 6 months . . .

I have *gained* a lot of weight (more than 5 kg or 11 lbs).	___ 0
I have *gained* quite a bit of weight (3-5 kg or 6-10 lbs).	___ 1
I have *gained* some weight (1-2 kg or 2-5 lbs).	___ 2
I have *gained* a little weight (less than 1 kg or 2 lbs).	___ 3
My weight has not changed.	___ 4
I have *lost* a little weight (less than 1 kg or 2 lbs).	___ 3
I have *lost* some weight (1-2 kg or 5 lbs).	___ 2
I have *lost* quite a bit of weight (3-5 kg or 6-10 lbs).	___ 1
I have *lost* a lot of weight (more than 5 kg or 11 lbs).	___ 0
I don't know if I have lost or gained weight.	___ 0
Item 1 Score	___

2. **Fruits and Vegetables**
Each day, I usually eat fruits or vegetables . . .
(canned, fresh, frozen, or juice)

five or more times.	___ 4
four times.	___ 3
three times.	___ 2
two times.	___ 1
less than two times.	___ 0
Item 2 Score	___

Figure 43-6 Sample items from SCREEN for nutrition screening of seniors. **Source:** From Keller, H. H., Hedley, M. R., & Brownlee, S. W. (2000). The development of seniors in the community: Risk evaluation for eating and nutrition (SCREEN). *Canadian Journal of Dietetic Practice and Research, 61*(2), 72. SCREEN©. Seniors in the Community: Risk Evaluation for Eating and Nutrition. *Note:* this is only a sample from the tool and cannot be used on its own.

laboratory tests used to study nutritional status include measures of plasma proteins such as albumin, transferrin, prealbumin, retinol-binding protein, total iron-binding capacity, and hemoglobin. After feeding, the response time for changes in these proteins ranges from hours to weeks. The metabolic half-life of albumin is 21 days; transferrin, 7 days; prealbumin, 2 days; and retinol-binding protein, 12 hours. This range demonstrates why albumin level, for example, is not an accurate short-term indicator of serum protein status (Corbett, 2008). Serum albumin levels are affected by the following factors: hydration; hemorrhage; renal or hepatic disease; acquired immune deficiency syndrome (AIDS); high-output drainage of wounds, drains, burns, or the gut; steroid administration; albumin infusions; age; pregnancy; and trauma, burns, stress, or surgery. In summary, albumin level is a better indicator of chronic illnesses, whereas prealbumin level is a preferred indicator of acute conditions.

Nitrogen balance is important to establish serum protein status (see "Proteins" section). Nitrogen intake is calculated by dividing 6.25 into the total grams of protein ingested in a 24-hour period (Schlenker & Long, 2007). The output of nitrogen is established through laboratory analysis of a 24-hour urinary urea nitrogen level. For clients with diarrhea or fistula drainage, a further addition of 2 to 4 g of nitrogen output is estimated. Nitrogen balance is found by subtracting the nitrogen output from the nitrogen intake. A positive (more nitrogen taken in than put out) 2- to 3-g nitrogen balance is ideal for anabolism. In contrast, negative (more nitrogen put out than taken in) nitrogen balance is present when catabolic states exist, such as in starvation or physiological stress.

Dietary History and Health History

In addition to the general nursing health history, you need to obtain a diet history to assess the client's needs (Table 43–5). The dietary history focuses on the client's habitual intake of foods and liquids, as well as information about preferences, allergies, and other relevant areas, such as ability to obtain food. Gather information about the client's illness or activity level to determine energy needs and compare that information with food intake. Nursing assessment of nutrition includes health status; age; cultural background (see Box 43–3); religious food patterns (see Table 43–4); socioeconomic status; personal food preferences; psychological factors; use of alcohol or illegal drugs; use of vitamin, mineral, or herbal supplements or prescription or over-the-counter drugs; and the client's general nutrition knowledge. Polypharmacy, the number of medications taken, is a significant predictor of nutritional status in older adults and requires careful assessment (Chen et al., 2007).

Outpatient clients may keep a 3- to 7-day food diary, which will enable you to calculate nutritional intake and to compare it with *Eating Well with Canada's Food Guide* and DRIs to see if dietary habits are adequate. Culturally sensitive food-frequency questionnaires may also be used to establish patterns over time.

Clinical Observation and Physical Examination

Clinical observation is key to nutritional assessment. Observe the client for signs of nutritional alterations. Because improper nutrition affects all body systems, clues to malnutrition can be picked up during physical assessment (see Chapter 32). When the general physical assessment of the body systems is complete, you can recheck pertinent areas to evaluate the client's nutritional status. The clinical signs of nutritional status (Table 43–6) provide guidelines for observation during physical assessment.

You need to assess for aspiration (choking) risk and dysphagia. Those at risk of aspiration have decreased levels of alertness, decreased gag or cough reflexes, difficulty managing saliva, or a wet, gurgling voice. You should assess ability to swallow before giving food or medications. To check swallow adequacy, place your fingers at the level of the client's larynx, and ask the person to swallow. You should be able to palpate the movement of the larynx. Clients at risk of aspiration need specialized assistance with feeding.

The warning signs of dysphagia (difficulty when swallowing) include coughing during eating; change in voice tone or quality after swallowing; abnormal movements of the mouth, tongue, or lips; slow, weak, imprecise, inconsistent, or uncoordinated speech; abnormal gag reflex; delayed swallowing; incomplete oral clearance or pocketing of food or medications; regurgitation; and pharyngeal pooling. Clients with dysphagia often do not show overt signs such as coughing when food enters the airway. "Silent aspiration" occurs in clients with neurological problems that lead to decreased sensation (Ramsey et al., 2005). Silent aspiration accounts for most of the aspiration in clients with dysphagia following stroke (Westergreen, 2006), and approximately 20% of dysphagic clients die of aspiration pneumonia

TABLE 43-5 Obtaining a Dietary History

Components of a Dietary History	Areas to Assess and Questions to Ask
Diet	
Number, type, and location of meals eaten per day	How many meals do you eat? At what times do you usually eat? Are these scheduled meals or snacks? Where do you usually eat meals and snacks?
Food preferences	What types of food do you like?
Food-preparation practices	Who prepares the food?
Food-purchasing practices	Who purchases the food?
Unpleasant symptoms	
Indigestion, heartburn, gas	What foods cause indigestion, gas, or heartburn? Does this occur each time you eat the food?
Relief practices	What relieves the symptoms?
Allergies	Are you allergic to any foods? Specify these foods. What happens when you eat these foods? Specify the type of allergic response (e.g., hives, itching, anaphylaxis). What is done to treat allergies (e.g., EpiPen, oral antihistamines)?
Taste	Have you noticed any changes in taste? Did these changes occur with medications or following an illness?
Chewing and swallowing	Do you wear dentures? Are the dentures comfortable? Assess the condition of the client's teeth. Do you experience mouth pain or sores (e.g., cold sores, canker sores)? Do you have difficulty swallowing? Do you cough or gag when you swallow?
Appetite	Have you had a change in appetite? Have you noticed a change in weight? Was this change an anticipated change (e.g., were you following a weight-reduction diet)?
Elimination patterns	How often do you have bowel movements? Do you experience diarrhea with meals or specific foods? If yes, how do you manage the diarrhea? Do you experience constipation? If yes, how do you manage it?
Use of medications	What medications do you take? Do you take any over-the-counter medications that your doctor does not prescribe? If yes, specify them. Describe any nutritional or herbal supplements you use.

within a year of their stroke (Paintal & Kuschner, 2007; Shariatzadeh et al., 2006). Dysphagia often leads to dehydration, inadequate food intake, possibly resulting in malnutrition and weight loss. Early screening with a formal dysphagia protocol can be used to identify problems with swallowing, help you initiate referrals for more in-depth assessment (Skill 43–1), and significantly decrease risk of aspiration pneumonia.

Client Expectations

Because clients rely on nurses and other health care professionals to identify problems, nurses must be knowledgeable about nutrition and nutritional screening, assessment, and referral to meet client expectations and needs.

❖Nursing Diagnosis

Assessment enables you to determine any actual or potential nutrition problems (Box 43–5). A problem may occur when overall intake is significantly decreased or increased, or when one or more nutrients are not ingested, completely digested, or completely absorbed. Specific diagnoses are related to the actual nutritional problem (e.g., inadequate intake) but may also involve problems that place the client at risk for nutritional deficiencies, such as oral trauma, severe burns, or infections.

The nursing diagnostic statement is based on defining characteristics present in the assessment database. The suspected health problem related to the nursing diagnosis is stated. The following are examples of nursing diagnoses of clients with nutritional problems:

- *Risk for aspiration*
- *Constipation*
- *Diarrhea*
- *Deficient fluid volumes*
- *Excess fluid volume*
- *Health maintenance, ineffective*
- *Health-seeking behaviours (nutrition)*
- *Risk for infection*
- *Knowledge deficit (nutrition)*
- *Ineffective management of therapeutic regimen, individuals*
- *Imbalanced nutrition: less than body requirements*
- *Imbalanced nutrition: more than body requirements*
- *Risk for imbalanced nutrition: more than body requirements*
- *Feeding self-care deficit*

❖Planning

The planning for enhanced, optimal nutritional status requires a higher level of care than simply correcting problems. You will need to synthesize information from multiple sources to devise an individualized approach to care that is relevant to the client's needs (Figure 43–7). All data sources are considered when developing a nursing care plan (Box 43–6). It is crucial that you refer to published standards that are based on scientific findings.

In clinical situations, clients have multiple related problems. The concept map in Figure 43–8 (on p. 1068) shows the relationship of nursing diagnoses in a client with myasthenia gravis.

TABLE 43-6 Clinical Signs of Nutritional Status

Body Area	Signs of Good Nutrition	Signs of Poor Nutrition
General appearance	Alert; responsive	Listless, apathetic, cachectic appearance
Weight	Weight normal for height, age, body build	Obese or underweight appearance (special concern for underweight)
Posture	Erect posture; straight arms and legs	Sagging shoulders; sunken chest; humped back
Muscles	Well-developed, firm muscles; good tone; some fat under skin	Flaccid appearance, poor tone, underdeveloped tone; tenderness; edema; wasted appearance; inability to walk properly
Nervous system control	Good attention span; lack of irritability or restlessness; normal reflexes; psychological stability	Inattention; irritability; confusion; burning and tingling of hands and feet (paresthesia); loss of position and vibratory sense; weakness and tenderness of muscles (may result in inability to walk); decrease or loss of ankle and knee reflexes; absent vibratory sense
Gastrointestinal function	Good appetite and digestion; normal regular elimination; no palpable organs or masses	Anorexia; indigestion; constipation or diarrhea; liver or spleen enlargement
Cardiovascular function	Normal heart rate and rhythm; lack of murmurs; normal blood pressure for age	Rapid heart rate (above 100 beats/minute), enlarged heart; abnormal rhythm; elevated blood pressure
General vitality	Endurance; energy; good sleep habits; vigorous appearance	Easily fatigued; lack of energy; falling asleep easily; tired and apathetic appearance
Hair	Shiny, lustrous appearance; firmness; strands not easily plucked; healthy scalp	Stringy, dull, brittle, dry, thin, and sparse, depigmented appearance; strands that can be easily plucked
Skin (general)	Smooth and slightly moist skin with good colour	Rough, dry, scaly, pale, pigmented, irritated appearance; bruises; petechiae; subcutaneous fat loss
Face and neck	Uniform colour; smooth, pink, healthy appearance; lack of swelling	Greasy, discoloured, scaly, swollen appearance; dark skin over cheeks and under eyes; lumpiness or flakiness of skin around nose and mouth
Lips	Smoothness; good colour; moist (not chapped or swollen) appearance	Dry, scaly, swollen appearance; redness and swelling (cheilosis); angular lesions at corners of mouth; fissures or scars (stomatitis)
Mouth, oral membranes	Reddish pink mucous membranes in oral cavity	Swollen, boggy oral mucous membranes
Gums	Good pink colour; healthy and red appearance; lack of swelling or bleeding	Spongy gums that bleed easily; marginal redness, inflammation; receding gums
Tongue	Good pink or deep reddish colour; lack of swelling; smoothness, presence of surface papillae; lack of lesions	Swelling, scarlet, and raw appearance; magenta colour, beefiness (glossitis); hyperemic and hypertrophic papillae; atrophic papillae
Teeth	Lack of cavities and pain; bright, straight appearance; lack of crowding; well-shaped jaw; clean appearance with no discoloration	Unfilled caries; absent teeth; worn surfaces; mottling (fluorosis); malpositioned appearance
Eyes	Bright, clear, shiny appearance; lack of sores at corner of membranes; eyelids moist and healthy pink colour; prominent blood vessels or lack of mound of tissue or sclera; lack of fatigue circles beneath eyes	Pale eye membranes (pale conjunctivae); redness of membrane (conjunctival infection); dryness; signs of infection; buildup of keratin debris in the conjunctiva (Bitot's spots), redness and fissuring of eyelid corners (angular palpebritis); dryness of eye membrane (conjunctival xerosis); dull appearance of cornea (corneal xerosis); soft cornea (keratomalacia)
Neck (glands)	Lack of enlargement	Thyroid enlargement
Nails	Firm, pink appearance	Spoon shape (koilonychia); brittleness; ridges
Legs, feet	Lack of tenderness, weakness, or swelling; good colour	Edema; tender calves; tingling; weakness
Skeleton	Lack of malformation	Bowlegs; knock-knees; chest deformity at diaphragm; prominent scapulae and ribs

From Schlenker, E. D., & Long, S. (2007). *William's essentials of nutrition and diet therapy* (9th ed., p. 12). St. Louis, MO: Mosby Elsevier.

➤ SKILL 43-1 Aspiration Precautions

Delegation Considerations

The assessment of a client's risk for aspiration and determination of positioning cannot be delegated to unregulated care providers (UCPs). However, UCPs may feed clients after receiving instructions about aspiration precautions. It is important to instruct the unregulated care provider about the following:

- To position the client appropriately to decrease aspiration risk
- To report any onset of coughing, gagging, or pocketing of food

Equipment

- Chair or electric bed (to allow client to sit upright)
- Thickening agents as needed (rice, cereal, yogurt, gelatin, commercial thickening agent)
- Tongue blade
- Penlight

STEPS	RATIONALE
1. Perform nutritional screening.	• Clients at risk for aspiration from dysphagia often alter their eating patterns or choose foods that do not provide adequate nutrition (Matheny, 2006).
2. Assess clients who are at increased risk of aspiration for signs and symptoms of dysphagia (e.g., cough, pharyngeal pooling, change in voice after swallowing).	• Clients at risk include those who have neurological or neuromuscular diseases and those who have had trauma to or surgical procedures of the oral cavity or throat.
3. Observe client during mealtime for signs of dysphagia and allow client to attempt to feed self. Observe client eat various consistencies of foods and drink liquids. Note at the end of the meal if client becomes tired.	• Helps detect abnormal eating patterns such as frequent clearing of throat or prolonged eating time. Fatigue increases risk of aspiration.
4. Ask client about any difficulties with chewing or swallowing various foods with different textures.	• Certain types of food are more easily aspirated
5. Report signs and symptoms of dysphagia to the health care professional.	• Signs or symptoms associated with aspiration indicate the need for further evaluation of swallowing by a radiologist or speech pathologist, such as a fluoroscopic swallow study (Canadian Stroke Network, 2006).
6. Place identification on client's chart or Kardex indicating that dysphagia is present.	• Identifying the client as having dysphagia alerts the health care team to the problem and helps the team to develop and implement an individualized plan of care (Nowlin, 2006).
7. Explain to the client why you are observing him or her while the client eats.	• Increases client cooperation.
8. Perform hand hygiene.	• Reduces transmission of microorganisms.
9. Using a penlight and tongue blade, gently inspect mouth for pockets of food.	• Pockets of food in the mouth often indicate difficulty swallowing.
10. Elevate head of client's bed so that hips are flexed at a 90-degree angle and the head is flexed slightly forward, or help client to the same position in a chair.	• Reduces risk of aspiration (Metheny, 2004).
11. Observe client consume various consistencies of foods and liquids.	• Referral to a dietitian is appropriate if a client has difficulty with a particular consistency.
12. Add thickener to thin liquids to create the consistency of mashed potatoes, or serve client pureed foods.	• Thin liquids such as water and fruit juice are difficult to control in the mouth and are more easily aspirated (Canadian Stroke Network, 2006; Metheny, 2004).
13. Place 1/2 to 1 teaspoon of food on unaffected side of the mouth, allowing utensil to touch the mouth or tongue.	• Provides client with tactile cues to begin eating.
14. Place hand on throat to gently palpate swallowing event as it occurs. Swallowing twice is often necessary to clear the pharynx.	• Helps evaluate swallowing effort.
15. Provide verbal coaching and positive reinforcement while feeding client. **A.** Feel the food in your mouth. **B.** Chew and taste the food. **C.** Raise your tongue to the roof of your mouth. **D.** Think about swallowing. **E.** Close your mouth and swallow. **F.** Swallow again. **G.** Cough to clear airway.	• Verbal cueing keeps client focused on swallowing. Positive reinforcement enhances client's confidence in ability to swallow.
16. Observe for coughing, choking, gagging, and drooling of food; suction airway as necessary.	• These are indications that suggest dysphagia and risk for aspiration.
17. Provide rest periods as necessary during meal to avoid rushed or forced feeding.	• Avoiding fatigue decreases the risk of aspiration.
18. Ask client to remain sitting upright for at least 30 minutes after the meal.	• Reduces the risk of gastroesophageal reflux, which causes aspiration (Nowlin, 2006).

Continued

SKILL 43-1 Aspiration Precautions *continued*

STEPS	RATIONALE
19. Help client to perform hand hygiene and perform mouth care.	• Mouth care after meals helps prevent dental caries and reduces colonization of bacteria, which reduces the risk of pneumonia (Nowlin, 2006).
20. Return client's tray to appropriate place, and perform hand hygiene.	• Reduces spread of microorganisms.
21. Observe client's ability to ingest foods of various textures and thickness.	• Indicates whether aspiration risk is increased with thin liquids.
23. Weigh client weekly at the same time on the same scale.	• Determines if weight is stable and reflects adequate caloric level.
24. Observe client's oral cavity after meal to detect pockets of food.	• Determines client's ability to swallow.

Unexpected Outcomes and Related Interventions

Coughs, Gags, Food "Stuck in Throat," or Left in Mouth

- Client may require a swallowing evaluation.
- Initiate consultation with a speech therapist for swallowing exercises and techniques to improve swallowing and reduce risk of aspiration.
- Notify health care professional and speech pathologist of any symptoms that occurred during meal and which foods caused the symptoms.

Avoidance of Certain Textures of Food

- Change consistency and texture of food.

Weight Loss

- Discuss findings with health care professional, speech pathologist, or registered dietitian.

Recording and Reporting

- Document the following in the client's chart: client's tolerance of various food textures, amount of assistance required, position during meal, absence or presence of any symptoms of dysphagia, and amount eaten.
- Report any coughing, gagging, choking, or swallowing difficulties to the nurse in charge or the health care professional.

Goals and Outcomes

Goals and outcomes and priorities of care reflect the client's physiological, therapeutic, and individualized needs. Mutually planned goals negotiated between the client, dietitian, and nurse help ensure success. An overall goal for an obese client might be "to achieve appropriate BMI height–weight range or be within 10% of ideal body weight (IBW)." To this end, establishing regular obtainable goals of moderate weight loss rather than one large overwhelming goal is crucial (Costain & Croker, 2005). The following smaller goals or outcomes can help the client achieve the goal:

- Daily nutritional intake meets the minimal DRIs
- Daily nutritional fat intake is less than 30%
- Sugared beverages are removed from diet
- Client refrains from eating between meals and after dinner
- Client loses 0.5 to 1 kg per week

BOX 43-5 NURSING DIAGNOSTIC PROCESS

Imbalanced Nutrition: More Than Body Requirements

Assessment Activities	***Data and Defining Characteristics***
Obtain height and weight	52-year-old man Height: 180 cm Weight: 122 kg Body mass index (BMI) = 37.7
Obtain 24-hour food history	Lack of satiety High fat and carbohydrate intake, three meals plus a large evening snack/day, 3–4 beers/day
Fluid	Fluid intake is cola, beer, and juice, all high caloric
Physical assessment	Short of breath on walking Large abdomen Blood pressure: 158/88 mm Hg Pulse: 102 beats/minute Respirations: 32 breaths/minute
Laboratory values	Cholesterol and triglycerides elevated. All others within normal limits.
Medication	None
Social	Wife and family eat out 2 or 3 times a week.

Knowledge	Experience
• Role of dietitians and nutritionists in caring for clients with altered nutrition • Impact of community support groups and resources in assisting clients to manage nutrition • Impact of bad diets on clients' nutritional status	• Previous client responses to nursing interventions for altered nutrition • Personal experiences with dietary change strategies (what worked and what did not)

Planning

- Select nursing interventions to promote optimal nutrition
- Select nursing interventions consistent with therapeutic diets
- Consult with other health care professionals (e.g., dieticians, nutritionists, physicians, pharmacists, physiotherapists, and occupational therapists) to adopt interventions that reflect the client's needs
- Involve family when designing interventions

Standards	Qualities
• Individualize therapy according to client needs • Select therapies consistent with established standards of normal nutrition • Select therapies consistent with established standards for therapeutic diets	• Display confidence when selecting interventions • Creatively adapt interventions for the client's physical limitations, culture, personal preferences, budget, and home care needs

Figure 43-7 Critical thinking model for nutrition planning.

The setting of goals and outcomes requires interdisciplinary input. A satisfactory care plan requires accurate exchange of information between disciplines.

Setting Priorities

By identifying clients at risk for nutritional problems, health professionals can help prevent or minimize those problems through timely interventions. Although changes in the client's weight are often gradual, improving nutritional intake is a priority. With acute illness or surgery, food intake is often altered in the perioperative period. The priority of care may be to provide optimal preoperative nutrition support for clients with malnutrition. The priority for the resumption of food intake postoperatively depends on the return of bowel function, the extent of the surgical procedure, and whether or not complications exist (Chapter 49).

Sometimes other priorities take precedence. For example, clients who have had throat surgery must be out of pain and comfortable before nutritional priorities can be addressed.

Note also that it is important to collaborate with the client and family when setting care priorities. The purchase of food and its preparation may involve the family, and the care plan may not succeed without their commitment to, involvement in, and understanding of the nutritional priorities.

Continuity of Care

In any health care setting, continuity of care is essential, including continuity of nutritional interventions. Hospital discharge planning should extend nutritional interventions to the home or long-term care facility. In extended settings, the dietitian monitors the client's nutritional status and intake and makes recommendations for changes.

When clients require long-term care or care at home, occupational therapists can help them to choose assistive devices, such as large-handled utensils and cups with a space for the nose. They can also help rearrange food preparation areas to maximize the client's function. Speech therapists recommend appropriate dietary textures and feeding strategies and assist clients with swallowing exercises and techniques to reduce aspiration risk.

❖Implementation

Health Promotion

Nurses are in a key position to educate clients about proper nutritional habits. When clients incorporate knowledge of nutrition into their lifestyle they may prevent the development of many diseases. Early identification of potential or actual problems is the best way to avoid more serious problems. Outpatient and community-based settings are key locations for nursing assessment of nutritional practices and status. Clients with nutritional problems such as obesity may require help with menu planning and compliance strategies. Frequently you will be in a position to educate families about nutrition, tell them about community resources, and provide contact information for a dietitian or nurse so that families can direct questions to him or her.

Insufficient income is the most significant barrier to healthy eating (Raine, 2005). Food selection and quantity are positively associated with income. For example, the degree to which adequate amounts of thiamine and vitamins A and C are consumed correlates with level of income (Ricciuto & Tarasuk, 2006). Higher intake of fruits and vegetables among children has been associated with better nutritional education of parents and with parental knowledge of health, both of which relate to income status (Riediger et al., 2007). At the same time, lower socioeconomic status is associated with physical inactivity in Canadian adolescents (Janseen et al., 2006).

Approximately 3.7 million (15%) Canadians rely on food banks that are unable to supply recommended amounts of fresh fruits, vegetables, dairy products, and meats and alternatives (Irwin et al., 2007). In Atlantic Canada, low-income lone mothers and their older children have poor diet quality (Glanville & McIntyre, 2006). The problem is worsened when such children cannot access nutritional programs at schools (Henry et al., 2003). Mandatory fortification of staple foods with micronutrients has helped to reduce income-related disparities (Ricciuto & Tarasuk, 2006).

Interventions to counter the threat to good nutrition and health from lack of purchasing power are needed at individual and collective levels. For those on limited budgets, food preparation can be modified for substances that need to be used sparingly. Substitutes can be used; for example, bean or cheese dishes can often replace meat. Menu planning a week in advance helps clients comply with a specific diet, eat nutritiously, and stay within their budget. A nurse or dietitian may check menus for content. Often, simple tips can help, such as baking rather than frying to reduce fat intake, using lemon juice or spices to add flavour to low-sodium diets, and avoiding grocery shopping when hungry because it can lead to

BOX 43-6 NURSING CARE PLAN

Imbalanced Nutrition: Less Than Body Requirements

Assessment

Belinda Wong, a nurse practitioner in a community health centre, is seeing 68-year-old Mrs. Cooper, who has a history of congestive heart failure. Recently, Mrs. Cooper noticed a weight loss (15%). She has been taking an antidepressant (sertraline) for 3 months for an initial episode of depression related to the loss of her husband 6 months ago. Mrs. Cooper was referred for counselling 3 months ago for help with grief and depression. When Belinda inquired about Mrs. Cooper's financial situation, Mrs. Cooper responded that it was difficult living on an income from the Canada Pension Plan but she was able to manage.

Assessment Activities	*Data and Defining Characteristics*
Ask Mrs. Cooper about her food intake during the last 2 days.	She says she drinks one glass of juice in the morning and two or three cups of coffee. She may eat a sandwich in the late afternoon. "I'm just not interested in food. It has no taste."
Assess Mrs. Cooper's knowledge base by asking her what she sees as strengths of her diet, about areas in which her diet is ineffective, and what resources she uses in guiding her meal planning.	She says she does not need to worry about being overweight and believes her diet is adequate for her needs, as she does not feel hungry. She says she thinks she should be eating more vegetables and drinking more milk. Her meal preparation is "quick and easy," which pleases her. She says she is "too tired to fuss over food."
Assess her use of medication.	She takes the following prescribed medications as instructed on a daily basis: sertraline, digoxin (cardiac glycoside), chlorothiazide (diuretic), and captopril (antihypertensive).
Ask Mrs. Cooper about social interaction.	Mrs. Cooper says she is lonely and does not get out much, although her psychologist recommended more socializing. Her friends at church call to ask her to come back to meetings, but she is not ready. She says she tires easily.
Weigh Mrs. Cooper and assess her posture.	This weight loss occurred over 6 months, down 11 kg. She has stooped posture. She has a low BMI of 17.
Observe Mrs. Cooper for signs of poor nutrition.	Dull, thinning hair Dry, scaling skin Pale conjunctivae and mucous membranes
Palpate her muscles and extremities.	2+ bilateral pitting ankle edema Generalized poor muscle tone

Nursing Diagnosis: *Imbalanced nutrition:* less than body requirements related to a decreased ability to ingest food as a result of depression and loss of appetite associated with antidepressant use.

Planning

*Goals (Nursing Outcomes Classification)**	*Expected Outcomes*
	Weight Control
Mrs. Cooper will progressively gain weight.	Client will gain 1/2 to 1 kg/month until goal of 59 kg is reached.
	Nutritional Status: Nutrient Intake
Mrs. Cooper will consume adequate nourishment each day.	Client will ingest 1900 kcal/day, including 50 g of protein per day.
Mrs. Cooper will exhibit no signs of malnutrition.	Physical assessment and laboratory values will be within normal limits.

*Outcome classification labels are from Wilkinson, J. M., & Ahern, N. R. (2009). *Nursing Diagnosis Handbook* (9th ed.). Upper Saddle River, NJ: Pearson Prentice Hall.

Interventions (Nursing Interventions Classification)†	**Rationale**
Nutritional Counselling	
Coordinate a plan of care with Mrs. Cooper, her family doctor, her therapist, and her dietitian.	Successful nutrition care planning involves an interdisciplinary approach (Brauer et al., 2006).
Individualize menu plans.	Encourages client to eat by incorporating her food preferences into her diet (Paquet et al., 2003).
Teach Mrs. Cooper about the value associated with consulting *Eating Well with Canada's Food Guide.*	Health Canada (2007b) recommendations for food selections provide optimal nutrition.
Nutritional Monitoring	
Monitor Mrs. Cooper monthly for weight gain, anemia, serum albumin level, and total lymphocyte count (TLC).	Weight gain should be slow and progressive. Serum albumin of 40 g/L and TLC of 1500/mm^3 are within normal limits (Corbett, 2008).
Perform physical assessment of hair, eyes, mouth, skin, and muscle tone.	Provides progressive monitoring for improved nutritional status.

BOX 43-6 NURSING CARE PLAN *continued*

Interventions (Nursing Interventions Classification)†	Rationale
Nutritional Management	
Encourage Mrs. Cooper to eat small meals and to increase dietary intake to help offset anorexia secondary to use of sertraline.	Sertraline is a selective serotonin reuptake inhibitor (SSRI) medication; diminished taste and anorexia are common effects of SSRIs. Frequent small meals help to reduce anorexia-associated weight loss.
Encourage fluid intake.	Older adults need eight 250-mL glasses per day of fluid from beverage and food sources. Concentrating intake in the morning and early afternoon prevents nocturia (Meiner & Lueckenotte, 2006).
Encourage fibre intake.	Fibre helps prevent constipation.
Encourage Mrs. Cooper to have congregate meals (lunch at senior centre) five times per week.	Eating with others encourages good nutrition and promotes socialization with peers. Encouragement from health professionals and from family and friends is helpful for women of ages 55–74 who do not exercise and eat nutritiously (Tannenbaum & Shatenstein, 2007).

†Intervention classification labels from Dochterman, J. M., & Bulechek, G. M. (Eds.). (2004). *Nursing Interventions Classification (NIC)* (4th ed.). St. Louis, MO: Mosby.

Evaluation

Nursing Actions	*Client Response and Finding*	*Achievement of Outcome*
Ask Mrs. Cooper to keep a food diary for 3 days.	Her diary reflects that she ate her main meal at the senior centre, has fruit and grain fibre for breakfast, and has either soup or a sandwich with fruit in the evening.	Mrs. Cooper is selecting more nutritionally rich foods, consistent with current guidelines.
Observe Mrs. Cooper's appearance.	Her skin is less pale, hair appears to be in better condition and styled. Ankle edema is present, but less than 1+.	Mrs. Cooper has improved physical parameters of nutrition; still needs follow-up.
Weigh Mrs. Cooper.	Weight gain of 2 kg in 4 weeks.	Weight gain is steady; the client is still below ideal body weight.
Ask Mrs. Cooper about appetite and energy level.	Mrs. Cooper responds that on days when she eats at the senior centre, her appetite seems better and she "wants to do more things." She notes that weekends are very lonely.	Weekday support for nutritional status appears effective. Mrs. Cooper needs to increase activity status and nutritional intake during weekends.

spontaneous purchases of foods not included in meal plans. Strategies to help financially disadvantaged groups improve their nutrition include collective kitchens and gardens (Engler-Stringer & Berenbaum, 2005), coalitions with community-based organizations, antipoverty advocacy, and political commitment to policies of full employment (Power, 2005). Also important are public-awareness forums (Chapman, 2006) and a rights-based approach to food security at federal and provincial levels (Rideout et al., 2007) with support to families that have inadequate resources to meet their daily nutritional needs (Kurtz Landy, 2007). See Box 43–7 for an example of an innovative program that aims to increase food security for children and their families and communities.

safety alert Food safety is also an important public health issue. Food-borne illnesses can occur from poor hygiene practices and improper food storage or preparation. Nurses should educate clients about reducing the risks of food-borne illnesses (Table 43–7; Box 43–8).

Acute Care

Many factors influence nutritional intake in acute care settings. Ill or debilitated clients often have loss of appetite (**anorexia**). The ketosis that accompanies starvation can further suppress appetite, as can the pain that results from surgical procedures and trauma. You can help clients to understand the factors that cause anorexia and use creative approaches to stimulate appetite.

During hospitalizations, mealtimes are often interrupted or the client is too fatigued or uncomfortable to eat. Clients worried about families, finances, employment, or illnesses are often not able to eat an adequate diet. Diagnostic testing also disrupts many mealtimes or requires a nothing by mouth (NPO) status before tests. Clients who are NPO and receive only standard IV fluids for more than 7 days are at nutritional risk. Both physiological stress and emotional stress influence dietary need and intake. Medications may interfere with taste, cause nausea, interfere with absorption, or affect metabolism.

You must continuously assess the client's nutritional status and plan interventions that promote normal dietary intake, digestion, and metabolism of nutrients. Clients may have a gradual progression of dietary intake or need therapeutic diets to manage their illnesses (Box 43–9). For inpatients, a physician will order a therapeutic diet and the dietetic services department will prepare it.

Promoting Appetite. In providing an environment that promotes a client's appetite it is important to eliminate unpleasant odours, to provide oral hygiene as needed to remove unpleasant tastes, and to maintain client comfort. In addition, certain medications can affect dietary and nutrient intake. For example, insulin, glucocorticoids,

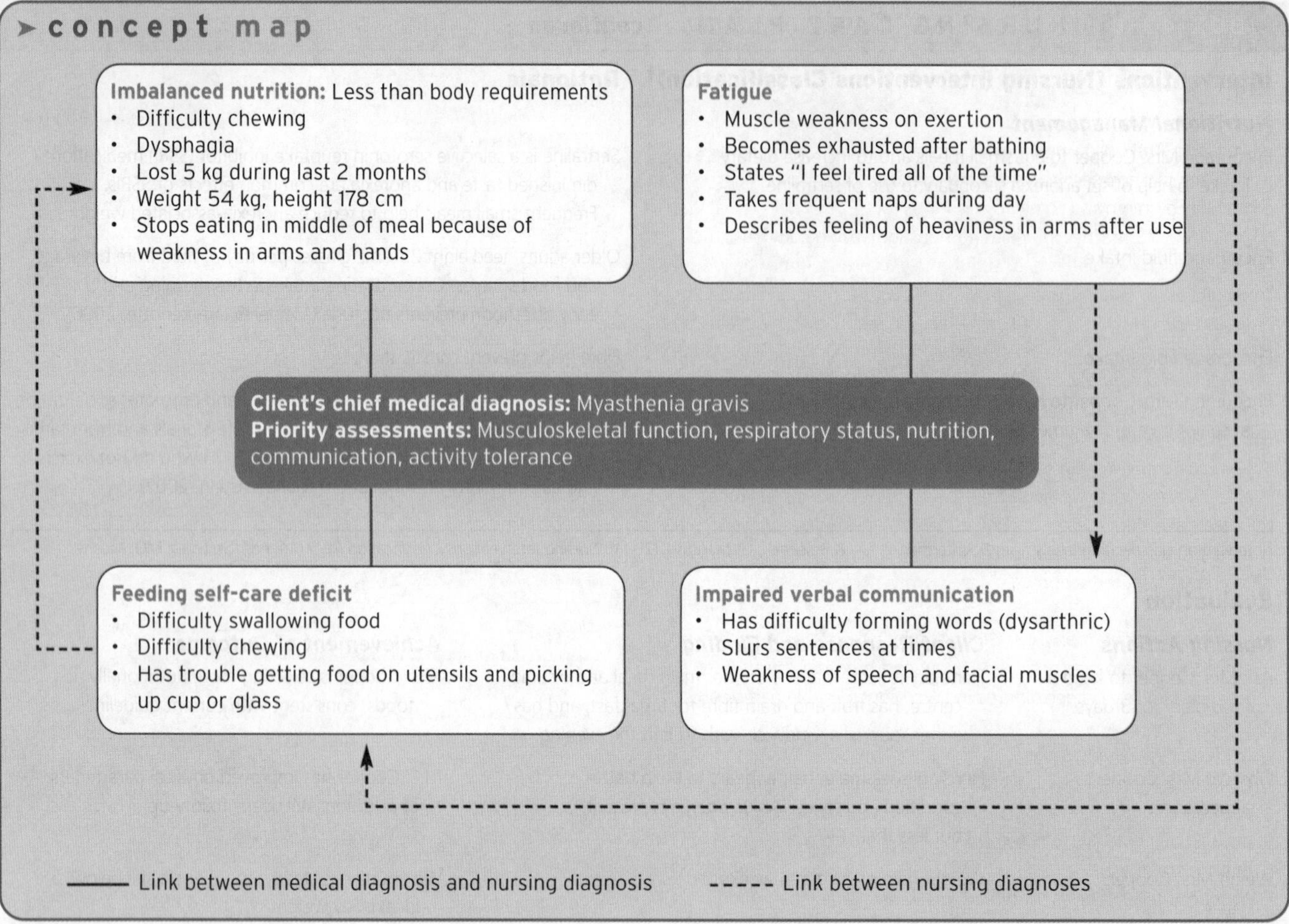

Figure 43-8 Concept map for client with myasthenia gravis.

and thyroid hormones affect metabolism. Other medications, such as antifungal agents, can affect taste. Some of the psychotropic medications affect appetite, cause nausea, and may alter taste. Sometimes you and the dietitian can help the client select foods to reduce the altered taste sensations or the nausea. In other situations, medication may need to be changed. Physicians may order pharmacological agents to stimulate appetite (e.g., cyproheptadine [Periactin], megestrol [Megace]) or to manage symptoms that interfere with nutrition.

Assisting Clients With Feeding

When helping clients to eat, you must protect their safety, independence, and dignity. Glasses, hearing aids, and dentures should be functioning and in place. You will need to assess the client's risk of aspiration (see "Assessment" section in this chapter and Skill 43–1). Risk factors for aspiration are decreased alertness, decreased gag or cough reflexes, and difficulty managing saliva.

Clients with dysphagia need help with feeding. You can collaborate with the speech pathologist, who evaluates clients at risk for dysphagia and provides recommendations to improve swallowing. Interventions also include postural changes, feeding strategies, and dietary changes (Lindsay et al., 2008). The client may be ordered a diet of thickened fluids because these are safer to swallow than thin liquids. The client should sit upright at a 75- to 90-degree angle and may be supported by pillows, foam wedges, or rolled towels. Do not feed a client while he or she is lying back or has his or her neck arched or hyperextended because these positions create an open airway susceptible to aspiration. Small bites of food should be placed and chewed on the stronger side of the client's mouth. Turning the head to the affected side may ease swallowing. Assess swallowing during feeding and give clients with dysphagia enough time to chew. Observe for two completed swallows between mouthfuls. The client's Adam's apple should move up and down. When a client with bite reflexes needs to be fed, a metal teaspoon is usually the best utensil to use. After each meal, the client should rinse the mouth and perform oral hygiene.

Clients with visual deficits also need special assistance. Those with poor vision may be able to feed themselves if adequate care and information is given. If the client wears glasses or contact lenses, they should be clean and in place. Identify the location of the food on the plate as if it were a clock (e.g., meat at 9 o'clock and vegetable at 3 o'clock). Tell the client where the beverage is located in relation to the plate. Position food within the client's visual field. Clients with decreased motor skills may retain more independence by using large-handled adaptive utensils, which are easier to grip and manipulate.

Small measures can help promote comfort and a sense of independence in many clients. Provide opportunities for clients to direct the order and speed at which they want to eat. When food intake is less than usual because of illness or fatigue, nutrient-dense items should be provided first. Small frequent meals, five to six per day, may be required for those who eat slowly. When possible, try to heed special requests, such as a request for the food to be warmed up. Clothing and bedding should be protected with napkins, towels, or aprons, and these items should not be called "bibs." Because mealtime is usually a social activity, it is important that nurses and other

BOX 43-7 FOCUS ON PRIMARY HEALTH CARE

Case Study

In Saskatoon, an innovative program is aiming to eradicate child hunger and malnutrition. The Child Hunger and Education Program (CHEP) takes a primary health care approach to disease prevention and health promotion in the community by improving access to good food for all. The goal is to facilitate collaborative approaches in achieving nonstigmatizing solutions to child hunger that enhance self-reliance and dignity for children, their families, and communities. CHEP's philosophy is that food is a basic right, and inadequate nutrition adversely affects a child's development, learning ability, health, and participation in the community. Targeting children at risk, CHEP supports community groups in the operation of programs for children at schools and community centres. CHEP's partners include the provincial government, Public Health Services, the Community Clinic, the University of Saskatchewan Kinesiology and Nutrition faculties, Aboriginal organizations, and school boards. Kinesiologists, dietitians, public health nurses, teachers, parents, and volunteers all work together on various aspects of the program:

- *Meal programs:* Breakfast, lunch, snack, and supper programs are offered at targeted schools. The goal is to provide one third of a child's daily nutrition needs at each meal.
- *Collective cooking programs:* Groups of people pool resources and come together to plan and prepare low-cost nutritious meals in bulk for their families. Leadership training workshops enable participants to lead other collective kitchen groups and champion healthy lifestyles in the community.
- *Community gardening programs:* Together families plan and support each other in planning and tending gardens and harvesting the produce. Educational workshops on topics such as composting and jam making are offered.
- *Nutritious food choices programs:* These programs bring good nutrition into the whole school community. Classroom and school activities, staff events, fundraising projects, and meal programs all focus on good nutrition and creating healthy food environments.
- *The Good Food Box:* This food distribution system provides fresh, nutritious foods at affordable prices. Families, as part of neighbourhood-based groups, each with a volunteer coordinator, pay for and order food boxes ahead of time. The CHEP program worker purchases foods in bulk from local producers and wholesalers. Volunteers and staff pack the boxes and deliver them to the neighbourhood depots.
- *Food security programs:* In addition to the Good Food Box, other food-related activities for families with infants and preschoolers include workshops on making homemade baby food and on cooking with kids.
- *Health promotion program:* This program seeks to prevent type 2 diabetes among Aboriginal families by improving access to good food and encouraging active living. Groups of adults and youth meet for discussions about health and related issues, to cook meals, to order Good Food Boxes, and to take part in physical activities.
- *Linking with farms:* Through a link with producers, city families pool their orders for meat and purchase directly from producers.
- *Food coalition:* Groups and individuals, including producers, Social Services, and community food action organizations, meet at workshops and events to work at improving the food system for the Saskatoon region. CHEP also hosts educational and community-building workshops. The CHEP program works to ensure food security for all residents by researching and advocating for policies that will support access to an equitable, healthy, sustainable food system.

From Child Hunger and Education Program (n.d.). Retrieved April 28, 2008, from http://www.chep.org

TABLE 43-7 Food Safety

Food-Borne Disease	Organism	Food Source	Symptoms*
Botulism	*Clostridium botulinum*	Improperly home-canned foods, smoked and salted fish, ham, sausage, shellfish	Symptoms vary from mild discomfort to death in 24 hours, initial nausea and dizziness progressing to motor (respiratory) paralysis
Escherichia coli	*Escherichia coli 0157:H7*	Undercooked meat (ground beef)	Severe cramps, nausea, vomiting, diarrhea (may be bloody), renal failure. Appears 1–8 days after eating, lasts 1–7 days
Listeriosis	*Listeria* species *L. monocytogenes*	Soft cheese, meat (hot dogs, pâté, lunch meats), unpasteurized milk, poultry, seafood	Severe diarrhea, fever, headache, pneumonia, meningitis, endocarditis, appears 3–21 days after infection
Perfringens enteritis	*Clostridium* species *C. perfringens*	Cooked meats, meat dishes held at room or warm temperature	Mild diarrhea, vomiting. Appears 8–24 hours after eating, lasts 1–2 days
Salmonellosis	*Salmonella* species *S. typhi* *S. paratyphi*	Milk, custards, egg dishes, salad dressing, sandwich fillings, polluted shellfish	Mild to severe diarrhea, cramps, vomiting. Appears 12–24 hours after ingestion, lasts 1–7 days
Shigellosis	*Shigella* species *S. dysenteriae*	Milk, milk products, seafood, salads ingestion, lasts 3–14 days	Mild diarrhea to fatal dysentery. Appears 7–36 hours after
Staphylococcus	*Staphylococcus* species *S. aureus*	Custards, cream fillings, processed meats, ham, cheese, ice cream, potato salad, sauces, casseroles	Severe abdominal cramps, pain, vomiting, diarrhea, perspiration, headache, fever, prostration. Appears 1–6 hours after ingestion, lasts 1–2 days

*Symptoms are generally most severe for youngest and oldest age groups.

From Nix, S. (2005). *Williams' basic nutrition and diet therapy* (12th ed.). St. Louis, MO: Mosby.

BOX 43-8 CLIENT TEACHING

Food Safety

Objectives

- Client will be able to verbalize measures to prevent food-borne illness.
- Client will understand the primary types of illness and how they are transmitted.
- Client will not experience food-borne illness.

Teaching Strategies

Food safety has become an important public health issue in recent years. Populations particularly at risk are older and younger people and immunosuppressed individuals. Instruct clients on the following:

- Wash hands with warm, soapy water before touching or eating food.
- Cook meat, poultry, fish, and eggs until they are well done.
- Wash fresh fruits and vegetables thoroughly.
- Do not eat raw meats or drink unpasteurized milk.
- Do not buy or consume food that has passed the expiration date.
- Keep foods properly refrigerated at 4°C and frozen at −18°C.
- Wash dishes and cutting boards with hot, soapy water or use a bleach sanitizer using 5 mL bleach in 750 mL water.
- Do not save leftovers for more than 4 days in the refrigerator.
- Wash dishcloths, towels, and sponges regularly, or use paper towels.
- Clean the inside of the refrigerator and microwave regularly to prevent microbial growth.

Evaluation

- Ask client to describe measures to prevent food-borne illnesses.
- Observe the client at home for safe practices, if making a home visit.

"Teaching strategies" from Canadian Food Inspection Agency. (2007). *Food safety tips*. Retrieved April 30, 2008, from http://canadaonline.about.com/gi/dynamic/offsite.htm?zi=1/XJ/Ya&sdn=canadaonline&cdn=newsissues&tm=31&gps=419_536_1000_458&f=00&tt=14&bt=0&bts=0&zu=http%3A//www.inspection.gc.ca/english/fssa/concen/tipcone.shtml

health care professionals talk to clients during meals. Use this opportunity to educate clients about therapeutic diets, medications, or adaptive devices.

Restorative and Continuing Care

Clients discharged from a hospital with dietary prescriptions often need dietary education to plan meals that meet specific therapeutic requirements. Restorative care includes both immediate postsurgical care and routine medical care, and is thus pertinent to hospitalized and home care clients.

❖Evaluation

Care plans should reflect achievable goals and outcomes. You will need to evaluate outcomes of nursing actions and be alert for signs that goals are being met. Allow adequate time for testing each nursing approach to a problem.

Client Care

The effectiveness of nutritional interventions is best measured by meeting the client's expected outcomes and goals of care (Figure 43–9). Nutrition therapy does not always produce rapid results. Ongoing comparisons may be made with baseline measures of weight, serum albumin or prealbumin, and protein and kilocalorie intake. Medications may produce unwanted side effects. If gradual weight gain is not observed, or if weight loss continues, the prescription may need to

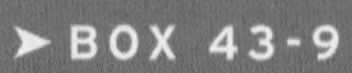

➤ BOX 43-9 Diet Progression and Therapeutic Diets

Clear Liquid

This diet is limited to broth, bouillon, coffee, tea, carbonated beverages, clear fruit juices, gelatin, or Popsicles.

Thickened Liquid

Fruits thickened with rice flakes or thickening agents are used when thin fluids cannot be safely swallowed and may be aspirated.

Full Liquid

To a clear- or thickened-liquid diet can be added smooth-textured dairy products, custards, refined cooked cereals, vegetable juice, pureed vegetables, or any fruit juices.

Pureed

This diet includes all of above with the addition of scrambled eggs, pureed meats, vegetables, fruits, or mashed potatoes and gravy.

Mechanical Soft

This diet includes all of above with the addition of ground or finely diced meats, flaked fish, cottage cheese, cheese, rice, potatoes, pancakes, light breads, cooked vegetables, cooked or canned fruits, bananas, soups, or peanut butter.

Soft or Low Residue

Low-fibre, easily digested foods, such as pastas, casseroles, moist tender meats, canned cooked fruits and vegetables, desserts, cakes, and cookies without nuts or coconut, can be added.

High Fibre

This diet includes fresh uncooked fruits, steamed vegetables, bran, oatmeal, and dried fruits.

Low Sodium

A low-sodium diet is limited to 4 g (no added salt), 2 g, 1 g, or 500 mg sodium. These diets vary from no added salt to severe sodium restriction (500-mg sodium diet), requiring selective food purchases.

Low Cholesterol

This diet is restricted to <200 mg/day cholesterol, in keeping with the National Cholesterol Education Program (NCEP) recommendations (Grundy et al., 2004).

Diabetic

In general, people with diabetes should follow a healthy diet recommended for the general population in *Eating Well with Canada's Food Guide* (Canadian Diabetes Association, 2003; Health Canada, 2007b). This includes consuming a variety of foods from the four food groups (grain products, vegetables and fruits, milk products, meat and alternatives), attaining and maintaining a healthy body weight, decreasing total fat intake to >30% of calories, and ensuring an adequate intake of carbohydrate, protein, essential fatty acids, vitamins, and minerals.

Regular

Dietary restrictions are not necessary unless specified.

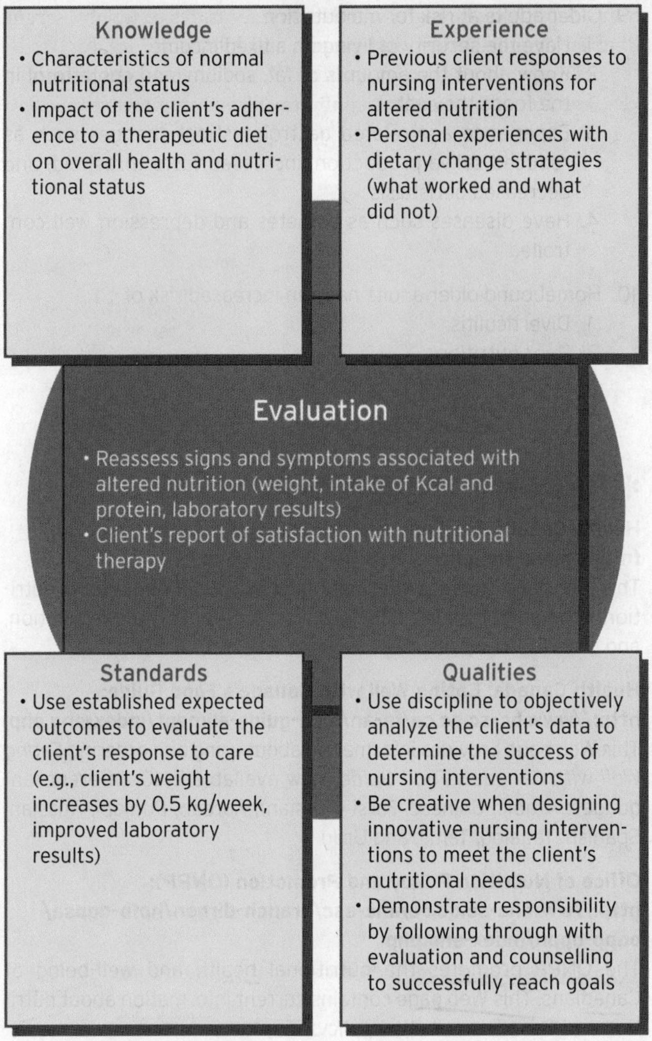

Knowledge
- Characteristics of normal nutritional status
- Impact of the client's adherence to a therapeutic diet on overall health and nutritional status

Experience
- Previous client responses to nursing interventions for altered nutrition
- Personal experiences with dietary change strategies (what worked and what did not)

Evaluation
- Reassess signs and symptoms associated with altered nutrition (weight, intake of Kcal and protein, laboratory results)
- Client's report of satisfaction with nutritional therapy

Standards
- Use established expected outcomes to evaluate the client's response to care (e.g., client's weight increases by 0.5 kg/week, improved laboratory results)

Qualities
- Use discipline to objectively analyze the client's data to determine the success of nursing interventions
- Be creative when designing innovative nursing interventions to meet the client's nutritional needs
- Demonstrate responsibility by following through with evaluation and counselling to successfully reach goals

Figure 43-9 Critical thinking model for nutritional evaluation.

be increased or adjusted. Changes in condition may also indicate a need to change the nutritional care plan. Interdisciplinary members of the health care team should be consulted, and the client should be an active participant whenever possible. The client's ability to incorporate dietary changes into his or her lifestyle with the least amount of stress or disruption will ensure that outcome measures are met. When expected outcomes are not met, revise the interventions or expected outcomes on the basis of the clients' needs and preferences.

Client Expectations

Clients expect competent and accurate care. If outcomes of nutritional therapies are unsuccessful, clients expect nurses to alter the care plan. Your expectations and health care values may differ from those held by clients. By working closely with clients, you can get to know your clients' expectations and try to meet these expectations within the limits of their conditions and treatments.

* KEY CONCEPTS

- Nurses must have current, culturally sensitive nutritional knowledge to apply to the complexities of health care and illness and to the changing needs of diverse populations and demographics.
- A balanced diet featuring carbohydrates, fats, proteins, vitamins, and minerals provides the essential nutrients to carry out the body's normal physiological functioning throughout the lifespan.
- Through digestion, food is broken down into its simplest form for absorption. Digestion and absorption occur mainly in the small intestine.
- Dietary reference intakes (DRIs) provide a range of values that address the needs of groups (estimated average requirement) and individuals (adequate intakes, recommended dietary allowances, and tolerable upper intake level).
- Guidelines for dietary change advocate reduced saturated and trans fat, reduced sodium, and reduced refined sugars, as well as an increased intake of complex carbohydrates and fibre.
- Nutritional screening helps to identify clients at risk of malnourishment. Because improper nutrition can affect all body systems, nutritional assessment includes total physical assessment.
- Interdisciplinary collaboration is essential to helping a client achieve optimal nutrition.
- Special diets alter the composition, texture, digestibility, and residue of foods to suit the client's particular needs.

* CRITICAL THINKING EXERCISES

1. Charlene MacDonald, a 63-year-old accountant, is overweight with a sedentary lifestyle, uses alcohol infrequently, consumes restaurant food for most meals, and takes 400 IU of vitamin D daily. She wants to undergo cataract surgery to improve her vision; however, the surgeon has advised her to take off at least 10 kg of weight before the operation. Ms. MacDonald weighs 90 kg and has a height of 156 cm. Her waist circumference is 100 cm. What indications would lead you to believe Ms. MacDonald is adequately caring for her health? What additional laboratory tests and dietary and health history information are needed to perform a comprehensive nutritional assessment? What conclusions can you draw from the information available about Ms. MacDonald's weight status? Using *Eating Well with Canada's Food Guide*, what suggestions would you make to Ms. MacDonald to help her achieve weight loss?
2. Corey Green, a 32-year-old mother, is considering switching her entire family to a vegan diet because she believes it will make her 3-year-old twin daughters healthier. What nutritional concerns should you watch for? How would you assess the family's nutritional needs and monitor for such concerns? What advice would you offer to Corey to enhance her family's health while following a vegan diet? Plan one day of meals for this family, indicating food servings for the twins that would meet their protein needs and respect the vegan food diet.
3. Roberta, a junior-high-school student, is unhappy with her shape and weight. Using tools she found on the Internet, she calculated her BMI as 29 one month ago. "I am the smallest person in my family, but I am too fat!" she thought. So she began to skip breakfast and lunch and to exercise for more than 2 hours a day to "tone up." Her skin, lips, and hair are becoming dry. She denies having lost weight even though her clothes look loose and baggy. Roberta's friends have told the homeroom teacher that Roberta goes to the bathroom immediately after eating any food. Her teacher requests that you plan a session with Roberta to increase her understanding of her daily nutritional requirements and of healthy eating patterns. What will you discuss with Roberta?

* REVIEW QUESTIONS

1. The nutrient that provides the body's most preferred energy source is
   1. Fat
   2. Protein
   3. Vitamin
   4. Carbohydrate
2. The nutrient needed for tissue repair is
   1. Fat
   2. Protein
   3. Vitamin
   4. Carbohydrate
3. Positive nitrogen balance would occur in
   1. Infection
   2. Starvation
   3. Burn injury
   4. Pregnancy
4. The major determinant of healthy eating is
   1. Educational level
   2. Income
   3. Food preferences
   4. Vitamin supplementation
5. Hypervitaminosis can result from
   1. Women over the age of 50 taking a vitamin D supplement of 10 micrograms (400 IU)
   2. Megadoses of supplemental fat- or water-soluble vitamins
   3. Decreasing the amount of vitamin-fortified food ingested
   4. Limiting intake of fish oils
6. A nutrient content claim of *light* means
   1. The food may be light in colour
   2. The food has no added sugar or salt
   3. The food is reduced in calories or fat by 10%
   4. The levels of saturated and trans fatty acids are restricted
7. When a mother tells you that she would like to switch her 15-month-old toddler from whole to skim milk so the child will not get "too fat," you encourage her to continue with the whole milk because
   1. Whole milk has more calcium than skim
   2. Whole milk has a longer refrigerated storage life
   3. Whole milk costs the same as skim milk
   4. Whole milk contains fatty acids needed for the toddler's brain development
8. Which of the following interventions is appropriate for the client experiencing dysphagia?
   1. Encourage the client to rest lying down for at least 30 minutes after a meal
   2. Offer thin liquids to make swallowing easier
   3. Place the food on the strong side of the client's mouth
   4. Leave the client with all food items within easy reach and tell the client when you will come back to take away the tray.
9. Older adults at risk for malnutrition
   1. Have the security of living on a fixed income
   2. Know about the amounts of fat, sodium, and cholesterol in the foods they eat
   3. Experience age-related gastrointestinal changes such as reduced saliva production, increased taste threshold, and decreased peristalsis
   4. Have diseases such as diabetes and depression well controlled
10. Homebound older adults have an increased risk of
    1. Diverticulitis
    2. Poor nutrition
    3. Food intolerances
    4. Peptic ulcers

* RECOMMENDED WEB SITES

Health Canada Food and Nutrition: http://www.hc-sc.gc.ca/fn-an/index-eng.php

This Web page provides information for the public about food, nutrition, food safety issues, allergy alerts, food policy and legislation, and other nutrition issues.

Health Canada: Eating Well with Canada's Food Guide: http://www.hc-sc.gc.ca/fn-an/food-guide-aliment/index-eng.php

This Web page provides information about using and ordering *Eating Well with Canada's Food Guide*, now available in 10 different languages: Arabic, Chinese, Farsi (Persian), Korean, Punjabi, Russian, Spanish, Tagalog, Tamil, and Urdu.

Office of Nutrition Policy and Promotion (ONPP): http://www.hc-sc.gc.ca/ahc-asc/branch-dirgen/hpfb-dgpsa/onpp-bppn/index-eng.php

The ONPP promotes the nutritional health and well-being of Canadians. This Web page contains current information about nutrition and Canadian nutrition policy.

Ontario Public Health Association (OPHA): http://www.opha.on.ca/programs/nrc.shtml

Ontario Public Health Association has a Nutrition Resource Centre that provides support for nutrition promotion programming and offers other resources to support healthy eating.

Dieticians of Canada: http://www.dieticians.ca/

Dieticians of Canada is an association of food and nutrition professionals committed to the health and well-being of Canadians. This Web page contains numerous nutritional resources and links to other resources and research abstracts.

National Eating Disorder Information Centre: http://www.nedic.ca

This Web site provides information, resources, and support for individuals, families, and professionals regarding eating disorders and weight preoccupation.

National Heart, Lung, and Blood Institute: The DASH Eating Plan: http://www.nhlbi.nih.gov/health/public/heart/hbp/dash/

The Dietary Approaches to Stop Hypertension (DASH) is an eating plan low in total fat, saturated fat, and cholesterol, and rich in fruits, vegetables, and low fat dairy products. The DASH eating plan is developed for clients with hypertension and is based on clinical studies that showed how elevated blood pressure levels can be reduced with specific eating habits.

44

Urinary Elimination

Original chapter by Judith Ann Kilpatrick, RN, MSN, DNSc

Canadian content written by Jill Milne, RN, PhD

and Kathleen F. Hunter, RN, NP, PhD, GNC(C)

objectives

Mastery of content in this chapter will enable you to:

- Define the key terms listed.
- Describe the process of urination.
- Identify factors that commonly influence urinary elimination.
- Compare common alterations in urinary elimination.
- Identify two modalities of renal replacement therapy.
- Obtain a nursing health history for a client with urinary elimination problems.
- Identify nursing diagnoses appropriate for clients with alterations in urinary elimination.
- Obtain urine specimens.
- Describe characteristics of normal and abnormal urine.
- Describe the nursing implications of common diagnostic tests of the urinary system.
- Discuss nursing measures to promote normal micturition and to reduce episodes of incontinence.
- Insert a urinary catheter.
- Discuss nursing measures to reduce urinary tract infection.
- Irrigate a urinary catheter.

media resources

evolve Web Site

- Animations
- Audio Chapter Summaries
- Glossary
- Multiple-Choice Review Questions
- Skills Performance Checklists
- Student Learning Activities
- Video Clips
- Weblinks

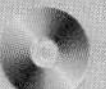

Companion CD

- Glossary
- Interactive Learning Activities
- Fluids and Electrolytes Tutorial
- Test-Taking Skills

key terms

Normal elimination of urinary wastes is a basic function that most people take for granted. When the urinary system fails to function properly, virtually all organ systems will be affected eventually. Clients with alterations in urinary elimination also may suffer emotionally from changes in body image. It is important that you be understanding and sensitive to all of your clients' needs. Understanding the reasons for urinary elimination problems and finding acceptable solutions are essential nursing functions.

Scientific Knowledge Base

Urinary elimination depends on the functioning of the kidneys, ureters, bladder, and urethra. Kidneys remove wastes from the blood to form urine. Ureters transport urine from the kidneys to the bladder. The bladder stores urine until the urge to urinate develops. Urine then leaves the body through the urethra. All organs of the urinary system must be intact and functional for successful removal of urinary waste (Figure 44–1).

Upper Urinary Tract

Kidneys. The kidneys lie on either side of the vertebral column behind the peritoneum and against deep muscles of the back. The kidneys extend from the twelfth thoracic vertebra to the third lumbar vertebra. Normally, the left kidney is higher than the right one because of the anatomical position of the liver.

Waste products of metabolism that collect in the blood are filtered in the kidneys. Blood reaches each kidney by a renal (kidney) artery that branches from the abdominal aorta. Approximately 20% to 25% of the cardiac output circulates each minute through the kidneys. The nephron, the functional unit of the kidney, forms the urine. The **nephron** is composed of the glomerulus, Bowman's capsule, proximal convoluted tubule, loop of Henle, distal tubule, and collecting duct (Figure 44–2). Each kidney contains approximately 1 million nephrons (Sherwood, 2007).

A cluster of blood vessels forms the capillary network of the glomerulus, which is the initial site of filtration of the blood and the beginning of urine formation. The glomerular capillaries permit filtration of water, glucose, amino acids, urea, creatinine, and major electrolytes into Bowman's capsule. Large proteins and blood cells normally do not filter through the glomerulus. The presence of large proteins in urine (**proteinuria**) is a sign of glomerular injury.

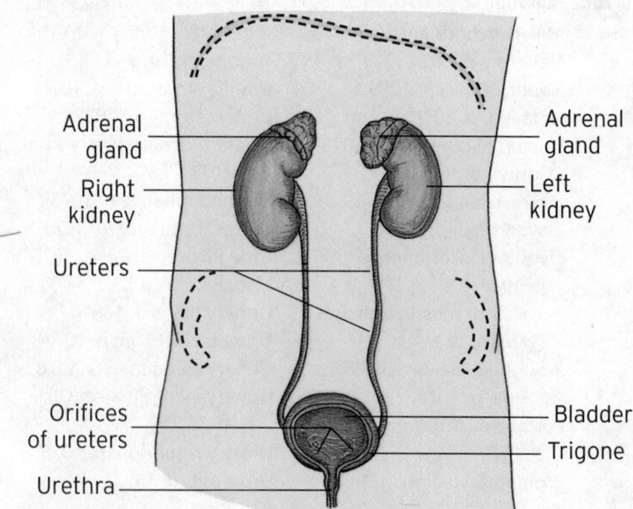

Figure 44-1 Organs of the urinary system.

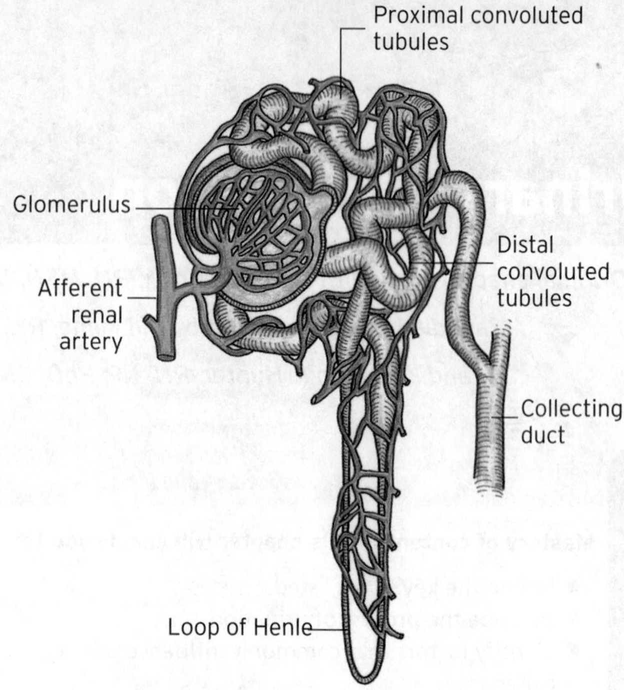

Figure 44-2 Renal nephron.

The glomerulus filters approximately 125 millilitres of plasma per minute (180 litres per day). Most (99%) of the filtrate is reabsorbed into the plasma, with the remaining 1% excreted as urine (Sherwood, 2007). The kidneys play a key role in fluid and electrolyte balance (see Chapter 40). Although output does depend on intake, normal adult urine output is 1500 to 1600 mL/day. An output of less than 30 mL/hour may indicate renal alterations.

The kidneys produce several substances vital to the production of red blood cells (RBCs), blood pressure regulation, and bone mineralization. The kidneys are responsible for maintaining a normal RBC volume by producing **erythropoietin**, a hormone that functions within the bone marrow to stimulate RBC production and maturation and that prolongs the life of mature RBCs (Sherwood, 2007). Clients with chronic alterations in kidney function cannot produce sufficient quantities of this hormone and are therefore prone to anemia.

Renin is another hormone produced by the kidneys. Its major role is the regulation of blood flow in times of renal ischemia (decreased blood supply). Renin is released from the juxtaglomerular cells (Figure 44–3) and functions as an enzyme to convert angiotensinogen (a substance synthesized by the liver) into angiotensin I. Angiotensin I is converted to angiotensin II in the lungs. Angiotensin II causes vasoconstriction and stimulates aldosterone release from the adrenal cortex. Aldosterone causes retention of water, which increases blood volume. Both of these mechanisms increase arterial blood pressure and renal blood flow (Sherwood, 2007). The kidneys also produce prostaglandin E2 and prostacyclin, which are important in maintaining renal blood flow through vasodilation.

The kidneys play a role in calcium a nd phosphate regulation by producing a substance that converts vitamin D into its active form. Clients with chronic alterations in kidney function do not make sufficient amounts of active vitamin D. They are prone to develop renal bone disease resulting from the demineralization of bone caused by impaired calcium absorption.

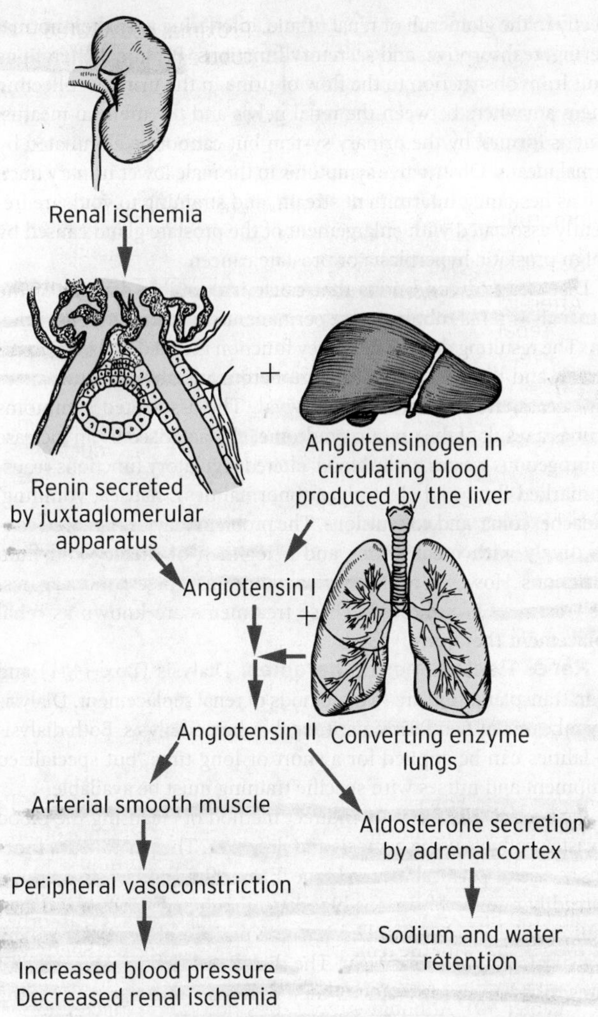

Figure 44-3 Physiological effects of renin–angiotensin mechanism.

Ureters. Urine enters the **renal pelvis** from the collecting ducts and travels to the bladder through the ureters. The ureters are tubular structures that enter the urinary bladder obliquely through the posterior wall, at the **ureterovesical junction** (the juncture of the ureters and the bladder). This arrangement normally results in compression of the ureter at the junction during **micturition** (urination) to prevent the reflux of urine.

Peristaltic waves cause urine to enter the bladder in spurts rather than steadily. An obstruction within a ureter, such as a kidney stone (**renal calculus**), results in strong peristaltic waves that attempt to move the obstruction into the bladder. These strong peristaltic waves often result in pain known as *renal colic.*

Lower Urinary Tract

Bladder. The urinary bladder is a hollow, distensible muscular organ that stores and excretes urine. When empty, the bladder lies behind the symphysis pubis in the pelvic cavity. It rests against the anterior wall of the rectum in men and against the anterior walls of the cervix and vagina in women (Figure 44–4).

The bladder expands as it becomes filled with urine. Pressure increases only minimally during bladder filling because the relaxed bladder is normally highly compliant (Fry et al., 2005). When the bladder is full, it expands and extends above the symphysis pubis. A very distended bladder may reach the umbilicus. In a pregnant woman, the developing fetus pushes against the bladder, reducing its capacity and causing a feeling of fullness. This effect is more likely to occur in the first and third trimesters.

The main muscle of the bladder is the **detrusor muscle.** Contraction of the detrusor expels urine from the body. The **trigone** is a triangular area of smooth muscle at the base of the bladder. An opening exists at each of the trigone's three angles, two for the ureters and one for the urethra.

Urethra. Urine travels from the bladder through the urethra (a fibromuscular tube) and passes outside of the body through the **urethral meatus.** In women, the urethra is approximately 4 cm long. This short length predisposes women and girls to infection. The male urethra is about 20 cm long and serves as both a urinary canal and a passageway for cells and secretions from reproductive organs. The male urethra has three sections: the prostatic urethra, the membranous urethra, and the penile urethra. The prostatic urethra pierces the anterior portion of the **prostate gland** (see Figure 44–4A).

The ability of the urethra to maintain adequate closure pressure between voids is critical to retaining urine in the bladder (Ashton-Miller & DeLancey, 2007), particularly because intra-abdominal pressure increases during coughing, lifting, laughing, and sneezing. This task is accomplished through a combination of factors known collectively as the **urethral closure mechanism.** Detrusor muscle surrounds the urethra at the level of the **bladder neck,** helping to constrict the opening. Circular smooth muscle as well as striated sphincter muscle (also known as the external sphincter, or **rhabdosphincter**) comprise

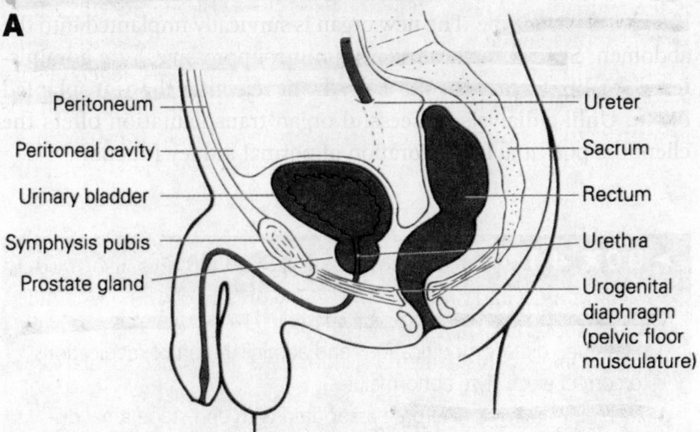

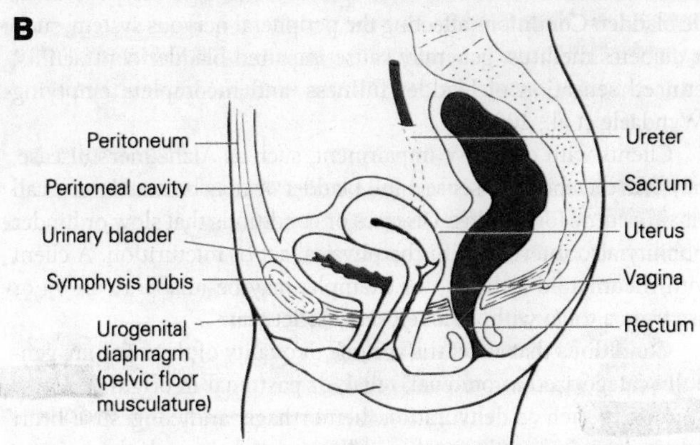

Figure 44-4 Anatomical location of bladder and pelvic organs. A, In men. B, In women. **Source:** From Getliffe, K., & Dolman, M. (1997). Normal and abnormal bladder function. In K. Getliffe & M. Dolman (Eds.); *Promoting continence* (pp. 22–67). London: Bailliere Tindall.

the proximal two thirds of the urethra and play an important role in sustaining tone. In addition, a highly vascular mucosal surface helps to maintain a watertight seal (Ashton-Miller & DeLancey, 2007). The striated musculature of the pelvic floor surrounds the urethra and provides additional closure pressure. Finally, increases in intra-abdominal pressure, such as those that occur during coughing and sneezing, are normally transmitted to the bladder neck, enhancing closure of the proximal urethra during stress (Griffiths et al., 2005).

Act of Urination

The act of urination relies on the coordinated effort of the bladder and the urethral closure mechanism. The adult bladder normally holds approximately 500 mL of urine and empties, on average, five to seven times per day. As the bladder becomes distended and as it is deemed appropriate to urinate, the detrusor (bladder muscle) contracts and the urethral sphincter mechanism relaxes to allow expulsion of urine (Morrison et al., 2005).

Several brain structures influence urination. As the bladder fills, sensory impulses are sent to the sacral spinal cord and relayed to the **pontine micturition centre**. If a person is ready to void, the pontine micturition centre relays the impulses back to initiate detrusor contraction, sphincter relaxation, and bladder emptying. If a person chooses not to void, the impulses are relayed to the cerebral cortex for voluntary inhibition of a detrusor contraction. If the urge to void has been ignored repeatedly, bladder capacity may be reached and the resulting pressure on the sphincter may make continued voluntary control impossible (Morrison et al., 2005).

Factors Influencing Urination

Many factors influence the volume and quality of urine and the client's ability to urinate. Some pathophysiological conditions may be acute and reversible (urinary tract infection), whereas others may be chronic and irreversible (slow, progressive development of renal dysfunction).

Disease Conditions. The complex role that the nervous system plays in urinary elimination suggests that any disruption to the central or peripheral pathways can affect urination. Between 40% and 60% of individuals admitted to hospital after a cerebrovascular accident experience urinary incontinence, and 15% remain incontinent 1 year later (Thomas et al., 2008). Between 30% and 50% of clients with multiple sclerosis experience urgency, frequency, and urge incontinence, which can be complicated by urinary retention if the urethral sphincter fails to relax as the bladder contracts (Wyndaele et al., 2005). Deficiencies in neurotransmission that occur with Parkinson's disease can lead to overactive bladder symptoms or to a hypocontractile bladder. Conditions affecting the peripheral nervous system, such as diabetes mellitus, generally cause impaired bladder contractility, reduced sensation of bladder fullness, and incomplete emptying (Wyndaele et al., 2005).

Clients with cognitive impairment, such as Alzheimer's disease, may lose the ability to sense a full bladder or may be unable to recall the procedure for voiding. Diseases or conditions that slow or hinder mobility also interfere with the physical act of micturition. A client with rheumatoid arthritis, for example, may be unable to sit on or rise from a toilet without an elevated toilet seat.

Conditions that affect the volume or quality of the urine are generally categorized as prerenal, renal, or postrenal in origin. Prerenal alterations such as dehydration, hemorrhage, and congestive heart failure decrease circulating blood flow to and through the kidneys and can lead to **oliguria** (diminished capacity to form urine) or, less commonly, **anuria** (inability to produce urine). Renal alterations result from conditions such as diabetes mellitus that cause injury directly to the glomeruli or renal tubule, interfering with their normal filtering, reabsorptive, and secretory functions. Postrenal alterations result from obstruction to the flow of urine in the urinary collecting system anywhere between the renal pelvis and the urethral meatus. Urine is formed by the urinary system but cannot be eliminated by normal means. Obstructive symptoms in the male lower urinary tract, such as hesitancy, intermittent stream, and straining to void, are frequently associated with enlargement of the prostate gland caused by benign prostatic hyperplasia or prostate cancer.

Diseases and conditions that cause irreversible damage to the glomeruli or renal tubules cause permanent alterations in renal function. The resulting decline in kidney function is called end-stage renal disease, and the client manifests numerous metabolic disturbances that necessitate treatment for survival. The associated symptoms occur as a result of the **uremic syndrome**, characterized by an increase in nitrogenous wastes in the blood, altered regulatory functions (causing marked fluid and electrolyte abnormalities), nausea, vomiting, headache, coma, and convulsions. The problem may be managed conservatively with medications and a regimen of dietary and fluid restrictions. However, as the uremic symptoms worsen, more aggressive treatment is indicated. These treatments are known as **renal replacement therapies.**

Renal Replacement Therapies. Dialysis (Box 44–1) and organ transplantation are two methods of renal replacement. Dialysis may take one of two forms: peritoneal or hemodialysis. Both dialysis modalities can be applied for a short or long time, but specialized equipment and nurses with specific training must be available.

Peritoneal dialysis is an indirect method of cleansing the blood of waste products using osmosis and diffusion. The peritoneum functions as a semi-permeable membrane. Excess fluid and waste products are readily removed from the bloodstream when a sterile electrolyte solution (dialysate) is instilled into the peritoneal cavity by gravity via a surgically placed catheter. The dialysate is left in the cavity for a prescribed time interval and then drained out by gravity, taking accumulated wastes and excess fluid and electrolytes with it.

Hemodialysis involves using a machine equipped with a semi-permeable filtering membrane (artificial kidney) that removes accumulated waste products and excess fluids from the blood. In the dialysis machine, dialysate fluid is pumped through one side of the filter membrane (artificial kidney) while the client's blood passes through the other side. The processes of diffusion, osmosis, and ultrafiltration cleanse the client's blood, which is returned through a specially placed vascular access device (Gore-Tex graft, arteriovenous fistula, or hemodialysis catheter).

Organ transplantation is the replacement of a client's diseased kidney with a healthy one from a living or cadaver donor of compatible blood and tissue type. The new organ is surgically implanted into the abdomen. Special medications (immunosuppressives) are administered for life to prevent the body from rejecting the transplanted organ. Unlike dialysis, successful organ transplantation offers the client the potential for restoration of normal kidney function.

➤ BOX 44-1 Indications for Dialysis

Renal failure that can no longer be controlled by conservative management (i.e., dietary modifications and administration of medications to correct electrolyte abnormalities)

Worsening of uremic syndrome associated with end-stage renal disease (i.e., nausea, vomiting, neurological changes, pericarditis)

Severe electrolyte or fluid abnormalities that cannot be controlled by simpler measures (i.e., hyperkalemia, pulmonary edema)

Fluid Balance. Fluid balance directly affects the quantity of urine produced. The kidneys maintain a sensitive balance between retention and excretion of fluids (see Chapter 40). If fluids and the concentration of electrolytes and solutes are in equilibrium, an increase in fluid intake causes an increase in urine production. Ingested fluids increase the body's circulating plasma and thus increase the volume of urine excreted. In a healthy person, the intake of water in food and fluids balances the output of water in urine, feces, and insensible losses through perspiration and respiration. An excessive output of urine is known as **polyuria**, a common symptom of diabetes mellitus and diabetes insipidus.

Ingestion of certain fluids directly affects urine production and excretion. Coffee, tea, cocoa, and cola drinks that contain caffeine promote increased urine formation (**diuresis**). Alcohol inhibits the release of antidiuretic hormone (ADH), resulting in increased water loss in urine.

Febrile conditions also affect urine production. The client who becomes diaphoretic (sweats profusely) loses a large amount of fluid through insensible water loss, which decreases urine production. However, the increased body metabolism associated with fever increases accumulation of body wastes. Although urine volume may be reduced, it is highly concentrated.

Medications. Medications may interfere with the production of urine and affect the act of urination. Diuretics prevent reabsorption of water and certain electrolytes, resulting in a sudden increase in urine output that can challenge continence. Drugs with anticholinergic side effects such as tranquilizers or tricyclic antidepressants, antiarrythmics, sedating antihistamines, antiparkinsonian agents, and antispasmodics relax the bladder and can contribute to incomplete emptying and urinary retention (Mostwin et al., 2005). The drug-induced cough associated with angiotension converting enzyme (ACE) inhibitors can precipitate stress incontinence. You must be aware of any prescribed and over-the-counter medications a client is taking and how these medications may affect bladder function. Clients with altered kidney function require dosage modifications in any medications excreted by the kidneys.

Diagnostic Examination. Examination of the urinary system can influence micturition. Procedures such as an intravenous pyelogram may necessitate that the client limit fluid intake before the test. A restriction in fluid intake commonly lowers urine output. A laxative used to cleanse the bowel also may limit fluid available for urine production. Diagnostic examinations (i.e., cystoscopy) that involve direct visualization of urinary structures may cause localized edema of the urethral passageway and spasm of the striated muscle. The client often has urinary retention after such a procedure and may pass red or pink urine because of trauma to the urethral or bladder mucosa.

Surgical Procedures. The stress of surgery initially triggers the general adaptation syndrome (see Chapter 30). The surgical client is often in an altered state of fluid balance before surgery due to the disease process or preoperative fasting, which aggravates the reduction in urine output. The stress response releases an increased amount of ADH, which increases water reabsorption. Stress also elevates the level of aldosterone, causing retention of sodium and water. Both of these substances reduce urine output in order to maintain circulatory volume. The decreased blood pressure after surgery releases renin and thus increases angiotensin II to increase vascular tone. This aids in counteracting the effects of ADH and aldosterone.

Anaesthetics and narcotic analgesics may alter the glomerular filtration rate (generally 125 mL/minute), reducing urine output. These pharmacological agents also impair sensory and motor impulses travelling between the bladder, spinal cord, and brain. Clients recovering from anaesthesia and deep analgesia are often unable to sense bladder fullness and unable to initiate or inhibit micturition. Spinal and epidural anaesthetics, in particular, may cause urinary retention because the client cannot feel the need to void and the bladder muscle and sphincter may not respond (Sherwood, 2007).

angiotensin II releases aldosterone??

Surgery involving lower abdominal and pelvic structures can impair urination because of local trauma to surrounding tissues. The edema and inflammation may obstruct the flow of urine from the kidneys to the bladder or from the bladder or urethra, interfere with relaxation of pelvic and sphincter muscles, or cause discomfort during voiding. After returning from surgery involving the ureters, bladder, and urethra, clients routinely have catheters.

The surgical formation of a **urinary diversion** temporarily or permanently bypasses the bladder and urethra as the exit routes for urine. Permanent urinary diversions may be needed in the client with cancer of the bladder. The client with a urinary diversion has a **stoma** (artificial opening) on the abdomen through which urine is drained.

Psychological Factors. Anxiety and emotional stress may cause a sense of urgency and increased frequency of urination. Anxiety also may prevent a person from being able to urinate completely; as a result, the urge to void may return shortly after urinating. Emotional tension makes it difficult to relax the abdominal and perineal muscles. If the sphincter is not completely relaxed, voiding may be incomplete.

Attempting to void in a public restroom also may result in a temporary inability to urinate. Privacy and adequate time to urinate are important to most people, and some may need distractions to help them relax (e.g., reading). The possibility that incomplete voiding may result from physiological abnormalities, however, must always be considered.

Common Alterations in Urinary Elimination

Most clients with urinary problems have disturbances in the act of micturition that involve a failure to store urine, a failure to empty urine, or both. Disturbances may be acute or chronic and result from infection, impaired bladder function, obstruction to urine outflow, or inability to control micturition voluntarily.

Urinary Tract Infections. Urinary tract infections (UTIs) are responsible for more than 500,000 visits to Canadian doctors every year (Kidney Foundation of Canada, 2004). If left untreated, UTIs can spread to the kidneys, causing kidney infection (**pyelonephritis**) and possibly long-term kidney damage.

Etiology. Although several different microorganisms may cause UTIs, *Escherichia coli* is the most frequent causative pathogen, accounting for 80% of uncomplicated infections. Between 10% and 20% of UTIs are caused by *Staphylococcus saprophyticus*, and approximately 5% are caused by *Klebsiella*, *Proteus*, and *Enterobacter* organisms.

Bacteria in the urine (**bacteriuria**) may lead to the spread of organisms into the kidneys and the bloodstream, leading to **urosepsis.** Bacteria usually enter the urinary tract by ascending the urethra. They inhabit the distal urethra, external genitalia, and vagina in women. Organisms enter the urethral meatus easily and travel up the inner mucosal lining to the bladder. Women are more susceptible to infection because of the short urethra and the proximity of the vaginal vestibule and rectum to the urethral meatus (Nguyen, 2004).

Infection depends on the virulence of the bacteria and the presence of host defence mechanisms. In a healthy person with good bladder function, organisms are flushed from the body during voiding. Normal urine has a low pH, which inhibits bacterial growth.

Although the short length of the female urethra makes women more susceptible to UTIs, organisms such as *Lactobacillus* that occur naturally in the periurethral area inhibit colonization of pathogenic bacteria. In addition, mucus-secreting glands found in the distal two thirds of the female urethra impede bacterial ascension. In men, the length of the urethra and the presence of zinc, a powerful antimicrobial substance found in prostatic secretions, reduce susceptibility (Nguyen, 2004).

Alterations in any of these defence mechanisms can contribute to a UTI. For example, if the client cannot empty the bladder when voiding or the free flow of urine is impeded, **residual urine** (urine left in the bladder after voiding) becomes more alkaline and is an ideal site for microorganism growth. Therefore, a kinked, obstructed, or clamped catheter or any condition resulting in urinary retention increases the risk of bladder infection. Risk factors for urinary infection in women include sexual activity, pregnancy, diaphragm or spermicide use, and pelvic organ prolapse. UTIs are less common in men and risk factors include the introduction of instruments into the urinary tract (instrumentation) and congenital abnormalities (Nguyen, 2004). Older adults, clients using antibiotics, and clients with progressive underlying disease or decreased immunity are also at increased risk. Changes associated with aging, including **prostatic hypertrophy** and diminished bacteriocidal activity of prostatic secretions in men, and diminished estrogen in women, predispose older adults to bacteriuria (Juthani-Mehta, 2007). Prostatic hypertrophy, the enlargement of the prostate gland, is particularly troubling, as it can lead to obstruction of the urethral outlet and affects approximately 80% of men in their eighties. Clients with diabetes mellitus are especially susceptible to UTIs because increased glucose in the urine is a good medium for bacterial growth.

One of the most common causes of UTI, however, is instrumentation. UTIs account for nearly half (40%) of nosocomial, or hospital-acquired, infections (Saint et al., 2008). The introduction of a catheter through the urethra provides a direct route for microorganisms. Bacteria ascend along the outside of an in-dwelling catheter on the urethral wall or travel up the catheter's lumen, and bacteriuria is generally inevitable within two days. One hundred percent colonization can be expected after 30 days. Local irritation to the urethra or bladder also predisposes tissues to bacterial invasion. Catheter-related bacteriuria has been associated with a twofold to threefold increase in risk of death among hospitalized clients (Cottenden et al., 2005).

Signs and Symptoms. Clients with lower UTIs may experience pain or a burning sensation during urination **(dysuria)** as urine flows over inflamed tissues. Fever, chills, nausea, vomiting, and malaise may develop as the infection worsens. Inflammation of the bladder **(cystitis)** causes a frequent and urgent sensation of the need to void, and may cause **incontinence**. Irritation to bladder and urethral mucosa results in blood-tinged urine **(hematuria)**. The urine appears concentrated and cloudy because of the presence of white blood cells (WBCs) or bacteria. If infection spreads to the upper urinary tract (i.e., to the kidneys, causing pyelonephritis), rapid onset of flank or lower back pain, tenderness, fever, and chills can occur.

Lower UTIs also can be asymptomatic, particularly in pregnant women, children, and older adults. Asymptomatic UTIs generally are not treated in older adults, in part because no evidence of short-term or long-term adverse effects or impact on survival exists (Juthani-Mehta, 2007).

Urinary Incontinence. **Urinary incontinence** (UI) is the involuntary loss of urine (Abrams et al., 2002). It is a prevalent condition experienced by more than 3 million Canadians of all ages (Canadian Continence Foundation, 2007). Psychosocial impact ranges from minor lifestyle changes to self-imposed social isolation.

Urinary incontinence may present as any of the following types (Registered Nurses Association of Ontario, 2005):

- **Transient incontinence**: urine loss resulting from causes outside of or affecting the urinary system that resolves when the underlying causes are treated. Causes include *d*ementia or acute confusion, *i*nfection (symptomatic UTI), *a*trophic urethritis or vaginitis in women, *p*harmaceuticals (medications), *e*ndocrine disorders, *r*estricted mobility, and *s*tool impaction (DIAPERS).*
- **Urge incontinence**: urine loss associated with or immediately preceded by a sudden and urgent need to void that cannot be postponed. Individuals with urge incontinence generally present with **urinary frequency** (need to void more often than every 2 hours) and **nocturia** (voiding overnight). Causes include nervous system disorders (cerebrovascular accident, multiple sclerosis) and outflow obstruction, particularly in men with an enlarged prostate, but urge incontinence also may be idiopathic (of unknown origin).
- **Stress incontinence**: generally small-volume (<50 mL) urine loss resulting from increased intra-abdominal pressure (e.g., coughing, sneezing, laughing, lifting). Stress incontinence is most common in women and in men after radical prostatectomy. Weak pelvic floor muscles and supportive tissue, obesity, and lifestyle factors such as heavy lifting are often contributing factors.
- **Mixed incontinence**: urine loss that has features of both stress and urge incontinence.
- **Functional incontinence**: urine loss that is caused by alterations in cognitive or physical function or by environmental factors. The person has bladder control but is unable to reach the toilet. Causes may include confusion, difficulty removing clothing, or immobility. Older clients with restricted mobility are at high risk of this type of incontinence.
- **Overflow incontinence**: small or large amounts of urine loss associated with overdistension of the bladder. The person may feel as if the bladder is never completely empty. Overflow incontinence may be associated with bladder outlet obstruction, fecal impaction, diabetes, spinal cord injury, prostate enlargement, or severe uterine prolapse.
- **Reflex incontinence**: involuntary urine loss that occurs at somewhat predictable intervals. The person is unaware that the bladder is filling and does not feel the urge to void, but the bladder contracts spontaneously. Reflex incontinence may be caused by spinal cord dysfunction (either inhibition of cerebral awareness or impairment of the reflex arc).
- **Total incontinence**: continuous and unpredictable loss of urine caused by damage to the nerves that control the bladder. It may be a result of spinal deformities such as spina bifida or scoliosis, spinal cord injury, or advanced disease such as multiple sclerosis or Alzheimer's disease. Repeated pelvic surgery also may cause total incontinence if it causes scarring of the urethra.

safety alert Continued episodes of incontinence create the potential for skin breakdown. The immobilized client who experiences frequent incontinence is especially at risk for pressure ulcers (see Chapter 47). Timely and meticulous skin care is essential.

---

*The acronym DIAPERS was coined to help clinicians remember the causes, but it is not used in medical notes.

Overactive Bladder Syndrome. **Overactive bladder syndrome** (OAB) is a symptom-based syndrome characterized predominantly by the presence of urgency, the sudden and compelling desire to void that is difficult to postpone (Abrams et al., 2002). Approximately 16% to 18% of adults experience OAB; one third of these adults also experience urge incontinence. Similar to urge incontinence, OAB can be idiopathic but is commonly attributed to changes associated with nervous system disorders and outflow obstruction. OAB may be aggravated by caffeinated beverages, although effects appear to be dose-dependent (Arya et al., 2000).

Nocturia. Nocturia has been defined as waking at night to void (Fonda et al., 2005). It is associated with aging and an overactive bladder, as well as with an enlarged prostate in men. Clients with peripheral edema (e.g., caused by circulatory problems associated with venous insufficiency) may experience nocturia because lying down facilitates reabsorption of pooled fluid and leads to increased urinary output overnight (Mostwin et al., 2005). Causes are generally categorized as **diurnal polyuria** (excessive production of urine during the day, as can occur with diabetes mellitus or diabetes insipidus), **nocturnal polyuria** (at least one third of total daily urine production occurs overnight), or low bladder capacity (Appell & Sand, 2008). The latter may be due to an overactive bladder or a compromised urethral closure that affects urine storage, or to reduced functional capacity.

Regardless of the cause, it is important to learn whether a client wakes at night to void, or voids because he or she is awake. Treatment options include reducing fluid intake in the evening, elevating the feet for 1 to 2 hours before bedtime to encourage return of fluid from the lower extremeties, medication to reduce the volume of urine produced overnight, or medication to relax the bladder muscle.

Urinary Retention. **Urinary retention** is the marked accumulation of urine in the bladder as a result of the bladder's inability to empty. Normally, urine production slowly fills the bladder and prevents activation of stretch receptors until the bladder distends to a certain extent. The micturition reflex then occurs, and the bladder empties. With urinary retention, the bladder becomes unable to respond to the micturition reflex and thus is unable to empty. Urine continues to collect in the bladder, causing feelings of pressure, discomfort, tenderness over the symphysis pubis, restlessness, and diaphoresis. As retention progresses, overflow incontinence may occur. Pressure in the bladder builds to a point at which the urethral sphincter is unable to hold back urine and a small volume escapes (<75 mL). The client may void small amounts of urine two or three times an hour with little relief of discomfort.

Urinary retention results from an underactive or acontractile detrusor muscle, urethral obstruction (more common in men and usually related to prostatic enlargement), surgical or childbirth trauma, alterations in motor and sensory innervation of the bladder, medication side effects (e.g., anticholinergics), or fecal impaction. **Urethral stricture**, a narrowing of the urethral canal that can be congenital or acquired as a result of infection or trauma, is also a more common cause of urinary retention in men.

You should be aware of the volume and frequency of voiding to assess this condition in the client. Key signs of urinary retention are absence of urine output over several hours, bladder distension, restlessness, diaphoresis, and moderate to extreme abdominal discomfort. A client under the influence of anaesthetics or analgesics may feel only pressure, but an alert client experiences severe pain as the bladder distends beyond its normal capacity. In severe urinary retention, the bladder may hold as much as 2000 to 3000 mL of urine. Intermittent catheterization may be needed to empty the bladder and reduce the risk of overflow incontinence and UTI.

Urinary Diversions. A urinary **stoma** to divert the flow of urine from the kidneys directly to the abdominal surface is created for several reasons, including cancer of the bladder, trauma, radiation injury to the bladder, fistulas, and chronic cystitis. A urinary diversion may be temporary or permanent. The client with an incontinent urinary diversion must wear an ostomy appliance continuously because no sphincter control exists to regulate urine flow. Local irritation and skin breakdown occur when urine comes in contact with the skin for long periods. Figure 44–5 illustrates several approaches to urinary diversion.

The ileal loop or conduit involves separating a loop of intestinal ileum with its blood supply intact. The ureters are implanted into the isolated segment of ileum. The remaining ileum is reconnected to the rest of the digestive tract. The ileal segment can then be used as a conduit for continuous urine drainage or fashioned into a continent reservoir (Carroll et al., 2004). The continent pouch is constructed to provide urinary storage in a leak-proof pouch. The portion of the ileum connected to the abdominal wall acts as a continent nipple, and intermittent catheterization is therefore needed for emptying. The disadvantage of an ileal conduit or reservoir is that if urine outflow becomes obstructed, irreversible damage to the kidneys can occur secondary to chronic infections or hydronephrosis.

A **ureterostomy** involves bringing the end of one or both ureters to the abdominal surface. To avoid the need for two collecting devices, a transureteroureterostomy connects the ureters and brings one out through the abdominal wall. In some cases, a tube may need to be placed directly into the renal pelvis to provide urinary drainage. This procedure is called a **nephrostomy**.

It is essential that stoma appliances fit correctly, that the client (or caregiver) is capable of changing the appliance easily, and that skin around the stoma remains protected and intact. Unprotected skin that comes in contact with urine will quickly become macerated and break down, causing pain, infection, increased hospital stays, and potential breakdown of the stoma. All clients must be referred to an

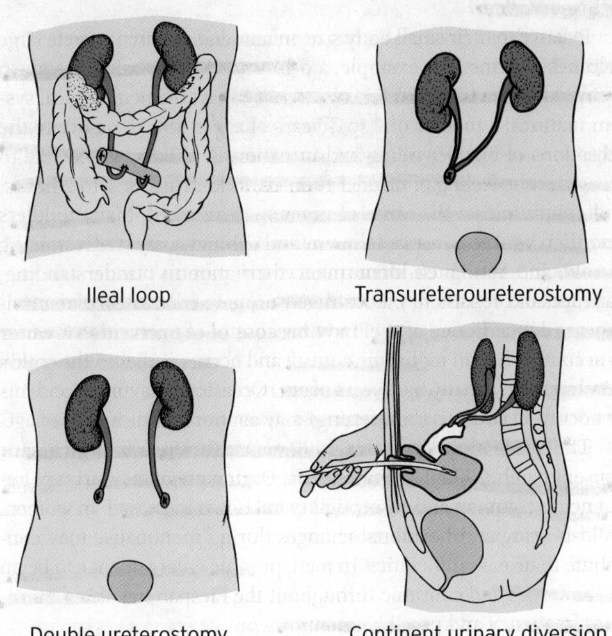

Figure 44-5 Types of urinary diversions.

enterostomal nurse for preoperative stoma siting and assessment and should be followed closely for several months postoperatively. The client should also be referred to the United Ostomy Association of Canada, an invaluable source of advice and networking.

A urinary diversion poses threats to a client's body image, and adjustment to it takes time. Although a normal lifestyle is possible with a stoma, adjustment can be difficult and each person will cope differently.

Nursing Knowledge Base

Urinary elimination is a basic human function that is usually a private process. Nurses are often the first to become aware that a client has elimination problems and must be alert to cues, prepared to discuss relevant assessment and treatment options, and able to provide counselling and support. These skills require a sound base of scientific knowledge related to anatomy and physiology, as well as an understanding of concepts such as infection control and hygiene, normal growth and development, and psychosocial and cultural considerations.

Infection Control and Hygiene

The urinary tract is considered to be sterile. You must use infection-control principles to help prevent the development and spread of UTIs, as well as to treat existing infections (see Chapter 33). Hospital-acquired UTIs are often related to poor hand hygiene, improper catheter care, or faulty catheterization technique (Nguyen, 2004). Knowledge of both medical and surgical asepsis must be applied meticulously when providing care involving the urinary tract and external genitalia. Any invasive procedure of the urinary tract such as catheterization necessitates sterile technique. Procedures such as perineal care or examination of the genitalia necessitate medical asepsis.

Growth and Development

Growth and development factors determine the client's ability to control the act of urination during the lifespan. Infants and young children cannot concentrate urine effectively. Their urine appears light yellow and clear.

Relative to their small body size, infants and children excrete large volumes of urine. For example, a 6-month-old infant who weighs 6 to 8 kg excretes 400 to 500 mL of urine daily. As the neurological system matures, a toddler of 2 to 3 years of age is able to associate the sensations of bladder filling and urination. A child must be able to recognize the feeling of bladder fullness, hold urine for 1 to 2 hours, and communicate the sense of urgency to an adult. Many toddlers may then be able to control the urethral sphincter, and toilet training can begin. Young children need their parents' understanding, patience, and consistency. A child may not gain full control of micturition until 4 or 5 years of age. Daytime control of micturition is easier to accomplish than nighttime control and occurs earlier in the child's development, usually by 2 years of age. Occasional daytime accidents or nocturnal enuresis (bedwetting) may continue until 5 years of age.

The adult normally voids 1500 to 1600 mL of urine daily, or approximately 500 mL every 4 hours. During pregnancy, urinary frequency is common and susceptibility to UTIs is increased. In women, child-bearing and hormonal changes during menopause may contribute to urinary difficulties. In men, prostate enlargement can begin in the forties and continue throughout the lifespan, resulting in urinary frequency and possibly retention.

Changes in kidney and bladder function also occur with aging. The kidney's ability to concentrate urine or reabsorb water and sodium declines. Alterations in kidney function include a reduction in glomerular filtration rate, from 125 mL per minute in younger adults to 60 to 70 mL per minute in adults 80 years of age. The older adult often experiences nocturia, due in part to age-related changes in vasopressin secretion (Fonda et al., 2005). The functional capacity of the bladder decreases, resulting in increased urinary frequency. Detrusor contractility also decreases, contributing to less effective emptying, elevated postvoid residuals (the volume remaining in the bladder after a void), and increased susceptibility to UTIs. A decrease in urethral closure pressure in women, which is generally associated with a decline in estrogen levels, can contribute to an increase in incontinence (Fonda et al., 2005). Older men commonly experience incomplete bladder emptying associated with prostatic enlargement.

Psychosocial and Cultural Considerations

You must consider that urinary elimination problems may result in alterations of sexuality and self-concept (which includes body image, self-esteem, roles, and identity). The embarrassment associated with elimination problems may delay or prevent help-seeking. Individuals with incontinence often blame themselves for their condition and go to great lengths, including self-imposed social isolation, to keep others from finding out about it. Nurses must therefore initiate discussion by asking clients if they are experiencing any issues related to urinary elimination or bladder control as a routine part of care. It is also important to determine how bothersome symptoms are for each client before planning care. Although men tend to feel greater distress about incontinence than women do (Gray, 2003), clients who are not overly bothered by their symptoms are less likely to adhere to therapies. Understanding a client's goals and expectations for treatment will help to ensure that interventions are realistic.

Sociocultural factors may influence the client's expectation of the degree of privacy and location for attending to urinary needs. Your approach to a client's elimination needs must consider cultural, social, and gender habits. If a client prefers privacy, try to prevent interruptions as the client voids. A client with less need for privacy should also be treated with understanding and acceptance. Ensure that the client is comfortable when he or she is trying to void. In some cultures, people prefer to squat over a receptacle rather than sit on one. Culture dictates when and where it is appropriate to urinate. In some cultures, a woman with urinary needs should be assisted only by another woman.

Critical Thinking

Critical thinking during assessment of urinary elimination requires the integration of evidence-informed knowledge from nursing and other disciplines, experiential knowledge, and an understanding of the client's perceptions of the alterations in elimination and their impact. Critical thinking also involves an understanding of relevant cultural, environmental, and personal factors, including the unique goals of every client. Empathy, teaching, and ongoing support are needed to assist the client in meeting these goals and maintaining improvement.

Professional standards provide valuable directions for treatment and management of elimination problems. When planning and implementing care for the client with alterations in urinary elimination, use the standards developed by professional organizations such as the Canadian Nurses Association, the Canadian Continence Foundation, the United Ostomy Association of Canada, and the Urology Nurses of Canada. You should also follow clinical care guidelines for management of urinary incontinence as developed by a multidisciplinary team of health care professionals (Canadian Continence Foundation, 2001).

Nursing Process and Alterations in Urinary Function

❖Assessment

To identify a urinary elimination problem and gather data for a care plan, you obtain information by collecting a health history, performing a focused physical assessment, assessing the client's urine, and reviewing information from diagnostic tests and examinations. Use critical thinking to synthesize this information as assessment proceeds (Figure 44–6). Adequate assessment should result in the formulation of nursing diagnoses appropriate for alterations in urinary elimination. You should be alert to individual needs related to normal aging that predispose older adults to certain elimination problems (Box 44–2).

Health History

The nursing health history includes a review of the client's urinary elimination patterns and symptoms of urinary alterations and an assessment of factors that may affect the ability to urinate normally.

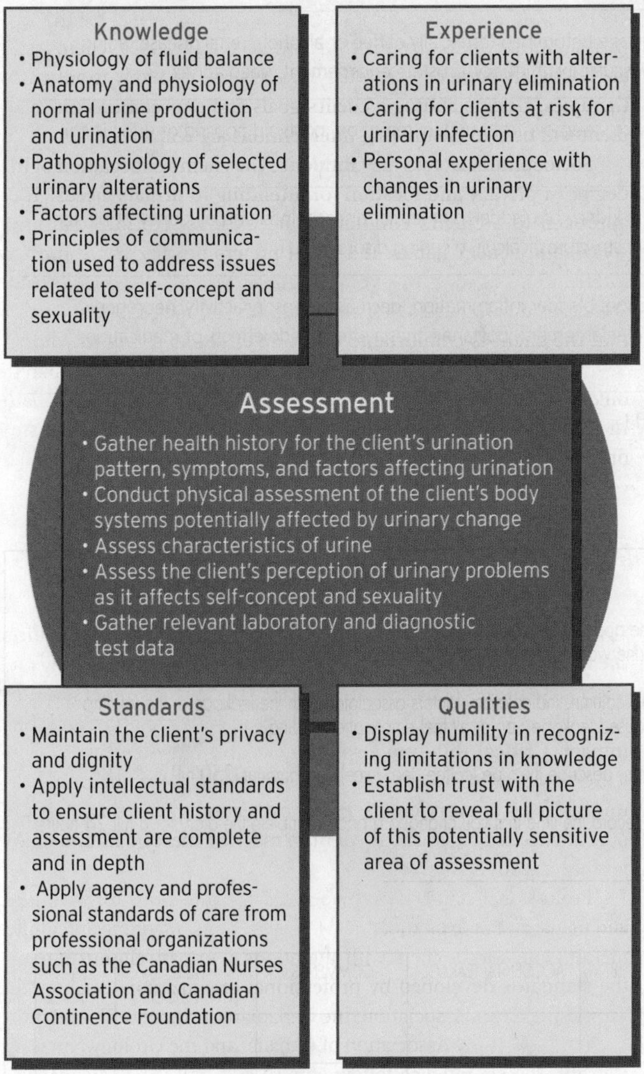

Knowledge
- Physiology of fluid balance
- Anatomy and physiology of normal urine production and urination
- Pathophysiology of selected urinary alterations
- Factors affecting urination
- Principles of communication used to address issues related to self-concept and sexuality

Experience
- Caring for clients with alterations in urinary elimination
- Caring for clients at risk for urinary infection
- Personal experience with changes in urinary elimination

Assessment
- Gather health history for the client's urination pattern, symptoms, and factors affecting urination
- Conduct physical assessment of the client's body systems potentially affected by urinary change
- Assess characteristics of urine
- Assess the client's perception of urinary problems as it affects self-concept and sexuality
- Gather relevant laboratory and diagnostic test data

Standards
- Maintain the client's privacy and dignity
- Apply intellectual standards to ensure client history and assessment are complete and in depth
- Apply agency and professional standards of care from professional organizations such as the Canadian Nurses Association and Canadian Continence Foundation

Qualities
- Display humility in recognizing limitations in knowledge
- Establish trust with the client to reveal full picture of this potentially sensitive area of assessment

Figure 44-6 Critical thinking model for urinary elimination assessment.

BOX 44-2 FOCUS ON OLDER ADULTS

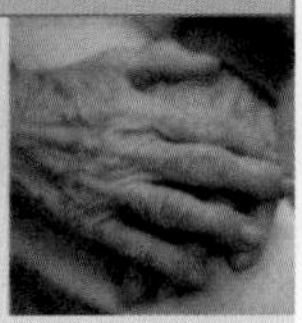

- Physiological changes in the lower urinary tract occur in continent as well as incontinent older adults.
- Dilute urine discourages bacterial growth; therefore, older adults should be encouraged to increase their fluid intake to at least six glasses a day, unless medically contraindicated (Gray & Krissovich, 2003).
- Fluids that promote an acidic urine (e.g., cranberry juice) should be made available as part of the client's fluid intake because an acidic urine also helps to inhibit bacterial growth and may prevent UTIs (Nguyen, 2004).
- Restriction of fluids 2 hours before sleep, combined with elevating the legs to allow for venous return and bladder emptying before bedtime (leg elevation for at least 1 hour) may decrease the incidence of nocturia (Gray & Krissovich, 2003).
- In-dwelling catheters should not be used routinely in older adults unless other options have been tried. The risk of infection increases dramatically for catheterized clients (Juthani-Mehta, 2007).
- Treating asymptomatic bacteriuria in older adults is not recommended.
- Incontinence is not a normal part of aging, and efforts should be made to assess incontinence and provide interventions to promote return to continence.

Pattern of Urination. Ask the client about usual daily voiding patterns and any recent changes. Information about voiding symptoms such as hesitancy (Table 44–1) and the overall pattern of urination, including average time between voids and episodes of urgency and incontinence, is important to a nursing assessment and establishes a baseline for comparison.

A **urinary diary** is an important diagnostic tool (Figure 44–7), particularly because many adults are not aware of how often they void throughout the day. A diary is kept by the client or the caregiver; it records approximate times of urination, times of leakage and estimates of the amount lost (dribbled, wet pad, wet clothing), and types and amount of fluids ingested. Measuring two or more voids (not including the first void of the morning) will provide useful information about the volume of urine that a client generally stores. Recording factors that precipitated urination or leakage, such as a strong urge or a cough, is particularly helpful. The number of pad changes per day is also useful information. Three-day (72-hour) diaries provide more reliable information than 24-hour diaries, but ensuring completion can be more difficult (Schick et al., 2003). The diary should be adjusted to whatever format the client finds most practical.

Factors Affecting Urination. It is important to summarize the factors associated with the client's medical history, surgical history, and current environment that may affect urination. Medical history includes disease conditions that can affect elimination, such as multiple sclerosis, spinal cord injury, stroke, and diabetes. Another factor to consider is the client's bowel elimination pattern. Constipation often interferes with normal urine elimination. Medication history, including the name, amount, and frequency of each prescription and over-the-counter medication, should also be noted as part of the medical history.

Relevant surgical history (e.g., urological and gynecological interventions and pelvic radiation) should be considered because surgery may cause scarring and disruption of neurological pathways. The presence or history of an in-dwelling catheter should be noted because of

TABLE 44-1 Common Symptoms of Urinary Alterations

Symptom	Description	Common Causes or Associated Factors
Incontinence	Involuntary loss of urine	Multiple factors: urethral hypermobility, loss of pelvic floor muscle tone, fecal impaction, neurological impairment, pelvic organ prolapse
Urgency	Sudden and compelling urge to void that cannot be postponed	Overactive bladder syndrome that is neurogenic, sensory, or idiopathic; calculi or tumour; urinary tract infection (UTI)
Dysuria	Painful or difficult urination	Bladder inflammation; urethral trauma; UTI; inflammation of urethra, sphincter, or both
Frequency	Voiding more than 8 times in 24 hours	Increased fluid intake, bladder infection or inflammation, increased pressure on bladder (pregnancy, psychological stress), incomplete emptying, small bladder capacity, overactive bladder syndrome, polyuria
Hesitancy	Difficulty initiating urination	Hypotonic bladder, anxiety, urethral stricture, obstruction associated with prostate enlargement
Polyuria	Voiding large amounts of urine	Excess fluid intake, diabetes mellitus or diabetes insipidus, use of diuretics, postobstructive diuresis
Oliguria	Diminished urinary output relative to intake (usually 400 mL/24 hours)	Dehydration, renal failure, increased antidiuretic hormone (ADH) secretion, congestive heart failure
Nocturia	Getting up at night to void	Excessive fluid intake before bed (especially coffee or alcohol), renal disease, aging process, cardiovascular insufficiency, prostate enlargement, sleep apnea
Dribbling	Leakage of urine despite voluntary control of urination	Stress incontinence, overflow from urinary retention, postvoid pooling of urine in the urethra (men)
Hematuria	Blood in the urine	Neoplasms of the kidney or bladder, glomerular disease, infection of kidney or bladder, trauma to urinary structures, calculi, bleeding disorders, UTI
Retention	Accumulation of urine in the bladder, with inability of bladder to empty fully	Urethral obstruction, bladder inflammation, decreased sensory activity, neurogenic bladder, prostate enlargement, postanaesthesia effects, side effects of medications (e.g., anticholinergics, antidepressants)
Elevated postvoid residual urine	Elevated volume of urine remaining after voiding (>100 mL)	Neurogenic bladder, prostate enlargement, trauma, inflammation of urethra, inflammation or irritation of bladder mucosa from infection

Instructions:

- ❒ Mark the time in the appropriate column each time you void in a toilet or accidentally leak urine. Note how much urine was leaked (a small, moderate, or large amount).
- ❒ In the COMMENTS column, indicate any factors associated with the leakage or the voiding (e.g., "coughing caused leakage," or "don't feel empty after voiding").
- ❒ In the FLUIDS column, describe the type (coffee, tea, juice) and amount (250 mL).
- ❒ In the last column, record the time that you changed a pad. Complete the diary for a full 24 hours.

NAME: ____________________

DAY/DATE: ____________________

TIME	VOIDED IN TOILET	ACCIDENTAL LEAKAGE	COMMENTS	FLUIDS (TYPE, AMOUNT)	PAD CHANGE

Figure 44-7 Sample urinary diary. **Source:** Adapted from Women's Continence Center, University of California. (2001). *Urinary diary.* San Francisco, CA: Author. Retrieved February 22, 2005, from http://www.ucsf.edu/wcc/print_diary.html

the potential for infection, catheter blockage, or skin care problems. Environmental barriers in the home or health care setting also should be evaluated. The client's mobility and ability to dress or undress and use the toilet independently should be assessed. Such aids as elevated toilet seats, grab bars, or a portable commode may be needed.

One of the most important parts of the assessment is the impact of alterations in elimination on the client's lifestyle and quality of life. The impact of urinary incontinence in particular can be substantial and it is important to discuss changes the client has made to cope with the condition. It is also important to note whether the client has previously seen a health care professional for help with or advice on urination.

Physical Assessment

A physical examination (see Chapter 32) provides you with data with which you can determine the presence and severity of urinary elimination problems. The primary structures reviewed include the skin and mucosal membranes, kidneys, bladder, and perineum.

Skin and Mucosal Membranes. Assess the condition of the skin and mucosal membranes. Problems with urinary elimination are often associated with fluid and electrolyte disturbances. By assessing skin turgor and the oral mucosa, you assess the client's hydration status. Urinary incontinence increases the risk of skin breakdown (see Chapter 47).

Kidneys. Flank pain usually develops if the kidneys become infected or inflamed. Assess for flank tenderness early in the disease by percussing the costovertebral angle (the angle formed by the spine and the twelfth rib). Auscultation is also performed to detect the presence of a renal artery bruit (sound resulting from turbulent blood flow through a narrowed artery).

Nurses with advanced examination skills learn to palpate the kidneys during abdominal examination. The kidneys' position, shape, and size can reveal renal swelling.

Bladder. In adults, the bladder rests below the symphysis pubis and is difficult to palpate. When distended, the bladder rises above the symphysis pubis at the midline of the abdomen and may extend to just below the umbilicus. On inspection, you may note a swelling or convex curvature of the lower abdomen. You should lightly palpate the lower abdomen. The partially filled bladder normally feels smooth and rounded. As you apply light pressure to the bladder, the client may feel the urge to urinate, tenderness, or even pain. Percussion of a full bladder yields a dull note.

The Female Perineum. When examining the female client, request that she assume a dorsal recumbent position to provide full exposure of the genitalia. Inspect the perineum for skin integrity and for the presence of a rash associated with incontinence and the use of containment pads. The rash may be monilial (maculopapular, red rash) or an ammonia-contact perineal dermatitis (papular with macerated skin).

Assess the vaginal vault for signs of vaginitis, a common result of estrogen depletion after menopause (Mostwin et al., 2005). Signs include dry, thin, pale mucosa; erosions; and tenderness or sensitivity to touch. Inspect the vaginal orifice carefully for signs of inflammation and describe any drainage.

Also, assess the urethral meatus and note the presence of any discharge, inflammation, or lesions. Normally the meatus is pink and appears as a small, slitlike opening below the clitoris and above the vaginal orifice. It may recede well into the vaginal vault with aging, making catheterization difficult. Discharge from the meatus is normally not present. If it is present, specimens of urethral discharge should be obtained before the client voids.

Pelvic floor muscle strength can be digitally assessed in women by gently inserting a gloved finger into the vagina. Ask the client to squeeze around your finger as firmly as possible, and then hold the contraction (generally for three to five seconds). Digital assessment is very useful in helping the client to identify the pelvic floor muscles correctly.

The Male Perineum. The male urethral meatus normally appears as a small opening at the tip of the penis. You should inspect the meatus for any discharge, inflammation, or lesions. If the foreskin needs to be retracted in uncircumcised men to see the meatus, it must be replaced to avoid constriction of the glans. Disposable gloves should be worn when retracting the foreskin. Pelvic floor muscle strength can be digitally assessed in men by gently inserting a gloved finger into the rectum and asking the client to squeeze around it.

Assessment of Urine

Assessment of urine involves measuring the client's fluid intake and urine output and observing characteristics of the urine.

Intake and Output. It is important to assess the client's average daily fluid intake. If an accurate measurement of fluid intake is needed from the client who is at home, ask him or her to show a commonly used glass or cup on which the intake estimate is based. In a health care setting, measure a client's fluid intake either when the physician orders intake and output measurements or when nursing judgement warrants a more precise measurement (see Chapter 40). A change in urine volume is a significant indicator of fluid alterations or kidney disease. While caring for the client, assess urine volume by measuring output with each voiding (using plastic receptacles, bedpans, or urinals). Special receptacles (urimeters) attach between in-dwelling catheters and drainage bags and are a convenient means of accurately measuring urine volume. A urimeter holds 100 to 200 mL of urine. After measuring urine with a urimeter, you can drain the cylinder into the urinary drainage bag or into a receptacle for disposal. Urimeters are indicated when precise hourly measurements of urine are needed.

When urine from a drainage bag is measured, the urine should be drained into a plastic graduated receptacle for more precise measurement of output (Figure 44–8). Each client should have a graduated receptacle for his or her exclusive use to prevent potential cross-contamination.

You should report any extreme increase or decrease in urine volume. An hourly output of less than 30 mL for more than 2 hours is cause for concern. Similarly, consistently high volumes of urine (polyuria), over 2000 to 2500 mL daily, should be reported to a physician.

Characteristics of Urine. You will inspect the client's urine for colour, clarity, and odour.

Colour. Normal urine ranges from a pale, straw colour to amber, depending on its concentration. Urine is usually more concentrated in the morning or with fluid volume deficits. As a person drinks more fluids, urine becomes less concentrated.

Bleeding from the kidneys or ureters causes urine to become dark red; bleeding from the bladder or urethra causes urine to become bright red. Various medications and foods also change urine colour and will cause a false positive on a urinalysis. For example, phenazopyridine, a urinary analgesic, colours the urine bright orange. Eating beets, rhubarb, or blackberries may cause red urine. Special dyes used in intravenous diagnostic studies also discolour urine. Dark

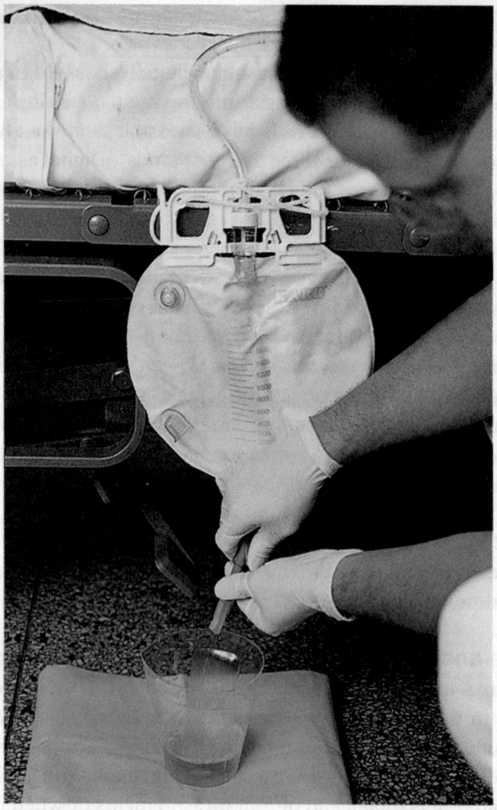

Figure 44-8 Urine drainage bag.

amber urine may result from high concentrations of bilirubin caused by liver dysfunction or vitamin B. Document and report any abnormal colour or sediment, especially if the cause is unknown.

Clarity. Normal urine appears transparent at voiding. Urine that stands for several minutes in a container becomes cloudy. Freshly voided urine in clients with renal disease may appear cloudy or foamy because of high protein concentrations. Urine also will appear thick and cloudy as a result of bacteria.

Odour. Urine has a characteristic odour. The more concentrated the urine, the stronger the odour. Stagnant urine has an ammonia odour, which is common in clients who are repeatedly incontinent. A sweet or fruity odour occurs from acetone or acetoacetic acid (by-products of incomplete fat metabolism) seen with diabetes mellitus or starvation.

Urine Testing. It is common to collect urine specimens for laboratory testing (Table 44–2). The type of test being done determines the method of collection. All specimens are labelled with the client's name, the date, and the time of collection. Specimens should be transported to the laboratory quickly to ensure accuracy of test results. Agency infection control policies require adherence to standard precautions or routine practices by all personnel during the handling of specimens (see Chapter 33).

Specimen Collection. You will collect random, clean-voided or midstream (Skill 44–1), sterile (Figure 44–9), and timed specimens.

Urine Collection in Children. Collecting specimens from infants and children is often difficult. School-age children and adolescents are usually able to cooperate, although they may be embarrassed. Preschool children and toddlers have difficulty voiding on request. Offering a young child fluids 30 minutes before requesting a specimen may help. You must use terms for urination that the child can understand. A young child may be reluctant to void in unfamiliar receptacles. A potty-chair or specimen hat placed under the toilet seat is usually effective. You must use special collection devices for infants and toddlers who are not toilet trained. Clear plastic, single-use bags with self-adhering material can be attached over the child's urethral meatus. Specimens should not be obtained by squeezing urine from the diaper material because test results may be inaccurate.

➤ TABLE 44-2 Urine Testing

Collection Type (Use of Specimen)	Nursing Considerations
Random specimen (routine urinalysis)	Can be collected during normal voiding, from an in-dwelling catheter or a urinary diversion collection bag. Collected in a clean specimen cup.
Clean-voided or midstream specimen (culture and sensitivity)	See Skill 44–1. Collected in a sterile specimen cup.
Sterile specimen (culture and sensitivity)	If the client has an in-dwelling catheter, a sterile specimen can be collected using the aseptic technique through the special port (see Figure 44–9) found on the side of the catheter. If the catheter has been in situ for more than three days, it should be changed before the specimen is collected to avoid contamination by organisms in the catheter lumen. Clamp the tubing below the port, allowing fresh, uncontaminated urine to collect in the tube. After wiping the port with an antimicrobial swab, insert a sterile syringe needle and withdraw at least 3 to 5 mL of urine. Using the sterile aseptic technique, transfer the urine to a sterile container (see Chapter 33).
Timed urine specimens (for measuring levels of adrenal cortical steroids or hormones, creatinine clearance, or protein quantity tests)	Time required between collections may be 2, 12, or 24 hours. The timed period begins after the client urinates and ends with a final voiding at the end of the time period. The client voids into a clean receptacle, and the urine is transferred to the special collection container, which may contain special preservatives. Each specimen must be free of feces and toilet tissue. Missed specimens make the entire collection inaccurate. Check agency policy and with the laboratory for specific instructions.

➤ SKILL 44-1 Collecting a Midstream (Clean-Voided) Urine Specimen

video

Delegation Considerations

Collecting a midstream (clean-voided) urine specimen may be delegated to unregulated care providers (UCPs). If appropriate, an alert client who is physically able may be instructed to collect the specimen. It is your responsibility to ensure that this specimen is obtained correctly and in a timely manner. Be aware of agency policy regarding specimen collection.

Instruct the UCP to inform you of the following:

- When the specimen was obtained
- Whether the client was unable to initiate a stream or had pain or burning on urination
- Whether the collected specimen is dark, bloody, or cloudy; is odorous; or contains mucus

Equipment

- Soap or cleansing solution, washcloth, towel, and handwashing basin
- Commercial kit for clean-voided specimen or individual supplies as listed
- Sterile cotton balls or sterile gauze pads
- Antiseptic solution (e.g., providone-iodine); check for client allergy, and if allergy exists, provide an alternative
- Sterile water
- Sterile specimen collection cup or jar
- Sterile and nonsterile (disposable) gloves
- Bedpan, bedside commode, or specimen hat
- Completed specimen label

Procedure

STEPS	RATIONALE
1. Assess voiding status of client:	
A. When client last voided	• May indicate readiness to void.
B. Level of awareness or developmental stage	• Reveals client's ability to cooperate during procedure.
C. Mobility, balance, and physical limitations	• Determines level of assistance in acquiring specimen.
2. Assess client's understanding of purpose of test and method of collection.	• Information allows for clarification and promotes client cooperation.
3. Explain procedure to client:	
A. Reason midstream specimen is needed	
B. Ways client and family can assist	• Helps client understand the procedure.
C. Ways to obtain specimen free of feces	• Feces change characteristics of urine and may cause abnormal values.
4. Provide fluids to drink a half-hour before collection unless contraindicated (i.e., fluid restriction) if client does not feel urge to void.	• Improves likelihood of client being able to void.
5. Provide privacy for client by closing door or bed curtain.	• Privacy allows client to relax and produce specimen more quickly.
6. Give client or family members soap, washcloth, and towel to cleanse perineal area.	• Client may prefer to wash own perineal area.
7. Perform hand hygiene and apply nonsterile gloves and assist nonambulatory clients with perineal care. Assist female client onto bedpan.	• Prevents transmission of microorganisms to nurse, provides easy access to perineal area to collect specimen.
8. Change gloves if necessary.	• Reduces transfer of infection.
9. Using surgical asepsis, open sterile kit (see Step 9 illustration) or prepare sterile supplies. Apply sterile gloves after opening sterile specimen cup, placing cap with sterile inside surface up; do not touch inside of container or cap (see Chapter 33).	• The sterile technique is essential to maintain sterility of equipment and specimen. Sterile gloves prevent the transmission of microorganisms. A contaminated specimen is the most frequent reason for inaccurate reporting of urine cultures and sensitivities.
10. Pour antiseptic solution over cotton balls or gauze pads unless kit contains prepared gauze pads in antiseptic solution.	• Cotton balls or gauze pads will be used to further cleanse the perineum.

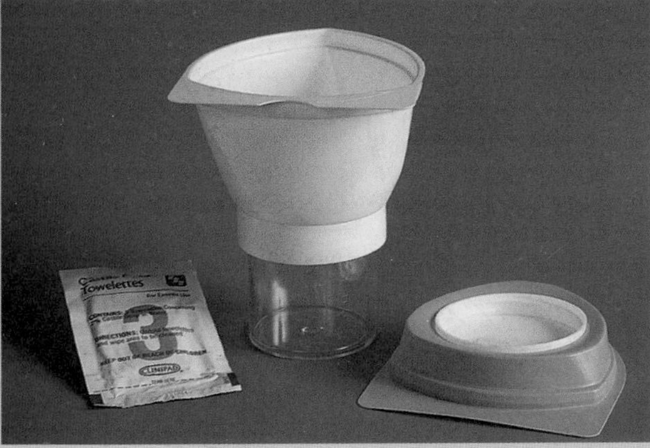

Step 9 Commercial midstream urine collection kit.

Continued

➤ SKILL 44-1 Collecting a Midstream (Clean-Voided) Urine Specimen *continued*

STEPS	RATIONALE
11. Assist or allow client to independently cleanse perineum and collect specimen:	
A. Female client	
(1) Spread labia with thumb and forefinger of nondominant hand.	• Provides access to urethral meatus.
(2) Cleanse area with cotton ball or gauze, moving from front (above urethral orifice) to back (toward anus; see Step 11A(2) illustration).	• Cleanse from area of least contamination to area of greatest contamination to decrease bacterial levels.
(3) If agency policy indicates, rinse area with sterile water, and dry with cotton ball or gauze.	• Prevents contamination of specimen with antiseptic solution.
(4) While you continue holding client's labia apart, client should initiate stream; after stream is achieved, pass container into stream and collect 30 to 60 mL (see Step 11A(4) illustration).	• Initial stream flushes out microorganisms that accumulate at the urethral meatus and prevents transfer into specimen.
B. Male client	
(1) Hold client's penis with one hand; using circular motion and antiseptic swab, cleanse end of penis, moving from centre to outside (see Step 11B(1) illustration). In uncircumcised men, the foreskin should be retracted before cleansing.	• Cleanse from area of least contamination to area of greatest contamination to decrease bacterial levels.
(2) If agency procedure indicates, rinse area with sterile water, and dry with cotton ball or gauze.	• Prevents contamination of specimen with antiseptic solution.
(3) After client has initiated urine stream, pass specimen collection container into stream and collect 30 to 60 mL (see Step 11B(3) illustration).	• Initial stream flushes out microorganisms that accumulate at the urethral meatus and prevents transfer into specimen.
12. Remove specimen container before flow of urine stops and before releasing labia or penis. Client finishes voiding in bedpan or toilet. If foreskin was retracted for specimen collection, it must be replaced over the glans.	• Prevents contamination of specimen with skin flora. If foreskin is not replaced, swelling and constriction may occur, causing pain and possible obstruction of urine flow.

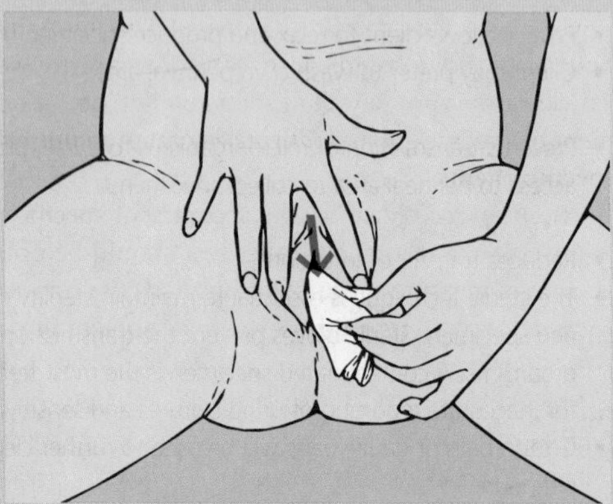

Step 11A(2) Cleansing technique (female).

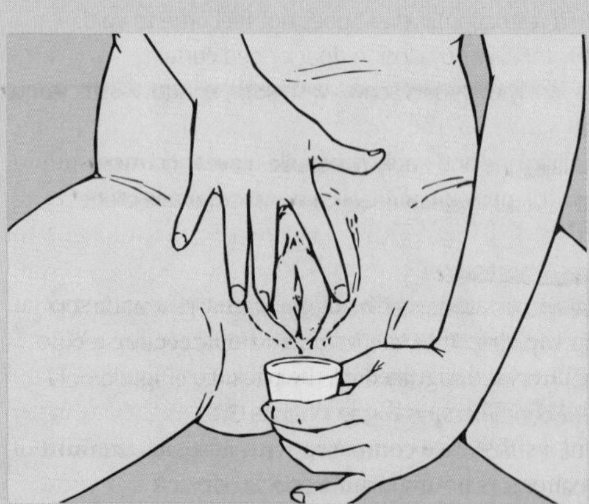

Step 11A(4) Specimen collection (female).

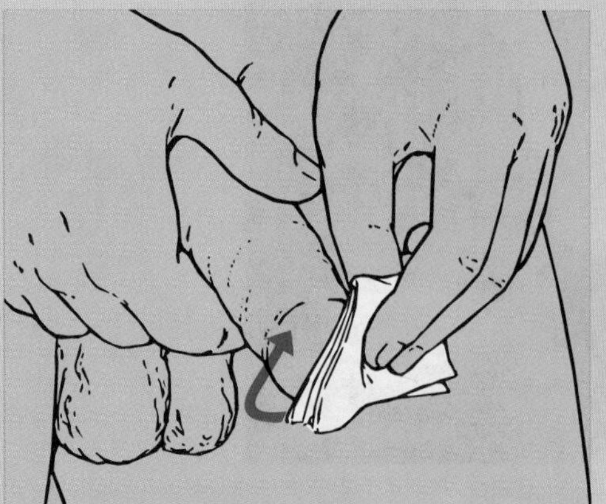

Step 11B(1) Cleansing technique (male).

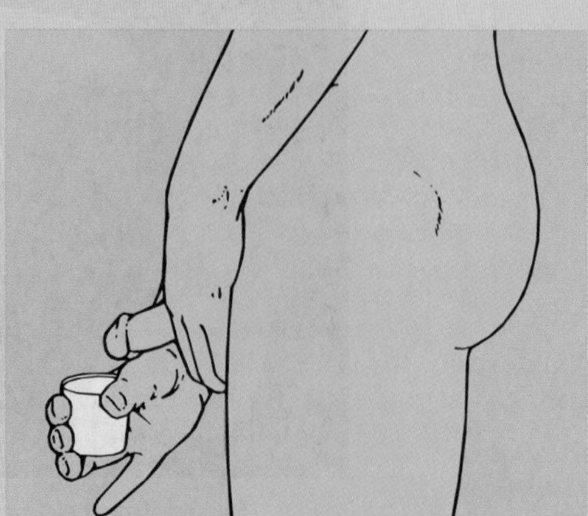

Step 11B(3) Specimen collection (male).

➤ SKILL 44-1 Collecting a Midstream (Clean-Voided) Urine Specimen *continued*

STEPS	RATIONALE
13. Replace cap securely on specimen container (touch outside only).	• Retains sterility of inside of container and prevents spillage of urine.
14. Cleanse any urine from exterior surface of container, and place in a plastic specimen bag.	• Prevents transfer of microorganisms to others.
15. Remove bedpan (if applicable), assist client to comfortable position, and provide handwashing basin if needed.	• Promotes relaxing environment.
16. Label specimen, and attach laboratory requisition.	• Prevents inaccurate identification that could lead to errors in diagnosis or treatment.

Critical Decision Point: If client is menstruating, indicate this information on the laboratory requisition.

17. Remove gloves, dispose of them in proper receptacle, and perform hand hygiene.	• Reduces transmission of infection.
18. Transport specimen to laboratory within 15 minutes or refrigerate immediately.	• Bacteria grow quickly in urine, and specimen should be analyzed immediately to obtain correct results.

Unexpected Outcomes and Related Interventions

Urine Specimen Is Contaminated With Feces or Toilet Paper

- Repeat instruction to client or assist client in obtaining a new specimen.
- Obtain a new specimen.
- Consider using a straight catheterization to obtain specimen.

Specimen Is Accidentally Discarded

- Repeat specimen collection.

Recording and Reporting

- Record date and time urine specimen was obtained in nurses' notes.
- Notify physician of any significant abnormalities.

Home Care Considerations

- If client is required to collect specimen as an outpatient, a clean technique may be used. Provide proper instruction for collection.
- Appropriate equipment must be given to the client and family.
- Information on storing the specimen until time of delivery to doctor's office or hospital laboratory must be provided.

Common Urine Tests

Urinalysis. The laboratory performs a **urinalysis** on a specimen obtained through any of the previously described methods. Table 44–3 lists normal values for a urinalysis. The specimen should be examined as soon as possible after it is collected, preferably within 2 hours. It should be the first voided specimen in the morning to ensure a uniform concentration of constituents. For a quick screening, you can perform certain portions of the urinalysis with special reagent strips. Dip the strip into the urine and observe for a colour change in the time interval designated on the package (Figure 44–10).

Specific Gravity. The **specific gravity** is the weight or degree of concentration of a substance compared with an equal amount of water. A urine specimen is poured into a special dry, clean cylinder. The weighted urinometer is suspended in the cylinder of urine. The concentration of dissolved substances in the urine aids in the determination of a client's fluid balance. This measurement is always done as part of a complete urinalysis. If you are working in a critical care unit you may be responsible for doing periodic measurement of specific gravity of urine as part of a complete assessment of specific clients.

If questions regarding the accuracy of specific gravity measurements arise, a urine osmolality test should be obtained. Although both tests measure urine concentration, the osmolality test is more accurate because it measures the total number of particles in a solution (see Chapter 40).

Urine Culture. For a urine culture, a sterile or clean-voided sample of urine is required. Early-morning specimens should be obtained when possible because bacterial counts are highest at that time (Fischbach, 2004). Because urine is an excellent medium for bacterial growth and bacteriological changes may alter test results,

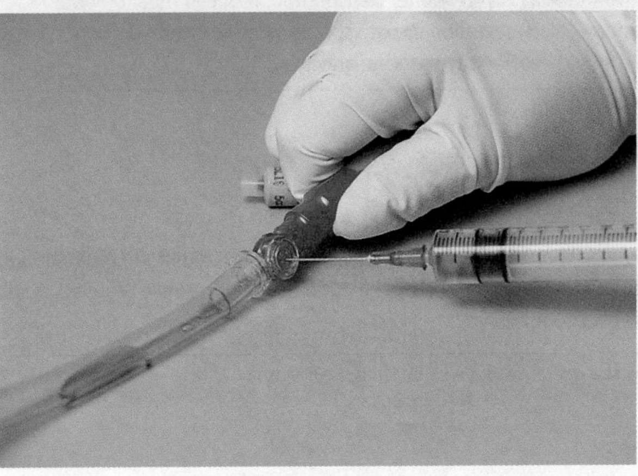

Figure 44-9 Urine specimen collection: aspiration from a collection port in drainage tubing on an in-dwelling catheter.

facilities may require that urine samples for culture and sensitivity be stored in a refrigerator until pickup.

It will be approximately 24 to 48 hours before the laboratory can report findings of bacterial growth. While results are awaited, a broad-spectrum antibiotic may be ordered as soon as a culture has been obtained. The test for sensitivity determines which specific antibiotics are effective. The results of a urine culture may show that another antibiotic would be more effective. In this case, a new antibiotic is ordered.

Diagnostic Examinations

The urinary system is amenable to accurate diagnostic study by several radiographic techniques. The two approaches for visualization of urinary structures, direct and indirect techniques, can be quite simple or very complex, necessitating extensive nursing intervention. These procedures are further subdivided into invasive or noninvasive categories (Table 44–4). One noninvasive procedure involves computed tomography (CT), shown in Figure 44–11 (see p. 1089).

Many of the nursing responsibilities related to diagnostic examinations of the urinary tract are common to more than one type of procedure. Common responsibilities before an examination include the following:

- Witnessing a signed consent (if agency policy).
- Assessing the client for history of shellfish (iodine) allergy, which predicts allergy to the dye used in specific studies (intravenous pyelogram [IVP] and renal arteriogram).
- Administering bowel-cleansing medications (check agency policy).
- Ensuring that the client receives the appropriate pretest diet (clear liquids) or nothing by mouth (NPO), as needed.

Common postprocedure interventions may include the following:

- Assessing intake and output.
- Observing characteristics of urine (colour, clarity, presence of blood).

Client Expectations

Clients depend on their caregivers to recognize and promptly meet their needs. Nurses need to use a skilled and caring approach, be creative in using a variety of assessment techniques, and serve as a client advocate. A caring nurse will meet the client's needs in a way that is acceptable and individualized to the client and the family situation. Clients with alterations in urinary elimination expect you to be respectful of privacy needs and sensitive to the impact of urinary impairments on sexuality and self-concept. You and your client should develop the care plan together whenever possible and establish goals that are mutually acceptable. Cultural practices and personal preferences also must be considered.

➤ TABLE 44-3 Routine Urinalysis

Measurement (Normal Value)	Interpretation
Routine Laboratory Value	
pH (4.6–8.0, average 6.0)	pH indicates acid–base balance. Urine that stands for several hours becomes alkaline. An acid pH helps protect against bacterial growth.
Protein (none or up to 8 mg/100 mL)	Protein is not normally present in urine. It is seen in renal disease because damage to glomeruli or tubules allows protein to enter urine.
Glucose (none)	Diabetic clients have glucose in their urine as a result of inability of tubules to reabsorb high glucose concentrations (180 mg/100 mL). Ingestion of high concentrations of glucose may cause some glucose to appear in the urine of healthy people.
Ketones (none)	Clients whose diabetes mellitus is poorly controlled experience breakdown of fatty acids. Ketones are end products of fat metabolism. Clients with dehydration, starvation, or excessive aspirin usage also may have **ketonuria.**
Blood (up to 2 red blood cells [RBCs])	Damage to glomeruli or tubules may allow RBCs to enter the urine. Trauma, disease, or surgery of the lower urinary tract also may cause blood to be present. In women, blood in a routine urine specimen may indicate contamination with menstrual fluid.
Specific gravity (1.010–1.025)	Specific gravity measures concentration of particles in urine. High specific gravity reflects concentrated urine, and low specific gravity reflects diluted urine. Dehydration, reduced renal blood flow, and increased antidiuretic hormone (ADH) secretion elevate specific gravity. Overhydration, early renal disease, and inadequate ADH secretion reduce specific gravity.
Microscopic Examination	
White blood cells (WBCs) (0–4 per low-power field)	Greater numbers may indicate urinary tract infection (UTI).
Bacteria (none)	Bacteria indicate UTI. (Client may or may not have symptoms.)
Casts (none)	Casts are cylindrical bodies whose shapes take on the likeness of objects within the renal tubule. Types include hyaline, WBCs, RBCs, granular cells, and epithelial cells. Their presence is always an abnormal finding and indicates renal alterations.

Data from Pagana, K. D., & Pagana, T. J. (2007). *Mosby's diagnostic and laboratory test reference* (8th ed.). St. Louis, MO: Mosby.

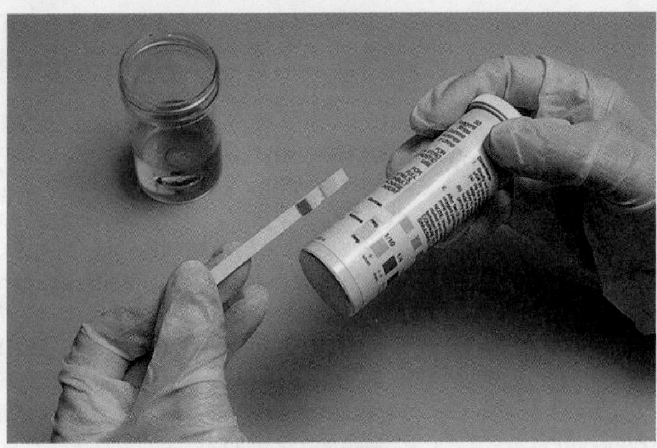

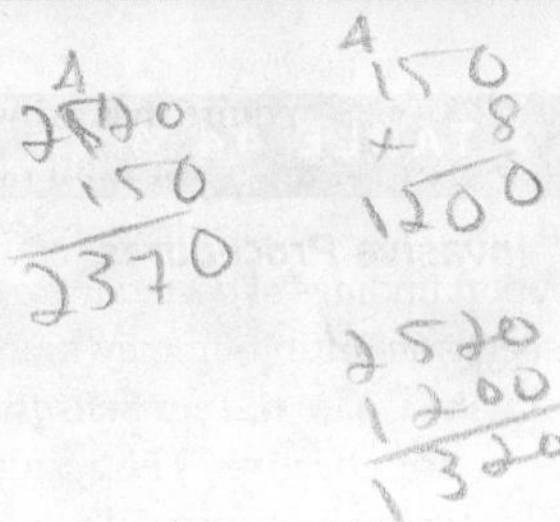

Figure 44-10 Checking results of a chemical reagent strip dipped in urine.

TABLE 44-4 Diagnostic Examinations

Name of Procedure	Purpose and Method of Procedure	Special Nursing Considerations
Noninvasive Procedures		
Abdominal roentgenogram (plain film; kidney, ureter, bladder [KUB], or flat plate)	To determine the size, shape, symmetry, and location of the kidneys; diagnose urinary calculi; preliminary X-ray imaging before intravenous pyelogram (IVP).	No special preparation or precautions; bowel preparation is required if preliminary X-ray imaging before IVP.
Computerized axial tomographic (CT) scan (see Figure 44–11)	A computerized X-ray procedure used to obtain detailed images of structures within a selected plane of the body. The computer reconstructs a cross-sectional image and thus allows the physician to view pathological conditions such as tumours and obstructions.	Bowel cleansing as per agency or physician preference. Assess client for shellfish (iodine) allergy if a CT scan with contrast material is ordered. Prepare client for the procedure (e.g., client will be placed into a large machine and need to lie still, feelings of claustrophobia occur in some clients).
Intravenous pyelogram (IVP)	To view the collecting ducts and renal pelvis and outline the ureters, bladder, and urethra with the use of dye, which is excreted through the urine. A special dye is injected intravenously. The client's ability to empty the bladder is assessed through a postvoiding X-ray film	Bowel cleansing will be completed as per agency or physician preference. Only clear liquids are permitted until after test is completed. Assess client for shellfish (iodine) allergy before test. After test, fluid intake is encouraged to dilute and flush dye from client. Observe for late symptoms of allergic reaction (rash, throat tightness, difficulty breathing, etc.).
Retrograde pyelogram	Series of X-ray films that provide detailed anatomical views of the ureter, ureteropelvic junction, renal pelvis, and calyces. A ureteral catheter is placed in the lower ureteral segment, and contrast material is injected or infused into the upper urinary tract.	Same as for IVP.
Retrograde urethrogram (RUG)	To obtain oblique X-ray films of the male urethra by instilling a small volume of iodine-bound contrast material into the urethra from a retrograde direction.	Assess client for shellfish (iodine) allergy before test.
Renal (kidney) scan	To determine renal blood flow, anatomical structure of the kidneys, and excretory function using a radioisotope.	Usually no bowel cleansing is needed, but check agency policy. After test, only precaution is rinsing bedpan or urinal after use and flushing the urine, as urine will contain a minute amount of radioisotope. Rinse fluid carefully using a double flush.
Renal ultrasonography	To identify gross renal structures and structural abnormalities in the kidney using high-frequency, inaudible sound waves.	No bowel cleansing is needed.
Bladder ultrasonography	To identify structural abnormalities of bladder or lower urinary tract. Also used to estimate the volume of urine in the bladder and to measure postvoid residual volume.	Client may be asked to drink fluids before the ultrasonography to cause bladder distension for better results. To measure postvoid residual volume, ultrasonography should be performed within 15 minutes of void. No special care is necessary after either study.

Continued

➤TABLE 44-4 Diagnostic Examinations *continued*

Invasive Procedures		
Endoscopy	Use of an endoscope allows for direct visualization, specimen collection, or treatment of the interior of the kidney (nephroscopy), ureter (ureteroscopy), bladder (cystosopy), and urethra (cystourethroscopy). Although this procedure may be accomplished using local anaesthesia, it is more commonly performed using general anaesthesia or conscious sedation to avoid unnecessary anxiety and trauma for the client.	Signed consent is obtained. If ordered, a bowel cleansing is completed. Follow agency policy for preoperative preparation and checklist (see Chapter 49). After client's return, assess the vital signs and the characteristics of urine, monitor intake and output, encourage ingestion of fluids, and observe for fever, dysuria, and pain in the suprapubic region.
Arteriogram (angiography)	Used primarily to visualize the renal arteries or their branches to detect narrowing or occlusion. A catheter is placed in one of the femoral arteries and introduced up to the level of the renal arteries. Radiopaque contrast is injected through the catheter while X-ray images are taken in rapid succession.	Signed consent is required. Assess for shellfish (iodine) allergy. Follow agency preprocedure checklist. After the procedure, monitor vital signs frequently until stable; bed rest is maintained for prescribed time interval; fluids are encouraged to flush the contrast from the system. Also monitor the affected extremity for neurocirculatory function (pulse, skin temperature, sensation, and movement), and observe catheter site for bleeding, swelling, increased tenderness, or hematoma formation. Physician must be notified immediately of any postprocedure abnormality.
Urodynamic testing (cystometrogram)	Determines bladder and sphincter function in the case of urinary obstruction or urinary incontinence. A catheter is inserted, the urine is drained, and sterile water or contrast liquid is used to fill the bladder. Pressure readings are taken and compared with the client's reported sensations.	Explain the need for the client to report all sensations during the test. After the test, assess the client for sensations of sweating, pain, nausea, bladder fullness, or a strong urge to void.

Adapted from Malarkey, L. M., & McMorrow, M. E. (2005). *Saunders' nursing guide to laboratory and diagnostic tests*. St. Louis, MO: Saunders.

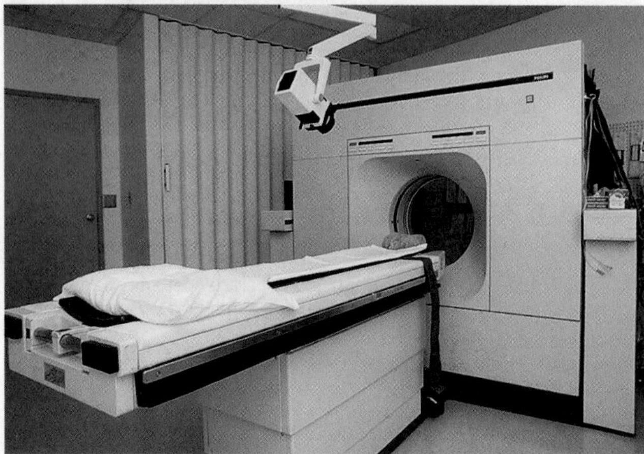

Figure 44-11 Equipment for computed tomography. **Source:** From Brundage, D. J. (1992). *Renal disorders*. St. Louis, MO: Mosby.

❖Nursing Diagnosis

A thorough assessment of the client's urinary elimination function reveals patterns of data that allow you to make relevant and accurate nursing diagnoses. The diagnosis may focus on a specific alteration or an associated problem such as *impaired skin integrity related to urinary incontinence*. Identification of defining characteristics leads you to select an appropriate diagnosis. Specifying related factors for each diagnosis allows selection of individualized nursing interventions (see Chapter 14). A sample of diagnostic reasoning is found in Box 44–3. Nursing diagnoses common to clients with alterations in urine elimination include the following:

- *Disturbed body image*
- *Pain (acute, chronic)*
- *Self-care deficit, toileting*
- *Impaired skin integrity*
- *Impaired urinary elimination*
- *Urinary incontinence (transient, urge, stress, mixed, functional, overflow, reflex, total)*
- *Urinary retention*

Common symptoms that contribute to a nursing diagnosis of impaired urinary elimination, such as frequency, urgency, and nocturia, were described in Table 44–1. Each of these symptoms is associated with multiple underlying disorders. You assimilate what has been learned from personal history taking, physical assessment, and diagnostic tests to determine a nursing diagnosis and an appropriate care plan.

❖Planning

During planning, you need to integrate the knowledge gained from assessment and the knowledge related to resources and available therapies to develop an individualized care plan (Box 44–4). The client's needs should be matched with clinical and professional standards

➤ BOX 44-3 NURSING DIAGNOSTIC PROCESS

Assessment Activities	Defining Characteristics	Nursing Diagnosis
Have client describe situations that accompany urine leakage.	Client states that she "loses a little urine" whenever she sneezes, coughs, or laughs. Client states that she has been having problems for several years.	*Stress urinary incontinence related to decreased pelvic muscle tone and urethral sphincter trauma*
Observe client behaviour.	Client is wearing a menstrual minipad continuously. Client is reluctant to interact with others and tries not to cough or laugh.	
Review medical history.	Client is menopausal after three vaginal births.	

➤ BOX 44-4 NURSING CARE PLAN

Mixed Urinary Incontinence

Assessment

Kay, a home care nurse, is seeing Mrs. Grayson, a 75-year-old widow, at her home. Mrs. Grayson was referred by her physician because of arthritis. She lives alone, but her daughter lives less than a 10-minute drive away. Kay's assessment included a discussion of Mrs. Grayson's current health problems.

Assessment Activities	Findings and Defining Characteristics
Ask Mrs. Grayson about how she is coping with her arthritis.	She responds, "It slows me down. The pain medication is helping, but it takes me longer to get out of my chair and get anywhere." Mrs. Grayson begins to cry and states, "You can see the plastic cover on my chair. I'm so embarrassed; sometimes I can't get out of the chair fast enough and I lose my water. I've beenwearing those diapers lately."
Ask Mrs. Grayson to describe how long she has had trouble controlling her urine and whether she has ever sought help.	Mrs. Grayson says that she has had trouble with dribbling for more than 10 years, but she really didn't think anything could be done about it because of her age. Over the past few years it has gotten worse. With little warning she has to rush to the bathroom and is often wet on the way.
Ask Mrs. Grayson about any changes, such as new medication, that may have contributed to her worsening symptoms. Ask Mrs. Grayson to complete a bladder diary for three days when she is likely to be at home most of the time, and provide a receptacle so that she can measure several of her voids. Establish diary format she understands and can work with.	Mrs. Grayson completes the diary for only two days because she finds it difficult to write everything down.
Assess bladder diary findings and discuss patterns with Mrs. Grayson so she becomes aware of her usual bladder routines and is more able to participate in her care planning.	The diary findings discussed are as follows: 1. Largest volume void is 200 mL and longest interval between voids is 1.25 hours. Mrs. Grayson is up 3 to 4 times at night to void. 2. Two episodes of incontinence occur on the way to the bathroom. Mrs. Grayson records that she gets a sudden urge to void but is "very wet" on the way to the bathroom. 3. Mrs. Grayson also records that she can feel herself dribbling while coughing. 4. Fluid intake is low, averaging 800 mL per 24 hours.

Nursing Diagnosis: *Mixed incontinence.* Mrs. Grayson has symptoms of urge incontinence: frequency, incontinence associated with severe urgency, and nocturia. She also describes episodes of stress incontinence. Her impaired mobility makes it more difficult to get to the bathroom in time. Mrs. Grayson also may be at risk for a urinary tract infection (UTI) due to reduced fluid intake.

Planning

Goals (Nursing Outcomes Classification)*	Expected Outcomes
Client will review bladder diary and think about aspects of her elimination pattern that may be amenable to change	Enhanced understanding of bladder function
Client will report reduced episodes of incontinence within 1 month and longer intervals between voids	Reduced episodes of urinary incontinence
Client will increase fluid intake to help ensure adequate hydration and prevent urinary tract infection	Adequate hydration

*Outcome classification labels from Moorhead, S., Johnson, M., & Maas, M. L. (Eds.). (2004). *Nursing Outcomes Classification (NOC)* (3rd ed.). St. Louis, MO: Mosby.

Continued

➤ BOX 44-4 NURSING CARE PLAN *continued*

Interventions (Nursing Interventions Classification)

Urinary Incontinence Care	*Rationale*
Discuss "normal" bladder habits with client as well as her actual patterns of intake and output, based on bladder diary.	The success of conservative therapies for urinary incontinence (UI) such as pelvic floor muscle exercises (PFMEs) requires motivation and ongoing commitment and self-care, meaning that the client must be an active part of assessment and care planning.
Assess client's pelvic floor strength digitally to establish baseline and to teach client appropriate muscle to tighten. Instruct client to practise PFMEs at least twice a day (see Box 44–12).	Cognitively intact and motivated older adults can learn PFMEs when able to identify the correct musculature. Growing evidence supports the positive impact of PFMEs in women with stress UI and overactive bladder syndrome (OAB), including the reflex inhibition of involuntary detrusor contractions (Hay-Smith & Dumoulin, 2007).
Work with client to establish a manageable program of bladder training, asking the client to void at regular, prespecified intervals throughout the day based on maximum intervals in bladder diary (1.25 hours). Gradually increase the interval by 15 to 30 minutes per week as tolerated, until acceptable pattern is achieved.	Bladder training reduces frequency and urgency in women with OAB (Subak et al., 2002) but may be more successful when pelvic floor muscle strength has improved.
Discuss safety issues related to the client's nocturia and the possibility of acquiring a bedside commode.	Older adults who get up at night to urinate are more likely to experience a fall. Because older adults are also at increased risk for bone fractures, it is important to identify those with nocturia and to ensure that appropriate safety precautions are taken.
Encourage client to increase noncaffeinated fluid intake gradually to approximately 1500 mL, with fluid intake restricted 2 hours before bedtime.	Adequate hydration will help prevent urinary tract infection (UTI) and maintain dilute urine. Avoiding fluids before bedtime may reduce nocturia.

Evaluation

Nursing Action	*Client Response and Finding*	*Achievement of Outcome*
Ask Mrs. Grayson to complete a bladder diary at regular intervals (monthly or every 2 months) to compare to the baseline diary.	Three months after initiating conservative treatment, client responds, "I'm dry most of the time now."	Mrs. Grayson has reduced her episodes of incontinence and increased the interval between voids. She is now voiding every 3 hours on average and is up one or two times at night. She reports that she feels better because she is getting more sleep.

recommended in the literature (Figure 44–12). Building a relationship of trust with the client is important because implementing the care plan involves interaction of a very personal nature.

Goals and Outcomes

The care plan for alterations in urinary elimination must include realistic and individualized goals along with relevant outcomes. You and your client must collaborate in setting goals and outcomes. A general goal might be normal urinary elimination, but the individual goal may differ depending on the problem. The goals may be short term or long term. For example, for a client with urinary retention after surgery, the short-term goal may be "Client will have normal voiding with complete bladder emptying within 24 hours." Relevant expected outcomes for this goal may include the following:

- Client will void within 8 hours.
- Urinary output of 300 mL or greater will occur with each voiding.
- Client's bladder will not be distended on palpation.
- Client will not continually feel an urge to void.

Conversely, the client with stress incontinence may have a long-term goal that involves weeks of pelvic floor muscle exercise (PFMEs; also known as Kegel exercises) to achieve urinary control: "Client will achieve improved urinary continence within 12 weeks after start of exercise program (Kegel)." Goals must be reasonably achievable for the client and be relevant to the client's situation.

Setting Priorities

Urinary elimination is a personal and intimate activity. You must establish a relationship with the client that promotes open discussion. A supportive and collaborative environment allows the client's priorities to become apparent and fosters mutual understanding of realistic goals.

When a client has multiple nursing diagnoses (Figure 44–13), you must recognize the primary health problem and its influence on other problems. In the example of the client with chronic confusion, the resultant incontinence creates several risks. Focusing on the management of incontinence will often help to resolve more than one nursing diagnosis. Although physical care needs may appear to have

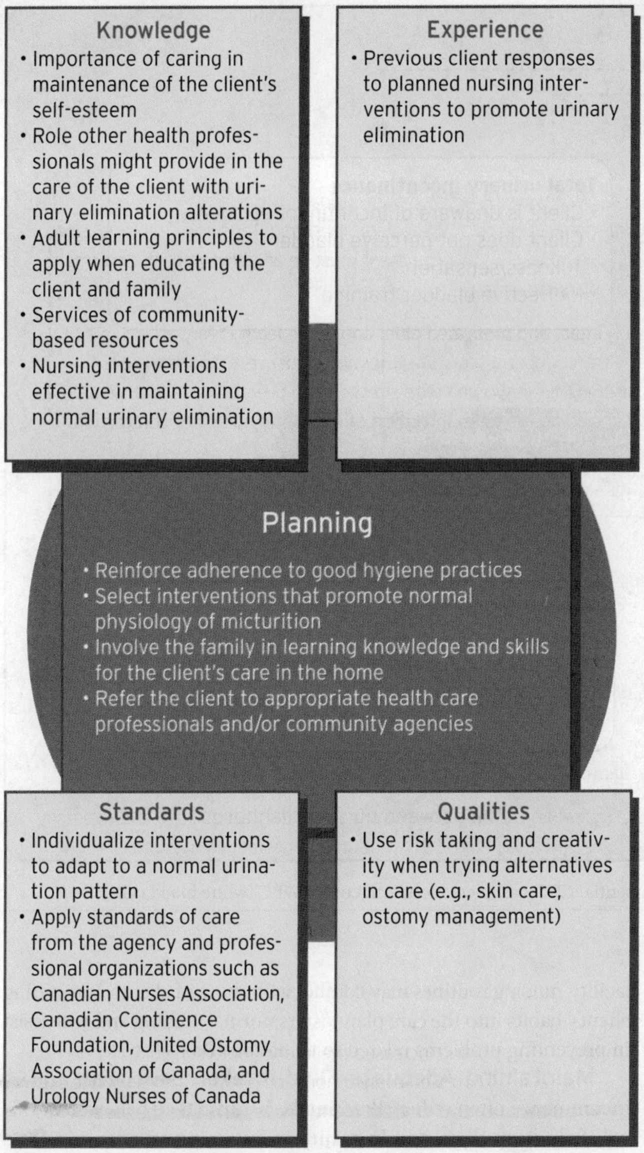

Knowledge
- Importance of caring in maintenance of the client's self-esteem
- Role other health professionals might provide in the care of the client with urinary elimination alterations
- Adult learning principles to apply when educating the client and family
- Services of community-based resources
- Nursing interventions effective in maintaining normal urinary elimination

Experience
- Previous client responses to planned nursing interventions to promote urinary elimination

Planning
- Reinforce adherence to good hygiene practices
- Select interventions that promote normal physiology of micturition
- Involve the family in learning knowledge and skills for the client's care in the home
- Refer the client to appropriate health care professionals and/or community agencies

Standards
- Individualize interventions to adapt to a normal urination pattern
- Apply standards of care from the agency and professional organizations such as Canadian Nurses Association, Canadian Continence Foundation, United Ostomy Association of Canada, and Urology Nurses of Canada

Qualities
- Use risk taking and creativity when trying alternatives in care (e.g., skin care, ostomy management)

Figure 44-12 Critical thinking model for urinary elimination planning.

higher priority, the psychological needs related to self-esteem or sexuality may be of higher priority to the client. Attention to the client's perceived needs may be the most satisfactory and successful approach to accomplishing all of the goals. Reinforcement and praise of good health habits improve compliance with the care plan.

Continuity of Care

The care plan incorporates health promotion activities and therapeutic interventions for clients. Preventive interventions may be required for clients at risk for urinary problems. It is important to consider the client's home environment and normal elimination routines when planning therapies. Consultation with other health care professionals and with the client's family is often necessary. For example, the physiotherapist can design an exercise plan to increase strength and endurance so that the client will be able to ambulate to the bathroom. The need for home care services should be explored and appropriate referrals made. The family may need to alter the home environment to make it easier and safer for the client to use the bathroom.

❖Implementation

Implementation is the action phase of the nursing process. You will carry out the independent and collaborative activities needed to assist the client in achieving the desired outcomes and goals. Independent activities are those in which nurses use their own judgement. An example of these is teaching self-care activities to the client. Collaborative activities are those prescribed by the physician that you carry out, such as medication administration.

Health Promotion

The focus of health promotion is to assist the client in understanding and participating in self-care practices that will preserve and protect healthy urinary system function (Box 44–5). This can be achieved through several means.

Client Education. Success of therapies aimed at solving or minimizing urinary elimination problems depends in part on successful client education. Although many clients may need to learn about all aspects of urinary elimination, you should first focus the teaching on the client's specific elimination problems. For example, clients who practise poor hygiene benefit most from learning about the normal sterility of the urinary tract and ways to prevent infection. Clients also learn the significance of symptoms of urinary alterations so that early preventive health care can be initiated.

Nurses can easily incorporate teaching while providing nursing care. For example, when attempting to increase the client's fluid intake, a good time to discuss the benefits of this action is while giving fluids with medications or meals. Teaching about perineal hygiene may be appropriate while giving a bath or performing catheter care.

Promoting Regular Micturition. Maintaining regular patterns of urinary elimination can help prevent many urination problems. Clients with urinary incontinence commonly void frequently throughout the day to avoid accidental urine loss. However, frequent voiding (e.g., at hourly intervals) may contribute to small-capacity bladders. Conversely, clients who hold their urine for long periods (more than eight hours) may develop a hypotonic bladder with incomplete emptying. You should reinforce the importance of voiding regularly (approximately every three to four hours) to help maintain a normal bladder capacity (400 to 500 mL). Because constipated stool in the rectum may compress the urethra and impede emptying, you should emphasize the importance of regular bowel movements and encourage measures to enhance regularity, including diets rich in fibre (see Chapter 45).

Many nursing measures have been designed to promote normal voiding in clients at risk for urination difficulties and in clients with established urination problems. You can initiate many of these measures independently.

Stimulating Micturition Reflex. The client's ability to void depends on feeling the urge to urinate, being able to control the urethral sphincter, and being able to relax during voiding. You can help a client learn to relax and stimulate the micturition reflex by enabling the client to assume the normal position for voiding. A woman is better able to void in a squatting or sitting position. If the woman is unable to use toilet facilities, you can help her into a sitting position on a bedpan (see Chapter 45) or bedside commode. A man voids more easily in a standing position. If the man cannot reach toilet facilities, he may stand at the bedside and void into a urinal (a metal or plastic receptacle for urine; Figure 44–14). At times, it may be necessary for one or more nurses to assist a man in standing.

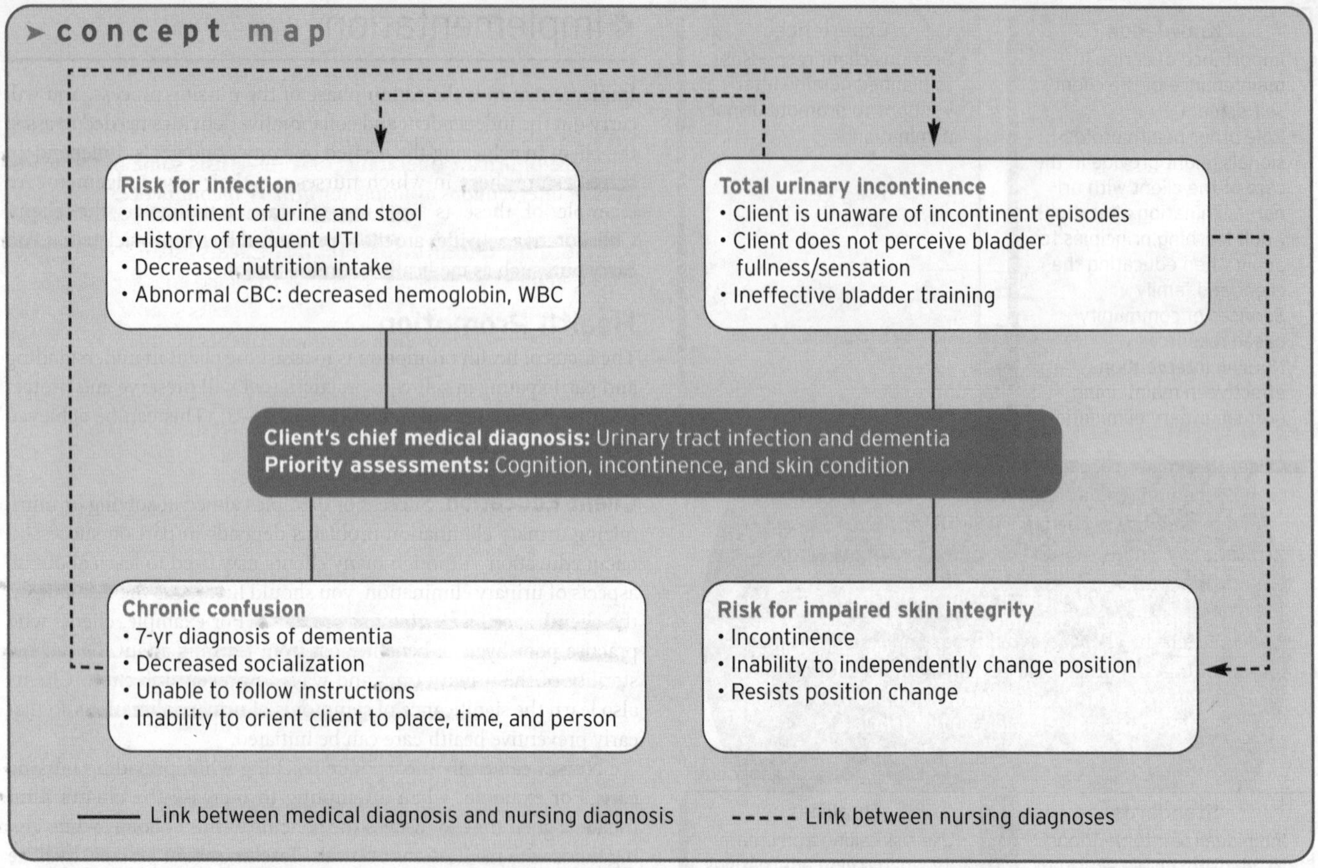

➤ concept map

Risk for infection
- Incontinent of urine and stool
- History of frequent UTI
- Decreased nutrition intake
- Abnormal CBC: decreased hemoglobin, WBC

Total urinary incontinence
- Client is unaware of incontinent episodes
- Client does not perceive bladder fullness/sensation
- Ineffective bladder training

Client's chief medical diagnosis: Urinary tract infection and dementia
Priority assessments: Cognition, incontinence, and skin condition

Chronic confusion
- 7-yr diagnosis of dementia
- Decreased socialization
- Unable to follow instructions
- Inability to orient client to place, time, and person

Risk for impaired skin integrity
- Incontinence
- Inability to independently change position
- Resists position change

—— Link between medical diagnosis and nursing diagnosis ----- Link between nursing diagnoses

Figure 44-13 Concept map for client with urinary tract infection (UTI) and dementia. CBC, complete blood cell count; WBC, white blood cells.

Providing certain sensory stimuli also may promote relaxation and voiding. The sound of running water helps many clients void. Stroking the inner thigh may stimulate sensory nerves and promote the micturition reflex. You can also pour warm water over the client's perineum to create the urge to urinate. If urine output is being measured, you must first measure the volume of water that will be poured over the perineal area.

Maintaining Elimination Habits. Many clients follow routines to promote normal voiding. In a hospital or long-term care facility, nursing routines may conflict with those of clients. Integrating clients' habits into the care plan fosters normal voiding and will assist in preventing problems related to urination (Box 44–6).

Maintaining Adequate Fluid Intake. Clients with urinary incontinence often reduce fluid intake because they believe that this will help keep them dry. In reality, maintaining an adequate fluid intake of 1500 to 2000 mL promotes continence because concentrated urine can irritate the bladder mucosa. Fluid intake should not include caffeinated beverages, which have a diuretic effect. Remind

BOX 44-5 FOCUS ON PRIMARY HEALTH CARE

Urinary Incontinence

People with urinary incontinence often attempt to manage the condition on their own and do not seek professional help because they are embarrassed, they believe that incontinence is a normal part of aging, or they are not aware of the treatment options. Consequently, routine screening for incontinence at the primary health care level should be a fundamental aspect of care provided by all nurses. Such routine screening demonstrates that it is acceptable to discuss elimination problems and provides a forum for teaching about bladder health. Health promotion topics that should be taught include the following:

- Basic education about lower urinary tract function.
- Education about promoting good bladder and bowel habits.
- Education about risk factors, including smoking, caffeine, weight gain, and fluid restriction.
- Education about preventing UTIs.

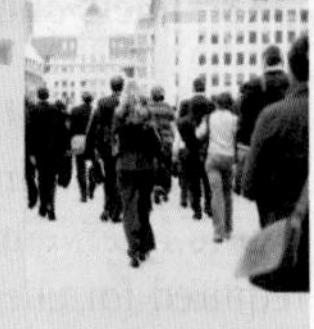

In the case of clients who are already experiencing urinary incontinence, nurses at the primary health care level provide information about common causes, goals and expectations of treatment, and absorbent products available. You should communicate with other health care professionals (particularly the client's family physician) and be aware of how to access additional care at the secondary or tertiary levels. You should also able to perform a focused assessment that includes obtaining relevant medical and surgical history, conducting a physical examination, conducting urinalysis, and completion of a 24- to 72-hour bladder diary. You would then initiate behavioural interventions that are relevant to the nursing diagnosis.

Adapted from Canadian Continence Foundation. (2001). *Promoting a collaborative consumer-focused approach to continence care in Canada*. Peterborough, ON: Author. Retrieved June 16, 2004, from http://www.continence-fdn.ca

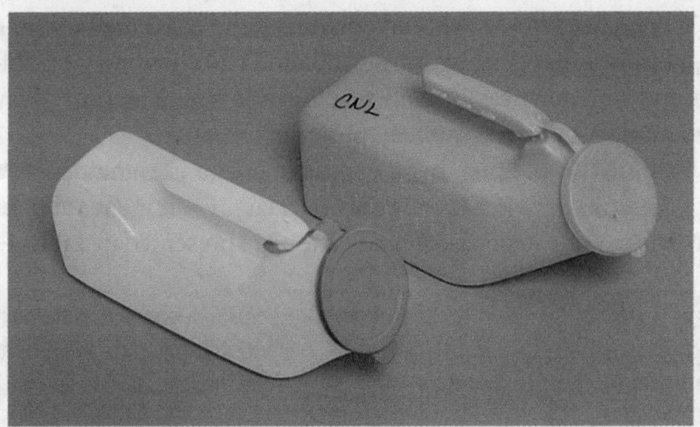

Figure 44-14 Types of male urinals.

the client that many vegetables and fruits have a high fluid content and can contribute to daily fluid intake. At the client's home, it may be helpful to establish a schedule for drinking fluids (e.g., with meals or medications). Fluids should be avoided two hours before bedtime to minimize nocturia.

Avoiding Food and Fluids That Can Irritate the Bladder Mucosa. Teach the client to avoid foods and fluids that may cause symptoms of urgency and frequency, including the following:

- Tobacco
- Alcohol
- Substances containing caffeine, such as coffee, tea, and chocolate
- Carbonated beverages
- Aspartame (artificial sweetener)
- Citrus fruits or juices
- Tomatoes or tomato-based products
- Greasy or spicy foods (Nygaard et al., 2008)

Promoting Complete Bladder Emptying. Under normal circumstances, a small amount of urine (50 mL) remains in the bladder after voiding (residual urine) because the urinary sphincters close. Thus, people normally remain continent and dry. People with residual urine are able to remain dry when their urethral closure pressure is sufficient to prevent leakage. However, urinary incontinence may occur when too much residual urine is in the bladder or when the urinary sphincters are too weak to maintain closure pressure. As well as contributing to incontinence, residual urine can be a medium for bacterial growth.

Clients should be encouraged to take their time while voiding and to try again when they feel they have not emptied their bladders fully. Those with consistently elevated postvoid residual volumes (>100 mL) may require intermittent catheterization. Portable bladder scanners offer a noninvasive means of assessing postvoid residual volumes.

Preventing Infection. One of the most important considerations for a client with alterations in urinary elimination is the need to prevent infection of the urinary system. Good perineal hygiene that includes cleaning the urethral meatus after each voiding or bowel movement is essential. Clients with limited dexterity due to conditions such as arthritis or stroke can benefit from the use of a squirt bottle filled with warm water to rinse the perineum after defecation.

Maintaining an adequate daily intake of fluids (1500 to 2000 mL) dilutes urine and promotes regular micturition. In contrast, very concentrated or excessively diluted urine can impair host defence mechanisms (Gray & Krissovich, 2003). Urine is normally acidic and tends to inhibit growth of microorganisms. Meats, eggs, whole-grain breads, cranberries, and prunes increase urine acidity. Cranberry juice has been shown to lower urine pH and decrease bacterial adherence to the bladder wall (Gray & Krissovich, 2003).

Acute Care

Many measures can be used in the acute care setting to decrease the incidence of urinary alterations. Box 44–7 lists some of the many types of interventions available for urinary incontinence.

Maintaining Elimination Habits. Clients usually require time to void. Requesting a urine specimen on demand does not contribute to relaxation and normal voiding habits. Clients should be given at least 30 minutes to provide a specimen. Clients normally void upon

BOX 44-6 NURSING STORY

Motivated to Promote Continence

It is impossible to know how the seemingly isolated decisions we make will continue to affect us as we go forward. I had recently started working as a registered nurse in long-term care when the opportunity arose to enter the world of research. The proposed project would involve the assessment and treatment of 50 older adults with urinary incontinence. I knew as little about research as I did about incontinence, but my eyes were quickly opened. Interested residents and families lined the length of the hallway to attend the project's information session. What still stands out to me today is the fact that not one resident I spoke with that night had known before arriving at the facility that his or her urinary incontinence could be treated. The phrase "suffering in silence" had never been more true.

Assessment included much of what you are now familiar with: completing a bladder diary (by the resident or by a clinician as necessary), a focused history, conducting blood work, and obtaining postvoid residual. Treatment was generally noninvasive: only one woman underwent surgery. The other participants initiated dietary modifications, bladder training, pelvic floor muscle exercises, or medication, or a combination of these. A regimen of prompted voiding was undertaken with residents who were cognitively impaired.

When assessment, intervention, and follow-up were complete approximately 1 year later, few of the 50 study participants were totally continent (i.e., dry). The majority, however, had at least 50% fewer episodes of incontinence. Of equal importance, these men and women understood that they were not alone and did not have to accept their incontinence as part of the aging process.

The differences that I witnessed in the participants' quality of life continue to motivate me in my work to this day. One resident who voided large volumes of urine each time she stood up, and who slept in her chair because she was afraid of soaking her bed, was able to leave the nursing home for the first time in years to visit with her brother before he died. Her treatment involved changing the medication that had contributed to her condition and ensuring that she had assistance to reach the toilet at appropriate times, as dictated by findings in her bladder diary.

On the downside, many of the participants' lifestyle improvements were not permanent. For a variety of reasons that included staffing shortages, supportive strategies such as prompted voiding and scheduled toileting were not well maintained after the project was completed, and several residents who required toileting assistance regressed despite earlier successes. As a result of my participation in this incontinence project, I was left with a determination to teach those with urinary incontinence how to help themselves, and to teach caregivers that despite heavy workloads it is their ongoing responsibility to ask patients about urinary leakage, to direct them to the appropriate resources, and, above all, to ensure the dignity of those who are unable to help themselves by offering toileting assistance .

➤ BOX 44-7 Urinary Incontinence Treatment Options

For Transient Incontinence
- Address underlying cause of incontinence (e.g., treat for infection or manage for constipation, as necessary)

For Urge Incontinence and Overactive Bladder
- Anticholinergic medications
- Bladder training
- Scheduled toileting
- Pelvic floor muscle exercises
- Biofeedback
- Lifestyle modifications (e.g., selected dietary and fluid modifications)

For Stress Incontinence
- Biofeedback
- Lifestyle modifications (e.g., weight loss, smoking cessation)
- Medications (i.e., estrogen replacement)
- Surgery
- Artificial sphincter

For Mixed Incontinence
- Interventions as for stress incontinence and urge incontinence

For Functional Incontinence
- Habit retraining
- Environmental alterations
- Scheduled toileting
- Condom catheter (men)
- Protective undergarments

For Overflow Incontinence
- Intermittent catheterization
- Surgery (i.e., for treatment of obstruction)
- In-dwelling or condom catheter

For Reflex Incontinence
- Anticholinergic medications
- Surgery
- Intermittent catheterization
- In-dwelling or condom catheter

For Total Incontinence
- Artificial sphincter
- Surgery (e.g., sling procedure)
- Urinary diversion

awakening or before meals; therefore, you should offer them the opportunity to use toilet facilities then. Also important is the need to respond promptly to clients' urges to urinate. Delays in assisting clients to the bathroom may interfere with normal micturition and contribute to incontinence. This is particularly the case with clients who have overactive bladders.

safety alert Many falls by older adults are related to the urge to urinate. Anticipate an older adult's need to urinate and provide scheduled bathroom visits. Make sure that the pathway between the bed and the toilet facility is clear of any barriers.

Privacy is essential to normal voiding. If the client cannot reach the bathroom, make sure that the bedside curtain is closed. The debilitated client at home may prefer to use a bedside commode screened by a partition or room divider. Young children are often unable to void in the presence of people other than their parents.

When possible, you should encourage the continued use of special measures that the client uses to void. The client may be able to relax and void more easily while reading or listening to music. Having a cup or glass of fluids also may promote urination.

Medications. Drug therapy, either alone or in combination with other therapies, can help problems of urinary incontinence and retention. The major categories of medication are presented in Table 44–5.

safety alert a-Adrenergic blockers may cause postural hypotension and increase the client's risk of falling and injury. Instruct clients taking these medications to plan their nighttime toileting and to get out of bed slowly.

Catheterization. Catheterization of the bladder involves introducing a narrow tube through the urethra and into the bladder to allow a continuous flow of urine into a drainage receptacle. Indications for urethral catheterization are numerous in acute, community, and long-term care settings (Box 44–8). In acute care, catheterization is particularly useful for careful monitoring of output in hemodynamically unstable clients. Because bladder catheterization carries the risk of UTI, blockage, and trauma to the urethra, it is preferable to rely on other measures for either specimen collection or management of incontinence (Getliffe, 2003).

Types of Catheterization. Catheters may be intermittent or in-dwelling (retention). With the intermittent technique, a single-use straight catheter (Figure 44–15A) is introduced for 5 to 10 minutes, just long enough to drain the bladder. The straight catheter has a single lumen with a small opening about 1.3 cm from the tip. Urine drains from the tip, through the lumen, and into a receptacle. Intermittent catheterization is performed by the client or by a nurse and is common in clients who have incomplete bladder emptying due to neurogenic conditions (e.g., spinal cord injury). In hospital, intermittent catheterization is sterile to reduce the risk of nosocomial infections. In the community, clients use the clean intermittent

➤ BOX 44-8 Indications for Catheterization

Short-Term In-Dwelling Catheterization
- When urine outflow is obstructed (e.g., prostate enlargement)
- When bladder, urethra, and surrounding structures have been surgically repaired
- When seeking to prevent urethral obstruction from blood clots
- When measuring urinary output in critically ill clients
- When continuous or intermittent bladder irrigations are required

Long-Term In-Dwelling Catheterization
- When chronic urinary retention is not manageable by intermittent catheterization
- When skin rashes, ulcers, or wounds become irritated by contact with urine
- In those with a terminal illness when bed linen changes or toileting is painful

Intermittent Catheterization
- When seeking to relieve discomfort due to bladder distension, provision of decompression
- When required to obtain a sterile urine specimen
- When required to assess residual urine after urination
- When managing urethral strictures
- When engaging in the long-term management of clients with spinal cord injuries, neuromuscular degeneration, or incompetent bladders

➤ TABLE 44-5 Medications Used to Treat Urinary Incontinence and Retention

Classification	Action	Generic Name	Side Effects	Contraindications or Alerts
Anticholinergics or antimuscarinics	Inhibit effect of acetylcholine on smooth muscle: antispasmodic	Oxybutynin Oxybutynin XL Tolterodine Tolterodine LA Propantheline bromide	Constipation Dry mouth Blurred vision Confusion and decreased cognition in older adults Retention	Narrow-angle glaucoma Gastrointestinal obstruction Ulcerative colitis Myasthenia gravis Retention elevated residual (can be used in conjunction with intermittent catheterization)
α-Adrenergic blockers	Block α receptors to relax bladder neck or proximal urethra and reduce symptoms of obstructive voiding	Terazosin Doxazosin Tamsulosin	Postural hypotension Syncope fainting, especially first dose	Clients taking antihypertensives will require dosage titration
α-Adrenergic agents	Stimulate α receptors at bladder neck or proximal urethra to increase tone and reduce stress incontinence	Pseudophedrine	Hypertension Insomnia Tremor Agitation	Monoamine oxidase inhibitors Hypertension Narrow-angle glaucoma Older clients
Low-dose, topical hormone replacement therapy	Reduces irritation and atrophic vaginitis. Can reduce symptoms of overactive bladder and stress incontinence	Premarin vaginal cream Estradiol ring Vagifem tab	Sore breasts Spotting (rare with very low dose	History of endometrial, ovarian, or breast cancer

Adapted from Reiss, B., Evans, M., & Broyles, B. (2002). *Pharmacological aspects of nursing care* (6th ed.). Clifton Park, NY: Delmar Learning. © Delmar Learning, a part of Cengage Learning, Inc. Reproduced by permission.

catheterization technique and reuse their catheters many times. Catheters are washed with soap and water and left to air-dry until the next use. No evidence exists to confirm that UTIs are increased in people who use the clean technique rather than the sterile technique (Moore et al., 2007).

The coude catheter is a type of catheter that has a curved tip and is used for male clients who have enlarged prostates that partly obstruct the urethra. It is less traumatic during insertion because it is stiffer and easier to control than the straight-tip catheter.

An in-dwelling or Foley catheter (see Figure 44–15B) is retained for longer periods in the bladder by means of a small balloon that anchors it against the bladder neck. The catheter remains in place until the client is able to void completely and voluntarily or for as long as accurate measurements are needed. In-dwelling catheters are either two lumen (the most common type; one lumen drains urine and the other carries sterile water to inflate or deflate the balloon) or three lumen (the third lumen allows for irrigation). They can be used on a short-term or long-term basis.

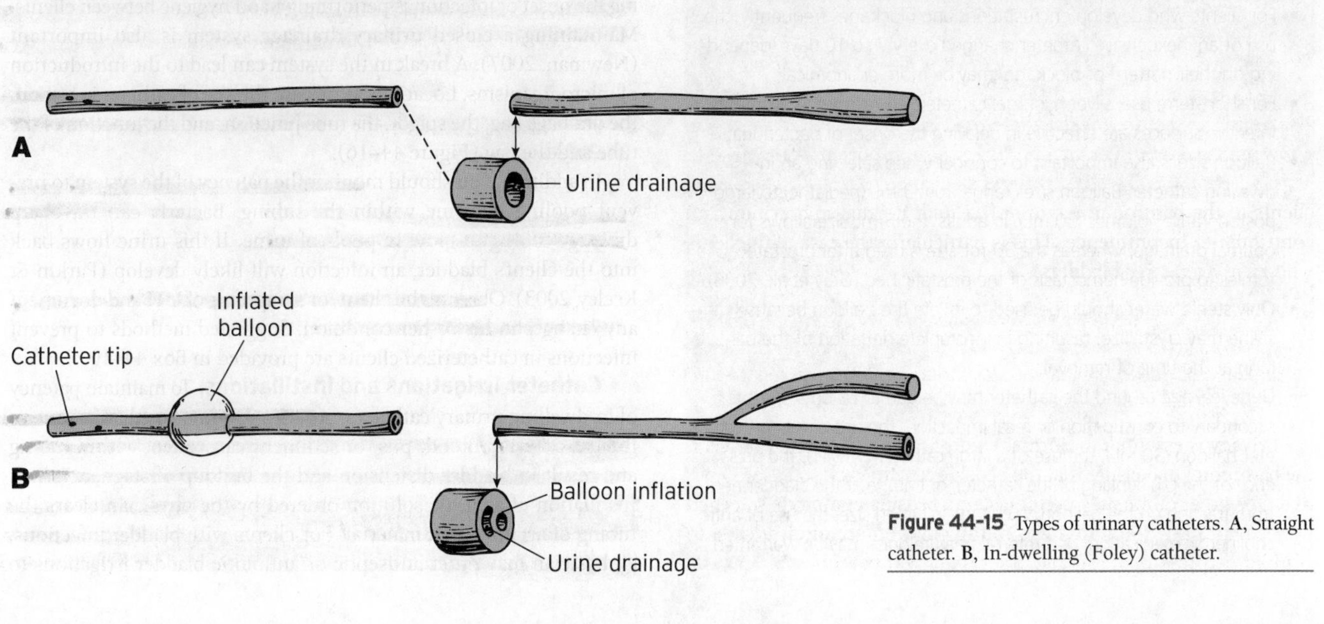

Figure 44-15 Types of urinary catheters. A, Straight catheter. B, In-dwelling (Foley) catheter.

Catheters are manufactured in many different materials (latex, silicone, Teflon) and come in many different diameters. Guidelines on how to make appropriate decisions regarding catheter selection are provided in Box 44–9.

Catheter Insertion. For urethral catheterization of any type, a physician's order is required. You must use the strict aseptic technique (see Chapter 33). Organizing equipment before beginning the procedure prevents interruptions. The steps for inserting in-dwelling and single-use straight catheters are basically the same. The difference lies in the procedure taken to inflate the in-dwelling catheter balloon and secure the catheter. Skill 44–2 lists the steps for inserting in-dwelling and single-use straight catheters in both men and women.

Closed Drainage Systems. After inserting an in-dwelling catheter, maintain a closed urinary drainage system to minimize the risk of infection. Urinary drainage bags are plastic and can hold about 1000 to 1500 mL of urine. The drainage bag should never be raised above the level of the client's bladder. The bag should hang on the bed frame or wheelchair without touching the floor. Urine in the bag and tubing can become a medium for bacteria, and infection is likely to develop if urine flows back into the bladder. Therefore, do not hang the bag on the bed's side rails because in that location it can be raised above the level of the bladder accidentally. When the client ambulates, the drainage bag must be held below the client's waist.

If the catheter must be disconnected from the drainage tubing, both tips should be cleansed with an alcohol swab before being reconnected to minimize the transfer of microorganisms into the tubing.

Most drainage bags contain an antireflux valve to prevent urine in the bag from re-entering the drainage tubing and contaminating the client's bladder. A spigot at the base of the bag is used to empty the bag. The spigot should always be clamped, except during emptying, and tucked into the protective pouch on the side of the bag (see agency policy). To ensure that the drainage system remains unobstructed, check for kinks or bends in the tubing, avoid positioning the client on the drainage tubing, and observe for clots or sediment that may occlude the collecting tubing.

Routine Catheter Care. Clients with in-dwelling catheters have a number of special care needs. Nursing measures are directed at maintaining client comfort, preventing infection, and maintaining an unobstructed flow of urine.

Perineal Hygiene. Buildup of secretions or **encrustation** at the catheter insertion site is a source of irritation and potential infection. You should provide perineal hygiene (see Chapter 38) at least twice daily, after a bowel movement, or as needed for a client with an in-dwelling catheter. Soap and water or skin cleansers are effective in reducing the number of microorganisms around the urethra and help to maintain skin health and client comfort. Be careful not to accidentally advance the catheter upward into the bladder during cleansing; if you do, you risk introducing bacteria into the bladder.

Catheter Care. In addition to routine perineal hygiene, many institutions recommend that clients with catheters receive special care three times a day and after defecation or bowel incontinence to help minimize discomfort and infection (Skill 44–3, p. 1107).

Fluid Intake. All clients with catheters should have a daily fluids intake of 2000 to 2500 mL if permitted. This can be met through oral intake or intravenous infusion. A high fluid intake produces a large volume of urine that flushes the bladder and keeps the catheter tubing free of sediment.

Preventing Infection. The most important strategy in preventing the onset of infection is performing hand hygiene between clients. Maintaining a closed urinary drainage system is also important (Newman, 2007). A break in the system can lead to the introduction of microorganisms. Locations at risk are the site of catheter insertion, the drainage bag, the spigot, the tube junction, and the junction of the tube and the bag (Figure 44–16).

In addition, you should monitor the patency of the system to prevent pooling of urine within the tubing. Bacteria can travel up drainage tubing to grow in pools of urine. If this urine flows back into the client's bladder, an infection will likely develop (Parkin & Keeley, 2003). Observe the client for symptoms of UTI and document any changes in his or her condition. Suggested methods to prevent infections in catheterized clients are provided in Box 44–10.

Catheter Irrigations and Instillations. To maintain patency of in-dwelling urinary catheters, at times you may need to irrigate or flush a catheter. Blood, pus, or sediment can collect within tubing and result in bladder distension and the buildup of stagnant urine. Instillation of a sterile solution ordered by the physician clears the tubing of accumulated material. For clients with bladder infections, a physician may order antiseptic or antibiotic bladder irrigations to

➤ BOX 44-9 Guidelines for Appropriate Catheter Selection

- The catheter size should be determined by the size of the client's urethral canal. When the French system is used, the larger the gauge number, the larger the catheter size. In general, an 8 to 10 Fr gauge is required for children, and a 14 to 16 Fr gauge is required for adults (Gray et al., 2006). The smallest effective catheter size is preferred to prevent trauma.
- After urologic procedures (prostatectomy), a 20 to 24 Fr three-lumen catheter is used to allow clot drainage and irrigation.
- The expected time required for catheterization will determine the catheter material selection (Teflon- or silicone-coated latex, 100% silicone, hydrophilic-coated latex).
- Plastic catheters are suitable only for intermittent use because of their inflexibility.
- Latex and rubber catheters are recommended for use up to three weeks. Be aware of client allergies to either of these materials.
- Pure silicone or Teflon catheters are best suited for long-term use (two to three months) because they cause less encrustation at the urethral meatus.
- Silicone catheters have larger interior lumens than those of other catheters of the same size and may allow for more efficient urine drainage.
- Hydrophilic-coated catheters may be more comfortable and less likely to inflame urethral tissue than are nonhydrophilic catheters; encrustation may develop more slowly (Gray, 2006).
- For clients who develop encrustations and blockages frequently, the use of an inexpensive catheter changed every 7 to 10 days (depending on their pattern of blockage) may be more economical.
- For short-term use, silver-hydrogel catheters and catheters with anti-infective surfaces are effective in delaying the onset of bacteriuria.
- Balloon size is also important to consider when selecting an in-dwelling catheter. Balloon sizes range from 3 mL (pediatric) to large postoperative volumes (30 mL). In adults, the 5-mL size allows for optimal drainage, whereas the 30-mL size is used after prostatectomies to provide hemostasis of the prostatic bed (Gray et al., 2006).
- Only sterile water should be used to inflate the balloon because saline may crystallize, resulting in incomplete deflation of the balloon at the time of removal.
- Urine leakage around the catheter may be due to bladder spasms secondary to constipation or fecal impaction, the use of a large catheter balloon (30 mL), the use of a large catheter (>18 Fr), the presence of the UTI, kinking of the catheter, or trauma at the bladder neck from traction on the balloon. A change in lumen size, the use of anticholinergic medication, or a referral to a urologist may be warranted.

➤ SKILL 44-2 Inserting a Straight or In-Dwelling Catheter

video

Delegation Considerations

Catheterization is usually not delegated to unregulated care providers (UCPs). However, in some settings, agency policy may permit this skill to be delegated to UCPs who have been properly instructed. UCPs routinely assist with positioning the client and maintaining client privacy and comfort, empty urine from the collection bag, and provide perineal care. If using an UCP, instruct him or her to inform you of the following:

- Client discomfort or fever
- Abnormal colour, odour, or amount of urine in drainage bag

Equipment

Catheterization kit containing the following sterile items:

- Gloves (extra pair optional)
- Drapes, one fenestrated
- Lubricant
- Antiseptic cleansing solution
- Cotton balls
- Forceps
- Prefilled syringe with sterile water to inflate the balloon of an in-dwelling catheter
- Catheter of correct size and type for procedure (i.e., intermittent or in-dwelling)
- Sterile drainage tubing with collection bag and multi-purpose tube holder or tape, safety pin, and elastic band for securing tubing to bed if client is bed bound (for an in-dwelling catheter)
- Receptacle or basin (usually bottom of catheterization tray)
- Specimen container
- Blanket

Procedure

STEPS	RATIONALE
1. Review client's medical record, including physician's order and nurses' notes.	• Determines purpose of inserting catheter: preparation for surgery, urinary irrigations, collection of sterile specimens, measurement of residual urine, and size and style of catheter. Assess for previous catheterization, including catheter size, response of client, and time of last catheterization.
2. Close bedside curtain or door.	• Offers privacy, reduces embarrassment, and aids in relaxation during procedure.
3. Assess status of client:	
A. Ask client when he or she last voided, or check intake and output flow sheet, or palpate bladder.	• Determines time of last voiding or potential for bladder fullness.
B. Level of awareness or developmental stage	• Reveals the client's ability to cooperate and the level of explanation needed.
C. Mobility and physical limitations of client	• Affects the way that the client is positioned.
D. Client's gender and age	• Determines catheter size: 8 to 10 Fr is generally used for children, 14 to 16 Fr is indicated for adults, 12 Fr may be considered for young girls.
E. Distended bladder	• Causes pain. Can indicate need to insert catheter if client is unable to void independently.
F. Perform hand hygiene. Apply clean gloves. Inspect perineum for erythema, drainage, and odour.	• Reduces infection. Determines condition of the perineum.
G. Any pathological condition that may impair passage of catheter (e.g., enlarged prostate in men)	• Obstruction prevents passage of catheter through urethra into the bladder. Use of coude catheter may be required.
H. Allergies	• Procedure risks exposure to antiseptic, tape, latex, and lubricant. Betadine allergies are common; if the client is unaware of allergy, ask if allergic to shellfish.
4. Assess client's knowledge of the purpose for catheterization.	• Reveals need for client instruction.
5. Explain procedure to client.	• Promotes cooperation.
6. Arrange for extra nursing personnel to assist as necessary.	• Client may be unable to assume positioning for procedure.
7. Perform hand hygiene.	• Reduces transmission of microorganisms.
8. Raise bed to appropriate working height.	• Promotes use of proper body mechanics.
9. Facing client, stand on left side of bed if right-handed (on right side of bed if left-handed). Clear the bedside table and arrange equipment.	• To insert catheter successfully, you must assume a comfortable position with all equipment easily accessible.
10. Raise side rail on opposite side of bed, and lower side rail on working side.	• Promotes client safety.
11. Place waterproof pad under client.	• Prevents soiling of bed linens.
12. Position client:	
A. Female client	
(1) Assist to dorsal recumbent position (supine with knees flexed). Ask client to relax thighs so that the hips can be rotated externally.	• Provides good visualization of perineal structures. Legs may be supported with pillows to reduce muscle tension and promote comfort.

Continued

➤ SKILL 44-2 Inserting a Straight or In-Dwelling Catheter *continued*

STEPS	RATIONALE
(2) Assist to side-lying (Sims') position with upper leg flexed at hip if unable to assume dorsal recumbent position. If this position is used, you must take extra precautions to cover rectal area with drape to reduce chance of cross-contamination.	• This alternative position is used if client cannot abduct legs at hip joint (e.g., if client has arthritic joints). Support client with pillows if necessary to maintain position.
B. Male client	
(1) Assist to supine position with thighs slightly abducted.	• Comfortable position for client that aids in visualization.
13. Drape client:	• Avoids unnecessary exposure of body parts and maintains client's comfort.
A. Female client (see Step 13A illustration)	
(1) Drape with bath blanket. Place blanket in diamond fashion over client, with one corner at client's midsection, side corners over each thigh and abdomen, and last corner over perineum.	
B. Male client (see Step 13B illustration)	
(1) Drape upper trunk with bath blanket and cover lower extremities with bedsheets, exposing only genitalia.	
14. Wearing disposable gloves, wash perineal area with soap and water as needed; dry thoroughly. Remove and discard gloves; perform hand hygiene.	• Reduces microorganisms near urethral meatus and allows further opportunity to visualize perineum and landmarks.
15. Position lamp to illuminate perineal area. (If you use a flashlight, have an assistant hold it.)	• Permits accurate identification and good visualization of urethral meatus.
16. Open package containing drainage system; place drainage bag over edge of bottom bed frame, and bring drainage tube up between side rails and mattress.	• Prepares system for eventual connection with catheter.

Critical Decision Point: This step is necessary only when an in-dwelling catheter is being inserted and a drainage system is not part of the catheterization kit.

STEPS	RATIONALE
17. Open catheterization kit according to directions, keeping bottom of container sterile.	• Prevents transmission of microorganisms from table or work area to sterile supplies. The materials in the kit are arranged in sequence of use.

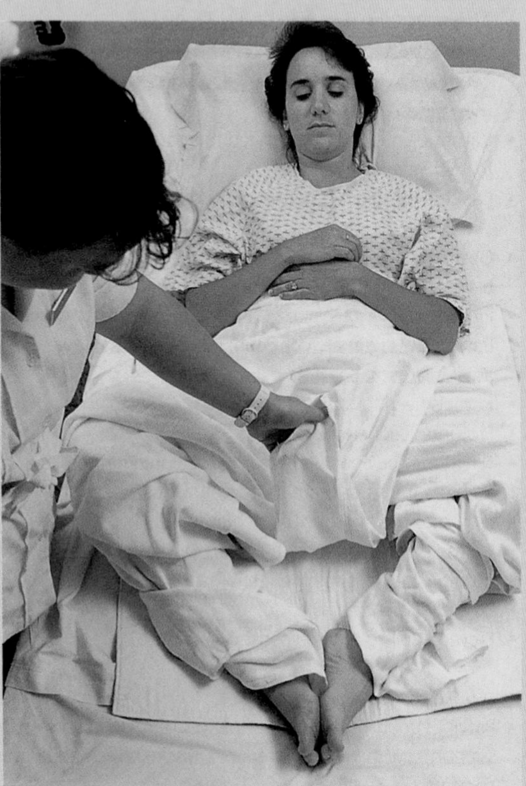

Step 13A Draping technique (female).

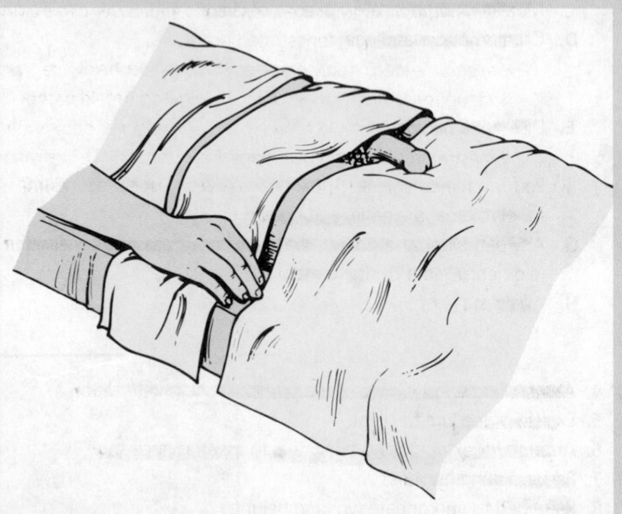

Step 13B Draping technique (male).

➤ SKILL 44-2 Inserting a Straight or In-Dwelling Catheter *continued*

STEPS	RATIONALE
18. Place plastic bag that contained kit within reach of work area to use as a waterproof bag in which used supplies can be disposed.	• Allows you to handle sterile supplies without contamination.
19. Apply sterile gloves (see Chapter 33).	

Critical Decision Point: If underpad is the first item in the catheterization kit, place pad plastic side down under client, touching only the edges so as to maintain sterility. Then apply sterile gloves.

STEPS	RATIONALE
20. Organize supplies on sterile field. Open inner sterile package containing catheter. Pour sterile antiseptic solution into correct compartment containing sterile cotton balls. Open packet containing lubricant. Remove specimen container (lid should be placed loosely on top) and prefilled syringe from collection compartment of tray, and set them aside on sterile field.	• Maintains principles of surgical asepsis and organizes work area. • Note: Pretesting of balloon is no longer recommended because catheters are pretested during manufacturing and inflation may distort the balloon, leading to increased trauma (Smith, 2006).
21. Before inserting an in-dwelling catheter, test balloon by injecting fluid from prefilled syringe into balloon port.	• Checks integrity of balloon. Do not use the catheter if the balloon does not inflate or leaks.
22. Lubricate 2.5 to 5 cm of catheter for women and 12.5 to 17.7 cm for men.	• Makes insertion of the catheter easier by decreasing friction.

Critical Decision Point: Some catheters have plastic sheaths over them that must be removed before lubrication. In some cases, the physician may order local anaesthetic lubricant.

STEPS	RATIONALE
23. Apply sterile drape:	
A. Female client	
(1) Allow top edge of drape to form a cuff over both gloved hands. Place drape on bed between client's thighs. Slip cuffed edge just under buttocks, taking care not to touch contaminated surface with gloves.	• Outer surface of drape covering hands remains sterile. Sterile drape against sterile gloves is sterile.
(2) Pick up fenestrated sterile drape and allow it to unfold without touching any unsterile objects. Apply drape over perineum, exposing labia and being sure not to touch contaminated surface.	• Maintains sterility of work surface.
B. Male client	
(1) Two methods are used for draping, depending on preference. *First method:* Apply drape over thighs and under penis without completely opening fenestrated drape. *Second method:* Apply drape over thighs just below penis. Pick up fenestrated sterile drape, allow it to unfold without touching any unsterile objects, and drape it over penis with fenestrated slit resting over penis (see Step 23B(1) illustration).	• Maintains sterility of work surface.

Step 23B(1) Draping male with fenestrated drape.

Continued

➤ SKILL 44-2 Inserting a Straight or In-Dwelling Catheter *continued*

STEPS	RATIONALE
24. Place sterile tray and contents on sterile drape. Open specimen container.	• Provides easy access to supplies during catheter insertion. Maintains aseptic technique during procedure.
25. Cleanse urethral meatus:	
A. Female client	
(1) With nondominant hand, carefully retract labia to fully expose urethral meatus. Maintain position of nondominant hand throughout procedure.	• Full visualization of urethral meatus is provided. Full retraction prevents contamination of urethral meatus during cleansing.
(2) Using forceps held in sterile dominant hand, pick up cotton ball saturated with antiseptic solution and clean perineal area, wiping from clitoris toward anus (front to back). Using a new cotton ball for each area, wipe along the far labial fold, near labial fold, and directly over centre of urethral meatus (see Step 25A(2) illustration).	• Cleansing reduces number of microorganisms at urethral meatus. Use of a single cotton ball for each wipe prevents transfer of microorganisms. Cleansing for each of the three areas proceeds from area of least contamination to that of most contamination. Dominant hand remains sterile.

Critical Decision Point: If the labia close during cleansing, then the cleansing procedure must be repeated because the area has become contaminated.

STEPS	RATIONALE
B. Male client	
(1) If client is not circumcised, retract foreskin with nondominant hand. Grasp penis at shaft just below glans. Retract urethral meatus between thumb and forefinger. Maintain nondominant hand in this position throughout procedure.	• If foreskin is accidentally released or if penis is dropped during cleansing, the process must be repeated because the area has become contaminated.
(2) With sterile dominant hand, pick up cotton ball with forceps and clean penis. Move in a circular motion from urethral meatus down to base of glans. Repeat cleansing three more times, using a clean cotton ball each time (see Step 25B(2) illustration).	• Cleansing reduces number of microorganisms at urethral meatus and proceeds from area of least contamination to that of most contamination. Dominant hand remains sterile.

Critical Decision Point: If the foreskin does not remain retracted during cleansing, then the cleansing procedure must be repeated because the area has become contaminated.

STEPS	RATIONALE
26. Pick up catheter with gloved dominant hand, 7.5 to 10 cm from catheter tip. Hold end of catheter loosely coiled in palm of dominant hand. (Optional: May grasp catheter with forceps.)	• Use the dominant hand so that you can manipulate the catheter more readily.
27. Insert catheter:	
A. Female client	
(1) Ask client to bear down gently as if voiding, and slowly insert catheter through urethral meatus (see Step 27A(1) illustration).	• Relaxation of urethral sphincter and pelvic floor muscle aids in insertion of catheter.

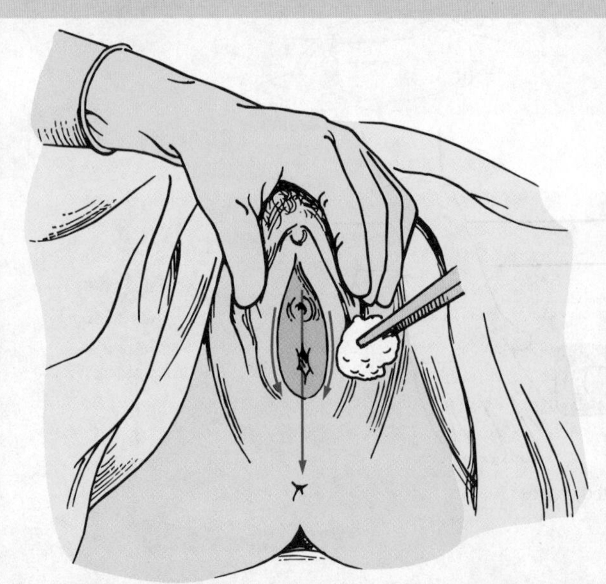

Step 25A(2) Cleansing technique (female).

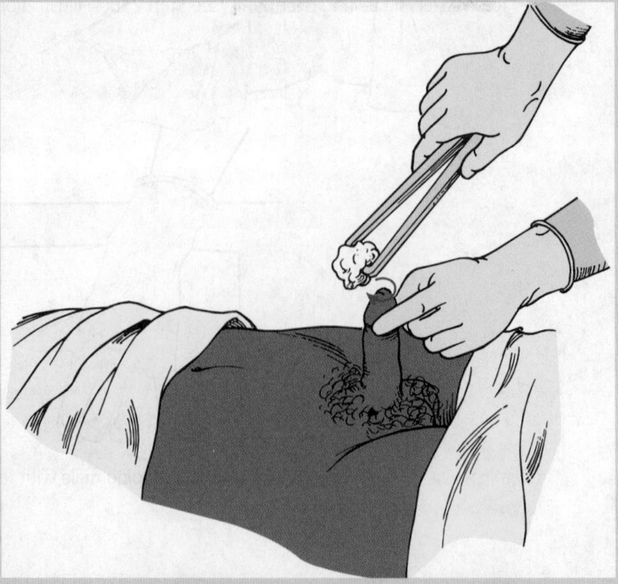

Step 25B(2) Cleansing technique (male).

➤ SKILL 44-2 Inserting a Straight or In-Dwelling Catheter *continued*

STEPS	RATIONALE
(2) Advance catheter a total of 5 to 7.5 cm in adult female or until urine flows out of catheter's end. When urine appears, advance catheter another 2.5 to 5 cm. *Do not force against resistance.*	• Female urethra is short. Appearance of urine indicates that the catheter tip is in bladder or lower urethra. Further advancement of catheter ensures bladder placement.
(3) Release labia and hold catheter securely with nondominant hand. Slowly inflate balloon if in-dwelling catheter is being used (see Step 27A(3) illustrations; see Step 30).	• Catheter may be expelled accidentally by bladder or sphincter contraction.

Critical Decision Point: If no urine appears, check whether catheter is in vagina. If misplaced, leave catheter in vagina as landmark indicating where not to insert, and insert another through urethral meatus.

STEPS	RATIONALE
B. Male client	
(1) Lift penis to position perpendicular to client's body and apply light traction (see Step 27B(1) illustration).	• Straightens urethral canal to ease catheter insertion.
(2) Ask client to bear down as if voiding, and slowly insert catheter through urethral meatus.	• Relaxation of urethral sphincter and pelvic floor muscle aids in insertion of catheter.
(3) Advance catheter 17 to 22.5 cm in adult male or until urine flows out of catheter's end. If resistance is felt, withdraw catheter; do not force it through urethra. When urine appears, advance catheter another 2.5 to 5 cm. *Do not use force against resistance.*	• The adult male urethra is long. It is normal to meet resistance at the prostate. When resistance is felt, you should hold the catheter firmly without forcing it. After a few seconds, the muscle relaxes and the catheter is advanced. Appearance of urine indicates that the catheter tip is in bladder or urethra. Advancement of the catheter to the bifurcation ensures proper placement.
(4) Lower penis and hold catheter securely in nondominant hand. Place end of catheter in urine tray. Inflate balloon if in-dwelling catheter is being used (see step 30).	• Catheter may be expelled accidentally by bladder or urethral contraction. Collection of urine prevents soiling and provides output measurement.
(5) Reduce (or reposition) the foreskin.	• Paraphimosis (retraction and constriction of the foreskin behind the glans penis) secondary to catheterization may occur if foreskin is not reduced.

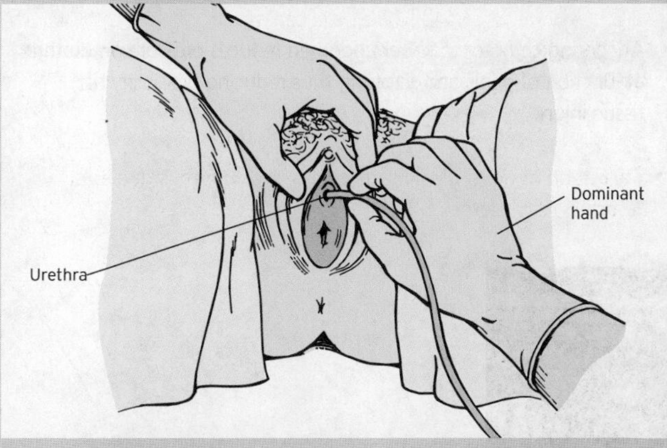

Step 27A(1) Inserting the catheter.

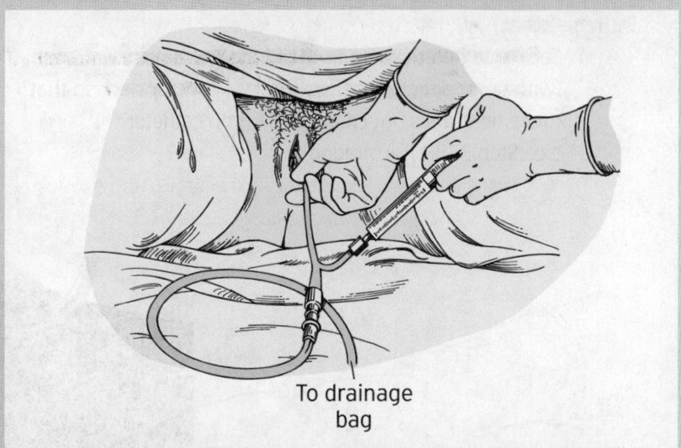

Step 27A(3) **A,** Inflating the balloon (in-dwelling catheter).

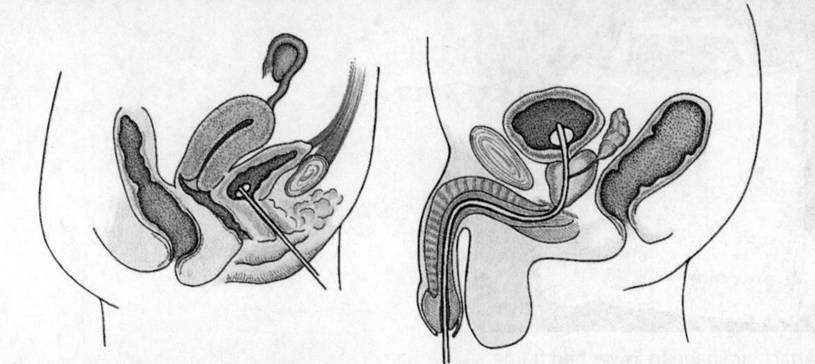

Step 27A(3) **B,** Placement of inflated balloon in bladder.

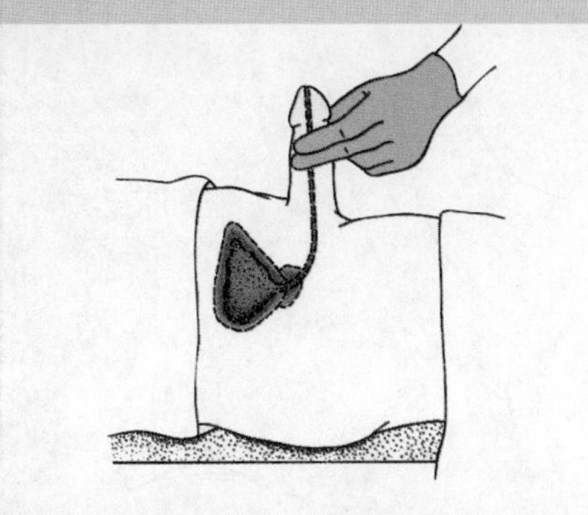

Step 27B(1) Position penis perpendicular to body for catheter insertion.

Continued

➤ SKILL 44-2 Inserting a Straight or In-Dwelling Catheter ***continued***

STEPS	RATIONALE
28. Collect urine specimen as needed. Fill specimen cup or jar to desired level (20–30 mL) by holding end of catheter over cup with your dominant hand.	• Allows sterile specimen to be obtained for culture analysis.
29. Allow bladder to empty fully (about 800 to 1000 mL) unless institution policy restricts maximal volume of urine to drain with each catheterization. Check institution policy before beginning catheterization.	• As always, you should monitor the client's condition; if the vital signs change or bleeding occurs, temporarily stop the flow of urine and continue when the client's condition warrants. Retained urine may serve as a reservoir for growth of microorganisms.

Critical Decision Point: If a single-use straight catheter was inserted, withdraw it slowly but smoothly until it is removed.

STEPS	RATIONALE
30. Inflate balloon fully per manufacturer's recommendation and then release catheter with nondominant hand and pull gently.	• Inflation of balloon anchors the catheter tip in place above the bladder outlet to prevent the catheter's removal. Note size of balloon on catheter. Most commonly, a 5-mL balloon is used, but a 30-mL balloon may be ordered in some cases. A prefilled syringe may be included with the kit. Use only the amount included. Do not overinflate the balloon. A 5-mL balloon should be inflated with the supplied amount (10 mL) to allow symmetrical expansion (Smith, 2006).

Critical Decision Point: If resistance to inflation is noted or if client complains of pain, the balloon may not be entirely within the bladder. Stop inflation, aspirate the fluid injected into the balloon, and advance the catheter a little more before attempting to inflate the balloon again.

STEPS	RATIONALE
31. Attach end of in-dwelling catheter to collecting tube of drainage system. Drainage bag must be below level of bladder. Attach bag to bed frame; do not place bag on bed's side rails (see Step 31 illustration).	• In-dwelling catheters drain the bladder by gravity. Attaching to the bed frame prevents accidental pulling of the catheter when a bed rail is lowered.
32. Anchor catheter:	
A. Female client	
(1) Secure catheter tubing to inner thigh or abdomen with a strip of nonallergenic tape (or multi-purpose tube holders with a Velcro strap). Allow for slack so that movement of thigh does not create tension on catheter (see Step 32A(1) illustration).	• Anchoring catheter to inner thigh reduces pressure on urethra, thus reducing possibility of tissue injury.
B. Male client	
(1) Secure catheter tubing to top of thigh or lower abdomen (with penis directed toward chest). Allow for slack so that movement does not create tension on catheter (see Step 32B(1) illustration).	• Anchoring catheter to lower abdomen reduces pressure on urethra at junction of penis and scrotum, thus reducing possibility of tissue injury.

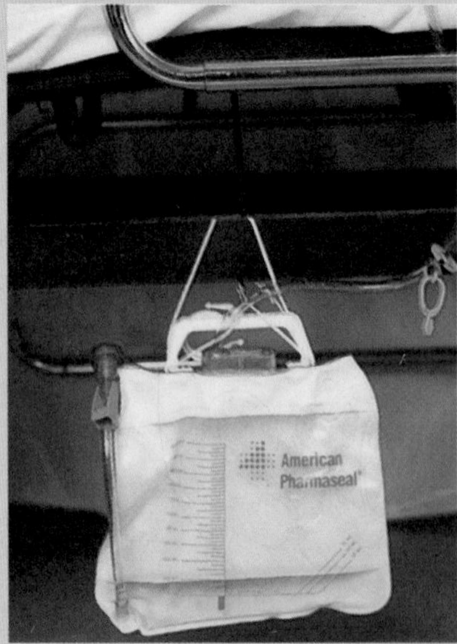

Step 31 Attach drainage to lower bed frame.

➤ SKILL 44-2 Inserting a Straight or In-Dwelling Catheter *continued*

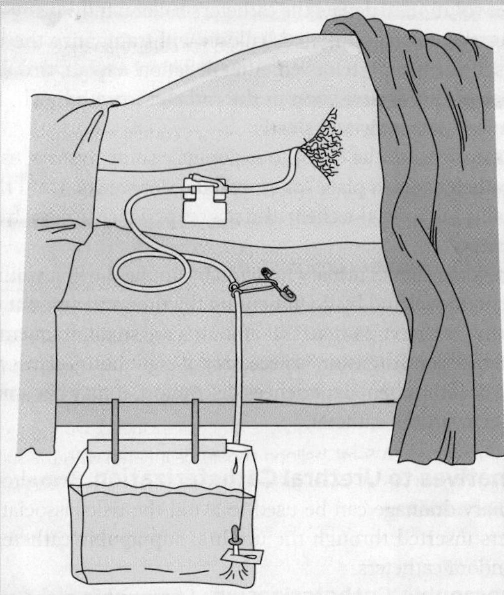

Step 32A(1) Tape catheter to inner thigh (female) and coil extra tubing on bed and attach to sheet. **Source:** From Sorrentino, S. A., Wilk, M. J., & Newmaster, R. (2008). *Mosby's Canadian textbook for the support worker* (2nd ed., p. 592, Figure 31–11A). Toronto: Elsevier.

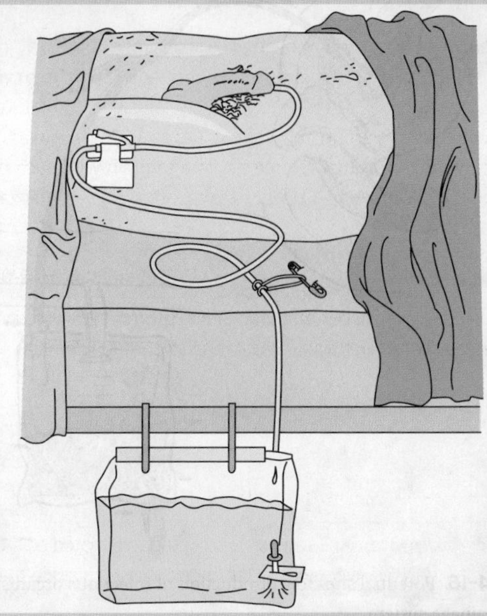

Step 32B(1) Tape catheter to lower thigh (male) and coil extra tubing on bed and attach to sheet. **Source:** From Sorrentino, S. A., Wilk, M. J., & Newmaster, R. (2008). *Mosby's Canadian textbook for the support worker* (2nd ed., p. 592, Figure 31–11B). Toronto: Elsevier.

Critical Decision Point: Be sure that the tubing has no obstructions. Coil excess tubing on bed and fasten it to the bottom sheet with clip from kit, or use rubber band and safety pin.

STEPS	RATIONALE
33. Assist client to comfortable position. Wash and dry perineal area as needed.	• Maintains comfort and security.
34. Remove gloves and dispose of equipment, drapes, and urine in proper receptacles.	• Reduces transmission of microorganisms.
35. Perform hand hygiene.	• Reduces transmission of microorganisms.
36. Palpate bladder.	• Determines whether distension has been relieved.
37. Ask about client's comfort.	• Determines whether client's sensation of discomfort or fullness has been relieved.
38. Observe character and amount of urine in drainage system.	• Determines whether urine is flowing adequately.
39. Ensure that no urine is leaking from catheter or tubing connections.	• Prevents injury to client's skin.

Unexpected Outcomes and Related Interventions

Urethral or Perineal Irritation

- Observe for leaking catheter; replace if necessary.
- Assess whether in-dwelling catheter is anchored properly.
- Perform perineal hygiene and catheter care more frequently.

Fever or Odour, or Small Frequent Voidings, Burning Sensations, or Bleeding on Voiding

- Obtain clean voided urine specimen.
- Notify physician.

Urinary Retention and Inability to Void After Catheter Is Removed

- Provide adequate fluid intake and ensure client privacy.
- If client is unable to void six to eight hours after catheter removal, notify physician.

Recording and Reporting

- Report and record type and size of catheter inserted, amount of fluid used to inflate the balloon, characteristics of urine, amount of urine, reasons for catheterization, specimen collection if appropriate, and client's response to procedure and teaching concepts.
- Initiate intake and output record.
- If catheter is definitely in bladder and no urine is produced within 1 hour, absence of urine should be reported to physician immediately.

Home Care Considerations

- Clients who are at home may use a leg bag during the day and switch to a large-volume bag at night so that sleep can be uninterrupted.
- Clients may catheterize themselves at home, using a clean technique.

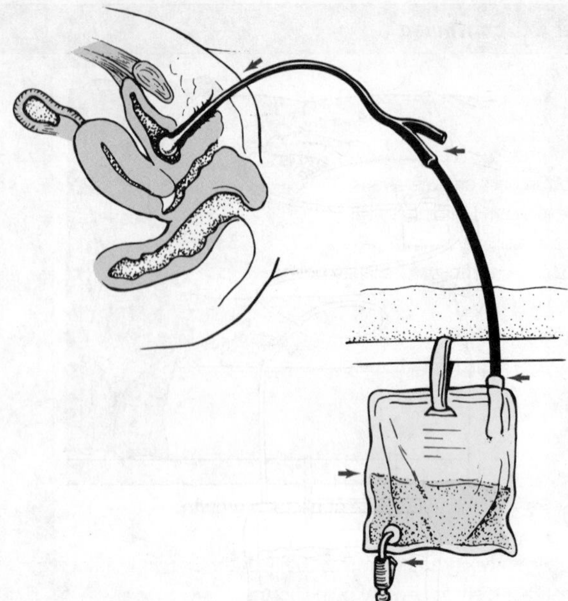

Figure 44-16 Potential sites for introduction of infectious organisms into a urinary drainage system.

wash out the bladder or treat local infection. In both types of irrigation, the sterile aseptic technique is followed.

Before performing catheter irrigation, assess the catheter for blockage. If the amount of urine in the drainage bag is less than the client's intake or less than the output during the previous shift, blockage can be expected. If urine does not drain freely, you may milk the tubing. Milking is done by gently squeezing and then releasing the drainage tube, starting from the client's body and working toward the drainage bag so that a clot or sediment will not be forced back into the catheter.

Maintenance of a closed system is recommended during intermittent irrigations or instillations. This technique is effective for irrigating a partially blocked catheter or for bladder instillations. A single intermittent irrigation is safer and less likely to introduce infections into the urinary tract than repeated irrigations. Two additional methods for catheter irrigation exist. The first is a closed bladder irrigation 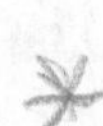 system (Skill 44–4), which provides for frequent intermittent irrigations or continuous irrigation without disruption of the sterile catheter system through use of a three-way catheter. This method is used most often in clients who have had genitourinary surgery and are at risk for blood clots and mucus fragments occluding the catheter. The second system involves opening the closed drainage system to instill bladder irrigations (see Skill 44–4). This technique poses greater risk of infection. However, it may be needed when a catheter becomes blocked and it is undesirable to change the catheter (e.g., after recent bladder or prostate surgery).

Removal of In-Dwelling Catheter. When removing an in-dwelling catheter, you promote normal bladder function and prevent trauma to the urethra.

To remove a catheter, you need a clean, disposable towel; a discard receptacle; a sterile syringe that is the same size as the volume of solution within the catheter's inflated balloon; and disposable gloves. The end of the catheter contains a label that denotes the volume of solution (5 to 30 mL) within the balloon.

Assist the client into the same position as during catheterization. Some institutions recommend collecting a sterile urine specimen at this time or sending the catheter tip for culture and sensitivity tests. After removing the tape that holds the catheter in place, put a towel between a female client's thighs or over a male client's thighs. Insert the syringe into the injection port. Most ports are self-sealing and require that only the tip of the syringe be inserted. Slowly withdraw all of the solution to deflate the catheter's balloon fully. If any solution remains, the partially inflated balloon will traumatize the urethral canal as the catheter is removed. After deflation, explain that the client may feel a burning sensation as the catheter is withdrawn. Pull the catheter out smoothly and slowly.

It is normal for the client to experience some dysuria, especially if the catheter was in place for several days or weeks. Until the bladder regains full tone, the client also may experience urinary frequency or retention.

Assess the client's urinary function by noting the first voiding after catheter removal and by documenting the time and amount of voiding during the next 24 hours. If amounts are small, frequent assessment of bladder distension is necessary. If eight hours elapse without voiding or if the client experiences discomfort, it may become necessary to reinsert the catheter.

Alternatives to Urethral Catheterization. Two alternatives for urinary drainage can be used to avoid the risks associated with catheters inserted through the urethra: suprapubic catheterization and condom catheters.

Suprapubic Catheterization. Suprapubic catheterization involves surgical placement of a catheter through the abdominal wall above the symphysis pubis and into the urinary bladder. A physician performs the procedure under local or general anaesthesia. The catheter is anchored in place with sutures, a commercially prepared body seal, or both. Urine drains into a urinary drainage bag. Maintenance of the tubing and drainage bag is the same as for an in-dwelling catheter. The suprapubic catheter is relatively painless and reduces the incidence of infection commonly seen with in-dwelling catheters. Studies comparing the use of this method of

➤ BOX 44-10 Preventing Infection in Catheterized Clients

- Use appropriate hand-hygiene techniques (see Chapter 33).
- Do not allow the spigot on the drainage system to touch a contaminated surface.
- Use only the sterile technique to collect specimens from a closed drainage system.
- If the drainage tube becomes disconnected, wipe the ends of both the tubing and the catheter with an antimicrobial solution before reconnecting.
- Ensure that each client has his or her own separate receptacle for measuring urine to prevent cross-contamination.
- Ensure that urine does not pool in the tubing and cause reflux of urine into the bladder.
- If it is necessary to raise the bag during transfer of the client to a bed or stretcher, clamp the tubing until the transfer is complete.
- Ensure drainage of urine from the tubing to the bag by proper positioning the tubing.
- Ensure that prolonged kinking or clamping of the tubing does not occur.
- Empty the drainage bag at least every eight hours and record output. If large outputs are noted, empty the bag more frequently.
- Encourage the client to maintain fluid intake (if not contraindicated).
- Remove the catheter as soon as clinically warranted (Fernandez & Griffiths, 2006).
- Tape or secure the catheter appropriately for the client (see Skill 44–2).
- Perform routine perineal hygiene per agency policy and after defecation or bowel incontinence (see Skill 44–3).

➤ SKILL 44-3 In-Dwelling Catheter Care

video

Delegation Considerations

Perineal care is often part of routine hygiene care that is delegated to unregulated care providers (UCPs). Proper assessment and care of the perineal area requires professional clinical judgement. If the client has had trauma or surgical procedures that involve the perineal area, care of this area should not be delegated.

- Instruct the UCP to report any client discomfort, perineal pain, perineal discharge, or odour to a nurse.

Equipment

- Catheter care kit or individual supplies
- Disposable gloves
- Cotton balls or large swabs
- Clean washcloth and towel
- Warm water and soap
- Antibiotic ointment (if agency policy)
- Bath blanket
- Waterproof absorbent pad

Procedure

STEPS	RATIONALE
1. Assess for episode of bowel incontinence or client discomfort or provide care as per agency routine regarding hygiene measures (see Chapter 38).	• Accumulation of secretions or feces causes irritation to perineal tissues and acts as a source of bacterial growth.
2. Explain procedure to client. Offer the able client an opportunity to perform self-care.	• Reduces anxiety and promotes cooperation. Embarrassment may motivate client to perform own hygiene.
3. Close door or bedside curtain.	• Maintains client privacy.
4. Perform hand hygiene.	• Reduces transmission of infection.
5. Position client: A. Female client (1) Dorsal recumbent position B. Male client (1) Supine or Fowler's position	• Ensures easy access to perineal tissues.
6. Place waterproof pad under client.	• Prevents soiling of bed linens.
7. Drape bath blanket over client so that only perineal area is exposed.	• Prevents unnecessary exposure of body parts.
8. Apply gloves.	
9. Remove anchor device to free catheter tubing.	
10. With nondominant hand: A. Female client (1) Gently retract labia to expose urethral meatus and catheter insertion site fully, maintaining position of hand throughout procedure.	• Provides full visualization of urethral meatus. Full retraction prevents contamination of urethral meatus during cleansing.
B. Male client (1) Retract foreskin if not circumcised, and hold penis at shaft just below glans, maintaining position throughout procedure.	• If foreskin is accidentally released or penis is dropped during cleansing, the process must be repeated because the area has become contaminated.
11. Assess urethral meatus and surrounding tissue for inflammation, swelling, and discharge. Note amount, colour, odour, and consistency of discharge. Ask client if any burning or discomfort has been experienced.	• Determines presence of local infection and status of hygiene.
12. Cleanse perineal tissue: A. Female client (1) Use clean cloth and perineal cleanser. Cleanse around urethral meatus and catheter. Moving from pubis toward anus, clean labia minora. Use a clean side of the cloth for each wipe. Finally, clean around anus. Dry each area well.	• Reduces the number of microorganisms at the urethral meatus. Use of a clean cloth prevents transfer of microorganisms.
B. Male client (1) While spreading urethral meatus, cleanse around catheter first, and then wipe in circular motion around meatus and glans.	• Cleansing moves from area of least contamination to that of most contamination.
13. Reassess urethral meatus for discharge.	• Determines whether cleansing is complete.
14. With towel and perineal cleanser, wipe in a circular motion along length of catheter for 10 cm.	• Reduces presence of secretions or drainage on exterior surface of catheter.
15. In male client, reduce (or reposition) the foreskin.	• Prevents trauma to the head of the penis.
16. Reanchor catheter tubing.	• Prevents trauma to the urethra.
17. Place client in a safe, comfortable position.	• Promotes comfort.
18. Dispose of contaminated supplies, remove gloves, and perform hand hygiene.	• Prevents spread of infection.

Continued

➤SKILL 44-3 In-Dwelling Catheter Care *continued*

Unexpected Outcomes and Related Interventions

Urethral Discharge

- Increase frequency of in-dwelling catheter care.
- Apply topical antibiotic ointment per agency policy.
- Notify physician.
- Assess for urethral trauma.
- Monitor urine output.

Recording and Reporting

- Report and record the presence and characteristics of drainage, the condition of the perineal tissue, and any discomfort reported by the client.
- If infection is suspected, report your findings to a physician.

Home Care Considerations

- If client is discharged with an in-dwelling catheter in place, the client and family should be taught catheter care as well as educated about the signs and symptoms that should be reported to a nurse or physician.

urinary drainage have shown mixed results. While infection rates may be slightly lower, the long-term complications are similar (Doughty, 2006). Sediment, clots, encrustations, or the abdominal wall itself can block the suprapubic catheter. Adequate fluid intake will help minimize the risk of blockage by sediment or infection due to stagnation. The suprapubic catheter must remain patent at all times. You must monitor the client's intake and output carefully, monitor the appearance of urine, and observe for signs of infection (e.g., fever and chills). You also should administer skin care around the insertion site.

Condom Catheters. The second alternative to catheterization is the condom catheter (external urinary catheter; Box 44–11), which may be suitable for incontinent or comatose men who still have complete and spontaneous bladder emptying. The condom is a soft, pliable, rubber sheath that slips over the penis. It may be worn at night only or continuously, depending on the client's needs. One method used to secure the condom catheter involves a strip of elastic tape or rubber that encircles the top of the condom to hold it in place. An alternative is to use a self-adhesive condom sheath. Care must be taken to ensure that whatever type or size of condom is used, blood supply to the penis is not impaired. Standard adhesive tape should never be used to secure a condom catheter because this tape does not expand with changes in penis size and is painful to remove.

The end of the condom is attached to plastic drainage tubing that can be attached to the side of the bed or strapped to the client's leg. The condom catheter itself poses little risk of infection. Infections usually result from buildup of secretions around the urethra, trauma to the urethral meatus, or buildup of pressure in the outflow tubing. Condom catheters must be applied and changed according the manufacturers' directions to prevent abrasion, dermatitis, ischemia, necrosis, edema, and maceration of the penis. Frequent skin assessment is vital.

If the condom catheter is made of opaque material, you should remove it daily to check for skin irritation. Some new condom catheters are transparent, and the skin may be observed through them more easily. During each catheter change, thoroughly clean the urethral meatus and penis. The drainage tubing must be checked often for patency.

For a man with a retracted penis, maintaining a conventional condom catheter may prove difficult. Special devices are available to help alleviate this problem (Figure 44–17). Manufacturer's guidelines for product application should be consulted.

No collection devices for women are as effective as the condom catheter is for men; usually the only incontinence devices used are pads and protective clothing. To maintain the client's dignity, pads and protective clothing should not be referred to as adult diapers, and they should be changed frequently to control odour. These devices should be used only temporarily to minimize or prevent episodes of incontinence while treatment is ongoing. Clients should be monitored frequently and good skin care should be provided to prevent irritation caused by urine.

Maintenance of Skin Integrity. Urine is irritating to skin and when in continuous contact with the skin becomes alkaline, causing dermatitis and skin breakdown. Continuous exposure of the perineal area or skin around an ostomy leads to gradual maceration and excoriation (see Chapter 47). Washing with pH-balanced soap and warm water is the best way to remove urine. Body lotion keeps skin moisturized and petroleum-based ointments provide a barrier to urine. Clients who soil their clothing should receive partial baths and dry clothing and bed linens immediately after voiding. If the skin becomes irritated or inflamed, the physician may prescribe a cream or spray containing steroids to reduce inflammation. If fungal growth develops, the antifungal drug nystatin, available in cream or powder, is effective.

Promotion of Comfort. Clients with urinary alterations become uncomfortable as a result of the symptoms of urinary problems. Frequent or unpredictable voiding, dysuria, and painful distension are all sources of discomfort.

If the client has local discomfort, a warm sitz bath may soothe inflamed tissues near the urethral meatus by improving blood supply. The client is often relaxed after a sitz bath, and voiding occurs easily. Pain due to distension cannot be relieved unless the client is able to empty the bladder. Interventions that stimulate micturition or intermittent catheterization may be the only sources of pain relief.

Conservative Therapies to Restore Bladder Control and Promote Continence

The following therapies can help incontinent clients of all ages to maintain and regain control over urination:

- Pelvic floor muscle exercises to strengthen the pelvic floor.
- Initiating a voiding schedule.
- Using methods to initiate voiding (e.g., running water and stroking the inner thigh).
- Using relaxation techniques to aid complete bladder emptying (e.g., reading and deep breathing).
- Never ignoring the urge to void (if urinary problem involves infrequent voidings that result in retention).
- Minimizing ingestion of tea, coffee, other caffeinated drinks, and alcohol.
- Taking prescribed diuretic medication or fluids that increase diuresis (such as tea or coffee) early in the morning.
- Progressively lengthening or shortening periods between voiding as appropriate for control of specific cause of incontinence.
- Offering protective undergarments to contain urine and to reduce the client's embarrassment (not diapers).
- Following a weight-control program if obesity is a problem.

➤ SKILL 44-4 Closed and Open Catheter Irrigation

Delegation Considerations

Although closed catheter irrigation poses less risk of infection, neither closed nor open catheter irrigation is usually delegated to unregulated care providers (UCPs). Catheter irrigation is usually done in clients with complications such as UTIs or after a prostatectomy.

- UCPs may assist with other aspects of client care, such as positioning the client and measuring intake and output.
- Instruct the UCP to report any complaints of pain, discomfort, or fever to a nurse.
- Instruct the UCP to report the presence of clots in the output or a change in output to a nurse.

Equipment

- When using the closed intermittent method:
  - Sterile irrigation solution at room temperature
  - Sterile graduated container
  - Sterile 30- to 50-mL syringe
  - Sterile 19- to 22-gauge 2.5-cm needle
  - Antiseptic swab
  - Clamp for catheter or tubing
  - Bath blanket
- When using the closed continuous method:
  - Sterile irrigation solution at room temperature
  - Irrigation tubing and clamp (with or without Y connector)
  - IV pole
  - Y connector (optional)
  - Antiseptic swab
  - Bath blanket
- When using the open method:
  - Sterile irrigation set with tray
  - Bulb syringe or 60-mL piston-type syringe
  - Sterile collection basin
  - Waterproof drape
  - Sterile solution container
  - Antiseptic swabs
  - Sterile gloves
  - Sterile correct irrigation solution at room temperature
  - Tape or elastic band to resecure catheter
  - Bath blanket

Procedure

STEPS	RATIONALE
1. Assess physician's order for type of irrigation and irrigation solution to use.	• Ensures proper selection of equipment.
2. Assess colour of urine and presence of mucus or sediment.	• Determines whether client is bleeding, has infection, or is sloughing tissue.
3. Determine type of catheter in place:	
A. Triple lumen (one lumen to inflate balloon, one to instill irrigation solution, one to allow outflow of urine).	• Triple lumen is for closed continuous irrigation.
B. Double lumen (one lumen to inflate balloon, one to allow outflow of urine).	• Double lumen is for closed intermittent or open irrigation.
4. Determine patency of drainage tubing.	• Ensures that drainage tubing is not kinked, clamped incorrectly, or looped.
5. Assess amount of urine in drainage bag (may want to empty drainage bag before irrigation).	• If drainage bag is not empty, you will need to subtract urine volume from the amount drained to determine whether all irrigant has returned.
6. Explain procedure and purpose to client.	• Helps client relax and cooperate during procedure.
7. Perform hand hygiene and apply disposable gloves for closed methods.	• Prevents transmission of microorganisms.
8. Provide privacy by pulling bed curtains closed. Fold back covers so that the catheter is exposed. Cover client's upper torso with bath blanket.	• Promotes client comfort.
9. Assess lower abdomen for bladder distension.	• Detects whether catheter is malfunctioning or blocking urinary drainage.
10. Position client in dorsal recumbent or supine position.	• Promotes client comfort and provides easy access to catheter. • Promotes flow of irrigating solution into bladder.
11. *Closed intermittent irrigation (with double-lumen catheter):*	
A. Prepare prescribed sterile solution in sterile graduated cup.	• Ensures that irrigating fluid remains sterile.
B. Draw sterile solution into syringe by using aseptic technique.	

Critical Decision Point: Avoid cold solution as irrigant because it may cause bladder spasm and discomfort.

STEPS	RATIONALE
C. Clamp in-dwelling catheter just distal to soft injection (specimen) port.	• Occlusion of catheter provides resistance against which irrigant can be forcefully instilled into catheter.
D. Cleanse injection port with antiseptic swab (same port used for specimen collection).	• Reduces transmission of infection.
E. Insert needle of syringe through port at 30-degree angle toward bladder.	• Ensures that needle tip enters lumen of catheter and flow is directed into bladder.

Continued

➤SKILL 44-4 Closed and Open Catheter Irrigation *continued*

STEPS	RATIONALE
F. Slowly inject fluid into catheter and bladder.	• Slow, continuous pressure dislodges clots and sediment without traumatizing the bladder wall.

Critical Decision Point: If catheter does not irrigate easily, the tip may be incorrectly placed in the urethra and not in the bladder. Use slow pressure when injecting fluid. Too much pressure may traumatize the urethal or bladder wall.

G. Withdraw syringe, remove clamp, and allow solution to drain into drainage bag. If ordered by physician, keep clamped to allow solution to remain in bladder for a short time (20 to 30 minutes).	• Allows drainage by gravity.

Critical Decision Point: If solution is to remain in bladder, do not forget to unclamp tubing at the end of the instillation period.

12. *Closed continuous irrigation (with triple-lumen catheter)* (see Step 12 illustration):

A. Using the aseptic technique, insert tip of sterile irrigation tubing into bag of sterile irrigating solution.	• Prevents entrance of microorganisms.
B. Close clamp on tubing and hang bag of solution on IV pole.	
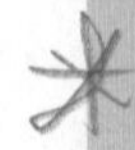 C. Open clamp and allow solution to flow through tubing, keeping end of tubing sterile. Close clamp.	• Removes air from tubing.
D. Wipe off irrigation port of triple-lumen catheter, or attach sterile Y connector to double-lumen catheter and then attach to irrigation tubing.	• Third lumen or Y connector provides means for irrigation solution to enter bladder. System must remain sterile.
E. Be sure that drainage bag and tubing are securely connected to drainage port of triple-lumen catheter or other arm of Y connector.	• Ensures that urine and irrigation solution will drain from bladder.
F. For intermittent flow, clamp tubing on drainage system, open clamp on irrigation tubing, and allow prescribed amount of fluid to enter bladder (100 mL is normal for adults). Close irrigation clamp and then open drainage tubing clamp. (Optional: Leave clamp closed for 20 to 30 minutes if ordered. See previous critical decision point.)	• Fluid instills through catheter into bladder, flushing system. Fluid drains out after irrigation is completed.

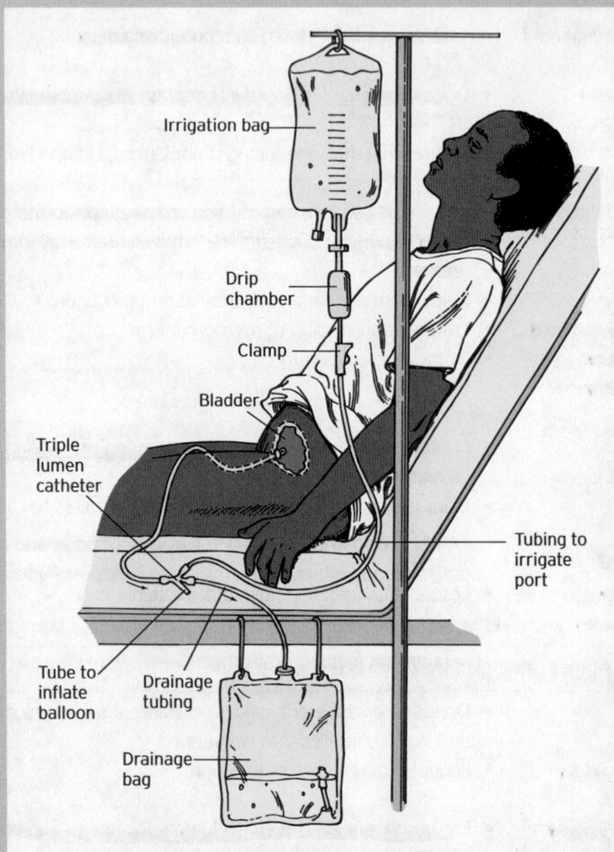

Step 12 Closed continuous bladder irrigation.

➤ SKILL 44-4 Closed and Open Catheter Irrigation *continued*

STEPS	RATIONALE
G. For continuous drainage, calculate drip rate and adjust clamp on irrigation tubing accordingly. Be sure that clamp on drainage tubing is open and check volume of drainage in drainage bag. Ensure that drainage tubing is patent, and avoid kinks.	• Ensures continuous, even irrigation of catheter system. • Prevents accumulation of solution in bladder, which may cause bladder distension and possible injury.
13. *Open irrigation (with double-lumen catheter):*	
A. Open sterile irrigation tray, establish sterile field, pour required volume of sterile solution into sterile container, and replace cap on large container of solution.	• Adheres to principles of surgical asepsis (see Chapter 33).
B. Apply sterile gloves.	• Reduces transmission of infection.
C. Position sterile waterproof drape under catheter.	• Prevents soiling of bed linens.
D. Aspirate 30 mL of solution into sterile irrigating syringe.	• Prepares irrigant for instillation into catheter.
E. Move sterile collection close to client's thighs.	• Prevents soiling of bed linens and prohibits reaching over sterile field.
F. Disconnect catheter from drainage tubing, allowing urine from catheter to flow into collection basin. Allow urine in tubing to flow into drainage bag. Cover end of tubing with sterile protective cap. Position tubing in a safe place.	• Maintains sterility of inner aspect of catheter and drainage tubing and reduces potential of introducing pathogens into bladder.
G. Insert tip of syringe into catheter lumen, and gently instill solution.	• Gentle instillation reduces incidence of bladder spasm but clears catheter of obstruction.

Critical Decision Point: If resistance is noted, do not force the irrigation.

STEPS	RATIONALE
H. Withdraw syringe, lower catheter, and allow solution to drain into basin. Repeat instillation until prescribed solution has been used or until drainage is clear (will depend on purpose of irrigation).	• Allows drainage to flow by gravity. Provides for adequate flushing of catheter.
I. If solution does not return, have client turn onto his or her side facing you. If changing position does not help, reinsert syringe and gently aspirate solution.	• Change of position may move catheter tip in bladder, increasing likelihood that instilled fluid will flow out.
J. After irrigation is complete, remove protector cap from tubing, cleanse end with alcohol swab (or recommended agency solution), and re-establish drainage system.	• Reduces entrance of microorganisms into system.
14. Reanchor catheter to client with tape or elastic tube holder.	• Prevents trauma to urethral tissue.
15. Assist client to comfortable position.	• Promotes relaxation and rest.
16. Lower bed to lowest position. Raise side rails if appropriate.	• Promotes client safety.
17. Dispose of contaminated supplies, remove gloves, and perform hand hygiene.	• Prevents spread of infection.
18. Calculate fluid used to irrigate bladder and catheter and subtract from total output.	• Determines accurate urinary output.
19. Assess characteristics of output: viscosity, colour, and presence of matter (e.g., sediment, clots, blood).	• Evaluates results of irrigation.

Unexpected Outcomes and Related Interventions

Irrigating Solution Does Not Return or Is Not Flowing at Prescribed Rate, Possible Occlusion of Catheter

- Examine tubing for kinks, clots, or urine sediment.
- Notify physician if irrigant is retained, if client complains of pain, or if bladder is distended.

Cloudy or Foul Urine, Fever

- Monitor fever.
- Notify physician.
- Obtain sterile urine specimen if ordered by physician.

Increase in Bladder Spasms, Possible Occlusion of Catheter With Foreign Object (e.g., Blood Clot)

- Notify physician.
- May be instructed to perform intermittent irrigations until clots clear.

Recording and Reporting

- Record type and amount of irrigation solution used, amount returned as drainage, and the character of drainage.
- Record and report any findings such as complaints of bladder spasms, inability to instill fluid into bladder, or presence of blood clots.

Home Care Considerations

- If client is discharged with an in-dwelling catheter and requires bladder irrigations, either the client or the client's family must be properly instructed on how to perform this task.
- In the home, it is most likely that open irrigation will be required. Because this method poses the highest risk of contamination, you must assess the level of understanding of surgical asepsis by the client and his or her family.

Numerous therapies can help restore normal urinary voiding function, including surgical, pharmacological, and behavioural options. Conservative therapies should be the first line of treatment because they generally are noninvasive and have few side effects, and are feasible for older as well as younger adults (Box 44–12). Conservative therapies include lifestyle modification, pelvic floor muscle exercises, bladder training, habit retraining, and prompted voiding (Registered Nurses Association of Ontario, 2005). Because the success of all of these therapies necessitates changes in daily lifestyle and ongoing adherence, it is important that you provide support and follow-up to enhance motivation. If conservative therapies do not eliminate the urinary alteration, then self-catheterization may restore a measure of control to the client.

Lifestyle Modification. Several lifestyle factors have been associated with urinary incontinence. Smoking has been associated with increased risk of moderate to severe incontinence, likely due to the chronic cough experienced by smokers (Dallosso et al., 2003; Hannestad et al., 2000). Increased weight, particularly in obese and moderately obese individuals, is believed to increase intrapelvic pressure; in one study, women who lost an average of 15 kg experienced a 51% reduction in incontinent episodes (Subak, et al., 2002).

➤ BOX 44-11 Procedural Guidelines

Condom Catheter

Delegation Considerations: The application of a condom catheter can be delegated to unregulated care providers (UCPs). The registered nurse is responsible for assessing the condition of the penis over time and should inform the UCP to notify the registered nurse of any signs of skin irritation or tissue swelling.

Equipment

- Condom catheter (may be self-adhesive or provided with elastic adhesive)
- Collection bag
- Basin with warm water
- Towel and washcloth
- Disposable gloves
- Scissors

Procedure

1. Check physician's order.
2. Perform hand hygiene.
3. Assess urinary elimination patterns, the client's ability to urinate voluntarily, and continence.
4. Assess the client's mental status to determine appropriate teaching related to condom catheter care.
5. Assess condition of penis and scrotum. Ensure that the foreskin of the uncircumcised male is not retracted.
6. Assess the client's knowledge of the purpose of the condom catheter.
7. Explain procedure to client.
8. Raise bed to working height and raise far upper side rail.
9. Using sheet, drape client so that only genitals are exposed.
10. Prepare condom catheter and drainage system (see manufacturer's directions).
11. Apply gloves and provide perineal care.
    A. If necessary, clip hair at base of penile shaft.
12. Apply skin preparation to penile shaft and allow to dry.
13. Holding penis in nondominant hand, apply condom by rolling smoothly onto penis. *Note:* Leave a 2.5-cm to 5-cm space between tip of penis and end of catheter (see Step 13 illustration).
14. Secure condom catheter:
    A. If elastic adhesive is used, wrap the strip of adhesive over the condom catheter to secure it in place, using a spiral technique (see Step 14A illustration). *Note:* Adhesive tape must never be used.
    B. If self-adhesive catheter is used, follow the manufacturer's directions.
15. Attach catheter to drainage bag and attach drainage bag to lower bed frame.
16. Make client comfortable.
17. Observe urinary drainage, drainage tube patency, condition of penis, and tape placement.

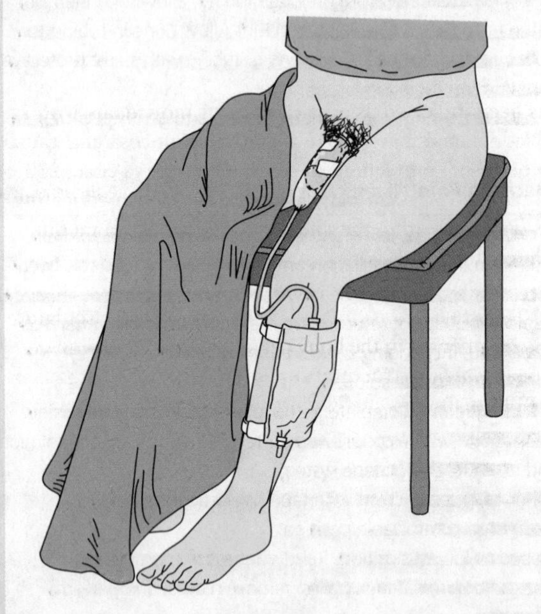

Step 13 Distance between end of penis and tip of catheter.

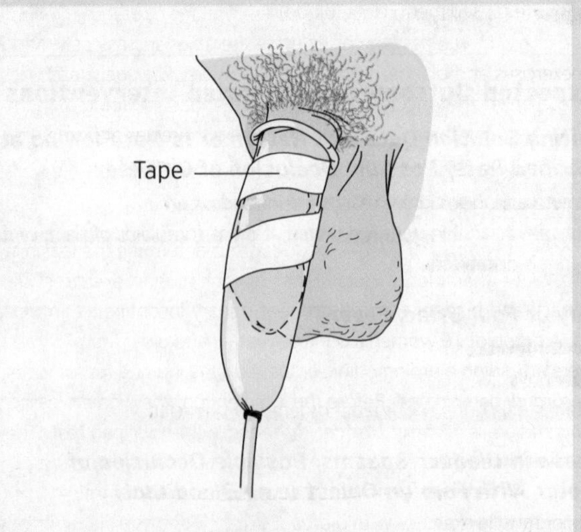

Step 14A Elastic tape is applied in spiral fashion to secure the condom catheter to the penis.

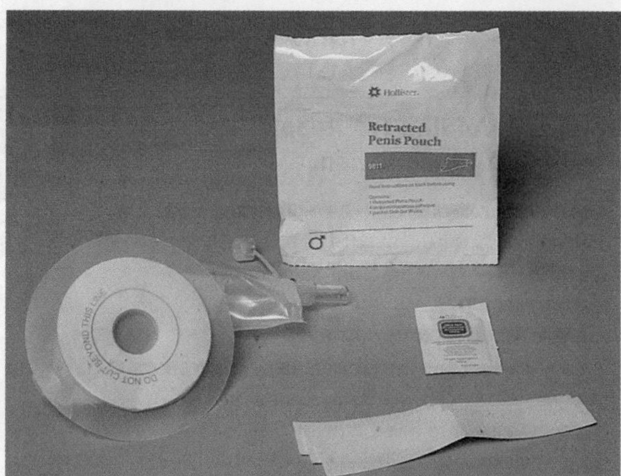

Figure 44-17 Retracted penis pouch external urinary device.

Caffeine has been indicated as a risk factor for individuals with an overactive bladder, and may irritate the bladder mucosa and cause involuntary detrusor contractions in some clients (Arya et al., 2000; Bryant et al., 2002). You can play an important role in educating, counselling, and supporting the client to enable lifestyle modification that reduces the risk factors for incontinence.

Pelvic Floor Muscle Exercises. The pelvic floor musculature (PFM) spans the opening in the bony pelvis and combines with connective tissue to provide structural support for the pelvic organs. A well-toned PFM maintains the bladder neck in position to ensure that any increase in intra-abdominal pressure, as occurs with coughing, is transmitted not only to the bladder but also to the bladder neck to maintain closure. Contraction of the PFM results in urethral compression as the urethra is pulled forward toward the symphysis pubis (Ashton-Miller & Delancey, 2007). Weakened PFMs can result from muscle wasting caused by prolonged immobility, frequent straining in association with urinary or fecal elimination, stretching of muscles during childbirth, menopausal muscle atrophy, or traumatic damage.

Pelvic floor muscle exercises (PFMEs), also known as **Kegel exercises,** improve the strength of PFMs through hypertrophy and recruitment of additional muscle fibres associated with repetitive contractions (Thompson & Smith, 2002). These exercises have demonstrated effectiveness in treating stress incontinence, overactive bladders, and mixed causes of urinary incontinence (Sampselle, 2003). Clients begin these exercises during voiding to learn the technique: if they are able to slow the urinary stream, they are contracting the proper muscles. The exercises are then practised at nonvoiding times (Box 44–13). Clients should be alert and motivated to perform the exercises. They also should be aware that it may take 12 to 16 weeks to notice appreciable change, but that maintaining the exercises is important in terms of obtaining a positive outcome.

Bladder Training. The goal of bladder training is to increase gradually the interval between voids and to decrease voiding frequency during waking and sleeping hours (Sampselle, 2003). The overall purpose is to restore a normal pattern of voiding. For bladder training to be successful, clients must be alert, motivated, and physically able to follow a training program. The program includes education, scheduled voiding, and positive reinforcement.

BOX 44-12 RESEARCH HIGHLIGHT

Promoting Conservative Therapies for Older Adults

Research Focus

The incidence of urinary incontinence rises with age, affecting 30% to 40% of middle-aged women and 30% to 50% of older women. The least invasive treatments are recommended as the first line of therapy, yet little is known about how older women tolerate therapies such as pelvic floor muscle exercises and bladder training. It is possible that ageist attitudes, including a belief that incontinence is a normal part of aging and that older adults are not able to learn and apply new therapies at home, continue to affect the ability of older adults to obtain appropriate care.

Research Abstract

The purpose of Perrin et al.'s (2006) study was to determine the feasibility of conservative therapies, including pelvic floor muscle exercises with biofeedback and bladder training, to treat urinary incontinence in older women. A group of 10 women (cognitively intact and older than 75 years) who were attending a urology clinic or were on the waiting list for incontinence surgery participated. Before the intervention, the women learned how to complete a 72-hour bladder diary and a 24-hour pad test. They then met with a physiotherapist at the clinic six times, over a period of 6 to 9 weeks. All received a combined approach of bladder training and pelvic floor muscle exercises with biofeedback included as a learning tool. The women were asked to carry out the exercise program three times each day at home and to record their progress.

Three women did not complete the study, one because of the demands of the study and two because of comorbidities. All seven women who completed the program said that they were comfortable with the intervention. Although some thought the exercises were difficult at first, they improved their techniques with practice. Most were also comfortable with the manual vaginal examination and the use of the vaginal probe. Some noted difficulty with completing the bladder diary, but a 95% compliance rate was reported. Three of the seven women completed the home therapy program three times a day as advised; the other four were compliant 67.5% of the time. Episodes of leakage decreased by 39%, a decrease that correlated with an improvement in reported quality of life. All of the women reported that they would recommend the treatment to a friend. The researchers concluded that physical therapies and even biofeedback with vaginal probes are feasible in women older than 75 years.

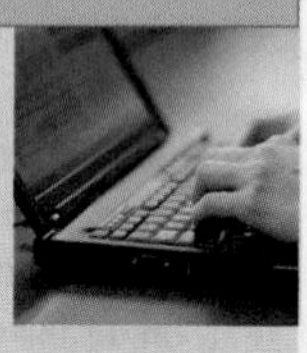

Evidence-Informed Practice

- Incontinence, frequency, or both, are experienced by adults of all ages, educational levels, economic status, and health status.
- Many adults wrongly believe that urinary incontinence and frequency are an expected part of the aging process.
- The use of biofeedback and conservative therapies is generally well tolerated by older adults.
- Nurses can support the use of conservative, inexpensive nonpharmacological interventions to enhance comfort in community-based and some institutionalized older adults.

References: Perrin, L., Dauphinee, S., Corcos, J., Hanley, J., & Kuchel, G. (2006). Pelvic floor muscle training with biofeedback and bladder training in elderly women. *Journal of Wound, Ostomy, and Continence Nursing, 32*(3), 186–199.

BOX 44-13 CLIENT TEACHING

Pelvic Floor Muscle Exercises (Kegels)

Objectives

The client who is cognitively alert and motivated will achieve continence or experience fewer episodes of incontinence as a result of increased pelvic floor muscle tone and strength.

Teaching Strategies

- Explain the method used to identify proper muscle contraction: a female client sits on the toilet with knees apart and tightens muscles to stop the flow of urine; a male client tries to stop the flow of urine midstream.
- After muscle is identified, instruct the client to lie down with knees bent and apart, or to sit.
- Instruct the client to contract the pelvic floor muscle gradually and hold the contraction for 3 to 10 seconds without tensing the muscles of the legs, buttocks, back, or abdomen. Remind the client to breathe during the exercise.
- Instruct the client to relax the muscle gradually for an equal time period between each contraction.
- The client should repeat this exercise at least two or three times, and work up to 10 repetitions as it becomes easier. The client should do this exercise two or three times a day, or as often as possible.

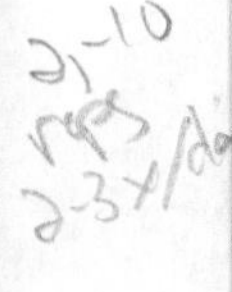

- Explain that within the first week of exercises, the client and nurse can assess whether proper muscle contraction is occurring by the client placing two fingers in the vagina (or, for men, one finger in the rectum) while contracting the pelvic floor muscle. The client should feel tightening in the vagina or anus during the contraction.
- Teach the client and the caregiver to keep a 24- to 72-hour urinary diary to identify changes in patterns of urinary elimination.

Evaluation

- Ask the client if he or she has identified the pelvic floor muscle via finger insertion (into the vagina or rectum).
- During vaginal or rectal (male) bimanual examination, ask the client to perform the exercises; then assess muscle tone.
- Monitor the client's urinary diary.
- Ask the client and the caregiver about degree of satisfaction related to the control achieved over urinary elimination.

BOX 44-14 EVIDENCE-INFORMED PRACTICE GUIDELINE

Prompted Voiding for People with Urinary Incontinence

- Approach the client at scheduled prompted voiding times.
- Wait five seconds for the client to initiate a request to toilet.
- Ask the client if he or she is wet or dry.
- Physically assess the client to determine continence status.
- Provide positive feedback if the client is dry.
- Prompt the client to toilet.
- Offer assistance with toileting.
- Provide feedback.
- Inform the client of the next scheduled prompted voiding session.
- Encourage the client to self-initiate requests to toilet.
- Record the result of the prompted voiding session.

Adapted from Wyman, J. (2008). Prompted voiding. In B. Ackley, B. Swan, G. Ludwig, & S. Tucker (Eds.), *Evidence-based nursing care guidelines. Medical–surgical interventions* (pp. 696–698). St. Louis, MO: Mosby.

The first step in bladder training is establishing a baseline. The client or caregiver completes a urinary diary to assess maximum voiding intervals. It is not uncommon for the client with frequency or an overactive bladder to void small amounts hourly or more often. An initial training schedule for such a client might involve a voiding schedule of every 75 minutes while awake, increasing every 1 to 3 weeks by 15-minute increments toward a 3-hour schedule. The rate of incremental changes will depend on the client's progress and on his or her ability to adhere to a rigid schedule. Urge-suppression techniques, such as counting backward from 100 when the urge to void is felt and performing pelvic floor muscle contractions, are helpful. You must be aware that the client who has experienced an episode of incontinence in public will be particularly hesitant to deter voiding for even brief periods.

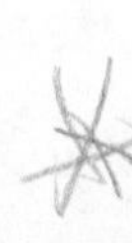

Habit Retraining and Prompted Voiding. Habit retraining and **prompted voiding** are useful strategies for clients with cognitive or physical impairment, or both, who rely on caregiver assistance. Habit retraining involves assessment of a client's normal pattern of voiding to establish a toileting schedule that pre-empts incontinence (Ostaszkiewicz et al., 2008). Such individualized toileting schedules have demonstrated effectiveness but are labour-intensive. You should help the client to the bathroom before episodes of incontinence occur. Fluids and medications are timed to prevent interference with the toileting schedule. When combined with positive reinforcement, this approach is also called prompted voiding (Box 44–14).

Self-Catheterization. Some clients with chronic disorders such as spinal cord injury learn to perform self-catheterization. The client must be physically able to manipulate equipment and assume a position for successful catheterization. You must teach the client the structure of the urinary tract, the clean versus sterile technique, the importance of adequate fluid intake, and the frequency of self-catheterization. In general, the goal is to have clients perform self-catheterization every six to eight hours, but the schedule should be individualized.

❖Evaluation

Client Care

The client is the best source of evaluation of outcomes and responses to nursing care (Figure 44–18). However, you will also evaluate the effectiveness of nursing interventions through comparisons with baseline data. You should evaluate for changes in the client's voiding pattern, the presence of urinary tract alteration, and the client's physical condition. Actual outcomes are compared with expected outcomes to determine the client's health status. Continuous evaluation allows you to determine whether new or revised therapies are required or if any new nursing diagnoses have developed.

Client Expectations

If you have developed a trust relationship with the client, indications of the client's degree of satisfaction with his or her care will be evident. The client may smile or nod in appreciation. However, you need to confirm whether the client's expectations have been met to

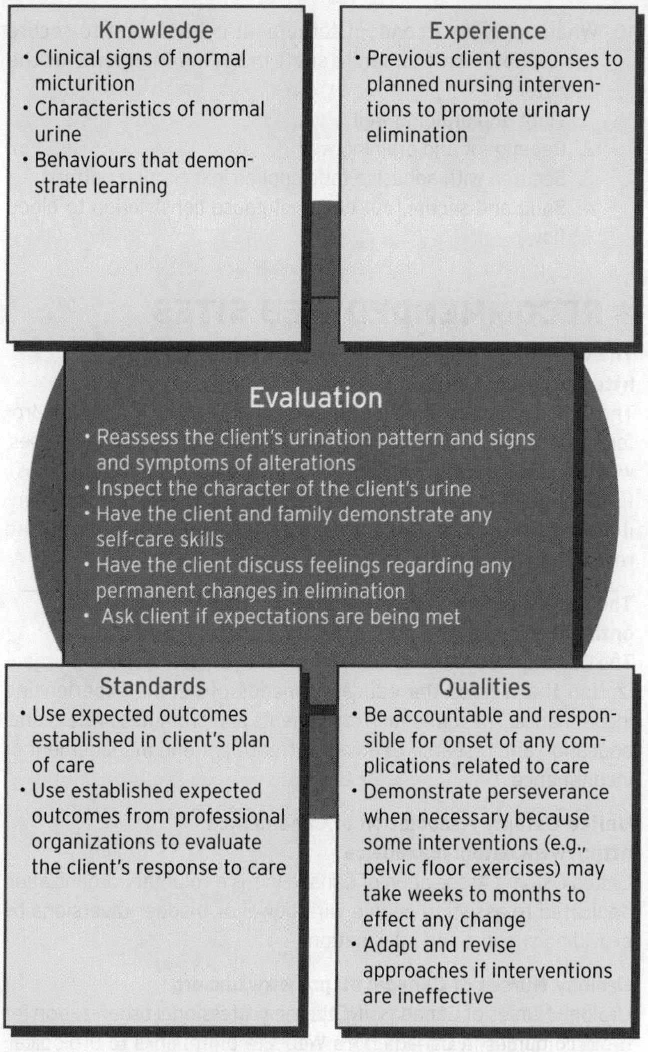

Figure 44-18 Critical thinking model for urinary elimination evaluation.

full satisfaction. You may need to ask specifically about the client's degree of urinary control and comfort. If simply asked, "How are you feeling today?" the client may reply with a noncommittal "Okay." However, you need specific information about how well an intervention has met the client's need in order to continue or to revise the care plan. You can also assist the client in redefining unrealistic expectations when impairment in function is not likely to be altered as completely as he or she might like.

* KEY CONCEPTS

- The act of micturition, or voiding, is influenced by voluntary control from higher brain centres and involuntary control from the spinal cord.
- Symptoms common to urinary disturbances include urgency, frequency, dysuria, polyuria, oliguria, and difficulty in starting the urinary stream.
- When collected properly, a clean-voided urine specimen does not contain bacteria from the urethral meatus.
- Methods of promoting the micturition reflex assist clients in sensing the urge to urinate and in controlling urethral sphincter relaxation.
- An increased fluid intake results in increased diluted urine formation that reduces the risk of urinary tract infections.
- An in-dwelling urinary catheter remains in the bladder for an extended period, making the risk of infection greater than with intermittent catheterization.
- Catheter irrigation is necessary when the catheter becomes occluded with sediment or blood clots.
- A catheter drainage system should be a closed system positioned to allow free drainage of urine by gravity.
- Incontinence is classified as transient, urge, stress, mixed, functional, overflow, reflex, or total. Each type has specific nursing interventions.
- Specific guidelines for catheter selection should be followed so that the catheter does not cause harm.

* CRITICAL THINKING EXERCISES

1. Mrs. Rodriquez is 77 years old and has had problems with urgency for the past two years. The episodes are becoming increasingly frequent. She has been attempting to deal with the problem by using an absorbent pad in her underwear, but she feels as though everyone knows about her incontinence. The embarrassment of urinary odours often keeps her at home. She has given up attending daily mass at church.
   a. How can you help Mrs. Rodriquez regain control of her urinary elimination?
   b. What actual nursing diagnoses apply to Mrs. Rodriquez?
   c. For one of the diagnoses, provide one goal or outcome and two nursing interventions.
2. Mrs. Brownell is 37 years old and has been admitted with back pain radiating downward into her groin. She has also noticed blood in her urine for a week, but she was hoping it would go away. She is scheduled to undergo an intravenous pyelogram (IVP) in four hours.
   a. What is the purpose of the IVP?
   b. What nursing care is needed before Mrs. Brownell goes to the radiography department?
   c. Provide at least two nursing responsibilities for care of a client who has undergone an IVP.
3. Mrs. Fenton is 70 years old and has physical limitations related to rheumatoid arthritis. Her daughter, with whom she lives, has brought her to her family practitioner's office. You are the family nurse practitioner in the practice. As you assess Mrs. Fenton, you ask her how she is coping. She begins to answer but then starts to cry and says, "I know when I have to go to the bathroom, but I often don't make it in time." Her daughter asks you for suggestions on how to manage, as she has noticed that her mother's perineal skin is reddened and sore. What assessments need to be completed before planning interventions for Mrs. Fenton's care?

* REVIEW QUESTIONS

1. The normal adult urine output is
   1. 1000 mL/day
   2. 1500 to 1600 mL/day
   3. 3000 to 3200 mL/day
   4. 4000 mL/day
2. Renal alterations result from factors that cause injury directly to the glomeruli or renal tubule, interfering with their normal filtering, reabsorptive, and secretory functions. Selected causes include
   1. Transfusion reactions
   2. Dehydration
   3. Hemorrhage
   4. Congestive heart failure

3. Postrenal alterations result from obstruction to the flow of urine in the urinary collecting system caused by
   1. Dehydration
   2. Calculi
   3. Hemorrhage
   4. Diabetes mellitus

4. Which of the following is NOT a risk factor for UTI?
   1. Catheterization
   2. Antibiotic use
   3. Acidic urine
   4. Spermicide use

5. Hospital-acquired UTIs are often related to poor hand hygiene and
   1. Urinary drainage bags
   2. Poor perineal hygiene
   3. Poor catheterization technique
   4. Poor urinary output

6. The urine appears concentrated and cloudy because of the presence of white blood cells (WBCs) or
   1. Bacteria
   2. Urinary drainage bags
   3. Blood clots
   4. Poor perineal hygiene

7. Prompted voiding is most appropriate for
   1. Clients with cognitive disorders
   2. Clients with small-capacity bladders
   3. Clients with urinary obstruction
   4. Male clients after prostatectomy

8. A client with stress incontinence
   1. Is incontinent after a strong urge to void
   2. Is unaware of the need to void
   3. Loses small amounts of urine with increased intra-abdominal pressure (e.g., coughing)
   4. Exhibits a small-capacity bladder

9. Ensuring that an in-dwelling catheter drainage bag is lower than the bladder prevents
   1. Urine flowing back into the bladder, which will likely cause an infection
   2. Urinary retention
   3. Reflex incontinence
   4. Urinary incontinence

10. When applying a condom catheter, it is important to secure the catheter on the penile shaft in such a manner that the catheter is
    1. Tight and draining well
    2. Dependent and draining well
    3. Secured with adhesive tape applied in a circular pattern
    4. Snug and secure, but does not cause constriction to blood flow

* RECOMMENDED WEB SITES

The Canadian Association for Enterostomal Therapy: http://www.caet.ca

The Canadian Association for Enterostomal Therapy (CAET) is a professional organization that represents enterostomal therapy nurses, who provide services for clients with abdominal stomas (openings), fistulae, draining wounds, or selected skin, gastrointestinal, and genitourinary disorders. CAET promotes education, standards, and research for enterostomal practice.

The Canadian Continence Foundation: http://www.ontinence-fdn.ca

The Canadian Continence Foundation is a national, nonprofit organization that serves the education needs of people experiencing incontinence. The foundation implements and promotes professional education and research to advance treatment and management of incontinence.

United Ostomy Association of Canada Inc.: http://www.ostomycanada.ca

United Ostomy Association of Canada Inc. is a voluntary organization dedicated to assisting people with bowel or bladder diversions by providing support and information.

Urology Nurses of Canada: http://www.unc.org

Urology Nurses of Canada (UNC) is the professional organization for urologic nurses in Canada. This Web site offers links to urological-related information, including the UNC's professional standards.

45

Bowel Elimination

Original chapter by Lori Klingman, RN, MSN

Canadian content written by

Jo-Ann E. T. Fox-Threlkeld, RN, BN, MSc, PhD

objectives

Mastery of content in this chapter will enable you to:

- Define the key terms listed.
- Discuss the role of gastrointestinal organs in digestion and elimination.
- Describe the integrated processes of oral pharyngeal swallowing and breathing.
- Describe the functions of the large intestine.
- Explain the physiological aspects of normal defecation.
- Discuss the psychological and physiological factors that influence the elimination process.
- Describe the common physiological alterations in elimination.
- Assess a client's pattern of elimination.
- List the nursing diagnoses related to alterations in elimination.
- Describe the nursing implications for common diagnostic examinations of the gastrointestinal tract.
- List the nursing measures that promote normal elimination.
- List the nursing measures included in bowel training.
- Discuss the nursing measures required for clients with a bowel diversion.
- Use critical thinking in the provision of care to clients with alterations in bowel elimination.

key terms

Bolus, p. 1118
Bowel training, p. 1157
Cathartics, p. 1123
Chyme, p. 1119
Colitis, p. 1123
Colostomy, p. 1126
Constipation, p. 1124
Crohn's disease, p. 1123
Defecation, p. 1121
Diarrhea, p. 1125
Effluent, p. 1146
Endoscopy, p. 1123
Enema, p. 1141
Enterostomal therapist (ET), p. 1146
Excoriation, p. 1146
Fecal incontinence, p. 1125
Fecal occult blood testing (FOBT), p. 1131
Feces, p. 1121
Fibre, p. 1122
Flatulence, p. 1125
Flatus, p. 1120
Gastrocolic reflex, p. 1120
Hemorrhoids, p. 1126
Ileostomy, p. 1126
Impaction, p. 1124
Lactose intolerance, p. 1122
Laxatives, p. 1123
Masticate, p. 1118
Paralytic ileus, p. 1123
Peristalsis, p. 1120
Peristaltic contractions, p. 1119
Polyps, p. 1126
Stoma, p. 1126
Valsalva manoeuvre, p. 1121

media resources

evolve Web Site

- Animations
- Audio Chapter Summaries
- Glossary
- Multiple-Choice Review Questions
- Skills Performance Checklists
- Student Learning Activities
- Video Clips
- Weblinks

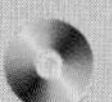

Companion CD

- Glossary
- Interactive Learning Activities
- Fluids and Electrolytes Tutorial
- Test-Taking Skills

Food enters the gastrointestinal tract, is dissolved by intraluminal water, and is broken down by mechanical and chemical digestion. Nutrients and water are absorbed from the lumen, and the remaining contents are propelled along by contractions of the smooth muscle layers. The material that reaches the colon is further dehydrated and expelled from the anus as stool.

Regular elimination of bowel waste is essential for normal body functioning. Alterations in bowel elimination are often early indications of problems within either the gastrointestinal tract or another body system. Because bowel function depends on the balance of several factors, bowel elimination patterns and habits vary among individuals.

To manage the bowel elimination problems of clients, you must understand the normal elimination process and the factors that promote, impede, or cause alterations in elimination. Supportive nursing care respects the client's privacy and emotional needs. Measures designed to promote normal elimination should also minimize discomfort for the client.

Scientific Knowledge Base

The gastrointestinal (GI) tract is a series of hollow, multilayered, muscular organs that are lined with mucous membranes. The GI tract begins at the mouth and continues through to the anus. The mucosal and muscle layers are innervated by the intrinsic enteric nervous system comprising sensory, interneuronal, and motor fibres. The rate of rhythmic contractions is specific to each organ and is controlled by the pacemaker cells in the muscle layers. The mucosa contains neurons; mucous, endocrine, and immune cells; and the crypt ion-secreting cells that mature into the absorptive enterocytes of the villus tip. The central nervous system receives input from the gastrointestinal tract through sensory fibres, which travel in the vagus and sympathetic nerves. Extrinsic sympathetic and parasympathetic motor nerves terminate on the enteric nervous system and act to modulate the activity of the intrinsic enteric nervous system. The gastrointestinal tract's specialized immune system prevents bacteria and viruses of the nonsterile lumen from entering the bloodstream. In addition, blood from the gastrointestinal tract passes through the portal venous vessels to the liver for further passage through the immune cells in the liver sinusoids (i.e., the Kupfer cells) before entering the vena cava. The liver secretes bile; regulates the metabolism of carbohydrates, lipids, and proteins; synthesizes proteins; degrades hormones; and inactivates drugs and toxins. Some toxins are secreted into the bile and re-enter the gastrointestinal tract through the gallbladder (Berne et al., 2004).

The purposes of the GI tract are to ingest (take in) food, break down the ingested food into absorbable forms (digestion), absorb fluid and nutrients, prepare food for both absorption and use by the body's cells, and provide temporary storage of feces (Figure 45–1). The volume of fluids absorbed by the GI tract is high. Oral fluid intake is approximately 1.2 L per day; an additional 7 L of fluid enters from the blood as the result of the secretion of digestive enzymes by the mucosa, liver, gallbladder, and pancreas, and by osmosis as the numbers of molecules in the lumen increase by digestion. Absorption from the small and large intestine amounts to 8.1 L per day, leaving 100 mL to be excreted in the feces. Therefore, maintaining fluid and electrolyte balance is a key function of the GI system. Another function of the gastrointestinal tract is the elimination of toxic substances from the upper GI tract by vomiting.

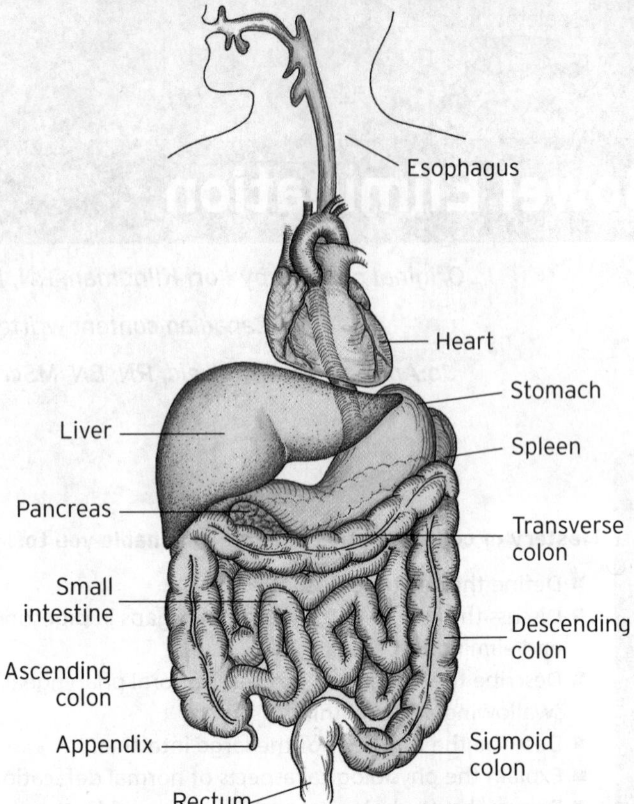

Figure 45-1 Organs of the gastrointestinal tract (with the heart as a reference point).

Mouth

The mouth mechanically and chemically breaks down nutrients into usable sizes and forms. The teeth **masticate** food, breaking it down into a soft, moist ball (a **bolus**) suitable for swallowing. Saliva, which is produced by the salivary glands in the mouth, dilutes and softens the food in the mouth for easier swallowing and commences digestion of carbohydrates with the enzyme ptyalin. (Saliva also contains growth factors, antibacterial agents, and antibodies that are necessary to maintain the integrity of the gums and teeth.) In addition, mucus from the salivary glands lubricates the passage of the bolus through the pharynx and down the esophagus during swallowing, and in the reverse direction during vomiting.

Swallowing begins with the lips closing and the tongue curling with its tip and then the back being pressed to the roof of the mouth (Figure 45–2; to demonstrate, put the tip of your tongue behind your lower teeth, open your mouth, and then try to swallow). The action of swallowing tips the bolus into the pharynx. The pharyngeal cavity is common to both the gastrointestinal tract and the respiratory tract. To prevent aspiration, the vocal cords in the glottis close, and the epiglottis moves downward to seal off the trachea. The swallowed bolus must cross the nasopharynx, and the soft palate must elevate toward the nasopharynx to prevent material from entering the back of the nose. To prevent aspiration, the vocal cords in the glottis close, the epiglottis moves downward to seal off the trachea, and breathing is inhibited in the central nervous system. The bolus enters the esophagus through the relaxed upper esophageal sphincter. This complex process is under striated muscle control and requires an intact nervous system. Anaesthesia, strokes, and high blood alcohol levels inhibit

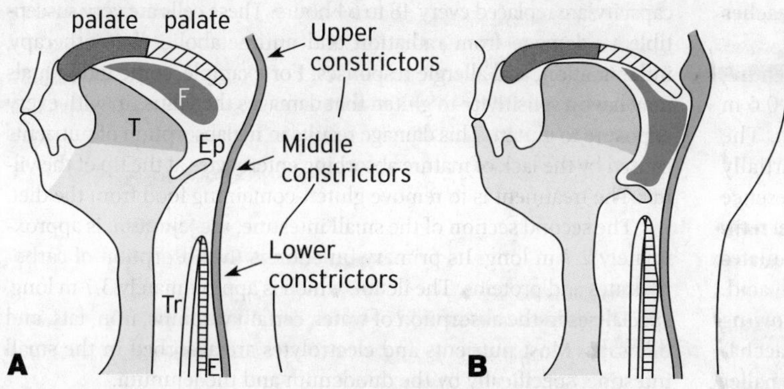

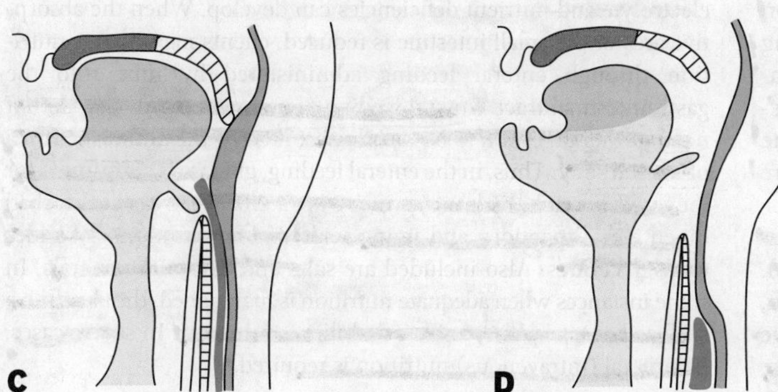

Figure 45-2 Oral and pharyngeal events during swallowing. A, The bolus (F) is propelled into the pharynx by placement of the tongue (T) on the roof of the hard palate. B, Further propulsion is caused by movement of the more distal regions of the tongue against the palate. Contraction of the upper constrictors of the pharynx and the soft palate separate the oropharynx from the nasopharynx. C, Contraction of the pharynx and relaxation of the cricopharyngeal muscle propels the bolus through the upper esophageal sphincter. Upward movement of the glottis and downward movement of the epiglottis (EP) seal off the trachea (Tr), and the respiratory drive is inhibited in the central nervous system. D, The bolus is now in the esophagus (E) and is propelled into the stomach by a peristaltic contraction. **Source:** From Johnson, L. R. (2001). *Gastrointestinal physiology* (6th ed., Figure 3–1, p. 28). St. Louis, MO: Mosby.

this close regulation and can lead to the aspiration of either food or vomited gastric contents into the trachea and lungs.

Esophagus

The esophagus provides a conduit through the chest cavity, which it shares with the lungs, heart, and the large blood vessels. The esophagus enters the abdominal cavity through the diaphragm at the lower esophageal sphincter, which maintains a barrier against the acid-proteolytic contents of the stomach. When persons age, the esophageal sphincter frequently herniates into the chest cavity to produce a hiatus hernia and regurgitation of gastric contents into the esophagus.

The bolus travels down the relaxed esophagus mainly by gravity to the lower esophageal sphincter, which is opened by the initiation of swallowing in the pharynx and upper esophageal sphincter. A wave of **peristaltic contractions** propels the bolus into the stomach. Peristaltic contractions relax over the bolus and contract behind the bolus, thus moving contents through the length of the GI tract. If the bolus moves slowly or is stuck, a local reflex will relax the area ahead of the bolus and produce a powerful contraction behind the bolus. In the esophagus, this action is known as secondary peristalsis. Tertiary contractions of the esophagus are frequently simultaneous and are produced by irritation of the mucosa by gastric contents. These contractions can be extremely painful and may mimic cardiac chest pain. During vomiting, which is controlled by the vomiting centre in the brain, reverse peristalsis forces intestinal contents into the stomach through the open pyloric sphincter, where forceful contractions of the stomach open the esophageal sphincters forcing the vomitus up into the esophagus and out into the pharynx, while the vocal cords close, the glottis closes, and respiration is inhibited.

Stomach

The stomach performs several tasks: storage of swallowed food and liquid, mixing of food with liquid and gastric digestive juices, and the controlled emptying of its contents through the pyloric sphincter into the small intestine. The stomach produces and secretes hydrochloric acid (HC1), mucus, the enzyme pepsin, the intrinsic factor, and gastrointestinal hormones, such as gastrin and somatostatin. Pepsin and HC1 facilitate the digestion of protein and are antibacterial. Mucus protects the stomach mucosa from acidity and enzyme activity. The intrinsic factor is essential in the absorption of vitamin B_{12}. Gastrin and somatostatin regulate the secretion of acid and pepsin in the stomach.

The rate of emptying of the stomach depends on the content of the dissolved and partially digested bolus (**chyme**). Water diffuses from both the stomach and the small intestine and is emptied rapidly. Carbohydrates are emptied only slightly more slowly, particularly if they are not strongly acidic. Proteins empty even more slowly and in smaller amounts as determined by the acidity of the chyme. Fats are emptied the slowest of all. The controlled emptying allows the pancreatic secretions and bile to neutralize the chyme and secrete enzymes for luminal digestion.

Small Intestine

Propulsion of contents along the small intestine occurs by segmentation, which facilitates both digestion and absorption (Figure 45–3). Chyme mixes with secretions from the gallbladder (i.e., bile) and pancreatic enzymes (i.e., amylases, proteolytic enzymes, and lipases) and is exposed to the absorbing surfaces of the mucosa. Reabsorption in the small intestine is so efficient that by the time the chyme reaches the end of the small intestine, it is pastelike in consistency.

The small intestine is divided into three sections: the duodenum, the jejunum, and the ileum. The duodenum is approximately 0.6 m long and continues to process the chyme from the stomach. The chyme that enters the duodenum is acidic and contains partially digested protein, carbohydrates, and unemulsified fats. The presence of these substances stimulates the release of the hormones secretin and cholecystokinin from the duodenal mucosa. Secretin stimulates the pancreas to secrete bicarbonate to neutralize the acid. Cholecystokinin stimulates the pancreas to secrete the following enzymes: (1) amylases, which convert carbohydrates to disaccharides; (2) proteases, which further hydrolyze proteins into smaller peptides; and (3) lipases, which hydrolyze triglycerides into fatty acids and monoglycerides. The presence of fats in the duodenum further stimulates cholecystokinin release, which causes the gallbladder to contract, which in turn releases bile to emulsify the fats. Any blockage of the release of these enzymes prevents the digestion of fats and proteins and results in large, fatty, and foul-smelling stools. This is the case in clients who have cystic fibrosis: the metabolic error in chloride pumping produces a thick mucus that prevents emptying of the pancreatic and biliary ducts into the duodenum. Undigested fats and proteins reach the colon and are responsible for the changes in fecal appearance.

The cells at the base of the villus are secretory and can be stimulated to produce massive volumes of fluid (e.g., from cholera toxins). These cells migrate to the villus tip, lose their secretory function, and mature into absorptive cells. Thus, in the presence of massive secretion, absorption can be stimulated by a solution of glucose, sodium chloride, and other ions, in a process known as oral rehydration therapy (Rehydration Project, 2008). The mature enterocytes at the tip of the villi, along with their digestive enzymes and absorptive capacity, are replaced every 48 to 64 hours. These cells are very susceptible to damage from radiation and antimetabolic chemotherapy, inflammation, and allergic responses. For example, some individuals may have a sensitivity to gluten that damages the villus tip with every exposure to gluten. This damage results in malabsorption of nutrients caused by the lack of mature absorbing enterocytes at the tip of the villus. The treatment is to remove gluten-containing food from the diet.

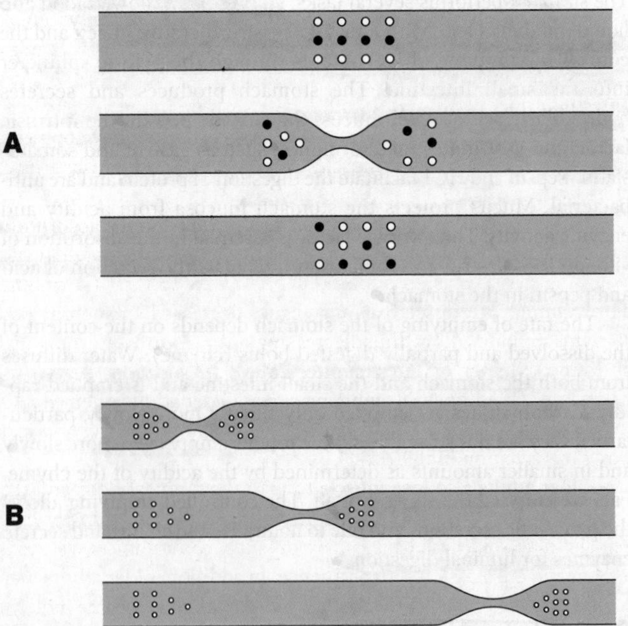

Figure 45-3 The influence of contractions on the contents within a region of the intestine. A, A contraction that is neither preceded by nor followed by other contractions serves to mix and locally circulate the intestinal contents. B, Contractions that have an orad to aborad sequence (left to right) serve to propel contents in an aborad direction. **Source:** From Johnson, L. R. (2001). *Gastrointestinal physiology* (6th ed., Figure 5–3, p. 50). St. Louis, MO: Mosby.

The second section of the small intestine, the jejunum, is approximately 2.7 m long. Its primary function is the absorption of carbohydrates and proteins. The ileum, which is approximately 3.7 m long, specializes in the absorption of water, certain vitamins, iron, fats, and bile salts. Most nutrients and electrolytes are absorbed in the small intestine, specifically by the duodenum and the jejunum.

If the small intestine function is impaired, the digestive process is greatly altered. For example, conditions such as inflammation, surgical resection, or obstruction can disrupt contractile activity, reduce the area of absorption, or block the passage of chyme. As a result, electrolyte and nutrient deficiencies can develop. When the absorptive area of the small intestine is reduced, clients may receive nutrition through enteral feeding administered by tube into the gastrointestinal tract. Enteral feeding contains nutrients that do not need further digestion to be rapidly absorbed by the diminished area of the intestine. Thus, in the enteral feeding, glucose is substituted for longer-chain carbohydrates, proteins are a mix of the easily absorbed dipeptides, tripeptides, and amino acids, and fats are monoglycerides or triglycerides. Also included are salts and essential minerals. In some instances when adequate nutrition is maintained, the absorptive surface hypertrophies, and an oral diet can resume. In severe cases, parenteral (intravenous) nutrition is required.

Large Intestine

The lower GI tract is called the large intestine because it is larger in diameter than the small intestine; however, at 1.5 to 1.8 m in length, it is much shorter. The large intestine is the primary organ of bowel elimination and is divided into the cecum, the colon, and the rectum (Figure 45–4).

Chyme from the terminal ileum enters the cecum of the large intestine, propelled by waves of peristalsis through the ileocecal sphincter, a circular muscle layer that regulates ileal emptying and prevents regurgitation of fecal contents. After a meal, the gastroilieal reflex causes the terminal ileum to contract regularly, and the sphincter opens with each contraction, thereby pushing the ileal contents into the colon.

The colon is divided into the ascending, transverse, descending, and sigmoid colons. The colon's muscular tissue allows it to accommodate and eliminate large quantities of waste and gas (**flatus**). The colon has three functions: absorption, secretion, and elimination. Each day, a large volume of water and significant amounts of sodium and chloride are absorbed by the colon (Doughty, 2006).

Two types of muscle contractions occur in the colon: slow-mixing contractions (similar to segmentation, but slower) and mass **peristalsis** (or mass movement). Slow-mixing contractions move contents through the colon and expose the chyme to the mucosa, where active absorption of sodium and chloride causes water absorption and dries the chyme to feces. Intestinal content is the main stimulus for the slow-mixing contractions. Mass peristalsis movements then push the feces toward the rectum. The ingestion of food is the main stimulus for mass peristalsis, which is known as the **gastrocolic reflex.** In adults, these mass movements occur only three or four times each day.

When the slow-mixing contractions increase and the mass peristalsis diminishes, water continues to be absorbed and the feces dry out, resulting in constipation. Conversely, when the mixing movements

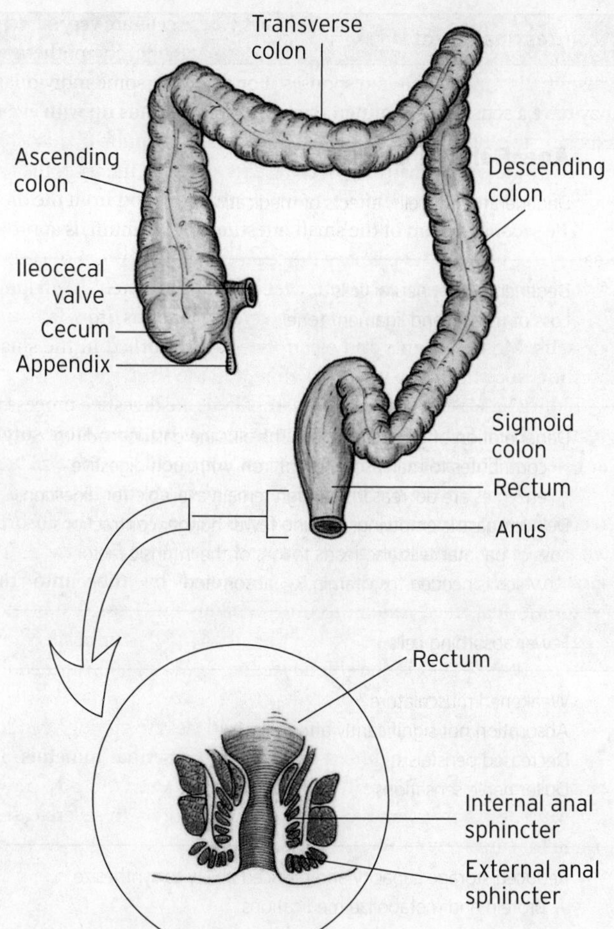

Figure 45-4 Divisions of the large intestine.

are decreased and the mass peristalsis is increased, the water has less time to be absorbed, and the stool will be watery (diarrhea).

The secretory function of the colon aids in electrolyte balance. Bicarbonate is secreted in exchange for chloride. Approximately 4 to 9 mmol of potassium is also excreted daily. Extreme alterations in colon function (e.g., diarrhea) can cause severe electrolyte disturbances.

The rectum is the final portion of the large intestine. Normally, the rectum is empty of waste products, or **feces**, until just before defecation. The rectum contains vertical and transverse folds of tissue that may help to temporarily hold fecal contents during **defecation**. Each fold contains an artery and vein that can become distended from pressure during straining. This distension can result in the formation of hemorrhoids.

Anus

Feces and flatus are expelled from the rectum through the anal canal and the anus. Contraction and relaxation of the internal anal sphincter is under autonomic (unconscious) control, whereas the external anal sphincter is under somatic neural (conscious) control. The anal canal is richly supplied with sensory and motor nerve fibres to help control continence.

Defecation

The physiological factors critical to bowel function and defecation include normal GI tract function, sensory awareness of rectal distension and rectal contents, voluntary sphincter control, and adequate rectal capacity and compliance (Doughty, 2006). Normal defecation is painless, resulting in the passage of a soft, formed stool.

Defecation begins with contractions in the left colon, moving the stool toward the anus. When a stool reaches the rectum, the distension causes relaxation of the internal anal sphincter and signals an awareness of the need to defecate. At the time of defecation, the external sphincter relaxes and abdominal muscles contract to increase intrarectal pressure and force the stool out (Doughty, 2006). Pressure can be exerted to expel feces through a voluntary contraction of the abdominal muscles and the diaphragm while maintaining forced expiration against a closed airway. This action is termed the **Valsalva manoeuvre.** Use of the Valsalva manoeuvre will assist in stool passage but affects the return of blood up the inferior vena cava. (For example, take your pulse while holding your breath and bearing down. Your pulse will grow weak and thready and then speed up because the diaphragm has occluded the return of the blood through the inferior vena cava. When you exhale, the pulse will feel very full and bounding as the blood return surges up the vena cava). When clients who have cardiovascular disease, glaucoma, increased intracranial pressure, or a new surgical wound use this manoeuvre, they are at risk of cardiac irregularities and elevated blood pressure and should therefore be cautioned to avoid straining to pass a stool.

Nursing Knowledge Base

Factors Affecting Bowel Elimination

Many factors influence the process of bowel elimination. Knowledge of these factors enables you to anticipate measures required to maintain a normal pattern of bowel elimination.

Age. Developmental changes that affect bowel elimination occur throughout life. An infant has a small stomach capacity and secretes fewer digestive enzymes than an adult. Some foods, such as complex starches, are tolerated poorly. Food passes quickly through an infant's intestinal tract because of rapid peristalsis. The infant is unable to control defecation because of a lack of neuromuscular development. The development of these muscles usually does not take place until 2 to 3 years of age.

Systemic changes in the function of digestion and the absorption of nutrients result from alterations in older clients' cardiovascular and neurological systems, as opposed to alterations to their GI system. For example, arteriosclerosis may cause decreased splanchnic and mesenteric blood flow, thus decreasing absorption from the small intestine (Meiner & Lueckenotte, 2006). In addition, peristalsis decreases and esophageal emptying slows. Older adults often experience changes in their GI system that impair normal digestion and bowel elimination (Table 45–1).

Older adults also lose muscle tone in the perineal floor and the anal sphincter. Although the integrity of the external sphincter may remain intact, older adults may have difficulty controlling bowel evacuation and are at risk for incontinence. In addition, older adults may have a slowing of the nerve impulses to the anal region: some individuals are less aware of the need to defecate and, as a result, develop irregular bowel movements and are at risk for constipation.

Older women, particularly those who have borne children, frequently develop loss of tone and weakening of the ligaments and muscles of the anterior and posterior vaginal walls. This condition can lead to cystocele (the dropping of the bladder into the vagina), rectocele (the pouching of the feces-filled rectum into the vagina),

TABLE 45-1 Normal Age-Related Changes in the Gastrointestinal Tract

Portion of Gastrointestinal Tract	Functional or Physiological Change	Age-Related Causes
Mouth	Decreased chewing and decreased salivation, including oral dryness	Degeneration of cells, effects of medication
Esophagus	Reduced motility, especially in the lower third Herniation of the lower esophageal sphincter and gastric fundus into the chest cavity above the diaphragm	Degeneration of neural cells Loss of muscle and ligament tone
Stomach	Decrease in acid secretions	Degeneration of gastric mucosa. The alkaline gastric medium contributes to malabsorption of iron. Although digestive enzymes are decreased, enough remain available for digestion.
	Decrease in motor activity	Delayed gastric emptying, causing fewer hunger contractions
	Decrease in mucosal thickness	Loss of parietal cells also leads to loss of the intrinsic factor, which is needed for vitamin B_{12} absorption.
Small intestine	Decreased nutrient absorption	Fewer absorbing cells
Large intestine	Increase in pouches on the weakened intestinal wall Constipation Missed defecation signal Increasing risk for fecal incontinence	Weakened musculature Absorption not significantly affected Decreased peristalsis Duller nerve sensations
Liver	Size decreased	Reduced storage capacity and reduced ability to synthesize protein and metabolize medications

Data from Meiner, S. & Lueckenotte, A. G. (2006). *Gerontologic nursing* (3rd ed.). St. Louis, MO: Mosby.

and sometimes complete prolapse of the uterus out of the vagina. Various surgical repairs for rectoceles have been shown to be not completely successful. Continence nurses (i.e., nurses who are specially trained in continence care) treat these problems by adjusting diet and promoting pelvic floor exercises, such as Kegel exercises (Skelly et al., 2006).

Diet. The food a person eats influences bowel elimination. Regular daily food intake helps to maintain a routine pattern of peristalsis in the colon. **Fibre**, the indigestible residue in the diet, provides the bulk of fecal material. Bulk-forming foods, such as grains, fruits, and vegetables, absorb fluids and increase stool mass. The bowel walls are stretched, which creates peristalsis and initiates the defecation reflex. Because they stimulate peristalsis, bulk-forming foods pass quickly through the intestines and keep the stool soft. Ingestion of a high-fibre diet or taking a fibre supplement can improve the likelihood of a regular bowel elimination pattern if other factors are normal. However, because fibre retains fluid in the GI tract, when additional fibre is injested, adequate fluid intake is essential; inadequate fluid intake can lead to serious constipation or impaction.

Gas-producing foods, such as onions, cauliflower, and beans, stimulate peristalsis. The gas that forms acts to distend the intestinal walls and increase colon motility. Some spicy foods can increase peristalsis but can also cause indigestion and watery stools.

The enzyme lactase converts the nonabsorable lactose to absorbable galactose and glucose in the small intestine; however, because lactase is genetically programmed to decrease or disappear in childhood, 75% of the world's population do not drink milk or milk products in adulthood. Only persons of Northern European ancestry—mainly those in North America, Australia, and New Zealand—are able to digest large quantities of milk and milk products as adults because of a mutation in the enzyme some 10,000 years ago. As a result of globalization and immigration, many new residents of North America cannot tolerate the milk and milk products common to many diets. These persons are deemed to have **lactose intolerance**, or the inability to digest lactose, the predominant sugar in milk. When lactose cannot be absorbed, it acts as an osmotic laxative, resulting in diarrhea, gaseous distension, and cramping (Lomer et al., 2008). Persons who have lactose intolerance must learn how much lactose their body can tolerate. For example, some persons can drink one glass of milk without effect, but not two. However, young children with lactose intolerance should not eat any foods with lactose (Lomer et al., 2008).

Fluid Intake. An inadequate fluid intake or disturbances that result in fluid loss (such as vomiting) can affect the character of feces. Fluid liquefies intestinal contents to ease their passage through the colon. Reduced fluid intake slows the passage of food through the intestine and can result in hardening of the stool. Unless a medical contraindication exists, an adult should drink six to eight glasses (1400 to 2000 mL) of noncaffeinated fluid daily. An increase in the intake fruit juices softens the stool and increases peristalsis; however, too much fruit juice, especially in children, can lead to diarrhea. In very young children, too much fruit juice can also delay toilet training of the bowels.

Older adults are at risk of insufficient intake of fluids and are thus predisposed to constipation. Sometimes, older adults reduce their fluid intake in an attempt to reduce micturition (see Chapter 44). In addition, in some persons, an increased ingestion of milk or milk products may slow peristalsis and cause constipation (Registered Nurses' Association of Ontario [RNAO], 2005).

Physical Activity. Physical activity promotes peristalsis, whereas immobilization depresses peristalsis. Thus, early ambulation is encouraged as a client's illness begins to resolve or as soon as possible after surgery to promote maintenance of peristalsis and thereby normal bowel elimination. Maintaining the tone of skeletal muscles used during defecation is important. Weakened abdominal and pelvic floor muscles impair the ability to increase intra-abdominal pressure and to control the external sphincter. Muscle tone may be weakened or lost as a result of long-term illness or neurological disease that impairs nerve transmission. Clients who experience these changes in the abdominal and pelvic floor muscles are at increased risk for constipation.

Psychological Factors. The function of almost all body systems can be impaired by prolonged emotional stress (see Chapter 30). When an individual becomes anxious, afraid, or angry, the stress response is initiated to allow the body to restore its defences. The digestive process accelerates and peristalsis increases. The side effects of increased peristalsis are diarrhea and gaseous distension. When a person becomes depressed, the autonomic nervous system slows impulses and peristalsis can decrease, resulting in constipation. Stress exacerbates several diseases of the GI tract, including ulcerative **colitis**, gastric and duodenal ulcers, and **Crohn's disease**.

Personal Habits. Personal bowel elimination habits can affect bowel function. Most persons benefit from being able to use their own toilet facilities at a time that, for them, is both most effective and most convenient. A busy work schedule may prevent a person from going to the bathroom in response to the urge to defecate, thus disrupting regular habits and possibly causing constipation. A person should establish a regular time for bowel elimination. The gastrocolic reflex is initiated by eating food and frequently leads to the need to defecate after a meal.

Chronically ill and hospitalized clients may not be able to maintain privacy during defecation. In a hospital or long-term care setting, bathroom facilities are often shared with a roommate whose hygienic habits might be very different. In addition, a chronic illness may limit a client's balance, activity tolerance, or physical activity; therefore, the client may require the use of a bedpan or a bedside commode. The sights, sounds, and odours associated with sharing toilet facilities or using bedpans are often embarrassing. Embarrassment prompts clients to ignore the urge to defecate, which can begin a vicious cycle of constipation and discomfort.

Position During Defecation. Squatting is the normal position during defecation. Toilets are designed to facilitate this posture, by allowing the person to lean forward, exert intra-abdominal pressure, and contract the thigh muscles. For clients who are immobilized in bed, defecation is often difficult. In a supine position, it is impossible to contract the muscles used during defecation. If the client's condition permits, raise the head of the bed; this action assists the client to a more normal sitting position on a bedpan, enhancing the ability to defecate.

Pain. Normally, the act of defecation is painless. However, several conditions can result in discomfort, including hemorrhoids, rectal surgery, rectal fistulas, and abdominal surgery. In these instances, to avoid pain, the client often suppresses the urge to defecate. As a result, constipation and impaction may develop.

Pregnancy and Labour. As pregnancy advances, the size of the fetus increases and pressure is exerted on the rectum. A temporary obstruction created by the fetus impairs the passage of feces. Slowing of peristalsis during the third trimester often leads to constipation. A pregnant woman's frequent straining during defecation or delivery can result in the formation of permanent hemorrhoids. Damage to the perineum extending to the anal sphincters during labour can also alter sphincter integrity.

Surgery and Anaesthesia. The general anaesthetic agents used during surgery cause temporary cessation of peristalsis (see Chapter 49). Inhaled anaesthetic agents block the parasympathetic impulses to the enteric nervous system, and the stress of surgery stimulates the sympathetic nervous system. The anaesthetic's action slows or stops the integrated contractions. Pain control medication that contains opioids has the side effects of slowing mass peristalsis (or mass movement) and increasing the slow-mixing contractions and fluid absorption from the colon. Thus, following surgery, abdominal discomfort from intraluminal gas and constipation are frequent, and the surgeon's postoperative orders typically include bowel routine with laxatives and enemas if bowel movements do not occur within 2 to 3 days. Thus, you need to note whether and when the first bowel movement postsurgery occurs because the client may require treatment for constipation. Early postoperative ambulation stimulates the evacuation of flatus, stimulates peristalsis, and alleviates abdominal pain.

The client who receives local or regional anaesthesia is less at risk for bowel elimination alterations because bowel activity may be affected minimally or not at all. Any surgery that involves direct manipulation of the bowel temporarily stops peristalsis. This condition, called **paralytic ileus**, usually lasts 24 to 48 hours. If the client remains inactive or is unable to eat after surgery, return of normal bowel function may be further delayed.

Medications. Medication may have certain expected actions on the bowel; for example, some medications promote defecation and others control diarrhea. In addition, medications prescribed for acute and chronic conditions may have secondary effects on the client's bowel elimination patterns (Table 45–2). **Laxatives** are defined as products that stimulate evacuation of the formed stool from the rectum, whereas **cathartics** are defined as products that evacuate unformed and usually watery fecal material from the entire colon. Laxatives are thus milder in action than cathartics. When used correctly, laxatives and cathartics safely maintain normal bowel elimination patterns; however, chronic use of cathartics causes the large intestine to lose muscle tone and to become less responsive to stimulation by laxatives. Laxative overuse can also cause serious diarrhea that can lead to dehydration and electrolyte depletion. Mineral oil, a common laxative, decreases fat-soluble vitamin absorption. Laxatives can influence the efficacy of other medications by altering the transit time (i.e., the time the medication remains in the GI tract and is available for absorption).

Diagnostic Tests. Diagnostic examinations that involve visualization of GI structures often require that portions of the bowel be empty. The client receives a prescribed bowel preparation before the test. Usually, the client is asked to drink a large volume (4 L) of a solution containing a nonabsorbable inert molecule, such as polyethylene glycol. Other medications, cathartics, or enemas may also be used. In addition, the client is not allowed to eat or drink after midnight of the day preceding examinations such as a colonoscopy, **endoscopy**, or other testing that requires visualization of the lower GI tract. Following the diagnostic procedure, the client may experience changes in bowel elimination, such as increased gas or loose stools. These changes will stop when the client resumes a normal eating pattern.

Common Bowel Elimination Problems

You might care for clients who have or are at risk for bowel elimination problems because of emotional stress (anxiety or depression), inflammatory diseases, prescribed therapy, disorders impairing defecation, or physiological changes in the GI tract, such as surgical alteration of intestinal structures.

Constipation. Constipation is a symptom, not a disease (Box 45–1). The signs of constipation vary among clients, but usually include infrequent bowel movements (fewer than three per week), difficult evacuation of feces, inability to defecate at will, and hard feces (Ginsberg et al., 2007). Common signs are abdominal pain and distension and a sensation of fullness and pressure in the rectum. Straining during defecation is also an associated sign. When intestinal motility slows, the fecal mass becomes exposed over time to the intestinal walls and most of the fecal water is absorbed. Little water is left to soften and lubricate the stool. Passage of a dry, hard stool may cause rectal pain.

Constipation can be a significant hazard to health. Straining during defecation may cause problems to the client who has recently undergone abdominal, gynecological, or rectal surgery. The effort to pass a stool can cause sutures to separate, thereby reopening the wound. Clients who have a history of cardiovascular disease, diseases causing elevated intraocular pressure (glaucoma), and increased intracranial pressure should prevent constipation and avoid using the Valsalva manoeuvre. The Valsalva manoeuvre can be avoided by exhaling through the mouth during straining. Clients

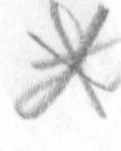

may experience constipation as a result of medications they are taking. Medications that cause constipation include acetylsalicylic acid (Aspirin), antihistamines, diuretics, tranquilizers, hypnotics, antacids with aluminum or calcium, opiates, and drugs used to control Parkinson's disease. Constipation can also occur in conjunction with the treatment of urinary conditions, as a side effect of the medication but also because individuals with urinary incontinence may reduce their fluid intake to reduce the frequency of their need to urinate (Ginsberg et al., 2007).

Constipation in children can be a particularly difficult problem. Because the passage of hard, dry stools is painful for the child, the child may voluntarily withhold the feces, which leads to impaction and subsequent fecal soiling. In most cases, this situation can be described as functional constipation; it is also known as idiopathic constipation, functional retention, and fecal withholding. A detailed family and dietary history is essential to rule out organic causes. To commence treatment, the impaction must be emptied by using stool softeners and increasing the intake of fluids, particularly fruit juices containing sorbital, such as pear, prune, and apple juices. Long-term treatment must include regular physical activity and a diet including sources of dietary fibre, such as whole grains, fruits, and vegetables (see North American Society for Pediatric Gastroenterology, Hepatology and Nutrition [NASPGHN] Constipation Guideline Committee, 2006).

Impaction. Fecal impaction results from unrelieved constipation. Fecal impaction is a collection of hardened feces that are wedged in the rectum and cannot be expelled. In cases of severe impaction, the mass can extend into the sigmoid colon. Clients who are debilitated, confused, or unconscious are most at risk for impaction. They are too weak or are unaware of the need to defecate, or they

➤ TABLE 45-2 Medications and the Gastrointestinal System

Medication	Action
Dicyclomine HC1 (Bentyl)	Suppresses peristalsis and can decrease gastric emptying.
Narcotic analgesics	Increase the mixing action of segmentation contractions and slow the propulsive contractions, often resulting in constipation (McKenry et al., 2006).
Anticholinergic drugs, such as atropine or glycopyrrolate (Robinul)	Inhibit gastric acid secretion and depress gastrointestinal motility (McKenry et al., 2006). Although anticholinergics are useful in treating hyperactive bowel disorders, they can cause constipation.
Antibiotics	Frequently produce diarrhea by disrupting the normal bacterial flora in the gastrointestinal tract. Antibiotic use has been shown to promote infection with the highly contagious *Clostridium difficile* (*C. difficile*), which has a high mortality rate in older adults. Concurrently taking a probiotic acidophilus supplement has been shown to reduce the incidence of diarrhea and to reduce the risk of *C. difficile* infections (McFarland, 2006).
Nonsteroidal anti-inflammatory drugs (Motrin, ibuprofen, and Cox-2 inhibitors)	Prostaglandin inhibitors are used to treat arthritic pain but can also promote gastrointestinal irritation that can range from dyspepsia to life-threatening hemorrhage (Scheiman, 2008). These drugs also appear to promote *C. difficile* (Todd, 2006) and have been implicated in sudden death from cardiovascular disease.
Aspirin	A prostaglandin inhibitor. It can interfere with the formation and production of protective mucus and can predispose clients to gastritis.
Histamine₂ (H_2) antagonists	Suppress the secretion of hydrochloric acid and may interfere with the digestion of some foods (Abrams et al., 2007).
Proton pump inhibitors	Suppress gastric acid secretion and may also promote *C. difficile* infection (Todd. 2006).
Iron	Can cause blackening of the stool and can lead to constipation (McKenry et al., 2006).

> **BOX 45-1 Common Causes of Constipation**
>
> - Irregular bowel habits and ignoring the urge to defecate
> - Chronic illnesses (e.g., Parkinson's disease, multiple sclerosis, rheumatoid arthritis, chronic bowel diseases, depression, eating disorders) (Ginsberg et al., 2007)
> - A low-fibre diet high in animal fats (e.g., meats, dairy products, eggs) and refined sugars (e.g., rich desserts)
> - A low fluid intake (it slows peristalsis) (RNAO, 2005).
> - Situational stress (e.g., illness of a family member, death of a loved one, divorce) (Dosh, 2002)
> - Lengthy bed rest or lack of regular exercise
> - Heavy laxative use causes loss of the normal defecation reflex. In addition, laxatives completely empty the lower colon, and the lower colon requires time to refill with bulk (Ginsberg et al., 2007).
> - Older adults experience slowed peristalsis, loss of abdominal muscle elasticity, and reduced intestinal mucous secretion. Also, older adults often eat low-fibre foods.
> - Neurological conditions that block the nerve impulse to the colon (e.g., spinal cord injuries, tumours)
> - Organic illnesses such as hypothyroidism, hypocalcemia, or hypokalemia (Ginsberg et al., 2007)

may be so dehydrated that the stool is too hard and too dry to pass. High intake of fibre or cellulose without accompanying fluids can increase the risk of impaction.

An obvious sign of impaction is the inability to pass a stool for several days, despite the repeated urge to defecate. A continuous oozing of diarrhea stool may develop when the liquid portion of feces located higher in the colon seeps around the impacted mass. Loss of appetite (anorexia), nausea or vomiting, abdominal distension and cramping, and rectal pain may accompany the condition. If you suspect an impaction, you can gently perform a digital examination of the rectum and palpate for the impacted mass.

Diarrhea. Diarrhea is an increase in the number of stools (several bowel movements per day) and the passage of liquid, unformed feces. Diarrhea is associated with disorders affecting digestion, absorption, and secretion in the GI tract. Intestinal contents pass through the small and large intestine too quickly to allow the usual absorption of fluid and nutrients. Irritation within the colon can result in an increased mucus secretion. As a result, feces become watery and the client may be unable to control the urge to defecate.

Excess loss of colonic fluid can result in serious fluid, electrolyte, or acid-base imbalances. Infants and older adults are particularly susceptible to complications associated with diarrhea (see Chapter 40). Because repeated passage of diarrhea stools exposes the skin of the perineum and the buttocks to irritating intestinal contents, meticulous skin care and containment of fecal drainage is needed to prevent skin breakdown (see Chapter 38).

Many conditions cause diarrhea. Antibiotic administered by any route may cause diarrhea because these medications alter the normal flora in the gastrointestinal tract (Bartlett, 2002). To counteract this effect of antibiotics, the client may be advised to eat active-culture yogurt or to take a lactobacillus supplement to reintroduce the normal flora of the colon. Clients receiving enteral nutrition are also at risk for diarrhea, which may be due to the GI response to the enteral feeding's nutritional components, frequency, or volume. Food allergies and intolerances increase peristalsis and cause diarrhea. Diarrhea can also be caused by diseases, surgeries, laxatives, chemotherapy, radiotherapy, and diagnostic testing of the lower gastrointestinal tract. The aims of treatment are to remove the precipitating conditions and to slow peristalsis.

Communicable food-borne pathogens can also cause diarrhea. The risk of food-borne illnesses can be greatly reduced by handwashing after using the bathroom and before and after preparing foods, and by properly storing and preparing of fresh produce and meats. When diarrhea is the result of a food-borne virus, the goal is usually to rid the system of the pathogen, not to slow peristalsis.

Outbreaks of the highly contagious Norwalk virus are common in Canadian schools, hospitals, day care centres, and nursing homes. The Norwalk virus has been described as "the winter vomiting disease" and rapidly spreads to staff, students, and clients (Conly & Johnston, 2003). When the Norwalk virus is detected, standard infection-control procedures need to be implemented rapidly, accompanied by further precautions, such as isolation of the affected units, strict handwashing protocols, the wearing of gloves and gowns, and a thorough washing down of the affected units. When an outbreak occurs, the institution is frequently closed to visitors, and infected staff are required to remain off-duty until they are symptom free for 48 hours. In healthy individuals, symptoms last from 12 to 60 hours. The very young, older adults, and ill clients are at danger from dehydration and electrolyte imbalance.

Infections with *Clostridium difficile* (*C. difficile*) have become more frequent in the past decade, and the infections are more severe, sometimes leading to severe colitis, toxic megacolon, and an increased mortality rate (Todd, 2006). The bacteria recently mutated to a more virulent strain (known as the Quebec strain) that produces more toxins. Increased susceptibility is associated with antibiotic use, particularly the fluoroquinolones (i.e., ciprofloxacin [Cipro]), which may actually promote the widespread emergence of infections. The use of nonsteroidal anti-inflammatory drugs for treatment of arthritic diseases is frequently accompanied by gastric acid inhibition with proton pump inhibitors, both of which appear to increase susceptibility to *C. difficile*. You should be alert for the possibility that diarrhea may be caused by *C. difficile*. As soon as *C. difficile* is suspected, isolation and appropriate cleaning procedures must be initiated. Because the bacteria produce spores, *C. difficile* is difficult to eliminate from the surroundings. Alcohol does not kill the spores, so hands must be washed with soap and water. Cleaning and disinfection of the room requires the addition of hypochlorite (bleach) to inactivate the spores. In many areas, *C. difficile* has become a reportable disease.

Incontinence. Fecal incontinence is the inability to control the passage of feces and gas from the anus. Incontinence can harm a client's body image (see Chapter 26). In many situations, the client is mentally alert but is physically unable to avoid defecation. Because incontinence can occur in a variety of settings, the possible embarrassment of soiling clothes can lead to self-imposed social isolation (Skelly et al., 2006). Physical conditions that impair anal sphincter function or control can cause incontinence. Conditions that create frequent, loose, large-volume, watery stools are predispositions for fecal incontinence (Box 45–2).

Flatulence. In most healthy individuals, 100 to 200 mL of gas is present in the GI tract. Gas in the upper GI tract may increase from the swallowing of air. Gas production in the colon occurs from bacteria digesting cellulose in the colon.

As gas accumulates in the lumen of the intestines, the bowel wall stretches and distends, resulting in flatulence. Flatulence is a common cause of abdominal fullness, pain, and cramping. Normally, intestinal gas escapes through the mouth (belching) or the anus (passing of

BOX 45-2 RESEARCH HIGHLIGHT

Factors Associated With Fecal Incontinence

Research Focus

Identifying the causes of fecal incontinence of clients in acute care settings is difficult. Nurses care for many clients who are incontinent. Incontinence is embarrassing for the client; however, it also increases the client's risk of complications secondary to incontinence, such as impaired skin integrity or prolonged hospital stays.

Research Abstract

The purpose of the study by Bliss et al. (2000) study was to determine the presence of fecal incontinence in hospitalized clients who were acutely ill and to determine whether a relationship exists between fecal incontinence and stool consistency, and between two well-known nosocomial or iatrogenic causes of diarrhea: *Clostridium difficile* and enteral tube feedings. Data from 152 clients were collected on fecal incontinence, stool frequency and consistency, presence of tube feedings and medications, severity of illness, and nutritional information. Rectal swabs and stool specimens were obtained weekly and cultured for nosocomial infections.

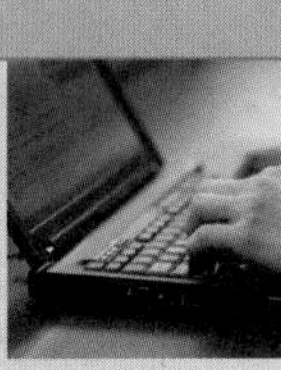

Evidence-Informed Practice

- The presence of diarrhea was more frequently associated with incontinence.
- Clients who were incontinent with loose, watery diarrhea had little or no warning prior to the incontinence episode.
- Diarrhea was __________ present without a positive stool culture.
- Controlling the diarrhea proves to be beneficial because the more formed a stool becomes, the less frequent is the incontinence.
- When clients have organism-related diarrheas, as with *C. difficile*, treatments that slow intestinal transit should be avoided.

References: Bliss, D. Z., Johnson, S., Savik, K., Clabots, C., & Gerding, D. (2000). Fecal incontinence in hospitalized patients who are acutely ill. *Nursing Research, 49*, 101–108.

flatus). For a person eating a normal diet, 50 to 500 mL of gas is passed 10 to 15 times a day. However, if intestinal motility is reduced as a result of the effects of opiates, general anaesthetics, abdominal surgery, or immobilization, flatulence can become severe enough to cause abdominal distension and severe, sharp pain.

Hemorrhoids. **Hemorrhoids** are dilated, engorged veins in the lining of the rectum. They are either external or internal. External hemorrhoids are clearly visible as protrusions of skin. If the underlying vein is hardened, a purplish discoloration (i.e., thrombosis) may be visible. This condition causes increased pain, and the hemorrhoid may need to be excised. Internal hemorrhoids have an outer mucous membrane. Increased venous pressure as a result of pregnancy, heart failure, chronic liver disease, or straining at defecation can cause hemorrhoids. The presence of hemorrhoids is frequently accompanied by fecal soiling of undergarments and irritation of the distended veins by overly vigorous cleaning of the anus. The use of baby wipes for cleaning following a bowel movement may reduce the possibility of irritation.

Bowel Diversions

Certain diseases cause conditions that prevent the normal passage of feces through the rectum. The treatment for these disorders may result in the need for a **stoma**, which is a temporary or permanent artificial opening in the abdominal wall. The opening may be either an **ileostomy**, a surgical opening in the ileum, or a **colostomy**, a surgical opening in the colon. The ends of the intestine are brought through the abdominal wall to create the stoma. The Canadian Association for Enterostomal Therapy's Web site provides regularly updated information handbooks in addition to resources and information on educational programs for nurses (Canadian Association for Enterostomal Therapy [CAET], 2008a, 2008b).

The standard bowel diversion creates a stoma, or the client can undergo reconstructive surgery that uses the native sphincter for bowel continence. The reconstructive surgery includes either a continent stoma procedure, which is now rarely done, or the ileoanal pouch anastomosis, which is described later (CAET, 2008).

Ostomies. The location of the ostomy determines the consistency of the stool. An ileostomy bypasses the entire large intestine. As a result, stools are frequent and liquid. The same is true for a colostomy of the ascending colon. A colostomy of the transverse colon, in general, results in a more solid, formed stool. The sigmoid colostomy emits a near-normal stool. The location of a colostomy is determined by the client's medical problem and general condition. Colostomies have three types of construction: loop colostomy, end colostomy, and double-barrel colostomy.

Loop Colostomy. A loop colostomy is usually performed in a medical emergency when closure of the colostomy is anticipated. Loop colostomies are usually temporary large stomas constructed in the transverse colon (Figure 45–5A–D). The surgeon pulls a loop of bowel onto the abdomen (Figure 45–5E). An external supporting device, such as a plastic rod, bridge (Figure 45–5C and D), or rubber catheter is temporarily placed under the bowel loop to keep it from slipping back (Figure 45–5A). The surgeon then opens the bowel and sutures it to the skin of the abdomen (Figure 45–5F). A communicating wall remains between the proximal and distal bowel. The loop ostomy has two openings through the one stoma (Figure 45–5D and G). The proximal end drains stool, whereas the distal portion drains mucus. Within 7 to 10 days, the external supporting device is removed.

End Colostomy. The end colostomy consists of one stoma formed from one end of the bowel with the distal portion of the GI tract either removed or sewn closed (known as Hartmann's pouch) and left in the abdominal cavity. For many clients, end colostomies are a result of surgical treatment for colorectal cancer. In such cases, the rectum might also be removed. Clients with diverticulitis who are treated surgically often have a temporary end colostomy with a Hartmann's pouch (Figure 45–6).

Double-Barrel Colostomy. In a double-barrel colostomy (as opposed to the loop colostomy), the bowel is surgically severed (Figure 45–7A) and the two ends are brought out onto the abdomen (Figure 45–7B). The double-barrel colostomy consists of two distinct stomas: the proximal functioning stoma and the distal nonfunctioning stoma.

Alternative Procedures

Ileoanal Pouch Anastomosis. The ileoanal pouch anastomosis is a surgical procedure that may be used in clients who require a colectomy for treatment of ulcerative colitis or familial **polyps** (a projecting growth of mucous membrane). In this procedure, the colon is removed, a pouch (or reservoir) is created from the end of the small intestine, and the pouch is attached to the client's anus (Figure 45–8).

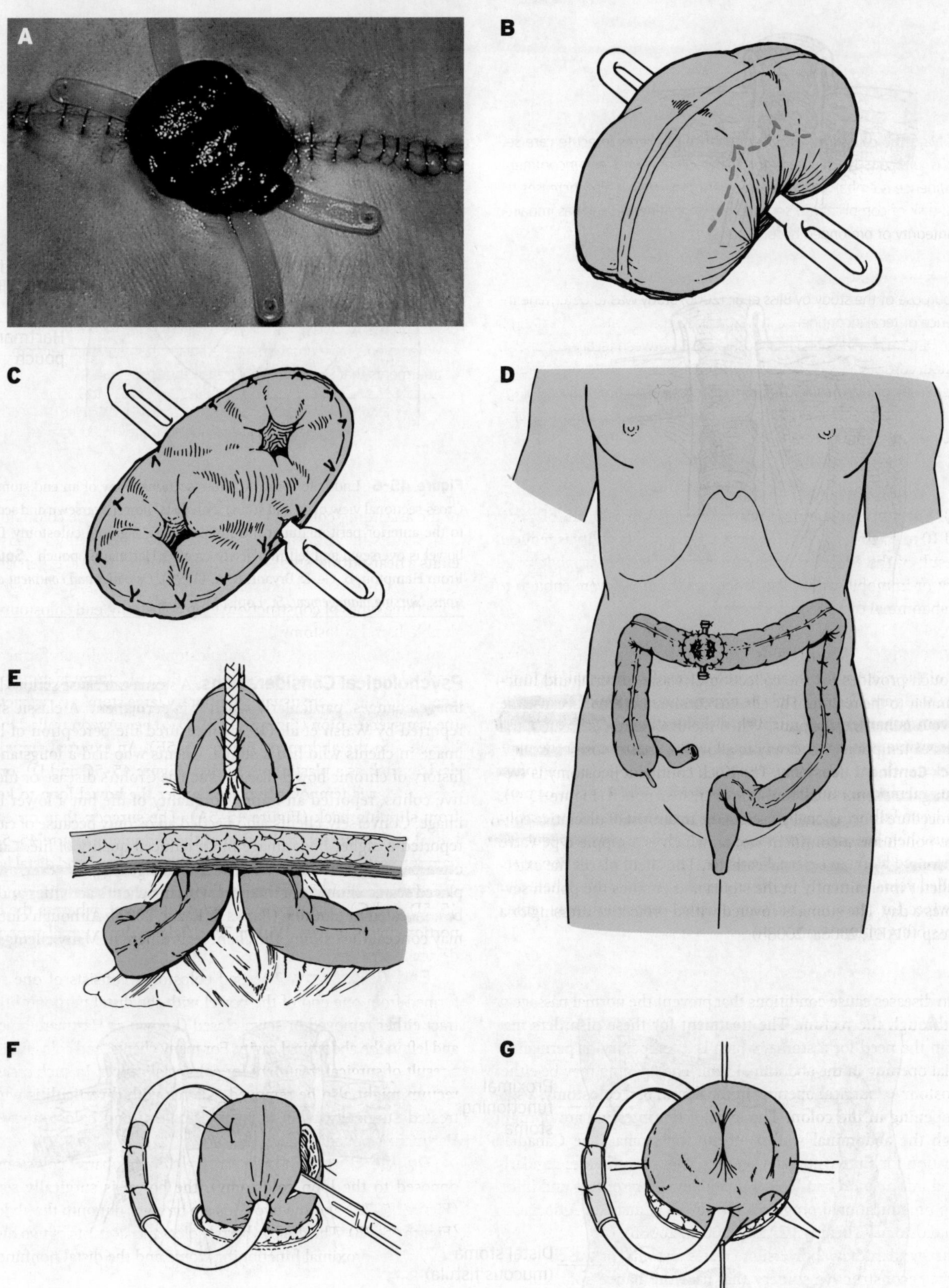

Figure 45-5 A, Transverse loop colostomy supported with a flexible red rubber catheter. A, B, Abdominal view of a loop colostomy in the transverse colon. C, Loop colostomy construction is much the same as the construction of a loop ileostomy. The stoma is created with a longitudinal incision through sacculations in the colon. D, Loop colostomy matured. E, Loop ostomy construction showing loop of bowel exteriorized. F, Support device placed to maintain position of the bowel on the abdominal surface. The distal bowel of the ileum is incised. A stitch is placed to designate the proximal bowel. G, Loop ileostomy matured with protruding functional limb. **Source:** A, Courtesy Hollister, Inc., Libertyville, IL; B to G, From Hampton, B. G., & Bryant, R. A. (1992). *Ostomies and continent diversions: Nursing management*. St. Louis, MO: Mosby.

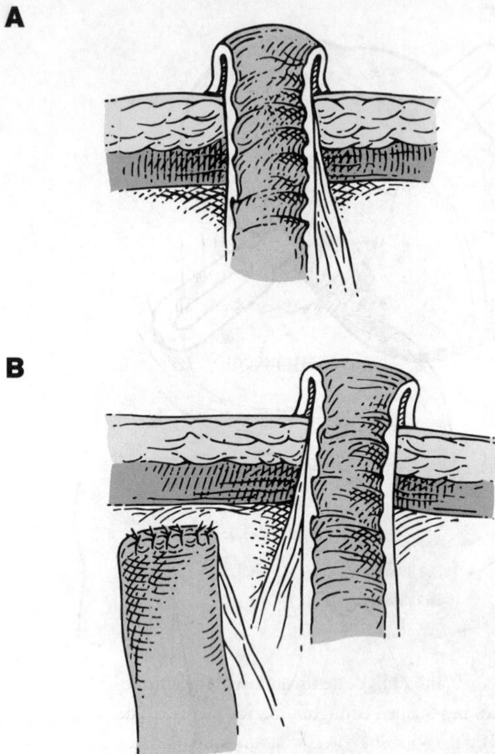

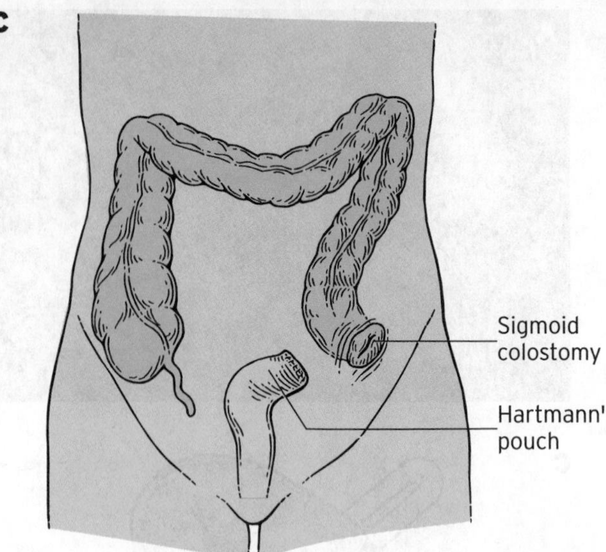

Figure 45-6 End colostomy. A, Cross-sectional view of an end stoma. B, Cross-sectional view of an end stoma with distal bowel oversewn and secured to the anterior peritoneum at the stoma site. C, Sigmoid colostomy. Distal bowel is oversewn and left in place to create a Hartmann's pouch. **Source:** From Hampton, B. G., & Bryant, R. A. (1992). *Ostomies and continent diversions: Nursing management*. St. Louis, MO: Mosby.

This pouch provides for the collection of waste material and functions similar to the rectum. The client is continent of stool because the stool is evacuated via the anus. When the ileal pouch is created, the client has a temporary ileostomy to allow the anastomosis to heal.

Kock Continent Ileostomy. The Kock continent ileostomy is created using the client's small intestine to create a pouch (Figure 45–9). This procedure is occasionally used in the treatment of ulcerative colitis. The pouch has a continent stoma, which is a nipple-type valve that is drained with an external catheter. The client places the external catheter intermittently in the stoma and empties the pouch several times a day. The stoma is covered with a protective dressing or a stoma cap (CAET, 2008a, 2008b).

Psychological Considerations. A stoma can cause serious body image changes, particularly when it is permanent. A classic study reported by Walsh et al. (1995) measured the perception of body image in clients who had a stoma. Clients who had a longstanding history of chronic bowel disease, such as Crohn's disease or ulcerative colitis, reported an improved quality of life but a lower body image. Conversely, clients who needed an ostomy because of cancer reported a higher body image but a reduced quality of life. Clients often perceive a stoma as invasive and disfiguring; however, a well-placed stoma should not interfere with the client's activities and can be concealed by clothing (Banks & Razor, 2003). Although clothing may conceal the ostomy, the client feels different. Many clients have

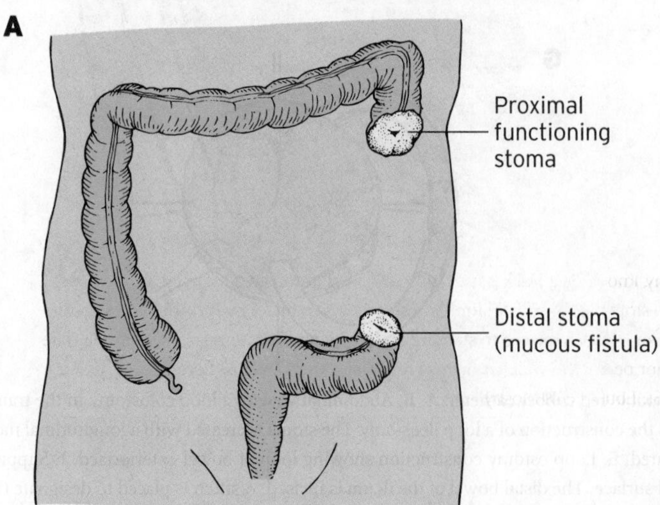

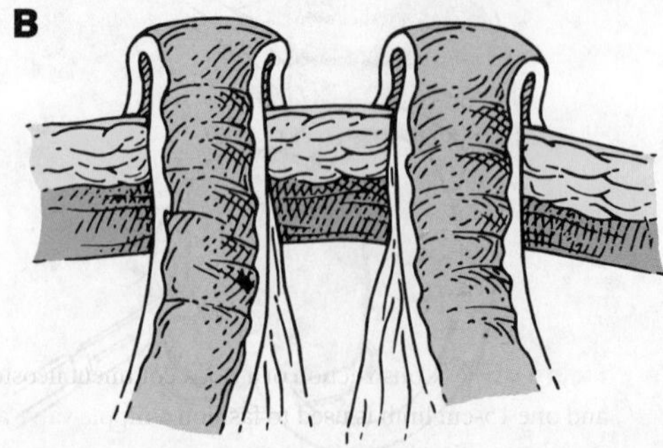

Figure 45-7 Double-barrel colostomy. A, Double-barrel colostomy in the descending colon. B, Cross-sectional view of a double-barrel stoma. **Source:** From Hampton, B. G., & Bryant, R. A. (1992). *Ostomies and continent diversions: Nursing management*. St. Louis, MO: Mosby.

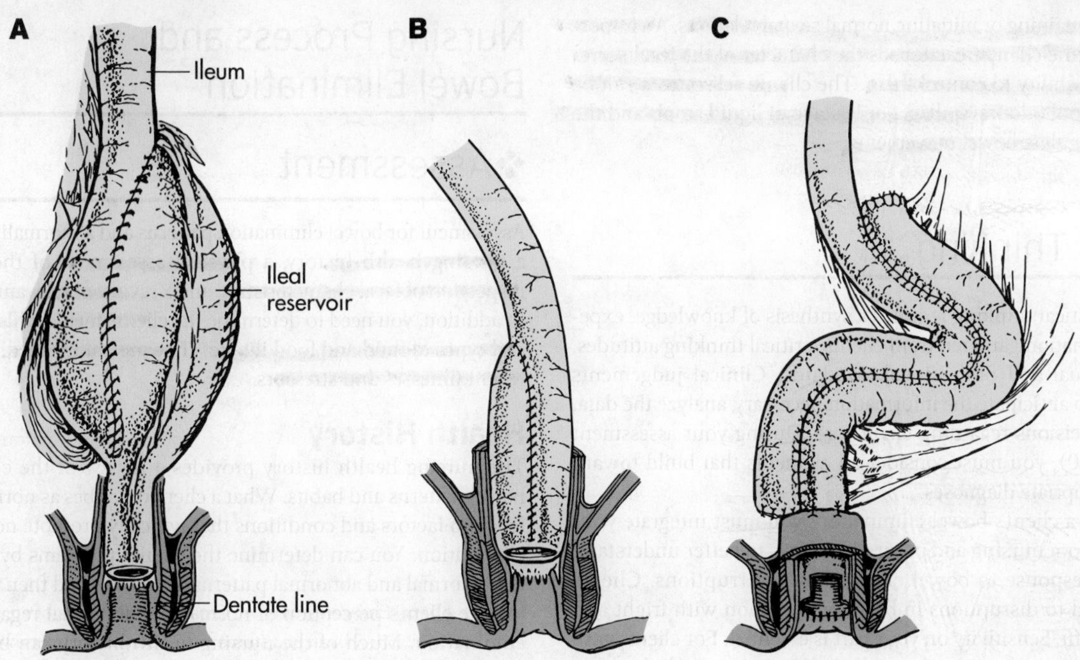

Figure 45-8 Ileoanal reservoirs (IARs). A, S-shaped configuration for the IAR. Three 10-cm limbs of ileum are used, the antimesenteric surface of each limb is opened, and the adjacent bowel walls are anastomosed. B, J-shaped configuration for the IAR. The distal ileum is aligned in a J shape; the antimesenteric surface of the J shape is opened, and the adjacent bowel walls are anastomosed. A side-to-end anastomosis of the bowel to the dentate line is evident. C, Lateral or side-by-side ileoanal pouch configuration. **Source:** From Hampton, B. G., & Bryant, R. A. (1992). *Ostomies and continent diversions: Nursing management*. St. Louis, MO: Mosby.

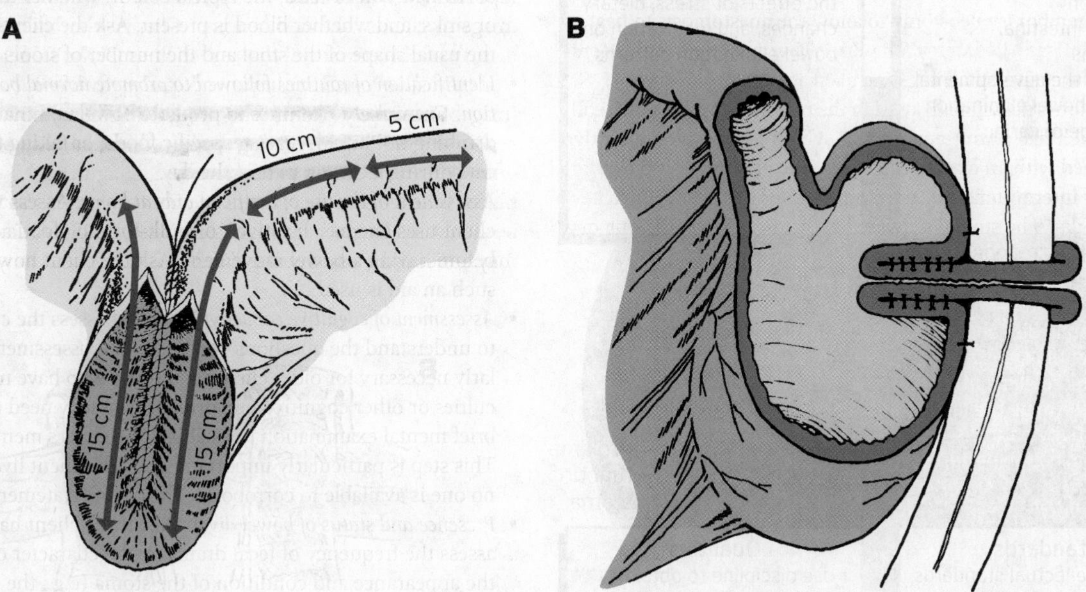

Figure 45-9 Construction of a Kock continent ileostomy, known as a Kock pouch. A, Two 15-cm limbs are used to create the pouch, and one 15-cm limb is used to fashion a nipple valve and stoma. B, The distal limb is intussuscepted into a reservoir to create a one-way valve and accomplish continence. Sutures or staples, or both, are placed to stabilize and maintain the intussuscepted nipple. The anterior surface of the reservoir is anchored to the anterior peritoneal wall. **Source:** From Hampton, B. G., & Bryant, R. A. (1992). *Ostomies and continent diversions: Nursing management*. St. Louis, MO: Mosby.

difficulty maintaining or initiating normal sexual relations. An important factor in the client's reactions is the character of the fecal secretions and the ability to control them. The client's self-esteem can be impaired by foul odours, spillage, or leakage of liquid stools and the inability to regulate bowel movements.

Critical Thinking

Successful critical thinking requires a synthesis of knowledge, experience, information gathered from clients, critical thinking attitudes, and intellectual and professional standards. Clinical judgements require you to anticipate the information necessary, analyze the data, and make decisions regarding client care. During your assessment (Figure 45–10), you must consider all elements that build toward making appropriate diagnoses.

To assess a client's bowel elimination, you must integrate your knowledge from nursing and other disciplines to better understand the client's response to bowel elimination interruptions. Clients often respond to disruptions in bowel elimination with fright and embarrassment. Sensitivity on your part is essential. For clients with significant interruptions, such as a bowel diversion, include information from an enterostomal specialist as an important part of the care plan.

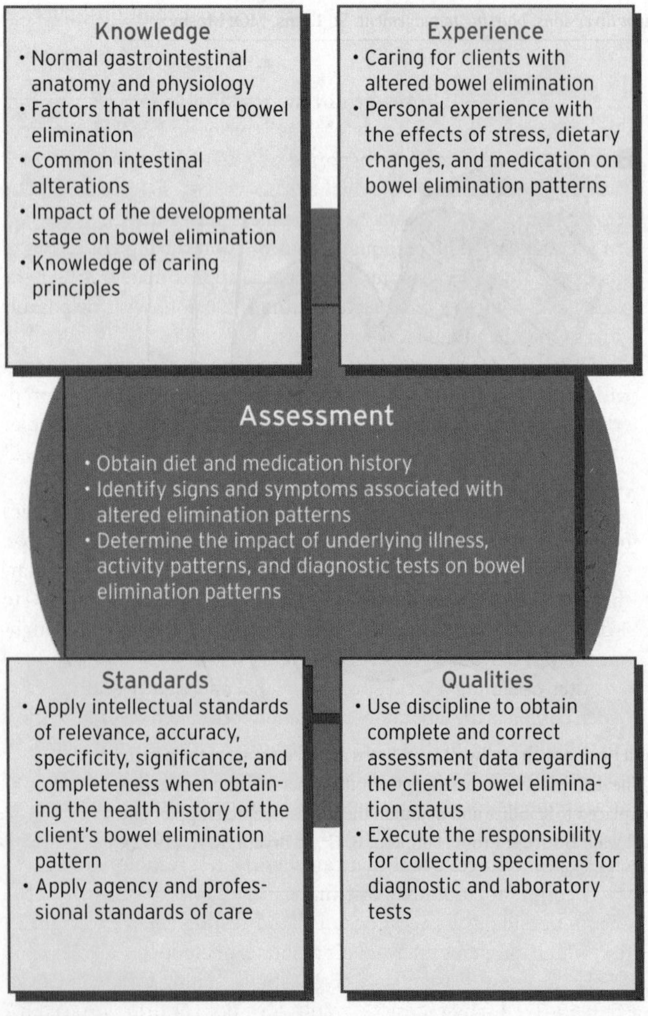

Knowledge
- Normal gastrointestinal anatomy and physiology
- Factors that influence bowel elimination
- Common intestinal alterations
- Impact of the developmental stage on bowel elimination
- Knowledge of caring principles

Experience
- Caring for clients with altered bowel elimination
- Personal experience with the effects of stress, dietary changes, and medication on bowel elimination patterns

Assessment
- Obtain diet and medication history
- Identify signs and symptoms associated with altered elimination patterns
- Determine the impact of underlying illness, activity patterns, and diagnostic tests on bowel elimination patterns

Standards
- Apply intellectual standards of relevance, accuracy, specificity, significance, and completeness when obtaining the health history of the client's bowel elimination pattern
- Apply agency and professional standards of care

Qualities
- Use discipline to obtain complete and correct assessment data regarding the client's bowel elimination status
- Execute the responsibility for collecting specimens for diagnostic and laboratory tests

Figure 45-10 Critical thinking model for bowel elimination assessment.

Nursing Process and Bowel Elimination

❖Assessment

Assessment for bowel elimination patterns and abnormalities includes a nursing health history, a physical assessment of the abdomen, inspection of fecal characteristics, and a review of relevant test results. In addition, you need to determine the client's medical history, pattern and types of fluid and food intake, chewing ability, medications, and recent illnesses and stressors.

Health History

The nursing health history provides a review of the client's usual bowel patterns and habits. What a client describes as normal may differ from factors and conditions that typically promote normal bowel elimination. You can determine the client's problems by first identifying normal and abnormal patterns and habits and then understanding the client's perception of normal and abnormal regarding bowel elimination. Much of the nursing health history can be organized around the factors that affect bowel elimination:

- *Determination of the client's usual bowel elimination pattern:* The frequency and time of day of the client's bowel eliminations should be noted. Have the client or caregiver complete a bowel elimination diary for a week to enable an accurate assessment of the typical bowel elimination pattern.
- *The client's description of the usual stool characteristics:* The client's description should indicate whether the stool is normally watery or formed, soft or hard; the typical colour; whether the stool floats or sinks; and whether blood is present. Ask the client to describe the usual shape of the stool and the number of stools per day.
- *Identification of routines followed to promote normal bowel elimination:* Examples of routines to promote bowel elimination are drinking hot liquids, eating specific foods, or taking time to defecate during a certain part of the day.
- *Assessment of the use of artificial aids at home:* Assess whether the client uses enemas, laxatives, or bulk-forming food additives before having a bowel movement. Ask the client how often an such an aid is used.
- *Assessment of cognitive capacity:* You must assess the client's ability to understand the questions you pose. This assessment is particularly necessary for older clients and those who have memory difficulties or other cognitive impairment. You may need to conduct a brief mental examination to establish the client's mental status. This step is particularly important when the client lives alone and no one is available to corroborate the client's statements.
- *Presence and status of bowel diversions:* If the client has an ostomy, assess the frequency of fecal drainage, the character of the feces, the appearance and condition of the stoma (e.g., the colour, the presence of swelling, and signs of irritation), the type of fecal collection device used, and the methods used to maintain the ostomy's function.
- *Changes in appetite:* Note any changes in the client's normal eating patterns and any change in weight (i.e., the amount lost or gained). If a change of weight has occurred, ask whether the weight change was planned, such as weight loss as a result of a low-calorie diet.
- *Diet history:* Determine the client's dietary preferences for a day or a week. Assess the intake of fruits, vegetables, cereals, and breads and whether mealtimes are regular or irregular. In the

case of the frail, older client living alone, determine whether acquiring food requires assistance (e.g., financial help, food preparation assistance, or transportation to a grocery store with a full selection of fresh fruits and vegetables).

- *Description of daily fluid intake:* Determine the type and amount of fluid consumed in a typical day. The client might need to estimate the amount by using common household measurements.
- *History of surgery or illnesses affecting the GI tract:* This information can help to explain symptoms and to assess the client's potential for maintaining or restoring a normal bowel elimination pattern. A client's family history of gastrointestinal cancer is also relevant to your assessment.
- *Medication history:* Ask for a list of the client's current medications. The medication history must include both prescribed and over-the-counter medications (e.g., laxatives, antacids, iron supplements, and analgesics) that might alter defecation or fecal characteristics. The community nurse should ask to see the medications.
- *Emotional state:* The client's emotional state can significantly alter the frequency of defecation. During assessment, observe the client's emotions, tone of voice, and mannerisms, which can reveal significant behaviours that indicate the presence of stress.
- *History of exercise:* Ask the client to describe the type and amount of daily exercise.
- *History of pain or discomfort:* Ask whether the client has a history of abdominal or anal pain. The type, frequency, and location of pain may help to identify the source of the problem.
- *Social history:* Clients have many different living arrangements. Where clients live may affect their toileting habits. If the client is sharing living quarters, how many bathrooms are available? Does the client have his or her own bathroom, or does the client need to share the facilities and thus adjust the time the bathroom is used to accommodate other persons? If the client lives alone, is he or she capable of ambulating to the toilet safely? If the client is not independent in bowel management, who assists the client and how?
- *Mobility and dexterity:* The client's mobility and dexterity need to be evaluated to determine whether the client needs assistive devices or personal assistance.

Physical Assessment

Your physical assessment (see Chapter 32) evaluates a client's body systems and functions that are likely to be affected by the presence of bowel elimination problems.

Mouth. Your inspection of the mouth includes examining the client's teeth, tongue, and gums. Poor dentition or poorly fitting dentures influence the ability to chew (see Chapter 43). Sores in the mouth can make eating not only difficult but also painful. A dry mouth may indicate dehydration.

Abdomen. Inspect all four abdominal quadrants for contour, shape, symmetry, and skin colour. Note masses, peristaltic waves, scars, venous patterns, stomas, and lesions. Normally, peristaltic waves are not visible; however, observable peristalsis can be a sign of intestinal obstruction.

Abdominal distension appears as an overall outward protuberance of the abdomen. Distension may be caused by intestinal gas, large tumours, or fluid in the peritoneal cavity. A distended abdomen feels tight, like a drum, and the skin appears taut, as if stretched.

Use percussion to detect lesions, fluid, or gas in the abdomen. Familiarity with the five percussion notes (see Chapter 32) permits identification of the underlying abdominal structures. Gas or flatulence creates a tympanic note. Masses, tumours, and fluid are dull to percussion.

Auscultate the abdomen with the stethoscope to assess bowel sounds in each quadrant (see Chapter 32). Normal bowel sounds occur every 5 to 15 seconds and last from one second to several seconds. While auscultating, note the character and frequency of the bowel sounds. An increase in pitch or a tinkling sound may be heard when the abdomen is distended. The lack of bowel sounds or the presence of hypoactive sounds (fewer than five sounds per minute) occur when the client has a paralytic ileus, such as after abdominal surgery. High-pitched and hyperactive bowel sounds (35 or more sounds per minute) occur when the small intestine is obstructed or when inflammatory disorders are present.

Gently palpate the abdomen for masses or areas of tenderness (see Chapter 32). During this procedure, encourage the client to relax. Tensing of the abdominal muscles interferes with palpating underlying organs or masses.

Rectum. Inspect the area around the anus for lesions, discolorations, inflammation, and hemorrhoids. Abnormalities should be carefully recorded (see Chapter 32).

Laboratory Tests

Laboratory and diagnostic examinations yield useful information concerning bowel elimination problems (Table 45–3). Laboratory analysis of fecal contents can detect pathological conditions, such as tumours, bleeding, and infection.

Fecal Specimens. You are directly responsible for ensuring that fecal specimens are accurately obtained, properly labelled in appropriate containers, and transported to the laboratory on time. Institutions provide special containers for fecal specimens. Some tests require specimens to be placed in chemical preservatives.

Medical aseptic technique should be used during collection of stool specimens (see Chapter 33). Because approximately 25% of the solid portion of a stool is bacteria from the colon, wear disposable gloves when handling fecal specimens.

Hand hygiene is necessary for anyone who might come in contact with the specimen. The client can often obtain the specimen if properly instructed. Explain that feces cannot be mixed with urine or water. For this reason, the client must defecate into a clean, dry bedpan or a special container placed under the toilet seat.

Tests performed by the laboratory for occult (microscopic) blood in the stool and stool cultures require only a small sample. Collect about 2.5 cm of formed stool or 15 to 30 mL of liquid diarrhea stool. Tests for measuring the output of fecal fat require a 3- to 5-day collection of stool. All fecal material must be saved throughout the test period.

After obtaining a fecal specimen, label and tightly seal the container, complete the laboratory requisition forms, and record the specimen collections in the client's medical record. Avoid delays in sending specimens to the laboratory because some tests, such as measurements for ova and parasites, require the stool to be warm. When stool specimens are allowed to stand at room temperature, bacteriological changes occur that can alter the test results.

A common laboratory test that can be done at home or at the client's bedside is the **fecal occult blood testing (FOBT)**, or guaiac test, which measures microscopic amounts of blood in the feces (Box 45–3). This test is useful as a diagnostic screening for colon cancer (Box 45–4). A single positive result does not confirm GI bleeding. The test should be repeated at least three times while the client

TABLE 45-3 Laboratory and Diagnostic Tests for Bowel Function

Measurement and Normal Values	Interpretation
Laboratory Tests	
Total bilirubin: 0.1–1.0 mg/dL	Increased levels of bilirubin may result from hepatobiliary diseases, obstructions in the bile duct, certain anemias, and reactions to blood transfusions.
Alkaline phosphatase: 30–85 ImU/mL	Elevated levels of alkaline phosphatase may indicate obstructive hepatobiliary diseases, hepatobiliary carcinomas, bone tumours, or healing fractures.
Amylase: 56–190 IU/L	Elevated levels of amylase may indicate abnormalities of the pancreas, such as inflammation, tumours, cholecystitis, necrotic bowel, and diabetic ketoacidosis.
Carcinoembryonic antigen: (CEA): <5 ng/mL	The carcinoembryonic antigen is elevated in the presence of cancer, inflammation of the GI tract, or hepatobiliary organs.
Direct Visualization	
Endoscopy	A colonoscopy is a routine examination for persons 50 years of age and older. Normally the GI tract is free of polyps, tumours, inflammation, ulcers, hernias, obstruction, and ulcerations. If a lesion, such as a polyp, is identified, the physician removes the growth or a portion of the growth and sends it to pathology for analysis. If bleeding is present, the physician may attempt to coagulate the source. In some cases, the identification of an abnormality may indicate the need for follow-up surgery for the client.
Indirect Visualization	
X-ray with contrast medium	An X-ray may identify the presence of abnormalities in the GI tract. A series of X-rays will allow for indirect visualization of the entire tract. The presence of tumours, ulcerations, inflammation, or other abnormalities may indicate the need for further diagnostic testing and medical or surgical intervention.

From Pagana, K. D., & Pagana, T. J. (2006). *Mosby's diagnostic and laboratory test reference* (8th ed.). St. Louis, MO: Mosby.

refrains from ingesting foods and medications that can cause false-positive results. For example, during the test period, the client should avoid ingesting red meat, poultry, fish, some raw vegetables, vitamin C, Aspirin, or other nonsteroidal anti-inflammatory medications that can cause false-positive results (Colon Cancer Check, 2008). Clients who receive anticoagulants or who have a bleeding disorder or a GI disorder known to cause bleeding (e.g., intestinal tumours, bowel inflammation, or ulcerations) should be regularly screened for fecal occult blood.

Fecal Characteristics. Inspection of fecal characteristics (Table 45–4) reveals information about the nature of bowel elimination alterations. Several factors can influence each characteristic. A key to assessment is knowing whether any recent changes have occurred. The client can best provide this information during the health history assessment.

Diagnostic Examinations

A variety of radiological and diagnostic tests may be ordered for the client who experiences altered bowel elimination (Box 45–5). Visualization of GI structures may be made by either a direct or indirect approach. Each test has a prescribed preparation routine to empty the GI area under study to facilitate visualization. Many facilities use conscious sedation during these procedures. Midazolam (Versed) is often the sedative drug of choice, which may be augmented with Demerol or morphine. Be sure you understand the safety precautions involved in the use of this form of anaesthesia. In many institutions, special training is required. A crash cart must be present at the bedside, and the client must be monitored continuously with pulse oximetry and frequent vital signs, usually every 15 minutes during and immediately following the procedure. Check the agency policy regarding the use of sedation for these examinations.

Client Expectations

Clients expect you to answer all their questions regarding diagnostic tests and the preparation for those tests. Clients will be concerned about discomfort and exposure. Fear of losing control of their bowel elimination is especially worrisome. Clients need reassurance that their needs will be met and that you are supportive. Constipation becomes more of a problem as persons age. Some older clients may fail to recognize their bowel elimination needs; you will need to monitor their bowel elimination patterns to avoid negative consequences. Remember that the client brings to any situation an individual perception of what is right for them. Clients expect a knowledgeable nurse who can teach them methods of promoting and maintaining a normal bowel elimination pattern.

❖Nursing Diagnosis

Your assessment of the client's bowel function reveals data that may indicate an actual or potential bowel elimination problem or a problem resulting from bowel elimination alterations. The concept map in Figure 45–11 depicts how the nursing diagnosis of constipation may be related to other diagnoses. In this example, a client with cancer has developed constipation as a result of activity intolerance and imbalanced nutrition. Both conditions are a result of the client's pain. Diagnoses that may apply to clients with bowel elimination problems include the following:

- *Bowel incontinence*
- *Constipation*
- *Constipation, risk for*
- *Constipation, perceived*
- *Diarrhea*

➤ BOX 45-3 Procedural Guidelines

Measuring Fecal Occult Blood

Delegation Considerations: This skill can be delegated to unregulated care providers. You assess the significance of the findings.

Equipment
- Hemoccult test paper
- Hemoccult developer
- Wooden applicator (see illustration).

Procedure
1. Explain to the client the purpose of the test and how the client can assist. Clients can collect their own specimens if possible.
2. Perform hand hygiene.
3. Apply clean disposable gloves.
4. Use the tip of the wooden applicator (see illustration of equipment) to obtain a small portion of a stool specimen. Ensure the specimen is free of toilet paper.
5. Perform the Hemoccult slide test.
   A. Open the flap of the slide. Using the wooden applicator, thinly smear the stool in the first box of the guaiac paper. Apply a second fecal specimen from a different portion of the stool to the slide's second box (see Step 5A illustration).
   B. Close the slide cover and turn the packet to the reverse side (see Step 5B illustration). Open the cardboard flap and apply two drops of developing solution on each box of guaiac paper. A blue colour indicates a positive guaiac, or presence of fecal occult blood.
   C. Assess the colour of the guaiac paper after 30–60 seconds.
   D. Dispose of the test slide in the proper receptacle.
6. Wrap the wooden applicator in a paper towel. Remove gloves and discard in the proper receptacle.
7. Perform hand hygiene.
8. Record results of the test and note any unusual fecal characteristics.

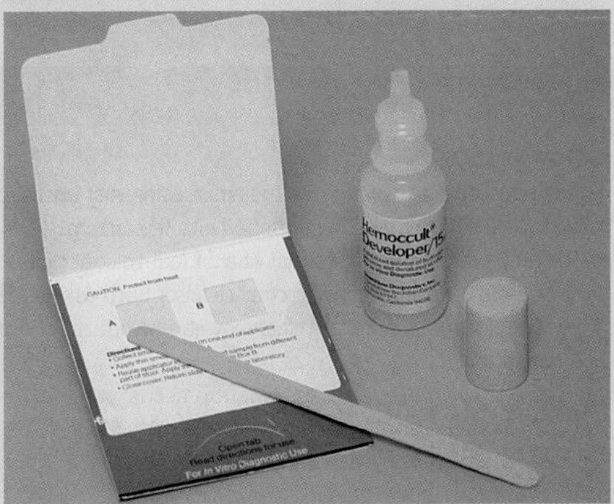

Equipment for performing fecal occult blood testing.

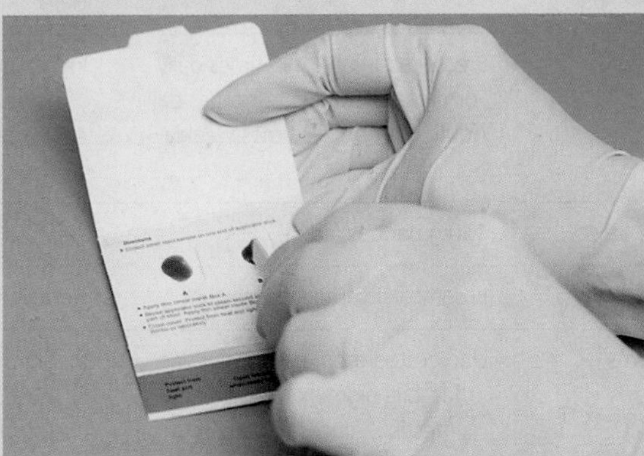

Step 5A Application of the fecal specimen on guaiac paper.

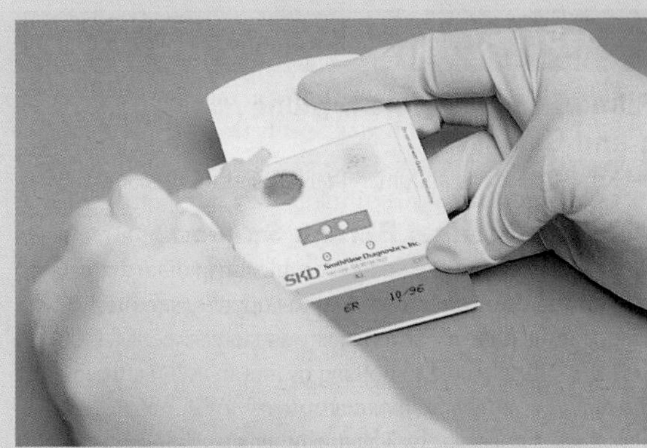

Step 5B Application of the Hemoccult developing solution on the guaiac paper on the reverse side of the test kit.

➤ BOX 45-4 Screening for Colon Cancer

Risk Factors
- Age: older than 50 years of age
- Family history: colon polyps or colorectal cancer
- History of inflammatory bowel disease (e.g., colitis or Crohn's disease)
- Personal history of polyps
- Diet: high intake of animal fats and low fibre intake
- Obesity and inactivity
- Heavy alcohol consumption or smoking

Warning Signs
- Change in bowel habits for no apparent reason
- Blood in or on the stool
- Sensation of incomplete bowel evacuation

Screening Tests
- Digital rectal examination every year after age 40
- Fecal occult blood test (FOBT) at least every 2 years after age 50
- A positive FOBT should be followed up with a colonoscopy, sigmoidoscopy, and double-contrast barium enema

From Colon Cancer Check. (2008). *Prevention and screening.* Retrieved April 5, 2008, from http://www.coloncancercheck.ca/prevention and screening.html

TABLE 45-4 Fecal Characteristics

Characteristic	Normal	Abnormal	Cause of Abnormality
Colour	Infant: yellow Adult: brown	White or clay Black or tarry (i.e., melena) Red Pale with fat Translucent mucus Bloody mucus	Absence of bile Iron ingestion or upper gastrointestinal bleeding Lower gastrointestinal bleeding, hemorrhoids Malabsorption of fat Spastic constipation, colitis, excessive straining Blood in feces, inflammation, infection
Odour	Pungent; affected by food type	Noxious change	Blood in feces or infection
Consistency	Soft, formed	Liquid Hard	Diarrhea, reduced absorption Constipation
Frequency	Breast-fed infant: 4–6 times daily Formula-fed infant: 1–3 times daily Adult: daily or 2–3 times weekly	Infant: more than six times daily or less than once every 1–2 days Adult: more than three times a day or less than once a week	Hypomotility or hypermotility
Amount	150 g per day (adult)		
Shape	Resembles diameter of rectum	Narrow, pencil shaped	Obstruction, rapid peristalsis
Constituents	Undigested food, dead bacteria, fat, bile pigment, cells lining intestinal mucosa, water	Blood, pus, foreign bodies, mucus, worms Excess fat	Internal bleeding, infection, swallowed objects, irritation, inflammation Malabsorption syndrome, enteritis, pancreatic disease, surgical resection of intestine

BOX 45-5 Radiologic and Diagnostic Tests

Plain Film of the Abdomen, Kidneys, Ureter, and Bladder

- A simple X-ray film of the abdomen that requires no preparation.

Upper Gastrointestinal Barium Swallow

- An X-ray examination uses an opaque contrast medium (e.g., barium) to examine the structure and motility of the upper gastrointestinal tract, including the pharynx, esophagus, and stomach.
- The client must be restricted to nothing by mouth (NPO) after midnight the night before the examination.
- The client must remove all jewellery and other metallic objects.
- After the test, the client must increase fluids to facilitate passage and elimination of the barium.

Upper Endoscopy

- An endoscopic examination of the upper gastrointestinal tract allows a more direct visualization via a lighted fibre-optic tube that contains a lens, forceps, and brushes for biopsy.
- The preparation is similar to that of the upper gastrointestinal barium swallow.
- A light sedation is required.

Barium Enema

- An X-ray examination uses an opaque contrast medium to examine the lower gastrointestinal tract.
- The preparation includes NPO after midnight; a bowel preparation, such as magnesium citrate; and, in some instances, enemas to empty any remaining stool particles.

Ultrasound Imaging

- High-frequency sound waves echo off body organs to create a picture.
- The preparation depends on the organ to be visualized and may include either NPO or no preparation.

Colonoscopy

- An endoscopic examination of the entire colon that uses a long, flexible tube (i.e., a colonoscope) inserted into the rectum.
- The preparation is similar to that of a barium enema: clear liquids the day before are followed by a bowel cleanser, such as GoLYTELY. Enemas until the bowels are clear may also be ordered. Light sedation is required.

Flexible Sigmoidoscopy

- An examination of the interior of the sigmoid colon uses a flexible or rigid lighted tube.
- Preparation is similar to that of a barium enema or colonoscopy.
- Light sedation is required.

Computerized Tomography Scan

- An X-ray examination of the body from many angles uses a scanner and is analyzed by a computer.
- The preparation may be either NPO or no preparation.
- The client must be informed of the need to lie very still. If claustrophobia is a problem, light sedation may be used.

Magnetic Resonance Imaging

- A noninvasive examination uses magnetic and radio waves to produce a picture of the inside of the body.
- The preparation is NPO 4–6 hours before examination.
- No metallic objects are allowed in the room, including metal objects on clothes.

Enteroclysis

- The introduction of contrast material to the jejunum allows the entire small intestine to be studied.
- Preparation is 24 hours of clear liquid diet and colon cleansing (e.g., GoLYTELY) or enemas until the bowels are clear.

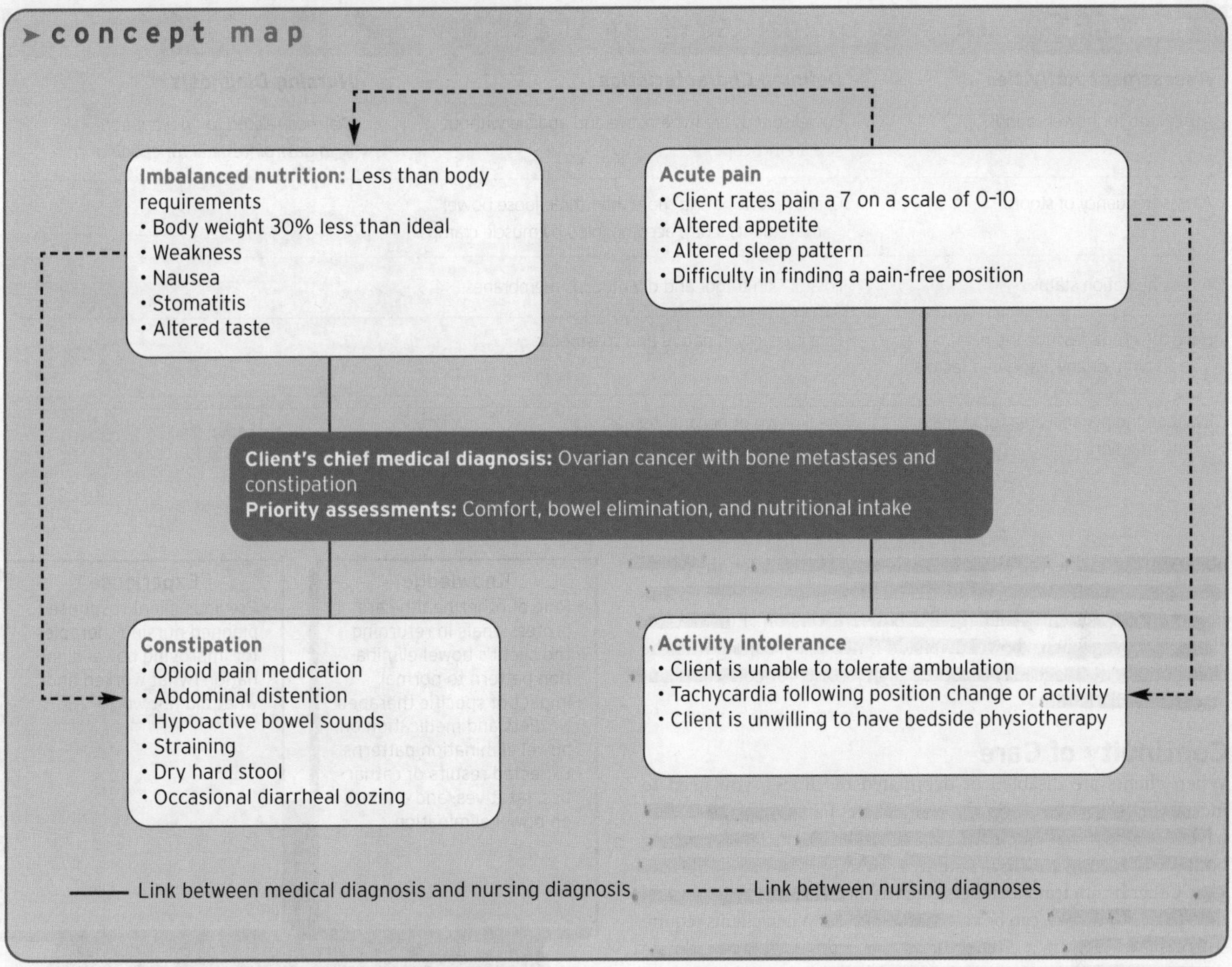

➤ concept map

Figure 45-11 Concept map for a client who has ovarian cancer with bone metastases and constipation.

A client's associated problems, such as body-image changes or skin breakdown, require interventions unrelated to bowel function impairment. In some instances, however, you need to direct as much attention to the associated problem as to the bowel elimination problem.

Your ability to identify the correct nursing diagnosis depends not only on the thoroughness of assessment but also on recognition of defining characteristics and factors that can impair bowel elimination (Box 45–6). You need to determine the client's risk, then institute measures to ensure maintenance of normal bowel function.

❖Planning

During the planning of care, you synthesize information from multiple resources (Figure 45–12). Critical thinking ensures that the plan of care integrates all you know about the client and the clinical problem. You must rely on professional standards. The guidelines on incontinence (see Chapter 44) can assist you in protecting the client's skin, promoting continence, and reducing the embarrassment associated with incontinence. In addition, the Agency for Health Care Policy and Research (AHCPR), the Registered Nurses Association of Ontario (RNAO), and the Canadian Association of Wound Care (CAWC) have guidelines on the reduction of pressure ulcers that also assist in developing care for clients with bowel incontinence (see Chapter 47).

Goals and Outcomes

You and the client establish goals and outcomes by incorporating the client's bowel elimination habits or routines as much as possible and by reinforcing routines that promote health. You also consider pre-existing health concerns. For example, if the client is at risk for the worsening of heart failure, an outcome of increased fluid intake must be tailored to the client's cardiac function and ability to safely handle the increased fluid. For another example, if the client's bowel habits caused the elimination problem, you can help the client to learn new bowel habits. The overall goal of returning the client to a normal bowel elimination pattern may include the following outcomes:

- The client practises regular defecation habits.
- The client lists the proper fluid and food intake needed to achieve regular bowel elimination.
- The client implements a regular exercise program.
- The client reports daily passage of soft, formed brown stool.
- The client does not report any discomfort associated with defecation.

Setting Priorities

Defecation patterns vary among individuals. For this reason, you and client must work together closely to plan effective interventions (see Box 45–7). A realistic time frame to establish a normal defecation pattern for one client might differ for another client. For the client who

BOX 45-6 NURSING DIAGNOSTIC PROCESS

Assessment Activities	Defining Characteristics	Nursing Diagnosis
Auscultate for bowel sounds.	Bowel sounds are hyperactive and audible without a stethoscope.	*Diarrhea related to an alteration in gastrointestinal functioning*
Assess frequency of stools.	Client reports having more than three loose bowel movements a day, accompanied by muscle cramps.	
Assess hydration status.	Loss of skin turgor and dry mucous membranes.	
Have the client describe the pain, cramping, or any associated factors.	Pain is colicky in nature and spasmodic.	
Evaluate the perianal area for redness and irritation.	Breakdown of perianal tissues.	

has a new ostomy as the result of newly diagnosed cancer, the priority of coping with cancer and its treatment may precede the client's need to independently manage the bowel diversion. For another client, however, when a bowel diversion is necessary, coping with the changes in body image may become a high priority for both the client and the client's family.

Continuity of Care

When clients are disabled or debilitated by illness, you need to include the client's family in the plan of care. Family members often have the same bowel elimination habits as the client. Thus, teaching both the client and the client's family is an important part of the care plan. Other health team members, such as dietitians and enterostomal therapist (ET) nurses, can be valuable resources. When clients require surgical intervention, a critical pathway may be used to coordinate the activities of the multidisciplinary health care team.

The client who has alterations in bowel elimination will require intervention from many members of the health care team. Certain tasks, such as assisting clients onto the bedpan or bedside commode, are appropriate to delegate to unregulated care providers (UCPs). Remind the UCP to report any abnormal findings or difficulties encountered during the bowel elimination process. Non-nursing personnel perform many of the diagnostic tests used to evaluate the gastrointestinal system. You must maintain ongoing communication with these caregivers to ensure that the client's safety, needs, wants, and concerns are addressed.

❖Implementation

The success of your interventions depends on improving the client's and the family members' understanding of bowel elimination. In the home, hospital, or long-term care facility, clients capable of learning can be taught effective bowel habits.

Teach the client and the client's family about proper diet, adequate fluid intake, and factors that stimulate or slow peristalsis, such as emotional stress. Your instruction can often best be done during the client's mealtime. The client should also learn the importance of establishing regular bowel routines, participating in regular exercise, and taking appropriate measures when bowel elimination problems develop.

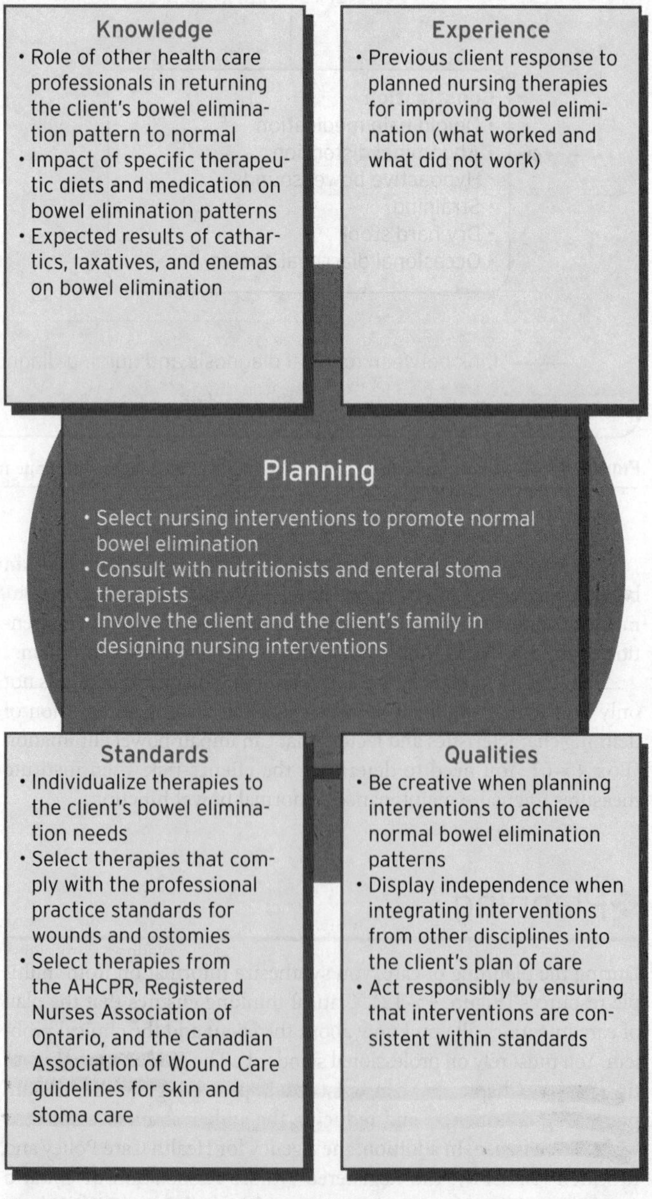

Knowledge
- Role of other health care professionals in returning the client's bowel elimination pattern to normal
- Impact of specific therapeutic diets and medication on bowel elimination patterns
- Expected results of cathartics, laxatives, and enemas on bowel elimination

Experience
- Previous client response to planned nursing therapies for improving bowel elimination (what worked and what did not work)

Planning
- Select nursing interventions to promote normal bowel elimination
- Consult with nutritionists and enteral stoma therapists
- Involve the client and the client's family in designing nursing interventions

Standards
- Individualize therapies to the client's bowel elimination needs
- Select therapies that comply with the professional practice standards for wounds and ostomies
- Select therapies from the AHCPR, Registered Nurses Association of Ontario, and the Canadian Association of Wound Care guidelines for skin and stoma care

Qualities
- Be creative when planning interventions to achieve normal bowel elimination patterns
- Display independence when integrating interventions from other disciplines into the client's plan of care
- Act responsibly by ensuring that interventions are consistent within standards

Figure 45-12 Critical thinking model for bowel elimination planning.

BOX 45-7 NURSING CARE PLAN

Constipation

Assessment

Javier is a nurse who visits Larry at his home on a cattle ranch. Larry lives 40 km from town. He is 22 years old and had surgery 6 days ago for repair of a broken right leg. Larry tells Javier "I just don't feel good."

Assessment Activities	*Findings and Defining Characteristics*
Ask Larry about his recent bowel elimination patterns over the last 5 days.	Larry has not had a bowel movement since he left the hospital 4 days ago and he feels like his abdomen is tight and sore.
Review Larry's medication.	Larry has been prescribed Lortabs for pain. He takes 1 tablet every 6 hours, up to 3 tablets a day.
Review Larry's dietary intake over the past day.	Larry has eaten eggs, bacon, and toast for breakfast and soup for lunch. For supper, Larry had chicken, rice, and corn. He drinks about 6 cups of coffee each day, no water, but will drink a cola.
Ask about any nausea or vomiting.	Larry has not felt nauseated.
Auscultate the abdomen.	Decreased bowel sounds are auscultated throughout all four abdominal quadrants.
Palpate the abdomen.	While Javier is palpating Larry's abdomen, Larry tells Javier, "It really hurts." On palpation, the left lower quadrant is tender and firm.

Nursing Diagnosis: Constipation related to opiate-containing pain medication and decreased fibre intake

Planning

*Goals (Nursing Outcomes Classification)**	*Expected Outcomes*
	Bowel Elimination
Larry will establish normal defecation.	Larry will drink at least 1500 mL of fluid over the next 8 hours.
Larry will voice relief from constipation.	Larry will report passage of soft stool without straining within 24 hours.
	Nutritional Status: Food and Fluid Intake
Larry will identify measures to prevent constipation.	Larry will increase the fibre content of his diet.
Larry will increase the amount of daily exercise.	

*Outcome classification labels from Moorhead, S., Johnson, M., & Maas, M. L. (Eds.). (2004). *Nursing Outcomes Classification (NOC)* (3rd ed.). St. Louis, MO: Mosby.

Interventions (Nursing Interventions Classification)†	**Rationale**
Constipation or Impaction Management	
Encourage fluid intake of fruit juice, water, and other appropriate fluids.	Adequate fluid intake is necessary to prevent hard, dry stool.
Encourage activity within the limits of Larry's mobility regimen.	Even minimal activity (such as leg lifts) increases peristalsis.
Add bran flakes or bran to the diet.	The number of bowel movements is increased with consumption of bran (Bliss et al., 2001).
Provide laxative or stool softeners as ordered.	Medications can soften the stool and prevent straining (McKenry et al., 2006).
Provide a private atmosphere for bowel elimination.	Clients should feel relaxed when moving their bowels.

†Intervention classification labels adapted from Dochterman, J. M., & Bulechek, G. M. (Eds.). (2004). *Nursing Interventions Classification (NIC)* (4th ed.). St. Louis, MO: Mosby.

Evaluation

Nursing Actions	*Client Response and Findings*	*Achievement of Outcome*
Ask Larry to identify foods high in fibre.	Larry is able to correctly identify high-fibre foods. Review of the 24-hour diet diary shows Larry is selecting high-fibre, low-fat foods.	Larry is making excellent progress in introducing high-fibre and low-fat foods into his diet.
Ask Larry to plan menus to increase fibre.	Review of the 24-hour diet diary shows meals planned with high-fibre content. Larry reviews his shopping list, which includes bran, oat, and fruit products.	Larry is knowledgeable about fibre content and purchases foods that are high in fibre.
Ask Larry about increased activity.	Larry states that he has not changed his level of activity.	Larry has not increased his level of activity and needs to continue to work on increasing his physical activity.
Observe Larry's subsequent stool for characteristics such as consistency and colour.	Stools are now every 24–48 hours. Larry states he does not "feel regular." The abdomen is soft and nondistended. Stools are formed and hard, and Larry reports straining.	Larry has not achieved passage of a regular, formed stool.

Health Promotion

One of the most important habits you can teach regarding bowel habits is to take time for defecation. To establish regular bowel habits, a client must know when the urge to defecate normally occurs. Advise the client to begin establishing a routine during a time when defecation is most likely to occur, usually an hour after a meal. Many evidenced-informed interventions are available to reduce the risk of constipation (Box 45–8). If a client is restricted to bed or requires assistance in ambulating, you can offer a bedpan or help the client to reach the bathroom in a timely manner.

Many clients have their established routines for defecation. In a hospital or long-term care facility, ensure that treatment routines do not interfere with the client's bowel elimination routine. The provision of privacy is important to maintain. When a client shares the room with other clients, pull the curtain around the area so the client can relax, with the knowledge that interruptions will not occur. The call light should always be placed within the client's reach. Bathroom doors should be closed, although you may stand close by in case the client needs assistance.

Promotion of Normal Defecation. Several interventions can stimulate the defecation reflex, affect the character of feces, or increase peristalsis to help clients evacuate bowel contents normally and without discomfort.

Sitting Position. You might need to assist clients who have difficulty sitting because of muscular weakness and mobility problems. Regular toilets are too low for clients who are unable to lower themselves to a sitting position because of joint- or muscle-wasting diseases. Elevated toilet seats require less effort to sit or stand. In many provinces and territories, elevated toilet seats can be acquired through a service agency for minimal or no cost. The community nurse must assess the client's capabilities in the home and the requirement for any additional equipment to facilitate daily living.

Positioning on Bedpan. Clients restricted to bed must use bedpans for defecation. Women use bedpans to pass both urine and feces, whereas men use bedpans only for defecation. Sitting on a bedpan can be extremely uncomfortable. You need to help clients to position themselves comfortably. Two types of bedpans are available (Figure 45–13). The regular bedpan, made of metal or hard plastic, has a curved, smooth upper end, a sharp-edged lower end, and is approximately 5 cm deep. A fracture pan, designed for clients with body or leg casts, has a shallow upper end and is approximately 1.3 cm deep. The upper end of the pan fits under the buttocks toward the sacrum, and the lower end fits just under the upper thighs. The pan should be high enough so that feces enter the pan. A metal bedpan should be warmed with water first, then dried.

When positioning a client on a bedpan, use the proper method to prevent muscle strain and discomfort. Never try to lift a client onto a bedpan. A client should never be placed on a bedpan and then left with the bed flat unless activity restrictions demand it. When the bed is flat, the hips remain hyperextended.

Figure 45–14 shows proper and improper positions on a bedpan. The best method is to ensure the client is positioned high in bed. Raise the client's head about 30 degrees to prevent hyperextension of the back and to provide support to the upper torso. The client then raises the hips by bending the knees and lifting the hips upward. Place your hand, palm up, under the client's sacrum; rest your elbow on the mattress and use it as a lever to help in lifting, while slipping the pan under the client. Clients who have had abdominal surgery are hesitant to exert strain on suture lines and may have difficulty positioning themselves on a bedpan. To prevent abrasions, do not force the pan along the client's skin. Always wear gloves when handling a bedpan.

If the client is immobile or if it is unsafe to allow the client to exert such effort, you can assist the client to roll onto the bedpan by using the following steps:

1. Lower the head of the bed flat and assist the client to roll onto one side, backside toward you.
2. Apply a little powder to the back and buttocks to prevent the skin from sticking to the pan.
3. Place the bedpan firmly against the buttocks, down into the mattress with the open rim toward the client's feet (Figure 45–15).
4. Keeping one hand against the bedpan, place your other hand around the client's far hip. Ask the client to roll back onto the pan, flat in bed. Do not shove the pan under the client.

BOX 45-8 EVIDENCE-INFORMED PRACTICE GUIDELINE

Management of Constipation

- Fluid intake of at least 1.5 L/day is recommended. The preferred fluid is water because it is sodium free and calorie free. The client may also benefit from drinking 1–2 glasses of fruit juice.
- Coffee, tea, and alcohol should be avoided because of their diuretic properties.
- A high-fibre diet (25–30 g/day) reduces constipation; fibre that passes though the colon acts as a sponge. As a result, bulkier and softer stools develop. In addition, the waste moves through the body more easily and results in more regular bowel movements. A high-fibre diet is not recommended for individuals who are immobile or who do not consume at least 1.5 L of fluid per day.
- The most beneficial means to prevent constipation is a combination of insoluble and soluble fibre (e.g., bran, fruits, and vegetables).
- Physical activity in combination with adequate fluid intake and a high-fibre diet is beneficial in the management of constipation. For clients who are fully mobile, walking once or twice a day for 15–20 minutes is sufficient.
- For individuals who are unable to walk, recommend chair or bed exercises, such as the pelvic tilt, low trunk rotation, and single leg lifts.
- Laxatives should be used with caution. If laxatives are necessary, a stepwise progression is recommended: first bulk-forming laxatives, followed by stool softeners, osmotics, stimulants, suppositories, and enemas as a last resort.

Adapted from Hinrichs, M., & Huseboe, J. (2001). Research-based protocol: Management of constipation. In M.G. Titler (Series Ed.). *Series on evidence-based practice for older adults*. Iowa City, IA: The University of Iowa College of Nursing Gerontological Nursing Interventions Research Center, Research Dissemination Core.

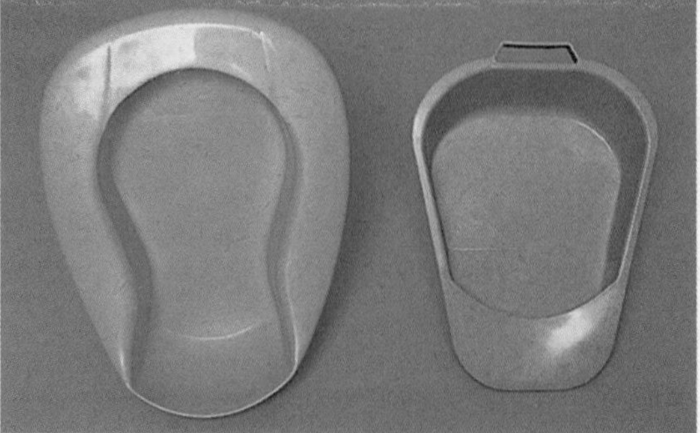

Figure 45-13 Types of bedpans. From left, regular bedpan and fracture bedpan.

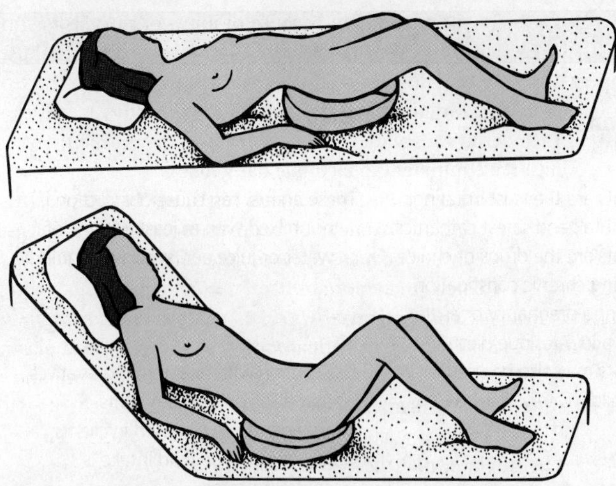

Figure 45-14 Positions on a bedpan. **Top**, Improper positioning of a client. **Bottom**, Proper positioning of the client reduces back strain.

5. When the client is positioned comfortably, raise the head of the bed 30 degrees.
6. Place a rolled towel or small pillow under the lumbar curve of the client's back for added comfort.
7. Raise the knee gatch or ask the client to bend the knees to assume a squatting position. Do not raise the knee gatch if contraindicated.

Privacy. Ensure that you maintain the client's privacy during bowel elimination. Privacy is especially important for a client using a bedpan. The call light and a supply of toilet paper should be within easy reach. When the client finishes, respond to the call signal immediately and remove the pan. The client might require assistance with wiping. To remove the pan, ask the client to roll off to the side or to raise the hips. Hold the pan steady to avoid spilling. Avoid pulling or shoving the pan from under the client's hips; these actions can pull the client's skin and cause tissue injury, such as shearing (see Chapter 47). After the pan is removed, while wearing gloves, clean the anal and perineal areas.

After assessing the stool, you should immediately empty the bedpan's contents into the toilet or in a special receptacle in the utility room. The bedpan should be rinsed thoroughly. Care must be taken to avoid splashing the contents or the rinse. Avoiding spillage is of critical importance when *C. difficile* or other infectious agents are suspected. The client uses the same bedpan each time. Chart the characteristics of the feces.

You should offer the bedpan or commode chair often. Clients may accidentally soil bedclothes if forced to wait. Many clients try to avoid using a bedpan because they find it embarrassing and uncomfortable.

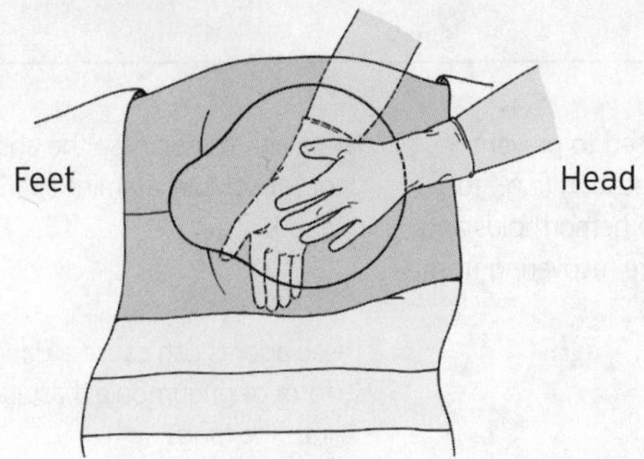

Figure 45-15 Positioning an immobilized client on a bedpan.

They may try to get to the bathroom even when their conditions prohibit ambulation. You must warn clients about the risk of falls or accidents.

Acute Care

The GI system may be affected by any acute illness. Changes in the client's fluid status, mobility patterns, nutrition, and sleep cycle can affect regular bowel habits. Surgical interventions on the GI tract affect bowel elimination, as will surgery on other systems, such as the musculoskeletal and cardiovascular systems. You must remain sensitive to the client's bowel elimination needs and intervene to assist the client to maintain as normal bowel elimination habits as possible.

Medications. Medications may be used to initiate and facilitate bowel elimination. Cathartics, laxatives, and occasionally an enema are used to control constipation, whereas antidiarrheal preparations assist the client in resolving diarrhea. All these medications are available over the counter; stronger preparations are available through prescriptions. Clients must be cautioned not to use these over-the-counter medications on a prolonged basis without consulting their health care professional.

safety alert Excessive use of laxatives, enemas, or bulk-forming agents increases the client's risk for diarrhea and abnormal bowel elimination and destroys the client's normal defecation reflex. In addition, the client may develop an altered absorption of nutrients, fluid and electrolyte imbalances, and generalized weakness. When these symptoms occur in chronically ill or older adult clients, they may result in an increased risk for falls and other injuries.

Cathartics and Laxatives. A client is often unable to defecate normally because of pain, constipation, or impaction. Cathartics and laxatives provide the short-term action of emptying the bowel. They are also used in bowel evacuation for clients undergoing GI tests and abdominal surgery. Although the terms *cathartic* and *laxative* are often used interchangeably, cathartics have a stronger effect on the intestines. Five types of laxatives and cathartics are available (Table 45–5).

Cathartics and laxatives are available in oral, tablet, and powder suppository dosage forms (see Chapter 34). Although the oral route is most commonly used, cathartics that are prepared as suppositories are more effective because of their stimulant effect on the rectal mucosa. Cathartic suppositories such as bisacodyl (Dulcolax) can act within 30 minutes. Older adults who use Dulcolax often have a strong, sudden urge to defecate.

Electrolyte Balance and Antidiarrheal Agents. For clients with diarrhea, frequent passage of liquid stools becomes a problem. When a person has secretory diarrhea, cells at the base of the villi secrete massive amounts of fluid into the lumen of the small intestine. However, the tip of the villi can still absorb sugars and fluids. Therefore, diarrhea can quickly lead to serious electrolyte imbalances, particularly in infants and children (see Chapter 40). Therefore, the first course of action is to immediately replace fluids by mouth. Fluids with adequate electrolyte content (e.g., Pedialyte and Gastrolyte) are a wise choice. In developing countries without a safe water supply or during epidemics of infectious diarrhea (e.g., cholera), millions of lives have been saved by using a cheap, safe, and simple method of replacing water and salts lost through diarrhea. This method, known as oral rehydration therapy (ORT), involves mixing a very low-cost package of salts (sodium, potassium chloride, citrate or bicarbonate, and glucose) with boiled water.

Many clients will use over-the-counter agents, such as Imodium, to relieve common diarrhea. However, the most effective antidiarrheal agents are prescriptive opiates, such as codeine phosphate, opium

TABLE 45-5 Common Types of Laxatives and Cathartics

Agents and Brand Names	Action	Indications	Risks
Bulk Forming			
Methylcellulose (Cologel, Hydrolose)	The high-fibre content absorbs water and increases solid intestinal bulk.	These agents are the least irritating, most natural, and safest cathartics. These agents are the drugs of choice for treating chronic constipation (e.g., during pregnancy or as the result of a low-residue diet).	These agents can cause obstruction if not mixed with at least 240 mL of water or juice and swallowed quickly.
Psyllium (Metamucil, Naturacil)	These agents stretch the intestinal wall to stimulate peristalsis.	These agents may also be used to relieve mild, watery diarrhea.	Use caution with bulk-forming laxatives that also contain stimulants. These agents are not used in clients for whom large fluid intake is contraindicated.
Emollient or Wetting			
Docusate sodium (Colace, Disonate) Docusate calcium (Surfak) Docusate potassium (Dialose)	Stool softeners are detergents that lower the surface tension of feces, allowing water and fat to penetrate. They may increase the secretion of water by the intestines.	These agents are used for short-term therapy to relieve straining on defecation. These agents would be beneficial for clients who have hemorrhoids, have undergone perianal surgery, are pregnant, or are recovering from myocardial infarction.	These agents are of little value for treatment of chronic constipation.
Saline			
Magnesium citrate or citrate of magnesia (Citroma)	These agents contain a salt preparation that is not absorbed by the intestines.	These agents are used only for acute emptying of the bowel (e.g., as a preparation for endoscopic examination, in cases of suspected poisoning, or to treat acute constipation).	These agents are not used for long-term management of constipation.
Magnesium hydroxide (Milk of Magnesia)	The osmotic effect increases pressure in the bowel to act as stimulant for peristalsis.		These agents are contraindicated for clients with kidney dysfunction (to avoid a toxic buildup of magnesium).
Sodium phosphate (Fleet Phospho-Soda, Fleet Enema)	These agents may also lubricate the feces.		Phosphate salts are not used for clients on fluid restriction.
Stimulant Cathartics			
Bisacodyl (Dulcolax)	These agents irritate the intestinal mucosa to increase motility.	These agents may be used to prepare the bowel for diagnostic procedures.	These agents may cause severe cramping.
Castor oil (Neoloid, Purge)	These agents decrease absorption in the small bowel and colon.		These agents are not for long-term use.
Casanthranol (Dialose Plus, Peri-Colace)			Chronic use may cause fluid and electrolyte imbalances.
Danthron (Modane Bulk)			The use of these agents should be avoided during pregnancy and lactation.
Phenolphthalein (Doxidan, Correctol, Ex-Lax)	Phenolphthalein and danthron may cause pink or red urine.		
Lubricants			
Mineral oil (Haley's M-O, Petrogalar Plain)	These agents coat the fecal contents, which allows easier passage of the stool.	These agents are used to prevent straining on defecation (e.g., for clients who have hemorrhoids and for those who are recovering from perianal surgery).	These agents decrease the absorption of fat-soluble vitamins (A, D, E, and K).
	These agents reduce water absorption in the colon.		These agents can cause a dangerous form of pneumonia if aspirated into the lungs. Mineral oil when taken with emollients can increase the risk for fat emboli.

tincture (Paregoric), and diphenoxylate (Lomotil). Opiates inhibit the peristaltic waves that move feces forward but also increase the segmental contractions that mix intestinal contents and expose the contents to the mucosal absorbing surface. The further effect of opiates on increasing the absorption of sodium and water also dries out the feces. As a result, more water is absorbed by the colonic mucosa. These antidiarrheal agents should be used with caution because opiates are habit forming.

Enemas. An **enema** is the instillation of a solution into the rectum and sigmoid colon. The primary reason for using an enema is to promote defecation by stimulating peristalsis. The volume of fluid instilled breaks up the fecal mass, stretches the rectal wall, and initiates the defecation reflex. Enemas are also used as a vehicle for administering medications that exert a local effect on rectal mucosa.

The most common use for an enema is temporary relief of constipation. Other indications include removing impacted feces; beginning a program of bowel training; and emptying the bowel before diagnostic tests, surgery, or childbirth.

Cleansing Enemas. Cleansing enemas promote the complete evacuation of feces from the colon. They act by stimulating peristalsis through the infusion of a large volume of solution or through local irritation of the colon's mucosa. Solutions used in cleansing enemas include tap water, normal saline, low-volume hypertonic saline, and soapsuds solution. Each solution exerts a different osmotic effect to move fluids between the colon and the interstitial spaces beyond the intestinal wall. Infants and children should receive only normal saline because they are at risk for fluid imbalance.

A physician may order a high or low cleansing enema. The terms *high* and *low* refer to the height from which, and hence the pressure with which, the fluid is delivered. High enemas are given to cleanse the entire colon. After the enema is infused, the client is asked to turn from the left lateral position to the dorsal recumbent position and to the right lateral position. The position change ensures that fluid reaches all of the large intestine. A low enema cleanses only the rectum and the sigmoid colon.

Tap Water. Tap water is hypotonic and exerts a lower osmotic pressure than that of fluid in interstitial spaces. After infusion into the colon, tap water escapes from the bowel lumen into the interstitial spaces. The net movement of water is low. The infused volume stimulates defecation before large amounts of water leave the bowel. Tap water enemas should not be repeated because water toxicity or circulatory overload can develop if large amounts of water are absorbed.

Normal Saline. Physiologically, normal saline is the safest solution to use because it exerts the same osmotic pressure as that of fluids in the interstitial spaces surrounding the bowel. The volume of infused saline stimulates peristalsis. Unlike tap water enemas, saline enemas do not create the danger of excess fluid absorption.

Hypertonic Solutions. Hypertonic solutions infused into the bowel exert osmotic pressure that pulls fluids out of the interstitial spaces. The colon fills with fluid, and the resultant distension promotes defecation. Clients unable to tolerate large volumes of fluid benefit most from this type of enema, which is, by design, low volume. Contraindications for this type of enema are clients who are dehydrated and young infants. A hypertonic solution of 120 to 180 mL is usually effective. The commercially prepared Fleet Enema is the most commonly used hypertonic solution.

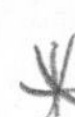

Soapsuds. Soapsuds may be added to tap water or saline to create the effect of intestinal irritation to stimulate peristalsis. Only pure castile soap is safe to use. A liquid form of castile soap is included in most soapsuds enema kits. Harsh soaps or detergents can cause serious bowel inflammation.

Oil-Retention Enemas. Oil-retention enemas lubricate the rectum and colon. The feces absorb the oil and become softer and easier to pass. To enhance the action of the oil, the client retains the enema for several hours if possible.

Other Types of Enemas. Carminative enemas provide relief from gaseous distension. Use of a carminative enema improves the ability to pass flatus. An example of a carminative enema is MGW solution, which contains 30 mL of magnesium, 60 mL of glycerine, and 90 mL of water.

Medicated enemas contain drugs. An example is sodium polystyrene sulphonate (Kayexalate), which is used to treat clients with dangerously high serum potassium levels. This drug contains a resin that exchanges sodium ions for potassium ions in the large intestine. Another medicated enema is neomycin solution, which is an antibiotic used to reduce bacteria in the colon before bowel surgery.

Enema Administration. Enemas are administered in either commercially packaged, disposable units or with reusable equipment prepared before use. Sterile technique is unnecessary because the colon normally contains bacteria; however, gloves should be worn to prevent the transmission of fecal microorganisms.

You should explain the procedure to the client, including the position to assume, precautions to take to avoid discomfort, and the length of time necessary to retain the solution before defecation. If the client is to receive the enema at home, explain the procedure to a family member.

Often the physician orders "enemas until clear." This order means that the enema is to be repeated until the client passes fluid that is clear and contains no fecal material. As many as three enemas may be necessary, but you should caution the client against more than three enemas. Excess enema use seriously depletes fluids and electrolytes. If the enema fails to return a clear solution after three times (check agency policy on the maximum number of enemas permitted) or if the client seems to not be tolerating the rigours of repeated enemas, notify the physician.

Giving an enema to a client who is unable to contract the external sphincter can pose difficulties. In these cases, give the enema with the client positioned on the bedpan. Giving the enema with the client sitting on the toilet is unsafe because the curved rectal tubing can abrade the rectal wall. Skill 45–1 outlines the steps for an enema administration.

Digital Removal of Stool. For clients with an impaction, the fecal mass may be too large to be passed voluntarily. If enemas fail, you must break up the fecal mass with your fingers and remove it in sections (Box 45–9) The procedure can be very uncomfortable for the client. Excess rectal manipulation may cause irritation to the mucosa, bleeding, and stimulation of the vagus nerve, which results in a reflex slowing of the heart rate. Because of the procedure's potential complications, a physician's order is necessary for you to remove a fecal impaction (Box 45–10).

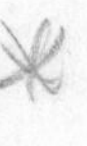

Inserting and Maintaining a Nasogastric Tube. A client's condition or situation may warrant special interventions to decompress the GI tract. Such conditions include surgery, infections of the GI tract, trauma to the GI tract, and the absence of peristalsis.

A nasogastric (NG) tube is a pliable tube that is inserted through the client's nasopharynx into the stomach. The tube has a hollow lumen that allows removal of gastric secretions and introduction of solutions into the stomach. Nasogastric intubation has several purposes (Table 45–6).

The Levin and Salem sump tubes are the most common tubes used for stomach decompression. The Levin tube is a single-lumen tube with holes near the tip. A sump tube may be connected to either a drainage bag or an intermittent suction device to drain stomach secretions.

➤ SKILL 45-1 Administering a Cleansing Enema

video

Delegation Considerations

The skill of administering an enema can be delegated to unregulated care providers (UCPs). You have the responsibility to assess the client for specific considerations, such as his or her safety, the need for alternative positioning and comfort, and the presence of stable vital signs prior to the procedure. In addition, you have the responsibility to determine the client's response to the enema. If delegating this task to a UCP:

- Inform and assist the UCP in the proper way to position clients who have mobility restrictions, such as clients with arthritis or severe fatigue.
- Instruct the UCP how to position clients who have therapeutic equipment present, such as drains, intravenous catheters, or traction.
- Instruct the UCP about the specific signs and symptoms that will appear in clients not tolerating the procedure and about when the procedure must be stopped. For example, these signs and symptoms may include abdominal pain more than a pressure sensation, abdominal cramping, abdominal distension, or rectal bleeding.

Equipment

- Disposable gloves
- Water-soluble lubricant
- Waterproof, absorbent pads
- Bath blanket
- Toilet tissue
- Bedpan, bedside commode, or access to toilet
- Washbasin, washcloths, towel, and soap
- Intravenous (IV) pole
- Enema bag administration
  - Enema container
  - Tubing and clamp (if not already attached to the enema container)
  - Appropriate size rectal tube:
    - *Adult:* 22–30 Fr
    - *Child:* 12–18 Fr
  - Correct volume of warmed solution:
    - *Adult:* 750–1000 mL
    - *Child:*
      150–250 mL, infant
      250–350 mL, toddler
      300–500 mL, school-age child
      500–750 mL, adolescent
- Prepackaged enema
  - Prepackaged enema container with rectal tip

STEPS	RATIONALE
1. Assess the status of the client: last bowel movement, normal bowel patterns, presence of hemorrhoids, mobility, external sphincter control, and abdominal pain.	• Your assessment determines the factors indicating a need for enema and influences the type of enema used.
2. Assess the client for presence of increased intracranial pressure, glaucoma, or recent rectal or prostate surgery.	• These conditions contraindicate the use of an enema.
3. Check the client's medical record to clarify the rationale for the enema.	• You need to determine the purpose of the enema administration: either as a preparation for a special procedure or for relief of constipation.
4. Review the physician's order for the enema.	• An order by a physician is required. The order determines the number and type of enemas to be given.
5. Determine the client's level of understanding of the purpose of the enema.	• The client's current level of understanding allows you to plan for appropriate teaching measures.
6. Perform hand hygiene. Collect appropriate equipment.	• Proper hand hygiene reduces the transmission of microorganisms.
7. Correctly identify the client and explain the procedure.	• Explaining the procedure promotes client cooperation and reduces anxiety.
8. Assemble the enema bag with the appropriate solution and rectal tube.	
9. Perform hand hygiene and apply gloves.	• Proper hand hygiene reduces the transmission of microorganisms.
10. Provide privacy by closing the curtains around the bed or by closing the door.	• Privacy reduces the embarrassment for the client.
11. Raise the bed to an appropriate working height; raise the side rail on the client's left side.	• Raising the bed and use of the side rail promote good body mechanics and client safety.
12. Assist the client into a position lying on the left side with right knee flexed (i.e., Sims' position). Children may instead be placed in a dorsal recumbent position.	• The Sims' position allows the enema solution to flow downward by gravity along the natural curve of the sigmoid colon and rectum, thus improving retention of the solution.

Critical Decision Point: Clients who have poor sphincter control will have difficulty retaining the enema solution. If the client is suspected of having poor sphincter control, position the client on a bedpan.

STEPS	RATIONALE
13. Place a waterproof pad under the hips and buttocks.	• A waterproof pad prevents soiling of the bed linen.
14. Cover the client with a bath blanket, exposing only the rectal area, with the anus clearly visible.	• The bath blanket provides warmth, reduces exposure of body parts, and allows the client to feel more relaxed and comfortable.
15. Place the bedpan or commode in an easily accessible position. If the client will be expelling contents in toilet, ensure the toilet is available. (If the client will be walking to the bathroom to expel the enema, place the client's slippers and bathrobe in an easily accessible position.)	• A bedpan or commode should be nearby in case the client is unable to retain the enema solution.

➤ SKILL 45-1 Administering a Cleansing Enema *continued*

STEPS	RATIONALE
16. Administer the enema:	
A. Enema bag	
(1) Add warmed solution to the enema bag: warm the tap water as it flows from faucet, place the saline container in a basin of hot water before adding saline to the enema bag, check the temperature of solution with a bath thermometer or by pouring a small amount of solution over your inner wrist.	• Hot water can burn intestinal mucosa. Cold water can cause abdominal cramping and is difficult to retain.
(2) Raise the container, release the clamp, and allow the solution to flow long enough to fill the tubing.	• Raising the container removes air from the tubing.
(3) Reclamp the tubing.	• Reclamping prevents further loss of the solution.
(4) Lubricate 6–8 cm of the tip of the rectal tube with lubricating jelly.	• The lubricating jelly allows smooth insertion of the rectal tube without risk of irritation or trauma to the mucosa.
(5) Gently separate the buttocks and locate the anus. Instruct the client to relax by breathing out slowly through the mouth.	• Exhaling promotes relaxation of the external anal sphincter.
(6) Insert the tip of the rectal tube slowly by pointing the tip in the direction of the client's umbilicus (see Step 16A(6) illustration). The length of the insertion varies: Adult: 7.5–10 cm Child: 5–7.5 cm Infant: 2.5–3.75 cm	• Careful insertion prevents trauma to the rectal mucosa from an accidental lodging of the tube against the rectal wall. Insertion beyond the proper limit can cause bowel perforation.

Critical Decision Point: If the tube does not pass easily, do not force it. Consider allowing a small amount of fluid to infuse and then try reinserting the tube slowly.

STEPS	RATIONALE
(7) Hold the tubing in the rectum constantly until the end of the fluid instillation.	• Bowel contractions can cause expulsion of the rectal tube.
(8) Open the regulating clamp and allow the solution to enter slowly with the enema container at the client's hip level.	• Rapid instillation can stimulate evacuation of the rectal tube.
(9) Raise the height of the enema container slowly to the appropriate level above the anus: 30–45 cm for a high enema, 30 cm for regular enema, 7.5 cm for a low enema (see Step 16A(6) illustration). Instillation time varies depending on the volume of solution administered.	• Raising the height slowly allows for continuous, slow instillation of the solution. Raising the container too high causes rapid instillation and possible painful distension of the colon. High pressure can cause rupture of the bowel in an infant.

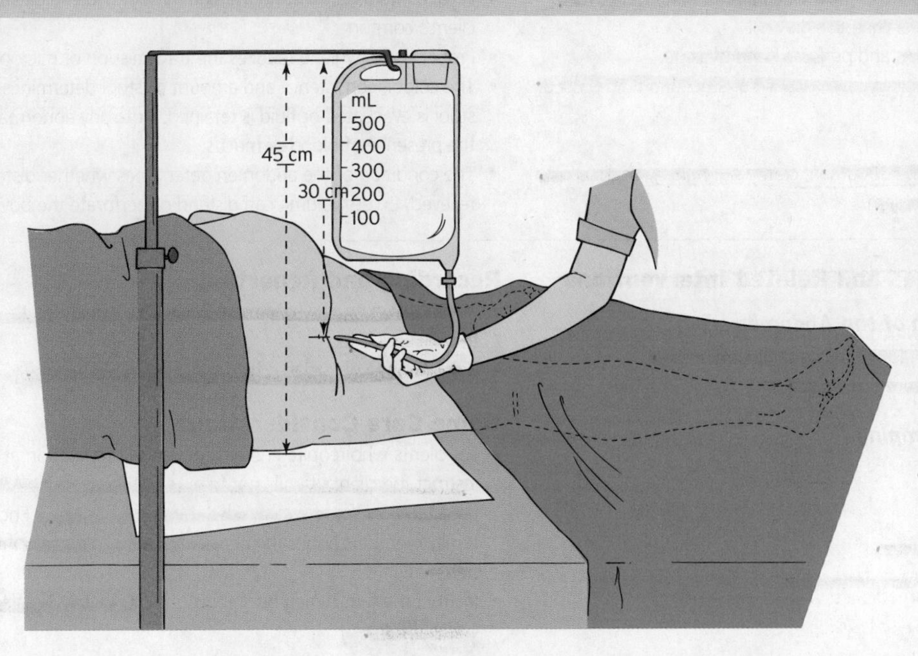

Step 16A(6) Insertion of a rectal tube into the rectum.

Continued

➤ SKILL 45-1 Administering a Cleansing Enema *continued*

STEPS	RATIONALE
(10) Lower the container or clamp tubing if the client complains of cramping or if fluid escapes around the rectal tube.	• Temporary cessation of instillation prevents cramping, but may prevent the client from retaining all the fluid, thus altering the effectiveness of the enema.
(11) Clamp the tubing after all solution is instilled.	• Clamping prevents entrance of air into the rectum.
B. Prepackaged disposable container	
(1) Remove the plastic cap from the rectal tip. The tip is already lubricated, but more jelly can be applied as needed.	• Lubrication provides for smooth insertion of rectal tube while avoiding rectal irritation or trauma.
(2) Gently separate the buttocks and locate the rectum. Instruct the client to relax by breathing out slowly through mouth.	• Breathing out promotes relaxation of the external rectal sphincter.
(3) Insert the tip of the bottle gently into the rectum. Adult: 7.5–10 cm Child: 5–7.5 cm Infant: 2.5–3.75 cm	• Gentle insertion prevents trauma to the rectal mucosa.
(4) Squeeze the bottle until all the solution has entered the rectum and colon. Instruct the client to retain the solution until the urge to defecate occurs, usually within 2–5 minutes.	• Hypertonic solutions require only small volumes to stimulate defecation.
17. Place layers of toilet tissue around the tube at the anus and gently withdraw the rectal tube.	• The use of toilet paper provides the client with comfort and cleanliness.
18. Explain to the client that the feeling of distension is normal. Ask the client to retain the solution for as long as possible while lying quietly in bed. (For an infant or young child, gently hold the buttocks together for a few minutes.)	• The enema solution distends the bowel. The length of retention varies depending on the type of enema and the client's ability to contract the rectal sphincter. Longer retention promotes more effective stimulation of peristalsis and defecation.
19. Discard the enema container and tubing in the proper receptacle; or rinse thoroughly with warm soap and water if the container is to be reused.	• Proper handling of the used enema container and tubing reduces the transmission and growth of microorganisms.
20. Assist the client to the bathroom or help to position the client on a bedpan.	• The normal squatting position promotes defecation.
 **21.** Observe the character of the feces and solution (caution the client against flushing the toilet until you can inspect the feces).	• The character of the expelled feces determines the efficacy of the enema.

Critical Decision Point: When enemas are ordered "until clear," observe the contents of the solution passed. Return is "clear" when no solid fecal material exists, but solution may be coloured.

STEPS	RATIONALE
22. Assist client as needed to wash the anal area with warm soap and water (if providing perineal care, use gloves).	• Fecal contents can irritate the skin. Proper hygiene promotes the client's comfort.
23. Remove and discard gloves and perform hand hygiene.	• Proper hand hygiene reduces the transmission of microorganisms.
24. Inspect the colour, consistency, and amount of stool and fluid passed.	• The colour, consistency and amount of stool determines whether the stool is evacuated or fluid is retained. Note any abnormalities, such as the presence of blood or mucus.
25. Assess the condition of the abdomen; cramping, rigidity, or distension can indicate a serious problem.	• The condition of the abdomen determines whether distension is relieved. Excess volume can distend or perforate the bowel.

Unexpected Outcomes and Related Interventions

Rigidity and Distension of the Abdomen

- Stop the enema administration if fluid is still being instilled.
- Notify the physician and obtain vital signs.

Abdominal Pain or Cramping

- Slow the rate of instillation.

Bleeding

- Stop the enema administration.
- Notify the physician and obtain vital signs.

Recording and Reporting

- Record the type and volume of the enema given and the characteristics of the results.
- Report to the physician if the client failed to defecate.

Home Care Considerations

- For clients who require enemas for bowel preparation at home, instruct the client's family not to exceed the recommended fluid volume levels or the recommended number of enemas. Encourage the family members about the need for slow administration of warmed fluid.
- Instruct the family members about the negative side effects of tap water enemas.

➤ BOX 45-9 Procedural Guidelines

Digital Removal of Stool

Delegation Considerations: The digital removal of stool procedure should not be delegated to unregulated care providers.

Equipment

- Bath blanket
- Waterproof pad
- Disposable gloves
- Lubricant
- Towel
- Washcloth
- Soap and water
- Bedpan

Procedure

1. Explain the procedure to the client.
2. Perform hand hygiene. Take baseline vital signs prior to the procedure. Help the client to lie on the left side with knees flexed and back toward you.
3. Drape the trunk and lower extremities with a bath blanket and place a waterproof pad under the buttocks. Keep a bedpan next to the client.
4. Apply disposable gloves and lubricate the index finger of your dominant hand with lubricating jelly.
5. Gently insert the gloved index finger into the rectum and advance the finger slowly along the rectal wall toward the umbilicus.
6. Gently loosen the fecal mass by massaging around it. Work the finger into the hardened mass.
7. Work the feces downward toward the end of the rectum. Remove small pieces at a time and discard into the bedpan.
8. Reassess the client's vital signs and look for signs of fatigue. Stop the procedure if the heart rate drops significantly or if the heart rhythm changes.
9. Continue to remove feces and allow the client to rest at intervals.
10. After completion, wash and dry the buttocks and anal area.
11. Remove the bedpan and dispose of the feces. Remove gloves by turning them inside out, and then discard.
12. Assist the client to the toilet or position the client on a clean bedpan if the urge to defecate develops.
13. Perform hand hygiene. Record results of the removal of the impaction by describing the fecal characteristics.
14. Follow the procedure with enemas or cathartics as ordered by physician.
15. Reassess the client's vital signs and level of comfort.

BOX 45-10 NURSING STORY

Disimpaction Is a Painful Stimulus

The first time I, as a newly hired nursing instructor, took fourth-year students to a clinical experience, we attended a small (8-bed) neurological intensive care unit. One client, a young man in his late teens who was conscious but still confused, was recovering from a motorbike accident. The student who was assigned to this client read the doctor's order for rectal disimpaction (the client's bowels had not moved since the accident five days previously). The student and I discussed in great detail the procedure and came to a disagreement about the highest priority for the client after safety. I said that the student required assistance, but she said no the greater need was for the client's privacy. As I hovered near the curtains, she explained the procedure to the young man, assessed his vital signs, prepared the bedpan, put on her gloves, lubricated her index finger, and drew the curtains ever tighter. She then attempted to insert her gloved, lubricated finger into the rectum. To the young man, this was a startling procedure (although it had been verbally explained to him). I heard a loud yell from the client and the clatter of a bedpan bouncing across the floor, and then a bedraggled nursing cap sailed under the curtains. I rushed behind the curtains to rescue the student from the flailing arms of the strong young man. No harm was done and the student gratefully accepted assistance from the orderly.

Lesson learned: disimpaction is a strong, noxious stimulus and the client's reactions may be unpredictable. In an older adult client, the reaction may even be pathological, such as a cardiovascular response or increased heart rate and blood pressure from sympathetic stimulation. In very ill clients, the crash cart should be present at the bedside because a cardiac arrest could ensue.

As a footnote to the story, this student and I had a several further disagreements that year. Several years later, however, I received a note from this woman, who was now teaching nursing herself. She apologized for her behaviour. She had taught several students who had reminded her of herself when she was a student, she said; and now she wondered how I ever put up with her behaviour.

➤ TABLE 45-6 Purposes of Nasogastric Intubation

Purpose	Description	Type of Tube
Decompression	Removal of secretions and gaseous substances from the gastrointestinal tract to prevent or relieve abdominal distension	Salem sump, Levin, Miller-Abbott
Feeding (i.e., gavage; see Chapter 43)	Instillation of liquid nutritional supplements or feedings into the stomach for clients unable to swallow fluid	Duo, Dobhoff, Levin
Compression	Internal application of pressure by means of an inflated balloon to prevent internal esophageal or gastrointestinal hemorrhage	Sengstaken-Blakemore
Lavage	Irrigation of the stomach in cases of active bleeding, poisoning, or gastric dilation	Levin, Ewald, Salem sump

The Salem sump tube is preferable for stomach decompression. This tube has two lumina: one for removal of gastric contents (Figure 45–16) and one to provide an air vent. A blue "pigtail" is the air vent that connects with the second lumen. When the sump tube's main lumen is connected to suction, the air vent permits free, continuous drainage of secretions. The air vent should never be clamped off, connected to suction, or used for irrigation.

Nasogastric tube insertion (Skill 45–2) does not require a sterile technique; you simply use a clean technique. The procedure is uncomfortable. The client experiences a burning sensation as the tube passes through the sensitive nasal mucosa. When the tube reaches the back of the pharynx, the client may begin to gag. You must help the client to relax, which makes tube insertion easier. Some institutions allow Xylocaine Jelly to be used when inserting the tube because it increases client comfort during the procedure.

One of the greatest problems in caring for a client with an NG tube is maintaining comfort. The tube is a constant irritation to the nasal mucosa. You must assess the condition of the nares and mucosa for inflammation and excoriation. The tape used to anchor the tube often becomes soiled. Change it every day to reduce skin irritation. Frequent lubrication of the nares also minimizes excoriation. With one naris occluded, the client may breathe through the mouth. Frequent mouth care (at least every 2 hours) helps to minimize dehydration. A glass of cool water for rinsing is useful; however, if the client is allowed nothing by mouth (NPO), the water should not be swallowed. The client will frequently complain of a sore throat. An ice bag applied externally to the throat may help. Gargling with topical Xylocaine Jelly or sucking on ice chips or throat lozenges may be used if ordered by the physician.

After the tube is inserted, you must maintain its patency. If the tip of the tubing rests against the stomach wall or if the tube becomes blocked with thick secretions, regular irrigation is necessary. Flushing the tube with normal saline by way of a catheter-tipped syringe clears blockage within the tube (see Skill 45–2). If an NG tube continues to drain improperly after irrigation, you must reposition it by either advancing or withdrawing it slightly. Any change in the tube position requires you to verify the placement of the tube in the client's GI tract (see Skill 45–2).

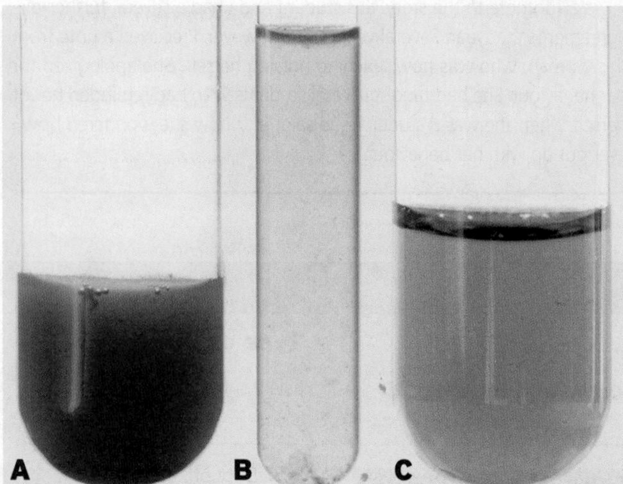

Figure 45-16 Gastric contents. A, Stomach. B, Stomach. C, Intestinal. **Source:** Courtesy Dr. Norma Metheny, St. Louis University, School of Nursing. St. Louis, MO.

The NG tube can cause distension. The presence of the tube causes many clients to swallow large volumes of air. Channels of gastric secretions also form along the walls of the stomach and bypass the suction holes. Turning the client regularly helps to collapse the channels and promote emptying of the stomach contents.

Continuing and Restorative Care

As the client recovers and is able to return home or to a long-term care facility, regular bowel elimination patterns must begin. When clients have a colostomy, they must learn to care for the ostomy. Other clients may require bowel training. Remember that ostomy care and bowel training may be initiated in the acute care setting; however, because these activities are long-term care needs, they are usually completed in the restorative care settings.

Care of Ostomies. Clients with temporary or permanent bowel diversions have unique bowel elimination needs. Persons with an ostomy wear a pouch or appliance to collect the **effluent** (the stool discharged from an ostomy) from the stomas (CAET, 2008a). These clients must use meticulous skin care to prevent liquid stool from irritating the skin around the stoma (Box 45–11).

Irrigating a Colostomy. Although this practice is not as common as it once was, some clients may be instructed to irrigate their left-sided colostomies in order to regulate colon emptying. Other clients do not want to spend the additional 60 to 90 minutes in the bathroom every day, and they empty their pouch only as necessary (CAET, 2008a).

Specific equipment for irrigating a colostomy should be used. An enema set should never be used to irrigate a colostomy. A special cone-tipped irrigator (Figure 45–17) is used. This device prevents both bowel penetration and backflow of the irrigating solution. Clients usually sit on the toilet and place an irrigating sleeve over the stoma. The end of this sleeve extends into the bowl of the toilet. The physician orders the amount and type of solution. For adults, the amount ranges from 500 to 700 mL of tap water. The solution is instilled slowly through the lubricated cone tip. Irrigation should take 5 to 10 minutes. The client then removes the cone tip and waits 30 to 45 minutes for the solution and feces to drain out of the irrigation sleeve. Once the drainage stops, the client applies a stoma cap or a pouch. If a client chooses to irrigate the colostomy, the timing of the irrigation can be individualized to the client's lifestyle.

Pouching Ostomies. Ostomies require a pouch to collect fecal material. An effective pouching system protects the skin, contains fecal material, remains odour-free, and is comfortable and inconspicuous. A person wearing a pouch should feel secure in participating in any activity.

Many pouching systems are available. To ensure that a pouch fits well and meets the client's needs, consider the location of the ostomy; the type and size of the stoma; the type and amount of the ostomy drainage; the size and contour of the abdomen; the condition of the skin around the stoma; the physical activities of the client; the client's personal preference, age, and dexterity; and the cost of the equipment. An **enterostomal therapist** (ET) is a nurse trained to care for wound and ostomy management. The staff nurse collaborates with the ET to ensure the correct pouching system is used. For example, a referral to an ET nurse would be appropriate to plan the care of a client who has a high-output ostomy that requires a pouch modification.

➤ SKILL 45-2 Inserting and Maintaining a Nasogastric Tube

video

Delegation Considerations

The skill of inserting and maintaining the nasogastric (NG) tube should not be delegated to unregulated care providers (UCPs). You are responsible for the proper function and drainage of the nasogastric tube, all relevant assessments, and determining the client's level of comfort. You may instruct the UCP to do the following tasks:

- Measure and record the drainage
- Provide oral and nasal hygiene
- Perform selected comfort measures

Equipment

- No. 14 or no. 16 Fr NG tube (smaller-lumen catheters are not used for decompression in adults because they must be able to remove thick secretions)
- Water-soluble lubricating jelly
- pH test strips (to measure gastric aspirate acidity)
- Tongue blade
- Flashlight
- Emesis basin
- Asepto bulb or catheter-tipped syringe
- 2.5-cm-wide hypoallergenic tape (7.5–10 cm long) or a commercial fixation device
- Safety pin and rubber band
- Clamp, or suction machine; or pressure gauge if wall suction is to be used
- Towel
- Glass of water with straw
- Facial tissues
- Normal saline
- Tincture of benzoin (optional)
- Suction equipment
- Disposable gloves

STEPS	RATIONALE
1. Perform hand hygiene. Inspect the condition of the client's nasal and oral cavities.	• The baseline condition of the nasal and oral cavities determines the need for special nursing measures for oral hygiene after tube placement.
2. Ask whether the client has a history of nasal surgery and note whether a deviated nasal septum is present.	• Insert the tube into an uninvolved nasal passage. This procedure may be contraindicated if surgery is recent.
3. Palpate the client's abdomen for distension, pain, and rigidity. Auscultate for bowel sounds.	• The baseline level of abdominal distension later serves as a comparison once the tube is inserted.
4. Assess the client's level of consciousness and ability to follow instructions.	• The ability to follow directions determines the client's ability to assist in the procedure.

Critical Decision Point: If the client is confused, disoriented, or unable to follow commands, obtain assistance from another staff member to insert the tube.

STEPS	RATIONALE
5. Check the medical record for the surgeon's order, the type of NG tube to be placed, and whether the tube is to be attached to suction.	• This procedure requires a physician's order. Adequate decompression depends on nasogastric suction.
6. Perform hand hygiene. Prepare equipment at the bedside. Cut a piece of tape approximately 10 cm long and split one end in half to form a V; or have the nasogastric tube fixator device available.	• Proper hand hygiene reduces the transmission of infection. Preparing the equipment ensures a well-organized procedure. The tape or fixator device will be used to hold the tube in place after insertion.
7. Identify the client and explain the procedure.	• Identification prevents the error of placing the tube in the wrong client. Explaining the procedure gains the client's cooperation and reduces the possibility that the client will remove the tube.
8. Apply disposable gloves.	• The use of gloves reduces the transmission of microorganisms.
9. Position the client in a high Fowler's position with pillows behind the head and shoulders. Raise the bed to a horizontal level that is comfortable for you.	• The high Fowler's position promotes the client's ability to swallow during the procedure. Good body mechanics prevent injury to both you and the client.
10. Place a bath towel over the client's chest; give facial tissues to the client. Place the emesis basin within reach.	• The bath towel prevents soiling of the client's gown. Tube insertion through the nasal passages may cause tearing and coughing accompanied by increased salivation.
11. Pull the curtain around the bed or close the room door.	• Privacy reduces the embarrassment for the client.
12. Stand on the client's right side if you are right-handed, on the left side if you are left-handed.	• Standing on the side that corresponds to your dominant hand allows for easier manipulation of the tubing.
13. Instruct the client to relax and breathe normally while occluding one naris. Repeat this action for the other naris. Select the nostril with the greater airflow.	• The tube passes more easily through the naris that is more patent.

Continued

➤ SKILL 45-2 Inserting and Maintaining a Nasogastric Tube *continued*

STEPS	RATIONALE
14. Measure the distance to insert the tube:	
A. Measure the distance from the tip of the client's nose to the earlobe to the xiphoid process (see Step 14A illustration).	
B. Mark the 50-cm point on the tube, then take a traditional measurement. The tube should be inserted to a midway point between 50 cm and the traditional mark.	• The measurement approximates the distance from the naris to the stomach. The tube should extend from the naris to the stomach; this distance varies with each client.
15. Mark the length of tube to be inserted by using a small piece of tape placed so that it can easily be removed.	• The tape marks the amount of tube to be inserted from the naris to the stomach.
16. Curve 10–15 cm of the end of the tube tightly around your index finger, then release.	• Curving the tube tip aids the insertion and decreases the stiffness of the tube.
17. Lubricate 7.5–10 cm of the end of the tube with water-soluble lubricating jelly.	• The lubricating jelly minimizes the friction against the nasal mucosa and aids insertion of the tube.
18. Alert the client that the procedure is to begin.	• Communicating the start of the procedure decreases client anxiety and increases client cooperation.
19. Instruct the client to extend the neck back against the pillow; insert the tube gently and slowly through the naris with the curved end pointing downward (see Step 19 illustration).	• The extended neck facilitates the initial passage of the tube through the naris and maintains a clear airway for the open naris.
20. Insert the tube slowly through the naris with the curved end pointing downward. Continue to insert the tube along the floor of the nasal passage aiming down toward the client's ear. If resistance is met, apply gentle downward pressure to advance the tube (do not force the tube past the area of resistance).	• A slow insertion along the floor of the nasal passage minimizes the discomfort of the tube rubbing against the upper nasal turbinates. Resistance is caused by the posterior nasopharynx. Downward pressure helps the tube to curl around the corner of the nasopharynx.
21. If resistance is met, try to rotate the tube to see whether it advances. If resistance continues, withdraw the tube, allow the client to rest, relubricate the tube, and insert the tube into the other naris.	• Forcing the tube against resistance can cause trauma to the mucosa. Removing the tube and using the other naris helps to relieve the client's anxiety.

Critical Decision Point: If you are unable to insert the tube in either naris, stop the procedure and notify the physician.

STEPS	RATIONALE
22. Continue insertion of tube by gently rotating the tube toward the opposite naris. Insert until the tube is just past the nasopharynx.	• A gentle rotation of the tube helps to prevent coiling of the tube in the oropharynx.
A. Stop the tube advancement, allow the client to relax. Provide the client with tissues.	• Allowing a period of relaxation relieves the client's anxiety; tissues are needed because tearing is a natural response to mucosal irritation, and excessive salivation may occur because of oral stimulation.
B. Explain to client that the next step requires that the client swallow. Give the client a glass of water unless contraindicated.	• Slipping of water aids passage of the nasogastric tube into the esophagus.

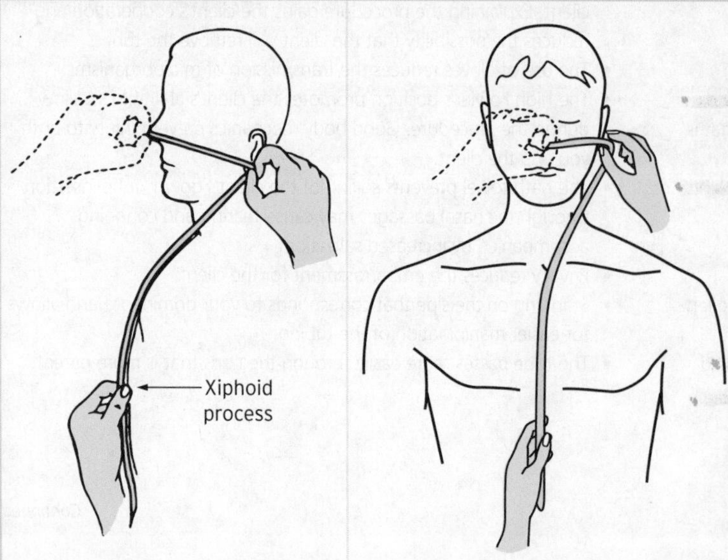

Step 14A Technique for measuring the distance to insert the nasogastric tube.

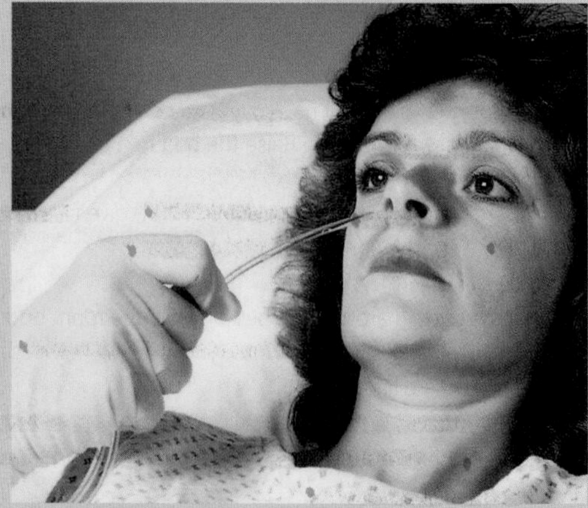

Step 19 Insert the nasogastric tube with the curved end pointing downward.

➤ SKILL 45-2 Inserting and Maintaining a Nasogastric Tube *continued*

STEPS	RATIONALE
23. With the tube just above the oropharynx, instruct the client to flex the head forward, while you place your hand at the back of the neck to support it. Have the client take a small sip of water, and swallow. Advance the tube 2.5–5 cm with each swallow of water. If client is not allowed fluids, instruct the client to dry swallow or to suck air through a straw.	• The flexed position closes off the upper airway to the trachea and opens the esophagus. Swallowing closes the epiglottis over the trachea and helps move the tube into the esophagus. Swallowing water reduces the gagging or choking reflex. Water can be removed later from stomach by suction.
24. If the client begins to cough, gag, or choke, withdraw the tube slightly (do not completely remove the tube) and stop tube advancement. Instruct the client to breathe easily and take sips of water.	• The tube may be displaced into the larynx and produce coughing. Swallowing water closes the epiglottis over the trachea and helps to move the tube into the esophagus. The risk for aspiration increases if vomiting occurs.

Critical Decision Point: If vomiting occurs, assist the client in clearing the airway; oral suctioning may be needed. Do not proceed until the airway is cleared.

STEPS	RATIONALE
25. If the client continues to gag and cough or if the client complains that the tube feels as though it is coiling in the back of the throat, check the back of the oropharynx using a tongue blade. If the tube has coiled, withdraw it until the tip is back in the oropharynx. Reinsert the tube with the client swallowing.	• The tube may coil around itself in the back of the throat and stimulate the gag reflex.
26. Continue to advance the tube with swallowing until the tape or mark is reached. Temporarily anchor the tube to the client's cheek with a piece of tape until the tube placement is checked.	• The tip of the tube must be well within the stomach to provide adequate decompression. The tube should be anchored before placement is verified.
27. Verify tube placement. Check agency policy for the preferred methods for checking nasogastric tube placement.	
A. Ask the client to talk.	• An inability to speak may indicate that tube advanced through client's vocal cords into the lungs.
B. Inspect the posterior pharynx for the presence of coiled tube.	• The tube is pliable and can coil in back of the pharynx instead of advancing into the esophagus.
C. Aspirate gently back on the syringe to obtain gastric contents. Note the colour and other characteristics.	• Gastric contents are usually cloudy and green, but may be off-white, tan, bloody, or brown. Aspiration of contents provides a means to measure the fluid pH and thus determine the tube tip placement in the gastrointestinal tract (see Figure 45–16). • Duodenal placement is indicated by yellow or bile-stained contents, and placement in the esophagus may or may not show saliva-appearing aspirate.
D. Measure the pH of the aspirate with colour-coded pH paper with a range of whole numbers 1 to 11 (see Step 27D illustration).	• Gastric aspirates have decidedly acidic pH values, preferably 4 or less, compared with intestinal aspirates, which are usually greater than 4, or respiratory secretions, which are usually greater than 5.5 (Metheny & Titler, 2001).
E. Have an X-ray examination performed of the chest or abdomen.	• Placement of the tube can be reliably verified by X-ray examination.

Critical Decision Point: Be sure to use a gastric (Gastroccult) pH test and not a Hemoccult test.

STEPS	RATIONALE
F. If the tube is not in the stomach, advance another 2.5–5 cm and repeat steps 27B, C, and D to check the tube position.	• The tube must be in the stomach to provide decompression.

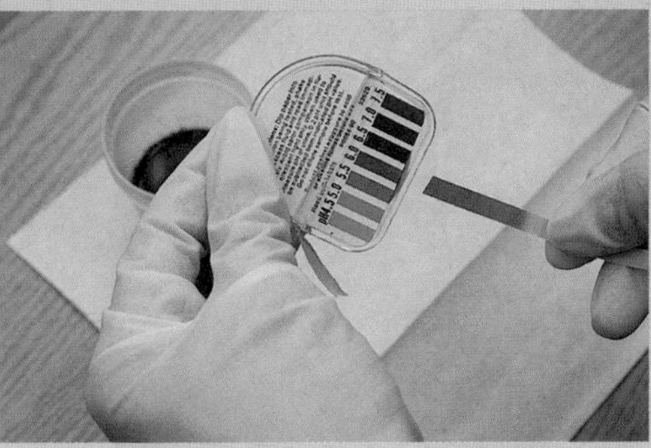

Step 27D Checking the pH of gastric aspirate.

Continued

➤ SKILL 45-2 Inserting and Maintaining a Nasogastric Tube *continued*

STEPS	RATIONALE
28. Anchor the tube:	
A. After the tube is properly inserted and positioned, either clamp the end or connect the end to the drainage bag or a suction machine.	• The drainage bag is used for gravity drainage. Intermittent, low suction is most effective for decompression. When the client is undergoing surgery, the tube is often clamped.
B. Tape the tube to the nose; avoid putting pressure on both nares.	• The use of tape anchors the tube securely. Avoidance of pressure prevents tissue necrosis.
(1) Before taping the tube to the nose, apply a small amount of tincture of benzoin to the lower end of the nose and allow it to dry (optional). Ensure the top end of the tape over the nose is secure.	
(2) Carefully wrap the two split ends of tape around the tube (see Step 28B(2) illustration).	
(3) Alternative: Apply the tube fixation device using a shaped adhesive patch (see Step 28B(3) illustration).	• The use of benzoin prevents the loosening of tape if the client perspires.
C. Fasten the end of the nasogastric tube to the client's gown by looping a rubber band around the tube into a slip knot. Pin the rubber band to the client's gown (to provide slack for movement).	• Fastening the tube to the gown by this method reduces pressure on the nares if the tube moves.
D. Unless the physician orders otherwise, the head of the bed should be elevated 30 degrees.	• Elevating the bed helps to prevent esophageal reflux and minimizes the irritation of the tube against the posterior pharynx.
E. Explain to the client that the sensation of the tube will decrease with time.	• Your explanation will ease the client's adaptation to the continued sensory stimulus.
F. Remove gloves and wash hands.	• Proper hand hygiene reduces the transmission of microorganisms.
29. Once placement is confirmed:	
A. Place a mark, either a red mark or tape, on the tube to indicate where the tube exits the nose.	
B. Alternatively, measure the length of the tube from the naris to the connector.	
C. Document the tube length in the client record.	• The mark or tube length is used as a guide to indicate whether displacement has occurred.
30. Tube irrigation:	
A. Wash hands and apply gloves.	• Proper hand hygiene reduces the transmission of microorganisms.
B. Check for tube placement in the stomach (see Step 27). Reconnect the nasogastric tube to the connecting tube.	• Correct placement of the tube prevents accidental entrance of irrigating solution into the lungs.
C. Draw up 30 mL of normal saline into Asepto or catheter-tipped syringe.	• Use of saline minimizes the loss of electrolytes from the stomach fluids.
D. Clamp the nasogastric tube. Disconnect from the connection tubing and lay the end of the connection tubing on a towel.	• Use of a towel reduces soiling of the client's gown and the bed linen.
E. Insert the tip of the irrigating syringe into the end of the nasogastric tube. Remove the clamp. Hold the syringe with the tip pointed at the floor and inject the saline slowly and evenly. Do not force the solution.	• The position of the syringe prevents introduction of air into the vent tubing, which could cause gastric distension. Solution that is introduced under pressure can cause gastric trauma.

Critical Decision Point: Do not introduce saline through the blue "pigtail" air vent of the Salem sump tube.

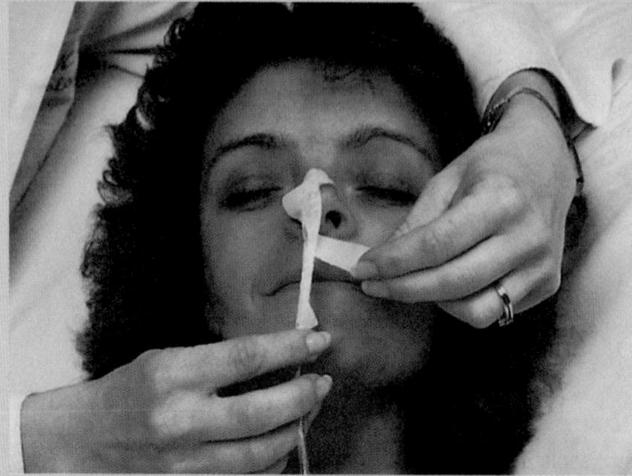

Step 28B(2) Tape is crossed over and around the nasogastric tube.

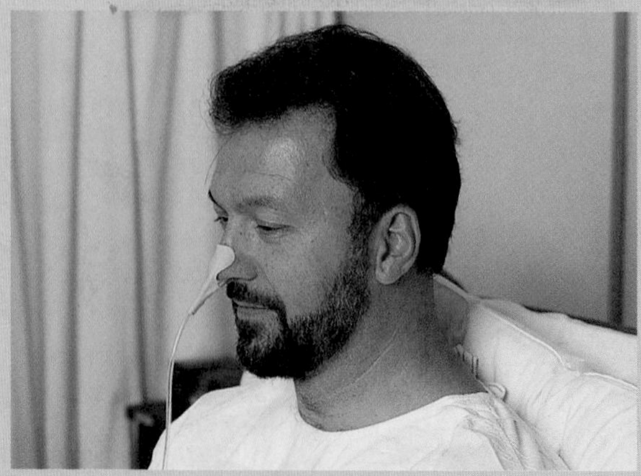

Step 28B(3) Client with a tube fixation device.

➤ SKILL 45-2 Inserting and Maintaining a Nasogastric Tube ***continued***

STEPS	RATIONALE
F. If resistance occurs, check for kinks in the tubing. Turn the client onto the left side. Repeated resistance should be reported to the physician.	• The tip of the tube may lie against the stomach lining. Repositioning the client to the left side may dislodge the tube away from the stomach lining. The buildup of secretions will cause distension.
G. After instilling saline, immediately aspirate or pull back slowly on the syringe to withdraw fluid. If the amount aspirated is greater than amount instilled, record the difference as output. If the amount aspirated is less than amount instilled, record the difference as intake.	• The irrigation process clears the tubing; the stomach should remain empty. Fluid remaining in the stomach is measured as intake.
H. Reconnect the nasogastric tube to the drainage bag or suction (if the solution does not return, repeat the irrigation.)	• This step re-establishes the drainage collection; repeat the irrigation or reposition the tube until the nasogastric tube drains properly.
I. Remove gloves and perform hand hygiene.	• Proper hand hygiene reduces transmission of microorganisms.
31. Observe the amount and character of the contents draining from the nasogastric tube. Ask whether the client feels nauseated.	• The amount and character of the contents and the client's presence of nausea determine whether the tube is decompressing the stomach of its contents.
32. Palpate the client's abdomen periodically, noting any distension, pain, or rigidity. Turn off the suction and auscultate for the presence of bowel sounds.	• Palpation determines the success of abdominal decompression and the return of peristalsis. The sound of the suction apparatus may transmit to the abdomen and be misinterpreted as bowel sounds.
33. Inspect the condition of the nares and the nose.	• Inspection of the nares and nose evaluates the onset of skin and tissue irritation.
34. Observe the position of the tubing.	• The tube positioning determines whether tension is being applied to nasal structures.
35. Ask whether the client has a sore throat or feels irritation in the pharynx.	• Questioning the presence of a sore throat or irritation evaluates the level of the client's discomfort.
36. Discontinuation of a nasogastric tube:	
A. Verify the order to discontinue the nasogastric tube.	• A physician's order is required to discontinue the nasogastric tube.

Critical Decision Point: Immediately prior to removing the nasogastric tube, verify the presence of bowel sounds.

STEPS	RATIONALE
B. Explain the procedure to the client and reassure the client that removal is less distressing than insertion.	• Explaining the procedure minimizes anxiety and increases cooperation.
C. Perform hand hygiene and apply disposable gloves.	• Proper hand hygiene reduces the transmission of microorganisms.
D. Turn off the suction and disconnect the nasogastric tube from the drainage bag or suction. Remove tape from the bridge of the nose and unpin the tube from the gown.	• Free the tube from all connections before removal.
E. Stand on the client's right side if you are right-handed, on the left side if you are left-handed.	• Standing on the side that corresponds to your dominant hand allows for easier manipulation of the tubing.
F. Hand the client a facial tissue; place a clean towel across the chest. Instruct the client to take a deep breath and to hold the breath.	• The client may wish to blow the nose after the tube is removed. Use of a towel reduces soiling of the client's gown and the bed linen. The airway will be temporarily obstructed during the tube removal.
G. While the client holds the breath, clamp or kink the tubing securely and then pull the tube out steadily and smoothly into a towel held in your other hand.	• Holding the breath helps to prevent aspiration. Clamping prevents the tube contents from draining into the oropharynx, reduces trauma to the mucosa, and minimizes the client's discomfort. The towel covers the tube, which can be an unpleasant sight.
H. Measure the amount of drainage and note the character of the contents. Dispose of the tube and drainage equipment into the proper container.	• Measuring the drainage amount provides an accurate calculation of the fluid output. Proper disposal reduces the transfer of microorganisms.
I. Clean the nares and provide mouth care.	• Cleaning the nares and checking the mouth promotes the client's comfort.
J. Position the client comfortably and explain the procedure for drinking fluids, if not contraindicated.	• Some clients are allowed nothing by mouth (NPO) for up to 24 hours. When fluids are allowed, the order usually begins with a small amount of ice chips each hour and increases as the client's toleration improves.
37. Clean the equipment and return to their proper place. Place soiled linen in the utility room or the proper receptacle.	• Proper disposal of equipment prevents the spread of microorganisms and ensures proper exchange procedures.
38. Remove gloves and perform hand hygiene.	• Proper hand hygiene reduces the transmission of microorganisms.
39. Inspect the condition of the nares and the nose.	• Inspection of the nares and nose is needed to evaluate the onset of skin and tissue irritation.
40. Ask whether the client has a sore throat or feels irritation in the pharynx.	• Questioning the presence of a sore throat or irritation evaluates the level of the client's discomfort.

Continued

➤ SKILL 45-2 Inserting and Maintaining a Nasogastric Tube *continued*

Unexpected Outcomes and Related Interventions

Distension of or Pain in the Abdomen

- Assess the patency of the tube and irrigate as needed.

Sore Throat Caused by Dry, Irritated Mucous Membranes

- Increase the frequency of oral hygiene.
- Ask the physician whether the client may suck on ice chips or throat lozenges.

Irritation of the Skin Around the Naris

- Provide skin care to the naris.
- Retape so the tube does not press against the naris.
- Consider switching the tube to the other naris.

Signs of Pulmonary Aspiration (Fever, Shortness of Breath, Pulmonary Congestion)

- Perform a respiratory assessment.
- Notify the physician.
- Obtain the chest X-ray examination as ordered.

Recording and Reporting

- Record in the nurses' notes the time and type of nasogastric tube inserted, the client's tolerance of the procedure, confirmation of the tube placement, character of the gastric contents, the pH value, whether the tube is clamped or connected to a drainage device, and the amount of suction applied.
- Record in the nurses' notes or flow sheet, or both, the amount and character of the contents draining from the nasogastric tube every shift, unless ordered more frequently by the physician.

BOX 45-11 CLIENT TEACHING

Stomal Care (Incontinent Ostomy)

Objective

- The client will demonstrate the correct procedure for stomal care.

Teaching Strategies

- Teach the client that the drainage from a stoma is very irritating to the skin and that contact of the skin with the drainage should be avoided. When contact does occur, the client should clean the area as soon as possible.
- Show the client how to inspect the appearance of the skin and the surrounding stoma. The stoma should be moist, shiny, and pink (Hyland, 2002). Bleeding should be minimal. The skin around the stoma, called the peristomal area, should be a normal skin tone.
- The peristomal area should be cleaned with mild soap and water or even plain water (CAET, 2008a). The client must dry the area thoroughly.
- Instruct the client to avoid the use of creams, ointments, baby wipes, or other moist towelettes on the peristomal skin, as these agents can prevent the pouch from adhering securely on the client's skin (CAET, 2008a).
- Instruct the client to report either to you or to the physician excess bleeding or prolonged oozing.
- Demonstrate to the client how to select and apply a skin barrier and pouch; instruct the client regarding the length of wear.
- Demonstrate to the client how to empty and change the pouching system.
- Instruct the client on how to reduce the odour that accompanies a stoma and the commercial agents to use.
- Assist the client in determining the ostomy supplies that should be carried at all times. Provide the client and the client's family with a list of resources from which to obtain supplies in the community.
- Instruct the client that if a yeast infection occurs, the client should thoroughly clean the area, pat dry, and apply a prescribed topical agent to the affected region, such as triamcinolone acetonide (Kenalog) spray or nystatin (Mycostatin).

Evaluation

- The client will correctly state the skin care procedures.
- The client will correctly perform the stoma skin care procedure.

A pouching system consists of a pouch and a skin barrier (Figure 45–18). Some pouching systems, such as those manufactured by Squibb-ConvaTec, Hollister, Coloplast, and Smith & Nephew, are attached to the client's skin from the product's adhesive surface, whereas other pouching systems, such as VIP, are nonadhesive systems. Pouches come in one- and two-piece systems that are disposable or reusable. Some pouches have the opening precut by the manufacturer; others require the stoma opening to be custom cut to the client's specific stoma size.

Skin barriers include wafers, pastes, powders, and liquid film that are applied to the skin around the stoma. Wafer skin barriers, which are permanently attached to the ostomy pouch, are called one-piece pouch systems. In a two-piece system, the pouch can be detached from the skin barrier for emptying or changing. This system allows the skin barrier to remain around the client's stoma for several days, thus minimizing the chance of skin damage from too-frequent removal of the skin barrier from the peristomal skin (Figure 45–19). When using a two-piece pouching system, the skin barrier and pouch must be the same corresponding size and from the same manufacturer. The pouch from one manufacturer will not fit correctly on the skin barrier from another manufacturer. Ensure the client understands to use an ostomy pouch made for collecting fecal matter (i.e., a pouch specifically for a colostomy or ileostomy) and not a pouch for collecting urine.

Instruct clients to measure the stoma size carefully when selecting and cutting out the opening on the wafer skin barrier. A good skin barrier protects the skin, prevents irritation from repeated removal of the pouch, and is comfortable for the client to wear. Skill 45–3 describes the steps for applying one type of pouch system.

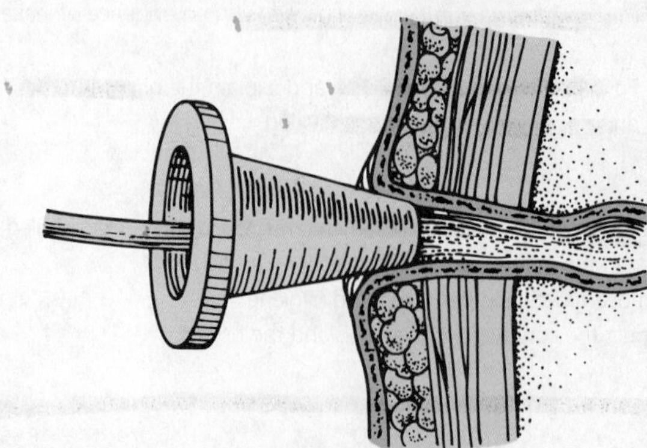

Figure 45-17 Ostomy irrigation cone inserted into the stoma.

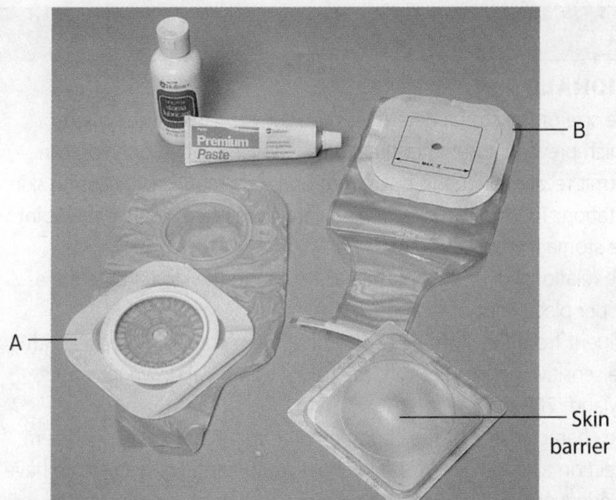

Figure 45-18 Ostomy pouches and skin barriers. **A,** Two-piece detachable system. (Note: The skin barrier needs to be custom cut to fit the stoma). The pouch opening is precut by the manufacturer to fit the size of the flange on the skin barrier. **B,** One-piece pouch with skin barrier attached. **Source:** Permission to use this copyrighted photo has been granted by the owner, Hollister Incorporated.

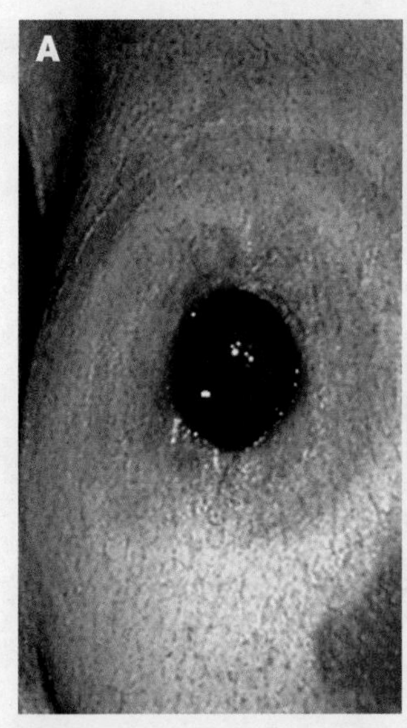

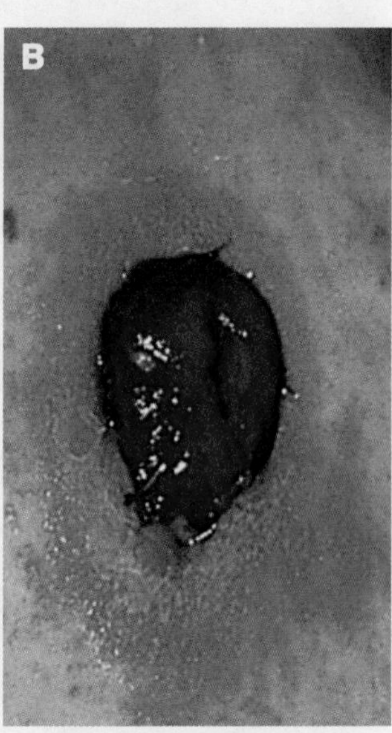

Figure 45-19 **A,** Mechanical injury to the peristomal skin. **B,** Candidiasis damage to the peristomal skin. **Source:** Permission to use these copyrighted photos has been granted by the owner, Hollister Incorporated.

➤ SKILL 45-3 Pouching an Ostomy

video

Delegation Considerations

The skill of pouching a newly established ostomy should not be delegated to unregulated care providers (UCPs). Pouching of a well-established ostomy can be delegated to a UCP. You must do the following:

- Assist the caregiver in selecting the appropriate pouch and skin barrier.
- Inform the caregiver of the signs of stomal and peristomal skin changes that should be reported to a nurse.
- Ask the caregiver to monitor and report the characteristics and volume of the ostomy output and report changes in volume or consistency to you for further assessment.

Equipment

- Clear drainable colostomy (or ileostomy) pouch in the correct size for a two-piece system or custom cut to fit a one-piece system with an attached skin barrier
- Pouch closure device, such as a clamp
- Disposable gloves
- Deodorant specific for an ostomy collection bag
- Gauze pads and washcloths
- Towel or disposable waterproof barrier
- Basin with warm tap water
- Scissors or pen
- Adhesive remover (optional)

STEPS	RATIONALE
1. Perform hand hygiene and auscultate for bowel sounds.	• Auscultation documents the presence of peristalsis.
2. Apply gloves. Observe the skin barrier and pouch for leakage and the length of time in place. Depending on the type of pouching system used (e.g., an opaque pouch), you may need to remove the pouch to fully observe the stoma. Clear pouches permit the viewing of the stoma without their removal.	• Leakage may indicate the need for a different type of pouch or sealant.

Critical Decision Point: Intact skin barriers with no evidence of leakage do not need to be changed daily and can remain in place for 3–5 days.

STEPS	RATIONALE
3. Observe the stoma for colour, swelling, trauma, and healing; the stoma should be moist and reddish-pink. Assess the type of stoma. Stomas can be flush with the skin or can be a bud-like protrusion on the abdomen (see Step 3 illustration).	• Stoma characteristics are one factor to consider when selecting an appropriate pouching system.

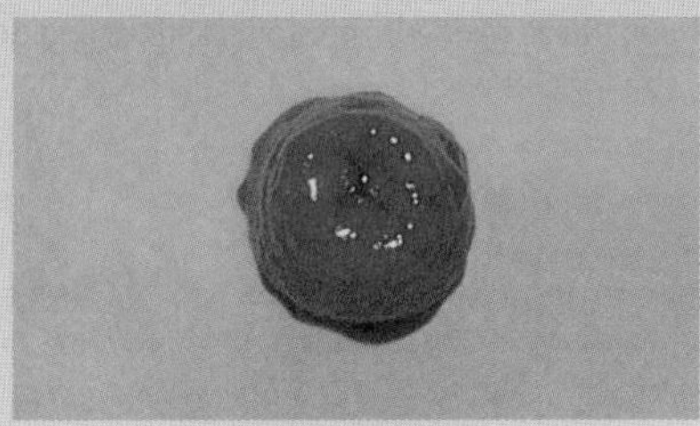

Step 3 Normal bud stoma. **Source:** Permission to use this copyrighted photo has been granted by the owner, Hollister Incorporated.

Continued

➤ SKILL 45-3 Pouching an Ostomy *continued*

STEPS	RATIONALE
4. Measure the stoma at each pouching change. Follow the pouch manufacturer's directions and measuring guide to determine which pouch to use on the basis of the client's stoma size. The opening around the appliance should be no greater than 2 mm larger than the stoma (Hyland, 2002).	• The size of the stoma determines the correct size of equipment, which prevents trauma to the stoma. Too large of an opening can permit fecal drainage to ooze from under the appliance, causing skin irritation. Too small of an opening can cause the appliance to cut into the stoma (Hyland, 2002).
5. Observe the abdominal incision (if present).	• The relationship of the abdominal incision to the stoma determines proper placement of the pouch.
6. Observe the effluent from the stoma and record the intake and output. Ask the client about skin tenderness. Remove gloves and perform hand hygiene.	• Effluent from the stoma is caustic. If effluent comes in contact with the sensitive peristomal skin, the risk of skin breakdown increases (Hyland, 2002).
7. Assess the abdomen for the best type of pouching system to use. Consider the following: A. Contour and peristomal plane B. Presence of scars, incisions C. Location and type of stoma	• The characteristics of the abdomen determine the pouching system selection and the need for additional equipment. For a stoma to have an adequate seal with an ostomy appliance, the stoma must be placed within the abdominal rectus muscle, away from abdominal creases and folds, away from the bony understructures, and surrounded by at least 5 cm of smooth surface on all sides (Banks & Razor, 2003).
8. Assess the client's self-care ability to determine the best type of pouching system to use.	• Clients who have difficulty using their hands or who have limited vision may find a one-piece system or a precut pouch and skin barrier more desirable to use; others prefer being able to keep the skin barrier in place for several days, changing just the pouch, and therefore prefer the two-piece system.
9. After removing the skin barrier and pouch, assess the skin around the stoma, noting scars, folds, skin breakdown, and the peristomal suture line, if present. Keep the pouch loosely attached to the stoma to collect any drainage while the system is being changed.	• Assessing the skin around the stoma determines the need for barrier paste to increase adherence of the pouch to the skin or to fill in irregularities.

Critical Decision Point: If the skin around the stoma is discoloured, weeping, itchy, or sore, refer the client to an ostomy specialist (Hyland, 2002).

STEPS	RATIONALE
10. Determine the client's emotional response, knowledge, and understanding of an ostomy and its care.	• Understanding the client's perspective assists in determining both the extent to which client is able to participate in care and the client's need for teaching and the clarification of information.
11. Explain the procedure to the client; encourage the client's interaction and questions.	• Explaining the procedure reduces the client's anxiety and promotes the client's participation.
12. Perform hand hygiene. Assemble the equipment and close the room curtains or door.	• Proper hand hygiene reduces the transmission of infection. Organizing the equipment optimizes the use of time and conserves the client's and nurse's energy. Privacy reduces the embarrassment for the client.
13. Position the client either standing or supine and draped. If seated, position the client either on or in front of the toilet.	• When the client is supine, fewer wrinkles ease the application of the pouching system; draping maintains the client's dignity.
14. Perform hand hygiene and apply disposable gloves.	• Proper hand hygiene reduces the transmission of microorganisms.
15. Place the towel or disposable waterproof barrier under the client.	• The towel or waterproof barrier protects the bed linen.
16. Completely remove the used pouch and skin barrier by gently pushing the skin away from the barrier. An adhesive remover may be used to facilitate removal of the skin barrier.	• Working gently reduces trauma; jerking irritates the skin and can cause tears.
17. Clean the peristomal skin gently with warm tap water using gauze pads or a clean washcloth; do not scrub the skin; dry completely by patting the skin with gauze or towel.	• Avoid the use of soap because it leaves a residue on the skin that interferes with pouch adhesion to the skin. Skin must be as dry as the skin barrier; the pouch does not adhere to wet skin. If blood appears on the gauze pad, do not be alarmed; the stoma, if rubbed, may ooze some blood from the cleaning process. The stoma's surface is a highly vascular mucous membrane. Bleeding into the pouch is abnormal.
18. Measure the stoma for the correct size of pouching system needed, using the manufacturer's measuring guide (see Step 18 illustration).	• Measuring the stoma ensures accuracy in determining the correct pouch size needed. The stoma shrinks and does not reach its usual size for 6–8 weeks.

➤ SKILL 45-3 Pouching an Ostomy ***continued***

STEPS	RATIONALE
19. Select the appropriate pouch for the client on the basis of your client assessment. For a custom cut-to-fit pouch, use an ostomy guide to cut an opening on the pouch 2 mm larger than the stoma before removing the backing (Hyland, 2002). Prepare the pouch by removing the backing from the barrier and adhesive (see Step 19 illustration). For an ileostomy, apply a thin circle of barrier paste around the opening in the pouch; allow to dry.	• The barrier paste facilitates the seal and protects the skin. The size of the pouch opening keeps drainage off the skin and reduces the risk of damage to the stoma during peristalsis or physical activity. The pouch and skin barrier are changed whenever leaking occurs. They can also be changed before or after a tub bath or shower. The stool is alkaline, which is an irritant on the skin; fecal bacteria can colonize on the skin and increase the risk of infection. Change the pouch and skin barrier when the client is comfortable; before a meal is better because this timing avoids increased peristalsis and the chance of evacuation during the pouch change.

Critical Decision Point: If client has a large volume of liquid stool from an ileostomy, consider using a high-output pouch that will contain the volume of effluent and reduce the frequency of pouch emptying.

20. Apply the skin barrier and pouch. If creases occur next to the stoma, use a barrier paste to fill in; let dry 1–2 minutes.

Critical Decision Point: If the client has a surgical incision near the stoma, the skin barrier may need to be trimmed to fit.

STEPS	RATIONALE
A. For a one-piece pouching system:	
(1) Use skin sealant wipes on the skin directly under the adhesive skin barrier or pouch; allow to dry. Press the adhesive backing of the pouch or skin barrier smoothly against the skin, starting from the bottom and working up and around the sides.	
(2) Hold the pouch by the barrier, centre it over the stoma, and press down gently on the barrier; the bottom of the pouch should point toward the client's knees (see Step 20A(2) illustration).	
(3) Maintain gentle finger pressure around the barrier for 1–2 minutes.	
B. For a two-piece pouching system:	
(1) Apply the flange (the barrier with adhesive) as in steps above for a one-piece system (see Step 20B(1) illustration). Then snap on the pouch and maintain finger pressure.	• The flange creates a wrinkle-free, secure seal and decreases irritation from the adhesive on skin.
C. For both pouching systems, gently tug on the pouch in a downward direction.	• Tugging on the pouch determines whether the pouch is securely attached.
21. Apply a nonallergic paper tape around the pectin skin barrier in a "picture frame" method. Half of the tape should be on the skin barrier and half on the client's skin. Some clients prefer a belt attached to the pouch for extra security in place of the tape.	• "Picture framing" the pectin skin barrier adds to the security of keeping the pouch system attached securely.

Critical Decision Point: If the client chooses to wear a belt, ensure it is not fastened too tightly by placing two fingers between the belt and the client's skin.

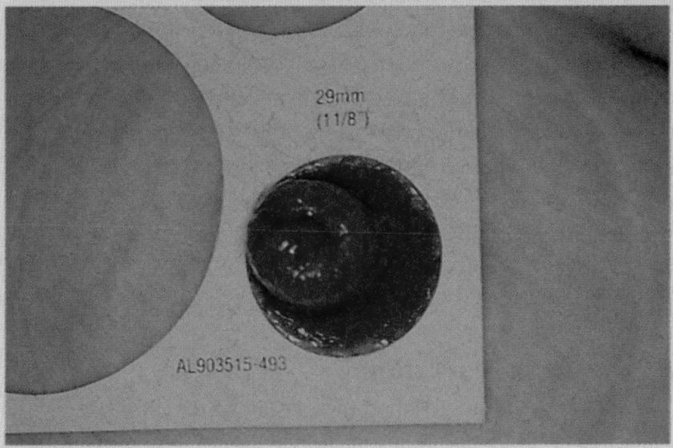

Step 18 Measuring a stoma.

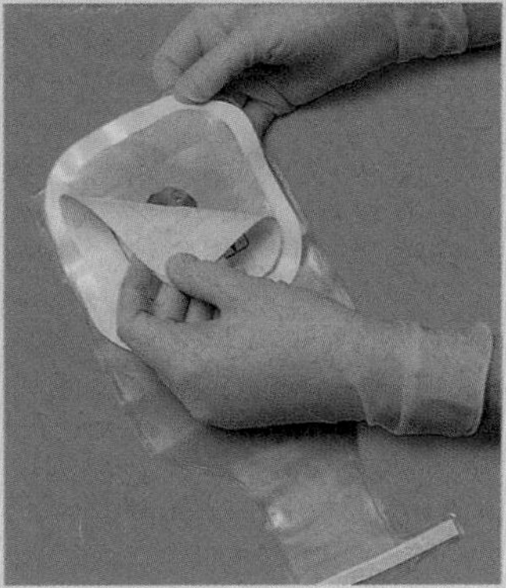

Step 19 Preparing an ostomy pouch.

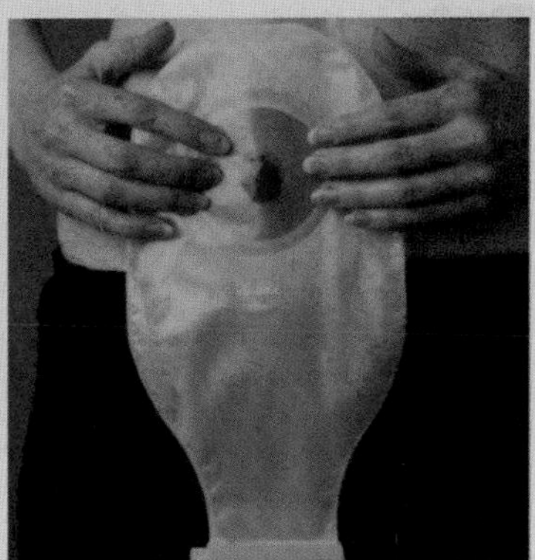

Step 20A(2) Applying a one-piece pouch.
Source: Courtesy ConvaTec, Princeton, NJ.

Continued

➤ SKILL 45-3 **Pouching an Ostomy** ***continued***

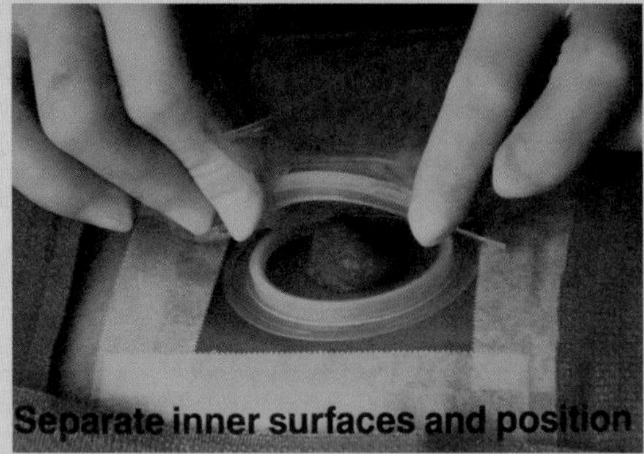

Step 20B(1) Application of a barrier-paste flange. **Source:** Courtesy ConvaTec, Princeton, NJ.

STEPS	RATIONALE
22. Although many ostomy pouches are odour-proof, some nurses and clients like to put a small amount of ostomy deodorant into the pouch. Do not use "home remedies," such as aspirin, to control the ostomy odour.	• Aspirin or other substances can harm the stoma.
23. Fold the bottom of drainable open-ended pouches up once and close using a closure device such as a clamp (or follow the manufacturer's instructions for closure).	• Proper closure maintains a secure seal to prevent leaking.
24. Properly dispose of the old pouch and the soiled equipment. Consider spraying deodorant in the room if needed.	• Deodorant spray can reduce the odours in the room.
25. Remove gloves and perform hand hygiene.	• Proper hand hygiene reduces the transmission of microorganisms.
26. Change a one- or two-piece pouch every 3–7 days unless it is leaking; a pouch can remain in place for tub bath or shower; after a bath or shower, pat the adhesive dry.	• Avoid unnecessary trauma to the skin from too frequent changes. Drying the adhesive ensures the adhesion of the pouch.
27. Ask whether the client feels discomfort around the stoma.	• The client's perception of discomfort determines the presence of skin irritation.
28. While the pouch is removed and the skin is being cleaned, note the appearance of the stoma around the skin and the existing incision (if present). Reinspect the condition of the skin barrier and adhesive.	• Assessing the skin and existing incision determines the condition of the tissues and the progress of healing. The condition of the skin barrier and adhesive can detect the presence of leaks.
29. Auscultate for bowel sounds and observe the characteristics of the stool.	• Bowel sounds and characteristics of the stool confirm the return of peristalsis and bowel elimination.
30. Observe the client's nonverbal behaviours as the pouch is applied. Ask whether the client has any questions about the pouching.	• Nonverbal behaviours indicate the client's emotional response to the stoma and the readiness for learning. The client's questions determine the level of understanding of the procedure.

Unexpected Outcomes and Related Interventions

Damage of the Peristomal Skin

- Assess for the following conditions and report their occurrence to the physician for treatment:
  - Mechanical damage (see Figure 45–19A) due to inappropriate skin care or incorrect tape removal
  - Chemical damage due to the effluent coming into contact with the peristomal skin or a skin reaction to the adhesive
  - Damage due to a fungus (e.g., candidiasis; see Figure 45–19B), usually caused by excessive skin moisture

Necrosis of Stoma (Purple or Black Discoloration, Dryness, Failure to Bleed, or Sloughing of Tissue)

- Assess the circulation to the stoma.
- Observe for excessive edema or tension on the bowel suture line (if present).
- Immediately report this finding to the physician.

Recording and Reporting

- Chart the type of pouch and skin barrier applied.
- Record the amount, appearance, and texture of the stool; the condition of the peristomal skin; and the condition of any sutures.
- Report any of the following to the charge nurse or the physician, or both:
  - Any abnormal appearance of the stoma, the suture line, the peristomal skin, the character of output, or the absence of bowel sounds
  - No flatus in 24–36 hours and no stool by the third day
- Document abdominal distension, excessive tenderness, and the nature of bowel sounds.
- Record the client's level of participation and need for instruction.

Home Care Considerations

- Evaluate the client's home toileting facilities. Note the presence of adequate toileting facilities, a flushable toilet, and the number and locations of toilets.
- Caution the client that most ostomy pouches and barriers cannot be flushed down the toilet; they clog the plumbing system. Dispose of used ostomy pouch according to agency policy and local sanitation regulations.

Nutritional Considerations for Clients with Ostomies. Nutritional therapy is important for clients with ostomies. During the first weeks after surgery, many physicians recommend low-fibre diets, particularly for ileostomy clients, because the small bowel requires time to adapt to the diversion. Low-fibre foods include bread, noodles, rice, cream cheese, eggs (not fried), strained fruit juices, lean meats, fish, and poultry. As ostomies heal, clients can eat almost any food. High-fibre foods, such as fresh fruits and vegetables, help to ensure a more solid stool, which is needed to achieve success at irrigation. Blockage must be avoided. The stoma's surgical construction can affect the likelihood of blockage.

Clients with an ileostomy should eat slowly and chew their food completely. Drinking 10 to 12 glasses of water daily also helps to prevent blockage. High-fibre foods that may cause problems include stringy meats; mushrooms; popcorn; some fruits, such as cherries; and some seafood, such as shrimp and crab. Ostomy clients may benefit from avoiding foods that cause gas and odour, including broccoli, cauliflower, dried beans, and Brussels sprouts.

Bowel Training. The client with incontinence is unable to maintain bowel control. A **bowel training** program can help some clients achieve normal defecation, especially those who still have some neuromuscular control.

The training program involves setting up a daily routine. By attempting to defecate at the same time each day and by using measures that promote defecation, the client gains control of the bowel reflexes. The program requires time, patience, and consistency. The physician determines the client's physical readiness and ability to benefit from bowel training. A successful program includes the following:

- Assessing the client's normal bowel elimination pattern and recording times when the client is incontinent.
- Incorporating principles of gerontologic nursing when providing bowel training programs for the older adult client (Box 45–12).
- Choosing a time in the client's pattern of effluent to initiate defecation-control measures.
- Giving stool softeners orally every day or a cathartic suppository at least half an hour before the selected defecation time (because the lower colon must be free of stool so that the suppository contacts the intestinal mucosa).
- Offering a hot drink (e.g., tea), fruit juice (e.g., prune juice), or another fluid that normally stimulates peristalsis for the client before the selected defecation time.
- Assisting the client to the toilet at the designated time
- Instructing the client to avoid medications such as analgesics, which may increase constipation.
- Providing privacy and setting a time limit for the defecation (15 to 20 minutes).
- Instructing the client to lean forward at the hips while sitting on the toilet, to apply manual pressure with the hands over the abdomen, and to bear down but not to strain to stimulate the colon to empty.
- Refraining from making critical remarks or conveying frustration if the client is unable to defecate.
- Providing regular meals with adequate fluids and fibre (Bliss et al., 2001).
- Maintaining normal exercise within the client's physical ability.

Clients with cognitive impairment present a special challenge when managing fecal incontinence. A team approach is required (Box 45–13).

Maintenance of Proper Fluid and Food Intake. In choosing a diet to promote normal bowel elimination, you need to consider the frequency of defecation, the characteristics of the feces, and the types of foods that impair or promote defecation. The client with frequent constipation or impaction requires an increased intake of high-fibre foods and more fluids. The client needs to understand that diet therapy provides only long-term relief of bowel elimination problems and may not give immediate relief from problems such as constipation. The community nurse should ascertain whether the client has both sufficient income to buy the foods recommended and a method of obtaining these foods. Community services, such as Meals on Wheels, can be arranged.

When diarrhea is a problem, you can recommend foods with a low-fibre content and discourage foods that typically cause gastric upset or abdominal cramping. Diarrhea caused by illness can be debilitating. If the client cannot tolerate foods or liquids orally, intravenous therapy (with potassium supplements) is necessary. The client returns to a normal diet slowly, often beginning with fluids. Excessively hot or cold fluids stimulate peristalsis, thereby causing abdominal cramps and further diarrhea. As the tolerance to liquids improves, solid foods are ordered. Following a severe diarrheal episode, milk products may need to be withheld until the enterocyte population has matured. Milk products may have the effect of perpetuating the diarrhea.

Promotion of Regular Exercise. A daily exercise program helps prevent bowel elimination problems. Walking, riding a stationary bicycle, or swimming stimulates peristalsis. Clients who are sedentary at work are most in need of regular exercise. For clients with mobility problems, such as arthritis, a passive exercise program may be helpful.

For a client who is temporarily immobilized, you should attempt ambulation of the client as soon as possible. If the condition permits, assist a postoperative client in walking to a chair on the evening of the day of surgery. The client should walk farther each day.

BOX 45-12 FOCUS ON OLDER ADULTS

- The energy needs of persons older than 50 years of age are considered to be lower because of the loss of metabolic tissue that accompanies the aging process. Protein needs do not decrease with aging.
- Maintaining a well-balanced diet that is high in fibre will assist in maintaining normal bowel elimination patterns (Bliss et al., 2001).
- Constipation is a common complaint in older clients. Contributing factors are impaired general health, use of medication, and decreased mobility and physical activity.
- If constipation is ignored, significant complications can arise. Instruct clients to establish a specific time for bowel elimination, which may assist in preventing constipation (Dosh, 2002).
- Clients need to feel at ease during bowel elimination. Lack of privacy may lead the client to ignore the urge to defecate.
- Older adults are known for their concern about their bowel elimination habits.
- Warm liquids and certain juices (e.g., prune juice) stimulate bowel motility.

Some clients have difficulty passing stool because of weak abdominal and pelvic floor muscles. Exercises can help bedridden clients to more comfortably use a bedpan. The client can practise the following exercises:

* Lie supine; tighten the abdominal muscles as though pushing them to the floor. Hold them tight to the count of three; relax. Repeat 5 to 10 times as tolerated.
* Flex and contract the thigh muscles by raising one knee slowly toward the chest. Repeat for each leg at least five times and increase the frequency as tolerated.

BOX 45-13 FOCUS ON PRIMARY HEALTH CARE

A Team Approach to Managing Fecal Continence in the Cognitively Impaired Client

* Before establishing an appropriate bowel control program for a cognitively impaired client, the physician or nurse must assess the musculoskeletal system for the level of activity the individual can attain, the rectum and anus for such problems as hemorrhoids or rectal prolapse, and the client's cognitive status so that the interventions can be matched to cognitive ability.
* Information concerning bowel habits may be provided by the client's family. If not, you and the unregulated care providers assess the client's frequency and consistency of bowel movements and the client's level of independence in toileting, including the amount of assistance required.
* The dietitian or nutritional staff should assess the client's diet.
* Adequate hydration (i.e., six to eight glasses of fluid daily) is an important part of normal bowel routine and is particularly difficult to achieve with cognitively impaired individuals. The team must come up with creative methods of delivering adequate nutrition and hydration.
* Caregivers should be made aware that individuals sometimes become impacted from the use of psyllium (Metamucil) when insufficient fluids do not accompany them. Gentle laxatives for a few days, rather than treatments that irritate the bowel, may be effective. However, a natural dietary cathartic (e.g., a mixture of applesauce, pureed prunes, and bran) or simply adding more high-fibre foods to the diet may be preferable to a pharmacological intervention.
* As with all individuals, appropriate exercise and fluid intake should be included in the care plan. A physiotherapist or occupational therapist may be involved in the exercise plan.
* Environmental cues, such as having the toilet visible and conducting gentle questioning may facilitate the client's independent functioning, but these cues may also be stressful for the client and cause belligerence.
* The individual with cognitive impairment may not respond appropriately to the urge to defecate. Caregivers should be aware that the urge to defecate is strongest the first hour after breakfast and should offer opportunities for toileting at that time.
* Assisted toileting procedures include stabilizing the client on the toilet or commode by placing a chair next to the toilet for stabilization. To facilitate bowel emptying, a glass of warm water may be given as a drink, a warm pack may be placed on the abdomen, or the abdomen may be gently massaged.
* For a client who is continually incontinent, provide appropriate continence products that will maintain the client's dignity.
* Severely cognitively impaired clients may smear the incontinent feces. Emptying the rectum regularly diminishes the problem; however, necessary interventions may include administering fleet enemas, increasing the bulk of the stool with psyllium (Metamucil), or stimulating the local peristalsis with glycerine suppositories to facilitate rectal emptying.

Hemorrhoids. Many clients experience discomfort from alterations in their bowel elimination. Pain results when hemorrhoid tissues are directly irritated. The primary goal for the client with hemorrhoids is to have soft-formed, painless bowel movements. Proper diet, fluids, and regular exercise improve the likelihood of the stools being soft. If the client becomes constipated, passage of hard stools may cause bleeding and irritation. Local heat provides temporary relief to swollen hemorrhoids. A sitz bath is the most effective means of heat application (see Chapter 47).

Maintenance of Skin Integrity. The client with diarrhea or fecal incontinence is at risk for skin breakdown when fecal contents remain on the skin. The same problem exists for the client with an ostomy that drains liquid stool. Liquid stool is usually acidic and contains digestive enzymes. Irritation from repeated wiping with toilet tissue aggravates the breakdown of skin. Bathing the skin after soiling helps but may result in more breakdown unless the skin is thoroughly dried.

When caring for a debilitated, incontinent client who is unable to ask for assistance, you should check often for defecation. The anal areas can be protected with petrolatum, zinc oxide, or another ointment that holds moisture in the skin to prevent drying and cracking. Yeast infections of the skin can develop easily. Several powdered antifungal agents are effective against yeast. Baby powder or cornstarch should not be used because they have no medicinal properties and they frequently cake on the skin, which makes them difficult to remove.

❖Evaluation

Client Care

The effectiveness of care depends on success in meeting the goals and expected outcomes of care. Optimally, the client will be able to have regular, pain-free defecation of soft, formed stools. The client is the only person who is able to determine whether the bowel elimination problems have been relieved and which therapies were the most effective (Figure 45–20). The client will also be able to demonstrate information learned regarding establishment of a normal bowel elimination pattern. The client will be able to demonstrate any skills learned, such as ostomy protocols and skin protection. The client will be able to accomplish normal defecation by manipulating components of daily living, such as diet, fluid intake, and exercise. The client will have minimal reliance on artificial means of defecation, such as enemas and laxative use.

Client Expectations

If you have been successful in establishing a therapeutic relationship with the client, the client will feel more comfortable in discussing the intimate details often associated with bowel elimination. The client will also not be as fearful of embarrassment as you assist the client with his or her bowel elimination needs. The client will relate a feeling of comfort and freedom from pain as bowel elimination needs are met within the limits of the client's condition and treatment.

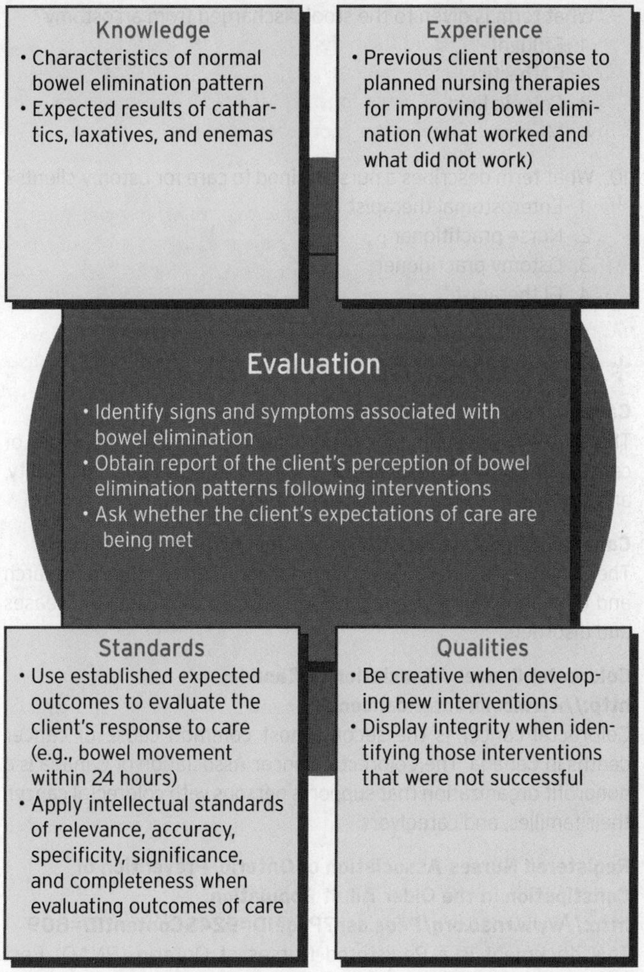

Figure 45-20 Critical thinking model for bowel elimination evaluation.

✻ KEY CONCEPTS

- The mechanical breakdown of food elements, gastrointestinal motility, and selective absorption and secretion of substances by the large intestine influence the character of feces.
- Food high in fiber content and an increased fluid intake keep feces soft.
- Ongoing use of cathartics, laxatives, and enemas affects and delays the reflexes of normal defecation.
- Vagal stimulation, which slows the heart rate, may occur during straining while defecating, receiving enemas, and during digital removal of an impacted stool.
- The greatest danger from diarrhea is developing an imbalance of fluids and electrolytes.
- The location of an ostomy influences the consistency of the stool.
- Assessment of bowel elimination patterns should focus on bowel habits, factors that normally influence defecation, recent changes in bowel elimination, and a physical examination.
- Indirect and direct visualization of the lower gastrointestinal tract requires cleansing of the bowel before the procedure.
- When selecting a diet to promote normal bowel elimination, consider the frequency of defecation, the fecal characteristics, and the effect of foods on the gastrointestinal function.
- Proper positioning on a bedpan allows the client to assume a position similar to squatting without experiencing muscle strain.
- Nasogastric intubation decompresses the gastric contents by removing secretions and gaseous products from the gastrointestinal tract.
- The purposes of gastric decompression are to keep the gastrointestinal tract free of secretions, to reduce nausea and gas, and to decrease the risk of vomiting and aspiration.
- Proper selection and use of an ostomy pouching system are necessary to prevent damage to the skin around the stoma.
- Dangers during digital removal of stool include traumatizing the rectal mucosa and promoting vagal stimulation.
- Skin breakdown can occur after repeated exposure to liquid stool.

✻ CRITICAL THINKING EXERCISES

1. A 19-year-old man with a history of good health and regular exercise is your client at the university health service facility where you work. He complains of increasing diarrhea and abdominal cramping; he has no weight loss. He states that on rare occasions he noticed blood on the toilet paper he used. What additional pieces of assessment data do you need?
2. A long-term care facility has invited you to present a talk on preventing bowel incontinence in their residents. What points of information do you include in your presentation?
3. A 22-year-old man is to undergo surgery for Crohn's disease. He will have a new pouching ileostomy. He and his mother need to learn what the ileostomy means for his future bowel elimination needs. What do you tell them?
4. Mrs. Edna Pidpahora is 82 years old and a resident in a long-term care facility. She has just been assessed for acute confusion in the Emergency Department and has been admitted to your ward. In her documentation, you see that she has become more confused and forgetful since she has moved into long-term care 4 months ago. She spends most of her time in bed or sitting in a chair in her room. She is occasionally incontinent of urine and has not had a bowel movement in 5 days. She is taking the following medications and supplements: levothyroxine (Synthroid), calcium carbonate, vitamin D, chlorothiazide, risperidone, chloral hydrate. What steps would you take to understand and address her apparent constipation (Neil et al., 2003; Robson et al., 2000; Spina & Scordo, 2002)?

✻ REVIEW QUESTIONS

1. Most nutrients and electrolytes are absorbed in which of the following areas?
   1. Colon
   2. Stomach
   3. Esophagus
   4. Small intestine
2. During the nursing assessment, the client reveals that he has diarrhea and cramping every time he eats ice cream. He attributes this reaction to the cold nature of the food. These symptoms might be associated with which of the following?
   1. Food allergy
   2. Irritable bowel syndrome
   3. Lactose intolerance
   4. Increased peristalsis

3. You are assessing a 55-year-old client who is in the clinic for a routine physical examination. Under which of the following scenarios would you instruct the client to obtain fecal occult blood testing (FOBT)?
   1. The client has a family history of polyps.
   2. The client reports rectal bleeding.
   3. A palpable mass is detected on digital examination.
   4. The client is due for a routine examination for colon cancer.
4. Which of the following agents decreases colonic propulsive contractions while increasing the mixing of contractions?
   1. Antidiarrheal opiate agents
   2. Hypertonics
   3. Cathartics
   4. Laxatives
5. Which of the following situations results in diarrhea that occurs with a fecal impaction?
   1. A clear liquid diet
   2. Irritation of the intestinal mucosa
   3. Seepage of stool around the impaction
   4. Inability of the client to form a stool
6. A cleaning enema is ordered for a 55-year-old client before intestinal surgery. What amount of solution should be instilled?
   1. 150 to 200 mL
   2. 200 to 400 mL
   3. 400 to 750 mL
   4. 750 to 1000 mL
7. During the enema, the client complains of pain. You note rectal bleeding and blood in the return fluid. What action do you take?
   1. Stop the instillation.
   2. Slow the rate of instillation.
   3. Stop the instillation, notify the physician, and obtain vital signs.
   4. Tell the client to breathe slowly and relax.
8. What is one of the greatest problems in caring for a client with a nasogastric tube?
   1. Dehydration
   2. Maintaining comfort
   3. Constipation
   4. Nutritional therapy
9. What term is given to the stool discharged from an ostomy?
   1. Effluent
   2. Cathartics
   3. Colonic fluid
   4. Mucosa
10. What term describes a nurse trained to care for ostomy clients?
    1. Enterostomal therapist
    2. Nurse practitioner
    3. Ostomy practitioner
    4. GI therapist

* RECOMMENDED WEB SITES

Canadian Cancer Society: http://www.cancer.ca

This Web site is a source for general information about all types of cancers, including Canadian statistics of the prevalence, mortality, and survival rates for specific cancers.

Canadian Digestive Health Foundation: http://www.cdhf.ca/

The Canadian Digestive Health Foundation (CDHF) supports research and education in the management and cure of digestive diseases and disorders.

Colorectal Cancer Association of Canada: http://www.colorectal-cancer.ca

Colorectal cancer is the second most common cause of cancer deaths in Canada. The Colorectal Cancer Association of Canada is a nonprofit organization that supports persons with colorectal cancer, their families, and caregivers.

Registered Nurses Association of Ontario, Prevention of Constipation in the Older Adult Population: http://www.rnao.org/Page.asp?PageID=924&ContentID=809

This document is a Registered Nurses of Ontario (RNAO) Best Practice Guideline and offers a professional nursing standard for reducing the frequency and severity of constipation among older adults. The guideline is relevant to all areas of clinical practice including acute care, community care, and long-term care.

Rehydration Project: http://rehydrate.org/index.html

The Rehydration Project is a private, nonprofit, international development group concerned with oral rehydration therapy (ORT). This Web site provides information on diarrhea in developing countries and how ORT can help. A wealth of information is available, including facts, resources, and links to current research.

46

Mobility and Immobility

Written by Jan Park Dorsay, RN, MN, NP, CON(C)
and Brett Sanderson, BScPT
Based on the original chapter by Ann Tritak, BS, MS, EdD

objectives

Mastery of content in this chapter will enable you to:

- Define the key terms listed.
- Describe the functions of the musculoskeletal (skeleton, skeletal muscles) and nervous systems in the regulation of movement.
- Discuss physiological and pathological influences on body alignment and joint mobility.
- Identify changes in physiological and psychosocial function associated with immobility.
- Assess for correct and impaired body alignment and mobility.
- State correct nursing diagnoses for impaired body alignment and mobility.
- Develop nursing care plans for clients with impaired body alignment and mobility.
- Describe essential techniques when assisting with active and passive range-of-motion (ROM) exercises, assisting a client to move up in bed, repositioning a client, assisting a client to a sitting position, and transferring a client from a bed to a chair or from a bed to a stretcher.
- Evaluate the nursing care plan for maintaining body alignment and mobility.

key terms

Activity tolerance, p. 1170
Anthropometric measurements, p. 1176
Atelectasis, p. 1165
Bariatric, p. 1197
Bed rest, p. 1164
Body alignment, p. 1162
Body mechanics, p. 1162
Chest physiotherapy (CPT), p. 1184
Crutch gait, p. 1210
Deconditioning, p. 1162
Disuse osteoporosis, p. 1166
Embolus, p. 1177
Exercise, p. 1170
Fracture, p. 1164
Footdrop, p. 1167
Friction, p. 1162
Gait, p. 1170
Gait belt, p. 1198
Hemiparesis, p. 1208
Hemiplegia, p. 1208
Hypostatic pneumonia, p. 1165
Immobility, p. 1164
Instrumental activities of daily living (IADLs), p. 1198
Joint contracture, p. 1167
Joints, p. 1162
Ligaments, p. 1162
Logroll, p. 1195
Mobility, p. 1164
Muscle atrophy, p. 1164
Negative nitrogen balance, p. 1165
Orthostatic hypotension, p. 1166
Osteoporosis, p. 1166
Pathological fractures, p. 1164
Posture, p. 1162
Pressure ulcer, p. 1168
Tendons, p. 1162
Thrombus, p. 1166
Transfer belt, p. 1198
Trapeze bar, p. 1189
Trochanter roll, p. 1188
Urinary stasis, p. 1167

media resources

evolve Web Site

- Animations
- Audio Chapter Summaries
- Glossary
- Multiple-Choice Review Questions
- Skills Performance Checklists
- Student Learning Activities
- Video Clips
- Weblinks

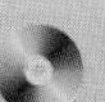
Companion CD

- Glossary
- Interactive Learning Activities
- Fluids and Electrolytes Tutorial
- Test-Taking Skills

Mobility refers to the ability to move easily and independently. To maintain optimal physical mobility, the musculoskeletal and nervous systems of the body must be intact and functioning. Illnesses, surgery, injuries, pain, and aging can temporarily or permanently impair mobility. Nurses need to know the many hazards created by immobility and how to prevent them. Nurses also need to know how to care for clients who are immobile. This care includes positioning the immobile client so that optimal body alignment is attained, and moving and transferring clients when they cannot do so independently. Clinical nursing practice related to mobility requires knowledge of body mechanics and of the basic structure and function of bones and muscles.

Scientific Knowledge Base

Physiology and Principles of Body Mechanics

Body mechanics are the coordinated efforts of the musculoskeletal and nervous systems to maintain balance, posture, and body alignment during lifting, bending, moving, and performing activities of daily living (ADLs; see Chapter 36). Use of proper body mechanics reduces risk of injury to the musculoskeletal system, facilitates mobility, and allows for efficient use of energy.

By using proper body mechanics, you help ensure the safety and well-being of both you and your client. For each nursing activity, such as walking during nursing rounds, administering medications, lifting and transferring clients, and moving objects, you use a variety of muscle groups. The physical forces of weight and friction can influence body movement. Correctly used, these forces can increase your efficiency. Incorrect use can impair your ability to lift, transfer, and position clients and can cause serious injury. Knowledge of the basic structures and functions of the neuromuscular and skeletal systems and knowledge of physiological and pathological influences on mobility and body alignment are important to a full understanding of body mechanics (see Box 36–3).

Alignment and Balance. The terms **body alignment** and **posture** are analogous and refer to the positioning of the **joints, tendons, ligaments,** and muscles while standing, sitting, and lying. *Body alignment* means that the individual's centre of gravity is stable and body strain is minimized. Correct body alignment reduces strain on musculoskeletal structures and risk for injury, aids in maintaining adequate muscle tone, and contributes to balance. Without balance control, the centre of gravity is displaced, creating a risk for falls and subsequent injuries. Balance is enhanced with a wide base of support and correct body posture and when the body's centre of gravity is kept low and within the base of support.

Balance is required for maintaining a static position such as sitting, for performing ADLs, and for moving freely. The ability to balance can be compromised by disease, injury, pain, physical development (e.g., age), life changes (e.g., pregnancy), medications (e.g., in which dizziness or drowsiness is a side effect), and prolonged immobility, which may cause **deconditioning**. Deconditioning is a clinical syndrome that results in reduced functioning of multiple body systems, especially the musculoskeletal system. Nurses must be alert to impaired balance because it is a major threat to physical safety. Impaired balance can also lead to a client's fear of falls and self-imposed restrictions on activity.

safety alert In Canada, falls are the sixth leading cause of death in older adults. Generalized weakness, impaired balance, and unsteady gait are risk factors for falls among older adults. Injuries from falls contribute to reduced quality of life and increased morbidity, mortality, and health care costs. Most falls in the hospital occur near the client's bedside while trying to transfer him or her. Nursing interventions should be aimed at a thorough assessment of client safety and implementing strategies to prevent a fall (Registered Nurses Association of Ontario [RNAO], 2005a).

Gravity and Friction. *Weight* is the force exerted on a body by gravity. To lift safely, the lifter must overcome the weight of the object to be lifted and know its centre of gravity. In a person, the centre of gravity is usually at 55% to 57% of standing height and is located in the midline. People who are unsteady can fall as their centres of gravity become unbalanced because of the gravitational pull of their weight when it moves outside their base of support.

Friction is a force that occurs in a direction to oppose movement. As you turn, transfer, or move a client up in bed, friction must be overcome. The larger the surface area of the object to be moved, the greater is the friction. A larger object produces greater resistance to movement. To decrease surface area and reduce friction when a client is unable to assist in moving up in bed, place the client's arms across the chest. This position decreases surface area and reduces friction.

Whenever possible, you should use some of the client's strength when lifting, transferring, or moving the client. Explain the procedure to the client and tell the client when and what body parts to move. The result should be a synchronized movement in which the client can participate and in which friction is decreased. By involving the client you may have the added bonus of increasing the client's participation in self-care, thus promoting his or her sense of accomplishment.

Lifting a client, rather than pushing or pulling, can also reduce friction. Lifting has an upward component and decreases the pressure between the client and the bed or chair. By placing the client on a drawsheet or friction-reducing device (e.g., slider board) and then pulling this sheet to move the client you can reduce friction, because the client is raised off of the surface and is more easily moved along the bed's surface.

Regulation of Movement

Coordinated body movement involves integrated functioning of the skeletal system, skeletal muscle, and nervous system. These three systems cooperate closely in mechanical support of the body. They are discussed as a single functional unit in Chapter 36.

Pathological Influences on Mobility

Many pathological conditions affect mobility. Although a complete description of each is beyond the scope of this chapter, an overview of four pathological influences are presented here: postural abnormalities, impaired muscle development, damage to the central nervous system, and direct trauma to the musculoskeletal system.

Postural Abnormalities. Congenital or acquired postural abnormalities affect the efficiency of the musculoskeletal system, as well as body alignment, balance, and appearance. During assessment, observe body alignment and range of motion (ROM; see Chapter 36). Postural abnormalities can cause pain, impair alignment or mobility, or both. Knowledge about the characteristics, causes, and treatment of common postural abnormalities (Table 46–1) is necessary for lifting, transfering, and positioning a client. Some postural abnormalities may limit ROM. Nurses intervene to maintain maximum ROM in

TABLE 46-1 Postural Abnormalities

Abnormality	Description	Cause	Possible Treatments*
Torticollis	Inclining of head to the affected side, in which the sternocleidomastoid muscle is contracted	Congenital or acquired condition	Surgery, heat, support, or immobilization, depending on cause and severity, gentle range of motion
Lordosis	Exaggeration of anterior convex curve of lumbar spine	Congenital condition Temporary condition (e.g., pregnancy)	Spine-stretching exercises (based on cause)
Kyphosis	Increased convexity in curvature of thoracic spine	Congenital condition Rickets, osteoporosis Tuberculosis of the spine	Spine-stretching exercises, sleeping without pillows, use of bed board, bracing, spinal fusion (based on cause and severity)
Kypholordosis	Combination of kyphosis and lordosis	Congenital condition	Similar to methods used in kyphosis or lordosis (based on cause) Immobilization and surgery (based on cause and severity)
Scoliosis	Lateral "S" curvature of spine, unequal heights of hips and shoulders	Congenital condition Poliomyelitis Spastic paralysis Unequal leg length	Immobilization and surgery (based on cause and severity)
Kyphoscoliosis	Abnormal anteroposterior and lateral curvature of spine	Congenital condition Poliomyelitis Cor pulmonale	Immobilization and surgery (based on cause and severity)
Congenital hip dysplasia	Hip instability with limited abduction of hips and, occasionally, adduction contractures (head of femur does not articulate with acetabulum because of abnormal shallowness of acetabulum)	Congenital condition (more common with breech deliveries)	Maintenance of continuous abduction of the thigh so that head of femur presses into the centre of acetabulum Abduction splints, casting, surgery
Knock-knee (genu valgum)	Legs curved inward so that knees come together as person walks	Congenital condition Rickets	Knee braces, surgery if not corrected by growth
Bowlegs (genu varum)	One or both legs bent outward at knee, which is normal until 2–3 years of age	Congenital condition Rickets	Slowing rate of curving if not corrected by growth With rickets, increase of vitamin D, calcium, and phosphorus intake to normal ranges
Clubfoot	95%: medial deviation and plantar flexion of foot (equinovarus) 5%: lateral deviation and dorsiflexion (calcaneovalgus)	Congenital condition	Casts, splints such as Denis–Browne splint, and surgery (based on degree and rigidity of deformity)
Footdrop	Inability to dorsiflex and evert foot because of peroneal nerve damage	Congenital condition Trauma Improper position of immobilized client	None (cannot be corrected) Prevention through physiotherapy Bracing with ankle–foot orthotic
Pigeon-toes	Internal rotation of forefoot or entire foot, common in infants	Congenital condition Habit	Growth, wearing reversed shoes

*Severity of the condition and its cause will dictate treatment, which must be individualized.

Data from McCance, K. L., & Huether, S. E. (2005). *Pathophysiology: The biologic basis for disease in adults and children* (5th ed.). St. Louis, MO: Mosby.

unaffected joints and then may design interventions to strengthen affected muscles and joints, improve the client's posture, and adequately use affected and unaffected muscle groups. Referral to or collaboration with a physiotherapist and occupational therapist may enhance your interventions for a client with a postural abnormality.

Impaired Muscle Development. Injury and disease can lead to numerous alterations in musculoskeletal function. The muscular dystrophies, for example, are a group of familial disorders that cause degeneration of skeletal muscle fibres. The most prevalent of the muscle diseases in childhood, the muscular dystrophies are characterized by progressive, symmetrical weakness and wasting of skeletal muscle groups, with increasing disability and deformity (McCance & Huether, 2005).

Damage to the Central Nervous System. Damage to any component of the central nervous system that regulates voluntary movement results in impaired body alignment and mobility. The motor strip in the cerebral cortex can be damaged by trauma from a head injury, ischemia from a stroke or brain attack (cerebrovascular accident), tumour, or bacterial infection such as meningitis. Motor impairment is directly related to the amount of destruction of the motor strip. For example, a person with a right-sided cerebral hemorrhage with complete necrosis will likely have destruction of the right motor strip and left-sided hemiplegia. Trauma to the spinal cord also impairs mobility. Common trauma includes transection of the spinal cord in which motor fibres are cut. A complete transection will likely result in a bilateral loss of voluntary motor control below the level of the trauma.

Direct Trauma to the Musculoskeletal System. Direct trauma to the musculoskeletal system can result in bruises, contusions, sprains, and fractures. A **fracture** is a disruption of bone tissue continuity. Fractures most commonly result from direct external trauma but can also occur as a consequence of some deformity of the bone (e.g., **pathological fractures** of osteoporosis, Paget's disease, metastatic cancer, or osteogenesis imperfecta). Young children are usually able to form new bone more easily than adults and, as a result, have few complications after a fracture. Treatment often includes positioning the fractured bone in proper alignment and immobilizing it to promote healing and restore function. Even this temporary immobilization can result in some **muscle atrophy**, loss of tone, and joint stiffness. After the fracture has healed, physiotherapy may be required to regain functional losses.

Nursing Knowledge Base

Mobility–Immobility

A full understanding of mobility requires more than an overview of body mechanics and of the regulation of movement by the musculoskeletal and nervous systems. You must also know how mobility and immobility affect the systems of the body and the psychosocial and developmental aspects of clients.

Mobility refers to a person's ability to move about freely, and **immobility** refers to the inability to move about freely. Mobility and immobility are best understood as the end points of a continuum, with many degrees of partial immobility in between. Some clients move back and forth on this continuum, but for other clients, immobility is absolute and continues indefinitely. The terms *bed rest* and *impaired physical mobility* are frequently used when discussing clients on the mobility–immobility continuum.

Bed rest is an intervention that restricts clients to bed for therapeutic reasons. Nurses and physicians most often prescribe this intervention. Clients with a wide variety of conditions are placed on bed rest. The general objectives of bed rest are as follows:

- To reduce physical activity and the oxygen needs of the body.
- To reduce pain, including postoperative pain, and the need for large doses of analgesics.
- To promote safety for clients recovering from effects of anaesthetics or who are sedated.
- To allow ill or debilitated clients to rest.
- To allow exhausted clients the opportunity for uninterrupted rest.

The duration of bed rest depends on the illness or injury and the client's prior state of health.

Impaired physical mobility is defined by the North American Nursing Diagnosis Association as a state in which the individual experiences or is at risk of experiencing limitation of physical movement (Ackley & Ladwig, 2006). Alterations in the level of physical mobility can result from prescribed restriction of movement in the form of bed rest, physical restriction of movement because of external devices (e.g., a cast or skeletal traction), voluntary restriction of movement, or impairment of motor or skeletal function.

The effects of muscular deconditioning associated with lack of physical activity may be apparent in a matter of days. The normal individual on bed rest loses muscle strength from baseline levels at a rate of 3% a day. Bed rest is also associated with cardiovascular, skeletal, and other organ changes. The term *disuse atrophy* has been used to describe the pathological reduction in normal size of muscle fibres after prolonged inactivity from bed rest, trauma, casting, or local nerve damage (McCance & Huether, 2005).

In a classic study, Deitrick and others (1948) found that even young, healthy men put on bed rest had physiological problems. Periods of immobility or prolonged bed rest can cause major physiological, psychological, and social effects. These effects can be gradual or immediate and vary from client to client. The greater the extent and the longer the duration of immobility, the more pronounced are the consequences. The client with complete mobility restrictions is continually at risk for hazardous system-wide effects.

Systemic Effects of Immobility. All body systems work more efficiently with some form of movement. Exercise has been shown to have positive outcomes for all major systems of the body. Therefore, when mobility is altered, each body system is at risk for impairment. The severity of the impairment depends on the client's overall health, degree and length of immobility, and age. For example, older adults with chronic illnesses develop pronounced effects of immobility more quickly than younger clients with the same immobility problem (Box 46–1).

Metabolic Changes. Endocrine metabolism, calcium resorption, and functioning of the gastrointestinal system are altered by changes in mobility.

The endocrine system, made up of hormone-secreting glands, helps to maintain and regulate vital functions such as response to stress and injury, growth and development, reproduction, ionic homeostasis, and energy metabolism. When injury or stress occurs, the endocrine system triggers a series of responses aimed at maintaining blood pressure and preserving life. The endocrine system is important in maintaining homeostasis. Tissues and cells live in an internal environment that the endocrine system helps regulate through maintenance of sodium, potassium, water, and acid–base balance. The endocrine system also helps regulate energy metabolism. The basal metabolic rate (BMR) is increased by thyroid hormone, and energy is

BOX 46-1 NURSING STORY

Client Rehabilitation

When Grace Lo was admitted to the inpatient rehabilitation unit, it was difficult for me to imagine her living independently in a condominium, driving her car, going out to lunch, shopping, or playing bridge with her friends. She looked so frail and tired, and she needed assistance with everything. Grace was a 66-year-old widow with a diagnosis of uterine cancer. After being diagnosed, Grace was started on chemotherapy to help shrink the size of the tumour before having surgery to remove it. She experienced side effects from the chemotherapy—anemia and neutropenia. Unfortunately, she also developed recurrent pneumonia, and had been immobilized in the intensive care and oncology units for over 5 weeks.

When Grace was admitted to the rehabilitation unit she was significantly deconditioned. She had never enjoyed exercising and was feeling regret about not maintaining her physical fitness before her cancer diagnosis. Her ability to complete her chemotherapy treatments depended on her regaining her strength, endurance, mobility, and independence for her ADLs. Grace was very motivated to work with the rehabilitation team, but she was also afraid. What if she couldn't get strong enough to finish her chemotherapy?

At the beginning of rehabilitation Grace needed assistance from two people for all of her transfers. She had a Foley catheter in place, and she fatigued quickly with minimal exertion. Her respiratory status had been compromised by recurrent pneumonia and her past behaviour of cigarette smoking. The first goal was to increase her upper and lower extremity strength for transferring from the bed to a commode at the bedside. It took a coordinated interdisciplinary approach to work on Grace's pace at exercising and her ability to practice ADLs independently. Once Grace was able to safely transfer from the bed with a one-person, minimally assisted standing pivot transfer, the team was able to focus on the goal of social urinary continence. Because she had been immobilized for an extended period of time, Grace often felt light-headed and dizzy when sitting at the bedside before a transfer. These experiences contributed to her feelings of apprehension about falling and to a loss of confidence. It was important to raise the head of Grace's bed in increments before attempting transfers to minimize postural hypotension. After 2 weeks of exercising and practice, Grace was socially continent, using the bathroom in her room. However, she still had a long way to go.

Four months after she had been discharged from rehabilitation I heard my name being called. A fit-looking woman was calling out to me—I barely recognized a radiant Grace. She had continued outpatient rehabilitation and was exercising regularly. Grace excitedly told me that she had finished her last cycle of chemotherapy. Her computerized tomography (CT) scan showed that the tumour in her uterus had decreased in size and she no longer needed surgery. Grace told me that while the diagnosis of cancer scared her, the experiences of being immobilized and dependent on others for all her ADLs had "terrified" her. Her story reminded me of the impact of immobility on all aspects of a person's life and of the importance of setting small, attainable goals in promoting independence and hope.

made available to cells through the integrated action of gastrointestinal and pancreatic hormones (Copstead-Kirkhorn & Banasik, 2005).

Immobility disrupts normal metabolic functioning by decreasing the metabolic rate; altering the metabolism of carbohydrates, fats, and proteins; causing fluid, electrolyte, and calcium imbalances; and causing gastrointestinal disturbances such as decreased appetite and slowing of peristalsis. However, in the presence of an infectious process, immobilized clients may have an increased BMR as a result of fever or wound healing. Fever and repair of wounds increase cellular oxygen requirements (Copstead-Kirkhorn & Banasik, 2005).

A deficiency in calories and protein is characteristic of clients with a decreased appetite secondary to immobility. Proteins are constantly being synthesized and broken down into amino acids in the body to be re-formed into other proteins. Amino acids that are not used are excreted. The body can synthesize certain nonessential amino acids but depends on ingested proteins to supply the eight essential amino acids. When more nitrogen (the end product of amino acid breakdown) is excreted than is ingested in proteins, the body is said to have a **negative nitrogen balance** (Figure 46–1). Weight loss, decreased muscle mass, and weakness result from tissue catabolism (tissue breakdown). Protein loss leads to muscle loss.

Another metabolic change is calcium resorption (loss) from bones. As a result, urinary excretion of calcium increases because immobility causes the release of calcium into the circulation. Normally, the kidneys can excrete the excess calcium. However, if the kidneys are unable to respond appropriately, hypercalcemia results (Copstead-Kirkhorn & Banasik, 2005).

Decreased mobility also leads to decreased gastrointestinal motility, which in turn can cause a variety of impairments to gastrointestinal functioning. Difficulty in passing stools (constipation) is a common symptom, although pseudodiarrhea may result from a fecal impaction (accumulation of hardened feces). You must be aware that this finding is not normal diarrhea, but rather liquid stool passing around the area of impaction (see Chapter 45). Left untreated, fecal impaction can result in a mechanical bowel obstruction that may partially or completely occlude the intestinal lumen, blocking normal propulsion of liquid and gas. The resulting fluid in the intestine produces distension and increases intraluminal pressure. Over time, intestinal function becomes depressed, dehydration occurs, absorption ceases, and fluid and electrolyte disturbances worsen.

Respiratory Changes. Regular aerobic exercise is known to enhance respiratory functioning. Lack of movement and exercise places clients at higher risk for respiratory complications. Postoperative and immobile clients are at high risk for developing pulmonary complications. The most common respiratory complications are **atelectasis** (collapse of alveoli) and **hypostatic pneumonia** (inflammation of the lung from stasis or pooling of secretions). Both

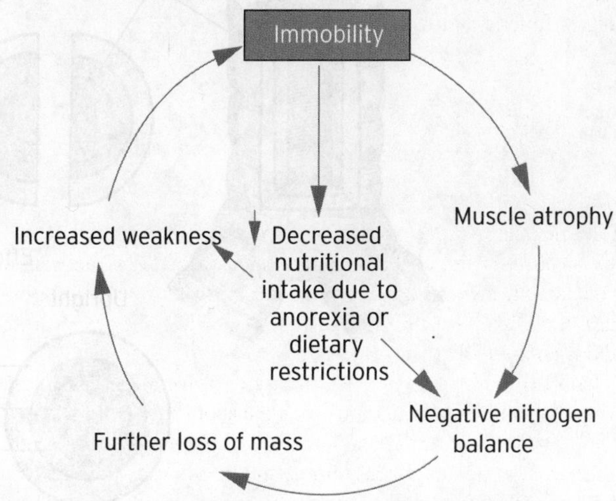

Figure 46-1 Factors contributing to negative nitrogen balance associated with immobility. **Source:** From Gröer, M. W., & Shekleton, M. E. (1989). *Basic pathophysiology: A holistic approach* (3rd ed.). St. Louis, MO: Mosby.

conditions decrease oxygenation, prolong recovery, and add to the client's discomfort (Black & Hawks, 2005). In atelectasis, secretions block a bronchiole or a bronchus, and the distal lung tissue (alveoli) collapses as the existing air is absorbed, producing hypoventilation. The site of the blockage determines the extent of atelectasis. A lung lobe or even a whole lung may collapse. At some point in the development of these complications, the client's ability to cough productively declines proportionately. Ultimately, the distribution of mucus in the bronchi increases, particularly when the client is in the supine, prone, or lateral position (Figure 46–2). Mucus accumulates in the dependent regions of the airways. Because mucus is an excellent medium for bacterial growth, hypostatic pneumonia may result.

Cardiovascular Changes. The cardiovascular system is also affected by immobilization. The three major changes are orthostatic hypotension, increased cardiac workload, and thrombus formation.

Orthostatic hypotension is a drop of 20 mm Hg or more in systolic blood pressure and of 10 mm Hg in diastolic blood pressure within 3 minutes when the client rises from a lying or sitting position to a standing position (Medow et al., 2008). In the immobilized client, decreased circulating fluid volume, pooling of blood in the lower extremities, and decreased autonomic response occur. These factors result in decreased venous return, followed by a decrease in cardiac output, which is reflected by a decline in blood pressure (McCance & Huether, 2005).

As the workload of the heart increases, its oxygen consumption does as well. The heart therefore works harder and less efficiently during periods of prolonged rest. As immobilization increases, cardiac output falls, further decreasing cardiac efficiency and increasing workload.

Clients are also at risk for thrombus formation. A **thrombus** is an accumulation of platelets, fibrin, clotting factors, and the cellular elements of the blood attached to the interior wall of a vein or artery, sometimes occluding the lumen of the vessel (Figure 46–3). Three factors contribute to venous thrombus formation: (1) loss of integrity of the vessel wall (e.g., injury), (2) abnormalities of blood flow (e.g., slow blood flow in calf veins associated with bed rest), and (3) alterations in blood constituents (e.g., a change in clotting factors or increased platelet activity). These three factors are sometimes referred to as *Virchow's triad* (McCance & Huether, 2005).

Musculoskeletal Changes. The effects of immobility on the musculoskeletal system can include temporary or permanent impairment. Restricted mobility may result in loss of endurance, strength, and muscle mass as well as decreased stability and balance. Other effects of restricted mobility affecting the skeletal system are impaired calcium metabolism and impaired joint mobility.

Muscle Effects. Because of protein breakdown, the client loses lean body mass, which is composed partially of muscle. The reduced muscle mass is unable to sustain activity without increased fatigue. If immobility continues and the muscles are not exercised, muscle mass decreases further. Muscle weakness always occurs with immobility. Prolonged immobility often leads to muscle atrophy (or loss of muscle tissue). Therefore, atrophy is widely observed in response to illness, decreased ADLs, and immobilization. Loss of endurance, decreased muscle mass and strength, and joint instability (see "Skeletal Effects" section) put clients at risk for falls.

Skeletal Effects. Immobilization causes two skeletal changes: impaired calcium metabolism and joint abnormalities. Because immobilization results in bone resorption, the bone tissue is less dense, or is atrophied, and **disuse osteoporosis** results. When disuse osteoporosis occurs, the client is at risk for pathological fractures. Immobilization and non-weight-bearing activities increase the rate of bone resorption. Bone resorption also causes calcium to be released in the blood, and hypercalcemia results.

Osteoporosis is a major health concern in Canada. Most affected are women; 25% of women and 12.5% of men have osteoporosis (Brown & Josse, 2002). A 50-year-old woman has a lifetime risk of 40% for an osteoporosis-related fracture. Fifty percent of women who fracture their hip do not return to their previous functional level (Brown & Josse, 2002). Although primary osteoporosis is different in origin from the osteoporosis that results from immobility, it is imperative for nurses to recognize that immobilized clients may be at high risk for accelerated bone loss if they have primary osteoporosis. Important interventions for preventing disability in clients with primary osteoporosis who become immobilized include early client

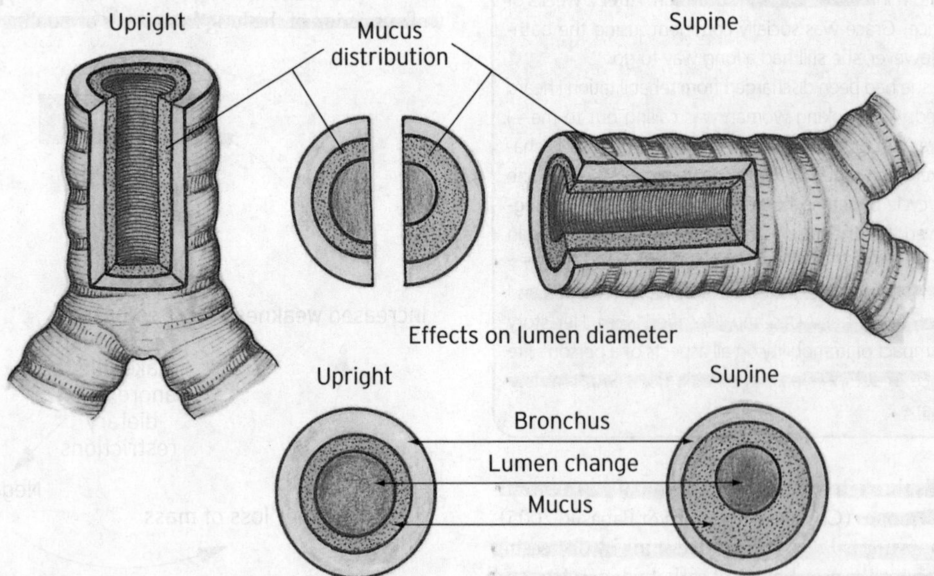

Figure 46-2 Effect of recumbency and gravity on distribution of respiratory tract and diameter of bronchiolar lumen. **Source:** From Gröer, M. W., & Shekleton, M. E. (1989). *Basic pathophysiology: A holistic approach* (3rd ed.). St. Louis, MO: Mosby.

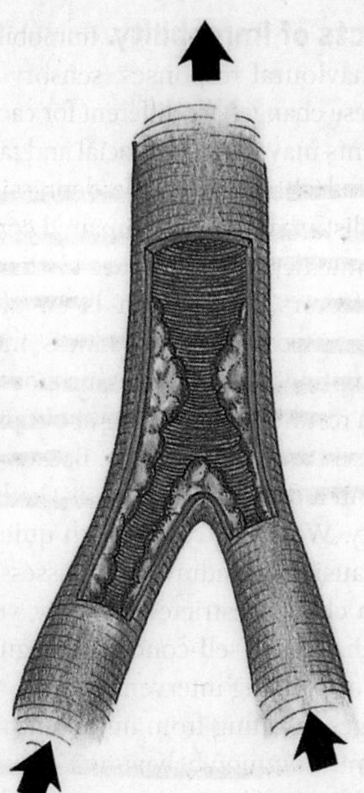

Figure 46-3 Thrombus formation in a vessel.

evaluation, and consultation with and referral to physicians, dietitians, occupational therapists, and physiotherapists. For the client with osteoporosis, the goal is to maintain independence with ADLs. Assistive ambulatory devices, adaptive clothing, and safety bars may assist the client with maintaining independence. Client teaching should focus on limiting the severity of the disease through diet and activity (Box 46–2).

Immobility can lead to joint contractures. A **joint contracture** is an abnormal and possibly permanent condition characterized by fixation of the joint. It is caused by disuse, atrophy, and shortening of the muscle fibres. When a contracture occurs, the joint cannot obtain full ROM. Contractures may leave a joint in a nonfunctional position (Figure 46–4). Early prevention of contractures is key; they can begin to form after only 8 hours of immobility in the older client (Fletcher, 2005).

One common and debilitating contracture is footdrop (Figure 46–5). When **footdrop** occurs, the foot is permanently fixed in plantar flexion. Ambulation is difficult with the foot in this position because the client cannot dorsiflex the foot. The client with footdrop is therefore unable to lift the toes off the ground. Clients who have suffered a cerebral vascular accident with resulting left- or right-sided paralysis (hemiplegia) are susceptible to footdrop.

Urinary Elimination Changes. The client's urinary elimination is altered by immobility. In the upright position, urine flows out of the renal pelvis and into the ureters and bladder because of gravitational forces. When the client is recumbent or flat, the kidneys and the ureters move toward a more level plane. Urine formed by the kidney must enter the bladder unaided by gravity. Because the peristaltic contractions of the ureters are insufficient to overcome gravity, the renal pelvis may fill before urine enters the ureters. This condition, called **urinary stasis**, increases the risk of urinary tract infection and renal calculi (see Chapter 44). Renal calculi are calcium stones that lodge in the renal pelvis and pass through the ureters. Immobilized clients are at risk for calculi because of altered calcium metabolism and the resulting hypercalcemia.

As the period of immobility continues, fluid intake can diminish, and this increases the risk for dehydration. As a result of decreased fluid intake, urinary output may decline around the fifth or sixth day after immobilization and the urine is often highly concentrated. This concentrated urine increases the risk for calculi formation and infection. An immobile client may also have less access to bathing equipment and be unable to perform adequate perineal hygiene, which may also increase the risk of urinary tract contamination by *Escherichia coli* bacteria. Another cause of urinary tract infections in immobilized clients is the use of an in-dwelling urinary catheter.

BOX 46-2 CLIENT TEACHING

Clients with Osteoporosis

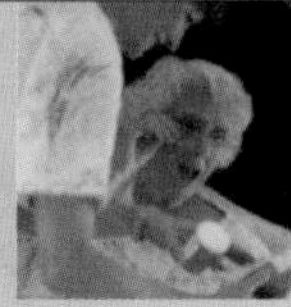

Objective

- Client will identify strategies to prevent or limit the severity of osteoporosis.

Teaching Strategies

- Instruct client (and caregiver, if present) on common risk factors and how to modify lifestyle (e.g., eliminating smoking, caffeine, alcohol).
- Teach client and caregiver the current recommended dietary allowances for calcium and vitamin D, and review foods high in calcium and vitamin D.
- Instruct client and caregiver to do appropriate types of weight-bearing exercises as recommended by the physician or physiotherapist to prevent injury or fractures.
- Teach client and caregiver about safety, fall prevention, and strategies to create a safe home environment.
- Instruct client and caregiver in self-administration of appropriate medication as ordered by the physician.
- Foster a positive self-image in the client by providing realistic yet optimistic and positive feedback about changes in the client's appearance and mobility.

Evaluation

- Client and caregiver identify strategies to modify the client's lifestyle, such as stopping smoking, reducing caffeine or alcohol intake, or increasing dietary calcium.
- Client and caregiver identify foods high in calcium and vitamin D.
- Client and caregiver demonstrate appropriate weight-bearing exercises.
- Client and caregiver identify safety strategies to prevent falls.
- Client and caregiver demonstrate appropriate knowledge about medications.
- Client and caregiver express positive but realistic feedback regarding the effects of disease.

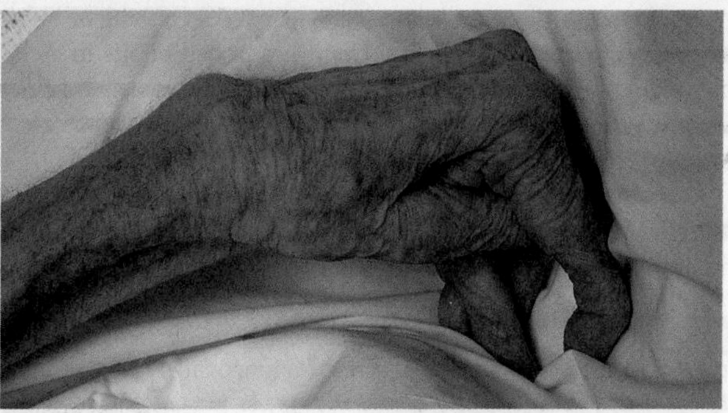

Figure 46-4 A contracture of the joints in the fingers. **Source:** From Sorrentino, S. A., Wilk, M. J., & Newmaster, R. (2008). *Mosby's Canadian textbook for the support worker* (2nd ed.). Toronto, ON: Elsevier.

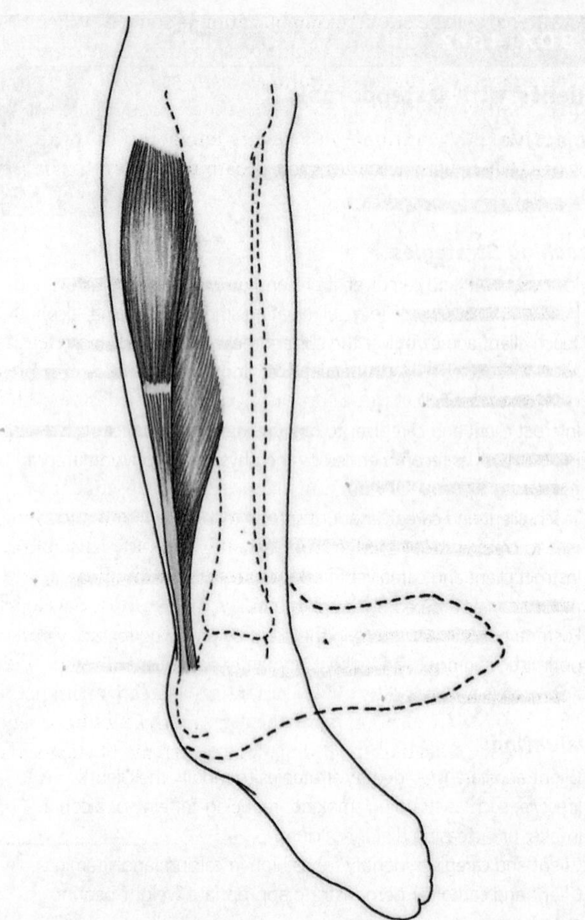

Figure 46-5 Footdrop. The ankle is fixed in plantar flexion. Normally, the ankle is able to flex (dotted line), which eases walking.

Integumentary Changes. The direct effect of pressure on the skin by immobility is compounded by the changes in metabolism that accompany immobility. Any break in the skin's integrity is difficult to heal in the immobilized client, thus immobility is a major risk for pressure ulcers. A **pressure ulcer** is an impairment of the skin as a result of prolonged ischemia (decreased blood supply to an area) in tissues (see Chapter 47). The ulcer is characterized initially by inflammation and usually forms over a bony prominence. Ischemia develops when the pressure on the skin is greater than the pressure inside the small peripheral blood vessels supplying blood to the skin.

Tissue metabolism depends on the body's receipt of oxygen and nutrients from the blood supply and on the elimination of metabolic wastes. Pressure affects cellular metabolism by decreasing or obliterating tissue circulation. When a client lies in bed or sits in a chair, the weight of the body is on bony prominences. The longer the pressure is applied, the longer the period of ischemia and, thus, the greater the risk of skin breakdown.

Preventing a pressure ulcer is much less expensive than treating one (RNAO, 2007). Thus preventive nursing interventions are imperative.

safety alert Implement a comprehensive skin care program to prevent skin breakdown in all clients, from neonates to older adults. Effective skin care programs include accurate and consistent assessment and documentation as well as interventions to protect the skin (e.g., turn the client every 2 hours and use mechanical devices such as lifts when you need to move the client; Butler, 2006).

Psychosocial Effects of Immobility. Immobilization may lead to emotional and behavioural responses, sensory alterations, and changes in coping. These changes are different for each client. In addition, immobilized clients may also have social and family difficulties.

Common emotional changes include depression, behavioural changes, sleep–wake disturbances, and impaired coping. The immobilized client can become depressed because of changes in role, self-concept, and other factors. Depression is an affective disorder characterized by exaggerated feelings of sadness, melancholy, dejection, worthlessness, emptiness, and hopelessness out of proportion to reality. Depression can result from worrying about present and future levels of health, finances, and family needs. Because immobilization removes the client from a daily routine, he or she has more time to worry about disability. Worrying can in turn quickly increase the client's depression, causing withdrawal. By assessing behavioural changes throughout a client's restricted mobility, you will be better equipped to identify changes in self-concept, recognize early signs of depression, and develop nursing interventions.

Behavioural changes resulting from immobilization vary widely, depending on the client. Common behavioural changes include hostility, belligerence, giddiness, fear, and anxiety. Early in the nursing process you should interview the client's family about normal behavioural patterns to gain baseline data. If unexpected behaviours are observed later, you can intervene to reduce the effects of immobilization on the client's behavioural patterns.

Sleep–wake alterations in the immobile client may occur from nursing care or changes in habit or environment. Disruption of normal sleeping patterns can further cause behavioural changes. Nursing interventions should be used to ensure that the client receives sufficient sleep (see Chapter 41). The client who is on bed rest and is able to change position during sleep does not require continuous physical nursing care. Unless other treatment activities are required during the night, the care plan for the physiologically stable client on bed rest should provide for uninterrupted sleep.

Long-term immobility or bed rest can affect usual coping patterns. Such a client may withdraw and become passive. The passive client allows nurses to provide care but is not interested in increasing independence or involvement in care. Early in the care of an immobilized client, you should assess the client's normal coping mechanisms in order to design a nursing care plan that will accommodate the client's coping abilities or help the client develop new ones.

Developmental Changes. Developmental changes associated with immobility tend to occur most commonly in very young children and in older adults. The immobilized young or middle-age adult who has been healthy may have experienced few, if any, developmental changes. However, exceptions exist, and clients must be fully assessed for developmental implications. One exception might be a mother who has complications at childbirth and as a result cannot interact with the newborn infant as expected.

Infants, Toddlers, and Preschoolers. The newborn infant's spine is flexed and lacks the anteroposterior curves of the adult (see Chapter 23). As the baby grows, musculoskeletal development permits support of weight for standing and walking. Posture is awkward because the head and upper trunk are carried forward. Because body weight is not evenly distributed along a line of gravity, posture is off balance, and falls occur often. When the infant, toddler, or preschooler is immobilized, it is usually because of trauma or the need to correct a congenital skeletal abnormality. Prolonged immobilization can delay the child's gross motor skills, intellectual development, or musculoskeletal development. Nurses caring for immobilized children should plan activities that provide physical and psychosocial stimuli.

Adolescents. The adolescence stage is usually initiated by a tremendous growth spurt (see Chapter 23). Growth is frequently uneven. Prolonged immobilization may alter adolescent growth patterns. In addition, the adolescent may lag behind peers in gaining independence. When immobilization occurs, social isolation will likely be a concern for this age group.

Adults. An adult who has correct posture and body alignment feels good, looks good, and generally appears self-confident. The healthy adult also has the necessary musculoskeletal development and coordination to carry out ADLs (see Chapter 24). When periods of prolonged immobility occur, however, all physiological systems are at risk. In addition, the role of the adult may change with regard to the family or social structure. The adult may lose identity associated with a job.

Older Adults. Aging is normally associated with a progressive loss of total bone mass, muscle strength, and aerobic capacity. Some of the possible causes of this loss include decreased physical activity, hormonal changes, and actual bone resorption. The effect of bone loss is weaker bones. Older adults may walk more slowly, take smaller steps, and appear less coordinated. Thus balance is impaired, and they are at greater risk for falls and injuries (see Chapter 25). The outcomes of a fall include not only possible injury but also hospitalization, loss of independence, and psychological effects.

Older adults may experience functional-status changes secondary to hospitalization and altered mobility status (Box 46–3). Those older adults who are immobilizd may become more physically dependent on others and suffer more functional losses. In some older adults, immobilization results from a degenerative disease, neurological trauma, or chronic illness. Immobilization can occur gradually and progressively in some individuals, whereas for others, especially those who have had a stroke, immobilization is sudden. When providing nursing care for an older adult, you should develop a care plan that encourages the client to perform as many self-care activities as possible, thereby maintaining the highest level of mobility. Nurses may inadvertently contribute to a client's immobility by providing unnecessary help with activities such as bathing and transferring.

> **BOX 46-3 Hazards of Immobility in Hospitalized Older Adults**
>
> For many older adults, admission to the hospital often results in functional decline. Older adults can quickly regress to a dependent state. Rapid intervention of an interdisciplinary health team is required to maintain the client's functional capacity.
>
> Usual aging is associated with decreased muscle strength and aerobic capacity. Ordering bed rest for clients without sufficient ambulation leads to a loss of mobility and functional decline. Immobility causes weakness, fatigue, and an increased risk for falls. It also results in shallow breathing, which may lead to pneumonia. Inadequate turning or repositioning of an immobile client can result in skin breakdown and pressure ulcers.
>
> Catheter use and improper pericare can lead to urinary tract infections. Older adults are prone to nosocomial infections (infections obtained in the health care environment) because they often have compromised immune systems. Infections, as well as medications, treatments, and translocation, often cause confusion in older adults.
>
> Hospitalization affects the nutritional status of the older adult. Limited access to fluids causes dehydration; conversely, fluid overload occurs from improper administration of intravenous (IV) fluids. Treatments and medications can cause fluid and electrolyte imbalances, contributing to confusion in the geriatric client.
>
> Finally, multiple interruptions and noise in the environment impair sleep, causing fatigue, depression, and confusion. Any of these factors may thrust vulnerable older adults into a state of irreversible functional decline.
>
> Adapted from Ebersole, P., Hess, P., Touhy, T., & Jett, K. (2005). *Geriatric nursing and healthy aging* (2nd ed.). St. Louis, MO: Elsevier Mosby.

Critical Thinking

Critical thinking requires you to combine knowledge, experiences, client data, critical thinking attitudes, and intellectual and professional standards. Each of these sources must be weighed for its validity and applicability to the client facing impaired mobility. The immobile client has multiple needs; by integrating these sources, you can best judge appropriate nursing diagnoses and subsequent care.

To understand the impact of immobility on the client and family, you must integrate knowledge from nursing and other disciplines, previous experiences, and information gathered from clients. A creative approach can also be helpful. Standards such as those developed by provincial nursing associations (e.g., Registered Nurses Association of Ontario [RNAO] Best Practice Guidelines) provide valuable guides for managing complications associated with immobility (Figure 46–6). In addition, many health care facilities have standards of practice related to the lifting and transferring of clients and to the prevention of falls and pressure sores.

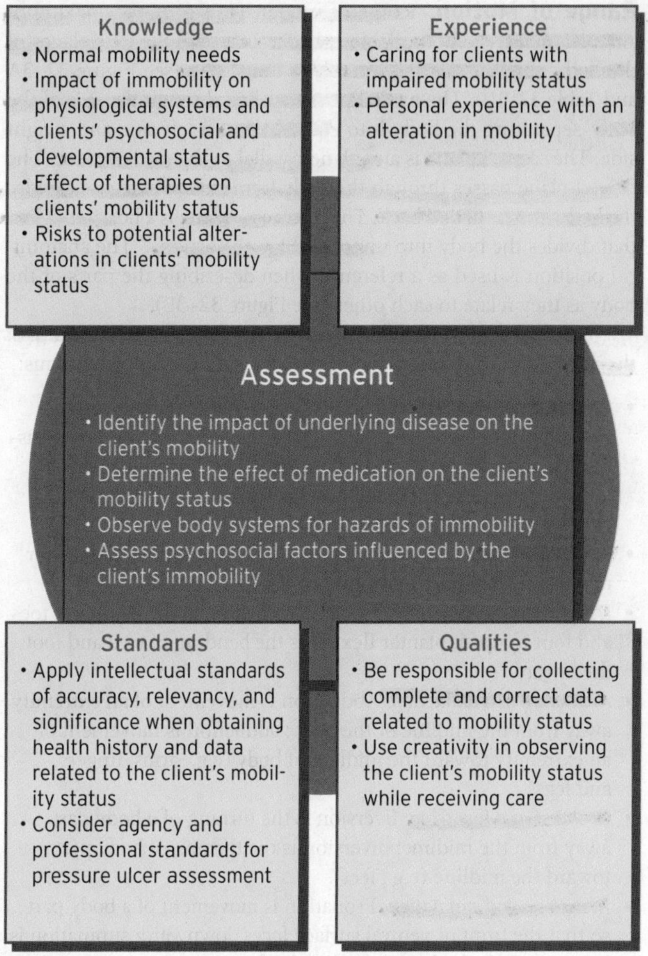

Figure 46-6 Critical thinking model for mobility assessment.

Nursing Process for Impaired Body Alignment and Mobility

By applying the nursing process and using a critical thinking approach, you can develop individualized care plans for clients with mobility impairments or risk for immobility. The aim of the care plan is to improve the client's functional status, promote self-care, maintain psychological well-being, and reduce the hazards of immobility.

❖Assessment

Nursing assessment is presented here in two sections: mobility and immobility. Both areas are usually assessed during the complete physical examination.

Mobility

Assessment of client mobility focuses on ROM, gait, exercise and activity tolerance, and body alignment. When unsure of the client's abilities, you should begin assessment of mobility with the client in the most supportive position and move to higher levels of mobility according to the client's tolerance. Generally, start assessing movement while the client is lying, then proceed to assessing sitting positions in bed, transfers to chair, and, finally, gait. This sequence of assessment helps to protect the client's safety.

Range of Motion. Range of motion (ROM) is the maximum amount of movement available at a joint in one of the four planes of the body: medial, sagittal, frontal, or transverse (see Figure 32–3A and Table 32–10). The medial plane is a line through the axis of the body, separating the body into equal halves, a left side and a right side. The sagittal plane is any plane parallel to the medial plane. The frontal plane passes through the body from side to side and divides the body into front and back. The transverse plane is a horizontal line that divides the body into upper and lower portions. The anatomical position is used as a reference when describing the parts of the body as they relate to each other (see Figure 32–3B).

Joint mobility is limited by ligaments, muscles, and the nature of the joint. Joint movements are described using the followng terms:

- *Flexion and extension:* Flexion is decreasing the angle between two adjoining bones (bending of the joint); extension is increasing the angle between two adjoining bones (extending the joint). Examples of affected body parts include the fingers, elbows, and knees.
- *Hyperextension:* This is movement of a body part beyond its normal resting extended position.
- *Dorsiflexion and plantar flexion:* Dorsiflexion is the flexion of toes and foot upward; plantar flexion is the bending of toes and foot downward.
- *Abduction and adduction:* Abduction is movement of an extremity away from the midline of the body; adduction is movement of an extremity toward the midline of body (e.g., arms, fingers, and legs).
- *Eversion and inversion:* Eversion is the turning of a body part away from the midline; inversion is the turning of body part toward the midline (e.g., feet).
- *Pronation and supination:* Pronation is movement of a body part so that the front or ventral surface faces downward; supination is movement of a body part so that the front or ventral surface faces upward (e.g., hands, forearm).
- *Internal and external rotation:* Internal rotation is rotation of the joint inward; external rotation is rotation of the joint outward (e.g., hip).
- *Circumduction:* This is the circular movement of a limb in a cone-shaped manner (e.g., shoulder).

When assessing ROM, physically examine the client for stiffness, swelling, pain, limited movement, and unequal movement, and ask the client whether any of these features are present. Chapter 36 describes specific techniques for measuring the degrees of motion in a joint. Assessment of ROM is important as a baseline measurement to compare and evaluate whether loss in joint mobility has occurred. Clients whose mobility is restricted require ROM exercises to reduce the hazards of immobility. Thus it is important to assess the type of ROM exercise a client can perform. ROM exercises may be active (the client is able to move all joints through their ROM unassisted), passive (the client is unable to move independently, and the nurse moves each joint through its ROM), or somewhere in between (Table 46–2). With a weak client, for example, you may provide support while the client performs most of the movement, or the client may be able to move some joints actively while you passively move others. First assess the client's ability to engage in active ROM exercises and the need for assistance, teaching, or reinforcement. In general, exercises should be as active as health and mobility allow. Contractures may develop in joints not moved periodically through their full ROM.

Gait. The term gait is used to describe a particular manner or style of walking. The gait cycle begins with the heel strike of one leg and continues to the heel strike of the other leg. Assessment of a client's gait helps you to draw conclusions about balance, posture, safety, and ability to walk without assistance. The mechanics of human gait involve coordination of the skeletal, neurological, and muscular systems of the human body.

Exercise and Activity Tolerance. Exercise is physical activity for conditioning the body, improving health, and maintaining fitness. It can be used as therapy to correct a deformity or to restore the overall body to a maximal state of health. When a person exercises, physiological changes occur in body systems (see Chapter 36).

Assessment of the client's energy level includes assessment of the physiological effects of exercise and activity tolerance. **Activity tolerance** is the type and amount of exercise or work that a person is able to perform. It is important to assess a client's activity tolerance when planning activities for the client such as walking or ROM exercises or ADLs such as bathing. To assess activity tolerance you will need data from physiological, emotional, and developmental domains (see Chapter 36). This assessment is applicable in all clinical settings and can be quickly completed.

When activity begins, you should monitor clients for symptoms such as dyspnea, fatigue, chest pain, or change in vital signs from baseline. Some clients may be unable to sustain activity because the energy needed to complete the activity creates fatigue and generalized weakness. Even simple tasks such as eating or moving in bed may need to be monitored. If you note decreased activity tolerance, carefully assess the time needed by the client to recover. A decreasing recovery time may indicate improved activity tolerance.

People who are depressed, worried, or anxious are frequently unable to tolerate exercise. Depressed clients are usually not motivated to participate. Clients who are worried or anxious tire easily because they expend a great deal of energy in states of worry and anxiety. Thus, they may experience physical and emotional exhaustion.

➤ TABLE 46-2 Range-of-Motion Exercises

Body Part	Type of Joint	Type of Movement	Range (Degrees)	Primary Muscles
Neck, cervical spine	Pivotal 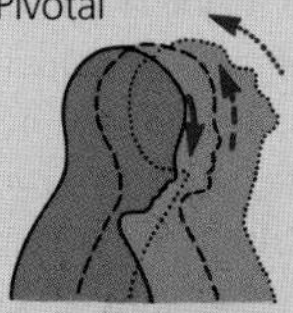	Flexion: Bring chin to rest on chest.	45	Sternocleidomastoid
		Extension: Return head to erect position.	45	Trapezius
		Hyperextension: Bend head back as far as possible.	10	Trapezius
	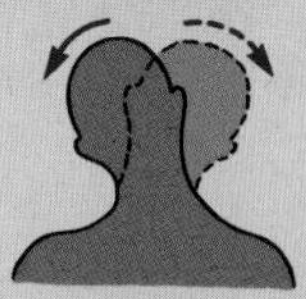	Lateral flexion: Tilt head as far as possible toward each shoulder.	40–45	Sternocleidomastoid
	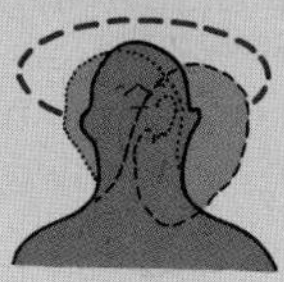	Rotation: Turn head as far as possible along transverse plane to each side.	70–90	Sternocleidomastoid, trapezius
Shoulder	Ball and socket 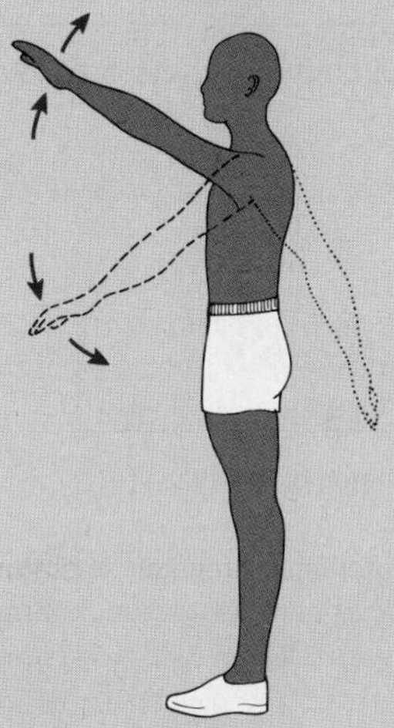	Flexion: Raise arm from side position forward to position above the head.	180 45–60	Coracobrachialis, biceps brachii, deltoid, pectoralis major
		Extension: Return arm to position at side of the body.	180	Latissimus dorsi, teres major, triceps brachii
		Hyperextension: Move arm behind body, keeping elbow straight.	45–60	Latissimus dorsi, teres major, deltoid
	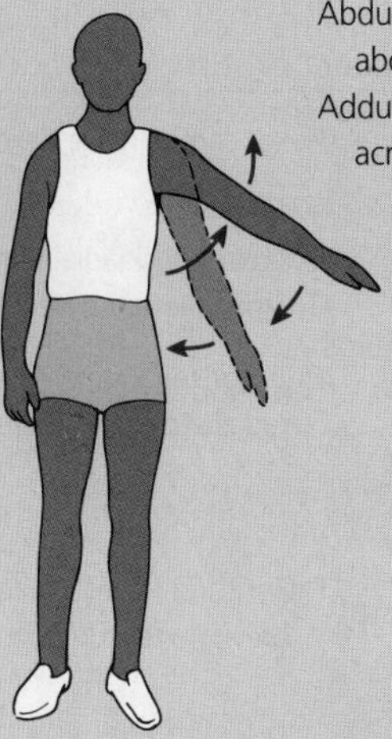	Abduction: Raise arm to side to position above head with palm away from head.	180	Deltoid, supraspinatus
		Adduction: Lower arm sideways and across body as far as possible.	320	Pectoralis major

Continued

➤ TABLE 46-2 Range-of-Motion Exercises *continued*

Body Part	Type of Joint	Type of Movement	Range (Degrees)	Primary Muscles
Shoulder	Ball and socket 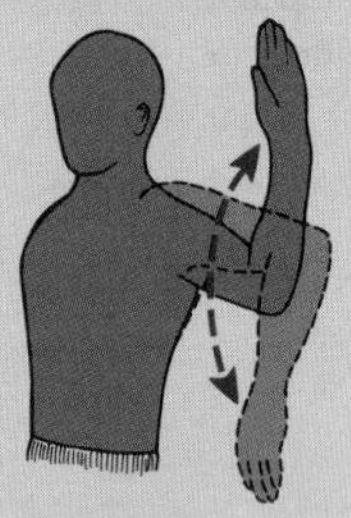	Internal rotation: With elbow flexed, rotate shoulder by moving arm until thumb is turned inward and toward back.	90	Pectoralis major, latissimus dorsi, teres major, subscapularis
		External rotation: With elbow flexed, move arm until thumb is upward and lateral to head.	90	Infraspinatus, teres major, deltoid
	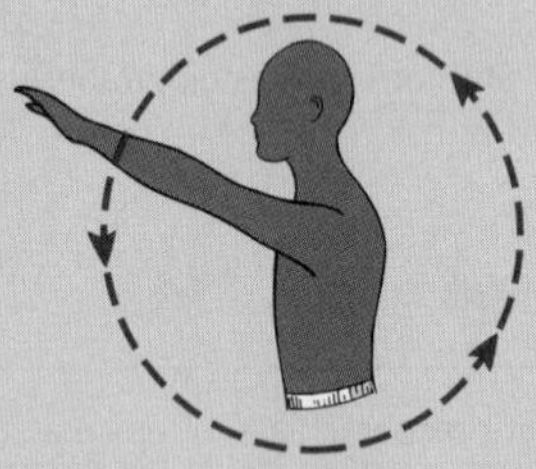	Circumduction: Move arm in full circle. (Circumduction is a combination of all movements of the ball-and-socket joint.)	360	Deltoid, coracobrachialis, latissimus dorsi, teres major
Elbow	Hinge 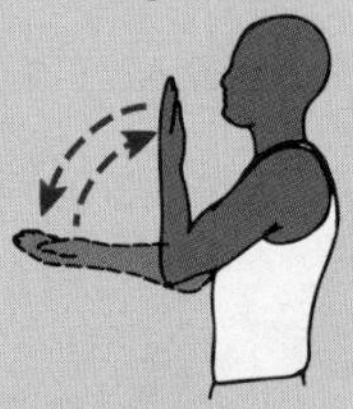	Flexion: Bend elbow so that lower arm moves toward its shoulder joint and the hand is level with the shoulder.	150	Biceps brachii, brachialis, brachioradialis
		Extension: Straighten elbow by lowering hand.	150	Triceps brachii
Forearm	Pivotal 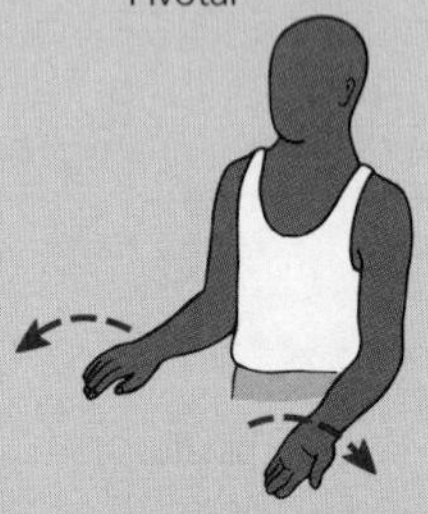	Supination: Turn lower arm and hand so that the palm is up.	70–90	Supinator, biceps brachii
		Pronation: Turn lower arm so that the palm is down.	70–90	Pronator teres, pronator quadratus
Wrist	Condyloid 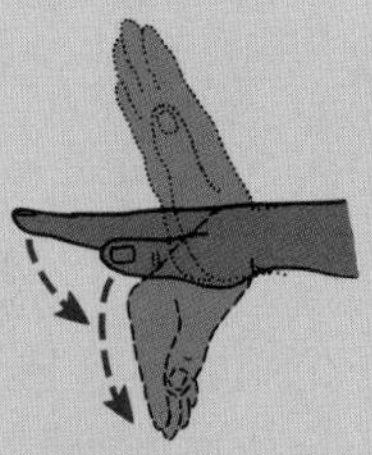	Flexion: Move palm toward inner aspect of forearm.	80–90	Flexor carpi ulnaris, flexor carpi radialis
		Extension: Move fingers and hand posterior to midline.	80–90	Extensor carpi radialis brevis, extensor carpi radialis longus, extensor carpi ulnaris
		Hyperextension: Bring dorsal surface of hand back as far as possible.	80–90	Extensor carpi radialis brevis, extensor carpi radialis longus, extensor carpi ulnaris
	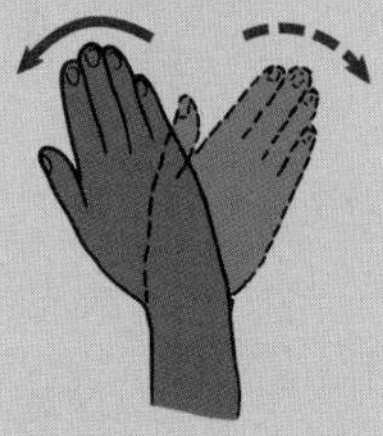	Abduction (radial deviation): Place hand with palm down and extend wrist laterally toward fifth finger.	Up to 30	Flexor carpi radialis, extensor carpi radialis brevis, extensor carpi radialis longus
		Adduction (ulnar deviation): Place hand with palm down and extend wrist medially toward thumb.	30–50	Flexor carpi ulnaris, extensor carpi ulnaris

➤ TABLE 46-2 Range-of-Motion Exercises *continued*

Body Part	Type of Joint	Type of Movement	Range (Degrees)	Primary Muscles
Fingers	Condyloid hinge	Flexion: Make a fist.	90	Lumbricales, interosseus volaris, interosseus dorsalis
	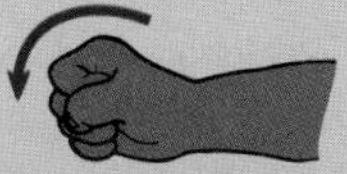	Extension: Straighten fingers.	90	Extensor digiti quinti proprius, extensor digitorum communis, extensor indicis proprius
	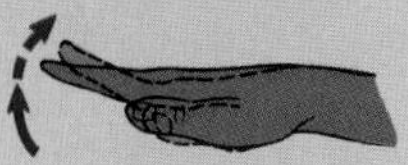	Hyperextension: Bend fingers back as far as possible.	30–60	
	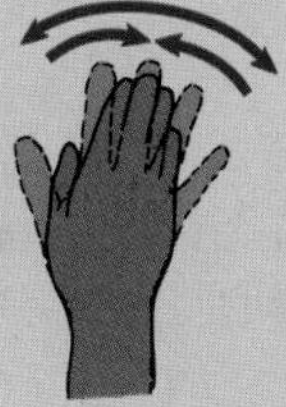	Abduction: Spread fingers apart.	30	Interosseus dorsalis
		Adduction: Bring fingers together.	30	Interosseus volaris
Thumb	Saddle	Flexion: Move thumb across palmar surface of hand.	90	Flexor pollicis brevis
	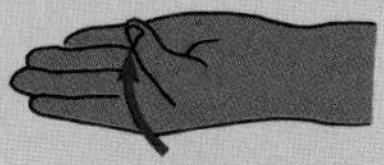	Extension: Move thumb straight away from hand.	90	Extensor pollicis longus, extensor pollicis brevis
		Abduction: Extend thumb laterally (usually done when placing fingers in abduction and adduction).	30	Abductor pollicis brevis
	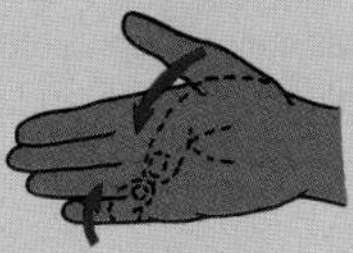	Adduction: Move thumb back toward hand.	30	Adductor pollicis obliquus, adductor pollicis transversus
		Opposition: Touch thumb to each finger of the same hand.		Opponeus pollicis, opponeus digiti minimi
Hip	Ball and socket	Flexion: Move leg forward and up.	90–120	Psoas major, iliacus, sartorius
	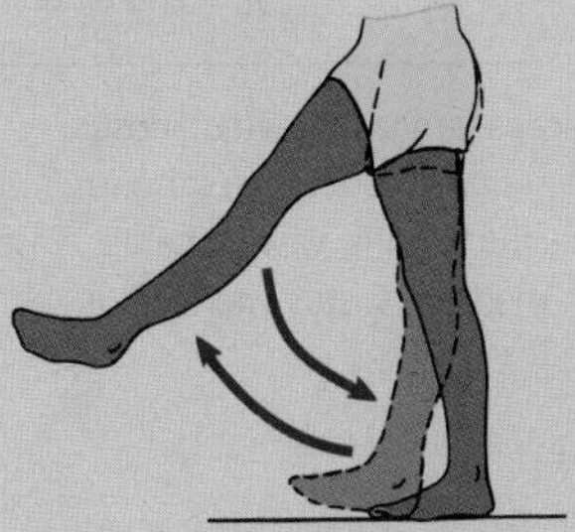	Extension: Move leg back beside other leg.	90–120	Gluteus maximus, semitendinosus, semimembranosus
	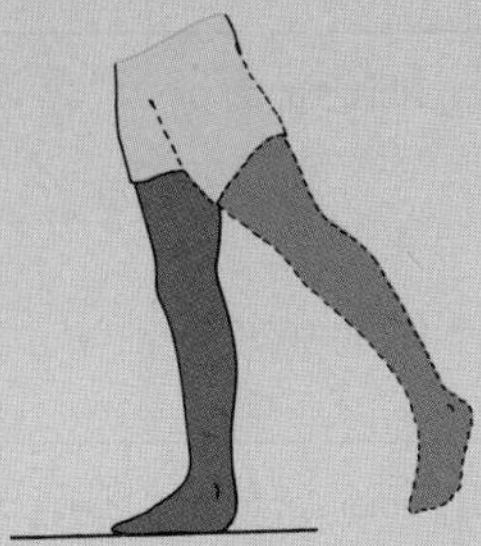	Hyperextension: Move leg behind the body.	30–50	Gluteus maximus, semitendinosus, semimembranosus

Continued

➤TABLE 46-2 Range-of-Motion Exercises *continued*

Body Part	Type of Joint	Type of Movement	Range (Degrees)	Primary Muscles
Hip	Ball and socket	Abduction: Move leg laterally away from the body.	30–50	Gluteus medius, gluteus minimus
		Adduction: Move leg back toward medial position and beyond, if possible.	30–50	Adductor longus, adductor brevis, adductor magnus
		Internal rotation: Turn foot and leg toward other leg.	90	Gluteus medius, gluteus minimus, tensor fasciae latae
		External rotation: Turn foot and leg away from other leg.	90	Obturatorius internus, obturatorius externus
		Circumduction: Move leg in a circle.		Psoas major, gluteus maximus, gluteus medius, adductor magnus
Knee	Hinge 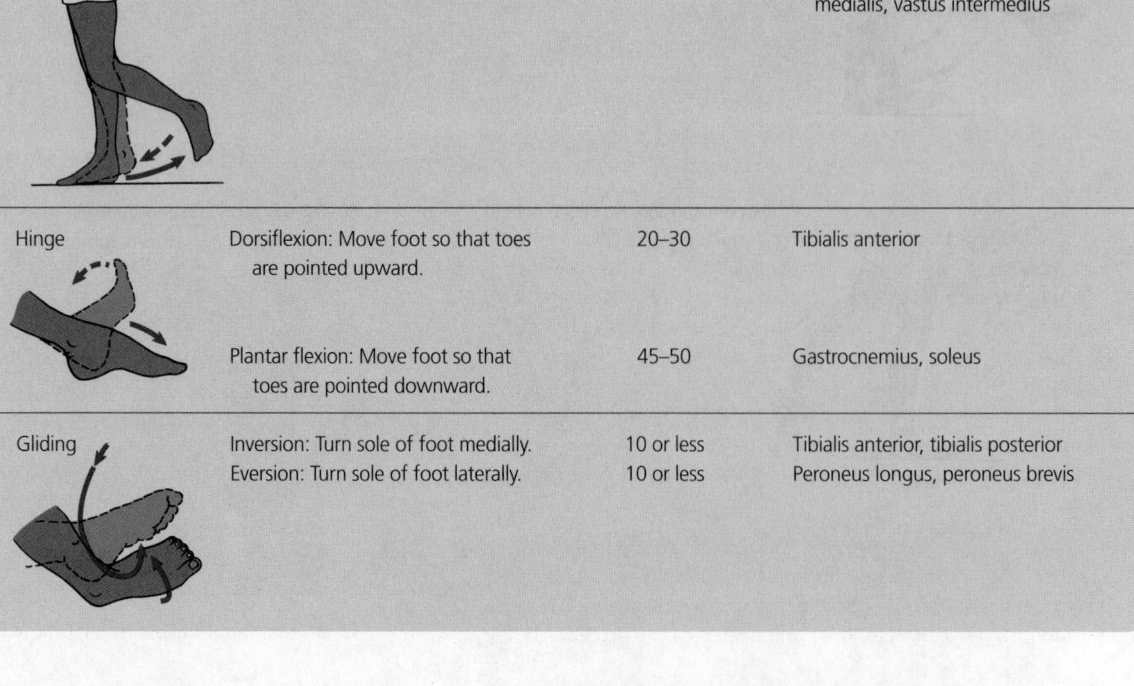	Flexion: Bring heel back toward back of thigh.	120–130	Biceps femoris, semitendinosus, semimembranosus, sartorius
		Extension: Return leg to the floor.	120–130	Rectus femoris, vastus lateralis, vastus medialis, vastus intermedius
Ankle	Hinge	Dorsiflexion: Move foot so that toes are pointed upward.	20–30	Tibialis anterior
		Plantar flexion: Move foot so that toes are pointed downward.	45–50	Gastrocnemius, soleus
Foot	Gliding	Inversion: Turn sole of foot medially.	10 or less	Tibialis anterior, tibialis posterior
		Eversion: Turn sole of foot laterally.	10 or less	Peroneus longus, peroneus brevis

TABLE 46-2 Range-of-Motion Exercises *continued*

Body Part	Type of Joint	Type of Movement	Range (Degrees)	Primary Muscles
Toes	Condyloid	Flexion: Curl toes downward.	30–60	Flexor digitorum, lumbricalis pedis, flexor hallucis brevis
		Extension: Straighten toes.	30–60	Extensor digitorum longus, extensor digitorum brevis, extensor hallucis longus
		Abduction: Spread toes apart.	15 or less	Abductor hallucis, interosseus dorsalis
		Adduction: Bring toes together.	15 or less	Adductor hallucis, interosseus plantaris

Developmental changes also affect tolerance for activity. As the infant enters the toddler stage, the activity level increases and the need for sleep declines. The child entering preschool or primary grades expends mental energy in learning and may require more rest after school or before strenuous play. The adolescent going through puberty may require more rest because much of the body's energy is expended for growth and hormone changes.

Changes may still occur through the adult years, but many of these changes are related to work and lifestyle choices. Pregnancy may decrease a woman's energy tolerance, especially during the first and third trimesters. Hormonal changes and fetal development use body energy, and the woman may be unable or unmotivated to carry out physical activities. During the last trimester, fetal development consumes a great deal of the mother's energy, and the size and location of the fetus may limit the mother's ability to take a deep breath, resulting in less oxygen being available for physical activities.

As the person grows older, activity tolerance changes. Muscle mass is reduced, posture changes, and the composition of bones is altered. Changes often occur in the cardiopulmonary system, such as decreased maximum heart rate and decreased lung compliance, that affect the intensity of exercise. The older adult may still exercise but will do so at a reduced intensity. The more inactive a client becomes, the more pronounced these activity changes are.

Body Alignment. Assessment of body alignment can be carried out with the client standing, sitting, or lying down. This assessment has the following objectives:

- To determine normal physiological changes in body alignment resulting from growth and development for each individual client.
- To identify deviations in body alignment caused by poor posture.
- To provide opportunities for clients to observe their posture.
- To identify learning needs of clients for maintaining correct body alignment.
- To identify trauma, muscle damage, or nerve dysfunction.
- To obtain information about other factors contributing to poor alignment, such as fatigue, malnutrition, and psychological problems.

The first step in assessing body alignment is to put clients at ease so that unnatural or rigid positions are not assumed. When assessing the body alignment of an immobilized or unconscious client, pillows and positioning supports should be removed from the bed and the client placed in the supine position.

Standing. When the client is standing, check for the following signs of good body alignment:

- The head is erect and midline.
- When observed posteriorly, the shoulders and hips are straight and parallel.
- When observed posteriorly, the vertebral column is straight.
- When the client is observed laterally, the head is erect and the spinal curves are aligned in a reversed "S" pattern. The cervical vertebrae are anteriorly convex, the thoracic vertebrae are posteriorly convex, and the lumbar vertebrae are anteriorly convex.
- When observed laterally, the abdomen is comfortably tucked in and the knees and ankles are slightly flexed. The person appears comfortable and does not seem conscious of the flexion of knees or ankles.
- The arms hang comfortably at the sides.
- The feet are placed slightly apart to achieve a base of support, and the toes are pointed forward.
- When the client is viewed anteriorly, the centre of gravity is in the midline, and the line of gravity is from the middle of the forehead to a midpoint between the feet. Laterally, the line of gravity runs vertically from the middle of the skull to the posterior third of the foot (Figure 46–7).

Sitting. Assess body alignment when the client is sitting in a chair or wheelchair by observing for the following (Figure 46–8):

- The head is erect, and the neck and vertebral column are in straight alignment.
- The body weight is evenly distributed on the buttocks and thighs.
- The thighs are parallel and in a horizontal plane.
- Both feet are supported on the floor or on wheelchair footrests. With short clients, a footstool is used and the ankles are comfortably flexed.
- A 2.5- to 5-cm space is maintained between the edge of the seat and the popliteal space on the posterior surface of the knee. This space ensures that no pressure is on the popliteal artery or nerve to decrease circulation or impair nerve function.
- The client's forearms are supported on the armrest, in the lap, or on a table in front of the chair.

It is particularly important to assess alignment when sitting if the

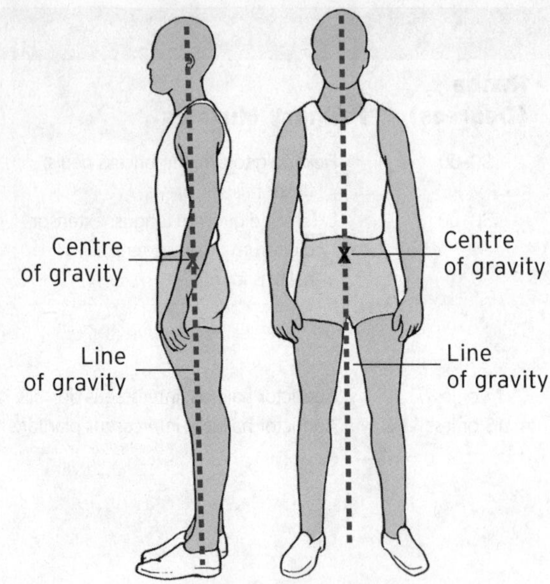

Figure 46-7 Correct body alignment when standing.

client has muscle weakness, muscle paralysis, or nerve damage. Because of these alterations, the client has diminished sensation in the affected area and is unable to perceive pressure or decreased circulation. Proper alignment while sitting reduces the risk of musculoskeletal system damage in such a client. The client with severe respiratory disease may assume a posture of leaning on the table in front of the chair in an attempt to breathe more easily.

Lying. People who are conscious have voluntary muscle control and normal perception of pressure. As a result, they usually assume a position of comfort when lying down. Because their ROM, sensation, and circulation are within normal limits, they change positions when they perceive muscle strain and decreased circulation.

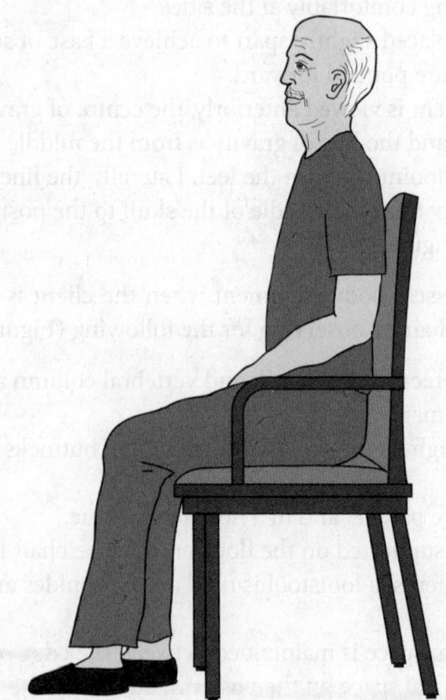

Figure 46-8 Correct body alignment when sitting. The client's feet are flat on the floor, the calves do not touch the chair, and the back is straight and against the back of the chair. **Source:** From Sorrentino, S. A. (2004). *Mosby's Canadian textbook for the support worker* (p. 287, Fig 21-23). Toronto, ON: Elsevier.

Assessment of body alignment in the lateral position is best done with the client who is restricted to bed and not able to move well. All positioning supports should be removed from the bed except for the pillow under the head, and the body should be supported by an adequate mattress (Figure 46–9). This position allows for full view of the spine and back and will help provide other baseline body alignment data, such as whether the client can remain positioned without aid. The vertebrae should be aligned, and the position should not cause discomfort. Conditions that create a risk of damage to the musculoskeletal system when lying down include impaired mobility, such as in clients in traction or those with arthritis; decreased sensation, such as in clients with hemiparesis (one-sided weakness) after stroke or brain attack; impaired circulation, such as in client with diabetes; and lack of voluntary muscle control, such as in clients with spinal cord injuries.

Immobility

Physiological Assessment. To assess the immobilized client for hazards of immobility, you will need to perform a head-to-toe physical assessment (see Chapter 32). The nursing assessment should focus on certain physiological areas, as well as on the client's psychosocial and developmental dimensions. The physiological hazards of immobility that may be identified during a nursing assessment are summarized below and in Table 46–3.

Metabolic System. When assessing metabolic functioning, use **anthropometric measurements** (measures of height, weight, and skinfold thickness) to evaluate muscle atrophy (see Chapter 32). In addition, you may need to analyze intake and output records for fluid balance. Does fluid intake equal output? Intake and output measurements assist in determining whether a fluid imbalance exists (see Chapter 40). Dehydration and edema can increase the rate of skin breakdown in an immobilized client. Monitoring laboratory data such as electrolytes, serum protein (albumin and total protein) levels, and blood urea nitrogen can help you determine metabolic functioning.

Assessment of wound healing and monitoring of food intake and elimination patterns will help to determine altered gastrointestinal functioning and potential metabolic problems. If an immobilized client has a wound, the rate of healing indicates how well nutrients are being delivered to tissues. Normal progression of healing indicates that metabolic needs of injured tissues are being met. Anorexia occurs commonly in immobilized clients. The client's food intake should be assessed before the meal tray is removed to determine the amount eaten. Nutritional imbalances can be avoided if you assess the client's dietary patterns and food preferences early in immobilization (see Chapter 43).

Respiratory System. A respiratory assessment should be performed at least every 2 hours for clients with restricted activity. Inspect chest wall movements during the full inspiratory–expiratory cycle. If a client has an atelectatic area, chest movement may be asymmetrical. In addition, auscultate the entire lung region to identify diminished breath sounds, crackles, or wheezes. Auscultation should focus on the dependent lung fields because pulmonary secretions

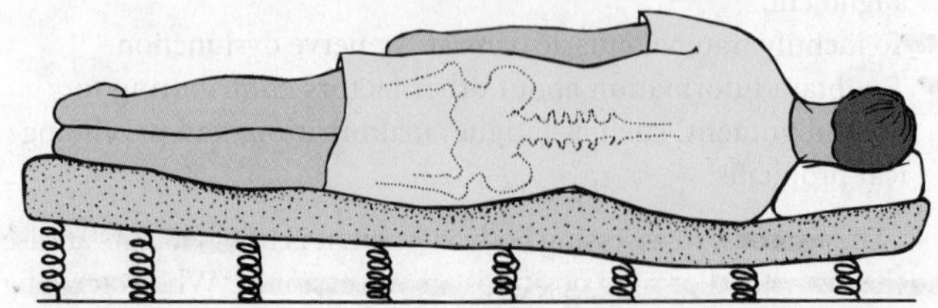

Figure 46-9 Correct body alignment when lying down.

TABLE 46-3 Physiological Hazards of Immobility

System	Assessment Techniques	Abnormal Findings
Metabolic	Inspection	Slowed wound healing, abnormal laboratory data
	Inspection	Muscle atrophy
	Anthropometric measurements (mid-upper arm circumference, triceps skinfold measurement)	Decreased amount of subcutaneous fat
	Palpation	Generalized edema
Respiratory	Inspection	Asymmetrical chest wall movement, dyspnea, increased respiratory rate
	Auscultation	Crackles, wheezes, decreased air entry
Cardiovascular	Auscultation	Orthostatic hypotension
	Auscultation, palpation	Increased heart rate, third heart sound, weak peripheral pulses, peripheral edema
Musculoskeletal	Inspection, palpation	Decreased range of motion, erythema, increased diameter in calf or thigh
	Palpation	Joint contracture
	Inspection	Activity intolerance, muscle atrophy, joint contracture
Elimination	Inspection	Decreased urine output, cloudy or concentrated urine, decreased frequency of bowel movements
	Palpation	Distended bladder and abdomen
	Auscultation	Decreased bowel sounds
Skin	Inspection, palpation	Break in skin integrity

tend to collect in these lower regions. Perform a complete respiratory assessment to identify the presence of secretions and to determine nursing interventions necessary for optimal respiratory function.

Cardiovascular System. Cardiovascular assessment of the immobilized client includes blood pressure monitoring, evaluation of apical and peripheral pulses, and observation for signs of venous stasis (e.g., edema and poor wound healing). All clients should have their vital signs monitored during the first few attempts at sitting or standing.

When getting the client from a supine position into a chair, move the client gradually. When performing this procedure, assess and document orthostatic changes. First obtain baseline blood pressure and pulse measurements with the client in the supine position, and then assist the client to a position sitting at the side of the bed. The client should remain sitting for 3 minutes before you take the blood pressure and pulse. Remain with the client in a sitting position and continually monitor the client for dizziness or light-headedness. If the client has no dizziness or drop in blood pressure (‡ 20 mm Hg systolic or 10 mm Hg diastolic), assist the client to a standing position and retake the blood pressure and pulse immediately when the client stands and again after 3 minutes of standing. The client should be monitored closely for dizziness throughout this procedure. The longer the period of immobility, the greater the risk of hypotension when the client stands (Copstead-Kirkhorn & Banaski, 2005).

You will also need to assess the apical and peripheral pulses. Recumbency increases cardiac workload and pulse rate. In some clients, particularly older adults, the heart may not tolerate the increased workload, and a form of cardiac failure may develop. A third heart sound, heard at the apex with the bell of the stethoscope, can be an early indication of congestive heart failure. Monitoring of peripheral pulses will enable you to evaluate the heart's ability to pump blood. The absence of a peripheral pulse in the lower extremities, particularly one that was previously present, should be documented and reported to the physician.

Edema may develop in clients who have had injury or whose heart is unable to handle the increased workload of bed rest. Because edema moves to dependent body regions, assessment of the immobilized client should include the sacrum, legs, and feet. If the heart is unable to tolerate the increased workload, peripheral body regions, such as the hands, feet, nose, and earlobes, will be colder than central body regions.

Finally, assess the venous system, because deep vein thrombosis (DVT) is a hazard of restricted mobility. A dislodged venous thrombus, called an **embolus**, may travel through the circulatory system to the lungs and impair circulation and oxygenation. Venous emboli that travel to the lungs may be life threatening. More than 90% of all pulmonary emboli begin in the legs or pelvis (Copstead-Kirkhorn & Banaski, 2005).

To assess for a DVT, remove the client's elastic stockings or sequential compression devices (SCDs) every 8 hours and observe the calves for redness, warmth, and tenderness. Homans' sign, or calf pain on dorsiflexion of the foot, was once used as an indicator of a probable thrombus, but this sign is not always present. Checking for Homans' sign may be contraindicated in a suspected DVT, as some investigators think that vigorous dorsiflexion may dislodge the thrombus. In addition, calf circumference should be measured daily. To do this, mark a point on each calf 10 cm from the midpatella. The circumference is measured each day using the mark for placement of the tape measure. Unilateral increases in calf diameter can be an early indication of thrombosis. Because DVTs can also occur in the thigh, you should measure the thighs daily if the client is prone to thrombosis. In many clients, DVTs can be prevented by active exercise and compression devices in conjunction with prescribed anticoagulant treatment.

Musculoskeletal System. Major musculoskeletal abnormalities that may be identified during nursing assessment include decreased muscle tone and strength, loss of muscle mass, and contractures. The anthropometric measurements described previously may indicate losses in muscle tone and muscle mass. Muscle atrophy is a common complication that arises from bed rest.

Early assessment of ROM is important as a baseline against which later measurements can be compared to evaluate whether a loss in joint mobility has occurred. ROM can be measured with a goniometer.

Disuse osteoporosis (generalized bone loss resulting from the lack of mechanical stress on bones) cannot be identified by physical assessment. However, clients on prolonged bed rest, postmenopausal women, clients taking steroids, and people with increased serum and urine calcium levels have a greater risk for bone demineralization. The risk of disuse osteoporosis should be considered when planning nursing interventions. Not only may falls result in injury but they may also occur because of pathological fractures secondary to osteoporosis. Clients who are at risk for osteoporosis should have their diet assessed for calcium intake. Some clients have lactose intolerance and need dietary teaching about alternative sources of calcium (Maher et al., 2002).

Elimination System. The client's elimination status should be evaluated on each shift, and total intake and output should be evaluated every 24 hours and compared over time. You should determine that the client is receiving the correct amount and type of fluids orally or parenterally (see Chapter 40). Inadequate intake and output or fluid and electrolyte imbalances can increase the risk for renal system impairment, ranging from recurrent infections to kidney failure. Dehydration can also increase the risk for skin breakdown, thrombus formation, respiratory infections, and constipation.

Assessment of elimination status should also include the adequacy of dietary choices, bowel sounds, and the frequency and consistency of bowel movements (see Chapter 45). With accurate assessment you will be able to intervene before constipation and fecal impaction occur.

Integumentary System. Continually assess the client's skin for breakdown and colour changes such as pallor or redness. The skin should be observed when the client is turned, during hygiene measures, and when elimination needs are provided for. At a minimum, assessment should occur every 2 hours (see Chapter 47).

Psychosocial Assessment. Many alterations in physiological, sociocultural, and developmental functioning are related to immobility. Often these problems are interrelated. Nursing care must focus on all dimensions, not just on physical problems (Box 46–4).

Abrupt changes in personality may have a physiological cause, such as surgery, a medication reaction, a pulmonary embolus, or an acute infection. For example, compromised older clients have confusion as their primary symptom when experiencing a pulmonary emboli or an acute urinary tract infection. Identifying confusion is an important component of the nurse's assessment. Acute confusion in older adults is not normal and should be thoroughly examined (Ebersole et al., 2005).

Common reactions to immobilization include boredom, feelings of isolation, depression, and anger. Observe for changes in a client's emotional status. Examples of change that may indicate psychosocial concerns are a cooperative client who becomes less cooperative or an independent client who asks for more help than is necessary. Try to determine the reasons for such alterations. Identify how the client usually copes with loss (see Chapters 29 and 30). A change in mobility status, whether permanent or not, may cause a grief reaction. Families are a key resource for information about behaviour changes.

Unexplained changes in the sleep–wake cycle must be recognized and corrected. Most can be prevented or minimized, such as those occurring because of nursing activities, a noisy environment, or discomfort. They may also occur because of the effects of medications such as analgesics, sleeping pills, or cardiovascular drugs (see Chapter 41).

Because psychosocial changes usually occur gradually, observe the client's behaviour on a daily basis. If behavioural changes occur, determine the causes and evaluate the changes as short or long term. Identification of the cause will help you to design appropriate nursing interventions. For example, a fear of falling often limits the bariatric client's mobility; fear may be related to past experiences of falling and not being able to get up (Dumas, 2001). Interventions include encouraging the client to lean forward before standing rather than standing straight up, and teaching the client how to get up and down from the floor, with assistance if needed (Dumas, 2001).

Developmental Assessment. Assessment of the immobilized client should include developmental considerations to ensure that the client's needs are identified. When caring for a young child, determine whether the child can meet developmental tasks and is progressing normally. The child's development may regress or be slowed because of immobilization. By identifying a child's overall

BOX 46-4 RESEARCH HIGHLIGHT

The Meaning of Mobility

Research Focus

It is widely known that decreased mobility contributes to physical and psychological impairment. Little is known, however, about the significance of mobility to other residents and to nurses in long-term care facilities. The purpose of this study was to determine nurses' and residents' perceptions of mobility in order to develop strategies that would support mobility in the institutionalized adult.

Research Abstract

In this exploratory, qualitative study by Bourret et al. (2002), residents and nursing staff comprised focus groups in three long-term care facilities. A total of 20 residents and 15 nurses participated in the study. When asked about the importance of mobility, both groups identified it as key to quality of life. Older adults equated mobility with freedom, choice, and independence. Nurses valued mobility and associated it with freedom and autonomy. Both nurses and residents viewed having to wait for assistance as an impediment to mobility. Nurses identified further obstacles such as heavy workload and lack of time. Residents focused on physical barriers such as steep ramps, crowded elevators, and the negative attitudes of staff.

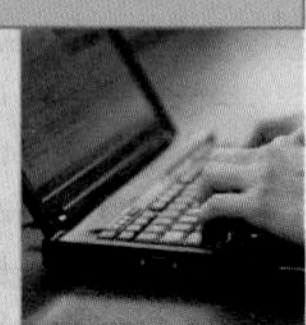

Evidence-Informed Practice

- Mobility is central to clients' quality of life and well-being.
- Nurses play a key role in assessing and assisting clients with their mobility needs.
- Nurses should focus on minimizing obstacles to mobility.
- Nurses should coordinate with other health care professionals to meet client's mobility needs.
- Nurses need to use creative strategies to encourage mobility in older adults.

References: Bourret, E., Bernick, L., Cott, C., & Kontos, P. (2002). The meaning of mobility for residents and staff in long-term care facilities. *Journal of Advanced Nursing, 37*(4), 338–345.

developmental needs, you can design nursing therapies to maintain normal development. You may also need to assure the parents that developmental delays are usually temporary.

Immobilization of a family member changes the family's functioning. The family's response to this change may lead to problems, stress, and anxieties. Children seeing parents who are immobile may have difficulty understanding what is occurring and may have difficulty coping.

Immobility can have a significant effect on the older adult's levels of health, independence, and functional status. Nursing assessment will enable you to determine the older client's ability to meet needs independently and to adapt to developmental changes such as declining physical functioning and altered family and peer relationships. A decline in developmental functioning needs prompt investigation to determine why the change occurred and what can be done to return the client to an optimal level of functioning as soon as possible. Activities that reduce immobility and promote participation in ADLs are vital to prevent functional decline (Kawamoto et al., 2006). Assessment should also include the client's home and community to identify factors that are risks to the client's mobility and safety (see Chapter 37).

Client Expectations

Clients may have unrealistic expectations of themselves or their caregivers. They may agree with the staff and understand their limitations, or they may set their expectations of themselves too high or too low. Some clients may expect to be waited on, and other clients may want to do as much as possible. Ask clients to explain what they know about their mobility status, what questions they and their families have, and how the immobility is affecting their goals.

❖Nursing Diagnosis

An immobilized or partially immobilized client may have one or more nursing diagnoses. The two diagnoses most directly related to mobility problems are *impaired physical mobility* and *risk for disuse syndrome*. The diagnosis of *impaired physical mobility* is used for the client who has some limitation but is not completely immobile. The diagnosis of *risk for disuse syndrome* should be considered for the client who is immobile and at risk for multisystem pathophysiology because of inactivity. The list of potential diagnoses is extensive, because immobility affects multiple body systems:

- *Activity intolerance*
- *Ineffective airway clearance*
- *Ineffective breathing pattern*
- *Ineffective individual coping*
- *Risk for disuse syndrome*
- *Risk for fluid volume deficit*
- *Impaired gas exchange*
- *Risk for infection*
- *Risk for injury*
- *Impaired physical mobility*
- *Impaired skin integrity*
- *Risk for impaired skin integrity*
- *Disturbed sleep pattern*
- *Social isolation*
- *Ineffective (peripheral) tissue perfusion*
- *Impaired urinary elimination*

Through assessment you should find clusters of data indicating whether a client is at risk or if an actual problem exists. Such clusters of data should include defining characteristics that support the diagnostic label and probable cause of the diagnosis. It is important to determine the probable cause of the diagnosis (on the basis of assessment data) in order to plan client-centred goals and subsequent nursing interventions.

Impaired physical mobility related to bed rest requires different interventions than those for *impaired physical mobility related to pain in the left shoulder*. Thus, you must identify and cluster defining characteristics that support the nursing diagnosis selected (Box 46–5). The diagnosis related to bed rest requires interventions aimed at keeping the client as mobile as possible and encouraging the client to do self-care and ROM exercises in bed. The diagnosis related to pain would require you to assist the client with comfort measures so that the client would subsequently be more willing and able to move. In both situations, you need to explain to the client the importance of activity to healthy body functioning.

Often the physiological dimension is the major focus of nursing care for clients with impaired mobility, and the psychosocial and developmental dimensions are neglected. However, all dimensions are important to health. For example, during immobilization, social interaction and stimuli tend to be decreased. Ultimately, the client may become isolated, withdrawn, and bored. Such clients may frequently use the call bell to request minor physical attention when their real need is greater socialization. Nursing diagnoses for health

BOX 46-5 NURSING DIAGNOSTIC PROCESS

Assessment Activities	Defining Characteristics	Nursing Diagnosis
Measure range of motion (ROM) during exercises of extremities	Client has limited ROM with left shoulder	*Impaired physical mobility related to left shoulder pain*
	Client has impaired coordination while attempting to perform ROM with left shoulder	
Observe client use left shoulder in activities of daily living	Client is reluctant to attempt movement with left shoulder	
Ask client about perception of pain	Client complains of sharp pain in shoulder	
Ask client about endurance and activity tolerance	Client reports decreased muscle strength in left shoulder	

needs in developmental areas reflect changes from the client's normal activities. Immobility can lead to a developmental crisis if the client is unable to resolve problems and continue to mature.

Immobility may also lead to complications such as pulmonary emboli or pneumonia. If these conditions develop, you will need to collaborate with the physician or nurse practitioner for prescribed therapy to intervene.

❖Planning

During planning, you will need to synthesize information from resources such as knowledge of the roles of respiratory therapy, occupational therapy, and physiotherapy; professional standards such as the RNAO (2005a, 2005b, 2007) guidelines for prevention of falls and pressure ulcers; qualities involving creativity and perseverance; and past experiences with immobilized clients (Figure 46–10).

Goals and Outcomes

Develop an individualized care plan for each nursing diagnosis (Box 46–6). You and the client should set realistic expectations for care. Goals are to be individualized, realistic, and measurable, focusing on prevention of problems or risks to body alignment and mobility. These goals are client centred and should be mutually set with the client and family.

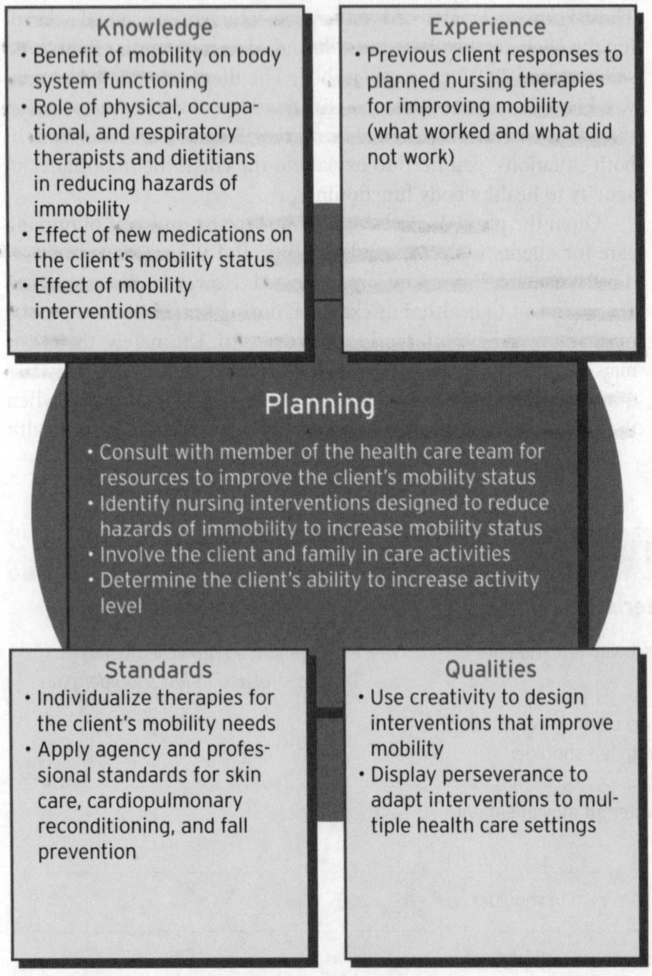

Knowledge
- Benefit of mobility on body system functioning
- Role of physical, occupational, and respiratory therapists and dietitians in reducing hazards of immobility
- Effect of new medications on the client's mobility status
- Effect of mobility interventions

Experience
- Previous client responses to planned nursing therapies for improving mobility (what worked and what did not work)

Planning
- Consult with member of the health care team for resources to improve the client's mobility status
- Identify nursing interventions designed to reduce hazards of immobility to increase mobility status
- Involve the client and family in care activities
- Determine the client's ability to increase activity level

Standards
- Individualize therapies for the client's mobility needs
- Apply agency and professional standards for skin care, cardiopulmonary reconditioning, and fall prevention

Qualities
- Use creativity to design interventions that improve mobility
- Display perseverance to adapt interventions to multiple health care settings

Figure 46-10 Critical thinking model for immobility planning.

The goals and expected outcomes are developed to assist the client in achieving his or her highest level of mobility. In addition, these goals may be written to reduce the hazards of immobility. For example, a client who has left-sided paralysis after a stroke may have two long-term goals. The first, directed toward improved mobility, may be "Client uses walker to ambulate around the home and grocery store." A parallel goal, directed toward the hazards of immobility, may be "Client's skin remains free of pressure." Both of these goals are essential to restoring maximal mobility for this client. Because sensation is impaired, both the client and caregivers must be aware of the client's need to have the skin free of pressure. Expected outcomes for the second goal could include the following:

- Client's skin colour and temperature return to normal baseline within 20 minutes of position change.
- Client's skin remains dry and intact.

Setting Priorities

In developing a care plan it is important to set priorities so that immediate needs are attended to first. This is particularly important when clients have multiple diagnoses (Figure 46–11). Plan therapies according to the severity of risks to the client. Individualize the plan according to the client's developmental stage, level of health, and lifestyle. The immediacy of any problem is determined by the effect the problem has on the client's mental and physical health.

Potential complications should not be overlooked. Many times, actual problems such as pressure ulcers and disuse osteoporosis get addressed only after they develop. Therefore, you must be vigilant in monitoring the client, reinforcing prevention techniques to both the client and other caregivers, and supervising unregulated care providers (UCPs) in carrying out activities aimed at preventing complications of impaired mobility.

Continuity of Care

The interventions planned for the client may be done directly by the nurse or delegated to UCPs. UCPs can reinforce leg exercises, use of the incentive spirometer, and coughing and deep breathing (see Chapter 39). They may also turn and position clients, apply elastic stockings, and assess leg circumferences and height and weight.

Because many of the skills associated with care of the immobile client can be delegated, you need to be vigilant in performing routine assessments to identify any developing complications early. It is also your responsibility to inform the UCP when clients are at risk for immobility hazards so that complications can be prevented. For example, although turning and positioning of a comatose client may be delegated, you must ensure that it is done correctly and that the position is changed frequently enough to reduce the risk of poor alignment and future injury to the skin and musculoskeletal system. The frequency of turning is based on client assessment for risk of pressure ulcer development (see Chapter 47).

Collaborate with other health team members such as physiotherapists or occupational therapists when considering a client's mobility needs. For example, physiotherapists are a resource for planning ROM or strengthening exercises, and occupational therapists are a resource for planning ADLs that clients need to modify or relearn. Discharge planning is begun when a client enters the health care system. In anticipation of the client's discharge from an institution, a referral may be made to help the client remain mobile or regain mobility at home. Therefore, consideration must be given to the client's home environment when planning therapies to maintain or improve body alignment and mobility.

BOX 46-6 NURSING CARE PLAN

Impaired Physical Mobility

Assessment

Ms. Barbara Adams, an 84-year-old client, has been admitted for rehabilitation after a total hip replacement for osteoarthritis. The wound is clean, dry, and intact. Staples are to be removed in 2 days. She is not able to safely transfer independently from a chair to the bed. She states that she is "afraid of falling" and frequently refuses to get out of bed. She rates her pain as a 2 on a scale of 0 to 10. Ms. Adams has a history of smoking. She states that she needs pain medication to help her sleep during the night but does not need any during the day.

Assessment Activities	***Findings and Defining Characteristics***
Assess Ms. Adams' pain level.	She rates her pain as a 2 on a scale of 0 to 10. She states that she needs pain medication at night to help her sleep, but does not need any during the day.
Assess Ms. Adams' ability to transfer.	She is not able to transfer without help from chair to bed.
Ask Ms. Adams how her surgery has affected her mobility.	She responds that she is "afraid of falling," and she frequently refuses to get out of bed.
Assess Ms. Adams' wound status.	Wound is clean, dry, and intact.

Nursing Diagnosis: Impaired physical mobility related to musculoskeletal impairment from surgery and a fear of falling

Planning

Goals (Nursing Outcomes Classification)*	***Expected Outcomes***
Ms. Adams will be free from skin breakdown by discharge.	**Tissue Integrity: Skin** Client's skin will remain intact. Client's skin will be free of erythema.
Ms. Adams will exhibit no evidence of deep vein thrombosis (DVT) by discharge.	**Tissue Perfusion: Peripheral** Client's calf diameters will remain within 1 cm of baseline through discharge. Client's lower extremity pulses will remain equal. Client will have no complaints of calf pain.
Ms. Adams will be able to safely transfer with assistance within 2 days.	**Mobility Level** Client will transfer with assistance three times per day within 2 days. Client will state fear of falling during transfer is less within 2 days.

*Outcome classification labels from Moorhead, S., Johnson, M., & Maas, M. L. (Eds.). (2004). *Nursing Outcomes Classification (NOC)* (3rd ed.). St. Louis, MO: Mosby.

Interventions (Nursing Interventions Classification)†	**Rationale**
Circulatory Care	
Administer low-dose heparin as ordered.	Administration of low-dose heparin has been shown to reduce risk for vein thrombosis (Nunnelee, 1997).
Apply graduated compression stockings (TED) as ordered and remove them each shift for hygiene.	Application increases venous tone, improving venous return and reducing venous stasis.
Reinforce antiembolic exercises while awake.	Exercises promote venous return.
Assist client out of bed slowly.	Moving slowly will decrease the likelihood of orthostatic hypotension. Moving the client slowly will also avoid the perception by the client of being rushed, which may cause the client to become fearful.
Skin Surveillance	
Instruct client to shift position every 1 to 1.5 hours while awake.	Position changes should occur every 1 to 1.5 hours or more frequently if needed. This reduces the risk of pressure ulcer development.
When recumbent, place client in 30-degree lateral position.	The 30-degree lateral position reduces pressure from the sacral area and reduces the risk of skin breakdown (RNAO, 2007).
Keep client's heels off of bed by placing a pad under the lower legs.	Use of a thin pad under the lower legs raises the heels just enough so that a paper can slide between the heels and the bed, thereby reducing the pressure on the heels so that tissue blood flow is maintained (RNAO, 2005b).
Positioning	
Explain positioning procedure to client.	Reduces anxiety.
Refer client to physiotherapy for transfer training.	Helps to strengthen muscles used in transfer.
Encourage client to assist in transfer and positioning.	Promotes independence.
Teach client safe positioning after total hip replacement, for example, no hip flexion >90 degress, do not cross legs, and when in bed use a pillow between the knees.	Minimizes risk of dislocation of hip. Client education is important for continued rehabilitation and healing.

†Intervention classification labels from Dochterman, J. M., & Bulechek, G. M. (Eds.). (2004). *Nursing Interventions Classification (NIC)* (4th ed.). St. Louis, MO: Mosby.

Continued

BOX 46-6 NURSING CARE PLAN *continued*

Evaluation

Nursing Actions	*Client Response and Finding*	*Achievement of Outcome*
Ask Ms. Adams if her mobility has improved postoperatively. Observe client transfer from bed to chair.	Client is able to transfer from the chair to the bed with assistance.	Client has achieved goal of transferring with assistance.
Observe Ms. Adams's skin integrity at each shift.	Client's wound remains clean, dry, and intact. No breakdown is noted on extremities.	Client has achieved outcome that skin will remain intact.
Perform circulatory assessment of extremities at every shift.	Client's calf diameters remain within 1 cm of baseline. Swelling, pain, redness, and warmth are not evident.	DVT is not evident.
Ask Ms. Adams to rate her fear of falling on a scale of 0 to 10.	Client rates fear of falling a 7 on a scale of 0 to 10.	Outcome of decrease in fear of falling has not been totally achieved.
	Client is getting out of bed every shift.	Continue to encourage client.

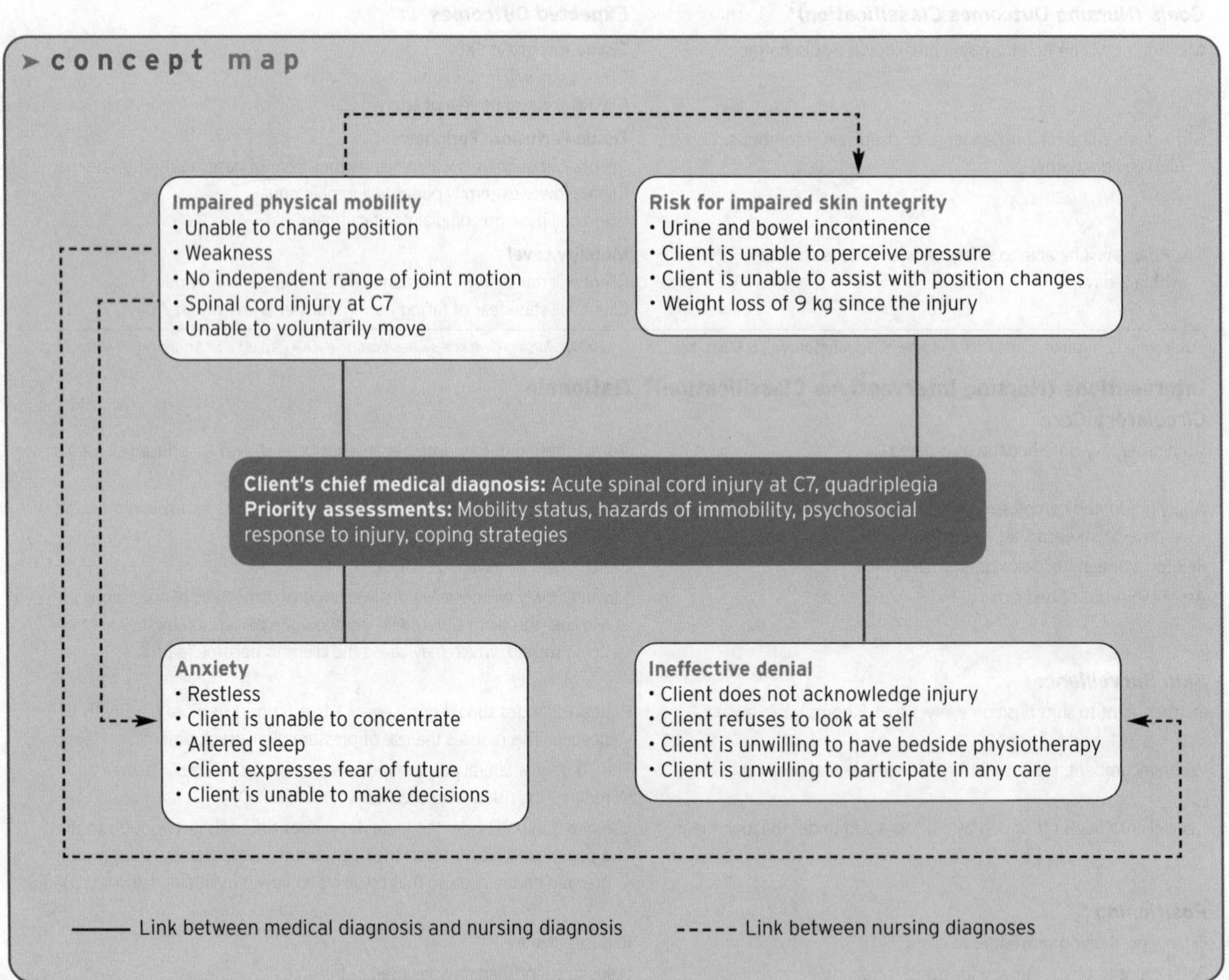

Figure 46-11 Concept map for client with acute spinal cord injury at C7 and quadriplegia.

❖Implementation

Health Promotion

Health promotion activities are an essential part of primary health care and include a variety of interventions that can be divided into education, prevention, and early detection. Encouragement of exercise should be a key health promotion strategy (Box 46–7). In promoting exercise, it is important to take into account different cultural views of what constitutes exercise (Box 46–8).

Lifting

Proper lifting techniques are important for preventing injury of clients and nurses. Musculoskeletal back injuries are a significant problem in health care, especially for nurses providing direct client care. In 1998, over 25% of occupational injuries were to the back (Association of Workers' Compensation Boards of Canada, 1999, cited in Occupational Health and Safety Agency for Healthcare in British Columbia, 2004). Back injuries are often the direct result of improper lifting and bending. The most common back injury is strain on the lumbar muscle group, which includes the muscles around the lumbar vertebrae. Injury to these areas affects the ability to bend forward, backward, and from side to side and limits the ability to rotate the hips and lower back.

Nurses and UCPs are especially at risk for injury to lumbar muscles when lifting, transferring, or positioning immobilized clients. Many health care agencies have a "no-lift" policy, in which manual lifting of the whole or a large part of the weight of the client by a health care worker is prohibited except for in exceptional or life-threatening situations. Therefore, do not attempt to lift a client without assistance unless the client is a young child or a light-weight adult who is able to help while being moved. Alternatives to manual lifting may include the use of mechanical lifts, drawsheets, friction-reduction devices, slide boards, and other handling aids (Health Care and Health & Safety Association of Ontario, 2003). Two or more people may be needed to turn or position a client.

Nurses need to be aware of good lifting techniques to protect themselves, those they supervise, and the clients being cared for. Before lifting, assess the weight to be lifted and what assistance is needed. If help is needed, determine if a second person or mechanical assistance is needed.

Once the amount of assistance is determined, the following steps should be followed:

1. Keep the weight to be lifted as close to the body as possible; this action places the object in the same plane as the lifter and close to the centre of gravity for balance.

✱ BOX 46-7 FOCUS ON PRIMARY HEALTH CARE

Promoting Exercise

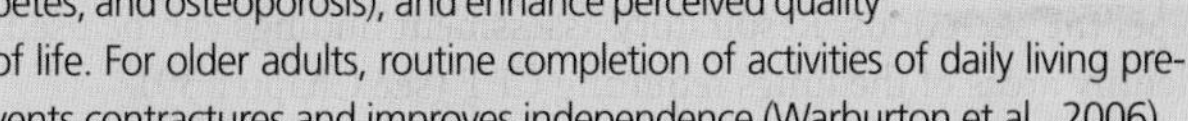

Exercise is known to increase mobility and strength, maintain functional performance, reduce the risk of many health problems (e.g., cardiovascular disease, diabetes, and osteoporosis), and enhance perceived quality of life. For older adults, routine completion of activities of daily living prevents contractures and improves independence (Warburton et al., 2006).

Functional decline from disuse is a major concern as aging occurs. Nurses can contribute to health improvement for many types of clients by encouraging or starting managed exercise programs. All people can enjoy and benefit from exercise. Even hospitalized clients can be encouraged to perform stretching, range-of-motion exercises, and light walking within the limits of their condition. However, older adults and people with mobility problems face some obstacles to physical activity (Schutzer & Graves, 2004). Nurses can do the following to help these clients participate in exercise:

- Educate clients about the importance of exercise in preserving health.
- Encourage clients to pace activities and increase speed and intensity gradually to avoid pain.
- Administer prescribed anti-inflammatory medications 1–2 hours before starting an exercise program.
- Encourage clients to balance rest and activity and to get plenty of sleep.
- Advise clients to avoid ingesting caffeine and alcohol before going to bed.
- Teach clients to use canes or walkers to assist with walking as needed.
- Encourage clients to choose smooth and even walking surfaces.
- Advise clients not to force joints past the point of resistance or pain.
- Teach clients to check legs and feet daily for redness, swelling, blisters, or broken skin.
- Teach clients to wear properly fitting shoes with non-slip soles.
- Encourage clients to walk with a companion or group so that exercise is socially rewarding.
- Consider cultural influences on choice of physical activity (see Box 46–8).

✱ BOX 46-8 CULTURAL ASPECTS OF CARE

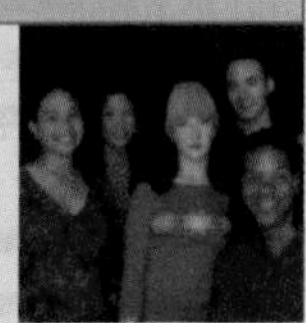

Cultural influences play an important role in defining exercise and physical activity. Often, exercise is described relative to White, middle-class values. Immigrants may be more sedentary and less likely to engage in recommended exercise activities such as joining a fitness club or golfing because they lack the financial means and social support or would not feel comfortable in fitness or golf club environments (Im & Choe, 2004). Certain cultures discourage involvement in organized recreational physical activities such as basketball, running, and aerobics. In some cultures, ethnic dancing is a more acceptable activity than organized sports (Jain & Brown, 2001). Other cultures emphasize exercise in terms of activities of daily living, such as walking, gardening, and prayer or meditation. As an example, people from Bangladesh view prayer as a structured form of exercise. Muslims value participation in community activities and may consider walking to the mosque as part of their weekly exercise regime.

Implications for Practice

- Nurses must evaluate patterns of daily living and culturally prescribed activities before suggesting specific forms of exercise to clients.
- Nurses must help clients plan physical activities that are culturally acceptable.
- Exercise programs must be flexible and accommodate the client's family, cultural, and community responsibilities.

Data from Andrews, M., & Boyle, J. (2002). *Transcultural concepts in nursing care* (4th ed.), Philadelphia: Lippincott; Cromwell, S., & Berg, J. (2006). Lifelong physical activity patterns of sedentary Mexican American women. *Geriatric Nursing, 27,* 209; Im, E., & Choe, M. (2004). Korean women's attitudes toward physical activity. *Research in Nursing and Health, 27*(1), 4–18; Lim, K., Kaiser-Jones, J., Waters, C., & Yoo, G. (2007). Aging, health and physical activity in Korean Americans. *Geriatric Nursing, 28*(2), 112; and Shin, Y., Yun, S., Jang, H., & Lim, J. (2006). A tailored program for the promotion of physical exercise among Korean adults with chronic diseases. *Applied Nursing Research, 19*(2), 88.

2. Bend at the knees; this helps to maintain the centre of gravity and uses the stronger leg muscles to do the lifting (Figure 46–12). Avoid twisting. Twisting can overload the spine and lead to serious injury.
3. Tighten abdominal muscles and tuck the pelvis; this provides balance and helps protect the back.
4. Maintain the trunk erect and knees bent so that multiple groups work together in a coordinated manner (see Chapter 36).

Nurse injuries are related not only to lifting. Many nursing activities involve bending and twisting and may cause injury. Examples of such activities include bathing, feeding, and dressing and undressing clients (Nelson et al., 2003a).

Acute Care

In the acute care setting, use interventions to reduce the hazards of immobility. You should also know proper positioning and transferring techniques to safely move clients.

Immobility Hazards. Clients in acute care settings may demonstrate some problems associated with prolonged immobility, such as impaired respiratory status, orthostatic hypotension, and impaired skin integrity. For these clients, nursing interventions are designed to reduce the impact of immobility on body systems and prepare the client for the restorative phase of care.

Metabolic System. The immobilized client requires a high-protein, high-calorie diet with vitamin B and C supplements. Protein is needed to repair injured tissue and rebuild depleted protein stores. A high-calorie intake provides sufficient fuel to meet metabolic needs and to replace subcutaneous tissue. Supplementation with vitamins C and B complex is needed for skin integrity and wound healing.

If the client is unable to eat, nutrition must be provided parenterally or enterally. Enteral feedings include delivery through a nasogastric, nasointestinal gastrostomy, or jejunostomy tube of high-protein, high-calorie solutions with complete requirements of vitamins, minerals, and electrolytes (see Chapter 43). Total parenteral nutrition refers to delivery of nutritional supplements through a central or peripheral intravenous catheter.

Respiratory System. Nursing interventions for the respiratory system are aimed at promoting expansion of the chest and lungs, preventing stasis of pulmonary secretions, maintaining a patent airway, and promoting adequate exchange of respiratory gases.

Promoting Expansion of the Chest and Lungs. Changing the position of the client at least every 2 hours allows the dependent lung regions to re-expand. Re-expansion maintains the elastic recoil property of the lungs and clears the dependent lung regions of pulmonary secretions.

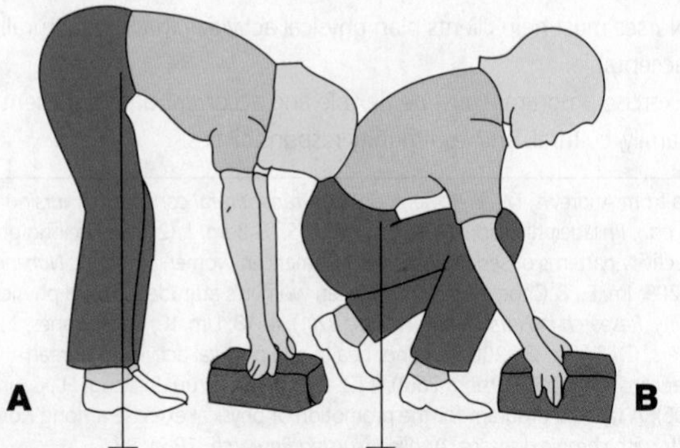

Figure 46-12 Body position for lifting. A, Incorrect. B, Correct.

Encourage the client to deep breathe and cough every 1 to 2 hours. Alert clients can be taught to deep breathe or yawn every hour or to use an incentive spirometer (see Chapter 39). Instruct the client to take in three deep breaths and cough with the third exhalation. This technique produces a more forceful, productive cough without excessive fatigue. These respiratory interventions will aid alveolar expansion and prevent atelectasis. Coughing reduces the stasis of pulmonary secretions.

If abdominal binders are required, they should be removed every 2 hours to allow the client to breathe deeply. Binders must be assessed for correct positioning and adjusted as necessary to prevent interference with respirations. Often clients will wear the binder only when ambulating. Specific physician instructions for the use of binders will vary.

Preventing Stasis of Pulmonary Secretions. Stagnant secretions accumulating in the bronchi and lungs may lead to growth of bacteria and subsequent development of pneumonia. Changing the client's position every 2 hours can reduce stagnation of secretions. This change rotates the dependent lung, mobilizing secretions.

The immobile client should take in a minimum of 2000 mL of fluid a day, if not contraindicated, to help keep mucociliary clearance normal. In clients free from infection and with adequate hydration, pulmonary secretions will appear thin, watery, and clear. The client can easily remove the secretions by coughing. Without adequate hydration, the secretions are thick and difficult to remove. Encouragement of fluid intake also benefits bowel and urine elimination and aids in maintaining circulation and skin integrity.

Chest physiotherapy (CPT; percussion and positioning) is an effective method for preventing pulmonary secretion stasis. CPT techniques help the client to drain secretions from specific segments of the bronchi and lungs into the trachea so that the client can cough and expel the secretions. Respiratory assessment findings can be used to identify areas of the lungs requiring CPT (see Chapter 39).

Maintaining a Patent Airway. Immobilized clients and those on bed rest are generally weakened. If weakness progresses, the cough reflex gradually becomes inefficient. The stasis of secretions in the lungs may be life threatening for an immobilized client because hypostatic pneumonia can easily develop. The dislodging and mobilizing of the stagnant secretions reduce the risk of pneumonia. Assessment findings that indicate this condition include productive cough with greenish yellow sputum; fever; pain on breathing; and crackles, wheezes, and dyspnea. You should actively work with the client to deep breathe and cough every 1 to 2 hours as described earlier in the section "Promoting Expansion of the Chest and Lungs."

In the immobilized client, an obstructed airway is usually a result of a mucous plug. You can implement several therapies (e.g., CPT) to reduce the risk of mucous plugs and to maintain a patent airway. Nasotracheal or orotracheal suction techniques may be used to remove secretions in the upper airways of a client who is unable to cough productively. This procedure must be performed aseptically. You can also suction secretions when clients have artificial airways such as an endotracheal or tracheal tube. Insert a catheter into the artificial airway using sterile technique. This can be used to remove pulmonary secretions from the upper and lower airways (see Chapter 39).

Cardiovascular System. The effects of bed rest or immobilization on the cardiovascular system include orthostatic hypotension, increased cardiac workload, and thrombus formation. Nursing therapies are designed to minimize or prevent these alterations.

Reducing Orthostatic Hypotension. After bed rest, clients usually have increased pulse rate and decreased pulse pressure and blood pressure. A large decrease in blood pressure when arising to a sitting or standing position (orthostatic hypotension) can result in light-headedness and fainting (Copstead-Kirkhorn & Banasik, 2005). When getting an immobile client up for the first time, you should be assisted by at least one other person. This is a precautionary step in case the client faints. The client will still be expected to do as much of the transfer as the condition allows.

Interventions should be directed toward reducing or eliminating the effects of orthostatic hypotension. Attempt to get the client moving as soon as the physical condition allows, even if this only involves sitting at the side of the bed (dangling) or moving to a chair. Changing position slowly and gradually helps to prevent orthostatic hypotension. Before the client gets up from the bed, slowly raise the head of the bed so that the client is sitting up for about 10 minutes before standing. Then help the client to sit on the side of the bed for a few minutes before the client stands up. This activity helps maintain muscle tone and increase venous return. Then help the client to stand. It is important to ask the client if he or she feels weak, dizzy, or sees spots before the eyes. If any of these symptoms occur, help the client sit down again.

Reducing Cardiac Workload. Cardiac workload is increased by immobility. A primary intervention is to discourage clients from holding their breath while bearing down (the Valsalva manoeuvre), as may occur when the client is moving up in bed or straining to defecate. The Valsalva manoeuvre increases intrathoracic pressure, thus decreasing venous return and cardiac output. When the strain is released, venous return and cardiac output immediately increase and systolic blood pressure and pulse pressure rise. These pressure changes produce a reflex bradycardia and a possible decrease in blood pressure that may cause sudden cardiac death in clients with heart disease. Remind the client to breathe out while moving or being lifted up in bed.

Preventing Thrombus Formation. The most cost-effective way to address the problem of deep vein thrombosis (DVT) is through prevention (prophylaxis). It begins with identifying clients at risk and continues throughout the time clients are immobile or otherwise at risk. This is clearly a collaborative venture between nurses and physicians. You can easily identify risk factors during an admission nursing assessment. Many interventions reduce the risk of thrombus formation in the immobilized client. Leg exercises, encouragement of fluids, position changes, and teaching of such preventive measures should begin when the client becomes immobile. Preoperative clients should be given this information before surgery (see Chapter 49). Other interventions such as intermittent pneumatic compression (IPC) and sequential compression devices (SCDs) require a physician's order. Maintenance and administration of prophylaxis is a nursing role, and nurses can determine when the client is fully mobile postoperatively, decreasing the continued risk for DVT.

Medications also require a physician's order. Heparin and low-molecular-weight heparin (LMWH) are the most widely used drugs in the prophylaxis of DVT. Standard heparin is considered the gold standard for treatment because it has been well studied and validated. Common dosage for heparin therapy is 5000 units given subcutaneously 2 hours before surgery and repeated every 8 to 12 hours until the client is fully mobile or discharged. Heparin is an anticoagulant, and it suppresses clot formation. Because of the action of this medication, you must continually assess the client for signs of bleeding, such as increased bruising, guaiac-positive stools, and bleeding gums. Common dosage of Lovenox (LMWH) to prevent DVT is 30 to 40 mg subcutaneously 2 hours before surgery and continued throughout the postoperative period. Although most clients receiving LMWH do not experience side effects, the risk of bleeding is present (Nunnelee, 1997).

SCDs and IPCs consist of sleeves or stockings made of fabric or plastic that are wrapped around the leg and secured with Velcro (Box 46–9). The sleeves are then connected to a pump that alternately inflates and deflates the stocking around the leg. A typical cycle is

➤ BOX 46-9 Procedural Guidelines

Application of Sequential Compression Stockings

Delegation Considerations: The skill of applying sequential compression stockings (SCSs) can be delegated to unregulated care providers (UCPs). The nurse is responsible for assessing circulation in the extremities; therefore, when application of the SCSs is delegated, it is important to instruct the UCP to do the following:

- Notify the nurse if the client complains of pain in the leg.
- Notify the nurse if discoloration develops in the extremities.

Equipment

Tape measure, sequential stockings, stockinette, hygiene supplies

Procedure

1. Assess the client for the need for sequential compression stockings.
2. Obtain baseline assessment data about the status of circulation, pulse, and skin integrity on the client's lower extremities before initiating application of sequential compression stockings.
3. Measure the client for proper-size stocking by measuring around the largest part of the client's thigh. Review the manufacturer's directions regarding measuring for proper fit.
4. Perform hand hygiene. Provide hygiene to lower extremities if needed.
5. Place a protective stockinette over the client's leg.
6. Wrap the stocking around the leg, starting at the ankle, with the opening over the patella (see Step 6 illustration).
   A. Attach the stockings to the insufflator and verify that the intermittent pressure is between 35 and 45 mm Hg.
7. Record date and time of stocking application, and stocking length and size in nurses' notes.
8. Record condition of skin and circulatory assessment.
9. Monitor skin integrity and circulation to the client's lower extremities as ordered or according to the manufacturer's guidelines.

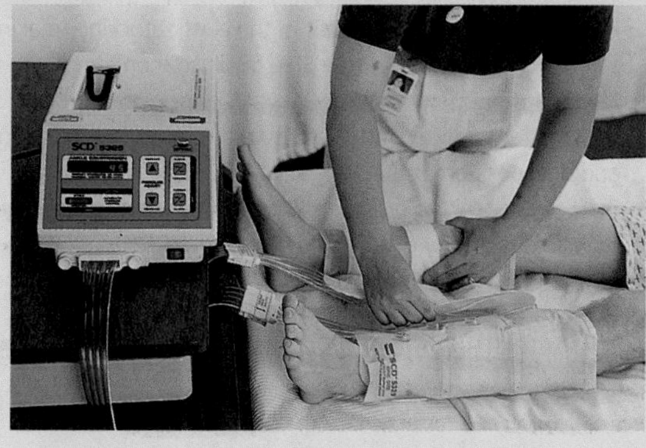

Step 6 Application of sequential compression stocking.

inflation for 10 to 15 seconds and deflation for 45 to 60 seconds. Inflation pressures average 40 mm Hg. Use of SCDs or IPCs on the legs decreases venous stasis by increasing venous return through the deep veins of the legs. For optimal results, use of SCDs or IPCs is begun as soon as possible and maintained until the client becomes fully ambulatory. Graded compression stockings can help prevent DVT, but clients must receive the right size, and the SCD or IPC must be used correctly.

Elastic stockings (sometimes called *thromboembolic device hose* [TED]) also aid in maintaining external pressure on the muscles of the lower extremities and thus may promote venous return (Box 46–10). When considering applying TED stockings, first assess the client's suitability for wearing them. The stockings should not be applied if any local condition affects the leg (e.g., any skin lesion, gangrenous condition, or recent vein ligation) because application may compromise circulation. You will need to measure the client's legs with a tape measure to determine proper stocking size. The stockings must be applied properly, and they must be removed and reapplied at least twice a day. Assess circulation at the toes to ensure that the hose are not too tight. In addition, the stockings should always be clean and dry; it may be useful for the client to have two pairs.

Positioning techniques aid in reducing compression of the leg veins. Proper positioning used with other therapies (e.g., heparin or TED stockings) aids in reducing the client's risk of thrombus formation. When positioning clients, use caution to prevent pressure on the posterior knee and deep veins in the lower extremities. Client teaching should include avoiding crossing the legs, not sitting for prolonged periods of time, not wearing clothing that constricts the legs or waist, not putting pillows under the knees, and avoiding massaging the legs.

Although ROM exercises are designed to reduce the risk of contractures, they may also aid in preventing thrombi. Activity causes contraction of the skeletal muscles, which in turn exerts pressure on the veins to promote venous return, thereby reducing venous stasis. Specific exercises that help prevent thrombophlebitis are ankle pumps, foot circles, and knee flexion. Ankle pumps, sometimes called

➤ BOX 46-10 Procedural Guidelines

Application of Thromboembolic Device Hose

Delegation Considerations: The skill of applying thromboembolic device (TED) hose can be performed by unregulated care providers (UCPs). The nurse is responsible for assessing circulation to the lower extremities; therefore, when application of the TED hose is delegated, it is important to instruct the UCP to report if the client develops leg pain or discoloration.

Equipment

Tape measure, TED hose, hygiene supplies

Procedure

1. Assess the need for elastic stockings and condition of the client's skin.
2. Observe for conditions that might contraindicate use of stockings.
3. Perform hand hygiene. Provide hygiene to lower extremities if needed.
4. Use tape measure to measure the client's legs to determine proper stocking size (measure according to manufacturer's directions). Elastic stockings come in two lengths: knee length and thigh length.
5. Apply stockings:
   A. Turn elastic stocking inside out up to the heel. Place one hand into the sock, holding heel. Pull top of sock with the other hand inside out over foot of sock.
   B. Place client's toes into the foot of the elastic stocking, making sure that sock is smooth (see Step 5B illustration).
   C. Slide remaining portion of sock over the client's foot, being sure that the toes are covered. Make sure the foot fits into the toe and heel position of the sock (see Step 5C illustration).
   D. Slide top of sock up over client's calf until sock is completely extended. Be sure sock is smooth and no ridges or wrinkles are present, particularly behind the knee (see Step 5D illustration).
6. Instruct client not to roll socks partially down.
7. Record date and time of stocking application, and stocking length and size in nurses' notes.
8. Record condition of skin and circulatory assessment.

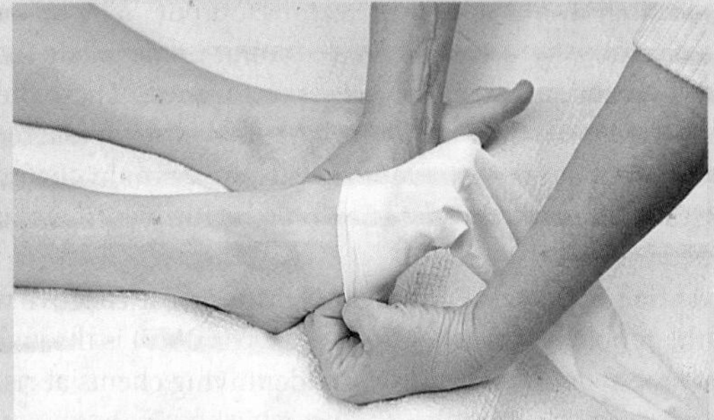

Step 5B

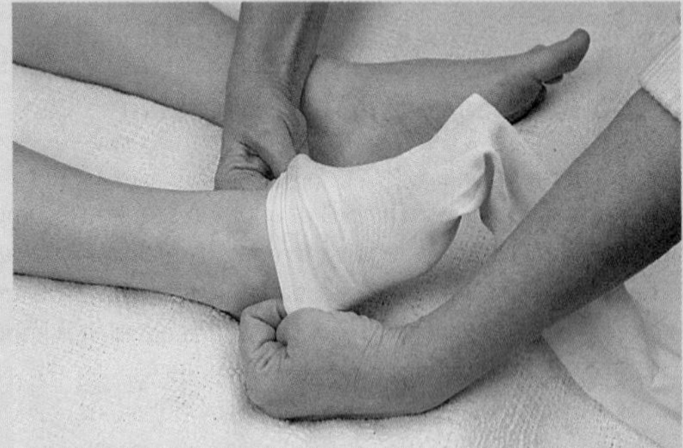

Step 5C

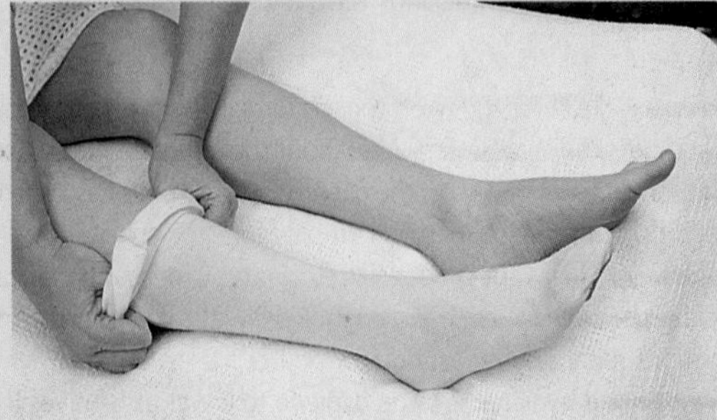

Step 5D

calf pumps, include alternating plantar flexion and dorsiflexion. To perform foot circles, the client rotates the ankle. Making the letters of the alphabet with their feet every 1 to 2 hours is a good exercise for clients. Knee flexion involves alternately extending and flexing the knee. These exercises are sometimes referred to as *antiembolic exercises* and should be done hourly while the client is awake.

When DVT is suspected, you should report it immediately. The leg should be elevated with no pressure on the thrombus. The family, client, and all health care personnel should be instructed to not massage the area because of the danger of dislodging the thrombus.

Musculoskeletal System. The immobilized client must receive some exercise to prevent or minimize muscle atrophy and joint contractures. If the client is unable to move part or all of the body, perform passive ROM exercises for all immobilized joints while bathing the client and at least two or three more times a day (see "Restorative Care" section). If one extremity is paralyzed, the client can be taught to put each joint independently through its ROM. Clients on bed rest should have active ROM exercises incorporated into their daily schedules. Nurses can teach clients to integrate exercises during ADLs. Some orthopedic conditions require frequent passive ROM exercises to restore the injured joint's function after surgery. Clients with such conditions may use automatic equipment (continuous passive motion [CPM]) for passive ROM exercises (Figure 46–13). The CPM machine moves an extremity to a prescribed angle for a prescribed period. This is beneficial when the client must gradually increase the degree and duration of flexion and extension. Researchers are currently investigating new uses for CPM. In one study, clients who had suffered a cerebrovascular accident (CVA) and who received CPM therapy to their affected shoulder had better joint stability than that of clients who received traditional ROM exercises (Lynch et al., 2005).

Active ROM exercises help maintain function of the musculoskeletal system. You should also plan interventions for the gradual return of mobility for clients who will be able to resume normal activity. The best nursing intervention is establishing an individualized progressive exercise program (Shin et al., 2006). A progressive exercise program gradually increases the client's physical activity to reverse the deconditioning associated with immobility. Progressive exercise programs are used for clients with musculoskeletal, neurological, cardiopulmonary, renal, and other chronic diseases.

When working with older adults, keep in mind gerontological principles that enhance the effectiveness of exercise programs and limit injuries (Box 46–11).

Teaching, referral, and interdisciplinary collaboration are important for clients with limited mobility. Depending on the setting and resources available, you may want to refer the client for physiotherapy. The therapist would set up the specific exercise program, and the nurse would reinforce it.

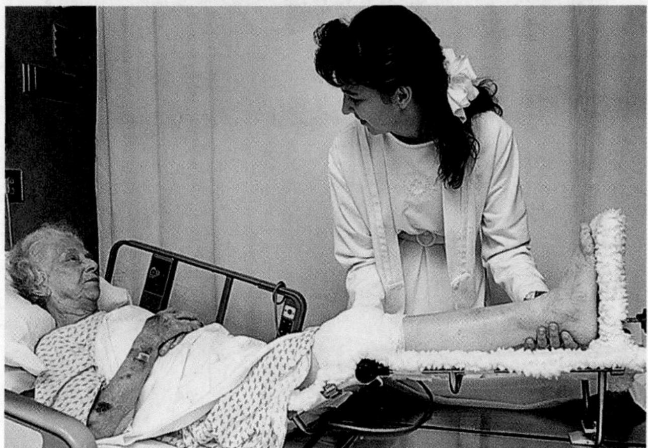

Figure 46-13 Continuous passive motion machine.

Elimination System. The nursing interventions for maintaining optimal urinary functioning are directed at keeping the client well hydrated and preventing urinary stasis, calculi, and infections without causing bladder distension.

Adequate hydration (i.e., 2000 to 3000 mL of fluids per day) helps prevent renal calculi and urinary tract infections. The well-hydrated client should void large amounts of dilute urine that are approximately equal to fluid intake. If the client is incontinent, modify the care plan to include toileting aids and a hygiene schedule so that the increased urinary output does not cause skin breakdown.

To prevent bladder distension, assess the frequency and amount of urinary output. A client who continually dribbles urine and whose bladder is distended may have overflow incontinence. If the immobilized client does not have voluntary control of bladder elimination, bladder training may be necessary. If the client experiences bladder distension, you may be required to insert a straight catheter or an indwelling Foley catheter (see Chapter 44).

The frequency and consistency of bowel movements must be recorded. A diet rich in fluids, fruits, vegetables, and fibre can facilitate normal peristalsis. If a client is unable to maintain regular bowel patterns, stool softeners, cathartics, or enemas may be needed (see Chapter 45).

Integumentary System. The major risk to the skin from restricted mobility is the formation of pressure ulcers. Early identification of high-risk clients and their risk factors can aid you in preventing pressure ulcers (see Chapter 47). Interventions aimed at prevention are positioning, skin care, and the use of therapeutic devices to relieve pressure. The immobilized client's position should be changed according to the client's activity level, perceptual ability,

BOX 46-11 FOCUS ON OLDER ADULTS

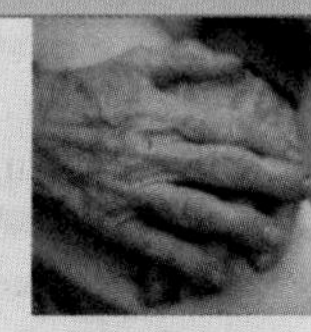

You should base an older client's exercise program on individual assessment data (underlying conditions, medications, present activity level). Before starting an exercise program, consult the physician for exercise restrictions. Modification of the exercise program is based on the individual's responses. Instruct the client to do the following:

- Use correct body mechanics, wear appropriate clothing and footwear, and maintain sufficient hydration.
- Perform a gradual, extended exercise warm-up (e.g., 15 minutes) to maximize flexibility and decrease muscle injury.
- Begin at a low level (40%–50% of predicted maximal heart rate; maximal heart rate is estimated as the number 220 minus client's age), and follow gentle exercise progression.
- Avoid sudden twisting movements, rapid movements, and rapid transitions from one movement to the next.
- Avoid exercises that tax vision and balance.
- Avoid sustained isometric contractions of >10 seconds.
- Avoid exercise during acute viral infections.
- Stop exercising if cardiac dysrhythmias, angina, or excessive breathlessness occurs.
- Perform cool-down exercises until the heart rate returns to resting level to decrease postural hypotension and cardiac dysrhythmias.

Adapted from Ebersole, P., Hess, P., Touhy, T., & Jett, K. (2005). *Geriatric nursing and healthy aging* (2nd ed.). St. Louis, MO: Elsevier Mosby.

treatment protocols, and daily routines. Although turning every 1 to 2 hours is recommended for preventing ulcers, it may also be necessary to use devices for relieving pressure. The amount of time that a client sits uninterrupted in a chair should be limited to 1 hour or less, although this time interval is individualized. The client should be repositioned frequently because uninterrupted pressure will cause skin breakdown. You should teach clients who are able to do so to shift their weight every 15 minutes. Chair-bound clients should have a device for the chair that reduces pressure; however, donut-shaped devices should not be used (RNAO, 2007).

Psychosocial Changes. Through assessment you can identify effects of prolonged immobilization on the client's psychosocial dimension. People who have a tendency toward depression or mood swings are at greater risk for developing psychosocial changes during bed rest or immobilization.

You should anticipate changes in the client's psychosocial status and provide routine and informal socialization. Nursing activities can be planned so that the client can talk and interact with staff. If possible, the client should be placed in a room with others who are mobile and interactive. If a private room is required, staff members and family should be asked to visit throughout the shift to provide meaningful interaction.

Provide stimuli to maintain a client's orientation. Maintaining a calendar and clock; providing a newspaper, books, radio, or television; and encouraging visits from significant others may reduce the risk of social isolation. Spending time in the room talking and listening to the client also helps reduce isolation.

An important part of nursing care for immobilized clients is encouraging them to perform as many ADLs as independently as possible. Clients should continue to perform personal grooming if they did so before their mobility was restricted. This type of activity preserves the client's dignity and gives the client a sense of accomplishment.

In institutional health care settings, nursing care given between 2200 hours and 0700 hours should be scheduled to minimize interruptions of sleep. For example, the nurse may administer medications and assess vital signs at the time when the client is turned or receives special skin care.

Observe the client's ability to cope with restricted mobility. If the nursing care plan is not improving coping patterns, a clinical nurse specialist, counsellor, social worker, spiritual adviser, or other consultant may be needed. Their recommendations should be incorporated into the care plan.

Developmental Changes in Children. Ideally, immobilized clients continue normal development; nursing interventions can help with this. Nursing care should provide mental and physical stimulation, particularly for a young child. Play activities can be incorporated into the care plan. Completing puzzles, for example, helps a child to develop fine motor skills, and reading helps the child to develop cognitively. Parents should be encouraged to stay with a child who is hospitalized. An immobilized child should be placed with children of the same age who are not immobilized, unless a contagious disease is present. You must watch for significant changes from normal behavioural patterns. If these changes continue, consult with a clinical nurse, counsellor, or other health care professional whose specialty is children.

Positioning Devices and Techniques. Clients with impaired function of the nervous, skeletal, or muscular system and with general weakness often require your help to attain proper body alignment while in bed or sitting. You must assess skin integrity regularly for pressure points or skin breakdown when using positioning devices.

Several positioning devices are available for maintaining good body alignment for clients:

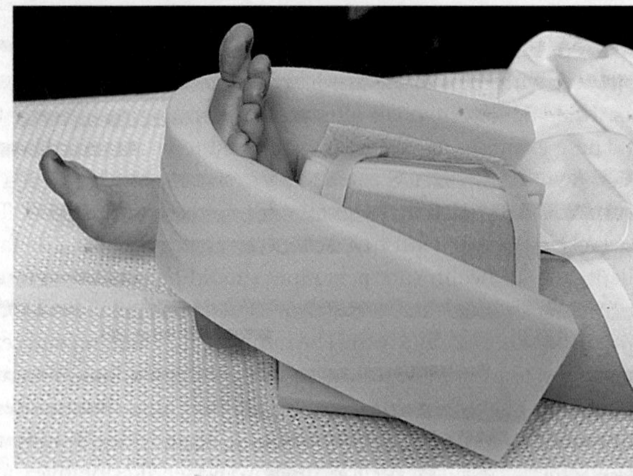

Figure 46-14 Foot boot.

- *Pillows:* These provide support, elevate body parts, and can splint incisional areas, reducing postoperative pain during activity or coughing and deep breathing. Before using a pillow, you should determine whether it is the proper size. A thick pillow under the client's head increases cervical flexion. A thin pillow under body prominences may be inadequate to protect skin and tissue from damage caused by pressure. When additional pillows are unavailable, or if they are an improper size, folded sheets, blankets, or towels can be used as positioning aids.
- *Wedge (or abductor) pillow:* This is a triangular-shaped pillow made of heavy foam used to maintain the legs in abduction after total hip replacement surgery.
- *Foot boot:* This maintains feet in dorsiflexion. Foot boots are made of rigid plastic or heavy foam (Figure 46–14). They keep the foot flexed at the proper angle and the weight of the bedsheets off the toes. Remove the foot boots two or three times a day to assess skin integrity and joint mobility.
- *Trochanter roll:* This prevents external rotation of the hips when the client is in a supine position. A **trochanter roll** is formed by folding a cotton bath blanket lengthwise to a width that will extend from the greater trochanter of the femur to the lower border of the popliteal space (Figure 46–15). The blanket is placed under the buttocks and then rolled counterclockwise until the thigh is in neutral position or in inward rotation. When correct alignment of the hip is achieved, the patella faces directly upward.

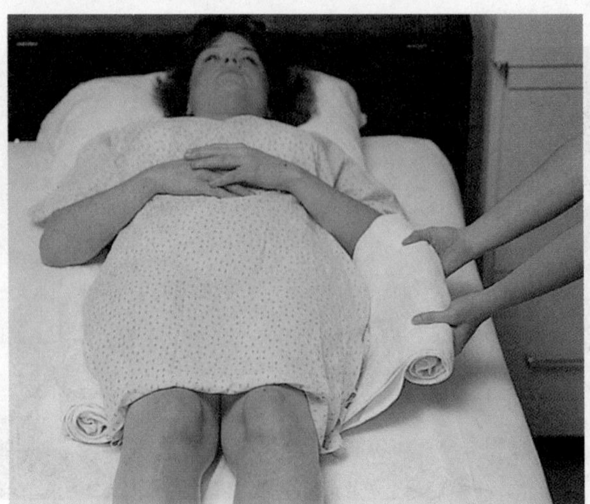

Figure 46-15 Trochanter roll.

- *Sandbags:* These are sand-filled plastic tubes or bags that can be shaped to body contours. Sandbags can be used in place of or in addition to trochanter rolls. They immobilize an extremity or maintain body alignment.
- *Hand rolls* maintain the thumb in slight adduction and in opposition to the fingers. A hand roll maintains the hand, thumb, and fingers in a functional position, thus preventing contractures (Figure 46–16). Evaluate the hand roll to make sure that the hand is indeed in a functional position. Hand rolls are most often used for clients whose arms are paralyzed or who are unconscious. Rolled washcloths should not be used as hand rolls, because they do not keep the thumb well abducted, especially in clients who have a spastic paralysis.
- *Hand–wrist splints:* These are individually moulded for the client to maintain proper alignment of the thumb (slight adduction) and the wrist (slight extention). These splints should be used only by the client for whom the splint was made (Figure 46–17).
- *Trapeze bar:* This is a triangular device that descends from a securely fastened overhead bar attached to the bed frame. A **trapeze bar** allows the client to use their upper extremities to raise their trunk off the bed, to assist in transfer from bed to wheelchair, or to perform arm exercises (Figure 46–18). It is a useful device for helping to increase independence, maintain upper body strength, and decrease the shearing action from sliding across or up and down in bed.

Although procedures for each position have specific guidelines, some universal steps should be followed for clients who require positioning assistance (Skill 46–1). By following the guidelines, you reduce the risk of injury to the musculoskeletal system. When joints are unsupported, their alignment is impaired. Joints must be positioned in a slightly flexed position or their mobility is decreased. During positioning, it is important to also assess bony prominences (pressure points; see Figure 47–2). When actual or potential pressure areas exist, nursing interventions involve removal of the pressure, thus decreasing the risk for development of pressure ulcers and further trauma to the musculoskeletal system. For clients at risk for pressure ulcers, the 30-degree lateral position should be used (see Chapter 47).

Supported Fowler's Position. In the supported Fowler's position, the head of the bed is elevated 45 to 60 degrees and the client's knees are slightly elevated without pressure; the client is sitting up in bed. Do not elevate the head of the bed more than 60 degrees because this would increase shearing force on the client's back and heels. The angle of head and knee elevation and the length of time that the client should remain in the supported Fowler's position vary depending on the client's illness and overall condition. Supports must permit flexion of the hips and knees and proper alignment of the normal curves in the cervical, thoracic, and lumbar vertebrae. The following are common trouble areas for the client in the supported Fowler's position (see Skill 46–1 for preventive measures):

- Excessive cervical flexion because the pillow at the head is too thick and the head thrusts forward.
- Hyperextension of the knees, allowing the client to slide to the foot of the bed.
- Pressure on the posterior aspect of the knees, decreasing circulation to the feet.
- External rotation of the hips.
- Arms hanging unsupported at the client's sides.
- Unsupported feet or pressure on the heels.
- Unprotected pressure points at the sacrum and heels.

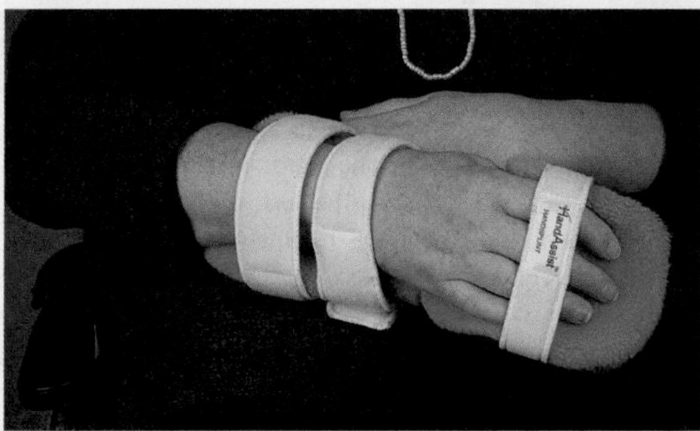

Figure 46-17 Hand–wrist splint. **Source:** From Sorrentino, S. A., Wilk, M. J., & Newmaster, R. (2008). *Mosby's Canadian textbook for the support worker* (2nd ed.). Toronto, ON: Elsevier.

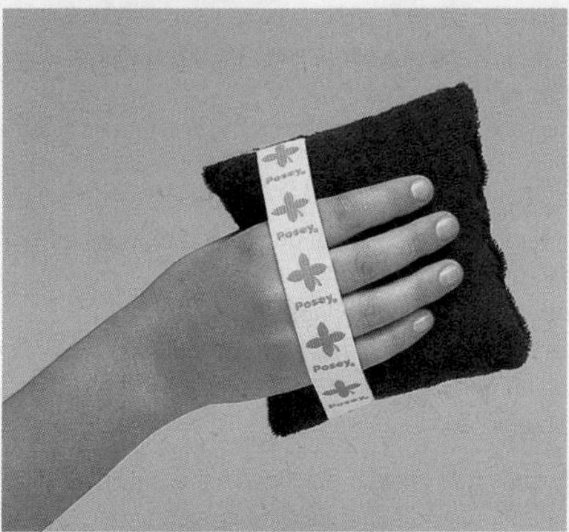

Figure 46-16 Hand roll. **Source:** Courtesy J. T. Posey, Arcadia, CA.

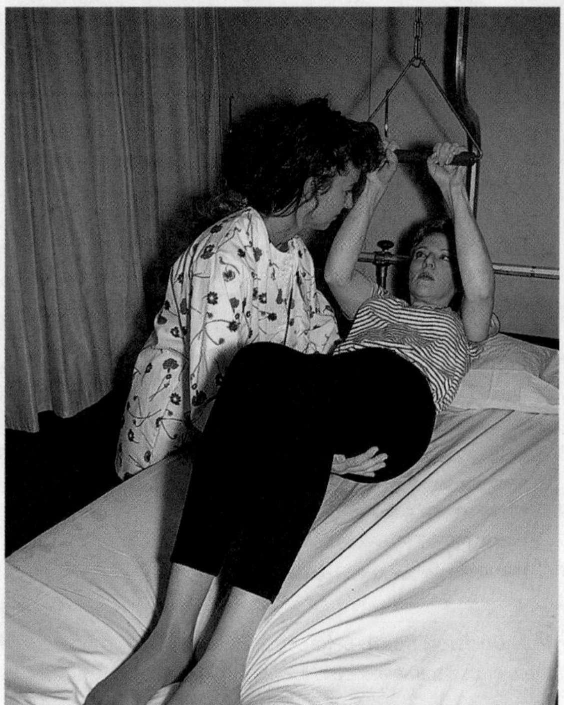

Figure 46-18 Client using a trapeze bar.

➤ SKILL 46-1 Moving and Positioning Clients in Bed

video

Delegation Considerations

The skills of moving and positioning clients in bed can be delegated to unregulated care providers (UCPs). The nurse is responsible for assessing the client's level of comfort and for any potential hazards. It is important to instruct the UCP on any limitations affecting movement and positioning of the client in bed.

Equipment

- Pillows
- Drawsheet or friction-reducing device
- Positioning devices as required (e.g., trochanter roll, extra pillows, hand rolls, etc.)

Procedure

STEPS	RATIONALE
1. Assess client's body alignment and comfort level while client is lying down.	• Provides baseline data for later comparisons. Determines ways to improve position and alignment.
2. Assess for risk factors that may contribute to complications of immobility:	• Increased risk factors require client to be repositioned more frequently.
A. Paralysis: Hemiparesis resulting from cerebrovascular accident; decreased sensation	• Paralysis impairs movement and causes muscle tone changes; sensation can be affected. Because of difficulty in moving and poor awareness of the involved body part, the client is unable to protect and position the affected body part.
B. Impaired mobility: Traction or arthritis or other contributing disease processes	• Traction or arthritic changes of affected extremity result in decreased range of motion (ROM).
C. Impaired circulation	• Decreased circulation predisposes the client to pressure sores.
D. Age: Very young, older adults	• Premature and young infants require frequent turning because their skin is fragile. Normal physiological changes associated with aging predispose older adults to greater risks for developing complications of immobility.
E. Level of consciousness and mental status	• Comatose or semicomatose clients are unable to convey areas of skin pressure, increasing the risk for skin breakdown.
F. Assess condition of client's skin.	• Provides a baseline to determine effects of positioning.
3. Assess client's physical ability to help with moving and positioning:	• Enables nurse to use client's mobility and strength. Determines need for additional help. Ensures client's and nurse's safety.
A. Age	• Older adult clients may move more slowly and with less strength.
B. Level of consciousness and mental status	• Determines need for special aids or devices. • Clients with altered levels of consciousness may not understand instructions and may be unable to help.
C. Disease process	• Cardiopulmonary disease may require the client to have the head of the bed elevated.
D. Strength, coordination	• Determines amount of assistance provided by client during position change.
E. ROM	• Limited ROM may contraindicate certain positions.
4. Assess physician's orders. Clarify whether any positions are contraindicated because of the client's condition (e.g., spinal cord injury; respiratory difficulties; certain neurological conditions; presence of incisions, drain, or tubing).	• Placing client in an inappropriate position could cause injury.
5. Perform hand hygiene.	• Reduces transfer of microorganisms.
6. Assess for the presence of tubes, incisions, and equipment (e.g., traction).	• Will alter positioning procedure and may affect client's ability to independently change positions.
7. Assess the ability and motivation of the client, family members, and primary caregiver to participate in moving and positioning the client in bed in anticipation of discharge to home.	• Determines ability of the client and caregivers to assist with positioning.
8. Raise level of bed to a comfortable working height, and get extra help if needed.	• Raises level of work to centre of gravity and provides for client's and nurse's safety.
9. Perform hand hygiene.	• Reduces transfer of microorganisms.
10. Explain procedure to client.	• Decreases anxiety and increases client cooperation.
11. Position client flat in bed if this is tolerated.	• Repositioning from a flat position decreases friction and possible shear on client's skin.

Critical Decision Point: Before flattening the bed, account for all tubing, drains, and equipment to prevent dislodgement or tipping if caught in the mattress or bed frame as bed is lowered.

➤ SKILL 46-1 Moving and Positioning Clients in Bed ***continued***

STEPS	RATIONALE
12. Position client in bed.	
A. Assist client in moving up in bed (one or two nurses). NOTE: Only a young child or a lightweight client requiring minimal assistance can be safely moved by one nurse.	
(1) Remove pillow from under the head and shoulders, and place pillow at head of bed. Ask client to cross arms across the chest.	• Prevents striking of client's head against head of the bed. • Reduces surface area and friction.
(2) Face head of bed.	• Facing the direction of movement prevents twisting of nurse's body while moving the client.
(a) Each nurse should have one arm under the client's shoulders and one arm under the client's thighs.	
(b) Alternative position: Position one nurse at the client's upper body. The nurse's arm nearest head of bed should be under the clients' head and opposite shoulder; the other arm should be under the client's closest arm and shoulder. Position the other nurse at client's lower torso. The nurse's arms should be under the client's lower back and torso.	• Prevents trauma to client's musculoskeletal system by supporting shoulder and hip joints and evenly distributing weight.
(3) Place feet apart, with foot nearest head of bed behind the other foot (forward–backward stance; see Step 12A(3) illustration).	• A wide base of support increases balance. This stance enables you to shift body weight as the client is moved up in bed, thereby reducing force needed to move load.
(4) Ask client to flex knees with feet flat on bed.	• Decreases friction and enables client to use leg muscles during movement.
(5) Instruct client to flex neck, tilting chin toward chest.	• Prevents hyperextension of neck when moving client up in bed.
(6) Instruct client to assist moving by pushing with feet on bed surface.	• Reduces friction. Increases client mobility. Decreases workload.
(7) Flex knees and hips, bringing forearms closer to the level of the bed.	• Increases balance and strength by bringing the centre of gravity closer to the client. Uses thighs instead of back muscles.
(8) Instruct client to push with heels and elevate trunk while breathing out, thus moving toward head of bed on a count of 3.	• Prepares client for move. Reinforces assistance in moving up in bed. Increases client cooperation. Breathing out avoids Valsalva manoeuvre.
(9) On count of 3, rock and shift weight from back to front leg. At the same time, the client pushes with heels and elevates trunk.	• Rocking enables you to improve balance and overcome inertia. Shifting weight counteracts the client's weight and reduces the force needed to move load. The client's assistance reduces friction and workload.
B. Move immobile client up in bed with drawsheet or friction-reducing device (two nurses are needed).	
(1) Adjust bed to appropriate height for caregiver's body mechanics. Place drawsheet or friction-reducing device under the client by turning side to side. Have sheet extend from shoulders to thighs. Return client to supine position.	• Supports client's body weight and reduces friction during movement. Reduces risk of injury to caregivers and maximizes leaverage to move the client safely.
(2) Position one nurse at each side of the client.	• Distributes weight equally between nurses.

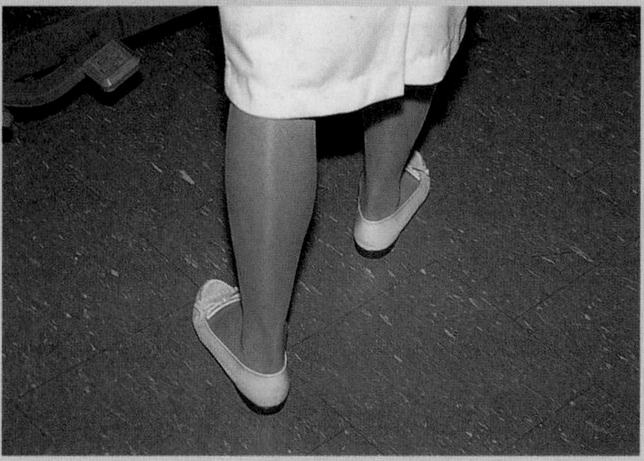

Step 12A(3) Position of feet: feet placed apart in a forward-to-backward stance.

Continued

➤ SKILL 46-1 **Moving and Positioning Clients in Bed** ***continued***

STEPS	RATIONALE
(3) Grasp drawsheet or friction-reducing device firmly near the client with palms facing up.	
(4) Place feet apart with forward–backward stance. Flex knees and hips. Shift weight from back to front leg, and move client and drawsheet or friction-reducing device to desired position in bed.	• Facing the direction of movement ensures proper balance. Shifting weight reduces the force needed to move load. Flexing knees lowers the centre of gravity and uses thighs instead of back muscles.
(5) Realign client in correct body alignment.	• Prevents injury to musculoskeletal system.
C. Position client in supported Fowler's position (see Step 12C illustration).	
(1) Elevate head of bed 45–60 degrees.	• Increases comfort, improves ventilation, and increases client's opportunity to socialize or relax.
(2) Rest client's head against mattress or on a small pillow.	• Prevents flexion contractures of cervical vertebrae.
(3) Use pillows to support arms and hands if the client does not have voluntary control or use of hands and arms.	• Prevents shoulder subluxation from effect of downward pull of unsupported arms, promotes circulation by preventing venous pooling, and prevents flexion contractures of arms and wrists.
(4) Position pillow at lower back.	• Supports lumbar vertebrae and decreases flexion of vertebrae.
(5) Place a small pillow under thigh.	• Prevents hyperextension of knee and occlusion of popliteal artery caused by pressure from body weight.
(6) Position client's heel in heel boots or other heel pressure relief devices.	• Heel pressure relief devices are more effective than pillows for consistently reducing pressure from the mattress on the heels. When pillows are used, they must be repositioned each time the client moves.

Critical Decision Point: A foot cradle may also be used in clients with poor peripheral circulation as a means of reducing pressure on the tips of a client's toes.

STEPS	RATIONALE
D. Position hemiplegic client in supported Fowler's position.	
(1) Elevate head of bed 45–60 degrees.	• Increases comfort, improves ventilation, and increases client's opportunity to relax.
(2) Position client in sitting position as straight as possible.	• Counteracts tendency to slump toward affected side. Improves ventilation and cardiac output, and decreases intracranial pressure. Improves client's ability to swallow and helps to prevent aspiration of food, liquids, and gastric secretions.
(3) Position head on a small pillow with the chin slightly forward. If client is totally unable to control head movement, hyperextension of the neck must be avoided.	• Prevents hyperextension of neck. Too many pillows under the head may cause or worsen neck flexion contracture.

Critical Decision Point: If the client has a paralyzed extremity, provide support for involved arm and hand on overbed table in front of client. Place arm away from the client's side and support elbow with pillow.

- Position *flaccid* hand in a normal resting position with the wrist slightly extended, arches of hand maintained, and fingers partially flexed. You may use a hand grip or section of rubber ball cut in half; clasp client's hands together.
- Position *spastic* hand with wrist in neutral position or slightly extended; fingers should be extended with palm down. It may be difficult to position spastic hands without the use of specially made splints for the client (discuss with occupational therapist).

STEPS	RATIONALE
(4) Flex client's knees and hips by using a pillow or folded blanket under the knees.	• Ensures proper alignment. Flexion prevents prolonged hyperextension, which could impair joint mobility.
(5) Support feet in dorsiflexion with firm pillow or therapeutic boots or splints.	• Prevents footdrop. Stimulation of ball of the foot by a hard surface has a tendency to increase muscle tone in a client with extensor spasticity of lower extremity. Therapeutic boots or splints are manufactured with thick padding to cushion the heel and prevent pressure ulcers.

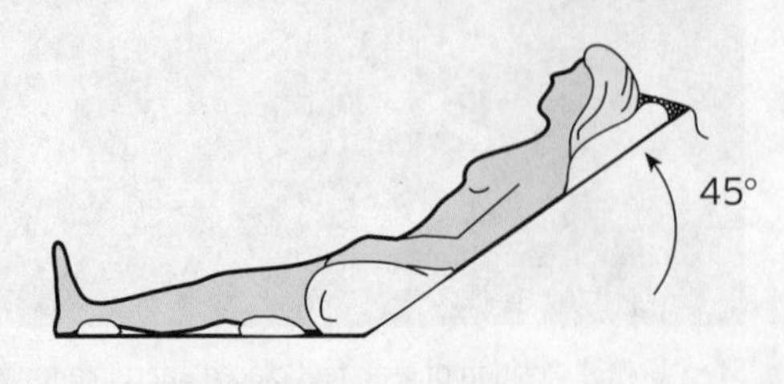

Step 12C Supported Fowler's position.

➤ SKILL 46-1 Moving and Positioning Clients in Bed ***continued***

STEPS	RATIONALE
E. Position client in supine position.	
(1) Be sure client is comfortable on back with head of bed flat.	• Some clients' physical conditions will not tolerate a supine position.
(2) Place a small rolled towel under the lumbar area of the back.	• Provides support for lumbar spine.
(3) Place a pillow under upper shoulders, neck, or head.	• Maintains correct alignment and prevents flexion contractures of cervical vertebrae.
(4) Place trochanter rolls or sandbags parallel to lateral surface of the client's thighs.	• Reduces external rotation of hip.
(5) Place a small pillow or roll under ankle to elevate heels (see Step 12C illustration).	• Reduces pressure on heels, helping to prevent pressure sores.
(6) Place firm pillows against bottom of client's feet.	• Maintains dorsiflexion and prevents footdrop.
(7) Place foot boots on client's feet, if necessary.	• Maintains feet in dorsiflexion. Prevents footdrop.
(8) Place pillows under pronated forearms, keeping upper arms parallel to client's body (see Step 12E(8) illustrations).	• Reduces internal rotation of shoulder and prevents extension of elbows. Maintains correct body alignment.
(9) Place hand rolls in client's hands. Consider occupational therapy referral for use of hand splints, if necessary.	• Reduces extension of fingers and abduction of thumb. Maintains thumb slightly adducted and in opposition to fingers.
F. Position hemiplegic client in supine position.	
(1) Place head of bed flat.	• Necessary for positioning in supine position.
(2) Place folded towel or small pillow under shoulder or affected side.	• Decreases possibility of pain, joint contracture, and subluxation. Maintains mobility in muscles around shoulder to permit normal movement patterns.
(3) Keep affected arm away from body with elbow extended and palm up. (An alternative is to place arm out to side, with elbow bent and hand toward head of the bed.)	• Maintains mobility in arm, joints, and shoulder to permit normal movement patterns. (The alternative position counteracts limitation of ability of arm to rotate outward at shoulder [external rotation]. External rotation must be present to raise arm overhead without pain.)

Critical Decision Point: Position the affected hand in one of the recommended positions for flaccid or spastic hand.

STEPS	RATIONALE
(4) Place a folded towel under the hip of client's involved side.	• Diminishes effect of spasticity in entire leg by controlling hip position.
(5) Flex affected knee 30 degrees by supporting it on a pillow or folded blanket.	• Slight flexion breaks up abnormal extension pattern of leg. Extensor spasticity is most severe when the client is supine.
(6) Support feet with soft pillows at a right angle to leg.	• Maintains foot in dorsiflexion and prevents footdrop. Pillows prevent stimulation to ball of foot by hard surface, which has a tendency to increase muscle tone in a client with extensor spasticity of lower extremity.
G. Position client in prone position: This requires two staff members to safely position client.	
(1) With drawsheet under client, move client toward one side of the bed. Ensure that side rail on opposite side is up for safety. With client supine, roll client over arm positioned close to body, with elbow straight and hand under hip. Position on abdomen in centre of the bed.	• Positions client correctly so that alignment can be maintained. • Diminishes effects of spasticity in entire leg by controlling hip position. Slight hip flexion breaks up abnormal extension pattern of leg; extensor spasticity is most severe when the client is supine.
(2) Turn client's head to one side and support head with a small pillow (see Step 12G(2) illustration).	• Reduces flexion or hyperextension of cervical vertebrae.

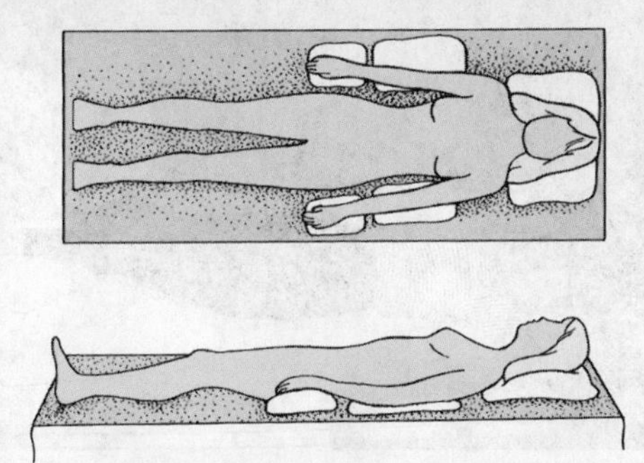
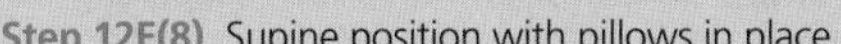
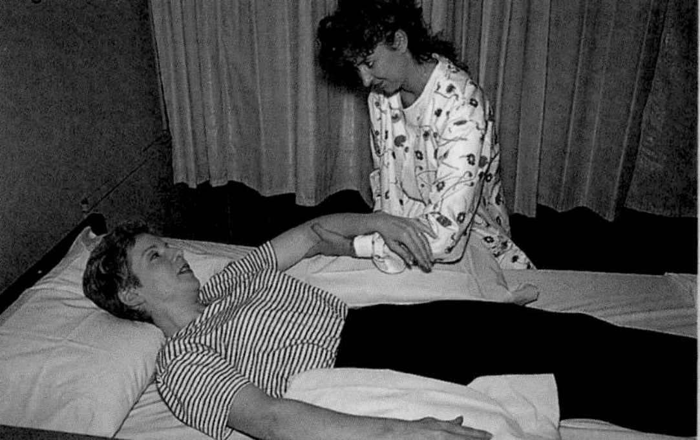

Step 12E(8) Supine position with pillows in place.

Continued

➤ SKILL 46-1 Moving and Positioning Clients in Bed *continued*

STEPS	RATIONALE
(3) Place small pillow under client's abdomen below level of diaphragm (see Step 12G(3) illustration).	• Reduces pressure on breasts of some female clients and decreases hyperextension of lumbar vertebrae and strain on lower back.
(4) Support arms in flexed position, level at shoulders.	• Maintains proper body alignment. Support reduces risk of joint dislocation.
(5) Support lower legs with pillows to elevate toes (see Step 12G(5) illustration).	• Prevents footdrop. Reduces external rotation of hips. Reduces mattress pressure on toes.
H. Position hemiplegic client in prone position.	

Critical Decision Point: Increase frequency of position changes if pressure areas begin to appear, joint mobility becomes impaired or worsened, or client complains of discomfort. Consult with physiotherapist and occupational therapist as needed. Use 30-degree lateral position (see Chapter 47) to help prevent pressure ulcers.

STEPS	RATIONALE
(1) Move client toward unaffected side.	• Creates room for proper client alignment in centre of bed when client is rolled onto abdomen.
(2) Roll client onto side.	• Prevents sagging of abdomen when client is rolled over; decreases hyperextension of lumbar vertebrae and strain on lower back.
(3) Place pillow on client's abdomen.	• Prevents injury to affected side.
(4) Roll client onto abdomen by positioning involved arm close to client's body, with elbow straight and hand under hip. Roll client carefully over arm.	• Promotes development of neck and trunk extension, which is necessary for standing and walking.
(5) Turn head toward involved side.	• Counteracts limitation of the arm's ability to rotate outward at the shoulder (external rotation). External rotation must be present to raise arm over head without pain.
(6) Position involved arm out to side, with elbow bent, hand toward head of bed, and fingers extended (if possible).	• Flexion prevents prolonged hyperextension, which could impair joint mobility.
(7) Flex knees slightly by placing pillow under legs from knees to ankles.	• Maintains feet in dorsiflexion.
(8) Keep feet at right angle to legs by using a pillow high enough to keep toes off mattress.	
I. Position client in lateral (side-lying) position.	
(1) Lower head of bed completely or as low as the client can tolerate.	• Provides position of comfort for client and removes pressure from bony prominences on back and buttocks.
(2) Position client to the side of the bed.	• Provides room for client to turn to side.
(3) Prepare to turn client onto side. Flex client's knee that will not be next to mattress. Place one hand on the client's hip and one hand on the client's shoulder.	• Positioning will set up leverage for easy turning.
(4) Roll client onto side toward you.	• Rolling client toward nurse decreases trauma to tissues. In addition, client is positioned so that leverage on hip makes turning easy.
(5) Place pillow under client's head and neck.	• Maintains alignment. Reduces lateral neck flexion. Decreases strain on sternocleidomastoid muscle.
(6) Bring shoulder blade forward.	• Prevents client's weight from resting directly on shoulder joint.
(7) Position both arms in a slightly flexed position. The upper arm is supported by a pillow level with the shoulder; the other arm, by the mattress.	• Decreases internal rotation and adduction of the shoulder. Supports both arms in a slightly flexed position.

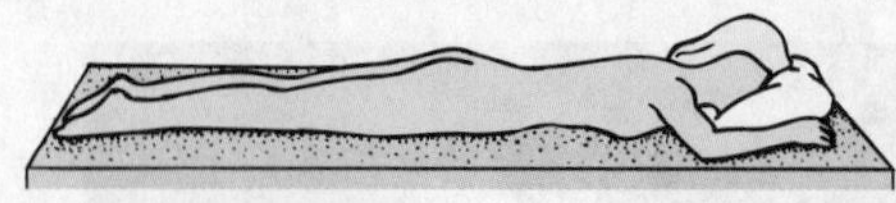

Step 12G(2) Prone position, head supported with pillow.

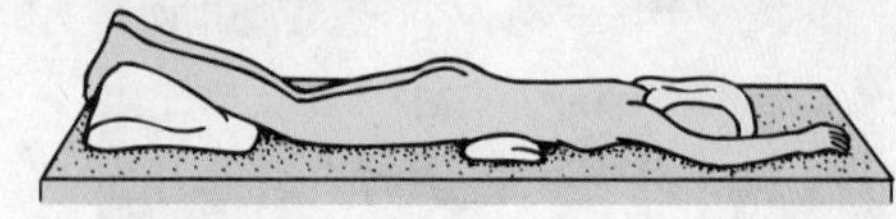

Step 12G(3) Prone position, pillow under client's abdomen and feet.

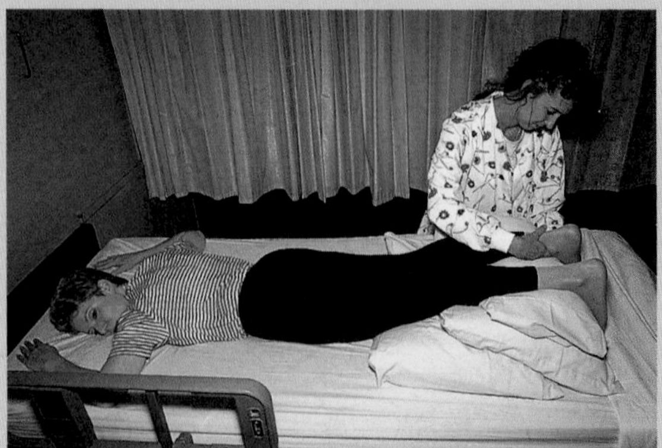

Step 12G(5) Prone position with pillows supporting lower legs.

➤ SKILL 46-1 Moving and Positioning Clients in Bed *continued*

STEPS	RATIONALE
(8) Place tuck-back pillow behind client's back. (Make by folding pillow lengthwise. The smooth area is slightly tucked under the client's back.)	• Provides support to maintain client on side.
(9) Place pillow under semiflexed upper leg level at hip from groin to foot (see Step 12I(9) illustrations).	• Maintains leg in correct alignment. Prevents pressure on bony prominence.
(10) Place sandbag parallel to plantar surface of dependent foot.	• Maintains dorsiflexion of foot. Prevents footdrop.
J. Position client in Sims' (semiprone) position.	
(1) Lower head of bed completely.	• Provides for proper body alignment while client is lying down.
(2) Be sure client is comfortable in supine position.	• Prepares client for position. Client is rolled partially onto abdomen.
(3) Position client in lateral position, with dependent arm straight along the client's body and with client lying partially on abdomen.	
(4) Carefully lift client's dependent shoulder and bring arm back behind the client.	
(5) Place a small pillow under client's head.	
(6) Place pillow under flexed upper arm, supporting arm level with shoulder.	• Maintains proper alignment and prevents lateral neck flexion. Prevents internal rotation of shoulder. Maintains alignment.
(7) Place pillow under flexed upper leg, supporting leg level with hip.	• Prevents internal rotation of hip and adduction of leg. Flexion prevents hyperextension of leg. Reduces mattress pressure on knees and ankles.
(8) Place sandbags or pillows parallel to plantar surface of foot (see Step 12J(8) illustration).	• Maintains foot in dorsiflexion. Prevents footdrop.
K. **Logroll** the client (this requires three nurses).	

Critical Decision Point: Supervise and aid UCPs when a physician's order is to logroll a client. Clients who have suffered from spinal cord injury or are recovering from neck, back, or spinal surgery often need to keep the spinal column in straight alignment to prevent further injury.

STEPS	RATIONALE
(1) Place pillow between client's knees.	• Prevents tension on the spinal column and adduction of the hip.
(2) Cross client's arms on chest.	• Prevents injury to arms.
(3) Position two nurses on side of bed to which the client will be turned. Position third nurse on the other side of bed (see Step 12K(3) illustration).	• Distributes weight equally among nurses.

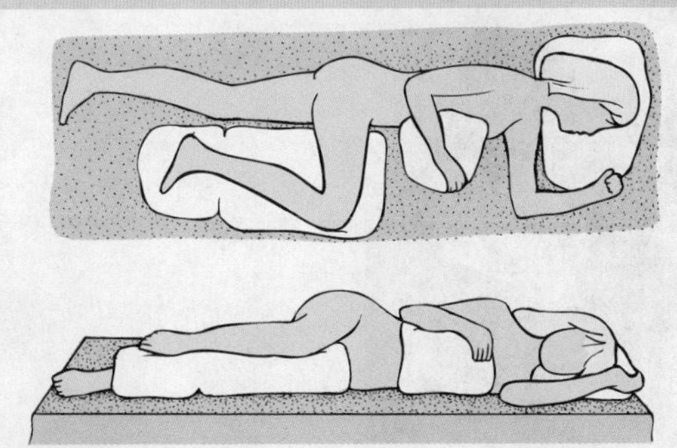

Step 12I(9) Side-lying position with pillows in place.

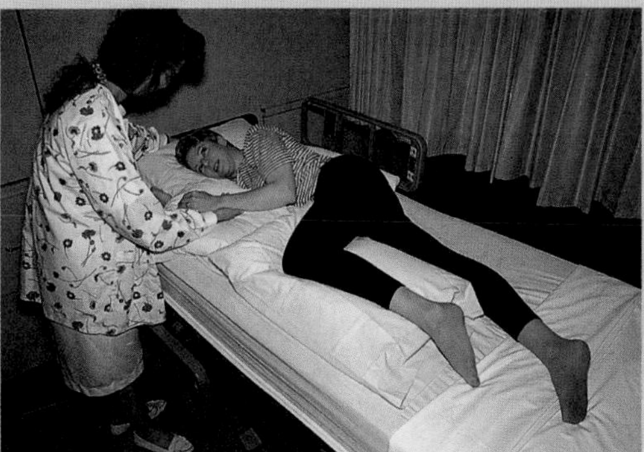

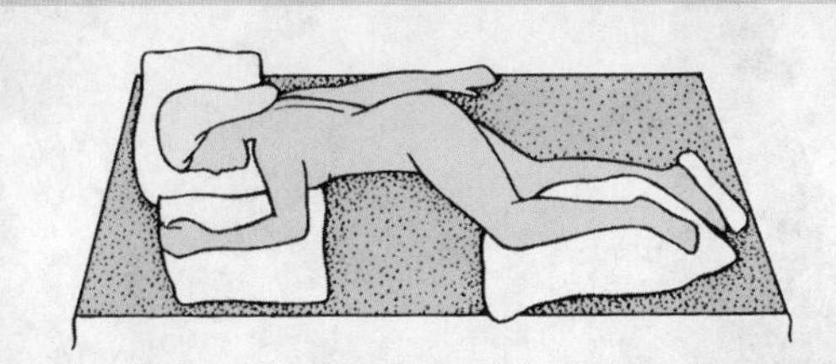

Step 12J(8) Sims' (semiprone) position with pillows in place.

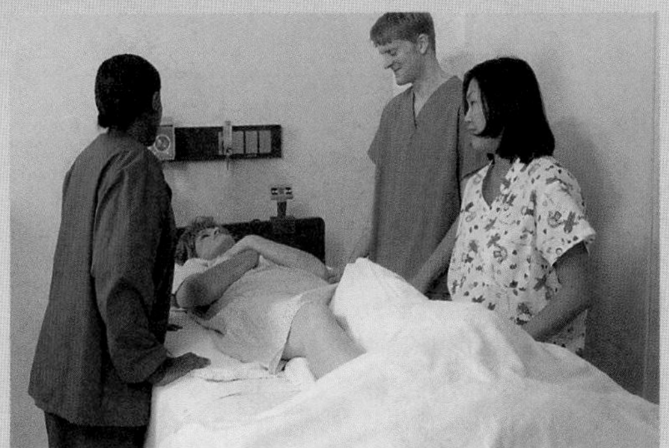

Step 12K(3) Position nurses on each side of client.

Continued

➤ SKILL 46-1 Moving and Positioning Clients in Bed *continued*

STEPS	RATIONALE
(4) Fanfold or roll the drawsheet or pull sheet.	• Provides strong handles to grip the drawsheet or pull sheet without slipping.
(5) Move the client as one unit in a smooth, continuous motion on the count of 3 (see Step 12K(5) illustration).	• Maintains proper alignment by moving all body parts at the same time, preventing tension or twisting of the spinal column.
(6) The nurse on the opposite side of the bed places pillows along the length of the client (see Step 12K(6) illustration).	• Pillows keep the client aligned.
(7) Gently lean the client as a unit back toward the pillows for support (see Step 12K(7) illustration).	• Ensures continued straight alignment of spinal column, preventing injury.
13. Perform hand hygiene.	• Reduces transmission of microorganisms.
14. Evaluate client's level of comfort and ability to assist in position change.	• Clients with reduced activity tolerance and increased levels of pain may find position changes very tiring and will need post-position change interventions to restore their level of comfort.
15. After each position change, evaluate client's body alignment and presence of any pressure areas. Observe for areas of erythema or breakdown involving skin.	• Prompt identification of poor alignment reduces risks to the client's skin and musculoskeletal systems.

Unexpected Outcomes and Related Interventions

Joint Contractures

- Improper positioning results in shortening of muscles.

Skin Erythema and Breakdown

- Frequency of repositioning is inadequate.
- Place turning schedule above client's bed.

Client Avoids Moving

- This indicates fear of pain.
- Medicate as ordered by the physician to ensure the client's comfort before moving the client.
- Allow pain medication to take effect before proceeding.

Recording and Reporting

- Record procedure and observations (e.g., condition of skin, joint movement, client's ability to assist with positioning).
- Report observations at change of shift and document in nurses' notes.

Home Care Considerations

- Teach the family about the importance of body mechanics for themselves and the client.
- Teach the client and family about the signs of skin breakdown and the importance of safety during positioning clients with decreased sensation or mobility.

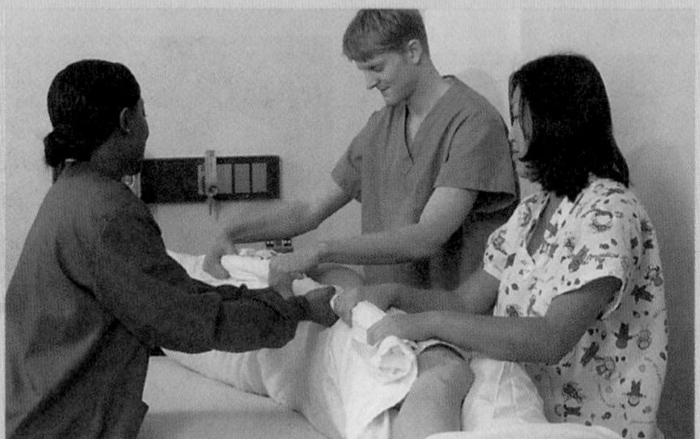

Step 12K(5) Move client as a unit, maintaining proper alignment.

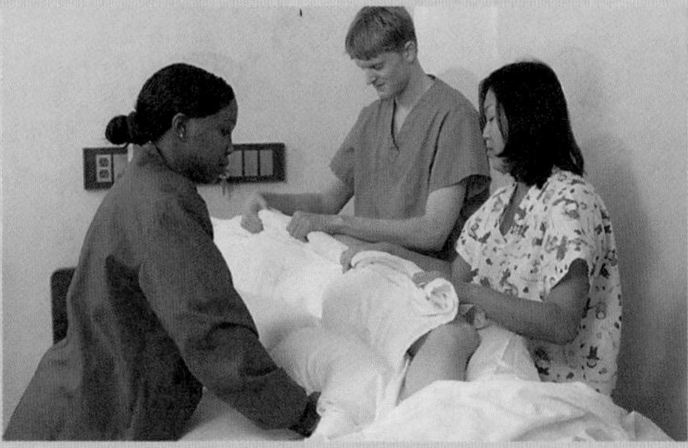

Step 12K(6) Place pillows along client's back for support.

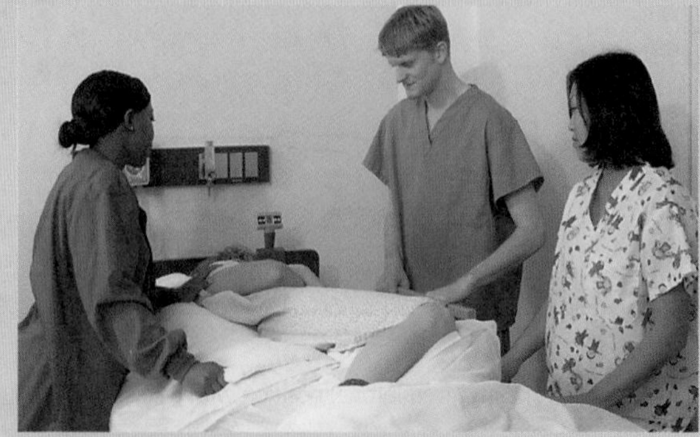

Step 12K(7) Gently lean client as a unit against pillows.

Supine Position. The supine position is a back-lying position. In the supine position, the relationship of body parts is essentially the same as in good standing alignment except that the body is in the horizontal plane. Pillows, trochanter rolls, and hand rolls or arm splints are used to increase comfort and reduce injury to the skin or musculoskeletal system. The mattress should be firm enough to support the cervical, thoracic, and lumbar vertebrae. Shoulders are supported, and the elbows are slightly flexed to control shoulder rotation. A foot support is used to prevent footdrop and maintain proper alignment. The following are some common trouble areas for clients in the supine position (see Skill 46–1 for preventive measures):

- Excessive cervical flexion because the pillow at the head is too thick and the head thrusts forward.
- Head flat on the mattress.
- Shoulders unsupported and internally rotated.
- Elbows extended.
- Thumb not in opposition to the fingers.
- Hips externally rotated.
- Unsupported feet.
- Unprotected pressure points at the occipital region of the head, vertebrae, coccyx, elbows, and heels.

Prone Position. The client in the prone position is lying chest down. Often the head is turned to the side. If a pillow is under the head, it should be thin enough to prevent cervical flexion or extension and maintain alignment of the lumbar spine. Placing a pillow under the lower leg permits dorsiflexion of the ankles and some knee flexion, which promotes relaxation. If a pillow is unavailable, the ankles should be in dorsiflexion over the end of the mattress. Although the prone position is seldom used in practice, nurses should consider this as an alternative, especially in clients who normally sleep in this position. The prone position may also have some benefits for clients with acute respiratory distress syndrom and acute lung injury (Marklew, 2006).

Assess for and correct any of the following potential trouble points for clients in the prone position (see Skill 46–1 for preventive measures):

- Neck hyperextension.
- Hyperextension of the lumbar spine.
- Plantar flexion of the ankles.
- Unprotected pressure points at the chin, elbows, hips, knees, and toes.

Side-Lying Position. In the side-lying (or lateral) position, the client is resting on the side with the major portion of body weight on the dependent hip and shoulder. A 30-degree lateral position is recommended for clients at risk for pressure ulcers (see Chapter 47). Trunk alignment should be the same as in standing. For example, the structural curves of the spine should be maintained, the head should be supported in line with the midline of the trunk, and rotation of the spine should be avoided. The following trouble points are common in the side-lying position (see Skill 46–1 for preventive measures):

- Lateral flexion of the neck.
- Spinal curves out of normal alignment.
- Shoulder and hip joints internally rotated, adducted, or unsupported.
- Lack of support for the feet.
- Lack of protection for pressure points at the ear, shoulder, anterior iliac spine, trochanter, and ankles.
- Excessive lateral flexion of the spine if the client has large hips and a pillow is not placed superior to the hips at the waist.

Sims' Position. Sims' position differs from the lateral position in the distribution of the client's weight. In Sims' position, the weight is placed on the anterior ilium, humerus, and clavicle. Trouble points common in Sims' position include the following (see Skill 46–1 for preventive measures):

- Lateral flexion of the neck.
- Internal rotation, adduction, or lack of support to the shoulders and hips.
- Lack of support for the feet.
- Lack of protection for pressure points at the ilium, humerus, clavicle, knees, and ankles.

Transfer Techniques. Nurses often provide care for immobilized clients whose position must be changed, who must be moved up in bed, or who must be transferred from a bed to a chair or from a bed to a stretcher. Use of proper body mechanics will enable you to position, move, or transfer clients safely and also protect you from injury to the musculoskeletal system. Although many transfer techniques are used, the following general guidelines should be followed in any transfer procedure:

- Raise the side rail on the side of the bed opposite you to prevent the client from falling out of bed.
- Elevate the level of the bed to a comfortable working height.
- Assess the client's mobility and strength to determine what assistance the client can offer during transfer.
- Determine the need for assistance from other care providers or mechanical lifts.
- Explain the procedure to the client and describe what is expected of the client.
- Assess for correct body alignment and pressure areas after each transfer.

safety alert Recognition of your own personal strengths and limits is crucial. Moving a completely immobilized client alone is dangerous and not allowed in many agencies. If you are attempting transfer or moving techniques for the first time, you should request help to reduce the risk of injury to yourself and to the client.

Moving Clients. Clients require various levels of assistance to move up in bed, move to the side-lying position, or sit up at the side of the bed. For example, a young, healthy woman may need only a little support as she sits at the side of the bed for the first time after childbirth, whereas an older person may need help from one or more nurses to do the same task 1 day after abdominal surgery.

Always enlist the client's help to the fullest extent possible. To determine what the client is able to do alone and how many people are needed to help move the client in bed, you need to assess the client to determine whether the illness contradicts exertion (e.g., cardiovascular disease).

Next, determine whether the client comprehends what is expected. For example, a client recently medicated for postoperative pain may be too lethargic to understand instruction. To ensure safety, two nurses would be needed to move the client in bed. You must then determine the comfort level of the client and evaluate personal strength and knowledge of the procedure.

Finally, determine whether the client is too heavy or immobile for you to complete the procedure alone (Nelson et al., 2003b; see Skill 46–1). If in doubt, always request assistance from another person. Collaborate with the physiotherapist, occupational therapist, and physician to plan for mobilizing the **bariatric** client (Box 46–12. Use of mechanical transfer devices may be warranted (Figure 46–19), and agency lifting and transferring policies must be followed.

➤ BOX 46-12 Mobilizing Bariatric Clients

Several measures are used to evaluate a client's weight status. One such measure, the body mass index (BMI), expresses the relative percentages of fat and muscle mass; weight in kilograms is divided by height in meters. The result is used as an index of obesity.

The World Health Organization uses the BMI to categorize weight status:

BMI 25–29.9: grade I, moderately overweight
BMI 30–39.9: grade II, severely obese
BMI >40: grade III, massively or morbidly obese

The Canadian Medical Association has declared obesity an "epidemic"(Katzmarzyk, 2002). A survey conducted in 2004 reported that 59% of the adult population is overweight (BMI 25–29.9) and 23% are obese (BMI 30–39.9) (Starky, 2005).

The first step in mobilizing bariatric clients is to ensure that they are surounded by a safe environment (Barr and Cunneen, 2001). You must assess both the bariatric client's ability to assist in the move and the environment where it will occur, including equipment, before mobilizing the client. Until you know that a bariatric client has the ability to move independently, even minimally, you will need to ensure that the sequence of activities is carried out in a safe manner. Specific assessment forms for the safe mobilization of the bariatric client have been developed (Muir and Gerlach, 2003). You will need to collaborate with the physiotherapist, occupational therapist, and physician to plan for mobilizing, and you may need to use a mechanical transfer device. Specially designed equipment needed for moving a bariatric client includes a hospital gown, blood pressure cuff, wheelchair, walker, commode, bed, chair, transfer device and lift, and over-bed trapeze and grab bar. An over-bed trapeze and grab bars enable the client to be more independent and to participate in mobilizing. For example, a stirrup and pulley system can be used by the client to elevate a leg, using the upper extremities, when you are assisting with perineal care (Dionne, 2002).

A fear of falling often limits bariatric clients' mobility. This fear may be related to past negative, unsafe, or humiliating experiences of falling and not being able to get up (Dumas, 2001). To help decrease the fear of falling, improve the client's sitting balance by, for example, encouraging the client to lean forward and learn where the centre of balance is. You can also assist the client in leaning forward to gain momentum before standing instead of attempting to lift straight up from sitting (Dumas, 2001).

When assisting the bariatric client to transfer from the bed to a chair, you can help reduce skin shear and friction resistance during positioning by inflating the air mattress and using devices such as a Gortex sheet (Dionne, 2002). Once the client is sitting at the edge of the bed, deflate the air mattress. Place a low footstool under the client's feet to position the client's thigh so that it is level with the hip joint. If the knee is down-sloping and the client begins to slide to the floor it will be impossible to stop the slide. If the client's knee is kept level with the hip joint, you may return the client to the centre of the bed by lowering the client's trunk (Dionne, 2002).

Assessment criteria and tools have been developed to help you gather data and to assess and plan for the safe transfer of clients. An example of a client mobility assessment form is shown in Table 46–4.

Transferring a Client From a Bed to a Chair. Transfer of a client from a bed to a chair by one nurse requires assistance from the client and should not be attempted with a client who cannot help (Skill 46–2). Explain the procedure to the client before the transfer. Moving obstacles out of the way also prepares the environment. The chair is placed next to the bed with the chair back in the same plane as the head of the bed. Placement of the chair allows you to pivot with the client and to transfer the client's weight in a controlled manner.

A safe transfer is the first priority. If you are doubtful about personal strength or the client's ability to help, you should request assistance. A **transfer belt** should be used with all clients being transferred for the first time and thereafter as deemed necessary. Use of a transfer belt (called a **gait belt** when used for walking with a client) helps prevent caregiver back injuries and aids in the safe transfer of the client. The belt encircles the client's waist and has handles attached for the nurse to hold. It is applied over the client's clothing, never over bare skin. The belt is tightened so that it is snug but does not cause discomfort or impair breathing, and the buckle is placed off-centre in the front or in the back. The buckle should not be over the spine.

The client should sit and dangle the feet at the side of the bed for a minute before standing. The client should then stand at the side of the bed for another minute so that he or she can quickly sit down on it in case of dizziness or fainting. When moving a client from a bed to a wheelchair, both nurses must use proper body mechanics. If a client has an immobile lower extremity from a cast or paralysis, the transfer should be toward the unaffected leg.

Transferring a Client From a Bed to a Stretcher. To transfer an immobilized client from a bed to a stretcher or from a bed to another bed, use of a drawsheet (lift sheet) or a friction-reducing device under the client is oftern required. In this technique, nurses need to be on opposite sides of the bed and holding on to the lift sheet or friction-reducing device when transferring the client to the stretcher. The stretcher and the bed are placed side by side so that the client can be transferred quickly and easily using the lift sheet. As with all procedures, safety is the priority. To increase safety, the lifters of the three-person team need to work together, with one person assuming the leadership role.

Exercise caution when transferring a client who has or is suspected of having spinal cord trauma. If the client must be moved, a transfer board should be placed under the client to maintain spinal alignment before transferring the client to a stretcher. The client should be prepared for the transfer and asked to help when possible (e.g., by folding the arms over the chest). The environment should be free from obstacles, and unnecessary equipment should be removed from the bed.

Restorative Care

The goal of restorative care for the client who is immobile is to maximize functional mobility and independence and reduce residual functional deficits such as impaired gait and decreased endurance. The focus in restorative care is on not only ADLs that relate to physical self-care but also **instrumental activities of daily living (IADLs)**. IADLs are activities that are necessary to be independent in society beyond eating, grooming, transferring, and toileting. They include such skills as shopping, preparing meals, banking, and taking medications.

Although you will use many of the interventions described in the "Health Promotion" and "Acute Care" sections, the emphasis here is on working collaboratively with clients and their significant others and with other health care professionals. The goal is to enhance the client's quality of life by helping the client return to maximal functional ability in both ADLs and IADLs.

Intensive specialized rehabilitation such as occupational or physiotherapy is common. If the client is in an institution, he or she will likely go to the therapy department two to three times a day. Your role is to work collaboratively with these professionals and reinforce

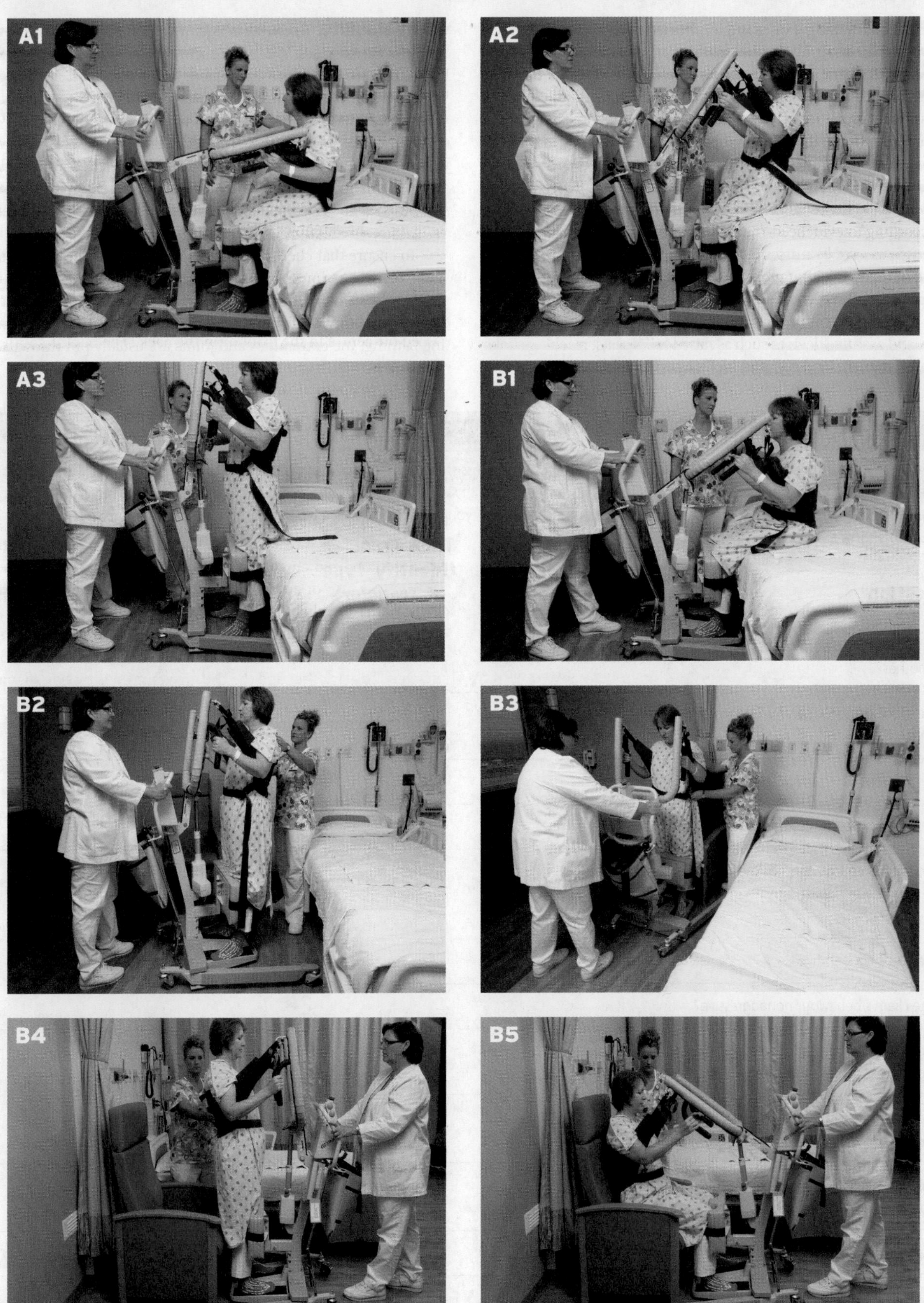

Figure 46-19 A1, Ensure that safety straps are secured appropriately when using a motorized lift to help a client move to standing position. A2, Client grasps handles as the nurse enables motorized lift. A3, Client is in standing position with feet on the floor and is ready to ambulate to a chair with nurses' help. B1, When the client is unable to walk, secure safety straps, and use platform of the motorized lift. B2, Client in upright position. B3, Position client in front of chair. B4, Explain to client the need to hold on to the handles as motorized lift begins to lower client into chair. B5, Guide client into chair.

exercises and teaching. For example, after a stroke, a client will likely receive gait training from a physiotherapist, speech rehabilitation from a speech therapist, and training from an occupational therapist on getting dressed and preparing food. Working with allied health professionals on an interdisciplinary plan of care, you can reinforce and further enhance the client's mobilization. The therapy may not be able to restore total functional health, but it may help the client adapt to limited mobility and related complications.

Restorative interventions are focused on the regaining of mobility. According to evidenced-informed protocols, common restorative interventions used by nurses include promotion of exercises for maintaining or regaining joint mobility and teaching of the use of assistive devices for walking (Box 46–13). Items frequently used to help a client adapt to mobility limitations include walkers, canes, wheelchairs, and assistive devices such as raised toilet seats, reaching sticks, special silverware, and adaptive clothing with Velcro closures.

Joint Mobility. To ensure adequate joint mobility, teach the client about ROM exercises. When the client does not have voluntary motor control, start the client on passive ROM exercises. Walking also increases joint mobility. Occasionally, clients need to use assistive devices such as crutches or walkers to help them walk.

Range-of-Motion Exercises. Clients with restricted mobility are unable to perform some or all ROM exercises independently. Such clients include those with limited movement in one extremity and those who are completely immobilized. Provide ROM exercises to maintain maximum joint mobility.

To ensure that clients routinely receive ROM exercises, schedule them at specific times, perhaps with another nursing activity, such as during the client's bath. Doing so will enable you to systematically reassess mobility while improving the client's ROM. In addition, during bathing, the extremities and joints are usually put through complete ROM.

TABLE 46-4 Client Mobility Assessment Summary Form

This assessment form helps caregivers to determine if it is appropriate to assist the client using a physical transfer or a mechanical lift. If the answer to any of the questions on the assessment form is "no," then a mecahnical lift should be used for the safety of the client and caregivers. After determining whether the type of assistance is a physical transfer or mechanical lift, you must decide which type of transfer is most appropriate (see Skill 46–2).

Question	If All Are "Yes"	Then Transfer (Identify Type of Transfer)	If Any Are "No"	Then Lift (Identify Type of Lift)
Can the client bear weight through one leg or both arms, to be moved from one surface to another?				
Is the client consistent and reliable in bearing weight?				
Can the client communicate with you?				
Can the client follow commands?				
Is the client free from pain or medical devices that may interfere with carrying out the procedure?				
Is the client cooperative?				
Is the client's behaviour nonaggressive?				
Is the client's range of motion suitable for performing transfer?				
Is the client's strength suitable for performing a transfer?				
Is the client's mobility and balance suitable for performing a transfer?				
Are all environmental factors suitable?				
Are all equipment factors suitable?				
Are all caregivers able to perform the task?				

From Health Care Health and Safety Association of Ontario (HCHSA). (2003). *Handle with care: A comprehensive approach to developing and implementing a client handling program. Resource manual* (p. 101, Table 16). Toronto: Author. Retrieved November 7, 2008, from http://www.osach.ca/products/resrcdoc/rerge320toc.pdf

➤ SKILL 46-2 Using Safe and Effective Transfer Techniques

video

Delegation Considerations

The skills of effective transfer techniques can be delegated to unregulated care providers (UCPs). Clients who are transferred for the first time after prolonged bed rest, extensive surgery, critical illness, or spinal cord trauma usually require supervision by professional nurses. When delegating this skill, it is important to instruct the UCP about the following:

- The need to seek assistance before moving or lifting a heavy client.
- Any client limitations that may affect safe transfer techniques.

Equipment

- Transfer belt, sling, or lapboard (as needed), nonskid shoes, bath blankets, pillows
- Wheelchair: Position chair at 45-degree angle to bed, lock brakes, remove footrests, lock bed brakes.
- Stretcher: Position at right angle (90 degrees) to bed, lock brakes on stretcher, lock brakes on bed.
- Mechanical or hydraulic lift: Use ceiling track or mechanical portable lift, and sling.

Procedure

STEPS	RATIONALE
1. Assess the client for the following:	• Provides information relative to the client's abilities, physical status, and ability to comprehend. The number of individuals needed to provide a safe transfer can then be determined.
A. Muscle strength (legs and upper arms)	• Immobile clients have decreased muscle strength, tone, and mass. Affects ability to bear weight or raise body.
B. Joint mobility and contracture formation	• Immobility or inflammatory processes (e.g., arthritis) may lead to contracture formation and impaired joint mobility.
C. Paralysis or paresis (spastic or flaccid)	• Client with central nervous system damage may have bilateral paralysis (requiring transfer by swivel bar, sliding bar, or mechanical lift) or unilateral paralysis, which requires belt transfer to "best" (unaffected) side. Weakness (paresis) requires stabilization of knee during transfer. Flaccid arm must be supported with sling during transfer.
D. Orthostatic hypotension	• Determines risk of fainting or falling during transfer. Immobile clients may have decreased ability for autonomic nervous system to equalize blood supply, resulting in drop of 20 mm Hg or more in systolic blood pressure or 10 mm Hg in diastolic blood pressure when rising from sitting position.
E. Activity tolerance	• Determines ability of client to assist with transfer.
F. Presence of pain	• Pain may reduce client's motivation and ability to be mobile. Pain relief before transfer enhances client participation.
G. Vital signs	• Vital sign changes such as increased pulse and respiration may indicate activity intolerance (see Chapter 31).
2. Assess client's sensory status:	
A. Adequacy of central and peripheral vision	
B. Adequacy of hearing	
C. Loss of sensation	• Determines influence of sensory loss on ability to make transfer. Visual-field loss may decrease client's ability to transfer safely. Clients with visual and hearing losses need transfer techniques adapted to deficits. Clients with cerebrovascular accident (CVA) may lose area of visual field, which profoundly affects vision and perception.

Critical Decision Point: Clients with hemiplegia also may "neglect" one side of the body (inattention to or unawareness of one side of body or environment), which distorts perception of the visual field.

STEPS	RATIONALE
3. Assess client's cognitive status.	• Determines client's ability to follow directions and learn transfer techniques.

Critical Decision Point: Clients with head trauma or CVA may have perceptual cognitive deficits that create safety risks. If client has difficulty in comprehension, simplify instructions and maintain consistency.

STEPS	RATIONALE
4. Assess client's level of motivation:	
A. Client's eagerness or unwillingness to be mobile	
B. Whether client avoids activity and offers excuses	• Altered psychological states reduce the client's desire to engage in activity.
5. Assess previous mode of transfer (if applicable).	• Determines mode of transfer and assistance required to provide continuity. Transfer belts should be used with all clients being transferred for the first time and thereafter as deemed necessary.

Continued

➤ SKILL 46-2 Using Safe and Effective Transfer Techniques *continued*

STEPS	RATIONALE
6. Assess client's specific risk of falling when transferred.	• Certain conditions increase the client's risk of falling or potential for injury. Neuromuscular deficits, motor weakness, calcium loss from long bones, cognitive and visual dysfunction, and altered balance increase the risk of falls.
7. Assess special transfer equipment needed for home setting. Assess home environment for hazards.	• Transfer ability at home is greatly enhanced by prior teaching of family and support people, and assessment of home for safety risks and functionality.
8. Perform hand hygiene.	• Reduces transmission of microorganisms.
9. Explain procedure to client.	• Increases client participation.
10. Transfer client:	
A. Assist client to sitting position.	
(1) Place client in supine position.	• Enables nurse to assess client's body alignment continually and to administer additional care, such as suctioning or hygiene needs.
(2) Face head of bed at a 45-degree angle and remove pillows.	• Proper positioning reduces twisting of nurse's body when moving the client. Pillows may cause interference when the client is sitting up in bed.
(3) Place feet apart with foot nearer bed behind other foot, continuing at a 45-degree angle to the head of the bed.	• Improves balance and allows transfer of body weight as client is sitting up in bed.
(4) Place hand farther from client under shoulders, supporting client's head and cervical vertebrae.	• Maintains alignment of head and cervical vertebrae and allows for even lifting of client's upper trunk.
(5) Place other hand on bed surface.	• Provides support and balance.
(6) Raise client to sitting position by shifting weight from front to back leg. Pivot feet as weight is shifted from front to back leg so that the upper body does not twist.	• Improves balance, overcomes inertia, and transfers weight in direction in which client is being moved.
(7) Push against bed with arm that is placed on bed surface.	• Divides activity between arms and legs and protects back from strain. By bracing one hand against the mattress and pushing against it as client is lifted, part of the weight that would be lifted by the back muscles is transferred through the arm onto the mattress.
B. Assist client to sitting position on side of bed with bed in low position.	
(1) Turn client to side facing you on side of bed on which client will be sitting (see Step 10B(1) illustration).	• Decreases amount of work needed by client and nurse to raise client to sitting position.
(2) Raise head of bed 30 degrees.	• Prepares client to move to side of bed and protects client from falling.
(3) Stand opposite client's hips. Turn diagonally so that you face client and far corner of foot of bed.	• Places nurse's centre of gravity nearer client. Reduces twisting of nurse's body by facing the direction of movement.
(4) Place feet apart with foot closer to head of bed in front of other foot.	• Increases balance and allows nurse to transfer weight as client is brought to sitting position on side of bed.
(5) Place arm nearer head of bed under client's shoulders, supporting head and neck.	• Maintains alignment of head and neck as nurse brings client to sitting position.
(6) Place other arm over client's thighs (see Step 10B(6) illustration).	• Supports hip and prevents client from falling backward during procedure.
(7) Move client's lower legs and feet over side of bed. Pivot toward rear leg, allowing client's upper legs to swing downward.	• Decreases friction and resistance. Weight of client's legs when off the bed allows gravity to pull down lower legs, and weight of legs assists in pulling upper body into sitting position.

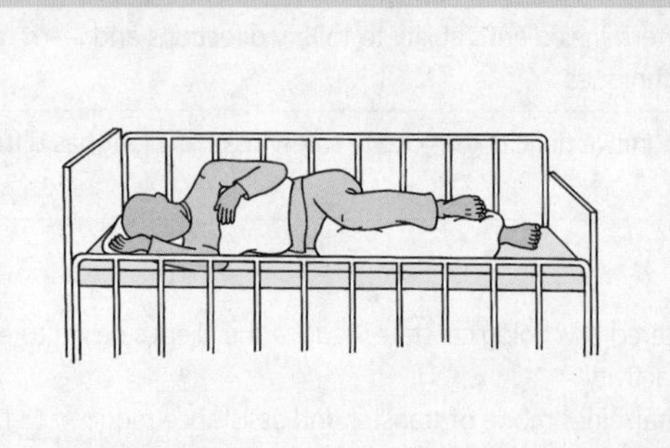

Step 10B(1) Side-lying position.

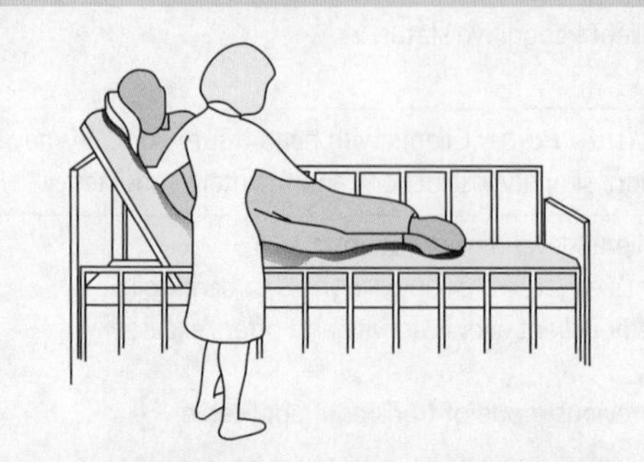

Step 10B(6) Nurse places arm over client's thighs.

➤SKILL 46-2 Using Safe and Effective Transfer Techniques *continued*

STEPS	RATIONALE
(8) At the same time, shift weight to rear leg and elevate client (see Step 10B(8) illustration). Pivot feet in the direction of movement to avoid twisting of upper body.	• Reduces client risk for falling. Immobilized clients may experience light-headedness or dizziness when assuming a sitting position.
C. Transfer client from bed to chair with bed in low position.	
(1) Assist client to sitting position on side of bed. Have chair in position at 45-degree angle to bed.	• Positions chair within easy access for transfer.
(2) Apply transfer belt or other transfer aids.	• Transfer belt maintains stability of client during transfer and reduces risk of falling (Owen et al., 1999). Client's arm should be in a sling if flaccid paralysis is present.
(3) Ensure that client has stable nonskid shoes. Weight-bearing or unaffected (strong) leg is placed back with the affected (weak) knee slightly forward or parallel.	• Nonskid soles decrease risk of slipping during transfer. Always have client wear shoes during transfer; bare feet increase risk of falls. Client will stand on unaffected (stronger, or weight-bearing) leg.
(4) Place feet shoulder-width apart.	• Ensures balance with wide base of support.
(5) Flex hips and knees, supporting client's weaker knee or leg with your knees (see Step 10C(5) illustration).	• Flexion of knees and hips lowers the centre of gravity to object to be raised; supporting knees with nurse's knees allows for stabilization of client's knee when the client stands.
(6) Grasp transfer belt from underneath.	• Transfer belt is grasped at client's side to provide movement of client at centre of gravity. Clients with upper extremity paralysis or paresis should never be lifted by or under the arms.

Critical Decision Point: A transfer belt or gait belt with handles should be used in place of the under-axilla technique. The under-axilla technique has been found to be physically stressful for nurses and uncomfortable for clients (Owen et al., 1999).

STEPS	RATIONALE
(7) Rock client up to standing position on count of 3 while straightening hips and legs and keeping knees slightly flexed (see Step 10C(7) illustration). Unless contraindicated, client may be instructed to use hands to push up if applicable.	• Rocking motion gives client's body momentum and requires less muscular effort for the nurse to lift client.
(8) Maintain stability of client's weak or paralyzed leg between your knees.	• Ability to stand can often be maintained in a paralyzed or weak limb with support of nurse's knees to stabilize it.
(9) Pivot on foot farther from chair. Instruct client to stand straight. Pivot body in direction of chair, instructing client to take small steps toward chair. Ask client to tell you when the chair touches the back of his or her knees.	• Maintains support of client while allowing adequate space for client to move.
(10) Instruct client to use armrests on chair for support and ease client into chair (see Step 10C(10) illustration).	• Increases client stability.

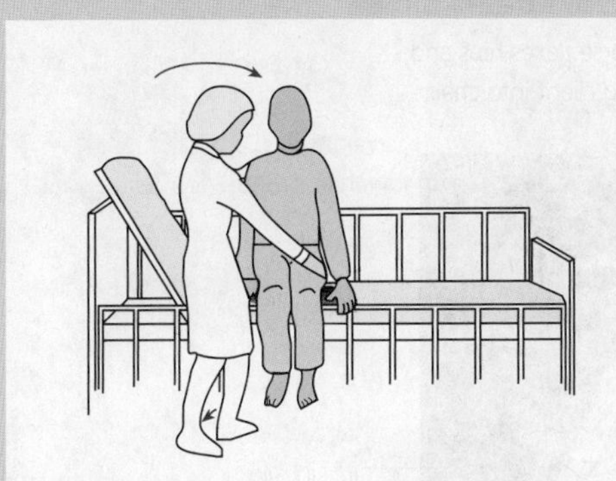

Step 10B(8) Nurse shifts weight to rear leg and elevates client.

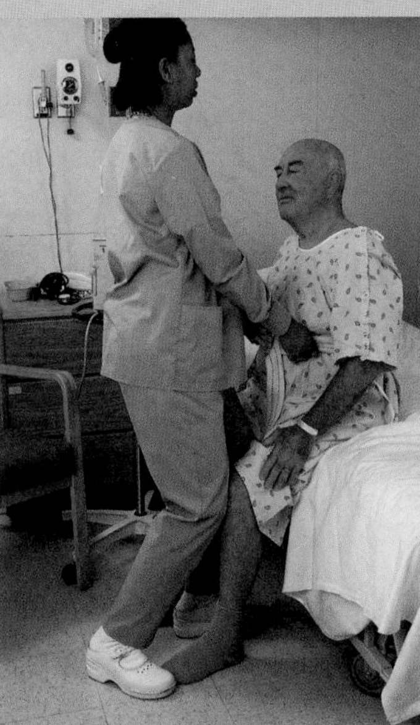

Step 10C(5) Nurse flexes hips and knees, supporting client's knee between nurse's knees.

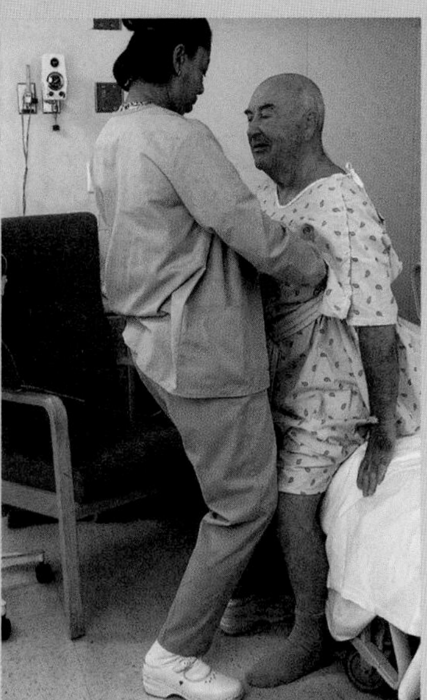

Step 10C(7) Nurse rocks client to standing position.

Continued

➤SKILL 46-2 Using Safe and Effective Transfer Techniques *continued*

STEPS	RATIONALE
(11) Flex hips and knees while lowering client into chair (see Step 10C(11) illustration).	• Prevents injury to nurse from poor body mechanics.
(12) Assess client for proper alignment for sitting position. Provide support for paralyzed extremities. Lapboard or sling will support flaccid arm. Stabilize leg with bath blanket or pillow.	• Prevents injury to client from poor body alignment.
(13) Praise client's progress, effort, or performance.	• Continued support and encouragement provide incentive for the client to persevere with these efforts.
D. Transfer client from bed to stretcher or other bed, using drawsheet or friction-reducing device.	
(1) Place bed flat, and position at same level as stretcher. Ensure that bed brakes are locked.	• Bed and stretcher need to be at the same level to allow client to slide from bed to stretcher.
(2) Lower side rails. Have two caregivers stand on the side where the stretcher will be, while the third caregiver stands on the other side.	• Minimizes caregiver's stretching. Prevents client from falling out of bed and promotes safety.
(3) Two caregivers help client roll onto side toward one caregiver.	• Positions client for friction-reducing lateral transfer device.
(4) Work together to position friction-reducing device properly under client's back (see Step 10D(4) illustration).	• Client needs to be placed on transfer device properly to enable safe transfer.

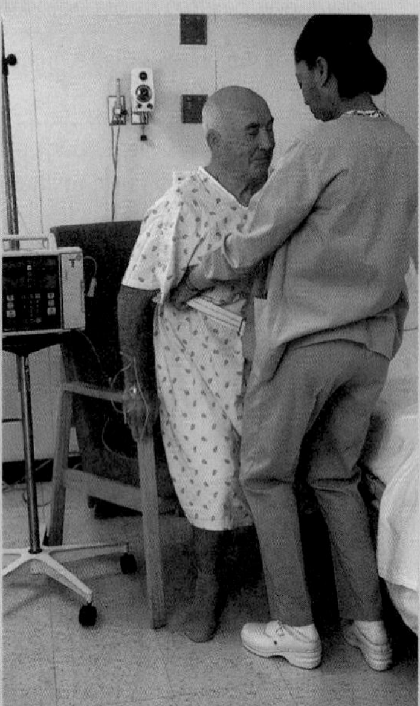

Step 10C(10) Client uses armrests for support.

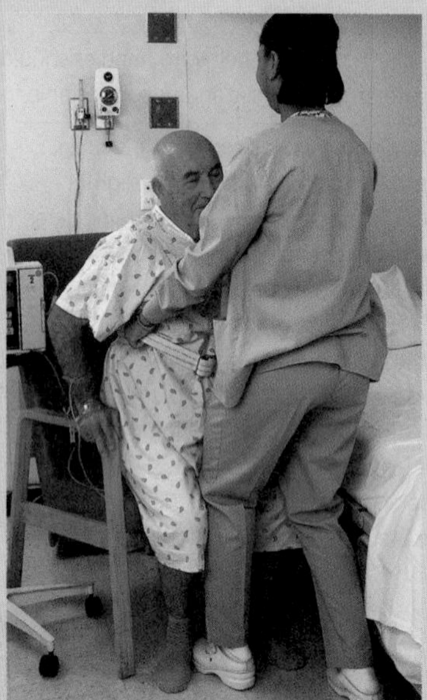

Step 10C(11) Nurse flexes hips and knees while easing client into chair.

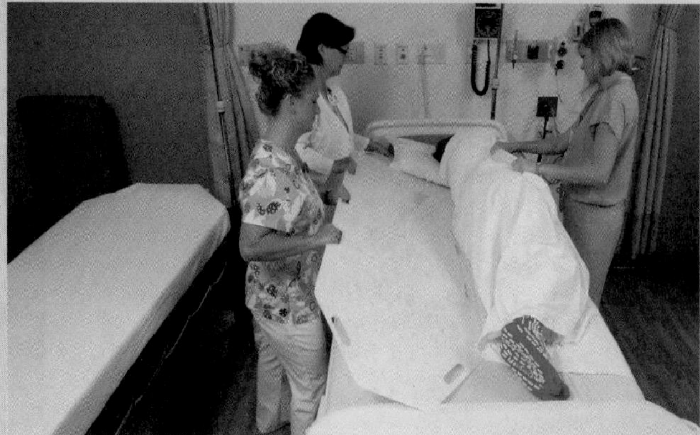

Step 10D(4) Two caregivers position sliding board under client.

➤ SKILL 46-2 Using Safe and Effective Transfer Techniques *continued*

STEPS	RATIONALE
(5) Roll stretcher along side of bed. Lock wheels of stretcher once it is in place. Instruct client to place arms across chest and not to move.	• Positions stretcher correctly for transfer and prevents client from falling out of bed.
(6) All three caregivers place feet widely apart with one foot slightly in front of the other, and grasp the friction-reducing device.	• Prepares for transfer. Wide base of support allows nurse to shift weight and minimizes back strain.
(7) On the count of 3, caregivers pull the client from the bed onto the stretcher, using the friction-reducing device and shifting weight appropriately (see Step 10D(7) illustration).	• Transfers client smoothly and efficiently to the stretcher.
(8) Put up side rail of stretcher on side where caregivers are, then roll stretcher away from side of bed and put siderails up on that side.	• Side rails prevent client from falling off stretcher.
E. Use mechanical or hydraulic lift to transfer client from bed to chair. Before using lift, be thoroughly familiar with its operation. Gather all necessary equipment and caregivers.	
(1) Choose the appropriate-size sling for client's weight and height. Position lift properly at bedside.	• Ensures safe elevation of client off bed.
(2) Position chair near bed, and allow adequate space to manoeuvre lift.	• Prepares environment for safe use of lift and subsequent transfer.
(3) Raise bed to a high position with mattress flat. Lower side rail.	• Maintains nurses' alignment during transfer.
(4) Keep bed side rail up on the side opposite you.	• Maintains client safety.
(5) Roll client on side away from you.	• Allows positioning of client on mechanical or hydraulic sling.
(6) Place sling under client. Place lower edge under client's knees (wide piece); upper edge fits under client's shoulders (narrow piece).	• Places sling under client's centre of gravity and greatest portion of body weight.
(7) Roll client to opposite side and pull sling through.	• Completes positioning of client on mechanical or hydraulic sling.
(8) Roll client supine onto sling.	• Sling should extend from shoulders to knees (hammock) to support client's body weight equally.
(9) Remove client's glasses, if present.	• Swivel bar is close to client's head and could break eyeglasses.
(10) If using transportable Hoyer lift, place lift's horseshoe bar under side of bed (on side with the chair).	• Positions lift efficiently and promotes smooth transfer.
(11) Lower horizontal bar to sling level by releasing hydraulic valve. Lock valve.	• Positions hydraulic lift close to client. Locking valve prevents injury to client.
(12) Attach hooks on strap to holes in sling. Short straps hook to top holes of sling; longer straps hook to bottom of sling.	• Secures hydraulic lift to sling.
(13) Elevate head of bed.	• Positions client in sitting position.
(14) Fold client's arms over chest.	• Prevents injury to paralyzed arms.
(15) Use lift to raise client off the bed and manoeuvre to chair (see Step 10E(15) illustration).	

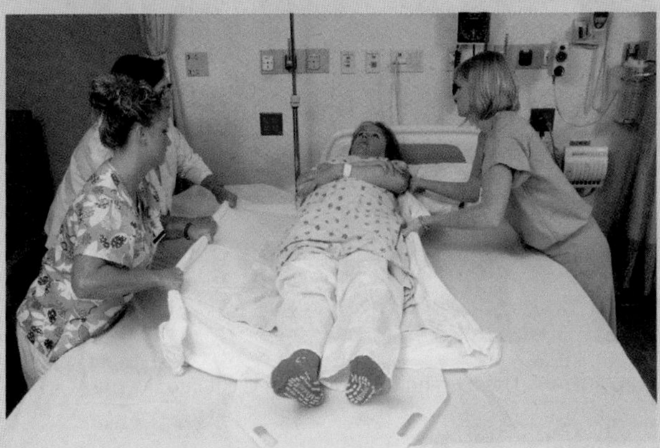

Step 10D(7) Transfer of client from bed to stretcher, using friction-reducing device.

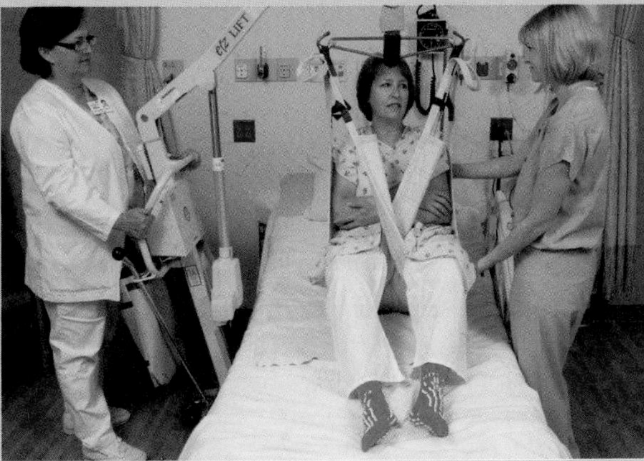

Step 10E(15) Use mechanical lift to raise client off the bed.

Continued

➤ SKILL 46-2 Using Safe and Effective Transfer Techniques *continued*

STEPS	RATIONALE
(16) Position client and lower slowly into chair (see Step 10E(16) illustration).	• Moves client from bed to chair.
(17) Close check valve as soon as client is down, and release straps.	• If valve is left open, boom may continue to lower and injure client.
(18) Remove straps and mechanical or hydraulic lift.	• Prevents damage to skin and underlying tissues from canvas or hooks.
(19) Check client's sitting alignment and correct it if necessary.	• Prevents injury from poor posture.
11. Perform hand hygiene.	• Reduces transmission of microorganisms.
12. With each transfer, evaluate client's tolerance and level of fatigue and comfort.	• Increased activity may result in symptoms associated with activity intolerance (e.g., increased pulse, changes in blood pressure, increased respirations, and decreased level of comfort). These clients may find transfer very tiring and will need post-transfer interventions to restore their level of comfort.
13. After each transfer, evaluate client's body alignment.	• Prompt identification of poor alignment reduces risks to the client's skin and musculoskeletal systems.

Not all clients require a fully mechanically assisted lift. Many types of lifts allow clients to partially weight bear. Benefits of these types of lifts include practice at standing, promotion of independence and control, and fostering of a sense of safety and confidence for clients who may have been immobile for a long period of time. An example of a lift that allows for partial weight-bearing is the SERA Lift. Before using any lift, you should receive instruction and practice this skill (see Figure 46–19).

Unexpected Outcomes and Related Interventions

Client Inability to Comprehend and Follow Directions
- Cognitive impairment affects learning and retention.
- Reassess continuity and simplicity.

Client Injury on Transfer
- This indicates that improper transfer technique was used.
- Evaluate the incident that caused the injury (e.g., assessment inadequate, change in client status, improper use of equipment).
- Complete an incident report according to health care facility's policy.

Client Too Weak for Active Transfer
- Physical impairments require increased assistance from nursing personnel.
- Increase client's bed activity and exercise to heighten tolerance.

Weight on Non-Weight-Bearing Limb
- Certain conditions (e.g., hip fractures that have not been surgically stabilized) need to be non–weight bearing through the healing process.
- Reassess client's understanding of weight-bearing status.

Uneven Client Ability for Transfer
- Transfers may be difficult when the client is fatigued or in pain. Assess the client's ability before transfer (allow for a rest period before transferring, or medicate for pain if indicated).
- Periodic confusion may also alter performance.

Inability to Stand During Transfer
- This results from increased fatigue, orthostatic hypotension, or pain.
- Provide for adequate assistance during transfer.

Localized Areas of Persistent Erythema
- Perform complete assessment of pressure ulcers and carry out appropriate interventions (see Chapter 47).

Recording and Reporting
- Record procedure, including the following pertinent observations: client's weakness, ability to follow directions, weight-bearing ability, balance, and ability to pivot; number of personnel needed to assist; and amount of assistance (muscle strength) required.
- Report any unusual occurrence to the nurse in charge. Report transfer ability and assistance needed to next shift or other caregivers. Report progress or remission to rehabilitation staff (physiotherapist or occupational therapist).

Home Care Considerations
- Teach family members about proper body mechanics for themselves and the client.
- Provide community resources for hospital equipment that can be used in the home setting (e.g., transfer belts, mechanical lifts) to assist in safe transfer techniques.

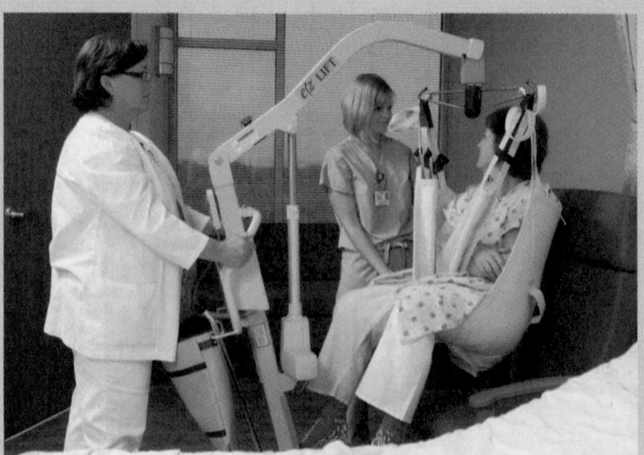

Step 10E(16) Use mecahnical lift to lower client into the chair.

Unless contraindicated, the care plan should include movement of the client's extremities through the fullest ROM possible. ROM exercises may be active, passive, or somewhere in between (active assisted). With a weak client, for example, you may support an extremity while the client performs the movement, or the client may be able to move some joints actively while you passively move others. In general, exercises should be as active as health and mobility allow. Passive ROM exercises should begin as soon as the client's ability to move the extremity or joint is lost. Movements are carried out slowly and smoothly, just to the point of resistance, and should not

✱ BOX 46-13 EVIDENCE-INFORMED PRACTICE GUIDELINE

Exercise Promotion: Reinitiating Exercise in the Previously Immobile Client

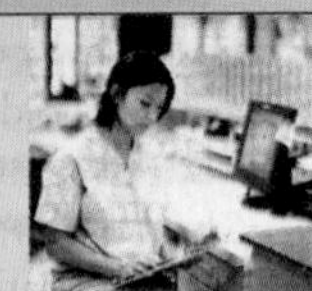

- Encourage client to contemplate change in activity level.
- Increase client's awareness of current activity levels.
- Provide information about the benefits of exercise.
- Determine any impediments to exercise.
- Provide choices of physical activities.
- Assist client in preparing for an activity program.
- Provide information about how to safely carry out the exercise (e.g., proper walking, safety considerations).
- Assist client in strengthening exercise tolerance and activity levels.
- Emphasize client's ability to become more active.
- Provide resources for social exercise groups (e.g., fitness groups, community walking programs, walking in local shopping malls).
- Assist client in establishing an activity program.
- Provide positive, constructive feedback.
- Increase physical activity as appropriate for client's mobility status.
- Assist client in developing a long-term exercise plan.
- Visit the client while he or she is participating in an exercise program.
- Assist client in maintaining an activity program.
- Recognize each success.
- If relapse occurs, remind client that it is okay and to continue with the exercise program.
- Maintain a supportive environment.
- Encourage family and friends to participate in the exercise program.

Adapted from Jitramontree, N. Evidence-based protocol: Exercise promotion: Walking in elders. In M. G. Titler (Series Ed.). (2001). *Series on evidence-based practice for older adults.* Iowa City, IA: The University of Iowa College of Nursing Gerontological Nursing Interventions Research Center, Research Dissemination Core.

cause pain. Never force a joint beyond its capacity. Each movement should be repeated five times during the session.

When performing passive ROM exercises, stand at the side of the bed closest to the joint being exercised. Passive ROM exercises are performed using a head-to-toe sequence and moving from larger to smaller joints. If an extremity is to be moved or lifted, place a cupped hand under the joint to support it (Figure 46–20), support the joint by holding the adjacent distal and proximal areas (Figure 46–21), or support the joint with one hand and cradle the distal portion of the extremity with the remaining arm (Figure 46–22). The following sections provide an overview of nursing considerations for ways to support major joints in the body. See Table 46–2 for detailed ROM exercises and illustrated motion for each joint.

Neck. A flexion contracture of the neck is a serious disability because the client's neck is permanently flexed with the chin close to or actually touching the chest. Ultimately, the client's body alignment is altered, the visual field is changed, and the level of independent functioning is decreased.

Shoulder. The shoulder is controlled by the deltoid muscle and rotator cuff muscles. When caring for a client with limited shoulder mobility, you may need to provide support devices for the shoulder, such as slings when the client is standing or sitting, or pillows when the client is in bed. Correctly positioning the shoulder prevents pain, joint subluxation, and further changes in body alignment.

Elbow. The elbow functions optimally at an angle of about 90 degrees. An elbow fixed in full extension is disabling and limits the client's independence.

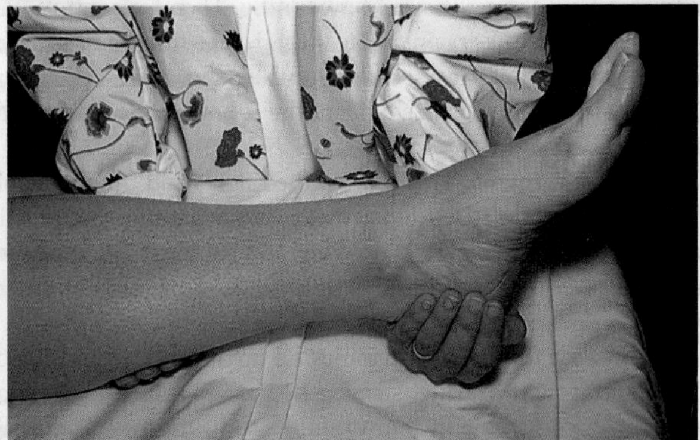

Figure 46-20 Using a cupped hand to support a joint.

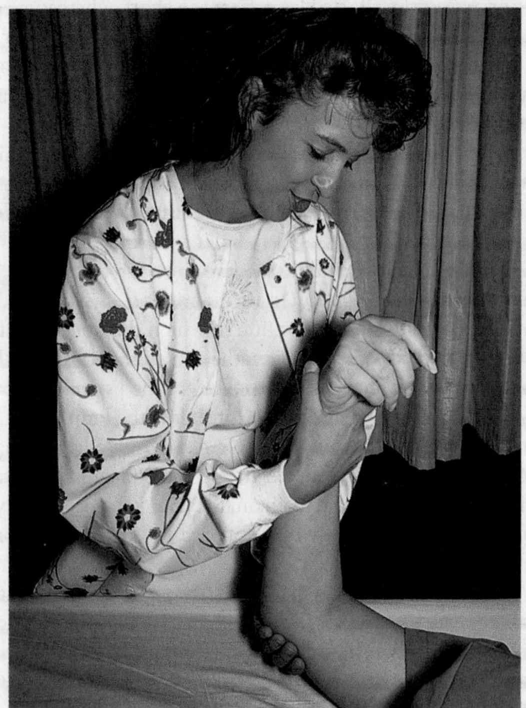

Figure 46-21 Supporting the joint by holding the distal and proximal areas adjacent to the joint.

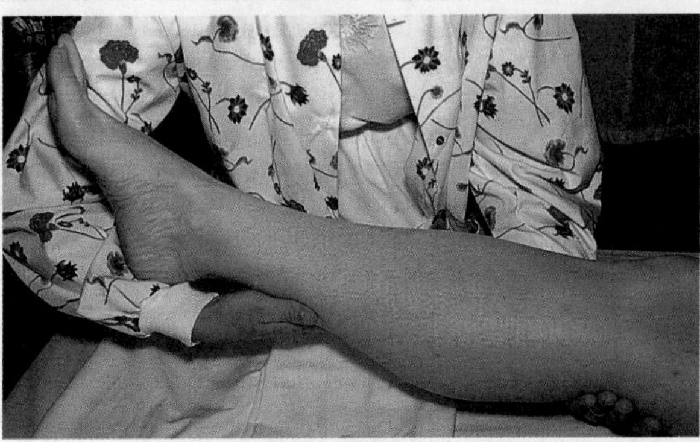

Figure 46-22 Cradling the distal portion of an extremity.

Forearm. Most functions of the hand are best carried out with the forearm in moderate pronation. When the forearm is fixed in a position of full supination, the client's use of the hand is limited.

Wrist. The primary function of the wrist is to place the hand in slight extention, the position of functioning. Therefore, full ROM is not as great a priority as maintaining the wrist in a functional position. When the wrist is fixed in even a slightly flexed position, the grasp is weakened. In the immobilized client, the functional position of the wrist can be achieved by using splints.

Fingers and Thumb. The ROM in the fingers and thumb enables the client to perform ADLs and activities requiring fine motor skills, such as carpentry, needlework, drawing, and painting. The functional position of the fingers and thumb is slight flexion of the thumb in opposition to the fingers.

Hip. Because the lower extremities are involved chiefly with locomotion and weight bearing, stability of the hip joint may be more important than its mobility. For example, if the hip has no mobility but is fixed in a neutral position and fully extended, it is possible to walk without a significant limp.

Contractures often fix the hip in positions of deformity. Excessive abduction makes the affected leg appear too short, whereas excessive adduction makes the affected leg appear too long. In either case, the client has limited mobility and walks with an obvious limp. Internal and external rotation contractures cause an abnormal and unbalanced gait.

Knee. A primary function of the knee is stability, which is achieved by ROM, ligaments, and muscles. However, the knees cannot remain stable under weight-bearing conditions unless quadriceps power is adequate for maintaining the knee in full extension. ROM exercises should include pulling the knee into full extension.

An immobile knee joint can result in serious disability. The degree of disability depends on the position in which the knee is stiffened. If the knee is fixed in full extension, the person must sit with the leg thrust out in front. When the knee is flexed, the person limps while walking. The greater the flexion, the greater is the limp.

Ankle and Foot. Without full ROM of the ankle, gait deviations will occur. If the joint is not stable, the person will fall. If joint mobility is diminished, you should maintain the joint in a position in which walking can be carried out with a forward rolling motion from the heel onto the forefoot.

When the person relaxes as in sleep or coma, the foot relaxes and assumes a position of plantar flexion. As a result, the foot may become fixed in plantar flexion (footdrop), which impairs the ability to walk. Inversion and eversion must also be avoided to allow the foot to rest flat on the floor.

Toes. Excessive flexion of the toes results in clawing. When this is a permanent deformity, the foot is unable to rest flat on the floor and the client is unable to walk properly. Flexion contractures are the most common foot deformity associated with reduced joint mobility.

Adequate ROM provides the necessary mobility to carry out ADLs and exercise. In addition, adequate ROM in the lower extremities allows walking.

Walking.

In the normal walking posture, the head is erect; the cervical, thoracic, and lumbar vertebrae are aligned; the hips and knees have appropriate flexion; and the arms swing freely with the legs. Illness or trauma can reduce activity tolerance, so that assistance in walking is required. In addition, temporary or permanent damage to the musculoskeletal and nervous systems may necessitate use of an assistive device for walking.

Helping a Client Walk. When a client's mobility has restricted the ability to walk, you must assess the client's activity tolerance, tolerance to the upright position (orthostatic hypotension), strength, level of pain, coordination, and balance to determine the amount of assistance needed.

Explain to the client how far the client should try to walk, who is going to help, when the walk will take place, and why walking is important. In addition, you and the client should determine how much independence the client can assume.

Check the walking environment to be sure that no obstacles are in the client's path. Clear chairs, overbed tables, and wheelchairs out of the way so that the client has ample room to walk safely. Before starting, establish rest points in case activity tolerance is less than estimated or the client becomes dizzy. For example, a chair might be placed in the hall for the client to rest, if needed.

Provide support at the waist so that the client's centre of gravity remains midline. This can be achieved by placing both hands at the client's waist or using a gait belt. While walking, the client should not lean to one side because this alters the centre of gravity, distorts balance, and increases the risk of falling. Walk to the side and slightly behind the client (Figure 46–23).

A client who at any point appears unsteady or complains of dizziness should be returned to a nearby bed or chair. If the client faints or begins to fall, assume a wide base of support with one foot in front of the other, thus supporting the client's body weight. Extend one leg and let the client slide against the leg, and gently lower the client to the floor, protecting the head. Although lowering a client to the floor is not difficult, you should practise this technique with a friend or classmate before attempting it in a clinical setting.

Clients with **hemiplegia** (one-sided paralysis) or **hemiparesis** (one-sided weakness) often need assistance to walk. Always stand on the client's affected side and support the client by holding one arm around the client's waist (or use a gait belt once the client's stability

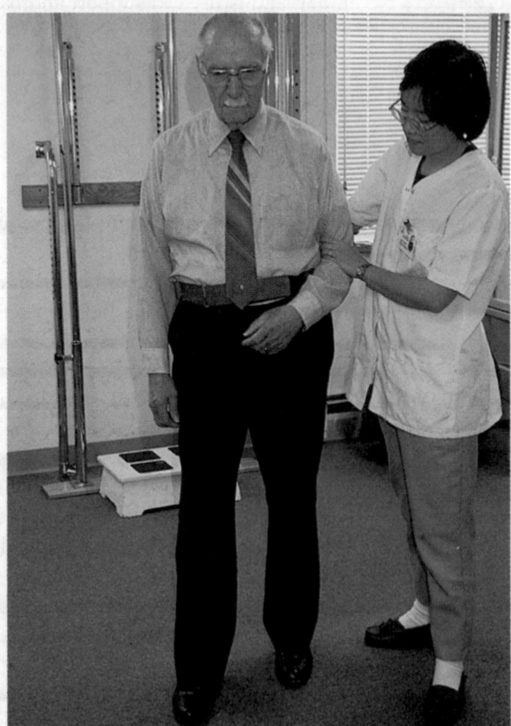

Figure 46-23 When helping a client walk, the nurse uses a gait belt and walks slightly behind the client's side. **Source:** From Sorrentino, S. A., Wilk, M. J., & Newmaster, R. (2008). *Mosby's Canadian textbook for the support worker* (2nd ed.). Toronto, ON: Elsevier.

is ensured) and the other arm around the inferior aspect of the client's upper arm so that your hand is under the client's axilla. Providing support by holding the client's arm is incorrect because you cannot easily support the client's weight to lower the client to the floor if he or she faints or falls. In addition, if the client falls while you are holding the client's arm, a shoulder joint may be injured.

If you do not have a lot of strength and are unable to ambulate a client alone, you should request help. The two-nurse method helps distribute the client's weight evenly. The two nurses stand on either side of the client. Each nurse's near arm is around the client's waist, and the other arm is around the inferior aspect of the client's arm so that both nurses' hands are supporting the client's axillae.

Using Assistive Devices for Walking. Clients recovering from a lengthy illness that required bed rest and whose mobility is impaired frequently require assistive devices to help them with ambulation. These devices include canes, walkers, and crutches. The client and family must be educated in the use of these devices.

Walkers. Walkers are extremely light, moveable devices that are about waist high and made of metal tubing (Figure 46–24). They have four widely placed, sturdy, rubber-tipped legs. The client holds the handgrips on the upper bars, moves the walker forward, takes a step with the weaker or painful leg, and then takes a step with the unaffected leg. Other metal-framed walkers (rollator walkers) have wheels, brakes, and a seat. These walkers are used with clients who have mild balance problems.

Canes. Canes are lightweight, easily moveable devices made of wood or metal. They provide less support than a walker and are less stable. A person's cane length is equal to the distance between the floor and the crease at their wrist when they are standing tall with their arm straight down at their side. Two common types of canes are the single straight-legged cane and the quad cane. The single straight-legged cane is more common and is used to support and balance a client with decreased leg strength. This cane should be kept on the stronger side of the body. For maximum support when walking, the client places the cane forward 15 to 25 cm, keeping the body weight on both legs. The weaker leg is moved forward to the cane so that the body weight is divided between the cane and the stronger leg. The stronger leg is then advanced past the cane so that the weaker leg and body weight are supported by the cane and weaker leg. During walking, the client continually repeats these three steps. The client must be taught that two points of support, such as both feet or one foot and the cane, are present at all times.

The quad cane provides the most support and is used when partial or significant leg paralysis or some hemiplegia is present. The same three steps used with the straight-legged cane are used with the quad cane and need to be taught to the client.

Crutches. Crutches are often needed to increase mobility. Begin crutch instruction with guidelines for safe use (Box 46–14). The use of crutches may be temporary, such as after ligament damage to the knee. A client with paralysis of the lower extremities, by contrast, may need crutches permanently. A crutch is a wooden or metal staff. The two types of crutches are the double adjustable Lofstrand, or forearm, crutch (Figure 46–25) and the axillary wooden or metal crutch. The forearm crutch has a handgrip and a metal band that fits around the client's forearm. The metal band and the handgrip are adjusted to fit the client's height. The axillary crutch has a padded curved surface at the top, which fits under the axilla. A handgrip in the form of a crossbar is held at the level of the palms to support the body. It is important that crutches be measured for the appropriate length and that clients be taught to use their crutches safely, to achieve a stable gait, to ascend and descend stairs, and to rise from a sitting position.

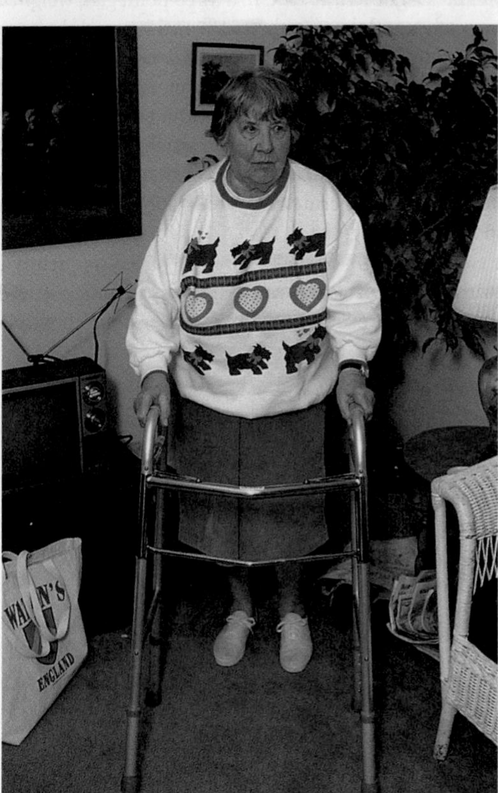

Figure 46-24 Client using a walker.

BOX 46-14 CLIENT TEACHING

Crutch Safety

Objective

- Client will describe and demonstrate safe crutch walking.

Teaching Strategies

- Teach client with axillary crutches about the dangers of pressure on the axillae, which occurs when leaning on the crutches to support body weight.
- Explain why the client must use crutches that were measured for him or her.
- Show the client how to routinely inspect crutch tips. Rubber tips should be securely attached to the crutches. When tips become worn out, they should be replaced. Rubber crutch tips increase surface friction and help prevent slipping.
- Explain that the crutch tips should remain dry. Water decreases surface friction and increases the risk of slipping.
- Show client how to inspect the structure of the crutches.
- Cracks in a wooden crutch decrease its ability to support weight. Bends in aluminum crutches can alter body alignment.
- Provide client with a list of medical supply companies in the community where repairs, new rubber tips, handgrips, and crutch pads can be obtained.
- Instruct client to have spare crutches and spare tips readily available.

Evaluation

- Client can describe principles of crutch safety.
- Client correctly demonstrates proper use of crutches.

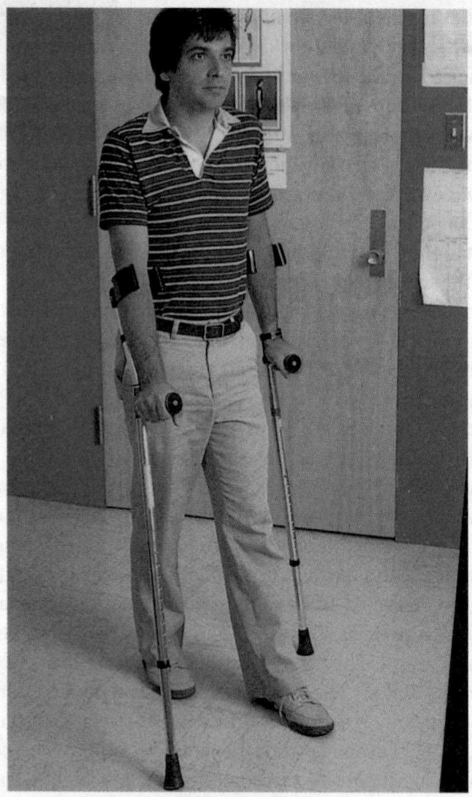

Figure 46-25 Double adjustable Lofstrand, or forearm, crutch.

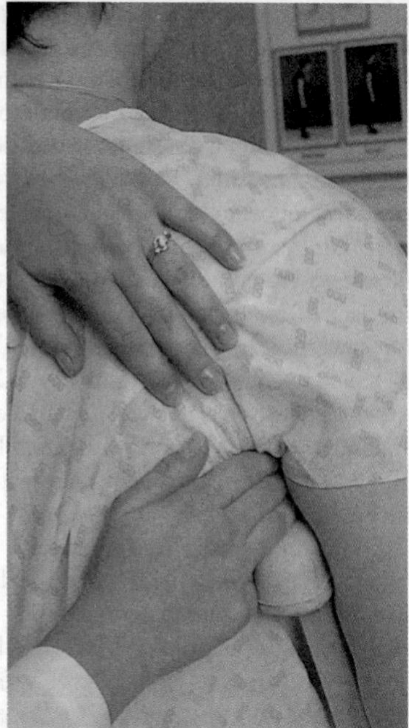

Figure 46-27 Verifying correct distance between crutch pads and axilla.

Measuring for Crutches. The axillary crutch is the more common crutch used. Measurements include the client's height, the angle of elbow flexion, and the distance between the crutch pad and the axilla. When crutches are fitted, the length of the crutch should be from three to four fingerwidths from the axilla to a point 15 cm lateral to the client's heel (Hoeman, 2008; Figure 46–26).

The handgrips should be positioned so that the client's body weight is not supported by the axillae. Pressure on the axillae increases risk to underlying nerves, which could result in partial paralysis of the arm. Correct position of the handgrips is determined with the client upright, supporting weight by the handgrips with the elbows slightly flexed at 30 degrees

When the height and placement of the handgrips have been determined, you should again verify that the distance between the crutch pad and the client's axilla is three to four fingerwidths (Figure 46–27).

Crutch Gait. The **crutch gait** is assumed by alternately bearing weight on one or both legs and on the crutches. The gait selected by the physician is determined by assessing the client's physical and functional abilities and the disease or injury that resulted in the need for crutches. This section summarizes the basic crutch stance and the four standard gaits: four-point alternating gait, three-point alternating gait, two-point gait, and swing-through gait.

The basic crutch stance is the tripod position, formed when the crutches are placed 15 cm in front of and 15 cm to the side of each foot (Figure 46–28). This position improves the client's balance by providing a wider base of support. The body alignment of the client in the tripod position includes an erect head and neck, straight vertebrae, and extended hips and knees. The tripod position is assumed before crutch walking.

Three-point alternating, or three-point, gait requires the client to bear all of the weight on one foot. In a three-point gait, weight is borne on both crutches and then on the unaffected leg, and the sequence is repeated (Figure 46–29). The affected leg does not touch the ground during the early phase of the three-point gait. Gradually, the client progresses to touchdown and full weight bearing on the affected leg.

The two-point gait requires at least partial weight bearing on each foot (Figure 46–30). The client moves a crutch at the same time as the opposing leg, so that the crutch movements are similar to arm motion during normal walking.

The swing-through, or swing-through gait, is frequently used by clients with paraplegia who wear weight-supporting braces on their legs. With weight placed on the supported legs, the client places the

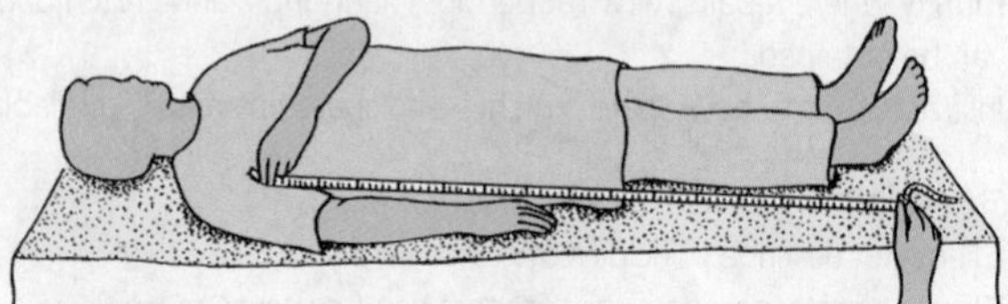

Figure 46-26 Measuring crutch length.

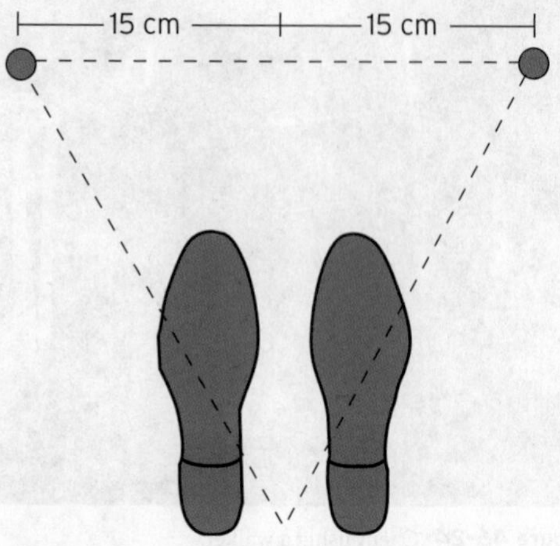

Figure 46-28 Tripod position, basic crutch stance.

crutches one stride in front and then swings to or through the crutches while they support the client's weight.

Crutch Walking on Stairs. When ascending stairs on crutches, the client usually uses a modified three-point gait (Figure 46–31). The client stands at the bottom of the stairs and transfers body weight to the crutches. The unaffected leg is advanced between the crutches to the stairs. The client then shifts weight from the crutches to the unaffected leg. Finally, the client aligns both crutches on the stairs. This sequence is repeated until the client reaches the top of the stairs.

To descend the stairs (Figure 46–32), a three-phase sequence is also used. The client transfers body weight to the unaffected leg. The crutches are placed on the stairs, and the client begins to transfer body weight to the crutches, moving the affected leg forward. Finally,

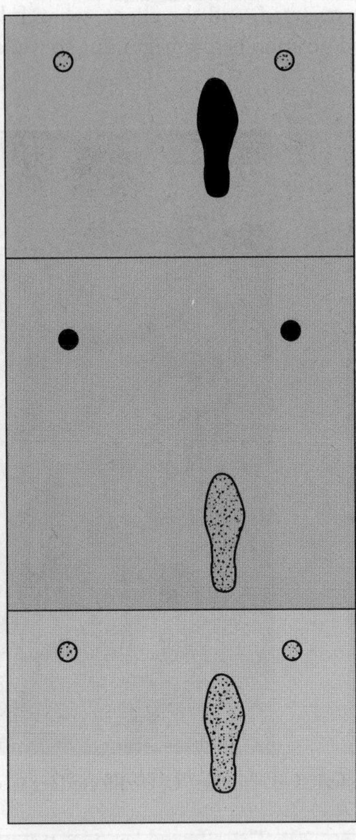

Figure 46-29 Three-point gait with weight borne on unaffected leg. Solid foot and crutch tips show weight bearing in each phase. (Read from bottom to top.)

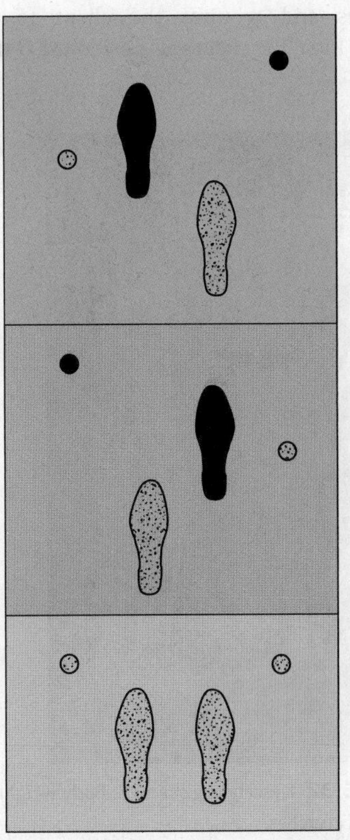

Figure 46-30 Two-point gait with weight borne partially on each foot and each crutch advancing with opposing leg. Solid areas indicate leg and crutch tips bearing weight. (Read from bottom to top.)

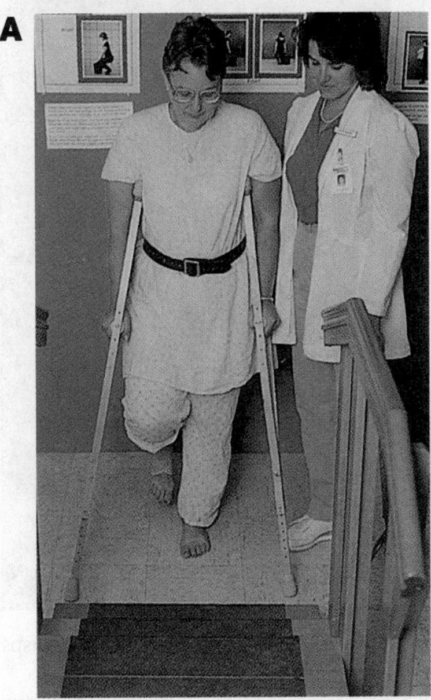

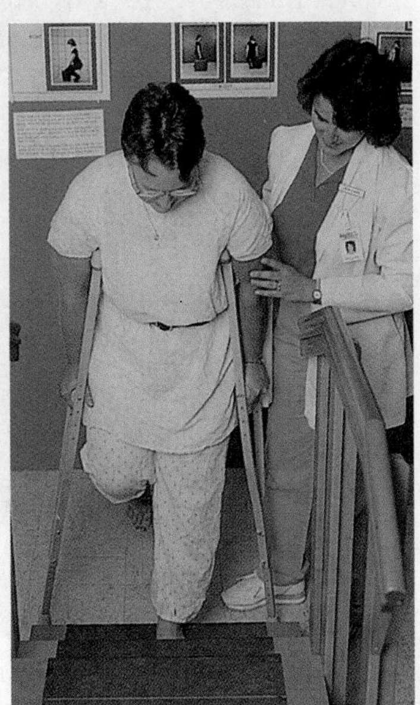

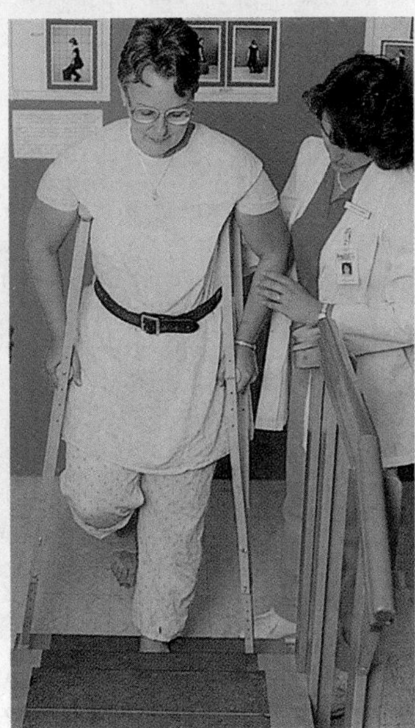

Figure 46-31 Ascending stairs. A, Weight is placed on crutch. B, Weight is transferred from crutches to unaffected leg on stairs. C, Crutches are aligned with unaffected leg on stairs.

the unaffected leg is moved to the stairs with the crutches. Again, the client repeats the sequence until reaching the bottom of the stairs.

Because in most cases clients will need to use crutches for some time, they should be adequately taught to use crutches on stairs before discharge. This instruction applies to all crutch-dependent clients, not just those who have stairs in their homes.

Sitting in a Chair With Crutches. As with crutch walking and crutch walking up and down stairs, the procedure for sitting in a chair involves phases and requires the client to transfer weight (Figure 46–33). First, the client gets positioned at the centre front of the chair with the posterior aspect of the legs touching the chair. Then the client holds both crutches in the hand opposite the affected leg. If both legs are affected, as with a client with paraplegia who wears weight-supporting braces, the crutches are held in the hand on the client's stronger side. With both crutches in one hand, the client supports body weight on the unaffected leg and the crutches. While still holding the crutches, the client grasps the arm of the chair with the remaining hand and lowers his or her body into the chair. To stand, the procedure is reversed, and the client, when fully erect, should assume the tripod position before beginning to walk.

A

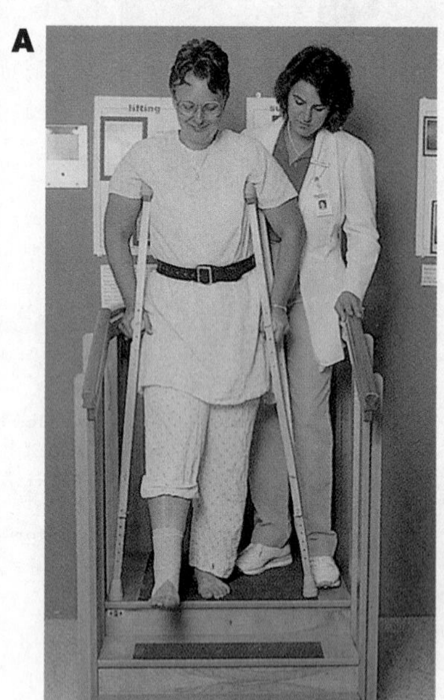

B

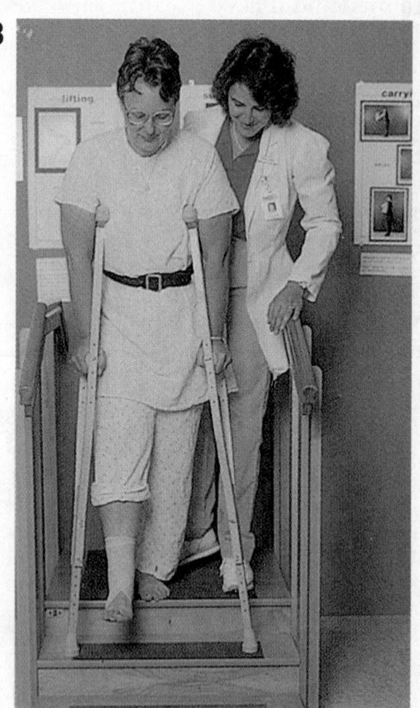

C

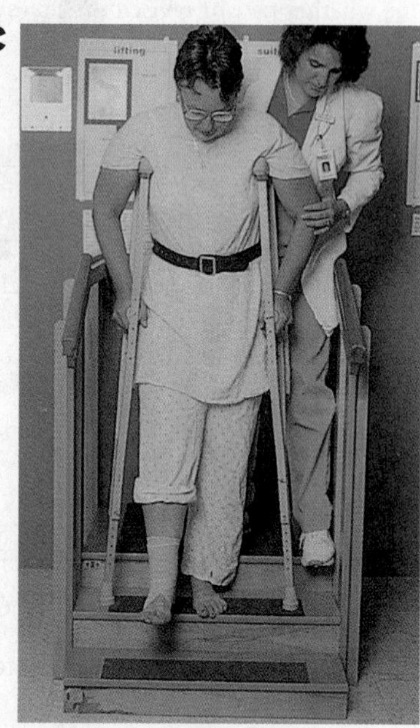

Figure 46-32 Descending stairs. A, Body weight is on unaffected leg. B, Body weight is transferred to crutches. C, Unaffected leg is aligned on stairs with crutches.

A

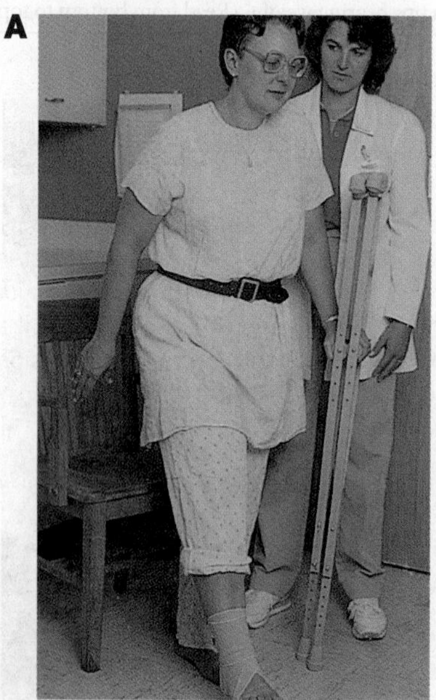

B

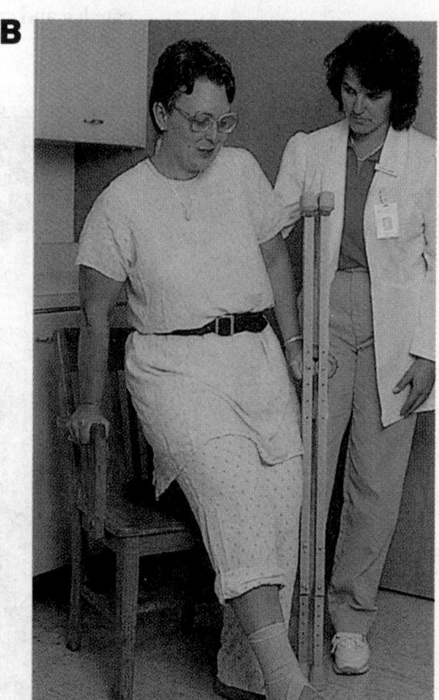

C

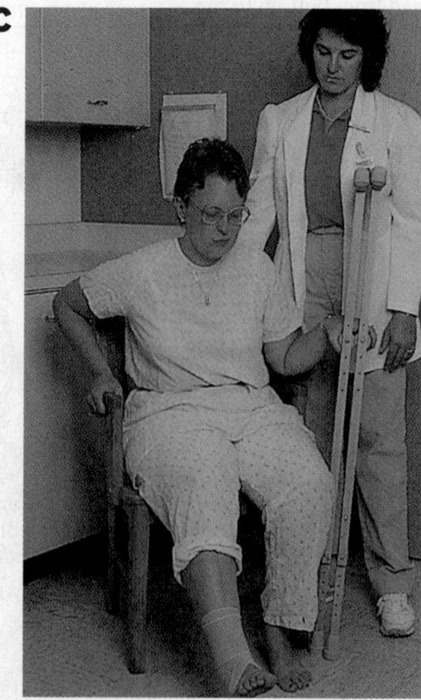

Figure 46-33 Sitting in a chair. A, Both crutches are held by one hand. Client transfers weight to crutches and unaffected leg. B, Client grasps arm of chair with free hand and begins to lower herself into chair. C, Client completely lowers herself into chair.

❖Evaluation

Client Care

To evaluate outcomes and response to nursing care, measure the effectiveness of all interventions. Compare the actual outcomes with the outcomes selected during planning. Evaluate specific interventions designed to promote body alignment, improve mobility, and protect the client from the hazards of immobility. Also evaluate client and family instruction to prevent future risks to body alignment and hazards of immobility (Figure 46–34). The evaluation enables you to determine whether new or revised therapies are required and if new nursing diagnoses have developed.

Client Expectations

Clients who are immobile and dependent on others for some or all of their needs can become overly dependent or try to do too much themselves too early. Finding the balance between independence and dependence is a difficult task. Clients will want control over mobility that is personally satisfactory. For the client who is completely dependent on others for care, control over how and when things are done may be very important. Do clients feel they are treated with dignity? Do caregivers treat them as adults? Are they given opportunities to make meaningful choices?

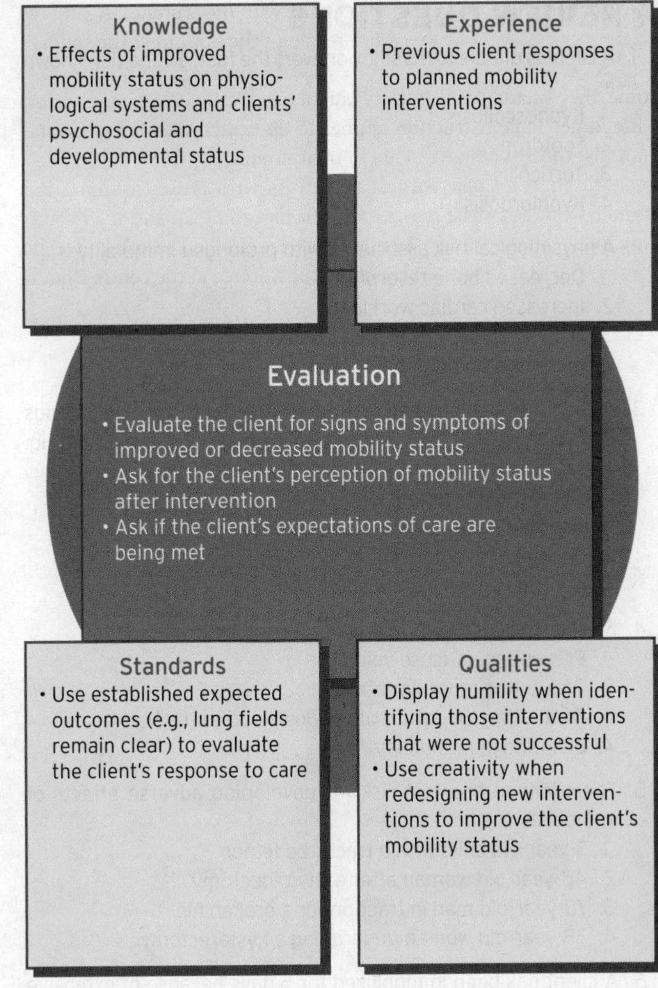

Figure 46-34 Critical thinking model for immobility evaluation.

✻ KEY CONCEPTS

- Body mechanics are the coordinated efforts of the musculoskeletal and nervous systems as the person moves, lifts, bends, stands, sits, lies down, and completes daily activities.
- Balance is assisted through nervous system control by the cerebellum and inner ear.
- Range-of-motion (ROM) exercises include one or all of the body joints and can be active or passive.
- Body alignment is the condition of joints, tendons, ligaments, and muscles in various body positions.
- Balance is achieved when a wide base of support is present, the centre of gravity falls within the base of support, and a vertical line falls from the centre of gravity through the base of support.
- Developmental stages influence body alignment and mobility; the greatest impact of physiological changes on the musculoskeletal system is observed in children and older adults.
- The risk of disabilities related to immobilization depends on the extent and duration of immobilization and the client's overall level of health.
- Immobility may result from illness or trauma or may be prescribed for therapeutic reasons (bed rest).
- Immobility presents hazards in the physiological, psychological, and developmental dimensions.
- Use the nursing process and critical thinking synthesis to provide care for clients who are experiencing or are at risk for the adverse effects of impaired body alignment and immobility.
- After identifying nursing diagnoses, plan and implement interventions to prevent or minimize the hazards and complications of impaired body alignment and immobilization.
- Clients with weakness and impaired function of the nervous, skeletal, or muscular system often require nursing assistance to attain proper body alignment while in bed or sitting and to transfer from a bed to a chair.
- Positioning devices help clients maintain good body alignment while lying or sitting.
- Assistive devices to promote walking include canes, walkers, and crutches.

✻ CRITICAL THINKING EXERCISES

1. You are caring for a 57-year-old man who had a bilateral total knee replacement for osteoarthritis 2 days ago. He is beginning to transfer to a chair with help. He is 45 kg overweight and has a history of deep vein thrombosis. He has compression stockings, continuous passive range of motion, and a heparin or saline lock. Make a list of potential nursing diagnoses.
2. When you are conducting a home visit for a 75-year-old woman, the client's granddaughter runs in and says, "Did you show the nurse the sore on your leg that you got from falling yesterday?" What questions about mobility are important to ask the client? How do you begin your assessment?
3. You are caring for a 75-year-old man who is immobilized after spinal cord trauma from a motor vehicle accident. What potential complications would you assess for in this client?

* REVIEW QUESTIONS

1. A client is unable to dorsiflex or evert the foot, a condition known as
   1. Kyphoscoliosis
   2. Footdrop
   3. Torticollis
   4. Kyphlordosis
2. A physiological risk associated with prolonged immobility is
   1. Decreased bone resorption
   2. Increased cardiac workload
   3. Decreased serum calcium levels
   4. Increased hemoglobin formation
3. A client has been on bed rest for several days. The client stands and you note that the client's systolic pressure drops 20 mm Hg. This is referred to as
   1. Orthostatic hypotension
   2. Rebound hypotension
   3. Positional hypotension
   4. Central venous hypotension
4. Elastic stockings help to prevent thrombus formation by
   1. Preventing varicose veins
   2. Preventing muscular atrophy
   3. Facilitating the return of venous blood to the heart
   4. Ensuring joint mobility
5. The client at greatest risk for developing adverse effects of immobility is a
   1. 3-year-old child with a fractured femur
   2. 48-year-old woman after a thyroidectomy
   3. 78-year-old man in traction for a broken hip
   4. 38-year-old woman undergoing a hysterectomy
6. A client has been immobilized for 5 days because of extensive abdominal surgery. When getting this client out of bed for the first time, a nursing diagnosis related to the safety of this client would be
   1. Pain
   2. Impaired skin integrity
   3. Altered tissue perfusion
   4. Risk for activity intolerance
7. Heparin and low-molecular-weight heparin are the most widely used drugs in the prophylaxis of deep vein thrombosis. Common dosage for heparin therapy is
   1. 5000 units given subcutaneously 2 hours before surgery and repeated every 8 to 12 hours
   2. 500 units given subcutaneously 2 hours before surgery and repeated every 8 to 12 hours
   3. 500 units given subcutaneously 8 hours before surgery and repeated every 8 to 12 hours
   4. 5000 units given subcutaneously 8 hours before surgery and repeated every 2 to 4 hours
8. The following device allows the client to pull with the upper extremities to raise the trunk off the bed, to assist in transfer from bed to wheelchair, or to perform upper arm exercises:
   1. Trapeze bar
   2. Trochanter roll
   3. Hand rolls
   4. Footboard
9. The client in this position is lying chest down:
   1. Supine
   2. Prone
   3. Fowler's
   4. Lateral
10. When positioning a client in the supported Fowler's position, you would place a small pillow under the client's thighs to
    1. Decrease intracranial pressure
    2. Support the lumbar vertebrae
    3. Prevent occlusion of popliteal artery
    4. Prevent pressure of mattress on heel

* RECOMMENDED WEB SITES

American Association of Rehabilitation Nurses: Related Sites: http://www.rehabnurse.org/sites/index.html

This Web page provides an extensive list of links to resources for nurses working with clients with actual or potential impairments or disabilities. It provides information about both prevention and treatment. Although the content has an American orientation, it is also useful to Canadian nurses.

Physical Activity Guide to Healthy Active Living: http://www.phac-aspc.gc.ca/pau-uap/paguide/older/index.html

This Web page is a general guide to physical activity and includes links to specific physical-activity guides for older adults and children. These guides are a good source of consumer education on the benefits of activity.

The Osteoporosis Society of Canada: Health Professionals Resource Links: http://www.osteoporosis.ca/english/For%20Health%20Professionals/Related%20Links/default.asp?s=1

The Osteoporosis Society of Canada is a national organization that works toward educating and supporting individuals and communities in the prevention and treatment of osteoporosis. This site provides numerous links to evidence-informed resources on osteoporosis.

The Registered Nurses Association of Ontario (RNAO) Best Practice Guidelines: Prevention of Falls and Injury in the Older Adult: http://www.rnao.org/Storage/12/617_BPG_Falls_rev05.pdf

The RNAO has developed a series of practice guidelines based on the consensus of nurse experts across a variety of practice, academic, and research agencies. This site provides information on client participation in ADLs, cognition, continence, strength, gait, and balance in relation to the risk for falls.

47

Skin Integrity and Wound Care

Written by Rosemary Kohr, RN, BA, BScN, MScN, PhD, ACNP(cert)

Based on the original chapter by Janice C. Colwell, RN, MS, CWOCN, FAAN

objectives

Mastery of content in this chapter will enable you to:

- Describe the key terms listed.
- Discuss the risk factors that contribute to pressure ulcer formation.
- Recognize the stages of pressure ulcers.
- Describe the etiology and key components of venous, arterial, diabetic, and malignant wounds.
- Discuss the normal process of wound healing.
- Describe the differences between wounds that heal by primary or secondary intention.
- Describe the complications of wound healing.
- Explain the factors that impede or promote wound healing.
- Describe the differences in nursing care for acute and chronic wounds.
- Describe the types of dressings appropriate for moist wound healing.
- Complete an assessment for a client with impaired skin integrity.
- List nursing diagnoses associated with impaired skin integrity.
- Develop a nursing care plan for a client with impaired skin integrity.
- List appropriate nursing interventions for a client with impaired skin integrity.
- State evaluation criteria for a client with impaired skin integrity.

key terms

media resources

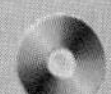 **Web Site**

- Audio Chapter Summaries
- Glossary
- Multiple-Choice Review Questions
- Skills Performance Checklists
- Student Learning Activities
- Video Clips
- Weblinks

Companion CD

- Glossary
- Interactive Learning Activities
- Fluids and Electrolytes Tutorial
- Test-Taking Skills

Skin, the body's largest organ, constitutes 15% of the total adult body weight (Wysocki, 2007). It protects against disease-causing organisms; senses pain, temperature, and touch; and synthesizes vitamin D. Injury to the skin poses risks to safety and triggers a complex healing response.

As a nurse, one of your most important responsibilities is to monitor skin integrity and prevent skin breakdown. Understanding normal wound healing helps in planning, implementing, and assessing interventions that maintain skin integrity and optimize wound healing.

Scientific Knowledge Base

Skin

The skin has two layers: the epidermis and the dermis (Figure 47–1). These two layers are separated by a membrane, often referred to as the dermal–epidermal junction. The epidermis, or top layer, also consists of several layers. The stratum corneum is the thin, outermost layer of the epidermis, consisting of flattened, dead, keratinized cells. The cells originate from the innermost epidermal layer, commonly called the basal layer. Cells in the basal layer divide, proliferate, and migrate toward the epidermal surface.

After cells reach the stratum corneum, they flatten and die. This constant movement ensures replacement of surface cells sloughed during normal desquamation or shedding. The stratum corneum protects underlying cells and tissues from dehydration and prevents the entrance of certain chemical agents. The stratum corneum allows the evaporation of water from the skin and permits the absorption of certain topical medications.

The dermis, the inner layer of the skin, provides tensile strength, mechanical support, and protection to the underlying muscles, bones, and organs. It differs from the epidermis in that it contains mostly connective tissue and few skin cells. Collagen (a tough, fibrous protein), blood vessels, and nerves are in the dermal layer. Fibroblasts, which are responsible for collagen formation, are the only distinctive cell type within the dermis.

Understanding skin structure helps you to maintain skin integrity and promote wound healing. Intact skin protects the client from chemical and mechanical injuries. When the skin is injured, the epidermis functions to resurface the wound and restore the barrier against invading organisms while the dermis responds to restore the structural integrity (collagen) and the physical properties of the skin. Age alters skin characteristics and makes skin more vulnerable to damage. Box 47–1 provides a summary of the changes in aging skin.

Pressure Ulcers

Pressure ulcer, pressure sore, decubitus ulcer, and *bedsore* are terms used to describe impaired skin integrity related to unrelieved, prolonged pressure. The most current terminology is *pressure ulcer*, which is consistent with the recommendations of the pressure ulcer guidelines developed by the Registered Nurses Association of Ontario (Assessment & Management of Stage I to IV Pressure Ulcers, revised 2007). A **pressure ulcer** is localized injury to the skin and other underlying tissue, usually over a bony prominence, as a result of pressure, or pressure in combination with shear or friction, or both (Figure 47–2).

Pressure ulcers have a high prevalence rate in all health care settings. It is estimated that one individual in four within the Canadian health care system has some issue with skin integrity (Woodbury & Houghton, 2004). The prevalence rate in acute care settings is 25%; nonacute care settings (including long-term care facilities), 30%; and community care and home care settings, 15% (Woodbury & Houghton, 2004).

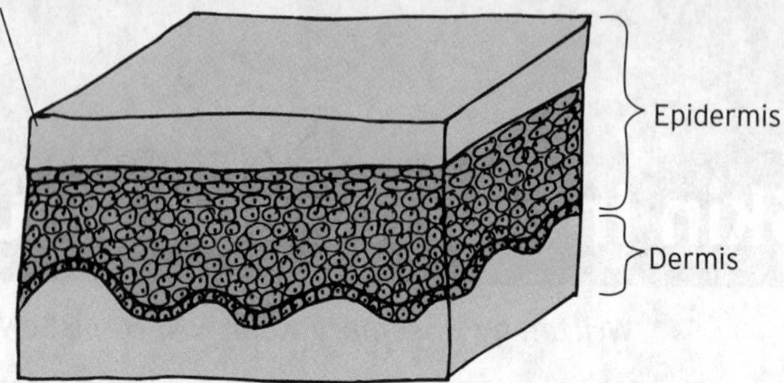

Figure 47-1 Layers of skin. **Source:** From Pires, M., & Muller, A. (1991). Detection and management of early tissue pressure indicators: A pictorial essay. *Progressions, 3*(3), 3.

The impact of pressure ulcers and other chronic wounds on quality of life is significant, as normal activities may be restricted because of pain, odour, or treatments. Costs associated with chronic wound care can substantially increase the burden on the health care system. It has been estimated that in the United States, an increase of 50% of nursing time along with treatments can cost from $10,000 to $86,000 (US$; in Canadian currency, $12,300 to $105,800) (Clarke et al., 2005).

Thus, it is essential that attention be paid to the causes of pressure ulcers as well as to the healing process of wounds. The focus of this text is on pressure ulcer prevention and treatment options, but other chronic wounds, such as diabetic, arterial, venous, and malignant wounds, will be briefly discussed and are important for you to recognize and treat. Additional resources are readily available on Web sites for the Canadian Association of Wound Care (CAWC), the Canadian Association of Enterostomal Therapists (CAET), and the Registered Nurses Association of Ontario (RNAO), which has produced a large number of evidence-informed best practice guidelines for pressure ulcers, venous leg ulcers, diabetic foot ulcers, continence and constipation, among others. These and other resources are provided for you at the end of this chapter.

BOX 47-1 FOCUS ON OLDER ADULTS

Skin-Associated Issues

- Age-related changes, such as reduced skin elasticity, decreased collagen, and thinning of underlying muscle and tissues, cause the older adult's skin to be easily torn in response to mechanical trauma, especially shearing forces (Wysocki, 2007).
- Concomitant medical conditions and polypharmacy, which is common in the older adult, are factors that interfere with wound healing.
- The attachment between the epidermis and dermis becomes flattened in older adults, which allows the skin to be easily torn in response to mechanical trauma (e.g., tape removal).
- Aging causes a diminished inflammatory response, resulting in slow epithelialization and wound healing (Doughty & Sparks-Defriese, 2007).
- The hypodermis decreases in size with age. Older clients have little subcutaneous padding over bony prominences, so they are more prone to skin breakdown (Wysocki, 2007).
- Reduced nutritional intake, commonly seen in older adults, increases the risk of pressure ulcer development and impaired wound healing (Posthauer & Thomas, 2004).

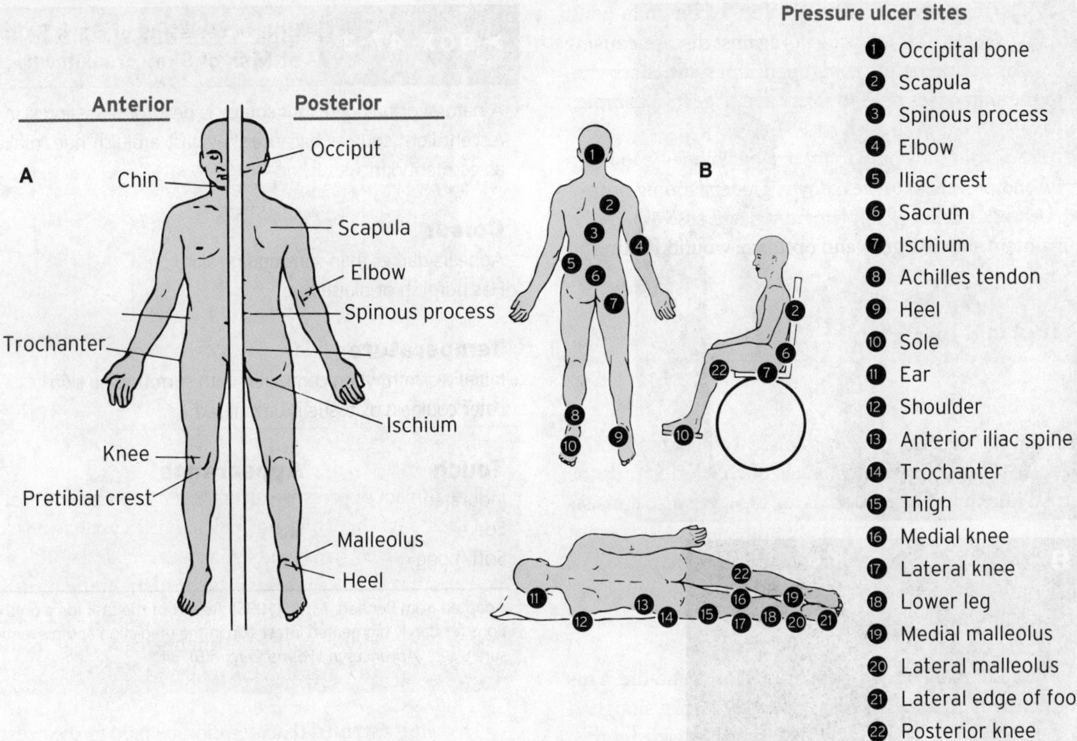

Figure 47-2 A, Bony prominences most frequently underlying pressure ulcers. B, Common pressure ulcer sites. **Source:** Adapted from Trelease, C. C. (1988). Developing standards for wound care. *Ostomy/Wound Management, 20*, 46.

Pathogenesis of Pressure Ulcers. Pressure is the major element in the cause of pressure ulcers. Three pressure-related factors contribute to pressure ulcer development: (1) pressure intensity, (2) pressure duration, and (3) tissue tolerance.

Pressure Intensity. A classic research study identified capillary closing pressure as the minimal amount of pressure required to collapse a capillary (e.g., when the pressure exceeds the normal capillary pressure range of 15–32 mm Hg) (Burton & Yamada, 1951). Therefore, if the pressure applied over a capillary exceeds the normal capillary pressure and the vessel is occluded for a prolonged period of time, **tissue ischemia**, or reduction in blood flow, can occur. If the client has decreased sensation and cannot respond to the discomfort of the ischemia, tissue ischemia and tissue death result. The clinical presentation of obstructed blood flow will occur when you evaluate areas of pressure. After a period of tissue ischemia, if the pressure is relieved and the blood flow returns, the skin turns red. The effect of this redness is vasodilatation (blood vessel expansion), called **hyperemia** (redness) (Figure 47–3*A*). Evaluate the area of hyperemia by pressing a finger over the affected area. If the area blanches (turns lighter in colour) (Figure 47–3*B*) and the erythema returns when you remove your finger, the hyperemia is transient and is an attempt to overcome the ischemic episode; thus, it is called blanching hyperemia (Pieper, 2007).

If, however, the erythematous area does not blanch (nonblanching erythema) (Figure 47–4) when you apply pressure, deep tissue damage is probable.

Blanching occurs when the normal red tones of the light-skinned client are absent. Blanching does not occur in clients with darkly pigmented skin. The Task Force on the Implications for Darkly Pigmented Intact Skin in the Prediction and Prevention of Pressure Ulcers (Bennett, 1995) defined **darkly pigmented skin** as skin that "remains unchanged (does not blanch) when pressure is applied over a bony prominence, irrespective of the client's race or ethnicity." Characteristics of intact dark skin that will alert you to the potential for pressure ulcers are found in Box 47–2.

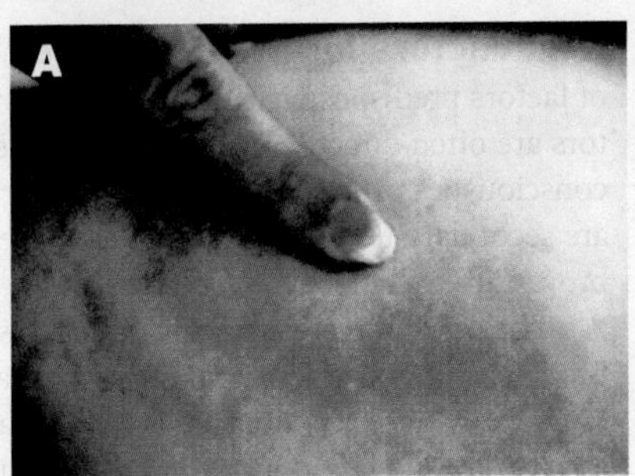

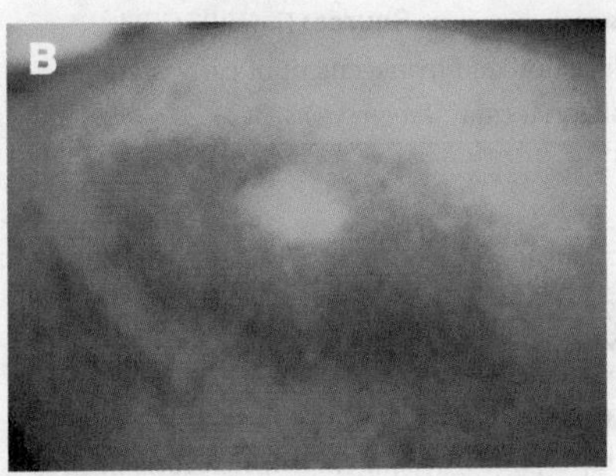

Figure 47-3 A, Reactive hyperemia. B, Blanching erythema: blanches with fingertip pressure.

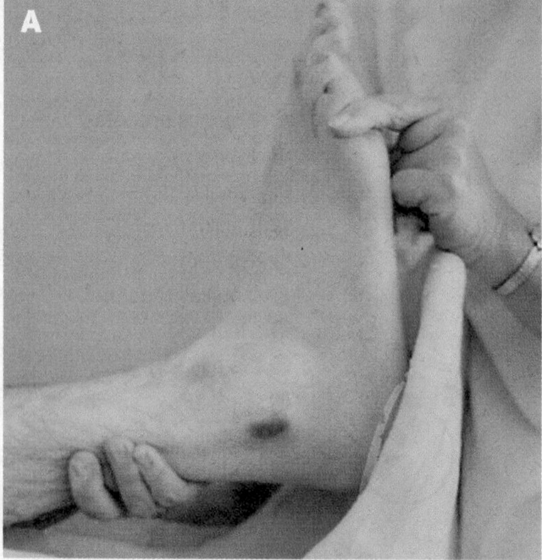

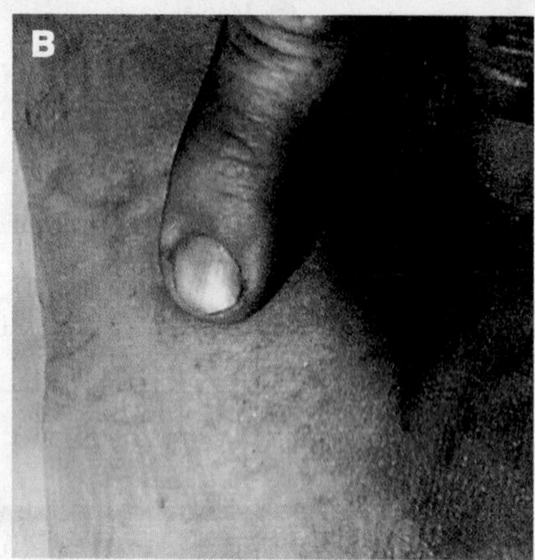

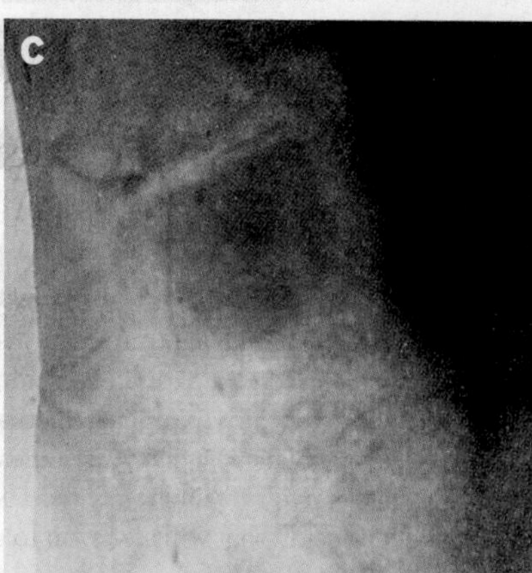

Figure 47-4 A, Reactive hyperemia. B and C, In nonblanching erythema, the area is much darker than the surrounding skin and does not blanch with fingertip pressure. **Source:** From Pires, M., & Muller, A. (1991). Detection and management of early tissue pressure indicators: A pictorial essay. *Progressions, 3*(3), 3.

BOX 47-2 Characteristics of Dark Skin at Risk of Skin Breakdown

A natural or halogen light source is best for assessing skin. Avoid fluorescent light sources because they cast a bluish hue, making accurate assessment difficult.

Colour
Appears darker than surrounding skin
Has purplish or bluish hue

Temperature
Initial warmth when compared with surrounding skin
Later coolness as tissue is devitalized

Touch	Appearance
Indurated	Taut
Edema	Shiny
Soft, boggy	Scaly

Adapted from Bennett, M. A. (1995). Report of the task force on the implications for darkly pigmented intact skin in the prediction and prevention of pressure ulcers. *Advances in Wound Care, 8*(6), 34.

Pressure Duration. Two considerations are related to the duration of pressure. Low pressures over a prolonged time period and high-intensity pressure over a short period of time both cause tissue damage. Extended pressure occludes blood flow and nutrients and contributes to cell death (Pieper, 2007). Clinical implications of pressure duration include evaluating the amount of pressure (check the skin for reactive hyperemia) and determining the amount of time that a client tolerates pressure (check to be sure after relieving pressure that the affected area blanches).

Tissue Tolerance. The ability of tissue to endure pressure depends on the integrity of the tissue and the supporting structures. The extrinsic factors of shear, friction, and moisture affect the ability of the skin to tolerate pressure: the greater degree to which the factors of shear, friction, and moisture are present, the more susceptible the skin will be to damage from pressure. Another factor related to tissue tolerance pertains to the ability of the underlying skin structures (blood vessels, collagen) to assist in redistributing pressure. Systemic factors such as poor nutrition, increased aging, and low blood pressure affect the tissue's tolerance to externally applied pressure.

Nursing Knowledge Base

Prediction and Prevention of Pressure Ulcers

A major aspect of nursing care is the maintenance of skin integrity. Consistent, planned skin care interventions are critical to ensuring high-quality care. You need to take every opportunity to observe and assess your clients' skin for impaired skin integrity.

Risk Factors for Pressure Ulcer Development. A variety of factors predispose a client to pressure ulcer formation. These factors are often directly related to disease, such as a decreased level of consciousness, the after-effects of trauma, or the presence of a cast, or are secondary to an illness, such as decreased sensation after a cerebrovascular accident.

The use of a pressure ulcer risk assessment tool, such as the Braden Risk Assessment Tool (described later in Table 47–2), is essential in providing an initial assessment that can be used to determine appropriate interventions as well as scheduled regular assessment that can evaluate ongoing skin status and treatment plans.

Impaired Sensory Perception. Clients with an altered sensory perception of pain and pressure are at more risk of impaired skin integrity than are clients with normal sensation. Clients with impaired sensory perception of pain and pressure are unable to feel when a portion of their body senses increased, prolonged pressure or pain. Thus, the client without the ability to feel or sense pain or pressure is at risk of developing pressure ulcers (Skill 47–1).

Impaired Mobility. Clients unable to independently change positions are at risk of pressure ulcer development. For example, clients with spinal cord injuries have decreased or absent motor and sensory perception and are unable to reposition themselves after lying on bony prominences for too long.

Alteration in Level of Consciousness. Clients who are confused or disoriented or who have changing levels of consciousness are unable to protect themselves from pressure ulcer development because they can sometimes feel pressure but are not always able to understand how to relieve it or communicate their discomfort. Clients in a coma cannot perceive pressure and are unable to move voluntarily to relieve pressure.

➤ SKILL 47-1 Assessment for Risk of Pressure Ulcer Development

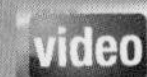

Delegation Considerations

Assessment of clients for the risk of pressure ulcers should not be delegated to unregulated care providers (UCPs). Check with your institution's policy in this regard.

Prevention

- Document any changes to the client's skin, such as redness, blistering, abrasions, or cuts.
- Keep the client's skin dry and provide hygiene after incontinence of urine or stool or exposure to other body fluids.
- Reposition the client according to the frequency established on the nursing care plan or agency policy.
- Avoid trauma to the client's skin from tape, pressure, friction, or shear.

Equipment

- Use a risk assessment tool: Braden Scale (used in this skill) or other tool, according to agency policy.
- Documentation record

Procedure

STEPS	RATIONALE
1. Identify at-risk individuals needing prevention and the specific factors placing them at risk.	• Identification determines factors that increase the client's risk of developing pressure ulcers (Braden, 2001).
A. Use a validated risk assessment tool (e.g., the Braden Scale)	• Consistent, reliable, comparable assessments are ensured (AHCPR, 1992a, 1992b; NPUAP, 2007a, 2007b; RNAO, 2007).
B. Assess the client on admission to the hospital, long-term care facility, home care program, or other health care facility.	• A baseline assessment is provided.
C. Inspect the condition of the client's skin at least once a day (see Box 47–4) and examine all bony prominences, noting skin integrity. (Check agency policy for reassessment and reassess at periodic intervals.) If redness or discoloration is noted, use thumb to gently palpate area of redness. The discoloration may vary from pink to deep red.	• Routine skin assessments will identify changes in client's risk of pressure ulcers. • Nonblanchable erythema or discoloration in the client's skin may be an early indicator of skin injury (Pieper, 2007).

Critical Decision Point: In dark-skinned clients, the discoloration appears as a deepening of the normal colour (see Box 47–2). Darkly pigmented skin does not always show direct changes in colour (Bennett, 1995; NPUAP, 1998).

STEPS	RATIONALE
D. Observe all assistive devices, such as braces or casts, and medical equipment, such as nasogastric and enteral tubes and catheters, for pressure points.	• Presence of medical equipment has the potential to cause pressure and skin breakdown in sensitive regions, such as the nares, ears, bony prominences, and other pressure areas.
2. Determine the client's ability to respond meaningfully to pressure-related discomfort (sensory perception).	• Clients with completely, very, or slightly limited ability to respond to pressure-related discomfort cannot communicate discomfort, will have a limited ability to feel pain and, thus, will have a risk of developing pressure ulcers.
3. Assess the degree to which the client's skin is exposed to moisture.	• A person whose skin is exposed to excessive moisture has an increased risk of skin breakdown due to changes in skin pH and maceration of skin.
4. Evaluate the client's activity level.	• The client who is bedfast, chairfast, or only walks occasionally will be at risk of developing pressure ulcers because of the degree of physical inactivity.
A. Determine the client's ability to change and control body position (mobility).	• Potential for friction and shear injury increases when the client is completely dependent on others for position change.
B. Determine client's preferred positions.	• The weight of the body will be placed on certain bony prominences, and the client may resist repositioning to different areas.

Continued

➤ SKILL 47-1 Assessment for Risk of Pressure Ulcer Development *continued*

STEPS	RATIONALE
5. Assess the client's usual food and fluid intake pattern (nutrition and hydration).	• A client who never eats a complete meal, rarely eats a complete meal, or has limited fluid intake is at risk of skin breakdown.
A. Review weight pattern and nutritional laboratory values.	• Decreased nutritional status is linked with pressure ulcer formation and poor wound healing (AHCPR, 1994; RNAO, 2007).
B. Complete a fluid intake assessment.	• Fluid imbalance, either dehydration or edema, can increase the client's risk of pressure ulcers.
6. Evaluate the presence of friction and shear.	• The client who has a problem in moving, requires maximum assistance in moving, or slides against sheets when moved is at an increased risk of skin damage.
7. Document the risk assessment on admission, on a regular basis according to institutional policy, and if any change in status occurs (Sibbald et al., 2006a).	• The documentation will provide a baseline for comparison of increased or decreased risk of development of pressure ulcers and allow planning of interventions.
A. Observe the Braden Scale scores: as they become lower, predicted risk becomes higher.	• Scores: 15–16, mild risk 13–14, moderate risk 10–12, high risk <10, very high risk
B. Link the risk assessment to preventive protocols.	• Prevention protocols will target problem areas to assist in prevention of skin breakdown (Braden, 2001).
C. Institute mild-risk interventions (score of 15–16). Plan of care should include frequent turning; maximum remobilization; off-load heel pressure; use of pressure-reducing support surface; manage moisture, nutrition, and friction and shear.	• The risk of skin breakdown is decreased.
D. Institute moderate-risk interventions (score of 13–14). Plan of care should include interventions for mild risk (step 7c), as well as use of foam wedges to position the client in the 30-degree lateral position.	• The increased risk of skin breakdown is decreased with appropriate interventions.
E. Institute high-risk interventions (score of 10–12). Plan of care should include interventions for moderate risk (step 7d), as well as instructions to turn the client with small shifts in weight.	• The factors that contribute to skin breakdown are addressed, and interventions to address the causative factors are planned.
F. Institute very high-risk interventions (score <10). Plan of care should include interventions for high-risk (step 7e) as well as use of a pressure-relieving surface if the client has uncontrolled pain or severe pain exacerbated by turning.	• Plan interventions to decrease the effects of immobility, decreased sensory perception, moisture, friction, shear, decreased activity, and nutritional issues in a high-risk individual.
8. Provide education to client and family regarding pressure ulcer risk and prevention.	• Clients and family understand the interventions designed to reduce pressure ulcer risk.
9. Evaluate measures to reduce pressure ulcer development	• Evaluation on a regular basis provides opportunity to assess interventions and adjust as required.
A. Observe client's skin for areas at risk.	• Client's response to risk-reduction interventions is determined over time.
B. Observe tolerance of client for positioning.	• Frequent change in position further reduces client's risk of pressure ulcer development.
C. Monitor the success of a toileting program or other measures to reduce the frequency of incontinence of urine or stool.	• Timeliness of a toileting program or schedule to assist the client in meeting elimination needs is determined.
D. Evaluate laboratory nutrition values.	• The success of nutritional supplements in improving nutritional status is determined.

Unexpected Outcomes and Related Interventions

No Blanching When Skin Is Firmly Pressed, Purple Discoloration, or Significant Colour Change

- Reassess frequency of turning schedule.
- Implement agency's skin care protocols.
- Consider support surface to reduce pressure ulcer risk.

Recording and Reporting

- Record client's risk score.
- Record appearance of skin under pressure.
- Describe position, turning intervals, pressure-relieving devices, and other prevention strategies.
- Report any need for additional consultations (e.g., wound care specialist or dietitian) for the high-risk client.

Home Care Considerations

- Instruct the caregiver to use the 30-degree lateral position. This position reduces pressure over the trochanter.
- Pressure-relief manoeuvres need to be individualized for client needs and the home environment. Provide the family with resources for hospital equipment.

Shear. **Shear** is the force exerted parallel to the skin and results from both gravity pushing down on the body and resistance (friction) between the client and a surface (Pieper, 2007). For example, shear force occurs when the head of the bed is elevated and the skeleton starts to slide but the skin is fixed because of friction with the bed (Figure 47–5). In addition, shear force occurs when you transfer a client from the bed to a stretcher and the client's skin is pulled across the bed. When shear is present, the skin and subcutaneous layers adhere to the surface of the bed, and the layers of muscle and the bones slide in the direction of body movement. The underlying tissue capillaries are stretched and angulated by the shear force. As a result, necrosis occurs deep within the tissue layers, causing undermining of the dermis.

Friction. The force of two surfaces moving across one another, such as the mechanical force exerted when skin is dragged across a coarse surface such as bed linens, is called **friction** (Wound, Ostomy, and Continence Nurses [WOCN], 2003). Unlike shear injuries, friction injuries affect the epidermis, or top layer of the skin. The denuded skin appears red and painful and is sometimes referred to as a "sheet burn." A friction injury occurs in a client who is dragged over the bed surface instead of being lifted slightly during position changes.

Moisture. The presence and duration of moisture on the skin increases the risk of ulcer formation. Moisture reduces the skin's resistance to other physical factors such as pressure and shear force. Prolonged moisture softens skin, which makes it more susceptible to damage. Immobilized clients, who are unable to take care of their own hygiene needs, depend on you to keep their skin dry and intact. Skin moisture originates from wound drainage, excessive perspiration, and fecal or urinary incontinence.

Nutrition. Adequate nutritional intake is essential for not only wound healing but also wound prevention (Stratton et al., 2005). In particular, high protein oral nutritional supplementation is necessary in clients whose prealbumin or albumin, hemoglobin, and serum zinc stores are low (RNAO, 2007).

For clients weakened or debilitated by illness, nutritional therapy is especially important. A client who has undergone surgery (see Chapter 49) and is well nourished still requires at least 1500 kcal/day for nutritional maintenance. Alternatives such as enteral feedings and parenteral nutrition (see Chapter 43) are available for clients unable to maintain normal food intake.

Normal wound healing requires proper nutrition (Table 47–1). Deficiencies in any of the nutrients result in impaired or delayed healing (Stotts, 2007a). Physiological processes of wound healing depend on the availability of protein, vitamins (especially A and C), and the trace minerals zinc and copper. **Collagen** is a protein formed from amino acids acquired by fibroblasts from protein ingested in food. Vitamin C is necessary for the synthesis of collagen, and vitamin A reduces the negative effects of steroids on wound healing. Trace elements such as zinc (used for epithelialization and collagen synthesis) and copper (for collagen fibre linking) are also necessary.

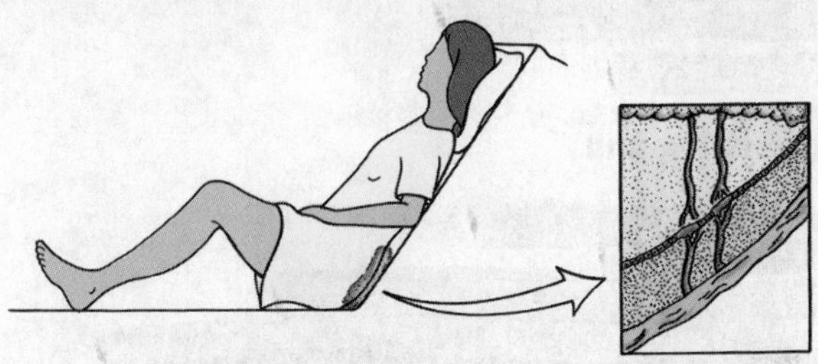

Figure 47-5 Sketch of shear force exerted against the sacral area.

Calories provide the material needed to support the cellular activity of wound healing, and protein needs, especially, are increased. A balanced intake of various nutrients is critical for wound healing and should include protein, fat, carbohydrates, vitamins, and minerals. Serum proteins are biochemical indicators of malnutrition (Stotts, 2007a). Serum albumin is probably the most frequently measured of these laboratory parameters, but albumin alone is not sensitive to rapid changes in nutritional status. Transferrin is also used to evaluate protein status, but alone it does not determine malnutrition. The best measure of nutritional status is prealbumin because it reflects not only what the client has ingested but also what the body has absorbed, digested, and metabolized (Stotts, 2007a).

Tissue Perfusion. Oxygen fuels the cellular functions essential to the healing process; therefore, the ability to perfuse the tissues with adequate amounts of oxygenated blood is critical to wound healing (Doughty & Sparks-Defriese, 2007). Clients with shock or peripheral vascular diseases, such as diabetes, are at risk of poor tissue perfusion due to poor circulation. Oxygen requirements depend on the phase of wound healing; for instance, chronic tissue hypoxia is associated with impaired collagen synthesis and reduced tissue resistance to infection.

Infection. Wound infection prolongs the inflammatory phase, delays collagen synthesis, prevents epithelialization, and increases the production of proinflammatory cytokines, which leads to additional tissue destruction (Stotts, 2007b). Indications that a wound infection is present include the presence of pus; a change in odour, volume, or the character of wound drainage; redness in the surrounding tissue; fever; or pain (Box 47–3).

Pain. Uncontrolled pain can affect the client's ability to tolerate movement and can decrease tissue perfusion because of rapid, shallow breathing and tensed muscles. In addition, the client's appetite may be diminished because of nausea from pain, and if the restorative powers of sleep are not accessible, the individual may feel hopeless and depressed from the unrelenting nature of both the wound and the persistent pain (Kohr & Gibson, 2008).

Age. Increased age affects all phases of wound healing. A decrease in the functioning of macrophages leads to a delayed inflammatory response, delayed collagen synthesis, and slower epithelialization.

Psychosocial Impact of Wounds. The client's psychological response to any wound is part of your assessment. Body image changes often impose a great stress on the client's adaptive mechanisms. In addition, body image changes influence self-concept (see Chapter 26) and sexuality (see Chapter 27). Make sure the client's personal and social resources for adaptation are a part of the assessment. Factors that affect the client's perception of the wound include the presence of scars, drains (drains are often necessary for weeks or even months after certain procedures), odour from drainage, and temporary or permanent prosthetic devices.

Critical Thinking

Successful critical thinking requires a synthesis of knowledge, experience, information gathered from clients, critical thinking attitudes, and intellectual and professional standards. Clinical judgement means you need to anticipate the information necessary, analyze the data, and make decisions regarding client care. Critical thinking is always changing. During assessment, consider all elements that build toward making appropriate nursing diagnoses (Figure 47–6).

When caring for clients who have impaired skin integrity and chronic wounds, you must integrate knowledge from nursing and

TABLE 47-1 Role of Selected Nutrients in Wound Healing

Nutrient	Role In Healing	Recommendations	Sources
Calories	Fuel for cell energy "protein protection"	35–40 kcal/kg/day, or enough to maintain positive nitrogen valance	
Protein	Fibroplasia, angiogenesis, collagen formation and wound remodelling, immune function	1.0–1.5 g/kg/day, or enough to maintain positive nitrogen balance	Poultry, fish, eggs, beef
Vitamin C (ascorbic acid)	Collagen synthesis, capillary wall integrity, fibroblast function, immunological function, antioxidant	100–1000 mg/day Need long time before clinical scurvy from vitamin C deficiency develops Low toxicity	Citrus fruits, tomatoes, potatoes, fortified fruit juices
Vitamin A	Epithelialization, wound closure, inflammatory response, angiogenesis, collagen formation Can reverse steroid effects on skin and delayed healing	1600–2000 retinol equivalents per day Supplement if deficient 20,000 units × 10 days	Green leafy vegetables (spinach), broccoli, carrots, sweet potatoes, liver
Vitamin E	No known role in wound healing, antioxidant	None	Fish, oysters, liver, dark meat, eggs, legumes
Zinc	Collagen formation, protein synthesis, cell membrane and host defenses	15–30 mg Correct deficiencies No improvement in wound healing with supplementation unless zinc deficient Use with caution: large doses can be toxic May inhibit copper metabolism and impair immune function	Vegetables, meats, legumes
Fluid	Essential fluid environment for all cell function	30–35 mL/kg/day Increase by another 10–15 mL/kg if client is on an air-fluidized bed	Use noncaffeine, nonalcoholic fluids without sugar Water is best: 6–8 glasses/day

Adapted from Ayello, E. A., Thomas, D. R., & Litchford, M. A. (1999). Nutritional aspects of wound healing. *Home Health Nurse, 17*(11), 719; and Stotts, N. A. (2007). Nutritional assessment and support. In R. A. Bryant & D. P. Nix (Eds.), *Acute and chronic wounds: Current management concepts* (3rd ed.). St. Louis: Mosby.

other disciplines, previous experiences, and information gathered from clients to understand the risks to skin integrity and wound healing. Knowledge of normal musculoskeletal physiology, the pathogenesis of pressure ulcers, normal wound healing, and the pathophysiology of underlying diseases provides you with a scientific basis for care. The CAWC (2006) and the RNAO (2007) provide evidence-derived guidelines for assessment of the risk of impaired skin integrity, prevention measures, and interventions to promote wound healing, as well as other standards of practice that you should use in planning care. Past experience with clients at risk of impaired skin integrity or with clients with wounds increases the experiential knowledge base helping you to identify interventions.

Finally, you need to ensure that you remain attentive during assessment to obtain comprehensive and correct assessment data. As identified previously, a *continuum* exists to wound healing that implies change over time. You need to be aware that the client and the skin or wound condition will not remain static, so you should reassess on a regular basis and adjust your plan of care accordingly. Knowledge and experience regarding wound healing will assist you in taking advantage of all the available and appropriate treatment options.

BOX 47-3 Classic Signs of Wound Infection

- Pain and tenderness at the wound site
- Erythema (reddening of the surrounding tissue)
- Edema (swelling), **induration** (increased firmness of the tissue)
- Inflammation of wound edges
- Purulent discharge
- Warmth in surrounding tissue
- Fever, chills
- Foul odour
- Elevated white blood cell count
- Delayed healing

Chronic Wounds

The above signs and symptoms as well as the following:

- Increased exudates
- Bright red discoloration of granulation tissue
- New areas of slough or breakdown on the wound surface
- Undermining (dead space under the edges of the wound)

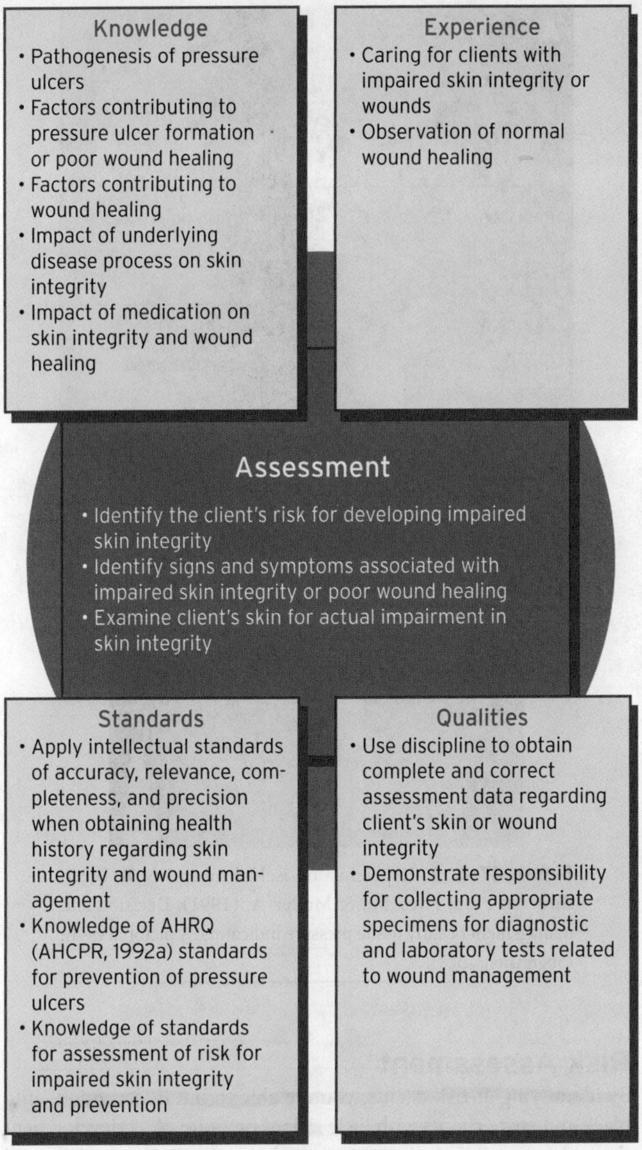

Knowledge
- Pathogenesis of pressure ulcers
- Factors contributing to pressure ulcer formation or poor wound healing
- Factors contributing to wound healing
- Impact of underlying disease process on skin integrity
- Impact of medication on skin integrity and wound healing

Experience
- Caring for clients with impaired skin integrity or wounds
- Observation of normal wound healing

Assessment
- Identify the client's risk for developing impaired skin integrity
- Identify signs and symptoms associated with impaired skin integrity or poor wound healing
- Examine client's skin for actual impairment in skin integrity

Standards
- Apply intellectual standards of accuracy, relevance, completeness, and precision when obtaining health history regarding skin integrity and wound management
- Knowledge of AHRQ (AHCPR, 1992a) standards for prevention of pressure ulcers
- Knowledge of standards for assessment of risk for impaired skin integrity and prevention

Qualities
- Use discipline to obtain complete and correct assessment data regarding client's skin or wound integrity
- Demonstrate responsibility for collecting appropriate specimens for diagnostic and laboratory tests related to wound management

Figure 47-6 Critical thinking for skin integrity and wound care assessment.

Nursing Process

❖Assessment

Baseline and continual assessment data provide critical information about the client's skin integrity and the increased risk of pressure ulcer development. When you focus on specific elements such as the client's level of sensation, movement, and continence status, you guide the skin assessment (Box 47–4).

Skin

You should ensure that ongoing assessment occurs to guard against skin breakdown, and you should treat any tears or ulcers promptly (Box 47–5). The neurologically impaired client, the chronically ill client in long-term care, the client with diminished mental status, and clients in the intensive care unit (ICU) or oncology, hospice, or orthopedic departments all have an increased potential of developing pressure ulcers.

> **BOX 47-4 Nursing Assessment Questions**
>
> **Skin Integrity**
>
> ***Sensation***
> - Do you have any decreased sensation in your extremities or any other region?
> - Do you have sensitivity to heat or cold?
>
> ***Mobility***
> - Do you have any physical limitations, injury, or paralysis that limits your mobility?
> - Can you easily change your position?
> - Is movement painful?
>
> ***Continence***
> - Do you have any problems with urine or bowel continence?
> - What assistance do you need using the toilet?
> - How often do you need to use the toilet? During the day? During the night?
>
> ***Presence of a Wound***
> - What caused the wound?
> - When did the wound occur? What is its location and size?
> - When did the client last receive a tetanus shot?
> - What happened to this wound since it occurred? What were the changes, and what caused them?
> - What treatments, activities, or care have slowed or helped the wound-healing process? Does the client have special needs that might impair wound healing?
> - Are there associated symptoms such as pain or itching? How are they being managed, and are the interventions effective?
> - What is the goal for the client, wound, and healing?

Assessment for tissue pressure damage includes visual and tactile inspection of the skin. You perform a baseline assessment to determine the client's normal skin characteristics and any potential or actual areas of breakdown. You need to individualize assessment characteristics of a client's skin, depending on the client's skin tone (Bennett, 1995; Henderson et al.,1997). Assessment characteristics of darkly pigmented skin appear in Boxes 47–2 and 47–5.

Pay particular attention to areas located over bony prominences or under casts, traction, splints, braces, collars, or other orthopedic devices. The frequency of pressure checks depends on the schedule of appliance application and the skin's response to the external pressure (Figure 47-7).

When you note hyperemia, document the location, size, and colour and reassess the area after 1 hour (Figure 47–8, *A*). When you suspect abnormal reactive hyperemia, outline the affected area with a marker to make reassessment easier. These signs are early indicators of impaired skin integrity, but damage to the underlying tissue is sometimes more progressive (Figure 47–8, *B*). Tactile assessment enables you to use palpation to acquire further data about induration and the damage to the skin and underlying tissues.

Gently palpate the reddened tissue, observing for blanching as normal skin tones return in clients with light-toned skin. In addition, palpate for induration, noting the size in millimetres or centimetres of the induration around the injured area. Also use palpation to note changes in the temperature of the surrounding skin and tissues.

Use visual and tactile inspection over the body areas most frequently at risk of pressure ulcer development (see Figure 47–2). For example, when clients lie in bed or sit in a chair, they place their

BOX 47-5 CULTURAL ASPECTS OF CARE

Skin Colour Impact

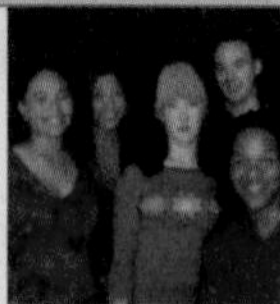

Your ability to detect cyanosis and other changes in skin colour in clients is an important clinical skill. However, this detection becomes a challenge in dark-skinned clients. Cyanosis is "a slightly bluish grayish slatelike or dark purple discoloration of the skin due to the presence of at least 5 grams of reduced hemoglobin in arterial blood." Colour differentiation of cyanosis varies according to skin pigmentation. In dark-skinned clients, you need to know the individual's baseline skin tone. You should not confuse the normal hyperpigmentation of mongolian spots that are seen on the sacrum of African, Native American, and Asian clients as cyanosis. Observe the client's skin in nonglare daylight. The Gaskin's Nursing Assessment of Skin Colour (GNASC) is a useful assessment tool for identifying changes in skin colour that increase the client's risk of pressure ulcers.

Implications for Practice

- Cyanosis is difficult but possible to detect in the dark-skinned client.
- Be aware of situations that produce changes in skin tone, such as inadequate lighting.
- Examine body sites with the least melanin, such as under the arm, for underlying colour identification.
- Evaluate pigmented skin for colour-specific changes in skin tone.

Adapted from Gaskin, F. C. (1986). Detection of cyanosis in the person with dark skin. *Journal of National Black Nurses' Association, 1,* 52; and Henderson, C. T., Ayello, E. A., Sussman, C., Leiby, D. M., Bennet, M. A., Dungog, E. F., et al. (1997). Draft definition of stage I pressure ulcers: Inclusion of persons with darkly pigmented skin. *Advances in Wound Care, 10*(5), 16.

body weight heavily on certain bony prominences. Body surfaces subjected to the greatest weight or pressure are at greatest risk of pressure ulcer formation.

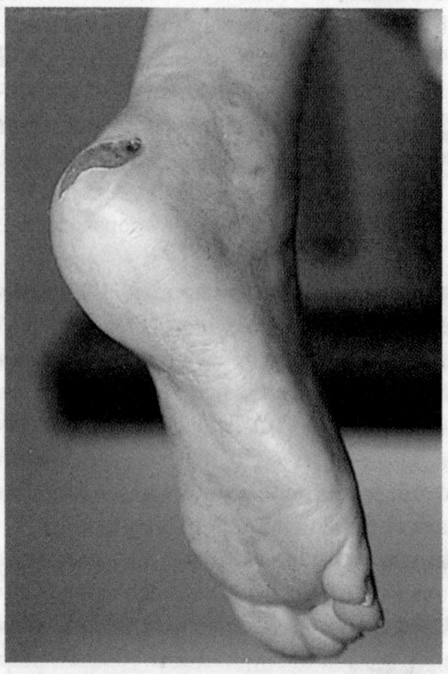

Figure 47-7 A pressure ulcer on the heel caused by pressure exerted by the mattress.

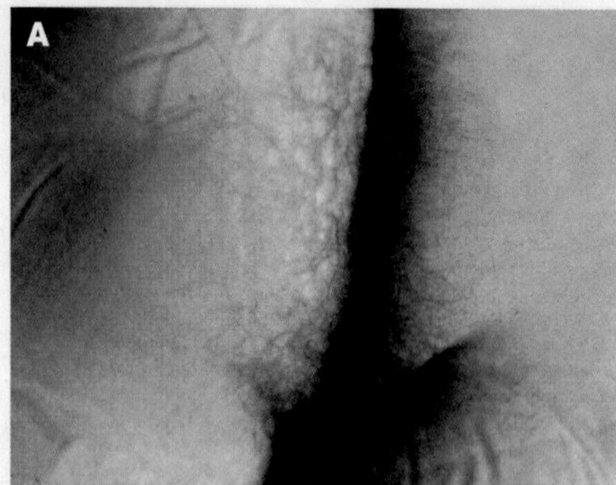

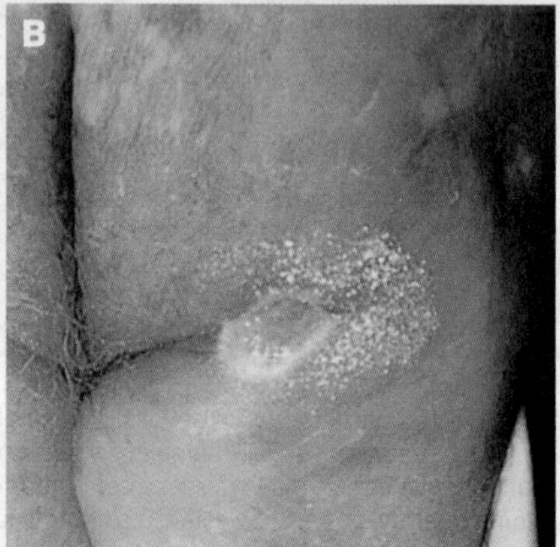

Figure 47-8 A, Hyperemia on ischial tuberosity. B, Ulcer. **Source:** From Pires, M., & Muller, A. (1991). Decision and management of early tissue pressure indicators: A pictorial essay. *Progressions,* 3(3), 3.

Risk Assessment

By identifying at-risk clients, you are able to put interventions into place and spare clients with little risk of pressure ulcer development the unnecessary and sometimes costly preventive treatments and related risks of complications. The prevention and treatment of pressure ulcers are major nursing priorities, no matter what the health care setting. The incidence of pressure ulcers in a facility or agency is an important indicator of quality of care. Evidence exists that a program of prevention guided by consistent risk assessment simultaneously reduces the institutional incidence of pressure ulcers by as much as 60% and decreases the costs of prevention at the same time (Braden, 2001). Several risk assessment tools have been validated in the research literature as reliable in predicting the risk of skin breakdown (Braden & Bergstrom, 1989; Norton et al., 1962). The Braden Scale has been identified by the CAWC and the RNAO Best Practice Guidelines as a reliable and valid risk assessment tool across all health care sectors (RNAO, 2007; Keast et al., 2006). However, an assessment tool is exactly that, a tool to assist you in planning intervention strategies and evaluation of your client's skin on an ongoing basis. No assessment tool can replace your clinical judgement as a nurse (RNAO, 2007).

Braden Scale

The Braden Scale (Table 47–2) was developed based on risk factors in a nursing home population (Bergstrom, Braden, et al., 1987). The Braden Scale comprises six subscales: sensory perception, moisture,

TABLE 47-2 Braden Scale for Predicting Pressure Sore Risk

Client's Name ______________ Evaluator's Name ______________ Date of Assessment ______________

Characteristic	Score: 1	Score: 2	Score: 3	Score: 4
Sensory Perception				
Ability to respond meaningfully to pressure-related discomfort	1. Completely limited Unresponsive (does not moan, flinch, or gasp) to painful stimuli due to diminished level of consciousness or sedation. OR Limited ability to feel pain over most of body surface.	2. Very limited Responds only to painful stimuli. Cannot communicate discomfort except by moaning or restlessness. OR Has a sensory impairment that limits the ability to feel pain or discomfort over half of body.	3. Slightly limited Responds to verbal commands but cannot always communicate discomfort or need to be turned. OR Has some sensory impairment that limits ability to feel pain or discomfort in 1 or 2 extremities.	4. No impairment Responds to verbal commands. Has no sensory deficit that would limit ability to feel or voice pain or discomfort.
Moisture				
Degree to which skin is exposed to moisture	1. Constantly moist Skin is kept moist almost constantly by perspiration, urine, etc. Dampness is detected every time client is moved or turned.	2. Moist Skin is often, but not always, moist. Linen must be changed at least once a shift.	3. Occasionally moist Skin is occasionally moist, requiring an extra linen change approximately once a day.	4. Rarely moist Skin is usually dry. Linen only requires changing at routine intervals.
Activity				
Degree of physical activity	1. Bedfast Confined to bed.	2. Chairfast Ability to walk severely limited or nonexistent. Cannot bear own weight or must be assisted into chair or wheelchair.	3. Walks occasionally Walks occasionally during day but for very short distances, with or without assistance. Spends majority of each shift in bed or chair.	4. Walks frequently Walks outside the room at least twice a day and inside room at least once every 2 hours during waking hours.
Mobility				
Ability to change and control body position	1. Completely immobile Does not make even slight changes in body or extremity position without assistance.	2. Very limited Makes occasional slight changes in body or extremity position but unable to make frequent or significant changes independently.	3. Slightly limited Makes frequent though slight changes in body or extremity position independently.	4. No limitations Makes major and frequent changes in position without assistance.
Nutrition				
Usual food intake pattern	1. Very poor Never eats a complete meal. Rarely eats more than one third of any food offered. Eats 2 servings or less of protein (meat or dairy products) per day. Takes fluids poorly. Does not take a liquid dietary supplement. OR Is NPO or maintained on clear liquids or IVs for more than 5 days.	2. Probably inadequate Rarely eats a complete meal and generally eats only about half of any food offered. Protein intake includes only 3 servings of meat or dairy products per day. Occasionally will take a dietary supplement. OR Receives less than optimum amount of liquid diet or tube feeding.	3. Adequate Eats over half of most meals. Eats a total of 4 servings of protein (meat, dairy products) each day. Occasionally will refuse a meal but will usually take a supplement if offered. OR Is on a tube feeding or total parenteral nutrition regimen that probably meets most nutritional needs.	4. Excellent Eats most of every meal. Never refuses a meal. Usually eats a total of 4 or more servings of meat and dairy products. Occasionally eats between meals. Does not require supplementation.

Continued

➤ TABLE 47-2 Braden Scale for Predicting Pressure Sore Risk *continued*

Friction and Shear	1. Problem Requires moderate to maximum assistance in moving. Complete lifting without sliding against sheets is impossible. Frequently slides down in bed or chair, requiring frequent repositioning with maximum assistance. Spasticity, contractures or agitation leads to almost constant friction.	2. Potential problem Moves feebly or requires minimum assistance. During a move, skin probably slides to some extent against sheets, chair, restraints, or other devices. Maintains relatively good position in chair or bed most of the time but occasionally slides down.	3. No apparent problem Moves in bed and in chair independently and has sufficient muscle strength to lift up completely during move. Maintains good position in bed or chair at all times.
			TOTAL SCORE

NPO, Nothing by mouth.

Copyright 1988. Used with permission of Barbara Braden, PhD, RN, Professor, Creighton University School of Nursing, Omaha, Nebraska; and Nancy Bergstrom, Professor, University of Texas-Houston, School of Nursing, Houston, Texas. Retrieved January 30, 2009, from http://www.bradenscale.com.

activity, mobility, nutrition, and friction and shear. The total score ranges from 6 to 23, and a lower total score indicates a higher risk of pressure ulcer development (Braden & Bergstrom, 1989). The cutoff score for onset of pressure ulcer risk with the Braden Scale in the general adult population is 18 (Ayello & Braden, 2002). Researchers have suggested a cutoff score of 18 for Black and Latino clients with darkly pigmented skin (Lyder et al., 2001). The Braden Scale is highly reliable when you use it to identify clients at greatest risk of pressure ulcers (Braden & Bergstrom, 1994; Bergstrom, Braden, et al., 1987; Keast et al., 2006).

Case Example. Your patient is Mrs. Hetje Lamont, an 85-year-old widow with a recent left-sided stroke who lives alone and who has been admitted to your acute care medical floor. She has obvious slurred speech and some facial drooping; her left arm is flaccid and she tells you she "can't feel it at all." She has been incontinent of urine since the stroke and is wearing an adult continence product. She seems alert (oriented to time, place, person) but has been noted to be "a bit confused and weepy at times." Her status has been NPO for the past 48 hours, in preparation for a swallowing assessment. (She is currently receiving only IV normal saline) Her daughter tells you that Mrs. Lamont "has been eating like a bird" for the past few weeks.

When you come to the bedside, she is lying on her right side and has difficulty moving without help. She is too weak to ambulate and needs assistance to sit in a chair.

Questions:

- What is her score on the Braden Risk Assessment Tool?
- From the subscore results, what interventions would be appropriate?
- How often would you reassess your patient for risk of skin breakdown?

Classification of Pressure Ulcers

You need to assess pressure ulcers at regular intervals using systematic variables to evaluate wound healing, plan appropriate interventions, and evaluate progress. Assessment includes depth of tissue involvement (staging), type and approximate percentage of tissue in the wound bed, wound dimensions, exudate description, and condition of the surrounding skin.

One method you can use for assessment of a pressure ulcer is a staging system. Staging systems for pressure ulcers are based on your description of the depth of tissue destroyed. Accurate staging requires knowledge of the skin layers, and a major drawback of a staging system is that you cannot stage an ulcer covered with necrotic tissue because the necrotic tissue is covering the depth of the ulcer (Figure 47–9). The necrotic tissue must be debrided or removed to expose the wound base to allow for assessment.

The National Pressure Ulcer Advisory Panel (NPUAP) (2007a) has proposed a four-stage classification system with an additional Deep Tissue Injury (DTI) descriptor (Table 47–3). Pressure ulcer staging describes the pressure ulcer depth at the point of assessment. Thus, once you have staged the pressure ulcer, this stage endures even as the pressure ulcer heals. Pressure ulcers do not progress from a stage III to a stage I; rather a stage III ulcer demonstrating signs of healing is described as a healing stage III pressure ulcer (Nix, 2007). In 2007, the NPUAP redefined the definition of a pressure ulcer and the stages of pressure ulcers, including the original four stages, by adding two stages on deep tissue injury and unstageable pressure ulcers (Box 47–6).

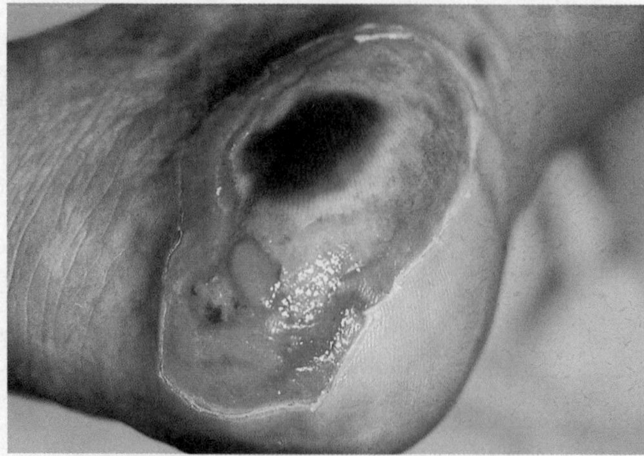

Figure 47-9 Pressure ulcer with tissue necrosis.

TABLE 47-3 Guidelines for Staging Pressure Ulcers

The following criteria can be used as a visual aid to help identify and appropriately stage pressure ulcers. The definitions were derived from work done by the National Pressure Ulcer Advisory Panel and published in February 2007.

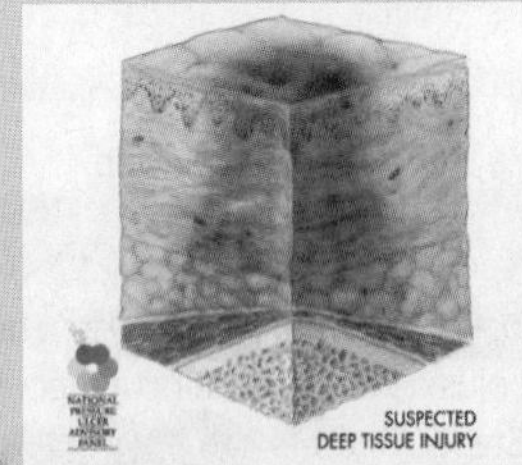

Suspected Deep Tissue Injury

Purple or maroon localized area of discoloured intact skin or blood-filled blister due to damage of underlying soft tissue from pressure or shear or both. The area may be preceded by tissue that is painful, firm, mushy, boggy, warmer or cooler as compared to adjacent tissue.

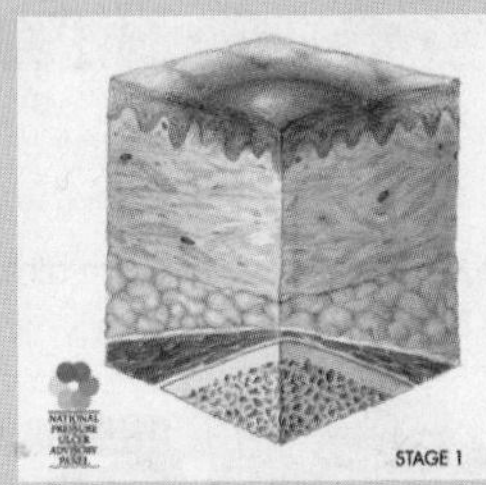

Stage I

Intact skin with nonblanchable redness of a localized area usually over a bony prominence. Darkly pigmented skin may not have visible blanching; its colour may differ from the surrounding area.

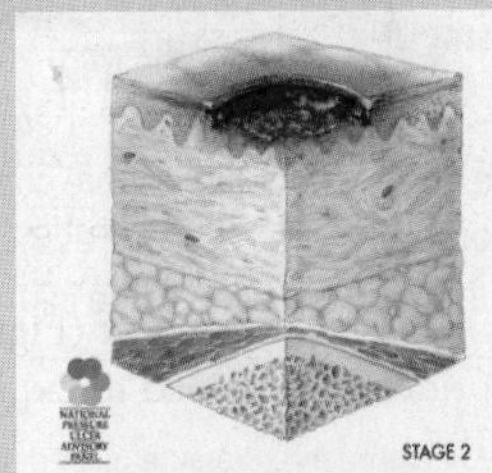

Stage II

Partial thickness loss of dermis presenting as a shallow open ulcer with a red pink wound bed, without slough. May also present as an intact or an open or ruptured serum-filled blister.

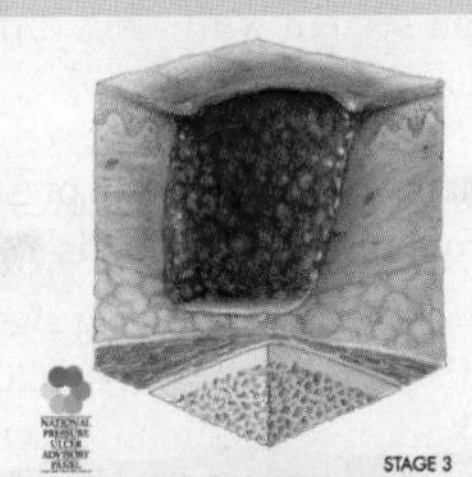

Stage III

Full thickness tissue loss. Subcutaneous fat may be visible, but bone, tendon, or muscle are not exposed. Slough may be present but does not obscure the depth of tissue loss. May include undermining and tunnelling.

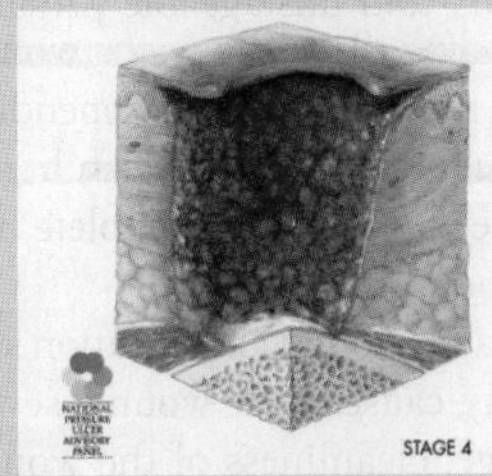

Stage IV

Full thickness tissue loss with exposed bone, tendon, or muscle. Slough or eschar may be present on some parts of the wound bed. Often includes undermining and tunnelling.

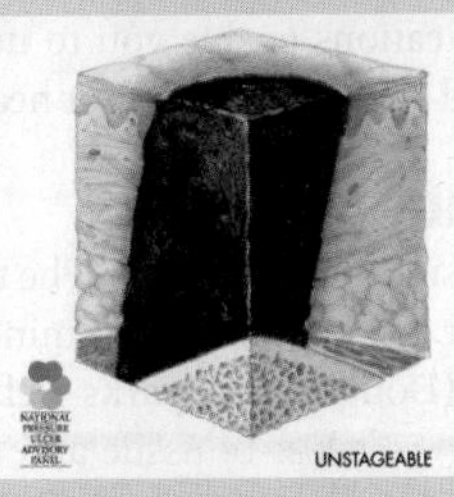

Unstageable

Full thickness tissue loss in which the base of the ulcer is covered by slough (yellow, tan, grey, green or brown) or eschar (tan, brown or black), or both, in the wound bed.

From National Pressure Ulcer Advisory Panel. (2007, February). Retrieved August 13, 2008, from http://www.hill-rom.com/usa/IPUP_Survey/SurveyTraining/page24.htm. Images from National Pressure Ulcer Advisory Panel. (2008). *Updated staging system*. Staging Illustrations. Retrieved February 19, 2009, from http://www.npuap.org/resources.htm.

BOX 47-6 National Pressure Ulcer Advisory Panel Staging Guidelines

Suspected Deep Tissue Injury

Please refer to Table 47–3 for a description of a suspected deep tissue injury.

Further Description

Deep tissue injury may be difficult to detect in individuals with dark skin tones. Evolution may include a thin blister over a dark wound bed. The wound may further evolve and become covered by thin eschar. Evolution may be rapid, exposing additional layers of tissue, even with optimal treatment.

Stage I

Please refer to Table 47–3 for a description of a stage I pressure ulcer.

Further Description

The area may be painful, firm, soft, warmer, or cooler as compared with adjacent tissue. Stage I may be difficult to detect in individuals with dark skin tones. The stage may indicate "at-risk" persons (a heralding sign of risk).

Stage II

Please refer to Table 47–3 for a description of a stage II pressure ulcer.

Further Description

The stage presents as a shiny or dry shallow ulcer without slough or bruising.* This stage should not be used to describe skin tears, tape burns, perineal dermatitis, maceration, or excoriation.

Stage III

Please refer to Table 47–3 for a description of a stage III pressure ulcer.

Further Description

The depth of a stage III pressure ulcer varies by anatomical location. The bridge of the nose, ear, occiput, and malleolus do not have subcutaneous tissue and stage III ulcers can be shallow. In contrast, areas of significant adiposity can develop extremely deep stage III pressure ulcers. The bone or tendon is not visible or directly palpable.

Stage IV

Please see Table 47–3 for a description of a stage IV pressure ulcer.

Further Description

The depth of a stage IV pressure ulcer varies by anatomical location. The bridge of the nose, ear, occiput, and malleolus do not have subcutaneous tissue and these ulcers can be shallow. Stage IV ulcers can extend into muscle or supporting structures (e.g., fascia, tendon, or joint capsule), or both, making osteomyelitis possible. Exposed bone or tendon is visible or directly palpable.

Unstageable

Please refer to Table 47–3 for a description of an unstageable pressure ulcer.

Further Description

Until enough slough or eschar is removed to expose the base of the wound, the true depth, and, therefore, stage cannot be determined. Stable (dry, adherent, intact without erythema or fluctuance) eschar on the heels serves as "the body's natural (biological) cover" and should not be removed.

The staging system was defined by Shea in 1975 and provides a name to the amount of anatomical tissue loss. The original definitions were confusing to many clinicians and led to inaccurate staging of ulcers associated with or due to perineal dermatitis and those due to deep tissue injury.

*Bruising indicates suspected deep tissue injury.

From National Pressure Ulcer Advisory Panel. (2007, February). Pressure ulcer definitions. Retrieved August 22, 2008, from http://www.npuap.org/documents/NPUAP2007_PU_Def_and_Descriptions.pdf.

In addition, Bennett (1995) suggested that when you assess clients with darkly pigmented skin, proper lighting is important to accurately assess the skin (see Box 47–2). Either natural light or a halogen light is recommended. This prevents the blue tones that fluorescent light sources produce on darkly pigmented skin, which interfere with accurate assessment.

For a wound with **nonviable tissue**, you will need to assess the type of tissue in the wound base because this information will be used to plan appropriate interventions. The assessment of tissue type includes the amount (percentage) and appearance (colour) of viable and nonviable tissue.

Granulation tissue is red, moist tissue composed of new blood vessels, the presence of which indicates progression toward healing. Soft yellow or white tissue is characteristic of **slough** (a stringy substance attached to the wound bed), and you will need to remove this before the wound is able to heal. Black or brown necrotic tissue is **eschar**, which will also need to removed before healing can proceed.

The measurement of the size of the wound provides overall changes in size, which is an indicator for wound healing progress (Nix, 2007). Use disposable wound-measuring devices to obtain measurements of width and length. Obtain depth by using a sterile cotton-tipped applicator to gently probe for tunnelling and undermining in the wound bed.

Wound **exudate** describes the amount, colour, consistency, and odour of wound drainage and is part of the wound assessment. Excessive exudate usually indicates the presence of an infection. You should also evaluate the condition of the skin surrounding the wound for redness, warmth, maceration, or edema (swelling). The presence of any of these factors on the skin surrounding the wound is indicative of wound deterioration.

Wound Classifications

A **wound** is a disruption of the integrity and function of tissues in the body (Baharestani, 1994). It is imperative that you understand that *all wounds are not created equal.* Understanding the etiology of a wound is important because the treatment for the wound varies depending on the underlying disease process. Some treatments are even harmful to certain wounds, so you always need to obtain a complete history, including the etiology of the wound.

You can classify wounds in many ways. Wound classification systems describe the status of skin integrity, cause of the wound, severity or extent of tissue injury or damage, cleanliness of the wound (Table 47–4), or descriptive qualities of the wound tissue such as colour (Figure 47–10). Wound classifications enable you to understand the risks associated with a wound and implications for healing.

Process of Wound Healing

Wound healing involves integrated physiological processes. The tissue layers involved and their capacity for regeneration determine the mechanism for repair of any wound (Doughty & Sparks-Defriese, 2007). Two types of wounds are those with loss of tissue and those without. A clean surgical incision is an example of a wound with little tissue loss. The surgical wound heals by **primary intention**. The skin edges are **approximated**, or closed, and the risk of infection is low.

TABLE 47-4 Wound Classification

Description	Causes	Implications for Healing
Onset and Duration		
Acute		
A wound that proceeds through an orderly and timely reparative process that results in sustained restoration of anatomical and functional integrity.	Trauma, a surgical incision	Wounds are usually easily cleaned and repaired. Wound edges are clean and intact.
Chronic		
Wound that fails to proceed through an orderly and timely process to produce anatomical and functional integrity.	Vascular compromise, chronic inflammation, or repetitive insults to the tissue (Doughty & Sparks-Defriese, 2007)	Continued exposure to insult impedes wound healing.
Healing Process		
Primary Intention		
Wound that is closed.	Surgical incision, wound that is sutured or stapled	Healing occurs by epithelialization; heals quickly with minimal scar formation.
Secondary Intention		
Wound edges are not approximated.	Pressure ulcers, surgical wounds that have tissue loss	Wound heals by granulation tissue formation, wound contraction, and epithelialization.
Tertiary Intention		
Wound is left open for several days, then wound edges are approximated.	Wounds that are contaminated and require observation for signs of inflammation	Closure of wound is delayed until risk of infection is resolved (Doughty & Sparks-Defriese, 2007).

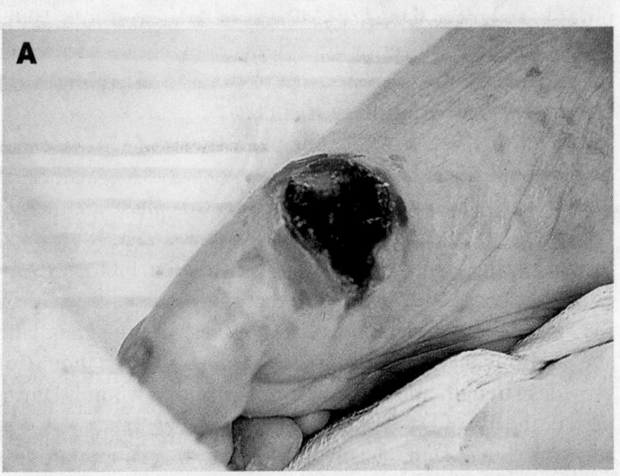

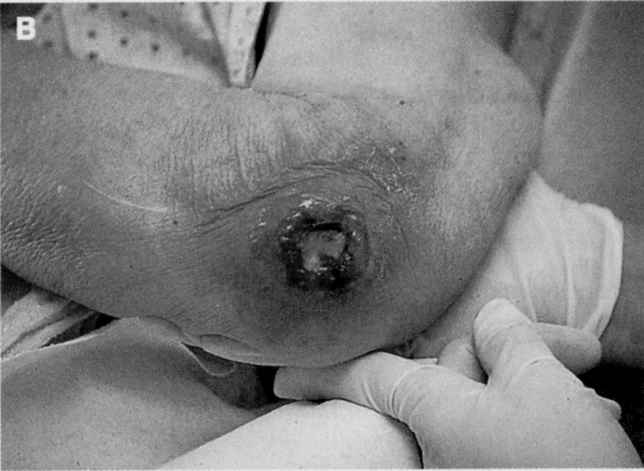

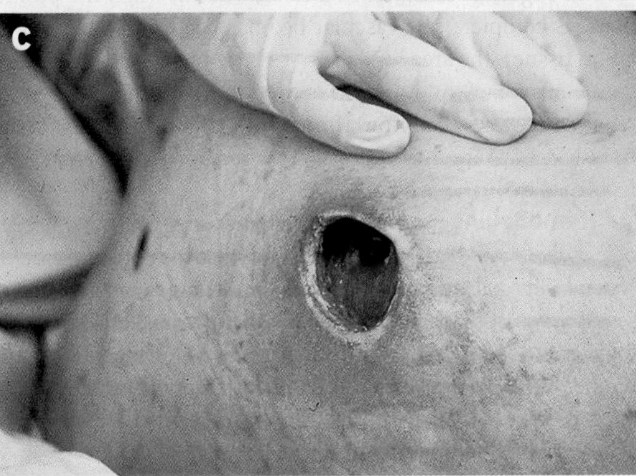

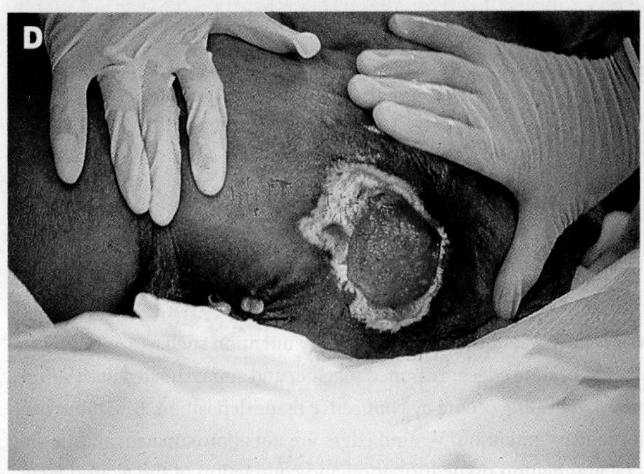

Figure 47-10 Wounds classified by colour assessment. A, Black wound. B, Yellow wound. C, Red wound. D, Mixed-colour wound. **Source:** Courtesy Scott Health Care—A Molnlycke Company. Philadelphia, PA.

Healing occurs quickly, with minimal scar formation, as long as infection and secondary breakdown is prevented (Doughty & Sparks-Defriese, 2007). In contrast, a wound involving loss of tissue, such as a burn, pressure ulcer, or severe laceration, heals by **secondary intention**. The wound is left open until it becomes filled by scar tissue. It takes longer for a wound to heal by secondary intention; thus, the chance of infection is greater. If scarring from secondary intention is severe, loss of tissue function is often permanent (Figure 47–11).

Wound Repair

Partial-thickness wounds are shallow wounds involving loss of the epidermis (top layer) and possibly partial loss of the dermis. Epidermal wounds, such as a clean surgical wound or an abrasion, heal by regeneration. However, full-thickness wounds extending into the dermis (involving both layers of tissue) heal by scar formation because deeper structures do not regenerate. Pressure ulcers are an example of full-thickness wounds.

Partial-Thickness Wound Repair. Three components comprise the healing process of a partial-thickness wound: inflammatory response, epithelial proliferation (reproduction) and migration, and re-establishment of the epidermal layers. Tissue trauma causes the *inflammatory response*, which, in turn, causes redness and swelling to the area, as well as a moderate amount of serous exudate. This response is generally limited to the first 24 hours after wounding. The epithelial cells begin to regenerate, which provides new cells to replace the lost cells. This *epithelial proliferation and migration* starts at both the wound edges and the epidermal cells lining the epidermal appendages, which allows for quick resurfacing. Epithelial cells begin to migrate across the wound bed soon after the wound occurs. *A wound left open to air can resurface within 6 to 7 days, whereas a wound that is kept moist can resurface in 4 days. The difference in the healing rate is related to the fact that epidermal cells only migrate across a moist surface.* In a dry wound, the cells migrate down into a moist level before migration can occur (Doughty & Sparks-Defriese, 2007). New epithelium is only a few cells thick and must undergo *re-establishment of the epidermal layers.* The cells slowly re-establish normal thickness and appear as dry pink tissue.

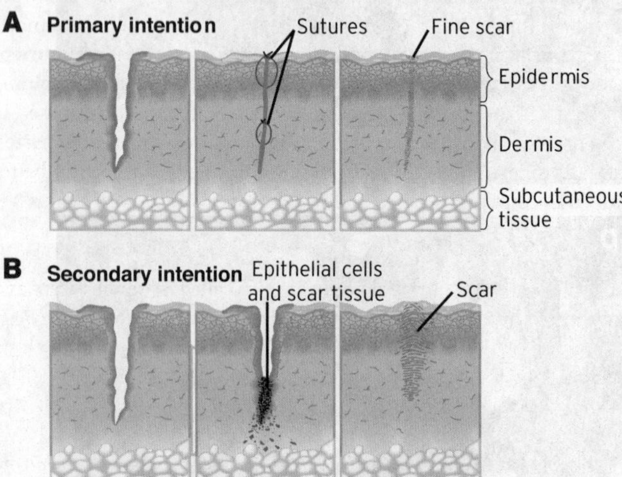

Figure 47-11 A, Wound healing by primary intention such as a surgical incision. Wound healing edges are pulled together and approximated with sutures or staples, and healing occurs by connective tissue deposition. B, Wound healing by secondary intention. Wound edges are not approximated, and healing occurs by granulation tissue formation and contraction of the wound edges. **Source:** Bryant, R. A., & Nix, D. P. (Eds.). (2007). *Acute and chronic wounds: Nursing management* (3rd ed.). St. Louis: Mosby. Used with permission.

Full-Thickness Wound Repair. Inflammatory, proliferative, and remodelling phases are involved in the healing process of a full-thickness wound.

Inflammatory Phase. The inflammation stage is the body's reaction to wounding, begining within minutes of injury and lasting approximately 3 days. During **hemostasis**, injured blood vessels constrict, and platelets gather to stop bleeding. Clots form a **fibrin** matrix that later provides a framework for cellular repair. Damaged tissue and mast cells secrete histamine, which results in vasodilation of surrounding capillaries and exudation of serum and white blood cells into damaged tissues. This results in localized redness, edema, warmth, and throbbing. The inflammatory response is beneficial, and attempting to cool the area or reduce the swelling has no value unless the swelling occurs within a closed compartment (e.g., ankle or neck).

Leukocytes (white blood cells) reach the wound within a few hours. The primary acting white blood cell is the neutrophil, which begins to ingest bacteria and small debris. The second important leukocyte is the monocyte, which transforms into macrophages.

The macrophages are the "garbage cells" that clean a wound of bacteria, dead cells, and debris by phagocytosis. Macrophages continue the process of clearing the wound of debris and release growth factors that attract fibroblasts, the cells that synthesize collagen (connective tissue). Collagen appears as early as the second day and is the main component of scar tissue.

In a clean wound, the inflammatory phase accomplishes control of bleeding and establishes a clean wound bed. The inflammatory phase is prolonged if too little inflammation occurs, as in debilitating diseases such as cancer or after the administration of steroids. Too much inflammation also decreases the speed of healing as arriving cells compete for available nutrients.

Proliferative Phase. The proliferative phase, in which new blood vessels appear as reconstruction progresses, begins, lasting from 3 to 24 days. The main activities during this phase are the filling of the wound with granulation tissue, contraction of the wound, and the resurfacing of the wound by epithelialization. Fibroblasts are present in this phase and are the cells that synthesize collagen, providing the matrix for granulation. Collagen mixes with the granulation tissue, and this matrix will support the re-epithelialization. Collagen provides strength and structural integrity to a wound. During this period, the wound contracts to reduce the area that requires healing (**wound contraction**). Lastly, the epithelial cells migrate from the wound edges to resurface. In a clean wound, when the proliferative phase is complete, the vascular bed has been re-established (granulation tissue), the area has been filled with replacement tissue (collagen, contraction, and granulation tissue), and the surface has been repaired (**epithelialization**). Impairment of healing during this stage usually results from systemic factors such as age, anemia, hypoproteinemia, and zinc deficiency.

Remodelling. Maturation, the final stage of healing, sometimes occurs for more than a year, depending on the depth and extent of the wound. The collagen scar continues to reorganize and gain strength for several months. However, a healed wound usually does not have the tensile strength of the tissue it replaces. Collagen fibres undergo remodelling or reorganization before assuming their normal appearance. Usually, scar tissue contains fewer pigmented cells (melanocytes) and has a lighter colour than normal skin.

All chronic wounds described in this chapter are discussed in detail in the RNAO Best Practice Guidelines, which are readily available to you online at www.rnao.org.

Skin Tears

Aging skin is at a greater risk of developing skin tears because of the thinning of the epidermis. Dehydration, poor nutrition, prolonged use of corticosteroids, impaired sensory perception, and cognitive impairment are all risk factors for skin breakdown. When moving older adult clients in bed or transferring them from bed to gurney for tests, for example, you need to be careful in your handling of the clients. Skin tears and bruising are common problems in this population (Figure 47–12). Any open area on the skin creates the potential for infection (portal of entry for bacteria). Using tape or adhesive dressings on fragile skin can also precipitate skin tears. The use of simple Telfa pads held in place with a woven cotton wrapped bandage (e.g., Kling wrap) or a soft silicone dressing that will not adhere to the skin is effective in protecting the area from further damage and supporting wound healing.

Venous and Arterial Wounds

Venous and arterial wounds are the result of poor circulation and occur in the lower extremities. Venous ulcers are the most common type of lower extremity wound and account for approximately 80% of leg wounds. In addition, these wounds have a recurrence rate of 70% (RNAO, 2007: Assessment & Management of Venous Ulcers).

Venous Ulcers. Venous ulcers are superficial and irregular in shape (Figure 47–13, *A*). The client may complain of these wounds as being very painful and frustrating because as one wound heals, another one may develop. These wounds usually have a large amount of exudate caused by the edema in the surrounding tissue. Venous insufficiency is related to weak vein walls in the legs; furthermore, limited range of motion in the ankle decreases the ability of the calf muscle to pump. Serum and red blood cells leak into the surrounding tissue, which causes the characteristic brownish hemosiderin staining of the tissue and skin. In chronic venous insufficiency, the edema in the tissue becomes firm and the lower legs develop a wooden-like appearance, called lipodermatosclerosis.

Treatment of Venous Leg Ulcers. It is important that you assess the ankle-brachial pressure index before using compression therapy to prevent, treat, or diminish edema in the lower legs (Vowden & Vowden, 2001). Because venous leg ulcers are often hard-to-heal wounds, clients may have tried a variety of products, such as lanolin in topical moisturizers, topical antibiotics, or others. These products may create allergic contact dermatitis, and it is best to avoid anything but the most simple, natural products to clean, debride, moisten, and cover. Use normal saline, autolytic debriding agents, preservative-free hydrogels, and soft silicone dressings. Avoid products with preservatives, chemicals in the dressing, and fragrances. Edema control is essential, but many clients are not willing to try or maintain compression therapy. A wound care specialist with training in compression therapy is helpful in assisting you to determine (1) whether the client has adequate blood flow to allow for compression and (2) different types of compression treatments that may be better suited to certain clients and their goals, especially as lifestyle modifications are usually required to heal venous ulcers.

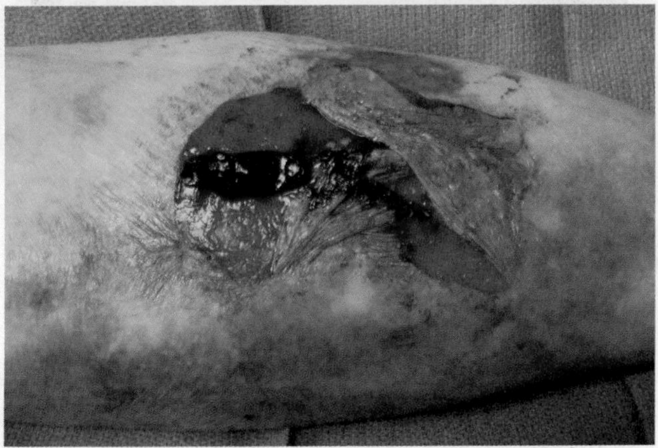

Figure 47-12 Skin tear. **Source:** From Cain, J. E. (2009). *Mosby's PDQ for wound care* (p. 18). St. Louis: Mosby.

A

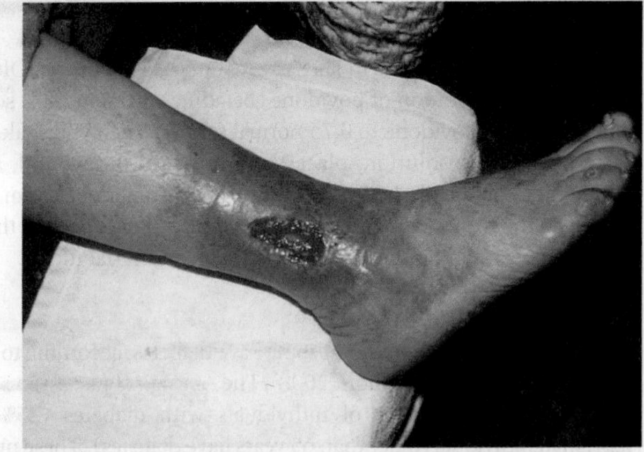

B

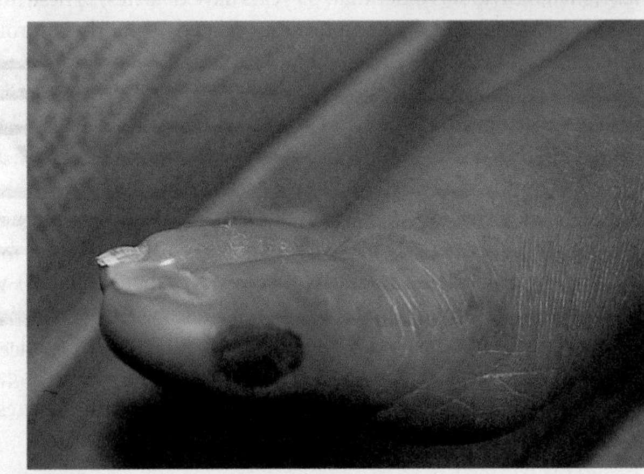

Figure 47-13 A, Venous leg ulcer. B, Arterial lower limb wound. **Source:** From Bryant, R., & Nix, D. (2007). *Acute and chronic wounds: Current management concepts* (3rd ed., Plates 34 and 35). St. Louis: Mosby.

Arterial Ulcers. Arterial ulcers are also called ischemic ulcers and are caused by inadequate blood flow to the lower extremity (unlike venous ulcers, which are caused by poor blood return). Arterial ulcers have a "punched out" appearance that is both deeper and smaller than venous ulcers. They are often located on the feet, over the tips of the toes, or the toe joints, but are also found on other locations on the lower leg (Figure 47–13, *B*). Arterial wounds may be necrotic (black, crusted) in appearance or have very pale wound beds. The legs of a client with arterial disease are thin and have shiny, taut, and hairless skin that has an almost translucent appearance. These wounds are often quite painful, and clients may tell you that dangling their feet over the side of the bed helps decrease the pain.

Because of the nature of this disease, arterial wounds are quite resistant to healing and could be considered as "maintenance" wounds, where the goal is to provide comfort and protection from infection. These wounds are *not* good candidates for debridement because, if opened, the wounds have a limited ability to heal. The best option for treatment is to keep the wounds clean and dry. Often, you can make a solution of povidone (Betadine) (10% in a 1% solution) using 0.25 povidone to 0.75 normal saline. When you soak the gauze pads in the solution, place them in or on the wound, and change them on a daily basis, you will provide some relief from the bacteria in the wound and promote drying of the tissue. Both of these results are useful in nonhealing wounds such as arterial ulcers.

Diabetic Ulcers

In Canada, more than 2 million people have diabetes, according to the Canadian Diabetes Association (2008). The Aboriginal population has much higher percentages of individuals with diabetes (25% of Aboriginal individuals older than 65 years have diabetes). These numbers are growing, and the complications related to poorly controlled diabetes affect health care resource utilization: diabetes leads to renal failure, which requires dialysis, diabetic neuropathy leads to limb amputation (Figure 47–14), and retinal neuropathy leads to blindness. People with diabetes have compromised healing potential, and any break in the skin can cause long-term problems because these wounds can resist healing. Forty-five percent of lower extremity amputations occur in individuals with diabetes. One lower limb amputation of a nontraumatic nature (e.g., diabetes-related) will result in a second limb amputation within 3 years and death within 5 years (Tentolouris et al., 2004). These are sobering statistics and reinforce how important it is for you to provide education as well as careful assessment and early intervention to your clients with diabetes.

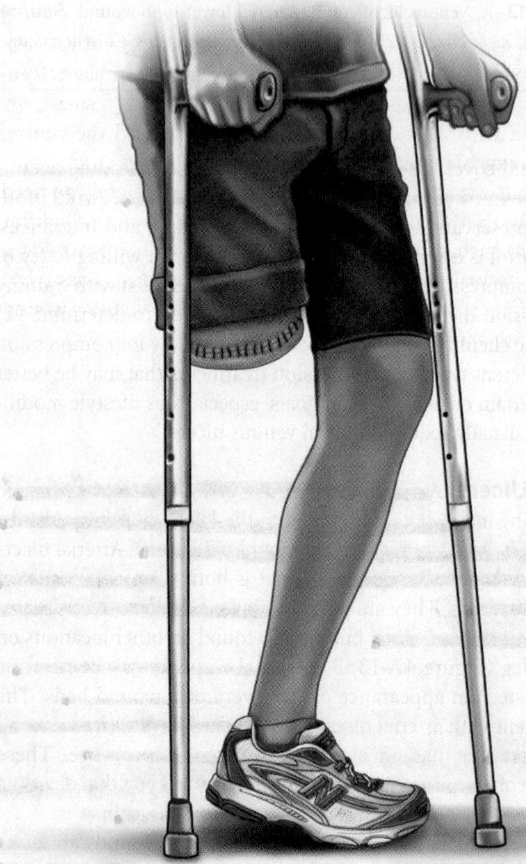

Figure 47-14 An amputee.

Diabetic ulcers occur because of neuropathic changes related to diabetes. They are most commonly over bony prominences located on the plantar surface of the foot, over the metatarsal heads, and beneath the heels. These changes include sensory neuropathy, which is the loss of protective sensation (e.g., a decrease in the ability to feel pain or temperature change); autonomic neuropathy, which leads to the absence of sweating that, in turn, causes dry skin with fissures, cracks, and calluses over pressure points such as the heels and the ball of the foot; and motor neuropathy, which results in changes in muscle contractions leading to high arches and cocked up "hammer" toes. These contribute to pressure points that create calluses (Figure 47–15).

Assessment. Assessment of the feet in clients with diabetes with a monofilament test (CAWC, 2006) will assist you in determining the extent of the neuropathy (Figure 47–16). However, in clients with diabetes, it is safe to assume that peripheral neuropathy is a risk, and you should conduct education and close inspection and palpation of the feet and lower legs. To reinforce the importance of preventive care, instruct clients on appropriate footwear, including the use of hard-soled shoes in the home environment, how to test the water before stepping into the bath or shower, and good foot care, including the involvement of a certified foot-care specialist such as a chiropodist.

Diabetic Wound Treatment. Once the healing potential of the wound has been established, necrotic tissue and callus build-up must be debrided to establish a clean wound bed and diminish pressure. Sharp or surgical debridement should only be performed by a qualified health care professional (RN or MD) who has obtained the appropriate skills and knowledge and is supported by the institution's policy regarding sharp and surgical debridement. Incorrect sharp or surgical debridement can significantly harm your client. Because of the potential for infection, diabetic wounds are often treated with some form of topical antimicrobial dressing. If the client complains of pain at the wound site, particularly persistent pain, you should suspect osteomyelitis (bone infection). Ensure that the physician or advanced practice nurse primarily responsible for the client is aware of this so appropriate action can be taken.

Malignant or Fungating Wounds

Cancer tumours may extrude through the skin as swollen masses with numerous fissures that drain purulent, often very malodourous exudate and that sometimes bleed when cleansed or touched. Typical sites for fungating wounds are the side of the face or neck and the breast or groin area (Figure 47–17). These wounds are not only

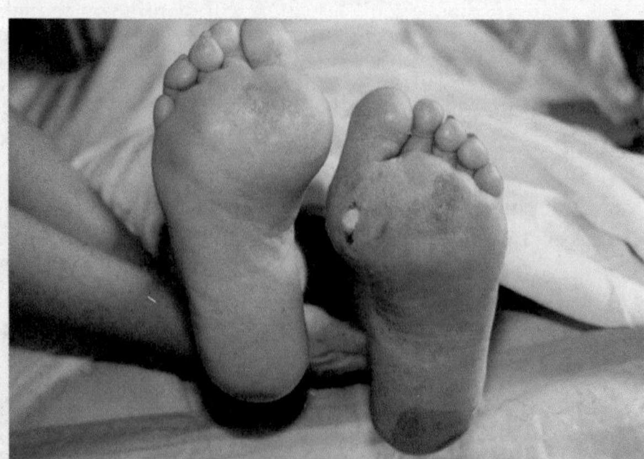

Figure 47-15 Diabetic foot with callus and packing in wound. **Source:** From Bryant, R., & Nix, D. (2007). *Acute and chronic wounds: Current management concepts* (3rd ed., Plate 38). St. Louis: Mosby. Reprinted with permission.

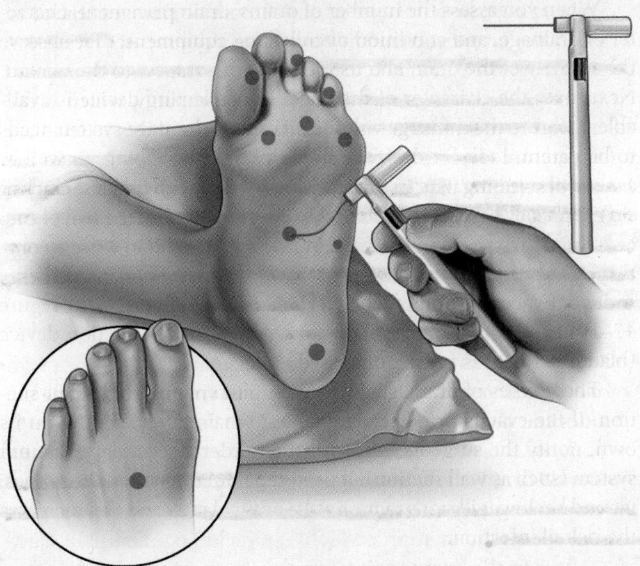

Figure 47-16 Monofilament test.

painful at dressing change but also often embarrass the client because of their odour and unsightliness. They are malignant wounds that will not heal, but the tumours may be reduced in size with radiation or chemotherapy.

Care of the malignant or fungating wound requires attention to environmental and extrinsic issues such as odour, drainage, and appearance of the wound. Odour control may be difficult and may require topical antifungal or antimicrobial dressings such as metronidazole (Flagyl) or a topical silver dressing. Various types of charcoal dressings are also available to provide odour management but are not always effective once they are wet. To avoid trauma to the wound bed, do not use adhesive dressings but use atraumatic dressings such as soft silicone, which will allow for moisture vapour transfer and decrease pain at dressing change. Barrier films and the use of silicone (dimethicone)-based creams will provide supportive care and protect the periwound skin. Minimizing the frequency of dressing changes as well as using "low profile" dressings will enhance quality of life.

Acute and Surgical Wounds

You may be in situations in which you are assessing a wound, either at the time of injury before treatment or after therapy, when the wound is relatively stable. Each situation will require you to make different observations and to take different actions. Regardless of the setting, it is important that you obtain information regarding the cause and history of the wound (see Box 47–4).

Emergency Setting, or Acute, Wounds. You will see wounds in any setting, including the clinic, emergency department, youth camps, or your own backyard. When you judge a client's condition to be stable because of the presence of spontaneous breathing, a clear airway, and a strong carotid pulse (see Chapter 39), inspect the wound for bleeding. The type of wound determines the criteria for inspection. For example, a client presenting with an abrasion would not likely require you to inspect for signs of internal bleeding, but you should do so in the event of a puncture wound.

An **abrasion** is superficial with little bleeding and is considered a partial-thickness wound. The wound often appears "weepy" because of plasma leakage from damaged capillaries. A **laceration,** which is a jagged, unintentional (ie, nonsurgical) wound, sometimes bleeds more profusely, depending on the wound's depth and location. For example, minor scalp lacerations tend to bleed profusely because of the rich blood supply to the scalp. Lacerations greater than 5 cm (2 inches) long or 2.5 cm (1 inch) deep cause serious bleeding. Puncture wounds bleed in relation to the depth and size of the wound; for example, a nail puncture does not cause as much bleeding as a knife wound. The primary dangers of puncture wounds are internal bleeding and infection.

Inspect the wound for foreign bodies or contaminate material. Most traumatic wounds are dirty. Soil, broken glass, shreds of cloth, and foreign substances clinging to penetrating objects sometimes become embedded in the wound.

Your next step is to assess the size (including depth) of the wound. A deep laceration requires suturing. A large, open wound may expose bone or tissue that needs to be protected.

When the injury is a result of trauma from a dirty penetrating object, determine when the client last received a tetanus toxoid injection. Tetanus bacteria reside in soil and in the gut of humans and animals. A tetanus antitoxin injection is necessary if the client's last one was more than 5 years ago.

Stable Setting, or Surgical, Wounds. When the client's condition is stabilized (e.g., after surgery or treatment), assess the wound to determine its healing progress. If the wound is covered by a dressing and the dressing is intact and not saturated with drainage, do not directly inspect the wound unless you suspect serious complications. In such a situation, inspect only the dressing and any external drains.

Change dressings contaminated with external drainage (e.g., feces or urine) and saturated dressings with leakage to periwound tissue. When doing so, take care to avoid accidental removal or displacement of underlying drains. Because removal of dressings may be painful, assess the client's need for an analgesic, and once ordered, make sure it is given at least 30 minutes before exposing the wound.

Wound Appearance. Observe whether wound edges are closed. A surgical incision healing by primary intention should have clean, well-approximated edges. A **puncture** wound is usually a small, circular wound with the edges coming together toward the centre. Crusts from exudate often form along the wound edges.

If a wound is open, the wound edges are separated, and you need to inspect the condition of tissue at the wound base. Also, look for complications such as dehiscence and evisceration. The outer edges of a wound normally appear inflamed for the first 2 to 3 days, but this slowly disappears. Within 7 to 10 days, a normally healing wound resurfaces with epithelial cells, and edges close.

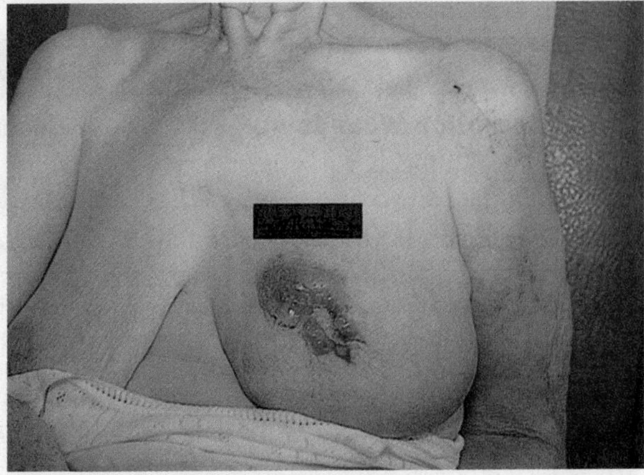

Figure 47-17 Malignant breast tumour. **Source:** From Bale, S., & Jones, V. (2005). *Wound care nursing: A patient-centred approach* (2nd ed., p. 195, Fig. 9-16). St. Louis: Mosby. Reprinted with permission.

Table 47–5 lists assessment characteristics for abnormal wound healing in primary and secondary wounds. If an infection develops, the area directly surrounding the wound becomes brightly inflamed and swollen.

Skin discoloration usually results from bruising of interstitial tissues or hematoma formation. Blood collecting beneath the skin first takes on a bluish or purplish appearance. Gradually, as the clotted blood is broken down, shades of brown and yellow appear.

Character of Wound Drainage. Note the amount, colour, odour, and consistency of drainage. The amount of drainage depends on the location and extent of the wound. For example, drainage is minimal after a simple appendectomy. In contrast, wound drainage is moderate for 1 to 2 days after drainage of a large abscess. When you need an accurate measurement of the amount of drainage within a dressing, weigh the dressing and compare it with the weight of the same dressing when clean and dry. The general rule is that 1 g of drainage equals 1 mL of drainage volume. Another method of quantifying wound drainage is to chart the number of dressings used and the frequency of changes. An increase or decrease in the number or frequency of dressings will indicate a relative increase or decrease in wound drainage.

The colour and the consistency of drainage vary depending on the components. Types of drainage include the following: **serous, sanguineous, serosanguineous,** and **purulent** (see Table 47–6). If the drainage has a pungent or strong odour, you should suspect infection.

Describe the wound's appearance according to the characteristics observed. An example of accurate recording follows:

Abdominal incision is 5 cm in width, in RLQ (right lower quadrant); wound edges well approximated without inflammation or exudate. 1.2-cm diameter circle of serous drainage present on one 4 × 4 gauze changed every 8 hours.

Drains. If a large amount of drainage is anticipated, a drain is often inserted in or near a surgical wound. Some drains are sutured in place. *Exercise caution when changing the dressing around drains, regardless of whether they are sutured, to prevent accidental removal.* A Penrose drain lies under a dressing; at the time of placement, a pin or clip is placed through the drain to prevent it from slipping farther into a wound (Figure 47–18). It is usually the nurse's responsibility to pull or advance the drain as drainage decreases to permit healing deep within the wound site.

When you assess the number of drains, drain placement, character of drainage, and condition of collecting equipment, first observe the security of the drain and its location with respect to the wound. Next, note the character of drainage. If a collecting device is available, measure the drainage volume. Because a drainage system needs to be patent, look for drainage flow through the tubing, as well as around the tubing. *A sudden decrease in drainage through the tubing may indicate a blocked drain, which may require surgical revision. Contact the physician in this case.* When a drain is connected to suction, assess the system to be sure that the pressure ordered is being exerted. Evacuator units such as a Hemovac or Jackson-Pratt (Figure 47–19) exert a constant low pressure as long as the suction device (bladder or bag) is fully compressed.

These types of drainage devices are often referred to as self-suction. If the evacuator device is unable to maintain a vacuum on its own, notify the surgeon, who will then order a secondary vacuum system (such as wall suction). If fluid accumulates within the tissues, wound healing will not progress at an optimal rate, and this increases the risk of infection.

Wound Closures. Surgical wounds are closed with staples, sutures, or wound closures. A frequent skin closure is the stainless steel staple. The staple provides more strength than nylon or silk sutures and tends to cause less irritation to tissue. However, you should look for irritation around staple or suture sites and note whether closures are intact. Normally, for the first 2 to 3 days after surgery, the skin around sutures or staples is edematous. Continued swelling indicates that the closures are too tight. The skin can be cut by overly tight suture material, which can lead to wound separation. Sutures that are too tight are also a common cause of wound dehiscence. Early suture removal reduces formation of defects along the suture line and minimizes chances of unattractive scar formation.

Tissue adhesive such as Dermabond forms a strong bond across apposed wound edges, which allows normal healing to occur below. It can be used to replace small sutures for incisional repair. The product is applied across the approximated wound edges, which are then held together until the solution dries, providing an adhesive closure. Although surgeons generally use it for small superficial lacerations, some may use it on larger wounds, where subcutaneous sutures are needed (Bruns & Worthington, 2000).

Palpation of the Wound. When inspecting a wound, observe swelling or separation of wound edges. Wearing sterile gloves, lightly press the wound edges to detect localized areas of tenderness or

➤ TABLE 47-5 Assessment of Abnormal Healing in Primary and Secondary Intention Wounds

Primary Intention Wounds	Secondary Intention Wounds
Incision line poorly approximated	Pale or fragile granulation tissue; granulation tissue bed is excessively dry or moist
Drainage present more than 3 days after closure	Exudate present
Inflammation decreased in first 3–5 days after injury	Necrotic or slough tissue present in wound base
No epithelialization of wound edges by day 4	Epithelialization not continuous
No healing ridge by day 9	Fruity, earthy, or putrid odour present
	Presence of fistula(s), tunnelling, undermining

Adapted from Stotts, N. A., & Cavanaugh, C. E. (1999). Assessing the client with a wound. *Home Healthcare Nurse, 17*(1), 27.

drainage collection. If pressure causes fluid to be expressed, note the character of the drainage. The client is normally sensitive to palpation of wound edges; however, extreme tenderness may be indicative of infection.

➤TABLE 47-6 Types of Wound Drainage

Type	Appearance
Serous	Clear, watery plasma
Purulent	Thick, yellow, green, tan, or brown
Serosanguineous	Pale, red, watery: mixture of clear and red fluid
Sanguineous	Bright red: indicates active bleeding

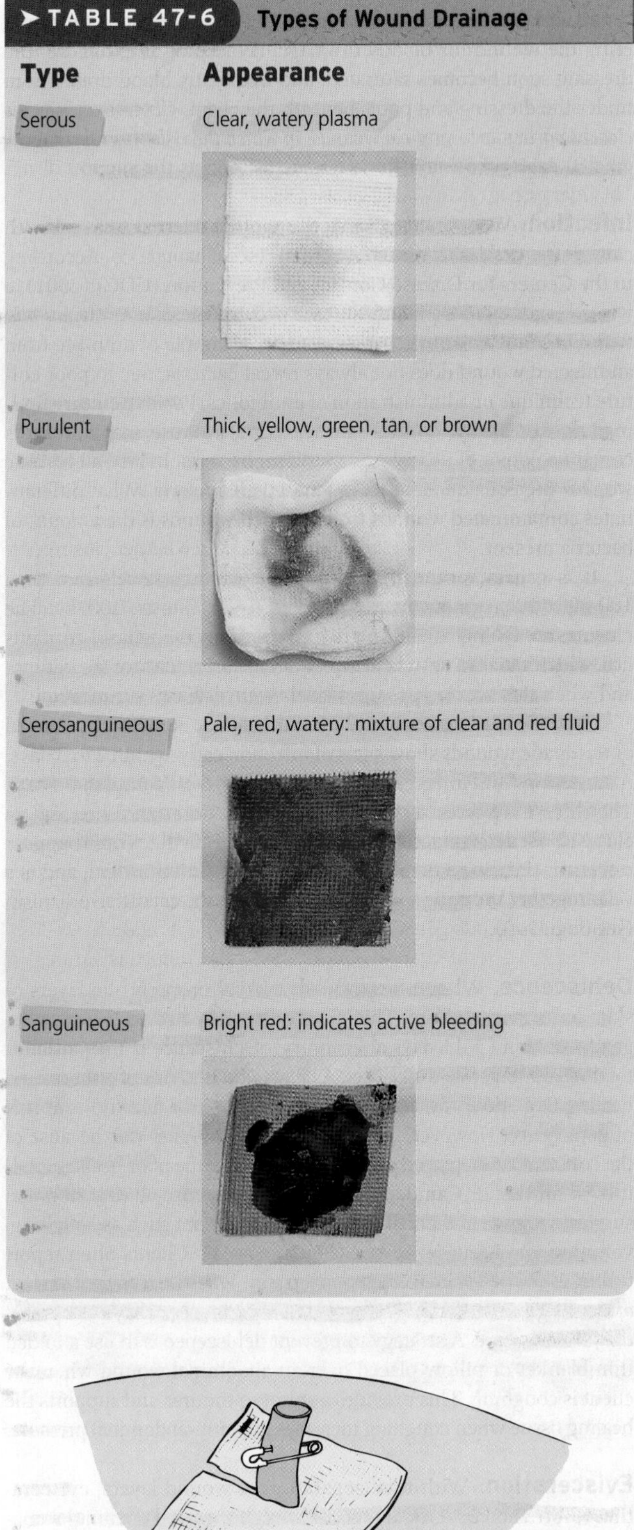

Figure 47-18 Penrose drain.

Wound Cultures. If you detect purulent or suspicious-looking drainage, you may need to obtain a specimen of the drainage for culture (see Chapter 33). Never collect a wound culture sample from old drainage. Resident colonies of bacteria from the skin grow within exudate and are not always the true causative organisms of a wound infection. Clean a wound first with normal saline to remove skin flora. Aerobic organisms grow in superficial wounds exposed to the air, and anaerobic organisms tend to grow within body cavities. Use a different method of specimen collection for each type of organism as per agency policy (Box 47–7).

Gram stains, which result in more appropriate treatment earlier in the course of infection than do cultures, are often also performed.

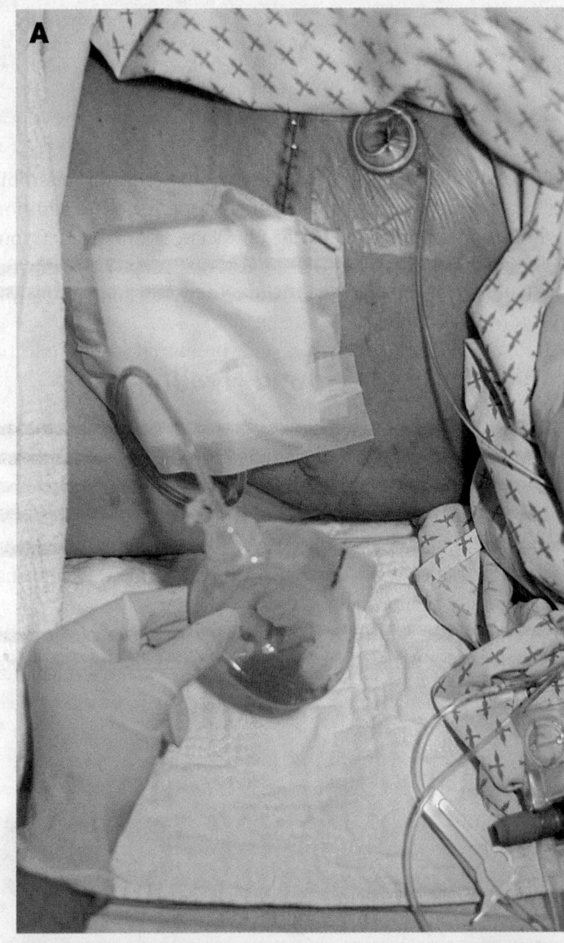

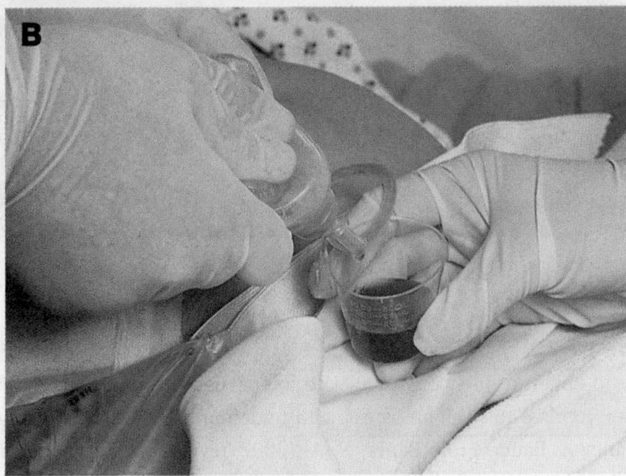

Figure 47-19 Jackson-Pratt drainage device. A, Drainage tubes and reservoir. B, Emptying drainage reservoir.

> **BOX 47-7 Recommendations for Standardized Techniques for Wound Cultures***
>
> **Quantitative Swab Procedure**
>
> - Clean the wound surface with a *nonantiseptic* (i.e., sterile water or normal saline) solution.
> - Use a sterile swab from a culturette tube.
> - Rotate the swab in 1 cm² of clean tissue in the open wound (Figure 47–20). Apply pressure to the swab to elicit tissue fluid. (Stotts, 2007b). Insert the tip of the swab into the appropriate sterile container, and transport to the laboratory.
>
> *Check agency policy to determine whether you need to obtain an order from a health care professional.
>
> Adapted from Stotts, N. A. (2007). Wound infection: Diagnosis and management. In R. A. Bryant, & D. P. Nix (Eds.), *Acute and chronic wounds: Current management concepts* (3rd ed.). St. Louis: Mosby.

No additional specimens are usually required, and the microbiology laboratory needs only to be notified to perform the additional test, which would be ordered by the physician or nurse practitioner. The gold standard of wound culture is tissue biopsy, which would be obtained by the physician or nurse with specialized training (Stotts, 2007b).

Complications of Wound Healing

Hemorrhage. **Hemorrhage**, or bleeding from a wound site, is normal during and immediately after initial trauma. Hemostasis occurs within several minutes unless large blood vessels are involved or the client has poor clotting function. Hemorrhages that occur after hemostasis indicate a slipped surgical suture, a dislodged clot, infection, or erosion of a blood vessel by a foreign object (e.g., a drain). Hemorrhage occurs externally or internally.

You detect internal bleeding by looking for distention or swelling of the affected body part, a change in the type and amount of drainage from a surgical drain, or signs of hypovolemic shock. A **hematoma** is a localized collection of blood underneath the tissues. It appears as a swelling, a change in colour, sensation, or warmth, or a mass that often takes on a bluish discoloration. A hematoma near a major artery or vein is dangerous because pressure from the expanding hematoma obstructs blood flow.

External hemorrhaging is obvious. You observe the dressings covering the wound for bloody drainage. If bleeding is extensive, the dressing soon becomes saturated, and frequently blood drains from under the dressing and pools beneath the client. *Observe all wounds closely, particularly surgical wounds, in which the risk of hemorrhage is greatest during the first 24 to 48 hours after surgery or injury.*

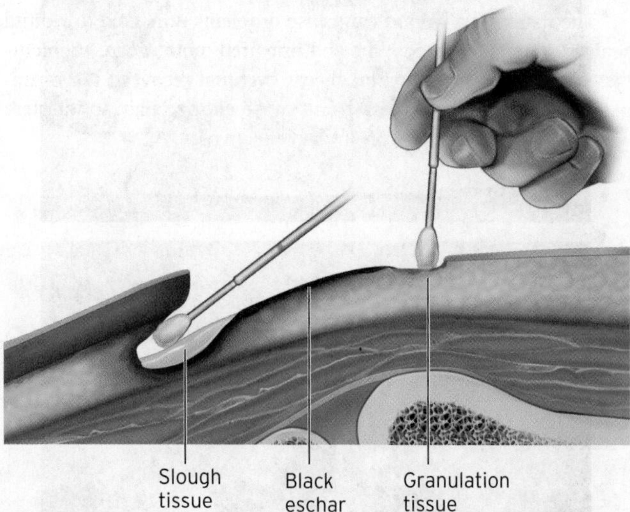

Figure 47-20 Swabbing technique. Swab wound from healthiest looking tissue to obtain results consistent with infectious condition of wound. It is also appropriate to swab any areas with undermining. **Source:** Illustration by Nancy A. Bauer. From Bauer, N. A. (2007, revised). *RNAO best practice guideline: Assessment and management of stage I–IV pressure ulcers* (p. 100). Toronto: RNAO.

Infection. Wound infection is the second most common health care–associated infection (nosocomial) (see Chapter 33). According to the Centers for Disease Control and Prevention (CDC) (2001), a wound is infected if purulent material drains from it, even if a culture is not taken or has negative results. A sample of drainage from an infected wound does not always reveal bacteria, due to poor culture technique or administration of antibiotics. Positive culture findings do not always indicate an infection because many wounds contain colonies of noninfective resident bacteria. In fact, all chronic wounds are considered contaminated with bacteria. What differentiates contaminated wounds from infected wounds is the amount of bacteria present.

It is generally agreed that infected wounds have more than 100,000 (10^5) organisms per gram of tissue (Stotts, 2007b). The chances of wound infection are greater when the wound contains dead or necrotic tissue, when foreign bodies are in or near the wound, and when the blood supply and local tissue defenses are reduced.

Bacterial infection inhibits wound healing. Some contaminated or traumatic wounds show signs of infection early, within 2 to 3 days. A surgical wound infection usually does not develop until day 4 or 5. The client has a fever, tenderness and pain at the wound site, and an elevated white blood cell count. The edges of the wound appear inflamed. If drainage is present, it is odorous and purulent, and is a yellow, green, or brown colour, depending on the causative organism (see Box 47–9).

Dehiscence. When a wound fails to heal properly, the layers of skin and tissue separate. This most commonly occurs before collagen formation (3–11 days after injury). **Dehiscence** is the partial or total separation of wound layers. A client who is at risk of poor wound healing (e.g., poor nutritional status, infection, or obesity) is at risk of dehiscence. However, obese clients have a higher risk because of the constant strain placed on their wounds and the poor healing qualities of fat tissue (Camden, 2007). Dehiscence involves abdominal surgical wounds and occurs after a sudden strain, such as coughing, vomiting, or sitting up in bed (Figure 47–21). Clients often report feeling as though something has given way. *When an increased amount of serosanguineous drainage from a wound occurs, be alert for the potential for dehiscence.* A strategy to prevent dehiscence is to use a folded thin blanket or pillow placed over an abdominal wound when the client is coughing. This provides a splint to the area and supports the healing tissue when coughing increases the intra-abdominal pressure.

Evisceration. With total separation of wound layers, **evisceration** (protrusion of visceral organs through a wound opening) sometimes occurs. It is an emergent condition that requires surgical repair. *When evisceration occurs, you need to quickly place sterile towels soaked in sterile saline over the extruding tissues to reduce the chance of bacterial invasion and drying of the tissues.* If the organs

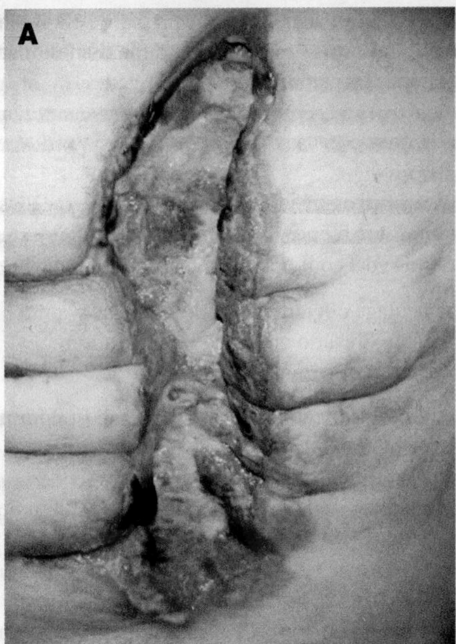

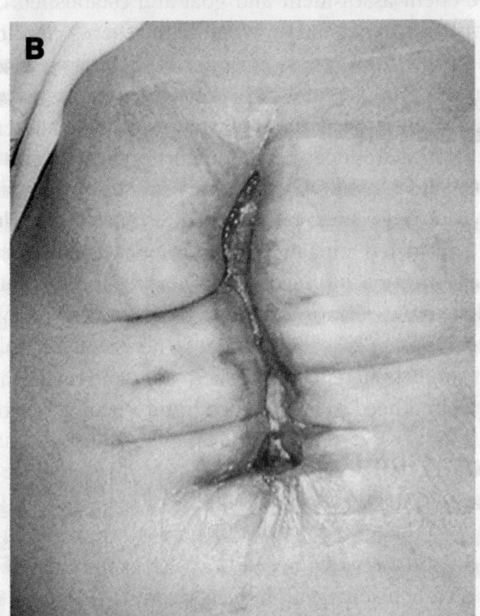

Figure 47-21 A, Dehisced wound before wound V.A.C. therapy. B, Dehisced wound after wound V.A.C. therapy. **Source:** Courtesy Kinetic Concepts, Inc. San Antonio, TX.

protrude through the wound, blood supply to the tissues is compromised. Do not allow the client anything by mouth (NPO), observe for signs and symptoms of shock, and prepare the client for emergency surgery.

Fistulas. A fistula is an abnormal passage between two organs or between an organ and the outside of the body. Most fistulas form as a result of poor wound healing or as a complication of disease, such as Crohn's disease. Trauma, infection, radiation exposure, and diseases such as cancer will prevent tissue layers from closing properly and will allow the fistula tract to form. Fistulas increase the risk of infection and fluid and electrolyte imbalances from fluid loss. Chronic drainage of fluids through a fistula also predisposes a client to skin breakdown (Box 47–8).

➤ BOX 47-8 Risk of Skin Breakdown From Body Fluids

Low Risk	Moderate Risk	High Risk
Saliva	Bile	Gastric drainage
Serosanguineous drainage	Stool	Pancreatic drainage
	Urine	
	Ascitic fluid	
	Purulent exudate	

❖Nursing Diagnosis

Through assessment, clusters of data reveal whether an actual or a risk of *impaired skin integrity* exists. In addition, the assessment data sometimes support more than one diagnostic label. For example, a postoperative client has purulent drainage from a surgical wound and reports tenderness around the area of the wound. These data support a nursing diagnosis of *impaired skin integrity related to a contaminated wound* (Box 47–9). After completing an assessment of the client's wound, you would identify nursing diagnoses that will direct supportive and preventive care. Multiple nursing diagnoses are associated with impaired skin integrity and wounds:

- *Risk of infection*
- *Imbalanced nutrition: less than body requirements*
- *Acute or chronic pain*
- *Impaired physical mobility*
- *Impaired skin integrity*
- *Risk of impaired skin integrity*
- *Ineffective tissue perfusion*
- *Impaired tissue integrity*

Some clients are at risk of poor wound healing because of previously defined factors that impair healing. Thus, even though the client's wound appears normal, you would identify nursing diagnoses, such as *impaired nutrition* or *ineffective tissue perfusion*, that direct nursing care toward support of wound repair.

The nature of a wound can cause problems unrelated to wound healing. Alteration in comfort and impaired mobility are problems that have implications for the client's eventual recovery. For example, a large abdominal incision can cause enough pain to interfere with the client's ability to turn in bed effectively.

➤ BOX 47-9 Impaired Skin Integrity Related to a Contaminated Wound

Assessment Activities That Define Characteristics

Inspect surface of skin: presence of wound, break in skin integrity
Yellow, foul-smelling drainage from wound
Edges of wound red and warm, not approximated
Sutures remain in place. Inspect wound for signs of healing
Brown-red drainage 5 days after surgery
Edges of wound not approximated
Obtain client's temperature, heart rate, white blood cell count, and serum albumin level
Client is febrile, heart rate is 125 beats per minute, leukocyte (white blood cell) count is 12,000/mm^3, and serum albumin level is less than 3.5 mg/100 mL.

❖Planning

After identifying nursing diagnoses, you develop a plan of care for the client who is at risk or who has actual impaired skin integrity. During planning, synthesize information from multiple resources (Figure 47–6). Critical thinking ensures that the client's plan of care integrates all that you know about the individual, as well as key critical thinking elements. Professional standards of practice are especially important to consider when developing your plan of care. Ask yourself what aspects of care you are able to perform without medical orders, what aspects of care you can delegate to other regulated health care professionals, and what are your obligations to the client.

For many of your clients, the wound is only a part of the story. For example, consider the following scenario:

You are caring for Mrs. Kathy Crane, a 65-year-old woman who lives with her recently retired husband and who has a 30-year history of diabetes mellitus. She currently takes insulin, but her diabetes is poorly controlled because of her inability to adhere to a 1200-calorie diabetic diet and her "hit or miss" approach to testing her serum glucose on a regular basis. She is 32 kg overweight.

For the last 10 years, she has reported decreased sensation in her lower extremities. She does not practice good foot care; she cuts her own toenails and, at home, goes barefoot or wears socks. She regularly soaks her feet in an Epsom-salt footbath because she "read this was good for your feet."

She was admitted to the hospital for elective repair of an abdominal aneurysm. The surgery went well, but postoperatively Mrs. Crane had difficulty ambulating and performing coughing and deep breathing exercises. On her second postoperative day she developed pneumonia, which required intravenous antibiotics. During the course of her pneumonia, Mrs. Crane stated she was "too tired" to walk or get up to use the commode or toilet. She required an adult continence product as she was now incontinent of urine and stool. She complained of pain when repositioned and would generally reposition herself on her back. Two weeks after her surgery, Mrs. Crane developed a large draining sacral wound, which is now 6 cm in diameter. The base of the wound can be visualized down to bone (stage IV). In addition, she has a smaller, stage III ulcer on her left heel. Skin assessment also reveals areas of prolonged redness over pressure points, especially on the right heel and over both hips.

When planning care for Mrs. Crane, you can use a concept map to individualize care for her, as she has multiple health problems and related nursing diagnoses (Figure 47–22). This map assists you in using critical thinking skills to organize complex client assessment data and related nursing diagnoses with the client's chief medical diagnosis. As you identify linkages between the nursing diagnoses and the chief medical diagnosis, the concept map also links potential interventions with the client's health care needs.

Goals and Outcomes

Nursing care is based on the client's identified needs and priorities. Your first job is to ensure you and the client are on the same path regarding the establishment of goals and expected outcomes. In addition, you need to determine whether the wound is likely to heal. For example, a pressure ulcer for which the pressure is unrelieved or coupled with poor nutritional status will not be a good candidate for healing. In addition, patients in terminal stages of illness may not have the physiological resources to heal, despite pressure off-loading and optimal dressings. Thus, it is important to plan interventions according to the risk of skin breakdown, the type and severity of the wound, and the presence of any complications, such as infection, poor nutrition, peripheral vascular diseases, or immunosuppression, that can affect wound healing.

A goal frequently identified when working with a client with a wound is to see wound improvement within a 2-week period. The outcomes of this goal could possibly include the following:

- Higher percentage of granulation tissue in the wound base
- No further skin breakdown in any body location
- An increase in caloric intake of 10%

These outcomes are reasonable if the overall goal for the client is to heal the ulcer. Other goals of care for clients with wounds include promoting wound hemostasis, preventing infection, promoting wound healing, maintaining skin integrity, gaining comfort, and health promotion.

Setting Priorities

You establish nursing care priorities in wound care based on the comprehensive client assessment and goal and established outcomes. These priorities also depend on whether the client's condition is stable or emergent. An acute wound needs immediate intervention, whereas in the presence of a chronic, stable wound, other factors, such as mobilization, may have a greater priority. No matter what the risk level of pressure ulcer development, preventive interventions such as skin care practices, appropriate positioning, and elimination of friction and shear are high priorities. Promotion of skin health should be considered a major nursing priority. Existing skin breakdown, from skin tears to large chronic wounds, also requires ongoing attention because it is frequently the reason for both hospitalization and a decrease in quality of life for clients, no matter what the setting. Client and family preferences, daily activities, and the healing potential of the wound need to be included in the setting of priorities.

Collaborative Care

Wound care is not the sole responsibility of the nurse. In fact, it is a team effort that includes the physiotherapist, occupational therapist, dietitian, pharmacist, and physician, as well as the client, family, and nurse. With early discharge from health care settings, it is important to consider what resources are required for the client's discharge plan. Anticipating the client's discharge wound care needs and related equipment and resources, such as referral to a home care agency or outpatient wound care clinic, assists in improving not only wound healing but also the client's level of independence.

Clients and their families often need to continue the objectives of wound management after discharge (Box 47–10). You need to consider the ability of the caregiver and the amount of time needed to change a particular dressing when selecting a dressing for the client to use after discharge. For example, in the home setting, the frequency of dressing changes is a key factor in resource management of home health agencies. In addition, clients, families, and caregivers need to be provided with education and knowledge so that they understand the importance of good nutrition, pressure off-loading (particularly when sitting in a recliner chair for long periods of time), and how different wound dressings are used. The nurse and client work together to establish ways of maintaining client involvement in nursing care and to promote wound healing, whether the client is in the hospital or at home.

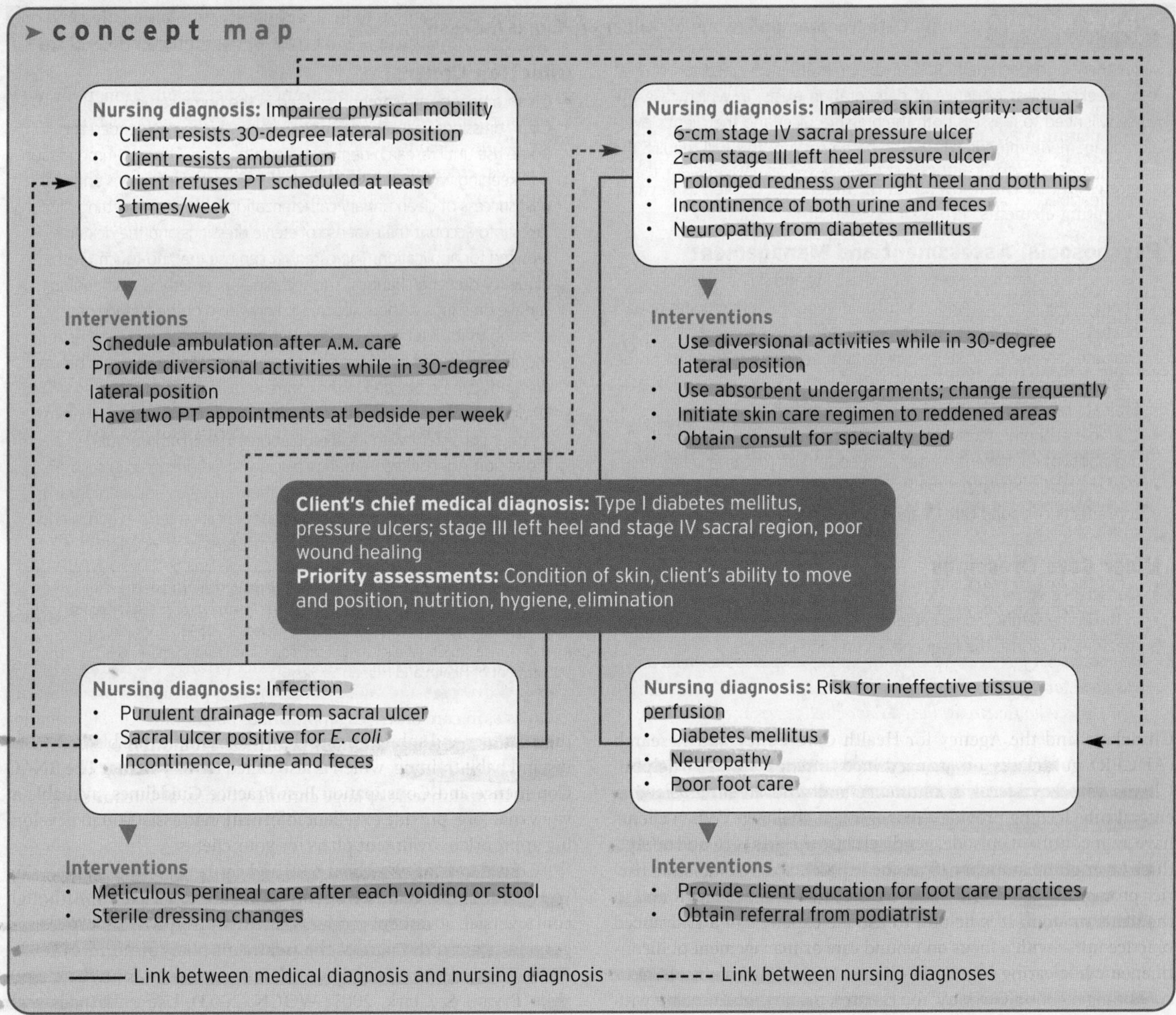

Figure 47-22 Concept map for a client with a chronic wound.

❖Implementation: Preventing Skin Breakdown

Health Promotion

The most effective intervention for problems with skin integrity and wound care is prevention. Prompt identification of high-risk clients and their risk factors aids in the prevention of pressure ulcers. Early identification of clients at risk and their risk factors will assist you in preventing pressure ulcers. The use of a risk assessment tool, such as the Braden Risk Assessment Tool (see Table 47–2) is a first step in identifying a client's risk of skin breakdown. Table 47–7 provides nursing interventions based on the risk factors identified in the Braden Tool. The three major areas of nursing interventions for prevention of skin breakdown are (1) skin care, which includes hygiene and skin care; (2) mechanical loading and support devices, which include proper positioning and the use of therapeutic surfaces; and (3) education (RNAO, 2007).

Topical Skin Care

You need to perform frequent skin assessments (see Box 47–4), at a minimum of once a day; however, high-risk clients will need more frequent skin assessments, such as every shift. In addition, ensure that the client's skin is clean and dry. Assessment and skin hygiene are two initial defenses for preventing skin breakdown. When you clean the skin, avoid soaps and hot water. Use cleansers with nonionic surfactants that are gentle to the skin (CAWC, 2006; RNAO 2007). Many types of products are available for skin care, and you need to match their use to the specific needs of your client.

After you cleanse the skin and make sure it is completely dry, apply moisturizer to keep the epidermis well-lubricated but not oversaturated. Make an effort to control, contain, or correct incontinence, perspiration, and wound drainage (Bryant & Clark, 2007).

> BOX 47-10 **Home Care Recommendations for Ulcer or Wound Assessment**

Assessment and documentation of the pressure ulcer need to occur at least weekly, unless evidence of deterioration exists, in which case the nurse will need to reassess both the pressure ulcer and the client's overall management immediately. In the home setting, this will require the assistance of the client and family because weekly assessment is not always feasible.

Psychosocial Assessment and Management

- Assess the client's resources (e.g., availability and skill of caregivers, finances, equipment). A successful treatment program requires adequate caregiver and equipment resources.
- Evaluate caregivers for their ability to comprehend and implement the treatment requirements.
- Evaluate caregivers for their level of strength and endurance.
- Consider economic factors because they often limit the supply and availability of equipment, as well as opportunities to relieve caregivers.
- Use an approach that focuses on the psychosocial and physical factors affecting wound care (Teare & Barrett, 2002).

Ulcer Care Dressings

- Consider caregiver time when selecting a dressing.
- In the home setting, some caregivers choose more expensive dressing materials to reduce the frequency of dressing changes.

Infection Control

- Clean dressings are sometimes used in the home setting.
- Clean dressings, as opposed to sterile ones, are recommended for home use until research demonstrates otherwise. This recommendation is in keeping with principles regarding nosocomial infections and with past success of clean urinary catheterization in the home setting, and it takes into account the expense of sterile dressings and the dexterity required for application. The caregiver can use the "no-touch" technique for dressing changes. This technique is a method of changing surface dressings without touching the wound or the surface of any dressing that might be in contact with the wound. Adherent dressings should be grasped by the corner and removed slowly, whereas gauze dressings can be pinched in the centre and lifted off.
- Disposal of contaminated dressings in the home should be done in a manner consistent with local regulations. The Environmental Protection Agency recommends placing soiled dressings in securely fastened plastic bags before adding them to other household trash. Local regulations vary, however, and home care agencies and clients need to follow procedures that are consistent with local laws.

Adapted from Agency for Health Care Policy and Research, Panel for the Treatment of Pressure Ulcers in Adults. (1994). *Treatment of pressure ulcers: Clinical practice guideline no. 15* (AHCPR Pub No. 95-0653). Rockville, MD: Agency for Health Care Policy and Research, Public Health Service, U.S. Department of Health and Human Services.

Clinicians find the Agency for Health Care Policy and Research (AHCPR) guidelines on urinary incontinence (1992b) helpful. Clients who have fecal incontinence and who are also receiving enteral tube feeding provide a management challenge. When clients have an incontinent episode, gently cleanse the area, dry, and apply a thick layer of moisture barrier to the exposed areas. A moisture barrier protects the skin from excessive moisture and bacteria found in the urine or stool. It is helpful to use the expertise of an advanced practice nurse with a focus on wound care or management of incontinence while caring for at-risk clients. Methods for controlling or containing incontinence vary. You can treat urinary incontinence with medication, surgery and behavioural techniques such as prompted voiding. Behavioural techniques help clients learn ways to control their bladder and sphincter muscles. Two examples are bladder training and habit training, which is also called timed voiding. The RNAO Continence and Constipation Best Practice Guidelines, available at www.rnao.org, provide excellent information to assist you in developing appropriate treatment plans for your clients.

Consider using absorbent pads and garments only after assessing your client's potential to respond to the above measures. Although controversial, absorbent products, such as absorptive underpads and garments, are often part of the treatment plan for an incontinent client. Use only products that wick moisture away from the client's skin (Bryant & Clark, 2007; WOCN, 2003). Use underpads with caution because some of these pads do not wick the drainage away from the client's skin and will cause skin damage. In addition, clients

> TABLE 47-7 **A Quick Guide to Pressure Ulcer Prevention**

Risk Factor	Nursing Interventions
Decreased sensory perception	Assess pressure points for signs of nonblanching reactive hyperemia. Provide a pressure-redistribution surface.
Moisture	Assess need for incontinence management. After each incontinent episode, cleanse area with no-rinse perineal cleanser and protect skin with a moisture-barrier ointment.
Friction and shear	Reposition client by using a drawsheet to lift the client off the surface. Provide a trapeze to facilitate movement. Position client at a 30-degree lateral turn and limit head elevation to 30 degrees.
Decreased activity or mobility	Establish and post an individualized turning schedule.
Poor nutrition	Provide adequate nutritional and fluid intake; assist with intake, as necessary. Consult dietitian for nutritional evaluation.

who are provided with specialty pressure relief or off-loading bed surfaces may require continence pads that are designed specifically for the bed surface.

Positioning

Positioning interventions reduce pressure and shearing force to the skin. Elevating the head of the bed to 30 degrees or less will decrease the chance of pressure ulcer development from shearing forces (RNAO, 2007). Given that it is important to change the immobilized client's position according to activity level, perceptual ability, and daily routines (Braden, 2001; RNAO, 2007), a standard turning interval of 1.5 to 2 hours does not always prevent pressure ulcer development in some clients. Regardless, clients need repositioning at least every 2 hours on a schedule. When repositioning, use positioning devices to protect bony prominences (RNAO, 2007). The RNAO guidelines (2007) recommend a 30-degree lateral position, which should prevent positioning directly over a bony prominence. To prevent shear and friction injuries, use a sheet to lift, rather than drag, the client when changing positions. Use the expertise of physiotherapists and occupational therapists, who are skilled at assessment and treatment modalities for both seating and positioning for beds, chairs, and wheelchairs.

safety alert Incorrect positioning of an immobile client can possibly create a shearing injury. When repositioning the client, place a flat folded sheet under the client's body. Obtain assistance for repositioning, and with at least one other caregiver, lift the sheet up and toward the new position. Dragging the client on the sheets will place the client at high risk of shearing and friction injuries.

Some clients are able to sit in a chair, but make sure to limit the time clients sit to 2 hours or less. Again, you should individualize the exact time, but it should not be longer than the recommended time that was calculated during assessment. Thus, if the interval is every 1.5 hours, the client should remain in a sitting position for less than 1.5 hours. In the sitting position, the pressure on the ischial tuberosities is greater than in the supine position. In addition, encourage clients in a sitting position who are also at risk of skin breakdown to shift weight every 15 minutes (RNAO, 2007). Shifting weight provides short-term relief on the ischial tuberosities. In addition, have clients sit on a foam, gel, or air cushion to redistribute weight away from the ischial areas, and engage assistance of the physical therapist or occupational therapist to ensure that cushions are correctly inflated and positioned. Rigid and doughnut-shaped cushions are contraindicated because they reduce blood supply to the area, which results in wider areas of ischemia (RNAO, 2007).

After repositioning the client, reassess the skin. See Box 47–2 for identifying characteristics that indicate early signs of tissue ischemia in darkly pigmented skin. In clients with light-toned skin, check for normal reactive hyperemia and blanching.

Never massage the reddened areas. Massaging reddened areas increases breaks in the capillaries in the underlying tissues and increases the risk of injury to those tissues and of pressure ulcer formation (RNAO, 2007).

Support Surfaces (Therapeutic Beds and Mattresses)

A support surface is a specialized device for pressure redistribution designed for management of tissue loads, microclimate, and other therapeutic functions (i.e., mattresses, integrated bed system, mattress replacement, overlay or seat cushion, or seat cushion overlay) (NPUAP, 2007b). A variety of support surfaces exist, including specialty beds and mattresses that reduce the hazards of immobility to the skin and musculoskeletal system. However, none eliminates the need for meticulous nursing care, and no single device eliminates the effects of pressure on the skin.

When selecting support surfaces, thoroughly assess the client's needs. Knowledge about support surface characteristics (Table 47–8) will assist you in clinical decision making, along with consultations with the physical therapist and occupational therapist. In selecting a support surface, know the client's risks, and the purpose of the support surface; a flow chart is often helpful.

Teach clients and families the reason for and proper use of the beds or mattresses (Box 47–11). Some common errors when support surfaces are used include placing the wrong side of the support surface toward the client, not plugging powered support surfaces into the electrical source, not turning on the power source for powered support surfaces, failing to do "hand checks," and improper inflation (too much or too little) for some support surfaces. Hand checks are done by placing your hand under the support surface, at the pressure point, with the palm facing up and fingers flat. If less than 2.5 cm (1 inch) of support surface exists between your client's pressure point and your hand, then the support cushion or bed surface does not provide adequate support. When used correctly, support surfaces assist in reducing pressure ulcers in clients at risk.

Education

Education of the client and caregivers is an important nursing function (Rolstad & Ovington, 2007). You can use a variety of educational tools, including Web-based learning, videotapes, and written materials, when teaching clients and caregivers or family to prevent and treat pressure ulcers. Written materials are available on many topics, including dressing changes; guides for measuring wounds and charts for positioning clients can also be found. Booklets and pamphlets are available from a variety of sources, including the AHCPR (1992a, 1994). What is important is that you individualize your teaching for each client, especially for older clients or those for whom English is not their first language. Many educational resources are available in various languages.

Understanding and assessment of the experience of the client and caregiver are also important dimensions in the treatment of clients with pressure ulcers (RNAO, 2007). Through research, clinicians are beginning to explore the caregiver's perspective of the concerns and issues faced by frail older spouses caring for their loved ones with pressure ulcers. You need to plan interventions to meet the identified psychosocial needs of clients and their caregivers (RNAO, 2007; CAWC, 2006).

Management of Pressure Ulcers

Treatment of clients with pressure ulcers requires a holistic, team approach (RNAO, 2007). Aspects of pressure ulcer treatment include local care of the wound and supportive measures such as adequate nutrients and redistribution of pressure (Skill 47–2), which may call for the expertise of other members of the interdisciplinary health care team, including the physician, physical therapist, occupational therapist, dietitian, pharmacist, and social worker.

When treating a pressure ulcer, reassess the wound for location, stage, size, tissue type and amount, exudate, and the surrounding skin condition (Nix, 2007). Optimizing wound healing requires monitoring of the wound, but unless infection is suspected or present, the wound will heal best when undisturbed. Many current wound dressings are designed to remain in place for up to a week or even longer, and this approach supports healing in chronic, noninfected wounds (RNAO, 2007; CAWC, 2006).

TABLE 47-8 Support Surfaces

Categories and Definitions	Mechanism of Action	Indications	Examples of Manufacturers' and Product Names
Low-Air-Loss			
Available in a mattress placed directly on the existing bed frame or an overlay placed directly on top of an existing surface	Pressure redistribution Provides a flow of air to assist in managing the heat and humidity of the skin	Prevention or treatment of skin breakdown	Hill-Rom; Flexair Kinetic Concepts, Inc.; First Step Select; Crown Therapeutics; Select Air Mattress
Nonpowered			
Any support surface not requiring or using external sources of energy for operation. Examples: foam, interconnected air-filled cells	Pressure redistribution Air moves to and from cells as body position changes	Prevention or treatment of skin breakdown	Crown Therapeutics Roho Dry Floatation Mattress Gaymar Industries/Sof-Care
Air-Fluidized Beds			
Surfaces that change load distribution properties when powered and when client is in contact with the surface	Provides pressure redistribution via a fluidlike medium created by forcing air through beads, as characterized by immersion and envelopement	Prevention or treatment of skin breakdown May also be used to protect newly flapped or grafted surgical sites and for clients with excessive moisture	Kinetic Concepts, Inc./FluidAir/ Hill-Rom/Clinitron
Lateral Rotation			
Provides passive motion to promote mobilization of respiratory secretions and provides low-air-loss therapy	Features a support surface that provides rotation about a longitudinal axis, as characterized by degree of client turn, duration, and frequency	Treatment and prevention of pulmonary complications associated with immobility	Hill-Rom/Total Care Sport/Kinetic Concepts, Inc./TriaDyne

The use and documentation of a systematic approach to the assessment of the actual pressure ulcers leads to better decision making and optimum outcomes (Nix, 2007). Several healing and documentation tools are available for you to use to document wound assessments over time. Using a tool helps link the assessment to outcomes so that an evaluation of the plan of care follows objective criteria (Nix, 2007). For example, the Pressure Ulcer Status Tool (PSST) (Bates-Jensen, 1995) addresses 15 wound characteristics. You score individual items and total them, providing an overall indication of wound status. The scoring assists in evaluating whether the goals of the wound management plan are effective. Tools such as the PSST may seem overly detailed and time consuming, but when you use them judiciously and regularly, they provide a method of ensuring reliable documentation of nursing actions.

Wound Management

Maintenance of a physiological local wound environment is the goal of effective wound management (Rolstad & Ovington, 2007). To maintain a healthy wound environment, you need to address the following directives: prevent and manage infection, cleanse the wound, remove nonviable tissue, manage exudate, maintain the wound in a moist environment, and protect the wound. A wound will not move through the phases of wound healing if the wound is infected. Prevention of wound infection includes wound irrigation, cleansing, and removal of nonviable tissue.

BOX 47-11 CLIENT TEACHING

Pressure-Redistribution Surfaces

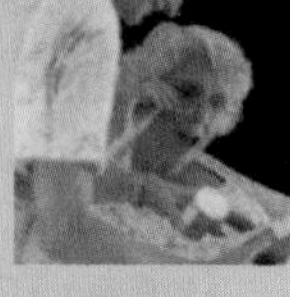

Objectives

- Client and family will describe their understanding of the purposes and basic operations of the pressure-redistribution surfaces.

Teaching Strategies

- Explain the reasons for the pressure-redistribution surface.
- Explain proper body mechanics while using the pressure redistribution surface.
- Educate client and family about the use and care of the pressure-redistribution surface.
- Explain additional pressure-redistribution measures.

Evaluation

- Client and family will state the basic purposes for the pressure-redistribution surface.
- Client and family will be able to describe the function of the pressure-redistribution surface.
- Client and family will be able to demonstrate proper use of the pressure-redistribution surface.

➤ SKILL 47-2 Treating Pressure Ulcers

video

Delegation Considerations

The skill of treating pressure ulcers cannot be delegated to unregulated care providers (UCPs). In some practice settings, you can delegate *non-sterile* dressing application for chronic, established wounds when a nurse has evaluated and designated the protocol. The *assessment* of the wound remains within the scope of the nurse, however, even if the dressing change is delegated. Instruct nursing assistive personnel to:

- Report changes in skin integrity to you immediately
- Report pain, fever, or wound drainage to you immediately
- Report any potential contamination to the existing dressing (e.g., client incontinence or other bodily fluids; dressing becomes dislodged)

Equipment

- Disposable gloves (clean)
- Plastic bag for dressing disposal
- Measuring device
- Cotton-tipped applicators
- Topical cleansing agent
- Dressing of choice (see Box 47–10)
- Hypoallergenic tape (if needed)
- Documentation record
- Scale for assessing wound healing

Procedure

STEPS	RATIONALE
1. Assess client's level of comfort using a scale of 1 to 10 and the need for pain medication.	• Clients tolerate dressing change procedures better if pain is controlled.
2. Determine if client has allergies to topical agents.	• Topical agents cause localized skin reactions.
3. Review order for topical agent or dressing.	• Administration of proper medication and treatment is ensured.
4. Close room door or bedside curtains. Position client to allow dressing removal.	• Privacy is provided, and the area is accessible for dressing change.
5. Perform hand hygiene, and apply clean gloves. Remove dressing, and place in plastic bag.	• Transmission of microorganisms is reduced and accidental exposure to body fluids is prevented.
6. Assess pressure ulcer(s). All pressure ulcers need individual assessments (see Step 6 illustration).	• Consistent assessment will provide the basis for evaluating wound progress (Nix, 2007).
A. Note colour, type, and percentage of tissue present in the wound base.	• Determining the tissue type will assist in the choice of dressing.
B. Measure width and length of the ulcer(s). Determine width by measuring the dimension from left to right and the length from top to bottom.	• Ulcer size will change as healing progresses; therefore, the longest and widest areas of the wound will change over time. Measuring the width and length by measuring the same area will provide a consistent measurement (Nix, 2007).
C. Measure depth of pressure ulcer using a sterile cotton-tipped applicator or other device that will allow measurement of wound depth (see Step 6 illustration).	• Depth measure is important for determining wound volume. Although surface area adequately represents tissue loss in stage II ulcers, volume more adequately represents tissue loss in stage III and IV wounds.
D. Measure depth of undermining using a cotton-tipped applicator to gently probe under skin edges (see Step 6 illustration).	• Undermining represents the loss of the underlying tissue (subcutaneous and muscle) to a greater extent than the skin. Undermining indicates progressive tissue loss and needs to be accommodated with an appropriate dressing.

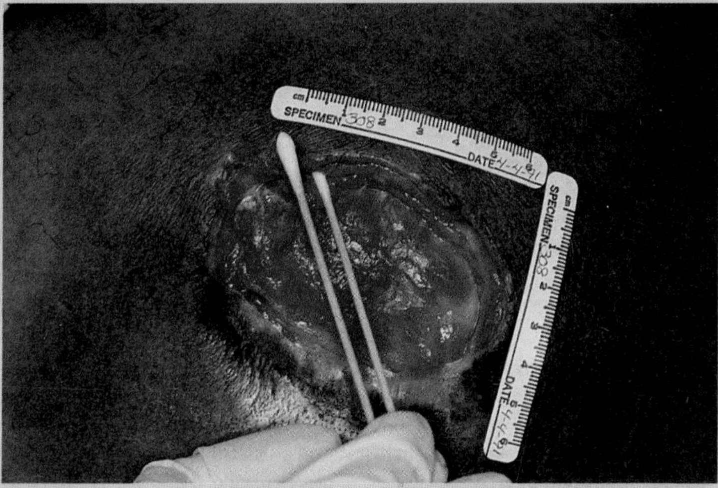

Step 6 Measuring wound depth (steps b, c, and d.)

Continued

➤ SKILL 47-2 Treating Pressure Ulcers *continued*

STEPS	RATIONALE
7. Assess the periwound skin; check for maceration, redness, and denuded area.	• Deterioration of the skin around a wound indicates infection, excessive wound exudate, or skin stripping from adhesive removal.
8. Change to sterile gloves (check agency policy).	• Aseptic technique needs to be maintained during cleansing and application of dressings. Refer to institutional policy regarding use of clean or sterile gloves.
9. Cleanse ulcer thoroughly with normal saline or cleansing agent. Use irrigating syringe for deep ulcers.	• Wound debris is removed.
10. Apply topical agents, as prescribed:	
A. Enzymes (where available)	
(1) Apply thin, even layer of ointment over necrotic areas of ulcer only. Do not apply enzyme to surrounding skin.	• A thick layer of ointment is not necessary; a thin layer absorbs and is more effective. Excess medication irritates surrounding skin (Rolstad & Ovington, 2007). Some enzymes cause burning, paresthesia, and dermatitis to surrounding skin. Check manufacturer's direction for frequency of application.
(2) Apply secondary nonadherent gauze dressing directly over ulcer.	• Wound is protected. Bacteria is prevented from entering wound.
(3) Tape securely in place.	• Dressing is kept in place. Use tape or adhesive that will not irritate skin.
B. Hydrogel	
(1) Cover surface of ulcer with thin layer of hydrogel using applicator or gloved hand.	• A moist wound environment is maintained.
(2) Apply secondary nonadherent gauze dressing or transparent dressing over wound, and adhere to intact skin.	• Wound base is covered and hydrogel–wound interface is maintained
C. Calcium alginate	
(1) Lightly pack wound with alginate using applicator or gloved fingers.	• Wound moisture is maintained while excess drainage is absorbed.
(2) Apply secondary dressing of nonadherent gauze, absorbent pad, or foam over alginate. Tape in place.	• Alginate is held against wound surface.
11. Remove gloves, and dispose of soiled supplies. Perform hand hygiene.	• Transmission of microorganisms is reduced.
12. Assess the pressure ulcer at each dressing change or sooner if the wound or client's condition deteriorates (Nix, 2007). Utilize the agency's tool for wound assessment.	• Not all clients with wounds will demonstrate quick wound healing because of other health issues. The wound assessment will provide a report of wound healing progress or the lack of healing.
13. Compare wound assessment to the identified plan of care, and if the wound is not progressing toward healing, as indicated by an increase in size, increased presence of pain, foul-smelling drainage, or increase in devitalized tissue, discuss findings with the health care team.	• Wound care is an interdisciplinary activity and requires the involvement of the team of health care professionals as well as the client and family.

Critical Decision Point: A clean pressure ulcer should show evidence of some healing within 2 to 4 weeks. Do *not* use the pressure ulcer staging system to measure pressure ulcer healing. The system measures depth of wound, not healing (WOCN, 2003).

14. Complete wound documentation required for one of the wound assessment instruments per agency's protocol.	• Assessments compared over time will determine progress toward wound healing.

Unexpected Outcomes and Related Interventions

Maceration of Skin Surrounding Ulcer

- Reduce exposure of surrounding skin to topical agents and moisture.
- Consider the use of a liquid skin barrier on periwound skin.
- Use a dressing that will wick exudate away from periwound skin.

Deepening of Ulcer and Increased Drainage

- Notify health care professional for possible change in pressure ulcer status.
- Obtain necessary wound cultures.
- Obtain additional consults (e.g., wound care specialist).

Recording and Reporting

- Record assessment of ulcer in client's record.
- Describe type of topical agent used, dressing applied, and client's response.
- Report any deterioration in ulcer appearance.

Home Care Considerations

- Clients need to dispose of contaminated dressings in the home in a manner consistent with local regulations (WOCN, 2003).
- Discuss the need for a home pressure-redistribution surface or bed.

Cleaning a Wound. Use only noncytotoxic wound cleansers, such as normal saline or commercial wound cleansers, to clean wounds. Noncytotoxic cleansers will not damage or kill fibroblasts and healing tissue (Rolstad & Ovington, 2007). Cytotoxic solutions to absolutely avoid are sodium hypochlorite solution (Dakin's solution—essentially bleach), acetic acid, povidone-iodine, and hydrogen peroxide. These are *not* to be used in clean granulating wounds because they inhibit wound healing (RNAO, 2007; CAWC, 2006).

Irrigation. Irrigation is a common method of delivering the wound cleansing solution to the wound. Studies have shown that an optimal effective range of irrigation pressures exists that ensure adequate removal of bacteria (RNAO, 2007; Rodeheaver, 2001). To ensure an irrigation pressure within the correct range, use a 35-mL syringe with a 19-gauge angiocatheter or a single 100-mL saline squeeze bottle. Both methods will enhance wound cleansing, but by delivering saline at a pressure between 4 and 15 psi (RNAO, 2007), you will avoid trauma to the wound bed.

Debridement. **Debridement** is the removal of nonviable, necrotic tissue, and is necessary to rid the ulcer of a source of infection, to enable visualization of the wound bed, and to provide a clean base for healing. However, a dry necrotic heel pressure ulcer is an exception. According to the RNAO guidelines (2007), stable, dry, black eschar on heels should not be debrided if no evidence of infection (e.g., pain, purulence, or erythema) appears. The method of debridement—mechanical, autolytic, chemical, or sharp or surgical—will depend on which is most appropriate to the client's condition and care goals (RNAO, 2007). During the debridement process, remember that increases in wound exudate, odour, and size are likely to be observed. You will need to assess and prevent or effectively manage pain that occurs with debridement (RNAO, 2007; CAWC, 2006).

Mechanical debridement, or a "wet-to-dry" saline gauze dressing, is *not* considered appropriate, as it is nonselective in its removal of both devitalized and viable tissue (RNAO 2007; CAWC, 2006). Biological debridement is the use of maggot therapy. Sterile maggots are used in a wound because they ingest the dead tissue and do not impede granulation (Thomas et al, 2001). Although chemical debridement is an option, topical enzyme preparations are not currently available in Canada. Topical enzymes induce changes in the substrate, resulting in the breakdown of necrotic tissue (Ramundo & Wells, 2000). Depending on the type of enzyme used, the preparation either digests or dissolves the tissue. Current best practice treatment options are autolytic and sharp or surgical debridement (the "gold standard").

Autolytic debridement uses synthetic dressings over a wound to allow the eschar and fibrinous slough within the wound to be self-digested by the action of enzymes that are present in wound fluids (CAWC, 2006). Dressings that support moisture at the wound surface (e.g., hydrogel) maintain a moist wound bed ("moist like your eyeball"), which allows the movement of epithelial cells and facilitates wound closure; however, a wound that has excessive wound exudate (drainage) provides an environment that supports bacterial growth, macerates the periwound skin, and slows the healing process (CAWC, 2006). If exudate is excessive, use an absorptive dressing (e.g., calcium alginate or foam) and evaluate the volume, consistency, and odour of the drainage to determine whether signs and symptoms of infection are present.

Surgical debridement with a scalpel, scissors, or other sharp instrument should only be used by those health care professionals who have the knowledge, skill, and competence to perform the procedure, usually physicians and advanced practice nurses (e.g., nurse practitioners). Your regulating authority (e.g., College of Nurses) and the policy of your health care agency or institution will mandate whether you are able to perform sharp or surgical debridement. It is the most efficient way to reach vitalized tissue at the base of a wound and is also used when sepsis can be localized and excised.

Remember, the wound will not heal, regardless of the use of topical therapy (Rolstad & Ovington, 2007), unless you control or eliminate the causative factors (e.g., shear, friction, pressure, and moisture). In addition, given the phases of wound healing, you will need to alter the treatment plan as the ulcer heals. For example, in the management of a necrotic and sloughy wound, you may initially use a hydrocolloid dressing to autolytically debride the wound. Because this process takes time, leave the dressing intact for up to 1 week. Once the wound is cleansed of necrotic, fibrinous tissue, you will discontinue the hydrocolloid dressing and choose another dressing after assessing the wound base characteristics. Continued reassessment is key to supporting the wound as it moves through the phases of wound healing.

Growth Factors. Growth factors regulate most of the key actions of cells during wound healing, and topical growth factors regulate the healing of chronic wounds (Schultz, 2007). Through extensive studies of the molecular regulation of healing, researchers now better understand the role of various growth factors involved in wound healing, including epidermal growth factor, platelet-derived growth factor, fibroblast growth factor, and transforming growth factor. Depending on the setting, you may be responsible for the use of this treatment modality.

Nutritional Status. Nutritional assessment and support of the client with a wound is based on the appreciation that nutrition is fundamental to normal cellular integrity and tissue repair (Stotts, 2007a). You need to correct inadequate nutrition and support healing through early intervention. The Joint Commission (2007) recommends nutritional assessment within 24 hours of admission. Assess the client's mouth and skin for signs of nutritional deficiencies (see Chapter 43). Reassessments reflect changes in status and effects of interventions (Stotts, 2007a). Box 47–12 defines parameters for clinically significant malnutrition (AHCPR, 1994).

Protein Status. Clients with a potential for or actual decreased serum albumin levels or poor protein intake need a nutritional evaluation to ensure proper caloric intake (AHCPR, 1994). A client can lose as much as 50 g of protein per day from an open, weeping pressure

➤ BOX 47-12 AHCPR* Recommendations for Nutritional Assessment and Management of Pressure Ulcers

Assessment of Clinically Significant Malnutrition

Serum albumin is less than 3.5 mg/100 mL.
Total lymphocyte count is less than 1800/mm^3.
Body weight has decreased more than 15%.

Interventions

- Involve dietitian to prevent malnutrition and ensure adequate dietary intake to the extent that is compatible with the client's wishes and ideal body weight.
- Maintain serum albumin level greater than 3.5 mg/100 mL.
- Maintain total lymphocyte count greater than 1800/mm^3.
- Perform an abbreviated nutritional assessment, according to institutional policy and as defined by the Nutritional Screening Initiative, at least every 3 months for clients who are unable to take food by mouth or who experience an involuntary change in weight.
- Encourage dietary intake or supplementation if a client with a pressure ulcer is malnourished. If dietary intake continues to be inadequate, impractical, or impossible, use nutritional support (usually tube feeding) to place the client into positive nitrogen balance (approximately 30–35 calories/kg/day and 1.25–1.50 g of protein/kg/day) according to the goals of care.
- Give vitamin and mineral supplements if you suspect or confirm deficiencies.

*AHCPR, Agency for Health Care Policy and Research.

Adapted from Agency for Health Care Policy and Research, Panel for Treatment of Pressure Ulcers in Adults. (1994). *Treatment of pressure ulcers: Clinical practice guideline no. 15.* (AHCPR Pub No. 95-0653). Rockville, MD: Agency for Health Care Policy and Research, Public Health Service, U.S. Department of Health and Human Services.

ulcer. Although the recommended intake of protein for adults is 0.8 g/kg/day, a higher intake of protein up to 1.8 g/kg/day is necessary for healing. Increased protein intake helps rebuild epidermal tissue. Increased caloric intake helps replace subcutaneous tissue. Vitamin C promotes collagen synthesis, capillary wall integrity, fibroblast function, and immunological function.

Hemoglobin. A low hemoglobin level decreases delivery of oxygen to the tissues and leads to further ischemia. When possible, maintain hemoglobin at 12 g/100 mL.

Dressings

For surgical wounds that heal by primary intention, it is common to remove dressings as soon as drainage stops. In contrast, when a wound is healing by secondary intention, the dressing material becomes a means for providing moisture to the wound or assisting in debridement.

Purposes of Dressings. A dressing serves several purposes:

- Protects a wound from microorganism contamination
- Aids in hemostasis
- Promotes healing by absorbing drainage and supports autolytic debridement
- Supports or splints the wound site
- Protects the client from seeing the wound (if perceived as unpleasant)
- Promotes thermal insulation of the wound surface
- Provides a moist environment for the wound bed

In a normally healing wound, when wound drainage is minimal, the healing process forms a natural fibrin seal that eliminates the need for a dressing. Wounds with extensive tissue loss always need a dressing.

A pressure dressing is applied with elastic bandages, exerts localized downward pressure over an actual or potential bleeding site, and eliminates dead space in underlying tissues so that wound healing progresses normally. Check pressure dressings to be sure that they do not interfere with circulation to a body part. Assess skin colour, pulses in distal extremities, the client's comfort, and changes in sensation. Pressure dressings are not routinely removed.

Specific dressings cover and protect certain types of wounds, such as large wounds, wounds with drainage tubes or suction catheters in the wound, wounds that need frequent changing, and fistulas. For these wounds, pouches or special wound collection systems cover the wound and collect the wound drainage. Some of these devices have a plastic flange on the front of the wound pouch that allow you to change the wound packing without removing the wound pouch from the skin.

Understanding the method of action and purpose of the dressing selection facilitates wound healing (Rolstad & Ovington, 2007). When you identify the objectives for care of the wound, the dressing choice becomes clear. For example, a wound requiring exudate management requires a different type of dressing than one that requires debridement.

A primary function of a dressing on a healing wound is to protect the fragile wound bed. Most traditional surgical dressings have three layers: a contact or primary layer, an absorbent layer, and an outer protective or secondary layer. The contact dressing covers the incision and part of the adjacent skin. Fibrin, blood products, and debris adhere to the contact dressing's surface. A dressing that does not adhere to the wound bed, such as a Telfa pad or soft silicone, will not cause the dressing to stick to the suture line. Use of dry gauze or improper removal of the dressing can cause disruption of the healing epidermal surface. If the gauze dressing is sticking to the surgical incision, the dressing needs to be moistened with saline solution. This will cause the dressing to become saturated, loosening it from the incisional area and preventing trauma to the wound bed.

Types of Dressings. Dressings vary by type of material and mode of application (wet or dry) (Skill 47–3). They need to be easy to apply, comfortable, and made of materials that promote wound healing. The RNAO guidelines (2007) should help you select dressings that respond to the need of the wound, based on the goal for the wound: to heal, to protect from infection, to provide comfort, or to maintain current status (nonhealing wound). A dressing designed to wick away exudate and avoid skin stripping from adhesives will protect the periwound skin. Protecting the wound bed requires a dressing that will maintain a moist wound bed (not too dry; not too wet), prevent contamination from external sources such as feces or urine, and be conformable to the wound and surrounding tissue (Box 47–13; see also Box 47–14 and Table 47–9). In addition, if the wound is deep, undermining, or has tunnelling or sinus tracts, ensure that no dead space remains to create an opportunity for an abscess to develop. In this situation, lightly pack the wound with appropriate dressing material (i.e., nonwoven gauze moistened with hydrogel in a dry wound, hypertonic sodium ribbon in a wet or contaminated wound, and silver or cadexomer iodine packing in an infected wound [Sibbald et al., 2006a]).

Woven Gauze Dressings. In the past, woven gauze dressings were commonly used to provide coverage for wounds; however, research has demonstrated their efficacy in wound healing is limited (CAWC, 2006). Providing the opportunity for a noninfected wound to heal using "moist wound healing" approaches and dressings does limit the use of gauze as an effective dressing. However, nonwoven gauze remains useful as packing material (e.g., Nu-gauze). Gauze is available in different textures and in various lengths and sizes; the 4 × 4 is the most common. Gauze can be saturated with solutions and used to cleanse and pack a wound. When used to pack a dry wound, the gauze should be lightly moistened with hydrogel (see p. 1251) to provide moisture to the wound bed. Use nonadherent gauze dressings such as Telfa over clean wounds with little or no drainage. Telfa gauze has a shiny, nonadherent surface that does not stick to incisions or wound openings but allows drainage to pass through to the gauze topper. Acute surgical wounds are most likely to be packed with saline-moistened nonwoven gauze and the dressing changed at frequent intervals, usually determined by the surgeon.

Transparent Film Dressings. Self-adhesive, transparent film dressings are occlusive and trap the wound's moisture over the wound, providing a moist environment. The transparent film dressing has been used for small, superficial wounds such as skin tears or for protection of high-risk skin. However, transparent film dressings can be difficult to remove and can cause unnecessary trauma to fragile periwound tissue. You must remove the transparent film with a "lateral pull" technique, in which you support the dressing with one hand while lifting (and breaking the adhesive seal) with the other, instead of just pulling off the dressing. Bearing these factors in mind, you can use transparent film dressing to affix gauze, and it can also function as a secondary dressing or provide autolysis for small wounds.

Transparent film dressing has the following characteristics:

- Adheres to undamaged skin
- Serves as a barrier to external fluids and bacteria but provides some moisture vapour transmission across the wound bed (depends on the particular film)
- Promotes a moist environment that speeds epithelial cell growth
- Can be removed without damaging underlying tissues when a lateral pull is used
- Permits a view of the wound
- Does not require a secondary dressing

➤ SKILL 47-3 Applying Dry and Moist Dressings

video

Delegation Considerations

The skill of applying dry and moist dressings to the new acute wound cannot be delegated to unregulated care providers (UCPs). In some settings, you can delegate aspects of wound care, such as changing of dressings using *clean* techniques for chronic wounds. The *assessment* of the wound remains within the scope of the nurse, however, even if the dressing change is delegated. Instruct nursing assistive personnel to:

- Report pain, fever, bleeding, or wound drainage to you immediately
- Report any potential contamination to the existing dressing (e.g., client incontinence or other bodily fluids; dressing becomes dislodged)

Equipment

- Sterile gloves
- Variety of gauze dressings and pads
- Irrigation kit
- Cleansing solution
- Sterile solution
- Clean, disposable gloves
- Tape, ties, or bandages, as needed
- Waterproof bag
- Extra gauze dressings, or ABD pads

Procedure

STEPS	RATIONALE
1. Perform hand hygiene. Obtain information about size and location of wound.	• Transmission of microorganisms is reduced. Plan for proper type and amount of supplies needed. Know when assistance is needed to hold dressings in place.
2. Assess client's level of comfort.	• Removal of a dry dressing is painful; some clients require pain medication.
3. Review orders for dressing change procedure.	• Orders indicate type of dressing or applications to use.
4. Explain procedure to client, and instruct client not to touch wound area or sterile supplies.	• Explanation decreases anxiety. Sudden, unexpected movement on client's part will result in contamination of wound and supplies.
5. Close room or cubicle curtains and windows.	• Privacy is provided, and airborne microorganisms are reduced.
6. Position client comfortably, and drape with bath blanket to expose only wound site.	• Wound is accessible yet unnecessary exposure is minimized.
7. Place disposable bag within reach of work area. Fold top of bag to make cuff (see Step 7 illustration).	• Soiled dressings can easily be disposed of. Bag's outer surface is not soiled.
8. Apply face mask and protective eyewear, if splashing occurs.	• Transmission of pathogens to exposed tissues is reduced. Mask and eyewear protects from splashes.
9. Put on clean, disposable gloves, and remove tape, bandage, or ties.	• Transmission of infectious organisms from soiled dressings to hands is prevented.
10. Remove tape: pull parallel to skin toward dressing; remove remaining adhesive from skin.	• Pulling tape toward dressing reduces stress on suture line or wound edges.
11. With gloved hand, carefully remove gauze dressings one layer at a time, taking care not to dislodge drains or tubes.	• Appearance of drainage is sometimes upsetting to client. Removal of one layer at a time reduces the chance of accidental removal of underlying drains.

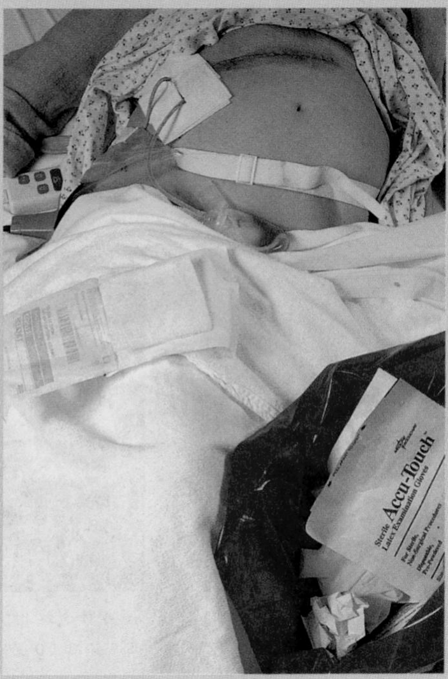

Step 7 Disposable waterproof bag placed near the dressing site.

Continued

➤ SKILL 47-3 Applying Dry and Moist Dressings *continued*

STEPS	RATIONALE
A. If dressing sticks on a wet-to-dry dressing, do not moisten it; instead gently free dressing, and alert client of potential discomfort.	• Wet-to-dry dressing should debride wound (Ramundo & Wells, 2000). Do not wet the dressing to remove it. It is supposed to be dry so that as it is removed from the wound it also removes necrotic tissue.

Critical Decision Point: Never use a wet-to-dry dressing in a clean granulating wound. Use only for debridement (Ramundo, 2007).

STEPS	RATIONALE
12. Observe character and amount of drainage on dressing and appearance of wound.	• Estimate of drainage amount and assessment of wound's condition are provided.
13. Fold dressings with drainage contained inside, and remove gloves inside out. With small dressings, remove gloves inside out over dressing (see Step 13 illustration). Dispose of gloves and soiled dressings in disposable bag. Perform hand hygiene.	• Transmission of microorganisms is reduced. Hands do not come into contact with material on gloves.
14. Open sterile dressing tray or individually wrapped sterile supplies. Place on bedside table (see Step 14 illustration).	• Sterile dressings remain sterile while on or within sterile surface. Preparation of supplies prevents break in technique during dressing change.
15. If ordered, cleanse or irrigate wound:	
A. Pour ordered solution into sterile irrigation container.	
B. Using syringe, gently allow solution to flow over wound.	
C. Continue until the irrigation flow is clear.	
D. Dry surrounding skin.	

Critical Decision Point: Some commercial cleansers come in a spray bottle. Spray the wound to loosen the debris.

STEPS	RATIONALE
16. Apply dressing:	
A. Dry dressing	
(1) Apply sterile gloves.	• Sterile supplies can be handled without contamination.
(2) Inspect wound for appearance, drains, drainage, and integrity.	• Wound healing status is indicated.
(3) Cleanse wound with solution:	
(a) Clean from least-contaminated area to most-contaminated area.	• Contamination of previously cleaned area is prevented.
(4) Dry area.	• Protection and absorption of wound drainage is provided.
(5) Apply sterile, dry dressing covering wound.	• Wound is protected from external environment.
(6) Apply topper dressing if indicated.	• Topper dressing prevents strikethrough of wound drainage and provides a surface to tape the dressing in place.
B. Moist dressing	
(1) Apply clean gloves.	
(2) Remove old dressings, discard.	
(3) Assess surrounding skin (see Step 16B(3) illustration). Discard gloves.	• Surrounding skin assessment provides an evaluation of wound management.
(4) Apply sterile gloves.	• Handling of sterile supplies can occur without contamination.
(5) Cleanse wound base with normal saline or commercially prepared wound cleanser. Assess wound base.	• Cleansing removes wound debris for adequate assessment.
(6) Moisten gauze with prescribed solution. Gently wring out excess solution. Unfold.	• Gauze needs to be moist to allow for absorption of wound debris.

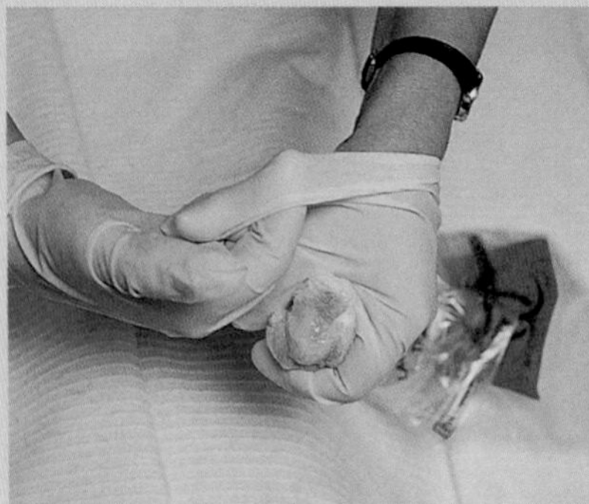

Step 13 Removal of disposable gloves over contaminated dressing.

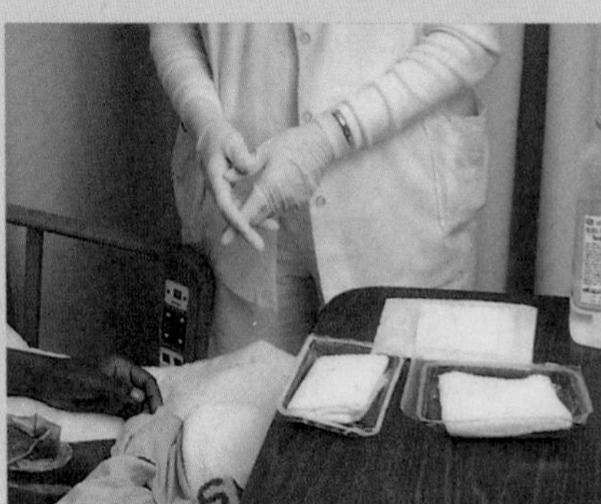

Step 14 Sterile dressing equipment.

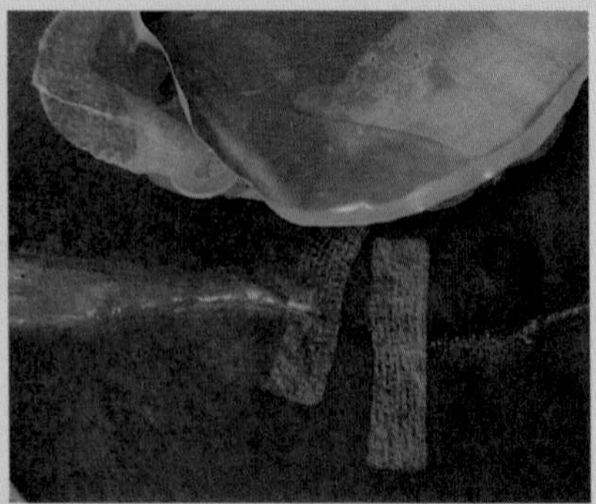

Step 16B(3) Exposure of wound facilitates assessment of wound and surrounding skin.

➤ SKILL 47-3 Applying Dry and Moist Dressings *continued*

STEPS	RATIONALE
(7) Apply gauze as a single layer (see Step 16B(7) illustration) directly onto the wound surface. If wound is deep, gently pack dressing into wound base by hand or with forceps until all wound surfaces are in contact with the gauze. If tunnelling is present, use a cotton-tipped applicator to place gauze into tunnelled area. Be sure gauze does not touch the surrounding skin (see Step 16B(7) illustration).	• Inner gauze needs to be moist, not dripping wet, to absorb drainage and adhere to debris. Excessively moist dressings result in moisture-associated skin damage (maceration) in the periwound skin (Gray & Weir, 2007). The wound needs to be loosely packed to facilitate wicking of drainage into absorbent outer layer of dressing.
(8) Cover with sterile dry gauze and topper dressing.	• Topper dressing prevents strikethrough of wound drainage and provides a surface to tape the dressing in place.
17. Secure dressing.	
A. Tape: Apply nonallergenic tape to secure dressing in place.	• The goal for securing a dressing is to keep the dressing in place and intact without causing damage to underlying and surrounding skin.
B. Montgomery ties (see Figure 47–23 on p. 1254)	
(1) Expose adhesive surface of tape on end of each tie.	
(2) Place ties on opposite sides of dressing.	
(3) Place adhesive directly on skin, or use skin barrier.	• Skin barrier (Stomahesive) protects intact skin from stretch and tension of adhesive tape.
C. For dressings on an extremity, secure dressing with rolled gauze or an elastic net (see Step 17C illustration)	
18. Remove gloves, and dispose of in bag. Remove any mask or eyewear.	• Transmission of infection is reduced.
19. Dispose of supplies, and perform hand hygiene.	• Transmission of infection is reduced.
20. Assist client to comfortable position.	• Client's sense of well-being is promoted. Comfort is enhanced.

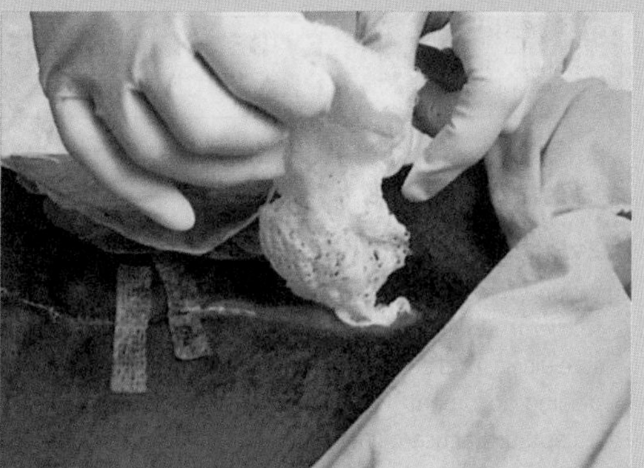

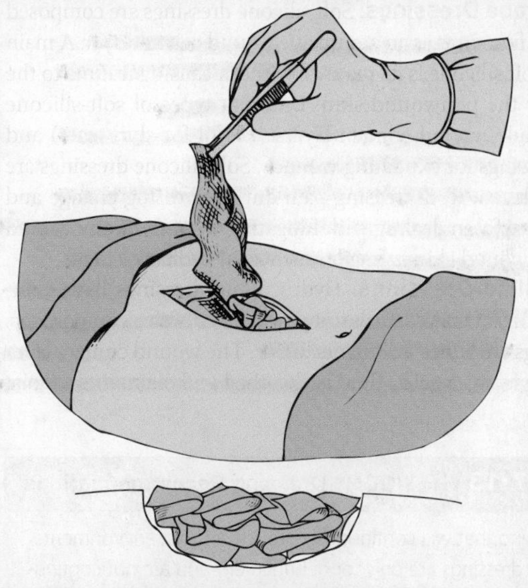

Step 16B(7) Packing wound with single layer of gauze.

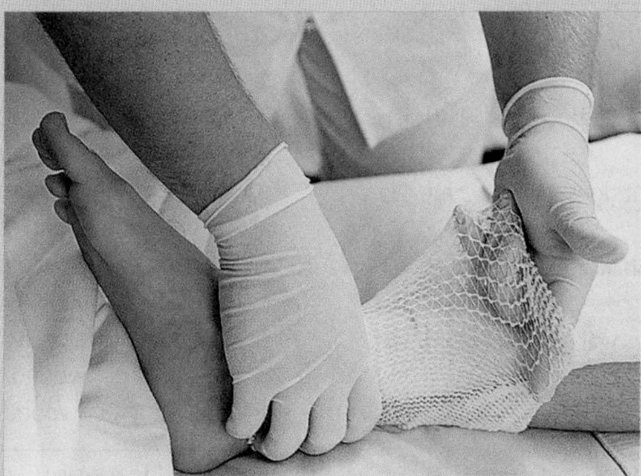

Step 17C Elastic net securing a lower extremity dressing.

Continued

➤ SKILL 47-3 Applying Dry and Moist Dressings *continued*

Unexpected Outcomes and Related Interventions

Wound Appears Inflamed, Tender, With or Without Drainage

- Monitor client for signs of infection (e.g., increased temperature or white blood cell count).
- Obtain wound culture.
- Notify health care professional.

Wound Drainage Increases

- Increase frequency of dressing changes.
- Notify health care professional, who may consider drain placement to facilitate wound drainage.

Wound Bleeds During Dressing Change

- Observe colour. If drainage is bright red and excessive, you will need to apply pressure.
- Inspect along dressing and underneath client to determine amount of bleeding.
- Obtain vital signs, as needed.
- Notify health care professional.

Sensation That "Something Has Given Way Under the Dressing"

- Observe wound for increased drainage or separation of sutures.
- Protect wound. Cover with sterile moist dressing.
- Instruct client to lie still.
- Notify health care professional.

Recording and Reporting

- Report brisk, bright-red bleeding or evidence of wound dehiscence or evisceration to health care professional immediately.
- Report wound and periwound tissue appearance, colour, and tissue type and presence and characteristics of exudate, type and amount of dressings used, and tolerance of client to procedure.
- Record client's level of comfort.
- Write date and time dressing applied on tape in ink (not marker).

Home Care Considerations

- More expensive specialty dressings are sometimes used because they decrease the frequency of dressing changes.
- Clean dressings may also be used in the home setting.
- Clients need to dispose of contaminated dressings in the home in a manner consistent with local regulations.

Soft Silicone Dressings. Soft silicone dressings are composed of silicone that functions as an atraumatic wound contact layer. A main advantage of soft silicone is its removal without causing trauma to the wound bed or the periwound skin. Different types of soft silicone dressings include wound contact layers (useful for skin tears) and absorbent dressings for exudating wounds. Soft silicone dressings are particularly relevant in decreasing pain during dressing change and are especially useful in dealing with fungating wounds or any wound where the periwound skin is fragile, such as in pediatric clients.

Hydrocolloid Dressings. Hydrocolloid dressings have complex formulations of colloidal, elastomeric, and adhesive components. These dressings are adhesive and occlusive. The wound contact layer of the dressing forms a gel as fluid is absorbed and maintains a moist

➤ BOX 47-13 WOCN* Dressing Recommendations

- Use a dressing that will continuously provide a moist environment. Wet-to-dry dressings are only for debridement and are not continuously moist saline dressings.
- Perform wound care using topical dressings as determined by a thorough assessment. No specific studies have proven an optimal dressing type for pressure ulcers.
- Choose a dressing that keeps the surrounding intact (periulcer) skin dry while keeping the ulcer bed moist.
- Choose a dressing that controls exudate but does not desiccate the ulcer bed.
- Consider caregiver time, ease of use, availability, and cost when selecting a dressing.
- Eliminate wound dead space by loosely filling all cavities with dressing material.

*WOCN, wound, ostomy, and continence nurses.

Adapted from Wound, Ostomy and Continence Nurses Society. (2003). *Guideline for prevention and management of pressure ulcers.* WOCN Clinical Practice Guidelines Series. Glenview, IL: Author.

✱ BOX 47-14 EVIDENCE-INFORMED PRACTICE GUIDELINE

Moisture-Associated Skin Damage From Dressings

Evidence Summary

Wound management and wound healing are critical to clients at risk for pressure ulcers, clients with pressure ulcers, or clients with other chronic wounds. The advances in wound healing document the benefit of a moist wound environment and the accepted practice of moist wound healing. However, a moist wound environment has the potential to macerate periwound skin: the tissues of the periwound skin soften, and the connective fibres are damaged. This condition is also classified as moisture-associated skin damage (MASD). Gray & Weir (2007) reviewed the existing literature to evaluate the effect of moist wound healing on the periwound skin. Although further research is needed to identify and evaluate the best strategy for managing existing periwound maceration, some clinical applications may help prevent or manage MASD.

Application to Nursing Practice

- Use of a skin protectant (no-sting barrier cream or pad or spray, dimethicone cream or zinc-based ointment) helps to prevent periwound skin maceration.
- Dressing selection needs to be individualized to the type of wound, the phase of wound healing, and the potential for wound healing.
- Selection of topical prescriptions such as BCT ointment (Xenaderm) helps to manage MASD to periwound skin.
- Use of negative pressure wound therapy (e.g., V.A.C.) may reduce the risk of periwound maceration by reducing local edema and exudate in the periwound tissue.

From Gray, M., & Weir, D. (2007). Prevention and treatment of moisture-associated skin damage (maceration) in the periwound skin. *Journal of Wound, Ostomy, and Continence Nurses, 34*(2), 153.

healing environment. Hydrocolloids support healing in clean granulating wounds, autolytically debride necrotic wounds, and are available in a variety of sizes and shapes.

Hydrocolloid dressing has the following characteristics:

- Has minimal absorption capabilities and is best for autolytically debriding a dry or slightly moist wound with fibrinous or necrotic debris
- Maintains wound bed moisture
- Slowly liquefies necrotic debris
- Is impermeable to external bacteria and other contaminants
- Is self-adhesive and conforms to the body well
- Acts as a preventive dressing for high-risk friction areas
- May be left in place for 5 to 7 days

This type of dressing is most useful on shallow to moderately deep wounds. Hydrocolloid dressings should not be used in heavily draining wounds or in full-thickness or infected wounds. Because of the manner in which hydrocolloids interact with the wound bed matter, when the dressing is removed, residue in the wound bed may be confused with pus (colour, odour) until the wound is cleansed. Hydrocolloids are quite adherent to the periwound skin and should be used with caution where the periwound tissue is fragile or friable.

Hydrogel Dressings. Hydrogel dressings donate moisture to the wound bed (hence, the term *hydro*, indicating water) and are gauze or sheet dressings impregnated with water- or glycerin-based amorphous gel. This type of dressing hydrates wounds and absorbs some smaller amounts of exudate. Hydrogel dressings are for partial-thickness and full-thickness wounds, deep wounds with minimal drainage, necrotic wounds, burns, and radiation-damaged skin. They are very useful in painful wounds because they are soothing to the client, do not adhere to the wound bed, and cause minimal trauma during dressing removal. Hydrogels should not be used on draining wounds; sheets should not be used on infected wounds. Hydrogels come in a sheet dressing or in a tube. When using hydrogel from a tube, do not squirt gel directly into the wound; rather, use a sterile gauze dressing or sterile implement (e.g., tongue depressor) to apply the gel so that potential contamination of the tube from matter in the wound is avoided.

Hydrogel has the following characteristics:

- Is soothing and reduces pain in the wound
- Provides a moist environment
- Debrides the wound (by softening the necrotic tissue)
- Does not adhere to the wound base and is easy to remove

Foam Dressings. Foam dressings are composed of nonadhesive or adhesive polyurethane foam, are provided as sheets or packing, and come in a variety of sizes and shapes. They are useful for wounds with large amounts of drainage or for autolytic debridement because they can be left intact for up to 7 days. Some foam dressings have a "fluid lock" to wick drainage off the wound and periwound skin, which prevents maceration. Furthermore, nonborder foam dressings can be cut to fit around drainage tubes.

Calcium Alginate Dressings. Calcium alginate dressings are manufactured from seaweed and are available in sheet and rope form. The alginate forms a thickened, stronger surface when it comes in contact with wound fluid. These highly absorbent dressings are useful in highly draining wounds and also provide hemostasis in friable tissue. Calcium alginate dressings are bioreabsorbable but should be removed from the wound.

Another type of dressing very useful for highly exudative wounds are hydrofibres, composed of sodium carboxymethylcellulose. These are available in sheets or ribbon and are used in similar situations to the calcium alginates. The main advantage of the hydrofibre dressing is that when exposed to fluid, it becomes a solid gel. This is particularly useful when the wound bed or wound edge is friable, for example, in malignant fungating wounds.

Neither of these dressings should be used on or in dry wounds. Secondary dressing (usually some form of absorbent pad) is required.

Composite Dressings. Composite dressings are a combination of two different dressing types. These multilayered dressings are designed to provide both absorption and autolysis. Composite dressings can remain in place for up to 3 days.

Topical Treatment for Infected Wounds. Superficially infected wounds require topical dressings to deal with the bacteria within the wound and surrounding tissue. Deep tissue infection requires the addition of antibiotic therapy, which can be determined from wound swab cultures (Sibbald et al, 2006b). Topical dressings range from hypertonic sodium solutions to silver antimicrobials.

Hypertonic Dressings. Hypertonic dressings contain a high concentration of sodium, which pulls out interstitial fluid, decreases edema to improve blood flow to the tissue surrounding the wound, and establishes a negative environment for bacterial growth. These dressings are available in ribbon, sheet, or gel form. Some clients find that the hypertonic dressings sting, and they should be changed once a day. Carefully monitor dressings with active ingredients on a daily basis.

Cadexomer Iodine. Cadexomer iodine dressings are available in sheets or a tube and provide the toxicity of iodine in a starch matrix. The iodine downloads into the wound bed in a controlled fashion, targeting only bacteria. The colour change of the dressing indicates its efficacy: it is brown when you apply it and gradually changes to cream-coloured as the iodine is absorbed. This process usually takes 72 hours, so the dressing should be left intact for 3 days. Changing the dressing more frequently will interfere with the effectiveness of the product. Use large amounts of cadexomer iodine with caution (see product monograph for limits), and do not use in breast-feeding women or clients with thyroid conditions.

Silver Dressings. Silver dressings have antimicrobial effects similar to cadexomer iodine, against approximately 150 different pathogens, including fungal infections, methicillin-resistant *Staphylococcus aureus* (MRSA), and vancomycin-resistant enterococci (VRE). You can use silver dressings in sheet, ribbon, rope, woven, and foam formats in a variety of sizes. The amount of silver in the dressing, which affects the kill rate (speed and sustainability), varies, and silver dressings require moisture to become activated—either from the wound bed exudate or with the use of a scant amount of hydrogel laid down in the base of the wound first. In addition, most silver dressings will require a secondary dressing, and their efficacy ranges from 3 to 7 days, depending on the product. No sensitivity to silver dressings has been reported, but clients do occasionally complain of stinging as the silver is activated. Be aware that some forms of silver dressings may leave a black stain around the periwound skin.

Negative Pressure Wound Therapy. Negative pressure wound therapy (NPWT) is another modality for dressings. The approach uses a machine that applies localized negative pressure to the surface and margins of the wound, pulling up the base of the wound and enhancing healing rates. It can be very effective, particularly in wounds in which rapid healing is viable, and will enhance patient quality of life. Although expensive, the method, in the appropriate situation, can significantly increase wound healing, thus decreasing the requirement for health care resources, including hospitalization. Usually these dressings are changed three times a week.

NPWT is also used to enhance the viability of split-thickness skin grafts. Placing it over the graft intraoperatively decreases the ability of the graft to shift and evacuates fluids that build up under the graft (Frantz et al, 2007).

TABLE 47-9 Wound Care Dressings

Class	Description	Local Wound Care* Tissue Debridement	Infection	Moisture Balance	Care Considerations Indications and Contraindications
1. Films and Membranes	Semipermeable adhesive sheet. Impermeable to H_2O molecules and bacteria	+	–	–	Moisture vapour transmission rate varies from film to film. Should not be used on draining or infected wounds.* Create occlusive barrier against infection.
2. Nonadherent	Sheets of low adherence to tissue. Nonmedicated tulles	–	–	–	Allow drainage to seep through pores to secondary dressing. Facilitate application of topicals.
3. Hydrogels	Polymers with high H_2O content. Available in gels, solid sheets, or impregnated gauze	++	–	+	Should not be used on draining wounds. Solid sheets should not be used on infected wounds.
4. Hydrocolloids	May contain gelatin, sodium, carboxymethylcellulose, polysaccharides, or pectin, or a combination of these. Sheet dressings are occlusive and have polyurethane film outer layer	+++	+/–	++	Should be used with care on fragile skin. Should not be used on heavily draining or infected wounds.* Create occlusive barrier to protect the wound from outside contamination. Characteristic odour may accompany dressing change and should not be confused with infection.
5. Calcium alginates	Sheets or fibrous ropes of calciumsodium alginate (seaweed derivative). Have hemostatic capabilities	++	+	+++	Should not be used on dry wounds. Avoid packing into narrow deep sinuses because of low tensile strength. Bioreabsorbable.
6. Composite dressings	Multilayered, combination dressings to increase absorbency and autolysis	+	–	+++	Use on wounds on which dressing may stay in place for several days.*
7. Foams	Nonadhesive or adhesive polyurethane foam. May have occlusive backing. Sheets or cavity packing. Some have fluid lock.	–	–	+++	Use on moderate to heavily draining wounds. Occlusive foams should not be used on heavily draining or infected wounds.*
8. Charcoal	Contains odour-absorbent charcoal within product	–	–	+	Some charcoal products are inactivated by moisture. Ensure that dressing edges are sealed.
9. Hypertonic	Sheet, ribbon, or gel impregnated with sodium concentrate.	+	+	++	Gauze ribbon should not be used on dry wounds. May be painful on sensitive tissue. Gel may be used on dry wounds.
10. Hydrophilic fibres	Sheet or packing strip of sodium carboxymethyl-cellulose. Converts to a solid gel when activated by moisture (fluid lock).	+	–	+++	Best for moderate amount of exudate. Should not be used on dry wounds. Avoid packing into narrow deep sinuses because of low tensile strength.

➤ TABLE 47-9 Wound Care Dressings *continued*

Class	Description	Tissue Debridement	Infection	Moisture Balance	Care Considerations: Indications and Contraindications
11. Antimicrobials	Silver or cadexomer iodine with vehicle for delivery: sheets, gels, alginates, foams, or paste.	+	+++	+	Broad spectrum against bacteria. Not to be used on patients with known hypersensitivities to any product components.
12. Other devices	NPWT applies localized negative pressure to surface and margins of wound. Dressings consist of polyurethane or polyvinyl alcohol materials.	–	+	+++	Pressure-distributing wound dressing actively removes fluid from the wound and promotes wound edge approximation. Advanced skill required for patient selection for this therapy.
13. Biological	Living human fibroblasts provided in sheets at ambient or frozen temperatures. Extracellular matrix. Collagen-containing preparations. Hyaluronic acid. Platelet-derived growth factor.	–	–	–	Should not be used on wounds with infection, sinus tracts, excessive exudate, or on patients known to have hypersensitivity to any of the product components. Cultural issues related to source. Advanced skill required for patient selection for this therapy.

"*+" indicates the appropriateness of the dressing for tissue debridement, infection, and moisture balance. "–" indicates the dressing is not considered beneficial in these areas. Use with caution if critical colonization is suspected.

From Registered Nurses Association of Ontario. (2007, revised). *RNAO Best Practice Guideline: Assessment and management of stage I–IV pressure ulcers* (pp. 102–103). Toronto, ON: Author.

Changing Dressings. When changing a dressing, keep in mind that the characteristics of the wound may have changed. However, be prepared with similar dressings as previously used and know the location of underlying drains or tubing and the type of supplies needed for care of the wound. Poor preparation can result in a break in aseptic technique (see Chapter 33), accidental dislodging of a drain, or unnecessary discomfort to the client as you search for supplies.

Your judgement in modifying a dressing change procedure is important during wound care. If the character of a wound changes, notify the physician or wound care specialist. Ensure open and clear communication with the physician or advanced practice nurse who documents your interventions, even though you do not require a medical order to change a dressing. If an order is written, then it is your responsibility to assess the current status of the wound in relation to the order. Has the wound changed? Would a different dressing be more effective? You will need to communicate this to the physician or advanced practice nurse.

An order to "reinforce dressing prn" (add dressings without removing the original one) is common immediately after surgery, when the surgeon does not want accidental disruption of the suture line or bleeding. The medical or operating room record usually indicates whether drains are present and from what body cavity they drain. After the first dressing change, describe the location of drains and the type of dressing materials and solutions to use in the client's care plan.

The CDC (2001) recommends the following during the dressing change procedure:

- Assess the skin beneath the tape.
- Perform thorough hand hygiene before and after wound care.
- Wear sterile gloves before directly touching an open or fresh wound (see Chapter 33).
- Remove or change dressings over closed wounds when they become wet or if the client has signs or symptoms of infection.

Clean or Sterile Technique. The body of literature about sterile versus clean dressing techniques is growing. The RNAO guidelines (2007) recommend sterile dressings, good handwashing, and clean gloves changed between wounds or when soiled. For surgical wounds, preliminary research indicates no difference in the healing rate of wounds when a clean rather than a sterile dressing change technique is used. Although aseptic or sterile technique is often used for surgical wound care, the most important aspects of this approach are to ensure as clean a field as possible with the use of sterile dressing packs, sterile scissors and forceps, and sterile dressings and gloves.

Preparing for Dressing Change (in Any Care Setting). To prepare a client for a dressing change, do the following:

- Administer required analgesics so that peak effects occur during the dressing change
- Describe steps of the procedure to lessen client anxiety
- Gather all supplies required for the dressing change

- Recognize normal signs of healing
- Answer questions about the procedure or the wound

You may often need to teach clients how to change dressings in preparation for home care. Demonstrate dressing changes to the client and family and then provide an opportunity for the client to practice changing a dressing independently or with assistance from a family member. By the time the client is ready to be discharged, wound healing has usually progressed past the point when complications such as dehiscence or evisceration might occur. The AHCPR guidelines (1994) regarding clean dressings in the home setting and disposal of contaminated dressings in the home can be found in Skill 47–3 (shown earlier), which outlines the steps for changing dry and moist dressings.

Packing a Wound. When packing a wound, first assess the size, depth, and shape of the wound, then assess for tunnelling and undermining of the wound. These wound characteristics will help you determine the size and type of dressing material needed to pack the wound. Many dressing materials, such as alginates, are used to pack wounds. If nonwoven gauze is the appropriate dressing material, saturate the gauze with the ordered solution, wring it out, unfold it, and lightly pack it into the wound. The entire wound surface needs to be in contact with part of the moist gauze dressing (see Skill 47–3). As stated in the RNAO guidelines (2007), "keeping the wound moist and the surrounding intact skin dry" (p. 43) will prevent maceration and help maintain a moist wound environment, and when using a dressing "loosely pack any sinus tract or cavity to eliminate dead space" (p. 77). Dead space (e.g., tunnelling) in the wound is not filled with dressing and will allow wound debris to accumulate in that area, which may cause an abscess.

Do not pack the wound too tightly. Overpacking the wound causes pressure on the tissue in the wound bed, decreasing blood flow to the area and preventing healing and wound closure. The packing material should never extend higher than the wound surface, because packing that overlaps onto the wound edges may cause maceration of the tissue surrounding the wound.

Securing Dressings. Use tape, ties, or a secondary dressing and cloth binders or gauze net to secure a dressing over a wound site. The choice of anchoring depends on the wound size and location, the presence of drainage, the frequency of dressing changes, and the client's level of activity. Of equal importance is the potential for skin stripping as tape is applied and removed frequently from the same area of skin. Clients with chronic wounds tend to have skin that is fragile and prone to breakdown. Thus, pay attention to the method used in affixing dressings.

If dressings without adhesive or other self-adhering borders are used, tape will secure dressings. Ensure that the periwound skin is not excoriated or at risk of breakdown. Make sure the client does not have an allergy or sensitivity to tape. Nonallergenic paper and silicone tapes are available to minimize skin reactions. Common adhesive tape adheres strongly to the skin's surface, whereas elastic adhesive tape compresses closely around pressure bandages and permits more movement of a body part. Skin sensitive to adhesive tape becomes severely inflamed and denuded and, in some cases, even sloughs when the tape is removed. Assess the skin under the tape at each dressing change. If the skin does not remain intact or is irritated, use an alternative solution (e.g., paper or silicone tapes).

Tape is available in various widths such as 1.3 cm (0.5 inch), 2.5 cm (1 inch), 5 cm (2 inches), and 7.6 cm (3 inches). Choose the size that sufficiently secures the dressing. Strips of 7.6 cm (3-inch) adhesive tape will likely ensure that a large dressing does not continually slip off. Other options, such as gauze wrap or burn-net dressings, may also be used.

When *applying tape*, ensure that the skin is dry so that the tape will adhere to several inches of skin on both sides of the dressing. Also place tape across the middle of the dressing. When securing the dressing, press the tape gently, exerting pressure away from the wound. With tension occurring in both directions away from the wound, skin distortion and irritation is minimized. Never apply tape over irritated or broken skin. Barrier film or spray can assist with adherence of the tape and protect the periwound skin from breakdown due to tape adhesives.

To remove tape *safely*, loosen the tape ends and gently pull the outer end parallel with the skin surface toward the wound. Apply light traction to the skin away from the wound as the tape is loosened and removed. The traction minimizes pulling of the skin. If tape covers an area of hair growth, the client experiences less discomfort if you pull the tape in the direction of hair growth. Adhesive remover can also be used to release the tape from the skin.

When frequent dressing changes are required, particularly for large abdominal or chest wounds, avoid repeated removal of tape from sensitive skin by using dressings secured with pairs of reusable Montgomery ties (Figure 47–23). Each section consists of a long strip; half contains an adhesive backing to apply to the skin, and the other half folds back and contains a cloth tie to fasten across a dressing and untie at dressing changes. Another method to protect the surrounding skin on wounds that need frequent dressing changes is to place strips of hydrocolloid dressings on either side of the wound edges, cover the wound with a dressing, and then apply the tape to the hydrocolloid dressing. To provide even support to a wound and

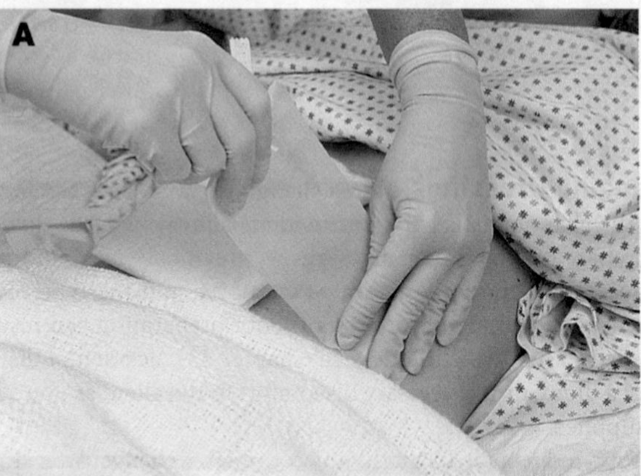

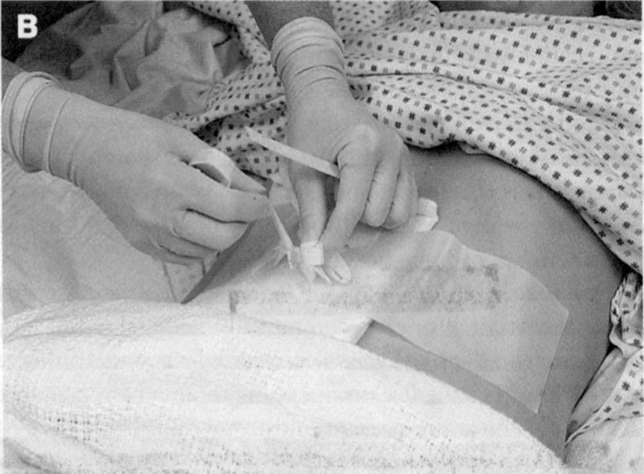

Figure 47-23 Montgomery ties. A, Each tie is placed at side of dressing. B, Securing ties encloses dressing.

immobilize a body part, apply elastic gauze or cloth bandages and binders over a dressing.

Comfort Measures. A wound is often painful, depending on the extent of tissue injury and the client's other medical health issues. Use several techniques to minimize discomfort during wound care. Administration of analgesic medications 30 to 45 minutes before dressing changes (depending on a drug's time of peak action) reduces discomfort. Careful removal of tape, gentle cleansing of wound edges, and careful manipulation of dressings and drains minimize stress on sensitive tissues. Often, propping and positioning the client with pillows or foam wedges can decrease positioning pain or discomfort, particularly in complex, time-consuming dressing changes.

Surgical or Traumatic Wound Considerations

Basic Skin Cleansing for Surgical or Traumatic Wounds.

Cleanse surgical or traumatic wounds by applying noncytotoxic solutions with sterile gauze or by irrigating. The following three principles are important when cleansing an incision or the area surrounding a drain:

1. Cleanse in a direction from the least contaminated area, such as from the wound or incision to the surrounding skin (Figure 47–24) or from an isolated drain site to the surrounding skin (Figure 47–25).
2. Use gentle friction when applying solutions locally to the skin.
3. When irrigating, allow the solution to flow from the least to most contaminated area (see Skill 47–5)

Never use the same piece of gauze to cleanse across an incision or wound twice. Use gauze to clean the skin, not the open wound. Open wound beds would be damaged by the abrasive contact of gauze.

Cleansing Skin and Drain Sites. In cases in which the open drain leaks onto surrounding skin, ensure that the drainage is removed from the skin to avoid maceration or excoriation of the tissue from possibly caustic drainage. You may also need to clean the drain itself on a regular basis to avoid a build-up of potentially contaminated material.

Drain sites are a source of contamination because moist drainage harbours microorganisms. If a wound has a dry incisional area and a moist drain site, use two separate swabs or gauze pads, one to cleanse from the top of the incision toward the drain and one to

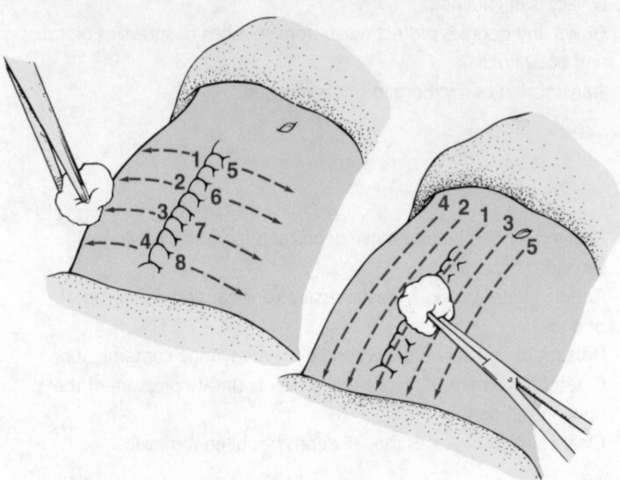

Figure 47-24 Methods for cleansing a wound site.

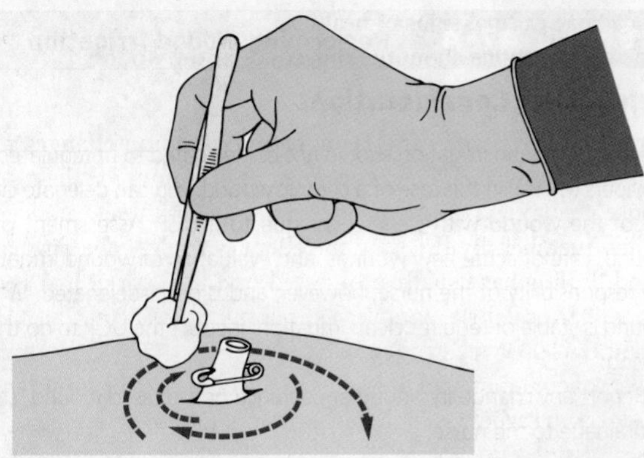

Figure 47-25 Cleansing a drain site.

cleanse from the bottom of the incision toward the drain. To cleanse the area of an isolated drain site, clean around the drain, moving in circular rotations outward from a point closest to the drain. In this situation, the skin near the site is more contaminated than the site itself. To cleanse circular wounds, use the same technique as in cleansing around a drain.

Irrigation. Irrigation is a special way of cleansing wounds. You use an irrigating syringe to flush the area with a constant low pressure flow of noncytotoxic solution (usually saline). The gentle washing action of the irrigation cleanses a wound of exudate and debris. Irrigations are particularly useful for open, deep wounds. *"Irrigate, irrigate, irrigate…and then irrigate some more"* However, make sure that the irrigant is not left pooled in the wound bed (usually by repositioning the client to allow gravity to assist in drainage).

Wound Irrigation. Irrigation of an open wound requires sterile technique. Use a 35-mL syringe with a 19-gauge angiocatheter (Rolstad & Ovington, 2007) or a single-use bottle of normal saline to deliver the solution, so as not to damage healing wound tissue. Never occlude a wound opening with a syringe, because this results in the introduction of irrigating fluid into a closed space. In this case, the pressure of the fluid causes tissue damage and discomfort. Always irrigate a wound with the syringe tip over but not in the drainage site. Make sure fluid flows directly into the wound and not over a contaminated area before entering the wound. Skill 47–4 lists steps for wound irrigation.

Sutures. A surgeon closes a wound by bringing the wound edges as close together as possible to reduce scar formation. Proper wound closure involves control of bleeding and minimal trauma and tension to tissues.

Sutures are threads or metal used to sew body tissues together. The client's history of wound healing, the site of surgery, the tissues involved, and the purpose of the sutures determine the choice of suture material. For example, if the client has had repeated surgery for an abdominal hernia, wire sutures may be used to provide greater strength for wound closure. In contrast, a small laceration of the face calls for the use of very fine polyester sutures to minimize scar formation.

Sutures are available in a variety of materials, including silk, steel, cotton, linen, wire, nylon, and polyester. Sutures come with or without sharp surgical needles attached. Steel staples are a common type of outer skin closure that cause less trauma to tissues than do sutures, while providing extra strength. Tape closures such as Steri-Strips applied over the wound to keep the edges closed are also common.

Sutures are placed within tissue layers in deep wounds as well as superficially, as the final means for wound closure. Deep sutures are

➤ SKILL 47-4 Performing Wound Irrigation

Delegation Considerations

The skill of wound irrigation should not be delegated to unregulated care providers (UCPs). In the case of a chronic wound, you can delegate cleansing of the wound with clean technique to a UCP. Assessment of any wound, care of acute new wounds, and evaluation of wound irrigation is the responsibility of the nurse, however, and is never delegated. When a wound is stable or requires clean irrigation, instruct the UCP to do the following:

- Report any change in wound appearance or increased wound drainage to the nurse.
- Use proper clean technique to avoid cross-contamination from irrigation syringes and equipment.

Equipment

- Irrigant or cleansing solution (volume 1.2–2 times the estimated wound volume)
- Irrigation delivery system, depending on amount of pressure desired:
  - Sterile 35-mL irrigation syringe with sterile soft angiocatheter or 19-gauge needle (AHCPR, 1994) or
  - Whirlpool or hand-held shower
- Disposable gloves and sterile gloves (check agency policy)
- Waterproof underpad, if needed
- Dressing supplies
- Disposable waterproof bag
- Gown, if risk of spray
- Goggles, if risk of spray

Procedure

STEPS	RATIONALE
1. Assess client's level of pain. Administer prescribed analgesic 30–45 minutes before starting wound irrigation procedure.	• Discomfort may be related directly to the wound or indirectly to muscle tension or immobility. Increased comfort permits client to move more easily and be positioned to facilitate wound irrigation.
2. Review medical record for physician's prescription for irrigation of open wound and type of solution to be used.	• Open wound irrigation requires medical order, including type of solution to use.
3. Assess recent recording of signs and symptoms related to client's open wound.	• Data are used as baseline to indicate change in condition of wound (Sibbald, et al, 2006a).
A. Condition of skin and wound	
B. Elevation of body temperature	• Elevated temperature may indicate response to infection.
C. Drainage from wound (amount, colour)	• Amount will decrease as healing takes place.
D. Odour	• Strong odour indicates infectious process.
E. Consistency of drainage	• Leukocytes produce thick drainage.
F. Size of wound, including depth, length, and width	• Size of the wound determines stage of healing.
4. Explain procedure of wound irrigation and cleansing.	• Information will reduce client's anxiety.
5. Perform hand hygiene.	• Transmission of microorganisms is reduced.
6. Position client comfortably to permit gravitational flow of irrigating solution through wound and into collection receptacle. Position client so that wound is vertical to collection basin.	• Directing solution from top to bottom of wound and from clean to contaminated area prevents further infection. Positioning client during planning stage provides bed surfaces for later preparation of equipment.
7. Warm irrigation solution to approximate body temperature.	• Warmed solution increases comfort and reduces vascular constriction response in tissues.
8. Form cuff on waterproof bag and place it near bed.	• Cuffing helps to maintain large opening, thereby permitting placement of contaminated dressing without touching refuse bag itself.
9. Close room door or bed curtains.	• Privacy is maintained.
10. Apply gown and goggles, if needed.	• Gown and goggles protect nurse from splashes or sprays of blood and body fluids.
11. Put on disposable gloves, remove soiled dressing, and discard in waterproof bag. Discard gloves.	• Transmission of microorganisms is reduced.
12. Prepare equipment; open sterile supplies.	
13. Put on sterile gloves (check agency policy).	
14. Irrigate wound with wide opening:	
A. Fill 35-mL syringe with irrigation solution.	• Flushing wound helps remove debris and facilitates healing by secondary intention.
B. Attach 19-gauge needle or angiocatheter.	• Angiocatheter provides ideal pressure for cleansing and removal of debris.
C. Hold syringe tip 2.5 cm above upper end of wound and over area being cleansed.	• Holding the tip above the wound prevents syringe contamination. Careful placement of the syringe prevents unsafe pressure of the flowing solution.
D. Using continuous pressure, flush wound; repeat steps 14A, 14B, and 14C until solution draining into basin is clear.	• Clear solution indicates that all debris has been removed.

➤ SKILL 47-4 Performing Wound Irrigation ***continued***

15. Irrigate deep wound with very small opening:
    A. Attach soft angiocatheter to filled irrigating syringe.
       - Catheter permits direct flow of irrigant into wound. Expect wound to take longer to empty when opening is small.
    B. Lubricate tip of catheter with irrigating solution; then gently insert tip of catheter and pull out about 1 cm.
       - Tip is not in fragile inner wall of wound.
    C. Using slow, continuous pressure, flush wound.

Critical Decision Point: Caution: Splashing may occur during this step.

    D. Pinch off catheter just below syringe while keeping catheter in place.
       - Sterile solution will not be contaminated.
    E. Remove and refill syringe. Reconnect to catheter and repeat until solution draining into basin is clear.
16. Cleanse wound with hand-held shower:
    - Method is useful for clients able to shower with assistance or independently. Shower may be accomplished at home. A shower table is helpful for bed-bound or acutely ill clients.
    A. With client seated comfortably in shower chair, adjust spray to gentle flow; water temperature should be warm.
    B. Cover showerhead with clean washcloth, if needed.
    C. Shower for 5–10 minutes with showerhead 30 cm from wound.

Critical Decision Point: Consider culturing a wound if it has a foul and purulent odour, if inflammation surrounds the wound, if a nondraining wound begins to drain, or if the client is febrile.

17. Obtain cultures, if needed, after cleansing with nonbacteriostatic saline.
    - Routine culturing of open wounds is not recommended in the AHCPR guidelines (1994). They recommend using quantitative bacterial cultures (tissue biopsy or wound fluid by needle aspiration) rather than swab cultures, which often detect only surface bacterial contaminants.
18. Dry wound edges with gauze; dry client, if shower or whirlpool is used.
    - Maceration of surrounding tissue is prevented if excess moisture is dried.
19. Apply appropriate dressing (see Skill 45–2 and Skill 45–4).
    - Protective barrier and healing environment for wound is maintained.
20. Remove gloves and, if worn, mask, goggles, and gown.
    - Transfer of microorganisms is prevented.
21. Dispose of equipment and soiled supplies. Perform hand hygiene.
    - Transmission of microorganisms is reduced.
22. Assist client to comfortable position.
23. Assess type of tissue in the wound bed.
    - Wound healing progress is identified and type of wound cleansing needed is determined.
24. Inspect dressing periodically.
    - Client's response to wound irrigation and need to modify plan of care are determined.
25. Evaluate skin integrity.
    - Whether extension of wound has occurred is determined.
26. Observe client for signs of discomfort.
    - Client's pain should not increase as a result of wound irrigation.
27. Observe for presence of retained irrigant.
    - Retained irrigant is a medium for bacterial growth, and subsequent infection may occur.

Unexpected Outcomes and Related Interventions

Wound Does Not Appear to Heal

- Obtain wound culture.
- Notify physician, who may change frequency of dressing, irrigation, or both.

Wound Drainage Increases

- Apply more absorbent gauze.
- Increase the frequency of irrigation.

Recording and Reporting

- Record wound irrigation and client response on progress notes.
- Immediately report to attending physician any evidence of fresh bleeding, sharp increase in pain, retention of irrigant, or signs of shock.
- At change of shift, report expected and unexpected outcomes that have occurred.

Home Care Considerations

- Teach client and caregiver how to make normal saline, especially if cost is an issue. Normal saline can be made by using 10 mL of salt in 1 L of boiling water (Barr, 1995).
- Tell client and caregiver that because normal saline has no preservatives, it should be discarded 24 to 48 hours after it is first opened or made (Barr, 1995).

usually an absorbable material that will disappear over time; however, sutures are foreign bodies and, thus, are capable of causing local inflammation. The surgeon tries to minimize tissue injury by using the finest suture possible and the smallest number necessary.

Suture Removal. Policies vary within institutions as to who is able to remove sutures. If it is appropriate for the nurse remove them, an order is required. Special scissors with curved cutting tips or special staple removers slide under the skin closures for suture removal (Figure 47–26). If the suture line appears to be healing better in certain locations than in others, the surgeon may choose to have only some sutures removed (e.g., every other one).

To remove staples, simply insert the tips of the staple remover under each wire staple. While slowly closing the ends of the staple remover together, you squeeze the centre of the staple with the tips, freeing the staple from the skin (see Figure 47–26).

To remove sutures, first check the type of suturing used (Figure 47–27). With intermittent suturing, the surgeon ties each individual suture made in the skin. Continuous suturing, as the name implies, is a series of sutures with only two knots, one at the beginning and one at the end of the suture line. Retention sutures are placed more deeply than skin sutures, and nurses may or may not remove them, depending on agency policy.

The manner in which the suture crosses and penetrates the skin determines the method for removal. Never pull the visible portion of a suture through underlying tissue. Sutures on the skin's surface harbour microorganisms and debris, but the portion of the suture beneath the skin is sterile. Pulling the contaminated portion of the suture through tissues may lead to infection. Clip suture materials as close to the skin edge on one side as possible and pull the suture through from the other side (Figure 47–28).

Drainage Evacuation. When drainage interferes with healing, you achieve drainage evacuation by using either a drain alone or a drainage tube with continuous suction. Apply special skin barriers, including hydrocolloid dressings, similar to those used with ostomies (see Chapter 45), around drain sites. The skin barriers are soft material applied to the skin with adhesive. Drainage flows on the barrier but not directly on the skin.

Drainage evacuators (Figure 47–29) are convenient, portable units that connect to tubular drains lying within a wound bed and exert a safe, constant, low-pressure vacuum to remove and collect drainage. Ensure that suction is exerted and that connection points between the evacuator and tubing are intact. After the evacuator collects drainage, assess for volume and character every shift and as needed. When the evacuator fills, measure output by emptying the contents into a graduated cylinder and immediately reset the evacuator to apply suction.

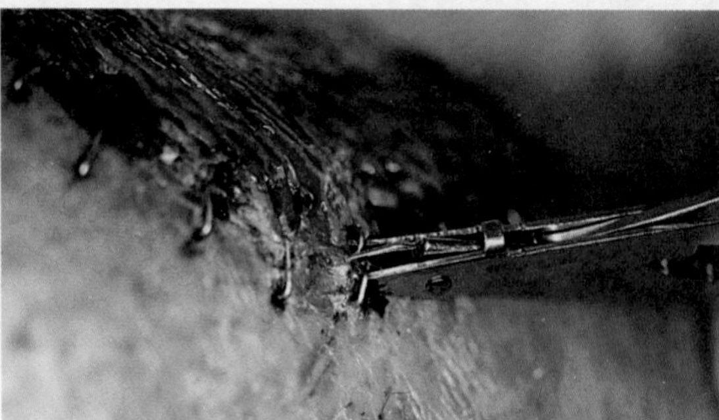

Figure 47-26 Staple remover.

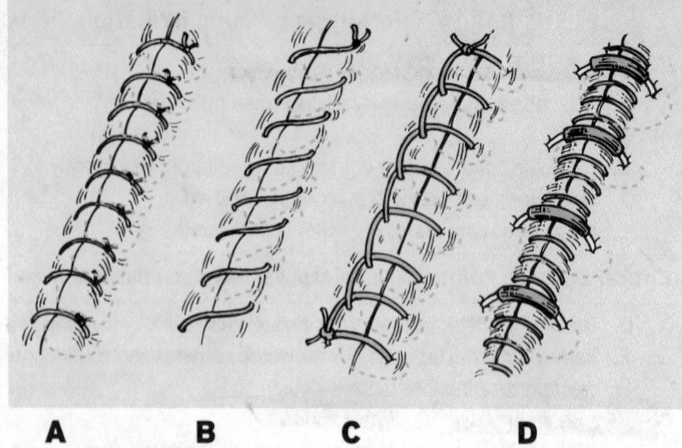

Figure 47-27 Examples of suturing methods. A, Intermittent. B, Continuous. C, Blanket continuous. D, Retention.

Bandages and Binders. A simple gauze dressing is often not enough to immobilize or provide support to a wound. Binders and bandages applied over or around dressings provide extra protection and therapeutic benefits by:

1. Creating pressure over a body part (e.g., an elastic pressure bandage applied over an arterial puncture site)
2. Immobilizing a body part (e.g., an elastic bandage applied around a sprained ankle)
3. Supporting a wound (e.g., an abdominal binder applied over a large abdominal incision and dressing)
4. Reducing or preventing edema (e.g., a well-supporting bra to minimize breast discomfort after delivery of a baby)
5. Securing a splint (e.g., a bandage applied around hand splints for correction of deformities)
6. Securing dressings (e.g., elastic webbing applied around leg dressings after a vein stripping)

Bandages are available in rolls of various widths and materials, including gauze, elasticized knit, elastic webbing, flannel, and muslin. Gauze bandages are lightweight and inexpensive, conform easily around contours of the body, and permit air circulation to prevent skin maceration. Elastic bandages conform well to body parts but also exert pressure.

Principles for Applying Bandages and Binders. Correctly applied bandages and binders do not cause injury to underlying and nearby body parts or create discomfort for the client. For example, a chest binder should not be so tight as to restrict chest wall expansion. Before applying a bandage or binder, the following are your responsibilities:

- Inspecting the skin for abrasions, edema, discoloration, or exposed wound edges
- Covering exposed wounds or open abrasions with a sterile dressing
- Assessing the condition of underlying dressings and changing them, if soiled
- Assessing the skin of underlying areas that will be distal to the bandage for signs of circulatory impairment (coolness, pallor or cyanosis, diminished or absent pulses, swelling, numbness, and tingling) to provide a means for comparing changes in circulation after bandage application.

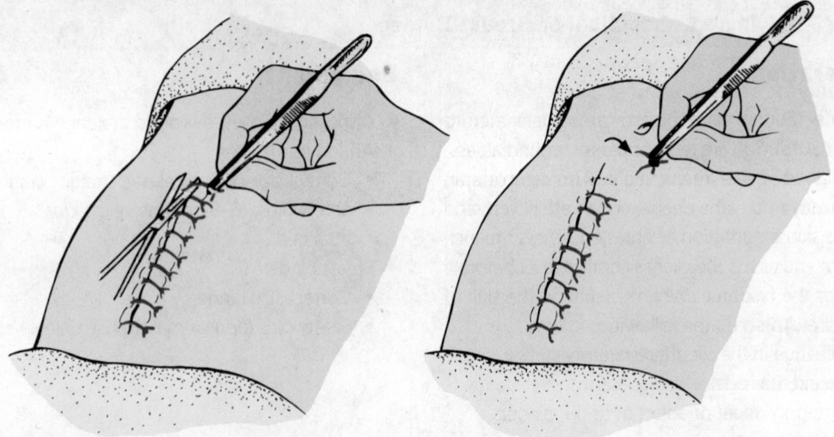

Figure 47-28 Removal of intermittent suture. A, Cut the suture as close to the skin as possible, away from the knot. B, Remove the suture and never pull the contaminated stitch through the tissues.

After applying a bandage, you need to assesses, document, and immediately report changes in circulation, skin integrity, comfort level, and body function (e.g., ventilation or movement). When you apply the bandage, readjust it, as necessary. Make sure you explain to the client that the binder may feel relatively firm or tight. Carefully assess a bandage to be sure that it is properly applied (according to the written order) and is providing therapeutic benefit. Replace any soiled bandages.

Binder Application. Binders are especially designed for the body part to be supported. Most binders are made of elastic or cotton. The most common types of binders are the abdominal binder and breast binder (Skill 47–5). Well-fitting bras are now replacing breast binders. Both provide support after breast surgery or exert pressure to reduce lactation in a woman after childbirth.

Abdominal Binders. An abdominal binder supports large abdominal incisions that are vulnerable to tension or stress as the client moves or coughs. Secure an abdominal binder with safety pins, Velcro strips, or metal stays.

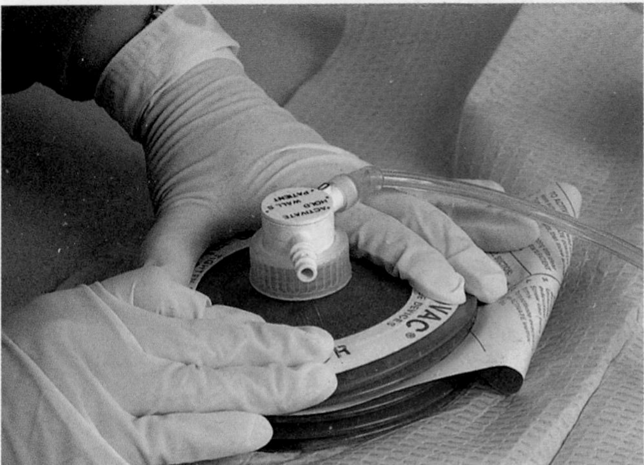

Figure 47-29 Setting the suction on a drainage evacuator. 1. With the drainage port open, the lever on the diaphragm is raised. 2. Push straight down on the lever to lower the diaphragm. 3. Closure of the port prevents escape of air and creates vacuum pressure.

Bandage Application. Rolls of bandage secure or support dressings over irregularly shaped body parts. Each roll has a free outer end and a terminal end at the centre of the roll. The rolled portion of the bandage is its body, and its outer surface is placed against the client's skin or dressing. Skill 47–6 describes the steps for applying an elastic bandage.

The Whole Person, the Whole Team

Skin management and wound care require the involvement of the health care team because the factors that create skin breakdown, from pressure to nutrition, are assessed and treated by experts within the health care team: physiotherapist, occupational therapist, dietitian, nurse, physician, social worker, and pharmacist. In addition, the wound belongs to the client and you need to recognize the impact of the individual on both the development and healing potential of a wound.

Case Study. Mr. John Purata is an 84-year-old gentleman who has returned to his home in a long-term care facility where you are looking after the ulcer on his sacrum, developed during his stay in Acute Care after hip replacement surgery. Mr Purata has been too tired to get up for meals, and you have noticed that his nutritional status is declining. Although he is on a pressure-relief surface, Mr. Purata tends to lie on his back. You have mentioned to him the importance of repositioning to assist in healing the wound, but he merely closes his eyes and tells you he is "fine" the way he is. When you and the other staff in the long-term care facility try to get him up to walk, Mr. Purata is hesitant and requires a great deal of coaching and encouragement to walk even a few steps. He then says he is too tired to go further and asks to go back to bed. He is frequently lying in bed, with eyes closed and the lights dim. His daughter and son are concerned that he seems to have lost his "get up and go" attitude. The wound is not improving, and you are concerned.

- What are the key issues that need to be addressed?
- What members of the health care team need to be involved?
- What would be realistic goals for Mr. Purata?
- How would you develop a plan of care for this client?

➤ SKILL 47-5 Applying an Abdominal or Breast Binder

Delegation Considerations

The skills of applying a binder (abdominal or breast) can be delegated to unregulated care providers (UCPs). You are responsible for wound assessment and the evaluation of wound care interventions. Also complete an assessment of the client's ability to breathe deeply, cough effectively, and move independently; assess skin for irritation or abrasion; assess the incision or wound and dressing; and assess the client's comfort level before a binder or sling is applied for the first time. When delegating the skill of applying a binder, instruct the UCP to do the following:

- Immediately report any change in the client's respiratory status.
- Report an increase in wound drainage.
- Report changes in skin integrity under or adjacent to the binder.
- Remove the binder at prescribed intervals.

Equipment

- Disposable gloves, if wound drainage is present
- Abdominal binder:
  - Correct size cloth or elastic straight binder
  - Safety pins, (6–8), unless Velcro closure or metal fasteners are attached
- Breast binder:
  - Correct size binder
  - Safety pins (approximately 12), unless Velcro closure is attached

Procedure

STEPS	RATIONALE
1. Observe client with need for support of thorax or abdomen. Observe ability to breathe deeply and cough effectively.	• Baseline assessment determines client's ability to breathe and cough. Impaired ventilation of lungs can lead to alveolar atelectasis and inadequate arterial oxygenation.
2. Review medical record, if medical prescription for particular binder is required, and reasons for application.	• Application of supportive binders may be used on nursing judgement. In some situations, physician input is required.
3. Inspect skin for actual or potential alterations in integrity. Observe for irritation, abrasion, skin surfaces that rub against each other, or allergic response to adhesive tape used to secure dressing.	• Actual impairments in skin integrity can be worsened with application of a binder. Binder can cause pressure and excoriation.
4. Inspect any surgical dressing.	• Dressing replacement or reinforcement precedes application of any binder.

Critical Decision Point: Dressing should be clean and dry, and incision or wound should be entirely covered by dressing.

STEPS	RATIONALE
5. Assess client's comfort level, using analogue scale of 0–10 (see Chapter 42), noting any objective signs and symptoms of pain.	• Data will determine effectiveness of binder placement.

Critical Decision Point: Expect client in moderate-to-severe pain to have diaphoresis, tachycardia, and elevated blood pressure.

STEPS	RATIONALE
6. Gather necessary data regarding size of client and appropriate binder.	• Proper fit of binder will be ensured.
7. Explain procedure to client.	• Client will understand and be more cooperative.
8. Teach skill to client or significant other.	• Anxiety is reduced and continuity of care after discharge is ensured.
9. Perform hand hygiene and apply gloves (if likely to contact wound drainage).	• Transmission of microorganisms is reduced.
10. Close curtains or room door.	• Client's comfort and dignity are maintained.
11. Apply binder.	
A. Abdominal binder:	
(1) Position client in supine position with head slightly elevated and knees slightly flexed.	• Muscular tension on abdominal organs is minimized.
(2) Fanfold far side of binder toward midline of binder.	• Client's time in uncomfortable position is reduced.
(3) Instruct and help client to roll away from you toward raised side rail while firmly supporting abdominal incision and dressing with hands.	• Pain and discomfort is reduced.
(4) Place fanfolded ends of binder under client.	• Placement and centring of binder is accomplished with minimal discomfort.
(5) Instruct or assist client to roll over folded ends.	
(6) Unfold and stretch ends out smoothly on far side of bed.	• Skin integrity and comfort is maintained.
(7) Instruct client to roll back into supine position.	• Chest expansion and adequate wound support is facilitated when binder is closed.
(8) Adjust binder so that supine client is centred over binder using symphysis pubis and costal margins as lower and upper landmarks.	• Support from binder is centred over abdominal structures, which reduces incidence of decreased lung expansion.

Critical Decision Point: Cover any exposed areas of an incision or wound with sterile dressing.

➤SKILL 47-5 Applying an Abdominal or Breast Binder ***continued***

Steps	Rationale
(9) Close binder. Pull one end of binder over centre of client's abdomen. While maintaining tension on that end of binder, pull opposite end of binder over centre and secure with Velcro closure tabs, metal fasteners, or horizontally placed safety pins.	• Continuous wound support and comfort is provided.
B. Breast binder:	
(1) Assist client in placing arms through binder's armholes.	• Binder placement process is made easier for client.
(2) Assist client to supine position in bed.	• Supine positioning facilitates normal anatomical position of breasts; facilitates healing and comfort.
(3) Pad area under breasts, if necessary.	• Skin contact with undersurface is prevented.
(4) Using Velcro closure tabs or horizontally placed safety pins, secure binder at nipple level first. Continue closure process above and then below nipple line until entire binder is closed.	• Horizontal placement of pins may reduce risk of uneven pressure or localized irritation.
(5) Make appropriate adjustments, including individualizing fit of shoulder straps and pinning waistline darts to reduce binder size.	• Support to client's breasts is maintained.
(6) Instruct and observe skill development in self-care related to reapplying breast binder.	• Self-care is an integral aspect of discharge planning. Skin integrity and comfort level goals are ensured.
12. Remove gloves and perform hand hygiene.	• Cross-infections are prevented.
13. Assess client's comfort level, using analogue scale of 0–10, noting any objective signs and symptoms.	• Effectiveness of binder placement is determined. Binders should not increase discomfort.
14. Adjust binder, as necessary.	• Comfort and chest expansion is promoted.
15. Observe site for skin integrity, circulation, and characteristics of the wound. (Periodically remove binder and surgical dressing to assess wound characteristics.)	• Binder should not result in complication to skin, wound, or underlying organs.
16. Assess client's ability to ventilate properly.	• Any impaired ventilation and potential pulmonary complications are identified.
17. Identify client's need for assistance with activities such as hair combing.	• Mobility of upper extremities may be limited, depending on severity and location of incision.

Unexpected Outcomes and Related Interventions

Client's Pain Increases

- Remove binder and assess wound.
- Reapply binder using less pressure.

Client's Respiratory Rate Decreases

- Remove binder.
- Encourage client to cough and deep breathe.
- Reapply binder using less pressure.

Client Develops Impaired Skin Integrity Under the Binder

- Remove binder.
- Initiate skin care measure to heal affected site.

Recording and Reporting

- Report any skin irritation at between-shift report.
- Record application of binder, condition of skin, circulation, integrity of dressing, and client's comfort level.
- Report ineffective lung expansion to physician immediately.

Home Care Considerations

- Abdominal and breast binders can be washed and hung to dry.
- Instruct caregiver to avoid excessive pressure with binder application.

➤ SKILL 47-6 Applying an Elastic Bandage

Delegation Considerations

The application of an elastic bandage can be delegated to UCPs. You are responsible for wound assessment and the evaluation of the wound. In addition, you should assess for adequate circulation to the extremity distal to the elastic bandage (e.g., pulse, skin temperature, capillary refill). When delegating this skill to a UCP, instruct about any restrictions that the client might have (e.g., unable to independently raise leg or independently roll over). Also instruct the UCP to report the following:

- Any change in the skin colour of the client's injured extremity
- Any increases in the client's pain

Equipment

- Correct width and number of bandages
- Safety pins, clips, or adhesive tape
- Disposable gloves, if wound drainage is present

Procedure

STEPS	RATIONALE
1. Perform hand hygiene and apply gloves, if needed. Inspect skin for alterations in integrity as indicated by abrasions, discoloration, chafing, or edema. (Look carefully at bony prominences.)	• Altered skin integrity contraindicates the use of elastic bandages.
2. Inspect surgical dressing. Remove gloves and perform hand hygiene.	• Surgical dressing replacement or reinforcement precedes application of any bandage.
3. Observe adequacy of circulation (distal to bandage) by noting surface temperature, skin colour, and sensation of body parts to be wrapped.	• Comparison of area before and after application of bandage is necessary to ensure continued adequate circulation. Impairment of circulation may result in coolness to touch when compared with opposite side of body, cyanosis or pallor of skin, diminished or absent pulses, edema or localized pooling, and numbness or tingling of part.
4. Review medical record for specific orders related to application of elastic bandage. Note area to be covered, type of bandage required, frequency of change, and previous response to treatment.	• Specific prescription may direct procedure, including factors such as extent of application (e.g., toe to knee, toe to groin) and duration of treatment.
5. Identify client's and primary caregiver's present knowledge level of skill, if bandaging will be continued at home.	• Planning and teaching should be individualized.
6. Explain procedure to client.	• Increased knowledge promotes cooperation and reduces anxiety.
7. Teach skill to client or primary caregiver.	• Anxiety is reduced and continuity of care after discharge is ensured.
8. Perform hand hygiene and apply gloves if drainage is present.	• Transmission of microorganisms is reduced.
9. Close room door or curtains.	• Client's comfort and dignity are maintained.
10. Help client to assume comfortable, anatomically correct position.	• Alignment is maintained, and musculoskeletal deformity is prevented.

Critical Decision Point: Bandages applied to lower extremities are applied before client sits or stands. Elevation of dependent extremities for 20 minutes before bandage application will enhance venous return.

STEPS	RATIONALE
11. Hold roll of elastic bandage in dominant hand and use other hand to lightly hold beginning of bandage at distal body part. Continue transferring roll to dominant hand as bandage is wrapped.	• Appropriate and consistent bandage tension is maintained.

Critical Decision Point: Toes or fingertips should be visible for follow-up circulatory assessment.

STEPS	RATIONALE
12. Apply bandage from distal point toward proximal boundary using variety of turns to cover various shapes of body parts.	• Bandage is applied in a manner that conforms evenly to body part and promotes venous return.
13. Unroll and very slightly stretch bandage.	• Uniform bandage tension is maintained.
14. Overlap turns by one-half to two-thirds width of bandage roll.	• Uneven bandage tension and circulatory impairment is prevented.
15. Secure first bandage with clip or tape before applying additional rolls.	
16. Apply additional rolls without leaving any uncovered skin surface. Secure last bandage applied.	• Wrinkling and loose ends are prevented.
17. Remove gloves, if worn, and perform hand hygiene.	• Transmission of microorganisms is reduced.
A. Assess distal circulation when bandage application is complete and at least twice during 8-hour period.	• Early detection and management of circulatory impairment ensures healthy neurovascular status.
B. Observe skin colour for pallor or cyanosis.	
C. Palpate skin for warmth.	
D. Palpate pulses and compare bilaterally.	
E. Ask if client is aware of pain, numbness, tingling, or other discomfort.	• Neurovascular changes indicate impaired venous return.
F. Observe mobility of extremity.	• Joint immobility is determined; if bandage is too tight, movement will be restricted.
18. Have client demonstrate bandage application.	• Return demonstration documents learning.

> SKILL 47-6 **Applying an Elastic Bandage** *continued*

Unexpected Outcomes and Related Interventions

Impaired Circulation Distal to Elastic Bandage

- Release bandage.
- Palpate extremity and assess pulse, temperature, and capillary refill.
- Reapply dressing with less pressure.

Break in Skin Under Elastic Bandage

- Remove bandage.
- Reapply bandage with less pressure.

Inability of Client to Change Dressing

- Reinstruct client on bandage application.
- Observe client apply bandage.

Recording and Reporting

- Document condition of the wound, integrity of dressing, application of bandage, circulation, and client's comfort level.
- Report any changes in neurological or circulatory status to the nurse in charge or physician.

Home Care Considerations

- Instruct client or caregiver not to secure bandages too tightly, which interferes with circulation.
- Elastic bandages that are used to reduce swelling are best applied to the feet in the morning, before getting out of bed.
- Always remove an elastic bandage daily and inspect the area.

❖Evaluation

You evaluate nursing interventions for reducing and treating pressure ulcers by determining the client's response to nursing therapies and whether the client achieved each goal (Figure 47–30). To evaluate outcomes and responses to care, you measure the effectiveness of interventions. The optimal outcomes are to prevent injury to the skin and tissues, reduce injury to the skin and underlying tissues, and restore skin integrity.

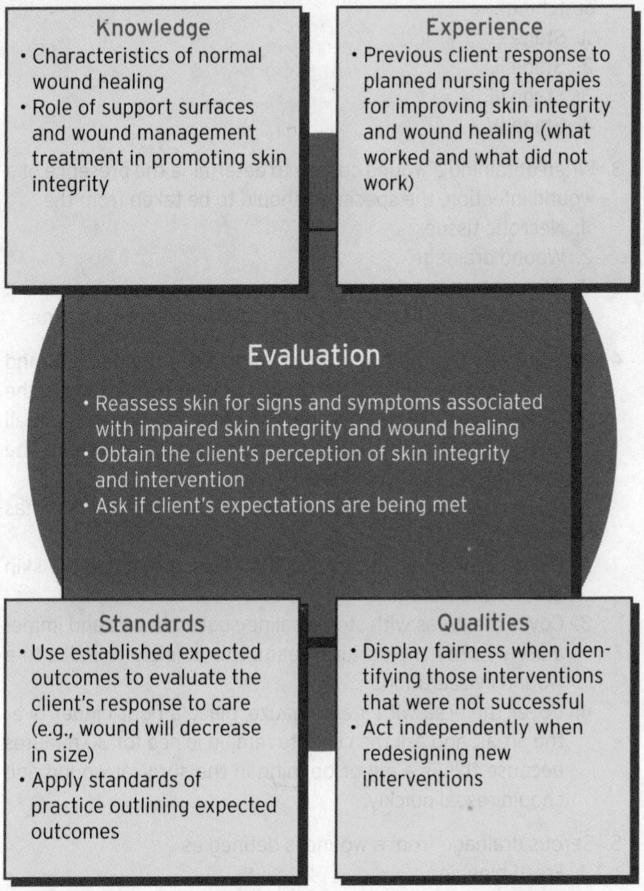

Knowledge
- Characteristics of normal wound healing
- Role of support surfaces and wound management treatment in promoting skin integrity

Experience
- Previous client response to planned nursing therapies for improving skin integrity and wound healing (what worked and what did not work)

Evaluation
- Reassess skin for signs and symptoms associated with impaired skin integrity and wound healing
- Obtain the client's perception of skin integrity and intervention
- Ask if client's expectations are being met

Standards
- Use established expected outcomes to evaluate the client's response to care (e.g., wound will decrease in size)
- Apply standards of practice outlining expected outcomes

Qualities
- Display fairness when identifying those interventions that were not successful
- Act independently when redesigning new interventions

Figure 47-30 Critical thinking model for skin integrity and wound care evaluation.

Because each client has different risk factors for impaired skin integrity, you need to individualize nursing interventions. Clients with minimal mobility impairments or relatively stable health status need only a few measures.

Clients with impaired skin integrity need assessment on an ongoing basis for factors that contribute to skin breakdown. This includes a comprehensive skin assessment and a wound assessment using a validated risk assessment tool. Assessment provides the foundation for the plan of care and is critical for monitoring the effectiveness of the plan (Nix, 2007).

Include the client and the caregiver in the assessment process. Determine what they know about impaired skin integrity, and develop a plan of care to provide education. Chronic wounds such as pressure ulcers take time to heal, and it is likely that the client will be in the home or long-term care setting with the pressure ulcer.

If the identified outcomes are not met for a client with impaired skin integrity, questions to ask include the following:

- Was the etiology of the skin impairment addressed? Were the pressure, friction, shear, and moisture components identified, and did the plan of care decrease the contribution of each of these components?
- Was wound healing supported by providing the wound base with a moist protected environment?
- Were issues such as nutrition assessed and a plan of care developed that provided the client with the calories to support healing?

Finally, evaluate the need for additional referrals to other experts in wound management, such as occupational therapists, dietitians, and wound care specialists. Care of the client with a pressure ulcer requires a multidisciplinary team approach.

✻ KEY CONCEPTS

- Prevention of skin breakdown is a major nursing focus for all clients, irrespective of their age or the health care setting.
- Clients should be assessed for risk of skin breakdown with the use of a validated risk assessment tool, such as the Braden Risk Assessment Tool, on admission to care and subsequently at least once per week.
- Alterations in mobility, sensory perception, level of consciousness, and nutrition, as well as the presence of moisture increase the risk of pressure ulcer development.

- Preventive skin care is aimed at controlling external pressure on bony prominences and keeping the skin clean, well-lubricated, hydrated, and free of excess moisture.
- Proper positioning (the 30-degree rule) reduces the effects of pressure and guards against shearing force.
- Wound assessment requires a description of the appearance of the wound base, size (length · width · depth), presence of exudate, and the periwound skin condition.
- Moist wound-healing approaches are based on evidence and support the healing cycle of wounds.
- Wounds require pressure off-loading, adequate nutrition and hydration, blood flow, and an absence of infection to heal.
- Arterial, venous, and diabetic wounds are often the result of impaired peripheral circulation to the extremities.
- Wound irrigation should be at room or body temperature and provide 4 to 15 psi of pressure to avoid damaging fragile granulating tissue.
- Therapeutic beds and mattresses redistribute the effects of pressure; however, base selection on assessment data to identify the best bed for individual needs.
- Cleansing and topical agents used to treat pressure ulcers vary according to the stage of the pressure ulcer and condition of the wound bed. Assessment of the ulcer will enable you to select proper skin care agents.
- Direct nutritional interventions at improving wound healing through increasing protein and calorie levels, as required.
- When extensive tissue loss occurs, a wound heals by secondary intention.
- The chances of wound infection are greater when the wound contains dead or necrotic tissue, when foreign bodies lie on or near the wound, and when the blood supply and tissue defences are reduced.
- The principles of wound first aid include control of bleeding, cleansing, and protection.
- The layers of a dry dressing absorb drainage and prevent the entrance of bacteria.
- A moist environment supports wound healing.
- When cleansing wounds or drain sites, clean from the least to most contaminated area, away from wound edges.
- Apply a bandage or binder in a manner that does not impair circulation or irritate the skin.

* CRITICAL THINKING EXERCISES

Mrs. Stein, who is 76 years of age, is at postoperative day 7 after a total hip replacement. She developed redness and oozing of foul-smelling tan-coloured drainage from the hip incision on postoperative day 4. Significant medical history includes arthritis and mild hypertension. Because of surgical pain at the incision site, she did not easily transfer from her bed to the chair. Now on day 7, she notes some pain at the incision and complains of a painful, burning sensation in the sacral region. She is continent of urine and stool but continues to "scoot" over to the side of the bed when preparing for bed-to-chair transfers.

1. The staples from the surgical incision were removed and an order was written for a moist saline gauze dressing to be applied to the area three times a day. Would this be the approach that best supports wound healing? Provide a rationale and suggest alternative approaches. When the dressing is removed, what are the critical factors to assess?
2. A head-to-toe skin assessment is done per institutional policy on a daily basis. At the most recent assessment, redness was noted over the sacral area, and on direct examination, a small area of denuded tissue was noted. The involved area has minimal depth and a red, moist base. How would you describe the impairment in skin integrity in your charting?
3. What will you include in your plan of care to address the impairment in skin integrity in the sacral area?
4. Mrs. Stein will be discharged tomorrow. What issues must be assessed regarding her care before discharge? Describe why those issues are of importance.

* REVIEW QUESTIONS

1. When repositioning an immobile client, you notice redness over a bony prominence. When the area is assessed, the red spot blanches with a fingertip touch, indicating
   1. A local skin infection requiring antibiotics.
   2. This client has sensitive skin and requires special bed linen.
   3. A stage III pressure ulcer needing the appropriate dressing.
   4. Reactive hyperemia, a reaction that causes the blood vessels to dilate in the injured area.
2. This type of pressure ulcer is an observable, pressure-related alteration of intact skin, whose indicators, compared with an adjacent or opposite area on the body, may include changes in one or more of the following: skin temperature (warmth or coolness), tissue consistency (firm or beefy feel), and sensation (pain or itching).
   1. Stage I.
   2. Stage II.
   3. Stage III.
   4. Stage IV.
3. When obtaining a wound culture to determine the presence of a wound infection, the specimen should to be taken from the
   1. Necrotic tissue.
   2. Wound drainage.
   3. Drainage on the dressing.
   4. Wound after it has first been cleansed with normal saline.
4. Postoperatively, the client with a closed abdominal wound reports a sudden "pop" after coughing. When you examine the surgical wound site, the sutures are open and pieces of small bowel are noted at the bottom of the now opened wound. The correct intervention would be to
   1. Allow the area to be exposed to air until all drainage has stopped.
   2. Place several cold packs over the areas, protecting the skin around the wound.
   3. Cover the areas with sterile saline-soaked towels and immediately notify the surgical team; this is likely to indicate a wound evisceration.
   4. Cover the area with sterile gauze, place a tight binder over the areas, and ask the client to remain in bed for 30 minutes because this is a minor opening in the surgical wound and should reseal quickly.
5. Serous drainage from a wound is defined as
   1. Fresh bleeding.
   2. Thick and yellow.
   3. Clear, watery plasma.
   4. Beige to brown and foul-smelling.

6. Before changing a dressing, you should
   1. Read the medical orders and follow them exactly.
   2. Gather together all the supplies that might be required for the dressing change and remove the dressing from the wound.
   3. Discuss the plan to change the dressing with the client, assess the need for analgesia, and provide it, if necessary.
   4. Tell the family to leave the room because dressings can be difficult for non-health care professionals to see.

7. Interventions to manage a client who is experiencing fecal and urinary incontinence include
   1. Keeping the buttocks exposed to air at all times.
   2. Use of large absorbent diapers that are changed when saturated.
   3. Utilization of an incontinence cleanser, followed by application of a moisture barrier ointment.
   4. Frequent cleansing, application of an ointment, and coverage of the areas with a thick, absorbent towel.

8. The best description of a hydrocolloid dressing is
   1. A seaweed derivative that is highly absorptive.
   2. Premoistened gauze placed over a granulating wound.
   3. A debriding enzyme that is used to remove necrotic tissue.
   4. A dressing that forms a gel that interacts with the wound surface.

9. A binder placed around a surgical client with a new abdominal wound is indicated for
   1. Collection of wound drainage.
   2. Reduction of abdominal swelling.
   3. Reduction of stress on the abdominal incision.
   4. Stimulation of peristalsis (return of bowel function) by direct pressure.

10. Clients with pressure ulcers require
    1. Repositioning every 4 to 6 hours.
    2. Bedrest and a quiet environment.
    3. Frequent dressing changes.
    4. Nutritional assessment from a dietitian.

✻ RECOMMENDED WEB SITES

Canadian Association for Enterostomal Therapy (CAET): http://www.caet.ca

CAET is an association of health care professionals (ET nurses) promoting education, research, and standards for enterostomal nursing practice. Nurses with the ET designation have obtained additional post-Baccalaureate level certification to offer care to clients with the following conditions: abdominal stomata (openings), fistulae, draining wounds, and selected disorders of the integumentary (skin), gastrointestinal, and genitourinary systems.

Canadian Association of Wound Care (CAWC): http://www.cawc.net

The CAWC is an interprofessional national organization dedicated to prevention, treatment, evaluation, and scholarship regarding wound care across the continuum of care. The CAWC Web site has quick reference guides and Best Practice articles available for downloading on all aspects of wound care practice, as well as information on upcoming seminars, conferences, and scholarship funding opportunities.

European Pressure Ulcer Advisory Panel: http://www.epuap.org

Created in 1996, this group of health care professionals and wound care experts works to lead and support all European countries in the efforts to prevent and treat pressure ulcers. The mission statement is "to provide the relief of persons suffering from or at risk of pressure ulcers, in particular through research and the education of the public." Numerous links to European wound care organizations appear on the Web site.

National Pressure Ulcer Advisory Panel (NPUAP): http://www.npuap.org

The NPUAP provides multidisciplinary leadership for improved client outcomes in pressure ulcer prevention and management through education, public policy, and research.

Registered Nurses' Association of Ontario (RNAO) Best Practice Guidelines: http://www.rnao.org/bestpractices/index.asp

This Web site provides links to the RNAO Best Practice Guidelines, including Risk Assessment and Prevention of Pressure Ulcers and Assessment and Management of Stage I to IV Pressure Ulcers, which can be downloaded as a pdf file or purchased through RNAO.

Wound, Ostomy, and Continence Nurses (WOCN) Society: http://www.wocn.org

The WOCN Society is a professional nursing society that supports the practice and delivery of expert health care to clients with wounds, ostomies, and incontinence.

World Wide Wounds: http://www.worldwidewounds.com

World Wide Wounds is an online, peer-reviewed journal with a focus on current research and evidence-informed practice issues.

Wound Care Management: http://www.lhsc.on.ca/wound

This Web site is a clinical resource, based on evidence-informed best practices for wound care. The site includes numerous links to online resources, and typical wounds and dressing options.

48

Sensory Alterations

Original chapter by Jill Weberski, RN, MSN, PCCN, CNS

Canadian content written by Marion Allen, RN, PhD

objectives

Mastery of content in this chapter will enable you to:

- Define the key terms listed.
- Differentiate among the processes of reception, perception, and reaction to sensory stimuli.
- Discuss the relationship of sensory function to an individual's level of wellness.
- Discuss common causes and effects of sensory alterations.
- Discuss common sensory changes that occur with aging.
- Identify factors important in the assessment of a client's sensory status.
- Identify nursing diagnoses relevant to clients with sensory alterations.
- Develop a plan of care for clients with sensory deficits.
- List interventions for preventing sensory deprivation and controlling sensory overload.
- Describe conditions in the health care agency or client's home that you can adjust to promote meaningful sensory stimulation.
- Discuss ways to maintain a safe environment for clients with sensory deficits.

key terms

Aphasia, p. 1274
Audiologist, p. 1270
Auditory, p. 1267
Conductive hearing loss, p. 1281
Expressive aphasia, p. 1274
Global aphasia, p. 1274
Gustatory, p. 1267
Hyperesthesia, p. 1281
Kinesthetic, p. 1267
Olfactory, p. 1267
Otolaryngologist, p. 1270
Ototoxic, p. 1274
Proprioceptive, p. 1270
Receptive aphasia, p. 1274
Refractive error, p. 1278
Sensory deficit, p. 1267
Sensory deprivation, p. 1269
Sensory overload, p. 1269
Stereognosis, p. 1267
Strabismus, p. 1278
Tactile, p. 1267
Tinnitus, p. 1268
Vertigo, p. 1268
Visual, p. 1267

media resources

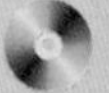

Web Site

- Animations
- Audio Chapter Summaries
- Glossary
- Multiple-Choice Review Questions
- Student Learning Activities
- Video Clips
- Weblinks

Companion CD

- Glossary
- Interactive Learning Activities
- Fluids and Electrolytes Tutorial
- Test-Taking Skills

Imagine the world without vision, sound, or the ability to feel objects, taste foods, or smell aromas. People rely on a variety of sensory stimuli to give meaning and order to events occurring in their environment. The senses help form the perceptual base of our world (Ebersole et al., 2005). Stimulation comes from many sources inside and outside the body, particularly through the senses of sight (**visual**), hearing (**auditory**), touch (**tactile**), smell (**olfactory**), and taste (**gustatory**). The body also has a **kinesthetic** sense that enables a person to be aware of the position and movement of body parts without seeing them. **Stereognosis** is a sense that allows a person to recognize an object's size, shape, and texture. The ability to speak, although not a sense, is similar to a sense in that without it the client may lose the ability to interact meaningfully with others. When sensory function is altered, the person's ability to relate to and function within his or her environment changes drastically. Meaningful stimuli allow a person to learn about the environment and are necessary for healthy functioning and normal development.

Many clients seeking health care have pre-existing sensory alterations (e.g., cataracts). Others may develop sensory alterations as a result of medical treatment (e.g., hearing loss from antibiotic use). The health care environment itself (e.g., a noisy intensive care unit [ICU]) can cause sensory alterations. A health care setting is often a place of unfamiliar sights, sounds, and smells, as well as a place that minimizes contact with family and friends. As a nurse, you must understand and help meet the needs of clients with sensory alterations, as well as recognize clients most at risk for developing sensory problems. You will help clients learn to interact and react safely and effectively in their environment.

Scientific Knowledge Base

Normal Sensation

The nervous system continuously receives thousands of bits of information from sensory nerve receptors, relays the information through appropriate channels, and integrates the information into a meaningful response. Sensory stimuli reach the sensory receptors and can elicit an immediate reaction or present information to the brain to be stored for future use. The nervous system must be intact for sensory stimuli to reach appropriate brain centres and for the individual to perceive the sensation. After interpreting the significance of a sensation, the person can then react to the stimulus (Table 48–1).

Reception, perception, and reaction are the three components of any sensory experience. Reception begins with stimulation of a nerve cell called a receptor, which is usually designed for only one type of stimulus, such as light, touch, or sound. In the case of special senses, the receptors are grouped close together or located in specialized organs (McCance & Huether, 2006), such as the taste buds of the tongue or the retina of the eye. When a nerve impulse is created, it travels along pathways to the spinal cord or directly to the brain. For example, sound waves stimulate hair cell receptors within the organ of Corti, which causes impulses to travel along the eighth cranial nerve to the acoustic area of the temporal lobe. Sensory nerve pathways usually cross over to send stimuli to opposite sides of the brain. The actual perception or awareness of unique sensations depends on the receiving region of the cerebral cortex, where specialized brain cells interpret the quality and nature of sensory stimuli. When the person becomes conscious of the stimuli and receives the information, perception takes place. Perception includes integration and interpretation of the stimuli on the basis of the person's experiences. A person's level of consciousness influences how well stimuli are perceived and interpreted. Any factors lowering consciousness impair sensory perception. If sensation is incomplete, such as blurred vision, or if past experience is inadequate for understanding stimuli such as pain, the person may react inappropriately to the sensory stimulus.

It is impossible to react to all of the multiple stimuli entering the nervous system. The brain prevents sensory bombardment by discarding or storing sensory information. A person will usually react to stimuli that are the most meaningful or significant at the time. After continued reception of the same stimulus, however, a person stops responding, and the sensory experience goes unnoticed. For example, a person concentrating on reading a good book may not be aware of music in the background.

The balance between sensory stimuli entering the brain and those actually reaching a person's conscious awareness maintains a person's well-being. If an individual attempts to react to every stimulus within the environment, or if the variety and quality of stimuli are insufficient, sensory alterations occur.

Sensory Alterations

The most common types of sensory alterations are sensory deficits, sensory deprivation, and sensory overload. When a client has more than one sensory alteration, the ability to function and relate effectively within the environment can be seriously impaired.

Sensory Deficits. A loss in the normal function of sensory reception and perception is a **sensory deficit**. In Canada, one in nine individuals will experience severe vision loss by the age of 65 years; this increases to one in four by age 75 (Canadian National Institute for the Blind [CNIB], 2004). Approximately 1 per 10 Canadians has a hearing loss—the most common sensory impairment in adults over age 65 (Public Health Agency of Canada, Division of Aging and Seniors, 2006).

When senses are impaired, the sense of self is impaired. Initially, a person may withdraw by avoiding communication or socialization with others in an attempt to cope with the sensory loss. It becomes difficult for the person to interact safely with the environment until new skills are learned. When a deficit develops gradually or when considerable time has passed since the onset of an acute sensory loss, the person learns to rely on unaffected senses. Some senses may even become more acute to compensate for an alteration. For example, blind clients may rely more on their sense of hearing for information about the world.

Clients with sensory deficits may change behaviour in effective or ineffective ways. For example, one client with a hearing impairment may turn the unaffected ear toward the speaker to hear better, whereas another client may shun people to avoid the embarrassment of not being able to understand their speech.

Many conditions and diseases cause sensory deficits (Box 48–1). Certain sensory deficits occur more commonly in some ethnic groups. For example, the frequency and severity of glaucoma are higher among Black Canadians (Adatia & Damji, 2005). Certain types of glaucoma are more prevalent among the Inuit and Asian-Canadian populations and less prevalent among people of European and African descent (Perrucio et al., 2007). Otitis media is more prevalent among Inuit, Métis, and First Nations populations, especially in northern Canada (Bowd, 2005). The prevalence of diabetes and diabetic retinopathy also is higher in Aboriginal communities (Hanley et al., 2005).

Sensory Deprivation. The reticular activating system in the brain stem mediates all sensory stimuli to the cerebral cortex. Even in deep sleep, clients are able to receive stimuli. Sensory stimulation must be of sufficient quality and quantity to maintain a person's awareness.

TABLE 48-1 Normal Hearing and Vision

Function	Anatomy and Physiology
The Ear	
Transmits to the brain an accurate pattern of all sounds received from the environment, the relative intensity of these sounds, and the direction from which they originate	Two ears provide stereophonic hearing to judge sound direction. The external ear canal shelters the eardrum (tympanic membrane) and maintains relatively constant temperature and humidity to maintain elasticity. The middle ear is an air-containing space between the eardrum and oval window. It contains three small bones (malleus, incus, and stapes) called ossicles. The eardrum and ossicles transfer sound to the fluid-filled inner ear. Movement of the stapes in the oval window creates vibrations in the fluid that bathes the membranous labyrinth, which contains the end organs of hearing and balance. The union of the vestibular (balance) and cochlear (hearing) portions of the labyrinth explains the combination of hearing and balance symptoms that may occur with inner ear disorders. Vibration of the eardrum is transmitted through the bony ossicles. Vibrations at the oval window are transmitted in perilymph within the inner ear to stimulate hair cells that send impulses along the eighth cranial nerve to the brain.
The Eye	
Transmits to the brain an accurate pattern of light reflected from solid objects in the environment and transformed into colour and hue	Light rays enter the convex cornea and begin to converge. Fine adjustment of light rays occurs as they pass through the pupil and through the lens. Change in the shape of the lens focuses light on the retina. The retina has a pigmented layer of cells to enhance visual acuity. The sensory retina contains the rods and cones—photoreceptor cells sensitive to stimulation from light. Photoreceptor cells send electrical potentials by way of the optic nerve to the brain.

BOX 48-1 Common Diseases and Conditions That Cause Sensory Deficits

Visual Deficits

Presbyopia: A gradual decline in the ability of the lens to accommodate or to focus on close objects. Individual is unable to see near objects clearly.

Cataract: Cloudy or opaque areas in part of or in the entire lens that interfere with passage of light through the lens. Cataracts usually develop gradually, without pain, redness, or tearing in the eye. Eventually leads to blurring, decreased vision, and glare. Although associated with aging, cataracts can also be caused by diabetes, injury, or medications, especially steroids.

Dry eyes: Results when tear glands produce too few tears. Common in older adults and results in itching, burning, or blurred vision.

Glaucoma: A condition of increased fluid pressure inside the eye that can eventually damage the optic nerve. Left untreated, can result in visual field loss, decreased visual acuity, a halo effect seen around objects, and blindness. Can be idiopathic in origin or may be caused by eye injury, inflammation, tumours, diabetes, or medications such as steroids.

Diabetic retinopathy: Long-term or poorly managed diabetes can lead to progressive damage to the blood vessels of the retina, resulting in decreased vision or blindness.

Macular degeneration: Condition in which the macula (specialized portion of the retina responsible for central vision) loses its ability to function efficiently. First signs may include blurring of reading matter, distortion or loss of central vision, and distortion of vertical lines. Is a common cause of blindness in people over age 50 but may also affect younger adults and children.

Hearing Deficits

Presbycusis: A common progressive hearing disorder in older adults.

Cerumen accumulation: Buildup of cerumen (earwax) in the external auditory canal. Cerumen becomes hard, collects in the canal, and causes conduction deafness. More common in older people.

Otosclerosis: The hardening of the ossicles in the middle ear, resulting in gradual and progressive hearing loss that is usually accompanied by **tinnitus** (background noises in the ear, hissing or ringing sounds, or discrete tones or pulses). Otosclerosis is a hereditary condition.

Menière's disease: A disorder of the inner ear characterized by hearing loss, tinnitus, and **vertigo** (sudden loss of balance). It likely is caused by increased fluid in the inner ear. This disorder usually begins in people between the ages of 20 and 50 years.

Otitis media: Infection of the middle ear; common in infants and children. Recurrent or chronic otitis media can cause damage to the eardrum or middle ear, resulting in permanent hearing loss.

Balance Deficit

Benign positional vertigo: Common condition in older adulthood, usually resulting from vestibular dysfunction. Frequently, episodes of vertigo or disequilibrium are precipitated by a change in the position of the head.

Taste Deficit

Xerostomia: Decrease in salivary production that leads to thicker mucus and dry mouth. Result of medications such as antihistamines. Can interfere with the ability to eat and leads to appetite and nutritional problems.

Taste alterations: Alterations, manifested by food aversions and decreased caloric intake, can occur frequently in clients with cancer.

> **BOX 48-1 Common Diseases and Conditions Causing Sensory Deficits** *continued*
>
> **Neurological Deficits**
>
> *Peripheral neuropathy:* Disorder of the peripheral nervous system. Commonly caused by diabetes, carpal tunnel syndrome, and neoplasms (Ebersole et al., 2005). Symptoms include loss of sensation, numbness and tingling of the affected area, and stumbling gait.
>
> *Stroke:* Cerebrovascular accident caused by clot, hemorrhage, or emboli disrupting blood flow to the brain. Creates altered proprioception with marked incoordination and imbalance. Loss of sensation, such as diminished response to superficial sensation, and loss of motor function in extremities controlled by the affected area of the brain also occurs. A stroke affecting the left hemisphere of the brain results in symptoms on the right side, such as difficulty with speech. A stroke in the right hemisphere will create symptoms on the left side, which may include visuospatial alterations, such as loss of half of a visual field. Perceptual issues may also occur, such as distorted body image and inability to recognize familiar objects (agnosia).

The sensory deprivation that clients experience may relate to the need for a comforting touch. Clients in health care settings, especially ICUs, are often exposed to physical touch, but it is often associated with technical intervention rather than with a personal, comforting touch (Henricson, et al., 2006). A decrease in stimuli can occur when clients are placed in isolation. This can reduce the number of people entering their room and contact with the outside world. As well, nurses are required to follow transmission-based precautions, which include the use of masks and gloves. Masks may prevent visualization of caregivers' faces, and gloves will alter the sense of touch.

When a person experiences an inadequate quality or quantity of stimulation, **sensory deprivation** occurs. Three types of sensory deprivation are reduced sensory input (e.g., caused by sensory deficit from visual or hearing loss), elimination of pattern or meaning from input (e.g., exposure to strange environments), and restriction of the environment (e.g., bedrest or reduced environmental variation) that produces monotony and boredom (Ebersole et al., 2005).

Sensory deprivation has many effects (Box 48–2). The symptoms can easily cause nurses and physicians to believe that a client is psychologically ill and confused, is suffering from severe electrolyte imbalance, or is under the influence of psychotropic drugs. Therefore, you must always be aware of the client's existing sensory function and the quality of stimuli within the environment.

Sensory Overload. When a person receives multiple sensory stimuli and cannot perceptually disregard or selectively ignore some stimuli, **sensory overload** occurs. Excessive sensory stimulation prevents the brain from appropriately responding to or ignoring certain stimuli. Because of the multitude of stimuli leading to overload, the person no longer perceives his or her environment in a way that makes sense. Overload prevents meaningful response by the brain; the person's thoughts race, attention moves in many directions, and anxiety and restlessness may occur. As a result, overload causes a state similar to that produced by sensory deprivation. However, in contrast to deprivation, overload is individualized. The amount of stimuli needed for healthy function varies with each individual. A person's tolerance to sensory overload may vary by level of fatigue, attitude, and emotional and physical well-being.

The acutely ill client may easily be affected by sensory overload. The client in constant pain or who undergoes frequent monitoring of vital signs is at risk. Multiple stimuli can combine to cause overload even if you offer a comforting word or provide a gentle back rub. Clients may not benefit from nursing interventions because their attention and energy are focused on more stressful stimuli. Another example is the client who is hospitalized in an ICU, where activity is constant. Lights are always on. Sounds can be heard from monitoring equipment, staff conversations, equipment alarms, and the activities of people entering the unit. Even at night, an ICU can be very noisy.

> **BOX 48-2 Effects of Sensory Deprivation**
>
> **Cognitive Effects**
>
> Reduced capacity to learn
> Inability to think or to problem solve
> Poor task performance
> Disorientation
> Bizarre thinking
> Increased need for socialization, altered mechanisms of attention
>
> **Affective Effects**
>
> Boredom
> Restlessness
> Increased anxiety
> Emotional lability (i.e., rapid mood swings)
> Panic
> Increased need for physical stimulation
>
> **Perceptual Effects**
>
> Alterations in
> - Visual–motor coordination
> - Colour perception
> - Apparent movement
> - Tactile accuracy
> - Ability to perceive size and shape
> - Spatial and time judgement
>
> Adapted from Ebersole, P., Touhy, T., Hess, P., & Jett, K. (2007). *Toward healthy aging: Human needs and nursing response* (7th ed.). St. Louis, MO: Mosby Elsevier.

The behavioural changes associated with sensory overload can easily be confused with mood swings or simple disorientation. You must look for symptoms such as racing thoughts, scattered attention, restlessness, and anxiety. Clients in ICUs sometimes resort to constantly fingering tubes and dressings. Constant reorientation, control of excessive stimuli, and, if possible, providing care in blocks of time become an important part of the client's care.

Nursing Knowledge Base

Factors Affecting Sensory Function

Many factors affect sensory function, including the client's age, the quantity and quality of stimuli, social interaction, and family and environmental factors. As the nurse delivering care, you must be aware of and address as many of these factors as possible.

Age. Infants are unable to discriminate sensory stimuli because nerve pathways are immature. Visual changes during adulthood include presbyopia, which leads to the need for reading glasses. These changes usually occur from ages 40 to 50 years. Changes normally associated with aging include reduced visual fields, increased glare sensitivity, impaired night vision, reduced accommodation and depth perception, and reduced colour discrimination.

Hearing changes include decreased hearing acuity, speech intelligibility, pitch discrimination, and hearing threshold. Older adults hear low-pitched sounds best but have difficulty hearing conversation over background noise. Speech sounds are garbled, and reception of and reaction to speech are delayed. Older adults have difficulty discriminating particular consonants (*z, t, f, g*) and high-frequency sounds (e.g., *s, sh, ph, k*). A problem with age-related hearing loss is that some individuals may not even be aware of their deficit, or what are thought of as age-related changes are, in fact, abnormal changes. A serious concern for those with a hearing deficit is that they may be inappropriately labelled as confused.

Gustatory and olfactory changes include a decrease in the number of taste buds in later years and a reduction in olfactory nerve fibres by the age of 50 years. Reduced taste discrimination and reduced sensitivity to odours are common.

Proprioceptive changes after the age of 60 years include increased difficulty with balance, spatial orientation, and coordination. Older adults experience tactile changes, including declining sensitivity to pain, pressure, and temperature.

Older adults are a high-risk group because of normal physiological changes involving sensory organs. However, you must be careful not to assume automatically that a client's sensory problem is related to advancing age. For example, adult sensorineural hearing loss can be caused by metabolic, vascular, and other systemic alterations or by exposure to excess and prolonged noise. Hearing loss may also be a side effect of medications, such as thiazide diuretics. A client may benefit from a referral to an **audiologist** or **otolaryngologist** if the assessment reveals a serious hearing problem.

Quality of Stimuli. Meaningful stimuli reduce the incidence of sensory deprivation. In a client's home or a long-term care facility, meaningful stimuli may include such things as pets, music, television, family photographs, a calendar, and a clock. In a health care setting, you note whether clients have roommates or visitors. The presence of others can offer positive stimulation. However, a roommate who constantly watches television, persistently tries to talk, or continuously keeps lights on can contribute to sensory overload. The presence or absence of meaningful stimuli influences alertness and the ability to participate in care. Too little stimulation, such as in a barren isolation room, may lead to disorientation.

Quantity of Stimuli. Excessive stimuli in an environment can cause sensory overload. The frequency of observations and procedures performed in an acute care setting may be stressful. If the client is in pain, has many tubes and dressings, or is restricted by casts or traction, overstimulation can be a problem. As well, the sounds of electrical monitors and equipment, bright lighting around the clock, and the odour of body fluids are other examples of stimuli that can contribute to overload. Also, a client's room may be near repetitive or loud noises (e.g., an elevator or a nurses' station).

Conversely, not enough meaningful stimuli can cause sensory deprivation. Living in a confined environment places people at risk for sensory deprivation. The individual who is confined to a wheelchair, has poor hearing or vision, has decreased energy, or avoids contact with others is at significant risk for sensory deprivation. If the environment creates monotony, the individual has a reduced capacity to learn and to think.

Social Interaction. Clients with hearing loss tend to decrease the time spent with social activities and verbal communication. Family members may notice a reluctance to use the telephone and that questions are being answered inappropriately. Children with hearing deficits may be inattentive, uncooperative, or easily bored. Often a client is too embarrassed to continually ask another person to repeat what has been said; instead, the person avoids communication. Clients who find their lifestyles influenced by a hearing loss may experience loneliness and lowered self-esteem.

Family Factors. The amount and quality of contact with supportive family members and significant others can influence the degree of isolation the client feels. The absence of visitors during hospitalization or residency in a long-term care facility can also affect sensory status. This is a common problem in hospital settings, where visitation is restricted. The ability to discuss fears or concerns with loved ones is an important coping mechanism for most people. Therefore, the absence of meaningful conversation can cause a person to become sensorially deprived, and you may not be alerted to this problem until behavioural changes occur.

Environmental Factors. A person's work environment can also increase the risk for sensory alterations. Individuals who are exposed to loud noises at work or who have occupations involving the risk of exposure to chemicals or flying objects should be screened for hearing and visual problems. Clients who use their hands in a repetitive fashion (e.g., computer programmers) are at risk for carpal tunnel syndrome, a condition characterized by swelling or inflammation of the wrists. This inflammation creates pressure on the nerve as it passes through the narrow area in the wrist. The client can experience numbness, tingling, pain, and weakness in the hand while performing fine hand movements.

A hospitalized client can be at risk for sensory alterations from exposure to environmental stimuli or a change in sensory input. Clients who are immobilized because of bedrest, disability, or physical encumbrances (e.g., casts or traction) are at risk because they are unable to move freely and to seek out meaningful interactions. Clients placed in isolation because they have a communicable disease are also at risk (see Chapter 33) because of a lack of interaction with visitors.

As a result of illness or hospitalization, a client is often confined to an unfamiliar environment. This does not mean that all hospitalized clients have sensory alterations. However, you must carefully assess clients who are subjected to continued sensory stimulation. The client's environment, within both the health care setting and the home, is carefully assessed, looking for factors that pose risks or that need adjustment to provide safety and more stimulation.

Critical Thinking

Critical thinking involves synthesizing knowledge and information gathered from clients, experience, and intellectual and professional standards. Required information is anticipated, data are analyzed, and decisions are made regarding client care. During assessment (Figure 48–1), you consider all critical thinking elements that help you make appropriate nursing diagnoses.

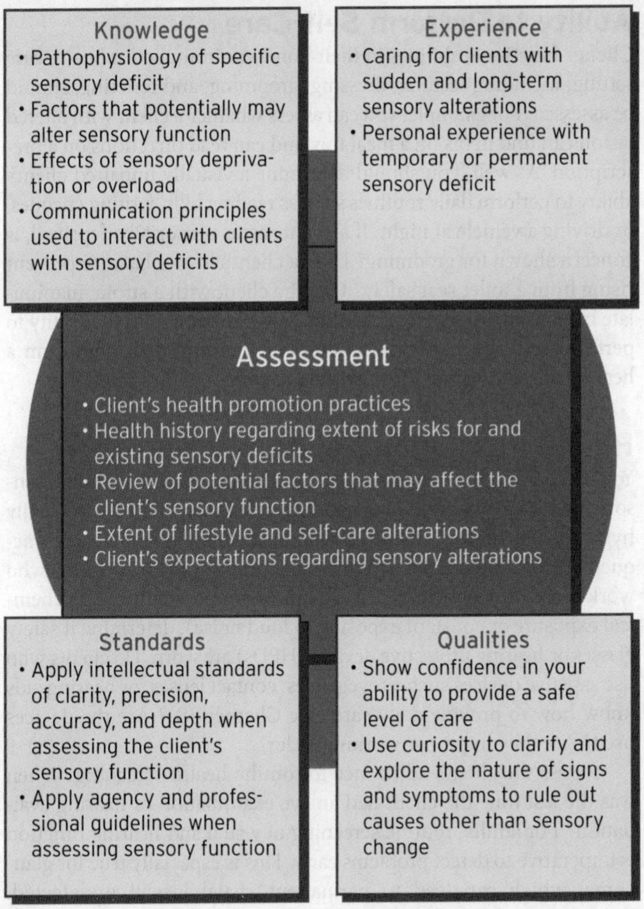

Knowledge
- Pathophysiology of specific sensory deficit
- Factors that potentially may alter sensory function
- Effects of sensory deprivation or overload
- Communication principles used to interact with clients with sensory deficits

Experience
- Caring for clients with sudden and long-term sensory alterations
- Personal experience with temporary or permanent sensory deficit

Assessment
- Client's health promotion practices
- Health history regarding extent of risks for and existing sensory deficits
- Review of potential factors that may affect the client's sensory function
- Extent of lifestyle and self-care alterations
- Client's expectations regarding sensory alterations

Standards
- Apply intellectual standards of clarity, precision, accuracy, and depth when assessing the client's sensory function
- Apply agency and professional guidelines when assessing sensory function

Qualities
- Show confidence in your ability to provide a safe level of care
- Use curiosity to clarify and explore the nature of signs and symptoms to rule out causes other than sensory change

Figure 48-1 Critical thinking model for sensory alterations assessment.

In caring for clients with sensory alterations, you must integrate knowledge from several areas: normal anatomy and physiology of the sensory and nervous systems, the pathophysiology of sensory deficits and factors that affect sensory function, and therapeutic communication principles. This information enables you to conduct appropriate assessments, anticipate what to recognize when a client describes a sensory problem, and recognize abnormalities. For example, knowing the normal symptoms of a cataract helps you recognize the pattern of visual changes a client with a cataract might report.

Previous experience in caring for clients with sensory deficits enables you to recognize limitations in function in each new client and how those limitations might affect the client's ability to carry out daily activities. For example, after caring for a client with a hearing impairment, you will be able to conduct a more effective assessment of the next client.

Critical thinking qualities and standards, when applied during assessment, ensure a thorough and accurate database from which to make decisions. For example, perseverance is needed to learn details as to how visual changes influence a client's ability to socialize. Standards of care and practice, such as those from the Canadian Ophthalmological Society, the Registered Nurses' Association of Ontario, the Canadian Gerontological Nursing Association, and CNIB provide criteria for screening sensory problems and for establishing standards for competent, safe, and effective care and practice. Using critical thinking, you can conduct a thorough assessment and then plan, implement, and evaluate care that will enable the client to function safely and effectively.

Nursing Process

❖Assessment

When assessing clients with or at risk for sensory alterations, you must consider how the client's particular illness may lead or has led to sensory changes. As well, all the factors that may influence sensory function must be considered. For example, if the client has a hearing impairment, communication style is adjusted and assessment is focused on relevant criteria related to hearing deficits. You collect a history that also assesses the client's current sensory status and the degree to which a sensory deficit affects the client's lifestyle, psychosocial adjustment, developmental status, self-care ability, and safety. The assessment must also focus on the quality and quantity of environmental stimuli.

Sensory Alterations History

The nursing health history includes assessment of the nature and characteristics of sensory alterations or any problem related to an alteration. When taking the sensory alterations history, you should consider the ethnic background of the client because certain alterations are higher in some ethnic groups (see "Sensory Deficits" section, earlier in the chapter). Begin by asking the client to describe the sensory deficit, as in the following examples:

- Describe your hearing loss.
- Describe how your vision is affected.
- Explain how use of your hands has changed.

Knowledge about the onset and duration of the sensory alteration can be helpful. You can learn how long the client has taken measures to adjust to the alteration by asking questions such as the following:

- How long have you had a visual problem?
- When did you begin to feel numbness in your hands? In your legs?
- How long have you noticed being unable to hear conversations clearly?

It is also useful to assess the client's self-rating for a sensory deficit. You can simply say, "Rate your hearing as excellent, good, fair, poor, or bad." Then, from the client's self-rating, explore more fully the client's perception of a sensory loss. This provides a more in-depth look at how the client's quality of life has been influenced. In the specific case of hearing problems, a screening tool developed by Ventry and Weinstein (1982) has been found to be effective in identifying clients needing audiological intervention. The screening version of the Hearing Handicap Inventory for the Elderly (HHIE-S) is a 5-minute, 10-item questionnaire designed to assess how a client perceives the emotional and social effects of hearing loss. The greater the handicapping effect from the hearing loss, the higher the score is (Stark & Hickson, 2004).

A health history can also reveal any recent changes in a client's behaviour. Often friends or family are the best resources for this information because the client may be unaware of any change. Asking the following questions may be helpful:

- Have you noticed any change in hearing (e.g., television being turned louder)?
- Has your family member or friend shown any recent mood swings (e.g., outbursts of anger, nervousness, fear, or irritability)?
- Have you noticed him or her avoiding social activities?

It is important to remember that many adults are sensitive about admitting losses and may hesitate to share information.

Mental Status

Mental status assessment is an important component of any evaluation of sensory function (Box 48–3). This is particularly important as visual impairment is a risk factor for cognitive decline (Whitson et al., 2007). Observing the client during history-taking, physical examination, and nursing care provides valuable data for evaluation of a client's mental status. An assessment of mental status is valuable particularly if you suspect sensory deprivation or overload. Observe the client's physical appearance and behaviour, measure the client's cognitive ability, and assess the client's emotional status. The Mini-Mental State Examination is an example of a tool that can be used to measure disorientation, altered conceptualization and abstract thinking, and change in problem-solving abilities (see Chapter 32). For example, a client with severe sensory deprivation may not be able to carry on a conversation, remain attentive, or display recent or past memory.

Physical Assessment

To identify sensory deficits and their severity, assess vision, hearing, olfaction, taste, and the ability to discriminate light touch, temperature, pain, and position. Chapter 32 describes assessment techniques in detail. Table 48–2 summarizes assessment techniques for identifying sensory deficits. The data will be more accurate if the examination room is private, quiet, and comfortable for the client.

You will also rely on personal observation of the client to detect sensory alterations. Some useful observations indicating hearing loss include the following: The client seems inattentive to others, responds with inappropriate anger when spoken to, believes people are talking about him or her, has trouble following clear directions, asks to have something repeated, has monotonous voice quality and speaks unusually loudly or softly, has the television unusually loud, and answers questions inappropriately (Ebersole et al., 2005).

The typical physical tests used to screen for hearing impairment rely on an examiner's whispered voice or a tuning fork. The Welch Allyn AudioScope is very effective for measuring hearing acuity. The hand-held instrument includes an ear speculum that is placed within the external ear canal. The examiner can view the tympanic membrane to ensure that cerumen is not blocking the canal. A tonal sequence is initiated by pressing a button on the audioscope. The instrument is highly sensitive to detecting hearing loss.

➤ BOX 48-3 Assessment of Mental Status

Physical Appearance and Behaviour

Assess motor activity, posture, facial expression, hygiene

Cognitive Ability

Assess level of consciousness, abstract reasoning, calculation, attention, judgement

Assess ability to carry on conversation; ability to read, write, and copy figures

Assess recent and remote memory

Emotional Stability

Assess agitation, euphoria, irritability, hopelessness, or wide mood swings

Assess auditory, visual, or tactile hallucinations; illusions; delusions

Ability to Perform Self-Care

Clients' functional abilities in their home environment or health care setting, including feeding, dressing, grooming, and toileting, should be assessed. For example, you can assess whether a client with altered vision can find items on a meal tray and can read directions on a prescription. As well, you should determine a visually impaired client's ability to perform daily routines such as reading bills, writing cheques, or driving a vehicle at night. If a client seems sensorially deprived, is concern shown for grooming? Does a client's loss of balance prevent rising from a toilet seat safely? Can the client with a stroke manipulate buttons or zippers for dressing? Any impairment in the ability to perform self-care has implications for planning discharge from a health care setting and for providing resources within the home.

Health Promotion Habits

You must assess the daily routines that clients follow to maintain sensory function. What type of eye and ear care is incorporated into daily hygiene? For those individuals who participate in sports (e.g., racquetball) or recreational activities (e.g., motorcycle riding) or who work in a setting where ear or eye injury is a possibility (e.g., chemical exposure or constant exposure to loud noise), determine if safety glasses or hearing protective devices (HPDs) are worn. Do clients who use assistive devices such as eyeglasses, contact lenses, or hearing aids know how to provide daily care (see Chapter 38)? Are the devices used? Are they in proper working order?

Assess the client's adherence to routine health screening. When was the last time the client had an eye examination or hearing evaluation? For adults, routine screening of visual and hearing function is imperative to detect problems early. This is especially true for glaucoma, which can lead to permanent visual loss if undetected. Recommended screening guidelines are usually structured according to age. When a client begins to show a hearing deficit, routine screening should be incorporated into regular examinations.

Hazards

A client with sensory alterations is at risk for injury if the living environment is unsafe. For example, a client with visual impairment cannot see potential hazards clearly. A client with proprioceptive problems may lose balance easily and fall. The condition of the home, the rooms, and the front and back entrances can be problematic for the client with sensory alterations. Some of the more common hazards include the following:

- Uneven, cracked walkways leading to front or back door
- Doormats with slippery backing
- Extension and telephone cords in the main route of walking traffic
- Loose area rugs and runners placed over carpeting
- Bathrooms without shower or tub grab bars
- Water faucets unmarked to designate hot and cold
- Bathroom floor with slippery surface
- Absence of smoke detectors in rooms
- Unlit stairways, lack of handrails
- Floors cluttered with material and excessive furniture, including footstools
- Kitchen equipment (e.g., ranges, irons, toasters) with hard-to-read settings

Visually impaired clients may also be unable to read medication labels and syringe gauges. Therefore, ask the client to read a label to determine whether he or she can adequately see the dosage and frequency instructions. If a client has a hearing impairment, check to

TABLE 48-2 Assessment of Sensory Function

Assessment	Behaviour Indicating Deficit (Children)	Behaviour Indicating Deficit (Adults)
Vision*		
Ask client to read newspaper, magazine, or lettering on menu. Measure visual acuity with Snellen chart (see Chapter 32). Assess visual fields and depth perception. Assess pupil size and accommodation to light. Ask client to identify colours on colour chart or crayons.	Self-stimulation, including eye rubbing, body rocking, sniffing or smelling, arm twirling; hitching (using legs to propel while in sitting position) instead of crawling	Poor coordination, squinting, underreaching or overreaching for objects, persistent repositioning of objects, impaired night vision, accidental falls
Hearing		
Perform conventional assessment, including whisper and tuning fork (see Chapter 32). Perform audiometry, if indicated. Observe client conversing with others. Compare client's ability to recognize consonants with ability to distinguish vowels. Assess client's perception of hearing ability and history of tinnitus. Inspect ear canal for hardened cerumen.	Frightened when unfamiliar people approach, no reflex or purposeful response to sounds, failure to be awakened by loud noise, slow or absent development of speech, greater response to movement than to sound, avoidance of social interaction with other children	Blank looks, decreased attention span, lack of reaction to loud noises, increased volume of speech, positioning of head toward sound, smiling and nodding of head in approval when someone speaks, use of other means of communication such as lip-reading or writing, complaints of ringing in ears
Touch		
Assess client for sensitivity to light touch and temperature (see Chapter 32). Check client's ability to discriminate between sharp and dull stimuli. Assess whether client can distinguish objects (coin or safety pin) in the hand with eyes closed. Ask whether client feels unusual sensations.	Inability to perform developmental tasks related to grasping objects or drawing, repeated injury from handling of harmful objects (e.g., hot stove, sharp knife)	Clumsiness, overreaction or underreaction to painful stimulus, failure to respond when touched, avoidance of touch, sensation of pins and needles, numbness
Smell		
Ask client to close eyes and identify several nonirritating odours (e.g., coffee, vanilla).	Difficult to assess until child is 6 or 7 years old, difficulty discriminating noxious odours	Failure to react to noxious or strong odour, increased body odour, decreased sensitivity to odours
Taste		
Ask client to sample and distinguish different tastes (e.g., lemon, sugar, salt). Have client drink or sip water and wait 1 minute between each taste. Ask client if recent weight change has occurred.	Inability to tell whether food is salty or sweet, possible ingestion of strange-tasting things	Change in appetite, excessive use of seasoning and sugar, complaints about taste of food, weight change
Position Sense		
Perform conventional tests for balance and position sense (see Chapter 32).	Clumsiness, extraneous movement, excessive arm swinging in those with hyperactivity or learning difficulty Inability to sit or stand as per expected milestones	Poor balance and spatial orientation, shuffling gait, reduced response to brace self when falling, more precise and deliberate movements

*Go to http://www.cnib.ca/en/about/publications/vision-health/lwvl/default.aspx to see pictures of what persons with varying visual impairments might see.

see whether the sounds of a doorbell, telephone, smoke alarm, and alarm clock are easy to discriminate.

In the hospital environment, caregivers often forget to rearrange furniture and equipment to keep paths from the bed and chair to the bathroom and entrance clear. Walking into a client's room and looking for safety hazards must be a routine part of your care. Check frequently for the following:

- Is the call light within easy, safe reach?
- Are intravenous (IV) poles on wheels and easy to move?
- Are footstools in the middle of the room?
- Are suction machines, IV pumps, or drainage bags positioned so that a client can rise from a bed or chair easily?

Communication Methods

To understand the nature of a communication problem, you must know whether a client has trouble speaking, understanding, naming, reading, or writing. Clients with existing sensory deficits often develop alternative ways of communicating. To interact with the client and to promote interaction with others, you must understand the client's method of communication (Figure 48–2). A deaf or hearing-impaired client may read lips, use sign language, listen with the help of a hearing aid, or read and write notes. For someone who is hearing impaired, speak clearly with a moderate rate of speech and pause to determine understanding.

Visually impaired clients may be unable to observe facial expressions and other nonverbal behaviours that clarify the content of spoken communication. Instead, they rely on voice tones and inflections to detect the emotional tone of communication. Clients with visual impairments often learn to read Braille, although decreased tactile acuity of the fingers may make this more difficult in older people. If the person has a visual impairment, speak normally from a reasonably close distance and ensure that lighting is sufficient.

Clients with **aphasia** may be unable to produce or understand language. **Expressive aphasia**, a motor type of aphasia, is the inability to name common objects or to express simple ideas in words or writing. For example, a client may understand a question but be unable to express an answer. Sensory or **receptive aphasia** is the inability to understand written or spoken language. The client may be able to express words but is unable to understand the questions or comments of others. **Global aphasia** is the inability to understand language or communicate orally.

The temporary or permanent loss of the ability to speak is extremely traumatic to an individual. It is important to assess a client's alternative communication method and whether it causes anxiety in the client. Clients who have undergone laryngectomies often write notes, use communication boards or laptop computers, speak with mechanical vibrators, or use esophageal speech. Clients with endotracheal or tracheostomy tubes have a temporary loss of speech. Most use a notepad to write their questions and requests. However, the client may become incapacitated and unable to write messages. You need to determine whether the client has developed a sign language or system of symbols to communicate needs. If not, you may need to assist the client in developing a meaningful one during the temporary loss.

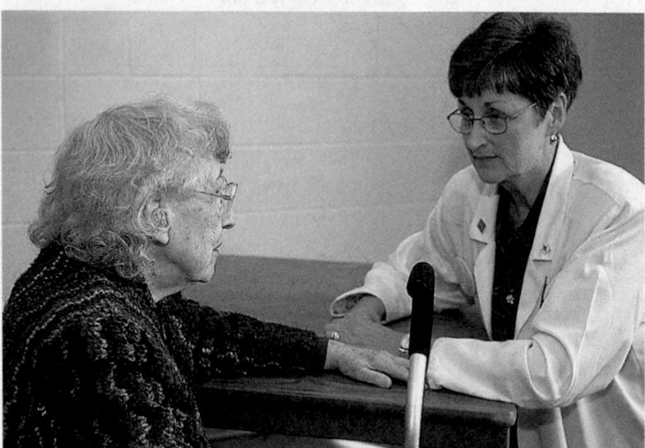

Figure 48-2 Nurse sits at eye level so that client with hearing impairment can communicate.

Social Support

It is important for you to know the client's social skills and level of satisfaction with the support given by family and friends. Is the client satisfied with the support made available from friends? Is the client able to solve problems with family members? Does the family offer the support needed when the client requires assistance as a result of a sensory loss? The long-term effects of sensory alterations can influence family dynamics and a client's willingness to remain active in society.

Use of Assistive Devices

Assess for the use of assistive devices (e.g., hearing aids or glasses) and the sensory effects for the client. This includes learning how often the devices are used daily, the client's or family caregiver's method for cleaning, and the client's knowledge of what to do when a problem develops. However, just because the client has an assistive device, do not assume that it works or that the client uses it or benefits from it.

Other Factors Affecting Perception

Factors other than sensory deprivation or overload may cause impaired perception (e.g., medications or pain). Assess the client's medication history, which includes prescribed and over-the-counter medications, as well as herbal products. This history includes gaining information regarding the frequency, dose, method of administration, and last time these medications were taken. Some antibiotics (e.g., streptomycin, gentamicin, and tobramycin) are **ototoxic** and can permanently damage the auditory nerve; chloramphenicol can irritate the optic nerve. Opioid analgesics, sedatives, and antidepressant medications can alter the perception of stimuli. Conduct a thorough pain assessment when pain is suspected to be causing perceptual problems (see Chapter 42). Also assess the use of caffeine and over-the-counter remedies.

Client Expectations

Clients depend on their senses to provide them with information so as to respond or react to a specific situation or problem. Therefore, clients may expect caregivers to recognize and appropriately manage and adjust their environment to meet their sensory needs. This would include assisting the client in adapting his or her lifestyle as a result of sensory impairment. You should determine from clients exactly what they expect to achieve and what interventions have been helpful in the past in the management of their limitations. Remember that clients with sensory alterations may have strengthened their other senses and expect caregivers to anticipate their needs (e.g., for safety and security).

❖Nursing Diagnosis

After assessment, you need to review all available data and look for patterns and trends suggestive of a health problem relating to sensory alterations (Box 48–4). For example, a client's advanced age, apathy, inattentiveness during conversations, and self-rating of hearing as "poor" are all defining characteristics for the nursing diagnosis of

BOX 48-4 NURSING DIAGNOSTIC PROCESS

Assessment Activities	Defining Characteristics	Nursing Diagnosis
Assess client's visual acuity.	Has reduced ability to see objects clearly. Needs brighter light to read. Has trouble distinguishing edges of stairs.	*Risk for injury related to visual impairment from cataract formation*
Visit home setting and inspect for any hazards that may pose risks to client.	Lighting in rooms, hallways, and stairwells is very dim. Carpet in living room is old, and edges are curled up. Steps lead up to front entrance of home.	
Review medical record from clinic visit.	Client has been diagnosed as having cataracts in both eyes.	

disturbed sensory perception (auditory). Validate your findings to ensure the accuracy of the diagnosis. For example, the diagnosis of disturbed thought processes could mistakenly be made if you do not confirm the client's hearing deficit and perception of poor hearing.

As well, determine the factor that likely causes the client's health problem. In the previous example, impacted cerumen is the cause of the client's hearing alteration. The etiology or related factor of a nursing diagnosis is a condition that can be affected by nursing interventions. The etiology must be accurate; otherwise, nursing therapies will be ineffective. For a client with impacted cerumen, regular irrigation of the ear canal has the potential to improve auditory perception (Barnett, 2007). In contrast, if the client's auditory alteration were related to hearing loss from nerve deafness, nursing interventions for alternative communication methods would be necessary.

The client may also have health care problems for which sensory alteration is the etiology, such as with the diagnosis of risk for injury. For example, people with visual impairment fall more frequently than those with normal sight (Campbell et al., 2005). You may also select nursing diagnoses by recognizing the way that sensory alterations affect a client's ability to function (e.g., self-care deficit). In addition, most clients present themselves to health care professionals with multiple diagnoses (Figure 48–3). In the example of the concept map, a client with retinal detachment has the nursing diagnosis of disturbed sensory perception, which can lead to risk for falls and fear. You must

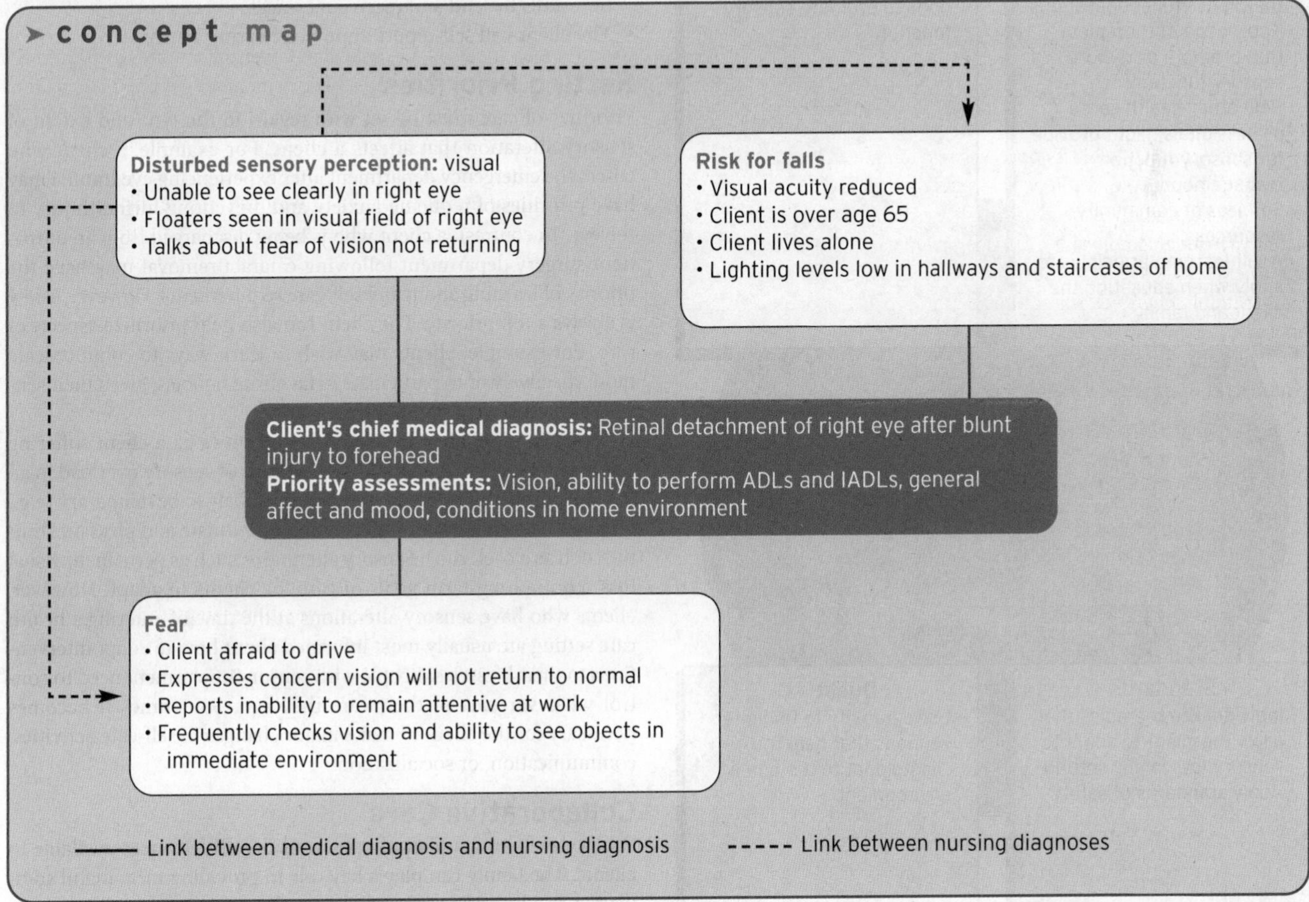

Figure 48-3 Concept map for client with retinal detachment of right eye after blunt injury to forehead. ADLs, activities of daily living; IADLs, instrumental activities of daily living.

recognize patterns of data that reveal health problems created by the client's sensory alteration. Examples of nursing diagnoses that might apply to clients with sensory alterations include the following:

- *Impaired adjustment*
- *Impaired verbal communication*
- *Risk for injury*
- *Impaired physical mobility*
- *Self-care deficit, including bathing or hygiene, dressing or grooming, or toileting*
- *Situational low self-esteem*
- *Disturbed sensory perception*
- *Social isolation*
- *Disturbed thought processes*
- *Altered socialization*

❖Planning

During planning, use your critical thinking skills to synthesize information from multiple resources (Figure 48–4), including knowledge gained from the assessment and knowledge of how sensory deficits affect normal functioning. In this way, you can recognize the extent of the client's deficit and know the type of interventions most likely to be helpful. Also consider the role that other health care professionals can play in planning care and the available community resources (e.g., CNIB) that may be useful. Previous experience in caring for clients with sensory alterations can be invaluable when planning nursing approaches.

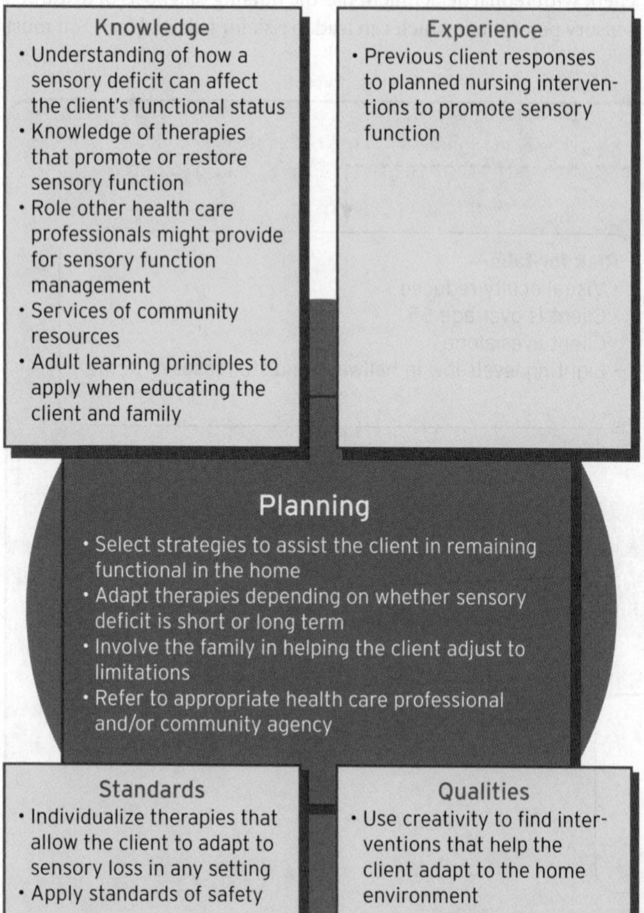

When applying critical thinking to planning care, professional standards can be particularly useful. These standards, in the form of clinical pathways or clinical practice guidelines, often recommend interventions based on research evidence for the client's condition. For example, clients who have visual deficits and are hospitalized may be placed on a fall prevention protocol that will incorporate research-based precautions to ensure client safety.

Knowledge
- Understanding of how a sensory deficit can affect the client's functional status
- Knowledge of therapies that promote or restore sensory function
- Role other health care professionals might provide for sensory function management
- Services of community resources
- Adult learning principles to apply when educating the client and family

Experience
- Previous client responses to planned nursing interventions to promote sensory function

Planning
- Select strategies to assist the client in remaining functional in the home
- Adapt therapies depending on whether sensory deficit is short or long term
- Involve the family in helping the client adjust to limitations
- Refer to appropriate health care professional and/or community agency

Standards
- Individualize therapies that allow the client to adapt to sensory loss in any setting
- Apply standards of safety

Qualities
- Use creativity to find interventions that help the client adapt to the home environment

Figure 48-4 Critical thinking model for sensory alterations planning.

Goals and Outcomes

During planning, you will develop an individualized plan of care for each nursing diagnosis (Box 48–5). With the client, develop a realistic plan that incorporates what you know about the client's sensory problems and the extent to which sensory function can be maintained or improved. If maintenance or improvement is not realistic, preventing injury and learning alternate ways of maintaining independence are key. Goals and outcomes should be realistic and measurable. A goal of care for a client with an actual or a potential sensory alteration may include this: "The client will regain improvement in hearing acuity within 2 weeks." Associated outcomes for this goal might include the following:

- The client will report using communication techniques for improved reception of messages within 2 weeks.
- The client will successfully demonstrate the technique for cleansing the hearing aid within 1 week.
- The client and family will be observed using proper communication skills to send and receive messages.
- The client will self-report improved hearing acuity.

Setting Priorities

Priorities of care must be set with regard to the type and extent of sensory alteration that affects a client. For example, a client who enters the emergency department after experiencing eye trauma may have priorities of reducing anxiety and preventing further injury to the eye. In contrast, a client who is being discharged from an outpatient surgery department following cataract removal may have the priority of learning about any self-care requirements. However, safety is always a top priority. The client can also help prioritize aspects of care. For example, clients may wish to learn ways to communicate more effectively or to participate in favourite hobbies, given their sensory limitation.

Some sensory alterations are short term (e.g., a client suffering sensory or perceptual alterations as a result of sensory overload in an ICU). Appropriate interventions are thus likely to be temporary (e.g., frequent reorientation or introduction of intimate and pleasant stimuli, such as a back rub). Sensory alterations such as permanent visual loss require long-term goals of care for clients to adapt. However, clients who have sensory alterations at the time of entering a health care setting are usually most informed about how to adapt interventions to their lifestyles. People with sensory impairment need to control whatever part of their care they can. Sometimes it becomes necessary for the client to make major changes in self-care activities, communication, or socialization.

Collaborative Care

When developing a plan of care, consider all resources available to clients. The family can play a key role in providing meaningful stimulation and learning ways to help the client adjust to any limitations. As part of a multidisciplinary health care team, you may also refer the client to other health care professionals. Early referrals to occupational

BOX 48-5 NURSING CARE PLAN

Disturbed Sensory Perception

Assessment

Judy Long, a 70-year-old retired receptionist, tells the community health nurse that her vision has become progressively blurred over the last several years. She comments that she is having her neighbour drive her places. Judy visited an ophthalmologist, and surgery is planned.

Assessment Activities	*Findings and Defining Characteristics*
Ask Judy to describe her vision changes.	Judy states, "My left eye seems to have a film over it that makes my vision blurred. I am having difficulty reading. I also have difficulty with night driving; the headlights are large and blurred."
Ask Judy to describe any life changes that have occurred since the change in vision.	Judy indicates that she has always managed her home and done volunteering. She says she is losing her independence because she has to have someone drive her, and she is now hesitant to use stairs at home.
Assess Judy's visual acuity.	Judy cannot read the Snellen chart with the left eye.
Ask Judy the results of the visit to the ophthalmologist.	Judy states that she was told she has a cataract in the left eye and a cataract beginning in her right eye; surgery is planned on her left eye.
Conduct a home hazard assessment.	The home is cluttered, the lighting is dim, and the stairs going into the house have no handrails.

Nursing Diagnosis: Disturbed sensory perception related to altered sensory reception of senile cataract

Planning

*Goals (Nursing Outcomes Classification)**	*Expected Outcomes*
	Safety Behaviour: Home Physical Environment
Judy will maintain independence in a safe home environment.	Judy will verbalize changes made to protect and maintain visual acuity for indoor and outdoor activities in 2 weeks. A safety check of her home will show removal of safety hazards in 1 week. Judy will explain plans for alternative transportation to work and social activities in 1 week.
	Sensory Function: Vision
Judy will make the best use of existing visual function.	Judy will use visual aid devices in 1 week.

*Outcome classification labels from Moorhead, S., Johnson, M., & Maas, M. L., (Eds.). (2004). *Nursing Outcomes Classification (NOC)* (3rd ed.). St. Louis, MO: Mosby.

Interventions (Nursing Interventions Classification)†	Rationale
Environmental Management	
Teach Judy how to improve the safety of her environment, such as making sure her home is free of clutter, footstools, and electrical cords, and to avoid rearranging furniture.	Keeping the area clutter free reduces the risk of injury (Campbell et al., 2005).
Instruct Judy to reduce glare by wearing dark-coloured sunglasses outside.	Clients have better visual acuity when they protect their eyes from bright light (Ebersole et al., 2007).
Teach Judy to use a light over the shoulder for reading and writing.	People with cataracts see better with wider illumination (Ebersole et al., 2007).
Provide magnifier for Judy to use to read newspaper and mail.	Devices will provide magnification to improve visual acuity.
Emotional Support	
Encourage Judy to express feelings regarding loss of vision and lifestyle changes.	People who experience visual loss grieve over loss of independence (Fourie, 2007).
Family Involvement	
Confer with Judy on selecting a family member, friend, or community resource person who can provide transportation until after the eye condition has been corrected.	An alternate means of transportation will foster safety.

†Intervention classification labels from Dochterman, J. M., & Bulechek, G. M. (Eds.). (2004). *Nursing Interventions Classification (NIC)* (4th ed.). St. Louis, MO: Mosby.

Continued

BOX 48-5 NURSING CARE PLAN *continued*

Evaluation

Nursing Actions	*Client Response and Finding*	*Achievement of Outcome*
Ask Judy to describe the changes that have made the home environment safer.	Judy responds that the family has removed the clutter and handrails have been placed at the entryway. Lighting has been placed behind her chair, and100-watt lights are in the living room.	Judy reports feeling safer walking the stairs and moving about in her home. The home hazards have been reduced.
During a home visit, observe the home environment for safety hazards.		
Observe Judy's verbal and nonverbal responses to the lifestyle adaptations.	Judy says, "I feel safer when walking in my home."	
As Judy uses a magnifier, have her read a medication label.	Judy is able to read the name of her medication and dosage correctly.	Better use is made of current vision.
Ask Judy if she is able to maintain a degree of independence with the environmental and lifestyle modifications.	Judy states, "I am more independent at home, and until surgery, I do not mind someone driving for me."	Judy has attained some degree of independence.
Ask Judy to identify source of transportation.	Judy says a family member has agreed to drive her shopping and for surgery.	Judy has transportation through the weeks required for the surgical experience.

or speech therapists, for example, can speed a client's recovery. If a client has experienced a major loss of sensory function and is also unable to manage medical needs, such as medication self-administration or dressing changes, referral to home care may be an option. Numerous community-based resources (e.g., CNIB, Canadian Association of Independent Living Centres, Canadian Hearing Society) are also available. You may be able to arrange a volunteer to visit a client or have printed materials made available that describe ways to help cope with sensory problems.

❖Implementation

Nursing interventions involve the client and family so that a safe, pleasant, and stimulating sensory environment can be maintained. The most effective interventions enable the client with sensory alterations to function safely with existing deficits and to continue a normal lifestyle. Learning to adjust to sensory impairments can occur at any age with proper support and resources. Use measures to maintain a client's sensory function at the highest level possible.

Health Promotion

Good sensory function begins with prevention. Almost everyone becomes exposed to risks in the environment that may cause sensory alterations. When clients enter primary health care settings, you can take the opportunity to review common-sense approaches for reducing the risk of sensory loss (Box 48–6).

Screening. Globally, more than 161 million people are visually impaired (World Health Organization, 2004). Preventable blindness is a worldwide health issue. Therefore, prevention of visual impairment begins with children and requires appropriate screening (Hockenberry & Wilson, 2007). Three recommended interventions are (a) screening for rubella or syphilis in women who are considering pregnancy; (b) adequate prenatal care to prevent premature birth (with the danger of exposure of the infant to excessive oxygen); and (c) periodic screening of all children, especially newborns through preschoolers, for congenital blindness and visual impairment caused by refractive errors, amblyopia (loss of visual acuity in the nondominant eye because of lack of use in childhood), and **strabismus** (misalignment of the eyes).

Visual impairment is common during childhood. The most common visual problem is a **refractive error** such as nearsightedness. Parents must know signs suggesting visual impairment (e.g., failure to react to light and reduced eye contact from the infant) and should be instructed to report these signs to a physician immediately. Vision

BOX 48-6 FOCUS ON PRIMARY HEALTH CARE

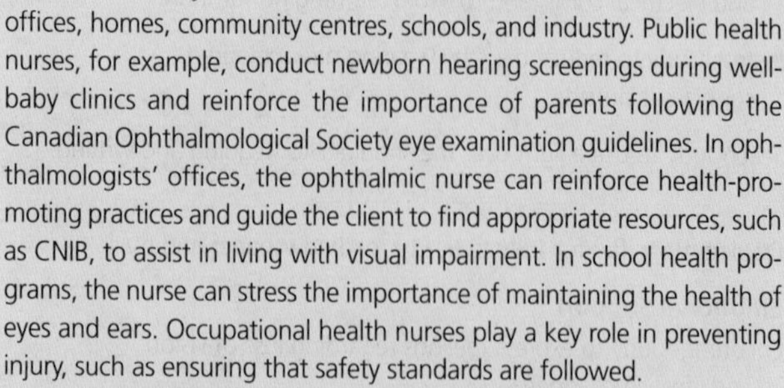

Sensory Alterations

The major goals in primary health care settings are health promotion, disease prevention, early detection, and referral. In the community, primary health care related to sensory alterations is delivered in doctors' offices, homes, community centres, schools, and industry. Public health nurses, for example, conduct newborn hearing screenings during well-baby clinics and reinforce the importance of parents following the Canadian Ophthalmological Society eye examination guidelines. In ophthalmologists' offices, the ophthalmic nurse can reinforce health-promoting practices and guide the client to find appropriate resources, such as CNIB, to assist in living with visual impairment. In school health programs, the nurse can stress the importance of maintaining the health of eyes and ears. Occupational health nurses play a key role in preventing injury, such as ensuring that safety standards are followed.

Nurses are often consulted for guidance when changes in vision and hearing occur. Consequently, your knowledge of screening techniques is important, such as the use of the Amsler grid for macular degeneration. This is a grid consisting of 5-mm squares with a black dot in the centre of the grid for fixation, used for testing the central 20 degrees of the field of vision. It is also important that you are familiar with the normal aging process, as well as the signs and symptoms of common diseases so that appropriate suggestions for referral can be made.

screening of school-age children and adolescents can detect problems early. The school nurse or public health nurse is usually responsible for vision testing. Their main role is one of detection and referral.

In Canada, glaucoma is the second leading cause of blindness and affects 1 in 100 Canadians over the age of 40 years. The risk is eight times higher among Black Canadians. It is important to recommend that clients between the ages of 40 and 64 years have an eye examination every 2 to 4 years. Examinations should occur every 1 to 2 years if the client's family has a history of glaucoma or if the client is of African ancestry, has had a serious eye injury in the past, is taking steroid medications, or is over 65 years of age (Smith & Neely, 2007).

Children at risk for hearing impairment include those with a family history of childhood hearing impairment, perinatal infection (rubella, herpes, cytomegalovirus), low birth weight, chronic ear infection, and Down syndrome. You should advise pregnant women of the importance of early prenatal care, avoidance of ototoxic drugs, and testing for syphilis or rubella.

Children with chronic middle ear infections, a common cause of impaired hearing, should receive periodic auditory testing. Parents must be warned of the risks (e.g., exposure to smoke, previous history of ear infections, siblings with otitis media, attending day care) and should seek medical care when the child has symptoms of earache or respiratory infection (Kerschner et al., 2005).

Many teenagers and young adults already have permanent hearing loss caused by exposure to excessive noise from such things as iPods, MP3 players, automobile stereo systems, and concerts. This hearing impairment results in loss of sound quality. Sounds are barrel-like, and consonants are hard to hear. According to provincial occupational health and safety legislation, workers must use HPDs to minimize or prevent hearing loss. As well, various provincial jurisdictions mandate occupational noise exposure limits. You should routinely teach parents and children to take precautions when involved in activities associated with high-intensity noise. As well, you should assess clients for noise exposure and participate in providing hearing conservation classes for teachers, students, and clients. Some "rules of thumb" are as follows: if someone standing a metre away has to shout to be understood, or if after the noise has stopped, the person experiences a temporary hearing loss or tinnitus, then the risk for hearing loss is increased. More seriously, if someone has to shout in a person's ear to be understood, the person is at risk for permanent hearing loss if exposed to this level of noise for just 5 minutes per day (Health Canada, 2006).

The guidelines for hearing screening for adults are less prescriptive. In general, if a client works or lives in an environment where the noise level is high, routine screening is highly recommended and may be mandated by occupational health and safety measures in the workplace. Nurses in occupational settings can assess for symptoms of tinnitus and make prompt referrals. Early detection may prevent hearing disabilities (Davis et al., 2007). Barnett (2007) recommends that, since aging is associated with degenerative changes, clients over 40 have a routine hearing assessment. However, adults must not accept hearing loss as a natural part of aging. If a hearing loss does occur, it is important to have regular hearing testing. Nurses should encourage clients to follow through with recommendations for hearing aids.

Preventive Safety. Trauma is a common cause of blindness in children. Penetrating injuries from propulsive objects such as firecrackers, slingshots, rubber bands, or rocks and penetrating wounds from sticks, scissors, or toys are just a few examples. Parents and children require counselling on ways to avoid eye trauma (Box 48–7). Safety equipment can easily be found in most sports shops and large department stores. In some Canadian jurisdictions, legislation or association bylaws mandate the wearing of protective equipment (e.g., visors in minor hockey).

Adults are at risk for eye injury while playing sports and working in jobs involving exposure to chemicals or flying objects. The Canadian Centre for Occupational Health and Safety has guidelines for safety in the workplace. Employers are required to have employees wear eye goggles or use equipment such as HPDs to reduce the risk of injury. Eyewash stations should be provided where a worker is exposed to potential contact with a biological or chemical substance (Canadian Centre for Occupational Health and Safety, 2005). Nurses in occupational health settings can reinforce use of protective devices and ensure that things such as eyewash stations are in close proximity to the risk for injury.

Preventing hearing loss requires individuals to avoid exposure to continuously high noise levels and brief, loud impulse noise. The potential for hearing loss increases as the decibel level rises. HPDs should be worn by clients who must work around noise. Earplugs and earphones are useful in blocking high-decibel sounds (Box 48–8).

Another means of prevention involves regular immunization of children against diseases capable of causing hearing loss (e.g., rubella, mumps, and measles). Public health nurses, nurse practitioners, and nurses who work in physicians' offices, schools, and community clinics should reinforce the importance of early and timely immunization. When a child or an adult develops any type of health problem, caution should be used in prescribing drugs that are ototoxic.

Use of Assistive Devices. Health promotion requires appropriate use of assistive aids and good, routine hygiene measures. Clients who wear corrective contact lenses, eyeglasses, or hearing aids should make sure that they are kept clean, accessible, and functional (see Chapter 38). It is critical for contact lens wearers to frequently clean lenses and use the appropriate solutions for cleaning and disinfection. With the rise in the use of soft contact lenses, particularly extended-wear lenses, some clients have become casual with regard to both the care and the wearing time of the contacts; as a result, the number of serious corneal infections has increased. Infrequent lens disinfection, contamination of lens storage cases and contact lens solutions, and

➤ BOX 48-7 Tips for Preventing Eye Injury in Children

Infants and Toddlers

Avoid toys with long, pointed projections.
Do not allow children to walk or run with pointed object in hand.
Keep pointed instruments and tools out of reach.

Preschoolers

Supervise use of sharp or pointed objects such as scissors.
Teach children to walk carefully when carrying pointed objects.
Keep children away from projectile activities.
Begin to teach respect for firearms and fireworks.

School-Age Children and Adolescents

Teach proper use of potentially dangerous equipment such as power tools, fireworks, and sports equipment (hockey sticks or pool cues).
Stress use of eye protection when playing hockey or ball and racquet sports, shooting, using power tools, or riding motorcycles.
Warn children not to look directly at the sun even when wearing sunglasses.
Be sure that corrective lenses are made of shatterproof glass.

BOX 48-8 RESEARCH HIGHLIGHT

Effectiveness of Computer-Based Tailoring Versus Targeting to Promote Use of Hearing Protection

Research Focus

The prevention of occupational hearing loss is a priority issue for health care practitioners and policymakers. Of particular concern is the noise-induced hearing loss among construction workers. Some evidence indicates that up to 74% of construction workers experience hearing loss. The focus of this research was to evaluate the effectiveness of two computer-based interventions and booster messages on construction workers' use of hearing protection. Targeted and tailored interventions have been shown to be more effective than generic approaches. However, further research is required to assess the components of effective hearing loss prevention programs and which messages and approaches are most effective.

Research Abstract

Using a theory-based intervention designed by integrating concepts from the Predictors of Use of Hearing Protection Model, Kerr et al. (2007) randomly assigned 343 construction workers to either a tailored education group (addressing individual characteristics) or to a targeted education group (addressing shared characteristics) with or without booster messages. The educational program made use of an interactive multimedia game-type format with an espionage storyline in which participants tried to foil the noise villain by using hearing protective devices (HPDs). The researchers found that participants improved their use of hearing protection from 42% to 50% of the time they were exposed to noise 1 year postintervention. Differences between intervention groups were not significant. The significant improvement in the use of hearing protection demonstrated that interventions can have a positive impact on preventing noise-induced hearing loss.

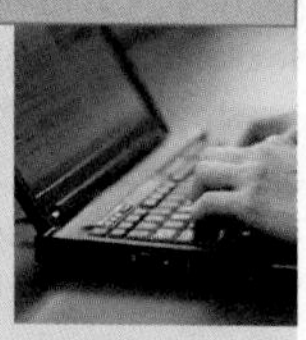

Evidence-Informed Practice

- Assess construction workers for noise-induced hearing loss.
- Design and evaluate teaching tools to educate workers exposed to high noise levels regarding the use of HPDs for prevention of hearing loss.
- Tailor interventions to the specific characteristics of the trade or work.
- Refer clients with suspected hearing impairment to a hearing clinic or to an audiologist for testing.

References: Kerr, M. J., Savik, K., Monsten, K. A., & Lusk, S. L. (2007). Effectiveness of computer-based tailoring versus targeting to promote use of hearing protection. *Canadian Journal of Nursing Research, 39*, 80–97.

use of homemade saline add to a client's risk. Swimming while wearing lenses also creates a serious risk of infection.

Many people are reluctant to wear a hearing aid. Several factors may determine a person's likelihood for wearing a hearing aid: perceived need for improved hearing, attitude toward the hearing problem, and motivation to seek solutions. Cost may also be a concern for having hearing assessed and for purchasing a hearing aid if the client is not covered by a provincial health plan. In some provinces, hearing aids must be purchased from an approved dispensor or dealer for the cost to be covered by the province's health program.

Acknowledging a need to improve hearing is a person's first step. You can give clients useful information on the benefits of wearing a hearing aid. A wide variety of aids not only successfully enhance a person's hearing but can also be cosmetically acceptable. Chapter 38 summarizes the types of hearing aids available and tips for proper care and use. It is also important to have a significant other available to assist with hearing aid adjustment (Box 48–9).

If a client has any of the following ear conditions, a hearing aid cannot be used: visible congenital or traumatic deformity of the ear, active drainage in the last 90 days, sudden or progressive hearing loss within the last 90 days, acute or chronic dizziness, unilateral sudden hearing loss within the last 90 days, visible cerumen accumulation or a foreign body in the ear canal, pain or discomfort in the ear, or an audiometric air–bone gap of 15 decibels or greater. All but the last of these can be detected on physical examination. Referrals to or recommendations that the client see an otolaryngologist or audiologist for further counselling should be made (Ebersole et al., 2007).

Another option for those with severe to profound hearing loss is a cochlear implant. This is a small, complex electronic device that can help provide a sense of sound to a person who is profoundly deaf or severely hard of hearing. The implant consists of an external portion that sits behind the ear and a second portion that is surgically placed under the skin. An implant does not restore normal hearing. Instead, it can give a deaf person a useful representation of sounds in the environment and help him or her understand speech.

Promoting Meaningful Stimulation. Life becomes more enriching and satisfying when meaningful and pleasant stimuli exist within a person's environment. You can help clients make adjustments to their environment in many ways so that it becomes more stimulating.

BOX 48-9 CLIENT TEACHING

Troubleshooting Hearing Aid Malfunction

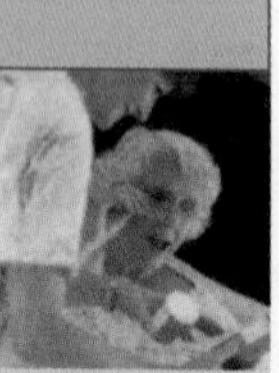

Objectives

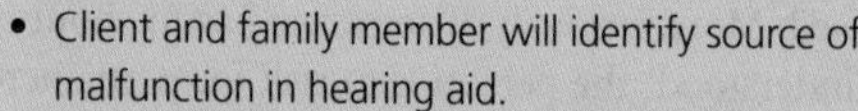

- Client and family member will identify source of malfunction in hearing aid.
- Client and family member will demonstrate hearing aid care.

Teaching Strategies

- Show client and family member locations on hearing aid device where damage (e.g., cracks, fraying) is likely to occur: ear mould or case, earphone, dials, cord, and connection plugs.
- Demonstrate battery replacement and stress the importance of having an extra set of unused batteries available.
- Review method to check volume: turn dial to maximum gain and then check. Is voice clear?
- Consult manufacturer's directions for specific care measures for cleaning battery case and ear mould.
- Review factors to report to hearing aid laboratory: static, distortion of sound, poor volume quality.

Evaluation

- Ask client and family member to describe types of common malfunctions with hearing aid.
- Ask client and family to demonstrate battery removal and cleaning of the device.

To do this, consider the normal physiological changes that accompany sensory deficits.

Vision. As a result of the normal changes of aging, the pupil's ability to adjust to light diminishes. As a result, older adults are often more sensitive to glare. You can suggest ways for the client to minimize glare by selecting satin and nongloss finishes for walls and countertops in the home, selecting a tile pattern for flooring, and choosing sheer curtains, tinted windows, or adjustable shades to reduce outdoor light. Wearing sunglasses outside can reduce the glare of direct sunlight.

The ability to read is important to everyone. Therefore, clients should be encouraged to use their glasses whenever possible (e.g., during procedures and client instruction), which helps clients remain oriented, maintain some control, and retain their dignity. Clients with reduced visual acuity may need more than corrective lenses. A pocket magnifier can help a client read most printed material. Telescopic lens eyeglasses are smaller, are easier to focus, and have a greater range. Books and other publications are also available in larger print. If a client has a legal or other important document he or she wishes to read, standard copying machines have enlarging capabilities. Closed-circuit television magnifying units or portable or desktop video magnifiers using solid-state digital technology enlarge written characters. Minimum and maximum magnification varies from 12 to 60 times the original, depending on the screen size. As well, many word processing programs allow print to be enlarged. Audio-recorded books are available on DVD or audiotape and can be readily purchased in book stores or borrowed from public libraries or CNIB. Described videos are also available.

With aging, a person experiences a change in colour perception. Perception of the colours blue, violet, and green usually declines. Brighter colours, such as red, orange, and yellow, are easier to see. You can offer suggestions of ways the client may decorate a room and paint hallways or stairwells so that differentiations can be made in surfaces and objects in a room.

Hearing. To maximize residual hearing function, you work closely with the client to suggest ways to modify the environment. Telephones and televisions can be amplified. Alarm clocks that shake the bed or activate a flashing light are useful devices. An innovative way to enrich the lives of those with a hearing impairment is recorded music. Some clients with severe hearing loss can hear music recorded in the low-frequency sound cycles. Closed captioning, in which audio content and nonspeech information, such as the identity of speakers and sound effects, are described using words or symbols, is available for many television programs.

One way to help an individual with a hearing loss is to ensure that the problem is not impacted cerumen. With aging, cerumen thickens and builds up in the ear canal. Excessive cerumen occluding the ear canal can cause a **conductive hearing loss**. Irrigation of the canal with tepid water in a 60-mL syringe (see Chapter 38) will remove cerumen. Removal of cerumen can significantly improve not only the client's hearing ability but also the client's mental status (Torchinsky & Davidson, 2006).

Taste and Smell. You can easily promote the sense of taste by using measures to enhance remaining taste perception. Good oral hygiene keeps the taste buds well hydrated. Taste perception is heightened if foods are well seasoned, differently textured, and eaten separately. Flavoured vinegar or lemon juice can add tartness to food. Ask the client what foods appeal most to taste. If taste perception is improved, food intake and appetite will also improve.

Stimulation of the sense of smell with aromas such as brewing coffee, cooking garlic, and baking bread can heighten taste sensation. The client needs to avoid blending or mixing foods because these actions make it difficult to identify tastes. Older adults should chew food thoroughly to allow more food to contact the remaining taste buds.

Smell can be improved by strengthening pleasant olfactory stimulation. A client's environment can be made more pleasant with smells such as cologne, mild room deodorizers, fragrant flowers, and sachets, although you must assess the client for allergies or sensitivities before using these items. Certain aromas may actually cause clients to lose their appetites.

Removal of unpleasant odours improves the quality of a person's environment. You should keep a client's room clean, empty bedpans or urinals, remove and dispose of soiled dressings, and keep bathroom doors closed.

Touch. Clients with reduced tactile sensation usually have the impairment over a limited portion of their bodies. You can stimulate existing function by providing touch therapy. If the client is willing to be touched, hair brushing and combing, a back rub, and touching of the arms or shoulders are ways of increasing tactile contact. When sensation is reduced, firm pressure may be necessary for the client to feel your hand. Turning and repositioning can also improve the quality of tactile sensation. When invasive procedures are being performed, it is important to use touch by holding the client's hands and keeping them warm and dry.

If a client is overly sensitive to tactile stimuli (**hyperesthesia**), you must minimize irritating stimuli. Keeping bed linens loose to minimize direct contact with the client and protecting the skin from exposure to irritants are helpful measures. If the client has numbness and tingling or pain in the hands, as with carpal tunnel syndrome, special wrist splints may be worn to dorsiflex the wrist to relieve the nerve pressure. For those clients who use computers, special keyboards and wrist pads are available to decrease the pressure on the median nerve, aid in relief of pain, and promote healing.

Establishing Safe Environments. When sensory function becomes impaired, individuals become less secure and the world around them becomes smaller. Older adults in particular find it important to feel secure about their immediate environment. Feeling safe allows a person to function within the home and helps provide a sense of independence. You can suggest various strategies to assist clients in making their living environment safer without restricting their independence. During a home visit or while completing an examination in the clinic, suggestions for home safety can be discussed. The nature of the actual or potential sensory loss determines the safety precautions taken.

Adaptations for Visual Loss. When a client experiences a decrease in visual acuity, peripheral vision, adaptation to the dark, and depth perception, safety becomes a concern. With reduced peripheral vision, a client cannot see panoramically because the outer visual field is less discrete. This creates a special hazard for driving or walking in crowded areas. Adults with reduced adaptation to the dark require three times as much light to see objects as they did as young adults. With reduced depth perception, a person cannot see how far away objects are located, making walking down stairs or over uneven surfaces dangerous.

safety alert To create a safe environment, the nurse begins by looking at the results of the home environment assessment (see Chapter 37).

Driving can also be a safety hazard. Reduced peripheral vision may prevent a driver from seeing a car in an adjacent lane. Reduced adaptation to the dark and sensitivity to glare make driving at night a significant risk. Although vision is a primary consideration for safety, other factors exist as well. In the case of older adults, decreased reaction time, reduced hearing, and decreased strength in the legs and arms may further compromise driving skills. Safety tips for those who continue to drive include driving in familiar areas, not driving during rush hour, avoiding major highways for local drives, using rear-view and side-view mirrors when changing lanes, avoiding driving at dusk or at night, keeping the car in good working condition, and carrying a cellular phone (but not using it while driving).

Visual alterations can make conducting normal activities of daily living more difficult. Because of reduced depth perception, clients can trip on throw rugs, runners, or the edge of stairs. Flooring or carpeting should be kept in good repair. Advise the client to use low-pile carpeting. Thresholds between rooms should be level with the floor. Clutter should be removed to ensure clear pathways for walking. Furniture should be arranged so that the client can move about easily without fear of tripping or running into objects. Any stairwell should have a securely fastened handrail extending the full length of the stairs.

Front and back entrances to homes, work areas, and stairwells need to be properly lit. Light fixtures need higher-wattage bulbs with wider illumination. Although less energy efficient, incandescent lighting may be preferred over fluorescent lighting because of the flickering of fluorescent lights. Compact fluorescent lighting, however, has eliminated some of these problems (Capezuti et al., 2007). A light switch should be located at the top and bottom of stairwells. It is also important that lighting on the stairs does not cast shadows. You should ensure that the client is able to see the edge of each step clearly, especially the first and last steps. When possible, steps inside and outside the home should be replaced with ramps.

When a client is unable to see visual contrasts, a number of interventions can be helpful. Sometimes settings on electrical appliances and equipment are only highlighted in black and white or shades of grey. Coloured tape, paint, nail polish, or raised label dots can be used to colour-code appliance dials. Colour can also be useful to highlight the edge of stairs. Applying a broad strip of coloured tape at the stair edge can help a person better see the edges. Tour the home with the client to find opportunities for colour-coding. Telephones with large numbers may be helpful.

You can also ensure that the client is able to self-administer medications safely. Labels on medication containers should be in large print. A friend or spouse should always be familiar with dosage schedules. People who are visually impaired may have some difficulty manipulating eyedroppers. Eye-drop dispensers are available and often allow older or visually impaired people to independently administer their drops.

Adaptations for Reduced Hearing. Important environmental sounds may best be heard if amplified or changed to a lower-pitched, buzzer-like sound. Lamps are available that respond with light to sounds such as doorbells, burglar alarms, smoke detectors, and babies crying. These lamps can be purchased from hearing aid dealers, telephone companies, and appliance stores. Signalling devices allow the deaf person greater independence. Family members or anyone who calls the client regularly should learn to let the telephone ring for longer periods. Amplified receivers for telephones and telephone communications devices use a computer and a printer to transfer words over the telephone for people who are hearing impaired. Both sender and receiver must have the special device to complete a call. Telecommunication relay services (TRS) are available from most telephone companies. A telephone operator service translates voice to text and vice versa. Video relay services (VRS) are also available. VRS enables persons with hearing disabilities who use American Sign Language to communicate with voice telephone users through video equipment rather than through typed text. Video equipment links the VRS user with an operator so that they can see and communicate with each other in signed conversation.

Adaptations for Reduced Olfaction. A reduced sensitivity to odours means that the client may be unable to smell leaking gas, a smouldering cigarette or fire, or spoiled food. The client should use smoke and carbon monoxide detectors and other alternative precautions, such as checking ashtrays or placing cigarette butts in water. A client can learn to check dates on food packages and the colour and texture of food. Leftovers should be kept in labelled containers with the preparation date. Pilot gas flames should be checked visually or professionally on a regular basis.

Adaptations for Reduced Tactile Sensation. When clients have reduced sensation in their extremities, they are at risk for injury from exposure to temperature extremes. You should caution them on the use of water bottles or heating pads (see Chapter 47). The temperature of bathwater should be checked routinely before stepping into the tub. The temperature setting on the home water heater should be no higher than 48.8°C.

Promoting Communication. A sensory deficit can cause a person to feel isolated because of an inability to communicate with others. It is important for individuals to be able to interact with people whom they encounter. The nature of the sensory loss influences the methods and styles of communication that you can use (Box 48–10). Communication methods can also be taught to family members and significant others.

When beginning a conversation with a client who has a hearing deficit, it helps to reduce any background noise by turning off or lowering the volume of any television, appliance, or radio. It is also helpful to have conversations in settings where the acoustics are better, which aids in controlling and muffling extraneous background noises. In a group setting, forming a semicircle in front of the client helps him or her see who is speaking next, thereby fostering group involvement. The client with a hearing impairment may be able to speak normally. However, the deaf client's inability to hear self-spoken words may cause serious speech alterations. Clients may use sign language (American or Quebec Sign Language), lip-read, write with a pad and pencil, or learn to use a computer for communication. Special communication boards that contain common terms used in nursing care (e.g., pain, bathroom, dizzy, or walk) help clients express their needs.

Client instruction is one aspect of communication. Teaching booklets are available in large print. The client who is blind may require more frequent and detailed verbal descriptions of information. This is particularly true if no instructional booklets are written in Braille. Visually impaired clients can learn by listening to audiotapes or the sound portion of a televised teaching session. Clients with hearing impairment may benefit from written instructional materials and visual teaching aids (e.g., posters and graphs). Demonstrations are very useful. Also, owing to a 1997 Supreme Court ruling, provinces must now pay for sign language interpreters for deaf clients when they receive medical treatment.

Acute Care

When clients enter acute care settings for therapeutic management of sensory deficits or as a result of traumatic injury, you should try to maximize sensory function existing at the time. Safety is an obvious priority until sensory status is either stabilized or improved. For example, clients with sensory deficits have a high risk for falls in the acute care environment. It also becomes very important to know the extent of any existing sensory impairment before the acute episode of illness so that you can reinforce what the client already knows about self-care or plan for more instruction before and following discharge.

Clients who are acutely ill are also at risk for developing sensory alterations from the constant activity around them and the frequent monitoring that may be required. Your main challenge becomes introducing regular, meaningful stimulation so that clients maintain

➤ BOX 48-10 Communication Methods

Clients With Aphasia

Listen to the client and wait for the client to communicate.

Do not shout or speak loudly (hearing loss is not the problem).

If the client has problems with comprehension, use simple, short questions and facial gestures to give additional clues.

Speak of things that are familiar and of interest to the client.

If the client has problems speaking, ask questions that require simple yes or no answers or blinking of the eyes. Offer pictures or a communication board so that the client can point to communicate.

Give the client time to understand, be calm and patient, and do not pressure or tire the client.

Avoid patronizing and childish phrases.

Make a note at the nursing station that the client is aphasic.

Clients With an Artificial Airway

Use pictures, objects, or word cards so that the client can point to communicate.

Offer a pad and pencil or Magic Slate for the client to write messages.

Do not shout or speak loudly.

Give clients time to write messages as they may be easily fatigued.

Provide an artificial voice box (vibrator) for the client with a laryngectomy to use to speak words or phrases.

Clients With Hearing Impairment

Get the client's attention. Do not startle the client when entering the room. Do not approach a client from behind. Be sure the client knows you wish to speak.

Face the client and stand or sit on the same level. Be sure your face and lips are illuminated to promote lip-reading. Keep hands away from the mouth.

If the client wears glasses, be sure they are clean so that your gestures and face can be seen.

If the client wears a hearing aid, make sure it is in place and working.

Speak slowly and articulate clearly. Older adults may take longer to process verbal messages.

Use a normal tone of voice and inflections of speech. Do not speak with something in your mouth.

When you are not understood, rephrase rather than repeat the conversation.

Use visible expressions. Speak with your hands, your face, and your eyes.

Do not shout. Loud sounds are usually higher pitched and may impede hearing by accentuating vowel sounds and concealing consonants. If it is necessary to raise your voice, speak in lower tones.

Speak toward the client's best or unaffected ear. Use written information to enhance the spoken word.

Do not restrict a deaf client's hands. Ensure that IV lines are not secured to both of the client's hands if the preferred method of communication is sign language.

Avoid speaking from another room or while walking away.

Make a note at the nursing station that the client has a hearing impairment or is deaf.

a clearer perception of their immediate environment. Ongoing explanations help orient the client to any new stimuli within their environment and reduce fear and disorientation.

Orientation to the Environment. The client with recent sensory impairment requires a complete orientation to the immediate environment. Reorientation to the institutional environment may be provided by ensuring that name tags on uniforms are visible, addressing the client by name, explaining where the client is (especially if clients are transported to different areas for treatment), and using conversational cues to time or location. Reduce the tendency for clients to become confused by offering short, simple, repeated explanations and reassurance. Family members and visitors can also help orient clients to the hospital surroundings.

Clients with serious visual impairment must feel comfortable in knowing the boundaries of the immediate environment. Blind or severely visually impaired clients may want to touch the boundaries of a room or objects to gain a sense of their surroundings. The client may need to walk through a room and feel the walls to establish a sense of direction. You can help by describing furniture or equipment within the room. As it takes time to absorb a room's arrangement, the client may need further reorientation, with the nurse explaining the location of key items (e.g., call light, telephone, and chair).

It is important to keep all objects in the same position and place. Simply moving a chair aside may create a dangerous safety hazard. Ensure that you ask the client if any item should be arranged to make ambulation easier. Traffic patterns should be kept clear, and use of furniture with sharp edges should be avoided. The client who is blind needs extra time to perform tasks and a detailed description of how to perform an activity.

Bedridden clients are at risk for sensory deprivation. Normally, movement gives an integrated awareness of the self through vestibular and tactile stimulation. A person's sensory perception is influenced by movement patterns. The limited movement of bedrest changes how a person interprets the environment; surroundings seem different, and objects seem to assume shapes different from normal. A person who is on bedrest requires routine stimulation through range-of-motion exercises, positioning, and participation in self-care activities (as appropriate). Comfort measures such as washing the client's face and hands and providing back rubs can help improve the quality of stimulation and lessen the chance of sensory deprivation. Planning time to talk with clients is also essential. Explain unfamiliar environmental noises and sensations. As well, a calm, unhurried approach during contact with a client gives you quality time to help reorient and familiarize the client with care activities. The client who is well enough to read will benefit from a variety of reading materials.

Communication. The most common language disorder following a stroke is aphasia. As a result of a disruption in blood flow to the brain, the speech centre becomes damaged, altering a person's ability to use or understand spoken words. Depending on the type of aphasia, the inability to communicate can be frustrating and frightening. You should initially establish very basic communication and recognize that aphasia does not indicate intellectual impairment or degeneration of personality. Explain situations and treatments that are pertinent to your client because he or she may be able to understand the spoken word (see Box 48–10). Because a stroke often causes partial or complete paralysis of one side of the client's body, an aphasic client may need special assistive devices. Communication boards have been developed for several levels of disability. Sensitive pressure switches, activated by the touch of an ear, the nose, or the chin, can control electronic communication boards (Ebersole et al., 2005). Clients who have had a stroke usually require referrals to speech therapists to develop appropriate rehabilitation plans.

In acute care hospitals or long-term care facilities, nurses often care for clients with artificial airways (see Chapter 39). For example, an endotracheal tube is inserted into the oropharynx and down through the vocal cords of the larynx into the upper bronchus. The placement of the tube prevents a client from speaking. In this case, you must use special communication methods to help the client express needs (see Box 48–10). The client may be completely alert and able to hear and see you normally. Giving the client time to convey needs and requests is very important. Communication techniques such as use of a communication board or a laptop computer can be used to foster clients' communication with those around them.

Controlling Sensory Stimuli. Excessive stimuli for clients at risk for sensory overload should be controlled. You can reduce sensory overload by organizing the care plan. Combining activities such as dressing changes, bathing, and vital sign measurement in one visit prevents the client from becoming overly fatigued. Coordination with laboratory and radiology departments may help minimize the number of procedures the client must undergo. Encourage, as appropriate, a family member to sit quietly with a client or involve the client in an undemanding, repetitive activity, such as combing hair. The client also needs scheduled time for rest and quiet. Planning for rest periods often requires cooperation from family, visitors, and health care colleagues. Many nursing care units have instituted a set time for rest periods.

When clients experience sensory overload or deprivation, the resultant behaviour can be difficult for family or friends to accept. Encourage the family not to argue with or contradict the confused client but to explain calmly the client's location and identity and the time of day. Engaging the client in a normal discussion about familiar topics may assist in reorientation. Prearranging tests and procedures with departments reduces the amount of time needed for tests and examinations. Anticipating client needs, such as voiding, helps reduce uncomfortable stimuli.

You can also try to control extraneous noise in and around the client's room. It may be necessary to ask a roommate to lower the volume on a television or to move the client to a quieter room. Equipment noise should be kept to a minimum. Bedside equipment not in use, such as suction and oxygen equipment, should be turned off. You also should try to avoid abrupt loud noises, such as suddenly causing the overbed table to adjust to the lowest level. Nursing staff should also try to control laughter or conversation at the nurses' station. Nurses should allow clients to close room doors.

When the client leaves an acute care setting for home, you should communicate with colleagues in the home care setting about the interventions that helped the client adapt to sensory problems. Similarly, information describing the client's existing sensory deficits should be reported. Continuity of care is achieved when the client is required to make only minimal changes to the plan of care in the home setting.

Safety Measures. The client with recent visual impairment often requires help with walking. The presence of an eye patch, frequently instilled eye drops, and the swelling of eyelid structures following surgery are just a few factors that cause a client to need more assistance than usual. A sighted guide can give confidence to the visually impaired person and ensure safe mobility. Ebersole et al. (2005) list four suggestions for a sighted guide:

- Ask the blind client if he or she wants a "sighted guide."
- If assistance is accepted, offer an elbow or arm. Instruct the client to grasp your arm just above the elbow. If necessary, physically assist the person by guiding his or her hand to your arm or elbow.
- Go one half-step ahead and slightly to the side of the blind person. The shoulder of the person should be directly behind your shoulder. If the person is frail, place his or her hand on your forearm.
- Relax and walk at a comfortable pace. Warn the client when you approach doorways or narrow spaces.

While walking the client, describe the course of movement and ensure that obstacles have been removed. A client with visual impairment should never be left standing alone in an unfamiliar area. For clients who undergo eye surgery, it is important to teach family members techniques for assisting with ambulation. For those clients who are blind, mobility training is available from CNIB. Guide dogs may also prove useful.

A visually impaired client who spends considerable time in bed should have a call light nearby. Necessary objects should be placed in front of the client to prevent falls caused by reaching over the bedside. Side rails may also be useful to provide added security. At night, a night light reduces the time required for the eyes to adapt to the dark and allows the client to see well enough to function without keeping the regular light on.

Nurses often rely on clients in health care settings to report unusual sounds, such as a suction apparatus running improperly or an IV pump alarm. However, the client with a hearing loss may not hear such sounds and thus requires careful monitoring by the nurse. The client can also benefit from learning to use vision to discover sources of danger. For example, you should face the client when speaking, use simple sentences, and speak more slowly and at a normal volume. It is wise to note on the intercom button and the client's chart if the client is deaf or blind. A client lacking the ability to speak cannot call out for assistance. Clients should have message boards or the call light easily available.

Clients with reduced tactile sensation risk injury when their conditions confine them to bed because they are unable to sense pressure on bony prominences or the need to change position. These clients rely on nurses for timely repositioning, moving tubes or devices they may be lying on, and turning them to avoid skin breakdown. When the client is less able to sense temperature variations, you should be extra cautious when applying heat and cold therapies and preparing bathwater. You must check the condition of the client's skin frequently.

Restorative and Continuing Care

Maintaining Healthy Lifestyles. After a client has experienced a sensory loss, it becomes important to understand the implications of the loss and to make the adjustments needed to continue a normal lifestyle. Sensory impairments need not prevent a person from leading an active, rewarding life. Many of the interventions applicable to health promotion, such as adapting the home environment, can be used after a client leaves an acute care setting.

Understanding Sensory Loss. Clients who have experienced a recent loss must understand how to adapt so that their living environments can be safe and appropriately stimulating. All family members should understand the way that a client's sensory impairment affects normal daily activities. Family and friends can be more supportive when they understand sensory deficits and the types of elements that worsen or lessen sensory problems. For example, family and friends need to learn how to communicate with the person with a hearing loss. Resources are available within a community that provide information that assists clients with personal management needs. For example, CNIB, the Canadian Hearing Society, and the Canadian Association of the Deaf offer resource materials and product information.

Socialization. The ability to communicate is gratifying. It tests our intellect, opens opportunities, and allows us to exchange the feelings we have about others. When interactions are hindered by sensory alterations, a person can feel ineffective and lose self-esteem. If clients feel socially unaccepted, they will perceive sensory losses as seriously impairing their quality of life.

Interacting with others can become a burden for many clients with sensory alterations. Asking people to continually repeat what they say is both embarrassing and exhausting for a client with hearing loss. Many clients lose the motivation to engage in social situations. As a person withdraws from interaction, a deep sense of loneliness can develop. You can introduce therapies to reduce loneliness, particularly for older clients (Box 48–11). In addition, family members need to learn to focus on a person's ability rather than on the disability. It should not be assumed, for example, that a person who is hard of hearing does not wish to speak. A blind person can still enjoy a walk through a park with a companion describing the sights around them.

Promoting Self-Care. The ability to perform self-care is essential for self-esteem. Frequently, family members and nurses believe that clients with sensory impairments require assistance when, in fact, they can help themselves. Useful guidelines are available to assist clients with visual or tactile impairment so that they can help themselves with daily living activities. For example, a meal tray can be set up as though food on the tray and condiments and drinks around the tray are numbers on the face of a clock (Figure 48–5). The visually impaired client can easily become oriented to the items after the nurse or family member explains each item's location.

The client with visual problems may need assistance in reaching toilet facilities safely. Safety bars should be installed near the toilet. It may be helpful to have the bar a different colour than the wall for easier visibility. Towels should never be placed on safety bars because they may interfere with a person's grasp. Toilet paper should be within easy reach. The use of sharply contrasting colours, especially red, on drawers and other places helps promote functional independence. Choosing clothes that match can be an issue, but techniques such as hanging clothes together on a hanger or marking them with similar labels often overcome this difficulty. The client's preference must always be considered when helping to arrange or buy clothes.

If tactile sense is diminished, the client can dress more easily with zippers or Velcro strips, pullover sweaters or blouses, and elasticized waists. If a client has partial paralysis and reduced sensation, the affected side should be dressed first. Dressing training, using a step-by-step process, is often useful to help a person relearn this skill following a stroke with resultant hemiplegia (Suzuki et al., 2006).

Clients with proprioceptive problems may lose balance easily. Floor mats should have rubberized, skid-proof bottoms. They should be checked and replaced as needed. Bathrooms should have nonskid surfaces in the tub and shower. Grab bars should be installed either vertically or horizontally in tubs and showers, depending on how the client is able to grasp or hold on to the bar. You can instruct family members to supervise ambulation and sitting, make frequent checks to prevent falls, and help caution the client against leaning forward.

Any sensory impairment has a significant influence on body image, and it is important for the client to feel well groomed and attractive. Some clients may need assistance with basic grooming. Others may need assistance with medication selection, clothing identification, and learning to manage routine procedures, such as blood pressure and glucose monitoring. A variety of aids are available to help persons with varying types of sensory deficits. It is important to assist clients in maintaining a degree of independence and in having as much control over the management of their care and lifestyle as possible.

BOX 48-11 FOCUS ON OLDER ADULTS

Interaction Strategies With a Focus on Older Adults

- Spend time with a person, either in silence or in conversation.
- Use physical contact—holding a hand, embracing a shoulder—to convey caring.
- Recommend alterations in living arrangements if physical isolation is a factor.
- Assist older adults to maintain contact with people important to them.
- Help obtain information about mutual help groups.
- Arrange for security escort services as needed.
- Suggest that the client obtain a pet that is easy to care for.
- Link the client with religious or other organizations attuned to the social needs of older adults.

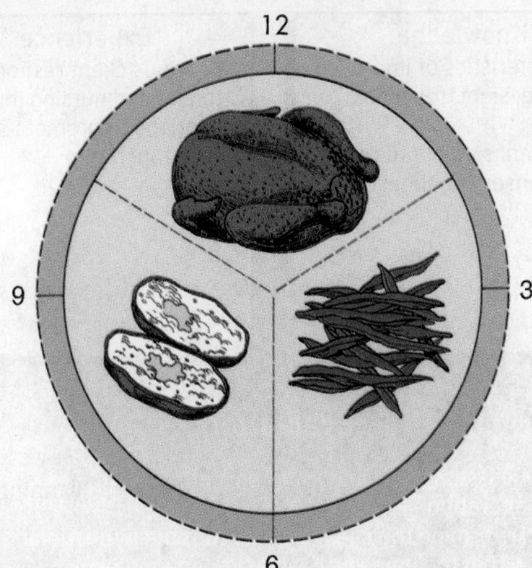

Figure 48-5 Location of food using the clock as a frame of reference.

❖Evaluation

Client Care

It is essential to determine whether care measures maintain or improve clients' ability to interact and function within their environment. Only clients themselves will know if their sensory abilities are improved and which interventions or therapies are the most successful (Figure 48–6). To evaluate the effectiveness of nursing interventions, you will use critical thinking and make comparisons with the baseline sensory assessment data to evaluate if sensory alterations have changed.

As the nurse, you determine if expected outcomes have been met. The nature of the sensory alteration influences the way you evaluate the outcome of care. For example, you use proper communication techniques with a client with a hearing deficit and then evaluate whether the client has gained the ability to hear or interact more effectively. When expected outcomes have not been achieved, it may be necessary to change interventions or alter the client's environment. Family members may need to be involved in support of the client. You may also consult with the multidisciplinary team (e.g., physician, occupational therapist, audiologist) for suggestions to achieve unmet needs. The client must be involved in all evaluation and planning activities.

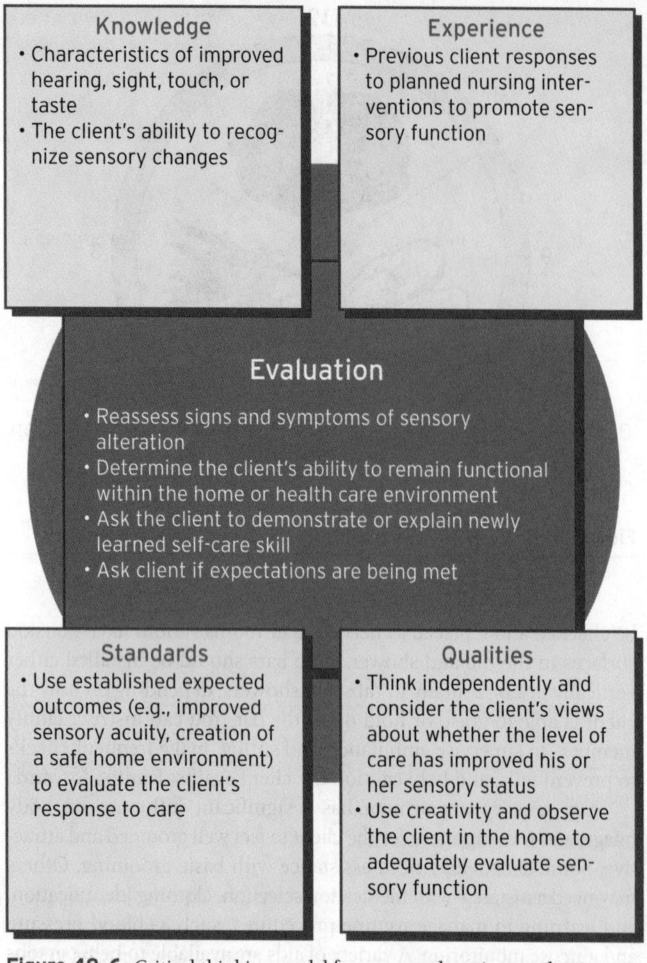

Figure 48-6 Critical thinking model for sensory alterations evaluation.

If nursing care has been directed at improving sensory acuity, evaluate the integrity of the sensory organs and the client's ability to perceive stimuli. Any interventions designed to relieve problems associated with sensory alterations are evaluated on the basis of the client's ability to function normally without injury. When you attempt to directly or indirectly (through education) alter the client's environment, evaluation is directed at observing whether the client makes environmental changes. When client teaching is designed to improve a client's sensory function, it is important to determine whether the client is following recommended therapies. Asking the client to explain or demonstrate self-care skills evaluates the level of learning that has occurred. It may be necessary to reinforce previous instruction if learning has not taken place.

Client Expectations

If you have successfully developed a good relationship with a client and have a therapeutic plan of care, subtle behaviours often indicate the level of the client's satisfaction. Note whether the client responds appropriately, such as by smiling. As well, observe whether the client interacts more and is not asking to have information repeated. However, it is important for you to ask the client if his or her sensory needs have been met. For example, you may ask the client, "Can you tell me if you feel we have done all we can do to help improve your ability to hear?" If the client's expectations have not been met, then you need to spend more time understanding the client's needs and specific preferences. Ask the client, "How can the health care team better meet your needs?" Working closely with the client and family will enable you to redefine expectations that can be realistically met within the limits of the client's condition and therapies. Interventions are effective when goals and expectations have been met.

* KEY CONCEPTS

- Sensory reception involves stimulation of sensory nerve fibres and transmission of impulses to higher centres within the brain.
- When sensory function is impaired, the sense of self is impaired and can affect one's ability to socialize.
- Sensory deprivation results from an inadequate quality or quantity of sensory stimuli.
- Aging usually results in a gradual decline of acuity in all senses.
- Clients who are older, immobilized, or confined in isolated environments are at risk for sensory alterations.
- Assessment of a client's health promotion habits helps reveal risks for sensory impairment.
- An older adult may not admit to a sensory loss.
- An assessment of hazards in the environment requires the nurse to tour living areas in the home and to look for conditions that increase the chances of accidents.
- The plan of care for clients with sensory alterations needs to include participation by family members. The extent of support from family members and friends can influence the quality of sensory experiences.
- The plan of care may differ if the sensory alteration is chronic or short term in nature.
- Clients with sensory deficits develop alternative ways of communicating that rely on other senses.
- Care of clients at risk for sensory deprivation includes introducing meaningful and pleasant stimuli for all senses.
- To prevent sensory overload, the nurse controls stimuli and orients the client to the environment.
- Clients with artificial airways can communicate effectively with communication boards, laptop computers, and written messages.

* CRITICAL THINKING EXERCISES

1. Mr. Tully is a 54-year-old farmer who is having a physical examination. Overall, his health is good. His wife reports that over the past year, he has lost interest in being involved in social gatherings, is more irritable, and often has asked her to repeat what was said. Recently, he has complained of a constant buzzing in his ears. What assessment data are needed? What specific interventions may be needed?

2. Mrs. Marfell, 79 years old, is visiting the outpatient cardiac centre for a routine checkup. You notice that she needed help reading the physical forms. She also told you she is having increased difficulty driving at night. What additional assessment data should you gather from Mrs. Marfell?

3. You have an opportunity to speak with a group of parents and students regarding the importance of hearing protection. What information would you share with this varied age group to promote healthy hearing?

✻ REVIEW QUESTIONS

1. The following sense enables a person to be aware of the position and movement of body parts without seeing them:
   1. Auditory
   2. Kinesthetic
   3. Tactile
   4. Gustatory
2. A sense that allows a person to recognize an object's size, shape, and texture is
   1. Stereognostic
   2. Kinesthetic
   3. Tactile
   4. Gustatory
3. A client who is in constant pain and undergoes frequent monitoring of vital signs is at risk for experiencing sensory
   1. Deprivation
   2. Deficits
   3. Overload
   4. Stimuli
4. Proprioceptive changes after 60 years of age include increased
   1. Hearing and vision impairment
   2. Difficulty with balance, spatial orientation, and coordination
   3. Hearing impairment and difficulty with balance and coordination
   4. Vision impairment and difficulty with spatial orientation
5. For a hearing-impaired client to hear a spoken conversation, the nurse should
   1. Approach a client quietly from behind
   2. Face the client when speaking and use a louder-than-normal tone of voice
   3. Select a public area to have a spoken conversation
   4. Face the client when speaking and speak slower and at a normal volume
6. When obtaining a history of the client's hearing loss, the nurse should ask,
   1. "How long have you been deaf?"
   2. "Do you also have vision problems?"
   3. "Why don't you pay attention to me while I speak?"
   4. "How does your hearing now compare with your hearing a year ago?"
7. A realistic goal for an older adult client who drives is to
   1. Drive very slowly all of the time
   2. Use rear-view and side-view mirrors when changing lanes
   3. Always drive at night to prevent sun glare
   4. Drive during rush hour when others are on the road
8. To prevent hearing impairment among children, a nursing intervention is to teach parents, schoolteachers, and children to
   1. Avoid activities in which crowds and loud noises occur
   2. Delay childhood immunizations until hearing can be verified
   3. Take precautions when involved in activities associated with high-intensity noises
   4. Administer antibiotics to reduce the risk of infections
9. A high priority in a home assessment for a client with diminished olfaction is the inclusion of
   1. A low-temperature water setting
   2. Extra lighting in hallways
   3. Smoke detectors on all levels
   4. Amplified telephone receivers
10. Sensory deficits happen when a problem with sensory reception or perception occurs. As a result, clients may
    1. Withdraw socially to cope with the loss
    2. Rely solely on one sense
    3. Respond normally to stimuli
    4. Function safely within their environment

✻ RECOMMENDED WEB SITES

The Canadian Hearing Society: http://www.chs.ca/
The Canadian Hearing Society provides services that prevent hearing loss and promote the independence of deaf and hearing-impaired people.

Canadian Helen Keller Centre: http://www.chkc.org/main/index.htm
The Canadian Helen Keller Centre (CHKC) provides training programs to individuals who are deaf-blind to help them increase and maintain their independence and autonomy, access services in the community, and decrease isolation. The Web site outlines links relevant to deaf-blindness and communicating with people who are deaf-blind.

Canadian National Institute for the Blind: http://www.cnib.ca/
CNIB is a national, voluntary organization that offers information and support to people with visual loss.

VoicePrint: http://www.voiceprintcanada.com
VoicePrint is a nonprofit audio newsstand that broadcasts international, national, regional, and local stories from over 600 Canadian newspapers and magazines.

49

Care of Surgical Clients

Original chapter by Lynn Schallom, MSN, CCRN, CCNS

Canadian content written by

Frances Fothergill-Bourbonnais, RN, BScN, MN, PhD

objectives

Mastery of content in this chapter will enable you to:

- Define the key terms listed.
- Understand the aspects of perioperative nursing care.
- Differentiate between classifications of surgery and types of anaesthesia.
- List factors to include in the preoperative, intraoperative, and postoperative assessment of a surgical client.
- Demonstrate postoperative exercises: diaphragmatic breathing, coughing, incentive spirometer use, turning, and leg exercises.
- Design a preoperative teaching plan.
- Prepare a client for surgery.
- Explain the nurse's role in the operating room.
- Describe the rationales for nursing interventions designed to prevent postoperative complications.
- Explain the differences and similarities in caring for ambulatory (outpatient) surgical clients versus inpatient surgical clients.

key terms

Abdominal gas, p. 1328
Ambulatory surgery, p. 1290
Antiembolism stockings, p. 1318
Atelectasis, p. 1295
Bariatric, p. 1295
Cholecystectomy, p. 1290
Circulating nurse, p. 1317
Clinical pathways, p. 1302
Conscious sedation, p. 1319
Convalescence, p. 1319
Dehiscence, p. 1295
Dermatomes, p. 1323
General anaesthesia, p. 1318
Informed consent, p. 1302
Latex sensitivity, p. 1314
Local anaesthesia, p. 1319
Malignant hyperthermia, p. 1323
Paralytic ileus, p. 1324
Perioperative nursing, p. 1289
Pneumatic compression devices, p. 1304
Postanesthesia Recovery Score (PARS), p. 1320
Postanesthesia Recovery Score for Ambulatory Patients (PARSAP), p. 1321
Preoperative teaching plan, p. 1300
Regional anaesthesia, p. 1318
Scrub nurse, p. 1317

media resources

evolve Web Site

- Audio Chapter Summaries
- Glossary
- Multiple-Choice Review Questions
- Skills Performance Checklists
- Student Learning Activities
- Video Clips
- Weblinks

Companion CD

- Glossary
- Interactive Learning Activities
- Fluids and Electrolytes Tutorial
- Test-Taking Skills

Perioperative nursing care includes care given before (preoperative), during (intraoperative), and after (postoperative) surgery. Surgical procedures generally take place in a hospital, although some minor surgical procedures can be conducted in a physician's office. Perioperative nursing is based on your understanding of several important principles, including the following:

- Excellence in perioperative practice
- Multidisciplinary teamwork
- Effective and therapeutic communication and collaboration with the client, the client's family, and the surgical team
- Effective and efficient client assessment and intervention in all phases
- Advocacy on behalf of the client and the client's family
- Understanding of cost containment

You must practise surgical asepsis, thoroughly document care, and emphasize client safety in all phases of care. The nursing process provides a basis for perioperative nursing, with you individualizing strategies so that the client receives continuity of care from admission into the health care system through convalescence. By using the nursing process, you can help to anticipate needs and minimize complications.

The continuing care of the surgical client has shifted from hospital-based convalescence to home-based convalescence, with the client and family assuming increased responsibility. As the length of hospital stays decreases, the educational needs of the clients and their families increase. Clients are sent home with complex medical or surgical conditions that require education and follow-up. Effective teaching and early discharge planning are essential to ensure positive surgical outcomes (Gershenson et al., 1999).

History of Surgical Nursing

Surgery gave physicians the means to treat conditions that were difficult or impossible to manage solely through medicinal applications. Early surgeons had little knowledge of the principles of asepsis, and anaesthesia techniques were primitive and unsafe. Indeed, the early surgeon's success was based on speed. The discovery of anaesthesia in the 1840s revolutionized surgery. Anaesthesia provided a combination of analgesia, muscle relaxation, and amnesia, which allowed the time for surgical procedure to be extended. The value of handwashing and the development of germ theory in the 1860s (Pasteur) and 1870s (Koch) triggered the study of aseptic technique, which reduced postoperative infections and mortality. Joseph Lister (1827–1912) was associated with antisepsis or listerism. Initially, antisepsis was one way to protect clients from pathogens in the environment. After experimenting with carbolic acid dressings and continuous carbolic acid sprays during surgical operations, in 1867 Lister described a reduced incidence of gangrene and mortality. He eventually abandoned carbolic acid by 1890, when Koch demonstrated heat to be more effective than chemicals for sterilizing instruments (Porter, 1997). Therefore, Pasteur, Lister, and Koch helped provide a scientific basis to prevent infection in hospitals.

Asepsis and the techniques associated with it ensured that the client did not acquire in-hospital infections. Germ theory influenced nursing practice through the creation of carefully delineated procedures designed to preserve asepsis (McPherson, 1996). Nurses working in the first operating rooms (ORs) cleaned the rooms and equipment, prepared the solutions and dressings, performed technical tasks such as obtaining supplies, administered anaesthetics as graduates, and occasionally accompanied clients to the surgical ward to deliver nursing care.

In Canada, OR nursing began to be part of training at Montreal General Hospital in 1890 ("Nurses life in the Montreal General Hospital," 1892). Toronto General Hospital, St. Michael's Hospital in Toronto, and Winnipeg General Hospital quickly followed suit. OR nursing in the early twentieth century became organized around the therapeutic technology of surgery. Nurses ensured that the aseptic conditions of the surgical environment were maintained by all personnel and, along with physicians, became the first specialists in anaesthesia. As sterile ORs developed, OR nursing became a specialty separate from anaesthesia and surgical nursing. Two roles emerged: the sterile scrub nurse, who handled the instruments and passed them to the surgeon, and the circulating nurse, who ensured that all sponges used in operations were accounted for outside the client's body and that aseptic conditions were maintained. OR nursing was confined to activities in and around the OR and was a well-established field of practice by the 1920s. During the Second World War, a proliferation of courses that focused on OR nursing developed. These postdiploma courses subsequently enabled nurses to join the military, where they were highly valued to work with trauma clients (Toman et al., 2006).

The trend of including OR experience in training continued into the 1960s. However, during the 1970s, a change occurred in nursing education, whereby nurses were expected to acquire a broad knowledge base. As a result, many schools eliminated OR experience from the curriculum, believing that it focused only on manual skills (Sandelowski, 2000). What was not recognized was the role that OR nurses play in ensuring clients' comfort and safety and continuity of care before, during, and after surgery.

In 1956 in the United States, the Association of Operating Room Nurses (AORN) was formed. The organization developed standards of nursing practice that outlined the perioperative nurse's scope of responsibility. AORN was the first nursing organization to develop structure, process, and outcome standards as defined by the American Nurses Association. AORN has since changed its name to the Association of Perioperative Registered Nurses; however, AORN is still used as its acronym. The organization continues to be a driving force for the practice of perioperative nursing and works closely with Canadian associations.

In Canada, the Operating Room Nurses Association of Canada (ORNAC) was founded in 1983. The mission of this professional organization is the promotion and advancement of excellence in the provision of perioperative care to patients and the professional growth and personal enhancement of perioperative registered nurses. It sets the standards for Canadian perioperative nursing practice. Specifically, ORNAC values are (1) knowledge—education and research are essential components that guide practice, (2) collaboration—with nurses within the specialty, organizations, agencies, and other disciplines, (3) respect—for worth, quality, diversity, and the importance of the clients and of each other, (4) professionalism—to advance the specialty, and (5) continuous improvement—to achieve excellence. Opportunities exist in conjunction with the Canadian Nurses Association for registered nurses to obtain perioperative nursing certification. In addition to the National Association of PeriAnesthesia Nurses of Canada (NAPAN), there are provincial associations. For example, the Ontario PeriAnesthesia Nurses Association (OPANA) was founded in 1985 to represent all nurses involved in the care of clients in the postanaesthetic phase. OPANA (2005) has developed standards of perianaesthesia nursing practice that are used in Ontario hospitals.

Ambulatory Surgery

A recent change in the surgical field is the advent of **ambulatory surgery**, also referred to as outpatient surgery, short-stay surgery, or same-day surgery. These services are provided within a hospital setting. More than half of all surgical procedures are conducted on an outpatient basis, including ophthalmic, gastroenterological, gynecological, otorhinolaryngologic, orthopedic, cosmetic and restorative, and general procedures. Same-day surgery, in which the client is admitted on the day of surgery and observed overnight (23-hour admission), has also increased in popularity.

There are distinct benefits for the client who has ambulatory surgery. Anaesthesia drugs that metabolize rapidly with few after-effects allow for shorter operative times. Nurses recognize the benefit of early postoperative ambulation and encourage clients to assume an active role in recovery. Ambulatory surgery also results in shorter hospital stays, as clients are frequently discharged the day of or the day after surgery. This reduces the possibility of acquiring nosocomial infections, which occur when clients become colonized with bacteria found in the hospital setting. Procedures such as tumour biopsies and gallbladder removal (**cholecystectomy**) can now be done using laparoscopic procedures. Because of the small incision required, a laparoscopic cholecystectomy involves a hospital stay of only a few to 24 hours and a recovery period of a week. In contrast, a traditional open cholecystectomy requires a large abdominal incision and involves a hospital stay of 3 to 5 days and a recovery period of at least 4 weeks. Thus, many surgeons use laparoscopic procedures for a variety of surgical interventions, thereby decreasing the length of surgery, hospitalization, and associated costs. Laparoscopic approaches are just one form of the increasingly used minimally invasive surgical techniques (MIS). For example, specialized instruments and cameras can be used for procedures such as pyeloplasty (Francis & Winfield, 2006) or total hip arthroplasty (Sculco et al., 2004). Construction of new operating room suites is increasingly providing dedicated rooms for MIS, and thus OR nurses are being educated regarding their role related to the techniques as well as intraoperative client care.

Ambulatory surgery requires that nurses provide extensive preoperative and postoperative teaching and assess the client's available support systems and readiness for self-care. For example, discharge education should include potential complications and what to do about them, instructions on care of incision sites and any drains, instructions on diet and activity, telephone numbers to contact, and managing pain. Surgical day care nurses frequently call clients at home on the day after surgery to inquire about how recovery is progressing. As well, home care nurses must refer the client to appropriate community agencies or services such as physiotherapy.

Scientific Knowledge Base

Classification of Surgery

Surgical procedures are classified according to seriousness, urgency, and purpose (Table 49–1). A procedure may fall into more than one classification. For example, surgical removal of a disfiguring scar is minor in seriousness, elective in urgency, and reconstructive in purpose. Frequently, the classes overlap. An urgent procedure is also considered major in seriousness. As well, the same operation may be performed for different reasons on different clients. For example, a gastrectomy may be performed as an emergency procedure to resect a bleeding ulcer or as an urgent procedure to remove a cancerous growth. The classification indicates to you the level of care a client might require. Hospitals have a system for prioritizing the booking of surgeries based on their classification.

The American Society of Anesthesiologists (ASA) assigns classification on the basis of a client's physiological condition, independent of the proposed surgical procedure (Table 49–2). Intraoperative difficulties occur more frequently with clients who have a poor physical status classification (Rothrock, 2003). ASA physical status class I and class II clients are acceptable for ambulatory surgery. Clients in classes IV and V require inpatient surgery because they are at higher risk for complications (e.g., cardiac or pulmonary complications). The ASA classification system is used in Canadian hospitals.

Nursing Knowledge Base

Nursing knowledge offers important contributions for the care of the perioperative client. For example, nursing research has shown the benefit of preoperative education in promoting positive client outcomes after surgery. Structured preoperative teaching that includes the AORN (2004) standards and return demonstration of postoperative exercises has been shown to improve outcomes such as pain severity, pulmonary function, length of stay, and clients' levels of anxiety.

Significant evidence-based knowledge is also available for proper wound care interventions. Nursing research has contributed to what is known about the characteristics of wound healing and the types of applications most likely to be beneficial (see Chapter 47).

Within the OR setting, knowledge has improved the standards for infection control and client safety. For example, surgical hand scrubs (see Chapter 33) can now be performed without the use of brushes as a result of research that has shown the efficacy of alcohol-based hand antiseptics in reducing bacteria on the skin (Hobson et al., 1998; Larson et al., 1990). Evidence-based practice changes within the OR improve the quality of care for surgical clients and ultimately improve client outcomes.

Critical Thinking

Successful critical thinking requires a synthesis of knowledge, information gathered from clients, experience, critical thinking qualities, and intellectual and professional standards. Clinical judgements require you to anticipate the information necessary, analyze the data, and make decisions regarding client care. A client's condition is always changing. During assessment (Figure 49–1), you must consider all of the elements that contribute to making appropriate nursing diagnoses.

When caring for the perioperative client, you make clinical care decisions by integrating knowledge of anatomy, physiology, pathophysiology, and the surgical stress response with previous experiences in caring for surgical clients and information gathered from the client, such as medical and surgical history, potential for surgical risk, and coping resources. Your use of critical thinking qualities such as perseverance is needed to develop a plan of care that provides successful perioperative care (e.g., airway management, infection control, pain management, and discharge planning). Professional standards and guidelines developed by, for example, AORN, NAPAN, and ORNAC, provide valuable information for perioperative management and evaluation of processes and outcomes. However, you should review guidelines within the context of new and emerging evidence-based practice and agency policies.

➤ TABLE 49-1 Classification of Surgical Procedures

Type	Description	Examples
Seriousness		
Major	Involves extensive reconstruction or alteration in body parts; poses great risks to well-being	Coronary artery bypass, colon resection, removal of larynx, resection of lung lobe
Minor	Involves minimal alteration in body parts; often designed to correct deformities; involves minimal risks compared with major procedures	Cataract extraction, facial plastic surgery, tooth extraction
Urgency		
Elective	Is performed on basis of client's choice; is not essential and may not be necessary for health	Bunionectomy, facial plastic surgery, hernia repair, breast reconstruction
Urgent	Is necessary for client's health; may prevent additional problems from developing (e.g., tissue destruction or impaired organ function); not necessarily emergency	Excision of cancerous tumour, removal of gallbladder for stones, vascular repair for obstructed artery (e.g., coronary artery bypass)
Emergency	Must be done immediately to save life or preserve function of body part	Repair of perforated appendix, repair of traumatic amputation, control of internal hemorrhaging
Purpose		
Diagnostic	Surgical exploration that allows physician to confirm diagnosis; may involve removal of tissue for further diagnostic testing	Exploratory laparotomy (incision into peritoneal cavity to inspect abdominal organs), breast mass biopsy
Ablative	Excision or removal of diseased body part	Amputation, removal of appendix, cholecystectomy
Palliative	Relieves or reduces intensity of disease symptoms; will not produce cure	Colostomy, debridement of necrotic tissue, resection of nerve roots
Reconstructive or restorative	Restores function or appearance to traumatized or malfunctioning tissues	Internal fixation of fractures, scar revision
Procurement for transplant	Removal of organs, tissues, or both from a person pronounced brain dead for transplantation into another person	Kidney, heart, or liver transplant
Constructive	Restores function lost or reduced as result of congenital anomalies	Repair of cleft palate, closure of atrial septal defect in heart
Cosmetic	Performed to improve personal appearance	Blepharoplasty to correct eyelid deformities; rhinoplasty to reshape nose

➤ TABLE 49-2 Physical Status (PS) Classification of the American Society of Anesthesiologists

Class	Description	Characteristics and Examples
PS-I	A normal, healthy client	No physiological, biological, or organic disturbance
PS-II	A client with a mild systemic disease	Disease imposes minimal restriction on activity; e.g., hypertension (HTN), obesity, diabetes mellitus
PS-III	A client with a severe systemic disease that limits activity but is not incapacitating	Disease limits activity (e.g., severe diabetes with systemic complications); history of myocardial infarction, angina pectoris, or poorly controlled HTN
PS-IV	A client with a severe systemic disease that is a constant threat to life	Severe cardiac, pulmonary, renal, hepatic, or endocrine dysfunction
PS-V	A moribund client who is not expected to survive without the operation	Surgery is done as a last recourse or as a resuscitative effort; e.g., major multi-system or cerebral trauma, ruptured aneurysm, or large pulmonary embolus
PS-VI	A client declared brain dead whose organs are being removed for donor purposes	

Note: The addition of an "E" to the physical status class indicates emergency surgery, such as PS-IE, PS-IIE, and so on.

Adapted from *Physical status (PS) classification*. (2008). Reprinted with permission of the American Society of Anesthesiologists (520 N. Northwest Highway, Park Ridge, IL, 60068-2573, http://asahq.org/clinical/physicalstatus.htm).

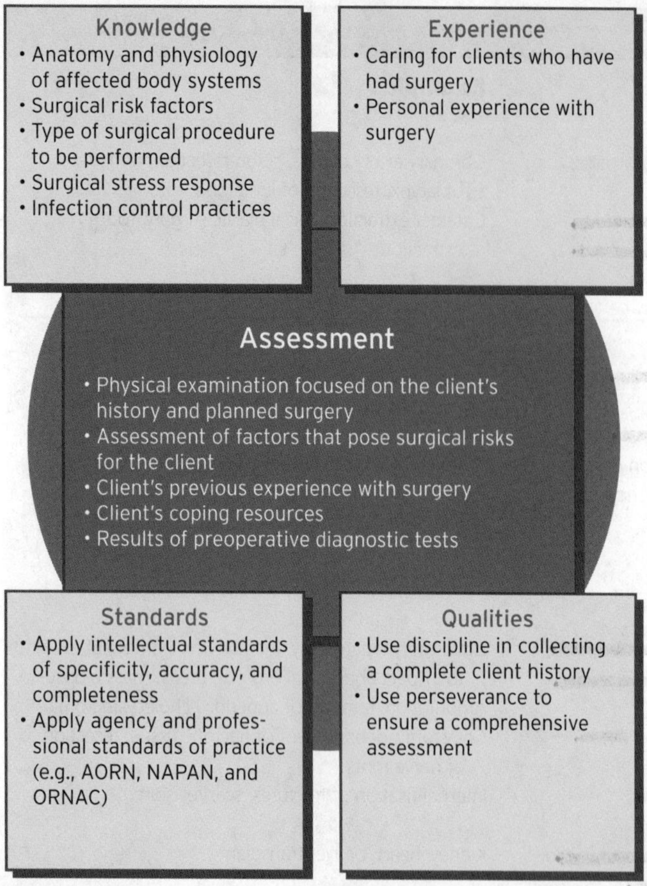

Figure 49-1 Critical thinking model for surgical client assessment.

The Nursing Process in the Preoperative Surgical Phase

Surgical clients enter the health care setting in different stages of health. A client may enter the hospital on a predetermined day feeling relatively healthy and prepared to face elective surgery. In contrast, a victim of a motor vehicle collision may face emergency surgery with no time to prepare. The ability to establish rapport and maintain a professional relationship with the client is an essential component of the preoperative phase. You must do this quickly but compassionately and effectively.

The surgical client may undergo tests and procedures to confirm or rule out problems requiring surgery. Most testing is performed before the day of surgery. Usually clients scheduled for ambulatory surgery have tests done several days before surgery. Testing done the day of surgery is usually limited to such tests as glucose monitoring for the client with diabetes. You must be familiar with the tests, their purpose, and how to monitor results.

The client meets many health care personnel, including surgeons, anaesthesiologists, physiotherapists, and nurses. All play a role in the client's care and recovery. Family members attempt to provide support through their presence but face many of the same stressors as the client. You must communicate effectively with the client and family because the nurse–client relationship is the foundation of care (see Chapter 18). You should assess the client's physical, emotional, and spiritual well-being and cultural heritage; recognize the degree of surgical risk; coordinate diagnostic tests; identify nursing diagnoses and nursing interventions; and establish outcomes in collaboration with the client and his or her family. Pertinent data and the care plan are communicated among the members of the surgical team.

❖Assessment

The assessment of the surgical client is intended to establish the client's baseline preoperative function to assist in preventing and recognizing possible postoperative complications. Assessment of the surgical client can be extensive. Ambulatory and same-day surgical programs require that client data be completed several days in advance. A multidisciplinary team approach is essential. Clients are admitted only hours before the surgical event; thus, you must organize and verify data obtained preoperatively to implement a perioperative care plan. This occurs not only with the ambulatory care client, but also with the client who will require a more prolonged hospital stay. Increasingly, clients are admitted on the day of surgery, even for such major procedures as open heart surgery and bowel surgery.

Most assessments begin in the physician's office or in a preadmission clinic before admission for surgery. Clients may answer a self-report inventory and you may complete an initial physical examination, draw or complete laboratory tests, begin teaching, identify potential risks, answer questions, and initiate paperwork. This streamlines the care required for the client on the day of surgery. In the immediate preoperative period, you assess the client's understanding of previous teaching and individualize client and family care.

The physician performs a comprehensive history and physical examination with follow-up by the preadmission nurse. In this case, you need to review assessments and testing already completed and to highlight significant information (e.g., the client being on diuretics). You focus on key measurements for all body systems to ensure that no obvious problems are overlooked and that the client has understood education previously provided. Even though the surgeon will screen the client before scheduling surgery, preoperative assessment occasionally reveals an abnormality that delays or cancels surgery. For example, the client may have a cough and low-grade fever on admission. This may indicate the onset of infection, and the surgeon will need to be notified immediately.

Nursing Health History

You should conduct an initial interview to collect a client history similar to that described in Chapter 32. If a client is unable to relate all of the necessary information, you should rely on family members as resources.

Medical History

A review of the client's medical history should include past illnesses and the primary reason for currently seeking medical care. The client's current medical record and medical records from past hospitalizations are excellent sources of data.

Pre-existing illnesses can influence the choice of anaesthetic agents used and the client's ability to tolerate surgery and reach full recovery (Table 49–3). Candidates for ambulatory surgery must be carefully screened for medical conditions that may increase the risk for complications during or after surgery. For example, a client who has a history of congestive heart failure may experience a further decline in cardiac function both intraoperatively and postoperatively. Intravenous (IV) fluids may need to be administered at a slower rate, or a diuretic may need to be given if blood transfusions are required.

TABLE 49-3 Medical Conditions That Increase the Risks of Surgery

Type of Condition	Reason for Risk
Bleeding disorders (thrombocytopenia, hemophilia)	Increase risk of hemorrhaging during and after surgery.
Diabetes mellitus	Increases susceptibility to infection and may impair wound healing due to altered glucose metabolism and associated circulatory impairment. Stress of surgery may cause increases in blood glucose levels.
Heart disease (recent myocardial infarction, dysrhythmias, congestive heart failure) and peripheral vascular disease	Stress of surgery causes increased demands on myocardium to maintain cardiac output. General anaesthetic agents depress cardiac function.
Obstructive sleep apnea	Administration of opioids increases risk of airway obstruction postoperatively. Clients will desaturate as revealed by drop in oxygen saturation by pulse oximetry.
Upper respiratory infection	Increases risk of respiratory complications during anaesthesia (e.g., pneumonia and spasm of laryngeal muscles).
Liver disease	Alters metabolism and elimination of drugs administered during surgery and impairs wound healing and clotting time because of alterations in protein metabolism.
Fever	Predisposes client to fluid and electrolyte imbalances and may indicate underlying infection.
Chronic respiratory disease (emphysema, bronchitis, asthma)	Reduces client's means to compensate for acid–base alterations (see Chapter 40). Anaesthetic agents reduce respiratory function, increasing risk for severe hypoventilation.
Immunological disorders (leukemia, acquired immune deficiency syndrome [AIDS], bone marrow depression, and use of chemotherapeutic drugs or immunosuppressive agents)	Increase risk of infection and delayed wound healing after surgery.
Abuse of street drugs	Clients who abuse drugs may have underlying disease (HIV, hepatitis), which can affect response to anaesthesia and surgery and the healing process.
Chronic pain	Regular use of pain medications may result in higher tolerance, a reduced effect from repeated doses of the same analgesic class (Ferrell & Coyle, 2001). Increased doses of analgesics may be required to achieve postoperative pain control.

Risk Factors

Various conditions and factors increase a person's risk when undergoing surgery. Knowledge of risk factors enables you to take necessary precautions in planning care.

Age. Very young clients are at risk during surgery because of their immature physiological status. During surgery, nurses and physicians are especially concerned with maintaining an infant's normal body temperature. The infant's shivering reflex is underdeveloped, and often wide temperature variations occur. Anaesthesia adds to the risk because anaesthetics can cause vasodilation and heat loss.

During surgery, an infant has difficulty maintaining a normal circulatory blood volume. The total blood volume of an infant is considerably less than that of an older child or an adult. Therefore, even a small amount of blood loss can be serious. A reduced circulatory volume makes it difficult for the infant to respond to increased oxygen demands during surgery. In addition, the infant is highly susceptible to complications associated with dehydration. However, if blood or fluids are replaced too quickly, overhydration may occur. Other important and unique aspects of a child's surgical care include airway management, treatment of seizures, management of temperature alterations, identification and treatment of emergence delirium and delayed emergence from anaesthesia, treatment of pain and agitation, and availability of age-appropriate emergency equipment and medications.

Older clients are also at risk for complications. With advancing age, a client's physical capacity to adapt to the stress of surgery is hampered because of deterioration in certain body functions. Despite the risk, the majority of clients undergoing surgery are older adults. Table 49–4 summarizes the physiological factors that place older clients at risk during surgery.

➤TABLE 49-4 Physiological Factors That Place the Older Adult at Risk During Surgery

Alterations	Risks	Nursing Implications
Cardiovascular System		
Degenerative change in myocardium and valves	Reduced cardiac reserve	Assess baseline vital signs. Recognize the longer time period required for heart rate to return to normal after stress on the heart and evaluate the occurrence of tachycardia accordingly (Eliopoulos, 2001).
Rigidity of arterial walls and reduction in sympathetic and parasympathetic innervation to heart	Alterations predispose client to postoperative hemorrhage and rise in systolic and diastolic blood pressure	Maintain adequate fluid balance to minimize stress to the heart. Ensure that blood pressure level is adequate to meet circulatory demands.
Increase in calcium and cholesterol deposits within small arteries; thickened arterial walls	Predispose client to clot formation in lower extremities	Instruct client on techniques for performing leg exercises and proper turning. Apply elastic stockings, sequential compression devices.
Integumentary System		
Decreased subcutaneous tissue and increased fragility of skin	Prone to pressure ulcers and skin tears	Assess skin every 4 hours; pad all bony prominences during surgery. Turn or reposition at least every 2 hours (see Chapter 47).
Pulmonary System		
Stiffening and reduction in size of the rib cage	Reduced vital capacity	Instruct client on proper technique for coughing, deep breathing, and use of spirometer.
Reduced range of movement in diaphragm	Residual capacity (volume of air left in lung after normal breath) increases, reducing amount of new air brought into lungs with each inspiration	When possible, have client ambulate and sit in chair frequently.
Stiffened lung tissue and enlarged air spaces	Alteration reduces blood oxygenation	Obtain baseline oxygen saturation; measure as indicated throughout perioperative period.
Renal System		
Reduced blood flow to kidneys	Increased risk of shock when blood loss occurs	For clients hospitalized before surgery, determine baseline urinary output for 24 hours.
Reduced glomerular filtration rate and excretory times	Limits ability to eliminate drugs or toxic substances	Assess for adverse response to drugs.
Reduced bladder capacity	Voiding frequency increases, and larger amount of urine stays in bladder after voiding. Sensation of need to void may not occur until bladder is filled.	Instruct client to notify nurse immediately when sensation of bladder fullness develops. Keep call light and bedpan within easy reach. Toilet every 2 hours, or more frequently if indicated.
Neurological System		
Sensory losses, including reduced tactile sense	Decreased ability to respond to early warning signs of surgical complications	Inspect bony prominences for signs of pressure that client may not sense. Orient client to surrounding environment. Observe for nonverbal signs of pain.
Decreased reaction time	Confusion after anaesthesia. Delirium postoperatively is an acute confusional state with rapid onset, disturbance in consciousness, and change in cognition (Hogan et al., 2006). Delirium can be caused by medications such as narcotics, or by physiological reasons such as infection or dehydration.	Allow adequate time to respond, process information, and perform tasks. Institute Best Practice Guidelines (BPGs) on screening for and on caregiving strategies for older adults with delirium, dementia, and depression (Registered Nurses' Association of Ontario [RNAO], 2004a, 2004b). Institute fall precautions (RNAO, 2002b).

TABLE 49-4 Physiological Factors That Place the Older Adult at Risk During Surgery *continued*

Metabolic System		
Lower basal metabolic rate	Reduced total oxygen consumption	Ensure adequate nutritional intake when diet is resumed, but avoid intake of excess calories.
Reduced number of red blood cells and hemoglobin levels	Ability to carry adequate oxygen to tissues is reduced	Administer necessary blood products. Monitor blood test results.
Change in total amounts of body potassium and water volume	Greater risk for fluid or electrolyte imbalance occurs	Monitor electrolyte levels and supplement as necessary.
Impaired thermoregulatory mechanisms	Cold operating rooms; exposure of body parts during procedure, IV fluids, medications	Ensure careful, close monitoring of client temperature; provide warm blankets; monitor cardiac function; warm IV fluids.

Nutrition. Normal tissue repair and resistance to infection depend on adequate nutrients. Surgery intensifies this need. After surgery, a client requires at least 1500 kcal/day to maintain energy reserves. Increased protein, vitamins A and C, and zinc facilitate wound healing (see Chapters 43 and 47). A malnourished client is prone to poor tolerance of anaesthesia, negative nitrogen balance, delayed blood clotting mechanisms, infection, poor wound healing, and the potential for multiple organ failure. If a client is having elective surgery, attempts to correct nutritional imbalances should be made before the surgery. However, if a malnourished client must undergo an emergency procedure, efforts to restore nutrients will occur after surgery.

Obesity. Obesity increases surgical risk by reducing respiratory and cardiac functions. Hypertension, coronary artery disease, diabetes mellitus, and congestive heart failure are common in the **bariatric** (obese) population. Embolus, **atelectasis** (partial or total collapse of the alveoli), and pneumonia are also more frequent postoperative complications in the obese client. The client may have difficulty resuming normal physical activity after surgery. The obese client is susceptible to poor wound healing and wound infection because of the structure of fatty tissue, which contains a poor blood supply. This slows delivery of essential nutrients, antibodies, and enzymes needed for wound healing (see Chapter 43). It is often difficult to close the surgical wound of an obese client because of the thick adipose layer. An obese client is also at risk for **dehiscence** (opening of the suture line).

Immunocompetence. For the client with cancer, radiation therapy may be given preoperatively to reduce the size of the cancerous tumour so that it can be removed surgically. Radiation has some unavoidable effects on normal tissue, such as excess thinning of skin layers, destruction of collagen, and impaired vascularization of tissue. Ideally, the surgeon waits 4 to 6 weeks after completion of radiation treatments to perform surgery. Otherwise, the client may face serious problems with wound healing. In addition, chemotherapeutic drugs used for cancer treatment, immunosuppressive medications used to prevent rejection after organ transplantation, and steroids used to treat a variety of inflammatory conditions increase the risk for infection.

Fluid and Electrolyte Imbalances. The body responds to surgery as if it is a form of trauma. As a result of the adrenocortical stress response, sodium and water are retained and potassium is lost within the first 2 to 5 days after surgery. The severity of the stress response influences the degree of fluid and electrolyte imbalances. The more extensive the surgery, the greater is the stress response. A client who is hypovolemic or who has serious preoperative electrolyte alterations is at significant risk during and after surgery. For example, an excess or depletion of potassium increases the chance of dysrhythmia during or after surgery. If the client has pre-existing renal, gastrointestinal, or cardiovascular abnormalities, the risk for fluid and electrolyte alterations is even greater.

Pregnancy. The perioperative care plan must address the needs of both the mother and the developing fetus. Surgery is performed on a pregnant client only on an emergency basis. All of the mother's major systems are affected during pregnancy. For example, cardiac output significantly increases, as does respiratory tidal volume to accommodate the increase in metabolic rate. Gastrointestinal motility decreases, hormone levels increase, and energy levels decrease with advancing pregnancy. Laboratory and hemodynamic values change. Fibrinogen levels increase, making pregnant clients more susceptible to the development of deep vein thrombosis because of increased coagulability. Hemoglobin and hematocrit levels decrease, mostly as a result of the effects of hemodilution (increased circulating volume). The white blood cell (WBC) count is elevated when the woman is near term and postpartum without the presence of infection. However, infection always must be ruled out in the presence of an elevated WBC count. General anaesthesia is administered with caution because of the increased risk for fetal death and preterm labour. Psychological considerations for mother and family are essential.

Previous Surgeries

A client's past experience with surgery can influence physical and psychological responses to a procedure. You should ask the client to recall the previous type of surgery, level of discomfort, extent of disability, and overall level of care provided are factors. Address any complications that the client experienced. It is also important to assess clients for motion sickness, nausea, and vomiting with previous surgeries (Gan, 2002; Tramer, 2001). These factors increase the risk for aspiration. Prior anaesthesia records may be a useful source of information if previous problems such as malignant hyperthermia occurred. This information helps you to anticipate the client's preoperative and postoperative needs.

Previous surgery also may influence the level of physical care required after a surgical procedure. For example, a client who has had a previous thoracotomy for resection of a lung lobe has a greater risk for postoperative pulmonary complications than does a client with intact, normal lungs.

Perceptions and Understanding of Surgery

The surgical experience affects not only the client, but also the entire family. You therefore must prepare both the client and the family for the surgical experience. Identifying a client's and family's knowledge, expectations, and perceptions allows you to plan teaching and to provide individualized emotional support measures.

Each client feels fearful when entering the surgical setting. Some fears are due to past hospital experiences, warnings received from friends and family, or lack of knowledge. You must assess the client's understanding of the planned surgery and its implications. For example, you need to determine whether the client recognizes that she will have a breast biopsy performed, not a mastectomy. You might ask questions such as "Tell me what you think will happen before and after surgery," or "Explain what you know about your surgery." If a client is misinformed or unaware of the reason for surgery, you must confer with the physician before the client is sent to the surgical suite. You also determine whether further explanations are needed related to routine preoperative and postoperative procedures. When a client is well prepared and knows what to expect, you reinforce the client's knowledge and maintain accuracy and consistency.

Medication History

If a client regularly uses prescription or over-the-counter medications, the surgeon or anaesthesiologist may temporarily discontinue the drugs before surgery or adjust the dosages. Certain medications have special implications for the surgical client, creating greater risks for complications or interacting negatively with anaesthetic agents (Table 49–5). For example, you instruct clients in a preadmission unit to ask the physician whether usual medications should be taken on the morning of surgery. Clients also should be asked whether any herbal preparations are used, because many clients do not view herbs as medications and may omit them from their medication history (see Chapter 35). Certain herbs may interfere with the action of other medications (a pharmacist must be consulted). In the preadmission clinic, you determine whether the client is taking any herbal medications. For hospitalized clients, prescription drugs taken preoperatively are automatically discontinued postoperatively unless the physician reorders them. It is important for you to be aware of the client's previous medications that likely will need to be resumed postoperatively (e.g., antihypertensives).

Allergies

You must assess for allergies to drugs that may be given during a phase of the surgical experience. In addition, it is critical to assess for latex, food, and contact allergies (e.g., allergies to tape, ointments, or solutions). A client may be too young or have too few exposures to drugs to know whether he or she has any allergies. The type of allergic response is also very important to assess. Allergies need to be delineated from unpleasant side effects. For example, the client may state that codeine causes nausea (a side effect), or that it causes hypotension and confusion (an allergy). When asking a client about allergies, realize that the term *allergy* can be confusing for some clients. Asking

TABLE 49-5 Drugs With Special Implications for the Surgical Client

Drug Class	Effects During Surgery
Antibiotics	Antibiotics can potentiate action of anaesthetic agents. For example, if taken within 2 weeks before surgery, aminoglycosides (gentamicin, tobramycin, neomycin) may cause mild respiratory depression due to depressed neuromuscular transmission.
Antidysrhythmics	Antidysrhythmics can reduce cardiac contractility and impair cardiac conduction during anaesthesia.
Anticoagulants	Anticoagulants alter normal clotting factors and thus increase risk of hemorrhaging. They should be discontinued at least 48 hours before surgery. Aspirin is a commonly used medication that can alter clotting mechanisms.
Anticonvulsants	Long-term use of certain anticonvulsants (e.g., phenytoin [Dilantin] and phenobarbital) can alter the metabolism of anaesthetic agents.
Antihypertensives	Antihypertensives may interact with anaesthetic agents to cause bradycardia, hypotension, and impaired circulation. They may inhibit synthesis and storage of norepinephrine in sympathetic nerve endings.
Corticosteroids	With prolonged use, corticosteroids cause adrenal atrophy, which reduces the body's ability to withstand stress. Before and during surgery, dosages may be temporarily increased.
Insulin	Diabetic clients' need for insulin after surgery is altered. Stress response and IV administration of glucose solutions can increase dosage requirements after surgery. Decreased nutritional intake can decrease dosage requirements.
Diuretics	Diuretics potentiate electrolyte imbalances (particularly potassium) after surgery.
Nonsteroidal anti-inflammatory drugs (NSAIDs)	NSAIDs inhibit platelet aggregation and may prolong bleeding time, increasing susceptibility to postoperative bleeding.
Herbal therapies: ginger, gingko, ginseng	Some herbal therapies have the ability to affect platelet activity and increase susceptibility to postoperative bleeding. Ginseng may increase hypoglycemia with insulin therapy.

a client whether he or she has ever "had a problem with a medication or substance" may be another helpful approach to questioning.

It is critical that the client be asked specifically about latex allergies because a latex-free environment must be provided for clients with latex allergies. You ensure that a list of the client's allergies is noted appropriately in his or her chart, the hospital computer system, or both, as well as in any other places designated by institutional policy, such as an allergy band.

Smoking Habits

The client who smokes is at greater risk for postoperative pulmonary complications than one who does not. The chronic smoker already has an increased amount and thickness of mucous secretions in the lungs. General anaesthetics increase airway irritation and stimulate pulmonary secretions, which are retained as a result of reduction in ciliary activity during anaesthesia. After surgery, the client who smokes has greater difficulty clearing the airways of mucous secretions and needs education on the importance of postoperative deep breathing and coughing (see Chapter 39). In addition, smoking can compromise blood flow to the heart, which can affect the response to surgery. Nurses play a key role in reducing smoking, and there are nursing Best Practice Guidelines (BPGs) on smoking cessation (RNAO, 2007). Nicotine replacement therapy may be required to support the client, who smokes, during the postoperative period.

Alcohol Ingestion and Substance Use and Abuse

Habitual use of alcohol and illegal drugs predisposes the client to adverse reactions to anaesthetic agents. The client also may experience a cross-tolerance to anaesthetic agents, necessitating higher-than-normal amounts. In addition, the physician may need to increase postoperative dosages of analgesics. Clients with a history of excessive alcohol ingestion also may be malnourished, which may contribute to delayed wound healing. These clients are also at risk for liver disease, portal hypertension, and esophageal varices (predisposing the client to bleeding disorders). The client who habitually uses alcohol and is required to remain in the hospital for longer than 24 hours is also at risk for acute alcohol withdrawal and its more severe form, delirium tremens.

Family Support

It is important for you to determine the extent of the client's support from family members or friends. Because blood relations do not always define family, it is best to have the client identify his or her sources of support (see Chapter 20). Surgery often results in temporary or permanent disability that requires added assistance during recovery. The client usually cannot immediately assume the same level of physical activity enjoyed before surgery. Often a client returns home with dressings to change or exercises to perform. With ambulatory surgery, clients and families assume responsibility for postoperative care. The family is an important resource for the client with physical limitations and provides the emotional support needed to motivate the client to return to a previous state of health. In addition, the family may better remember preoperative and postoperative teaching.

You should ask whether family members or friends could provide support. The client may want someone else present when you provide instructions or explanations. Family presence should be encouraged when feasible, especially for clients having ambulatory surgery. Often a family member can become the client's coach, offering valuable support during the postoperative period, when the client's participation in care is vital.

Occupation

Surgery may result in physical alterations that hinder or prevent a person from returning to work. You should assess the client's occupational history to anticipate the possible effects of surgery on recovery and eventual work performance. Explain any restrictions before a client returns to work, such as lifting, use of the extremities, or climbing stairs. When a client is unable to return to his or her job, you should confer with a social worker or occupational therapist to refer the client to job-training programs or to help the client seek economic assistance.

Preoperative Pain Assessment

Surgical manipulation of tissues, treatments, and positioning on the OR table may result in postoperative pain for the client. Pain is a very personal experience and requires an individualized care plan. Preoperatively, you should conduct a comprehensive pain assessment (see Chapter 42), including the client's and the family's expectations for pain management after surgery. You should begin education regarding pain management as soon as possible (Barnes, 2001). The preoperative assessment should introduce to the client the use of a pain instrument to rate the presence and severity of pain postoperatively (see Chapter 42). Several instruments for both pediatric and adult clients have shown reliability and validity (Summers, 2001). Frequent pain assessments with the client are necessary in terms of alerting you to treat the pain and assessing the adequacy (outcome) of pain interventions.

Review of Emotional Health

Surgery is psychologically stressful. The client may be anxious about the surgery and its implications. Clients often feel that they are powerless over their situation. Family members may perceive the client's surgery as a disruption of their lifestyle. Hospitalization and the recovery period at home may be lengthy. The family is usually concerned about the client returning to a normal, productive life. When the client has chronic illness, the family may be fearful that surgery will result in further disability or may be hopeful that it will improve their lifestyle. To understand the impact of surgery on a client's and a family's emotional health, you should assess the client's feelings about surgery, self-concept, body image, and coping resources.

It is often difficult to assess feelings thoroughly when ambulatory surgery is scheduled. You usually have less time to establish a relationship with the client. Box 49–1 describes a study that explored the needs of ambulatory surgery clients. In some outpatient surgical programs, you may visit with a client in the home or on the telephone before surgery. In a hospital room, you should choose a time for discussion after admitting procedures or diagnostic tests have been completed. Explain to the client that it is normal to have fears and concerns. The client's ability to share feelings partially depends on your willingness to listen, be supportive, and clarify misconceptions.

If the client feels powerless, you should attempt to determine the reason. The medical diagnosis may generate apprehension of increased dependence and loss of physical or mental function. The thought of being "put to sleep" under anaesthesia may create concern about loss of control. Many clients feel the need to retain the power to make decisions about treatment. You must assure clients of their right to ask questions and seek information.

A client may be angry about the need for surgery. For example, a young person may feel that it is unfair to have a disorder that typically affects older people. Surgery may occur at a time when it is inconvenient or potentially disruptive. The client occasionally may express anger verbally at you or the physician. Being argumentative or overly

BOX 49-1 RESEARCH HIGHLIGHT

Perceptions of Ambulatory Care Surgical Clients

Research Focus

Since the 1990s, the number of ambulatory surgical procedures has increased continually. Nursing care of the ambulatory surgery client must be condensed into shorter time periods in all phases of perioperative care. Ensuring that the needs of ambulatory surgery clients are met is imperative.

Research Abstract

The purpose of Costa's (2001) study was to explore the perceptions and views of ambulatory surgery clients. A study of 16 clients who underwent abdominal surgical procedures in an ambulatory surgery setting was conducted. Data were collected by intensive semi-structured interviews conducted in the surgeon's office at the time of the 1-week postoperative appointment. Topics in the interviews included clients' recall of how they felt the night before surgery, experiences on the day of surgery, whether the perioperative experience met their expectations, feelings regarding the discharge process, and the experience of recovering at home. The interviews were then analyzed. Three areas were identified: fear, knowing, and presence. This study supported the importance of the nurse's presence throughout the perioperative experience and provided the perioperative nurse with an understanding of the needs of the ambulatory surgery client.

Evidence-Informed Practice

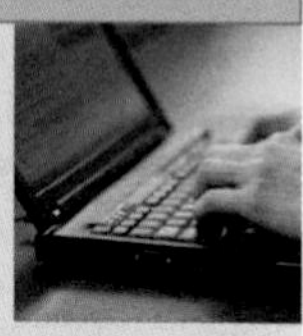

- Fear in general was expressed, and fear of anaesthesia was discussed most often. Frequently, clients discuss their fears indirectly. You must listen to clients for cues and provide them with an opportunity to express their fears.
- Clients often had insufficient knowledge about what to expect preoperatively and postoperatively despite a good understanding of the surgical procedure itself. Education and reinforcement of this type of education is important throughout all phases of the perioperative experience.
- Clients wanted to know that they mattered as an individual. You should address clients by name and listen to individual requests and concerns. Incorporate the individual and the support system into the care plan.
- Clients wanted to know that their nurse was truly there for them, both physically and emotionally.
- Connection with family members or significant others is important throughout the perioperative experience.

References: Costa, M. J. (2001). The lived perioperative experience of ambulatory surgery patients. *AORN Journal, 74*(6), 874–881.

demanding, refusing to cooperate, and criticizing your efforts to provide care are manifestations of the client's anger and anxiety.

Body Image. Surgical removal of any diseased body part often leaves permanent disfigurement, alteration in body function, or concern over mutilation. Loss of certain body functions (e.g., with a colostomy or ureterostomy) may compound a client's fears. You should assess for the body image alterations that clients perceive will result from surgery. Clients will respond differently depending on their culture, self-concept, and degree of self-esteem (see Chapter 26).

Often, surgery changes the physical or psychological aspects of clients' sexuality. Excision of breast tissue, colostomy, ureterostomy, hysterectomy, or removal of the prostate gland may affect the clients' perceptions of their sexuality. Some surgeries (e.g., hernia repairs) require the client to refrain from sexual intercourse temporarily, until the return to normal physical activity.

You should encourage clients to express their concerns about sexuality. The client facing even temporary sexual dysfunction requires understanding and support. Discussions about the client's sexuality should be held with the client's sexual partner so that both individuals can gain a shared understanding of how to cope with limitations in sexual function.

Coping Resources. Assessment of feelings and self-concept helps to reveal whether the client can cope with the stress of surgery. The physiological effects of stress are well documented. Activation of the endocrine system results in the release of hormones and catecholamines (epinephrine, norepinephrine), which results in increases in blood pressure, heart rate, and respiration. Platelet aggregation also occurs, along with many other physiological responses. You must be aware of these responses and assist with stress management (see Chapter 30). Ask the client about past stress management. If the client has had previous surgery, you should determine what behaviours helped to resolve any tension or nervousness. You may instruct the client on relaxation exercises that can help control anxiety.

When reviewing the client's coping resources, ask the client about specific family members and friends who may provide support. Once they are identified, you should include these individuals in any client teaching and interventions aimed at managing stress and anxiety.

Culture

Culture is a system of beliefs that have developed over time and subsequently been passed on through many generations (Lipson et al., 1996). Clients come from diverse cultural and religious backgrounds that affect the way they perceive and react to their surgical experience. If cultural, ethnic, and religious differences are not acknowledged and incorporated into the perioperative care plan, desired surgical outcomes may not be achieved. Therefore, learning about a client's cultural and ethnic heritage helps you provide effective perioperative care. Although it is important to recognize and plan for differences based on culture, you also must recognize that members of the same culture are individuals and may not hold these shared beliefs. Box 49–2 highlights cultural care aspects in the perioperative period.

Client Expectations

Clients rely on their caregivers for information, comfort, pain control, adequate monitoring, and performance of interventions that ensure their safety throughout the surgical experience. This requires you to have a caring attitude, advocate for the client, be skilled in surgical assessment and interventions, and anticipate the client's needs throughout the perioperative period. You must understand the client's expectations in order to develop an individualized care plan. Does the client expect full pain relief or simply to have pain reduced? Does the client expect to be independent immediately after surgery, or does he or she expect to be fully dependent on you or on family members? These are only a few of the questions that need to be asked of the surgical client to establish a care plan congruent with his or her needs and expectations.

Physical Examination

You should conduct a partial or complete physical examination, depending on the client's preoperative condition (see Chapter 32). Assessment focuses on findings related to the client's medical history and on body systems that likely will be affected by the surgery. The

BOX 49-2 CULTURAL ASPECTS OF CARE

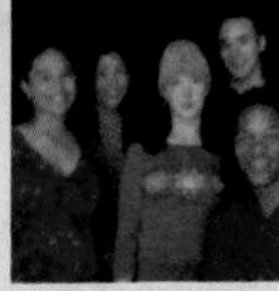

Providing individualized education and perioperative nursing care to clients of various cultural, religious, and ethnic groups can be challenging. Using a variety of resources available within a health care agency, both in the literature and from the Internet, will help you to provide culturally sensitive care.

Implications for Practice

- Preoperative assessment should include a cultural assessment with questions such as primary language spoken, feelings regarding surgery and pain, pain management, expectations, support system, and feelings toward self-care with postoperative implications (e.g., Does client relate to concept of pain? Does client have feelings about gender of caregiver? Does client follow custom that gives family members control over decisions?).
- Use a professional interpreter to communicate with a client whose language is different than yours.
- Use pictures or phrase cards with various languages to communicate with a client whose language is different than yours; these cards can be used to assess pain, comfort, temperature, and so forth.
- Provide preoperative and postoperative educational materials in a variety of languages.

Adapted from De Ruiter, H. P., & Larsen, K. E. (2002). Developing a transcultural patient care Web site. *Journal of Transcultural Nursing, 13*(1), 61–70; and Douglas, M. (1999). Pain as the fifth vital sign: Will cultural variations be considered? *Journal of Transcultural Nursing, 10,* 285.

nursing assessment should complement the surgeon's and anaesthesiologist's physical examination (Barnes, 2002).

General Survey. You should observe the client's general appearance. Gestures and body movements may reflect weakness caused by illness. The client may appear malnourished. Height, body weight, and history of recent weight loss are important indicators of nutritional status.

Preoperative vital signs, including blood pressure while sitting and standing, provide important baseline data with which alterations that occur during and after surgery can be compared. Some institutions request that blood pressure be obtained in both arms for comparison. Anxiety and fear commonly cause elevations in heart rate and blood pressure. As the effects of the anaesthesia diminish after surgery, compare vital sign findings with the preoperative baseline. Preoperative assessment of vital signs is also important to rule out fluid and electrolyte abnormalities (see Chapter 31).

An elevated temperature before surgery is a cause for concern. If the client has an underlying infection, the surgeon may choose to postpone surgery until the infection has been treated. An elevated body temperature increases the risk for fluid and electrolyte imbalances after surgery.

Head and Neck. The condition of oral mucous membranes is one indicator of the client's level of hydration. A dehydrated client is at risk for developing serious fluid and electrolyte imbalances during surgery. Inspection of the soft palate and nasal sinuses can reveal sinus drainage, indicative of respiratory or sinus infection. Cervical lymph node enlargement may reveal local or systemic infection.

You should inspect the jugular veins for distension. Excess fluid within the circulatory system or failure of the heart to contract efficiently may lead to jugular vein distension and reveal a risk for cardiovascular complications during surgery.

During the examination of the oral mucosa, loose or capped teeth must be identified because they could become dislodged during endotracheal intubation. Dentures must be noted so that they can be removed before surgery, especially if general anaesthesia is required.

Integument. You should carefully inspect the skin, especially over bony prominences, such as the heels, elbows, sacrum, and scapula. During surgery, a client must lie in a fixed position, often for several hours. As a result, the client may have an increased risk for pressure ulcers (see Chapter 47), especially if the skin is thin and dry and has poor turgor (Schoonhoven et al., 2002). Chronic use of steroids also increases the client's susceptibility to skin tears. In addition, the overall condition of the skin reveals the client's level of hydration. An older adult is at high risk for alteration in skin integrity from positioning on the OR table, causing pressure.

Thorax and Lungs. Assessment of the client's breathing pattern and chest excursion aids in assessing ventilatory capacity. A decline in ventilatory function places the client at risk for respiratory complications. For example, a client who has high abdominal surgery will have difficulty breathing deeply because of a painful abdominal incision. Auscultation of breath sounds will indicate whether the client has pulmonary congestion or narrowing of airways.

Existing atelectasis or moisture in the airways will be aggravated during surgery. Serious pulmonary congestion may cause postponement of the surgery. Certain anaesthetics can cause laryngeal muscle spasm; thus, if you auscultate wheezing in the airways preoperatively, the client is at risk for further airway narrowing during surgery and after extubation (removal of the endotracheal tube); therefore, the physician should be made aware of these findings.

Heart and Vascular System. You should assess the character of the apical, radial, and peripheral pulses; the capillary refill; and the colour and temperature of the client's extremities. If peripheral pulses are not palpable, a Doppler instrument should be used to assess their presence. Acceptable capillary refill occurs in less than 3 seconds. Measurement of capillary refill and assessment of peripheral pulses are particularly important for the client having vascular surgery or for the client who may have casts or constricting bandages applied to his or her extremities after surgery (see Chapter 32).

Abdomen. You should assess the abdomen for size, shape, symmetry, and presence of distension. Assessment of preoperative bowel sounds is useful as a baseline. You also should ask whether the client has regular bowel movements and inquire about the colour and consistency of stools.

Neurological Status. Preoperative assessment of neurological status is imperative for all clients who will be receiving general anaesthesia. The baseline neurological status assists with the assessment of ascent from anaesthesia. During the health history and physical assessment, observe the client's level of orientation, alertness, and mood, noting whether the client answers questions appropriately and can recall recent and past events. A client who will have surgery for neurological disease (e.g., brain tumour or aneurysm) may demonstrate an impaired level of consciousness or altered behaviour.

If the client is scheduled for spinal anaesthesia, preoperative assessment of gross motor function and strength is important. Spinal anaesthesia causes temporary paralysis of the lower extremities (see Chapter 42). You should be aware if a client enters surgery with weakness or impaired mobility of the lower extremities so that, when the spinal anaesthetic wears off, you will not expect full motor function to return.

Diagnostic Screening

Before a client has surgery, the surgeon may order diagnostic tests to screen for pre-existing abnormalities. The tests ordered are determined by the client's history and physical assessment. Table 49–6 lists common diagnostic tests performed preoperatively based on the client's medical history. The tests ordered are also determined by the procedure itself. For procedures where blood loss is expected (e.g., hip and knee replacements), a type and crossmatch would be indicated preoperatively. The surgeon will designate the number of blood units to have available during surgery. Table 49–7 outlines the purpose and normal values for the more common blood tests. If diagnostic tests reveal severe problems, the surgeon may cancel surgery until the condition stabilizes. You are responsible for the preparation of clients for diagnostic studies and for coordinating completion of the tests. You also review diagnostic results as they become available, not only to alert physicians to these findings and to assist with planning appropriate therapy, but also to integrate these findings into decisions related to client care.

If a client is over age 65 or has heart disease, an electrocardiogram (ECG) is mandatory. The ECG measures the electrical activity of the heart to assess the heart rate, rhythm, and other factors. A chest X-ray (an examination of the condition of the heart and lungs) is required for thoracic surgery or if the client has certain medical conditions.

Pulmonary function testing and arterial blood gas analysis may be performed on clients with pre-existing lung disease. Blood glucose levels are measured on diabetic clients.

Autologous infusions are an option for some clients who choose to donate their own blood before surgery to ease their anxiety over the risk of transfusion-related infections. Although Canadian Blood Services screens all blood donors and blood products for infections such as HIV and hepatitis, some clients are more comfortable donating their own blood. The donation usually must be made several weeks before the scheduled surgery. The client who self-donates may exhibit lower hemoglobin and hematocrit levels on the day of surgery. Autotransfusion via the use of a cell-saver device during surgery may be possible if physicians anticipate large blood loss (e.g., open heart surgery). The cell-saver device, although expensive, returns washed RBCs to the client and has created positive outcomes in terms of length of client stay (Rothrock, 2003). Autologous infusions are commonly used in orthopedic surgery.

➤ TABLE 49-6 Common Diagnostic Tests Performed Preoperatively Based on Client History

History	Tests
Hepatic disease	International normalized ratio (INR); partial thromboplastin time (PTT); liver enzymes, such as serum aspartate aminotransferase; alkaline phosphatase
Cardiovascular disease	BUN, creatinine, complete blood count (CBC), chest X-ray study, electrocardiogram (ECG)
Pulmonary disease	CBC, chest X-ray study, ECG
Central nervous system disease	White blood cell (WBC) count, electrolytes, BUN, creatinine, glucose, and electroencephalography (EEG)
Medications	
Diuretics	Blood urea nitrogen (BUN), creatinine, electrolytes
Steroids	Electrolytes, glucose
Anticoagulants	INR, PTT

❖Nursing Diagnosis

You will cluster patterns of defining characteristics gathered during assessment to identify nursing diagnoses for the surgical client (Box 49–3). The client with pre-existing health problems is likely to have a variety of risk diagnoses. For example, a client with pre-existing bronchitis who has abnormal breath sounds and a productive cough will be at risk for ineffective airway clearance. In addition, a client who undergoes a surgical procedure is at risk for developing infection at the surgical site, the IV site, or the bloodstream (sepsis). A diagnosis of risk for infection will require your attention from admission through convalescence.

The related factors for each diagnosis establish directions for nursing care that will be provided during one or all of the surgical phases. For example, the diagnosis of risk for infection related to an invasive procedure will require different interventions than if the related factor were inadequate immune response. Preoperative nursing diagnoses allow the nurse to take precautions and actions so that the care provided during the intraoperative and postoperative phases is consistent with the client's needs.

Nursing diagnoses made preoperatively will also focus on the potential risks a client may face after surgery. Preventive care is essential so that the surgical client can be managed effectively. The following are common nursing diagnoses relevant to the surgical client:

- *Ineffective airway clearance*
- *Risk for allergy response to latex*
- *Anxiety*
- *Disturbed body image*
- *Risk for imbalanced body temperature*
- *Ineffective breathing pattern*
- *Ineffective coping*
- *Fear*
- *Risk for deficient fluid volume*
- *Risk for infection*
- *Risk for perioperative-positioning injury*
- *Deficient knowledge (specify)*
- *Impaired physical mobility*
- *Acute pain*
- *Powerlessness*
- *Impaired skin integrity*
- *Disturbed sleep pattern*
- *Delayed surgical recovery*

❖Planning

During planning, you once again synthesize information from multiple resources (Figure 49–2). For example, knowledge pertaining to adult learning principles, coupled with the client's unique needs, will ensure a well-designed **preoperative teaching plan**. Critical thinking ensures that the client's care plan integrates your knowledge, previous experience, and established standards of care. Previous experience in caring for surgical clients helps you anticipate how to approach client care (e.g., complications to prevent and anticipate, and methods to reduce anxiety). Professional standards are especially important to

TABLE 49-7 Diagnostic Screening for Surgical Clients

Measurement and Normal Values	Interpretation
Complete blood count (CBC) *Red blood cells (RBCs):* Men: 4.7–5.14 × 10^{12}/L; Women: 4.2–4.87 × 10^{12}/L *Hemoglobin (Hgb):* Men: 132–173 g/L; Women: 117–155 g/L *Hematocrit (Hct):* Men: 0.43–0.49; Women: 0.38–0.44 *White blood cells (WBCs):* Adults and children >2 years: 4.5–11 × 10^9/L	Peripheral venous sample of blood measures RBCs, WBCs, Hgb, and Hct. May reveal infection, low blood volume, and potential for oxygenation problems. Surgeon may order blood replacement.
Serum electrolytes *Sodium (Na):* 136–145 mmol/L *Potassium (K):* 3.5–5.0 mmol/L *Chloride (Cl):* 98–106 mmol/L *Bicarbonate (HCO_3):* 22–26 mmol/L	Peripheral venous sample of blood reveals significant fluid and electrolyte imbalances preoperatively. Attention is given to Na, K, and Cl levels. Intravenous (IV) fluid replacement may be indicated preoperatively.
Coagulation studies *International normalized ratio (INR):* 0.76–1.27 *Activated partial thromboplastin time (APTT):* 30–40 seconds *Platelets:* 150–400 × 10^9	INR, APTT, and platelet counts reveal clotting ability of blood. Reveals clients at risk for bleeding tendencies and thrombus formation.
Serum creatinine *Men:* 53–106 µmol/L *Women:* 44–97 µmol/L	Ability of kidneys to excrete creatinine, a by-product of muscle metabolism, indicates renal function. Elevated level can indicate renal failure.
Blood urea nitrogen (BUN) 2.9–7.5 mmol/L	Ability of kidneys to excrete urea and nitrogen indicates renal function. BUN becomes elevated if client is dehydrated. Preoperative IV fluid replacement may be needed.
Glucose *Fasting:* 4.2–6.1 mmol/L	Finger stick or peripheral blood sample. Clients may require treatment of low or high levels preoperatively and postoperatively. Elevated blood sugar results from a deficiency in insulin secretion (type 1 diabetes), insulin action, or combination of both (type 2 diabetes).

Adapted from Pagana, K. D., & Pagana, T. J. (2007). *Mosby's diagnostic and laboratory test reference* (8th ed.). St. Louis, MO: Mosby; and Van Leeuwen, A. M., Kranpitz, T. R., & Smith, L. (2006). *Davis's comprehensive handbook of laboratory and diagnostic tests with nursing implications.* Philadelphia: F. A. Davis.

BOX 49-3 NURSING DIAGNOSTIC PROCESS

Assessment Activities	*Defining Characteristics*	*Nursing Diagnosis*
Ask client to describe previous surgical experiences.	Client mentions a traumatic prior experience with surgery	*Fear related to knowledge deficit and previous surgical experience*
Ask client about preoperative education and preparation before admission.	Unaware of preoperative testing	
Observe client's nonverbal behaviour.	Client's behaviour indicates fear and tension	
Assess vital signs.	Increased heart rate	

consider when you develop a care plan, as they often provide a scientific basis for selecting effective nursing interventions. You will develop an individualized care plan for each nursing diagnosis (Box 49–4). You and the client will set realistic expectations for care.

Successful planning requires the involvement of both the surgical client and the family in establishing the care plan. Early client involvement minimizes surgical risks and postoperative complications. A client who is well informed about the surgical experience is less likely to be fearful and can prepare to participate in the postoperative recovery phase so that outcomes can be met. Diagnosis, interventions, and outcomes are established to ensure recovery or maintenance of the preoperative state.

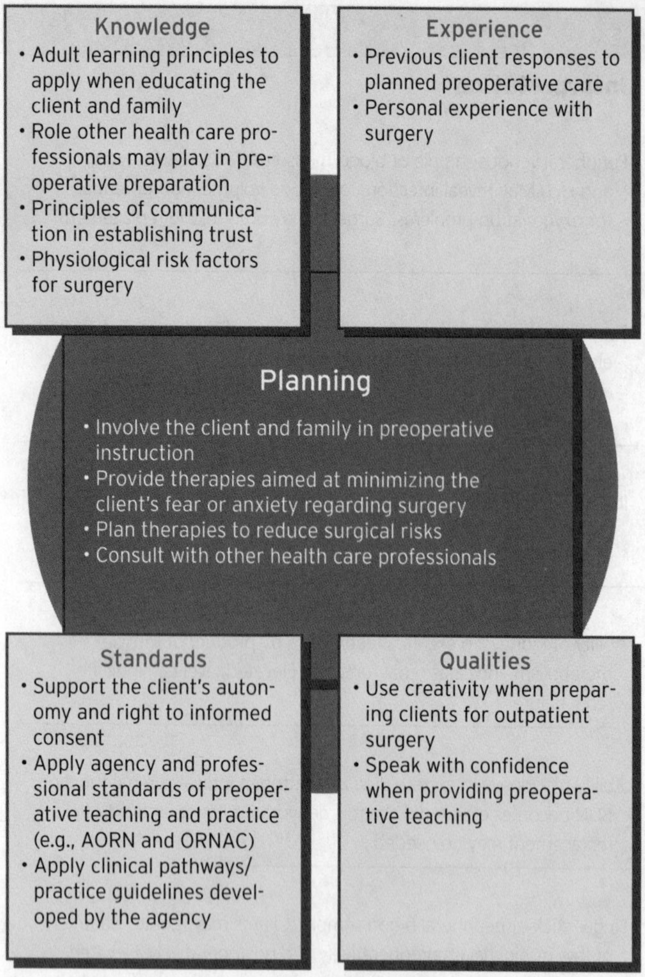

Knowledge
- Adult learning principles to apply when educating the client and family
- Role other health care professionals may play in preoperative preparation
- Principles of communication in establishing trust
- Physiological risk factors for surgery

Experience
- Previous client responses to planned preoperative care
- Personal experience with surgery

Planning
- Involve the client and family in preoperative instruction
- Provide therapies aimed at minimizing the client's fear or anxiety regarding surgery
- Plan therapies to reduce surgical risks
- Consult with other health care professionals

Standards
- Support the client's autonomy and right to informed consent
- Apply agency and professional standards of preoperative teaching and practice (e.g., AORN and ORNAC)
- Apply clinical pathways/ practice guidelines developed by the agency

Qualities
- Use creativity when preparing clients for outpatient surgery
- Speak with confidence when providing preoperative teaching

Figure 49-2 Critical thinking model for surgical client planning.

Goals and Outcomes

The preoperative care plan is based on individualized nursing diagnoses. This plan is reviewed and modified during the intraoperative and postoperative periods. Outcomes established for each goal of care provide measurable behavioural evidence to gauge the client's progress toward meeting the stated goals.

The following example provides a goal of care and expected outcomes relevant for the preoperative surgical client:

- Client is able to verbalize the significance of postoperative exercises.
- Client verbalizes prevention of lung congestion and pneumonia as reasons for deep breathing and coughing exercises and incentive spirometer.
- Client verbalizes promotion of blood flow to prevent leg clots as reason for postoperative leg exercises.
- Client verbalizes rationale for early ambulation, as it improves lung function, assists with return of bowel function, and promotes recovery.

Setting Priorities

Using clinical judgement, you should prioritize nursing diagnoses and interventions based on the assessed unique needs of each client. Clients who need emergency surgery may experience changes in their physiological status that require the nurse to reprioritize quickly. For example, if a client's blood pressure begins to drop, hemodynamic stabilization becomes a priority over education and stress management. Generally, when the preoperative situation is more controlled, the approach to each client must be thorough and reflect an understanding of the implications of the client's age, physical and psychological health, educational level, and cultural and religious practices. Increasingly, clients are preparing advanced medical directives to indicate their wishes should aggressive medical treatment be required after surgery.

Continuity of Care

For ambulatory surgery clients and clients admitted on the day of their scheduled surgeries, preoperative planning occurs days before admission to the hospital. Frequently, preoperative education begins in the physician's office, continues during the scheduled preadmission testing visit, and is reinforced by you on the day of admission. Preoperative instruction gives the client time to think about the surgical experience, make necessary physical preparations (e.g., altering diet or discontinuing medications), and question postoperative procedures. The ambulatory surgical client usually returns home on the day of surgery. Thus, well-planned preoperative care ensures that the client is well informed and able to be an active participant during recovery. The client's family or spouse can also play an active supportive role for the client.

❖Implementation

Preoperative nursing interventions provide the client with a complete understanding of the surgery and prepare the client physically and psychologically for surgical intervention.

Informed Consent

Surgery cannot be legally or ethically performed until a client understands the need for a procedure, the steps involved, the risks, the expected results, and alternative treatments. The surgeon is responsible for explaining the procedure and obtaining the **informed consent**. You may witness the client signing the consent form (see Chapter 9). You ensure that the completed form is placed in the client's medical record, which goes to the OR with the client.

Health Promotion

Health promotion activities during the preoperative phase focus on health maintenance, prevention of complications, and support of possible rehabilitation needs postoperatively.

Preoperative Teaching

Education is an important aspect of the client's surgical experience. Preoperative teaching concerning a client's expected postoperative behaviour, provided in a systematic and structured format with teaching and learning principles, has a positive influence on the client's recovery. Nurses in preadmission clinics may call clients up to 1 week before surgery to answer the client's questions and reinforce explanations. Preoperative information and instructions may include telephone calls, mailings from the physician's office or hospital, preoperative teaching guidelines and checklists, and the use of videotapes or **clinical pathways** (Figure 49–3).

Lookinland and Pool (1998) found that clients who received structured education before admission had better clinical outcomes and were more satisfied. However, despite education being provided to clients, retention of information after discharge is poor, especially

➤ BOX 49-4 **NURSING CARE PLAN**

Deficient Knowledge Regarding Preoperative and Postoperative Care Requirements

Assessment

Mrs. Campana is an 80-year-old woman scheduled to be admitted in 5 days for elective bowel resection. Joe Marrero is the nurse in the clinic surgery service assigned to prepare Mrs. Campana for surgery. During his initial discussion with Mrs. Campana, Joe observes her to be alert and oriented. Mrs. Campana has severely reduced visual acuity but is able to hear Joe's questions clearly.

Assessment Activities	*Findings and Defining Characteristics*
Ask Mrs. Campana about previous surgeries and her experience with them.	She responds, "I had surgery over 20 years ago, and I was in the hospital for 10 days."
Ask Mrs. Campana what she has been told regarding her surgery.	She states that her surgeon explained the procedure using a drawing of the bowel and indicating the location of the part to be removed.
Ask Mrs. Campana what she has been told regarding preoperative preparation and what to expect postoperatively.	She states that she received information from the surgeon's office regarding medicines to stop taking and those she should take on the morning of surgery, her diet before surgery and when to stop eating, and who to call with questions. She does not recall receiving information regarding what to expect postoperatively.
Assess Mrs. Campana's ability to read typical font type.	She is unable to read the text font on the newspaper; she can read the headlines with her glasses.
Assess Mrs. Campana's family and support system for preoperative and postoperative assistance.	She states that her daughter will be coming into town on the day of surgery to help her after surgery.

Nursing Diagnosis: Deficient knowledge regarding preoperative and postoperative care requirements related to lack of exposure to information.

Planning

*Goals (Nursing Outcomes Classification)**	*Expected Outcomes* **Knowledge of Treatment Procedures**
Client will understand the postoperative routines of surgical care by day before surgery.	Client will discuss monitoring routines after surgery by morning of surgery in the preoperative period. Client will be able to describe importance of postoperative exercises by morning of surgery, including turn, cough, and deep breathing; incentive spirometer; leg exercises. Client will be able to describe schedule for activity and nutritional management postoperatively by day 1 after surgery.
Client will participate actively in postoperative recovery activities by day 1 after surgery.	Client will successfully perform postoperative exercises by morning of surgery in the preoperative period.

*Outcome classification labels from Moorhead, S., Johnson, M., & Maas, M. L. (Eds.). (2004). *Nursing Outcomes Classification (NOC)* (3rd ed.). St. Louis, MO: Mosby.

Interventions (Nursing Interventions Classification)† *Teaching in the Preoperative Period*	**Rationale**
Provide client with audiotape program that explains preoperative and postoperative routines. Supply instruction booklet designed for the visually impaired. Make a follow-up call to client and to her daughter to give them an opportunity to ask questions and voice concerns. Document all phases of education—preoperative before admission, day of surgery, and postoperative—provided to client in her record.	Preadmission education can require less teaching time and better performance of exercises on admission. Education has a beneficial effect in reducing postoperative anxiety (Shuldham, 1999).
On admission to hospital, demonstrate to client and daughter the performance of postoperative exercises and how to get out of bed.	Demonstration is an effective method to reinforce didactic instruction.
Explain sensations to be expected postoperatively (e.g., incisional pain that will be controlled with medications, intravenous [IV], nasogastric tube, wound care, frequent vital signs assessments).	Teaching about sensory aspects (what the client sees, feels, smells) should be structured (Shuldham, 1999).
Give client opportunity to return demonstrate postoperative exercises before surgery.	Return demonstration measures client learning and provides an opportunity to reinforce instruction.
Correct any unrealistic expectations the client or daughter may have regarding surgery.	Unrealistic expectations, when unmet, can contribute to client's anxiety. Psychological preparation for surgery reduces anxiety.

†Intervention classification labels from Dochterman, J. M., & Bulecheck, G. M. (Eds.). (2004). *Nursing Interventions Classification (NIC)* (4th ed.). St. Louis, MO: Mosby.

Continued

➤ BOX 49-4 NURSING CARE PLAN *continued*

Evaluation

Nursing Actions	*Client Response and Finding*	*Achievement of Outcome*
Ask client to describe typical monitoring and care activities after surgery. Document evaluation of client's understanding and demonstration of learned activities in client's record.	She is able to verbalize typical monitoring and care after surgery. She states that the instruction booklet and audiotape were both helpful.	Mrs. Campana has a good understanding of the typical postoperative course.
Observe client's demonstration of postoperative exercises.	She is able to demonstrate leg exercises and deep breathing and coughing exercises but is having difficulty with incentive spirometer use.	Mrs. Campana is able to demonstrate most of the postoperative exercises but needs further teaching and practice on incentive spirometer use.
Explore with client and daughter if they have any remaining fears or concerns.	Both Mrs. Campana and her daughter deny any fears or concerns at the present time.	Informational and psychological needs of Mrs. Campana and her daughter have been met.

in the older adult population (Bean & Waldron, 1995). Lee et al. (1998) conducted postdischarge surveys of 206 clients hospitalized over a six-week period. Results from this study indicated that continuity of care was enhanced if education was provided before, during, and after discharge. The researchers found that half of the clients who were contacted requested additional education. Therefore, it seems ideal to attempt perioperative education before admission, during the hospital stay, and after discharge. Including family members in perioperative preparation is advised.

Often a family member is the coach for postoperative exercises when the client returns home from surgery. The family also may recognize untoward events that may unfold once the client is home. Therefore, family members need to be aware of the normal expectations after discharge from hospital. If anxious relatives do not understand routine postoperative events, their anxiety will likely heighten the client's fears and concerns. Preoperative preparation of family members can help to minimize anxiety and misunderstanding.

You should provide clients with information about sensations typically experienced after surgery. Preparatory information helps clients anticipate the steps of a procedure and thus helps them form realistic images of the surgical experience. When events occur as predicted, clients are better able to cope and attend to them. For example, in the OR, the anaesthesiologist may apply ointment to clients' eyes to prevent corneal damage. Warning clients about sensations of blurred vision will reduce their anxiety on awakening from surgery. Sensations that you may describe include expected pain at the surgical site, tightness of dressings, dryness of the mouth, or a sore throat resulting from an endotracheal tube.

Anxiety and fear are barriers to learning, and both emotions are heightened as surgery approaches. You should assess the surgical client's readiness and ability to learn. If the client is capable of and receptive to learning, present information in a logical sequence, beginning with preoperative events and advancing to intraoperative and postoperative routines. The following demonstrates a client's understanding of the surgical experience.

Client Cites Reasons for Preoperative Instructions and Exercises. If given a rationale for preoperative and postoperative procedures, the client is better prepared to participate in his or her care. Every preoperative teaching program includes explanation and demonstration of postoperative exercises: diaphragmatic breathing, incentive spirometry, coughing, turning, and leg exercises. These exercises are designed to prevent postoperative complications (Skill 49–1).

If the client is measured for elastic stockings or sequential **(pneumatic) compression devices,** you must teach about the purposes of these devices and the nursing care that will be required after their application (see Chapter 46).

After explaining each exercise, you should demonstrate it. You act as a coach, guiding the client through each exercise. For example, you assess whether the client is sitting properly and help the client place his or her hands in the proper position during breathing. You then allow the client time for independent practice and return to evaluate effectiveness before surgery.

Client States the Time of Surgery. The client and family should be told the approximate time that surgery will begin. If the hospital has a busy OR schedule, it is best to let them know whether other procedures are scheduled before the client's. The surgeon usually informs the client and family of the anticipated length of surgery. Unanticipated delays may occur for many reasons. The family needs to be aware that delays do not necessarily indicate a problem.

Client Knows Where the Postoperative Unit Is and Where the Family Will Be During Surgery and Recovery. The unit to which the client is admitted before surgery may be different from the postoperative unit. The family needs to know where the client will be taken after surgery. You also should explain where the family can wait, and where the surgeon will attempt to find family members after surgery. Many institutions have implemented programs in which the circulating nurse gives periodic reports to the family in the waiting room when prolonged surgeries are involved. If the client will be taken to a special unit postoperatively, it helps to orient the client and family members to the unit's environment before surgery. Programs designed to connect with the family also have been developed in the same-day admit and day-surgery areas. For example, Queen Elizabeth II Health Sciences Centre in Halifax, Nova Scotia, has created the role of the surgical liaison nurse to provide communication and support for families of surgical clients (Fowlie et al., 2000).

The Ottawa Hospital | L'Hôpital d'Ottawa

CLINICAL PATHWAY – PLAN CLINIQUE

Total Hip Arthroplasty, Primary and Revision
Arthroplastie totale de la hanche, primaire et réintervention

☐ Civic ☐ Gen.-Gén.

Addressograph/Plaque

INPATIENT 5 FLOW SHEET

PAU — Unité pré-admission	Day of Surgery Pre-op — SDA/SDCU — Jour de la chirurgie pré-opératoire
Date: yyaa ______ mm ______ dj ______	Date: yyaa ______ mm ______ dj ______
Critical Path	**Critical Path**
• **Assessment & teaching per PAU standard of care and procedure specific education material.** • **Pre-operative diagnostic testing as per PAU Medical Directive for Pre-Admission Diagnostic Testing for Elective Surgery.** **Tests** • PTT, INR • CBC • Type and screen to ensure minimum of 2 units pRBCs (including autologous blood) **Additional Orders** • X-ray: AP pelvis (top of film @ ASIS) and lateral of affected hip **Discharge Planning** • Discuss expected length of stay (LOS) • Discuss issues that could cause delay of discharge and discuss discharge preparation • Ensure patient has Total Hip Arthroplasty education booklet	• **Assessment and teaching per same day admission standard of care and procedure specific education material.** **Tests** • Glucose meter: for diabetic patient • PTT/INR: for patient normally taking warfarin (Coumadin) – Unless normal result obtained after warfarin discontinued per pre-op instructions • Electrolytes: for dialysis dependant patient unless acceptable post-dialysis results obtained within 24 h of surgery • CBC if autologous blood donor **Additional Orders** • IV NS at 50 mL/h if IV medications to be given in SDA/SDCU ***OR*** If patient is insulin-dependent diabetic: IV D5W @ 100 mL/h **Antibiotics:** • If No history of allergy to penicillin or to other beta-lactam antibiotics; *or* • History of non-life threatening reaction to penicillin or other beta-lactam antibiotics (eg. rash, diarrhea, stomach upset) **IV Cefazolin** on chart for administration in OR: • 1 g if weight < 60 kg • 2 g if weight ≥ 60 kg **Or** • If patient has a history of life threatening reaction (hypotension, bronchospasm, urticaria, angioedema) to penicillin or other beta-lactam antibiotics **IV Vancomycin:** • 1 g if weight < 90 kg (infuse over 60 minutes pre-op) • 1.5 g if weight ≥ 90 kg (infuse over 90 minutes pre-op)
Patient Outcomes	**Patient Outcomes**
Patient/Family Teaching • Understands pre-op instructions and events • Understands usual post-op course, plan for pain management, and usual self care measures to prevent post-op complications **Discharge Planning** • Understands usual LOS • Appropriate discharge plan in place or if no suitable discharge plan in place – social work has been consulted	**Patient Teaching** • Adherence with pre-op instructions • Understands usual events/expectations of operative day • Understands usual post-op course, plan for pain management, and usual self care measures to prevent post-op complications
Patient progress corresponds with clinical pathway	**Patient progress corresponds with clinical pathway**
Nursing: ☐ Yes ☐ No Signature: Time: ______ NTV – circle above, VC ______	**Nursing:** ☐ Yes ☐ No Signature: Time: ______ NTV – circle above, VC ______

Variance Codes (VC)

186 Activity variance	**510** Not discharged by end of pathway – non-medical reason
653 Consult not sent by Day 3	**NTV** Non-Tracked Variance
492 Not discharged by end of pathway – continued need for acute care	**OFF** Ordered off clinical pathway

CP 4A (REV 01–2008) (12–2006) CHART – DOSSIER © THE OTTAWA HOSPITAL – L'HÔPITAL D'OTTAWA

Figure 49-3 Preoperative client instructions for a clinical pathway for a total hip arthroplasty. The first day of a six-day pathway highlights what the client can expect before surgery. **Source:** Courtesy of The Ottawa Hospital, Ottawa, ON.

➤ SKILL 49-1 Demonstrating Postoperative Exercises

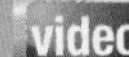

Delegation Considerations

The skill of demonstrating postoperative exercises should not be delegated to unregulated care providers (UCPs). However, other aspects of client care may be delegated. When using UCPs be sure to:

- Educate the UCP to encourage clients to practise exercises regularly, following instruction.
- Instruct the UCP to inform you if clients are unwilling to perform these exercises.

Equipment

- Pillow or wrapped blanket (used to splint surgical incision during coughing)
- Incentive spirometer
- Positive expiratory pressure (PEP) device and nose clip

Procedure

STEPS	RATIONALE
1. Assess the client's risk for postoperative respiratory complications. Review the medical history to identify presence of chronic pulmonary conditions (e.g., emphysema, chronic bronchitis, asthma), any condition that affects chest wall movement, history of smoking, and presence of reduced hemoglobin.	• General anaesthesia predisposes the client to respiratory problems because the lungs are not fully inflated during surgery and the cough reflex is suppressed, so that mucus collects within airway passages. After surgery, the client may have reduced lung volume and require greater efforts to cough and breathe deeply; inadequate lung expansion can lead to atelectasis and pneumonia. The client is at greater risk for developing respiratory complications if other chronic lung conditions are present. Smoking damages ciliary clearance and increases mucus secretion. Reduced hemoglobin level can lead to inadequate oxygenation.
2. Assess ability to cough and breathe deeply by having the client take a deep breath and observing movement of shoulders and chest wall. Measure chest excursion during deep breath. Ask client to cough after taking deep breath.	• Reveals maximum potential for chest expansion and ability to cough forcefully; serves as baseline to measure ability to perform exercises after surgery.
3. Assess risk for postoperative thrombus formation. (Older clients, those with active cancer, and those immobilized for more than 3 days are most at risk.) Observe for localized tenderness along the distribution of the venous system, swollen calf or thigh, calf swelling more than 3 cm compared with asymptomatic leg, pitting edema in symptomatic leg, and collateral superficial veins. If any of these signs are present, notify the physician.	• Venous stasis, hypercoagulability, and vein trauma exist simultaneously for thrombus formation to occur (Lewis et al., 2004). After general anaesthesia, circulation is slowed, thus increasing the risk for clot formation. Immobilization results in decreased muscular contraction in the lower extremities, which promotes venous stasis.

Critical Decision Point: A positive Homans' sign (calf pain when dorsiflexing the client's foot with knee flexed) has been found to have a low specificity for deep vein thrombosis (DVT) diagnosis and often is not present or may be present when no DVT exists (Anand et al., 1998; Tick et al., 2002).

STEPS	RATIONALE
4. Assess the client's ability to move independently while in bed.	• Determines existence of any mobility restrictions.
5. Explain postoperative exercises to the client, including their importance to recovery and physiological benefits.	• Information allows the client to understand the significance of exercises and can motivate learning. People tend to learn new skills when benefits can be gained.
6. Demonstrate exercises.	
A. Diaphragmatic breathing	
(1) Assist the client to a comfortable sitting position on side of bed or in chair or to standing position.	• Upright position facilitates diaphragmatic excursion.
(2) Stand or sit facing the client.	• Allows the client to observe the breathing exercise.
(3) Instruct the client to place palms of hands across from each other, down and along lower borders of anterior rib cage. Place tips of third fingers lightly together (see Step 6A(3) illustration). Demonstrate for the client.	• Position of hands allows the client to feel movement of the chest and abdomen as the diaphragm descends and lungs expand.
(4) Have the client take slow, deep breaths, inhaling through the nose and pushing abdomen against hands. Tell the client to feel the middle fingers separate during inhalation. Demonstrate.	• Taking slow, deep breaths prevents panting or hyperventilation. Inhaling through the nose warms, humidifies, and filters air.
(5) Explain that the client will feel normal downward movement of the diaphragm during inspiration. Explain that abdominal organs descend and the chest wall expands.	• Explanation and demonstration focus on normal ventilatory movement of the chest wall. The client develops understanding of how diaphragmatic breathing feels.
(6) Avoid using auxiliary chest and shoulder muscles while inhaling and instruct the client in same manner.	• Using auxiliary chest and shoulder muscles increases useless energy expenditure.

STEPS	RATIONALE
(7) Have the client hold a slow, deep breath for a count of three and then slowly exhale through the mouth as if blowing out a candle (with pursed lips). Tell the client that middle fingertips will touch as the chest wall contracts.	• Allows for gradual expulsion of all air and helps prevent airway collapse by facilitating the maintenance of positive airway pressure.
(8) Repeat breathing exercise three to five times.	• Allows the client to observe a slow, rhythmic breathing pattern.
(9) Have the client practise the exercise. Instruct the client to take 10 slow, deep breaths every hour while awake during the postoperative period until mobile.	• Repetition of the exercise reinforces learning. Regular deep breathing prevents postoperative complications.
B. Incentive spirometry	
(1) Perform hand hygiene.	• Reduces transmission of microorganisms.
(2) Instruct the client to assume semi-Fowler's or high-Fowler's position.	• Promotes optimal lung expansion during respiratory manoeuvre.
(3) Either set or indicate to the client on the device scale the volume level to be attained with each breath.	• Establishes goal of the volume level necessary for lung expansion.
(4) Demonstrate to the client how to place the mouthpiece of the spirometer so that the lips completely cover it (see Step 6B(4) illustration).	• Demonstration is a reliable technique for teaching psychomotor skills and enables the client to ask questions.
(5) Instruct the client to inhale slowly and maintain constant flow through the unit, attempting to reach goal volume. When maximal inspiration is reached, the client should hold breath for 2 to 3 seconds (see Step 6B(5) illustration) and then exhale slowly. Number of breaths should not exceed 10 to 12 per minute in each session.	• Maintains maximal inspiration and reduces risk of progressive collapse of individual alveoli. Slow breath prevents or minimizes pain from sudden pressure changes in chest.
(6) Instruct the client to breathe normally for a short period.	• Prevents hyperventilation and fatigue.
(7) Have the client repeat the manoeuvre until goals are achieved.	• Ensures correct use of spirometer.
(8) Perform hand hygiene.	• Reduces transmission of microorganisms.

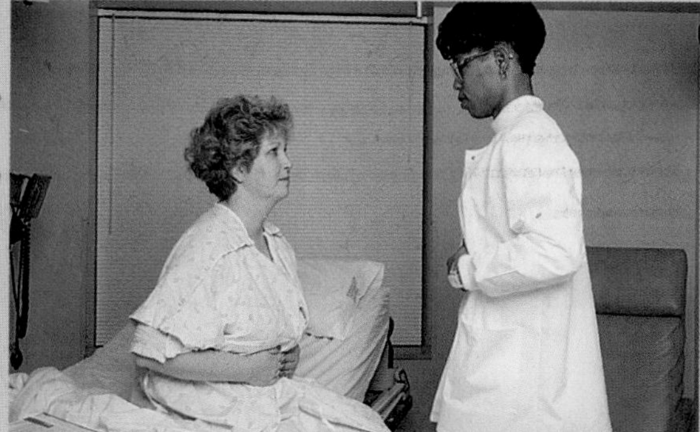

Step 6A(3) Client learns how to feel proper abdominal breathing.

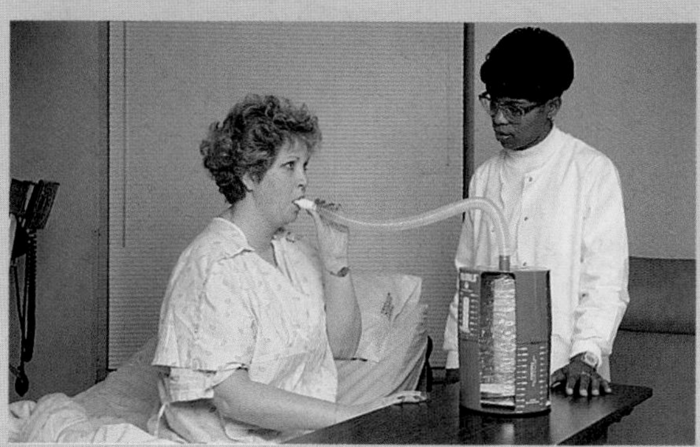

Step 6B(4) Client inhales using incentive spirometer.

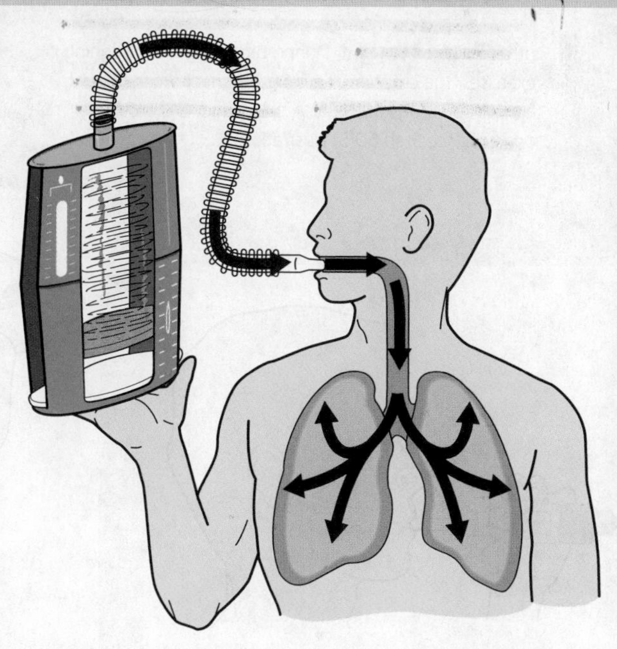

Step 6B(5) Incentive spirometer increases flow of air into lungs.

Continued

➤ SKILL 49-1 Demonstrating Postoperative Exercises *continued*

STEPS	RATIONALE
C. Positive expiratory pressure (PEP) therapy and "huff" coughing	
(1) Perform hand hygiene.	• Reduces transmission of microorganisms.
(2) Set PEP device to the setting ordered.	• The higher the setting, the more effort will be required by the client. Ideally, the device should deliver 10 to 20 cm of water during passive expiration (American Association for Respiratory Care [AARC], 2002).
(3) Instruct the client to assume semi-Fowler's or high-Fowler's position and place nose clip on the client's nose (see Step 6C(3) illustration).	• Promotes optimal lung expansion and expectoration of mucus (AARC, 2002).
(4) Have the client place lips around the mouthpiece. The client should take a full breath and then exhale two to three times longer than inhalation. Pattern should be repeated for 10 to 20 breaths.	• Ensures that all breathing is done through the mouth and that the device is used properly.
(5) Remove device from the mouth and have the client take a slow, deep breath and hold for 3 seconds.	• Promotes lung expansion before coughing.
(6) Instruct the client to exhale in quick, short, forced exhalations or "huffs."	• "Huff" coughing, or forced expiratory technique, promotes bronchial hygiene through increased expectoration of secretions.
D. Controlled coughing	
(1) Explain the importance of maintaining an upright position.	• Position facilitates diaphragm excursion and enhances thorax expansion.
(2) Demonstrate coughing. Take two slow, deep breaths, inhaling through the nose and exhaling through the mouth.	• Deep breaths expand the lungs fully so that air moves behind mucus and facilitates the effects of coughing.
(3) Inhale deeply a third time and hold breath to count of three. Cough fully for two or three consecutive coughs without inhaling between coughs. (Tell the client to push all air out of lungs.)	• Consecutive coughs help remove mucus more effectively and completely than one forceful cough.

Critical Decision Point: Coughing may be contraindicated after brain or eye surgery.

STEPS	RATIONALE
(4) Caution the client against simply clearing the throat instead of coughing. Explain that coughing will not cause injury to incision when done correctly.	• Clearing the throat does not remove mucus from deep in airways. Postoperative incisional pain makes it harder for the client to cough effectively.
(5) If surgical incision will be abdominal or thoracic, teach the client to place one hand over the incisional area and the other hand on top of it. During breathing and coughing exercises, the client presses gently against the incisional area to splint or support it. A pillow over the incision is optional (see Step 6D(5) illustration).	• Surgical incision cuts through muscles, tissues, and nerve endings. Deep breathing and coughing exercises place additional stress on the suture line and cause discomfort. • Splinting the incision with hands provides firm support and reduces incisional pulling. (Some clients prefer to have a pillow to place over the incision.)

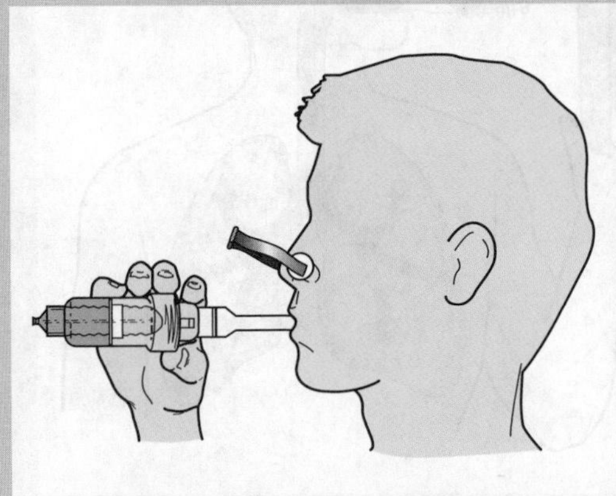

Step 6C(3) Positive expiratory pressure device.

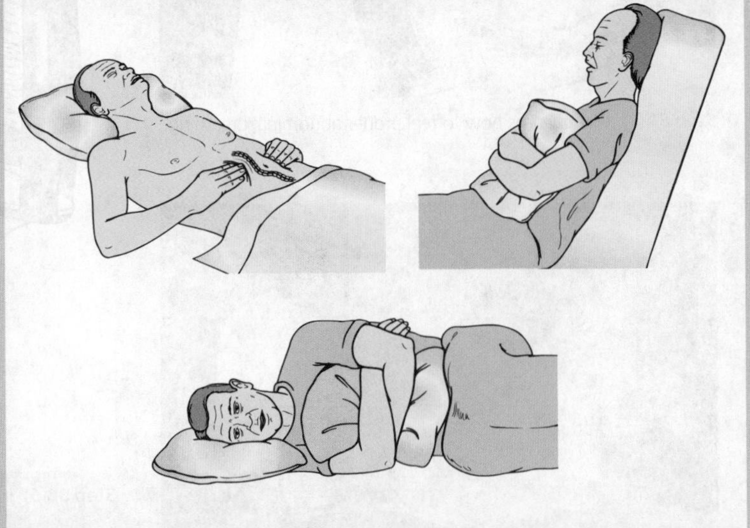

Step 6D(5) Techniques for splinting incision. **Source:** From Lewis, S. M., Heitkemper, M. M., & Dirksen, S. R. (2007). *Medical-surgical nursing: Assessment and management of clinical problems* (7th ed.). St. Louis, MO: Mosby.

➤ SKILL 49-1 Demonstrating Postoperative Exercises *continued*

STEPS	RATIONALE
(6) The client continues to practise coughing exercises, splinting imaginary incision. Instruct the client to cough two to three times every 2 hours while awake.	• Value of deep coughing with splinting is stressed to expectorate mucus effectively with minimal discomfort.
(7) Instruct the client to examine sputum for consistency, odour, amount, and colour changes.	• Sputum consistency, odour, amount, and colour changes may indicate presence of pulmonary complication, such as pneumonia.
E. Turning	
(1) Instruct the client to assume supine position and move to side of bed if permitted by surgery. Have the client move by bending knees and pressing heels against the mattress to raise and move buttocks (see Step 6E(1) illustration). Top side rails on both sides of the bed should be raised.	• Positioning begins on side of the bed so that turning to other side will not cause the client to roll toward the bed's edge.
(2) Instruct the client to place right hand over the incisional area to splint it.	• Supports and minimizes pulling on the suture line during turning.
(3) Instruct the client to keep right leg straight and flex left knee up (see Step 6E(3) illustration). If back or vascular surgery is being performed, client will need to logroll or will require assistance with turning.	• Straight leg stabilizes the client's position. Flexed left leg shifts weight for easier turning.
(4) Have the client grab the right side rail with left hand, pull toward right, and roll onto right side.	• Pulling toward side rail reduces effort needed for turning.
(5) Instruct the client to turn every 2 hours while awake.	• Reduces risk of vascular and pulmonary complications.
F. Leg exercises	
(1) Have the client assume supine position in bed. Demonstrate leg exercises by performing passive range-of-motion exercises and simultaneously explaining exercise.	• Provides normal anatomical position of lower extremities.
(2) Rotate each ankle in complete circle. Instruct the client to draw imaginary circles with big toe (see Step 6F(2) illustration). Repeat five times.	• Leg exercises maintain joint mobility and promote venous return to prevent thrombi.

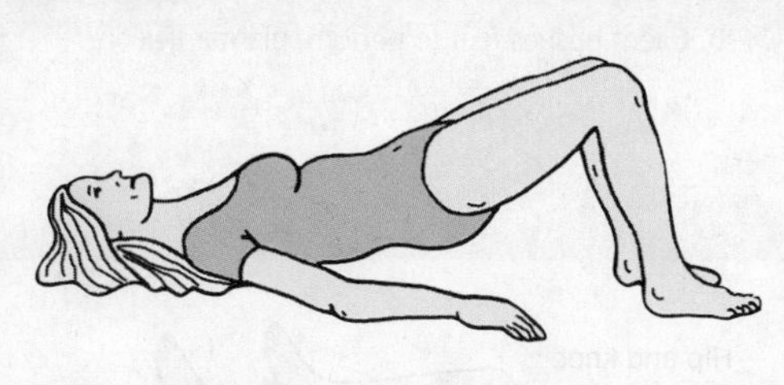

Step 6E(1) Buttocks lift.

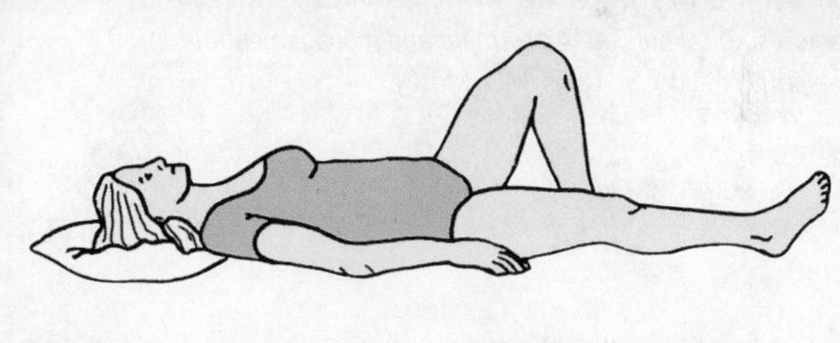

Step 6E(3) Leg position for turning.

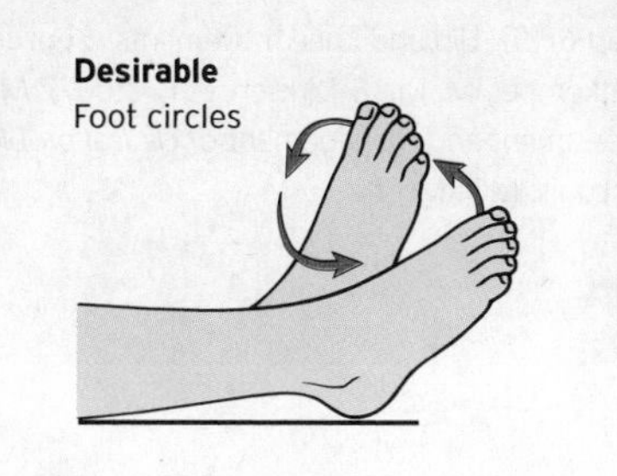

Step 6F(2) Foot circles. **Source:** From Lewis, S. M., Heitkemper, M. M., & Dirksen, S. R. (2007). *Medical-surgical nursing: Assessment and management of clinical problems* (7th ed.). St. Louis, MO: Mosby.

Continued

➤SKILL 49-1 Demonstrating Postoperative Exercises *continued*

STEPS	RATIONALE
(3) Alternate dorsiflexion and plantar flexion of both feet. Direct the client to feel calf muscles contract and relax alternately (see Step 6F(3) illustrations, parts A and B). Repeat five times.	• Stretches and contracts gastrocnemius muscles.
(4) Perform quadriceps setting by tightening thigh and bringing knee down toward mattress, then relaxing (see Step 6F(4) illustration). Repeat five times.	• Contracts muscles of upper legs, maintains knee mobility, and enhances venous return.
(5) Have the client alternately raise each leg straight up from the bed surface, keeping legs straight, and then have the client bend leg at hip and knee (see Step 6F(5) illustration). Repeat five times.	• Promotes contraction and relaxation of quadriceps muscles.
7. Have the client practise exercises at least every 2 hours while awake. Instruct the client to coordinate turning and leg exercises with diaphragmatic breathing, incentive spirometry, and coughing exercises.	• Repetition of sequence reinforces learning. Establishes routine for exercises that develops habit for performance. Sequence of exercises should be leg exercises, turning, breathing, incentive spirometry, and coughing.
8. Observe the client's ability to perform all five exercises independently.	• Ensures that the client has learned correct techniques. Documents the client's education and provides data for instructional follow-up.

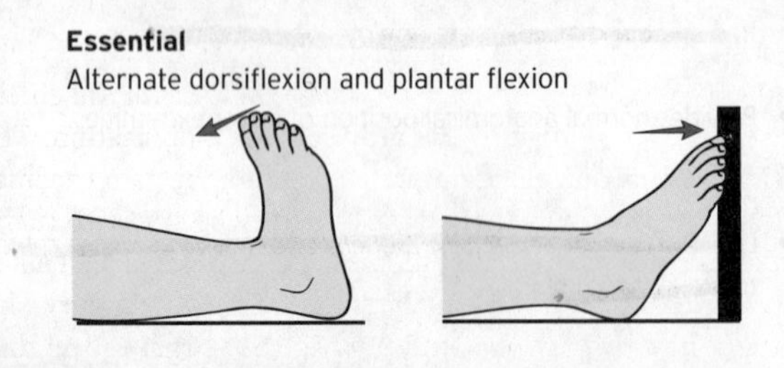

Step 6F(3) **A,** Alternate dorsiflexion and plantar flexion. **Source:** From Lewis, S. M., Heitkemper, M. M., & Dirksen, S. R. (2007). *Medical-surgical nursing: Assessment and management of clinical problems* (7th ed.). St. Louis, MO: Mosby.

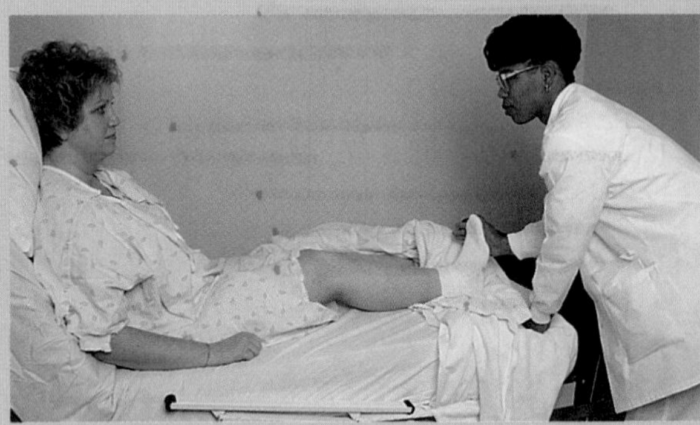

Step 6F(3) **B,** Client pushes feet to perform plantar flexion.

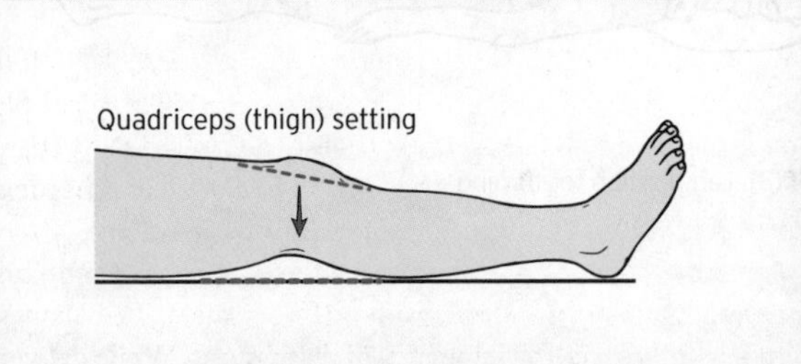

Step 6F(4) Quadriceps (thigh) setting. **Source:** From Lewis, S. M., Heitkemper, M. M., & Dirksen, S. R. (2007). *Medical-surgical nursing: Assessment and management of clinical problems* (7th ed.). St. Louis, MO: Mosby.

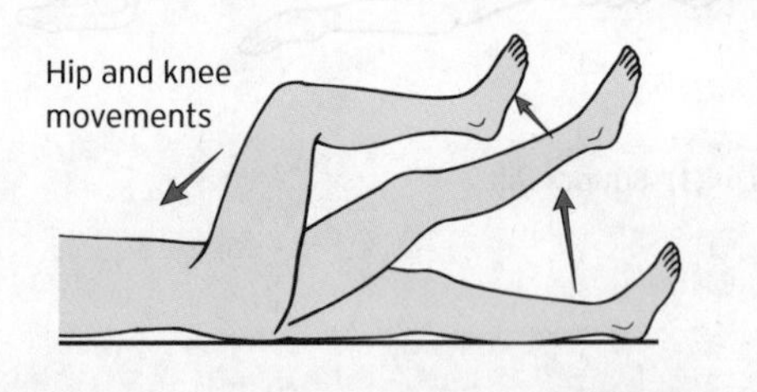

Step 6F(5) Hip and knee movements. **Source:** From Lewis, S. M., Heitkemper, M. M., & Dirksen, S. R. (2007). *Medical-surgical nursing: Assessment and management of clinical problems* (7th ed.). St. Louis, MO: Mosby.

➤ SKILL 49-1 Demonstrating Postoperative Exercises *continued*

Unexpected Outcomes and Related Interventions

Inability to Perform Exercises Correctly After Surgery

- Assess for the presence of anxiety, pain, and fatigue.
- Teach the client stress reduction techniques, pain management strategies, or both.
- Repeat the teaching using additional demonstration or re-demonstration at a time when family members or friends are present.

Unwillingness to Perform Exercises Postoperatively Because of Incisional Pain of Thorax or Abdomen (Deep Breathing, Coughing, and Turning) or Because of Surgery Involving Lower Abdomen, Groin, Buttocks, or Legs (Leg Exercises, Turning)

- Instruct the client to ask for pain medication 30 minutes before performing postoperative exercises or to use patient-controlled analgesia (PCA) immediately before exercising.
- Report to the surgeon inadequate pain relief and the need to change analgesic or increase dose.

Recording and Reporting

- Record the exercises demonstrated and whether the client can perform them independently.
- Report any problems the client has in practising exercises to the nurse assigned to the client on the next shift for follow-up.

Client Discusses Anticipated Postoperative Monitoring and Therapies. The client and family need to know about postoperative events. If they understand the frequency of postoperative vital sign monitoring before surgery occurs, they will be less apprehensive when nurses measure vital signs. You can also explain whether the client is likely to have IV lines, monitoring lines, dressings, or drainage tubes or whether he or she will require ventilator support.

Client Describes Surgical Procedures and Postoperative Treatment. After the surgeon has explained the basic purpose of the surgical procedure, the client may ask you additional questions to clarify any misunderstandings. Pre-established teaching standards, such as those integrated in clinical pathways for preoperative and postoperative care (Figure 49–4), give you an excellent guide for instruction. A good starting point is to ask what the client has been told. If the client has limited understanding about the surgery, you can provide additional explanations. If necessary, the surgeon can be asked to reinform the client.

Client Describes Postoperative Activity Resumption. The type of surgery a client undergoes affects the speed with which normal physical activity and regular eating habits can be resumed. You should explain that it is normal to progress gradually in both activity and eating. If the client tolerates activity and diet well, activity levels will progress more quickly.

Client Describes Pain-Relief Measures. Typically, one of the surgical client's fears is pain. The family is also concerned for the client's comfort. Pain after surgery is expected. You should inform the client and family of interventions available for pain relief (e.g., analgesics, positioning, splinting, and relaxation exercises; see Chapter 42). The client needs to know the schedule for analgesic drugs, their route of administration, and their effects.

Surgical clients may avoid taking pain-relief drugs for fear of becoming dependent on them. You should encourage the client to use analgesics as needed and explain to the client that the risks of becoming dependent are almost negligible. Explain to the client that unless the pain is controlled, it will be difficult for the client to participate in postoperative therapy such as mobilization. The client should be encouraged to inform you before the pain becomes a constant discomfort. If a client waits until pain becomes excruciating, an analgesic may not provide relief at the dose ordered. Clients who will have patient-controlled analgesia (PCA) after surgery should be taught how to push the button when they begin to feel discomfort and should understand that use of PCA will not cause overmedication (see Chapter 42). The client should also understand the length of time that it takes for the drug to begin working. Information from preoperative assessment will be helpful to you when teaching about pain-relief measures. Pain reporting and expectations regarding pain management based on a client's cultural beliefs are areas that need to be explored both individually and systematically through research (Douglas, 1999; Ramer et al., 1999).

Client Expresses Feelings Regarding Surgery. If the client is admitted to hospital during the preoperative surgical phase, frequent visits by staff, diagnostic testing, and physical preparation for surgery consume a lot of time; as a result, the client has few opportunities to reflect on the upcoming surgical experience. You must recognize the client as a unique individual. The client and family need time to express their feelings about the surgery. The client's level of anxiety influences the frequency of discussions. While delivering bedside care, you can encourage expression of concerns. Family members may wish to discuss their concerns without the client present so that their fears will not frighten the client, and vice versa. Establishing a trusting and therapeutic relationship with the client and family allows this to happen.

Acute Care

Acute care activities in the preoperative phase focus on interventions to prepare the client physically for surgery.

Patient(e) ______________ **Chart No. – Nº du dossier** ______________

Post-op Day 1 — Jour 1 post-opératoire

Date: yyaa ______ **mm** ______ **dj** ______

Critical Path	Patient Outcomes
Assessments/Treatments • VS, NVS, Pain q4h → q shift, SpO_2 • Monitor dressing / Hemovac • Monitor Intake & Output • Pain management as per APS – Discontinue APS modality as per weaning guideline if patient meets criteria – If single dose intrathecal only: discontinue from APS 24 hours following time of injection **Activity** • DB&C • Exercise program • Pivot transfer with walker • Comfirm weight bearing status • Up in chair x 2 ______ initial, ______ initial • Ambulate x 1 with assistance: ______ initial • Assistive devices, specify: ______ **Nutrition** • Diet as ordered **Elimination** • Catheter as ordered **Patient Teaching** • Reinforce exercise program • Proper pillow positioning • Hip precautions • If on Low Molecular Weight Heparin – start self injection teaching and provide booklet • Ensure patient has Total Hip Arthroplasty patient information booklet • Pain management	**Pain Control** • Adequate pain control achieved: Pain ≤ 3 rest, ≤ 5 activity; pain not preventing movement; satisfied with pain control **Activity** • Completes transfer with assistance • Performs exercises according to self directed exercise program **Prevention of DVT** • Demonstrates appropriate exercises & positioning for prevention of DVT • Verbalizes understanding of anticoagulant therapy **Patient Teaching** • Verbalizes understanding of "Total Hip Arthroplasty" instructions and exercise program • Understands basics of self injection if applicable • Demonstrates: – Proper positioning – Understanding of weight-bearing status

Patient progress corresponds with clinical pathway

Physiotherapy:

☐ Yes ☐ No Signature: ______________ Time: ______ NTV – circle above, VC ______

Nursing:

D ☐ Yes ☐ No Signature: ______________, Initial ______ Time: ______ NTV – circle above, VC ______

E ☐ Yes ☐ No Signature: ______________, Initial ______ Time: ______ NTV – circle above, VC ______

N ☐ Yes ☐ No Signature: ______________, Initial ______ Time: ______ NTV – circle above, VC ______

D = 8-12 h day shift **E** = evening shift, if applicable **N** = 8-12 h night shift

Variance Codes (VC)

186	Activity variance	**510**	Not discharged by end of pathway – non-medical reason
653	Consult not sent by Day 3	**NTV**	Non-Tracked Variance
492	Not discharged by end of pathway – continued need for acute care	**OFF**	Ordered off clinical pathway

© THE OTTAWA HOSPITAL – L'HÔPITAL D'OTTAWA CHART – DOSSIER CP 4A (3 – 7)

Figure 49-4 Postoperative client instructions for a clinical pathway for a total hip arthroplasty. Highlights what the client can expect on the first day after surgery. **Source:** Courtesy of The Ottawa Hospital, Ottawa, ON.

Physical Preparation. The degree of preoperative physical preparation depends on the client's health status and on the surgery to be performed. A seriously ill client receives more supportive care in the form of medications, IV fluid therapy, and monitoring than does a client facing a minor elective procedure. You should explain the purpose of all procedures.

Maintenance of Normal Fluid and Electrolyte Balances. The surgical client is vulnerable to fluid and electrolyte imbalances as a result of inadequate preoperative intake, excessive fluid losses during surgery, and the physiological effect of third spacing of fluid in the initial postoperative period (see Chapter 40). A client traditionally took nothing by mouth (NPO) after midnight on the morning of surgery to keep the stomach empty and thus reduce the risk of vomiting and aspiration. Recommendations for preoperative fasting have been published by the Canadian Anesthesiologists Society (2005) and by the American Society of Anesthesiologists (American Society of Anesthesiologists Task Force on Preoperative Fasting, 1999). They recommended fasting from intake of a light meal (e.g., toast and clear liquids) for 6 or more hours, and from clear liquids for 2 to 3 hours before elective procedures that require general anaesthesia, regional anaesthesia, or sedation.

Agencies vary as to the extent that these guidelines have been adopted. You will remove fluids and solid foods from the client's bedside and post a sign over the client's bed to alert hospital personnel and family members about fasting restrictions. The client may be instructed to take specific medications (e.g., cardiovascular medications, anticonvulsants, or antibiotics) with a sip of water. Although the parameters of preoperative fasting have changed, studies demonstrate that recent guidelines have not been fully implemented and that multidisciplinary improvement processes may be required (O'Callaghan, 2002; Williams, 1999).

A client who is at home on the evening before surgery must understand the importance of the specific fasting period that has been ordered. You can allow clients to rinse their mouths with water or mouthwash and brush their teeth immediately before surgery as long as they do not swallow water. You must notify the surgeon and anaesthesiologist if the client has eaten or drunk fluids during the fasting period.

During surgery, normal mechanisms for controlling fluid and electrolyte balances, including respiration, digestion, circulation, and elimination, are disturbed. The surgical procedure may cause extensive losses of blood and other body fluids. The surgical stress response aggravates any fluid and electrolyte imbalances. The client's preoperative diet should include foods high in protein, with sufficient carbohydrates, fat, and vitamins. If a client cannot eat because of gastrointestinal alterations or impairments in consciousness, an IV route for fluid replacement is started. The physician assesses serum electrolyte levels to determine the type of IV fluids and electrolyte additives to administer. Clients with severe nutritional imbalances may require supplements containing concentrated protein and glucose (see Chapter 43).

Reduction of Risk of Surgical Wound Infection. The risk of developing a surgical wound infection is determined by the amount and type of microorganisms contaminating a wound, the susceptibility of the host, and the surgical wound itself. All three factors interact to cause infection. Antibiotics may be ordered in the preoperative period. Risk of wound infection decreases when an antibiotic is present in sufficient concentrations at the wound site before incision (Polk & Christmas, 2000). Antibiotics given before surgery may be administered orally or intravenously. Increasingly, antibiotics are administered in the OR immediately before surgery (Dellinger et al., 1994).

Microorganisms grow and multiply on the skin. Without proper skin preparation, the risk of postoperative wound infection is high. Many surgeons instruct clients to bathe or shower the evening before surgery. Some physicians may request that clients bathe or shower more than once, whereas others may ask clients to give special attention to cleansing the proposed operative site. This attention could include the use of an antibacterial soap. Depending on the surgical procedure, a client may also shower on the morning of surgery. If the surgical procedure involves the head, neck, or upper chest area, the client may be required to shampoo his or her hair. Cleansing and trimming of fingernails and toenails also may be necessary.

The need for hair removal is less common now and depends on the amount of hair, the location of the incision, and the surgical procedure planned (AORN, 2002b). Hair removal can damage and cause breaks in the client's skin, which may allow for the entry of microorganisms. If required, hair is removed with a clipper or shaver as close to the time of surgery as possible. Short hospital stays are known to reduce the chance of a nosocomial (hospital-acquired) infection. Respiratory, urinary tract, and wound infections can all be acquired during hospitalization. This is one advantage of ambulatory surgical procedures, because the client usually returns home once the surgery has been completed.

Precautions for Client Requiring Infection Control Procedures. If a client requires surgery but also has an infectious process, the OR must be notified in advance to ensure appropriate preparation. For example, clients with tuberculosis would be placed in a reverse airflow OR suite and subsequently in a reverse airflow room in the postanaesthesia care unit (PACU). Clients with methicillin-resistant staphlococcus aureus (MRSA) may have their surgery performed at the end of the day so that the surgical suite can be cleaned afterward. These clients on transfer to the PACU are placed in an isolation room. Some hospitals now require that all "same-day admit" patients be screened for MRSA and vancomycin-resistant enterococci (VRE).

Prevention of Bowel and Bladder Incontinence. The client may receive a bowel preparation (e.g., a cathartic or enema) if the surgery involves the lower gastrointestinal system or lower abdominal organs. Manipulation of portions of the gastrointestinal tract during surgery results in absence of peristalsis for 24 hours or longer. Enemas and cathartics, such as GoLYTELY, cleanse the gastrointestinal tract to prevent intraoperative incontinence and postoperative constipation. An empty bowel reduces the risk for injury to the intestines and minimizes contamination of the operative wound if a portion of the bowel is incised or opened accidentally, or if colon surgery is planned. The surgeon's plan may read "give enemas until clear." This means that you must administer enemas until the enema return contains no solid fecal material (see Chapter 45). Too many enemas given over a short period of time, however, can cause serious fluid and electrolyte imbalances. Most agencies recommend a limit (usually three) to the number of enemas you may administer successively.

The bladder is not prepared until the morning of surgery.

Promotion of Rest and Comfort. Rest is essential for normal healing. Anxiety about the impending surgery can easily interfere with the client's ability to relax or sleep. As well, the underlying condition requiring surgery may be painful, further impairing rest.

If the client is admitted to hospital before the day of surgery, you should attempt to make the client's environment quiet and comfortable. Sometimes the client is ordered a sedative-hypnotic or anxiolytic agent for the night before surgery. Sedative-hypnotics (e.g., temazepam [Restoril]) affect and promote sleep. Anxiolytic agents (e.g., alprazolam [Xanax]) act on the cerebral cortex and limbic system to relieve anxiety.

An advantage of ambulatory surgery or same-day surgical admissions is that the client is able to sleep at home the night before surgery. He or she is likely to get more rest in a familiar environment. The nonhospitalized client also may have medication ordered by the physician if apprehension about surgery interferes with a good night's rest.

Preparation on the Day of Surgery. You must complete a number of interventions before releasing the client for surgery.

Hygiene. Basic hygiene measures provide additional comfort before surgery. The client may want to bathe before surgery. Because the client cannot wear personal nightwear to the OR, you must provide a clean hospital gown. If the client has been NPO for the last several hours, his or her mouth may be very dry. You may offer the client mouthwash and toothpaste, again with the caution not to swallow any water.

Hair and Cosmetics. During surgery with general anaesthesia, the client's head is positioned to introduce an endotracheal tube into the airway (see Chapter 39). This procedure may involve manipulation of the client's hair and scalp. To avoid injury, ask the client to remove hairpins or clips before leaving for surgery. Hairpieces or wigs also should be removed. Long hair can be braided. The client will wear a disposable hat before entering the OR.

During and after surgery, the anaesthesiologist and nurses will assess skin and mucous membranes to determine the client's level of oxygenation and circulation. Therefore, all makeup (lipstick, powder, blush, nail polish) should be removed to expose normal skin and nail colouring. Pulse oximetry is capable of recording accurate measurements through most nail polish colours, but removal is still considered good practice. Contact lenses, false eyelashes, and eye makeup also must be removed. The client's glasses can be stored or given to the family immediately before the client enters the OR.

Removal of Prostheses. It is easy for any type of prosthetic device to become lost or damaged during surgery. The client must remove all prostheses, including partial or complete dentures, artificial limbs, artificial eyes, and hearing aids. If a client has a brace or a splint, check with the physician to determine whether it should remain with the client.

Many clients are embarrassed at having to remove dentures, wigs, or other devices that enhance their personal appearance. Privacy should be offered as these personal items are removed. Clients may be allowed to keep personal items until they reach the preoperative area. For safekeeping, dentures must be placed in special containers labelled with the client's name and other identification required by the agency. In many institutions, nurses must make an inventory of all prosthetic devices or personal items and lock them away according to agency policy. It is also common practice for nurses to give prostheses to family members or to keep items like dentures at the client's bedside. Documentation in the nursing notes, the surgical checklist, or per agency policy should reflect these actions.

Safeguarding Valuables. If a client has any valuables, you should give them to family members or secure them for safekeeping. Many hospitals require clients to sign a release form that frees the institution of responsibility for any lost valuables. Valuables usually can be stored and locked in a designated location. Often clients are reluctant to remove wedding rings or religious medals. A wedding band can be taped in place. However, if there is a risk that the client will experience swelling of the hand or fingers (related to mastectomy, hand surgery, or fluid shifts), the wedding band should be removed. Many hospitals allow clients to pin religious medals to their gowns, although the risk of loss increases with this practice. For safety, other metal items, such as for pierced areas, should also be removed. The location of valuables is documented per hospital policy.

Preparing the Bowel and Bladder. The client may require an enema or cathartic on the morning of surgery to ensure that the colon is empty. If so, it should be given at least 1 hour before the client is scheduled to leave for surgery, allowing time for the client to defecate without rushing. You should instruct the client to void just before leaving for the OR and before giving preoperative medications. An empty bladder prevents a client from becoming incontinent during surgery. This is important during abdominal surgery, when it may be necessary for the surgeon to manipulate the bladder. An empty bladder also makes abdominal organs more accessible during surgery. The last time of voiding is charted. If the client is unable to void, this should be noted on the preoperative (preprocedure) checklist. An indwelling urinary catheter may be placed if the surgery is long or the incision will be in the lower abdomen.

Vital Signs. You must measure a final preoperative set of vital signs. The anaesthesiologist uses these values as a baseline during surgery. If preoperative vital signs are abnormal, surgery may need to be postponed. Notify the physician of any abnormalities before sending the client to surgery.

Documentation. Before the client goes to the OR, check the contents of the medical record to ensure that pertinent laboratory results are present. Any abnormal findings in laboratory results, such as low potassium, should be reported. Check consent forms for accuracy of information. A preoperative checklist (Figure 49–5) provides you with guidelines to ensure that nursing interventions are completed. You should also check the nursing notes to ensure that documentation of care is current. This is especially important if the hospitalized client experienced unpredicted problems on the night before surgery. The OR should be alerted through notation of any positioning challenges for the client, such as difficulty flexing knees, or of any sensory impairment.

Performing Special Procedures. A client's condition may warrant special interventions before surgery. The client may need IV infusions started or a nasogastric tube inserted before leaving for surgery. These procedures also may be done once the client is in the preoperative area, but are usually done in the OR.

Administering Preoperative Medications. The advent of ambulatory surgery has reduced the use of preoperative medications. However, the anaesthesiologist or surgeon may order preanaesthetic drugs ("on-call medications," "pre-ops") to reduce the client's anxiety, the amount of general anaesthesia required, the risk of nausea and vomiting and resultant aspiration, and respiratory tract secretions.

You should provide all nursing care measures before giving the client preoperative medications at the prescribed time. The consent form needs to be signed before the administration of these medications. In addition, the client should be helped to void. Because the drugs cause sedation, the client should not be allowed to leave the bed or stretcher until surgical personnel arrive to transport him or her to the OR. The client should be warned to expect drowsiness and a dry mouth.

> **safety alert** Explain to the client the effects of the preoperative medications. Remind the client to remain in bed or on the stretcher. Raise the side rails and keep the bed or stretcher in the low position. Place the call light within easy reach of the client.

Latex Sensitivity or Allergy. As the incidence and prevalence of **latex sensitivity** and allergy increases, the need to recognize potential sources of latex is critical. The Canadian Society of Hospital Pharmacists (2001) released new guidelines recommending procedures to prevent and treat occupational latex allergies. Guidelines

The Ottawa Hospital | L'Hôpital d'Ottawa

❑ Civic ❑ General

❑ Riverside

PRE PROCEDURE CHECKLIST
FEUILLE DE VÉRIFICATION
PRÉ-INTERVENTION

PART-PARTIE 1
To be completed prior to the patient leaving the Nursing Unit.
À être remplie avant le départ du patient de l'Unité des soins.

Patient is-Le(la) patient(e) est:
❑ **calm-calme** ❑ **anxious-anxieux(se)**
❑ **tearful-en larmes** ❑ **other-autre:**

CHART REVIEW-RÉVISION DU DOSSIER	Yes Oui	No Non	N/A S/O	CHART REVIEW-RÉVISION DU DOSSIER	Yes Oui	No Non	N/A S/O
❑ Allergies Allergies ❑ Allergy band Bracelet d'allergies ❑ Latex allergy Allergie au latex				Addressograph plate Plaque d'adressographe			
Caution sheet-Feuille de précaution Civic and Riverside only-seulement				Anesthesia record Fiche d'anesthésie			
Consent completed as per policy Consentement rempli d'après la politique				Medication record/MAR Fiche des médicaments/RAM			
Consult notes/Medical history Notes de consultation/Antécédents médicaux				Nursing History Histoire des soins infirmiers			
				Old chart if required Dossier antérieur si nécessaire			

ASSESSMENT-ÉVALUATION	Yes Oui	No Non	N/A S/O	ASSESSMENT-ÉVALUATION	Yes Oui	No Non	N/A S/O
Identity bracelet verified-Bracelet d'identité vérifié				Precautions - if yes, check-si oui, cocher: ❑ contact(es) ❑ total(es) ❑ airborne-aériennes ❑ droplet-gouttelettes			
Removed-Enlevé - Medic alert bracelet/necklace-collier				Communication barrier-Conflit de communication			
Teeth-Dents : ❑ capped-couronne ❑ loose-branlante				Interpreter present-Interprète présent			
Removed-Enlevé(s) : ❑ dentures-dentiers ❑ bridge-pont				Skin integrity problem-Problème de l'intégrité de la peau Site:			
❑ glasses-lunettes ❑ contacts-verres de contacts							
❑ hearing aid-appareil auditif				Surgical implants-Implants chirurgicaux Site:			
❑ jewellery/body piercing-bijoux/perçage corporel				Pacemaker/Internal defibrillator Stimulateur cardiaque/Défibrillateur interne			
Pregnancy possibility-Possibilité de grossesse				Antibiotics ordered-Antibiotiques ordonnés			
If yes, physician notified: (Name) Si oui, médecin avisé : (Nom)				Sent to OR with patient-Envoyés au bloc avec patient			

❑ Ate-Ingestion de nourriture last-dernière: ❑ Water-Ingestion d'eau last-dernière: ❑ Void-Miction last-dernière: ❑ Catheterized-Cathétérisé

DIAGNOSTIC TESTS ORDERED AND ON CHART EXAMENS DIAGNOSTIQUES DEMANDÉS ET AU DOSSIER	Yes Oui	N/A S/O	DIAGNOSTIC TESTS ORDERED AND ON CHART EXAMENS DIAGNOSTIQUES DEMANDÉS ET AU DOSSIER	Yes Oui	N/A S/O
ECG			Urinalysis-Analyse d'urine		
CBC			Type & Screen-Hémotypologie et dépistage		
PTT/INR			Autologus-Auto-transfusion-units-unités		
Electrolytes / BUN			Chest X-Ray-Radio pulmonaire		

CARE PLAN DE SOINS

Is the patient DNR-Est-ce que le(la) patient(e) est NPR : ❑ yes-oui ❑ no-non
If yes contact anesthesiologist for DNR consult-Si oui, avisez l'anesthésiologiste pour une consultation de NPR

Consult done-Consultation terminée ❑ yes-oui ❑ no-non

SIGNATURE (Nurse-Infirmière) Init.

SIGNATURE (Nurse transferring patient to OR-Infirmière transférant patient au bloc) Init. DATE

PART-PARTIE 2 To be completed by OR nurse-À être remplie par l'infirmière du bloc opératoire

1. ❑ Patient identified-Patient identifié
2. ❑ Patient chart reviewed-Dossier du patient révisé
3. ❑ Consent checked-Consentement vérifié
4. ❑ Surgical site identified as per policy-Site chirurgical identifié d'après la politique ❑ N/A-S/O
5. Positional problems-Problèmes de position : ❑ N/A-S/O ❑ Yes-Oui :

Verbal lab report obtained, physician notified Médecin avisé après l'obtention du rapport de lab Name-Nom Time-Heure

CARE PLAN DE SOINS

Signature Date (yyaa-mm-dj) Time-Heure

ORA 06 (03/2005) Cat.: 412550 **CHART-DOSSIER**

Figure 49-5 Preprocedure checklist. **Source:** Courtesy of The Ottawa Hospital, Ottawa, ON.

developed through Canadian and American health care organizations are also available for the management of latex allergies and safe latex use in health care facilities (Sussman & Gold, 2004).

The OR and PACU contain innumerable products that include latex. Some common sources are gloves, IV tubing, syringes, and rubber stoppers on bottles and vials. Latex is also present in objects that may be overlooked, including adhesive tape, disposable electrodes, endotracheal tube cuffs, protection sheets, and ventilator equipment. Those most at risk include people with a genetic predisposition to latex allergy, children with spina bifida, clients with urogenital abnormalities or spinal cord injury (because of a long history of catheter use), clients with a history of multiple surgeries, health care professionals, and workers who manufacture rubber products (Paquet, 1998). Symptoms of a latex reaction can include local effects ranging from urticaria and flat or raised red patches to vesicular, scaling, or bleeding eruptions. Acute dermatitis also may be present. Rhinitis and rhinorrhea are other common symptoms in both mild and severe latex reactions. Immediate hypersensitivity reactions can be life-threatening, with the client exhibiting focal or generalized urticaria, edema, bronchospasm, and mucous hypersecretion, which can compromise respiratory status. Vasodilatation compounded by increased capillary permeability can lead to circulatory collapse and eventual death. Because the client may be draped during surgery, any unexplained acute deterioration in a previously healthy client should be investigated for possible latex allergy (Shoup, 1998).

Protocols exist for clients with a latex allergy or sensitivity. Clients with this allergy are identified preoperatively. Latex-free kits are available; they include latex-free equipment (e.g., a latex-free ambu bag) and follow the clients throughout their hospitalization. A reference binder is kept that indicates supplies, medications, and appropriate care options for latex-sensitive clients. It is recommended that the client with a latex allergy be scheduled as the first case of the day in the OR. The room should be cleaned thoroughly, including all equipment, and all unnecessary items should be removed (Doepke, 1998). The client can then be safely accommodated by using appropriate latex-free items during the perioperative period and recovery. Box 49–5 lists precautions for clients with latex sensitivity or allergy.

Eliminating Wrong Site and Wrong Procedure Surgery. Whenever an invasive surgical procedure is to be performed, you and the surgeon must ensure that the site has been marked by the surgeon (see agency policy). Indelible ink may be used to mark left and right distinction, multiple structures (e.g., fingers), and levels of the spine. You also must verify the client and the procedure to be performed. In addition, once the client reaches the OR, he or she is introduced to the surgical team. The client is asked to describe what procedure is being performed and to indicate the site for the surgery. The consent form is verified.

BOX 49-5 EVIDENCE-INFORMED PRACTICE GUIDELINE

Latex Precautions

1. Survey the client care area and remove any products containing latex (e.g., examination gloves, rubber sheets, or blood pressure cuff).
2. Place a latex precautions label on the client's chart and latex precautions signs on the door to the client's room and on the transport cart.
3. Use only non-latex gloves. Order an adequate supply.
4. Review the supplies to be used for the client and substitute with latex-free supplies as necessary.
5. Review the medications to be administered and verify that they are latex-free. Include the following steps:
   a. Notify the pharmacy of the need for latex precautions.
   b. Verify that all prescribed medications are latex-free.
   c. Place a sign in the area where medications (including mixing solutions) are kept, indicating that the client is on latex precautions.
   d. Use latex-free syringes.
6. Review the intravenous supplies to be used and verify that they are latex-free. Include the following steps:
   a. Use latex-free solutions.
   b. Use latex-free tubing
   c. Use latex-free syringes, including those for patient-controlled analgesia.
   d. Use latex-free tape.
7. Verify that bedding and support garments are latex-free (e.g., mattress protectors, anti-embolism stockings, and binders).
8. Verify that dressings and tape are latex-free.
9. Notify the family and visitors of the use of latex precautions.
10. Routinely survey the client care area to verify that latex products are not present (e.g., examination gloves, balloons).
11. Before transfer to another area or agency, notify care professionals of the need for latex precautions.
12. Provide education programs about latex allergy to health care professionals, clients, and family or caregivers. This education should include the following:
    a. Definition of latex allergy
    b. Exposures to latex
    c. Latex avoidance
    d. Signs and symptoms of a reaction to latex
    e. Emergency treatment of a reaction to latex

Adapted from Sussman, G., & Gold, M. (2004). *Guidelines for the management of latex allergies and safe latex use in health care facilities.* Retrieved February, 2009, from http://www.accai.org/public/physicians/latex.htm; and Association of Operating Room Nurses (AORN). (2004). AORN latex guidelines. In *Standards, recommended practices and guidelines* (pp. 103–118). Denver, CO: Author.

❖Evaluation

Client Care

The nurse in the preoperative area will be the source for evaluating outcomes during the preoperative period (Figure 49–6). With regard to the preoperative client's care plan, limited time is available to evaluate the outcomes. The client's current status is compared with expected outcomes to determine whether new or revised interventions or nursing diagnoses need to be implemented.

Because interventions continue during and after surgery, evaluation of many goals and outcomes do not occur until after surgery. For example, you will not be able to evaluate the success in preventing postoperative wound infection or promoting return of normal physiological function until a few days after surgery. If the client is having ambulatory surgery, he or she will return home; therefore, the effectiveness of certain interventions may not be easily evaluated.

Client Expectations

Determining whether the client's expectations have been met regarding preoperative teaching may be difficult. You are evaluating the client in a hurried atmosphere because there are many things that need to be accomplished in a short amount of time. The client's surgery may be an emergency, or performance of various procedures may

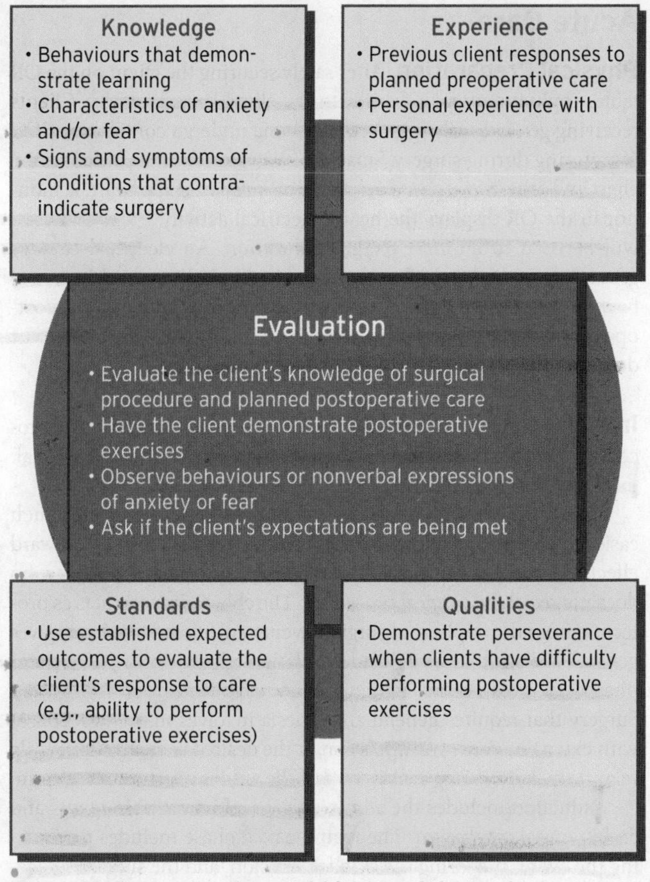

Knowledge
- Behaviours that demonstrate learning
- Characteristics of anxiety and/or fear
- Signs and symptoms of conditions that contraindicate surgery

Experience
- Previous client responses to planned preoperative care
- Personal experience with surgery

Evaluation
- Evaluate the client's knowledge of surgical procedure and planned postoperative care
- Have the client demonstrate postoperative exercises
- Observe behaviours or nonverbal expressions of anxiety or fear
- Ask if the client's expectations are being met

Standards
- Use established expected outcomes to evaluate the client's response to care (e.g., ability to perform postoperative exercises)

Qualities
- Demonstrate perseverance when clients have difficulty performing postoperative exercises

Figure 49-6 Critical thinking model for surgical client evaluation.

make it difficult for you to find time for evaluation. The client may feel somewhat depersonalized by the need to complete preoperative procedures. It is important that you remember to attend to the client's emotional needs (privacy, fear, anxiety), as well as to his or her physical needs. The client should be given an opportunity to state whether expectations have been met. If expectations have not been met, you will need to work closely with the client to redefine expectations that can be realistically met within the time limits imposed by the particular setting.

Transport to the Operating Room

Personnel in the OR notify the nursing division or ambulatory surgery area when it is time for the client's surgery. In many hospitals, a nursing orderly or transporter brings a stretcher for transporting the client. The transporter checks the client's identification bracelet against the client's chart to ensure that the right person is going to surgery. Because the client may have received preoperative drugs, the nurses and transporter assist the client when transferring from bed to stretcher to prevent falls. The ambulatory surgery client may ambulate to the OR if able to do so and not medicated. Provide the family with an opportunity to visit before the client is transported to the OR. Then direct the family to a waiting area. In some hospitals, the family may be allowed to wait with the client in the OR holding area until he or she is transported into the OR.

After the client leaves the nursing division, you should prepare the bed and the room for the client's return, if the client is returning to the same nursing division. A postoperative bedside unit should include the following:

- Sphygmomanometer, stethoscope, and equipment to take a temperature
- Emesis basin
- Clean gown
- Washcloth, towel, and facial tissues
- IV pole
- Suction equipment (if needed)
- Oxygen equipment (if needed)
- Extra pillows for positioning the client comfortably
- Bed pads to protect bed linens from drainage
- Bed raised to stretcher height with bed linens pulled back and furniture moved to accommodate the stretcher and equipment (such as IV lines)

Intraoperative Surgical Phase

Care of the client during surgery requires careful preparation and knowledge of the events that occur during the surgical procedure. The nurse usually functions in one of two roles in the OR: circulating nurse or scrub nurse. The **circulating nurse** must be a registered nurse. Responsibilities of this nurse include reviewing the preoperative assessment, establishing and implementing the intraoperative care plan, evaluating the care, and providing for continuity of care postoperatively. The circulating nurse assists with procedures, such as endotracheal intubation and blood administration, as needed. In addition, this nurse monitors sterile technique and a safe OR environment, assists the surgeon and surgical team by providing additional supplies, verifying sponge and instrument counts, and maintaining accurate and complete written records.

The **scrub nurse** may be a registered nurse or a registered practical nurse. This nurse maintains a sterile field during the surgical procedure, assists with applying sterile drapes, hands the surgeons instruments and other sterile supplies, and completes sponge and instrument counts.

Preoperative (Holding) Area

In most hospitals, the client enters a holding area outside the OR, also known as the PACU. As the nurse in the holding area, you should explain the steps that will be taken to prepare the client for surgery, verify that appropriate data have been obtained, assess a client's readiness both physically and emotionally, and reinforce teaching (Sullivan, 2000). Nurses in the holding area are members of the OR staff and wear surgical scrub suits, hats, and footwear in accordance with infection-control policies. In some ambulatory surgical settings, a perioperative primary nurse admits the client, circulates for the operative procedure, and manages the client's recovery and discharge.

In the preoperative area, you or the anaesthesiologist may insert an IV catheter into the client's arm to establish a route for fluid replacement and IV drugs. A large-bore (18-gauge) IV catheter is used for easy infusion of fluids and blood products if necessary. You also apply a blood pressure cuff. The cuff will remain in place throughout the surgery so that the anaesthesiologist can assess blood pressure readings. You usually review the preoperative checklist, and the anaesthesiologist may perform a client assessment at this time.

If any preoperative medications have been given, the client begins to feel drowsy. The temperature in the holding area and adjacent OR suites is usually cool, and the client should be offered an extra blanket. The client's stay in the holding area is usually brief.

Admission to the Operating Room

Nurses transfer the client to the OR via a stretcher. Usually the client is still awake and will notice nurses and physicians wearing complete surgical masks, gowns, and eyewear. The staff carefully transfers the client to the OR table, after ensuring that the stretcher and table are locked in place. After the client is on the table, fasten a safety strap around the client. Support the client by explaining procedures and encouraging the client to ask questions. Sights and sounds in the surgical suite can seem frightening to clients.

The Nursing Process in the Intraoperative Surgical Phase

❖Assessment

In the holding area, conduct a focused preoperative assessment to verify that the client is ready for surgery and to plan intraoperative care. Because clients will not be able to speak for themselves while under general anaesthesia, this preoperative assessment in the OR is important for the client's safety.

safety alert Verification of the client's name by client response compared with chart and ID bracelet is completed before sedation. The chart is reviewed for consent forms, allergies, medical history, physical assessment findings, test results, and verification of preoperative medications. You verify with the client the planned surgical procedure and the surgical site before anaesthesia is administered. Some agencies ask the client to mark the surgical site. You ensure that the client's prosthetic devices and valuables have been removed.

You review the preoperative care plan to establish an intraoperative care plan and assess the client's psychological comfort.

❖Nursing Diagnosis

You review preoperative nursing diagnoses and modify them to individualize the care plan in the OR.

❖Planning

Goals and Outcomes

Client-centred outcomes of preoperative care extend into the intraoperative phase. For example, one goal would be to maintain skin integrity. Expected outcomes include the following:

- Client will have intact skin and show no signs of redness.
- Client will be free of burns at the grounding pad.

❖Implementation

A primary focus of intraoperative care is to prevent injury and complications related to anaesthesia, surgery, positioning, and equipment used. The perioperative nurse serves as an advocate for the client during surgery and protects the client's dignity and rights at all times.

Acute Care

Physical Preparation. After safely securing the client on the OR table, apply monitoring devices to the client before surgery. Clients receiving general and regional anaesthesia undergo continuous ECG monitoring during surgery. Small plastic electrodes are placed on the chest and extremities to record electrical activity of the heart. A monitor in the OR displays the heart's electrical activity. Pulse oximetry will be used to monitor oxygen saturation. An electrical cautery grounding pad is applied to the skin. **Antiembolism stockings** may be applied intraoperatively (especially during long surgeries) or postoperatively according to agency policy (see Chapter 46). Document device application and client tolerance to procedures.

Introduction of Anaesthesia. Clients undergoing surgical procedures receive one of four types of anaesthesia: general, regional, local, or conscious sedation.

General Anaesthesia. Modern anaesthetic agents are much easier to reverse and allow the client to recover with fewer untoward effects. **General anaesthesia** results in an immobile, quiet client who does not recall the surgical procedure. The client's amnesia acts as protection from the unpleasant surgical events. An anaesthesiologist gives general anaesthetics by IV and inhalation routes through the three phases of anaesthesia: induction, maintenance, and emergence. Surgery that requires general anaesthesia involves major procedures with extensive tissue manipulation or the desire for analgesia, muscle relaxation, immobility, and control of the autonomic nervous system.

Induction includes the administration of anaesthetic agents and endotracheal intubation. The maintenance phase includes positioning the client, preparing the skin for incision, and the surgical procedure itself. Appropriate levels of anaesthesia are maintained during this phase. During emergence, anaesthetics are decreased and the client begins to awaken. Because of the short half-life of current medications, emergence often begins to occur in the OR.

The duration of anaesthesia depends on the length of surgery. The greatest risks from general anaesthesia are the side effects of anaesthetic agents, including cardiovascular depression or irritability, respiratory depression, and liver and kidney damage.

Regional Anaesthesia. Induction of **regional anaesthesia** results in loss of sensation in an area of the body. The method of induction influences the portion of sensory pathways that are anaesthetized. No loss of consciousness occurs with regional anaesthesia, but the client may be sedated. The anaesthesiologist gives regional anaesthetics by infiltration and local application. Administration techniques include nerve blocks and spinal or epidural anaesthesia, and IV regional anaesthesia.

Infiltrative anaesthetics do involve risks, particularly in the case of spinal anaesthesia. Because the level of anaesthesia may rise, which means that the anaesthetic agent moves upward in the spinal cord, breathing may be affected. This migration of the anaesthetic agent depends on the drug type, amount, and client position. If the level of anaesthesia rises, respiratory paralysis may develop, requiring resuscitation. Elevation of the upper body prevents respiratory paralysis. The client may experience a sudden fall in blood pressure, which results from extensive vasodilation caused by the anaesthetic block to sympathetic vasomotor nerves and pain and motor nerve fibres. The client requires careful monitoring during and immediately after surgery.

Because the client is responsive and capable of breathing voluntarily, it is not necessary for the anaesthesiologist to use an endotracheal tube. OR personnel can gain a false sense of security because of the client's relative alertness. Nurses must remember that burns and other trauma can occur on the anaesthetized part of the body without the client's being aware of these injuries. Therefore, nurses must observe the position of the extremities and the condition of the skin frequently.

Local Anaesthesia. Local anaesthesia involves loss of sensation at the desired site (e.g., a growth on the skin or the cornea of the eye). The anaesthetic agent (e.g., lidocaine) inhibits nerve conduction until the drug diffuses into the body's circulation. It may be injected locally or applied topically. The client experiences a loss in pain and touch sensation at the site. Local anaesthesia is commonly used for minor procedures performed in ambulatory surgery. Physicians may infiltrate the operative area with local anaesthetics to promote postoperative pain relief. For example, peripheral nerve blocks produce anaesthetic effect both at and distal to the site of injection (Turjanica, 2007).

Conscious Sedation. Conscious sedation is routinely used for procedures that do not require complete anaesthesia but rather a depressed level of consciousness. A client under conscious sedation must independently retain a patent airway and airway reflexes and must be able to respond appropriately to physical and verbal stimuli (Litwack, 1999). Short-acting IV sedatives, such as midazolam, are given.

Advantages of conscious sedation include adequate sedation and reduction of fear and anxiety with minimal risk, amnesia, relief of pain and noxious stimuli, mood alteration, elevation of pain threshold, enhanced client cooperation, stable vital signs, and rapid recovery. A variety of diagnostic and therapeutic procedures are appropriate for conscious sedation (burn dressing changes, some cosmetic surgery, pulmonary biopsy and bronchoscopy, colonoscopy, and many others (Litwack, 1999). Nurses assisting with the administration of local anaesthesia and conscious sedation must demonstrate competency in the care of these clients. Knowledge of anatomy, physiology, cardiac dysrhythmias, procedural complications, and pharmacological principles related to the administration of individual agents is essential. Nurses also must be able to assess, diagnose, and intervene in the event of untoward reactions and demonstrate skill in airway management and oxygen delivery. Resuscitation equipment must be readily available when local anaesthesia or conscious sedation is used (AORN, 2002a).

Positioning the Client for Surgery. When general anaesthesia is being used, the nursing personnel and surgeon often do not position the client until the stage of complete relaxation is achieved. The choice of position is usually determined by the surgical approach. Ideally, the client's position provides good access to the operative site and sustains adequate circulatory and respiratory function. It should not impair neuromuscular structures. The client's comfort and safety must be considered.

Normal range of joint motion is maintained in an alert person by pain and pressure receptors. If a joint is extended too far, pain stimuli provide a warning that muscle and joint strain is too great. In a client who is anaesthetized, normal defence mechanisms cannot guard against joint damage, muscle stretch, and strain. The muscles are so relaxed that it is relatively easy to place the client in a position the individual normally could not assume while awake. The client then remains in a given position, often for several hours. Although it may be necessary to place a client in an unusual position, attempt to maintain correct alignment and protect the client from pressure, abrasion, and other injuries. Attachments to the operating table allow protection and padding of extremities and bony prominences. Positioning should not impede normal movement of the diaphragm or interfere with circulation to body parts. If restraints are necessary, pad the area to be restrained to prevent skin trauma.

Documentation of Intraoperative Care. During the intraoperative phase, the nursing staff continues the preoperative care plan. For example, strict asepsis must be followed to minimize the risk of surgical wound infection. IV fluid infusion and monitoring of urinary and nasogastric output are examples of actions nurses will take to maintain the client's fluid balance. Throughout the surgical procedure, keep an accurate record of client care activities and procedures performed by OR personnel. Documentation of intraoperative care provides useful data for the nurse who will care for the client postoperatively.

❖Evaluation

Interventions implemented during the intraoperative phase are evaluated throughout the surgical procedure.

Client Care

Nurses perform intraoperative evaluation of the client. Vital signs and intake and output are monitored continuously. The client's body temperature is measured during the procedure and on completion of the surgical procedure. The skin is inspected under the grounding pad and at areas where pressure from positioning may have been exerted. Schoonhoven et al. (2002) conducted research related to the development of pressure ulcers during surgery that lasts more than 4 hours. Of the 208 clients in their study, 44 developed ulcers in the first 2 days after surgery. Therefore, careful monitoring and preventive measures must be taken during and after surgery.

Client Expectations

Nurses should frequently question clients not undergoing general anaesthesia regarding pain, numbness, perceived room temperature, and overall comfort. The circulating nurse provides updates to family members in the waiting room.

Postoperative Surgical Phase

After surgery, a client's care can become complex as a result of physiological changes that may occur. Clients who have undergone general anaesthesia are more likely to face complications than those who have had only local anaesthesia or conscious sedation. The client who has had general anaesthesia usually has undergone extensive surgery as well. In contrast, an ambulatory surgical client who has had local anaesthesia with no sedation and has stable vital signs may be discharged immediately. A client who has undergone regional or general anaesthesia usually is transferred to the PACU to be stabilized before discharge to the nursing unit or back to the ambulatory surgery area.

To assess a client's postoperative condition, you must apply critical thinking while relying on information from the preoperative nursing assessment, knowledge regarding the surgical procedure performed, and events occurring during surgery. This information helps you detect any changes and make decisions about the client's care. A variation from the client's norm may indicate the onset of surgery-related complications. Along with the anaesthesiologist, the circulating nurse may accompany the client to the PACU and report to the nurse to provide continuity of care.

A client's postoperative course involves two phases: the immediate recovery period and postoperative convalescence. For an ambulatory surgical client, recovery normally lasts only 1 to 2 hours, and **convalescence** occurs at home. For a hospitalized client, recovery may last a few hours, and convalescence occurs over 1 or more days, depending on the extent of the surgery and the client's response to it.

Immediate Postoperative Recovery

Before the client arrives in the PACU, the PACU nurse obtains data from the surgical team in the OR regarding the client's general status and the need for special equipment and nursing care. Careful planning allows the nursing staff to consider placement of clients in the PACU. For example, clients who have undergone spinal anaesthesia are aware of their surroundings and may benefit from being in a quieter part of the PACU, away from clients who need frequent monitoring. The client with a serious infection such as tuberculosis should be isolated from other clients. Standard precautions or routine practices for infection control are used for all clients (see Chapter 33). Nurses must be familiar with agency and professional protocols related to preventing respiratory infection transmission (Ontario Ministry of Health and Long-Term Care, 2004).

When the client is admitted to the PACU, the PACU personnel notify the client care area of the client's arrival. This allows the nursing staff to inform family members. Usually, nurses would advise family members to remain in the designated waiting area so that they can be found when the surgeon arrives to explain the client's condition. The surgeon is responsible for describing the client's status, the results of surgery, and any complications that may have been encountered. Nurses can be a valuable resource to the family if complications arose during the operative phase.

When the client enters the PACU (Figure 49–7), nurses and members of the surgical team confer about the client's status. The surgical team's report includes a review of anaesthetic agents administered so that nurses can anticipate both how quickly a client should regain consciousness and his or her analgesic needs. A report on IV fluids or blood products administered during surgery alerts nurses to the client's fluid and electrolyte balances. The surgeon often reports any special concerns (e.g., whether the client is at risk for hemorrhaging or infection). The anaesthesiologist discusses whether there were complications during surgery, such as excessive blood loss or cardiac irregularities. Frequently, this report takes place while PACU nurses are admitting the client. You will attach the client to monitoring equipment such as the noninvasive blood pressure monitor, ECG monitor, and pulse oximeter. Clients usually receive some form of oxygen in this immediate recovery period. Take vital signs when the client arrives and confirm these with the surgical team.

After reviewing events in the OR, make a complete assessment of the client's status. This assessment should be performed rapidly and thoroughly and be targeted to the needs of the postsurgical client. Standards of perianaesthetic nursing practice, such as those of OPANA (2005), function as a guide for agencies in outlining the urgent nature and components of the admission assessment as well as ongoing monitoring of client status. A systems approach to assessment is discussed in a later section outlining the nursing process in postoperative care. Nursing care in the PACU focuses on monitoring and maintaining respiratory, circulatory, neurological, and fluid and electrolyte status; assessing wound status; and assessing and managing pain (see "The Nursing Process in Postoperative Care" section).

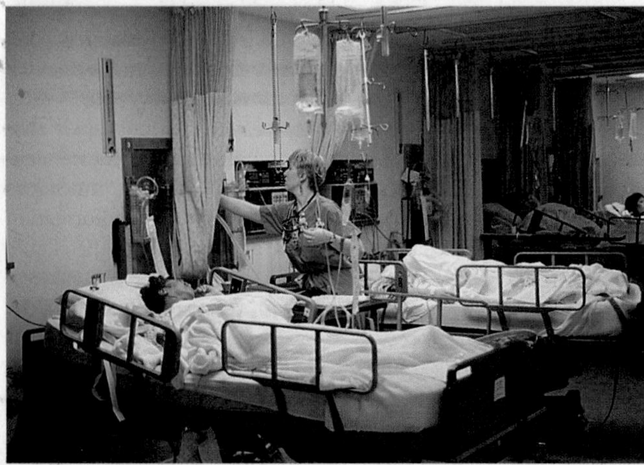

Figure 49-7 Postanaesthesia care unit.

Discharge From the Postanaesthesia Care Unit

Nurses evaluate readiness for discharge from the PACU by comparing vital sign stability with the preoperative data. Other outcomes for discharge include body temperature control, good ventilatory function, orientation to surroundings, absence of complications, minimal pain and nausea, controlled wound drainage, adequate urine output, and fluid and electrolyte balances. Clients who had more extensive surgery that required anaesthesia of longer duration usually recover more slowly. Many PACU staff use an objective scoring system that helps to delineate when clients may be discharged. The Aldrete score, or the **Postanesthesia Recovery Score (PARS)**, is the most widely used scoring tool (Table 49–8). The client must receive a composite score of 8 to 10 before discharge from the PACU. Some agencies have

TABLE 49-8 Modified Aldrete Score

Parameter	Task	Score
Activity	Able to move four extremities voluntarily or on command	2
	Able to move two extremities voluntarily or on command	1
	Unable to move extremities voluntarily or on command	0
Respiration	Able to breathe deeply and cough freely	2
	Dyspnea or limited breathing	1
	Apneic	0
Blood pressure	±20% of preanaesthetic level	2
	±20%–49% of preanaesthetic level	1
	±50% of preanaesthetic level	0
Consciousness	Fully awake	2
	Arousable on calling	1
	Not responding	0
Oxygen saturation	SpO_2 >92% on room air	2
	Needs O_2 inhalation to maintain SpO_2 >90%	1
	SpO_2 <90% even with extra O_2	0
Total		

Adapted from Aldrete, J. A., & Kroulik, D. (1970). A post-anesthetic recovery score. *Anesthesia and Analgesia, 49,* 924–934; and Aldrete, J. A. (1998). Modifications to the post-anesthesia score for use in ambulatory surgery. *Journal of Perianesthesia Nursing, 13*(3), 148.

modified this scoring system; for example, some remove movement of extremities and add presence of pain, and some agencies require that the client have a composite score of 10 before discharge from the PACU. If the client's condition is still poor after 2 to 3 hours, the stay in the PACU lengthens or the surgeon may transfer the client to an intensive care unit.

When the client is ready to be discharged from the PACU, you may call the nursing unit to report the client's status, including vital signs, respiratory status, the type of surgery and anaesthesia performed, any complications that occurred during surgery or in the PACU, blood loss, level of consciousness, general physical condition, type and amount of fluids received, and presence of IV lines, drainage tubes, and dressings. You also should review physician orders that require attention. Your report helps the nurse in the acute client care area to anticipate special client needs and obtain necessary equipment. Any outstanding family issues are also addressed.

Personnel, who may include nurses, transport the client on a stretcher. If the PACU nurse accompanies the client to the surgical unit, a report will be given to the acute care nurse at that time. Some institutions have policies related to which clients must be accompanied by a nurse, such as those who have experienced recent seizure activity or who have had upper airway surgery. Staff members assist in safely transferring the client to a bed (see Chapter 36). The PACU nurse, if helping to transport the client, shows the acute care nurse the recovery room record and reviews the client's condition and course of care.

Recovery in Ambulatory Surgery

The thoroughness and extent of postoperative recovery care depends on the ambulatory client's condition, type of surgery, and anaesthesia. There are two phases of postanaesthesia recovery. During phase I, you focus on helping the client safely transition from a totally anaesthetized state to one requiring less acute interventions. After clients become stable and no longer require such intensive monitoring, you transfer them to phase II recovery. During phase II, you focus on continuing the recovery process, addressing the client's needs, and preparing the client and family for discharge from phase II (OPANA, 2005).

With new anaesthetic agents and techniques, clients experience a more rapid awakening in the OR (Apfelbaum et al., 2002; Fredman et al., 2002; Saar, 2001). Therefore, some ambulatory surgery clients may bypass phase I. This is known as fast tracking (White et al., 2003). Phase II recovery may consist of a room equipped with medical recliner chairs, side tables, and footrests. Kitchen facilities for preparing light snacks and beverages are usually located in the area, along with bathrooms. Aldrete (1998) has added five more areas of functional assessment for the ambulatory surgery client, which constitute the **Postanesthesia Recovery Score for Ambulatory Patients** (**PARSAP**; Table 49–9). The phase II environment is designed to promote both the client's and the family's comfort and well-being until discharge. You continue to monitor clients but not at the same intensity as during phase I. In phase II recovery, you initiate postoperative teaching with clients and family members (Box 49–6).

Ambulatory surgical clients are discharged to home when they meet certain criteria. A client being monitored by PARSAP must achieve a score of 18 or higher before being discharged. An exception may be allowed if the client was unable to walk or move his or her extremities before surgery (Aldrete, 1998). Postoperative nausea and vomiting may occur once the client is home even if the symptoms were not present at the time of discharge. Options for therapy include the prophylactic use of the drug ondansetron (an orally disintegrating tablet), transcutaneous acupoint electrical stimulation, or a transdermal scopolamine patch (Gan, 2002).

➤ TABLE 49-9 Expanded Postanesthetic Recovery Score for Ambulatory Patients

Parameter	Task	Score
Activity	Able to move four extremities voluntarily or on command	2
	Able to move two extremities voluntarily or on command	1
	Unable to move extremities voluntarily or on command	0
Respiration	Able to breathe deeply and cough freely	2
	Dyspnea or limited breathing	1
	Apneic	0
Blood pressure	±20% of preanaesthetic level	2
	±20%–49% of preanaesthetic level	1
	±50% of preanaesthetic level	0
Consciousness	Fully awake	2
	Arousable on calling	1
	Not responding	0
Oxygen saturation	SpO_2 >92% on room air	2
	Needs O_2 inhalation to maintain SpO_2 >90%	1
	SpO_2 <90% even with extra O_2	0
Dressing	Dry and clean	2
	Wet but marked and not increasing	1
	Growing area of wetness	0
Pain	Pain-free	2
	Mild pain handled by oral medication	1
	Severe pain requiring parenteral medication	0
Ambulation	Able to stand up and walk straight*	2
	Vertigo when erect	1
	Dizziness when supine	0
Fasting or feeding	Able to drink fluids	2
	Nauseated	1
	Nausea and vomiting	0
Urine output	Has voided	2
	Unable to void but comfortable	1
	Unable to void and uncomfortable	0
Total		

Note: Total score must be at least 18 for client to be discharged to home.
*May be substituted by Romberg's test, or by picking up 12 clips in one hand.

Adapted from Aldrete, J. A., & Kroulik, D. (1970). A post-anesthetic recovery score. *Anesthesia and Analgesia, 49*, 924–934; and Aldrete, J. A. (1998). Modifications to the post-anesthesia score for use in ambulatory surgery. *Journal of Perianesthesia Nursing, 13*, 148.

BOX 49-6 CLIENT TEACHING

Postoperative Instructions for Ambulatory Surgical Clients

Objectives

- Client will verbalize resources to contact for assistance.
- Client will describe signs and symptoms of post-operative problems.
- Client will list the name and dose of medications to self-administer.
- Client will describe guidelines related to specific surgery.

Teaching Strategies

- Provide instruction sheet with physician's or nurse's telephone number, surgery centre's number, and follow-up appointment date and time. Allow client and family to ask questions.
- Explain to family members the signs and symptoms of infection for which to observe.
- Explain name, dose, schedule, and purpose of medications. Provide drug information leaflets.
- Explain activity restrictions, diet progression, and any special wound care related to specific surgery. Provide instruction sheet with clear, focused explanations.

Evaluation

- Ask client to describe signs indicating potential problems and normal convalescence.
- Ask client to explain when and how to call health care professionals such as the home care nurse.
- Ask client to recite date for follow-up appointment.
- Ask client and family members to describe the signs and symptoms of infection.
- Ask client to verbalize name of drug, dose, and when to take.
- Ask client to demonstrate proper activity or movement and wound care.

Written postoperative instructions and prescriptions are reviewed with the client and the family, and you should ensure that they verbalize understanding of these instructions. The client is discharged to the care of a responsible adult.

Postoperative Convalescence

Inpatient clients are kept in the PACU until their conditions stabilize; they are then transported to the postoperative nursing unit. Ambulatory surgery clients will return home. Nursing care focuses on returning the client to a relatively functional level of wellness as soon as possible. The speed of convalescence depends on the type or extent of surgery, the risk factors involved, and any postoperative complications.

The Nursing Process in Postoperative Care

Nursing care in the PACU focuses on managing pain and monitoring and maintaining respiratory, circulatory, fluid and electrolyte, and neurological status. Other important factors to assess include temperature control, skin and incision or wound status, and genitourinary and gastrointestinal function. However, these factors are not unique to the PACU setting. The nurse in the acute care unit continues to assess these critical factors on a less intensive basis until the client's discharge from the acute care facility.

❖Assessment

After assessment upon the client's arrival to the PACU, the PACU nurse repeats evaluation of vital signs and other key observations at least every 15 minutes or more frequently, depending on the client's condition and unit policy. This assessment usually continues until discharge from the PACU. Once the client is returned to the surgical unit, the nurse admitting the client takes vital signs immediately in order to compare them with the PACU findings. Vital sign monitoring in the postoperative nursing unit initially should be hourly for 4 hours and then every 4 hours, unless complications develop. Frequency of assessment should always be based on the client's current condition, which can change rapidly, especially during the postoperative period.

You thoroughly document your assessment, including vital signs, respiratory status, level of consciousness, condition of dressings and drains, comfort level, skin warmth and colour, ability to move extremities, IV fluid status, and urinary output measurements. Client data can be entered on flow sheets, a computerized client record, or written progress notes. The initial findings are a baseline for comparing any postoperative changes.

Once the client returns to the acute care area, you focus on completing the assessment, meeting the client's immediate needs, and providing an opportunity for the family to be with the client. The call light and emesis basin should be within the client's reach. You can explain the purpose of postoperative procedures or equipment and the client's status. The family should know that the client will fall in and out of sleep for most of the rest of the day due to the effects of general anaesthesia and pain medication. The family also should be reminded that frequent assessments are to be expected and that limited sensation and movement in the client's extremities may remain for a few hours if he or she had spinal or epidural anaesthesia.

Respiration

Certain anaesthetic agents may cause respiratory depression. Thus, you must be especially alert for shallow, slow breathing and a weak cough. You assess airway patency, respiratory rate, rhythm, depth of ventilation, symmetry of chest wall movement, breath sounds, and colour of mucous membranes. If breathing is unusually shallow, placing a hand near the client's nose or mouth allows you to feel exhaled air. Pulse oximetry should reflect 92% to 100% saturation. Some agencies now have directives that allow nurses to administer oxygen at 3 L/minute via nasal prongs if the client has a saturation of less than 92%.

The client often has an oral or nasal airway (see Chapter 39) inserted in the OR after removal of the endotracheal tube to maintain a patent airway until the client can protect his or her airway. As the client awakens in the PACU, he or she will spit out the airway or you will ask him or her to spit it out. The client's ability to do so signifies the return of a normal gag reflex.

One of your greatest concerns is airway obstruction. A number of factors can contribute to obstruction, including weak pharyngeal or laryngeal muscle tone from anaesthetics; secretions in the pharynx, bronchial tree, or trachea; and laryngeal or subglottic edema (Litwack, 1999). In the postanaesthetic client, the tongue causes the majority of airway obstructions. Ongoing assessment of airway patency is crucial. Clients are often kept in side-lying positions until airways are clear.

In the acute care area, you continue to assess respiratory status and breath sounds. Older clients, smokers, and clients with a history of respiratory disease are prone to developing complications such as atelectasis or pneumonia. The client is also assessed for any signs of shortness of breath with activity.

Circulation

The client is at risk for cardiovascular complications resulting from actual or potential blood loss from the surgical site, side effects of anaesthesia, electrolyte imbalances, and depression of normal circulatory regulating mechanisms. Careful assessment of heart rate and rhythm, along with blood pressure, reveals the client's cardiovascular status. A rhythm strip is usually obtained postoperatively, compared with preoperative ECG tracings, and mounted on the PACU record. The vital signs are monitored at least every 15 minutes throughout the PACU recovery phase. Preoperative vital signs are compared with postoperative values. The physician should be notified if the client's blood pressure drops progressively with each check or if the heart rate changes or becomes irregular.

You assess circulatory perfusion by noting capillary refill, pulses, and the colour and temperature of the nail beds and skin. If the client has had vascular surgery or has casts or constricting devices that may impair circulation, you should assess peripheral pulses and capillary refill distal to the site of surgery. For example, after surgery to the femoral artery, you assess posterior tibial and dorsalis pedis pulses. You also compare pulses in the affected extremity with those in the nonaffected extremity.

A common early circulatory problem is hemorrhage. Blood loss may occur externally through a drain or incision, or internally. Either type of hemorrhage may result in a fall in blood pressure; elevated heart and respiratory rates; thready pulse; cool, clammy, pale skin; and restlessness. Often, the first sign of hemorrhage is restlessness. Signs such as thready pulse and clammy skin are noted much later, after significant blood loss has occurred. The surgeon must be notified if these types of changes are noted. You maintain IV fluid infusion and may need to increase IV replacement fluids. Monitor the client's vital signs every 15 minutes or more frequently until his or her condition stabilizes. Oxygen may need to be continued. Volume replacement and medications to promote perfusion to vital organs such as the brain may be considered. Plasma expanders (colloids) may be used instead of blood transfusions. Colloids may be made from blood products (i.e., albumin), but artificial colloids, such as hetastarch, also exist (Diepenbrock, 2008). Blood counts and coagulation studies are drawn and sent to the laboratory. The potential for cardiovascular complications remains when the client is transferred to the acute care area. In that area, you continue to assess the same factors that were identified in the PACU.

Temperature Control

The OR and recovery room environments are kept extremely cool. The client's anaesthetically depressed level of body function results in a lowering of metabolism and a fall in body temperature. When clients begin to awaken, they complain of feeling cold and uncomfortable. The length of time spent in the OR and laminar flow rooms contributes to heat loss. Surgeries that require an open body cavity also contribute to heat loss. Older adults and pediatric clients are at higher risk for developing problems associated with hypothermia.

In rare instances, **malignant hyperthermia**, a genetically determined condition and a life-threatening complication of anaesthesia, develops. Malignant hyperthermia causes tachypnea, tachycardia, premature ventricular contractions, unstable blood pressure, cyanosis, skin mottling, and muscular rigidity. An elevated temperature occurs late. Although it is often seen during the induction phase of anaesthesia, symptoms may recur 24 to 72 hours postoperatively (Karlet, 1998). Without prompt detection and treatment, it can be fatal.

Temperature is monitored closely in the acute care area. Because an elevated temperature may be the first indication of an infection, you evaluate the client for a potential source of infection, including the IV site (if present), the surgical incision or wound, and the respiratory and urinary tracts. The physician must be notified, because further evaluation, including blood, sputum, and urinary cultures, likely will be needed. In elderly clients, fever may not be seen with infection (Litwack, 2006).

Fluid and Electrolyte Balances

Because of the surgical client's risk for fluid and electrolyte abnormalities, you assess the hydration status and monitor cardiac and neurological function for signs of electrolyte alterations (see Chapter 40). Laboratory values will be monitored and compared with the client's baseline values.

One of your important responsibilities is monitoring the rate and maintaining the patency of IV infusions. The client's only source of fluid intake immediately after surgery is through IV catheters. You must inspect the catheter insertion site to ensure that the catheter is properly positioned within a vein so that fluid flows freely. Accurate recording of intake and output helps assess renal and circulatory function. You record the intravenous infusions received as well as any sources of oral intake once peristalsis returns. You measure all sources of output, including urine, surgically placed drains, gastric drainage, and drainage from wounds, and note any insensible loss from diaphoresis. Daily weights may be assessed postoperatively if the client has a known cardiac or renal history (e.g., heart failure). It is important to compare preoperative and postoperative weights and to be consistent in the scale used, the amount of clothing worn by the client, and the time of day to obtain accurate weight measurement. Accurate recording of intake and output is crucial. It is also important to be aware of the amount of fluids received in the intraoperative and immediate postoperative period. For example, if large amounts of fluid were received during surgery, the client may exhibit signs of fluid retention such as pedal edema or abnormal breath sounds.

Neurological Functions

The client is often drowsy in the PACU. As anaesthetic agents are metabolized, the client's reflexes return, muscle strength is regained, and a normal level of orientation returns. A client should at least be oriented to self and to the hospital before discharge from the PACU. Assess gag reflexes (see Chapter 32), hand grips, and movement of the client's extremities. If the client has had surgery involving a portion of the neurological system, conduct a more thorough neurological assessment, including assessing pupil size and reaction.

Clients who had regional anaesthesia begin to experience a return in motor function before tactile sensation. You check the client's sensation along **dermatomes** (segmental skin areas innervated by specific segments of the spinal cord). Knowing where anaesthesia was introduced, you are able to check the distribution of the spinal nerves affected (see Chapter 32). Typically, you assess the dermatome level by touching the client bilaterally and documenting where he or she feels touch. The sense of touch can be tested using a paper clip, for example. Assessment of extremity strength, movement, and sensation continues to be important if spinal or epidural anaesthesia has been given, although the client should remain in the PACU until sensation and voluntary movement of the lower extremities have been re-established.

Skin Integrity and Condition of the Wound

In the PACU, nurses assess the condition of the client's skin, noting rashes, petechiae, abrasions, or burns. A rash may indicate a drug sensitivity or allergy. Abrasions or petechiae may result from a clotting disorder or from inappropriate positioning or restraining that injures skin layers. Burns may indicate that an electrical cautery grounding pad was incorrectly placed on the client's skin. Burns or serious injury to the skin should be documented in an incident report (see Chapter 16).You should also make a note if the client complains of any burning or pain in the eye that could indicate a corneal abrasion.

After surgery, most wounds are covered with a dressing that protects the site and collects drainage. You observe the amount, colour, odour, and consistency of drainage on dressings. Serosanguineous drainage is the most common type of drainage occurring immediately after surgery. You estimate the amount of drainage by noting the number of saturated gauze sponges. If drainage appears on the outer surface of a dressing, another way to assess drainage is by drawing a circle around the outer perimeter of the drainage and dating it with the time noted. This way, you can easily note if drainage is increasing (see Chapter 47).

Many physicians prefer to change surgical dressings the first time so that they can inspect the incisional area. The nurse on the surgical nursing unit usually will have the first opportunity to view and thoroughly assess and document the status of the incision or wound. Initially, it is important to note if wound edges are approximated and no active bleeding or drainage is present. Wound assessment is especially important because it forms the baseline for continued monitoring during the client's hospital stay.

It is also important to assess the client's mobility level. If the client is unable or unwilling to turn, pressure ulcer development is a concern. You should use the Braden Scale to determine the client's risk of developing pressure ulcers (RNAO, 2005). Preventive measures such as a turning schedule and pressure-reduction devices can be instituted (see Chapter 47).

Genitourinary Function

Depending on the surgery, a client may not regain voluntary control over urinary function for 6 to 8 hours after anaesthesia. An epidural or spinal anaesthetic may prevent the client from feeling bladder fullness. You should palpate the lower abdomen just above the symphysis pubis for bladder distension or you may use a bladder scanner to identify the amount of urine in the bladder. If the client has a urinary catheter, there should be a continuous flow of urine of 30 to 50 mL/hour in adults (Metheny, 2000). You observe the colour and the odour of the urine. Surgery involving portions of the urinary tract normally causes bloody urine for at least 12 to 24 hours, depending on the type of surgery. You will provide ongoing assessment of genitourinary function.

Gastrointestinal Function

Anaesthetics slow gastrointestinal motility and may cause nausea. Normally during the immediate recovery phase, faint or absent bowel sounds are auscultated in all four quadrants. You inspect the abdomen for distension that may be caused by an accumulation of gas. In a client who has had abdominal surgery, distension will develop if internal bleeding occurs; however, this is a late sign of bleeding. Distension also may occur in the client who develops a **paralytic ileus** as a result of handling of the bowel in surgery.

You closely monitor the client's initial oral intake for potential aspiration or the presence of nausea and vomiting. Assessment also includes checking for return of peristalsis every 4 to 8 hours. Routinely, you auscultate the abdomen to detect return of normal bowel sounds; 5 to 30 loud gurgles per minute over each quadrant indicates that peristalsis has returned. High-pitched tinkling sounds accompanied by abdominal distension suggest that the bowel is not functioning properly. You should ask if the client is passing gas (flatus). This is an important sign indicating normal bowel function. If a nasogastric tube is in place, assess the patency of the tube (see Chapter 45), the colour and amount of any drainage, and (if ordered) the level of suction required.

Comfort

Pain management is included in the overall aim of ensuring client comfort. Comfort is also achieved through nursing measures such as bathing and providing clean bedding. As clients awaken from general anaesthesia, the sensation of pain becomes prominent. Pain can be perceived before full consciousness is regained. Acute incisional pain causes clients to become restless and may be responsible for temporary changes in vital signs. It is difficult for clients to begin coughing and deep breathing exercises when they experience pain. The client who had regional or local anaesthesia may not experience pain initially because the incisional area is still anaesthetized.

Assessment of the client's discomfort and evaluation of pain-relief therapies are essential nursing functions. Pain scales are an effective method for nurses to assess postoperative pain, evaluate response to analgesics, and objectively document pain severity (see Chapter 42). By frequently assessing pain, you can evaluate the effectiveness of interventions (e.g., positioning, analgesics) throughout the client's recovery.

Client Expectations

The nurse assesses the client's and family's expectations and perceived progress in the recovery and convalescence phases. Ongoing assessment of expectations regarding pain control, comfort level, dietary intake, activity level, and readiness for discharge are also performed. You determine the client's and the family's expectations regarding needs at home and incorporate these into the care plan.

❖Nursing Diagnosis

You determine the status of problems identified from preoperative nursing diagnoses, and cluster new relevant data to identify new diagnoses. Previously defined diagnoses, such as *impaired skin integrity*, may continue as a postoperative problem. You may identify new risk factors leading to identification of nursing diagnoses. For example, an older client who has undergone major abdominal surgery and who has a pre-existing problem of reduced hip mobility resulting from arthritis will likely have the diagnosis of *impaired physical mobility*. The surgery itself may add risk factors for the client. You also consider the needs of a client's family when making diagnoses. For example, the inability of the family to cope with the client's condition requires your intervention. Early dialogue with the family can identify any challenges.

❖Planning

Because of the critical nature of the immediate postoperative period, the care plan in the PACU involves close monitoring of the client and frequent assessments to ensure a return to stable physiological function. During the convalescent phase, you use current physical assessment data and analysis of the preoperative nursing health history for planning the client's care. The surgeon's postoperative plan and the institution's clinical pathways also offer guidelines. Typical postoperative plans include the following:

- Frequency of vital sign monitoring and special assessments
- Types of IV fluids and rates of infusion
- Postoperative medications (especially those for pain and nausea)
- Resumption of preoperative medications as condition allows (some oral medications will be converted to the IV route with appropriate dose adjustment)
- Fluids and food allowed by mouth
- Level of activity that the client is allowed to resume
- Position that the client is to maintain while in bed
- Intake and output
- Laboratory tests and X-ray studies
- Special directions (e.g., surgical drains to suction, tube irrigations, dressing changes)
- Discharge planning

Goals and Outcomes

You consider the effects of the stress of surgery and the limitations it produces when establishing goals, expected outcomes, and interventions for the client. Measurable outcomes help to ensure timely and appropriate recovery from surgery. For example, the client at risk for impaired mobility should have specific outcomes that include targeted ambulation (e.g., steps to take and distance down hallway) and range of joint movement. After each outcome is met, the client ultimately will achieve the goal of independent mobility at a preoperative level or better. You carefully consider all goals of care established during the preoperative surgical phase. The following is an example of goals and expected outcomes for the postoperative period:

- Client achieves a return of normal physiological function after surgery.
- Client's vital signs return to preoperative baseline.
- Client's airway is patent and respirations are even and unlaboured.
- Client's temperature returns to baseline. Client's fluid and electrolyte levels remain balanced.
- Client returns to previous level of activity.

Setting Priorities

In the PACU, priorities of care include the assessment and stability of the client's airway; intervention for an impaired airway; assessment of the client's respiratory, circulatory, neurological, and fluid and electrolyte status; and pain control. As the client progresses on the acute care unit, priorities should focus on advancement of client activity to return the client to preoperative functioning or better. The client generally will have multiple nursing diagnoses (Figure 49–8). You may re-establish priorities several times as the client's health status changes.

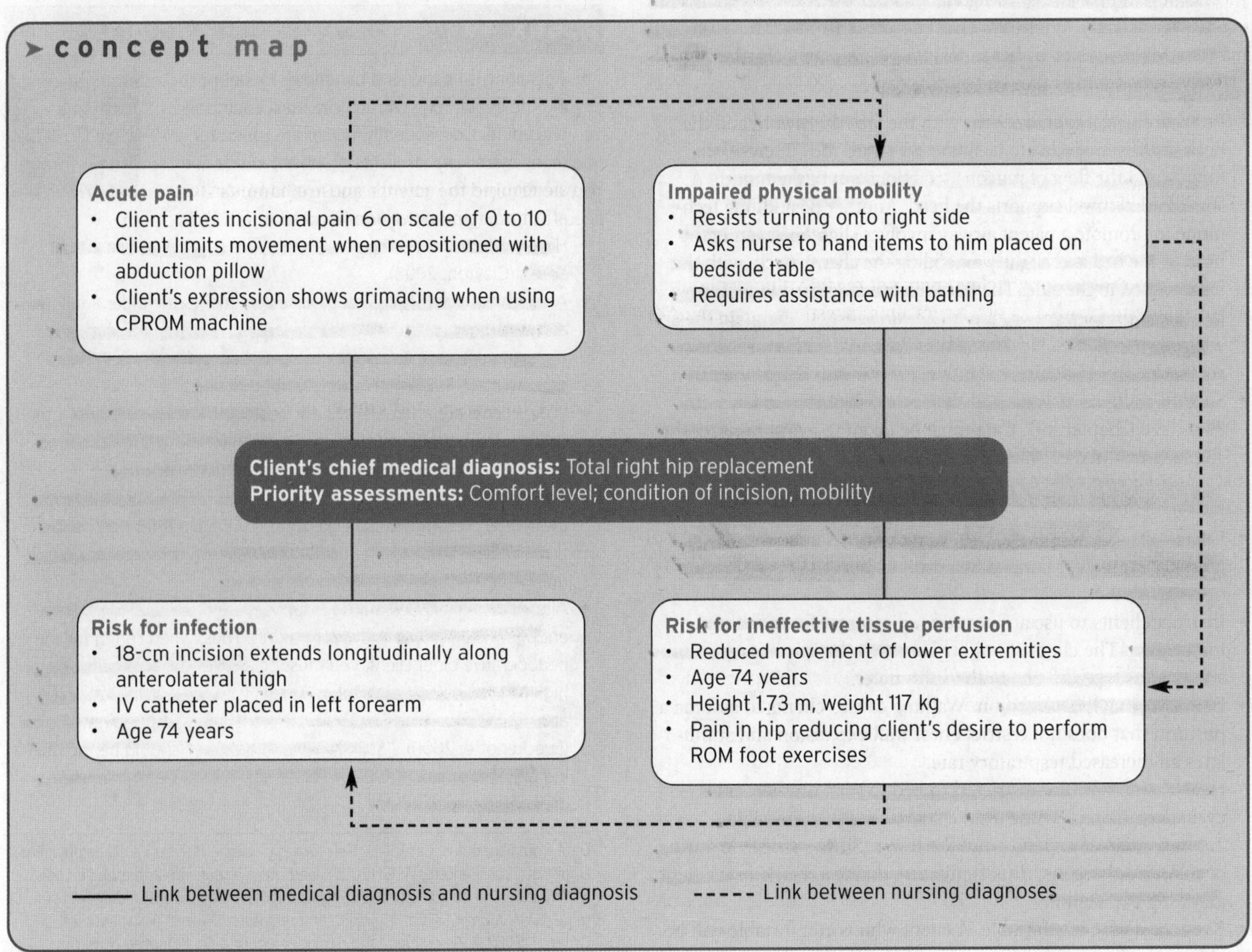

Figure 49-8 Concept map for surgical client with total hip replacement.

Continuity of Care

In the recovery phase, you collaborate on the care plan with staff from respiratory therapy, physiotherapy, occupational therapy, dietary, social work, home care, and other areas to meet the client's needs. The goal of all of these disciplines is to assist the client to return to the best possible level of functioning with a smooth transition to home. The family's role in the care plan to foster recovery is also essential.

❖Implementation

Health Promotion

Primary causes of postoperative complications include the surgical wound, the effects of prolonged immobilization during surgery and convalescence, preoperative risks such as age (Box 49–7), and the influence of anaesthesia and analgesics. Nursing interventions in the postoperative period are directed at preventing complications so that the client returns to the highest level of functioning possible. Failure of the client to become actively involved in recovery adds to the risk for complications (Table 49–10). Virtually any body system can be affected. You must consider the interrelationship of all systems and therapies provided.

Maintaining Respiratory Function. To prevent respiratory complications, begin pulmonary interventions early. The benefits of thorough preoperative teaching are realized when clients are able to participate actively. When the client awakens from anaesthesia, you may need to assist him or her in maintaining a patent airway. The following measures maintain airway patency:

- Position the client on one side with the face downward and the neck slightly extended to facilitate a forward movement of the tongue and the flow of mucous secretions out of the mouth. A small folded towel supports the head. Another positioning technique to promote a patent airway involves slightly elevating the head of the bed and slightly extending the client's neck, with the head turned to the side. The PACU nurse may need to perform a jaw thrust manoeuvre or chin lift continuously to maintain the airway in some clients. Never position the client with arms over or across the chest because this reduces maximum chest expansion.
- Suction artificial airways and the oral cavity for mucous secretions (see Chapter 39). Care must be taken to avoid eliciting the gag reflex, which could cause vomiting.

The following measures promote expansion of the lungs:

- Encourage diaphragmatic breathing exercises every hour while clients are awake. Maximal inspirations lasting 3 to 5 seconds open up alveoli.
- Instruct clients to use an incentive spirometer for maximum inspiration. The client should try to reach the inspiratory volume achieved preoperatively on the spirometer.
- Encourage early ambulation. Walking causes clients to assume a position that does not restrict chest wall expansion and stimulates an increased respiratory rate.
- Help clients who are restricted to bed to turn on their sides every 1 to 2 hours while awake and to sit when possible. Turning permits expansion of the lungs. Sitting causes lowering of abdominal organs, thus facilitating diaphragmatic movement and lung expansion.
- Keep the client comfortable. A client who is comfortable will be able to participate in the postoperative regimen. Assess, document, treat, and evaluate the client's pain on a regular basis.

The following measures promote removal of pulmonary secretions if they are present:

- Encourage coughing exercises every 2 hours while clients are awake and maintain pain control to promote a deep, productive cough. Coughing may be contraindicated for clients who have had eye or intracranial surgery because of the potential increase in intraocular or intracranial pressure.
- Provide oral hygiene to facilitate expectoration of mucus. The oral mucosa becomes dry when clients are NPO or are placed on limited fluid intake.
- Initiate orotracheal or nasotracheal suction for clients who are too weak or unable to cough (see Chapter 39).
- Administer oxygen as ordered and monitor oxygen saturation with a pulse oximeter.

Preventing Circulatory Complications. Measures directed at preventing circulatory complications avert circulatory stasis. Some clients are at greater risk of venous stasis because of the nature of their surgery or medical history. The following measures promote normal venous return and circulatory blood flow:

- Encourage clients to perform leg exercises at least every hour while awake. Exercise may be limited in an affected extremity involving vascular repair or realignment of fractured bones and torn cartilage.

BOX 49-7 FOCUS ON OLDER ADULTS

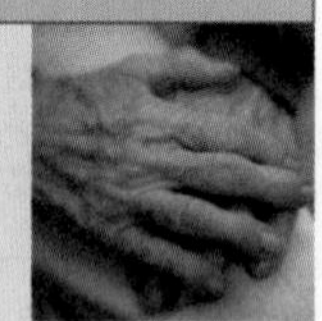

- Age alone is no longer a parameter for determining the benefit one can achieve from a surgical procedure. Consequently, nurses are caring for many more surgical clients of advanced age and are required to know the age-related factors that affect a surgical procedure (Eliopoulos, 2001).
- Hypothermia and postoperative embolism may be seen in older adults (Clayton, 2008).
- A smaller margin of physiological reserve makes the older adult less able to compensate during the perioperative period for changes that can occur due to infection, hemorrhage, alterations in blood pressure, and fluid and electrolyte abnormalities.
- Older clients are at greater risk for postoperative delirium after procedures such as hip replacement. A rapid decline in cognitive function, fluctuations in awareness and orientation, disturbed sleep–wake cycle, and personality and mood changes characterize the typical presentation (Lueckenotte, 2000). Delirium may be the first indicator of infection, fluid or electrolyte imbalances, or deteriorating respiratory or hemodynamic status.
- Altered and unexpected drug responses are often related to different pharmacokinetics in the older adult. Thus, when caring for the perioperative older client, you must be alert to the possibility of a high risk for adverse medication events with the administration of anaesthetic agents and postoperative analgesics, especially narcotics (Lueckenotte, 2000). "Start lower and go slow" should be the guiding principle when medicating older adults because of their slower drug-clearance capability.

Data from Eliopoulos, C. (2001). *Gerontologic nursing* (5th ed.). Philadelphia, PA: Lippincott; Lueckenotte, A. G. (2000). *Gerontologic nursing* (2nd ed.). St. Louis, MO: Mosby; Clayton, J. L. (2008). Special needs of older adults undergoing surgery. *AORN Journal, 87*(3), 557–570; and Registered Nurses' Association of Ontario. (2002a). *Assessment and management of pain.* Retrieved November 5, 2008, from http://www.rnao.org/Page.asp?PageID=924&ContentID=720

TABLE 49-10 Postoperative Complications

Complication	Cause
Respiratory System	
Atelectasis: Collapse of alveoli with retained mucous secretions. Signs and symptoms include elevated respiratory rate, dyspnea, fever, crackles auscultated over involved lobes of lungs, and productive cough.	Inadequate lung expansion. Anaesthesia, analgesia, and immobilized position prevent full lung expansion. There is greater risk in clients with upper abdominal surgery who have pain during inspiration and repress deep breathing.
Pneumonia: Inflammation of alveoli. It may involve one or several lobes of lung. Development in lower dependent lobes of lung is common in immobilized surgical client. Signs and symptoms include fever, chills, productive cough, chest pain, purulent mucus, and dyspnea.	Poor lung expansion with retained secretions or aspirated secretions.
Hypoxemia: Inadequate concentration of oxygen in arterial blood. Signs and symptoms include restlessness, dyspnea, high or low blood pressure, tachycardia or bradycardia, diaphoresis, and cyanosis.	Respirations are depressed by anaesthetics or analgesics. Increased retention of mucus with impaired ventilation occurs because of pain or poor positioning.
Pulmonary embolism: Embolus blocking pulmonary arterial blood flow to one or more lobes of lung. Signs and symptoms include dyspnea, sudden chest pain, cyanosis, tachycardia, and drop in blood pressure.	Same factors lead to formation of thrombus or embolus. Immobilized surgical client with pre-existing circulatory or coagulation disorders is at risk.
Circulatory System	
Hemorrhage: Loss of large amount of blood externally or internally in short period of time. Signs and symptoms include hypotension, weak and rapid pulse, cool and clammy skin, rapid breathing, restlessness, and reduced urine output.	Slipping of suture or dislodged clot at incisional site. Clients with coagulation disorders are at greater risk.
Hypovolemic shock: Inadequate perfusion of tissues and cells from loss of circulatory fluid volume. Signs and symptoms are same as for hemorrhage.	In surgical client, hypovolemic shock is usually caused by hemorrhage.
Thrombophlebitis: Inflammation of vein often accompanied by clot formation. Veins in legs are most commonly affected. Signs and symptoms include swelling and inflammation of involved site and aching or cramping pain. Vein feels hard, cordlike, and sensitive to touch.	Venous stasis is aggravated by prolonged sitting or immobilization. Trauma to vessel wall and hypercoagulability of blood increase risk of vessel inflammation.
Thrombus: Formation of clot attached to interior wall of a vein or artery, which can occlude the vessel lumen. Signs and symptoms include localized tenderness along distribution of the venous system, swollen calf or thigh, calf swelling more than 3 cm compared with asymptomatic leg, pitting edema in symptomatic leg, collateral superficial veins, and decrease in pulse below location of thrombus (if arterial).	Venous stasis (see discussion of thrombophlebitis) and vessel trauma. Venous injury is common after surgery of legs, abdomen, pelvis, and major vessels. Clients with pelvic and abdominal cancer or traumatic injuries to the pelvis or lower extremities are at high risk for thrombus formation.
Embolus: Piece of thrombus that has dislodged and circulates in bloodstream until it lodges in another vessel, commonly lungs, heart, brain, or mesentery.	Thrombi form with increased coagulability of blood (e.g., polycythemia and use of birth control pills containing estrogen).
Gastrointestinal System	
Paralytic ileus: Nonmechanical obstruction of the bowel caused by physiological, neurogenic, or chemical imbalance associated with decreased peristalsis.	Handling of intestines during surgery can lead to loss of peristalsis for a few hours to several days.
Abdominal distension: Retention of air within intestines and abdominal cavity during gastrointestinal surgery. Signs and symptoms include increased abdominal girth, tympanic percussion over abdominal quadrants, and client complaints of fullness and "gas pains."	Slowed peristalsis from anaesthesia, bowel manipulation, or immobilization. During laparoscopic surgeries, influx of air for procedure causes distension.
Nausea and vomiting: Symptoms of improper gastric emptying or chemical stimulation of vomiting centre. Client complains of gagging or feeling full or sick to stomach.	Abdominal distension, fear, severe pain, medications, eating or drinking before peristalsis returns, and initiation of gag reflex.
Genitourinary System	
Urinary retention: Involuntary accumulation of urine in bladder as a result of loss of muscle tone. Signs and symptoms include inability to void, restlessness, and bladder distension. It appears 6–8 hours after surgery.	Effects of anaesthesia and narcotic analgesics. Local manipulation of tissues surrounding bladder and edema interfere with bladder tone. Poor positioning of client impairs voiding reflexes.
Urinary tract infection: An infection of the urinary tract as a result of bacterial or yeast contamination. Signs and symptoms include dysuria, itching, abdominal pain, possible fever, cloudy urine, white blood cells and leukocyte esterase positive on urinalysis.	Most frequently a result of catheterization of the bladder.

Continued

➤ TABLE 49-10 Postoperative Complications *continued*

Complication	Cause
Integumentary System	
Wound infection: An invasion of deep or superficial wound tissues by pathogenic microorganisms. Signs and symptoms include warm, red, and tender skin around incision; fever and chills; and purulent material exiting from drains or from separated wound edges. Infection usually appears 3–6 days after surgery.	Infection is caused by poor aseptic technique or contaminated wound or surgical site before surgical exploration. For example, with a bowel perforation, the client is at increased risk for a wound infection because of bacterial contamination from the large intestine.
Wound dehiscence: Separation of wound edges at suture line. Signs and symptoms include increased drainage and appearance of underlying tissues. This usually occurs 6–8 days after surgery.	Malnutrition, obesity, preoperative radiation to surgical site, old age, poor circulation to tissues, and unusual strain on suture line from coughing or positioning cause dehiscence.
Wound evisceration: Protrusion of internal organs and tissues through incision. Incidence usually occurs 6–8 days after surgery.	See discussion of wound dehiscence. Client with dehiscence is at risk for developing evisceration.
Skin breakdown: Result of pressure or shearing forces. Surgical clients are at increased risk if alterations in nutrition and circulation are present, resulting in edema and delayed healing.	Prolonged periods on the operating room (OR) table and in the bed postoperatively can lead to pressure breakdown. Skin breakdown results from shearing during positioning on the OR table and improper pulling of the client up in bed.
Nervous System	
Complex pain situations: These might include situations in which pain is unresponsive to standard treatment or where there are multiple sources of pain (RNAO, 2002a).	The source may be related to, for example, surgical site or concomitant injuries or pathology.

- Apply elastic antiembolism stockings or pneumatic compression stockings as ordered by the physician (see Chapter 46). The antiembolism stockings should be removed every 8 hours and left off for 1 hour; in some agencies, they are left off overnight. Perform a thorough assessment of the skin of the lower extremities at this time.
- Encourage early ambulation. Some clients are expected to ambulate on the evening of surgery, depending on the severity of the surgery and their condition. Even if a client has an epidural catheter or a PCA device, ambulation should be encouraged. The degree of activity allowed progresses as the condition improves. Before ambulation, you should assess the client's vital signs. Abnormalities may contraindicate ambulation. If vital signs are at baseline, you first help the client to sit on the side of the bed. Client complaints of dizziness are a sign of postural hypotension. Rechecking the client's blood pressure will help you to determine whether ambulation is safe. You assist with ambulation by standing at the client's side and ensuring that he or she can stand safely and walk steadily. The first few times out of bed, clients may be able to walk only a few metres. This should improve each time. Evaluate tolerance to activity by periodically assessing the pulse rate as the client ambulates.
- Avoid positioning clients in a manner that interrupts blood flow to their extremities. While in bed, clients should not have pillows or rolled blankets placed under their knees. Compression of the popliteal vessels can cause thrombi. When clients sit in chairs, their legs should be elevated on footstools. A client should never be allowed to sit with one leg crossed over the other.
- Administer anticoagulant drugs as required. Physicians often order prophylactic doses of anticoagulants, such as heparin or Fragmin (dalteparin), for clients at greatest risk for thrombus formation.
- Promote adequate fluid intake. Adequate hydration prevents concentrated buildup of formed blood elements, such as platelets and red blood cells. When the plasma volume is low, these elements may gather and form small clots within blood vessels.

Achieving Rest and Comfort. A surgical client's pain increases as the effects of anaesthesia diminish. The client becomes more aware of the surroundings and more perceptive of discomfort. The incisional area may be only one source of pain. Irritation from **abdominal gas**, drainage tubes, tight dressings or casts, and the muscular strains caused from positioning on the OR table can cause discomfort.

It is common to administer narcotic analgesics immediately after surgery. Initial analgesic doses are usually given by IV infusion in the PACU and titrated to client comfort. After an anaesthetized client is awake and aware, PCA may be used. This is given by IV or subcutaneous infusion or via an epidural, often with dilaudid or morphine. The PCA system allows clients to administer their own analgesics from a specially prepared pump (see Chapter 42). If clients are able to gain a sense of control over their pain, they usually have fewer postoperative problems. Gagliese et al. (2000) found that both young and older adult surgical clients were able to use PCA to attain adequate levels of pain relief. One research study found that the use of subcutaneous PCA resulted in lower pain scores and less sleep disturbance from pain (Dawson et al., 1999). Many clients receive epidural analgesia that may be continued during the recovery period (see Chapter 42).

In the acute care area, you continue pain assessment and determine the effectiveness of interventions. If the client has a PCA system and is trying to use it more frequently than the amount programmed, you should investigate his or her pain further and contact the physician or the advanced practice nurse on the acute pain service to increase, for example, the amount of medication received. PCA provides you with a useful monitor of the effectiveness of pain medication. As oral intake is tolerated, you facilitate changing the client's pain medication from IV to oral administration. It is important to ensure adequate pain coverage when the client is switched from an IV to an oral route (Snell et al., 1997). Sometimes clients are given a subcutaneous injection of analgesia before transfer to the acute care area to ensure pain control over this time period. Although less common today, intramuscular injections of analgesics may be given at regular intervals in the acute care area.

The importance of nonpharmacological interventions should not be overlooked. You should assess which care measures may contribute to pain and use nonpharmacological measures to treat it. An example would be to lower the head of the bed and use a pillow for incisional splinting while turning a client with recent abdominal surgery. You can also use other methods of promoting pain relief, such as positioning, back rubs, distraction, or imagery. Pain can slow recovery significantly. The client becomes reluctant to cough, breathe deeply, turn, ambulate, or perform necessary exercises. You should assess the client's pain thoroughly (see Chapter 42). You should not assume that the pain is only incisional. When the client asks for pain medication, determine the location, intensity, and character of the pain. During the first 24 to 48 hours after surgery, you should provide analgesics on a regular basis around the clock to improve pain control (Agency for Health Care Research and Policy, 2002; RNAO, 2002a). If pain medications are not relieving discomfort, you should notify the physician or the acute pain service after completing a thorough assessment. Recognizing the potential complications of analgesics and knowing what to do if they occur is an important role of the postoperative nurse.

Acute Care

Temperature Regulation. Temperature regulation is important in the postoperative period. Clients are often cool after surgery, and the PACU nurse provides warmed blankets in the immediate postoperative period. If the client's temperature is 35.6°C or below, a warming device such as the Bair Hugger may be used. Increasing body warmth causes the client's metabolism to rise and circulatory and respiratory functions to improve.

Shivering may not be a sign of hypothermia but rather a side effect of certain anaesthetic agents. Meperidine (Demerol) may be given in small increments to decrease shivering. Deep breathing and coughing helps to expel retained anaesthetic gases.

Malignant hyperthermia is a potentially lethal condition that can occur in clients who receive general anaesthesia. It should be suspected when there is unexpected tachycardia and tachypnea; jaw muscle rigidity; body rigidity of limbs, abdomen, and chest; or hyperkalemia. Temperature elevation is a late sign. The PACU nurse will immediately administer dantrolene sodium ordered by the physician.

Infection is another possible cause of temperature elevation. The following interventions decrease the risk of postoperative infections: encouraging deep breathing and coughing, assisting with early ambulation, promptly removing in-dwelling urinary catheters and IV catheters, and providing aseptic care of the surgical wound. Cultures are obtained from clients suspected of having infections (see Chapter 47).

Maintaining Neurological Function. Orientation to the environment is important in maintaining the client's mental status. You reorient the client, explain that surgery has been completed, and describe procedures and nursing measures. The client who was properly prepared before surgery is less likely to be anxious when nurses provide care. Any change in level of consciousness should be promptly reported to a physician.

Maintaining Fluid and Electrolyte Balances. An important nursing responsibility is maintaining patency and prescribed rate of IV infusions and monitoring fluid and electrolyte balances in the postoperative period. As the client begins to take and tolerate oral fluids, the IV rate will be decreased. When an ambulatory surgical client awakens and is able to tolerate fluids by mouth without gastrointestinal upset, the IV catheter is removed. When the client no longer needs a continuous IV infusion, the IV line may be saline locked to preserve the site for antibiotics or other use (see Chapter 40). The client also may receive blood products or artificial volume expanders, depending on blood loss during and after surgery.

Promoting Normal Bowel Elimination and Adequate Nutrition. Normally a client who has had general anaesthesia does not receive fluids to drink in the PACU because of bowel sluggishness, the risk of nausea and vomiting, and grogginess from general anaesthesia. To minimize nausea, the client should avoid sudden movement. For clients identified as being at high risk for the development of nausea and vomiting or clients who must not vomit (e.g., eye surgery), a combination of antiemetics may be recommended (Gan, 2002; Tramer, 2001). If the client has a nasogastric tube, you check the position of the tube and ensure patency by observing for drainage. If suction is required, you verify that it is maintained at the required level (see Chapter 45). Occlusion of a nasogastric tube results in accumulation of gastric contents within the stomach.

The client likely will begin taking ice chips or sips of fluids once he or she is returned to the acute care unit. If these are tolerated, a clear liquid meal usually will be ordered. Interventions for preventing gastrointestinal complications promote return of normal elimination and faster return of normal nutritional intake. It takes several days for a client who has had surgery on gastrointestinal structures (e.g., a colon resection) to resume a normal diet. Normal peristalsis may not return for 2 to 3 days. In contrast, the client whose gastrointestinal tract is unaffected directly by surgery can resume dietary intake after recovering from the effects of anaesthesia. The following measures promote return of normal elimination:

- Maintain a gradual progression in dietary intake. For the first few hours after surgery, a client receives only IV fluids. If bowel sounds are active and the physician orders a normal diet for the first evening after surgery, begin by providing clear liquids, such as water, ginger ale, broth, or tea, after nausea subsides. Overloading the client with large amounts of fluids may lead to distension and vomiting. If the client tolerates liquids without nausea, advance the diet as ordered. Clients who have had abdominal surgery are usually NPO for the first 24 to 48 hours after the procedure. As peristalsis returns, provide clear liquids, followed by full liquids, a light diet of solid foods, and finally the client's usual diet. Encourage intake of foods high in protein and vitamin C.
- Promote ambulation and exercise. Physical activity stimulates a return of peristalsis. The client who suffers abdominal distension and "gas pain" may obtain relief while walking.
- Maintain an adequate fluid intake. Fluids keep fecal material soft for easy passage. Fruit juices and warm liquids are especially effective.
- Administer fibre supplements, stool softeners, and rectal suppositories such as Dulcolax (bisacodyl) as ordered. If constipation or distension develops, the physician may attempt to stimulate peristalsis with cathartics or enemas.
- Promote adequate food intake by stimulating the client's appetite:
  - Remove sources of noxious odours and provide small servings of nonspicy foods.
  - Assist the client to a comfortable position during mealtime. The client should sit if possible to minimize pressure on the abdomen.
  - Provide desired servings of food. For example, a client may be more willing to face his or her first meal when servings are not large.
  - Provide frequent oral hygiene. Adequate hydration and cleansing of the oral cavity eliminate dryness and bad tastes.

- Provide meals when the client is rested and free from pain. Often a client loses interest in eating if mealtime has been preceded by exhausting activities, such as ambulation, coughing and deep breathing exercises, or extensive dressing changes. When a client has pain, the associated nausea often causes a loss of appetite.

Promoting Urinary Elimination. The depressant effects of anaesthetics and analgesics impair the sensation of bladder fullness. If bladder tone is reduced, the client has difficulty starting urination. However, clients should void within 8 to 12 hours after surgery. Because a full bladder can be painful and often causes restlessness in recovery, it may become necessary to insert a catheter. If the client has an in-dwelling urinary catheter, the goal should be to have it removed as soon as possible because of the high risk for the development of a nosocomial bladder or urinary tract infection.

Clients who undergo surgery of the urinary system frequently have an in-dwelling urinary catheter inserted to maintain free urinary flow until voluntary control of urination returns. The following measures promote normal urinary elimination (see Chapter 44):

- Help the client to assume normal positions during voiding. The male client may need assistance to stand to void. Bedpans make voiding difficult. A female client will have better results if she is able to use a toilet or a bedside commode.
- Check the client frequently for the need to void. A surgical client restricted to bed needs assistance in handling and using bedpans or urinals. Often the client acquires a sudden feeling of bladder fullness and urgency to void and will need help quickly.
- Assess for bladder distension. If a client does not void within 8 hours of surgery or if bladder distension is present, it may be necessary to insert a straight urinary catheter. A physician's order is needed for this. Continued difficulty in voiding may require an in-dwelling catheter, although the risk for a urinary tract infection increases.
- Monitor intake and output. Urine output should be at least 30 mL/hour for adults. If the urine is dark, concentrated, and low in volume, the physician should be notified. A client can easily become dehydrated as a result of fluid loss from the surgical wound. Measure intake and output for several days after surgery until normal fluid intake and urinary output are achieved.

Promoting Wound Healing. A surgical wound undergoes considerable stress during convalescence. The stress of inadequate nutrition, impaired circulation, and metabolic alterations increases the risk for delayed healing (see Chapter 47). A wound also may undergo considerable physical stress. Strain on sutures from coughing, vomiting, distension, and movement of body parts can disrupt the wound layers. You protect the wound and promote healing. A critical time for wound healing is 24 to 72 hours after surgery, after which time a seal is established. If a wound becomes infected, it usually occurs 3 to 6 days after surgery. A clean surgical wound usually does not regain strength against normal stress for 15 to 20 days after surgery. You must use the aseptic technique during dressing changes and wound care (see Chapters 33 and 47). Surgical drains must remain patent so that accumulated secretions can escape from the wound bed. Ongoing observation of the wound identifies early signs and symptoms of infection.

Maintaining and Enhancing Self-Concept. The appearance of wounds, bulky dressings, and extruding drains and tubes threatens a client's self-concept. The effects of surgery, such as disfiguring scars, may create permanent changes in the client's body image. If surgery leads to impairment in body function, the client's role within the family can change significantly.

You should observe clients for alterations in self-concept. Clients may show revulsion toward their appearance by refusing to look at incisions, carefully covering dressings with bedclothes, or refusing to get out of bed because of tubes and devices. The fear of not being able to return to a functional role in their families may cause clients to avoid participating in the care plan.

The family becomes an important part of efforts to improve the client's self-concept. You explain the client's appearance to the family and suggest ways to avoid nonverbal expressions of revulsion or surprise. The family needs to be accepting of the client's concerns and encourage the client's independence. If the condition is permanent, the family and client will go through a grieving process. Coping strategies develop over time to manage the situation. The following measures help to maintain the client's self-concept:

- Provide privacy during dressing changes or inspection of the wound. Keep room curtains closed around the bed, and drape the client so that only the dressing or incisional area is exposed.
- Maintain the client's hygiene. Wound drainage and antiseptic solutions from the surgical skin preparation dry on the client's skin surface and cause irritation. When clients return to the unit, they should be given a postoperative bath and provided oral hygiene. In addition, a complete bath on the first day after surgery can make the client feel renewed. When the client's gown becomes soiled by wound drainage, offer a clean gown and washcloth. Keep the client's hair clean and neatly combed. Offer frequent oral hygiene. Room deodorizers may be useful if the odour from drainage seems particularly troublesome to the client and the family.
- Prevent drainage devices from overflowing. Contents of drainage collections are measured every 8 hours for output recording and are emptied as they become full. The client sometimes becomes preoccupied with observing the gradual collection of drainage, and some drainage devices can leak contents if they become too full.
- Maintain a pleasant environment. Self-concept is heightened by the client being in pleasant, comfortable surroundings. Store or remove unused supplies and keep the client's bedside orderly and clean.
- Offer opportunities for the client to discuss feelings about his or her appearance. A client who avoids looking at an incision may need to discuss fears or concerns. A client having surgery for the first time is often more anxious than one who has had multiple surgeries. When the client chooses to look at an incision for the first time, the area should be clean. Eventually, the client should be able to care for the incision site by applying simple dressings or cleaning the affected area.
- Provide the family with opportunities to discuss ways to promote the client's self-concept. Encouraging independence can be difficult for a family member who has a strong desire to assist the client in any way. By knowing about the appearance of a wound or incision, family members can be supportive during dressing changes. The topic or tone of a conversation can also help family members support a client who is dwelling on fears and concerns. Family members should not avoid discussing the future. However, they need help to know when it is appropriate to discuss future plans. Then the client and family can work together to discuss realistic plans for the client's return home.

Restorative and Continuing Care

You, the client, and the family work to prepare the client for discharge. Education regarding wound care, activity level, diet, medications, and specifics related to the type of surgery is an ongoing process throughout hospitalization. After discharge, some clients will need assistance from home care services with tasks such as wound care (Box 49–8). With ambulatory surgery clients, focused education within the limited time is essential. Including the family or a significant other person provides a resource for the client once he or she is at home (see Box 49–6). With both ambulatory and hospitalized surgical clients, nurses provide a wide variety of written educational materials. For example, educational materials with many pictures should be used with clients who do not speak your language or who have limited reading ability. Materials should be sensitive to various cultures and religions. However, the provision of materials does not ensure understanding. Verification, return demonstration, and ongoing clarification are required.

❖Evaluation

Client Care

You evaluate the effectiveness of care provided to the surgical client on the basis of expected outcomes after nursing interventions. In all surgical settings, you consult with the client and the family to gather evaluation data. You can evaluate the ambulatory surgical client's outcomes via a telephone call to the client's home, asking specific questions to determine whether complications have developed and whether the client understands restrictions or medications. This call is usually placed 24 hours after surgery, which allows you to evaluate the progress of recovery.

In an acute care setting, evaluation of a surgical client is ongoing. If a client fails to progress as expected, you revise the client's care plan according to the priorities of the client's needs. Every effort is made to assist the client in returning to as healthy and functional a state as possible. Your evaluation also includes determining the extent to which the client and the family have learned self-care measures.

BOX 49-8 FOCUS ON PRIMARY HEALTH CARE

Recovery at Home

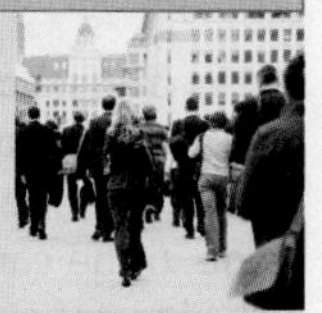

Regardless of the length of time the client spends in hospital, it is essential that you ensure that the client and family have the appropriate information and skills needed to continue a successful recovery at home. However, time is often very limited, especially with the move toward preadmission units and short hospital stays. A comprehensive approach is needed to ensure continuity of care from hospital to home. A client is often expected to continue dressing care, follow activity restrictions, continue medication therapy, and observe for signs and symptoms of complications upon returning home. In addition, the client needs someone to be present for the first 24 hours to ensure that no delayed reaction from the anaesthesia occurs, such as difficulty breathing. A referral to home care assists clients who are unable to perform self-care activities. Close association with home care services is required for some clients if dressing changes or physiotherapy is needed. It is useful to have a case management nurse in attendance at discharge to convey what tasks a client can perform effectively.

Client Expectations

With short hospital stays and ambulatory surgery, it is especially important to evaluate client expectations early in the postoperative process. Pain relief is usually a priority. Asking the client if everything possible has been done to alleviate pain, including nonpharmacological measures, can determine whether the client's needs have been met. Timeliness of response to the client's needs, such as scheduled times for pain medication and prompt answering of a call light, may increase satisfaction. The client usually wants to be discharged from acute care as soon as possible and when indicated by the physician. Ensuring that discharge plans are in place facilitates that process and enhances the client's satisfaction with care.

✻ KEY CONCEPTS

- Perioperative nursing is nursing care provided to the surgical client before, during, and after surgery.
- Surgery is classified by level of severity, urgency, and purpose.
- The preoperative period may be several days or only a few hours long.
- Preoperative assessment of vital signs and physical findings provides an important baseline with which to compare postoperative assessment data.
- Nursing diagnoses of the surgical client may pose implications for nursing care during one or all phases of surgery.
- Primary responsibility for obtaining informed consent rests with the client's surgeon.
- Structured preoperative teaching has a positive influence on a client's postoperative recovery.
- Basic to preoperative teaching is an explanation of all preoperative and postoperative routines and demonstration of postoperative exercises.
- In ambulatory surgery, nurses must use the limited time available to educate clients, assess their health status, and prepare them for surgery.
- A routine preoperative (preprocedure) checklist can be used as a guide for final preparation of the client before surgery.
- Many responsibilities of nurses within the OR focus on protecting the client from potential harm.
- All medications taken before surgery are automatically discontinued after surgery unless a physician reorders the drugs.
- Family members or other supportive networks are important in assisting clients with any physical limitations and in providing emotional support during postoperative recovery and ongoing care at home.
- Assessment of the postoperative client centres on the body systems most likely to be affected by anaesthesia, immobilization, and surgical trauma.
- Accurate pain assessment and intervention are necessary for healing.
- Nurses in the postoperative surgical unit provide the discharge education required so that the client and the family can manage at home.

* CRITICAL THINKING EXERCISES

1. An 82-year-old client is admitted for surgery on a fractured hip caused by a fall. What postoperative complications are typical in the older client undergoing this type of surgery?
2. Mr. B. is a 52-year-old client who will undergo thoracic surgery. He has smoked one pack of cigarettes per day for 30 years. What type of pulmonary preventive measures would you expect Mr. B to need postoperatively?
3. Mrs. C. was admitted for ambulatory surgery for an inguinal hernia repair. What discharge criteria would be used for Mrs. C., and what discharge instructions would she require?
4. Your client is scheduled for abdominal hysterectomy at 2:00 p.m. Based on NPO guidelines, what fasting schedule should you implement in collaboration with the surgeon and the anaesthesiologist?
5. You are doing preoperative teaching for a client undergoing a minimally invasive surgical technique. Identify one advantage of this type of surgery.

* REVIEW QUESTIONS

1. An obese client is at risk for poor wound healing and for wound infection postoperatively because
   1. Ventilatory capacity is reduced
   2. Fatty tissue has a poor blood supply
   3. Risk for dehiscence is increased
   4. Resuming normal physical activity is delayed
2. You should ask each client preoperatively for the name and dose of all prescription and over-the-counter medications taken before surgery because they
   1. May cause allergies to develop
   2. Are automatically ordered postoperatively
   3. May create greater risks for complications or interact with anaesthetic agents
   4. Should be taken on the morning of surgery with sips of water
3. A client who smokes two packs of cigarettes per day is most at risk postoperatively for
   1. Infection
   2. Pneumonia
   3. Hypotension
   4. Cardiac dysrhythmias
4. Family members should be included when you teach the client preoperative exercises so that they can
   1. Supervise the client at home
   2. Coach the client postoperatively
   3. Practise with the client while waiting to be taken to the operating room
   4. Relieve you by getting the client to do his or her exercises every 2 hours
5. In the postoperative period, measuring input and output helps assess
   1. Renal and circulatory function
   2. Client comfort
   3. Neurological function
   4. Gastrointestinal function
6. In the PACU, one measure taken to maintain airway patency is to
   1. Suction the pharynx and bronchial tree
   2. Give oxygen through a mask at 10 L/minute
   3. Position the client so that the tongue falls forward
   4. Ask the client to use an incentive spirometer
7. Which one of the following measures promotes normal venous return and circulatory blood flow?
   1. Suctioning artificial airways and the oral cavity
   2. Monitoring fluid and electrolyte status during every shift
   3. Having the client use incentive spirometry
   4. Encouraging the client to perform leg exercises at least once an hour while awake
8. A client with an international normalized ratio (INR) or an activated partial thromboplastin time (APTT) greater than normal is at risk postoperatively for
   1. Anemia
   2. Bleeding
   3. Infection
   4. Cardiac dysrhythmias
9. When the client is engaging in deep breathing and coughing exercises, it is important to have the client sitting because this position
   1. Is more comfortable
   2. Facilitates expansion of the thorax
   3. Increases the client's view of the room and is more relaxing
   4. Helps the client to splint with a pillow
10. In the postoperative period, if a client has unexpected tachycardia and tachypnea; jaw muscle rigidity; body rigidity of limbs, abdomen, and chest; or hyperkalemia, you should suspect
    1. Infection
    2. Hypertension
    3. Pneumonia
    4. Malignant hyperthermia

* RECOMMENDED WEB SITES

Canadian Anesthesiologists' Society: http://www.cas.ca
This Web site offers client information about and guidelines for using anaesthesia.

National Association of PeriAnesthesia Nurses of Canada: http://www.napanc.org
Perianaesthesia nurses are registered nurses with advanced knowledge in the care of clients during all phases of perianaesthesia, including, for example, nurses in postanaesthetic care units, same-day surgery, and diagnostic imaging.

Operating Room Nurses Association of Canada: http://www.ornac.ca
This Web site provides practice standards for Canadian operating room nurses, as well as information on certification with the Canadian Nurses Association (CNA).

Ontario PeriAnesthesia Nurses Association: http://www.opana.org
This Web site provides position statements on and standards of perianaesthesia nursing practice.

Appendix A Practical Nursing in Canada

Written by Vivian Lucas, RN, MEd

Revised by Barb Morrison, RN, HBScN, MEd

✻ Key Terms

acuity Level of sickness.

attrition The process of losing numbers from a group (such as people failing a course or retiring from or quitting jobs).

competence "The integration and application of knowledge, skills, attitude, and judgement required for safe, ethical, and appropriate performance in an individual's nursing practice" (Registered Nurses Association of British Columbia, 2003b, p. 26).

controlled act (reserved act) A clinical skill that may present a danger to the public if not performed properly and therefore may be performed only by certain health care professionals.

credentialling The process of officially acknowledging that a person is competent in an occupation or profession. Licensure and certification are two forms of credentialling.

creeping credentialism The trend toward higher entry-to-practice requirements.

delegation The transfer of authority to perform certain restricted activities.

educational laddering A process whereby a person progresses from one level of practice to another as a result of acquiring extra formal or informal education, or both.

environmental scan An analysis of the external and internal issues that can affect a person or an organization.

epidemiology The study of disease occurring in populations.

gatekeeper A person who monitors or oversees the actions of others.

jurisdiction A particular legal or geographic area of practice, such as Ontario or the Vancouver Island Health Authority.

LPN Licensed practical nurse.

practical nurse A nurse with the title of Licensed Practical Nurse in all provinces and territories except Ontario, where the title is Registered Practical Nurse.

paraprofessional A person who performs a particular skill that requires special training but whose required skill level is much less than that of a professional. (*Para* is a prefix from Greek with various meanings, including "beside," "near," and "like.")

proactive Thinking or planning ahead and anticipating change.

professionalization The process of developing into a profession.

protected title A title that can be used only by a person officially licensed in a profession or occupation in a particular area. For example, in Alberta, only a practical nurse registered with the College of Licensed Practical Nurses of Alberta can use the abbreviation or title LPN. The person can use this title only in Alberta. The person cannot use the title in British Columbia unless the person is also registered in British Columbia as an LPN.

registration Inclusion in a register. Once a person is licensed to practise a particular profession in a specific area, that person's name goes on an official register of practitioners.

RPN In Ontario, registered practical nurse; in the four western provinces, registered psychiatric nurse.

RN Registered nurse.

semiprofessional A synonym for *paraprofessional*, meaning partly professional.

specialization Development of expertise in a specific area of an occupation or profession (e.g., emergency nursing, mental health nursing, pediatric nursing).

speciation In biology, the development of a new species or subspecies from the original.

reactive Reacting to an observed problem or change that has already occurred.

scope of nursing practice The legal limits of nurses' professional role; the activities that nurses are educated and authorized to perform.

stakeholder An individual or group with a vested interest or share in an organization.

standard of practice Written statement describing the desired level of performance; actual performance is compared with the standard.

supervision The process of overseeing the performance of a person or group.

unregulated care provider (Also called *unlicensed care worker* [UCW], *unlicensed assistive personnel* [UAP], *unlicensed care personnel* [UCP].) A person, paid or volunteer, whose practice is not licensed under the law in a jurisdiction. such as ward aide, orderly, home care worker, or family member.

History of Practical Nursing in Canada

Practical nursing is the second largest regulated nursing group in Canada. It has a relatively short history, having become a profession only in the late 1930s. Initially beginning as a hands-on. hospital-based program with few common standards and little legislative control, practical nursing has evolved into a profession that requires a sound knowledge base and is publicly accountable under legislative control.

The Beginnings of Practical Nursing

In some respects, practical nursing has always existed. Whenever people have provided "hands-on" nursing care, they have been providing practical nursing care. Only since the 1970s, however, has practical nursing been recognized as a distinct profession that necessitates formal education. Until about the mid-1970s, only minimal high school preparation was necessary for entry into a practical nursing program, and the program was most often a short apprenticeship in a hospital setting. No licensure examination was required. Also, no official registration, protected title, or professional body existed.

The Evolution of Practical Nursing

Practical nursing has evolved in a similar way in most provinces. It has also followed a similar pattern that other occupations have followed when they are established as professions. Abbott (1988) studied 130 occupations and noted that as they evolve into professions, the following characteristics are developed:

1. A national professional association
2. Government-sponsored licensing legislation
3. Professional examinations
4. A professional school separate from schools for other professions
5. A university-based professional education
6. A code of ethics
7. A national-level journal
8. An accreditation program (in the United States) or a certification program (in the United Kingdom)

Except for university-based education requirements and a national-level journal, practical nursing has established all the other steps. Abbott (1988), however, did not note the series of name and designation changes that seem to be unique to practical nursing, nor did his list highlight the tendency to require increasing levels of education, which some authorities have termed "creeping credentialism."

Canada

As early as 1914, the Canadian National Association for Trained Nurses (called the Canadian Nurses Association [CNA] since 1924) recognized the value of practical nursing, especially for providing care to clients in the home (College of Licensed Practical Nurses of British Columbia [CLPNBC], 2003). The first practical nurses were usually called either nursing aides (if female) or orderlies (if male).

In 1931, practical nurses in Canada numbered 4700. By 1947, this statistic had increased to more then 7900, largely because of increased hospital service needs after the Second World War. The first formal education program specifically for practical nurses (as opposed to nursing aides or orderlies) began in Manitoba in 1945 (Canadian Institute for Health Information [CIHI], 2002; College of Licensed Practical Nurses of British Columbia [CLPNBC], 2003). The first legislative acts controlling the education, testing, licensing, regulation, and practice of practical nursing were introduced in the 1940s.

Over the years, practical nursing in Canada has undergone many changes in designation, as well as function. Practical nurses have struggled to achieve self-regulation, rather than government regulation, of their profession.

Many of the changes in the education of the practical nurse reflect the same changes that occurred earlier in the education of the registered nurse. Practical nurses are required to obtain higher levels of education. Education programs have become longer and more complex and have moved from hospital schools to postsecondary institutions, such as colleges. Rather than continuing to emphasize tasks and procedures, education programs began focusing more on holistic principles of nursing.

In the 1980s, most provinces developed regulations to govern practical nursing and were requiring graduates to write a licensing examination provided by what was then the Canadian Nurses Association Testing Service (CNATS). Graduates of practical nursing programs across Canada (except in Quebec) now must pass a national registration examination before they can begin professional practice. (Quebec has its own practical nursing examination.)

Table A–1 presents historical highlights in the evolution of practical nursing in selected provinces.

United States

In the United States, the first practical nurse program was started by the Ballard School in New York in 1893, with a 3-month course to train women in simple nursing care, emphasizing care of infants and children, older adults, and the disabled in their own homes (McLennan Community College, 2004).

US nurses were the first to use the term Licensed Practical Nurse (LPN), setting a precedent that many Canadian provinces and territories have since followed.

United Kingdom and Australia

Before the early 1990s, nursing education in the United Kingdom was provided in nursing schools attached to hospitals. Project 2000, started in the early 1990s in the United Kingdom, aimed to increase the professional stature of nursing by removing it from its hospital service base and placing it in postsecondary educational institutions. Today, nursing education in the United Kingdom, as in Canada and the United States, takes place in the postsecondary school system at the college or technical school level (Nursing Courses UK, n.d.). Courses in enrolled nursing (the closest equivalent to practical nursing) no longer officially exist. Therefore, practical nurses from other countries cannot be certified in nursing in the United Kingdom. They must first undergo extensive theoretical and clinical upgrading.

In Australia, the practical nurse is referred to as an Enrolled Nurse (EN) and is legally considered to be "the second level nurse in a 2-tier qualified nursing framework of professional care workers. By legislation . . . an enrolled nurse must work under the direction and supervision of a registered nurse" (Enrolled Nurses Professional Association of New South Wales, 2000). This situation is very similar to that in many Canadian provinces in that nursing is recognized as a profession that encompasses different categories of practitioners.

The Demand for Practical Nursing

In the late 1940s and early 1950s, demand for practical nurses increased significantly in most jurisdictions. A number of factors were responsible for this increased demand, including political and economic pressures, changes within the nursing profession, and ecological and sociological factors.

Political and Economic Pressures

As roles for women expanded after the Second World War and more opportunities were available in a range of occupations and professions, the numbers of nurses decreased. This shortage of registered nurses came at a time when clients' acuity (i.e., their level of sickness) was increasing in institutions. In addition, an increasing aged population was requiring more supportive care in communities and long-term care facilities, and private enterprise began exerting a greater economic influence on health care.

Because this public demand for safe and competent practice increased at the same time as economic and personnel challenges, practical nursing became more important within the health care system. Practical nursing offered an economical but highly competent workforce to meet the needs of clients in hospitals and those requiring long-term care.

Changes Within Nursing

Nursing Education

The changing methods of educating nurses also contributed to the personnel and economic challenges in the health care sector. For many years, hospitals and other health care agencies depended on nursing students for the free staffing of their institutions. When nursing education moved from a hospital base to a postsecondary base (beginning in the early 1970s), the numbers of available staff decreased suddenly. Institutions responded by employing greater numbers of poorly trained health care assistants (i.e., unregulated care providers) to provide basic care. This reliance on a less trained workforce has not always benefited the public, who now demand accountability and professionalism in health care. Increased public demand has resulted in higher standards and legal licensing requirements for all categories of nurse, including the practical nurse.

Registration Laws

The introduction of registration requirements for RNs also influenced the rise of the practical nurse. Nurse registration laws in the earlier part of the twentieth century protected the title of "registered

TABLE A-1

History of Practical Nursing in Selected Provinces

Province	Year	Significant Developments and Comments
British Columbia (BC)	1951	*Practical Nurse Act* passed
	1965	*Practical Nurses' Act* legally approved
		Council of LPNs established as the licensing body under auspices of Ministry of Health
	1977	BC practical nurses required to write Canada-wide licensing examination
	1989	Ministry of Advanced Education,Training, and Technology strongly supports future role of LPNs in health care
	1991	Council of LPNs becomes an independent regulatory body of the Ministry of Health
	1992–1993	Twelve-month college program piloted that differentiates LPN and RN roles on the basis of client's acuity and complexity of care required
	1996	Council becomes the College of LPNs of BC under *Health Professions Act*
Manitoba	1945	First official practical nurse education program in Canada
Prince Edward Island	1952	*Licensed Nursing Assistants Act* proclaimed
	1960	Training for nursing assistants centralized in one place
	1963	Association of Licensed Nursing Assistants incorporated
	1994	Training program moves from hospital to college
	2002	*Licensed Practical Nurses Act* affirms title of LPN
Alberta	1945	First school for nursing aides in Calgary, sponsored by Department of Veterans Affairs and Canadian Vocational Training
	1947	*Nurses Aide Act* passed, allowing licensing for certified nursing aide; training program is 40 weeks long
	1958	Department of Public Health takes over training of nurses aides
	1964	Entrance requirements for nurses aide program increased to Grade 10
	1967	Department of Education begins orderly program for male aides
	1972	Alberta Certified Nursing Aide Association becomes a founding member of the Canadian Association of Practical Nurses and Nursing Assistants
	1974	Certified nursing aides appeal to Alberta Human Rights Commission about pay inequities between them and orderlies; nursing aides win
	1978	*Nursing Assistant Registration Act* combines aide and orderly in one category of RNA (Registered Nursing Assistant)
	1979	*Health Occupation Act* becomes *Health Disciplines Act*
	1987	Professional Council of RNAs (PCRNA) becomes first health care discipline under *Health Disciplines Act* (council is regulating body for RNAs)
		Nursing assistant graduates required to write Canadian Practical Nurse Registration Examination (national licensing examination)
	1990	RNAs change title to LPNs
		Professional Council of RNAs becomes Professional Council of LPNs
	1998	Council changes its name to College of Licensed Practical Nurses of Alberta
	1999	*Health Disciplines Act* becomes *Health Professions Act,* which will eventually include all regulated health care professions under their separate provincial colleges
	2003	The College of Licensed Practical Nurses of Alberta is formally proclaimed
Saskatchewan	1955	Professional affairs of the Certified Nursing Assistant/Licensed Practical Nurse controlled by RNs under *Saskatchewan Registered Nurses Association Act*
	1988	*Certified Nursing Assistants Act* passed
	1992	*Certified Nursing Assistants Act* is amended to *Licensed Practical Nurses Act;* Saskatchewan Association of Licensed Practical Nurses (SALPN) has legal authority to regulate practice of LPNs
	2000	*Licensed Practical Nurses Act* amended to reflect independent role of the LPN; removed the phrase "works under the direction of a physician, registerd nurse or registered psychiatric nurse."

Continued

TABLE A-1

History of Practical Nursing in Selected Provinces *continued*

Province	Year	Significant Developments and Comments
Ontario	1938	Centres begin offering 6-month courses for nursing assistants
	1941–1945	With approval of Ontario Department of Health, Registered Nurses Association of Ontario (RNAO) sponsors eight 6-month training programs for nursing assistants
	1947	*Nurses Act* is amended to allow title of Certified Nursing Assistant (CNA)
	1953	Requirement for training is increased to 10 months
	1957	Part-time evening programs and high school programs (Grades 11 and 12) started
	1963	CNA title is changed to Registered Nursing Assistant (RNA)
	1990	RNA training programs moved to community colleges
	1993	RNA title is changed to Registered Practical Nurse (RPN)
	2002	College of Nurses of Ontario passes a regulation to require all RPNs to obtain their basic diploma through an enhanced 2-year program in a provincial college (Colleges of Applied Arts and Technology [CAATs]), beginning January 2005

Data from Canadian Institute for Health Information (CIHI, 2007), College of Licensed Practical Nurses of British Columbia (2003), College of Licensed Practical Nurses of Alberta (2008), Saskatchewan Association of Licensed Practical Nurses (2008), Prince Edward Island Licensed Practical Nurses (2008), Registered Practical Nurses Association of Ontario (2008).

nurse"; however, they could not control other forms of nonregistered nursing. As long as unregulated care providers did not claim to be registered, they could still practise many nursing activities. This enabled agencies to save money by hiring these less expensive but less qualified workers.

After the Second World War, the public began demanding more qualified practitioners. As a result, nurse registration laws were amended to allow the creation of another level within nursing practice. Most provinces now have two categories of nurses: (1) registered nurses, who are educated at a high level and are responsible for a complex client base (including nurse practitioners), and (2) practical nurses, who have less education and are responsible for the care of stable and predictable clients. A nurse in the practical nurse category can use the title "registered practical nurse" (RPN) or "licensed practical nurse" (LPN), depending on the provincial or territorial regulatory body. In the four western provinces, a third category exists: registered psychiatric nurses (also referred to as RPNs).

Development of Categories Within the Nursing Profession

As noted previously, Canadian nursing has evolved into two categories of professional practitioners (and in the four western provinces, three): registered nurses and practical nurses. In comparison with the nursing profession, the medical profession essentially has one level of practitioner (a medical doctor) and many subspecialties (e.g., pediatrics, ophthalmology, orthopedics, and so on). Medical doctors also cede limited activities to other professions while maintaining their own professional position. For example, ophthalmologists (medical doctors specializing in vision disorders) are authorized to measure vision and prescribe corrective lenses. However, their practice involves many more responsibilities than these two simple functions. Therefore, they cede these two functions to optometrists. Optometrists have a unique, limited scope of practice and make no claims to be medical doctors. In the United States, doctors also have physician's assistants to perform limited tasks. Like optometrists, these workers do not claim to be medical doctors.

Between the medical profession and its various offshoots, it can thus be seen that the boundaries of practice are quite distinct. Medicine has retained the central tasks of diagnosis and treatment of human disease states, functions that are clear in the public mind. Nursing, however, has developed a much less definitive practice, dividing the professional knowledge base and functions somewhat less clearly and neatly. Basic theory and practice are common to both categories of nurses, which are divided only by depth of knowledge and complexity of care required. However, client complexity, predictability, and stability are hardly absolute. They are easily changeable and can be difficult to define. As a result, practitioners and the public are sometimes unsure about the boundaries between registered and practical nurses. This blurring of boundaries is well supported in the Health Professions Regulatory Advisory Council (1996) report, which states that "the distinction between nurses (RPNs, RNs, and NPs [nurse practitioners]) are not publicly understood, and they are not as great as distinctions between professions regulated by the OMA [Ontario Medical Association] for instance" (p. 10).

Exploring the theories of ecology and sociology as they apply to nursing can offer further insights into the development of two categories of nursing. These theories consider reactions to change and competition among groups for functions, power, rewards, and even professional survival.

Ecological and Sociological Factors

Ecology Theory Applied to Nursing

Ecology theory in general describes changes in populations resulting from environment and evolution. Ecology theory originally referred only to plants and animals, but some authorities have expanded it to apply to social groups such as companies and professions (Wilson, 1992).

In order to survive, groups must (1) compete for niches (places or functions in any system) and (2) evolve to cope effectively with environmental changes. Groups that have too narrow a function or who fail to compete successfully lose their niche to other groups. Niches may also change; therefore, successful adaptation requires either competing for a new niche or acquiring the niche first and establishing a solid place in it.

Two concepts in biological evolution that can be applied to practical nursing are the concepts of speciation and hybridization. In *speciation,* the species divides into one or more subspecies, each with its own particular function or niche. In *hybridization,* the new species adopts characteristics of one or more of the ancestor species (Van House & Sutton, 1996).

If the concept of speciation is applied to nursing, it is apparent that the functions of the "species" of nurses have evolved. Out of the single species, two "subspecies" have arisen: the registered nurse (who usually has a university degree and is educated to cope with a wide variety of client [environmental] challenges) and the practical nurse (who has a college diploma and is educated to cope with a limited variety of client challenges). Some provinces also have a third "subspecies," the registered psychiatric nurse, who has a college education and is trained to provide care to clients with mental illness. The niche for the registered nurse is wider than that of the practical nurse, and the niche for the registered psychiatric nurse is the narrowest of all.

The concept of hybridization can also be applied to nursing. Nursing has adopted characteristics of other "species"; in particular, it has adopted ideas and technology that have previously been exclusively medical functions. For example, taking blood pressure, starting intravenous infusions, and making certain types of diagnoses are now nursing functions that used to be medical functions.

It is interesting that whereas nursing has developed speciation, medicine has avoided speciation and instead developed specialization. Where nurses share functions, doctors cede specific unwanted functions to different professionals. The sharing of functions among practical and registered nurses is what contributes to the public and professional confusion about the roles of the two levels of nurses.

Sociology Applied to Nursing

Sociology is the study of group roles, functions, and interactions. Abbott's (1988) unique theory about professions can be melded with ecology theory to provide more insight into the development of professions. According to Abbott, a profession attempts to keep certain tasks or problems for itself and shares them with others only if it can do so without endangering its own niche.

Abbott (1988) also believed that a profession protects itself and its niche position by possessing a sound knowledge base. In other words, acquiring knowledge is central to developing a strong professional identity. Abbott believed that knowledge sets a true profession apart from a mere occupation:

> *"Practical skill grows out of an abstract system of knowledge and control of the occupation lies in control of the abstractions that generate the practical techniques . . . . Any occupation can obtain licensure (e.g., beauticians) or develop an ethics code (e.g., real estate). But only a knowledge system governed by abstractions can redefine its problems and tasks, defend them from interlopers, and seize new problems . . . . Abstraction enables survival in the competitive system of professions."*

Professional tasks are either objective (knowledge and technology based) or subjective (culturally or legally based) in nature. Some objective tasks unique to nursing have been the development of the nursing process and nursing diagnoses. Subjective tasks are most clearly seen in the legal criteria for nursing defined in each province. For example, the Ontario *Regulated Health Professions Act* defines three authorized (controlled) acts that may be performed by nurses in that province: performing a procedure below the dermis or mucous membrane; placing an instrument, hand, or finger into a body opening; and administering a substance by injection or inhalation. Of course, much overlap exists; that is, the authorized nursing acts in Ontario are based on both knowledge and technology and are legally defined.

Objective tasks are more resistant to change than are subjective tasks. Environment often brings in new tasks, new knowledge, and new technology. The successful profession adopts the knowledge and new tasks it wants, strives to maintain current knowledge and tasks it considers worth keeping, and works to prevent other professions from intervening in its acquired knowledge and task base (its ecological niche). A successful profession is supported in this by subjective forces from the environment, such as legal sanctions, public opinion, and workplace practices and rules, all of which reflect the culture and the society.

Practical nursing has had mixed success in these areas. Most jurisdictions have enacted definitive legal supports (such as registration, licensing, and protected title) for a particular knowledge base and specified range of tasks. However, practical nurses still strive to clarify their role for both the public and the government. Their knowledge and practice are very similar to those of registered nurses (varying only in depth and skill level, as noted previously). The workplace in many provinces is also challenged to make appropriate use of the practical nurse's skills in many areas, avoiding either underuse or exploitation of the practical nurse's knowledge and skill set:

> *"Abbott's [1988] analysis also casts light on the debate raging in most professional schools—what is the perfect balance between theory and practice? A student focusing solely on theory (or the abstract knowledge base) lacks the skills and tools to practice the profession; however, Abbott [warned] that practice-based knowledge lacks abstraction. An exclusive focus on the tools and service models leaves the student with no ability to extend the underlying knowledge base to new niches. In times of rapid change in niches, a thorough understanding of the knowledge base, not simply the tools and skills, is most likely to provide safe passage to the new environment." (Van House & Sutton, 1996, p. 8)*

Practical nurses in Canada are striving to achieve a balance in both theory and practice. Basic education is increasing in complexity and promoting the concept of lifelong learning for the professional. In addition to basic education, many practical nurses complete credentialing in specialty areas after graduation, which enhances the individual's knowledge base and adaptive ability and increases professional credibility in the public mind.

Failure to adapt to changes can result in a loss of niche, role, and position. A profession could become like the panda, endangered because it has an extremely narrow niche in the ecosystem and is unable to adapt to the changing environment (Van House & Sutton, 1996). On the other hand, having a niche that is too broad could result in the profession's loss of political (public, governmental, and interprofessional) support. Too much knowledge or task sharing between specific niches (blurred boundaries) could also threaten survival of a professional species.

We have addressed some reasons for the development of practical nursing as a unique profession and provided some theoretical insights. However, why distinct levels (or species) have developed within nursing is still unanswered. It remains to be seen whether this division of professional nursing into two (and three) levels of practitioner will strengthen or weaken nursing as a profession and preserve its position in the health care system.

Practical Nursing Today: Issues and Trends

Like other evolving professions, practical nurses face many issues and trends pertaining to their educational requirements and clinical roles. Many of the same issues and trends are apparent across the country.

Educational Preparation

Clients' needs are becoming ever more complex. Practical nurses must respond to increased acuity, wide cultural and social variations among clients, and a continuing trend toward home and community care. As the practice environment for practical nurses changes, national entry-to-practice competencies are reviewed and revised (as of this writing, the most recent changes occurred in 2007; Assessment Strategies Inc., 2006). Practical nursing education has become more demanding as programs strive to prepare practical nurses to meet these changing requirements at the entry level. Most programs include strong theory and practical hands-on components, as well as clinical consolidation and preceptorship experiences before graduation.

Entry to a Practical Nurse Program

Entry requirements for practical nursing programs have become more stringent. At one time, only a Grade 9 or 10 level of education was required for entry into a practical nursing school. Now, Canadian practical nursing programs require that applicants have a high school diploma. Most require that they also have high marks in language and in one or two sciences. Many postsecondary institutions also admit mature students without a high school diploma if they can demonstrate equivalent learning through other forms of education or can successfully complete mature student testing.

Location and Length of Program

In most Canadian jurisdictions, practical nursing programs are diploma programs that run for 2 academic years (approximately four semesters) and are offered in postsecondary institutions. In order to facilitate student access to nursing education, some educational institutions are offering practical nursing programs by nontraditional delivery methods such as distance education and online learning. The CIHI (2007) reported that in 2006, 90% of practical nurses in all provinces and territories possessed an initial diploma level of education (p. 26). The programs require 2 years in order to address the complexity of the client base and the need for knowledgeable and flexible professional care.

Instructors in Practical Nurse Programs

Canadian nursing instructors are usually required to have clinical experience and educational preparation that is at least one level beyond that of their students. At one time, this meant that registered nurses taught aides and practical nurses. Today, almost without exception, registered nurses with baccalaureate degrees teach in practical nursing programs. Many have master's degrees or doctorates in nursing, education, or other related areas.

Registered nurses and practical nurses are most often involved with teaching students in the clinical area. These clinical teachers may be hired directly by a postsecondary institution or may be employees of the agency in which clinical practice takes place. Teaching models vary; some programs employ practical nurses as course instructors, and others employ them as assistants under the direction of a lead course instructor. Practising LPNs also serve as role models and support students educationally during preceptorship experiences.

Student Clinical Practice

The practical nurse can work in many clinical settings. Securing appropriate clinical placements for students is a challenge in some provinces, for two main reasons:

1. Many acute care areas (e.g., surgery, acute medicine, and pediatric wards) either do not use or limit the use of practical nurses in client care. Even though documented professional standards indicate that practical nurses are qualified to work in such areas, many institutional bureaucracies and individual staff either are unfamiliar with new standards or feel personally and legally uncomfortable with them.
2. Many areas are inundated with requests for clinical placements of students from various health care fields, often at the same time. This problem is especially prominent in the larger urban centres, at which many university and college health care students compete for clinical placements. Not having appropriate clinical placements is a serious issue for students. Practical nursing students need to be placed in clinical settings in which they can work to their full scope of practice. If they do not have this opportunity, their educational experience suffers. To address these challenges, practical nursing programs are incorporating innovative approaches to better prepare their students for clinical placements and to maximize the quality of their clinical experiences. Many schools are integrating the use of "computerized human patient simulators" and clinical simulations in order to increase student confidence and enhance readiness to practise before clinical practicum experiences. Clinical scheduling has extended beyond "banker's hours" to weekends and a variety of other shifts. Program delivery models have also been adjusted to allow for clinical placements during summer months, when units are more readily available.

Entry-to-Practice Requirements

The professional regulatory college is mandated by the government to set minimum entry-to-practice requirements in order to promote public safety and professional accountability. Usually, professional groups tell the regulatory college what these requirements should be. In most Canadian jurisdictions, entry-to-practice requirements for practical nursing include the following:

- Graduation from an approved postsecondary program for practical nursing, with the appropriate number of hours of theory and practice and with the appropriate courses taken.
- A clear result of a criminal record check.
- A sound knowledge base in all aspects of the nursing process (assessment, planning, implementing, and evaluating nursing care) for clients throughout the lifespan.
- Ability to function independently with clients in stable and predictable conditions and to function collaboratively under supervision of other health care professionals, especially registered nurses, with clients in more acute, unpredictable, or unstable conditions.
- Ability to work in a variety of settings with individuals, families, and groups.
- Ability to apply ethical practice standards.
- Ability to collaborate and communicate with others, including the client and other health care personnel (including health teaching).
- Ability to be accountable for own actions and to work within the scope of practice.
- Ability to be a lifelong learner.
- Ability to cope effectively with change.

Credentialling is performed by the professional registering body through its admission criteria, because the "government itself does not have the resources or expertise to ensure that professional competence, credibility and integrity are maintained in the numerous health professions" (May, 2003, p. 10).

It is important to note that these entry-to-practice requirements reflect minimal standards for practice (although that minimum appears to be increasing). Meeting these requirements is not a guarantee of safe practice. These standards may also vary among jurisdictions; for example, LPNs in Saskatchewan are not limited to practising solely with stable and predictable clients (Saskatchewan Association of Licensed Practical Nurses, 2008).

Trend to More Education

For some time, the entry-to-practice requirements have increased (this phenomenon is also called *creeping credentialism*). A number of factors are thought to be responsible for this trend, including new and rapid developments in technology, increased public expectations, professional competitiveness and turf protection, increased postsecondary education trends, and expanded markets.

These increases in entry-to-practice requirements have both positive and negative aspects for the individual professional, the professions, the workplace, the government, and society in general. The positive effects may include increases in employment opportunities, national and international mobility, and the quality of service to the public and enhancement of research potential and development. The negative effects may include increases in educational costs for the individual and society, delay of the professional's entry into the job market, problems in workplace collective agreements, exacerbation of job shortages, and creation of economic burdens for employers because people with more credentials tend to expect higher wages.

Continuing Education Issues

Laddering

Should health care aides be given the opportunity to become practical nurses? Should practical nurses be given the opportunity to become degree nurses? The concept of educational *laddering*, or *bridging*, recognizes prior learning and acknowledges that knowledge and expertise are acquired in various ways. It provides a means by which individuals can progress in their careers without being forbidden reasonable access to other levels or categories. Institutions across Canada are beginning to offer academic pathways that bridge health care aide and practical nursing programs, as well as practical nursing and registered nursing programs. The key phrase is "reasonable access." Because registered nurses and practical nurses aspire to different levels of practice, the applicant's previous experience must be carefully considered in order to protect the discipline of nursing.

Postgraduate Certification

Practical nurses can further their education and their contribution to the profession by specializing in specific fields.

Practical nurses have plentiful opportunities to obtain certification in specialty areas after graduation from the basic program. These certificates may be offered to practical nurses or to both registered and practical nurses. Such examples include, but are not limited to, certification in operating room technique and management, foot care, gerontology and geriatric nursing, dialysis, women's health, specialized mental health, and occupational nursing.

The Role of the Practical Nurse

Most jurisdictions recognize that practical nursing is a separate category within the wider field of professional nursing. Most jurisdictions also recognize that practical nurses follow the same nursing practice and theory as registered nurses but have a more basic understanding of the theory and care for clients with more stable and predictable conditions.

The main difference between registered nurses and practical nurses is their knowledge base. Although they study the same material, registered nurses study it for a longer time and in more depth. They therefore have a broader foundation in clinical practice, decision making, critical thinking, leadership, research, and resource management. Practical nurses, however, have a strong foundation in clinical practice, decision making, and critical thinking. Many practical nurses are employed in chronic care settings and in the fields of gerontology and geriatrics. Increasingly, however, health care agencies and institutions are hiring practical nurses in acute care and nontraditional settings. Consequently, practical nurse programs are teaching students to provide care for stable acute care clients and are providing training for skills needed in acute care settings (e.g., intravenous therapy, oxygen therapy).

Table A–2 lists the percentages of practical nurses in Canada employed in different areas of responsibility in 2006.

Many practical nurses are eager to assume these new roles and responsibilities in acute care settings, and they are legally entitled to do so. However, they may have difficulty obtaining employment and may be underutilized in these settings because many barriers arise from institutional culture, personal prejudices, and past practices.

As registered nurses continue to exert a large amount of control within the nursing profession, practical nurses may be restricted entry into certain aspects of the nursing niche. Most nursing managers are registered nurses with baccalaureate degrees or postgraduate degrees. They sometimes resist allowing practical nurses into certain clinical areas for a combination of reasons: lack of understanding regarding the latest changes in practical nursing and scope of practice, belief that clients' acuity is too extreme for practical nurses, and fear of litigation, bureaucratic pressures, or union pressures to maintain registered nurses' positions. Practical nurses themselves may encounter difficulties because of personal fears associated with role change. As staffing proportions change, it is imperative that institutions establish clear mechanisms and policies that support effective utilization of both registered nurses and practical nurses in providing client care.

Workplace Issues

The nursing profession currently has a high rate of attrition and frequent occurrences of stress and burnout in the workplace. Many factors create this climate of unease in the workplace:

- The pay is relatively poor for the work provided.
- Nurses face heavy workloads, and staffing patterns are complicated.
- Rates of overtime and sick time are high among nurses.
- Full-time nursing positions are decreasing and part-time positions are increasing as employers try to retrench and save money. Consequently, many part-time nurses have to be employed in more than one job in order to receive an adequate income.
- Clients are entering hospitals with a higher level of acuity.
- Care requirements are becoming more complex.
- Practice settings are shifting to community and long-term care, but full-time nursing positions are actually declining in the community, teaching facilities, and small institutions.
- Institutional support for nursing activities is either actually lacking or perceived to be lacking. Many practical nurses feel discouraged when the nursing system fails to recognize or fully use their abilities.
- Bed closures, downsizing, and use of unregulated care providers are increasing.

Workforce Issues

The numbers of practical nurses are increasing slowly, but an actual shortage is forthcoming as nurses reach retirement age, are downsized, are replaced by other personnel, or leave the nursing profession. Government and nursing bodies alike have identified the critical need for action to address the predicted nursing shortage through recruitment and retention strategies (Registered Nurses Association of Ontario & Registered Practical Nurses Association of Ontario, 2000).

The nursing workforce is aging, and high retirement rates are pending. In 2007, the average age of Canadian LPNs in direct care was 42.9 years, in administration it was 46.8 years, in education it was 45.5 years, and in research 47.8 years (CIHI, 2008). The highest proportion of LPNs in the workforce in 2007 also included nurses in the Baby Boomer generation between the ages of 43 to 61 (CIHI, 2008). As these veteran nurses age, it is expected that many will leave the workforce and retire. The loss of these practitioners will have a significant impact on practice settings.

Canada is having difficulty recruiting practical nurses from other jurisdictions. Fewer practical nurses are immigrating to Canada, largely because of actual or perceived diminished job opportunities. In addition, because of the concern about accountability and public safety—as well as a tendency to protect niche and turf—regulating authorities often are not quick to accept the credentials of a practical nurse from another jurisdiction. The "creeping credentialism" tendency may present significant barriers to the licensing of nursing professionals from other provinces or countries. According to some authorities, Canadian immigration policy often "fails to recognize the skills and qualifications that foreign-trained workers bring to Canada" (Access Issues for Regulators Workshop 2, 2001, p. 3).

TABLE A-2

Number and Percentage Distribution of LPNs Employed in Practical Nursing by Area of Responsibility

	Counts	%
Direct Care	**64,562**	**98.6**
Medicine and surgery	12,584	19.2
Psychiatry and mental health	3,422	5.2
Pediatrics	677	1.0
Maternity and newborn care	767	1.2
Geriatrics and long-term care	30,484	46.5
Critical care	363	0.6
Community health	2,023	3.1
Ambulatory care	1,133	1.7
Home care	1,147	1.8
Occupational health	146	0.2
Operating room and recovery room	656	1.0
Emergency room	582	0.9
Several clinical areas	2,503	3.8
Oncology	68	0.1
Rehabilitation	2,394	3.7
Palliative care	1,053	1.6
Other direct care	4,560	7.0
Administration	**583**	**0.9**
Nursing service	158	0.2
Nursing education	9	<0.1
Other administration	416	0.6
Education	**334**	**0.5**
Teaching: students	183	0.3
Teaching: employees	23	<0.1
Teaching: clients	16	<0.1
Other education	112	0.2
Research	**19**	**<0.1**
Research only	9	<0.1
Other research	10	<0.1
Total	**65,498**	**100.00**

Modified from Canadian Institute for Health Information (CIHI). (2007). *Workforce trends of licenced practical nurses in Canada, 2006* (p. 29, Table 8). Ottawa, ON: Author. Retrieved September 4, 2008 from http://secure.cihi.ca/cihiweb/products/Workforce_Trends_LPN_2006_e.pdf

Notes: Values less than 0.05% are displayed as "<0.1" to prevent displaying cells of 0.0 that are not true zero values. LPNs not stating area of responsibility (*n* = 1802) are excluded from this table. Data for Nunavut were not collected. CIHI data differ from provincial and territorial statistics because of the CIHI methods of collection, processing, and reporting.

Employment Trends

Practical nursing is one of the largest regulated health care professions in Canada, second only to registered nursing. In 2007, practical nurses represented 21% of the total regulated nursing workforce in Canada. CIHI estimated that in 2007, approximately 78,080 practical nurses existed in Canada. This represents an increase of 4.2% since 2006 and 10.9% since 2003 (CIHI, 2008).

Table A–3 summarizes the numbers of practical nurses in the workforce for each province and territory from 2003 to 2006.

Employment Status of Practical Nurses

The proportion of full-time positions in practical nursing is significantly lower than that of many other professional positions in Canada (Villeneuve & MacDonald, 2006). In 2006, slightly fewer than half (46.5%) of practical nurses in Canada worked full time; the remainder worked in part-time (35.6%) and casual (17.1%) positions (CIHI, 2007, Figure 8, p. 24). The proportion of full- and part-time nurses in the workforce varied among juristiction. The highest percentage of full-time practical nurses is in the Northwest Territories, where more than 80% of all practical nurses were employed full-time. Manitoba, in contrast, had the highest percentage of part-time practical nurses (53.2%) (CIHI, 2007, Figure 8, p. 24). In 2006, 16.5% of practical nurses were working for more than one employer, which reveals an interesting trend (CIHI, 2007, Figure 10, p. 26).

Workplace Settings

The proportion of practical nurses working in different settings currently varies across Canada. The public may think that practical nurses work exclusively in a long-term care setting. This was indeed a key area of employment for about 39% of practical nurses in 2006, but a greater number (about 45%) worked in hospitals. Only about 6% worked in the community, and approximately 6% worked in other areas (CIHI, 2007, p. 67). According to the CIHI (2007, p. 27), "other" places of employment include business, industry, occupational health care offices, private nursing agencies, private duty, physicians' offices, family practice units, self-employment, schools and other educational institutions, government, and volunteer associations.

These trends in workplace settings raise some concerns. If clients requiring nursing care are increasingly found in the community and not in institutions such as hospitals and nursing homes, then why

TABLE A-3

LPN Workforce by Province or Territory of Registration, Canada, 2003 to 2006

	2003	2004	2005	2006	Change 2003 to 2006
Newfoundland	2,719	2,710	2,696	2,639	-2.9%
Prince Edward Island	619	628	606	599	-3.2%
Nova Scotia	3,022	3,058	3,127	3,174	5.0%
New Brunswick	2,429	2,556	2,633	2,646	8.9%
Quebec	14,831	15,472	16,293	17,104	15.3%
Ontario	25,730	24,467	24,458	25,084	-2.5%
Manitoba	2,417	2,415	2,590	2,652	9.7%
Saskatchewan	2,056	2,131	2,194	2,224	8.2%
Alberta	4,766	5,051	5,313	5,614	17.8%
British Columbia	4,391	4,811	4,884	5,412	23.3%
Yukon Territory	60	53	56	60	0.0%
Northwest Territories	98	91	101	92	-6.1%
Canada	**68,138**	**63,443**	**64,951**	**67,300**	**6.6%**

From Canadian Institute for Health Information (CIHI). (2007). *Workforce trends of licenced practical nurses in Canada, 2006* (p. 10, Table 4). Ottawa, ON: Author. Retrieved February 12, 2009, from http://secure.cihi.ca/cihiweb/products/Workforce_Trends_LPN_2006_e.pdf
Notes: CIHI data differ from provincial and territorial statistics because of the CIHI methods of collection, processing, and reporting. Data for Nunavut were not collected. The Methodological Notes, available from CIHI provide more comprehensive information regarding the collection and comparability of the data in the Licensed Practical Nurses Database.

are the numbers of practical nurses in the community or "other" settings so low? Perhaps these statistics reflect reluctance on the part of other health care workers to permit practical nurses to function at the full scope of practice for which they are prepared.

Standards and Scope of Practice

Standards of Practice

As a regulated profession, practical nursing is responsible for establishing its own standards of practice. The professional regulatory body for practical nurses in each jurisdiction (e.g., the provincial college of practical nurses) has the authority to set standards of practice for its members. It also has the authority to ensure that members meet these standards.

Standards of practice are written statements that detail the level of performance expected of nurses in a particular jurisdiction. They provide general guidelines about several aspects of professional practice and performance. The practice of any nurse can be continually measured against these standards. They also demonstrate to the public that the profession of practical nursing is dedicated to protecting public safety and providing high-quality care.

Although they differ in details, most standards of practice for practical nurses in Canada offer performance guidelines for the following areas (among others): the nursing process (i.e., assessment, participation in nursing diagnoses, planning, implementation, evaluation), ethics, education, leadership, research, and collaboration with other professionals.

Each individual nurse and the regulatory body are responsible for standards: the nurse for knowing and using them, and the regulatory body for publishing and enforcing them. In addition, the professional association and employers must support these standards in practice and in theory. Finally, members of the public are responsible for being good consumers of the professional health care they receive.

Ethics in Nursing

Ethics refers to the moral principles or values that guide people when they decide what is right and what is wrong. Ethics influence behaviour and relationships with other people. Providing ethical nursing care means that the nurse forms a dynamic, caring, helping relationship with the client in order to help the client achieve and maintain optimal health.

Regulatory bodies for practical nursing are responsible for establishing and promoting codes of ethics. These codes of ethics guide practical nurses in ethical decision making. They also uphold ethical standards for practical nurses. The following values are promoted in most codes of ethics for practical nurses:

- Being accountable for one's actions.
- Upholding the client's rights to privacy and confidentiality.
- Providing care that maintains the client's dignity.
- Demonstrating respect for the client at all times.
- Promoting integrity by providing safe, competent, and ethical nursing care.
- Evaluating one's work and maintaining competency.

Continuing Education and Expanded Competencies

The practical nurse is expected to continue professional growth and acquire a range of knowledge, skill, and judgement beyond that of the minimal entry-to-practice standards. Many educational opportunities are available to the nurse from postsecondary institutions, professional organizations, employers, and charitable agencies (e.g., the Canadian Diabetic Association). Increasingly, nurses are encouraged to attend educational events offered by other health care professionals, such as respiratory therapists, pharmacists, physiotherapists, and gerontologists. This cross-professional education is also immensely valuable in encouraging greater understanding and collaboration among members of the health care team.

Inevitably, nurses in various areas develop different competencies. This presents individual and workplace challenges. As individual competencies are enhanced and scopes of practice are expanded, nurses and employers must continuously seek clarification of their roles. Nurses are accountable for their actions at all times. The employer needs to remain fully aware of the new competencies of nurses, both at entry level and beyond. Employers must also develop clear policies to address the expanded practices of all nursing staff.

Challenges to Working to Full Scope of Practice

Perhaps the best way to maintain competency is to continually use skills and training. Unfortunately, many employers do not allow practical nurses to work to their full scope of practice. For both personal and political reasons, the potential of practical nurses is often not recognized by the health care system. This results in a mismatch between the "scope of employment" and the "scope of practice" that practical nurses are prepared for.

In response to the changing health care system—including employer demand, client acuity levels, nursing shortages, and professional organizational efforts—many areas do make efforts to allow practical nurses to apply their full scope of practice. This shifts practical nurses from a task orientation to a competency base and, in the process, improves client care and professional job satisfaction. Optimizing and clearly defining roles for both categories of nurses can also lead to more cost-effective nursing care.

Collaboration

The practical nurse is a team member and thus should always be working in a collaborative manner with other health care personnel. Collaboration includes communicating with the client, the family, and other health care workers to define, implement, and evaluate the plan of care. Collaboration with the client and family includes focusing on real and perceived needs and wishes and how they intersect with medical and nursing plans. Good working relationships and collaboration between practical nurses and registered nurses in the team are essential in the delivery of quality client care. The practical nurse also makes suggestions and referrals to individual members of the health care team and in team meetings in which client care and concerns are discussed. Full understanding of all roles and clear and appropriate communication are integral to effective collaboration within a team.

Scope of Practice

Scope of practice refers to the legal limits of a professional role. Four categories of health care professionals provide nursing care: unregulated care providers (e.g., nurse's aides, support workers), practical nurses, registered nurses, and nurse practitioners. Each category of health care professional has its own scope of practice. These scopes of practice are different because each category of health care professional has different education, legal authority, and performance requirements.

In Table A–4, the scopes of practice for practical and registered nurses in New Brunswick are compared. (Each province and territory has a similar scope of practice requirements for nursing in its jurisdiction.) In Table A–4, notice that practical nurses have a more limited scope of practice in that they must assist a registered nurse or be closely supervised by a registered nurse when providing care for unstable clients. They may work independently only with clients who are in stable conditions. Registered nurses, however, may independently provide care for all clients.

Figure A–1 illustrates the expanding scopes of practice among the three categories of nursing care professionals. It shows that unregulated care providers have the most limited scope of practice, practical nurses have a more expanded scope of practice, and registered nurses have the largest scope of practice. Registered nurses are ultimately responsible for the direction of nursing care.

Notice that in Figure A–1, a solid line depicts the separation of each scope of practice. In reality, the boundaries between the scopes of practice vary. Between registered and practical nurses, the scopes of practice are much less definitive and the boundaries are sometimes blurred because both levels of nurses share a base knowledge and practice and develop new competencies during clinical practice. However, the boundaries between practical nurses and unregulated care providers are more definite because little of the basic knowledge or competencies are shared between the two roles. Indeed, the roles of practical and registered nurses are "separate and overlapping" (Nurses Association of New Brunswick & Association of New Brunswick Licensed Practical Nurses, 2003, p. 2).

Leadership: Supervising and Delegating

The practical nurse is often in a position to supervise or to delegate, as well as to be the recipient of supervision and delegation. In order to supervise and delegate, the practical nurse must have sufficient knowledge, skill, and judgement. Both supervision and delegation, although different skills, serve to protect the public and the profession by ensuring that a task is performed safely and competently. The same principles of supervision and delegation are applicable to both levels of nurse.

Supervision

Supervision is usually required by individuals who are new to a skill or role, such as students of a profession, new members of a profession, and professionals or nonprofessionals (such as family members or unregulated care providers). The person who is supervising usually has experience in that knowledge and skill, and he or she may or may not be a member of the same profession or occupational group.

Supervision is an intervention and usually an ongoing relationship. The purposes of supervision are (1) to enhance competent functioning of an inexperienced person and (2) to protect the public and the professional practice. Because supervision requires continual observation, monitoring, and evaluation, the supervisor must have a positive, collaborative relationship with the person being supervised. Both parties in the relationship must understand the roles each must play. The ongoing nature of most supervision allows the relationship to grow and develop. People should be supervised until they can safely perform the task alone. Supervision may occur in many forms, such as a one-on-one observation, an interview with the client who has received care, or an analysis of the written report of a task. The supervisor provides evaluative information about the task performed as soon as is feasible.

If supervision of a skill occurs in a more isolated instance, the development of a relationship and the analysis of progress are more difficult.

Delegation

In delegation, authority to perform a restricted task or function is transferred to another person or group. The nurse must make this decision carefully. The professional standards are quite clear in this matter. Before delegating a task to another, the nurse must ensure that the person has the required knowledge, skill, and judgement to perform that function. The nurse must consider numerous other factors before a function is delegated to someone else: the associated risks and benefits for the client, the need for another person to perform the task, the ability of the person to maintain competence in the procedure over time, and the ability to provide adequate supervision once the skill has been learned. The Massachusetts Board of Registration in Nursing (2000) provided a useful discussion of the "five rights of delegation": (1) the right task, (2) the right circumstances, (3) the right person, (4) the right direction or communication, and (5) the right

TABLE A-4

Scope of Practice Requirements for Practical and Registered Nurses in New Brunswick

	Practical Nurse	Registered Nurse
Education for entry to practice	College diploma or certificate Program length: 1–2 years	University baccalaureate degree (BScN or BN) Program length: 4 years
Legislated scope	Under RN supervision or direction, physician direction, or both* Greater independence in care of stable and predictable clients Under close direction of RN or assisting RN in care of unstable or unpredictable clients	Independent practice of nursing for all clients Collaboration with physicians and other health care personnel
Client	Individuals, families, and groups	Individuals, families, groups, communities, and populations
Application of nursing process	Participates in client assessment and developing a care plan Implements interventions and evaluates effectiveness	Determines client status; integrates, analyzes, interprets, implements care Evaluates care and makes independent judgements

*Supervision and direction need not always be carried out in person; it may be accomplished by agency policies and procedures and through a collaborative consultative relationship between the practical nurse and the registered nurse. For some functions, the practical nurse may function independently. For the sake of client and professional safety, collaboration must exist at all times in health care, regardless of the task or who is performing it.

supervision and evaluation. These rights are applicable to nurses working at all levels.

In addition, the nurse must know institutional policies and procedures about delegation and whether the particular function may be legally delegated. This is particularly crucial because of the increasing numbers of unregulated care providers with varied skill sets and functions within the health care system. Responsibility does not stop once a task is delegated to another person. The delegating nurse retains ultimate responsibility for the correct completion of the task. The College of Nurses of Ontario (2008) provided a useful decision tree to help the nurse decide whether a function can be delegated to another person (Figure A–2).

Clinical Skills

Although graduates of practical nursing programs are prepared to perform skills that are considered entry-to-practice competencies, many factors dictate their ability to do so in the workplace. Medication administration is one of the specific knowledge-based clinical skills that is within the scope of practical nursing in some jurisdictions but not in others. Even if it is part of the scope of practice, institutions may be reluctant to allow practical nurses to use this skill. In some areas, boundary issues arise with accompanying confusions about who may administer what medications, to whom, and when. In some jurisdictions, practical nurses may administer injections, monitor intravenous therapy and administer intravenous medications; in other jurisdictions, they may not. Practice related to clinical skills varies tremendously across the country, between institutions in a region, and even within an institution itself.

Additional Clinical Skills

In most cases, practical nurses can and do acquire other clinical skills beyond those needed for entry to practice. The restrictions on these skills are the same as those for the registered nurse; the practical nurse must usually take a specific postbasic course to acquire the needed knowledge and skill base and must usually be employed in an area allowing frequent enough application of these skills to maintain continued competency levels. For example, courses are available to learn about various types of dialysis, but entry into these courses is usually confined to those employed or soon to be employed in this area, in which they will require the skill and will be able to use it often enough to maintain competency.

Whether an added skill may be practised by a practical nurse is sometimes restricted by legislation, local institutional or regional health care policy, or both. Theoretically, any health care skill that a family member or layperson can be taught should be learned by a nurse, the parameters being the same: a proper knowledge base and demonstrated initial and continued competency and judgement in application of the skill. However, practical nurses need to be aware of the possible unique legal restrictions on their roles. Whether sensible or not, these legal restrictions do not apply in the same way to family members.

Because the situations necessitating nursing are increasingly complex, variation has arisen in the functions that can be assigned to practical nurses. Some of the more common added competencies for practical nurses in many jurisdictions include (but are not limited to) operating room techniques, special foot care, orthopedic care, gerontology, community care, and specialized mental health care.

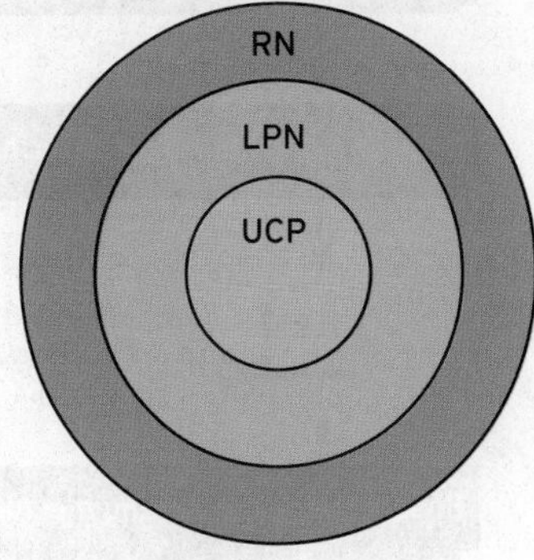

Figure A-1 Health care professionals' scope of practice. **Source:** Adapted from Nurses Association of New Brunswick & Association of New Brunswick Licensed Practical Nurses. (2003). *Working together: A framework for the registered nurse and the licensed practical nurse* (p. 4). Retrieved January 29, 2004, from http://www.nanb.nb.ca/pdf_e/Publications/General_Publications/RN-LPN%20(e)1.pdf

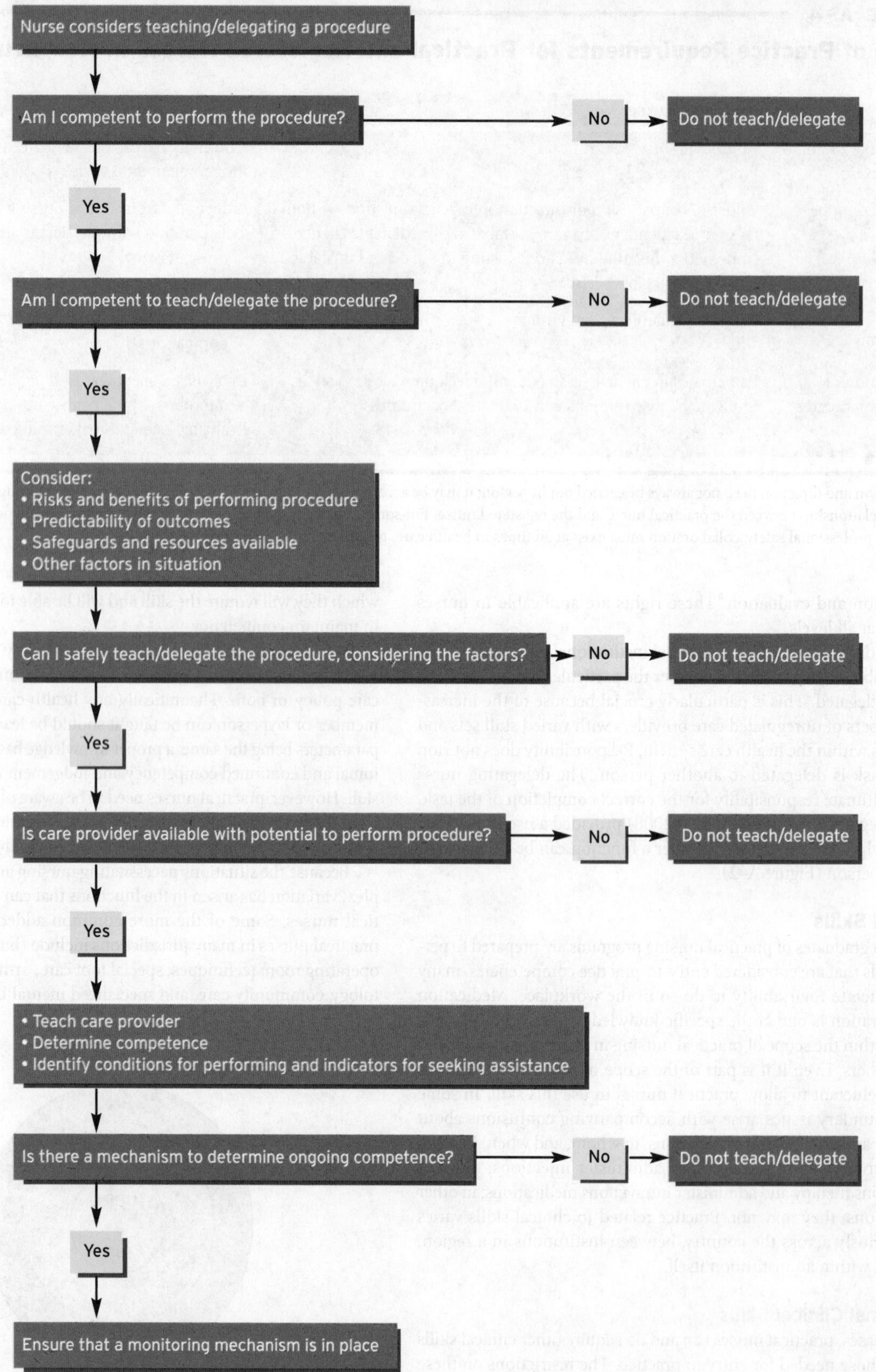

Figure A-2 Decision tree for teaching or delegating performance of a procedure. **Source:** From College of Nurses of Ontario. (2008). *Working with unregulated care providers* (p. 16). Retrieved February 12, 2009, from http://www.cno.org/docs/prac/41014_workingucp.pdf

The only commonality appears to be continued rapid change. The nurse must be careful never to assume that standards and scopes of practice are the same within or between institutions, between jurisdictions, or over time. One way to keep pace with change is to keep in close contact with a variety of sources: the professional association, the regulatory body, agency policies, and the ever-expanding body of health care knowledge.

Legislation, Regulatory Bodies, and Professional Associations

Legislation, regulatory bodies, and professional associations govern the practice of nursing. These have been created to protect public safety and promote ethical practice.

Legislation

In most provinces and territories, nursing practice has similar legal regulatory requirements (education, registration, and complaints and disciplinary processes) and professional standards (scope and standards of practice, and competency issues). Laws that govern regulated health care professions serve to protect the best interests of the public by regulating health care practitioners and determining how, what, and where they practise.

Acts That Govern Specific Health Care Professions

In all provinces and territories (except Ontario and British Columbia), each profession has its own governing law, called an *act.* For example, medical doctors, registered nurses, practical nurses, chiropractors, and so forth each are governed by a professional act. These acts list specific tasks that those professionals are allowed to perform because they have the required skills. However, the skills of one profession often overlap with those of another, which causes confusion for public and professionals alike.

Acts That Govern Multiple Health Care Professions

Some provinces have removed or are in the process of removing separate acts for individual health care professions and are replacing them with a single, generic act that applies to all health care professions. In Ontario, this act is called the *Regulated Health Professions Act,* and in British Columbia, it is called the *Health Professions Act.* This trend is occurring for several reasons:

- The public is demanding safe and accountable practice.
- New technology, which is increasingly complex and invasive, is potentially dangerous if improperly used. Trained professionals must, with great care, administer treatments such as radiation therapy, drugs for cancer, surgery, and even injections.
- People requiring health care have increasingly complex physical, emotional, and social needs.
- As many professions expand their scope of practice and acquire new knowledge and skill sets, significant overlap in knowledge and skills occurs between various groups. These general health care acts are an attempt to apply a regulatory structure common to all groups.
- Health care professionals are more mobile today (i.e., they move between jurisdictions) and may have wide variations in knowledge and competence.
- The number and variety of health care professions have increased.
- It is fundamentally just to have set standards and expectations that are applicable to all groups wanting to be regulated by the health care act. This also applies to foreign-trained professionals who apply to enter the profession in Canada (Registered Nurses Association of British Columbia, 2003a).

These generic health care acts list (1) professions that are regulated by the law and (2) activities that only members of certain professions are authorized to perform. These laws are called *reserved acts* (in British Columbia) and *controlled acts* (in Ontario); the restricted activities are as follows:

> *"[C]linical activities that may present a risk of harm and are therefore reserved for special professions only. Examples of reserved or controlled actions are diagnosing, prescribing medications, managing labour, ordering and applying hazardous forms of energy (including diagnostic ultrasound, electricity, laser and x-ray) and setting or casting a simple fracture." (Registered Nurses Association of British Columbia, 2003a, p. 4)*

Different health care professions are legally permitted to perform certain restricted activities. For instance, diagnosing a disease is a controlled act that is usually restricted to the medical profession. In Ontario, the *Regulated Health Professions Act* lists 13 controlled acts, 3 of which can be performed by nurses.

All the laws governing the actions of health care professionals, whether they are profession-specific acts or generic health care acts, include statements about the type of educational background necessary to enter a professional school and the type and length of education the professional schools must offer. The laws also require the profession to set up a governing body to monitor and regulate professional practice in the public interest.

These laws may seem excessively cumbersome and confusing. However, they are a reasonable attempt to establish uniform professional competencies and thereby protect the public.

Regulatory Bodies

According to the professional and health care acts, each profession must have a regulatory body that governs it. As the health care environment changes, regulatory bodies adapt by modifying practice standards and guidelines accordingly. Depending on the province or territory, this regulatory body may be called a *college,* a *council,* an *association,* or a *board.* Its primary mandate is to protect the public by controlling the activities of the professionals. In order to practise or use their professional title, all professionals must be members of their regulatory body.

Functions of the Regulatory Body

Each regulatory body uses many methods to protect the public. It ensures that its members have been properly educated; meet the minimum entry standards; maintain continued competence; and have the required knowledge, skill, and judgement to practise the particular profession. Almost all regulatory bodies perform the following functions:

- Ensuring that professionals have the necessary credentials to practise in the specific province or territory.
- Determining whether qualifying examinations are necessary.
- Registering the professional as a member of the profession once all criteria for membership have been met.

- Keeping a public register of the names, registration numbers, and business addresses of all members.
- Defining scope of practice and competency standards, according to professional standards and the existing laws.
- Ensuring that members renew or update registration and maintain competency criteria on a regular basis.
- Receiving complaints from the public or other professionals about personal practices of members, investigating these complaints, and disciplining members as necessary.
- Publishing disciplinary results regularly (i.e., name, registration number, offence, and disciplinary decision).

"The privilege of professional registration ensures that the registered members must meet the minimal education and competence requirements of the profession. For the public, registration also provides the expectation of professional service and ethical standards." (CLPNBC, n.d.)

Because the names, registration numbers, and business addresses of registered health care professionals are made public, some people have expressed concern that members' right to privacy is compromised. However, regulatory bodies and most provincial and territorial governments believe this information is necessary for public safety. Therefore, they consider that protecting the public safety supersedes the professional's right to privacy. In many areas, governments also permit the publication of disciplinary action against a health care professional, believing that doing so fulfills this mandate of serving the best interests of the public.

Protecting or Reserving Titles

Usually, regulatory bodies are also responsible for ensuring that the members' professional title (e.g., LPN, Dr.) is protected, or reserved. This means that only registered members are authorized to call themselves by the professional title. The protected title is usually related to the terms used in the jurisdiction, but protection is usually also extended to other, synonymous terms. For example, in Ontario, all the following related terms and abbreviations are protected: *nurse, registered practical nurse, RPN, LPN, PN,* and their variants.

The provincial or territorial college of licensed practical nurses is the provincial regulatory body responsible for superintending the profession of licensed practical nursing in the public interest. As such, the college sets the requirements for the privilege of using the professional titles related to licensed practical nurses. The professional title assures the public and other care professionals that the individual has met the minimal requirements for entry into the profession and maintains competence to practise as a professional licensed practical nurse (CLPNBC, n.d.).

In all provinces and territories (except Ontario), the official designation of the practical nurse is *licensed practical nurse* (LPN). In Ontario, the official designation is *registered practical nurse* (RPN).

Obtaining Criminal Record Checks

Because professionals have positions of power, concerns have inevitably arisen that they could take advantage of vulnerable people, especially young children and older adults. In response, some provinces and territories require people registering with a regulatory body to undergo a criminal record check.

Self-Regulation

To what extent should governments be involved in the regulation of a health care profession? Surely professionals are capable of regulating themselves and do not require paternalistic interference from government bureaucrats. The public good must be balanced with individuality, as must government laws with professional input. Professional self-regulation in nursing means that each nurse is expected to assume personal responsibility for maintaining competence and personal, physical, social, and emotional fitness to practise. Self-regulation also means that nurses establish standards of practice and an ethical framework for the nursing profession as a whole.

Self-regulation is a privilege that is entrusted to a regulating college in order to serve and protect the public interest:

"The college establishes requirements to enter the profession and assures the quality of the practice of LPNs through the development and enforcement of standards of practice and continuing competence programs." (College of Licensed Practical Nurses of Manitoba, 2008)

The Registration Process for the Practical Nurse (Credentialling)

In all territories and provinces of Canada, registration with the local regulatory body must proceed through a specific process. The regulatory body (also called a *registering body*) in each jurisdiction determines whether the applicant has sufficient educational background and competency for registration in the particular area. To be registered as practical nurses, applicants must prove that their education meets requirements for theoretical and clinical hours in specified topics and clinical areas. They also must provide evidence of competent practice by passing a licensing examination, providing evidence of recent competent work in the practical nursing field, or both. As already noted, in many jurisdictions, applicants must also pass a criminal record check before registering to practice.

Registering Locally

Successful graduates of a practical nursing school submit their names to the local licensing authority for permission to write the national certification examination, the Canadian Practical Nursing Registration Examination. As a general rule, students must write the certifying examination in the province or territory in which they received their education because their local registration body must recommend them to write the examination. The students are notified of where and when examinations will be written. After the examination is written, the student is notified of the results by mail. Usually, the school receives a summary of the passing and failing marks in that class and information about their success in relation to other schools in the jurisdiction. Privacy of examination marks is an issue in many areas. In Ontario, for instance, students must sign a waiver allowing their examination results to be included in the information sent to their educational institution. When the examination results are sent to the school, the student names are obscured.

After passing the licensing examination and (if required) completing a criminal record check, the new graduate then applies to the regulatory body to be registered as a practical nurse.

Registering in Another Province or Territory

Just as they would in their own jurisdictions, applicants wanting to register in a province or territory in which they have not been educated must formally apply for registration. This generally means the applicants must submit official transcripts from their school, indicating both hours and topics of theory and practice they completed in the basic program. They must show competent practice by submitting a record of success in the national certification examination or its equivalent from another country. If they are not recent graduates, they must also provide evidence of a sufficient amount of recent (within the previous 3 to 5 years) appropriate work in practical nursing. If they have not already done so, they may have to complete a criminal record check (at their own expense). If the certification examination, educational background, or recent nursing experience is not accepted by the regulatory body, then the applicant may be required to write the Canadian examination and take a theoretical or clinical nursing course to upgrade to Canadian standards.

Registering in Other Countries

The registration process for the United States, the United Kingdom, and Australia is very similar to the Canadian process. The applicants must prove to the foreign regulatory body that (1) they have successfully completed a basic nursing education program that includes a specified number and type of theoretical and clinical hours, and (2) they are capable of competent nursing practice (i.e., they have successfully written the examination, have recent practical experience, or both). Countries vary in how they accept marks on Canadian certification examinations and hours in clinical and theoretical basic nursing programs. In the United States and Australia, nurses are certified in the specific state or territory; in the United Kingdom, nurses are certified nationally.

Practical nurses planning to relocate to another jurisdiction (country, state, or province) should contact the new registering or licensing body well in advance because this body may have different requirements for professional practice. The procedure for attaining registration in a new jurisdiction can take up to 3 months in the absence of complications or deficiencies, but it can take much longer if problems exist.

Professional Associations

In Prince Edward Island and Ontario, the professional association is separate from the regulatory body (e.g., the College of Nurses of Ontario is the regulatory body, and the Registered Practical Nurses Association of Ontario is the professional association). However, in all other provinces and territories, they are the same body. The purpose of most professional associations is to advocate for and promote the particular profession they serve. The mandate of the Licensed Practical Nurses Association of Prince Edward Island (2008) is as follows:

- Foster public recognition and awareness of the profession.
- Encourage members to interact and take pride in their profession.
- Promote proficiency, continuing education, and career development among members.
- Represent members collectively in relations with other persons and organizations.
- Provide for services to members such as group liability insurance.
- Promote action and work for improvements in regard to health care issues.
- Pursue such other goals as the association may consider necessary to advance the profession and further the interest of its members.

The fundamental differences between a regulatory body and a professional association have been highlighted. Protection of the public is the distinct mandate of the regulatory body, whereas promoting professional development is the mandate of the professional association. Many nurse leaders and politicians believe that regulatory bodies and professional associations should not be combined because doing so may lead to public confusion and conflicts of interest. In the interests of both professional issues and public accountability, the professional association and regulatory body must remain in continuous, effective communication.

The provinces and territories that do not have a professional association separate from the regulatory body depend on the Canadian Practical Nurses Association (CPNA) for professional advocacy and promotion issues. The CPNA's mission is, in part, to promote education, research, and excellent nursing practice, and the association collaborates in the development of national practical nursing standards. Unlike membership in the regulatory body, membership in the professional association is usually voluntary.

The Canadian Association of Practical Nurse Educators, an affinity group of the nationwide Association of Canadian Community Colleges, offers educational and networking opportunities and holds yearly conferences for educators throughout Canada.

Benefits of Membership in the Professional Association

Members of professional associations enjoy the following benefits:

- Receiving emotional support from other professionals by sharing thoughts, feelings, and ideas.
- Enhancing a personal and collective knowledge base, thus contributing to individual and group growth.
- Being part of a strong force for change (groups often lobby for change more effectively than do individuals).
- Achieving some economic advantages (e.g., better insurance rates through a group plan).
- Having opportunities to network.

In summary, nursing is a complex profession that exists in a challenging environment under constant legal and professional changes. No nurse works alone; he or she is always in an environment with the public and other health care professionals. Each nurse must understand how legislation, regulatory bodies, and professional associations work together to inform safe and competent practice.

The Future of Practical Nursing in Canada

It is not possible to know the future of practical nursing definitively, but it is possible to make reasonable predictions on the basis of current and projected trends. The health care system in Canada is continually changing, and these changes have an effect on practical nursing. In order to cope effectively, nurses must be proactive and view change as a challenge and an opportunity rather than a threat. By doing so, nursing will maintain or advance its niche position in health care.

Both Abbott (1988) and Wilson (1992) believed that organisms and professions that do not respond to change lose their niche positions and either fade to unimportant entities controlled by others or die out completely. According to Wilson, "homogeneity means vulnerability" (p. 301). The *Romanow Report* repeated this idea: "In the face of uncertainty, the solution is not to sit back and wait for the outcomes of potential challenges" (Government of Canada, 2002, p. xxxiv).

General Health Care Trends

A number of current and projected changes can potentially affect practical nursing. The following issues each have an impact on the delivery of health care services in Canada:

- Rising costs of health care; the individual consumer will need to pay more.
- Increased privatization of health care with less government funding.
- Increased use of technology, including robotics for treatment and computer technology for communications and teaching.

- Expanded public access to information.
- Increased population diversity.
- Stronger public demands for a voice in health care and competent health care services.
- Increased medicolegal litigation.
- Higher percentage of older adults in the population.
- Trends toward post-acute care, rehabilitation, palliative care, long-term care, and chronic care in the home rather than in hospitals or other institutions.
- Increased acuity of admitted clients, so hospitals are becoming large intensive care units.
- Proliferating interprofessional models for health care.

In the report *Toward 2020: Visions for Nursing* (CNA, 2006), Villeneuve and MacDonald identified trends that will affect Canadian nurses of the future. They predicted that by 2020, chronic diseases and virulent infectious diseases would increase in number, health care would focus on wellness promotion, more health care would take place in homes and communities, interdisciplinary care would be the norm, technology would continue playing a major role in health care, foreign-trained nurses would be integrated into the Canadian workforce, and nursing credentials from different provinces and territories would be accepted across Canada.

Specific Health Care Issues in Canada

The *Romanow Report* (Government of Canada, 2002) offers several suggestions about the unique needs of Canadians that will affect practical nursing:

- Government should increase strategies that promote physical activity and reduce obesity.
- Efforts to reduce smoking should be expanded.
- Immunization programs should be given closer attention, especially in response to new infectious diseases and increased population mobility between countries.
- Services to new Canadians, visible minorities, people with disabilities, Aboriginal people, and rural and isolated populations should be given more attention and funding.
- Home care is one of the fastest-growing sectors of the health care system; investing more in home care will improve services and quality of life for home care clients and will also save the system money by keeping people out of hospitals and long-term care facilities.
- Better services should be provided in mental health care, post-acute care, rehabilitation, and palliative care.
- A national approach to human resources planning for health care should be developed so that one province does not "poach" scarce health care professionals from other provinces.

Implications for Practical Nursing

Continuous rapid change requires professionals to respond appropriately in order to cope effectively. Practical nurses need to be lifelong learners and develop increasingly broad-based competencies to adapt to changing occupational demands. This is not the time to focus solely on one narrow skill set or to cling stubbornly only to the knowledge base acquired in undergraduate school.

Modern technological treatment is increasingly expensive and time intensive. Practical nurses have the knowledge, abilities, and skills to contribute significantly to newly evolving primary health care models. Practical nurses of the future will likely need to have increased knowledge of epidemiology and to play a greater role in illness prevention, health promotion, and health teaching for clients throughout the lifespan. For instance, nurses will likely be required to provide information to reduce infectious and chronic lifestyle-related diseases such as cancer, diabetes, obesity, and heart–lung disorders. Health teaching for individuals and groups in the areas of diet, exercise, and reducing high-risk habits such as smoking will become increasingly important. Practical nurses will continue needing to focus on clients and empowering them to be active participants in their own health care. Because health care problems are often too complex to be addressed by any one person, practical nurses will need to focus more on working collaboratively in teams and networks of health care professionals. The trend toward interdisciplinary health care models will require nurses to be increasingly aware of scope of practice and of changes in scope of practice among all workers. Because of this emphasis on collaborative teamwork, outcome-based care frameworks (in the text, called *care maps* or *critical pathways*) will probably be emphasized over more narrow frameworks unique to only one profession (such as the nursing care plan). Having all health care team members work from the same model would simplify care issues and reduce the chance of error.

As more health care services are offered by the private sector, nurses will likely encounter different and challenging ethical issues. Nurses will need to be more aware of conflicts of interest. They may find that their professional values clash with corporate interests. In this regard, professional colleagues and the professional association will become increasingly important sources of information and support. Practical nurses will have to consider strengthening their national association and, in some provinces and territories, having more direct and local input in their provincial or territorial association.

The increased use of computers in health care is resulting in remarkable advances in health informatics systems. Computer use has become the norm rather than the exception in most health care institutions. Practical nurses will need to become skilled in the use of electronic medical health record systems, which can involve documentation and full access to current and past medical records, diagnostic test results, and digital radiographic images. New technologies are changing bedside care as nurses begin to use personal digital assistants (PDAs), mobile or cell phone pagers, computerized medication administration systems, online educational resources, and telemedicine systems. Computer literacy will be essential for practical nurses of the future. Nurses work with an increasingly diverse and multicultural population base. Practical nurses of the future will thus have to develop more knowledge and skill in applying concepts from the humanities and social sciences such as psychology, sociology, and anthropology.

Possible Evolution of the Practical Nurse Role

Changes in Educational Standards for Entry to Practice

In view of the likely expanding roles for the practical nurse, a high school diploma will continue to be the minimum requirement for entry into a practical nursing program. The applicant must have a firm grounding in communication skills (written and oral), as well as in advanced sciences to cope with the increased scientific base of nursing. Some knowledge of or fluency in a second language would be useful in this increasingly multicultural society.

Practical nurse education programs need to be at least 2 academic years in length and must occur in a postsecondary institution that meets general program standards for preparing professionals to meet entry-to-practice requirements. These programs must be academically sound and include components of pure science, social science, and humanities. The curricula must also incorporate interprofessional education. Should the practical nurse decide to continue with studies in registered nursing, the practical nursing program should be accepted in whole or in part toward a university baccalaureate program. Private postsecondary schools may present some issues about control of program standards and conflict of interest between profit taking and the public interest, although this need not be so if regulating authorities closely monitor these schools.

As noted in earlier in this appendix, "laddering" into registered nursing is not the only option for practical nurses to enhance their professional careers. Many opportunities exist for nurses to gain expertise in specific health care areas while retaining a practical nursing identity. Practical nurses with advanced skill sets become valuable members of the health care team.

Should a university degree in practical nursing be available? Some places in the United States offer degrees in practical nursing, but this raises some questions. If university degrees become common, what would be the difference between practical nursing and registered nursing? Would the levels of nurses and their currently separate scopes of practices become even more blurred, or would they merge? Does the public need two very similar practitioners with the same education?

If practical nursing required a degree, this would mean registered nurses would be required to have master's degrees. A master's degree might even become a requirement for entry to practice for the registered nurse. This is already happening in the United States and much of Canada, where a master's degree in nursing is required for almost all entry-level teaching or administrative positions and most nurse practitioner (registered nursing extended class) positions. This scenario may appeal to health care agencies because they could employ more practical nurses, presumably for less cost than the same number of registered nurses. However, if university degrees in practical nursing were required, professionals educated at this level would demand higher pay. Thus, the health care system would not be much further ahead economically.

Will practical nursing remain a recognized health care profession, or will it be swallowed up by professions on either side of it (the registered nurse with baccalaureate degrees on one side and the unregulated care providers on the other)? If practical nursing fails to maintain or expand the knowledge base, then unregulated care providers may begin to absorb nursing competencies into their own skill set.

Scope of Practice and New Competencies

The practical nursing profession faces an exciting future. The practical nursing scope of practice will continue to evolve in response to changes in the Canadian health care system. The *Toward 2020* report (CNA, 2006) proposed that the structure of the health care system and the delivery of nursing by regulated nursing professions will be very different in the future. They predicted that by 2020, registered nurses would undertake more of the primary care that is currently provided by general practitioners. If this becomes reality, how will it affect the role of practical nurses? The report also predicted that by 2020, the proportion of practical nurses would increase and that the majority of nurses would work in community settings and in multidisciplinary teams. It suggested that practical nurses would play a greater role in preoperative, preprocedure, and perioperative settings and would be primarily responsible for rehabilitation and long-term care, with the assistance of personel support workers. Acute care in 2020 was further envisioned as consisting of a combination of all categories of nurses (Villeneuve & MacDonald, 2006).

Practical nurses of the future will continue to acquire separate postgraduate competencies in specific areas through postbasic education and on-the-job training and experience. In the future, more of these competencies may involve community health care, consultations and advice by telephone ("Telehealth"), disease prevention (epidemiology), rehabilitation, palliative care, special needs populations, and health teaching opportunities for groups and individuals. Practical nurses will also probably have many opportunities to work with multicultural groups, including new immigrants, Aboriginal and other indigenous people, and rural populations, and they will continue to work in long-term and chronic care settings.

If professionals in acute care increase their use of the critical pathway (care map) system, practical nurses could have expanded roles in areas such as intensive care units. They would be able to work with less stable clients because the critical pathway system allows for more interdependence and collaboration, technological and personnel help, and distinct instructions for care and consultation. The registered nurse would continue with the role of case manager.

Currently, registered nursing requires a greater depth of knowledge and a broader practice base than does practical nursing, and it exerts great influence on scope of practice among all categories of nurses. Practical nursing associations of the future will persist in addressing strategies to challenge restrictions imposed by other nursing groups. As all categories of nursing professions face the future, it is imperative that they engage in dialogue and planning to ensure that their future roles and scopes of practice most effectively serve all stakeholders in the Canadian health care system.

What Is the Final Answer?

What will happen to practical nursing in the future? No one knows for certain, but ecological and sociological studies of professions indicate that individuals and groups—both animal and human—grow, develop, change, flourish, fade out, and disappear. According to Wilson (1992), "environment is the theatre and evolution is the play" (p. 82).

Practical nurses and registered nurses are likely to always maintain separate scopes of practice for survival reasons. But practical nursing can strengthen its position by developing more diverse and specialized competencies in this changing society. It must develop competencies that address the needs of the environment. It must change to meet health care demands. For nurses, health care—more specifically, nursing—is the theatre, and constant change is the play. If practical nurses wish to maintain their particular niche in the health care system, it is essential that they respond effectively in this environment of continued rapid change.

✻ References

Abbott, A. D. (1988). *The system of professions: An essay on the division of expert labor*. Chicago, IL: University of Chicago Press.

Access Issues for Regulators Workshop 2. (2001). *Panel discussion*. Retrieved January 25, 2004, from http://www.maytree.com/PDF_Files/AIRRisingStandards.pdf

Assessment Strategies Inc. (2006). *The Canadian PN exam prep guide* (3rd ed.). Ottawa, ON: Author.

Canadian Institute for Health Information. (2002). Workforce trends of licensed practical nurses in Canada. Retrieved January 25, 2004, from http://secure.cihi.ca/cihiweb/products/dispPage.jsp?cw_page=AR_365_E

Canadian Institute for Health Information. (2007). *Workforce trends of licensed practical nurses in Canada, 2006.* Ottawa, ON: Author. Retrieved September 6, 2008, from http://secure.cihi.ca/cihiweb/products/Workforce_Trends_LPN_2006_e.pdf

Canadian Institute for Health Information. (2008). Regulated Nurses: Trends, 2003 to 2007. Ottawa, ON: Retrieved February 19, 2009, from http://secure.cihi.ca/cihiweb/dispPage.jsp?cw_page=AR_365_E

College of Licensed Practical Nurses of Alberta. (2003). *Collaborative nursing practice in Alberta.* Retrieved January 15, 2004, from http://www.clpna.com/doc_collaborationdocument.pdf

College of Licensed Practical Nurses of Alberta. (2008). *History of Alberta LPNs.* Retrieved September 7, 2008, from http://www.clpna.com/AboutCLPNA/HistoryofAlbertaLPNs/tabid/61/Default.aspx

College of Licensed Practical Nurses of British Columbia. (n.d.). *Position statement: Use of protected titles for licensed practical nurses in British Columbia.* Retrieved February 15, 2004, from http://www.clpnbc.org/pdf/UseOfTitle.pdf

College of Licensed Practical Nurses of British Columbia. (2003). *History of LPNs in Canada.* Retrieved February 12, 2009, from http://www.clpnbc.org

College of Licensed Practical Nurses of Manitoba. (2008). [Home page]. Retrieved September 4, 2008, from http://www.clpnm.ca/content/

College of Nurses of Ontario. (2008). *Working with unregulated care providers.* Retrieved September 4, 2008, from http://www.cno.org/docs/prac/41014_workingucp.pdf

Enrolled Nurses Professional Association of New South Wales. (2000). *What is an enrolled nurse?* Retrieved January 20, 2004, from http://enpansw.org/whatis.htm

Government of Canada. (2002). *Building on values: The future of health care in Canada* [*Romanow Report*]. Ottawa, ON: Commission on the Future of Health Care in Canada. Retrieved February 20, 2004, from http://www.hc-sc.gc.ca/english/care/romanow/hcc0086.html

Health Professions Regulatory Advisory Council. (1996, June). *Advice to the Minister of Health: Separate college for registered practical nurses.* Retrieved April 22, 2004, from http://www.hprac.org/downloads/rpn/rpc2.pdf

Licensed Practical Nurses Association of Prince Edward Island. (2008). *Mandate.* Retrieved September 4, 2008, from http://www.lpna.ca/mandate.htm

Massachusetts Board of Registration in Nursing. (2000). *The five rights of delegation.* Retrieved April 19, 2004, from http://www.state.ma.us/reg/boards/rn/advrul/thefive.htm

May, D. (2003). *Changing entry level education requirements: Is the neoclassical model helpful?* [Economics 6030, MER Program, Memorial University]. Retrieved January 26, 2004, from http://www.nlhba.nf.ca/Web_Site_Files/LR/ETP.pdf

McLennan Community College. (2004, Spring). *Historical development of vocational nursing.* Retrieved January 23, 2004, from http://www.mclennan.edu/syllabi/VNSG/VNSG1119.html

Nurses Association of New Brunswick and Association of New Brunswick Licensed Practical Nurses. (2003). *Working together: A framework for the registered nurse and the licensed practical nurse.* Retrieved January 29, 2004, from http://www.nanb.nb.ca/pdf_e/Publications/General_Publications/ RN-LPN%20(e)1.pdf

Nursing Courses UK. (n.d.). *About nursing-training.* Retrieved January 23, 2004, from http://www.nursingcourses.co.uk/about_nursing/training.html

Registered Nurses Association of British Columbia. (2003a). *In touch: Keeping you informed.* Vancouver, BC: Author.

Registered Nurses Association of British Columbia. (2003b). *Standards for registered nursing practice in British Columbia* [Publication No. 128]. Vancouver, BC: Author.

Registered Nurses Association of Ontario & Registered Practical Nurses Association of Ontario. (2000). *Ensuring the care will be there: Report on nursing recruitment and retention in Ontario.* Retrieved October 25, 2008, from http://www.rnao.org/Page.asp?PageID=122&ContentID=1058&SiteNodeID=467

Registered Practical Nurses Association of Ontario. (2008). *History.* Retrieved February 17, 2009, from http://www.rpnao.org/about/history.asp

Saskatchewan Association of Licensed Practical Nurses. (2008). *A short history.* Retrieved October 25, 2008, from http://www.salpn.com/public/pdf/SALPNHistory_20080508.pdf

Van House, N. A., & Sutton, S. A. (1996). The panda syndrome: An ecology of LIS education [Electronic version]. *Journal of Education for Library and Information Science, 37,* 131–147.

Villeneuve, M., & MacDonald, J. (2006). *Toward 2020: Visions for nursing.* Ottawa, ON: Canadian Nurses Association. Retrieved October 25, 2008, from http://www.cna-aiic.ca/CNA/documents/pdf/publications/Toward-2020-e.pdf

Wilson, E. O. (1992). *The diversity of life.* Cambridge, MA: Harvard University Press.

Appendix B Laboratory Values

*Adapted by Jennifer E. Cooke**

The tables in this appendix list some of the most common tests, their normal values, and possible etiologies of abnormal values. Laboratory values are expressed in the Système Internationale d'Unités (SI units) that are used in Canada. Conventional units, used in the United States, are presented in parentheses after the SI units. Laboratory values may vary with different techniques or different laboratories. Possible etiologies are presented in alphabetical order. Abbreviations appearing in the tables are defined as follows:

<	less than	mm	millimetre	mcL	microlitre
>	greater than	g	gram	IU	international unit
≤	less than or equal to	mg	milligram (10^{-3})	mOsm	milliosmole
≥	greater than or equal to	mcg	microgram (one millionth	U	unit
L	litre		of a gram) (10^{-6})	mmol	millimole
mEq	milliequivalent	ng	nanogram (one billionth	mcmol	micromole
mL	millilitre		of a gram) (10^{-9})	nmol	nanomole
dL	decilitre	pg	picogram (one trillionth	pmol	picomole
mm Hg	millimetre of mercury		of a gram) (10^{-12})	kPa	kilopascal
fL	femtolitre	mcU	microunit	mckat	microkatal

TABLE B-1

Serum, Plasma, and Whole Blood Chemistry Profiles

	Normal Values		Possible Etiology	
Test	SI Units	Conventional Units	Higher	Lower
Acetone				
• Quantitative	<200 mcmol/L	<1.16 mg/dL	Diabetic ketoacidosis, high-fat diet, low-carbohydrate diet, starvation	
• Qualitative	Negative	Negative		
Albumin	35–50 g/L	3.5–5 g/dL	Dehydration	Burns, chronic liver disease, malabsorption syndrome, malnutrition, nephrotic syndrome, pregnancy
Aldolase	22–59 mU/L	3–8.2 Sibley-Lehninger U/dL	Infection, muscle trauma, skeletal muscle disease	Late-stage muscular dystrophy, renal disease
α_1-Antitrypsin	0.85–2.13 g/L	85–213 mg/dL	Acute and chronic inflammation and infection, arthritis, malignancy, stress syndrome, thyroid infections	Chronic lung disease (early onset of emphysema), malnutrition, nephrotic syndrome
α_1-Fetoprotein	<40 mcg/L	<40 ng/mL	Cancer of testes and ovaries, carcinoma of liver, neural tube defects in fetuses, or multiple pregnancies in pregnant women	Trisomy 21 or fetal distress or fetal death
Ammonia	6–47 mcmol/L	10–80 mcg/dL	GI hemorrhage, hepatic encephalopathy, portal hypertension, severe liver disease	Essential or malignant hypertension
Amylase	30–220 U/L	60–120 Somogyi U/dL	Acute and chronic pancreatitis, mumps (salivary gland disease), perforated ulcers	Acute alcoholism, cirrhosis of liver, extensive destruction of pancreas

Continued

*Adapted from Lewis, S. M., McLean Heitkemper, M., Dirksen, S. R., Goldworthy, S., & Barry, M.A. (2006). *Medical–surgical nursing in Canada* (1st Canadian ed.). Toronto, ON: Mosby.

TABLE B-1

Serum, Plasma, and Whole Blood Chemistry Profiles ***continued***

	Normal Values		Possible Etiology	
Test	SI Units	Conventional Units	Higher	Lower
Ascorbic acid	23–85 mcmol/L	0.4–1.5 mg/dL	Excessive ingestion of vitamin C	Connective tissue disorders, hepatic disease, renal disease, rheumatic fever, vitamin C deficiency
B-type natriuretic peptide	<100 ng/L	<100 pg/mL	Congestive heart failure, myocardial infarction, hypertension, cor pulmonale	
Bicarbonate	21–28 mmol/L	21–28 mmol/L	Chronic use of loop diuretics, compensated respiratory acidosis, metabolic alkalosis	Acute renal failure, compensated respiratory alkalosis, diarrhea, metabolic acidosis
Bilirubin				
• Total	5.1–17 mcmol/L	0.3–1.0 mg/dL	Biliary obstruction, hemolytic anemia, impaired liver function, pernicious anemia, prolonged fasting	
• Indirect	3.4–12 mcmol/L	0.2–0.8 mg/dL		
• Direct	1.7–5.1 mcmol/L	0.1–0.3 mg/dL		
Blood gases*				
• Arterial pH	7.35–7.45	Same as SI units	Alkalosis	Acidosis
• Venous pH	7.31–7.41	Same as SI units	Alkalosis	Acidosis
• Arterial PCO_2	35–45 mm Hg	Same as SI units	Compensated metabolic alkalosis, respiratory acidosis	Compensated metabolic acidosis, respiratory alkalosis
• Arterial PO_2	80–100 mm Hg	Same as SI units	Administration of high concentration of oxygen	Chronic lung disease, decreased cardiac output
• Venous PO_2	40–50 mm Hg	Same as SI units		
Calcium	2.25–2.75 mmol/L	9–10.5 mg/dL	Acute osteoporosis, hyperparathyroidism, multiple myeloma, vitamin D intoxication	Acute pancreatitis, hypoparathyroidism, liver disease, malabsorption syndrome, renal failure, vitamin D deficiency
Calcium, ionized	1.05–1.30 mmol/L	4.5–5.6 mg/dL		
Carbon dioxide (CO_2 content)	21–28 mmol/L	21–28 mmol/L	Chronic use of loop diuretics, compensated respiratory acidosis, metabolic alkalosis	Chronic diarrhea, chronic use of loop diuretics, renal failure, diabetic ketoacidosis, starvation
β-Carotene	1.4–4.7 mcmol/L	75–253 mcg/dL	Cystic fibrosis, hypothyroidism, pancreatic insufficiency	Dietary deficiency, malabsorption disorders
Chloride	98–106 mmol/L	98–106 mmol/L	Corticosteroid therapy, dehydration, excessive infusion of normal saline, metabolic acidosis, respiratory alkalosis, uremia	Addison's disease, congestive heart failure, diarrhea, metabolic alkalosis, overhydration, respiratory acidosis, SIADH, vomiting
Cholesterol	<5.2 mmol/L	<200 mg/dL	Biliary obstruction, cirrhosis, hypothyroidism, hyperlipidemia, idiopathic hypercholesterolemia, renal disease, uncontrolled diabetes	Corticosteroid therapy, extensive liver disease, hyperthyroidism, malnutrition
High-density lipoproteins (HDL)				
• Male	>0.75 mmol/L	>45 mg/dL		
• Female	>0.91 mmol/L	>55 mg/dL		
Low-density lipoproteins (LDL)	<3.37 mmol/L	<60–180 mg/dL		
Cholinesterase (RBC)	5–10 U/L	Same as SI units	Exercise, sickle cell disease	Acute infections, insecticide intoxication, liver disease, muscular dystrophy
Pseudocholinesterase (serum)	8–18 U/mL	Same as SI units		
Copper	11–22 mcmol/L	70–140 mcg/dL	Cirrhosis, female contraceptive use	Wilson's disease

TABLE B-1

Serum, Plasma, and Whole Blood Chemistry Profiles *continued*

	Normal Values		Possible Etiology	
Test	**SI Units**	**Conventional Units**	**Higher**	**Lower**
Cortisol	0800 hours: 138–635 nmol/L 2000 hours: <83–359 nmol/L	5–23 mcg/dL 3–13 mcg/dL	Adrenal adenoma, Cushing's syndrome, hyperthyroidism, pancreatitis, stress	Addison's disease, adrenal insufficiency, hypopituitary states, hypothyroidism, liver disease
Creatine	15.3–76.3 mcmol/L	0.2–1 mg/dL	Active rheumatoid arthritis, biliary obstruction, hyperthyroidism, renal disorders, severe muscle damage	Diabetes mellitus
Creatine kinase (CK)				
• Male	55–170 U/L	Same as SI units	Brain damage, exercise, musculoskeletal injury or disease, myocardial infarction, numerous intramuscular injections, severe myocarditis	
• Female	30–135 U/L	Same as SI units		
• CK-MB (CK-2)	Male: 2–6 mcg/L Female: 2–5 mcg/L	2–6 ng /mL 2–5 ng/mL	Acute myocardial infarction	
• CK mass fraction	<0.05 fraction of total CK	<5%	Myocardial infarction	
Creatinine				
• Male	53–106 mcmol/L	0.6–1.2 mg/dL	Severe renal disease	Diseases with decreased muscle mass (e.g. muscular dystrophy, myasthenia gravis)
• Female	44–97 mcmol/L	0.5–1.1 mg/dL		
Ferritin (serum)				
• Male	12–300 mcg/L	12–300 ng/mL	Anemia of chronic disease (infection, inflammation, liver disease), sideroblastic anemia	Iron-deficiency anemia, severe protein deficiency
• Female	10–150 mcg/L	10–150 ng/mL		
Folic acid (folate)	11–57 nmol/L	5–25 ng/mL	Hypothyroidism, pernicious anemia	Alcoholism, hemolytic anemia, inadequate diet, malabsorption syndrome, malnutrion, megaloblastic anemia
Gamma-glutamyl transpeptidase (GGT)	8–38 IU/L	Same as SI units	Cholestasis, CMV infection, Epstein-Barr virus infection, liver disease, MI, pancreatitis	
Glucose, fasting	4–6 mmol/L	70–110 mg/dL	Acute stress, cerebral lesions, Cushing's syndrome, diabetes mellitus, hyperthyroidism, pancreatic insufficiency	Addison's disease, hepatic disease, hypothyroidism, insulin overdosage, pancreatic tumour, pituitary hypofunction, postdumping syndrome
Oral glucose tolerance testing (OGTT) (2-hour)				
• Fasting	4–6 mmol/L	70–110 mg/dL	Diabetes mellitus	Hyperinsulinism
• 1 hour	<11.1 mmol/L	<200 mg/dL		
• 2 hours	<7.8 mmol/L	<140 mg/dL		
Haptoglobin	0.5–2.2 g/L	50–220 mg/dL	Acute MI, infectious and inflammatory processes, malignant neoplasms	Chronic liver disease, hemolytic anemia, mononucleosis, SLE, toxoplasmosis, transfusion reactions
Homocysteine	4–14 mcmol/L	0.54–1.9 mg/L	Cardiovascular disease, cerebrovascular disease, peripheral vascular disease, cystinuria, vitamin B_6 or B_{12} deficiency, folate deficiency, malnutrition	

Continued

TABLE B-1

Serum, Plasma, and Whole Blood Chemistry Profiles *continued*

	Normal Values		Possible Etiology	
Test	SI Units	Conventional Units	Higher	Lower
Insulin	43–186 pmol/L	6–26 mcU/mL	Acromegaly, adenoma of islet cells, obesity, untreated mild case of type 2 diabetes	Diabetes mellitus, obesity
Iron				
• Total	9–26.9 mcmol/L	50–150 mcg/dL	Excessive RBC destruction, hemochromatosis, massive transfusion	Anemia of chronic disease, iron-deficiency anemia
• Male	14–32 mcmol/L	80–180 mcg/dL		
• Female	11–29 mcmol/L	60–160 mcg/dL		
Total iron-binding capacity (TIBC)	45–82 mcmol/L	250–460 mcg/dL	Iron-deficient state, oral contraceptive use, polycythemia	Cancer, chronic infections, pernicious anemia, uremia
Lactic acid	0.6–2.2 mmol/L	5–20 mg/dL	Acidosis, congestive heart failure, severe liver disease, shock, tissue ischemia	
Lactate dehydrogenase (LDH)	100–190 U/L	Same as SI units	Congestive heart failure, hemolytic disorders, hepatitis, metastatic cancer of liver, myocardial infarction, pernicious anemia, pulmonary embolus and infarction, skeletal muscle damage	
Lactate dehydrogenase isoenzymes				
• LDH_1	0.17–0.27 of total	17%–27%	Myocardial infarction, pernicious anemia, strenuous exercise	
• LDH_2	0.27–0.37 of total	27%–37%	Exercise, pulmonary embolus, sickle cell crisis	
• LDH_3	0.18–0.25 of total	18%–25%	Malignant lymphoma, pulmonary embolus	
• LDH_4	0.03–0.08 of total	3%–8%	Systemic lupus erythematosus (SLE), pancreatitis, pulmonary infarction, renal disease	
• LDH_5	0.0–0.05 of total	0%–5%	Congestive heart failure, hepatitis, pulmonary embolus and infarction, skeletal muscle damage, strenuous exercise	
Lipase	0–160 U/L	Same as SI units	Acute and chronic pancreatitis, hepatic disorders, pancreatic disorder (cancer, pseudocyst), perforated peptic ulcer, salivary gland inflammation or tumour	
Magnesium	0.65–1.05 mmol/L	1.3–2.1 mmol/L	Addison's disease, hypothyroidism, renal failure	Chronic alcoholism, hyperparathyroidism, hyperthyroidism, hypoparathyroidism, malnutrition, severe malabsorption syndrome
Myoglobin	<90 mcg/L	Same as SI units	Myocardial infarction, myositis, malignant hyperthermia, muscular dystrophy, skeletal muscle ischemia or trauma, rhabdomyolysis, seizures	Polymyositis (at levels of <10 mcg/L)
Osmolality	285–295 mmol/kg	285–295 mOsm/kg H_2O	Chronic renal disease, dehydration, diabetes mellitus, hypernatremia, shock	Addison's disease, diuretic therapy, hyponatremia, overhydration

TABLE B-1

Serum, Plasma, and Whole Blood Chemistry Profiles *continued*

	Normal Values		Possible Etiology	
Test	SI Units	Conventional Units	Higher	Lower
Oxygen saturation				
• Arterial	≥95%	Same as SI units	Increased inspired oxygen, poly-cythemia vera	Anemia, cardiac decompensation, decreased inspired oxygen, respiratory disorders
• Venous	60%–80%	Same as SI units		
pH	See blood gases			
Phenylalanine	0–121 mcmol/L	0–2 mg/dL	Phenylketonuria	
Phosphatase, acid	2.2–10.5 U/L	0.13–0.63 U/L – Roy, Brower, Hayden 37°C	Advanced Paget's disease, cancer of prostate, hyperparathyroidism	
Phosphatase, alkaline (ALP)	0.5–2.0 mckat/L	30–120 U/L	Bone diseases, cirrhosis, malignancy of liver or bone, marked hyperparathyroidism, obstruction of biliary system, rickets	Excessive vitamin D ingestion, hypothyroidism, milk-alkali syndrome
Phosphorus, inorganic	0.97–1.45 mmol/L	3.0–4.5 mg/dL	Bone metastasis, healing fractures, hypoparathyroidism, hypocalcemia, renal disease, vitamin D intoxication	Chronic alcoholism, diabetes mellitus, hypercalcemia, hyperparathyroidism, vitamin D deficiency
Potassium	3.5–5.0 mmol/L	3.5–5.0 mmol/L	Acute or chronic renal failure, Addison's disease, dehydration, diabetic ketosis, excessive dietary or intravenous intake, massive tissue destruction, metabolic acidosis	Burns, Cushing's syndrome, deficient dietary or intravenous intake, diarrhea (severe), diuretic therapy, gastrointestinal fistula, insulin administration, pyloric obstruction, starvation, vomiting
Prostate-specific antigen (PSA)	<4 mcg/L	<4 ng/mL	Benign prostatic hypertrophy, prostate cancer, prostatitis	
Proteins				
• Total	64–83 g/L	6.4–8.3 g/dL	Burns, cirrhosis (globulin fraction), dehydration	Congenital agammaglobulinemia, increased capillary permeability, inflammatory disease, liver disease, malabsorption syndrome, malnutrition
• Albumin	35–50 g/L	3.5–5 g/dL		
• Globulin	23–34 g/L	2.3–3.4 g/dL		
• Albumin/globulin ratio	1.5:1–2.5:1	Same as SI units	Multiple myeloma (globulin fraction), shock, vomiting	Malnutrition, nephrotic syndrome, proteinuria, renal disease, severe burns
Renin				
• Upright position	0.03–1.2 ng/L/sec	0.1–4.3 mg/mL/hr	Renal hypertension, salt-losing GI disease (vomiting/diarrhea), volume decrease (e.g., hemorrhage)	Increased salt intake, primary aldosteronism
Sodium	135–145 mmol/L	135–145 mmol/L	Corticosteroid therapy, dehydration, impaired renal function, increased sodium intake in diet or intravenous infusion, primary aldosteronism	Addison's disease, decreased sodium intake in diet or intravenous infusion, diabetic ketoacidosis, diuretic therapy, excessive sodium loss from GI tract, excessive perspiration, water intoxication

Continued

TABLE B-1

Serum, Plasma, and Whole Blood Chemistry Profiles *continued*

	Normal Values		Possible Etiology	
Test	SI Units	Conventional Units	Higher	Lower
Testosterone				
• Male	9.75–38 nmol/L	280–1080 ng/dL	Adrenal hyperplasia, adrenal or pituitary tumours, testicular tumours	Primary and secondary hypogonadism
• Female	0.52–2.43 nmol/L	<70 ng/dL	Polycystic ovary, virilizing tumours	
Thyroxine (T_4), total	64–154 nmol/L	5–12 mcg/dL	Hyperthyroidism, thyroiditis	Cretinism, hypothyroidism, myxedema
T_4, free	10–36 pmol/L	0.8–2.8 ng/dL	Hyperthyroidism, metastatic neoplasms	Hypothyroidism, pregnancy
Triiodothyronine (T_3) uptake	24–34 AU	24%–34%		
T_3, total	1.2–3.4 nmol/L	70–205 ng/dL	Hyperthyroidism	Hypothyroidism
Thyroid-stimulating hormone (TSH)	2–10 mU/L	2–10 mcU/L	Graves' disease, myxedema, primary hypothyroidism	Secondary hypothyroidism
Transaminases	0–0.58 mkat/L	0–35 U/L	Acute hepatitis, liver disease, myocardial infarction, pulmonary infarction	
• Serum glutamic oxaloacetic transaminase (SGOT) or aspartate aminotransferase (AST)				
• Serum glutamate pyruvate transaminase (SGPT) or alanine aminotransferase (ALT)	4–36 U/L	Same as SI units	Liver disease, shock	
Triglycerides				
• Male	0.45–1.81 mmol/L	40–160 mg/dL	Diabetes mellitus, hyperlipidemia, hypothyroidism, liver disease	Hyperthyroidism, malabsorption syndrome, malnutrition
• Female	0.40–1.52 mmol/L	35–135 mg/dL		
Troponin T (cTnT)	<0.2 mcg/L	<0.2 ng/mL	Cardiac muscle damage (MI, myocarditis, or pericarditis), chronic renal failure, multi-organ failure, severe heart failure	
Troponin I (cTnI)	<0.03 mcg/L	<0.3 ng/mL		
Urea nitrogen (BUN)	3.6–7.1 mmol/L	10–20 mg/dL	Burns, dehydration, GI hemorrhage, increase in protein catabolism (fever, stress), renal disease, shock, urinary tract infection	Fluid overload, malnutrition, severe liver damage, SIADH
Uric acid				
• Male	0.24–0.51 mmol/L	4.0–8.5 mg/dL	Alcoholism, eclampsia, gout, gross tissue destruction, high-protein weight reduction diet, leukemia, multiple myeloma, renal failure	Administration of uricosuric drugs
• Female	0.16–0.43 mmol/L	2.7–7.3 mg/dL		
Vitamin A	0.52–2.09 mcmol/L	15–60 mcg/dL	Excess ingestion of vitamin A	Vitamin A deficiency
Vitamin B_{12}	118–701 pmol/L	160–950 pg/mL	Chronic myeloid leukemia	Malabsorption syndrome, pernicious anemia, strict vegetarianism, total or partial gastrectomy
Zinc	11.5–18.5 mcmol/L	75–120 mcg/dL	Alcoholic cirrhosis	

AU, arbitrary units; CMV, cytomegalovirus; GI, gastrointestinal; MI, myocardial infarction; PCO_2, partial pressure of carbon dioxide; PO_2, partial pressure of oxygen; RBC, red blood cell; SIADH, syndrome of inappropriate ADH; SLE, systemic lupus erythematosus.

*Because arterial blood gases are influenced by altitude, the value for PO_2 decreases as altitude increases. The lower value is normal for an altitude of 1 mile (1.6 km).

TABLE B-2

Hematology Profiles

	Normal Values		Possible Etiology	
Test	SI Units	Conventional Units	Higher	Lower
Bleeding time (IVY)	1–9 min	Same as SI units	Aspirin ingestion, clotting factor deficiency, defective platelet function, thrombocytopenia, vascular disease, von Willebrand's disease	–
Activated partial thromboplastin time (APTT)	30–40 sec*	Same as SI units	Deficiency of factors I, II, V, VIII, IX, and X, XI, XII; hemophilia; heparin therapy; liver disease	
Partial thromboplastin time (PTT)	60–70 sec	Same as SI units	Same etiology as for APTT	
Automated coagulation time or activated clotting time (ACT)	70–120 sec	Same as SI units	Same etiology as for APTT	
Prothrombin time (Protime, PT)	11–12.5 sec*	Same as SI units	Deficiency of factors I, II, V, VII, and X; liver disease; vitamin K deficiency; warfarin therapy	
International normalized ratio (INR)	0.81–1.2	Same as SI units	Same etiology as for PT	
Thrombin time	8–12 sec	Same as SI units	DIC, increased tendency to bleed	Burns (during first 36 hr), DIC, severe liver disease
Fibrinogen	2–4 g/L	200–400 mg/dL	Burns (after first 36 hr), inflammatory disease	
Fibrin split (degradation) products	<10 mg/L	<10 mcg/mL	Acute DIC, massive hemorrhage, massive trauma, primary fibrinolysis	
D-Dimer	<250 mcg/L	<250 ng/mL	Deep vein thrombosis, DIC, myocardial infarction, unstable angina	
Erythrocyte count† (altitude dependent)				
• Male	$4.7–6.1 \times 10^{12}$/L	$4.7–6.1 \times 10^6$/mcL	Dehydration, high altitudes, polycythemia vera, severe diarrhea	Anemia, leukemia, status post hemorrhage
• Female	$4.2–5.4 \times 10^{12}$/L	$4.2–5.4 \times 10^6$/mcL		
Mean corpuscular volume (MCV)	80–95 mm^3	Same as SI units	Folic acid and vitamin B_{12} deficiency, liver disease, macrocytic anemia	Microcytic anemia
Mean corpuscular hemoglobin (MCH)	27–31 pg	Same as SI units	Macrocytic anemia	Microcytic anemia
Mean corpuscular hemoglobin concentration (MCHC)	320–360 g/L	32–36 g/dL (32%–36%)	Intravascular hemolysis, spherocytosis	Hypochromic anemia
Erythrocyte sedimentation rate (ESR), Westergren				
• Male <50 yr	<15 mm/hr	Same as SI units	*Moderate increase:* acute hepatitis, myocardial infarction, rheumatoid arthritis *Marked increase:* acute and severe bacterial infections, malignancies, pelvic inflammatory disease	Malaria, severe liver disease, sickle cell anemia
• Male >50 yr	<20 mm/hr	Same as SI units		
• Female <50 yr	<20 mm/hr	Same as SI units		
• Female >50 yr	<30 mm/hr	Same as SI units		

Continued

TABLE B-2

Hematology Profiles *continued*

Test	Normal Values		Possible Etiology	
	SI Units	Conventional Units	Higher	Lower
Hematocrit (altitude dependent)†				
• Male	0.42–0.52 volume fraction	42%–52%	Dehydration, high altitudes, polycythemia	Anemia, bone marrow failure, hemorrhage, leukemia, overhydration
• Female	0.37–0.47 volume fraction	37%–47%		
Hemoglobin (altitude dependent)†				
• Male	8.7–11.2 mmol/L	14–18 g/dL	COPD, high altitudes, polycythemia	Anemia, hemorrhage
• Female	7.4–9.9 mmol/L	12–16 g/dL		
Hemoglobin, glycosylated or glycated (HbA1c [A1C])	Less than 6% (nondiabetic adult)	Same as SI units	Nondiabetic hyperglycemia, poorly controlled diabetes mellitus	Chronic blood loss, chronic renal failure, pregnancy, sickle cell anemia
RBC distribution width (RDW)	11%–14.5%		Anisocytosis, macrocytic anemia, microcytic anemia	
Platelet count (thrombocytes)	$150–400 \times 10^9$/L	150,000–400,000 mm^3	Acute infections, chronic granulocytic leukemia, chronic pancreatitis, cirrhosis, collagen disorders, polycythemia, status post splenectomy	Acute leukemia, cancer chemotherapy, DIC, hemorrhage, infection, SLE, thrombocytopenic purpura
Reticulocyte count (manual)	0.5%–2% of RBC	Same as SI units	Hemolytic anemia, polycythemia vera	Hypoproliferative anemia, macrocytic anemia, microcytic anemia
White blood cell (WBC) count†	$5–10 \times 10^9$/L	5000–10,000 mm^3	Inflammatory and infectious processes, leukemia	Aplastic anemia, autoimmune diseases, overwhelming infection, side effects of chemotherapy and irradiation
WBC differential				
• Segmented neutrophils	$2.5–7.5 \times 10^9$/L	62%–68%	Bacterial infections, collagen diseases, Hodgkin's disease	Aplastic anemia, viral infections
• Band neutrophils	$0–1 \times 10^9$/L	0%–9%	Acute infections	
• Lymphocytes	$0.1–0.4 \times 10^9$/L (1000–4000 mm^3)	20%–40%	Chronic infections, lymphocytic leukemia, mononucleosis, viral infections	Corticosteroid therapy, whole-body irradiation
• Monocytes	$0.02–0.07 \times 10^9$/L (100–700 mm^3)	2%–8%	Acute infections, Chronic inflammatory disorders, Hodgkin's disease, malaria, monocytic leukemia	
• Eosinophils	$0.01–0.04 \times 10^9$/L (50–100 mm^3)	1%–4%	Allergic reactions, eosinophilic and chronic granulocytic leukemia, Hodgkin's disease, parasitic disorders	Corticosteroid therapy
• Basophils	$0.0–0.01 \times 10^9$/L (25–100 mm^3)	0.5%–1%	Hypothyroidism, myeloproliferative diseases, ulcerative colitis	Hyperthyroidism, stress
Sickle cell solubility test	Negative	Negative	Sickle cell anemia	

*Values depend on reagent used

†Components of complete blood count (CBC)

COPD, Chronic obstructive pulmonary disease; DIC, disseminated intravascular coagulation; GI, gastrointestinal; RBC, red blood cell; SLE, systemic lupus erythematosus; WBC, white blood cell.

TABLE B-3

Serology-Immunology Profiles

Test	Normal Values		Possible Etiology	
	SI Units	Conventional Units	Higher	Lower
Antinuclear antibody (ANA)	Negative at 1:40 dilution	Same as SI units	Chronic hepatitis, rheumatoid arthritis, scleroderma, SLE	–
Anti-DNA antibody	Negative <70 U/mL	Same as SI units	SLE	
Anti-RNP	Negative	Negative	Mixed connective-tissue disease, scleroderma, rheumatoid arthritis, Sjögren syndrome, SLE	
Anti-Sm (Smith)	Negative	Negative	SLE	
Antistreptolysin-O (ASO)	≤160 Todd U/mL	Same as SI units	Acute glomerulonephritis, rheumatic fever, streptococcal infection	
C-reactive protein (CRP)	<10 mg/L	<1.0 mg/dL	Acute infections, any inflammatory condition (e.g., acute rheumatic fever/arthritis), widespread malignancy	
Carcinoembryonic antigen (CEA)	5 mcg/L	5 ng/mL	Carcinoma of colon, liver, pancreas; chronic cigarette smoking; inflammatory bowel disease; other cancers	
Complement assay components				
• Total	75–160 kU/L	75–160 U/mL		Acute glomerulonephritis, rheumatoid arthritis, serum sickness, subacute bacterial endocarditis, SLE
• C3	0.55–1.2 g/L	55–120 mg/dL		
• C4	0.2–0.5 g/L	20–50 mg/dL		
Direct antihuman globulin test (DAT) or direct Coombs	Negative (No agglutination)	Negative	Acquired hemolytic anemia, drug reactions, hemolytic disease of the newborn, transfusion reactions	
Fluorescent treponemal antibody absorption (FTAAbs)	Negative	Nonreactive	Syphilis	
Hepatitis A antibody	Negative	Negative	Hepatitis A	
Hepatitis B surface antigen (HB_sAg)	Negative	Negative	Hepatitis B	
Hepatitis C antibody	Negative	Negative	Hepatitis C	
Immunoglobulins				
• IgA	0.85–3.85 g/L	85–385 mg/dL	Autoimmune disorders, chronic infection, chronic liver disease, IgA myeloma, rheumatoid arthritis	Burns, hereditary telangiectasia, malabsorption syndromes
• IgD Minimal			Chronic infection, connective tissue disease	
• IgE Minimal			Anaphylactic shock, atopic disease (allergies), parasite infections	
• IgG	5.65–17.65 g/L	565–1765 mg/dL	Hepatitis, IgG monoclonal gammopathy, infections (acute and chronic), SLE	Acquired deficiencies, burns, congenital immune deficiencies, immunosuppression, nephrotic syndromes
• IgM	0.55–3.75 g/L	55–375 mg/dL	Acute infections, liver disease, rheumatoid arthritis	Congenital and acquired antibody deficiencies, lymphocytic leukemia, protein-losing enteropathies

Continued

TABLE B-3

Serology-Immunology Profiles *continued*

Test	Normal Values: SI Units	Normal Values: Conventional Units	Possible Etiology: Higher	Possible Etiology: Lower
Monospot or monotest	Negative	<1:28 titre	Infectious mononucleosis	
Rheumatoid (RA) factor	0.2 kU/L (Nephalometric method) <1:20 titre (Agglutination method)	0.2 U/mL	Rheumatoid arthritis, Sjögren's syndrome, SLE	
Rapid plasma reagin (RPR)	Negative or nonreactive	Same as SI units	Febrile diseases, IV drug abuse, leprosy, malaria, rheumatoid arthritis, syphilis, SLE	
VDRL or nonreactive	Negative	Same as SI units	Syphilis	
Thyroid antibodies	Titre <1:100	Same as SI units	Early hypothyroidism, Graves' disease, Hashimoto's thyroiditis, pernicious anemia, SLE, thyroid carcinoma	

IgA, IgD, IgE, IgG, and IgM, immunoglobulins A, D, E, G, and M; IV, intravenous; RNP, ribonucleoprotein; SLE, systemic lupus erythematosus; VDRL, Venereal Disease Research Laboratory test.

TABLE B-4

Urine Chemistry Profiles

Test	Speciman	Normal Values: SI Units	Normal Values: Conventional Units	Possible Etiology: Higher	Possible Etiology: Lower
Acetone (ketones)	Random	Negative	Negative	Diabetes mellitus, high-fat and low-carbohydrate diets, starvation states	–
Aldosterone	24 hr	6–72 nmol/24 hr (depends on urinary sodium)	2–26 mcg/24 hr	*Primary aldosteronism*: adrenocortical tumours *Secondary aldosteronism*: cardiac failure, cirrhosis, large dose of ACTH, salt depletion	ACTH deficiency, Addison's disease, corticosteroid therapy
Amylase	24 hr	Up to 5000 Somogyi U/24 hr *or* 6.5–48.1 U/hr	–	Acute pancreatitis	
Bence Jones protein	Random	Negative	Negative	Biliary duct obstruction, multiple myeloma	
Bilirubin	Random	Negative	Negative	Hepatitis	
Calcium	24 hr	6.2 mmol/day	<250 mg/day	Bone tumour, hyper-parathyroidism, milk-alkali syndrome	Hypoparathyroidism, malabsorption of calcium and vitamin D
Catecholamines	24 hr				
• Epinephrine		<109 nmol/day	<20 mcg/day	Heart failure, pheochromo-cytoma, progressive muscular dystrophy	
• Norepinephrine		<590 nmol/day	<100 mcg/day		

TABLE B-4

Urine Chemistry Profiles *continued*

Test	Speciman	Normal Values		Possible Etiology	
		SI Units	Conventional Units	Higher	Lower
Chloride	24 hr	110–250 mmol/day	110–250 mmol/day	Addison's disease	Burns, diarrhea, excess perspiration, menstruation, vomiting
		<0.5 mcmol/day	<30 mcg/day		
Copper	24 hr	0.6 mcmol/day	<40 mcg/day	Cirrhosis, Wilson's disease	
Coproporphyrin	24 hr	<300 nmol/day	<200 mcg/day	Lead poisoning, oral contraceptive use, poliomyelitis	
Creatine					
• Male	24 hr	<300 mcmol/day	<60 mg/day	Addison's disease, burns, carcinoma of liver, diabetes, hyperthyroidism, infections, muscular dystrophy, skeletal muscle atrophy	Hypothyroidism
• Female	24 hr	<600 mcmol/day	<80 mg/day		
Creatinine	24 hr	7.1–17.7 mmol/day	0.8–2 g/day	Anemia, leukemia, muscular atrophy, salmonellae	Renal disease
• Male		1.78–2.32 mL/sec	107–139 mL/min		
• Female		1.45–1.78 mL/sec	87–107 mL/min		
Estriol, female	24 hr				
• Ovulation peak		104–370 nmol/day	28–100 mcg/day	Gonadal or adrenal tumour	Agenesis of ovaries, endocrine disturbance, menopause, ovarian dysfunction
• Luteal peak		81–296 nmol/day	22–80 mcg/day		
• Pregnancy		≤166,455 nmol/day	≤45,000 mcg/day		
• Menopause		5.2–72.5 nmol/day	1.4–19.6 mcg/day		
Estriol, male		18–67 nmol/day	5–18 mcg/day		
Glucose	Random	Negative	Negative	Diabetes mellitus, low renal threshold for glucose resorption, physiological stress, pituitary disorders	
Hemoglobin	Random	Negative	Negative	Extensive burns, glomerulonephritis, hemolytic anemias, hemolytic transfusion reaction	
5-Hydroxyindoleacetic acid (5-HIAA)	24 hr	10–40 mcmol/day	2–8 mg/24 hr	Malignant carcinoid syndrome	
Ketone bodies	Random	Negative	Negative	Alcoholism, fasting, high-protein diets, marked ketonuria, poorly controlled diabetes mellitus, starvation	
Lead	24 hr	<0.40 mcmol/day	<80 mcg/day	Lead poisoning	
Metanephrine	24 hr	<7 mcmol/day	<1.3 mg/day	Pheochromocytoma	
Myoglobin	Random	Negative	Negative	Crushing injuries, electric injuries, extreme physical exertion	

Continued

TABLE B-4

Urine Chemistry Profiles *continued*

		Normal Values		Possible Etiology	
Test	**Speciman**	**SI Units**	**Conventional Units**	**Higher**	**Lower**
pH	Random	4.6–8 Average: 6	Same as SI units	Chronic renal failure, compensatory phase of alkalosis, salicylate intoxication, vegetarian diet	Compensatory phase of acidosis, dehydration, emphysema
Phenylpyruvic acid	Random	Negative	Negative	Phenylketonuria	
Phosphorus, inorganic	24 hr	29–42 mmol/day	0.9–1.3 g/day	Fever, hypoparathyroidism, nervous exhaustion, rickets, tuberculosis	Acute infections, nephritis
Porphobilinogen	Random	Negative	Negative	Acute intermittent porphyria, liver disorders	
	24 hr	0–8.8 mcmol/day	0–2 mg/24hr		
Potassium	24 hr	25–100 mmol/day	25–100 mmol/day	Chronic renal failure, starvation, Cushing's syndrome, hyperaldosteronism, alkalosis, diuretic therapy	Reduced intake, dehydration, Addison's disease, malnutrition, vomiting, diarrhea, acute renal failure
Protein (dipstick)	Random	Negative	Negative	Congestive heart failure, nephritis, nephrosis, physiological stress	
Protein (quantitative)	24 hr	<0.15 g/day	<150 mg/day	Cardiac failure, inflammatory processes of urinary tract, nephritis, nephrosis, toxemia of pregnancy	
Protein (qualitative)					
• At rest		0.05–0.08 g/day	<50–80 mg/day		
• During exercise		<0.25 g/day	<250 mg/day		
Sodium	24 hr	40–250 mmol/day	40–250 mmol/day	Acute tubular necrosis	Hyponatremia
Specific gravity	Random	1.005–1.030	Same as SI units	Albuminuria, dehydration, fever, GI losses (vomiting, diarrhea, or both), glycosuria, SIADH	Diabetes insipidus, diuresis, overhydration
Titratable acidity	24 hr	20–50 mmol/day	Same as SI units	Metabolic acidosis	Metabolic alkalosis
Uric acid	24 hr	1.48–4.43 mmol/day	250–750 mg/24 hr	Gout, leukemia	Nephritis
Urobilinogen	24 hr	0.0–6.8 mcmol/day	0.0–4.0 mg/24 hr	Hemolytic disease, hepatic parenchymal cell damage, liver disease	Complete obstruction of bile duct
	Random	<0.01–1 EU	Same as SI units		
Uroporphyrins					
• Male	24 hr	4–46 mcg/day	Same as SI units	Lead poisoning, liver disease, porphyria	
• Female	24 hr	3–22 mcg/day	Same as SI units		
Vanillylmandelic acid	24 hr	<35 mcmol/day	<6.8 mg/day	Pheochromocytoma, neuroblastomas	

ACTH, Adrenocorticotropic hormone; EU, ehrlich unit; GI, gastrointestinal; SIADH, syndrome of inappropriate ADH

TABLE B-5

Gastric Analysis

Test	Normal Values		Possible Etiology	
	SI Units	Conventional Units	Higher	Lower
Basal Measurements				
Free hydrochloric acid	0.3 mmol/L	0.3 mmol/L	Hypermotility of stomach	Pernicious anemia
Total acidity	15–45 mmol/L	15–45 mmol/L	Gastric and duodenal ulcers, Zollinger-Ellison syndrome	Gastric carcinoma, severe gastritis
Poststimulation Measurements				
Free hydrochloric acid	10–130 mmol/L	10–130 mmol/L	–	
Total acidity	20–150 mmol/L	20–150 mmol/L		

TABLE B-6

Fecal Analysis

Test	Normal Values		Possible Etiology	
	SI Units	Conventional Units	Higher	Lower
Fecal fat	7.21 mmol/day	2–6 g/day	Chronic pancreatic disease, cystic fibrosis, malabsorption syndrome, obstruction of common bile duct, short gut syndrome	
Urobilinogen	51–372 mcmol/ 100 g of stool	30–220 mg/100 g of stool	Hemolytic anemias	Complete biliary obstruction
Mucus	Negative	Negative	Mucous colitis, spastic constipation	
Pus	Negative	Negative	Chronic bacillary dysentery, chronic ulcerative colitis, localized abscesses	
Blood*	Negative	Negative	Anal fissures, hemorrhoids, inflammatory bowel disease, malignant tumour, peptic ulcer	
Colour				
• Brown	–	–	Various colours depending on diet	
• Clay	–	–	Biliary obstruction or presence of barium sulphate	
• Tarry	–	–	More than 100 mL of blood in GI tract	
• Red	–	–	Blood in large intestine	
• Black	–	–	Blood in upper GI tract or iron medication	

GI, gastrointestinal; N.A., not applicable.

*Ingestion of meat may produce false-positive results. Client may be placed on a meat-free diet for 3 days before the test.

TABLE B-7

Cerebrospinal Fluid Analysis

Test	Normal Values		Possible Etiology	
	SI Units	Conventional Units	Higher	Lower
Pressure	<20 cm H_2O	Same as SI units	Hemorrhage, intracranial tumour, meningitis	Head injury, spinal tumour, subdural hematoma
Blood				
Cell count (age-dependent)	Negative	Negative	Intracranial hemorrhage	–
• WBC	0–5 × 10^6/L	0–5 cells/μL	Inflammation or infections of CNS	
• RBC	Negative	Negative		
Chloride	115–130 mmol/L	115–130 mmol/L	Uremia	Bacterial infections of CNS (meningitis, encephalitis)
Glucose	2.8–4.2 mmol/L	50–75 mg/dL	Diabetes mellitus, viral infections of CNS	Bacterial infections and tuberculosis of CNS
Protein				
• Lumbar	0.15–0.45 g/L	15–45 mg/dL	Guillain-Barré syndrome, poliomyelitis, traumatic spinal tap	
• Cisternal	0.15–0.25 g/L	15–25 mg/dL	Syphilis of CNS	
• Ventricular	0.05–0.15 g/L	5–15 mg/dL	Acute meningitis, brain tumour, chronic CNS infections, multiple sclerosis	

CNS, central nervous system; RBC, red blood cell; WBC, white blood cell.

Chapter 1

Agency for Health Care Policy and Research, Panel for the Prediction and Prevention of Pressure Ulcers in Adults. (1992). Pressure ulcers in adults: Prediction and prevention (Clinical Practice Guideline No. 3, AHCPR Publication No. 92-0047). Rockville, MD: Author, U.S. Department of Health and Human Services.

Antonovsky, A. (1987). *Unraveling the mystery of health: How people manage stress and stay well.* San Francisco: Jossey-Bass.

Bartley, M., Ferrie, J., & Montgomery, S. (1999). Living in a high-unemployment economy: Understanding the health consequences. In M. Marmot & R.Wilkinson (Eds.), *Social determinants of health* (pp. 81–104). Oxford, UK: Oxford University Press.

Berkman, L. (1995). The role of social relations in health promotion. *Psychosomatic Medicine, 57,* 245–254.

Bryant, T. (2002). The role of knowledge in public health and health promotion policy change. *Health Promotion International, 17,* 89–98.

Bryant, T. (2004). Housing and health in Canada. In D. Raphael (Ed.), *Social determinants of health: Canadian perspectives* (pp. 217–232). Toronto, ON: Canadian Scholars' Press.

Canadian Centre for Justice Statistics (2005). *Family violence in Canada: A statistical profile.* Ottawa, ON: Statistics Canada, Minister of Industry.

Canadian Council on Social Development (2006). *The progress of Canada's children and youth 2006.* Ottawa, ON: Author.

Canadian Council on Social Development (2007). *Populations vulnerable to poverty: Urban poverty in Canada, 2000.* Ottawa, ON: Author.

Canadian Institute for Health Information. (2004). *Improving the health of Canadians.* Ottawa, ON: Author.

Canadian Institute of Child Health (2000). Low birth weight. Fact sheet. In *The health of Canada's children: A CICH profile* (3rd ed). Retrieved August 27, 2008, from http://www.cich.ca/PDFFiles/ProfileFactSheets/English/LBWEng.pdf

Canadian Nurses Association and Canadian Medical Association (2005). *Joint CNA/CMA position statement on environmentally responsible activity in the health sector.* Retrieved August 4, 2008, from http://www.cna-aiic.ca/CNA/documents/pdf/publications/PS33_Joint_Stat_Envir_Resp_Activity_Health_Sector_Feb_2006_e.pdf

Canadian Policy Research Networks (2008). *Workplace health.* Retrieved August 4, 2008, from http://www.jobquality.ca/indicators/environment/phy1.sHTML

Canadian Public Health Association. (1996a). *The health impacts of unemployment: A position paper.* Ottawa, ON: Author.

Canadian Public Health Association. (1996b). *Action statement for health promotion in Canada.* Ottawa, ON: Author.

Carpiano, R. M. (2007). Neighborhood social capital and adult health: An empirical test of a Bourdieu-based model. *Health & Place, 13,* 639–655.

Che, J., & Chen, J. (2001). Food insecurity in Canadian households [Electronic version]. *Health Reports, 12*(4), 11–22.

Cohen, B., & Reutter, L. (2007). Development of the role of public health nurses in addressing child and family poverty: A framework for action. *Journal of Advanced Nursing, 60*(1), 96–107.

Cohen, S. (1992). Stress, social support, and disorder. In H. Veiel & U. Baumann (Eds.), *The meaning and measurement of social support* (pp. 109–124). New York: Hemisphere.

Community Health Nurses Association of Canada. (2003). *Canadian community health nursing standards of practice.* Retrieved August 4, 2008, from http://www.chnac.ca/images/downloads/standards/chn_standards_of_practice_jun04_english.pdf

Craig, W., & Edge, H. (2008). Bullying and fighting. In *Healthy Settings for Young People in Canada* (chap. 5). Retrieved August 4, 2008, from http://www.phace-aspc.gc.ca/dca-dea/yjc/ch5_105_108-eng.php

Department of Justice Canada (2008). *Family violence: A fact sheet from the Department of Justice Canada.* Retrieved August 27, 2008, from http://canada.justice.gc.ca/eng/pi/fv-vf/facts-info/fv-vf.pdf

Duncan, S., Hyndman, K., Estabrooks, C. A., et al. (2001). Nurses' experience of violence in Alberta and British Columbia hospitals. *Canadian Journal of Nursing Research, 32*(4), 57–78.

Dunn, J. R. (2002). *Are widening income inequalities making Canada less healthy?* Retrieved August 4, 2008, from http://www.opha.on.ca/resources/incomeinequalities/summary.pdf

Engel, G. L. (1977). The need for a new medical model: A challenge for biomedicine. *Science, 196,* 129-136.

Epp, J. (1986). *Achieving health for all: A framework for health promotion.* Ottawa, ON: Health and Welfare Canada.

Federal, Provincial, and Territorial Advisory Committee on Population Health. (1994). *Strategies for population health: Investing in the health of Canadians.* Ottawa, ON: Minister of Supply and Services Canada.

Federal, Provincial, and Territorial Advisory Committee on Population Health. (1999). *Toward a healthy future: Second report on the health of Canadians.* Ottawa, ON: Minister of Public Works and Government Services Canada.

Frankish, C. J., Hwang, S., & Quantz, D. (2005). Homelessness and health in Canada. *Canadian Journal of Public Health, 96*(Suppl. 2), S23–S29.

Friendly, M. (2004). Early childhood education and care. In D. Raphael (Ed.), *Social determinants of health: Canadian perspectives* (pp. 109–123). Toronto, ON: Canadian Scholars' Press.

Galabuzi, G. (2004). Social exclusion. In D. Raphael (Ed.), *Social determinants of health: Canadian perspectives* (pp. 235–251). Toronto, ON: Canadian Scholars' Press.

Garriguet, D. (2007). Canadians' eating habits. *Health Reports, 18*(2), 17–32.

Gilmour, H. (2007). Physically active Canadians. *Health Reports, 18*(3), 45–65.

Gottleib, L., & Rowat, K. (1987). The McGill model of nursing: A practice-derived model. *Advances in Nursing Science, 9*(4), 51–61.

Hamilton, N., & Bhatti, T. (1996). *Population health promotion: An integrated model of population health and health promotion.* Ottawa, ON: Health Promotion Development Division, Health Canada.

Hancock, T., & Perkins, F. (1985). The mandala of health: A conceptual model and teaching tool. *Health Education, 24*(1), 8–10.

Health Canada. (1996). *Towards a common understanding: Clarifying the concepts of population health.* Ottawa, ON: Author.

Health Canada. (1998). *Taking action on population health: A position paper for health promotion and programs branch staff.* Ottawa, ON: Author.

Health Canada. (2007). *First Nations, Inuit, and Aboriginal health. Facts on smoking rates.* Retrieved August 4, 2008, from http://www.hc-sc.gc.ca/fnih-spni/substan/tobac-tabac/index_e.HTML#facts

Health Canada. (2008). *Canadian Tobacco Use Monitoring Survey (CTUMS) 2007.* Summary of results for the first half of 2007 (February–June). Retrieved August 27, 2008, from http://www.hc-sc.gc.ca/hl-vs/tobac-tabac/research-recherche/stat/_ctums-esutc_2007/wave-phase-1_summary-sommaire-eng.php

Health Council of Canada. (2006). *Their future is now: Healthy choices for Canada's children and youth.* Toronto, ON: Author.

Health Disparities Task Group of the Federal/Provincial/Territorial Advisory Committee on Population Health and Health Security. (2005). *Reducing health disparities—Roles of the health sector: Discussion paper.* Retrieved August 4, 2008, from http://www.phac-aspc.gc.ca/ph-sp/disparities/pdf06/disparities_discussion_paper_e.pdf

Healthy Aging and Wellness Working Group. (2006). *Healthy aging in Canada: A new vision, a vital investment. From evidence to action. A background paper prepared for the Federal, Provincial and Territorial Committee of Officials (Seniors).* Retrieved August 4, 2008, from http://www.phac-aspc.gc.ca/seniors-aines/pubs/haging_newvision/pdf/vision-rpt_e.pdf

House, J. (1981). *Work, stress, and social support.* Menlo Park, CA: Addison-Wesley.

International Council of Nurses. (2001). *Guidelines on shaping effective health policy.* Geneva, Switzerland: Author.

Jackson, A. (2004). The unhealthy Canadian workplace. In D. Raphael (Ed.), *Social determinants of health: Canadian perspectives* (pp. 79–94). Toronto, ON: Canadian Scholars' Press.

Jensen, L., & Allen, M. (1993). Wellness: The dialectic of illness. *Image—The Journal of Nursing Scholarship, 25,* 220–224.

Jones, P., & Meleis, A. (1993). Health is empowerment. *Advances in Nursing Science, 15*(3), 1–14.

Kawachi, I., & Kennedy, B. (1997). The relationship of income inequality to mortality: Does the choice of indicator matter? *Social Science and Medicine, 45,* 1121–1127.

Khandor, E., & Mason, K. (2007). *The Street Health Report 2007.* Retrieved August 4, 2008, from http://www.streethealth.ca/Downloads/SHReport2007.pdf

Kosteniuk, J., & Dickinson, H. (2003). Tracing the social gradient in the health of Canadians: Primary and secondary determinants. *Social Science & Medicine, 57,* 263–276.

Labonte, R. (1993). *Issues in health promotion series. 3. Health promotion and empowerment: Practice frameworks.* Toronto, ON: Centre for Health Promotion, University of Toronto, & ParticipACTION.

Laffrey, S., & Craig, D. (2000). Health promotion for communities and aggregates: An integrated model. In M. J. Stewart (Ed.), *Community nursing: Promoting Canadians' health* (2nd ed., pp. 105–125). Toronto, ON: W. B. Saunders.

Lalonde, M. (1974). *A new perspective on the health of Canadians.* Ottawa, ON: Government of Canada.

Lasser, K., Boyd, W., Woolhandler, S., Himmelstein, D. U., McCormick, D., & Bor, D. H. (2000). Smoking and mental illness: A population-based prevalence study. *JAMA 284,* 2606–2610.

Leavell, H., & Clark, A. (1965). *Preventive medicine for doctors in the community* (3rd ed.). New York: McGraw-Hill.

Ledrou, I., & Gervais, J. (2005). Food insecurity. *Health Reports, 16*(3), 47–51.

Lethbridge, L., & Phipps, S. (2005). Chronic poverty and childhood asthma in the Maritimes versus the rest of Canada. *Canadian Journal of Public Health, 96,* 18–23.

Makamowski Illing, E., & Kaiserman, M. (2004). Mortality attributable to tobacco use in Canada and its regions, 1998. *Canadian Journal of Public Health, 95*(1), 38–44.

Menendez, M., Benach, J., Muntaner, C., Amable, M., & O'Campo, P. (2007). Is precarious employment more damaging to women's health than men's? *Social Science & Medicine, 64,* 776–781.

Mitchell, I., & Laforet-Fliesser, Y. (2003). Promoting healthy school communities. *Canadian Nurse, 99*(8), 21–24.

Naidoo, J., & Wills, J. (1994). *Health promotion: Foundations for practice.* London: Bailliere Tindall.

National Council of Welfare. (2007). *Poverty profile 2004—Web-only data.* Retrieved August 27, 2008, from http://www.ncwcnbes.net/en/research/povertyprofile/webonly2004.HTML

Neuman, B. (1995). *The Neuman systems model: Applications to nursing education and practice* (2nd ed.). Norwalk, CT: Appleton & Lange.

Nutbeam, D. (1998). Health promotion glossary. *Health Promotion International, 13*(4), 349–364.

Orem, D. (1995). *Nursing: Concepts of practice* (5th ed.). New York: McGraw-Hill.

Pederson, A., & Raphael, D. (2006). Gender, race, and health inequalities. In D. Raphael, T. Bryant, & M. Rioux (Eds.), *Staying alive: Critical perspectives on health, illness, and health care.* (pp. 159-191). Toronto, ON: Canadian Scholars' Press.

Pender, N., Murdaugh, C., & Parsons, M. (2006). *Health promotion in nursing practice* (5th ed.). Upper Saddle River, NJ: Pearson–Prentice Hall.

Phipps, S. (2003). *The impact of poverty on health: A scan of research literature.* Ottawa, ON: Canadian Institute for Health Information and Canadian Population Health Initiative. Retrieved August 4, 2008, from http://dsp-psd.communication.gc.ca/Collection/H118-11-2003-1E.pdf

Physicians for a Smoke-Free Canada (2005). *Smoking in Canada: A statistical snapshot of Canadian smokers.* Retrieved August 4, 2008, from http://www.smoke-free.ca/pdf_1/SmokinginCanada-2005.pdf

Preyde, M. (2007). Mothers of very preterm infants: Perspectives on their situation and a culturally sensitive intervention. *Social Work in Health Care, 44*(4), 65–83.

Public Health Agency of Canada (2004). *What makes Canadians healthy or unhealthy?* Retrieved August 27, 2008, from http://www.phac-aspc.gc.ca/ph-sp/determinants/determinants-eng.php#income

Raeburn, J., & Rootman, I. (2007). A new appraisal of the concept of health. In M. O'Neill, A. Pederson, S. Dupere, & I. Rootman (Eds.), *Health promotion in Canada: Critical perspectives* (2nd ed., pp. 19–31). Toronto, ON: Canadian Scholars' Press.

Rains, J., & Barton-Kriese, P. (2001). Developing political competence: A comparative study across disciplines. *Public Health Nursing, 18,* 219–224.

Raphael, D. (2004). Introduction to the social determinants of health. In D. Raphael (Ed.), *Social determinants of health: Canadian perspectives* (pp. 1–18). Toronto, ON: Canadian Scholars' Press.

Raphael, D., Anstice, S., & Raine, K. (2003). The social determinants of the incidence and management of type II diabetes mellitus: Are we prepared to rethink our questions and redirect our research activities? *Leadership in Health Services, 16,* 10–20.

Raphael, D., Bryant, T., & Curry-Stevens, A. (2004). Toronto charter outlines future health policy directions for Canada and elsewhere [Electronic version]. *Health Promotion International, 19,* 269–273.

Raphael, D., & Farrell, E. (2002). Beyond medicine and lifestyle: Addressing the societal determinants of cardiovascular disease in North America. *Leadership in Health Services, 15,* 1–5.

Registered Nurses Association of British Columbia. (1994). *Creating the new health care: A nursing perspective.* Vancouver, BC: Author.

Reutter, L., Dennis, D., & Wilson, D. (2001). Young parents' understanding and actions related to the determinants of health. *Canadian Journal of Public Health, 92,* 335–339.

Reutter, L., & Duncan, S. (2002). Preparing nurses to promote health-enhancing public policies. *Policy, Politics, and Nursing Practice, 3,* 294–305.

Reutter, L., & Ogilvie (in press). Primary health care: Challenges and opportunities for the nursing profession. In J. Ross-Kerr & M. Wood (Eds.), *Canadian nursing: Issues and perspectives* (5th ed.). Toronto, ON: Elsevier.

Reutter, L., & Williamson, D. (2000). Advocating healthy public policy: Implications for baccalaureate nursing education. *The Journal of Nursing Education, 39*(1), 21–26.

Robertson, A. (1998). Shifting discourses on health in Canada: From health promotion to population health. *Health Promotion International, 13,* 155–166.

Rootman, I., & Ronson, B.(2005). Literacy and health research in Canada. *Canadian Journal of Public Health, 96*(Suppl. 2), S62–S77.

Saskatchewan Health, Population Health Branch. (2002) *A Population health promotion framework for Saskatchewan Regional Health Authorities.* Retrieved August 4, 2008, from http://www.health.gov.sk.ca/ic_pub_3793_skhlth framewk.pdf

Saskatchewan Public Health Association. (1994). *The determinants of health: Position paper.* Regina, SK: Author.

Shields, M. (2006). Overweight and obesity among children and youth. *Health Reports, 17*(3), 27–42.

Shields, M. (2007). Smoking-prevalence, bans and exposure to second-hand smoke. *Health Reports, 18*(3), 67–85.

Shields, M., & Martel, L. (2006). Healthy living among seniors. *Supplement to Health Reports, 16,* 7–20.

Simich, L., Beiser, M., & Mawani, F. (2003). Social support and the significance of shared experience in refugee migration and resettlement. *Western Journal of Nursing Research, 25,* 872–891.

Simich, L., Beiser, M., Stewart, M., & Makwarimba, E. (2005). Providing social support for immigrants and refugees in Canada: Challenges and directions. *Journal of Immigrant Health, 7,* 259–267.

Spitzer, D. (2005). Engendering health disparities. *Canadian Journal of Public Health, 96*(Suppl. 2), S78–S95.

Steinhauer, P. (1998). Developing resiliency in children from disadvantaged populations. In *Determinants of health: Children and youth: Vol. 1. Canada health action: Building on the legacy.* Papers commissioned by the National Forum on Health. Sainte-Foy, QC: MultiMondes.

Stewart, M. (2000). Social support, coping, and self-care as public participation mechanisms. In M. J. Stewart (Ed.), *Community nursing: Promoting Canadians' health* (2nd ed., pp. 83–104). Toronto, ON: W.B. Saunders.

Stewart, M., Kushner, K., Spitzer, D., Letourneau, N., Greaves, L., & Boscoe, M. (2004). *Support intervention for low income women smokers: Phase I public report.* Retrieved August 4, 2008, from http://www.ssrp.ualberta.ca/projects_women_smokers.HTML

Stewart, M., Reutter, L., Makwarimba, E., Veenstra, G., Love, R., & Raphael, D. (2008). Left out: Perspectives on social exclusion and inclusion across income groups. *Health Sociology Review, 17*(1), 78–94.

Stroick, S., & Jenson, J. (1999). *What is the best policy mix for Canada's young children?* (CPRN Study No. F/09). Ottawa, ON: Canadian Policy Research Networks.

Tarasuk, V. (2004). Health implications of food insecurity. In D. Raphael (Ed.), *Social determinants of health: Canadian perspectives* (pp. 187–200). Toronto, ON: Canadian Scholars' Press.

Tjepkema, M. (2006). Adult obesity. *Health Reports, 17*(3), 9–25.

Tomaka, J., Thompson, S., & Palacios, R. (2006). The relation of social isolation, loneliness, and social support to disease outcomes among the elderly. *Journal of Aging and Health, 18,* 359–383.

Tompa, E., Scott-Marshall, H., Dolinschi, R., Trevithick, S., & Bhattacharyya, S. (2007). Precarious employment experiences and their health consequences: Towards a theoretical framework. *Work: A Journal of Prevention, Assessment, and Rehabilitation, 28,* 209–224.

US Department of Health and Human Services. (2006). *The health consequences of involuntary exposure to tobacco smoke: A report of the surgeon general—Executive summary.* A. Rockville, MD: Public Health Service, Office of the Surgeon General, Centers for Disease Control and Prevention.

US Department of Health and Human Services. (2004). *2004 Surgeon General's report—The health consequences of smoking.* Atlanta, GA: US Department of Health and Human Services, Centers for Disease Control and Prevention, National Center for Chronic Disease Prevention and Health Promotion,

Office on Smoking and Health. Retrieved August 27, 2008, from http://www.cdc.gov/tobacco/data_statistics/sgr/sgr_2004/index.htm

Villeneuve, M., & MacDonald, J. (2006). *Toward 2020: Visions for nursing.* Ottawa, ON: Canadian Nurses Association.

Wallerstein, N. (1992). Powerlessness, empowerment, and health: Implications for health promotion programs. *American Journal of Health Promotion, 6*(3), 197–205.

Wilkins, K. (2007). Work stress among health care providers. *Health Reports, 18*(4), 33–36.

Wilkins, K., & Mackenzie, S. (2007). Work injuries. *Health Reports, 18*(3), 1–17.

Wilkins, R., Berthelot, J., & Ng, E. (2002). Trends in mortality by neighbourhood income in urban Canada from 1971 to 1996. *Health Reports, 13*(Suppl.), 1–28.

Wilkinson, R. (1996). *Unhealthy societies: The afflictions of inequality.* London: Routledge.

Wilkinson, R., & Marmot, M. (1998). *Social determinants of health: The solid facts.* Copenhagen, Denmark: World Health Organization. Retrieved August 4, 2008, from http://www.euro.who.int/document/e81384.pdf

World Health Organization. (1947). *World Health Organization Act 1947. Constitution of the World Health Organization. Section 3.* Retrieved August 27, 2008, from http://www.austlii.edu.au/au/legis/cth/consol_act/whoa1947273/sch1.html

World Health Organization. (1984). *A discussion document on the concept and principles of health promotion.* Copenhagen, Denmark: European Office of the World Health Organization.

World Health Organization. (1986). *Ottawa charter for health promotion.* Ottawa, ON: Canadian Public Health Association.

World Health Organization. (1997). *The Jakarta declaration on health promotion into the 21st century.* Retrieved August 4, 2008, from http://www.who.int/healthpromotion/conferences/previous/jakarta/declaration/en/print.HTML

World Health Organization (2005). *The Bangkok charter for health promotion in a globalized world.* Retrieved August 4, 2008, from http://www.who.int/healthpromotion/conferences/6gchp/hpr_050829_%20BCHP.pdf

World Health Organization (2006). *Commission on the social determinants of health.* Geneva: Author. Retrieved August 4, 2008, from http://www.who.int/social_determinants/resources/csdh_brochure.pdf

Chapter 2

Alvarez, R. C. (2005, November 14). It's time to modernize our health information systems. *The Globe and Mail,* Primary Health Care Section (special edition).

Annapolis Valley Health. (2007). *Strengthening primary health care: Renovation report 2004–2007.* Retrieved September 10, 2008, from http://www.avdha.nshealth.ca/newsroom/Downloads/AVH_Strengthening_PHC.pdf

Armstrong, P. (1999). *The impact of health reform on women: A cautionary tale.* Retrieved August 6, 2008, from http://www.fedcan.ca/francais/fromold/breakfast-armstrong0299.cfm

Baker, G. R., & Norton, P. (2004). *Patient safety and healthcare error in the Canadian health care system—a systematic review and analysis of leading practices in Canada with reference to key initiatives elsewhere.* Retrieved August 5, 2008, from http://www.hc-cs.gc.ca/hcs-sss/pubs/qual/2001-patient-securi-rev-exam/index-eng.php

Baker, G. R., Norton, P. G., Flintoft, V., Blais, R., Brown, A., Cox, J., et al. (2004). The Canadian Adverse Events Study: The incidence of adverse events among hospital patients in Canada. *Canadian Medical Association Journal, 170,* 1678–1686.

Bassendowski, S., Petrucka, P., Debs-Ivall, S., Hall, A., & Shand, S. (2008, May). Longitudinal study on the use of technology in the academic and clinical practice of nursing students as they transition from the undergraduate program into practice roles. *Canadian Nurse, 104*(5), 33.

Building the future: An integrated strategy for nursing human resources in Canada—Research synthesis report (2005). Retrieved September 10, 2008, from http://www.buildingthefuture.ca http://www.hhrchair.ca/images/CMSImages/Building%20the%20future%20Research-Synthesis-Report.pdf

Caiger, B. (2006). *Walking alongside: The essence of parish nursing.* Victoria, BC: Trafford.

Canadian Association for Parish Nursing Ministry. (2007). *Parish nurse fact sheet.* Retrieved August 6, 2008, from http://www.capnm.ca/fact_sheet.htm

Canadian Health Services Research Foundation. (2005). *Interdisciplinary teams in primary healthcare can effectively manage chronic illness.* Retrieved August 6, 2008, from http://www.chsrf.ca/mythbusters/HTML/boost3_e.php

Canadian Institute for Health Information. (2004a). *Health personnel trends in Canada, 1993–2002.* Ottawa, ON: Author.

Canadian Institute for Health Information. (2004b). *Health spending in Canada, 1993–2003.* Ottawa, ON: Author.

Canadian Institute for Health Information. (2006). National health expenditure trends: 1975–2006. Retrieved September 10, 2008, from http://secure.cihi.ca/cihiweb/dispPage.jsp?cw_page=PG_592_E&cw_topic=592&cw_rel=AR_31_E

Canadian Institute for Health Information. (2007a). *Workforce trends of licensed practical nurses in Canada, 2006.* Ottawa, ON: Author.

Canadian Institute for Health Information. (2007b). *Workforce trends of registered nurses in Canada, 2006.* Ottawa, ON: Author.

Canadian Institute for Health Information. (2007c). *Workforce trends of registered psychiatric nurses in Canada, 2006s.* Ottawa, ON: Author.

Canadian Nurses Association. (2002). *Planning for the future: Nursing human resource projections.* Ottawa, ON: Author.

Canadian Nurses Association. (2003). Primary health care—The time has come. *Nursing Now, 16,* 1–4.

Canadian Nurses Association. (2005). *Primary health care: A summary of the issues.* Retrieved September 10, 2008, from http://www.cna-nurses.ca/CNA/documents/pdf/publications/BG7_Primary_Health_Care_e.pdf

Canadian Nursing Informatics Association. (2008). *Introduction: Nursing informatics.* Retrieved August 6, 2008, from http://cnia.ca/intro.htm

Canadian Occupational Health Nurses Association. (2008). *Our scope.* Retrieved August 6, 2008, from http://www.cohna-aciist.ca/pages/content.asp?CatID=2&CatSubID=8

Canadian Patient Safety Institute. (2005). *Patient safety matters.* Retrieved August 6, 2008 from http://www.patientsafetyinstitute.ca/

Chui, T., Tran, K., & Maheux, H. (2007). *Immigration in Canada: A portrait of the foreign-born population, 2006 census: Findings.* Retrieved August 8, 2008, from http://www12.statcan.ca/english/census06/analysis/immcit/index.cfm

Clemen-Stone, S., McGuire, S. L., & Eigsti, D. G. (2002). *Comprehensive community health nursing: Family, aggregate, and community practice* (6th ed.). St. Louis, MO: Mosby.

Conference Board of Canada. (2007). *How Canada Performs: A Report Card on Canada.* Ottawa, ON: Author.

Corbella, L. (2008). *Oh baby, Canada's aging population needs more babies.* Retrieved August 7, 2008, from http://www.canada.com/calgaryherald/news/theeditorialpage/story.HTML?id=3ade5ffd-666e-4ccd-b2eb-1f6e1ba511aa&p=2

Department of Justice Canada. (2003). *Indian Act.* Retrieved August 7, 2008, from http://laws.justice.gc.ca/en/I-5/73349.HTML

Falk-Rafael, A. (2005). Speaking truth to power: Nursing's legacy and moral imperative. *Advances in Nursing Science, 28,* 212–223.

Hart, C. (2004). *Nurses and politics: The impact of power and practice.* New York: Palgrave MacMillan.

Harvey, P. W. (2005). Approaches to population health care: The emerging context! *Australian Journal of Primary Health, 11*(2), 45–53.

Health Canada. (1992). *Canada Health Act.* Retrieved March 31, 2008, from http://www.hc-sc.gc.ca/hcs-sss/medi-assur/index-eng.php

Health Canada. (2003). *First Nations, Inuit and Aboriginal health: Ten years of health transfer First Nation and Inuit control.* Retrieved September 10, 2008, from http://www.hc-sc.gc.ca/fniah-spnia/pubs/finance/_agree-accord/10_years_ans_trans/2_intro-eng.php

Health Canada. (2006a). *Canada's health care system.* Retrieved August 7, 2008, from http://www.hc-sc.gc.ca/hcs-sss/medi-assur/index-eng.php

Health Canada. (2006b). *About primary health care.* Retrieved August 7, 2008, from http://www.hc-sc.gc.ca/hcs-sss/prim/about-apropos_e.HTML

Health Canada. (2006c). *Building a stronger foundation: A framework for planning and evaluating community-based services in Canada.* Retrieved August 7, 2008, from http://www.hc-sc.gc.ca/hcs-sss/pubs/hhrhs/1995-build-plan-commun/index_e.HTML

Health Canada. (2006d). *Family/informal caregivers.* Retrieved March 31, 2008, from http://www.hc-sc.gc.ca/hcs-sss/home-domicile/caregiv-interven/index-eng.php

Health Canada. (2007a). *Canada Health Act annual report.* Ottawa, ON: Author.

Health Canada. (2007b). *Interprofessional education for collaborative patient-centred practice strategy.* Retrieved August 7, 2008, from http://www.hc-sc.gc.ca/hcs-sss/hhr-rhs/strateg/interprof/index_e.HTML

Health Canada. (2007c). *Canada Health Act: Introduction.* Accessed March 31, 2008, from http://www.hc-sc.gc.ca/hcs-sss/pubs/cha-lcs/2006-cha-lcs-ar-ra/intro-eng.php

Health Consumer Powerhouse AB & Frontier Centre for Public Policy. (2008). *Canada at the bottom in 30 country health-care survey.* Retrieved March 30, 2008, from http://www.fcpp.org/main/publication_detail.php?PubID=2020

Health Council of Canada. (2008). *Fixing the foundation: An update on primary health care and home care renewal in Canada*. Ottawa, ON: Author.

Hollander, M. J., & Chappell, N. L. (2001). *Final report of the study on the comparative cost analysis of home care and residential care services*. Victoria, BC: National Evaluation of the Cost-Effectiveness of Home Care.

Indian and Northern Affairs Canada. (2004). *Interpreting Treaty Six*. Retrieved September 10, 2008, from http://www.ainc-inac.gc.ca/pr/trts/hti/t6/int_e.HTML

Indian and Northern Affairs Canada. (2008). *Aboriginal self-government. The Government of Canada's approach to implementation of the inherent right and the negotiation of Aboriginal self-government*. Retrieved August 7, 2008, from http://www.ainc-inac.gc.ca/pr/pub/sg/plcy_e.HTML

International Society for Quality in Health Care. (2007). *ISQua: Improving healthcare worldwide*. Retrieved September 10, 2008, from http://www.isqua.org/isquaPages/General.HTML

Kirby, M. J. L. (2002). *The health of Canadians—The federal role. Vol. 6: Recommendations for reform*. Ottawa, ON: Standing Senate Committee on Social Affairs, Science and Technology. Retrieved August 8, 2008, from http://www.parl.gc.ca/37/2/parlbus/commbus/senate/ com-e/soci-e/rep-e/repoct02vol6-e.htm

Lalonde, M. (1974). *A new perspective on the health of Canadians*. Ottawa, ON: Government of Canada.

Lalonde, M. (1986). *Ottawa charter for health promotion: An international conference on health promotion*. Ottawa, ON: Author.

Law, S., Flood, C., & Gagnon, D. (2007). *Listening for Direction III* (unpublished work). Ottawa, ON: Listening for Direction III.

Lewis, S., & Kouri, D. (2004). Regionalization: Making sense of the Canadian experience. *Healthcare Papers, 5*(1), 12–31.

MacKinnon, J. (2004). The arithmetic of health care. *Canadian Medical Association Journal, 171*, 603–604.

Mang, R. A. (2005, November 14). Critical care: Canada's movement towards primary health care. *The Globe and Mail*, Primary Health Care Section (special edition).

Mansell, D. (2004). *Forging the future: A history of nursing in Canada*. Ann Arbor, MI: Thomas Press.

Marchildon, G.P. (2006). *Health systems in transition*. Toronto, ON: University of Toronto Press.

Meiner, S.E., & Lueckenotte, A. (2006). *Gerentologic Nursing* (3rd ed.). St. Louis, MO: Mosby.

Melnyk, B. M., & Fineout-Overholt, E. (2005). *Evidence-based practice in nursing and healthcare: A guide to best practice*. Philadelphia: Lippincott Williams & Wilkins.

National Coalition on Health Care. (2008). *Facts about healthcare—Health insurance costs*. Retrieved August 7, 2008, from http://www.nchc.org/facts/cost.sHTML

National Primary Health Care Awareness Strategy. (2006a). *Primary health care*. Retrieved September 10, 2008, from http://www.hc-sc.gc.ca/hcs-sss/prim/about-apropos-eng.php

National Primary Health Care Awareness Strategy. (2006b). *Canadians more aware of primary health care*. Retrieved May 15, 2008, from http://www.hc-sc.gc.ca/hcs-sss/pubs/prim/2007-initiatives/2007-initiatives-2-eng.php

Natural Resources Canada. (2003). *Historical Indian treaties* [map]. Retrieved September 10, 2008, from http://atlas.gc.ca/site/english/maps/historical/indiantreaties/historicaltreaties

Ontario Health Services Restructuring Commission. (2000). *Looking back, looking forward: A legacy report from the Ontario Health Services Restructuring Commission, 1996–2000*. Toronto, ON: Author.

Petrucka, P. (2005). Impacts and implications of health reform/renewal on select Saskatchewan and Manitoba rural women. *Dissertation Abstracts International*, AAT NR08715.

Public Health Agency of Canada (2006). *Canadian pandemic influenza plan for the health sector*. Retrieved August 8, 2008, from http://www.phac-aspc.gc.ca/cpip-pclcpi/

Rachlis, M. (2005). *Prescription for excellence*. Toronto, ON: Harper Collins.

Romanow, R. J. (2002). *Building on values: The future of health care in Canada—Final report*. Ottawa, ON: Commission on the Future of Health Care in Canada.

Royal Commission on Health Services. (1964). *Hall commission report* (Vol 1). Ottawa, ON: Author

Royal Commission on Health Services. (1965). *Hall commission report* (Vol 2). Ottawa, ON: Author

Schoen, C., Osborn, R., Huynh, P.T., Doty, M., Zapert, K., Peugh, J., et al. (2005). Taking the pulse of health care systems: Experiences of patients with health problems in six countries. *Health Affairs*. Retrieved September 10, 2008, from http://content.healthaffairs.org/cgi/content/abstract/hlthaff.w5.509

Smadu, M. (2005, November 14). Team model puts client at centre. *The Globe and Mail*, Primary Health Care Section (special edition).

Smadu, M. (2006). *A healthy nation is a wealthy nation*. Ottawa, ON: Canadian Nurses Association. Retrieved August 8, 2008, from http://www.cna-aiic.ca/CNA/documents/pdf/publications/Standing_Committee_Submission-2006_e.pdf

Statistics Canada. (2007). *Canada's population by age and sex, July 1, 2007 (preliminary)*. Retrieved September 3, 2008, from http://www.statcan.ca/Daily/English/071129/d071129c.htm

Statistics Canada. (2008). *Survey of household spending—2006*. Retrieved August 8, 2008, from http://www.statcan.ca/Daily/English/080226/d080226a.htm

Storch, J. (2006). Canadian health care system. In M. McIntyre, E. Thomlinson, & C. McDonald (Eds.), *Realities of Canadian nursing: Professional, practice, and power issues* (pp. 29–53). Philadelphia: Lippincott Williams & Wilkins.

Sutherland, R. W., & Fulton, M. J. (1992). *Health care in Canada*. Ottawa, ON: The Health Group.

Vårdguiden. (2007). European Union–regulated health care Web site. Retrieved August 8, 2008, from http://www.vardguiden.se

Villeneuve, M., & MacDonald, J. (2006). *Towards 2020: Visions for nursing*. Ottawa, ON: Canadian Nurses Association.

Wayland, S. V. (2006). *Unsettled: Legal and policy barriers for newcomers to Canada*. Retrieved August 8, 2008, from http://www.canada.metropolis.net/publications/pf_9_ENG_Immigration.pdf

Wilson, D. M. (1995). *The Canadian health care system*. Edmonton, AB: Health Canada.

World Health Organization. (1978). *Declaration of Alma-Ata: International conference on primary health care, Alma-Ata, USSR, 6–12 September 1978*. Geneva: Author.

Yalnizyan, A., & Macdonald, D. (2005). *CHC cost effectiveness literature*. Toronto, ON: Author.

Chapter 3

Allemang, M. M. (1974). *Nursing education in the United States and Canada, 1873–1950: Leading figures, forces, views on education*. Unpublished doctoral dissertation, University of Washington, Seattle.

Bonin, M. A. (1976). *Trends in integrated basic degree nursing programs in Canada: 1942–1972*. Unpublished doctoral dissertation, University of Ottawa, Ottawa, ON.

Brown, C. (2002). *The illustrated history of Canada*. Toronto, ON: Key Porter. Retrieved August 10, 2008, from http://canadian-settlement.suite101.com/article.cfm/hbert_the_first_french_family

Canadian Institute for Health Information. (2006). *Measuring the retention of registered nurses in Canada: A study of 2000–2004 registration data*. Ottawa, ON: Author. Retrieved August 10, 2008, from http://www.cihi.ca/cihiweb/products/Measuring_RN_Retention_e.pdf

Canadian Medical Association, Canadian Nurses Association, Canadian Pharmacists Association, & Canadian Healthcare Association. (2004). Common vision for the Canadian health system. Retrieved September 10, 2008, from http://www.cna-nurses.ca/CNA/documents/pdf/publications/G4vision-e.pdf

Canadian Nurses Association. (1965). *Report on the Canadian Nurses Association School Improvement Program*. Ottawa, ON: Author.

Canadian Nurses Association. (1968). *The leaf and the lamp*. Ottawa, ON: Author.

Canadian Nurses Association. (1991). NB for BN: Province joins nurses' call for degree. *Edufacts, 1*(2), 1.

Canadian Nurses Association. (2004). *Helping to sustain Canada's health system: Nurse practitioners in primary health care*. Ottawa, ON: Author.

Canadian Nurses Association. (2006). 2005 Workforce Profile of Registered Nurses in Canada. Retrieved August 10, 2008, from http://www.cna-nurses.ca/CNA/documents/pdf/publications/workforce-profile-2005-e.pdf

Canadian Nurses Association. (2008a). Certification program continues to grow. *Canadian Nurse, 104*(4), 22.

Canadian Nurses Association. (2008b). *Code of ethics for registered nurses*. Ottawa, ON: Author.

Canadian Nurses Association. (2008c). *Position statement: Clinical nurse specialist*. Retrieved August 10, 2008, from http://www.cna-aiic.ca/CNA/documents/pdf/publications/PS65_Clinical_Nurse_Specialist_March_2003_e.pdf

Canadian Nurses Association. (2008d). *Position statement: Promoting nursing history*. Retrieved August 10, 2008, from http://www.cahn-achn.ca/pdf/PS72_Promoting_nursing_history_March_2004_e.pdf

Canadian Nurses Association. (2008e). *Vision and mission*. Ottawa, ON: Author. Retrieved August 10, 2008, from http://www.cna-nurses.ca/CNA/about/mission/default_e.aspx

Canadian Nurses Association & Canadian Association of Schools of Nursing. (2004). *Joint position statement: Educational preparation for entry to the practice of nursing.* Ottawa, ON: Author.

Canadian Red Cross Society. (1962). The role of one voluntary organization in Canada's health services: A brief presented to the Royal Commission on Health Services. Toronto, ON: Author.

Chapman, M. E. (1969). *Nursing education and the movement for higher education for women: A study of interrelationship, 1870–1900.* Unpublished doctoral dissertation, Columbia University, New York.

College of Nurses of Ontario. (2002). *Professional standards, revised 2002.* Toronto, ON: Author. Retrieved August 10, 2008, from http://www.cno.org/docs/prac/41006_ProfStds.pdf

Gates, M.G. (2007). *Demographic diversity, value congruence, and workplace outcomes in acute care.* Unpublished doctoral dissertation, University of North Carolina, Chapel Hill.

Gibbon, J. M., & Mathewson, M. S. (1947). *Three centuries of Canadian nursing.* Toronto, ON: Macmillan.

Gunn, J. I. (1933, March). Educational adjustments recommended by the survey. *Canadian Nurse, 29,* 139–145.

Healey, P. (1990). *The Mack training school for nurses.* Unpublished doctoral dissertation, University of Texas, Austin.

Henderson, V. (1966). *The nature of nursing.* New York: Macmillan.

McDonald, L. (2008). *The collected works of Florence Nightingale.* Guelph, ON: Wilfrid Laurier University Press. Retrieved August 10, 2008, from http://www.sociology.uoguelph.ca/fnightingale/review/index.htm

MacDonald, M., Screiber, R., & Davis, L. (2005). *Exploring new roles for advanced nursing practice: A discussion paper.* Ottawa, ON: Canadian Nurses Association.

Nightingale, F. (1979). *Cassandra.* New York: The Feminist Press of the City University of New York (Original work published 1872).

O'Lynn, C., & Tranbarger, R. (2006). *Men in nursing: History, challenges and opportunities.* New York: Springer.

Paul, P. (1998). Nursing education becomes synonymous with nursing service: The development of training schools. In J. C. Ross-Kerr (Ed.), *Prepared to care: Nurses and nursing in Alberta* (pp. 133–134). Edmonton, AB: The University of Alberta Press.

Paul, P., & Ross-Kerr, J. (in press). Nursing in Canada, 1600 to the present: A brief account. In J. C. Ross-Kerr & M. J. Wood (Eds.), *Canadian nursing: Issues and perspectives.* Toronto, ON: Elsevier Science.

Riegler, N. (1997). *Jean I. Gunn, nursing leader.* Markham, ON: Associated Medical Services with Fitzhenry and Whiteside.

Ross-Kerr, J. (in press). The Canadian health care system. In J. C. Ross-Kerr & M. J. Wood (Eds.), *Canadian nursing: Issues and perspectives.* Toronto, ON: Elsevier Science.

Royal Commission on Aboriginal Peoples. (1996). From time immemorial: A demographic profile. In *Report of the Royal Commission on Aboriginal Peoples: Vol. 1. Looking forward looking back* (Chap. 2). Ottawa, ON: Indian and Northern Affairs Canada. Retrieved August 10, 2008, from http://www.ainc-inac.gc.ca/ch/rcap/sg/sg3_e.HTML#10

Royal Commission on Health Services. (1964). *Report.* Ottawa, ON: Queen's Printer.

Schreiber, R., & MacDonald, M. (2008). A closer look at the "supervision" and "direction" of certified registered nurse anesthetists. *Canadian Nurse, 104*(3), 28–33.

Service Employees International Union Local 333 v Nipawin District Staff Nurses Association et al., (1973) Carswell, SK 120[1974] 1 W.W.R. 653, 41 D.L.R. (3d) 6, 73 C.L.L.C. 14,193, 1 S.C.R. 382 (1975).

Tunis, B. L. (1966). *In caps and gowns.* Montreal, QC: McGill University Press.

Villeneuve, M.J. (2002–2003). Healthcare, race and diversity: Time to act. *Hospital Quarterly, 6*(2), 67–73.

Weir, G. M. (1932). *Survey of nursing education in Canada.* Toronto, ON: University of Toronto Press.

Wood, M. J. (in press). Monitoring standards in nursing education. In J. C. Ross-Kerr & M. J. Wood (Eds.), *Canadian nursing: Issues and perspectives.* Toronto, ON: Elsevier Science.

Young, S. L. (1994) *Standards in diploma nursing education: The involvement of the University of Alberta, 1920–1970.* Unpublished master's thesis, University of Alberta, Edmonton.

Chapter 4

Ayers, M., Bruno, A. A., & Langford, R. W. (1999). *Community-based nursing care: Making the transition.* St. Louis, MO: Mosby.

Baas, L. S., Bell, B., Stuebbe, S. D., Giesting, R., & Wagoner, L. E. (2002). The challenge of managing the care of older heart transplant recipients. *AACN Clinical Issues, 13,* 114–131.

Barr, R. G., Somers, S., Speizer, F. E., & Camargo, C. A. (2002). Patient factors and medication guidline adherence among older women with asthma. *Archives of Internal Medicine, 162,* 1761–1768.

Beiser, M., & Stewart, M. (2005). Reducing health disparities. *Canadian Journal of Public Health, 96,* S4–S5.

Brighty, K. (1942). *Collection of facts for a history of nursing in Alberta: 1864–1942.* Edmonton, AB: Alberta Association of Registered Nurses,

Brighty Colley, K. (1970). *While rivers flow: Stories of early Alberta.* Saskatoon, SK: The Western Producer.

Canadian Nurses Association. (2006). *Community health nursing certification.* Ottawa, ON: Author.

Canadian Population Health Initiative. (2004). *Summary report: Improving the health of Canadians.* Ottawa, ON: Canadian Institute for Health Information.

Canadian Public Health Association. (1990, November). *Community health–public health nursing in Canada: Preparation and practice.* Ottawa, ON: Author.

Canadian Public Health Association. (1994). *Violence in society: A public health perspective.* Ottawa, ON: Author.

Canadian Public Health Association. (2008). *Mission statement.* Retrieved August 12, 2008, from http://www.cpha.ca/en/about.aspx

Ceci, C. (2006). Impoverishment of practice: Analysis of effects of economic discourses in home care case management practice. *Nursing Leadership, 19,* 56–68.

Chalmers, K. I., & Bramadat, I. J. (1996). Community development: Theoretical and practical issues for community health nursing in Canada. *Journal of Advanced Nursing, 24,* 719–726.

Chalmers, K. I., Bramadat, I. J., & Andrusyszyn, M. A. (1998). The changing environment of community health practice and education: Perceptions of staff nurses, administrators, and educators. *Journal of Nursing Education, 37,* 109–117.

Community Health Nurses Association of Canada. (2008, March). *Canadian community health nursing standards of practice.* Retrieved November 3, 2008, from http://www.chnac.ca/images/downloads/standards/chn_standards_of_practice_mar08_english.pdf

Community Health Nurses Association of Canada. (2003, May). *Canadian community health nursing standards of practice.* Retrieved August 12, 2008, from http://www.chnac.ca/images/downloads/standards/chn_standards_of_practice_mar08_english.pdf

Cooke, H. (2002). Empowerment. In G. Blakeley & V. Bryson (Eds.), *Contemporary political concepts* (pp. 162–178). London: Pluto Press.

Cradduck, G. R. (2000). Primary health care practice. In M. J. Stewart (Ed.), *Community nursing: Promoting Canadians' health* (2nd ed., pp. 352–369). Toronto, ON: W. B. Saunders.

Craig, D. M. (2000). Health promotion with older adults. In M. J. Stewart (Ed.), *Community nursing: Promoting Canadians' health* (2nd ed., pp. 283–295). Toronto, ON: W. B. Saunders.

Crowe, C. (2007). *Dying for a home: Homeless activists speak out.* Toronto, ON: Between the Lines.

DiCenso, A., & Van Dover, L. (2000). Prevention of adolescent pregnancy. In M. J. Stewart (Ed.), *Community nursing: Promoting Canadians' health* (2nd ed., pp. 262–282). Toronto, ON: W. B. Saunders.

Diekemper, M., SmithBattle, L., & Drake, M. A. (1999). Bringing the population into focus: A natural development in community health nursing practice. Part I. *Public Health Nursing, 16,* 3–10.

Duncan, S., & Reutter, L. (2006). A critical policy analysis of an emerging agenda for home care in one Canadian province. *Health and Social Care in the Community, 14,* 242–253.

Edwards, N. C., & Moyer, A. (2000). Community needs and capacity assessment: Critical component of program planning. In M. J. Stewart (Ed.), *Community nursing: Promoting Canadians' health* (2nd ed., pp. 420–442). Toronto, ON: W. B. Saunders.

Falk-Rafael, A. (2001). Empowerment as a process of evolving consciousness: A model of empowering care [Electronic version]. *Advances in Nursing Science, 24*(1), 1–16.

Farrell, S., Huff, J., MacDonald, S., Middlebro, A., & Walsh, S. (2005). Taking it to the street: A psychiatric outreach service in Canada. *Community Mental Health Journal, 41,* 737–746.

Fulford, A., & Ford-Gilboe, M. (2004). An exploration of the relationships between health promotion practices, health work, and felt stigma in families headed by adolescent mothers. *Canadian Journal of Nursing Research, 36*(4), 47–72.

Geduld, J., & Gatali, M. (2003). Estimates of HIV prevalence and incidence in Canada, 2002 [Electronic version]. *Canada Communicable Disease Report, 29*, 197–207.

Gillis, A. J. (2000). Adolescent health promotion: An evolving opportunity for community health nurses. In M. J. Stewart (Ed.), *Community nursing: Promoting Canadians' health* (2nd ed., pp. 241–261). Toronto, ON: W. B. Saunders.

Gray, B. (1989). *Collaborating: Finding common ground for multiparty problems*. San Francisco: Jossey-Bass.

Griffiths, H. (2002). Dr. Peter Centre: Removing barriers to health care services. *Nursing BC, 34*(5), 10–14.

Hamilton, N., & Bhatti, T. (1996). *Population health promotion: An integrated model of population health and health promotion*. Ottawa, ON: Health Promotion Development Division, Health Canada.

Health Canada. (1998). *Taking action on population health*. Ottawa, ON: Author.

Health Canada. (1999). *Toward a healthy future*. Ottawa, ON: Author.

Health Canada. (2002). *A report on mental illnesses in Canada*. Ottawa, ON: Author.

Hilton, B. A., Thompson, R., & Moore-Dempsey, L. (2000). Evaluation of the AIDS Prevention Street Nurse Program: One step at a time. *Canadian Journal of Nursing Research, 32*, 17–38.

Hilton, B. A., Thompson, R., Moore-Dempsey, L., & Hutchinson, K. (2000). AIDS prevention on the streets. *Canadian Nurse, 96*(8), 24–28.

Hilton, B. A., Thompson, R., Moore-Dempsey, L., & Hutchinson, K. (2001). Urban outpost nursing: The nature of nurses' work in the AIDS Prevention Street Nurse Program. *Public Health Nursing, 18*, 273–280.

Hilton, B. A., Thompson, R., Moore-Dempsey, L., & Janzen, R. (2001). Harm reduction theories and strategies for control of human immunodeficiency virus: A review of the literature. *Journal of Advanced Nursing, 33*, 357–370.

Hunt, R. (1998). Community-based nursing: Philosophy or setting? *American Journal of Nursing, 98*(10), 44–47.

Hunt, R., & Zurek, E. L. (1997). *Introduction to community based nursing*. Philadelphia: Lippincott.

Hwang, S. (2000). Mortality among men using homeless shelters in Toronto, Ontario. *Journal of the American Medical Association, 283*, 2152–2157.

Kotler, P., & Roberto, E. (1989). *Social marketing*. New York: Free Press.

Labonte, R. (1993). *Health promotion and empowerment: Practice frameworks*. Toronto, ON: Centre for Health Promotion, University of Toronto, & ParticipACTION.

Laverack, G. (2004). *Health promotion practice: Power and empowerment*. Thousand Oaks, CA: Sage.

Leipert, B. (1999). Women's health and the practice of public health nurses in Northern British Columbia. *Public Health Nursing, 16*, 280–289.

Leipert, B., & Reutter, L. I. (2005). Developing resilience: How women maintain their health in northern geographically isolated settings. *Qualitative Health Research, 15*, 49–65.

Maurer, F.A., & Smith, C. M. (2005). *Community/public health nursing practice: Health for families and populatoins* (3rd ed.). St. Louis, MO: Elsevier.

McKay, M. (2008). The origins of community health nursing in Canada. In L. L. Stamler & L. Yiu (Eds.), *Community health nursing: A Canadian perspective* (pp. 1–19). Toronto, ON: Pearson Prentice Hall.

Meagher-Stewart, D., Aston, M., Edwards, N., Smith, D., Young, L., Woodford, E., et al. (2005). *The study of public health nurses primary health care practice. Fostering citizen participation and collaborative practice: Tapping the wisdom and voices of public health nurses in Nova Scotia*. Retrieved August 12, 2008, from http://preventionresearch.dal.ca/pdf/PHN_study_Nov25.pdf

Ogden Burke, S, Kauffmann, E., Wiskin, N. M. W., & Harrison, M. B. (2000). Children with chronic conditions and their families in the community. In M. J. Stewart (Ed.), *Community nursing: Promoting Canadians' health* (2nd ed., pp. 211–240). Toronto, ON: W. B. Saunders.

Pauly, B., Goldstone, I., McCall, J., Gold, F., & Payne, S. (2007). The ethical, legal and social context of harm reduction. *Canadian Nurse, 103*(8), 19–23.

Public Health Agency of Canada. (2007). *Core competencies for public health in Canada Release 1.0*. Ottawa, ON: Author.

Racher, F. (2007). The evolution of ethics for community practice. *Journal of Community Health Nursing, 24*, 65–76.

Reutter, L. I., & Ford, J. S. (1996). Perceptions of public health nursing: Views from the field. *Journal of Advanced Nursing, 24*, 7–15.

Reutter, L. I., & Ford, J. S. (1998). Perceptions of changes in public health nursing practice: A Canadian perspective. *International Journal of Nursing Studies, 35*, 85–94.

Rew, L., Taylor-Seehafer, M., Thomas, N. Y., & Yockey, R. D. (2001). Correlates of resilience in homeless adolescents. *Journal of Nursing Scholorship, 33*(1), 33–40.

Ross-Kerr, J. C. (1996). The growth of community health nursing in Canada. In J. Ross-Kerr & J. MacPhail (Eds.), *An introduction to issues in community health nursing in Canada* (pp. 1–15). Toronto, ON: Mosby.

Sebastian, J. G. (2006). Vulnerability and vulnerable populations: An introduction. In M. Stanhope & J. Lancaster (Eds.), *Foundations of nursing in the community: Community-oriented practice* (2nd ed., pp. 403–417). St. Louis, MO: Mosby.

Shah, C. P. (2003). *Public health and preventive medicine in Canada* (3rd ed). Toronto, ON: Elsevier.

Shoveller, J., & Johnson, J. (2006). Risky groups, risky behaviour, and risky persons: Dominating discourses on youth sexual health. *Critical Public Health, 16*, 47–60.

SmithBattle, L., Diekemper, M., & Leander, S. (2004). Moving upstream: Becoming a public health nurse, part 2. *Public Health Nursing, 21*(2), 95–102.

Stamler, L. L., & Yiu, L. (Eds.) (2008). *Community health nursing: A Canadian perspective*. Toronto, ON: Pearson Prentice Hall.

Stanhope, M., Lancaster, J., Jessup-Falcioni, H., & Viverais-Dresler, G. (2008). *Community health nursing in Canada*. Toronto, ON: Elsevier.

Steenbeek, A. (2004). Empowering health promotion: A holistic approach in preventing sexually transmitted infections among First Nations and Inuit adolescents in Canada. *Journal of Holistic Nursing, 22*, 254–266.

Stewart, M. J., & Leipert, B. (2000). Community health nursing in the future. In M. J. Stewart (Ed.), *Community nursing: Promoting Canadians' health* (2nd ed., pp. 602–632). Toronto, ON: W. B. Saunders.

Thibaudeau, M. F., & Denoncourt, H. (2000). Nursing practice in outreach clinics for the homeless in Montreal. In M. J. Stewart (Ed.), *Community nursing: Promoting Canadians' health* (2nd ed., pp. 443–460). Toronto, ON: W. B. Saunders.

Toofany, S. (2007). Empowering older people. *Nursing Older People, 19*(2), 12–14.

Vollman, A. R., Anderson, E. T., & McFarlane, J. (2008). *Canadian community as partner*. Toronto, ON: Lippincott Williams & Wilkins.

Wood, R. A., Zettel, P., & Stewart, W. (2003). The Dr. Peter Centre: Harm reduction nursing. *Canadian Nurse, 99*(5), 20–24.

Zotti, M. E., Brown, P., & Stotts, R. C. (1996). Community-based nursing versus community health nursing: What does it all mean? *Nursing Outlook, 44*, 211–217.

Chapter 5

Anderson, B. L. (1993). Predicting sexual and psychologic morbidity and improving the quality of life for women and gynecologic cancer. *Cancer, 7* (Suppl. 4), 1678–1690.

Anderson-Hanley, C., Sherman, M. L., Riggis, R., Agocha, V. B., & Compas, B. E. (2003). Neuropsychological effects of treatments for adults with cancer: A meta-analysis and review of the literature. *Journal of the International Neuropsychological Society, 9*, 967–982.

Aziz, N. M., & Rowland, J. H. (2003). Trends and advances in cancer survivorship research: Challenge and opportunity. *Seminars in Radiation Oncology, 13*, 248.

Barton-Burke, M. (2006). Cancer-related fatigue and sleep disturbances. *American Journal of Nursing, 106*(Suppl. 3), 72.

Blum, D. (2006, July 13–15), *State of the science: Social well-being and survivorship*. Paper presented at Survivorship Education for Quality Cancer Care conference, Pasadena, CA.

Brown, K. W., Levy, A. R., Rosberger, Z., & Edgar, L. (2003). Psychological distress and cancer survival: A follow-up 10 years after diagnosis. *Psychosomatic Medicine, 65*, 636–643.

Brown-Saltzman, K. (2006, July 13–15). *Spiritual well-being and survivorship*. Paper presented at Survivorship Education for Quality Cancer Care conference. Pasadena, CA.

Canadian Cancer Society. (2005). *Living with cancer: A guide for people with cancer and their caregivers*. Toronto, ON: Author.

Canadian Cancer Society. (2007). *Canadian cancer statistics 2007*. Toronto, ON: Author.

Ferrell, B. R. (2006). *Introduction to cancer survivorship strategies for success: Survivorship education for quality cancer care*. Pasadena, CA: City of Hope National Medical Center.

Ganz, P. A., Coscarelli, A., Fred, C., Kahn, B., Polinsky, M. L., & Petersen, L. (1996). Breast cancer survivors: Psychosocial concerns and quality of life. *Breast Cancer Research and Treatment, 38*, 183–189.

Ganz, P. A. (2004, July 27). *Understanding the late effects of cancer treatment: Making the case for systematic follow-up*. Paper presented at the meeting of the Institute of Medicine Committee on Cancer Survivorship, Woods Hole, MA.

Holtzman, J., Schmitz, K., Babes, G., Kane, R. L., Duval, S., Wilt, T. J., et al. (2004). *Effectiveness of behavioral interventions to modify physical activity behaviors in general populations and cancer patients and survivors* [Summary, Evidence Report/Technology Assessment No. 102, prepared by the University of Minnesota Evidence-based Practice Center, under Contract No. 290-02-0009; AHRQ Publication No. 04-E027-1]. Rockville, MD: Agency for Healthcare Research and Quality.

Institute of Medicine & National Research Council. (2006). *From cancer patient to cancer survivor: Lost in transition* (M. Hewitt, S. Greenfield, & E. Stovall, Eds.). Washington, DC: National Academies Press.

Jacobsen, P. (2006, July 13–15). *State of science: Psychological well-being and survivorship.* Paper presented at Survivorship Education for Quality Cancer Care conference, Pasadena, CA.

Kwekkebboom, L. L., & Seng, J. S. (2002). Recognizing and responding to post-traumatic stress disorder in people with cancer. *Oncology Nursing Forum, 29,* 643–650.

Leigh, S. (2006). Cancer survivorship: A first-person perspective. *American Journal of Nursing, 106*(Suppl. 3), 12.

Lewis, F. M. (2006). The effects of cancer survivorship on families and caregivers. *American Journal of Nursing, 106*(Suppl. 3), 20–25.

Lorig, K. (2003). Self-management education: More than a nice extra. *Medical Care, 41,* 699–701.

Mellon, S., Northouse, L. L., & Weiss, L. K. (2006). A population-based study of the quality of life of cancer survivors and their family caregivers. *Cancer Nurse, 29,* 120–131

Nail, L. M. (2006). Cognitive changes in cancer survivors. *American Journal of Nursing, 106*(Suppl. 3), 48.

Pelusi, J. (2006). Sexuality and body image. *American Journal of Nursing, 106*(Suppl. 3), 32–38.

Polomano, R. C., & Farrar, J. T. (2006). Pain and neuropathy in cancer survivors. *American Journal of Nursing, 106*(Suppl. 3), 39–47.

President's Cancer Panel. (2004). *Living beyond cancer: finding a new balance.* Bethesda, MD: National Cancer Institute.

Satia, J. A., Campbell, M. K., Galanko, J. A., James, A., Carr, C., & Sandler, R. S. (2004). Longitudinal changes in lifestyle behaviors and health status in colon cancer survivors. *Cancer Epidemiology Biomarkers & Prevention, 13,* 1022–1031.

Shimozuma, K., Ganz, P., Petersen, L., & Hirji, K. (1999). Quality of life in the first year after breast cancer surgery: Rehabilitation needs and patterns of recovery. *Breast Cancer Research and Treatment, 56,* 45–57.

Spelten, E. R., Sprangers, M. A., & Verbeek, J. H. (2002). Factors reported to influence the return to work of cancer survivors: a literature review. *Psycho-Oncology, 11,* 124–141.

Stetz, K. M., & Brown, M. (2004). Physical and psychosocial health in family caregivers: A comparison of AIDS and cancer caregivers. *Public Health Nursing, 21,* 553–540.

Strang, V. R., & Koop, P. M. (2003). Factors which influence coping: Home-based family caregiving of persons with advanced cancer. *Journal of Palliative Care, 19,* 107–114

Vachon, M. (2006). Psychosocial distress and coping after cancer treatment. *Cancer Nursing, 29*(Suppl. 2), 26–31.

Wilkes, G. (2003). Depression. *Cancer Source RN.*

Yabroff, K. R., Lawrence, W. F., Clauser, S., Davis, W. W., & Brown, M. L. (2004). Burden of illness in cancer survivors: Findings from a population-based national sample. *Journal of the National Cancer Institute, 96,* 1322–1330.

Yehuda, R. (2003). Hypothalmic–pituitary–adrenal alterations in PTSD: Are they relevant to understanding cortisol alterations in cancer? *Brain Behavior and Immunity, 17*(Suppl 1), S73.

Zahlis, E. H., & Lewis, F. M. (1998). The mother's story of the school-age child's experience with the mother's breast cancer. *Journal of Psychosocial Oncology, 16,* 25–43.

Chapter 6

Adam, E. (1979). *Être infirmière.* Montréal, QC: Editions HRW Ltée.

Adam, E. (1991). *To be a nurse* (2nd ed.). Philadelphia, PA: W. B. Saunders.

Alfaro-LeFevre, R. (2004). *Critical thinking in nursing: A practical approach* (3rd ed.). Philadelphia: W. B. Saunders.

Barnum, B. J. S. (1998). *Nursing theory: Analysis, application, evaluation* (5th ed.). Philadelphia, PA: J. B. Lippincott.

Barnum, B. J. S. (1994). *Nursing theory: Analysis, application, evalutation* (4th ed.). Philadelphia, PA: J. B. Lippincott.

Beckstrand, J. (1978). The notion of a practice theory and the relationship of scientific and ethical knowledge to practice. *Research in Nursing & Health, 1,* 131–136.

Benner, P., & Tanner, C. (1987). Clinical judgment: How expert nurses use intuition. *American Journal of Nursing, 87,* 23–31.

Benner, P., Tanner, C. A., & Chesla, C. A. (1996). *Expertise in nursing practice: Caring, clinical judgment, and ethics.* New York: Springer.

Brenwick, J. M., & Webster, G. A. (2000). *Philosophy of nursing: A new vision for health care.* Albany, NY: State University of New York Press.

Campbell, J. C., & Bunting, S. (1991). Voices and paradigms: Perspectives on critical and feminist theory in nursing. *ANS. Advances in Nursing Science, 13*(3), 1–15.

Campbell, M. A. (1987). *The UBC model for nursing: Directions for practice.* Vancouver: The University of British Columbia School of Nursing.

Campbell, M. A., Cruise, M. J., & Murakami, T. R. (1976). A model for nursing: University of British Columbia School of Nursing. *Nursing Papers, 8*(2), 5–9.

Carnevali, D. L., & Thomas, M. D. (1993). *Diagnostic reasoning and treatment decision making in nursing.* Philadelphia, PA: Lippincott.

Carper, B. A. (1978). Fundamental patterns of knowing in nursing. *ANS. Advances in Nursing Science, 1*(1), 13–23.

Chinn, P. L., & Kramer, M. K. (2004). *Integrated knowledge development in nursing* (6th ed.). St. Louis, MO: Mosby.

Clarke, B., James, C., & Kelly, J. (1996). Reflective practice: Reviewing the issues and refocussing the debate. *International Journal of Nursing Studies, 33,* 171–180.

Cody, W. K. (1995). About all those paradigms: Many in the universe, two in nursing. *Nursing Science Quarterly, 8,* 144–147.

Coppa, D. F. (1993). Chaos theory suggests a new paradigm for nursing science. *Journal of Advanced Nursing, 18,* 985–991.

Cull-Wilby, B. L., & Peppin, J. I. (1987). Towards a coexistence of paradigms in nursing knowledge development. *Journal of Advanced Nursing, 12,* 515–521.

Dean, H. (1995). Science and practice: The nature of knowledge. In A. Omery, C. E. Kasper, & G. G. Page (Eds.), *In search of nursing science* (pp. 275–290). Thousand Oaks, CA: Sage.

Donaldson, S. K. (1995). Nursing science for nursing practice. In A. Omery, C. E. Kasper, & G. G. Page (Eds.), *In search of nursing science* (pp. 3–12). Thousand Oaks, CA: Sage.

Durand, M., & Prince, R. (1966). Nursing diagnosis: Process and decision. *Nursing Forum, 4,* 50–64.

Ellis, R. (1968). Characteristics of significant theories. *Nursing Research, 17,* 217–222.

Engebretson, J. (1997). A multiparadigm approach to nursing. *ANS. Advances in Nursing Science, 20*(1), 21–33.

Fawcett, J. (1992). Contemporary conceptualizations of nursing: Philosophy or science. In J. F. Kikuchi & H. Simmons (Eds.), *Philosophic inquiry in nursing* (pp. 55–63). Newbury Park, CA: Sage.

Fawcett, J. (2005). *Contemporary nursing knowledge: Analysis and evaluation of nursing models and theories* (2nd ed.). Philadelphia, PA: F. A. Davis.

Fawcett, J., Watson, J., Neuman, B., Walker, P. H., & Fitzpatrick, J. J. (2001). On nursing theories and evidence. *Journal of Nursing Scholarship, 33,* 115–119.

Feeley, N., & Gerez-Lirette, T. (1992). Development of professional practice based on the McGill model of nursing in an ambulatory care setting. *Journal of Advanced Nursing, 17,* 801–808.

Feeley, N., & Gottlieb, L. N. (1998). Classification systems for health concerns, nursing strategies, and client outcomes: Nursing practice with families who have a child with a chronic illness. *Canadian Journal of Nursing Research, 30,* 45–49.

Field, P. A. (1987). The impact of nursing theory on the clinical decision making process. *Journal of Advanced Nursing, 12,* 563–571.

Fitzpatrick, J. J. (1990). Conceptual basis for the organization and advancement of nursing knowledge: Nursing diagnosis/taxonomy. *Nursing Diagnosis, 1,* 102–106.

Fry, S. T. (1995). Science as problem solving. In A. Omery, C. E. Kasper, & G. G. Page (Eds.), *In search of nursing science* (pp. 72–80). Thousand Oaks, CA: Sage.

George, J. B. (Ed.). (1995). *Nursing theories: The base for professional nursing practice.* Norwalk, CT: Appleton Lange.

Gleick, J. (1987). *Chaos: Making a new science.* New York: Penguin.

Gottlieb, L. N., & Feeley, N. (1999). Nursing intervention studies: Issues related to change and timing in children and families. *Canadian Journal of Nursing Research, 30,* 193–212.

Gottlieb, L. N., & Rowat, K. (1987). The McGill model of nursing: A practice-derived model. *ANS. Advances in Nursing Science, 9*(4), 51–61.

Grubbs, J. (1980). An interpretation of the Johnson behavioral system model for nursing practice. In J. P. Riehl & C. Roy (Eds.), *Conceptual models for nursing practice* (2n ed., pp. 217–254). New York: Appleton-Century-Crofts.

Harbour, L. S., Creekmur, T., DeFelice, J., Doub, M. S., Hodel, A., Tomey, A. M., et al. (2002). Evelyn Adam: Conceptual model for nursing. In A. Marriner-Tomey (Ed.), *Nursing theorists and their work* (4th ed., pp. 516–528). St. Louis, MO: Mosby.

Harmer, B., & Henderson, V. (1955). *Textbook of the principles and practice of nursing* (5th ed). New York: Macmillan.

Henderson, V. (1966). *The nature of nursing*. New York: Macmillan.

Henderson, V. (1982). The nursing process: Is the title right? *Journal of Advanced Nursing, 7*, 103–109.

Holden, R. J. (1990). Models, muddles and medicine. *International Journal of Nursing Studies, 27*, 223–234.

Johnson, D. E. (1974a). Development of theory: A requisite for nursing as a primary health profession. *Nursing Research, 23*, 372–377.

Johnson, D. E. (1974b). The behavioral system model for nursing. In J. P. Riehl & C. Roy (Eds.), *Conceptual models for nursing practice* (pp. 160–196). New York: Appleton-Century-Crofts.

Johnson, D. E. (1980). The behavioral system model for nursing. In J. P. Riehl & C. Roy (Eds.), *Conceptual models for nursing practice* (2nd ed., pp. 207-216). New York: Appleton-Century-Crofts.

Johnson, J. L. (1991). Nursing science: Basic, applied, or practical? Implications for the art of nursing. *ANS. Advances in Nursing Science, 14*(1), 7–16.

Jones, M. (1997). Thinking nursing. In S. E. Thorne & V. E. Hayes (Eds.), *Nursing praxis: Knowledge and action* (pp. 125–139). Thousand Oaks, CA: Sage.

Kikuchi, J. F. (1999). Clarifying the nature of conceptualizations about nursing. *Canadian Journal of Nursing Research, 30*, 115–128.

Kikuchi, J. F., & Simmons, H. (1999). Practical nursing judgment: A moderate realist conception. *Scholarly Inquiry for Nursing Practice, 13*, 43–55.

King, I. M., & Fawcett, J. (1997). *The language of nursing theory and metatheory*. Indianapolis, IN: Sigma Theta Tau International Center Nursing Press.

Kuhn, T. S. (1962). *The structure of scientific revolutions*. Chicago: University of Chicago Press.

Lee, J., Chan, A. C., & Phillips, D. R. (2006). Diagnostic practise in nursing: A critical review of the literature. *Nursing and Health Sciences, 8*, 57–65.

Levine, M. E. (1995). The rhetoric of nursing theory. *Image—The Journal of Nursing Scholarship, 27*, 11–14.

Liaschenko, J. (1997). Knowing the patient? In S. E. Thorne & V. E. Hayes (Eds.), *Nursing praxis: Knowledge and action* (pp. 23–38). Thousand Oaks, CA: Sage.

Liaschenko, J., & Fisher, A. (1999). Theorizing the knowledge that nurses use in the conduct of their work. *Scholarly Inquiry for Nursing Practice, 13*, 29–41.

Maslow, A. H. (1954). *Motivation and personality*. New York: Harper & Row.

McKay, R. (1969). Theories, models, and systems for nursing. *Nursing Research, 18*, 393–400.

Meleis, A. I. (1987). ReVisions in knowledge development: A passion for substance. *Scholarly Inquiry for Nursing Practice, 1*, 5–19.

Meleis, A. I. (2007). *Theoretical nursing: Development and progress* (4th ed.). Philadelphia, PA: Lippincott Williams & Wilkins.

Mitchell, G. J. (1995). Reflection: The key to breaking with tradition. *Nursing Science Quarterly, 8*, 57.

Nagle, L. M., & Mitchell, G. J. (1991). Theoretic diversity: Evolving paradigmatic issues in research and practice. *ANS. Advances in Nursing Science, 14*(1), 17–25.

Neuman, B. M. (1982). *The Neuman systems model: Application to nursing education and practice*. Norwalk, CT: Appleton-Century-Crofts.

Newman, M. A. (1972). Nursing's theoretical evolution. *American Journal of Nursing, 20*, 449–453.

Newman, M. A. (1992). Prevailing paradigms in nursing. *Nursing Outlook, 40*, 10–13, 32.

Nightingale, F. (1946). *Notes on nursing: What it is and what it is not*. Philadelphia, PA: Lippincott. (Original work published 1859)

Orem, D. E. (2001). *Nursing: Concepts of practice* (6th ed.). New York: McGraw Hill.

Orem, D. E., & Parker, K. S. (1964). *Nursing content in preservice nursing curriculums*. Washington, DC: Catholic University of America Press.

Orem, D. E. (1971). *Nursing: Concepts of practice*. New York: McGraw Hill.

Orlando, I. J. (1961). *The dynamic nurse–patient relationship: Function, process, and principles*. New York: GP Putnam's Sons.

Parse, R. R. (1981). *Man–living–health: A theory of nursing*. New York: Wiley.

Parse, R. R. (1987). *Nursing science: Major paradigms, theories, and critiques*. Philadelphia, PA: W. B. Saunders.

Parse, R. R. (1997). The human becoming theory: The was, is, and will be. *Nursing Science Quarterly, 10*(1), 32–38.

Parse, R. R. (1999). Nursing science: The transforming of practice. *Journal of Advanced Nursing, 30*, 1383–1387.

Parse, R. R. (2004). The many meanings of unitary: A plea for clarity. *Nursing Science Quarterly, 17*, 293.

Peplau, H. E. (1952). *Interpersonal relations in nursing*. New York: G. P. Putnam's Sons.

Raudonis, B. M., & Acton, G. J. (1997). Theory-based nursing practice. *Journal of Advanced Nursing, 26*, 138–145.

Ray, M. A. (1998). Complexity and nursing science. *Nursing Science Quarterly, 11*, 91–93.

Reed, J., & Ground, I. (1997). *Philosophy for nursing*. London: Arnold.

Reed, P. G. (1995). A treatise on nursing knowledge development for the 21st century: Beyond postmodernism. *ANS. Advances in Nursing Science, 17*(3), 70–84.

Rodgers, B. L. (1991). Deconstructing the dogma in nursing knowledge and practice. *Image—The Journal of Nursing Scholarship, 23*, 177–181.

Rogers, M. E. (1970). *An introduction to the theoretical basis of nursing*. Philadelphia, PA: F. A. Davis.

Roy, C. (1970). Adaptation: A conceptual framework for nursing. *Nursing Outlook, 18*, 42–45.

Roy, C. (1974). The Roy adaptation model. In J. P. Riehl & C. Roy (Eds.), *Conceptual models for nursing practice* (pp. 135–144). New York: Appleton-Century-Crofts.

Roy, C. (1982). Historical perspective of the theoretical framework for the classification of nursing diagnosis. In M. J. Kim & D. A. Moritz (Eds.), *Classification of nursing diagnoses: Proceedings of the third and fourth national conferences held in St. Louis, MO, in 1978 and 1980* (pp. 235–246). New York: McGraw-Hill.

Roy, C. (1984). *Introduction to nursing: An adaptation model* (2nd ed.). Englewood Cliffs, NJ: Prentice-Hall.

Roy, C., & Andrews, H. A. (1999). *The Roy adaptation model: The definitive statement* (2nd ed.). East Norwalk, CT: Appleton & Lange.

Sarter, B. J. (1990). Philosophical foundations of nursing theory: A discipline emerges. In N. L. Chaska (Ed.), *The nursing profession: Turning points* (pp. 223–229). St. Louis, MO: Mosby.

Silva, M. C., Sorrell, J. M., & Sorrell, S. C. (1995). From Carper's patterns of knowing to ways of being: An ontological philosophical shift in nursing. *ANS. Advances in Nursing Science, 18*(1), 1–13.

Starzomski, R., & Rodney, P. (1997). Nursing inquiry for the common good. In S. E. Thorne & V. E. Hayes (Eds.), *Nursing praxis: Knowledge and action* (pp. 219–236). Thousand Oaks, CA: Sage.

Tanner, C. A. (1993). Rethinking clinical judgment. In N. L. Diekelman & M. L. Rather (Eds.), *Transforming RN education: Dialogue and debate* (2nd ed., Publication No. 14-2511, pp. 15–41). New York: National League for Nursing.

Thorne, S., Jillings, C., Ellis, D., & Perry, J. (1993). A nursing model in action: The University of British Columbia experience. *Journal of Advanced Nursing, 18*, 1259–1266.

Thorne, S. E. (1997). Introduction: Praxis in the context of nursing's developing inquiry. In S. E. Thorne & V. E. Hayes (Ed.), *Nursing praxis: Knowledge and action* (pp. xi–xxiii). Thousand Oaks, CA: Sage.

Torres, G. (1974). Curriculum process and the integrated curriculum. In National League for Nursing (Ed.), *Unifying the curriculum: The integrated approach* (Publication No. 15-1522, pp. 15–31). New York: National League for Nursing.

Torres, G. (1986). *Theoretical foundations of nursing*. Norwalk, CT: Appleton-Century-Crofts.

Travelbee, J. (1971). *Interpersonal aspects of nursing*. Philadelphia: F. A. Davis.

Varcoe, C. (1996). Disparagement of the nursing process: The new dogma? *Journal Advanced Nursing, 23*, 120–125.

von Bertalanffy, L. (1968). *General systems theory: Foundations, development, application*. New York: George Braziller.

Wald, F. S., & Leonard, R. C. (1964). Toward development of nursing practice theory. *American Journal of Nursing, 13*, 309–313.

Warren, J. J., & Hoskins, L. M. (1990). The development of NANDA's nursing diagnosis taxonomy. *Nursing Diagnosis, 1*, 162–168.

Watson, J. (1979). *Nursing: The philosophy and science of caring*. Boston: Little, Brown.

Watson, J. (1990). Caring knowledge and informed moral passion. *ANS. Advances in Nursing Science, 13*(1), 15–24.

Watson, J. (1999). *Postmodern nursing and beyond*. Edinburgh, Scotland: Churchill Livingstone.

White, J. (1995). Patterns of knowing: Review, critique, and update. *ANS. Advances in Nursing Science, 17*(4), 73–86.

Yeo, M. (1989). Integration of nursing theory and nursing ethics. *ANS. Advances in Nursing Science, 11*(3), 33–42.

Yura, H., & Walsh, M. B. (1973). *The nursing process: Assessing, planning, implementing, evaluating* (2nd ed.). New York: Appleton-Century-Crofts.

Chapter 7

Arthur, H. M., Gunn, E., Thorpe, K. E., Ginis, K. M., Mataseje, L., McCartney, N., et al. (2007). Effect of aerobic vs combined aerobic-strength training on 1 year post–cardiac rehabilitation outcomes in women after a cardiac event. *Journal of Rehabilitation Medicine, 39*, 730–735.

Boudreaux, E. D., Francis, J. S., & Loyacano, T. (2002). Family presence during invasive procedures and rescusitations in the emergency department: A critical review and suggestions for further research. *Annals of Emergency Medicine, 40*, 193–205.

Canadian Association of Schools of Nursing. (1997). *Canadian nursing research priorities: Results of Phase III of National Nursing Research Symposium.* Ottawa, ON: Author.

Canadian Institutes of Health Research, the Natural Sciences and Engineering Research Council of Canada, & the Social Sciences and Humanities Research Council of Canada. (2003). *Tri-Council policy statement: Ethical conduct for research involving humans, 1998* (with 2000, 2002, and 2005 amendments). Retrieved August 20, 2008, from http://www.pre.ethics.gc.ca/english/policy statement/policystatement.cfm

Canadian Nurses Association. (2002). *Policy statement: Evidence-based decision-making and nursing practice.* Ottawa, ON: Author.

Canadian Nurses Association. (2008). *Code of ethics for registered nurses.* Ottawa, ON: Author.

Carper, B. A. (1978). Fundamental patterns of knowing in nursing. *ANS. Advances in Nursing Science, 1*(1),13–23.

Chinn, P. L., & Kramer, M. K. (2008). *Integrated theory and knowledge development in nursing.* St. Louis, MO: Mosby/Elsevier.

Glaser, B., & Strauss, A. (1967). *The discovery of grounded theory.* Chicago: Aldine.

Good, S. R. (1969). *Submission to the study of support of research in universities for the Science Secretariat of the Privy Council.* Ottawa, ON: Canadian Nurses Association and Canadian Nurses Foundation.

Husserl, E. (1962). *Ideas: General introduction to pure phenomenology.* New York: Collier. (Original work published 1931)

International Council of Nurses. (2007). *Nursing research: ICN position statement.* Geneva: Author.

Jeffers, B. R. (1998). The surrogate's experience during treatment decision making. *Medsurg Nursing, 7*, 357–363.

Kuhn, T. (1970). *The structure of scientific revolutions* (2nd ed.). Chicago: University of Chicago Press.

Lauzon Clabo, L. M. (2008). An ethnography of pain assessment and the role of social context on two postoperative units. *Journal of Advanced Nursing, 61*, 531–539.

Lysaught, J. P. (1970). *An abstract for action.* New York: McGraw-Hill.

McCaughan, D., Thompson, C., Cullum, N., Sheldon, T. A., & Thompson, D. R. (2002). Acute care nurses' perceptions of barriers to using research information in clinical decision-making. *Journal of Advanced Nursing, 39*(1), 46–60.

McGahey-Oakland, P. R., Lieder, H. S., Young, A., & Jefferson, L. S. (2007). Family experiences during resuscitation at a Childrens' Hospital emergency department. *Journal of Pediatric Health Care, 21*, 217–225.

Medical Research Council of Canada. (1985). *Report to the Medical Research Council of Canada by the Working Group on Nursing Research.* Ottawa, ON: Author.

Melnyk, B. M., & Fineout-Overholt, E. (2005). *Evidence-based practice in nursing and health care. A guide to best practice.* Philadelphia, PA: Lippincott Williams & Wilkins.

Mills, J., Francis, K., & Bonner, A. (2007). Live my work: Rural nurses and their multiple perspectives of self. *Journal of Advanced Nursing, 59*, 583–590.

National Center for Nursing Research/International Council of Nurses. (1990). *Nursing research worldwide: Report of the Task Force on International Nursing Research.* Geneva, Switzerland: Author.

Nightingale, F. (1858). *Notes on matters affecting the health, efficiency, and hospital administration of the British army. Founded chiefly on the experience of the late war.* Presented by request to the Secretary of State for War. Privately printed for Miss Nightingale. London: Harrison and Sons.

Nightingale, F. (1863). *Notes on hospitals.* London, UK: Longman, Green, Roberts & Green.

Polit, D. F., & Beck, C. T. (2004). *Nursing research: Principles and methods* (7th ed.). Philadelphia, PA: Lippincott Williams & Wilkins.

Registered Nurses Association of Ontario (RNAO). (2008). Best Practice Guidelines. Retrieved August 31, 2008, from http://www.rnao.org/Page.asp?PageID=1110&SiteNodeID=190&BL_Ex:

Stetler, C. B., Brunell, M., Giuliano, K. K., Morsi, D., Prince, L., & Newell-Stokes. V. (1998). Evidence-based practice and the role of nursing leadership. *Journal of Nursing Administration, 28*, 45–53.

Speziale, H. J. S., & Carpenter, D. R. (2006). *Qualitative research in nursing: Advancing the humanistic imperative.* Philadelphia, PA: Lippincott Williams & Wilkins.

Titler, M. G., Kleiber, C., Steelman, V. J., Rakel, B. A., Budreau, G., Everett, L. Q., et al. (2001). The Iowa model of evidence-based practice to promote quality care. *Critical Care Nursing Clinics of North America, 13*, 497–509.

Tripepi-Bova, K. A., Woods, K. D., & Loach, M. C. (1997). A comparison of transparent polyurethane and dry gauze dressings for peripheral i.v. catheter sites: Rates of phlebitis, infiltration, and dislodgment by patients. *American Journal of Critical Care, 6*, 377–381.

Wood, M., & Ross-Kerr, J. (2006). *Basic steps in planning nursing research, from question to proposal.* Sudbury, MA: Jones and Bartlett.

Chapter 8

Aiken, L., Clarke, S., Sloane, D., Sochalski, J., & Silber, J. (2002). Hospital nurse staffing and patient mortality, nurse burnout, and job dissatisfaction. *Journal of the American Medical Association, 288*, 1987–1993.

Austin, W., Bergum, V., & Goldberg, L. (2003). Unable to answer the call of our patients: Mental health nurses' experiences of moral distress. *Nursing Inquiry, 10*, 177–183.

Beauchamp, T., & Childress, J. (2001). *Principles of biomedical ethics* (5th ed.). New York: Oxford University Press.

Bennett Jacobs, B., & Taylor, C. (2005a). Medical futility in the natural attitude. *ANS Advances in Nursing Science, 28*, 288–305.

Bennett Jacobs, B., & Taylor, C. (2005b). Seeing artificial hydration and nutrition through an ethical lens. *Home Healthcare Nurse, 23*, 749–743.

Bergum V. (2004). Relational ethics in nursing. In J. Storch, P. Rodney, & R. Starzomski, (Eds.), *Toward a moral horizon: Nursing ethics for leadership and practice.* Toronto, ON: Pearson Education.

Bergum, V., & Dossetor, J. (2005). *Relational ethics: The full meaning of respect.* Hagerstown, MD: University Publishing Group.

Boutain, D. (2005). Social justice in nursing: A review of the literature. In M. de Chesney (Ed.). *Caring for the vulnerable: Perspectives in nursing theory, practice, research.* Mississauga, ON: Jones & Barlett Publications.

Callahan, D. (1991). Medical futility, medical necessity: The-problem-without-a-name. *Hastings Center Report, 21*(4), 30–35.

Canadian Health Services Research Foundation. (2006). *What's ailing our nurses? A discussion of the major issues affecting nursing human resources in Canada.* Ottawa, ON: Author.

Canadian Nurses Association. (1998). *Advance directives: The nurses' role.* Ottawa, ON: Author.

Canadian Nurses Association. (2001, May). Futility presents many challenges for nurses. *Ethics in Practice*, ISSN issue 1480-9990. Ottawa, ON: Author. Retrieved August 23, 2008, from http://www.cna-nurses.ca/cna/documents/pdf/publications/Ethics_Pract_Futility_challenges_May_2001_e.pdf

Canadian Nurses Association. (2008). *Code of ethics for registered nurses.* Ottawa, ON: Author.

Curtin, L., & Flaherty, M. J. (1982). *Nursing ethics: Theories and pragmatic.* Bowie, MD: Brady.

Drevdahl, D., Kneipp, S., Canales, M., & Dorcy, K. (2001). Reinvesting in social justice: A capital idea for public health nursing. *ANS. Advances in Nursing Science, 24*, 19–31.

Ganzini, L. (2006). Artificial nutrition and hydration at the end of life: Ethics and evidence. *Palliative and Supportive Care, 4*, 135–143.

Gilligan, C. (1982). *In a different voice.* Cambridge, MA: Harvard University Press.

Hardingham, L. (2004). Integrity and moral residue: Nurses as participants in a moral community. *Nursing Philosophy, 5*, 127–134.

Hartrick Doane, G., & Varcoe, C. (2007). Relational practice and nursing obligations. *ANS. Advances in Nursing Science, 30*, 192–205.

International Council of Nurses. (2006). *ICN code of ethics for nurses.* Geneva, Switzerland: Author.

Johnstone, M.-J. (2004). *Bioethics: A nursing perspective.* Melbourne, Australia: Churchill Livingstone.

Kohlberg, L. (1981). *Essays on moral development (Vols. 1–3).* San Francisco: Harper & Row.

Lindemann, H. (2006). *An invitation to feminist ethics.* New York: McGraw-Hill
Lindemann Nelson, H. L. (2000). Feminist bioethics: Where we've been, where we're going. *Metaphilosophy, 31,* 492–508.
Oberle, K., & Raffin Bouchal, S. (in press). *Nursing ethics in Canadian practice.* Toronto, ON: Pearson.
Peter, E., Lunardi, V., & Macfarlane, A. (2004). Nursing resistance as ethical action: Literature review. *Journal of Advanced Nursing, 46,* 403–416.
Rodney, P., Hartrick Doane, G., Storch, J., & Varcoe, C. (2006). Ethics in action: Strengthening nurses' enactment of their moral agency within the cultural context of health care delivery. *Canadian Nurse, 102*(8), 25–26.
Sherwin, S. (1992). *No longer patient: Feminist ethics and health care.* Philadelphia, PA: Temple University Press.
Taylor, C. (1995). Medical futility and nursing. *Image: Journal of Nursing Scholarship, 27,* 301–306.
Webster, G., & Baylis, F. (2000). Moral residue. In S. Rubin & L. Zoloth (Eds.), *Margin of error: The ethics of mistakes in the practice of medicine.* Hagerstown, MD: University Publishing Group.
Wolf, S. M. (Ed.). (1996). *Feminism and bioethics.* New York: Oxford University Press.

Chapter 9

Assisted Human Reproduction Act, S.C., c.2 (2004).
Black, H. C. (1999). *Black's law dictionary* (7th ed.). St. Paul, MN: West Publishing.
Canadian Nurses Association. (2008). *Code of ethics for registered nurses.* Ottawa, ON: Author.
Canadian Nurses Protective Society. (1997, September). Telephone advice. *infoLAW Bulletin, 6*(1).
Canadian Nurses Protective Society. (1998, April). Vicarious liability. *infoLAW Bulletin, 7*(1).
Canadian Nurses Protective Society. (2004a, May). Patient restraints. *infoLAW Bulletin, 13*(2).
Canadian Nurses Protective Society. (2004b, December). Consent for the incapable adult. *infoLAW Bulletin, 13*(3).
Canadian Nurses Protective Society. (2007a, January). Quality documentation: Your best defence. *infoLAW Bulletin, 1*(1).
Canadian Nurses Protective Society. (2007b, February). Nursing students' FAQ. Available to members only at http://cnps.ca/members/students/students_e.HTML
College of Registered Nurses of British Columbia. (2007). *Practice standard: Duty to provide care.* Vancouver, BC: Author.
College of Registered Nurses of Nova Scotia. (2006). *Emergency preparedness plan.* Halifax, NS: Author.
Controlled Drugs and Substances Act, S.C., c. 19 (1996).
Criminal Code, R.S.C., c. C-46 (1985).
Dessauer v. Memorial General Hospital and Glorious Bourque, 96 N.M. 92; 628 P.2d 337; N.M (1981).
Downey v. Rothwell, 5 W.W.R. 311, 49 D.L.R. (3d) 82 (Alta. S.C. 1974).
Downie, J. (2004). *Dying justice: A case for decriminalizing euthanasia and assisted suicide in Canada.* Toronto, ON: University of Toronto Press.
Emergency Medical Aid Act, R.S.N.W.T., c.E-4 (2000).
Food and Drugs Act, R.S.C., c. F-27 (1985).
Fridman, G. H. L. (2003). *Introduction to the Canadian law of torts* (2nd ed.). Markham, ON: LexisNexis.
Granger v. Ottawa General Hospital, O.J. No. 2129 (Gen. Div. 1996).
Guido, G. (2006). *Legal and ethical issues in nursing* (4th ed.). Upper Saddle River, NJ: Prentice Hall.
Health Canada. (1997, May). Canadian national report on immunization, 1996. In *Canada Communicable Disease Report* (Suppl., Vol. 23 S4). Ottawa, ON: Public Health Agency of Canada.
Keatings, M., & Smith, O. (2000). *Ethical and legal issues in Canadian nursing* (2nd ed.). Toronto, ON: W.B. Saunders.
Kolesar v. Jeffries, 9 O.R. (2d) 41, 59 D.L.R. (3d) 367 (S.C.C. 1976).
Malette v. Shulman, CarswellOnt 642, 2 C.C.L.T. (2d), 1, 72 O.R. (2d), (1990).
McIntyre, M., Thomlinson, E., & McDonald, C. (2006). *Realities of Canadian nursing: Professional, practice, and power issues* (2nd ed.). Philadelphia, PA: Lippincott Williams & Wilkins.
Mental Health and Consequential Amendments Act, S.M., c. 36 (1998).
Meyer v. Gordon, 17 C.C.L.T. 1 (B.C. S.C. 1981).
Morris, J. J., Ferguson, M., & Dykeman, M. J. (1999). *Canadian nurses and the law* (2nd ed.). Toronto, ON: Butterworths.
Nancy B. v. Hôtel-Dieu de Québec, R.J.Q. 361, 86 D.L.R. (4th) 385, 69 C.C.C. (3d) 450 (S.C. 1992).
Osborne, P. H. (2003). *Essentials of Canadian law: The law of torts* (2nd ed.). Toronto, ON: Irwin Law.
Phillips, E. (1999a). The author responds to: If it's not charted it's not done? *The Canadian Nurse, 95*(5), 12.
Phillips, E. (1999b). Is there a risk in being a Good Samaritan? *The Canadian Nurse, 95*(8), 43–44.
Phillips, E. (2002). Managing legal risks in preceptorships. *The Canadian Nurse, 98*(9) 25–26.
R. v. Morgentaler, 37 C.C.C. (3d) 449 (S.C.C. 1988).
Regulated Health Professions Act, S.O., Chapter 18 (1991). Retrieved September 16, 2008, from http://www.e-laws.gov.on.ca/html/statutes/english/elaws_statutes_91r18_e.htm
Roberts v. Cape Breton Regional Hospital 162 N.S.R. (2d) 342 (S.C.) (1997).
Sneiderman, B., Irvine, J., & Osborne, P. (2003). *Canadian medical law* (3rd ed.). Scarborough, ON: Thompson.
Tapp, A. (1996). Release of confidential information to the police. *The Canadian Nurse, 92*(3), 49–50.
Tapp, A. (2001). The legal risks of e-mail. *The Canadian Nurse, 97*(3), 35–36.
Tapp, A. (2003). New developments in privacy law. *The Canadian Nurse, 99*(3), 32.
The Protection of Persons in Care Act, C.C.S.M. c. P144 (2000). Retrieved September 16, 2008, from http://web2.gov.mb.ca/laws/statutes/ccsm/p144e.php
Vital Statistics Act, R.S.M., c. V60, s. 2 (1987).

Chapter 10

Adams, M. (2007). *Unlikely utopia: The surprising triumph of Canadian pluralism.* Toronto, ON: Viking.
Anderson, J., Perry, J., Blue, C., Browne, A., Henderson, A., Khan, K. B., et al. (2003). "Rewriting" cultural safety within the postcolonial and postnational feminist project: Toward new epistemologies of healing. *ANS. Advances in Nursing Science, 26,* 196–214.
Andrews, M. M., & Boyle, J. S. (2003). *Transcultural concepts in nursing care* (4th ed.). Philadelphia, PA: Lippincott Williams & Wilkins.
Baker, C. (2007). Globalization and the cultural safety of an immigrant Muslim community. *Journal of Advanced Nursing, 57,* 296–305.
Barton, S. S. (2004). Narrative inquiry: Locating Aboriginal epistemology in a relational methodology. *Journal of Advanced Nursing, 45,* 519–526.
Barton, S. S., Anderson, N., & Thommasen, H.V. (2005a). The diabetes experience of Aboriginal people living in a rural Canadian community. *Australian Journal of Rural Health, 13,* 242–246.
Barton, S. S., Thommasen, H. V., Tallio, B., Zhang, W., & Michalos, A. C. (2005b). Health and quality of life of Aboriginal residential school survivors, Bella Coola Valley, 2001. *Social Indicators Research, 73,* 295–312.
Browne, A. J., & Fiske, J. (2001). First Nations women's encounters with mainstream health care services. *Western Journal of Nursing Research, 23,* 126–147.
Browne, A., & Varcoe, C (2006). Critical cultural perspectives and health care involving Aboriginal peoples. *Contemporary Nurse, 22,* 155–167.
Campinha-Bacote, J. (2002). The process of cultural competence in the delivery of healthcare services: A model of care. *Journal of Transcultural Nursing, 13,* 181–184.
Canadian Nurses Association. (2004). *Promoting culturally competent care.* Ottawa, ON: Author.
Canadian Nurses Association (2008). *Code of ethics.* Ottawa, ON: Author.
College of Registered Nurses of British Columbia. (2006). *Competencies in the context of entry-level registered nurse practice in British Columbia* (Publication No. 375-1). Vancouver, BC: Author.
Cowan, D. T., & Norman, J. (2006). Cultural competence in nursing: New meanings. *Journal of Transcultural Nursing, 17,* 82.
Davidhizar, R. E., & Giger, J. N. (Eds.). (1998). *Canadian transcultural nursing: Assessment and intervention.* St. Louis, MO: Mosby.
Dickason, O. P. (2006). *A concise history of Canada's First Nations.* Toronto, ON: Oxford University Press.
Dion Stout, M., & Downey, B. (2006). Nursing, indigenous peoples and cultural safety: So what? Now what? *Contempory Nurse, 22,* 327–332.
Foster, G. (1976). Disease etiologies in non-Western medical systems. *American Anthropologist, 78,* 773–782.
Giger, J. N., & Davidhizar, R. E. (Eds.). (2004). *Transcultural nursing: Assessment and intervention* (4th ed.). St. Louis, MO: Mosby.
Glittenberg, J. (2004). A transdisciplinary, transcultural model for health care. *Journal of Transcultural Nursing, 15,* 6–10.
Gustafson, D. L. (2005). Transcultural nursing theory from a critical cultural perspective. *ANS. Advances in Nursing Science, 28,* 2–16.

Hartrick Doane, G. H., & Varcoe, C. (2005). Family nursing as relational inquiry: Developing health-promoting practice. Philadelphia, PA: Lippincott Williams & Wilkins.

Hartrick Doane, G. H., & Varcoe, C. (2007). Relational practice in nursing obligations. *ANS. Advances in Nursing Science, 30,* 192–205.

Health Canada. (2003). *Aboriginal diabetes initiative.* Retrieved September 16, 2004, from http://www.hc-sc.gc.ca/fniah-spnia/diseases-maladies/diabete/moauipp-ppmahrimu-eng.php

Health Canada. (2008a). *First Nations, Inuit and Aboriginal health: Tuberculosis in First Nations communities.* Retrieved September 16, 2008, from http://www.hc-sc.gc.ca/fniah-spnia/diseases-maladies/tuberculos/tb_fni-pni_commun-eng.php

Health Canada (2008b). *First Nations, Inuit and Aboriginal health: Substance use and treatment of addictions.* Retrieved September 11, 2008, from http://www.hc-sc.gc.ca/fniah-spnia/substan/index-eng.php

Helsel, D., Mochel, M., & Bauer, R. (2005). Chronic illness and Hmong shamans. *Journal of Transcultural Nursing, 16,* 150–154.

Hunter, L., Logan, J., Barton, S., & Goulet, J. (2004). Linking Aboriginal healing traditions to holistic nursing practice. *Journal of Holistic Nursing, 22,* 267–285.

Indian and Northern Affairs Canada. (2004). *Status—Most often asked questions.* Retrieved September 16, 2004, from http://www.ainc-inac.gc.ca/pr/pub/ywtk/index-eng.asp

Kemp, C. (2004). Promoting healthy partnerships with refugees and immigrants. In A. R. Vollman, E. T. Anderson, & J. McFarlane (Eds.), *Canadian community as partner: Theory and practice in nursing* (pp. 407–430). Philadelphia, PA: Lippincott Williams & Wilkins.

Kirkham, S. (2003). The politics of belonging and intercultural health care. *Western Journal of Nursing Research, 25,* 762–780.

Korean health beliefs. (2003). Retrieved September 3, 2008, from http://www.hawcc.hawaii.edu/nursing/RNKorean00.htm

Leininger, M. (2002a). Essential transcultural nursing care concepts, principles, examples and policy statements. In M. Leininger & M. R. McFarland (Eds.), *Transcultural nursing: Concepts, theories, research and practice* (3rd ed., pp. 45–69). New York: McGraw-Hill.

Leininger, M. (2002b). Culture care theory: A major contribution to advance transcultural nursing knowledge and practices. *Journal of Transcultural Nursing, 13,* 189–192.

Leininger, M., & McFarland, M. R. (2002). *Transcultural nursing: Concepts, theories, research and practice* (3rd ed.). New York: McGraw-Hill.

Lo, H., & Pottinger, A. (2007). Mental health practice. In R. H. Srivastava (Ed.), *The healthcare professional's guide to clinical cultural competence* (pp. 247–263). Toronto, ON: Elsevier.

Majumdar, B. B., Chambers, T. L., & Roberts, J. (2004). Community-based, culturally sensitive HIV/AIDS education for Aboriginal adolescents: Implications for nursing practice. *Journal of Transcultural Nursing, 15,* 69–73.

Mill, J., Astle, B., Ogilvie, L., & Opare, M. (2005). Global health and equity. Part I: Setting the context. *Canadian Nurse, 101*(5), 22–24.

Minuk, G. Y., & Uhanova, J. (2003). Viral hepatitis in the Canadian Inuit and First Nations populations. *Canadian Journal of Gastroenterology, 17,* 707–712.

Narayanasamy, A. (2002). The ACCESS model: A transcultural nursing practice framework. *British Journal of Nursing, 11,* 643–650.

Narayanasamy, A., & White, E. (2005). A review of transcultural nursing. *Nurse Education Today, 25,* 102–111.

National Aboriginal Health Organization. (2008). *Cultural competency and safety: A guide for health care administrators, providers and educators.* Retrieved September 3, 2008, from http://www.naho.ca/publications/culturalcompetency.pdf

Ogilvie, L., Astle, B., Mill, J., & Opare, M. (2005). Global health and equity. Part II: Exploring solutions. *Canadian Nurse, 101*(6), 25–28.

Pacquiao, D. F. (2002). Ethics and cultural diversity: A framework for decision-making. *Bioethics Forum, 17*(3–4), 12–17.

Pacquiao, D. F. (2003). Cultural competence in ethical decision-making. In M. M. Andrews & J. S. Boyle (Eds.), *Transcultural concepts in nursing care* (pp. 503–532). Philadelphia, PA: Lippincott Williams & Wilkins.

Polaschek, N. R. (1998). Cultural safety: A new concept in nursing people of different ethnicities. *Journal of Advanced Nursing, 27,* 452–457.

Racher, F. E., & Annis, R. C. (2008). Honouring culture and diversity in community practice. In A. R. Vollman, E. T. Anderson, & J. McFarlane (Eds.), *Canadian community as partner: Theory & multidisciplinary practice* (2nd ed., pp. 164–189). Philadelphia, PA: Lippincott Williams & Wilkins.

Ramsden, I. M. (2002). *Cultural safety and nursing education in Aotearoa and Te Waipounamu.* Unpublished doctoral dissertation, Victoria University of Wellington, New Zealand. Retrieved September 3, 2008, from http://culturalsafety.massey.as.nz/thesis.htm

Smith, D. (2003). Maternal–child health care in Aboriginal communities. *Canadian Journal of Nursing Research, 35,* 143–152.

Smith, D., Edwards, N., Martens, P. J., & Varcoe, C. (2007). "Making a difference": A new care paradigm for pregnant and parenting Aboriginal people. *Canadian Journal of Public Health, 98,* 321–325.

Smith, D., Edwards, N., Varcoe, C., Martens, P. J., & Davis, B. (2006). Bringing safety and responsiveness into the forefront of care for pregnant and parenting aboriginal people. *ANS. Advances in Nursing Science, 29,* E27–E44.

Spector, R. E. (2004). *Cultural diversity in health & illness* (6th ed.). Upper Saddle River, NJ: Prentice Hall Health.

Srivastava, R. H. (2007a). Culture: Perspectives, myths, and misconceptions. In R. H. Srivastava (Ed.), *The healthcare professional's guide to clinical cultural competence* (pp. 28–52). Toronto, ON: Elsevier.

Srivastava, R. H. (Ed.). (2007b). *The healthcare professional's guide to clinical competence.* Toronto, ON: Elsevier.

Statistics Canada. (2007a). *Census snapshot—Immigration in Canada: A portrait of the foreign-born population, 2006 Census* (Statistics Canada Catalogue No. 97-557-XIE). Ottawa, ON: Author. Retrieved September 16, 2008, from http://www.statcan.ca/bsolc/english/bsolc?catno=11-008-X200800110556

Statistics Canada. (2007b). *Population by knowledge of official language, by province and territory (2006 Census).* Retrieved September 3, 2008, from http://www40.statcan.ca/101/cst01/demo15.htm

Statistics Canada. (2008a). *Aboriginal identity population, 2006 counts, percentage distribution, percentage change for both sexes, for Canada, provinces and territories—20% sample data. Aboriginal peoples highlight tables. 2006 Census* (Statistics Canada Catalogue No. 97-558-XWE2006002). Ottawa, ON: Author. Retrieved September 3, 2008, from http://www12.statcan.ca/english/census06/data/highlights/Aboriginal/pages/Print.cfm?Lang=E&Geo=CSD&Code=47&Table=2&Data=Count&Sex=1&Abor=1&StartRec=1&Sort=2&Display=Page&CSDFilter=250

Statistics Canada. (2008b). *Canada's ethnocultural mosaic, 2006 census: Findings.* (Statistics Canada Catalogue No. 97-562-X). Ottawa, ON: Author. Retrieved September 16, 2008, from http://www.12.statcan.ca/english/census06/analysis/ethnicorigin/index.cfm

Statistics Canada. (2008c). *Aboriginal peoples in Canada in 2006: Inuit, Métis and First Nations, 2006 Census: Findings* (Statistics Canada Catalogue No. 97-558-XIE). Ottawa, ON: Author. Retrieved September 16, 2008, from http://www12.statcan.ca/english/census06/analysis/aboriginal/index.cfm

St. Hill, P., Lipson, J. G., & Meleis, A. I. (2003). *Caring for women cross-culturally.* Philadelphia, PA: F. A. Davis.

Suh, E. E. (2004). The model of cultural competence through an evolutionary concept analysis. *Journal of Transcultural Nursing, 15,* 93–102.

Tarlier, D. S., Browne, A. J., & Johnson, J. (2007). The influence of geographical and social distance on nursing practice and continuity of care in a remote First Nations community. *Canadian Journal of Nursing Research, 39,* 126–148.

Vollman, A. R., Anderson, E. T., & McFarlane, J. (2008). *Canadian community as partner: Theory & multidisciplinary practice* (2nd ed.). Philadelphia, PA: Lippincott Williams & Wilkins.

Waldram, J. B., Herring, D. A., & Young, T. K. (2006). *Aboriginal health in Canada: Historical, cultural, and epidemiological perspectives* (2nd ed.). Toronto, ON: University of Toronto Press.

Wasekeesikaw, F. H. (2006). Challenges for the new millennium: Nursing in First Nations. In M. McIntyre, E. Thomlinson, & C. McDonald (Eds.), *Realities of Canadian nursing: Professional, practice, and power issues* (2nd ed., pp. 415–433). Philadelphia, PA: Lippincott Williams & Wilkins.

Watts, N., & McDonald, C (2007). The beginning of life (the perinatal period). In R. H. Srivastava (Ed.), *The healthcare professional's guide to clinical cultural competence* (pp. 203–226). Toronto, ON: Elsevier.

Chapter 11

A century of progress—Overview of significant themes and issues. (2005, September). *Canadian Nurse (Centennial Edition), 101*(7), 22–28.

Aiken, L., Clarke, S., Sloane, D., Sochalski, J., Busse, R., Clarke, H., et al. (2001). Nurses reports on hospital care in five countries. *Health Affairs, 20*(3), 43–53.

Aiken, L. H., Clarke, S. P., Sloane, D. M. Sochalski, J., & Silber, J. H. (2002). Hospital nurse staffing and patient mortality, nurse burnout, and job dissatisfaction. *Journal of the American Medical Association, 288,* 1987–1993.

Anders, R. L., & Hawkins, J .A. (2006). *Mosby's nursing leadership and management online.* St. Louis, MO: Mosby.

Canadian Association of Schools of Nursing. (2006). *Position statement: Patient safety and nursing education.* Ottawa, ON: Author.

Canadian Council on Health Services Accreditation. (2003). *2003 Accreditation recognition guidelines.* Ottawa, ON: Author.

Canadian Nurses Association. (2002). *Nursing leadership—Position statement.* Ottawa, ON: Author.

Canadian Nurses Association. (2003a). *Scopes of practice—Joint position statement.* Ottawa, ON: Author.

Canadian Nurses Association. (2003b). *Staffing decisions for the delivery of safe nursing care—Position statement.* Ottawa, ON: Author.

Canadian Nurses Association. (2005a). *Nursing leadership development in Canada.* Ottawa, ON: Author. Retrieved March 15, 2008, from http://www.cna-aiic.ca/CNA/documents/pdf/publications/Nursing_Leadership_Development_Canada_e.pdf

Canadian Nurses Association. (2005b, January). Nursing staff mix: A key link to patient safety. *Nursing Now: Issues and trends in Canadian Nursing, 19,* 1–6.

Canadian Nursing Advisory Committee. (2008). *Our health, our future: Creating quality workplaces for Canadian nurses. Final report.* Ottawa, ON: Advisory Committee on Health Human Resources.

Canadian Patient Safety Institute. (2007). *The safety competencies—Enhancing patient safety across the health professions.* Retrieved September 5, 2008, from http://www.patientsafetyinstitute.ca/education/safetycompetencies.HTML

Case Management Society of America. (2008). *Member benefits: Why you should join.* Retrieved September 5, 2008, from http://www.cmsa.org/LinkClick.aspx?fileticket=Gt%2fhLsKRbeg%3d&tabid=271

College of Nurses of Ontario. (2004). *Quality assurance practice consultation program.* Toronto, ON: Author.

College of Registered Nurses of British Columbia. (2005). *Practice standard: Delegating tasks to unregulated care providers.* Vancouver, BC: Author.

College of Registered Nurses of British Columbia. (2006). *Competencies in the context of entry-level registered nurse practice in British Columbia. Leadership and management practices for healthy work environments.* Vancouver, BC: Author.

Cott, C.A., Falter, L., Gignac, M., & Badley, E. (2008). Helping networks in community home care for the elderly: Types of team. *Canadian Journal of Nursing Research, 40*(1), 19–37.

Cullum, N., Ciliska, D. L., Marks, S., & Haynes, B. (2008). An introduction to evidence-based nursing. In N. Cullum, D. Ciliska, R. B. Haynes, & S. Marks (Eds.), *Evidence-based nursing* (pp. 1–8). Oxford, UK: Blackwell.

Cummings, G. G. (2004). Investing relational energy: The hallmark of resonant leadership. *Canadian Journal of Nursing Leadership, 17,* 76–87.

Dadich, K. A. (2003). Care delivery strategies. In P. S. Yoder-Wise (Ed.), *Leading and managing in nursing* (3rd ed., pp. 253–274). St. Louis, MO: Mosby.

Davidson, D., Weisbrod, L., Gregory, D., & Neudorf, K. (2006). Case study: On the leading edge of new curricula concepts: Systems and safety in nursing education. *Canadian Journal of Nursing Leadership, 19,* 34–42.

Ellis, J. R., & Hartley, C. L. (2005). *Managing and coordinating nursing care* (4th ed). Philadelphia, PA: Lippincott Williams & Wilkins.

Estabrooks, C., Midodzi, W., Cummings, G., Ricker, K., & Giovannetti, P. (2005). The impact of hospital nursing characteristics on 30-day mortality. *Nursing Research, 54*(2), 74–84.

Gardner, D. B. (2005). Ten lessons in collaboration. *Online Journal of Issues in Nursing, 10*(1), manuscript 1. Retrieved September 5, 2008, from http://www.nursingworld.org/MainMenuCategories/ANAMarketplace/ANAPeriodicals/OJIN/TableofContents/Volume102005/No1January31/tpc26_116008.aspx

Gifford, W. A., Davies, B., Edwards, N., & Graham, I. D. (2006). Leadership strategies to influence the use of clinical practice guidelines. *Canadian Journal of Nursing Leadership, 19,* 72–88.

Gokenbach, V. (2007). Professional nurse councils: A new model to create excitement and improve value and productivity. *Journal of Nursing Administration, 37,* 440–443.

Graham, I. D., & Harrison, M. B. (2008). Appraising and adapting clinical practice guidelines. In N. Cullum, D. Ciliska, R.B. Haynes & S. Marks (Eds.), *Evidence-Based Nursing* (pp. 219–230). Oxford, UK: Blackwell.

Health Canada. (n.d.). *Office of Nursing Policy.* Retrieved September 5, 2008, from http://www.hc-sc.gc.ca/ahc-asc/branch-dirgen/hbp-dgps/onp-bpsi/index_eng.php

Hendry, C., & Walker, A. (2004). Priority setting in clinical nursing practice: Literature review. *Journal of Advanced Nursing, 47*(4), 427–436.

...erd, J. M., Smith, D. L., & Wylie, D. M. (2006). Leadership and leaders. In J. M. Hibberd & D. L. Smith (Eds.), *Nursing leadership and management in Canada* (pp. 369–394). Toronto, ON: Elsevier.

Hicks, F. (2003). Collective action. In P. S. Yoder-Wise (Ed.), *Leading and managing in nursing* (3rd ed., pp. 155–171). St. Louis, MO: Mosby.

Hinshaw, S. (2008). Navigating the perfect storm: Balancing a culture of safety with workforce challenges. *Nursing Research, 57*(1 Suppl.), S4–S10.

Keeling, B., Adair, J., Seider, D., & Kirksey, G. (2000). Appropriate delegation. *American Journal of Nursing, 100*(12), 24A, 24C–24D.

Kimball, B., Joynt, J., Cherner, D., & O'Neil, E. (2007). The quest for innovative care delivery models. *Journal of Nursing Administration, 9,* 392–398.

Manojlovich, M., Barnsteiner, J., Bolton, L. B., Disch, J., & Saint, S. (2008). Nursing practice and work environment issues in the 21st century: A leadership challenge. *Nursing Research, 57,* S11–S14.

Marriner Tomey, A. (2004). *Guide to nursing management and leadership* (7th ed.). St. Louis, MO: Mosby.

McGillis Hall, L. (Ed.). (2004). *Quality nurse environmenst for nurse and patient safety.* Sudbury, MA: Jones and Bartlett.

Neufeld, K. (2008, September 8). *Exercise your voice—Your right, your responsibility* [Open letter from the CNA president]. Retrieved September 30, 2008, from http://23072.vws.magma.ca/CNA/documents/pdf/publications/Open_Election_Letter_2008_e.pdf

Ogilvie, L., & Reutter, L. (2003). Primary health care: Complexities and possibilities from a nursing perspective. In J. C. Ross-Kerr & M. J. Wood (Eds.), *Canadian nursing: Issues and perspectives* (4th ed., pp. 441–465). Toronto, ON: Mosby.

Peters, D. A. (1995). Outcomes: The mainstay of a framework for quality care. *Journal of Nursing Care Quality, 10*(1), 61–69.

Quality Worklife Quality Health Care. (n.d.). *About us.* Retrieved September 30, 2008, from http://www.qwqhc.ca/about.aspx

Registered Nurses Association of British Columbia. (2003). *Quality practice environment program.* Vancouver, BC: Author.

Registered Nurses Association of Ontario. (2003). *A phenomenal journey: The Nursing Best Practice Guidelines Project: Shaping the future of nursing.* Toronto, ON: Author.

Registered Nurses Association of Ontario. (2006a, June). *Healthy work environments best practices guidelines: Developing and sustaining nursing leadership.* Toronto, ON: Author.

Registered Nurses Association of Ontario. (2006b, November). *Healthy work environments best practice guidelines: Collaborative practice among nursing teams.* Toronto, ON: Author.

Registered Nurses Association of Ontario. (2007a). *National Collaborative on Falls in Long-Term Care.* Retrieved September 30, 2008, from http://www.rnao.org/Storage/35/3013_Call_to_Action.pdf

Registered Nurses Association of Ontario. (2007b, January). *Falls prevention—Building the foundations for patient safety. Self-learning package.* Retrieved September 30, 2008, from http://www.rnao.org/Storage/26/2035_168_Falls_Self-LearningPackage_FINAL.pdf

Ritter-Teitel, J. (2002). The impact of restructuring on professional nursing practice. *Journal of Nursing Administration, 32*(1), 31–41.

Scott, J. G., Sochalski, J., & Aiken, L. (1999). Review of magnet hospital research: Findings and implications for professional nursing practice. *Journal of Nursing Administration, 29*(1), 9–19.

Senge, P. (2006). *The fifth discipline: The art and practice of the learning organization.* New York: Doubleday.

Silas, L. (2007). From promise to practice: Getting healthy work environments in health workplaces. *Healthcare Papers, 7,* 46–51.

Smith, D. L., Smith, J. E., Boechler, V., Giovannetti, P., & Lendrum, B. (2006). Structure and organization of nurses' work. In J. M. Hibberd & D. L. Smith (Eds.), *Nursing leadership and management in Canada* (pp. 199–237). Toronto, ON: Elsevier.

Sorrentino, S. (2004). *Mosby's Canadian textbook for the support worker.* Toronto, ON: Elsevier.

Spenceley, S. M., Reutter, L., & Allen, M. (2006). The road less traveled; Nursing advocacy at the policy level. *Policy, Politics and Nursing Practice, 7,* 180–194.

Tourangeau, A., Giovannetti, P., Tu, J., & Wood, M. (2002). Nursing-related determinants of 30-day mortality for hospitalized patients. *Canadian Journal of Nursing Research, 33*(4), 71–88.

Tschannen, D. (2004). The effect of individual characteristics on perceptions of collaboration in the work environment. *Medical Surgical Nursing, 13,* 312.

Vancouver Coastal Health Authority. (November, 2007). *Vancouver Acute Nursing Collaborative practice resource guide* [Unpublished resource guide]. Vancouver, BC: Author.

Wendt, D. A., & Vale, D. J. (2003). Managing quality and risk. In P. S. Yoder-Wise (Ed.), *Leading and managing in nursing* (3rd ed., pp. 173–189). St. Louis, MO: Mosby.

Wywialowski, E. (2004). *Managing client care* (3rd ed.). St. Louis, MO: Mosby.

Chapter 12

Benner, P. (1984). *From novice to expert: Excellence and power in clinical nursing practice.* Menlo Park, CA: Addison-Wesley.

Bilinski, H. (2002). The mentored journal. *Nursing Educator, 27,* 37–41.

Brunt, B. A. (2005a). Critical thinking in nursing: An integrated review. *Journal of Continuing Education in Nursing, 36,* 60–67.

Brunt, B. A. (2005b). Models, meaurement, and strategies in developing critical thinking skills. *Journal of Continuing Education in Nursing, 36,* 255–262.

Canadian Nurses Association. (2008). *Code of ethics for registered nurses.* Ottawa, ON: Author.

Di Vito-Thomas, P. (2005). Nursing student stories on learning how to think like a nurse. *Nurse Education, 30*(3), 133–136.

Facione, P. (1990). *Critical thinking: A statement of expert consensus for purposes of educational assessment and instruction. The Delphi report: Research findings and recommendations prepared for the American Philosophical Association* (ERIC Doc No. ED 315-423). Washington, DC: Educational Resources Information Center (ERIC).

Facione, N., & & Facione, P. (1996). Externalizing the critical thinking in knowledge development and clinical judgement. *Nursing Outlook, 44,* 129–136.

Ferrario, C. G. (2004). Developing nurses' critical thinking skills with concept mapping. *Journal for Nurses in Staff Development, 20,* 261–267.

Glaser, E. (1941). *An experiment in the development of critical thinking.* New York, NY: Bureau of Publications, Teachers College, Columbia University.

Hill, C. (2006). Integrating clinical experiences into the concept mapping process. *Nurse Educator, 31,* 36–39.

Ironside, P. M. (2005). Teaching thinking and reaching the limits of memorization: Enacting new pedagogies. *Journal of Nursing Education, 44,* 441–449.

Kataoka-Yahiro, M., & Saylor, C. (1994). A critical thinking model for nursing judgment. *Journal of Nursing Education, 33*(8), 351–356.

Kessler, P. D., & Lund, C. H. (2004). Reflective journalling: Developing an online journal for distance education. *Nurse Educator, 29,* 20–24.

Miller, M. A., & Malcolm, N. S. (1990). Critical thinking in the nursing curriculum. *Nursing and Health Care, 11,* 66–73.

Nielsen, A., Stragnell, S., & Jester, P. (2007). Guide for reflection using the clinical judgment model. *Journal of Nursing Education, 46,* 513–516.

Paul, R. W. (1993). The art of redesigning instruction. In J. Willsen & A. J. A. Blinker (Eds.), *Critical thinking: How to prepare students for a rapidly changing world.* Santa Rosa, CA: Foundation for Critical Thinking.

Perry, W. (1979). *Forms of intellectual and ethical development in the college years: A scheme.* New York, NY: Holt, Rinehart, & Winston.

Profetto-McGrath, J. (2003). The relationship of critical thinking skills and critical thinking dispositions of baccalaureate nursing students. *Journal of Advanced Nursing, 43*(6), 569–577.

Registered Nurses Association of Ontario. (n.d.). *Nursing best practice guidelines.* Retrieved September 9, 2008, from http://www.rnao.org/bestpractices/

Roche, J. P. (2002). A pilot study of teaching clinical decision making with the clinical educator model. *Journal of Nursing Education, 41,* 365–367.

Schuster, P. M. (2003). *Concept mapping: A critical thinking approach to care planning.* St. Louis, MO: Mosby.

Settersten, L., & Lauver, D. R. (2004). Critical thinking, perceived health status, and participation in health behaviors. *Nursing Research, 53,* 11–18.

Smith Higuchi, K. A., & Donald, J. G. (2002). Thinking processes used by nurses in clinical decision making. *Journal of Nursing Education, 41,* 145–153.

Tanner, C. (2006). Thinking like a nurse: A research-based model of clinical judgment in nursing. *Journal of Nursing Education, 45,* 204–211.

Tanner, C. A., Benner, P., Chesla, C., & Gordon, D. R. (1993). The phenomenology of knowing the patient. *Image: Journal of Nursing Scholarship, 25,* 273–280.

Watson, G., & Glaser, E. (1980). *Watson-Glaser critical thinking appraisal manual.* New York, NY: Macmillan.

White, A. H. (2003). Clinical decision making among fourth year nursing students: An interpretive study. *Journal of Nursing Education, 42,* 113–120.

Chapter 13

Benner, P., & Wrubel, J. (1989). *The primacy of caring.* Menlo Park, CA: Addison-Wesley.

Bulechek, G. M., Butcher, H. K., & Dochterman, J. M. (2008). *Nursing interventions classification (NIC)* (5th ed.). St. Louis, MO: Mosby.

Canadian Nurses Association. (2008). *Canadian registered nurse examination: Competencies.* Retrieved on September 12, 2008, from http://www.cna-aiic.ca/CNA/nursing/rnexam/competencies/default_e.aspx

Carpenito-Moyet, L. J. (2005). *Nursing diagnosis: Application to clinical practice* (11th ed.). Philadelphia, PA: Lippincott Williams & Wilkins.

Dochterman, J. M., & Jones, D. A. (2003). *Unifying nursing languages: The harmonization of NANDA, NIC, NOC.* Washington, DC: American Nurses Association.

Ferrario, C. G. (2004). Developing nurses' critical thinking skills with concept mapping. *Journal for Nurses in Staff Development, 20,* 261–267.

Fontana, D. (1993). *Managing time.* Leicester, UK: British Psychological Society.

Hendry, C., & Walker. A. (2004). Priority setting in clinical nursing practice: Literature review. *Journal of Advanced Nursing, 47,* 427–436.

Hinck, S. M., Webb, P., Simms-Giddens, S., Helton, C., Hope, K. L., Utley, R., et al. (2006). Student learning with concept mapping of care plans in community-based education. *Journal of Professional Nursing, 22*(1): 23–29.

Hsu, L., & Hsieh. S. (2005). Concept maps as an assessment tool in a nursing course. *Journal of Professional Nursing, 21,* 141–149.

Iowa Intervention Project. (1993). The NIC taxonomy structure. *Image—The Journal of Nursing Scholarship, 25,* 187–192.

King, M., & Shell, R. (2002). Teaching and evaluating critical thinking with concept maps. *Nurse Educator, 27,* 214–216.

Lunney, M. (1998). Accuracy of nurses' diagnoses: Foundation of NANDA, NIC, and NOC. *Nursing Diagnosis, 9*(2), 83–85.

Lunney, M. (2006). Helping nurses use NANDA, NOC, and NIC: Novice to expert. *Journal of Nursing Administration, 36*(3), 118–125.

McCaffery, M., & Pasero, C. (1999). *Pain: Clinical manual* (2nd ed.). St. Louis, MO: Mosby.

McCloskey, J. C., & Bulechek, G. M. (1994). Standardizing the language for nursing treatments: An overview of the issues. *Nurs Outlook, 42*(2), 56–63.

Moody, L. E., Slocumb, E., Berg, B., & Jackson, D. (2004). Electronic health records documentation in nursing: Nurses' perceptions, attitudes, and preferences. *Computers, Informatics, Nursing: CIN, 22,* 337–344.

Mueller, A., Johnston, M., & Bligh, D. (2002). Joining mind mapping and care planning to enhance student critical thinking and achieve holistic nursing care. *Nursing Diagnosis, 13*(1), 24–27.

NANDA International. (2007). *NANDA-I nursing diagnoses: Definitions and classification, 2007–2008,* Philadelphia, PA: Author.

Potter, P., Wolf, L., Boxerman, S., Grayson, D., Sledge, J., Dunagan, C., et al. (2005). Understanding the cognitive work of nursing in the acute care environment, *Journal of Nursing Administration, 35,* 327–335.

Redman, B. K. (2005). *The practice of patient education* (10th ed.). St. Louis, MO: Mosby.

Registered Nurses Association of Ontario. (2008). *Nursing best practice guidelines.* Retrieved September 19, 2008, from http://www.rnao.org/Page.asp?PageID=861&SiteNodeID=133

Schuster, P. M. (2003). *Concept mapping: A critical thinking approach to care planning.* St. Louis, MO: Mosby.

Seidel, H. M., Ball, J. W., Dains, J. E., & Benedict, S. W. (2003). *Mosby's guide to physical examination* (5th ed.). St. Louis, MO: Mosby.

University of Iowa College of Nursing. (2008). *Nursing Outcomes Classification.* Retrieved September 26, 2008, from http://www.nursing.uiowa.edu/excellence/nursing_knowledge/clinical_effectiveness/nocoverview.htm

White, L. (2003). *Documentation and the nursing process.* Clifton Park, NY: Delmar Learning.

Chapter 15

Bulechek, G. M., Butcher, H. K., & Dochterman, J. M. (2008). *Nursing Interventions Classification (NIC)* (5th ed.). St. Louis, MO: Mosby.

Canadian Pain Society. (2008). Retrieved October 8, 2008, from http://canadianpainsociety.ca/

Donabedian, A. (1980). Methods for deriving criteria for assessing the quality of medical care. *Medical Care Review, 37,* 653.

Moorhead, S., Johnson, M., & Maas, M. (2008). *Nursing outcomes classification (NOC)* (4th ed.). St. Louis, MO: Mosby.

NANDA International. (2007). *NANDA-I nursing diagnoses: Definitions and classification 2007–2008.* Philadelphia, PA: Author.

Registered Nurses Association of Ontario. (2008). *Nursing best practice guidelines.* Retrieved September 19, 2008, from http://www.rnao.org/Page.asp?PageID=861&SiteNodeID=133

Chapter 16

Canada Health Infoway. (2007). *Electronic health records: Transforming health care, improving lives* [Corporate Business Plan 2007-08]. Retrieved September 24, 2008, from http://www.infoway-inforoute.ca/Admin/Upload/Dev/Document/Business%20Plan_2007-08_EN.pdf

Cheevakasemsook, A., Chapman, Y., Francis, K., & Davies, C. (2006). The study of nursing documentation complexities. *International Journal of Nursing Practice, 12,* 366–374.

College of Nurses of Ontario. (2005). *Documentation* [Publication No. 41001]. Retrieved September 24, 2008, from http://www.cno.org/docs/prac/41001_documentation.pdf

Dy, S.M., Garg, P., Dawson, P. B., Pronovost, P. J., Morlock, L., Rubin, H., et al. (2005). Critical pathway effectiveness: Assessing the impact of patient, hospital care, and pathway characteristics using qualitative comparative analysis. *Health Services Research, 40,* 499–515.

Graves Ferrell, K. (2007). Documentation, Part 2: The best evidence of care. *American Journal of Nursing, 107*(7), 61–64.

Health Canada. (2007). *Electronic health record (EHR).* Retrieved September 24 2008, from http://www.hc-sc.gc.ca/hcs-sss/ehealth-esante/ehr-dse/index_e.HTML

Hebda, T. L., Czar, P., & Mascara, C. M. (2005). *Handbook of informatics for nurses & health care professionals.* New York: Pearson Prentice Hall.

Institute for Safe Medication Practices. (2007). *ISMP's list of error-prone abbreviations, symbols, and dose designations,* 8(24). Retrieved September 24, 2008, from http://www.ismp.org/PDF/ErrorProne.pdf

Karch, A. M. (2004). What's wrong with U? JCAHO places limits on abbreviations used in practice. *American Journal of Nursing, 104*(6), 65–66.

Leonard, M., Graham, S., & Bonacum, D., (2004). The human factor: The critical importance of effective teamwork and communication in providing safe care. *Quality and Safety in Health Care, 13,* 85–90.

Monarch, K. (2007). Documentation, Part 1: Principles for self protection. *American Journal of Nursing, 107*(7), 58–60.

Mosby's surefire documentation: How, what, and when nurses need to document. (2006). St. Louis, MO: Mosby.

Nurses Service Organization. (2008). *8 Common charting mistakes to avoid.* Retrieved September 24, 2008, from http://www.nso.com/nursing-resources/article/16.jsp

Scordo, K. A., Yeager, S., & Young, L. (2003). Use of personal digital assistants with acute care nurse practitioner students. *AACN Clinical Issues, 14,* 350–362.

Wolfstadt, J., Gurwitz, J., Field, T., Lee, M., Kalkar, S., Wu, W., et al. (2008). The effect of computerized physician order entry with clinical decision support on the rates of adverse drug events: A systematic review. *Journal of General Internal Medicine, 23,* 451–458.

Chapter 17

Alberta Association of Registered Nurses. (1994). *Client status, nursing intervention, and client outcome taxonomies: A background paper.* Edmonton, AB: Author.

Alvarez, D. (1993). Health information strategy. In Canadian Nurses Association (Ed.), *Papers from the Nursing Minimum Nursing Data Set Conference* (pp. 16–20). Ottawa, ON: Canadian Nurses Association.

American Nurses Association. (1994). *The scope of practice for nursing informatics.* Washington, DC: Author.

American Nurses Association Council on Computer Applications in Nursing. (1992). *Report on the designation of nursing informatics as a nursing specialty* [Congress of Nursing Practice unpublished report]. Washington, DC: American Nurses Association.

Ball, M. J., & Hannah, K. J. (1984). *Using computers in nursing.* Reston, VA: Reston Publishing.

Ball, M. J., Hannah, K. J., Newbold, S. K., & Douglas, J. V. (Eds.). (2000). *Nursing informatics: Where caring and technology meet* (3rd ed.). New York: Springer.

Canada Health Infoway (2004). *Electronic health record (EHR): Standards needs analysis.* Toronto, ON: Author.

Canada Health Infoway. (2007). *Infoway Standards Collaborative.* Retrieved October 3, 2008, from http://www.infoway-inforoute.ca/en/WhatWeDo/SCOverview.aspx

Canada Health Infoway. (2008a). 2015 advancing Canada's next generation of healthcare. Retrieved December 9, 2008, from http://www2.infoway-inforoute.ca/Documents/Vision_2015_Advancing_Canadas_next_generation_of_healthcare[1].pdf

Canada Health Infoway. (2008b). *Standards Collaborative: Enabling solutions, enhancing health outcomes . . . together.* Toronto, ON: Author.

Canadian Institute for Health Information. (2001, June). *Final report of the Canadian Enhancement of ICD-10 [International Statistical Classification of Diseases and Related Health Problems, tenth revision].* Ottawa, ON: Author.

Canadian Institute for Health Information. (2007). *CIHI—Taking health information further.* Retrieved October 3, 2008, from http://secure.cihi.ca/cihiweb/dispPage.jsp?cw_page=profile_e

Canadian Nurses Association. (2000). *Collecting data to reflect nursing impact: Discussion paper.* Ottawa, ON: Author.

Canadian Nurses Association. (2001a, September). What is nursing informatics and why is it so important? *Nursing Now, 11.* Retrieved October 5, 2008, from http://www.cna-nurses.ca/CNA/documents/pdf/publications/NursingInformaticsSept_2001_e.pdf

Canadian Nurses Association. (2001b). *Position statement: Collecting data to reflect the impact of nursing practice.* Ottawa, ON: Author.

Canadian Nurses Association. (2006a). *Nursing information and knowledge management.* Ottawa, ON: Author. Retrieved October 5, 2008, from http://cna-aiic.ca/CNA/documents/pdf/publications/PS87-Nursing-info-knowledge-e.pdf

Canadian Nurses Association (2006b). *E-nursing strategy for Canada.* Ottawa, ON: Author. Retrieved October 5, 2008, from http://www.cna-nurses.ca/CNA/documents/pdf/publications/E-Nursing-Strategy-2006-e.pdf

Canadian Nurses Association (2006c). *NurseONE.* Retrieved October 7, 2008, from http://www.cnaaiic.ca/CNA/documents/pdf/publications/Portal_Overview_2_e.pdf

Canadian Nurses Association. (2008a). *The code of ethics for registered nurses.* Ottawa, ON: Author.

Canadian Nurses Association. (2008b). *Mapping Canadian clinical outcomes in ICNP.* Ottawa, ON: Author.

Canadian Nursing Informatics Association. (2000, November 17). [November Board minutes.] Retrieved October 5, 2008, from http://www.cnia.ca/Minutes/minutes_nov_17_2000.doc

Canadian Organization for Advancement of Computers in Health. (2007). *Health informatics professional core competencies.* Retrieved October 5, 2008, from http://www.coachorg.com/default.asp?ID=822

Canadian Organization for Advancement of Computers in Health. (2008). *COACH: Canada's health informatics association.* Retrieved October 5, 2008, from http://www.coachorg.com/default.asp?ID=367

Clark, J. (1999). A language for nursing. *Nursing Standard, 13*(31), 42–47.

Clark, J., & Lang, N. M. (1992). Nursing's next advance: An international classification system for nursing practice. *International Nursing Review, 39*(4), 109–112, 128.

Giovannetti, P., Smith, D., & Broad, E. (1999). Structuring and managing health information. In J. Hibberd & D. Smith (Eds.), *Nursing management in Canada* (2nd ed., pp. 297–318). Toronto, ON: W.B. Saunders.

Goodwin, S., Matthews, S., Carr, H., Holubiec, I, Hitsman, C, & Cleator, N. (2008). Transforming home and community care. *Canadian Nurse, 104*(5), 30–31.

Government of Canada. (1983). *The Privacy Act. Bill C-21.* Retrieved October 7, 2008, from http://laws.justice.gc.ca/en/ShowFullDoc/cs/P-21///en

Government of Canada (2004). *Personal Information Protection and Electronic Documents Act.* Bill C-6. Retrieved December 2, 2008 from http://www.parl.gc.ca/PDF/36/2/parlbus/chambus/house/bills/government/C-6_4.pdf

Graves, J. R., & Corcoran, S. (1989). The study of nursing informatics. *Image: Journal of Nursing Scholarship, 21,* 227–231.

Hannah, K. J. (2005). Health informatics and nursing in Canada. *Healthcare Information Management and Communications, 19*(3), 45–51.

Hannah, K. J., Ball, M. J., & Edwards, M. J. A. (1994). *Introduction to nursing informatics.* New York: Springer-Verlag.

Hannah, K. J., Ball, M. J., & Edwards, M. J. A. (2006). *Introduction to nursing informatics* (3rd ed.). New York: Springer-Verlag.

International Council of Nurses. (2005). *International Classification for Nursing Practice®, Version 1.0.* Geneva, Switzerland: Author.

International Medical Informatics Association. (1998). *IMIA working groups. SIG NI nursing informatics.* Retrieved December 9, 2008, from http://www.imia.org/working_groups/WG_Profile.lasso?-Search=Action&-Table=CGI&-MaxRecords=1&-SkipRecords=15&-Database=organizations&-KeyField=Org_ID&-SortField=workgroup_sig&-SortOrder=ascending&type=wgsig

International Medical Informatics Association. (2004). *IMIA-NI is a supporting organisation for the HIMSS AsiaPac 2009 conference.* Retrieved October 7, 2008, from http://www.imiani.org/index.php?option=com_frontpage&Itemid=1

Kennedy, M. A. (2005). *Packaging nursing as politically potent: A critical reflexive cultural studies approach to nursing informatics.* Unpublished doctoral dissertation, University of South Australia, Adelaide, Australia.

Kennedy, M. A. (2008). *Mapping clinical outcomes in ICNP®. Version 1.0: The C-HOBIC project* (final report). Merigomish, NS: Kennedy Health Informatics Inc.

Kennedy, M. A., Hannah, K. J., & White, P. (2008). C-HOBIC: Mapping a path for Canada in nursing documentation. *Canadian Nurse, 104*(5), 27–29.

Marck, P. (1994). The problem with good nursing care . . . it is often invisible. *Alberta Association of Registered Nurses Newsletter, 50*(5), 10–11.

Marek, K., & Lang, N. (1993). Nursing sensitive outcomes. In Canadian Nurses Association (Ed.), *Papers from the Nursing Minimum Data Set Conference* (pp. 100–120). Ottawa, ON: Canadian Nurses Association.

McGee, M. (1993). Response to V. Saba's paper on nursing diagnostic schemes. In Canadian Nurses Association (Ed.), *Papers from the Nursing Minimum Data Set Conference* (pp. 64–67). Ottawa, ON: Canadian Nurses Association.

Mercer, C. (2008). The five Ws of clinical engagement. *Canadian Nurse, 104*(5), 9–10.

National Task Force on Health Information. (1991). Health information for Canada. In M. Wilk (Ed.), *Wilk report* [Unpublished report]. Ottawa, ON: National Health Information Council, Health Canada.

Norwood, S. (2001). NP education: The invisibility of advanced practice nurses in popular magazines. *Journal of the American Academy of Nurse Practitioners, 13*(3), 129–134.

O'Brien-Pallas, L., & Giovanetti, P. (1993). Nursing intensity. In Canadian Nurses Association (Ed.), *Papers from the Nursing Minimum Data Set Conference* (pp. 68–76). Ottawa, ON: Canadian Nurses Association.

Powers, P. (2001). The image of nursing in hospital promotional materials: A discourse analysis. *Scholarly Inquiry for Nursing Practice, 15*(2), 91–107.

Roch, J. (2008). Protecting health information is of paramount importance. *Canadian Nurse, 104*(5), 8.

Saba, V. K., & McCormick, K. A.(1986). *Essentials of computers for nurses.* Philadelphia, PA: Lippincott.

Saba, V. K., & McCormick, K. A. (Eds.). (1996). *Essentials of computers for nurses.* New York: McGraw-Hill.

Schwirian, P. (1986). The NI pyramid: A model for research in nursing informatics. *Computers in Nursing, 4*(3), 134–136.

Staggers, N., & Bagley Thompson, C. (2002). The evolution of definitions of nursing informatics: A critical analysis and revised definitions. *Journal of the American Medical Informatics Association, 9*(3), 255–262.

Tracey, P. (2008). Integrating a standardized assessment into acute care settings: One LHIN's approach. *Canadian Nurse, 104*(5), 25–26.

Turley, J. P. (1996). Toward a model of nursing informatics. *Image: Journal of Nursing Scholarship, 28*(1), 309–313.

Werley, H. H. (1988). Introduction to the nursing minimum data set and its development. In H. H. Werley & N. M. Lang (Eds.), *Identification of the nursing minimum data set* (pp. 1–15). New York: Springer.

Weyrauch, B. (2002). President's message: DNA joins alliance to increase nursing's visibility. *Dermatology Nursing, 14*(6), 356.

Zielstorff, R., Abraham, L., Werley, H., Saba, V. K., & Schwirian, P. (1990). Nursing information systems. *Computers in Nursing, 7*(5), 203–208.

Chapter 18

Adler, B., Towne, N., & Rolls, J. (2004). *Looking out: Looking in* (2nd Canadian ed.). Toronto, ON: Harcourt.

Apker, J., Propp, K. M., & Zabava Ford, W. (2006). *Journal of Professional Nursing,* 22, 130–189.

Arnold, E., & Boggs, K. (2007). *Interpersonal relationships: Professional communication skills for nurses* (5th ed.). St. Louis, MO: Saunders.

Balzer Riley, J. (2004). *Communication in nursing* (5th ed.). St. Louis, MO: Mosby.

Beebe, S. A., Beebe, S. J., Redmond, M. V., & Geerinck, T. B. (2004). *Interpersonal communication: Relating to others* (3rd Canadian ed.). Toronto, ON: Prentice Hall.

Burkhardt, M. A. & Nagai-Jacobson, M. G. (2002). *Spirituality: Living our connectedness.* Albany, NY: Delmar.

Canadian Association of Speech–Language Pathologists and Audiologists. (n.d.). *Speech, language and hearing fact sheet.* Retrieved October 8, 2008, from http://www.caslpa.ca/PDF/fact%20sheets/speechhearingfactsheet.pdf

Chauvet, S., & Hofmeyer, A. (2006). Humor as a facilitative style in problem-based learning environments for nursing students. *Nurse Education Today,* 27, 286–292.

Devito, J., Shimoni, R., & Clark, D. (2005). *Messages: Building interpersonal communication skills.* Toronto, ON: Pearson.

Doenges, M. E., Moorhouse, M. F., & Murr, A. C. (2005). *Nursing diagnosis manual: planning, individualizing, and documenting client care.* Philadelphia, PA: Davis.

Dubrin, J., & Geerinck, T. (2006). *Human relations: Interpersonal, job-oriented skills* (2nd Canadian ed.). Toronto, ON: Pearson.

Dziegielewski, S. F., Jacinto, G. A., Laudadio, A., & Legg-Rodriguez, L. (2004). Humor: An essential communication tool in therapy. *International Journal of Mental Health, 32*(3), 74–90.

Fahrenwald, N. L., Boysen, R. Fischer, C., & Maurer, R. (2001). Developing cultural competence in the baccalaureate nursing student: A population-based project with the Hutterites. *Journal of Transcultural Nursing, 12,* 48–55.

Feldman-Stewart, D., Brundage, M., & Tishelman, C. (2005). A conceptual framework for patient-professional communication: an application to the cancer context. *Psychooncology, 14,* 801–809.

Gleeson, M., & Timmins, F. (2004). Touch: a fundamental aspect of communication with older people experiencing dementia. *Nursing Older People, 16*(2), 13–21.

Goldfarb, R., & Santo Pietro, M. J. (2004). *Journal of Ambulatory Care Management, 27.* 356–365.

Grover, S. M. (2005). Shaping effective communication skills and therapeutic relationships at work: The foundation of collaboration. *American Association of Occupational Health Nurses Journal, 53,* 177–182.

Iezzoni, L. I., O'Day, B. L., Killeen, M., & Harker, H. (2004). Communicating about health care: Observations from persons who are deaf or hard of hearing. *Annals of Internal Medicine, 140,* 356–363.

Lane, M. R. (2006). Arts in health care: A new paradigm for holistic nursing practice. *Journal of Holistic Nursing, 24*(1), 70–75.

Larson, E. B., & Yao, X. (2005). Clinical empathy as emotional labor in the patient–physician relationship. *Journal of the American Medical Association, 293,* 1100–1106.

McCaffrey, R., & Fowler, N. L. (2003). Qigong practice: A pathway to health and healing. *Holistic Nursing Practice, 14,* 110–116.

Meador, H. E., & Zazove, P. (2005). Health care interactions with deaf culture. *The Journal of the American Board of Family Practice, 18,* 218–222.

Paul, R., & Elder, L. (2001). Critical thinking: Tools for taking charge of your learning and your life (2nd ed.). Upper Saddle River, NJ: Prentice Hall.

Shattell, M., & Hogan, B. (2005). Facilitating communication: How to truly understand what patients mean. *Journal of Psychosocial Nursing, 43*(10), 29–32.

Sheldon, L. K., Barrett, R., & Ellington, L. (2006). Difficult communication in nursing. *Journal of Nursing Scholarship, 38,* 141–147.

Shulman, N., & Haugo, Z. (2003). An overview of the science and practice of humor—HA! *Primary Care Reports, 9*(1), 1–7.

Spence, D. G. (2001). Prejudice, paradox, and possibility: Nursing people from cultures other than one's own. *Journal of Transcultural Nursing, 12,* 100–106.

Stanhope, M., & Lancaster, J. (2004). *Community and public health nursing* (6th ed.). St. Louis, MO: Mosby.

Stewart, J., & Logan, C. (2005). *Together: Communicating interpersonally* (5th ed.). Boston, MA: McGraw-Hill.

Stuart, G., & Laraia, M. (2005). *Principles and practice of psychiatric nursing* (8th ed.). St. Louis, MO: Mosby.

Sully, P., & Dallas, J. (2005). *Essential communication skills for nursing.* St. Louis, MO: Mosby.

Taylor, E. J. (2002). *Spiritual care. Nursing theory, research, and practice.* Upper Saddle River, NJ: Prentice Hall.

Townsend, M. (2005). *Psychiatric mental health nursing: Concepts of care* (5th ed.). Philadelphia, PA: Elsevier.

Wanzer, M., Booth-Butterfield, M., & Booth-Butterfield, S. (2005). "If we didn't use humor, we'd cry": Humorous coping communication in health care settings. *Journal of Health Communication, 10,* 105–125.

Williams, A. M., & Irurita, V. F. (2006). Emotional comfort: The patient's perspective of a therapeutic context. *International Journal of Nursing Studies, 43,* 405–415.

Williams, K., Kemper, S., & Hummert, L. (2004). Enhancing communication with older adults: Overcoming elderspeak. *Journal of Gerontological Nursing, 30*(10), 17–25.

Chapter 19

Attree, M. (2001). Patients' and relatives' experiences and perspectives of "good" and "not so good" quality care. *Journal of Advanced Nursing, 33,* 456–466.

Benner, P. (1984). *From novice to expert.* Menlo Park, CA: Addison-Wesley.

Benner, P. (2004). Relational ethics of comfort, touch, and solace—Endangered arts? *American Journal of Critical Care, 13,* 346–349.

Benner, P., & Wrubel, J. (1989). *The primacy of caring: Stress and coping in health and illness.* Menlo Park, CA: Addison Wesley.

Bernick, L. (2004). Caring for older adults: Practice guided by Watson's care-healing model. *Nursing Science Quarterly, 19,* 128–134.

Boyek, K., & Watson, R. (1994). A touching story. *Elderly Care, 3,* 20–21.

Boykin, A., Schoenhofer, S. O., Smith, N., St. Jean, J., & Aleman, D. (2003). Transforming practice using a caring-based nursing model. *Nursing Administration Quarterly, 27,* 223–230.

Bulfin, S. (2005). Nursing as caring theory: Living caring in nursing practice. *Nursing Science Quarterly, 18,* 313–319.

Campo, R. (1997). *The poetry of healing: A doctor's education in empathy, identification, and desire.* New York: W. W. Norton.

Canadian Nurses Association. (1997). *The code of ethics for registered nurses.* Ottawa, ON: Author.

Canadian Nurses Association. (2002). *Quality of worklife indicators for nurses in Canada: Workshop Report.* Ottawa, ON: Author.

Canadian Nurses Association. (2008). *The code of ethics for registered nurses.* Ottawa, ON: Author.

Cara, C. (2003). A pragmatic view of Jean Watson's caring theory. *International Journal for Human Caring,* 7(3), 51–61.

Chang, Y., Lin, Y. P., Chang, H. J., & Lin, C. C. (2005). Cancer patient and staff ratings of caring behaviors: Relationship to pain intensity, *Cancer Nursing, 28,* 331–339.

Cohen, M. Z., Hausner, J., & Johnson, M. (1994). Knowledge and presence: Accountability as described by nurses and surgical patients. *Journal of Professional Nursing, 3,* 177–185.

Cook, P. R., & Cullen, J. A. (2003). Caring as an imperative for nursing education, *Nursing Perspectives, 24,* 192–197.

Fareed, A. (1996). The experience of reassurance: Patients' perspectives. *Journal of Advanced Nursing, 23,* 272–279.

Frank, A. W. (1998). Just listening: Narrative and deep illness. *Family, Systems and Health, 16,* 197–212.

Fredriksson, L. (1999). Modes of relating in a caring conversation: A research synthesis on presence, touch, and listening. *Journal of Advanced Nursing, 30,* 1167–1196.

Gerteis, M., Edgman-Levitan, S., Walker, J. D., Stoke, D. M., Cleary, P. D., & Delbanco, T. L. (1993). What patients really want. *Health Management Quarterly, 15,* 2–6.

Gilje, F. (1997). Presence: US–Norway nursing research perspectives. In J. K. Hummelvoll & U. A. Lindström (Eds.), *Nordiska perspektiv på psykiatrisk omvårdnad [Nordic perspectives on psychiatric nursing].* Lund, Sweden: Studentlitteratur.

Hoover, J. (2002). The personal and professional impact of undertaking an educational module on human caring. *Journal of Advanced Nursing, 37,* 79–86.

Kemper, B. J. (1992). Therapeutic listening: Developing the concept. *Journal of Psychosocial Nursing and Mental Health Services, 7,* 21–23.

Lamb, G. S., & Stempel, J. E. (1994). Nurse case management from the client's view: Growing as insider-expert. *Nursing Outlook, 42*(7), 7–13.

Leininger, M. (1978). *Transcultural nursing: Concepts, theories and practices.* New York: John Wiley & Sons.

Leininger, M. (1988). *Care: The essence of nursing and health.* Detroit, MI: Wayne State University Press.

Lesniak, R. (2005). Caring through technological competency. *Journal of School Nursing, 21*(4), 194–195.

Mayer, D. K. (1986). Cancer patients' and families' perceptions of nurse caring behaviors. *Topics in Clinical Nursing, 8*(2), 63–69.

Mayer, D. K. (1987). Oncology nurses' versus cancer patients' perceptions of nurse caring behaviors: A replication study. *Oncology Nursing Forum, 14*(3), 48–52.

Pederson, C. (1993). Presence as a nursing intervention with hospitalized children. *Maternal-Child Nursing Journal, 3,* 75–81.

Pusari, N. D. (1998). Eight "Cs" of caring: A holistic framework for nursing terminally ill patients. *Contemporary Nurse, 7,* 156–160.

Radwin, L. (1995). Knowing the patient: A process model for individualized interventions. *Nursing Research, 44,* 364–370.

Radwin, L. (2000). Oncology patients' perceptions of nursing care. *Research in Nursing & Health, 23,* 179–190.

Radwin, L., Farquhar, S., Knowles, M., & Virchick, B. (2005). Cancer patients' descriptions of their nursing care. *Journal of Advanced Nursing, 50,* 162–169.

Registered Nurses Association of Ontario (2006). *Client centred care* (rev. suppl.). Toronto, ON: Author.

Roach, S. (1992). *The human act of caring. A blueprint for the health professions.* Ottawa, ON: Canadian Hospital Association.

Roach, S. (1997). *Caring from the heart: The convergence of caring and spirituality.* Mahwah, NJ: Paulist Press.

Storch, J. L. (2007). Enduring values in changing times: The CNA codes of ethics. *Canadian Nurse, 103*(4), 29–34.

Swanson K. (1991). Empirical development of a middle-range theory of caring. *Nursing Research, 40,* 161–166.

Swanson, K. (1999). Effects of caring, measurement, and time on miscarriage impact and women's well being. *Nursing Research, 48,* 288–298.

Tarlier D. S. (2004). Beyond caring: The moral and ethical bases of responsive nurse–patient relationships. *Nursing Philosophy, 5,* 230–241.

Tanner, C., Benner, P., Chesla, C., & Gordon, D. R. (1993). The phenomenology of knowing the patient. *Image—The Journal of Nursing Scholarship, 25,* 273–280.

Tommasini, N. R. (1990). The use of touch with the hospitalized psychiatric patient. *Archives of Psychiatric Nursing, 4,* 213–220.

Watson, J. (1979). *Nursing: The philosophy and science of caring.* Boston: Little, Brown.

Watson, J. (2006a). Can an ethic of caring be maintained? *Journal of Advanced Nursing, 15,* 125.

Watson, J. (2006b). Caring theory as an ethical guide to administrative and clinical practices. *Nursing Administration Quarterly, 30,* 48–55.

Watson, J. (2008). *Nursing: The philosophy and science of caring* (rev. ed.). Boulder, CO: University of Colorado Press.

Watson, J., & Foster, R. (2003). The Attending Nurse Caring Model: Integrating theory, evidence and advanced caring–healing therapeutics for transforming professional practice. *Journal of Clinical Nursing, 12,* 360–365.

Watson, M. J. (1988). New dimensions of human caring theory. *Nursing Science Quarterly, 1,* 175–181.

Williams, S. A. (1997). The relationship of patients' perceptions of holistic nurse caring to satisfaction with nursing care. *Journal of Nursing Care Quality, 11*(5), 15–29.

Wolf, Z. R., Miller, P. A., & Devine, M. (2003). Relationship between nurse caring and patient satisfaction in patients undergoing invasive cardiac procedures. *Medsurg Nursing, 12,* 391.

Chapter 20

Astedt-Kurki, P., Tarkka, M. D., Paavilainen, E., & Lehti, K. (2002). Development and testing of a family nursing scale. *Western Journal of Nursing Research, 24,* 567–579.

Baumann, S. L. (2006). The researcher–person–family process. *Nursing Science Quarterly, 19*(1), 14–18.

Bell, J. M., Swan, N. K. W., Taillon, C., McGovern, G., & Dorn, J. (2001). Learning to nurse the family [Editorial]. *Journal of Family Nursing, 7,* 117–126.

Black, K., & Lobo, M. (2008). A conceptual review of family resilience factors. *Journal of Family Nursing, 14,* 33–55.

Bohn, U., Wright, L. M., & Moules, N. J. (2003). A family systems nursing interview following a myocardial infarction: The power of commendations. *Journal of Family Nursing, 9,* 151–165.

Canadian Nurses Association. (1997, September). The family connection. *Nursing Now* (No. 3). Retrieved October 20, 2008, from http://cna-aiic.ca/CNA/documents/pdf/publications/FamilyConnection_Sept1997_e.pdf

Carruth, A. K. (1996). Development and testing of the Caregiver Reciprocity Scale. *Nursing Research, 45,* 92–97.

Carter, B., & McGoldrick, M. (Eds.). (1999). *The expanded family life cycle: Individual, family and social perspectives* (3rd ed.). Boston: Allyn & Bacon.

Castellano, M. B. (2002). Aboriginal family trends: Extended families, nuclear families, families of the heart. Ottawa, ON: Vanier Institute of the Family. Retrieved on October 20, 2008, from http://www.vifamily.ca/library/cft/aboriginal.HTML

Dryburgh, H. (2000). Teenage pregnancy. *Health Reports, 12*(1), Catalogue No. 82-003. Retrieved October 20, 2008, from http://www.statcan.ca/english/kits/preg/preg3.htm

Feeley, N., & Gottlieb, L. N. (2000). Nursing approaches for working with family strengths and resources. *Journal of Family Nursing, 6,* 9–24.

Ford-Gilboe, M. (2002). Developing knowledge about family health promotion by testing the developmental model of health and nursing. *Journal of Family Nursing, 8,* 140–156.

Hartrick, G. (2000). Developing health-promoting practice with families: One pedagogical experience. *Journal of Advanced Nursing, 3,* 27–34.

Harvey, E. (1999). Short-term and long-term effects of early parental employment on children: The National Longitudinal Survey of Youth. *Developmental Psychology, 35,* 445–459.

Hill, R. (2003). Generic features of families under stress. In P. Boss & C. Milligan (Eds.), *Family stress: Classic and contemporary readings* (pp. 177–190). Thousand Oaks, CA: Sage (Original work published 1958).

Hougher Limacher, L. (2003). *Commendations: The healing potential of one family systems nursing intervention.* Unpublished doctoral thesis, University of Calgary, Calgary, AB.

Hougher Limacher, L., & Wright, L. M. (2003). Commendations: Listening to the silent side of a family intervention. *Journal of Family Nursing, 9,* 130–135.

Hunt, C. K. (2003). Concepts in caregiver research. *Journal of Nursing Scholarship, 35,* 27–32.

Isaksen, A. S., Thuen, F., & Hanestad, B. (2003). Patients with cancer and their close relatives: Experiences with treatment, care, and support. *Cancer Nursing, 26,* 68–74.

Leahey, M., & Harper-Jaques, S. (1996). Family-nurse relationships: Core assumptions and clinical implications. *Journal of Family Nursing, 2,* 133–151.

Leahey, M., Harper-Jaques, S., Stout, L., & Levac, A. M. (1995). The impact of a family systems nursing approach: Nurses' perceptions. *Journal of Continuing Education in Nursing, 26,* 219–225.

Levac, A. M. C., Wright, L. M., & Leahey, M. (2002). Children and families: Models for assessment and intervention. In J. Fox (Ed.), *Primary health care of infants, children, and adolescents* (2nd ed., pp. 10–19). St. Louis, MO: Mosby.

McCubbin, M. A., McCubbin, H. I., & Thompson, A. I. (1996). Family Hardiness Index (FHI). In H. I. McCubbin, A. I. Thompson, & M. S. McCubbin (Eds.), *Family assessment: Resiliency, coping, and adaptation, inventories for research and practice.* Madison, WI: University of Wisconsin Press.

McGoldrick, M., & Carter, E. (1982). The stages of the family life cycle. In Walsh, F. (Ed.), *Normal family processes.* New York: Guilford Press.

McLeod, D. L. (2003). *Opening space for the spiritual: Therapeutic conversations with families living with serious illness.* Unpublished doctoral dissertation, University of Calgary, Calgary, AB.

Moules, N. J. (2002). Nursing on paper: Therapeutic letters in nursing practice. *Nursing Inquiry, 9*(2), 104–113.

Neabel, B., Fothergill-Bourbonnais, F., & Dunning, J. (2000). Family assessment tools: A review of the literature from 1978–1997. *Heart & Lung, 29,* 196–209.

Nichols, M. P. (1995). *The lost art of listening.* New York: Guilford Press.

Picot, S. J. F., Youngblut, J., & Zeller, R. (1997). Development and testing of a measure of perceived caregiver rewards in adults. *Journal of Nursing Measurement, 5,* 33–52.

Robinson, C. A. (1998). Women, families, chronic illness, and nursing interventions: From burden to balance. *Journal of Family Nursing, 4,* 271–290.

Schober, M., & Affara, F. (2001). *The family nurse: Frameworks for practice.* Geneva, Switzerland: International Council of Nurses.

Statistics Canada. (2002). *Canadian families and households.* Retrieved October 20, 2008, from http://www12.statcan.ca/english/census01/Products/Analytic/companion/fam/canada.cfm

Statistics Canada. (2003a, December 9). Grandparents and grandchildren: 2001. *The Daily* (Catalogue No. 11-001-XIE). Retrieved October 20, 2008, from http://www.statcan.ca/Daily/English/031209/d031209b.htm

Statistics Canada. (2003b). *Income of Canadian families.* Retrieved October 20, 2008, from http://www12.statcan.ca/english/census01/Products/Analytic/companion/inc/canada.cfm

Statistics Canada. (2004, May 4). Divorces: 2001 and 2002. *The Daily* (Catalogue No. 11-001-XIE). Retrieved October 20, 2008, from http://www.statcan.ca/Daily/English/040504/d040504a.htm

Statistics Canada. (2007a, July 17). 2006 Census: Age and sex. *The Daily.* Retrieved on October 20, 2008, from http://www.statcan.ca/Daily/English/070717/d070717a.htm

Statistics Canada. (2007b, September 12). 2006 Census: Families, marital status, households and dwelling characteristics. *The Daily.* Retrieved on October 20, 2008, from http://www.statcan.ca/Daily/English/070912/d070912a.htm

Statistics Canada. (2007c, January 15). Aboriginal peoples in Canada in 2006: Inuit, Métis and First Nations, 2006 census. *The Daily.* Retrieved on October 20, 2008, from http://www.statcan.ca/Daily/English/080115/d080115a.htm

Statistics Canada. (2007d). *Aboriginal peoples in Canada in 2006: Inuit, Métis and First Nations, 2006 census.* Retrieved on October 20, 2008, from http://www12.statcan.ca/English/Census06/analysis/aboriginal/children.cfm

Statistics Canada. (2007e, May 29). Family income: 2005. *The Daily.* Retrieved October 20, 2008, from http://www.statcan.ca/Daily/English/070529/d070529e.htm

Stuart, M. (1991). An analysis of the concept of family. In A. Whall & J. Fawcett (Eds.), *Family theory development in nursing: State of the science and art* (pp. 31–42). Philadelphia, PA: F. A. Davis.

Svavarsdottir, E. K., McCubbin, M. A., & Kane, J. H. (2000). Well-being of parents of young children with asthma. *Research in Nursing & Health, 23,* 346–358.

Tapp, D. M. (2001). Conserving the vitality of suffering: Addressing family constraints to illness conversations. *Nursing Inquiry, 8,* 254–263.

Tomm, K. (1987). Interventive interviewing: Part II. Reflexive questioning as a means to enable self-healing. *Family Process, 26,* 167–183.

Tomm, K. (1988). Interventive interviewing: Part III. Intending to ask lineal, circular, strategic or reflexive questions? *Family Process, 27,* 1–15.

The Vanier Institute of the Family. (2000). *Profiling Canada's families II.* Nepean, ON: Author.

Wright, L. M. (2004). *Spirituality, suffering, and illness: Ideas for healing.* Philadelphia, PA: F. A. Davis.

Wright, L. M., & Leahey, M. (2005). *Nurses and families: A guide to family assessment and intervention* (4th ed). Philadelphia, PA: F. A. Davis.

Wright, L. M., & Nagy, J. (1993). Death: The most troublesome family secret of all. In E. I. Black (Ed.), *Secrets in families and family therapy* (pp. 121–137). New York: W. W. Norton.

Wright, L. M., Watson, W. L., & Bell, J. M. (1996). *Beliefs: The heart of healing in families and illness.* New York: Basic Books.

Chapter 21

Bandura, A. (1997). *Self-efficacy: The exercise of control.* New York: W. H. Freeman.

Bandura, A. (2001). Social cognitive theory: An agentic perspective. *Annual Review of Psychology, 52,* 1–26.

Bastable, S. (2003). *Nurse as educator: Principles of teaching and learning for nursing practice.* Sudbury, MA: Jones & Bartlett.

Bastable, S. (2006). *Essentials of patient education.* Sudbury, MA: Jones & Bartlett.

Bloom, B. S. (Ed.). (1956). *Taxonomy of educational objectives: The classification of educational goals: Vol. 1. Cognitive domain.* New York: Longman.

Canadian Nurses Association. (2003, September). Primary health care—The time has come. *Nursing Now: Issues and Trends in Nursing, 16,* 1–4.

Canadian Nurses Association. (2008). *Code of ethics for registered nurses.* Ottawa, ON: Author.

Cutilli, C. C. (2005). Do your patients understand? Determining your patients' health literacy skills. *Orthopaedic Nursing, 24,* 372–379.

Cutilli, C. C. (2006). Do your patients understand? Providing culturally congruent patient education. *Orthopaedic Nursing, 25,* 218–226.

Demir, F., Ozsaker, E. & Ilce, A. O. (2008). The quality and suitabilty of written materials for patients, *Journal of Clinical Nursing, 17,* 259–265.

DiClemente, D., Prochaska, J., Velicer, W., Fairhurst, S., Rossi, J., & Velasquez, M. (1991). The process of smoking cessation: An analysis of precontemplation, contemplation and preparation stages of change. *Journal of Consulting and Clinical Psychology, 59,* 295–304.

Edelman, C. L., & Mandle, C. L. (2006). *Health promotion throughout the life-span* (6th ed.). St. Louis, MO: Mosby.

Falvo, D. R. (2004). *Effective patient teaching: A guide to increased compliance* (3rd ed.). Sudbury, MA: Jones & Barlett.

Heading, G. (2008). Rural obesity, healthy weight and perceptions of risk: Struggles, strategies and motivation to change. *Australian Journal of Rural Health, 16*(2), 86–91.

Krathwohl, D. R., Bloom, B. S., & Masia, B. B. (1964). *Taxonomy of educational objectives: The classification of educational goals: Handbook 2. Affective domain.* New York: David McKay.

Kübler-Ross, E. (1969). *On death and dying.* New York: Macmillan.

Kutzleb, J., & Reiner, D. (2006). The impact of nurse-directed patient education on quality of life and functional capacity in people with heart failure. *Journal of the American Academy of Nurse Practitioners, 18*(3), 116–123.

Learning Disabilities Association of Canada. (2002). *Official definition of learning disabilities.* Retrieved October 23, 2008, from http://www.ldac-taac.ca/Defined/defined_new-e.asp

Mennies, J. (2001). Teaching adult patients with learning disabilities. *Nursing Spectrum, 14*(21), 20.

Pender, N. J., Murdaugh, C. L., & Parsons, M. A. (2006). *Health promotion in nursing practice* (5th ed.). Upper Saddle River, NJ: Prentice Hall.

Prochaska, J. C., & DiClemente, C. C. (1992). Stages of change in the modification of problem behaviors. In M. Hersen, R. M. Eisler, & P. M. Miller (Eds.), *Progress in behaviour modification* (pp. 184–218). Newbury Park, CA: Sage.

Rankin, S. M., & Stallings, K. D. (2005). *Patient education in health and illness* (5th ed.). Philadelphia, PA: Lippincott Williams & Wilkins.

Redman, B. K. (2005). The ethics of self-management preparation for chronic illness. *Nursing Ethics, 12,* 360–369.

Redman, B. K. (2007). *The practice of patient education* (10th ed.). St. Louis, MO: Mosby.

Saarmann, L., Daugherty, J., & Riegel, B. (2002). Teaching staff a brief cognitive–behavioral intervention. *Medsurg Nursing, 11*, 144–151.

Sand-Jecklin, K. (2007). The impact of medical terminology on readability of patient education materials. *Journal of Community Health Nursing, 24*, 119–129.

Statistics Canada & Organisation for Economic Co-operation and Development. (2005). *Learning a living: First results of the Adult Literacy and Life Skills Survey.* Ottawa, ON: Statistic Canada. Retrieved October 23, 2008, from http://www.statcan.ca/english/freepub/89-603-XIE/2005001/pdf/89-603-XWE-part1.pdf

Wendell, I., Durso, S. C., Zable, B., Loman, K., & Remsburg, R. E. (2003). Group diabetes patient education: A model for use in a continuing care retirement community. *Journal of Gerontological Nursing, 29*(2), 37–44.

Wingard R. (2005). Patient education and the nursing process: Meeting the patient's needs. *Nephrology Nursing, 32*, 211–215.

Chapter 22

Ainsworth, M. D. S. (1979). Infant–mother attachment. *American Psychologist, 34*, 932–937.

Berk, L. (2006). *Child development* (7th ed.). Boston, MA: Allyn & Bacon.

Berk, L. (2008). *Exploring lifespan development*. Boston, MA: Allyn & Bacon.

Bukatko, D., & Daehler, M. (2004). *Child development: A thematic approach* (5th ed.). Boston, MA: Houghton Mifflin.

Bornstein, M., & Lamb, M. (1999). *Developmental psychology: An advanced textbook* (4th ed.). Hillsdale, NJ: Lawrence Erlbaum.

Cavanaugh, J. C., & Blanchard-Fields, F. (2006). *Adult development and aging* (5th ed.). Boston, MA: Wadsworth.

Chess, S., & Thomas, A. (1995). *Temperament in clinical practice*. New York: Guilford Press.

Cicchetti, D. (Ed.) (2007). Gene–environmental interactions [Special issue]. *Development and Psychopathology, 19*(4), 957-1195.

Cicchetti, D., & Curtis, W. J. (Eds.). (2007). A multilevel approach to resilience [Special issue]. *Development and Psychopathology, 19*(3), 627-955.

Crain, W. (2005). *Theories of development: Concepts and applications* (5th ed.). Englewood Cliffs, NJ: Prentice Hall.

Crittenden, P. (2008). *Raising parents: Attachment, parenting and child safety*. Portland, OR: Willan Publishing.

Crittenden, P., & Clausen, A. (Eds.). (2003). *The organization of attachment relationships. Maturation, culture, and context.* Philadelphia, PA: Cambridge University Press.

Cynader, M., & Frost, B. (1999). Mechanisms of brain development: Neuronal sculpting by the physical and social environment. In D. Keating & C. Hertzman (Eds.), *Developmental health and the wealth of nations: Social, biological, and educational dynamics* (pp. 153–185). New York: Guilford Press.

Drummond, J., Kysela, G. M., McDonald, L., Alexander, J., & Fleming, D. (1996–1997). Risk and resiliency in two samples of Canadian families. *Health and Canadian Society, 4*(1), 117–152.

Edelman, C., & Mandle, C. (2006). *Health promotion throughout the lifespan* (6th ed.). St. Louis, MO: Mosby.

Erikson, E. (1993). *Childhood and society*. New York: W. W. Norton.

Erikson, E. (1997). *The lifecycle completed*. New York: W. W. Norton.

Gesell, A. (1948). *Studies in child development*. New York: Harper.

Gilligan, C. (1982). *In a different voice: Psychological theory and women's development*. Cambridge, MA: Harvard University Press.

Gould, R. L. (1972). The phases of adult life: A study in developmental psychology. *American Journal of Psychiatry, 129*, 521–531.

Hartup, W. (2002). *Growing points in developmental science: An introduction*. New York: Psychology Press.

Hockenberry, M. J., & Wilson, D. (2007). *Wong's nursing care of infants and children* (8th ed.). St. Louis, MO: Mosby.

Kail, R. (2002). *Advances in child development and behaviour* (Vol. 32). Burlington, MA: Elsevier.

Keating, D., & Hertzman, C. (1999). *Developmental health and the wealth of nations: Social, biological, and educational dynamics*. New York: Guilford Press.

Kliegman, R., Behrman, R., Jensen, H., & Stanton, B. (2007). *Nelson textbook of pediatrics* (18th ed.). Philadelphia, PA: W. B. Saunders.

Kohlberg, L. (1981). *The philosophy of moral development: Moral stages and the idea of justice*. San Francisco: Harper & Row.

Letourneau, N., Drummond, J., Fleming, D., Kysela, G., McDonald, L., & Stewart, M. (2001). Supporting parents: Can intervention improve parent–child relationships? *Journal of Family Nursing, 7*, 159–187.

McCain, M., Mustard, F., & Shanker, S. (2007). *Early years study 2: Putting science into action*. Toronto, ON: Council for Early Child Development.

Middlebrooks, J., & Audage, N. C. (2008). *The effects of childhood stress on health across the lifespan*. Atlanta, GA: US Department of Health and Human Services, Centers for Disease Control and Prevention.

Mustard, J. F. (2006). *Early child development and experience-based brain development: The scientific underpinnings of the importance of early child development in a globalized world.* Toronto, ON: The Brookings Institute.

Nelson, C., de Haan, M., & Thomas, K. (2006). *Neuroscience of cognitive development: The role of experience and the developing brain*. Hoboken, NJ: John Wiley & Sons.

Salkind, N. (2004). *An introduction to theories of human development*. Thousand Oaks, CA: Sage.

Singer, D. G., & Revenson, T. A. (1996). *A Piaget primer: How a child thinks*. New York: Penguin Books.

Smylie, J. (2000). A guide for health professionals working with Aboriginal peoples: The sociocultural context of Aboriginal peoples in Canada. *Journal SOGC*, 22, 1070–1081.

Smylie, J. (2001, January). A guide for health professionals working with Aboriginal peoples: Health issues affecting Aboriginal peoples. *Journal SOGC* (100), 1–15.

Sumner, G. (1995). Keys to caregiving: A new NCAST program for health care providers and parents of newborns. *Zero to Three, 5*, 33–35.

Thomas, R. M. (1997). *Moral development theories: Secular and religious—A comparative study*. Westport, CT: Greenwood Press.

Chapter 23

Behrman, R., Kliegman, R., & Jenson, H. (2008). *Nelson textbook of pediatrics* (18th ed.). Philadelphia, PA: W. B. Saunders.

Campaign 2000. (2007). *2007 Report card on child and family poverty in Canada: It takes a nation to raise a generation: Time for a national poverty reduction strategy.* Retrieved October 30, 2008, from http://www.campaign2000.ca/rc/rc07/2007_C2000_NationalReportCard.pdf

Canadian Centre on Substance Abuse. (2007). *Substance abuse in Canada: Youth in focus*. Ottawa, ON: Author.

Canadian consensus statement. (2007, Revised). Comprehensive school health. Retrieved December 21, 2008, from http://www.safehealthyschools.org/CSH_Consensus_Statement2007.pdf

Canadian Paediatric Society (1996). *Clinical practice guidelines.Neonatal circumcision revisited* (Ref. No. FN96-01). Retrieved October 30, 2008, from http://www.cps.ca/english/statements/ FN/fn96-01.htm

Edelman, C., & Mandle, C. (2006). *Health promotion throughout the life span* (6th ed.). St. Louis, MO: Mosby Elsevier.

Erikson, E. H. (1963). *Childhood and society* (2nd ed.). New York: W. W. Norton.

Erikson, E. H. (1968). *Identity: Youth and crises*. New York: W. W. Norton.

Gilligan, C. (1982). In a different voice: Psychological theory and women's development. Cambridge, MA: Harvard University Press.

Greaves, L., Johnson, J., Bottorff, J., Kirkland, S., Jategaonkar N., McGowan, M., et al. (2006). What are the effects of tobacco policies on vulnerable populations? A better practice review. *Canadian Journal of Public Health, 97*, 310–315.

Health Canada. (1999). *Nutrition for a healthy pregnancy—National guidelines for the childbearing years* (Catalogue No. H39-459/1999E). Ottawa, ON: Author. Retrieved October 30, 2008, from http://www.hc-sc.gc.ca/fn-an/nutrition/prenatal/national_guidelines_cp-lignes_directrices_nationales_pc-eng.php

Health Canada. (2001). *Folic acid: A preconceived notion* [Pamphlet]. Retrieved October 30, 2008, from http://www.phac-aspc.gc.ca/fa-af/pamphlet-eng.php

Health Canada. (2002). *A report on mental illness in Canada*. Ottawa, ON: Author.

Health Canada. (2004). *Exclusive breastfeeding duration: 2004 Health Canada recommendation* (Catalogue No. H44-73/2004E). Ottawa, ON: Author. Retrieved October 30, 2008, from http://www.hc-sc.gc.ca/fn-an/nutrition/child-enfant/infant-nourisson/excl_bf_dur-dur_am_excl-eng.php

Health Canada. (2006). *Is your child safe? Consumer product safety*. Retrieved April 17, 2008 from http://www.hc-sc.gc.ca/home-accueil/contact/pubs-eng.php

Health Canada. (2007). *Eating well with Canada's food guide* (Catalogue No. H164-38/1-2007E). Ottawa, ON: Author.

Herman, M., & Le, A. (2007). The crying infant. *Emergency Medicine Clinics of North America, 25*, 1137–1159.

Hockenberry, M. J., & Wilson, D. (2007). *Wong's nursing care of infants and children* (8th ed.). St. Louis, MO: Mosby.

KidsHealth. (2007). *Backpack safety*. Retrieved October 30, 2008, from http://kidshealth.org/parent/positive/learning/backpack.HTML

Kingston, D., Dennis, C-L., & Sword, W. (2007). Exploring breast-feeding self-efficacy. *Journal of Perinatal and Neonatal Nursing, 21*, 207–215.

Kohlberg, L. (1964). Development of moral character and moral ideology. In M. L. Hoffman & L. N. W. Hoffman (Eds.), *Review of child development research* (Vol. 1). New York: Russell Sage Foundation.

Knowledge Network (n.d.) *Making it happen: Healthy eating at school*. Burnaby, BC: Author. Retrieved October 29, 2008, from http://www.knowledgenetwork.ca/news/2005/feb2005/Making%20It%20Happen.pdf

Leitch, K. (2007). *Reaching for the top: A report by the advisor on healthy children and youth* (Catalogue No. H21-296/207E). Ottawa, ON: Health Canada.

MacNeil, M. S. (2008). An epidemiologic study of aboriginal adolescent risk in Canada: The meaning of suicide. *Journal of Child and Adolescent Psychiatric Nursing, 21*, 3–12.

Mitchinson, W. (2002). *Giving birth in Canada 1900–1950*. Toronto, ON: University of Toronto Press.

Murray, S., & McKinney, E.S. (2006). *Foundations of maternal-newborn nursing* (4th ed.). Philadelphia, PA: Saunders

Pan, S. Y., Desmeules, M., Morrison, H., Semenciw, R., Ugnat, A. M., Thompson, W., et al. (2007). Adolescent injury deaths and hospitalization in Canada: Magnitude and temporal trends (1979–2003). *Journal of Adolescent Health, 41*, 84–92.

Petch, J., & Halford, W.K. (2008). Psycho-education to enhance couples' transition to parenthood. *Clinical Psychology Review, 28*, 1125–1137

Piaget, J. (1952). *The origins of intelligence in children*. New York: International Universities Press.

Pickett, W., Molcho, M., Simpson, K., Janssen, I., Kuntsche, E., Mazur, J., et al. (2005). Cross national study of injury and social determinants in adolescents. *Injury Prevention, 11*, 213–218.

Public Health Agency of Canada. (2002). *Sudden infant death syndrome (SIDS)*. Retrieved on December 21, 2008, from http://www.phac-aspc.gc.ca/dca-dea/prenatal/sids-js-eng.php

Public Health Agency of Canada. (1999b). *Healthy development of children and youth: The role of the determinants of health* (Catalogue No. H39-501/1999E). Ottawa, ON: Author. Retrieved October 30, 2008, from http://www.phac-aspc.gc.ca/dca-dea/publications/healthy_dev_overview_e.HTML

Public Health Agency of Canada. (2006). *Canadian immunization guide: Seventh edition—2006*. Retrieved October 30, 2008, from http://www.phac-aspc.gc.ca/publicat/cig-gci/index-eng.php

Public Health Agency of Canada. (2007). Human papillomavirus (HPV). Retrieved December 21, 2008, from http://www.hc-sc.gc.ca/hl-vs/iyh-vsv/diseases-maladies/hpv-vph-eng.php

Safe Kids Canada (n.d.). *Children's rural safety* [Pamphlet]. Retrieved October 20, 2008, from http://www.sickkids.ca/SKCForPartners/custom/NewRuralSafetyFactsheetENG.pdf

Santock, J. W. (2007). *Child development* (11th ed.). Boston, MA: McGraw-Hill.

Sex Facts in Canada. (2006). Retrieved on October 30, 2008, from http://www.sexualityandu.ca/

Transport Canada. (2006). *Keep kids safe: Car time 1-2-3-4* (Catalogue No. TP13511E -03/2006) [Brochure]. Ottawa, ON: Minister of Public Works and Government Services,. Retrieved October 30, 2008, from http://www.tc.gc.ca/roadsafety/tp/tp13511/menu.htm

Trocmé, N., Fallon, B., MacLaurin, B., Daciuk, J., Feistiner, C. Black, T., et al. (2005). *The Canadian incidence study of reported child abuse and neglect—2003: Major findings*. Ottawa, ON: Ministry of Public Works and Government Services Canada.

Ward, L., Gaboury, I., Ladhani, M., & Zlotkin, S. (2007). Vitamin D–deficiency rickets among children in Canada. *Canadian Medical Association Journal, 177*(2), 161–166.

Wardle, J., & Cooke, L. (2005). The impact of obesity on psychological well-being. *Best Practices and Research Clinical Endocrinology and Metabolism, 19*, 421–440.

Chapter 24

Breslin, E. T., & Lucas, V. A. (2003). *Women's health nursing: Toward evidence-based practice*. St. Louis, MO: W. B. Saunders.

Canadian Cancer Society. (2008). *Canadian cancer statistics for 2008*. Retrieved November 3, 2008, from http://www.cancer.ca/Canada-wide/About%20cancer/Cancer%20statistics/~/media/CCS/Canada%20wide/Files%20List/English%20files%20heading/pdf%20not%20in%20publications%20section/Canadian%20Cancer%20Society%20Statistics%20PDF%202008_614137951.ashx

Canadian Institute for Health Information. (2004). *Overweight and obesity in Canada: A population health perspective*. Retrieved November 10, 2008, from http://secure.cihi.ca/cihiweb/products/CPHIOverweightandObesityAugust2004_e.pdf

Cancer Care Ontario. (2006). *Cancer in young adults in Canada*. Retrieved on November 3, 2008, from http://www.cancercare.on.ca/pdf/CYAC2006E.pdf

Campbell, D. A., Lake, M. F., Falk, M., & Backstrand, J. R. (2006). A randomized control trial of continuous support in labor by a lay doula. *Journal of Obstetric, Gynecologic and Neonatal Nursing, 35*, 456–464.

Condon, M.C. (2004). *Women's health: An integrated approach to wellness and illness*. Upper Saddle River, New Jersey: Prentice Hall.

Domian, E. (2001). Cultural practices and social support of pregnant women in a northern New Mexico community. *Journal of Nursing Scholarship, 33*, 331–336.

Dunn, S., Davies, B., McCleary, L., Edwards, N., & Gaboury, I. (2006). The relationship between vulnerability factors and breastfeeding outcomes. *Journal of Obstetric, Gynecologic and Neonatal Nursing, 35*, 87–97.

Edelman, C., & Mandle, C. (2002). *Health promotion throughout the lifespan* (5th ed.). St. Louis, MO: Mosby.

Elliott, J., Berman, H., & Kim, S. (2002). A critical ethnography of Korean Canadian women's menopause experience. *Health Care for Women International, 23*, 377–388.

Erikson, E. (1963). *Childhood and society* (2nd ed.). New York: W. W. Norton.

Erikson, E. (1968). *Identity: Youth and crisis*. New York: W. W. Norton.

Erikson, E. (1982). *The life cycle completed: A review*. New York: W. W. Norton.

Fortinash, K., & Holoday Worret, P. (2004). *Psychiatric Mental Health Nursing* (3rd Ed.). St. Louis: Mosby.

Gilligan, C. (1993). *In a different voice*. Cambridge, MA: Harvard University Press.

Gould, R.L. (1972). The phases of adult life: A study in developmental psychology. The American Journal of Psychiatry, 129, 521-531.

Havighurst, R. (1972). Successful aging. In R. H. Williams, C. Tibbits, & W. Donahue (Eds.), *Process of aging* (Vol. 1). New York: Atherton.

Lemone, P., & Burke, K. (2004). *Medical surgical nursing: Critical thinking in client care* (3rd ed.). Upper Saddle River, NJ: Pearson Prentice Hall.

Lowdermilk, D., & Perry, S. (2003). *Maternity nursing* (6th ed.). St. Louis, MO: Mosby.

McManus, A., Hunter, L.P., & Renn, H. (2006). Lesbian experiences and needs during childbirth: Guidelines for health care providers. *Journal of Obstetric, Gynecologic and Neonatal Nursing, 35*, 13–23.

Public Health Agency of Canada. (2007). *Reported cases of notifiable STI from January 1 to December 31, 2006 and January 1 to December 31, 2007 and corresponding rates for January 1 to December 31, 2006 and 2007*. Retrieved November 3, 2008, from http://www.phac-aspc.gc.ca/std-mts/stdcases-casmts/cases-cas-08-eng.php

Registered Nurses Association of Ontario. (2003). *Breastfeeding best practice guidelines for nurses*. Toronto, ON: Author.

Society of Obstetricians and Gynaecologists of Canada. (2006). *Sex facts in Canada 2006*. Retrieved November 3, 2008, from http://www.sexualityandu.ca/media-room/fact-sheets-1.aspx

Somers-Smith, M. J. (1999). A place for the partner? Expectations and experiences of support during childbirth. *Midwifery, 15*, 101–108.

Statistics Canada. (2008a). *Health*. Retrieved November 3, 2008, from http://cansim2.statcan.ca/cgi-win/cnsmcgi.pgm?Lang=E&SP_Action=Theme&SP_ID=2966

Statistics Canada. (2008b). *Population and demography*. Retrieved November 3, 2008, from http://cansim2.statcan.ca/cgi-win/cnsmcgi.pgm?Lang=E&SP_Action=Theme&SP_ID=3867

Statistics Canada. (2008c). *Women in Canada: Work chapter updates*. Retrieved November 3, 2008, from http://www.statcan.ca/english/freepub/89F0133XIE/89F0133XIE2006000.htm

University of Toronto. (2007, Fall). Making babies [whole issue]. *Edge, 8*(3). Retrieved November 3, 2008, from http://www.research.utoronto.ca/edge/fall2007/1.HTML

Chapter 25

Alzheimer Society of Canada. (2008). *Alzheimer disease: Related dementias*. Retrieved November 5, 2008, from http://www.alzheimer.ca/english/disease/dementias-intro.htm

Amella, E. J. (2004). Presentation of illness in older adults. *American Journal of Nursing, 104*(10), 40–51.

Atkinson, P. J. (2006). Intimacy and sexuality. In S. Meiner & A. Lueckenotte (Eds.)., *Gerontologic nursing* (3rd ed.). St. Louis, MO: Mosby.

Beers, M., & Berkow, R. (2000). *The Merck manual of geriatrics* (3rd ed.). Whitehouse Station, NJ: Merck.

Bolla, L., Filley, C., & Palmer, R. (2000). Dementia DDx: Office diagnosis of the four major types of dementia. *Geriatrics, 55*(1), 34–37, 41–42, 45–46.

Buijs, R., Ross-Kerr, J., Cousins, S. O., & Wilson, D. (2003). Promoting participation: Evaluation of a health promotion program for low income seniors. *Journal of Community Health Nursing, 20*(1), 93–107.

Canadian Cancer Society. (2008). *Prostate cancer stats.* Retrieved November 6, 2008, from http://www.cancer.ca/ccs/internet/standard/0,3182,3172_14471__langId-en,00.HTML

Canadian Coalition for Seniors' Mental Health. (2008). *The CCSMH National Guidelines for Seniors' Mental Health Project.* Retrieved November 6, 2008, from http://www.ccsmh.ca/en/natlGuidelines/initiatives.cfm

Canadian Continence Foundation. (2007, May). Incontinence: A Canadian perspective. Retrieved November 6, 2008, from http://www.continence-fdn.ca/pdf/Research_paper_August2007.pdf

Canadian Council on Social Development for the Division of Aging and Seniors, Public Health Agency of Canada (2004). *Canadian seniors at a glance.* Retrieved November 6, 2008, from https://www.mysudbury.ca/Seniors/Publications/Canadian+Seniors+At+a+Glance/

Canadian Gerontological Nursing Association. (1996). *Standards of practice for the Canadian Gerontological Nursing Association.* Retrieved November 6, 2008, from http://www.cgna.net/index.php?action=viewContents&id=5

Canadian Network for the Prevention of Elder Abuse. (2008). *What is abuse of seniors?* Retrieved November 6, 2008, from http://www.cnpea.ca/what_is_abuse.htm

Chasteen, A., Schwarz, N., & Park, D. (2002). The activation of aging stereotypes in younger and older adults. *Journals of Gerontologicy, Series B, Psychological Sciences and Social Sciences, 57*(6), P540–P547.

Chochinov, H. (2007). Dignity and the essence of medicine: The A, B, C and D of dignity conserving care. *British Medical Journal, 335,* 184–187.

Conn, D. (2001). Cholinesterase inhibitors: Comparing the options for mild-to-moderate dementia. *Geriatrics, 56*(9), 56–57.

Cummings, E., & Henry, W. (1961). *Growing old: The process of disengagement.* New York: Basic Books.

Davidhizar, R., Eshleman, J., & Moody, M. (2002). Health promotion for aging adults. *Geriatric Nursing, 23*(1), 28–34.

Division of Aging and Seniors, Public Health Agency of Canada. (2008). *Medication matters: How you can help seniors use medication safely.* Retrieved November 5, 2008, from http://www.phac-aspc.gc.ca/seniors-aines/pubs/med_matters/intro_e.htm

Dowling-Castronovo, A., & Bradway, C. (2003). Urinary incontinence. In M. Mezey, T. Fulmer, & I. Abraham (Eds.), *Geriatric nursing protocols for best practice* (2nd ed., pp. 83–98). New York: Springer.

Duggleby, W., Degner, L., Williams, A., Wright, K., Cooper, D., Popkin, D. (2007). Living with hope: Initial evaluation of a psychosocial hope intervention for older palliative home care patients. *Journal of Pain and Symptom Management, 33,* 247–257.

Duggleby, W., & Wright, K. (2005). Transforming hope: How elderly palliative patients live with hope. *Canadian Journal of Nursing Research, 37*(2), 70–84.

Ebersole, P., Hess, P., Touhy, T., Jett, K., & Luggen, A. (2008). *Toward healthy aging: Human needs and nursing response* (7th ed.). St. Louis, MO: Mosby.

Filiatrault, J., Parisien, M., Laforest, S., Genest, C., Gauvin, L, Fournier, M, et al. (2007). Implementing a community-based falls-prevention program: From drawing board to reality. *Canadian Journal of Aging, 26,* 213–226.

Flaherty, E. (2007). Pain assessment for older adults. *Try This: Best Practices in Nursing Care to Older Adults* (Issue No. 7). New York: Hartford Foundation for Geriatric Nursing. Retrieved November 19, 2008, from http://consultgerirn.org/uploads/File/trythis/issue07.pdf

Flaherty, E., Fulmer, T., & Mezey, M. (Eds.). (2003). *Geriatric nursing review syllabus: A core curriculum in advanced practice geriatric nursing.* New York: American Geriatrics Society.

Forbes, D. A. (2004). Cognitive stimulation therapy improves cognition and quality of life in dementia. *Evidence-Based Nursing, 7,* 54.

Gillis, A. J., & MacDonald, B. (2006). Unmasking delirium. *Canadian Nurse, 102*(9), 19–24.

Gomolin, I., & Kathpalia, R. (2002). Influenza: How to prevent and control nursing home outbreaks. *Geriatrics, 57*(1), 28–30, 33–34.

Hadjistavropoulos, T., & Fine, P. G. (2006). Chronic pain in older persons: Prevalence, assessment and management. *Reviews in Clinical Gerontology, 16,* 231–241.

Havens, B., Hall, M., Sylvestre, G., & Jivan, T. (2004). Social isolation and loneliness: Differences between older rural and urban Manitobans. *Canadian Journal of Aging, 23,* 129–140.

Hawranik, P., Johnston, P., & Deatrich, J. (2008). Therapeutic touch and agitation in individuals with Alzheimer's disease. *Western Journal of Nursing Research, 30,* 417–434.

Health Canada. (2007). *Eating well with Canada's food guide* (Catalogue No. H164-38/1-2007E). Ottawa, ON: Author.

Hess, T. M. (2006). Attitudes toward aging and their effects on behavior. In J. E. Birring & K. S. Shaie (Eds.), *Handbook of the psychology of aging* (6th ed., pp. 379–406). San Diego, CA: Elsevier Academic Press.

King, T. (2005). The escalating demand for long term care. *Canadian Nurse, 101*(6), 11–15.

Kresevic, D. M., & Mezey, M. (2003). Assessment of function. In M. Mezey, T. Fulmer, & I. Abraham (Eds.), *Geriatric nursing protocols for best practice* (2nd ed., pp. 31–46). New York: Springer.

Lemon, B., Bengston, V., & Peterson, J. (1972). An exploration of the activity theory of aging: Activity types and life satisfaction among in-movers to a retirement community. *Journal of Gerontology, 27,* 511–523.

Meiner. S. E., & Lueckenotte, A. G. (2006). Overview of gerontologic nursing. In S. E. Meiner & A. G. Lueckenotte (Eds.), *Gerontologic nursing* (3rd ed., pp. 1–19) St. Louis, MO: Mosby.

Menec, V. H., Black, C., MacWilliam, L., & Aoki, F. Y. (2003). The impact of influenza-associated respiratory illnesses on hospitalizations, physicians visits, emergency room visits, and mortality. *Canadian Journal of Public Health, 94,* 59–64.

Miller, C. (in press). *Nursing for wellness in older adults. Theory and practice* (5th ed.). Philadelphia, PA: Lippincott.

National Advisory Council on Aging. (2006). *Seniors in Canada: Report card 2006.* Retrieved November 5, 2008, from http://dsp-psd.pwgsc.gc.ca/Collection/HP30-1-2006E.pdf.

Neugarten, B. (1964). *Personality in middle and late life.* New York: Atherton.

Osteoporosis Canada. (2008). *About osteoporosis.* Retrieved November 6, 2008, from http://www.osteoporosis.ca/english/about%20osteoporosis/default.asp?s=1

Pender, N. J., Murdaugh, C. L., & Parsons, M. A. (2002). *Health promotion in nursing practice* (4th ed.). Upper Saddle River, NJ: Prentice Hall.

Rantz, M., Popejoy, L., & Zwygart-Stauffacher, M. (2001). *The new nursing homes: A 20-minute way to find great long-term care.* Minneapolis, MN: Fairview Press.

Registered Nurses Association of Ontario. (2002a). *Prevention of falls and fall injuries in the older adult.* Retrieved November 6, 2008, from http://www.rnao.org/Page.asp?PageID=924&ContentID=810

Registered Nurses Association of Ontario. (2002b). *Promoting continence using prompted voiding.* Retrieved November 6, 2008, from http://www.rnao.org/Page.asp?PageID=924&ContentID=813

Registered Nurses Association of Ontario. (2003). *Screening for delirium, dementia and depression in the older adult.* Retrieved November 6, 2008, from http://www.rnao.org/Page.asp?PageID=924&ContentID=818

Resnick, B. (2003). Health promotion practices of older adults: Testing an individualized approach. *Journal of Clinical Nursing, 12*(1), 46–55.

Robson, S., Edwards, J., Gallagher, E., & Baker, D. (2003). Steady As You Go (SAYGO): A falls-prevention program for seniors living in the community. *Canadian Journal on Aging, 22,* 207–216.

Saskatoon Health Region. (2006). *Older Adult Wellness Program: Annual report.* Saskatoon, SK: Author.

Spector, A., Thorgrimsen, L., Woods, B., Royan, L., Davis, S., Butterworth, M., et al. (2003). Efficacy of an evidence-based cognitive stimulation therapy programme for people with dementia: Randomised control trial. *British Journal of Psychiatry, 183,* 248–254.

Statistics Canada. (2008). *A portrait of seniors in Canada.* Retrieved November 6, 2008, from http://www.statcan.ca/english/ads/89-519-XPE/index.htm

Waszynski, C. M. (2007). The Confusion Assessment Method (CAM). *Try This: Best Practices in Nursing Care to Older Adults* (Issue No. 13). New York: Hartford Foundation for Geriatric Nursing. Retrieved November 19, 2008, from http://consultgerirn.org/uploads/File/trythis/issue13_cam.pdf

Chapter 26

Beck, C. T. (2008). State of the science on postpartum depression: What nurse researchers have contributed—Part 1. *MCN: The American Journal of Maternal Child Nursing, 33*(2), 121–126.

Birndorf, S., Ryan, S., Auinger, P., & Aten, M. (2005). High self-esteem among adolescents: Longitudinal trends, sex differences, and protective factors. *Journal of Adolescent Health, 37,* 194–201.

Biro, F. M., Streigel-Moore, R. H., Franco, D. L., Padgett, J., & Bean, J. A. (2006). Self-esteem in adolescent females. *Journal of Adolescent Health, 39,* 501–507.

Bowlby, J. (1982). *Attachment and loss: Vol 1. Attachments* (2nd ed.). New York: Basic Books.

Christie-Mizell, C. A. (2003). Bullying: The consequences of interparental discord and child self-concept. *Family Process, 42,* 237–251.

Coloroso, B. (2002). *The bully, the bullied, and the bystander.* Toronto, ON: HarperCollins.

Eliopoulos, C. (2005). *Gerontologic nursing* (6th ed.). Philadelphia, PA: Lippincott.

Erikson, E. (1963). *Childhood and society* (2nd ed.). New York: W. W. Norton.

Gomez, R., & McLaren, S. (2006). The inter-relations of mother and father attachment, self-esteem and aggression during late adolescence. *Aggressive Behavior, 33,* 160–169.

Good, M., & Willoughby, T. (2007). The identity formation experiences of church-attending rural adolescents. *Journal of Adolescent Research, 22,* 387–412.

MacPhee, A. R., & Andrews, J. J. W. (2006). Risk factors for depression in adolescence. *Adolescence, 41,* 435–466.

Meadus, R. J., & Twomey, J. C. (2007). Men in nursing: Making the right choice. *Canadian Nurse, 103*(2), 13–16.

Park, J. (2003). Adolescent self-concept and health into adulthood [Catalogue 82-003]. *Health Reports, 14,* 41–52.

Pedro, L. W. (2001). Quality of life for long-term survivors of cancer: Influencing variables. *Cancer Nursing, 26,* 1–11.

Robins, R. W., Trzesniewski, K. H., Tracy, J. L., Gosling, S. D., & Potter, J. (2002). Global self-esteem across the life span. *Psychology and Aging, 17,* 423–434.

Rosenberg, M. (1965). *Society and the adolescent self-image.* Princeton, NJ: Princeton University Press.

Ruiz, S. Y., Roosa, M. W., & Gonzales, N. A. (2002). Predictors of self-esteem for Mexican American and European American youths: A reexamination of the influence of parenting. *Journal of Family Psychology, 16,* 70–80.

Schmatz, D. L., Deane, G. D., Birch, L. L., & Davison, K. K. (2007). A longitudinal assessment of the links between physical activity and self-esteem in early adolescent non-Hispanic females. *Journal of Adolescent Health, 41,* 559–565.

Sinclair, J., & Milner D. (2005). On being Jewish: A qualitative study of identity among British Jews in emerging adulthood. *Journal of Adolescent Research, 20,* 91–117.

Smith, C. (2003a). Religious participation and network closure among American adolescents. *Journal for the Scientific Study of Religion, 42,* 259–267.

Smith, C. (2003b). Theorizing religious effects among American adolescents. *Journal for the Scientific Study of Religion, 42,* 17–30.

Strahan, E. J., Lafrance, A., Wilson, A. E., Ethier, N., Spencer, S. J., & Zanna, M. P. (2008). Victoria's dirty little secret: How sociocultural norms influence adolescent girls and women. *Personality and Social Psychology Bulletin, 34,* 288–301.

Strahan, E. J., Wilson, A. E., Cressman, K. E., & Buote, V. M. (2006). Comparing to perfection: How cultural norms for appearance affect social comparisons and self-image. *Body Image, 3,* 211–227.

Strong, W. B., Malina, R. M., & Blimkie, C. J. R., Daniels, S. R., Dishman, R. K., Gutin, B., et al. (2005). Evidence based physical activity for school-age youth. *Journal of Pediatrics, 146,* 732–737.

Stuart, G. W., & Laraia, M. T. (2005). *Principles and practice of psychiatric nursing* (8th ed.). St. Louis, MO: Mosby.

Trzesniewski, K. H., Donnellan, M. B., Moffitt, T. E., Robins, R. W., Poulton, R., & Caspi, A. (2006). Low self-esteem during adolescence predicts poor health, criminal behavior and limited economic prospects during adulthood. *Developmental Psychology, 42,* 381–390.

Twenge, J. M., & Crocker, J. (2002). Race and self-esteem: Meta-analyses comparing Whites, Blacks, Hispanics, Asians, and American Indians. *Psychology Bulletin, 128,* 371–408.

Van Baarsen, B. (2002). Theories on coping with loss: The impact of social support and self-esteem on adjustment to emotional and social loneliness following a partner's death in later life. *Journals of Gerontology, Series B, Psychological Sciences and Social Sciences, 57*(1), S33–S42.

Vickery, C. D., Sepehri, A., & Evans, C. C. (2008). Self-esteem in an acute stroke rehabilitation sample: A control group comparison. *Clinical Rehabilitation, 22,* 179–187.

Wilburn, V. R., & Smith, D. E. (2005). Stress, self-esteem, and suicidal ideation in late adolescents. *Adolescence, 40*(157), 33–45.

Wild, L. G., Flisher, A. J., Bhana, A., & Lombard, C. (2004). Associations among adolescent risk behaviours and self-esteem in six domains. *Journal of Child Psychology & Psychiatry, 45,* 1454–1467.

Chapter 27

Albaugh, J., & Kellog-Spadt, S. (2003). Sexuality and sexual health: The nurse's role and initial approach to patients. *Urologic Nursing, 23,* 227–228.

American Psychiatric Association. (in press). *Diagnostic and statistical manual of mental disorders* (5th ed.). Washington, DC: Author.

Annon, J. S. (1976). The PLISSIT model: A proposed conceptual scheme for the behavioral treatment of sexual problems. *Journal of Sex Education and Therapy, 2,* 1–15.

Anttila, T., Saikku, P., Koskela, P., Bloigu, A., Dillner, J., Ikäheimo, I., et al. (2001). Serotypes of *Chlamydia trachomatis* and risk for development of cervical squamous cell carcinoma. *Journal of the American Medical Association, 285,* 47–51.

Auld, R. B., & Brock, G. (2002). Sexuality and erectile dysfunction: Results of a national survey. *Journal of Sexual & Reproductive Medicine, 2,* 50–54.

Bartlik, B., Rosenfeld, S., & Beaton, C. (2005). Assessment of sexual functioning: Sexual history taking for health care practitioners. *Epilepsy & Behavior 7,* S15–S21.

Barton, D., Wilwerding, M., Carpenter, L., & Loprinzi, C. (2004). Libido as part of sexuality in female cancer survivors. *Oncology Nursing Forum, 31,* 599–609.

Basson, R. (2005). Women's sexual dysfunction: Revised and expanded definitions. *Canadian Medical Association Journal, 172,* 1327–1333.

Beitz, J. M. (1998). Sexual health promotion in adolescents and young adults: Primary prevention strategies. *Holistic Nursing Practice, 12,* 27–37.

Bernhard, L. A. (2002). Sexuality and sexual health care for women. *Clinical Obstetrics and Gynecology, 45,* 1089–1098.

Beutner, K. R., Reitano, M. V., Richwald, G. A., & Wiley, D. J. (1998). External genital warts: Report of the American Medical Association Consensus Conference. AMA Expert Panel on External Genital Warts. *Clinical Infectious Diseases, 27,* 796–806.

Birley, H., Duerden, B., Hart, C. A., Curless, E., Hay, P. E., Ison, C. A., et al. (2002). Sexually transmitted diseases: Microbiology and management. *Journal of Medical Microbiology, 51,* 793–807.

Burd, I., Nevadunsky, N., & Bachmann, G. (2006). Impact of physician gender on sexual history taking in a multispecialty practice. *Journal of Sexual Medicine 3,* 194–200.

Butcher, J. (1999a). ABC of sexual health: Female sexual problems. I: Loss of desire—What about the fun? *British Medical Journal, 318,* 41–43.

Butcher, J. (1999b). ABC of sexual health: Female sexual problems. II: Sexual pain and sexual fears. *British Medical Journal, 318,* 110–112.

Canadian Abortion Rights Action League. (2003). *Protecting abortion rights in Canada.* Ottawa, ON: Author.

Canadian Institute of Health Information. (2004). *Teen pregnancy, by outcome of pregnancy and age group, count and rate per 1,000 women aged 15 to 19, Canada, provinces and territories, 1998.* Retrieved November 14, 2004, from http://www.statcan.ca/english/freepub/82-221-XIE/01201/tables/HTML/P411.htm

Centers for Disease Control and Prevention. (2008). *HPV vaccine information for young women.* Retrieved November 15, 2008, from http://www.cdc.gov/std/hpv/STDFact-HPV-vaccine.htm

Centre for Infectious Disease Prevention and Control, Population and Public Health Branch, Health Canada. (2002). *Condoms, sexually transmitted infections, safe sex and you.* Ottawa, ON: Health Canada.

Centre for Infectious Disease Prevention and Control, Population and Public Health Branch, Health Canada. (2003). Estimates of HIV prevalence and incidence in Canada, 2002. *Canada Communicable Disease Report, 29,* 197–206.

de Marquiegui, A., & Huish, M. (1999). ABC of sexual health: A woman's sexual life after an operation. *British Medical Journal, 318,* 178–181.

Dickinson, L. M., deGruy, F. V. III, Dickinson, W. P., Candib, L. M. (1999). Health-related quality of life and symptom profiles of female survivors of sexual abuse. *Archives of Family Medicine, 8,* 35–43.

Division of STD Prevention and Control, Bureau of HIV/AIDS, STI and TB, Centre for Infectious Disease Prevention, Health Canada. (2000). 1998/1999 Canadian sexually transmitted diseases (STD) surveillance report. *Canada Communicable Disease Report, 26*(S6), 1–36.

Duncan, P., Dixon, R. R., & Carlson, J. (2003). Childhood and adolescent sexuality. *Pediatric Clinics of North America, 50,* 765–780.

Engender Health. (2004). *Sexuality and sexual health* [Online minicourse]. Retrieved November 14, 2004, from http://www.engenderhealth.org/res/onc/sexuality/index.HTML

Finan, S. F. (1997). Promoting healthy sexuality: Guidelines for the school-age child and adolescent. *The Nurse Practitioner, 22*(11), 62, 65–67, 71–72.

Glass, C., & Soni, B. (1999). ABC of sexual health: Sexual problems of disabled patients. *British Medical Journal*, 318, 518–521.

Gott, C. M. (2001). Sexual activity and risk-taking in later life. *Health & Social Care in the Community, 9*, 72–78.

Guthrie, C. (1999). Nurses' perceptions of sexuality relating to patient care. *Journal of Clinical Nursing* 8, 313–321.

Haboubi, N. H., & Lincoln, N. (2003). Views of health professionals on discussing sexual issues with patients. *Disability and Rehabilitation, 25*, 291–296.

Haroian, L. (2000, February 1). Child sexual development. *Electronic Journal of Human Sexuality*. Retrieved November 14, 2008, from http://www.ejhs.org/volume3/Haroian/body.htm

Health Canada. (2008). *Sexually transmitted infections (STIs)*. Retrieved November, 2008, from http://www.hc-sc.gc.ca/dc-ma/sti-its/index-eng.php

Heiman, J. R. (2002). Sexual dysfunction: Overview of prevalence, etiological factors, and treatments. *Journal of Sex Research, 39*, 73–78.

Herson, L., Hart, K. A., Gordon, M. J., & Rintala, D. H. (1999). Identifying and overcoming barriers to providing sexuality information in the clinical setting. *Rehabilitation Nursing, 24*, 148–151.

Huang, C. (1999). Discussing sex with disabled patients. *Western Journal of Medicine, 171*(2), 76–77.

Jewell, D., Tacchi, J., & Donovan, J. (2000). Teenage pregnancy: Whose problem is it? *Family Practice, 17*, 522–528.

Johnson, O. S. (2004). *The sexual spectrum: Exploring human diversity*. Vancouver, BC: Raincoast Books.

Kaplan, H. S. (1979). *Disorders of sexual desire*. New York: Simon & Schuster.

Keller M., Duerst, B. L., & Zimmerman, J. (1996). Adolescents' views of sexual decision-making. *Image—The Journal of Nursing Scholarship, 28*, 125–130.

Kenney, J. W., Reinholtz, C. O., & Angelini, P. O. (1998). Sexual abuse, sex before age 16, and high-risk behaviors of young females with sexually transmitted diseases. *Journal of Obstetric, Gynecologic, and Neonatal Nursing, 27*, 54–63.

Liao, L. M. (2003). Learning to assist women born with atypical genitalia: Journey through ignorance, taboo and dilemma. *Journal of Reproductive and Infant Psychology, 21*, 229–238.

Lueckenotte, A. G. (2000). *Gerontologic nursing* (2nd ed.). St. Louis, MO: Mosby.

Magnan, M. A., Reynolds, K. E., & Galvin, E. A. (2005). Barriers to addressing patient sexuality in nursing practice. *Medsurg Nursing, 14*, 282–289.

Masters, W. H., & Johnson, V. E. (1966). *Human sexual response*. Boston: Little, Brown.

Mayo Foundation for Medical Education and Research. (2004). *Sex during pregnancy: What's OK, what's not*. Retrieved November 14, 2004, from http://www.mayoclinic.com/invoke.cfm?id=HO00140

McCabe, M. P., & Matic, H. (2008). Erectile dysfunction and relationships: Views of men with erectile dysfunction and their partners. *Sexual and Relationship Therapy, 23*(1), 51–60.

McIlhaney, J. S. (2000). Sexually transmitted infection and teenage sexuality. *American Journal of Obstetrics and Gynecology, 183*, 334–338.

NANDA International. (2007). *NANDA-I nursing diagnoses: Definitions and classification, 2007–2008*, Philadelphia, PA: Author.

National Institute of Allergy and Infectious Diseases, National Institutes of Health, US Department of Health and Human Services. (2003). *Sexually transmitted infections*. Retrieved November 14, 2008, from http://www3.niaid.nih.gov/topics/sti/

Nusbaum, M. R., Hamilton, C., & Lenahan, P. (2003). Chronic illness and sexual functioning. American Family Physician, 67, 347–354.

Palacios, S., Tobar, A. C., & Menendez, C. (2002). Sexuality in the climacteric years. *Maturitas, 43*(Suppl. 1), S69–S77.

Planned Parenthood Federation of America. (2008a). *Female condom*. Retrieved November 14, 2004, from http://www.plannedparenthood.org/health-topics/birth-control/female-condom-4223.htm

Planned Parenthood Federation of America. (2008b). *Gonorrhea*. Retrieved November 14, 2004, from http://www.plannedparenthood.org/health-topics/stds-hiv-safer-sex/gonorrhea-4269.htm

Public Health Agency of Canada. (2004). *2004 Canadian sexually transmitted infections surveillence report*. Retrieved November 14, 2008, from http://www.phac-aspc.gc.ca/publicat/ccdr-rmtc/07pdf/33s1_e.pdf

Public Health Agency of Canada. (2006). *Frequently asked questions on emergency contraception*. Retrieved November 14, 2008, from http://www.phac-aspc.gc.ca/std-mts/ec_cu_e.HTML

Riley, A. (1999). Sex in old age: Continuing pleasure or inevitable decline? *Geriatric Medicine, 29*(3), 25.

Ross, M. W., Channon-Little, L. D., & Rosser, B. R. (2000). *Sexual health concerns: Interviewing and history taking for health practitioners* (2nd ed.). Philadelphia, PA: F. A. Davis.

Running, A., & Berndt, A. (2003). *Management guidelines for nurse practitioners working in family practice*. Philadelphia, PA: F. A. Davis.

Society for Human Sexuality. (2004). *Guide to safe sex*. Retrieved November 14, 2008, from http://www.sexuality.org/safesex.HTML

Statistics Canada. (2004, June 15). *Canadian community health survey*. Retrieved November 14, 2008, from http://www.statcan.ca/Daily/English/040615/d040615b.htm

van der Riet, P. (1998). The sexual embodiment of the cancer patient. *Nursing Inquiry, 5*, 248–257.

Vilain, E. (2004, April 19). Commentary: Gender blender: Intersexual? Transsexual? Male, female aren't so easy to define. *Los Angeles Times*, p. B-11.

von Sydow, K. (1999). Sexuality during pregnancy and after childbirth: A meta-content analysis of 59 studies. *Journal of Psychosomatic Research, 47*, 27–49.

Wagner, G., Bondil, P., Dabees, K., Dean, J., Fourcroy, J., Gingell, C., et al. (2005). Ethical aspects of sexual medicine. *Journal of Sexual Medicine, 2*, 163–168.

World Health Organization. (2004). *Sexual health*. Retrieved November 14, 2008, from http://www.who.int/reproductive-health/gender/sexualhealth.HTML.

Chapter 28

Aaron, K. F., Levine, D., & Burstin, H. R. (2003). African American church participation and health care practices. *Journal of General Internal Medicine, 18*, 908–913.

Adegbola, M. (2006). Spirituality and quality of life in chronic illness. *Journal of Theory Construction and Testing, 10*(2), 42–46.

Andrews, M. M., & Boyle, J. S. (2007). *Transcultural concepts in nursing care* (5th ed.). Philadelphia, PA: Lippincott.

Banks-Wallace, J., & Parks, L. (2004). It's all sacred: African American women's perspectives on spirituality. *Issues in Mental Health Nursing, 25*, 25–45.

Barnum, B. S. (2003). *Spirituality in nursing: From traditional to new age* (2nd ed.). New York: Springer.

Barry, L. C., Kerns, R. D., Guo, Z., Duong, B. D., Iannone, L. P., & Reid, M. C. (2004). Identification strategies used to cope with chronic pain in older persons receiving primary care from a Veterans Affairs medical center. *Journal of the American Geriatric Society, 52*, 950–956.

Benner, D. G. (1985). *Baker encyclopedia of psychology*. Grand Rapids, MI: Baker Book House.

Benner, P. (1984). *From novice to expert*. Menlo Park, CA: Addison-Wesley.

Benner, P., & Wrubel, J. (1989). *The primacy of caring*. Menlo Park, CA: Addison-Wesley.

Bibby, R. (2002). *Restless gods: The renaissance of religion in Canada*. Toronto, ON: Stoddart.

Bibby, R. W. (2006). *The boomer factor: What Canada's most famous generation is leaving behind*. Toronto, ON: Bastian Books.

Burnard, P. (1988). The spiritual needs of atheists and agnostics. *Professional Nurse, 4*, 130–132.

Bradshaw, A. (1994). *Lighting the lamp: The spiritual dimension of nursing care*. Middlesex, UK: Scutari Press.

Browne, A. J.,& Fiske, J. (2001). First Nations women's encounters with mainstream health care services. *Western Journal of Nursing Research, 23*, 126–147.

Canadian Association for Parish Nursing Ministry. (2008). *Parish nurse*. Retrieved November 17, 2008, from http://www.capnm.ca/

Canadian Nurses Association. (2008). *The code of ethics for registered nurses*. Ottawa, ON: Canadian Nurses Association. Retrieved November 21, 2008, from http://www.cna-aiic.ca/CNA/documents/pdf/publications/Code_of_Ethics_2008_e.pdf

Cavendish, R., Konecny, L., Luise, B. K., & Lanza, M. (2004). Nurses enhance performance through prayer [Electronic version]. *Holistic Nursing Practice, 18*, 26–31.

Chiu, L. (2001). Spiritual resources of Chinese immigrants with breast cancer in the USA. *International Journal of Nursing Studies, 38*, 175–184.

Clark, C. C., Cross, J. R., Deane, D. M., & Lowry, L. W. (1991). Spirituality: Integral to quality care. *Holistic Nursing Practice, 5*(3), 67–76.

Clark, M. B., & Olson, J. K. (2000). *Nursing within a faith community: Promoting health in times of transition*. Thousand Oaks, CA: Sage.

Como, J. M. (2007). Spiritual practice: A literature review related to spiritual health and health outcomes. *Holistic Nursing Practice, 21*(5), 224–236.

Davidhizar, R. E., & Giger, J. N. (1998). *Canadian transcultural nursing*. Toronto, ON: Mosby.

Delgado, C. (2005). A discussion of the concept of spirituality. *Nursing Science Quarterly, 18*, 157–162.

Draper, P., & McSherry, W. (2002). A critical view of spirituality and spiritual assessment. *Journal of Advanced Nursing, 39*, 1–2.

Ebersole, P., Hess, P., & Luggen, A. S. (2004). *Toward healthy aging* (6th ed.). St. Louis, MO: Mosby.

Elkins, M., & Cavendish, R. (2004). Developing a plan for pediatric spiritual care. *Holistic Nursing Practice,18,* 179–184.

Emblen, J. D. (1992). Religion and spirituality defined according to current use in nursing literature. *Journal of Professional Nursing, 8,* 41–47.

Emblen, J. D., & Halstead, L. (1993). Spiritual needs and interventions: Comparing the views of patients, nurses, and chaplains. *Clinical Nursing Specialist, 7,* 175–182.

Friedemann, M. L., Mouch, J., & Racey, T. (2002). Nursing the spirit: The framework of systemic organization. *Journal of Advanced Nursing, 39,* 325–332.

Fryback, P. B. (1993). Health for people with a terminal diagnosis. *Nursing Science Quarterly, 6*(3), 147–149.

Grant, D. (2004). Spiritual interventions: How, when and why nurses use them [Electronic version]. *Holistic Nursing Practice, 18*(1), 36–41.

Gray, J. (2006). Measuring spirituality: Conceptual and methodological considerations. *Journal of Theory Construction and Testing, 10*(2), 58–64.

Griffith, J., Caron, C. D., Desrosiers, J., & Thibeault, R. (2007). Defining spirituality and giving meaning to occupation: The perspective of community-dwelling older adults with autonomy loss. *Canadian Journal of Occupational Therapy, 74*(2), 78–90.

Griffith, J. K. (1996). *The religious aspects of nursing care.* Vancouver, BC: Author.

Grypma, S. (2001). *Lived experience of cross-cultural nurses: A phenomenological study.* Unpublished master's thesis, University of Calgary, Calgary, AB. Retrieved November 17, 2008, from https://dspace_ucalgary.ca/bitstreatm/1880/40823/1/64937Grypma.pdf

Grypma, S. (2008). *Healing Henan: Canadian nurses at the North China Mission, 1888–1947.* Vancouver, BC: University of British Columbia Press.

Hall, B. A. (1998). Patterns of spirituality in persons with advanced HIV disease. *Research in Nursing & Health, 21,* 143–153.

Heliker, D. (1992). Reevaluation of a nursing diagnosis: Spiritual distress. *Nursing Forum, 27*(4), 15–20.

Henderson, V. (1966). *The nature of nursing: A definition and its implications for practice, research, and education.* New York: Macmillan.

Holstad, M. K. M., Pace, J. C., De, A. K., & Ura, D. R. (2006). Factors associated with adherence to antiretroviral therapy. *Journal of the Association of Nurses in AIDS Care, 17*(2), 4–15.

Hungelmann, J., Kenkel-Rossi, E., Klassen, L., & Stollenwerk, R. (1996). Focus on spiritual well-being: Harmonious interconnectedness of mind–body–spirit—Use of the JAREL Spiritual Well-Being Scale. *Geriatric Nursing, 17,* 262–266.

Isaia, D., Parker, V., & Murrow, E. (1999). Spiritual well-being among older adults. *Journal of Gerontological Nursing, 26*(8),15–21.

Jackson, C. (2004). Healing ourselves, healing others: First in a series. *Holistic Nursing Practice, 18*(2), 67–81.

Koenig, H. G., George, L. K., & Titus, P. (2004). Religion, spirituality and health in medically ill hospitalized older patients. *Journal of the American Geriatric Society, 52,* 554–562.

Krebs, K. (2003). Complementary healthcare practices: The spiritual aspect of caring—an integral part of health and healing. *Gastroenterological Nursing, 26* (5), 212–214.

Kulig, J. C., Hall, B. L., Babcock, R., Campbell, R., & Wall, M. (2004). Childbearing practices in Kanadier Mennonite women. *Canadian Nurse, 100*(8), 34–37.

Labun, E., & Emblen, J. (2007). Spirituality and health in Punjabi Sikh. *Journal of Holistic Nursing, 25*(3), 141–148.

Lin, H. R., & Bauer-Wu, S. M. (2003). Psycho-spiritual well-being in patients with advanced cancer: An integrative review of the literature. *Journal of Advanced Nursing, 44,* 69–80.

Lindberg, D. A. (2005). Integrative review of research related to meditation, spirituality, and the elderly. *Geriatric Nursing, 26* (6), 372–377.

Louis, A., & Alpert, P. (2000). Spirituality for nurses and their practice. *Nursing Leadership Forum, 5*(2), 43–51.

Macrae, J. A. (2001). *Nursing as a spiritual practice: A contemporary application of Florence Nightingale's views.* New York: Springer.

Mauk, K. L., & Schmidt, N. K. (2004). *Spiritual care in nursing practice.* Philadelphia, PA: Lippincott Williams & Wilkins.

Mazanec, P., & Tyler, M. K. (2004). Cultural considerations in end-of-life care: How ethnicity, age, and spirituality affect decisions when death is imminent. *Home Healthcare Nurse, 22,* 317–326.

McEvoy, M. (2003). Culture and spirituality as an integrated concept in pediatric care. *MCN American Journal of Maternal Child Nursing, 28*(1), 39–44.

McSherry, W. (1998). Nurses' perceptions of spirituality and spiritual care. *Nursing Standard 13*(4), 36–40.

McSherry, W. (2001). Spiritual crisis? Call a nurse. In H. Orchard (Ed.), *Spirituality in health care contexts* (pp. 107–117). London: Jessica Kingsley.

McSherry, W., & Ross, L. (2002). Dilemmas of spiritual assessment: Considerations for nursing practice. *Journal of Advanced Nursing, 38,* 479–488.

McSherry, W., Cash, K., & Ross, L. (2004). Meaning of spirituality: Implications for nursing practice. *Journal of Clinical Nursing, 13,* 934–941.

Meyerhoff, H., Van Hofwegen, L., Harwood, C. H., Drury, M., & Emblen, J. (2002). Spiritual nursing interventions. *Canadian Nurse, 98*(3), 21–24.

Miller, W. R., & Thoresen, C. E. (2003). Spirituality, religion and health: An emerging research field [Electronic version]. *The American Psychologist, 58,* 24–35.

Miner-Williams, D. (2006). Putting a puzzle together: Making spirituality meaningful for nursing using an evolving theoretical framework. *Journal of Clinical Nursing, 15,* 811–821.

Morse, J. M., & Doberneck, B. (1995). Delineating the concept of hope. *Image: The Journal of Nursing Scholarship, 27,* 277–285.

Mosgrove, J. (2007). Nurse to know: Joanne Olson: A leader in academia and the parish community. *Canadian Nurse, 103*(6), 28–29.

NANDA International (2007). *NANDA-I Nursing diagnoses: Definitions and classification 2007–2008.* Philadelphia, PA: Author.

Narayanasamy, A. (2004). Spiritual coping mechanisms in chronic illness: A qualitative study. *Journal of Clinical Nursing, 13,* 116–117.

Narayanasamy, A., Clissett, P., Parumal, L., Thompson, D., Annasamy, S., & Edge, R. (2004). Responses to the spiritual needs of older people. *Journal of Advanced Nursing, 48,* 6–16.

Neuman, B. (1982). *The Neuman systems model: Application to nursing education and practice.* Norwalk, CT: Appleton-Century-Crofts.

O'Brien, M. E. (2003). *Parish nursing: Healthcare ministry within the church.* Sudbury, MA: Jones & Bartlett.

Olson, J., Simington, J. A., & Clark, M. B. (1998). Educating parish nurses. *Canadian Nurse, 98*(8), 40–44.

Paley, J. (2008). Spirituality in nursing: A reductionist approach. *Nursing Philosophy, 9,* 3–18.

Paul, P. (2000). The history of the relationship between nursing and faith traditions. In M. B. Clark & J. K. Olson (Eds.), *Nursing within a faith community: Promoting health in times of transition* (pp. 147–159). Thousand Oaks, CA: Sage.

Perry, D. J. (2004). Self-transcendence: Lonergan's key to integration of nursing theory, research, and practice. *Nursing Philosophy, 5,* 67.

Pesut, B. (2006). Fundamental or foundational obligation?: Problematizing the ethical call to spiritual care in nursing. *ANS. Advances in Nursing Science, 29,* 125–133.

Pesut, B. (2008). A philosophic analysis of the concepts of spirituality and spiritual care in nursing fundamentals textbooks. *Journal of Nursing Education, 47,* 167–173.

Pesut, B., Fowler, M., Taylor, E. J., Reimer Kirkham, S., & Sawatzky, R. (2008). Conceptualising spirituality and religion for healthcare. *Journal of Clinical Nursing, 17*(21), 2803–2810.

Pesut, B., & Sawatzky, R. (2006). To describe or prescribe: Assumptions underlying a prescriptive nursing process approach to spiritual care. *Nursing Inquiry, 13,* 127–134.

Pincharoen, S., & Congdon, J. G. (2003). Spirituality and health in older Thai persons in the United States. *Western Journal of Nursing Research, 25,* 93–108.

Sawatzky, J. E., & Fowler-Kerry, S. (2003). Impact of caregiving: Listening to the voice of informal caregivers. *Journal of Psychiatric and Mental Health Nursing, 10,* 277–286.

Sawatzky, R., & Pesut, B. (2005). Attributes of spiritual care in nursing practice. *Journal of Holistic Nursing, 23,* 19–33.

Semenic, S. E., Callister, L. C., & Feldman, P. (2004). Giving birth: The voices of Orthodox Jewish women living in Canada. *Journal of Obstetric, Gynecologic and Neonatal Nursing, 33,* 80–87.

Sessanna, L., Finnell, D., & Jezewski, M. A. (2007). Spirituality in nursing and health related literature: A concept analysis. *Journal of Holistic Nursing, 25,* 252–262.

Skalla, K. A., & McCoy, P. (2006). Spiritual assessment of patients with cancer: The moral authority, vocational, aesthetic, social and transcendent model. *Oncological Nursing Forum, 33,* 745–751.

Smith, A. R. (2006). Using the synergy model to provide spiritual nursing care in critical care settings. *Critical Care Nurse, 26*(4), 41–47.

Spurlock, W. R. (2005). Spiritual well-being and caregiver burden in Alzheimer's caregivers. *Geriatric Nursing, 26,* 154–161.

Tanyi, R. A., & Werner, J. S. (2008). Women's experience of spirituality within end-stage renal disease and hemodialysis. *Clinical Nursing Research, 17,* 32–49.

Taylor, E. J. (2002). *Spiritual care: Nursing theory, research, and practice.* Upper Saddle River, NJ: Prentice Hall.

Taylor, E. J. (2003a). Spiritual needs of patients with cancer and family caregivers. *Cancer Nursing, 26,* 260–266.

Taylor, E. J. (2003b). Prayer's clinical issues and implications. *Holistic Nursing Practice, 17,* 179–188.

Travelbee, J. (1966). *Interpersonal aspects of nursing.* Philadelphia: F.A. Davis.

Vance, D. L. (2001). Nurses' attitudes towards spirituality and spiritual care. *Medsurg Nursing, 10,* 264–268.

Van Dover, L., & Bacon-Pfeiffer, J. (2007). Spiritual care in Christian parish nursing. *Journal of Advanced Nursing, 57,* 213–221.

Van Dover, L. J., & Bacon, J. M. (2001). Spiritual care in nursing practice: A close-up view. *Nursing Forum, 36,* 18–30.

Van Leeuwen, R., Tiesinga, L. J., Jochemasen, H., & Post, D. (2007). Aspects of spirituality concerning illness. *Scandinavian Journal of Caring Sciences, 21,* 482–489.

Watson, J. (1979). *Nursing: The philosophy and science of caring.* Boston: Little, Brown.

Wright, L. M. (2005). *Spirituality, suffering, and illness: Ideas for healing.* Philadelphia, PA: F.A. Davis.

Chapter 29

Allan, D. E., Stajduhar, K. I., & Reid, R. C. (2005). The uses of provincial administration health databases for research on palliative care: Insights from British Columbia, Canada. *BMC Palliative Care, 4*(2). Retrieved November 21, 2008, from http://www.biomedcentral.com/1472-684x/4/2

Benner, P., Kerchner, S., Corless, I. B., & Davies, B. (2003). Attending death as a human passage: Core nursing principles for end-of-life care. *American Journal of Critical Care, 12,* 558–561.

Bowlby, J. (1980). *Attachment and loss: Vol. 3. Loss, sadness, and depression.* New York: Basic Books.

Canadian Hospice Palliative Care Association Nursing Standards Committee. (2002). *Hospice palliative care nursing standards of practice.* Ottawa, ON: Canadian Hospice Palliative Care Association.

Canadian Nurses Association. (1994). *Joint statement on advance directives* [Position statement]. Ottawa, ON: Author.

Canadian Nurses Association. (1998). *Advance directives: The nurse's role, ethics in practice.* Ottawa, ON: Author.

Canadian Nurses Association. (2000). *Fact sheet: Palliative care.* Ottawa, ON: Author.

Canadian Nurses Association. (2008). *Code of ethics for registered nurses.* Ottawa, ON: Author.

Chochinov, H.M. (2006). Dying, dignity, and new horizons in palliative end-of-life care. *CA: A Cancer Journal for Clinicians, 56,* 84–103.

Davies, B., Collins, J. B., Steele, R., Pipke, I., & Cook, K. (2003). The impact on families of a children's hospice program. *Journal of Palliative Care, 19*(1), 15–26.

Davies, B., & Oberle, K. (1990). Dimensions of the supportive role of the nurse in palliative care. *Oncology Nursing Forum, 17*(1), 87–94.

Egan, K. A., & Arnold, R. L. (2003). Grief and bereavement care. *American Journal of Nursing, 103*(9), 42–52.

Ferris, F. D., Balfour, H. M., Bowen, K., Farley, J., Hardwick, M., Lamontagne, C., et al. (2002). A model to guide patient and family care: Based on nationally accepted principles and norms of practice. *Journal of Pain and Symptom Management, 24,* 106–123.

Grassi, L. (2007). Bereavement in families with relatives dying of cancer. *Current Opinion in Supportive and Palliative Care, 1,* 43–49

Gray, K., & Lassance, A. (2003). *Grieving reproductive loss: The healing process.* Amityville, NY: Baywood.

Hasler, K. (1996). Understanding and managing bereavement. *Nursing Standard, 10*(24), 51–54.

Kagawa-Singer, M. (1998). The cultural context of death rituals and mourning practices. *Oncology Nursing Forum, 25*(10), 1752–1756.

Kirk, P., Kirk, I, & Kristjanson, L. (2004). What do patients receiving palliative care for cancer and their families want to be told? A Canadian and Australian qualitative study. *British Medical Journal, 328,* 1343–1349.

Kouch, M. (2006). Managing symptoms for a good death. *Nursing, 36*(11), 58–63.

Kübler-Ross, E. (1969). *On death and dying.* New York: Macmillan.

Lund, D. A. (1989). Conclusions about bereavement in later life and implications for interventions and future research. In D. A. Lund (Ed.), *Older bereaved spouses: Research with practical application* (pp. 217–231). New York: Hemisphere.

Parkes, C. M. (1972). *Bereavement: Studies of grief in adult life.* London: Tavistock.

Perry, A, (2005). *Clinical nursing skills and techniques* (6th ed.). St. Louis, MO: Mosby.

Senate of Canada. (2000). *Quality end-of-life care: The right of every Canadian* [Final report of the Subcommittee to Update "Of Life and Death" of the Standing Senate Committee on Social Affairs, Science and Technology]. Retrieved November 21, 2004, from http://www.parl.gc.ca/36/2/parlbus/commbus/senate/com-e/upda-e/rep-e/repfinjun00-e.htm

Smith, A., & Kautz, D. (2007). A day with Blake: hope on a medical-surgical unit. *Medsurg Nursing, 16,* 378–382.

Tilden, V. P., Tolle, S. W., Nelson, C. A., & Fields, J. (2001). Family decision-making to withdraw life-sustaining treatments from hospitalized patients. *Nursing Research, 50,* 105–115.

Tolle, S., Tilden, V. P., Rosenfeld, A. G., & Hickman, S. E. (2000). Family reports of barriers to optimal care of the dying. *Nursing Research, 49,* 310–317.

van Bommel, H. (2006). *Family hospice care: Pre-planning and care guide.* Scarborough, ON: Resources Supporting Family and Community Legacies.

Verosky, D. (2006). Good grief: assisting patients and their loved ones in dealing with death. *Academy of Medical-Surgical Nurses Newsletter, 15*(6), 1, 14–15.

Waldrop, D. (2007). Caregiver grief in terminal illness and bereavement: A mixed methods study. *Health and Social Work, 32,* 197–206.

Worden, J. W. (1991). *Grief counseling and grief therapy: A handbook for the mental health practitioner* (2nd ed.). New York: Springer.

World Health Organization. (2008). *WHO definition of palliative care.* Retrieved November 21, 2008, from http://www.who.int/cancer/palliative/definition/en/

Chapter 30

Adshead, G. (2000). Psychological therapies for post-traumatic stress disorder. *British Journal of Psychiatry, 177*(2), 144–148.

Aguilera, D. C. (1998). *Crisis intervention: Theory and methodology* (8th ed.). St. Louis, MO: Mosby.

Aldwin, C. (1992). Aging, coping, and efficacy: Theoretical framework for examining coping in life-span developmental context. In M. Wykle, E. Kahava, & J. Kowal (Eds.), *Stress and health among the elderly* (pp. 96–115). New York: Springer.

Aldwin, C. M. (2000). *Stress, coping, and development: An integrative perspective.* New York: Guilford Press.

Aldwin, C. M., Sutton, K. J., Chiara, G., & Spiro, A., III. (1996). Age differences in stress, coping, and appraisal: Findings from the Normative Aging Study. *Journals of Gerontology, Series B, Psychological Sciences and Social Sciences, 51*(4), P179–P188.

American Psychiatric Association. (2000). *Diagnostic and statistical manual of mental disorders* (4th ed.). Washington, DC: Author.

Andersen, S. L., & Teicher, M. H. (2008). Stress, sensitive periods and maturational events in adolescent depression. *Trends in Neuroscience, 31,* 183–191.

Bauman, A., O'Brien-Pallas, L., Armstrong-Sassen, M., Blythe, J., Bourbonnais, R., Cameron, S., et al. (2001). *Commitment and care: The benefits of a healthy workplace for nurses, their patients and the system. A policy synthesis.* Ottawa, ON: Canadian Health Services Research Foundation.

Blackburn-Munro, G., & Blackburn-Munro, R. E. (2001). Chronic pain, chronic stress & depression: Coincidence or consequence? *Journal of Neuroendocrinology, 13,* 1009–1023.

Breslau, N., & Kessler, R. C. (2001). The stressor criterion in *DSM-IV* posttraumatic stress disorder: An empirical investigation. *Biological Psychiatry, 50,* 699–704.

Brunello, N., Davidson, J. R., Deahl, M., Kessler, R. C., Mendlewicz, J., Racagni, G., et al. (2001). Posttraumatic stress disorder: Diagnosis and epidemiology, comorbidity and social consequences, biology and treatment. *Neuropsychobiology, 43,* 150–162.

Butcher, S. K., & Lord, J. M. (2004). Stress responses and innate immunity: Aging as a contributing factor. *Aging Cell, 3,* 151–160.

Canadian Nurses Association. (2008). *Code of ethics for registered nurses.* Ottawa, ON: Author.

Caplan, G. (1981). Mastery of stress: Psychosocial aspects. *American Journal of Psychiatry, 138,* 413–420.

Chapman, D. P., & Perry, G. S.(2008). Depression as a major component of public health for older adults. *Prevalent Chronic Diseases, 5*(1), A22.

Chiriboga, D. A. (1992). Paradise lost: Stress in the modern age. In M. Wykle, E. Kahava, & J. Kowal (Eds.), *Stress and health among the elderly* (pp. 35–72). New York: Springer.

Chrousos, G. P., Loriaux, L., & Gold, P. W. (1988). The concept of stress and its historical development. In G. P. Chrousos, L. Loriaux, & P. W. Gold (Eds.), *Mechanisms of physical and emotional stress* (pp. 3–10). New York: Plenum Press.

Davis, M. C., Matthews, K. A., & Twamley, E. W. (1999). Is life more difficult on Mars or Venus? A meta-analytic review of sex differences in major and minor life events. *Annals of Behavioral Medicine, 21,* 83–97.

Desbonnet, L., Garrett, L., Daly, E., McDermott, K. W., & Dinan, T. G. (2008). Sexually dimorphic effects of maternal separation stress on corticotrophin-releasing factor and vasopressin systems in the adult rat brain. *International Journal of Developmental Neuroscience, 26,* 259–268.

Dochterman, J. M., & Bulechek, G. M. (Eds.). (2004). *Nursing Interventions Classification (NIC)* (4th ed.). St. Louis, MO: Mosby.

Dunn, A. J. (1989). CRF as mediator of stress responses neurochemical and behavioral aspects. In L. Bueno, S. Collins, & J.-L. Junien (Eds.), *Stress and digestive mobility* (pp. 13–22). London: John Libbey.

Engelmann, M., & Ludwig, M. (2004). The activity of the hypothalamo-neuro-hypophysial system in response to acute stressor exposure: Neuroendocrine and electrophysiological observations. *Stress, 7*(2), 91–96.

Etters, L., Goodall, D., & Harrison, B. E. (2008). Caregiver burden among dementia patients caregivers: A review of the literature. *Journal of the Academy of Nurse Practitioners, 20,* 423–428.

Foster, J. (1997). Successful coping, adaptation and resilience in the elderly: An interpretation of epidemiological data. *The Psychiatric Quarterly, 68,* 189–219.

Graham, J. E., Christian, L. M., & Kiecolt-Glaser, J. K. (2006). Stress, age, and immune function: Towards a lifespan approach. *Journal of Behavioral Medicine, 29,* 389–400.

Guendelman, S., Malin, C., Herr-Harthorn, B., & Vargas, P. N. (2001). Orientations to motherhood and male partner support among women in Mexico and Mexican-origin women in the United States. *Social Sciences in Medicine, 52,* 1805–1813.

Hyer, L. A., & Sohnle, S. J. (2001). *Trauma among older people.* Ann Arbor, MI: Taylor & Francis.

Joy, D., Probert, R,, Bisson J. I., & Shephard, J. P. (2000). Post-traumatic stress reactions after injury. *Journal of Trauma, 48,* 490–494.

Kasl, S. V. (1992). Stress and health among the elderly: An overview of issues. In M. Wykle, E. Kahava, & J. Kowal (Eds.), *Stress and health among the elderly* (pp. 5–35). New York: Springer.

Kimerling, R., Clum, G. A., & Wolfe, J. (2000). Relationships among trauma exposure, chronic posttraumatic stress disorder symptoms, and self-reported health in women: Replication and extension. *Journal of Trauma Stress, 13,* 115–128.

Lazarus, R. (1999). *Stress and emotion: A new synthesis.* New York: Springer.

Le Moal, M. (2007). Historical approach and evolution of the stress concept: A personal account. *Psychoneuroendocrinology, 32*(Suppl. 1), S3–S9.

Lupien, S. J., Fiocco, A., Wan, N., Maheu, F., Lord, C., Schramek, T., et al. (2005). Stress hormones and human memory function across the lifespan. *Psychoneuroendocrinology, 30,* 225–242.

Magri, F., Cravello, L., Barili, L., Sarra, S., Cinchetti, W., Salmoiraghi, F., et al. (2006). Stress and dementia: The role of the hypothalamic–pituitary–adrenal axis. *Aging: Clinical and Experimental Research, 18,* 167–170.

Matthews K. A., Gump, B. B., & Owens, J. F. (2001). Chronic stress influences cardiovascular and neuroendocrine responses during acute stress and recovery, especially in men. *Health Psychology, 20,* 403–410.

Manning, G., Curtis, K., & McMillen, S. (1999). *Stress: Living and working in a changing world.* Duluth, MN: Whole Person Associates.

McEwen, B. (2007). Physiology and neurobiology of stress and adaptation: Central role of the brain. *Physiology Reviews, 87,* 873–904.

Mollica, R. F., Sarajlic, N., Chernoff, M., Lavelle J., Vukovic, I. S., & Massagli, M. P. (2001). Longitudinal study of psychiatric symptoms, disability, mortality, and emigration among Bosnian refugees. *JAMA: The Journal of the Medical Association, 286,* 546–554.

Monat, A., & Lazarus, R. (1991). *Stress and coping: An anthology.* New York: Columbia University Press.

Moorhead, S., Johnson, M., & Maas, M. (Eds.). (2004). *Nursing outcomes classification (NOC)* (3rd ed.). St. Louis, MO: Mosby.

Neuman, B. (1995). *The Neuman systems model* (3rd ed.). Stamford, CT: Appleton & Lange.

O'Farrell, P., Murray, J., & Hotz, S. B. (2000). Psychologic distress among spouses of patients undergoing cardiac rehabilitation. *Heart & Lung, 29*(2), 97–104.

Pender, N. J., Murdaugh, C., & Parsons, M. A. (2002). *Health promotion in nursing practice* (4th ed.). Upper Saddle River, NJ: Haworth Press.

Selye, H. (1974). *Stress without distress.* New York: J. B. Lippincott.

Selye, H. (1991). History and present status of the stress concept. In A. Monat & R. Lazarus (Eds.), *Stress and coping: An anthology* (pp. 21–35). New York: Columbia University Press.

Shalev, A. Y., Bonne, O., & Eth, S. (1996). Treatment of posttraumatic stress disorder: A review. *Psychosomatic Medicine, 58,* 165–182.

Shen, B. J., & Takeuchi, D. T. (2001). A structural model of acculturation and mental health status among Chinese Americans. *American Journal of Community Psychology, 29,* 387–418.

Shontz, F. (1975). *The psychological aspects of physical illness and disability.* New York: Macmillan.

Skultety, K. M., & Rodriguez, R. L. (2008). Treating geriatric depression in primary care. *Current Psychiatry Reports, 10,* 44–50.

Solomon, P., & Draine, J. (1995). Adaptive coping among family members of persons with serious mental illness. *Psychiatric Services, 46,* 1156–1160.

Stuart, G., & Wright, L. (1995). Applying the Neuman systems model to psychiatric nursing practice. In B. Neuman (Ed.), *The Neuman systems model* (3rd ed.). Stamford, CT: Appleton & Lange.

Varcarolis, E. M. (2002). *Foundations of psychiatric mental health nursing: A clinical approach* (4th ed.). St. Louis, MO: W. B. Saunders.

Chapter 31

Canadian Hypertension Education Program. (2008). *Recommendations for the management of hypertension: Hypertension as a public health risk in BP Measurement Slides.* Retrieved January 7, 2009, from http://www.hypertension.ca/chep/educational-resources/slides/

Chobanian, A. V., Bakris, G. L., Black, H. R., Cushman, W. C., Green, L. A., Izzo, J. L., Jr., et al. (2003). National Heart, Lung, and Blood Institute; National Institutes of Health: The seventh report of the Joint National Committee on Detection, Evaluation, and Treatment of High Blood Pressure. *Journal of the American Medical Association, 289,* 2560–2571.

Ebersole, P., Hess, P., & Luggen, A. S. (2004). *Toward healthy aging: Human needs and human response* (6th ed). St. Louis, MO: Mosby.

Health Canada. (2007). *Mercury: Your health and the environment.* Environmental & Workplace Health. Retrieved December 4, 2008, from http://www.hc-sc.gc.ca/ewh-semt/pubs/contaminants/mercur/q18-q27-eng.php

Henker, R., & Carlson, K. K. (2007). Fever. *Advances in Critical Care, 18*(1), 76.

Hockenberry, M. J., & Wilson, D. (2007). *Wong's nursing care of infants and children* (8th ed.). St. Louis, MO: Mosby.

Holtzclaw, B. J. (2003). *Use of thermoregulatory principles in patient care: Fever management.* Retrieved December 4, 2008, from http://www.esrnexus.com/displayArticle.aspx?codedarticleid=350169

Jones, D. W., Appel, L. J., Sheps, S. G., Roccella, E. J., & Lenfant, C. (2003). Measuring blood pressure accurately: New and persistent challenges. *Journal of the American Medical Association, 289,* 1027–1030.

Jones, H., Atkinson, G., Leary, A., George, K., Murphy, M., & Waterhouse, J. (2006). Reactivity to ambulatory blood pressure to physical activity varies with time of day. *Hypertension, 47,* 778–784. Retrieved December 4, 2008, from http://hyper.ahajournals.org/cgi/content/full/47/4/778

Maxton, F. J., Justin, L., & Gillies, D. (2004). Estimating core temperature in infants and children after cardiac surgery: A comparison of six methods. *Journal of Advanced Nursing, 45,* 214–222. Retrieved January 22, 2009, from http://www.blackwell-synergy.com/links/doi/10.1046/j.1365-2648.2003.02883.x

Redon, J. (2004). The normal circadian pattern of blood pressure: Implications for treatment. *International Journal of Clinical Practice, 58*(Suppl. 145), 3.

Schell, K., Lyons, D., Bradley, E., Bucker, L., Seckel, M., Wakai, S., et al. (2006). Clinical comparison of automatic, noninvasive measurements of blood pressure in the forearm and upper arm with the patient supine or with the head of the bed raised 45 degrees: A follow-up study. *American Journal of Critical Care, 15,* 196–205.

Chapter 32

American Cancer Society. (2008). *Cancer prevention and early detection facts and figures 2008.* Retrieved April 27, 2008 from http://www.cancer.org/docroot/NWS/content/NWS_1_1x_ACS_Report_Calls_For_Greater.

Barton, M. B., Harris, R., & Fletcher, S. W. (1999). Does this patient have breast cancer? The screening clinical breast examination: Should it be done? How? *Journal of the American Medical Association, 282,* 1270–1280.

Bickley, L. S., & Szilagyi, P. G. (2007). *Bates guide to physical examination and history taking* (9th ed.). Philadelphia, PA: Lippincott Williams & Wilkins.

Boyd, N. F., Guo, H., & Martin, L. J. (2007). Mammographic density and the risk and detection of breast cancer. *New England Journal of Medicine, 356,* 227–236.

Canadian Breast Cancer Foundation. (2006). *Established risk factors in breast cancer.* Retrieved November 25, 2008, from http://www.cbcf.org/breastcancer/bc_risk_er.asp

Canadian Cancer Society. (2008a). *Get to know your breasts*. Retrieved November 15, 2008, from http://www.cancer.ca

Canadian Cancer Society. (2008b). *Early detection and screening*. Retrieved November 15, 2008, from http://www.cancer.ca/Canada-wide/Prevention/Get%20screened/Early%20detection%20and%20screening%20for%20breast%20cancer.aspx?sc_lang=en

Canadian Cancer Society. (2007). *Canadian cancer statistics 2007*. Toronto, ON: Author.

Canadian Cancer Society/Alberta/NWT Division. (2002). *Breast self-examination: You're worth it* [Brochure]. Calgary, AB: Author.

Canadian Nurses Association. (2008). *Code of ethics for registered nurses*. Ottawa, ON: Author.

Folstein, M. F., Folstein, S., & McHugh, P. R. (1975). "Mini-mental state": A practical method for grading the cognitive state of patients for the clinician. *Journal of Psychiatric Research, 12*, 189–198.

Hardy, M. A. (1996). What can you do about your patient's dry skin? *Journal of Gerontological Nursing, 22*(5), 10–18.

Health Canada. (2007). *First Nations comparable health indicators*. Retrieved April 25, 2008, from http://www.hc-sc.gc.ca/fnih-spni/pubs/gen/2005-01_health-sante_indicat/index_e.html

Health Canada. (2003). *Canadian guidelines for body weight classification in adults*. Ottawa, ON: Author.

Health Canada. (1999). Routine practices and additional precautions for preventing the transmission of infection in health care. *Canada Communicable Disease Report, 25*(Suppl. 4), 1–142. Retrieved November 15, 2008, from http://www.phac-aspc.gc.ca/publicat/ccdr-rmtc/99vol25/25s4/

Hockenberry, M. J., & Wilson, D. (2007). *Wong's nursing care of infants and children* (8th ed.). St. Louis, MO: Mosby.

Jackson, M. (2002). *Pain: The fifth vital sign*. Toronto, ON: Random House of Canada.

Jarvis, C. (2004). *Physical examination and health assessment* (4th ed.). St Louis, MO: Elsevier Science.

Kahn, R. L., Goldfarb, A. I., Pollack, M., & Peck, A. (1960). Brief objective measures for the determination of mental status of the aged. *American Journal of Psychiatry, 117*, 326–328.

Kearney, A. J., & Murray, M. (2006). Commentary—evidence against breast self examination is not conclusive: What policymakers and health professionals need to know. *Journal of Public Health Policy, 27*, 282–292.

Kennedy-Malone, L., Fletcher, K. R., & Plank, L. M. (2000). *Management guidelines for gerontological nurse practitioners*. Philadelphia, PA: F. A. Davis.

Miller, C. A. (2009). *Nursing for wellness in older adults. Theory and practice* (4th ed.). Philadelphia, PA: Lippincott.

Rogers, B. (2003). *Occupational and environmental health nursing: Concepts and practice* (2nd ed). Philadelphia, PA: W. B. Saunders.

Seidel, H. M., Ball, J. W., Dains, J. E., & Benedict, G. W. (2006). *Mosby's guide to physical examination* (6th ed.). St. Louis, MO: Mosby.

Stuart, G., & Laraia, M. (Eds.).(2003). *Principles and practice of psychiatric nursing* (8th ed.). St. Louis, MO: Mosby.

Swartz, M. H. (2005). *Textbook of physical diagnosis: History and examination* (5th ed.). Philadelphia, PA: W. B. Saunders.

Talbot, L., & Curtis, L. (1996). The challenges of assessing skin indicators in people of color. *Home Healthcare Nurse, 14*, 167–171.

Chapter 33

Association of Perioperative Registered Nurses. (2004). Hand antisepsis, surgical. In *Standards, recommended practices, and guidelines*. Denver, CO: Author.

Boyce, J. M., & Pittet, D. (2002). Guideline for hand hygiene in health-care settings. Recommendations of the Healthcare Infection Control Practices Advisory Committee and the HIPAC/SHEA/APIC/IDSA Hand Hygiene Task Force. *American Journal of Infection Control, 30*(8), S1–S46.

Canadian Needle Stick Surveillance Network. (2003, December 15). Update—Surveillance of health care workers exposed to blood, body fluids and blood-borne pathogens in Canadian hospital settings: 1 April 2000, to 31 March 2002. *Canada Communicable Disease Report, 29*(34). Retrieved May 13, 2004, from http://www.phac-aspc.gc.ca/ publicat/ccdr-rmtc/03vol29/dr2924ea.html

Centers for Disease Control and Prevention. (2002). *Guideline for hand hygiene in health-care settings*. Retrieved January 4, 2008, from http://www.cdc.gov/mmwr/preview/mmwrhtml/rr5116a1.htm

Centers for Disease Control and Prevention. (2004). Guidelines for preventing health-care–associated pneumonia—United States, 2003. Recommendations of the CDC and the Healthcare Infection Control Practices Advisory Committee. *MMWR. Morbidity and Mortality Weekly Report*, 53(RR-13).

Community and Hospital Infection Control Association—Canada. (2004). *Home page*. Retrieved January 4, 2008, from http://www.chica.org

Forster, A. J., Asmis, T. R., Clark, H. D., Al Saied, G., Code, C. C., Caughey, S. C., et al. (2004). Ottawa Hospital Patient Safety Study: Incidence and timing of adverse events in patients admitted to a Canadian teaching hospital. *Canadian Medical Association Journal, 170*, 1235–1240.

Gantz, N. M., Tkatch, L. S., & Makris, A. T. (2000). Geriatric infections. In J. A. Pfeiffer (Ed.), *APIC text of infection control and epidemiology* (pp. 35.1–35.13). Washington, DC: Association for Professionals in Infection Control and Epidemiology.

Garner, J. S. (1996). Guideline for isolation precautions in hospitals. The Hospital Infection Control Practices Advisory Committee. *Infection Control and Hospital Epidemiology, 17*(1), 54–80.

Girou, E., Loyeau, S., Legrand, P., Oppein, F., & Brun-Buisson, C. (2002). Efficacy of handrubbing with alcohol based solution versus standard handwashing with antiseptic soap: Randomized clinical trial. *British Medical Journal, 325*, 362–365.

Green, J. N. (1996). The microbiology of colonization, including techniques for assessing measuring colonization. *Infection Control and Hospital Epidemiology, 17*, 114–118.

Grimes, D., & Grimes, R. (1994). *AIDS and HIV infections*. St. Louis, MO: Mosby.

Gruendeman, B. J., & Mangum, S. S. (2001). *Infection prevention in surgical settings*. Philadelphia, PA: WB Saunders Co.

Gupta, C., Czubatyj, A. M., Briski, L. E., & Malani, A. K. (2007). Comparison of two alcohol-based surgical scrub solutions with an iodine-based scrub brush for presurgical antiseptic effectiveness in a community hospital. *Journal of Hospital Infection, 65*, 277–278.

Health Canada. (1997). Infection control guidelines: Preventing the spread of vancomycin-resistant enterococci (VRE) in Canada. *Canada Communicable Disease Report, 23*(Suppl. 8), i–iv, 1–16.

Health Canada. (1998). Infection control guidelines: Hand washing, cleaning, disinfection and sterilization in health care. *Canada Communicable Disease Report, 24*(Suppl. 8). Retrieved January 24, 2005, from http://www.hc-sc.gc.ca/pphb-dgspsp/publicat/ccdr-rmtc/98pdf/cdr24s8e.pdf

Health Canada. (1999). Infection control guidelines: Routine practices and additional precautions for preventing the transmission of infection in health care. *Canada Communicable Disease Report, 25*(Suppl. 4), 83–111.

Hedderwick, S. A., McNeil, S. A., Lyons, M. J., & Kauffman, C. A. (2000). Pathogenic organisms associated with artificial fingernails worn by healthcare workers. *Infection Control and Hospital Epidemiology, 21*, 505–509.

Ignatavicius, D., & Workman, M. L. (2002). *Medical–surgical nursing: Critical thinking for collaborative care*. Philadelphia, PA: Saunders.

Jernigan, J. A., Siegman-Igra, Y., Guerrant, R. C., & Farr, B. M. (1998). A randomized crossover study of disposable thermometers for prevention of *Clostridium difficile* and other nosocomial infections. *Infection Control and Hospital Epidemiology, 19*, 494–499.

Keroack, M. A., & Rosen-Kotilainen, H. (1996). Microbiology/laboratory diagnostics. In N. R. Olmsted (Ed.), *APIC infection control and applied epidemiology: Principles and practice* (pp. 7.1–7.32). St. Louis, MO: Mosby.

Larson, E. (1996). APIC guideline for handwashing and hand antisepsis in health-care settings. In R. N. Olmsted (Ed.), *APIC infection control and applied epidemiology: Principles and practice, Appendix G* (pp. G1–G17). St. Louis, MO: Mosby.

Louie, T. J., & Meddings, J. (2004). *Clostridium difficile* infection in hospitals: Risk factors and responses. *Canadian Medical Association Journal, 171*(1), 45–46.

Maki, D. G., Alvarado, C., & Hassemer, C. (1986). Double-bagging of items from isolation rooms is unnecessary as an infection control measure: A comparative study of surface contamination with single- and double-bagging. *Infection Control, 7*, 535–537.

Meeker, M. H., & Rothrock, J. C. (1999). *Alexander's care of the patient in surgery* (11th ed.). St. Louis, MO: Mosby.

Operating Room Nurses Association of Canada. (2003). *Recommended standards, guidelines and position statements for perioperative registered nursing practice* (5th ed.). Ottawa, ON: Author.

Parienti, J. J., Thibon, P., Heller, R., Le Roux, Y., von Theobald, P., Bensadoun, H., et al. (2002). Hand-rubbing with an aqueous alcoholic solution vs traditional surgical hand-scrubbing and 30-day surgical site infection rates: A randomized equivalence study. *Journal of the American Medical Association, 288*, 722–727.

Parker, J. (Ed.). (1998). *Contemporary nephrology nursing. American Nephrology Nurses' Association*. Pitman, NJ: Anthony J. Jannetti, Inc.

Pittet, D., Hugonnet, S., Harbarth, S., Mourouga, P., Sauvan, V., & Touveneau, S., et al. (2000). Effectiveness of a hospital-wide programme to improve compliance with hand hygiene. Infection Control Programme. *Lancet, 356,* 1307–1312.

Siegel, J. D., Rhinehart, E., Jackson, M., Chiarello, L., & the Healthcare Infection Control Practices Advisory Committee. (2007). *Guideline for isolation precautions: Preventing transmission of infectious agents in healthcare settings 2007.* Retrieved January 4, 2008, from http://www.cdc.gov/ncidod/dhqp/pdf/guidelines/Isolation2007.pdf

Sorrentino, S. A. (2004). *Mosby's Canadian textbook for the support worker.* Toronto, ON: Elsevier Canada.

Weinstein, S. A., Gantz, N. M., Pelletier, C., Hibert, D. (1989). Bacterial surface contamination of patient's linen: Isolation precautions versus standard care. *American Journal of Infection Control, 17,* 264–267.

Wilson, J. (2006). *Infection control in clinical practice* (3rd ed.). London, UK: Bailliere Tindall.

Chapter 34

American Diabetes Association. (2004). Insulin administration: Position statement. *Diabetes Care, 27*(Suppl. 1), S106.

Annersten, M., & Willman, A. (2005). Performing subcutaneous injections: A literature review. *Worldviews on Evidence-Based Nursing, 2,* 122–130.

Bastable, S. (2003). *Nurse as educator: Principles of teaching and learning for nursing practice.* Sudbury, MA: Jones & Bartlett.

Brager, R., & Soland, E. (2005). The spectrum of polypharmacy. *Nurse Practitioner, 30*(6), 44–50.

Canadian Centre for Occupational Health and Safety. (2005). *Needlestick injuries.* Retrieved May 1, 2008, from http://www.ccohs.ca/oshanswers/diseases/needlestick_injuries.html

Canadian Diabetes Association. (2008). [Home page]. Retrieved January 23, 2009, from http://www.diabetes.ca/

Canadian Lung Association. (n.d.). Retrieved January 23, 2009, from http://www.lung.ca/search-cherchez/index.php?index=411663&query=Inhalers&SEARCH=Search&opt=ALL

Capriotti, T. (2005). Changes in inhaler devices for asthma and COPD. *Medsurg News, 14,* 185–194.

Cook, I. F., & Murtagh, J. (2006). Ventrogluteal area: A suitable site for intramuscular vaccination of infants and toddlers. *Vaccine, 24,* 2403–2408.

Ebersole, P., Hess, P., & Schmidt Luggen, A. (2004). *Toward healthy aging: Human needs and nursing response* (6th ed.). St. Louis, MO: Mosby.

Health Canada. (1997). Preventing the transmission of bloodborne pathogens in health care and public service settings. *Canada Communicable Disease Report,* 23(Suppl. 3), 1–43.

Health Canada. (1999). Routine practices and additional precautions for preventing the transmission of infection in health care [Electronic version]. *Canada Communicable Disease Report,* 25(Suppl. 4), 1–142.

Hockenberry, M. J., & Wilson, D. (2007). *Wong's nursing care of infants and children* (8th ed.). St. Louis, MO: Mosby.

Hughes, R., & Ortiz, E. (2005). Medication errors: Why they happen, and how they can be prevented. *American Journal of Nursing, 105*(3), 14–24.

Institute for Safe Medication Practices. (2002, January 23). ISMP quarterly action agenda: October–December, 2001. *ISMP Medication Safety Alert!* Retrieved January 14, 2009, from http://www.ismp.org/Newsletters/acutecare/articles/A1Q02Action.asp

Institute for Safe Medication Practices. (2006a). *ISMP list of error-prone abbreviations, symbols, and dosage designations.* Retrieved November 12, 2008, from http://www.ismp.org/Tools/errorproneabbreviations.pdf

Institute for Safe Medication Practices. (2006b). *Preventing errors with tablet splitting.* Retrieved January 14, 2009, from http://www.accessdata.fda.gov/scripts/cdrh/cfdocs/psn/transcript.cfm?show=54#7

Institute for Safe Medication Practices. (2007). Patches: What you can't see can harm patients. *Nurse Advise-ERR, 5*(4), 1.

Institute of Medicine. (2003). *Report brief. To err is human: Building a safer health system.* Retrieved November 12, 2008, from http://www.iom.edu/?id=12735

The Joint Commission. (2007). *National patient safety goals.* Retrieved January 14, 2009, from http://www.jointcommission.org/PatientSafety/NationalPatientSafetyGoals/

Karch, A. M., & Karch, F. E. (2003). Not so fast! *American Journal of Nursing, 103*(8), 71.

Manno, M. S. (2006). Preventing adverse drug events. *Nursing, 36*(3), 56–61.

MayoClinic.com. (2007). *Asthma.* Retrieved January 23, 2009, from http://www.mayoclinic.com/health/asthma/DS00021

McKenry, L. M., Tessier, E., & Hogan, M. A. (2006). *Mosby's pharmacology in nursing* (22nd ed.). St. Louis, MO: Mosby.

Meiner, S., & Lueckenotte, A. (2006). *Gerentologic nursing* (3rd ed.). St. Louis, MO: Mosby.

Metheny, N. A. (2006). Preventing aspiration in older adults with dysphagia. *Medsurg Nursing, 15,* 110–111.

Mills, P. D., Neily, J., Mims, E., Burkhardt, M. E., & Bagian, J. (2006). Improving the bar-coded administration system at the Department of Veteran Affairs. *American Journal of Health Systems and Pharmacy, 63,* 1442–1447.

Morris, H. (2006). Managing dysphagia in older people. *Primary Health Care, 16*(6), 34–36.

National Coordinating Council for Medication Error Reporting and Prevention. (2006). *Council recommendations to recude medication errors associated with verbal medication orders and prescriptions.* Retrieved January 14, 2009, from http://www.nccmerp.org/council/council2001-02-20html?USP_Print=true&frame=lowerfrm

National Institute for Occupational Safety and Health (NIOSH). (1999, November). *NIOSH alert: Preventing needle-stick injuries in health care settings* (U.S. Department of Health and Human Services [NIOSH] Publication No. 2000-108). Cincinnati, OH: Author.

Nicoll, L. H., & Hesby, A. (2002). Intramuscular injection: An integrative research review and guideline for evidence-based practice. *Applied Nursing Research, 15,* 149–162.

Paoletti, R. D., Suess, T. M., Lesco, M. G., Feroli, A. A., Kennel, J. A., Mahler, J. M. et al. (2007). Using bar-code technology and medication observation methodology for safer meducation administration. *American Journal of Health Systems Pharmacy, 64,* 536–543.

Pape, T. M., Guerra, D. M., Muzquiz, M., Bryant, J. B., Ingram, M., Schranner, B. et al. (2005). Innovative approaches to reducing nurses' distractions during medication administration. *Journal of Continuing Nursing Education, 36,* 108–116.

Ptasinski, C. (2007). Develop a medication reconciliation process. *Nurse Manager, 38*(3), 18.

Rushing, J. (2004). Clinical do's and don'ts. How to administer a subcutaneous injection. *Nursing, 34*(6), 32.

Sanofi-Aventis. (2006). *Lovenox prescribing information.* Retrieved January 14, 2009, from http://products.sanofi-aventis.us/lovenox/lovenox.html#Dosage%20and%20Administration

Skibinski, K. A., White, B. A., Lin, L., Dong, Y., & Wu, W. (2007). Effects of technological interventions on the safety of a medication-use system. *American Journal of Health Systems Pharmacy, 64,* 90–96.

Small, S. P. (2004). Preventing sciatic nerve injury from intramuscular injections: Literature review. *Journal of Advanced Nursing, 47,* 287–296.

Stein, H. G. (2006). Glass ampules and filter needles: An example of implementing the sixth "R" in medication administration. *Medsurg Nursing, 15,* 290–294.

Vella, C., & Grech, V. (2005). Assessment of use of spacer devices for inhaled drug delivery to asthmatic children. *Pediatric Allergy and Immunology, 16,* 258–261.

VisionRx. (2005). *Encyclopedia: Eye drops.* Retrieved November 12, 2008, from http://www.visionrx.com/library/enc/enc_eyedrops.asp

Willburn, S. Q., & Eijkemans, G. (2004). Preventing needlestick injuries among healthcare workers: A WHO–OCN Collaboration. *International Journal of Occupational and Environmental Health, 10,* 451–456.

World Health Organization. (2005). *Safe Injection Global Network (SIGN): Report of the global injection safety and infection control meeting* [13–15 October, 2008, Moscow, Russian Federation]. Retrieved January 23, 2009, from http://www.who.int/injection_safety/Final-SIGNHanoiReport22March06.pdf

Chapter 35

Andrews, G. J., & Boon, H. (2005). CAM in Canada: Places, practice, research. *Complementary Therapies in Clinical Practice, 11,* 21–27.

Bardia, A., Nisly, N. L., Zimmerman, B., Gryzlak, B. S., & Wallace, R. B. (2007). Use of herbs among adults based on evidence-based indications: Findings from the National Health Survey. *Mayo Clinic Proceedings, 82,* 561–566.

Beliveau, R., & Gingras, D. (2006). *Cooking with foods that fight cancer.* Toronto, ON: McClelland and Stewart.

Benson, H. (1975). *The relaxation response.* New York: Avon.

Berkow, S. E., Barnard, N. D., Saxe, G., & Ankerberg-Nobis, T. (2007). Diet and survival after prostate cancer diagnosis. *Nutrition Reviews, 65,* 391–403

Bonakdar, R. A. (2003). Herb–drug interactions: What physicians need to know. *Patient Care, 37*(1), 58–69.

Bragdon, M. S., & Scroggs, S. (2006). Cancer prevention. *Clinical Journal of Oncology Nursing, 10,* 649–655.

Brazier, A., Mulkins, A., & Verhoef, M. (2006). Evaluating a yogic breathing and meditation intervention for individuals living with HIV/AIDS. *American Journal of Health Promotion, 20*(3), 192–195.

Breuhl, S., & Chung, O. Y. (2006). Psychological and behavioral aspects of complex regional pain syndrome management. *Clinical Journal of Pain, 22,* 430–437.

Brown, R. P., & Gerbarg, P. L. (2005). Sudarshan Kriya Yogic breathing in the treatment of stress, anxiety, and depression. II. Clinical applications and guidelines. *Journal of Alternative and Complementary Medicine, 11,* 711–717.

Canadian Cancer Society. (2007). *Phytochemicals and antioxidants.* Retrieved January 15, 2009, from http://www.old.cancer.ca/ccs/internet/standard/0,,3278_1736569999_1739704552_langId-en,00.html

Canadian Holistic Nurses Association. (2006). *Standards of practice.* Retrieved January 18, 2009, from http://chna.ca/standards-of-practice/

Chan, J. M., Holick, C. N., Leitamann, M. F., Stampfer, M. J., & Giovannucci, E. L. (2006). Diet after diagnosis and the risk of prostate cancer progression, recurrence and death (United States). *Cancer Causes Control, 17,* 199–208.

Chiarioni, G., Salandini, L., & Whitehead, W. E. (2005). Biofeedback benefits only patients with outlet dysfunction, not patients with isolated slow transit constipation. *Gastroenterology, 129,* 86–97.

Cristea, C. M., Ptito, A., & Levin, M. F. (2006). Feedback and cognition in arm motor skill reacquisition after stroke. *Stroke, 37,* 1237–1242.

College of Registered Nurses of Nova Scotia. (2005). *Complementary and alternative therapies: A guide for registered nurses.* Halifax, NS: Author. Retrieved January 24, 2009, from http://www.crnns.ca/documents/Complementary%20and%20Alternative%20Therapies%202005.pdf

Damen, L., Bruijn, J., Koes, B. W., Berger, M. Y., Passchier, J., & Verhagen, A. P. (2006). Prophylactic treatment of migraine in children. Part 1. A Systematic review of non-pharmacological trials. *Cephalalgia, 26*(4), 373–383.

de Jong, A. E., & Gambel, C. (2006). Use of a simple relaxation technique in burn care: Literature review. *Journal of Advanced Nursing, 54,* 710–721.

Dinkova-Kostova, A. T. (2007). Chemoprotection against cancer: An idea whose time has come. *Alternative Therapies in Health and Medicine, 13*(2), S122–S127.

Dossey, B., Keegan, L., & Guzzetta, C. (2005). *Holistic nursing: A handbook for practice* (4th ed.). Sudbury, MA: Jones & Bartlett.

Esposito, K., Marfella, R., Ciotola, M., Di Palo, C., Giugliano, G., Giugliano, G. et al. (2004). Effect of a Mediterranean style diet on endothelial dysfunction and markers of vascular inflammation in the metabolic syndrome: A randomized trial. *Journal of the American Medical Association, 292,* 1440–1446.

Fontaine, K. (2005). *Healing practices: Alternative therapies for nursing* (2nd ed). Upper Saddle River, NJ: Prentice Hall.

Galvin, J. A., Benson, H., Deckro, G. R., Fricchione, G. L., & Dusek, J. A. (2006). The relaxation response: Reducing stress and improving cognition in healthy aging adults. *Complementary Therapies in Clinical Practice, 12,* 186–191.

Gawain, S. (2002). *Creative visualization.* Novato, CA: New World Library.

Gustavsson, C., & von Koch, L. (2006). Applied relaxation in the treatment of long-lasting neck pain: A randomized controlled pilot study. *Journal of Rehabilitation Medicine, 38,* 100–107.

Hui, P. N., Wan, M., Chan, W. K., & Yung, P. M. (2006). An evaluation of two behavioral rehabilitation programs, Qigong versus progressive relaxation, in improving the quality of life in cardiac patients. *Journal of Alternative and Complementary Medicine, 12,* 373–378.

Kane, K. E. (2006). The phenomenology of meditation for female survivors of intimate partner violence. *Violence Against Women, 12,* 501–518.

Kanji, N., White, A. R., & Ernst, E. (2006). Autogenic training for tension type headaches: A systematic review of controlled trials. *Complementary Therapies in Medicine, 14,* 144–150.

Katzmarzyk, P. T., & Ardern, C. I. (2004). Physical activity levels of Canadian children and youth: Current issues an recommendations. *Canadian Journal of Diabetes, 28,* 67–78.

Kaushik, R. M., Kaushik, R., Mahajan, S. K., & Rajesh, V. (2006). Effects of mental relaxation and slow breathing in essential hypertension. *Complementary Therapies in Medicine, 14,* 120–126.

Keegan, L., & Shames, K. H. (2005). Touch: Connecting with the healing power. In B. M. Dossey, L. Keegan, & C. E. Guzzeta (Eds.), *Holistic nursing: A handbook for practice* (pp. 643–666). Sudbury, MA: Jones & Bartlett.

Kempainnen, J. K., Eller, L. L., Bunch, E., Hamilton, M. J., Dole, P., Holzemer, W. et al. (2006). Strategies for self-management of HIV-related anxiety. *AIDS Care, 18,* 597–607.

Krieger, D. (1975). Therapeutic touch: The imprimatur of nursing. *American Journal of Nursing, 75,* 784–787.

Krieger, D., Peper, E., & Ancoli, S. (1979). Therapeutic touch: Searching for evidence of physiological change. *American Journal of Nursing, 79,* 660–662.

Kuhn, M., & Winston, D. (2001). *Herbal therapy and supplements: A scientific and traditional approach.* New York: Lippincott, Williams & Wilkins.

Larden, C. N., Palmer, M. L., & Janssen, P. (2004). Efficacy of therapeutic touch in treating pregnant women inpatients who have a chemical dependency. *Journal of Holistic Nursing, 22,* 320–332.

Linde, K., Berner, M. M., & Kriston, L. (2008). St. John's wort for major depression. *Cochrane Database of Systematic Reviews* (4), CD000448.

McKeown, N. M., Meigs, J. B., Liu, S., Saltzman, E., Wilson, P. W. F., & Jacques, P. F. (2004). Carbohydrate nutrition, insulin resistance and the prevalence of the metabolic syndrome in the Framingham Offspring cohort. *Diabetes Care, 27,* 538–546.

Medlicott, M. S., & Harris, S. R. (2006). A systematic review of the effectiveness of exercise, manual therapy, electrotherapy, relaxation training, and biofeedback in the management of temporomandibular disorder. *Physical Therapy, 86,* 955–973.

Mehling, W. E., Hamel, K. A., Acree, M., Byl, N., & Hecht, F. M. (2005). Randomized, controlled trial of breath therapy for patients with chronic low-back pain. *Alternative Therapies in Health and Medicine, 11*(4), 44–52.

Milner, J. A. (2006). Diet and cancer: Facts and controversies. *Nutrition and Cancer, 56,* 216–224.

Movaffaghi, Z., Hasanpoor, M., Farsi, M., Hooshmand, P., & Abrishami, F. (2006). Effects of therapeutic touch on blood hemoglobin and hematocrit level. *Journal of Holistic Nursing, 24,* 41–48.

Mulkins, A., Verhoef, M., Eng, J., Findlay, B., & Ramsum, D. (2003). Evaluation of the Tzu Chi Institute for Complementary and Alternative Medicine's Integrative Care Program. *Journal of Alternative and Complementary Medicine, 9,* 585–592.

Norrbrink, B. D., Kowalski, J., & Lundeberg, T. (2006). A comprehensive pain management programme comprising educational, cognitive, and behavioral interventions for neuropathic pain following spinal cord injury. *Journal of Rehabilitation Medicine, 38,* 172–180.

Ornish, D., Scherwitz, L. W., Billings, J. H., Gould, L., Merritt, T. A., Sparler, S. et al. (1998). Intensive lifestyle changes for reversal of coronary artery disease. *Journal of the American Medical Association, 289,* 2001–2007.

Parkin, D. M., Pisani, P., & Ferlay, J. (1999). Estimates of the worldwide incidence of 25 major cancers in 1990. *International Journal of Cancer, 80,* 827–841.

Patterson, C., Kaczorowski, J., Arthur, H., Smith, K., & Mills, D. A. (2003). Complementary therapy practice: Defining the role of advanced nurse practitioners. *Journal of Clinical Nursing, 12,* 816–823.

Paul-Labrador, M., Polk, M., Dwyer, J., Velasquez., I., Nidich, S., Rainforth, M. et al. (2006). Effects of a randomized controlled trial of transcendental meditation on components of the metabolic syndrome in subjects with coronary heart disease. *Archives of Internal Medicine, 166,* 1218–1284.

Peeters, P. H., Keinen-Boker, Y. T., van der Schouw, Y. T., & Grobbee, D. E. (2003). Phytoestrogens and breast cancer risk. *Breast Cancer Research and Treatment, 77,* 171–183

Rakel, D. P., & Faass, N. (2006). *Complementary medicine in clinical practice.* Sudbury, MA: Jones & Bartlett.

Stapleton, J. A., Taylor S., & Asmundson, G. J. (2006). Effects of three PTSD treatments on anger and guilt: Exposure therapy, eye movement desensitization and reprocessing, and relaxation training. *Journal of Trauma and Stress, 19,* 19–28.

Steele, T., Rogers, C. J., & Jacob, S. E. (2007). Herbal remedies for psoriasis: What are our patients taking? *Dermatology Nursing, 19,* 448–463.

Stewart, B., Ashby, P., Bailey, P., Bourque, P., Boyle, C., Bril, V. et al. (2002). *Statement of concern to the Canadian public from Canadian neurologists regarding the debilitating and fatal damage manipulation of the neck may cause to the nervous system.* Retrieved June 2008, from http://www.chirobase.org/15News.neurol.html

The Fraser Institute. (2007). *More Canadians choosing alternative health therapies despite having to pay their own way.* Retrieved January 15, 2009, from http://www.fraserinstitute.org/newsandevents/news/4188.aspx

Thorogood, M., Simera, I., Dowler, E., Summerbell, C., & Brunner, E. (2007). A systematic review of population and community dietary interventions to prevent cancer. *Nutrition Research Reviews, 20,* 74–88.

Troppmann, L., Johns, T., & Gray-Donald, K. (2002). Natural health product use in Canada. *Canadian Journal of Public Health, 93,* 426–430.

University of York Department of Health Sciences. (2008). *Complementary and alternative medicine.* Retrieved March 13, 2008, from http://www.york.ac.uk/healthsciences/research/comaltmed.htm

Walton, K. G., Schneider, R. H., Nidich, S. I., Salemo, J., W., Nordstrom, C. K., & Bairey Merz, C. N. (2002). Psychosocial stress and cardiovascular disease.

Part 2: Effectiveness of the transcendental meditation program in treatment and prevention. *Behavioral Medicine, 28,* 106–123.

Webb, A. L., & McCullough, M. L. (2005). Dietary lignans: Potential role in cancer prevention. *Nutrition and Cancer, 51*(2), 117–131.

Willison, L., & Andrews, G. J. (2004). Complementary medicine and older people: Past research and future directions. *Complementary Therapies in Nursing and Midwifery, 10,* 40–91.

Zaza, C., Sellick, S. M., & Hillier, L. M. (2005). Coping with cancer: What do patients do? *Journal of Psychosocial Oncology, 23*(1), 5–73.

Chapter 36

Ackley, B. J., & Ladwig, G. B. (2008). *Nursing diagnosis handbook: An evidence-based guide to planning care* (8th ed.). St. Louis, MO: Mosby.

Active Healthy Kids Canada. (2007). *Older but not wiser: Canada's future at risk. Canada's report card on physical activity for children & youth—2007.* Toronto, ON: Author.

Adler, P. A., & Roberts, B. L. (2006). The use of Tai Chi to improve health in older adults. *Orthopaedic Nursing, 25*(2), 122.

Anonymous. (1965). The nurse's load [Editorial]. *Lancet, 286,* 422–423.

Beers, M. H. (Ed.) (2000). *Merck manual of geriatrics* (3rd ed.). Whitehouse Station, NJ: Merck Research Laboratories.

Bloomfield, S. A. (2005). Contributions of physical activity to bone health over the lifespan. *Topics in Geriatric Rehabilitation, 21*(1), 68–76.

Canadian Association for Health, Physical Education, Recreation and Dance. (2008). *Quality daily physical education: About QDPE* . Retrieved April 15, 2008, from http://www.cahperd.ca/eng/physicaleducation/about_qdpe.cfm

Canadian Centre for Occupational Health and Safety. (2004). *OSH answers: Ergonomics/human factors.* Retrieved April 12, 2008, from http://www.ccohs.ca/oshanswers/ergonomics/

Canadian Diabetes Association. (2003). *2003 Clinical practice guidelines.* Retrieved April 12, 2008, from http://www.diabetes.ca/cpg2003/download.aspx

Canadian Fitness and Lifestyle Research Institute. (2005). *2005 Physical activity monitor.* Retrieved April 17, 2008, from http://www.cflri.ca/eng/statistics/surveys/pam2005.php

Canadian Fitness and Lifestyle Research Institute. (2006). *Capacity study. Increasing physical activity: Building active workplaces.* Retrieved April 17, 2008, from http://www.cflri.ca/eng/statistics/surveys/capacity2006.php

Conroy, M. B., Cook, N. R., Manson, J. E., Buring, J. E., & Lee, I. (2005). Past physical activity, current physical activity, and risk of coronary heart disease. *Medicine and Science in Sports and Exercise, 37,* 1251–1256.

Dacey, M. L. (2005). A client-centered counseling approach for motivating older adults toward physical activity. *Topics in Geriatric Rehabilitation, 21,* 194–205.

Dingle, M. (2003). Role of dangling when moving from supine to standing position. *British Journal of Nursing, 12,* 346.

Fahlman, M. M., Topp, R., McNevin, N., Morgan, A. L., & Boardley, D. J. (2007). Structured exercise in older adults with limited functional ability: Assessing the benefits of an aerobic plus resistance training program. *Journal of Gerontological Nursing, 33,* 32.

Flynn, M. A. T., McNeil, D. A., Maloff, B., Mutasingwa, D., Wu, M., et al. (2006). Reducing obesity and related chronic disease risk in children and youth: A synthesis with 'best practice' recommendations. *Obesity Reviews, 7*(Suppl. 1), 7–66.

Gillespie, H. O. (2006). Exercise. In C. L. Edelman & C. L. Mandle (Eds.), *Health promotion throughout the lifespan* (5th ed.), St. Louis, MO: Mosby.

Hamilton, M. T., Hamilton, D. G., & Zderic, T. W. (2007). Role of low energy expenditure and sitting in obesity, metabolic syndrom, type 2 diabetes, and cardiovascular disease. *Diabetes, 56,* 2655.

Health Canada. (2002). *Handbook to Canada's physical activity guide to healthy active living* [Electronic version]. Ottawa, ON: Author.

Health Canada. (2003a). *Canada's physical activity guide to healthy active living* [Electronic version]. Ottawa, ON: Author.

Health Canada. (2003b). *Physical activity guide for older adults* [Electronic version]. Ottawa, ON: Author.

Health Canada. (2003c). *Public Health Agency of Canada, Healthy Living Unit.* Retrieved April 16, 2008, from http://www.phac-aspc.gc.ca/pau-uap/fitness/about.html

Health Canada. (2004). *The business case for active living at work.* Retrieved April 14, 2008, from http://www.phac-aspc.gc.ca/pau-uap/fitness/work/main_a_e.html

Health Canada. (2005a). *Family guide to physical activity for children* [Electronic version]. Ottawa, ON: Author.

Health Canada. (2005b). *Family guide to physical activity for youth* [Electronic version]. Ottawa, ON: Author.

Hockenberry-Eaton, M., & Wilson, D. (2008). *Wong's essentials of pediatric nursing* (7th ed.). St. Louis, MO: Mosby.

Hoeman, S. P. (2008). *Rehabilitation nursing: Process, application, and outcomes* (4th ed.). St. Louis, MO: Mosby.

Huddleston, J. S. (2006). Exercise. In C. L. Edelman & C. L. Mandle (Eds.), *Health promotion throughout the lifespan* (6th ed.). St. Louis, MO: Mosby.

Huether, S. E., & McCance, K. L. (2008). *Understanding pathophysiology* (4th ed.). St. Louis, MO: Mosby.

Hyman, I. (2004). Setting the stage: Reviewing current knowledge on the health of Canadian immigrants. *Canadian Journal of Public Health, 95,* 4–8.

Katula, J. A., Sipe, M., Rejeski, W. J., & Focht, B. C. (2006). Strength training in older adults: An empowering intervention. *Medicine and Science in Sports and Exercise, 38*(1), 106–111.

Lewis, S. M., Heitkemper, M. M., Ruff Dirksen, S., Graber O'Brien, P., & Bucher, L. (2007). *Medical-surgical nursing (single volume): Assessment and management of clinical problems* (7th ed.). St. Louis, MO: Mosby.

Lloyd, C. E., & Barnett, A. H. (2008). Physical activity and risk of diabetes. *The Lancet, 371,* 5.

Lu, C. (2006). *East meets West: Chinese-Canadians' perspectives on health and fitness.* Retrieved April 29, 2008, from http://www.brocku.ca/brockinternational/files/eastmeetswest.pdf

McCance, K. L., & Huether, S. E. (2005). *Pathophysiology: The biologic basis for disease in adults and children* (5th ed.). St. Louis, MO: Mosby.

Monohan, F. D., Sands, J. K., Neighbors, M., Marek, J., & Green-Nigro, C. J. (2007). *Phipps' medical-surgical nursing: Health and illness perspectives* (8th ed.). St. Louis, MO: Mosby.

Myers, T. (Ed.). (2006). *Mosby's dictionary of medicine, nursing and health professions* (7th ed.). St. Louis, MO: Mosby.

Nelson, A., & Baptiste, A. (2004). Evidence-based practices for safe patient handling and movement. *Online Journal of Issues in Nursing, 9*(3), 4. Retrieved January 11, 2009, from http://www.nursingworld.org/MainMenuCategories/ANAMarketplace/ANAPeriodicals/OJIN/TableofContents/Volume92004/No3Sept04/EvidenceBasedPractices.aspx

Occupational Health & Safety Agency for Healthcare in British Columbia. (2003). *Reference guidelines for safe patient handling.* Retrieved April 14, 2008, from http://www.ohsah.bc.ca/index.php?section_id=309§ion_copy_id=1155

Robitaille, Y., Laforest, S., Fournier, M., Gauvin, L., et al. (2004). Moving forward in fall prevention: An intevention to improve balance among older adults in real-world settings. *American Journal of Public Health, 95,* 2049–2056.

Rockwood, K., Howlett, S. E., MacKnight, C., Beattie, B. L., et al. (2004). Prevalence, attributes, and outcomes of fitness and frailty in community-dwelling older adults: Report from the Canadian Study of Health and Aging. *The Journals of Gerontology, 59A,* 1310.

School of Physical and Health Education. (2004). *Psychological benefits of sport and exercise* [class notes]. Retrieved April 14, 2008, from http://www.phe.queensu.ca/courses/phed165/

Sigal, R. G., Kenny, G. P., Wasserman, D. H., Castaneda-Sceppa, C., & White, R. D. (2006). Physical activity/exercise and type 2 diabetes: A consensus statement from the American Diabetes Association. *Diabetes Care, 29,* 1433.

Smeltzer, S., & Bare, B. (2003). *Brunner and Suddarth's textbook of medical-surgical nursing* (10th ed.). Philadelphia, PA: Lippincott Williams & Wilkins.

South Asian Dietary Resource Working Group. (2007). *Background information for health professionals.* Toronto, ON: Author. Retrieved April 29, 2008, from http://www.diabetes.ca/Files/south-asian-background-info.pdf

Thibodeau, G. A., & Patton, K. T. (2007). *Anatomy and physiology* (6th ed.). St. Louis, MO: Mosby.

Veterans Affairs Canada. (2003). Understanding normal aging. Retrieved April 14, 2008, from http://www.vac-acc.gc.ca/providers/sub.cfm?source=caregivrmanual/sect4/module2/workshop2#agingbody

Villareal, D. T., Miller, B.V. III, Banks, M., Fontana, L., Sinacore, D. R., & Klein, S. (2006). Effect of lifestyle intervention on metabolic coronary heart disease risk factors in obese older adults. *American Journal of Clinical Nutrition, 84,* 1317–1323.

Walker, J. (2008). Osteoporosis: Pathogenesis, diagnosis, and management. *Nursing Standard, 22,* 48–56.

Warburton, D. E. R., Katzmarzyk, P. T., Rhodes, R. E., & Shephard, R. J. (2007). Evidence-informed physical activity guidelines for Canadian adults. *Canadian Journal of Public Health, 98*(Suppl. 2), S16–S68.

Warburton, D. E. R., Nicol, C. W., & Bredin, S. D. (2006). Health benefits of physical activity: The evidence. *Canadian Medical Association Journal, 174,* 801–809.

Waters, T., Collins, J., Galinsky, T., & Caruso, C. (2006). NIOSH efforts to prevent musculoskeletal disorders in the healthcare industry. *Orthopaedic Nursing, 25,* 380–389.

Wilson, S. F., & Giddens, J. F. (2005). *Health assessment for nursing practice* (3rd ed.). St. Louis, MO: Mosby.

Workers Health and Safety Centre. (2003, Summer). Patient lifting: Getting a handle on it. *Resource Lines.* Retrieved April 12, 2008, from http://www.whsc.on.ca/pubs/res_lines2.cfm?resID=52

Chapter 37

American Academy of Pediatrics. (2004). *Don't treat swallowed poison with syrup of ipecac says AAP* [News release].

American Geriatrics Society (2001). Guideline for the prevention of falls in older persons. *Journal of the American Geriatrics Society, 49,* 664–672.

Baker, G. R., Norton, P. G., Flintoft, V., Blais, R., Brown, A., Cox, J., et al. (2004). The Canadian Adverse Events Study: The incidence of adverse events among hospital patients in Canada. *Canadian Medical Association Journal, 170,* 1678–1686.

Black, J. M., & Hawks, J. H. (2005). *Medical–surgical nursing: Clinical management for positive outcomes.* St. Louis, MO: Saunders.

Canada Safety Council. (2006). *Every home needs a fire escape plan.* Retrieved August 9, 2004, from http://www.safety-council.org/info/home/escape.html

Canadian Institute for Health Information. (2004). *National trauma registry report: Injury hospitalizations.* Retrieved April 15, 2008, from http://secure.cihi.ca/cihiweb/products/NTRInjuryHosp2004.pdf

Canadian Institute for Health Information. (2006). *National trauma registry report: Major injury in Canada.* Retrieved April 16, 2008, from http://secure.cihi.ca/cihiweb/products/NTR_Major_Injury_in_Canada_2006.pdf

Canadian Institute for Health Information. (2007). *Patient safety in Canada: An update.* Retrieved April 15, 2008, from http://secure.cihi.ca/cihiweb/en/downloads/Patient_Safety_AIB_EN_070814.pdf

Canadian Nurses Association & University of Toronto Faculty of Nursing. (2004). *Nurses and patient safety: A discussion paper.* Retrieved April 16, 2008, from http://www.cna-aiic.ca/CNA/documents/pdf/publications/patient_safety_discussion_paper_e.pdf

Canadian Pediatric Society. (2004). *Position statement: Recommendations for safe sleeping environments for infants and children.* Retrieved April 15, 2008, from http://www.cps.ca/english/statements/CP/cp04-02.pdf

Christian, M. D., Kollek, D., & Schwartz, B. (2005). Emergency preparedness: What every health care worker needs to know. *Canadian Journal of Emergency Medicine, 7,* 330–337.

College of Nurses of Ontario. (2005). *Practice standard: Restraints.* Toronto, ON: Author.

DriveABLE. (2007). *Worried about someone's driving?* Retrieved June 4, 2008, from http://www.driveable.com/resources/Worried%20lo.pdf

Ebersole, P., Hess, P., & Luggen, A. (2004). *Toward healthy aging: Human needs and nursing response* (6th ed.). St. Louis, MO: Mosby.

Edelman, C. L., & Mandle, C. L. (2006). *Health promotion throughout the lifespan* (6th ed.). St. Louis, MO: Mosby.

Epilepsy Canada. (2005). *First aid for seizure treatment.* Retrieved April 15, 2008, from http://www.epilepsy.ca/eng/mainSet.html

Etchells, E., Juurlink, D., & Levinson, W. (2008). Medication errors: the human factor. *Canadian Medical Association Journal, 178*(1), 63–64.

Government of Saskatchewan. (2008). Nitrate [Fact sheet]. Retrieved June 3, 2008, from http://www.saskh20.ca/PDF-WaterCommittee/nitrate.pdf

Health Canada. (2004). *Hepatitis: A fact sheet.* Retrieved April 16, 2008, from http://www.phac-aspc.gc.ca/hcai-iamss/bbp-pts/hepatitis/hep_a_e.html

Health Canada. (2005). *Proper use and disposal of medication.* Retrieved June 12, 2008, from http://www.hc-sc.gc.ca/hl-vs/iyh-vsv/med/disposal-defaire-eng.php

Health Canada. (2008a). *Lead information package: Some commonly asked questions about lead and human health.* Retrieved April 14, 2008, from http://www.hc-sc.gc.ca/ewh-semt/contaminants/lead-plomb/exposure-exposition_e.html

Health Canada. (2008b). *Workplace Hazardous Materials Information System.* Retrieved April 14, 2008, from http://www.hc-sc.gc.ca/ewh-semt/occup-travail/whmis-simdut/about-a_propos_e.html

Hynes-Gay, P., Bennett, J., Sarjoo-Devries, A., Jones, H., & McGeer, A. (2003). Severe acute respiratory syndrome: The Mount Sinai experience. *Canadian Nurse, 99*(5), 17–19.

Kollek, D. (2003). Canadian emergency department preparedness for a nuclear, biological or chemical event. *Canadian Journal of Emergency Medicine, 5*(1), 18–26.

McCullagh, M. C. (2006). Home modification: How to help patients make their homes safer and more accessible as their abilities change, *American Journal of Nursing, 106*(10), 54.

Meiner, S., & Lueckenotte, A. (2006). *Gerontologic nursing* (3rd ed.). St. Louis, MO: Mosby.

National Steering Committee on Patient Safety. (2002). *Building a safer system: A national integrated strategy for improving patient safety in Canadian health care.* Retrieved April 16, 2008, from http://rcpsc.medical.org/publications/building_a_safer_system_e.pdf

Nix, S. (2005). *Williams' basic nutrition and diet therapy* (1st ed.). St. Louis, MO: Mosby.

Public Health Agency of Canada. (2004). *Leading causes of death and hospitalization in Canada.* Retrieved April 14, 2008, from http://www.phac-aspc.gc.ca/publicat/lcd-pcd97/table1-eng.php

Registered Nurses Association of Ontario. (2005). *Nursing best practice guideline: Prevention of falls and fall injuries in the older adult* (Revised). Retrieved April 16, 2008, from http://www.rnao.org/Storage/12/617_BPG_Falls_rev05.pdf

Safe Kids Canada. (2007). *Child and youth unintentional injury: 10 years in review* [Electronic version]. Retrieved June 11, 2008, from http://www.sickkids.ca/SKCForPartners/custom/NationalReportUpdatedENG.pdf

SMARTRISK. (1998). *The economic burden of unintentional injury in Canada* [Electronic version]. Retrieved April 16, 2008, from http://smartrisk.ca/uploads/cf127134791602109375.pdf

Technical Standards and Safety Authority. (2004). *Danger! Carbon monoxide: What you need to know to protect you and your family from the "silent killer."* Retrieved May 25, 2004, from http://www.safetyinfo.ca/home_safety/articles/co_more.asp

Trinkoff, A., Geiger-Brown, J., Brady, B., Lipscomb, J., & Muntaner, C. (2006). How long and how much are nurses working? *American Journal of Nursing, 106*(4), 60–71.

Vanier Institute of the Family. (2004). *Profiling Canada's families III.* Nepean, ON: Author.

Zusman, J. (2001). *Restraint and seclusion: Understanding the JCAHO standards and federal regulations* (3rd ed.). Marblehead, MA: Opus Communications.

Chapter 38

Bauroth, K., Charles, C. H., Mankodi, S. M., Simmons, K., Zhao, Q., & Kumar, L. D. (2003). The efficacy of an essential oil antiseptic mouthwash vs. dental flossing in controlling interproximal gingivitis: A comparative study. *Journal of the American Dental Association, 134,* 359–365.

Bennett, M. A. (1995). Report of the task force on the implications for darkly pigmented intact skin in the prediction of pressure ulcers. *Advances in Wound Care, 8*(6), 34–35.

Berry, A. M., Davidson, P. M., Masters, J., & Rolls, K. (2007). Systematic literature review of oral hygiene practices for intensive care patients receiving mechanical ventilation. *American Journal of Critical Care, 16,* 552–562.

Canadian Dental Association. (2005). *Your oral health—caring for your teeth.* Retrieved January 16, 2009, from http://www.cda-adc.ca/en/oral_health/cfyt/index.asp

Canadian Diabetes Association. (2003). *2003 clinical practice guidelines for the prevention and management of diabetes in Canada.* Retrieved May 26, 2004, from http://www.diabetes.ca/cpg2003/chapters.aspx

Canadian Diabetes Association. (2006a). *Foot care: a step toward good health.* Retrieved January 16, 2009, from http://www.diabetes.ca/about-diabetes/living/complications/foot-care/

Canadian Diabetes Association. (2006b). *Skin problems.* Retrieved January 16, 2009, from http://www.diabetes.ca/about-diabetes/living/complications/skin-problems

Ebersole, P., Hess, P., Touhy, T.A., Jett, K., & Schmidt-Luggen, A. (2008). *Toward healthy aging: Human needs and nursing response* (7th ed.). St. Louis, MO: Mosby.

Estes, M. E., & Buck, M. (2008). *Health assessment and physical examination* (1st Canadian ed.). Toronto, ON: Thomson Nelson.

Galanti, G. A. (2004). *Caring for patients from different cultures* (3rd ed.). Philidelphia, PA: University of Pennsylvania Press.

Gaskin, F. C. (1986). Detection of cyanosis in person with dark skin. *Journal of National Black Nurses, Association, 1,* 52–60.

Gulanick, M., & Myers, J. L. (2007). *Nursing care plans: Diagnosis and intervention* (6th ed.). St. Louis, MO: Mosby.

Health Canada. (2006). *It's your health: Contact lenses* (Catalogue No. 0-662-35396-X). Retrieved January 16, 2009, from http://www.hc-sc.gc.ca/hl-vs/iyh-vsv/med/lenses-lentilles-eng.php

Henderson, C. T., Ayello, E. A., Sussman, C., Leiby, D. M., Bennett, M. A., Dungog, E. F., et al. (1997). Draft definition of stage I pressure ulcers: Inclusion of persons with with darkly pigmented skin. *Advances in Wound Care, 10*(5), 16–19.

Hockenberry, M. J. (2005) *Wong's essentials of pediatric nursing* (7th ed.). St. Louis, MO: Mosby.

Hockenberry, M. J., & Wilson, D. (2007) *Wong's nursing care of infants and children* (8th ed.). St. Louis, MO: Mosby.

Infectious Diseases and Immunization Committee, Canadian Pediatric Society. (2003). *Head lice infestations: A clinical update.* Accessed January 16, 2009, from http://www.cps.ca/ENGLISH/statements/ID/id08-06.htm

Larsen, E. L., Ciliberti, T., Chantler, C., Abraham, J., Lazaro, E. M. Venturanza, M., et al. (2004). Comparison of traditional and disposable bed baths in critically ill patients. *American Journal of Critical Care, 13,* 235–241.

Meiner, S., & Lueckenotte, A. G. (2006). *Gerontologic nursing* (2nd ed.). St. Louis, MO: Mosby.

Miller, C. A. (2009). *Nursing for wellness in older adults* (5th ed.). Philadelphia, PA: Lippincott Williams & Wilkins.

Moulik, P., Mtonga, R., & Gill, G. V. (2003). Amputation and mortality in new-onset diabetic ulcers stratified by etiology. *Diabetes Care, 26,* 491–494.

Munro, C. L., Grap, M. M., Elswick, R. K., Jr., McKinney, J., Sessler, C., & Hummel, R. S. (2006). Oral health status and development of ventilator-associated pneumonia: A descriptive study. *American Journal of Critical Care, 15,* 453–460.

Neil, J. A. (2002). Assessing foot care knowledge in a rural population with diabetes. *Ostomy/Wound Management, 48*(1), 50–56.

Pender, N., Murdaugh, C. L., & Parsons, M. A. (2006). *Health promotion in nursing* (5th ed.). Upper Saddle River, NJ: Pearson Prentice Hall.

Smeltzer, S. C., & Bare, B. (2004). *Brunner and Suddarth's textbook of medical–surgical nursing* (10th ed.). Philadelphia, PA: Lippincott Williams & Wilkins.

Zullino, D. F., Krenz, S., Resard, E., Cancela, E., & Khazall, Y. (2005). Local back massage an automated massage chair: general muscle and psychophysiologic relaxing properties. *Journal of Alternative and Complementary Medicine, 11,* 1103–1106.

Zurlinden, J. (2003). Drug news: New warnings for Lindane shampoo and lotion. *Nursing Spectrum—Midwestern Edition, 40*(6), 10.

Chapter 39

Akgul, S., & Akyolcu, N. (2002). Effects of normal saline on endotracheal suctioning. *Journal of Clinical Nursing, 11,* 826–830.

Akgul, S., & Kanan, N. (2006). A current conflict use of isotonic sodium chloride on endotracheal suctioning in critically ill patients. *Dimensions of Critical Care Nurse, 25*(1), 11–14.

Allibone, L. (2003). Nursing management of chest drains. *Nursing Standard, 17*(22), 45–54.

American Association of Respiratory Care (AARC). (2004). Clinical practice guideline, nasotracheal suction. *Respiratory Care, 49,* 1080–1084.

American Heart Association. (2003). *CPR and AEDs.* Retrieved December 18, 2004, from www.AHA.org

American Heart Association. (2005). 2005 American Heart Association guidelines for cardiopulmonary resuscitation and emergency cardiovascular care. *Circulation, 112*(24 Suppl.), IV1–IV203.

American Heart Association. (2006). Community lay rescuer automated external defibrillator programs, *Circulation, 113,* 1260.

Black, J. M., & Hawks, J. H. (2005). *Medical surgical nursing clinical management for positive outcomes* (7th ed.). St, Louis, MO: Elsevier.

Bourgault, A. M., Brown, C. A., Hains, S. M. J., & Parlow, J. L. (2006). Effects of endotracheal tube suctioning on arterial oxygen tension and heart rate variability. *Biological Research For Nursing, 7,* 268–278.

Canadian Cancer Society. (2007). *About cancer.* Retrieved June 11, 2008, from http://www.cancer.ca/ccs/internet/standard/0,3182,3172_14459_371459_langld-en,00.html

Carroll, P. (2002). A guide to mobile chest drains. *RN, 65*(5), 56–60.

Carroll, P. (2005). Keeping up with mobile chest drains. *RN, 68*(10), 26–32.

Centres for Disease Control and Prevention. (2006). *Adult immunization schedule, national immunization program.* Retrieved April 27, 2008, from http://www.cdc.gov/vaccines/recs/schedules/adult-schedule.htm#print

Cerfolio, R. J. (2005). Recent advances in the treatment of air leaks. *Current Opinion in Pulmonary Medicine, 11*(4)319–23.

Chambers, T. A., Bagai, A., & Ivascu, N. (2007). Current trend in coronary artery disease in women. *Current Opinion in Anaesthesiology, 20*(1), 75–82.

Cuvelier, A., et al. (2002). Refillable oxygen cylinders may be an alternative for ambulatory oxygen therapy in COPD. *Chest, 122*(2), 451–456.

Day, T., Farnell, S., Haynes, S., Wainwright, S., & Wilson-Barnett, J. (2002). Tracheal suctioning: An exploration of nurses' knowledge and competence in acute and high dependency ward areas. *Journal of Advanced Nursing, 39*(1), 35–45.

Denke, M. A. (2001). Primary prevention of heart disease in women. *Current Atherosclerosis Reports, 3*(2):136–138.

Fujimoto, K., Matsuzawa, Y., Yamaguchi, S., Koizumi, T., & Kubo, K. (2002). Benefits of oxygen on exercise performance and pulmonary hemodynamics in patients with COPD with mild hypoxemia. *Chest, 12*(2), 457–463.

Granger, B. B., & Miller, C. M. (2001). Acute coronary syndrome: Putting the new guidelines to work. *Nursing, 31*(11), 36–42.

Health Canada. (2007). *Go smokefree!* Retrieved April 27, 2008, from http://www.hc-sc.gc.ca/hecs-sesc/tobacco/index.html

Health Canada. (2005). *Influenza (The "flu")* Retrieved April 28, 2008, from http://www.hc-sc.gc.ca/iyh-vsv/diseases-maladies/flu-grippe_e.html

Health Canada. (2008). *Smoking and your body.* Retrieved June 11, 2008, from http://www.hc-sc.gc.ca/hl-vs/tobac-tabac/body-corps/index-eng.php

Hess, D. R. (2005). Tracheostomy tubes and related appliances. *Respiratory Care, 50,* 497–510.

Halm, M. A. (2007). To strip or not to strip? Physiological effects of chest tube manipulation. *American Journal of Critical Care, 16,* 609–612.

Hockenberry, M. J., & Wilson, D. (2007). *Wong's nursing care of infants and children* (8th ed.). St. Louis, MO: Mosby.

Jevon, P., & Ewens, B. (2001). Assessment of a breathless patient. *Nursing Standard, 15*(16), 48–53.

Joint National Committee on Prevention, Detection, Evaluation and Treatment of High Blood Pressure. (2003). *The seventh report of the Joint National Committee on Prevention, Detection, Evaluation and Treatment of High Blood Pressure (JNC VII).* Bethesda, MD: US Department of Health and Human Services, National Heart, Lung, and Blood Institute. Retrieved December 18, 2004, from www.nhlbi.nih.gov/guidelines/hypertension/express.pdf

Kerr, M. E., Weber, B. B., Sereika, S. M., Darby J., Marion D. W., & Orndoff, P. A. (1999). Effect of endotracheal suctioning on cerebral oxygen in traumatic brain injured patients. *Critical Care Medicine, 27*(2), 2776–2781.

Lawrence, V. A., Cornell, J. E., & Smetana, G. W. (2006). Strategies to reduce postoperative pulmonary complications after noncardiothoracic surgery; systematic review for the American college of physicians. *Annals of Internal Medicine, 144,* 596–608.

Lewarski, J. S. (2005). Long-term care of the patient with a tracheostomy. *Respiratory Care, 50,* 534–537.

Lewis, S. M., Heitkemper, M. M., & Dirksen, S. R. (2000). *Medical-surgical nursing: Assessment and management of clinical problems* (5th ed.). St. Louis, MO: Mosby.

Lewis, S. M., Heitkemper, M. M., & Dirksen, S. R. (2006). *Medical-surgical nursing: Assessment and management of clinical problems* (1st Canadian ed.). Toronto, ON: Elsevier Mosby.

McCance, K. L., & Huether, S. E. (2005). *Pathophysiology: The biologic basis for disease in adults and children* (5th ed.). St. Louis, MO: Mosby.

Meiner, S., & Lueckenotte, A. G. (2006). *Gerontologic nursing* (3rd ed.). St. Louis, MO: Mosby.

Moore, T. (2003). Suctioning techniques for the removal of respiratory secretions. *Nursing Standard, 18*(9), 47–53.

National Cancer Institute of Canada. (2008). *Canadian cancer statistics 2008.* Toronto, ON: Author. Retrieved April 30, 2008, from http://www.ncic.cancer.ca/vgn/images/portal/cit_86751114/14/35/195991821ncic_stats2004_en.pdf

Oh, H., & Seo, W. (2003). A meta-analysis of the effects of various interventions in preventing endotracheal suction-induced hypoxemia. *Journal of Clinical Nursing, 12,* 912–924.

Potter, P. A., & Weilitz, P. B. (2003). *Health assessment pocket guide series* (5th ed.). St. Louis, MO: Mosby.

Pruitt, W., & Jacobs, M. (2003). Breathing lessons basics of oxygen therapy. *Nursing, 33*(10), 43–45.

Rhoads, J., & Meeker, B. J. (2008). *Davis guide to clinical nursing skills.* Philadelphia, PA: F. A. Davis Company.

Roman, M., & Mercado, D. (2006). Review of chest tube use. *Medical Surgical Nursing, 15*(1), 41.

Shaw, L. J., Merz, C. N., Pepine, C. J., Reis, S. E., Bittner, V., Kip, K. E., et al. (2006). The economic burden of angina in women with suspected ischemic heart disease. *Circulation, 114,* 894–904.

Snow, V., Lascher, S., & Mottur-Pilson, C. (2001). The evidence base for management of acute exacerbations of COPD: Clinical practice guideline, part 1. *Chest, 119,* 1185–1189.

Thomson, A., Webb, D., Maxwell, S., & Grant, I. (2002). Oxygen therapy in acute medical care: The potential dangers of hyperoxia need to be recognised. *British Medical Journal, 324,* 1406–1407.

Chapter 40

Barrett, B. J. (2003). Applying multiple interventions in chronic kidney disease. *Seminars in Dialysis, 16*, 157–164.

Brungs, S. M., & Render, M. L. (2006). Using evidence-based practice to reduce central line infections. *Clinical Journal of Oncology Nursing, 10*, 723–725.

Burgess, R. (2006). Blood transfusion in A & E. *Emergency Nursing, 13*(10), 18–22.

Casey, A. L., & Elliott, T. S. (2007a). Infection risks associated with needleless intravenous access devices. *Nursing Standard, 22*(11), 38–44.

Casey, A. L., & Elliott, T. (2007b). IV nursing. The usability and acceptability of a needleless connector system. *British Journal of Nursing, 16*, 267–268, 270–271.

Chapelhow, C., & Crouch, S. (2007). Applying numeracy skills in clinical practice: Fluid balance. *Nursing Standard, 21*(27), 49–56, 58, 60.

Chavin, G., & Chow, G. (2008). Maintaining proper fluid balance in the postoperative urologic patient. *Contemporary Urology, 20*(1), 30–35.

Chukhraev, A. M., & Grekov, I. G. (2000). Local complications of nursing interventions on peripheral veins. *Journal of Intravenous Nursing, 23*, 167–169.

Clancy, J., & McVicar, A. (2007a). Clinical education. Short-term regulation of acid-base homeostasis of body fluids. *British Journal of Nursing, 16*, 1016–1021.

Clancy, J., & McVicar, A. (2007b). Intermediate and long-term regulation of acid-base homeostasis. *British Journal of Nursing, 16*, 1076–1079.

Coulter, K. (2004). The older adult patient. In D. Macklin & C. Chernecky (Eds.), *Real world nursing survival nursing guide: IV therapy*. St. Louis. MO: Saunders.

Curtis, B. M., Levin, A., & Parfrey, P. S. (2005). Multiple risk factor intervention in chronic kidney disease: Management of cardiac disease in chronic kidney disease patients. *Medical Clinics of North America, 89*, 511–523.

Davidhizar, R., Dunn, C. L., & Hart, A. N. (2004). A review of the literature on how important water is to the world's elderly population. *International Nursing Review, 51*, 159–166.

Davis, K., Hui, C. H., & Quested, B. (2005–2006). Transfusing safely: A 2006 guide for nurses. *Australian Nursing Journal, 13*(6), 17–20.

Day, R., Paul, P., Williams, B., Smeltzer, S. C., & Bare, B. (2007). *Medical-surgical nursing*. Philadelphia: Lippincott Williams & Wilkins.

Dochterman, J. M., & Bulechek, G. M. (2004). *Nursing interventions classification (NIC)* (4th ed.). St. Louis, MO: Mosby.

Goertz, S. (2006). Eye on diagnostics. Gauging fluid balance with osmolality. *Nursing, 36*(10), 70–71.

Grandjean, A. C., Reimers, K. J., & Buyckx, M. E. (2003). Hydration: Issues for the 21st century. *Nutrition Reviews, 61*, 261–271.

Hamilton, H. (2004). Intravenous therapy. Central venous catheters: Choosing the most appropriate access route. *British Journal of Nursing, 13*, 862–870.

Hamilton, H. (2006a). Complications associated with venous access devices: Part one... first of two. *Nursing Standard, 20*(26), 43.

Hamilton, H. (2006b). Complications associated with venous access devices: Part two. *Nursing Standard, 20*(27), 59.

Hartling, L., Bellemare S, Wiebe, N., Russell K., Klassen, T. P., & Craig, W. (2006). Oral versus intravenous rehydration for treating dehydration due to gastroenteritis in children. *Cochrane Database of Systemic Reviews*, (3), CD004390.

Heitz, U. E., & Horne, M. M. (2005). *Mosby's pocket guide series: Fluid, electrolyte, and acid-base balance* (5th ed.). St. Louis, MO: Mosby.

Hindley, G. (2004). Infection control in peripheral cannulae. *Nursing Standard 18*(27), 37–40.

Hockenberry, M. J., & Wilson, D. (2007). *Wong's essentials of pediatric nursing* (7th ed.). St. Louis, MO: Mosby.

Ignatavicius, D., & Workman, M. J. (2005). *Medical-surgical nursing* (5th ed.). Philadelphia: Saunders.

Infusion Nurses Society. (2006). Infusion nursing standards of practice. *Journal of Infusion Nursing, 29*(1 Suppl), S1–S92.

International Council of Nurses. (2002). Universal access to clean water. *International Council of Nurses Position Statement*. Accessed June 6, 2008, from http://www.icn.ch/pswater.htm

Kaler, W., & Chinn, R. (2007). Successful disinfection of needleless access ports: A matter of time and friction. *Journal of the Association for Vascular Access, 12*, 140–143.

Lehne, R. A. (2007). *Pharmacology for nursing care* (7th ed.). Philadelphia: Saunders Elsevier.

Martini, F. H., & Nath, J. L. (2009). *Fundamentals of anatomy and physiology* (8th ed.). San Francisco: Pearson Benjamin Cummings.

McKenry, L. Tessier, E., & Hogan, M. A. (2006). *Mosby's pharmacology in nursing* (22nd ed.). St. Louis, MO: Mosby.

Millam, D. A., & Hadaway, L. C. (2003). On the road to successful I.V. starts. *Nursing, 33*(5), 1–14.

Monahan, F. D., Sands, J. K., Neighbors, M., Marek, J. F., Green, C. J., & Green-Nigro, C. J. (2007). *Phipps' medical-surgical nursing: Health and illness perspectives* (8th ed.). St. Louis, MO: Mosby.

Nicholls, C., & Sani, M. (2004). Diuretics and their use with older people. *Nursing Older People, 15*(10), 31–33.

O'Grady, N. P., Alexander, M., Dellinger, E. P., Gerberding, J. L., Heard, S. O., Maki, D. G., et al. (2002). Guidelines for the prevention of intravascular catheter-related infections. Centers for Disease Control and Prevention. *MMWR Recommendations and Reports, 51*(RR-10), 1–29.

Phillips, L. D. (2005). *Manual of I.V. therapeutics* (4th ed.). Philadelphia: Davis.

Porth, C. M. (2005). *Pathophysiology: Concepts of altered health states* (7th ed.). Philadelphia: Lippincott Williams & Wilkins.

Registered Nurses Association of Ontario. (2005). *Nursing Best Practice Guideline: Care and maintenance to reduce vascular access complications*. Toronto: Author.

Registered Nurses Association of Ontartio. (2008). Care and maintenance to reduce vascular access complications: Guideline supplement. Toronto: Author. Retrieved June 10, 2008, from http://www.rnao.org/Storage/39/3380_Care_and_Maintenance_to_Reduce_Vascular_Access_Complications_Supplement_FINAL.pdf

Rosenthal, K. (2005). Tailor your IV insertion techniques to special populations. *Nursing, 35*(5):36–42.

Schelper, R. (2003). The aging venous system. *Journal of the Association for Vascular Access, 7*(1), 8–10.

Woodrow, P. (2003a). Assessing blood results in older people: Cardiac enzymes and biochemistry. *Nursing Older People, 15*(4), 31–33.

Woodrow, P. (2003b). Assessing fluid balance in older people: Fluid replacement. *Nursing Older People, 14*(10), 29–30.

Chapter 41

Attarian, H. P. (2000). Helping patients who say they cannot sleep: Practical ways to evaluate and treat insomnia. *Postgraduate Medicine, 107*, 127–130, 133–137, 140–142.

Basner, R. (2005). Shift work sleep disorder: The glass is more than half empty. *New England Journal of Medicine, 353*, 519–521.

Benca, R. M., & Schenck, C. H. (2005). Sleep and eating disorders. In M. H. Kryger, T. Roth, & W. C. Dement (Eds.), *Principles and practice of sleep medicine* (4th ed., pp. 1337–1344). Philadelphia, PA: Elsevier.

Blachowicz, E., & Letizia, M. (2006). The challenges of shift work. *Medsurg Nursing, 15*, 274–280.

Buysse, D. J. (2005). Diagnosis and assessment of sleep and circadian rhythm disorders. *Journal of Psychiatric Practice, 11*, 102–115.

Buysse, D. J., Schweitzer, P. K., & Moul, D. E. (2005). Clinical pharmacology of other drugs used as hypnotics. In M. H. Kryger, T. Roth, & W. C. Dement (Eds.), *Principles and practice of sleep medicine* (4th ed., pp. 452–467). Philadelphia, PA: Elsevier.

Canadian Nurses Association. (2007). *Framework for the practice of registered nurses in Canada*. Ottawa, ON: Author.

Chasens, E. R., Williams, L. L., & Umlauf, M. G. (2008). Excessive sleepiness. In E. Capezuti, D. Zwicker, M. Mezey, & T. Fulmer (Eds.), *Evidence-based geriatric nursing protocols for best practice*. (3rd ed., pp. 459–476). New York: Springer.

Cmiel, C. A., Karr, D. M., Gasser, D. M., Oliphant, L. M., & Neveau, A. J. (2004). Noise control: A nursing team's approach to sleep promotion. *American Journal of Nursing, 104*(2), 40–48.

Cohen, F. L. (2004). Measuring sleep. In M. Frank-Stromborg, & S. J. Olsen (Eds.), *Instruments for clinical-healthcare research*, (3rd ed., pp. 264–285). Boston, MA: Jones & Bartlett.

Cote, K. (2003). *Normal sleep and sleep hygiene* [Brochure]. Montreal, QC: Canadian Sleep Society

Craig, T., McCann, J., Gurevich, F., & Davies, M. (2004). The correlation between allergic rhinitis and sleep disturbance. *Journal of Allergy and Clinical Immunology, 114*, S139–S145.

Cullen, D. F. (2001). Obstructive sleep apnea and postoperative analgesia—A potentially dangerous combination. *Journal of Clinical Anesthesia, 13*(2), 83–85.

Dines-Kalinowski, C. M. (2002). Nature's nurse: Promoting sleep in the ICU. *Dimensions of Critical Care Nursing, 21*, 32–34.

Driver, H. S. (2003). *Unusual behaviors during sleep: the parasomnias* [Brochure]. Montreal, QC: Canadian Sleep Society.

Driver, H. S. (2005). *Sleep in women* [Brochure]. Montreal, QC: Canadian Sleep Society.

Dochterman, J. M., & Bulechek, G. M. (Eds.). (2004). *Nursing interventions classification (NIC)* (4th ed.). St. Louis, MO: Mosby.

Edinger, J. D., & Means, M. K. (2005). Overview of insomnia: Definitions, epidemiology, differential diagnosis, and assessment. In M. H. Kryger, T. Roth, & W. C. Dement (Eds.), *Principles and practice of sleep medicine* (4th ed., pp. 702–713). Philadelphia, PA: Elsevier.

Elliott, A. C. (2001). Primary care assessment and management of sleep disorders. *Journal of the American Academy of Nurse Practitioners, 13,* 409–417.

Ferebee, L. (2006). Sleep and activity. In S. E. Meiner, & A. G. Lueckenotte (Eds.), *Gerontologic nursing* (3rd ed., pp. 229–244). St. Louis, MO: Elsevier.

Gangwisch, J. E., Heymsfield, S. B., Boden-Albala, B., Buijs, R. M., Kreier, F., Pickering, T. G., et al. (2007). Sleep duration as a risk factor for diabetes incidence in a large US sample. *Sleep, 30,* 1667–1673.

Gibson, E. S., & Trajanovic, N. (2005). *Adolescents and sleep: A guide to the sleep-deprived world of teenagers.* Montreal, QC: Canadian Sleep Society.

Groth, M. (2005). Sleep apnea in the elderly. *Clinics of Geriatric Medicine, 21,* 701–712.

Guilleminault, C., & Bassiri A. (2005). Clinical features and evaluation of obstructive apnea. In M. H. Kryger, T. Roth, & W. C. Dement (Eds.), *Principles and practice of sleep medicine* (4th ed., pp. 1043–1052). Philadelphia, PA: Elsevier.

Guilleminault, C., & Fromberz, S. (2005). Narcolepsy: Diagnosis and management. In M. H. Kryger, T. Roth, & W. C. Dement (Eds.), *Principles and practice of sleep medicine* (4th ed., pp. 780–790). Philadelphia, PA: Elsevier.

Hockenberry, M. J., & Wilson, D. (2007). *Wong's nursing care of infants and children* (8th ed.). New York: Mosby.

Hoffman, S. (2003). Sleep in the older adult: Implications for nurses. *Geriatric Nursing, 24,* 210–216.

Holman, M. L. (2005). Obstructive sleep apnea syndrome: Implications for primary care. *Nurse Practitioner, 30*(9), 38–43.

Honkus, V. L. (2003). Sleep deprivation in critical care units. *Critical Care Nursing Quarterly, 26,* 179–191.

Irwin, M. R., Cole, J. C., & Nicassio, P. M. (2006). Comparative meta-analysis of behavioral interventions for insomnia and their efficacy in middle-aged adults and in older adults 55+ years of age. *Health Psychology, 25*(1), 3–14.

Izac, S. M. (2006). Basic anatomy and physiology of sleep. *American Journal of Electroneurodiagnostic Technology, 46,* 18–38.

Jones, B. (2005). Basic mechanisms of sleep-wake states. In M. H. Kryger, T. Roth, & W. C. Dement (Eds.), *Principles and practice of sleep medicine* (4th ed., pp. 136–153). Philadelphia, PA: Elsevier.

Malow, B. A. (2005). Approach to the patient with disordered sleep. In M. H. Kryger, T. Roth, & W. C. Dement (Eds.), *Principles and practice of sleep medicine* (4th ed., pp. 589–593). Philadelphia, PA: Elsevier.

Maur, K. L. (2005). Promoting sound sleep habits in older adults. *Nursing, 35*(2), 22–25.

McCance, K. L., & Huether, S. E. (2006). *Pathophysiology: The biologic basis for disease in adults and children* (5th ed.). St. Louis, MO: Mosby.

McKenry, L. M., & Salerno, E. (2003). *Mosby's pharmacology in nursing* (21st ed.). St. Louis, MO: Mosby.

Mendelson, W. B. (2005). Hypnotic medications: Mechanisms of action and pharmacologic effects. In M. H. Kryger, T. Roth, & W. C. Dement (Eds.), *Principles and practice of sleep medicine* (4th ed., pp. 444–451). Philadelphia, PA: Elsevier.

Mendez, J. L., & Olson, E. J. (2006a). Obstructive sleep apnea syndrome. Part I: Identifying the problem. *Journal of Respiratory Diseases, 27,* 144–157.

Mendez, J. L., & Olson, E. J. (2006b). Obstructive sleep apnea syndrome. Part II: Reviewing the treatment options. *Journal of Respiratory Diseases, 27,* 222–224.

Mignot, E. (2005). Narcolepsy: Pharmacology, pathophysiology, and genetics. In M. H. Kryger, T. Roth, & W. C. Dement (Eds.), *Principles and practice of sleep medicine* (4th ed., pp. 761–779). Philadelphia, PA: Elsevier.

Morin, A. K., Jarvis, C. I., & Lynch, A. M. (2007). Therapeutic options for sleep-maintenance and sleep-onset insomnia. *Pharmacotherapy, 27,* 89–110.

Morin, C. M. (2003). *Insomnia* [Brochure]. Montreal, QC: Canadian Sleep Society.

National Heart, Lung, and Blood Institute Working Group on Restless Legs Syndrome. (2000). Restless leg syndrome: Detection and management in primary care. *American Family Physician, 62,* 108–114.

National Sleep Foundation. (2002a). *Sleep apnea.* Retrieved October 30, 2008, from http://www.sleepfoundation.org/site/c.huIXKjM0IxF/b.2464479/apps/nl/content3.asp?content_id={3E9E479E-4C8E-4C35-9564-363A6918C391}¬oc=1 National Sleep Foundation. (2002b). *When you can't sleep: ABCs of ZZZs.* Retrieved October 30, 2008, from http://www.sleepfoundation.org/site/apps/nlnet/content3.aspx?c=huIXKjM0IxF&b=2462647&content_id={1636C27B-B123-4CEE-BE7D-FABE706709E7}¬oc=1

National Sleep Foundation. (2003). *Let sleep work for you.* Retrieved October 30, 2008, from http://www.sleepfoundation.org/site/c.huIXKjM0IxF/b.2421185/k.7198/Let_Sleep_Work_for_You.htm

National Sleep Foundation. (2006a). *How sleep changes.* Retrieved October 31, 2008, from http://www.sleepfoundation.org/site/c.huIXKjM0IxF/b.2419263/k.9F61/How_Sleep_Changes.htm

National Sleep Foundation. (2006b). *2006 sleep in America poll highlights and key findings.* Retrieved from http://sleepfoundation.org

Olson, D. M., Borel, C. O., Laskowitz, D. T., Moore, D. T., & McConnell, E. S. (2001). Quiet time: A nursing intervention to promote sleep in neurocritical care units. *American Journal of Critical Care, 10,* 74–78.

Orr, W. C. (2005). Gastrointestinal physiology. In M. H. Kryger, T. Roth, & W. C. Dement (Eds.), *Principles and practice of sleep medicine* (4th ed., pp. 283–291). Philadelphia, PA: Elsevier.

Redline S. (2005). Genetics of obstructive sleep apnea. In M. H. Kryger, T. Roth, & W. C. Dement (Eds.), *Principles and practice of sleep medicine* (4th ed., pp. 1013–1022). Philadelphia, PA: Elsevier.

Reishtein, J. L., Pack, A., Maislin, G., Dinges, D., Bloxham, T., George, C., et al. (2006). Sleepiness and relationships in obstructive sleep apnea. *Issues in Mental Health Nursing, 27,* 319–330.

Richardson, S. (2003). Effects of relaxation and imagery on the sleep of critically ill adults. *Dimensions of Critical Care Nursing, 22,* 182–187.

Robinson, S. B., Weitzel, T., and Henderson, L. (2005). The sh-h-h-h project: Nonpharmacological interventions. *Holistic Nursing Practice, 19,* 263–266.

Santos, C., Pratt, E., Hanks, C., McCann, J. & Craig, T. (2006). Allergic rhinitis and its effect on sleep, fatigue, and daytime somnolence. *Annals of Allergy, Asthma & Immunology, 97,* 579–587.

Scheer, F. A., Cajochen, C., Turek, F. W., & Czeisler, C. A. (2005). Melatonin in the regulation of sleep and circadian rhythms. In M. H. Kryger, T. Roth, & W. C. Dement (Eds.), *Principles and practice of sleep medicine* (4th ed., pp. 395–404). Philadelphia, PA: Elsevier.

Schwab, R. (2005). Genetic determinants of upper airway structures that predispose to obstructive sleep apnea. *Respiratory Physiology & Neurobiology, 147,* 289–298.

Schweitzer, P. K. (2005). Drugs that disturb sleep and wakefulness. In M. H. Kryger, T. Roth, & W. C. Dement (Eds.), *Principles and practice of sleep medicine* (4th ed., pp. 499–518). Philadelphia, PA: Elsevier

Scott, L. D., Hwang, W., Rogers, A. E., Nysse, T., Dean, G. E., & Dinges, D. F. (2007). The relationship between nurse work schedules, sleep duration, and drowsy driving. *Sleep, 30,* 1801–1807.

Shen, J., Botly, L., Chung, S., Gibbs, A., Sabanadzovic, S. & Shapiro, C. (2006). Fatigue and shift work. *Journal of Sleep Research, 15,* 1–5.

Sitzman, K. (2005). Avoid sleepiness while driving. *Home Healthcare Nurse, 23,* 260.

Spilsbury, J. C., Storfer-Isser, A., Drotar, D., Rosen, C. L., Kirchner, L. H., Benhan, H. et al. (2004). Sleep behavior in an urban US sample of school aged children. *Archives of Pediatric and Adolescent Medicine, 158,* 988–994.

Stickgold, R. (2005). Why we dream. In M. Kryger, T. Roth, & W. C. Dement (Eds.), *Principles and practice of sleep medicine* (4th ed., pp. 579–588). Philadelphia, PA: Elsevier.

Tsai, W. H. (2003). *Obstructive sleep apnea* [Brochure]. Montreal, QC: Canadian Sleep Society.

Van Dongen, H. (2006). Shift work and inter-individual differences in sleep and sleepiness. *Chronobiology International, 23,* 1139–1147.

Verrier, R. L., & Josephson, M. E. (2005). Cardiac arrhythmogenesis during sleep: Mechanisms, diagnosis, and therapy. In M. Kryger, T. Roth, & W. C. Dement (Eds.), *Principles and practice of sleep medicine* (4th ed., pp. 1171–1179). Philadelphia, PA: Elsevier.

Walsh, J. K., Dement, W. C., & Dinges, D. F. (2005). Sleep medicine, public policy and public health. In M. Kryger, T. Roth, & W. C. Dement (Eds.), *Principles and practice of sleep medicine* (4th ed., pp. 648–656). Philadelphia, PA: Elsevier

Weiss, S. (2005). *Sleep in children* [Brochure]. Montreal, QC: Canadian Sleep Society.

White, D. P. (2005). Central sleep apnea. In M. Kryger, T. Roth, & W. C. Dement (Eds.), *Principles and practice of sleep medicine* (4th ed., pp. 969–982). Philadelphia, PA: Elsevier.

Wolfson, A. R., & Lee, K. P. (2005). Pregnancy and the postpartum period. In M. Kryger, T. Roth, & W. C. Dement (Eds.), *Principles and practice of sleep medicine* (4th ed., pp. 1278–1286). Philadelphia, PA: Elsevier.

Chapter 42

Agency for Health Care Policy and Research, Acute Pain Management Guideline Panel. (1992). *Acute pain management: Operative or medical procedures and trauma. Clinical Practice Guideline* (AHCPR Publication No. 92-0032). Rockville, MD: Agency for Health Care Policy and Research, Public Health Service, U.S. Department of Health and Human Services.

American Geriatrics Society. (2002). The management of persistent pain in older persons. *Journal of the American Geriatrics Society, 50*(Suppl. 6), 205–224.

American Pain Society. (2003). *Principles of analgesic use in the treatment of acute and cancer pain* (4th ed.). Glenview, IL: Author.

American Society for Pain Management Nursing. (n.d.) *Position papers* [Web page]. Retrieved February 5, 2009, from http://www.aspmn.org/Organization/position_papers.htm

Anand, K. J. S., & Craig, K. (1996). New perspectives on the definition of pain. *Pain, 67*, 3–6.

Anand, K. J. S., & Scalzo, F. M. (2000). Can adverse neonatal experiences alter brain development and subsequent behavior? *Biology of the Neonate, 77*(2), 69–82.

Anand, K. J. S., Sippell, W. G., & Aynsley-Green, A. (1987). Randomized trial of fentanyl anesthesia in preterm babies undergoing surgery: Effects on the stress response. *Lancet, 1*, 243–248.

Aubrun, F. (2005). Management of postoperative analgesia in elderly patients. *Regional Anesthesia and Pain Medicine, 30*, 363–379.

Avancen. (2006). *Improving patient care at the bedside.* Ormond Beach, FL: Author. Retrieved January 28, 2009, from http://www.avancen.com.

Beyer, J. E., Denyes, M. J., & Villarruel, A. M. (1992). The creation, validation, and continuing development of the Oucher: A measure of pain intensity in children. *Journal of Pediatric Nursing, 7*, 335–346.

Canadian Pain Society. (2001). *Patient pain manifesto.* Retrieved February 19, 2005, from http://www.canadianpainsociety.ca/cont-ang/4nouvelles-manifeste.htm

Carroll, D., & Seers, K. (1998). Relaxation for the relief of chronic pain: A systematic review. *Journal of Advanced Nursing, 27*, 476–487.

Cassileth, B., & Vickers, A. (2004). Massage therapy for symptom control: Outcome study at a major cancer center. *Journal of Pain Symptom Management, 28*, 244.

Chambers, C. T., von Baeyer, C. L., Montgomery, C., Court, C. & Hardial, J. (2003). *Self-report measures for pediatric pain assessment: Impact of scale format on nurses' ratings of clinically significant pain.* Poster presented at the Canadian Pain Society Annual Conference, Toronto, ON.

Cox, F. (2001). Clinical care of patients with epidural infusions. *Professional Nurse, 16*, 1429–1432.

D'Arcy, Y. (2006). Hot topics in pain management: Using NSAIDs safely. *Nursing, 35*(2), 22.

Donahue, P. (1989). *Nursing: The finest art.* St. Louis, MO: Mosby.

Douglass, A., Maxwell, T., & Whitecar, P. (2005). Principles of palliative care medicine. I. Patient assessment, *Advanced Studies in Medicine, 4*(1), 15.

Du Pen, S. L., & Williams, A. R. (1992). Management of patients receiving combined epidural morphine and bupivacaine for the treatment of cancer pain. *Journal of Pain and Symptom Management, 7*(2), 125–127.

Eksterowicz, N. (2003). *Meperidine—using evidence-based rationale, 12*(1), 4.

Ersek, M., Cherrier, M. M., Overman, S. S., & Irving, G. A. (2004). The cognitive effects of opioids. *Pain Management Nursing, 5*(2), 75–93.

Feldt, K. S. (2000). The checklist of nonverbal pain indicators (CNPI). *Pain Management Nursing, 1*(1), 13–21.

Ferrell, B., & Coyle, N. (2001). *Textbook of palliative nursing.* London, UK: Oxford Press.

Ferrini, R., & Paice, J. (2004). How to initiate and monitor infusional lidocaine for severe and/or neuropathic pain. *Journal of Supportive Oncology, 2*(1), 91.

Fernandez, E. (2002). *Anxiety, depression, and anger in pain: Research findings and clinical options.* San Antonio, TX: Advanced Psychological Resources.

Fick, D., Cooper, J. W., Wade, W. E., Waller, J. L., Maclean, J. R., & Beers, M. H. (2003). Updating the Beers criteria for potentially inappropriate medication use in older adults: Results of a U.S. consensus panel of experts. *Archives of Internal Medicine, 163*, 2716–2724.

Finnerup, N., & Jensen, R. (2004). Spinal cord injury pain—Mechanisms and treatment. *European Journal of Neurology, 11*(2), 73.

Fitzgerald, M. (1995). Pain in infancy: Some unanswered questions. *Pain Reviews, 2*(2), 77–91.

Fowler-Kerry, S., & Lander, J. R. (1987). Management of injection pain in children. *Pain, 30*, 169–175.

Fuchs-Lacelle, S., & Hadjistavropoulos, T. (2004). Development and preliminary validation of the Pain Assessment Checklist for Seniors with Limited Ability to Communicate (PACSLAC). *Pain Management Nursing, 5*, 37–49.

Gil, K. (1990). Psychologic aspects of acute pain. *Anesthesiology Reports, 2*(2), 246.

Gordon, D., & Love, G. (2004). Pharmacologic management of neuropathic pain. *Pain Management Nursing, 5*(4, S1), 19.

Grant, M. S., Cordis, G. A., & Doberman, D. J. (2007). Acute pain management in hospitalized patients with current opioid abuse. *Topics in Advanced Practice Nursing eJournal, 7*(1).

Grealish, L., Lomasney, A., & Whiteman, B. (2000). Foot massage: A nursing intervention to modify the distressing symptoms of pain and nausea in patients hospitalized with cancer. *Cancer Nursing, 23*, 237–243.

Gruener, D., & Lande, S. (2006), *Pain control in the primary care setting.* Glenview, IL: American Pain Society.

Grunau, R. V., & Craig, K. (1987). Pain expression in neonates: Facial action and cry. *Pain, 28*, 395–410.

Grunau, R. V. E., Whitfield, M. F., Petrie, J. H., & Fryer, E. L. (1994). Early pain experience, child and family factors, as precursors of somatization: A prospective study of extremely premature and full-term children. *Pain, 56*, 353–359.

Grunfeld, E., Coyle, D., Whelan, T., Clinch, J., Reyno, L., Earle, C. C., et al. (2004). Family caregiver burden: results of a longitudinal study of breast cancer patients and their principal caregivers. *Canadian Medical Association Journal, 170*, 1795-1801.

Haythornthwaite, J. A., Menefee, L. A., Heinberg, L. T., & Clark, M. R. (1998). Pain coping strategies predict perceived control over pain. *Pain, 77*, 33–39.

Herr, K. (2002a). Chronic pain: Challenges and assessment strategies. *Journal of Gerontological Nursing, 28*(1), 20–27.

Herr, K. (2002b). Chronic pain in the older patient: Management strategies. *Journal of Gerontological Nursing, 28*, 28–34.

Herr, K., Coyne, P. J., Key, T., Manworren, R., McCaffery, M., Merkel, et al. (2006). Pain assessment in the nonverbal patient: Position statement with clinical practice recommendations. *Pain Management Nursing, 7*, 44–52.

Hockenberry, M. J., & Wilson, D. (2007). *Wong's nursing care of infants and children* (8th ed.). St. Louis, MO: Mosby.

International Association for the Study of Pain, Subcommittee on Taxonomy. (1979). Pain terms: A list with definitions and notes on usage. *Pain, 6*, 249.

Jacox, A., Carr, D., Payne, R., Berde, C., Breitbart, W., Cain, J., et al. (1994). *Management of cancer pain. Clinical practice guideline no. 9* (AHCPR Publication No. 94-0592). Rockville, MD: Agency for Health Care Policy and Research, Public Health Service, U.S. Department of Health and Human Services.

Jensen, M. P., Turner, J. A., Romano, J. M., & Karoly, P. (1991). Coping with chronic pain: A critical review of the literature. *Pain, 47*, 249–283.

Johnston, C. C., Stevens, B. J., Franck, L. S., Jack, A., Stremler, R., & Platt, R. (1999). Factors explaining lack of response to heel stick in preterm newborns. *Journal of Obstetric, Gynecologic, and Neonatal Nursing, 28*, 587–594.

Johnston, C. C., Collinge, J. M., Henderson, S. J., & Anand, K. J. S. (1997). A cross-sectional survey of pain and pharmacological analgesia in Canadian neonatal intensive care units. *Clinical Journal of Pain, 13*, 308–312.

The Joint Commission. (2008, September 24). Preventing errors relating to commonly used anticoagulants. *Sentinel Event Alert*, Issue 41. Retrieved, February 5, 2009, from http://www.jointcommission.org/SentinelEvents/SentinelEventAlert/sea_41.htm

The Joint Commission. (2009). *National Patient Safety Goals, 2009.* Retrieved October 30, 2008, from http://www.jointcommission.org/patientsafety/nationalpatientsafetygoals/

Jovey, R. D., Ennis, J., Gardner-Nix, J., Goldman, B., Hayes, H., Lynch, M., et al. (2003). Use of opioid analgesics for the treatment of chronic noncancer pain: A consensus statement and guidelines from the Canadian Pain Society. *Pain Research & Management, 8*(Suppl A), 3A–14A.

Kelly, A. (2003). *Geriatric pain assessment: Self-directed learning module.* Pensacola, FL: American Society of Pain Management Nurses (ASPMN).

King, S., & Walsh K. (2007) I think PCA is great, but . . .—Surgical nurses' perceptions of patient-controlled analgesia. *International Journal of Nursing Practice, 13*, 276–283.

Kotani, N., Hashimoto, H., Sato, Y., Sessler, D. I., Yoshioka, H., Kitayama, M., et al. (2001). Preoperative intradermal acupuncture reduces postoperative pain, nausea and vomiting, analgesic requirements, and sympathoadreanal responses. *Anesthesiology, 95*, 349–356

LaMontagne, L. L., Hepworth, J. T., & Salisbury, M. H. (2001). Anxiety and postoperative pain in children who undergo major orthopedic surgery. *Applied Nursing Research, 14*, 119–124.

Lansbury, G. (2000). Chronic pain management: A qualitative study of elderly people's preferred coping strategies and barriers to management. *Disability and Rehabilitation, 22*, 2–14.

Lawler, K. (1997). Pain assessment. *Professional Nurse Study Supplement, 13*(Suppl. 1), S5–S8.

Lehne, R. (2001). *Pharmacology for nursing care* (4th ed.). Philadelphia, PA: W. B. Saunders.

MacDonald, N., Ayoub, J., Farley, J., Foucault, C., Lesage, P., & Mayo, N. (2002). A Quebec survey of issues in cancer pain management. *Journal of Pain and Symptom Management, 23*(1), 39–47.

Manworren, R. (2006). A call to action to protect range orders. *American Journal of Nursing, 106*(7), 65.

Maxwell, T., Brouch, M., & Jungquist., C. (2005). *Palliative and end-of-life pain management: self-directed learning module.* Pensacola, FL: American Society for Pain Management Nursing.

McCaffery, M. (1979). *Nursing management of the patient with pain* (2nd ed.). Philadelphia, PA: Lippincott.

McCaffery, M., Ferrell, B. R., & Pasero, C. (2000). Nurses' personal opinion about patients' pain and their effect of recorded assessments and titration of opioid doses. *Pain Management Nursing, 1*(3), 79–87.

McCaffery, M., & Pasero, C. (1999). *Pain: Clinical manual* (2nd ed.). St. Louis, MO: Mosby.

McGrady, A., Wauquier, A., McNeil, A., & Gerard, G. (1994). Effect of biofeedback-assisted relaxation on migraine headache and changes in cerebral blood flow velocity in the middle cerebral artery. *Headache, 34,* 424–428.

McGrath, P. J., & Finley, G. A. (Eds.). (1999). *Chronic and recurrent pain in children and adolescents.* Seattle, WA: IASP Press.

McMillan, S. C. (1996). Pain and pain relief experienced by hospice patients with cancer. *Cancer Nursing, 19,* 298–307.

Meek, S. S. (1993). Effects of slow-stroke back massage on relaxation in hospice clients. *Image: The Journal of Nursing Scholarship, 25*(1), 17–21.

Mehta, V., & Langford, R. (2006). Acute pain management for opioid dependent patients. *Anaesthesia, 61,* 269.

Melzack, R., & Wall, P. D. (1965). Pain mechanisms: A new theory. *Science, 150,* 971–979.

Melzack, R., & Wall, P. D. (2003). *Handbook of pain management.* London, UK: Churchill Livingstone.

Miaskowski, C. (2005). The next step to improving cancer pain management. *Pain Management Nursing, 6*(1), 1.

Nightingale, F. (1969). *Notes on nursing: What it is and what it is not.* New York: Dover (Original work published 1859).

Oberlander, T. F., O'Donnell, M. E., & Montgomery, C. J. (1999). Pain in children with significant neurological impairment. *Journal of Developmental & Behavioral Pediatrics, 20,* 235–243.

O'Mathuna, D. (2000). Evidence-based practice and reviews of therapeutic touch. *Journal of Nursing Scholarship, 32,* 279–285.

Otis-Green, S., Sherman, R., Perez, M., & Baird, P. (2002). An integrated psychosocial–spiritual model for cancer pain management. *Cancer Practice, 10*(Suppl. 1), 58–65.

Paice, J. A. (1994). *The physiology and pharmacologic management of pain: Physiology of pain: Unraveling the mystery.* Baltimore, MD: Williams & Wilkins.

Paice, J. A., Noskin, G. A., Vanagunas, A., & Shott, S. (2005). Efficacy and safety of scheduled dosing of opioid analgesics: a quality improvement study. *Journal of Pain, 6,* 639–643.

Pasero, C. (2000). Continuous local anesthetics. *American Journal of Nursing, 100*(8), 22–23.

Pasero, C. (2003). *Intravenous patient-controlled analgesia for acute pain management: Self-directed learning module.* Pensacola, FL: American Society of Pain Management Nurses (ASPMN).

Pasero, C., & McCaffery, M. (2002). Monitoring sedation. *American Journal of Nursing, 102*(2), 67–69.

Passik, S., Kirsh. K., & Portenoy, R. (2003). Substance abuse issues in palliative care. In A. Berger, R. Portenoy, & D. Weissman (Eds.), *Principles and practice of palliative care and supportive oncology* (pp. 457–466). Philadelphia, PA: Lippincott Williams & Wilkins.

Popp, B., & Portenoy, R. (1996). Management of chronic pain in the elderly: Pharmacology of opioids and other analgesics. In B. A. Ferrell & B. R. Ferrell (Eds.), *Pain in the elderly* (pp. 21–34). Seattle, WA: IASP Press.

Porter, F. L., Wolf, C. M., Gold, J., Lotsoff, D., & Miller, J. P. (1997). Pain and pain management in newborn infants: A survey of physicians and nurses. *Pediatrics, 100,* 626–632.

Puntillo, K. A., White, C., Morris, A. B., Perdue, S. T., Stanik-Hutt, J., Thompson, C. L., et al. (2001). Patients' perceptions and responses to procedural pain: Results from Thunder Project II. *American Journal of Critical Care, 10,* 238–251.

Registered Nurses Association of Ontario. (2002). *Assessment and management of pain.* Retrieved October 30, 2008, from http://www.rnao.org/Page.asp?PageID=924&ContentID=720

Reiff, P., & Nizolek, M. (2001). Troubleshooting tips for PCA. *RN, 64*(4), 33–37.

Roman, M., & Cabaj, T. (2005). Epidural analgesia, *Medsurg Nursing, 14,* 257.

Ruda, M. A., Ling, Q.-D., Hohmann, A. G., Peng, Y. B., & Tachibana, T. (2000). Altered nociceptive neuronal circuits after neonatal peripheral inflammation. *Science, 289,* 628–630.

Salerno, E., & Willens, J. S. (1996). *Pain management handbook: An interdisciplinary approach.* St. Louis, MO: Mosby.

Schumacher, K. L., Koresawa, S., West, C., Hawkins, C., Johnson, C., Wais, E., et al. (2002). Putting cancer pain management regimens into practice at home. *Journal of Pain and Symptom Management, 23,* 369–382.

Stallard, P. I., Williams, L., Lenton, S., & Velleman, R. (2001). Pain in cognitively impaired, non-communicating children. *Archives of Disease in Childhood, 85,* 460–462.

Stevens, B. (1998a). Composite measures of pain. In G. A. Finley & P. J. McGrath (Eds.), *Progress in pain research and management: Vol. 10. Measurement of pain in infants and children* (pp. 161–178). Seattle, WA: IASP Press.

Stevens, B., & Koren, G. (1998b). Evidence-based pain management for infants. *Current Opinion in Pediatrics, 10,* 203–207.

The SUPPORT Principal Investigators. (1995). A controlled trial to improve care for seriously ill hospitalized patients: The Study to Understand Prognoses and Preferences for Outcomes and Risks of Treatments (SUPPORT). *Journal of the American Medical Association, 274,* 1591–1598.

Taylor, E. M., Boyer, K., & Campbell, F. A. (2008). Pain in hospitalized children: A prospective cross-sectional survey of pain prevalence, intensity, assessment and management in a Canadian pediatric teaching hospital. *Pain Research Management, 13*(1), 25–32.

Tesler, M. D., Wilkie, D. J., Holzemer, W. L., & Savedra, M. C. (1994). Postoperative analgesics for children and adolescents: Prescription and administration. *Journal of Pain and Symptom Management, 9,* 85–95.

Thompson, W. (2000). Placebos: A review of the placebo response. *American Journal of Gastroenterology, 95,* 1637–1643.

Titler, M., & Rakel, B. (2001). Nonpharmacological treatment of pain. *Critical Care Nursing Clinics of North America, 13,* 221–232.

Tucker, K. (2001). Deceptive placebo administration. *American Journal of Nursing, 101,* 55–56.

Vila H., Smith, R. A., Augustyniak, M. J., Nagi, P. A., Soto, R. G., Ross, T. W., et al. (2005). The efficacy and safety of pain management before and after implementation of hospital-wide pain management standards: Is patient safety compromised by treatment based solely on numerical pain ratings? *Anesthesia and Analgesia, 101,* 474.

Vitetta, L., Kenner, D., & Sali, D. (2005). Sedation and analgesia-prescribing patterns in terminally ill patients at the end of life. *American Journal of Hospice & Palliative Care, 22,* 465–473.

Wall, P., & Melzack, R. (1999). *Textbook of pain* (4th ed.). London, UK: Churchill Livingstone.

Warnock, F. F. (2003). An ethogram on neonatal distress related pain behavior (newborn male circumcision). *Infant Behavior and Development, 26,* 398–420.

Warnock, F., & Sandrin, D. (2004). Comprehensive description of newborn distress behavior in response to acute pain (newborn male circumcision). *Pain, 107,* 242–255.

Wheeler, M., Oderda, G. M., Ashburn, M. A., & Lipman, A. G. (2002). Adverse events associated with postoperative opioid analgesia: A systemic review. *Journal of Pain, 3,* 159–180.

Whelan, T. J., Mohide, E. A., William, A. R., Arnold, A., Tew, M., Sellick, S., et al. (2000). The supportive care needs of newly diagnosed cancer patients attending a regional cancer center. *Cancer, 80,* 1518–1524.

Whitecar, P., Maxwell, T., & Douglass, A.B. (2004). Principles of palliative care medicine. II. Pain and symptom management. *Advanced Studies in Medicine, 4,* 88–99.

Willens, J. (2006). Consumer group urges food and drug administration to ban drug Darvon. *Pain Management Nursing, 7*(2), 43.

Williams, G. (2005). Determining the appropriate use of COX-2 inhibitors in pain management. *Clinical Advisor,* 9.

Williams, H. (2006). Assessing, diagnosing and managing neuropathic pain. *Nursing Times, 102*(16), 22–24.

Wirth, J. H., Hudgins, J. C., & Paice, J. A. (2005). Use of herbal therapies to relieve pain: a review of efficacy and adverse effects. *Pain Management Nursing, 6,* 145–167.

Wong, D. L., & Baker, C. M. (1988). Pain in children: Comparison of assessment scales. *Oklahoma Nurse, 33*(1), 8.

World Health Organization. (1990). *Cancer pain relief and palliative care: Report of a WHO expert committee* (WHO Tech Rep Series No. 804). Geneva, Switzerland: Author.

Yoon, S., & Schaffer, S. (2006). Herbal, prescribed, and over-the-counter drug use in older women: Prevalence of drug interactions. *Geriatric Nursing, 27,* 118.

Chapter 43

Active Healthy Kids Canada. (2008). Making the grade: Canada's report card on physical activity for children and youth. Retrieved January 18, 2009, from http://www.activehealthykids.ca/Ophea/ActiveHealthyKids_v2/programs_2008 reportcard.cfm

Adolescent Health Committee, Canadian Pediatric Society. (2004) Dieting in adolescence. *Pediatrics & Child Health, 9,* 487–491. Retrieved April 13, 2008, from http://www.cps.ca/english/statements/AM/AH04-01.htm

Alberta Health and Wellness. (2008). *Feeding baby solid foods: From 6 to 12 months of age.* Retrieved July 16, 2008, from http://www.health.alberta.ca/documents/Infant-feeding-guide.pdf

Amarat, T. F., Matos, L. C., Tavares, M. M., Subtil, A., Martins, R., Nazare, M., & Pereira, N. S. (2007). The economic impact of disease-related malnutrition at hospital admission. *Clinical Nutrition, 27,* 778–784.

American Diabetes Association. (2000). Type 2 diabetes in children and adolescents. *Diabetes Care, 23*(3), 381–389.

Anonymous. (2005). Alphabet soup: Nutrition and literacy for preschoolers and parents. *Canadian Journal of Dietetic Practice and Research, 66*(4), A1–A2.

Beaton, G. H. (2006). When is an individual and individual versus a member of a group? An issue in the application of the Dietary Reference Intakes. *Nutrition Reviews, 64,* 211–225.

Brauer, P., Dietrich, L., & Davidson, B. (2006). Nutrition in primary health care: Using a Delphi process to design new interdisciplinary services. *Canadian Journal of Dietetic Practice and Research,* Fall (Suppl.), S14–S29.

Brown, J. E., Isaacs, J., Krinke, B., Murtaugh, M., & Sharbaugh, C. (2005). *Nutrition through the life cycle* (2nd ed.). Belmont, CA: Thompson Wadson.

Brownie, S. (2006). Why are elderly individuals at risk of nutritional deficiency? *International Journal of Nursing Practice, 12*(2), 110–118.

Cabré, E. (2004). Fibre supplementation of enteral formula-diets: A look to the evidence. *Clinical Nutrition Supplements, 1,* 63–71.

Canadian Dental Association. (2005). *Dental care for children.* Retrieved July 16, 2008, from http://www.cda-adc.ca/en/oral_health/cfyt/dental_care_children/index.asp

Canadian Diabetes Association. (2003). *Evidence-based best practices for the nutritional management of diabetes: Nutritional management of diabetes mellitus in the new millennium: A position statement of the Canadian Diabetes Association.* Retrieved January 18, 2004, from http://www.diabetes.ca/Files/nutritional_guide_eng.pdf

Canadian Diabetes Association. (2005). *The glycemic index.* Retrieved July 16, 2008, from http://www.diabetes.ca/files/Diabetes_GL_FINAL2_CPG03.pdf

Canadian Diabetes Association. (2008). *Clinical practice guidelines for the prevention and management of diabetes in Canada.* Retrieved January 6, 2009, from http://www.diabetes.ca/for-professionals/resources/2008-cpg/

Canadian Paediatric Society. (2005). Risk reduction for type 2 diabetes in Aboriginal children in Canada *Paediatric Child Health, 10*(1), 49–52.

Canadian Society of Intestinal Research. (2002–2008). *Inflammatory bowel disease.* Retrieved April 12, 2008, from www.badgut.com/index.php?content File=ibdndex&title=Inflammatory%20Bowel%20Disease

Canadian Stroke Network. (2006). Acute stroke management. Dysphagia assessment. In *Canadian best practice recommendations for stroke care: 2006* (pp. 56–58). Ottawa, ON: Author. Retrieved January 19, 2009, from http://www.guideline.gov/summary/summary.aspx?doc_id=12166&nbr=006263&string=stroke

Chapman, K. (2006). Food insecurity in Canada. *Canadian Journal of Dietetic Practice and Research, 67,* 170.

Chen, C. C., Bai, Y-Y., Huang, G-H., & Tang, S. T. (2007). Revisiting the concept of malnutrition in older people. *Journal of Clinical Nursing, 16,* 2015–2026.

College of Family Physicians of Canada (2007). *Anemia—When low blood iron is the cause.* Retrieved July 16, 2008, from http://www.cfpc.ca/English/cfpc/programs/patient%20education/anemia/default.asp?s=1

Contento, I. R., Williams, S. S., Michela, J. L., & Franklin, A. B. (2006). Understanding the food choice process of adolescents in the context of family and friends. *Journal of Adolescent Health, 38,* 575–582.

Cooper, M. J., Cockell, K. A., & L'Abbe, M. R. (2006). The iron status of Canadian adolescents and adults: Current knowledge and practical implications. *Canadian Journal of Dietetic Practice and Research, 67,* 130–138.

Corbett, J. V. (2008). *Laboratory test and diagnostic procedures with nursing diagnoses* (7th ed), Upper Saddle River, NJ: Pearson Prentice Hall.

Costain, L., & Croker, H. (2005). Helping individuals to help themselves. *Proceedings of the Nutrition Society, 64,* 89–96.

Croll, J. K., Neumark-Sztainer, D., Story, M., Wall, M., Perry, C., & Harnack, L. (2006). Adolescents involved in weight-related and power team sports have better eating patterns and nutrient intakes than non-sport-involved adolescents. *Journal of the American Dietitian Association, 105,* 717–718.

CTV National News with Lloyd Robertson. (2003, January 23). *Food portion sizes growing with our waistlines.* Retrieved April 14, 2008, from http://www.ctv.ca/servlet/ArticleNews/story/CTVNews/1043184903876_38594103/?hub=CTVNewsAT11

Enger-Stringer, R., & Berenbaum, S. (2005). Collective kitchens in Canada: A review of the literature. *Canadian Journal of Dietetic Practice and Research, 66,* 246–251.

Food and Nutrition Board. (1997). *Dietary reference intakes for calcium, phosphorus, magnesium, vitamin D, and fluoride.* Washington, DC: National Academy Press.

Glanville, N. T., & McIntyre, L. (2006). Diet quality of Atlantic families headed by single mothers. *Canadian Journal of Dietetic Practice and Research, 67*(1), 28–35.

Green, S. M., & Watson, R. (2005). Nutritional screening and assessment tools for use by nurses: Literature review. *Journal of Advanced Nursing, 50*(1), 69–83.

Grundy, S. M., Cleeman, J. I., Merz, C. N., Brewer, H. B., Jr., Clark, L. T., Hunninghake, D. B., et al. (2004). Implications of recent clinical trials for the National Cholesterol Education Program Adult Treatment Panel III Guidelines. *Circulation 110,* 227–239. Retrieved April 17, 2008, from http://www.circulationaha.org

Hassan, T., Marchessault, G., Campbell, M., & Huhmann, B. (2007). Messages about calcium and weight in Canadian women's magazines. *Canadian Journal of Dietetic Practice and Research, 68,* 103–106.

He, M., & Beynon, C. (2006). Prevalence of overweight and obesity in school-aged children. *Canadian Journal of Dietetic Practice and Research, 67,* 125–129.

Health Canada. (1999). *Nutrition for a healthy pregnancy: National guidelines for the childbearing years.* Ottawa: Minister of Public Works and Government Services Canada. Retrieved April 12, 2008, from http://www.hc-sc.gc.ca/fnan/nutrition/prenatal/national_guidelines_cp-lignes_directrices_nationales_pc-eng.php

Health Canada. (2002). *Nutrition for health: An agenda for action.* Retrieved January 6, 2009, from http://www.hc-sc-gc.ca/fn-an/nutrition/pol/nutrition_health_agenda_nutrition_virage_sante-eng.php

Health Canada. (2003a). *Caffeine and your health.* Retrieved April 27, 2008, from http://www.hc-sc.gc.ca/fn-an/securit/facts-faits/caffeine_e.html

Health Canada (2003b). *Canadian guidelines for body weight classification in adults.* Retrieved January 6, 2009, from http://www.hc-sc.gc.ca/fn-an/nutrition/weights-poids/guide-ld-adult/weight_book-livres_des_poids-14_e.html

Health Canada. (2004a). *Exclusive breastfeeding duration—2004 Health Canada recommendation.* Retrieved April 8, 2008, from http://www.hc-sc.gc.ca/fn-an/nutrition/child-enfant/infant-nourisson/excl_bf_dur-dur_am_excl-eng.php

Health Canada. (2004b). *Vitamin D supplementation for breastfed infants.* 2004 Health Canada recommendation (Catalogue No.: H44-74/2004 E-HTML, HC Publication No.: 4828). Retrieved July 16, 2008, from http://www.hc-sc.gc.ca/fn-an/nutrition/child-enfant/infant-nourisson/vita_d_supp-eng.php

Health Canada. (2005a). *Transition to solid foods.* Retrieved January 18, 2009, from http://www.hc-sc.gc.ca/fn-an/pubs/infant-nourrisson/nut_infant_nourrisson_term_6- eng.php

Health Canada. (2005b). *What is early childhood tooth decay (ECTD)?* Retrieved April 30, 2006, from http://www.hc-sc.gc.ca/hl-vs/oral-bucco/care-soin/child-enfant-eng.php

Health Canada. (2006). *Dietary reference intakes tables.* Retrieved April 30, 2006, from http://www.hc-sc.gc.ca/fn-an/nutrition/reference/table/index_e.html

Health Canada. (2007a). *Breastfeeding.* Retrieved July 16, 2008, from http://www.hc-sc.gc.ca/fn-an/pubs/infant-nourrisson/nut_infant_nourrisson_term_3-eng.php

Health Canada. (2007b). *Eating well with Canada's food guide.* Retrieved January 6, 2009, from http://www.hc-sc.gc.ca/fn-an/alt_formats/hpfb-dgpsa/pdf/food-guide-aliment/print_eatwell_bienmang-eng.pdf

Health Canada. (2007c). *Eating well with Canada's food guide—First Nations, Inuit and Métis* (Catalogue no. H34-159/2007-PDF). Ottawa, ON: Author. Retrieved January 19, 2009, from http://www.hc-sc.gc.ca/fn-an/food-guide-aliment/fnim-pnim/index-eng.php

Health Canada. (2007d). *First Nations, Inuit & Aboriginal health diseases & health conditions.* Retrieved July 16, 2008, from http://www.hc-sc.gc.ca/fniah-spnia/diseases-maladies/index-eng.php

Health Canada. (2007e). *Interactive nutrition label: Get the facts.* Retrieved April 9, 2008, from http://www.hc-sc.gc.ca/fn-an/label-etiquet/nutrition/cons/inl_main_e.html

Health Odyssey International. (2008). *Neonatal nutritional intervention for mothers who cannot breast-feed. Choosing the formula for optimal infant growth and development* (HO08-001E ML). Retrieved July 16, 2008, from http://www.healthodyssey.ca/R_NeonatalNutrition.htm

Heart and Stroke Foundation of Canada. (2008). *Weighing in on BMI.* Retrieved April 30, 2008, from http://ww2.heartandstroke.ca/Page.asp?PageID=1562&ArticleID=3732&Src=& From=SubCategory

Henry, C. J., Allison, D. J., & Garcia, A. C. (2003). Child nutrition programs in Canada and the United States: Comparisons and contrasts. *Journal of School Health, 73*(2), 83–85.

Hobbie, C., Baker, S., & Bayerl, C. (2000). Parental understanding of basic infant nutrition: Misinformed feeding choices. *Journal of Pediatric Health Care, 14,* 26–31.

Hockenberry, M. (2004). *Wong's essential of pediatric nursing* (7th ed.). Philadelphia, PA: Mosby Elsevier.

Irwin, J. D., Ng, V. K., Rush, T. J., Nguyen, C., & He, M. (2007). Can food banks sustain nutrient requirements? A case study in southwestern Ontario. *Canadian Journal of Public Health, 98*(1), 17–19.

Janseen, I., Boyce, W. F., Simpson, K., & Pickett, W. (2006). Influence of individual- and area-level measures of socioeconomic status on obesity, unhealthy eating, and physical inactivity in Canadian adolescents. *American Journal of Clinical Nutrition, 83*(1), 139–145.

Joint Working Group: Canadian Paediatric Society, Dietitians of Canada, Health Canada. (1998). *Nutrition for healthy term infants.* Ottawa, ON: Minister of Public Works and Government Services Canada.

Katamay, S. W., Esslinger, K. A., Vigneault, M., Johnston, J. L., Junkins, B. A., Robbins, L. G., et al. (2007). Eating well with Canada's food guide (2007): Development of the food intake pattern. Nutrition Reviews, 65, 155–166.

Kim, Y.-I. (2007). Folic acid fortification and supplementation—Good for some but not so good for others. *Nutrition Reviews, 65*(11), 504–511.

Kramer, M. S., Platt, R. W., Wen, S. W., Joseph, K. S., Allen, A., Abrahanomowicz, M., et al., for the Fetal/Infant Health Study Group of the Canadian Perinatal Surveillance System. (2001). A new and improved population-based Canadian reference for birth weight for gestational age. *Pediatrics, 108*(2), e35. Retrieved April 25, 2008, from http://www.pediatrics.org/cgi/content/full/108/2/e35

Kubrak, C., & Jensen, L. (2007). Malnutrition in acute care patients: A narrative review. *International Journal of Nursing Studies, 44,* 1036–1054.

Kuperberg, K., & Evers, S. (2006). Feeding patterns and weight among First Nations children. *Canadian Journal of Dietetic Practice and Research, 67*(2), 79–84.

Kurtz Landy, C. (2007). Children who had experienced family food insufficiency were more likely to be overweight at 4.5 years of age [Commentary]. *Evidence Based Nursing, 10,* 58.

LaForest, S., Goldin, B., Nour, K., Roy, M-A., & Payette, H. (2007). Nutrition risk in home-bound older adults: Using dietician-trained and supervised nutrition volunteers for screening and intervention. *Canadian Journal of Aging, 26,* 305–315.

Latner, J. D., & Stunkard, A. J. (2003). Getting worse: The stigmatization of obese children. *Obesity Research, 11,* 452–456.

Lindsay, P., Bayley, M., Hellings, C., Hill, M., Woodbury, E., Phillips, S. (2008). Canadian best practice recommendations for stroke care (updated 2008). *Canadian Medical Association Journal, 179* (12), S1–S25. Retrieved January 19, 2009, from http://www.cmaj.ca/cgi/content/full/179/12/S1

Mangels, A. R., Messina, V., & Melina, V. (2003). Position of the American Dietitic Association and Dieticians of Canada: Vegetarian diets. *Journal of the American Dietetic Association, 103,* 748–765.

Masse, P. G., Mahuren, J.D., Trannchant, C., & Dosy, J. (2004). B-6 vitamers and 4-pyridoxic acid in the plasma, erythrocytes, and urine of postmenopausal women. *American Journal of Clinical Nutrition, 80,* 946–951.

Meiner, S. E., & Lueckenotte, A. (2006). *Gerontologic nursing.* St. Louis, MO: Mosby.

Mendelson, R. (2007). Think tank on school-aged children: Nutrition and physical activity to prevent the rise in obesity. *Applied Physiology, Nutrition, & Metabolism, 32,* 495–499.

Merchant, A. T., Kelemen, L. E., de Koning, L., Lonn, V., Vuksan, V., Jacobs, R., et al. (2008). Interrelation of saturated fat, trans fat, alcohol intake, and subclinical atherosclerosis. *American Journal of Clinical Nutrition, 87,* 168–174.

Messina, V., Melina, V, & Mangels, A. R. (2003). A new food guide for North American vegetarians. *Canadian Journal of Dietetic Research and Practice, 64*(2), 82–86.

Metheny, N. A. (2004, Fall). Preventing aspiration in older adults with dysphagia. *Try This: Best Practices in Nursing Care to Older Adults,* Fall(20). Retrieved January 6, 2009, from https://login.proxy.hil.unb.ca/login?url=http://search.ebscohost.com/login.aspx?direct=true&db=cin20&AN=2009241217&site=ehost-live

Metheny, N. A. (2006). Preventing respiratory complications of tube feedings: Evidence-based practice. *American Journal of Critical Care, 15,* 360–369.

Millar, W., & Maclean, H. (2005). Breastfeeding practices. *Health Report, 16,* 23–31.

Murphy, S. P., & Barr, S. I. (2007). Food guides reflect similarities and difference in dietary guidance in three countries (Japan, Canada, and the United States). *Nutrition reviews, 65,* 141–148.

Murphy, S. P., Guenther, P. M., & Kretsch, M. J. (2006). Using the dietary reference intakes to assess intakes of groups: Pitfalls to avoid. *Journal of the American Dietetic Association, 106,* 1550–1553.

Myr, R. (2004). Promoting, Protecting, and supporting breastfeeding in a community with a high rate of tobacco use. *Journal of Human Lactation, 20,* 415–416.

Nightingale, F. (1858). *Notes on nursing: What it is and what it is not.* London: Hanson & Son.

Nowlin, A. (2006). The dysphagia dilemma: How you can help. *RN, 69*(6), 44–48, 50.

Paintal, H. S., & Kuschner, W. G. (2007). Aspiration syndromes: 10 Clinical pearls every physician should know. *International Journal of Clinical Practice, 61,* 846–852.

Paisley, J., Greenberg, M., & Haines, J. (2005). Cultural relevance of a fruit and vegetable food frequency questionnaire. *Canadian Journal of Dietetic Practice and Research, 66,* 231–236.

Paquet, C., St. Arnaud-McKenzie, D., Ferland, G., & Dubé, L. (2003). A blueprint-based case study analysis of nutrition services provided in a midterm care facility for the elderly. *Journal of the American Dietetic Association, 103,* 363–368.

Payette, H., & Shatenstein, B. (2005). Determinants of healthy eating in community-dwelling elderly. *Canadian Journal of Public Health, 96,* S27–S31.

Perry, & McClaren, (2003).

Plourde, G. (2006). Preventing and managing pediatric obesity. *Canadian Family Physician, 52,* 322–328.

Power, E. (2005). Individual and household food insecurity in Canada: Position of dieticians of Canada. *Canadian Journal of Dietetic Practice and Research, 66*(1), 43–46.

Public Health Agency of Canada. (2008). *The sensible guide to a healthy pregnancy.* Ottawa, ON: Author. Retrieved January 6, 2009, from http://www.healthycanadians.gc.ca/hp-gs/pdf/hpguide-eng.pdf

Qureshi, S., & Mink, R. (2003). Aspiration of fruit gel snacks. *Pediatrics, 111,* 693–695.

Raine, K. D. (2005). Determinants of healthy eating in Canada: An overview and synthesis. *Canadian Journal of Public Health, 96*(Suppl. 3), S8–S14.

Ramsey, D., Smithard, D., & Kalra, L. (2005). Silent aspiration: What do we know? *Dysphagia, 20,* 218–225.

Ricciuto, L. E., & Tarasuk, V. S. (2006). An examination of income-related disparities in the nutritional quality of food selections among Canadian households from 1986–2001. *Social Science & Medicine, 64,* 186–198.

Richardson, S. A., Goodman, N., Hastorf, A. H., & Dornbusch, S. M. (1961). Cultural uniformity in reaction to physical disabilities. *American Sociological Review, 26,* 241–247.

Rideout, K., Riches, G., Ostry, A., Buckingham, D., & MacRae, R. (2007). Bringing home the right to food in Canada: Challenges and possibilities for achieving food security. *Public Health Nutrition, 10,* 566–573.

Riediger, N. D., Shooshtari, S., & Moghadasian, M. H. (2007). The influence of sociodemographic factors on patterns of fruit and vegetable consumption in Canadian adolescents. *Journal of the American Dietetic Association, 107,* 1511–1518.

Salmerón, J., Hu, F. B., Manson, J. E., Stampfer, M. J., Colditz, G. A., Rimm, E. B., et al. (2001). Dietary fat intake and risk of type 2 diabetes in women. *American Journal of Clinical Nutrition, 73,* 1019–1026.

Saylor, K. First Nations and Inuit Health Committee, Canadian Paediatric Society (CPS). (2005). Risk reduction for type 2 diabetes in Aboriginal children in Canada. *Paediatrics & Child Health,10*(1), 49–52. Reaffirmed by CPS May 2008. Retrieved July 19, 2008, from http://www.cps.ca/English/statements/II/FNIH05-01.htm#Committee%23Committee

Scheier, L. M. (2004). School health report cards attempt to address the obesity epidemic. *Journal of the American Dieteticians Association, 104,* 341–344.

Schlenker, E. D., & Long, S. (2007). *Williams' essentials of nutrition & diet therapy* (9th ed). St. Louis, MO: Mosby Elsevier.

Shariatzadeh, M. R., Huang, J., & Marrie, T. J. (2006). Differences in the features of aspiration pneumonia according to site of acquisition: Community or continuing care facility. *American Geriatrics Society, 54,* 298–302.

Stabler, S. P., & Allen, R. H. (2004). Vitamin B12 deficiency as a worldwide problem. *Annual Review of Nutrition, 24,* 299–326.

Starky, S. (2005). The obesity epidemic in Canada. Library of Parliament. Retrieved October 10, 2006, from http://www.parl.gc.ca/information/library/PRBpubs/prb0511-e.htm

Statistics Canada. (2003). *Canada's ethnocultural portrait: The changing mosaic.* Ottawa: Author.

Statistics Canada. (2004, June 15). Canadian Community Health Survey. Retrieved January 18, 2009, from http://www.statcan.gc.ca/daily-quotidien/040615/dq040615b-eng.htm

Statistics Canada. (2006). *Health Reports, 17*(3, Catalogue no. 82-003-XIE). Retrieved January 18, 2009, from http://www.statcan.gc.ca/pub/82-003-x/82-003-x2005003-eng.pdf

Statistics Canada. (2007). *Families, households and housing.* Retrieved January 19, 2009, from http://www41.statcan.gc.ca/2007/40000/ceb40000_000_e.htm

Stratton, R. J., & Elia, M. (2006). Deprivation linked to malnutrition risk and mortality in hospital. *British Journal of Nutrition, 96,* 870–876.

Stratton, R. J., King, C. L., Stroud, M. A., Jackson, A. A., & Elia, M. (2006)."Malnutrition Universal Screening Tool" predicts mortality and length of hospital stay in acutely ill elderly. *British Journal of Nutrition, 95,* 325–330.

Tannenbaum, C., & Shatenstein, B. (2007). Exercise and nutrition in older Canadian women: Opportunities for community intervention. *Canadian Journal of Public Health, 98,* 187–193.

Taylor, J. P., Timmons, V., Larsen, R., Walton, F., Bryanton, J., Critchley, K., & McCarthy, M. J. (2007). Nutritional concerns in Aboriginal children are similar to those in Non-Aboriginal children in Prince Edward Island, Canada. *Journal of the American Dietetic Association, 107,* 951–955.

Tonn, S. (2007, April). *Trans fat-free.* Retrieved March 18, 2008, from http://www.alive.com/6008a15a2.php?subject_bread_cramb=192

Tontisirin, K., & de Haen, H. (2001). *Human energy requirements: Report of a Joint FAO/WHO/UNU Expert Consultation* [Food and Nutrition Technical Report Series 1]. Rome, Italy: Food and Agriculture Organizations of the United Nations, October 17–24.

Touz, R. M., Campbell, N. R., Logan, A., Gledhill, N., Petrella, R., & Padwal, R. (2004). The Canadian recommendations for the management of hypertension: Part III—Lifestyle modifications to prevent and control hypertension. *Canadian Journal of Cardiology, 20*(1), 55–59.

Tremblay, M. S. (2003). *The evolution of Canada's "supersize" generation.* Presentation at the Continuing Medical Education and Professional Development Conference: "Obesity: New Prescriptions for the Canadian Epidemic," October 17, 2003. Retrieved January 18, 2009, from http://www.usask.ca/cme/articles/supersize.shtml

Tremblay, M. S., & Willms, J. D. (2003). Obesity in Canadian children. *The Canadian Medical Association Journal, 164,* 1564–1565.

Trumbo, P., Schlicker, S., Yates, A., & Poos, M. (2002). Dietary reference intakes for energy, carbohydrate, fiber, fat, fatty acids, cholesterol, protein and amino acids. *Journal of the American Dietetic Association, 102,* 1621–1630.

Tucker, P., Irwin, J. D., He, M., Sangter Bouch, M., & Pollett, G. (2006). Preschoolers' dietary behaviours: Parents' perspectives. *Canadian Journal of Dietetic Practice and Research, 67*(2), 67–71.

Van Dillen, S. M. E., Hiddink, G. J., Koelen, M. A., de Graaf, C. & van Woerkum, C. M. J. (2008). Exploration of possible correlates of nutrition awareness and the relationship with nutrition-related behaviours: Results of a consumer study. *Public Health Nutrition, 11,* 478–485.

Verkman, A. S. (2005). More than just water channels: Unexpected cellular roles of aquaporins. *Journal of Cell Science, 118,* 3225–3232.

Watson, L., Leslie, W., & Hankey, C. (2006). Under-nutrition in old age: Diagnosis and management. *Reviews in Clinical Gerontology, 16,* 23–34.

Weaver, K. (2008). Eating disorders. In W. Austin & M. A. Boyd (Eds.), *Psychiatric nursing for Canadian practice* (pp. 463–496). Philadelphia: Lippincott Williams & Wilkins.

Westergreen, A. (2006). Detection of eating difficulties after stroke: A systematic review. *International Nursing Review, 53,* 143–149.

Willms, J. D., Tremblay, M. S., & Katzmarzyk, P. T. (2003). Geographic and demographic variation in the prevalence of overweight Canadian children. *Obesity Research, 11,* 668–673.

Willows, N. D. (2005). Determinants of healthy eating in Aboriginal peoples in Canada. *Canadian Journal of Public Health, 96*(Suppl. 3), S32–S36.

World Health Organization. (2001). *Global strategy for infant and young child feeding: The optimal duration of exclusive breastfeeding.* Geneva. Retrieved January 18, 2009, from http://www.paho.org/english/ad/fch/ca/GSIYCF_infantfeeding_eng.pdf

World Health Organization. (2008). *Risks to oral health and intervention.* Retrieved January 18, 2009, from http://www.who.int/oral_health/action/risks/en/print.html

Young, T. K., Reading, J., Elias, B., & O'Neil, J. D. (2000). Type 2 diabetes mellitus in Canada's First Nations: Status of an epidemic in progress. *Canadian Medical Association Journal, 163,* 561–566.

Chapter 44

Abrams, P., Cardozo, L., Fall, M., Griffiths, D., Rosier, P., Ulmsten, U., et al. (2002). The standardization of terminology of lower urinary tract function: Report from the standardization sub-committee of the International Continence Society. *Neurourology and Urodynamics, 21,* 167–178.

Appell, R., & Sand, P. (2008). Nocturia: Etiology, diagnosis, and treatment. *Neurourology and Urodynamics, 27,* 34–39.

Arya, L., Myers, D., & Jackson, N. (2000). Dietary caffeine intake and the risk for detrusor instability: A case control study. *Obstetrics and Gynecology, 96,* 85–89.

Ashton-Miller, J., & DeLancey, J. (2007). Functional anatomy of the female pelvic floor. *Annals of the New York Academy of Science, 1101,* 266–296.

Bryant, C., Dowell, C., & Fairbrother, G. (2002). Caffeine reduction education to improve urinary symptoms. *British Journal of Nursing, 11,* 560–565.

Canadian Continence Foundation. (2001). *Promoting a collaborative consumer-focused approach to continence care in Canada.* Retrieved March 21, 2008, from http://www.continence-fdn.ca

Canadian Continence Foundation (2007). *Incontinence: A Canadian perspective.* Retrieved March 20, 2008, from http://www.continence-fdn.ca/consumers/index.html

Carroll, P., Grossfeld, G., & Barbour, S. (2004). Urinary diversion and bladder substitution. In E. Tanagho & J. McAninch (Eds.), *Smith's general urology* (pp. 400–415). New York: McGraw-Hill.

Cottenden, A., Bliss, D., Fader, M., Getliffe, K., Herrera, H., Paterson, J., et al. (2005). Management with continence products. In P. Abrams, L. Cardoza, S. Khoury, & A. Wein (Eds), *Incontinence* (pp. 151–254). Paris, France: Health Publication Ltd.

Dallosso, H., McGrother, C., Matthews, R., & Donaldson, M. (2003). The association of diet and other lifestyle factors with overactive bladder and stress incontinence: A longitudinal study in women. *BJU International, 92,* 69–77.

Doughty, D. B. (2006). *Urinary and fecal incontinence: Current management concepts* (3rd ed.). St. Louis, MO: Mosby.

Fernandez, R. S., & Griffiths, R. D. (2006). Duration of short-term indwelling catheter: A systematic review of the evidence. *Journal of Wound, Ostomy and Continence Nursing, 33,* 145–153.

Fischbach, F. (2004). A manual of laboratory and diagnostic tests. Philadelphia, PA: Lippincott Williams & Wilkins.

Fonda, D., DuBeau, C., Harari, D., Ouslander, J., Palmer, M., & Roe, B. (2005). Incontinence in the frail elderly. In P. Abrams, L. Cardoza, S. Khoury, & A. Wein (Eds), *Incontinence* (pp. 1165–1239). Paris, France: Health Publication Ltd.

Fry, C., Brading, A., Hussain, M., Lewis, S., Takeda, M., Tuttle, J., et al. (2005). Cell biology. In P. Abrams, L. Cardoza, S. Khoury, & A. Wein (Eds.), *Incontinence* (pp. 313–362). Paris, France: Health Publication Ltd.

Getliffe, K. (2003). Managing recurrent urinary catheter blockage: Problems, promises, and practicalities. *Journal of Wound, Ostomy, and Continence Nursing, 30,* 146–151.

Gray, M. (2003). Gender, race, and culture in research on UI. *American Journal of Nursing, 103*(Suppl. 3), 20–25.

Gray, M. (2006). Does the construction material affect outcomes in long-term catheterization? *Journal of Wound, Ostomy and Continence Nursing, 33,* 116–121.

Gray, M., & Krissovich, M. (2003). Does fluid intake influence the risk for urinary incontinence, urinary tract infection, and bladder cancer? *Journal of Wound, Ostomy, and Continence Nursing, 30,* 126–131.

Gray, M., Newman, D. K., Einhorn, C. J., & Reid Czarapata, B. J. (2006). Expert review: Best practices in managing the indwelling catheter. *Perspectives, 7*(1, Special ed.). Burlington, VT: Saxe Healthcare Communications. Retrieved January 20, 2009, from http://www.perspectivesinnursing.org/pdfs/Perspectives25.pdf

Griffiths, D., Kondo, A., Bauer, S., Diamant, N., Liao, L., Lose, G., et al. (2005). Dynamic testing. In P. Abrams, L. Cardoza, S. Khoury, & A. Wein (Eds), *Incontinence* (pp. 585–673). Paris, France: Health Publication Ltd.

Hannestad, Y., Rortveit, G., Sandvik, H., & Hunskaar, S. (2000). A community-based epidemiological survey of female urinary incontinence: The Norwegian EPINCONT study. *Journal of Clinical Epidemiology, 53,* 1150–1157.

Hay-Smith, J., & Dumoulin, C. (2007). Pelvic floor muscle training versus no treatment, or inactive control treatments, for urinary incontinence in women. *Cochrane Database of Systematic Reviews,* (1), CD005654.

Juthani-Mehta, M. (2007). Asymptomatic bacteriuria and urinary tract infection in older adults. *Clinics in Geriatric Medicine, 23,* 585–594.

Kidney Foundation of Canada, Northern Alberta and the Territories Branch. (2004). *Urinary tract infections (UTIs).* Retrieved November 23, 2004, from http://www.kidney.ab.ca/kidneys/utis.html

Moore, K. N., Fader, M., & Getliffe, K. (2007). Long-term bladder management by intermittent catheterisation in adults and children. *Cochrane Database of Systematic Reviews,* (4), CD006008.

Morrison, J., Birder, L., Craggs, M., De Groat, W., Downie, J., Drake, M., et al. (2005). Neural control. In P. Abrams, L. Cardoza, S. Khoury, & A. Wein (Eds), *Incontinence* (pp. 363–422). Paris, France: Health Publication Ltd.

Mostwin, J., Bourcier, A., Haab, F., Koelbl, H., Rao, S., Resnick, N., et al. (2005). Pathophysiology of urinary incontinence, fecal incontinence, and pelvic organ prolapse. In P. Abrams, L. Cardoza, S. Khoury, & A. Wein (Eds), *Incontinence* (pp. 423–484). Paris, France: Health Publication Ltd.

Newman, D. K. (2007). The indwelling urinary catheter: Principles for best practice. *Journal of Wound, Ostomy, and Continence Nursing, 34,* 655–661.

Nguyen, H. (2004). Bacterial infections of the genitourinary tract. In E. Tanagho & J. McAninch (Eds.), *Smith's general urology* (pp. 203–227). New York: McGraw-Hill.

Nygaard, I., Bryant, C., Dowell, C., & Wilson, P. (2008). Lifestyle interventions for the treatment of urinary incontinence in adults. *Cochrane Database of Systematic Reviews,* (1), CD003505.

Ostaszkiewicz, J., Chestney, T., & Roe, B. (2008). Habit retraining for the management of urinary incontinence in adults. *Cochrane Database of Systematic Reviews,* (1), CD002801.

Parkin, J., & Keeley, F. X. (2003). Indwelling catheter-associated urinary tract infections. *British Journal of Community Nursing, 8*(4), 166.

Perrin, L., Dauphinee, S., Corcos, J., Hanley, J., & Kuchel, G. (2006). Pelvic floor muscle training with biofeedback and bladder training in elderly women. *Journal of Wound, Ostomy, and Continence Nursing, 32,* 186-199.

Registered Nurses Association of Ontario. (2005). *Promoting continence using prompted voiding* (Revised). Retrieved April 7, 2005, from http://www.rnao.org/bestpractices/completed_guidelines/BPG_Guide_C1_Promote_Continence.asp

Saint, S., Kowalski, C., Kaufman, S., Hofer, T., Kauffamn, C., Olmsted, R., et al. (2008). Preventing hospital-acquired urinary tract infection in the United States: A national study. *Clinical Infectious Diseases, 46,* 243–250.

Sampselle, C. M. (2003). Behavioral interventions in young and middle-age women. *American Journal of Nursing, 103*(Suppl. 3), 9–19.

Schick, E., Jolviet-Tremblay, M., DuPont, C., Bertrand, P., & Tessier, J. (2003). Frequency-volume chart: The minimum number of days required to obtain reliable results. *Neurourology and Urodynamics, 22,* 92–96.

Sherwood, L. (2007). *Human physiology: From cells to systems.* Belmont, CA: Thomson, Brooks/Cole.

Smith, J. M. (2006). Current concepts in catheter management. In D. B. Doughty (Ed.), *Urinary and fecal incontinence: Current management concepts* (3rd ed., pp. 269–308). St. Louis, MO: Mosby.

Subak, L., Johnson, C., Johnson, C., Whitcomb, E., Boban, D., Saxton, J., et al. (2002). Does weight loss improve incontinence in moderately obese women? *International Urogynecology Journal, 13,* 40–43.

Subak, L., Quesenberry, C., Posner, S., Cattolica, E., & Soghikian, K. (2002). The effect of behavioral therapy on urinary incontinence: A randomized controlled trial. *Obstetrics and Gynecology, 100,* 63–67.

Thomas, L., Cross, S., Barrett, J., French, B., Leathley, M., Sutton, C., et al. (2008). Treatment of urinary incontinence after stroke in adults. *Cochrane Database of Systematic Reviews,* (1), CD004462.

Thompson, D. L., & Smith, D. A. (2002). Continence nursing: A whole person approach. *Holistic Nursing Practice, 16*(2), 14–31.

Wyndaele, J., Castro, D., Madersbacher, H., Chartier-Kastler, E., Igawa, Y., Kovindha, A., et al. (2005). Neurologic urinary and faecal incontinence. In P. Abrams, L. Cardoza, S. Khoury, & A. Wein (Eds.), *Incontinence* (pp. 1061–1162). Paris, France: Health Publication Ltd.

Chapter 45

Abrams, A. C., Lammon, C. B., & Pennington, S. S. (2007). *Clinical drug therapy: Rationales for nursing practice* (8th ed.). Philadelphia, PA: Lippincott Williams & Wilkins.

Banks, N., & Razor, B. (2003). Preoperative stoma site assessment and marking: Trained RNs can improve ostomy outcomes. *American Journal of Nursing, 103*(3), 64A–64D.

Bartlett, J. G. (2002). Antibiotic-associated diarrhea. *New England Journal of Medicine, 346,* 334–349.

Berne, R. M., Levy M. N., Koeppen, B. M., & Stanton B. A. (2004). *Physiology* (5th ed.). St. Louis, MO: Mosby.

Bliss, D. Z., Jung, H.-J., Savik, K., Lowry, A., LeMoine, M., Jensen, L., et al. (2001). Supplementation with dietary fiber improves fecal incontinence. *Nursing Research, 50,* 203–213.

Canadian Association for Enterostomal Therapy. (2008a). *A guide to living with a colostomy.* Retrieved April 5, 2008, from http://www.caet.ca/booklet_colostomy1.htm

Canadian Association for Enterostomal Therapy. (2008b). *A guide to living with an ileostomy.* Retrieved April 5, 2008, from http:/www.caet.ca/booklet_ileostomy1.htm

Colon Cancer Check. (2008). *What health care providers need to know about the fecal occult blood test.* Retrieved April 5, 2008, from http://www.coloncancercheck.ca/docs/ccc_fobtinstructions.pdf

Conly, J. M., & Johnston, B. L. (2003). Norwalk virus: Off and running. *Canadian Journal of Infectious Diseases, 14,* 11–13.

Dosh, S. A. (2002). Evaluation and treatment of constipation. *Journal of Family Practice, 51,* 555–559.

Doughty, D. (2006). *Urinary and fecal incontinence: Current management concepts* (3rd ed.). St. Louis, MO: Mosby.

Ginsberg, D. A., Phillips, S. F., Wallace, J., & Josephson, K. L. (2007). Evaluating and managing constipation in the elderly. *Urologic Nursing, 27,* 191–200.

Hyland, J. (2002). Basics of ostomies. *Gastroenterology Nursing, 25,* 241–244.

Lomer, M. C. E., Parkes, G. C., & Sanderson, J. D. (2008). Review article: Lactose intolerance in clinical practice—Myths and realities. *Alimentary Pharmacology and Therapeutics, 27,* 93–103.

McFarland, L.V. (2006). Meta-analysis of probiotics for the prevention of antibiotic associated diarrhea and the treatment of *Clostridium difficile* disease. *American Journal of Gastroenterology, 101,* 812–822.

McKenry, L., Tessier, E., & Hogan, M. (2006). *Pharmacology in nursing* (2nd ed.). St. Louis, MO: Mosby.

Meiner, S. E., & Lueckenotte, A. G. (2006). *Gerontologic nursing* (3rd ed.). St. Louis, MO: Mosby.

Metheny, N. A., & Titler, M. G. (2001). Assessing placement of feeding tubes. *American Journal of Nursing, 101*(5), 36–46.

Neil, W., Curran, S., & Wattis, J. (2003). Antipsychotic prescribing in older people. *Age and Aging, 32,* 475–483.

North American Society for Pediatric Gastroenterology, Hepatology and Nutrition Constipation Guideline Committee. (2006). Evaluation and treatment of constipation in children and infants: Recommendations of the North American Society for Pediatric Gastroenterology, Hepatology and Nutrition. *Journal of Pediatric Gastroenterology and Nutrition, 43*(3), e1–e13.

Registered Nurses Association of Ontario. (2005). *Prevention of constipation in the older adult.* Retrieved April 3, 2008, from www.rnao.org//Page.asp?PageID=924&ContentID=809

Rehydration Project. (2008). *Oral rehydration therapy.* Retrieved January 21, 2008, from http://www.rehydrate.org/ors/ort.htm

Robson, K. M., Kiely, D. K., & Lembo, T. (2000). Development of constipation in nursing home residents. *Diseases of the Colon and Rectum, 45,* 940–945.

Scheiman, J. M. (2008). Prevention of NSAID-induced ulcers. *Current Treatment Options in Gastroenterology, 11,* 125–134.

Skelly, J., Carr, M., Cassel, B., Robbs, B., & Whytock, S. (2006). *Promoting continence care: A bladder and bowel handbook for care providers,* P. Eyles (Ed.). [Custom courseware]. Hamilton, ON: McMaster University Press.

Spina, E., & Scordo, M. G. (2002). Clinically significant drug interactions with antidepressants in the elderly. *Drugs and Aging, 19,* 299–320.

Todd, B. (2006). Emerging infections: *Clostridium difficile*—Familar pathogen, changing epidemiology. *American Journal of Nursing, 106*(5), 33–36.

Walsh, B. A., et al. (1995, May). *Psychometric evaluation of body image and quality of life following ostomy surgery.* Oral abstract presented at the Wound, Ostomy, Continence Nurses (WOCN) Society 27th Annual Conference, Denver, CO.

Chapter 46

Ackley, B., & Ladwig, G. (2006). *Nursing diagnosis handbook: A guide to planning care* (7th ed.). St. Louis, MO: Mosby.

Association of Workers' Compensation Boards of Canada. (1999). *Work injuries and diseases, 1996–1998* (pp. 20–27). Ottawa, ON: Author.

Barr, J., & Cunneen, J. (2001). Understanding the bariatric client and providing a safe hospital environment. *Clinical Nurse Specialist, 15,* 219–223.

Black, J., & Hawks, J. (2005). *Medical-surgical nursing: Clinical management for positive outcomes* (7th ed.). Philadelphia, PA: Saunders.

Brown, J., & Josse, R. (2002). 2002 Clinical practice guidelines for the diagnosis and management of osteoporosis in Canada. *Canadian Medical Association Journal, 167*(Suppl. 10), S1–S34.

Butler, C. (2006). Pediatric skin care guidelines for assessment, prevention and treatment. *Pediatric Nursing, 32,* 443.

Copstead-Kirkhorn, L., & Banasik, J. (2005). *Pathophysiology* (3rd ed.). Philadelphia, PA: Saunders.

Deitrick, J. E., Whedon, G. D., & Shorr, E. (1948). Effects of immobilization upon various metabolic and physiological functions of normal men. *American Journal of Medicine, 4,* 3–36.

Dionne, M. (2002). 10 tips for safe mobility in the bariatric population. *Rehab Management, 15*(8), 28.

Dumas, C. (2001). Rehab and the bariatric patient. *Rehab Management, 14*(9), 44–45.

Ebersole, P., Hess, P., Touhy, T., & Jett K. (2005). *Gerontologic nursing and health aging* (2nd ed.) St. Louis, MO: Mosby.

Fletcher, K. (2005). Immobility: Geriatric self-learning module. *Medsurg Nursing, 14*(1), 35.

Health Care Health & Safety Association of Ontario. (2003). *Handle with care: A comprehensive approach to developing and implementing a client handling program. Resource manual* (2nd ed.). Retrieved April 16, 2008, from http://www.oha.com/client/OHA/OHA_LP4W_LND_WebStation.nsf/resources/Handle+with+Care/$file/HCHSAHandleWithCare.pdf

Hoeman, S. (2008). *Rehabilitation nursing: prevention, intervention and outcomes* (4th ed.). St. Louis, MO: Mosby.

Im, E., & Choe, M. (2004). Korean women's attitudes toward physical activity. *Research in Nursing and Health,* 27(1), 4–18.

Jain, S., & Brown, D. (2001). Cultural dance: An opportunity to encourage physical activity and health in communities. *American Journal of Health Education, 32,* 216–222.

Katzmarzyk, P. (2002). The Canadian obesity epidemic: An historical perspective. *Obesity Research, 10,* 666–674.

Kawamoto, R., Tomita, H., Oka, Y., & Ohtsuka, N. (2006). Predictors of functional status in Japanese community-dwelling older persons during a 2-year follow up. *Geriatrics and Gerontology International, 6,* 116–123.

Lynch, D., Ferraro, M., Krol, J., Trudell, C. Christos, P., & Volpe, B. (2005). Continuous passive motion improves shoulder joint integrity following stroke. *Clinical Rehabilitation, 19,* 594–599.

Maher, A., Salmond, S., & Pellino, T. (2002). *Orthopedic nursing* (3rd ed.). Philadelphia, PA: Saunders.

Marklew, A. (2006). Body positioning and its effect on oxygenation: A literature review. *Nursing Critical Care,* 11(1), 16.

McCance, K. L., & Huether, S. E. (2005). *Pathophysiology: The biologic basis for disease in adults and children* (5th ed.). St. Louis, MO: Mosby.

Medow, M., Stewart, J., Sanyal, S., Mumtaz, A., Sica, D., & Frishman, W. (2008). Pathophysiology, diagnosis, and treatment of orthostatic hypotension and vasovagal syncope. *Cardiology in Review, 16*(1), 4–20.

Muir, M., & Gerlach, S. (2003). Reducing the risks in bariatric patient handling. *The Canadian Nurse, 99*(8), 29–33.

Nelson, A., Fragala, G., & Menzel, N. (2003a). Myths and facts about back injuries. *American Journal of Nursing, 103*(2), 32–40.

Nelson, A., Owen, B., Lloyd, J., Fragala, G., Matz, M., Amato, M., et al. (2003b). Safe patient handling movement, *American Journal of Nursing, 103*(3), 32–43.

Nunnelee, J. (1997). Low molecular-weight heparin. *Journal of Vascular Nursing, 15*(3), 94–96.

Occupational Health and Safety Agency for Healthcare in British Columbia. (2004). *Trends in workplace injuries, illnesses and policieis in healthcare across Canada.* Retrieved April 16, 2008, from http://www.ohsah.bc.ca/media/17-Trends-Workplace-Injuries-Canada-FinalReport.pdf

Owen, B., Welden, N., & Kane, J. (1999). What are we teaching about lifting and transferring patients? *Research in Nursing and Health, 22,* 3–13.

Registered Nurses Association of Ontario. (2005a). *Prevention of falls and fall injuries in the older adult.* Retrieved April 20, 2008, from http://www.rnao.org/Storage/26/2035_168_Falls_Self-LearningPackage_FINAL.pdf

Registered Nurses Association of Ontario. (2005b). *Risk assessment and prevention of pressure ulcers.* Retrieved November 7, 2008, from http://www.rnao.org/Storage/12/638_BPG_Pressure_Ulcers_v2.pdf

Registered Nurses Association of Ontario. (2007). *Assessment and management of stage I to IV pressure ulcers (revised).* Retrieved April 20, 2008, from http://www.rnao.org/Storage/29/2371_BPG_Pressure_Ulcers_I_to_IV.pdf

Schutzer, K., & Graves, S. (2004). Barriers an motivations to exercise in older adults. *Preventive Medicine, 39,* 1056–1061.

Shin, Y., Yun, S., Jang, H., & Lim, J. (2006). A tailored program for the promotion of physical exercise among Korean adults with chronic diseases. *Applied Nursing Research, 19*(2), 88.

Sorrentino, S. A. (2004). *Mosby's Canadian textbook for the support worker.* Toronto, ON: Elsevier.

Starky, S. (2005). *The obesity epidemic in Canada.* Ottawa, ON: Library of the Parliament, Parliamentary Information and Research Service. Retrieved January 21, 2009, from http://www.parl.gc.ca/information/library/PRBpubs/prb0511-e.htm

Warburton, D., Whitney Nicol, C., & Bredin, S. (2006) Health benefits of physical activity: The evidence. *Canadian Medical Association Journal, 174,* 801–809.

Chapter 47

Agency for Health Care Policy and Research, Panel for the Prediction and Prevention of Pressure Ulcers in Adults. (1992a). *Pressure ulcers in adults: prediction and prevention: Clinical practice guideline no. 3* (AHCPR Pub No. 92-0047). Rockville, MD: Agency for Health Care Policy and Research, Public Health Service, U.S. Department of Health and Human Services.

Agency for Health Care Policy and Research, Panel for Urinary Incontinence Guideline. (1992b). *Urinary incontinence in adults: Clinical practice guideline* (AHCPR Pub No. 92-0038). Rockville, MD: Agency for Health Care Policy and Research, Public Health Service, U.S. Department of Health and Human Services.

Agency for Health Care Policy and Research, Panel for Treatment of Pressure Ulcers in Adults. (1994). *Treatment of pressure ulcers: Clinical practice guideline no. 15* (AHCPR Pub No. 95-0653). Rockville, MD: Agency for Health Care Policy and Research, Public Health Service, U.S. Department of Health and Human Services.

Ayello, E. A., & Braden, B. (2002). How and why to do pressure ulcer risk assessment. *Advances in Skin & Wound Care, 15*(13), 125.

Baharestani, M. M. The lived experience of wives caring for their frail, homebound, elderly husbands with pressure ulcers. *Advances in Wound Care* 7(3), 40.

Barr, J. E. (1995). Principles of wound cleansing. *Ostomy/Wound Management,* August 41 (7A Suppl), 15S–21S, discussion 22S.

Bates-Jensen, B. M. (1995). Toward an intelligent wound assessment system. *Ostomy/Wound Management,* 41(Suppl 7A), 80S.

Bennett, M. A. (1995). Report of the task force on the implications for darkly pigmented intact skin in the prediction and prevention of pressure ulcers. *Advances in Wound Care,* 8(6), 34.

Bergstrom, N., Braden, B. J., Laguzza, A., & Holman, V. (1987). The Braden Scale for predicting pressure sore risk. *Nursing Ressearch,* 36, 205–210.

Braden, B. J. (2001). Risk assessment in pressure ulcer prevention. In D. L. Krasner, G. T. Rodeheaver, & R. G. Sibbald (Eds.). *Chronic wound care: a clinical source book for healthcare professionals.* Wayne, PA: HMP Communications.

Braden, B. J., & Bergstrom, N. (1994). Predictive validity of the Braden Scale for pressure sore risk in a nursing home population. *Research in Nursing & Health,* 17, 459.

Braden, B. J., & Bergstrom, N. (1989). Clinical utility of the Braden Scale for predicting pressure sore risk. *Decubitus,* 2(3), 50.

Bruns, T. B., & Worthington, J. M. (2000). Using tissue adhesive for wound repair: a practical guide to Dermabond. *American Family Physician, 61,* 1383.

Bryant, R. A., & Clark, R. A. F. (2007). Skin pathology and types of damage. In R. A. Bryant & D. P. Nix (Eds.). *Acute and chronic wounds: current management concepts* (3rd ed.). St. Louis, MO: Mosby.

Burton, A. C., & Yamada, S. (1951). Relation between blood pressure and flow in the human forearm. *Journal of Applied Physiology, 4,* 329.

Camden, S. G. (2007). Skin care needs of the obese patient. In R. A. Bryant & D. P. Nix (Eds.). *Acute and chronic wounds: current management concepts,* (3rd ed.). St. Louis, MO: Mosby.

Canadian Association of Wound Care. (2006). Special issue: Best practice recommendations. *Wound Care Canada* 4(1).

Canadian Diabetes Association. (2008). *Clinical practice guidelines 2008.* Retrieved November 1, 2008, from http://www.diabetes.ca/for-professionals/resources/2008-cpg/

Centers for Disease Control and Prevention. (2001). Feeding back surveillance data to prevent hospital acquired infections. *Emerging Infectious Diseases,* 7, 295.

Clarke, H. F., Bradley, C., Whytock, S., Handfield, S., van der Wal, R., & Gundry, S. (2005). Pressure ulcers: implementation of evidence-based nursing practice. *Journal of Advanced Nursing, 49,* 578–90.

Doughty, D. B., & Sparks-Defriese, B. (2007). Wound-healing physiology. In R. A. Bryant & D. P. Nix (Eds.). *Acute and chronic wounds: current management concepts* (3rd ed.). St. Louis, MO: Mosby.

Frantz, R. A., Broussard, C.L., Mendez-Eastman, S. & Cordrey, R. (2007). Devices and technology in wound care. In R. A. Bryant & D. P. Nix (Eds.). *Acute and chronic wounds: current management concepts* (3rd ed.). St. Louis: Mosby.

Gray M., & Weir, D:. (2007). Prevention and treatment of moisture-associated skin damage (maceration) in the periwound skin., *Journal of Wound, Ostomy and Continence Nursing, 34*(2), 153.

Henderson, C. T., Ayello, E. A., Sussman, C., Leiby, D. M., Bennett, M. A., Dungog, E. F., et al. (1997). Draft definition of stage I pressure ulcers: inclusion of persons with darkly pigmented skin. *Advances in Wound Care, 10*(5), 16–19.

The Joint Commission. (2007). *Comprehensive accreditation manual for hospitals: the official handbook (CAMH).* Chicago, IL: The Joint Commission.

Keast. D., Parslow, N., Houghton, P., Norton, L., & Fraser C. (2006). Best practice guidelines for the prevention and treatment of pressure ulcers: Update 2006. *Wound Care Canada* 4(1), 31–43.

Kohr, R., & Gibson, M. (2008). Doing the right thing: using hermeneutic phenomenology to understand management of wound pain. *Ostomy/Wound Management, 54*(4), 52–60.

Lyder, C. H., Preston, J., Grady, J. N., Scinto, J., Allman, R., Bergstrom, N., et al. (2001). Quality of care for hospitalized Medicare patients at risk for pressure ulcers. *Archives of Internal Medicine, 161,* 1549–1554.

National Pressure Ulcer Advisory Panel. (1998). *Position statement on stage I assessment in darkly pigmented skin.* Retrieved August, 2008, from http://www.NPUAP.org/position4/htm.

National Pressure Ulcer Advisory Panel. (2007a). *Pressure ulcer definitions.* Retrieved August, 2008, from http://www.npuap.org/documents/NPUAP2007_PU_Def_and_Descriptions.pdf.

National Pressure Ulcer Advisory Panel. (2007b). *Terms and definitions related to support surfaces.* Retrieved August, 2008, from http://www.npuap.org/pdf/NPUAP_S3I_TD.pdf.

Nix, D. (2007). Patient assessment and evaluation of healing. In R. A. Bryant & D. P. Nix (Eds.). *Acute and chronic wounds: current management concepts* (3rd ed.). St. Louis, MO: Mosby.

Norton, D., McLaren, R., Exon-Smith, A.N.(1962). *An investigation of geriatric nursing problems in hospital.* Edinburgh: Churchill Livingstone.

Pieper, B. (2007). Mechanical forces: pressure, shear and friction. In R. A. Bryant & D. P. Nix (Eds.). *Acute and chronic wounds: current management concepts* (3rd ed.).St. Louis, MO: Mosby.

Posthauer, M. E., & Thomas, D. R. (2004). Nutrition and wound care. In S. Baranoski & E. A. Ayello (Eds.). *Wound care essentials: practice principles.* Philadelphia: Lippincott Williams and Wilkins.

Ramundo, J., & Wells. J. (2000). Wound debridement. In R. A. Bryant (Ed.). *Acute and chronic wounds: nursing management* (2nd ed., pp. 157–175). St. Louis, MO: Mosby.

Registered Nurses Associaton of Ontario. (2007, revised). *Assessment & management of stage I to IV pressure ulcers.* Toronto, ON: Author.

Rodeheaver, G. T. (2001). Wound cleansing, wound irrigation, wound disinfection. In D. L. Krasner, G. T. Rodeheaver, & R. G. Sibbald (Eds.). *Chronic wound care: a clinical source book for healthcare professionals.* Wayne, PA: HMP Communications.

Rolstad, B. S., & Ovington, L. (2007). Principles of wound management. In R. A. Bryant & D. P. Nix (Eds.) *Acute and chronic wounds: current management concepts* (3rd ed.). St. Louis, MO: Mosby.

Schultz, G. (2007). Molecular regulation of wound healing. In R A. Bryant & D. P. Nix (Eds.). *Acute and chronic wounds: current management concepts* (3rd ed.). St. Louis: Mosby.

Sibbald, R. G., Orsted, H. L., Coutts, P. M., & Keast, D. H. (2006a). Best practice recommendations for preparing the wound bed: Update 2006. *Wound Care Canada,* 4, 15–29.

Sibbald, R. G., Woo, K., & Ayello, E. A. (2006b). Increased bacterial burden and infection: The story of NERDS and STONES. *Advances in Skin & Wound Care, 19,* 447–461.

Shea, J.D. (1975). Pressure sores: Classification and management. *Clinical Orthopedics and Related Research,* Oct(112), 189-100.

Stotts, N. A. (2007a). Nutritional assessment and support. In R. A. Bryant & D. P. Nix (Eds.). *Acute and chronic wounds: current management concepts* (3rd ed.). St. Louis, MO: Mosby.

Stotts, N. A. (2007b). Wound infection: diagnosis and management. In R. A. Bryant & D. P. Nix (Eds.). *Acute and chronic wounds: current management concepts* (3rd ed.). St. Louis, MO: Mosby.

Stratton, R. J., Elk, A.-C., Engfer, M., Moore, Z., Rigby, P., Wolfe, R., & Elia, M. (2005). Enteral nutritional support in prevention and treatment of pressure ulcers: A systematic review and meta-analysis. *Ageing Research Reviews, 4,* 422–450.

Teare, J., & Barrett, C. (2002). Using a quality of life assessment in wound care. *Nursing Standard, 17*(6), 67.

Tentolouris, N., Al-Sabbagh, S., Walker, M., Boulton, A., & Jude, E. (2004). Mortality in diabetic and nondiabetic patients after amputations performed from 1990 to 1995: A 5-year follow-up study. *Diabetes Care, 27,* 1598–1604.

Thomas, S., Jones, M., Wynn, K., & Fowler, T. (2001) The current status of maggot therapy in wound healing. *British Journal of Nursing,* 10 (22), Suppl, S5–S12.

Vowden, P., & Vowden, K. (2001). Dopper assessment & ABPI: Interpretation in the management of leg ulceration. *World Wide Wounds.* Retrieved May 27, 2008, from http://www.worldwidewounds.com/2001/march/Vowden/Doppler-assessment-and-ABPI.html.

Woodbury, M. G., & Houghton, P. E. (2004). Prevalence of pressure ulcers in Canadian healthcare settings. Ostomy/Wound Management, 50 (10), 22–38.

Wound, Ostomy and Continence Nurses Society. *Guideline for prevention and management of pressure ulcers* (WOCN clinical practice guidelines series). Glenview, IL: Author.

Wysocki, A. B. (2007). Anatomy and physiology of skin and soft tissue. In R. A. Bryant & D. P. Nix (Eds.) *Acute and chronic wounds: current management concepts* (3rd ed.). St. Louis, MO: Mosby.

Chapter 48

Adatia, F. A., & Damji, K. F. (2005). Chronic open-angle glaucoma: Review for primary care physicians. *Canadian Family Physician, 51,* 1229–1237.

Barnett, T. O. (2007). Problems of the ear. In F. Monahan, J. Sands, M. Neighbors, J. Marek, & C. Green-Nigro (Eds.), *Phipps' medical-surgical nursing: Health and illness perspectives* (8th ed.). St. Louis, MO: Mosby.

Bowd, A. D. (2005). Otitis media: Health and social consequences for Aboriginal youth in Canada's north. *International Journal of Circumpolar Health, 64*(1), 5–15.

Campbell, A. J., Robertson, M. C., La Grow, S. J., Kerse, N. M., Sanderson, G. F., Jacobs, R. J., et al. (2005). Randomised controlled trial of prevention of falls in people aged >75 with severe visual impairment: The VIP trial. *British Medical Journal, 331,* 817–828.

Canadian Centre for Occupational Health and Safety. (2005). *Emergency shower and eye wash stations.* Hamilton, ON: Author. Retrieved April 12, 2008, from http://www.ccohs.ca/oshanswers/safety_haz/emer_showers.html

Canadian National Institute for the Blind. (2004). *A clear vision. Solutions to Canada's national vision loss crisis.* Toronto, ON: Canterbury Communications. Retrieved April 9, 2008, from http://www.costofblindness.org/

Capezuti, E., Siegler, E., & Mezey, M. (Eds.). (2007). *Encyclopedia of elder care.* New York: Springer.

Davis, A., Smith, P., Ferguson, M., Stephens, D., & Gianopoulos, I. (2007). Acceptability, benefit and costs of early screening for hearing disability: A study of potential screening tests and models. *Health Technology Assessment, 11,* 1–294.

Dochterman, J. M., & Bulecheck, G. M. (Eds.). (2004). *Nursing interventions classification (NIC)* (4th ed.). St. Louis, MO: Mosby.

Ebersole, P., Hess, P., Touhy, T., & Jett, A. (2005). *Geriatric nursing and healthy aging.* St. Louis, MO: Mosby.

Ebersole, P., Touhy, T., Hess, P., & Jett, K. (2007). *Toward healthy aging: Human needs and nursing response* (7th ed.). St. Louis, MO: Mosby Elsevier.

Fourie, R. J. (2007). A qualitative self-study of retinitis pigmentosa. *British Journal of Visual Impairment, 25,* 217–232.

Hanley, A. J. G., Harris, S. B., Mamakeesick, M., Goodwin, K., Fiddler, E., Hegele, R. A., et al. (2005). Complications of type 2 diabetes among Aboriginal Canadians: Prevalence and associated risk factors. *Diabetes Care, 28,* 2054–2057.

Health Canada. (2006). *It's your health: Hearing loss and leisure noise.* Ottawa: Author. Retrieved November 12, 2008, from http://www.hc-sc.gc.ca/hl-vs/iyh-vsv/environ/leisure-loisirs-eng.php

Henricson, M., Berglund, A. L., Määtä, S., & Segeston, K. (2006). A transition from nurse to touch therapist—A study of preparation before giving tactile touch in an intensive care unit. *Intensive and Critical Care Nursing, 22,* 239–245.

Hockenberry, M. J., & Wilson, D. (2007). *Wong's nursing care of infants and children* (8th ed.). St. Louis, MO: Mosby.

Kerschner, J. E., Lindstrom, D. R., Pomeranz, A., & Rohloff, B. (2005). Comparison of caregiver otitis media risk factor knowledge in suburban and urban primary care environments. *International Journal of Pediatric Otorhinolaryngology, 69,* 49–56.

McCance, K. L., & Huether, S. E. (2006). *Pathophysiology: The biologic basis for disease in adults and children* (5th ed.). St. Louis, MO: Elsevier Mosby.

Moorhead, S., Johnson, M., & Maas, M. (Eds.). (2004). *Nursing outcomes classification (NOC)* (3rd ed.). St. Louis, MO: Mosby.

Perrucio, A. V., Badley, E. M., & Trope, G. E. (2007). Self-reported glaucoma in Canada: Findings from population based surveys, 1994-2003. *Canadian Journal of Ophthalmology, 42,* 219–226.

Public Health Agency of Canada, Division of Aging and Seniors. (2006). *Hearing loss Info-sheet for seniors.* Ottawa, ON: Minister of Public Works and Government Services Canada. Retrieved April 9, 2008, from http://www.phac-aspc.gc.ca/seniors-aines/pubs/info_sheets/hearing_loss/index.htm

Smith, S. C., & Neely, S. (2007). Nursing management: Visual and auditory problems. In S. L. Lewis, M. Heitkemper, S. Dirksen, P. G. O'Brien, & L. Bucher (Eds.), *Medical-surgical nursing: Assessment and management of clinical problems* (7th ed.). St. Louis, MO: Mosby Elsevier.

Stark, P., & Hickson, L. (2004). Outcomes of hearing aid fitting for older people with hearing impairment and their significant others. *International Journal of Audiology, 43,* 390–398.

Suzuki, M., Omori, M., Hatakeyama, M., Yamada, S., Matsushita, K., & Iijima, S. (2006). Predicting recovery of upper body dressing ability after stroke. *Archives of Physical Medicine and Rehabilitation, 87,* 1496–1502.

Torchinsky, C., & Davidson, T. M. (2006). Cerumen impaction. In K. Calhoun & D. E. Eibling (Eds.), *Geriatric otolaryngology* (pp. 43–58). London, UK: Informa Healthcare.

Ventry, I. M., & Weinstein, B. E. (1982). The hearing handicap inventory for the elderly: A new tool. *Ear Hear, 3,* 128–134.

Whitson, H. E., Cousins, S. W., Burchett, B. M., Hybels, C. F., Pieper, C. F., & Cohen, H. J. (2007). The combined effect of visual impairment and cognitive impairment om disability in older people. *Journal of the American Geriatrics Society, 55,* 885–891.

World Health Organization. (2004). *Magnitude and causes of visual impairment.* Geneva, Switzerland: Author. Retrieved April 12, 2008, from http://www.who.int/mediacentre/factsheets/fs282/en/

Chapter 49

Agency for Health Care Policy and Research. (2002). *Acute pain management: Operative or medical procedures and trauma* (Clinical Practice Guideline No. 1, AHCPR Publication No. 92-0032). Rockville, MD: Public Health Service, U.S. Department of Health and Human Services.

Aldrete, J. A. (1998). Modifications to the post anesthesia score for use in ambulatory surgery. *Journal of Perianesthesia Nursing, 13,* 148–155.

American Association for Respiratory Care. (2002). *AARC Clinical Practice Guideline: Use of positive airway pressure adjuncts to bronchial hygiene therapy.* Retrieved October 31, 2008, from http://www.rcjournal.com/cpgs/papcpg.html

American Society of Anesthesiologists Task Force on Preoperative Fasting. (1999). Practice guidelines for preoperative fasting and the use of pharmacologic agents to reduce the risk of pulmonary aspiration: Application to healthy patients undergoing elective procedures. *Anesthesiology, 90,* 896–905.

Anand, S. S., Wells, P. S., Hunt, D., Brill-Edwards, P., Cook, D., & Ginsberg, J. S. (1998). Does this patient have deep vein thrombosis? *Journal of the American Medical Association, 279,* 1094–1099.

Apfelbaum, J. L., Walawander, C. A., Grasela, T. H., Wise, P., McLeskey, C., Roizen, M. F., et al. (2002). Eliminating intensive postoperative care in same-day surgery patients using short-acting anesthetics. *Anesthesiology, 97*(1), 66–74.

Association of Operating Room Nurses. (2002a). Recommended practices for managing the patient receiving moderate sedation/analgesia. *AORN Journal, 75,* 642–651.

Association of Operating Room Nurses. (2002b). Recommended practices for skin preparation of patients. *AORN Journal, 75*(1), 184–187.

Association of Operating Room Nurses. (2004). *Standards, recommended practices, and guidelines.* Denver, CO: Author.

Barnes, S. (2001). Pain management: What do patients need to know and when do they need to know it? *Journal of Perianesthesia Nursing, 16*(2), 107–108.

Barnes, S. (2002). Patient preparation: The physical assessment. *Journal of Perianesthesia Nursing, 17*(1), 46–47.

Bean, P., & Waldron, K. (1995). Readmission study leads to continuum of care. *Nursing Management, 26,* 65–68.

Canadian Anesthesiologists Society (2005). *Guidelines for the practice of anesthesia. The pre-anesthetic period.* Retrieved January 29, 2009, from http://www.cas.ca/members/sign_in/guidelines/practice_of_anesthesia/default.asp?load=preanesthetic

Canadian Society of Hospital Pharmacists. (2001). *Guidelines for preparing medications for natural rubber latex (NRL) sensitive/allergic patients.* Ottawa, ON: Author.

Clayton, J. L. (2008). Special needs of older adults undergoing surgery. *AORN Journal, 87,* 557–570.

Costa, M. J. (2001). The lived perioperative experience of ambulatory surgery patients. *AORN Journal, 74,* 874–884.

Dawson, L., Brockbank, K., Carr, E. C., & Barrett, R. F. (1999). Improving patients' postoperative sleep: A randomized control study comparing subcutaneous with intravenous patient-controlled analgesia. *Journal of Advanced Nursing, 30,* 875–881.

Dellinger, E. P., Gross, P. A., Barrett, T. L., Krause, P. J., Martone, W. J., McGowan, J. E., Jr., et al. (1994). Quality standard for antimicrobial prophylaxis in surgical procedures. *Clinical Infectious Diseases, 18,* 422–427.

Diepenbrock, N. H. (2008). *Quick reference to critical care* (3rd ed.). New York: Lippincott, Williams & Wilkins.

Doepke, S. (1998). Identifying the risk. *Seminars in Perioperative Nursing, 7,* 226–238.

Douglas, M. (1999). Pain as the fifth vital sign: Will cultural variations be considered? *Journal of Transcultural Nursing, 10,* 285.

Eliopoulos, C. (2001). *Gerontologic nursing* (5th ed.). Philadelphia, PA: Lippincott.

Ferrell, B. R., & Coyle, N. (2001). *Textbook of palliative nursing.* Oxford, UK: Oxford University Press.

Fowlie, P., Francis, H., & Russell, S. (2000). The surgical liason nurse: A perioperative communication with families. *Canadian Nurse, 96*(8), 30–33.

Francis, P., & Winfield, H. N. (2006). Care of the patient undergoing robotic-assisted laparoscopic pyeloplasty. *Urologic Nursing, 26,* 110–115.

Fredman, B., Sheffer, O., Zohar, E., Paruta, I., Richter, S., Jedeikin, R., et al. (2002). Fast-track eligibility of geriatric patients undergoing short urologic procedures. *Anesthesia and Analgesia, 94,* 560–564.

Gagliese, L., Jackson, M., Ritvo, P., Wowk, A., & Katz, J. (2000). Age is not an impediment to effective use of patient-controlled analgesia by surgical patients. *Anesthesiology, 93,* 601–610.

Gan, T. J. (2002). Postoperative nausea and vomiting—Can it be eliminated? *Journal of the American Medical Association, 287,* 1233–1236.

Gershenson, T. A., Quon, H., Somerville, S., & Cohn, E. (1999). Tilling the soil: Nurturing the seeds of patient and family education. *Journal of Nursing Care Quality, 13*(6), 83–91.

Hobson, D. W., Woller, W., Anderson, L., & Guthery, E. (1998). Development and evaluation of a new alcohol-based surgical hand scrub formulation with persistent antimicrobial characteristics and brushless application. *American Journal of Infection Control, 26,* 507–512.

Hogan, D., McCabe, L., Bruto, V., Burne, D., Chan, P., Malach, F., et al. (2006). National guidelines for seniors mental health: The assessment and treatment of delirium. *Canadian Journal of Geriatrics, 9*(Suppl. 2), S42–S51.

Karlet, M. C. (1998). Malignant hyperthermia consideration for ambulatory surgery. *Journal of Perianesthesia Nursing, 13,* 304–312.

Larson, E. L., Butz, A. M., Gullette, D. L., & Laughon, B. A. (1990). Alcohol for surgical scrubbing? *Infection Control and Hospital Epidemiology, 11,* 139–143.

Lee, N. C., Wasson, D. R., Anderson, M. A., Stone, S., & Gittings, J. A. (1998). A survey of patient education postdischarge. *Journal of Nursing Care Quality, 13*(1), 63–70.

Lewis, S. M., Heitkemper, M. M., & Dirksen, S. R. (2004). *Medical-surgical nursing: Assessment and management of clinical problem* (6th ed.). St. Louis, MO: Mosby.

Lipson, J., Dibble, S., & Minarik, P. (1996). *Culture and nursing care: A pocket guide.* San Francisco, CA: UCSF Nursing Press.

Litwack, K. (1999). *Core curriculum for perianesthesia nursing practice* (4th ed.). Philadelphia, PA: Saunders.

Litwack, K. (2006). Adjusting post surgical care for older patients. *Nursing 2006, 36*(1), 66–67.

Lookinland, S., & Pool, M. (1998). Study on effect of methods of preoperative education in women. *AORN Journal, 67*(1), 203–213.

Lueckenotte, A. G. (2000). *Gerontologic nursing* (2nd ed.). St. Louis, MO: Mosby.

McPherson, K. (1996). *Bedside matters: The transformation of Canadian nursing, 1900–1990.* Toronto, ON: Oxford University Press.

Metheny, N. M. (2000). *Fluid and electrolyte balance: Nursing considerations* (4th ed.). Philadelphia, PA: Lippincott.

Nurse's life in the Montreal General Hospital. (1892, October). *Dominion Monthly Magazine,* 541–550.

O'Callaghan, N. (2002). Pre-operative fasting. *Nursing Standard, 16*(36), 33–37.

Ontario Ministry of Health and Long-Term Care. (2004, April 15). *Standard for all Ontario health care facilities/settings for high-risk respiratory procedures under nonoutbreak conditions.* Toronto, ON: Author.

Ontario Perianesthesia Nurses Association. (2005). *Standards of perianesthetic nursing practice.* Toronto, ON: Author.

Paquet, J. (1998). Latex hypersensitivity: The IgE response. *Seminars in Perioperative Nursing, 7,* 203–205.

Polk, H. C., & Christmas, A. B. (2000). Prophylactic antibiotics in surgery and surgical wound infections. *American Surgeon, 66,* 105–111.

Porter, R. (1997). *The greatest benefit to mankind: A medical history of humanity.* New York: W. W. Norton.

Ramer, L., Richardson, J. L., Cohen, M. Z., Bedney, C., Danley, K. L., & Judge, E. A. (1999). Multimeasure pain assessment in an ethnically diverse group of patients with cancer. *Journal of Transcultural Nursing, 10,* 94–101.

Registered Nurses Association of Ontario. (2002a). *Assessment and management of pain.* Retrieved November 5, 2008, from http://www.rnao.org/Page.asp?PageID=924&ContentID=720

Registered Nurses Association of Ontario. (2002b). *Prevention of falls and fall injury in the older adult population.* Retrieved September 1, 2004, from http://www.rnao.org/bestpractices/index.asp

Registered Nurses Association of Ontario. (2004a). *Caregiving strategies for older adults with delirium, dementia asnd depression.* Retrieved May 22, 2008, from http://www.rnao.org/bestpractices/index.asp

Registered Nurses Association of Ontario. (2004b). *Screening for delirium, dementia asnd depression in older adults.* Retrieved May 22, 2008, from http://www.rnao.org/bestpractices/index.asp

Registered Nurses Association of Ontario. (2005). *Risk assessment and prevention of pressure ulcers* (Revised). Retrieved October 31, 2008, from http://www.rnao.org/Storage/12/638_BPG_Pressure_Ulcers_v2.pdf

Registered Nurses Association of Ontario. (2007). *Smoking cessation.* Retrieved June 23, 2008, from http://www.rnao.org/bestpractices/index.asp

Rothrock, J. C. (2003). *Alexander's care of the patient in surgery* (12th ed.). St. Louis, MO: Mosby.

Saar, L. (2001). Use of a modified postanesthesia recovery score in phase II perianesthesia period of ambulatory surgery patients. *Journal of Perianesthesia Nursing, 16*(2), 82–89.

Sandelowski, M. (2000). *Devices and desires: Gender, technology and American nursing.* Chapel Hill, NC: The University of North Carolina Press.

Schoonhoven, L., Defloor, T., & Grypdonck, M. (2002). Incidence of pressure ulcers due to surgery. *Journal of Clinical Nursing, 11,* 479–487.

Sculco, T. P., Jordan, L. C., & Walter, W. L. (2004). Minimally invasive total hip arthroplasty: The Hospital for Special Surgery experience. *Orthopedic Clinics of North America, 35,* 137–142.

Shoup, A. (1998). Why latex allergy now? *Seminars in Perioperative Nursing, 7,* 222–225.

Shuldham, C. (1999). A review of the impact of pre-operative education on recovery from surgery. *International Journal of Nursing Studies, 36,* 171–177.

Snell, C. C., Fothergill-Bourbonnais, F., & Durocher-Hendriks, S. (1997). Patient controlled analgesia and intramuscular injections: A comparison of patient pain experiences and postoperative outcomes. *Journal of Advanced Nursing, 25,* 681–690.

Sullivan, E. E. (2000). Preoperative holding areas. *Journal of Perianesthesia Nursing, 15,* 353–354.

Summers, S. (2001). Evidence-based practice. II. Reliability and validity of selected acute pain instruments. *Journal of Perianesthesia Nursing, 16*(1), 35–40.

Sussman, G., & Gold, M. (2004). *Guidelines for the management of latex allergies and safe latex use in health care facilities.* Retrieved September 1, 2004, from http://www.acaai.org/public/physicians/latex.htm

Tick, L. W., Ton, E., van Voorthuizen, T., Hovens, M. M., Leeuwenburgh, I., Lobatto, S., et al. (2002). Practical diagnostic management of patients with clinically suspected deep vein thrombosis by clinical probability test, compression ultrasonography, and D-dimer test. *American Journal of Medicine, 113,* 630–635.

Toman, C., Heap, R., & Frize, M. (2006). Canadian women in engineering and science: Historical and contemporary perspectives. *Scientia Canadiensis, 29,* 155–175.

Tramer, M. R. (2001). A rational approach to the control of postoperative nausea and vomiting: Evidence from systematic reviews. II. Recommendations for prevention and treatment, and research agenda. *Acta Anaesthesiologica Scandinavica, 45,* 14–19.

Turjanica, M. A. (2007). Postoperative continuous peripheral nerve blockade in the lower extremity total joint arthroplasty population. *MEDSURG Nursing, 16,* 151–154.

White, P. F., Rawal, S., Nguyen, J., & Watkins, A. (2003). PACU fast-tracking: An alternative to "bypassing" the PACU for facilitating the recovery process after ambulatory surgery. *Journal of Perianesthesia Nursing, 18,* 247–253.

Williams, J. R. (1999). Pre-operative fasting: Putting research into practice. *Nursing Standard, 13*(39), 33–35.

Review Question Answers

For answers with rationales, see answer key beginning on p. 1415.

Chapter 1

1. The correct answer is 1
2. The correct answer is 4
3. The correct answer is 1
4. The correct answer is 1
5. The correct answer is 2
6. The correct answer is 3
7. The correct answer is 2
8. The correct answer is 3
9. The correct answer is 2
10. The correct answer is 2

Chapter 2

1. The correct answer is 2
2. The correct answer is 4
3. The correct answer is 2
4. The correct answer is 1
5. The correct answer is 3
6. The correct answer is 1
7. The correct answer is 4
8. The correct answer is 1
9. The correct answer is 2
10. The correct answer is 3

Chapter 3

1. The correct answer is 2
2. The correct answer is 3
3. The correct answer is 4
4. The correct answer is 3
5. The correct answer is 1
6. The correct answer is 2
7. The correct answer is 2
8. The correct answer is 1
9. The correct answer is 2
10. The correct answer is 3

Chapter 4

1. The correct answer is 1
2. The correct answer is 2
3. The correct answer is 3
4. The correct answer is 4
5. The correct answer is 4
6. The correct answer is 2
7. The correct answer is 2
8. The correct answer is 3
9. The correct answer is 1
10. The correct answer is 1

Chapter 5

1. The correct answer is 2
2. The correct answers are 1, 2, 3
3. The correct answer is 1
4. The correct answers are 3, 4
5. The correct answer is 4

Chapter 6

1. The correct answer is 4
2. The correct answer is 3
3. The correct answer is 1
4. The correct answer is 1
5. The correct answer is 3
6. The correct answer is 1
7. The correct answer is 1
8. The correct answer is 2
9. The correct answer is 2
10. The correct answer is 2
11. The correct answer is 2

Chapter 7

1. The correct answer is 4
2. The correct answer is 4
3. The correct answer is 1
4. The correct answer is 3
5. The correct answer is 2
6. The correct answer is 1
7. The correct answer is 2
8. The correct answer is 3
9. The correct answer is 3
10. The correct answer is 4

Chapter 8

1. The correct answer is 3
2. The correct answer is 4
3. The correct answer is 3
4. The correct answer is 1
5. The correct answer is 4
6. The correct answer is 2
7. The correct answer is 3
8. The correct answer is 3
9. The correct answer is 1
10. The correct answer is 2

Chapter 9

1. The correct answer is 1
2. The correct answer is 1
3. The correct answer is 2
4. The correct answer is 4
5. The correct answer is 2
6. The correct answer is 4
7. The correct answer is 4
8. The correct answer is 4
9. The correct answer is 3

Chapter 10

1. The correct answer is 1
2. The correct answer is 2
3. The correct answer is 1
4. The correct answer is 2
5. The correct answer is 1
6. The correct answer is 1
7. The correct answer is 4
8. The correct answer is 3
9. The correct answer is 1
10. The correct answer is 4

Chapter 11

1. The correct answer is 3
2. The correct answer is 3
3. The correct answer is 1
4. The correct answer is 4
5. The correct answer is 3
6. The correct answer is 2
7. The correct answer is 1
8. The correct answer is 1
9. The correct answer is 4
10. The correct answer is 3

Chapter 12

1. The correct answer is 1
2. The correct answer is 3
3. The correct answer is 2
4. The correct answer is 3

Chapter 13

1. The correct answer is 4
2. The correct answer is 4
3. The correct answer is 4
4. The correct answers are 1, 3, 5
5. The correct answer is 3
6. The correct answer is 4
7. The correct answer is 4
8. The correct answer is 4
9. The correct answer is 2
10. The correct answer is 1
11. The correct answer is 3
12. The correct answer is 4
13. The correct answers are 1, 2

Chapter 14

1. The correct answers are 2, 3
2. The correct answer is 1
3. The correct answers are 1, 2
4. The correct answer is 4
5. The correct answer is 4
6. The correct answer is 3
7. The correct answer is 2
8. The correct answer is 1
9. The correct answer is 2

Chapter 15

1. The correct answer is 3
2. The correct answers are 2, 4
3. The correct answer is 4
4. The correct answer is 4
5. The correct answer is 2
6. The correct answers are 1, 2

Chapter 16

1. The correct answer is 1
2. The correct answer is 4
3. The correct answer is 3
4. The correct answer is 4
5. The correct answer is 1
6. The correct answer is 4
7. The correct answer is 3
8. The correct answer is S = 2, O = 4, A = 3, P = 1

Chapter 17

Six review questions appear at the end of Chapter 17, however, they are short answer questions. For answers to those six short answer questions, see answer key on p. 1420.

Chapter 18

1. The correct answer is 4
2. The correct answer is 3
3. The correct answer is 1
4. The correct answer is 3
5. The correct answer is 1
6. The correct answer is 3
7. The correct answer is 4
8. The correct answer is 2
9. The correct answer is 2
10. The correct answer is 2

Chapter 19

1. The correct answer is 4
2. The correct answer is 4
3. The correct answer is 2
4. The correct answer is 4
5. The correct answer is 3
6. The correct answer is 1
7. The correct answer is 4
8. The correct answer is 3
9. The correct answer is 1

Chapter 20

1. The correct answer is 4
2. The correct answer is 2
3. The correct answer is 4
4. The correct answer is 4
5. The correct answer is 3
6. The correct answer is 2
7. The correct answer is 1
8. The correct answer is 4
9. The correct answer is 1
10. The correct answer is 3

Chapter 21

1. The correct answer is 3
2. The correct answer is 2
3. The correct answer is 3
4. The correct answer is 4
5. The correct answer is 3
6. The correct answer is 1
7. The correct answer is 3
8. The correct answer is 1
9. The correct answer is 2
10. The correct answer is 1

Chapter 22

1. The correct answer is 4
2. The correct answer is 1
3. The correct answer is 1
4. The correct
5. The correct
6. The correct
7. The correct
8. The correct
9. The correct
10. The correc

Chapter 2

1. The corre
2. The corre
3. The corre
4. The corr
5. The corr
6. The corr
7. The corr
8. The cor
9. The cor
10. The co

Chapter

1. The co
2. The co
3. The c
4. The c
5. The
6. The
7. The
8. The
9. The
10. The

Chapt

1. The correct answer is
2. The correct answer is 3
3. The correct answer is 3
4. The correct answer is 2
5. The correct answer is 1
6. The correct answer is 3
7. The correct answer is 1
8. The correct answer is 1
9. The correct answer is 4
10. The correct answer is 1

Chapter 26

1. The correct answer is 2
2. The correct answer is 2
3. The correct answer is 4
4. The correct answer is 3
5. The correct answer is 1
6. The correct answer is 4
7. The correct answer is 3
8. The correct answer is 1
9. The correct answer is 3
10. The correct answer is 1

Chapter 27

1. The correct answer is 3
2. The correct answer is 2
3. The correct answer is 4
4. The correct answer is 1
5. The correct answer is 2
6. The correct answer is 1
7. The correct answer is 2
8. The correct answer is 2
9. The correct answer is 3
10. The correct answer is 1

Chapter 28

1. The correct answer is 3
2. The correct answer is 2
3. The correct answer is 4
4. The correct answer is 4
5. The correct answer is 4
6. The correct answer is 1
7. The correct answer is 1
8. The correct answer is 4
9. The correct answer is 2
10. The correct answer is 1

Chapter 29

1. The correct answer is 1
2. The correct answer is 2
3. The correct answer is 3
4. The correct answer is 4
5. The correct answer is 4
6. The correct answer is 2
7. The correct answer is 3
8. The correct answer is 4
9. The correct answer is 2
10. The correct answer is 3

Chapter 30

1. The correct answer is 1
2. The correct answer is 4
3. The correct answer is 3
4. The correct answer is 3
5. The correct answer is 2
6. The correct answer is 4
7. The correct answer is 2
8. The correct answer is 4
9. The correct answer is 1

Chapter 31

1. The correct answer is 3
2. The correct answer is 1
3. The correct answer is 1
4. The correct answer is 2
5. The correct answer is 3
6. The correct answer is 1
7. The correct answer is 2
8. The correct answer is 1
9. The correct answer is 3
10. The correct answer is 1

Chapter 32

1. The correct answer is 4
2. The correct answer is 4
3. The correct answer is 2
4. The correct answer is 3
5. The correct answer is 3
6. The correct answer is 4
7. The correct answer is 2
8. The correct answer is 3
9. The correct answer is 3
10. The correct answer is 2

Chapter 33

1. The correct answer is 1
2. The correct answer is 1
3. The correct answer is 4
4. The correct answer is 2
5. The correct answer is 2
6. The correct answer is 2
7. The correct answer is 4
8. The correct answer is 2
9. The correct answer is 2
10. The correct answer is 1

Chapter 34

1. The correct answer is 4
2. The correct answer is 2
3. The correct answer is 1
4. The correct answer is 1
5. The correct answer is 4
6. The correct answer is 3
7. The correct answer is 1
8. The correct answer is 2
9. The correct answer is 4
10. The correct answer is 1

Chapter 35

1. The correct answer is 3
2. The correct answer is 4
3. The correct answer is 1
4. The correct answer is 1
5. The correct answer is 1
6. The correct answer is 1
7. The correct answer is 3
8. The correct answer is 1
9. The correct answer is 2
10. The correct answer is 2

Chapter 36

1. The correct answer is 3
2. The correct answer is 1
3. The correct answer is 1
4. The correct answer is 1
5. The correct answer is 4
6. The correct answer is 2
7. The correct answer is 2
8. The correct answer is 2

Chapter 37

1. The correct answer is 3
2. The correct answer is 2
3. The correct answer is 2
4. The correct answer is 1
5. The correct answer is 2
6. The correct answer is 2
7. The correct answer is 3
8. The correct answer is 3
9. The correct answer is 4

Chapter 38

1. The correct answer is 1
2. The correct answer is 3
3. The correct answer is 3
4. The correct answer is 2
5. The correct answer is 3
6. The correct answer is 2
7. The correct answer is 2
8. The correct answer is 1
9. The correct answer is 3
10. The correct answer is 4

Chapter 39

1. The correct answer is 1
2. The correct answer is 2
3. The correct answer is 1
4. The correct answer is 3
5. The correct answer is 1
6. The correct answer is 1
7. The correct answer is 2
8. The correct answer is 1
9. The correct answer is 3
10. The correct answer is 4

Chapter 40

1. The correct answer is 1
2. The correct answer is 4
3. The correct answer is 2
4. The correct answer is 4
5. The correct answer is 1
6. The correct answer is 1
7. The correct answer is 1
8. The correct answer is 3
9. The correct answer is 2
10. The correct answer is 4

Chapter 41

1. The correct answer is 4
2. The correct answer is 2
3. The correct answer is 4
4. The correct answer is 4
5. The correct answer is 1
6. The correct answer is 3
7. The correct answer is 1
8. The correct answer is 3
9. The correct answer is 4
10. The correct answer is 4

Chapter 42

1. The correct answer is 1
2. The correct answer is 2
3. The correct answer is 3
4. The correct answer is 1
5. The correct answer is 4
6. The correct answer is 3
7. The correct answer is 2
8. The correct answer is 1
9. The correct answer is 3
10. The correct answer is 3

Chapter 43

1. The correct answer is 4
2. The correct answer is 2
3. The correct answer is 4
4. The correct answer is 2
5. The correct answer is 2
6. The correct answer is 4
7. The correct answer is 4
8. The correct answer is 3
9. The correct answer is 3
10. The correct answer is 2

Chapter 44

1. The correct answer is 2
2. The correct answer is 1
3. The correct answer is 2
4. The correct answer is 3
5. The correct answer is 3
6. The correct answer is 1
7. The correct answer is 1
8. The correct answer is 3
9. The correct answer is 1
10. The correct answer is 4

Chapter 45

1. The correct answer is 4
2. The correct answer is 3
3. The correct answer is 4
4. The correct answer is 1
5. The correct answer is 3
6. The correct answer is 4
7. The correct answer is 3
8. The correct answer is 2
9. The correct answer is 1
10. The correct answer is 1

Chapter 46

1. The correct answer is 2
2. The correct answer is 2
3. The correct answer is 1
4. The correct answer is 3
5. The correct answer is 3
6. The correct answer is 4
7. The correct answer is 1
8. The correct answer is 1
9. The correct answer is 2
10. The correct answer is 3

Chapter 47

1. The correct answer is 4
2. The correct answer is 1
3. The correct answer is 4
4. The correct answer is 3
5. The correct answer is 3
6. The correct answer is 3
7. The correct answer is 3
8. The correct answer is 4
9. The correct answer is 3
10. The correct answer is 4

Chapter 48

1. The correct answer is 2
2. The correct answer is 1
3. The correct answer is 3
4. The correct answer is 2
5. The correct answer is 4
6. The correct answer is 4
7. The correct answer is 2
8. The correct answer is 3
9. The correct answer is 3
10. The correct answer is 1

Chapter 49

1. The correct answer is 2
2. The correct answer is 3
3. The correct answer is 2
4. The correct answer is 2
5. The correct answer is 1
6. The correct answer is 3
7. The correct answer is 4
8. The correct answer is 2
9. The correct answer is 2
10. The correct answer is 4

Review Question Rationales

Chapter 1

1. **The correct answer is 1.** The Lalonde Report shifted emphasis from a medical to a behavioural approach to health. It concluded that the traditional medical approach to health care was inadequate and that "further improvements in the environment, reductions in self-imposed risks, and a greater knowledge of human biology" are necessary to improve the health status of Canadians.
2. **The correct answer is 4.** The *Ottawa Charter for Health Promotion* supported a socioenvironmental approach to health. It identified prerequisites for health: peace, shelter, education, food, income, a stable ecosystem, sustainable resources, social justice, and equity.
3. **The correct answer is 1.** Labonte (1993) categorized the major determinants of health in a socioenvironmental approach as psychosocial risk factors and socioenvironmental risk conditions. Political, social, and cultural forces affect health and well-being directly and indirectly through their influence on personal health behaviours. Socioenvironmental risk conditions can contribute to psychosocial risk factors, which can then result in unhealthy behaviours
4. **The correct answer is 1.** Given that the determinants of health are broad, healthy public policy must extend beyond traditional health care agencies and government health care departments to other sectors such as agriculture, education, transportation, labour, social services, energy, and housing. Therefore, policy-makers in all government sectors and organizations should know the health consequences of their policies.
5. **The correct answer is 2.** Primary prevention includes activities that protect against a disease before signs and symptoms occur. Examples include immunization (to prevent infectious diseases) and reduction of risk factors (such as inactivity, smoking, and exposure to air pollution).
6. **The correct answer is 3.** Rather than focusing only on helping people develop healthy behaviours, health promotion seeks to create healthy public policy, supportive environments, community action, and personal skill. Health promotion is committed to empowerment and community-based health planning and addresses health issues within the context of the social, economic, and political environment. It therefore is political.
7. **The correct answer is 2.** The belief that health is primarily an *individual* responsibility is most congruent with the behavioural approach to health. The behavioural approach places responsibility for health on the individual, thereby favouring health promotion strategies such as education. Strategies are often based on the assumption that if people know the risk factors of disease, then they will engage in healthy behaviours.
8. **The correct answer is 3.** Rather than focusing primarily on interventions at the societal level, the population health promotion model advocates that interventions be implemented toward individuals and families, communities, individual sectors of society (such as health care or environmental sectors), and society as a whole.
9. **The correct answer is 2.** Income and social status are the greatest determinants of health. Canadians who live in poverty have poorer health and are more likely to die earlier and to suffer more illnesses than those with higher incomes, regardless of age, sex, race, culture, and place of residence.
10. **The correct answer is 2.** Health promotion is directed toward increasing the level of well-being and self-actualization.

Chapter 2

1. **The correct answer is 2.** Canada contributes 10.3% of its gross domestic product to health care, whereas the United States contributes 16%.
2. **The correct answer is 4.** A number of target groups (e.g., Royal Canadian Mounted Police [RCMP], Aboriginal peoples, members of military services) are covered directly by the Canadian government. People who are moving between provinces or territories are covered under the Canadian Health Act.
3. **The correct answer is 2.** Public health care is focused on preventive measures and programs that ensure conditions and circumstances to keep people healthy through appropriate screening, assessment, development, monitoring, and support (i.e., public policy).
4. **The correct answer is 1.** The five principles of the Canadian Health Act are public administration, comprehensiveness, universality, portability, and accessibility.
5. **The correct answer is 3.** Community services are directed at primary and secondary care, located where they live, work, play, and interact. An adult day care centre is a community agency.
6. **The correct answer is 1.** The five levels of health care services are promotive, preventive, curative (diagnosis and treatment), rehabilitative, and supportive (including home care, long-term care, and palliative care).
7. **The correct answer is 4.** Hospitals and health care institutions account for the largest share of total health care expenditures (30%) in comparison with retail drug sales (17%) and physician services (13%). In 2005, this translated to hospital expenditures of $40.35 billion (CAD), drug expenditures of $23.34 billion (CAD), and physician services expenditures of $18.34 billion (CAD), in contrast to $8.46 billion (CAD) for public health care and $15.21 billion (CAD) for other health care professionals' services.
8. **The correct answer is 1.** Health care cost accelerators include new technology, new pharmaceuticals, an increase in chronic and new diseases, and changing demographics and expectations.
9. **The correct answer is 2.** Disease prevention services help clients, families, and communities reduce risk factors for disease and injury. Prevention strategies include clinical (screening, immunization), behavioral (lifestyle change, support groups), or environmental (societal pressure for a healthy environment).
10. **The correct answer is 3.** Secondary care involves provision of a specialized medical service by a physician specialist or a hospital on referral from a primary care practitioner. Secondary care deals with clients seeking definitive diagnosis or requiring further diagnostic review.

Chapter 3

1. **The correct answer is 2.** Florence Nightingale, considered to be the founder of modern nursing, spearheaded the movement to improve standards of nursing care in the mid-19th century.
2. **The correct answer is 3.** Marguerite d'Youville formed the Sisters of Charity of Montreal, a Canadian order of nuns, in 1737. They began as a small group of women who pooled their possessions to form a refuge for the poor and needy and eventually became the first visiting nurses in Canada.

3. **The correct answer is 4.** The first doctoral nursing program was established at the University of Alberta on January 1, 1991.
4. **The correct answer is 3.** As a result of a movement that began in the 1960s, nursing legislation has recently been developed in most provinces and territories to regulate the practice of nurse practitioners.
5. **The correct answer is 1.** A code of ethics defines the principles by which nurses function. The first code of ethics for nursing was developed by the International Council of Nurses (ICN) in 1953 and was adopted by the Canadian Nurses Association (CNA) in 1954. The CNA Code of Ethics was updated most recently in 2008.
6. **The correct answer is 2.** Professional nursing organizations establish education and practice standards for nurses, carry out the regulatory functions of registration and licensure, and discipline members who do not meet the standards. They also serve as the voice of nurses on matters of professional interest and concern, help their members maintain competence through continuing education and collaborate with other health care professional organizations on matters of mutual interest. They do not monitor unregulated care providers.
7. **The correct answer is 2.** In all provinces and territories, nursing practice acts regulate licensure and the practice of nursing. Each province or territory defines for itself the scope of nursing practice because consitutional responsibility for education and health care rests with individual provinces and territories.
8. **The correct answer is 1.** Because health care is a provincial and territorial responsibility, each professional nursing organization is responsible for developing the standards for nursing practice in its particular jurisdiction. The standards provided by the College of Nurses of Ontario for nurses in Ontario include accountabilty, continuing competence, ethics, knowledge, knowledge application, leadership and relationships.
9. **The correct answer is 2.** In all provinces except Ontario and Quebec, provincial nursing associations assume responsibility for defining and monitoring standards.
10. **The correct answer is 3.** Nursing unions are primary participants as the representatives of nurses in particular provinces or territories when new contracts are negotiated.

Chapter 4

1. **The correct answer is 1.** The overall goals of a population health approach are to maintain and improve the health of the entire population and to eliminate health disparities. The population health approach provides a framework for thinking about health and for taking action to improve the health of populations. Action is directed primarily at community levels.
2. **The correct answer is 2.** Public health nursing merges knowledge from the public health sciences with professional nursing theories to safeguard and improve the health of populations in the community.
3. **The correct answer is 3.** Community-based nursing involves acute, chronic, and palliative care of clients and families that enhances their capacity for self-care and promotes autonomy in decision making.
4. **The correct answer is 4.** Vulnerable populations of clients are those who are likely to develop health problems as a result of excess risks, who experience barriers when trying to access to health care services, or who are dependent on others for care.
5. **The correct answer is 4.** Competent care of vulnerable populations does not include offering financial or legal advice.
6. **The correct answer is 2.** Physical, emotional, and sexual abuse, as well as neglect, are major public health problems affecting older adults, women, and children.
7. **The correct answer is 2.** A successful community health nursing practice requires an ability to build relationships with the community and to be responsive to changes within the community.
8. **The correct answer is 3.** Perinatal classes, infant care, child safety, and cancer screening are just some of the health education programs in which a nurse in community practice may participate as a nurse educator.
9. **The correct answer is 1.** The nurse as consultant provides information and supports participation in health activities. In this role, the nurse responds to inquiries about and makes referrals to community resources.
10. **The correct answer is 1.** The community can be viewed as having three components: locale or structure, the social systems, and the people.

Chapter 5

1. **The correct answer is 2.** Older clients in the advanced stage of their disease tend to experience more treatment-related problems because their stamina to withstand advanced treatments can be physically exhausting. Younger clients tend to handle treatment for their cancer better because of their ability to heal faster.
2. **The correct answers are 1, 2, and 3.** It is important to obtain a comprehensive assessment of the client's medical history because the number and type of past cancer therapies, as well as current medical conditions, may affect current and future treatment options. In addition, establishing a therapeutic relation approach between the nurse and client may enable the client to freely express his or her feelings in a safe and respectful environment; otherwise, it may be difficult for a cancer survivor to readily express what he or she is experiencing.
3. **The correct answer is 1.** The client who is at most risk for post-treatment symptoms after cancer treatment is the mother who is dealing with a late- to end-stage cancer diagnosis. This client not only must deal with her diagnosis and prognosis but also must manage a household and care for children. The combination of these two factors in this scenario is known to be particularly stressful for such a client. In the other three scenarios, although the clients have a cancer diagnosis and will experience stress in some form, the disease is not in an advanced stage, and they do not have the additional stress of caring for children.
4. **The correct answers are 3 and 4.** Altered vision, such as blurred vision, and impaired cognitive function are examples of possible residual effects of brain surgery. Intestinal obstruction is a late effect more commonly seen in clients after abdominal surgery. Difficulty breathing is a late effect more commonly seen in clients after a lung resection.
5. **The correct answer is 4.** This assessment question requires the client to focus on providing a description of the activities and functions in his or her daily life, which may better reveal cognitive difference because of the detailed information required over a period of time. The other assessment questions require more short-answer responses and do not require the client to think about a situation over a long period of time.

Chapter 6

1. **The correct answer is 4.** A theory is a purposeful set of assumptions or propositions that show relationships between concepts. Theories are useful because they provide a systematic view of explaining, predicting and prescribing phenomena.
2. **The correct answer is 3.** The drive for early theorizing about nursing practice came from nursing educators, who noted that traditional ways of preparing professional nurses were becoming outdated.
3. **The correct answer is 1.** The nursing process originally involved four steps: assessment, planning, intervention, and evaluation.
4. **The correct answer is 1.** Each conceptual framework attempted to define nursing by creating a theoretical definition for the substance and structure of the key bodies of knowledge needed to understand clinical situations. This knowledge was called the metaparadigm concepts and included person, environment, health care, and nursing care.
5. **The correct answer is 3.** The question confronting early theorists about nursing practice remained as follows: How does a nurse organize and make sense of all available knowledge and apply it intelligently to the challenges that arise in an individual clinical case?
6. **The correct answer is 1.** Kuhn challenged the traditional notion of science as a logical progression of discoveries. He argued that major scientific developments occurred when scientists thought about problems in radically new and different ways.
7. **The correct answer is 1.** The main features of the McGill model were "a focus on health rather than illness and treatment, on all family members rather than the patient alone, on family goals rather than on the nurse's, and on family strengths rather than their deficits."
8. **The correct answer is 2.** Peplau defined the essence of nursing as the interpersonal relationship between the nurse and the client. She viewed this relationship as interactive and therapeutic, in which the goal was to support the client to achieve independent living.
9. **The correct answer is 2.** Canadian theorist Evelyn Adam articulated the essence of nursing as a helping process. From her perspective, the nurse played a complementary–supplementary role in supporting the client's strength, knowledge, and will.
10. **The correct answer is 2.** Systems theory accounted for the whole of an entity (the system) and its component parts (subsystems), as well as the interactions between the parts and the whole.
11. **The correct answer is 2.** Parse's nursing model does not articulate goals for nursing in the traditional sense of defining health; instead, it relies on the notion of people in a continuous process of making choices and changing health care priorities.

Chapter 7

1. **The correct answer is 4.** The first provincially approved doctoral nursing program was established at the University of Alberta Faculty of Nursing in 1991.
2. **The correct answer is 4.** Carper (1978) described empirics as "knowledge that is systematically organized into general laws and theories for the purpose of describing, explaining and predicting phenomena of special concern to the discipline of nursing."
3. **The correct answer is 1.** The scientific method is characterized by systematic, orderly procedures that seek to limit the possibility of error and minimize the likelihood that any bias or opinion by the researcher might influence the results of research and, thus, the knowledge gained.
4. **The correct answer is 3.** Ethnography is chosen if the research question leads to the study of behaviour within a specific group or culture. Ethnography involves the observation and description of behaviour in social settings. It is derived from anthropology, in which it provides the means to study the culture of groups of people.
5. **The correct answer is 2.** Subjectivity from the participants' perspective is sought in qualitative research. Because of the nature of the data, rich with personal experience and example, the research is usually reported in a literary style, similar to storytelling.
6. **The correct answer is 1.** The grounded theory is "discovered," developed, and verified through a rigorous process of data collection and analysis. Glaser and Strauss (1967) advocated that researchers not review the literature before carrying out the study because they might be influenced by what others have found. The strength of the grounded theory approach comes from examining the situation afresh and opening up the possibility of a new perspective on an old problem.
7. **The correct answer is 2.** The sample in a survey design should be representative of the population so that generalizations can be made on the basis of the sample data.
8. **The correct answer is 3.** Naming other participants is not required for informed consent. The consent form must describe the purpose of the study, the role of the subjects, types of data that are to be obtained, how the data are obtained, the duration of the study, subject selection, procedures, risks to the subject, potential benefits, alternatives to participation, and contact information.
9. **The correct answer is 3.** A quasi-experimental research design is one in which groups are formed and the conditions are controlled, but the subjects are not randomly assigned to a control group or treatment conditions.
10. **The correct answer is 4.** As well as using knowledge based on systematic research studies, evidence-informed practice also takes into account a nurse's clinical experience, practice trends, and client preferences.

Chapter 8

1. **The correct answer is 3.** By understanding their personal values, nurses better understand their clients' and colleagues' values. In "value conflict," personal values are at odds with those of a client, a colleague, or an institution. Values clarification plays a major role in resolving these dilemmas.
2. **The correct answer is 4.** *Justice* refers to fairness. The term is often used during discussions about resources. The question in this situation is how to determine the just distribution of resources. What constitutes a fair distribution of resources may not always be clear.
3. **The correct answer is 3.** *Maleficence* refers to harm or hurt; thus, *nonmaleficence* is the avoidance of harm or hurt. In health care ethics, ethical practice involves not only the will to do good but also the equal commitment to do no harm.
4. **The correct answer is 1.** *Beneficence* refers to taking positive actions to help other people. Commitment to beneficence helps to guide difficult decisions wherein the benefits of a treatment may be challenged by risks to the client's well-being or dignity.

5. **The correct answer is 4.** *Autonomy* refers to a person's independence. Autonomy represents an agreement to respect another person's right to determine a course of action. Respect for a client's autonomy is fundamental to the practice of health care. It is why clients are included in all aspects of decision making regarding their care.
6. **The correct answer is 2.** The value of autonomy is to respect a client's choice or self-determination.
7. **The correct answer is 3.** Advocacy calls for the nurse to allow clients' opinions to be heard (give clients a voice) and to speak out for those who cannot speak.
8. **The correct answer is 3.** The nurse does not make decisions for the client. Advocating for the client includes protecting the client's right to choice by providing information, obtaining informed consent for all nursing care, and respecting clients' decisions.
9. **The correct answer is 1.** Relational ethics explores the notion of relationships as a central activity of human behaviour. Scholars who write about relational ethics maintain that relationship is central to everything that nurses do and reflects a way of "being," displayed in everyday interactions rather than a mode of decision making.
10. **The correct answer is 2.** Each step in the processing of an ethical dilemma resembles steps in critical thinking. The nurse begins by gathering information and moves through assessment and identification of the problem, planning a solution, implementation of a solution, and evaluation of the results.

Chapter 9

1. **The correct answer is 1.** Statute law is created by elective legislative bodies such as Parliament and provincial or territorial legislatures. Examples of provincial statutes are the nursing practice acts throughout the country, which describe and define nursing practice within each province.
2. **The correct answer is 1.** Any intentional physical contact such as treating a client without the client's consent is considered battery.
3. **The correct answer is 2.** The inappropriate or unjustified use of restraints (e.g., by confining a person to an area, using physical or chemical restraints) may be viewed as false imprisonment.
4. **The correct answer is 4.** Negligence in nursing is conduct that falls below a standard of care established by law. No intent is needed for negligence to occur. It is characterized chiefly by inadvertence, thoughtlessness, or inattention. Therefore, failing to raise the side rails when they are ordered is negligence.
5. **The correct answer is 2.** Obtaining informed consent is part of the physician–client relationship. If a nurse suspects that a client does not understand a procedure for which he or she is being asked to give consent or has consented to, the nurse must notify the physician or nursing supervisor.
6. **The correct answer is 4.** If a client is harmed as a direct result of a nursing student's actions or lack of action, the liability is generally shared by the student, the instructor, the hospital or health care facility, and the university or educational institution.
7. **The correct answer is 4.** A nurse providing emergency assistance at an accident scene would not be covered by an employer's insurance policy because the care given would not be the responsibility of the employer. However, some provinces have passed "Good Samaritan" laws (e.g., Alberta's *Emergency Medical Aid Act,* 1988) that prevent voluntary rescuers from being sued for wrongdoing unless it can be proved that they displayed gross negligence.
8. **The correct answer is 4.** The physician is responsible for directing medical treatment. Nurses are obligated to follow physicians' orders unless they believe the orders are in error, violate hospital policy, or would harm clients.
9. **The correct answer is 3.** Whenever information is requested on a client by any third parties, including insurance companies or employers, nurses must obtain a signed release by the client before releasing confidential information.

Chapter 10

1. **The correct answer is 1.** The processes of enculturation and acculturation facilitate cultural learning. Socialization into one's primary culture during childhood is known as *enculturation.*
2. **The correct answer is 2.** In Canada, rather than assimilation, the preferred outcome is multiculturalism, in which immigrants and other people maintain their cultures and different people of diverse cultures interact peacefully within the nation. Canadians believe, as enshrined in the multiculturalism policy, that citizens should be able to retain their unique ethnic cultures and traditions within a Canadian context.
3. **The correct answer is 1.** Cultural awareness is being aware of one's own background, and it involves an in-depth self-examination to recognize biases, prejudices, and assumptions about other people.
4. **The correct answer is 2.** Culturally competent care is a process whereby nursing care is based on knowledge of the client's cultural heritage, beliefs, and attitudes. It requires the practitioner to bridge cultural gaps in care, work with cultural differences, and enable clients and families to receive meaningful care.
5. **The correct answer is 1.** Ethnocentrism is the root of stereotypes, biases, and prejudices against other people who are perceived to be different from the valued group.
6. **The correct answer is 1.** When a person acts on his or her prejudices, discrimination—treating people unfairly on the basis of their group membership—occurs.
7. **The correct answer is 4.** The dominant value orientation in North American society is individualism and self-reliance in achieving and maintaining health. Caring approaches generally promote the client's independence and ability for self-care.
8. **The correct answer is 3.** Disparities in health outcomes between rich and poor clients illustrate the influence of socio-economic factors on morbidity and mortality. Social factors such as poverty and lack of access to health resources compromise the health status of poor and unemployed clients.
9. **The correct answer is 1.** Clients may suffer cultural pain when their valued way of life is disregarded by practitioners.
10. **The correct answer is 4.** The high value that Western society places on individual autonomy and self-determination may be in direct conflict with the values of diverse groups. Advance directives, informed consent, and consent for hospice are examples of mandates that may violate clients' values.

Chapter 11

1. **The correct answer is 3.** The functional nursing model of care delivery is task focused, not client focused. Tasks are divided, with one nurse assuming responsibility for certain tasks, such as hygiene and dressing changes, and another nurse assuming responsibility for other tasks, such as medication administration.

2. **The correct answer is 3.** The collaborative practice model is the most inclusive of client participation in care, and client centredness is foundational to this model.
3. **The correct answer is 1.** Case management is a care management approach that coordinates and links health care services to clients and their families while streamlining costs and maintaining quality.
4. **The correct answer is 4.** Working in a decentralized structure has the potential for greater collaborative effort, increased staff competency, and a greater sense of professional accomplishment and satisfaction.
5. **The correct answer is 3.** Accountability means being answerable for one's actions. It involves follow-up and reflection on one's decisions to evaluate effectiveness.
6. **The correct answer is 2.** Research shows that the staffing model is an important determinant of a high-quality work life and patient safety.
7. **The correct answer is 1.** It is most important to value the experiences and perspectives of the UCPs and to seek input before setting up educational and support systems.
8. **The correct answer is 1.** First-order priority needs represent an immediate threat to a client's survival or safety, such as an obstructed airway, loss of consciousness, or an anxiety attack.
9. **The correct answer is 4.** UCPs should not be assigned sole responsibility for client care. The nurse in charge of client care decides which activities the UCP can perform independently and which activities must be performed by the nurse and UCP in partnership. UCPs are trained to bathe clients.
10. **The correct answer is 3.** A nurse-sensitive outcome reveals whether interventions are effective, whether clients progress or remain safe, how well standards are being met, and whether changes are necessary. A client outcome is a measure of the client's health status as a result of implementing best practice guidelines for preventing falls.

Chapter 12

1. **The correct answer is 1.** An important aspect of critical thinking is reflection: the process of purposefully thinking back or recalling a situation to discover its purpose or meaning. Nurses should think back on a client situation, make sense of the experience, and thus gain insight into the meaning of the situation.
2. **The correct answer is 3.** At the basic level of critical thinking, a learner trusts that experts have the right answers for every problem. Thinking is concrete and based on a set of rules or principles. For example, a nurse uses an institution's procedures manual to confirm how complete a specific procedure.
3. **The correct answer is 2.** The nursing process consists of five steps: assessment, nursing diagnosis, planning, implementation, and evaluation. During the evaluation phase, the nurse evaluates whether the nursing action has been effective.
4. **The correct answer is 3.** The nurse's knowledge base is an important component of critical thinking. It varies according to a nurse's educational experience, including basic nursing education, continuing education courses, and additional university degrees. In addition, it includes the initiative a nurse shows in reading the nursing literature to remain current in nursing science.

Chapter 13

1. **The correct answer is 4.** The other answers relate to diagnosis and intervention, rather than assessment.
2. **The correct answer is 4.** Only factual information is recorded during assessment.
3. **The correct answer is 4.** Documenting nursing care and reviewing data with other health care professionals are part of intervention, not assessment. Making inferences is the step after data clustering.
4. **The correct answers are 1, 3, and 5.** These symptoms are related to the respiratory system and adequate oxygen intake. The others relate to other body systems.
5. **The correct answer is 3.** Diagnosis and treatment of clients' responses describes the entire nursing process; a common nursing language refers to the process of developing nursing diagnoses; identification of a disease refers to evaluation. A nursing diagnosis for an individual client is the clinical judgement about responses to actual and potential health problems or life processes.
6. **The correct answer is 4.** Data collection, clustering, and interpretation are part of assessment.
7. **The correct answer is 4.** Evaluating nursing care is evaluation, gathering client information is assessment, and helping nurses focus on their role refers to the entire nursing process.
8. **The correct answer is 4.** A wellness nursing diagnosis describes levels of wellness in an individual, family, or community that can be enhanced. A risk nursing diagnosis describes human responses to health conditions or life processes that may develop in a vulnerable individual. An actual nursing diagnosis describes responses to health conditions or life processes that exist in an individual, family, or community. A potential nursing diagnosis is one under consideration during data interpretation.
9. **The correct answer is 2.** A wellness nursing diagnosis describes levels of wellness in an individual, family, or community that can be enhanced. A risk nursing diagnosis describes human responses to health conditions or life processes that may develop in a vulnerable individual. An actual nursing diagnosis describes responses to health conditions or life processes that exist in an individual, family, or community. A potential nursing diagnosis is one under consideration during data interpretation
10. **The correct answer is 1.** Risk factors are evidence considered during assessment; related factors are those contributing to the diagnosis; the complete statement is the nursing diagnosis.
11. **The correct answer is 3.** The other answers are related not to data collection but rather to other aspects of assessment.
12. **The correct answer is 4.** *"Diarrhea related to intestinal colitis"* refers to a medical condition not responsive to nursing care.
13. **The correct answers are 1 and 2.** The other answers are related factors but do not define the primary diagnosis.

Chapter 14

1. **The correct answers are 2 and 3.** Controlling pain and monitoring vital signs are important direct care priorities for safe and effective care for a patient who has just returned from the recovery room. Family visits and end-of-shift reports are important, but they are not high priorities in the immediate recovery period.
2. **The correct answer is 1.** Maintaining proper drainage of the wound is a high priority for this patient immediately after surgery. The condition of the intravenous dressing, the client's comfort, and obtaining more intravenous fluids are important, but they do not have the highest priority in this situation.

3. **The correct answers are 1 and 2.** The descriptions "afebrile until discharge" and "without phlebitis by the third postoperative day" reflect the actual condition or state of the patient.
4. **The correct answer is 4.** Rating pain acuity on a scale is the only report of the expected outcome in measurable terms.
5. **The correct answer is 4.** *Collaboration* means that a number of health care professionals are involved in care.
6. **The correct answer is 3.** Assessment, diagnosis, and planning must be performed before implementation of care or intervention to give care.
7. **The correct answer is 2.** Recording vital sign measurements is an indirect care measure because it takes place away from the patient.
8. **The correct answer is 1.** Client safety always comes first.
9. **The correct answer is 2.** An out-of-date or incorrect care plan compromises the quality of nursing care. Without review and modification of the care plan, the nurse cannot provide timely nursing and effective interventions to meet the client's needs.

Chapter 15

1. **The correct answer is 3.** Auscultation of lung sounds is an evaluation of the effectiveness of suctioning, which is the nursing intervention being evaluated.
2. **The correct answers are 2 and 4.** Evaluative criteria must relate to the intervention (suctioning) that is intended to clear the client's airway and lungs to promote normal breathing. Drinking water and reporting abdominal pain are not directly associated with breathing.
3. **The correct answer is 4.** Evaluating the client's response to interventions is the entire evaluation process; selecting a response that reflects goal achievement is the determination of expected outcomes; reviewing diagnoses and establishing goals and outcomes reflect the establishment of criteria and standards.
4. **The correct answer is 4.** The other actions take place during assessment, diagnosis, and intervention.
5. **The correct answer is 2.** Fever is not necessarily related to infection in the incision; administration of antibiotics and dressing are related to medical care prescribed by the physician.
6. **The correct answers are 1 and 2.** The care plan is discontinued when all goals are met or when it has been determined to be ineffective through evaluation. Gathering assessment data about a different nursing diagnosis is unrelated to this question. Comparing one client's responses with those of another client is not part of the evaluation process.

Chapter 16

1. **The correct answer is 1.** This information about a fellow nursing student is confidential. You cannot share it with classmates or visit him because you learned of his admission accidentally in the course of your work. You have no right to access his EHR because you are not caring for him.
2. **The correct answer is 4.** Enter only objective descriptions of client's behaviour, not opinions or judgements. Do not write retaliatory or critical comments about a client; such comments can be used as evidence of nonprofessional behaviour or poor quality of care in a court of law.
3. **The correct answer is 3.** Subjective data is what the patient says, and this is often his or her own words in quotation marks.
4. **The correct answer is 4.** Enter only objective descriptions of client's behaviour, not opinions or judgements. Do not write retaliatory or critical comments about client; such comments can be used as evidence of nonprofessional behaviour or poor quality of care in a court of law.
5. **The correct answer is 1.** Clients frequently request copies of their health records, and they have the right to do so. Each institution has policies for controlling the manner in which records are shared. In most situations, clients are required to give written permission for release of medical information.
6. **The correct answer is 4.** Use complete, concise descriptions of care so that documentation is objective and factual. Avoid using empty phrases such as "well tolerated," which is too generalized and has no meaning.
7. **The correct answer is 3.** Acuity records (also known as workload measurement systems) provide a method of determining the hours of care and staff required for a given group of clients. A client's acuity level is based on the type and number of nursing interventions required for providing care in a 24-hour period.
8. **The correct answers are as follows:** S = 2, O = 4, A = 3, P = 1. S stands for *subjective:* "The pain increases every time I try to turn on my left side." O stands for *objective:* Left lower abdominal surgical incision, 3 inches in length, closed, sutures intact, no drainage. Pain noted on mild palpation. A stands for *assessment:* Acute pain related to tissue injury from surgical incision. P stands for *plan:* Repositioned client on right side. Encouraged client to use patient-controlled analgesia.

Chapter 17

1. **Open-ended answer is as follows:** Changes in the health care system have led to an increased need for high-quality comparable, aggregated data to support effective decision making, whether decisions are made at the clinical level, the local or regional level, or the system level. Nurses recognize the value of adopting technology to support evidence-informed professional practice, innovation, and nursing data collection and representation.
2. **Open-ended answer is as follows:** The field of nursing needs standardized documentation to facilitate aggregation of nursing data, to support comparison and analysis, and to enhance communication among nurses, and to improve representation regarding nursing contributions.
3. **Open-ended answer is as follows:** The CNA formally adopted the ICNP® as the nomenclature of choice for professional nursing practice. Standardized nursing terminology reflecting the ICNP® is being implemented through the C-HOBIC project. In this project, nursing-sensitive outcomes are examined and compared across various clinical settings. Because all outcomes are coded according to the ICNP®, this comparison will improve the quality of documentation and allow for more accurate analysis.
4. **Open-ended answer is as follows:** Although all nurses must practise in accordance with both the provincial standards of care and the CNA's Code of Ethics, all nurses must be aware of both pieces of federal legislation governing the privacy of health information in Canada: the *Privacy Act* and the *Personal Information Protection and Electronic Documents Act (PIPEDA)*, which prohibit nurses from disclosing personal health information about any patient, with very limited exceptions.
5. **Open-ended answer is as follows:** You can enact the e-nursing strategy by advocating for access and participation and by engaging in developing your competencies. In addition, you should work toward the seven key outcomes identified by the CNA:
   a. Nurses will integrate ICT into their practice to achieve desirable client outcomes.

b. Nurses will have the required information and knowledge to support their practice.
c. Human resources planning will be facilitated.
d. New models of nursing practice and health services delivery will be supported.
e. Nursing groups will be well connected.
f. ICT will improve the quality of nurses' work environments.
g. Canadian nurses will contribute to the global community of nursing.

6. **Open-ended answer is as follows:** Many professional and informal nursing communities are available to foster nurses' engagement in the informatics communities. Canada Health Infoway solicits clinician engagement in support of development of the pan-Canadian EHR. You can be a voluntary member of any one or more Standards Collaborative Working Groups (SCWGs), and you can contribute to specific aspects of EHR development. The CNIA is a national group that all nurses are welcome to join. In addition, many provinces have special interest groups that are dedicated to nursing informatics. COACH is also another Canadian organization that nurses may join. International opportunities include AMIA, IMIA-SIGNI, and HISA. You may also consider other informal communities such as listservs, wikis, blogs, and other social networks such as Facebook. You must remember, however, that most informal communities are not held to the professional content standards as those of more formal organizations, and you should consider their content with caution.

Chapter 18

1. **The correct answer is 4.** Assessment of a client's ability to communicate includes gathering data about the many contextual factors that influence communication. These include the participants' internal factors and characteristics, the nature of their relationship, the situation prompting communication, the environment, and the sociocultural elements present. Assessing these contextual factors helps you make sound decisions during the communication process.
2. **The correct answer is 3.** Active listening means to be attentive to what the client is saying both verbally and nonverbally. The acronym *SOLER* represents facilitative skills for attentive listening: S (sit facing the client); O (observe an open posture; that is, keep arms and legs uncrossed); L (lean toward the client); E (establish and maintain intermittent eye contact); R (relax).
3. **The correct answer is 1.** A helping relationship between nurse and client does not just happen; it is created with care and skill and is built on the client's trust in the nurse. During the orientation phase of a relationship, the nurse sets the tone for the relationship by adopting a warm, empathic, and caring demeanour. During this phase, the relationship is often superficial, uncertain, and of a social nature. The phase is a period of getting to know each other and establishing trust.
4. **The correct answer is 3.** Interacting with clients who have conditions that impair communication requires sensitivity and creativity. Communication techniques must be adapted to the client's unique circumstances and sensory, motor, and cognitive needs. The nurse must be patient, ask simple questions, encourage the client to converse, and allow sufficient time for the client to understand and respond. Visual cues and communication aids may be useful in communicating with aphasic clients.
5. **The correct answer is 1.** Nurses function in roles that require interaction with multiple members of the health care team. Many elements of the nurse–client helping relationship are also applied in these collegial relationships, which are focused on accomplishing the work and goals of the clinical setting. It is especially important to involve the client and family in decisions about the plan of care to determine whether suggested methods are acceptable.
6. **The correct answer is 3.** *Clarifying* means checking whether understanding is accurate, as in restating an unclear or ambiguous message to elicit the sender's meaning. Instead of restating the message, you can also ask the other person to rephrase it, explain further, or give an example of what he or she means.
7. **The correct answer is 4.** Focusing is used to centre on key elements or concepts of a message. If conversation is vague or rambling, or if clients begin to repeat themselves, focusing is a useful technique.
8. **The correct answer is 2.** Intrapersonal communication, or self-talk, is a powerful communication tool. It strongly influences perceptions, feelings, self-concept, and behaviour and can replace negative thoughts with positive assertions.
9. **The correct answer is 2.** A tip for improved communication with older adults is to stick to one topic at a time.
10. **The correct answer is 2.** In the zones of personal space and touch, the personal zone (45 cm to 1 m) includes nursing activities such as sitting at a client's bedside and documenting the client's nursing history.

Chapter 19

1. **The correct answer is 4.** Touch is one way to offer comfort and communicate concern and support. Touch leads to a connection between nurse and client. However, touch can convey many messages; it must be used with discretion.
2. **The correct answer is 4.** To know a client means that the nurse avoids assumptions, focuses on the client, and engages in a caring relationship with the client that reveals information and cues that facilitate critical thinking and clinical judgements. Knowing the client is at the core of the process by which nurses make clinical decisions.
3. **The correct answer is 2.** Enabling is the caring process that helps the new mother's passage through the life transition of birthing. This process is accomplished by preserving dignity, explaining, supporting, focusing, and providing treatment alternatives.
4. **The correct answer is 4.** Spiritual health is achieved when people find a balance between their own life values, goals, and belief systems and those of others. Research has shown a link between spirit, mind, and body. An individual's beliefs and expectations can and do have effects on the person's physical well-being.
5. **The correct answer is 3.** Strategies to enable nurses to demonstrate more caring behaviours include introducing greater flexibility into the work environment structure, rewarding experienced nurse mentors, improving nurse staffing, and providing nurses with autonomy over their practice.
6. **The correct answer is 1.** A nurse demonstrates caring by helping family members become active participants in a client's care.
7. **The correct answer is 4.** Listening includes not only "taking in" what a client says but also interpreting and understanding what is said and reflecting that understanding to the person talking.
8. **The correct answer is 3.** Presence involves a person-to-person encounter that conveys closeness and a sense of caring that involves "being there" and "being with" clients.

9. **The correct answer is 1.** Knowing the behaviours that clients perceive as caring helps nurses to understand what clients expect of them as caregivers. Establishing a reassuring presence, recognizing an individual as unique, and being attentive to the client are recurrent caring behaviours identified by researchers. Each client has a unique background of experiences, values, and cultural perspectives; however, understanding common behaviours that clients associate with caring will help you learn to express caring in practice.

Chapter 20

1. **The correct answer is 4.** The nurse must think of family as defined by each individual. In other words, the nurse can think of the family as a set of relationships that the client identifies as family or as a network of individuals who influence each other's lives, whether the ties actually are biological or legal.
2. **The correct answer is 2.** The blended family is formed when both parents bring children from previous relationships into a new, joint living situation or when children from the current union and children from previous unions are living together.
3. **The correct answer is 4.** The proportion of teenagers giving birth has been declining steadily since the 1980s, probably as a result of increased sexual education, the availability of contraceptives, and the use of abortion.
4. **The correct answer is 4.** The family is the primary social context in which health promotion and disease prevention take place. The family's beliefs, values, and practices also strongly influence health-promoting behaviours of its members.
5. **The correct answer is 3.** Health promotion researchers have focused on the stress-moderating effect of hardiness and resiliency as factors that contribute to long-term health. Family hardiness is the internal strengths and durability of the family unit. Family resiliency is the ability to cope with expected and unexpected stressors.
6. **The correct answer is 2.** When the family as client is the approach, you focus on the entire family: its processes and relationships (e.g., parenting or family caregiving).
7. **The correct answer is 1.** *Internal structure* refers to the people who are included in the family and how they are connected to each other. Specifically, this question assesses family composition, a subcategory of internal structure. *Family composition* refers to the individual members who form the family. The family composition is not limited to the traditional nuclear family; instead, it may include any of the various family forms.
8. **The correct answer is 4.** *Expressive functioning* refers to the ways in which people communicate. Emotional communication is a subcategory of expressive functioning and encompasses the range and types of feelings that are expressed by the family.
9. **The correct answer is 1.** Circular questions facilitate change by inviting the family to discover their own answers; they help explain a problem.
10. **The correct answer is 3.** In an effective family interview, the nurse can engage a family to assess, explore, and identify strengths and problems. The nurse can also decide to intervene or refer the family to another health professional.

Chapter 21

1. **The correct answer is 3.** Psychomotor learning involves acquiring skills that require the integration of mental and muscular activity; therefore, teaching a client to use a walker requires the use of the psychomotor domain. The client masters skills by manipulating equipment and practising manual skills.
2. **The correct answer is 2.** If a client's learning ability is impaired or if distractions are present, the nurse should modify or postpone teaching activities. Any physical condition (e.g., pain, fatigue, or hunger) that depletes energy also impairs the ability to learn. Therefore, the nurse should teach the client when pain medications are working.
3. **The correct answer is 3.** Readiness to learn is related to the grieving stage. Clients cannot learn when they are unwilling or unable to accept the reality of illness. However, properly timed teaching can help a client to adjust to illness or disability. When a client is in denial or disbelief, you should teach in the present tense (e.g., explain what client needs to know to be discharged).
4. **The correct answer is 4.** As a child matures, intellectual growth moves from concrete to abstract. By developing topics for discussion that require problem solving, the nurse is considering the adolescents' level of development and will engage the students in learning about nutrition.
5. **The correct answer is 3.** Behavioural objectives are measurable and observable and indicate how learning will be evidenced. An objective is more precise when it describes the conditions or timing under which the behaviour occurs (e.g., the client will perform breast self-examination correctly before the end of the teaching session).
6. **The correct answer is 1.** The telling approach is useful when limited information must be taught (e.g., preparing a client for an emergency diagnostic procedure).
7. **The correct answer is 3.** Role-play helps teach new ideas and attitudes. During role-play, clients play themselves or someone else and rehearse a desired behaviour.
8. **The correct answer is 1.** Learning disabilities are disorders that may impair ability to acquire, organize, remember, understand, or apply information. When teaching clients with learning disabilities or other barriers to learning, a recommended technique is to demonstrate procedures such as measuring dosages and then ask for return demonstrations (provides opportunity to clarify instructions and time to review procedures).
9. **The correct answer is 2.** In general, teaching and learning begin when a person identifies a need for knowing or acquiring an ability to do something.
10. **The correct answer is 1.** Demonstrations help teach psychomotor skills such as preparing a syringe. The client is able to observe a skill before practising it.

Chapter 22

1. **The correct answer is 4.** Growth is the quantitative, or measurable, aspect of an individual's increase in physical measurements. Measurable growth indicators include changes in height, weight, teeth, skeletal structures, and sexual characteristics.
2. **The correct answer is 1.** Moral development is the ability of an individual to distinguish right from wrong and to develop ethical values on which to base his or her actions.
3. **The correct answer is 1.** Organicism is a theoretical focus on the organism itself. According to theories in this tradition, development is a result of biologically driven behaviour and the person's adaptation to the environment.
4. **The correct answer is 1.** Three major categories of factors influence human growth and development: genetics, environment, and the interaction between these two. The family is an example of an environmental factor. Family influences through its values, beliefs, customs, and specific patterns of interaction and communication.

5. **The correct answer is 4.** Psychiatrist Roger Gould believed his findings described a sequential process that takes place between the internal life (personality) of adults and their outer world (culture, lifestyle).
6. **The correct answer is 2.** The fourth theme, identified in individuals in their 40s, "The die is cast," is indicative of resignation and the belief that possibilities are limited. The personality is believed to be set. Changes in career are believed to be less likely to be successful. Parents are blamed for their lack of choices. Mistakes made in raising children are regretted.
7. **The correct answer is 1.** During formal operations, the individual's thinking moves to abstract and theoretical subjects. Thinking can venture into such subjects as achieving world peace, finding justice, and seeking meaning in life. Adolescents can organize their thoughts in their minds. New cognitive powers allow the adolescent to achieve more far-reaching problem solving.
8. **The correct answer is 2.** The microsystem consists of the immediate settings, activities, and personal relationships of the individual. Examples of microsystems include family, classroom, workplace, or recreation group.
9. **The correct answer is 3.** According to Keating and Hertzman's (1999) population health approach, human development is a population phenomenon. They referred to the strong association between the health of a population, developmental outcomes, and the social and economic forces affecting the larger society. Therefore, improving community housing would be an attempt to improve the health of the population.
10. **The correct answer is 4.** According to resilience theory, protective processes shield people from adversity and include social supports, such as high-quality day care.

Chapter 23

1. **The correct answer is 1.** Maternal risk factors associated with preterm labour include physiological stresses such as renal and cardiovascular disease, diabetes mellitus, and uterine and cervical abnormalities.
2. **The correct answer is 3.** In the tonic neck reflex, the newborn's head is turned to one side, the arm and leg on that side are extended, and the opposite leg and arm are in a flexed position. Eliciting reflex activity helps in the assessment of the infant's neurological status. It is important to note the presence and the strength of the various reflexes in the newborn.
3. **The correct answer is 2.** Healthy infants begin their routine immunization schedule at 2 months of age so that they may be protected against infectious diseases as early as possible.
4. **The correct answer is 4.** According to Piaget (1952), during the preoperational thought stage of cognitive development, toddlers recognize that they are separate beings from their mothers, but they are unable to assume another person's viewpoint. They use symbols to represent objects, places, and people. This function is demonstrated when children imitate the behaviour of another person that they viewed earlier (e.g., pretend to shave like their daddy).
5. **The correct answer is 3.** The play of preschool children becomes more social after the third birthday as it shifts from parallel to associative play. Most 3-year-old children are able to play with one other child in a cooperative manner in which they make something or play designated roles such as mother and baby. By the age of 4 years, children play in groups of two or three, and by 5 years, the group has a temporary leader for each activity.
6. **The correct answer is 2.** Preschoolers average 12 hours of sleep a night and take infrequent naps.
7. **The correct answer is 1.** Motor development in the school-aged child (aged 8–10 years) includes learning to floss teeth effectively and be independent in tooth care.
8. **The correct answer is 1.** Obesity has become the most common nutritional disturbance in childhood. You can help children avoid this problem by teaching about and encouraging a balanced healthy diet, promoting physical exercise and limiting inactivity, and promoting a healthy body image.
9. **The correct answer is 3.** Good communication skills are critical for overcoming peer pressure and unhealthy behaviours. The following are some hints for communicating with adolescents: do not avoid discussing sensitive issues, ask open-ended questions, look for the meaning behind their words or actions, be alert to clues to their emotional state, and involve other individuals and resources when necessary.
10. **The correct answer is 3.** Injuries, including self-inflicted injuries and injuries caused by motor vehicle accidents and poisoning, are the leading cause of death in adolescents.

Chapter 24

1. **The correct answer is 2.** Most young adults have completed physical growth by the age of 20 years.
2. **The correct answer is 1.** Your role in health promotion is to identify lifestyle risk factors and provide education and support to reduce unhealthy behaviours.
3. **The correct answer is 4.** When determining the amount of information the individual needs to make decisions about the prescribed course of therapy, you should consider factors that may affect the individual's compliance with the regimen, including educational level, socioeconomic factors, motivation, and desire to learn.
4. **The correct answer is 4.** A common physiological change in the second trimester is quickening, which is the sensation of fetal movements as experienced by the pregnant woman.
5. **The correct answer is 2.** Accidents are the leading causes of accidental injury for young adults.
6. **The correct answer is 2.** Close friends and associates of the single young adult may also be viewed as the individual's "family."
7. **The correct answer is 3.** A family history of a disease may put a young adult at risk for developing that disease in the middle or older adult years. For example, if a young man's father and paternal grandfather had myocardial infarctions (heart attacks) in their 50s, his risk for a future myocardial infarction is increased.
8. **The correct answer is 3.** In the middle adult years, as children depart from the household, the family enters the post-parental family stage. Time and financial demands on the parents decrease, and the couple faces the task of redefining their relationship.
9. **The correct answer is 3.** Health teaching and health counselling are often directed at improving health habits.
10. **The correct answer is 3.** The physiological response to stress can be avoided. You use relaxation techniques, imagery, and biofeedback to recondition the client's response to stress.

Chapter 25

1. **The correct answer is 4.** Two factors contribute to the projected increase in the number of older adults: the aging of the baby boom generation and the growth of the population segment older than 85 years. The baby boomers are the adults born between 1946 and 1964.

2. **The correct answer is 3.** Various theorists have attempted to describe the complex biopsychosocial process of aging. Although many theories have been developed, no single universally accepted theory predicts and explains the complexities of the aging process.
3. **The correct answer is 3.** The three common conditions affecting cognition are delirium, dementia, and depression. The nurse may find that distinguishing among these three conditions is challenging but essential.
4. **The correct answer is 2.** Sexuality is increasingly recognized as an important factor in the lives of older adults. All older adults, whether healthy or frail, need to express sexual feelings. Sexuality involves love, warmth, sharing, and touching, not just the act of intercourse.
5. **The correct answer is 1.** The libido does not decrease in older adults, although frequency of sexual activity may decline. An older woman who does not understand physical changes affecting sexual activity may be concerned that her sex life is nearly over. The older man may feel the same when he discovers a change in the firmness of his erection, a decreased need for ejaculation with each orgasm, or a longer recovery period between episodes of intercourse.
6. **The correct answer is 3.** Presbyopia (the gradual decline in the ability to focus on near objects) is common in older adults.
7. **The correct answer is 1.** Presbycusis, common in older adults, is a decrease in the ability to hear high-pitched sounds and sibilant consonants such as "s," "sh," and "ch."
8. **The correct answer is 1.** Taste buds atrophy and lose sensitivity. Older adults are less able to discern among salty, sweet, sour, and bitter tastes.
9. **The correct answer is 4.** The anteroposterior diameter of the thorax increases. The incidence of osteoporosis is increased in older adults; vertebral changes caused by osteoporosis lead to dorsal kyphosis, the curvature of the thoracic spine sometimes called "dowager's hump."
10. **The correct answer is 1.** Frontotemporal dementia has an insidious onset and progresses slowly. Early symptoms include poor hygiene, lack of social tact, hyperorality, and sexual disinhibition. Incontinence is an early symptom in frontotemporal dementia, whereas it is a late symptom in the more common Alzheimer's disease.

Chapter 26

1. **The correct answer is 2.** Self-concept is how a person thinks about himself or herself. It is a subjective sense of the self and a complex mixture of unconscious and conscious thoughts, attitudes, and perceptions. Mastectomy is a surgical procedure that alters the appearance and function of the body. Although the changes may not be apparent to other people when the individual is dressed, these bodily changes have a significant impact on the individual.
2. **The correct answer is 2.** One of the self-concept developmental tasks of 1- to 3-year-olds is developing self through modelling, imitation, and socialization.
3. **The correct answer is 4.** Identity involves the internal sense of individuality, wholeness, and consistency of a person over time and in various circumstances.
4. **The correct answer is 3.** Body image depends only partly on the reality of the body. Body image involves attitudes related to the body, including physical appearance, structure, or function. Feelings about body image include those related to sexuality, femininity and masculinity, youthfulness, health, and vitality. These mental images are not always consistent with a person's actual physical structure or appearance.
5. **The correct answer is 1.** Through the process of reinforcement–extinction, certain behaviours become common or are avoided, depending on whether they are approved and reinforced or are discouraged and punished.
6. **The correct answer is 4.** Through the process of identification, an individual internalizes the beliefs, behaviour, and values of role models into a personal, unique expression of self.
7. **The correct answer is 3.** An individual's identity is affected by stressors throughout life but is particularly vulnerable during adolescence, a time characterized by many changes.
8. **The correct answer is 1.** Identity confusion results when a person does not maintain a clear, consistent, and continuous consciousness of personal identity.
9. **The correct answer is 3.** By asking clients how they feel about themselves, the nurse is seeking information about their self-esteem.
10. **The correct answer is 1.** Increasing the client's self-awareness is achieved through establishing a trusting nurse–client relationship that allows the client to openly explore thoughts and feelings.

Chapter 27

1. **The correct answer is 3.** *Gender identity* refers to the degree to which a person identifies as male, female, or some combination. It begins in early childhood as the child becomes aware of the differences of the sexes and perceives that he or she is male or female.
2. **The correct answer is 2.** *Sexual health* means that a person has freedom from physical and psychological impairment, awareness of and positive attitudes toward sexual functioning, and accurate knowledge about sexuality.
3. **The correct answer is 4.** Sexual dysfunction is the absence of complete sexual functioning.
4. **The correct answer is 1.** A major problem in dealing with STIs is that symptoms are absent or go unnoticed. Finding and treating the people who have them can be difficult. Some people who are infected may not even know that they are.
5. **The correct answer is 2.** The most common bacterial STI is genital chlamydia. (HIV infection and AIDS are viral STIs.) A chlamydial infection may cause an abnormal genital discharge and burning with urination. There are many serious complications of genital chlamydia in women, including chronic pelvic pain, infertility, and ectopic pregnancy.
6. **The correct answer is 1.** Contraceptive methods that require a health care professional's intervention include hormonal contraception, intrauterine devices (IUDs), the diaphragm, the vaginal contraceptive ring, the cervical cap, and surgical procedures (vasectomy and tubal ligation).
7. **The correct answer is 2.** Effectiveness rates are as follows: for birth control pills, 98% to 99%; for the contraceptive sponge, 80% to 91%; for vaginal spermicides, 78% to 90%; and for the female condom, 79% to 85%.
8. **The correct answer is 2.** The most valuable tool that you can use when providing care in areas of sexuality is effective, nonjudgemental communication. A perceptive and educated approach to talking about sexuality can offer the support that many clients require. Effective communication about sexuality requires caring, sensitivity, tact, compassion, the use of appropriate language, and nondiscriminatory attitudes.

9. **The correct answer is 3.** When caring for older adults, you may adjust your assessment approach. When gathering a sexual history from an older adult, it is important to keep in mind that the client may have difficulty discussing intimate details with health care providers. You are responsible for helping maintain the sexuality of older adults by offering the opportunity to discuss any concerns. Often, asking questions on the topic of sexuality in a comfortable, relaxed manner facilitates older adults' discussion of their sexual needs.
10. **The correct answer is 1.** A useful framework to guide planning is the PLISSIT model developed by Annon (1976). P stands for "permission giving." During assessment, you can bring up the topic of sexuality and can give the individual permission to talk about sexual concerns. LI stands for "limited information," which is basic information regarding sexuality and sexual functioning. SS stands for "specific suggestions," whereby you provide specific suggestions regarding a sexual concern or issue. If you are not equipped to address a particular concern, you should refer the client to another health care professional. IT stands for "intensive therapy." At this level of intervention, your role is to refer the client to a qualified practitioner, such as a social worker or a sex counsellor, for individualized therapy.

Chapter 28

1. **The correct answer is 3.** Caring for a client's spiritual needs means caring for the whole person, accepting his or her beliefs and experiences, and helping the client with issues surrounding meaning and hope.
2. **The correct answer is 2.** Atheists do not believe in the existence of God. Agnostics believe that any ultimate reality is unknown. This does not mean that spirituality is not an important concept for the atheist or agnostic. Atheists search for meaning in life through their work and their relationships with other individuals.
3. **The correct answer is 4.** When a person has the attitude of something to live for and look forward to, hope is present. Hope is a multidimensional concept that provides comfort while people endure life threats and personal challenges.
4. **The correct answer is 4.** Canadian Hutterites believe that it is not appropriate to pray for good health; rather, prayers may be for wisdom to live a healthy life or bear suffering without complaint.
5. **The correct answer is 4.** A ritual can provide the client with structure and support during difficult times. If rituals are important to the client, the nurse should account for them as part of nursing intervention.
6. **The correct answer is 1.** The ability to establish presence is part of the art of nursing. It is not simply being in the same room with a client while performing procedures or sharing information. Being present involves "being with" a client, as opposed to "doing for" a client. It involves offering a closeness with the client: physically, psychologically, and spiritually.
7. **The correct answer is 1.** Some sects of Hinduism are vegetarians. The belief is not to kill any living creature.
8. **The correct answer is 4.** Some members of Jehovah's Witnesses may avoid food prepared with or containing blood.
9. **The correct answer is 2.** Members of the Mormon faith abstain from alcohol, caffeine, and tobacco.
10. **The correct answer is 1.** Clients who experience terminal illness or who have been recently disabled by disease or injury require the nurse's support in grieving over and coping with their loss. Supporting a client during times of grief can be enhanced by a spiritual relationship with the client.

Chapter 29

1. **The correct answer is 1.** An actual loss is any loss of a person or object that can no longer be felt, heard, known, or experienced by the individual. Lost objects that have been valued by a client include any possession that is worn out, misplaced, stolen, or ruined.
2. **The correct answer is 2.** A perceived loss is any loss that is uniquely defined by the grieving client. It may be less obvious to others.
3. **The correct answer is 3.** Situational loss includes any sudden, unpredictable external event.
4. **The correct answer is 4.** During Bowlby's phase of disorganization and despair, an individual may constantly examine how and why the loss occurred.
5. **The correct answer is 4.** During Kübler-Ross's stage of depression, the person finally realizes the full impact and significance of the loss and may feel overwhelmingly lonely and withdraw from interpersonal interaction.
6. **The correct answer is 2.** Worden's task 3 is to adjust to the environment in which the deceased is missing. According to Worden, a person does not realize the full impact of a loss for at least 3 months. At this point, many friends and associates make less frequent contact, and the person is left to ponder the full impact of loneliness.
7. **The correct answer is 3.** Loneliness and problems associated with completing the tasks of daily living are two of the most common and difficult adjustments for older bereaved spouses.
8. **The correct answer is 4.** Expression of hopefulness is an expected outcome for clients experiencing a loss.
9. **The correct answer is 2.** For transplantation of organs, ventilatory and circulatory support must be maintained until the organs are harvested. The family must clearly understand that the client is "brain dead" and that the equipment (i.e., ventilator and vasopressor medications) is not keeping the client alive but keeping the physical body in a state so that the organs will not be damaged before being harvested.
10. **The correct answer is 3.** Palliative care allows clients to make more informed choices, achieve better alleviation of symptoms, and have more opportunity to manage unfinished business.

Chapter 30

1. **The correct answer is 1.** The medulla oblongata controls vital functions necessary for survival, including heart rate, blood pressure, and respiration.
2. **The correct answer is 4.** The general adaptation syndrome is a three-stage reaction to stress. During the alarm reaction, rising hormone levels result in increases in blood volume, blood glucose levels, epinephrine and norepinephrine levels, heart rate, blood flow to muscles, oxygen intake, and mental alertness.
3. **The correct answer is 3.** Post-traumatic stress disorder (PTSD) can develop after a traumatic injury or event.
4. **The correct answer is 3.** Situational stress can arise from the person's current circumstances, such as moving, changing jobs, and adjusting to a chronic illness or condition.
5. **The correct answer is 2.** The nurse uses the interview to determine the client's perception of the stressor by asking the client what is of the most concern at this time.
6. **The correct answer is 4.** Three primary modes of coping with stress are to decrease exposure to stress-producing situations,

increase resistance to stress by increasing action-oriented coping strategies, and learn skills that reduce physiological response to stress. A support group can provide information about a wide range of coping strategies, guidance about reducing exposure to stressful situations, and shared training sessions on techniques to reduce physiological responsiveness.

7. **The correct answer is 2.** In the presence of anxiety-provoking thoughts and events, a common physiological symptom is muscle tension. Physiological tension will be diminished through a systematic approach of relaxing major muscle groups.
8. **The correct answer is 4.** Rapid changes in health care technology, diversity in the workforce, organizational restructuring, and changing work systems can place stress on nurses.
9. **The correct answer is 1.** A crisis creates a turning point in a person's life because it changes the direction of a person's life in some way. The precipitating event usually occurs from 1 to 2 weeks before the individual seeks help, but it may have occurred within the past 24 hours. In general, a crisis is resolved in some way within approximately 6 weeks.

Chapter 31

1. **The correct answer is 3.** Bradycardia is a slow heart rate, slower than 60 beats per minute in adults. Bradypnea is an abnormally slow rate of breathing, slower than 12 breaths per minute.
2. **The correct answer is 1.** An inefficient contraction of the heart that fails to transmit a pulse wave to the peripheral pulse site creates a pulse deficit. To assess a pulse deficit, the nurse and a colleague assess radial and apical rates simultaneously and then compare rates. The difference between the apical and radial pulse rates is the pulse deficit.
3. **The correct answer is 1.** The normal temperature range gradually drops as individuals approach older adulthood. Older adults have a narrower range of body temperatures than do younger adults. Oral temperatures of 35°C are not unusual for older adults in cold weather. However, the average body temperature of older adults is approximately 36°C.
4. **The correct answer is 2.** Blood pressure measurements are not accurate unless the blood pressure cuff is the correct size. If the cuff is too small, it tends to become loose if inflated; this results in false high headings.
5. **The correct answer is 3.** Apnea is the cessation of breathing. It may occur during sleep, in which it is most often caused by obstruction from relaxed tissues. With respiratory effort, it can be followed by normal breathing.
6. **The correct answer is 1.** The blood pressure measurements indicate that the client has orthostatic hypotension. If orthostatic hypotension is assessed, the client is assisted to a supine position, and the physician or nurse in charge is then notified. While obtaining orthostatic measurements, the nurse observes for other symptoms of hypotension, such as fainting, weakness, or light-headedness.
7. **The correct answer is 2.** If the nurse detects an abnormal rate while palpating a radial pulse, the next step is to assess the apical rate. The apical rate requires auscultation of heart sounds, which provides a more accurate assessment of cardiac contraction.
8. **The correct answer is 1.** Conduction is the transfer of heat from one object to another with direct contact. Heat is conducted through contact with solids, liquids, and gases. When the warm skin touches a cooler object, heat is lost. Conduction normally accounts for a small amount of heat loss. The nurse increases conductive heat loss when bathing a client with a cool cloth.
9. **The correct answer is 3.** Diseases causing poor oxygenation, such as asthma or chronic obstructive pulmonary disease (COPD), cause an increase in pulse rate.
10. **The correct answer is 1.** The basic techniques of inspection, palpation, and auscultation are used to measure vital signs.

Chapter 32

1. **The correct answer is 4.** The nursing diagnosis is made after completion of both the health history and the physical examination and after any necessary diagnostic or laboratory tests. The quality, intensity, and location of the symptom or sign are 3 of the 10 characteristics of a symptom/sign analysis by nurses. Information about the 10 characteristics provides the nurse with comprehensive information about the symptom or sign.
2. **The correct answer is 4.** Recent memory involves the recall of events that occurred within the previous 24 hours, such as what was eaten for breakfast. Immediate recall is the ability to recall information such as a telephone number that has been learned within the last few minutes. Remote memory is the ability to recall significant information learned in the past, such as birthdays or historical events.
3. **The correct answer is 2.** When you conduct an otoscopic examination, you straighten the ear canal, use the largest ear speculum that fits the ear canal without touching the skin, and move the otoscope slowly to visualize the ear structures, including the ear canal and the integrity of the tympanic membrane. The client is sitting without being asked to change the head position.
4. **The correct answer is 3.** You assess the consistency of the nodes, the delineation (demarcation) of the node borders, the mobility or fixation of a node, and the presence of node tenderness. These are just four of the characteristics that you need to assess when palpating lymph nodes. You would also assess enlargement, location, size, shape, and surface characteristics of the nodes. During palpation of lymph nodes, you do not assess turgor, moisture, temperature, or colour, which are all characteristics of skin. Configuration is a characteristic of skin lesions.
5. **The correct answer is 3.** Adventitious breath sounds are unexpected. When you hear crackles, rhonchi, wheezes or friction rubs, you need to identify their location in the lungs, determine when they occur in inspiration and expiration, and confirm that they do not clear with coughing or after several deep inspirations. Measuring the ratio of inspiratory phase to expiratory phase is one way of determining the type of expected breath sound as vesicular, bronchovesicular, or bronchial.
6. **The correct answer is 4.** If the apical impulse is palpated 4 cm to the left of the left midclavicular line, you would suspect the presence of an enlarged left ventricle. Expect to palpate the apical impulse only at about the fifth left interspace and to detect it during the first two thirds of systole, and expect it to feel like a brisk tap against your palpating finger.
7. **The correct answer is 2.** To ensure accurate comparison for percussion of symmetrical areas, you always keep the force of your percussion blow consistent between sides. During percussion, use a brisk, arclike, but relaxed wrist motion; apply your pleximeter finger firmly to the skin surface; and use the lightest percussion blow to achieve clear percussion notes.
8. **The correct answer is 3.** You palpate the paravertebral muscles bilaterally for symmetry of bulk and to detect tenderness or spasm, but you do not assess the attachments of the paravertebral

muscles to the 24 vertebrae. When inspecting the spine, you assess curvatures, alignment, and range of motion of the spine.

9. **The correct answer is 3.** The testicles of a young adult male are smooth and slightly rubbery. An elderly male client is expected to demonstrate age-related changes that include diminished and grey pubic hair, a more pendulous scrotal sac because of dartos muscle relaxation, and a small penis, whether circumcised or uncircumcised.
10. **The correct answer is 2.** Clients should be able to perform point-to-point testing accurately whether eyes are closed or open. When a client can perform the test accurately with eyes open but not with eyes closed, the client has lost position sense because of the lack of visual cues. Vision aids accuracy. Without visual cues, the test cannot be performed with accuracy when position sense is lost.

Chapter 33

1. **The correct answer is 1.** If an infection can be transmitted from one person to another either directly or indirectly, it is a communicable (infectious, contagious) disease.
2. **The correct answer is 1.** Hepatitis A is transmitted by direct and indirect contact. Hepatitis A can be transmitted person to person by the fecal–oral route. It can also be transmitted indirectly via contaminated water or infected food handlers.
3. **The correct answer is 4.** The interval when a client manifests signs and symptoms specific to the type of infection (e.g., common cold manifested by sore throat, sinus congestion, or rhinitis) is the illness stage.
4. **The correct answer is 2.** Hand hygiene is the most important and most basic technique in preventing the transmission of infections. Hand hygiene includes using an instant alcohol hand antiseptic before and after providing client care, handwashing with soap and water when hands are visibly soiled, and performing a surgical scrub when necessary. The components of good handwashing include using an adequate amount of soap, rubbing the hands together to lather the soap and create friction, and rinsing under a stream of water.
5. **The correct answer is 2.** Washing times of at least 15 seconds are needed to remove most transient microorganisms from the skin. If the hands are visibly soiled, more time may be needed.
6. **The correct answer is 2.** Before isolation measures are instituted, the client must understand the nature of the disease or condition, the purposes of isolation, and the steps for carrying out specific precautions. You also take measures to improve the client's sensory stimulation during isolation.
7. **The correct answer is 4.** Gowns or cover-ups protect health care workers and visitors from coming in contact with infected material, blood, or body fluid, or contaminated surfaces or objects in the environment.
8. **The correct answer is 2.** Gloves should be removed promptly after use and hand hygiene performed before touching non-contaminated items and environmental surfaces, before moving from a contaminated body site to a clean body site on the same patient, and before going to another client.
9. **The correct answer is 2.** Contact precautions are needed when standard precautions or routine practices are not sufficient to prevent transmission. *C. difficile* spores have a high potential for environmental contamination and can be spread to other patients via health care workers' hands and contaminated equipment.
10. **The correct answer is 1.** When you are doing a surgical scrub, you must keep your hands above your elbows.

Chapter 34

1. **The correct answer is 4.** Right reason has been added to the six rights of medication administration. Knowing the right reason about why a client is receiving a particular medication enhances client safety. Ordered medications should be consistent with the client's diagnosis and health deviations. Awareness of the reason why a client is receiving a particular medication can help you to evaluate the client's response and effectiveness of medication therapy.
2. **The correct answer is 2.** A medication order is required for any medication to be administered. To protect client safety, you should ensure the medication order contains all of the elements (e.g., medication name, dose, route). If the medication order is incomplete, you should inform the prescriber and ensure completeness before carrying out the medication order. Incomplete transcriptions are a source of medication errors.
3. **The correct answer is 1.** The primary contraindications to administering oral medications include the presence of gastrointestinal alterations, the inability of a client to swallow foods or fluids, the risk of aspiration in clients with impaired ability to swallow, and the use of gastric suction.
4. **The correct answer is 1.** A medication error is any event that could cause or lead to a client either receiving inappropriate medication therapy or failing to receive appropriate medication therapy. Most medication errors occur when you fail to follow routine procedures, such as checking dose calculations, deciphering illegible handwriting, and recording the names of or administering medications with which you are unfamiliar.
5. **The correct answer is 4.** Apply the following formula for solid dose forms of medications:
   Dose ordered/Dose on hand × Amount on hand = Amount to administer
   500 mg/250 mg × 1 tablet = 2 tablets
   Therefore, if the physician orders 500 mg orally (PO) of Keflex and the medication is only available in tablets containing 250 mg, 2 tablets should be administered.
6. **The correct answer is 3.** Subcutaneous injections involve placing medications into the loose connective tissue under the dermis. Because subcutaneous tissue is not as richly supplied with blood as the muscles, absorption is commonly slower than intramuscular injections.
7. **The correct answer is 1.** You are responsible for following legal provisions when administering controlled substances (drugs that alter the mind or behaviour patterns), which can be only be dispensed with a prescription. Violations of the *Narcotic Control Act* are punishable by fines, imprisonment, and loss of nurse licensure or registration.
8. **The correct answer is 2.** Pharmacokinetics is the study of how medications enter the body, reach their site of action, are metabolized, and exit the body. Use your knowledge of pharmacokinetics when timing medication administration, judging the client's risk for alterations in medication action, and observing the client's response.
9. **The correct answer is 4.** Official publications, such as the *British Pharmacopoeia* and the *Canadian Formulary*, set standards for drug strength, quality, purity, packaging, safety, labelling, and dosage form. Physicians, nurses, and pharmacists depend on these standards to ensure that clients receive pure drugs in safe and effective dosages.

10. **The correct answer is 1.** Administration of the *Food and Drugs Act* and the *Controlled Drugs and Substances Act* is carried out by the Health Protection Branch (HPB) of the federal government. Before a new drug can be marketed in Canada, an application for approval must be made to the HPB. After intensive testing, the HPB reviews the application. When sufficient information has been accumulated to ensure its safety, the drug is released for general use.

Chapter 35

1. **The correct answer is 3.** Despite the success of allopathic medicine (traditional Western medicine), many health conditions are difficult to treat: for example, arthritis, chronic back pain, gastrointestinal problems, allergies, headaches, and insomnia. Many clients with these health conditions choose to explore alternative methods to relieve their symptoms.
2. **The correct answer is 4.** Many complementary therapies, such as acupuncture, require diagnostic and therapeutic methods specific to their field, whereas other complementary therapies, such as guided imagery and breathwork, are, in general, easily learned and applied.
3. **The correct answer is 1.** One study reported that half of the Canadians surveyed had used alternative therapies in the previous year. Of these, 88% stated the care they received was either somewhat helpful or very helpful. Most respondents (81%) reported using alternative therapies to prevent illness or to maintain wellness.
4. **The correct answer is 1.** Holistic nursing regards and treats the mind, body, and spirit of the client. Nurses can use holistic interventions such as relaxation therapy, guided imagery, music therapy, simple touch, massage, and prayer. Such interventions affect the whole person (mind–body–spirit) and are economical, noninvasive, nonpharmacological complements to traditional medical care.
5. **The correct answer is 1.** Some complementary and alternative medicine therapies and techniques use natural processes, such as breathing, concentration, and simple touch, to help clients feel better and cope with chronic conditions. You can learn these techniques with minimum preparation, and many of these procedures can be used with clients as part of your independent nursing practice (Dossey et al., 2005). Adequate assessment and the client's permission are prerequisites for implementing a complementary medicine therapy.
6. **The correct answer is 1.** According to one of the principles of complementary and alternative medicine therapies, the individual must be actively involved in the treatment. Clients achieve better responses if they practise the techniques or exercises daily. The client must commit to implementing and maintaining the therapy until a desired outcome is achieved.
7. **The correct answer is 3.** St. John's Wort is effective as a mild antidepressant and sedative and offers some protection against viruses. Clinical trials have begun to investigate the effectiveness of St. John's wort in treating AIDS.
8. **The correct answer is 1.** Meditation can augment the effects of certain drugs. For example, individuals taking antihypertensive, thyroid-regulating, antidepressant, or antianxiety medications should be monitored. Prolonged practice of meditation techniques may, in some cases, lead to the reduced need for certain medications, and some doses of medications may need to be adjusted.
9. **The correct answer is 2.** Biofeedback techniques are frequently used in addition to relaxation interventions to assist individuals in learning how to control specific autonomic nervous system responses.
10. **The correct answer is 2.** Therapeutic touch is a training-specific therapy that was developed in the 1970s by a nurse, Dr. Dolores Krieger. Although the philosophical and religious assumptions of therapeutic touch differ from those of other Eastern healing modalities, both practices involve trained practitioners who attempt to direct their own balanced energies in an intentional and motivated manner toward the client.

Chapter 36

1. **The correct answer is 3.** To reduce the risk of injury to you and the client, you must understand and practise techniques for safe lifting, positioning, and transfer. This includes knowledge of the actions of various muscle groups, understanding the factors involved in the coordination of body movement, and familiarity with the integrated functioning of the skeletal, muscular, and nervous systems, as well as the correct use of lifting and positioning equipment.
2. **The correct answer is 1.** Proprioception is the awareness of the position of the body and its parts. Proprioception is monitored by proprioceptors located on nerve endings in muscles, tendons, and joints. Posture is regulated by the nervous system and requires coordination of proprioception and balance.
3. **The correct answer is 1.** A client with a right-sided cerebral hemorrhage and damage to the right motor strip may have left-sided hemiplegia. However, a client with a right-sided head injury may have only cerebral edema (but not destruction) of the motor strip.
4. **The correct answer is 1.** Older adults may walk more slowly and appear less coordinated. They also may take smaller steps, keeping their feet closer together, which decreases their base of support. Thus, body balance may become unstable, and they are at greater risk for falls and injuries.
5. **The correct answer is 4.** Clients are more open to developing an exercise program if they are at the stage of being ready to change their behaviour. Information on the benefits of regular exercise may be helpful to the client who has not yet reached the stage of being ready to act.
6. **The correct answer is 2.** It is increasingly clear that children are becoming less active, resulting in an increase in childhood obesity. Children and adolescents spend a great deal of their time in school, yet most Canadian children currently do not receive the recommended five periods of physical activity per week. Physical education has become an optional subject in most secondary schools, and only 18 percent of Canadian teenagers are accumulating enough daily activity to meet the international guidelines for optimal growth and development.
7. **The correct answer is 2.** If the client has a syncopal episode or begins to fall, you should assume a wide base of support with one foot in front of the other, thus supporting the client's body weight. You can then extend your front leg and slide the client against this leg to lower him or her gently to the floor, protecting the head.

Chapter 37

1. **The correct answer is 3.** Noise pollution occurs when the noise level in an environment becomes uncomfortable to the inhabitants of the environment. A health care facility can be polluted by noise. The sounds of machines, persons talking, intercoms, and paging systems can result in increased noise levels. This

may produce a syndrome called *sensory overload,* which is a marked increase in the intensity of auditory and visual stimuli.

2. **The correct answer is 2.** In Canada, accidental injuries are the leading cause of death for persons between the ages of 1 and 34 years.
3. **The correct answer is 2.** Adolescents are at greatest risk for injury from motor vehicle accidents, suicide, and substance abuse.
4. **The correct answer is 1.** Advancing age and the concurrent physiological changes in vision, hearing, mobility, reflexes, circulation, and the ability to make quick judgements predispose older adults to falls.
5. **The correct answer is 2.** WHMIS consists of three main elements: worker education programs, cautionary labelling of products, and the provision of MSDSs.
6. **The correct answer is 2.** Procedure-related accidents occur during therapy. They include medication and fluid administration errors, the improper application of external devices, and accidents related to the improper performance of procedures (e.g., improper Foley catheter insertion).
7. **The correct answer is 3.** Restraints are *not* considered a long-term intervention. Restraints are used only after other alternatives have been tried, and the least-restrictive method of restraint is used. The use of restraints must be part of the client's medical treatment. Restraints are considered a short-term intervention; once they have been applied, regular assessments are needed to determine whether they should be continued.
8. **The correct answer is 3.** The poison control centre phone number should be visible on the telephone in homes with young children. In all cases of suspected poisoning, this number should be called immediately, before any intervention.
9. **The correct answer is 4.** Having a family member with the client at all times is an unrealistic expectation; a trained sitter may be used if constant observation is required. Attending to personal needs, offering diversionary activities, and camouflaging IV lines may help to avoid the need for a restraint.

Chapter 38

1. **The correct answer is 1.** As clients with diabetes often have decreased sensation in their feet, feet should be inspected daily for signs of skin breakdown or infection; changes in colour, temperature and sensation; and any discoloration or thickening of toenails. Daily inspection can help decrease the development of foot ulcers and subsequent complications.
2. **The correct answer is 3.** Psoriasis is a chronic inflammatory skin condition, the exact cause of which is unknown, and there is currently no cure. It is thought to be an immune-mediated disease whereby the person's immune system reacts against its own cells. It is not contagious and cannot be passed from one person to another. It is not related to poor hygiene.
3. **The correct answer is 3.** With her chronic disease, she may have decreased sensation and circulation, and an increased healing time. She is at a higher risk of developing infection and foot ulcers, which are difficult to treat and slow to heal.
4. **The correct answer is 2.** The skin holds information about the body's circulation, nutritional status, and signs of systemic disease.
5. **The correct answer is 3.** Pallor in a client of African American decent appears ashen, grey, or dull.
6. **The correct answer is 2.** Inflammation is not easily recognized, and it is often necessary to palpate the skin for increased warmth, taut surfaces that may indicate edema, and induration (hardening of the tissue) as redness at the site of the inflammation is not be seen in a dark-skinned client.
7. **The correct answer is 2.** The anchoring device on the nasogastric tube should be changed daily to prevent skin maceration and to provide an opportunity to inspect the surface of the naris to prevent ulceration from the tube.
8. **The correct answer is 1.** The client should always be included in the care plan. Cultural preferences should always be considered. If the client is unconscious, the family can provide information on hair care preferences.
9. **The correct answer is 3.** This action prevents secretions from entering the nasolacrimal duct.
10. **The correct answer is 4.** It is important to do all these actions.

Chapter 39

1. **The correct answer is 1.** Anemia, a lower than normal hemoglobin level, is a result of decreased hemoglobin production, increased red blood cell destruction, blood loss, or a combination of these factors. Clients will have complaints of fatigue, decreased activity tolerance, and increased breathlessness, as well as pallor (especially seen in the conjunctiva of the eye) and an increased heart rate.
2. **The correct answer is 2.** Carbon monoxide is the most common toxic inhalant that decreases the oxygen-carrying capacity of blood. The affinity for hemoglobin to bind with carbon monoxide is greater than 200 times its affinity to bind with oxygen, creating a functional anemia. Because of the bond's strength, carbon monoxide is not easily dissociated from hemoglobin, making the hemoglobin unavailable for oxygen transport.
3. **The correct answer is 1.** Hypovolemia is caused by conditions such as shock and severe dehydration resulting from extracellular fluid loss and reduced circulating blood volume. With a significant fluid loss, the body tries to adapt by increasing the heart rate and peripheral vasoconstriction to increase the volume of blood returned to the heart and, in turn, increase the cardiac output.
4. **The correct answer is 3.** Fever increases the tissues' need for oxygen, and as a result, carbon dioxide production also increases. If the febrile state persists, the metabolic rate remains high and the body begins to break down protein stores, resulting in muscle wasting and decreased muscle mass. Respiratory muscles such as the diaphragm and intercostal muscles are also wasted.
5. **The correct answer is 1.** Left-sided heart failure is an abnormal condition characterized by impaired functioning of the left ventricle as a result of elevated pressures and pulmonary congestion. If left ventricular failure is significant, the amount of blood ejected from the left ventricle drops greatly, resulting in decreased cardiac output.
6. **The correct answer is 1.** Right-sided heart failure results from impaired functioning of the right ventricle characterized by venous congestion in the systemic circulation. Right-sided heart failure more commonly results from pulmonary disease or is a consequence of long-term left-sided failure. Right-sided heart failure results from impaired functioning of the right ventricle, characterized by venous congestion in the systemic circulation. Right-sided heart failure more commonly results from pulmonary disease or from long-term left-sided failure. As the failure continues, the amount of blood ejected from the right ventricle declines, and blood begins to "back up" in the systemic circulation. Clinically, the client has weight gain, distended neck veins, hepatomegaly and splenomegaly, and dependent peripheral edema.

7. **The correct answer is 2.** Cyanosis, blue discoloration of the skin and mucous membranes caused by the presence of desaturated hemoglobin in capillaries, is a late sign of hypoxia. The presence or absence of cyanosis is not a reliable measure of oxygenation status.
8. **The correct answer is 1.** A person who starts smoking in adolescence and continues to smoke into middle age has an increased risk for cardiopulmonary disease and lung cancer.
9. **The correct answer is 3.** Frequent changes of position are simple and cost-effective methods for reducing the risks of stasis of pulmonary secretions and decreased chest wall expansion.
10. **The correct answer is 4.** The most effective position for clients with cardiopulmonary diseases is the 45-degree semi-Fowler's position, using gravity to assist in lung expansion and reduce pressure from the abdomen on the diaphragm.

Chapter 40

1. **The correct answer is 1.** Hypokalemia is one of the most common electrolyte imbalances, in which an inadequate amount of potassium circulates in extracellular fluid (ECF). When severe, hypokalemia can affect cardiac conduction and function. Because the normal amount of serum potassium is so small, fluctuations are poorly tolerated. The most common cause of hypokalemia is the use of potassium-wasting diuretics such as thiazide and loop diuretics.
2. **The correct answer is 4.** An infant's proportion of total body water (70% to 80% total body weight) is greater than that of children or adults. Infants are not protected from fluid loss because they ingest and excrete a relatively greater daily water volume than do adults. Therefore, they are at a greater risk for FVD and hyperosmolar imbalance because body water loss is proportionately greater per kilogram of weight. In addition, infants are dependent on others for fluid intake.
3. **The correct answer is 2.** Older adults experience a number of age-related changes that can affect fluid, electrolyte, and acid–base balances. They have a decreased thirst sensation, which may affect their oral intake of fluids. The kidneys have a decrease in the glomerular filtration rate and in the number of filtering nephrons. These changes can mean that in the presence of sodium depletion or overload, the older adult may be unable to maintain homeostasis, and the imbalance is instead worsened.
4. **The correct answer is 4.** For clients in health care settings, measurement of intake and output is a nursing intervention routinely used for clients following a procedure, clients who are febrile, clients with restricted fluids, or clients who receive diuretic or intravenous therapy. Output includes urine, diarrhea, vomitus, gastric suction, and drainage from postsurgical wounds or other tubes.
5. **The correct answer is 1.** Health promotion activities in the area of fluid, electrolyte, and acid–base imbalances focus primarily on client teaching. Clients and caregivers need to recognize risk factors for these imbalances and implement appropriate preventive measures.
6. **The correct answer is 1.** Under no circumstances should potassium chloride (KCl) be given by intravenous push. A direct intravenous infusion of KCl can be fatal. If an intravenous fluid is to have additives, a physician's order must be obtained that includes the required additives.
7. **The correct answer is 1.** The client's microflora and contamination by insertion are initially controlled for in the procedure for intravenous insertion. However, the other factors are controlled through conscientious use of infection control principles. This begins with thorough hand hygiene before and after the nurse handles any component of the intravenous system.
8. **The correct answer is 3.** An infiltration occurs when intravenous fluids enter the surrounding space around the venipuncture site. This is manifested as swelling (from increased tissue fluid) and pallor and coolness (caused by decreased circulation) around the venipuncture site.
9. **The correct answer is 2.** Phlebitis may be prevented by the routine removal and rotation of intravenous sites. The RNAO recommends replacing peripheral venous catheters and rotating sites at least every 72 hours.
10. **The correct answer is 4.** Although tachycardia and possibly some dyspnea with acute hemolytic and anaphylactic reactions will occur, the most common symptoms of circulatory overload related to blood administration are cough, dyspnea, and tachycardia. In other reactions, fever, chills, or both also occur.

Chapter 41

1. **The correct answer is 4.** Excessive daytime sleepiness (EDS) is the most common complaint of people with obstructive sleep apnea (OSA). People with severe OSA may report experiencing a disruption in their daily activities because of sleepiness.
2. **The correct answer is 2.** In hospitals and long-term care facilities, clients may have difficulty finding the time they need to rest and sleep. You should plan care to avoid awakening clients for nonessential tasks. You should schedule assessments, treatments, procedures, and routines for times when clients are awake. For example, you should not wake a stable client to check vital signs.
3. **The correct answer is 4.** The use of nonprescription sleeping medications is not advisable. Clients should learn the risks of such drugs. Over the long term, these drugs can lead to further sleep disruption even when they initially seemed to be effective. Older adults should be cautioned about using over-the-counter antihistamines because of their long duration of action that can cause confusion, constipation, urinary retention, and increased risk of falls.
4. **The correct answer is 4.** Clients should be cautioned about the dosage and use of herbal compounds because active ingredients can vary from product to product. Herbal compounds may interact with prescribed medication, and concurrent use should be avoided.
5. **The correct answer is 1.** Although dreams occur during both nonrapid eye movement (NREM) and rapid eye movement (REM) sleep, the dreams of REM sleep are more vivid and elaborate and are believed to be functionally important to learning, memory processing, and adaptation to stress.
6. **The correct answer is 3.** Alcohol can initially make a person feel drowsy; however, it can also cause a person to awaken during the night and can cause difficulty returning to sleep.
7. **The correct answer is 1.** Limiting alcohol, caffeine, and nicotine and decreasing fluids 2 to 4 hours before sleep may promote sleep for older adults.
8. **The correct answer is 3.** The Canadian Paediatric Society recommends that apparently healthy infants be placed in the supine position during sleep because of an association between the prone position and the occurrence of sudden infant death syndrome (SIDS).
9. **The correct answer is 4.** Narcolepsy is a dysfunction of mechanisms that regulate the sleep and wake states. Excessive daytime

sleepiness (EDS) is the most common complaint associated with this disorder. Brief daytime naps no longer than 20 minutes help reduce subjective feelings of sleepiness. During the day, the person may suddenly feel an overwhelming wave of sleepiness and fall asleep; REM sleep can occur within 15 minutes of falling asleep.

10. **The correct answer is 4.** Sleep needed during the school years is individualized because of varying activity and health levels. Six-year-olds average 11 to 12 hours of sleep nightly, whereas 11-year-olds sleep 9 to 10 hours. Six- or 7-year-olds can usually be persuaded to go to bed by encouraging quiet activities.

Chapter 42

1. **The correct answer is 1.** In the past, pain was viewed simply as a symptom of an illness or condition. Pain itself is now considered to be a separate disease.
2. **The correct answer is 2.** Chronic pain is generally defined as pain that has been present for at least 6 months, persists beyond the normal time of healing, may not have an identifiable cause, serves no biological benefit, and leads to great personal suffering.
3. **The correct answer is 3.** One of the common misconceptions about pain management is that regular administration of analgesics will lead to drug addiction.
4. **The correct answer is 1.** Cognitively, toddlers and preschoolers are often unable to recall explanations about pain, or associate pain with experiences that can occur in various situations.
5. **The correct answer is 4.** You can only make an accurate diagnosis of pain after you have performed a complete client assessment. You will consider the client's withdrawal from communication, grimacing, moaning, and verbalizations of discomfort.
6. **The correct answer is 3.** Descriptive scales are used both to assess pain severity and to evaluate changes in a client's condition. A rating of 7 or more on a 0 to 10 scale requires immediate attention. The dose was insufficient.
7. **The correct answer is 2.** Teaching clients about pain reduces anxiety and helps them to achieve a sense of control. When a client is anticipating pain, you need to explain procedures and any associated discomfort. A confident explanation of the procedure helps you to gain a client's trust. When clients are informed about an upcoming painful experience, they often perceive the actual experience as less unpleasant.
8. **The correct answer is 1.** Nonpharmacological interventions include cognitive-behavioural and physical approaches. The goals of cognitive-behavioural interventions are to change pain perceptions, alter pain behaviour, and provide a greater sense of control. Relaxation and guided imagery are examples.
9. **The correct answer is 3.** One way to maximize pain relief while minimizing drug toxicity is to administer medication on a regular around-the-clock (ATC) basis rather than on an as-needed (prn) basis. The Canadian Pain Society, the American Pain Society, and the AHCPR all have stated that if pain is anticipated for the majority of the day, ATC administration should be considered. This is to prevent breakthrough pain, which is hard to control once it appears.
10. **The correct answer is 3.** A drug delivery system called patient-controlled analgesia (PCA) is a safe method for postoperative and cancer pain management that most clients prefer. The client gains control over his or her pain, and pain relief does not depend on nurse availability. Small doses of medications are delivered at short intervals, stabilizing serum drug concentrations for sustained pain relief.

Chapter 43

1. **The correct answer is 4.** Carbohydrates are the main source of energy in the diet.
2. **The correct answer is 2.** Proteins are essential for synthesis (building) of body tissue in growth, maintenance, and repair.
3. **The correct answer is 4.** When the intake of nitrogen exceeds the output, the body is in positive nitrogen balance, which is required for growth, normal pregnancy, maintenance of lean muscle mass and vital organs, and wound healing.
4. **The correct answer is 2.** Income as the major determinant is positively correlated with food selection and quantity.
5. **The correct answer is 2.** Hypervitaminosis can result from megadoses of supplemental fat- or water-soluble vitamins, excessive amounts in fortified food, and large intake of fish oils.
6. **The correct answer is 4.** The nutrient content claim *light* is permitted only on foods reduced in fat or reduced in calories. The percent of reduction in calories or fat has not been established for the claim *light*.
7. **The correct answer is 4.** Whole milk helps ensure adequate intake of fatty acids necessary for brain and neurological development.
8. **The correct answer is 3.** Turning the head toward the weaker side closes the weaker *side* and directs the food down the stronger side, which can do the work of chewing and swallowing.
9. **The correct answer is 3.** Age-related factors affect appetite, comfort, and digestion of food.
10. **The correct answer is 2.** Homebound older adults with chronic illness have an increased risk of poor nutrition.

Chapter 44

1. **The correct answer is 2.** The normal adult urine output is 1500 to 1600 mL/day.
2. **The correct answer is 1.** Renal alterations result from factors that cause injury directly to the glomeruli or renal tubule, interfering with their normal filtering, reabsorptive, and secretory functions. Selected causes include transfusion reactions, diseases of the glomeruli, and systemic diseases such as diabetes mellitus.
3. **The correct answer is 2.** Postrenal alterations result from obstruction to the flow of urine in the urinary collecting system anywhere between the renal pelvis and the urethral meatus. Urine is formed by the urinary system but cannot be eliminated by normal means. Urinary obstruction can be caused by calculi (stones), blood clots, or tumours.
4. **The correct answer is 3.** The urine is normally acidic, which inhibits bacterial growth and may prevent UTIs. Residual urine left in the bladder becomes alkaline and is an ideal medium for microbial growth.
5. **The correct answer is 3.** Hospital-acquired UTIs are often related to poor hand hygiene and urinary catheterization. The introduction of a catheter through the urethra provides a direct route for microorganisms to enter the bladder.
6. **The correct answer is 1.** The urine appears concentrated and cloudy because of the presence of white blood cells (WBCs) or bacteria.
7. **The correct answer is 1.** Prompted voiding is a useful strategy for clients with cognitive and/or physical impairment who rely on caregiver assistance.

8. **The correct answer is 3.** With stress incontinence, urine loss results from increased intra-abdominal pressure (e.g., coughing, sneezing, laughing, lifting). It usually involves a small volume of urine loss (less than 50 mL), and usually occurs in women or in men following radical prostatectomy. Pregnancy and delivery, weak pelvic floor muscles, heavy lifting, and obesity are sometimes contributing factors.
9. **The correct answer is 1.** The drainage bag should never be raised above the level of the client's bladder. It should hang on the bed frame or wheelchair without touching the floor. Urine in the bag and tubing can become a medium for bacteria, and infection is likely to develop if urine flows back into the bladder.
10. **The correct answer is 4.** Care must be taken to ensure that whatever type or size of condom is used, blood supply to the penis is not impaired. Therefore, the condom catheter should be snug and secure but should not cause constriction of blood flow.

Chapter 45

1. **The correct answer is 4.** Most nutrients and electrolytes are absorbed in the small intestine, specifically in the duodenum and jejunum.
2. **The correct answer is 3.** Lactose intolerance is the inability to digest lactose, which is the predominant sugar in milk and milk products. Lactose intolerance is caused by a shortage of the enzyme lactase. Lactase is normally produced by the cells that line the small intestine and is needed to digest lactose; however, lactase is genetically programmed to disappear in adulthood in everyone except in persons of northern European ancestry. As a result, many adults cannot digest lactose, which results in diarrhea, gaseous distension, and cramping.
3. **The correct answer is 4.** Fecal occult blood testing (FOBT), or the guaiac test, is a common laboratory test that can be done at home or at the client's bedside. This test measures microscopic amounts of blood in the feces. FOBT is useful as a diagnostic screening test for colon cancer.
4. **The correct answer is 1.** Antidiarrheal opiate agents decrease intestinal muscle tone to slow the passage of feces. Opiates inhibit the peristaltic waves that move feces forward but they also increase segmental contractions that mix the intestinal contents and expose them to the mucosal-absorbing surface.
5. **The correct answer is 3.** An obvious sign of impaction is the inability to pass a stool for several days, despite the repeated urge to defecate. When a continuous oozing of diarrhea stool develops, impaction should be suspected. The diarrhea is the result of the liquid portion of feces, located higher in the colon, seeping around the impacted mass.
6. **The correct answer is 4.** Cleansing enemas promote the complete evacuation of feces from the colon. The amount of solution to be instilled in an adult is 750 to 1000 mL.
7. **The correct answer is 3.** The specific signs and symptoms of intolerance to an enema include abdominal pain that is greater than a pressure sensation, abdominal cramping, abdominal distension, or rectal bleeding. The enema must be stopped. Notify the physician and obtain vital signs.
8. **The correct answer is 2.** One of the greatest problems in caring for a client with a nasogastric tube is maintaining comfort. The tube is a constant irritation to nasal mucosa. The nurse must assess the condition of both nares and mucosa for inflammation and excoriation.
9. **The correct answer is 1.** The stool discharged from an ostomy is called *effluent*.
10. **The correct answer is 1.** A nurse trained to care for ostomy clients is an enterostomal therapist (ET).

Chapter 46

1. **The correct answer is 2.** Footdrop is the inability to dorsiflex and invert the foot because of peroneal nerve damage. The foot is permanently fixed in plantar flexion and the person is therefore unable to lift the toes off the ground.
2. **The correct answer is 2.** The effects of bed rest or immobilization on the cardiovascular system include orthostatic hypotension, increased cardiac workload, and thrombus formation.
3. **The correct answer is 1.** After bed rest, clients usually have increased pulse rate and decreased pulse pressure and blood pressure. A large decrease in blood pressure when arising to a sitting or standing position (a drop of 20 mm Hg or more in systolic blood pressure and of 10 mm Hg in diastolic blood pressure) is known as orthostatic hypotension, and can result in light-headedness and fainting.
4. **The correct answer is 3.** Elastic stockings (sometimes called thromboembolic device hose, or TED) help to maintain external pressure on the muscles of the lower extremities and thus may promote venous return.
5. **The correct answer is 3.** Immobility can have a significant effect on the older adult's levels of health, independence, and functional status.
6. **The correct answer is 4.** Increased activity may result in symptoms associated with activity intolerance (e.g., increased pulse, changes in blood pressure, increased respirations, and decreased level of comfort). This can jeopardize the client's safety.
7. **The correct answer is 1.** Heparin and low-molecular-weight heparin (LMWH) are the most widely used drugs in the prophylaxis of deep vein thrombosis (DVT). Standard heparin is considered the gold standard for treatment because it has been well studied and validated. Common dosage for heparin therapy is 5000 units given subcutaneously 2 hours before surgery and repeated every 8 to 12 hours until the client is fully mobile or discharged.
8. **The correct answer is 1.** The trapeze bar is a triangular device that descends from a securely fastened overhead bar attached to the bed frame. It allows the client to use the upper extremities to raise the trunk off the bed, to assist in transfer from the bed to a wheelchair, or to perform upper arm exercises.
9. **The correct answer is 2.** The client in the prone position is lying face or chest down.
10. **The correct answer is 3.** When a client is in supported Fowler's position, placement of a small pillow or roll under the thigh prevents occlusion of the popliteal artery from pressure from body weight. It also prevents hyperextension of the knee.

Chapter 47

1. **The correct answer is 4.** When the skin is being compressed, blood flow is slowed and the skin becomes pale. After the pressure is relieved, the skin in the affected area turns red (erythema), which is a result of the blood vessels expanding (vasodilation) to allow more blood into the area to overcome the ischemic episode. This process is called *normal reactive hyperemia*. Assess the reddened area by pressing a fingertip over it. If the area blanches (turns white or a pale colour) and the erythema returns when the finger is removed, the reactive hyperemia is likely transient. If, however, the reddened area

does not blanch when finger pressure is applied (abnormal reactive hyperemia), suspect deep tissue damage.

2. **The correct answer is 1.** A stage I pressure ulcer is an observable pressure-related alteration of intact skin, whose indicators, as compared with an adjacent or opposite area on the body, may include changes in skin temperature (warmth or coolness), tissue consistency (firm or beefy feel), and sensation (pain or itching).
3. **The correct answer is 4.** If purulent or suspicious-looking wound drainage is present or there is a change in a previously healing chronic wound, obtaining a specimen of the drainage for culture may be necessary. The wound culture sample should never be collected from old drainage. Resident colonies of bacteria from the skin grow within exudate and may not be the true causative organisms of a wound infection. Before culturing a wound, clean the base of the wound with normal saline to remove superficial slough and debris. Select the cleanest part of the wound bed (granulating tissue is optimal), press the swab into a 1-cm-square area of this cleanest part of the wound, and rotate fully, pressing to express fluid beneath the surface of the wound bed.
4. **The correct answer is 3.** When evisceration occurs, place sterile towels soaked in sterile saline over the extruding tissues to reduce chances of bacterial invasion and drying of the tissues. If the organs protrude through the wound, blood supply to the tissues is compromised. The client should be allowed nothing by mouth (NPO), observed for signs and symptoms of shock, and prepared for emergency surgery.
5. **The correct answer is 3.** Serous drainage is clear, watery plasma.
6. **The correct answer is 3.** Ensuring the client understands the plan of care will decrease anxiety and increase the client's feeling of control. Pain can also have a negative impact on wound healing; thus, assessing the need for analgesia and providing it before the dressing change supports optimal healing and patient comfort and control.
7. **The correct answer is 3.** Exposure to fecal and urinary incontinence creates a caustic environment on the skin that leads to excoriation and further breakdown, once the skin is no longer intact. An incontinence cleanser and a moisture barrier ointment will remove urine and feces from the skin, leaving a protective (usually silicone-based) barrier that repels moisture.
8. **The correct answer is 4.** Hydrocolloid dressings are dressings with complex formulations of colloidal, elastomeric, and adhesive components that are both adhesive and occlusive. The wound contact layer of this dressing forms a gel as fluid is absorbed and maintains a moist healing environment.
9. **The correct answer is 3.** An abdominal binder will support the wound and reduce stress on large abdominal incisions that are vulnerable to tension or stress as the client moves or coughs.
10. **The correct answer is 4.** The body requires additional energy to heal pressure ulcers. Dietitians are trained in thorough assessment of caloric requirements and intake for effective wound healing and, thus, are essential members of the health care team looking after clients with skin breakdown. In addition, dietitians are knowledgeable about different sources of nutrition, including supplements or tube feeding, if required.

Chapter 48

1. **The correct answer is 2.** A kinesthetic sense enables a person to be aware of the position and movement of body parts without seeing them.
2. **The correct answer is 1.** Stereognosis is a sense that allows a person to recognize an object's size, shape, and texture.
3. **The correct answer is 3.** When a person receives multiple sensory stimuli and cannot perceptually disregard or selectively ignore some stimuli, sensory overload occurs. The client in constant pain or who undergoes frequent monitoring of vital signs is at risk. Multiple stimuli can combine to cause overload.
4. **The correct answer is 2.** Proprioceptive changes after the age of 60 years include increased difficulty with balance, spatial orientation, and coordination.
5. **The correct answer is 4.** For a client with hearing impairment, you should face the client when speaking, use simple sentences, and speak more slowly and at a normal volume.
6. **The correct answer is 4.** The nursing health history includes assessment of the nature and characteristics of sensory alterations or any problem related to an alteration. The nurse begins by asking the client to describe the sensory deficit. For example, "How does your hearing now compare with your hearing a year ago?"
7. **The correct answer is 2.** Advise older adults as follows: Do not drive during rush hour. Use rear-view and side-view mirrors when changing lanes. Avoid driving at dusk or at night. Drive slowly, but not too slowly. Keep your car in good working condition.
8. **The correct answer is 3.** Hearing loss caused by noisy environments was once thought to affect primarily older individuals; however, recent research has observed this loss in youth. As a nurse, you should routinely teach parents and children to take precautions when involved in activities associated with high-intensity noise. You should assess clients for noise exposure and participate in providing hearing conservation classes for teachers, students, and clients.
9. **The correct answer is 3.** Olfaction is the sense of smell. A client who cannot smell smoke may not know that something is burning. A smoke detector would be essential.
10. **The correct answer is 1.** When senses are impaired, the sense of self is impaired. Initially, a person may withdraw by avoiding communication or socialization with others in an attempt to cope with the sensory loss.

Chapter 49

1. **The correct answer is 2.** The obese client is susceptible to poor wound healing and to wound infection because of the structure of fatty tissue, which contains a poor blood supply. This slows delivery of essential nutrients and enzymes needed for wound healing.
2. **The correct answer is 3.** If a client regularly uses prescription or over-the-counter medications, the surgeon or anaesthesiologist may temporarily discontinue the drugs before surgery or adjust the dosages. Certain medications have special implications for the surgical client, creating greater risks for complications or interacting negatively with anaesthetic agents.
3. **The correct answer is 2.** The client who smokes is at greater risk for postoperative pulmonary complications than a client who does not.
4. **The correct answer is 2.** The family is an important resource for a client with physical limitations and provides the emotional support needed to motivate the client to return to a previous state of health. Often, a family member can become the client's coach, offering valuable support during the postoperative period.

5. **The correct answer is 1.** Accurate recording of intake and output helps assess renal and circulatory function. For example, you measure all sources of output, including urine, surgically placed drains, gastric drainage, and drainage from wounds, and note any insensible loss from diaphoresis.
6. **The correct answer is 3.** Position the client on one side with the face downward and the neck slightly extended to facilitate a forward movement of the tongue and the flow of mucous secretions out of the mouth.
7. **The correct answer is 4.** To promote normal venous return and circulatory blood flow, encourage clients to perform leg exercises at least every hour while awake. Other measures include applying elastic stockings or pneumatic compression stockings as ordered, encouraging early ambulation, positioning the client so that blood flow is not interrupted, administering anticoagulant drugs as ordered, and promoting adequate fluid intake.
8. **The correct answer is 2.** International normalized ratio (INR) and activated partial thromboplastin time (APTT) indicate the clotting ability of blood, which if greater than normal reveal clients at risk for bleeding tendencies.
9. **The correct answer is 2.** Maintaining an upright position facilitates diaphragm excursion and enhances expansion of the thorax.
10. **The correct answer is 4.** Malignant hyperthermia is a potentially lethal condition that can occur in clients who received general anaesthesia. It should be suspected when there is unexpected tachycardia and tachypnea; jaw muscle rigidity; body rigidity of limbs, abdomen, and chest; or hyperkalemia. Temperature elevation is a late sign.

Index

Page numbers followed by "f" denote figures; those followed by "t" denote tables; those followed by "b" denote boxes

A

B

C

D

F

G

I

M

N

Q

R

T

U

V

W

X

Y

Z

Special Features

CLIENT TEACHING

CONCEPT MAPS

RESEARCH HIGHLIGHTS

NURSING CARE PLANS